Vascular Medicine

A Textbook of Vascular Biology and Diseases

Vascular Medicine

A Textbook of Vascular Biology and Diseases

Second Edition

Edited by **JOSEPH LOSCALZO, M.D., Ph.D.**
Distinguished Professor of Medicine and Biochemistry
Director, Whitaker Cardiovascular Institute
Vice Chairman, Department of Medicine
Chief, Cardiovascular Medicine
Boston University School of Medicine
Boston

MARK A. CREAGER, M.D.
Associate Professor of Medicine
Harvard Medical School
Medical Director, Vascular Center
Cardiovascular Division
Department of Medicine
Brigham and Women's Hospital
Boston

VICTOR J. DZAU, M.D.
Arthur L. Bloomfield Professor and Chairman
Department of Medicine
Stanford University School of Medicine
Director, Falk Cardiovascular Research Center
Stanford Medical Center
Stanford, California

Foreword by **ARAM CHOBANIAN, M.D.**
Dean and Professor of Medicine
Boston University School of Medicine
Boston

Little, Brown and Company
Boston New York Toronto London

To our wives and children
for their patience, understanding, and
support throughout this and many other
endeavors

Second Edition

Library of Congress Cataloging-in-Publication Data

Vascular medicine: a textbook of vascular biology and diseases / edited by Joseph Loscalzo, Mark A. Creager, Victor J. Dzau; foreword by Aram Chobanian.—2nd ed.

p. cm.

Includes bibliographical references and index.

ISBN 0-316-53400-5 (clothbound)

1. Blood-vessels—Diseases. 2. Blood-vessels—Physiology. 3. Blood-vessels—Pathophysiology. I. Loscalzo, Joseph. II. Creager, Mark A. III. Dzau, Victor J.

[DNLM: 1. Vascular Diseases. WG 500 V3323 1996]

RC691.V39 1996

616.1'3—dc20

DNLM/DLC

for Library of Congress 95-39262

CIP

Printed in the United States of America

MV-NY

Editorial: Nancy E. Chorpenning, Kristin Odmark
Production Editor: Katharine S. Mascaro
Production Services: Books By Design, Inc.
Production Supervisor: Michael A. Granger
Cover Designer: Linda Dana Willis

Contents

Foreword vii
Preface ix
Contributing Authors xi

I
Biology of the Vasculature

1. Physiologic Functions of Normal Endothelial Cells 3
Mary E. Gerritsen

2. Connective Tissues of the Subendothelium 39
Jerome M. Seyer and Andrew H. Kang

3. The Vascular Smooth Muscle Cell 69
Jonathan S. Stamler, Victor J. Dzau, and Joseph Loscalzo

4. Vascular Pharmacology 117
Stephen T. O'Rourke and Paul M. Vanhoutte

5. Rheology, Transport, and Thrombosis in the Circulation 141
Vincent T. Turitto and Harry L. Goldsmith

6. Arterial Stiffness and Vascular/Ventricular Interaction in Humans 185
Raymond P. Kelly, David E. Gallagher, Lina L. Lee, and Michael F. O'Rourke

7. Normal Mechanisms of Hemostasis and Fibrinolysis 207
Douglas E. Vaughan, Andrew I. Schafer, and Joseph Loscalzo

II
Pathophysiology of Vascular Disease

8. Vascular Injury 219
Stephen M. Schwartz

9. Endothelial Dysfunction in Vascular Disease 245
Joseph A. Vita, John F. Keaney, Jr., and Joseph Loscalzo

10. Pathophysiology of Thrombosis 265
Andrew I. Schafer

11. Pathogenesis of Atherosclerosis: Cell Biology 289
Russell Ross

12. Pathogenesis of Atherosclerosis: Cellular Interactions 297
Peter Libby

13. Pathogenesis of Atherosclerosis: Lipid Metabolism 307
David P. Via, John R. Guyton, and Antonio M. Gotto, Jr.

14. Pathophysiology of Ischemic Syndromes 333
Antonio Fernandez-Ortiz and Valentin Fuster

15. Pathogenesis of Essential Hypertension 349
Jeffrey C. Webber and Allen J. Naftilan

16. Pathophysiology of Vasospasm 369
John P. Cooke and Victor J. Dzau

17. Pathophysiology of Vasculitis 387
Kenneth M. Pariser and Sheldon M. Wolff

III
Diagnostic Methods in Vascular Disease

18. Examination of the Patient with Vascular Disease 397
John W. Joyce

19. Noninvasive Vascular Testing 415
Mark A. Creager, Daniel H. O'Leary, and Peter M. Doubilet

20. Magnetic Resonance Imaging of Vascular Disease 445
Joseph F. Polak, Mary K. Adamis, and Mahesh R. Patel

21. Vascular Nuclear Medicine 467
Finn Mannting and Joseph F. Polak

22. Principles of Angiography 493
Michael A. Bettmann and Michael F. Meyerovitz

23. Computed Tomography in Vascular Disorders 519
Sabah S. Tumeh, Steven E. Seltzer, and Ay-Ming Wang

IV
General Principles of Therapy

24. Epidemiology of Risk-Factor Reduction 569
J. Michael Gaziano

25. The Atherogenic Dyslipoproteinemias 587
Allan D. Sniderman and Katherine Cianflone

26. Hypertension: Evaluation and Management 609
Peter Rudd and Victor J. Dzau

27. Anticoagulants, Antiplatelet Agents, and Fibrinolytics 639
Joseph Loscalzo and Andrew I. Schafer

28. Future Molecular Approaches to the Treatment of Cardiovascular Disease: Gene Therapy 665
Heiko E. von der Leyen and Victor J. Dzau

29. Principles of Vascular Surgery 675
Anthony D. Whittemore and John A. Mannick

30. Assessment and Reduction of Cardiac Risk in Peripheral Vascular Surgery 703
Khether E. Raby

31. Percutaneous Revascularization in Peripheral Arterial Disease 717
Kenneth Rosenfield, Robert Schainfeld, and Jeffrey M. Isner

32. Selective Intra-arterial Thrombolytic Therapy in Peripheral Arterial Disease 765
Krishna Kandarpa

V

Specific Disorders

A. Arterial Disorders

33. Cerebrovascular Disease 781
Frances E. Jensen

34. Coronary Artery Disease 797
Thomas C. Andrews and Gilbert H. Mudge, Jr.

35. Arterial Obstructive Diseases of the Extremities 825
Jonathan L. Halperin and Mark A. Creager

36. Renovascular Hypertension 853
Thomas G. Pickering

37. Visceral Ischemic Syndromes 869
Kimberley J. Hansen, Stephen P. Murray, and Ronald J. Stoney

38. Vasculogenic Impotence 885
Irwin Goldstein

39. Aneurysmal Disease of the Aorta and Its Branches 901
Mark A. Creager, Jonathan L. Halperin, and Anthony D. Whittemore

40. Aortic Dissection 927
Patrick T. O'Gara and Roman W. DeSanctis

41. Pulmonary Hypertension 951
Lewis J. Rubin, Harold I. Palevsky, and Alfred Fishman

B. Vasospastic Disorders and Vasculitis

42. Raynaud's Phenomenon and Other Vascular Disorders Related to Temperature 965
Mark A. Creager, Jonathan L. Halperin, and Jay D. Coffman

43. The Clinical Spectrum of Vasculitis 999
Sheldon M. Wolff and Kenneth M. Pariser

44. Thromboangiitis Obliterans (Buerger's Disease) 1033
Jeffrey W. Olin and J. T. Lie

C. Venous Thromboembolism and Chronic Venous Disorders

45. Venous Thrombosis 1051
Russell D. Hull and Graham F. Pineo

46. Pulmonary Embolism 1069
Samuel Z. Goldhaber

47. Chronic Venous Disorders 1081
Magruder C. Donaldson

D. Miscellaneous Disorders of the Vasculature

48. Vascular Infection 1103
Paul F. Kamitsuka

49. Lymphedema 1133
John P. Cooke and Thom W. Rooke

50. Vascular Trauma 1147
James O. Menzoian, Nancy L. Cantelmo, J. Gordon Wright, Michael Belkin, and Jeanne E. Doyle

51. Vascular Ulcers 1173
Ronald L. Dalman, E. John Harris, Jr., and Christopher K. Zarins

52. Neurovascular Compression Syndromes of the Thoracic Outlet 1187
Herbert I. Machleder

53. Reflex Sympathetic Dystrophy 1209
Robert J. Schwartzman

54. Congenital Malformations of the Vasculature 1223
Renu Virmani and Allen P. Burke

55. Iatrogenic Vascular Injuries 1253
Renu Virmani, Andrew Farb, and Allen P. Burke

56. Neoplastic Diseases of the Blood Vessels 1269
Janina A. Longtine

Index *1285*

Foreword

The field of vascular medicine has experienced explosive growth during the past decade. In contrast to beliefs first introduced by William Harvey that blood vessels are inactive tubes that serve only to distribute blood to tissues, the vasculature has turned out to be an extremely dynamic organ that plays a critical role in the regulation of blood flow. It also acts as a first line of defense against infection and tissue injury and participates actively in the processes of inflammation and thrombosis.

The endothelium is particularly important in mediating these vascular responses. It possesses sensors that detect changes in stretch, pressure, flow, and ambient oxygen concentration. It produces a number of vasoactive agents including nitric oxide, bradykinin, prostaglandins, and angiotensin. It also synthesizes most of the proteins involved in coagulation and fibrinolysis, and has specific surface receptors that are involved in the initiation and termination of thrombosis. Recent studies have demonstrated the importance of the endothelium in the inflammatory process, which appears to develop in response to any form of injury to the arterial wall and which appears responsible for some of the adverse consequences of such injury.

Emerging data would suggest a high level of integration between the responses of endothelial, smooth muscle, and periadventitial cells of the vessel wall. These cells appear to interact with one another and with the intervening extracellular matrix by an intricate network of autocrine and paracrine factors. Such interactions are involved in the structural remodeling that occurs as part of many pathological processes in both the macrovasculature and microvasculature. The vascular responses to hypertension and diabetes and the arterial changes associated with atherosclerosis include major changes in cellular growth and restructuring of the extracellular matrix, which can lead to additional pathological consequences associated with arterial occlusion and reduced organ blood flow.

Major advances are being made at an accelerating pace to understand the mechanisms involved in the development of vascular diseases. The new knowledge has led to improved methods for the noninvasive imaging of both arterial and venous diseases and to earlier recognition of vascular disorders. It also has provided exciting new approaches for the prevention or amelioration of vascular diseases and their complications. The advances have relevance not only to the problems of atherosclerosis, hypertension, ischemic heart disease, pulmonary vascular disease, and diabetes, but to other fields as well. For example, inhibition of angiogenesis can result in inhibition of tumor growth and therefore holds promise for the treatment of malignant disorders. Understanding the vascular responses to inflammation also may become important in the treatment of diseases resulting from excessive tissue fibrosis.

In view of these spectacular advances, it is not surprising that vascular medicine has achieved a position of prominence in both research and clinical arenas. The National Institutes of Health have established specific initiatives to enrich research in this field including the introduction of the Vascular Medicine Academic Award and specifically-targeted program project grants for the study of vascular disorders. Sections of vascular medicine have proliferated in departments of medicine and cardiology units throughout the country as have new medical journals dealing with the vasculature.

This new edition of *Vascular Medicine* provides an in-depth and up-to-date summary of the current status of scientific and clinical knowledge on the biology, pathophysiology, diagnosis, and treatment of vascular diseases. It offers much new information and an outstanding bibliography. Drs. Loscalzo, Creager, and Dzau are uniquely qualified to present this treatise because of their outstanding expertise in both research and clinical aspects of vascular diseases. They again have produced a superlative reference text that will be of value to a wide array of individuals interested in vascular medicine.

Aram Chobanian, M.D.

Preface

The vasculature represents the largest organ in the body. Composed of endothelial cells, smooth muscle cells, and adventitial fibroblasts, blood vessels are more than mere conduits for the delivery of oxygen and nutrients to metabolizing tissue. Vascular cells regulate the flow of blood, resist thrombus formation, maintain blood fluidity, interact dynamically with motile cells, and respond to injury in a predictable pattern. The substantial growth of the field of vascular biology in recent years supports these concepts and has led to the continued evolution of the basic tenets of this paradigm.

Vascular medicine has continued to develop as an important and dynamic medical discipline, well poised to facilitate the transfer of information acquired at the bench to the bedside of patients with vascular diseases. From the perspective of the second edition of this textbook, we continue to believe that diseases of the blood vessels should be considered under a single rubric. Atherosclerosis, thromboembolism, hypertension, vasculitis, vasospasm, and venous and lymphatic disorders are responsible for the majority of disabilities and death in Western society. Recent technological achievements in areas like magnetic resonance angiography and potential therapeutic modalities, such as vascular gene therapy, provide a continued impetus for this integrated view of the vascular system and vascular diseases.

This second edition of the textbook has, accordingly, been written to integrate a contemporary understanding of vascular biology with a detailed and thorough review of clinical vascular diseases. In this second edition, we have expanded significantly both the section devoted to basic vascular biology—with the newly added chapters on arterial stiffness, the pathophysiology of ischemic syndromes, and vascular gene therapy—and the section devoted to specific vascular disorders—with newly added chapters on thromboangiitis obliterans, vasculogenic impotence, vascular infections, and vascular ulcers. All of the clinical chapters have been updated to reflect recent developments in diagnosis and treatment.

We feel that this textbook will continue to be useful both for scientists and for clinicians caring for patients with vascular disease. We also hope that it will continue to serve as an important resource for medical students and trainees. We have attempted to present the information in a manner that will enable readers to understand the relevant concepts of vascular biology and to use these concepts in a rational approach to the broad range of vascular diseases that confront them frequently in their daily practice. The vasculature is an organ system in its own right, and we believe that the approach presented in the revised version of this textbook will place physicians in a better position to evaluate patients with a broad and complex range of vascular diseases, and to implement appropriate diagnostic and therapeutic strategies in the care of these patients.

J.L.
M.A.C.
V.J.D.

Contributing Authors

Mary K. Adamis, M.D.
Instructor of Radiology, Harvard Medical School; Assistant Director, MRI, Department of Radiology, Beth Israel Hospital, Boston
20. Magnetic Resonance Imaging of Vascular Disease

Thomas C. Andrews, M.D.
Assistant Professor of Medicine, Department of Cardiology, Uniformed Services University of the Health Sciences, F. Edward Hébert School of Medicine, Bethesda, Maryland; Director of Research, Department of Cardiology, Wilford Hall U.S. Air Force Medical Center, San Antonio
34. Coronary Artery Disease

Michael Belkin, M.D.
Assistant Professor of Surgery, Harvard Medical School; Staff Surgeon, Brigham and Women's Hospital, Boston
50. Vascular Trauma

Michael A. Bettmann, M.D.
Professor of Radiology, Dartmouth Medical School, Hanover; Director, Cardiovascular and Interventional Radiology, Dartmouth-Hitchcock Medical Center, Lebanon, New Hampshire
22. Principles of Angiography

Allen P. Burke, M.D.
Staff Pathologist, Department of Cardiovascular Pathology, Armed Forces Institute of Pathology, Washington
54. Congenital Malformations of the Vasculature, 55. Iatrogenic Vascular Injuries

Nancy L. Cantelmo, M.D.
Associate Professor of Surgery, Boston University School of Medicine; Associate Chief, Surgical Service, Boston Veterans Administration Medical Center, Boston
50. Vascular Trauma

Katherine Cianflone, M.D.
Assistant Professor of Medicine, Department of Cardiology, McGill University Faculty of Medicine, Montreal, Quebec Canada
25. The Atherogenic Dyslipoproteinemias

Jay D. Coffman, M.D.
Professor of Medicine, Boston University School of Medicine; Chief, Peripheral Vascular Medicine, Boston University Medical Center, Boston
42. Raynaud's Phenomenon and Other Vascular Disorders Related to Temperature

John P. Cooke, M.D., Ph.D.
Associate Professor of Medicine, Division of Cardiovascular Medicine, Stanford University School of Medicine; Director, Section of Vascular Medicine, Stanford Hospital, Stanford, California
16. Pathophysiology of Vasospasm, 49. Lymphedema

Mark A. Creager, M.D.
Associate Professor of Medicine, Harvard Medical School; Medical Director, Vascular Center, Cardiovascular Division, Department of Medicine, Brigham and Women's Hospital, Boston
19. Noninvasive Vascular Testing, 35. Arterial Obstructive Diseases of the Extremities, 39. Aneurysmal Disease of the Aorta and Its Branches, 42. Raynaud's Phenomenon and Other Vascular Disorders Related to Temperature

Ronald L. Dalman, M.D.
Assistant Professor, Division of Vascular Surgery, Stanford University School of Medicine, Stanford; Chief, Vascular Surgery Service, Palo Alto Veterans Administration Medical Center, Palo Alto, California
51. Vascular Ulcers

Roman W. DeSanctis, M.D.
Professor of Medicine, Harvard Medical School; Physician and Director, Clinical Cardiology, Cardiac Unit, Massachusetts General Hospital, Boston
40. Aortic Dissection

Magruder C. Donaldson, M.D.
Associate Professor of Surgery, Harvard Medical School; Surgeon, Brigham and Women's Hospital, Boston
47. Chronic Venous Disorders

Peter M. Doubilet, M.D., Ph.D.
Associate Professor of Radiology, Harvard Medical School; Co-Director, Ultrasound, Department of Radiology, Brigham and Women's Hospital, Boston
19. Noninvasive Vascular Testing

Jeanne E. Doyle, B.S., R.N.
Executive Director, Society for Vascular Nursing, Norwood, Massachusetts
50. Vascular Trauma

Victor J. Dzau, M.D.
Arthur L. Bloomfield Professor and Chairman, Department of Medicine, Stanford University School of Medicine; Director, Falk Cardiovascular Research Center, Stanford Medical Center, Stanford, California
3. The Vascular Smooth Muscle Cell, 16. Pathophysiology of Vasospasm, 26. Hypertension: Evaluation and Management, 28. Future Molecular Approaches to the Treatment of Cardiovascular Disease: Gene Therapy

Andrew Farb, M.D.
Staff Cardiologist, Department of Cardiovascular Pathology, Armed Forces Institute of Pathology, Washington
55. Iatrogenic Vascular Injuries

Antonio Fernandez-Ortiz, M.D., Ph.D.
Research Fellow in Cardiology, Harvard Medical School and Massachusetts General Hospital, Boston; Interventional Cardiologist, San Carlos University Hospital, Complutense University, Madrid, Spain
14. Pathophysiology of Ischemic Syndromes

Alfred Fishman, M.D.
William Maul Measey Professor of Medicine and Attending Physician, Department of Medicine, University of Pennsylvania School of Medicine, Philadelphia
41. Pulmonary Hypertension

Valentin Fuster, M.D., Ph.D.
Professor of Medicine, Mount Sinai School of Medicine of the City University of New York; Director, Cardiovascular Institute, Mount Sinai Medical Center, New York
14. Pathophysiology of Ischemic Syndromes

David E. Gallagher, M.B.
Research Fellow, Medical Professorial Unit, St. Vincent's Hospital; Visiting Medical Officer, Department of Cardiology, Liverpool Hospital, Sydney, Australia
6. Arterial Stiffness and Vascular/Ventricular Interaction in Humans

J. Michael Gaziano, M.D., M.P.H.
Assistant Professor of Medicine, Harvard Medical School; Director, Cardiovascular Epidemiology, Department of Medicine, Brigham and Women's Hospital, Boston
24. Epidemiology of Risk-Factor Reduction

Mary E. Gerritsen, Ph.D.
Principal Staff Scientist and Section Head, Inflammation Research, Institute of Bone and Joint Disease and Cancer, Bayer Corporation, West Haven, Connecticut
1. Physiologic Functions of Normal Endothelial Cells

Samuel Z. Goldhaber, M.D.
Associate Professor of Medicine, Harvard Medical School; Staff Cardiologist, Department of Medicine, Brigham and Women's Hospital, Boston
46. Pulmonary Embolism

Harry L. Goldsmith, Ph.D.
Professor of Medicine, McGill University Faculty of Medicine; Research Investigator, Montreal General Hospital Research Institute, Montreal, Quebec Canada
5. Rheology, Transport, and Thrombosis in the Circulation

Irwin Goldstein, M.D.
Professor of Urology, Boston University School of Medicine, Boston
38. Vasculogenic Impotence

Antonio M. Gotto, Jr., M.D., D.Phil.
Chairman and Distinguished Service Professor of Medicine, Baylor College of Medicine; Chief, Internal Medicine Service, The Methodist Hospital, Houston
13. Pathogenesis of Atherosclerosis: Lipid Metabolism

John R. Guyton, M.D.
Associate Professor of Medicine and Director, Duke Lipid Clinic, Duke University Medical Center, Durham, North Carolina
13. Pathogenesis of Atherosclerosis: Lipid Metabolism

Jonathan L. Halperin, M.D.
Professor of Medicine, Mount Sinai School of Medicine of the City University of New York; Director, Clinical Services, The Cardiovascular Institute, Mount Sinai Medical Center, New York
35. Arterial Obstructive Diseases of the Extremities,
39. Aneurysmal Disease of the Aorta and Its Branches,
42. Raynaud's Phenomenon and Other Vascular Disorders Related to Temperature

Kimberley J. Hansen, M.D.
Associate Professor of Surgery and Director, Clinical Vascular Laboratory, Department of General Surgery, Bowman Gray School of Medicine of Wake Forest University, Winston-Salem, North Carolina
37. Visceral Ischemic Syndromes

E. John Harris, Jr., M.D.
Assistant Professor, Division of Vascular Surgery, Stanford University School of Medicine, Stanford; Attending Vascular Surgeon, Palo Alto Veterans Administration Medical Center, Palo Alto, California
51. Vascular Ulcers

Russell D. Hull, M.D.
Professor of Medicine, University of Calgary Faculty of Medicine; Director, Clinical Trials Unit, Foothills Provincial General Hospital, Calgary, Alberta Canada
45. Venous Thrombosis

Jeffrey M. Isner, M.D.
Professor of Medicine and Pathology, Tufts University School of Medicine; Chief, Cardiovascular Research, Department of Medicine and Cardiology, St. Elizabeth's Medical Center, Boston
31. Percutaneous Revascularization in Peripheral Arterial Disease

Frances E. Jensen, M.D.
Assistant Professor of Neurology, Harvard Medical School; Division of Neurology, Brigham and Women's Hospital and the Children's Hospital, Boston
33. Cerebrovascular Disease

John W. Joyce, M.D.
Professor of Medicine, Division of Cardiovascular Disease and Internal Medicine, Mayo Medical School, Rochester, Minnesota
18. Examination of the Patient with Vascular Disease

Paul F. Kamitsuka, M.D.
Assistant Clinical Professor, University of North Carolina School of Medicine; Infectious Disease Consultant, Wilmington Health Associates, Wilmington, North Carolina
48. Vascular Infection

Krishna Kandarpa, M.D., Ph.D.
Associate Professor of Radiology, Harvard Medical School; Co-Director, Cardiovascular and Interventional Radiology, Brigham and Women's Hospital, Boston
32. Selective Intra-arterial Thrombolytic Therapy in Peripheral Arterial Disease

Andrew H. Kang, M.D.
Goodman Professor of Medicine, University of Tennessee, Memphis, College of Medicine, Memphis, Tennessee
2. Connective Tissues of the Subendothelium

John F. Keaney, Jr., M.D.
Assistant Professor of Medicine, Boston University School of Medicine; Staff Physician, Department of Medicine, Boston University Medical Center, Boston
9. Endothelial Dysfunction in Vascular Disease

Raymond P. Kelly, M.D.
Physician and Cardiologist, St. Vincent's Hospital, Darlinghurst, New South Wales, Australia
6. Arterial Stiffness and Vascular/Ventricular Interaction in Humans

Lina L. Lee, M.Sc.
St. Vincent's Hospital, Darlinghurst, New South Wales, The University of New South Wales Medical Professional Unit, Sydney, Australia
6. Arterial Stiffness and Vascular/Ventricular Interaction in Humans

Peter Libby, M.D.
Associate Professor of Medicine, Harvard Medical School; Director, Vascular Medicine and Atherosclerosis Unit, Brigham and Women's Hospital, Boston
12. Pathogenesis of Atherosclerosis: Cellular Interactions

J. T. Lie, M.D.
Professor of Medical Pathology, University of California, Davis, School of Medicine, Davis; Director, Anatomic Pathology, University of California, Davis, Medical Center, Sacramento, California
44. Thromboangiitis Obliterans (Buerger's Disease)

Janina A. Longtine, M.D.
Assistant Professor of Pathology, Harvard Medical School; Department of Pathology, Brigham and Women's Hospital, Boston
56. Neoplastic Diseases of the Blood Vessels

Joseph Loscalzo, M.D., Ph.D.
Distinguished Professor of Medicine and Biochemistry, Director, Whitaker Cardiovascular Institute, Vice Chairman, Department of Medicine, Chief, Cardiovascular Medicine, Boston University School of Medicine; Chief, Cardiovascular Medicine, Boston University Medical Center, Boston
3. The Vascular Smooth Muscle Cell, 7. Normal Mechanisms of Hemostasis and Fibrinolysis, 9. Endothelial Dysfunction in Vascular Disease, 27. Anticoagulants, Antiplatelet Agents, and Fibrinolytics

Herbert I. Machleder, M.D.
Professor of Surgery, University of California, Los Angeles, School of Medicine; Professor and Vascular Surgeon, Vascular Disease Section, University of California, Los Angeles, Medical Center, Los Angeles
52. Neurovascular Compression Syndromes of the Thoracic Outlet

John A. Mannick, M.D.
Moseley Distinguished Professor of Surgery, Harvard Medical School; Surgeon, Division of Vascular Surgery, Brigham and Women's Hospital, Boston
29. Principles of Vascular Surgery

Finn Mannting, M.D., Ph.D.
Associate Professor of Radiology, Harvard Medical School; Director, Nuclear Medicine Division, Brigham and Women's Hospital, Boston
21. Vascular Nuclear Medicine

James O. Menzoian, M.D.
Professor of Surgery, Boston University School of Medicine; Chief, Section of Vascular Surgery, Boston University Medical Center, Boston
50. Vascular Trauma

Michael F. Meyerovitz, M.D.
Associate Professor of Radiology, Harvard Medical School; Co-Director, Cardiovascular and Interventional Radiology, Brigham and Women's Hospital, Boston
22. Principles of Angiography

Gilbert H. Mudge, Jr., M.D.
Associate Professor of Medicine, Harvard Medical School; Director, Cardiac Transplantation, Cardiovascular Division, Brigham and Women's Hospital, Boston
34. Coronary Artery Disease

Stephen P. Murray, M.D.
Assistant Clinical Professor of Surgery, Uniformed Services University of the Health Sciences, F. Edward Hébert School of Medicine, Bethesda, Maryland; Assistant Chief, Vascular Surgery, Brooke Army Medical Center, Fort Sam, Houston; Lieutenant Colonel, U.S. Army Medical Corps
37. Visceral Ischemic Syndromes

Allen J. Naftilan, M.D., Ph.D.
Assistant Professor of Medicine and Pharmacology, Vanderbilt University School of Medicine, Nashville, Tennessee
15. Pathogenesis of Essential Hypertension

Patrick T. O'Gara, M.D.
Assistant Professor of Medicine, Harvard Medical School; Director, Clinical Cardiology, Brigham and Women's Hospital, Boston
40. Aortic Dissection

Daniel H. O'Leary, M.D.
Professor of Radiology, Tufts University School of Medicine; Chairman, Department of Radiology, New England Medical Center Hospitals, Boston
19. Noninvasive Vascular Testing

Jeffrey W. Olin, D.O.
Associate Professor of Medicine, Ohio State University College of Medicine, Columbus; Co-Director, Vascular Laboratory, Cleveland Clinic Foundation, Cleveland, Ohio
44. Thromboangiitis Obliterans (Buerger's Disease)

Michael F. O'Rourke, M.D.
Professor of Medicine, University of New South Wales; Physician, St.Vincent's Hospital, New South Wales, Sydney, Australia
6. Arterial Stiffness and Vascular/Ventricular Interaction in Humans

Stephen T. O'Rourke, Ph.D.
Assistant Professor of Pharmaceutical Sciences, North Dakota State University College of Pharmacy, Fargo, North Dakota
4. Vascular Pharmacology

Harold I. Palevsky, M.D.
Associate Professor of Medicine, Pulmonary and Critical Care Division, University of Pennsylvania School of Medicine; Medical Director, Lung Transplant Program and Director, Pulmonary Vascular Disease Program, Hospital of the University of Pennsylvania, Philadelphia
41. Pulmonary Hypertension

Kenneth M. Pariser, M.D.
Associate Professor of Medicine, Tufts University School of Medicine; Chief, Division of Rheumatology, Faulkner Hospital, Boston
17. Pathophysiology of Vasculitis, 43. The Clinical Spectrum of Vasculitis

Mahesh R. Patel, M.D.
Instructor in Radiology, Harvard Medical School; Staff Radiologist, Beth Israel Hospital, Boston
20. Magnetic Resonance Imaging of Vascular Disease

Thomas G. Pickering, M.D., D.Phil.
Professor of Medicine, Cornell University Medical College; Attending Physician, Department of Medicine, New York Hospital, New York
36. Renovascular Hypertension

Graham F. Pineo, M.D.
Professor of Medicine, University of Calgary; Director, Clinical Trials Unit, Department of Medicine, Calgary General Hospital, Calgary, Alberta Canada
45. Venous Thrombosis

Joseph F. Polak, M.D.
Associate Professor of Radiology, Harvard Medical School; Attending Radiologist and Director, Division of Interventional Radiology, Brigham and Women's Hospital, Boston
20. Magnetic Resonance Imaging of Vascular Disease, 21. Vascular Nuclear Medicine

Khether E. Raby, M.D.
Clinical Assistant Professor of Medicine, Boston University; Attending Physician, Cardiac Catheterization Laboratory, University Hospital, Boston
30. Assessment and Reduction of Cardiac Risk in Peripheral Vascular Surgery

Thom W. Rooke, M.D.
Associate Professor of Medicine and Director, Gonda Vascular Center, Department of Cardiovascular Disease and Internal Medicine, Johns Hopkins; Consultant, Department of Cardiovascular Diseases and Internal Medicine, St. Mary's and Rochester Methodist Hospitals, Mayo Medical Center, Rochester, Minnesota
49. Lymphedema

Kenneth Rosenfield, M.D.
Assistant Professor of Medicine, Tufts University School of Medicine; Cardiologist, Division of Cardiovascular Medicine and Research, St. Elizabeth's Medical Center, Boston
31. Percutaneous Revascularization in Peripheral Arterial Disease

Russell Ross, Ph.D.
Professor of Pathology, University of Washington School of Medicine, Seattle
11. Pathogenesis of Atherosclerosis: Cell Biology

Lewis J. Rubin, M.D.
Professor of Medicine and Physiology, University of Maryland School of Medicine; Head, Division of Pulmonary and Critical Care Medicine, University of Maryland Medical System, Baltimore
41. Pulmonary Hypertension

Peter Rudd, M.D.
Professor of Medicine, Stanford University School of Medicine, Stanford, California
26. Hypertension: Evaluation and Management

Andrew I. Schafer, M.D.
The W.A. and Deborah Moncrief Professor of Medicine and Vice-Chairman, Department of Medicine, Baylor College of Medicine; Chief, Medical Service, Veterans Affairs Medical Center, Houston
7. Normal Mechanisms of Hemostasis and Fibrinolysis, 10. Pathophysiology of Thrombosis, 27. Anticoagulants, Antiplatelet Agents, and Fibrinolytics

Robert Schainfeld, D.O.
Assistant Professor of Medicine, Tufts University School of Medicine; Director, Non-Invasive Vascular Laboratory, Division of Cardiovascular Medicine and Research, St. Elizabeth's Medical Center, Boston
31. Percutaneous Revascularization in Peripheral Arterial Disease

Stephen M. Schwartz, M.D., Ph.D.
Professor of Pathology, University of Washington School of Medicine, Seattle
8. Vascular Injury

Robert J. Schwartzman, M.D.
Professor and Acting Chairman, Department of Neurology, Medical College of Pennsylvania and Hahnemann University School of Medicine, Philadelphia
53. Reflex Sympathetic Dystrophy

Steven E. Seltzer, M.D.
Associate Professor of Radiology, Harvard Medical School; Co-Director, Abdominal Imaging and Director, CT Scanning, Department of Radiology, Brigham and Women's Hospital, Boston
23. Computed Tomography in Vascular Disorders

Jerome M. Seyer, Ph.D.
Professor of Biochemistry, University of Tennessee, Memphis, College of Medicine; Research Career Scientist, Department of Research Services, Veterans Administration Medical Center, Memphis, Tennessee
2. Connective Tissues of the Subendothelium

Allan D. Sniderman, M.D.
Edwards Professor of Cardiology and Professor of Medicine, McGill University; Director, McGill Unit for the Prevention of Cardiovascular Disease, Royal Victoria Hospital, Montreal, Quebec Canada
25. The Atherogenic Dyslipoproteinemias

Jonathan S. Stamler, M.D.
Associate Professor of Medicine, Departments of Medicine and Cell Biology, and Pulmonary and Cardiovascular Divisions, Duke University School of Medicine, Durham, North Carolina
3. The Vascular Smooth Muscle Cell

Ronald J. Stoney, M.D.
Professor of Surgery, University of California, San Francisco, School of Medicine; Faculty, Department of Vascular Surgery, Moffitt and Long Hospital, San Francisco
37. Visceral Ischemic Syndromes

Sabah S. Tumeh, M.D.
Professor of Radiology, Eastern Virginia Medical School of the Medical College of Hampton Roads, Norfolk; Vice Chairman, Department of Radiology, General Hospital of Virginia Beach, Virginia
23. Computed Tomography in Vascular Disorders

Vincent T. Turitto, D.Engr.Sci.
Professor and Chair of Excellence, Biomedical Engineering Department, University of Tennessee, Memphis, College of Medicine, Memphis, Tennessee
5. Rheology, Transport, and Thrombosis in the Circulation

Paul M. Vanhoutte, M.D., Ph.D.
Vice-President for Research, Institut de Recherches Internationales Servier, Courbevoie, France
4. Vascular Pharmacology

Douglas E. Vaughan, M.D.
Associate Professor of Medicine and Pharmacology, Vanderbilt University School of Medicine; Staff Physician, Department of Cardiology, Vanderbilt University and Veterans Administration Medical Center, Nashville, Tennessee
7. Normal Mechanisms of Hemostasis and Fibrinolysis

David P. Via, Ph.D.
Assistant Professor of Medicine, Baylor College of Medicine, Houston
13. Pathogenesis of Atherosclerosis: Lipid Metabolism

Renu Virmani, M.D.
Professor of Pathology, Vanderbilt University School of Medicine, Nashville, Tennessee; Chairperson, Department of Cardiovascular Pathology, Armed Forces Institute of Pathology, Washington
54. Congenital Malformations of the Vasculature, 55. Iatrogenic Vascular Injuries

Joseph A. Vita, M.D.
Associate Professor of Medicine, Boston University School of Medicine; Associate Director, Cardiac Catheterization Laboratory, Department of Medicine, Boston University Medical Center, Boston
9. Endothelial Dysfunction in Vascular Disease

Heiko E. von der Leyen, M.D.
Instructor, Division of Cardiovascular Medicine, Stanford University School of Medicine, Stanford, California
28. Future Molecular Approaches to the Treatment of Cardiovascular Disease: Gene Therapy

Ay-Ming Wang, M.D.
Clinical Professor of Radiology, University of Missouri—Kansas City School of Medicine, Kansas City, Missouri; Co-Chief, Neuroradiology, Department of Diagnostic Radiology, William Beaumont Hospital, Royal Oak, Michigan
23. Computed Tomography in Vascular Disorders

Jeffrey C. Webber, M.D.
Former Cardiology Fellow in Internal Medicine, Vanderbilt University School of Medicine; Staff Cardiologist, Department of Medicine, Centennial Medical Center, Nashville, Tennessee
15. Pathogenesis of Essential Hypertension

Anthony D. Whittemore, M.D.
Professor of Surgery, Harvard Medical School; Chief, Vascular Surgery, Brigham and Women's Hospital, Boston
29. Principles of Vascular Surgery, 39. Aneurysmal Disease of the Aorta and Its Branches

†Sheldon M. Wolff, M.D.
Endicott Professor and Chairman, Department of Medicine, Tufts University School of Medicine; Physician-in-Chief, Department of Medicine, New England Medical Center, Boston
17. Pathophysiology of Vasculitis, 43. The Clinical Spectrum of Vasculitis

J. Gordon Wright, M.D.
Assistant Professor of Surgery, Division of Vascular Surgery, Ohio State University College of Medicine, Columbus, Ohio
50. Vascular Trauma

Christopher K. Zarins, M.D.
Chidester Professor of Surgery, Division of Vascular Surgery, Stanford University School of Medicine; Chairman, Division of Vascular Surgery, Stanford University Medical Center, Stanford, California
51. Vascular Ulcers

†Deceased

I

Biology of the Vasculature

Physiologic Functions of Normal Endothelial Cells

Mary E. Gerritsen

The endothelium forms a continuous lining of the cardiovascular system, strategic positioned as a biologic interface between the blood and all other tissues. Endowed with a rich array of receptors and enzymes, the endothelium is ideally positioned to monitor bloodborne or locally produced stimuli and respond with appropriate adaptive responses in function. The endothelium is both a target and a source of autocoids, growth factors, cytokines, oxygen radicals, and hemostatic factors. In this chapter, the roles of the endothelial cell in barrier function, hemostasis, regulation of vascular tone, inflammation, wound healing, and angiogenesis will be discussed.

Barrier Functions

PERMEABILITY

As the principal barrier between blood and tissues, endothelial cells play a central role in regulating the exchange of water and solutes. Water and small lipid-soluble substances (oxygen, nitrogen, carbon dioxide) can directly penetrate the cell surface, whereas large water-insoluble lipid molecules are thought to diffuse laterally within the lipid bilayer [1]. Cations (Na^+, K^+), anions (Cl^-, HCO_3^-), and small solutes (amino acids, glucose) permeate the intercellular junctions. The mechanisms whereby large macromolecules traverse endothelial cells remain controversial; pathways through large pores (thought to be some site at the intercellular junctions) or via plasmalemmal vesicles have been proposed [2–8].

The endothelial cells of exchange vessels (capillaries and pericytic, nonmuscular venules) exhibit remarkable variability in structure and permeability, leading to their classification as continuous, fenestrated, or discontinuous [9,10].

Endothelium of the continuous type is the most abundant and widespread. Found in the chambers of the heart; the walls of arterioles, capillaries, and venules in skeletal, smooth, and cardiac muscle; mesentery; skin; connective tissue; the lungs; and neural tissue (brain, retina, and spinal cord), continuous endothelia are characterized by occluding (tight) junctions (Fig. 1-1a). These occluding junctions act as a physical link between two adjoining cells and are instrumental in the electronic coupling and intercellular exchange of ions and small solutes. There are organ-specific structural modulations within the general class of continuous endothelia, for example, in the frequency of plasmalemmal vesicles, which range from 1,000/μm^3 in myocardial endothelia to 130/μm^3 in the lung to far fewer in brain capillaries. Additionally, a third level of structural heterogeneity, longitudinal, occurs. Vesicle numerical density is greatest in the endothelium of true capillaries [11,12].

Fenestrated endothelium is found in the exchange vessels of secretory and excretory organs (exocrine and endocrine glands), gastrointestinal mucosa, the kidneys (glomerular and peritubular capillaries), synovia, and the choroid plexus of the brain. Although much of the surface of this endothelial type is similar to continuous endothelium (50%–95% of the cell surface), the remainder bears numerous fenestrae, small transcellular circular openings 50–80 nm in diameter (Fig. 1-1b). At the level of the electron microscope, fenestrae may appear as open perforations or closed by thin membranous diaphragms. Fenestrae may occur in clusters, and their frequency varies from one vascular bed to another. Fenestrae lack a lipid bilayer, but they do contain heparan sulfate proteoglycan, imparting to those structures a high net negative charge [13]. The functional significance of fenestrae is still problematical; fenestrated capillaries show no greater permeability to plasma proteins than continuous capillaries, but they are more permeable to water, ions, and small solutes [2,3].

Discontinuous endothelia have a limited distribution and are found in the sinusoids of the liver, spleen, and bone marrow. Thin-walled vessels with an irregular outline and caliber, discontinuous endothelia are usually molded on the neighboring epithelial cells. In the liver, endothelial cells have an attenuated cytoplasm that is highly fenestrated. The majority of the fenestrae are 100–150 nm in diameter and tend to be clustered to form sieve plates; none of the fenestrae is closed with a diaphragm [14,15]. The endothelial fenestrae are not fixed but rather are dynamic structures whose diameter can be altered by luminal blood pressure, vasoactive substances, drugs, and toxins [16–22]. It has been proposed that the fenestrae of the hepatic endothelial cells regulate the passage of large substances such as chylomicron remnants while allowing the free exchange of plasma and large proteins [23]. The size and distribution of the fenestrae also vary longitudinally; at the portal end, the fenestrae are larger, although they make up less of the endothelial-cell surface area than they do in the pericentral region [23]. Discontinuous endothelia may be subject to more complex modulations than other types of endothelia because of continual interactions generated by cellular and humoral factors, including cell passage through the intercellular clefts.

As already discussed, exchange vessels of different vascular beds demonstrate a wide range of solute and protein permeabilities, and the mechanisms whereby larger macromolecules traverse the endothelial cells are not clearly understood. Serum albumin, perhaps because of its central role in microvascular exchange, has been the most widely studied macromolecule in transendothelial transport. Some suggest that serum albumin crosses through the endothelium via the extensive vesicular system of endothelia [24,25]. Others contend that albumin (as well as other macromolecules) is carried by convection through "large pores" that represent junctions between endothelial cells [26–29]. Specific and nonspecific binding sites of albumin to endothelial-cell surfaces have been demonstrated [30–37]. Recent data from several laboratories indi-

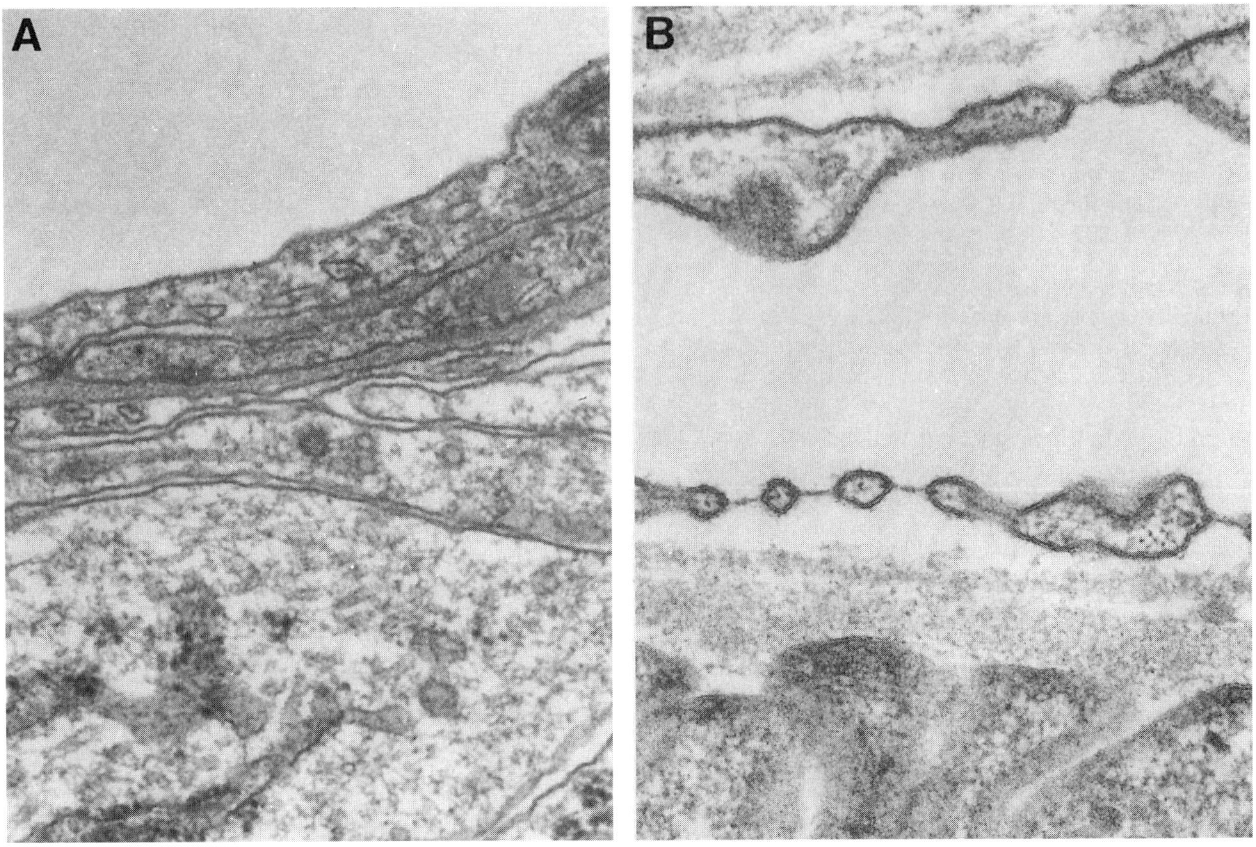

Fig. 1-1. Transverse section of **A.** continuous capillary endothelial cell from mouse brain and **B.** fenestrated endothelial cell from mouse peritubular capillaries. (Photographs kindly provided by Dr. A. J. Milici.)

cate that there may be several specific endothelial albumin receptors [34–36], with differential specificity for native versus modified albumin [36].

In response to local tissue injury or inflammation, additional transport pathways may become available. The mechanisms whereby this increase in permeability occurs are complex and also vary from one vascular bed to another. Endothelial cells in pericytic venules can contract, opening micron-wide gaps similar to those seen in fenestrated endothelium [38,39] and facilitate the extravasation of plasma proteins, up to 50-fold. Much of the leakage is localized to these venular gaps [38], and the conspicuous nature of these gaps initially led to the assumption that this is the only source of altered protein flux. However, augmented extravasation can occur in the absence of visible gaps [39], and increased permeability persists long after closure of the gaps [40,41]. In fenestrated vascular beds, changes in the number and the diameter of fenestrae may also contribute to increased permeability. A number of vasoactive mediators will directly increase permeability, including bradykinin, histamine, leukotrienes (LTC_4, LTD_4), reactive oxygen intermediates, and platelet activating factor (PAF). Other mediators, such as the prostaglandins PGI_2 and PGE_2, do not directly increase permeability, but by increasing blood flow they augment the permeability increases elicited by other mediators such as bradykinin. Cytokines such as interleukin-1 (IL-1), IL-2, and tumor necrosis factor (TNF) and endotoxins such as lipopolysaccharide (LPS) also increase vascular permeability through a variety of mechanisms, including increased production of vasoactive mediators and cytoskeletal rearrangements.

TRANSPORT AND METABOLISM

In organs such as the brain and the retina, the diffusion of solutes between the blood and the organ is highly restricted and is achieved by two principal features: (1) tight junctions between endothelial cells and (2) a paucity of pinocytotic vesicles. This anatomical barrier is fortified further by an enzymatic barrier, including aminopeptidases, choline esterases, butyrylcholine esterase, dihydrophenylalanine decarboxylase, gamma-glutamyltranspeptidase, monoamine oxidase, and 5′-nucleotidase. These activities are not unique to endothelial cells of the blood-brain barrier and may also be expressed in endothelial cells of other vascular beds. Specific transporters for the uptake and export of glucose, albumin, adenosine, amino acids, and other macromolecules provide a means for transcytosis and may be differentially expressed in different vascular beds [42–48]. Endothelial cells can methylate histamine to its competitive inhibitor, methylhistamine, or inactivate histamine by decarboxylation [49]. Adenosine triphosphate (ATP) is rapidly catabolized by vascular endothelial ectonucleotidases: adenosinetriphosphatase (ATPase), adenosinediphosphatase (ADPase), and 5′ nucleotidase. These ectoenzymes can thus sequentially hydrolyze ATP to adenosine and thus terminate the actions of ATP and adenosine diphosphate (ADP) [50,51]. Adenosine is removed by a specific uptake mechanism also expressed by vascular endothelial cells [47,48].

Angiotensin-I converting enzyme (ACE), (dipeptidyl dipeptidase A) is widely distributed in the circulation both as an endothelial ectoenzyme and in a soluble plasma form. The two principle substrates of ACE are angiotensin I (Ang I) and bradykinin [52,53]. ACE converts Ang I to the vasopressor and aldosterone-stimulating peptide Ang II by removal of a carboxyterminal dipeptide. By the cleavage of two carboxy terminal peptides from bradykinin, ACE suppresses the biologic effects of this peptide. The circulating form of ACE is found at relatively high concentrations (10^{-9} M) [54]; however, the membrane-bound endothelial enzyme is thought to be the most important contributor to blood pressure regulation [54,55]. In view of the high circulating and local ACE concentrations, it has been speculated that bradykinin might be generated locally, on the surface of endothelial cells. High-molecular-weight (HMW) kininogen, the precursor to bradykinin, can bind human vascular endothelial cells in a specific and saturable manner [56], although the nature of the HMW kininogen receptor has not been elucidated at this time. It has been speculated that vascular endothelium is normally saturated with HMW kininogen, allowing for the local generation of bradykinin by plasma or tissue kallikreins. Neutral endopeptidase (NEP) is another important endothelial peptidase, responsible for the degradation of a number of vasoactive peptides, including atrial natriuretic peptide, substance P, and enkephalins [57,58].

ADHESION PROTEINS AND CYTOSKELETAL ANCHOR PROTEINS

Because of their anatomic location as a blood-tissue interface, endothelial cells have the potential for differential adhesive interactions on their apical, lateral, and basal surfaces. Apical adhesion proteins mediate interactions with circulating blood cells and are discussed in detail in the section "Integrated Responses to Stress and Injury," later in this chapter. Lateral adhesive proteins mediate endothelial cell–endothelial cell interactions, playing important roles in the regulation of permeability to macromolecules as well as the egress of cells from blood to tissue. The basal adhesion proteins, that is, integrins, play a critical role in the adhesion of endothelial cells to the underlying basement membranes and are important in endothelial migration, proliferation, realignment, and responses to physical forces.

Lateral Adhesive Proteins. A number of junction-associated proteins have been identified, including cluster designation (CD) 31 (platelet-endothelial cell adhesion molecule, or PECAM) [59,60], E- and V-cadherins [61-63], integrins $\alpha_2\beta_1$ and $\alpha_5\beta_1$, and zona occludins (ZO-1) [64–66]. Elevations in cyclic adenosine 5′-monophosphate (cAMP) correlate with a decreased junctional permeability and increased electrical resistance [64], suggesting that cAMP protein kinase may phosphorylate one or more proteins associated with the tight junction. Addition of antibodies to $\alpha_2\beta_1$ or $\alpha_5\beta_1$ will disrupt the monolayer integrity and create large gaps, implying roles for integrins in the regulation of permeability and also in the diapedesis of leukocytes from blood to tissue. Cadherins, a family of transmembrane glycoproteins characterized by an extracellular domain with characteristic repeat sequences, a transmembrane domain, and a highly conserved cytoplasmic domain, bind cells via homotypic interactions in a Ca^{++} dependent manner. The cytoplasmic domain of cadherins, which associates with catenins and with actin, is crucial for binding. Recent studies suggest that cadherin-mediated adhesion is required for the development of other cell-to-cell interactions, such as the formation of gap junctions and the organization of the cytoskeleton [67]. Gap junctions between neighboring endothelial cells comprise hexameric assemblies of connexins in the plasma membranes of adjacent cells. The intercellular channels thus formed are permeable to small molecules (<1200–2000 Daltons) and are believed to play an important role in cell-to-cell communication. Gap-junctional communication has been demonstrated to occur in situ and in vitro between endothelial cells and endothelial cells, pericytes, and vascular smooth muscle cells [68–70].

Basal Adhesive Proteins (Integrins). Integrins constitute a large family of heterodimeric proteins, expressed on virtually all cell types. Integrins comprise two noncovalently linked subunits, a larger alpha chain and a smaller beta chain. Each subunit is an integral membrane protein with a short cytoplasmic tail. A number of different alpha subunits (to date, 15) and beta subunits (to date, 8) have been identified, but different cell types assemble and express different alpha, beta complexes. The integrins identified in large-vessel- and microvessel-derived endothelial cells are listed in Table 1-1. The combination of alpha and beta

Table 1-1. Endothelial cell integrins

Subunit	In large vessels	In microvessels	Ligands
$\alpha_1\beta_1$	—	+	Laminin, collagen
$\alpha_2\beta_1$	+	+	Laminin, collagen fibronectin
$\alpha_3\beta_1$	+	+	Fibronectin, collagen, laminin
$\alpha_5\beta_1$	+	+	Fibronectin
$\alpha_6\beta_1$	+	+	Laminin
$\alpha_6\beta_4$	?	+	Unknown
$\alpha_v\beta_1$	?	+	Unknown
$\alpha_v\beta_3$	+	+	Vitronectin, fibrinogen, vWF, thrombospondin, laminin, thrombin
$\alpha_v\beta_5$	?	+	Vitronectin

subunits determines ligand specificity, although considerable redundancy is evident; for example $\alpha_2\beta_1$, $\alpha_3\beta_1$, $\alpha_5\beta_1$, and $\alpha_v\beta_3$ all bind to fibronectin. Although the reason for this redundancy is unknown, it may reflect requirements for multiple interactions or binding to distinct sites on the same ligand.

As evidenced by the ligands for the endothelial integrins shown in Table 1-1, these heterodimers play a major role in cell adhesion, spreading, and migration. For example, when endothelial cells initially attach to a substratum, the basal surface of the cell makes focal contacts with the substrate [71]. Integrins cluster at these sites of focal contacts [72,73], although the type of integrins that organize in these adhesion plaques is dictated by the composition of the substratum. For example, if the substratum is vitronectin, $\alpha_v\beta_3$ accumulates; if fibronectin, only $\alpha_5\beta_1$ clusters [71].

Matrix adhesion is a requirement for the proliferation and survival of endothelial cells, and high cell density leads to growth arrest. Although the molecular mechanisms for adhesion-mediated signal transduction are unknown, the various molecules associated with the cytoplasmic domains of these adhesions (actin, alpha-actinin, paxillin, talin, vinculin) and tyrosine kinases (e.g., p125 focal adhesion kinase) are thought to be critical in this process [74]. The various junctional receptors at the adherens' junction bind and locally immobilize enzymes involved in signal transduction and their substrates; the assembly of the adherens' junction (or focal adhesion plaque) is required to bring the entities together. The clustering of various receptor tyrosine kinases could lead to cross-phosphorylation and activation of other elements in the signal transduction cascade. In endothelial cells, early responses of integrin binding to extracellular matrix have been shown to be similar to those triggered by growth factors, for example, calcium flux, cytoplasmic alkalinization, and protein tyrosine phosphorylation [75,76]. Another mechanism for altered integrin-ligand affinity is the induction of a conformational change in the external domain; this mechanism has been demonstrated in the platelet, where platelet activators induce GPIIb-IIIa ($\alpha_{IIb}\beta_3$) binding to fibrinogen (reviewed in [74]), and in the leukocyte, where various immune or inflammatory mediators activate $beta_2$ integrins (reviewed in [77]).

Hemostasis and Hemostatic Effectors

As the single-cell-thick lining of the circulatory system, the vascular endothelium constitutes a functionally dynamic focal interface. Anticoagulant, procoagulant, and fibrinolytic activities must be integrated to prevent coagulation and maintain blood fluidity, yet they also must rapidly respond to injury to prevent blood loss. The nonthrombogenic nature of vessel walls was originally thought to be a result of a passive role of the "nonreactive" endothelial cells. The efforts of many investigators have led to the demonstration that endothelial cells actively participate in the processes of hemostasis as a source or a site of anticoagulant, antiplatelet, procoagulant, platelet-activating, and fibrinolytic activities (Table 1-2). These activities are counterbalanced such that the hemostatic/thrombotic lever normally tips toward the antithrombotic activities contributing to blood fluidity. However, an important physiologic role of the endothelial cell is the ability to rapidly shift the balance to the prothrombotic side, activating coagulation factors leading to the generation of fibrin and to platelet adhesion. It is important that this shift in balance is limited to the site of injury, thus not allowing the coagulation process to be disseminated downstream.

Table 1-2. Properties of endothelial cells contributing to hemostasis

Hemostasis	
Anticoagulant activities	**Procoagulant activities**
Thrombomodulin	Tissue factor
Antithrombin III	Factor V
Protein C	von Willebrand factor
Protein S	Factor IX
Protease nexin	Factor X
Heparan sulfate	Factor XIII
Tissue factor pathway inhibitor	Thrombospondin
Antiplatelet activities	**Platelet-activating activities**
PGI_2, PGE_2	Platelet-activating factor
Endothelial-derived relaxing factor	von Willebrand factor
13-Hydroxyoctadeanoic acid	Subendothelial matrix
Fibrinolysis	
Fibrinolytic activities	**Antifibrinolytic activities**
Urokinase	Plasminogen activator inhibitor-1
Tissue plasminogen activator	Protease nexin

ANTICOAGULANTS

Thrombomodulin. Thrombomodulin is an intrinsic 65-kDa membrane glycoprotein, found on most endothelial cells, trophoblasts, some tumor cells, and some megakaryocytes. Thrombomodulin is not present on endothelium in lymph-node postcapillary high endothelial venules, sinusoidal capillaries of the liver, or cerebral microvessels [78]. Human umbilical-vein endothelial cells have been reported to express 30,000–100,000 thrombomodulin molecules/cell accounting for 50–60 percent of the thrombin-binding sites on the endothelial-cell surface [79]. Thrombomodulin has dramatic inhibitory influences on thrombin catalytic activity, converting thrombin from a procoagulant to an anticoagulant protease. By a high-affinity interaction between thrombin and the endothelial-cell surface, thrombomodulin effectively removes thrombin from solution and concentrates it on the surface of endothelial cells downstream from the site of an injury. Additionally, after binding thrombin, the thrombomodulin-thrombin complex is internalized, enabling the degradation of thrombin; the thrombomodulin is recycled to the cell surface [79]. Thrombomodulin also initiates reactions that prevent further activation of the coagulation system by altering thrombin substrate specificity, leading to the activation of protein C [80]. Thrombomodulin activity is suppressed by hypoxia, LPS, IL-1, and TNF [81–83], most likely by suppression of transcription [84]. It is of interest to note that these same stimuli increase tissue-factor activity (see coagulation). Homocysteine, an atherogenic and thrombotic stimulus, also inhibits thrombomodulin surface expression and protein C activation [85]. The complementary DNA (cDNA) for thrombomodulin has been cloned, and the gene for thrombomodulin has been mapped to chromosome 20. Thrombomodulin is structurally homologous to the low-density lipoprotein (LDL) receptor [86] with a lectin-like N-terminal region of 223 amino acids [87], a cysteine-rich EGF-like domain (residues 238–481), followed by a serine-threonine-rich region (residues 481–516) with O-linked sugars, a transmembrane domain (amino acids 517–537), and a short cytoplasmic tail of 38 amino acids. The protein C–activating cofactor activity resides in the last three EGF-like domains [88,89], while the glycosylated regions of thrombomodulin may modulate substrate specificity [90].

Protein C. Protein C is a vitamin-K-dependent protein synthesized by the liver. The protein-C pathway comprises two steps: (1) zymogen activation followed by (2) protease inactivation by cellular or plasma inhibitors. Activation of protein C by the thrombin-thrombomodulin complex is divalent cation dependent, with Ca^{++} as the most effective cation [90]. Interestingly, in the absence of thrombomodulin, Ca^{++} inhibits protein-C activation by thrombin [91]. Thrombin-thrombomodulin increases the rate of protein-C activation approximately 20,000-fold. Protein C inactivates factors Va and VIIIa by proteolytic cleavage of the heavy-chain subunits [92–95]. The critical role of protein C in vivo is exemplified by the severe and often fatal thrombotic disorders associated with protein-C deficiency [96–99].

Protein S. Protein S, also a vitamin-K-dependent protein, is another component of the endothelial anticoagulant armamentarium. Although protein S has no known enzymatic activity, it acts as a cofactor, binding activated protein C to phospholipid at a 1 : 1 stoichiometry and greatly accelerating the rate of inactivation of factors Va and VIIIa. Factor Va bound to factor Xa appears to be protected from inactivation by protein C, although the protective effect is lost in the presence of protein S [100,101]. Protein S is synthesized and secreted by endothelial cells, binding to the surface of endothelial cells, where it forms a macromolecular complex with protein C. Protein C is inactivated by a circulating plasma protein inhibitor [102].

Antithrombin III. Antithrombin III provides another important endothelial-dependent protective mechanism that limits the hemostatic plug-forming activity of thrombin. Antithrombin III is a 58-kDa serine protease normally present in plasma that inactivates thrombin as well as the coagulation factors IXa, VIIa, and Xa. Although antithrombin III itself can inhibit thrombin, this activity is dramatically accelerated by binding to heparan sulfate (HS) present on the endothelial-cell surface or the subendothelial matrix [103–107].

Protease Nexin. Protease nexin, a 40-kDa protease inhibitor secreted by endothelial cells [108–109] inactivates thrombin by forming a covalent complex, a complex whose formation is greatly accelerated by endothelial and subendothelial HS [110]. Bound thrombin–protease nexin complex is internalized and subjected to lysosomal degradation [108,111]. Protease nexin also binds and inactivates plasmin [111].

Glycosaminoglycans. Endothelial cells contain, as do all adherent cells, glycosaminoglycans at the cell surface, the most ubiquitous of which is HS. Structurally related to the more familiar heparin, HS has been implicated in diverse cellular processes, primarily because of the well-characterized inhibitory effects of heparin on morphogenesis, retroviral replication, cell growth, and coagulation. HS proteoglycans can interact via their core proteins with inositol phosphate [112] or putative receptors [113], whereas integral HS proteoglycans are bound to the cell surface via linkage with membrane phospholipids [114]. Transmembrane HS proteoglycans include the syndecan family, betaglycan, and CD 44 [115–117]. Endothelial cells have been shown to express syndecans 1 and 4 as well as CD 44 [118–120]. On endothelial cells, heparin-like glycosaminoglycans promote anticoagulation by interacting with proteases of the intrinsic coagulation cascade and thrombin, as well as with protein C and serpins (including antithrombin III) [120,121]. A specific pentasaccharide sequence found in HS binds to antithrombin III, facilitating the formation of an enzymatically inactive complex with several coagulation enzymes [121]. As discussed previously, a similar interaction also occurs with protease nexins.

The properties of HS isoforms with anticoagulant activity exhibit heterogeneity between vascular endothelial cells of diverse sites; for example, rat-fat-pad microvascular endothelial cells produce 5- to 10-fold more anticoagulant HS than do bovine aortic endothelial cells [118]. While only a small proportion of total HS, anticoagulant HS is preferentially localized to the abluminal surface [118].

Tissue Factor Pathway Inhibitor. Tissue factor pathway inhibitor (TFPI) is a novel Kunitz-type of coagulation inhibitor. Initially identified as a serum-derived inhibitor of tissue factor in 1947 [120,121], TFPI was later isolated and identified as a single protein [122,123]. TFPI inhibits tissue factor activity in a two-step manner: TFPI first binds to and inactivates factor Xa [124,125]; the TFPI-FXa complex in turn binds to and inhibits the activity of the tissue factor–factor VIIa complex [122,123,126,127]. TFPI, as predicted from the cDNA sequence, is a protein of 276 amino acids, with a molecular weight of 32 kDa, and comprises an acidic amino terminal, three Kunitz-type inhibitory domains, and a basic carboxy terminus [128,129]. Endothelial cells [130], monocytic cells [131], and a number of transformed cells [132] have been reported to produce TFPI. Cultured endothelial cells constitutively produce TFPI, and stimulation with thrombin, TNF, IL-1, or endotoxin results in little or no increase in TFPI synthesis [133–135]. Together, the endothelium, plasma, and platelets make up the three major intravascular pools of TFPI. Heparin injection releases the intravascular, predominantly endothelial, pool of TFPI, resulting in levels 2 to 10 times the amount in normal plasma [136]. Immunohistochemical studies of normal tissue have demonstrated TFPI in megakaryocytes and in the endothelium of capillaries and of venules, but not in large blood vessels [137].

INHIBITORS OF PLATELET FUNCTION

Platelets provide a first line of defense to vascular injury by adhering to the subendothelium, aggregating, and stimulating further platelet recruitment. However, endothelial cells are normally nonthrombogenic with at least three thromboprotective mechanisms: eicosanoids, endothelial-derived relaxing factor (EDRF), and ectonucleotidase / ADPase.

Several products (eicosanoids) of arachidonic acid metabolism contribute to antiplatelet activity. PGI_2 (prostacyclin), the major eicosanoid produced by most large-vessel-derived endothelial cells [138,139], is a strong inhibitor of platelet activation, shape change, aggregation, and adhesion [140–142]. The inhibitory activities of PGI_2 mediated via activation of specific G-protein-linked platelet membrane receptors lead to increased formation of cAMP [143,144]. In contrast, PGE_2, a major prostanoid produced by most microvascular endothelial cells [145,146], is a poor inhibitor of platelet aggregation. PGI_2 and PGE_2 production can be rapidly increased in an acute, protein synthesis–independent manner by agonists such as ATP / ADP, PAF, histamine, leukotrienes C_4 and D_4, thrombin, and bradykinin [146–153]. Moreover, cytokines and growth factors can greatly increase the capacity of endothelial cells to synthesize eicosanoids, probably by inducing cyclooxygenase II, a novel inducible PGG / H synthase [154–159]. Greater quantities of prostanoid production also may be facilitated by the process of transcellular metabolism. For example, platelet-derived PGH_2 can be converted to PGI_2 when platelets and endothelial cells are co-incubated [160,161].

The rapid release of PGI_2 and PGE_2 by most agonists is mediated by a Ca^{++} dependent acylhydrolase (probably phospholipase A_2, although other phospholipases may be involved, depending on the stimulus and the source of the endothelial cell) culminating in the release of arachidonic acid from membrane phospholipids. Arachidonate is then metabolized by one or more pathways, depending on the cellular milieu: cyclooxygenase, leading to prostanoid production; lipoxygenase, resulting in the formation of various hydroxyeicosatetaraenoic acids (HETEs); or cytochrome P450, leading to the formation of epoxide and diHETEs. Transcellular metabolism can also lead to additional products; for example, LTA_4 (which could be supplied by various granulocytes) can be metabolized by endothelial cells to LTC_4 and LTD_4 [162,163]. Another inhibitor of platelet adhesion, aggregation, and thromboxane production is 13-hydroxyoctadeanoic acid (13-HODE), an endothelial lipoxygenase metabolite of linoleic acid (18 : 2) [164,165]. 13-HODE is found in granular structures of cultured EC and also has been reported to be localized to the subendothelial basement membrane in vivo [166,167].

PROCOAGULANT ACTIVITIES

Tissue Factor. The predominant procoagulant expressed by a variety of cells is tissue factor (TF), a protein embedded in the phospholipid bilayer. Normal endothelial cells express little or no TF activity [168–171], although TF is present on the surface of pericytes and fibroblasts and thus is revealed at sites of vascular damage [172–174]. Perturbation of endothelial cells by various agents, including endotoxin, thrombin, interferon-γ (IFN-γ), IL-1, hypoxia, TNF, or bacterial cell walls, results in an induction of TF and subsequent activation of the procoagulant pathway [83,172,174–180].

TF has been cloned and sequenced [181–183] and can occur as a 261- or 263-amino acid polypeptide chain, depending on the site of cleavage of a leader peptide. With the exception of a 21-residue cytoplasmic tail and a 22-residue transmembrane domain, the remainder of the molecule is located on the outer surface of the membrane. TF exposure, whether because of disruption of the endothelial cell barrier or an induced expression on an activated endothelial cell, results in binding of plasma factor VII to TF. Factor VII is activated to factor VIIa by factor Xa, a reaction that occurs only when factor VII is bound to TF and that is accelerated by factors VIII and IX. Factor VIIa functions as a physiological enzyme bound to TF, where it in turn activates two substrates, factors X and IX (reviewed in [184,185]).

Prothrombin and Factor V. Prothrombin activation by factor Xa is accelerated by factor V, a product of endothelial cells [186] and hepatocytes [187]. Endothelial production of factor V is increased by mechanical injury [188]. In addition to producing factor V, endothelial cells also bind factor V (K_D 2 nM, Bmax 20,000–25,000 molecules / cells), and the bound factor V is active in coagulation assays [189,190].

Von Willebrand Factor. Von Willebrand factor (vWF) is a large multimeric glycoprotein, produced by platelets and endothelial cells [191,192] that promotes platelet adhesion and thrombus formation at sites of vascular injury [193,194]. vWF also serves as a carrier for factor VIII in the blood. Endothelial cells demonstrate two pathways of vWF synthesis: constitutive and regulated [195]. The majority of vWF synthesized by endothelial cells is secreted via the constitutive pathway and occurs bidirectionally: luminally into the circulating blood and abluminally into the subendothelial matrix. The constitutively secreted vWF is dimeric, consisting of precursor vWF and mature subunits [196–198] and is synthesized at a steady-state rate not altered by stimulation [199]. Additionally, vWF is stored in granules, the rod-shaped Weibel Palade bodies [200,201] in endothelial cells, and the alpha granules in platelets and megakaryocytes. Weibel Palade bodies are unique to endothelium and presumably are derived from the Golgi apparatus. Weibel Palade bodies are not a universal feature of all endothelial cells, however; while frequent in endothelia of large veins, they may be rare or absent in endothelia of small arterioles and capillaries [202,203]. At the level of the electron microscope, Weibel Palade bodies appear as membrane-bound longitudinally oriented tubules; these tubules actually represent multimeric vWF organized in a longitudinal array. Regulated secretion of vWF occurs in response to agonists such as histamine, thrombin, and fibrin and is the result of release from the Weibel Palade bodies [204,205]. Short-term release of vWF also can be elicited by fibrin, glucose, complement, estradiol, irradiation, mechanical injury, calcium ionophores, and various cytokines, effects thought to reflect release of vWF from preformed stores in Weibel Palade bodies [204–211]. However, long-term exposure to IL-1, interferon-γ, phorbol myristate acetate, or thrombin reduces vWF synthesis, release, and incorporation into the extracellular matrix [212–214]. The vWF in Weibel Palade bodies consists of the largest multimeric species, which is relevant since the largest oligomers are the most effective in promoting platelet adhesion and aggregation. The large oligomers preferentially bind to the subendothelial matrix and fibrin [215,216].

vWF present in the subendothelial matrix or plasma vWF that is rapidly adsorbed onto exposed structures of a damaged vessel interacts with the GPIb-IX-V as well as with GPIIb-IIIa receptor on platelets, initiating platelet adhesion, signaling, and activation of the platelet GPIIb-IIIa complex [217–220]. This activated receptor complex promotes platelet spreading at sites of injury and irreversible adhesion. Additional platelets are recruited into the growing thrombus, a process mediated at least in part by circulating vWF and vWF acutely released in situ by platelets and endothelial cells.

Mature vWF subunits contain 2,050 amino acids and a variable number (as many as 22) carbohydrate side chains, such that the estimated carbohydrate content of vWF varies from 10–19 percent of the total mass (~278 kDa). The gene for vWF is approximately equal to 180 kilobases, contains 52 exons, and has been mapped to the tip of the short arm of chromosome 12 [221,222]. The high cysteine content of vWF plays an essential role in the linking of subunits of vWF into higher-order structures. In endothelial cells, after translation of the mRNA, pro-vWF undergoes extensive posttranslational processing, initiated by association of pro-vWF monomers to form dimers through intermolecular disulfide bridges within the carboxyl terminal region. This is subsequently followed by the association of dimers into higher-order structures linked through cysteine residues in the amino terminal domain [223]. The noncovalent association of vWF with the coagulation factor VIII is apparent after endothelial-derived vWF is released into the circulation. The principal sites of factor VIII synthesis are unknown at present, although mRNA for this factor has been detected in the liver, spleen, and kidney. Factor VIII and vWF are not co-localized, implicating association of the two proteins following release from the respective cells [224].

The physiological importance of vWF is demonstrated by the diminished platelet adhesion to subendothelium observed in patients with von Willebrand's disease [225], an abnormality that is corrected by exogenous vWF [226]. Desamino-[Arg^8]-vasopressin, used to treat mild to moderate von Willebrand's disease and hemophilia, stimulates the release of vWF into the subendothelial matrix, but not into the media [227]. A second, although antigenically unrelated protein, vWFII is also absent or deficient in patients with von Willebrand's disease [228]. vWFII is also synthesized by endothelial cells and is localized to the Weibel Palade bodies [229]. vWFII is a cleavage product of precursor vWF [230,231] and is cleaved after vWF multimerization and is thought to mediate vWF multimer assembly [232].

Factors IX and X. Endothelial cells bind both factor IXa and factor Xa in a specific, saturable manner [233–236]. Endothelial-bound factor IXa is more active than soluble factor IXa [233]. The binding of factors IXa and Xa serves to localize the coagulation process to the endothelial-cell surface and to reduce the circulating concentration of activated coagulation factors.

Thrombospondin. Thrombospondin (TSP) is a large (450-kDa) trimeric glycoprotein that can occur in a number of isoforms and that is secreted by many cell types, including endothelial cells [237–239]. TSP interacts with components of the extracellular matrix, proteins involved in coagulation and fibrinolysis, and integrins mediating cell-TSP interactions [237,238]. TSP has many proposed functions, including the promotion of smooth muscle-cell and fibroblast proliferation [240,241]. The actions of TSP on cell growth may be mediated by an EGF-like domain on the molecule [242] or may be due to TSP-bound growth factors such as TGF-β [243]. In view of its activities on cell migration and proliferation as well as immunohistochemical studies localizing TSP to wound sites [244–246], it is likely that TSP plays an important role in the wound-healing response.

TSP plays many roles in the coagulation process, including interacting with and acting as a substrate for factors IXa and Xa [247]. TSP forms complexes with fibrinogen and copolymerizes with fibrin in clots [248]. Platelet-bound TSP binds HMW kininogen, supporting procoagulant activities of the platelet [249]. TSP also supports second-phase platelet aggregation [250,251]. TSP plays a role in fibrinolysis, forming a ternary complex with plasminogen and tissue-type plasminogen activator (tPA), catalyzing the activation of plasminogen into plasmin [252,253]. In solution, TSP also acts as an inhibitor of urokinase (uPA) activation [254].

Platelet Activating Factor. Platelet activating factor (PAF) (1-O-alkyl-2-acetyl-sn-glycero-3-phosphocholine) was initially identified as a factor that stimulated platelet activation and aggregation. PAF was later shown to be a potent vasoactive agent as well as an activator of neutrophils [255] and made by many cell types, including neutrophils, macrophages, monocytes, mast cells, mesangial cells, eosinophils, basophils, and platelets. PAF is rapidly synthesized and expressed by stimulated endothelial cells, and surface expression of PAF plays an important role in the microcirculation, increasing vascular permeability and stimulating the adhesion of neutrophils [256].

Endothelial synthesis of PAF is not constitutive but occurs rapidly following stimulation with thrombin, bradykinin, histamine, ATP, LTC_4, LTD_4, oxidants, and bacterial toxins [257–261] and is inhibited by PGI_2 [262]. The "remodeling" pathway represents the predominant pathway for endothelial PAF synthesis [263]. Phospholipase A_2–mediated hydrolysis of the fatty acid from the sn-2 position of phosphatidylcholine containing a long-chain fatty alcohol ether linkage at the sn-1 position produces 1-O-alkyl-2-lyso-sn-glycero-3-phosphocholine. Active PAF is produced by subsequent alkylation at the sn-2 position by a specific acetylhydrolase. PAF is degraded by hydrolysis of the acetate from the sn-2 position mediated by PAF acetylhydrolase, a specific phospholipase A_2 [264]. The accumulation of PAF is transient, representing the balance between synthesis and degradation, and the time course of expression is agonist dependent [263].

Fibrinolysis

The temporary hemostatic plug formed to prevent blood loss at a site of vessel injury contains two principal structural elements: platelets and a cross-linked fibrin matrix. This plug also contains other large fibrous proteins, such as fibronectin, and provides a matrix for cells to invade the wound and to rebuild the tissue. A precise timing of fibrin matrix dissolution must occur in context with restoration of normal intact tissue. If the timing is too rapid, vascular leakage and bleeding will ensue; if too slow, scar tissue will form.

Lysis of fibrin is mediated by the protease plasmin which is cleaved from the zymogen plasminogen by plasminogen activators (PA). Endothelial cells synthesize two forms of PA: tPA (tissue type PA) and uPA (urokinase) [265–268]. Both uPA and tPA are highly specific serine proteinases that cleave plasminogen at the same peptide bond [269]. tPA requires a cofactor, such as fibrin, for its activity [253]. tPA has a high affinity for fibrin, but not fibrinogen. tPA and plasminogen both bind to fibrin, markedly lowering the K_m of tPA for plasminogen [270]. tPA also can function efficiently on TSP or histidine-rich glycoproteins [253].

tPA is present in plasma and can be isolated in one- and two-chain forms. Native tPA has a molecular radius approximately equal to 72 kDa and 527 amino acids [271]. Plasmin cleaves tPA into two distinct portions. A heavy chain (36 kDa) embodies the NH_2-terminal structure, two kringle domains, and an EGF domain. The light chain (32 kDa) originating from the COOH terminal contains the active-site region and demonstrates considerable homology with other serine proteases [272–276]. Double-chain tPA more actively cleaves plasminogen in the absence of fibrin [277], which may enable preferential plasminogen activation on the endothelial-cell surface.

In contrast to tPA, uPA has no affinity for fibrin [269]. Plasma uPA is found in two forms, 33 kDa and 54 kDa; the smaller form results from the larger via proteolytic processing [269,278,279]. Because of its lack of affinity for fibrin, uPA was long thought not to exhibit clot specificity. However, the single-chain form of uPA (sc-uPA) is dissociated from its inhibitor by fibrin and can, albeit inefficiently, activate plasminogen [280]. Plasmin formed from this initial reaction can convert scuPA into two-chain uPA, which is a more effective activator of plasminogen. The scuPA gene also demonstrates a growth factor domain, a kringle domain with high homology to the kringle structures in tPA and plasminogen, and an active-site domain [281]. The major role for endothelial-derived uPA is probably in the control of local extracellular matrix proteolysis and remodeling (see angiogenesis).

Regulation of the "fibrinolytic" system of endothelial cells is principally dependent on the plasminogen activation inhibitor (PAI) PAI-1 [282,283]. The roles for PAI-2 and protease nexin, although expressed in endothelial cells, are unclear at this time [284]. PAI-1 is a single-chain glycoprotein, Mr approximately equal to 50 kDa, and can selectively neutralize the activity of both uPA and tPA [285–287]. The cDNA for PAI-1 has been cloned and sequenced; mature PAI-1 is 379 amino acids and has approximately equal to 30 percent homology with alpha-1PI and antithrombin III [288–290]. The gene for PAI-1 maps to chromosome 7 [291]. PAI-1 forms a strong and rapid complex with tPA (K_D 10^{-13} M) [290]. An unusual feature of PAI-1 is its exceptional sensitivity to inactivation by oxidants [290,291]. In conditioned media and purified forms, PAI-1 is present primarily in an inactive form. PAI-1 can be activated by denaturants such as sodium dodecyl sulfate, guanidine HCl, and urea, probably as a result of a conformational change in the molecule [286,290,292]. In view of the recognized role of surfaces in coagulation and fibrinolysis, it is possible that a biologic surface may act as the equivalent of the denaturant required for PAI-1 activation. Cultured endothelial cells secrete PAI-1 bidirectionally, that is, into the medium and the underlying subendothelium. Vitronectin, present in the subendothelial matrix, binds and stabilizes PAI-1 [293,294]. PAI-1 plays other roles in hemostasis in addition to inhibition of PAs. For example, PAI-1 inactivates factor XIa [295] and, by forming a complex with Protein C, loses inhibitory activity [296–298]. PAI-2 is a more effective inhibitor of uPA than tPA, but most endothelial PAI-2 is nonglycosylated and not secreted. IL-1α and TNFα upregulate endothelial-cell-associated PAI-2 levels [299]. PAI-2 may be released from damaged endothelial cells.

The balance of tPA and PAI-1 activity expressed by endothelial cells can be modulated by a number of mediators central to hemostasis. Thrombin, for example, increases both tPA and PAI-1 expression [300–303]. Other stimuli (histamine; shear stress; basic fibroblast growth factor, or bFGF; bradykinin; PAF) seem to be more selective in increasing tPA production than PAI-1 [304–306]. Cytokines such as endotoxin, IL-1, and TNF-α as well as TGF-β reduce tPA expression while increasing PAI-1 expression [307–313]. Treatment of endothelial cells with lipoprotein (a), a low-density lipoprotein-like particle associated with atherosclerosis, also selectively induces an increase in PAI-1 [314]. These observations clearly indicate that, under most circumstances, tPA regulation and PAI-1 expression in endothelial cells are not interdependent.

Plasmin-generating systems may assemble on the endothelial cell surface, facilitating formation of the active protease. Plasminogen (PLG) binds to endothelial cells and in so doing is converted to a truncated noncirculating form (Lys-PLG) following the proteolytic cleavage of 76 amino acids from the N-terminus [315]. Lys-PLG is 10- to 120-fold more efficiently activated by uPA or tPA [316,317], providing an explanation for the observation that the efficiency of plasmin generation at the cell surface is 12-fold greater than the same reaction in the fluid phase [318,319]. On human endothelial cells, a 40-kDa protein has been identified that specifically binds plasminogen or tPA (but not uPA) [320–323]. This receptor may act to colocalize enzyme and substrate in a manner that enhances the efficiency of plasmin activation. Studies of tPA binding to human umbilical-vein endothelial cells has demonstrated two binding sites, one of high affinity (K_D 29 pM) and one of lower affinity (K_D 18 nM) [324]. The high-affinity binding site may represent matrix-associated PAI-1 [325], whereas the lower-affinity binding site appears to have a separate binding domain for plasminogen [323].

Regulation of Vascular Tone

Endothelial cells play multiple roles in the regulation of vascular tone, activating or inactivating various circulating vasoactive substances and serving as a source of numerous local as well as systemic vasodilator and vasoconstrictor mediators. The metabolic roles of the endothelial cell were discussed in the subsection "Transport and Metabolism."

VASODILATORS

Eicosanoids. PGI_2 (prostacyclin) is a potent vasodilator and its principal source is the endothelial cell [138,326,327]. Endothelial cells also synthesize other vasoactive eicosanoids (e.g., PGE_2 and PGD_2); these products may act as vasodilators or vasoconstrictors, depending on the dose, the vascular bed, and the species tested. The agonists that elicit prostanoid release from endothelial cells were discussed in the subsection "Inhibitors of Platelet Function." In addition to the vasodilator and antiplatelet activities of PGI_2, this prostanoid also exhibits potent "cytoprotective" effects, down-regulates tissue factor expression, and increases smooth muscle cholesterol ester metabolism [reviewed in 328].

Endothelial-Derived Relaxing Factor. Initially identified as a labile, endothelial-derived relaxing factor (EDRF) [329] mediates the vasorelaxant effects of acetylcholine. Subsequent studies have shown that EDRF is either nitric oxide (NO) or a labile nitroso-compound [330–335] produced from L-arginine by NO-synthase. Several NO-synthases have been cloned and sequenced, resulting in the identification of at least three distinct NO-synthase genes. In endothelial cells, both a soluble and a particulate isoform of NO synthase are present [336]. The endothelial forms of NO synthase are constitutive and regulated by calcium and calmodulin. A variety of agonists can elicit EDRF release, including acetylcholine, bradykinin, calcium ionophores, adenine nucleotides, thrombin, substance P, neurokinins, vasopressin, oxytocin, uridine triphosphate (UTP), histamine, and $PGF_{2\alpha}$, although the responsiveness to this list of agonists exhibits some heterogeneity between vascular endothelial cells derived from different species and vascular beds. EDRF/NO has a number of important biological functions. NO activates soluble guanylate cyclase, leading to an increase in cyclic guanosine monophosphate (cGMP) levels [337], a mechanism responsible for vascular smooth muscle relaxing [330–338] and platelet aggregation [339] and adhesion [340] inhibitory effects of this mediator. EDRF/NO may also play a role in the regulation of neutrophil chemotaxis [341] and in the inhibition of vascular smooth muscle proliferation [342]. It also has been suggested that NO may serve as a physiological scavenger to cytotoxic superoxide anions continuously produced from all cells [343–345].

Endothelial-Derived Hyperpolarizing Factor. Endothelial-derived hyperpolarizing factor (EDHF) is an as yet unidentified EDRF that causes hyperpolarization of vascular smooth muscle. Initially described as an endothelium-dependent membrane hyperpolarizing factor elicited by acetylcholine in guinea pig mesenteric arteries [346], EDHF activity was later described in a number of isolated artery and vein preparations [347]. Although EDHF activity often co-occurs with agonists that release EDRF, this is not always the case [348]. It is unlikely that NO is the EDHF, because exogenous NO does not hyperpolarize most vascular smooth muscle preparations [349–359]. Furthermore, inhibitors of L-arginine-NO production (nitro-L-arginine, hemoglobin, methylene blue) do not reduce EDHF activity despite effectively inhibiting EDRF activity [352–358].

EDHF activity can be transferred in bioassay experiments [353,359,360], supporting the contention that EDHF is a soluble factor of endothelial origin. EDHF activity is not blocked by inhibitors of cyclooxygenase [353], indicating that EDHF probably is not a prostanoid. EDHF appears to act by activation of K^+ channels, although the subtype activated is not clear at this time [348,351,353,361–363].

VASOCONSTRICTORS

Endothelin. Endothelin was initially described as a slow-developing, long-lasting vasoconstrictor substance present in the conditioned media of bovine aortic endothelial cells [364]. The factor was later isolated, purified, and identified to be a 21-amino-acid peptide-termed endothelin [365]. Endothelin contains two intrachain disulfide bonds and is part of a larger family of vasoconstrictor peptides, the products of three distinct genes: endothelin ET-1, ET-2, and ET-3. ET-1 is found primarily in endothelium, whereas ET-2 and ET-3 are present in nonvascular tissues [366]. Like most peptides, ET-1 is processed from a larger (203-amino-acid) precursor (prepro-ET-1) through the formation of a 38- or 39-residue intermediate form called "Big ET-1." Big ET-1 is then further processed to the mature ET-1 by an unusual proteolytic cleavage between tryptophan (Trp) 21 and valine (Val) 22 residues by a putative enzyme, "endothelial converting enzyme" [365]. Big ET-1 has only one one-hundredth the potency of ET-1, but it is rapidly converted to ET-1 in the presence of endothelial cells or when administered in vivo [367,368]. Very little ET-1 or Big ET-1 can be identified intracellularly in endothelial cells, which suggests that ET-1 is synthesized constitutively and not stored [369]. A variety of stimuli can stimulate ET-1 production, including interleukin-1, thrombin, TGF-β, phorbol esters, calcium ionophores, arginine vasopressin, hypoxia, and shear stress

[370–373], although the detection of stimulated levels requires 3 to 6 hours, consistent with alterations in gene expression. Endothelins bind to cell-surface receptors in a rapid, specific, and saturable manner, although the dissociation rate is slow. The major signal-transduction systems appear to involve inositol 1,4,5-triphosphate and diacyglycerol generation, intracellular second messengers that can in turn activate processes such as the release of Ca^{++} from intracellular stores, enzyme activation, and cellular contractile mechanisms. Endothelins also influence the opening of ion channels, membrane potential, and the influx of Na^{+} and Ca^{++} [374–377]. Two ET receptors have been identified: ET_A, which exhibits a higher affinity for ET-1 than ET-3, and ET_B, which is nonselective [378,379]. Endothelins can contract all types of smooth muscle, but they may also relax some, either directly via activation of receptors or indirectly by releasing relaxing factors such as EDRF and eicosanoids [380–383]. Endothelins are also potent mitogens [384].

Endothelial-Derived Contractile Factors. Vascular endothelial cells can produce other vasoconstrictor substances, including angiotensin II and possibly other cyclooxygenase products or superoxide anion [385].

Integrated Responses to Stress and Injury

In addition to the regulation of the responses to injury though various functional alterations in the components contributing to hemostasis, permeability, and vascular tone, the endothelial cell integrates other important, complex, and interdependent processes. The endothelial cell alters the expression of various adhesion proteins that facilitate leukocyte rolling, adhesion, and diapedesis; produces chemotactic factors for neutrophils, monocytes, and lymphocytes; and synthesizes cytokines and growth factors modulating the proliferation of leukocytes, fibroblasts, and smooth muscle cells. Additionally, the endothelial cell contributes to wound healing through processes involving the synthesis and remodeling of matrix components and angiogenesis.

ENDOTHELIAL CELL STRESS AND INJURY

Endothelial cells sense and respond to both biomechanical and humoral sources of stress; extreme or prolonged exposure to either or both may lead to chronic changes in endothelial gene expression, morphology, and function.

Mechanical Stress. Although virtually all cell types can sense and respond to mechanical stress, the vascular endothelium is functionally unique. In addition to pressure, stretch, and associated mechanical forces, endothelial cells also are continuously exposed to fluid shear stresses. The functional role of endothelial responses to mechanical stress is demonstrated by the endothelial-dependent alterations in vascular tone in response to acute changes in blood flow and in vascular wall-cell and matrix composition in response to chronic changes in blood flow.

Studies with cultured endothelial cells have facilitated understanding of both acute and chronic responses of the endothelium to mechanical forces. Acute changes in shear stress, for example, can elicit K^{+} channel activation and hyperpolarization [386]; elevations in inositol triphosphate [387] and intracellular Ca^{++} [388–390]; decreases in intracellular pH [391]; and release of PGI_2 [392,393], endothelin [371], tPA [394], and EDRF [395]. Longer-term responses to shear stress include induction of platelet-derived growth factor (PDGF) [396], tPA [397], tissue factor [398], and intercellular adhesion molecule-1 (ICAM-1) [399]. Exposure to shear stress, cyclic strain, or hydrostatic pressure induces rearrangement of cell cytoskeletal elements and focal contacts [400–404]. Exposure of endothelial cells to mechanical forces such as hydrostatic pressure can also elicit the release of autocrine growth factors and stimulate cell proliferation [404].

How the endothelial cell perceives and transduces mechanical forces is not clear; however, cytoskeletal elements must play a central role. F-actin microfilaments are one likely candidate; indeed, disruption of actin microfilaments inhibits adenylate-cyclase activation and ion-channel activation elicited by stretch [405]. The redistribution of focal-adhesion plaques, cell-shape change, and realignment in the direction of flow are all inhibited by drugs that disrupt microfilaments. The microfilaments, through their network of connections to focal adhesions, intercellular adhesion proteins, integral membrane proteins of the integrin family, and the nuclear membrane, are ideally positioned to confer tension to the cell and to act as mechanotransducers at diverse sites within the cell. As already discussed in the subsection "Adhesion Proteins and Cytoskeletal Anchor Proteins," the integrins are also an important source of biochemical signals.

Recent studies have identified a shear-stress response element (SSRE) in the promoter of a number of genes (ICAM, PDGF, IL-8, NOS, MCP-1) whose expression is altered by shear stress [406]. This element has been demonstrated to be functional for PDGF expression [406]. The corresponding transactivating proteins have not been elucidated at this time.

Reactive Oxygen Intermediates (ROIs). Oxidant-induced endothelial injury can follow exposure of endothelial cells to oxidants such as hyperoxia, peroxides, or free radical species, which in turn can produce peroxidation of membrane lipids, oxidation of protein sulfhydryl groups, DNA damage, altered membrane fluidity, and cytoskeletal protein derangements. Protection from oxidant-induced stress is achieved by various intracellular and extracellular mechanisms, including various scavenger pathways and alterations in gene expression, although the precise nature of the response probably depends on the ROI species and the endothelial-cell type. Oxidant stress, modeled with tert-butyl hydroperoxide results in altered Ca^{++} signaling, inhibiting agonist-stimulated Ca^{++} influx and release of Ca^{++} from intracellular stores, as well as initiating a progressive increase in resting Ca^{++} [407].

Endothelial cells, like virtually all aerobic cells, generate a constitutive flux of superoxide anions, hydrogen peroxide, and perhaps hydroxyl radicals through both enzymatic and nonenzymatic reactions. Additionally, cytokines such as TNF and IL-1 and tumor promoters can increase the production of ROIs in endothelial and other cells [408–412]. Normally the abundant antioxidant defense mechanisms prevent the ROIs from causing cell injury. However, exposure of endothelial cells to cytokines or cytokine combinations, proteinases, neutrophil-derived ROIs, or oxidized lipids may result in a rate of formation of ROIs that exceeds the capacity of the antioxidant defense. For example, reduced glutathione (GSH) is an important scavenger of ROIs; however, cytokines such as TNF can reduce intracellular GSH levels [413].

An important response to oxidative stress is the increase in the cellular capacity to prevent O_2^- toxicity, and at least one major ROI-scavenging pathway is altered by cytokines and ROIs. Superoxide dismutases (SOD) are metalloenzymes that accelerate the dismutation of O_2^- to H_2O_2 and O_2. In endothelial cells, two forms have been described: a cytosolic Cu,Zn-SOD and a mitochondrial Mn-SOD. TNF-α and IL-1 have been reported to selectively induce endothelial Mn-SOD messenger RNA (mRNA) without affecting the levels of Cu,Zn-SOD, catalase, or GSH peroxidase mRNA [414–418]. However, measurements of Cu,Zn-SOD protein levels indicate that the levels of this enzyme may exhibit a delayed increase (>24 hours) following exposure to ROIs, endotoxins, TNF, or IL-1 [419].

ROIs may play a pivotal role in the adaptive responses of endothelial cells to various stimuli, including cytokines, ischemia-reperfusion, and ultraviolet radiation. It is now recognized that these diverse stimuli activate a similar profile of endothelial stress-related genes [420]. Common elements in the promoter regions of these genes include putative sites for the transcription factors NF-κB and AP-1. Cytokines and ROIs have been shown to activate NF-κB in endothelial cells [421,422]. Antioxidants will inhibit cytokine-stimulated vascular cell adhesion molecule-1 (VCAM-1) expression in endothelial cells [422], and it has been suggested that VCAM-1 expression is regulated by NF-κB [420–422,423]. Activation of NF-κB is strongly inhibited by N-acetyl cysteine (which directly inactivates oxidants and increases intracellular GSH) [424–426] and other thiols [427–429].

ENDOTHELIAL CELL RESPONSES TO INJURY

Leukocyte-Endothelial Interactions. Our current understanding of leukocyte interactions with the vessel wall has a history that can be traced back as far as 1839, when Rudolph Wagner [430] first used the technique of intravital microscopy to study leukocyte behavior in vivo. Cohnheim [431] was the first to document the behavior of leukocytes in induced inflammation in vivo describing several different adhesive states of leukocyte activity in the microvasculature: no detectable interactions with the vessel surface, slow rolling along the vessel walls, firm adhesion, and diapedesis into the vascular space. In that early study, Cohnheim postulated that these phenomena were due to molecular changes on the vessel surface. Today, more than a century later, many of the molecular mechanisms underlying these cell–vessel wall interactions have been elucidated.

The earliest visible adhesive event in vivo is rolling, characterized by a constant formation and breakage of adhesive bonds. This phenomenon keeps marginated leukocytes in contact with endothelial cells and slows considerably their velocity relative to the blood stream. Rolling is usually exclusively observed in venules, not arterioles [432,433], and is mediated by members of the selectin supergene family (Table 1-3) [434–439]. Selectins are single-chain glycoproteins with an N-terminal, Ca^{++} dependent lectin-like domain, a variable number of complement regulatory domains (2, 6, and 9 consensus repeats in L-selectin, E-selectin, and P-selectin, respectively), a transmembrane domain, and a short cytoplasmic tail [440–446]. L-selectin is found on leukocytes, whereas E-selectin is expressed exclusively by endothelial cells. P-selectin is expressed by endothelial cells, platelets, and megakaryocytes [442].

Conversion of rolling neutrophils to firmly attached cells appears to require additional activating signals originating from either the intra- or extravascular space or at the endothelial-cell surface [437] and also is mediated by members of the immunoglobulin supergene family (Table 1-4). At a site of localized bacterial infection, release of bacterial-derived lipopolysaccharides and formyl peptides can provide weak chemotactic stimuli. Mast cells and tissue macrophages can also participate, supplying mediators such as histamine and thrombin. PAF, a signaling molecule that is coexpressed with P-selectin, may also play an important role in activating neutrophils tethered on P-selectin [447]. Additionally, cytokines (IL-1, TNF) stimulate the endothelial cell to synthesize chemokines (e.g., IL-8) [448–450] and additional ligands, including E-selectin, ICAM, and possibly an as yet undefined L-selectin ligand [451,452]. Activation of the neutrophil upregulates CD11b(Mac-1) from an intracellular pool and can occur following stimulation of neutrophils with the leukotriene LTB_4, IL-8, or n-formyl-met-leu-phe (fMLP) [453–455]. Anti-ICAM-1 or anti-CD18 blocking monoclonal antibodies prevent the firm adhesion but not the rolling of neutrophils in vitro and in vivo [435,456,457]. Monocytes, in contrast to neutrophils, appear to utilize very late antigen (VLA) 4 : VCAM to mediate firm attachment to endothelial cells [458].

Transmigration of leukocytes appears to involve CD11a / CD18 : ICAM-1 and also CD31 (PECAM, Endo-CAM). In contrast to VCAM-1, which is confined to the apical surface of endothelium, ICAM-1 is found on apical and basal surfaces of endothelial cells and in the intercellular junctions [459], suggesting that the continuous distribution of ICAM-1 may provide an "adhesive pathway" for the CD18 integrins of activated leukocytes. Specific monoclonal antibodies against CD11a block transendothelial migration more effectively than CD11b [460,461]; anti-ICAM-1 antibodies also reduce leukocyte transmigration [460]. Diapedesis may also involve homotypic adhesion of CD31 expressed on both leukocytes and endothelium [462].

P-Selectin. P-selectin (also known as PADGEM, GMP-140, and CD62) is a glycoprotein of approximately 140 kDa associated with the Weibel Palade body of endothelial cells [463]. P-selectin is also found in the alpha and dense granules of platelets [464,465]. P-selectin is directed to secretory granule membranes by a sorting signal in the cytoplasmic domain [466,467]. Several lines of evidence

Table 1-3. The selectin family of endothelial adhesion proteins

	Molecular mass (kDa)	Ligand	Stimulus	Maximal expression	Leukocyte population binding
E-selectin	115	Sialylated Lewis X	IL-1, TNF LPS	4–6 hr	Neutrophils, monocytes, memory T-cells, eosinophils, basophils
P-selectin	140	Lewis X Sialylated Lewis X Cluster designation15 P-selectin glucoprotein ligand-1	Thrombin Histamine H_2O_2 Complement	<10 min	Neutropils, monocytes

suggest that posttranslational modifications of the cytoplasmic domain could be important in regulation of P-selectin trafficking. The single cysteine in the cytoplasmic tail is acylated with palmitic and stearic acids [468], and serine and threonine residues can be phosphorylated by a protein kinase C–dependent mechanism [469]. Following stimulation with various mediators, P-selectin is rapidly mobilized to the endothelial cell surface (see Table 1-3) [447,470–472]. P-selectin surface expression is short-lived, although recent data from canine and rodent models suggest that endotoxin can induce new P-selectin synthesis [473,474]. P-selectin will bind to different types of leukocytes, including neutrophils and monocytes [472,475]. The importance of P-selectin in leukocyte rolling was recently demonstrated in a P-selectin knock-out mouse. In this mouse model, leukocytes failed to roll in mesenteric venules subjected to stimuli (e.g., A23187), which normally elicited a profound rolling response [476]. Anti-P-selectin antibodies have been found to protect against neutrophil-dependent acute lung injury elicited by intravenous activation of cobra venom factor [477]. A ligand for P-selectin, P-selectin glycoprotein ligand-1 (PSGL-1), was recently identified and cloned [478]. PSGL is a mucin-like transmembrane protein. PSGL-1 can also serve as ligand for E-selectin [478]. PSGL-1 most likely bears the sialylated Lewis X (sLex) moiety that can mediate E-selectin binding.

E-selectin. E-selectin (also known as endothelial leukocyte adhesion molecule-1 (ELAM-1) is a 115-kDa protein expressed exclusively by activated endothelial cells [446,479,480]. Not present constitutively, E-selectin requires de novo synthesis, with detectable surface expression as early as 1 to 2 hours after treatment with cytokines such as TNF or IL-1 [479–481]. Peak levels are observed at 4 to 6 hours, after which E-selectin expression declines toward basal levels at 24 to 48 hours. In vivo studies suggest that E-selectin expression may be more prolonged following systemic cytokine activation [482]; the mediators and mechanism of this prolonged response are not clear at this time. E-selectin supports neutrophil and monocyte adhesion [446,452,483–486] and binds to as yet unidentified glycoproteins or glycolipids bearing a carbohydrate group, sLex [487,488]. Anti-E-selectin antibodies have demonstrated protective effects in neutrophil-mediated lung injury [489] and in a primate asthma model [490].

ICAM-1. ICAM-1 (intercellular adhesion molecule-1, CD54) was originally defined as the ligand for CD11a/CD18 leukocyte function antigen-1 (LFA-1) in homotypic lymphocyte aggregation [491]. ICAM-1, a 90-kDa single-chain glycoprotein, is a member of the immunoglobulin supergene family. ICAM-1 has five immunoglobulin domains; ICAM-1 binding to CD11a/CD18 occurs at the N-terminal domain 1 [492,493], while CD11b/CD18 binding occurs at domain 3 [494]. Unlike many of the vascular adhesion molecules, ICAM-1 is constitutively expressed on endothelial cells [481]. ICAM-1 also demonstrates constitutive and regulated expression on many other nonvascular cells, including epithelium, fibroblasts, and keratinocytes [495]. In endothelial cells, marked upregulation of ICAM occurs following stimulation with proinflammatory cytokines; detectable increases are observed as early as 3 to 4 hours with maximal expression observed at 6 to 12 hours [481,495]. The regulation of endothelial ICAM-1 expression may be organ specific. For example,

Table 1-4. Immunoglobulin-related endothelial cell adhesion molecules

	Molecular mass (kDa)	Ligand	Stimulus	Maximal expression	Leukocyte population binding
ICAM-1	90	CD11a/CD18 CD11b/CD18	IL-1, TNF LPS, IFN-gamma	12–24 hr	All
ICAM-2		CD11a/CD18	Unknown		Neutrophils, lymphocytes (all?)
VCAM-1	110	VLA4	IL-1, TNF IL-4, LPS	12–24 hr	Lymphocytes, monocytes, eosinophils, basophils
CD31	130	CD31	Unknown		Neutrophils, lymphocytes

while TNF or IL-1 will greatly increase ICAM-1 expression in human umbilical vein and dermal microvessel endothelium [496], these cytokines are relatively ineffective stimuli for synovial microvascular endothelial cells [497]. Upregulation of synovial endothelial ICAM-1 expression appears to require co-stimulation of IFN-γ with TNF or IL-1 [497].

Numerous studies support the concept that CD11/CD18 : ICAM-1 interactions play critical roles in acute and chronic inflammatory disease. Blocking studies with anti-ICAM-1 antibodies in various animal models have suggested important roles for this adhesion molecule in arthritis, ischemia-reperfusion injury, autoimmune diseases, and transplant rejection [498–503].

ICAM-2. ICAM-2 is structurally similar to ICAM-1 but contains only two immunoglobulin domains with considerable homology to the first two N-terminal domains of ICAM-1 [504]. In contrast to ICAM-1, ICAM-2 is not readily upregulated by cytokines, but appears to be constitutively expressed at or near maximal levels [505]. The functional role of ICAM-2 is not clear; it may play an initial role in early leukocyte adhesion and margination prior to upregulation of other adhesion molecules. In contrast to ICAM-1, ICAM-2 apparently binds to only CD11a/CD18 (LFA-1) [504].

VCAM-1. VCAM-1 (vascular cell adhesion molecule-1) is a 110-kDA single-chain glycoprotein, containing seven Ig domains, including an alternatively spliced fourth domain [506–510]. The N-terminal domain (domain 1) and domain 4, which are highly homologous in amino acid sequence [508-510], appear to function in leukocyte adhesion [511]. Endothelial cells treated with IL-1, TNF, or IL-4 will upregulate the expression of VCAM-1 with maximal activity reached by 6 to 12 hours. VCAM-1 is expressed on other, nonvascular cells, including dendritic cells of lymph nodes and skin, vascular smooth muscle, cardiac muscle, bone marrow stromal cells, and synovial lining cells and fibroblasts [512–516].

VCAM-1 supports the adhesion of lymphocytes, monocytes, eosinophils, and basophils (but not neutrophils) by binding to VLA4 (CD49d/CD29, $\alpha_4\beta_1$) [506,516,517]. Blocking antibodies to VCAM-1 are beneficial in experimental autoimmune encephalomyelitis, an animal model with similarities to human multiple sclerosis [518]. Upregulation of VCAM-1 may be an early response of dysfunctional endothelium at sites of high shear; recent studies in a rabbit model of atherosclerosis have demonstrated focal upregulation of VCAM-1 at various branch points of the thoracic and abdominal aorta [519]. Whether similar events occur in human disease is unclear at this time.

CD31. CD31 (PECAM, EndoCAM) is constitutively expressed on endothelial cells as well as on platelets and most leukocytes [520]. CD31 is a member of the immunoglobulin supergene family [521,522] and may play a role in endothelial cell-cell adhesion [60,522]. CD31 has a relatively large, 108–amino acid, cytoplasmic domain, with putative sites for phosphorylation, lipid modification, and possibly other posttranslation events. Recent studies have demonstrated that platelet CD31 becomes highly phosphorylated in response to cell activation and, coincident with phosphorylation, becomes associated with the cytoskeleton [523,524]. Neutralizing monoclonal antibodies to CD31 prevent the association of endothelial cells into a "cobblestone" monolayer appearance [522]. CD31 localizes to the cell-cell borders of contact-inhibited endothelial cells at confluence; however, CD31 is diffusely distributed in proliferating endothelium. A role for CD31 in leukocyte diapedesis was recently suggested by the observation that neutralizing monoclonal antibodies to CD31 inhibit leukocyte transmigration [462].

Vascular Addressins. A central event in the immune response is the regulation of lymphocyte trafficking from the blood to tissue by vascular endothelial cells. A phenomenon noted by immunologists for many years was the efficient migration of antigen-specific lymphocytes (memory and effector cells) back to the site of stimulation as well as to sites of inflammation. As already discussed, there are many potential molecular players in these interactions, which in the appropriate combination and sequence could conceivably account for this selective extravasation (homing). However, based on the observations that monoclonal antibodies to L-selectin selectively inhibited lymphocyte binding to peripheral lymph node high endothelial venules (HEV) in vitro and inhibited homing to peripheral lymph nodes in vivo, L-selectin was suggested to be the primary leukocyte ligand involved in the mediation of lymphocyte homing. Other studies have suggested that the putative HEV ligand (addressin) was a sulfated, glycosylated protein, and studies are still in progress to identify the molecules in the addressin family. Recent studies using L-selectin immunoglobulin chimeras to purify putative ligands have identified two sulfated, glycosylated, and sialated proteins 50 and 90 kDa, from mouse lymph nodes [525–528]. These putative L-selectin ligands are new members of the MUCIN family of glycoproteins. A mucosal vascular addressin, selectively expressed on endothelial cells of HEVs and lamina propria venules, was identified as a 58- to 66-kDa glycoprotein adhesion receptor for lymphocytes. Recently cloned [529], the mucosal addressin was demonstrated to be a novel immunoglobulin family member, mucosol addressin cell adhesion molecule-1 (MAdCAM-1). MAdCAM-1 has two amino terminal domains with strong homology to ICAM-1 and VCAM-1. In addition to the immunoglobulin domains, MAdCAM-1 has a serine-threonine-rich region proposed to serve as the backbone for presentation of carbohydrate ligands.

Leukocyte Adhesion Molecule Interactions Tumor Cells. Several studies have shown that some nonlymphoid tumor cells (e.g., carcinoma, melanoma) may utilize endothelial-leukocyte adhesion molecules to successfully metastasize. Cytokine-activated endothelial cells demonstrate a greater adhesiveness to tumor cells [530], and melanoma adhesion to activated endothelial cells is mediated by VCAM-1 inducible cell adhesion molecule (INCAM-110) interactions with VLA4 [531,532]. E-selectin may support adhesion of colon cancer cells [533–535], an observation in keeping with the abundant expression of the carbohydrate structures sialyl Lewis X (sLex) and sialyl Lewis A (sLea) on human colon cancer cells.

Synthesis of Cytokines and Growth Factors

In addition to the upregulation of adhesive receptors for leukocytes, endothelial cells increase the expression of a number of cytokines and growth factors that can influence leukocyte migration, activation, and proliferation.

Chemokines. Chemokines consist of two related gene families, members that exhibit sequence homology and structural similarities, the most striking of which is the positioning of four conserved cysteine residues. Expressed locally by many cell types, including endothelium, in response to inflammatory cytokines, chemokines are thought to play a role in the amplification of the inflammatory response. Various members of the chemokine family exhibit potent leukocyte chemoattractant and activating activities, and the production of these chemokines is closely associated with a number of human diseases and animal models of disease [536].

The endothelial expression of IL-8, a potent neutrophil chemoattractant and activator, is markedly upregulated by cytokines such as TNF-alpha, IL-1, and LPS [537–539]. In cell culture systems, the accumulation of IL-8 in culture supernatants actually inhibits polymorphonuclear neutrophil (PMN) adhesion [540]. The leukocyte inhibitory actions of IL-8 are not a consequence of the downregulation or loss of relevant adhesion molecules (E-selectin, L-selectin, ICAM-1, CD11b/CD18) on either the neutrophil or the endothelial cell. Intravenous injection of IL-8 reduces neutrophil recruitment into dermal inflammatory sites in vivo [541]. Direct in vivo observations by intravital microscopy of the exteriorized rabbit mesentery have demonstrated that intravenous injection of IL-8 inhibited granulocyte emigration. This inhibitory effect was observed in the presence of near-control levels of granulocyte rolling and surface expression of L-selectin. In the same preparation, extravascular application of IL-8 next to small venules induced mass adhesion and transmigration of leukocytes [542]. These observations may suggest that in the local microenvironment of "activated" or "inflamed" endothelial cells, endothelial-derived IL-8 may play a protective role, limiting leukocyte-endothelial interactions and possible deleterious consequences. Many investigators have noted that cytokine-activated endothelial cells are more susceptible to neutrophil-mediated injury; however, IL-8 has been shown to reduce morphological indices of neutrophil-mediated endothelial injury (i.e., cell detachment, monolayer retraction, cytolysis) [540]. IL-8 production by activated endothelial cells is somewhat delayed and sustained [538] compared to the surface expression of E-selectin [481]; thus, the antiadhesive actions of IL-8 could potentially contribute to the downregulation of an acute inflammatory response. Paradoxically, increased IL-8 levels in various body fluids and tissue sites appear to promote neutrophil diapedesis [542].

In addition to producing IL-8, cytokine-activated endothelial cells produce a factor that is selectively chemotactic for monocytes [543,544]. Monocyte chemoattractant protein-1 (MCP-1) a product of the JE gene, is secreted by endothelial cells treated with IL-1, TNF, IFN-γ, or IL-4 [543–547].

Granulocyte-Macrophage Colony Stimulating Factor (GM-CSF) and Granulocyte Colony Stimulating Factor (G-CSF). The observation that conditioned media derived from cultured endothelial cells contain a granulocyte-macrophage colony–stimulating activity led to the concept that endothelial cells might provide hematopoietic growth factors [548]. GM-CSF and G-CSF are glycoproteins that contribute to the differentiation and proliferation of endothelial cells. Through the production of GM-CSF and G-CSF, the endothelium plays a role in the regulation of granulopoiesis, the proliferation of primitive hematopoietic progenitor cells and phagocyte priming [549–552].

Normal endothelial cells constitutively produce little to undetectable amounts of GM-CSF or G-CSF; however, exposure to IL-1, TNF, LPS, acetylated LDL, viruses, and phorbol esters promotes the synthesis of both growth factors [553–559], primarily through posttranscriptional stabilization of the normally short half-life of GM-CSF and G-CSF mRNAs [559,560].

GM-CSF and G-CSF stimulate angiogenesis in vivo [561] and endothelial proliferation and migration in vitro [562]. Other reported activities of GM-CSF and G-CSF on endothelial cells include stimulating the synthesis and secretion of plasminogen activator [563], lymphocyte adhesion to HEVs [564,565], and upregulation of class-I major histocompatability complex (MHC) antigens [566]. In endothelial and other cells, the receptor for GM-CSF is a dimer with an alpha subunit of about 80 kDA and a beta chain of 130–135 kDa [567].

Interleukin-6 (IL-6). IL-6 is a pleiotropic lymphokine produced by many cell types, including endothelial cells. The ability of endothelial cells to produce IL-6 was first demonstrated by the observation that an endothelial-cell-conditioned medium could replace feeder cells in hybridoma growth [568]. IL-6 exhibits a broad spectrum of biological activities, including the stimulation of acute-phase protein production by hepatocytes [569], modulation of T-cell activation [570,571], and promotion of the differentiation of B-cells for immunoglobulin synthesis [572].

Endothelial production of IL-6 is stimulated by TNF, IL-1, lymphotoxin, IFN-γ, LPS [573–576], and hypoxia-reoxygenation [577]. Several products of the IL-6 gene are produced by human umbilical vein endothelial cells with masses of 23–25, 27–30, and 45 kDa [578], suggesting that the cells extensively modify the primary IL-6 translation product. IL-6 has no effect on endothelial production of PAI-1, tPA, or leukocyte adhesion proteins; procoagulant activity; or prostacyclin production [576]. Production of cytokine-stimulated IL-6 is blocked by glucocorticoids [579].

Angiogenesis

Under normal conditions, capillary growth, morphogenesis, and regression occur only during embryonic development, menses, and wound healing. However, under certain pathological conditions, for example, solid-tumor growth, diabetic retinopathy, rheumatoid arthritis, and some other chronic inflammatory diseases, angiogenesis plays a significant role in the progression of the disease state. The process of angiogenesis occurs in four sequential and mechanistic steps: (1) endothelial-mediated proteolytic degradation of the vascular basement membrane and interstitial matrix, (2) migration of endothelial cells, (3) proliferation of endothelial cells, and (4) formation of capillary loops. The factors that regulate matrix degradation and endothelial proliferation are discussed next.

MATRIX DEGRADATION AND ENDOTHELIAL MIGRATION

The basement membrane and surrounding extracellular matrix imposes a mechanical barrier to the migration of endothelial cells and subsequent formation of new blood vessels. Endothelial cells breach these barriers by limited proteolytic matrix degradation mediated by various proteases including urokinase and matrix metalloproteinases which either directly degrade matrix components or activate other matrix-degrading enzymes.

Plasminogen Activators. The production of plasminogen activators, particularly uPA, appears to be important in matrix degradation. uPA activation of plasminogen activation to plasmin results in two levels of activity: (1) direct proteolytic effects of plasmin on matrix components and (2) plasmin-mediated activation of latent matrix metalloproteinases, which may be coproduced or already present in the extracellular matrix. Human endothelial cells normally produce little or no uPA [580,581]. Serial subcultivation [267,284], TNF-α [582,583], endotoxin [582], IL-1 [582], TGF$_\beta$ [584], bFGF [585], and IL-4 [584] induce uPA mRNA, protein, and activity in cultured human endothelial cells. This may have in vivo correlates in view of recent studies immunolocalizing uPA to microvascular endothelial cells of inflamed appendices [586] and rheumatoid synovium [587]. In vitro, induced uPA release is vectorial, predominantly basolateral [582], supporting the concept that this form of PA has a primary function in matrix proteolysis. The spatial restriction of uPA activity is limited by the binding of uPA to PAI-1, which is bound to certain basement-membrane components [298,305,586,589]. PAI-1, a member of the serpin serine protease inhibitor superfamily, readily decays to an inactive form in solution, but it is stabilized by binding to extracellular matrix proteins such as vitronectin [590].

Extracellular uPA activity can also be modulated through conversion of the inactive single-chain zymosan form, sc-uPA, to the proteolytic, active two-chain form of uPA [591]. The predominant uPA secreted by cytokine-activated endothelial cells is the two-chain form [592]. Modulation of uPA activity is further regulated by a coordinate production of PAI-1; for example, LPS, IL-1, and TNF increase PAI-1 mRNA and protein in addition to the effects of these cytokines on uPA production [23,308,310–313,582].

Specific high-affinity urokinase receptors (uPARs) on endothelial cells provide an additional mechanism for the localization of uPA activity. The endothelial uPAR binds the EGF-like domain of uPA, maintaining uPA catalytic activity [592–596]. Receptor-bound uPA can thus function as a plasma-membrane-associated enzyme, generating plasmin in close proximity to the cell surface. uPAR may also play an important role in stimulating the conversion of sc-uPA to the enzymatically active form and in protecting uPA from PAI-1. Studies of the regulation of uPAR expression on endothelial cells are limited; however, it has been reported that elevation of intracellular cAMP levels leads to a modest increase in uPAR [597]. Treatment of endothelial cells with tumor promoters, such as phorbol myristate acetate (PMA), and with acidic and basic fibroblast growth factors (FGFs) also increases uPAR expression [573,594].

Table 1-5. Matrix metalloproteinases and inhibitors produced by endothelial cells

Enzyme	Other names	Substrate	Inducers
MMP-1	Interstitial collagenase	Collagens I, II, III	PMA VEGF
MMP-2	Gelatinase A 72 kD type IV collagenase	Collagens IV, V Fibronectin Proteoglycans	Unknown
MMP-3	Stromelysin	Collagen IV Fibronectin Proteoglycans Laminin	PMA TNF-alpha IL-1
MMP-9	Gelatinase B 92 kD gelatinase 92 kD type IV collagenase	Collagens IV, V Gelatin Elastin	PMA TNF IL-1
TIMP-1		All MMPs	PMA
TIMP-2		All MMPs	PMA

Matrix Metalloproteinases (MMPs) and Tissue Inhibitors of Matrix Metalloproteinases (TIMPs). Similar to the uPA-plasmin system, matrix metalloproteinases degrade proteins of the extracellular matrix (Table 1-5). Endothelial cells derived from macro- and microvascular origins have been demonstrated to express various MMPs after stimulation with tumor promoters, cytokines, or forskolin [598]. However, increased MMP expression does not necessarily translate to increased MMP activity, since these enzymes are secreted as latent enzymes and the same stimuli may also regulate the production of endogenous MMP inhibitors such as TIMP-1 and TIMP-2 [599].

ENDOTHELIAL PROLIFERATION

There are numerous regulators of endothelial-cell proliferation, both positive and negative (Table 1-6). Some positive regulators are true mitogens, while others act to facilitate proliferation or migration of endothelial cells.

Positive Regulators of Endothelial Cell Proliferation

FIBROBLAST GROWTH FACTOR (FGF). bFGF (basic FGF), originally isolated from bovine pituitary [600], is a single-chain protein, 146 aa, with an apparent Mr of approximately 16 kDa. bFGF has a high (basic) isoelectric point, is sensitive to acid and elevated temperatures, and exhibits a

Table 1-6. Positive and negative regulators of angiogenesis

Positive regulators	Negative regulators
MITOGENS	
aFGF	TSP
bFGF	Interferon-γ
VEGF	TGF-β
PDGF	TNF-α
Insulin	Platelet factor 4
IGF-1	
IL-4	
ANGIOGENIC PEPTIDES	
Angiogenin	
TGF-β	
IL-8	
Scatter factor	
ANGIOGENIC NONPEPTIDES	
Prostaglandins	
12-(R) HETE	
AMPLIFIERS	
Heparin	
HS proteoglycans	

strong affinity for heparin. Acidic FGF (aFGF) also was originally isolated from bovine pituitary [601]. aFGF is a single-chain protein, 140 amino acids, with an apparent Mr of 15–17 kDa. aFGF also binds with high affinity to heparin [601]. aFGF and bFGF exhibit 53% homology [601] as well as demonstrate high-sequence homology with three oncogene products, hst/ks, int-2, and FGF-5 [602–604].

Relevant to angiogenesis and wound healing, arterial and capillary endothelial cells, vascular smooth muscle cells, and fibroblasts are all capable of synthesizing both forms of FGF [605–609]. Neither protein expresses an obvious signal sequence, suggesting that they might be secreted as a complex with carrier proteins or extracellular matrix proteins [610]. Four FGF receptor subtypes have been described [611–613]; all are single-chain polypeptides, with Mr 110–150 kDa, and most exhibit more avid binding to bFGF than aFGF. The FGF receptors contain an extracellular domain with two or three immunoglobulin-like domains, a transmembrane domain, and a cytoplasmic tyrosine kinase domain. The four receptor subtypes are classified as type 1 (also known as flg), type 2 (also known as bek), type 3 (cek2), and type 4.

The high affinity of FGFs for heparin and other sulfated glycosaminoglycans (GAGs) is an important feature of FGF interactions with cells. HS is a major scaffolding GAG of the extracellular matrix and can serve to protect FGFs from degradation [608,614,615] as well as a releasable storage depot [615]. FGFs can be released from the matrix by proteolytic enzymes such as collagenase, plasmin, or heparinase [616–618]. HS binding sites on the endothelial-cell surface play a pivotal role in regulating the binding of FGFs to their membrane receptors.

The actual physiological roles of the FGFs with respect to the vascular endothelium are not clear at this time. However, treatment of cultured endothelial cells with bFGF or aFGF stimulates mitogenesis [605,607,610,619], synthesis, and deposition of extracellular matrix proteins and proteoglycans [610,620]; prostaglandin synthesis (in microvascular endothelial cells [158]); uPA, tPA, and PAI-1 expression [582,621]; and MMP and TIMP production [598,622]. In three-dimensional culture models, FGF elicits tube formation and capillary sprouting in vivo and in vitro [623,624]

VASCULAR ENDOTHELIAL GROWTH FACTOR (VEGF). VEGF (also known as vascular permeability factor, or VPF) is a secreted peptide (Mr 45 kDa), produced by various tumor cells, skeletal muscle, fibroblasts, and cardiac myocytes [625–629]. VEGF binds to specific endothelial receptors flt-1 (flk-1 in the mouse) [630,631] and KDR tyrosine kinase [632], two immunoglobulin superfamily members characterized by a cytoplasmic tyrosine kinase domain with significant homology to the tyrosine kinase domains of the bFGF, PDGF, stem cell factor, and CF receptors. VEGF is a potent endothelial mitogen [625,633] that potentiates the mitogenic effects of bFGF [634] and induces the expression of MMP-1 [599]. VEGF, in contrast to most other endothelial mitogens (see Table 1-6), appears to be selective for endothelial cells, lacking any demonstrable activity on epithelial cells, fibroblasts, lymphoid cells, or a variety of tumor cells. This selectivity is probably due to the endothelial-cell-restricted expression of VEGF receptors [635–638].

Functionally, VEGF may be a critical endothelial growth factor in the angiogenesis associated with tumors [639], pannus formation in rheumatoid arthritis [640], and other sites of hypoxia-initiated angiogenesis [629].

PLATELET DERIVED GROWTH FACTOR (PDGF). In addition to platelets, endothelial cells, like many diploid cells (e.g., vascular smooth muscle cells [641,642] and monocytes/macrophages [642,643]), produce PDGF [644–646]. PDGF (Mr 28–35 kDa) is composed of two homologous but distinct polypeptide chains (A and B) linked by disulfide bonds and can occur in various dimers (PDGF-AA, PDGF-BB, PDGF-AB). In normal blood vessels, PDGF-A chain transcripts are primarily associated with medial smooth muscle, whereas PDGF-B chain transcripts are expressed in the adventitia, localized to macrophages and the endothelial cells of the vasa vasorum [645,647,648]. Cultured endothelial cells can express both A and B chains, and all three possible dimers of PDGF have been identified in endothelial-cell culture supernatants [649–653].

Constitutive endothelial PDGF secretion is reduced by some modified LDLs, fish oil, and forskolin [650–653]. PDGF is transiently induced by TGF-β, IL-1, TNF-α, thrombin, and activated factor X [654,655]. PDGF receptors are homo- or heterodimers, comprised of alpha and beta subunits. The alpha subunit can bind A or B chains, whereas the beta subunit binds only B chains [656]. PDGF receptors generally are not found on endothelial cells, although some microvascular endothelial cells have been reported to express PDGF receptors [657,658]. Smooth muscle cells do express PDGF receptors, and the numbers and type(s) of receptor vary with development and disease. PDGF interactions with its receptor tyrosine kinase results in a number of signaling events, including receptor dimerization and phosphorylation, activation of protein kinase C-γ, phosphatidylinositol-3-kinase, ras-GAP and other kinases, protein kinase C activation, Na^+/H^+ exchange, and elevations in intracellular Ca^{++} [659].

PDGF has many diverse actions on vascular cells. It is a chemotactic and mitogenic agent for vascular smooth muscle cells [660,661], a mitogen for microvascular endothelium [657,658], and a stimulus for MMP and TIMP secretion [661].

INSULIN AND INSULIN-LIKE GROWTH FACTORS (IGF). Endothelial cells from all levels of the vasculature have been demonstrated to express specific receptors for insulin [661–667] and insulin-like growth factors I (IGF-I) and II (IGF-II) [663,668]. Insulin stimulates microvascular-, but not large-vessel-, derived endothelial-cell glucose transport and metabolism [48,669–671]. Insulin has been reported to stimulate small- and large-vessel-derived endothelial-cell proliferation [671]. Endothelial cells can take up and store or transport insulin and IGF-I, and it has been proposed that endothelial cells can act as a temporary storage site for these peptides [672–675]. Endothelial cells have been reported to express IGF-I mRNA [676], although they apparently synthesize and secrete little, if any, de novo IGF-I [677]. Cultured endothelial cells produce the IGF binding proteins (IGFBPs) IGFBP-2, IGFBP-3, and IGFBP-4 [678–680] and may contribute to the circulating and tissue levels of specific IGFBPs in vivo. IGFBPs can either inhibit [680] or promote [681] the effects of IGFs on vascular smooth muscle and endothelial cells. IGFs have been suggested to play roles in restenosis following vessel injury [682–684] and in angiogenesis [685,686].

SCATTER FACTOR. Scatter factor (SF) was initially described as a cytokine secreted by fibroblasts and vascular smooth muscle cells that dispersed cohesive epithelial colonies and stimulated cell motility [687]. SF is identical to hepatocyte growth factor and is a heparin-binding glycoprotein dimer comprised of heavy (58-kDa) and light (31-kDa) subunits [688–690]. SF exhibits 38% homology with plasminogen and is related to the blood coagulation group of proteases. SF stimulates endothelial-cell chemotaxis, random cell migration, and formation of capillary tubes, as well as the production of uPA [688,691,692]. Recent studies have shown that SF can be identified in areas surrounding new blood vessel formation in psoriatic skin [693].

INTERLEUKIN-8. Elevated levels of IL-8 are associated with a number of angiogenic disease states, including psoriasis and rheumatoid arthritis. In addition, IL-8 will bind to heparin, which is characteristic of many angiogenesis factors. IL-8 will stimulate endothelial chemotaxis and cell proliferation, and, when incorporated into Hydron pellets and implanted in the rat cornea, amounts as low as 10 ng will induce a corneal angiogenic response [694].

12(R) HYDROXYEICOSATRIENOIC ACID (12(R)HETE). Initially identified as a novel cytochrome P450 metabolite of arachidonic acid in corneal epithelial cells, 12(R)HETE was later demonstrated to exhibit potent neutrophil chemotactic activity in vitro and to stimulate angiogenesis in vivo [695]. It is unclear at this time if 12(R)HETE acts directly as an endothelial mitogen.

HEPARIN AND OTHER SULFATED PROTEOGLYCANS. Heparin, HS, and related polysaccharides are involved in many steps of the angiogenic process. Heparin binds to and stabilizes FGFs [608,695–700], potentiates the mitogenic effect of aFGF on endothelial cells [701], and increases the binding of aFGF to its receptor [702]. Specific sequences of HS have been found in the cell nucleus, and a role for heparin as a shuttle to chaperone FGF into the nucleus has been proposed [703]. FGFs may bind to HS in the extracellular matrix, resulting in a stabilized storage pool of these growth factors [615,617]. PDGF, TGF-β_1, and TSP also bind to HS [704–706]. Endothelial cells synthesize HS [707] and can metabolize heparin [708]. The mast cell is an important in vivo source of heparin, possibly demonstrated by the observation that mast cells accumulate at the site of tumor angiogenesis prior to capillary ingrowth [709].

Negative Regulators of Endothelial Cell Proliferation

TRANSFORMING GROWTH FACTOR β_1(TGFβ_1). TGFβ_1 is a disulfide-linked dimer (Mr $\approx$ 25 kDa) consisting of two identical 112-aa chains [710]. TGF-β_1 is secreted as an inactive, latent complex unable to interact with cell-surface receptors [711,712], although latent TGF-β_1 can bind to a cell-surface cation-independent mannose-6-phosphate/IGF II receptor [713,714], which appears to be critical for its activation. Although the mechanisms responsible for activation of TGF-β_1 in vivo are poorly understood, in vitro TGF-β_1 can be activated by acidification, alkalinization, proteolytic processing, or treatment with endoglycosidases or sialidases [711,715–717]. Local acidic environments could potentially occur at sites of wound healing or necrotic areas of atherosclerotic plaques. Plasmin or cathepsin D may be an important protease involved in TGF-β_1 activation [715] and could be supplied by activated endothelial cells or macrophages. Once activated, TGF-β_1 may bind to specific cell-membrane receptors or, alternatively, to various extracellular matrix proteins [705] that serve to protect TGF-β_1 from degradation. Stored extracellular matrix TGF-β_1 provides a repository for sustained release or rapid release of this growth factor when liberated by extracellular matrix degradation.

There are at least three distinct classes of TGF-β_1 receptors: I, II, and III. TGF-β_1 class I and class II receptors are glycoproteins [718–720], whereas the more abundant class-III form is a proteoglycan [721–723]. The precise roles played by these different receptors is poorly defined. TGF-β_1 stimulates the synthesis of extracellular matrix proteins (collagens I, III, IV, and V, TSP, tenascin, elastin, chondroitin/dermatin sulfates) produced by vascular smooth muscle and endothelial cells and fibroblasts [724–732]. Endothelial-derived TGF-β_1 stimulates the synthesis of glycosaminoglycans by vascular smooth muscle cells [733]. TGF-β_1 displays a diverse array of other biologic activities, including stimulation of PAI-1 and uPA secretion [308,584,733], the expression of alpha and beta subunits of fibronectin receptors [734,735], and stimulation or inhibition of cell proliferation [736,737]. In vivo,

TGF-β_1 is angiogenic, whereas in vitro the proliferation of endothelial cells cultured on plastic, laminin, type-IV collagen or fibronectin is inhibited by TGF-β_1 [716,736,737].

THROMBOSPONDIN (TSP). Exogenous TSP will inhibit endothelial proliferation [738,739] and tube formation [740], as well as inhibit endothelial adhesion [741] and formation of focal-adhesion plaques [742]. The effects of TSP on cell motility are controversial; both inhibitory [743] and supportive [739] effects have been reported. TSP will also inhibit angiogenesis in vivo [743].

Summary

This chapter discussed the various regulatory roles of the vascular endothelium in barrier and exchange functions, hemostasis, and vasoregulation, as well as endothelial contributions to the local and systemic inflammatory response and angiogenesis. These processes typically proceed in balance, contributing to the adaptive responses of organs and tissues to stress and nutritional requirements. However, various pathological stimuli can result in nonadaptive, dysfunctional changes in the properties of the vascular endothelium, contributing to disease etiology and progression. For example, the increased permeability to plasma lipoproteins, increased cytokine and growth-factor production, altered hemostatic balance, and increased leukocyte adhesiveness are manifestations of dysfunctional endothelial cells that are important to the initiation, progression, and clinical complications of atherosclerotic disease. There are numerous other disease states in which endothelial dysfunction contributes to the clinical manifestations. As our understanding of the causes and consequences of endothelial dysfunction progresses, improved diagnoses and treatment should follow.

References

1. Scow RO, Blanchette-Mackie EJ, Smith IC. Role of capillary endothelium in the clearance of chylomicrons: a model for lipid transport from blood by lateral diffusion in cell membranes. Circ Res 1976; 39:149–162.
2. Renkin EM. Multiple pathways of capillary permeability. Circ Res 1977; 41:735–743.
3. Palade GE. Transport in quanta across the endothelium of blood capillaries. Anat Rec 1960;136:254 (Abstr).
4. Taylor AE, Granger DN. Exchange of macromolecules across the circulation. In EM Renkin, CC Michel, eds. Handbook of Physiology. Sec 2: The cardiovascular system. Vol IV: The microcirculation. Bethesda: American Physiological Society, 1984. Pp 462–520.
5. Crone C, Levitt DG. Capillary permeability to small solutes. In EM Renkin, CC Michel, eds. Handbook of Physiology. Section 2: The cardiovascular system. Vol IV: The microcirculation. Bethesda: American Physiological Society, 1984. Pp 411–466.
6. Simionescu M, et al. How plasma macromolecules cross the endothelium. New Physiol Sci 1987; 2:135–138.
7. Renkin EM. Capillary transport of macromolecules: pores and other endothelial pathways. J Appl Physiol 1985; 58:315–325.
8. Michel CC. The transport of albumin: a critique of the vesicular system in transendothelial transport. Am Rev Resp Dis 1992; 146:532–536.
9. Majno G. Ultrastructure of the vascular membrane. In WF Hamilton, ed. Handbook of Physiology. Circulation. Sec 2, vol II. Washington DC: American Physiological Society, 1965. Pp 2293–2375.
10. Majno G, Joris I. Endothelium 1977; a review. In AB Chandler et al., eds. Advances in Experimental Medicine and Biology. The Thrombotic Process in Atherogenesis, New York: Plenum, 1977; vol 104. Pp 169–227.
11. Simionescu M, Simionescu N, Palade GE. Morphometric data on the endothelium of blood capillaries. J Cell Biol 1974; 60:128–152.
12. Simionescu M, Simionescu N, Palade GE. Structural basis of permeability in sequential segments of the microvasculature. I. Bipolar microvascular fields in the diaphragm. Microvasc Res 1978; 15:1–16.
13. Simionescu M, Simionescu N, Palade GE. Differentiated microdomains on the luminal surface of the capillary endothelium. I. Partial characterization of their anionic sites. J Cell Biol 1981; 90:614–621.
14. Wisse E, et al. Scanning electron microscopy observations on the structure of portal veins, sinusoids and central veins. Scanning Electron Misc 1983; 3:1441–1452.
15. Wisse E, et al. The liver sieve: considerations concerning the structure and function of endothelial fenestrae, the sinusoidal well and the space of Disse. Hepatology 5:683–692, 1985.
16. Boler RK, Bibighaus AJ. Ultrastructural alterations of dog livers during endotoxin shock. Lab Invest 1987; 17:537–561.
17. Fraser F, et al. High pressure perfusion damages the sieving ability of sinusoidal endothelium in rat livers. Br J Exp Pathol 1980; 61:222–228.
18. Frenzel H, Kremer B, Hucker H. The liver sinusoids under various pathological conditions. In E Wisse, DL Knook, eds. Kupffer Cells and Other Sinusoidal Cells. Amsterdam: Elsevier/North Holland, 1977. Pp 213–222.
19. McCuskey RS, Vonahme FJ, Grun M. In vivo and electron after portacaval anastomoses. Hepatology 1983; 3:96–104.
20. Napanitaya W, et al. Effect of venous outflow obstruction on pores and fenestrations in sinusoidal endothelium. Br J Exp Pathol 1976; 57:604–609.
21. Oda M, et al. Some dynamic aspects of the hepatic microcirculation—demonstration of sinusoidal endothelial fenestrae as a possible regulatory factor. In M Tsuchiya, et al., eds. Intravital Observation of Organ Microcirculation. Amsterdam: Excerpta Medica 1983. Pp 105–138.
22. Oda M, et al. Hepatic sinusoidal endothelium—its functional implications in the regulation of sinusoidal blood flow. In M Tsuchiya, et al., eds. Microcirculation—an Update, vol 2. Amsterdam; Excerpta Medica, 1983. Pp 317–320.
23. Simionescu M, Simionescu N. Ultrastructure of the microvascular wall: functional considerations. In EM Renkin, CC Michel, eds. Handbook of physiology. Section 2: The cardiovascular system. Vol IV: The microcirculation. Bethesda: American Physiological Society, 1984. Pp 41–101.
24. Milici AJ, et al. Transcytosis of albumin in capillary endothelium. J Cell Biol 1987; 105:2603–2612.
25. Wagner R, Chen S-C. Transcapillary transport of solute by the endothelial vesicular system: evidence from thin serial section analysis. Microvasc Res 1991; 42:139–150.
26. Crone C. The function of capillaries. In PF Baker, ed. Recent advances in physiology. Edinburg: Churchill-Livingstone, 1984. Pp 125–162.
27. Bundgaard M, Frøkjaer-Jensen J, Crone C. Endothelial plasmalemmal vesicles as elements in a system of branching invaginations from the cell surface. Proc Natl Acad Sci USA 1979; 76:6439–6442.
28. Bundgaard M, Hagman P, Crone C. The three dimensional organization of plasmalemmal vesicular profiles in the endo-

thelium of rat heart capillaries. Microvasc Res 1983; 25:358–368.
29. Frøkjaer-Jensen J. Three dimensional organization of plasmalemma vesicles in endothelial cells; an analysis by serial sectioning of frog mesenteric capillaries. J Ultrastruc Res 1980; 73:9–20.
30. Schneeberger EE, Hamelin M. Interaction of circulating proteins with pulmonary endothelial glycocalyx and its effect on endothelial permeability. Am J Physiol 1984; 247:H206–217.
31. Ghitescu L, et al. Specific binding sites for albumin restricted to plasmalemmal vesicles of continuous capillary endothelium: receptor-mediated transcytosis. J Cell Biol 1986; 102:1304–1311.
32. Schnitzer JE, Carley WW, Palade GE. Albumin interacts specifically with a 60-kDa microvascular endothelial glycoprotein. Proc Natl Acad Sci USA 1988; 85:6773–6777.
33. Schnitzer JE, Carley WW, Palade GE. Specific albumin binding to microvascular endothelium in culture. Am J Physiol 1988; 254:H425–437.
34. Ghinea N, et al. Identification of albumin-binding proteins in capillary endothelial cells. J Cell Biol 1988; 107:231–239.
35. Schnitzer JE. gp60 is an albumin-binding glycoprotein expressed by continuous endothelium involved in albumin transcytosis. Am J Physiol 1992; 262:H246–H254.
36. Schnitzer JE, et al. Preferential interaction of albumin-binding proteins gp30 and gp18 with conformationally modified albumins. J Biol Chem 1992; 267:24544–24553.
37. Ghinea N, et al. Endothelial albumin binding proteins are membrane associated components exposed on the cell surface. J Biol Chem 1989; 264:4755–4758.
38. Svensjö E, Arfors K-E, Grega GJ. Morphological and physiological correlation of bradykinin-induced macromoleular efflux. Am J Physiol 1979; 236:H600–606.
39. Carter RD, Joyner WL, Renkin EM. Effect of histamine and some other substances on molecular selectivity of the capillary wall to plasma proteins and dextran. Microvasc Res 1974; 7:31–48.
40. Curry FE, Joyner WL, Rutledge JC. Graded modulation of frog microvessel permeability to albumin using ionophore A23187. Am J Physiol 1990; 258:H587–598.
41. Svensjö E. Joyner WL. The effects of intermittent and continuous stimulation of microvessels in the cheek pouch of hamsters with histamine and bradykinin on the development of venular leaky sites. Microcirc Endothelium Lymphatics 1984; 1:381–396.
42. Banos G, Daniel PM, Pratt OE. Saturation of a shared mechanism which transports L-arginine and L-lysine into the brain of the living rat. J Physiol 1974; 236:29–41.
43. Betz AL, Goldstein GW. Polarity of the blood brain barrier-neutral amino acid transport into isolated brain capillaries. Science 1978; 202:225–227.
44. Pardridge WM, Boado RJ, Farrell CR. Brain-type glucose transporter (GLUT 1) is selectively localized to the blood brain barrier. Studies with quantitative Western blotting and in situ hybridization. J Biol Chem 1990; 265:18035–18040.
45. Dick APK, et al. Identification and characterization of the glucose transporter of the blood brain barrier by cytochalasin B binding and immunological reactivity. Proc Natl Acad Sci USA 1984; 81:7233–7237.
46. Dieterle Y, et al. Metabolism and uptake of adenosine triphosphate and adenosine by porcine aortic and pulmonary endothelial cells and fibroblasts in culture. Circ Res 1978; 42:869–876.
47. Pearson JD, et al. Uptake and metabolism of adenosine by pig aortic endothelial and smooth muscle cells in culture. Biochem J 1978; 170:265–271.
48. Gerritsen ME, Burke T, Allen L. Glucose starvation is required for insulin stimulation of hexose uptake and metabolism in coronary microvascular endothelial cells. Microvascular Research 1988; 35:153–166.
49. Haddock RC, et al. Role of receptors in metabolic interaction of histamine with human vascular endothelial cells and skin fibroblasts. J Biol Chem 262:10220–10228.
50. Pearson JD, Carleton JS, Gordon JL. Metabolism of adenine nucleotides by ectoenzymes of vascular endothelial and smooth muscle cells in culture. Biochem J 1990; 190:421–429.
51. Pearson JD, Coade SB, Cusack NJ. Characterization of ectonucleotidases on vascular smooth muscle cells. Biochem J 1985; 230:503–507.
52. Skeggs LTP Jr, Kahn JR, Shumway NP. The preparation and function of the hypertensin-converting enzyme. J Exp Med 1956; 103:295–299.
53. Erdös EG, Yang HYT. An enzyme in microsomal fraction of the kidney that inactivates bradykinin. Life Sci 1967; 6:569–574.
54. Alhenc-Gelas F, et al. Measurement of human converting enzyme level by direct radioimmunoassay. J Lab Med 1983; 101:83–96.
55. Erdös EG. Angiotensin I converting enzyme and the changes in our concept through the years. Lewis K Dahl Memorial Lecture. Hypertension 1990; 16:363–370.
56. Kaplan AP, et al. Studies of the activation and inhibition of the plasma kallikrien-kinin system. In H Fritz, et al., eds. Recent Progress on Kinins, Basel: Birkhäuser, 1992. Pp 317–328.
57. Kerr MA, Kenny AJ. The purification and specificity of neutral endopeptidase from rabbit kidney brush border. Biochem J 1974; 134:477–488.
58. Graf K, et al. Bradykinin degrading activity in cultured human endothelial cells. J Cardiovasc Pharmacol 1992; 20[Suppl 9]; S16–S20.
59. Muller WA, et al. A human endothelial cell-restricted basal externally disposed plasmalemmal protein enriched in intercellular junctions. J Exp Med 1989: 170:399–414.
60. Albelda SM, et al. EndoCAM: a novel endothelial cell–cell adhesion molecule. J Cell Biol 1990; 110:1227–1237.
61. Heimark RI, Degner M, Schwartz SM. Identification of a Ca^{2+}-dependent cell–cell adhesion molecule in endothelial cells. J Cell Biol 1990; 110:1745–1756.
62. Lampugnani MG, et al. A novel endothelial-specific membrane protein is a marker of cell–cell contacts. J Cell Biol 1992; 118:1511–1522.
63. Liaw CW, et al. Identification and cloning of two species of cadherins in bovine endothelial cells. EMBO J 1990; 9:2701–2708.
64. Lampughani MG, et al. The role of integrins in the maintenance of endothelial monolayer integrity. J Cell Biol 1991; 112:479–490.
65. Stevenson BR, et al. Identification of ZO-1: a high molecular weight polypeptide associated with the tight junction (zona occludens) in a variety of epithelial cells. J Cell Biol 1986:103:755–766.
66. Watson PM, et al. The tight junction specific protein ZO-1 is a component of the human and rat blood-brain barriers. Neurosci Lett 1991; 129:6–10.
67. Gumbiner B, Stevenson B, Grimaldi A. The role of the cell adhesion molecule uvomorulin in the formation and maintenance of the epithelial junctional complex. J Cell Biol 1988; 107:1575–1587.
68. Larson DM, Haudenschild CC. Junctional transfer in wounded cultures of bovine aortic endothelial cells. Lab Invest 1988; 59:373–379.
69. Larson DM, Carson MP, Haudenschild CC. Junctional transfer of small molecules in cultured bovine brain micro-

vascular endothelial cells and pericytes. Microvasc Res 1987; 34:184–199.
70. Larson DM, Haudenschild CC, Beyer EC. Gap junction messenger RNA expression by vascular wall cells. Circ Res 1990; 66:1074–1080.
71. Dejana E, et al. Fibronectin and vitronectin regulate the organization of their respective arg-gly-asp adhesion receptors in cultured human endothelial cells. J Cell Biol 1988; 107:1218–1223.
72. Burridge K. Substrate adhesions in normal and transformed fibroblasts: organization and regulation of cytoskeletal, membrane and extracellular matrix components at focal contacts. Cancer Rev 1986; 4:18–78.
73. Burridge K, et al. Focal adhesions: transmembrane junctions between the extracellular matrix and the cytoskeleton. Ann Rev Cell Biol 1988; 4:487–525.
74. Ginsberg MH, Du X, Plow EF. Inside-out integrin signalling. Curr Opin Cell Biol 1992; 4:766–771.
75. Schwartz MA. Spreading of human endothelial cells on fibronectin or vitronectin triggers elevation of intracellular free calcium. J Cell Biol 1993; 120:1003–1010.
76. Leavesly DI, et al. Integrin beta 1- and beta 3-mediated endothelial cell migration is triggered through distinct signaling mechanisms. J Cell Biol 1993; 121:163–170.
77. Landis RC, Bennett RI, Hogg N. A novel LFA-1 activation epitope maps to the I domain. J Cell Biol 1993; 120:1519–1527.
78. Maruyama I, Bill CE, Majerus PW. Thrombomodulin is found on endothelium of arteries, veins, capillaries and lymphatics and on syncytioblast of human placenta. J Cell Biol 1985; 101:363–371.
79. Maruyama I, Majerus PW. The turnover of thrombin-thrombomodulin complex in cultured human endothelial cells and A549 lung cancer cells. Endocytosis and degradation of thrombin. J Biol Chem 1985; 260:15432–15438.
80. Esmon CT. The roles of protein C and thrombomodulin in the regulation of blood coagulation. J Biol Chem 1989; 264:4743–4746.
81. Ogawa S, et al. Hypoxia modulates the barrier and coagulant function of cultured bovine endothelium. Increased monolayer permeability and induction of procoagulant properties. J Clin Invest 1990; 1090–1098.
82. Nawroth PP, et al. Interleukin 1 induces endothelial cell procoagulant while suppressing cell-surface anti-coagulant activity. Proc Natl Acad Sci USA 1986; 83:3460–3464.
83. Nawroth PP, Stern DM. Modulation of endothelial cell hemostatic properties by tumor necrosis factor. J Exp Med 1986; 163:740–745.
84. Conway EM, Rosenberg RD. Tumor necrosis factor suppresses transcription of the thrombomodulin gene in endothelial cells. Mol Cell Biol 1988; 8:5588–5592.
85. Rodgers GM, Conn MT. Homocysteine, an atherogenic stimulus, reduces protein C activation by arterial and venous endothelial cells. Blood 1990; 75:895–901.
86. Jackman RW, et al. Characterization of thrombomodulin cDNA reveals structural similarity to the low density lipoprotein receptor. Proc Natl Acad Sci USA 1986; 85:8834–8838.
87. Petersen TE. The amino terminal of thrombomodulin and pancreatic stone protein are homologous with lectins. FEBs Let 1988; 231:51–53.
88. Stearns D, Kurosawa S, Esmon CT. Microthrombomodulin, residues 310-486 from the epidermal growth factor precursor homology domain of thrombomodulin will accelerate protein C activation. J Biol Chem 1989; 264:3352–3356.
89. Suzuki K, et al. A domain composed of epidermal growth-factor like structures of human thrombomodulin is essential for thrombin binding and for protein C activation. J Biol Chem 1989; 264:4872–4876.
90. Esmon NL, Owen WG, Esmon CT. Isolation of membrane-bound cofactor for thrombin catalyzed activation of protein C. J Biol Chem 1983; 258:5548–5553.
91. Esmon NL, DeBault L, Esmon CT. Proteolytic formation and properties of gamma-carboxyglutamic acid domainless protein C. J Biol Chem 1983; 258:5548–5553.
92. Walker FJ, Sexton PW, Esmon CT. The inhibition of blood coagulation by activated protein C through the selective inactivation of activated factor V. Biochim Biophys Acta 1979; 571:333–342.
93. Stern DM, et al. Cultured bovine aortic endothelial cells promote activated protein C-protein S-mediated inactivation of factor Va. J Biol Chem 1986; 261:713–718.
94. Kisiel W, et al. Anticoagulant properties of bovine plasma protein C following activation by thrombin. Biochemistry 1977; 16:5824–5831.
95. Marlar RA, Kleiss AJ, Griffin JH. Mechanism of action of human activated protein C, a thrombin-dependent anticoagulant enzyme. Blood 1982; 59:1067–1072.
96. Griffin JH, et al. Deficiency of protein C in congenital thrombotic disease. J Clin Invest 1981; 68:1370–1373.
97. Broekmans AW, Veltkamp JJ, Bertina RM. Congenital protein C deficiency and venous thromboembolism. N Engl J Med 1983; 309:340–344.
98. Branson HE, et al. Inherited protein C deficiency and coumarin-responsive chronic relapsing purpura fulminans in a newborn infant. Lancet 1983; 2:1165–1168.
99. Seligsohn U, et al. Homozygous protein C deficiency manifested by massive venous thrombosis in the newborn. N Eng J Med 1984; 310:559–562.
100. Nesheim ME, et al. Studies of the capacity of factor Xa to protect factor Va from inactivation by activated protein C. J Biol Chem 1982; 257:1443–1447.
101. Solymoss S, Tucker MM, Tracy PB. Kinetics of inactivation of membrane bound factor Va by activated protein C. Protein S modulates factor Xa production. J Biol Chem 1988; 263:14884–14890.
102. Suzuki K, Nishioka J, Hashimoto S. Protein C inhibitor: purification from human plasma and characterization. J Biol Chem 1983; 258:163–168.
103. Marcum JA, McKinney JB, Rosenberg RD. Acceleration of thrombin-antithrombin complex formation in rat hindquarters via heparin-like molecules bound to the endothelium. J Clin Invest 1984; 74:341–350.
104. Busch C, Owen WG. Identification in vitro of an endothelial cell surface cofactor for antithrombin III. Parallel studies with isolated perfused rat hearts and microcarrier cultures of bovine endothelium. J Clin Invest 1982; 69:726–729.
105. Stern D. Interaction of antithrombin III with bovine aortic segments: role of heparin in binding and enhanced coagulant activity. J Clin Invest 1985; 75:272–279.
106. Rosenberg RD. Biochemistry of heparin antithrombin interactions, and the physiologic role of this natural anticoagulant mechanism. Am J Med 1987; 87:25–95.
107. Marcum JA, Rosenberg RD. Heparin-like molecules with anti-coagulant activity are synthesized by cultured endothelial cells. Biochem Biophys Res Comm 1985; 126:365–372.
108. Knauer DJ, Cunningham DD. Protease nexins: cell secreted proteins which regulate extracellular serine proteases. Trends Biochem Sci 1984; 9:231–233.
109. Shuman MA, et al. Endothelial cell and platelet binding sites for thrombin. Ann NY Acad Sci 1981; 370:57–66.
110. Leroy-Viard K, et al. Covalent binding of human thrombin to a human endothelial cell-associated protein. Exp Cell Res 1989; 181:1–10.
111. Hiramoto SA, Cunningham DD. Effects of fibroblasts and endothelial cells on inactivation of target proteases by prote-

ase nexin-1, heparin cofactor II and C1-inhibitor. J Cell Biochem 1988; 36:199–207.
112. Gallegher JT. The extended family of proteoglycans: social residents of the pericellular zone. Curr Opin Cell Biol 1989; 1:1201–1218.
113. Clement B, et al. Identification of a cell surface-binding protein for the core protein of the basement membrane proteoglycan. J Biol Chem 1989; 264:12467–12471.
114. David G, et al. Molecular cloning of a phosphatidylinositol anchored membrane heparan sulftate proteoglycan from human lung fibroblasts. J Cell Biol 1990; 111:3165–3176.
115. Kjellen L, Pettersson I, Höök, M. Cell surface heparan sulfate: an intercalated membrane proteoglycan. Proc Natl Acad Sci USA 1981; 78:5371–5375.
116. Wang X, et al. Expression cloning and characterization of the TGFβ type III receptor. Cell 1991; 67:797–805.
117. Lopez-Casellas F, et al. Structure and expression of the membrane proteoglycan betaglycan, a component of the TGFβ receptor system. Cell 1991; 67:785–795.
118. Kojima T, Shworak NW, Rosenberg R. Molecular cloning and expression of two distinct cDNA-encoding heparan sulfate proteoglycan core proteins from a rat endothelial cell line. J Biol Chem 1992; 267:4870–4877.
119. Lose E, Bernfield M. Pulmonary artery endothelial cells produce syndecan, a cell surface proteoglycan and possibly low affinity bFGF receptor. J Cell Biol 1991; 115:417a.
120. Thomas L. Studies of the intravascular thromboplastic effect of tissue suspension in mice II. A factor in normal rabbit serum which inhibits the thromboplastic effect of the sedimental tissue component. Bull John Hopk Hospital 1947; 81:26–42.
121. Schneider CL. The active principal placental toxin: thromboplastin; its inactivation in blood: antithromboplastin. Am J Physiol 1947; 149:123–129.
122. Broze GJ, Miletich JP. Characterization of inhibition of tissue factor in serum. Blood 1987; 69:150–155.
123. Rao LVM, Rapaport SI. Studies of a mechanism inhibiting the initiation of the intrinsic pathway of coagulation. Blood 1987; 69:645–651.
124. Broze GJ, et al. The lipoprotein associated coagulation inhibitor that inhibits the Factor VIIa-tissue factor complex, also inhibits Factor Xa: insight into its possible mechanisms of action. Blood 1988; 71:335–343.
125. Warn-Cramer B, et al. Modifications of extrinsic pathway inhibitor (EPI) and Factor Xa that affect their ability to interact and to inhibit Factor VIIa/tissue factor: evidence for a two-step model of inhibition. Thromb Haemostasis 1988; 60:454–456.
126. Hubbard AR, Jennings CA. Inhibition of tissue thromboplastin-mediated blood coagulation. Thromb Res 1986; 46:527–537.
127. Hubbard AR, Jennings CA. Inhibition of the tissue factor-factor VII complex: involvement of factor Xa and lipoproteins. Thromb Res 1987; 46:527–537.
128. Wun TC, et al. Cloning and characterization of a cDNA coding for the lipoprotein associated coagulation inhibitor shows it consists of three tandem Kunitz-type inhibitory domains. J Biol Chem 1988; 263:6001–6004.
129. Girard TJ, et al. Identification of the 1.4 kb and 4.0 kb messages for the lipoprotein associated coagulation inhibitor and expression of the encoded protein. Thromb Res 1989; 55:37–50.
130. Wam-Cramer BJ, Almus FE, Rapaport SI. Studies of the Factor Xa-dependent inhibitor of Factor VII/tissue factor (extrinsic pathway inhibitor) from cell supernatants of cultured human umbilical vein endothelial cells. Thromb Haemostas 1989; 61:101–105.
131. Rana SV, et al. Expression of tissue factor and Factor VIIa-tissue factor inhibitory activity in endototoxin, phorbol ester stimulated U937 monocyte-like cells. Blood 1988; 71:259–262.
132. Wun TC, et al. Immunoaffinity purification and characterization of lipoprotein-associated coagulation inhibitor from Hep G2 Hepatoma, Chang liver and SK hepatoma cells. J Biol Chem 1990; 265:16096–16101.
133. Bajaj MS, et al. Expression of tissue factor (TF) and suppression of Factor VIIa-TF inhibitor production by endotoxin or phorbol ester stimulated endothelial cells. Circulation 1988;78:315D (Abstr).
134. Bajaj MS, et al. Cultured normal human hepatocytes do not synthesize lipoprotein-associated coagulation inhibitor: evidence that the endothelium is the principal site of its synthesis. Proc Natl Acad Sci USA 1990; 87:8869–8873.
135. Sandstet PM, Abildgaard U. Extrinsic pathway inhibitor—the key to feedback control of blood coagulation initiation by tissue thromboplastin. Haemostasis 1991; 21:219–239.
136. Sandstet PM, Abilgaard U, Larsen ML. Heparin induces release of extrinsic pathway inhibitor (EPI). Thromb Res 1988; 50:803–813.
137. Werling RW, et al. Distribution of tissue factor pathway inhibitor (TFPI, EPI, LACI) in normal and pathological human tissues. Blood 1991; 78 [Suppl 1]:72 (Abstr).
138. Marcus AJ, Weksler BB, Jaffe EA. Enzymatic conversion of prostaglandin H_2 and arachidonic acid to prostacyclin by cultured human endothelial cells. J Biol Chem 1978; 253:7138–7141.
139. Weksler BB, Marcus AJ, Jaffe EA. Synthesis of prostaglandin I_2 (prostacyclin) by cultured human and bovine endothelial cells. Proc Natl Acad Sci USA 1977; 74:3922–3926.
140. Moncada S, et al. An enzyme isolated from arteries transforms prostaglandin endoperoxides to an unstable substance that inhibits platelet aggregation. Nature 1976; 263:663–665.
141. Gryglewski R, et al. Arterial walls are protected against deposition of platelet thrombi by a substance (prostaglandin X) which they make from prostaglandin endoperoxides. Prostaglandins 1976; 12:685–714.
142. Bunting S, et al. Arterial walls generate from prostaglandin endoperoxides a substance which relaxes strips of mesenteric and coeliac arteries and inhibits platelet aggregation. Prostaglandins 1976; 12:897–913.
143. Best LC, et al. Prostacyclin increases cyclic AMP levels and adenylate cyclase activity in platelets. Nature 1977; 267:850–852.
144. Marcus AJ, Safier LB. Thromboregulation: multicellular modulation of platelet reactivity in hemostasis and thrombosis. Faseb J 1993; 7:516–522.
145. Gerritsen ME, Cheli CD. Arachidonic acid and prostaglandin endoperoxide metabolism in isolated rabbit coronary microvessels and isolated cultivated coronary microvessel endothelial cells. J Clin Invest 1983; 72:1658–1671.
146. Charo IF, et al. Prostaglandin I_2 is not a major metabolite of arachidonic acid in cultured endothelial cells from human foreskin microvessels. J Clin Invest 1984; 74:914–919.
147. Pearson JD, Slakey LL, Gordon JL. Stimulation of prostaglandin production through purinergic receptors on endothelial cells and macrophages. Biochem J 1983; 214:273–276.
148. Mannix RJ., et al. A novel nucleotide receptor in rabbit microvascular endothelial cells. Am J Physiology 1993; 265:H675–H680.
149. D'Humieres S, Russo-Marie F, Vargaftig BB. PAF-acether-induced synthesis of prostacyclin by human endothelial cells. Eur J Pharmacol 1986; 131:13–19.
150. Baenziger NL, Force LE, Becherer PR. Histamine stimulates prostacyclin synthesis in cultured human endothelial cells. Biochem Biophys Res Commun 1980; 92:1435–1440.

151. Cramer EB, et al. Leukotriene C_4 promotes prostacyclin synthesis by human endothelial cells. Proc Natl Acad Sci USA 1983; 80:4109–4113.
152. Weksler BB, Ley CW, Jaffe EA. Stimulation of endothelial prostacyclin production by thrombin, trypsin, and the ionophore A23187. J Clin Invest 1978; 62:923–930.
153. Hong SL. Effect of bradykinin and thrombin on prostacyclin synthesis in endothelial cells from calf and pig aorta and human umbilical vein. Thromb Res 1980; 18:787–795.
154. Rossi V, et al. Prostacyclin synthesis induced in vascular cells by interleukin-1. Science 1985; 229:174–176.
155. Endo H, Akahoshi T, Kashiwazaki S. Additive effects of IL-1 and TNF on induction of prostacyclin synthesis in human vascular endothelial cells. Biochem Biophy Res Commun 1988; 156:1007–1014.
156. Zavoico GB, et al. IL-1 and related cytokines enhance thrombin-stimulated PGI_2 production in cultured endothelial cells without affecting thrombin-stimulated von Willebrand factor secretion or platelet-activating factor biosynthesis. J Immunol 1989; 142:3993–3999.
157. Eldor A, et al. Interferon enhances prostacyclin production by cultured vascular endothelial cells. J Clin Invest 1984; 73:251–257.
158. Moatter T, Gerritsen ME. Fibroblast growth factor upregulates PGG/H synthase in rabbit microvascular endothelial cells by a glucocorticoid independent mechanism. J Cell Physiol 1992; 151:571–578.
159. Moatter TM, Gerritsen ME. Acidic fibroblast growth factor induction of cyclooxygenase II in rabbit cardiac muscle microvessel endothelial cells: mediation by protein kinase C. Microcirculation 1994; 1:79–88.
160. Marcus AJ, et al. Synthesis of prostacyclin from platelet-derived endoperoxides by cultured human endothelial cells. J Clin Invest 1980; 66:979–986.
161. Schafer AI, Crawford DD, Gimbrone MA, Jr. Unidirectional transfer of prostaglandin endoperoxides between platelets and endothelial cells. J Clin Invest 1984; 73:1105–1112.
162. Feinmark SJ, Cannon PJ. Endothelial cell leukotriene C_4 synthesis results from intercellular transfer of leukotriene A_4 synthesized by polymorphonuclear leucocytes. J Biol Chem 1986; 261:16466–16472.
163. Ibe BO, Campbell WB. Synthesis and metabolism of leukotrienes by human endothelial cells: influence on prostacyclin release. Biochim Biophys Acta 1988; 960:309–321.
164. Yamaja Setty BN, Berger M, Stuart MJ. 13-hydroxyoctadeca-9,11-dienoic acid (13-HODE) inhibits thromboxane A_2 synthesis, and stimulates 12-HETE production in human platelets. Biochem Biophys Res Commun 1987; 148:528–533.
165. Buchanan MR, et al. Endothelial cells produce a lipoxygenase-derived chemo-repellent which influences platelet/endothelial cell interactions—effect of aspirin and salicylate. Thromb Haemost 1985; 53:306–311.
166. Aznar Salatti J, et al. Differential localization of von Willebrand factor, fibronectin and 13-HODE in human endothelial cell cultures. Histochemistry 1990; 93:507–511.
167. Buchanan MR, et al. The basement membrane underlying the vascular endothelium is not thrombogenic: in vivo and in vitro studies with rabbit and human tissue. Thromb Haemost 1987; 58:698–704.
168. Drake TA, Morrissey JH, Edgington TS. Selective cellular expression of tissue factor in human tissues. Implications for disorders of hemostasis and thrombosis. Am J Pathol 1989; 134:1087–1097.
169. Wilcox JN, et al. Localization of tissue factor in the normal vessel and in the atherosclerotic plaque. Proc Natl Acad Sci USA 1989; 86:2839–2843.
170. Maynard JR, et al. Tissue-factor coagulant activity of cultured human endothelial and smooth muscle cells and fibroblasts. Blood 1977; 50:387–396.
171. Colucci M, et al. Cultured human endothelial cells generate tissue factor in response to endotoxin. J Clin Invest 1983; 71:1893–1896.
172. Drake TA, Morrissey JH, Edginton TS. Selective cellular expression of tissue factor in human tissues: implications for disorders of hemostasis and thrombosis. Am J Pathol 1989; 134:1087–1097.
173. Wilcox JN, et al. Localization of tissue factor in the normal vessel wall and in the atherosclerotic plaque. Proc Natl Acad Sci USA 1989; 86:2839–2843.
174. Brox JH, et al. Production and availability of thromboplastin in endothelial cells: the effects of thrombin, endotoxin and platelets. Br J Haematol 1984; 57:239–246.
175. Carlsen E, Stinessen MB, Prydz H. Differential effect of alpha-interferon and gamma-interferon on thromboplastin response in monocytes and endothelial cells. Clin Exp Immunol 1987; 70:471–478.
176. Bevilacqua MP, et al. Interleukin-1 (IL-1) induces biosynthesis and cell surface expression of procoagulant activity in human vascular endothelial cells. J Exp Med 1984; 160:618–623.
177. Bevilacqua MP, et al. Recombinant tumor necrosis factor induces procoagulant activity in cultured human vascular endothelium: characterization and comparison with the actions of interleukin 1. Proc Natl Acad Sci USA 1986; 83:4533–4537.
178. Ogawa S, et al. Hypoxia modulates the barrier and coagulant function of cultured bovine endothelium. Increased monolayer permeability and induction of procoagulant properties. J Clin Invest 1990; 85:1090–1098.
179. Edgington TS, et al. Cellular immune and cytokine pathways resulting in tissue factor expression and relevance to septic shock. Nouv Rev Fr Hématol 1992; 34:S15–S27.
180. Geelen S, Bhattacharyya C, Tuomanen E. Induction of procoagulant activity on human endothelial cells by streptococcus pneumoniae. Infection and Immunity 1992; 60:4179–4183.
181. Morrisey JH, Fakhrai H, Edginton TS. Molecular cloning of the cDNA for tissue factor, the cellular receptor for the initiation of the coagulation protease cascade. Cell 1987; 50:129–135.
182. Spicer EM, et al. Human tissue factor: cDNA sequence and chromosome localization of the gene. Biochemistry 1987; 26:5234–5238.
183. Fisher K, et al. Cloning and expression of human tissue factor cDNA. Thromb Res 1987; 48:89–99.
184. Edgington TS, et al. The structural biology of expression and function of tissue factor. Thromb Haemost 1991; 66:67–79.
185. Rapaport SI, Rao LVM. Initiation and regulation of tissue factor-dependent blood coagulation. Arteriosclerosis Thrombosis 1992; 12:1111–1121.
186. Cerveny TJ, Fass DN, Mann KG. Synthesis of coagulation factor V by cultured aortic endothelium. Blood 1984; 63:1467–1474.
187. Wilson DB, et al. Biosynthesis of coagulation factor V by a human hepatocellular carcinoma cell line. J Clin Invest 1984; 73:654–658.
188. Annamalai AE, et al. Expression of factor V on human umbilical vein endothelial cells is modulated by cell injury. Arteriosclerosis 1986; 6:196–202.
189. Maruyama I, Salem HH, Majerus PW. Coagulation factor Va binds to human umbilical vein endothelial cells and accelerates protein C activation. J Clin Invest 1984; 74:224–230.
190. Rodgers GM, Shuman MA. Characterization of the interaction between factor Xa and bovine aortic endothelial cells. Biochim Biophys Acta 1985; 844:320–329.

191. Jaffe EA, Hoyer LW, Nachman RL. Synthesis of antihemophilic factor antigen by cultured human endothelial cells. J Clin Invest 1973; 52:2757–2764.
192. Jaffe EA, Hoyer LW, Nachman RL. Synthesis of von Willebrand factor by cultured human endothelial cells. Proc Natl Acad Sci USA 1974; 71:1906–1909.
193. Turitto VT, et al. Factor VIII/von Willebrand factor in subendothelium mediates platelet adhesion. Blood 1985; 65:823–831.
194. Meyer D, Baumgartner HR. Role of von Willebrand factor in platelet adhesion to the subendothelium. Br J Haematol 1983; 54:1–9.
195. Wagner DD. Storage and secretion of von Willebrand factor. In TS Zimmerman, ZM Ruggeri, eds. Coagulation and Bleeding Disorders. The Role of Factor VIII and von Willebrand Factor. New York: Marcel Dekker, 1989. Pp 161–180.
196. Sporn LA, Marder VJ, Wagner DD. Inducible secretion of large, biologically potent von Willebrand factor multimers. Cell 1986; 46:185–190.
197. Tsai HM, et al. Multimeric composition of endothelial cell-derived von Willebrand factor. Blood 1989; 73:2074–2076.
198. Wagner DD, Olmsted JB, Marder VJ. Immunolocalization of von Willebrand protein in Weibel-Palade bodies of human endothelial cells. J Cell Biol 1982; 95:355–360.
199. Mayadas T, Wagner DD, Simpson PJ. von Willebrand factor biosynthesis and partitioning between constitutive and regulated pathways of secretion after thrombin stimulation. Blood 1989; 73:706–711.
200. Warhol MJ, Sweet JM. The ultrastructural localization of von Willebrand factor in endothelial cells. Am J Pathol 1984; 117:310–315.
201. Wagner DD, Marder VJ. Biosynthesis of von Willebrand protein by human endothelial cells: processing steps and their intracellular localization. J Cell Biol 1984; 99:2123–2130.
202. Fuchs A, Weibel ER. Morphometrische untersuchung der verteilung einer spezifischen cytoplasmatischen organelle in endothelzellen der ratte. Zeitschrift für Zellforschung 1966; 73:1–9.
203. Weibel ER, Palade GE. New cytoplasmic components in arterial endothelia. J Cell Biol 1964; 23:101–110.
204. Ribes JA, Francis CW, Wagner DD. Fibrin induces release of von Willebrand factor from endothelial cells. J Clin Invest 1987; 79:117–1233.
205. Levine JD, et al. Thrombin-mediated release of factor VIII antigen from human umbilical vein endothelial cells in culture. Blood 1982; 60:531–534.
206. Harrison RL, McKee PA. Estrogen stimulates von Willebrand factor production by cultured endothelial cells. Blood 1984; 63:657–664.
207. Sporn LA, et al. Irradiation induces release of von Willebrand protein from endothelial cells in culture. Blood 1984; 64:567–570.
208. Mordes DB, et al. Elevated glucose concentrations increase factor VIIIR: Ag levels in human umbilical vein endothelial cells. Diabetes 1983; 32:876–878.
209. Hattori R, et al. Complement proteins C5b-9 induce secretion of high molecular weight multimers of endothelial von Willebrand factor and translocation of granule membrane protein GMP-140 to the cell surface. J Biol Chem 1989; 264:9053–9060.
210. Reidy MA, et al. Injury induces increase of von Willebrand factor in rat endothelial cells. Am J Pathol 1989; 134:857–864.
211. Schorer AE, Moldow CF, Rick ME. Interleukin 1 or endotoxin increases the release of von Willebrand factor from human endothelial cells. Br J Haematol 1987; 67:193–197.
212. Giddings JC, Shall L. Enhanced release of von Willebrand factor by human endothelial cells in culture in the presence of phorbol myristate acetate and interleukin 1. Thromb Res 1987; 47:259–267.
213. Paleolog EM, et al. Differential regulation by cytokines of constitutive and stimulated secretion of von Willebrand factor from endothelial cells. Blood 1990; 75:688–695.
214. Reinders JH, et al. Perturbation of cultured human vascular endothelial cells by phorbol ester or thrombin alters the cellular von Willebrand factor distribution. J Cell Physiol 1987; 133:79–87.
215. Sporn LA, Marder VJ, Wagner DD. von Willebrand factor released from Weibel-Palade bodies binds more avidly to extracellular matrix than that secreted constitutively. Blood 1987; 69:1531–1534.
216. Ribes JA, Francis CW. Multimer size dependence of von Willebrand factor binding to crosslinked or noncrosslinked fibrin. Blood 1990; 75:1460–1465.
217. Weiss HJ, et al. Fibrinogen-independent platelet adhesion and thrombus formation on subendothelium mediated by glycoprotein IIb-IIIa complex at high shear rate. J Clin Invest 1989; 288–297.
218. Ikeda Y, et al. The role of von Willebrand factor and fibrinogen in platelet aggregation under varying shear stress. J Clin Invest 1991; 87:1234–1240.
219. Ruggeri ZM, et al. Platelets have more than one binding site for von Willebrand factor. J Clin Invest 1983; 72:1–12.
220. Savage B, Shattil SJ, Ruggeri ZM. Modulation of platelet function through adhesion receptors: a dual role for glycoprotein IIb-IIIa (integrin $\alpha IIB\beta 3$) mediated by fibrinogen and glycoprotein Ib-von Willebrand factor. J Biol Chem 1992; 267:11300–11306.
221. Mancuso DJ, et al. Structure of the gene for human von Willebrand factor. J Biol Chem 264:19514–19527.
222. Ginsburg D, et al. Human von Willebrand factor (vWF): isolation of complementary DNA (cDNA) clones and chromsomal localization. Science 1985; 228:1401–1406.
223. Mayadas TN, Wagner DD. von Willebrand Factor biosynthesis and processing. Ann NY Acad Sci 1991; 614:153–166.
224. Wion KL, et al. Distribution of factor VIII mRNA and antigen in human liver and other tissues. Nature (London) 1985; 317:726–728.
225. Tschopp TB, Weiss HJ, Baumgartner HR. Decreased adhesion of platelets to subendothelium in von Willebrand's disease. J Lab Clin Med 1974; 83:296–300.
226. Weiss HJ, et al. Correction by factor VIII of the impaired platelet adhesion to subendothelium in von Willebrand's disease. Blood 1978; 51:267–279.
227. Takeuchi M, Nagura H, Kaneda T. DDAVP and epinephrine-induced changes in the localization of von Willebrand factor antigen in endothelial cells of human oral mucosa. Blood 1988; 72: 850–854.
228. Montgomery RR, Johnson J. Specific factor VIII-related antigen fragmentation: an in vivo and in vitro phenomenon. Blood 1982; 68:930–939.
229. McCarroll DR, Levin EG, Montgomery RR. Endothelial cell synthesis of von Willebrand antigen II, von Willebrand factor, and von Willebrand factor/von Willebrand antigen II complex. J Clin Invest 1985; 75:1089–1095.
230. Fay PJ, et al. Propolypeptide of von Willebrand factor circulates in blood and is identical to von Willebrand antigen II. Science 1986; 232:995–998.
231. Wise RJ, et al. The propeptide of von Willebrand factor independently mediates the assembly of von Willebrand multimers. Cell 1988; 52:229–236.
232. Wagner DD, et al. Divergent fates of von Willebrand factor and its propolypeptide (von Willebrand antigen II) after secretion from endothelial cells. Proc Natl Acad Sci USA 1987; 84:1955–1959.

233. Stern DM, et al. Binding of factors IX and IXa to cultured vascular endothelial cells. Proc Natl Acad Sci USA 1983; 80:4119–4123.
234. Heimark RL, Schwartz SM. Binding of coagulation factors IX and X to the endothelial surface. Biochem Biophys Res Commun 1983; 111:723–731.
235. Rimon S, et al. Identification of a factor IX/IXa binding protein on the endothelial cell surface. J Biol Chem 1987; 262:6023–6031.
236. Stern DM, et al. Activation of factor IX bound to cultured bovine aortic endothelial cells. Proc Natl Acad Sci USA 1984; 81:913–917.
237. Mosher DF. Physiology of thrombospondin. Annu Rev Med 1990; 41:85–97.
238. Frazier WA. Thrombospondins. Curr Opin Cell Biol 1991; 3:792–799.
239. Wight TN, et al. Light microscopic immunolocation of thrombospondin in human tissues. J Histochem Cytochem 1985; 33:295–302.
240. Majack RA, Goodman LV, Dixit VM. Cell surface thrombospondin is functionally essential for vascular smooth muscle proliferation. J Cell Biol 1988; 106:415–422.
241. Phan SH, et al. Stimulation of fibroblast proliferation by thrombospondin. Biochem Biophys Res Commun 1989; 163:55–63.
242. Engel J. EGF-like domains in extracellular matrix proteins: localized signals for growth and differentiation? Febs Lett 1989; 251:1–7.
243. Sage H, et al. SPARC, a secreted protein associated with cellular proliferation, inhibits cell spreading in vitro and exhibits Ca^{2+} dependent binding to the extracellular matrix. J Cell Biol 1989; 109:341–356.
244. Raugi GJ, Olerud JE, Gown AM. Thrombospondin in early human wound tissue. J Invest Dermatol 1987; 89:551–554.
245. Raugi GJ, et al. Thrombospondin deposition in rat carotid artery. Am J Pathol 1990; 137:179–185.
246. Munjal ID, Blake DA, Sabet MD. Thrombospondin: biosynthesis, distribution and changes associated with wound repair in corneal endothelium. Eur J Cell Biol 1990; 52:252–263.
247. Lawler J. The structural and functional properties of thrombospondin. Blood 1986; 67:1197–1209.
248. Murphy-Ulrich JE, Mosher DF. Localization of thrombospondin in clots formed in situ. Blood 1985; 66:1098–1104.
249. De la Cadena RA, et al. Structural determinants of the binding of human high molecular weight kininogen to platelet thrombospondin. Thromb Haemost 1991; 65:699.
250. Lahav J, Lawler J and Gimbrone MA Jr.Thrombospondin interactions with fibronectin and fibrinogen. Mutual inhibition in binding. Eur J Biochem 1984; 145:151–156.
251. Leung LLK. Role of thrombospondin in platelet aggregation. J Clin Invest 1984; 74:1764–1772.
252. Dardek R, Lahav J. Enzyme specific and conformation dependent degradation of thrombospondin by plasminogen activators. Blood 1991; 78:70a.
253. Silverstein RL, et al. Activation of immobilized plasminogen by tissue activator. Multimolecular complex formation. J Biol Chem 1985; 260:10346–10352.
254. Hogg PJ, Stenflo J, Mosher DF. Thrombospondin is a slow tight-binding inhibitor of plasmin. Biochemistry 1992; 31:265–269.
255. Benveniste J, Henson PM, Cochrane CG. Leukocyte-dependent histamine release from rabbit platelets. The role of IgE, basophils and a platelet activating factor. J Exp Med 1972;1356–1377.
256. McManus LM, et al. Pathobiology of the intravenous infusion of acetyl glycerol ether phosphorylcholine (AGEPC) infusion in the rabbit. Immunopharmacology 1980; 5:197–207.
257. Bjork J, et al. Paf-acether (platelet activating factor) increases microvascular permeability and affects endothelium granulocyte interaction in microvascular beds. Acta Physiol Scand 1983; 119:305–308.
258. Camussi G, et al. The release of platelet activating factor from endothelial cells in culture. J Immunol 1983; 131:2397–2403.
259. Prescott SM, Zimmerman GA, McIntyre TM. Human endothelial cells in culture produce platelet activating factor (1-alkyl-2-acetyl-sn-glycero-3-phosphocholine) when stimulated with thrombin. Proc Natl Acad Sci 1984; 81:3534–3538.
260. McIntyre TM, Zimmerman GA, Prescott SM. Leukotrienes C_4 and D_4 stimulate human endothelial cells to synthesize platelet activating factor and bind neutrophils. Proc Natl Acad Sci USA 1986; 83:2204–2208.
261. McIntyre TM, et al. Cultured endothelial cells synthesize both platelet activating factor and prostacyclin in response to histamine, bradykinin and adenosine triphosphate. J Clin Invest 1985; 76:271–280.
262. Zimmerman GA, McIntyre TM, Prescott SM. Production of platelet-activating factor by human vascular endothelial cells: Evidence for a requirement for specific agonists and modulation by prostacyclin. Circulation 1985; 72:718–727.
263. Whatley RE, et al. Lipid metabolism and signal transduction in endothelial cells. Prog Lipid Res 1990; 29:45–63.
264. Blank ML, et al. Metabolism of platelet activating factor (1-alkyl-2-acetyl-sn-glycero-3-phosphocholine) and 1-alkyl-2-acetyl-sn-glycerol by human endothelial cells. Biochim Biophys Acta 876:373–378.
265. Loskutoff DJ, Edgington TS. Synthesis of a fibrinolytic activator and inhibitor by endothelial cells. Proc Natl Acad Sci USA 1977; 74:3903–3907.
266. Levin EG, Loskutoff DJ. Cultured bovine endothelial cells produce both urokinase and tissue-type plasminogen activators. J Cell Biol 1982; 94:631–636.
267. Booyse FM, et al. Isolation and characterization of a urokinase-type plasminogen activator (Mr = 54,000) from cultured human endothelial cells indistinguishable from urinary urokinase. J Biol Chem 1984; 259:7198–7205.
268. Bykowska K, et al. Characterization of a plasminogen activator secreted by cultured bovine aortic endothelial cells. Biochim Biophys Acta 1982; 703:113–115.
269. Wallen P. Activation of plasminogen with urokinase and tissue activator. In R Paoletti, S Sherry, eds. Thrombosis and Urokinase. New York: Academic Press, 1977. Pp. 91.
270. Hoylaerts M, et al. Kinetics of the activation of plasminogen by human tissue plasminogen activator. Role of fibrin. J Biol Chem 1982; 257:2912–2919.
271. Bachman F, Kruithof EKO. Tissue plasminogen activator: chemical and physiological aspects. Semin Thromb Haemostasis 1984; 10:6–17.
272. Patthy L, et al. Kringles: modules specialized for protein binding. Homology of the gelatin binding region of fibronectin with the kringle structure of proteases. FEBS Lett 1984; 171:131–136.
273. Patthy L. Evolution of the proteases of blood coagulation and fibrinolysis by assembly from modules. Cell 1985; 41:657–663.
274. Pennica D, et al. Cloning and expression of human tissue-type plasminogen activator cDNA in E. Coli. Nature (London) 1983; 301:214–221.
275. Banyai L, Varadi A, Patthy L. Common evolutionary origin of the fibrin binding structures of fibronectin and tissue type plasminogen activator. FEBS Lett 1983; 163:37–41.
276. Ny T, Elgh F, Lund B. The structure of human tissue type plasminogen activator gene: correlation of intron and exon structures to functional and structural domains. Proc Natl Acad Sci USA 1984; 81:5355–5359.

277. Tate KM, et al. Functional role of proteolytic cleavage at arginine 275 of human tissue plasminogen activator as assessed by site-directed mutagenesis. Biochem 1987; 26: 338–343.
278. Collen D. On the regulation and control of fibrinolysis. Thromb Haemostasis 1980; 43:77–89.
279. Wun TC, Schleuning WD, Reich E. Isolation and characterization of urokinase from human plasma. J Biol Chem 1982; 277:3276–3283.
280. Collen D, et al. Activation of plasminogen by pro-urokinase II. Kinetics. J Biol Chem 1989; 261:1259–1266.
281. Verde P, et al. Identification and primary sequence of an unspliced human urokinase poly (A) + RNA. Proc Natl Acad Sci USA 1984; 81:4727–4731.
282. Crutchley DJ, Conanan LB. Endotoxin induction of an inhibitor of plasminogen activator in bovine pulmonary artery endothelial cells. J Biol Chem 1986; 261:154–159.
283. van Hinsbergh VW, et al. Production of plasminogen activators and inhibitor by serially propagated endothelial cells from adult human blood vessels. Arteriosclerosis 1987; 7:389–400.
284. Schleef RR, Wagner NV, Loskutoff DJ. Detection of both type 1 and type 2 plasminogen activator inhibitors in human cells. J Cell Physiol 1988; 134:269–274.
285. Loskutoff DJ, et al. Detection of an unusually stable fibrinolytic inhibitor produced by bovine endothelial cells. Proc Natl Acad Sci USA 1983; 80:2956–2960.
286. Hekman CM, Loskutoff DJ. Endothelial cells produce a latent inhibitor of plasminogen activators that can be activated by denaturants. J Biol Chem 1985; 260:11581–11587.
287. van Mourik JA, Lawrence DA, Loskutoff DJ. Purification of an inhibitor of plasminogen activator (antiactivator) synthesized by endothelial cells. J Biol Chem 1984; 259:14914–14921.
288. Ny T, et al. Cloning and sequence of a cDNA coding for the human beta-migrating endothelial-cell-type plasminogen activator inhibitor. Proc Natl Acad Sci USA 1986; 83:6776–6780.
289. Ginsburg D, et al. cDNA cloning of human plasminogen activator-inhibitor from endothelial cells. J Clin Invest 1986; 78:1673–1680.
290. Podor TJ, Curriden SA, Loskutoff DJ. The fibrinolytic system of endothelial cells. In US Ryan, ed. Endothelial Cells. Vol 1. Boca Raton, FL: CRC Press, 1988. Pp 128–148.
291. Lawrence DA, Loskutoff DJ. Inactivation of plasminogen activator inhibitor by oxidants. Biochemistry 1986; 25:6351–6355.
292. Lambers JWJ, et al. Activation of human endothelial cell-type plasminogen activator inhibitor (PAI-1) by negatively charged phospholipids. J Biol Chem 1987; 26:17492–17496.
293. Mimuro J, Loskutoff DJ. Purification of a protein from bovine plasma that binds to type 1 plasminogen activator inhibitor and prevents its interaction with extracellular matrix. Evidence that the protein is vitronectin. J Biol Chem 1989; 264:936–939.
294. Seiffert D, Wagner NN, Loskutoff DJ. Serum-derived vitronectin influences the pericellular distribution of type 1 plasminogen activator inhibitor. J Cell Biol 1990; 111:1283–1291.
295. Berrettini M, et al. Interaction of type 1 plasminogen activator inhibitor with the enzymes of the contact activation system. J Biol Chem 1989; 264:11738–11743.
296. van Hinsbergh VWM, et al. Activated protein C decreases plasminogen activator-inhibitor activity in endothelial cell-conditioned medium. Blood 1985; 65:444–451.
297. Sakata Y, et al. Activated protein C stimulates the fibrinolytic activity of cultured endothelial cells and decreases antiactivator activity. Proc Natl Acad Sci USA 1985; 82:1121–1125.
298. Sakata Y, et al. Mechanism of protein C-dependent clot lysis: role of plasminogen activator inhibitor. Blood 1986; 68:1218–1223.
299. Zoellner H, et al. Cytokine regulation of the synthesis of plasminogen activator inhibitor-2 by human vascular endothelial cells. Comparison with plasminogen activator inhibitor-1 synthesis. Thromb Haemost 1993; 69:135–140.
300. Levin EG, et al. Thrombin stimulates tissue plasminogen activator release from cultured human endothelial cells. J Clin Invest 1984; 74:1988–1995.
301. Gelehrter TD, Sznycer-Laszuk R. Thrombin induction of plasminogen activator-inhibitor in cultured human endothelial cells. J Clin Invest 1986; 77:165–169.
302. van Hinsberg VW, Sprengers ED, Kooistra T. Effect of thrombin on the production of plasminogen activators and plasminogen activator inhibitor-1 by human foreskin microvascular endothelial cells. Thromb Haemost 1987; 57:148–153.
303. Dichek D, Quertermous T. Thrombin regulation of mRNA levels of tissue plasminogen activator and plasminogen activator inhibitor-1 in cultured human umbilical vein endothelial cells. Blood 1989; 74:222–228.
304. Diamond SL, Eskin SG, McIntire LV. Fluid flow stimulates tissue plasminogen activator secretion by cultured human endothelial cells. Science 1989; 243:1483–1485.
305. Levin EG, Santell L. Stimulation and desensitization of tissue plasminogen activator release from human endothelial cells. J Biol Chem 1988; 263:9360–9365.
306. Hanss M, Collen D. Secretion of tissue-type plasminogen activator and plasminogen activator inhibitor by cultured human endothelial cells: modulation by thrombin, endotoxin, and histamine. J Lab Clin Med 1987; 109:97–104.
307. Medina R, et al. Interleukin-1, endotoxin or tumor necrosis factor/cachetin enhance the level of plasminogen activator inhibitor messenger RNA in bovine aortic endothelial cells. Thromb Res 1989; 54:41–52.
308. Sawdey M, Podor TJ, Loskutoff DJ. Regulation of type 1 plasminogen activator inhibitor gene expression in cultured bovine aortic endothelial cells. Induction by transforming growth factor beta, lipopolysaccharide, and tumor necrosis factor-alpha. J Biol Chem 1989; 264:10396–10401.
309. Van den Berg, EA, et al. Regulation of plasminogen activator-inhibitor-1 mRNA in human endothelial cells. Thromb Haemostasis 1988; 60:63–67.
310. van Hinsbergh VWM, et al. Tumor necrosis factor increases the production of plasminogen activator inhibitor in human endothelial cells in vitro and rats in vivo. Blood 1988; 72:1467–1473.
311. Colucci M, Paramo JA, Collen D. Generation in plasma of a fast-acting inhibitor of plasminogen activator in response to endotoxin stimulation. J Clin Invest 1985; 75:818–824.
312. Emeis JJ, Kooistra T. Interleukin 1 and lipopolysaccharide induce an inhibitor of tissue-type plasminogen activator in vivo and in cultured endothelial cells. J Exp Med 1986; 163:1260–1266.
313. Bevilacqua MP, et al. Regulation of the fibrinolytic system of cultured human vascular endothelium by interleukin 1. J Clin Invest 1986; 78:587–591.
314. Etingen OR, et al. Lipoprotein(a) regulates plasminogen activator inhibitor expression in endothelial cells. A potential mechanism in thrombogenesis. J Biol Chem 1990; 266:2459–2465.
315. Hoylaerts M, et al. Kinetics of the activation of plasminogen by human tissue plasminogen activator. J Biol Chem 1982; 257:2912–2919.
316. Markus G, Evers JL, Hobika GH. Comparison of some properties of native (Glu) and modified (Lys) human plasminogen. J Biol Chem 1978; 253:733–739.

317. Markus G, Priore RL, Wissler FC. The binding of tranexamic acid to native (Glu) and modified (Lys) human plasminogen and its effect on conformation. J Biol Chem 1979; 254:1211–1216.
318. Hajjar KA, Nachman RL. Endothelial cell-mediated conversion of Glu-plasminogen. Further evidence for assembly of the fibrinolytic system on the endothelial cell surface. J Clin Invest 1988; 82:1769–1778.
319. Schafer AI, et al. Inhibition of vascular endothelial cell prostacyclin synthesis by plasmin. Blood 1989; 74:1015–1020.
320. Hajjar KA, et al. Binding of plasminogen to cultured endothelial cells. J Biol Chem 1986; 261:11656–11662.
321. Hajjar KA. The endothelial cell tissue plasminogen activator receptor: specific interactions with plasminogen. J Biol Chem 1991; 266:21962–21970.
322. Hajjar KA, Hamel NH. Identification and characterization of human endothelial cell membrane binding sites for tissue plasminogen activator and urokinase. J Biol Chem 1990; 265:2908–2916.
323. Barnathan ES, et al. Characterization of human endothelial urokinase-type plasminogen activator receptor protein and messenger RNA. Blood 1990; 76:1795–1806.
324. Hajjar KA, et al. Binding of tissue plasminogen activator to cultured human endothelial cells. J Clin Invest 1987; 80:1712–1719.
325. Barnathan ES, et al. Tissue-type plasminogen activator binding to human endothelial cells. Evidence for two distinct sites. J Biol Chem 1988: 263:7792–7799, 1988.
326. Moncada S, et al. Differential formation of prostacyclin (PGX or PGI_2) by layers of the arterial wall. An explanation for the antithrombotic properties of the vascular endothelium. Thromb Res 1977; 11:323–344.
327. Gryglewski RJ, Botting RM, Vane JR. Mediators produced by the vascular endothelial cell. Hypertension 1988; 12:530–548.
328. Willis AL, Smith DL. Therapeutic impact of eicosanoids in atherosclerotic disease. Eicosanoids 1989; 2:69–99.
329. Furchgott RF, Zawadzki JV. The obligatory role of endothelial cells in the relaxation of arterial smooth muscle by acetylcholine. Nature 1980; 288:373–376.
330. Palmer RMJ, Ferrige AG, Moncada S. Nitric oxide release accounts for the biological activity of endothelium-derived relaxing factor. Nature 1987; 327:524–526.
331. Palmer RMJ, Ashton DS, Moncada S. Vascular endothelial cells synthesize nitric oxide from L-arginine. Nature 1988; 333:664–666.
332. Moncada S, Palmer RMJ, Higgs EA. Nitric oxide: physiology, pathophysiology and pharmacology. Pharmac Rev 1991; 43:109–142.
333. Furchgott RF, Vanhoutte PM. Endothelium-derived relaxing and contracting factors. Faseb J 1989; 3:2007–2018.
334. Ignarro LJ. Biological action and properties of endothelium-derived nitric oxide formed and released from artery and vein. Circ Res 1989; 65:1–21.
335. Myers PR, et al. Vasorelaxant properties of the endothelium-derived relaxing factor more closely resemble nitrocystein than nitric oxide. Nature 1990; 345:161–164.
336. Forstermann U, et al. Isoforms of nitric oxide synthase. Biochem Pharmacol 1991;42:1849–1857.
337. Craven PA, DeRubertis FR. Restoration of the responsiveness of purified guanylate cyclase to nitroguanidine, nitric oxide and related activators by heme and hemeproteins. J Biol Chem 1978; 253:8433–8443.
338. Ignarro LJ, et al. Endothelium-derived relaxing factor produced and released from artery and vein is nitric oxide. Proc Natl Acad Sci USA 1987; 84:9265–9269.
339. Mellion BT, et al. Evidence for the inhibitory role of guanosine 3′,5′ monophosphate in ADP-induced human platelet aggregation in the presence of nitric oxide and related vasodilators. Blood 1981; 57:946–955.
340. Radomski MW, Palmer RMJ, Moncada S. Endogenous nitric oxide inhibits human platelet adhesion to vascular endothelium. Lancet 1987; 2:1057–1058.
341. Kaplan SS, et al. Inhibition of chemotaxis with N- monomethyl-L-arginine: a role for cyclic GMP. Blood 1989; 74:1885–1887.
342. Garg UC, Hassid A. Nitric oxide-generating vasodilators and 8-bromo-cyclic guanosine monophosphate inhibit mitogenesis and proliferation of cultured rat vascular smooth muscle cells. J Clin Invest 1989; 83:1774–1777.
343. Feigl EO. EDRF-a protective factor? Nature (London) 1988; 331, 490–491.
344. Rubanyi GM, et al. Cytoprotective function of nitric oxide: inactivation of superoxide radicals produced by human leukocytes. Biochem Biophys Res Commun 1991;81:1392–1397.
345. Wolin MS. Activated oxygen metabolites as regulators of vascular tone. Klin Wochenschr 1991; 69; 1046–1049.
346. Bolton TB, Lang RJ, Takewaki T. Mechanism of action of noradrenaline and carbachol on smooth muscle of guinea-pig anterior mesenteric artery. J Physiol 1984; 351:549–572.
347. Nagao T, Vanhoutte PM. Membrane hyperpolarization contributes to endothelium-dependent relaxation induced by acetylcholine in the femoral vein of the rat. Am J Physiol 1991; 261:H1034–H1038.
348. Komori K, Suzuki H. Electrical responses of smooth muscle cells during cholinergic vasodilation in the rabbit saphenous artery. Circ Res 1987; 61:586–593.
349. Komori K, Lorenz RR, Vanhoute PM. Nitric oxide, acetylcholine and electrical and mechanical properties of canine arterial smooth muscle. Am J Physiol 1988; 255:H207–H212.
350. Bény J-L, Brunet PC. Neither nitric oxide nor nitroglycerin accounts for all of the characteristics of endothelial mediated vasodilatation of pig coronary arteries. Blood Vessels 1988; 25:308–311.
351. Brayden JE. Membrane hyperpolarization is a mechanism of endothelium dependent cerebral vasodilation. Am J Physiol 1990; 259:H668–H673.
352. Nagao T, Vanhoutte PM. Membrane hyperpolarization contributes to endothelium-dependent relaxations induced by acetylcholine in the femoral vein of the rat. Am J Physiol 1991; 261:H1034–H1038.
353. Chen GY, et al. Hyperpolarization of arterial smooth muscle induced by endothelial humoral substances. Am J Physiol 1991; 260:H1888–H1892.
354. Komori K, Lorenz RR, Vanhoutte PM. Nitric oxide, acetylcholine, and electrical and mechanical properties of canine arterial smooth muscle. Am J Physiol 1988; 255:H207–H212.
355. Chen G, Suzuki H, Weston AH. Acetylcholine releases endothelial-derived hyperpolarizing factor and EDRF from rat blood vessels. Br J Pharmacol 1988; 95:1165–1174.
356. Huang AH, Busse R, Bassenge E. Endothelium-dependent hyperpolarization of arterial smooth muscle is not mediated by EDRF. Naunyn Schmiedebergs Arch Pharmacol 1988; 338:438–442.
357. Nishiyi E, et al. Factors inducing endothelium dependent relaxation in the guinea pig basilar artery as estimated from the actions of haemoglobin. Brit J Pharmacol 1989; 96: 645–655.
358. Flavahan NA, Shimokawa H, Vanhoutte PM. Pertussis toxin inhibits endothelium dependent relaxation to certain agonists in porcine coronary arteries. J Physiol 1989; 408: 549–560.
359. Feletou M, Vanhoutte PM. Endothelium-dependent hyperpolarization of canine coronary smooth muscle. Br J Pharmacol 1989; 93:515–524.

360. Kauser K, et al. Mechanism of action of EDRF on pressurized arteries: effect on K^+ conductance. Circ Res 1989; 65:199–204.
361. Kuriyama H, Suzuki H. The effects of acetylcholine on the membrane and contractile properties of smooth muscle cells of the rabbit superior mesenteric artery. Br J Pharmacol 1978; 64:431–501.
362. Chen G, Suzuki H. Some electrical properties of the endothelium-dependent hyperpolarization recorded from rat arterial smooth muscle cells. J Physiol 1989; 410:91–106.
363. Nagao T, Vanhoutte PM. Hyperpolarization as a mechanism for endothelium-dependent relaxations in porcine coronary arteries. J Physiol 1992; 445:355–368.
364. Hickey KA, et al. Characterization of a coronary vasoconstrictor produced by endothelial cells in culture. Am J Physiol 1985; 248:C550–C556.
365. Yanagisawa M, et al. A novel potent vasoconstrictor peptide produced by vascular endothelial cells. Nature (London) 1988; 332:411–415.
366. Inoue A, et al. The human endothelin pathway: three structurally distinct isopeptides predicted by three separate genes. Proc Natl Acad Sci USA 1989; 86:2863–2867.
367. Kimura S, et al. Conversion of big endothelin-1 to 21 residue endothelin-1 is essential for expression of full vasoconstrictor activity: structure activity relationships of big endothelin-1. J Cardiovasc Pharmacol 1989; 13:S5–S7.
368. Sawamura T, et al. Analysis of endothelin related peptides in culture supernatant of porcine aortic endothelial cells: evidence for biosynthetic pathway of endothelin-1. Biochem Biophys Res Comm 1989; 162:1287–1294.
369. Hexum TD, et al. Characterization of endothelin secretion by vascular endothelial cells. Biochem Biophys Res Comm 1990; 167:294–300.
370. Yoshizumi M, et al. Interleukin-1 increases the production of endothelin-1 by cultured endothelial cells. Biochem Biophys Res Comm 1990; 166:324–329.
371. Yoshizumi M, et al. Hemodynamic shear stress stimulates endothelin production by cultured endothelial cells. Biochem Biophys Res Comm 1989; 161:859–864.
372. Kurihara H, et al. Transforming growth factor-β stimulates the expression of endothelin mRNA by vascular endothelial cells. Biochem Biophys Res Comm 1989; 159:1435–1440.
373. Kourembanas S, et al. Hypoxia induces endothelin gene expression and secretion in cultured human endothelium. J Clin Invest 1991; 88:1054–1057.
374. Vigne P, et al. Endothelin stimulates phosphatidylinositol hydrolysis and DNA synthesis in brain capillary endothelial cells. Biochemistry 1990; 266:415–420.
375. Bousso Mittler D, et al. Functional endothelin/sarafotoxin receptors in the rat uterus. Biochem Biophys Res Comm 1989; 162:952–957.
376. Inoue A, et al. The human endothelin family: Three structurally and pharmacologically distinct isopeptides predicted by three separate genes. Proc Natl Acad Sci USA 1989; 86:2863–2867.
377. Haynes WG, Webb DJ. Venoconstriction to endothelin-1 in humans: role of calcium and potassium channels. Am J Physiol 1993; 265:H1676–1681.
378. Sakurai T, et al. Cloning of a cDNA encoding a nonisopeptide-selective subtype of the endothelin receptor. Nature (London) 1990; 348:732–735.
379. Arai H, et al. Cloning and expression of a cDNA encoding an endothelin receptor. Nature (London) 1990; 348:730–732.
380. Rubanyi GM. Maintenance of "basal" vascular tone may represent a physiological role for endothelin. J Vasc Med Biol 1989; 1:315–316.
381. De Nucci G, et al. Pressor effects of circulating endothelin are limited by its removal in the pulmonary circulation and by the release of prostacyclin and endothelium-derived relaxing factor. Proc Natl Acad Sci USA 1988; 85:9797–9800.
382. Lidbury PS, et al. Interactions of endothelins with the endothelium. J Vasc Med Biol 1990; 2:178.
383. Boulanger C, Luscher TF. Release of endothelin from the porcine aorta: inhibition by endothelium-derived nitric oxide. J Clin Invest 1990; 85:587–590.
384. MacCumber MW, Ross CA, Snyder S. Endothelin in brain: receptors, mitogenesis and biosynthesis in glial cells. Proc Natl Acad Sci USA 1989; 87:2359–2363.
385. Rubanyi GM. Endothelium-derived vasoconstrictor factors. In US Ryan, ed. Endothelial Cells Vol 3. Boca Raton FL: CRC Press, 1988. Pp 61–74.
386. Olesen SP, Clapham DE, Davies PF. Hemodynamic shear stress activates a K^+ current in vascular endothelial cells. Nature 1988; 331:168–170.
387. Nollert MU, Eskin SG, McIntire LV. Shear stress increases inositol triphosphate levels in human endothelial cells. Biochem Biophys Res Comm 1990; 170:281–287.
388. Schwarz G, Droogmans G, Nilius B. Shear stress induced membrane currents and calcium transients in human vascular endothelial cells. Biochem Biophys Res Comm 1990; 170:281–287.
389. Shen J, et al. Fluid shear stress modulates cytosolic free calcium in vascular endothelial cells. Am J Physiol 1992; 262:C384–C390.
390. Shen J, et al. Fluid flow modulates vascular endothelial cytosolic calcium responses to adenine nucleotides. Microcirculation 1994; 1:67–78.
391. Ziegelstein RC, Cheng L, Capogrossi MC. Flow dependent cytosolic acidification of vascular endothelial cells. Science 1992; 258:656–659.
392. Frangos JA, et al. Flow effects on prostacyclin production by cultured endothelial cells. Science 1985; 227:1477–1479.
393. Grabowski EF, Jaffe EA, Weksler BB. Prostacyclin production by cultured human endothelial cells exposed to step increases in shear stress. J Lab Clin Med 1985; 105:36–43.
394. Diamond SL, Eskin SG, McIntire LV. Fluid flow stimulates tissue plasminogen activator secretion by cultured human endothelial cells. Science 1989; 243:1483–1485.
395. Cooke JP, et al. Flow stimulates endothelial cells to release a nitrovasodilator that is potentiated by reduced thiol. Am J Physiol 1990; 259:H804–H812.
396. Hsieh H, Li N, Frangos J. Shear stress increases endothelial platelet-derived growth factor mRNA levels. Am J Physiol 1991; 260:H642–H646.
397. Diamond SL, et al. Tissue plasminogen activator messenger RNA levels increase in cultured human endothelial cells exposed to laminar shear stress. J Cell Physiol 1990; 143:364–371.
398. Gemmell CH, Turrito VT, Nemerson Y. Flow as a regulator of the activation of factor X by tissue factor. Blood 1988; 72:1404–1406.
399. Nagel T, et al. Shear stress upregulates functional ICAM-1 expression in cultured vascular endothelial cells. FASEB J 1993; 7:A7 (Abstr).
400. Dewey CF, Jr, et al. The dynamic response of vascular endothelial cells to fluid shear stress. J Biomech Eng 1981; 103:177–181.
401. Levesque MJ, Nerem PR. The elongation and orientation of cultured endothelial cells in response to shear stress. J Biomech Eng 1985; 176:341–347.
402. Helmlinger G, et al. Effects of pulsatile flow on cultured vascular endothelial cell morphology. J Biomech Eng 1991; 113:123–131.
403. Robotewskyj A, et al. Dynamics of focal adhesion site remodelling in living endothelial cells in response to shear stress

forces using confocal image analysis. FASEB J 1991; 5:A527 (Abstr).
404. Acevedo AD, et al. Morphological and proliferative responses of endothelial cells to hydrostatic pressure: role of fibroblast growth factor. J Cell Physiol 1993; 157:603–614.
405. Watson PA. Function follows form: generation of intracellular signals by cell deformation. FASEB J 1991; 5:2013–2019.
406. Resnick N, et al. Platelet-derived growth factor B chain promoter contains a cis-acting shear-stress-responsive element. Proc Natl Acad Sci USA 1993; 90:4591–4595.
407. Elliot SJ, Messaros JG, Schilling WP. Effect of oxidant stress on calcium signalling in vascular endothelial cells. Free Radical Biology and Medicine 1992; 13:635–650.
408. Klebanoff SJ, et al. Stimulation of neutrophils by tumor necrosis factor. J Immunol 1986; 136:4220–4225.
409. Larrick JW, Wright SC. Cytotoxic mechanism of tumor necrosis factor-α. FASEB J 1990; 4:3215–3224.
410. Friedl HP, et al. Mediator-induced activation of xanthine oxidase in endothelial cells. FASEB J 1989; 3:2512–2518.
411. Yamauchi N, et al. Intracellular hydroxyl radical production induced by recombinant human tumor necrosis factor and its implication in the killing of tumor cells in vitro. Cancer Res 1989 49:1671–1675.
412. Radeks HH, et al. Interleukin 1-alpha and tumor necrosis factor-alpha induce oxygen radical production in mesangial cells. Kidney Int 1990 37:767–775.
413. Ishii Y, et al. Tumor necrosis factor-α mediated decrease in glutathione increases the sensitivity of pulmonary vascular endothelial cells to H_2O_2. J Clin Invest 1992; 89:794–802.
414. Masuda A, et al. Induction of mitochondrial manganese superoxide dismutase by interleukin 1. FASEB J 1988; 2:3087–3091.
415. Shaffer JB, Treanor CP, Del Vecchio PJ. Expression of bovine and mouse endothelial cell antioxidant enzymes following TNFα exposure. Free Rad Biol Med 1990; 8:497–502.
416. Shiki Y, et al. Endotoxin increases superoxide dismutase in cultured bovine pulmonary endothelial cells. Am J Physiol 1989; 252:C436–C440.
417. Visher GA, et al. Regulation of manganese superoxide dismutase by lipopolysaccharide, interleukin-1 and tumor necrosis factor. J Biol Chem 1990; 265:2856–2864.
418. Wong GHW, Goeddel DV. Induction of manganese superoxide dismutase by tumor necrosis factor: possible protective mechanism. Science 1988; 242:941–944.
419. Kong X-J, Fanburg BL. Regulation of Cu,Zn-superoxide dismutase in bovine pulmonary artery endothelial cells. J Cell Physiol 1992; 153:491–497.
420. Gerritsen ME, Bloor CM. Endothelial gene regulation in response to injury. FASEB J 1993; 7:523–532.
421. Read MA, et al. NF-kappa B and I kappa B alpha: an inducible regulatory system in endothelial activation. J Exp Med 1993; 179:503–512.
422. Marui N, et al. Vascular cell adhesion molecule-1 (VCAM-1) gene transcription and expression are regulated through an antioxidant-sensitive mechanism in human vascular endothelial cells. J Clin Invest 1993; 92:1866–1874.
423. Collins T, et al. A common theme in endothelial activation. Insights from the structural analysis of the genes for E-selectin and VCAM-1. Trends Cardiovasc Med 1993; 3:92–97.
424. Roederer M, et al. Cytokine-stimulated human immunodeficiency virus replication is inhibited by N-acetyl-L-cysteine. Proc Natl Acad Sci USA 1990; 87:4884–4888.
425. Aruoma OI, et al. The antioxidant action of N-acetyl cysteine: its reaction with hydrogen peroxide, hydroxyl radical, superoxide and hypochlorous acid. Free Rad Biol Med 1989; 6:593–597.
426. Burgunder JM, Varriale A, Lauterburg BH. Effect of N-acetyl cysteine on plasma cysteine and glutathione following paracetamol administration. Eur J Clin Pharmacol 1989; 36:127–131.
427. Toledano MB, Leonard WJ. Modulation of transcription factor NF-κB binding activity by oxidation-reduction in vitro. Proc Natl Acad Sci USA 1991; 88:4328–4332.
428. Staal FJT, et al. Intracellular thiols regulate activation of nuclear factor κB and transcription of human immunodeficiency virus. Proc Natl Acad Sci USA 1990; 87:9943–9947.
429. Shreck R, Rieber P, Baeuerle PA. Reactive oxygen intermediates as apparently widely messengers in the activation of the NF-κB transcription factor and HIV-1. EMBO J 10:2247–2258.
430. Wagner R. Erläuterungstafeln zur Physiologie und Entwicklungsgeschichte. Leipzig: Leopold Voss, 1839. Pp. xiv.
431. Cohnheim J. Lectures on General Pathology. A Handbook for Practitioners and Students. London: The New Sydenhan Society, 1889.
432. Atherton A, Born GVR. Quantitative investigations of the adhesiveness of circulating polymorphonuclear leukocytes to blood vessel walls. J Physiol (Lond) 1972; 222:447–474.
433. Atherton A, Born GVR. Relationship between the velocity of rolling granulocytes and that of the blood flow in venules. J Physiol 1973; 233:157–165.
434. Ley K, Gaehtgens P. Endothelial, not hemodynamic differences are responsible for preferential leukocyte rolling in venules. Circ Res 1991; 69:1034–1041.
435. Lawrence MB, Springer TA. Leukocytes roll on a selectin at physiologic flow rates: distinction from and prerequisite for adhesion through integrins. Cell 1991; 65:859–873.
436. Ley K, et al. Lectin-like cell adhesion molecule 1 mediates leukocyte rolling in mesenteric venules in vivo. Blood 1991; 77:2553–2555.
437. von Adrian UH, et al. L-selectin function is required for beta-2 integrin mediated neutrophil adhesion at physiological shear rates in vivo. Am J Physiol 1992; 263:1024–1044.
438. Zimmerman GA, Prescott SM, McIntyre TM. Endothelial cell interactions with granulocytes: tethering and signaling molecules. Immunol Today 1992;13:93–99.
439. Springer TA. Adhesion receptors of the immune system. Nature 1990;346:425–434.
440. Johnston GI, Cook RG, McEver RP. Cloning of GMP-140, a granule membrane protein of platelets and endothelium: sequence similarity to proteins involved in cell adhesion and inflammation. Cell 1989; 56:1033–1044.
441. McEver RP, et al. GMP-140, a platelet alpha granule membrane protein, is also synthesized by vascular endothelial cells and is localized in Weibel-Palade bodies. J Clin Invest 1989; 84:92–99.
442. Bevilacqua M, et al. Selectins: a family of adhesion receptors. 1991; Cell 67:233.
443. Tedder TF, et al. Expression of the human leukocyte adhesion molecule, LAM-1. Identity with TQ1 and Leu8 differentiation antigens. J Immunol 1990; 144:532–540.
444. Camerini D, et al. Leu-8/TQ1 is the human equivalent of the Mel-14 lymph node homing receptor. Nature 1989; 342:78–82.
445. Tedder TF, et al. Isolation and chromosomal localization of cDNAs encoding a novel human lymphocyte cell surface molecule, LAM-1. J Exp Med 1989; 170:123–133.
446. Bevilacqua MP, et al. Endothelial leukocyte adhesion molecule 1: An inducible receptor for neutrophils related to complement regulatory proteins and lectins. Science 1989; 243:1160–1165.
447. Lorant DE, et al. Coexpression of GMP-140 and PAF by endothelium stimulated by histamine or thrombin. A juxtacrine system for adhesion and activation of neutrophils. J Cell Biol 1991; 115:223–243.

448. Kuijpers TW, et al. Neutrophil migration across monolayers of cytokine-prestimulated endothelial cells: A role for platelet activating factor and IL-8. J Cell Biol 1992; 117:565–572.
449. Huber AR, et al. Regulation of transendothelial neutrophil migration by endogenous interleukin-8. Science 1991; 99–105.
450. Smith CW, et al. Chemotactic factors regulate lectin adhesion molecule-1 (LECAM-1)-dependent neutrophil adhesion to cytokine-stimulated endothelial cells in vitro. J Clin Invest 1991; 87:609–618.
451. Spertini O, et al. Leukocyte adhesion molecule-1 (LAM-1, L-selectin) interacts with an inducible endothelial cell ligand to support leukocyte adhesion. J Immunol 1991; 147:2565–2573.
452. Luscinskas FW, et al. Cytokine activated human endothelial monolayers support enhanced neutrophil transmigration via a mechanism involving both endothelial-leukocyte adhesion molecule-1 and intercellular adhesion molecule-1. J Immunol 1991; 146:1617–1625.
453. Smith CW, Hollers JC. Motility and adhesiveness in human neutrophils; Redistribution of chemotactic factor induced adhesion sites. J Clin Invest 1980; 65:804–812.
454. Hughes BJ, et al. Recruitment of CD11b/CD18 to the neutrophil surface and adherence dependent cell locomotion. J Clin Invest 1992; 90:1687–1696.
455. Tonnesen MG, et al. Mac-1 glycoprotein family mediates adherence of neutrophils to endothelial cells stimulated by leukotriene B4 and platelet activating factor. Fed Proc 1986; 45:379A (Abstr).
456. von Adrian UH, et al. A two step model of leucocyte-endothelial interaction in inflammation: distinct roles for LECAM-1 and the leucocyte $\beta 2$ integrins in vivo. Proc Natl Acad Sci USA 1991; 88:7538–7542.
457. Lawrence MB, et al. Effect of venous shear stress on CD18-mediated neutrophil adhesion to cultured endothelium. Blood 1990;75:227–237.
458. Spertini O, et al. Monocyte attachment to activated human vascular endothelium in vitro is mediated by leukocyte adhesion molecule-1 (L-selectin) under nonstatic conditions. J Exp Med 1992; 175:1789–1792.
459. Oppenheimer-Marks N, et al. Differential utilization of ICAM-1 and VCAM-1 during the adhesion and transendothelial migration of human T lymphocytes. J Immunol 1991; 147:2913–2921.
460. Furie MB, Tancino MCA, Smith CW. Monoclonal antibodies to leukocyte integrins CD11a/CD18 and CD11b/CD18 or intercellular adhesion molecule-1 (ICAM-1) inhibit chemoattractant-stimulated neutrophil transendothelial migration in vitro. Blood 1991; 78:2089–2097.
461. Smith CW, et al. Cooperative interactions of LFA-1 and Mac-1 with intercellular adhesion molecule-1 in facilitating adherence and transendothelial migration of human neutrophils in vitro. J Clin Invest 1989; 83:2008–2017.
462. Vaporciyan AA, et al. Involvement of platelet-endothelial cell adhesion molecule-1 in neutrophil recruitment in vivo. Science 1993; 262:1580–1582.
463. Bonfanti R, et al. PADGEM (GMP-140) is a component of Weibel-Palade bodies of human endothelial cells. Blood 1989; 73:1109–1112.
464. Hsu-Lin SC, et al. A platelet membrane protein expressed during platelet activation and secretion. Studies using a monoclonal antibody specific for thrombin-activated platelets. J Biol Chem 1984; 259:9121–9126.
465. Stenberg PE, et al. A platelet alpha granule membrane protein (GMP-140) is expressed on the plasma membrane after activation. J Cell Biol 1985; 101:880–886.
466. Koedam JA, et al. P-selectin, a granule membrane protein of platelets and endothelial cells, follows the regulated secretory pathway in AT-20 cells. J Cell Biol 1992; 617–625.
467. Disdier M, et al. Cytoplasmic domain of P-selectin (CD62) contains the signal for sorting into the regulated secretory pathway. Mol Biol Cell 1992; 3:309–321.
468. Fujimoto T, et al. P-selectin is acylated with palmitic acid and stearic acid at cysteine 766 through a thioester linkage. J Biol Chem 1993; 268:11394–11400.
469. Fujimoto T, McEver RP. The cytoplasmic domain of P-selectin is phosphorylated on serine and threonine residues. Blood 1993; 82:1758–1766.
470. Patel KD, et al. Oxygen radicals induce human endothelial cells to express GMP-140 and bind neutrophils. J Cell Biol 1991; 112:749–759.
471. Geng JH, et al. Rapid neutrophil adhesion to activated endothelium mediated by GMP-140. Nature 1990; 343:757–760.
472. Hattori R,et al. Stimulated secretion of endothelial von Willebrand factor is accompanied by rapid redistribution to the cell surface of the intracellular granule membrane protein GMP-140. J Biol Chem 1989; 264:7768–7771.
473. Manning AM, et al. Regulation of GMP-140 mRNA in a canine model of inflammation. FASEB J 1992; 6:A1060.
474. Weller A, Isenmann S, Westweber D. Cloning of the mouse endothelial selectins. Expression of both E- and P-selectin is inducible by tumor necrosis factor. J Biol Chem 267:15176–15183.
475. McEver RP. Leukocyte interactions mediated by selectins. Thromb Haemost 1991; 66:80–87.
476. Mayadas TN, et al. Leukocyte rolling and extravasation are severely compromised in P-selectin deficient mice. Cell 1993; 74:541–554.
477. Mulligan MS, et al. Neutrophil dependent acute lung injury: requirement for P-selectin (GMP-140). J Clin Invest 1992; 90:1600–1607.
478. Sako D, et al. Expression cloning of a functional glycoprotein ligand for P-selectin. Cell 1993; 75:1179–1186.
479. Bevilacqua MP, et al. Identification of an inducible endothelial-leukocyte adhesion molecule. Proc Natl Acad Sci USA 1987; 84:9238–9242.
480. Pober JS, et al. Two distinct monokines, interleukin-1 and tumor necrosis factor, each independently induce biosynthesis of the same antigen on the surface of cultured human vascular endothelial cells. J Immunol 1986; 136:1680–1687.
481. Pober JS, et al. Overlapping patterns of activation of human endothelial cells by interleukin 1, tumor necrosis factor and immune interferon. J Immunol 1986; 137:1893–1896.
482. Fries JWU, et al. Expression of VCAM-1 and E-selectin in an in vivo model of endothelial activation. Am J Pathol 1993; 143:725–737.
483. Bochner BS, et al. Adhesion of human basophils, eosinophils, and neutrophils to interleukin 1 activated human vascular endothelial cells: contributions of endothelial cell adhesion molecules. J Exp Med 1991; 173:1553–1556.
484. Weller PF, et al. Human eosinophil adherence to vascular endothelium mediated by binding to vascular cell adhesion molecule-1 and endothelial leukocyte adhesion molecule-1. Proc Natl Acad Sci USA 1991; 88:7430–7433.
485. Carlos T, et al. Human monocytes bind to two cytokine-induced adhesive ligands on cultured human endothelial cells: endothelial-leukocyte adhesion molecule-1 and vascular cell adhesion molecule-1. Blood 1991; 77:2266–2271.
486. Hakkert BC, et al. Neutrophil and monocyte adherence to and migration across monolayers of cytokine-activated endothelial cells: the contibution of CD18, ELAM-1 and VLA-4. Blood 1991; 78:2721–2726.
487. Walz G, et al. Recognition by ELAM-1 of the sialyl-Lex deter-

minant on myeloid and tumor cells. Science 1990; 250:1132–1135.

488. Phillips ML, et al. ELAM-1 mediates cell adhesion by recognition of a carbohydrate ligand sialyl-Lex. Science 1990; 250:1130–1132.
489. Mulligan MS, et al. Role of endothelial-leukocyte adhesion molecule-1 (ELAM-1) in neutrophil mediated lung injury in rats. J Clin Invest 1991; 88:1396–1406.
490. Gundel RH, et al. Endothelial leukocyte adhesion molecule-1 mediates antigen-induced acute airway inflammation and late-phase airway obstruction in monkeys. J Clin Invest 1991; 88:1407–1411.
491. Rothlein R, et al. A human intercellular adhesion molecule (ICAM-1) distinct from LFA-1. J Immunol 1986; 137:1270–1274.
492. Staunton DE, et al. Primary structure of ICAM-1 demonstrates interaction between members of the immunoglobulin and integrin supergene families. Cell 1988; 52:925–933.
493. Staunton DE, et al. The arrangement of the immunoglobulin-like domains of ICAM-1 and the binding sites for LFA-1 and rhinovirus. Cell 1990; 61:243–254.
494. Diamond MS, et al. Binding of the integrin Mac-1 (CD11b/CD18) to the third immunoglobulin-like domain of ICAM-1 (CD54) and its regulation by glycosylation. Cell 1991; 65:961–971.
495. Dustin ML, et al. Induction by IL-1 and interferon-γ: tissue distribution, biochemistry, function of a natural adherence molecule (ICAM-1). J Immunol 1986; 137:245–254.
496. Swerlick RA, et al. Studies of the modulation of MHC antigens and cell adhesion molecule expression on human dermal microvascular endothelial cells. J Invest Dermatol 1991; 97:190–196.
497. Gerritsen ME, et al. Regulation of the expression of intercellular adhesion molecule-1 (ICAM-1) in cultured human endothelial cells derived from rheumatoid synovium. Arth Rheum 1993; 36:593–602.
498. Iigo Y, et al. ICAM-1 dependent pathway is critically involved in the pathogenesis of adjuvant arthritis in rats. J Immunol 1991; 147:4167–4171.
499. Kakimoto K, et al. The effect of anti-adhesion molecule antibody on the development of collagen-induced arthritis in rats. Cellular Immunol 1992; 142:326–337.
500. Yamazaki T, et al. Expression of intercellular adhesion molecule-1 in rat heart with ischemia/repefusion and limitation of infarct size by treatment with antibodies against cell adhesion molecules. Am J Pathol 1993; 143:410–418.
501. Harning R, et al. Reduction in the severity of graft versus host disease and increased survival in allogenic mice by treatment with monoclonal antibodies to cell adhesion antigens LFA-1 and MALA-2. Transplantation 1991; 52:842–845.
502. Archelos JJ, et al. Inhibition of experimental autoimmune encephalomyelitis by an antibody to the intercellular adhesion molecule ICAM-1. Ann Neurol 1993; 34:145–54.
503. Isobe M, et al. Specific acceptance of cardiac allograft after treatment with antibodies to ICAM-1 and LFA-1. Science 1992; 255:1125–1127.
504. Staunton DE, Dustin ML, Springer TA. Functional cloning of ICAM-2, a cell adhesion ligand for LFA-1 homologous to ICAM-1. Nature 1989; 339:61–64.
505. Nortamo P, et al. The expression of human intercellular adhesion molecule-2 is refractory to inflammatory cytokines. Eur J Immunol 1991; 21:2629–32.
506. Rice GE, Munro JM, Bevilaqua MP. Inducible cell adhesion molecule 110 (INCAM-110) is an endothelial receptor for lymphocytes. A CD11/CD18 independent adhesion mechanism. J Exp Med 1990; 171:1369–1374.
507. Osborn L, et al. Direct expression cloning of vascular cell adhesion molecule 1, a cytokine induced endothelial protein that binds to lymphocytes. Cell 1989; 59:1203–1211.
508. Cybulsky MI, et al. Gene structure, chromosomal location, basis for alternative mRNA splicing of the human VCAM 1 gene. Proc Natl Acad Sci USA 1991; 88:7859–7863.
509. Cybulsky MI, et al. Alternative splicing of human VCAM-1 in activated vascular endothelium. Am J Pathol 1991; 138:815–820.
510. Hession C, et al. Cloning of an alternate form of vascular cell adhesion molecule-1 (VCAM-1) J Biol Chem 1991; 266:6682–6685.
511. Osborn L, et al. Activated endothelium binds lymphocytes through a novel binding site in the alternatively spliced domain of vascular cell adhesion molecule-1. J Exp Med 1992; 176:99–107.
512. Rice GE, Munro JM, Bevilacqua MP. Inducible cell adhesion molecule 110 (INCAM-119) is an endothelial receptor for lymphocytes. A CD11/CD18-independent adhesion mechanism. J Exp Med 1990; 171:1369–1374.
513. Rice GE, et al. Vascular and nonvascular expression of INCAM-110. A target for mononuclear leukocyte adhesion in normal and inflamed human tissues. Am J Pathol 1991; 138:385–393.
514. Marlor CW, et al. Expression of vascular cell adhesion molecule-1 in fibroblast like synoviocytes after stimulation with tumor necrosis factor. Am J Pathol 1990; 140:1055–1060.
515. Koch AE, et al. Immunolocalization of endothelial and leukocyte adhesion molecules in human rheumatoid and osteoarthritic synovial tissues. Lab Invest 1991; 64:313–320.
516. Carlos TM, et al. Vascular cell adhesion molecule-1 lymphocyte adherence to cytokine activated cultured human endothelial cells. Blood 1990; 76:965–970.
517. Schleimer RP, et al. IL-4 induces adherence of human eosinophils and basophils but not neutrophils to endothelium. J Immunol 1992; 148:1086–1092.
518. Yednock TA, et al. Prevention of experimental autoimmune encephalomyelitis by antibodies against $\alpha 1\beta 4$ integrin. Nature 1991; 356:63–68.
519. Cybulsky MI, Gimbrone MA, Jr. Endothelial expression of a mononuclear leukocyte adhesion molecule during atherogenesis. Science 1991; 251:788–791.
520. Newman PJ, Albelda SM. Cellular and molecular aspects of PECAM-1. Nouv Rev Fr Hématol 1992; 34:S7–S11.
521. Newman PJ, et al. PECAM-1 (CD31) cloning and relation to adhesion molecules of the immunoglobulin gene superfamily. Science 1990; 247:1219–1222.
522. Albelda SM, et al. Molecular and cellular properties of PECAM-1 (endoCAM/CD31): a novel vascular cell–cell adhesion molecule. J Cell Biol 1991; 119:1059–1068.
523. Newman PJ, et al. Activation-dependent changes in human platelet PECAM-1: phosphorylation, cytoskeletal association and surface membrane redistribution. J Cell Biol 1992; 199:239–246.
524. Zehnder JL, et al. The cell adhesion molecule CD31 is phosphorylated after cell activation. J Biol Chem 1992; 267:5243–5249.
525. Gallatin WM, Weissman IL, Butcher EC. A cell-surface molecule involved in organ-specific homing of lymphocytes. Nature 1983; 304:30–34.
526. Kishimoto TK, Jutila MA, Butcher EC. Identification of a human peripheral lymph node homing receptor: A rapidly down-regulated adhesion molecule. Proc Natl Acad Sci USA 1990; 87:2244–2248.
527. Imai Y, et al. Identification of a carbohydrate-based endothelial ligand for a lymphocyte homing receptor. J Cell Biol 1991; 113:1213–1221.
528. Berg EL, et al. The human peripheral lymph node vascular

addressin is a ligand for LECAM-1, the peripheral lymph node homing receptor. J Cell Biol 1991; 1213–1221.
529. Briskin MJ, McEvoy LM, Butcher EC. MAdCAM-1 has homology to immunoglobulin and mucin-like receptors and to IgA1. Nature 1993; 363:461–463.
530. Rice GE, Gimbrone MA, Jr, Bevilacqua MP. Tumor cell-endothelial interactions. Increased adhesion of human melanoma cells to activated vascular endothelium. Am J Pathol 1988; 133:204–210.
531. Rice GE, Bevilacqua MP. An inducible endothelial cell surface glycoprotein mediates melanoma adhesion. Science 1989; 246:1303–1306.
532. Rice GE, Munro JM, Bevilaqua MP. Inducible cell adhesion molecule 110 (INCAM-110) is an endothelial receptor for lymphocytes. A CD11/CD18 independent adhesion mechanism. J Exp. Med 1990; 171:1369–1374.
533. Takada A, et al. Adhesion of human cancer cells to vascular endothelium mediated by carbohydrate antigen sialyl Lewis A. Biochem Biophys Res Comm 1991; 179:713–719.
534. Kojima N, Handa K, Newman W. Inhibition of selectin-dependent tumor cell adhesion to endothelial cells and platelets by blocking O-glycosylation of these cells. Biochem Biophys Res Commun 1992; 182:1288–1295.
535. Majuri ML, Mattila P, Renkonen R. Recombinant E-selectin protein mediates tumor cell adhesion via sialyl-Lea and sialyl-Lex. Biochem Biophys Res Comm 1992; 182:1376–1382.
536. Oppenheim JJ, et al. Properties of the novel proinflammatory supergene "intercrine" cytokine family. Ann Rev Immunol 1991; 9:617–648.
537. Sica A, et al. IL-1 transcriptionally activates the neutrophil chemotactic factor/IL-8 gene in endothelial cells. Immunol 1990; 69:548–553.
538. Strieter RM, et al. Endothelial gene expression of neutrophil chemoattractant factor by TNFα, LPS and IL-1β. Science 1989; 242:1467–1469.
539. Schroder JM, Christophers E. Secretion of novel and homologous neutrophil-activating peptides by LPS-stimulated human endothelial cells. J Immunol 1989; 142:244–251.
540. Gimbrone MA, Jr, et al. Endothelial interleukin-8: a novel inhibitor of leukocyte-endothelial interactions. Science 1989; 246:1601–1603.
541. Hechtman DH, et al. Intravascular IL-8. Inhibitor of polymorphonuclear leukocyte accumulation at sites of inflammation. J Immunol 1991; 147:883–892.
542. Ley K, et al. Intravenous interleukin-8 inhibits granulocyte emigration from rabbit mesenteric venules without altering L-selectin expression or leukocyte rolling. J Immunol 1993; 151:6347–6357.
543. Huber AR, et al. Regulation of transendothelial neutrophil migration by endogenous interleukin-8. Science 1991; 254:99–102.
544. Dixit VM, et al. Tumor necrosis factor-α induction of novel gene products in human endothelial cells including a macrophage-specific chemotaxin. J Biol Chem 1990; 265:2973–2978.
545. Sica A, et al. Monocyte chemotactic and activating factor gene expression induced in endothelial cells by IL-1 and TNF. J Immunol 1990; 144:1229–1233.
546. Rollins BJ, et al. Cytokine activated human endothelial cells synthesize and secrete a monocyte chemoattractant, MCP-1/JE. Am J Pathol 1990; 136:1229–1233.
547. Rollins BJ, Pober JS. Interleukin-4 induces the synthesis and secretion of MCP-1/JE by human endothelial cells. Am J Pathol 1991; 138:1315–1319.
548. Quesenberry PJ, Gimbrone MA, Jr. Vascular endothelium as a regulator of granulopoiesis: production of colony stimulating activity by cultured human endothelial cells. Blood 1980; 56:1060–1067.
549. Sullivan R, et al. Effects of recombinant human granulocyte macrophage colony-stimulating factors on signal transduction pathways in human granulocytes. J Immunol 1987; 139:2422–3430.
550. Peters WP. The myeloid colony-stimulating factors: introduction and overview. Semin Hematol 1991; 28:1–5.
551. Gasson JC. Molecular physiology of granulocyte-macrophage colony stimulating factors. Blood 1991; 77:1131–1145.
552. Toner GC, Jakubowski AA, Crown JPL. Colony stimulating factors and neutrophil migration. Ann Int Med 1989; 110:846–847.
553. Broudy VC, et al. Interleukin 1 stimulates human endothelial cells to produce granulocyte-macrophage colony stimulating factor granulocyte colony stimulating factor. J Immunol 1987; 139:464–468.
554. Malone DG, et al. Production of granulocyte-macrophage colony stimulating factor by primary cultures of rat microvascular endothelial cells. Blood 1988; 71:684–689.
555. Rajavashisth TB, et al. Induction of endothelial cell expression of granulocyte and macrophage-colony stimulating factors by modified low density lipoproteins. Nature 1989; 344:254–257.
556. Segal G, McCall E, Bagby GC, Jr. Erythroid burst-promoting activity produced by interleukin-1 stimulated endothelial cells is granulocyte-macrophage colony stimulating factor. Blood 1988; 72:1364–1367.
557. Sieff CA, et al. Interleukin-1, tumor necrosis factor stimulate the production of colony stimulating factors by cultured mesenchymal cells. Blood 1988; 72:1316–1323.
558. Zsebo KM, et al. Vascular endothelial cells and granulopoiesis: interleukin-1 stimulates release of G-CSF and GM-CSF. Blood 1988; 71:399–403.
559. Bagby GC, Jr, Heinrich MC. Vascular endothelial cells and hematopoiesis: regulation of gene expression of human vascular endothelial cells. Hematol Pathol 1991; 5:93–99.
560. Bagby GC, Jr, et al. Interleukin-1 stimulation stabilizes GM-CSF mRNA in human vascular endothelial cells; preliminary studies of the role of the 3′ AU rich motif. Prog Clin Biol Res 1990; 352:223–239.
561. Bussolino F, et al. In vitro and in vivo activation of endothelial cells by colony stimulating factors. J Clin Invest 1991; 87:986–995.
562. Bussolino F, et al. Granulocyte and granulocyte macrophage-colony stimulating factors induce human endothelial cells to migrate and proliferate. Nature 1989; 337:471–473.
563. Kojima S, et al. Enhancement of plasminogen activator activity in cultured endothelial cells by granulocyte colony stimulating factor. J Cell Physiol 1989; 138:192–196.
564. Fu Y-X, et al. Regulation of leukocyte binding to endothelial cells by tumor derived GM-CSF. Int J Cancer 1992; 50:585–588.
565. Chin Y-C, Cai J-P, Johnson K. Lymphocyte adhesion to cultured Peyer's patch high endothelial venule endothelial cells is mediated by organ specific homing receptors and can be regulated by cytokines. J Immunol 1990; 145:3669–3677.
566. Leszczynski D, Hayry P. Effect of granulocyte-macrophage colony stimulating factor on endothelial antigenicity. Hum Immunol 1990; 28:175–178.
567. Bocchietto E, et al. Proliferative and migratory response of murine microvascular endothelial cells to granulocyte colony stimulating factor. J Cell Physiol 1993; 155:89–95.
568. Astaldi GCB, et al. Human endothelial culture supernatant (HECS): a growth factor for hybridomas. J Immunol 1980; 125:1411–1414.
569. Gauldie J, et al. Interferon β2/B-cell stimulatory factor type 2 share identity with monocyte-derived hepatocyte-stimulator

factor and regulates the major acute phase protein response in liver cells. Proc Natl Acad Sci USA 1987; 84:7251–7255.
570. Lotz M, et al. B cell stimulatory factor 2/interleukin 6 is a costimulant for human thymocytes and T-lymphocytes. J Exp Med 1988; 167:1253–1258.
571. Houssiau FA, et al. Synergistic activation of human T cells by interleukin 1 and interleukin 6. Eur J Immunol 1988; 18:653–656.
572. Poupart P, et al. B cell growth modulating and differentiating activity of recombinant human 26 kD protein. (BSF-2, Hu-IFN-beta 2, HPGF) EMBO J 1987; 6:1219–1224.
573. Jirik FR, et al. Bacterial lipopolysaccharide and inflammatory mediators augment IL-6 secretion by human endothelial cells. J Immunol 1989; 142:144–147.
574. Shalaby MR, Waage A, Espevik T. Cytokine regulation of interleukin 6 production by human endothelial cells. Cell Immunol 1989; 121:372–382.
575. Sironi M, Brevario F, Prosperpio P. Interleukin 1 stimulates IL-6 production in endothelial cells. J Immunol 1989; 142:549–553.
576. Podor TJ, et al. Human endothelial cells produce IL-6. Lack of responses to exogenous IL-6. Ann NY Acad Sci 1989; 557:374–385.
577. Ala Y, et al. Hypoxia-reoxygenation stimulates endothelial cells to promote interleukin-1 and interleukin-6 production. Effects of free radical scavengers. Agents Actions 1989 37:134–139.
578. May LT, et al. Interleukin-6 gene expression in human endothelial cells. RNA start site, multiple IL-6 proteins and inhibitor of proliferation. Biochem Biophys Res Comm 1989; 159:991–998.
579. Hettmannsperger U, et al. Cytokine stimulated human dermal microvascular endothelial cells produce interleukin 6-inhibition by hydrocortisone, dexamethasone and calcitrol. J Invest Dermatol 1992; 99:531–536.
580. van Hinsbergh VWM. Regulation of the synthesis and secretion of plasminogen activators by endothelial cells. Hemostasis 1988; 18:307–327.
581. Niedbala MJ. Cytokine regulation of endothelial cell extracellular proteolysis. Agents Actions Suppl 1993; 43:179–183.
582. van Hinsbergh VWM, et al. Tumor necrosis factor induces the expression of urokinase-type plasminogen activator by human endothelial cells. Blood 1990; 75:1991–1998.
583. Niedbala MJ, Stein M. Tumor necrosis factor induction of urokinase-type plasminogen activator in human endothelial cells. Biomed Biochem Acta 1991; 50:427–436.
584. Pepper MS, Belin D, Montesano R et al. Transforming growth factor-beta 1 modulates basic fibroblast growth factor-induced proteolytic and angiogenic properties of endothelial cells in vitro. J Cell Biol 1990; 111:743–755.
585. Wojta J, et al. Interleukin-4 stimulates expression of urokinase type plasminogen activator in cultured human foreskin microvascular endothelial cells. Blood 1993; 81:3285–3292.
586. Grondahl-Hansen J, et al. Urokinase type plasminogen activator in endothelial cells during acute inflammation of the appendix. Am J Pathol 1989; 135:631–636.
587. Weinberg JB, Pippen AM, Greenberg CS. Extravascular fibrin formation and dissolution in synovial tissue of patients with osteoarthritis and rheumatoid arthritis. Arthritis Rheum 1991; 34:996–1005.
588. Erikson LA, Hekman CM, Loskutoff DJ. The primary plasminogen activator inhibitors in endothelial cells, serum and plasma are immunologically related. Proc Natl Acad Sci USA 1988; 82:8710–8714.
589. Loskutoff DJ, et al. Fibrinolytic system of cultured endothelial cells. Regulation by plasminogen activator inhibitor. J Cell Biochem 1986; 32:273–280.
590. Seiffert D, Wagner NN, Loskutoff DJ. Serum derived vitronectin influences the pericellular distribution of type 1 plasminogen activator inhibitor. J Cell Biol 1990; 111:1283–1291.
591. Stump DC, Thienpont M, Collen D. Urokinase-related proteins in human urine. Isolation and characterization of single chain urokinase (pro-urokinase) and urokinase-inhibitor complex. J Biol Chem 1985; 261:1267–1273.
592. Fibbi G, et al. Interactions of urokinase with specific receptors stimulates mobilization of bovine adrenal capillary endothelial cells. Exp Cell Res 1988; 179:385–389.
593. Miles LA, et al. Plasminogen receptors, urokinase receptors and their modulation on human endothelial cells. Blood 1988; 72:628–635.
594. Barnathan ES, et al. Interaction of single-chain urokinase type plasminogen activator with human endothelial cells. J Biol Chem 1990; 265:2865–2872.
595. Mignatti P, Mazzieri R, Rifkin DB. Expression of urokinase receptor in vascular endothelial cells is stimulated by basic fibroblast growth factor. J Cell Biol 1992; 113:1193–1202.
596. Haddoch RC, et al. Urokinase binding and receptor identification in cultured endothelial cells. J Biol Chem 1986; 266:21466–21473.
597. Langer DJ, et al. Regulation of the endothelial cell urokinase-type plasminogen activator receptor. Evidence for cyclic AMP dependent and protein kinase-C dependent pathways. Circ Res 1993; 72:330–340.
598. Hanemaaijer R, et al. Regulation of matrix metalloproteinase expression in human vein and microvascular endothelial cells. Biochem J 1993; 296:803–809.
599. Unemori EN, et al. Vascular endothelial growth factor induces interstitial collagenase expression in human endothelial cells. J Cell Physiol 1992; 153:557–562.
600. Lemmon SK, Bradshaw RA. Purification and partial characterization of bovine pituitary fibroblast growth factor. J Cell Biochem 1983; 21:194–208.
601. Esch F, et al. Primary structure of bovine pituitary basic fibroblast growth factor (FGF) and comparison with the amino terminal sequence of bovine brain acidic FGF. Proc Natl Acad Sci USA 82:6507–6511.
602. Yoshida T, Miyagawa K, Odagiri H. Genomic sequence of hst, a transforming gene encoding a protein homologous to fibroblast growth factors and the int-2 encoding protein. Proc Natl Acad Sci USA 1987; 84:7305–7309.
603. Dickson C, Peters G. Potential oncogene product related to growth factors. Nature (London) 1987; 326:833.
604. Zhan X, et al. The human FGF-5 oncogene encodes a novel protein related to fibroblast growth factors. Mol Cell Biol 1988; 8:3487–3495.
605. Bensaid M, et al. Autocrine regulation of bovine retinal capillary endothelial cell (BREC) proliferation by BREC-derived basic fibroblast growth factor. Exp Eye Res 1989; 48:801–813.
606. Yu Z-X, et al. Localization of basic fibroblast growth factor in bovine endothelial cells. Immunohistochemical and biochemical studies. Exp Cell Res 1993; 204:247–259.
607. Schweigerer LG, et al. Capillary endothelial cells express basic fibroblast growth factor, a mitogen that promotes their own growth. Nature (London) 1987; 325:257–259.
608. Winkles JA, et al. Human vascular smooth muscle cells both express and respond to heparin binding growth factor 1 (endothelial cell growth factor). Proc Natl Acad Sci USA 1987; 84:7124–7128.
609. Burgess WH, Maciag T. The heparin binding (fibroblast) growth factor family of proteins. Annu Rev Biochem 1989; 58:575–606.
610. Vlodavsky I, et al. Endothelial cell-derived basic fibroblast growth factor; synthesis and deposition into subendothelial

extracellular matrix. Proc Natl Acad Sci USA 1987; 84:2292–2296.

611. Dionne CA, et al. Cloning and expression of two distinct high affinity receptors cross-reacting with acidic and basic fibroblast growth factors. EMBO J 1990; 2685–2692.
612. Keegan K, et al. Isolation of an additional member of the fibroblast growth factor receptor family, FGFR-3. Proc Natl Acad Sci 1991; 88:1095–1099.
613. Partanen J, et al. FGFR-4, a novel acidic fibroblast growth factor with a distinct expression pattern. EMBO J 1991; 10:1347–1354.
614. Gospodarowicz D, Cheng J. Heparin protects basic and acidic FGF inactivation. J Cell Physiol 1986; 128:475–484.
615. Folkman J, et al. A heparin binding angiogenic protein-fibroblast growth factor—is stored within basement membrane. Am J Pathol 1988; 130:393–400.
616. Saksela O, Rifkin DB. Release of fibroblast growth factor-heparan sulfate complexes from endothelial cells by plasminogen activator-mediated proteolytic activity. J Cell Biol 1990; 110:767–775.
617. Nakajima M, et al. Heparan sulfate degradation: relation to tumor invasive and metastatic properties of mouse B16 melanoma sublines. Science 1985; 220:611–613.
618. Vlodavsky I, et al. Lymphoma cell-mediated degradation of sulfated proteoglycans in the subendothelial extracellular matrix: relationship to tumor cell metastasis. Cancer Res 1983; 43:2704–2711.
619. Sato Y, Rifkin DB. Autocrine activities of basic fibroblast growth factor: regulation of endothelial cell movement, plasminogen activator synthesis and DNA synthesis. J Cell Biol 1988; 107:1199–1205.
620. Tseung S, et al. Fibroblast growth factor modulates synthesis of collagen in cultured vascular endothelial cells. Eur J Biochem 1982; 122:355–362.
621. Saksela O, Moscatelli D, Rifkin DB. The opposing effects of basic fibroblast growth factor and transforming growth factor on the regulation of plasminogen activator activity in capillary endothelial cells. J Cell Biol 1987; 105:957–963.
622. Banda MJ, et al. Regulation of metalloproteinase activity by microvascular endothelial cells. In DB Rifkin, M Klagsburn, eds. Angiogenesis, Mechanisms and Pathophysiology. New York: Cold Spring Harbor Laboratory, 1987. Pp 101–109.
623. Madri JA, Willimas SK. Capillary endothelial cultures: phenotypic modulation by matrix components. J Cell Biol 1983; 97:153–165.
624. Montesano R, et al. Basic fibroblast growth factor induces angiogenesis in vitro. Proc Natl Acad Sci USA 1986; 83:7297–7301.
625. Keck PJ, et al. Vascular permeability factor, an endothelial mitogen related to PDGF. Science 1989; 246:1309–1312.
626. Leung DW, Cachianes G, Kuang WJ. Vascular endothelial growth factor is a secreted angiogenic mitogen. Science 1989; 246:1306–1309.
627. Rosenthal RA, et al. Conditioned medium from mouse sarcoma 180 cells contains vascular endothelial growth factor. Growth Factors 1990; 4:53–59.
628. Phillips HS, et al. Vascular endothelial growth factor is expressed in rat corpus luteum. Endocrinol 1990; 127:965–967.
629. Shweiki D, et al. Vascular endothelial growth factor induced by hypoxia may mediate hypoxia-initiated angiogenesis. Nature 1992; 359:843–845.
630. Quinn TP, et al. Fetal liver kinase 1 is a receptor for vascular endothelial growth factor and is selectively expressed in vascular endothelium. Proc Natl Acad Sci USA 1993; 90:7533–7537.
631. De Vries C, et al. The fms-like tyrosine kinase, a receptor for vascular endothelial growth factor. Science 1992; 255:989–991.
632. Terman BI, et al. Identification of the KDR tyrosine kinase as a receptor for vascular endothelial cell growth factor. Biochem Biophys Res Comm 1993; 187:1579–1586.
633. Connolly DT, et al. Tumor vascular permeability factor stimulates endothelial cell growth and angiogenesis. J Clin Invest 1989; 84:1470–1478.
634. Pepper MS, et al. Potent synergism between vascular endothelial growth factor and basic fibroblast growth factor in the induction of angiogenesis in vitro. Biochem Biophys Res Commun 1992; 189:824–831.
635. Jakeman LB, et al. Binding sites for vascular endothelial growth factor are localized to endothelial cells in adult rat tissues. J Clin Invest 1992; 89:244–253.
636. Kaipainen A, Korhonen J, Pajusolak K. The related FLT4, FLT1 KDR receptor tyrosine kinases show distinct expression patterns in human fetal endothelial cells. J Exp Med 1993; 178:2077–2088.
637. Korhonen J, et al. Enhanced expression of tie tyrosine kinase in endothelial cells during neovascularization. Blood 1992; 80:2548–2555.
638. Yamaguchi TP, et al. flk-1, an flt-related receptor tyrosine kinase is an early marker for endothelial cell precursors. Development 1993; 118:489–498.
639. Dvorak HF. Distribution of vascular permeability factor (vascular endothelial growth factor) in tumors: concentration in tumor blood vessels. J Exp Med 1991; 174:1275–1278.
640. Koch AE, et al. Vascular endothelial growth factor: a cytokine mediating angiogenesis in rheumatoid arthritis. Arth Rheum 1993; 36:S175 (Abstr).
641. Seifert RA, Schwartz SM, Bowen-Pope DF. Developmentally regulated production of platelet derived growth factor-like molecules. Nature (London) 1984; 311:669–671.
642. Shimokado K, et al. A significant part of macrophage-derived growth factor consists of at least two forms of PDGF. Cell 1985; 43:277–286.
643. Martinet Y, et al. Activated human monocytes express the c-sis protooncogene and release a mediator showing PDGF-like activity. Nature 1986; 319:158–160.
644. DiCorleto PE, Bowen-Pope DF. Cultured endothelial cells produce a platelet-derived growth factor-like protein. Proc Natl Acad Sci USA 1983; 80:1919–1923.
645. Collins T, et al. Cultured human endothelial cells express platelet derived growth factor B chain; cDNA cloning and structure analyses. Nature 1985; 316:748–750.
646. Starksen NF, et al. Regulated expression of the platelet-derived growth factor-A chain gene in microvascular endothelial cells. J Biol Chem 1987; 262:14381–14384.
647. Barrett TB, Benditt EP. Platelet-derived growth factor gene expression in human atherosclerotic plaques and normal artery wall. Proc Natl Acad Sci USA 1988; 85:2810–2814.
648. Barrett TP, Benditt EP. sis (platelet-derived growth factor β-chain) gene transcript levels are elevated in human atherosclerotic lesions compared to normal artery. Proc Natl Acad Sci USA 1987; 84:1099–1103.
649. Bowen-Pope DF, Hart CE, Siefert RA. Sera and conditioned media contain different isoforms of platelet derived growth factor (PDGF) which bind to different classes of PDGF receptor. J Biol Chem 1989; 264:2502–2508.
650. Fox PL, DiCorleto PE. Modified low density lipoproteins suppress production of a platelet derived growth factor-like protein by cultured endothelial cells. Proc Natl Acad Sci 1986; 83:4774–4778.
651. Fox PL, DiCorleto PE. Fish oils inhibit endothelial cell production of platelet-derived growth factor-like protein. Science 1988; 241:453–456.

652. Fox PL, Chisholm GM, DiCorleto PE. Lipoprotein-mediated inhibition of endothelial cell production of platelet derived growth factor like protein depends on a free radical lipid peroxidation. J Biol Chem 1987; 262:6046–6054.
653. Daniel TO, et al. Agents that increase cAMP accumulation block endothelial c-sis induction by thrombin and transforming growth factor-B. J Biol Chem 1987; 262:11893–11896.
654. Harlan JM, et al. α-Thrombin induces release of PDGF-like molecule(s) by cultured human endothelial cells. J Cell Biol 1986; 1129–1133.
655. Gadjusek C, et al. Activation of coagulation releases endothelial cell mitogens. J Cell Biol 1986; 103:419–428.
656. Seifert RA, et al. Two different subunits associate to create isoform-specific platelet-derived growth factor receptors. J Biol Chem 1989; 264:8771–8778.
657. Smits A, et al. Rat brain capillary endothelial cells express functional PDGF B-type receptors. Growth Factors 1989; 2:1–8.
658. Bar RS, et al. The effects of platelet derived growth factor in cultured microvessel endothelial cells. Endocrinol 1989; 124:1841–1848.
659. Satoh T, et al. Platelet derived growth factor mediates activation of ras through different signalling pathways in different cell types. Mol Cell Biol 1993; 13:3706–3713.
660. Grotendorst GR, et al. Platelet-derived growth factor is a chemoattractant for vascular smooth muscle cells. J Cell Physiol 1982; 113:261–266.
661. Circolo A, et al. Differential regulation of the expression of proteinases/antiproteinases in fibroblasts. Effects of interleukin-1 and platelet derived growth factor. J Biol Chem 1991; 266:12283–12288.
662. Chua CC, et al. Induction of collagenase secretion in human fibroblast cultures by growth promoting factors. J Biol Chem 1985; 260:5213–5216.
663. Bar RS, et al. Actions of insulin and insulin-like growth factors I and II in cultured microvessel endothelial cells from bovine adipose tissue. Metabolism 1988; 37:714–720.
664. Vinters HV, et al. Insulin stimulates DNA synthesis in cerebral microvessel endothelium and smooth muscle. Diabetes 1985; 34:964–969.
665. Bar RS, et al. Differential binding of insulin to human arterial and venous endothelial cells in primary culture. Diabetes 1980; 29:991–995.
666. Haskell JF, Meezan E, Pillion DJ. Identification and characterization of the insulin receptor of bovine retinal microvessels. Endocrinol 1984; 115:698–704.
667. Gerritsen ME, Burke T. Insulin binding and effects of insulin on glucose metabolism and 2-deoxyglucose uptake in isolated rabbit coronary microvessel endothelial cells. Proc Soc Exp Biol Med 1985; 180:17–23.
668. Bar RS, Boes M. Distinct receptors for IGFI, IGFII and insulin are present on bovine capillary endothelial cells and large vessel endothelial cells. Biochem Biophys Res Comm 1984; 124:203–209.
669. Corkey RF, Corkey BE, Gimbrone MA, Jr. Hexose transport in normal and SV-40 transformed endothelial cells in culture. J Cell Physiol 1981; 106:425–431.
670. King GL, et al. Differential responsiveness to insulin of endothelial and support cells from macro and microvessels. J Clin Invest 1983; 71:974–979.
671. King GL, et al. Receptors and growth promoting effects of insulin and insulin-like growth factors on cells from bovine retinal capillary and aorta. J Clin Invest 1985; 75:1028–1036.
672. Dernovsek KD, et al. Rapid transport of biologically intact insulin through cultured endothelial cells. Endocrinol 1984; 58:761–763.
673. Jailal I, et al. Processing of insulin by bovine endothelial cells in culture: internalization without degradation. Diabetes 1984; 33:794.
674. King GL, Johnson SM. Receptor-mediated transport of insulin across endothelial cells. Science 1985; 227:1583–1586.
675. Bar RS, Boes M, Yorek M. Processing of insulin-like growth factors I and II by capillary and large vessel endothelial cells. Endocrinol 1986; 118:1972–2080.
676. Delafontaine P, Bernstein KE, Alexander RW. Insulin-like growth factor 1 gene expression in vascular cells. Hypertension 1991; 17:693–699.
677. Gajdusek CM, Luo Z, Mayberg MR. Sequestration and secretion of insulin-like growth factor-1 by bovine aortic endothelial cells. J Cell Physiol 1993; 154:192–198.
678. Moser DR, et al. Endothelial cells express insulin-like growth factor binding proteins 2 to 6. Mol Endocrinol 1992; 6:1805-1814.
679. Bar RS, et al. Production of IGF-binding proteins by vascular endothelial cells. Biochem Biophys Res Comm 1988; 148:734–739.
680. Gopinath R, Walton PE, Etherton TD. An acid stable insulin-like growth factor (IGF)-binding protein from pig serum inhibits binding of IGF-I and IGF-II to vascular endothelial cells. J Endocrinol 1989; 120:231–236.
681. Elgin RG, Busby WH, Clemmons DR. An insulin-like growth factor (IFG) binding protein enhances the biological response to IGF-I. Proc Natl Acad Sci USA 1987; 84:3254–3258.
682. Bar RS, et al. Insulin-like growth factor-binding proteins from vascular endothelial cells: purification, characterization, and intrinsic biological activities. Endocrinol 1989; 125:1910–1920.
683. Cercek B, Fishbein MC, Forrester JS. Induction of insulin-like growth factor 1 messenger RNA in rat aorta after balloon denudation. Circ Res 1990; 66:1755–1760.
684. Hannson H-A, Jennische E, Skottner A. Regenerating endothelial cells express insulin-like growth factor-1 immunoreactivity after arterial injury. Cell Tissue Res 1987; 250:499–505.
685. Hannson H-A, et al. Transient expression of insulin-like growth factor-1 immunoreactivity by vascular cells during angiogenesis. Exp Mol Pathol 1989; 50:125–138.
686. Nakao-Hayashi J, et al. Stimulatory effects of insulin and insulin-like growth factor on migration and tube formation by vascular endothelial cells. Atherosclerosis 1992; 92:141–149.
687. Stoker M, Perryman M. An epithelial scatter factor released by embryo fibroblasts. J Cell Sci 1985; 77:209–213.
688. Rosen EM, et al. Purification and migrating-stimulating activities of scatter factor. Proc Soc Exp Biol Med 1990; 195:34–43.
689. Gherardi E, et al. Purification of scatter factor, a fibroblast-derived protein that modulates epithelial interactions and movement. Proc Natl Acad Sci USA 1989; 86:5844–5848.
690. Weidner KM, et al. Scatter factor: molecular characteristics and effect on invasiveness of epithelial cells. J Cell Biol 1990; 111:2097–2108.
691. Rosen EM, et al. Scatter factor stimulates migration of vascular endothelium and capillary-like tube formation. In ID Goldberg, ed. Cell Motility Factors. Basel: Birkhäuser, 1991. Pp 76–88.
692. Grant DS, Kleinman HK, Goldberg ID. Scatter factor induces blood vessel formation in vivo. Proc Natl Acad Sci 1993; 90:1937–1941.
693. Rosen EM, et al. Scatter factor stimulates migration of vascular endothelium and capillary-like tube formation. EXS 1992; 59:76–88.
694. Koch AE, et al. Interleukin-8 as a macrophage derived mediator of angiogenesis. Science 1992; 258:1798–1801.

695. Masferrer JL, et al. 12 (R) hydroxyeicosatrienoic acid, a potent chemotactic and angiogenic factor produced by the cornea. Exp Eye Res 1991; 52:417–424.
696. Shing Y, et al. Heparin-affinity purification of a tumor-derived capillary endothelial cell growth factor. Science 1984; 223:1926–1929.
697. Klagsburn M, Shing Y. Heparin affinity of anionic and cationic capillary endothelial growth factors: analysis of hypothalamus-derived growth factors and fibroblast growth factors. Proc Natl Acad Sci USA 1985; 82:805–809.
698. Gospodarowicz D, Cheng J. Heparin protects basic and acidic FGF inactivation. J Cell Physiol 1986; 128:474–484.
699. Rosengurt TK, et al. Heparin protects heparin-binding growth factor from proteolytic degradation in vivo. Biochem Biophys Res Comm 1988; 152:432–440.
700. Saksela O, et al. Endothelial cell-derived heparan sulfate binds basic fibroblast growth factor and protects it from proteolytic degradation. J Cell Biol 1988; 107:743–751.
701. Thornton S, Mueller S, Levine E. Human endothelial cells: use of heparin in cloning and long-term serial cultivation. Science 1983; 222:623–625.
702. Schreiber A, et al. Interaction of endothelial cell growth factor with heparin: characterization by receptor and antibody recognition. Proc Natl Acad Sci USA 1985; 82:6138–6142.
703. Fedarko N, Conrad E. A unique heparan sulfate in the nuclei of hepatocytes: structural changes with the growth state of the cells. J Cell Biol 1986; 102:587–599.
704. Fager G, Camejo G, Bondjers G. The PDGF A-chain contains an amino acid sequence that specifically binds to heparin causing inactivation of the growth factor. Scan J Clin Lab Invest 1990; 199:33–36.
705. Andres J, et al. Membrane-anchored and soluble forms of beta-glycan, a polymorphic proteoglycan that binds transforming growth factor-β. J Cell Biol 1989; 109:3137–3145.
706. McKeon-Longo PJ, Hanning R, Mosher DF. Binding and degradation of platelet thrombospondin by cultured fibroblasts. J Cell Biol 1984; 98:22–28.
707. Nader H, et al. Heparin sequences in the heparan sulfate chains of an endothelial proteoglycan. Proc Natl Acad Sci USA 1987; 84:3565–3569.
708. Vannucchi S, et al. Internalization and metabolism of endogenous heparin by cultured endothelial cells. Biochem Biophys Res Comm 1986; 120:294–301.
709. Kessler D, et al. Mast cells and tumor angiogenesis. Int J Cancer 1976; 18:703–709.
710. Derynck R, et al. Human transforming growth factor-complementary DNA sequence and expression in normal and transformed cells. Nature (London) 1985; 316:701–705.
711. Lawrence D, Pircher R, Jullien P. Conversion of a high molecular weight latent beta-TGF from chicken embryo fibroblasts into a low molecular weight active beta-TGF under acidic conditions. Biochem Biophys Res Comm 1985; 133:1025–1034.
712. Pircher R, Jullien P, Lawrence DA. β-Transforming growth factor is stored in human blood platelets as a latent high molecular weight complex. Biochem Biophys Res Comm 1986; 135:30–37.
713. Purchio AF, Cooper JA, Brunner JA. Identification of mannose-6-phosphate in two asparagine-linked sugar chains in recombinant transforming growth factor-β1-precursor. J Biol Chem 1988; 263:14211–14215.
714. Kovaccina KS, et al. Interactions of recombinant platelet transforming growth factor-β1-precursor with the insulin-like growth factor / mannose-6-phosphate receptor. Biochem Biophys Res Comm 1989; 160:393–403.
715. Lyons RM, Keskioja J, Moses HL. Proteolytic activation of latent transforming growth factor-β from fibroblast conditioned medium. J Cell Biol 1988; 106:1659–1663.
716. Sato Y, et al. Characterization of the activation of latent transforming growth factor beta by co-cultures of endothelial cells and pericytes or smooth muscle cells: a self regulating system. J Cell Biol 1990; 111:757–763.
717. Miyanzo K, Heldin CH. Role for carbohydrate structures in transforming growth factor β latency. Nature (London) 1989; 338:158–160.
718. Frolik CA, et al. Characterization of a membrane receptor for transforming growth factor-β in normal rat kidney fibroblasts. J Biol Chem 1984; 100:1041–1049.
719. Massagúe J, Like B. Cellular receptors for type beta transforming growth factor. J Biol Chem 1985; 260:2636–2645.
720. Wakefield LM, et al. Distribution and modulation of the cellular receptor for transforming growth factor-beta. J Cell Biol 1987; 105:965–975.
721. Seagarini PR, Seyedin SM. The high molecular weight receptor to transforming growth factor-β contains glycosaminoglycan chains. J Biol Chem 1988; 263:8366–8370.
722. Cheifetz S, Res JL, Massagúe J. The transforming growth factor-β receptor type III is a membrane proteoglycan. Domain structure of the receptor. J Biol Chem 1988; 263:16984–16991.
723. Cheifetz S, et al. The transforming growth factor-β system, a complex pattern of cross reactive ligands and receptors. Cell 1987; 48:409–415.
724. Ignotz RA, Massagúe J. Transforming growth factor-β stimulates the expression of fibronectin and collagen and their incorporation into extracellular matrix. J Biol Chem 1986; 261:4337–4345.
725. Ignotz RA, Endo T, Massagúe J. Regulation of fibronectin and type I collagen mRNA levels by transforming growth factor-β. J Biol Chem 1987; 262:6443–6446.
726. Roberts AB, et al. Transforming growth factor-type β: rapid induction of fibrosis and angiogenesis in vivo and stimulation of collagen formation in vitro. Proc Natl Acad Sci USA 1986; 83:4167–4171.
727. Vorga J, Rosenbloom J, Himenez SA. Transforming growth factor-β (TGF-β) causes a persistent increase in steady state amounts of type I and type III collagen and fibronectin mRNAs in normal human dermal fibroblasts. Biochem J 1987; 247:597–604.
728. Madri JA, Pratt BM, Tucker A. Phenotypic modulation of endothelial cells by transforming growth factor-β depends upon the composition and organization of the extracellular matrix. J Cell Biol 1988; 106:1375–1384.
729. Penttinen PR, Kobayashi S, Bornstein P. Transforming growth factor-β increases mRNA for matrix proteins both in the presence and absence of changes in mRNA stability. Proc Natl Acad Sci USA 1988; 85:1105–1108.
730. Pearson CA, Pearson D, Shibahara S. Tenascin: cDNA cloning and induction by transforming growth factor-β. EMBO J 1988; 7:2677–2681.
731. Lui JM, Davidson JM. The elastogenic effect of recombinant transforming growth factor-β in porcine aortic smooth muscle cells. Biochem Biophys Res Comm 1988; 154:895–901.
732. Chen J-K, Hoshi H, McKeehan WL. Transforming growth factor-β specifically stimulates synthesis of proteogyclans in human arterial smooth muscle cells. Proc Natl Acad Sci USA 1987; 84:5287–5291.
733. Merrilees MJ, Scott L. Endothelial cell stimulation of smooth muscle glycosaminoglycan synthesis can be accounted for by transforming growth factor-beta activity. Atherosclerosis 1990; 81:255–265.
734. Reilly CF, McFall RC. Platelet derived growth factor-beta

regulates plasminogen activator inhibitor-1 synthesis in vascular smooth muscle cells. J Biol Chem 1991; 266:9419–9423.

735. Roberts CJ, et al. Transforming growth factor-β stimulates the expression of fibronectin and of both subunits of the human fibronectin receptor by cultured human lung fibroblasts. J Biol Chem 1988; 263:4586–4592.

736. Roberts AB, et al. Type beta transforming growth factor; a bifunctional regulator of cellular growth. Proc Natl Acad Sci USA 1985; 81:119–123.

737. Roberts AB, et al. Transforming growth factor type-beta: rapid induction of fibrosis and angiogenesis in vivo and stimulation of collagen formation in vitro. Proc Natl Acad Sci USA 1986; 83:4167–4171.

738. Bagavandoss P, Wilks JW. Specific inhibition of endothelial proliferation by thrombospondin. Biochem Biophys Res Commun 1990; 170:867–872.

739. Tarabolotti G, et al. Platelet thrombospondin modulates endothelial cell adhesion, motility and growth: a potential angiogenesis regulatory factor. J Cell Biol 1990; 111:765–772.

740. Iruela-Arispe ML, Bornstein P, Sage H. Thrombospondin exerts an anti-angiogenic effect on cord formation by endothelial cells in vitro. Proc Natl Acad Sci USA 1991; 88:5026–5030.

741. Lahav J, Pardik R, Stein O. Endothelial thrombospondin and its possible role in cell adhesion. Sem Throm Haemostasis 1987; 13:352–360.

742. Murphy-Ullrich JE, Hook M. Thrombospondin modulates focal adhesion in endothelial cells. J Cell Biol 1989; 109:1309–1319.

743. Good DJ, et al. A tumor suppressor-dependent inhibitor of angiogenesis is immunologically and functionally indistinguishable from a fragment of thrombospondin. Proc Natl Acad Sci 1990; 87:6624–6628.

Connective Tissues of the Subendothelium

Jerome M. Seyer
Andrew H. Kang

General Characteristics and Composition

The subendothelium, composed of connective tissue, provides mechanical strength and elasticity to the blood vessel and maintains the vessel's structural integrity. It may play a role in hemostasis and in thrombotic processes. Like all connective tissues, the subendothelium consists of cells and extracellular protein fibers with an amorphous ground substance occupying the extracellular, interfibrillar space. Three kinds of fibers have been described histologically: collagen, elastin, and reticulin, but reticulin has been shown chemically to be a form of collagen. The amorphous ground substance consists of acidic-glycosaminoglycans, glycoproteins such as fibronectin and laminin, and other less well-characterized matrix components.

At least 19 genetically distinct types of collagen have been identified so far in various mammalian connective tissues (Table 2-1), and undoubtedly more will be discovered in the future [1]. In blood vessels, nine types of collagen have been described (types I, III, IV, V, VI, VII, VIII, XII, and XIV). Type I and type III collagens, referred to as interstitial collagens, are the major collagens in the blood vessel wall. They form the mixed striated fibrils and are responsible for the high tensile strength [2]. Type IV collagen is found exclusively in the basement membrane [3]. Type V collagen appears with type I and type III in striated fibrils; its function in the mixed-fibril assembly remains unknown [2]. Type VI collagen has been isolated from the aortic intima [4], and type VIII collagen from endothelial cell cultures in vitro [5]. Type XII and type XIV collagens occupy positions along the striated fibril and may limit the fibril diameter or link extracellular matrix component [6]. Type VII collagen has been identified as the anchoring fibrils of the basement membranes in various organs [7], and type XVII collagen has been identified as the 180-kDa bullous pemphigoid antigen in the hemidesmosome structures [8]. Little is known about types XIII, XV, XVI, XVIII, and XIX collagens, except that they are minor constituents whose primary structure was initially identified by cDNA cloning [9–13].

Variations in the Vasculature

The vascular system consists of a massive network of tubular channels that are designed to carry blood throughout the body. The walls of these channels are considered specialized connective tissues, with collagen and elastin as their major structural protein constituents. The size and composition of individual blood vessels vary with their specific functional requirements. The major arteries that carry blood directly from the heart must be relatively thick and elastic. Their walls, therefore, contain a relatively large amount of elastin, which allows for elastic expansion and contraction in response to contractions of the heart. In this fashion, the large arteries contribute to a more continuous blood flow.

The smaller arteries are more rigid and hence contain a larger proportion of collagen. Their function is to regulate blood flow into the tissue. This regulation is achieved by the contractile activity of smooth muscle cells, which control the size of the vessel lumen based on the required blood flow.

The capillary contains only one layer of endothelial cells with an underlying basement membrane. This thin-walled tube permits a rapid exchange of water, nutrients, and metabolic products between blood and interstitial fluids. Capillaries deliver blood to the venous system at reduced pressure. Thus, the venules have thinner walls, less-dense connective tissue, and a larger lumen than their arterial counterparts. They have far fewer smooth muscle cells and are equipped with valves to prevent reversal of blood flow due to hydrostatic forces.

The walls of the large elastic arteries contain three identifiable tissue layers. The tunica intima is the internal layer and contains a single layer of polygonal endothelial cells joined by gap junctions. This cell layer rests on a basement membrane, which in turn is supported by a network of collagen fibrils, predominantly type III collagen, as indicated by immunohistochemistry [2]. The remainder of the intimal layer contains a few smooth muscle cells, a large amount of elastic microfibrils, and a few type I collagen fibers. The middle layer, or tunica media, is distinguished by elastic fibers in a fenestrated plate called the elastica interna. The tunica media, which represents the bulk of the vessel wall, contains elastic fibers and spaces filled with smooth muscle cells, their long axes perpendicular to the lumen axis [14]. The extracellular space contains collagen fibers in a continuous sheath adjacent to the elastic fibers. Fibers contain a variable mixture of types I, III, and V collagens, the more rigid containing a higher proportion of type I, whereas the smaller, more pliable fibers contain larger amounts of type III. The level of type V collagen remains relatively constant in all fibers. Smooth muscle cells synthesize types I, III, V, VI, XII and XIV collagen. The tunica adventitia is a thin, tough network of collagen fibers containing primarily type I collagen. This tissue layer merges with adjacent connective tissue [14].

The walls of smaller arteries are intermediate in size. The tunica intima is relatively thin, as is the medial layer. The tunica adventitia is usually much thicker than those of large arteries, with more densely packed collagen fibers arranged longitudinally along the vessel axis. Arterioles have simple walls. Smooth muscle cells surround the endothelial layer, and the adventitia is smaller and more pliable than that in larger arteries [2]. The capillaries adjoining the arterioles are surrounded by a few smooth muscle cells, which control the amount of blood passing

Table 2-1. Distribution of the collagens

Collagen	Tissue
Type I	Bone, cornea, dentin, tendon (> 95%) Dermis, gingiva, heart valve (85%) Intestine, large vessel, fibrocartilage (50–60%)
Type II	Articular cartilage, vitreous cartilage (> 90%) Fibrocartilage (40–50%)
Type III	Intestine, large vessel, and uterine wall (35–45%) Dermis, gingiva, heart valve (10–15%)
Type IV	Endothelial and epithelial basement membrane (> 95%)
Type V	Cornea, placental membrane, large vessel wall (5%) Bone, gingiva, heart valve, hyaline cartilage (< 5%)
Type VI	Placenta, aorta, neurofibroma (< 1%) Dermis, nucleus pulposus (< 1%)
Type VII	Dermal-epidermal junction, amnionic epithelium (< 1%)
Type VIII	Endothelial cell product, Descemet's membrane
Type IX	Articular cartilage (5–20%)
Type X	Hypertrophic cartilage only
Type XI	Articular cartilage (5%)
Type XII	Tendon, skin, peridontal ligament (< 1%)
Type XIII	Product of fibroblasts, tendon (trace)
Type XIV	Tendon, skin (< 1%)
Type XV	Many tissues (unknown)
Type XVI	Fibroblasts, keratinocytes (unknown)
Type XVII	Skin, hemidesmosomes (180-kDa bullus pemphigoid antigen)
Type XVIII	Liver, kidney, placenta (unknown)
Type XIX	Rhabdomyosarcoma cells (cDNA only)

Numbers in parentheses indicate approximate percentage of specified collagen type found in tissue's total collagen.

through. The walls of arterial and venous capillaries consist of flat endothelial cells surrounded by a basement membrane, to which are attached pericapillary cells called pericytes. These cells form a discontinuous sheath of reticulum fibers that are primarily type III collagen [14].

The walls of venules in the venous system contain a reticular network of collagen fibers derived from type III collagen along with smaller quantities of type I collagen fibers. As the vessel size increases, the relative proportions of type I collagen, smooth muscle cells, and elastic fibers also increase. The larger veins contain paired semilunar flaps, which consist of collagen fiber bundles covered by a layer of endothelial cells.

The Chemistry and Structure of Collagens

Collagens are by far the major molecules of most connective tissues and the most abundant proteins of the vasculature. Collagens play a dominant role in maintaining the structural integrity of the parent tissue and is also involved in development, organogenesis, cell attachment, chemotaxis, platelet aggregation, and as a filtration barrier in basement membranes. They have been defined as extracellular components that have a triple helical conformation in at least a portion of their structure. A unique feature of collagens is that they undergo extensive posttranslational modifications essential for the performance of their major function, namely to provide mechanical strength. These modifications are necessary for stabilization of the collagen molecule and maturation of fibils via lysine-derived covalent cross-links.

THE COLLAGEN MOLECULE

The collagen molecule, which represents the basic unit of collagen fibers or structures, has a highly asymmetric, rodlike structure in which triple helical features are present. Each molecule is composed of three polypeptide chains, called alpha chains. Because of the high content of imino acids (proline and hydroxyproline) and their stereochemistry, each alpha chain assumes a left-handed helical conformation (minor helix) (Fig. 2-1). Three alpha chains then wind around a common axis to form a right-handed superhelix (triple helix) to form the collagen molecule. Because of the complexity of the different collagens in blood vessels, they will be discussed in three groups: group 1 collagens have an alpha chain size with an approximate molecular weight of 95 kDa and a continuous uninterrupted helical domain of approximately 300 nm in the molecule (types I, III, and V); group 2 collagens have an alpha-chain size greater than 95 kDa with helical regions that are interrupted by short nonhelical segments (types IV and VII collagens). Group 3 collagens have triple helical domains less than 95 kDa but have large globular domains sometimes making their size even greater than the group 1 collagens (Fig 2-2). As in the case of the group 2 collagens, the gobular endpieces remain with the original chain in the extracellular matrix. In most cases, the globular domains may have vital functions with respect to tissue architecture. This is in contrast to the collagens of group 1, which shed their globular endpieces when they are incorporated into the extracellular matrix. To this group 3 belong types VI, VII, VIII, XII, XIII, XIV, XV, XVI, XVII, XVIII, and XIX. The remaining collagens, types II, IX, X, and XI, are excluded from this discussion because they are present only in cartilageous tissues.

Group 1 molecules consist of an uninterrupted triple-helical domain of approximately 300 nm (see Fig. 2-2). These collagen alpha chains have a repeating $[Gly\text{-}X\text{-}Y]_n$ structure: 338 triplets, or 1,014 amino acid residues, in type I chains and 341 triplets, or 1,023 amino acid residues, in type III chains. Their genomeic structure suggests that the collagen chains may have evolved by duplication and rearrangement from a primordial gene of 54 base pairs. Exons generally begin with coding a Gly residue at the intron-exon junction. At both the NH_2 and COOH ends of each alpha chain are short segments of nonhelical sequences of approximately 15 to 20 residues where glycine is not at every third residue. These nonhelical segments are referred to as telopeptides. The complete amino acid sequences of the alpha chains of type I and type III collagens and the $\alpha1[V]$ and $\alpha2[V]$ collagen chains have now been established. Clearly, type I and type III collagens are quantitatively the major collagens in the blood vessel and

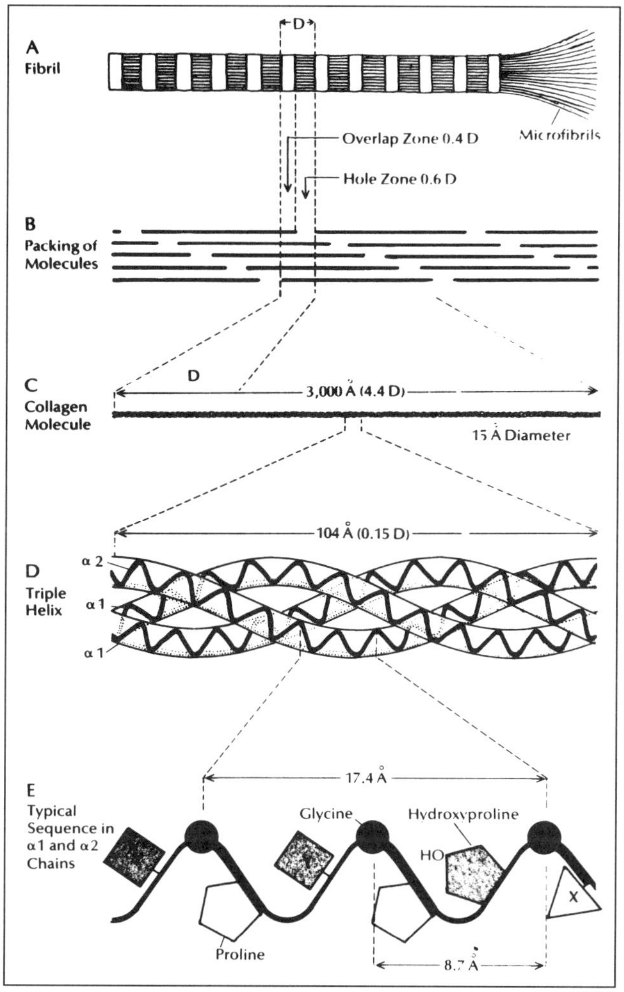

Fig. 2-1. Diagramatic representation of the collagen triple-helical structure: **A.** a large fibril of collagen exhibiting a dense packing of microfibrils with characteristic cross-striations and a regular repeat period (D) of approximately 68 nm and **B.** a two-dimensional representation of the packing arrangement of the collagen molecule in the microfibril. Each collagen molecule has a large number of dark staining bands, five of which are separated by a regular distance of 68 nm and which account for the repeat period in the microfibril. **C.** The collagen molecule consists of three alpha chains in a rigid rod, 300 nm in length and 15 angstroms in diameter with a 4.4-D spacing. **D.** The three alpha chains are in a left-handed helix with approximately three residues per turn. **E.** Glycine occurs at every third position and is mandatory. The X and Y positions in the Gly-X-Y triplet can be any amino acid but proline and hydroxyproline each occur approximately 10 percent of the time in the X and Y positions, respectively. (Taken with permission from DJ Prockop and NA Guzman. Collagen diseases and the biosynthesis of collagen. Hospital Practice, December 1977, pp. 61–68.)

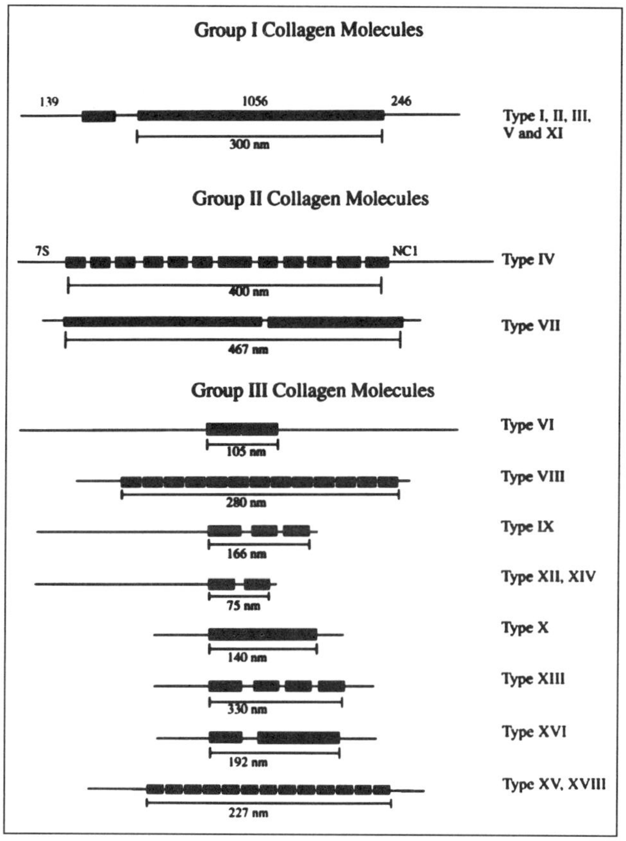

Fig. 2-2. Groups of collagen molecules in vertebrate tissues. The group 1 molecules represent the major fibril-forming collagens that account for the striated fibers in interstital tissues. The group 2 molecules are arbitrarily placed because they have a triple-helical domain much larger than the 300 nm of the group 1 collagens. Group 3 collagens all have triple-helical domains smaller than 300 nm. In some cases, however, the group 3 combined triple-helix and globular domains at the NH_2 and COOH ends may be greater than the collagens of groups 1 and 2. All the collagens in groups 2 and 3 have interruptions in their triple-helical domains. The thin lines in the figure represent globular domains, and the thick lines indicate the triple-helical domains. The lengths of the lines provide an estimate of their theoretical sizes (where known).

together form the striated fibrils. Type V collagen also contains a 300-nm uninterrupted helical domain, but less is known about its telopeptide segments. Current evidence suggests that they may be much longer and hence may interfere with or regulate striated-fibril formation.

The collagens of group 2 do not participate in striated-fiber formation. Characteristically, they contain interruptions in their triple-helical domain, generally 5 to 20 amino acids in length. These nonhelical segments provide a greater amount of flexibility, a property that would be beneficial for their proposed role of connecting extracellular matrix components. Unlike the fibril-forming collagens of group 1, the collagens of groups 2 and 3 evolved from a much different primordial gene, perhaps as small as nine nucleotides. The exon-intron junctions appear to occur almost at random, in some cases even splitting the Gly codon. The type IV collagens, which are found exclusively in basement-membrane structures, are the best characterized of the group. Three molecular forms have been identified, the most abundant being (α1[IV])2 (α2[IV]), which is present in all basement membranes. The molecules have a long collagenous domain (400 nm) with multiple interruptions in the triple helix. They are assembled in a lattice structure with head-to-head and tail-to-tail association via lysine-derived and cysteine-derived cross-linkages. The type VII collagen molecule is distinguished by its extraordinary length, nearly 467 nm, in which all but a very small portion is triple helical. Although the exact nature of the aggregate formed by type VII is not known, this collagen is found in the anchoring fibrils of basement membranes described by morphologists. The molecule extends from the basement membrane to the papillary dermis. Recent studies have defined mutations in the α1[VII] gene that are responsible for dystrophic forms of epidermolysis bullosa. One case has been localized to a single base substitution converting a residue of Met to Lys at the COOH-terminal nonhelical domain.

The third group of collagens are a heterogeneous group with variability in size and function. Type IV collagen was initially identified in this group from pepsin extracts of aorta. It was initially referred to as "short-chain collagen" because of its small pepsin-resistant, triple-helical domain. In contrast, the globular domains of the type VI collagen chains, which flank the 336-residue triple-helical regions, are quite large. Type VI monomers contain three distinct alpha chains, α1[VI], α2[VI], and α3[VI], with molecular weights of 150, 140, and 300 kDa, respectively. Each chain has regions similar to the type A repeats found in the von Willebrand factor. The α3[VI] collagen chain is much larger because it contains 11 repeats of this type A domain. It also has a 73-residue segment analogous to the platelet glycoprotein Ib. This region in the COOH-terminus is also flanked by a type III repeat of fibronectin and a Kunitz-type proteinase inhibitor. The type III domain suggests a role of type VI collagen in cell adhesion and type I collagen binding. The α3[VI] messenger RNA (mRNA) is present as several species that are generated by alternate splicing of an additional exon. Immunolocalization of type VI collagen has identified it as a component of microfibrils in cultured cells. The precise localization in tissue, however, is more difficult to define.

Another member of this mixed collagen group is type VIII collagen. It was originally described as a product of endothelial cells in culture. Now it has been characterized as the sheet-like structures found in Descemet's membrane. Descemet's membrane separates the corneal epithelial cells from the corneal stoma. It consists of stacks of collagen lattices made up of type VIII collagen. Type VIII collagen has a small triple-helical domain but also two small globular domains. Type XII and type XIV collagens have been more extensively characterized. Based on their nearly identical amino acid sequence and size, these two collagens have been assumed to be a unique family within the group 3 family. Most of the properties are very similar to a much better characterized collagen, type IX, from cartilageous tissue. These three collagens are unique in that they all contain a single chondroitin sulfate polysaccharide chain. Two other collagens also form another apparent family: type XV and type XVIII. They have short helical domains with similarities much like that found between types I and III and types XII and XIV. The distribution of type XV and type XVIII varies in tissues; for instance, liver contains type XVIII collagen but no type XV, while skin has both. The role of these latter collagens in tissues remains uncertain.

Type XVII collagen was identified initially through cDNA sequencing. This mRNA product was later identified as the protein of hemidesmosomes previously referred to as the 180-kDa bullous pemphigoid antigen. Type XIII collagen has also been characterized from the deduced amino acid sequence. It is now recognized as occurring in many tissues, and at least four mRNA species are present in varying amounts, depending on developmental state and specific tissue. The remaining collagens, types XVI and XIX, have been identified only through cDNA sequence analysis. Their structures revealed the short triple-helical domains with characteristic interruptions in the Gly-X-Y sequence akin to the other members of the group 3 family.

STRUCTURE AND PROPERTIES OF INTERSTITIAL (TYPE I AND TYPE III) COLLAGENS

Because of their similarities, type I and type III collagens are discussed together here. The type I collagen molecule is a heterotrimer of two identical alpha chains, α1(I) and a different alpha chain, α2(I), and has the chain structure $[\alpha 1(I)]_2\ \alpha 2(I)$. The type III collagen molecule is a homotrimer of three identical alpha chains, α1(III), and has the chain structure $[\alpha 1(III)]_3$.

The helical domain of the alpha chain contains a repeating triplet sequence of $[\text{Gly-X-Y}]_n$, where X and Y may be any amino acid but are most frequently proline or hydroxyproline. Together, these imino acids constitute approximately 20 to 25 percent of the total amino acid content in most mammalian collagens with nearly equal amounts in the X and Y positions. The imino acid residues in the Y position are nearly always hydroxylated (4-hydroxyproline) to variable extents. The stereochemical configuration of the amino acids forces the alpha chains to assume a left-handed helix. Gly, which occurs at every third residue in the helical domain, is critical since it contains no bulky side chain and will occupy the center position within the triple helix. Substitution of Gly for any other amino acid is not tolerated because of the space restriction. The triple helix is stabilized by interchain hydrogen bonding contributed by hydroxyproline. Thus, the collagen molecule is a long cylindrical rod with the dimensions of 1.5 nm × 300 nm (see Fig. 2-1). Under physiologic conditions of ionic strength, pH, and temperature, collagen molecules are not soluble and spontaneously aggregate into striated fibrils of the type seen in tissues. The fibril formation occurs by lateral aggregation of the collagen molecules, in which each neighboring row of molecules is displaced along the long axis of the molecule by a distance of 68 nm. In addition, within the same row, there is a gap, or "hole," of approximately 40 nm between the end of one molecule and the beginning of the next (see Fig. 2-1).

Each alpha chain contains, in addition to the 338 Gly-X-Y triplets, short nonhelical sequences (telopeptides) at the NH_2 and COOH ends. These telopeptides are located in the gap or hole zone of the fibril and are, therefore, accessible to various enzymes, including lysyl oxidase. Specific residues of lysine and hydroxylysine in the telopeptides are enzymatically deaminated to form the interchain cross-link precursors allysine and hydroxyallysine (see the subsection "Extracellular Maturation"), which can undergo a series of reactions to form the cross-links.

Metabolism of Collagen

BIOSYNTHESIS OF COLLAGEN

The collagen chains are synthesized on polyribosomes as linear precursor chains, or prepro-α chains. The hydrophobic leader sequence is removed from the prepro-α chains intracellularly prior to secretion, and the procollagen molecules, consisting of pro-α chains, are secreted into the extracellular space. The pro-α1(I) chain contains, in addition to the α1(I) chain domain, an NH_2 propeptide and a COOH propeptide. The NH_2 propeptide (pN) consists of a 139-residue sequence, most of which is nonhelical, but there is a short (16-triplet) helical segment ending five residues from the α1(I) chain domain. The α1(I) chain domain contains a 17-residue sequence of nonhelical NH_2 telopeptide, followed by 1,014 residues (338 triplets) of helical sequence and by a 26-residue sequence of nonhelical COOH telopeptide. The COOH telopeptide is followed by the COOH propeptide (pC), which is a 262-residue nonhelical sequence. The structures of pro-α2(I) and pro-α1(III) chains are similar except for minor variations in the number of amino acid residues.

As for all proteins, the amino acid sequence of pro-α chains is determined by genes. Since each pro-α chain contains approximately 1,500 residues, it requires a 6-kilobase mRNA molecule and a large polyribosome unit. Nineteen types of collagen molecules containing 30 different types of pro-α chains have been identified thus far in mammalian systems; therefore, there must be a minimum of 30 collagen genes. Each procollagen chain has been shown to be coded by a single procollagen gene. Surprisingly, procollagen genes identified so far have been widely distributed on different chromosomes, with the exception of α1(III) and α2(V), which are located on the same region of chromosome 2 [15]. However, no coordinate regulation has been found in the synthesis of these two procollagen chains. The pro-α2(I) gene is composed of a large, 40-kilobase genome (Fig. 2-3). The coding information of the pro-α chain is divided into approximately 50 coding segments (exons), which are separated by large sequences (introns). Each exon is a multiple of nine base pairs (bp), the minimum required for a single Gly-X-Y triplet. The length of the exon varies from 45 to 108 bp; seven thus far identified contain 54 bp each, and two contain 108 bp (a multiple of 54), indicating a possible primordial gene structure of 54 bp ($[Gly\text{-}X\text{-}Y]_6$). Growth of the primordial gene may have proceeded through duplication and recombination of this 54-bp unit [16]. Each exon within the triple-helical domain begins with a Gly codon.

There is no definite exon-intron junction separating the triple helical region, the telopeptides, or the initial segments of the propeptides. For example, a single exon codes for the COOH terminus of the NH_2 propeptide, the telopeptide, and the NH_2 terminus of the helical region. These inclusions within a single exon suggest a high degree of constraint with all the segments. The introns, or intervening sequences, are much larger (86–2000 bp) for the pro-α2(I) chain, but much smaller introns are present in other procollagen genes [17]. The pro-α1(I) gene contains approximately 18 kb, indicating a lack of evolutionary constraint on the gene size as opposed to the polypeptide size.

The molecular events for procollagen synthesis (DNA to RNA transcription and splicing of transcript RNA, leading to mRNA formation) are essentially identical to other eukaryotic systems and will not be discussed here. The mechanism for coordinate synthesis of two pro-α1(I) chains per pro-α2(I) chain is not understood, however, since a single gene codes for each separate chain. Likewise, most cells that produce type I collagen also produce type III collagen in variable amounts, depending on the specific type of tissue, the age, and the physiologic and pathologic situations. How the relative production of these procollagens is controlled remains unknown, but regulation most likely occurs at the transcriptional level.

Collagen synthesis is regulated closely by a variety of factors at several levels. Transforming growth factor beta (TGF-β) is a potent stimulater of collagen synthesis at the transcriptional level and stabilizes the mRNA in some cases. This cytokine is most likely the major driving force for elevated collagen production during wound healing and in fibrotic tissues. Tumor necrosis factor alpha (TNF-α) inhibits collagen production at the transcriptional level, while interleukin-1 beta (IL-1β) can be inhibitory or stimulatory, depending on the cell type and condition. Glucocorticosteroids are inhibitory to collagen synthesis. Nuclear regulatory proteins such as nuclear factor-1 (NF-1), activator protein-1 (AP-1), and SP-1 have been suggested to interact with their corresponding cis-elements in the 5′ upstream region, the promoter, and the first intron of the type I collagen gene and to enhance gene expression[18–21]. Feedback regulation of procollagen chain synthesis occurs with select peptide fragments from the NH_2-terminal and COOH-terminal propeptides [22,23]. Many other modulators of procollagen synthesis will most likely be found soon. Agents that cause an elevation in the intracellular cyclic adenosine 5′-monophosphate (cAMP) increase intracellular degradation and, consequently, decrease collagen deposition by lung or skin fibroblasts. This appears to be selective for type I collagen to a much greater extent than for type III collagen. In this manner, the intracellular degradation may be an additional mechanism by which cells regulate both the quality and the quantity of collagen secreted in normal or abnormal states [24].

The cell-free translation of procollagen chains by isolated mRNA specific for the pro-α1(I) chain has confirmed that the translated product is a linear chain with 1,440 amino acid residues and a leader sequence of 22 amino acid residues. Major posttranslational modifications occur during polypeptide chain elongation [2]. 4-proline hydroxylation occurs with the participation of ketoglutarate, oxygen, ferrous ion, and ascorbate as cofactors, the last being a nonspecific reducing agent and the others being specific and absolute. The enzyme 4-prolyl hydroxylase is ubiquitous, and the levels found in tissues tend to reflect the level of procollagen production. Inhibition of prolyl hydroxylase activity results in the synthesis of an underhydroxylated procollagen. Underhydroxylated procolla-

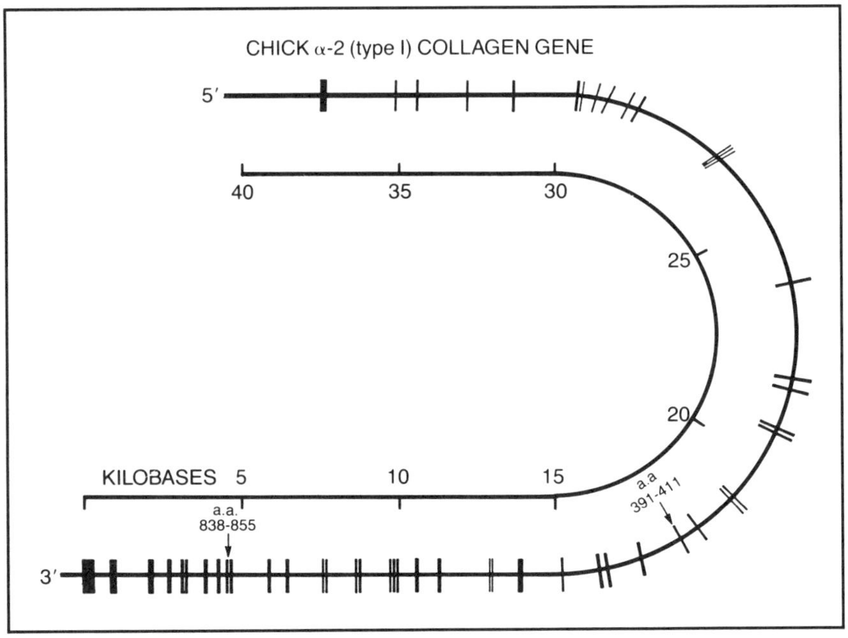

Fig. 2-3. Graphic representation of measurements of coding and intervening sequences of the chicken $\alpha 2$(I) gene, based on electronmicroscopic pictures of DNA-mRNA hybrids. Each vertical band represents the coding sequence of exon, and the lines between the bars correspond to intervening sequences, or introns. Note that the coding information of the $\alpha 2$(I) collagen chain is divided into approximately 50 coding segments, which are separated by intervening sequences of various lengths. The length of the noncoding sequences varies but in general is much greater than the coding sequences. (Reproduced from H Ohkubo, et al. Proc Natl Acad Sci USA 1980; 77:7061.)

gen, as in vitamin C deficiency, accumulates in the cell and is secreted at a greatly reduced rate. In addition, underhydroxylated collagen is considerably less stable than normal collagen and undergoes rapid degradation. A second enzyme, lysyl hydroxylase, adds a hydroxyl group to the L-carbon of lysine. This enzyme requires the same cofactors as prolyl hydroxylase and reacts only with a lysine residue in the Y position of the Gly-X-Y triplets. It also hydroxylates the lysine residue found in the NH_2-terminal telopeptide, which has no resemblance to a helical structure. The functional significance of lysine hydroxylation is not entirely clear, but hydroxylation of lysine residues that eventually become involved in the cross-link formation imparts significantly greater stability to the cross-link. Patients with an inherited deficiency of lysine hydroxylase (Ehlers-Danlos syndrome type VI) display a wide variety of connective tissue malfunctions, including skeletal deformities, tissue fragility, and vascular malformations [25]. Only a small percentage of the total lysine residues become hydroxylated in type I and type III collagen, whereas in all other collagens, almost all the lysine residues in the Y position become hydroxylated.

A third hydroxylation reaction involves the formation of 3-hydroxyproline by the action of a prolyl hydroxylase distinct from the prolyl 4-hydroxylase. Only one proline residue is hydroxylated in the $\alpha 1$(I) collagen chain, none in the type III collagen chain, and one to four residues in type IV collagen chains. In every case so far identified, the proline residue must be in the X position. At present, we have no indication of the significance of 3-hydroxyproline formation.

As hydroxylation of lysine residues proceeds during nascent procollagen chain synthesis, certain hydroxylysine residues become glycosylated. The enzyme UDP-galactose : hydroxylysine galactosyltransferase adds a galactose residue to the hydroxyl group of hydroxylysine. The UDPglucose : galactosylhydroxylysine glucosyltransferase then transfers a glucose residue to some of the hydroxylysine-linked galactose residues. Both enzymes require a divalent cation, and they act in sequence such that galactose is added first, with glucose added only to galactose.

Glycosylation occurs during nascent chain synthesis and before the formation of triple helices, since the triple-helical collagen cannot act as a substrate [2]. Only two of seven hydroxylysine residues of $\alpha 1$(I), $\alpha 2$(I), and $\alpha 1$(III) contain the disaccharide. However, all or nearly all the hydroxylysine in other collagens are glycosylated. Glycosylation of specific hydroxylysine that later becomes involved in collagen cross-linking imparts greater stability to the cross-link.

After completion of nascent chain synthesis, the procollagen chains are assembled into triple-helical molecules. This process is directed by the COOH-terminal propeptide with the formation of interchain disulfide bonds. Noteworthy is the high degree of conservation of the covalent structure within the propeptides of different species. The conservation of the disulfide bonds has thus far been absolute within the same collagen type of different

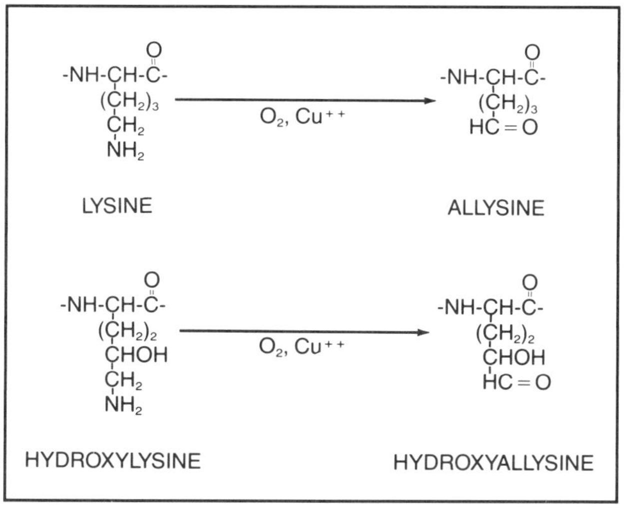

Fig. 2-4. Reactions catalyzed by peptidyl lysine oxidase.

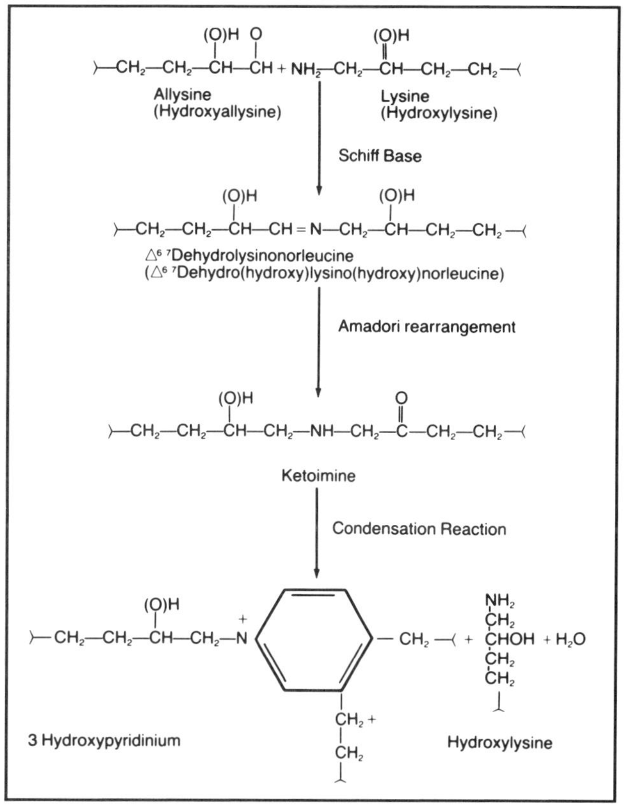

Fig. 2-5. Aldamine cross-links of collagen. Natural reduction of the double bond between N and C of the dehydro compounds apparently does not occur in collagen. In elastin, both dehydrolysinonorleucine and its reduced form lysinonorleucine are found. Hydroxylysine-containing cross-links in collagen are stabilized by the formation of ketoimine structures by Amadori rearrangement. The proposed condensation of two ketoimine structures yields a hydroxypyridinium residue and free hydroxylysine.

species [26]. A similarly high degree of homology of prosegments occurs among types I, III, and V collagen of the same species. In fact, a larger amount of covalent structure preservation occurs in these propeptide domains than occurs within the helical region of these collagens. This conservation of structure in the propeptide domains suggests the importance of these regions in directing triple-helix formation. Following the completion of its assembly, the procollagen molecule is secreted into the extracellular space. The exact form in which procollagen molecules are transported is not known. There is evidence that they are packaged in some type of aggregate during the transit, but the precise arrangement of the procollagen molecules in the aggregates is not understood [27]. Once secreted, however, the NH_2 and COOH propeptides are proteolytically removed by the action of procollagen peptidases to yield the collagen molecule. The procollagen peptidases are a group of proteases, each specific for the type of procollagen and for either the NH_2 or the COOH propeptides [2]. Recent studies suggest that fragments of the propeptides can specifically suppress procollagen biosynthesis by fibroblasts by means of feedback inhibition of procollagen mRNA translation [22,23].

EXTRACELLULAR MATURATION

During the period of extracellular collagen fibril formation, an enzyme, lysyl or hydroxylysyl oxidase, catalyzes the oxidative deamination of specific lysine or hydroxylysine residues in the NH_2- or COOH-terminal telopeptides (Fig. 2-4) to yield allysine or hydroxyallysine, respectively [28]. The enzyme utilizes molecular oxygen for the reaction. These reactive aldehydes, being located in the hole zone of the fibril, are free to react with the ε-amino group of lysine or hydroxylysine residues on adjacent chains to form a Schiff base, which can rearrange to a ketoimine via Amadori rearrangement, a more stable interchain cross-link (Fig. 2-5). With time, two ketoimine structures condense to form a trivalent cross-link named 3-hydroxypyridinium. At any given time, all three cross-linkages may be found in a specific connective tissue despite the fact that they are not in equilibrium with each other [29].

A second basic type of cross-link compound found in collagen originates from the condensation of two aldehydes in allysine or hydroxyallysine on adjacent chains with the formation of a dehydrated aldol condensate (Fig. 2-6). This aldol condensate has a free aldehyde that could react with other ε-amino groups of lysine or histidine to form, potentially, the tri- and tetra-functional cross-links—dehydrohydroxymerodesmosine, aldolhistidine, and histidinohydroxymerodesmosine—which link three or four collagen chains [30].

Once the aldehydes of allysine and hydroxyallysine are formed, subsequent aldamine and aldol condensation reactions proceed spontaneously but slowly in the tissue. The cross-linking results in an enormous complex of macromolecules, covalently linked, and gives rise to the high tensile strength and insolubility of the collagen fibrils. These reactions depend on the high degree of organization imparted by the specific aggregation of collagen molecules in the fibril itself. The particular stagger of the collagen molecules in the fibrils allows nonhelical allysine or hy-

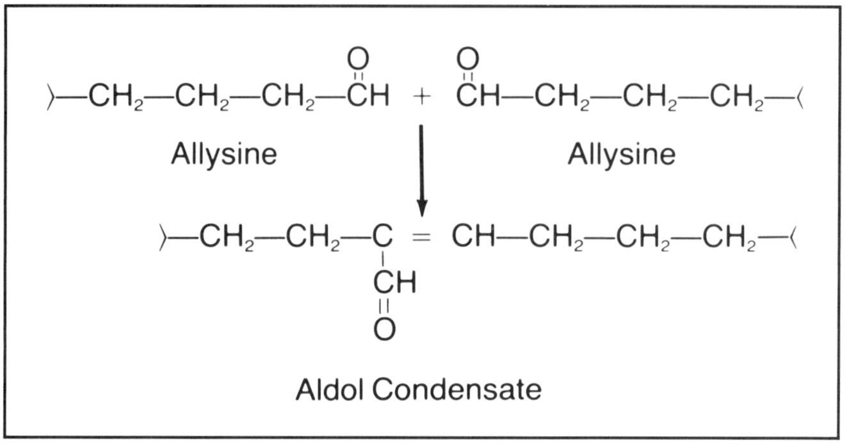

Fig. 2-6. Aldol condensation product between two residues of allysine. This cross-link is found in both collagen and elastin.

droxyallysine in the NH_2 and COOH telopeptides to form a cross-link at potentially four areas in the helical domain of the adjacent collagen molecules (see Fig. 2-1).

TURNOVER OF COLLAGEN

The metabolic turnover of interstitial collagen, as measured in a whole animal or in a tissue such as the blood vessel wall or tendon, is extremely low; the half-life is measured in years. In specific physiologic and pathologic situations, such as tissue remodeling and inflammation, however, a very rapid breakdown and synthesis of collagen must take place. The mechanism of degradation of the interstitial collagens (types I, II, III, V, and XI) has been the subject of considerable interest because these collagens in the native state are resistant to the action of general proteases, although they are readily degraded by a wide variety of proteases once the molecules are denatured (or the helical structures disrupted). In contrast, the collagens with interruptions in their triple helices, such as types VI to X and types XII to XIX, have noncollagenous regions that may be susceptible to a variety of proteases. At this time, little information is available on their degradation or turnover. After cleavage of the nonhelical segments, the short triple-helical domains would become unstable, denature at 37°C and also be susceptible to nonspecific proteases, such as gelatinases and stromolysin. Physiologic breakdown of the interstitial collagens is accomplished by the action of very specific interstitial collagenases [31–33]. These enzymes cleave the native collagen molecule at a single position within the triple helix (between residues 775 and 776), resulting in a bisection of the molecule into fragments representing approximately 75 percent and 25 percent, respectively, of the intact molecule (Fig. 2-7). The resulting products are unstable and denature spontaneously at body temperature and pH. The unraveled polypeptides are now susceptible to the action of gelatinases and are degraded further.

METALLOPROTEINASES

The interstitial collagenases and gelatinases that degrade collagens belong to a family of enzymes referred to as matrix metalloproteinases [34,35]. They require Ca^{++} and have a common Zn^{++} binding region. They are synthesized as proenzymes and activated by a variety of proteases, chemicals (HOCl, mercurials), or physical (chaotropic) agents. The gene expression of the metalloproteinases is regulated by a variety of agents, generally in the opposite direction of collagen gene expression. TNF-α and IL-1β stimulate enzyme production by signal transduction through the AP-1 proteins, c-fos and c-jun. The activator complex of these leucine-zipper proteins bind to the consensis AP-1 site in their promoter. Once activated, they stimulate gene expression of the enzymes [36].

Fig. 2-7. Diagrammatic illustration of sharing of type I collagen (TC) by collagenase at 25°C. Two helical fragments, TC_A and TC_B, three-fourths and one-fourth as long as the original molecule, respectively, are produced. (Adapted from DE Wooley. Mammalian collagenases. In KA Piez and AH Reddi, eds. Extracellular Matrix Biochemistry. New York: Elsevier, 1984. Pp. 119–157.)

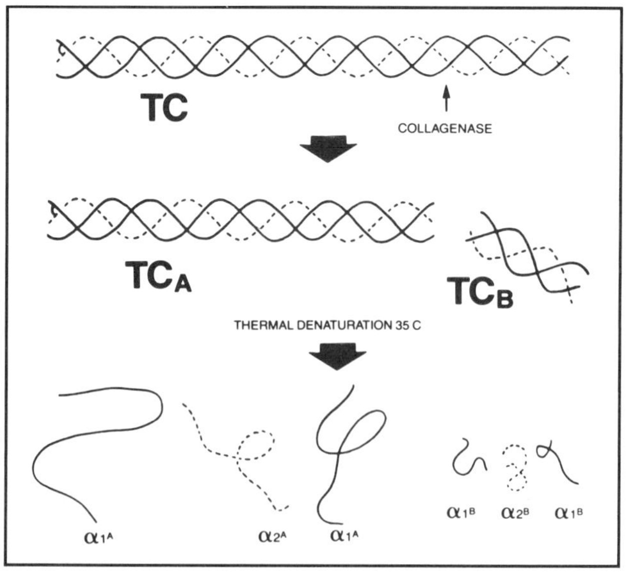

Table 2-2. Matrix metalloproteinases

Group	Names	Molecular weight		Matrix substrate
		Active form	Latent form	
I	Interstitial collagenase (MMP-1)	52	57	Collagens I, II, III, VII, and X
	Neutrophil collagenase (MMP-8)	65	85	Collagens I, II, and III
II	Type IV collagenase/72-kDa gelatinase (MMP-2)	66	72	Gelatins, collagens IV, V, VII, X, XI, fibronectin, and elastin
	Type I collagenase/92-kDa gelatinase (MMP-9)	84	92	Gelatins, collagens IV and V
III	Stromolysin/transin-1 (MMP-3)	52	57	Proteoglycans, link proteins, fibronectin, laminin, gelatins
	Stromolysin-2/transin-2 (MMP-10)	47	53	Fibronectin, gelatins

This table uses the common names of matrix metalloproteinases (MMPs) and their numerical names. The potential substrates in vivo also are listed. The term *collagen* assumes a triple-helical structure, while *gelatin* refers to the denatured state of collagen. The enzyme molecular weights are listed before and after activation.

Two species of interstitial collagenases exist, one produced by mesenchymal cells such as fibroblasts, macrophages, and synovial cells and the second produced by neutrophils (Table 2-2). In the latter case, the enzyme is packaged in specific granules during the early stages of cell maturation, then secreted when the cells are induced to degranulate. The two collagenases, referred to as matrix metalloproteinase (MMP)-1 and MMP-8, respectively, have enzymatic activity only with native triple-helical collagen but vary slightly in their specific activity against individual collagen types. After the initial cleavage of the collagen molecule into the two fragments, they denature at body temperature and are further degraded by gelatinases and possibly stromolysins (the latter enzymes also degrade proteoglycans and other matrix components). Two gelatinases exist in mammalian tissue, though not neccesarily in the same tissue. One is a 72-kDa enzyme (MMP-2) originally described as a type IV collagen-degrading enzyme; the other is a 92-kDa enzyme [MMP-9], which was described as a type V collagen-degrading enzyme, although it can also degrade type IV collagen. The two gelatinase structures differ from the interstitial collagenases and stromolysin structures in that they contain an additional amino acid segment corresponding to three repeats of a 58-amino acid segment constituting the fibronectin-like domain. This may be an important factor for binding to and digesting denatured collagens.

Two additional matrix-degrading enzymes present in mammalian tissues are referred to as stromelysin-1 and -2 [MMP-3 and MMP-10]. Although they have limited activity against gelatin peptides, they are more important in proteoglycan degradation. It should be emphasized that a concerted action by all these metalloproteinases may be neccesary for optimum tissue destruction.

The activity of matrix metalloproteinases must be carefully regulated not only at their level of synthesis but also as they reside within the tissue itself. This is achieved primarily with two metalloproteinase-specific inhibitors, referred to as tissue inhibitor of metalloproteinase 1 and 2 [TIMP-1 and TIMP-2]. Inhibitor levels are regulated transcriptionally, generally in the same direction as collagen gene expression. For instance, TGF-β stimulates both collagen transcription and TIMP-1 synthesis. The 28-kDa inhibitor molecule stoichiometrically binds to the enzyme noncovalently and noncompetitively inhibits the metalloproteinase activity. The balance between collagenase and TIMP undoubtedly plays a crucial role in the regulation of collagenolysis.

The Minor Collagens

The interstitial collagens (types I, II, III, V, and XI) were the first to be characterized, so more is known about their chemistry and biology. In addition, they represent the majority of collagen present in the body. Other types of collagens are present in much smaller quantities than the interstitial collagens and are, therefore, referred to as minor collagens. Although accurate in a quantitative sense, the term is not appropriate in a biologic sense—there is nothing functionally minor about the biologically important role these collagens play. Classifying or grouping the collagens has become an increasingly difficult task because of their heterogeneity in size and function. We have chosen to use their size, since in some cases this is all that is known, although in the two examples discussed next, this is clearly not the case.

THE BASEMENT-MEMBRANE COLLAGEN, TYPE IV

The type IV collagens are molecules with helical domains greater than 95,000 kDa_r with nonhelical segments interspersed within the helical domains. Rather than a quarter-stagger, side-by-side alignment of the individual molecules, as in the interstitial collagens, type IV collagen forms supramolecular structures by end-to-end associations with stabilization, quite often by both lysine-derived cross-links and interchain disulfide bonds (Fig. 2-8). This association occurs through globular domains located at the NH_2 and COOH ends of the molecules, which are not removed during procollagen processing [36,37].

The covalent structure of the six alpha chains have now been identified (see Fig 2-8); they contain approximately 1,700 amino acid residues [3]. The amino and carboxyl ends, represented as propeptides in interstitial collagens, remain as integral parts of the molecules when deposited in the tissue. The globular domains of the NH_2 terminus

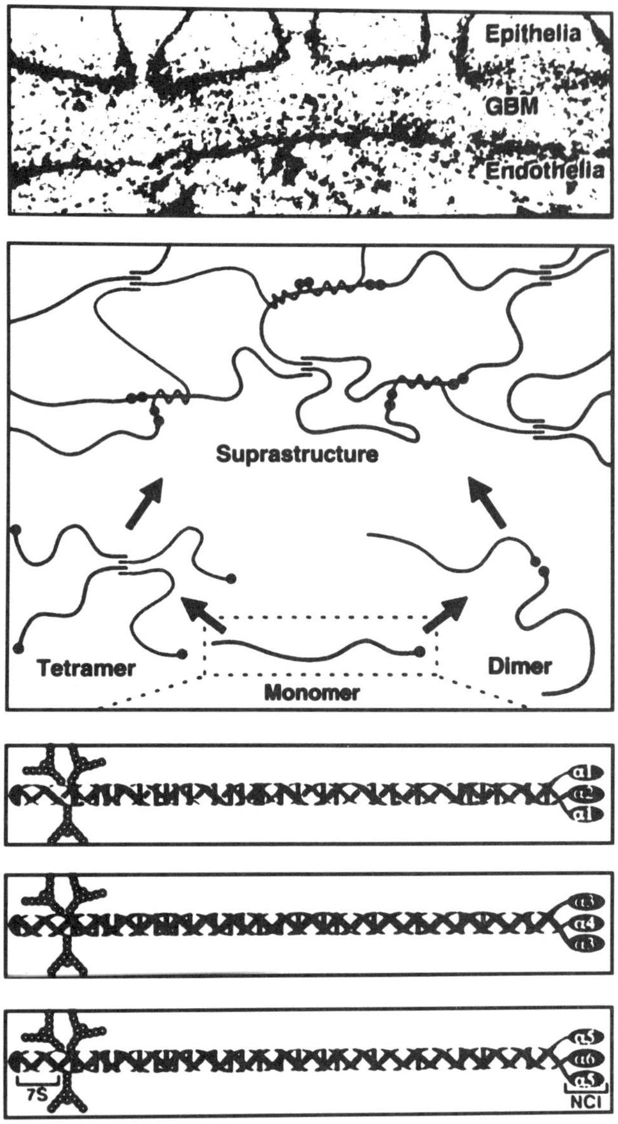

Fig. 2-8. Schematic illustration of the superstructure of type IV collagen molecules of renal glomeruli basement membrane (GBM). (*Top panel*) Electron micrograph shows GBM positioned between the fenestrated capillary endothelium and the foot processes of the epithelium (podocytes). (*Second panel*) The building block of the type IV collagen network in GBM is a triple-helical monomer. These monomers self-associate, forming a suprastructure in which they associate at the carboxyl termini, where they form dimers, and at the amino termini, where they form tetramers. The triple-helical domains intertwine and interact with the NCi domains, forming supercoiled structures. (*Lower panels*) Monomers are composed of three alpha chains that are assembled from six genetically distinct alpha chains ($\alpha1$–$\alpha6$), forming several triple-helical isoforms. These isoforms are exemplified by the ($\alpha1$)2($\alpha2$) isoform, the ($\alpha3$)2($\alpha4$) isoform, and the ($\alpha5$)2($\alpha6$) isoform. The triple-helical domain is interrupted at several sites by short noncollagenous sequences (vertical bars), which presumably confers flexibility. The N-linked oligosaccharide (Y-shaped circles) is known for the ($\alpha1$)2($\alpha2$) isoform and is hypothetical for isoforms composed of other chains. (Taken with permission from JNS Hudson, et al., Type IV collagen: structure, gene organization and role in human diseases. J Biol Chem 268:26033–26036, 1993.)

(7S segment) and the COOH terminus (NC1) participate in the intermolecular cross-links. The triple-helical domain between the two globular ends is 330 nm long and contains 12 interruptions in the Gly-X-Y triplet sequence (see Fig. 2-2). These interruptions impart a high degree of flexibility, which can be observed with rotary shadowing as kinks in the molecule in an electron micrograph. Four triple-helical molecules are joined at their amino-terminal globular ends to form a 7S region, while two carboxyl globular domains are joined to form the NC1 region [36]. The two-dimensional network thus formed is depicted in Fig. 2-8. Surprisingly, little homology exists between the $\alpha1$(IV) and $\alpha2$(IV) chains [37]. The significance of this is not known, but it is in strong contrast to type I collagen, which has greater than 80 percent homology between the $\alpha1$(I) and $\alpha2$(I) chains. Two other molecular species, $[\alpha3(IV)]_2\,\alpha4(IV)$ and $[\alpha5(IV)]_2\,\alpha6(IV)$, are present together with the predominant type IV collagen molecule. The distribution of these latter two are more restricted, primarily being described only in the kidney.

The genomic structure of the type IV collagen genes is somewhat unusual [3]. The $\alpha1$ and $\alpha2$ gene are paired head to head on the same chromosome and are transcribed in opposite directions. Whether they share nuclear transcription factors and how they are coordinately expressed remain unknown. The $\alpha3$ and $\alpha4$ and the $\alpha5$ and $\alpha6$ are arranged in an identical manner except they are located on two different chromosomes, suggesting they evolved through inversion and duplication. The type IV collagen genes are very large and complex, the $\alpha1$ and $\alpha5$ genes exceeding 100 kilobases.

The NH_2 terminus, or 7S domain, of the $\alpha1$(IV) chain contains a nonhelical segment of 20 amino acid residues followed by a helical segment of 108 amino acid residues and a nonhelical 13-residue segment (see Fig. 2-2). Twelve alpha chains from four molecules are cross-linked within the 7S region [36]. The COOH-terminal NC1 domain contains 229 amino acid residues, is nonhelical, and has a large quantity of cysteine, similar to the COOH propeptide of interstitial collagens. Surprisingly, greater homology exists between these COOH-nonhelical propeptide regions of $\alpha1$(IV) and interstitial collagen than any other segment [38].

MICROFIBRILLAR COLLAGEN, TYPE VI

Type VI collagen was initially isolated from pepsin digests of aortic intima [4]. It is a highly unusual collagen consisting of collagenous and noncollagenous domains, as in type IV collagen. It is widely distributed in many connective tissues in relatively small amounts. The functional role and precise location are not fully understood. Immunolocalization studies have led to an association with microfibrils in placenta and aorta [39]. Microfibrils of 5 to 20 nm in diameter are found in the extracellular matrix of many different organs, and these most likely represent type VI collagen. Smaller aggregates or microfibrils in the vicinity of smooth muscle cells, in neurofibromas, in nucleus pulposi, and in fibroblast cultures also are thought to be composed of this collagen [40].

The type VI collagen molecule is a 400-kDa triple-helical molecule containing large globular domains at both the

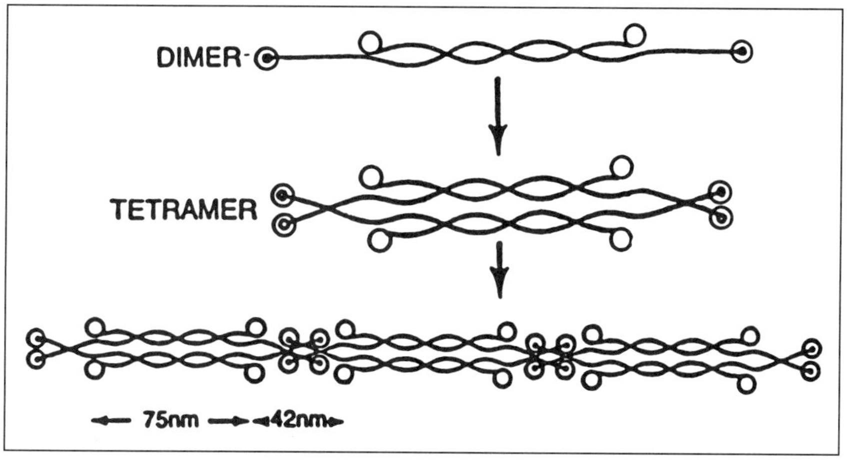

Fig. 2-9. Model of the assembly of type VI monomers to dimers, tetramers, and microfibrils. The globular domains are indicated by circles of a diameter of 7 nm, corresponding to a molar mass of 150,000 for each domain. (Adapted from J Engel, et al. Structure and macromolecular organization of type VI collagen. Ann NY Acad Sci 1985; 460:25–37, and RR Bruns. Beaded filaments and long-spacing fibrils: relation to type VI collagen. J Ultrastruct Rec 1984; 89:136–145.)

NH_2 and COOH ends. By electron microscopy, the helical domain has been estimated at 105 nm in length, corresponding to a mass of approximately 105 kDa for the three chains together. The globular domain at the COOH end has a mass of approximately 150 kDa, and that at the NH_2 end is estimated to be nearly as large as the COOH domain. The intact molecule has been difficult to isolate due to its exquisite sensitivity to nonspecific proteases. Its molecular structure consists a heterotrimer of three different alpha chains, such as [α1(VI) α2(VI) α3(VI)] [40].

The aggregates that type VI collagen forms are relatively unusual, as depicted in Fig. 2-9. Triple-helical monomeric units form dimers in an antiparallel fashion. These staggered aggregates contain 75-nm overlap regions and are held together in a supratwist by disulfide bonds. Tetrameres are formed from dimers and held together by disulfide bonds in the scissorlike regions. The inner globular domains remain pointed away from the axis of the fibers. Subsequent growth into multistranded, beaded filaments occurs by lateral and head-to-head or tail-to-tail aggregation. Structures containing cross-striations of 110 nm periodically have been observed in chick tendon fibroblast cultures, a finding that agrees well with the predicted periodicity of type VI microfibrils [41].

The function of type VI collagen remains unknown. Ultrastructural studies suggest a meshwork of fibrils oriented perpendicularly to the direction of major collagenous and elastic fibers. Possible interactions with cells, fibronectin, and other components need to be investigated using intact type VI collagen molecules.

THE FACIT COLLAGENS

The types IX, XII, and XIV collagens are another subfamily of collagens in the group 3 family of short-chain collagens. The best-characterized of this subfamily is type IX collagen, which has been the model for predicting the structure-functional relationships of type XII and XIV collagens. These collagens often are referred to as FACIT (fibril-associated collagens with interrupted triple helices) collagens. Their structures may be divided into triple-helical (COL) and non-triple-helical (NC) domains. The triple-helical domain nearest the COOH terminus (COL-1) associates with collagen fibrils, type II in the cartilagenous tissues or the mixed type I and type III in noncartilagenous tissues (Fig. 2-10). The second triple-helical domain (COL-2) appears like a rigid arm extending out into the matrix. This is made possible by the short interruption in the triple helix between COL-1 and COL-2, which acts like a hinge providing mobility in the area. Type IX collagen has an extra COL region between these two triple-helical domains; hence, COL-2 of type XII collagen is analogous to COL-3 in type IX collagen in the cartilagenous tissues. The NH_2 terminus of the collagen molecules in these subfamilies are large globular domains that extend into the extracellular matrix and react freely with cells or matrix molecules. In this manner, fibrils may become attached to type IX collagen and presumably type XII and type XIV collagen with interstitial fibrils stabilized through lysine-derived cross-linkages.

Type IX collagen consists of three alpha chains, α1(IX)-α2(IX)α3(IX), while type XII and type XIV collagens are homotrimers, $[\alpha(XII)]_3$ and $[\alpha1(XIV)]_3$. The α2(IX) contains a Ser recognition sequence for xylose-protein-transferase, the same enzyme that initiates glycosaminoglycan synthesis on the core protein of chondroitin sulfate. A chondroitin polysaccharide chain has been identified on the α2 chain and extends into the extracelluar space, thereby providing an additional site for components to attach ultimately to the collagen fibrils. Type XII and type XIV collagens likewise contain a glycosaminoglycan chain, although their exact location remains to be determined. In summary, the FACIT collagens appear to have a specific role in providing linkages of cells or extracellular matrix components to the interstitial collagen fibrils. As stated previously, type IX collagen is located only in cartilagenous tissues and vitreous humor, while type XII colla-

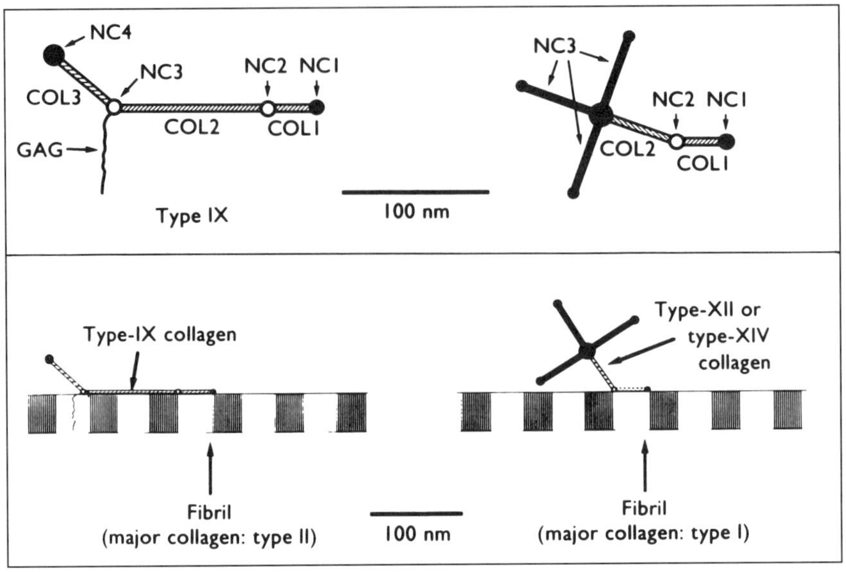

Fig. 2-10. Type IX, type XII, and type XIV collagen molecules (upper panel) contain triple-helical (COL) domains (indicated by dashed boxes) interrupted by short non-triple-helical (NC) domains (indicated by open circles). The large N-terminal domains (243 residues for $\alpha1$(IX) chain and the 190 kDa fragments for type XII and type XIV collagens) are indicated in black. The much smaller C-terminal domains are indicated as black circles. Type IX collagen binds to the surface of fibrils containing type II collagen (*lower panel, left side*). The relative orientation of the molecule has not been defined yet and is represented here parallel to type II collagen. The globular NC4 domain and the triple-helical COL3 domain project out of the fibril. The assembly of type XII and type XIV with the type I collagen, presented for comparison on the right side of the lower panel, is still largely hypothetical. (Taken with permission from van der Rest, et al. Structure and function of the fibril-associated collagen. Biochem Soc Trans 19:820–826, 1992.)

gen has been identified in skin tendon and periodontal ligament and type XIV has been located in skin and tendon. Undoubtedly, these latter two FACIT collagens will be found in all tissues that contain type I and type III collagen fibrils.

Elastin

Large arteries possess the property of elastic recoil, essential for their physiologic function. This physical property is due in large part to the presence of elastic fibers in the extracellular matrix. The large arteries contain as much as 50 percent elastin by dry weight. Lesser amounts are present in the smaller arteries and veins [42,43]. Elastin fiber has properties of an elastomer with a high extensibility (i.e., the degree of elongation without irreversible changes per unit force applied to unit cross-sectional areas is high). Elastic recoil is similar to the mechanical properties of rubber and is consistent with the function of elastin in relation to its distribution in the media of arterial walls. From considerations of its mechanical properties, together with the ultrastructural and wide-angle x-ray diffraction studies showing no evidence of any repeating fine structure, it has been suggested that elastin is a three-dimensional network of randomly coiled polypeptides joined together by covalent cross-links [44].

ELASTIN STRUCTURE

Elastin usually appears amorphous in electron micrographs. It is one of the most apolar and insoluble proteins in nature, which is evident from its amino acid composition (330 glycine, 128 proline, 174 alanine, 177 valine, and 52 leucine per 1,000 amino acid residues). Strong denaturants, hot alkali treatment, and repeated autoclaving all fail to dissolve the highly cross-linked polymer [41]. Generally, "pure" elastin preparations are defined operationally as the insoluble product remaining after exhaustive extraction procedures and containing a constant amino acid content. The glycine and proline content of elastin is similar to collagen, but elastin contains no hydroxyproline or hydroxylysine. It also contains very small amounts of polar amino acids.

Physicochemical studies to characterize the molecular structure have been impossible to obtain, because solubilization can be achieved only by partial hydrolysis with specific enzymes, such as pancreatic elastase or weak acids. Generally, such treatment yields two major groups of peptides with distinct amino acid composition and sequence [45]. The fact that a limited number of peptides can be obtained has led to the suggestion that a large number of interchain cross-links must exist and that these must occur within a repeating amino acid sequence in the polypeptide chain. This conclusion is not surprising, since a rubberlike elastomer must contain a reasonable number of cross-links in its structure. These cross-links impose a mechanical restriction on the elastomer so that, while stretching under stress, one chain does not slip completely past another, thus preserving the ability of the elastomer to return to its original size when the stress is removed [44].

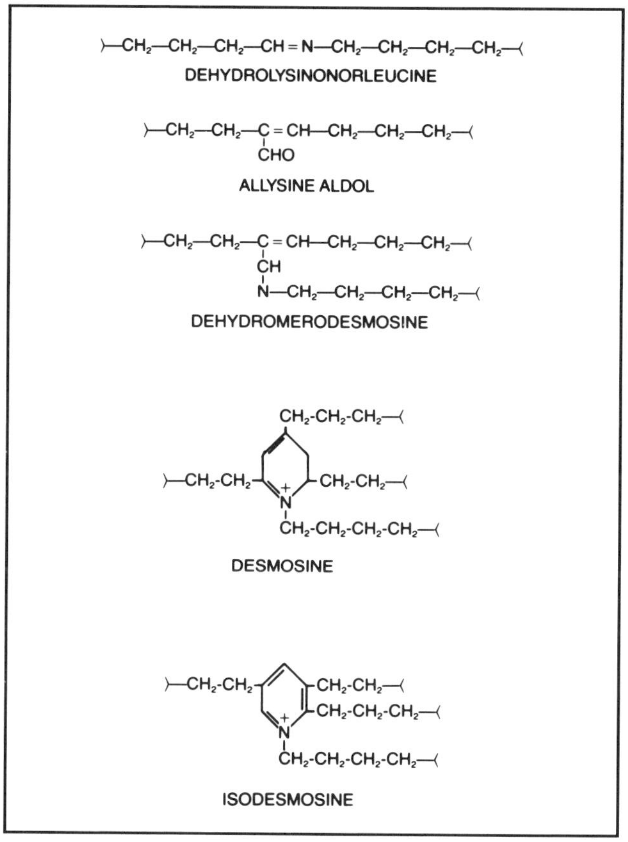

Fig. 2-11. The structures of cross-links found in elastin. The desmosine and isodesmosine represent final products of the lysine-derived cross-links.

ELASTIN CROSS-LINK

As in collagen cross-linking, the first step in the elastin cross-link formation is the oxidative deamination of the epsilon-amino group of lysine following polypeptide chain synthesis. In fact, the same lysyl oxidase reacts with both proteins. Since no hydroxylysine is present in elastin, only the allysine aldehyde becomes involved [46]. In contrast to collagen, however, reduction of the double bonds in the elastin cross-link occurs spontaneously by some unknown mechanism, and the quantity of lysine involved in cross-linking is much larger in elastin than in collagen. There may be as many as 40 residues of lysine deaminated per 1,000 amino acid residues in elastin, whereas collagen contains only 1 or 2 deaminated lysine residues per 1,000 residues. Four basic types of cross-link compounds have been identified in elastin: dehydrolysinonorleucine and its reduced form, lysinonorleucine; the aldol condensation product of two residues of allysine; dehydromerodesmosine and its reduced form, merodesmosine; and desmosine and isodesmosine (Fig. 2-11) [47].

Biosynthetically, all the cross-links are derived from lysyl residues through allysine [48]. The mechanism of formation of the aldol condensate and dehydrolysinonorleucine in elastin is identical to that described for collagen. The biosynthetic origin of dehydromerodesmosine appears to be through aldamine-bond formation between residues of lysine and the aldol condensate. The precise biosynthetic pathway for the formation of desmosine has not been well characterized. It should be noted that cross-linking in elastin occurs frequently, not only between peptide chains but also within the same polypeptide chain, producing kinks within the polypeptide chain.

ELASTIN PRECURSOR, TROPOELASTIN

Soluble precursors of elastin are not found in extracts of normal tissue. This provides a clue as to the rapid formation of mature, highly cross-linked elastin fibers and the low rate of synthesis. In experimental conditions such as copper deficiency or lathyrism (β-aminopropionitrile administration), which inhibit lysyl oxidase activity and cross-link formation, a soluble protein of 72 kDa, referred to as tropoelastin molecule, can be extracted from the aorta [49]. Apparently, the same tropoelastin molecule is present in lung and cartilage tissue. It is also apparent that a number of endothelial cells and a variety of mesenchymal cells are capable of tropoelastin synthesis.

Tropoelastin undergoes posttranslational modifications before its assembly into elastin fibers. Oxidative deamination of lysine residues followed by subsequent condensation reactions provides a family of unusual cross-links (see Fig. 2-11). Pulse-chase experiments with radiolabeled lysine indicate rapid incorporation of the labels into desmosine and isodesmosine such that the rate of formation of these cross-links parallels the rate of elastin synthesis. As stated previously, 40 lysine residues per 1,000 amino acids become incorporated into cross-links. The relative proportions reported for lung elastin are as follows: 6 to 9 lysine equivalent in desmosine; 3 to 5 in isodesmosine; 0.5 to 2.0 each for lysinonorleucine, allysine, and aldol condensation products; 0.2 to 0.5 as dehydrolysinonoleucine; and the remaining unaccounted for [49].

The amino acid sequences of human, bovine, and chicken elastin have been deduced from copy-DNA (cDNA) sequences. Significant portions of the 3′ and 5′ regions of both human and bovine genes have been characterized [49 and references therein]. Collectively, these analyses suggest that functionally distinct cross-linking and hydrophobic domains of elastin are encoded in separate exons. The segregation of these functionally distinct domains of the protein is a feature of the complete tropoelastin gene. The polypeptide chain contains approximately 800 residues of amino acids, the variability due to extensive alternate splicing. Short segments rich in alanine and lysine appear to cluster together, apparently to compose the cross-link region. They are in alpha-helical configuration, and each begins with tyrosine followed by either Ala-Ala-Lys or Ala-Ala-Ala-Lys. Their sequences are shown in Fig. 2-12. The clustering of alanyl residues adcent to desmosine is noteworthy. Space-filling atomic models indicate that lysines separated by two or three alanyl residues in alpha-helical conformation protrude on the same side of the helix. Hence, the sequence Lys-Ala-Ala-Lys allows the formation of dehydrolysinonorleucine, whereas the sequence Lys-Ala-Ala-Ala-Lys accommodates either aldol condensate or dehydrolysinonorleucine. Condensation of the two intrachain cross-links could result in the formation of the interchain desmosine cross-linkages [45].

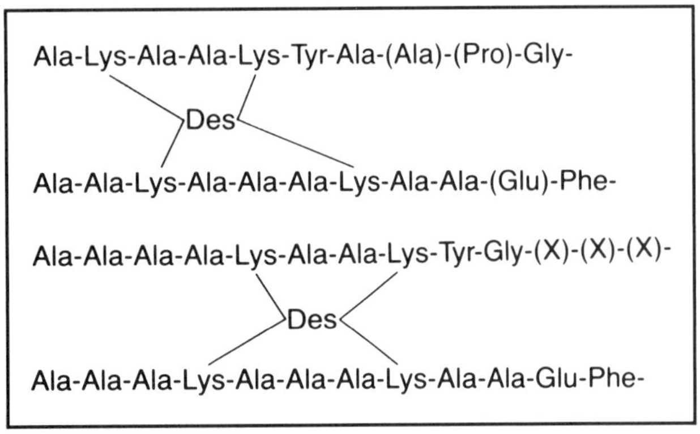

Fig. 2-12. Amino acid sequence of two desmosine cross-linked peptides from mature elastin. Lys connected to the desmosine (Des) is used to denote the lysine-derived desmosine cross-links. (See Fig. 3-14 for desmosine structure.) Tentative assignments are given for amino acids in parentheses and (X) denotes that the residue is unknown. (Adapted from JA Foster, et al. Isolation and characterization of cross-linked peptides from elastin. J Biol Chem 1974; 249:6191–6196.)

The alanine- and lysine-rich cross-linking segments are separated by large hydrophobic segments of 6 to 8 kDa (Fig. 2-13), which are in a beta spiral structure with elastomeric properties [49]. Within the hydrophobic segments, a repeating pentapeptide (Pro-Gly-Val-Gly-Val) is present, which would impart some unusual folding properties to the molecule. A collagenlike sequence (Gly-Val-Pro-Gly) occurs rather frequently, which would explain certain collagenlike properties of tropoelastin, such as its limited susceptibility to bacterial collagenase (Pro-Gly-X-Y) and the small amounts of hydroxyproline found in tropoelastin. The sequence Gly-X-Pro-Gly is recognized by the collagen enzyme prolylhydroxylase [49].

ELASTIN METABOLISM

The expression of the elastase gene is modulated by a variety of factors, including TGF-β, IL-1β, TNF-α, insulinlike growth factor, glucocorticosteroids, vitamin D_3, and cyclic nucleotides [50]. Most of this regulation occurs transcriptionally, although TGF-β has the additional property of stabilizing the elastin messenger RNA (mRNA). Elastin is initially synthesized as a 72-kDa polypeptide encoded by a 3.5-kb mRNA. The complete elastin gene spans a 45-Kb genomic DNA segment with a 5-Kb 5′ flanking DNA. During posttranslational processing, a considerable amount of alternate splicing results in synthesis of elastin isoforms. These isoforms are incorporated into the extracellular fibers, as evidenced from monoclonal studies.

The mechanism for the assembly of elastin fibers has been proposed to include secretion of the soluble precursor tropoelastin, which, together with a 67-kDa chaperone protein, finds its way through the extracellular space to the growing elastic fiber, where it interacts with glycoprotein microfibrils and becomes oriented in the proper alignment for cross-linking. The elastin-assembly process is mediated by an elastin-binding complex that contains three proteins, two being integral membrane proteins and a third being a detachable 67-kDa elastin-binding protein [50]. A transgenic mouse has been developed with a 5.2-Kb human 5′-flanking DNA, linked to the chloramphenicol acetyl transferase (CAT) reporter gene to aid in studying tissue-specific and developmentally dependent expression of the elastin gene. Lung and aorta had the highest level of expression; the lung was greatest in the 15-day embryo and declined rapidly 5 days after birth. The aorta had the highest level of gene expression at 5

Fig. 2-13. Hydrophilicity-hydrophobicity analysis of human tropoelastin. The hydrophilic peaks correspond for the most part to potential cross-linking domains. Amino acid sequences of potential cross-links are given, and cross-linking exons, where known, are numbered. Exons subject to alternate splicing are indicated by brackets [ ]. The bar (—) indicates position of the tyrosine-rich segment. (Taken with permission from Indik, et al., Proc Natl Acad Sci 1987; 84:5680–5864.)

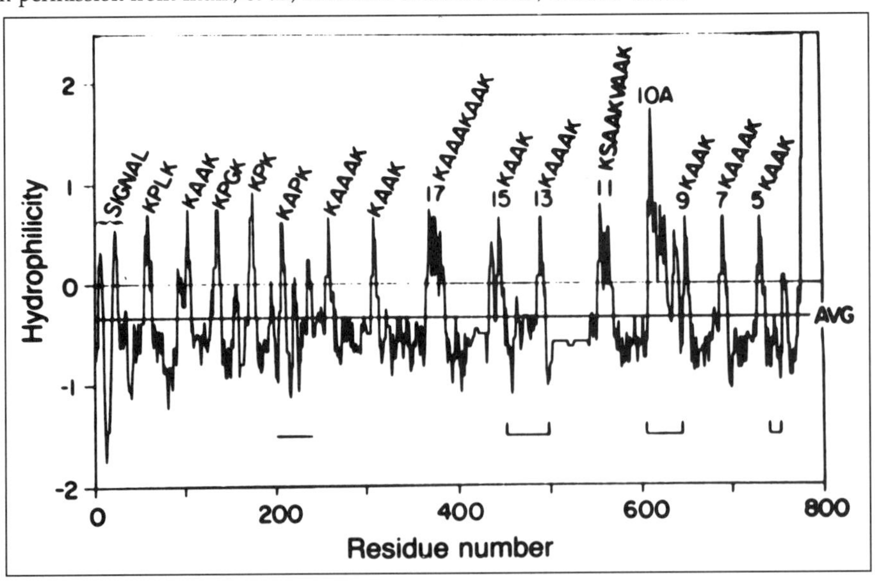

days after birth and continued high until 30 days. The skin had a peak at 30 days after birth and declined thereafter.

Tropoelastin is produced by a variety of fibroblast or fibroblastlike cells, but smooth muscle cells are responsible for elastin synthesis in the arterial wall [51]. The relative amount of elastin mRNA, as measured by cDNA hybridization, correlates well with the functional elastin mRNA measured by cell-free translation. Age-dependent changes in elastin synthesis also correlate with elastin mRNA content of the aorta [52,53].

Very little is known about the mechanism of elastin turnover. The half-life in normal humans has been estimated in years. Urine excretion of desmosine is normally 40 to 50 μg, which is equivalent to the turnover of 1 percent of the total body elastin per year, but the specific enzyme system involved in the elastin turnover is not well understood [54]. Although elastases capable of degrading elastin have been isolated from cells extrinsic to connective tissues, such as polymorphonuclear leukocytes, macrophages, and pancreatic acinar cells, no elastolytic enzyme has been detected in the connective tissue proper. Thus, in inflamed tissues, it is assumed that the elastases derived from the neutrophils or macrophages are responsible for elastolysis. The mechanism of elastin degradation in physiologic tissue remodeling, however, remains unclear.

Although the mechanism for the regulation of elastin turnover is unknown, there is evidence that the hereditary defect in the circulating elastase inhibitors is associated with the development of destructive pulmonary disorder. Affected individuals show progressive destruction of the alveolar wall, which is rich in elastin, resulting in premature emphysema. Furthermore, experimental instillation of elastase into the lungs of animals causes destruction of the lung similar to that seen in patients with the alpha-1-proteinase-inhibitor deficiency. However, no large-blood-vessel abnormalities have been shown to occur in this disorder [49].

Fibronectin

Fibronectin represents the best characterized of an increasing number of glycoproteins that have been identified in the extracellular matrix [55,56]. These glycoproteins are primarily known as cell-adhesion molecules with an ability to interact specifically with a number of extracellular molecules as well as different types of cells. Their potential role in the control of cellular functions such as replication, motility, and differentiation has stimulated extensive studies from a variety of scientific disciplines. Cell migration on fibronectin-containing matrices occurs primarily through interactions with the cell-recognition sequence Arg-Gly-Asp (RGD) with specific cell-surface integrin receptors [57–58]. Two other recognition sites, Leu-Asp-Val (LDV) and Arg-Glu-Asp-Val (REDV), located in the alternately spliced regions of fibronectin are involved in cell-type-specific adhesion by neural crest cells and certain lymphocytes [59].

It is now known that fibronectin is present in relatively large quantities in most, if not all, connective-tissue matrices, including the blood vessels. In addition, a soluble form of glycoprotein, termed plasma fibronectin, is also present in blood. Analyses of the multiple binding properties of fibronectin have led to the identification of specific binding domains within different areas of the polypeptide structure. Thus, information on fibronectin function has been rapidly expanded in cell adhesion, connective-tissue-matrix formation, opsonization, blood coagulation, and malignant transformation.

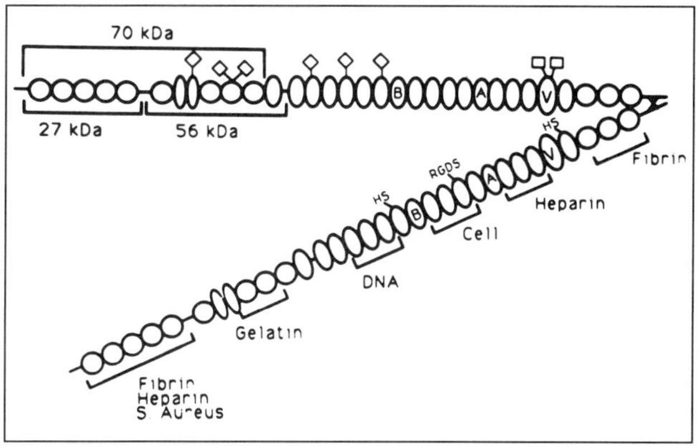

Fig. 2-14. Model of protomeric fibronectin. A model of fibronectin illustrating the location of the three types of homologous repeats and the functional binding domains is shown. Fibronectin is a dimeric glycoprotein consisting of two similar 250-kDa subunits held together by disulfide bonds. Type 1 repeats are shown as circles, type II repeats as smaller ovals, and type III repeats as larger ovals. Both the differentially spliced type III sequence (III-8 or B and III-13 or A) and the differentially spliced variable (V) region are also shown. Glycosylation sites (diamonds) and locations of the various binding domains, free cysyeins (-SH), and the Arg-Gly-Asp-Ser (RGDS) cell-adhesion sequence are shown for half the molecule. Also shown are the locations of the 27-, 56-, and 70-kDa fragments. (Reproduced with permission from DF Mosher, ed. Fibronectin. New York: Academic Press, 1989.)

FIBRONECTIN STRUCTURE

Fibronectin exists as a disulfide-linked dimer of 450 kDa in plasma and tissue. With reduction of the disulfide bonds, two nearly identically sized polypeptide chains of 220 kDa are apparent. Peptide maps of each chain are indistinguishable, leading to the conclusion that the two chains were closely related monomers [57]. In fact, the second chain is now known to result from alternate splicing of the original mRNA transcript [58].

Fibroblasts, endothelial cells and other cell types secrete, bind, and assemble fibronectin into fibrils in the extracellular matrix [59]. Fibroblasts contain discrete sites on the cell surface, termed matrix assembly sites, that bind soluble or serum fibronectin in a saturable and reversible manner. After initial binding, fibronectin interacts with other fibronectin molecules to form disulfide-stabilized multimers that represent extracellular matrix-associated fibronectin. This process requires the amino-terminal 70-kDa fragment for initiation of fibril assembly. The disulfide cross-links are located in the carboxyl end.

Three types of repeating sequences or modules are present in the large dimeric molecule. The amino-terminal 70-kDa segment contains nine repeats of a type I domain (45 amino acids each) and two type II domains (60 amino acids each) (Fig. 2-14). The middle region contains 15 to

17 type III domains (90 amino acids each), depending on alternate splicing. Three additional type I domains are found at the carboxyl terminus followed by 53 amino acids with no sequence homology to other regions of the fibronectin molecule. The two cysteines in this region participate in disulfide formation and the formation of dimeric molecules through interchain disulfide bonds.

THE FIBRONECTIN GENE

The fibronectin gene has distinctive regions in the gene structure that could account for the individual functional domains. The amino acid sequence of fibronectin shows a striking series of repeating polypeptide sequence units of the same size as the exon structure of the gene. From the available data, it appears that fibronectin probably evolved by a series of duplications of one or a few primordial genes, followed by evolutionary differentiation into the present functional domains [57]. Comparison of the covalent structure of fibronectin from several species by DNA or protein sequencing reveals a high degree of homology (over 95%) in specific regions that correspond to functional domains involved in interactions with target molecules. For example, a 97-percent identity between bovine and human fibronectin occurs in the 29,000-dalton amino-terminal domain, which has several specific binding activities. The amino-terminal region of the collagen-binding domain contains a 90-percent homology, but, in a separate region, a 95-percent identity was found in chicken and bovine structures. One may infer that in specific active site regions, greater sequence conservation was required during evolution.

FUNCTIONAL DOMAINS OF FIBRONECTIN

Fibronectin can be viewed as a multifunctional molecule with a series of specialized binding sites that mediate its function (see Fig. 2-14). The specific binding regions or domains have been isolated by covalently attaching the ligand to inert beads to produce affinity supports. Next, the fibronectin molecule is dissected into large fragments that are passed through the affinity column. Domains having binding affinity for the specific ligands are bound to the affinity column, yielding the type of information about the domain structures of fibronectin shown in Fig. 2-14.

The Amino-Terminal Domain. The amino-terminal domain binds to a surprisingly large number of ligands [57]. The highest-affinity site for fibrin (see fibrin I in Fig. 2-13) is located here. This domain also specifically binds several gram-positive bacteria such as *Staphylococcus aureus*, *Streptococcus pyogenes* and *Streptococcus pneumoniae*. Fibronectin on the mucosal cell surface serves as a receptor for the lipoteichoic acid moiety of group A *Streptococci*. The binding is mediated through the lipid region of lipoteichoic acid of the bacteria and a fatty-acid binding site on fibronectin [60]. The binding of bacteria to fibronectin has been shown to enhance opsonization and phagocytosis by phagocytic cells. Gram-negative bacteria do not bind to fibronectin, but, interestingly, *Escherichia coli* does bind to laminin, the fibronectin counterpart of basement-membrane tissue. The NH_2-terminal domain is also the primary site for covalent cross-linking of fibronectin to fibrin through the action of the enzyme transglutaminase. It has been proposed that fibronectin bound to the fibrin clot could provide an adhesive temporary matrix for cells to grow on. This would then provide a scaffold for early wound healing. This domain also contains the weaker binding site for heparin (see heparin in Fig. 2-14).

Collagen-Binding Domain. The collagen-binding domain mediates the binding of collagen to fibronectin [61,62]. It is enriched with disulfide bonds, which have been shown to be essential for collagen-binding activity, and is heavily glycosylated. All genetic types of collagen investigated so far have been shown to bind to fibronectin [63]. Interestingly, the first component of complement, C1q, which contains a collagen-like structure, has been shown to have an affinity for fibronectin. Surprisingly, denatured collagen has a much greater affinity for fibronectin than does native collagen. Although the biologic significance of this is unclear, the observation has allowed investigation of the structure of collagen involved in this interaction. From studies utilizing various enzymatically and chemically degraded collagen peptides, several binding sites along the collagen chain have been found, but the one with the greatest affinity is located in the precise region of the molecule cleaved by interstitial collagenases.

The Cell-Binding Domain. The domain that continues to gain the most attention is the cell-attachment site. This area of research has expanded further with the identification of multiple cell-receptor proteins, or integrins, that are used to bind fibronectin and other matrix components. An integrin consists of two proteins, generally alpha and beta subunits; at present, there are at least 14 alpha subunits and 8 beta subunits. The most commonly used receptor for fibronectin is the $\alpha 5\beta 1$ adhesion-cell-recognition receptor, although other integrin combinations are available and may be used by other cell types or to obtain other responses in the same cell type. It should be emphasized that when integrin receptors bind to extracellular matrix components, such as fibronectin and collagen, a signal is transmitted to the cell, which in turn integrates all the integrin signals before the appropriate response is taken [64].

The smallest fragment of fibronectin to provide 100 percent of the cell attachment properties is a 37-kDa recombinant peptide. Through use of site-directed mutagenesis, the requirement for the cell-recognition sequence RGD was confirmed. For other peptides in this fragment, LDV and REDV are used as other cell-type-specific cell-adhesion recognition sequences. Monoclonal antibodies to specific sites in the 37-kDa fragment pinpointed two additional sites, referred to as subregions A and B, required for optimum cell-binding activity. These sites are located in the eighth and ninth type III repeats in the fibronectin molecule [65].

Heparin-Binding Domain. The heparin-binding domain is clearly devoid of carbohydrates and yet is protease resistant [57]. Several polyanionic macromolecules, such as heparin, heparan sulfate, dextran sulfate, and DNA, compete with each other for binding to the fibronectin molecule, suggesting that they all share the same binding site. Other polyanionic macromolecules, such as chondroitin sulfates and dermatan sulfate, however, do not bind, demonstrating a certain degree of specificity.

The binding of a class of macromolecules to one of the fibronectin domains influences the binding of other macromolecules to another domain. Addition of polyanionic glycosaminoglycans, such as heparan sulfate or hyaluronic acid, to fibronectin-coated gelatin-Sepharose enhances the stability of fibronectin-gelatin binding. Similarly, gelatin-coated beads can be agglutinated by the addition of fibronectin and glycosaminoglycans. In the presence of heparin, fibronectin causes precipitation of type I or type III collagen in solution, whereas neither alone is effective. The cooperative effect of utilizing two distinct binding domains on the fibronectin molecule with enhancement of the binding is responsible for this phenomenon. This kind of combined interaction of the three major classes of extracellular matrix components—fibronectin, collagen, and glycosaminoglycans—may serve as a model for the formation of connective matrix as an insoluble matrix [55].

A similar situation occurs with fibrinogen. The addition of heparin to a solution of fibrinogen and fibronectin causes precipitation at low temperatures. Since fibrinogen occupies a site on the fibronectin molecule similar to that of collagen, a similar mechanism presumably operates. Therefore, the trimolecular complex may be a more physiologic situation to examine in the study of the biologic role of fibronectin in tissue matrix.

Fibrin-Binding Domain. The carboxyl-terminal domain binds weakly to fibrin, and it also contains one of the two free-sulfhydryl groups in fibronectin. This is the domain that may contain two different subunits on differing chains. The human fibronectin molecule contains a fibrin-binding domain at the carboxyl end of each chain, but hamster fibronectin is reported to have fibrin binding on only one chain. There also exist differences demonstrated by changes in proteolytic cleavages near this domain. It has been postulated that these differences may provide a recognition site of subunits and assist in the assembly of dimeric fibronectin molecules from monomers [57].

Functional Relationships between Domains. The functional characteristic of fibronectin with its multiple domains on two subunits leads to the concept that simultaneous interactions with multiple, different macromolecules may indeed be the physiologic role of this protein. Cell-cell interactions appear to require both subunits intact, whereas purified binding domains inhibit the binding of intact fibronectin to a specific ligand.

The circulating plasma fibronectin has been assigned a variety of roles in the cascade of wound-healing events. It promotes adhesion and spreading of platelets on exposed collagen surfaces, binding of circulating cells to the fibrin clot and exposed collagen, nonimmune opsonization for phagocytic cells by binding to cell debris, and fibroblast chemotaxis to the demand area for repair [61].

Fibronectin may play a role in directing the differentiation and morphogenesis of certain cells. Myoblasts, for example, lose their ability to produce fibronectin prior to fusion into myotubules. Chondrocytes also fail to produce this protein, but the addition of exogenous fibronectin to the culture medium causes the cells to dedifferentiate, and assume a fibroblastic phenotype with lowered production of proteoglycans and cartilage-specific type II collagen, and induces the synthesis of endogenous fibronectin [65].

There has been little conclusive information on abnormalities of fibronectin in diseased connective tissues. Skin lesions of scleroderma contain increased amounts of fibronectin, as judged by immunofluorescent microscopy. Changes in fibronectin distribution are seen in various diseases affecting the skin. It has been reported that fibronectin renders collagen resistant to degradation by interstitial collagenases. Whether this phenomenon plays a role in the pathogenesis of any of these conditions remains conjectural.

Laminin

Laminin is a large-molecular-weight glycoprotein present only in basement membranes. It consists of one A chain (M_r., 200 kDa) and two B chains (M_r., 200 kDa). Three types of B chains (B1, B2, and B3) and at least two A chains (A and Am) account for four different isoforms having the chain compositions of B1B2A, B3B2A, B1B2Am, and B3B1Am (Fig. 2-15). More isoforms will no doubt be identified in the future. Current evidence suggests that the triple-helical structure is formed by addition of the A chain to an already formed dimer consisting of two B chains in a coil structure [66]. The triple-stranded coil structure takes on an asymmetric crosslike molecular configuration seen by electron microscopy. Disulfide bonds at the cross section hold the three chains together, and at that point the two B chains separate to form the perpendicular arms seen in electron micrographs [67].

A number of biological activities have been attributed to laminin, including cell attachment, neurite outgrowth, and interactions with other matrix components. An accumulating body of data indicates that the various component chains can mediate different specific activities and also that different isoforms of the laminin molecule may vary with respect to tissue distribution and developmental expression [67].

Laminin is an adhesive glycoprotein specific to epithelial and endothelial cells and their basement membrane (type IV) collagen. Laminin, like fibronectin, alters cell morphology, growth, differentiation, and migration in vitro during tissue development and wound healing. Laminin, by its interaction with collagen and proteoglycans, also takes an active part in formation of the extracellular matrix itself. Distinct domains within the molecule recognize type IV collagen, epithelial-cell-surface receptors, and heparin. It also binds to ganglioside and to the basement-membrane-associated heparan sulfate proteoglycan [68]. Immunofluorescent studies with antibodies directed against laminin have confirmed its localization in the basement membrane, specifically in the lamina rara. The localization of laminin in the lamina rara suggests that laminin may play a role in the attachment of epithelial

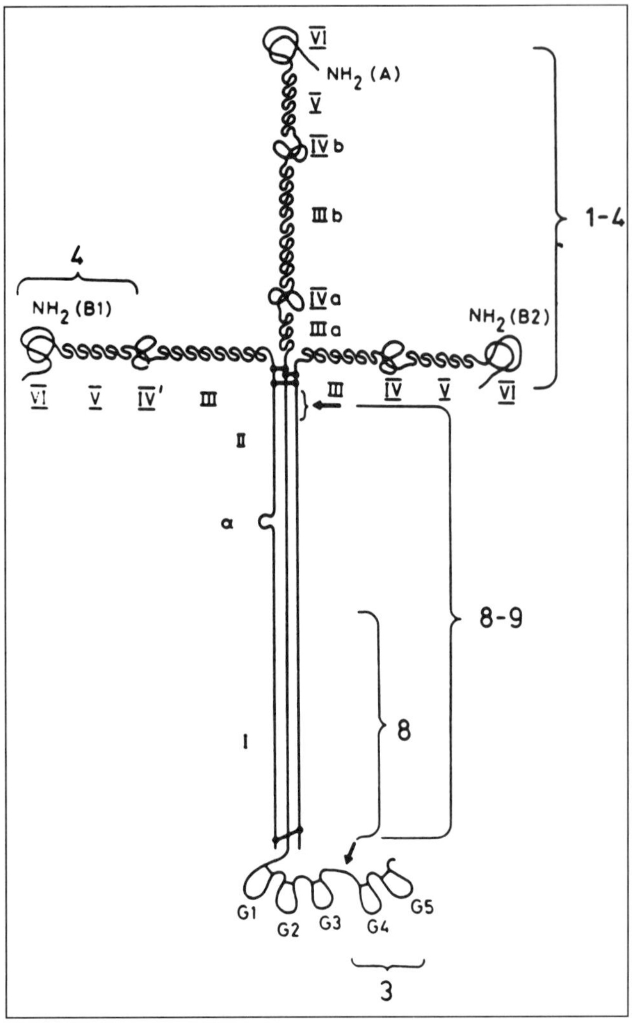

Fig. 2-15. Structural model of laminin. The A chain in the center represents the longest molecule and is joined by disulfide bonds to the B1 and B2 chains. The two B chains separate to form the characteristic cross-like structure of laminin. The domains are designated by roman numerals, and the regions of the molecule that can be isolated as fragments are indicated by numbers. (Taken with permission from K Beck, I Hunter, J Engel. Structure and function of laminin: anatomy of a multidomain protein. FASEB J 1990; 4, 148–160.)

cells to type IV collagen, the major constituent of the lamina densa. Indeed, a large body of evidence now indicates that certain epithelial cell lines adhere preferentially to the type IV collagen–coated substratum, and the adhesion is mediated by small amounts of laminin but not fibronectin. Laminin does not mediate attachment to substrates containing type I, III, or V collagen, nor does laminin promote fibroblast attachment to collagen-coated substrates. Although the specificity for the requirement of laminin is clear, some cells such as hepatocytes and human embryonic skin fibroblasts have separate receptors for fibronectin and laminin [69].

Laminin also binds to type IV collagen preferentially over the other collagen types. It binds to proteoglycans, with heparin having the highest affinity, followed by heparan sulfate; to lesser degrees, dermatan sulfate and chondroiton 6-sulfate; and, very minimally, hyaluronic acid and chondroitin 4-sulfate. Since the lamina rara consists primarily of laminin and heparan sulfate, this binding may be physiologically important.

Laminin has been shown to promote the attachment of tumor cells to type IV collagen, and some evidence has been presented that correlates the metastatic potential of a cell with this binding affinity. Uropathogenic *E. coli* also binds to laminin via the lectinlike activity of their pili specific to terminal α-D-galactose. No binding affinity can be detected with *S. aureus*, but the latter specifically binds to fibronectin [65].

In summary, although fibronectin and laminin represent the major adhesive glycoproteins in connective-tissue matrices, several other less well characterized adhesive glycoproteins may also be present. Fibroblasts synthesize Gp250, Gp190, Gp170, and Gp140 (the number represents molecular weight in thousands) in variable amounts along with fibronectin. Chondronectin is a serum glycoprotein that promotes the interaction between chondroblasts and type II collagen. It has a molecular weight of 180 kDa with two subunits of 80 kDa each. Entactin is a sulfated glycoprotein of 158 kDa and is localized in subendothelial and vascular basement membranes. It is interesting to note that entactin shares some antigenic determinants with laminin, although its functional role remains to be identified. Other adhesive glycoproteins, perhaps specific to their resident tissues, will undoubtedly be identified in the near future [67].

Glycosaminoglycans

The major macromolecular components of the amorphous ground substance in the extracellular, interfibrillar space are glycosaminoglycans. Histologically, they stain metachromatically with appropriate dyes. The metachromasia is due to the high density of anionic charges on the polysaccharide chain. Formerly, this class of compounds was called acid mucopolysaccharides, to describe the mucinous or viscous nature of the polysaccharide material [70–79]. More recently, Jeanloz proposed *glycosaminoglucuronoglycan* as a chemically more appropriate term to designate these long, unbranched chains of carbohydrate polymers (-glycans) composed of repeating disaccharide units, one of which is a hexosamine (glycosamino-) and the other a hexuronic acid (glucurono-). However, keratan sulfate contains galactose instead of hexuronic acid and, therefore, is not a glycosaminoglucuronoglycan. Nonetheless, a shortened version of the term, glycosaminoglycan (GAG), has been universally accepted in the field and is used currently in the literature.

In tissues, most of the GAGs are covalently bound to a specific core protein. The exception is hyaluronan, which is an extremely long polysaccharide chain that in most cases exists alone in the tissue. Aggrecan and versican are two large GAG molecules that interact with special link proteins and a hyaluronan polysaccharide chain to form much larger aggregates. The GAG-protein complexes are generally referred to as proteoglycans, although as many newer ones are identified, they are being given trivial

Table 2-3. Components of the glycosaminoglycan portion of proteoglycans

Current nomenclature (old nomenclature)	Approximate M_r of glycosaminoglycan	Disaccharide unit	Location of sulfate
Hyaluronic acid (hyaluronic acid)	5–50 × 10^5	*N*-acetylglucosamine β1,4 Glucuronic acid β1,3	—
Chondroitin 4-sulfate (chondroitin sulfate A)	2–5 × 10^4	*N*-acetylgalactosamine β1,4 Glucuronic acid β1,3	4
Chondroitin 6-sulfate (chondroitin sulfate C)	2–5 × 10^4	*N*-acetylgalactosamine β1,4 Glucuronic acid β1,3	6
Dermatan sulfate (chondroitin sulfate B)	2–5 × 10^4	*N*-acetylgalactosamine β1,4 Iduronic acid α1,3 or Glucuronic acid β1,3	4 2
Heparan sulfate (heparitin sulfate, heparin monosulfate)	1–5 × 10^4	*N*-acetylgalactosamine α 1,4 Iduronic acid α1,4 *N*-sulfoglucosamine α1,4 Glucuronic acid β1,4	2 N
Heparin (heparin)	0.5–4.0 × 10^4	*N*-sulfoglucosamine α1,4 Iduronic acid α1,4 *N*-sulfoglucosamine α1,4 Glucuronic acid β1,4	N 2 N
Keratan sulfate (keratosulfate)	4–19 × 10^3	*N*-acetylglucosamine β1,3 Galactose β1,4	—

names to represent the complex. For instance, aggrecan is the major proteoglycan component of cartilage [71].

STRUCTURE AND DISTRIBUTION OF GLYCOSAMINOGLYCANS

Seven GAGs have been identified and characterized: hyaluronic acid (HA), chondroitin 4- and chondroitin 6-sulfates (CS), dermatan sulfate (DS), heparan sulfate (HS), heparin, and keratan sulfate (KS) (71–75). The current nomenclature, which has evolved as the chemistry of these GAGs has become known, and their old synonyms are shown in Table 2-3. The structural characteristics of GAGs are similar in all tissues. They consist of unbranched polymers of repeating disaccharide units, of which one sugar is invariably a hexosamine, either a glucosamine or a galactosamine, and the other sugar a hexuronic acid (either a glucuronic or an L-iduronic acid) in all cases except keratan sulfate, which contains a galactose in the place of the hexuronic acid. Hexosamine is, as a rule, *N*-acetylated except in HS, where it may be *N*-sulfated. The structures of the repeating units of GAGs are presented in Fig. 2-16. These polyanions are highly charged because of the presence of sulfate groups, carboxyl groups, or both along the chains.

The uronic-acid linkage in chondroitin sulfates and the hyaluronate is β1,3, whereas it is α1,3 in DS because of the presence of L-iduronic acid in the latter as the hexuronyl group. The hexosaminidic linkage in all of these is β1,4. The disaccharide unit of KS has a different structure, β-galactosyl (1,4)-*N*-acetylglucosamine. It is polymerized by a β1,3 glucosaminidic bond. The structure of HS is more complex. It contains some disaccharide units composed of D-glucosamine and D-glucuronic acid and others of D-glucosamine and L-iduronic acid. Unlike other GAGs, the uronyl linkage is α1-4 rather than β1-3, and the hexosaminidic linkage is α1-4 rather than β1-4. The glucosamine residues are partly *N*-sulfated as well as *O*-sulfated. HS is closely related structurally to the anticoagulant heparin. The repeating unit of heparin contains a higher content of sulfate than does HS. In addition to the *N*-sulfate and *O*-sulfate groups of the glucosamine moiety, additional sulfate is present in the two positions of some of the iduronic moieties. Heparin, however, is synthesized by and stored in mast cells and does not appear to be a structural component of connective tissue.

The GAG chains are linear polymers of disaccharide units (15 to 5,000) with molecular weights ranging from several thousand to several million daltons. All hexosamine residues are N-substituted with either acetyl or sulfate groups. In addition, most GAGs have ester O-sulfate on one or both sugars of the disaccharide unit.

PROTEOGLYCANS

Proteoglycans are a complex and diverse group of macromolecules in connective tissues (Table 2-4). Although it is beyond the scope of this text to review all the proteoglycans, a representative few will be discussed. Except for hyaluronat (HA), they all contain a protein core to which the GAG chains are attached. Proteoglycans such as CS (aggrecan) and the fibroblast counterpart (vesican) bind additionally to HA chains with the help of link proteins to form extremely large aggregates. Most of the other proteoglycans have their own unique core protein, contain only one to three GAG chains, and do not form aggregates with HA. The exception is intracellular heparin, which contains 15 or more CS GAG chains on its core protein, serglycin, but it does not interact with HA.

The proteoglycan monomer of CS (referred to as the aggrecan) consists of a core protein approximately 223

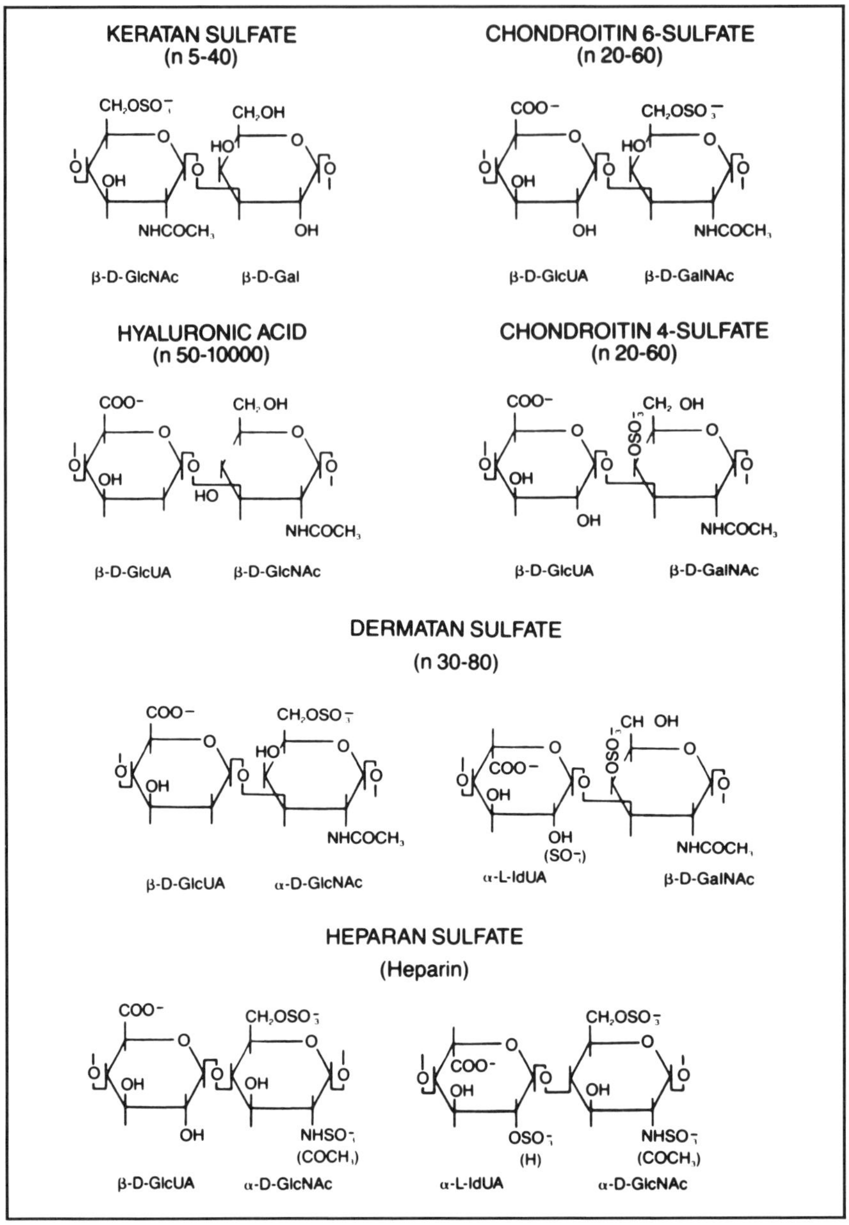

Fig. 2-16. Structures of repeating disaccharide units of the glycosaminoglycans. The letter *n* denotes number of disaccharide units in the chains. GlcNAc = *N*-acetylglucosamine; GalNAc = *N*-acetylagalactosamine; Gal = Galactose. (Adapted from D Heinegard and M Paulson. Structure and metabolism of proteoglycans. In KA Piez, AH Reddi, eds. Extracellular Matrix Biochemistry. New York: Elsevier, 1984. Pp. 227–328.)

kDa (2,109 amino acids) deduced from cDNA-sequence analysis [76]. The proposed core-protein structure contains three unique globular domains (Fig. 2-17) labeled G-1, G-2, and G-3. G-1 and G-2 are located at the NH_2 terminus and G-3 at the COOH terminus of aggrecan. The G-1 domain has three disulfide-bonded loop structures homologous to link protein, which are believed to assist in noncovalent interaction between link protein and HA. The G-2 domain has two of the same globular motifs as G-1 but does not participate in binding to the HA or link protein. The function of G-2 remains uncertain. The G-3 domain, located at the COOH terminus of aggrecan, contains an epidermal growth factor (EGF)–like, lectin-like, and complement regulatory–like domain. A lethal genetic mutation in aggrecan in chickens (referred to as nanomelia) contains a single G-to-T nucleotide switch at position 4553. This converts the GAA codon to a TAA stop codon and results in a shortened core protein (M_r. 158 kDa). This truncated core protein is not processed beyond the endoplasmic reticulin (ER), which suggests that the G-3 domain is required for processing and secretion [76].

Alternate splicing of the RNA yields at least three species of aggrecan, which accounts for some of the polydis-

Table 2-4. Proteoglycans

Nomenclature	Old nomenclature	Glycosaminoglycans	Protein-core size (number of amino acids)
Aggrecan	Chondroitin sulfate-4, -6	Chondroitin sulfate, keratan sulfate	2,109
Biglycan (DSPG-1)	Dermatan sulfate	Dermatan sulfate, chondroitin sulfate	370
Decorin (DSPG-2)	Dermatan sulfate	Dermatan sulfate, chondroitin sulfate	370
Perlecan	Heparin sulfate, basement-membrane associate	Heparan sulfate	3,707
Syndecan I	Heparin sulfate, cell surface	Heparan sulfate	310
Fibrocan (syndecan III)	Heparin sulfate, cell surface	Heparan sulfate	558
Serglycin	Intercellular	Chondroitin sulfate	

persity of the core protein. The region between G-2 and G-3 contains 117 Ser-Gly-X-Gly sequences that provide for up to 100 CS chains covalently attached to Ser and at least some KS chains (see Fig. 2-17). Surprisingly, CS chains are adjacent to the G-3 domain, together with some KS chains, but no CS chains are present in the KS domain. KS is the only GAG that is not linked to the core protein via Gal-Gal-Xly-Ser (Fig. 2-18); rather, it is linked to the protein through N-acetylgalactosamine-Thr-protein. An N-acetylneuraminic (sialic acid)–galactose disaccharide

Fig. 2-17. Schematic representation of proteoglycan structures: (*a*) serglycin, a small-molecular-weight intracellular proteoglycan; (*b*) syndecan I, a membrane-associated HS proteoglycan; (*c*) decorin, a DS proteoglycan; (*d*) aggrecan, a large cartilage proteoglycan. The aggrecan has three globular domains referred to as G1, G2, and G3 going from the amino terminus, with G3 being the COOH terminus. (Reproduced with permission from E Ruoslohti. Structure and biology of proteoglycans. Ann Rev Cell Biol 4:229–255, 1988.)

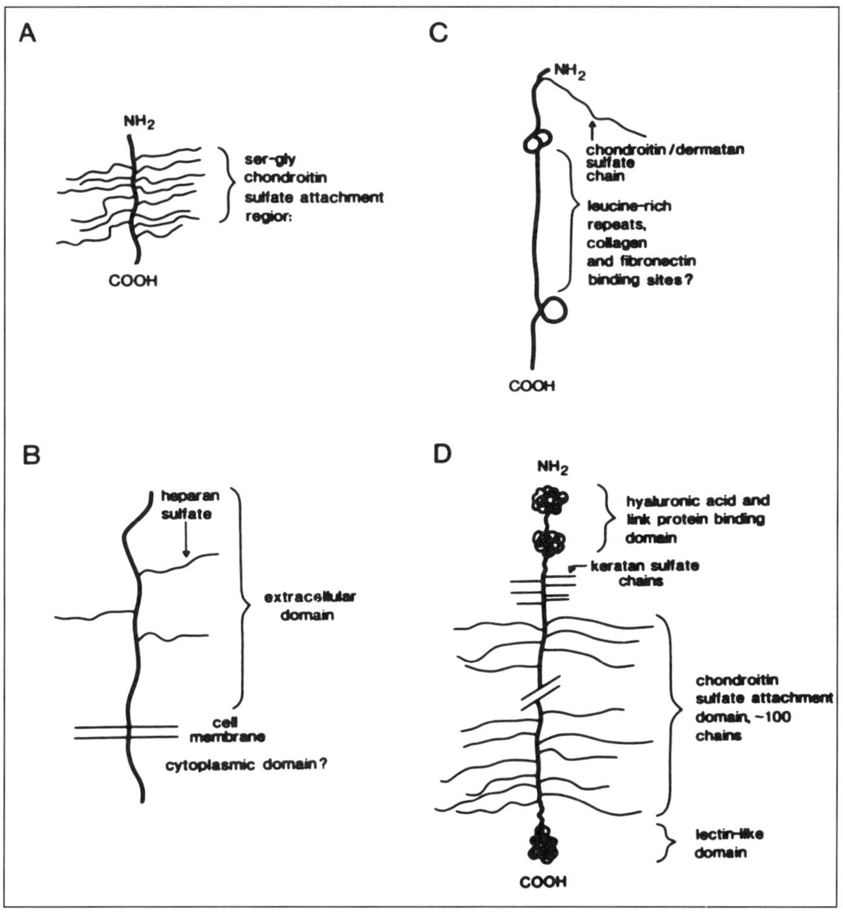

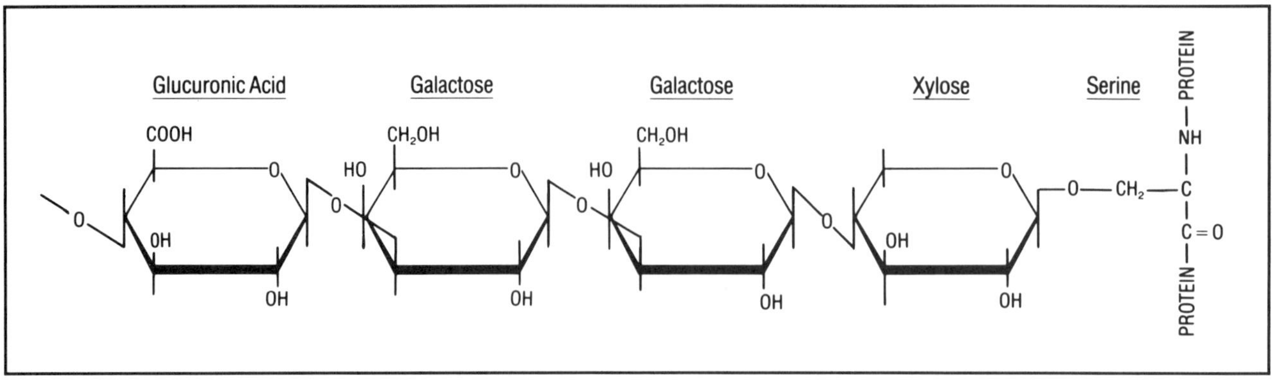

Fig. 2-18. Oligosaccharide linkage between glycosaminoglycans and protein core. (Reproduced with permission from JE Silber. Structure and metabolism of proteoglycans and glycosaminoglycans. J Invest Dermatol 79:31–37. Copyright by Williams & Wilkins, 1982.)

also is attached to the KS linking N-acetylgalactosamine. The CS chains contain 40 to 60 disaccharide units, while the KS chains have 10 to 20 disaccharide units. The molecular structure conceivably resembles a bottle brush, with bristles radiating from the central protein core. The repelling forces of thousands of negative charges from either the sulfate or the COOH groups would force this type of structure.

The CS proteoglycan monomer forms as a large aggregate as illustrated in Fig. 2-19. This occurs on a central single filament of HA. The G-1 domain of aggrecan recognizes a pentasaccharide of HA and binds at regular intervals from opposite sides of the chain. These noncovalent associations are stabilized by link proteins together with the G-1 domain of aggrecan [75].

Analyses of the biochemical nature of link protein were hampered by its apparent insolubility in physiological solutions. However, removal of trace amounts of divalent cations, notably zinc, has now made these studies possible. Alone in solution, link protein exists as a hexamer but disassociates into a monomer when it binds to G-1. The secondary structure of link protein contains three globular loops very much like the three loops (A, B, and B′) found in the G-1 domain of aggrecan. Although aggrecan is found only in cartilage, link protein identical to the one in cartilage can be isolated from other tissues, notably aorta [77,78].

The molecular weight of CS varies with tissue, age, and species. A typical CS molecule contains a full aggrecan (M_r, 220 kDa; length, 300 nm) with approximately 100 CS chains (M_r, 20–30 kDa each; length, 50–60 nm), 10 or more KS chains (M_r, 5–10 kDa; length, 10–20 nm), with a total molecular weight of 2–3 million. More than 100 of these aggrecan molecules are attached to a single HA chain (M_r 1.2 million; length, 4,000 nm). This together with one link protein (M_r, 37 kDa) per aggrecan brings its size to well over 200 million (see Fig. 2-19). The mechanical properties of different proteoglycan aggregates are related to size and hence to the number of proteoglycan monomers, the length of the aggrecan, and the density of GAG chains. It was formerly thought that limited proteolytic activity was responsible for the heterogeneity found in CS, but now we understand that much of that heterogeneity can be attributed to alternate splicing of the protein-core pre-mRNA or the use of different transcription start sites.

The second most abundant proteoglycan in tissue is DS. DS is a mixed GAG composed of two disaccharide units; glucuronic acid and *N*-acetylgalactosamine, as in CS; and iduronic acid and *N*-acetylgalactosamine. The two forms present are referred to as biglycan (DSPG-1) and decorin (DSPG-2). Their identity is defined by their core proteins. DSPG-1 contains Ser at residues 5 and 11 that provides attachment sites for its two GAG chains. DSPG-2 contains a Ser at position 4 that contains its single GAG. The two core proteins are highly homologous except for the NH_2 terminus. Their molecular weights are approximately 37 kDa and their GAG chains approximately 30 kDa; hence, their total sizes are 67 and 97 kDa. Another small component of this family has been referred to as fibromodulin, which has a core protein very similar to DSPG-1 and DSPG-2 but different in that it contains at least one KS chain for its GAG component.

Biglycan and fibromodulin core proteins, but not decorin or aggrecan core proteins, bind to type I collagen and inhibit fibrillogenesis. The decorin-collagen binding is very specific; when radiolabeled, it can be visualized at discrete points along the cross-striated fibril of collagen. The core proteins of decorin and biglycan likewise bind to the cell-binding region of fibronectin and thus prevent cell attachment. Another potentially important function of DS is to bind large quantities of cytokine and growth factors such as TGF-β, possibly serving as a reservoir for biologically active compounds where they can be rapidly released into the local tissue.

The third rapidly growing family of proteoglycans are the heparan sulfates, a highly diverse group of core proteins that contain at least one HS chain. Although they are widely distributed, heparan sulfates can be primarily divided into two groups: those that are associated with plasma membranes and those that bind to basement membranes. The disaccharide component of HS is glucuronic acid-N-acetylglucosamine, thus distinguishing it from CS (see Fig. 2-16). The unique feature of the HS GAG is that regions or domains of their polysaccharide chains have

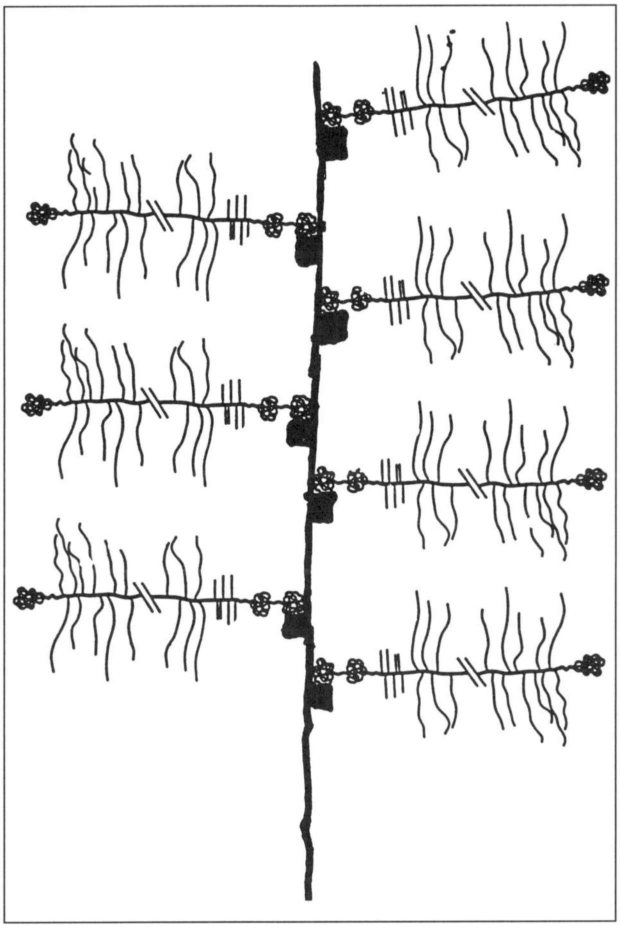

Fig. 2-19. Schematic representation of the large-molecular-weight aggregate of proteoglycans in cartilage. Multiple units of aggrecan are noncovalently associated with a single hyaluronic chain through the G1 globular domain. This association is stabilized by link proteins (solid squares), which bind both the aggrecan and the hyaluronic acid. Approximately 100 units of aggrecan and link protein are present on a single hyaluronic-acid chain. (Modified with permission from E. Ruoslohti, 1988. Structure and biology of proteoglycans. Ann Rev Cell Biol 1988; 4:229–255.)

their acetyl groups removed from the hexosamine and replaced with an N-sulfate group. Subsequent modifications that occur in these regions are epimerization of glucuronic acid, 2-O-sulfation of iduronic acid, and 6-O-sulfation of glucosamine. These clumps of modified disaccharides occur in discrete areas throughout the polysaccharide chain and presumably are important in the biologic functions of these HS chains. The biochemical signals that restrict these modifications to localized areas remain unknown. We also do not understand the function of these changes. In one case, though, 3-O-sulfated glucosamine is an absolute requirement for the highly specific binding of heparin to antithrombin III, a key component in the anticoagulant properties of heparin. In another case, 2-O-sulfated glucuronic acid is enriched in the fraction of HS that traffics to the nucleus of some cells.

Syndecan is the most abundant proteoglycan of the plasma-membrane-associated HS family. It associates with plasma membranes through its core protein. Syndecan I (there are four members) has a 310–amino acid core protein, which is intercalated into the cell membrane to provide a 35-residue intracellular cytoplasmic domain. Both HS and CS GAG units are linked to the core protein. Syndecan has been proposed to provide a link between extracellular matrix organization and intracellular cytoskeletal organization. Fibrocan (or syndecan III) is another HS proteoglycan that intercalates through a cell membrane. The predicted core protein contains 201 amino acids, a transmembrane domain, and only HS as its GAG. Another membrane-associated proteoglycan that has been identified is glypican, a 558–amino acid core protein that is anchored to the membrane via a glycosylphosphatidylinositol moiety. This proteoglycan is synthesized by a variety of cells and has little homology with syndecan or fibrocan.

The typical number of HS proteoglycans on the cell surface ranges between 10,000 and 100,000 per cell [79]. Given the length of the HS chain of 50 nm [30 kDa], when extended in a mobile fashion from the core protein as proposed, it would provide a network of polyanions that would encompass the entire cell surface. It is not surprising, then, that HS proteoglycans are involved in many cell-cell and cell-matrix interactions, and the ability of HS to bind cytokines and various growth factors could be a way for gathering large quantities in a restricted space. The HS molecules on the cell membrane have an estimated half-life of 3–8 hours, and degradation occurs through a combination of endocytosis and intracellular degradation (approximately 70%) and proteolytic cleavage of the core protein with shedding into the extracellular spaces (30%).

The second family of heparan sulfates are those associated with basement membranes. One member, referred to as perlecan, contains three HS GAGs linked to a large core protein of 3,707 amino acids [80]. The amino-terminal-172 amino acids contain three Ser-Gly-Asp sequences, which are most likely the attachment sites for the HS GAGs. When visualized by electron microscopy, the core protein contains a series of globular regions separated by rods and resembling a string of pearls; hence, the core protein was given the name *perlecan* (see Fig. 2-16). The protein has been divided into five clearly distinct domains. The amino terminus, domain I, contains the HS carbohydrate moiety, while domain II is very similar to the LDL receptor. Domain III has homology with the short arm of the laminin A chain, and domain IV contains 14 repeats of the immunoglobulin superfamily. Domain V contains three repeats of the G domain of the laminin A chain. Since laminin and perlecan bind to the same region of type IV collagen in basement membranes, it is possible that the shared sequences are involved in binding. It has been suggested that perlecan is inserted unidirectionally in the basement membrane with the HS chains toward the cell surface in the lamina rara interna and the molecule extending down through the lamina densa. The length of the molecule (80 nm) is sufficient to span the width of most basement membranes. This location of polyanionic charges on the surface of basement membranes could account for their molecular impermeability. Additionally, HS proteoglycans are involved in the sequestration of cytokines, growth factors, and heparan sulfate–specific endoglycosidases, which have been implicated in the process of basement-membrane degradation during tumor metastasis [81].

The final family of proteoglycans to be discussed are the heparins [81]. Heparin shares the same GAG as HS but is noticeably different in its higher level of *N*-sulfation (78%), higher overall sulfation, and higher iduronic acid content. A specific pentasaccharide found in heparin is required for binding to antithrombin III, which contributes to heparin's antithrombogenic properties. Tissue localization of heparin is limited to mast cells, where it is synthesized on a small core protein referred to as serglycin (see Fig. 2-17). The mature proteoglycan is localized in storage granules with 15 heparin chains per serglycin (M_r, 100 kDa).

HA is the largest GAG and occurs in all connective-tissue extracellular matrices [72]. It is an unbranched chain with 500 to several thousand disaccharide repeating units. The primary role of this large GAG, at least in some tissues, is to retain and regulate water flow. It is abundant in embryonic matrices and is replaced by other proteoglycans during development. In fact, rapid elevation of tissue hyaluronidase has been used as a marker of differentiation [82]. Finally, hyaluronate participates in proteoglycan aggregation and influences phagocytosis by white blood cells.

BIOSYNTHESIS OF PROTEOGLYCANS

The biosynthesis of all proteoglycans appears to occur through a similar pathway, and the rate-limiting step appears to be the synthesis of the core-protein molecule [74]. The core-protein molecule, like all protein molecules, is synthesized on a ribosomal template, and the sugar chains are assembled posttranslationally, one sugar at a time, starting with the linkage of xylose to Ser in a specific part of the core-protein molecule (see Fig. 2-18). Sulfation occurs after the appropriate monosaccharide has been linked to the growing GAG chain. Elongation of the chain and sulfation take place in the endoplasmic reticulum and the Golgi complex as the core-protein molecules progress to the exterior of the cell.

Proteoglycan synthesis begins in the late endoplasmic reticulum and the Golgi complex with the addition of xylose to the hydroxyl group of serine in the protein-core molecule by the action of xylosyltransferase. This enzyme recognizes Ser in the sequence Glu/Asp-X-Ser-Gly of the core protein [75]. The transfer of galactose from uridine diphosphate galactose (UDPgalactose) to xylose depends on galactosyl transferase, which does not discriminate between protein-bound xylose and other xylose derivatives, such as xylose-serine and xylose-DNP (see Fig. 2-18). The second galactose residue is also transferred via UDPgalactose to galactosyl-xylose by a second, distinct galactosyl transferase. Again, the core protein is not necessary for this addition reaction, and galactosyl-xylose alone may be the accepting molecule. This is followed by the addition of the first glucuronic acid moiety by the action of UDPglucuronic acid transferase. Growth of the GAG chain, then, occurs by alternating transfer of hexosamine and uronic acid residues from their respective UDP derivatives by the action of their specific transferases. Thus, the UDP derivatives of *N*-acetylglucosamine and glucuronic acid are precursors for HA, heparin, and HS, whereas *N*-acetylgalactosamine and glucuronic acid are precursors for CS and DS. The decision to add *N*-acetylglucosamine for an HS molecule or *N*-acetylgalactosamine for a CS molecule is decided by the protein core and the specificity of the tranferase. After addition of the first hexosamine, elongation occurs by the same *N*-acetylhexosaminyltransferase and glucuronosyltransferase regardless of which chain is being synthesized. The respective chains are variably modified by pathway-specific epimerization and sulfation reactions to yield iduronic acid and sulfation.

Sulfation occurs by direct transfer of the sulfate group from 3-phosphoribosyl phosphoadenosine-5 phosphoribosylphosphosulfate (PAPS) to the appropriate site on the GAG by a nonspecific sulfotransferase. This sulfotransferase and the glycosyl transferases involved in GAG synthesis are particulate enzymes, and the complex serves as a primer during polysaccharide-chain elongation and posttranslational modification. Sulfation may occur during synthesis or on completely synthesized chains by an all-or-none phenomenon. No partial sulfation occurs, thereby leading to the suggestion that the GAG may become attached to the primer and completely sulfated before release.

Heparin and HS contain an *N*-sulfate that is unique, since all others are in an *O*-sulfate linkage. The synthesis of this *N*-sulfate linkage proceeds through the *N*-acetylglucosamine addition to the GAG chain, deacetylation, and replacement of the acetyl group by sulfate. Iduronic-acid formation in heparin, HS, and DS takes place after polysaccharide synthesis by an epimerization reaction of glucuronic acid.

Variation in the size of the proteoglycan monomers has been well documented. Specific subpopulations are now recognized in the tissue; cartilage contains a large and a small subpopulation of KS-CS proteoglycans. Aorta contains both large and small CS-DS proteoglycans. Additionally, nonaggregating states of both heparin proteoglycan and HS proteoglycan (basement membrane-derived) are present. The size of the proteoglycan, in many cases, appears to be related to the length of the core protein [83].

DEGRADATION

The half-life of HA has been estimated to be 2 to 5 days in young rabbit skin; CS 7 to 14 days; and DS 7 to 10 days [84]. Although the half-lives may be somewhat longer in older tissues, these values indicate a relatively rapid turnover rate of proteoglycans compared with collagen or elastin. The mechanism of degradation remains incompletely understood. Degradation of the proteoglycans involves proteolysis of the core protein by nonspecific proteases such as stromolysin (see Table 2-2), breakdown of the sugar chain, and desulfation of the sugars. The dramatic loss of cartilage matrix that results from experimental intravenous injection of papain illustrates the importance of the protein core to the structural integrity of the proteoglycan. All connective-tissue cells have the ability to produce a variety of proteolytic enzymes that can degrade proteoglycans at the neutral pH. Macrophages and granulocytes also produce proteases that degrade proteoglycan. The activity of these neutral proteases appears to be controlled by tissue inhibitors of proteases [85].

Degradation of the sugar chains occurs principally intracellularly in lysosomes [86]. Perhaps the best-characterized GAG-degrading enzyme is testicular hyaluronidase, which is an endo-*N*-acetyl-β-hexosaminidase and which degrades hyaluronic acid, chondroitin sulfates, and dermatan sulfates to oligosaccharides. A similar enzyme has been demonstrated in a variety of mammalian tissues, including liver, skin, and synovium. Other glycosidases are required to complete the breakdown of the oligosaccharides to monosaccharides. Lysosomes contain glucuronidase and *N*-acetylhexosaminidases, which are exoenzymes capable of removing terminal glucuronic acid and hexosamine residues, respectively. Lysosomes also contain β-xylosidase, β-galactosidase, and α-iduronidase, which are required to complete the breakdown. Lysosomal sulfatases are responsible for the removal of the sulfate groups from the oligosaccharides.

Inherited defects in the activity of various GAG-degrading enzymes are associated with the intracellular accumulation of GAG fragments that cannot be further degraded. These storage diseases, called mucopolysaccharidoses, involve faulty catabolism of one or another type of GAGs [87].

Biological Considerations

In addition to their readily appreciable structural function, connective-tissue macromolecules are involved in a variety of interactions that may be just as important biologically. That subject is a large one, however, and cannot be covered comprehensively in this chapter. Only selected topics pertinent to the biology of the blood vessel are discussed here.

BIOLOGICAL INTERACTIONS OF GLYCOSAMINOGLYCANS

In addition to their structural and morphogenetic roles, GAGs appear to be involved in a variety of interactions [88]. Perhaps the best-known interaction involves heparin. Heparin binds to a serine protease inhibitor (serpin) and antithrombin III and accelerates the formation of the antithrombin-thrombin complex by 2,000-fold, thereby neutralizing the enzyme activity. Other serine proteases in the coagulation system (factors IXa, Xa, XIa, XIIa) are similarly inactivated by antithrombin in processes also greatly enhanced by heparin. Since heparin is not consumed during the process, it is available again for binding to another molecule of antithrombin on release from the antithrombin-protease complex. Thus, heparin exerts an anticoagulant effect. The antithrombin-binding region of heparin contains an octasaccharide with a unique glucosamine-O-sulfate group that is not present in other regions of the heparin molecule. Despite the ability of exogenous heparin to inhibit blood clotting, the function of endogenous heparin in anticoagulation under physiologic conditions remains unclear, since the endogenous heparin possesses only about 10 percent of the anticoagulant activity of the exogenous heparin.

Proteoglycans may additionally be involved in the regulation of blood clotting. Platelets contain platelet factor 4 (PF4) in the cytoplasmic granules, where it is complexed with chondroitin 4 sulfate proteoglycan. When released, PF4 has the ability to neutralize the anticoagulant effect of heparin. The proteoglycan-PF4 complex can be dissociated by high ionic strength and by GAGs. Thus, HS and DS present in blood vessel walls could serve to control the complex's deposition locally by dissociating PF4 from proteoglycan-PF4 complex.

GAGs from blood vessels such as the aorta also bind low-density lipoproteins (LDLs) and very low-density lipoproteins (VLDLs) [89]. The binding occurs more strongly with iduronic-acid-containing GAGs, such as HS, DS, and heparin. Binding is mediated by interactions between the apoproteins of LDL and VLDL and the anionic groups of the GAG chains. DS-proteoglycan isolated from arterial walls binds LDL, suggesting a possible role in the formation of atherosclerotic lesions. More work is needed to clarify the issue.

The HS and DS proteoglycans on the endothelial-cell surface are also able to bind lipoprotein lipase [90,91], which is the primary extrahepatic enzyme that hydrolyzes the circulating plasma triglycerides of VLDL and chylomicrons. The enzyme is synthesized by subendothelial cells, such as the adipocytes, and is secreted and transported to the vascular compartment, where it binds to the luminal surface of the endothelial cell [92]. Treatment of endothelial cells with proteases such as trypsin or pronase, which would degrade the HS proteoglycan, reduces binding of lipoprotein lipase by 80 to 90 percent. Similarly, treatment of endothelial cells with platelet endoglucuronidase, which would degrade HS chains, inhibits the binding of lipoprotein lipase almost completely [93]. The bound enzyme can be readily released by heparin into the circulation. The possible physiologic significance of these observations remains to be explored further.

CELL-MATRIX INTERACTIONS

The interaction of endothelial cells and their underlying matrix poses a complex question that can be answered only when all the players have been identified. Cells derived from large-vessel endothelium respond differently than do capillary endothelial cells. Cells cultured on glass or plastic behave differently than cells on biological matrices. The behavior of cells on biological supports differs depending on whether the substrata contain interstitial connective tissue components, basement-membrane components of the same or different tissue origin, or their own basement membranes synthesized by the cells in culture. The matrix components or some specific organization of the basement membrane may contain information that the overlying cells are able to receive and respond to by attempting to modify the surrounding matrix. The synthetic potential of endothelial cells with respect to collagen production appears to vary considerably, depending on both the cell-passage number and the external environment. Early-passage cells are more stable, producing primarily type IV and type V collagen, but when these cells are released from contact inhibition and induced to undergo sheet migration, they first express a type V collagen phenotype and only later express type IV collagen synthesis [94–96]. Viral transformation also changes their synthetic products to only type I and type III collagen synthesis [97]. Such a change in an endothelial-cell matrix layer would increase the potential platelet aggregability.

The composition of the extracellular matrix may also produce varying effects on endothelial-cell proliferation, migration, spreading, and multicellular organization. This is not surprising, since the endothelial cell may encounter a variety of matrix components during normal and pathologic conditions. Some components, such as fibronectin, allow rapid attachment and spreading and also tend to inhibit migration, whereas laminin allows a rapid migration rate but a lower level of attachment and spreading. Collagen types I, III, and IV, on the other hand, tend to promote cell attachment, spreading, and migration. The effect of matrix on endothelial-cell behavior was more dramatically tested when both sides of human amnionic membrane were used as biologic substrata for the cells. The cells on the basement-membrane side, containing types IV and V collagen and laminin, took on a flattened appearance with highly organized cytoskeletons similar to their appearance in situ. The cells on the opposite side, which contained interstitial collagens of type I and III, primarily appeared as plump cells with a high cell density. These cells appeared to produce their own basal-laminalike substrata over the interstitial surfaces on which they resided [95].

The capillary endothelial cells are also affected by the underlying matrix. Specifically, cells cultured on basement membrane have a slow proliferation rate, similar to their quiescent state when they are on basement-membrane structures in situ. When they are released from this constraint, they come into intimate contact with the interstitial matrix and undergo marked proliferation, as in angiogenesis. When these cells are placed on interstitial-collagen substrates in culture, cell proliferation is increased, and they form a confluent multilayer of flattened cells [95].

The concept that the matrix may influence the differentiated state of capillary endothelial cells is further demonstrated by the changes in collagen phenotypes of these cells. When grown on plastic, they produce mainly interstitial collagens (88% as opposed to 10% type V and 2% type IV). However, cells grown on collagenous substrates produce less interstitial collagen (58%) but more basement-membrane collagen (42%) [95]. Tubelike structures are produced by cells grown on basement-membrane collagen in short-term culture. These tubelike structures form only after long-term culture of capillary endothelial cells grown on interstitial collagen, suggesting that the cells produced their own basement-membrane components prior to undergoing morphologic changes [93]. This further demonstrates that the interstitial-collagen matrix may provide a supporting layer for the basement-membrane components synthesized by the endothelial cells and allow for the organization of these structures. This result would be in accord with studies of soft-tissue injury and wound healing: the capillary cells are quiescent when invested in their basement membrane, but, as with induction of protease activity, the cells are released from the restraints of basement membrane and actively proliferate and migrate through interstitial stroma. Ultimately, the capillary cells form new vessels and once again become surrounded by their basement-membrane matrix and are restrained.

In summary, the local, preexisting matrix and the newly synthesized matrix function as modulators of endothelial-cell behavior. These matrix components can effect changes in cytoskeletal organization, attachment, spreading, and migration of the cells. The cells, in turn, respond to specific matrices and produce variable types of collagens to form their own matrix components. Perhaps endothelial cells have receptors for specific matrix components, and any interaction or lack of interaction with these receptors may govern the endothelial-cell function.

COLLAGEN-PLATELET INTERACTION

One of the earliest events in hemostasis is the formation of a platelet plug at the site of injury. Following disruption of the endothelial surface, platelets adhere to the exposed subendothelium and aggregate, releasing several biologically active substances, including adenosine diphosphate (ADP) and thromboxane A_2, which in turn stimulate other platelets to aggregate [97]. The identity and nature of the specific reacting components on the platelet membrane and the subendothelium have been the subject of intense interest because of obvious implications for normal hemostasis and thrombosis.

Results obtained from several laboratories clearly indicate that the subendothelial component responsible for platelet adhesion and aggregation is the collagen fibril. Fibrils derived from purified types I, II, and III collagen can induce platelet aggregation in vitro. The specific ligands on collagen involved in this interaction have not been definitively established. There is evidence that hydroxylysine glycosides (glucosylgalactosyl hydroxylysine) in type I collagen [98] and a nonapeptide (Gly-Lys-Hyp-Gly-Glu-Hyp-Gly-Pro-Lys) region in type III collagen [99] may be involved in this interaction.

Specific collagen-binding receptor proteins for type I and type III collagens have been isolated and characterized from platelet membranes. The purified receptor for type I collagen is a glycoprotein with M_r of 65 kDa, while the receptor for type III collagen has an M_r of 47 kDa. Their biological activities are completely destroyed by treatment with proteases. When added to platelet suspension, the purified receptors inhibit platelet aggregation mediated by the corresponding collagens, presumably by competing with platelets for the available collagen for binding. Both polyclonal and monoclonal antibodies against the receptor proteins have been prepared. When platelets are pretreated with these antibodies, they block the corresponding collagen-induced platelet aggregation. These observations indicate that specific receptors on the platelet surface mediate the aggregation reaction [100].

The transduction mechanism that follows collagen-receptor binding in platelets remains unclear. It has been shown that exposure of platelets to collagen causes endogenous phosphorylation of several platelet-surface proteins. Phosphorylated platelets show enhanced sensitivity and responsiveness to collagen [101]. Dephosphorylation of the platelet membrane by the use of phosphatase reverses this phenomenon. In view of recent data that show increased hydrolysis of phospholipids into inositol phosphates and diacylglycerol in platelets exposed to collagen, it is tempting to speculate that protein kinase C may be involved in this process [102].

It should be pointed out that one of the substances released during platelet aggregation is platelet-derived growth factor (PDGF) [102]. PDGF has been shown to be an effective chemotactic factor as well as a growth factor for the mesenchymal cells. It also stimulates a markedly increased production of extracellular macromolecules by arterial smooth muscle cells in vitro. These observations suggest a potentially important role for platelet aggregation or thrombosis in the pathogenesis of atherosclerotic lesions.

References

1. Mayne R, Burgeson RE, eds. Structure and Function of the Collagen Types. Orlando: Academic, 1987. Pp. 1–317.
2. Fleishmajer R, Olsen B, Kuhn K, eds. Structure, molecular biology, and pathology of collagens. Ann NY Acad Sci 1990; 580:1–592.
3. Hudson BG, Reeders ST, Trygvason K. Type IV collagen: Structure gene organization and role in human diseases. J Biol Chem 1993; 268:26033–26036.
4. Chung E, Rhodes RK, Miller EJ. Isolation of three collagenous components of probable basement membrane origin from several tissues. Biochem Biophys Res Commun 1976; 71:1167–1174.
5. Muragaki Y, et al. The complete primary structure of the human a1(VIII) chain and assignment of its gene [collagen α1(VIII)] to chromosome 3. Eur J Biochem 1991; 197:615–622.
6. van der Rest M., et al. Structure and function of the fibril-associated collagen. Biochem Soc Trans 1992; 19:820–826.
7. Parente MG, et al. Human type VII collagen: cDNA cloning and chromosomal mapping of the gene. Proc Nat Acad Sci USA 1991; 88:6931–6935.
8. Li K, et al. Genomic organization of the collagenous domains and chromosomal assignment of human 180kDa bullous pemphigoid antigen-2, a novel collagen of stratified squamous epithlium. J Biol Chem 1991; 266:24064–24069.
9. Chu ML, et al. Amino acid sequence of the triple-helical domain of human collagen type VI. J Biol Chem 1988; 263:18601–18606.
10. Tikka L, et al. Gene structure for the α-1 chain of a human short-chain collagen (type XIII) with alternately spliced transcripts and translation termination codon at the 5′ end of the last exon. Proc Natl Acad Sci USA 1988; 85:7491–7495.
11. Pan TC, et al. Cloning and chomosomal location of human a1(XVI) collagen. Proc Natl Acad Sci USA 1992; 89:6565–6569.
12. Kivirikko S, et al. Primary structure of the a1 chain of human type XV collagen and exon-intron organization in the 3′ region of the corresponding gene. J Biol Chem 1994; 269: 4773–4779.
13. Rehn M, et al. Primary structure of the a1 chain of mouse type XVIII collagen, partial structure of the corresponding gene, and the comparison of the a1(XVIII) chain with its homologue, the a(XV) collagen chain. J Biol Chem 1994; 269:13929–13935.
14. Madri JA, et al. The collagenous components of the subendothelium. Correlation of structure and function. Lab Invest 1983; 43:303–315.
15. Emanuel BS, et al. Human α-1(III) and α-2(V) procollagen genes are located on the long arm of chromosome 2. Proc Natl Acad Sci USA 1985; 82:3385–3389.
16. Vuorio E, de Crombrugghe B. The family of collagen genes. Annu Rev Biochem 1990; 59:837–872.
17. Ramirez F, et al. Isolation and characterization of the human fibrillar collagen genes. Ann NY Acad Sci 1985; 460:117–129.
18. Liska DJ, et al. Elements in the first intron of the a1(I) collagen gene interacts with SP-1 to regulate gene expression. Gene Expression 1992; 4:379–389.
19. Jimenez SA, et al. Functional analysis of human a1(I) procollagen gene promoter. J Biol Chem 1994; 269:12684–12691.
20. Katai K, et al. An AP-1 like motif in the first intron of human Pro a1(I) collagen gene is a critical determinant of its transcriptional activity. Mol Cell Biochem 1992; 118:119–129.
21. Ritzenthaler JD. Transforming growth factor-b activator elements in the distal promoter regions of the rat a1 type I collagen gene. Biochem J 1991; 280:157–162.
22. Bornstein P, Horlein D, McPherson J. Regulation of collagen synthesis. In P Berk, H Castro-Malaspina, LR Wasserman, eds. Myelofibrosis and the Biology of Connective Tissue. New York: Alan R. Liss, 1984. Pp. 61–80.
23. Aycock RS, et al. Posttranscriptional inhibition of collagen and fibronectin synthesis by a synthetic homolog of a portion of the carboxyl propeptide of type I collagen. J Biol Chem 1986; 261:14355–14360.
24. Ramirez F, di Liberto M. Complex and diversified regulation programs control the expression of vertebrate collagen genes. FASEB J 1990; 4:1616–1623.
25. Byers PH, Holbrook KA. Molecular basis of clinical heterogeneity in the Ehlers-Danlos syndrome. Ann NY Acad Sci 1985; 460:298–310.
26. Myers JC, et al. Complete primary structure of the human α2 type V procollagen COOH-terminal propeptide. J Biol Chem 1986; 260:11216–11222.
27. Birk DE, Trelstad RL. Fibroblasts create compartments in the extracellular space where collagen polymerizes into fibrils and fibrils associate into bundles. Ann NY Acad Sci 1985; 460:258–273.
28. Tanzer ML. Cross-linking (of collagen). In GN Ramachandran, AH Reddi, eds. Biochemistry of Collagen. New York: Plenum Press, 1976. Pp. 192–229.
29. Fujimoto D, et al. The structure of pyridinoline: a collagen crosslink. Biochem Biophys Res Commun 1978; 84:52–59.
30. Bernstein PH, Mechanic GL. A natural histidine-based imminium crosslink in collagen and its location. J Biol Chem 1980; 255:10414–10421.
31. Harris ED, Krane SM. Collagenases. N Engl J Med 1974; 291:557–563, 605–609, 652–661.
32. Wooley D. Mammalian collagenases. In KA Piez, AH Reddi, eds., Extracellular Matrix Biochemistry. New York: Elsevier, 1984. Pp. 119–157.
33. Harris ED, Jr, Cartwright EC. Mammalian collagenase. In AJ Barrett, ed., Proteinases in Mammalian Cells and Tissues. Amsterdam: Elsevier, 1977. Pp. 249–283.
34. Woessner TF. Metalloproteinases and their inhibitors in connective tissue remodeling. FASEB J 1992; 5:2145–2154.
35. Matrisian LM. Metalloproteinases and their inhibitors in matrix remodeling. Trends Genet 1990: 6:121–125.
36. Timpl R, et al. Structure and biology of the globular domain of basement membrane type IV collagen. Ann NY Acad Sci 1985; 460:58–72.
37. Babel W, Glanville RW. Structure of human basement membrane (type IV) collagen: complete amino acid sequence of a 915 residue long pepsin fragment from the α1(IV) chain. Eur J Biochem 1984; 143:545–556.
38. Hudson BG, Reeders ST, Trygvason K. Type IV collagen: Structure, gene organization and role in human diseases. J Biol Chem 1993; 268:26033–26036.
39. Jander R, Troyer D, Rauterberg J. A collagen-like glycopro-

tein of the extracellular matrix is the undegraded form of type VI collagen. Biochemistry 1984; 23:3675–3681.
40. Bruns RR. Beaded filaments and long-spacing fibrils: relation to type VI collagen. J Ultrastruct Rec 1984; 89:136–145.
41. Bentz H, et al. Isolation and partial characterization of a non-human collagen with an extended triple-helical structural domain. Proc Natl Acad Sci USA 1983; 80:3168–3172.
42. Uitto J, et al. Elastin in Biochemistry and Physiology of Skin, 2nd ed., L. Goldsmith, ed. New York: Oxford University Press, 1991.
43. Urry DW. Molecular perspectives of vascular wall structure and disease–elastic component. Perspect Biol Med 1978; 21:265–295.
44. Sandberg LB, Soskel NJ, Wolt MS. Structure of the elastic fiber: an overview. J Invest Dermatol 1982; 79:128–135.
45. Foster JA, et al. Isolation and characterization of cross-linked peptides from elastin. J Biol Chem 1974; 249:6191–6196.
46. Siegel RC. Lysyl oxidase. Int Rev Conn Tissue Res 1980; 8:73–118.
47. Partridge SM, Elsden DF, Thomas J. Biosynthesis of the desmosine and isodesmosine cross-bridges in elastin. Biochem J 1964; 93:30–33.
48. Miller EJ, Martin GR, Piez KA. The utilization of lysine in the biosynthesis of elastin crosslinks. Biochem Biophys Res Commun 1964; 17:248–253.
49. Bashir MM, et al. Characterization of the complete human elastin gene. J Biol Chem 1989; 264:8887–8891.
50. Hsu-Wong S, et al. Tissue-specific and developmentally regulated expression of human elastin promoter activity in transgenic mice. J Biol Chem 1994; 269:18072–18075.
51. Foster JA, Rick CB, Karr SR. Elastin gene expression. Int Rev Conn Tiss Res 1983; 10:65–99.
52. Indik Z, et al. Structure of the elastin gene and alternate splicing of elastin mRNA: implications for human disease. Am J Med Genet 1989; 34:81–90.
53. Burnett W, et al. Control of elastin synthesis. J Invest Dermatol 1982; 79:138–151.
54. Lieberman J. Elastase, collagenase, emphysema and α-antitrypsin deficiency. Chest 1976; 70:1–13.
55. Hynes RO. Fibronectins. New York: Springer, 1990.
56. Hay ED, ed. Cell Biology of Extracellular Matrix. 2nd ed. New York: Plenum, 1991.
57. Ginsberg MH, Loftus JC, and Plow EF. Throm Hemostasis 1988; 59:1–6.
58. Mosher DF, ed. Fibronectin, New York: Academic Press, 1989.
59. Sottile J, Wiley S. Assembly of amino-terminal fibronectin dimers into the extracellular matrix. J Biol Chem 1994; 269:17192–17198.
60. Simpson WA, et al. Fibronectin mediates the binding of streptococci to human polymorphonuclear leukocytes. Infect Immun 1982; 37:805–812.
61. Kleinman HK, Klebe RJ, Martin GR. Role of collagenous matrices in the adhesion and growth of cells. J Cell Biol 1982; 88:473–486.
62. Klebe RJ. Isolation of a collagen-dependent cell attachment factor. Nature 1974; 250:248–249.
63. Engvall E, Ruoslahti E, Miller EJ. Affinity of fibronectin to collagen of different genetic types. J Exp Med 1978; 147:1584–1593.
64. Hynes RO. Integrins; versatility, modulation, and signaling in cell adhesion. Cell 1992; 69:11–25.
65. Aota S, et al. Fibronectin and integrins in cell adhesion and migration. Biochem Soc Trans 1991; 19:830–835.
66. Utani A, et al. Laminin chain assembly. J Biol Chem 1994; 269:19167–19175.
67. Beck K, Hunter I, Engel J. Structure and function of laminin: anatomy of a multidomain glycoprotein. FASEB J 1990; 4:148–160.
68. Rao CN, et al. Isolation of a subunit of laminin and its role in molecular structure and tumor cell attachment. J Biol Chem 1982; 257:9740–9744.
69. Otto U, et al. Protease resistance and conformation of laminin. Eur J Biochem 1982; 123:63–72.
70. Timpl R, Martin GR. Components of basement membranes. In H Furthmayr, ed., Immunochemistry of collagen, vol. 2. Cleveland, Ohio: CRC Press, 1982. Pp. 119–150.
71. Wright TN, Heinegard DK, Hascall VC. Proteoglycan Structure and Function in Cell Biology of Extracellular Matrix, 2nd ed., Elizabeth G Hay, ed. New York: Plenum, Pp. 45–78.
72. Heinegard D, Paulson M. Structure and metabolism of proteoglycans. In KA Piez, AH Reddi, eds., Extracellular Matrix Biochemistry. New York: Elsevier, 1984. Pp. 227–328.
73. Roden L. Structure and metabolism of connective tissue glycoproteins. In W Lennarz, ed., The Biochemistry of Glycoproteins and Proteoglycans. New York: Plenum, 1980. Pp. 271–371.
74. Kjellen L, Lindahl U. Proteoglycans: Structures and interactions. Ann Rev Biochem 1991; 60:443–475.
75. Ruoslohti E. Structure and biology of proteoglycans. Ann Rev Cell Biol 1988; 4:229–255.
76. Li H, Schartz NB, Vertel BM. cDNA cloning of the chick cartilage chondroitin sulfate (aggrecan) core protein and identification of a stop codon if the aggrecan gene associated with the chondrodystrophy, nanomelia. J Biol Chem 1993; 268:23504–23511.
77. Gardell S, et al. Link protein and a hyaluronic acid-binding region as components of aorta proteoglycan. Biochem Biophys Res Commun 1980; 95:1823–1831.
78. Baker JR, Caterson B. The isolation and characterization of the link proteins from the proteoglycan aggregate of bovine nasal cartilage. J Biol Chem 1979; 254:2387–2393.
79. Yanagishita M, Hascall VC. Cell surface heparin sulfate proteoglycans. J Biol Chem 1992; 267:9451–9454.
80. Noonan DM, et al. The complete sequence of perlecan, a basement membrane heparan sulfate proteoglycan, reveals extensive similarity with lamjinin A chain, low density lipoprotein-receptor, and the neural cell adhesion molecule. J Biol Chem 1991; 266:22939–22948.
81. Kjellin L, Oldberg A, Hook M. Cell-surface heparan sulfate. Mechanisms of proteoglycan-cell association. J Biol Chem 1980; 255:10407–10413.
82. Toole BP, et al. Hyaluronic cell interactions. In RL Trelstad, ed., The Role of Extracellular Matrix in Development. New York: Alan R. Liss, 1984. Pp. 43–66.
83. Fellini SA, Kimura JH, Hascall VC. Polydispersity of proteoglycans synthesized by chondrocytes from the swarm rat chondrosarcoma. J Biol Chem 1981; 256:7883–7889.
84. Schiller S, et al. The metabolism of mucopolysaccharides in animal. III: Further studies on skin utilizing ^{14}C-acetate and ^{35}S-sulfate. J Biol Chem 218:139–145.
85. Walton EA, et al. The role of serine protease inhibitors in normal and osteoarthritic human articular cartilage. Semin Arth Rheum 1981; 11:73–74.
86. Truppe W, Kresse H. Uptake of proteoglycans and sulfated glycosaminoglycans by cultured skin fibroblasts. Eur J Biochem 1978; 85:351–356.
87. Fluharty AL. The mucopolysaccharidosis: a synergism between clinical and basic investigation. J Invest Dermatol 1982; 79:38–44.
88. Comper WD, Laurent TC. Physiological function of connective tissue polysaccharides. Physiol Rev 1978; 58:255–315.
89. Iverius PH. Possible role of the glycosaminoglycans in the genesis of atherosclerosis. In R Porter, J Knight, eds., A Ther-

ogenesis: Initiating Factors. Amsterdam: Associated Scientific Publisher, Ciba Foundation Symposium 12, 1973.
90. Cheng CF, et al. Binding of lipoprotein lipase to endothelial cells in culture. J Biol Chem 1981; 256:12893–12898.
91. Shimada K, et al. Involvement of cell surface heparan sulfate in the binding of lipoprotein lipase to cultured bovine endothelial cells. J Clin Invest 1981; 68:995–1002.
92. Nilsson-Ehle P, Garfinkel AS, Schotz MC. Lipolytic enzyme and plasma lipoprotein metabolism. Annu Rev Biochem 1980; 49:667–693.
93. Madri JA, Stemm KS. Aortic endothelial cells migration. I: Matrix requirements and composition. Am J Pathol 1982; 106:180–186.
94. Madri JA, Williams SK. Capillary endothelial cell cultures: phenotypic modulation by matrix components. J Cell Biol 1983; 97:153–155.
95. Pratt BM, Form D, Madri JA. Endothelial cell–extracellular matrix interactions. Ann NY Acad Sci 1985; 460:274–288.
96. Madri JA. Endothelial cell-matrix interactions in hemostasis. In TH Spacet, ed., Progress in Hemostasis and Thrombosis, vol. 6. New York: Grune & Stratton, 1982.
97. Spaet TH, Zuker MB. Mechanism of platelet plug formation and role of adenosine diphosphate. Am J Physiol 1964; 206:1267–1274.
98. Kang AH, Beachey EH, Katzman RL. Interaction of an active glycoprotein from chick skin collagen $\alpha 1$(I) chain of chick skin collagen. J Immunol 1974; 133:872–876.
99. Legrand YJ, et al. Evidence that a collagen-derived nanopeptide is a specific inhibitor of platelet collagen interaction. Biochem Biophys Res Commun 1980; 96:1579–1585.
100. Chiang TM, et al. Immunological studies of the purified human platelet receptor for the $\alpha 1$(I) chain of chick skin collagen. J Immunol 1984; 133:872–876.
101. Siess W. Inositol phospholipid metabolism and platelet function. Biochem Pharmacol 1986; 35:3184–3187.
102. Bowen-Pope DF, et al. Platelet-derived growth factor in vivo: levels, activity, and rate of clearance. Blood 1984; 64:458.

The Vascular Smooth Muscle Cell

Jonathan S. Stamler
Victor J. Dzau
Joseph Loscalzo

As evidenced by the impressive list of publications in the latter half of the twentieth century alone, the vascular smooth muscle cell has been the subject of intensive investigation. Its structure, physiology, pharmacology, biochemistry, biophysics, and pathology have been extensively reviewed by a number of distinguished investigators [1–7]. It is beyond the scope of this chapter to review all aspects of vascular cellular function and pathology; in truth, it would be a difficult task to improve on some of these classic reviews, despite the new findings to which we are privy. Thus, we refer the interested reader to the above selected works, recognizing that other important contributors might easily have been added to this list. In this chapter, we attempt to provide an updated understanding of the fundamental aspects of vascular smooth muscles. Recognizing the individuality of different vascular beds and even of consecutive sections of the vasculature, we will diverge from this paradigm as necessary to incorporate information relevant to vascular smooth muscle heterogeneity [8,9].

In a general, simplified model, the smooth muscle response can be thought of as occurring in a three-step process: (1) a change in membrane characteristics resulting from activation of surface receptors through interactions with agonists or changes in the inherent electrical properties of the membrane; (2) signal transduction, that is, coupling of receptor activation with a functional response by changes in ion fluxes and via second messengers; and (3) functional response. Conservatively thought of as a contractile response alone, the diverse cellular functions of vascular smooth muscle also include proliferation, chemotaxis, adhesion, secretion, and various metabolic functions. That many of these responses may be mediated by a common receptor-agonist interaction further underscores the complexity of this multifaceted cell. We approach this review by addressing each component of the vascular smooth muscle response in a corresponding section of this chapter (Table 3-1).

MEMBRANE ACTIVATION

Surface Receptor Systems

ALPHA-ADRENERGIC RECEPTORS

Receptor Classification. The contraction of vascular smooth muscle by alpha-adrenergic agonists, in particular norepinephrine and epinephrine, is a biologic phenomenon that extends across species lines and heterogeneous vascular beds. It is a fundamental excitatory response, mediated by the alpha-adrenoreceptor, of all vascular smooth muscle. Alpha-receptor classification has been based on pharmacologic responses to receptor agonists and antagonists [4–10]. Early labeling experiments with tritiated haloethylamines [11,12] were unsuccessful owing to extensive "nonspecific" binding of these alpha blockers, and claims of isolation of alpha receptors to certain phospholipid fractions met with critical rebuttal [12]. More recently, assays of radioligand binding have been used successfully to determine affinities of various drugs for alpha-adrenoreceptors, the number of receptors in a given tissue, and alpha-receptor subtypes [13]. Implicit in pharmacologic methods for receptor identification are certain limitations. Pharmacologic differentiation of receptor subtypes depends on agonist or antagonist specificity; therefore, changes in the receptor microenvironment or functional changes that result in exposure of different binding sites on the same receptor cannot be easily distinguished from new and distinct receptor populations. In addition, because most smooth muscle preparations also include endothelium, connective tissue, and neuronal elements, these structures may indirectly influence pharmacologic responses to exogenous agents [10]. For these reasons, the final classification of alpha-adrenergic receptors awaits methodologic advances in receptor isolation and molecular analysis.

In 1948, Alquist classified adrenergic receptors into alpha and beta subtypes. The subsequent demonstration of alpha-receptor populations on nerve terminals (prejunctional) that could be pharmacologically distinguished from smooth muscle (postjunctional) surface receptors resulted in these receptors being subclassified into $alpha_1$ and $alpha_2$, respectively [14]. For example, phenylephrine more selectively activates $alpha_1$ receptors, and clonidine activates $alpha_2$ receptors. Similarly, $alpha_1$ receptors can be distinguished from $alpha_2$ receptors by the relative affinity of the antagonists prazosin ($alpha_1 > alpha_2$) and yohimbine ($alpha_2 > alpha_1$).

$Alpha_2$ receptors have since been localized to smooth muscle as well and are generally less abundant than $alpha_1$ receptors. Given this additional and important anatomic localization, the **prejunctional** and **postjunctional** terminology has fallen into disfavor. Accordingly, $alpha_1$ and $alpha_2$ receptors are distinguished solely by their affinity for a variety of agonists and antagonists [15]. In some vascular smooth muscle, pharmacologic analyses of alpha-adrenoreceptor interactions suggest that the receptor has both $alpha_1$ and $alpha_2$ properties. These atypical alpha-adrenergic receptors characterize rat vascular smooth muscle in particular [10,16], but they are not unique to this species [17,18]. In human digital arteries and veins, Stevens and Moulds concluded that a firm classification of alpha-adrenergic receptor subtyping was not possible [19,20]. Other investigators have more recently argued for the presence of a mixed population of postjunctional $alpha_1$ and $alpha_2$ receptors as an alternative interpretation of the atypical alpha-adrenoceptor data [21,22].

In 1980, Hirst demonstrated that the excitatory junc-

Table 3-1. Regulation of smooth muscle contractile response

- I. Membrane activation
  - A. Surface receptor system
    1. α-adrenergic
    2. β-adrenergic
    3. Angiotensin
    4. Muscarinic
    5. Serotoninergic
    6. Histaminergic
    7. Bradykinin
    8. Purinergic
    9. Dopaminergic
    10. Other peptides
        - a. Neuropeptide Y (NPY)
        - b. Calcitonin gene-related peptide (CGRP)
        - c. Tachykinin
        - d. Vasoactive intestinal polypeptide (VIP)
        - e. Vasopressin
        - f. Oxytocin
    11. Prostanoid
    12. Leukotriene
    13. Growth factor protein-tyrosine kinases
        - a. Platelet-derived growth factor (PDGF)
        - b. Epidermal growth factor (EGF)
        - c. Transforming growth factor (TGF)
        - d. Fibroblastic growth factor (FGF)
        - e. Insulinlike growth factor (IGF) I
  - B. Intrinsic electrical activity
    1. Myogenic
    2. Rhythmic
    3. Other
- II. Signal transduction
  - A. Guanine nucleotide regulatory protein (G protein)
  - B. Phosphoinositide metabolism
  - C. Cyclic adenosine monophosphate (cAMP)
  - D. Cyclic guanosine monophosphate (cGMP)
  - E. Calcium
- III. Functional response
  - A. Contraction
    1. Excitation-contraction coupling
    2. Sources of calcium
    3. Force generation
        - a. Overview
        - b. Ultrastructure of contractile apparatus
        - c. Regulatory mechanisms
  - B. Proliferation (as a model for other functional response)
    1. Platelet-derived growth factors (PDGFs)
    2. Fibroblast growth factors (FGFs)
    3. Transforming growth factors (TGFs)
    4. Endothelins

tional potential (EJP) evoked by sympathetic nerve stimulation of the submucosal arteriole in the guinea pig small intestine was not inhibited by alpha blockers [23]. The authors interpreted their results as evidence for a new class of adrenoreceptor, termed the **gamma receptor** [24], but this proposal has not met with universal acceptance [10]. Resolution of the gamma-receptor controversy and final classification of alpha-adrenoreceptor subtypes both await nonpharmacologic advances in receptor study.

Distribution and Location. The differential effectiveness of $alpha_1$ and $alpha_2$ antagonists at inhibiting nerve-stimulated pressor responses has furthered the concept that $alpha_1$ receptors are part of the synapse and that $alpha_2$ receptors lie in the extrajunctional membrane [15,25]. Thus, $alpha_1$ receptors appear to be the preferential receptors for neural responses, located at the medial-adventitial border, where noradrenergic terminals reside, whereas $alpha_2$ receptors are located mainly in proximity to the intima and as such are more susceptible to regulation by bloodborne substances [15,25]. Most vascular smooth muscle contains both $alpha_1$ and $alpha_2$ receptor subtypes; with the exception of the cerebral circulation, where $alpha_2$ is prevalent, the $alpha_1$ receptor usually predominates [15]. There appears to be no set rule a priori that predicts location of vascular smooth muscle alpha-receptor subtype, although $alpha_2$ receptors are generally more prevalent in large arteries than in small resistance vessels [10]. Bulbring and Tomita [10] and Langer and Hicks [15] have each methodically reviewed the localization and distribution of alpha-adrenoreceptor subtypes in various vascular beds of different species.

Mechanism of Action. Intracellular calcium availability is fundamental to smooth muscle contraction, and alpha-adrenoreceptors are linked to membrane channels that regulate this availability. Two calcium channels have been described: one operated by a surface receptor and independent of membrane voltage (receptor-operated channel, or ROC) and the other a voltage-sensitive channel (voltage-operated channel, or VOC) that is particularly sensitive to calcium channel blockers [26,27]. Whereas the VOC (opened by norepinephrine) is sensitive to calcium antagonists, the sensitivity of the ROC varies widely with the extent of tissue activation and the specific vessel under study [27]. Interestingly, $alpha_1$-mediated contraction is less strongly suppressed by calcium antagonists than that mediated by $alpha_2$, arguing for possible selective involvement of ROCs and VOCs [10]. To confuse matters, however, the receptor subtype responsible for membrane depolarization is both vessel- and species-specific [10,26], and the response to calcium-entry blockade may depend on the efficacy of either agonist-receptor interaction or stimulus-response coupling [28]. It follows that depolarization is not obligatory for calcium influx and that contraction can occur independently of voltage change. The latter occurrence has been termed **pharmacomechanical coupling** to distinguish it from electromechanical coupling, which describes contractions associated with membrane depolarization [29].

There are differences in the source of activator calcium generated by alpha-adrenoreceptor subtypes. $Alpha_2$ contractile responses are more dependent on extracellular calcium influx, whereas $alpha_1$ receptors mediate mobilization of intracellularly sequestered calcium in addition to augmenting permeability of the plasmalemma to calcium [10,25]. The extracellular calcium pool has been linked to the tonic (slow) component of the contractile response, and intracellular calcium has been linked to the phasic (fast) component. Consequently, $alpha_1$ receptors have been implicated in causing the phasic component of contraction, and $alpha_2$ the tonic component [10]. Alpha-adrenergic receptors also affect membrane permeability

Table 3-2. Characterization of vascular smooth muscle alpha-adrenoreceptor

	$Alpha_1$	$Alpha_2$
Anatomic location	Neuronal synapse/ medial-adventitial border	Extrajunctional/ intima
Calcium channel*	ROC > VOC	Unknown
Source of activator calcium	Intracellular + extracellular	Extracellular
Signal transduction	Phosphatidylinositol metabolism	Tonic (slow)
Contractile response	Phasic (fast)	

ROC = receptor-operated channel; VOC = voltage-operated channel.
* A limited distinction based on responses to calcium channel blockers; tissue and species variation exists [10].

of ions other than calcium. Specifically, ROCs influence permeability of sodium, potassium, and chloride [4,8,26].

$Alpha_2$ receptors differ from $alpha_1$ in their mechanism of signal transduction. $Alpha_2$ receptors are regulated by guanine nucleotides coupled to adenylate cyclase [25,30,31]. Guanosine triphosphate (GTP), sodium, and other divalent cations are important in receptor coupling to this enzyme, and they determine $alpha_2$-receptor affinity [25,31]. Activation of the receptor results in inhibition of adenylyl cyclase and a fall in cyclic adenosine monophosphate (cAMP) levels [25,30,31]. In contrast, guanine nucleotide regulatory protein (G-protein) coupling of the $alpha_1$ adrenoreceptor is still a point of interest and conjecture. There is growing evidence to support the involvement of phosphoinositides in the calcium-mediated sequence of events that follows $alpha_1$-receptor activation [10,32]. Mechanisms of signal transduction pertaining to this receptor system (in particular, the phosphoinositol pathway) are discussed in detail in the section "Signal Transduction," later in this chapter. The characteristics of vascular alpha-adrenoreceptors are summarized in Table 3-2.

Catecholamines also have important trophic effects on vascular smooth muscle cells that remain poorly delineated [33]. Cellular events regulated by alpha-adrenoreceptors that have been associated with mitogenic activity include calcium mobilization and modulation of adenylyl cyclase [10,34]. The recent observation that norepinephrine enhances the proto-oncogene, c-myc, expression provides a potential molecular mechanism for regulating DNA synthesis [35,36].

Heterogeneity. Although all blood vessels constrict on activation of membrane $alpha_1$ and $alpha_2$ receptors, the responsiveness of different vessels to agonists varies greatly. Moreover, the relative contributions of $alpha_1$ and $alpha_2$ receptors to the vasoconstrictor response differ among species, arteries, and veins; among vessels of varying size; and even between consecutive segments of the vasculature. Heterogeneous responsiveness is a complex phenomenon eloquently addressed in previous reviews [8,9], which constitute the basis for this discussion. Relevant factors include the thickness of smooth muscle in contact with the nerve varicosity, degree of penetration of nerve endings into smooth muscle, geometry of the vessel under consideration, density of alpha-adrenoreceptors, receptor subtype, inherent electrical excitability (myogenic tone), width of the synaptic cleft, and modifying influences such as bloodborne vasoactive substances and indirect control by the endothelium [8–10]. With regard to this final point, it has been demonstrated that exogenous norepinephrine induces vasodilation by an $alpha_2$-directed endothelium-dependent mechanism when $alpha_1$ and beta receptors are blocked [10]. General statements regarding sensitivities of vessels to catecholamines include the following [9]:

- At the level of the microvasculature, there is decreasing sensitivity from the precapillary sphincter to the larger arteries and muscular venules.
- Venules and small-capacity vessels are less reactive than precapillary vessels in visceral organs, but the reverse is true of the skin.
- Smaller blood vessels are less reactive than large conduit vessels.
- Cranial-vessel adrenergic receptors are less sensitive than their counterparts in systemic vessels.

BETA-ADRENERGIC AGONISTS

Receptor Classification. Beta receptors are distinguished from alpha-adrenergic receptors by an order of sympathomimetic agonist potency in which isoproterenol is greater than epinephrine, which in turn is greater than or equal to norepinephrine, and by susceptibility to blockade by propranolol [37]. The demonstration by Lands and coworkers that the receptors responsible for bronchodilation ($beta_2$) could be differentiated from those responsible for cardiac actions led to subclassification of the beta receptor into $beta_2$ and $beta_1$ subtypes, respectively [38,39]. Using a similar order-of-potency approach for sympathomimetic amines, beta-receptor subtyping has been performed on systemic vessels. Interestingly, a unifying argument has been made for a single beta receptor that assumes a different configuration depending on the activity and the metabolism of the surrounding tissue [9].

The seminal work of Frielle and colleagues has resulted in the cloning and characterization of the beta-adrenergic receptor. The $beta_1$ and $beta_2$ subtypes reveal significant sequence homology and a characteristic design feature of seven hydrophobic transmembrane domains, which contribute to the determination of subtype selectivity [40]. The construction of chimeric receptors and the development of receptor reconstitution techniques in lipid vesicles have aided greatly in the assessment of receptor functionality [40].

Distribution and Location. Like $alpha_2$ receptors, $beta_2$ receptors have been located on adrenergic nerve endings. Both $beta_1$ and $beta_2$ subtypes are present in postjunctional membranes, however; thus, a subclassification cannot be made by synaptic location [10,25]. Also like $alpha_1$ and $alpha_2$ adrenoreceptor location, $beta_1$ receptors are more likely to be present on the postjunctional membrane in close proximity to norepinephrine release from the nerve terminals, and $beta_2$ receptors are found extrajunctionally, with greater exposure and susceptibility to bloodborne substances such as epinephrine [25].

Beta-receptor presence has been demonstrated both in large arteries and veins and at the microcirculatory level in arterioles and venules of various vascular beds [4,9,10,41]. $Beta_1$ receptors predominate in coronary smooth muscle and $beta_2$ receptors in systemic vessels. The pharmacology of intracranial beta receptors resembles that of coronary vascular smooth muscle [9].

Mechanism of Action. With the possible exception of the basilar artery of the neonatal rat [42], beta receptors invariably induce relaxation of vascular smooth muscle [4,10,26]. This relaxation is achieved primarily by reducing the availability of ionized calcium for contraction. Reduction of calcium influx [43] and sequestration of intracellular calcium by the sarcoplasmic reticulum [10,26,44–46] have been promoted as predominant mechanisms in different blood vessels, with the latter mechanism more common [10,44,45]. Hyperpolarization that occurs with beta activation [10,47] is variably ascribed to increases in potassium permeability [3,10,26], activation of an electrogenic sodium pump [3], and secondary effects of cAMP [10], but the importance of hyperpolarization in mediating beta relaxation is not clear. Moreover, hyperpolarization probably is not obligatory for relaxation, because beta inhibition has been reported in association with depolarization [48]. Generally accepted concepts of beta-receptor-mediated action on smooth muscle include (1) modulation of the calcium economy of the cell without great effect on surface membrane permeability [26], (2) receptor coupling via G protein to adenylyl cyclase, and (3) regulation of intracellular actions at least partly by increasing levels of the cAMP second messenger [10,26,31]. There is, however, conflicting data on the correlation between increases in cyclic guanosine monophosphate (cGMP) induced by beta receptors and vascular smooth muscle relaxation [10].

Heterogeneity. Epinephrine is a more potent $beta_2$ agonist than norepinephrine, and the reverse holds true for $beta_1$ receptors [12]. Accordingly, epinephrine's effect predominates in systemic vessels and norepinephrine's in the coronary and cerebral circulations [9]. Both of these endogenous catecholamines are also potent alpha agonists; therefore, the ultimate contractile response of any given vascular bed depends on the relative densities of these two receptor populations. Thus, epinephrine dilates the $beta_2$-rich (systemic) precapillary vessels of skeletal muscle and constricts vessels in the skin and viscera in which alpha receptors predominate [9,37]. Similarly, the beta-adrenoreceptor action of norepinephrine predominates in cerebral and coronary vessels rich in $beta_1$ receptors while inducing vasoconstriction elsewhere. Vanhoutte has eloquently reviewed the thesis of adrenoreceptor modulation, in which the metabolic environment is thought to account for adrenoreceptor properties [9]. By this account, metabolically active tissue develops beta-receptor properties that explain the vasodilatory effects of catecholamines on vascular beds in skeletal and cardiac muscle and cutaneous vessels in hypotensive crises.

ANGIOTENSIN II

Receptor Classification. Early pharmacologic analyses of angiotensin-receptor interaction reflected the presence of more than one receptor type [49,50]. More recently, radioligand-binding studies in rat liver preparations identified two classes of angiotensin II receptors with different biochemical features and mechanisms of action [51]. Angiotensin receptors have been isolated and characterized from liver, adrenal, and uterus [52–54], but attempts to isolate the vascular smooth muscle receptor have been unsuccessful [54,55].

In the vessel wall, the binding of angiotensin II is highly specific, reversible, saturable, and of high affinity, which is characteristic of classical receptor-hormone interaction [56]. These same high-affinity sites also bind angiotensin I (57), but this peptide elicits a weaker biologic response [58,59]. The binding of angiotensin II is influenced by divalent cations and guanine nucleotides, although to a different degree in muscular resistance–type vessels (such as the rat mesenteric artery [58]) than in fibroelastic conduit vessels [56]. These modulating factors probably influence the coupling of the receptor with an inhibitory G protein similar to that described for $alpha_2$ adrenoreceptors. In both receptor systems, the regulatory protein regulates inhibition of adenylyl cyclase [31,58].

Distribution and Location. In a series of eloquent experiments, Schultz and co-workers demonstrated contraction of aortic smooth muscle to a membrane-impermeable analogue of angiotensin II, thus suggesting that the receptors are located on the plasma membrane [60]. Vasoconstriction to angiotensin II has been confirmed in many venous and arterial beds, with the implication that the receptors are present on most vascular smooth muscle [4,9,58]. Notably, vascular angiotensin receptors remain difficult to analyze directly, and a detailed description of their distribution and spatial localization is not available.

Mechanism and Action. Angiotensin II is one of the most potent endogenous pressor substances characterized to date. On a molar basis, it is approximately 40 times more potent than norepinephrine [58]. Central to its direct vasoconstrictor action on smooth muscle is its capacity to increase intracellular ionized calcium levels. Angiotensin II also indirectly influences smooth muscle tone via the facilitation of sympathetic neurotransmission [26,58].

The contractile action of angiotensin II is independent of its membrane-depolarizing effect [58]. Angiotensin II mobilizes calcium by increasing calcium influx from the extracellular compartment and by releasing calcium sequestered intracellularly [58,61]. The former event may occur via voltage-sensitive calcium channels and the latter in association with phosphoinositide turnover [58,61]. Sequestered calcium is responsible for the rapid change in calcium concentration that correlates with an initial fast (phasic) contractile response to the hormone [61]. Slower (tonic) contraction depends on extracellular calcium [61]. Accordingly, the relationship between calcium mobilization and the contractile response has similarities to that mediated by alpha adrenoreceptors. Calcium-dependent efflux is also regulated by angiotensin binding [58] and may play a role in the vasodilatory response to the hormone observed in some smooth muscle. Eicosanoid production stimulated by angiotensin II may also play a role in angiotensin II–mediated vasodilation [58,61].

The sodium/hydrogen antiporter system is but one of several means by which sodium transport is regulated through angiotensin II–receptor interaction. A sodium/calcium antiporter, a sodium-potassium-chloride transporter, and a sodium-ion channel also have been described [4,26,58]. Sodium and other divalent cations influence angiotensin II binding and thereby modulate hormone-receptor signaling [59]. Experiments addressing angiotensin II–induced changes in membrane permeability in greater detail have been summarized by Bolton [26].

Angiotensin II has been reported to enhance proliferation and hypertrophy of vascular smooth muscle [62–64]. The activation of the sodium/hydrogen antiport and calcium mobilization are two mitogenic signals regulated by angiotensin II [34]. Alkalinization of the cell microenvironment, possibly by the sodium/hydrogen antiport system, has been associated with induction of expression of the proto-oncogenes c-fos and c-myc and cell growth [34]. Moreover, angiotensin II can stimulate expression of both proto-oncogenes and the platelet-derived growth factor (PDGF) A chain [34,35].

Heterogeneity. The regional sensitivities and blood flow responses to angiotensin II vary greatly. The vascular beds of the gut, liver, kidney, and skin are particularly sensitive to the hormone, whereas the pulmonary and skeletal muscle vasculature are relatively resistant [4,58]. The uterine blood flow response to angiotensin II is variable, and in coronary vessels vasodilation has been reported [58]. Vanhoutte has offered the following observations [9]:

1. The effect of angiotensin II on the venous circulation pales in comparison to its effect on small resistance vessels.
2. Exceptions to the first statement exist: the rat vein is exquisitely sensitive to the octapeptide, and its arteriolar constrictor action also varies among vascular beds.

Explaining this heterogeneous responsiveness is a more difficult matter. In vivo, the precapillary vasoconstrictor effect of the hormone may regulate its access to the venous circulation. In addition, since vascular smooth muscle contains enzyme systems that convert renin substrate and angiotensin I to angiotensin II [9], both modulation of microcirculatory flow and local enzyme activity may influence responsiveness. The further contribution to the variability in vascular responsiveness made by biologically active peptide fragments, generated from angiotensins by other intracellular peptidases [58], is not known. The observation that metabolic conditions modify the constrictor effect of angiotensin II [9] is in keeping with the influence of pH [56], temperature [56], and redox state [65] on receptor responsiveness and likely also contributes to the thesis of heterogeneity. Underlying intrinsic myogenic activity, the availability of calcium, and the above data supporting the notion that the angiotensin receptor does not comprise a homogeneous population of molecules or that it exists in different conformational states are other factors that may contribute to differences in angiotensin sensitivity [45].

Finally, some smooth muscle becomes tachyphylactic to angiotensin II. This phenomenon is related to the relative dependence of smooth muscle on extracellular calcium for contraction and possibly to its ability to convert angiotensin II to angiotensin III [58,66]. In rabbit aorta, resistance to tachyphylaxis relates to a pressor response that is mediated by the intracellular calcium pool and high aminopeptidase activity capable of converting angiotensin II to angiotensin III [66].

MUSCARINIC RECEPTORS

Receptor Classification. Acetylcholine receptors of the muscarinic type are distinguished from the nicotinic variety by the antagonism of atropine [67], but the small variations in affinity constants for equilibrium binding of this and other classic muscarinic antagonists hindered initial attempts to subclassify these receptors further. The relatively recent discovery of heterogeneity of binding to the muscarinic antagonist piperazine has led to the now widely used classification of muscarinic receptors by their affinity for this antagonist. Receptors with high affinity are designated M_1 and those with low affinity, M_2 [68,69]. The use of the subscripts 1 and 2 is in keeping with a previous designation [70] of ganglionic receptors (M_1) and effector smooth muscle receptors (M_2) that were subsequently distinguished by their high and low affinities for piperazine, respectively [69]. The demonstration that the cDNA of cloned pig-brain M_1 receptor failed to hybridize with poly (A)+ RNA from tissue rich in M_2 receptors represents strong confirmatory evidence that M_1 and M_2 are different receptors [71]. Five distinct molecular forms of the muscarinic receptor have thus far been identified [72]. The muscarinic receptors belong to the family of seven-helix receptors (see the section "Beta-Adrenergic Agonists," earlier in this chapter), in which seven transmembrane hydrophobic domains contribute to subtype selectivity [72].

Several investigators have proposed other classification schemes for muscarinic receptors. The original data of Hammer and colleagues revealed an intermediate-affinity binding site for piperazine in addition to sites with high and low affinities [68]. A number of investigators have since proposed receptor subclassifications according to three or more sites [67]. Goyal proposes parallel nomenclatures for muscarinic receptors based on pharmacologic characteristics and molecular forms [72]. Mitchelson concludes that the "original suggestion of two subtypes is no longer satisfactory," and, based on evidence from functional studies, he proposes at least five different tissue-dependent receptor subtypes [67]. Ultimately, molecular receptor cloning promises to clarify receptor classification data, mostly based on differences in affinity for receptor antagonists with relatively limited specificity.

Distribution and Location. Postjunctional muscarinic receptors are present in both arteries and veins, but their exact location in vascular tissues is still in doubt [67]. Nonetheless, studies of autoradiographic and radioligand binding have demonstrated receptor presence on vascular myocytes [73–75]. By inference from vasodilatory responses in intact animals and in humans, vascular muscarinic receptors exist in intracranial, mesenteric, skeletal-muscle, renal, cardiac, and pulmonary vascular beds [9,76–79] and at the microcirculatory level in arterioles and venules [9]. Although the vasodilatory response to acetylcholine is mediated by the endothelium, in its absence vessels still respond to acetylcholine, albeit with constriction. This implies coexistence of smooth muscle and endothelial muscarinic receptors in blood vessels [78,80].

The distribution of M_1 and M_2 receptors in the vasculature is not known. In many of the receptor classification schemes, the M_2 designation for smooth muscle in general is not well substantiated for vascular smooth muscle in particular [67]. In support of this designation, however, the binding of piperazine in the rabbit ear artery both before and after removal of endothelium exhibited the low affinity characteristic of M_2 receptors [81]. Similarly, Furchgott and Cherry found that the receptor responsible for relaxation of rabbit aorta demonstrated affinity values that resembled the de-endothelialized smooth muscle [82]. These data support the notion that M_2 receptors are present on vascular smooth muscle and that the vascular endothelium receptor should receive a similar designation. Recently, Vanhoutte discovered postjunctional M_1 receptors in canine saphenous vein, representing the first demonstration of this subtype in vascular smooth muscle [83]. The implications are clear: First, M_1 receptors may exist elsewhere on vascular smooth muscle, and, second, given that M_2 receptors have been described in other canine vessels [67], smooth muscle receptor populations are not necessarily homogeneously distributed in individual species.

Mechanism and Action. The discrepancy between cholinergic vasodilatory responses in vivo and vasoconstrictor responses in isolated smooth muscle strips has baffled established investigators for over a quarter of a century [1,4,9,26]. The serendipitous discovery of the obligatory role of endothelium in mediating vasodilation to acetylcholine [80] has brought clarity to the fields of muscarinic vascular-receptor physiology and pharmacology where little previously existed. With the endothelium removed, muscarinic smooth muscle receptors induce vasoconstriction in virtually all large and small arteries and veins in a manner that extends across species lines [9,26,67,80,84]. Even in the presence of endothelium, high concentrations of acetylcholine can overcome the inhibitory effect of endothelium-derived relaxing factor(s) (EDRFs) and constrict the underlying smooth muscle [77,84]. This observation explains the biphasic cholinergic response often reported in the literature [4,26,67,77,84]. Rare exceptions to this dictum exist. In rabbit intrapulmonary artery, contraction by acetylcholine is endothelium dependent [85], and in canine splenic vein, acetylcholine has a direct vasodilatory effect on smooth muscle [86].

The cellular mechanisms responsible for constrictor cholinergic responses in vascular smooth muscle are not well established, and mechanisms proffered here have frequently been deduced from experiments in other cell lines. Contraction of smooth muscle by acetylcholine is usually associated with membrane depolarization [26], but rabbit mesenteric artery contracts while hyperpolarizing, which suggests that depolarization is not obligatory for calcium mobilization [87]. Both phasic and tonic contractile responses to acetylcholine, dependent on intracellular and extracellular calcium mobilization, respectively, are regulated by muscarinic receptors [88]. Concomitant cell-permeability changes to ions other than calcium in response to receptor occupation are also well described [26,67]. In several isolated cell lines, muscarinic agonists reduce cAMP levels and stimulate cGMP production [67]. Muscarinic receptors with low affinity for piperazine potently inhibit adenylyl cyclase, as in the alpha$_2$ adrenergic receptor system [67]. The direct stimulation of acetylcholine on cGMP production is a more variable and less potent effect that may play an inhibitory feedback role during contraction [67], as suggested by the vasodilatory properties of cGMP [89]. Alterations in cyclic nucleotides cannot explain the muscarinic receptor–coupled effect on calcium-ion mobilization. Thus, in part by default, current evidence overwhelmingly supports the role of phosphatidylinositol turnover in calcium-mobilization mechanisms, possibly via coupling of muscarinic receptors to G protein [67] (see the section "Signal Transduction," later in this chapter, for detailed discussion). Confirmation is needed for much of these data in vascular smooth muscle.

Heterogeneity. Much of the observed heterogeneity in vascular response to acetylcholine has now been accounted for: "Paradoxical" vasodilatory responses are explained by the observations of two series of investigators [85,90]. Vanhoutte first revealed that adrenergic neurotransmission in vascular smooth muscle was inhibited by acetylcholine and that this inhibitory effect was mediated by muscarinic (M_2) [83] receptors located on postganglionic sympathetic nerve terminals [90,91]. Prejunctional muscarinic modulation of adrenergic neurotransmission is probably most important in small resistance arteries and in veins where nerve terminals penetrate beyond the adventitia-media junction. This finding has been overshadowed by the work of Furchgott and Zawadzki, however, which describes the obligatory role of endothelium in mediating cholinergic vasodilation [80]. Consequently, much of the duality described in the literature and the heterogeneity in vascular responsiveness to acetylcholine can be explained by these observations. Metabolic factors, disease states affecting endothelial function, and innate differences between veins and arteries, all of which affect release of EDRF, influence the ultimate response of the vessel to acetylcholine [77–79,92].

Additional factors that potentially influence the smooth muscle response to acetylcholine include the concentration to which the vessel has access [91] and the receptor subtype [67]. In bovine cerebral arteries, high- and low-affinity receptor sites mediate contraction and relaxation, respectively [93]. However, the physiologic importance of receptor subclassification remains poorly appreciated [67].

SEROTONINERGIC RECEPTORS

Receptor Classification. With the advent of specific 5-hydroxytryptamine (5HT) receptor antagonists, the original D (dibenzyline-sensitive) and M (morphine-sensitive) classification of Gaddum and Picarelli [94] has been superseded by $5HT_1$ and $5HT_2$ nomenclature [95–99]. However, neither classification scheme encompasses all categories of the 5HT receptor. Moreover, in the absence of an established link between $5HT_1$ binding sites and a pharmacologic effect, these sites cannot be categorized with certainty as receptors [95].

$5HT_2$ receptor sites exhibit many pharmacologic similarities to D receptors (those blocked by methysergide and ketanserin), and in a critical review Humphrey concluded that in the vasculature they are probably one and the same [95]. A second receptor mediating neuronal depolarization is selectively blocked by cocaine and demonstrates similarities to the original M receptor but probably is not identical to it [95]. The prejunctional 5HT receptor responsible for inhibition of noradrenergic neurotransmission represents another receptor population that may be equated with the $5HT_1$ receptor by its affinity for agonists [95–97]. Also, 5HT receptors mediating smooth muscle relaxation (by an endothelium-dependent mechanism) have distinct characteristics, although they have not received an official designation [95]; Vanhoutte suggests that they may be $5HT_1$ receptors [96, discussion]. Clearly, at the present time, based on binding data alone, 5HT receptors have not been fully characterized.

Distribution and Location. $5HT_2$ receptors predominate on smooth muscle of arteries and veins of large conduits and smaller vessels. The receptor mediates vasoconstriction directly on interaction with agonist [4,95–100], and this response extends uniformly across species lines [4,9,95–99]. The pharmacology of canine basilar artery and saphenous vein is more consistent with the presence and involvement of $5HT_1$ receptors [97]. Although this remains a point of fair controversy [91,97], it indicates that $5HT_1$ receptors may have functional relevance elsewhere in the vasculature.

Mechanism of Action. The effect of serotonin in intact animals represents an integrated response of its excitatory and inhibitory actions. The direct contractile action of serotonin in isolated smooth muscle is masked in vivo by an endothelium-dependent mechanism mediating vasodilation [101,102]. Additional sympathetic inhibitory responses are modulated by prejunctional serotonin receptors that may be equated with $5HT_1$ binding sites [95,96,103]. In contrast, heterogeneous serotonin receptor populations that stimulate noradrenalin release have been located on sympathetic neurons in both pre- and postganglionic locations [103]. Furthermore, a nonspecific facilitative effect of serotonin on contraction induced by other vasoactive substances bespeaks a nonreceptor-mediated interaction by which serotonin can influence vascular response [4,9,94,96,104]. This amplifying effect of serotonin is also true of its mitogenic action, and it has been attributed to growth stimuli induced by inositol lipid derivatives [105,106].

Under experimental conditions, denervated, de-endothelialized vascular smooth muscle contracts on exposure to serotonin with accompanying depolarization; serotonin exerts much of its influence on membrane potential by affecting the permeabilities for potassium and chloride [107]. The mechanisms responsible for these electrophysiologic effects have not been established but are thought to be effected primarily through changes in passive ion permeability [107]. Depending on the vessel, the contraction may be sustained or transient, monophasic or biphasic. In bovine coronary arteries phasic and tonic contractions are primarily associated with release of intracellularly bound calcium, presumably induced by phosphoinositide turnover [32,105]. A time-dependent decline in calcium release accounts for the transient response observed [108]. In rabbit thoracic aorta, the dependence on extracellular calcium is far greater and the response more sustained [108]. These experiments allude to a relationship between the nature of the contractile response induced by serotonin, the source of activator calcium, and the kinetics of the calcium transient.

Heterogeneity. Many of the alleged discrepancies and observed differences in vascular sensitivity to serotonin can be explained by its differing actions, mediated directly via heterogeneous receptor populations and indirectly by the endothelium and autonomic neurotransmission [95–97,99,104,109]. Metabolic conditions and physiologic factors also influence vascular sensitivity to serotonin [9,26]. Hypothermia sensitizes the microcirculation and cutaneous vessels, and pressure profoundly increases vascular responsiveness. Under these conditions, serotonin's regulatory role in vivo may be particularly important. Although innate variation exists in smooth muscle of different species and among various vascular beds, two consistent patterns emerge. First, intracranial vascular smooth muscle is invariably more sensitive than extracranial [97]. Second, at the microcirculatory level, the direct constrictor effect on venules predominates over the effect on arterioles [9].

HISTAMINERGIC RECEPTORS

Receptor Classification. Two distinct classes of histamine receptors (H_1 and H_2) have been defined in receptor-binding studies with agonists and antagonists [110,111]. An H_3 receptor subtype has been proposed but has not yet been identified in the vasculature [110,111]. Interestingly, temperature interconversion of H_1 and H_2 receptors is proposed as a means of unifying the scheme for histamine-receptor classification [110]. The characterization of histamine receptors in vascular smooth muscle has been problematic, and certain experimental inconsistencies suggest that vascular receptors may be different from their nonvascular counterparts [110].

Distribution and Location. H_1 and H_2 receptors have been identified in the arterial and venous circulations [4,9,111], but the two receptors have different spatial distributions in blood vessels. H_1 receptors are located preferentially along the inner layers of the vessel wall [112,113] and on the vascular endothelium of systemic vessels [110,111,114,115]. In contrast, H_2 receptors are preferentially located within the outer smooth muscle layers [112,113], with the exception of cerebral vessels, where they are also present on the inner vessel wall and the endothelium but are absent from veins [112]. There are many species differences and notable regional differences in response to histamine, suggesting that the receptor subpopulations are not uniformly distributed among and within species [4,9,110,112,116,117].

Mechanism of Action. In most isolated vessels, histamine induces contraction of smooth muscle that is blocked by H_1 receptor antagonists [110,118]. However, in vivo the predominant effect is vasodilation. Intra-arterial infusions of histamine have a vasodepressor effect that is mediated by both H_1 and H_2 receptors [111,117]. At low concentrations, H_1 antagonists prevent vasodilation, but at higher concentrations the sustained depressor response cannot be prevented without added H_2 receptor antagonism [110,111,117]. One can conclude that H_1 receptors generally mediate vasoconstriction, and both H_1 and H_2 receptors play important roles in histamine-induced vasodilation. Pulmonary blood vessels of many species represent an exception in that vasodilation is the consequence of H_2 receptor activation alone [111,117].

Contraction and relaxation by H_1 receptors are associated with depolarization and hyperpolarization of vascular smooth muscle, respectively, but membrane voltage changes are not obligatory for a response [26]. During contraction, membrane permeability to sodium and calcium increase and potassium efflux is facilitated [110]. Phosphatidylinositol turnover is associated with calcium influx [110,119].

The characteristics of the multiple affinity states of H_1 agonist-receptor interaction are consistent with the notion of receptor regulation by guanine nucleotides [118]. Activation of H_1 receptors with contraction of bovine arteries causes at first decreased and then increased levels of cAMP [26]. These data, therefore, support G-protein coupling of the H_1 receptor to adenylyl cyclase (see the section "Signal Transduction," later in this chapter, for detailed discussion of G-protein regulation); additional experiments are required to clarify these assumptions. H_1 histaminergic receptors also mediate cGMP elevations via release of an EDRF [110]. Elevations of cGMP observed during vessel contraction may represent a direct effect of the receptor on smooth muscle designed for regulatory feedback purposes [110]; alternatively, it may be the consequence of cAMP elevations induced by either H_1 [26] or H_2 receptors [116]. In the case of H_2 receptors, the cGMP pathway appears to be the most plausible second-messenger system accountable for receptor action [111,116,119].

Heterogeneity. Despite the general vasodilatory properties of histamine in vivo, the sensitivities of blood vessels to this agent are far from uniform. At the microcirculatory level, it dilates arterioles more than precapillary sphincters [9,112]. In the brain, capacitance vessels do not respond to histamine [112], but veins are sensitive to it elsewhere [110,117]. In systemic vessels, vasodilation does not occur equally or uniformly in regional beds; this is well exemplified in cats, where vasodilation is reported in heart, stomach, kidney, and mesentery, and vasoconstriction in liver, spleen, and skin [117]. In pulmonary vessels, a constrictor response is almost uniformly observed [110]. Multiple factors contribute to this heterogeneity. The density, location, and type of receptor vary among organs [110–112,117]. Differential spatial organization of receptors may also affect responsiveness. Consequently, receptors on endothelium and in luminal proximity are most affected by blood histamine, and those on the abluminal surface by mast cell and perivascular histamine. The modulatory effect of the endothelium varies with endothelial integrity. In addition, sympathetic tone can affect histamine responses, which in turn can feed back to inhibit sympathetic neurotransmission by an H_2-mediated process [9]. The histaminergic regulation of sympathetic neurotransmission is complex, occurring at ganglionic and postganglionic nerve terminals [120]; H_1 receptors are facilitatory, and H_2 receptors are inhibitory [111,120]. Finally, it is important to note that the response to endogenous histamine may be quite different from the response to exogenous histamine under experimental conditions. Interestingly, one month of oral cimetidine did not affect blood pressure in humans under resting conditions or during exercise [121]. From this discussion, it might have been assumed otherwise.

BRADYKININ AND OTHER RELATED KININS

Receptor Classification. Of the naturally occurring kinins, bradykinin is the most illustrious, though not the most potent kinin receptor agonist [122]. Its receptors are classified as B_1 and B_2. The B_2 designation is used to define the receptor population that is different from B_1 and may include any number of as yet uncharacterized receptor subtypes. Thus, specific competitive B_2 antagonists are not available [122]. Designations of S (for *swelling*) and P (for *pain*) also have been proposed, but this distinction is not based on strict pharmacologic criteria [123].

Distribution and Location. The current state of knowledge does not permit a full, detailed description of the spatial location and distribution of kinin receptors. Moreover, a peculiar feature of B_1 receptors is their relative scarcity under normal conditions and their generation under noxious circumstances [122], suggesting that they have a role in pathologic conditions of vascular smooth muscle. Bradykinin receptors of either type can exist on smooth muscle of arteries and veins, and in some vessels both subtypes are present [122]; the distribution is species specific. The demonstrations by Couture and colleagues [124] that B_2 receptors mediate canine relaxations and by Cherry and colleagues that canine relaxations are endothelium dependent suggest that B_2 receptors exist on endothelium [125,126]. The role of endothelium in bradykinin responses of vascular smooth muscle have been summarized by Furchgott [127].

Mechanism of Action. Kinins are implicated in vasodilatory and vasoconstrictor responses that vary with the species and the organ under investigation. In veins, both B_1 and B_2 receptors cause vasoconstriction [128]. In arteries, B_1 receptors are generally associated with pressor responses, and B_2 receptors with vasodilation that is most likely endothelium dependent [122,127,128]. Under noxious circumstances (where endothelial integrity may be compromised) and in species without an endothelium-dependent vasodilatory mechanism, such as the rabbit, B_1 constrictor responses often predominate [110]. In most mammals, infusions of bradykinin are associated with dose-dependent hypotension, and in humans, specifically, bradykinin is inhibitory in all arteries studied to date, with the exception of the umbilical artery [122,128].

Kinins' actions are mediated through the activation of surface receptors and membrane enzymes [122]. The activation of membrane phospholipase A_2 results in arachidonate release and its conversion to prostaglandins, which have been implicated in vasodilatory and vasoconstrictor responses [122,123]; vasodilation occurs in association with activation of adenylyl cyclase [122,129]. In umbilical arteries, bradykinin was reported to stimulate cGMP production [130,131], but whether or not this effect is endothelium dependent is not known.

Heterogeneity. We have alluded to the various hemodynamic effects of bradykinin that are species-specific and dependent on the organ bed under investigation. Vascular sensitivity also depends on the dose of kinin and the duration of exposure [122,128]. Tachyphylaxis to B_2 responses occurs, but B_1 responses are facilitated with increasing exposure to bradykinin [128]. Factors potentially responsible for or contributing to heterogeneous responsiveness include the possibility of different B_2 receptor populations, a variable and as yet uncharacterized receptor distribution, a highly active heterogeneous kinin degradation mechanism, an intracellular protease system that can generate biologically active kinin metabolites, differing pharmacologic features of the three naturally occurring kinins, and the multiple variable influences of prostaglandins generated through kinin-receptor interaction [122,128,129].

PURINERGIC RECEPTORS

Receptor Classification. Purinoreceptors have been subdivided into P_1 and P_2 by Burnstock [131]. P_1 receptors are defined by agonist potency (adenosine > AMP > adenosine diphosphate [ADP] > adenosine triphosphate [ATP]), by their antagonism by methylxanthines, and by their capacity to induce changes in intracellular cAMP levels. P_2 purinoreceptors have an order-of-agonist potency as follows: ATP greater than ADP greater than AMP greater than adenosine. P_2 purinoreceptors are not inhibited by methylxanthines, and they do not modulate cAMP levels. The P_1 purinoreceptor has been subsequently divided into A_1 and A_2 subpopulations [132] (Ri/Ra classification of Londos et al. [133]), by pharmacologic order-of-agonist potency, and by biochemical effect on adenylyl cyclase. The A_1 receptor is regulated by GTP, and its activation is associated with inhibition of adenylyl cyclase. In contrast, A_2 activation results in increased activity of adenylyl cyclase and elevated cAMP levels. A basis for distinguishing two types of P_2 receptor by rank order-of-agonist potency of structural analogues of ATP and by the activity of P_2 receptor antagonism likewise has been proposed [134]. Subtypes 1 and 2 are designated P_{2x} and P_{2y}, respectively. In addition, an intracellular P site responsive to adenosine binding has been identified that is insensitive to methylxanthines [135].

Location and Distribution. From binding experiments, putative adenosine receptors on the surface of cultured aortic smooth muscle are distinguished from intracellular methylxanthine-insensitive P sites for adenosine [135–137]. The data accumulated to date suggest that the direct postjunctional (inhibitory) effects of adenosine on vascular smooth muscle are mediated by A_2 purinoreceptors [137–139]; these receptors also have been localized to endothelium [138]. Prejunctional modulation of noradrenergic neurotransmission can be affected by both P_1 purinoreceptors [139]. P_2 receptor subtypes have been identified in various vessels [134,140]. In most cases, ATP causes endothelium-dependent vasodilation via the P_{2y} purinoreceptor, but vasodilation also is induced by these purinoreceptors located on smooth muscle [140–143]. P_{2x} receptors are responsible for the excitatory responses demonstrated in rat femoral artery, rabbit central ear artery, and rat isolated perfused pancreas vascular bed [134].

Mechanism of Action. With the notable exceptions of the intact kidney vascular bed and the portal vein [3,9], adenosine is a vasodilator. This has been demonstrated in isolated strips of basilar, coronary, mesenteric, and renal arteries and portal and mesenteric veins [9]. Adenosine increases cerebral blood flow in rabbits and dilates splanchnic and skeletal muscle beds [138]. In humans, systemic administration of adenosine causes a rapid fall in blood pressure [138]. This vasodilatory effect is exerted by activation of A_2 cell-surface receptors and may also be mediated via adenosine's interactions with an intracellular site [137]. A_2 purinoreceptors stimulate adenylyl cyclase in the facilitatory presence of guanine nucleotides, suggesting that guanine-binding proteins couple the receptor to the enzyme [144]. An excellent correlation between relaxation and accumulation of cAMP strongly suggests a causal relationship [138], but this mechanism recently has been called into question [137]. Inhibition of cAMP phosphodiesterase by *S*-adenosylhomocysteine and *S*-adenosylmethionine, formed due to adenosine's interference with their hydrolysis, might contribute to the accumulation of cAMP [137].

The regulation of cAMP by adenosine plays an intriguing role in cell proliferation. Elevations in this cyclic nucleotide have been associated with inhibition of DNA synthesis and the lowering of its levels, with a mitogenic effect [145]. Consequently, A_1 and A_2 cell-surface receptors on smooth muscle may mediate bidirectional changes in cAMP and thereby modulate cell proliferation [145].

The excitatory action of purines on vascular smooth muscle is most pronounced for ATP and ADP, but dual effects of these adenosine nucleotides are well documented [4]. Vasoconstriction by ADP has been described in various isolated arteries and veins and in the pulmonary circulation. This is probably caused by an influx of calcium signaled by activation of P_{2x} purinoreceptors, indicating their strong dependence on the availability of extracellular calcium. The importance of cell depolarization in this mechanism remains to be elucidated fully. The inhibitory component of ATP and ADP has been attributed to the P_{2y} purinoreceptor subtype [134]; this mechanism is often, but not exclusively, endothelium dependent [140–143]. Vasodilation is demonstrated in isolated vessels, and hypotension results from the intravenous administration of ATP [138]. The endothelium-dependent aspect has been attributed both to release of an EDRF and to prostacyclin production [140,142].

Recent advances also have been made in the transduction mechanisms of vascular P_2 purinoreceptors. P_2-mediated phosphoinositide hydrolysis occurs in rat aortic smooth muscle, and receptor coupling to a GTP-binding protein is suggested [146]. In other very recent work, a receptor-operated calcium current evoked by ATP revealed an order-of-agonist efficacy characteristic of P_2 receptors [147]. This channel is selective for calcium, resistant to nifedipine, provides an excitable smooth muscle current that is independent of other second messengers, and, by depolarizing the cell, promotes activator calcium entry via voltage-dependent channels [147]. It is not known whether ATP-induced ion channels and inositolphosphate accumulations relate to P_{2x} or P_{2y} purinoreceptor activation.

Heterogeneity. Adenine nucleotides exert effects on vascular smooth muscle that depend on tissue concentrations of ATP, adenosine, and other purine intermediates. Consequently, in metabolically active tissue and under ischemic conditions, changes in the energy state lead to a marked increase in adenosine formation [138]. Adenosine has been implicated in cerebral hyperemia of hypoxic brain and in exercise hyperemia of skeletal muscle [9]. Paradoxically, high concentrations of adenosine have excitatory effects on portal veins [9]. Sensitivity to adenine nucleotides also depends on vascular tone, and ATP relaxes contracted rabbit aorta and contracts atonic strips (9). In rabbit pulmonary circulation, the vasoconstricting effect of ATP is reversed in the preconstricted bed. Likewise, the inhibitory effects of adenosine are influenced by smooth muscle tone and are most evident in well-contracted vessels [9]. The actions of purines on smooth muscle may be enhanced or moderated by prostaglandin-mediated effects on platelet aggregation and adrenergic neurotransmission [9,138,141]. In the latter instance, high concentrations of adenosine release norepinephrine from cutaneous veins, and an inhibitory prejunctional effect on neurotransmission is well documented [9,139]. Although a case for intrinsic heterogeneity of smooth muscle responsiveness has not been made, the kidney vascular smooth muscle may represent an exception [9,138]. Alternatively, the variable response of the renal vasculature might be a consequence of released prostaglandins or the potentiating effects of adenosine on renin-related actions [9,138].

DOPAMINERGIC RECEPTORS

Receptor Classification. In light of the importance of dopamine in diseases of the central nervous system, its receptors have been best characterized in the brain. The Kebabian and Calne classification distinguishes D_1 receptors, which are linked to adenylate cyclase, from D_2 receptors, which are not [148]. An extrapolation from the central nervous system to the less well investigated peripheral vasculature may represent an oversimplification, but, for lack of a better classification, it is proffered here. Vascular smooth muscle and endothelium are endowed with D_1 receptors, and D_2 receptors are present in prejunctional locations in the periphery [149,150]. It is significant that alpha [151], beta$_2$ [152], and serotonin [153] receptors also bind dopamine and therefore represent potential sites for dopamine action on peripheral blood vessels.

Location and Distribution. Dopamine receptors have been identified in renal, mesenteric, coronary, cerebral, and splenic vascular beds of different species [9,149,154]. The existence of a dopamine receptor in canine femoral smooth muscle is controversial [154]. In young rat aorta, dopamine induces vasodilation, suggesting the presence of its receptor [154]. Postjunctional D_1 receptors are presented on smooth muscle and endothelium [149], and receptor density may be greater in small resistance vessels than in large arteries [154].

Mechanisms of Action. Dopamine receptors mediate vasodilation. A dilator response has been documented in isolated arteries (renal, mesenteric, cerebral, splenic, and aortic) [9,154,155] and following infusions into those vascular beds [154]. The mechanism underlying vasorelaxation is thought to be an elevation of cAMP [156], possibly contributed to by endothelium. cAMP rises preceding dopamine-mediated relaxation of rabbit splenic arteries, and it induces a dose-dependent relaxation of pial arteries in accordance with a cause-effect relationship [155].

Contraction of large arteries, veins, venules, and capillaries is attributed mostly to dopamine's interaction with adrenergic and serotoninergic receptors [9,151]. A direct constrictor action has also been suggested [151].

Heterogeneity. The response to dopamine most clearly depends on the presence and the density of specific postjunctional dopaminergic receptors (D_1). Accordingly, the particular sensitivity of small arteries is suggestive of high receptor density. In more sparsely populated regions and in the absence of its receptor, dopamine acts on other postjunctional receptors (serotonin, beta$_2$, and alpha-adrenergic) and on ganglionic and prejunctional alpha and D_2 receptors that inhibit adrenergic neurotransmission [9,149–151]. The distribution of dopaminergic neurons and local concentrations of circulating free dopamine and its sulfate conjugate are additional plausible contributors to the variable physiologic response [157].

OTHER PEPTIDE RECEPTOR SYSTEMS

Advances in immunocytochemistry, histochemistry, and ultrastructural techniques have furthered our understanding of cardiovascular innervation and resulted in the identification of several important regulatory peptides. These diverse systems are summarized in relatively recent reviews [158–160].

Neuropeptide Y. Neuropeptide Y (NPY) binding sites have been reported in vascular smooth muscle of rabbit and guinea pig kidney [161]. Moreover, NPY immunoreactivity is the most abundant of all the peptides in the mammalian vasculature. It is distributed throughout the cardiovascular system, which reflects its coexistence with norepinephrine in sympathetic terminals [158,159]; NPY is probably also located in nonadrenergic neurons [159]. Not all adrenergic nerves contain NPY, and in those that do, differential release may be effected from distinct subcellular neuronal locations [158]. NPY exerts a calcium-dependent vasoconstrictor response that has been demonstrated in coronary, cerebral, submandibular, mesenteric, and renal arteries and veins from a number of species, including humans [158,159]. In addition to its direct postjunctional effect, NPY potentiates the effect of norepinephrine and exerts a prejunctional inhibitory action on neurotransmission [158,159].

Calcitonin Gene-Related Peptide. Calcitonin gene-related peptide (CGRP) binding sites have been demonstrated on cerebral, coronary, and peripheral blood vessels in a number of species, including humans [158]. The sites are located in the intima and media of arteries [162], which supports claims for both endothelium-dependent and -independent vasodilatory actions of CGRP, the latter mediated by adenylate cyclase [158]. As a contributing mechanism to vasodilation, CGRP induces release of prostaglandin and substance P; substance P coexists with CGRP in neuronal stores [158].

Tachykinins. Tachykinins are a family of at least three biologically active peptides that possess a common C-terminal amino acid sequence [158]. Substance P, NKA, and NKB have preferential affinities for their own receptors, designated NK1, NK2, and NK3, respectively [158]. The distribution of tachykinin receptors is species specific [158,163]. Unlike substance P, which causes vasodilation by an endothelium-dependent mechanism [127], NKA and NKB directly contract vascular smooth muscle [163].

Vasoactive Intestinal Polypeptide. Specific receptor sites for vasoactive intestinal polypeptide (VIP) have been identified in the media of mammalian vessels from several species; they mediate vasodilation of cerebral, pulmonary, coronary, and other peripheral vessels by stimulating adenylate cyclase [158]. VIP is presumed to reside in postganglionic parasympathetic neurons with another closely related human peptide termed PHM (peptide with N-terminal histamine and C-terminal methionine) [164], but the relative importance of these substances in the physiologic response is unknown.

Opioid Peptides. The subclassification of opiate receptors is based on the various actions of opioids in the chronic spinal injury model in the dog (mu, kappa, and sigma), rodent vas deferens (delta), and guinea pig ileum (epsilon) [165–169]. This subclassification is tentative, even in the central nervous system, and a more reliable estimation of the location, distribution, and physiologic role in the vasculature is required. The endogenous opiate peptides (leucine-enkephalin, methionine-enkephalin, and beta endorphin) coexist in vagal and sympathetic fibers, and enkephalin has been documented immunohistochemically in the perivasculature [159]. In isolated and perfused organ beds, opiate receptors mediate vasodilation by presynaptic delta and kappa attenuation of norepinephrine release [159,169,170] and possibly by a direct postsynaptic effect [159,169]. These actions are to be distinguished from a centrally mediated excitatory mechanism that is common to other neuropeptides, including bradykinin, substance P, and CGRP [159]. Because vasodilator peptides are typically endothelium dependent, acting via a cGMP messenger, this mechanism needs to be excluded in peripheral vessels [127]. In this regard, a rise in opiate-receptor-mediated calcium-dependent cGMP has been observed in vascular smooth muscle [171–173]. The hyperpolarizing effect of opiates seen in the myenteric plexus is another potential mechanism for the postsynaptic reversal of depolarization observed in blood vessels [170]. The importance of opiate peptides may be in the fine regulation of vascular perfusion, particularly by modulation of autonomic neurotransmission.

Atrial Natriuretic Peptide. High-affinity receptors have been demonstrated by both biochemical and autoradiographic techniques in peripheral vascular smooth muscle [174,175]. The correlation of atrial natriuretic peptide (ANP) binding with the accumulation of intracellular cGMP demonstrates that many tissues, including vascular smooth muscle and endothelium, possess two types of receptor populations [90]. The receptor designated ANP_1 is coupled to activation of particulate guanylate cyclase and cGMP synthesis, but ANP_2 is not coupled to production of cGMP and its function is unknown. It is of interest that ANP inhibits adenylate cyclase in certain tissues, but the physiologic relevance of this action remains to be determined [90]. In the kidney, both high- and low-affinity receptors have been identified, adding further complexity to the ANP classification scheme [175]. Regional differences in receptor density exist [174], and ANP can self-regulate the distribution and cellular processing of its own receptors [176]. ANP is a direct smooth muscle relaxant, inducing hypotension by intravenous infusions in humans [175]. In aorta, carotid, mesenteric, and renal arteries and in some veins, ANP counteracts vasoconstrictor responses [174,175], particularly those that are renin induced [158,177]. Heterogeneity in responsiveness to ANP in isolated artery and vein preparations is well recognized. ANP is ineffective in relaxing substantially depolarized smooth muscle (such as rat portal vein), is more effective in relaxing larger arteries than smaller resistance vessels, and has pronounced effects on the renal vasculature [174]. Variations in receptor density and distribution do not fully explain this heterogeneity [174].

Vasopressin. The synthesis of neurohypophyseal peptide analogues has been used extensively to study the structural-activity relationships and characteristics of neurohypophyseal peptide receptors [4,178]. V_1 receptors, present on vascular smooth muscle (and hepatocytes), have been distinguished from renal tubule V_2 receptors. Although V_2 receptors have not been identified on vascular smooth muscle, there are recent data to support their presence on these cells [179]. Moreover, the Alturas have made strong arguments for the existence of vasopressin receptor subtypes on vascular smooth muscle [180,181]. The determination of the distribution of receptor subtypes in blood vessels awaits their better characterization.

Vasopressin produces potent vasoconstrictor responses in most vessels, but response varies with species and the vessel under study [4,181]. Inositol-lipid turnover and calcium mobilization contribute to V_1-receptor-mediated contraction [182,183]. The critical receptor dependence on magnesium [4] may reflect G-protein regulation of vasopressin contraction [182]. The occasional vasodilatory response [4,181] may be mediated by V_2 receptors coupled to adenylate cyclase [180]. Alternatively, vasodilation may result from counter-regulatory cardiovascular effects [180,184], secondary effects on autonomic neurotransmission [4,179], or the effects of vasodilatory prostaglandins formed from V_1-induced arachidonate release [182]. The sensitivity of vascular smooth muscle to vasopressin reveals marked heterogeneity. In most species, vasopressin contracts splanchnic, skeletal, renal, carotid, and umbilical arteries and umbilical but not hepatic or pulmonary veins [181]. Vasopressin exerts little effect on cerebral and pulmonary arteries (although the pulmonary response is variable in humans [4]) and usually dilates coronary arteries [181]. In the microvasculature, there is a general predilection for contraction of muscular venules and other small venous vessels [181]. Mesenteric, intestinal, and skeletal muscle arterioles contract to vasopressin, but the cerebral arteriolar microvasculature is unresponsive [181]. Physiologic factors contributing to this heterogeneity include age, ionic milieu, temperature, tissue metabolism, indirect influence of local hormones and neurotransmitters, species differences, receptor heterogeneity, and vessel integrity [181].

Oxytocin. Studies of vascular oxytocin receptor binding are not available, and the characterization of the vascular oxytocin receptor has not been performed. Although there is support for the concept of an oxytocin receptor different from the vascular vasopressin receptor, this has not been proved [181]; clearly, specific V_1 and V_2 antagonists also potently antagonize oxytocin responses [178].

Oxytocin elicits both vasodilator and vasoconstrictor responses that depend on species differences, regional variation, and diverse physiologic factors [4,181]. There are also regional and species differences between the effects of oxytocin and vasopressin [181]. With the exception of its more potent constrictor action on placental and uterine vessels, oxytocin is a weaker constrictor than vasopressin in large vessels and in the microvasculature [181]. Furthermore, oxytocin generally relaxes hepatic, splanchnic, and skeletal artery tone, whereas vasopressin constricts those vessels [181]. Bolton has reviewed the biochemical and electrophysiologic actions of oxytocin in uterine smooth muscle [26]. By contrast, these aspects of the diverse response to oxytocin in vascular smooth muscle have not been investigated. In an effort to begin to characterize the contractile action of oxytocin, Barrigón and Tamargo recently demonstrated that contraction in rat isolated aorta is in part attributed to calcium influx through receptor-operated channels and to calcium release from intracellular stores [185].

The aforementioned physiologic factors that contribute to the heterogeneous oxytocin response have been well reviewed [4,181]. In particular, sex hormones can modify the actions of oxytocin on vascular smooth muscle. In a number of species, including humans, vasodilator actions of oxytocin are converted to constrictor responses by sex steroids [4].

PROSTANOID RECEPTORS

The identification of vascular prostanoid receptor sites and their tissue distribution is still in progress. Current classification schemes are based on rank-potency studies. Gardiner and Collier have suggested X and Y designations for contractile and relaxant activity, respectively [186]. Kennedy and colleagues have provided evidence for the existence of distinct smooth muscle receptors for prostaglandin E_2 (PGE_2), prostaglandin $F_{2,a5,a,a1}$ ($PGF_{2,a5,a,a1}$), and thromboxane A_2 (TXA_2), and they propose that specific receptors exist for each of the naturally occurring 2-series prostanoids [187]. In their nomenclature, prostanoid receptors are designated by a P and preceded by a letter signifying the most potent natural prostanoid agonist at that site. Accordingly, DP, EP, FP, IP, and TP represent the receptors that are most sensitive to prostaglandins D_2, E_2, $F_{2,a5,a,a1}$, I_2, and TXA_2, respectively. Published radiolabeled eicosanoid-binding studies support the evidence in favor of specific receptor sites for prostaglandins of a different series [188], but a subdivision may be required within a receptor group, and receptors common to prostaglandins of different series exist [187]. PGI_2 and PGE_1 interact with the same vascular smooth muscle receptor [189], and it appears that $PGF_{2,a5,a,a1}$ and TXA_2 also share receptors in some vascular smooth muscle [190]. Significantly, the strictest criteria for determination of distinct prostanoid receptor sites in vascular smooth muscle often have not been realized; the TXA_2 endoperoxide receptor in particular has undergone little biochemical or pharmacologic characterization [191].

The effects of prostaglandins on vascular smooth muscle are variable, and they depend on the type of prostaglandin, species, and vascular bed under study as well as the segment of blood vessel and age of the animal [187,192–196]. It is fair to say that PGI_2 almost exclusively causes vasorelaxation and that TXA_2 mediates only vasoconstriction [4,26,189,193–198]. The effects of other prostaglandins and prostaglandin endoperoxides are much more variable. The infusion of prostaglandins $PGF_{2,a5,a,a1}$, A_1, A_2, B_1, E_1, and E_2 in human brachial artery induces vasodilation [199], and intravenous infusion of PGI_2 induces hypotension in humans [196].

The immediate postreceptor binding events of the various prostanoids are poorly characterized. PGI_2 and PGF_1 regulate the synthesis of cAMP [189], and TXA_2 and PGH_2 endoperoxide modulate calcium availability directly through interaction with the vascular smooth muscle receptor [198,200]. These second messengers may regulate both vasoactive and proliferative responses [34,201]. Peroxide and hydroxy radical arachidonate derivatives also stimulate guanylate cyclase [89,202], but the relationship between cGMP formation and prostaglandin-mediated physiologic functions is not clear.

Reasons for vascular heterogeneity in vivo include the presence of different prostanoid receptors on the same vascular segment, the effects of prostaglandins on sympathetic discharge, the modulation of prostaglandin synthesis by other vasoactive substances, and the state of tissue injury [9,187,192,196].

LEUKOTRIENE RECEPTORS

The evidence, based on rank potencies of agonists and radioligand-binding studies, favors distinct smooth muscle surface receptors for the cysteinyl-containing leukotrienes LTC_4, LTD_4, and LTE_4 [188,193,203]. Additionally, there are data supporting the existence of high- and low-affinity sites, receptor populations that are both tissue and species specific, and binding sites on intracellular as well as surface-membrane fractions [193,203,204]. The full characterization and distribution of these receptors in the vasculature remain to be elucidated.

The vasoactive leukotrienes demonstrate marked species differences and organ specificity. In vitro, cysteinyl-leukotrienes are generally powerful vasoconstrictors with a rank-of-order potency of LTC_4 greater than LTD_4 greater than LTE_4 [205–207]. In vivo, the response depends on the vessel under investigation and the rapidity and duration of injection. Brief injections in small amounts induce pressor responses in most species; with time, however, a regulatory "escape" mechanism comes into effect. Large doses injected rapidly invariably cause hypotension [206,207]. In humans, cutaneous and pulmonary vessels intrinsically vasodilate to in vivo infusions, but cerebral and uterine vessels constrict [206,207]. Although untested in humans, coronary vasoconstriction has been demonstrated in all species tested to date [206]. Other actions of cysteinyl-leukotrienes on blood vessels include an increase in vascular permeability [206,207] and mitogenic effects [208]; both effects are shared by leukotriene B_4.

The constrictor response of leukotrienes requires mobilization of intracellular calcium and may be regulated in part by activation of G-protein inhibitory subunit leading to reduction of adenylate cyclase activity [203]. Leukotriene-induced contraction may result indirectly from TXA_2 generation [203,205]. The mechanism by which vasoconstriction is converted over time to vasodilation involves leukotriene-induced release of a platelet-derived vasodilator [207].

Much is still unknown about leukotriene receptor activity, and the mechanism of its heterogeneity requires further study. Other factors that might contribute to the variable responsiveness of different vascular beds also require elucidation.

GROWTH FACTOR PROTEIN-TYROSINE KINASE RECEPTOR SYSTEMS

Growth factor receptor–associated protein-tyrosine kinases (PTKs) are characterized by ligand-stimulated protein-tyrosine kinase activity that is intrinsic to the receptor [209–211]. Included in this discussion are the following PTKs (they receive additional individual attention later in this chapter):

- platelet-derived growth factor (PDGF)
- epidermal growth factor (EGF)
- transforming growth factor (TGF)
- fibroblastic growth factor (FGF)
- insulinlike growth factor (IGF) 1

Because ligand-stimulated autophosphorylation specific for tyrosine is a distinctive common feature of PTKs, it is useful to group these receptors conceptually. In further support of this grouping, all PTKs reveal a receptor presence on the plasma membrane, share a common platelet repository (PDGF, EGF, TGF), demonstrate contractile as well as mitogenic functions, and show an interactive interdependence for desired functional responses [212–216].

PDGF generally is considered to be the mitogen most important in the atherosclerotic proliferative response and is therefore the selected representative for more detailed consideration. It is important to note that not all growth factor receptors (e.g., IGF II, interleukin II, nerve growth factor) have protein kinase activity [211]. Receptors for PDGF have been identified on cells of mesenchymal origin, of which the vascular myocyte is no exception [217,218]. Two classes of PDGF receptor that recognize different isoforms of PDGF (AA, BB, AB) have been identified [219], and the common primary structural features of the receptor have been determined [220]. The B receptor binds the BB isoform of PDGF alone, whereas the AB receptor binds all three isoforms indiscriminately [219]. The location, distribution, and biologic functional differences of the two classes of receptor remain to be studied.

PDGF has important mitogenic activity. It regulates progression of the cell through its cell cycle independently of other promoters, and it is required to "prime" the cell (render it competent) for mitogenic response to other growth factors [34,221]. Within minutes of binding to its surface receptor, complex membrane and cytosolic signals initiate cellular and nuclear responses, eventually leading to DNA synthesis and cell growth [34]. The activation of a Na^+/H^+ antiport mechanism mediates cellular alkalinization that is thought to stimulate mitogenesis and secondarily regulate membrane permeability to other ions [34]. An influx of calcium contributes to the messenger pool of cytosolic calcium released from intracellular stores that is central to the growth response [34,201,213]. PDGF has been shown to stimulate phosphoinositide breakdown [222,223], thus generating intracellular second messengers (inositol 1,4,5-triphosphate and diacylglycerol) with important mitogenic effects (discussed in detail in the section "Signal Transduction," later in this chapter). In the cytoplasm, PDGF induces cAMP accumulations, while at the nuclear level, c-fos and c-myc are expressed in response to this stimulus [34]. Although the role of cAMP in vascular smooth muscle proliferation is controversial [224], c-fos and c-myc are postulated to play an important role in transduction of the mitogenic signal to the nucleus [34,201]. PDGF is also an important stimulus for vascular smooth muscle migration.

In much the same way that many vasoactive substances demonstrate mitogenic effects, PDGF is a powerful vasoactive substance that mediates vasoconstriction even more potently than angiotensin [213]. Accordingly, many mitogenic factors enhance contractile responsiveness and vice versa. During contraction, activator calcium is mobilized through influx and intracellular release [213], but the signal-transducing mechanisms of the contractile response require further elucidation.

Surface receptors for other PTKs have been identified on vascular smooth muscle cells [221,222,225–231], and mitogenic and contractile responses analogous to those of PDGF have been demonstrated [34,201,213,214,221]. In addition, certain unique characteristics of individual growth factors have been identified, and further studies undoubtedly will expand on these differences and elaborate on their physiologic significance.

Membrane Activation

MYOGENIC ACTIVITY

Changes in membrane permeability and the voltage difference across the membrane occur with activation of cell-surface receptors. Alternatively, these changes can be an inherent spontaneous property of certain smooth muscle cells and independent of external chemical influences [3,4,9]. It is this intrinsic property of membranes that is responsible for basal smooth muscle tone, otherwise known as **myogenic**, or stretch-dependent, tone. Myogenic activity is essential for maintaining a blood pressure compatible with human life and is important in local autoregulation of blood flow.

Myogenic tone is not a universal property of all vascular smooth muscle, and different types have been recognized, but certain characteristics hold true for myogenic tone in general. First, extracellular calcium and stretch are obligatory for the generation of myogenic tone [232,233]. Second, myogenic tone usually is resistant to calcium-channel blockers, suggesting that calcium is made available by a mechanism independent from the receptor-operated and voltage-dependent calcium channels [232]. Third, myogenic tone is present after denervation (by definition), but the magnitude of response to stretch is modified by neurotransmitters and other agonists [232]. Fourth, temperature [234] and pH [235] influence myogenic tone, implying that conditions and external factors affecting membrane fluidity and function are of physiologic importance.

One form of myogenic tone—spontaneous rhythmic contractions—was first described in pulsatile veins of bat wings [3] and has since been studied in detail in portal veins [3,232]. These spontaneous rhythmic depolarizations are associated with action potentials leading to phasic contractions that depend on the rate of stretch (Fig. 3-1) [232]. Myogenic propagation of electrical activity serves to synchronize tonic contractions, resulting in the classification of such smooth muscle as **single unit** [3]. The development of rhythmic tone is more characteristic of some large veins [3] and of smaller resistance vessels in the microcirculation, particularly those smaller than 20 μm [232].

Maintained tone describes a form of myogenic tone that is maintained as long as stretch is applied to the vessel [232]. The phenomenon is more commonly encountered than its rhythmic counterpart and predominates in small resistance vessels (> 20 μM) [232]. Maintained tone is generated without spike activity, in the absence of phasic contractions, and at low levels of stretch [232]. Ross has described another form of myogenic tone in human coronary arteries that is characterized by slow, regular oscillations [236], and Bevan has observed certain irregular tonic patterns that may occur more frequently in vessels from older individuals [232,237].

Fig. 3-1. Patterns of myogenic tone. **A.** Spontaneous rhythmic activity in small resistance artery (internal diameter 50 μM) from rabbit ear. Note that tone was maintained and then reversed by papaverine (10^{-5} M). **B.** Spontaneous rhythmic activity in longitudinal muscle of rabbit portal vein. **C.** Spontaneous rhythmic activity in human omental arteria. Left: female, normotensive, aged 20 years. Right: female, normotensive, aged 58 years.

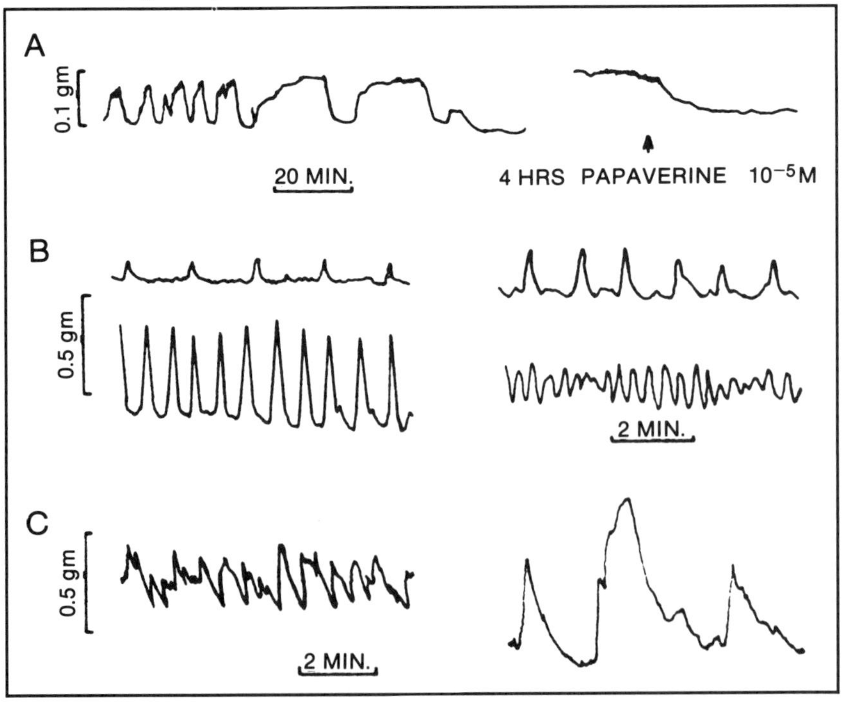

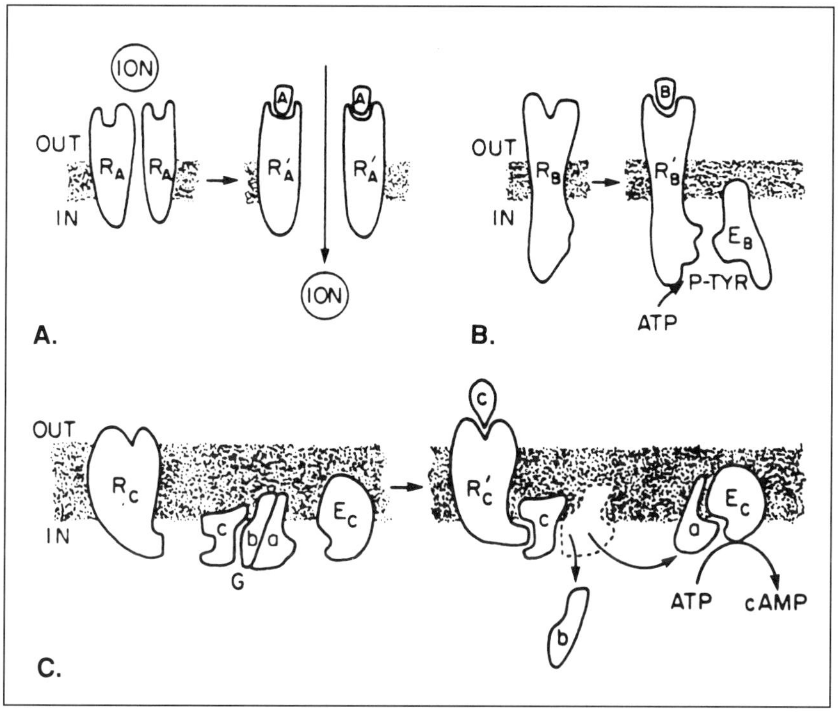

Fig. 3-2. Hypothetical models of ligand-activated transmembrane signaling using three basic mechanisms. **A.** Ligand-regulated ion channel, like the nicotinic cholinergic receptor. **B.** Ligand-regulated enzyme activity. receptor tyrosine kinase is used as the example, wherein phosphorylation of a membrane effector, E_B, plays a role in signaling. **C.** Ligand-modulated release of crytpic mediators. Upon interaction with a ligand-occupied receptor, a hypothetical guanine nucleotide regulatory complex (G) is shown to release an effector-stimulatory component (a) and at least one other regulatory protein (b). In this instance, adenylate cyclase is depicted as the effector (E_c). In principle, any other membrane process (ion channel, phosphodiesterase, phospholipase) could be similarly regulated. Models are shown for receptors in either the absence (R_A, R_B, R_C) or presence (R'_A, R'_B, R'_C) of their regulatory ligands (A, B, C). None of the components are drawn to scale. The extracellular (out) domains of the receptors face the top of the page; the intracellular (in) receptor domains, anchored in the membrane (stippled areas) face the bottom of the page. (Reproduced with permission from A Yanagisawa, et al.. Mechanism of antagonism of thromboxane receptors in vascular smooth muscle. Eur J Pharmacol 1987; 133:89–96.)

SIGNAL TRANSDUCTION

The process by which cell-surface receptors convert external stimuli into appropriate cellular responses is termed **signal transduction**. This discriminatory capacity of a cell is a complex and elusive property of its surface membrane. Although we are relatively ignorant of how limited numbers of intracellular signal transducers (second messengers) bring about a multitude of diverse responses, three basic ligand-operated receptor mechanisms for signal transduction have been elucidated: the receptor with intrinsic ion channel, the receptor with intrinsic enzymatic activity, and the receptor with ligand-dependent catalytic activity (Fig. 3-2). For each mechanism a series of reactions, designated **signal cascades**, convert the external stimulus into a regulated response [209,238].

Three structural regions are common to transmembrane glycoprotein receptors: an external ligand-specific region, a hydrophobic anchor traversing the membrane, and a submembranous region that is important in expression of activity [239] (see Fig. 3-2). The physical contiguity between external and internal receptor domains that is essential for generation of transmembrane signals can also result from communication via an ionic channel [209,240]. The ligand-modulated receptor with an intrinsic ionic channel represents the first mechanism (of the three mentioned) whereby the transmembrane receptor complex mediates an intracellular signal [209,240]. Alternatively, the cytoplasmic region of the receptor can interact specifically with the submembranous regulatory system, like the G protein, or express its own ligand-dependent enzymatic activity, as in the case of receptors with intrinsic tyrosine kinase catalytic activity, and in these ways transmit signals intracellularly (see Fig. 3-2) [209,239].

The amplification, regulation, and termination of signal transmission occur at various stages of the signal cascades, and these elaborate reactions are integrated into the overall response. For example, changes in ion flux in response to receptor activation may amplify a signal by depolarizing the membrane. This initiates long-range signals in the form of electrical potentials, with resulting effects on

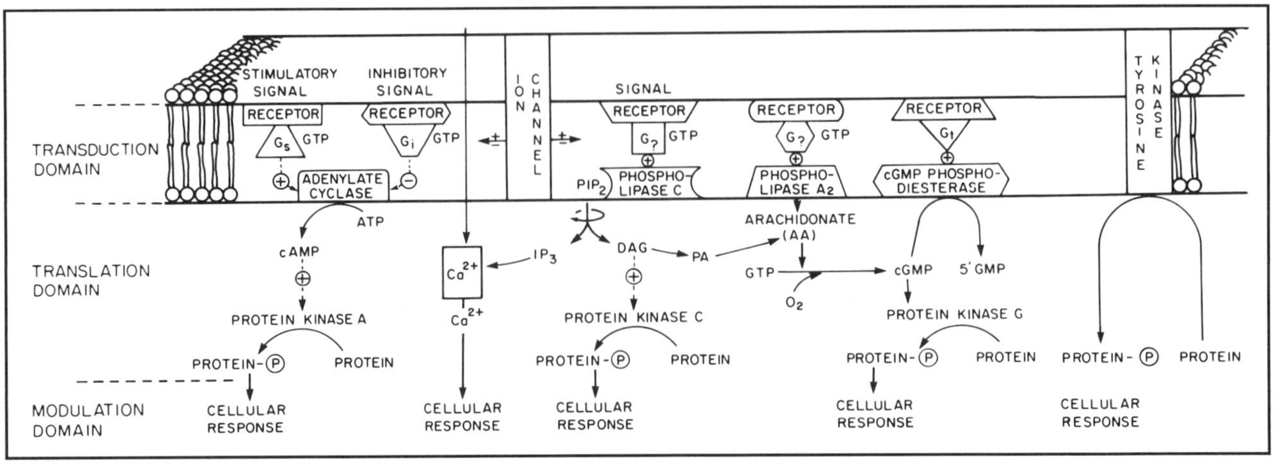

Fig. 3-3. A schematic representation of some established and less well established (potential) signal cascades used by vascular and smooth muscle cell-surface receptors. In the transduction domain, receptors controlling membrane-bound enzymes via G-protein coupling lie alongside receptors possessing intrinsic ion channels and intrinsic tyrosine kinase activity. (Adapted from MJ Mooibroek and JH Wang. Integration of signal-transduction processes. Biochem Cell Biol 1988; 66:557–566, and RH Mitchell. How do receptors at the cell surface send signals to the cell interior? Br Med J 1987; 295:1320–1323.)

calcium availability and protein orientation and function [209,241] (Fig. 3-3). Ultimately, proteins targeted by the signal for phosphorylation may include the ion channel itself, thereby regulating its permeability, and the receptor protein, thus rendering it insensitive to activation [209,238]. This is a case in point for receptors regulating the production of cAMP, where amplification reactions involve cAMP-dependent protein kinases that have additional regulatory functions in feedback inhibition of the receptor [215,238]. In noting that signal target proteins include receptors, coupling proteins, ion-channel proteins, ion pumps, enzymes, calcium-binding proteins, and other cytosolic and membrane-bound proteins, we can appreciate the complexity of the signal-transduction process and the many opportunities for regulation and integration of messages.

In the well-established transmembrane signal cascades, certain compounds have received particular attention in the transmission of information intracellularly and are referred to as second messengers. Figure 3-3 reveals a highly simplified overview of the established regulatory cascades: adenylate cyclase-cAMP; phospholipase-phosphotidylinositol 4, 5 biphosphate; phosphodiesterase-cGMP; receptor with intrinsic ion channel; and receptor with intrinsic enzyme catalytic activity. For receptors with intrinsic ion channels, such as the nicotinic acetylcholine receptor of skeletal muscle and ganglia and the gamma-aminobutyric acid receptor present on vascular smooth muscle [242], the ion itself is the messenger. But not all ionic fluxes transfer "primary" information. In some circumstances, other messengers may activate ion channels secondarily as part of an amplification or termination process. For ligand-regulated enzyme activity, the intrinsic catalytic activity of the receptor is the messenger. By phosphorylating tyrosine residues on proteins in receptor proximity with important metabolic functions, signal cascades are set in motion. The adenylate cyclase-cAMP, phospholipase-phosphotidylinositol, and phosphodiesterase-cGMP cascades are similar in design. At the membrane domain, second-messenger enzymes (adenylate cyclase, phospholipase, phosphodiesterase) are modulated by ligand-activated receptors coupled to G proteins that confer specificity on external stimuli [210]. Membrane enzyme activity is translated into modulation of inositol 1,4,5-triphosphate (IP_3), 1,2 diacylglycerol (DAG), cAMP, and cGMP. These second messengers perform signal regulatory functions mediated by messenger-binding proteins such as protein kinases [238,240] (see Fig. 3-3).

The mechanisms by which vascular smooth muscle receptors transfer information intracellularly were described for each receptor system individually in the section "Surface Receptor Systems," earlier in this chapter. Some examples of these mechanisms for signal transmission are provided in Table 3-3. Accordingly, the G-protein regulatory complex cyclic nucleotides (cAMP and cGMP), inositol lipids (IP_3 and DAG), and calcium all play important roles in the signal-transduction processes of vascular smooth muscle; consequently, their regulatory functions will be addressed individually in detail. It is important to recognize, however, that many neurotransmitters and hormones utilize a number of messengers in concert in the transmission of their signals (for example, calcium, DAG, and IP_3). Furthermore, a great deal of cross talk among signal cascades occurs, indicating that these cascades should not be considered as isolated entities [238].

G Proteins

G proteins function as intermediaries between extracellular receptors and intracellular effector proteins (enzymes

Table 3-3. Examples of mechanisms of signal transduction used by vascular smooth muscle receptor systems

Receptors modulating adenylate cyclase activity (stimulatory [+]; inhibitory [−])	
Adrenergic (alpha$_2$ [−]; beta$_2$ [+])	Vasopressin (V$_2$; [+])?
Histaminergic (H$_1$ [+] and [−]; H$_2$ [+])	Prostaglandin (I$_2$, E$_2$ [+])
Dopaminergic (D$_1$ [+])	Leukotriene (C$_4$, D$_4$, E$_4$ [−])?
Calcitonin gene-related peptide	Platelet-derived growth factor (+)
Vasoactive intestinal polypeptide (+)	
Receptors modulating guanylate cyclase activity (stimulatory [+]; inhibitory [−])	
Muscarinic (M$_{2i}$ [+])	Atrial natriuretic peptide (ANP$_1$ [+])
Histaminergic (H$_2$ [+])	
Kinin?	
Purinergic (A$_1$ [−]; A$_2$ [+])	
Opiate (+)?	
Receptors inducing phosphoinositol lipid turnover	
Adrenergic (alpha$_1$)	Vasopressin (V$_1$)
Angiotensinergic	Thromboxane A$_2$
Muscarinic (M$_2$)	
Serotoninergic (5HT$_2$)	
Histaminergic (H$_1$)	
Purinergic (P$_2$)	
Receptors with intrinsic protein kinase activity	
Platelet-derived growth factor	
Epidermal growth factor	
Transforming growth factor	
Fibroblastic growth factor	
Insulinlike growth factor I	

Source: Modified from RH Mitchell. How do receptors at the cell surface send signals to the cell interior? Br Med J 1987; 295:1320–1323.

and ion channels) for a variety of neurotransmitters [243] and hormones, thus controlling intracellular concentrations of signal molecules such as cyclic nucleotides, calcium, and inositol phosphates [244]. G-protein involvement has been conclusively demonstrated in the regulatory events following receptor activation by smooth muscle agonists modulating the effector enzyme adenylate cyclase [234,235]. G-protein involvement also is likely, as supported by indirect evidence, for receptor mechanisms mediated by phosphoinositide hydrolysis [10,236], and G proteins are plausible but unsubstantiated smooth muscle intermediaries for the cGMP-phosphodiesterase effector cascade. Thus, retinal light-sensitive G-protein activation of cGMP phosphodiesterase may well be representative of similar G-protein regulation of cGMP in vascular smooth muscle [240,244,245], but this is unproven. The general features of G-protein receptor-effector coupling have much in common, and yet a remarkable heterogeneity among this family of proteins confers signal specificity to individual receptor-ligand interactions. Recent reviews form the basis of the following discussion [30,244–253].

STRUCTURE

The G proteins are a family of heterotrimeric membrane proteins composed of alpha, beta, and gamma subunits, named in order of decreasing mass [245]. Alpha subunits demonstrate heterogeneity and serve to diversify uniquely the various G proteins. They also possess GTPase activity required for protein activation and a site, variably susceptible to ADP ribosylation by bacterial enzymes, that is used to subclassify G proteins into four groups. Accordingly, G proteins are amenable to ADP ribosylation by cholera toxin or pertussis toxin alone, both toxins, or neither toxin [244,247]. This modification of the alpha subunit has functional importance in signal transmission by impairing or enhancing the interaction of G protein with its receptor [245]. The characterization of the major classes of G proteins and the multiple forms within each class, which are a revelation of molecular cloning, is beyond the scope of this chapter. We will mention briefly the G$_s$ and G$_i$ subclassification because it is the most basic, exemplifies the concept of G (alpha) protein diversity, and is of particular relevance to vascular smooth muscle regulation by adenylate cyclase.

G proteins that stimulate adenylyl cyclase (G$_s$) were initially distinguished from those that inhibit the enzyme (G$_i$) by the alpha subunit susceptibility to cholera and pertussis toxins [244,245,247]. This division is now recognized as generally pertinent for other G-protein effector functions, although it is an oversimplification that masks the many small structural differences among alpha$_s$- and alpha$_i$-like proteins [244,245,247]. A single receptor can interact with more than one G protein (e.g., alpha$_2$ adrenoreceptors with alpha$_i$-beta-gamma and alpha$_0$-beta-gamma), and conversely, many receptors can stimulate adenylate cyclase via G$_s$, thus adding to signal diversification [247].

Heterogeneity of beta and gamma subunits is evident but less remarkable. Beta and gamma subunits are closely associated, and heterogeneity may be imparted by the formation of combinations of similar beta units with different gamma units and vice versa [244,245,347]. The functional relevance of this heterogeneity requires further

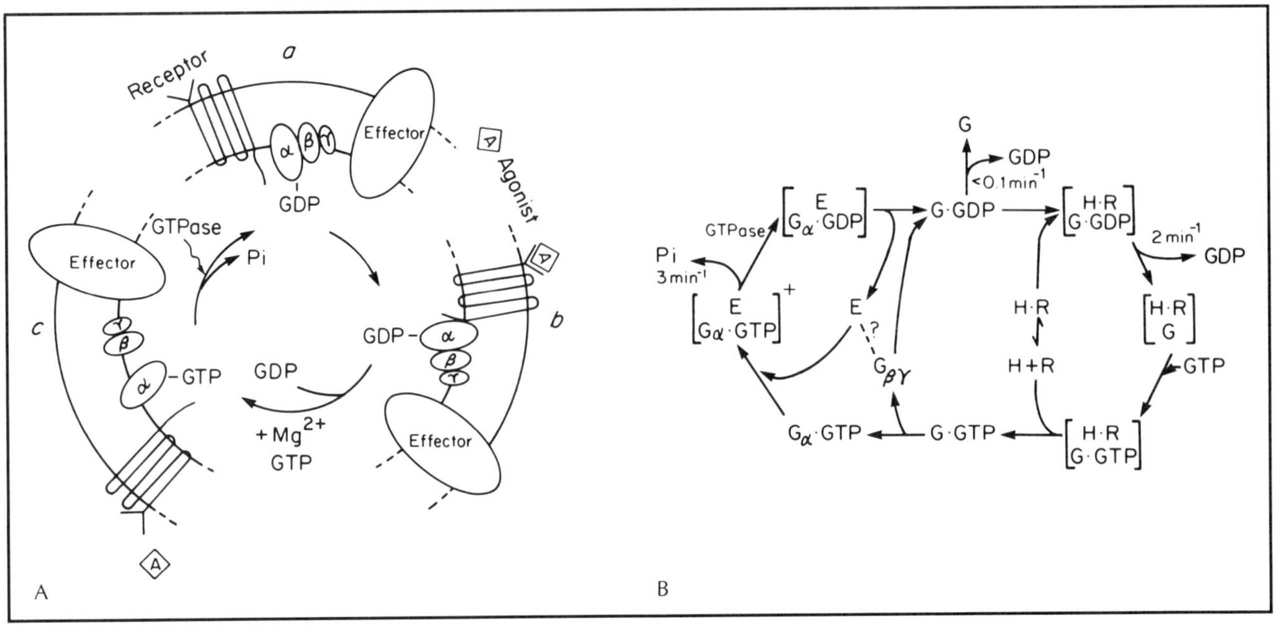

Fig. 3-4. **A.** Simple scheme for G-protein signal transduction. From the unliganded state (a), receptor binds agonist A (e.g., epinephrine, acetylcholine), which produces a change (b) in receptor–G protein interaction, allowing GTP, in the presence of Mg_{2+}, to replace GDP on the alpha subunit. The activated alphaGTP subunit and the beta-gamma subunits dissociate, and one or both interact with effectors (e.g., adenylyl cyclase). Alternatively, free beta-gamma may bind other alpha subunits. The intrinsic GTPase activity of the alpha subunit hydrolyzes GTP to GDP, releasing inorganic phosphate (p_i), and alphaGDP recombines with beta-gamma (c), ending the activation cycle. (Reproduced from EJ Neer and DE Clapham. Roles of G protein subunits in transmembrane signalling. Nature 1988; 333:129–134. Copyright 1988 Macmillan Magazines Limited.) **B.** Interactions of receptor, G protein, guanine nucleotide, and effector. G = G protein oligomer (alpha-beta-gamma); $[G_\alpha.GTP.E]^+$ = activated form of effector; H = ligand; R = receptor; HR = liganded receptor. (Reproduced with permission from PJ Casey and AG Gilman. G protein involvement in receptor-effector coupling. J Biol Chem 19968; 263(6):2577–2580.)

investigation, but it suggests that receptor recognition of a unique selective alpha-beta-gamma complex is important in the achievement of signal specificity [244,247].

MECHANISM

The G-protein regulatory cycle diagrammed in Fig. 3-4 explains the interactions among receptor, G-protein, guanine nucleotide, and effector protein on ligand binding. In Fig. 3-4A, a simplified scheme provides an overview of G-protein signal transduction [245], and the detailed interactions are outlined in Fig. 3-4B. In the resting state, G proteins exist bound to guanosine diphosphate (GDP), which readily dissociates from the alpha subunit of the G protein during ligand-receptor interaction. The resulting complex of ligand-receptor-G protein is a stable intermediate in the absence of GTP. GTP binding at the available guanine nucleotide site of the G protein in the complex lessens the affinity of ligand for receptor and consequently the receptor for GTP, allowing the receptor to recycle. GTP binding simultaneously induces the G protein to interact with its effector protein (E). This reaction is accompanied by dissociation of activated alphaGTP (alpha$_s$ or alpha$_i$ subunit) from the beta-gamma complex. The beta-gamma dimer is then free to interchange among the many G proteins of a given cell, with the potential to modulate further signal activity. For example, alpha$_i$GTP inhibition of effector protein (or enzyme) may be the consequence of direct inhibition by activated G_i. Alternatively, enzyme activity may be regulated by reassociation of excess beta-gamma with the alpha$_s$ subunit, thereby attenuating its stimulatory action [30,244]. Abundant free beta-gamma may, in addition, interact with alpha subunits of other systems [30,253] to regulate their activity independently. Thus, in certain systems, there is evidence to implicate the beta-gamma dimer in effector-protein modulation. GTPase activity is responsible for termination of the signal by hydrolysis of GTP to GDP, resulting in reassociation of alphaGDP with beta-gamma dimer. After purification, G proteins can be activated by GTP analogues and a magnesium cofactor in a process that is ligand independent, yielding G proteins composed of unique alphaG nucleotide complexes and beta/gamma dimers [254,255].

FUNCTIONS OF G PROTEIN

Modulation of Adenylyl Cyclase. G proteins function to activate and inhibit adenylate cyclase. Stimulatory G_s and inhibitory G_i proteins exist as distinct entities, with the former consistently coupled to the effector enzyme in vivo

[256] and fully accountable for its activation [244]. In contrast, the capacity of G_i to inhibit adenylate cyclase does not fully account for the inhibitory activity of the enzyme in vivo; G_i also serves as a reservoir for beta-gamma dimer, which reassociates with G_{alpha_s} to mediate hormonal inhibition of adenylate cyclase. The data on which these observations are based are reviewed in detail by Gilman [244]. This mechanism for receptor-effector coupling is pertinent to a variety of vascular smooth muscle receptor systems, including the adrenergic (alpha$_2$), muscarinic (M_2), adrenergic (beta$_2$), histaminergic (H_1 and H_2), purinergic (A_2), dopaminergic (D_1), prostaglandins (PGI_2 and PGE_1), and PDGF receptors, all of which modulate cAMP levels.

Phosphoinositide Hydrolysis. By analogy with the regulation of adenylate cyclase by G protein, a series of observations are consistent with G-protein regulation of phosphatidylinositol 4,5-bisphosphate (PIP_2) hydrolysis. First, hormone binding governing the phosphodiesteric cleavage of PIP_2 to IP_3 and DAG regulates an effector enzyme, phosphodiesterase (phospholipase C), that is guanine nucleotide dependent [250,257]. Second, hormone binding stimulates GTPase activity [250,257]. Third, the variable effect of pertussis toxin on PIP_2 breakdown by different agonists suggests participation by different G proteins [250,257]. Fourth, the activation of phospholipase C by fluoride is again analogous to the case for adenylate cyclase [258]. Although these data support the involvement of G proteins in this regulatory scheme [244,250], a single regulatory G-protein candidate that co-purifies with a receptor coupled to phospholipase C has not been identified. Consequently, the participation of G proteins in signal transduction by virtue of phospholipase C activation remains hypothetical for the many vascular smooth muscle agonists utilizing the phosphoinositide pathway (see Table 3-2).

Regulation of Ion Channels. Ion channels of excitable membranes are of three major types, classified by their gating mechanism [251]: ligand-gated channels sensitive to specific ligands, voltage-gated channels sensitive to membrane potential, and G protein–gated channels sensitive to signal-transducing membrane-confined G proteins. The nicotinic acetylcholine, gamma-aminobutyric acid, and glycine receptors are well-studied examples of ligand-gated ion channels characterized by an ion channel intrinsic to the receptor molecule, but they are a less well appreciated design feature of the cardiovascular system [242,252]. Other pertinent examples of ligand gating include the calcium-activated K^+ channels and the nucleotide-gated channels [251]. The voltage-gated (Ca^{++}, Na^+, K^+) channel is primarily regulated by membrane potential, but it can be modulated **indirectly** by surface-membrane receptors coupled to G proteins. In response to hormones and neurotransmitters, these G proteins control concentrations of cytosolic second messengers such as cAMP, which mediates channel phosphorylation, thereby influencing channel sensitivity to changes in membrane potential [249]. Calcium and potassium ion channels gated by G proteins (G protein–gated) have recently been uncovered in cardiac smooth muscle [259–261] and represent a **direct** G-protein regulatory mechanism by which receptor occupancy is coupled to an ionic signal. In that case, the effector protein is the receptor molecule, and the activator subunit of G protein mediates channel opening in the manner characteristic of the regulatory cycle of G protein [251]. Both direct G-protein gating and indirect G-protein control of ion channels appear to be widespread regulatory mechanisms that also undoubtedly pertain to voltage-dependent and receptor-operated ion-channel regulation of vascular smooth muscle.

Phosphoinositides

There has been much progress recently in our understanding of the relationships among receptor occupation, inositol-lipid turnover, and calcium mobilization in the stimulus response pathway. Many advances have been made from experiments in a variety of nonsmooth muscle tissues. However, as discussed next, the general findings are likely to pertain specifically to vascular smooth muscle.

PIP_2 is an important constituent of all plasma membranes, and its phosphodiesteric cleavage to IP_3 and DAG has been linked to M_2 [26,67,91], H_1 [110,119], angiotensinergic [61], alpha$_1$ [10], serotoninergic [28,257,262–264], TXA_2 [28,257], purinergic (P_2) [138], and vasopressin (V_1) [182,183] receptor activation. Moreover, the calcium-mobilizing properties of IP_3 have been verified in isolated porcine coronary smooth muscle [265] and rabbit pulmonary artery preparations [266]. Based on those observations, Somlyo has proposed that IP_3 is the physiologic coupler of excitation to pharmacomechanical contraction in vascular smooth muscle [267]. Other significant advances have been made in platelets, which demonstrate many ultrastructural and mechanistic similarities with the vascular smooth muscle cell. Thus, phosphotidylinositol (PI) hydrolysis seems in no way specific to activation of any one receptor or cell type but rather represents a common response to a wide range of stimuli, mediated by a variety of receptor systems in different cells types [26]. Accordingly, we will review the subject without limiting ourselves to observations made in the vascular smooth muscle cell, acknowledging that verification in this cell type may be lacking.

PI undergoes two-stage phosphorylation in the inner plasma membrane to form PIP_2, which is the precursor for receptor activation by external stimuli [268] (Fig. 3-5). Receptor occupation stimulates a calcium-dependent phospholipase C–type phosphodiesterase regulated by G protein that hydrolyzes PIP_2 to produce IP_3 and DAG [268]. The latter compound is immediately phosphorylated to phosphatidic acid (PA) by a kinase using ATP [268]. IP_3 is the proposed intracellular mediator of calcium release from internal stores by hormones and neurotransmitters such as vasopressin, noradrenalin, angiotensin II, and acetylcholine, and DAG is the membrane-associated activator of protein kinase C [268]. A synergistic interaction between these two independent pathways of information transmission may be observed in a physiologic response [32,105,257]. The intracellular levels of IP_3 and DAG are closely regulated by the rate of hydrolysis of PIP_2, and the active resynthesis of PI from inositol and

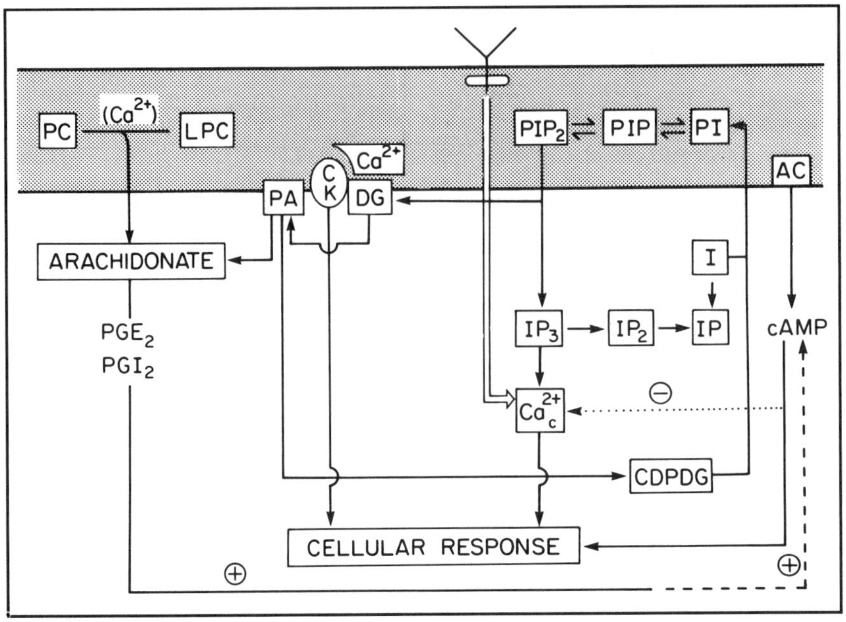

Fig. 3-5. The phosphatidylinositol cycle, the arachidonate acid cascade, the adenylate cyclase-cAMP pathway, and their participation in the calcium messenger system of vascular smooth muscle. The shaded area represents the plasma membrane. The interaction of hormone with its receptor (at top), results in an increase in the Ca^{2+} influx rate (hollow arrow), and the activation of a phospholipase C that catalyzes the hydrolysis of phosphatidylinositol 4,5-bisphosphate (PIP_2) to produce diacylglycerol (DG) and inositol triphosphate (IP_3). (Reproduced from H Rasmussen. The calcium messenger system (first of two parts). N Engl J Med 1986; 314(17):1094–1101. Reprinted by permission of the New England Journal of Medicine.)

cytidine diphosphate (CDP) diacylglycerol in the inositol-lipid cycles. The former precursor compound is the product of phosphatase action on IP_3 and the latter the product of phosphatidic acid priming by cytosine triphosphate (CTP) [105,269] (see Fig. 3-5).

MECHANISM OF ACTION OF IP_3

Second-messenger functions of calcium are critical to excitatory responses of vascular smooth muscle [270]. Calcium requirements are met by increasing membrane permeability to extracellular calcium and by its release from intracellular pools. IP_3 has been implicated in selectively inducing the release of calcium from endoplasmic reticulum without affecting the mitochondrial pool [271]. Moreover, recent observations have confirmed the existence of this mechanism for calcium release in vascular smooth muscle [10,267], which may entail specific binding of IP_3 to endoplasmic reticulum by an as yet uncharacterized receptor [272].

There is evidence that IP_3 also may be involved in promoting calcium entry by indirect means. Whereas a receptor target for IP_3 exists on endoplasmic reticulum but not on surface membranes, its phosphorylated metabolite IP_4 might interact with the plasma membrane to increase its permeability to calcium [273].

MECHANISM OF ACTION OF DAG

The work of Nishizuka and colleagues demonstrates that DAG, acting within the plane of the membrane, activates a calcium- and phospholipid-dependent protein kinase C [32,274,275]. The increased affinity of the enzyme for calcium in the presence of phospholipids and DAG (positive-sensitivity modulation) obviates the need for an increase in intracellular calcium concentration for enzyme activity and renders this pathway independent of IP_3 [32]. Vascular smooth muscle contraction and relaxation are among the many potential roles of protein kinase C [275,276]. The 20 kDa myosin light chain [277] and actin-binding proteins viniculin, filamin, and caldesmon of smooth muscle [278,279] are phosphorylated by protein kinase C, the light chain at a specific threonine site different from that regulated by myosin light-chain kinase. However, these effects have been demonstrated only in vitro, and their functional significance in contractile regulation is uncertain [267].

The appearance of DAG in membranes is transient, since it is recycled immediately to phosphoinositol or further degraded to arachidonate. In the latter instance, it may be shunted to form prostaglandins or involved in the activation of guanylate cyclase [32] (see Fig. 3-3).

SYNERGISM AND CROSS TALK IN INOSITOL-LIPID METABOLISM

The phosphotidylinositol signal cascade integrates the effects of calcium mobilization by IP_3, protein kinase C activation by DAG, and cGMP formation by arachidonate's induction of guanylate cyclase (see Fig. 3-3). The prostaglandins formed secondarily from arachidonate may elevate levels of cAMP, which serves as a feedback modulator of the initial cellular response [32,238]. Moreover, the achievement of a full physiologic response requires an interaction between the IP_3 and DAG arms of inositol-lipid metabolism. In platelets, calcium mobilization by IP_3, through activation of a calmodulin-dependent protein kinase, and protein kinase C activity can be monitored separately by measurement of the phosphorylation of a myosin light chain and a 40-K protein, respectively; individually, each is associated with a submaximal response. During platelet activation by agonists, both proteins are phosphorylated, and a full functional response (release reaction) is observed [32,268]. Synergistic interaction between protein kinase C and calmodulin-dependent protein kinase has been proposed as a mechanism for cellular responses in other systems [32,268], including the vascular smooth muscle cell [266,280,281]. In this instance, a temporally integrated cellular response leads to contraction [282].

FUNCTIONAL IMPORTANCE

Phosphoinositide turnover is an important transducing event in the coupling of cell excitation to contraction (excitation-contraction coupling). The hydrolysis of PIP_2 is stimulated by many vasoactive hormones and neurotransmitters and parallels the development of smooth muscle tone [283–285]. The relationship among phosphatidylinositol turnover, intracellular calcium concentration, and smooth muscle contraction is not straightforward, and both the IP_3 and DAG reaction cascades are involved in temporal integration of the cellular response [269]. IP_3-induced release of calcium from endoplasmic reticulum temporarily raises intracellular calcium concentrations, which is important in the early phase of contraction [286]. The rapid and sustained increases in agonist-induced calcium-influx rates are then matched by a highly efficient calcium-efflux mechanism that achieves calcium homeostasis [269]. The sustained response, observed after calcium homeostasis is achieved, depends on extracellular calcium entry and is modulated by protein kinase C [286,287]. Because DAG increases the calcium affinity of protein kinase C (modulation sensitivity) [32], the enzyme is activated in spite of resting intracellular calcium concentrations achieved as a consequence of this homeostatic mechanism [269].

Inositol-lipid turnover is also promoted by a variety of mitogenic stimuli. Certain growth-promoting vasoactive hormones, as well as cells transformed with src, ros, and abl oncogenes, initiate the bifurcating signal pathway of PIP_2 hydrolysis [106]. Both DAG and IP_3 are important mediators of cellular proliferation [106]. IP_3 releases intracellular sequestered calcium, which is an important transducer of the mitogenic response [30,201], and the DAG cascade has several growth-promoting functions mediated largely by protein kinase C [106,275,288]. The activation of a sodium-hydrogen exchanger by protein kinase C is thought to stimulate DNA synthesis by increasing cell pH, and the enzyme also enhances the formation of growth-promoting prostaglandins. These prostaglandins are generated by two means: (1) the inactivation of lipocortin protein, which functions to inhibit phospholipase A_2-mediated release of arachidonate, and (2) the hydrolysis of DAG by lipase, releasing arachidonate, which is then converted to prostaglandins [106]. These intracellular mechanisms are reviewed in detail elsewhere [30,105,106,275,288–296].

Cyclic Nucleotides

CYCLIC AMP

Cyclic AMP (cAMP) is formed from Mg^{2+}-ATP or Mn^{2+}-ATP in a reaction catalyzed by the enzyme adenylyl cyclase, which is located on the plasma membrane. The modulation of adenylyl cyclase by hormone- and neurotransmitter-receptor binding, is regulated by a unique and receptor-specific guanine nucleotide–binding protein (G protein) that couples the receptor to the effector enzyme (see Fig. 3-3) [244,245,247]. G proteins exist in stimulatory (G_s) and inhibitory (G_i) forms (see the section "G Proteins," earlier in this chapter) that control activation and inhibition of adenylate cyclase, respectively [244,245,247,282]. The alpha subunit (the protein is heterotrimeric; see the section "G Proteins") provides identity for each unique G protein, serves to divide G proteins into major classes by its heterogeneity, and accounts for the activity of the G_s nucleotide complex. In contrast, the capacity to inhibit adenylate cyclase is shared by $alpha_i$ and the beta-gamma complex [245]: G $alpha_i$ directly inhibits adenylyl cyclase, while the dissociated abundant free beta-gamma dimer, on receptor activation, binds G $alpha_s$ to prevent activation of adenylyl cyclase [245].

The levels of intracellular cAMP are also regulated by phosphodiesterase, which cleaves the 3′-bond of cAMP, yielding 5′-AMP. Cyclic nucleotide phosphodiesterase occurs in at least two isoforms and possibly up to five isoforms in vascular smooth muscle, with one isoform demonstrating a preference for cAMP over cGMP [297,298]. In light of the general calcium-lowering effects of cAMP in vascular smooth muscle, it is pertinent that the "with a high Michaelis constant (Km) for substrate" form of the enzyme is regulated by the calcium-dependent activating protein, calmodulin [299].

cAMP has an established role in vascular smooth relaxation. The extensive literature supporting this notion has been well reviewed [45,299–302]. Data supporting this general concept largely are derive from the study of beta-adrenergic vasorelaxation, and extrapolation to other receptor systems has been made without vigorous scientific scrutiny [299,302]. This is not to discount the importance of a generalized cAMP mechanism in mediating vasodilation but rather to underscore that discrepancies exist between cAMP levels and physiologic responses. cAMP also has been implicated in regulation of the vascular smooth muscle-cell growth cycle and cellular proliferation [230], but the role it plays is not at all clear. cAMP has been associated with both proliferation and inhibition of proliferation of vascular smooth muscle [303,304], and its levels in proliferating atherosclerotic plaques have been variable [305]. It is likely that in different instances the smooth muscle cell may be inhibited or stimulated in its cell cycle, depending on its needs. Friedman explains this concept by assuming that "cyclic AMP is not an inherent regulator of the cell cycle, but rather that regulation by cyclic AMP has been superimposed upon the primitive cell cycle, just as it was apparently appended to preexisting metabolic pathways" [305].

The actions of cAMP are mediated by the catalytic unit of cAMP-dependent protein kinase. As a result of the binding of cAMP to the regulatory unit of protein kinase, it dissociates from the activated enzyme subunit, which then catalyzes the transfer of phosphate from ATP to a protein substrate, thereby altering its function or activity [45,299,302]. In the smooth muscle cell, the phosphorylated proteins accelerate relaxation by antagonizing the effects of calcium and directly modifying contractile proteins [45,302]. cAMP facilitates calcium sequestration by the sarcoplasmic reticulum [45], regulates calcium entry into the cell [306], and stimulates calcium extrusion from smooth muscle [307]. These actions are accomplished by a calcium-sodium exchange system [302] and by the depression of membrane excitability by abolition of action potentials, thereby decreasing voltage-dependent calcium flux [308]. cAMP also antagonizes the mechanism of contraction by modifying the sensitivity of myosin light-chain kinase to activation by calcium [302] and, potentially, by myosin heavy-chain phosphorylation [309].

The role of cAMP in the regulation of proliferative and other noncontractile functions of smooth muscle has been alluded to, but these processes are far less well investigated. In light of the association of cellular alkalinization with growth [34,201], a recent report of a cAMP-sensitive bicarbonate-chloride antiport in vascular smooth muscle is noteworthy [310].

CYCLIC GMP

The enzymatic conversion of guanosine triphosphate to cyclic GMP (cGMP) is catalyzed by guanylyl cyclase [311]. In vascular smooth muscle, both cytosolic (soluble) and membrane-associated (particulate) isoenzyme forms of guanylate cyclase are prevalent [89]. Although these isoenzymes are regulated quite differently, activation of either manifests as an elevation in intracellular cGMP [89]. The metabolism of cGMP by the phosphodiesteric cleavage of its 3′ bond is analogous to cAMP, except for the substrate preference of the phosphodiesterase [297,298].

The literature regarding the role of cGMP in vascular physiology is marked by controversy [45,302,311–320]. At first, opposite roles were postulated for cAMP and cGMP in the regulation of vascular smooth muscle tone [45]. This yin-yang hypothesis was based on observations of cGMP accumulations, coincident with unaltered cAMP levels, accompanying contractions induced by vasoconstricting hormones, and neurotransmitters [45,302,311]. Through better characterization of the soluble form of guanylate cyclase [311–314], these observations were reconciled with contradictory studies in which cGMP attenuated the actions of vasoconstrictors and accumulated preceding vasodilation induced by nitric oxide and related compounds [315–320]. The detailed study of nitrate biochemistry [303,315,316] and, more recently, of an EDRF that induces accumulations of cGMP in vascular smooth muscle [77,80,127] have led to our current appreciation of cGMP as a mediator of vasodilation.

The soluble form of guanylyl cyclase is activated independently of calcium by free radicals such as nitric oxide [321,322], superoxide [323], and peroxy- and hydroxyradicals [202] and is modulated by the effects of cellular pH [315]. The activation of guanylyl cyclase is critically dependent on the redox state of the vicinal dithiols at the activator site, and a heme moiety in the activation site participates in enzyme activation [324]. On activation by nitric oxide–generating agents, nitric oxide is bound to the heme group; sulfhydryl oxidase and thiol alkalating agents rapidly inactivate the enzyme [321,325].

Although the precise mechanism whereby guanylate cyclase activation occurs is not understood, the lack of a calcium requirement for enzyme activation is clearly evident. A feedback regulatory role for cGMP in the vasoconstrictor response is proposed to explain the earlier observation of calcium-dependent accumulations of cGMP accompanying but not preceding contraction [279]. At the biochemical level, calcium mobilization during contraction may activate phospholipase A_2 to release arachidonate, which presumably undergoes oxidated conversion to compounds that stimulate guanylate cyclase. In support of this theory, the soluble enzyme is activated by prostaglandin endoperoxides and fatty acid hydroperoxides [202]. cGMP also plays a direct vasodilatory role in endothelium-dependent relaxation mediated by an EDRF [77,80,127]. This factor has been identified as nitric oxide [77], and a causal role for cGMP in its mechanism of action has been described [80,127].

In retina, a G protein is coupled to a cGMP phosphodiesterase, interacting to convert a light signal into a decrease in cGMP levels [326]. This raises the possibility of a similar transducing mechanism in vascular smooth muscle (see Fig. 3-3); a common membrane regulatory mechanism modulated by specific phosphodiesterase might therefore exist for both cyclic nucleotides.

cGMP-dependent protein kinases are present in soluble and particulate fractions of vascular smooth muscle cells and are the major receptor proteins for cGMP [89,302,327]. By activation of protein kinases, the phosphorylation of certain proteins is favored that then act to prevent calcium accumulation and possibly to inhibit contractile function directly; this mechanism thus facilitates smooth muscle relaxation. cGMP-dependent protein kinases stimulate the efflux of calcium by the plasma membrane calcium ATPase pump [327–329], prevent phosphatidylinositol hydrolysis [330], abolish calcium-dependent action potentials in aortic smooth muscle [308], and enhance the dephosphorylation of myosin light-chain kinase [89,299]. The spectrum of proteins phosphorylated by cGMP-dependent kinases in smooth muscle is distinct from those phosphorylated by cAMP, although some overlap does exist [299,331]. This evidence points to different regulatory functions for these cyclic nucleotides, despite their common vasoinhibitory effect on vascular smooth muscle.

The Calcium Messenger System

Calcium appears to have a nearly universal role in stimulus-response coupling of vascular smooth muscle, and its messenger function is intimately related to the other major intracellular transducing cascades rather than serving as an independent regulatory mechanism [282] (see Fig. 3-5). To initiate flow of information, a change must occur either in transmembrane calcium flux or in calcium concentration within the local microenvironment of an effector protein or transiently throughout the cell [269,282,289]. The central role of the sarcoplasmic reticulum in this regard has already received brief mention in the overview of phosphoinositide hydrolysis and will be covered in greater detail in the discussion of excitation-contraction coupling (see the next section, "Functional Response: Biochemistry and Molecular Events"). Furthermore, the modulation of calcium availability as it critically pertains to phosphoinositide turnover and the cyclic nucleotides is addressed in the context of those respective discussions and will not be reviewed again here.

Calcium also enters the cell directly via potential-sensitive or receptor-operated channels [26,310]. Potential-sensitive calcium channels are ubiquitous in all smooth muscle cells, although they tend to be sparser in electrically inexcitable vascular smooth muscle (i.e., tissue that does not generate an action potential with depolarization) [290]. Receptor-operated channels may sensitize the cell by shifting membrane potential closer to the threshold for activation by potential-sensitive channels [290], but the relative importance of these channels in facilitating calcium entry is receptor system specific.

Plasmalemma phospholipids are an additional candidate source for activator calcium. Phosphotidylserine molecules avidly bind calcium under resting conditions and release calcium on cell depolarization [291]. Along the inner membrane, calcium binding to acidic phosphotidylinositol moieties is sensitive to changes in the physical properties of the membrane, particularly those mediated by activation of specific surface receptors [291]. Thus, intracellular organelles, gated calcium channels, and the plasmalemma are all potential sources of activator calcium, and the relative contributions made by each need to be established for different physiologic responses. For the coupling between excitation and contraction, the major source of activator calcium remains controversial. Somlyo strongly favors the sarcoplasmic reticulum as the principal cellular site of calcium regulation [267,292,293], despite its small volume in smooth muscle, but support for other candidate sources exists as well [45,291].

Inside the cell, the site of calcium action is its receptor protein calmodulin. Calcium binding induces conformational and functional changes in calmodulin that are directly determined by the degree of calcium-ion saturation of the four binding sites on the protein, with at least three calcium ions required for target protein activation [294]. A variety of calmodulin-regulated enzymes with different proposed functions have been described [295]. The activation of protein kinases and phosphatases by the association of calcium with calmodulin is considered a central theme in calcium signal processing. The ATP-dependent phosphorylation by kinases and the dephosphorylation of cell-specific substrate proteins by phosphatases, which alters their structural and kinetic functions, is the major means by which calcium translates its biochemical signal into a physiologic response [269]. An example of this biochemical regulation in smooth muscle is the activation of calmodulin-dependent myosin light-chain kinase, resulting in a phosphorylated form of myosin that can interact with actin to cause smooth muscle contraction [269]. Calcium can also activate other kinases, such as the phospholipid-dependent protein kinase C, independent of calmodulin [45].

Complex changes in intracellular calcium metabolism tend to be transient and subtle due to highly proficient mechanisms acting to maintain calcium homeostasis [269,296]. When calcium concentrations change, compensatory mechanisms militate against it. Although the feedback mechanisms are diverse, the calcium-calmodulin complex has an important autoregulatory role in this process [269,296].

FUNCTIONAL RESPONSE: BIOCHEMISTRY AND MOLECULAR EVENTS

Contraction

EXCITATION-CONTRACTION COUPLING

The first section of this chapter described the mechanisms of cell excitation by receptor systems located on the cell surface and via the intrinsic electrical properties of the plasmalemma. The maintenance of a resting ionic gradient is a fundamental property of all cells that facilitates propagation and transmission of messages by electrical conduction. In smooth muscle, electrical modulation of cell force generation is referred to as electromechanical coupling. Although spike generation is involved in triggering contraction, tension may be regulated by depolarizations in quiescent smooth muscle that does not generate action potentials. It is also clear that contraction can occur by processes that are independent of cell depolarization; this is referred to as pharmacomechanical coupling [332]. Thus, pharmacologic contractions may be elicited by electromechanical (variable-frequency spike electrogenesis and graded depolarizations) and pharmacomechanical means [332], and it is likely that under physiologic conditions both processes contribute to activation simultaneously [107].

Comprehensive reviews of the electrophysiology of cell excitation are cited here for the interested reader [29,45,107]. It is remarkable that detailed mechanisms responsible for pharmacologic modulation of membrane potential are to a large extent unknown. The available evidence favors mechanisms acting primarily through regulation of passive-ion permeabilities and, occasionally, electrogenic ion transport; changes in ion binding to fixed-membrane charges represent a less well established proposal [107]. Similarly, the recent evidence in favor of IP_3 as an intracellular messenger in pharmacomechanical coupling of vascular smooth muscle notwithstanding [265,266,333], the molecular details of voltage-independent events as influenced by various excitatory agents are not known. What generally is agreed on is that neither mechanism triggers contraction directly but acts through the calcium mediator [107]. Moreover, the influx of calcium resulting directly from an electrochemical gradient or induced by pharmacologic agents, without a concomitant change in membrane potential (i.e., via receptor-operated channels), cannot account alone for contraction,

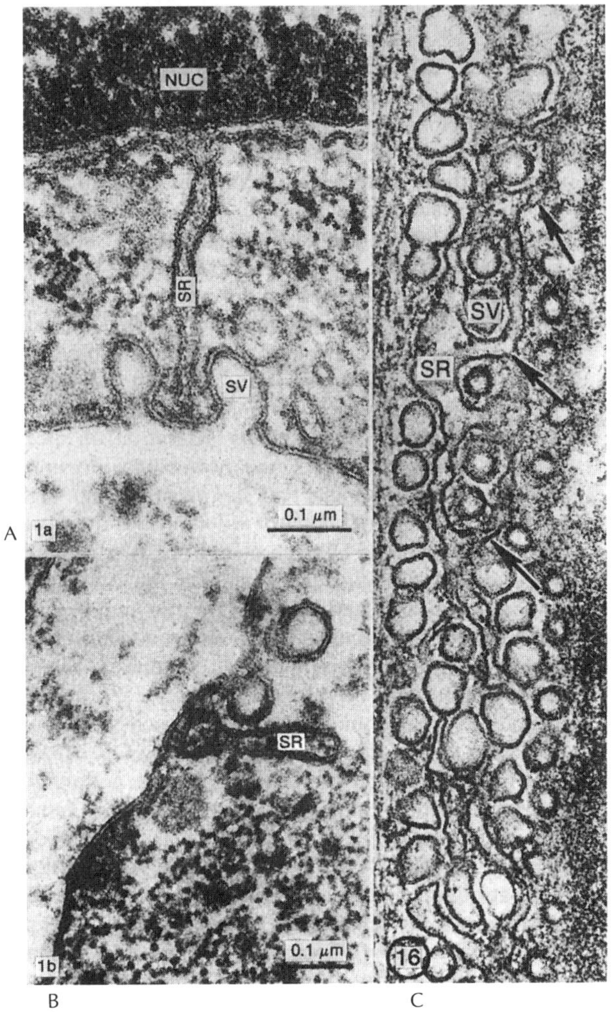

Fig. 3-6. A portion of a transversely sectioned smooth muscle cell from the portal anterior mesenteric vein showing an element of sarcoplasmic reticulum (SR), the lumen of which is continuous with the perinuclear space is shown **A.,** and an SR surface coupling with an approximately 12- to 20-nm junctional gap between the SR and the plasma membrane **B.** The SR also forms a fenestrated network running between and sometimes encircling (arrows) the surface vesicles **C.** NUC = nucleus; SR ⇒q sarcoplasmic reticulum; SV = surface vesicles. (Photos A and B reprinted with permission from AV Somlyo and C Franzini-Armstrong. New views of smooth muscle structure using freezing, deep-etching and rotary shadowing. Experientia 1985; 41:841–856. C reprinted with permission from AP Somlyo and AV Somlyo. Ultrastructure of smooth muscle. In EE Daniel, DM Paton, eds. Methods in Pharmacology, vol. 3. New York: Plenum, 1975. Pp. 3–43.)

because calcium does not enter in sufficient quantities [107,267]. Therefore, the calcium influx is probably most important in other intracellular regulatory events [29,267]. These considerations aside, the cellular process by which calcium links the excitatory events of the plasma membrane to activation of contractile proteins in the cell cytoplasm is known as excitation-contraction coupling.

SOURCES OF CALCIUM

There is no dispute over the requisite rise in intracellular ionized calcium for generation of force that resides in the interaction between actin and myosin filaments of smooth muscle [334]. There are four potential candidate pools of activator calcium: (1) the extracellular space, (2) calcium bound to the plasmalemma, (3) the sarcoplasmic reticulum, and (4) the mitochondria [45,107,267]. Excitatory surface events, whether or not associated with changes in membrane potential, trigger the influx of calcium and also facilitate its release from intracellular sources. The contributions of each of these pools to contractile activation during physiologic contraction is a matter of considerable controversy [267,291]. The following discussion reviews the ultrastructural aspects of the membrane systems regulating these sources of calcium and summarizes their contributory roles in physiologic contraction.

Plasma Membrane. Transmission electron micrographs demonstrate the trilaminar appearance of smooth muscle surface membranes characteristic of eukaryotic cells [267]. The membrane can be arbitrarily divided into three structural domains: invaginated caveolae, regions specialized for coupling to intracellular organelles, and the so-called nonspecialized membrane [267]. Invaginated caveolae are surface vesicles that aggregate in a linear fashion along the longitudinal axis of the cell and exist in direct contact with the extra cellular space [335] (Fig. 3-6). These vesicles also form elongated aggregates resembling beads on a string [336,337]; they are believed to represent the functional smooth muscle equivalent of the T tubules of striated muscle. As such, they have been implicated in ion transfer between intracellular organelles [45]. The surface vesicles are also coupled to adjacent sarcoplasmic reticulum across narrow (12-20 nm) spaces by small, electron-dense structures [267,336]. These specializations are known as surface couplings and are thought to represent sites of calcium release during action potentials [45,336] (Fig. 3-7). The possibility that calcium stores in the sarcoplasmic reticulum can be directly replenished from the extracellular space via channels within these bridging structures, rather than indirectly via the cytoplasm, requires verification [267,335]. The nonspecialized surface membrane is occupied by dense bodies that are made up of actin-binding proteins and that serve as attachment sites for actin filaments [267].

The plasma membrane regulates two of the four potential sources of activator calcium: the extracellular pool and membrane-bound calcium. In the latter instance, sialic acid residues on glycoproteins and glycolipids composing the external lamina of the membrane [45] and particular phospholipids [338] have each been proposed as sites of calcium binding. The functional aspects of the participation of the plasma membrane in calcium regulation have been studied by the use of agents that selectively alter transmembrane calcium flux [45]. Some agents used for this purpose are calcium-chelating agents; lanthanum, which blocks calcium transmembrane flux while displacing superficially bound and extracellular calcium; calcium channel blockers; and neuraminidase, which removes si-

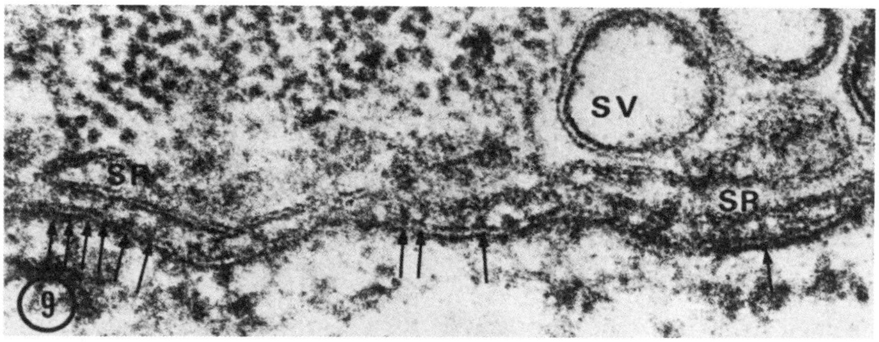

Fig. 3-7. High-magnification view of an SR-surface membrane coupling. Electron-opaque material (arrows) is present between the SR membrane and the plasma membrane. SV = surface vesicle. Trialdehyde with DMSO/osmium fixation. Portal anterior mesenteric vein: × 249,500. (Reproduced with permission from AP Somlyo and AV Somlyo. Ultrastructure of smooth muscle. In EE Daniel, DM Paton, eds. Methods in Pharmacology, vol. 3. New York: Plenum, 1975. Pp. 3–43.)

alic acid residues [45]. These studies have been complemented by electron probe analyses of calcium content in rapidly frozen tissue, which permits the intracellular localization of calcium and the measurement of calcium content with high sensitivity [292].

There is extensive evidence that excitatory agents increase calcium influx across the plasma membrane [107,267], but studies indicate that agents utilize plasmalemma-regulated calcium to differing extents in the generation of contraction [45]. Moreover, the increase in calcium contraction induced by an action potential is about 5 μM, and the requirement for maximal contraction is 40 to 50 times this amount [267]. Thus, variable degrees of calcium influx are observed under different experimental conditions in association with contraction, and the calcium requirement for contraction significantly exceeds the transmembrane contribution. These findings have led Somlyo to question the contribution of extracellular calcium to activation of contraction and to propose, instead, its role as a charge carrier in the depolarizing current [267]. Alternatively, calcium influx may play an indirect facilitatory role in contraction by activation of calmodulin-stimulated effector proteins that are sensitive to small rises in intracellular calcium in the range observed during cell depolarization [294].

The contribution of membrane-bound calcium to excitation-contraction coupling has not been resolved. The fundamental requirement that this calcium be amenable to mobilization by excitatory events initiating physiologic contraction has experimental backing. Certain membrane phospholipids lose their affinity for calcium in response to depolarization [339] and to receptor-mediated changes in the physical properties of the membrane [340,341]. In contrast, the likelihood that only small amounts of calcium are bound relative to the total requirement for contraction is in conflict with a major role for this calcium in contractile protein activation [267]. Membrane-bound calcium may indirectly influence the intracellular calcium concentration by its involvement in mechanisms that modulate membrane permeability [267]. This area of investigation requires further attention.

Sarcoplasmic Reticulum. The sarcoplasmic reticulum is a true intracellular system of tubules that functions in calcium uptake, release, and storage [336]. The smooth endoplasmic reticulum is in continuity with the rough endoplasmic reticulum and with the perinuclear space; it also forms a fenestrated network between caveolae that are in contact with the extracellular space (see Figs. 3-6 and 3-7) and in close proximity to mitochondria [336]. Surface couplings between plasma membrane and the sarcoplasmic reticulum are formed by bridging structures, and elements of sarcoplasmic reticulum may further intersperse between mitochondria and caveolae [336]. These ultrastructural associations suggest a functional association in regulation of calcium transfer.

The volume occupied by the sarcoplasmic reticulum in smooth muscle varies from 1.5 to 7.5 percent and directly correlates with the ability of smooth muscle to contract in a calcium-free medium [267,335]. However, the calcium content of the sarcoplasmic reticulum occupying even very small volumes is sufficient for contraction [342,343], and therefore its relative sparsity in vascular smooth muscle does not appear to detract from its contractile role [267]. On the other hand, the volume it occupies may have functional significance. Phasic smooth muscle that generates action potentials contains more sarcoplasmic reticulum than tonic smooth muscle that responds to excitation by graded depolarizations [45].

The release of calcium from sarcoplasmic reticulum by excitatory stimuli has been well documented in calcium-free and depolarized cell systems [342]. These experiments have provided supportive evidence that pharmacomechanical coupling is independent of extracellular calcium and mediated by calcium release from sarcoplasmic reticulum. Two factors implicate IP_3 in pharmacomechanical calcium release [267]: the demonstration in tracheal smooth muscle that chemically mediated PIP_2 hydrolysis is voltage independent [333] and, in pulmonary and coronary artery, that IP_3 induces release of calcium from sarcoplasmic reticulum in association with contractions [265,266]. The analogous electromechanical events preceding calcium efflux from sarcoplasmic reticulum are unknown.

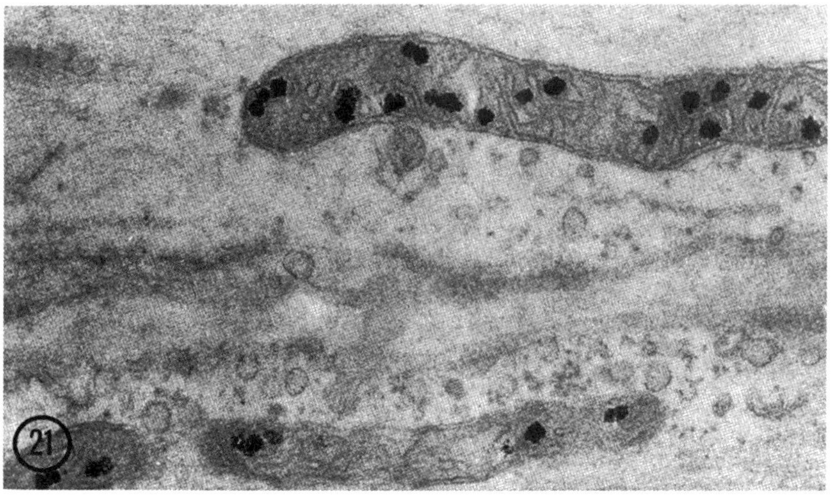

Fig. 3-8. High-magnification view of a longitudinal section from portal anterior mesenteric vein after 2-hour incubation in a Krebs solution containing 10 mM barium acetate. The two surrounding mitochondrial membranes and internal cristae are readily apparent. Dense deposits of barium can be seen in the mitochondria. No uranyl or lead stain. Primary osmium fixation. × 61,400. (Reproduced with permission from AP Somlyo and AV Somlyo. Ultrastructure of smooth muscle. In EE Daniel, DM Paton, eds. Methods in Pharmacology, vol. 3. New York: Plenum, 1975. Pp. 3–43.)

The sarcoplasmic reticulum plays an active role in smooth muscle relaxation. Marsh's early discovery that crude homogenates of skeletal muscle inhibit tension development [344] has since been attributed to the active microsomal component derived from sarcoplasmic reticulum [345]. Additional work confirmed that the relaxing effect is mediated by calcium sequestration [346]. The experiments that likewise demonstrate the energy-dependent calcium uptake capabilities of sarcoplasmic reticulum of smooth muscle are reviewed elsewhere [45,267].

Mitochondria. The mitochondria are oval intracellular organelles surrounded by two membranes (Fig. 3-8). The inner membrane system is highly convoluted, forming internal ridges known as cristae, which function in the respiratory cycle. Most of the important cellular biochemical reactions take place in the compartment bounded by the inner membrane called the matrix [347]. Whereas the inner membrane is intrinsically impermeable to most small molecules, the outer membrane is permeable to most ions that enter into the intermembrane space [347]. Mitochondria appear to be coupled functionally to other cellular systems. Surface membrane caveolae are found in close proximity to mitochondria (Fig. 3-9), and sarcoplasmic reticulum may intersperse between caveolae and mitochondria [336]. The formation of linear networks of surface caveolae may serve an ion-transfer purpose between mitochondria and sarcoplasmic reticulum [45].

Calcium in the mitochondrial matrix of vascular smooth muscle can be mobilized, although the efflux pathway is poorly understood [348,349]. Somlyo and colleagues have questioned the relevance of mitochondrial calcium release to contractile events [267]. By their calculations, the total mitochondrial calcium content of healthy smooth muscle is in the range to regulate mitochondrial enzymes but not sufficient to account for observed increases in intracellular calcium during contraction. They argue that the massive accumulations sometimes observed in mitochondria are characteristic of damaged cells and are not representative of physiologic contractions in situ [267]. These assumptions may be true, and yet they do not exclude a potential role for mitochondrial calcium in contractile events of atherosclerotic vasculature and in other pathologic conditions.

FORCE GENERATION

Smooth muscle shortens substantially during isotonic conditions. This remarkable feat is accomplished by the shortening of individual cells and is accompanied by rearrangement of the surface membrane and contractile apparatus [334,350]. Accordingly, geometric constraints are important considerations in the degree of shortening [334]. Active contraction that develops without a change in the length of the muscle is referred to as **isometric**, and knowledge of the structural rearrangements that occur is limited [334].

The development of tension concomitant with shortening resides in the interaction between actin and myosin filaments [334,350]. In the prevailing view of the contraction mechanism, myofilament length remains constant; thus, the myofilaments slide past one another during active shortening while changing their orientation to the cell axis [334]. The force generated during contraction is transmitted from the contractile apparatus to the cell membrane via actin insertions into membrane-dense bodies (Fig. 3-10). These insertion sites are distributed over

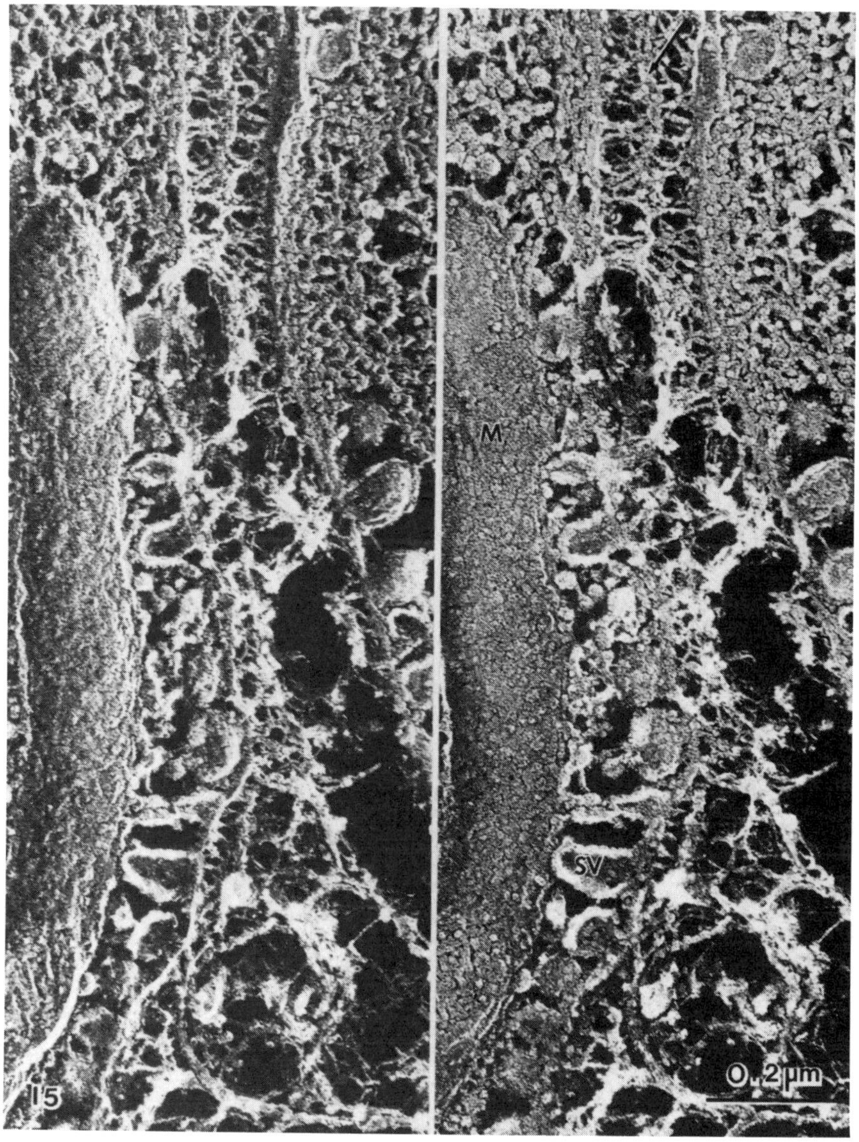

Fig. 3-9. Stereo ± 7% from rabbit portal anterior mesenteric vein showing mitochondria (M) and surface vesicles (SV) in close proximity. An intermediate junction or attachment plaque (arrow) is also shown. Tissue prepared by deep etching and rotary shadowing. The basement-membrane fibrils are attached to the cell membrane at right angles. (Reproduced with permission from AV Somlyo and C Franzini-Armstrong. New views of smooth muscle structure using freezing, deep-etching and rotary shadowing. Experientia 1985; 41:841–856.)

the length of the cell membrane, thereby dispersing myofilament pull over the entire cell [334]. Intermediate filaments generally are attached to dense bodies and may play a role in force transmission from contractile apparatus to the surface cytoskeleton [334] (see Fig. 3-10). These filaments are not continuous with either actin or myosin, however, and their exact function is unknown [336,351]. The cell-to-cell propagation of electrical depolarization via gap junctions results in recruitment of additional cells in the contractile response [267]. The transmission and coordination of contractile force from cell to cell occur through other sites of direct adherence, namely, intermediate and adherence-type junction and other nonspecialized regions [336,352]. Connections via the glycoprotein fibronectin may mediate the transmission of force from the cell to the surrounding stroma [334]. Fibronectin is found in the close vicinity of the vascular smooth muscle cell [353] and has a strong affinity for both intracellular actin [354] and extracellular collagen [355]; further cross-linkage details remain to be established.

An increase in cellular ionized calcium triggers the interaction between myosin and actin—thus, the "coupling" role of calcium. The intracellular calcium transient correlates directly with phosphorylation of the light chain of myosin and the maximal shortening velocity of the muscle [309,350] (Fig. 3-11). Whereas speed of contraction

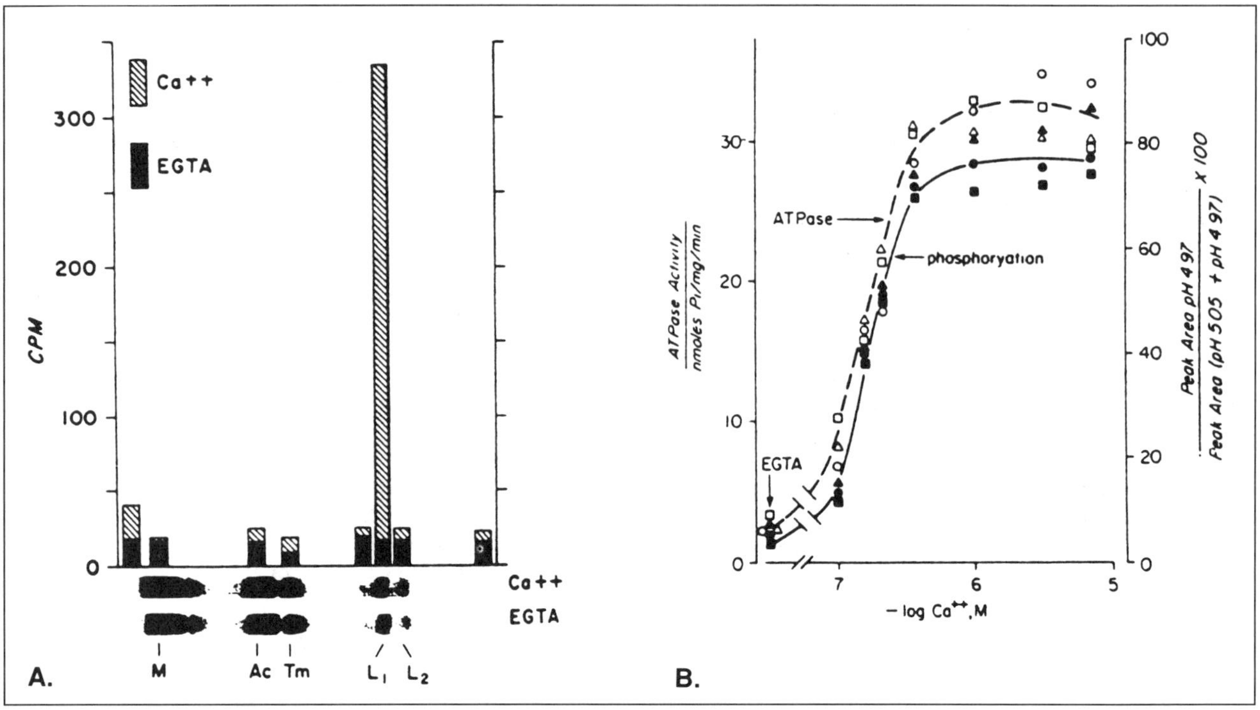

Fig. 3-10. **A.** Incorporation of ^{32}P from ATP. ^{32}P (cpm, ordinate) is shown for different regions of SDS gels (shown at bottom) prepared from reaction mixtures containing 1 mg actomyosin/ml. Striped bars show incorporation of ^{32}P in the presence of 10^{-5} M Ca^{2+}, whereas solid bars show incorporation in the presence of 1 mM EGTA. Major bands and corresponding molecular weights (daltons) are M (myosin 200,000), Ac (actin 45,000), Tm (Tropomyosin 37,000), L_1 (first light chain 15,000), and L_2 (second light chain 13,000). **B.** Relationships are shown between the concentration of Ca^{2+} in the reaction mixture (abscissa) and specific activity of Mg^{++}-stimulated actomyosin ATPase (left ordinate), and between Ca^{2+} and phosphorylated peptide detected during isoelectric focusing (right ordinate). Results are given for three different preparations identified by different symbols. The extent of phosphorylation is expressed as the ratio of the peak area of the phosphorylated polypeptide (pH 4.97) to the sum of the parent nonphosphorylated band (pH 5.05) plus the phosphorylated band (pH 4.97). (Reproduced with permission from J DiSalvo, E Gruenstein, and P Silver. Ca^{2+}-dependent phosphorylation of bovine aortic actomyosin. Proc Soc Exp Biol Med 1978; 158:410–414.)

is therefore a function of myosin ATPase activity [356], force of contraction is a function of the number and arrangement of force-generating interactions between mysoin and actin and can be maintained at low energy cost [357–359]. Tonic contractions of smooth muscle are explained by a "latch-bridge" mechanism between myosin and actin in which tension is maintained at relatively low ATP cost, calcium consumption, and myosin phosphorylation [358,359].

The conversion of chemical energy into mechanical force is a process intimately related to and dependent on high-energy phosphate metabolism. ATP, ADP, AMP, and phosphocreatine (PCr) are the major high-energy phosphate constituents of vascular smooth muscle [360]. ATP, however, is the sole phosphagen utilized directly in the course of mechanochemical force transduction, during which the energy released from ATP hydrolysis is stored in the heavy meromyosin molecule [45,269]. It is assumed that this energy powers the sliding mechanism of contraction resulting from actin-myosin interaction [361]. The conformational change in myosin occurring with this movement presumably exposes a site where ATP binds, which in turn causes myosin detachment from actin [361]. Thus, ATP is not a requirement for linkage of myosin to actin but rather for their dissociation. In light of the critical role of ATP in the transformation of chemical energy into mechanical force, the biochemistry of this event centers around ATP synthesis and consumption.

Vascular smooth muscle cells utilize carbohydrates, proteins, and lipids as substrates for energy generation [362]. Under stimulated conditions, free fatty acids are the preferred substrates to support basal energy processes [363]. The concept that oxidative phosphorylation is specifically coupled to tension generation and maintenance has now been substantiated. ATP utilization by myosin ATPase increases rapidly before declining to steady-state levels that are contributed to by ATP production via oxidative phosphorylation [363]. The degradation of glycogen in coordination with muscle activation suggests that it is an oxidative substrate in the early stages of tension generation and maintenance [363]. Other high-energy phosphates represent potential short-term ATP reserves

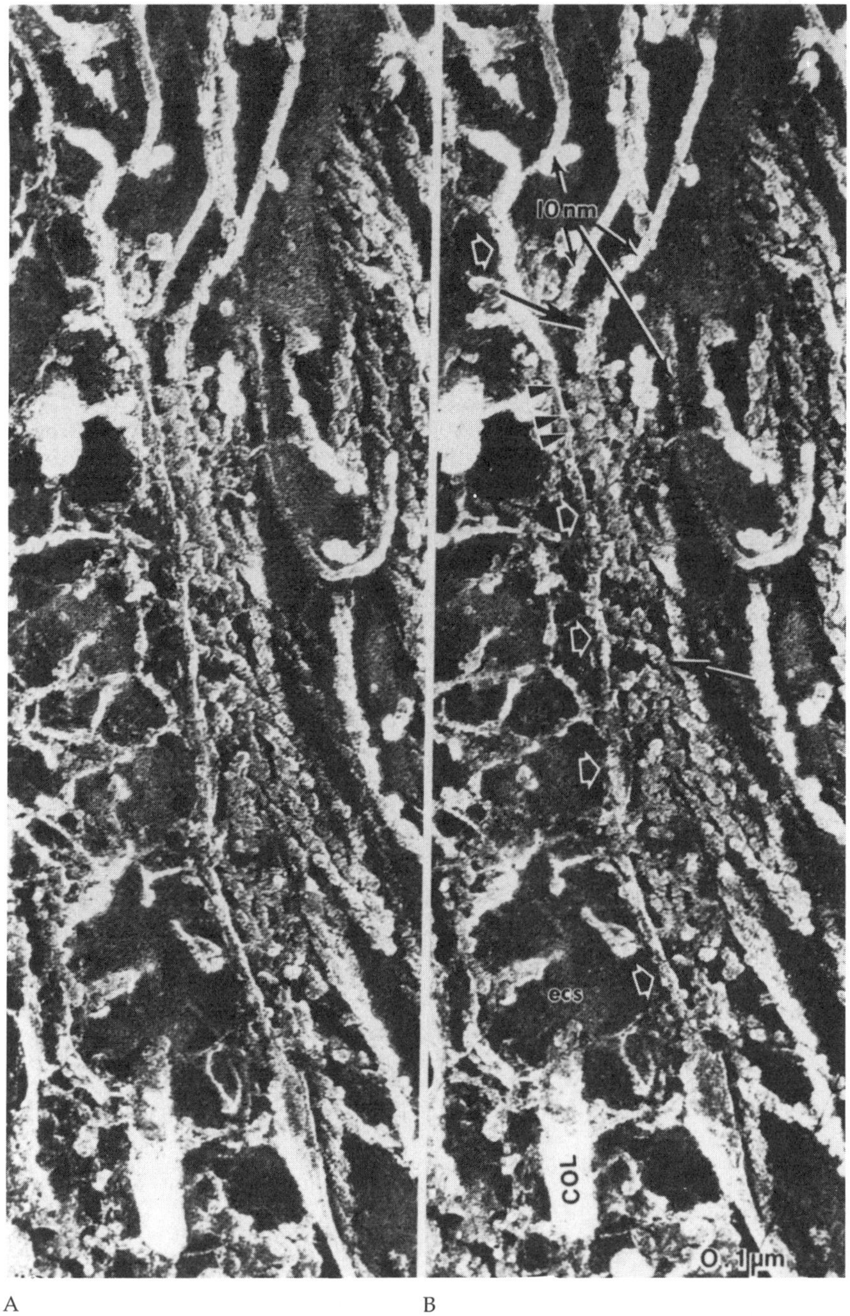

Fig. 3-11. Stereo tilt pair ±7-degree longitudinal view of a portion of two cells (**A.** and **B.**) and the intervening extracellular space (ECS) from rabbit vas deferens, showing another cell membrane–associated dense body where the inserting filaments lie parallel to the long axis of the cell. The extent of the dense body is indicated by the five open white arrows, the actin S_1-decorated filaments terminate in granular material (large arrow), which appears attached to the cell membrane (arrowheads). 10-nm filaments (small arrows) are, in general, associated with smooth muscle dense bodies. The middle 10-nm filament shown at the top of the print has remained within the fracture plane and can be followed until it terminates in granular material at the cell membrane. The actin associated with the dense body is decorated with myosin-S_1 fairly close to its region of insertion on the membrane. Extracellular fibrils insert on the outer aspect of the cell membrane and are attaching to collagen (COL) fibers. (Reproduced with permission from AV Somlyo and C Franzini-Armstrong. New views of smooth muscle structure using freezing, deep-etching and rotary shadowing. Experientia 1985; 41:841–856.)

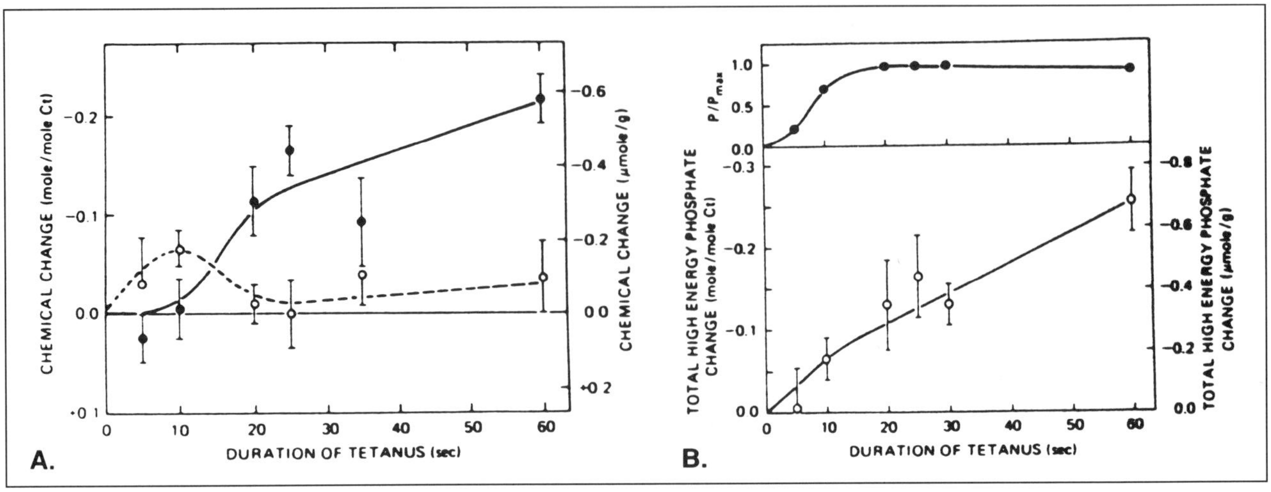

Fig. 3-12. **A.** ATP and PCr changes during isometric tetani of different durations in rabbit taeniae coli at 18°C. Muscles were frozen immediately on cessation of stimulus and compared to paired unstimulated controls. (●) = △ PCr; (○) = △ ATP. n = 5 for 5-, 25-, and 60-s tetani, and 6 for all others. **B.** Total high-energy phosphate and active force development during isometric tetani in rabbit taeniae coli at 18°C. (○) = △ ATP + △ PCr − △ AMP. Standard errors for P/P_{max} (●) are 0.01 for 20 and 25 s; 0.02 for 5, 10, and 35 s; and 0.04 for 60 s; n = 7. (Reproduced with permission from TM Butler et al. Chemical energetics of single isometric tetani in mammalian smooth muscle. Am J Physiol 1978; 235:C1–C7.)

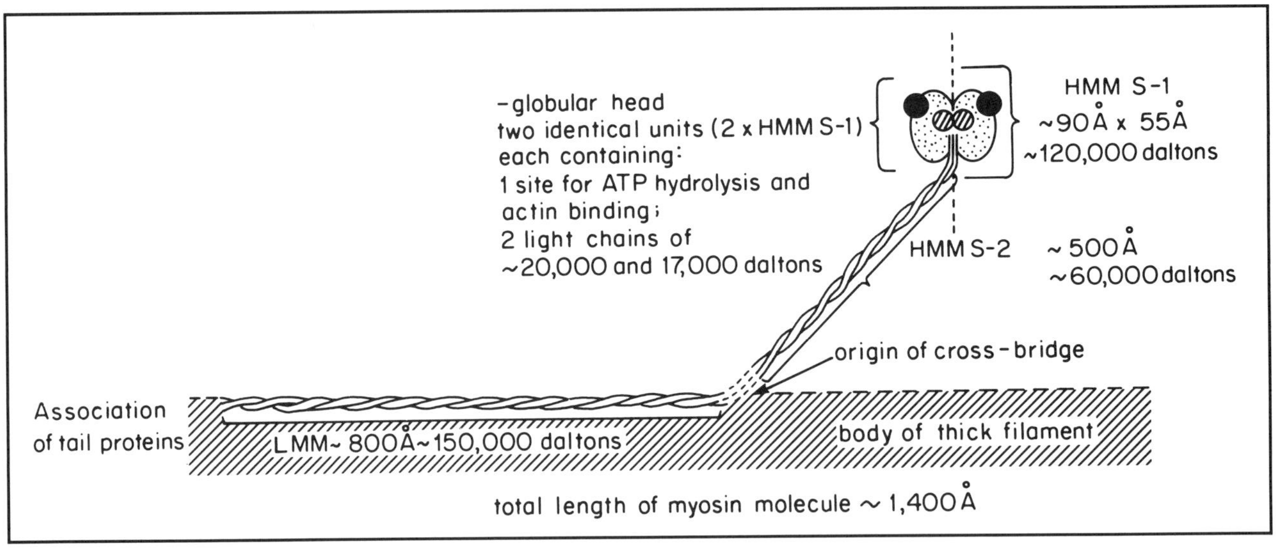

Fig. 3-13. Diagrammatic representation of the myosin molecule. Coiled-coil alpha-helical portion of the molecule is depicted as a ropelike structure. At the origin of the cross-bridge, that is, at one end of the heavy meromyosin subfragment 2 (HMM S-2) molecule, it is now known whether the alpha-helical structure is retained (dashed line). The position of the four light chains (shown as the smaller circles in the globular head) is completely arbitrary. Conformation of the globular head differs from the rest of the molecule in that it is not predominantly an alpha-helix, and this difference is presented diagrammatically. LMM = light meromyosin; HMM S-1 = heavy meromyosin subfragment 1. (Reproduced with permission from DJ Hartshorne and A Gorecka. Biochemistry of the contractile proteins of smooth muscle. In DF Bohr, AP Somlyo, HV Sparks, eds. The Handbook of Physiology: Section 2, The Cardiovascular System, Vascular Smooth Muscle. New York: Oxford University Press, 1980. Pp. 93–120.)

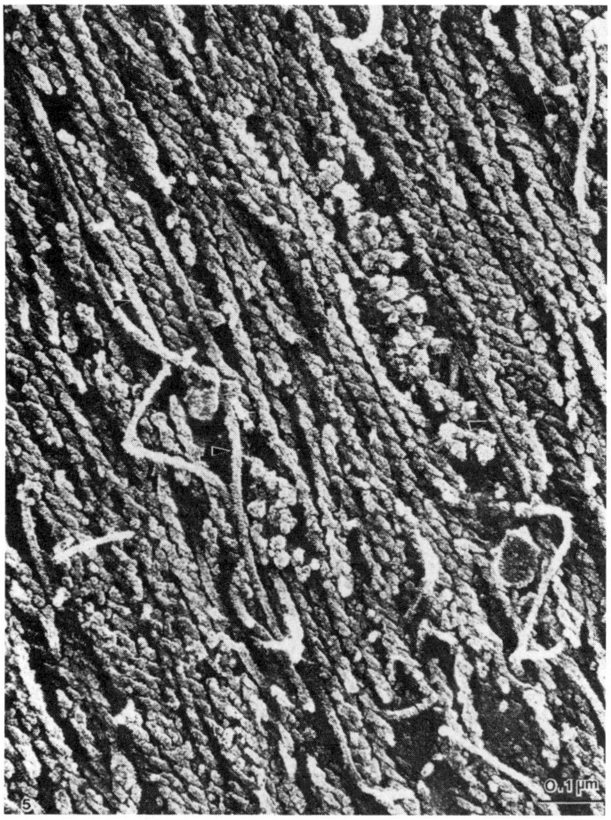

Fig. 3-14. Longitudinal section of saponin-skinned rabbit portal anterior mesenteric vein portion of a smooth muscle cell, incubated with a skeletal muscle myosin subfragment (S_1) prior to fixation, freezing, deep-etching, and rotary shadowing. The ropelike structures are myosin S_1–decorated actin, which shows a strong 38-nm half repeat. Smooth 10-nm filaments are indicated by arrowheads. (Reproduced with permission from AV Somlyo and C Franzini-Armstrong. New Views of smooth muscle structure using freezing, deep-etching and rotary shadowing. Experientia 1985; 41:841–856.)

by acting as reactants in ATP-recovery reactions. As in skeletal muscle, reactions catalyzed by creatinine kinase (PCr + ADP ⇄ ATP + Cr) and myokinase (2ADP ⇄ ATP + AMP) provide a means for ATP generation in activated muscle [360,362]. The PCr content of smooth muscle is approximately one-fifteenth the amount found in skeletal muscle, and most smooth muscle ADP is bound to actin; thus, the reserve potential of the recovery pathways in smooth muscle is limited [362]. To compensate for a less efficient ATP-generating mechanism, vascular smooth muscle contraction is characterized by slower-maintained contractions at low ATP cost, in sharp contrast to the fast, brief, high-energy contractions of skeletal muscle. Accordingly, levels of high-energy phosphates bear a relationship to the **rate** of force development. ATP content should not, however, be confused with maximal force-generating capacity, which is a function of the number of interactions between actin and myosin acting in parallel and sarcomere length [334,336]. Consequently, the maximal force generated by smooth muscle is comparable to that developed by skeletal muscle [334,336].

The accurate determination of ATP and PCr requirements during activation of contraction, force development, force maintenance, and relaxation of skeletal muscle are well documented. Unfortunately, a similarly detailed accounting of smooth muscle energetics has not been easy to come by. This area of investigation is poorly studied, fraught with technical difficulties, and full of inconsistencies [360]. Despite these limitations, the following important conclusions have been reached:

1. The ATP and PCr contents of smooth muscle in the resting state and during isometric contraction are lower than those of skeletal muscle [360,362].
2. The ATP content of vascular smooth muscle is not sufficient to sustain mechanical activity for more than a brief period [363].
3. During isometric tetanus, ATP levels decline initially, with subsequent resynthesis and normalization of levels within 25 seconds from the onset of contraction. In this time frame, PCr content at first remains constant, falling rapidly thereafter [364]. PCr usage then continues at a slower rate over the first minute [364] (Fig. 3-12A). These data demonstrate that changes in ATP content signal the onset of contraction and that ATP resynthesis heralds the recruitment of ATP recovery reactions (i.e., PCr hydrolysis) [364].
4. The average rate of energy used during muscle activation and force development is much greater than that required for force maintenance [364] (Fig. 3-12B).
5. The energy usage during muscle relaxation is small in comparison with stimulation requirements [360].
6. The rigor state of vascular smooth muscle, characterized by increased stiffness (resistance to stretch) of muscle in association with depleted ATP stores, bears a strong resemblance to the rigor state of skeletal muscle [360]. In both, in the absence of ATP, actin and myosin bind tightly without means for dissociation [360,361]. The importance of this concept of rigor state lies in the ability of (smooth) muscle to generate substantial force in an energy-depleted state [360,361].

Molecular Components of the Contractile Apparatus

MYOSIN. Myosin molecules are long fibrous structures composed of an alpha-helical portion that comprises two coiled subunits and two globular heads [350] (Fig. 3-13). The shape and size of myosin from different molecules is uniform, and the molecular weight is approximately 470,000 daltons [350]. Enzymatic treatment of myosin with trypsin separates it into heavy and light meromyosin. The former fibroprotein makes up the protruding bridge portion of myosin and is separated from the tail portion of the molecule by a functional "hinge" [350]. The association of approximately 200 myosin tails form the body of the thick filament [45]. Heavy meromyosin is further divided into an alpha-helical S2 segment (HMM S-2) and globular S1 heads (HMM S-1). The globular heads represent the operational site of myosin, and each contains an attachment site for actin, an enzymatic site for ATP

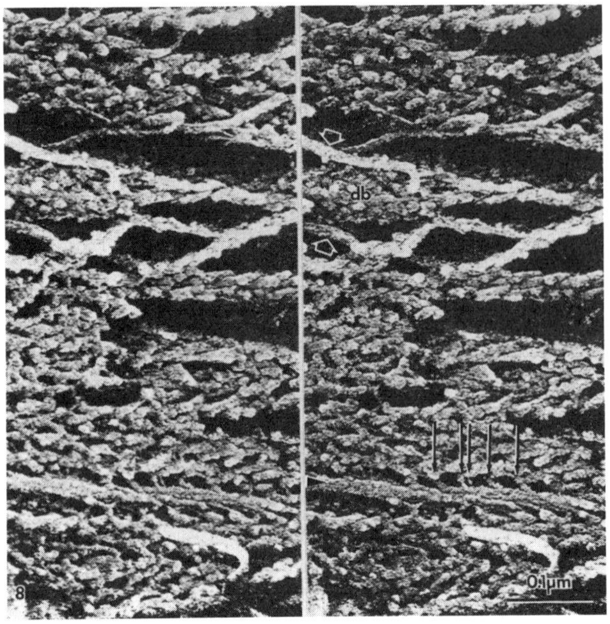

Fig. 3-15. Stereo pair ± 7 degree tilt of a portion of a frozen, deep-etched, rotary-shadowed smooth muscle cell from rabbit vas deferens. A longitudinally oriented myosin filament (arrowhead) is shown running across the lower portion of the print, with its cross-bridges (arrows) attached to adjacent S_1-decorated actin. A portion of cytoplasmic dense body (db) shown in the upper part of the print with its accompanying 10-nm filaments (white arrows) has a rather granular appearance. S_1-decorated actin appears to emerge from the right end of the dense body. (Reproduced with permission from AV Somlyo and C Franzini-Armstrong. New views of smooth muscle structure using freezing, deep-etching and rotary shadowing. Experientia 1985; 41:841–856.)

hydrolysis to provide energy for contraction, and two classes of myosin light chains with molecular weights of 17,000 and 20,000 Daltons [350]. The 20,000-Daltons light chain undergoes phosphorylation in the initiation of the contractile process; the function of the smaller light chain is not known.

ACTIN. Filamentous actin (F-actin) is a double-stranded, helical filament formed by noncovalent polymerization of single-chain G-actin monomers of molecular weight 42,000 [336] (Fig. 3-14). Actin from different sources is remarkably similar, but minor differences do exist [350]. The functional roles of actin in the contractile process include (1) its ability to activate the magnesium ATPase of HMM S-1 [45,350], (2) the ability to bind tropomyosin [336], and (3) the transmission of force generated by the sliding heavy meromyosin to the dense bodies of the cell membrane [334]. Actin is the major component of the thin filament.

TROPOMYOSIN. Tropomyosin is composed of two similar subunits arranged in an alpha-helical configuration [350]. In contrast to its thin-filament cohabitant, however, tropomyosin's subunit composition is not identical in all smooth muscle [350]. Thus, the molecular weight of tropomyosin varies from 70,000 to 80,000 Daltons. Significantly, these minor variations, which probably result from coding by similar but not identical genes [365], appear to have no functional relevance [350].

Tropomyosin lies within the two grooves of the actin filament and shifts position during activation [350]. In smooth muscle, the functional significance of this movement is unknown. Calcium-sensitive troponin, which regulates tropomyosin movement in skeletal muscle to expose the active site of actin for interaction with HMM S-1 [366,367], is absent from the smooth muscle thin filament [366]. Furthermore, the evidence supporting a facilitatory role of tropomyosin in smooth muscle contraction by stimulation of ATPase activity [368] directly contrasts with the inhibitory role of its skeletal-muscle counterpart.

DENSE BODIES AND DENSE BANDS. Membrane-associated electron-dense material measuring up to 2 μ in length is distributed over the entire cytoplasmic side of the cell surface [334]. During contraction, these regions of the plasma membrane retract, supporting their purported role in the transmission of force from contractile proteins to the cell surface [334]. The term **dense band**, used to describe this material, is to be distinguished from **dense body**, which refers to similar free-floating dense material in the cell cytoplasm [334,336]. Actin filaments are seen to insert into both types of dense material, and intermediate 10-nm filaments are associated with both, suggesting a common function [369,370] (Fig. 3-15; also see Fig. 3-10). In addition, both the membrane-apposed and free forms contain the protein alpha actinin (molecular weight 100,000), which acts to cross-link actin filaments, further supporting the notion of a common function [371]. On the other hand, vinculin, a 130,000-molecular-weight protein involved in binding actin to the cell membrane, may be absent from dense bodies [372]. Thus, the degree of similarity in composition and function between dense bands and dense bodies remains to be clarified.

RELATIONS OF CONTRACTILE PROTEINS. Under resting conditions, actin and myosin lie parallel to one another [334]. In vascular smooth muscle, actin filaments outnumber myosin filaments approximately 15 to 1 and are arranged in rosettes around myosin [373–375] (Fig. 3-16). In cell cross sections, the ratio of myosin to dense bodies is 5 to 1 [369]. The interaction of the myosin head with actin points away from the membrane dense body into which the actin filaments insert, which is evidence for actin filament polarization [334]. Tropomyosin molecules are located in the two grooves of the actin filament in a ratio of actin to tropomyosin of approximately 7 to 1 [45,336]. It has been suggested that the ordering of contractile proteins as they relate to a common discrete dense body represents a contractile unit. But strong evidence in favor of such organization in smooth muscle does not exist [334,336].

Regulatory Mechanisms. We do not fully understand the exact mechanism(s) by which smooth muscle contraction is regulated. It now appears that a variety of complex regulatory pathways modulate smooth muscle tone, with no single mechanism accountable for all smooth muscle behavior. On the basis of the fundamental principle that the development of tension resides in an interaction between actin and myosin, regulatory proteins necessarily effect control by influencing this interaction. As contraction is regulated by free intracellular calcium [267], molecular regulatory events often demonstrate a functional calcium dependence that may be generally classified as residing in thick filaments (myosin regulated) or thin filaments (actin regulated) [45]. More specifically, three types of regulatory proteins exist that act by an actin- or myosin-linked mechanism [376]: (1) calcium-binding receptors, such as calmodulin and leiotonin, which confer calcium sensitivity on smooth muscle actomyosin; (2) calcium-dependent protein kinases, which effect contraction by covalent protein modification; and (3) proteins such as caldesmon, which, through their own interaction with calmodulin or other calcium-binding proteins, modulate contraction by phosphorylation.

Fig. 3-16. Transverse section of a smooth muscle cell of the portal anterior mesenteric vein (PAMV). Thick filaments (large arrows) have a diameter of 15.5 ± 2.0 nm and the center-thick to center-thick spacing is approximately 60–70 nm. Thin filaments (small arrows) have a mean diameter of 6.4 ± 0.8 nm. Intermediate filaments (arrowhead) have a mean diameter of 9.7 ± 1.0 nm and are usually associated with dense bodies. PAMV × 96,000. Inset: High-magnification view of the intermediate filaments, which have an electron-lucent core (circles) in transverse section. × 204,800. (Reproduced with permission from AP Somlyo and AV Somlyo. Ultrastructure of smooth muscle. In EE Daniel, DM Paton, eds. Methods in Pharmacology, vol. 3. New York: Plenum, 1975. Pp. 3–43.)

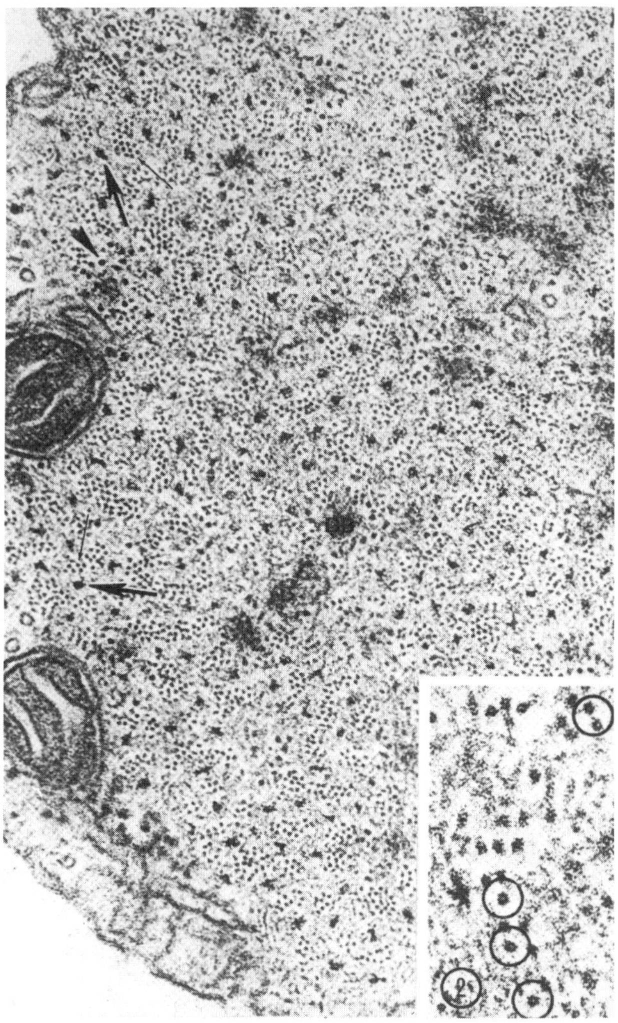

MYOSIN LIGHT-CHAIN KINASE. The phosphorylation and dephosphorylation of the myosin light chain is the most extensively investigated regulatory contractile mechanism in vascular smooth muscle and is purported to be the most important for isotonic contraction. The evidence supporting this statement has been reviewed in detail [45,350]. Myosin light-chain kinase of smooth muscle is responsible for myosin light-chain phosphorylation, which is assumed critical for its activation by actin [45,350]. Thus, phosphorylation is a prerequisite for myosin ATPase activity [377], which in turn is directly related to both the degree of phosphorylation [357] and the maximal speed of contraction [356]. The enzyme has a molecular weight between 130,000 and 150,000 daltons and is calmodulin-dependent [376]. The calcium-calmodulin complex activates the kinase, which then selectively phosphorylates the 20,000-dalton light chain in each globular head of myosin [377] (see Fig. 3-13). The same phosphorylation event regulates myosin filament conformational changes that are suggested to optimize the interaction of myosin with actin filaments [378] by altering the structure of the myosin head [379].

As is often the case in these regulatory schemes, the activating enzyme is also a potential site for regulation. The phosphorylation of myosin light-chain kinase reduces its affinity for the calcium-calmodulin complex, thereby decreasing its activity [45]. This result is brought about by the catalytic unit of the cAMP-dependent protein kinase [380–382], but the overall importance of this modification is disputed [309]. Smooth muscle phosphatase activity prevails to dephosphorylate the myosin light chain, inducing relaxation when the light-chain kinase is thereby inactivated [45,350].

MYOSIN HEAVY-CHAIN PHOSPHORYLATION. Phosphorylation of myosin heavy chain in vascular smooth muscle is a newly proposed mechanism by which the interaction between actin and myosin is regulated [309]. Naturally, in the determination of the importance of this reaction as a regulatory event, aspects of the more established regulatory mechanisms have been questioned.

From the preceding discussion, it is evident that myosin light-chain kinase is critically dependent on calcium and calmodulin for its activation. The enzyme also contains two peptides amenable to phosphorylation that modulate its activity [309]. It has been proposed that this mechanism deactivates the enzyme by the catalytic subunit of cAMP-dependent protein kinase [380–382], but recent evidence calls this notion into question. Whereas the phosphorylation of peptide 1 alone does not measurably affect the calmodulin requirement for maximal activation, the phosphorylation of both peptides results in a 20-fold calmodulin requirement for maximal activation in saturating calcium [309]. As it turns out, peptide 2 is a very poor substrate for cAMP-dependent protein kinase [309]. Thus,

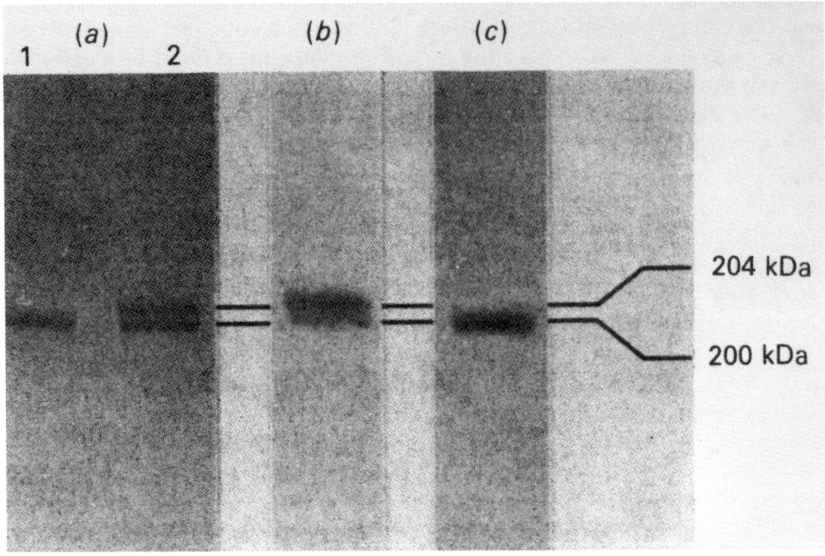

Fig. 3-17. Phosphorylation of vascular smooth muscle myosin heavy chain by protein kinase C and Ca^{2+}-calmodulin kinase II. **A.** Sodium dodecyl sulphate/polyacrylamide-gel electrophoresis of (1) rabbit skeletal muscle myosin heavy chain (200 kDa) and (2) bovine aortic myosin heavy chain (204 kDa and 200 kDa). In both cases, approximately 1 μg of protein was loaded on the gels. **B.** Autoradiogram of bovine aortic myosin phosphorylated with protein kinase C. Protein kinase C was purified from guinea pig brain. The incubation conditions included 10 mM-Mops, pH 7.2, 50 mM − KCL, 2 mM − $MgCl_2$, 0.5 mM-$CaCl_2$, 1 mM-[^{32}P]ATP, 1 mM-dithiothreitol, 50 g phosphatidylserine/ml, 10 μg diolein/ml and 1 mg myosin/ml. The reaction was started by adding 5 μg protein kinase C/ml and terminated at 60 min. **C.** Autoradiogram of bovine aortic myosin phosphorylated with Ca_{2+}-calmodulin kinase II. The latter was purified from rat liver. Incubation conditions were similar to those described for protein kinase C except that 10^{-6} M-calmodulin was included in place of the phospholipids. (Reproduced with permission from DR Hathaway et al. Myosin light chain and heavy chain phosphorylation in smooth muscle: potential regulatory roles for calcium phospholipids and cyclic nucleotides. Biochem Soc Trans 1988; 16:499–501.)

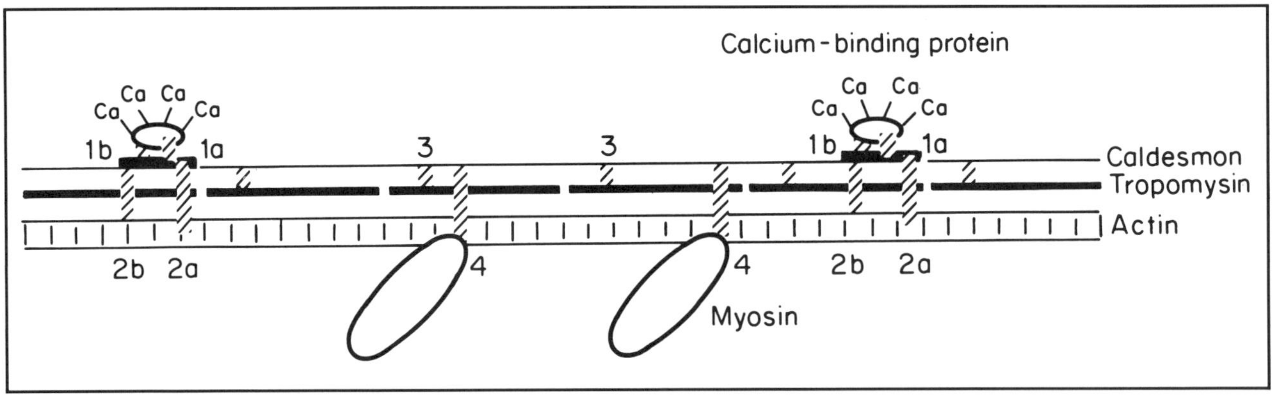

Fig. 3-18. A scheme for the structure of aorta thin filament and its regulation by calmodulin. The diagram represents one of the two actin strands that form a 38-nm pitch helix in the native thin filament. Key to interactions: 1, caldesmon (CD)-calcium binding protein (CBP) inactivates 2a when Ca^{2+} is bound; 1b, CD-CBP binding contact, independent of Ca^{2+}; 2a, CD-actin binding with inhibition of up to 28 actins; 2b, CD-actin binding contact only; Ca^{2+} independent; 3, CD-tropomyosin, located in CD tail; 4 CD-myosin binding contact only (?). (Reproduced with permission from S Marston et al. Ca^{2+} regulation of the thin filaments: biochemical mechanism and physiological role. Biochem Soc Trans 1988; 16:494–497.)

the regulation of myosin light-chain kinase activity by cAMP-dependent protein kinase may not be a relevant biologic mechanism, and regulation by phosphorylation of other sites has been sought.

The phosphorylation of the heavy chain of myosin has been reported to modulate its self-assembly and enzymatic activity [383,384]. These regulatory mechanisms are poorly understood, however, and have not been described in vascular smooth muscle. In bovine aorta, the selective phosphorylation of a 200,000-Dalton component of myosin heavy chain is mediated by calcium-calmodulin kinase II [309] (Fig. 3-17). Although a functional correlate of this phosphorylation has not been identified, phosphorylation of myosin heavy chain offers novel insight into a potential regulatory pathway modulated by calmodulin-dependent enzymes and provides supportive evidence for this mechanism at large. Similarly, the selective phosphorylation of the 204,000-Dalton component of vascular smooth muscle myosin heavy chain by protein kinase C (see Fig. 3-17) must be considered a potential independent mechanism of thick-filament regulation [309].

CALDESMON. Caldesmon is a 120,000-Dalton protein that inhibits actin-activated myosin ATPase [385–387]. The protein binds to both calmodulin and actin, thereby providing yet another mechanism for calcium regulation of thin filaments [387,388]. Through interaction with calcium, calmodulin-dependent phosphorylation of caldesmon reverses the inhibitory effect exerted on the myosin ATPase [386]. Thus, in smooth muscle, thin- as well as thick-filament regulatory mechanisms are operated by distinct calmodulin-dependent kinases that mediate phosphorylation of regulatory proteins.

The structural composition of the caldesmon thin-filament regulatory system is schematically diagrammed in Fig. 3-18. The major components are actin, tropomyosin, and caldesmon in molar ratios of 28 : 4 : 1 and a calcium binding protein that is required for calcium regulation [388]. Caldesmons are long, 150-nm randomly coiled molecules stretched out along the length of the thin filament surface, occupying the grooves between the actin double helix in intimate contact with tropomyosin. Their elongated structure accounts for the ability of a single molecule to modulate the activity of 28 actins [388]. Caldesmon binds to actin at two sites on the compact head of the molecule, only one of which induces inhibition of myosin ATPase. Caldesmon binding sites for tropomyosin are located in its tail [388].

The functional significance of this regulatory mechanism in vivo is a matter of conjecture. It is evident that the activity of the myosin light-chain kinase accounts well for isotonic-force development but not for isometric force, which is sustained at low calcium concentrations and levels of phosphorylation [45,358,359]. This so-called latch state of smooth muscle is responsible for maintaining tonic contracture through slow cycling of formed cross-bridges at reduced energy consumption. Caldesmon may play a regulatory role in this poorly understood mechanism, but this hypothesis remains to be proven [388].

LEIOTONIN. It has been almost 15 years since Ebashi and co-workers reported on a calcium-sensitive regulatory protein that was associated with thin filaments [389]. The importance of this regulatory protein in regulation of vascular smooth muscle contraction has since been confirmed [45]. Leiotonin comprises an 80,000-Dalton protein and a smaller protein of 17,000 molecular weight that resembles calmodulin [389,390]. These two components are named leiotonin A and C, respectively. The presence of leiotonin was deemed essential for full activation of the myosin ATPase and proposed as a viable alternative regulatory mechanism to the myosin light-chain kinase [391]. Although strong proponents of each regulatory mechanism exist, there is now a growing consensus that smooth muscle regulation involves modification of both thick and thin filaments [45,350,376,379]. In light of the recent discovery of caldesmon as a thin-filament-linked calcium-regulatory mechanism, early enthusiasm for leiotonin has waned. Nevertheless, leiotonin remains a viable candidate for regulatory protein with potential physiologic significance.

FILAMIN. Filamin is a 240,000-Dalton protein that binds to F-actin independently of calcium [392,393]. Filamin acts to inhibit actin-dependent activation of myosin ATPase, but its overall importance as a regulatory mechanism is not known [394]. Interestingly, filamin is among the actin-binding proteins phosphorylated by protein kinase C [278], but it is still too early to comment on the role of this enzyme in the contractile process [275].

TROPOMYOSIN. The evidence in favor of a troponin-tropomyosin regulatory mechanism in smooth muscle, mimicking its skeletal-muscle counterpart, is not convincing [350]. In fact, troponin is not present in smooth muscle at all [45,350], and tropomyosin appears to act as a cofactor for actin activation of myosin ATPase [368], which stands in marked contrast to its inhibitory role in skeletal muscle [366,367]. Thus, the actin-tropomyosin complex more efficiently activates myosin ATPase than does actin alone [350]. Independent observations suggest that this regulatory function is associated with a positional shift of tropomyosin within the groove of the actin double helix [395].

SMOOTH MUSCLE PROLIFERATION

An extensive literature dedicated to smooth muscle contraction has been discussed. The critical importance of vascular tone in sustaining the life of the organism notwithstanding, our bias to focus on this specific cellular response is based on two points. First, this body of work represents the most studied example of **stimulus-response coupling** in the vascular smooth muscle cell. Second, it is now accepted that different cellular functions share common extracellular signals, surface receptor systems, and intracellular regulatory mechanisms. Therefore, the contractile response provides certain well-studied concepts that are representative of other functional responses, such as proliferation, chemotaxis, adhesion, secretion, development, repair and rearrangement of structural apparatus, and various metabolic functions.

Unfortunately, because of space constraints, it is not possible to provide an overview of each of the different, albeit less well understood, functional responses. The following paragraphs endeavor to highlight the common components of the stimulus-response paradigm, using the proliferative response as another important example.

Table 3-4. Surface-receptor systems sharing contractile and proliferative functions

Norepinephrine
Angiotensin II
Serotonin
Bradykinin
Prostaglandins
Leukotrienes
Vasopressin
Platelet-derived growth factor (PDGF)
Epidermal growth factor (EGF)
Fibroblast growth factor (FGF)
Transforming growth factor (TGF)

Source: Modified from S Moncada, J Vane. Pharmacology and endogenous roles of prostaglandin endoperoxides, thromboxane A_2, and prostacyclin. Pharmacol Rev 1979; 30:293–331.

Many vasoactive substances mediate growth responses as well as contraction [34,201]. Growth may be expressed as differentiation of the vascular smooth muscle cell through the entire cell cycle to division, as in hyperplasia, or by a modified response in which protein synthesis or DNA content increases without division (ploidy), as in hypertrophy [201]. Surface-receptor systems sharing proliferation and contractile functions are listed in Table 3-4. The stimulation of quiescent cells in the G_0/G_1 phase of the cell cycle depends on the synergistic effects among mitogenic factors and is preceded by the obligatory expression of cellular oncogenes c-fos and c-myc [34,201]. The induction of oncogene expression has been corroborated in the case of catecholamines [36,396], bradykinin [36], prostaglandins [36], PDGF [30,36], and angiotensin [63,64]. Additional strong evidence supports mitogenic roles for vasopressin [62], serotonin [397], leukotrienes [208], and other vasoactive growth factors [30,212,216,227,231]. The means by which a single high-affinity surface receptor mediates the determination of proliferation versus contraction is not known.

Contractile and proliferative responses also share common signal-transducing mechanisms that are receptor mediated (Table 3-5). Thus, ion fluxes are recognized as important early membrane signals modulated by agonist-receptor interaction. These ion movements are involved in the propagation of both contractile and proliferative responses [4,10,26,139]. In this context, calcium deserves particular attention. Its presence is of paramount importance for contraction; furthermore, calcium is considered an important regulator of cellular proliferation [30,223,288,398,399]. In the vascular smooth muscle cell, increased levels of calcium rapidly increase c-fos and c-myc mRNA expression [400], and the modulation of extracellular as well as cytoplasmic calcium influences vascular smooth muscle proliferation [401]. Accordingly, the mobilization of intracellular calcium by IP_3 may be a relevant mitogenic transducing event for many vasoactive hormones, neurotransmitters, and growth factors that stimulate PIP_2 hydrolysis [105,240,402]. The phosphoinositide pathway can also influence cell proliferation by generating DAG, which activates protein kinase C (see discussion in the section "Signal Transduction"). This enzyme is a receptor for tumor promoters of the phorbol ester family and has several growth-promoting activities [268,288]. Its function as a second messenger in the proliferative response has already been reviewed (see "Functional Importance" in the section "Phosphoinositides"). These two signal cascades may act in concert or synergistically to promote DNA synthesis [403] in a manner analogous to their role in contraction.

Table 3-5. Signal-transduction mechanisms involved in contractile and proliferative responses

Ion flux
Calcium mobilization
Phosphoinositide turnover
Protein kinase C activation
Inositol 1,4,5-triphosphate generation
Adenylate cyclase activation

Sources: Modified from ER Weiss, et al. Receptor activation of G proteins. FASEB J 1988; 2:2841–2848; S Moncada, J Vane. Pharmacology and endogenous roles of prostaglandin endoperoxides, thrombane A_2, and prostacyclin. Pharmacol Rev 1979; 30:293–331.

The controversial role of cAMP in the regulation of cell growth has also been addressed (see the section "Cyclic AMP"). PDGF and the vasoinhibitory prostaglandins are among the mitogenic factors to raise intracellular cAMP levels; cause and effect, however, have not been established. In fact, most evidence suggests that the accumulation of this cyclic nucleotide does not represent a primary mitogenic signal in vascular smooth muscle. The vascular smooth muscle cell exhibits diversity in its functional response to common excitatory stimuli and intracellular signals. The mechanism by which specific high-affinity receptors mediate different cellular functions through common signal cascades remains a major unresolved issue in smooth muscle biology.

Recent parallels have been drawn between the normal development of blood vessels and the pathophysiologic aspects of blood vessel growth associated with remodeling and angiogenesis. The recent focus on restenosis in the setting of angioplasty has further highlighted the importance of vascular-derived growth factors such as PDGF, FGF, and TGF-β, to mention a few, in the proliferative responses, changes in cellular composition and modifications of extracellular matrix and ultrastructure smooth muscle that follow injury. Other vascular-derived cytokines such as interleukin-1, colony-stimulating factors, and the vasoconstrictor peptides, endothelin(s) and angiotensin II, also play influential roles [406]. The cellular biology of several important vascular smooth muscle factors is reviewed next.

Platelet-Derived Growth Factor. Platelet-derived growth factor (PDGF), named for the discovery that mitogenic activity of whole-blood serum is principally platelet-derived [407,408], is actually produced by many diploid cells, including endothelial cells, macrophages, and vascular smooth muscle. The protein is composed of two homologous polypeptide chains, A and B, which are linked by disulfide bridges. Various combinations of the dimeric PDGF molecule (PDGF-AA, PDGF-BB, PDGF-AB) have been identified. The multiple molecular-weight forms range from 28,000 to 35,000 Daltons [406]. Interestingly, the B chain of PDGF shows significant homology with $p28^{SIS}$, the proto-oncogene derived from simian sarcoma virus [409]. In the normal blood vessel wall, PDGF-B chain transcripts are expressed in adventitial macrophages and the endothelium of the vasovasorum, whereas PDGF-A transcripts are found in microvascular endothelial cells and the smooth muscle itself [406]. Shortly after (catheter-induced) vessel-wall injury, smooth muscle cells secrete much higher levels of PDGF into the medium and express high levels of both A- and B-chain mRNA [406,410]. Expression of PDGF activity can be further modulated by several atherogenic factors, including modified LDL, thrombin, and activated factor X. Each has been shown to regulate some aspect of the pathway from PDGF transcription through its secretion from cystolic storage pools [406]. Taken together, these data suggest that the expression processing and release of PDGF is tightly regulated; upregulation of expression is often seen in diseased vessels due to the presence of atherogenic stimuli.

PDGF transduces its signal through interactions with high-affinity receptors ($K_D 10^{-9}$-10^{-11}M) [411]. The receptor, like the protein itself, is a dimer of subunits. The alpha subunit can bind either A or B chains, whereas the beta subunit can bind only B chains. Three dimeric receptors have been isolated; alpha-alpha, alpha-beta, and beta-beta. Alpha-alpha binds PDGF-AA, PDGF-AB, and PDGF-BB; alpha-beta binds PDGF-AB and PDGF-BB; and beta-beta recognizes PDGF-BB [406,411,412]. When PDGF binds to its receptor, ligand-induced dimerization takes place, leading to signaling via an intracellular tyrosine kinase domain. Although the number and the proportion of the two receptor subunits vary from cell to cell and in response to physiologic stresses, the significance of this finding is less well understood. We know, for example, that the A chain is less efficient at inducing transformation in certain cell lines, but the secretory and mitogenic properties of the two chains are cell specific [406,412]. Further complicating this matter, positive and negative interactions with other mitogens appear to influence the proliferative response.

PDGF has several important actions on vascular cells. It is a potent chemotactic agent for smooth muscle and a mitogen at the same concentrations [406,412]. In selected muscle beds, PDGF has contractile effects as well [413]. In response to PDGF, several proteins involved in cell-matrix interactions are synthesized. Further, PDGF causes a decrease in smooth muscle alpha-actin, indicative of a phenotypic change in muscle from a contractile to a synthetic state [406]. In accordance with its diverse effects on vascular cells, PDGF has been implicated in angiogenesis, wound repair, hypertension, atherosclerosis, neoplasia, vascular hypertrophy, and intimal thickening [406,412].

Fibroblast Growth Factors. Fibroblast growth factors (aFGFs and bFGFs) are small proteins that promote growth of cultured fibroblasts [414,415]. Other truncated and extended forms also have been identified; however, their physiologic functions are not known [406]. FGFs show high-sequence homology with several oncogene products [406]. Fibroblasts, endothelial cells, and vascular smooth muscle cells are capable of synthesizing both aFGFs and bFGFs. Although the proteins are products of different genes, close similarities suggest evolution from a common ancestorial gene. The regulation of FGF expression and secretion is poorly understood.

High-affinity receptors for FGFs have been identified on endothelial cells, vascular smooth muscle, and fibroblasts [406,416]. Four FGF-receptor subtypes have been identified that, with one exception, bind bFGF more avidly than aFGF. The receptors are composed of an extracellular domain containing immunoglobulinlike regions and a cytoplasmic tyrosine kinase [417]. In addition to the their surface receptors, FGFs exhibit high affinity for heparin and related sulfated glycosaminoglycans [418]. This binding serves both to protect FGFs from degradation and as a storage repository. Indeed, the avid binding of FGFs to heparan sulfate on the cell surface may act to localize the molecule at its site of action [406]. Thus, following spontaneous FGF release, or facilitated by the actions of cell-derived heparinases or related proteolytic enzymes capable of degrading the extracellular matrix, the protein becomes available to the smooth muscle cell. The susceptibility of FGFs to proteolytic degradation once released from binding sites imparts an additional level of regulation to the response. The binding of FGFs by heparin may be one important mechanism by which such sulfated proteoglycans act to prevent neointimal thickening of vessels.

The individual functions of the different FGFs remain to be defined. However, as a family, FGFs generally are capable of stimulating mitogenesis of vascular smooth muscle, possess chemotactic activity, and are reported to regulate cell differentiation [406]. Moreover, many important effects on vascular smooth muscle appear to relate to the ability of FGFs to influence phenotypic expression of endothelial cells [414,415]. The phenomenon of contact inhibition by endothelial cells and the full-expression antithrombotic functional properties are FGF dependent [406,414,415]. Cells grown in the absence of FGF show altered morphological characteristics. These actions of FGF are related to the control of the synthesis of extracellular matrix proteins, cell surface polarity, and gene expression. It perhaps is not surprising, therefore, that FGF has been implicated in restenosis of arteries following balloon angioplasty. Several lines of evidence also suggests that FGF may play a role in the development of vascular hypertrophy and atherosclerosis. Despite the discovery of the multifunctional properties of FGF [406,414,415], its exact role in the pathophysiologic regulation of blood-vessel growth remains to be fully elucidated.

Transforming Growth Factor β. The transforming activity in conditioned media of murine sarcoma virus-transformed mouse fibroblasts was initially attributed to a combination of TGF-α and TGF-β [419,420]. The two proteins actually are structurally unrelated [419]. TGF-α closely resembles EGF (epidermal growth factor), to the extent that its actions are mediated by the EGF receptor. TGF-β is a dimer that comprises two identical 112–amino acid chains and belongs to a superfamily of factors implicated in cell growth and differentiation [406,419]. Indeed, TGF-β-1 through 5 are differentially expressed in various tissues. These factors are products of different genes sharing homology ranging from 64 to 82 percent [406]. In this context, rat vascular smooth muscle expresses TGF-β-1, TGF-β-2, and TGF-β-3 [406].

Expression of activity of TGF-βs is tightly controlled. Gene transcription is subject to control by phorbol esters and the transcription factor AP1 [421]. Regulation of the gene by angiotensin II, endothelin I, and TGF-β is thought to be mediated via protein kinase C (i.e., a phorbol ester–responsive pathway) [406,419]. The protein actually is released from vascular smooth muscle cells (endothelial cells and fibroblasts) as an inactive latent complex [1,14]. The pro-region of the inactive protein contains mannose-six phosphate, allowing it to bind to a cell-surface cation–independent IGF II (insulinlike growth factor 2) receptor on both endothelial and vascular smooth muscle [422]. The same pro-region contains an RGD (Arg-Gly-Asp) sequence by which the protein can bind certain cell-adhesion receptors of the integrin class [406,419]. The binding of TGF in latent form through the pro-region appears to be critical to its subsequent activation. The mechanism of activation is presumed to involve proteolysis; however, it is not well understood [406,419].

Three distinct classes of membrane receptors bind TGF-βs in the picomolar range [419]. The class 3 receptor is the most prevalent of the three [406] and is relatively unselective toward the various TGFs. The affinities of the different TGF-β family members differ for the receptor subtypes. Certain growth inhibitory effects specific to TGF-β-1 are thought to be mediated by the class 1 receptor. The class 2 receptor is a serine-threonine kinase of unknown function. That the effects of the various TGFs are markedly influenced by the state of cell differentiation, growth conditions, and the interactions with other growth factors has made the precise roles played by the different receptor classes difficult to define.

TGF-βs have many distinct pharmacologic actions. They profoundly affect the composition of the extracellular matrix by stimulating vascular smooth muscle cells, fibroblasts, and endothelial cells to synthesize collagen types I, III, IV, and V, thrombospondin, sulfated proteoglycans, and elastin [406,419]. TGF-β-1 also has been implicated in the increases in fibronectin and collagen subtypes produced in the neointima of balloon injured vessels [423]. Upregulation of cell-adhesion receptors, increased fibronectin expression, and cell adhesion suggest that TGF-β also contributes to increases in blood-vessel-wall stiffness. Taken with the induced expression of plasminogen activator-inhibitor by endothelial cells, further predisposing to a thrombotic tendency, TGF-β is an attractive target in programs aimed at preventing restenosis and hypertension-induced remodeling through pharmacologic manipulations.

The proliferative actions of TGF-β on vascular endothelial cells and smooth muscle are incompletely characterized. It is clear that TGF-β has angiogenic properties in vivo [424,425]. However, in vitro, the stimulation of endothelial-cell proliferation by TGF-β is subject to experimental conditions [424,425]. Thus, both stimulation and inhibition of endothelial-cell growth have been reported. The presence of specific receptor subtypes for TGF-β may account for some of these contrasting effects. Further, stimulation of vascular smooth muscle can occur both by the direct effects of TGF-β and though indirect effects on endothelial-cell function. TGF-β activates the expression of PDGF-A, PDGF-B, and FGF in endothelial cells [406]. Additional reports that TGF-β-1 can inhibit or potentiate the mitogenic properties of other growth factors is probably related to system-specific expression of TGF-β receptor phenotypes. TGF-β also has been reported to affect smooth muscle structure, size, and migratory ability.

Peptide Vasoconstrictors: Endothelins. Several vascular-derived cytokines (IL-1, IL-4, IL-6, and IL-8), colony-stimulating factors (i.e., G-CSF and GM-CSF), peptide vasoconstrictors (i.e., endothelins and angiotensin II), and peptide growth factors (i.e., IGFs) have been implicated in the development of atherosclerosis, hypertension, and the remodeling of injured vessels. Detailed reviews on these growth-influencing factors are beyond the scope of this chapter. Because the unique structure and pharmacologic properties of the endothelins have attracted significant attention in various biological fields, their vascular actions will be reviewed briefly. The endothelins (ETs) are designated 1, 2, and 3 [426,427]. ET-1 is the most potent vasopressor peptide characterized to date. The 21–amino acid active product is processed from an approximately 200–amino acid residue precursor, pre-proendothelin-1 through an intermediate "big endothelin" (proendothelin) by the actions of an ET-converting metalloendopeptidase [428]. ET-2 and ET-3 are products of different mammalian genes and differ from ET-1 in two and six amino acids, respectively [406].

The diverse responses of the ETs are mediated by different receptors [428,429]. The first insight into receptor heterogeneity was derived from the observations that ETs can elicit a vasodepressor effect and that the propensity for vasoconstriction and vasodepression differs for ET-1 and ET-3 [406,428]. Later it was shown that the ET-1 receptor mediating vasoconstriction is present on vascular smooth muscle, whereas a separate receptor present on endothelial cells mediates the release of EDRF in response to ET-3 [430]. Based on molecular cloning studies and pharmacologic agonist potencies, two receptors have been classified [427–429]. The first receptor is designated ET_A and shows the following order of affinity: ET-1 is greater than ET-2 is much greater than ET-3. The second receptor, designated ET_B, is nonselective, showing the affinity profile ET-1 equals ET-2 equals ET-3. ET_A is present on vascular smooth muscle and ET_B on endothelial cells. Both receptors exhibit sequence similarity of approximately 60 percent, and both appear to be coupled to phospholipase C by G proteins [406]. The vasodepressor effect of ET-3 is ascribed to its activation of ET_B receptors, which mediate phosphoinositide breakdown via pertussis toxin–

sensitive G proteins. This, in turn, triggers release of intracellular calcium, thereby activating the calcium-calmodulin–independent nitric-oxide synthase in endothelial cells [430]. Although ET-1 is a potent vasoconstrictor, activation of ET_B results in release of EDRF [406,430]. ET-1 also stimulates vascular smooth muscle cells to proliferate and synthesize DNA [406]. These mitogenic effects are, in part, sensitive to pertussis toxin, implicating the involvement of heterotrimeric G proteins. ET-1, ET-2, and ET-3 all are effective in potentiating PDGF-BB stimulation of DNA synthesis consistent with direct effects on the nonspecific ET_B receptor on endothelial cells [406]. However, it has been demonstrated that the mitogenic properties of ET-1 are mediated by the G protein–ET_A receptor on vascular smooth muscle [406]. Thus, these data speak to the dynamic interplay between the endothelium and the vascular smooth muscle, which is further coordinated by the ETs through receptor-specific pathways.

References

1. Furchgott RF. The pharmacology of vascular smooth muscle. Pharmacol Rev 1955; 7:183–265.
2. Bohr DF. Vascular smooth muscle updated. Circ Res 1973; 32:665–672.
3. Somlyo AP, Somlyo AV. Vascular smooth muscle. I: normal structure, pathology, biochemistry, and biophysics. Pharmacol Rev 1968; 20:197–272.
4. Somlyo AP, Somlyo AV. Vascular smooth muscle. II: pharmacology of normal and hypertensive vessels. Pharmacol Rev 1970; 22:251–353.
5. Altura BM. Pharmacology of venular smooth muscle. Bibl Anat 1977; 16:284–286.
6. Holman ME. Electrophysiology of vascular smooth muscle. Ergeb Physiol 1969; 61:137–177.
7. Fleish JH. Pharmacology of the rat aorta: A brief review. Blood Vessels 1974; 11:193–211.
8. Bohr DF. Individualities among vascular smooth muscles. In E Bajusz, ed. Electrolytes and Cardiovascular Diseases. Basel: Karger, 1986. Pp. 342–355.
9. Vanhoutte PM. Heterogeneity in vascular smooth muscle. In G Kaley, BM Altura, eds. Microcirculation, Vol. 2. University Park Press, 1978. Pp. 181–309.
10. Bulbring E, Tomita T. Catecholamine action on smooth muscle. Pharmacol Rev 1987; 39(1):49–96.
11. Dikstein S, Sulman FG. Interaction of Dibenamine with phospholipids of the aorta. Biochem Pharmacol 1965; 14:881–885.
12. Lewis JE, Miller JW. The use of tritiated phenoxybenzamine for investigating receptors. J Pharmacol Exp Ther 1966; 154:46–55.
13. Hoffman BB, Lefkowitz RJ. Alpha–adrenergic receptor subtypes. N Engl J Med 1980; 90.
14. Langer SZ. Presynaptic regulation of catecholamine release. Biochem Pharmacol 1974; 23:1793–1800.
15. Langer SZ, Hicks PE. Alpha–adrenoreceptor subtypes in blood vessels: physiology and pharmacology. J Cardiovasc Pharmacol 1984; S547–S558.
16. Randriantsoa A, Heitz C, Stoclet JC. Functional characterization of postjunctional alpha-adrenoceptors in rat aorta. Eur J Pharmacol 1981; 75:57–60.
17. Holck MI, Jones CHM, Haeusler G. Differential interactions of clonidine and methoxamine with postsynaptic alpha-adrenoceptor of rabbit main pulmonary artery. J Cardiovasc Pharmacol 1983; 5:240–248.
18. Hieble JP, Woodward DF. Different characteristics of post-junctional alpha-adrenoceptors on arterial and venous smooth muscle. Arch Pharmacol 1984; 328:44–50.
19. Stevens MJ, Moulds RF. Heterogeneity of post-junctional alpha-adrenoreceptors in human vascular smooth muscle. Arch Int Pharmacodyn Ther 1981; 254:43–57.
20. Stevens MJ, Moulds RF. Are the pre- and postsynaptic alpha-adrenoreceptors in human vascular smooth muscle atypical? J Cardiovasc Pharmacol 1982; 4:S129–S133.
21. Flavahan NA, et al. Human postjunctional $alpha_1$ and $alpha_2$ adrenoreceptors: differential distribution in arteries of the limbs. J Pharmacol Exp Ther 1987; 241:361–365.
22. Flavahan NA, McGrath JC. Are human vascular alpha-adrenoceptors atypical? J Cardiovasc Pharmacol 1984; 6:208–210.
23. Hirst GDS, Neild TO. Evidence for two populations of excitatory receptors for noradrenaline on arteriolar smooth muscle. Nature 1980; 283:767–768.
24. Hirst GDS, Neild TO, Siverberg GD. Noradrenaline receptors in the rat basilar artery. J Physiol 1982; 328:351–360.
25. Timmermans PB, van Zwieten PA. $Alpha_2$ adrenoceptors: classification, localization, mechanisms, and targets for drugs. J Med Chem 1982; 25(12):1389–1401.
26. Bolton TB. Mechanisms of action of transmitters and other substances on smooth muscle. Physiol Rev 1979; 59(3): 606–718.
27. Cauvin C, et al. Theoretical bases for vascular selectivity of Ca^{2+} antagonists. J Cardiovasc Pharmacol 1984; 6:S630–S638.
28. Cooke JP, et al. Nimodipine and inhibition of alpha adrenergic activation of the isolated canine saphenous vein. J Pharmacol Exp Ther 1985; 234:598–602.
29. Casteels R. Electro- and pharmacomechanical coupling in vascular smooth muscle. Chest 1980; 78:150–156.
30. Weiss ER, et al. Receptor activation of G proteins. FASEB J 1988; 2:2841–2848.
31. Lefkowitz RJ, Caron MG. Adrenergic receptors. Models for the study of receptors coupled to guanine nucleotide regulatory proteins. J Biol Chem 1988; 263(11):4993–4996.
32. Nishizuka Y. Turnover of inositol phospholipids and signal transduction. Science 1984; 225:1365–1370.
33. Blaes N, Boissel JP. Growth stimulating effect of catecholamines on rat aortic smooth muscle cells in culture. J Cell Physiol 1983; 116:167–172.
34. Rozengurt E. Early signals in the mitogenic response. Science 1986; 234:161–166.
35. Coughlin SR, et al. C-myc gene expression is stimulated by agents that activate protein kinase C and does not account for the mitogenic effect of PDGF. Cell 1985; 43:243–251.
36. Naftilan A, Pratt RE, Dzau VJ. Induction of platelet-derived growth factor A-chain and c-myc gene expressions by angiotensin II in cultured rat vascular smooth muscle cells. J Clin Invest 1989; 83:1419–1424.
37. Westfall DP. Adrenoreceptor antagonists. In CR Craig, RE Stitzel, eds. Modern Pharmacology. Boston: Little, Brown, 1982. Pp. 141–156.
38. Lands AM, et al. Differentiation of receptor systems activated by sympathomimetic amines. Nature 1967; 214:597–598.
39. Lands AM, Luduena FP, Buzzo HJ. Differentiation of receptors responsive to isoproterenol. Life Sci 1967; 6:2241–2249.
40. Frielle T, Caron MG, Lefkowitz RJ. Properties of the $beta_1$ and $beta_2$ adrenergic receptor subtypes revealed by molecular cloning. Clin Chem 1989; 35:721–725.
41. Shepherd JT, Vanhoutte PM. Veins and Their Control. Philadelphia: Saunders, 1975. Pp. 1–69.
42. Byrne NG, Hirst GDS, Large WA. Electrophysiological analysis of the nature of adrenoceptors in the rat basilar artery during development. Br J Pharmacol 1985; 86:217–227.

43. Meisheri KD, Van Breeman C. Effects of beta-adrenergic stimulation on calcium movements in rabbit aortic smooth muscle: relationship with cyclic AMP. J Physiol 1982; 331:429–441.
44. Baudouin-Legros M, Meyer P. Effects of angiotensin, catecholamines and cyclic AMP on calcium storage in aortic microsomes. Br J Pharmacol 1973; 47:377–385.
45. Webb RC, Bohr DF. Regulation of vascular tone, molecular mechanisms. Prog Cardiovasc Dis 1981; XXIV(3):213–242.
46. van Breeman C, et al. Ca^{2+} movements in smooth muscle. Chest 1980; 78:157–165.
47. Holman ME, et al. Some properties of the smooth muscle of rabbit portal vein. J Physiol 1968; 196:111–132.
48. Johansson B, et al. Electrical and mechanical characteristics of vascular smooth muscle response to norepinephrine and isoproterenol. Circ Res 1967; 21:619–633.
49. Papadimitriou A, Worcel M. Further evidence for the existence of different types of angiotensin II receptors. In E Betz, ed. Vascular Smooth Muscle. International Symposium on Vascular Smooth Muscle, Tubingen. Berlin, NY: Springer, 1971.
50. Moore AF, Hall MM, Khairallah PA. Comparison of the effects of angiotensin II and heptapeptide on smooth muscle (vascular and uterine). J Pharmacol 1976; 39:101–107.
51. Gunther S. Characterization of angiotensin II receptor subtypes in rat liver. J Biol Chem 1984; 259(12):7622–7629.
52. Capponi AM, Catt KJ. Solubilization and characterization of adrenal and uterine angiotensin II receptors after photo affinity labeling. J Biol Chem 1979; 255(24):12081–12086.
53. Sen I, Bull HG, Soffer RL. Isolation of an angiotensin II-binding protein from liver. Proc Natl Acad Sci 1984; 81:1679–1683.
54. Guillmette G, Escher E. Analysis of the adrenal angiotensin II receptor with photoaffinity labeling method. Biochemistry 1983; 22:5591–5596.
55. Catt KJ, Aguilera G. Angiotensin II receptors. In D Schuster, A Levitzki, eds. Cellular Receptors for Hormones and Neurotransmitters. New York: Wiley, 1980.
56. Devynck MA, Meyer P. Angiotensin II receptors in smooth muscle—a biochemical approach. Clin Exp Pharmacol Physiol 1975; 2:93–97.
57. Turker RK, et al. Competitive antagonism of 8-ALA-angiotensin II to angiotensin I and II on isolated rabbit aorta and rat ascending colon. Eur J Pharmacol 1971; 15:285–291.
58. Peach MJ. Renin-angiotensin system: biochemistry and mechanism of action. Physiol Rev 1977; 57(2):313–370.
59. Catt KJ, et al. The role of angiotensin II receptors in vascular regulation. J Cardiovasc Pharmacol 1984; 6:S575–S586.
60. Shultz GS, Galardy RE, Jamieson JD. Biological activity of angiotensin II-ferritin conjugate on rabbit aortic smooth muscle cells. Biochemistry 1981; 20:3412–3418.
61. Smith JB. Angiotensin-receptor signaling in cultured vascular smooth muscle cells. Am J Physiol 1986; 250:F759–F769.
62. Campbell-Boswell M, Robertson AL. Effects of angiotensin II and vasopressin on human smooth muscle cells in vitro. Exp Mol Pathol 1981; 35:265–276.
63. Geisterfer AAT, Owens GK. Hypertrophic response of cultured vascular smooth muscle cells to angiotensin II. Fed Proc 1986; 45:584.
64. Naftilan AJ, Pratt RE, Dzau VJ. Angiotensin II induction of c-fos, c-myc and platelet derived growth factor in vascular smooth muscle cells. Clin Res 1988; 36:303A.
65. Aguilera G, Catt KJ. Regulation of vascular angiotensin II receptors in the rat during altered sodium intake. Circ Res 1981; 49:751–758.
66. Khairallah PA, et al. Angiotensin tachyphylaxis and its reversal. Circ Res 1966; 19:247–254.
67. Mitchelson F. Muscarinic receptor differentiation. Pharmacol Ther 1988; 37:357–423.
68. Hammer R, et al. Pirenzepine distinguishes between different subclasses of muscarinic receptors. Nature 1980; 283(2):90–92.
69. Hammer R, Giachetti A. Muscarinic receptor subtypes: M1 and M2 biochemical and functional characterization. Life Sci 1982; 31:2991–2998.
70. Goyal RK, Rattan S. Neurohumoral, hormonal, and drug receptors for the lower esophageal sphincter. Gastroenterology 1978; 74:598–619.
71. Kubo T, et al. Cloning, sequencing and expression of complementary DNA coding the muscarinic acetylcholine receptor. Nature 1986; 323:411–416.
72. Goyal RK. Muscarinic receptor subtypes. Physiology and clinical implications. N Engl J Med 1989; 321:1022–1029.
73. Peach MJ, Singer HA, Loeb AL. Mechanisms of endothelium-dependent vascular smooth muscle relaxation. Biochem Pharmacol 1985; 34:1867–1874.
74. Stephenson JA, Summers RJ. Audioradiographic analysis of receptors on vascular endothelium. Eur J Pharmacol 1987; 134:35–43.
75. Yamanaka K, Hashimoto S, Muramatsu I. Species difference in the muscarinic receptors of thoracic aorta. J Pharmacol Exp Ther 1986; 237:980–986.
76. Cherry PD, Gillis CN. Evidence for the role of endothelium-derived relaxing factor in acetylcholine-induced vasodilation in the intact lung. J Pharmacol Exp Ther 1987; 241(2):516–520.
77. Ignarro LJ, et al. Endothelium-derived relaxing factor from pulmonary artery and vein possess pharmacologic and chemical properties identical to those of nitric oxide radical. Circulation 1987; 61:866–879.
78. Ludmer PL, et al. Paradoxical vasoconstriction induced by acetylcholine in atherosclerotic coronary arteries. N Engl J Med 1986; 315:1046–1051.
79. Vanhoutte PM. The endothelium control of coronary arterial tone. Hosp Pract 1988; 67–84.
80. Furchgott RF, Zawadzki JV. The obligatory role of endothelial cells in the relaxation of arterial smooth muscle by acetylcholine. Nature 1980, 288:373–376.
81. Hynes MR, et al. Characterization of muscarinic receptors of the rabbit ear artery smooth muscle and endothelium. J Pharmacol Exp Ther 1986; 238:100–105.
82. Furchgott RF, Cherry PD. The muscarinic receptor of vascular endothelium that subserves vasodilation. Trends Pharmacol Sci 1984; [Suppl]:45–48.
83. O'Rourke ST, Vanhoutte PM. Subtypes of muscarinic receptors on adrenergic nerves and vascular smooth muscle of the canine saphenous vein. J Pharmacol Exp Ther 1987; 241(1):64–67.
84. Furchgott RF, Zawadski JV, Cherry PD. Role of endothelium in the vasodilator response to acetylcholine. In PM Vanhoutte, I Leusen, eds. Vasodilation. New York: Raven, 1981. Pp. 49–72.
85. Altiere RJ, Kritsy-Roy JA, Catravas JD. Acetylcholine-induced contractions in isolated rabbit pulmonary arteries: role of thromboxane A_2. J Pharmacol Exp Ther 1986; 236:535–541.
86. De May JG, Vanhoutte PM. Heterogeneous behavior of the canine arterial and venous wall. Circ Res 1982; 51:439–447.
87. Kuriyama H, Suzuki H. Effects of acetylcholine on the membrane contractile properties of smooth muscle cells of the rabbit superior mesenteric artery. Br J Pharmacol 1978; 64:493–501.
88. Jones LM, Kirk ChJ, Mitchell RH. Molecular events following activation of muscarinic receptors: the role of inositol phospholipids. Scand J Gastroenterol 1982; 72[Suppl]:33–41.

89. Murad F. Cyclic guanosine monophosphate as a mediator of vasodilation. J Clin Invest 1986; 78:1–5.
90. Vanhoutte PM, Levy MN. Prejunctional cholinergic modulation of adrenergic neurotransmission in the cardiovascular system. Am J Physiol 1980; 7:H275–H281.
91. Vanhoutte PM. Inhibition by acetylcholine of adrenergic neurotransmission in vascular smooth muscle. Circ Res 1974; 50:317–326.
92. Rubanyi GM, Vanhoutte PM. Superoxide anions and hyperoxia inactivate endothelium-derived relaxing factor. Am J Physiol 1986; 250:H822–H827.
93. Estrada C, Krause DN. Muscarinic cholinergic receptor sites in cerebral blood vessels. J Pharmacol Exp Ther 1982; 221:85–90.
94. Gaddum JH, Picarelli ZP. Two kinds of tryptamine receptor. J Pharmacol 1957; 12:323–328.
95. Humphrey PPA. Peripheral 5-hydroxytryptamine receptors and their classification. Neuropharmacology 1984; 23(12B): 1503–1510.
96. Van Nueten JM, et al. Serotonergic receptor subtypes and vascular reactivity. J Cardiovasc Pharmacol 1984; 6:S564–S574.
97. Peroutka SJ. $5HT_1$ receptor sites and functional correlates. Neuropharmacology 1984; 23(12B):1487–1492.
98. Leysen JE, et al. Serotonin-S_2 receptor binding sites and functional correlates. Neuropharmacology 1984; 23(12B):1493–1501.
99. Bradley PB. The characterization of 5-HT receptors. Neuropharmacology 1984; 23(12B):1465–1466.
100. Cohen ML, Fuller RW, Wiley KS. Evidence for 5-HT_2 receptors mediating contraction in vascular smooth muscle. J Pharmacol Exp Ther 1981; 218(2):421–425.
101. Cohen RA, Shepherd JT, Vanhoutte PM. 5-hydroxytryptamine can mediate endothelium-dependent relaxation of coronary arteries. Am J Physiol 1983; 245:H1077–H1080.
102. Cohen RA, Shepherd JT, Vanhoutte PM. Inhibitory role of the endothelium in the response of isolated coronary arteries to platelets. Science 1983; 221:273–274.
103. Fozard JR. Neuronal 5-HT receptors in the periphery. Neuropharmacology 1984; 23(12B):1473–1486.
104. Van Nueten JM, et al. Interaction between S_2-serotonergic and alpha$_1$-adrenergic receptor activities at vascular sites. J Cardiovasc Pharmacol 1988; 11[Suppl I]:S10–S15.
105. Berridge MJ, Irvine RF. Inositol triphosphate, a novel second messenger in cellular signal transduction. Nature 1984; 312:315–321.
106. Berridge MJ. Inositol lipids and cell proliferation. Biochem Biophys Acta 1987; 907:33–45.
107. Johansson B, Somlyo AP. Electrophysiology and excitation-contraction coupling. In DF Bohr, AP Somlyo, HV Sparks, eds. The Handbook of Physiology: Section 2, The Cardiovascular System, Vascular Smooth Muscle. New York: Oxford University Press, 1984. Pp 301–324.
108. Ratz PH, Flaim SF. Mechanism of 5-HT contraction in isolated bovine ventricular coronary arteries. Evidence for transient receptor-operated calcium influx channels. Circ Res 1984; 54:135–143.
109. Luscher TF, Vanhoutte PM. Are there interactions between S_2-serotonergic and alpha$_1$-adrenergic receptors in isolated canine arteries? J Cardiovasc Pharmacol 1988; 11[Suppl I]:S16–S21.
110. Tsuru H. Histamine receptors in the cardiovascular system. Bibl Cardiol 1984; 38:70–80.
111. Marshall I. Characterization and distribution of histamine H_1- and H_2-receptors in precapillary vessels. J Cardiovasc Pharmacol 1984; 8:S587–S597.
112. Gross PM. Histamine H_1- and H_2-receptors are differentially and spatially distributed in cerebral vessels. J Cereb Blood Flow 1981; 1:441–446.
113. Powell JR, Brody MJ. Participation of H_1 and H_2 histamine receptors in physiological vasodilator responses. Am J Physiol 1976; 231:1002–1009.
114. Carrier GO, White RE, Kirby ML. Histamine-induced relaxation of rat aorta. Importance of H_1 receptor and vascular endothelium. Blood Vessels 1984; 21:180–183.
115. Haddock RC, et al. Role of receptors in metabolic interaction of histamine with human vascular endothelial cells and skin fibroblasts. An ordered sequence of enzyme action. J Biol Chem 1987; 262(21):10220–10228.
116. Hirschowitz BI. H-2 histamine receptors. Ann Rev Pharmacol Toxicol 1979; 19:203–244.
117. Owen DAA. Histamine receptors in the cardiovascular system. Gen Pharmac 1977; 8:141–156.
118. Carman-Krzan M. Characterization of vascular histamine H_1-receptors: multiple affinity states of aortic histamine H_1-receptor. Agents and Actions 1985; 16(3/4):179–182.
119. Berridge MJ. Phosphotidylinositol hydrolysis: a multifunctional transducing mechanism. Mol Cell Endocrinol 1981; 24:115–140.
120. Marshal I. Histamine modulation of neurotransmission in the sympathetic nervous system. J Auton Pharmacol 1981; 1:235–250.
121. Saltissi S, et al. The effects of oral cimetidine therapy on the cardiovascular system in man. Br J Clin Pharmacol 1981; 11:497–503.
122. Regoli D, Barabe J. Pharmacology of bradykinin and related kinins. Pharmacol Rev 1980; 32(1):1–46.
123. Rocha E, Silva M. Kinin Hormones. Springfield, Ill: Thomas, 1970.
124. Couture R, et al. The dog common carotid artery: a sensitive bioassay for studying vasodilator effects of substance P and of kinins. Can J Physiol Pharmacol 1980; 58:1234–1244.
125 Cherry PD, Furchgott RF, Zawadski JV. The indirect nature of bradykinin relaxation of isolated arteries: endothelial dependent and independent components (abstr). Fed Proc 1981; 40:689.
126. Cherry PD, et al. The role of endothelial cells in the relaxation of isolated arteries by bradykinin. Proc Natl Acad Sci USA 1982; 79:2106–2110.
127. Furchgott RF. Role of endothelium in responses of vascular smooth muscle. Circ Res 1983; 53:557–573.
128. Regoli D. Pharmacology of bradykinin and related kinins. Adv Exp Med Biol 1983; 156:569–583.
129. Roscher AA, et al. Autoregulation of bradykinin receptors and bradykinin-induced prostacyclin formation in human fibroblasts. J Clin Invest 1984; 74:552–558.
130. Burnstock G. A basis for distinguishing two types of purinergic receptor. In RW Straub, L Bolis, eds. Cell Membrane Receptors for Drugs and Hormones: A Multidisciplinary Approach. New York: Raven, 1978. Pp. 107–118.
131. Clyman RI, et al. Guanosine 3, 5′-monophosphate content of human umbilical artery. J Clin Invest 1975; 72:1020–1025.
132. Van Calker D, Muller M, Hamprecht B. Adenosine regulates via two different types of receptors, the accumulation of cyclic AMP in cultured brain cells. J Neurosci 1979; 33:999–1005.
133. Londos C, Cooper DMF, Woolf J. Subclasses of external adenosine receptors. Proc Natl Acad Sci USA 1980; 77:2551–2554.
134. Burnstock G, Kennedy C. Is there a basis for distinguishing two types of P_2-purinoceptor? Gen Pharmacol 1985; 16(5): 433–440.
135. Londos C, Wolf J. Two distinct adenosine sensitive sites on

adenylate cyclase. Proc Natl Acad Sci USA 1977; 74:5482–5486.
136. Ghai G, Mustafa J. Demonstration of a putative adenosine receptor in rabbit aorta. Blood Vessels 1982; 19:117–125.
137. Collis MG, Brown CM. Adenosine relaxes the aorta by interacting with an A_2 receptor and an intracellular site. Eur J Pharmacol 1983; 96:61–69.
138. Fredholm BB, Sollevi A. Cardiovascular effects of adenosine. Clin Physiol 1986; 6:1–21.
139. Kennedy C, Burnstock G. Evidence for an inhibitory prejunctional P_1-purinoreceptor in the rat portal vein with characteristics of the A_2 rather than the A_1 subtype. Eur J Pharmacol 1984; 100:363–368.
140. Pearson JD. Purine nucleotides as regulators of vessel tone. Biochem Soc Trans 1988; 16:480–482.
141. Mathieson JJI, Burnstock G. Purine-mediated relaxation and constriction of isolated rabbit mesenteric artery are not endothelium-dependent. Eur J Pharmacol 1985; 221–229.
142. Needham L, et al. Characteristics of the P_2 purinoreceptor that mediates prostacyclin production by pig endothelial cells. Eur J Pharmacol 1987; 134:199–209.
143. Chapal J, Loubatieres-Mariani M. Evidence for purinergic receptors on vascular smooth muscle in rat pancreas. Eur J Pharmacol 1983; 87:423–430.
144. Anand-Srivastava MB, et al. Presence of "Ra" and "P"-site receptors for adenosine coupled to adenylate cyclase in cultured vascular smooth muscle cells. Biochem Biophys Res Commun 1982; 108(1):213–219.
145. Jonzon B, Nilsson J, Fredholm BB. Adenosine receptor-mediated changes in cyclic AMP production and DNA synthesis in cultured arterial smooth muscle cells. J Cell Physiol 1985; 83:451–456.
146. Tsuda T, et al. Stimulation of phospholipase C mediated hydrolysis of phosphoinositides by adenosine 5′triphosphate via P_2 purinoreceptors in cultured rat aortic smooth muscle. JPN Circ J 1988; 52(6):570–579.
147. Benham CD, Tsien RW. A novel receptor-operated Ca^{++} permeable channel activated by ATP in smooth muscle. Nature 1987; 328:275–278.
148. Kebabian JW, Calne DB. Multiple receptors for dopamine. Nature 1979; 277:93–96.
149. Berkowitz BA, Ohlstein EH. Cardiovascular dopamine receptors: recent advances in agonists and antagonists of the DA_1-receptor. J Cardiovasc Pharmacol 1984; 6:S559–S563.
150. Buylaert WA, Willems JL, Bogaert MG. Peripheral prejunctional dopamine receptors. In PM Vanhoutte, I Leusen, eds. Vasodilation. New York: Raven, 1981. Pp. 125–130.
151. McNay JL, Goldberg LI. Comparison of the effects of dopamine isoproterenol, norepinephrine and bradykinin on canine renal and femoral blood flow after POB. J Pharmacol Exp Ther 1966; 151:23–31.
152. Goldberg LI. Cardiovascular and renal actions of dopamine: potential clinical applications. Pharmacol Rev 1972; 24:1–29.
153. Gilbert JC, Goldberg LI. Cyproheptadine blockade of dopamine-induced renal vasodilation in the dog. Circulation 1974; 50[Suppl III]:III–36A.
154. Goldberg LI, Kohli JD. Specific dopamine receptors in vascular smooth muscle. In PM Vanhoutte, I Leusen, eds. Vasodilation. New York: Raven, 1981. Pp. 161–175.
155. Owman C, Hardebo JE. Mechanisms of cerebral vasodilation: amines, peptides, and the blood-brain barrier. In PM Vanhoutte, I Leusen, eds. Vasodilation. New York: Raven, 1981. Pp. 161–175.
156. Murthy VV, et al. Dopamine sensitive adenylate cyclase in canine renal artery. J Pharm Pharmacol 1976; 28:567–571.
157. Fredholm BB. Sources and actions of dopamine. In PM Vanhoutte, I Leusen, eds. Vasodilation. New York: Raven, 1981. Pp. 117–125.
158. Wharton J, Gulbenkian S. Peptides in the mammalian cardiovascular system. Experentia 1987; 43:821–832.
159. Ganten D, et al. Peptidergic systems: effects on blood vessels. J Cardiovasc Pharmacol 1984; 6:S598–S607.
160. Krieger DT, Martin JB. Brain peptides, parts I and II. N Engl J Med 1981; 304:876–885, 944–951.
161. Leys K, Schachter M, Sever P. Autoradiographic localization of NPY receptors in rabbit kidney: comparison with rat, guinea pig and human. Eur J Pharmacol 1987; 134:233–237.
162. Sigrist S, et al. Specific receptor and cardiovascular effects of calcitonin gene-related peptide. Endocrinology 1986; 119:381–389.
163. Regoli D, et al. Pharmacological receptors for substance P and neurokinins. Life Sci 1987; 40:109–117.
164. Itoh N, et al. Human preprovasoactive intestinal polypeptide contains a novel PHI^{27}-like peptide, PHM^{27}. Nature 1983; 304:547–549.
165. Lord JAH, et al. Endogenous opioid peptides: multiple agonists and receptors. Nature 1977; 267:495–499.
166. Simon EJ, Hiller JM. Opiate receptors. Ann Rev Pharmacol Toxicol 1978; 18:371–394.
167. Schulz R, Wuster M, Herz A. Pharmacological characterization of the epsilon-opiate receptor. J Pharmacol Exp Ther 1980; 216:604–606.
168. Martin WR. History and development of mixed opioid agonists, partial agonists and antagonists. Br J Clin Pharm 1979; 7[Suppl 3]:273–279.
169. Cox BM. Peripheral actions mediated by opioid receptors. In GW Pasternak, ed. Opiate Receptors. Clifton, N.J.: Humana, 1988.
170. Beaumont A, Hughes J. Biology of opioid peptides. Ann Rev Pharmacol Toxicol 1979; 19:245–267.
171. Gullis R, Traber G, Hamprecht B. Morphine elevates levels of cyclic GMP in neuroblastoma X glioma hybrid cell line. Nature 1975; 256:57–59.
172. Brandt M, et al. Enkephalin regulates the levels of cyclic nucleotides in neuroblastoma X glioma hybrid cells. Nature 1976; 262:311–313.
173. Minneman K, Iversen LL. In HW Kosterlitz, et al., eds. Opiates and Endogenous Opioid Peptides. Amsterdam: North-Holland, 1976. Pp. 137–142.
174. Winquist RJ. The relaxant effects of atrial natriuretic factor on vascular smooth muscle. Life Sci 1985; 37:1081–1087.
175. Anderson JV, Bloom SR. Atrial natriuretic peptide: What is the excitement all about? J Endocr 1986; 110:7–17.
176. Hughes RJ, et al. Reaction of the atrial natriuretic peptide receptor on a smooth muscle cell. Am J Physiol 1987; 253:C809–C816.
177. Atlas SA, Laragh JH. Atrial natriuretic peptide: a new factor in hormonal control of blood pressure and electrolyte homeostasis. Ann Rev Med 1986; 37:397–414.
178. Manning M, Sawyer WH. Synthesis and receptor specificities of vasopressin antagonists. J Cardiovasc Pharmacol 1986; 8[Suppl 7]:S29–S35.
179. Liard J-F. Cardiovascular effects of vasopressin: some recent aspects. J Cardiovasc Pharmacol 1986; 8[Suppl 7]:S61–S65.
180. Altura BM. Dose-response relationships for arginine vasopressin and synthetic analogs on three types of rat blood vessels: possible evidence for regional differences in vasopressin receptor sites within a mammal. J Pharmacol Exp Ther 1975; 193(3):413–423.
181. Altura BM, Altura BT. Actions of vasopressin, oxytocin, and synthetic analogs on vascular smooth muscle. Fed Proc 1984; 43:80–86.

182. Crooke ST, et al. Vasopressin V_1 receptors and inter-receptor regulation in vascular smooth muscle cells. Biochem Pharmacol 1988; 37(11):2105–2108.
183. Doyle VM, Ruegg UT. Vasopressin induced production of inositol triphosphate and calcium efflux in a smooth muscle cell line. Biochem Biophys Res Commun 1985; 131:469–476.
184. Bennett T, Gardiner SM. Vasopressin and the cardiovascular system: physiology or pharmacology. J Cardiovasc Pharmacol 1986; 8[Suppl 7]:S44–S49.
185. Barrigón S, Tamargo J. The effect of oxytocin on contractile responses and ^{45}Ca movements in rat isolated aortic strips. Br J Pharmac 1986; 87:763–770.
186. Gardiner PJ, Collier HOJ. Specific receptors for prostaglandins in airways. Prostaglandins 1980; 19:819–841.
187. Kennedy I, et al. Studies on the characterization of prostanoid receptors: a proposed classification. Prostaglandins 1982; 24(5):667–689.
188. Robertson PR. Characterization and regulation of prostaglandin and leukotriene receptors: an overview. Prostaglandins 1986; 31(3):395–411.
189. Oliva D, Nicosia A. PGI_2-receptors and molecular mechanisms in platelets and vasculature: state of the art. Pharmacol Res Commun 1987; 19(11):735–769.
190. Darius H, Smith JB, Lefer AM. Beneficial effects of a new potent and specific thromboxane receptor antagonist (SQ-29,548) in vitro and in vivo. J Pharmacol Exp Ther 1985; 235:274–281.
191. Hanasaki K, et al. Specific receptors for thromboxane A_2 in cultured vascular smooth muscle cells of rat aorta. Biochem Biophys Res Commun 1988; 150(3):1170–1175.
192. Moncada S, Vane J. Pharmacology and endogenous roles of prostaglandin endoperoxides, thromboxane A_2, and prostacyclin. Pharmacol Rev 1979; 30:293–331.
193. Wendelberger KJ. Prostaglandin and leukotriene receptors in pulmonary, vascular, and uterine smooth muscle. Sem Perinatol 1987; 11(1):1–11.
194. Hatano Y, et al. Interactions between different prostaglandins and other relaxing agents on isolated vascular smooth muscle. In B Samuelson, PW Ramwell, R Paoletti, eds. Advances in Prostaglandin and Thromboxane Research, vol 7. New York: Raven, 1980. Pp. 683–686.
195. Kadowitz PJ, et al. Differential actions of the prostaglandins on the pulmonary vascular bed. In B Samuelson, PW Ramwell, R Paoletti, eds. Advances in Prostaglandin and Thromboxane Research, vol. 7. New York: Raven, 1980. Pp. 731–743.
196. Wennmalm A. Participation of prostaglandins in the regulation of peripheral vascular resistance. In JA Oates, ed. Prostaglandins and the Cardiovascular System. New York: Raven, 1982. Pp. 303–331.
197. Ogletree ML. Overview of physiological and pathophysiological effects of thromboxane A_2. Fed Proc 1987; 46:133–138.
198. Dorn GW, et al. Cultured human vascular smooth muscle cells with functional thromboxane A_2 receptors: measurement of U46619-induced ^{45}calcium efflux. Circ Res 1987; 60:952–956.
199. Robinson BF, et al. Effect of prostaglandins A_1, B_1, E_2, and F_2 on forearm arterial bed and superficial hand vein in man. Clin Sci 1973; 44:367–376.
200. Yanagisawa A, et al. Mechanism of antagonism of thromboxane receptors in vascular smooth muscle. Eur J Pharmacol 1987; 133:89–96.
201. Dzau VJ, Gibbons GH. Cell biology of vascular hypertrophy in systemic hypertension. Am J Cardiol 1988; 62:30G–35G.
202. Graff G, et al. Activation of soluble splenic cell guanylate cyclase by prostaglandin endoperoxides and fatty acid hydroperoxides. J Biol Chem 1978; 253(21):7662–7676.
203. Bray MA. Leukotriene receptors. In Leukotrienes in Cardiovascular and Pulmonary Function. New York: Alan R. Liss, 1985. Pp. 17–29.
204. Sun FF, Chau LY, Austen KF. Binding of leukotriene C_4 by glutathione transferase: a reassessment of biochemical and functional criteria for leukotriene receptors. Fed Proc 1987; 46:204–207.
205. Piper PJ, et al. Leukotrienes in the cardiovascular system. Biochem Soc Trans 1988; 16:482–483.
206. Feuerstein G. Cardiac and vascular effects of leukotrienes. In U Zor, et al., eds. Advances in Prostaglandin, Thromboxane, and Leukotriene Research. New York: Raven, 1986. Pp. 299–308.
207. Letts LG, Cirino M. Vascular actions of leukotrienes. Leukotrienes in Cardiovascular and Pulmonary Function. New York: Alan R. Liss, 1985. Pp. 47–58.
208. Palmberg L, Claesson H-E, Thyberg J. Leukotrienes stimulate initiation of DNA synthesis in cultured arterial smooth muscle cells. J Cell Sci 1987; 88:151–159.
209. Hollenberg MD. Mechanisms of receptor-mediated transmembrane signaling. Experientia 1986; 42:718–727.
210. Kenakin T. Are receptors promiscuous? Intrinsic efficacy as a transduction phenomenon. Life Sci 1988; 43:1095–1101.
211. Hunter T, Cooper JA. Protein-tyrosine kinases. Ann Rev Biochem 1985; 54:897–930.
212. Bowen-Pope DF, Ross R, Seifert RA. Locally acting growth factors for vascular smooth muscle cells: endogenous synthesis and release from platelets. Circulation 1985; 72(4):735–740.
213. Berk BC, et al. Vasoconstriction: a new activity for platelet-derived growth factor. Science 1986; 232:87–90.
214. Berk BC, et al. Epidermal growth factor, a vascular smooth muscle mitogen, induces rat aortic contraction. J Clin Invest 1985; 75:1083–1086.
215. Pfeifle B, Boeder H, Ditschuneit H. Interaction of receptors for insulin-like growth factor I, platelet-derived growth factor, and fibroblast growth factor in rat aortic cells. Endocrinology 1986; 120(6):2251–2258.
216. Clemmons DR. Interaction of circulating cell-derived and plasma growth factors in stimulating cultured smooth muscle cell replication. J Cell Physiol 1984; 121:425–430.
217. Bowen-Pope DF, Ross R. Platelet-derived growth factor. II: Specific binding to cultured cells. J Biol Chem 1982; 257:5167–5171.
218. Williams LT, Tremble P, Antoniades HN. Platelet-derived growth factor binds specifically to receptors on vascular smooth muscle cells and binding becomes non-dissociable. Proc Natl Acad Sci USA 1982; 79:5067–5070.
219. Hart CE, et al. Two classes of PDGF receptor recognize different isoforms of PDGF. Science 1988; 240:1529–1531.
220. Yarden Y, et al. Structure of the receptor for platelet-derived growth factor helps define a family of closely related growth factor receptors. Nature 1986; 323:226–232.
221. Gaspodarowitcz D. Growth factors and their action in vivo and in vitro. J Pathol 1983; 141:201–233.
222. Berridge MJ, et al. Inositol triphosphate formation and calcium mobilization in Swiss 3T3 cells in response to platelet-derived growth factor. Biochem J 1984; 222:195–201.
223. Habnicht AJR, et al. Early changes in phosphatidylinositol and arachidonate acid metabolism in quiescent Swiss 3T3 cells stimulated to divide by platelet-derived growth factor. J Biol Chem 1981; 256:12329–12335.
224. Namm DH. The role of cyclic nucleotides in the vasculature. In JW Kebabian, JA Nathanson, eds. Handbook of Experimental Pharmacology, Cyclic Nucleotides II. New York: Springer, 1981. Pp. 683–690.

225. Pfeifle B, Ditschuneit H. Two separate receptors for insulin and insulin-like growth factors on arterial smooth muscle cells. Exp Clin Endocrinol 1983; 81(3):280–286.
226. Bornfeldt KE, et al. Receptors for insulin-like growth factor-I in plasma membranes isolated from bovine mesenteric arteries. Acta Endocrinol 1988; 117:428–434.
227. Pfeifle B, Ditschuneit H. The effect of insulin and insulin-like growth factors on cell proliferation of human smooth muscle cells. Artery 1980; 8(4):336–341.
228. King GL, et al. Receptors and growth-promoting effects of insulin and insulinlike growth factors on cells from bovine retinal capillaries and aorta. J Clin Invest 1985; 75:1028–1036.
229. Pfeifle B, Ditschuneit H. Regulation of receptors for insulin-like growth factors in cultured arterial smooth muscle cells by thyroid hormone. J Endocrinol 1983; 98:373–379.
230. Adamson ED, Rees AR. Epidermal growth factor receptors. Mol Cell Biochem 1981; 34:129–152.
231. Bhargava G, Rifas L, Makman MH. Presence of epidermal growth factor receptors and influence of epidermal growth factor on proliferation and aging in cultured smooth muscle cells. J Cell Physiol 1979; 100:356–374.
232. Bevan JA. Vascular myogenic or stretch-dependent tone. J Cardiovasc Pharmacol 1985; 7[Suppl 3]:S129–S136.
233. Winquist RJ, Bevan JA. In vitro model of maintained myogenic vascular tone. Blood Vessels 1981; 18:134–138.
234. Prehn JL, Bevan JA. Facial vein of the rabbit. Intracellularly recorded hyperpolarization of smooth muscle cells induced by beta-adrenergic receptor stimulation. Circ Res 1983; 52:465–470.
235. Siegel G, Kampe CH, Ebeling BJ. pH-dependent myogenic control in cerebral vascular smooth muscle. In J Cervos-Navarro, E Fritschka, eds. Cerebral Microcirculation and Metabolism. New York: Raven, 1981. Pp. 213–226.
236. Ross G, et al. Spontaneous phasic activity of isolated human coronary arteries. Cardiovasc Res 1980; 14:613–618.
237. Bevan JA. Autonomic pharmacologist's guide to the cerebral circulation. Trends Pharm Sci 1984; 5:234–236.
238. Mooibroek MJ, Wang JH. Integration of signal-transduction processes. Biochem Cell Biol 1988; 66:557–566.
239. Yip CC. Cell-membrane hormone receptors: some perspectives on their structure and function relationship. Biochem Cell Biol 1988; 66:549–556.
240. Mitchell RH. How do receptors at the cell surface send signals to the cell interior? Br Med J 1987; 295:1320–1323.
241. Zierler K, Rogus EM. Effects of peptide hormones and adrenergic agents on membrane potentials of target cells. Fed Proc 1981; 40:121–124.
242. Anwar N, Mason DF. Two actions of gamma-aminobutyric acid on the response of the isolated basilar artery from the rabbit. Br J Pharmacol 1982; 75:172–181.
243. Stevens CF. Channel families in the brain. Nature 1987; 328:198–199.
244. Gilman AG. G proteins: transducers of receptor-generated signals. Ann Rev Biochem 1987; 56:615–649.
245. Casey PJ, Gilman AG. G protein involvement in receptor-effector coupling. J Biol Chem 1968; 263(6):2577–2580.
246. Litosch I, Fain JN. Regulation of phosphoinositide breakdown by guanine nucleotides. Life Sci 1986; 39:187–194.
247. Neer EJ, Clapham DE. Roles of G protein subunits in transmembrane signalling. Nature 1988; 333:129–134.
248. Stryer L, Bourne HR. G proteins: a family of signal transducers. Ann Rev Cell Biol 1986; 2:391–419.
249. Rosenthal W, et al. Control of voltage-dependent Ca^{2+} channels by G protein-coupled receptors. FASEB J 1988; 2:2784–2790.
250. Fain JN, Wallace MA, Wojcikiewicz JH. Evidence for involvement of guanine nucleotide-binding regulatory proteins in the activation of phospholipases by hormones. FASEB J 1988; 2:2569–2574.
251. Brown AM, Birnbaumer L. Direct G protein gating of ion channels. Am J Physiol 1988; 254:H401–H410.
252. Suzuki Y, et al. Gamma-aminobutyric acid-induced contraction of the dog basilar artery. Pharmacology 1984; 29:24–30.
253. Limbird LE. Receptors linked to inhibition of adenylate cyclase: additional signalling mechanisms. FASEB J 1988; 2:2686–2695.
254. Codina JJ, et al. Pertussis toxin substrate, the putative N_i of adenylate cyclases, is an alpha/beta heterodimer regulated by guanine nucleotide and magnesium. Proc Natl Acad Sci USA 1983; 80:4276–4280.
255. Codina JJ, et al. N_s and N_i: the stimulatory and inhibitory regulatory components of adenyl cyclases. Purification of the human erythrocyte proteins without the use of activating regulatory ligands. J Biol Chem 1984; 259:5871–5886.
256. Arad H, Rosenbusch JP, Levitski A. Stimulatory GTP regulatory N_s and the catalytic unit of adenylate cyclase are tightly associated: mechanistic consequences. Proc Natl Acad Sci USA 1984; 81:6579–6583.
257. Lapetina EG. The role of GTP-binding proteins in receptor activation of phospholipase C. Adv Exp Med Biol 1987; 221:95–100.
258. Blackmore PF, et al. Role of guanine nucleotide-binding regulatory protein in the hydrolysis of hepatocyte phosphatidylinositol 4,5-bisphosphate by calcium-mobilizing hormones and the control of cell calcium. Studies utilizing aluminum fluoride. J Biol Chem 1986; 260:14477–14483.
259. Codina J, et al. The alpha subunit of the G_k opens atrial potassium channels. Science 1987; 236:442–445.
260. Yatani A, et al. Direct activation of mammalian atrial muscarinic K channels by a human erythrocyte pertussis toxin-sensitive G protein G_k. Science 1987; 235:207–211.
261. Yatani A, et al. Direct regulation of mammalian cardiac calcium channels by a G protein. Science 1987; 238:1288–1292.
262. Michell RH, et al. The possible involvement of phosphatidylinositol breakdown in the mechanism of the stimulus-response coupling at receptors which control cell-surface calcium gates. Adv Exp Med Biol 1977; 83:447–464.
263. Berridge MJ. Rapid accumulation of inositol triphosphate reveals that agonists hydrolyse phosphoinositides instead of phosphatidylinositol. Biochem J 1983; 212:849–858.
264. Berridge MJ, Buchan PB, Heslop JP. Relationship of phosphoinositide metabolism to the hormonal activation of the insect salivary gland by 5-hydroxytryptamine. Mol Cell Endocr 1984; 36:37–42.
265. Suematsu E, et al. Inositol 1,4,5-triphosphate-releases Ca^{2+} from intracellular store sites in skinned single cells of porcine coronary arteries. Biochem Biophys Res Commun 1983; 120:481–492.
266. Somlyo AV, et al. Inositol triphosphate-induced calcium release and contraction in vascular smooth muscle. Proc Natl Acad Sci USA 1985; 82:5231–5235.
267. Somlyo AP. Excitation-contraction coupling and the ultrastructure of smooth muscle. Circ Res 1985; 57(4):497–507.
268. Hirasawa K. Phosphatidylinositol turnover in receptor mechanism and signal transduction. Ann Rev Pharmacol Toxicol 1985; 25:147–170.
269. Rasmussen H. The calcium messenger system (first of two parts). N Engl J Med 1986; 314(17):1094–1101.
270. Pomerantz KB, Hajjar DP. Eicosanoids in regulation of arterial smooth muscle cell phenotype, proliferative capacity and cholesterol metabolism. Arteriosclerosis 1989; 9:413–429.
271. Streb H, et al. Effect of inositol-1,4,5-triphosphate on isolated subcellular fractions of rat pancreas. J Membr Biol 1984; 312:374–376.

272. Smith JB, Smith L, Higgins BL. Inositol triphosphate opens an intracellular calcium channel by a ligand-binding mechanism. J Biol Chem 1985; 260:14413–14416.
273. Putney JW, Jr. Formation and actions of calcium-mobilizing messenger inositol 1,4,5-triphosphate. Am J Physiol 1987; 252(15):G149–G157.
274. Takai Y, et al. Studies on cyclic nucleotide-independent protein kinase and its proenzyme in mammalian tissues. J Biol Chem 252:7603–7609.
275. Nishizuka Y. Studies and perspectives of protein kinase C. Science 1986; 233:305–312.
276. Matsumoto H, Sasaki Y. Staurosporine, a protein kinase C inhibitor, interferes with proliferation of arterial smooth muscle cells. Biochem Biophys Res Comm 1989; 158(1): 105–109.
277. Nishikawa M, et al. Protein kinase C modulates in vitro phosphorylation of the smooth muscle heavy meromyosin by myosin light chain kinase. J Biol Chem 1984; 259:8808–8814.
278. Kawamoto S, Hidaka H. Ca^{2+}-activated, phospholipid-dependent protein kinase catalyses the phosphorylation of actin-binding proteins. Biochem Biophys Res Commun 1984; 118:736–742.
279. Umekawa H, Hidaka H. Phosphorylation of caldesmon by protein kinase C. Biochem Biophys Res Commun 1985; 132:56–62.
280. Forder J, Scriabine A, Rasmussen H. Plasma membrane calcium flux, protein kinase C activation and smooth muscle contraction. J Pharmacol Exp Ther 1985; 235:267–273.
281. Park S, Rasmussen H. Activation of tracheal smooth muscle contraction: synergism between Ca^{2+} and C-kinase activators. Proc Natl Acad Sci USA 1985; 82:8835–8839.
282. Rasmussen H. The calcium messenger system (second of two parts). N Engl J Med 1986; 314:1164–1170.
283. Egawa K, Sacktor B, Takenawa T. Ca^{2+}-dependent and Ca^{2+}-independent degradation of phosphatidylinositol in rabbit vas deferens. Biochem J 1981; 194:129–136.
284. Takenawa T, Masaki T, Goto K. Increase in norepinephrine-induced formation of phosphatidic acid in rat vas deferens after denervation. J Biochem 1983; 93:303–306.
285. Salmon DM, Honeyman TW. Proposed mechanism of cholinergic action in smooth muscle. Nature 1980; 284:344–345.
286. Morgan JP, Morgan KG. Stimulus-specific patterns of intracellular calcium levels in smooth muscle of ferret portal vein. J Physiol 1984; 351:155–167.
287. Silver PJ, Stull JT. Regulation of myosin light chain and phosphorylase phosphorylation in tracheal smooth muscle. J Biol Chem 1982; 257:6145–6150.
288. Takai Y, et al. Role of protein kinase C in transmembrane signaling. J Cell Biochem 1985; 29:143–155.
289. Hermsmeyer K, Sturek M. Membrane potential, Ca^{2+} influx and Ca^{2+} release in single vascular muscle cells. J Cardiovasc Pharmacol 1986; 8[Suppl 8]:S38–S41.
290. Bolton TB, et al. Calcium channels in smooth muscle cells. Biochem Soc Trans 1988; 16:492–493.
291. Lullmann H, Ziegler A. Calcium, cell membrane, and excitation-contraction coupling. J Cardiovasc Pharmacol 1987; 10[Suppl I]:S2–S8.
292. Somlyo AP, Somlyo AV. Electron probe analysis of calcium content and movements in sarcoplasmic reticulum, endoplasmic reticulum, mitochondria, and cytoplasm. J Cardiovasc Pharmacol 1986; 8[Suppl 8]:S42–S47.
293. Somlyo AP. Cellular site of calcium regulation. Nature 1984; 309:516–517.
294. Cox JA. Calcium-calmodulin interaction and cellular function. J Cardiovasc Pharmacol 1986; 8[Suppl 8]:S48–S51.
295. Klee CB, et al. Different modes of interaction of calmodulin with its target enzymes. J Cardiovasc Pharmacol 1986; 8[suppl 8]:S52–S56.
296. Borle AB. Control modulation and regulation of cell calcium. Rev Physiol Biochem Pharmacol 1981; 90:130–153.
297. Beavo JA, et al. Identification and properties of cyclic nucleotide phosphodiesterases. Mol Cell Endocrinol 1982; 28:387–410.
298. Keravis TM, Wells JN, Hardman JG. Cyclic nucleotide phosphodiesterase activity from pig coronary arteries: lack of interconvertability of major forms. Biochem Biophys Acta 1980; 613:116–129.
299. Hardman JG. Cyclic nucleotides and smooth muscle contraction: some conceptual experimental considerations. In E Bulbring, et al., eds. Smooth Muscle: An Assessment of Current Knowledge. Edward Arnold, 1981. Pp. 249–262.
300. Ross EM, Gilman AG. Biochemical properties of hormone sensitive adenylate cyclase. Ann Rev Biochem 1980; 49:553–564.
301. Kramer GL, Hardman JG. Cyclic nucleotides and blood vessel contraction. In DF Bohr, SP Somlyo, HV Sparks, eds. Handbook of Physiology: Section 2, The Cardiovascular System, Vascular Smooth Muscle. New York: Oxford University Press, 1980. Pp. 179–199.
302. Hardman JG. Cyclic nucleotides and regulation of vascular smooth muscle. J Cardiovasc Pharmacol 1984; 6:639–645.
303. Owen NE. Effect of prostaglandin E-1 on DNA synthesis in vascular smooth muscle cells. Am J Physiol 1986; 250:C584–C588.
304. Sjolund M, et al. Phenotype modulation in primary culture arterial smooth muscle cells: dual effect of prostaglandin E-1. Differentiation 1984; 27:158–162.
305. Friedman DL. Regulation of the cell cycle and cellular proliferation by cyclic nucleotides. In JW Kebabian, JA Nathanson, eds. Handbook of Experimental Pharmacology, vol. 2. Cyclic Nucleotides. New York: Springer, 1982. Pp. 151–188.
306. Meisheri KD, Van Breemen C. Effects of beta-adrenergic stimulation on calcium movements in rabbit aortic smooth muscle: relationship with cyclic AMP. J Physiol 1982; 331:429–441.
307. Scheid CR, Fay FS. Beta adrenergic effects on transmembrane ^{45}Ca fluxes in isolated smooth muscle cells. Am J Physiol 1984; 246:C431–C438.
308. Ousterhout JM, Sperelakis N. Cyclic nucleotides depress action potentials in cultured aortic smooth muscle cells. Eur J Pharmacol 1987; 144:7–14.
309. Hathaway DR, et al. Myosin light chain and heavy chain phosphorylation in smooth muscle: potential regulatory roles for calcium phospholipids and cyclic nucleotides. Biochem Soc Trans 1988; 16:499–501.
310. Vigne P, et al. Dual control of intracellular pH in aortic smooth muscle cells by a cAMP-sensitive HCO_3^-/CL^- antiporter and a protein kinase C-sensitive Na^+/H^+ antiporter. J Biol Chem. 1988; 263(34):18023–18029.
311. Ignarro LJ, Kadowitz PJ. The pharmacological and physiological role of cyclic GMP in smooth muscle relaxation. Ann Rev Pharmacol Toxicol 1985; 25:171–191.
312. Kimura H, Mittal CK, Murad F. Activation of cyclase from rat liver and other tissues by sodium azide. J Biol Chem 1975; 250:8016–8022.
313. Mittal CK, Kimura H, Murad F. Purification and properties of a protein required for sodium azide activation of guanylate cyclase. J Biol Chem 1977; 252:4384–4390.
314. Katsuki S, et al. Stimulation of guanylate cyclase by sodium nitroprusside nitroglycerin and nitric oxide in various tissue preparations and comparison to the effects of sodium azide and hydroxylamine. J Cyclic Nucleotide Res 1977; 3:23–25.
315. Ignarro LJ, et al. Mechanisms of vascular smooth muscle

relaxation by organic nitrates, nitrites, nitroprusside, and nitric oxide: evidence for the involvement of S-nitrosothiols as active intermediates. J Pharmacol Exp Ther 1981; 218(3):739–749.
316. Gruetter CA, et al. Relationship between cyclic guanosine 3′:5′-monophosphate formation and relaxation of coronary arterial smooth muscle by glyceryl trinitrate, nitroprusside, nitrite and nitric oxide: effects of methylene blue and methemoglobin. J Pharmacol Exp Ther 1981; 219(1):181–186.
317. Schultz K-D. Effects of 8-Br-cGMP on tonus of rat ductus deferens and aorta. Naunyn-Schmiedeberg Arch Pharmacol 1977; 297:R12.
318. Axelsson KL, Wikberg JES, Andersson RGG. Relationship between nitroglycerin, cyclic GMP and relaxation of vascular smooth muscle. Life Sci 1979; 24:1779–1786.
319. Kukovetz WR, et al. Evidence for cyclic GMP-mediated relaxant effects of nitro-compounds in coronary smooth muscle. Naunyn-Schmiedeberg Arch Pharmacol 1979; 310:129–138.
320. Napoli SA, et al. Relaxation of bovine coronary arterial smooth muscle by cyclic GMP, cyclic AMP and analogs. J Pharmacol Exp Ther 1980; 212:469–473.
321. Braughler JM. Soluble guanylate cyclase activation by nitric oxide and its reversal. Involvement of sulfhydryl group oxidation and reduction. Biochem Pharmacol 1983; 32(5):811–818.
322. Braughler JM, Mittal CK, Murad F. Effects of thiols, sugars, and proteins on nitric oxide activation of guanylate cyclase. J Biol Chem 1979; 254(24):12450–12454.
323. Veseley DL, Watson B, Levey GS. Activation of liver guanylate cyclase by paraquat: possible role of superoxide anion. J Pharmacol Exp Ther 1979, 209(1):162–164.
324. Ignarro LJ, Kadowitz PJ, Baricos WH. Evidence that regulation of hepatic guanylate cyclase activity involves interactions between catalytic site -SH groups and both substrate and activator. Arch Biochem Biophys 1981; 208(1):75–86.
325. Ignarro LJ, et al. Activation of soluble guanylate cyclase by NO-hemoproteins involves NO-heme exchange. J Biol Chem 1986; 261:4997–5002.
326. Spiegel AM, et al. Clinical implications of guanine nucleotide-binding proteins as receptor-effector couplers. N Engl J Med 1985; 312:26–33.
327. Lincoln TM, et al. Mechanism of cyclic-GMP-dependent relaxation in vascular smooth muscle. Biochem Soc Trans 1988; 16:497–499.
328. Kobayashi S, Kanaide H, Nakamura M. Cytosolic-free calcium transients in cultured vascular smooth muscle cells: microfluorometric measurements. Science 1985; 229:553–556.
329. Furukawa K-I, Tawada Y. Shigekawa M. Regulation of the plasma membrane Ca^{2+} pump by cyclic nucleotides in cultured vascular smooth muscle. In RE Decetzel, ed. Modern Pharmacology. Boston: Little, Brown, 1982. Pp. 141–156.
330. Lands AM, et al. Differentiation of receptor systems activated by sympathomimetic amines. Nature 1967; 214:597–598.
331. Lands AM, Luduena FP, Buzzo HJ. Differentiation of receptors responsive to isoproterenol. Life Sci 1967; 6:2241–2249.
332. Frielle T, Caron MG, Lefkowitz RJ. Properties of the $beta_1$ and $beta_2$ adrenergic receptor subtypes revealed by molecular cloning from smooth muscle. J Pharmacol Exp Ther 1968; 159(1):129–145.
333. Baron CB, et al. Pharamcomechanical coupling in smooth muscle may involve phosphotidylinositol metabolism. Proc Natl Acad Sci USA 1984; 81:6899–6903.
334. Gabella G. Structural apparatus for force transmission in smooth muscle. Physiol Rev 1984; 64(2):455–477.
335. Devine CE, Somlyo AV, Somlyo AP. Sarcoplasmic reticulum and excitation-contraction coupling in mammalian smooth muscle. J Cell Biol 1972; 52:690–718.
336. Somlyo AV. Ultrastructure of vascular smooth muscle. In DF Bohr, AP Somlyo, HV Sparks, eds. The Handbook of Physiology: Section 2, The Cardiovascular System, Vascular Smooth Muscle. New York, Oxford University Press, 1980. Pp. 33–67.
337. Forbes MS, Rennels L, Nelson E. Caveolar systems and sarcoplasmic reticulum in coronary smooth muscle cells of the mouse. J Ultrastruct Res 1979; 65:325–339.
338. Philipson KD, Bers DM, Nishimoto AY. The role of phospholipids in the Ca^{2+} binding of isolated cardiac sarcolemma. J Mol Cell Cardiol 1980; 12:1159–1173.
339. Lüllman H, Peters T. Plasmalemmal calcium in cardiac excitation-contraction coupling. Clin Exp Pharmacol Physiol 1977; 4:49–57.
340. Masters SB, Quinn MT, Brown JH. Relationships between phosphoinositide and calcium responses to muscarinic agonists in astrocytoma cells. Mol Pharmacol 1984; 26:149–155.
341. Campbell MD, et al. Phospoinositide hydrolysis is correlated with agonist-induced calcium flux and contraction in the rabbit aorta. Eur J Pharmacol 1985; 116:129–136.
342. Bond M, et al. Total cytoplasmic calcium in relaxed and maximally contracted rabbit portal vein smooth muscle. J Physiol 1984; 355:677–695.
343. Kaworski D, et al. Calcium released by norepinephrine from central sarcoplasmic reticulum in rabbit main pulmonary artery smooth muscle. J Physiol 1985; 366:153–175.
344. Marsh BB. Factor modifying muscle fibre synaeresis. Nature 1951; 167:1065–1066.
345. Muscatello U, Anderson-Cedergren E, Azzone GF. The mechanism of muscle-fiber relaxation adenosine triphosphatase and relaxing activity of the sarcotubular system. Biochim Biophys Acta 1962; 63:55–74.
346. Weber A, Herz R, Reiss I. On the mechanism of the relaxing effect of fragmented sarcoplasmic reticulum. J Gen Physiol 1963; 46:679–702.
347. Stryer L. Biochemistry, 2nd ed. San Francisco: Freeman, 1981. Pp. 307–308.
348. Zelck V, Karnstedt ZV, Albrecht E. Calcium uptake and calcium release by subcellular fractions of smooth muscle. II: Kinetics of calcium uptake by microsomes and mitochondria from pig coronary artery and guinea pig ileum. Acta Biol Med Germ 1975; 34:981–986.
349. Bond M, et al. Total cytoplasmic calcium in relaxed and maximally contracted rabbit portal vein smooth muscle. J Physiol 1984; 357:185–201.
350. Hartshorne DJ, Gorecka A. Biochemistry of the contractile proteins of smooth muscle. In DF Bohr, AP Somlyo, HV Sparks, eds. The Handbook of Physiology: Section 2, The Cardiovascular System, Vascular Smooth Muscle. New York: Oxford University Press, 1980. Pp. 93–120.
351. Somlyo AP, Somlyo AV. Ultrastructural aspects of activation and contraction of vascular smooth muscle. Fed Proc 1976; 35:1288–1293.
352. Henderson RM. Cell-to-cell contacts. In EE Daniel, DM Paton, eds., Methods in Pharmacology, vol. 3, Smooth Muscle. New York: Plenum, 1975. Pp. 47–77.
353. Stenman S, Vaheri A. Distribution of a major connective tissue protein, fibronectin, in normal human tissues. J Exp Med 1978; 147:1054–1064.
354. Keski-Oja A, Sen A, Todaro GJ. Direct association of fibronectin and actin molecules in vitro. J Cell Biol 1980; 85:527–533.

355. Engvall E, Ruoslahti E, Miller EJ. Affinity of fibronectin to collagens of different genetic types and to fibrinogen. J Exp Med 1978; 147:1584–1595.
356. Barany M. ATPase activity of myosin correlated with speed of muscle shortening. J Gen Physiol 1967; 50:197–218.
357. Dillon PF, et al. Myosin phosphorylation and the cross-bridge cycle in arterial smooth muscle. Science 1981; 211:495–497.
358. Kamm SE, Still JT. The function of myosin and myosin light chain kinase phosphorylation in smooth muscle. Ann Rev Toxicol 1985; 25:593–620.
359. Murphy RA. Myosin phosphorylation and cross-bridge regulation in arterial smooth muscle. State-of-the-art review. Hypertension 1982; 4[Suppl II]:3–7.
360. Butler TM, Davies RE. High-energy phosphates in smooth muscle. In DF Bohr, AP Somlyo, HV Sparks, eds. The Handbook of Physiology: Section 2, The Cardiovascular System, Vascular Smooth Muscle. New York: Oxford University Press, 1980. Pp. 227–252.
361. Guyton AC. Contraction of skeletal muscle. In Textbook of Medical Physiology, 6th ed. Philadelphia: Saunders, 1981. Pp. 122–137.
362. Paul RJ. Chemical energetics of vascular smooth muscle. In DF Bohr, AP Somlyo, HV Sparks, eds. Handbook of Physiology: Section 2, The Cardiovascular System, Vascular Smooth Muscle. New York: Oxford University Press, 1980. Pp. 227–252.
363. Lynch RM, Paul RJ. Energy metabolism and transduction in smooth muscle. Experientia 1985; 41(8):970–977.
364. Butler TM, et al. Chemical energetics of single isometric tetani in mammalian smooth muscle. Am J Physiol 1978; 235:C1–C7.
365. Fine RE, Blitz AL. A chemical comparison of tropomyosins from muscle and non-muscle tissues. J Mol Biol 1975; 95:447–454.
366. Bremel RD, Weber A. Cooperation within actin filament in vertebrate striated muscle. Nature New Biol 1972; 238:97–101.
367. Huxley HE. Structural changes in the actin- and myosin-containing filaments during contraction. Cold Spring Harbor Symposium on Quantitative Biology, 1973; 37:361–376.
368. Sobieszek A, Small JV. Regulation of the actin-myosin interaction in vertebrate smooth muscle: activation via a myosin light-chain kinase and the effect of tropomyosin. J Mol Biol 1977; 112:559–576.
369. Ashton FT, Somlyo AV, Somlyo AP. The contractile apparatus of vascular smooth muscle: intermediate high voltage stereo electron miscroscopy. J Mol Biol 1975; 98:17–29.
370. Cooke P. A filamentous cytoskeleton in vertebrate smooth muscle fibers. J Cell Biol 1976; 48:539–556.
371. Jockusch BM, Isenberg G. Interaction of alpha-actin and vinculin with actin: opposite effects on filament network formation. Proc Natl Acad Sci USA 1981; 78:3005–3009.
372. Geiger B, et al. Vinculin, an intracellular protein localized at specialized sites where microfilament bundles terminate at cell membrane. Proc Natl Acad Sci USA 1980; 77:4127–4131.
373. Devine CE, Somlyo AP. Thick filaments in vascular smooth muscle. J Cell Biol 1971; 49:636–649.
374. Murphy RA, Herlihy JT, Megerman J. Force-generating capacity and contractile content of arterial smooth muscle. J Gen Physiol 1974; 64:691.
375. Somlyo AP, et al. Filament organization in vertebrate smooth muscle. Philos Trans R Soc London [Biol] 1973; 265:223–229.
376. Schaub MC, Kunz B. Regulation of contraction in cardiac and smooth muscles. J Cardiovasc Pharmacol 1986; 8[Suppl 8]:S117–S123.
377. DiSalvo J, Gruenstein E, Silver P. Ca^{2+}-dependent phosphorylation of bovine aortic actomyosin. Proc Soc Exp Biol Med 1978; 158:410–414.
378. Cross RA, Citi S, Hendrick-Jones J. How phosphorylation controls the self-assembly of vertebrate smooth and non-muscle myosins. Biochem Soc Trans 1988; 16:501–503.
379. Johansson B. Calcium and regulation of contraction: a short review. J Cardiovasc Pharmacol 1987; 10[Suppl 1]:S9–S13.
380. Silver PJ, DiSalvo J. Adenosine 3′ : 5′-monophosphate-mediated inhibition of myosin light chain phosphorylation in bovine aortic actomyosin. J Biol Chem 1979; 254:9951–9954.
381. Bhalla RC, Sharma RV, Gupta RC. Isolation of two myosin light chain kinases from bovine carotid artery and their regulation by phosphorylation mediated by cyclic AMP-dependent protein kinase. Biochem J 1982; 203:583–592.
382. Conti MA, Adelstein RS. Phosphorylation by cyclic adenosine 3′ : 5′-monophosphate-dependent protein kinase regulates myosin light chain kinase. Fed Proc 1980; 39:1569–1573.
383. Albanesi J, Fujisaki H, Korn ED. A kinetic model for the molecular basis of contractile activity of Acanthamoeba myosins IA and IB. J Biol Chem 1985; 260:11174–11179.
384. Trotter JA, Nixon CS, Johnson MA. The heavy chain of macrophage myosin is phosphorylated at the tip of the tail. J Biol Chem 1985; 260:14374–14378.
385. Kakiuchi R, et al. Caldesmon, a calmodulin-binding, F actin-interacting protein, is present in aorta, uterus, and platelets. FEBS Lett 1983; 154:351–356.
386. Ngai PK, Walsh MP. Inhibition of smooth muscle actin-activated myosin Mg^{2+}-ATPase activity by caldesmon. J Biol Chem 1984; 259:13656–13659.
387. Marston SB, Smith CW. The thin filaments of smooth muscles. J Muscle Res Cell Motil 1985; 6:669–708.
388. Marston S, et al. Ca^{2+} regulation of the thin filaments: biochemical mechanism and physiological role. Biochem Soc Trans 1988; 16:494–497.
389. Ebashi S, Toyo-oka, T, Nonmura Y. Gizzard troponin. J Biochem 1975; 78:859–861.
390. Mikawa T, et al. Involvement of an acidic protein in regulation of smooth muscle contraction by the tropomyosin-leiotonin system. J Biochem (Tokyo) 1978; 84:1633–1636.
391. Nonomura Y, Ebashi S. Calcium regulatory mechanism in vertebrate smooth muscle. Biochem Res 1980; 1:1–14.
392. Shizuta Y, et al. Purification and properties of filamin, an actin binding protein from chicken gizzard. J Biol Chem 1976; 251:6562–6567.
393. Wang K, Singer SJ. Interaction of filamin with F-actin in solution. Proc Natl Acad Sci USA 1977; 74:2021–2025.
394. Davies P, Bechtel P, Pastan I. Filamin inhibits actin activation of heavy meromysin ATPase. FEBS Lett 1977; 77:228–232.
395. Vibert PJ, et al. Structural changes in actin-containing filament of muscle. J Mol Biol 1972; 71:757–767.
396. Starksen NF, et al. Cardiac myocyte hypertrophy is associated with c-myc protooncogene expression. Proc Natl Acad Sci USA 1986; 83:8348–8350.
397. Nemecek GM, et al. Stimulation of aortic smooth muscle cell mitogenesis by serotonin. Proc Natl Acad Sci USA 1986; 83:674–678.
398. Sawyer ST, Cohen S. Enhancement of calcium uptake and phosphatidylinositol turnover by epidermal growth factor in A-431 cells. Biochemistry 1981; 20:6280–6286.
399. Hazelton BJ, Tupper JT. Intracellular ionic changes in normal transformed human fibroblasts after extracellular Ca^{2+} deprivation. Biochem J 1981; 194:707–711.
400. Komuro I, et al. Endothelin stimulates c-fos and c-myc expression proliferation of vascular smooth muscle cells. Eur J Biochem 1988; 238(2):249–252.

401. Rokosova B, Bentley JP. Effect of calcium on cell proliferation and extracellular matrix synthesis in arterial smooth muscle cells and dermal fibroblasts. Exp Mol Pathol 1986; 44:307–317.
402. Michell RH. Inositol phospholipids and cell surface receptor function. Biochim Biophys Acta 1975; 415:81–147.
403. Nishizuka Y. Perspectives on the role of protein kinase C in stimulus-response coupling. JNCI 1986; 76(3):363–370.
404. Somlyo AV, Franzini-Armstrong C. New views of smooth muscle structure using freezing, deep-etching and rotary shadowing. Experientia 1985; 41:841–856.
405. Somlyo AP, Somlyo AV. Ultrastructure of smooth muscle. In EE Daniel, DM Paton, eds. Methods in Pharmacology, vol. 3. New York: Plenum 1975. Pp. 3–43.
406. Bobik A, Campbell, JH. Vascular derived growth factors: Cell biology, pathophysiology, and pharmacology. Pharm Rev 1993; 45:1–42.
407. Heldin CH, Westermark B, Wasteson A. Demonstration of an antibody against platelet-derived growth factor. Exp Cell Res 1981; 136:255–261.
408. Heldin CH, Wateson A, Westermark B. Partial purification and characterization of platelet factors stimulating the multiplication of human glial cells. Exp Cell Res 1977; 109:429–437.
409. Doolittle RF, et al. Simian sarcoma virus oncogene, v-sis is derived from the gene (or genes) encoding a platelet-derived growth factor. Science 1983; 221:275–277.
410. Walker LN, et al. Production of platelet-derived growth factor-like molecules by cultured arterial smooth muscle cells accompanies proliferation after arterial injury. Proc Natl Acad Sci USA 1986; 83:7311–7315.
411. Williams LT, Tremble P, Antoniades HN. Platelet-derived growth factor binds specifically to receptors on vascular smooth muscle cells and the binding becomes nondissociable. Proc Natl Acad Sci 1982; 79:5867–5870.
412. Ross R, et al. The platelet-derived growth factor and plasma control cell proliferation. In Hormones in Cell Culture. Cold Spring Harbor Conferences on Cell Proliferation, vol 6. New York: Cold Spring Harbor, 1979. P.27.
413. Berk BC, et al. Vasoconstriction: a new activity for platelet-derived growth factor. Science 1986; 232:87–90.
414. Gospodarowicz D. Growth factors and their action in in vivo and in vitro. J Pathol 1983; 141:201–233.
415. Gospodarowicz D. Fibroblast growth factor. In CH Li, ed. Hormonal Proteins and Peptides, vol. 12. New York: Academic, 1985. Pp. 205–230.
416. Huang SS, et al. Platelet-derived growth factor: specific binding to target cells. J Biol Chem 1982; 257:8130–8136.
417. Huang SS, Huang JS. Association of bovine brain-derived growth factor receptor with protein kinase activity. J Biol Chem 1986; 261:9568–9571.
418. Baird A, et al. Receptor and heparin-binding domains of basic fibroblast growth factor. Proc Natl Acad Sci 1988; 85:2324–2328.
419. Massague J. The transforming growth factor-family. Annu Rev Cell Biol 1990; 6:597–641.
420. Sporn MB, et al. Some recent advances in the chemistry and biology of transforming growth factor-beta. J Cell Biol 1987; 105:1039–1045.
421. Kim SJ, et al. Characterization of the promoter region of the human transforming growth factor-$\beta 1$ gene. J Biol Chem 1989; 264:402–408.
422. Purchio AF, et al. Identification of mannose-6-phosphate in two asparagine-linked sugar chains on recombinant transforming growth factor-$\beta 1$ precursor. J Biol Chem 1988; 263:14211–14214.
423. Majewsky MW, et al. Production of transforming growth factor 1 during repair of arterial injury. J Clin Invest 1991; 49:904–910.
424. Madri JA, Bell L, Merwin JR. Modulation of vascular cell behavior by transforming growth factors β. Mol Rep and Dev 1992; 32:121–126.
425. Roberts AB, et al. Transforming growth factor type-beta: rapid induction of fibrosis and angiogenesis in vivo and stimulation of collagen formation in vitro. Proc Natl Acad Sci 1986; 83:4167–4171.
426. Simonson MS, Dunn MJ. Endothelin: Pathways of transmembrane signaling. Hypertension 1990; 15:I-5–I-12.
427. Regoli D, et al. Vasoactive peptide and characterization of their receptors. Reg Pep 1993; 45:323–340.
428. Sakurai T, Yanagisawa M, Masaki T. Molecular characterization of endothelin receptors. TIPS 1992; 13:103–108.
429. Hay Douglas WP, Henry PJ, Goldie RG. Endothelin and the respiratory system. TIPS 1993; 14:29–32.
430. Hirata Y, et al. Endothelin receptor subtype B mediates synthesis of nitric oxide by cultured bovine endothelial cells. J Clin Invest 1993; 91:1367–1373.

Vascular Pharmacology

Stephen T. O'Rourke
Paul M. Vanhoutte

This chapter briefly outlines the major aspects of the pharmacology of the blood vessel wall. The first section describes the function of the major components that govern active changes in vascular diameter (vascular smooth muscle, adrenergic nerves, and endothelium) and discusses the drugs that directly affect the cell type under consideration. The second section focuses on the most important neurohumoral mediators, which, by acting on vascular smooth muscle, adrenergic nerves, and endothelial cells, change the tone of the blood vessel wall.

THE EFFECTOR SYSTEMS

Function of Vascular Smooth Muscle

Alterations in the degree of contraction of vascular smooth muscle permit active changes in diameter and wall tension of blood vessels. In the aorta and large arteries, vascular smooth muscle mainly adjusts the compliance of the vessel wall, which, together with variations in peripheral resistance, contributes to the impedance of the vascular circuit and thus the afterload of the heart. At the precapillary level, active changes in vessel diameter regulate blood flow to specific tissues and, by altering total peripheral resistance, contribute to arterial blood pressure. Changes in the degree of contraction of vascular smooth muscle in the venous wall, in particular the splanchnic area, control the capacity of the cardiovascular system and thus the filling pressure (preload) of the heart. Active changes in diameter of the cutaneous veins contribute mainly to the thermoregulatory function of the skin circulation.

Contraction of Vascular Smooth Muscle

The contractile apparatus of vascular smooth muscle closely resembles that of skeletal and cardiac muscle. The major contractile proteins are actin and myosin, and it is the interaction between these proteins that results in contraction.

As is the case with most cells, calcium ions play a central role in the activation of vascular smooth muscle. The contractile process is initiated when the concentration of free calcium within the cytoplasm rises to levels greater than 10^{-7} M. Calcium binds to calmodulin, an intracellular calcium-binding protein, and the resultant complex binds to the catalytic subunit of myosin light-chain kinase. The Ca^{2+}-calmodulin-activated enzyme phosphorylates the myosin light chain, permitting adenosinetriphosphatase (ATPase) activation of myosin cross-bridges by actin. Conformational changes occur in the cross-bridges when adenosine triphosphate (ATP) is hydrolyzed, and contraction ensues. Thus, the contractile state of vascular smooth muscle is governed by the activity of myosin light-chain kinase, which is itself regulated by calcium ions.

The increase in cytoplasmic Ca^{2+} concentration, which activates the contractile process in vascular smooth muscle cells, can be due either to an increased permeability of the cell membrane for extracellular calcium (i.e., calcium influx) or to mobilization of Ca^{2+} from cellular stores (e.g., sarcoplasmic reticulum and superficial binding sites). The source of the activator ion differs depending on the anatomic origin of the vascular smooth muscle, the contractile stimulus, or the experimental conditions to which the tissues are exposed.

At rest, the plasma membrane of vascular smooth muscle cells is relatively impermeable to Ca^{2+}. On activation, however, Ca^{2+} channels in the plasma membrane are opened, thereby allowing Ca^{2+} to flow down its concentration gradient into the cell. Two types of calcium channels have been proposed: potential, or voltage-operated, channels, which are regulated by changes in membrane potential, and receptor-operated channels, which are governed by drug-receptor interactions. Modulation of these channels by various pharmacologic agents markedly affects the contractile capability of vascular smooth muscle.

Ca^{2+} release from intracellular organelles also may play an important role in contraction of vascular smooth muscle. Indeed, in the absence of extracellular calcium, certain agonists (e.g., norepinephrine) can evoke contractions in some blood vessels. Although a small component of Ca^{2+} release may derive from the inner plasmalemmal surface, it is apparent that the major component originates from the sarcoplasmic reticulum.

At least two pathways have been proposed for the release of Ca^{2+} from subcellular stores. One pathway involves agonist-induced release of small amounts of Ca^{2+} from the inner plasmalemmal surface, resulting in transient increases in the concentration of Ca^{2+} near the superficial sarcoplasmic reticulum. This small increase in Ca^{2+} concentration may initiate the release of Ca^{2+} from the sarcoplasmic reticulum by a process known as Ca^{2+}-induced Ca^{2+} release.

Another potential pathway mediating intracellular Ca^{2+} release involves the breakdown of membrane phospholipids following agonist-receptor interaction. The initial event following binding of agonists to specific plasma membrane receptors is the activation of phospholipase C, which catalyzes the breakdown of inositol lipids. The action of phospholipase C on phosphatidylinositol 4,5-bisphosphate results in the formation of 1,2-diacylglycerol and inositol 1,4,5-triphosphate, which is responsible for a rapid mobilization of intracellular Ca^{2+} by activating Ca^{2+} efflux from the sarcoplasmic reticulum.

Relaxation of Vascular Smooth Muscle

Direct relaxation of vascular smooth muscle may occur by one or more of the following mechanisms: (1) hyperpolarization of the smooth muscle cell membrane; (2) inhibition of Ca^{2+} entry; (3) increased cytoplasmic concentration of cyclic 3′,5′-adenosine monophosphate (cAMP); and (4) increased formation of cyclic 3′,5′-guanosine monophosphate (cGMP).

HYPERPOLARIZATION

In most blood vessels, there is a tight coupling between membrane potential and tension. Thus, depolarization results in contraction of vascular smooth muscle, and hyperpolarization elicits relaxation. Lowering the membrane potential may affect the gating of calcium channels in the plasma membrane, which require depolarization above a certain threshold potential for activation and thereby reduce the entry of extracellular calcium.

Na^+,K^+-ATPase. Sodium, potassium-adenosinetriphosphatase (Na^+,K^+-ATPase) is responsible for the electrogenic pumping of Na^+ and K^+. This enzyme is localized in the cell membrane and contributes to the resting membrane potential of vascular smooth muscle cells. Three Na^+ are moved out of the cell in exchange for two K^+ pumped in per molecule of ATP hydrolyzed. Stimulation of Na^+,K^+-ATPase leads to hyperpolarization of vascular smooth muscle cells; endothelium-derived hyperpolarizing factor (EDHF) (see "Nonprostanoid Endothelium-Derived Relaxing Factor(s)," later in this chapter) may produce relaxation by this mechanism. Alternatively, cardiac glycosides such as ouabain produce contraction of isolated blood vessels due, in part, to inhibition of Na^+,K^+-ATPase.

K^+ Channels. Increased membrane K^+ permeability via specific K^+ channels serves to stabilize the cell membrane, because the outward movement of K^+ shifts the membrane potential toward more negative values. A new class of pharmacologic agents that increase membrane K^+ conductance (i.e., net efflux of K^+ from the cell) has recently been described. These substances, known as K^+-channel openers, produce vasodilation by hyperpolarizing vascular smooth muscle cells. Because of their vasodilator effects, these agents hold potential for the treatment of vascular disorders such as hypertension, angina, cerebrovascular disease, and peripheral vascular disease. In addition, the K^+-channel openers have become important pharmacologic tools in elucidating the role of K^+ channels in controlling blood vessel diameter.

The K^+-channel openers are a chemically diverse group with considerable structural differences. A number of novel compounds with K^+-channel-opening properties have been synthesized in recent years, including cromakalim, pinacidil, and nicorandil; nicorandil has nitrovasodilator properties as well (see below). Moreover, it is now recognized that the vasodilator effects of two antihypertensive drugs, diazoxide and minoxidil sulfate, are due to the opening of K^+ channels in vascular smooth muscle cells. In addition to these synthetic agents, it has been proposed that an endogenous K^+-channel opener, EDHF, released by endothelial cells plays a role in regulating vasomotor tone.

In isolated vascular preparations, the K^+-channel openers are able to inhibit spontaneous tone, as well as contractions evoked by vasoconstrictors such as norepinephrine, angiotensin II, and serotonin. Unlike some vasodilators, such as acetylcholine, the inhibitory effects of the K^+-channel openers are not dependent on the presence of an intact endothelium. The K^+-channel openers have in common three general characteristics in isolated tissues. First, K^+-channel openers induce an outward K^+ current, resulting in hyperpolarization of the cell membrane and a net efflux of $^{42}K^+$ or $^{86}Rb^+$. Second, K^+-channel openers cause relaxation of preparations contracted with low (< 30 mM) but not high (> 50 mM) concentrations of KCl. This behavior would be expected of substances that act simply by opening K^+ channels, since in the presence of high external K^+ concentrations, the actual membrane potential approaches the Nernst equilibrium potential for K^+, thereby reducing the achievable degree of hyperpolarization. Under these conditions (i.e., high external K^+ concentrations), the Nernst potential may be more positive than the threshold potential needed to interfere with calcium handling by the cell, thus abolishing the ability of the K^+-channel openers to interfere with these processes. Third, the mechanical and electrophysiologic effects of the K^+-channel openers can be antagonized by sulfonylureas, such as glyburide.

The molecular mechanism(s) by which K^+-channel openers cause relaxation of vascular smooth muscle have not yet been fully elucidated. The initial hypothesis put forth suggested that the K^+-channel openers act indirectly as Ca^{2+} channel antagonists. According to this scheme, increased membrane permeability to K^+ causes hyperpolarization, which in turn inhibits Ca^{2+} entry through voltage-dependent calcium channels, thereby causing vasorelaxation. However, it is clear from several studies that the inhibitory effects of the K^+-channel openers cannot be explained solely by the indirect closure of voltage-dependent calcium channels. Other mechanisms that have been proposed include (1) interference with refilling of intracellular Ca^{2+} stores, (2) inhibition of the synthesis of inositol 1,4,5-trisphosphate, and (3) decreased Ca^{2+} sensitivity of the contractile elements in vascular smooth muscle cells.

Several different types of K^+ channels have been identified in both arteries and veins; however, the nature of the specific channel activated by the K^+-channel openers in vascular smooth muscle has yet to be defined. Since glyburide, which is known to selectively block ATP-sensitive channels (K_{ATP}) in pancreatic beta cells, inhibits vascular responses to K^+-channel openers, it has been suggested that the K^+-channel openers exert their effects by activating K_{ATP} channels in vascular smooth muscle. This view is reinforced by the ability of K^+-channel openers to inhibit insulin release from isolated pancreatic islets and to increase the opening probability of K_{ATP} channels in cardiac muscle. Moreover, in rabbit mesenteric artery, a K^+ channel opened by cromakalim, closed by ATP, and inhibited by glyburide has been identified. Other laboratories, however, report that delayed rectifier and large conductance calcium-activated K^+ channels are targets for K^+-channel openers in vascular smooth muscle. Thus, there currently is no clear consensus concerning the site of action of these agents.

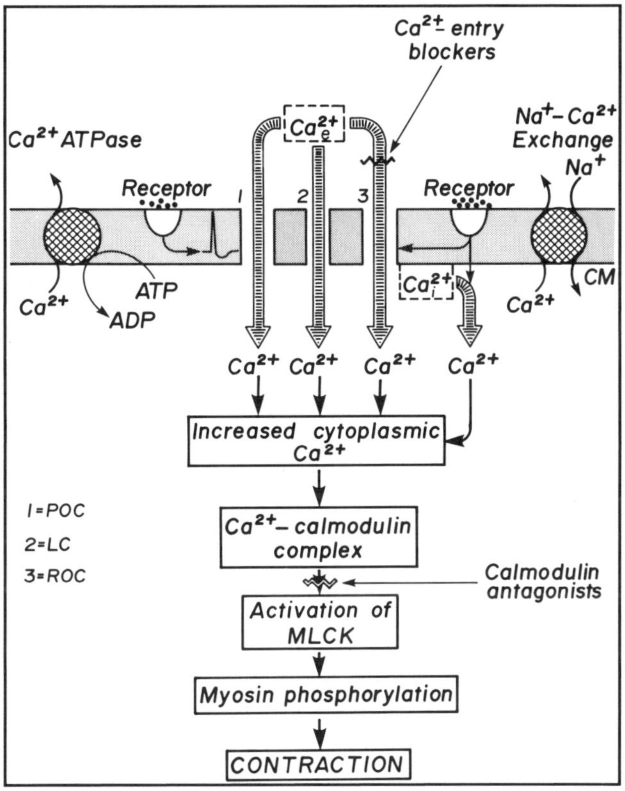

Fig. 4-1. Calcium-dependent regulation of contractile activity in vascular smooth muscle. Cytoplasmic calcium (Ca^{2+}) levels are increased by calcium influx through potential-operated calcium channels (1), a passive calcium leak pathway (2) (calcium entry that occurs under resting conditions), and receptor-operated calcium channels (3). Receptor occupation by a specific agonist may also induce release of calcium from intracellular storage sites or may depolarize the cell membrane and activate the potential-operated channel. Calcium activates myosin light-chain kinase (MLCK) by binding to calmodulin. Activated MLCK catalyzes the phosphorylation of myosin, which increases actin-myosin interactions, resulting in contraction. Cytoplasmic calcium levels are reduced through the operation of cell membrane pumps, including Ca^{2+}-ATPase (far left) and a Na^+/Ca^{2+} antiport (far right) that promote calcium efflux. (Reproduced with permission from TJ Rimele and PM Vanhoutte. Differential effects of calcium entry blockers on vascular smooth muscle. Int Angiol 1984; 3:17–23.)

INHIBITION OF CA^{2+} ENTRY

In light of the importance of Ca^{2+} in vascular smooth muscle contraction, it is not surprising that a host of compounds have been designed for the purpose of interfering with the entry of calcium through specific channels in the cell membrane. These so-called calcium antagonists inhibit contractions induced by a wide variety of agents, but they differ in their ability to interfere with the function of vascular smooth muscle from different anatomic origins or under different experimental conditions.

Substantial evidence now exists to support the hypothesis that the organic calcium antagonists (cinnarizine, diltiazem, flunarizine, nifedipine, nimodipine, and verapamil) inhibit smooth muscle contraction by blocking stimulated (receptor activation or membrane depolarization) calcium influx (Fig. 4-1). For example, in the presence of cinnarizine, diltiazem, flunarizine, and nifedipine, the inhibition of potassium-stimulated unidirectional calcium influx in various vascular smooth muscle preparations is highly correlated with the inhibition of potassium-induced contraction. In concentrations considered to correspond to therapeutic doses, the organic calcium antagonists do not (1) inhibit intracellular calcium release induced by specific agonists (cellular mobilization), (2) reduce passive calcium entry (calcium leak), or (3) stimulate calcium extrusion mechanisms (Ca^{2+}-ATPase and Na^+/Ca^{2+} antiport system) (see Fig. 4-1).

Site(s) of Action of Calcium Antagonists. Although the organic calcium antagonists can be subdivided into several distinct classes based on their chemical structures, in general their pharmacologic selectivity and potency suggest that specific sites exist for these compounds. The molecular and biochemical nature of these sites can be identified with radiolabeled compounds (e.g., ^{3}H-flunarizine, ^{3}H-nitrendipine, ^{3}H-nimodipine) in vascular and nonvascular preparations. The binding of ^{3}H-nitrendipine (and other labeled compounds) to isolated cell membranes from smooth muscle satisfies the requirements for specific receptor binding (i.e., high affinity, saturation, stereoselec-

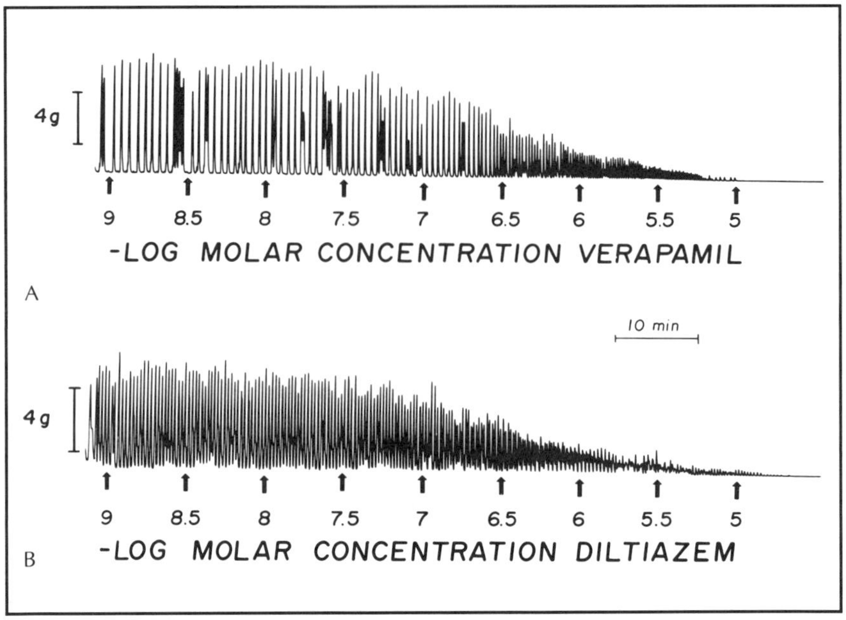

Fig. 4-2. Verapamil (A) and diltiazem (B) cause concentration-dependent inhibition of the myogenic activity in canine portal-mesenteric vein. (Reproduced with permission from TJ Rimele and PM Vanhoutte. Differential effects of calcium entry blockers on vascular smooth muscle. Int Angiol 1984; 3:17–23.)

tivity, and pharmacologic specificity that correlates with functional response). The binding sites for the structurally dissimilar calcium antagonists are not identical, but they do interact. This helps to explain how the various classes of calcium antagonists can act in a similar fashion functionally but still have specific sites of action. Data from binding as well as functional studies suggest that the synthetic calcium antagonists probably do not interact with the site at which inorganic cations, such as lanthanum, bind to block calcium entry. It is more likely that the various calcium-entry blockers specifically bind to other components within the calcium channel, thus causing their inactivation.

Calcium Antagonists and the Contractile Response of Vascular Smooth Muscle. In certain vascular preparations, most notably the portal-mesenteric vein of various species (Fig. 4-2) and the human coronary artery, spontaneous rhythmic (myogenic) contractions can be observed under control conditions. This myogenic activity depends on the availability of extracellular calcium and is presumably the result of spontaneous depolarization of the cell membrane, which then opens potential-operated calcium channels (see Fig. 4-1). Calcium antagonists inhibit the myogenic activity of portal-mesenteric veins with varying potencies, with the dihydropyridines (e.g., nifedipine) being the most potent. Since myogenic tone in the arterioles also depends on the entry of extracellular calcium, it is not surprising that the calcium antagonists that are the most potent in inhibiting the myogenic activity of portal-mesenteric veins also appear to cause the greatest reduction in peripheral vascular resistance in the intact organism and, hence, are the most likely candidates for use as antihypertensive agents.

Depolarization of the vascular smooth muscle cell membrane, for example, by increasing the extracellular potassium ion concentration, opens potential-operated calcium channels and accelerates the entry of extracellular calcium (see Fig. 4-1). Hence, the contractions of isolated blood vessels caused by potassium depolarization can be inhibited by all available calcium-entry blockers. In general, for a given calcium-entry blocker (e.g., diltiazem; Fig. 4-3), the sensitivity of the potassium-induced contraction is relatively constant throughout the vasculature. On the other hand, the potency of the various agents varies widely, which are ranked here from most to least potent: dihydropyridines, verapamil, diltiazem, flunarizine. The time of onset and the duration of the inhibitory effect of the calcium antagonists on potassium-induced contractions in given blood vessels also vary widely, reflecting the differing pharmacokinetic properties of these substances.

Heterogeneous Response to Calcium Antagonists. When comparing the responses of vascular smooth muscle preparations from different species and anatomic origin, a wide range of sensitivity to a variety of vasoactive agents is observed. Many factors have been proposed to account for this heterogeneity, including local ambient conditions (pH, temperature, osmolarity), differences in innervation, endothelial influences, and differences intrinsic to smooth muscle. Although external factors may also help to explain the heterogeneous responses of various vascular smooth muscle preparations to calcium antagonists, this discussion will focus only on differences intrinsic to the smooth muscle.

In addition to the differences seen in the potency among the various calcium antagonists, the following factors have been proposed to account for the heterogeneous

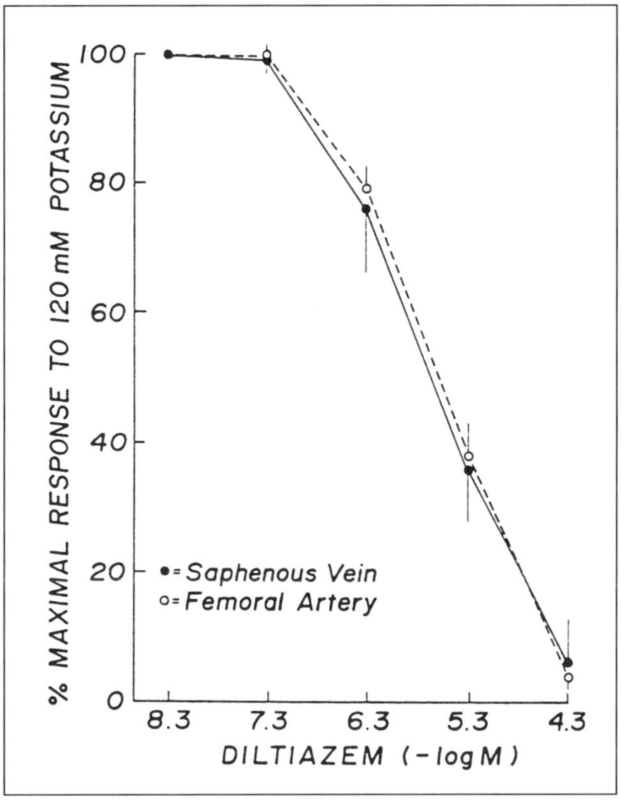

Fig. 4-3. Diltiazem and responsiveness of canine saphenous vein and femoral artery to potassium. Responses were obtained in the presence of phentolamine (3×10^{-5} M) and propranolol (3×10^{-6} M) to mask the effects of norepinephrine released by potassium. (Reproduced with permission from TJ Rimele and PM Vanhoutte. Differential effects of calcium entry blockers on vascular smooth muscle. Int Angiol 1984; 3:17–23.)

behavior of the calcium-entry blockers in various vascular smooth muscle preparations: (1) differences in calcium-influx pathways, (2) differing degrees of agonist-induced depolarization, (3) agonist-induced release of intracellular calcium, and (4) multiple activated states or types of calcium channels.

In general, the calcium antagonists are more selective for potential- than receptor-operated channels, but the inverse may be true in mesenteric resistance vessels. The ability of a given calcium antagonist to inhibit a given agonist-induced contraction may vary among different tissues from the same species. Therefore, there may be both distinct types of potential-operated channels, operating to different degrees in various smooth muscle cells, and various receptor-operated channels being activated by various agonists (see Fig. 4-1). Receptor-operated calcium channels may exist in different activated states that are characterized by different sensitivities to the calcium antagonists.

The ability of a given agonist to induce membrane depolarization (and thereby activate the potential-operated channel, which is more sensitive to calcium-entry blockade) or to release intracellularly bound calcium (which is insensitive to calcium-entry blockers) in different blood vessels are other factors influencing the ability of calcium-entry blockers to inhibit the contractile response in various blood vessels (see Fig. 4-1).

cAMP

Stimulation of a number of plasma membrane receptors (e.g., beta-adrenergic receptors) promotes the conversion of intracellular ATP to cAMP by the enzyme adenylate cyclase. Adenylate cyclase is coupled to the plasma membrane receptor by a guanine nucleotide–binding protein. Within the cell, cAMP binds to and activates cAMP-dependent protein kinase. The activated protein kinases catalyzes phosphorylation of specific enzymes, thus stimulating or inhibiting their activities. In vascular smooth muscle, increasing the cytoplasmic concentration of cAMP accelerates the removal of Ca^{2+} from the cytoplasm. This cAMP-mediated decrease in cytoplasmic Ca^{2+} probably accounts for the relaxation of vascular smooth muscle by beta-adrenergic receptor agonists (e.g., epinephrine, isoproterenol) and prostaglandins (e.g., prostacyclin, prostaglandin I_2).

Intracellular cAMP is metabolized rapidly by cyclic nucleotide phosphodiesterase. Thus, inhibitors of phosphodiesterase increase cytoplasmic cAMP levels. Inhibitors of phosphodiesterase, such as papaverine, dipyridamole, and methylxanthines (e.g., theophylline), are believed to relax vascular smooth muscle primarily by this mechanism.

cGMP

The cellular effects of cGMP are not as well understood as those of cAMP, but there are a number of similarities between the two nucleotides. cGMP is formed by the action of guanylate cyclase on guanosine triphosphate, and its effects are mediated by cGMP-dependent protein kinases. In addition, cGMP is metabolized by cyclic GMP phosphodiesterase. The activation of guanylate cyclase and the subsequent elevation of cGMP in vascular smooth muscle is associated with relaxation.

Several possibilities have been put forth to explain cGMP-mediated relaxation of vascular smooth muscle. Increased accumulation of cGMP is associated with dephosphorylation of the myosin light chain. Possible calcium-specific effects include the inhibition of a sarcolemmal calcium channel to inhibit Ca^{2+} influx or the activation of a sarcolemmal calcium-extrusion pump, both secondary to activation of cGMP-dependent protein kinases. The intracellular liberation of calcium may be impaired following inhibition of phosphatidylinositol hydrolysis, and the intracellular sequestration or binding of calcium may be increased. In addition, recent evidence indicates that cGMP-dependent protein kinase activates a large conductance Ca^{2+}-activated K^+ channel in vascular smooth muscle, thus increasing K^+ conductance and hyperpolarizing the cell membrane.

Guanylate cyclase can be activated by reactive free radicals such as nitric oxide (NO), which bind to the heme moiety of the enzyme. The term **nitrovasodilators** has been used to describe agents that can lead to the formation of NO and increase the synthesis of cGMP. These agents include the organic nitrates such as nitroglycerin and isosorbide dinitrate (which release NO inside cells), the inorganic compound sodium nitroprusside, and SIN-1, the active metabolite of molsidomine (the latter two release NO outside the cells). Treatment with these agents produces dilatation of both arteries and veins, resulting in decreased peripheral vascular resistance and venous return. The vasodilator hydralazine is thought to act by a cGMP-dependent mechanism, but it acts only on the arterial circulation.

Adrenergic-Nerve Endings

Anatomy. The sympathetic outflow to peripheral blood vessels originates in neurons located in the lateral parts of the reticular formation in the bulbar area of the brain stem, the vasomotor center. The activity of the vasomotor center is governed by the solitary tract nucleus, which relays information from arterial and cardiopulmonary mechanoreceptors (baroreceptors) and other afferents. The axons from neurons of the vasomotor center form the bulbospinal tract and descend in the intermediolateral column to the preganglionic neurons of the spinal cord, located in the anterolateral column. The neurons of the bulbospinal tract consist of both excitatory and inhibitory neurons, which innervate the preganglionic sympathetic neurons. The interplay between these pressor and depressor neurons determines the sympathetic outflow to the periphery. The cholinergic preganglionic neurons interconnect with the adrenergic postganglionic neurons in the sympathetic ganglia. The adrenergic postganglionic neurons innervate the heart and the peripheral blood vessels.

With the exception of the umbilical and placental vasculature, blood vessels contain smooth muscle cells that are innervated by postganglionic sympathetic nerves. The density of innervation varies widely, however, and may reflect the contribution of individual vascular beds to centrally controlled responses. The postganglionic sympathetic-nerve terminals form a network of unmyelinated slender processes that widen at regular intervals into varicosities. The varicosities are in close apposition to the smooth muscle cells they innervate; there is a minimal distance of 50 nm between the two types of cells, but in certain blood vessels this junctional cleft is much larger. In most arteries, the nerves are restricted to the adventitial-medial border; in veins, they usually penetrate into the media. Both in animals and in humans, the density of adrenergic innervation of the blood vessels decreases progressively with age. The adrenolytic agent, 6-hydroxydopamine, exerts its effect by destroying adrenergic-nerve endings. This effect depends on uptake of 6-hydroxydopamine by the biogenic amine pump located in the plasma membrane of adrenergic-nerve endings.

ORIGIN AND STORAGE OF THE ADRENERGIC NEUROTRANSMITTER

Synthesis. The postganglionic adrenergic neurons actively take up tyrosine from the extracellular fluid and transform it to dopamine by successive enzymatic reactions in the neuroplasm. Dopamine is then incorporated into the storage vesicles, where it is converted to norepinephrine by the enzyme dopamine β-hydroxylase, which is present in both the membrane and the content of the vesicles (Fig. 4-4). The antihypertensive drugs methyldopa and reserpine act at these points in the neurotransmitter synthetic pathway. Methyldopa is also converted to α-methylnorepinephrine, a potent alpha$_2$-adrenoreceptor agonist that inhibits sympathetic outflow from the central nervous system. Reserpine inhibits adrenergic neurotransmission by depleting norepinephrine stores within adrenergic-nerve endings. This effect most likely is due to inhibition of biogenic amine uptake into storage vesicles. An increased neuroplasmic concentration of norepinephrine exerts an end-product inhibition on the enzyme tyrosine hydroxylase, which is the rate-limiting step in the synthesis of the neurotransmitter. Increased activity of the adrenergic neuron or depletion of the catecholamine stores, on the other hand, stimulate the activity of the blood vessel wall decreases with age.

Storage. Most of the norepinephrine, whether synthesized or taken up from the extracellular space, is held in the storage vesicles as a complex with proteins, of which chromogranin A is the most important. The storage of adrenergic transmitter is reflected by the electron-dense core of the storage vesicles. The norepinephrine content of the blood vessel wall varies with the degree of innervation and decreases with age and after sympathectomy, reserpine treatment, and inhibition of tyrosine hydroxylase and dopamine β-hydroxylase.

Release of Transmitter. The norepinephrine stored in the adrenergic-nerve endings may be released by three different mechanisms; (1) leakage of the neurotransmitter to

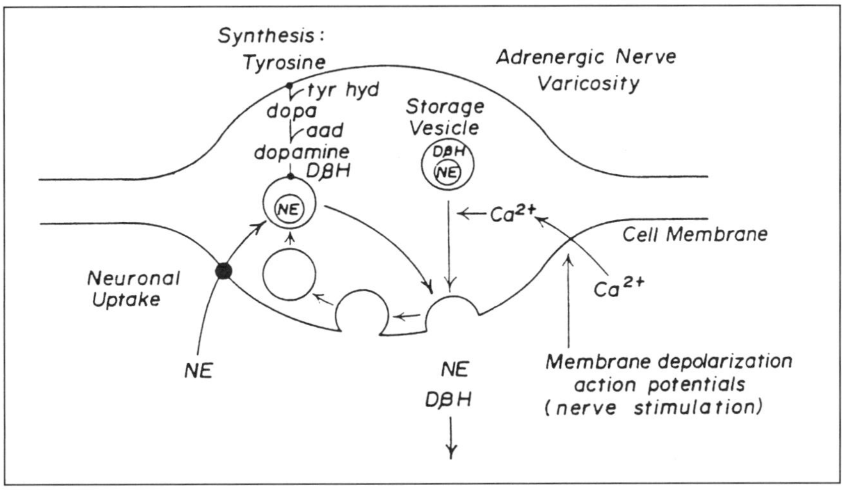

Fig. 4-4. Synthesis and exocytotic release of norepinephrine and recycling of the storage vesicles at the sympathetic (adrenergic) nerve varicosities. NE = norepinephrine; tyr hyd = tyrosine hydroxylase; aad = aromatic L-amino decarboxylase; DβH = dopamine-β-hydroxylase. (Reproduced with permission from PM Vanhoutte. Introductory remarks: alpha- and beta-adrenergic receptors and the cardiovascular system. J Cardiovasc Pharmacol 1981; 3:S1–S13.)

the neuroplasm and toward the extracellular space; (2) pharmacologic displacement by other substances such as tyramine, amphetamine, or ephedrine, which have a higher affinity for the storage proteins in the vesicles (indirect sympathomimetic effect); or (3) exocytotic release initiated by action potentials generated in the ganglionic cell body.

When action potentials are generated, they invade the adrenergic-nerve endings and activate in succession (**en passant synapse**) the different varicosities. The action potentials initiate an influx of Na^+ and Ca^{2+} into the neuroplasm by opening ion channels in the cell membrane. As a consequence of the increased intraneuronal Ca^{2+} concentration, the vesicles migrate toward and fuse with the neuronal cell membrane, emptying their content of norepinephrine, dopamine β-hydroxylase, and chromogranin A into the junctional cleft (exocytotic release; see Fig. 4-4). The exocytotic emptying of the vesicles creates the concentration gradient of norepinephrine between the nerve terminal and the innervated smooth muscle cells; this is the driving force for the diffusion of the adrenergic transmitter and thus for the activation of the effector tissue. When norepinephrine reaches the smooth muscle cells, it binds to and activates adrenoceptors on the cell membrane.

Norepinephrine release may be impaired by several pharmacologic agents. Guanethidine is taken up into adrenergic-nerve endings by the same mechanism responsible for transport of norepinephrine. It accumulates in and displaces norepinephrine from intraneuronal storage granules, thereby depleting norepinephrine stores. Guanethidine may also produce local blockade of membrane electrical activity in nerve endings. Bretylium tosylate is structurally similar to guanethidine and also inhibits norepinephrine release from adrenergic-nerve terminals.

The puffer fish poison, tetrodotoxin, selectively blocks sodium channels in nervous tissue, thereby inhibiting the inward sodium current. By suppressing the generation of action potentials, tetrodotoxin inhibits the release of norepinephrine from adrenergic nerve endings. Although the exocytotic release of norepinephrine depends on the entry of Ca^{2+}, calcium antagonists, except at very high concentrations, do not seem to inhibit it. This implies that Ca^{2+} does not enter the neuronal membrane through slow Ca^{2+} channels.

The secretory activity of the adrenergic-nerve ending may also be modulated by substances released into the junctional cleft during the exocytotic process and by other substances present in the junctional cleft (Fig. 4-5).

Disposition of the Released Transmitter. Norepinephrine is removed from the junctional cleft by several mechanisms (Fig. 4-6): (1) uptake by the neuronal cell membrane (uptake 1) and subsequent storage or intraneuronal deamination by the enzyme monoamine oxidase; (2) overflow to the extracellular space—part of the liberated neurotransmitter leaves the junctional cleft by diffusion and may overflow into the capillaries to constitute the most important fraction of circulating norepinephrine; (3) nonspecific binding to collagen structures and uptake by nonmuscle cells (e.g., fat cells); and (4) extraneuronal uptake by vascular smooth muscle cells (uptake 2) and subsequent enzymatic degradation. Postjunctional cell membrane sites, as distinct from receptor sites, can actively incorporate the norepinephrine into the smooth muscle cells.

NEURONAL UPTAKE. The cell membrane of the adrenergic neuron can take up norepinephrine and a number of other substances that can interact with adrenergic sites. This is an active process mediated by a carrier linked to Na^+,K^+-ATPase. The norepinephrine is either stored in the storage vesicles or deaminated by monoamine oxidase to 3,4-dihydroxyphenylglycol (DOPEG) before it reaches the storage sites (see Fig. 4-6); the DOPEG then diffuses to the extracellular space. The available evidence indicates that there is a temporal dissociation between the activation

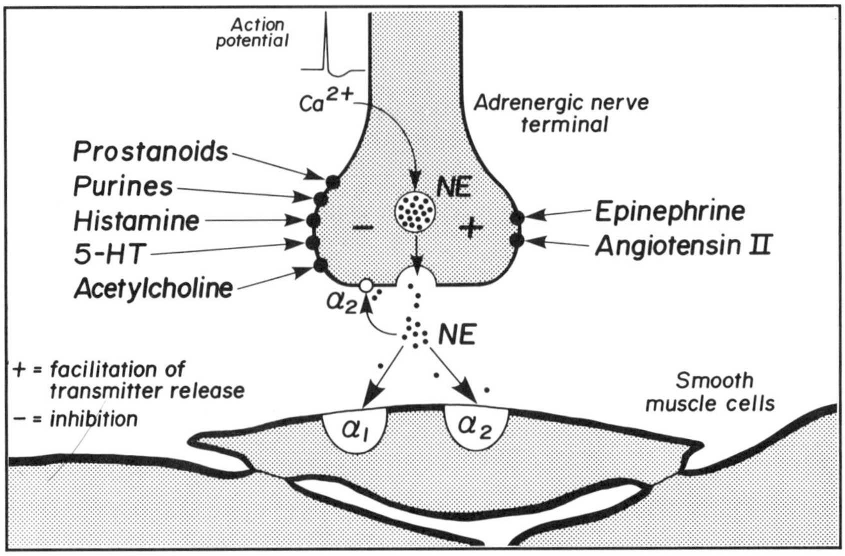

Fig. 4-5. Transmitter release at the sympathetic neuroeffector junction in vascular smooth muscle can be modulated by various substances that activate prejunctional receptors. For example, acetylcholine, 5-hydroxytryptamine (5-HT), histamine, purines, prostanoids, or norepinephrine can reduce the amount of neurotransmitter. Vasoactive substances such as epinephrine or angiotensin II can activate receptors on the sympathetic nerve endings, increasing the output of neurotransmitter. NE = norepinephrine. (Reproduced with permission from PM Vanhoutte and TF Lüscher. Peripheral mechanisms in cardiovascular regulation: transmitters, receptors and the endothelium. In RC Tarazi and A Zanchetti, eds. Handbook of Hypertension, vol. 8. Amsterdam: Elsevier Science Publishers, 1986.)

of the nerve terminal and the neuronal uptake process, with uptake operating only when the neuronal cell membrane is polarized. Thus, neuronal uptake normally plays a small role in determining the effector-response amplitude to sympathetic-nerve stimulation.

The norepinephrine taken up by nerve endings originates either from the terminals themselves or from the blood flowing through the blood vessel. Recapture of circulating norepinephrine by the adrenergic nerve endings of the blood vessel wall is particularly important when the media are innervated throughout and when the blood vessel wall is relatively thin, for example, in the case of densely innervated veins. By contrast, arteries, where the innervation is limited to the adventitial-medial border, do not easily recapture circulating catecholamines.

Inhibitors of neuronal uptake, such as cocaine, tricyclic antidepressants, and high concentrations of alpha-adrenoceptor antagonists (e.g., phenoxybenzamine), have the following effects on the response of the blood vessel wall to sympathetic-nerve stimulation:

1. There is little or no augmentation of the efflux of norepinephrine, particularly at low stimulation frequencies; with cocaine, this effect may be partially obscured by the local anesthetic properties of the compound.
2. A moderate augmentation of the contractile response to low-frequency stimulation occurs; this effect may be partially obscured by the alpha-adrenolytic properties of the drugs used (e.g., with desipramine) or by nonspecific augmentation of the responsiveness of the vascular smooth muscle cells (e.g., with cocaine).
3. The contractile response is prolonged, and relaxation is delayed.

Neuronal uptake inhibitors also reduce the response to indirect sympathomimetic amines (such as tyramine or amphetamines) but augment the response to exogenous catecholamines. In vessels where the adrenergic innervation is limited to the medial-adventitial border, these effects are particularly prominent when the adrenergic amines reach the blood vessel wall from the outside but are reduced when they are administered intraluminally. At high concentrations, inhibitors of neuronal uptake may cause the pharmacologic displacement of adrenergic transmitter.

DEAMINATION. A portion of the norepinephrine taken up by the adrenergic-nerve terminal is enzymatically destroyed by intraneuronal monoamine oxidase (Fig. 4-7). Inhibitors of monoamine oxidase (such as pargyline and tranylcypromine) have the following effects on the response to sympathetic-nerve stimulation: (1) decreased appearance of deaminated metabolites and moderate augmentation of the overflow of intact transmitter, (2) moderate (or no) augmentation of the contractile response, and (3) moderate (or no) prolongation of the contractile response and delayed relaxation. In addition, inhibitors of monoamine oxidase augment and prolong the response to indirect sympathomimetic amines and to exogenous norepinephrine, although the latter effect usually is not pronounced.

EXTRANEURONAL UPTAKE. Vascular smooth muscle cells possess an active carrier process for the uptake of norepi-

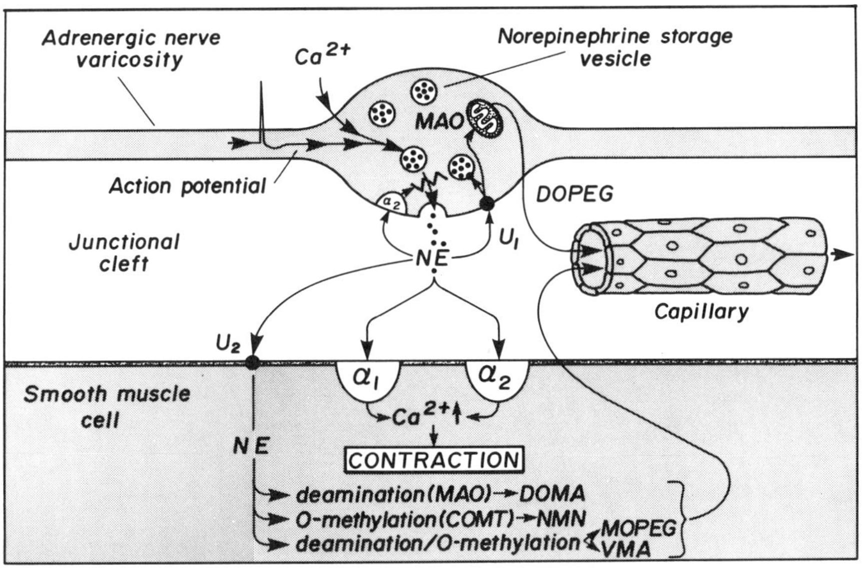

Fig. 4-6. Release and disposal of the sympathetic neurotransmitter. The nerve impulse (action potential) activates the entry of Ca^{2+} ions into adrenergic nerve varicosities. This causes the norepinephrine-containing vesicles to migrate and fuse with the neuronal membrane, then to rupture and release norepinephrine into the junctional cleft. The norepinephrine activates α_1- or α_2-adrenoceptors (or both) on the smooth muscle cells. It may also activate α_2-adrenoceptors on the sympathetic endings and thereby reduce its own release. It is removed (1) by uptake into the neerve endings (U_1), where part of it is enzymatically degraded by the intraneuronal monoamine oxidase (MAO) to 3,4-dihydroxyphenylglycol (DOPEG), but most is recycled to the storage vesicles; (2) by uptake by the effector cells (U_2) and enzymatic degradation by the enzymes MAO and catechol-O-methyltransferase (COMT) to 3,4-dihydroxymandelic acid (DOMA), normetanephrine (NMN), 3-methoxy, 4-dihydroxyphenylglycol (MOPEG), and 3-methoxy,4-hydroxymandelic acid (VMA); and (3) by diffusion to the capillaries. The metabolites of norepinephrine are inactive and diffuse to the extracellular fluid and the capillaries. (Reproduced with permission from JT Shepherd and PM Vanhoutte. The circulation in the limbs: normal function and effects of disease. In W Parmely and K Chatterjee, eds. Handbook of Cardiology. Philadelphia: Lippincott, 1987.)

nephrine. The extraneuronal uptake of norepinephrine is followed by enzymatic inactivation of the amine by catechol-O-methyltransferase, monoamine oxidase, or both. Certain steroids (hydrocortisone and estradiol-17β) can inhibit extraneuronal uptake and have the following effects on the response of the blood vessel wall to sympathetic-nerve stimulation: (1) no (or modest) increases in the overflow of transmitter, (2) reduced appearance of extraneuronal metabolites of norepinephrine, (3) augmentation of the contractile response, and (4) moderate prolongation of the contractile response and delayed relaxation. Inhibitors of extraneuronal uptake can sometimes, but not always, augment the contractile responses to exogenous norepinephrine.

The relative importance of the different pathways for the disposition of released norepinephrine varies from blood vessel to blood vessel and depends on factors such as density of adrenergic innervation, anatomic arrangement of the adrenergic-nerve terminals within the vessel wall, presence of nonspecific binding sites and fat cells, and the width of the junctional cleft. If the junctional cleft is narrow, neuronal uptake plays a prominent role. If it is wide, overflow to the capillaries and extraneuronal uptake become more important.

Endothelium

The vascular endothelium is the layer of squamous epithelial cells that is in direct contact with the blood. As such, the endothelium is ideally situated to perform a number of important functions. These include the transfer of nutrients and waste products between blood and tissue; the control of hemostasis; and the activation, inactivation, or production of several vasoactive substances that can affect the underlying vascular smooth muscle cells.

ACTIVATION AND INACTIVATION OF CIRCULATING SUBSTANCES

Endothelial cells, in particular those of the pulmonary vasculature, are capable of many metabolic functions (Fig. 4-8). Pulmonary endothelial cells take up norepinephrine and 5-hydroxytryptamine and subsequently degrade them via monoamine oxidase or catechol-O-methyltransferase; uptake is the rate-limiting step in this process. The pharmacologic evidence available suggests that the uptake sites for norepinephrine and 5-hydroxytryptamine are distinct; epinephrine, dopamine, and isoproterenol are not taken up. Studies with cultured porcine aortic endothelial cells demonstrate that although these cells contain monoamine oxidase, they

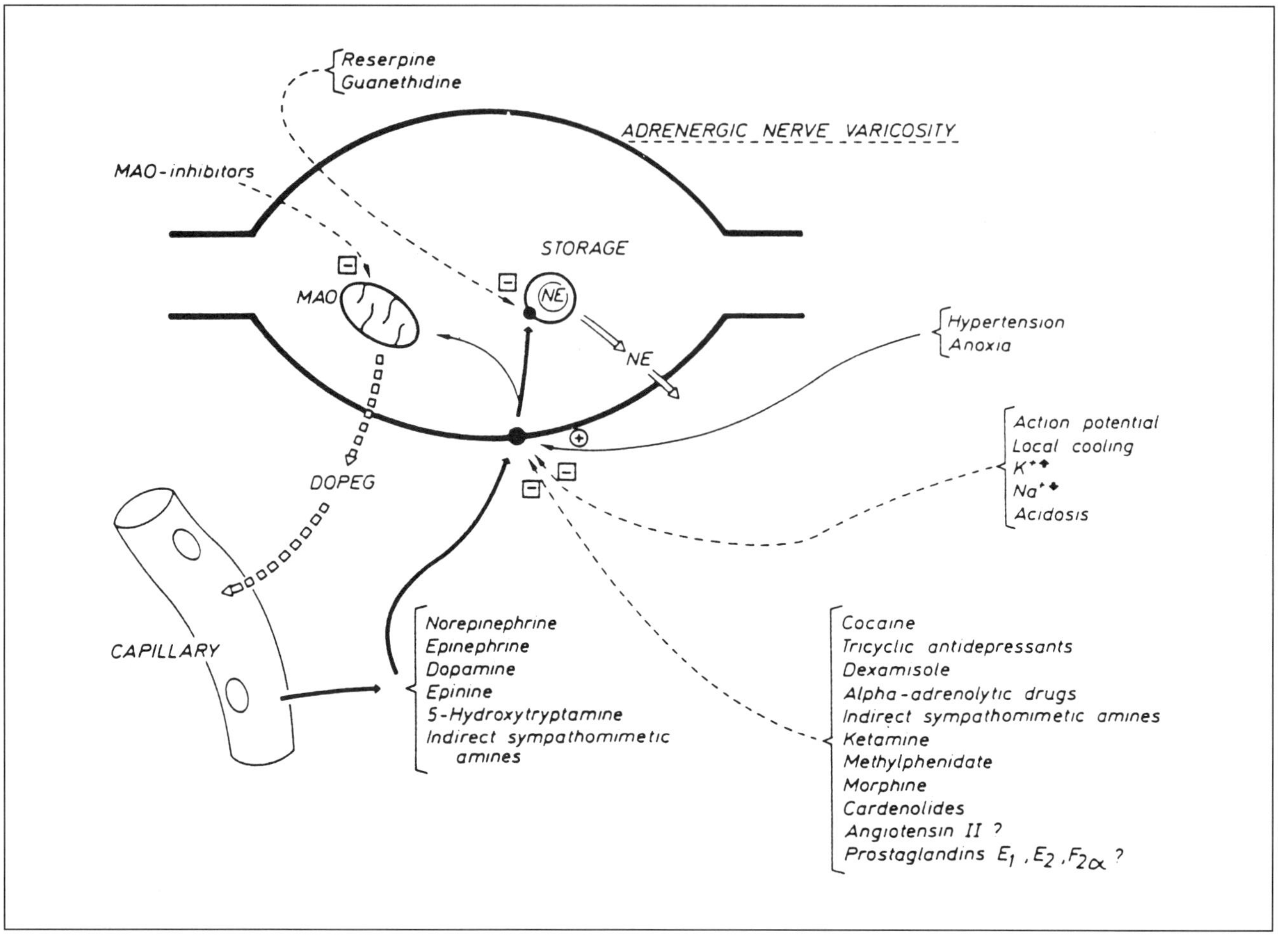

Fig. 4-7. Schematic representation of neuronal uptake process and intraneuronal deamination. DOPEG = 3,4-dihyroxyphenylglycol; MAO = monoamine oxidase; NE = norepinephrine; + = facilitation; dashed line = inhibitory effect; O = active carrier. (Reproduced with permission from PM Vanhoutte, TJ Verbeuren, and RC Webb. Local modulation of adrenergic neuroeffector interaction in the blood vessel wall. Physiol Rev 1981; 62:151–247.)

do not possess the amine-transport process present in the lung.

Angiotensin I, enkephalins, and bradykinin are substrates for converting enzyme that is located at the luminal surface. Products of this enzymatic conversion are angiotensin II and peptide fragments of bradykinin and enkephalins.

Vascular endothelial cells in culture also possess specific mechanisms for the uptake, metabolism, and release of ATP, adenosine diphosphate (ADP), and AMP.

Prostaglandins of the E and F series are also extensively metabolized by pulmonary endothelium; prostaglandin A and prostacyclin are not metabolized in vivo. Thus, endothelial cells can influence the amounts of vasoactive substances reaching vascular smooth muscle by activation, inactivation, and specific uptake. Furthermore, the ability of the endothelium to alter the concentration of various vasoactive agents that affect blood platelet function may also be important in hemostasis and thrombosis.

Prostacyclin. The endothelium forms a barrier, which, because of its surface characteristics and secretion of prostacyclin, prevents aggregation of platelets on the collagen and smooth muscle of the blood vessel wall. Prostacyclin is the major product of arachidonic acid metabolism through the cyclooxygenase pathway in blood vessels, with the endothelial layer having the greatest capacity for synthesis when compared with the media and adventitia. Endoperoxides released from platelets may also provide a substrate for the formation of prostacyclin by endothelial cells. Prostacyclin is a potent endogenous inhibitor of platelet aggregation and has profound vasodilator effects in several vascular beds. Classically, the action of prostacyclin opposes that of thromboxane A_2, which is the major metabolite of arachidonic acid in platelets; it stimulates platelet aggregation and can cause vasoconstriction. Thus, the balance between the production of prostacyclin and thromboxane A_2 may be critical in the regulation of both local vascular tone and hemostasis.

NONPROSTANOID ENDOTHELIUM-DERIVED RELAXING FACTOR(S)

The evidence for an obligatory role of arterial endothelial cells in the responses of smooth muscle was provided by

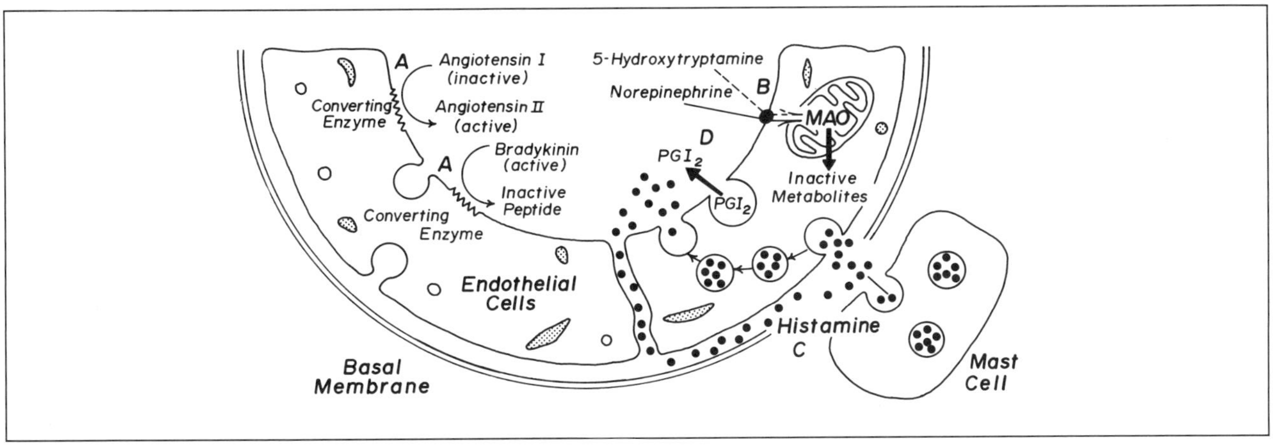

Fig. 4-8. The handling of bioactive substances by the endothelium of pulmonary capillaries. **A.** Substances such as angiotensin I and bradykinin are transformed "on" the endothelium by converting enzymes, with resulting formation of active and inactive components, respectively. **B.** Substances such as norepinephrine and 5-hydroxytryptamine are actively taken up and degraded enzymatically by monoamine oxidase (MAO). Other substances metabolically degraded by the lung capillaries include certain prostaglandins. **C.** During allergic and anaphylactic reactions, substances such as histamine can overflow into the capillary lumen. **D.** It is likely that the lung capillaries can produce certain prostaglandinlike substances such as prostacyclin (PGI_2) and release them into the bloodstream. (Reproduced with permission from TJ Rimele and PM Vanhoutte. Differential effects of calcium entry blockers on vascular smooth muscle. Int Angiol 1984; 3:17–23.)

Furchgott and Zawadzki in 1980, when they demonstrated that arteries denuded of endothelium failed to relax when exposed to acetylcholine. The arterial endothelium also accounts, at least in part, for the relaxation of smooth muscle caused by alpha$_2$-adrenergic agonists, arachidonic acid (when the relaxation it causes is not due to metabolization to prostacyclin), ADP, ATP, bradykinin, histamine, oxytocin, substance P, thrombin, and vasopressin. These substances are believed to interact with specific receptors on endothelial cells. Except for arachidonic acid, which causes endothelium-dependent relaxation after its conversion to prostacyclin by the endothelium, these agents stimulate the release of one or more endothelium-derived relaxing factors (EDRFs). By comparison, agents such as adenosine, isoproterenol, and nitrates, as a rule, do not depend on the endothelium for their effect but act directly on the smooth muscle.

EDRF is not a prostanoid, because blockers of cyclooxygenase do not modify endothelium-dependent relaxation. EDRF has a very short half-life (5–10 seconds) in physiologic salt solution. It is released from endothelial cells and diffuses to the underlying vascular smooth muscle. Endothelium-dependent relaxation is associated with a rise in cGMP in vascular smooth muscle and is inhibited by methylene blue, an inhibitor of soluble guanylate cyclase. EDRF is destroyed by superoxide anions and protected by scavengers of oxygen-derived free radicals such as superoxide dismutase. In addition, endothelium-dependent relaxation can be inhibited by hemoglobin, which binds to EDRF and prevents it from gaining entrance into vascular smooth muscle cells.

The release of EDRF appears to be a Ca^{2+}-activated process, since it is stimulated by calcium ionophores (e.g., A23187) and calcium-channel activators (e.g., Bay K 8644); it is not due to activation of Ca^{2+} channels sensitive to verapamil or dihydropyridines. Although endothelium-dependent relaxations are impaired in the absence of external Ca^{2+}, the release of EDRF still can be stimulated in an attenuated manner, suggesting that both extracellular and intracellular sources of Ca^{2+} participate in EDRF release. Activation of the phosphatidylinositol pathway may underly the release of Ca^{2+} from intracellular stores.

It is likely that agonist binding to endothelial-cell receptors is linked by several regulatory G proteins to the release of EDRF. Pertussis toxin, an inactivator of certain G proteins, inhibits endothelium-dependent relaxations evoked by the alpha$_2$-adrenergic agonist, UK 14304, 5-hydroxytryptamine, thrombin, and aggregating platelets. In addition, fluoride ions, which can activate G proteins directly, induce pertussis toxin–sensitive endothelium-dependent relaxations. Pertussis toxin–insensitive G proteins mediate EDRF release caused by activation of bradykinin and ADP receptors.

Although the chemical nature of EDRF remained elusive for several years, it is now apparent that, in many instances, the endothelial mediator is NO or a closely related molecule derived from the metabolism of L-arginine. The physicochemical and biologic properties of EDRF and NO are indistinguishable, and the release of nitric oxide from endothelial cells in quantities sufficient to relax vascular smooth muscle has been demonstrated.

The enzyme that initiates the conversion of L-arginine to nitric oxide by the endothelium, termed nitric oxide synthase, has been characterized partially in endothelial cells and other tissues and cloned in brain tissues. The activation of the nitric oxide synthase in endothelial cells is initiated by an increase in cytosolic Ca^{2+} and requires calmodulin. Two types of enzyme are present in cultured and native endothelial cells: a cytosolic isoform and a particulate one. The latter is responsible for 95 percent of the EDRF-NO-synthesizing activity. The membrane-associated enzyme possesses a molecular mass of 135 kDa, is sensitive to the reduced form of nicotinamide-adenine dinucleotide phosphate (NADPH) and to 5,6,7,8-tetrahydrobiopterin, and is Ca^{2+}-calmodulin dependent. This is in agreement with the calcium dependency of endothelium-dependent relaxations. The characteristics of the soluble endothelial enzyme are similar.

Besides the constitutive nitric oxide synthase, vascular endothelial cells may express an inducible form in response to endotoxin and cytokines, which will evoke a long-lasting release of large amounts of NO, resulting in cytotoxic activities. Activated endothelial cells express a cytosolic enzyme (of 150-kDa molecular mass) independent of Ca^{2+}-calmodulin with a rank order of potency similar to that of cytokine-activated macrophages. This form of nitric oxide synthase can also be induced in vascular smooth muscle cells and can produce high concentrations of NO for prolonged periods of time during immunologic and inflammatory reactions. Such events may play a role in the irreversible phase of septic shock, which is characterized by peripheral vascular paralysis.

The discovery of the role of 1-arginine in endothelium-dependent relaxation led the way for the use of specific inhibitors of EDRF production. Arginine analogs, such as N^G-monomethyl-L-arginine and L-N^G-nitro-arginine, act as inhibitors of NO production by competing with L-arginine for nitric oxide synthase. These compounds have become important pharmacologic tools for investigating the role of EDRF-NO in regulating vasomotor tone under normal and pathologic conditions.

Evidence from several laboratories demonstrates that not all endothelium-dependent relaxations are prevented by inhibitors of the L-arginine-NO-cGMP pathway, suggesting the existence of more than one EDRF. Moreover, many endothelium-dependent relaxations are accompanied by hyperpolarization of the vascular smooth muscle, and most studies indicate that NO does not mediate endothelium-dependent hyperpolarization. Bioassay experiments have shown that endothelium-dependent hyperpolarization is due to a diffusable substance called EDHF (endothelium-derived hyperpolarizing factor). The exact identity of this substance is unknown, but the data available suggest that EDRF-NO and EDHF are separate compounds, and that EDHF is a labile metabolite of arachidonic acid, presumably formed through the P-450 epoxygenase pathway.

Unlike NO, which is continuously produced by the constitutive nitric oxide synthase, there is probably no ongoing basal release of EDHF. However, the release of EDHF can be initiated by many of the same substances that stimulate the release of NO, including acetylcholine, bradykinin, adenine nucleotides, histamine, thrombin, and substance P. In the case of bradykinin, endothelium-dependent hyperpolarizations are potentiated by converting enzyme inhibitors. Like NO, the release of EDHF is a Ca^{2+}-dependent process and thus can be triggered by the Ca^{2+} ionophore, A23187. EDHF release is likely to be dependent on calmodulin, since it is prevented by several calmodulin inhibitors.

Most data suggest that EDHF acts on vascular smooth muscle by opening K^+ channels. Although the exact type of K^+ channel involved still is unclear, it appears to be different from the one activated by the synthetic K^+-channel openers, because glyburide has little or no effect on endothelium-dependent hyperpolarizations in most blood vessels. Alternatively, a role for activation of Na^+/K^+ ATPase has been proposed, because the action of EDHF can be prevented by ouabain in some vascular preparations.

CYCLOOXYGENASE-DEPENDENT ENDOTHELIUM-DERIVED CONTRACTING FACTOR(S)

The first evidence that the endothelium can generate a vasoconstrictor substance was obtained by De Mey and Vanhoutte in 1982. They reported that in systemic and pulmonary veins of the dog arachidonic acid causes endothelium-dependent contraction; the same is true in cerebral arteries of the same species. In the latter, endothelium-dependent contractions are also observed with the Ca^{2+}-ionophore A23187 and with acetylcholine. Since these responses are prevented by indomethacin, the endothelium-derived contracting factor appears to be a product of or to depend on the activity of cyclooxygenase. Thus far, three potential mediators of cyclooxygenase-dependent endothelium-dependent contraction have been identified: (1) superoxide anions, generated by hydroperoxidase activity of cyclooxygenase; (2) thromboxane A_2; and (3) prostaglandin H_2. These mediators act directly on vascular smooth muscle to cause contraction, as well as interact chemically with NO to remove the inhibitory influence of the endothelium. Because arachidonic acid probably is generated whenever cell membranes are perturbed, these observations may imply that, under a number of physiologic and pathologic conditions that result in deformation of the cell membrane, endothelial cells may become a source of vasoconstrictor signals. The obvious example is provided by the observation that in cerebral arteries, rapid stretch evokes a contraction, which depends on the presence of endothelial cells; the formation of the contracting substance again requires the activity of cyclooxygenase (Fig. 4-9). These observations suggest that the endothelium may contribute to the still unsolved phenomenon of autoregulation.

CYCLOOXYGENASE-INDEPENDENT ENDOTHELIUM-DERIVED CONTRACTING FACTOR(S)

Endothelial cells produce a potent vasoconstrictor peptide that has been isolated and named **endothelin** (ET). The ET family consists of three vasoconstrictor peptides, termed ET-1, ET-2, and ET-3. ET-1 is the only member of the family to be synthesized by endothelial cells. Since there are no known endothelial storage sites for ET, the peptide is apparently produced on demand with the messenger RNA (mRNA) for its production being rapidly inactivated. Factors that induce mRNA production and release of ET include thrombin, arginine-vasopressin, angiotensin II, epinephrine, prolonged (12–24 hours) hyp-

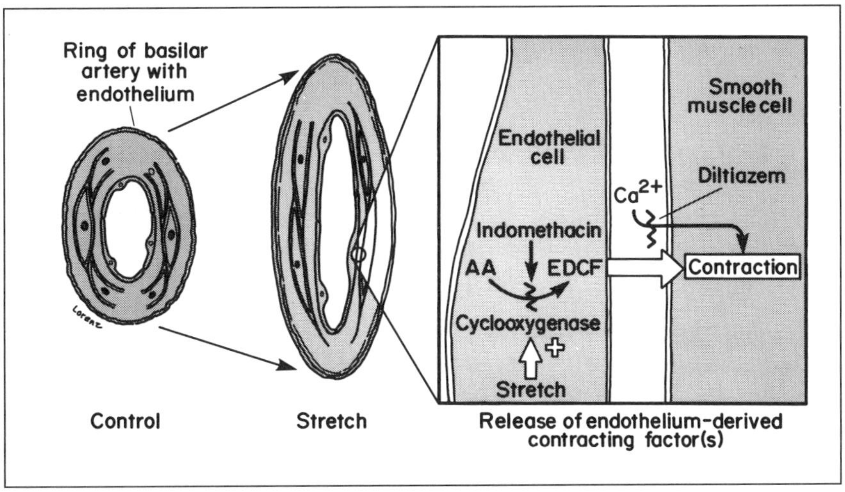

Fig. 4-9. Role of endothelium in response of basilar arteries to stretch. In isolated cerebral arteries of the dog, sudden stretch causes release from endothelium of vasoconstrictor prostanoids that activate entry of Ca^{2+} into vascular smooth muscle, thus tending to counteract stretch. If this were to occur in the intact organism, it could help to explain autoregulation. EDCF = endothelium-derived contracting factor; AA = arachidonic acid. (Reproduced with permission from PM Vanhoutte. Endothelium and the control of vascular tissue. News Physiol Sci 1987; 2:18–22.)

oxia, the calcium ionophore A23187, phorbol esters, and shear stress. ET is synthesized by endothelial cells initially as a 203-residue peptide named **pre-proendothelin**. After subsequent processing, it becomes the 39–amino acid termed **big endothelin** (**proendothelin**). Big endothelin is transformed by ET-converting enzyme to the potent 21–amino acid peptide ET.

ET interacts with endothelial cells to stimulate the release of EDRF; alternatively, endothelium-derived NO inhibits the stimulated release of ET. Under basal conditions, an intact endothelium reduces the contractile response to ET; this could be due both to basally released EDRF and stimulated release by endothelin. Moreover, NO released by the endothelium markedly inhibits the constrictor response to the peptide.

ET-1 binds to a single class of sites (ET_A receptors) on most vascular smooth muscle cell membranes. In certain blood vessels, activation of ET_B receptors contributes to the constrictor effect of the peptide. Dihydropyridines do not interfere with ET binding, which indicates that ET-1 is not an agonist for the dihydropyridine-binding site on voltage-dependent, L-type calcium channels.

The vasoconstrictor effects of ET result from a rise in intracellular calcium within the vascular smooth muscle cells. The available evidence suggests that ET activates the phosphoinositide cascade to generate inositol trisphosphate, which releases calcium from intracellular stores. The entry of extracellular calcium may play a role in the contraction elicited by ET in some, but not all, blood vessels; this most likely reflects the heterogeneity in extracellular calcium requirements of vascular smooth muscle from different sites.

Infusion of ET in vivo induces a transient vasodilation, which likely is due to the release of vasodilator prostaglandins (e.g., prostacyclin), of endothelium-derived NO, and of EDHF. The depressor response to ET is followed by a sustained and long-lasting increase in blood pressure resulting from an increase in peripheral vascular resistance that is best explained by the direct constrictor effect of the peptide on vascular smooth muscle. Endothelin is a more potent constrictor of arterioles than large arteries and a more potent constrictor of veins than arteries.

The slow onset and prolonged action of ET, coupled with its relatively slow rate of production (requiring de novo protein synthesis), suggests that the peptide is more likely to play a physiologic role in mid- or long-term regulation rather than to contribute to moment-to-moment changes in vascular tone. In addition, ET may play a role in a variety of cardiovascular disorders, since the circulating blood levels of ET in patients are increased in several disease states, including hypertension, heart failure, acute myocardial infarction, and ischemic heart disease. The recent availability of relatively selective ET-receptor antagonists (e.g., BQ123, bosentan) will help to determine whether the peptide plays a causal role under those pathologic conditions or must be regarded as an epiphenomenon.

In a variety of systemic, cerebral, coronary, and pulmonary blood vessels, acute anoxia augments the contraction evoked by constrictor agents such as norepinephrine and serotonin. These anoxic contractions are reduced markedly, even abolished, if the endothelial cells are removed. To judge from experiments in isolated blood vessels, a contracting factor is released by the anoxic ET, which then diffuses to and causes contraction of the smooth muscle cells by activating the entry of Ca^{2+} (Fig. 4-10). This endothelium-derived contracting factor is different from that released by arachidonic acid, stretch, or acetylcholine, because the endothelium-dependent hypoxic contractions are not prevented by inhibitors of cyclooxygenase. The rapid onset and reversal of the contraction and the inability to bioassay the contracting factor in cascade superfu-

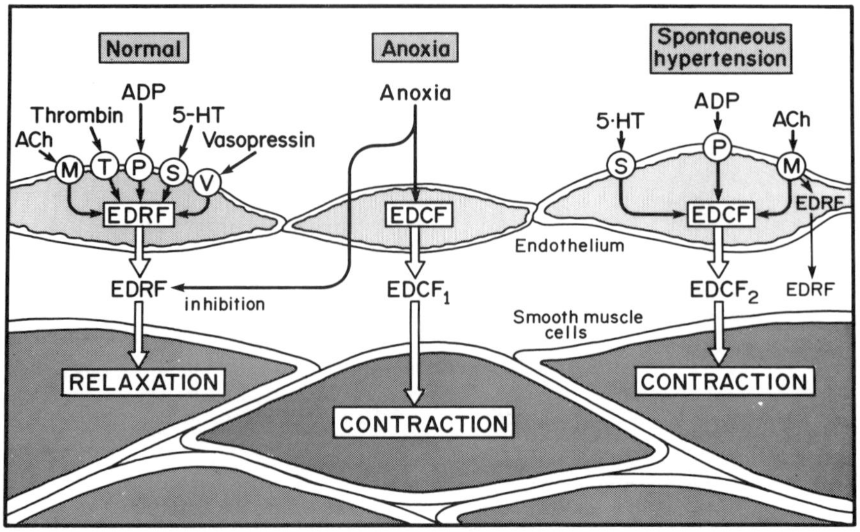

Fig. 4-10. Beside producing endothelium-derived relaxing factor (EDRF), endothelial cells can release at least two different constrictor substances (EDCF). One is released when the cells are anoxic; it is not a metabolite of arachidonic acid. The others can be released by several neurohumoral mediators or by stretch, particularly in hypertensive blood vessels; it is a product of cyclooxygenase. ACh = acetylcholine; 5-HT = serotonin. (Reproduced with permission from PM Vanhoutte. Endothelium and the control of vascular tissue. News Physiol Sci 1987; 2:18–22.)

sion experiments make it unlikely that the vasoconstrictor peptide ET mediates this response. An alternative mechanism contributing to endothelium-dependent hypoxic contractions may be reduced basal production of NO by the hypoxic endothelial cells.

In the pulmonary circulation, the production of endothelium-derived contracting factor could help to explain hypoxic pulmonary vasoconstriction. In the coronary, cerebral, and systemic circulations, endothelium-dependent constrictions evoked by anoxia would tend to prolong rather than attenuate, as one would expect under anoxic conditions, vasospastic episodes leading to ischemia.

THE NEUROHUMORAL MEDIATORS

Catecholamines

In the periphery, catecholamines such as norepinephrine and epinephrine are stored and released from two primary sites. Postganglionic adrenergic neurons are the major source of norepinephrine, whereas epinephrine is predominantly released into the bloodstream from the adrenal medulla.

Norepinephrine and epinephrine produce their physiologic effects by activating alpha- and beta-adrenoreceptors (or adrenoceptors) on target tissues. These receptors can be further subdivided into $alpha_1$, $alpha_2$, $beta_1$, and $beta_2$, based on their affinities for selective agonists and antagonists. Alpha- and beta-adrenoreceptors are found on adrenergic nerve endings, vascular smooth muscle, and endothelial cells.

VASCULAR SMOOTH MUSCLE

In most blood vessels innervated by sympathetic neurons, norepinephrine activates postjunctional alpha-adrenoceptors. This process, by increasing the cytoplasmic Ca^{2+} concentration, triggers the contractile process, thus causing contraction of the vascular smooth muscle cells and vasoconstriction. In addition, most vascular smooth muscle contains beta-adrenoceptors, which mediate relaxation of the vascular smooth muscle and, thus, vasodilatation.

Postjunctional Alpha-Adrenoceptors. Not all postjunctional vascular alpha-adrenoceptors belong to the same subtype. Most large arteries, when studied in vitro, respond with contraction to selective $alpha_1$-adrenergic agonists (such as phenylephrine) but are relatively insensitive to selective $alpha_2$-adrenergic agonists (e.g., clonidine, tramazoline, BHT-920, UK-14,307). The contractile response of these arteries to norepinephrine is competitively antagonized by specific $alpha_1$-adrenergic antagonists such as prazosin and by nonselective alpha-adrenolytic agents such as phentolamine, whereas selective $alpha_2$-adrenergic antagonists such as yohimbine and rauwolscine are less effective. This pattern of responsiveness allows the classification of the postjunctional receptors involved as $alpha_1$-adrenoceptors.

Postjunctional alpha-adrenoceptors of the smooth muscle cells in resistance vessels do not necessarily belong to the $alpha_1$-adrenoceptor subtype. The postjunctional alpha-adrenoceptors of certain veins differ from those of most larger arteries in that they respond to selective $alpha_2$-adrenergic agonists; in those veins the $alpha_1$-adrenergic antagonist prazosin is not a competitive antagonist of the response to norepinephrine, whereas yohimbine and rauwolscine are. These findings demonstate that, in addition to postjunctional $alpha_1$-adrenoceptors, venous smooth muscle cells may also contain postjunctional adrenoceptors with pharmacologic properties resembling those of the $alpha_2$-adrenoceptors involved in the prejunctional feedback inhibition of neurotransmitter release. The finding that postjunctional alpha-adrenoceptors are not a homogeneous pharmacologic group is illustrated also by the difference in responsiveness of systemic and cerebral arteries to alpha-adrenergic activation.

Postjunctional Beta-Adrenoceptors. Most vascular smooth muscle responds to beta-adrenergic activation with relaxation. With the exception of the coronary artery in certain species, the receptors involved belong to the beta$_2$-subtype, which is more sensitive to isoproterenol and epinephrine but relatively insensitive to norepinephrine. Under normal physiologic conditions, nerve-released norepinephrine primarily activates postjunctional alpha-adrenoceptors in most blood vessels. Concomitant activation of postjunctional beta-adrenoceptors may attenuate the vasoconstrictor response to sympathetic-nerve stimulation. Alpha-adrenergic blockade may unmask a beta-adrenoceptor–mediated dilator effect of exogenous norepinephrine, whereas beta-adrenergic blockade augments its constrictor effect. Neurogenically induced relaxation of vascular smooth muscle due to activation of postjunctional beta-adrenergic receptors, in the absence of alpha-adrenergic blockade, is observed only in certain facial veins and in coronary arteries.

In spontaneous hypertension, arterial smooth muscle is less sensitive to the relaxing effects of beta-adrenergic agonists, particularly in more mature animals. Similarly, a decreased beta-responsiveness related to age, blood pressure, and plasma catecholamines has been reported in essential human hypertension. This, together with the increase in alpha$_1$-adrenergic–mediated vasoconstriction, could contribute to the maintenance of blood pressure elevation in chronic hypertension.

ADRENERGIC NERVES

Prejunctional Alpha$_2$-Adrenergic Inhibition. The adrenergic neuronal membrane senses the concentration of transmitter present in the junctional cleft by means of alpha-adrenergic receptors on the sympathetic-nerve endings (prejunctional or presynaptic alpha-adrenoceptors) (see Fig. 4-5). Receptors that exert a negative feedback on the exocytotic process belong to the alpha$_2$-adrenergic subtype and are sensitive to alpha$_2$-adrenergic agonists, of which clonidine is the prototype. If these receptors are activated on a background of sympathetic-nerve stimulation, the release of norepinephrine is decreased. Conversely, alpha$_2$-adrenergic antagonists, such as rauwolscine, yohimbine, and phentolamine (in descending order of selectivity), but not selective alpha$_1$-adrenergic antagonists, such as prazosin, enhance the overflow of adrenergic transmitter during activation of the exocytotic process. Inhibitory prejunctional alpha$_2$-adrenoceptors are present in a number of isolated blood vessels from various species, including humans. In experimental hypertension, prejunctional inhibition of adrenergic neurotransmission becomes less effective as arterial pressure rises; thus, a defect in prejunctional modulation of adrenergic neurotransmission may contribute to the development of high blood pressure.

Beta-Adrenoceptors. Experiments performed mainly on isolated blood vessels indicate that beta$_2$-adrenergic agonists, in particular, isoproterenol and epinephrine, can augment the evoked release of norepinephrine in the blood vessel wall by activating prejunctional beta$_2$-adrenoceptors (see Fig. 4-5). This prejunctional beta$_2$-adrenergic facilitation is more pronounced in human than in animal blood vessels. Cardioselective beta$_1$-receptor antagonists are less effective in blocking prejunctional excitatory beta-receptors than are nonselective agents.

In at least some hypertensive individuals, plasma epinephrine levels are increased. It has been postulated that the primary abnormality in essential hypertension might be an increased adrenal secretion of epinephrine, which in turn, by facilitation of junctional norepinephrine release, might lead to the development of essential hypertension. Whether the prejunctional beta-adrenoceptors indeed play a role under normal conditions and, in particular, in essential hypertension, is still uncertain, however. If they do, beta-adrenergic antagonists also may act at this site and cause a decrease in neurotransmitter release, which could help to explain their antihypertensive properties.

ENDOTHELIUM

Norepinephrine and selective alpha$_2$-adrenergic agonists can cause relaxation of canine and porcine coronary and systemic arteries and canine pulmonary arteries and veins if the endothelium is present. In the canine pulmonary artery and femoral vein, which are chronically exposed to low oxygen tension, the inhibitory effects of endothelial alpha$_2$-adrenergic stimulation are masked in part by the contractions induced by stimulation of alpha$_2$-adrenoceptors on the vascular smooth muscle. The expression of the alpha$_2$-adrenergic relaxations of the femoral vein can be augmented when that vessel is chronically exposed to high flow and high arterial levels of oxygen tension by the creation of an arteriovenous fistula between the femoral artery and vein.

In canine coronary artery, the relaxing effects of beta-adrenergic agonists, in particular, norepinephrine and isoproterenol, are reduced following removal of the endothelium. It is uncertain whether the greater responsiveness to beta-adrenergic agonists in the presence of endothelial cells is due to the continuous (basal) release of an EDRF or to activation of beta-adrenoceptors on the endothelial cells, resulting in an augmented production of cAMP in the endothelial cells, which in turn facilitates the basal release of EDRF(s).

The presence of inhibitory alpha$_2$-adrenoceptors on the endothelial cells and the augmented beta-adrenergic relaxations that these cells provide may help to explain the vasodilator effects of catecholamines in certain vascular beds. Conversely, the absence of the endothelium favors vasoconstriction due to activation by catecholamines of alpha-adrenergic receptors on vascular smooth muscle cells. Therefore, contractions evoked by nonselective alpha-adrenergic agonists, in particular, epinephrine and norepinephrine, are augmented following removal of the endothelium.

BETA BLOCKERS AND TREATMENT OF HYPERTENSION

Beta-adrenergic–blocking drugs are well established in the treatment of essential hypertension. A reduction in cardiac output and in the rate of change of generated pressure might contribute to the decrease in arterial blood pressure that they cause, but their full antihypertensive effect is delayed and is related to a decrease in peripheral vascular resistance. Since activation of beta-adrenoceptors causes relaxation of vascular smooth muscle cells, the decrease of peripheral resistance caused by these agents is difficult to explain. It may be due to one or several of the following: (1) inhibition of renin secretion and in turn reduced activity of the renin-angiotensin-aldosterone system; (2) blockade of facilitatory prejunctional beta-adrenoceptors and, in turn, inhibition of adrenergic neurotransmission; (3) reduction of tyrosine hydroxylase and dopamine β-hydroxylase in sympathetic ganglia; (4) blockade of central beta-adrenoceptors; (5) interference with trophic effects of epinephrine and, in turn, prevention or reversal of structural vascular changes; (6) nonspecific vasodilator or alpha-adrenergic–blocking properties seen with some compounds, such as labetalol and bucindolol; (7) recovery of adenylate cyclase–induced relaxation in response to other vasodilator stimuli due to beta-adrenoceptor occupancy; (8) inhibitory effects on the binding of serotonin to the serotonergic receptors of vascular smooth muscle; (9) intrinsic sympathomimetic activity, resulting in stimulation of postjunctional vascular beta$_2$-adrenoceptors; and (10) facilitation of endothelium-dependent relaxations, in particular, those due to alpha$_2$-adrenergic activation.

Acetylcholine

Cholinergic nerves are the major source of acetylcholine, and several blood vessels are innervated by cholinergic neurons. In addition, certain endothelial cells contain the enzyme choline acetyltransferase, thus raising the possibility that these cells could synthesize and release acetylcholine. Acetylcholine is not present in significant amounts in plasma, however, which suggests that the effects of acetylcholine would be very localized.

Tissue responses to acetylcholine are mediated by activation of muscarinic or nicotinic receptors. Nicotinic receptors are found predominantly in autonomic ganglia and skeletal muscle. Muscarinic receptors are found on numerous end organs, including vascular smooth muscle, adrenergic-nerve endings, and endothelial cells. Recent work has shown that muscarinic receptors may now be divided into three subtypes based on their affinity for a novel series of antagonists. The three pharmacologically defined muscarinic receptors are M_1, which has a high affinity for pirenzepine; M_2, which has a high affinity for AFDX-116 or gallamine; and M_3, which has a high affinity for 4-diaphenyl acetoxyn-methylpiperidine methoidide (4-DAMP) or hexahydrosiladifenidol (HHSD). The classic muscarinic receptor antagonist, atropine, is nonselective.

ACETYLCHOLINE AND VASCULAR SMOOTH MUSCLE

When the endothelial cells are removed and the sympathetic nerve endings are quiescent, the only obvious effect of acetylcholine on certain, but not all, systemic arteries and veins is contraction. Acetylcholine activates muscarinic receptors on the membrane of the smooth muscle cells, which in turn trigger the entry of extracellular Ca^{2+}. Both M_1 and M_3 receptors have been identified in vascular smooth muscle.

ACETYLCHOLINE AND ADRENERGIC NERVES

Exogenous acetylcholine exerts a potent prejunctional inhibitory effect on the exocytotic release of norepinephrine in a wide variety of systemic arteries and veins from different species, including humans. Vagal-nerve stimulation causes inhibition of the release of norepinephrine in the heart and in the gastric circulation. Both exogenous and endogenous acetylcholine inhibit the release of norepinephrine in canine coronary artery.

The inhibitory effect of acetylcholine is due to activation of muscarinic receptors, which presumably causes hyperpolarization of the adrenergic-nerve endings. The prejunctional muscarinic receptor located on adrenergic-nerve endings has been characterized as an M_2 receptor. In higher concentrations, acetylcholine can activate nicotinic receptors on adrenergic-nerve endings; nicotine itself can facilitate or initiate the release of adrenergic neurotransmitter in the blood vessel wall.

ENDOTHELIUM

Acetylcholine applied to the luminal side of the blood vessel wall causes the release of EDRF and EDHF from the endothelial cells, which diffuse to the vascular smooth muscle. The release of these factors results from the activation of muscarinic receptors on the endothelial cells, since it can be blocked by muscarinic antagonists such as atropine. Depending on the experimental conditions, both M_1 and M_3 receptors may play a role in mediating the response to acetylcholine. Thus, the release of hyperpolarizing factor has been linked to activation of M_1 receptors, and the release of the factor causing activation of guanylate cyclase may be mediated by M_3 muscarinic receptors.

The endothelium-dependent inhibitory effect of acetylcholine is much less pronounced in veins than in arteries. The differences in magnitude of the endothelium-dependent relaxation to acetylcholine observed between arteries and veins could result from the presence of more muscarinic receptors on venous smooth muscle, which, when triggered by acetylcholine, accelerate the entry of calcium into the smooth muscle and thus activate the contractile process. Alternatively, the signal or signals generated by the endothelial cells may cause relaxation by inhibiting (as with calcium entry) or activating (as with Na^+,K^+-ATPase) cellular events that play a more prominent role in arterial than in venous smooth muscle. Although most of the preparations studied have been large conduit arteries, experiments carried out in smaller arteries and in vascular beds indicate that acetylcholine may induce endothelium-mediated relaxations in resistance vessels as well.

Purines

Most blood vessels are rich in receptors for circulating or locally released purine derivatives. Purinergic receptors have been classified into two groups, P_1 and P_2. For the P_1 purinoceptor, the potency order of adenosine greater than ADP greater than ATP has been proposed. Methylxanthines, such as theophylline, are believed to be selective antagonists of the P_1 purinoceptor, and activation of this receptor is accompanied by changes in intracellular levels of cAMP. For the P_2 purinoceptor, the agonist potency order is reverse (ATP > ADP > adenosine), methylxanthines are not antagonists, and receptor activation is not associated with changes in intracellular cAMP.

Activation of purinergic receptors can elicit either relaxation or contraction of vascular smooth muscle. Stimulation of P_1 purinoceptors results in relaxation of vascular smooth muscle; thus, adenosine acts primarily as a vasodilator. In particular, adenosine, released from ischemic myocardial cells, has been proposed as a mediator of hypoxic vasodilation in coronary vessels. Activation of P_2 purinoceptors by ADP or ATP can have either contractile or relaxant effects in different blood vessels.

Adrenergic nerve stimulation causes release of purine compounds in several vascular beds. These purines can inhibit adrenergic neurotransmission at the prejunctional level. The inhibitory effect of ATP on noradrenergic neurotransmission is caused by ATP's rapid breakdown to adenosine. Because the inhibition is antagonized by theophylline, the receptor on the adrenergic-nerve ending mediating the effect of adenosine can be classified as a P_1-purinergic receptor.

In all blood vessels studied, ADP and ATP cause endothelium-dependent relaxations that do not depend on the metabolism of arachidonic acid. These relaxations are mediated by P_2-purinergic receptors on the endothelial cells. In cerebral arteries, the endothelium-dependent effect of ADP is accompanied by an important endothelium-independent relaxation, which is not observed in systemic and coronary arteries. In pulmonary and systemic veins, the endothelium-dependent relaxation caused by adenosine nucleotides is masked partially by their direct excitatory effect on venous smooth muscle.

During platelet aggregation, large quantities of ADP and ATP are released. In the coronary artery, for example, purines released from aggregating platelets reach the endothelial cells first, where they cause the release of EDRF. This response protects against vasospasm at the site of a beginning thrombus and helps to "flush away" the early aggregate. With trauma and damage to the endothelial layer, however, the platelet-released ATP and ADP gain access to the smooth muscle, where they can promote vasoconstriction.

Serotonin

With the exception of some areas of the cerebral circulation, most blood vessels are not innervated by serotonergic neurons. Most of the circulating serotonin originates in the enterochromaffin cells of the gastrointestinal tract, which synthesize and release it into the portal circulation. Serotonin is inactivated by the liver or by endothelial cells (mainly in the lungs); the remaining part is taken up and stored by the platelets. As a consequence, very little, if any, serotonin is present in the plasma. Hence, levels of serotonin sufficient to affect the blood vessel wall probably occur only at sites of endothelial damage where platelet aggregation occurs.

Serotonin causes both vasoconstriction and vasodilatation by interacting with a variety of autonomic receptors in the blood vessel wall located either on smooth muscle cells, endothelial cells, or adrenergic-nerve endings. Several subtypes of serotonergic receptors are involved.

In 1957, Gaddum and Picarelli made the first major attempt to classify serotonergic receptors. They described D and M receptors in guinea pig ileum, according to whether the responses to the monoamine were blocked by phenoxybenzamine or morphine. More recently, binding sites for serotonin in brain tissues have been subclassified into 5-HT_1 and 5-HT_2 serotonergic binding sites. The former have a greater affinity for agonists and can be characterized by binding of ^{3}H-5-hydroxytryptamine; the latter have a higher affinity for antagonists and can be labeled with ^{3}H-spiroperidol. Ketanserin is a selective ligand for the 5-HT_2-serotonergic receptor. Most other classic serotonergic antagonists, such as methysergide, show some affinity for both 5-HT_1 and 5-HT_2 sites.

In certain tissues, including the adrenergic nerves to the heart of rabbit, serotonin is excitatory rather than inhibitory; the receptor mediating this effect is of yet another subtype (5-HT_3) and is specifically blocked by MDL 72222.

SEROTONIN AND VASCULAR SMOOTH MUSCLE

In most systemic arterial smooth muscle, serotonin induces contractions that are antagonized competitively by ketanserin. In other blood vessels, however, such as the coronary and cerebral arteries, ketanserin acts as a noncompetitive antagonist. This may indicate the presence of multiple serotonergic-receptor subtypes on arterial smooth muscles. In cerebral and coronary arteries, the receptors mediating serotonin-induced contraction may correspond to 5-HT_1-binding sites. In some blood vessels, methysergide, which is less selective for 5-HT_2-serotonergic receptors, acts as a competitive antagonist. In others, methysergide has partial agonistic properties and thus causes contraction, which further illustrates the complex characteristics of serotonergic receptors in vascular smooth muscle.

Besides acting on specific serotonergic receptors, serotonin may stimulate adrenergic receptors. Thus, in canine saphenous veins, for example, contractile responses to serotonin may be mediated by atypical alpha-adrenoceptors.

In addition to its direct contractile effects on vascular smooth muscle, serotonin amplifies the effects of other vasoconstrictor agonists such as histamine, angiotensin II, prostaglandin $F_{2\alpha}$, and noradrenaline (Fig. 4-11). In vascular smooth muscle endowed with 5-HT_2-serotonergic receptors, this action of serotonin is antagonized by ketanserin, suggesting that the amplification effect is mediated by receptors similar to those responsible for the direct effects of the monoamine. It is not known whether serotonin can cause amplification by acting on other subtypes of serotonergic receptors.

In some smooth muscle, including vascular smooth muscle, such as cat saphenous vein and dog femoral vein, serotonin causes relaxation. These effects are mediated by 5-HT_1-like serotonergic receptors. In addition, in cerebral arteries, serotonin can cause relaxations apparently mediated by beta-adrenoceptors.

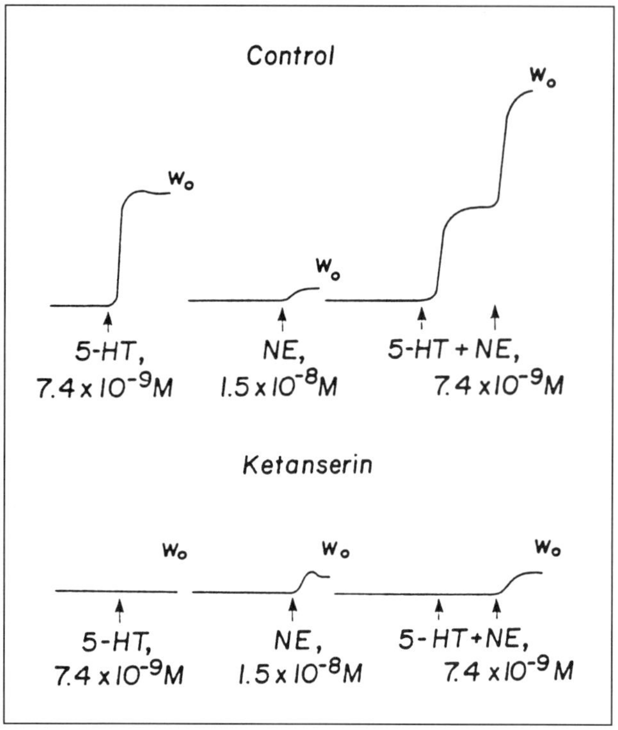

Fig. 4-11. Amplifying effect of serotonin. Traces represent recordings of isotonic contraction of rat caudal-artery strips. Serotonin (5-HT) augments the shortening caused by noradrenaline (NE = norepinephrine). The presence of ketanserin (1.6 nmol/L) abolishes the contraction to serotonin and its amplifying effect. (Reproduced with permission from JM Van Nueten, WJ Janssens, and PM Vanhoutte. Serotonin and vascular smooth muscle. In PM Vanhoutte, ed., Serotonin and the Cardiovascular System. New York: Raven, 1985.)

SEROTONIN AND ADRENERGIC NERVES

The release of norepinephrine from vascular adrenergic nerve varicosities can be inhibited by serotonin. This action of serotonin explains best the observations that the monoamine causes vasodilatation when sympathetic tone is high but vasoconstriction when it is low: in the latter case, the direct activation of the smooth muscle by serotonin predominates. The prejunctional inhibitory action of serotonin is mediated by receptors with pharmacologic similarities to the 5-HT_1-serotonergic subtype.

At high concentrations, serotonin can act as an indirect sympathomimetic amine by displacing norepinephrine from sympathetic-nerve endings—an effect that can be blocked by inhibitors of neuronal uptake. The serotonin taken up by adrenergic nerve endings can be released on stimulation of the nerves.

SEROTONIN AND ENDOTHELIUM

In some blood vessels, the contraction induced by serotonin is diminished in the presence of endothelium. In addition, in certain blood vessels, serotonin can produce endothelium-dependent relaxations during contractions with prostaglandin $F_{2\alpha}$. The exact mechanism underlying these observations still is obscure, although it has been established that the signal from the endothelial cells to the smooth muscle is carried by a diffusable mediator in the form of EDRF(s).

The endothelium-dependent relaxation evoked by serotonin is inhibited by the 5-HT_1- and 5-HT_2-serotonergic antagonist methiothepin but not by the selective 5-HT_2 antagonist ketanserin. This suggests that the endothelium-dependent relaxation to serotonin may be mediated by a 5-HT_1-like serotonergic receptor on endothelial cells. The demonstration of endothelium-dependent effects of serotonin is complicated by the direct activation of the smooth muscle that it causes.

SEROTONIN AND VASCULAR DISEASE

Aggregating platelets release enough serotonin to affect smooth muscle cells, adrenergic nerves, and endothelium. Serotonin plays a role in disease only if exaggerated amounts of it are released, if the removal of the monoamine from the plasma is deficient, or if the vascular wall is hyperresponsive to its constrictor effect. The last instance occurs mainly when the endothelial cells become dysfunctional.

Augmented vascular responsiveness to serotonin appears to characterize the blood vessel wall chronically exposed to an abnormally high blood pressure. A number of intriguing observations, in humans and in animals, suggest that in hypertension, greater than normal amounts of serotonin may be available to the vascular smooth muscle cells of the arterioles (Fig. 4-12). Augmented levels of serotonin could cause exaggerated vasoconstriction not only because the vascular smooth muscle cells are more responsive to the monoamine but also because serotonin markedly amplifies their response to other vasoconstrictor agents, in particular catecholamines and angiotensin II. In the aorta of the spontaneously hypertensive rat, serotonin causes endothelium-dependent contractions. If serotonin is involved in the maintenance of the increased peripheral resistance in hypertensive patients, this could help to explain the antihypertensive properties of the serotonergic antagonist ketanserin, although this compound also can inhibit postjunctional alpha$_1$-adrenoceptors.

The potent contractile effect of serotonin may also play a role in vasospastic disorders. In arteries with regenerated endothelium, for example, and certainly in atherosclerotic arteries, there may be significant dysfunction of the endothelial cells. Exposure of subendothelial structures could initiate platelet aggregation and the subsequent release of serotonin from platelet granules. Release of serotonin at sites with dysfunctional endothelium could result in powerful contractions of the underlying vascular smooth muscle.

Histamine

Histamine is stored primarily in mast cells and basophils. In large arteries and veins, histamine is also stored in a nonmast cell pool, presumably the smooth muscle cells.

Based on the relative potencies of several antagonists, two classes of histamine receptors are known to exist. Classic histamine-receptor antagonists, such as mepyramine and diphenhydramine, are selective for H_1-histamine receptors. The more recently introduced H_2-

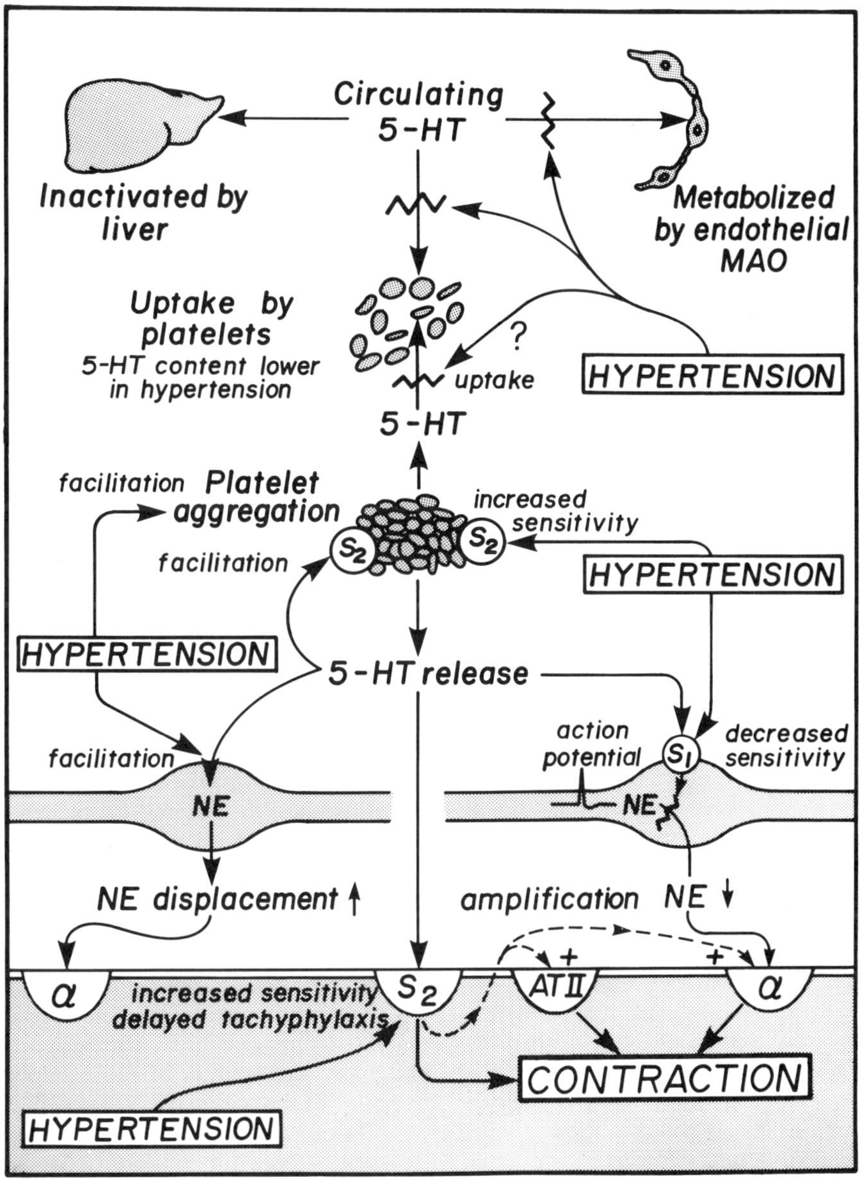

Fig. 4-12. Effects of high arterial blood pressure on the handling of serotonin (5-HT) by platelets and the blood vessel wall α = α-adrenoreceptor; AT II = angiotensin II; MAO = monoamine oxidase; NE = norepinephrine; S_2 = serotonergic receptor. (Reproduced with permission from PM Vanhoutte. Peripheral serotonergic receptors and hypertension. In PM Vanhoutte, ed., Serotonin and the Cardiovascular System. New York: Raven, 1985.)

histamine receptor antagonists include metiamide, cimetidine, and ranitidine. Functional histamine receptors are present in vascular smooth muscle, adrenergic-nerve endings, and endothelial cells.

The predominant effect of histamine in humans is to reduce peripheral vascular resistance and lower systemic blood pressure. Depending on the vessel, species, and concentration, however, histamine can elicit either contractions or relaxations by virtue of its direct effect on vascular smooth muscle. The contractions are mediated by H_1 receptors, since they are attenuated by H_1-receptor antagonists; in some vessels, the contractions are reversed to relaxations by such antagonists. These relaxations are inhibited by H_2-receptor antagonists. Thus, H_1 and H_2 receptors can be found in vascular smooth muscle; contractions are mediated by H_1 receptors, and relaxation is mediated by H_2 receptors. The observed response to histamine depends on the relative dominance of H_1- and H_2-receptor activation.

In isolated canine vessels, the relaxation caused by histamine during sympathetic-nerve activation is paralleled by a decreased overflow of norepinephrine; histamine reduces the release of transmitter evoked by high K^+ but not its displacement evoked by tyramine. Thus, it has been concluded that histamine causes prejunctional inhibition of adrenergic neurotransmission. The effects of histamine during sympathetic-nerve stimulation of canine blood vessels can be mimicked by H_2-receptor agonists:

they are inhibited by H_2-receptor antagonists but not by H_1-receptor-blocking drugs. Thus, the prejunctional inhibiting effect of histamine is caused by activation of H_2 receptors on the neuronal cell membrane. The prejunctional effect of histamine probably contributes to the vasodilator properties it has in certain vascular beds and, in particular, helps explain why the vasodilator effect it causes is prolonged: the direct dilator effect of histamine on the vascular smooth muscle cells is unopposed by norepinephrine released from sympathetic-nerve endings.

In isolated preparations contracted with prostaglandin $F_{2\alpha}$ or potassium, histamine relaxes numerous vessels, including resistance vessels. The relaxations are mediated by H_2 receptors on the vascular smooth muscle and by H_1 receptors on the endothelium. The endothelium-dependent relaxations to histamine are mediated by prostacyclin or EDRF (or both) released from the endothelial cells. In most cases, combined treatment with H_1- and H_2-receptor antagonists abolishes the relaxation to histamine.

Histamine is an important mediator of the vasodilatation accompanying inflammatory reactions, presumably because of its combined action on smooth muscle, adrenergic nerves, and endothelial cells.

Peptides

VASOPRESSIN

The neurohypophyseal peptide vasopressin promotes water reabsorption by the kidney, vasoconstriction in most peripheral vascular beds, and dilatation of large cerebral arteries. Vasopressin exerts its peripheral effects by activating two subtypes of receptors: (1) V_1-vasopressinergic receptors located in the blood vessel wall and (2) V_2-vasopressinergic receptors in the renal tubules. The V_2-vasopressinergic receptors are closely linked to adenylate cyclase formation, which increases the water permeability of the luminal membrane in the distal portions of the nephron.

Receptors for vasopressin in systemic vascular smooth muscle mediate vasoconstriction by increasing cytosolic Ca^{2+} concentration. Besides its direct vasoconstrictor effects, vasopressin also interacts with pre- and postjunctional adrenergic sites to facilitate both the indirect and direct effects of adrenergic agonists.

In cerebral arteries, vasopressin induces an endothelium-dependent relaxation. The relaxations can be prevented by the V_1-vasopressinergic antagonist $d(CH_2)_5Tyr(Me)AVP$, suggesting that effects of the neuropeptide are mediated by activation of V_1-vasopressinergic receptors on endothelial cells. Inhibitors of cyclooxygenase and lipoxygenase do not affect the inhibitory effect of vasopressin, which rules out a major role of prostacyclin in the phenomenon. The endothelium-dependent relaxations of the basilar artery to vasopressin are prevented by inhibitors of Na^+,K^+-ATPase; it is uncertain whether the inhibition of Na^+,K^+-ATPase affects the endothelial or smooth muscle cells of the basilar artery.

The differential effects of vasopressin on cerebral and peripheral arteries (vasodilation and vasoconstriction, respectively) favors the redistribution of blood from the periphery to the cerebral circulation during hemorrhage and shock.

ANGIOTENSIN II

The renin-angiotensin system plays an important role in regulating blood pressure and water and electrolyte balance. The primary mediator of this system is the octapeptide angiotensin II. Besides stimulating the synthesis and secretion of aldosterone by the adrenal cortex, angiotensin II is also a potent vasoconstrictor. The synthesis of angiotensin II is initiated when the enzyme renin, which is secreted from the kidney, acts on angiotensinogen in the plasma to release the decapeptide angiotensin I. This decapeptide has minimal pharmacologic activity. In the pulmonary circulation, angiotensin I is cleaved by angiotensin-converting enzyme to generate angiotensin II. The octapeptide in turn may be further cleaved by aminopeptidase to form angiotensin III. Although angiotensin I and angiotensin III are pharmacologically active, they are considerably less potent than angiotensin II. The conversion of angiotensinogen to angiotensin I by renin is the rate-limiting step in the biosynthesis of angiotensin II. Inhibitors of angiotensin-converting enzyme, such as captopril and enalapril, inhibit the biosynthesis of angiotensin II, thus limiting the amount of octapeptide available for receptor activation.

Angiotensin II causes contraction of most arterial and arteriolar and of certain venous smooth muscle cells. It also augments the vasoconstrictor responses to sympathetic-nerve stimulation by enhancing local synthesis of norepinephrine, inhibiting neuronal uptake of catecholamines, and facilitating the exocytotic release of norepinephrine. The stimulation of adrenergic neurotransmission caused by the octapeptide, combined with the activation of central angiotensin-receptor sites and the facilitation of transmission at the sympathetic ganglia, can augment the amount of norepinephrine present in the vicinity of the vascular effector cells.

A number of angiotensin II–receptor antagonists have been synthesized by modifying the amino acid composition of the octapeptide. Saralasin is the best studied of these antagonists. It is a weak partial agonist that behaves as a competitive antagonist at angiotensin II receptors.

In contrast to its direct vasoconstrictor effect, angiotensin II can induce endothelium-dependent relaxation of renal and cerebral arteries; this effect is apparently mediated by the production of prostacyclin.

To judge from animal data, renovascular hypertension may be accompanied by an augmented responsiveness to angiotensin II at a time when the resistance vessels respond normally to other vasoconstrictor agonists, particularly catecholamines. Thus, angiotensin-receptor antagonists and converting-enzyme inhibitors lower blood pressure in certain forms of hypertension.

BRADYKININ

Bradykinin is a nonapeptide formed in plasma and other biologic fluids by cleavage of precursors known as kininogens. The cleavage of kininogens is effected by enzymes, referred to as kallikreins, produced by the liver and by the exocrine glands. The synthesis of bradykinin is activated by Hageman factor when blood comes into contact with negatively charged surfaces such as glass or collagen, which is readily exposed by tissue damage. Bradykinin is inactivated by the same enzyme responsible for the conversion of angiotensin I to angiotensin II, namely, angiotensin-converting enzyme.

The biologic actions of bradykinin are thought to be mediated by specific receptors on the cell surface. Based on the order of potency of a series of structurally related peptides, at least two different receptors for bradykinin may exist. These receptors have been designated B_1 and B_2 bradykinin receptors.

Bradykinin is a potent vasodilator in vivo. Depending on their anatomic origin and species, however, isolated blood vessels may relax, contract, or show no response at all to bradykinin. Contractions to bradykinin are most prominent in veins. The stimulatory action of bradykinin on vascular smooth muscle is independent of the endothelium and may be mediated by both B_1 and B_2 receptors.

Relaxation of vascular smooth muscle by bradykinin appears to be an indirect effect mediated by the release of other vasoactive substances. Bradykinin-induced relaxations of cat and rabbit arteries are independent of the endothelium. These relaxations are suppressed by inhibitors of cyclooxygenase, suggesting that vasodilator prostaglandins, such as PGE_2 and prostacyclin, may play a role in mediating the response to bradykinin in these vessels.

Bradykinin depresses the response of isolated arteries to electrical stimulation of the adrenergic nerves; a similar depression is reported in the perfused kidney during sympathetic-nerve activation. In isolated pulmonary arteries, bradykinin reduces the overflow of norepinephrine evoked by electrical impulses. The decrease of the vasoconstrictor response in the kidney and the reduction of the overflow of transmitter in the pulmonary artery are accompanied by an augmented production of prostaglandinlike material, as shown by modulation of these effects by inhibitors of prostaglandin synthesis. Thus, the prejunctional inhibitory effect exerted by bradykinin in blood vessels apparently is secondary to the enhanced biosynthesis of prostanoids that it causes.

In canine and human blood vessels, the relaxation elicited by bradykinin is endothelium dependent. This response is probably due to the release of NO and EDHF, since it is not affected by the presence of inhibitors of cyclooxygenase. Whether the endothelium-dependent response to bradykinin contributes to the local regulation of blood flow under normal or pathologic conditions is now known. Potentiation of the endothelium-dependent relaxing effect of endogenous bradykinin may contribute to the vasodilator effect of inhibitors of converting enzyme.

The physiologic role of bradykinin is not well understood, but it has long been associated with defense and repair responses, particularly inflammatory reactions.

ATRIAL NATRIURETIC FACTOR

Atrial natriuretic factor (ANF) is a peptide hormone stored in specific granules located in atrial cardiocytes. ANF is intimately involved in the regulation of renal and cardiovascular homeostasis. The peptide is capable of exerting potent effects on fluid and electrolyte balance and on blood pressure. Circulating levels of ANF are low under basal conditions but may be increased by atrial stretch caused by volume expansion or constrictor agents that elevate atrial pressure.

ANF is a potent vasorelaxant peptide. Relaxation mediated by ANF is due to a direct effect on vascular smooth muscle and is independent of the vascular endothelium. The biochemical mechanism by which ANF produces vasodilatation most likely is related to its effect on guanine nucleotide metabolism. ANF stimulates the particulate form of guanylate cyclase, which leads to an elevation of cGMP within vascular smooth muscle cells. A strong correlation exists between changes in vascular levels of cGMP and ANF-induced vascular relaxation. ANF does not alter vascular levels of cAMP.

Several conditions under which ANF might play a significant pathophysiologic role have been identified. Plasma ANF levels are elevated in patients with chronic renal failure and in patients with congestive heart failure. The plasma concentrations of ANF appear to be directly related to the severity of the disease. Because of its potent diuretic effects, ANF may be a potentially useful therapeutic agent as well.

SUBSTANCE P

Substance P is widely distributed in sensory nerve endings localized to the adventitia of large and small blood vessels. It is a potent vasodilator, although in high doses the peptide has been shown to cause constriction of some vessels. The relaxation elicited by substance P is endothelium dependent, which raises the possibility that endothelial cells may contribute to the vasodilatation that accompanies axon reflexes.

VASOACTIVE INTESTINAL POLYPEPTIDE

Vasoactive intestinal polypeptide (VIP) is present in postganglionic cholinergic neurons innervating many tissues. It also is a potent vasodilator and may be the mediator of the atropine-resistant vasodilatation observed during parasympathetic-nerve stimulation. In some blood vessels, relaxations induced by VIP may be endothelium dependent.

CALCITONIN GENE-RELATED PEPTIDE

Calcitonin gene-related peptide (CGRP) is localized in sensory neurons, often together with substance P, and has strong vasodilator properties. It is present in perivascular nerves of the brain and several peripheral organs. Depending on the vascular bed, CGRP exerts its relaxing effect either through direct action on the vascular smooth muscle or through an endothelium-dependent mechanism. Additionally, CGRP may inhibit neurogenic vasoconstriction via a prejunctional effect on adrenergic neurons. The relaxant effects of CGRP appear to be closely linked to K^+-channel activation and to increased production of cAMP within vascular smooth muscle cells.

Bibliography

THE EFFECTOR SYSTEMS

Vascular Smooth Muscle

Bolton TB. Mechanisms of action of transmitter and other substances on smooth muscle. Physiol Rev 1979; 59:606–718.

Cook NS. The pharmacology of potassium channels and their therapeutic potential. Trends Pharmacol Sci 1988; 9:21–28.

Godfraind T, Miller R, Wibo M. Calcium antagonism and calcium entry blockade. Pharmacol Rev 1986; 38:321–415.

Ignarro, LJ. Heme-dependent activation of soluble guanylate cyclase by nitric oxide: Regulation of enzyme activity by porphorins and metalloporphyrins. Semin Hematol 1989; 26:63–76.

Kukovetz WR, Poch G, Holzman S. Cyclic nucleotides and relaxation of vascular smooth muscle. In PM Vanhoutte and I Leusen, eds. Vasodilatation. New York: Raven, 1981.

Murad F. Cyclic guanosine monophosphate as a mediator of vasodilatation. J Clin Invest 1986; 78:1–5.

Quast U. Do the K+ channel openers relax smooth muscle by opening K+ channels? Trends Pharmacol Sci 1993; 14:332–337.

Rasmussen H, Barrett PQ. Calcium messenger system: an integrated view. Physiol Rev 1984; 64:938–984.

Rimele TJ, Vanhoutte PM. Differential effects of calcium entry blockers on vascular smooth muscle. Int Angiol 1984; 3:17–23.

Shepherd JT, Vanhoutte PM. The Human Cardiovascular System: Facts and Concepts. New York: Raven, 1979.

Somlyo AP. Excitation-contraction coupling and the ultrastructure of smooth muscle. Circ Res 1985; 57:497–507.

Standen NB, et al. Hyperpolarizing vasodilators activate ATP-sensitive K+-channels in arterial smooth muscle. Science 1989; 245:177–180.

Van Breeman C, et al. Calcium activation of vascular smooth muscle. Hypertension 1986; 8 [Suppl II]:95.

Weston AH, Hamilton TC. Potassium Channel Modulators. Oxford, UK.: Blackwell, 1992. Pp 1–501.

Williamson JR. Role of inositol lipid breakdown in the generation of intracellular signals. Hypertension 1986; 8 [Suppl II]: 140–156.

Adrenergic-Nerve Endings

Axelrod J. Noradrenaline: fate and control of its biosynthesis. Science 1971; 173:598–606.

Bevan JA, Bevan RD, Duckles SP. Adrenergic regulation of vascular smooth muscle. In DF Bohr, AP Somlyo, HV Sparts, Jr., eds. Handbook of Physiology, The Cardiology System, vol. 2. Bethesda, Md.: American Physiology Society, 1980. Pp. 515–566.

Katusic ZS, Shepherd JT, Vanhoutte PM. Endothelium-dependent contractions to calcium ionophore A23187, arachidonic acid and acetylcholine in canine basilar arteries. Stroke 1988; 19:476–479.

Shepherd JT, Vanhoutte PM. The circulation in the limbs: normal function and effects of disease. In W Parmley, K Chatterjee, eds. Handbook of Cardiology. Philadelphia: Lippincott, 1987.

Trendelenberg U. The metabolizing systems involved in the inactivation of catecholamines. Naunyn-Schmiedeberg: Arch Pharmacol 1986; 332:201–207.

Vanhoutte PM. Introductory remarks: alpha- and beta-adrenergic receptors and the cardiovascular system. J Cardiovasc Pharmacol 1981; 3:S1–S13.

Vanhoutte PM, Verbeuren TJ, Webb RC. Local modulation of the adrenergic neuroeffector interaction in the blood vessel wall. Physiol Rev 1981; 61:151–247.

Endothelium

Furchgott RF. Role of endothelium in response of vascular smooth muscle. Circ Res 1983; 53:557–573.

Furchgott RF, Zawadzki JV. The obligatory role of endothelial cells in the relaxation of arterial smooth muscle by acetylcholine. Nature 1980; 288:373–376.

Furchgott RF, Vanhoutte PM. Endothelium-derived relaxing and contracting factors. FASEB J 1989; 3:2007–2017.

Griffith TM, et al. Endothelium-derived relaxing factor. J Amer Coll Cardiol 1988; 12:797–806.

Ignarro LJ. Biological actions and properties of endothelium-derived nitric oxide formed and released from artery and vein. Circ Res 1989; 65(1):1–21.

Lüscher TF, Vanhoutte PM. The Endothelium: Modulator of Cardiovascular Function. Boca Raton, Fl.: CRC Press, 1990. Pp. 1–228.

Masaki T, et al. Role of endothelin in mechanisms of local blood pressure control. J Hypertension 1990; 8 [Suppl. 7]:S107–S112.

Moncada S, Palmer RMJ, Higgs EA. Nitric oxide: physiology, pathophysiology, and pharmacology. Pharmacol Rev 1991; 43:109–142.

Moncada S. Biological importance of prostacyclin. Br J Pharmacol 1982; 76:3–31.

Nagao T, Vanhoutte PM. Endothelium-derived hyperpolarizing factor and endothelium-dependent relaxations. Am J Respir Cell Mol Biol 1993; 8:1–6.

Pearson PJ, Vanhoutte PM. Vasodilator and vasoconstrictor substances produced by the endothelium. Rev Physiol Biochem Pharmacol 1993; 122:1–67.

Schini VB, Vanhoutte PM. Endothelin-1: A potent vasoactive peptide. Pharmacol Toxicol 1991; 69:1–7.

Simonson MS, Dunn MJ. Endothelin: pathways of transmembrane signaling. Hypertension 1990; 15(2):S5–S12.

Vane JR, Anggard EE, Botting RM. Regulatory functions of the vascular endothelium. N Engl J Med 1990; 323(1):27–36.

Vanhoutte PM, et al. Modulation of vascular smooth muscle contraction by the endothelium. Ann Rev Physiol 1986; 48:307–320.

Yanagisawa M, et al. A novel potent vasoconstrictor peptide produced by vascular endothelial cells. Nature 1988; 332:411–415.

THE NEUROHUMORAL MEDIATORS

Catecholamines

Langer SZ. Presynaptic regulation of the release of catecholamines. Pharmacol Rev 1980; 32:337–362.

Ruffolo RR. The Alpha-1 Adrenergic Receptors. Clifton, N.J.: Humana, 1987.

Starke K. Alpha-adrenoceptor subclassification. Rev Physiol Biochem Pharmacol 1981; 88:199–236.

Vanhoutte PM, Lüscher TF. Peripheral mechanisms in cardiovascular regulation: transmitters, receptors and the endothelium. In RC Tarazi, A Zanchetti, eds. Handbook of Hypertension, vol. 8. Amsterdam: Elsevier Science Publishers B.V., 1986. Pp. 96–123.

Acetylcholine

Duckles SP. Vascular muscarinic receptors: pharmacological characterization in the bovine coronary artery. J Pharmacol Exp Ther 1988; 246:929–934.

Goyal RK. Muscarinic receptor subtypes: physiology and clinical implications. N Engl J Med 1989; 321:1022–1029.

Komori K, Suzuki H. Heterogeneous distribution of muscarinic receptors in the rabbit saphenous artery. Br J Pharmacol 1987; 92:657–664.

O'Rourke ST, Vanhoutte PM. Subtypes of muscarinic receptors on adrenergic nerves and vascular smooth muscle of the canine saphenous vein. J Pharmacol Exp Ther 1987; 241:64–67.

Vanhoutte PM. Endothelium and the control of vascular tissue. News Physiol Sci 1987; 2:18–22.

Vanhoutte PM, Levy MN. Prejunctional cholinergic modulation of adrenergic neurotransmission in the cardiovascular system. Am J Physiol 1990; 238:H275–H281.

Purines

Burnstock G. Local purinergic regulation of blood pressure. In PM Vanhoutte, ed. Vasodilatation: Vascular Smooth Muscle, Peptides, Autonomic Nerves, and Endothelium. New York: Raven, 1988. Pp. 1–14.

Vanhoutte PM, Houston DS. Platelets, endothelium and vasospasm. Circulation 1985; 72:728–734.

Serotonin

Cohen RA. Serotonin and the blood-vessel wall. J Hypertension 1986; 4 [Suppl. 5]:S116–S118.

Fozard JR. Neuronal 5-HT receptors in the periphery. Neuropharmacology 1984; 23:1473–1486.

Gaddum JH, Picarelli ZP. Two kinds of tryptamine receptors. Br J Pharmacol 1957; 12:323–328.

Houston DS, Vanhoutte PM. Serotonin and the vascular system: role in health and disease, and implications for therapy. Drugs 1986; 32:149–163.

Van Nueten JM, Janssens WJ, Vanhoutte PM. Serotonin and vascular smooth muscle. In PM Vanhoutte, ed. Serotonin and the Cardiovascular System. New York: Raven, 1985. Pp. 95–103.

Vanhoutte PM. Peripheral serotonergic receptors and hypertension. In PM Vanhoutte, ed. Serotonin and the Cardiovascular System. New York: Raven, 1985. Pp. 123–133.

Vanhoutte PM. Serotonin and vascular wall. Int J Cardiol 1987; 14:189–203.

Histamine

Leusen I, Van de Voorde J. Endothelium-dependent responses to histamine. In PM Vanhoutte, ed. Vasodilatation: Vascular Smooth Muscle, Peptides, Autonomic Nerves, and Endothelium. New York: Raven, 1988. Pp. 469–474.

McGrath MA, Shepherd JT. Histamine and 5-hydroxytryptamine-inhibition of transmitter release mediated by H_2- and 5-hydroxytryptamine receptors. Federation Proc 1978; 37:195–198.

Toda N. Heterogeneous responses to histamine in blood vessels. In PM Vanhoutte, ed. Vasodilatation: Vascular Smooth Muscle, Peptides, Autonomic Nerves, and Endothelium. New York: Raven, 1988. Pp. 531–535.

Peptides

Marshall I, Craig RK. The cardiovascular effects and mechanism of action of the calcitonin gene-related peptides. In PM Vanhoutte, ed. Vasodilatation: Vascular Smooth Muscle, Peptides, Autonomic Nerves, and Endothelium. New York: Raven, 1988. Pp. 81–87.

Needleman P, Greenwald JE. Atriopeptin: A cardiac hormone intimately involved in fluid, electrolyte and blood-pressure homeostasis. N Engl J Med 1986; 314:828–834.

Ohlstein EH, Berkowitz BA. Atrial natriutetic factor and production of cyclic GMP. In PM Vanhoutte, ed. Vasodilatation: Vascular Smooth Muscle, Peptides, Autonomic Nerves, and Endothelium. New York, Raven, 1988; Pp. 113–117.

Regoli D, Barabai J. Pharmacology of bradykinin and related kinins. Pharmacol Rev 1980; 32:1–46.

Vanhoutte PM. Interactions between nerves, smooth muscle and endothelium in vascular responses. In A Nobin, C Owman, B Arneklo-Nobin, eds. Neuronal Messengers in Vascular Function. Amsterdam: Elsevier, 1987. Pp. 295–304.

Vanhoutte PM, Katusic ZS. Endothelium-dependent responses in cerebral blood vessels. In C Owman, JE Hardebo, ed. Neural Regulation of Brain Circulation. Amsterdam: Elsevier, 1986. Pp. 19–25.

Vanhoutte PM, Verbeuren TJ, Webb RC. Local modulation of adrenergic neuroeffector interaction in the blood vessel wall. Physiol Rev 1981; 62:151–247.

Rheology, Transport, and Thrombosis in the Circulation

Vincent T. Turitto
Harry L. Goldsmith

Transport in the Circulation

The process of thrombosis involves the interaction in the flowing blood of the corpuscles and surrounding plasma with the surface of a vessel, either vascular or prosthetic. To describe this interaction, we must deal with the transport of solutes and suspended corpuscles from one site to another in the circulation. Transport occurs predominantly through convection in bulk flow and, to a lesser extent, at the local level, by diffusion due to Brownian motion. The aim of this chapter is to give a physical description of the two transport processes and to relate them to the rheology of the blood on the one hand and to blood-vessel interactions on the other.

From a rheological point of view, the bulk flow is that of a concentrated suspension of deformable erythrocytes in an aqueous solution of salts and proteins undergoing pulsatile motion through a continuously branching network of vessels from over 30 mm down to 0.005 mm diameter. The mechanics of the flow and the flow regimes in the major arteries and veins [1,2], in which mean velocities are greater than 100 mm/s, differ markedly from those in small vessels (mean velocities < 50 mm/s) [3] and in the microcirculation (velocities ~ 0.5 mm/s) [4]. Considering the enormous numbers of cells in the flow, a quantitative, complete description of the mechanics of transport is a formidable task. That problem can be circumvented by ignoring the particulate nature of blood and regarding it as a homogeneous liquid. Such an approximation is valid if, as in the domain of macrorheology, the scale of the observation is larger than that of the cells. In our discussion of thrombosis, however, we are not concerned with an overall description of the fluid mechanics of blood in either the arterial or the venous circulation. Rather, we seek the role of flow in events that occur locally on a scale of the same dimension as that of the corpuscles. For example, we may wish to study the effect of local flow patterns on the interactions between the corpuscles and the vessel wall in the presence of coagulation factors that lead to the formation of aggregates and their adherence to the vessel wall. To understand such events, we must know the flow behavior of the individual corpuscles and surrounding plasma in bulk flow as well as in the immediate vicinity of the vessel wall. To study motions at the cellular level is to approach the problem in the domain of microrheology [5–8], the aim of which is to predict the macroscopic flow properties of the suspension from a detailed description of its constituents.

Before dealing with the flow properties of blood cells, we consider some basic aspects of flow and transport in a vessel and how they apply in the circulation. For more comprehensive discussions of blood macro- and microrheology, the reader is referred to several reviews of the subject [4,9–11].

FLOW THROUGH A CIRCULAR TUBE

We begin with the simple case of Poiseuille flow, the steady laminar flow of a viscous liquid through a rigid circular tube of radius R, since it provides the basis for describing the flow behavior of suspended particles and blood cells in real vessels.

As illustrated in Fig. 5-1 [12], Poiseuille flow can be likened to telescoping cylinders sliding over each other. The elements of the liquid at the wall are at rest since there is no slip of fluid at the interface. As one proceeds from the wall to the axis along the radial coordinate r, adjacent layers, or laminae, slide over each other at progressively increasing linear velocities u, a function of r, given by

$$u(r) = \frac{\Delta P}{4\eta L}(R^2 - r^2), \tag{1}$$

where ΔP is the pressure difference between two points separated by the distance L (pressure gradient), and η is the viscosity of the liquid. Equation 1 is that of a parabola, as shown by the dashed line in Fig. 5-1. By normalizing the local velocity, $u(r)$, with the maximum velocity at the tube center, $u_{max} = u(0) = \Delta PR^2/4\eta L$, the following simplified expression for the velocity distribution is obtained:

$$\frac{u(r)}{u(0)} = 1 - \left(\frac{r}{R}\right)^2. \tag{2}$$

The integration of Equation 1 over the entire cross section of the tube gives the following pressure-flow relation, known as the Hagen-Poiseuille law:

$$Q = \frac{\pi R^4 \Delta P}{8\eta L}, \tag{3}$$

where Q is the volume flow rate through the tube.

While the linear fluid velocity, $u(r)$, decreases parabolically with increasing r, the gradient in velocity, or **shear rate**, $\gamma(r)$, increases linearly with increasing r, being zero at the tube center and a maximum at the tube wall:

$$\gamma(r) = -\frac{du}{dr} = \frac{\Delta P}{4\eta L}r = \frac{4Q}{\pi R^4}r. \tag{4}$$

Because of the gradient in velocity, work must be done to overcome the friction between adjacent layers of fluid sliding over each other. A measure of this work is given by the fluid **shear stress**, $\tau(r)$, defined as the tangential force per unit area exerted in the direction of flow on a layer of fluid at a radial distance r by fluid at a radial distance $r + dr$. In the case of a liquid obeying Newton's

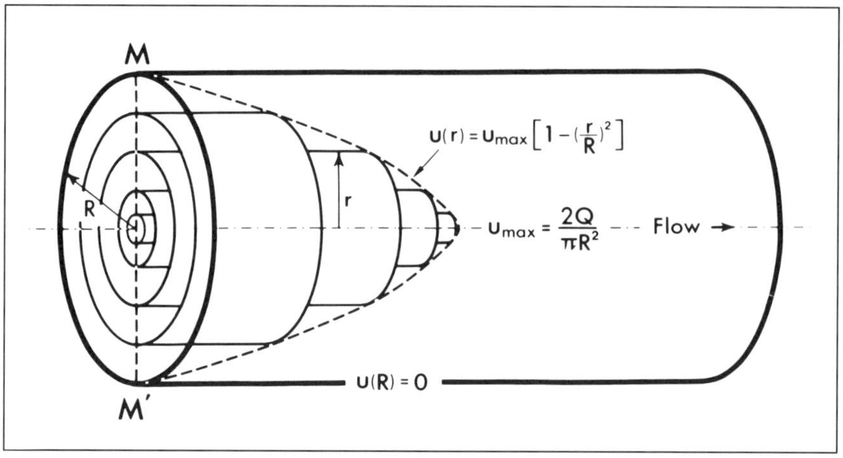

Fig. 5-1. Poiseuille, or laminar, viscous flow of a Newtonian liquid through a rigid circular tube. The motion of the liquid is pictured as the telescopic sliding of cylinders over each other. The layer at the wall is at rest—$u(R) = 0$—and the velocity $u(r)$ in the axial direction increases parabolically with increasing radial distance, r, reaching a maximum at the tube axis. (Reproduced with permission from HL Goldsmith. The flow of model particles and blood cells and its relation to thrombosis. In TH Spaet, ed. Progress in Hemostasis and Thrombosis, vol. 1. New York: Grune & Stratton, 1972. Pp. 97–139.)

second law, the shear stress is directly proportional to the shear rate, the constant of proportionality being the viscosity, η, or coefficient of internal friction:

$$\tau(r) = \eta\gamma(r). \tag{5}$$

Thus, the viscosity is the force per unit area required to maintain unit gradient in velocity.

REYNOLDS NUMBER

In the larger vessels of the circulation, where the velocities during the cardiac cycle are high, work is also required to accelerate and decelerate the fluid, so-called inertial work. The relative importance of liquid friction and liquid inertia in a vessel is given by a dimensionless ratio known as the Reynolds number (Re). In tube flow, the magnitude of the inertial force is proportional to the kinetic energy per unit volume, $m\bar{U}^2/\text{volume} = \rho\bar{U}^2$, where $\bar{U}$ is the mean velocity ($= Q/\pi R^2$) and ρ the liquid density. The magnitude of the viscous force is proportional to the shear stress, $\eta\gamma$, where γ is a representative shear rate in the tube equal to $\bar{U}/2R$. Hence, the tube Reynolds number, Re_t, is

$$\text{Re}_t = \frac{\rho\bar{U}^2}{\eta\bar{U}/2R} = \frac{2R\bar{U}\rho}{\eta}. \tag{6}$$

Using Eq. 1 through Eq. 6, valid for Poiseuille flow, representative values of Reynolds number, wall shear rate, γ_w, and shear stress, τ_w, in various parts of the vascular system can be calculated from the known vessel diameters and volume-flow rates. These values are given in Table 5-1 on page 147, where it can be seen that, in the human circulation, mean linear velocities over one cycle decrease from over 800 to less than 1 mm/s and the mean Re_t from over 6,000 to less than 10^{-3}, in going from the heart to the microcirculation [1,2,13–16], where viscous effects dominate the flow. The corresponding mean wall shear rate, and hence the shear stress, increases in going to the small vessels, reaching a maximum in the arterioles. It is evident, however, that wall shear rates at peak systole in some large arteries can be as large as those in small vessels.

FLOW IN THE CIRCULATION

Poiseuille flow represents a simplified picture of blood flow in vessels and does not strictly apply to the real circulation for various reasons, some of which relate to the occurrence and localization of thrombosis.

Entrance Effects. In large vessels, where Reynolds numbers are high, there is a region between the entrance and a point downstream, called the **entrance length,** where the velocity profile is in the process of being established. Figure 5-2 shows the entrance length for a fluid entering a tube with a uniform velocity. The layer of liquid in contact with the wall becomes stationary (no-slip condition), and laminae inside this layer slide against it, subject to internal friction, and form a **boundary layer,** in which the velocities are reduced from those at the entrance. The boundary layer grows thicker until it occupies the whole tube, and a steady, viscous flow is established. In steady flow, the entrance length, L_e, is given by $L_e = 0.07R\,(\text{Re}_t)$ [17]. This means that in the human aorta, with R approximately 13 mm and a mean Re_t over 3,000, the entrance length is more than 0.26 m, that is, it greatly exceeds the length available before branching occurs. It should also be noted that the velocity gradient near the wall in the entrance region is greater than that farther downstream. Thus, the vessel wall and the blood cells in the entrance region near the wall are subject to shear stresses higher than those in fully developed Poiseuille flow.

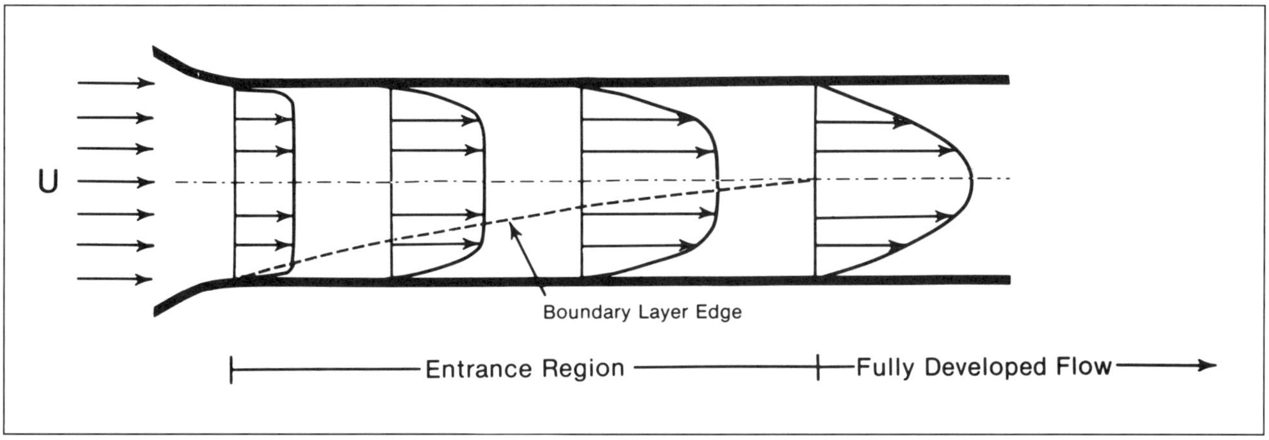

Fig. 5-2. The entrance length (L_e) required to establish a fully developed Poiseuille flow when a liquid enters a circular tube from a large reservoir. Note that the slope of the velocity with radial distance near the wall, the wall shear rate, γ_w, is very steep near the tube entry and decreases as the Poiseuille velocity distribution becomes established. (Reproduced with permission from HL Goldsmith and VT Turitto. Rheological aspects of thrombosis and haemostasis: basic principles and applications. Thromb Haemost 1986; 55:415.)

Pulsatile Flow. Flow is not steady but pulsatile down to the level of the arterioles and even in capillaries, where residual pulsations have been recorded. Within a given vessel, not all parts of the blood move in phase with each other. Near the wall, where the shear rate, now dependent on both radial distance and time, is high and wall-friction forces predominate, the liquid elements are almost in phase with the pulsatile pressure gradient. In the center of the stream, however, the kinetic energy is high, and inertia of the liquid results in its lagging increasingly behind the pressure gradient. The resulting velocity profiles are significantly blunted in the vessel center over much of the cycle. Flow reversal at the wall occurs before that in the vessel center, and the mean wall shear rates over the whole cycle are greater than those in Poiseuille flow [2].

Disturbed Flows: Effect of Vessel Geometry. Of considerable importance in the occurrence and localization of thrombosis are the flow patterns encountered at stenoses, branches, and curved segments of the vessels, where blood is subjected to sudden changes in direction and velocity. Here, we use the term **disturbed flow** to distinguish the regime from that in laminar or turbulent flow [18]. Laminar flow, as exemplified by Poiseuille flow (see Fig. 5-1), is characterized by the steady motion of the fluid in layers or streamlines parallel to a wall. Turbulent flow occurs at much higher flow rates beyond a certain critical value of the Reynolds number (Eq. 6), when fluid elements begin to exhibit irregular or random motions with respect to time and space. Disturbed flow, which is not observed in uniform-diameter straight tubes, is seen in branching and nonuniform-diameter vessels in the circulation. In those vessels, there are secondary fluid motions in directions away from that of the primary flow, and often the streamlines separate from the vessel wall, forming a vortex or a recirculation zone between the forward-flowing mainstream and the wall.

The way in which such disturbed flows are generated can be illustrated by the case of a sudden change in velocity, using the concept of the boundary layer. In fluid mechanics, an ideal fluid is defined as one that has no internal tangential stress, that is, no internal friction or viscosity ($\eta = 0$). As a consequence, the fluid is able to flow past a solid surface and maintain a slip velocity at the very interface. A real fluid has internal friction to a greater or lesser degree (as in plasma), and a true slip velocity is impossible. If the fluid has a low viscosity and is subjected to flow at a high velocity (i.e., the Reynolds number Re_t is large), the flow of a real fluid past a solid body can be pictured as being composed of two zones. The first zone is confined to a thin layer near the solid boundary, where, under the influence of viscosity, frictional forces retard the fluid motion. The velocity increases from zero at the interface to the full value in the mainstream. The mainstream is the second zone and is regarded as an ideal frictionless fluid, in which there is no velocity gradient. The first zone is known as the boundary layer, and its thickness can be calculated as inversely proportional to the square root of a Reynolds number, Re_y, defined by $Re_y = \bar{U}y\rho/\eta$, where y is a characteristic distance perpendicular to the edge of the solid body. This approach is strictly applicable to gases and liquids of low kinematic viscosity (defined as the dynamic viscosity divided by the fluid density) flowing past streamlined bodies (e.g., an airplane wing). The analysis should not be extended to liquids subjected to laminar flow in tubes at high Reynolds numbers. The concept of the boundary layer in explaining flow separation, however, is a useful one, as the following qualitative considerations show.

Consider the sudden tubular expansion shown in Fig. 5-3. A liquid flowing through the tube at a constant driv-

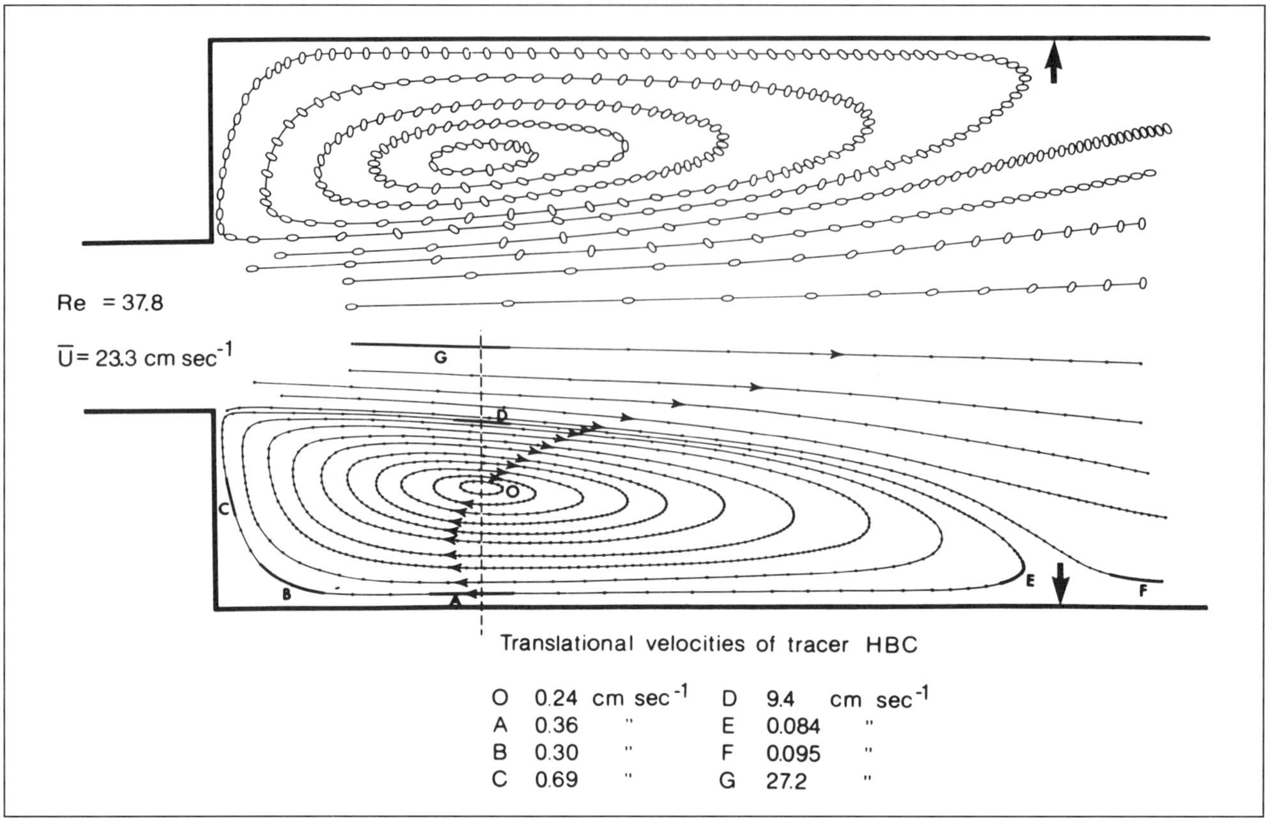

Fig. 5-3. Flow separation occurs as a suspension of hardened red blood cells (HBC) enters a sudden concentric expansion of vessel lumen from 150 to 500 μm, where it is rapidly decelerated, leading to a positive adverse gradient in pressure in the direction of flow. Suspension near the wall, unable to overcome the pressure gradient, is forced to a standstill and flows backward, finally leading to the formation of a vortex, the mainstream being pushed away from the wall, where it is separated from the beginning of the expansion until it reattaches at the point indicated by the large arrows. The region of flow separation is an annular vortex whose size depends on the inflow Reynolds number and the degree of expansion of the lumen. The streamlines and red cell orientations in the orbits of the annular vortex are shown in the lower and upper halves, respectively. The letters O and A to G indicate the positions at which the cell linear velocities listed were measured. (Reproduced with permission from T Karino and HL Goldsmith. Flow behaviour of blood cells and rigid spheres in an annular vortex. Phil Trans Roy Soc (London) 1977; B279:413.)

ing pressure in the axial direction is suddenly decelerated as it enters the expansion, due to the sudden increase in cross-sectional area. Assuming that the mainstream is an ideal fluid, we can apply Bernoulli's equation relating pressure, P, to linear velocity, u, of an ideal fluid:

$$\frac{P}{\rho} + gh + \frac{1}{2}u^2 = constant, \tag{7}$$

h being the height the liquid has traveled from a reference level. If the tube is horizontal (h is constant), differentiation of Eq. 7 with respect to flow distance x yields

$$\frac{1}{\rho}\frac{dP}{dx} + u\frac{du}{dx} = 0. \tag{8}$$

This equation shows that during deceleration on entry into the expansion, the gradient of flow has decreased ($du/dx < 0$), hence the pressure gradient, dP/dx, must increase to satisfy the equation, which is to say that there is a positive, adverse pressure gradient attempting to drive the fluid in the reverse direction. In the "frictionless layer" (mainstream), the kinetic energy of the fluid is sufficient to overcome this pressure gradient. However, the fluid within the boundary layer, which comes under the influence of the same pressure field, consumes its much smaller kinetic energy before having moved very far. It is eventually forced to a standstill and caused to flow backward by the external pressure. Fresh fluid arrives and experiences the same retardation, and the decelerated portion of the stream rapidly increases in volume, pushing the mainstream away from the boundary: flow separation has occurred [20]. The fluid in the reverse-flow regions coils, and a vortex is formed (see Fig. 5-3). It is evident from Eq. 8 that the decrease in u as well as the rate of deceleration, $-du/dx$, influences the size of the effect.

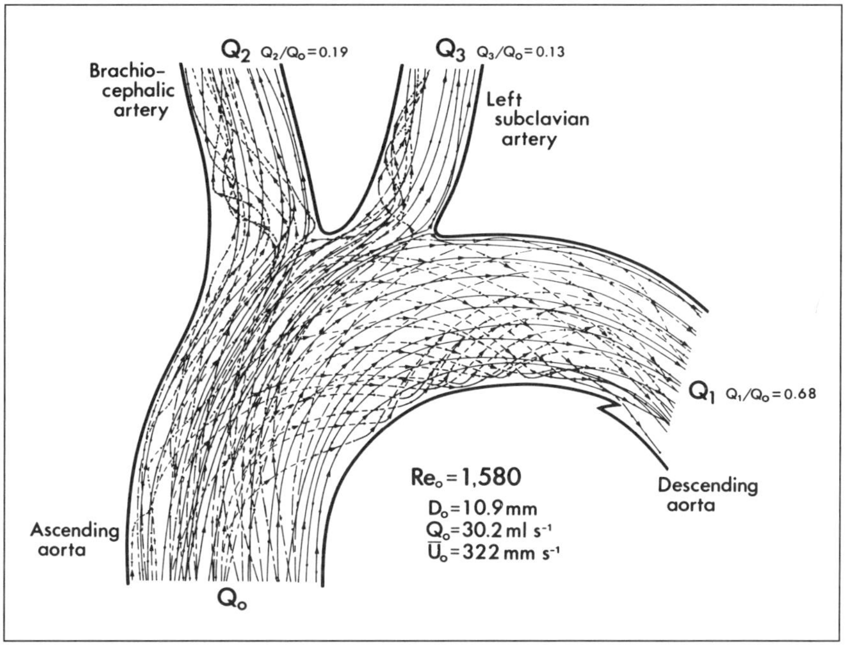

Fig. 5-4. Disturbed flow as a result of curvature in a vessel segment. Shown are the detailed flow patterns in dog aortic arch at an inflow Reynolds number Re_o = 1,500, obtained using an isolated transparent dog arterial tree, containing the whole heart, the aortic arch, and the descending aorta [21]. The figure shows the fluid streamlines traced from an analysis of cine films of the paths of 200–250 μm polystyrene spheres suspended in oil. It demonstrates the existence of three major flow components: a quasi-parallel undisturbed flow located close to the common median plane of the ascending aorta and two daughter branches (solid lines), a single clockwise spiral helicoidal secondary flow near the ventral periphery of the aorta and branches (dashed lines), and secondary flows generated at the flow dividers of the side branches (dashed lines). (Reproduced with permission from Y Sohara and T Karino. Secondary flows in the dog aortic arch. In M Harada, ed. Fluid Control and Measurement. New York: Pergamon, 1985. Pp. 143–147.)

When there is a change in the direction of flow, as at a bend or bifurcation (Fig. 5-4 and Fig. 5-5, respectively), a fluid experiences a transverse pressure gradient across the tube, forcing it to change direction. The elements of fluid with the highest kinetic energy continue to move to the outside of the bend, while fluid with low kinetic energy moves to the inside under the action of the pressure gradient. This gives rise to a secondary cross-flow. If the fluid enters the bend with a parabolic velocity distribution, the elements having high kinetic energy are situated in the tube center surrounded by elements with low kinetic energy at the periphery. In the bend, a secondary flow consisting of two semicircles is set up. In the case of a bend, as illustrated by dog aortic arch (see Fig. 5-4) [21,22], the mainstream fluid moves to the outside of the bend, and flow separation with a spiral secondary flow (but no recirculation zone) does occur at the inner (lower) wall of the arch. In the case of a bifurcation (see Fig. 5-5), low-velocity fluid at the top and the bottom of the parent tube moves across the upper and lower regions of the daughter tube to form a double-helical flow near the outside wall. The high velocity fluid in the center of the parent tube moves on without being appreciably diverted. Fluid coming from the side wall of the parent tube may separate at the corner of the bifurcation, and the streamlines from the top and bottom fill in the separated region. Figure 5-5 also shows that the velocity profile in the diametric plane of the daughter tube is skewed toward the flow divider. This is because relatively high velocity fluid at the center of the parent vessel is brought into close proximity to the wall of the flow divider.

The value of the Reynolds number in the parent tube at which secondary flow patterns and flow separation are first seen depends very much on the geometry of the bifurcation: the bifurcation angle θ, the area ratio defined as the sum of the cross-sectional area of the daughter branches to the cross-sectional area of the parent branch, and the radii of curvature of the outer walls (see Fig. 5-5).

In arterial bifurcations, θ varies from 30 degrees to 120 degrees, but the radii of curvature are large (i.e., the bends are gentle, as shown in Fig. 5-5). This, together with area ratios that are generally under 1.25 (i.e., there is not a marked decrease in blood velocity), minimizes the secondary flow. One notable exception to this rule exists in the circulation: the carotid bifurcation. There is a pronounced secondary flow and flow separation in the sinus of the internal carotid artery, due in large part to the sudden increase in vessel cross-sectional area. The flow patterns have been studied in a transparent arterial segment prepared from a human subject postmortem [14,23] as well

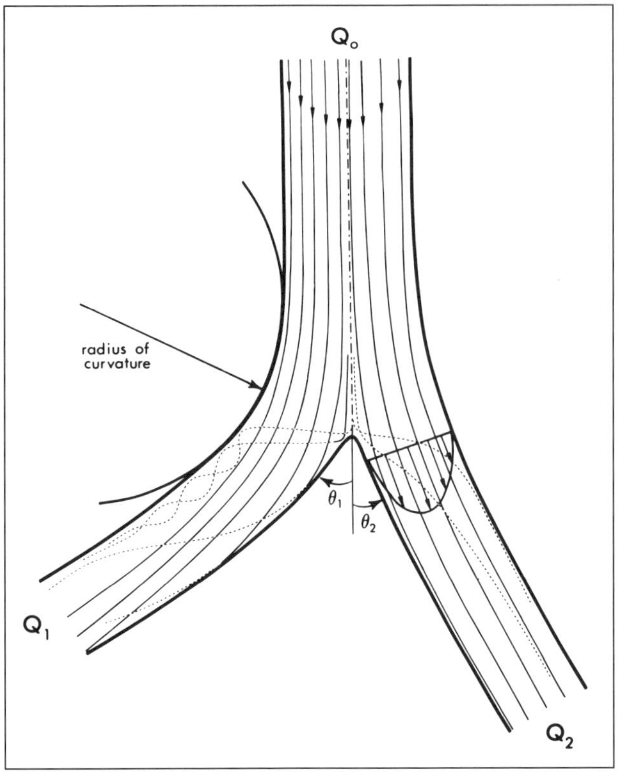

Fig. 5-5. Schematic representation of flow through a bifurcation showing the streamlines of the main flow in the median plane (solid lines), which move toward the inner wall of the daughter tubes, causing a secondary flow of low-velocity fluid (dashed lines). This fluid moves across the upper and lower regions of the entry into the daughter tube to form a double-helicoidal flow near the outside wall. The large radius of curvature of the outer walls of the bifurcation are typical of those found in the arterial circulation. The extent of secondary flow increases with increasing inflow Reynolds number, bifurcation angle, and the ratio of total cross-sectional area of daughter tubes to that of the parent tube. The velocity profile in the median plane of one of the daughter tubes also is shown. (Reproduced with permission from HL Goldsmith and VT Turitto. Rheological aspects of thrombosis and haemostasis: basic principles and applications. Thromb Haemost 1986; 55:415.)

as in casts of the bifurcation [24,25]. As shown in Fig. 5-6, a standing recirculation zone forms in the carotid sinus over a wide range of inflow Reynolds numbers and flow-rate ratio (internal: common carotid artery). The recirculation zone consists of a pair of complex spiral secondary flows, located symmetrically on both sides of the common median plane of the bifurcation. Particles are deflected at the flow divider and travel laterally and very slowly along the walls above and below the common median plane, almost at right angles to and encircling the mainstream. They then change direction, move back along the outer wall of the internal carotid artery at the site of the sinus, describing spiral orbits in the recirculation zone before rejoining the mainstream. Downstream from the reattachment point (R) in Fig. 5-6, a strong counterrotating double-helicoidal flow develops.

Similar considerations apply at T junctions such as those in the aorta. There, as illustrated in Fig. 5-7 [26] for a model glass T junction, two vortices or recirculation zones can exist: a main vortex just distal to the junction in the parent vessel, due to a sudden decrease in fluid velocity as a portion of the flow is drawn off into the side tube, and a corner vortex at the entry of the side tube due to fluid moving to the outside of the bend and vacating the inside corner, which is filled by a secondary flow. In aortic T junctions, however, as shown by work on transparent segments of dog descending aorta [27] (Fig. 5-8), the bend opposite the flow divider is gentle, so that there is no corner vortex, and the bend at the flow divider is sharp, thereby reducing the size of the main vortex.

NON-NEWTONIAN FLOW PROPERTIES OF BLOOD

Blood is not a Newtonian fluid; that is, the dynamic viscosity calculated from measurements of the shear stress at a known shear rate (Eq. 5), using a concentric cylinder or a cone-and-plate viscometer, is not a constant but decreases with increasing shear rate [9,28]. Similarly, the viscosity calculated from the pressure gradient and flow rate in a capillary tube using Eq. 3 is not a constant but decreases with increasing flow rate [29]. Hence, it is called an **apparent viscosity**.

The non-Newtonian flow properties of whole human and other mammalian blood are due to the presence of the red cells. These properties can be accounted for by the ability of red cells to (1) form linear and branched-chain aggregates (rouleaux), thought to be due to cross-linking of cell surfaces by fibrinogen [30] but more likely due to membrane adhesion because of polymer exclusion [31] and (2) deform under the influence of both fluid stresses in shear flow and cell crowding at normal hematocrit [3,4].

At shear rates under 50 s^{-1}, the decrease in apparent viscosity is due in part to the breakup of rouleaux (Fig. 5-9). At higher shear rates, it is due to the deformation of the cells and their increasing alignment in the direction of flow. When red cells are washed and suspended in physiologic saline, the non-Newtonian behavior at low shear rates is substantially reduced.

Effect on Velocity Distribution. As described next, in small vessels the high concentration of red cells at normal hematocrits leads to velocity distributions that are blunted from the parabolic. The degree of blunting decreases with increasing flow rate as the cells become increasingly deformed. As a result of blunting, the shear rate at the wall is greater than that in Poiseuille flow of homogeneous solutions at the same volume flow rate (see Fig. 5-13).

Aggregation and Thrombosis. As shown in Table 5-1, in the circulation, values of the wall shear rate, based on the mean linear flow rate over a cardiac cycle assuming Poiseuille flow, increase from about 300 s^{-1} in the largest arteries and reach a maximum greater than 10^3 s^{-1} in arterioles. The wall shear rate then decreases across the capillary bed, falling to between 500 and 800 s^{-1} in post-capillary venules (based on values obtained in cat mesentery) [16], and then gradually decreases to about 200 s^{-1}

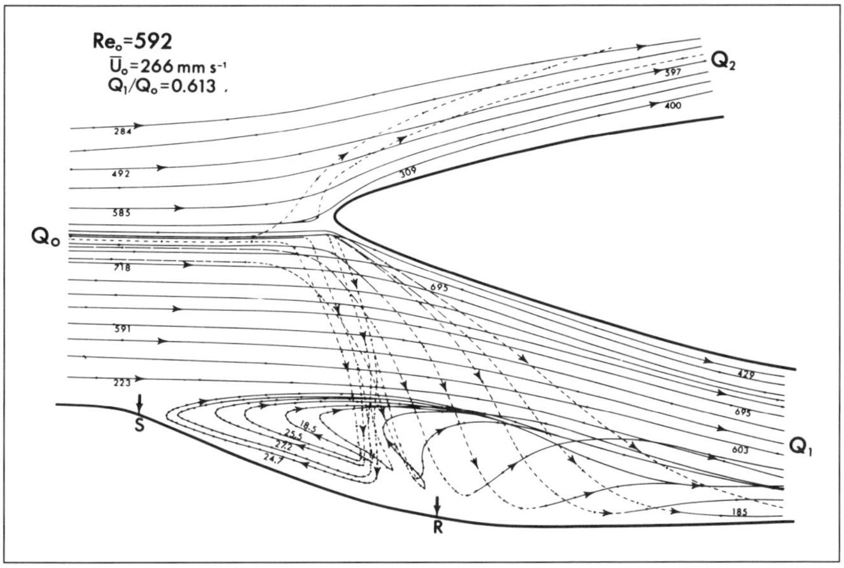

Fig. 5-6. Detailed flow patterns in the human carotid-artery bifurcation in steady flow at an inflow Reynolds number Re_o = 592 and flow-rate ratio (internal:common carotid) of 0.61. The streamlines were obtained from an analysis of cine films of the paths of 15-, 32- and 100-μm polystyrene spheres suspended in oil flowing through an isolated transparent arterial segment from a subject postmortem. The figure shows the formation of a recirculation zone (paired spiral secondary flows) and a counter-rotating double-helicoidal flow, both located symmetrically on either side of the common median plane in the internal carotid artery. The solid lines are the paths of particles in or close to the common median plane, and the dashed lines are paths that are far away from the common median plane (the projection of the particle paths on the common median plane). The arrows at S and R denote the separation and stagnation points, respectively. The numbers on the streamlines (particle paths) indicate the particle translational velocities in millimeters per second. (Reproduced from M Motomiya and T Karino. Flow patterns in the human carotid artery bifurcation. Stroke 1984; 15:50. Reproduced by permission of the American Heart Association, Inc.)

Table 5-1. Physiologic flow parameters in the human circulation

Vessel	Diameter mm	Linear velocity $\overline{U}$ mm/s Min.	Max.	Mean	Reynolds number $Re_t = \frac{\overline{U} \times 2R \times \text{density}}{\text{viscosity}}$ Mean	Wall shear rate[a] $\gamma_w = 8\overline{U}/2R$ s^{-1} Min.	Max.	Mean	Wall shear × stress[b] $\tau_w = \gamma(R) \times$ viscosity N/m^2 Min.	Max.	Mean
Ascending aorta[c]	23.0–43.5	—	—	245–876	3,210–6,075	—	—	45–305	—	—	0.16–1.07
Femoral artery[d]	5.0	−350	1175	188	283	−560	1885	302	1.96	6.59	1.06
Common carotid[d]	5.9	99	388	187	332	134	526	253	0.47	1.84	0.89
Carotid sinus[e]	5.2	85	325	156	244	130	500	240	0.46	1.69	0.84
External carotid[e]	3.8	83	327	157	180	175	687	331	0.61	2.41	1.16
Small arteries	0.3	—	—	50	2.3	—	—	1,335	—	—	4.67
Arterioles	0.025	—	—	5	3.8×10^{-2}	—	—	1,600[b]	—	—	5.60
Capillaries[f]	0.012	0.39–1.74		0.84	1.5×10^{-3} to 6.6×10^{-3}	260	1290	560	0.91	4.5	1.96[b]
Venules[g]	0.050	—	—	7–10		—	—				
Thoracic inferior Vena cava[c]	20.0	—	—	107–160	323–482	—	—	43–64	—	—	0.15–0.22

[a] Assuming Poiseuille flow.
[b] Assuming an asymptotic, high-shear-rate apparent viscosity for blood of 3.5 mPa/s.
[c] Mean systolic (aorta) and mean values (vena cava) from McDonald [2].
[d] Values obtained in vivo by Anliker et al. [13].
[e] Values calculated assuming 65% of flow into the internal carotid. Measured wall shear rates from ex vivo studies in steady flow at Re_t = 592 by Motomiya and Karino [14] show that at the outer wall of the sinus there is recirculating flow with $\gamma(R)$ varying from −135 to +530 s^{-1}. At the inner wall, $\gamma_w > 2000$ s^{-1}. At the inner wall of the external carotid, $\gamma_w > 1000$ s^{-1}.
[f] Values from Bollinger et al. [15] from red-cell velocities in human nailfold capillaries of large diameter. Calculations of wall shear rate would correspond to that in plasma flow. In bolus flow of a train of red cells, much higher wall shear rates and stresses would occur in the plasma layer surrounding the cells.
[g] Values from Lipowski et al. [16] from red-cell velocities in cat mesentery.

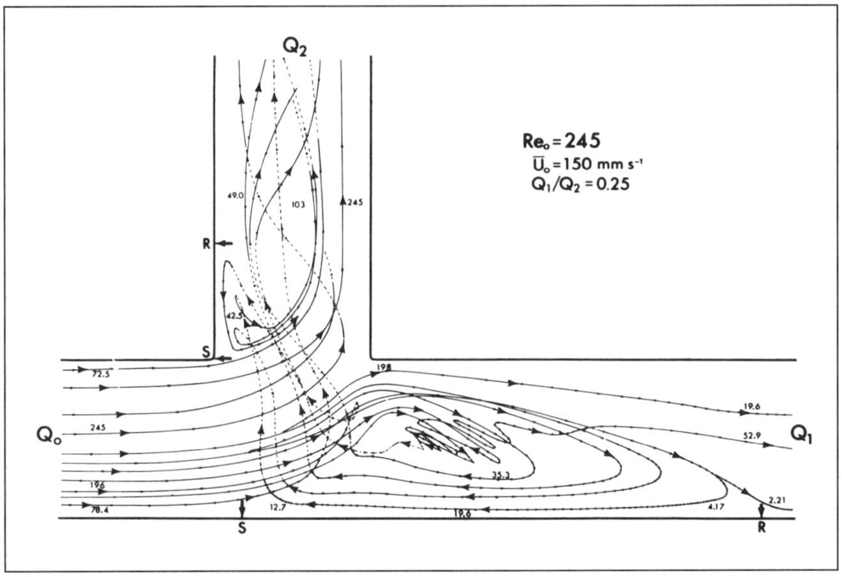

Fig. 5-7. Flow patterns in the common median plane of a model 3-mm-diameter glass T junction, as indicated by the paths of tracer 50-μm polystyrene spheres in aqueous glycerol. The suspension enters at the left with mean velocity $\overline{U}_0$ (tube Reynolds number = Re_0), and 80 percent of the flow leaves through the side tube. The T junction, made by fitting and gluing together two pieces of glass tubing, has a very low radius of curvature at the corner opposite the flow divider, as well as at the flow divider. This results in a small vortex in the corner at the entry of the side tube filled with fluid from the main large vortex in the parent vessel. The points are experimental, showing particle positions at intervals of 22 ms; the numbers indicate velocities in millimeters per second. The solid lines represent particles traveling in or close to the median plane; the dashed lines show those closer to the tube wall. The arrows at S and R indicate where flow first separates (S) and then reattaches (R) to the wall. (Reproduced with permission from T Karino, HM Kwong and HL Goldsmith. Particle flow behavior in models of branching vessels. I: Vortices in 90°-T junctions. Biorheology 1979; 16:231.)

in the largest veins [2]. The shear rate also varies across the vessel cross section, being zero at the tube center and a maximum at the wall in steady flow (see Figs. 5-12 and 5-13). Thus, when blood is subjected to a slow laminar flow through a straight circular vessel, red cells form aggregates near the tube axis and move as a solid core in a partial plug flow [12,32], resulting in a blunted velocity distribution in the diametrical plane [1]. Such a velocity profile also occurs in the venous circulation, though under normal circumstances it would not be expected to lead to any thrombotic disorders or detrimental effects on the circulation. There are situations, however, where local elevation of blood viscosity can result in a stoppage of flow, thrombosis, and ischemia. Such is the case in shock, when the sudden drop in blood pressure and hence in flow rate causes red cells to form aggregates. This results in an elevation of blood viscosity and a higher resistance to flow, possibly leading to stasis in small arteries and in the microcirculatory bed not only in the myocardium but also in other tissues. This makes reperfusion of the vessels and hence the recovery of the normal function of the heart and the circulatory system more difficult, since it requires a higher driving pressure to break up the formed aggregates and restore normal flow. Local variation in flow patterns may also favor the formation of red-cell aggregates in some areas of the circulation. This enhances the stagnation of the flow in regions of separated flow, such as downstream of severe stenoses and venous valves and at the entrances to branching vessels partially or totally occluded through the development of atherosclerotic plaques.

The importance of a shear rate–dependent blood viscosity is that it can exert much greater local effects on both the blood cells and the vessel wall (by elevating local fluid viscosity, enhancing stasis, and retarding mass transport in regions of low shear rate) than those expected with simple Newtonian fluids, such as saline and plasma, whose viscosities do not vary with shear rate.

CONVECTIVE AND DIFFUSIVE TRANSPORT

In convective transport within blood vessels, both solutes and cells are carried by the plasma at velocities essentially equal to those of the fluid (provided the ratio of cell to vessel diameter is much less than 1 [33]) given by a velocity distribution such as that in Poiseuille flow (Eq. 1). The mean velocities over one cycle in the human circulation range from about 300 mm/s in the major arteries down to 50 mm/s in small arteries and 0.5 mm/s in capillaries [1,2]. By contrast, diffusive transport, characterized by the translational Brownian diffusion coefficient,

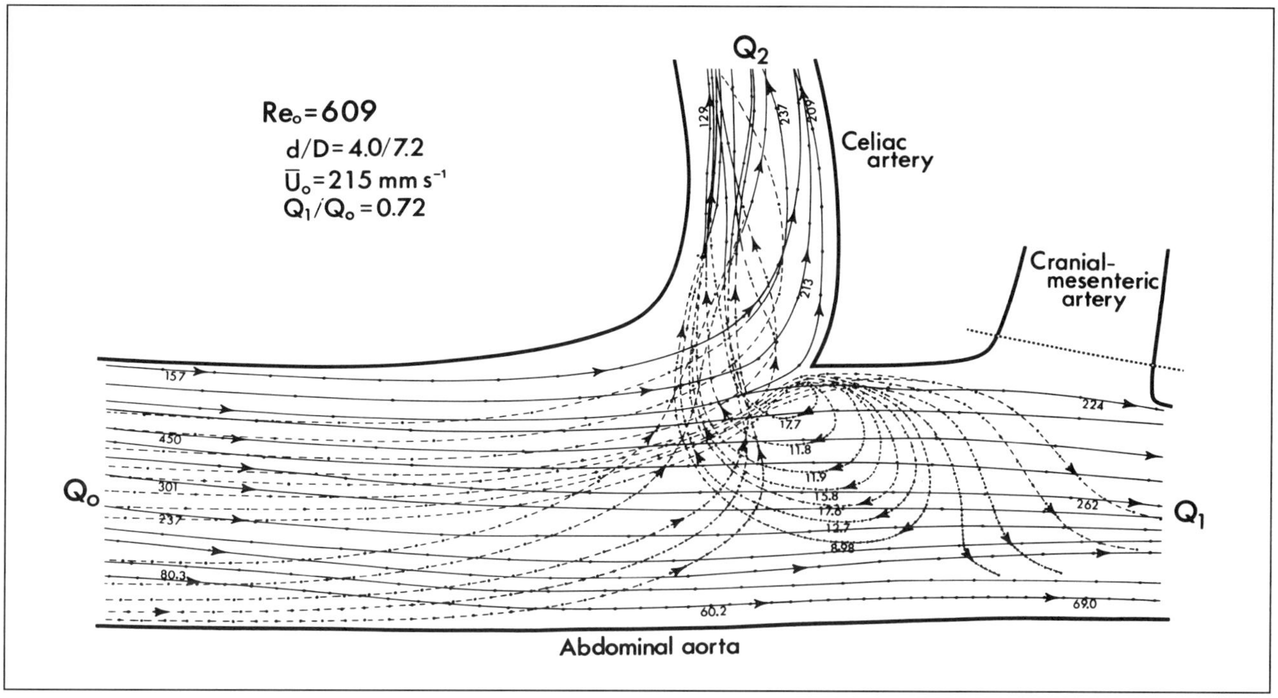

Fig. 5-8. Flow patterns at the aortoceliac artery junction of isolated transparent dog abdominal aorta, obtained from the analysis of cine films of the paths of polystyrene spheres, as in Fig. 5-4 and Fig. 5-6. Unlike the model T junction of Fig. 5-7, curvature of the wall opposite the flow divider is very high, and that at the flow divider is very low. This minimizes the flow disturbance and results in the formation of paired, thin-layered recirculation zones on both sides of the common median plane, adjacent to the vessel wall wrapped around the undisturbed mainstream. Numbers on the streamlines indicate polystyrene sphere velocities in millimeters per second. (Reproduced with permission from T Karino, M Motomiya, and HL Goldsmith. Flow patterns at the major T-junctions of the dog descending aorta. J Biomech 1990; 23:537.)

D_t, is relatively unimportant for the corpuscles and all but the smallest solute molecules in regions where convection is appreciable. The diffusion coefficient is given by the Stokes-Einstein equation [34]:

$$D_t = \frac{kT}{F}, \tag{9}$$

where k is the Boltzmann constant, T the absolute temperature, and F the friction coefficient related to the drag force opposing movement of the particle. For a sphere of radius b, $F = 6\pi\eta b$, η being the suspending-medium viscosity. Values of the diffusion coefficient for various solutes of increasing molecular weight and for the corpuscles are given in Table 5-2.

We are concerned with transport of the corpuscles to the vessel wall. Since most flow in the body is laminar (or streamline) in the absence of cell-cell interactions, solutes or suspended cells are expected to travel along paths parallel to the vessel walls and can approach the endothelium or underlying areas only through the random motion of Brownian translational diffusion. (In fact, in the absence of cell interactions, the corpuscles actually migrate *away* from the vessel wall in flow [12].) An estimate of the distance that the corpuscles can travel in a direction normal to flow in a tube in a time interval Δt is given by the mean square diffusion distance $\overline{\Delta x^2}$, where [34]

$$\overline{\Delta x^2} = 2D_t\,\Delta t. \tag{10}$$

Table 5-2 gives values of the root-mean-square diffusion distances over a time interval, Δt, of 1 s for some solute molecules in plasma and corpuscles. A measure of the relative magnitude of convective and diffusive transport is given by the particle Peclet number, Pe, defined as

$$\text{Pe} = \frac{u(r)b}{D_t}, \tag{11A}$$

which for radial distances $(R - r)$ close to the wall may be approximated by

$$\text{Pe} = \frac{\gamma_w(R - r)b}{D_t}, \tag{11B}$$

where γ_w and b are the wall shear rate and the particle radius, respectively.

At the vessel wall, both convective and diffusive transport are zero, the former because there is no slip at the interface, and the latter because the friction coefficient

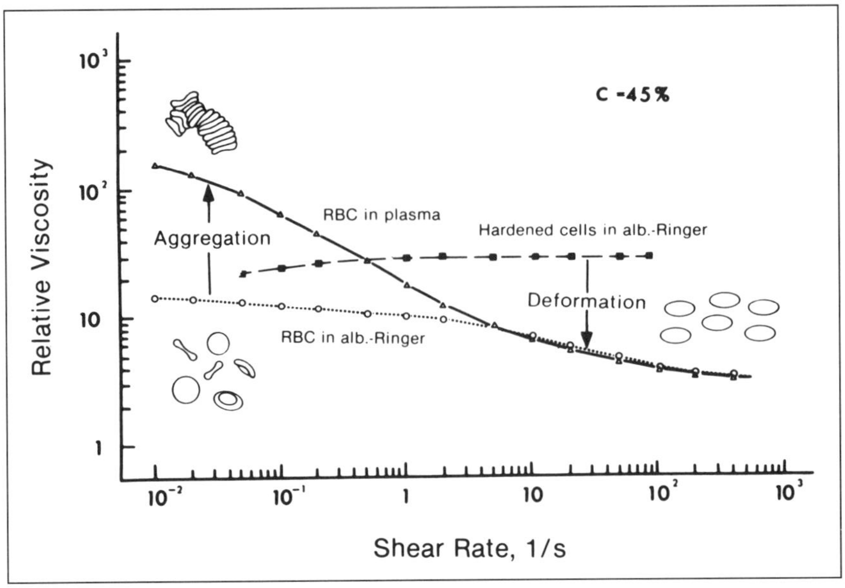

Fig. 5-9. Logarithmic plot of the relation between relative apparent viscosity (= apparent viscosity of suspension ÷ viscosity of suspending medium) and shear rate of suspensions of normal deformable and glutaraldehyde-fixed rigid human red cells at 45 percent hematocrit. Normal cells in plasma exhibit non-Newtonian behavior at low shear rates due to progressive breakup of rouleaux and at high shear rates due to cell deformation and alignment with the flow. Normal cells in albumin-Ringer's solution exhibit non-Newtonian behavior mainly at high shear rates, where they also deform and align with the flow. By contrast, suspensions of fixed cells exhibit almost Newtonian behavior, and their apparent viscosity at shear rates greater than 1 s^{-1} is markedly greater than that of suspensions of normal cells. Actually, there is a small increase in apparent viscosity with increasing shear rate (so-called dilatant flow) at high concentrations. (Reproduced with permission from S Chien. Biophysical behavior of red cells in suspensions. In D MacN Surgenor, ed. The Red Blood Cell, vol. 2. New York: Academic, 1975. Pp. 1026–1032.)

(Eq. 9) becomes infinitely large at $(R - r)$ close to one particle radius from the wall. Here, when surfaces are closer than 50 nm, van der Waals and electrostatic forces dominate the interactions between the blood elements and the endothelium. At distances of 100 nm or more, the convective and diffusive flux can be compared. This is shown in Table 5-2, which gives values of the Peclet number for solute molecules at $(R - r) = 100$ nm and for cells whose membranes approach to within 100 nm of the wall. Two cases are given: a large artery of 6-mm diameter,

Table 5-2. Diffusion as a function of molecular and particle size

Molecule or cell	Molecular weight	Molecular or particle radius b (nm)	D_t[a] 37°C ($m^2\ s^{-1}$)	$\sqrt{\overline{\Delta x^2}}$[b] ($\Delta t$ = 1 s) (μm)	$Pe = \frac{\gamma_w(R-r)b}{D_t}$[c] R = 0.3 mm	R = 6.0 mm
Water	18	0.15	1.26×10^{-9}	50.2	3.1×10^{-6}	1.6×10^{-5}
Oxygen	32		2.75×10^{-9}	74.2		
Sodium chloride	58.5	0.23	8.22×10^{-10}	40.5	8.4×10^{-6}	3.6×10^{-5}
Glucose	180	0.37	5.11×10^{-10}	32.0	2.2×10^{-5}	9.4×10^{-4}
Sucrose	342	0.48	3.94×10^{-10}	28.1	3.7×10^{-5}	1.6×10^{-4}
Serum albumin	67,000	3.6	5.25×10^{-11}	10.3	2.1×10^{-3}	8.9×10^{-3}
Fibrinogen	330,000	9.5	2.00×10^{-11}	6.3	1.4×10^{-2}	6.2×10^{-4}
Platelet	—	1,200	1.58×10^{-13}	0.56	3.0×10^{3}	1.3×10^{4}
Red cell	—	2,800	6.75×10^{-14}	0.37	3.6×10^{4}	1.6×10^{5}

[a] Calculated from Eq. 9 using molecular or particle radius, and plasma viscosity η = 1.2 mPa · S at 37°C.
[b] Root mean square distance moved in 1 second, calculated from Eq. 10.
[c] Peclet number calculated for a molecule at 100 nm from the vessel wall and blood cell whose membrane is 100 nm from the wall; the respective wall shear rates are 300 and 1,300 s^{-1} in the 6-mm and 0.3-mm vessels.

$\gamma_w = 300\ s^{-1}$, and a small artery of 0.3-mm diameter, $\gamma_w = 1{,}300\ s^{-1}$ (see Table 5-1). It is evident that, for the corpuscles, convection is much more important than diffusion in both vessels. By contrast, for both small and large solute molecules, diffusion is much more important than convection. Thus, for the corpuscles in dilute suspensions, wall interactions are not expected to be significant. This becomes more apparent in considering the observed inward radial migration of blood cells described in the next section, "Flow Properties of Blood Cells." However, two mechanisms facilitate cell-wall encounters in whole blood within the circulation [35]: (1) red cell–induced dispersion of blood elements, giving rise to cell-wall collisions (see "Erythrocyte-Induced Dispersion in Flowing Blood," later in this chapter) and (2) convective transport to the wall along curved streamlines, having pronounced radial velocity components such as are found in regions of disturbed flow (see Figs. 5-4 through 5-8). The effect of such flows on blood corpuscles is considered in "Disturbed Flow and Thrombogenesis," later in this chapter. It also should be noted that in disturbed flows there are stagnation points at the wall where blood cells in the vicinity have velocities of the order of 1 μm/s, resulting in Peclet numbers under 10, meaning that diffusive transport is important. Stagnation points occur at the flow divider in Y and T bifurcations, and where there is flow separation, it occurs at the separation and reattachment points of the flow.

Flow Properties of Blood Cells

Basic to all considerations of thrombus formation is the fact that a velocity gradient in the plasma carrying the corpuscles is necessary for aggregation of platelets, the primary constituents of a thrombus, to occur. The velocity gradient brings cells traveling at different velocities along adjacent streamlines in laminar flow into close proximity to each other, causing them to collide and, under certain conditions, to form aggregates. Even though activation of the cells must occur as the aggregating agent diffuses through the fluid, adding a chemical stimulus, such as adenosine diphosphate (ADP) or thrombin, to a stationary suspension of platelet-rich plasma produces only microaggregation [36,37]. For platelets to aggregate, the suspension must be stirred and, as users of the platelet aggregometer know, the angular velocity of the small stir bar in the cuvette affects the rate of aggregation [38,39]. Therefore, we first consider briefly the effects of flow on the suspended blood cells.

ROTATION, DEFORMATION, AND WALL MIGRATION OF BLOOD CELLS

When a particle is immersed in a liquid undergoing Poiseuille flow, it experiences stresses at its surface, there being no slip at the particle-fluid boundary. If the particle is rigid, the stresses cause it to rotate while it is carried by the flow along the tube. Thus, as shown in Fig. 5-10, a sphere located at a fixed radial distance, *r*, rotates with uniform angular velocity, given by half the value of the shear rate at that location. A disk rotates with periodically varying angular velocity, being at a maximum when oriented across the flow and at a minimum when aligned with the flow [33]. By contrast, if the particle is deformable, the external fluid stresses distort it. An emulsion droplet is deformed from a sphere into an ellipsoid, which is oriented at a constant angle to the direction of flow (see Fig. 5-10). The fluid stresses are transmitted across the droplet interface, and fluid at the surface and in the interior circulates about the particle center.

At hematocrits under 1 percent, single human red cells in plasma can be shown to behave as rigid disks, provided the shear stress is less than $10^{-2}\ N/m^2$ [40]. At higher shear stresses and in media more viscous than plasma (e.g., isotonic solutions of low-molecular-weight dextran or Ficoll), the cells exhibit fluid-droplike behavior, being oriented at a constant angle to the flow with the membrane circulating around the interior [40,41]. By contrast, platelets and white cells, having highly viscous interiors, remain undeformed in dilute suspensions and rotate as rigid disks and rigid spheres, respectively.

In dilute suspensions, radial migration of particles away from the wall in Poiseuille flow is a well-documented phenomenon [42]. Two mechanisms are responsible for such migration:

1. Lateral movement to the tube axis of deformable particles, which occurs at very low Reynolds numbers and in high-viscosity fluids but which also persists at much higher Re_t [33,43]. In the case of deformable liquid drops, this movement has been shown to be caused by an inwardly directed force arising from the interaction of the flow field with the tube wall around the deformed drop [42].
2. Two-way migration to an eccentric radial equilibrium position of rigid particles initially located either near the wall or near the axis—the so-called tubular pinch effect—at much higher Reynolds numbers [44]. The effect can be likened to the curve of a spinning tennis ball (Magnus effect), although it must be emphasized that nonrotating particles also migrate at these Reynolds numbers and that the presence of the tube wall is a cardinal feature of two-way migration. In the case of rigid spheres, the tubular pinch effect has been treated theoretically [45,46].

Both experiment and theory have shown that the rate of inward migration depends on the square of the mean flow rate and on the fourth power of the ratio of particle to tube diameter in the case of deformable drops and on the third power in the case of rigid spheres. The two mechanisms also apply in pulsatile flow [47]. Deformable normal red cells migrate rapidly away from the tube wall in Poiseuille flow; glutaraldehyde-fixed rigid cells migrate more slowly and exhibit the tubular pinch effect (Fig. 5-11) [48]. Inward lateral migration of the relatively rigid white cells [49] and the much smaller platelets in plasma [50,51] also has been observed, but the rate of migration is appreciably lower than that of normal red cells. Nevertheless, in the absence of particle interactions, one would not expect to find any platelets close to the vessel wall, where, at low Reynolds numbers in small vessels, the ratio of particle to vessel diameter is relatively large, and, at high Reynolds numbers in large vessels, the mean linear

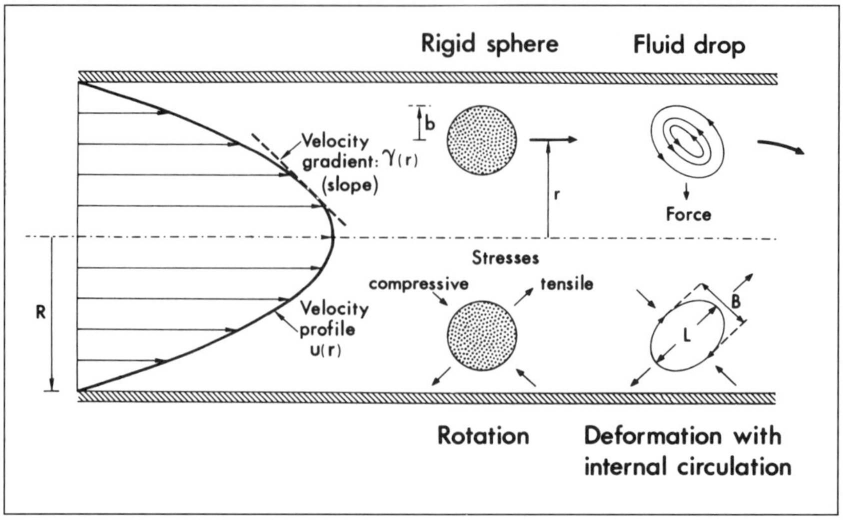

Fig. 5-10. The effect of fluid mechanical stresses on rigid and deformable spheres suspended in a liquid undergoing Poiseuille flow. The parabolic velocity profile and the linearly varying velocity gradient are shown in the median, MM′ plane (see Fig. 5-1) of the tube. The rigid sphere rotates with uniform angular velocity, whereas the liquid drop is distorted into an ellipsoid by the fluid stresses acting on its surface and aligns itself at a constant angle to the flow. The fluid in the liquid drop circulates around the interior. As a result of a net inwardly directed force acting on the deformed drop, the particle migrates to the tube axis. (Reproduced with permission from HL Goldsmith. The flow of model particles and blood cells and its relation to thrombosis. In TH Spaet, ed. Progress in Hemostasis and Thrombosis, vol. 1. New York: Grune & Stratton, 1972. Pp. 97–139.)

velocities are high. What alters the situation markedly in whole blood at normal hematocrits is the presence of very large numbers of red cells, so many that they continually interact with each other, greatly affecting the motions of the less numerous platelets and white cells.

AGGREGATION DUE TO CELL-CELL COLLISIONS

Two-Body Collision Model. The velocity gradient in shear flow determines the rate at which blood cells collide with each other. A simple model is provided by considering two-body collisions between equal-sized rigid spheres of radius b in a suspension containing n particles per milliliter undergoing Poiseuille flow, as shown in Fig. 5-12A. The collision frequency, f_s (number of collisions suffered by a given sphere per second), at radial distance r and shear rate $\gamma(r)$, are given by [52]

$$f_s = \frac{32}{3}\gamma(r)nb^3 \tag{12}$$

$$= \frac{8\gamma(r)c}{\pi}, \tag{13}$$

since the volume concentration $c = 4\pi b^3 n/3$. Thus, the total number of two-body collisions per second per milliliter of the suspension, $F_s = f_s n/2$, is greater at the tube periphery, where $\gamma(r)$ is larger, and is greatly affected by the size of the particle. In very dilute suspensions at the same number concentration and shear rate, the two-body collision frequency for red cells of equivalent sphere radius $b = 2.78$ μm (calculated from a mean cell volume of 90 μm^3) is more than 11 times greater than that of platelets whose equivalent sphere radius $b = 1.24$ μm (mean cell volume = 8 μm^3). Equations 12 and 13 may be applied to platelet-rich plasma, where it can be shown that, for $n = 3 \times 10^5$ cells/μl ($c = 0.3\%$) and at shear rates of 200 s^{-1}, typical of the mean values in arteries of about 2-mm diameter, $f_s = 1.5$ collisions/cell/s and $F_s = 2.2 \times 10^5$ two-body collisions/s/μl. However, the simple equations no longer apply to red cells at hematocrits over 10 percent, since there are now multibody collisions that result in larger, continuous radial fluctuations of cell paths than those shown in Fig. 5-12B [53].

Red Cells and Platelets. In the presence of interaction forces between cells, such collisions can lead to the formation of aggregates, as can readily be demonstrated with normal red cells in plasma flowing through a circular tube at mean shear rates less than 50 s^{-1}. Collisions between cells result in the formation of rouleaux in the presence of fibrinogen in plasma or in suspensions containing high-molecular-weight dextran [54,55]. Because of their deformation in the flow [40], these cells migrate to the axis, where they combine into larger stable aggregates in the low-shear region [12,32]. The kinetics of platelet aggregation in Poiseuille flow at mean tube shear rates from 40–2,000 s^{-1} (shear stresses from 0.07 to 3.5 N/m^2 in plasma at 23°C) has been studied by activation of platelets in citrated plasma with low (0.2 and 1 μM) concentrations of ADP. It was shown that the rate of aggregation increases with increasing flow rate, reaching a maximum at a mean tube shear rate of about 300 s^{-1} [56,57]. In the absence of

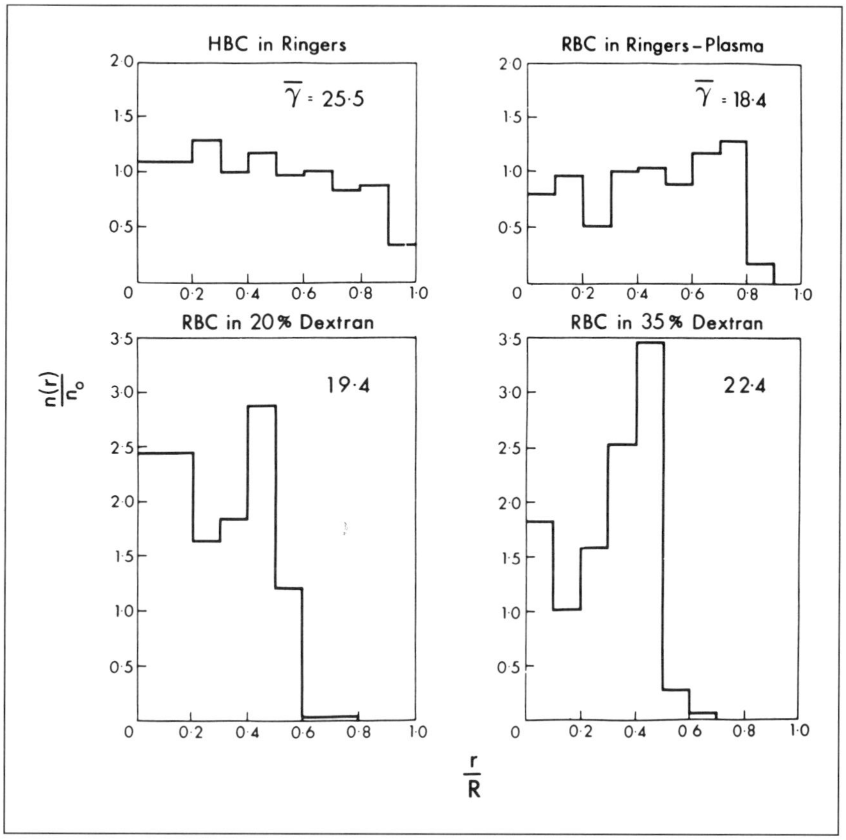

Fig. 5-11. Radial migration of normal deformable erythrocytes (RBC) and rigid glutaraldehyde-hardened erythrocytes (HBC) at low Reynolds numbers in an 83-μm-diameter tube measured 10 mm downstream from its entry from a reservoir. Shown are the concentration distributions of erythrocytes across the tube, plotted as the number of cells per milliliter of suspension, $n(r)$, at intervals of one-tenth the tube radius, divided by the number per milliliter in the reservoir, n_o, against the relative radial distance, r/R. If the distribution were uniform across the tube, $n(r)/n_o$ = 1 at all r/R. The figure shows that the deformable erythrocytes undergo appreciable inward migration, especially in the viscous dextran solutions, in contrast to the rigid erythrocytes, the distribution of which is fairly uniform across the tube. The values of the mean tube shear rate $\bar{\gamma} = 2\bar{U}/R$ are given in each panel. (Reproduced with permission from HL Goldsmith. Red cell motions and wall interactions in the tube flow. Fed Proc 1971; 30:1578.)

red cells and at 1 μM ADP, microaggregates first form near the tube wall. As they grow in size through collisions with other singlets and aggregates in flow along the tube, they migrate toward the axis because their rotation is physically impeded by the wall. Eventually they form a large, stable, but loosely bound aggregate at the tube center [56]. In the presence of red cells, one would predict that this is unlikely to occur because of the continuous collisions between the large numbers of red cells. The resulting lateral fluctuations of red cell paths (see Fig. 5-15), while increasing the frequency of platelet-platelet collisions, also disturb the motions of the platelet aggregates and might be expected to impede their growth. In fact, the contrary appears to be the case: when platelet aggregation in tube flow was studied in citrated whole blood, both the rate and the extent of aggregation were significantly higher than in platelet-rich plasma [58]. Increased aggregation is believed to be due in part to a physical effect of the red cells (increased collision rate, increased time spent by the platelets in close proximity while colliding) and in part to a chemical effect, in that some shear-induced release of ADP from red cells occurs [59]. In the circulation, therefore, red cells may enhance the growth of freely flowing platelet aggregates. Equally important, however, is the pronounced effect of the erythrocytes on both the distribution and the flow behavior of platelets near the vessel wall, considered in the section "Redistribution of Leukocytes and Platelets."

Effect of Shear on Platelet Activation and Aggregation. There have been extensive studies of shear-induced "spontaneous" platelet aggregation in the absence of added agonist, mostly using rotational viscometers. The range of shear stresses ($\tau = \eta\gamma$) covered in these studies encompasses the physiologic range (0–7 N/m^2) and beyond. In plasma, it appears that shear rates less than 2,000 s^{-1}

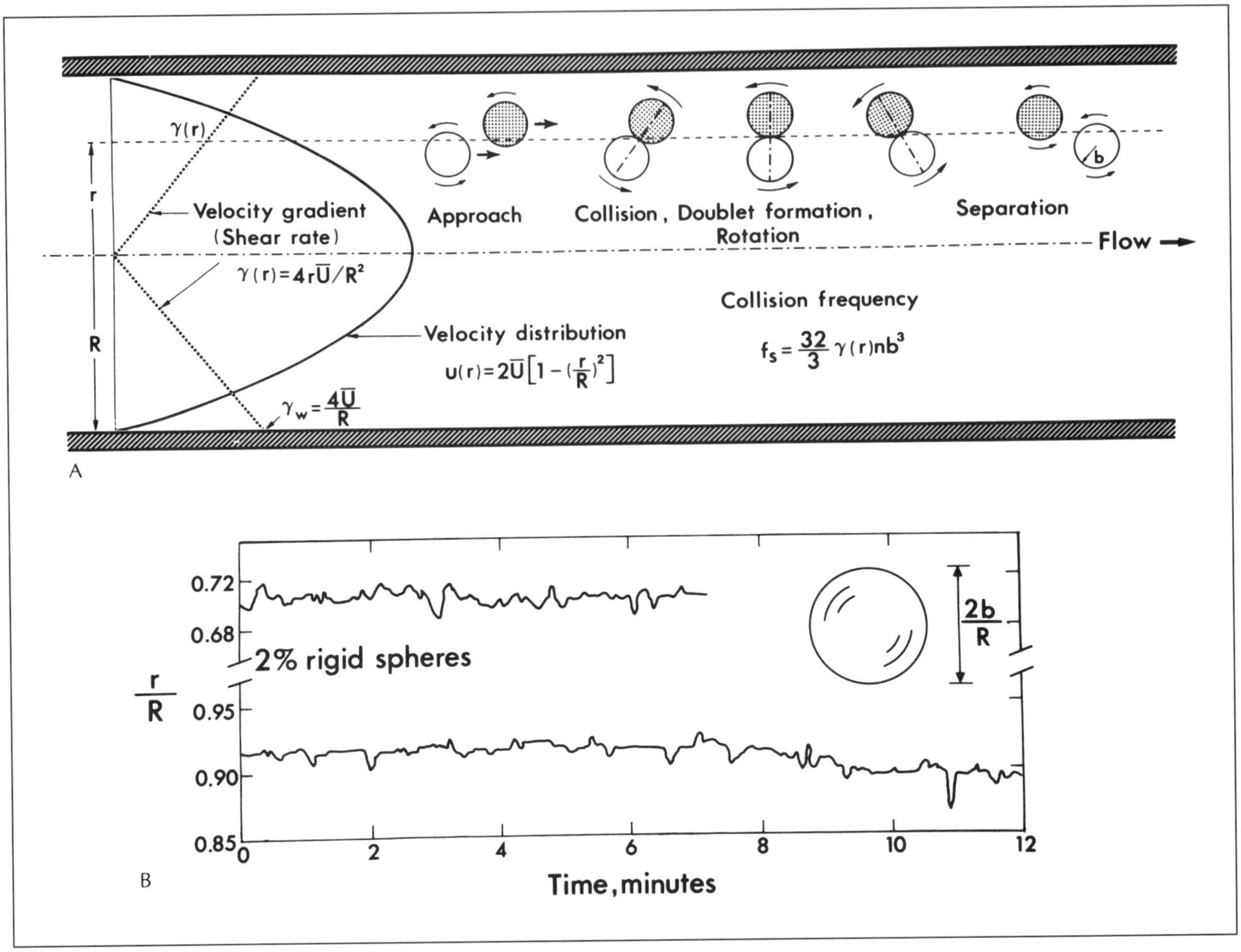

Fig. 5-12. **A.** A two-body, symmetric collision between rigid spheres of radius *b* in Poiseuille flow in the absence of interaction forces. The particles, traced from cine photomicrographs of 2-mm-diameter polystyrene spheres in a viscous oil in an 8-mm-diameter tube [48,52] are shown during approach, doublet formation and rotation, and separation, the final radial positions and velocities being the same as those before collision. (Reproduced with permission from M Anliker et al. [13].) **B.** The fluctuations, due to two-body collisions, in relative radial position r/R with time of the center of rotation of a single sphere being tracked in flow in a suspension of 2 percent by volume. Relative to the sphere diameter (shown), these fluctuations are small, but they increase markedly with increasing particle concentration (see Fig. 5-14). (Reproduced with permission from A Karnis, HL Goldsmith and SG Mason. The kinetics of flowing dispersions. I: Concentrated suspensions of rigid particles. J Colloid Interface Sci 1966; 22:531.)

($\tau < 2.4$ N/m^2 at 37°C) do not induce aggregation. An initial report of spontaneous aggregation using a cone-and-plate rotational viscometer [60] has not been supported by similar studies using cone-and-plate viscometers [61,62], cylindrical [36], or parallel-plate [63] Couette devices or steady laminar flow through tubes [56,57,64]. In the presence of red cells, however, there is some aggregation, probably due to release of ADP from the red cells [58,59]. Spontaneous aggregation in plasma also was absent in oscillatory flow in tubes, although the platelets were hypersensitive to postshear, thrombin-induced release [65].

The shear-induced aggregation of platelets in plasma at high shear stress follows progressive changes in the degree of platelet activation, lysis, and fragmentation in proportion to the level of fluid shear stress. Such effects, however, are highly dependent on the time of exposure to the shear field and the proximity of platelets to solid surfaces. Again, work using rotational viscometers has shown that unstable aggregates are formed at shear stresses τ greater than 3.5 N/m^2 ($\gamma > 2000$ s^{-1} at 25°C) through the shear-induced release of platelet ADP and serotonin [62,66]. Platelet lysis is detectable after 5 minutes of exposure to shear stresses over 10 N/m^2, in which case aggregation is essentially irreversible, while overt single-cell fragmentation and aggregate disintegration begin at τ greater than 25 N/m^2. Much higher shear stresses are required to produce similar results within 30 seconds of exposure to the shear field. Aggregation is completely reversible at $\tau = 10\ N/m^2$, and stresses greater than 20 N/m^2 are required to induce significant aggregation, with lysis occurring only at τ greater than 60 N/m^2. Impairment of normal platelet function also requires very high shear stresses after only 30 seconds in the shear field.

At extremely short exposure times (< 5 ms) to high shear stresses in narrow-bore capillary tubes, aggregation and fragmentation do not occur below $\tau = 2000\ N/m^2$, although serotonin release and platelet lysis begin at $\tau =$ 700 and 1500 N/m^2, respectively [67].

Experiments carried out in Couette viscometers in the absence of extrinsic activators have shown that, at shear stress greater than 8 N/m^2, washed platelets aggregate in the absence of exogenously added fibrinogen or activators such as ADP [68,69]. However, this aggregation requires the presence of von Willebrand factor (vWF) either added or released from the platelets [68–70], and there is some evidence that shear-induced ADP release occurs [70]. It appears that high-molecular-weight forms of vWF, such as found in the alpha granules of platelets are the most effective [69,70]. Significant ADP-induced aggregation in the absence of exogenous fibrinogen has been observed in washed platelet suspensions undergoing Poiseuille flow at shear stress as low as 3.5 N/m^2 and is believed to be mediated by vWF [71].

The response of whole blood to high shear stress is similar to that of platelet-rich plasma, although the aggregates in whole blood are larger and platelet adhesion to the viscometer surface probably complicates the results [72]. After shearing, platelets in whole blood exhibit impaired aggregation in response to ADP in a manner similar to that found with platelet-rich plasma.

FLOW BEHAVIOR OF BLOOD CELLS AT NORMAL HEMATOCRITS

When the hematocrit exceeds 20 percent, there is marked change in the flow regime, due primarily to crowding of the erythrocytes and the resulting cell-cell collisions. The following effects are obtained.

1. The velocity profile in the tube is no longer parabolic, as in Poiseuille flow, but is blunted with a region of partial plug flow in the tube center, in which all cells move with uniform and maximum velocity, lower than the centerline velocity, $u(0)$, in Poiseuille flow at the same volume flow rate (Fig. 5-13).
2. Deformation of red cells in blood occurs to a degree that is not attributable to shear alone (Fig. 5-14).
3. The blood-cell paths exhibit erratic displacements in a direction normal to the flow. This is of particular importance with regard to the motions of platelets and their interactions with the vessel wall (Fig. 5-15).

Blunting of the velocity distribution and the displacements of the particle paths occur in many concentrated suspensions. These have been studied by using photooptical methods in which the systems are made transparent to transmitted light and a small quantity of visible particles are added to serve as tracers of the particle movements in the interior of the flowing system. In model suspensions of rigid spheres or disks and in emulsions of oil droplets, transparency is achieved by matching refractive indices of the suspending phase to that of the particles [53,73]. In blood, transparency is achieved by use of reconstituted biconcave ghost cells in plasma [3,6,48]. Particles of the same size and shape but of different refractive index serve as tracers in the model suspensions. Normal erythrocytes, leukocytes, platelets, or microspheres serve as tracers in the ghost-cell suspensions.

Particle deformation due to crowding at high concentrations is observed in emulsions and in ghost-cell suspensions and is responsible for the low relative viscosities (viscosity of suspension divided by viscosity of suspending phase) compared to those in rigid-particle suspensions at the same concentrations [48,74]. The remarkable deformation of erythrocytes that is seen at concentrations over 30 percent (see Fig. 5-14) occurs at shear rates less than 7 s^{-1}, which corresponds to shear stresses under 0.03 N/m^2 (i.e., values at which an isolated erythrocyte in plasma would rotate as a rigid disk [40]). The erythrocytes are deformed into continually changing shapes and rotate only irregularly. At ghostcrits over 50 percent, the cells are continuously squeezed and no longer rotate as a whole; instead, the membrane probably moves around the cell interior in an irregular fashion.

Erythrocyte-Induced Dispersion in Flowing Blood. The presence of erythrocytes at volume concentrations from 40 to 50 percent considerably disturbs the motion of the formed elements in the plasma. One might expect that in such a concentrated suspension the erythrocytes would actually impede the diffusion of other cells and solutes. This is true when blood is stationary, but the opposite is observed in flow. The continued collisions and deformation of the erythrocytes in flowing blood actually lead to a continual radial displacement of their paths and an alternate method of solute mixing, similar on a macroscopic scale to the intermolecular collisions that result in Brownian motion. In fact, for particles as large as the erythrocytes, the movement induced by this mixing results in radial dispersion, or effective diffusion coefficients that are two to three orders of magnitude greater than those due to Brownian motion. This mixing motion becomes a major mechanism for permitting cells and possibly certain of the larger proteins to interact with the vascular surface.

The radial displacement of the cells in blood at normal hematocrits has been investigated using the model of the transparent ghost-cell suspensions. Measurements of the paths of tracer erythrocytes, 2-μm-diameter latex spheres, polymorphonuclear granulocytes, and platelets have been carried out over a range of ghostcrits, c, from 10 to 70 percent [3,48,75]. The magnitude of the particle radial displacements at first increases with c and then decreases at c greater than 50 percent, due to the pronounced cell deformation brought about by particle crowding at the high ghostcrits. As illustrated in Fig. 5-16, at a given c, the erythrocyte displacements are greatest at radial distances between 0.5 R and 0.8 R. Close to the wall, radial excursions of the cell paths are inhibited by the presence of the boundary. The amplitude of the displacements appears to be related both to particle deformability and to size, being somewhat greater for red cells, 2-μm spheres, and platelets than for the leukocytes.

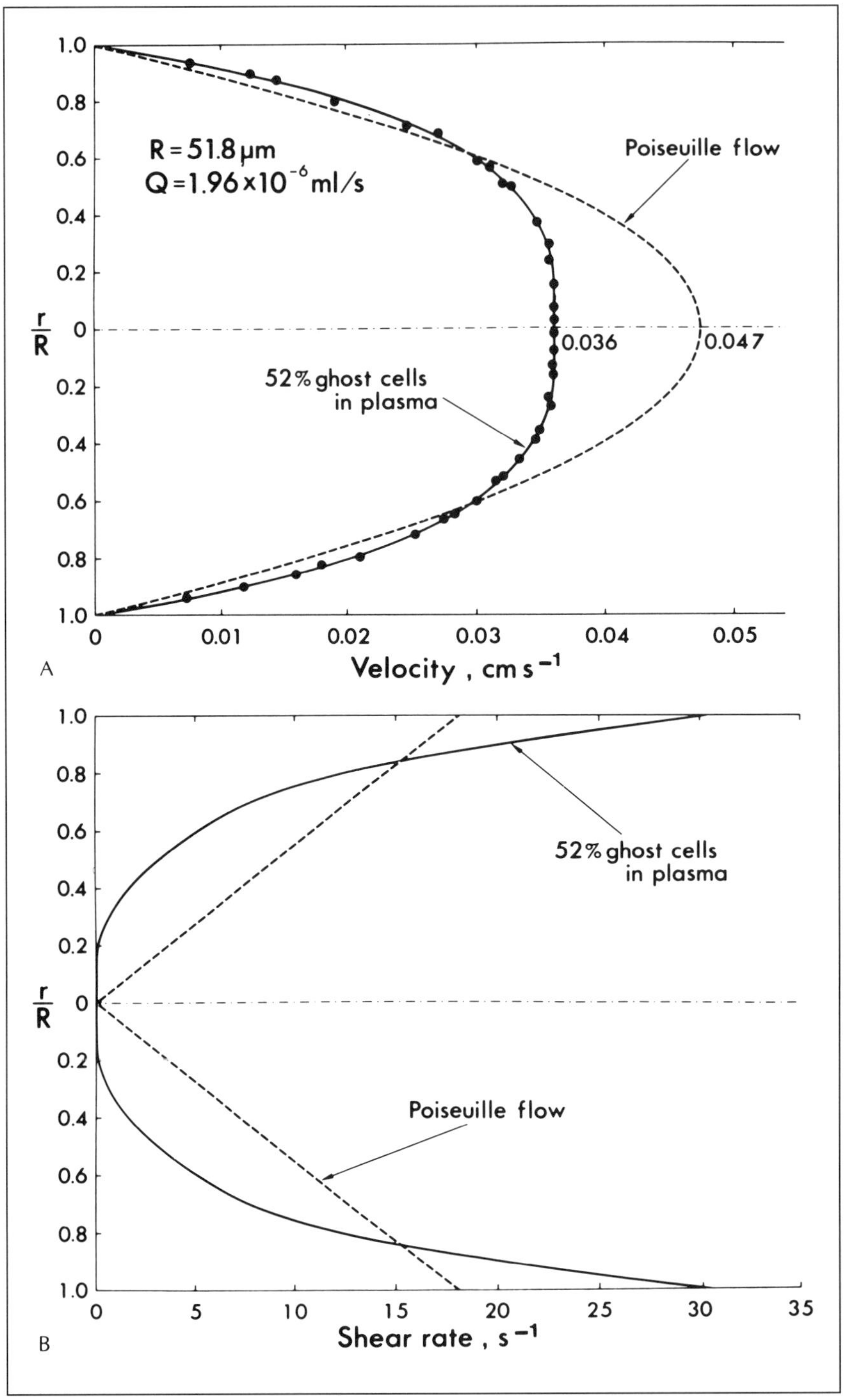

Fig. 5-13. Distribution of velocity **A.** and shear rate **B.** as a function of the relative radial position in a 52 percent (vol/vol) suspension of ghost cells in plasma containing tracer erythrocytes flowing through a 103.6-μm-diameter tube. The points represent the measured translational velocities of the erythrocytes. The line is the best fit drawn by eye. The solid line in B was obtained from measurements of the slope of the velocity distribution curve. The dashed lines represent the calculated velocity distribution and shear rate in a Poiseuille flow at the same volume flow rate as in the ghost-cell suspension. The graph illustrates the blunting of the velocity distributions from the parabolic, which occurs at ghostcrits above 20 percent, and results in a region of higher shear rate near the wall but zero shear rate close to the tube axis, where there is a partial plug flow. (Reproduced with permission from HL Goldsmith and VT Turitto. Rheological aspects of thrombosis and haemostasis: basic principles and applications. Thromb Haemost 1986; 55:415.)

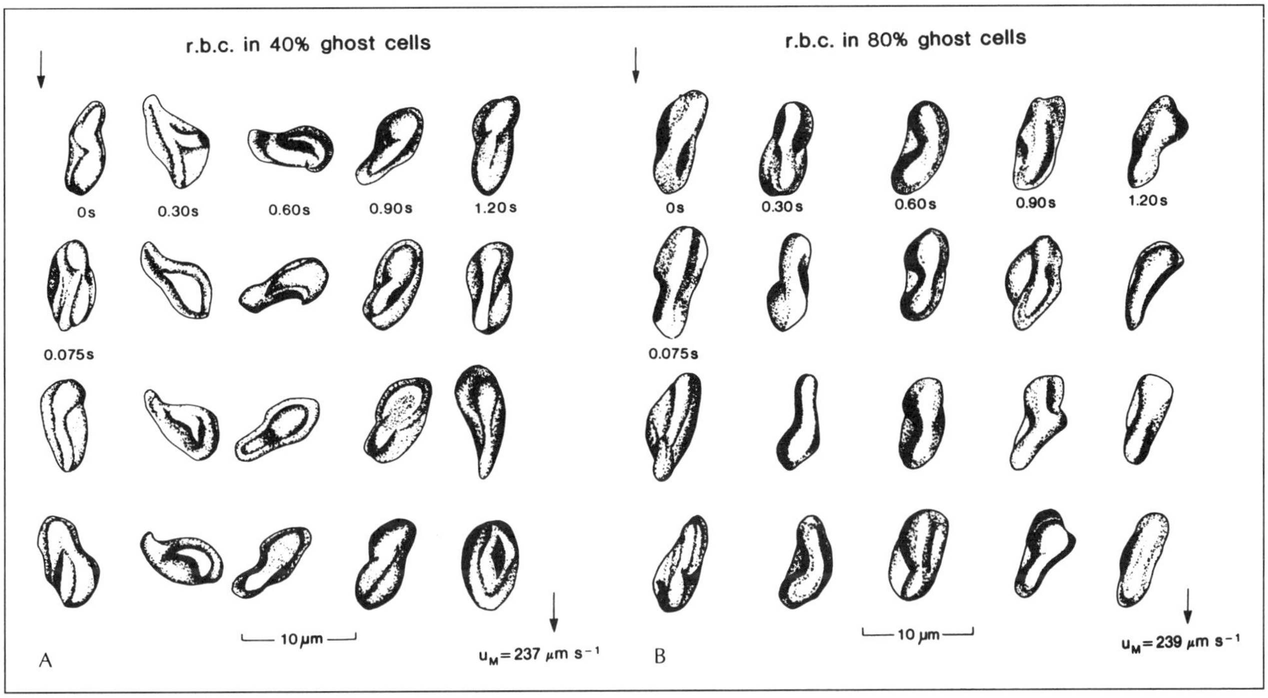

Fig. 5-14. Tracings from photomicrographs of the successive deformation of a tracer erythrocyte at 0.075-s intervals in a 40-percent (vol/vol) ghost-cell suspension **A.** and an 80-percent ghost-cell suspension **B.** flowing through a 109-μm-diameter tube with the maximum centerline velocity u_M = 238 μm/s. The cells, situated at a radial position $r \cong 0.7\ R$, undergo continuous changes in shape. At 40-percent ghostcrit, the cell still rotates as a whole, although erratically; at 80-percent ghostcrit, the cell is always aligned with the direction of flow. (Reproduced with permission from HL Goldsmith and J Marlow. Flow behavior of erythrocytes. II: Particle motions in concentrated suspensions of ghost cells. J Colloid Interface Sci 1979; 71:383.)

By analogy with Brownian translational diffusion (Eq. 10), a radial dispersion coefficient, D_r, obtained from the mean square radial distance $\overline{\Delta r^2}$ traveled by the particle in a time interval Δt,

$$\overline{\Delta r^2} = 2D_r\,\Delta t, \tag{14}$$

can be calculated. This does not imply that the motions are considered random, as in Brownian diffusion, even though the paths in Fig. 5-15 and Fig. 5-16 have the appearance of erratic random traces. The fluctuations in r are due to multibody collisions determined by the local velocity gradient, cell concentration, and cell deformation.

At local shear rates varying from 5 to 20 s^{-1} and ghostcrits from 20 to 70 percent, the values of the calculated radial dispersion coefficients ranged from 10^{-12} to 2×10^{-11} m^2/s for red cells and 2-μm microspheres [3]. These values are one to two orders of magnitude greater than the translational Brownian diffusion coefficients for the blood cells (see Table 5-2).

As a consequence of the radial dispersion of the erythrocytes, leukocytes, and platelets, the frequency of wall encounters of the corpuscles increases with increasing hematocrit. For platelets, this has been correlated with the observed increased adhesion to subendothelium [76,77] and other surfaces [78,79] as the hematocrit is increased. As might be expected from the observations in ghost-cell suspensions, wall adhesion of platelets is affected by red cell size and deformability [80,81]. The measured increase in diffusivity of platelets in blood as compared with that in plasma [82] and the resulting increased cell-wall interactions are of considerable importance in thrombotic processes. Values of the effective platelet diffusion constant in whole blood have been estimated to range from 3×10^{-11} to 8.6×10^{-10} m^2/s, as the shear rate is increased from 50 to 10^4 s^{-1} [77]. The extent to which erythrocyte deformation or size may affect the increase in the effective diffusion constant of cells and solute has also been studied. The transport of a molecular solute was found to increase slightly with both cell size and rigidity [83]. From the values of D_t given in Table 5-2, one would predict that only for large protein molecules such as fibrinogen and vWF (molecular weight > 10^6) would the dispersion or effective diffusion constant be appreciably greater than the Brownian translational diffusion constant. Indeed, the diffusion of low-molecular-weight solutes, such as oxygen and urea, in blood has been shown to be unaffected by the presence of erythrocytes [84,85].

Redistribution of Leukocytes and Platelets. In addition to disturbing the motion of the other formed elements in blood, erythrocytes appear to affect the distribution of leukocytes

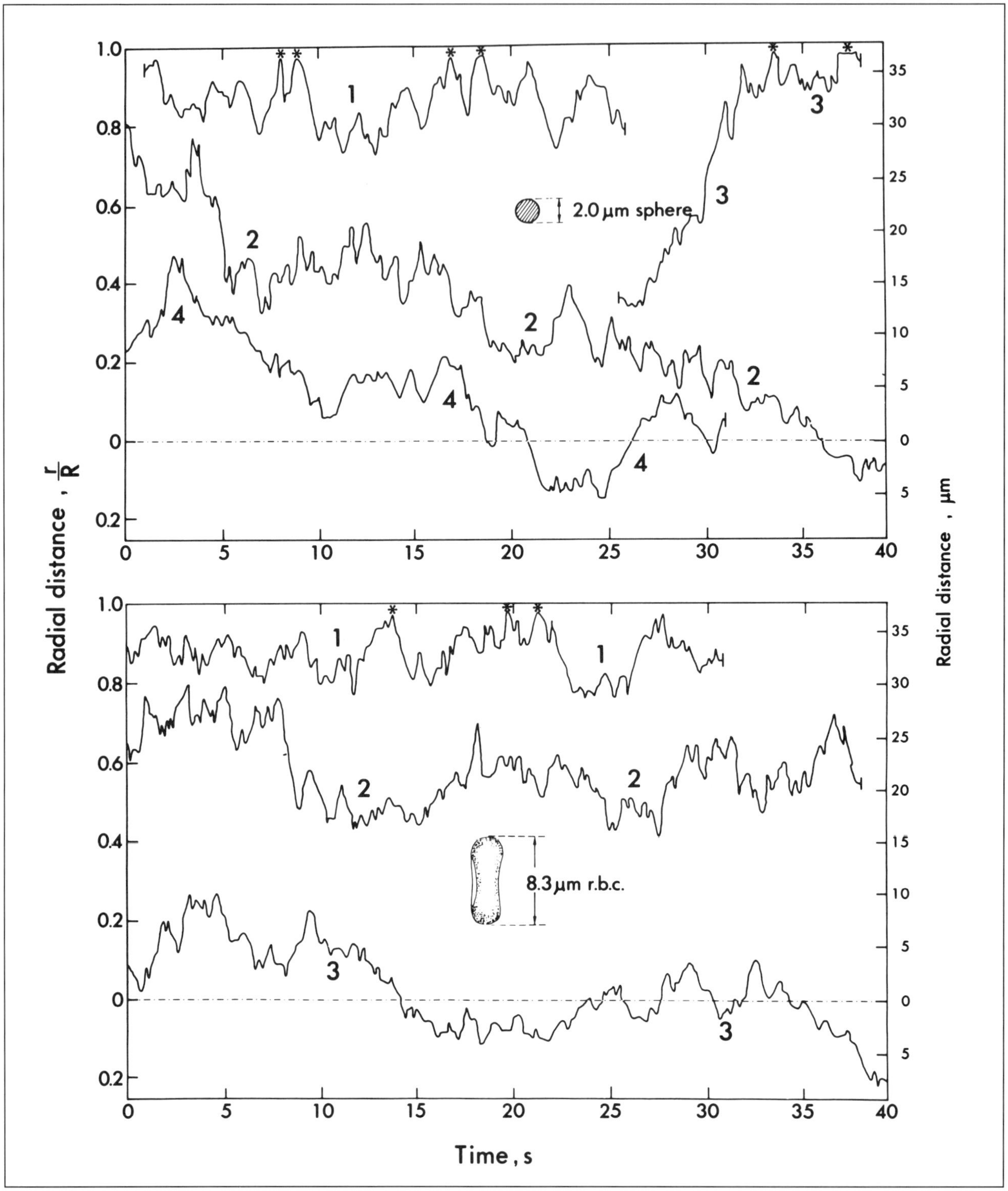

Fig. 5-15. Paths of tracer red cells (lower graph) and 2.0-μm latex spheres (upper graph) in a 40-percent (vol/vol) suspension of ghost cells in plasma flowing through a tube of 74-μm diameter at a mean velocity, $\overline{U}$, of 300 μm/s. The plot of relative radial distance from the tube axis against time shows that there is marked convective dispersion of the particles and cells, effectively increasing their diffusivity and inducing frequent collisions with the wall, as shown at the times marked with an asterisk. The particle diameter relative to that of the tube is shown. (Reproduced with permission from T Karino and HL Goldsmith. Rheological factors in haemostasis and thrombosis. In AL Bloom, DP Thomas, eds. Haemostasis and Thrombosis. Edinburgh: Churchill-Livingstone, 1987. Pp. 735–759.)

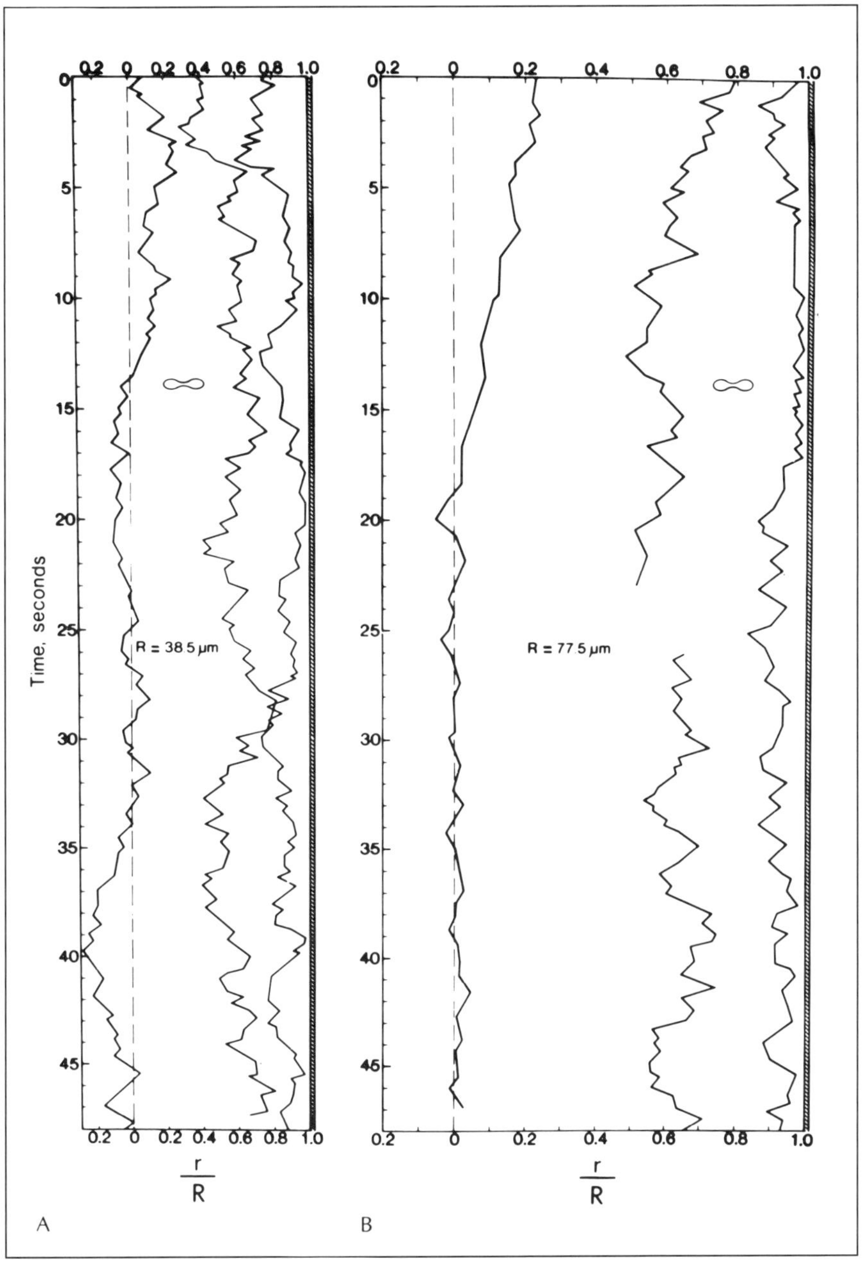

Fig. 5-16. Radial displacements of tracer erythrocytes in a 40-percent ghost-cell suspension in 77-μm- and 155-μm-diameter tubes (**A.** and **B.**, respectively). The cells situated in the region between $r = 0.4\ R$ and $0.8\ R$ appear to undergo the largest radial displacements. In the smaller tube, for the cell near the center at a mean $\bar{r} = 0.092\ R$, the root-mean-square radial displacement, $\sqrt{\overline{\Delta r^2}}$, is 2.00 μm; in the larger tube, for $\bar{r}$ of $0.076\ R$, $\sqrt{\overline{\Delta r^2}}$ is 1.62 μm. The respective values of $\bar{r}/R$ and $\sqrt{\overline{\Delta r^2}}$ for the cells at the intermediate radial position were 0.583 and 3.32 μm in the 77-μm tube and 0.662 and 3.84 μm in the 155-μm tube. For the cells near the tube wall, the values were 0.830 and 2.96 μm in the 77-μm tube and 0.952 and 1.97 μm in the 155-μm tube. (Reproduced with permission from HL Goldsmith and J Marlow. Flow behavior of erythrocytes. II: Particle motions in concentrated suspensions of ghost cells. J Colloid Interface Sci 1979; 71:383.)

and platelets because of their radial migration away from the wall and aggregation in the core of the vessel, where shear rates are very low. The extent to which the hematocrit is reduced near the endothelial wall and how far inward the erythrocyte-depleted zone extends are uncertain. The only in vivo measurements of the peripheral layer stem from sections of quick-frozen rabbit femoral arteries [86]. From that work and from the analysis of cine films of steady and pulsatile blood flow in glass tubes less than 100 μm in diameter [87], it appears unlikely that at normal hematocrits and physiologically representative flow rates the plasma-rich zone can be much larger than

4 μm. It should be noted, however, that inward migration of only a few microns in a vessel smaller than 150 μm in diameter brings about a significant decrease in the average red-cell concentration in the tube (Fahraeus effect) [88,89], resulting in a significant decrease in apparent blood viscosity (Fahraeus-Lindqvist effect) [90,91].

By contrast, the redistribution of platelets in whole blood occurs toward the vessel periphery: their concentration at a radial distance greater than 0.7 *R* in 25-μm-diameter arterioles is found to be twice that at the vessel center [92,93]. Similar results have been obtained in 100-μm-diameter glass tubes using latex microspheres as models of platelets [51,94–96] and in a parallel-flow chamber [97]. The effect is believed to be due in part to the differences in the inward migration rates between red cells and platelets and in part to the aggregation of red cells near the vessel center.

The aggregation of red cells is responsible for the so-called margination of white blood cells, a well-documented phenomenon in the microcirculation associated with low-blood-flow states such as occur in shock and in inflammation [98]. At high flow rates, leukocytes are found to be axially distributed in tube flow [99,100], although not to the same extent as the erythrocytes [49]. When red cells are caused to aggregate, however, by the addition of fibrinogen [99] or a high-molecular-weight dextran or by the reduction of the flow rate [49,99], leukocytes accumulate at the vessel periphery. Cine films taken in 100-μm-diameter tubes clearly show that the effect is due to the outward displacement of white cells by the inwardly migrating network of packed red-cell rouleaux, which push plasma containing both white cells and platelets toward the periphery. Margination of leukocytes is no longer found when the experiments are carried out in washed-erythrocyte suspensions in which rouleau formation is totally suppressed [49].

A different mechanism has been advanced to explain leukocyte margination in postcapillary venules [101]. Due to their larger volume and lower deformability, leukocytes travel more slowly than erythrocytes through the capillaries. As they enter the postcapillary venules, they are displaced to the wall by the more rapidly moving and deformable erythrocytes. The leukocytes adhere to or roll along the wall until they are displaced inward by the greater shear forces in the larger venules [101,102].

Disturbed Flow and Thrombogenesis

For some time, investigators from the biomedical as well as the physical and engineering sciences have postulated a connection between the occurrence of localized arterial wall injury, notably at branches and curved segments of vessels, and the disturbed patterns of flow at those sites [103]. Rapid changes in the rate or direction or both of the flow have been held responsible for bringing about alterations and injury, not only to the endothelium [104–107] and the media [108] but also to the corpuscles [109,110]. This, in turn, could lead to the aggregation and adhesion of the cells to the injured vessel wall. Indeed, atheromatous plaques and platelet thrombi have been observed at bifurcations and stenoses [111–113]. Do such disturbed patterns of flow lead to increased numbers of localized interactions with the vessel wall? We have obtained some answers to this question from our microrheologic studies of the flow behavior of blood cells in idealized models of stenoses [19,114] and T junctions [26] as well as in fixed transparent segments of natural arteries [14,21,23,27,115] and veins [116].

BLOOD CELLS IN AN ANNULAR VORTEX

A series of studies has described the flow behavior of human blood cells and model particles in an annular vortex distal to the sudden expansion of a 150- into a 500-μm-diameter glass tube [19,117,118]. For this geometry, fluid mechanical theory [119] predicts that particles flow in the closed orbits of a captive annular ring vortex.

Erythrocytes. The paths and orientations of hardened erythrocytes in the median plane of the tubular expansion are shown in Fig. 5-3. During a single orbit, the measured particle paths and velocities, as well as the locations of the vortex center and the reattachment point, agreed with those predicted by the theory applicable to the fluid [19,119]. Over longer periods, however, single cells and small aggregates less than 20 μm in diameter migrated outward across the closed streamlines of the vortex predicted by the theory and left the vortex after describing a series of spiral orbits of continually increasing diameter, until they rejoined the mainstream. In contrast, aggregates of cells over 30 μm in diameter remained trapped in the vortex, assuming equilibrium orbits or staying at the center. In pulsatile flow (a sinusoidal, oscillatory flow superimposed in parallel with the steady flow), the observed phenomena were qualitatively similar to those described in steady flow. The vortex varied periodically in size and intensity; the axial location of the vortex center and the reattachment point oscillated in phase with the upstream fluid velocity between maximum and minimum positions about a mean corresponding to that measured in the absence of the component of oscillatory flow. At higher hematocrits, from 15 to 45 percent, migration of single cells persisted and resulted in the lowering of the hematocrit in the vortex region in both steady and pulsatile flow [19].

The mechanism underlying the particle migration phenomenon is not a simple one, but a partial cause is probably the dilution effect of the cell-poor plasma taken into the vortex from the fluid layer adjacent to the vessel wall proximal to the expansion. The mechanism for the trapping of large aggregates in the vortex has been qualitatively explained by using existing fluid mechanics theories [42,46] concerned with lateral particle migration near a tube wall and by the operation of a mechanical wall effect [120].

Platelet Aggregation. The flow behavior and interactions of human platelets in the annular vortex were studied at 37°C, using heparinized or citrated platelet-rich plasma (PRP) as well as washed platelets in Tyrode's albumin solutions. It was demonstrated that the vortex provided favorable conditions for the spontaneous aggregation of normal human platelets through shear-induced collisions of particles circulating in its orbits [117]. In a given suspen-

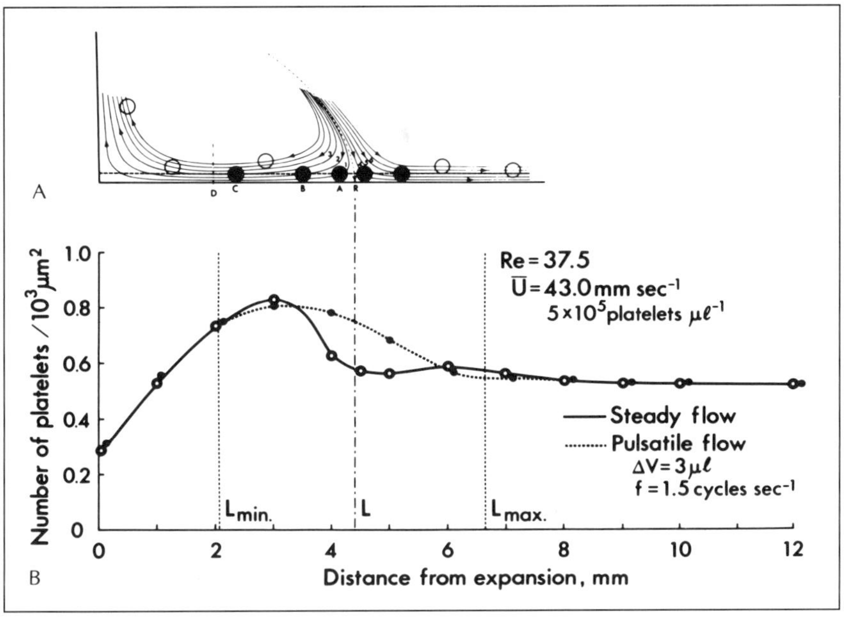

Fig. 5-17. **A.** Schematic representation of fluid streamlines near the tube wall downstream of a sudden concentric expansion, showing the convective transport of particles in bulk flow to the vessel wall along the radially directed curved streamlines on either side of the reattachment point, R. The black circles represent the particles carried by the flow along the streamlines 1 to 6 to within the critical distance for collision with the wall at points A to C in the vortex and the corresponding points downstream. The open circles represent particles that do not come close enough to collide with the wall. The adhesion density is maximal between the reattachment point and D, where the streamlines begin to be directed radially away from the wall. **B.** Plot of the measured number density of adhering platelets obtained from an experiment carried out with a suspension of washed human platelets in Tyrode's albumin solution containing no erythrocytes. The plot shows the relation between the flow pattern and the degree of platelet adhesion in and downstream from the vortex in steady and in pulsatile flow, the latter an oscillatory flow at 1.5 cycles/s and displacement of 0.3 μl, superimposed on a steady flow. The vortex reattachment point oscillated between the positions L_{min} and L_{max}. (Reproduced with permission from T Karino and HL Goldsmith. Role of blood cell-wall interactions in thrombogenesis and artherogenesis: a microrheological study. Biorheology 1984; 21:587.)

sion, the formation and growth of platelet aggregates could be observed only in a narrow range of tube Reynolds numbers, Re_t (based on mean suspension linear velocity in the 150-μm tube), which varied from suspension to suspension. Thus, in heparinized PRP, containing many sphered platelets with pseudopods and some microaggregates of two to six cells, the rate and extent of aggregation were the highest: large, elongated floating aggregates (> 100 μm in length) formed in less than 1 minute and within the widest range of Re_t, between 4.5 and 17. In citrated PRP and washed-platelet suspensions, in which no microaggregates were seen prior to flow, the degree of aggregation was much reduced. When platelets in these suspensions were activated with subthreshold concentrations of ADP or thrombin, however, the large aggregates seen in heparinized PRP were again formed. In pulsatile flow, there was a marked decrease in the number and the size of the aggregates that formed in the vortex. Presumably, this was due to the continually changing orbits of particles during the alternate expansion and contraction of the vortex, which shortened their residence times, as well as to the large variation in the shear rate in each cycle beyond the range favorable for platelet aggregation.

These results suggest that formation of platelet aggregates in vortices or recirculation zones is more likely to occur in the venous circulation, where the flow is steadier and Re_t is lower than in the arterial circulation.

Platelet Wall Adhesion. The effects of disturbed flow on initial platelet adhesion to the vessel wall were studied using a large-scale expansion flow tube (0.92- into 3.00-mm diameter), whose inner wall was coated with collagen fibers, and suspensions of washed human platelets containing washed erythrocytes at hematocrits from 0 to 50 percent [118]. As illustrated in Fig. 5-17, platelet adhesion was localized within the vortex and downstream on either side of the reattachment point with a local minimum at the reattachment point itself. Furthermore, platelet adhesion increased and both adhesion peaks become more pronounced as the hematocrit increased. Surprisingly, though, the adhesion peak in the vortex decreased and flattened out as the Reynolds number increased. These results are inconsistent with a diffusion-controlled platelet adhesion (when the rate-determining step in adhesion is the rate at which cells are brought to the vessel surface), which should show an increase in adhesion-number density with increasing shear rate [103,121]. It appears that the particular flow pattern in the vortex is responsible for this localization. Thus, as illustrated in Fig. 5-17A, only those cells carried by the curved streamlines to within one-particle radius of the surface interact with the vessel wall and adhere to it on both sides of the reattachment point, which is also a stagnation point [118,122].

BLOOD CELLS IN OTHER DISTURBED FLOWS

If the mechanism just described applies to other patterns of disturbed flow in the circulation, platelet adhesion onto the vessel wall, whether it be the natural endothelium or an artificial surface, should be localized wherever there is a stagnation point (or a reattachment point, if it is a result of flow separation) where blood cells are carried by the flow toward the vessel wall along the curved streamlines having a pronounced radial velocity component. If this mechanism operates in the circulation, a relatively higher adhesion of platelets, and hence a higher risk of platelet-mediated thrombus formation, is predictable, not only in regions of disturbed flow (adhesion peaks on either side of the reattachment point), such as downstream of aortic and venous valves, mural thrombi, and stenoses, but also in all the branching arteries at the flow divider where there is a stagnation point (see Fig. 5-6 through Fig. 5-8). Although the flow patterns illustrated in Fig. 5-4, Fig. 5-6, and Fig. 5-8 were obtained in fixed and rigid-walled segments of natural vessels, the fact that spiral secondary flows and recirculation zones were formed at Reynolds numbers equal to and even much lower than those prevailing in vivo makes it plausible that such disturbed flows exist under normal physiologic conditions. The regions of disturbed flow observed at flow dividers of aortic T junctions and the outer wall of the carotid sinus generally agree with the preferred sites of thrombosis and atherosclerosis clinically found in humans [25,123,124], which lends support to the mechanisms proposed above for cell-wall interaction. Clearly, in such disturbed flows, corpuscles and lipids are constantly carried to the vessel wall along the curved streamlines, and, because of the much lower local translational velocities and shear stress, they are able to interact with the vessel wall for longer periods than elsewhere in the circulation. One would therefore expect an enhanced deposition of platelets and leukocytes on the vessel wall and possibly an increased uptake of lipids by the endothelial cells in such regions.

In that regard, it must be remembered that the endothelial cells are affected by the variation in local shear stress at sites of disturbed flow. Cells exhibit morphologic changes that correspond to the direction of flow and, where spiral secondary flows and recirculation zones likely form and the shear stress is much lower, are not elongated but are oriented in a random fashion [107,108,125]. It is important, therefore, to ascertain whether there are differences in biologic, especially metabolic, function in these morphologically different cells. It is also necessary to investigate further the effect of the local flow pattern on the transport of oxygen, the uptake of plasma proteins and lipids by the endothelial cells, and the generation of procoagulant moieties either at or near the vessel wall. Only then can we arrive at a full explanation for the localization of thrombosis and atherosclerosis in the circulation and the role of the formed elements in those diseases.

Basic Concepts of Transport Processes Influencing Blood–Vessel Wall Interaction

BLOOD FLOW AND SURFACE INTERACTION

Two basic processes determine the *maximum* rate at which blood elements can interact with the vessel wall. The first of these, fluid convection, is the process by which blood elements (cells, proteins, or molecular species) are brought to various sites in the vasculature, be it the kidney for excretion, the lung for oxygenation, or a damaged vessel wall for repair. The supply of reactants and, implicitly, the removal of nonadherent elements by convective flow are the major mechanisms of transport, completely dominating the second process, diffusion, everywhere except very near the blood-vascular interface. At the vessel wall, both convective and diffusive transport are zero. Very close to the wall, however, diffusion, which is a random process induced by the thermal motion of the molecules, is the major mechanism of transport for the noncellular elements (see Table 5-2) and even for the corpuscles in areas of stagnant flow. Moreover, translational diffusion of blood elements does not have a preferred direction; thus, motion transverse to the fluid streamlines is as likely as that in the direction of flow. This latter phenomenon permits the direct collision of blood elements with the wall; without it, no reactive process could occur.

The study of velocity profiles and fluid streamlines is the subject of fluid mechanics, whereas the reaction of materials with solid interfaces is known as **heterogeneous reaction rate kinetics**. These two disciplines are linked (coupled) by diffusive processes, so that an understanding of the behavior of heterogeneous kinetics requires previous knowledge of the local fluid conditions in addition to the local reaction kinetics. The overall process of convective and diffusive flow coupled to heterogeneous reaction kinetics is known as convective-diffusive transport. In the case of blood–vessel wall interactions, mass transport is complicated by the complexity of the elements that can interact as well as the size of reactive elements, such as cells and proteins. Size imposes additional mechanisms that do not occur at the molecular level; thus, adaptations of classical concepts of transport mechanisms must be considered. We will discuss such modifications in transport processes after presenting the classic theory of molecular processes; these principles are applied in our discussion of certain cellular and proteinaceous interactions with vessel walls.

CLASSIC THEORY OF CONVECTIVE-DIFFUSIVE TRANSPORT

An approximation method frequently used in describing fluid-surface interactions is known as **boundary layer theory** [17,20,126]. The boundary layer is the fluid lying between the mainstream and a solid boundary in which velocity, under the influence of viscosity, decreases but does not become zero until the wall is reached. This concept simplifies the equations describing pressure and motion within the fluid boundary layer so that they can be solved. As applied to mass transport, the definition of the boundary layer is even more restricted. Since diffusion is a slow process compared to viscous flow, the thickness of the layer over which changes in local concentration occur (the mass transfer boundary layer) is much smaller than the thickness over which velocity changes occur (the fluid dynamic boundary layer). Thus, in general, one needs to know only the velocity within the mass transfer boundary layer; the remaining flow is unimportant for determining surface interactions. It is as if most of the blood elements that pass through the vessel never realize that there is a vessel wall and do not participate in surface interactions. (This obviously is not true of the smallest vessels in the microcirculation, whose dimensions approach the size of cellular species; for them, a very different type of analysis must be employed.) The thickness of the mass transfer boundary layer increases with distance, but growth is slow, again relative to the fluid boundary layer, so that often the transport process may be considered steady state and occurring within a well-developed fluid velocity profile (Fig. 5-18). The thinness of the mass transfer boundary layer has another important consequence: effects due to curvature of the flow field can be neglected. Thus, because curvature of the wall is small compared to the distance over which concentration changes occur, one can assume a linear increase in velocity with radial distance from the wall and a constant velocity gradient equal to the wall shear rate, γ_w (see Fig. 5-18). This not only simplifies the equations describing flow and mass transport, it also results in similar solutions for a variety of perfusion systems that have been developed to study blood–vessel wall interactions. Thus, the mathematic solutions for planar parallel-plate, tubular, and annular flow systems are all similar. The main reason for selecting a particular flow system, therefore, has less to do with the mathematics of convective-diffusive transport than with a particular experimental advantage (Table 5-3).

The theory for mass transport in tubular flow is presented here because it most closely approximates the vascular system in vivo. All theories used to describe flow and, especially, mass transport in vivo, are essentially gross approximations in that many of the finer details of the vasculature are completely ignored. However, such theories do incorporate many of the essential elements of the flow and are adequately able to predict the dependence of transport processes on selected variables. The main point is not that the theory be rigorous in incorporating all the finer aspects of the flow problem but that it identify the importance of critical parameters and consequently the relative unimportance of others. Lack of correlation between theory and experiment leads to modification of theory, that is, alteration of certain initial simplifying assumptions and inclusion of previously omitted details to better conform to experimental observation. Such "bootstrapping" leads to more refined analysis, which is essentially verified by additional experimentation.

Mass Transport in Tubular Flow. A number of authors have studied heterogeneous reactions in tubular flow [17,126,158], starting with Leveque [158]. The theory utilizes a number of assumptions, which are discussed in Table 5-4. Using these assumptions, the mass flux (mass of particles or solute crossing unit area per unit time) can be obtained for the case where the reaction at the surface is very fast compared to the ability of reactant to diffuse to the surface:

$$j = 0.84 \left(\frac{\gamma_w D_w^2}{x}\right)^{1/3} C_o. \qquad (15)$$

Fig. 5-18. Thickness of the fluid-dynamic and mass-transfer boundary layers as a function of distance from the inlet. The mass-transfer boundary layer, defined as the distance over which changes in the concentration of a specific reactant or product occurs, increases with increasing distance but at a much slower rate than that of the fluid-dynamic boundary layer. For many situations, the fluid-dynamic profile can be considered fully developed and the mass-transfer concentration gradient constant.

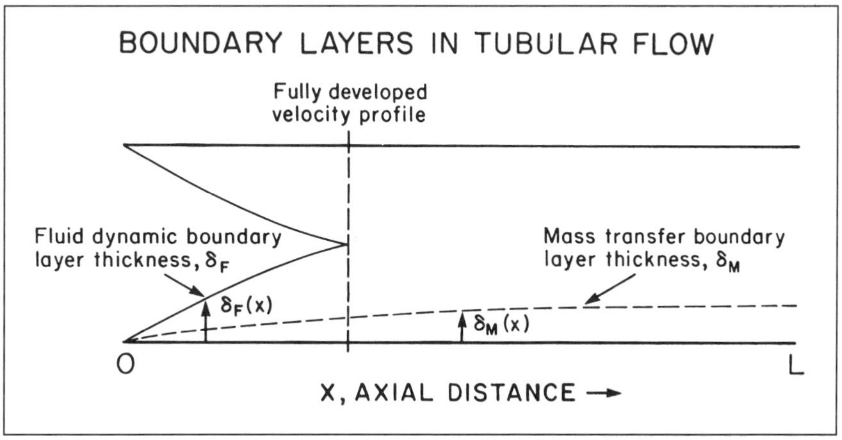

Table 5-3. Flow chambers for studying blood–vessel wall interaction

Type of chamber	Perfusate	Source of blood	Source of vessel	Comments
Annular[a]	Blood, plasma, reconstituted blood	Rabbit, rat, human	Rabbit aorta, human umbilical and renal	Convenient for exposing vascular surfaces, but chamber dimensions must match vascular dimensions
Tubular[b]	Blood	Pig	Pig aorta	Chamber not restricted by vascular dimensions; also advantageous for studying biomaterials
Rotating rod[c]	Blood, reconstituted blood	Human	Rabbit	Studies restricted to very low shear conditions due to flow instabilities; vessel dimensions important for mounting on rod

[a] Introduced by Baumgartner [127] and studied by numerous other investigators, a partial listing of whom follows: [76,77,80,81,127–152].
[b] Introduced by Badimon [153–156].
[c] Introduced by Feuerstein [78] and utilized by Cazenave [157].

In this case, γ_w is the wall shear rate, D_w is the diffusion coefficient of the reactant near the wall, x is the axial distance from the tube entrance, and C_o is the average concentration of reactant in the fluid. Thus, the analytic solution indicates that the reaction rate per unit area for diffusion-controlled transport (where reaction kinetics are fast compared to movement through the fluid) is most dependent on the concentration of reactant, less dependent on the diffusion coefficient, and weakest on the wall shear rate and axial position. When movement through the fluid is very rapid compared to surface kinetics, the mass flux equals the actual reaction-rate kinetics at the surface without any fluid-phase considerations (reaction rate–controlled transport). For a first-order reaction rate, this process can be defined as

$$j = kC_o, \tag{16}$$

in which the reaction rate per unit area now depends only on average fluid concentration and reaction-rate coefficient. (The simplest reaction kinetics have been selected for illustrative purposes). Such kinetics result in an analytic solution to the equations describing mass transport. Obviously, more complex kinetics may pertain to particular applications, especially those dealing with coagulation enzymes, but, in such cases, the solution usually must be generated by numeric modeling and computation.

For the general case of intermediate controlled transport, in which both reaction kinetics and fluid-phase movements influence the overall reaction product, the mass flux becomes [153]

$$j = \frac{C_o}{\dfrac{1}{k} + 0.84\left(\dfrac{x}{D_w^2\gamma_w}\right)^{1/3}}. \tag{17}$$

This equation reduces either to diffusion-controlled ($k \to \infty$) or to reaction rate–controlled ($D_w\gamma_w/x \to \infty$) transport under the appropriate conditions. In such a case, the dependency on physical parameters varies from 0 to the ⅓ power (⅔ power for D_w), depending on the relative magnitudes of the reaction and flow coefficients (Fig.

Table 5-4. Mass transport in blood: simplifying assumptions

Assumption	Remarks
Incompressible fluid (constant density)	Good assumption for blood.
No slip condition at vessel wall	Good assumption for blood.
Fully developed velocity profile	Entrance length (L_e) is generally short for fluids, varying from 1 to 100 times the diameter of the tube, depending on the flow (L_e/D = 0.03 RE_t), but many blood vessels are not long relative to their diameter. Also, blunting of velocity profile may occur at high hematocrits.
Constant (Newtonian) fluid viscosity	At wall shear rates > 100 s^{-1}, this is a good assumption; below this value, viscosity gradually increases with decreasing wall shear rate.
Fluid behaves as a continuum	In large vessels (diameter much greater than that of the red cell size), this is a good approximation; it becomes progressively poorer as vessel size decreases.
Steady, laminar flow	Flow is not generally steady in the major vessels but may be so in smaller conduits. In resting individuals, flow is probably laminar in all normal vessels except perhaps at systole in the aorta.
Rigid, straight, nonpermeable tube	Vessels are elastic, curved, and often permeable to certain elements. The effects of such properties on the mass transport of cells have never been fully considered.

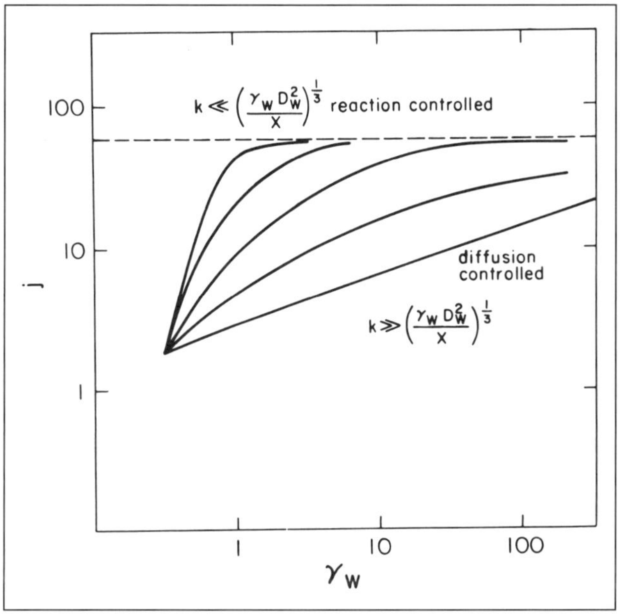

Fig. 5-19. Dependence of mass flux on wall shear rate (logarithmic coordinates). Depending on the relative magnitudes of $D_w^2\gamma_w/x$ and k (Eq. 17), the reaction can be in the diffusion- or the reaction rate–controlled regime. The wall shear rate can be varied so as to move from one regime to another. In the diffusion-controlled regime, flux is proportional to the ⅓ power of wall shear rate, whereas in the reaction-controlled regime, flux is independent of wall shear rate.

5-19). The relative magnitudes of the coefficients are determined from the experimental system under investigation, but in theory it is always possible to proceed from diffusion-controlled to reaction rate–controlled transport by increasing the wall shear rate to high-enough values. The other coefficients, such as D_w and x, are less amenable to variation.

Applicability to Vessel Wall Interactions. The use of Eq. 17 to describe *intravascular* blood–vessel wall interactions has never been attempted directly. While it is reasonable to suppose that, as a first-order approximation, the equation applies to a wide range of vessels, few experiments have been designed to test its validity (and, indirectly, the suitability of the assumptions in Table 5-4). What has been tested in a variety of in vitro and ex vivo perfusion systems is the interaction of blood platelets with aortic vessel wall denuded of its endothelial lining. More specifically, the short-term response of a high-flow (relatively low wall shear rate) vessel to an extensive vascular injury has been compared with the response of a similarly treated vessel mounted in a perfusion chamber and exposed to controlled flow conditions [127]. The responses, both with respect to platelet adhesion to the vessel wall and thrombus formation on top of adherent platelets, were quite comparable in both perfusion systems [127,128]. The sequence of events in rabbit is similar to that seen in other species following balloon-catheter denudation [159,160]. Within 30 to 60 seconds, platelets already have begun to attach to the subendothelium. These platelets are few in number, have undergone shape change, and are attached primarily by pseudopodic extension of the cellular membrane. Under normal arterial flow conditions (mean wall shear rates of 100–400 s^{-1}), platelets rapidly form a continuous layer on the surface. Platelet-platelet cohesion (mural thrombi) reaches a maximum after 5 to 10 minutes of blood flow, but disappears within 40 minutes of flow, leaving only a single layer of platelets adhering to the vessel wall. These platelets have secreted most of their alpha granules and serotonin-storage organelles. Under such flow conditions, electron microscopy can detect no evidence of fibrin [77,127,128]. A review of the process clearly depicts these initial interactions [77]. Such basic studies have led to the development of perfusion chambers that can simulate the full range of flow conditions existing in the vasculature using vessels or vascular components and whole blood or a suitable substitute (see Table 5-1). Table 5-3 lists some of these chambers. Such perfusion studies have become the basis for determining the importance of blood, vascular, and rheologic factors in influencing various mechanisms related to thrombosis. We have detailed the rheologic characteristics of blood; now we will document how such fluid dynamic factors interact with various elements in the blood and in the vessel wall to contribute to the process of thrombosis.

Influence of Flow on Blood–Vessel Wall Interactions

Two major systems are involved in the initiation of thrombosis in blood: platelets and the coagulation proteins. The role of platelets in thrombosis, with particular emphasis on the effects of flow, has been most studied. We have achieved major advances in our understanding of the dynamics of platelet thrombosis. Less well understood is the role of flow in the events leading to fibrin formation. Here, platelet deposition is considered first, then coagulation events that are influenced by flow, and the extent to which platelets and fibrin interact in the generation of thrombus mass. The emphasis is on physical factors influencing blood–vessel wall events rather than on biochemical mechanisms of adhesion. Such biochemical mechanisms are the subject of several chapters in this volume and have been reviewed elsewhere [77,161].

PHYSICAL FACTORS INFLUENCING CONVECTIVE-DIFFUSIVE TRANSPORT IN IN VITRO STUDIES

According to the classically derived theory for convective-diffusive transport, wall shear rate, platelet diffusivity, platelet concentration, and axial position all should influence the overall deposition rate on subendothelium.

Wall Shear Rate. Numerous studies have demonstrated that increases in flow rate (which, in chambers of constant cross-sectional area, imply increases in wall shear rate) lead to increased platelet deposits on vessel walls. Baumgartner's original studies [127] in vivo and in vitro in rabbit demonstrated decreased platelet adhesion (platelet–vessel wall attachment) and platelet thrombus formation (platelet-platelet interaction) with decreasing arterial

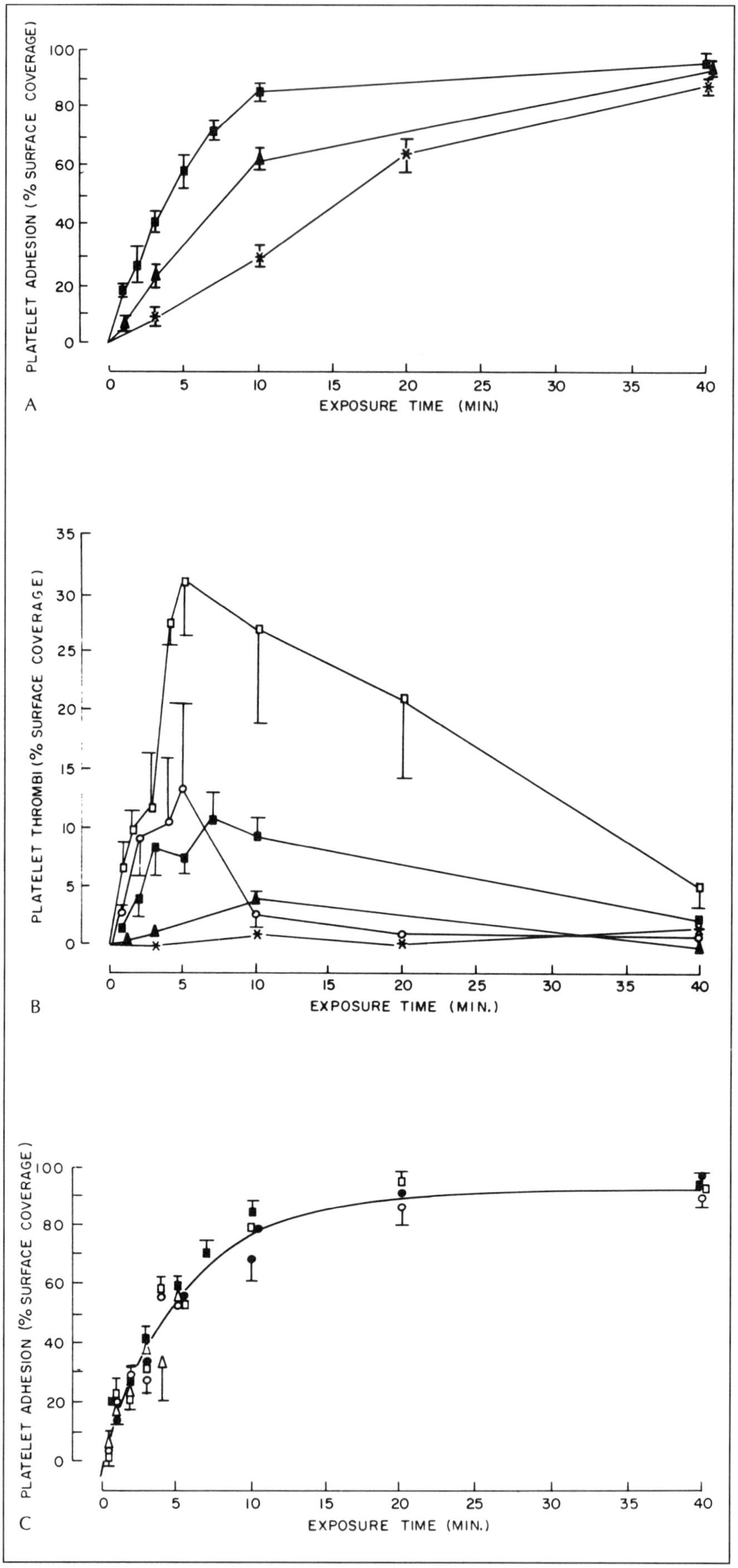
PLATELET ADHESION (% SURFACE COVERAGE)
EXPOSURE TIME (MIN.)
A
PLATELET THROMBI (% SURFACE COVERAGE)
EXPOSURE TIME (MIN.)
B
PLATELET ADHESION (% SURFACE COVERAGE)
EXPOSURE TIME (MIN.)
C

flow rates. Turitto et al. [129–132] have extensively analyzed the dependence of adhesion and thrombus formation on flow rate in citrated rabbit and human blood (Fig. 5-20). Those authors demonstrated experimentally in chambers of various dimensions that the important parameter influencing platelet deposition was not the total volume flow, the volume flow rate, or the local average velocity, but the wall shear rate (Fig. 5-21). Moreover, they demonstrated the existence of a transition region in which platelet adhesion (but not thrombus formation) became independent of wall shear rate (see Fig. 5-20C). This latter finding is in accord with the behavior predicted by classic theory because mass transport becomes less dependent on physical variables (diffusion-controlled) and more dependent on reaction kinetics (reaction rate–controlled). Similar findings about the increase in platelet adhesion with wall shear rate are reported by Sakariassen et al. [154] in an annular perfusion system modified to investigate the interaction of blood components (washed platelets inhibited with aspirin) with human vessels. More recent studies—utilizing an ex vivo perfusion system in swine, in which platelets are labeled with 111-In, and the total deposition (both adhesion and aggregation) is determined by radiometric evaluation—are consistent with the findings reported above; that is, the deposition rate increases with increasing wall shear rate up to values of 1,690 s^{-1}. No evidence that the total deposition reaches a plateau as wall shear rate increases is apparent, which supports findings that thrombus formation, in contrast to platelet adhesion, continues to increase with wall shear rate (see Fig. 5-20B) [132,153].

Direct comparison of either platelet adhesion rate (platelet–vessel wall attachment) or deposition rate (total platelet mass associated with the vessel wall) with those predicted by classic analysis indicates a much stronger dependence of platelet deposition on wall shear rate than predicted by the ⅓ power (Eq. 15). The dependence is considerably enhanced when total deposition is considered, compared with adhesion alone, as indicated by the slope determined from double logarithmic plots (1.4 and 0.62, respectively) [132,153] (Fig. 5-22). The enhanced contribution of shear rate on platelet deposition is in part indirect (rather than a direct effect on platelet reactivity); that is, the wall shear rate is influencing such physical parameters as the platelet diffusivity and the local concentration of platelets at the wall. These effects are nonclassic, since normally neither diffusion coefficient nor concentration gradient for small molecules is influenced by local flow factors. Conversely, part of the enhanced dependence may be related to direct effects of flow on platelets (see "Direct Effect of Flow on Platelet Reactivity," later in this chapter).

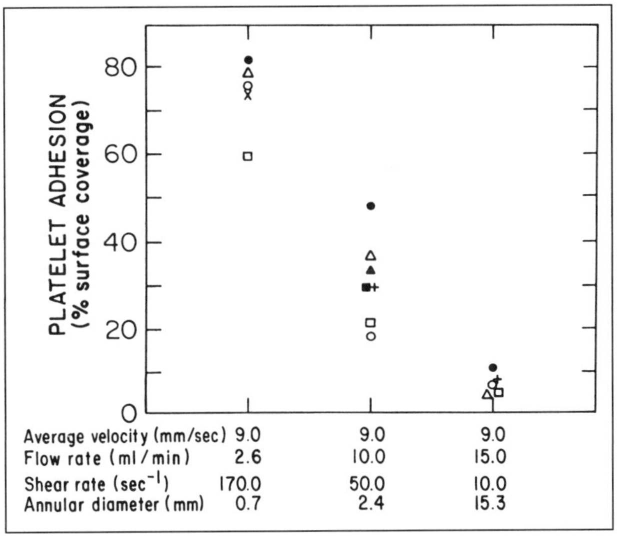

Fig. 5-21. Influence of average velocity, volumetric flow rate, and wall shear rate on platelet adhesion to subendothelium. Perfusions were conducted in three annular chambers of different diameter, such that average fluid velocity was constant. Deposition correlated with the wall shear rate, as expected from theoretical considerations, Eq. 15.

Platelet Diffusivity. Red cells have a major influence on the mobility of platelets in blood, especially near vessel walls. Brownian translational motion is very small for the size range of most cells (see Table 5-2), as indicated by the platelet diffusion coefficient (on the order of 10^{-13} m^2/s). In the presence of red cells, however, platelets exhibit a diffusion-like motion (termed **platelet diffusivity**), which is two to three orders of magnitude greater than their Brownian motion. The influence of the red cells on platelet adhesion is dramatically demonstrated when rates of platelet adhesion in plasma versus whole blood are compared (Fig. 5-23). The 50-fold increase in platelet adhesion in whole blood relative to plasma suggests a several-hundredfold increase in platelet diffusivity (D_w is raised to the ⅔ power, Eq. 15), an increase compatible with previous measurements of platelet diffusivity in the absence of reaction [18,75,82,133] and as estimated from measurements on biologic surfaces [76].

The effect of red cells over the full physiologic range of wall shear rate and a broad range of hematocrits indicates that red cells may not only contribute to the physical movements of platelets in blood but also provide certain chemical components that directly influence the platelet–vessel wall interaction [76,134]. The rationale for a dual mechanism derives from studies in which platelet adhe-

Fig. 5-20. Interaction of human platelets with rabbit subendothelium exposed for various times to citrated blood over the physiologic range of wall shear rate in an annular perfusion chamber. **A.** Platelet adhesion (direct platelet–vessel wall interaction) at low shear rates. **B.** Thrombus formation (platelet-platelet interaction, resulting in platelet microthrombi exceeding 5 μm in height). **C.** Platelet adhesion at high shear rates. Wall shear rates are 50 (*), 200 (▲), 650 (△), 800 (■, ●), 2,600 (○), and 10,000 (□) s^{-1}. (Reproduced with permission from VT Turitto, H Weiss, and HR Baumgartner. The effect of shear rate on platelet interaction with subendothelium exposed to citrated human blood. Microvasc Res 1980; 19:352.)

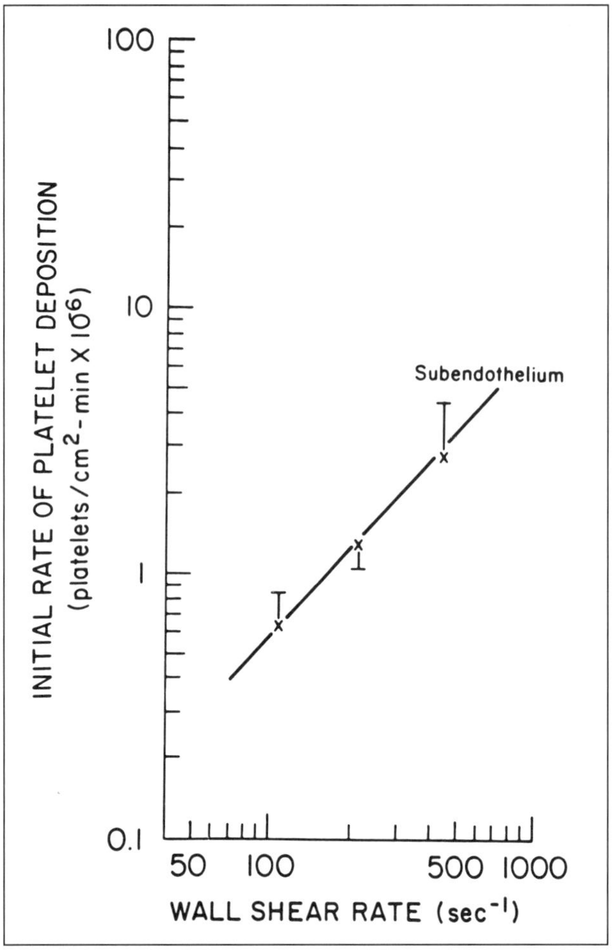

Fig. 5-22. Rate of platelet deposition on subendothelium exposed to 111-In-labeled platelets in a tubular flow chamber for a range of wall shear rates. The slope of the regression line (m = 1.41) is markedly greater than the maximum (m = 0.33) expected from theoretical considerations, Eq. 15. (Reproduced with permission from L Badimon et al. Platelet deposition in von Willebrand factor deficient vessels. Extracorporeal perfusion studies in von Willebrand's diseased swine utilizing native and heparinized blood. J Lab Clin Med 1987; 110:634.)

sion is observed at selected hematocrits over widely varying ranges of wall shear rate [162] (Fig. 5-24).

As seen in Fig. 5-24 and as indicated by earlier studies of platelet adhesion versus wall shear rate (see Fig. 5-20), at physiologic hematocrit between 38 and 45 percent, platelet adhesion undergoes a transition from strong dependence on to independence of wall shear rate. This behavior is analogous to that expected classically as the reaction (adhesion) undergoes a transition from diffusion- to reaction-controlled transport kinetics. In the region of reaction-controlled transport, increases in adhesion would be due primarily to changes in the reactivity of platelets (with the vessel wall), whereas in the diffusion-controlled regime, changes in adhesion are due primarily to alterations in convective-diffusive transport. Figure 5-24 shows that platelet adhesion is very sensitive to the red cell concentration at high shear rates for all values of hematocrit. Since this is the reaction rate–limiting regime, it follows that red cells are contributing to the platelet–vessel wall interaction through chemical rather than physical mechanisms. At lower shear rates, the strong dependence of platelet adhesion on the magnitude of the shear rate reinforces the importance of the red cell as a physical mediator of platelet adhesion. Thus, there are two mechanisms by which red cells contribute to platelet adhesion: (1) a physically induced motion predominant at low shear rates and hematocrits greater than 20 percent and (2) a chemically related activation maximal at high shear rates and hematocrits. The mechanism that seems to be limiting at low hematocrits is of a chemical nature, as determined by the relative lack of dependence of adhesion on wall shear rate under these conditions. Conversely, convective-diffusive events appear to be limiting at high hematocrits. Therefore, increases in hematocrit tend to shift the platelet–vessel wall interaction from a reaction-controlled to a diffusion-controlled transport kinetics, whereas increases in wall shear rate have the opposite effect. Obviously, the relative importance of the wall shear rate and hematocrit will vary in a complex fashion, depending on the magnitude of the two parameters.

The nature of the biochemical factor that induces enhanced platelet–vessel wall interactions at high hematocrits and shear rates is not certain. The obvious candidate for such an effect is ADP, which is contained in relatively large amounts in the red cell and which may be released as a result of stress-related lysis [163] and even appears to be released at low shear stress [59]. ADP is a well-known stimulant for platelet aggregation and has been implicated recently as a mediator of platelet adhesion on subendothelium [135].

In addition to red cell number, two other physical aspects of red cells—size and deformability [80,81]—have been shown to contribute to platelet–vessel wall interactions. An additional physical effect of red cells is their potential ability for inducing changes in local concentration of platelets near the vessel wall [92–96].

Platelet Concentration. The interchange of platelets with the vessel wall depends on the local cell concentration gradient in the radial direction perpendicular to the surface. Classically, this gradient is determined from a balance between reaction (attachment) at the surface and resupply of platelets by convective and diffusive motion. For example, a high rate of resupply relative to the rate of reaction is a qualitative description of reaction-controlled transport, which possesses a zero concentration gradient at the wall (local wall concentration equals bulk concentration). Conversely, a low rate of resupply relative to reaction results in a diffusion-limited transport for which the concentration gradient is maximal and the cell concentration at the wall is zero. A zero wall reaction rate is an extreme example of a reaction-controlled transport for which the radial concentration gradient should be zero. Recent experimental evidence indicates that radial concentration gradients near surfaces may not be uniform in the absence of platelet deposition [51,93–96,164,165]; that is, a nonuniform, heterogeneous concentration profile for platelets may exist in flowing blood. Since classic theory

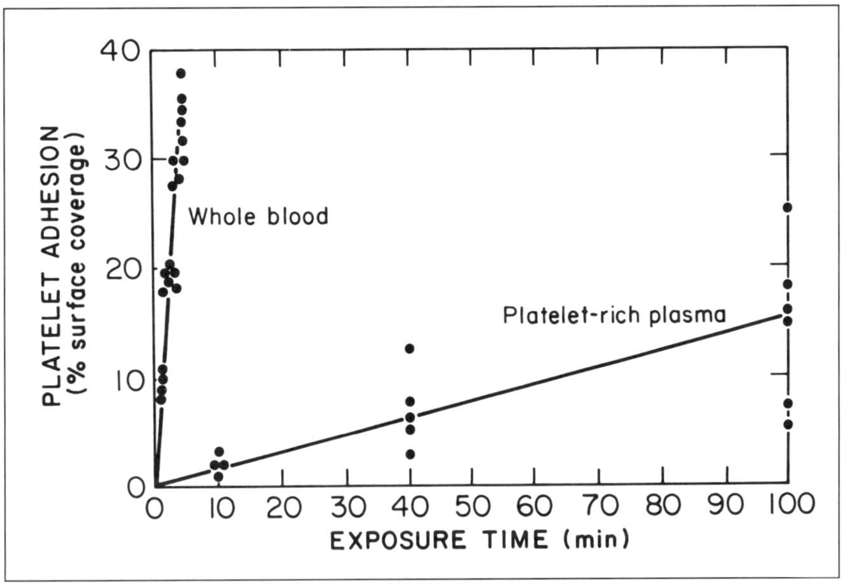

Fig. 5-23. Influence of red cells on platelet adhesion to rabbit subendothelium exposed for various times to blood flowing in an annular perfusion chamber at a wall shear rate of 800 s^{-1}. The initial rate of deposition of platelets is more than 50-fold greater when whole blood (H = 35–42%) is perfused, compared with PRP (H = 0%).

predicts a strong (linear) dependence of platelet deposition on concentration, variations in local platelet concentration near the wall could have a significant influence on the overall deposition. Early studies [94] suggested that in long, narrow tubes (length-to-diameter ratios ≅ 1 : 10^4) platelets suspended in plasma migrated away from the tube wall, thus producing a local depletion near the surface. When red cells were added, an excess of platelets at the surface was measured, implying that the platelets had migrated radially outward, toward the wall. Recent measurements using latex microspheres similar in size to platelets indicate a maximum in particle concentration in a region within 10 μm from the wall [95]. Depending on hematocrit and wall shear rate, the maximum concentration can reach a value of five times that of the bulk concentration. Generally, the maximum value increases with both hematocrit and wall shear rate. More extensive discussion of the near-wall excess of platelets, as well as a consideration of the physical mechanism by which particles are preferentially transported to the vicinity of the surface, has been considered recently [96]. At present, the nature of the fluid-particle interaction forces that initiate and maintain such a heterogeneous gradient of platelet and platelet-like particles in the presence of red cells is not certain. The importance of such a gradient compared with enhanced platelet diffusivity also is currently unknown, although it is likely that the relative importance varies with changes in both shear rate and hematocrit.

Axial Position. The variation in deposition of platelets with axial distance has been measured primarily by use of a morphometric evaluation technique in which platelet adhesion at selected distances from the proximal edge of vessel segments was evaluated. At a wall shear rate of 800 s^{-1}, the slope of a double-logarithmic plot of adhesion versus distance from the vessel origin was significantly less (0.18) than predicted by a diffusion-controlled reaction (0.33). However, the slope was consistent with a transport mechanism that was intermediate between theoretical predictions for diffusion- and reaction rate–controlled adhesion (slope = 0). These results were, therefore, consistent with previous findings that platelet adhesion under such shear conditions is controlled by both diffusive and kinetic parameters [131,134] and that shear rates in the range of 650 to 1,000 s^{-1} are a transition zone for platelet adhesion in which the overall transport is influenced by physical and chemical factors.

Additional studies have been conducted at 200 and 2,600 s^{-1} [136]. In accord with theoretical expectations, at low wall shear rates the dependence of adhesion is stronger and at high wall shear rates weaker than those observed at 800 s^{-1}. Interestingly, when a more thrombogenic substrate than subendothelium (such as a collagenous matrix) is utilized, the axial dependence is enhanced significantly. These findings indicate that the upstream depletion of the boundary layer can have a major influence on subsequent events downstream. Highly reactive substrates tend to acquire significantly greater deposits proximal rather than distal to the inlet [137] (Fig. 5-25). The mechanism facilitating such deposition has not been studied extensively but is probably related to the direct impact of cells on the upstream aggregates, enhancing their growth rate and in turn depleting the platelet boundary layer downstream. The mechanisms by which such growth and depletion occur may be important to the overall process of thrombosis at sites distant from vascular injury and in fact may be related to the thrombotic deposits that are observed on vascular grafts (grafts are often

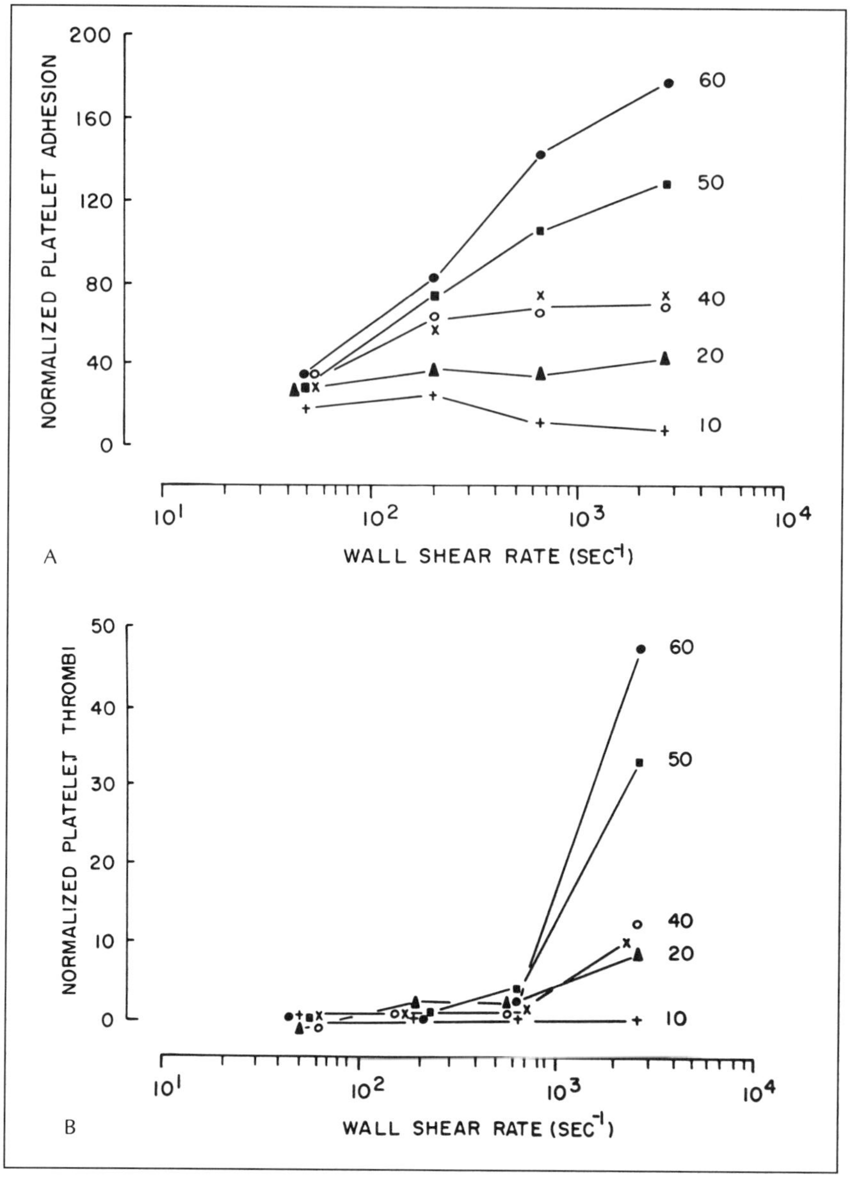

Fig. 5-24. Average values of platelet-platelet adhesion to and thrombus formation on subendothelium exposed in annular perfusion chamber to citrated human blood, reconstituted to various hematocrits. Wall shear rates ranged from 50 to 2,600 s^{-1}. Experimental results are normalized by exposure time and multiplied by a factor of 10 to yield hypothetical values at an exposure time of 10 minutes for purposes of comparison. **A.** Platelet adhesion. **B.** Thrombus formation. (Reproduced with permission from VT Turitto and HJ Weiss. Platelet and red cell involvement in mural thrombogenesis. Ann NY Acad Sci 1983; 416:363.)

located distal to an anastomotic vessel injury). Translocation of platelets from sites of active deposition and upstream activation of platelets [138] are events that have been described but not fully studied. It is clear that such events may be influenced significantly by fluid dynamic forces.

Direct Effect of Flow on Platelet Reactivity. It is generally assumed that flow and the associated fluid dynamic stresses have no direct effect on the chemical reactivity of solute molecules. For cells and large proteins, that assumption may not be valid, and there is growing evidence that platelets may be modified directly, in addition to having their physical interactions with surfaces affected by shear forces. It is well known that at an appropriate level of shear stress, platelet aggregation, secretion, and lysis may be observed [166]. Generally, the shear levels necessary to produce such changes are higher than those encountered intravascularly, but they may occur in artificial valves [67,166] or stenotic lesions [167–169]. Exposure time also contributes to the influence of shear stress, however, such that at physiologic shear stresses, times on the

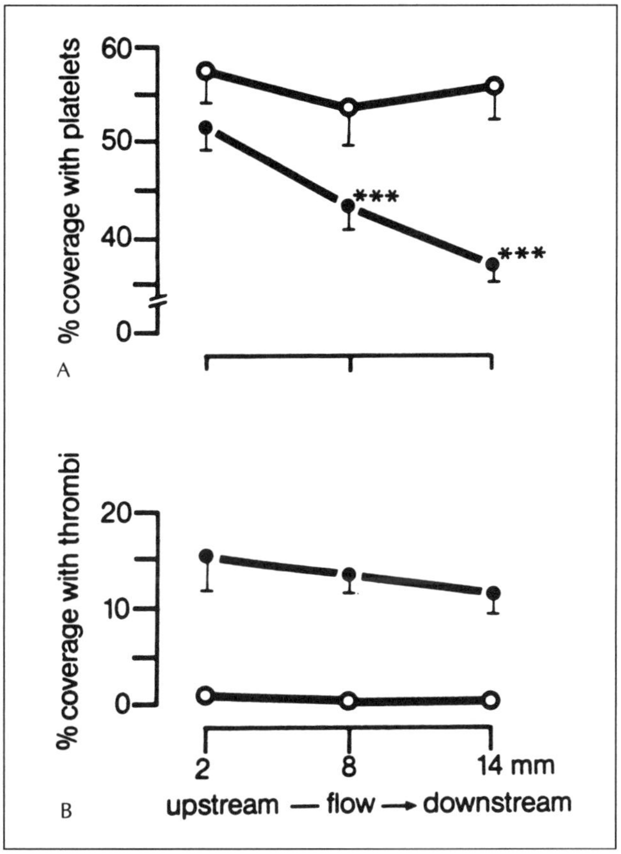

Fig. 5-25. Axial dependence of platelet adhesion **A.** and platelet thrombi **B.**, shown as percent-surface coverage. Human umbilical artery subendothelium (○) and collagen-coated coverslips (●) were exposed to human citrated blood flowing at a wall shear rate of 650 s^{-1} for 5 minutes. Platelet adhesion and thrombi were determined at three axial positions from the proximal end (0 mm) of the exposed thrombotic surface. Values at 8 and 14 mm were compared statistically with that at 2 mm. *** indicates p less than 0.001. (Reproduced with permission from HR Baumgartner and KS Sakariassen. Axial dependence of platelet-collagen interactions in flowing blood: upstream thrombus growth impairs downstream platelet adhesion. Arteriosclerosis 1989; 9:33.)

order of minutes can produce incipient lysis of platelets [170] (Fig. 5-26). While average transit times through the microcirculation—where wall shear rates are high—are short compared to the exposure required for lysis, two factors must be considered. First, platelets that interact with the vessel wall are those contained within the boundary layer where transit times are longest (due to the low fluid velocities near the wall). For instance, at a wall shear rate of 1,000 s^{-1}, a cell traveling with its center at an average distance of 1 μm from the vessel wall, where the average fluid velocity is 1,000 μm/s, moves only 6 cm/min. In general, the cell, except in bolus flow within capillaries [7], remains near the wall during its entire transit through the small vessels due to the lack of mixing at low Reynolds numbers (see Table 5-1), even where vessel branching occurs. Thus, individual cell residence times could well exceed the minimally required combination of shear and exposure times, especially in pathologic situations. Second, little is currently known about additional factors to which the platelets are exposed that might alter the relationship among shear stress, time, and lysis.

Several studies have suggested that shear stress may alter the procoagulant activity of platelets [171,172]. It is quite logical to suppose that biochemical mediators, perhaps released lysozymes from the platelets themselves or procoagulant moieties could facilitate the activation of platelets in a shear field. No studies of note have yet been performed in this area, and the interplay between chemical and physical factors resulting in alterations in platelet function is relatively unexplored.

PHYSICAL FACTORS AND BLOOD–VESSEL WALL INTERACTION IN NONANTICOAGULATED BLOOD IN EX VIVO STUDIES

Few controlled flow studies have been conducted in which both platelet–vessel wall interaction and coagulation occur simultaneously. In fact, few controlled studies have been conducted to determine the influence of flow on various aspects of the coagulation mechanism. The coagulation and platelet systems are difficult to study simultaneously because, although the systems are activated in parallel in the process of thrombosis, there are several key interlocking mechanisms. For instance, platelets or a phospholipid substitute enhance, by a factor of 10^4 to 10^5, the rate of activation of prothrombin by factor Xa, a critical

Fig. 5-26. The locus of incipient shear-related release of serotonin by platelets and hemolysis of red cells. Also shown are estimates of stress levels in cardiac valves and the normal circulation. (Reproduced with permission from Hellums et al. Studies on the mechanisms of shear stress-induced platelet aggregation. In A Hartmann, W Kuchinsky, eds. Cerebral Ischemia and Hemorheology. New York: Springer, 1987. Pp. 80–87.)

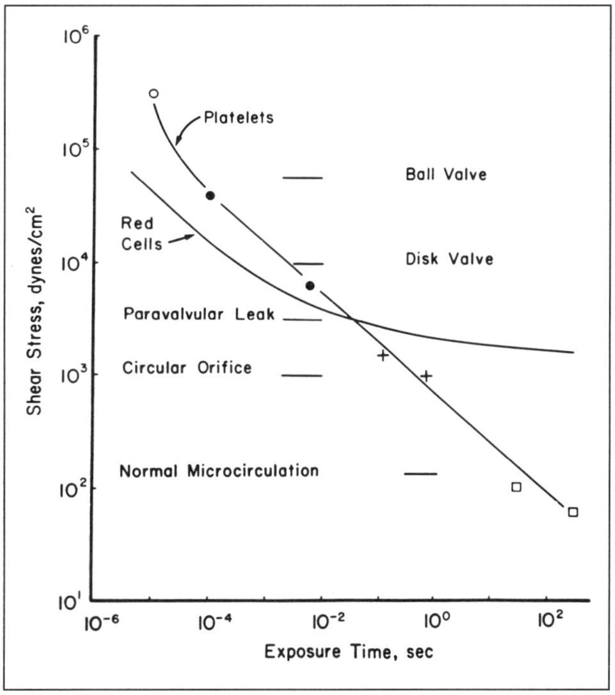

step in the production of thrombin [173]. Thrombin, whose primary enzymatic activity results in the conversion of fibrinogen to fibrin monomer, also acts as a powerful stimulant of platelet secretion and aggregation [174]. A major difficulty with the investigation of an active platelet and coagulation system is that each component, but especially the blood coagulation system, is sensitive to initiation by extraneous factors. For example, in most perfusion systems for exposing native blood to vascular substrates, blood must be drawn directly from the vessel through a venipuncture needle or catheter into the perfusion chamber. During this passage, blood can be activated by exposure to nonvascular materials, as demonstrated in the annular perfusion system by the generation of significant amounts of fibrinopeptide A (FPA) in the absence of any vessel wall [139,140]. In appropriately designed systems the activation is minor compared to that observed in the presence of a vessel wall [140], but the possibility exists that alternative or accelerated pathways for coagulation, and thrombosis in general, are generated separately from those developed intravascularly. As mentioned previously, the generation of certain procoagulant factors can indirectly influence the ensuing deposition of platelets.

Next, we will discuss studies performed with nonanticoagulated rabbit and human blood exposed to subendothelium from rabbit aorta in an annular perfusion system. The perfusion system is basically a model of simultaneous activation of both coagulation and platelet thrombosis, not necessarily an exact duplication of events that occur intravascularly. In fact, although platelet deposition appears somewhat comparable in the in vitro (citrate) and in vivo (native) systems [127,136], both platelet deposition and fibrin formation are somewhat enhanced on vessels exposed ex vivo [139,140], compared with intravascular studies of intact damaged vessels [153]. As in the previous sections, we consider primarily the physical aspects of platelet and fibrin deposition on vascular walls and the extent to which fluid dynamic factors influence the overall deposition.

Wall Shear Rate. Levels of platelet adhesion and thrombus formation obtained with native blood increase with increasing wall shear rate, as with citrated blood. In contrast, fibrin formation on the vessel wall, as measured by a morphometric technique, or FPA generation measured in outflow blood by radioimmunoassay, both decrease in value with increasing wall shear rate (Fig. 5-27). The platelet results indicate that the supply of platelets to the vessel wall by convective diffusion is favored over any potential removal mechanisms due to shear forces over the complete physiologic range of shear rate. However, the mechanisms underlying the decrease in fibrin on the wall and FPA in the blood with increasing shear rate are not understood. It is likely that removal of activated coagulation factors by flowing blood diminishes the activation rate of subsequent enzymes in the coagulation cascade. Thus, an increase in local shear rate (due to an increase in flow rate) brings more reactant (e.g., prothrombin) to the vicinity of the surface. The total amount of product that is formed at the vessel wall (thrombin) would be expected to increase according to some fractional power (0 to ⅓) of the wall shear rate (Eq. 17). Under such conditions, the bulk concentration of product in the fluid would actually decrease as the fractional power (⅔ to 1) of the wall shear rate due to the dilutional effect of flow rate. Thus, this reduced level of product (enzyme) may be less able to catalyze any subsequent activation reactions. Although this is a probable explanation, it has never been tested with coagulation reactions that occur primarily at surfaces (platelets and vessel wall), where the effects of dilution on local reaction product formation might be less important. Other mechanisms also could be postulated, such as a direct inhibition of enzyme-substrate reactivity, as has been reported for certain immobilized reactions [175–178], or a direct effect of shear forces on the ability of enzymes to bind to certain surfaces. More studies are needed to obtain a better understanding of the physical mechanisms influencing blood coagulation.

A comparison of platelet–vessel wall interactions in native blood versus citrated blood reveals several major distinctions between the two systems. With respect to platelet adhesion, levels in native blood are considerably lower than those observed in citrated blood at low shear rates but increase monotonically with wall shear rate to comparable levels in native and citrated blood at high shear rates (Fig. 5-28). It is interesting to note that the rate of adhesion does not diminish with increasing shear rate in native blood, as it does in citrated blood, but in fact appears to increase. Thus, the transition in citrated blood to a reaction rate–limited adhesion at high values of wall shear rate is not observed in native blood. The reason for this difference is probably related to the magnitude of thrombus formation induced in nonanticoagulated blood. In native blood, thrombi quite rapidly grow to considerable heights, compared to citrated blood (see Fig. 5-27), where thrombi rarely grow to more than 30 μm high [136,141]. This rapid growth of thrombus into the lumen creates valleys among the peaks of platelet thrombi into which platelets must be transported to adhere to the exposed subendothelium. Thus, increases in blood flow, by increasing the thrombus size (height), make it more difficult for the platelets to get to the vessel wall and so make it more likely that cells will attach to the growing thrombus rather than to the vessel wall. In addition, it is probable that a recirculation zone forms distal to the thrombus, as in Fig. 5-29, which shows a model of mural obstruction in a circular tube [114]. In such a region of disturbed flow, fluid velocity is very low near the base of the thrombus and in the reverse flow close to the wall. One would therefore expect the reduced adhesion rate in native blood noted at lower shear rates.

The continued attachment of platelets to the vessel wall at high shear rates, such that platelet adhesion in native blood may surpass that in citrated blood, is probably related to an alternate mechanism, namely, the deformability of platelet thrombi by high shear forces. As thrombi grow, the shear stresses on them are considerably enhanced. Analysis suggests that the shear stress acting to remove the mass is proportional to the local shear rate but that a clockwise torque develops, tending to detach the thrombus mass at the proximal edge. This torque is proportional not only to the shear stress but also to the

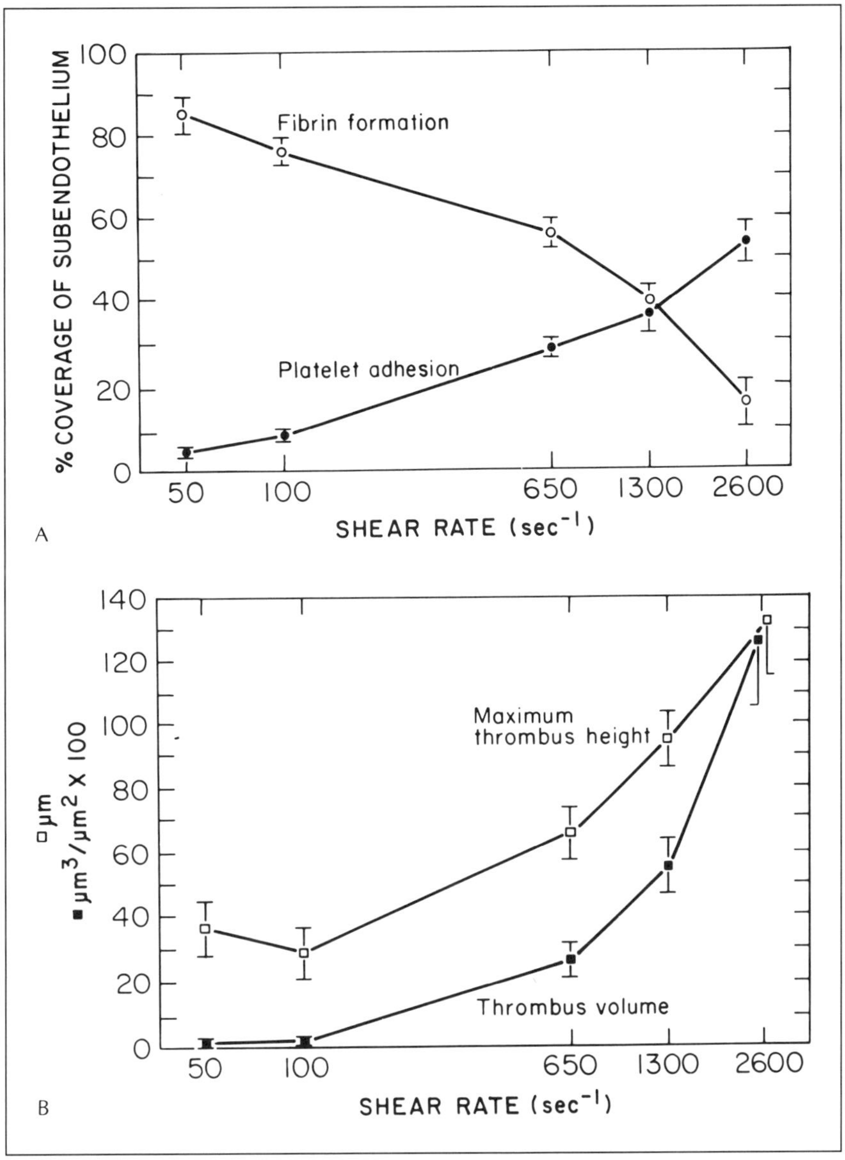

Fig. 5-27. Fibrin and platelet deposition on subendothelium exposed in an annular perfusion chamber to blood from normal subjects. Everted vessel segments were exposed to nonanticoagulated venous blood for 5 minutes at selected wall shear rates. **A.** The percent subendothelial coverage with adherent platelets (●) and fibrin (○). **B.** Dimensions of platelet thrombi, shown as the average height of the three tallest thrombi (□) and thrombus volume per μm^2 of vessel surface (■). (Reproduced with permission from HJ Weiss, VT Turitto, and HR Baumgartner. Shear-dependent role of platelets in promoting fibrin formation on blood vessels: studies utilizing patients with quantitative and qualitative platelet defects. J Clin Invest 1986; 78:1072.)

thrombus height to the third power [179]. This torque's strong dependence on thrombus shape may have important implications for determining the nature of thrombus growth patterns on vascular walls. Sakariassen et al. [142] have shown that cell deformability, at least on a collagenous substrate, can lead to a local bending of the thrombus peak toward the surface, thus generating additional platelet adhesion through a process that is related in part to platelet-platelet interactions. Although such deformation has never been directly demonstrated in native blood (aggregates on fibrillar collagen grow to great heights in citrated blood), it may well be that such a process of deformation can occur in vivo [143].

Other Physical Factors. Platelet diffusivity, platelet concentration, and axial position in native blood have not been much studied. Platelet diffusivity and platelet concentration cannot be manipulated easily in native blood experi-

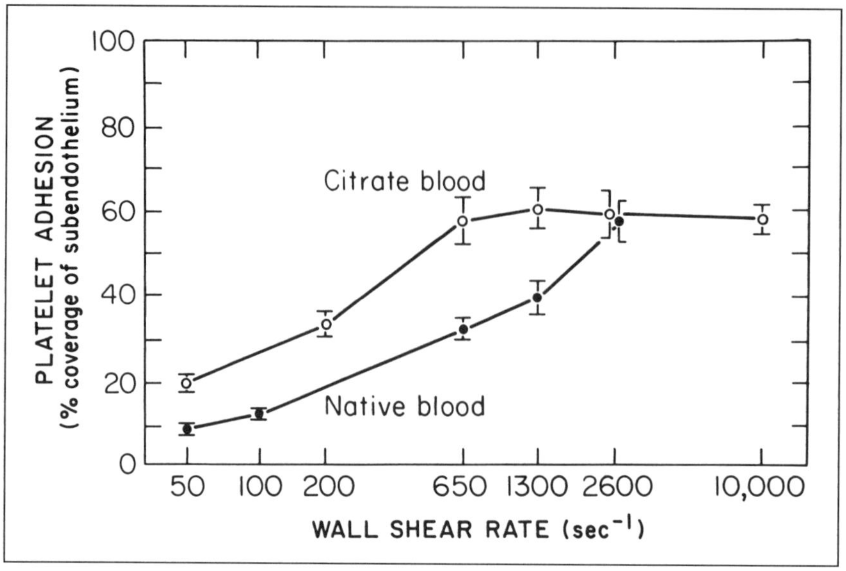

Fig. 5-28. Comparison of platelet adhesion on subendothelium in citrated and native (noncoagulated) blood. Vessels were exposed in an annular perfusion chamber for 5 minutes to human blood flowing at selected wall shear rates. Values of platelet adhesion were determined by a morphometric technique.

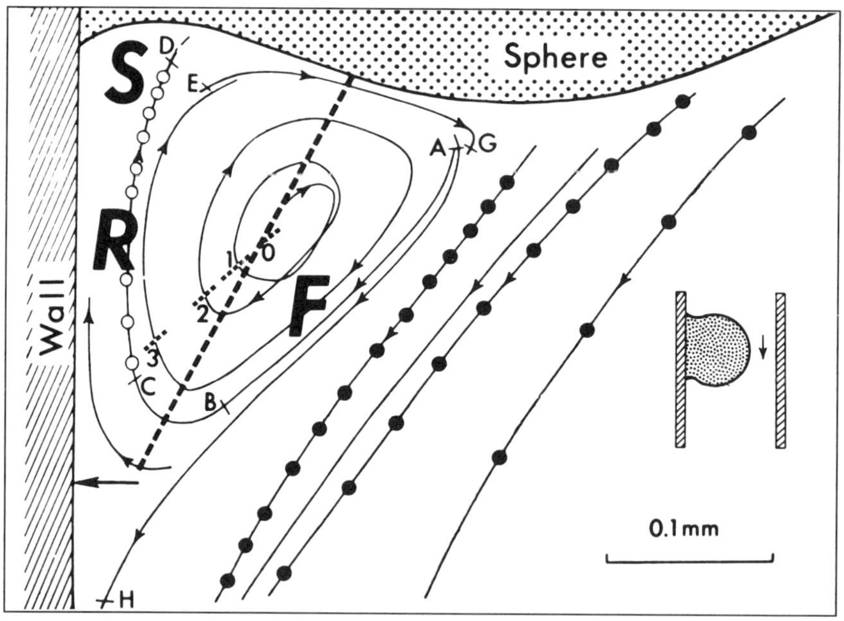

Fig. 5-29. A model of mural thrombus demonstrating disturbed flow distal to the obstruction. The model was made by fusing a polystyrene sphere of 0.65-mm diameter onto the wall of a glass tube of 1.05-mm diameter. A vortex forms downstream of the sphere. The spiral orbits traced by 30-μm microspheres are shown with the forward (F), reverse (R), and stagnation (S) regions. Particles spent long times circulating through the vortex: the times for the particles at positions 0, 1, 2, and 3 were 0, 0.8, 2.0, and 4.2 seconds, respectively. The mean linear flow rate was 31 mm/second, corresponding to a wall shear rate far from the obstruction of 240 s^{-1}. (Reproduced with permission from SK Yu and HL Goldsmith. Behavior of model particles and blood cells at spherical obstructions in tube flow. Microvasc Res 1973; 6:5.)

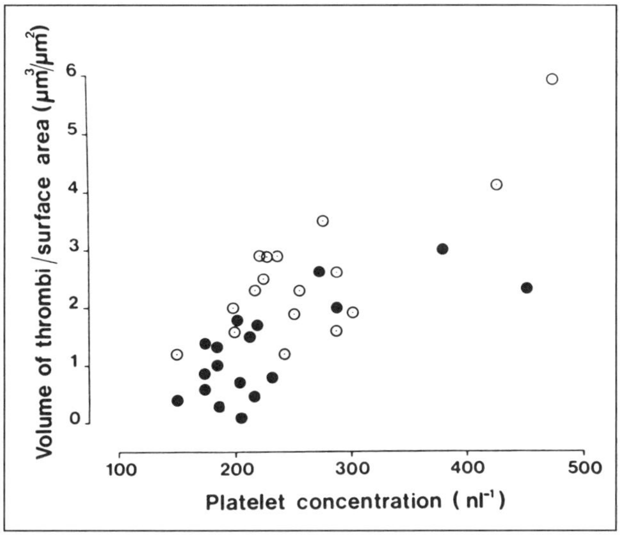

Fig. 5-30. Relationship between platelet concentration and total thrombus volume per unit area of subendothelium perfused in an annular chamber at 20 ml/minute (wall shear rate of 1,300 s^{-1}) for 3 minutes with native (○) or citrated (●) human blood. Values of platelet count are within the normal physiologic range. (Reproduced with permission from HR Baumgartner, VT Turitto, and HJ Weiss. Effect of shear rate on platelet interaction with subendothelium in citrated and native blood. II: Relationships among platelet adhesion, thrombus dimensions and fibrin formation. J Lab Clin Med 1980; 95:208.)

ments; thus, only naturally occurring abnormalities of platelet diffusivity (most likely related to red-cell abnormalities) or platelet concentration can be studied. (Such abnormalities, which are generally pathologic, are discussed in "Bleeding and Thrombotic Disorders," later in this chapter.) Direct dependence of platelet–vessel wall interaction on platelet concentration over the range found in the normal population has been demonstrated. As in citrated blood [144], the volume of platelet thrombi increased significantly with increasing platelet concentration (Fig. 5-30). Neither platelet adhesion nor the maximum height of platelet thrombi increased in this range of concentration, which suggests that heights of platelet thrombi may be limited under certain flow conditions, perhaps due to the level of the shear force acting at the peak of the growing thrombus.

No such correlation has been noted for the normal range of hematocrit (Fig. 5-31), but it must be remembered that the inability to control adequately for extraneous factors in native blood, such as the platelet concentration, may preclude the observation of any such dependence on hematocrit. (Variations of hematocrit beyond the normal range are considered in the next section.)

The existence of a radial concentration gradient of platelets or red cells in native blood has not been fully addressed experimentally, although in vivo there is evidence of red-cell depletion [86] and of platelet excess [93] near the vessel wall. It is logical to assume that the native-blood situation parallels the observations performed in vitro, but since the forces determining such a gradient are not well understood, it is difficult to say with certainty how a distensible vessel wall or the generation of procoagulant enzymes may influence this process.

Axial dependence of platelet deposition also has not been extensively considered with vessels exposed to native blood. Preliminary analysis indicates that the proximal-to-distant gradient may be steeper than that observed in citrated blood (Fig. 5-32). Such a finding would be consistent with the increased growth of platelet thrombi in native blood: larger aggregates could act more efficiently to intercept incoming platelets, leaving a local depletion downstream. The extent to which downstream effects persist requires additional study, as does the dependence of platelet deposition on axial position and the extent to which deposition may be influenced by either proximal or distal disturbances, such as would occur at sites of stenosis or intimal hyperplasia.

Interdependence of Platelets and Coagulation Factors. The interaction between platelets and the coagulation system becomes even more complex when local shear conditions are considered. Platelet deposition may be substantially enhanced when blood is exposed to subendothelium in the presence of an intact coagulation system (see Fig. 5-27B), but this enhancement varies with wall shear rate such that little deposition is observed at low shear rates, where fibrin formation is maximal, but deposition is maximal at high shear rates in the presence of minimal fibrin formation. Thus, although procoagulant moieties are probably responsible for the increased platelet deposition in native blood, the concentration of procoagulant material alone (as indicated by fibrin deposition or FPA generation) is not sufficient to explain the magnitude of the platelet deposition. Local shear conditions are also a major determinant in the growth and stability of these aggregates. The precise role of the shear rate in enhancing

Fig. 5-31. Relationship between hematocrit and total thrombus volume per unit area of subendothelium perfused in an annular chamber at 20 ml/minute (1,300 s^{-1}) for 3 minutes with native blood. Values of hematocrit are within the normal physiologic range.

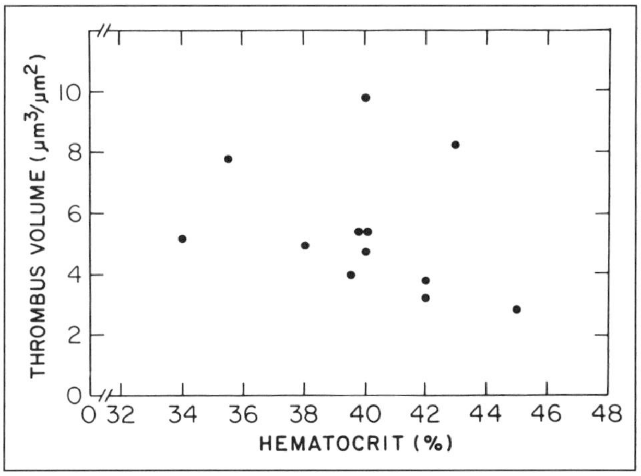

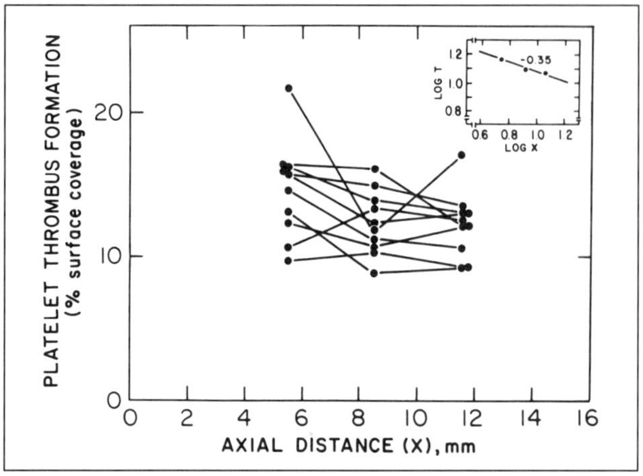

Fig. 5-32. Axial dependence of platelet-thrombus formation. Rabbit subendothelium was exposed to human native (nonanticoagulated) blood in an annular chamber at a wall shear rate of 1,300 s^{-1} for 3 minutes. Platelet adhesion values were determined at three axial positions: 5.5, 8.5, and 11.5 mm from the proximal end of the vessel segment. Inset: the dependence of thrombus formation on axial position in logarithmic coordinates (slope $m = -0.35$) using the mean values of the percent surface coverage.

platelet deposition in the presence of actively generated procoagulant material is unknown at present. One possibility, which is entirely untested, is that the magnitude of the shear rate alters the basic responsiveness of the platelet to certain agonists such as thrombin or ADP [65,180]. Laboratory investigations of platelet aggregation have generally been of the low shear–type (aggregometer cuvette) studies, which cannot address this question. Moreover, studies that have attempted to control the shear rate directly by studying platelet responses in various types of viscometers [67,72,166,167,181] have been conducted mostly at physiologically high shear rates and have not been directed at measuring the simultaneous effects of shear rate level and agonist concentration. Investigations in tube flow carried out at shear rates covering the physiologic range have, to some extent, addressed this question [56–58]. Nevertheless, more refined studies in this area are necessary to determine the influence of shear rate on thrombosis in vivo.

Also, little is known about the influence of platelets on the generation of procoagulant moieties. Platelets are a well-known accelerator for the generation of thrombin from prothrombin [174,182]. The mechanism for such an effect is thought to involve the binding of activated factors V and X to the platelet surface [183], but the precise importance of this mechanism in thrombogenesis is not known, and the extent to which platelets contribute to fibrin and other procoagulant enzyme formation has been studied primarily in static, closed–test tube systems. The importance of the platelet surface as a catalytic site for coagulation reactions is reinforced by the appearance of a mild bleeding disorder in a patient with abnormal binding of activated factors V and X to the platelet surface [183].

Bleeding and Thrombotic Disorders Related to Abnormalities in Platelet–Vessel Wall Interaction

The best evidence for the importance of a particular plasma protein or cell receptor in thrombosis comes from experiments of nature; that is, specific abnormalities in patients with either bleeding or thrombotic disorders have revealed much about thrombosis. Chronic bleeding disorders are more often encountered in the population at large (thrombotic episodes tend to be more acute due to often fatal consequences and are thus more difficult to study over time). The deficiencies observed in such disorders have served as the basic model for thrombosis, although abnormalities in the formation of a hemostatic plug, which is more often related to microvascular events, are not necessarily the same as large vessel thrombosis. The extent to which the abnormalities in various bleeding disorders can be characterized by use of perfusion flow systems helps to validate the use of a particular flow system and to define the importance of flow characteristics in thrombosis. More important, the precise control of flow and blood and vascular components permits detailed investigation of thrombotic mechanisms, which cannot be attained in static systems. Over the past 15 years, much has been learned about the importance of flow parameters in various bleeding disorders. In this section, we will detail patient abnormalities as they relate to the parameters listed in the previous section, "Influence of Flow on Blood–Vessel Wall Interactions." Little detail on biochemical mechanisms is presented, except for clarification or in cases where the mechanisms seem to be flow sensitive. (Such mechanisms have been reviewed [77,161].)

ABNORMALITIES IN PLATELET FUNCTION WITH RESPECT TO SHEAR RATE

The most studied blood-flow abnormality is von Willebrand's disease (vWD), a bleeding disorder characterized by abnormal or deficient levels of vWF in the plasma, platelets, and vessel wall [184,185]. Patients with classically severe vWD, who are deficient in vWF in the plasma and platelets, show reduced levels of both platelet adhesion [145,147] and thrombus formation [143,148,149] at high wall shear rates. The precise value of the shear rate at which the adhesion abnormality is observed differs slightly in citrated and native blood (Fig. 5-33) [186]. This difference is not completely understood, but it is probably related to the stability of initial interaction of the platelet with the vessel wall, a vWF-dependent interaction [150] that may be more stable in native blood than in citrated blood. Recently, the stability of platelet-platelet interactions at high shear stresses has been shown to depend on large-molecular-weight forms of vWF or platelet vWF [69,70,187]. These findings agree with earlier results suggesting a role of vWF in thrombus growth (platelet-platelet interactions), as distinct from platelet–vessel wall interaction [143,151].

A defect in platelet deposition in vWD in pigs also has been described [156,188]. The results are consistent with previous observations in human blood, with one exception: the total platelet deposition obtained in an ex vivo perfusion system in which heparin was used as an antico-

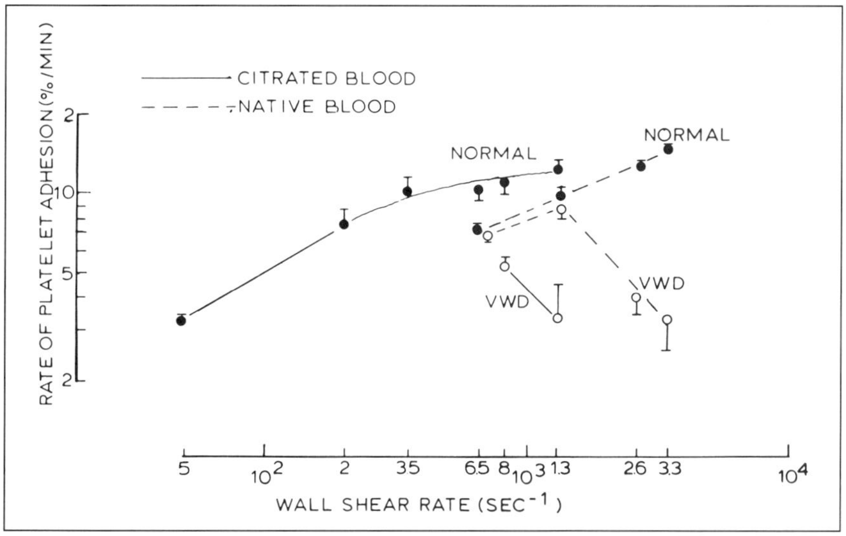

Fig. 5-33. Shear dependence of platelet adhesion in von Willebrand's disease (VWD). Initial rates of platelet adhesion are plotted versus wall shear rate, obtained when subendothelium is exposed to citrated blood or blood drawn directly from the veins without the use of anticoagulant (native). (Reproduced with permission from Turitto et al. Fluid dynamics, the Factor VIII-VWF complex and thrombosis on vessel walls. In A Hartmann, W Kuchinsky, eds. Cerebral Ischemia and Hemorheology. New York: Springer, 1987. Pp. 102–112.)

agulant is decreased in vWD even at low shear rates (200–400 s^{-1}). Although the precise mechanism is not clear, the defect in deposition is probably related to platelet-platelet interaction rather than platelet–vessel wall events [156]. Further investigation in these animals indicates that the nature of the perfusion system may be quite important in determining the precise values of the wall shear rate at which platelet interactions are inhibited. In vitro systems appear to be somewhat less sensitive than ex vivo systems for the observation of differences in platelet deposition between normal and vWD animals [155]. These findings are of some importance because the defect in platelet–vessel wall interactions, which is observed primarily at high shear rates, does not explain the protection afforded vWD animals from developing atherosclerosis of the abdominal aorta [189,190]. Mean wall shear rates in this area of the vasculature are on the order of 200 to 400 s^{-1} and thus should not be influenced by a defect in platelet adhesion or thrombus formation specific to high shear rates. In vivo studies are necessary to help determine the importance of platelets and vWF to the intravascular initiation and development of atherosclerosis.

A number of other bleeding disorders have been described in which platelet adhesion is abnormal [152,191] (Table 5-5). The deficiencies are comparable in vWD, thrombasthenia, and storage-pool disease but may be somewhat greater in Bernard-Soulier syndrome. Of course, such a comparison is limited to the conditions under which values are available. At different shear rates, relative levels may differ, which reemphasizes that certain abnormalities in platelet function may be more dominant in some locations of the vasculature than in others due to the local flow conditions.

Abnormalities in thrombus formation are also compared in Table 5-5. The abnormality in vWD is related to both platelet–vessel wall and platelet-platelet roles for vWF. The extent to which platelet-platelet abnormalities are distinct from platelet–vessel wall defects in Bernard-Soulier syndrome and storage-pool disease is not currently known. It can be observed that thrombasthenics fail to form thrombi under all shear and blood conditions studied thus far [135,139]. Of note is the absence of any defect in either platelet adhesion or thrombus formation in a patient with afibrinogenemia over a wide variety of flow conditions, indicating that, at least in those perfusion systems, fibrinogen is not an absolute requirement for thrombosis [143,146,151].

ABNORMALITIES OF PLATELET DIFFUSION

No direct tests of abnormal platelet diffusion have been conducted. The disorder in which an abnormality in platelet diffusion (which is directly related to platelets rather than red cells) is likely to contribute to the bleeding diathesis is Bernard-Soulier syndrome. This syndrome is characterized by platelets with a significantly larger diameter than normal platelets [191]. The enhanced size of the platelet could result in reduced mobility of the platelets through the blood (either by altering the platelet diffusivity or the radial concentration gradient for platelets). In fact, Aarts and colleagues have shown that when platelets and red cells are of comparable size little enhanced adhesion of platelets due to the red cells is observed [80].

An alternative possibility that has been little explored is that alterations in red-cell number, size, or shape (as observed in polycythemia, sickle cell anemia, iron deficiency, and red-cell disorders such as spherocytosis and other anemias) could play a role in the pathologic events associated with these diseases. For example, incidents of

Table 5-5. Platelet–vessel wall interaction

Blood condition	Wall shear rate (s^{-1})	Exposure time (min)	Normal subjects	Afibrinogenemia (AF)	von Willebrand's disease (vWD)	Benard-Soulier syndrome (BSS)	Storage-pool disease (SPD) δ[a]	$\alpha\delta$[b]	Thrombasthenia (TBA)
PLATELET ADHESION—% SURFACE COVERAGE									
Citrate	800	5	50	85	33	3[c]	50	20[c]	25[c]
Citrate	2,600	5	45	54	16[c]	2[c]	31	27	18[c]
Native	650	5	28	24	27	12[c]	42	25	27
Native	2,600	2	32	29	15[c]	4[c]	36	23	31
MAXIMUM THROMBUS HEIGHT—μM									
Native	650	5	76	78	59	25[c]	37[c]	27[c]	0[c]
Native	2,600	2	62	44	22	17[c]	26[c]	14[c]	0[c]

[a] Reduced contents of dense granules.
[b] Reduced contents of both dense and alpha granules.
[c] Significantly different from normal controls, $p < 0.05$.

both thrombosis and bleeding are a frequent occurrence in polycythemia [192]. In such patients, phlebotomy alone can significantly reduce the blood cell–vessel wall interaction (Table 5-6), suggesting that the treatment's ameliorative effect may be related to the reduced cell number. Conversely, bleeding is a frequent observation in uremia and can be corrected simply by infusing red cells [193]. The degree to which red cells can correct or bypass the variously reported platelet defects is currently under investigation in uremia as well as in bleeding disorders such as vWD, storage-pool deficiency, and thrombasthenia. Red-cell infusion or withdrawal may offer an alternative approach to therapeutic treatment in certain bleeding or thrombotic disorders.

ABNORMALITIES OF AXIAL DEPENDENCE

Studies of the axial dependence of platelet deposits as related to naturally occurring abnormalities of platelet function have not yet been conducted. However, several studies have demonstrated an altered (reduced) slope of platelet deposition on collagen surfaces versus distance when platelet function is inhibited with aspirin [137,194]. It is to be expected that disorders involving altered thrombus stability or platelet-secretion mechanisms are likely to produce reduced deposition and distance profiles. In fact, altered axial-dependence profiles may be a potential method for quantifying the extent of release reaction in perfusion systems.

Table 5-6. Blood–vessel wall interaction in polycythemia

Patient[a]	Hematocrit (%) Pre[b]	Post[b]	Platelet adhesion (% surface coverage) Pre	Post	Platelet thrombi (% surface coverage) Pre	Post
1	50	41	85.6	56.9	20.2	0
2	52	44	21.2	14.9	2.0	0.3
3	63	47	41.5	37.0	11.3	12.0
4	58	43	40.2	8.3	23.9	2.6
5	57	43	17.7	26.7	0.4	0.0
Mean	56	44	41.3	29.3	11.6	2.9

Citrated blood exposed in an annular chamber for 5 minutes at a wall shear of 2,600 s^{-1}.
[a] Patients were supplied by the Polycythemia Study Group, Dr. L. Wasserman.
[b] Blood samples obtained pre- and postphlebotomy.

FIBRIN FORMATION AND ITS ASSOCIATION WITH PLATELETS

The deposition of fibrin on subendothelium, with the concomitant production of FPA in the bulk fluid, depends heavily on the extrinsic coagulation system in flowing blood, perhaps operating through the factor-VIII and -IX pathway for activating factor X. At wall shear rates of 650 s^{-1}, for which moderate quantities of fibrin and platelets normally are deposited, the level of fibrin and FPA can be shown to depend on the presence of factors IX, VIII, X, and V but to depend much less on factors XI and XII [140] (Fig. 5-34). More recently, direct studies of the extrinsic system have shown that factor VII is also important for normal fibrin production and that treatment of human umbilical vessels with an antibody to tissue factor produces a dose-dependent inhibition of fibrin and FPA formation in the perfusion system [146]. At lower shear rates (50–100 s^{-1}), the requirement for factor VIII appears less evident, suggesting that pathways for the activation of coagulation may be modulated by the local flow conditions. The mechanism by which flow might affect such a control is currently under investigation.

Recent investigations have also demonstrated the complex effect of flow on platelet-induced coagulation. In studies conducted at 650 s^{-1}, the level of fibrin produced was shown to depend on the platelet number and the nature of the platelet membrane (Table 5-7). In thrombocytopenia, reduction in fibrin formation was observed only in patients whose platelet counts were below 5,000/μl (1–2% of normal). Thus, only a small fraction of the plate-

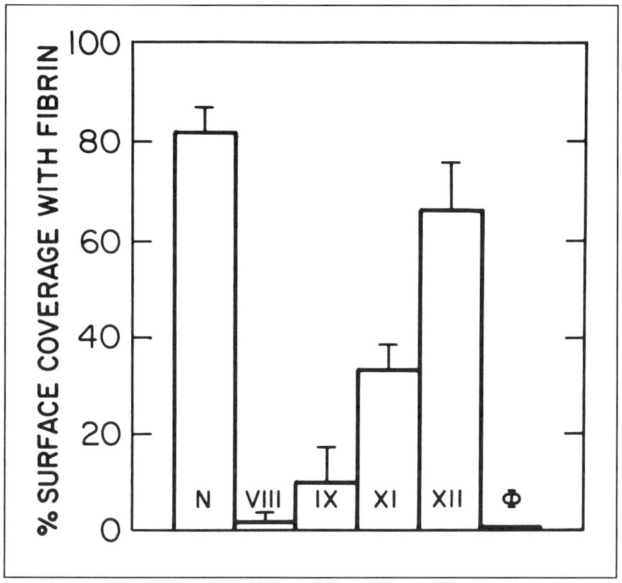

Fig. 5-34. Interaction of native blood with subendothelium in normal and coagulation factor–deficient subjects. Fibrin values obtained on rabbit subendothelium exposed for either 5 or 10 minutes to blood flowing in an annular chamber at a wall shear rate of 650 s^{-1} are shown for normal subjects and for patients with deficiencies of factors VIII, IX, XI, and XII and a single patient with fibrinogen (Φ) deficiency. For all subjects, the larger of the 5- and 10-minute-exposure time value was used to calculate group averages. (Reproduced with permission from HJ Weiss et al. Fibrin formation, fibrinopeptide A release, and platelet thrombus dimensions on subendothelium exposed to flowing native blood: greater in factor XII and XI than in factor VIII and IX deficiency. Blood 1984; 63:1004.)

lets need to be present to generate normal levels of surface-bound fibrin [139]. A patient with defective factor V_a-X_a binding to platelets showed reduced levels of fibrin formation on subendothelium under these conditions, which indicates a role for the platelet membrane in surface-generated fibrin formation. Interestingly, with this patient, as the deposition of platelets on the surface increased, the fibrin formation decreased. It appears that such a membrane defect in platelets may actually inhibit the production of fibrin by physically blocking activation sites on the vessel wall [139,146]. At lower shear rates (50 s^{-1}), the abnormality in fibrin formation is much less dependent on both platelet number and membrane characteristics. Thus, there appear to be three distinct flow regimes in which fibrin and platelet deposition may occur at different rates and perhaps through different mechanisms. At low shear rates typical of the low flow states in larger veins, such as in valve pockets [116], fibrin is deposited primarily through a tissue-factor mechanism, which is relatively independent of platelet-related factors. At intermediate wall shear rates, typical of the medium-sized arteries (650 s^{-1}), both fibrin and platelets deposit relatively quickly. The platelet component is enhanced by the number of platelets, but fibrin formation requires only a small number of platelets. Finally, at high shear rates typical of the microvasculature (1,300 s^{-1}), platelets are the primary thrombotic component. Fibrin formation is inhibited, but little is known about the mechanism of inhibition.

Summary

This chapter has attempted to present the fluid mechanical and mass transport mechanisms involved in thrombosis on vascular surfaces. The patterns of flow are complex and as yet incompletely understood, as are the biochemical mechanisms involved in the overall process of thrombosis. The systems developed to study such biochemical and fluid dynamic mechanisms are simple. They are in no way fully representative of the intravascular events, but they do represent major advances over previously used static or closed-flow systems. A great deal of information has been generated through the use of perfusion systems of various geometries that appears to be applicable to intravascular events. The evolution in the design of suitable systems is only in its initial stages, however, and is

Table 5-7. Fibrin deposition on subendothelium

Subject	*n*	Total (F_t)	On SE (F_{SE})	On platelets (F_{plt})	FPA (ng/ml)
		% Coverage			
Normal	24	76 ± 4	56 ± 3	20 ± 2	456 ± 34
Thrombocytopenia					
< 4%*	4	12 + 4	12 ± 4	0	498 ± 76
> 4%	6	82 ± 8	72 ± 3	10 ± 2	479 ± 87
Defective (FV_a–X_a) binding	1	14	12	2	196
Bernard-Soulier	2	50	47	3	274
Thrombasthenia	3	99 ± 1	74 ± 6	25 ± 5	620 ± 124

F = fibrin; SE = subendothelium; FPA = fibrinopeptide A formation in plasma. Everted vessel segments exposed in an annular chamber to native blood for 5 minutes at a wall shear rate of 650 s^{-1}.

* Patients grouped according to whether platelet adhesion (% surface coverage) on subendothelium was less or greater than 4%. Normal values of adhesion under these conditions are 80–90%.

Source: Reproduced with permission from HJ Weiss, VT Turitto, HR Baumgartner. Shear-dependent role of platelets in promoting fibrin formation on blood vessels: studies utilizing patients with quantitative and qualitative platelet defects. J Clin Invest 1986; 78:1072.

far from complete. Systems for incorporating additional complexities must be developed. For example, it is unlikely that significant clinical thrombosis ever occurs in laminar, streamline flow in which local shear conditions can be precisely defined. Areas of thrombosis are generally located at sites of vascular branching or in the vicinity of advanced stenotic lesions. Considerable information is available concerning the flow patterns and fluid dynamic stresses in the vicinity of such areas, but direct correlation with thrombotic events is less well documented [115,195]. Such areas are known to be characterized by low and high shear stresses in close proximity to each other, an event that is rarely found in streamline flow. The finding that very different thrombotic mechanisms dominate at these different shear conditions suggests that communication between the two activated systems (platelet and coagulation) may synergistically lead to pathologic results. Controlled experiments that define the relative importance of platelets and coagulation factors are prerequisites for a better understanding of the physical and chemical mechanisms involved in thrombosis. Rheologic modulation of the events involved in thrombosis is a relatively old concept that is only recently being supported by experimental findings. The pace has been slow, but current research promises a lasting influence.

References

1. Goldsmith HL, Turitto VT. Rheological aspects of thrombosis and haemostasis: basic principles and applications. Thromb Haemost 1986; 55:415.
2. McDonald DA. Blood Flow in Arteries, 2nd ed. Baltimore, Md: Williams & Wilkins, 1974. Also: McDonald's Blood Flow in Arteries, Theoretic, Experimental and Clinical Principles, 3rd ed. WW Nichols, MF O'Rourke, eds. Philadelphia: Lea & Febiger, 1990.
3. Goldsmith HL, Marlow J. Flow behavior of erythrocytes. II: Particle motions in concentrated suspensions of ghost cells. J Colloid Interface Sci 1979; 71:383.
4. Goldsmith HL, Skalak R. Hemodynamics. Ann Rev Fluid Mech 1975; 7:213.
5. Frojmovic MM, Newton M, Goldsmith HL. The microrheology of mammalian platelets: studies of rheological transients and flow in tubes. Microvasc Res 1976; 11:203.
6. Goldsmith HL. The microrheology of red blood cell suspensions. J Gen Physiol 1968; 52:5s.
7. Goldsmith HL, Mason SG. The microrheology of dispersions. In FR Eirich, ed. Rheology: Theory and Applications, vol. 4. New York: Academic, 1967. Pp. 85–250.
8. Goldsmith HL, Mason SG. Some model experiments in hemodynamics. V: Microrheological techniques. Biorheology 1975; 12:181.
9. Chien S. Biophysical behavior of red cells in suspensions. In D MacN Surgenor, ed. The Red Blood Cell, vol. 2. New York: Academic, 1975. Pp. 1026–1032.
10. Cokelet GR. The rheology of human blood. In YC Fung, N Perrone, M Anliker, eds. Biomechanics, Its Foundations and Objectives. Englewood Cliffs, N.J.: Prentice-Hall, 1972. Pp. 63–103.
11. Schmid-Schönbein H. Microrheology of erythrocytes, blood viscosity, and the distribution of blood flow in the microcirculation. In AC Guyton, AW Cowley, Jr., eds. Cardiovascular Physiology, vol. 2. International Review of Physiology. Baltimore, Md.: University Park Press, 1976. Pp. 1–62.
12. Goldsmith HL. The flow of model particles and blood cells and its relation to thrombosis. In TH Spaet, ed. Progress in Hemostasis and Thrombosis, vol. 1. New York: Grune & Stratton, 1972. Pp. 97–139.
13. Anliker M, et al. Noninvasive measurement of blood flow. In NHC Hwang, NA Normann, eds. Cardiovascular Flow Dynamics and Measurements. Baltimore, MD: University Park Press, 1977. Pp. 43–88.
14. Motomiya M, Karino T. Flow patterns in the human carotid artery bifurcation. Stroke 1984; 15:50.
15. Bollinger A, et al. Red blood cell velocity in nailfold capillaries of man, measured by a television microscopy technique. Microvasc Res 1974; 7:61.
16. Lipowsky HH, Kovalchek S, Zweifach BW. The distribution of blood rheological parameters in the microvasculature of cat mesentery. Circ Res 1978; 43:738.
17. Bird RB, Stewart WE, Lightfoot EN. Transport Phenomena. New York: Wiley, 1960.
18. Karino T, Goldsmith HL. Rheological factors in haemostasis and thrombosis. In AL Bloom, DP Thomas, eds. Haemostasis and Thrombosis. Edinburgh: Churchill-Livingstone, 1987. Pp. 735–759.
19. Karino T, Goldsmith HL. Flow behaviour of blood cells and rigid spheres in an annular vortex. Phil Trans Roy Soc (London) 1977; B279:413.
20. Schlichting H. Boundary Layer Theory, 7th ed. New York: McGraw-Hill, 1979.
21. Karino T. Microscopic structure of disturbed flows in the arterial and venous systems, and its implication in the localization of vascular diseases. Int Angiology 1986; 4:297.
22. Sohara Y, Karino T. Secondary flows in the dog aortic arch. In M Harada, ed. Fluid Control and Measurement. New York: Pergamon, 1985. Pp. 143–147.
23. Karino T, Motomiya M. Flow visualization in isolated transparent natural blood vessels. Biorheology 1985; 22:87.
24. Bharavdvaj BK, Mabon RF, Giddens DP. Steady flow in a model of human carotid bifurcation. Part 1: Flow visualization. Biomech J 1982; 15:349.
25. Zarins CK, et al. Carotid bifurcation atherosclerosis. Quantitative correlation of plaque localization with flow velocity profiles and shear stresses. Circ Res 1983; 53:502.
26. Karino T, Kwong HM, Goldsmith HL. Particle flow behavior in models of branching vessels. I: Vortices in 90°-T junctions. Biorheology 1979; 16:231.
27. Karino T, Motomiya M, Goldsmith HL. Flow patterns at the major T-junctions of the dog descending aorta. J Biomech 1990; 23:537.
28. Chien S. Present state of blood rheology. In K Messmer, H Schmid-Schönbein, eds. Hemodilution, Theoretical Basis and Clinical Application. Basel: Karger, 1972. Pp. 1–40.
29. Replogle RL, Meiselman HJ, Merrill EW. Clinical implications of blood rheology studies. Circulation 1967; 36:148.
30. Brooks DE, Greig RG, Janzen J. Mechanisms of erythrocyte aggregation. In GR Cokelet, HJ Meiselman, DE Brooks, eds. Erythrocyte Mechanics and Blood Flow. New York: Alan R. Liss, 1980. Pp. 119–140.
31. Evans EA, Needham D. Attraction between lipid bilayer membranes in concentrated solutions of nonadsorbing polymers: comparison of mean-field theory with measurements of adhesion energy. Macromolecules 1988; 21:1822.
32. Cokelet GR, Goldsmith HL. Decreased hydrodynamic resistance in the two-phase flow of blood through small vertical tubes at low flow rates. Circ Res 1991; 68:1.
33. Goldsmith HL, Mason SG. The flow of suspensions through tubes. I: Single spheres, rods and discs. J Colloid Sci 1962; 17:448.
34. Einstein A. The Theory of the Brownian Movement. New York: Dover, 1956.

35. Goldsmith HL, Karino T. Interactions of human blood cells with the vascular endothelium. Ann NY Acad Sci 1987; 516:468.
36. Chang HN, Robertson CR. Platelet aggregation by laminar shear and Brownian motion. Ann Biomed Eng 1976; 4:151.
37. Longmire K, Frojmovic M. Long range interactions in mammalian platelet aggregation I: Evidence from kinetic studies in Brownian diffusion. Biophys J 1990; 58:299.
38. Born GVR, Cross MJ. The aggregation of blood platelets. J Physiol (London) 1963; 168:178.
39. Frojmovic MM. Rheooptical studies of platelet structure and function. In TH Spaet, ed. Progress in Hemostasis and Thrombosis, vol. 4. New York: Grune & Stratton, 1979. P. 279.
40. Goldsmith HL, Marlow J. Flow behaviour of erythrocytes. I: Rotation and deformation in dilute suspensions. Proc Roy Soc (London) 1972; B182:351.
41. Fischer TM, Stöhr M, Schmid-Schönbein H. Red blood cell (RBC) microrheology: comparison of the behavior of single RBC and liquid droplets in shear flow. AI Ch E Symp Ser 1978; 74:38.
42. Brenner H. Hydrodynamic resistance of particles at small Reynolds numbers. In TB Drew, JW Hooper, T Vermeulen, eds. Advances in Chemical Engineering, vol. 6. New York: Academic, 1966. Pp. 287–438.
43. Karnis A, Goldsmith HL, Mason SG. The flow of suspensions through tubes. V: Inertial effects. Can J Chem Eng 1966; 44:181.
44. Segré S, Silberberg A. Behaviour of macroscopic rigid spheres in Poiseuille flow. II: Experimental results and interpretation. J Fluid Mech 1962; 14:136.
45. Cox RG, Mason SG. Suspended particles in fluid flow through tubes. Ann Rev Fluid Mech 1971; 3:291.
46. Cox RG, Hsu SK. The lateral migration of solid particles in a laminar flow near a plane wall. Int J Multiphase Flow 1977; 3:201.
47. Takano M, Goldsmith HL, Mason SG. The flow of suspensions through tubes. VIII: Radial migration of particles in pulsatile flow. J Colloid Interface Sci 1968; 27:253.
48. Goldsmith HL. Red cell motions and wall interactions in tube flow. Fed Proc 1971; 30:1578.
49. Goldsmith HL, Spain S. Margination of leucocytes in blood flow through small tubes. Microvasc Res 1984; 28:204.
50. Palmer AA. Platelet and leukocyte skimming. Bibliotheca Anat 1967; 9:300.
51. Eckstein EC. Rheophoresis—a broader concept of platelet dispersity. Biorheology 1982; 19:717.
52. Goldsmith HL, Mason SG. The flow of suspensions through tubes. III: Collisions of small uniform spheres. Proc Roy Soc (London) 1964; A282:569.
53. Karnis A, Goldsmith HL, Mason SG. The kinetics of flowing dispersions. I: Concentrated suspensions of rigid particles. J Colloid Interface Sci 1966; 22:531.
54. Brooks DE. The effect of neutral polymers on the electrokinetic potential of cells and other charged particles. III: Experimental studies on the dextran / erythrocyte system. J Colloid Interface Sci 1973; 43:700.
55. Chien S, Jan K-M. Ultrastructural basis of the mechanism of rouleaux formation. Microvasc Res 1973; 5:155.
56. Bell DN, Goldsmith HL. Platelet aggregation in Poiseuille flow. II: Effect of shear rate. Microvasc Res 1984; 27:316.
57. Bell DN, Spain S, Goldsmith HL. Adenosine diphosphate-induced aggregation of human platelets in flow through tubes. II: Effect of shear rate, donor sex and ADP concentration. Biophys J 1989; 56:829.
58. Bell DN, Spain S, Goldsmith HL. The effect of red blood cells on the ADP-induced aggregation of human platelets in flow through tubes. Thromb Haemost 1990; 63:112.
59. Goldsmith HL, et al. Physical and chemical effects of red cells in the shear-induced aggregation of human platelets. Submitted to Biophys J 1994. Published in October 1995 issue.
60. Klose JJ, Rieger H, Schmid-Schönbein H. A rheological method for the quantitation of platelet aggregation in vitro and its kinetics under defined flow conditions. Thromb Res 1975; 7:261.
61. Belval T, Hellums JD. The analysis of shear-induced platelet aggregation with population balance mathematics. Biophys J 1986; 50:479.
62. Belval T, Hellums JD, Solis T. The kinetics of platelet aggregation induced by shear. Microvasc Res 1984; 28:279.
63. Yung W, Frojmovic MM. Platelet aggregation in laminar flow. I: Adenosine diphosphate concentration, time and shear rate dependence. Thromb Res 1982; 28:367.
64. Gear ARL. Rapid reactions of platelets studied by a quenched flow approach: aggregation kinetics. J Lab Clin Med 1982; 100:866.
65. Goldsmith HL, Marlow JC, Yu SK. The effect of oscillatory flow on the release reaction and aggregation of human platelets. Microvasc Res 1976; 11:335.
66. Brown CH, et al. Morphological, biochemical, and functional changes in human blood platelets subjected to shear stress. J Lab Clin Med 1975; 86:462.
67. Hellums JD, Hardwick RA. Response of platelets to shear stress—a review. In DR Gross, NHC Hwang, eds. The Rheology of Blood, Blood Vessels and Associated Tissues. Rockville, Md.: Sitjhoff and Noordhoff, 1981. Pp. 160–183.
68. Ykeda Y, et al. The role of von Willebrand factor and fibrinogen in platelet aggregation under varying shear stress. J Clin Invest 1991; 87:1234.
69. Moake JL, et al. Involvement of large plasma von Willebrand Factor (vWF) multimers and unusually large vWF forms derived from endothelial cells in shear stress-induced platelet aggregation. J Clin Invest 1986; 78:1456.
70. Moake JL, et al. Shear-induced platelet aggregation can be mediated by vWF released from platelets, as well as by exogenous large or unusually large vWF multimers, requires adenosine diphosphate and is resistant to aspirin. Blood 1988; 71:1366.
71. Goldsmith HL, et al. Adenosine diphosphate-induced aggregation of human platelets in flow through tubes. III. Modulation by extrinsic fibrinogen. Thromb Haemost 1994; 71:78.
72. Dewitz TS, et al. Microaggregate formation in whole blood exposed to shear stress. Microvasc Res 1978; 16:263.
73. Vadas E, Goldsmith HL, Mason SG. The microrheology of colloidal dispersions. III: Concentrated emulsions. Trans Soc Rheol 1976; 20:373.
74. Chien S. Shear dependence of effective cell volume as a determinant of blood viscosity. Science 1970; 168:977.
75. Goldsmith HL, Karino T. Microscopic considerations: the motions of individual particles. Ann NY Acad Sci 1977; 283:241.
76. Turitto VT, Baumgartner H. Platelet interaction with subendothelium in a perfusion system: physical role of red cells. Microvasc Res 1975; 9:335.
77. Turitto VT, Baumgartner HR. Platelet-surface interactions. In R Coleman, et al., eds. Hemostasis and Thrombosis: Basic Principles and Clinical Practice, 2nd ed. Philadelphia: Lippincott, 1987. Pp. 555–571.
78. Feuerstein IA, Brophy BM, Brash JL. Platelet transport and adhesion to reconstituted collagen and artificial surfaces. Trans Am Soc Artif Intern Organs 1975; 21:427.
79. Grabowski EF, Friedman LI, Leonard EF. Effects of shear rate on the diffusion and adhesion of blood platelets to a foreign surface. Ind Eng Chem Fund 1972; 11:224.
80. Aarts PAMM, et al. Red blood cell size is important for

adhesion of blood platelets to artery subendothelium. Blood 1983; 62:214.
81. Aarts PAMM, Heethaar RM, Sixma JJ. Red blood cell deformability influences platelet-vessel wall interaction in flowing blood. Blood 1984; 64:1228.
82. Turitto VT, Benis AM, Leonard EF. Platelet diffusion in flowing blood. Ind Eng Chem Fund 1972; 11:216.
83. Wang NH, Keller KH. Solute transport induced by erythrocyte motions in shear flow. Trans Am Soc Artif Intern Organs 1979; 25:14.
84. Collingham RE. Mass transfer in flowing suspensions. [Ph.D. thesis, University of Minnesota, 1968.]
85. Walton CK, et al. Diffusion of urea in flowing blood. Am Inst Chem Eng J 1971; 17:800.
86. Phibbs RH. Orientation and distribution of erythrocytes in blood flowing through medium-sized arteries. In AL Copley, ed. Hemorheology: Proceedings of the First International Conference. New York: Pergamon, 1967. Pp. 617–630.
87. Bugliarello G, Sevilla J. Velocity distribution and other characteristics of steady and pulsatile flow in glass tubes. Biorheology 1971; 7:85.
88. Cokelet GR. Macroscopic rheology and the tube flow of human blood. In J Grayson, W Zingg, eds. Microcirculation, vol. 1. New York: Plenum, 1976. Pp. 9–31.
89. Fahraeus R. The suspension stability of blood. Physiol Rev 1929; 9:241.
90. Barbee JH. The flow of human blood through capillary tubes with inside diameters between 8.7 and 221 microns. [Ph.D. thesis, California Institute of Technology, 1970.]
91. Thomas HW. The wall effect in capillaries: an improved analysis suitable for application to blood and other particulate suspensions. Biorheology 1962; 1:41.
92. Tangelder GJ, et al. Localization within thin optical sections of fluorescent blood platelets flowing in a microvessel. Microvasc Res 1982; 23:214.
93. Tangelder GJ, et al. Distribution of blood platelets flowing in arterioles. Am J Physiol 1985; 248:H318.
94. Corattiyl V, Eckstein EC. Regional platelet concentration in blood flow through capillary tubes. Microvasc Res 1986; 32:261.
95. Tilles AW, Eckstein EC. The near-wall excess of platelet-sized particles in blood flow: its dependence on hematocrit and wall shear rate. Microvasc Res 1987; 33:211.
96. Eckstein EC, Belgacem F. Model of platelet transport in flowing blood with drift and diffusion terms. Biophys J 1991; 60:53.
97. Blackshear PH, Bartelt KW, Forstrom RJ. Fluid dynamic factors affecting particle capture and retention. Ann NY Acad Sci 1977; 283:270.
98. Grant L. The sticking and emigration of white blood cells in inflammation. In BW Zweifach, L Grant, RT McCluskey, eds. The Inflammatory Process. New York: Academic, 1973. Pp. 205–249.
99. Nobis V, Fries AR, Gaehtgens P. Rheological mechanisms contributing to WBC-margination. In U Bagge, GVR Born, P Gaehtgens, eds. White Blood Cells: Morphology and Rheology Related to Function. The Hague / Boston: Martinus Nijhoff, 1982. Pp. 57–65.
100. Vejlens G. The distribution of leukocytes in the vascular system. Acta Path Microbiol Scand [Suppl] 1938; 33:11.
101. Schmid-Schönbein GW, et al. The interaction of leukocytes and erythrocytes in capillary and postcapillary vessels. Microvasc Res 1980; 19:45.
102. Schmid-Schönbein GW, Fung Y-C, Zweifach BW. Vascular endothelium-leukocyte interaction: sticking force in venules. Circ Res 1975; 36:173.
103. Goldsmith HL, Karino T. Mechanically induced thromboemboli. In NHC Hwang, DR Gross, DJ Patel, eds. Quantitative Cardiovascular Studies: Clinical and Research Applications. Baltimore, Md.: University Park Press, 1978. Pp. 289–351.
104. Caro CG, Fitz-Gerald JM, Schroter RC. Arterial wall shear, observation, correlation and proposal of a shear-dependent mass transfer mechanism for artherogenesis. Proc Roy Soc (London) 1971; B177:109.
105. Fry DL. Hemodynamic forces in atherogenesis. In P Scheinberg, ed. Cardiovascular Diseases. New York: Raven, 1976. Pp. 77–95.
106. Glagov S. Hemodynamic risk factors: mechanical stress, mural architecture, medial nutrition and the vulnerability of arteries to atherosclerosis. In RW Wissler, JC Geer, eds. The Pathogenesis of Atherosclerosis. Baltimore, Md.: Williams & Wilkins, 1972. Pp. 164–199.
107. Reidy MA, Bowyer DE. Scanning electron microscopy of arteries. The morphology of aortic endothelium in hemodynamically stressed areas associated with branches. Atherosclerosis 1977; 26:181.
108. Roach MR. The effect of bifurcations and stenoses on arterial disease. In NHC Hwang, NA Normann, eds. Cardiovascular Flow Dynamics and Measurements. Baltimore, Md.: University Park Press, 1977. Pp. 489–593.
109. Mustard JF, et al. Factors influencing thrombus formation in vivo. Am J Med 1962; 33:621.
110. Mustard JF, Packham MA. The role of blood and platelets in atherosclerosis and the complications of atherosclerosis. Thromb Diathes Haemorrh 1975; 33:444.
111. Geissinger HD, Mustard JF, Rowsell HC. The occurrence of microthrombi on the aortic endothelium of swine. Can Med Assoc J 1962; 87:405.
112. Mitchell JRA, Schwartz CJ. The relationship between myocardial lesions and coronary artery disease. II: A select group of patients with massive cardiac necrosis or scarring. Brit Heart J 1963; 25:1.
113. Packham MA, et al. Localized protein accumulation in the wall of the aorta. Exp Mol Path 1967; 7:214.
114. Yu SK, Goldsmith HL. Behavior of model particles and blood cells at spherical obstructions in tube flow. Microvasc Res 1973; 6:5.
115. Karino T, et al. Flow patterns in vessels of simple and complex geometries. Ann NY Acad Sci 1987; 516:422.
116. Karino T, Motomiya M. Flow through a venous valve and its implication in thrombogenesis. Thromb Res 1984; 36:245.
117. Karino T, Goldsmith HL. Aggregation of human platelets in an annular vortex distal to a tubular expansion. Microvasc Res 1979; 17:217.
118. Karino T, Goldsmith HL. Adhesion of human platelets to collagen on the wall distal to a tubular expansion. Microvasc Res 1979; 17:238.
119. Macagno EO, Hung TK. Computational and experimental study of a captive annular eddy. J Fluid Mech 1967; 28:43.
120. Karnis A, Mason SG. The flow of suspensions through tubes. VI: Meniscus effects. J Colloid Interface Sci 1967; 23:120.
121. Turitto VT. Viscosity, transport and thrombogenesis. In TH Spaet, ed. Progress in Hemostasis and Thrombosis, vol. 6. New York: Grune & Stratton, 1982. Pp. 139–201.
122. Karino T, Goldsmith HL. Role of blood cell-wall interactions in thrombogenesis and artherogenesis: a microrheological study. Biorheology 1984; 21:587.
123. Cornhill JF, Roach MR. A quantitative study of the localization of atherosclerotic lesions in the rabbit aorta. Atherosclerosis 1976; 23:498.
124. Flaherty JT, et al. Localization factors in experimental atherosclerosis. In W Likoff, et al. eds. Atherosclerosis and Coronary Heart Disease. New York: Grune & Stratton, 1972. Pp. 40–104.

125. Reidy MA. Arterial endothelium around rabbit aortic ostia: a SEM study using vascular casts. Exp Mol Path 1979; 30:327.
126. Levich VG. Physicochemical Hydrodynamics. Englewood Cliffs, N.J.: Prentice-Hall, 1962.
127. Baumgartner HR. The role of blood flow in platelet adhesion, fibrin deposition and formation of mural thrombi. Microvasc Res 1973; 5:167.
128. Baumgartner HR, Muggli R. Adhesion and aggregation: morphological demonstration and quantitation in vivo and in vitro. In RL Gordon, ed. Platelets in Biology and Pathology. Amsterdam: Elsevier-North Holland Biomedical Press, 1976. Pp. 23–60.
129. Turitto VT, Baumgartner HR. Effect of physical factors on platelet adherence to subendothelium. Thromb Diath Haem [Suppl] 1974; 60:17.
130. Turitto VT, Baumgartner HR. Platelet deposition on subendothelium exposed to flowing blood: mathematical analysis of physical parameters. Trans Am Soc Artif Intern Organs 1975; 21:593.
131. Turitto VT, Baumgartner HR. Platelet interaction with subendothelium in flowing rabbit blood: effect of blood shear rate. Microvasc Res 1979; 17:38.
132. Turitto VT, Weiss HJ, Baumgartner HR. The effect of shear rate on platelet interaction with subendothelium exposed to citrated human blood. Microvasc Res 1980; 19:352.
133. Leonard EF, Turitto VT, Grabowski EF. The role of convection and diffusion on platelet adhesion and aggregation. Ann NY Acad Sci 1972; 201:329.
134. Turitto VT, Weiss HJ. Red cells: their dual role in thrombus formation. Science 1980; 207:541.
135. Weiss HJ, Turitto VT, Baumgartner HR. Platelet adhesion and thrombus formation on subendothelium in platelets deficient in glycoproteins IIb-IIIa, Ib and storage granules. Blood 1986; 67:322.
136. Baumgartner HR, Sakariassen KS. Factors controlling thrombus formation on arterial lesions. Ann NY Acad Sci 1985; 454:162.
137. Sakariassen KS, Baumgartner HR. Axial dependence of platelet-collagen interactions in flowing blood: upstream thrombus growth impairs downstream platelet adhesion. Arteriosclerosis 1989; 9:33.
138. Baumgartner HR, et al. Platelet adhesion: effect on surface properties and blood factors. Thromb Diath Haem 1976; 35:124.
139. Weiss HJ, Turitto VT, Baumgartner HR. Shear-dependent role of platelets in promoting fibrin formation on blood vessels: studies utilizing patients with quantitative and qualitative platelet defects. J Clin Invest 1986; 78:1072.
140. Weiss HJ, et al. Fibrin formation, fibrinopeptide A release, and platelet thrombus dimensions on subendothelium exposed to flowing native blood: greater in factor XII and XI than in factor VIII and IX deficiency. Blood 1984; 63:1004.
141. Baumgartner HR, Turitto VT, Weiss HJ. Effect of shear rate on platelet interaction with subendothelium in citrated and native blood. II: Relationships among platelet adhesion, thrombus dimensions and fibrin formation. J Lab Clin Med 1980; 95:208.
142. Sakariassen KS, et al. Growth and stability of thrombi in flowing citrated blood: assessment of platelet-surface interactions with computer-assisted morphometry. Thromb Haemost 1988; 60:392.
143. Turitto VT, Weiss HJ, Baumgartner HR. Platelet interaction with subendothelium in von Willebrand's disease: altered thrombus formation distinct from defective platelet adhesion. J Clin Invest 1984; 74:1730.
144. Turitto VT, Baumgartner HR. Effect of temperature on platelet interaction with subendothelium exposed to flowing blood. Haemostasis 1974; 3:224.
145. Baumgartner HR, Tschopp TB, Meyer D. Shear rate dependent inhibition of platelet adhesion and aggregation on collagenous surfaces by antibodies to human factor VIII/von Willebrand factor. Brit J Haem 1980; 44:127.
146. Weiss HJ, Baumgartner HR, Turitto VT. Regulation of platelet-fibrin thrombi on subendothelium. Ann NY Acad Sci 1987; 516:380.
147. Weiss HJ, Turitto VT, Baumgartner HR. Effect of shear rate on platelet interaction with subendothelium in citrated and native blood. I: Shear-dependent decrease of adhesion in von Willebrand's disease and the Bernard-Soulier syndrome. J Lab Clin Med 1978; 92:750.
148. Turitto VT, et al. Factor VIII/von Willebrand factor in subendothelium mediates platelet adhesion. Blood 1985; 65:823.
149. Weiss HJ, Turitto VT, Baumgartner HR. The role of factor VIII/wVF in the interaction of platelets with the vessel wall. In W Oates, J Hawiger and R Ross, eds. Interaction of Platelets with Vessel Walls. Baltimore: Waverly Press, 1985. Pp. 139–146.
150. Turitto VT, Weiss HJ, Baumgartner HR. Decreased platelet adhesion on vessel segments in von Willebrand's disease: a defect in initial platelet attachment. J Lab Clin Med 1983; 102:551.
151. Weiss HJ, et al. Fibrinogen-independent platelet adhesion and thrombus formation on subendothelium mediated by glycoprotein IIb-IIIa complex at high shear rate. J Clin Invest 1989; 83:288.
152. Weiss HJ et al. Interaction of platelets with subendothelium: a new method for identifying and classifying abnormalities of platelet function. Ann NY Acad Sci 1977; 283:293.
153. Badimon L, et al. Characterization of a tubular flow chamber for studying platelet interaction with biologic and prosthetic materials. Deposition of Indium-111-labelled platelets on collagen, subendothelium and expanded polytetrafluoroethylene. J Lab Clin Med 1987; 110:706.
154. Sakariassen KS, Bolhuis PA, Sixma JJ. Platelet adherence to subendothelium of human arteries in pulsatile and steady flow. Thromb Res 1980; 19:547.
155. Badimon L, et al. Role of von Willebrand factor in mediating platelet-vessel wall interaction at low shear rate: the importance of ex vivo perfusion conditions. Blood 1989; 73:961.
156. Badimon L, et al. Platelet deposition in von Willebrand factor deficient vessels. Extracorporeal perfusion studies in von Willebrand's diseased swine utilizing native and heparinized blood. J Lab Clin Med 1987; 110:634.
157. Cazenave J-P. Quantitative radioisotopic measurement and scanning electron microscopic study of platelet adherence to a collagen-coated surface and to subendothelium with a rotating probe device. J Lab Clin Med 1979; 93:60.
158. Leveque J. Les lois de la transmission de chaleur par convection. Ann Mines ser. 12, 1928; memoires 13:201.
159. Nam SC, et al. Rapid production of advanced atherosclerosis in swine by a combination of endothelial injury and cholesterol feeding. Exp Mol Pathol 1973; 18:369.
160. Stemerman MB, Ross R. Experimental arteriosclerosis. I: Fibrous plaque formation in primates, an electron microscope study. J Exp Med 1972; 136:769.
161. George JN, Nurden AT, Phillips DR. Molecular defects in interactions of platelets with the vessel wall. New Engl J Med 1984; 311:1084.
162. Turitto VT, Weiss HJ. Platelet and red cell involvement in mural thrombogenesis. Ann NY Acad Sci 1983; 416:363.
163. Reimers R, Sutera SP, Joist JH. Potentiation by red blood cells of shear-induced platelet aggregation: relative importance of chemical and physical mechanisms. Blood 1984; 64:1200.

164. Beck MR, Eckstein EC. Preliminary report on platelet concentration in capillary tube flow of whole blood. Biorheology 1980; 17:455.
165. Blasberg P, Wurzinger LJ, Schmid-Schönbein H. Micro-rheology of thrombocyte deposition: effect of stimulation, flow direction and red cells. In G Schettler, et al., eds. Fluid Dynamics as a Localizing Factor for Atherosclerosis. Berlin: Springer, 1983. Pp. 103–115.
166. Roschke EJ, Harrison EC. Fluid shear stress in prosthetic heart valves. J Biomech 1977; 10:299.
167. Anderson GH, et al. Platelet response to shear stress: changes in serotonin uptake, serotonin release and ADP induced aggregation. Thromb Res 1978; 13:1039.
168. Lee J, Fung Y. Flow in non-uniform small blood vessels. Microvasc Res 1971; 3:272.
169. Tiederman WG, et al. Turbulent shear stress from prosthetic heart valves. Trans Am Soc Artif Intern Organs 1985; 31:479.
170. Hellums JD, et al. Studies on the mechanisms of shear stress-induced platelet aggregation. In A Hartmann, W Kuchinsky, eds. Cerebral Ischemia and Hemorheology. New York: Springer, 1987. Pp. 80–87.
171. Wurzinger LJ, et al. Platelet and coagulation parameters following millisecond exposure to laminar shear stress. Thromb Haemost. 1985; 54:381.
172. Wurzinger LJ, et al. Shear-induced platelet activation—a critical re-appraisal. Biorheology 1985; 22:399.
173. Jackson CM. Mechanisms of prothrombin activation. In RW Coleman, et al., eds. Thrombosis and Hemostasis: Basic Principles and Clinical Practice, 2nd ed. Philadelphia: Lippincott, 1987. Pp. 135–147.
174. Mann KG, Lundblad RL. Biochemistry of thrombin. In RW Coleman, et al., eds. Thrombosis and Hemostasis: Basic Principles and Clinical Practice, 2nd ed. Philadelphia: Lippincott, 1987. Pp. 148–161.
175. Charm SE, Lai CJ. Comparison of ultrafiltration systems for concentration of biologicals. Biotech Bioeng 1971; 13:185.
176. Charm SE, Wong BL. Enzyme inactivation with shearing. Biotech Bioeng 1970; 12:1103.
177. Hsuanyu Y, Landler KJ. Flow kinetics of immobilized β-glucosidase. Biochem Cell Biol 1986; 64:139.
178. Tirrell M, Middleman S. Shear modification of enzyme kinetics. Biotech Bioeng 1975; 17:299.
179. Hyman WA. Shear flow over a protrusion from a plane wall. J Biomech 1972; 5:45.
180. Goldsmith HL, Yu S, Marlow J. Fluid mechanical stress and the platelet. Thromb Diath Haem 1975; 34:32.
181. Colantuoni G, et al. The response of human platelets to shear stress at short exposure times. Trans Am Soc Artif Int Org 1977; 23:626.
182. Bevers EM, Rosing J, Zwaal RF. Platelets and coagulation. In LV McIntire, RL Gordon, eds. Platelets in Biology and Pathology, vol. 3. New York: Elsevier, 1987. Pp. 127–158.
183. Miletich JP, et al. Deficiency of Factor-Xa Factor Va binding sites on the platelets with a bleeding disorder. Blood 1979; 54:1015.
184. Coller B. Von Willebrand disease. In RW Coleman, et al., eds. Hemostasis and Thrombosis: Basic Principles and Clinical Practice, 2nd ed. Philadelphia: Lippincott, 1987. Pp. 60–96.
185. Holmberg L, Nilsson IM. Von Willebrand disease. Clin Hematol 1985; 14:461.
186. Turitto VT, et al. Fluid dynamics, the Factor VIII-VWF complex and thrombosis on vessel walls. In A Hartmann, W Kuchinsky, eds. Cerebral Ischemia and Hemorheology. New York: Springer, 1987. Pp. 102–112.
187. Peterson DM, et al. Shear-induced platelet aggregation requires von Willebrand factor and platelet membrane glycoprotein Ib and IIb-IIIa. Blood 1987; 69:625.
188. Badimon L, et al. Influence of arterial damage and wall shear rate on platelet deposition. Ex vivo study in swine model. Arterioscler 1986; 6:312.
189. Fuster V, et al. Resistance to arteriosclerosis in pigs with von Willebrand's disease. Spontaneous and high cholesterol diet-induced arteriosclerosis. J Clin Invest 1978; 61:722.
190. Fuster V, et al. Arteriosclerosis in normal and von Willebrand pigs. Long term prospective study and aortic transplantation study. Circ Res 1982; 512:587.
191. George JN, Nurden AT. Inherited disorders of the platelet membrane: Glanzman's thrombasthenia and Bernard-Soulier syndrome. In RW Coleman, et al., eds. Thombosis and Hemostasis: Basic Principles and Clinical Practice, 2nd ed. Philadelphia: Lippincott, 1987. Pp. 726–740.
192. Wasserman LR. The treatment of polycythemia vera. Sem Hematol 1976; 13:57.
193. Goudable FF, et al. Low hematocrits and prolonged bleeding time in uraemic patients: effect of red cell transfusions. Brit J Haem 1985, 59:139.
194. Adams GA, Feuerstein IA. Platelet accumulation on collagen: drugs which inhibit arachidonic acid metabolism and affect intracellular AMP levels. Thromb Haemost 1984; 52:45.
195. Asakura T, Karino T. Flow patterns and spatial distribution of atherosclerotic lesions in human coronary arteries. Circ Res 1990; 66:1045.

Arterial Stiffness and Vascular/Ventricular Interaction in Humans

Raymond P. Kelly • David E. Gallagher
Lina L. Lee • Michael F. O'Rourke

The arterial system has two functions: the first is to act as a conduit, transmitting blood efficiently to tissues according to need; the second is to act as a cushion, smoothing the pulsations imposed by intermittent cardiac ejection so that flow through the tissues occurs in a steady, continuous stream [1,2]. The bulk of this book is directed at the first function and to the properties of blood vessels responsible for the transfer of blood. Disorders of conduit function result in ischemia to tissues downstream. This chapter is directed at the cushioning function of arteries and the disturbances that occur when that cushioning function is impaired by aging or disease. Because such disturbances have their main effect upstream on the heart, this chapter must properly consider ventricular-vascular interaction, that is, interaction between the whole arterial system and the intermittently contracting heart, together with therapeutic strategies for application in disease states. Thus, this chapter deals with the pulsations generated by the heart and cushioned by the elastic properties of arteries.

Recent studies of systolic blood pressure have drawn attention away from the resistance properties of small peripheral arteries, to the capacitative properties, or stiffness, of large central arteries [3,4]. The Framingham Study [5] has continued to show a more robust association between cardiovascular events and systolic rather than diastolic pressure. The European Working Party on Hypertension in the Elderly showed a consistent association between cardiovascular events and systolic blood pressure but no relationship between such events and diastolic pressure [6]. In the Systolic Hypertension in the Elderly Project (SHEP), there was a strong association between carotid plaque and low rather than high diastolic pressure. This has been confirmed in other studies [7]. SHEP showed that treatment of patients with high systolic (but normal diastolic) pressure reduces cardiovascular events [8]. High systolic pressure usually is caused by arterial stiffening; increased stroke volume is a less common cause [4,7].

Interest in arterial stiffening is by no means new, and recent studies showing the importance of systolic pressure are a return to the emphasis on arterial stiffening found in the literature early this century. Certainly in recent times, the preoccupation seems to have been with the diastolic pressure as obtained by the conventional sphygmomanometer, which appears to have distracted attention from systolic pressure [9,10]. The simplistic notion that diastolic pressure is a manifestation of arteriolar tone, with systolic pressure a manifestation of cardiac strength, has been attributed erroneously to Sir James Mackenzie [10]; in fact, that idea was slipped into the last edition of Mackenzie's classic textbook by his literary executor. Thomas Young (after whom the standard elastic modulus is named) was interested, as a physician, in arterial stiffening and described the relationship between pulse wave velocity and arterial stiffness in 1808 [11,12]. Richard Bright referred to arterial stiffening in his classic work on hypertension some 20 years later [13], while C. S. Roy in 1880 described the beneficial effects of compliant arteries in the young and the abnormalities that occur with age: "Only in the case of young children do we find that the elasticity of arteries is so perfectly adapted to the requirements of the organism as it is in the case of the lower animals" [14]. Nobel laureate A. V. Hill, with J. C. Bramwell, measured increase in arterial stiffness with age as pulse-wave velocity and described arterial stiffness (rather than peripheral resistance) as the major determinant of myocardial oxygen requirement as follows: "The amount of energy expended by the heart as measured by its oxygen consumption or carbon dioxide output has been shown to be proportional to the pressure developed . . . hence the amount of energy which the heart has to expend per beat other things being equal varies inversely with the elasticity of the arterial system" [15].

Physicians are not comfortable with arterial stiffness and usually prefer to discuss it in terms of systolic pressure. Certainly there are difficulties with the concepts and terminology used to describe arterial stiffness. Complexities are increased by the recent findings of differential effects of age and of drugs on larger, elastic arteries versus smaller, more muscular arteries [2,16–20] and by the recognition that altered arterial stiffness has major indirect effects (through altered wave reflection) as well as direct effects on arterial pressure [1,2,7]. It has long been recognized that arterial stiffness differs at different sites throughout the arterial tree, being lowest near the heart and highest at the periphery and that arterial stiffness varies with the level of intravascular pressure [1,2].

These same problems and related ones are germane to the consideration of systolic pressure. Systolic pressure depends not only on arterial stiffness but on stroke volume as well, which may be reduced in an elderly person with stiffened arteries and heart failure, even though systolic pressure remains normal or high. Under many conditions, systolic pressure is quite different in the brachial artery (where it is usually measured), compared to the left ventricle and the central arteries, where it has its major ill effects [2,16]. Still, clinicians have recoiled from detailed consideration of arterial stiffness and have settled with systolic blood pressure. Recent studies, however, provide a clearer understanding of arterial stiffness and its relevance to the circulation in health and disease. These studies are especially relevant in formulating strategies for treatment of older adult humans with hypertension, ischemic heart disease, and cardiac failure [3,21,22].

Definition of Arterial Stiffness

Arterial stiffness can be defined in terms of the mechanics of the material properties of the arterial wall or in terms of the capacitative function of the vessel as a whole. The mechanistic material properties of the arterial wall are measured by the **elastic modulus**. The term **distensibility** refers to the in vivo estimation of wall stiffness, while arterial **compliance** is a measure of vessel function. Such terms often are used loosely and interchangeably, resulting in confusion. The use of poorly defined terms such as **elasticity** further complicates attempts to define large-artery function.

The stiffness of any material can be quantified by Young's modulus of elasticity, **E**. The use of a physical quantity such as elastic modulus sits uncomfortably with many physicians, although Young's original work was performed on biologic materials such as the ligamentum nuchae [11,12]. Young's elastic modulus is defined as the relationship between stress (the deforming force) and strain (the resulting deformation). Stress is the force applied per unit area and hence has units of millimeters of mercury (mm Hg) or of dynes per square centimeter (dyn/cm^2). Strain is dimensionless, because it is a ratio that describes a relative change in dimension, for example, the increase in length from resting length, L_0, to a new length, L_1, or $(L_1 - L_0)/L_0$. Thus, elastic modulus has the same dimensions as stress. A readily deformable material has a low elastic modulus. Values of Young's elastic modulus range from $0.5–1.0 \times 10^8$ dyn/cm^2 for collagen, $0.4–1.0 \times 10^7$ dyn/cm^2 for elastin, to 1.0×10^5 dyn/cm^2 for maximally contracted smooth muscle, with arteries in the range of $5.5–31.0 \times 10^6$ dyn/cm^2 [23–25]. By comparison, most solids have values of elastic modulus of the order of 10^{10} to 10^{11} dyn/cm^2 [2].

The use of a material constant, E, in the evaluation of properties of the arterial wall in vivo introduces some assumptions and limitations. The arterial wall is not a flat sheet but rather a curved wall forming a tubular structure of a certain wall thickness. In vivo studies of arterial-wall stiffness have used a "pressure-strain" elastic modulus, E_p [26], with strain measured from the relative change in diameter. Thus, $E_p = D\Delta P/\Delta D$, where ΔP and ΔD are pulse pressure and pulse diameter, respectively, and D is the end diastolic diameter. Care should be taken in comparing published values of elastic modulus, since such pressure-strain measurements do not take into account possible changes in wall thickness. Other terms derived from Young's modulus to assess arterial stiffness are elastic modulus defined as the pressure increment required for a theoretic 100-percent stretch from resting length of a material; his **volume elastic modulus** is defined as the pressure step required for a theoretic 100-percent increase in volume (Table 6-1).

In seeking to explain the capacitative properties of arteries, physiologists have used the Windkessel model of the arterial vasculature. From that perspective, arteries are described as having a **storage** function that can be demonstrated by the pressure-volume relations within a given vessel. Related to the Windkessel approach has been the use of the term **compliance** to describe the capacitative function of an artery. Physicians are familiar with compliance defined as the change in volume for a given pressure change. Since arterial length remains constant over the period of measurement, arterial compliance is defined in terms of volume change per unit length, namely diameter or area change. Compliance is thus defined as the absolute change in diameter or cross-sectional area of an artery for a given pressure increment (see Table 6-1). As such, it describes the overall function of an artery but is at a level removed from the physical properties of the arterial wall. A change in arterial compliance may or may not signify a change in arterial-wall properties.

The distensibility of an artery comes closer than compliance to a direct measure of arterial-wall stiffness. Distensibility describes the in vivo function of the arterial wall due to its material properties. While it is not possible to measure precisely arterial distensibility noninvasively, it can be estimated by drawing on the capacitative model

Table 6-1. Indices of arterial stiffness

Elastic modulus*	Pressure step required for (theoretic) 100% stretch from resting diameter at fixed vessel length: $(P\Delta.D)/\Delta D$ in mm Hg
Arterial distensibility*	Relative diameter (or area) change for a pressure increment; inverse of elastic modulus: $\Delta D/(P\Delta.D)$ in mm Hg^{-1}
Arterial compliance*	Absolute diameter (or area) change for a given pressure step at fixed vessel length: $\Delta D/\Delta P$ in cm/mm Hg or cm^2/mm Hg
Volume elastic modulus*	Pressure step required for (theoretic) 100% increase in volume: $\Delta P/\Delta V/V = \Delta P/2\Delta D/D$ in mm Hg
Young's modulus*	Elastic modulus per unit area; pressure step per square centimeter required for (theoretic) 100% stretch from resting length: $\Delta P.D/(\Delta D.h)$ in mm Hg/cm where h is wall thickness
Pulse wave velocity*	Speed of travel of pulse along an arterial segment: *distance*/Δt in cm/s
Characteristic impedance*	Relationship between pressure change and flow velocity in the absence of wave reflections: $\Delta P/\Delta v$ in mm Hg/cm/s^{-1} where v is the flow velocity
Stiffness index	Ratio of logarithm (systolic/diastolic pressures) to relative change in diameter: $\beta = \frac{\ln(P_s/P_d)}{(D_s - D_d)/D_d}$ nondimensional
Capacitive compliance	Relationship between pressure fall and volume fall in arterial tree during exponential component of diastolic-pressure decay: $\Delta V/\Delta P$ in cm^3/mm Hg
Oscillatory compliance	Relationship between the oscillating-pressure change and oscillating-volume change around exponential pressure decay during diastole: $\Delta V/\Delta P$ in cm^3/mm Hg

* Site-specific indices that vary with distending pressure.

of arterial function. Distensibility is thus defined as the **relative** change in diameter or cross-sectional area of an artery for a given pressure increment. It is the inverse of the pressure-strain elastic modulus. Being a relative measure, distensiblity takes into account the resting volume of the artery. Distensibility comes close to being a measure of the material properties of the arterial wall, although there are still some limitations to this extrapolation [27]. A change in arterial distensibility with drug treatment, for example, may be interpreted as a change in material properties of the arterial wall, assuming other parameters such as wall thickness have not changed. A change in compliance also may indicate a true change in wall properties if the resting volume (or diameter) is the same for the control and intervention conditions.

The mechanics of the intact arterial wall are complex and difficult to measure. They are complex because an elastic modulus must be defined for radial, circumferential, and longitudinal directions as well as consideration of wall thickness. They are difficult because precise in vivo measurements of dynamic diameter changes are needed. Reading of the literature and interpretation of study results should be done carefully so as not to confuse the compliance of a vessel, the distensibility of the vessel wall, or the material properties of the wall as measured by its elastic modulus.

Following Young's definition of material stiffness, physicists set out to define an ideal "Hookean" material, that is, a material that has a linear stress-strain relationship over a given range, because of its homogeneous composition, and that is isotropic, having the same stress-strain relationship in any direction of deformation. The arterial wall, however, is nonhomogeneous (due to its collagen, elastic fiber, and smooth muscle components) and anisotropic (i.e., it has different elastic moduli in axial and radial directions [28,29]. Smooth muscle tone shifts the arterial stress-strain curve with a resultant change in elastic modulus at any given level of strain [30,31]. Arterial walls describe a curvilinear stress-strain relationship in the radial direction that is due to the variation of wall tension as a function of radius [28] as well as the nonhomogenous composition of the arterial wall [32]. Hence, arterial stiffness is a function of the vessel radius, which in turn is a function of arterial pressure. It is important, therefore, to define the operating pressure at which measurements of elastic modulus and distensibility are made [33]. Because of the curvilinear arterial stress-strain relationship, stiffness has been measured as the incremental elastic modulus over small increments of strain [34].

Because the stiffness of the arterial wall determines the speed of propagation of a pulse wave [2,11,23,35], arterial stiffness can be defined in terms of the pulse-wave velocity. Newton first determined that the velocity of wave propagation in a compressible fluid, such as air, was determined by the stiffness and density of the medium. That principle was subsequently applied to wave propagation in an elastic tube containing an incompressible fluid (or liquid) [2]. Since blood behaves as an incompressible medium enclosed within distensible arterial walls, the energy is propagated predominantly along the walls. The relationship between pulse-wave velocity and elastic modulus of the wall is described by the Moens-Korteweg equation:

$$c_o^2 = (Eh/2R\rho)$$

where c_o is the pulse-wave velocity, E is the elastic modulus, h is the wall thickness, R is the radius of the tube, and ρ is the density of the fluid in the tube. In a modification of the Moens-Korteweg equation, pulse-wave velocity can be related to the volume compliance of an artery by the Bramwell-Hill equation:

$$c_o^2 = (VdP/\rho dV)$$

where V is the arterial volume, dP is the pulse pressure, and dV is the change in arterial volume.

These equations assume a thin-walled tube filled with an ideal incompressible fluid with the absence of the effects of wave reflections and blood viscosity [36]. The errors in applying the Moens-Korteweg equation to large arteries filled with blood are small, and various modifications of the formula have not proved to be more accurate [2]. In smaller arteries, the effect of blood viscosity is to retard the true velocity of pulse propagation. The predominant variable influencing wave velocity in vivo is elastic modulus, with wall thickness, fluid density, and diameter remaining either constant or fluctuating to a lesser extent. In turn, elastic modulus is influenced by blood pressure [36], and changes in pulse-wave velocity track changes in mean arterial pressure [37]. In the absence of a concomitant change in mean pressure, a change in pulse-wave velocity is an index of change in arterial stiffness. Pulse-wave velocity measures the propagation velocity of the energy pulse imparted to the arterial tree by cardiac contraction and, like arterial impedance, is a pure measure of arterial properties, not of cardiac properties. The speed of propagation along the vessel wall (500–1,500 cm/s) is much faster than the velocity of blood flow within the vessel lumen (80–150 cm/s). The latter is a measure of cardiac function.

Techniques of measuring the pulse wave velocity are described below. Since measurements must be made in the absence of wave reflection, such techniques rely on the ability to measure a high-frequency component of the pulse wave given that there exists a frequency-dependent attenuation of wave propagation and hence wave reflection due to the viscosity of the arterial wall [38]. Wave reflections are an indirect effect of arterial stiffening and are discussed further in a subsequent section. The foot and the ascending portion of the pulse wave contain the high-frequency (>5 Hz) components of the pulse, which are free of reflected waves and can therefore be used for estimation of wave velocity. The foot-to-foot wave velocity is the most commonly used technique [35,39]. The time delay between two simultaneously recorded pulse waves is divided into the distance between the two measuring sites to obtain the pulse-wave velocity (see Table 6-1).

Arterial stiffness also can be defined in terms of parameters of arterial impedance. **Impedance** is a measure of the pulsatile pressure-flow relations in an artery, just as resistance describes the mean pressure-flow relation. Impedance plots are obtained from Fourier analysis of simultaneous measurements of arterial pressure and flow velocity expressed in the frequency domain [1]. The value of impedance at zero frequency is the total peripheral resistance, and impedance values at higher frequencies measure the pulsatile arterial load. **Characteristic impedance**, the average value of impedance at higher frequencies, is another index of arterial stiffness.

Another in vivo definition of arterial stiffness is the beta index (β) [40–42], which is based on the observed in vivo linear relation [43] between the logarithmic value of the relative pressure (P_s/P_d) and the distension ratio ($D_s - D_d/D_d$), where P is pressure, D is diameter, s is systole, and d is diastole. The slope of this relation is called the beta index. Since the beta index is based on relative values, it is dimensionless and describes, independent of pressure, the deformation behavior of the arterial wall during the cardiac cycle.

Finally, a modified Windkessel model of the vasculature, incorporating inductance terms, has been used to define **capacitative** and **oscillatory compliance** components of the arterial vasculature. This approach is based on contour analysis of the arterial-pressure-wave and cardiac-output measurements, to determine to distal compartment compliance [44,45]. Capacitative compliance describes the relationship between the fall in pressure and the fall in volume during the exponential component of diastolic pressure decay. Oscillatory compliance describes the relationship between the oscillating-pressure change and the oscillating-volume change around the exponential relation.

Measurements of Arterial Stiffness

Three general approaches are followed to measure arterial stiffness in vivo: measurement of arterial diameter and pressure change during the cardiac cycle, measurement of wave transmission along an arterial segment, and assessment of chamber distensiblity using diastolic pressure waveform analysis and a modified Windkessel model.

In the first approach, techniques have been used that measure either arterial diameter or volume change. Change in arterial volume traditionally has been easier to measure in vivo than change in arterial diameter. Plethysmographic techniques have been most commonly employed [46–50]. By necessity, the arteries most amenable to these techniques are found in the limbs and the digits. These techniques measure change in volume of the underlying segment and as such provide an indirect measure of change in arterial volume. Techniques to measure arterial-diameter change have included angiography [51], magnetic resonance imaging [52], ultrasound scanning using either Doppler or B-mode scanning [42,53–55], and phase-locked wall tracking using radio frequency signals [56,57]. To measure stiffness, these volume or diameter measurements are coupled with blood-pressure data obtained invasively [46,51] or noninvasively using, in the latter case, either brachial sphygmomanometry or more recently volume clamping techniques [57]. In most cases, blood pressure is recorded at a site apart from the vessel being investigated. Under those circumstances, it is assumed that the difference in pressure values between sites is small and can be neglected [57], an assumption that may not be valid in all situations.

When either pressure or volume data are discontinuous (i.e., only systolic and diastolic values for diameter, volume, and/or pressure changes are available), then results are expressed in the form of the pressure-strain elastic modulus, E_p. Attempts to normalize these values by comparing data at different levels of wall stress by varying external transmural pressure also have been performed [46,49,58]. When continuous diameter, volume, and pressure data are obtained, then results may be displayed as pressure-volume loops [46,59] or as compliance plotted against arterial pressure [57,60].

The second approach in measuring arterial stiffness is to assess arterial stiffness from the velocity of pulse-wave propagation along an arterial segment. Pulse-wave velocity can be measured directly in the time domain. Alternatively, characteristic impedance and phase velocity can be measured in the frequency domain and the pulse-wave velocity and elastic modulus subsequently determined from known formulas [23,36]. One difference between pulse-wave-velocity techniques and those based on local diameter-pressure measurements is that propagative techniques estimate the distensibilty of a given segment, while diameter-pressure measurements provide values for a particular site. It may be expected that pulse-wave-velocity measurements are less susceptible to local variation in wall properties [61,62].

Pulse-wave velocity traditionally is measured by the foot-to-foot delay of waveforms recorded a known distance apart. Pressure, flow, and diameter waveforms have been used, the velocity of propagation along the arterial wall being the same for each. Techniques for identification of the wavefront include the intersection of tangents between the late diastolic portion of the pressure wave and the ascending limb of the pressure wave and identification of the point of maximum rate of pressure rise on the ascending limb [63]. Both noninvasive [35,37,39,41,64] and invasive techniques [65,66] have been used to measure the time delay between two pulses. Invasive techniques have measured pulse-wave velocity directly through the use of a series of catheter-mounted transducers or indirectly by derivation of apparent phase velocity and values of characteristic impedance from the high-frequency components of the input impedance [67–69]. More recently, techniques have been described that assess input impedance noninvasively from the ascending aorta [70] and the femoral [71] arteries using a combination of applanation tonometry and Doppler ultrasound.

Given the blood pressure dependence of pulse-wave velocity, techniques have been devised to measure wave velocity after adjusting transmural pressure in a pressurized chamber [72,73]. This technique is suitable only for limb measurements. Other investigators have relied on population studies in which groups with similar blood pressures were compared [39,74].

The third method of estimation of arterial stiffness uses the contour of the aortic-pressure wave together with a lumped parameter model of the circulation such as the Windkessel model or a modification of it. Analysis of the arterial-pressure wave generally assumes an exponential diastolic pressure decay [44–46]. Mathematical techniques have been developed to overcome this assumption [75]. The development of high-fidelity transcutaneous pulse recorders [76] has allowed compliance estimates to be made noninvasively in combination with echo-Doppler derived estimates of cardiac output.

Structure and Function

The mechanical properties of arteries depend on the structure of the media that composes that part of the artery between the internal elastic lamella to which intimal cells are attached and the external elastic lamella [32,77–80]. The main components of the arterial media are elastic fibers, collagen fibers, and smooth muscle. Normally, all these components are arranged in a series of musculoelastic fascicles [79]. Most sections of arteries with which physicians are familiar show the elastic fibers as corrugated wavy lines, but that is not how they exist in life. When arteries are fixed at normal distending pressure of around 100 mm Hg, the elastic fibers are straight and run circumferentially around the artery; the intevening collagenous fibers are arranged in a more irregular fashion, together with thinner connecting fibers among the smooth muscle cells [79]. The principal feature of stress-strain relationships in arteries described here is a consequence of this two-phase arrangement of elastic and collagen fibers in the arterial wall [32,77,78]. At low levels of pressure in the artery, and thus of stress in the wall, the load is borne predominantly by the elastic fibers, and elastic modulus is low. As pressure and wall stretch increase, the collagen fibers are progressively recruited, and elastic modulus increases. At high pressure, the collagen fibers are fully recruited, and the artery behaves as though it were composed of collagen alone; it is very stiff [80].

The two-phase structure of arteries is of substantial importance to arterial function and structural integrity. At normal levels of pressure and in young healthy subjects, elastic fibers are stretched with minimal involvement of collagen [80]. The elastic fibers thus are responsible for normal arterial distensibility. The role of the collagen fibers is to prevent excessive stretch and to prevent sudden rupture of the artery if arterial pressure momentarily rises to very high levels. Acute arterial rupture occurs only when the collagenous protecting network gives way.

These paragraphs apply to an artery that is exposed to variable intraluminal pressure, and when it behaves passively in accord with the known properties of its collagenous and elastic components. Such features are seen in the many in vitro studies of arteries after removal from the body [2,31,33]. In vivo, the mechanical properties of elastic and collagenous fibers are modified by smooth muscle in the arterial wall. Studies of arterial distensibility and stiffness in vivo often have given quite different results to those obtained in vitro; the difference can be attributed to effects of smooth muscle tone [81]. It has been well established that an artery of a fixed muscular tone in vitro always becomes stiffer when its diameter is increased passively [31]. In contrast, an artery such as the brachial, radial or femoral, which dilates under the influence of a drug such as nitroglycerin, becomes more compliant [20,82–85]. Such an effect is a consequence of smooth muscle relaxation in the vessel wall. When there is a change in the contractility of vascular smooth muscle, the mechanical properties of the arterial wall also change, and the arterial wall behaves like one composed of different materials [31]. In that case, it is explained on the basis of alignment and interconnection of muscle cells with collagen and elastic fibers in the vessel wall [2,86]. From a functional viewpoint, it appears that the muscle cells behave as though in series with the collagenous fibers but in parallel with the elastic fibers. Hence, muscle contraction and increased tone transfer stress from the elastic to the collagenous fibers, making the arterial wall stiffer, whereas decrease in muscular tone unloads the collagen fibers and transfers stresses back to the elastic fibers so that the artery appears to the more compliant and less stiff [87].

Table 6-2. Comparison of properties of large elastic arteries and smaller muscular arteries

	Elastic arteries	Muscular arteries
SITE	Aorta, carotid, brachiocephalic	All others
DILATATION	~10%	~3%
MEDIAL DEGENERATION	+++	+
VASODILATOR EFFECT	+	+++

All arteries contain smooth muscle, even the ascending aorta. But the smooth muscle in the aorta and the large proximal arteries (brachiocephalic, carotid) appears to be relatively inactive. These vessels are minimally affected by vasodilator agents; there is little effect of such drugs on their caliber or distensibility [2,20,84,88–92]. In contrast, peripheral arteries leading down to the arterioles have a media that is almost exclusively muscular without significant amounts of elastic or collagen (Table 6-2). These arteries are more influenced by vasomotor influences [2,20,46,84,87,93,94]. Properties of the arterioles themselves are dominated by smooth muscle, whose tone regulates arterial flow and controls peripheral resistance. In the larger conduit arteries, smooth muscle tone modulates arterial distensibility. Its major role, however, appears to be a local one: to contract vigorously to prevent massive blood loss in the event of traumatic disruption.

The major large conduit arteries are often spoken of as being elastic or muscular, even though they all contain a mixture of collagen and elastic fibers and muscle. But the distinction is useful in structural and functional terms. The predominantly elastic arteries (aorta, brachiocephalic, carotid) normally, in young persons, dilate by 10–15 percent with each pulsation (see Table 6-2) [2,17]. They are predominantly responsible for the cushioning function of the arterial tree. Stiffness increases progressively along the abdominal aorta and in the peripheral arteries. The lower abdominal aorta, femoral artery, and brachial artery pulsate by around 5 percent in young subjects and the radial artery by only around 2 percent, despite increase

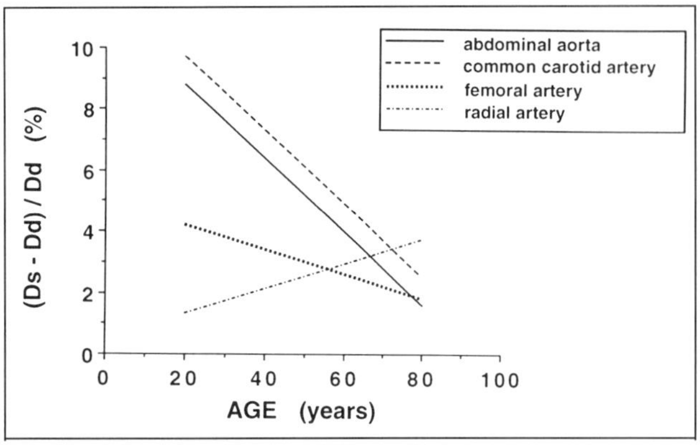

Fig. 6-1. The effects of age on the relative diameter change along the arterial tree. There is a decrease in the relative diameter change with age in the larger, more elastic arteries such as the common carotid artery and abdominal aorta. In the more muscular arteries, this reduction in relative diameter change is less pronounced (as observed in the femoral artery) or shows an opposite trend (as observed in the radial artery) with age. There is no significant change in the brachial artery, where relative diameter change lies around 5 percent. Ds = end-systolic diameter, Dd = end-diastolic diameter. Graph drawn from the data presented in P Boutouyrie, et al. Opposing effects of ageing on distal and proximal large arteries in hypertensives. J Hypertens 1992; 10[Suppl 6]:S87–S91.

of pulse pressure in the peripheral arteries [2,17,95–97]. Their major role is as a conduit, to transport blood to the peripheral arterioles and capillaries. They play a minor direct role in the arterial cushioning function.

An important physiologic modulator of arterial smooth muscle tone is the function of the intact endothelium [98–105]. A full discussion of the influence of endothelial-derived factors on arterial smooth muscle function is beyond the scope of this chapter. It is clear, however, that mechanical stretch and receptor-mediated release of endothelial vasoconstrictor and dilator substances provide an important local control mechanism that is modulated by reflex and hormonal influences and that changes with age and disease states. The net result is the integrated level of arterial function and stiffness, which this chapter addresses.

Effects of Age in Humans

With aging in humans, the aorta and predominantly elastic central arteries dilate and stiffen [1,2,15,39,106–108]. These changes are progressive from adolescence. Changes in peripheral muscular arteries are far less marked (Fig. 6-1) [17,95–97,106]. These aging changes are not apparent in experimental animals [1,2], although they recently have been observed in older birds whose history of cumulative cylic stresses approximates that in older humans [109]. The surface area of the aorta (Fig. 6-2) [108] and the pulse-wave velocity [106] double between 18 and 80 years of age (Fig. 6-3). In childhood and adolescence, pulse-wave velocity in the aorta is approximately half that in the brachial artery, whereas by the eighth decade, wave velocity is much the same, at around 13 m/second in the aorta and in the arterial system of upper and lower limbs [39,106]. Progressive dilation of the aorta, but not of iliac arteries, results in decrease in the ratio of daughter-to-parent-vessels cross-sectional areas at the aortic bifurcation with advancing years [110]. That and the relatively great dilation of the thoracic compared to abdominal aorta with age [111] can explain relatively high wave reflection in the aortic region of older human subjects [65]. It also may be relevant to the the predilection for the development of atherosclerotic aneurysms at that site [2].

Stiffening and dilation of the aorta and elastic arteries with age in humans is associated with and doubtless due to progressive breakdown in the orderly arrangement of musculo-elastic fascicles in the media of the vessel wall [112,113]. These changes occur quite independently of atherosclerosis and are seen in the absence of significant atherosclerosis in Oriental populations [39]. The primary changes appear to be in the elastin fibers and lamellae, which are thin and which fray and fracture. The vessel walls certainly thicken with age, but that is due mainly to intimal hyperplasia; the width of the load-bearing media remains relatively constant with age [113]. Elastic arteries in older subjects show the same number of musculo-elastic fascicles, but the elastin fibers are thinned and fracture. There is an increase in collagen and other fibers together with an increase in intercellular matrix [112,113]. In older human subjects, areas of cystic and medial necrosis frequently are seen in the arterial wall, with complete breakdown in the orderly structural arrangement seen in youth [114]. As with physical stiffening and dilation, these structural changes are not seen to any extent in human muscular peripheral arteries, nor are they seen in the aorta and elastic arteries in experimental animals [2]. Such animals rarely live more than 14 years, whereas animals most often studied for aging change, such as rats, rabbits, and guinea pigs, live considerably less. All these differences—between central and peripheral arteries and between humans and experimental animals—appear to be related to the extent and cumulative number of physical strains [1,2]. The arteries of older humans are exposed in a normal lifetime to far more cycles of stress than are the arteries of experimental animals, even when allowance is made for faster heart rate in the smaller mammals.

The aging effects in humans can be attributed to the fatiguing effects of cyclic stress on the nonliving elastin fibers and lamellae in the arterial wall [1,2,115–118]. Elastin is the most inert substance in the whole body, far more so than collagen or bone [119,120]. Once laid down, the elastin fibers remain constant and chemically unchanged for decades, if not for the whole of life [119,120]. More elastin may be added with growth and as age advances, but that which exists is not turned over or degraded chemically to any extent, though its physical structure may change. Material fatigue and fracture is a well-established branch of engineering science and can reasonably be applied to such a component of the human body [115–118]. Indeed, it would be fatuous to suggest that such principles are irrelevant, even if they have been overlooked in the past, except in relation to fatigue of tissue and prosthetic heart valves [121]. Materials exposed to repetitive stretch undergo changes in their crystalline mollecular structure, such that with time they become more brittle and eventu-

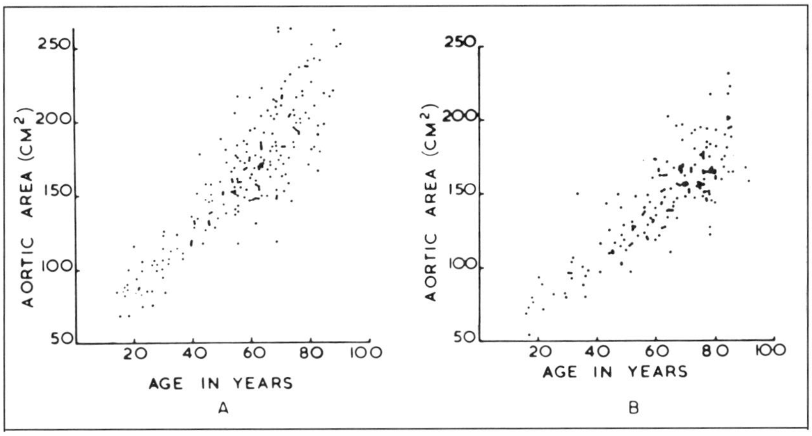

Fig. 6-2. Increase in cross-sectional area of aorta with age in men **A.** and in women **B.**, from the unselected autopsy study of Mitchell and Schwartz. (Reproduced with permission from JRA Mitchell, CJ Schwartz. Arterial Diseases. Oxford: Blackwell, 1965.)

ally fracture under a stress that they were previously able to tolerate [115,116]. Time to fracture is related to the extent of stretch and the number of stressing cycles [117]. Rubber, which has mechanical properties similar to those of elastin, fractures at a median of around 10^9 cycles when stretched repetitively by 10 percent of its initial length [118]. At a heart rate of 70 beats per minute, this point is reached after 25 or 30 years in humans. Thus, the principles of material fatigue and fracture can readily explain fracture of elastin fibers and lamellae in the elastic arterial wall, just as they have explained fatigue and fracture of wing spars, bulkheads, and other structural components of aircraft [115,116]. These principles are now routinely applied in the maintenance of aircraft, with replacement of key structural items well before the predicted time of fracture, even when the component appears perfectly sound.

Progressive dilation and stiffening of the aorta and central elastic arteries can be explained on the basis of fatigue and fracture of the structurally supported elastin fibers and lamellae in the media. These fibers fracture progressively in different parts of the arterial wall, causing stretch of the wall with progressive dilation and with transfer of stress to the stiffer collagenous fibers from the more extensible elastin [1,2]. Histological changes seen in the arterial wall are completely consistent with this concept [112,113]. The elastin-fiber breakdown with age appears to be the primary event. Other changes either are degener-

Fig. 6-3. Effects of age on the aortic pulse-wave velocity in a cohort of apparently normal human subjects with low prevalence of atherosclerosis. Increase in pulse-wave velocity is attributable to degeneration with progressively increasing aortic stiffness as age advances. (Reproduced with permission from AP Avolio et al. Effects of ageing on changing arterial compliance and left ventricular load in Northern Chinese urban community. Circulation 1983; 68:50–58. Copyright American Heart Association.)

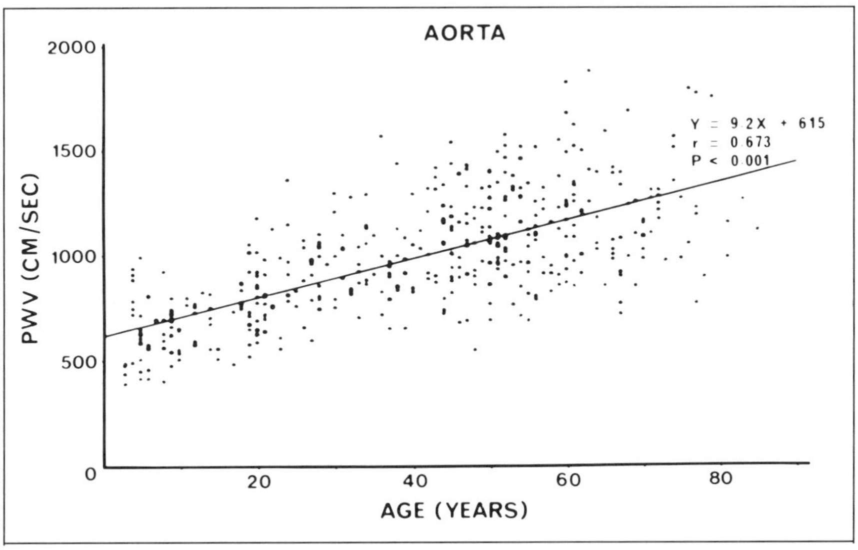

ative (such as cystic medial necrosis) or represent a remodeling process activated by the smooth muscle cells and other living components in the arterial wall.

The greater effects of age on elastic than on muscular arteries can be attributed to the lesser stretch of these latter arteries with each beat of the heart. The femoral and brachial arteries dilate by about 5 percent with each pulse (compared to the carotid's 10 percent) in youth, while the radial artery dilates by only around 2 percent [17,95–97]. Rubber, with a composition similar to that of elastin and when exposed to repetitive 5-percent stretch, does not fracture until over 3×10^9 cycles, which corresponds to 80–90 years in a human with an average heart rate of 70 beats per minute. The absence of such change in the elastic arteries of experimental animals can be attributed to the smaller cumulative number of pulses in a full life span. Dogs rarely live beyond 14 years and in that time would have fewer than 10^9 pulsations at 10-percent dilation of the proximal aorta, as required for elastin fiber fracture. Rabbits and rats would have considerably fewer, since even though their heart rate is faster, their life span usually is only 2–4 years.

We recently have had the opportunity to examine the hearts and arteries of birds that have lived over 20 years with heart rate similar to that in these experimental animals and with calculated cumulative life cycles well in excess of 10^9. These birds showed the same aortic elastin-fiber fracture and arterial dilation as seen in older humans and as predicted from theoretic engineering principles.

Progressive dilation and stiffening with age of the aorta and the elastic arteries of humans is associated with and due to degeneration of the media, consequent on elastin-fiber fracture. This occurs from childhood and is well established in adult humans. Similar changes are not seen in the muscular peripheral arteries. This difference in aging change between central and peripheral arteries contrasts with the difference in response to vasodilator drugs, where central arteries are little affected, whereas peripheral muscular arteries are substantially affected. Hopes have been held that arterial stiffening of older adults may be offset or antagonized by drugs. Such hopes have not been realized for the important central arteries and the aorta. Since the changes responsible for arterial stiffening are structural and degenerative, there is little basis for such hope; in addition, smooth muscle in these vessels is far less affected by vasomotor drugs than smooth muscle in the peripheral vessels. As will be explained later, ill effects of aortic degeneration of the heart are due largely to an indirect effect, wave reflection from peripheral sites, which certainly can be reduced substantially by drug therapy [1–3].

Effects of Hypertension

Hypertension has two effects on arterial stiffness: the first is functional and reversible, the second structural and irreversible [1,2]. The first effect affects all arteries, elastic and muscular, while the second, as with aging, has its greatest effect on the aorta and the central, predominantly elastic arteries, which pulsate greatly and are principally responsible for the cushioning function of the arterial tree.

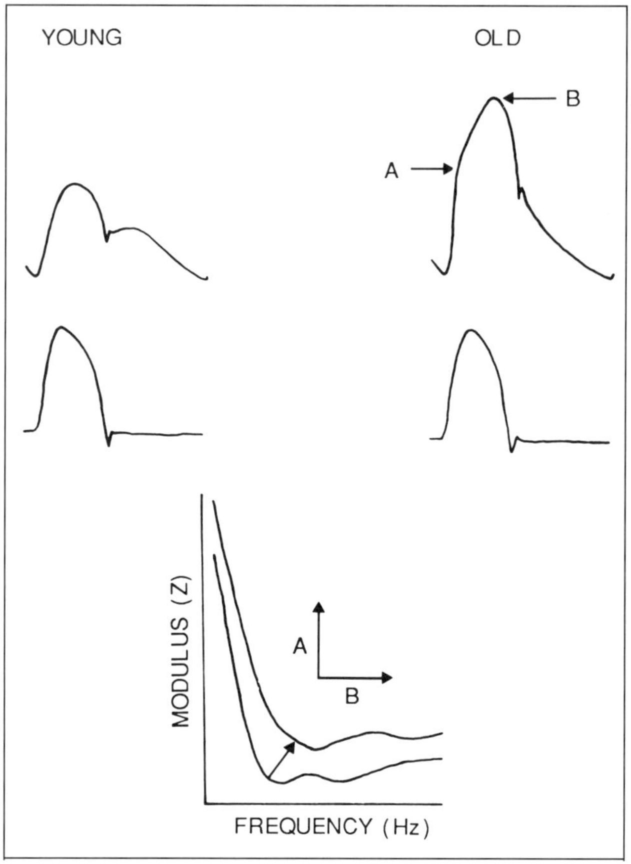

Fig. 6-4. Diagrammatic illustration of hypertensive and aging effects on the ascending aortic pressure wave with the same ascending aortic flow wave (top panels) and on the modulus of ascending aortic impedance (bottom panel). Increased peripheral resistance explains increased mean pressure (top) and increased impedance modulus at zero frequency (bottom). Increased proximal aortic stiffness, **A.**, explains a more rapid rate of rise of pressure in a high anacrotic "shoulder" (top) and increased characteristic impedance (bottom), whereas the earlier return of wave reflection explains, **B.** the late systolic peak of pressure (top) and shift of impedance curves to the right (bottom). (Reproduced with permission from MF O'Rourke, R Kelly, A Avolio. The Arterial Pulse. Philadelphia: Lea & Febiger, 1992.)

Elevation of arterial pressure, from whatever cause, results in arterial dilation accompanied by greater wall tension. This is a passive effect and is always seen unless there is simultaneous increase in arterial smooth muscle tone, offsetting the passive effect. Central, predominantly elastic arteries, such as the aorta, always dilate passively when distending pressure increases [1–3]. Passive dilation of an artery recruits collagenous fibers to the elastin fibers already bearing tension in the wall, such that the artery operates on a different part of the stress-strain curve and appears to be more stiff [1–3]. For the same (or greater) pulsatile pressure applied, diameter change is reduced. The major changes in pressure-wave contour in hypertension, first described in 1874 by Mahomed [122], are explicable on this basis, as are the characteristic changes in ascending aortic impedance (Fig. 6-4) [67,123–125]. Pressure-wave contour and impedance changes similar to those seen in hypertension can be seen in normal subjects during infusion of vasoconstrictor agents, which elevate blood pressure [1,2]. In hypertensive patients, a decrease in arterial pressure with antihypertensive therapy may normalize pressure-wave contour and ascending aortic impedance [67].

Long-standing hypertensive disease accelerates arterial degeneration. The aging changes previously described occur prematurely in hypertensive subjects and are attributable to the same process. High stresses and strains on the arterial wall result in fracture occurring at an earlier age than in normotensive subjects. Cystic medial necrosis—an extreme form of arterial degeneration—is far more common in elderly hypertensive than in elderly normotensive humans [114]. The aorta and elastic arteries of patients with chronic hypertension are stiffer than in normotensive controls, even when measured at the same distending pressure [66]. Long-standing hypertension also predisposes patients to intimal atherosclerosis; when it is widespread, and especially when it involves the medial layer of an artery, it must contribute to increased arterial stiffness [2].

There has been debate on the relative importance of functional (passive) and structural (degenerative) influences on arterial-wall stiffness in hypertensive disease [27,60,72,126,127]. Structural degenerative changes take time to develop and may not be apparent in persons whose blood pressure has been elevated for a relatively short period or indeed in animals with genetic hypertension that live for 2–3 years. There is general agreement that structural degenerative changes with increased stiffness are present in the aorta and elastic arteries in most patients with long-standing poorly controlled hypertension. Most of the controversy relates to peripheral muscular arteries. Some investigators have found that arterial stiffness of limb arteries in hypertensive patients is normal at physiologic distending pressure, but others have not [27,60,72,126,127]. More recent works on this subject, using phase-locked echo-tracking systems for the measurement of arterial diameter, have shown definite differences between elastic and peripheral arteries [17,95,128]. In the aorta and carotid artery, pulsatile diameter change was less in the hypertensive patients than in normotensive controls, at least up to age 60, whereas in the peripheral arteries, pulsatile diameter change was of similar amplitude in both hypertensive patients and normal controls. Also, caliber of the aorta and the carotid artery was significantly greater in the hypertensive patients compared to normal controls, whereas caliber was not significantly different in the femoral, brachial, or radial arteries. These findings are consistent with the thesis previously advanced, that structural degenerative changes are most marked in central elastic arteries, not apparent in peripheral muscular arteries, and not apparent in peripheral muscular arteries, where pulsatile cyclic strain is far less.

All findings are compatible with the idea that elevated blood pressure passively increases arterial stiffness in all arteries, while structural degenerative changes are usually found only in long-standing hypertension and, as with age, in the central vessels only.

Effects of Disease

It is often assumed that increased arterial stiffness in older subjects is due to atherosclerosis. This cannot be true, because aging changes seen in Western populations are also seen in Chinese and Japanese groups, whose blood pressure is similar to those in the West but who have virtually no atherosclerotic disease [39,129]. It is hard to believe that generalized atherosclerosis has no significant effect on arterial stiffness. It must, but we have not found measurements of pulse-wave velocity or other indices useful for separating patients with atherosclerosis from those without at any given age. There are many reports in the literature on increased arterial stiffness in patients with atherosclerosis [51,130,131]. Some of those reports, but by no means all, are flawed by methodologic problems that were not appreciated by the authors [2,130].

Arterial stiffness, measured as pulse-wave velocity, is generally increased in patients with Marfan's syndrome [132,133] and in other connective-tissue disorders [134]. In such diseases, the aorta often is considerably dilated, and measurements of arterial stiffness based on absolute diameter changes (i.e., compliance) may erroneously suggest that stiffness is normal or reduced.

In diabetic subjects, arterial stiffness appears to be increased [135–137]. However, earlier studies on this subject have not been consistently reproduced. Hypercholesterolemia has been reported as being associated with increased and with decreased arterial stiffness [135,137]. We have found no change [138].

An increasing number of reports on arterial stiffness are presented at scientific meetings. Many conflict with those presented before or with material published in the literature. Most do not reach journal publication, presumably because of methodological objections. Many reports have compared diameter change in one artery to pressure fluctuation in another artery, ignoring the difference in pressure-wave amplitude between the two sites and the effects of diseases or of an intervention on such difference in pressure [2]. Many reports are now appearing on changes in arterial diameter in the peripheral muscular arteries, using phase-locked echo-tracking systems. In the interpretation of the data obtained, it is important to take into account the spontaneous diameter changes that occur in such arteries [139] and to appreciate that apparent change in stiffness in these vessels cannot be extrapolated to the other arteries, especially to the large central arteries, which behave in a different and even opposite fashion [17].

Arterial stiffness is increased in congestive heart failure [22,124,140]. Changes appear to be most marked in the peripheral vessels [140], where they can be attributed to change in smooth muscle tone with consequent recruitment of collagenous fibers, as previously described. This doubtless is a factor in the increased wave reflection seen in patients with severe cardiac failure [22,124]. In congestive cardiac failure, increased aortic as well as peripheral arterial stiffness has been reported [22,124].

Effects of Drugs

The stiffness of arteries depends on their elastin collagenous components and on how properties of those components are modulated by smooth muscle tone [2,141]. The effects of drugs must result from their effects on smooth muscle, since no drug can have any direct pharmacologic effect on the structural properties of elastin or collagen [2,141,142]. One might expect, then, that drug effects would be more marked on the peripheral, predominantly muscular arteries than on the central, predominantly elastic arteries. That is the case, but the difference in effect is far more marked than one might expect (see Table 6-2). The central arteries show little direct effect [2,88–90,92], whereas the peripheral muscular arteries show substantial effect [46,87,94]. For the aortic characteristic impedance and pulse-wave velocity, we and others have shown little or no effect from nitroglycerin [88–90]. Slørdahl et al. [92] have shown no direct effect of nitroglycerin on the elastic modulus of pig thoracic aorta but a definite effect on the lower abdominal aorta. Laurent et al. [20] have shown no effect of isosorbide dinitrate on carotid distensibility but a very substantial effect on distensibility of the brachial artery. In the brachial artery, with nitroglycerin pulsatile diameter change increased from 3.6 percent to 6.5 percent, and elastic modulus decreased by over 50 percent. Similar changes in elastic modulus for small peripheral arteries have been shown for nitrates by others [46,59,87,94].

These and other findings [18,19,84,85,143–145] argue against any substantial effect of any drug on capacitance or Windkessel function of the large elastic arteries. Yet these vasodilator drugs do reduce systolic pressure and pulse pressure for the same output from the heart [18,143,145–147]. Their beneficial effects can be understood only when another factor is considered: the substantial changes in wave shape that are attributable to reduction in peripheral-wave reflection [2,21,143]. Such reduction in wave reflection is due to the effect of these drugs on the caliber and distensibility of the peripheral muscular arteries.

Direct and Indirect Effects of Arterial Stiffness on Pulse Waves

As mentioned previously, arterial stiffness has both a direct effect on the local capacitative function of an artery and an indirect effect through change in the propagative transmission of reflected waves. These two effects produce characteristic changes in the arterial pressure-pulse contour. The first clinical description of hypertension was based on the appreciation of this alteration in the pressure-wave contour [122]. The arterial pulse, of course, refers to any pulsation in an artery, although "pulse," as used by clinicians, refers to the pressure fluctuation in a large accessible artery. There are also flow and diameter pulse waves that are affected by arterial stiffening.

The effects of arterial stiffness have been most extensively studied by measurement of arterial pressure waves. Arterial pulsation is a consequence of cardiac contraction. The shape of the arterial pressure pulse, therefore, depends on the pattern of ventricular contraction and on the properties of the arterial system and arterioles. Despite a fairly constant pattern of ventricular ejection, the arterial pressure pulse shows a wide range of patterns. Different patterns of arterial pressure are seen in different arteries, in the same artery under varying physiologic conditions, in the same artery at different ages, and in corresponding arteries of different mammals [93].

In any given individual, the arterial pressure pulse shows progressive changes in amplitude and contour between the ascending aorta and the peripheral arteries. There is a substantial increase in pulse pressure mainly attributed to the increase in systolic pressure. In addition, the diastolic wave becomes more prominent. The change between central and peripheral-limb pressure pulses is best seen in young humans but becomes less marked with age (Fig. 6-5). With age, there are dramatic changes in the contour of the ascending aortic pressure pulse despite little change in the pattern of ejection from the left ventricle, other than a slight reduction in peak flow (see Fig. 6-4). With aging, there is an increase in the aortic pulse pressure associated with a change in wave contour. The change in contour is characterized by the presence of a late systolic peak and a reduction in fluctuation following the incisura. Similar changes are seen in patients with hypertension, although to a more marked degree. An individual with hypertension tends to have an older-looking aortic pressure waveform than one would expect for the subject's age [93].

One important consequence of the effect of arterial stiffness on arterial pressure wave contour is the difference in systolic pressure between central and peripheral sites. As noted, there is amplification in pulse pressure between the aortic root and peripheral arterial sites. This difference reduces with age as the arterial tree undergoes a generalized stiffening process (see Fig. 6-2). The important clinical implication is that brachial sphygmomanometric pressure may not accurately assess left ventricular pressure load. As discussed below, brachial sphygmomanometric pressure correlates poorly with measures of left ventricular mass [148]. Because of pressure-wave amplification in youth, brachial systolic pressure may overestimate the aortic pressure with which the heart interacts. In older subjects, while there is less difference in resting brachial and aortic pressure, the response to vasoactive drugs may be significantly underestimated by reliance on brachial systolic pressure. An example is shown in Fig. 6-6. In a middle-aged subject, administration of 0.3 mg of sublingual nitroglycerin results in up to a 20-mm-Hg fall in ascending aortic pressure with no change in brachial systolic pressure. This underestimation by peripheral-pressure measurement of central pressure changes in response to vasodilator drugs has been documented in both invasive and noninvasive studies [149–152].

These changes in arterial pressure pulse contour with age, hypertension, and anatomic location are due to both the direct and the indirect effects of arterial stiffening. The direct effect of arterial stiffening is that for any given stroke volume there will be a greater rise in pressure in the arterial system due to a reduction in capacitative function (Fig. 6-7). The indirect effect of arterial stiffening alters the timing and the intensity of wave reflection from peripheral vascular beds, due to a more rapid pulse-wave velocity (see Fig. 6-4). It is beyond the scope of this chapter to go into detailed explanation of peripheral-wave reflection, and the reader is directed to several reference sources on the subject [2,21]. The explanation for wave reflection

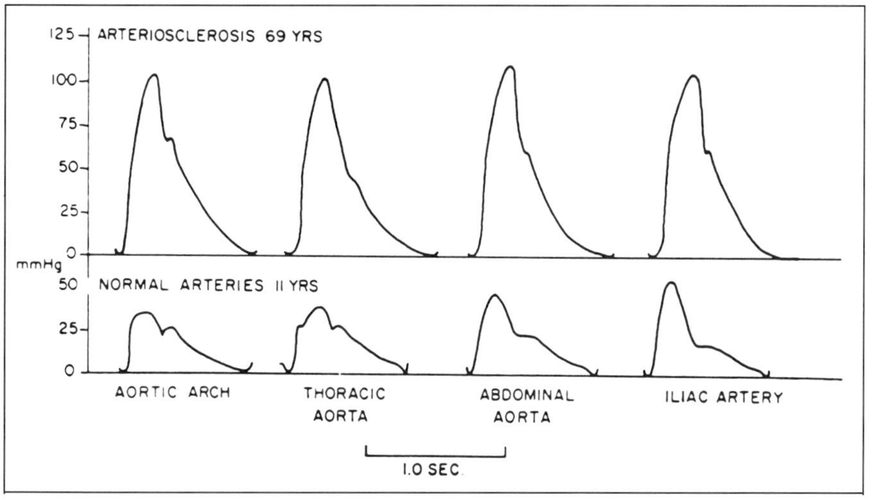

Fig. 6-5. Change in amplitude and contour of the pressure wave between the aortic arch and iliac artery of a young human subject (lower panel) and of a patient with arteriosclerosis (upper panel). (Reproduced with permission from MF O'Rourke. Arterial Function in Health and Disease. Edinburgh: Churchill Livingstone, 1982.)

comes from consideration of the anatomy of the arterial tree and its relation to the peripheral arteriolar bed [1,93,153]. The conduit function of the aorta and the large arteries provides a low-resistance pathway for blood between the heart and the peripheral capillaries. There is little fall in mean pressure through this arterial pathway to the periphery. However, just upstream from the capillaries, there is a dramatic fall in mean pressure over a short distance within the high-resistance arteriolar bed. It is at that junction, between the efficiently conducting arterial system and the high-resistance arteriolar bed, that substantial wave reflection occurs [21]. This reflection can be almost abolished by the intra-arterial injection of drugs that dilate peripheral arterioles. Normally, some 80 percent of the incident wave is reflected from arterioles in the periphery of the body [154]. Of course, there are numerous pathways between the heart and the periphery within the body. However, it appears that the wave reflections from these numerous sites summate and have their impact on the arterial pressure wave as a single pressure undulation. The timing of this reflected wave depends on the degree of arterial stiffness. Hence, in youth, the net effect of wave

Fig. 6-6. Pressure waves recorded directly in the ascending aorta (top) and brachial artery (bottom) under control conditions (left) and following 0.3-mg nitroglycerin (right) in an older human adult. X = pressure rise to first "shoulder"; R = reflected wave creating a late systolic peak in the central aortic pulse but a secondary wave on the downstroke of pressure in the brachial pulse. After nitroglycerin, R is reduced at both sites but causes a fall in systolic pressure in the aortic pulse only. (Reproduced with permission from RP Kelly, et al. Nitroglycerin has more favorable effects on left ventricular afterload than apparent from measurement of pressure in a peripheral artery. Eur Heart J 1990; 11:138–144.)

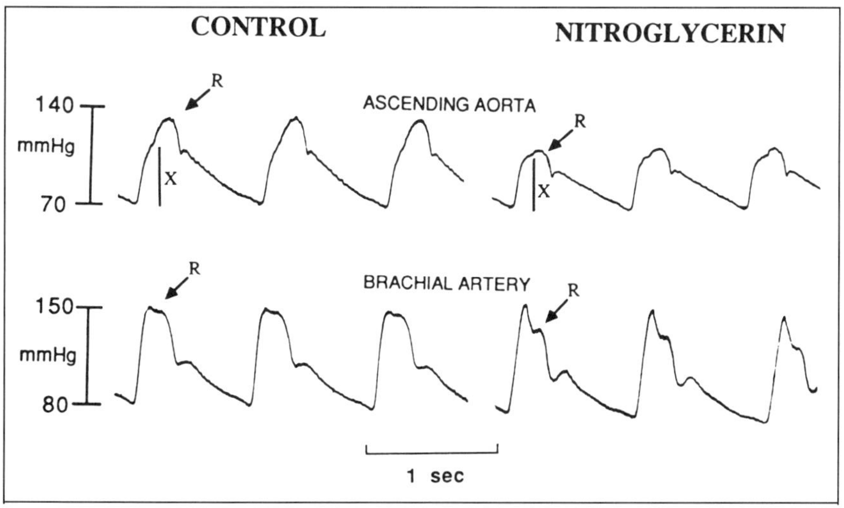

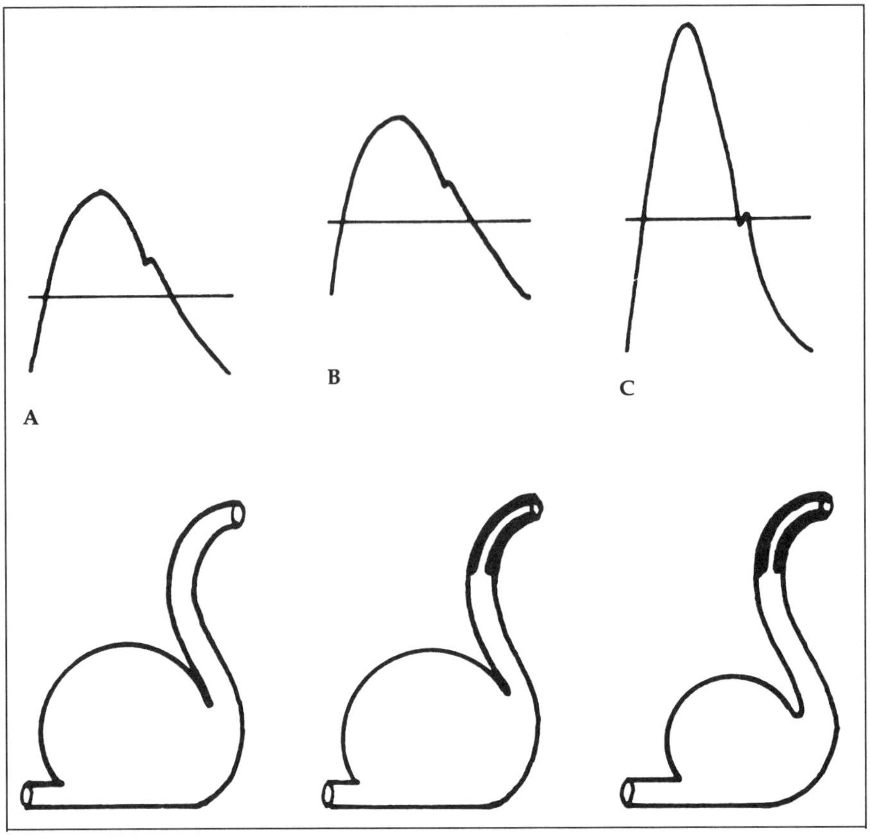

Fig. 6-7. Effects of increased resistance and decreased compliance on arterial pressure waves (top) in three Windkessel models of the arterial system (bottom). **A.** Normal compliance, normal resistance; **B.** normal compliance, increased resistance; **C.** reduced compliance, increased resistance. Mean arterial pressure is represented by the solid line. (Reproduced with permission from MF O'Rourke. Arterial Function in Health and Disease. Edinburgh: Churchill-Livingstone, 1982.)

reflection from all parts of the body is seen in the aortic root as a diastolic wave occurring after the incisura of the aortic pressure pulse contour (see Fig. 6-4 and Fig. 6-5) [74,155]. As arteries stiffen with age, there is an increase in velocity with which pulse waves travel. This increase in pulse-wave velocity with age has been documented in large-scale epidemiologic studies in both Western and Eastern societies (see Fig. 6-3) [74,155]. As a result of the increasing pulse-wave velocity with age, there is an alteration in the timing of wave reflection. For example, as recorded at the aortic root, the reflected wave is now seen to occur in late systole rather than during diastole. Hence, the characteristic late systolic peak that one sees in the aortic pressure pulse with age and with hypertension is explained by the indirect effects of arterial stiffening on pulse-wave velocity and timing of wave reflection (see Fig. 6-4) [21,156]. The characteristic changes in the pressure pulse contour that occur with change in anatomic site and various disease states can be explained similarly by alteration in timing and intensity of wave reflection [93].

The effects of arterial stiffness also may be seen in changes in flow contour. Pulsatile flow can be recorded in an artery with an electromagnetic flow meter applied around the outside of an artery or incorporated into an endoluminal catheter. More commonly, a Doppler ultrasonic probe can be applied over the artery to record flow-velocity profile. In the ascending aorta, the flow pulsation has a triangular shape during systole with tiny or no flow during diastole. The contour of this flow wave changes in two important ways as one moves downstream to the stiffer, more muscular arteries. First, the amplitude of flow is greatest in the large elastic arteries close to the heart. In peripheral arteries, the amplitude of flow is reduced as a consequence of both the cushioning effect of arteries on arterial pulsations and the distribution of blood volume into the large number of branches from peripheral arteries [2]. Second, as one moves from the heart to the periphery, the contour of the flow wave changes from the simple triangular shape to one that has multiple secondary fluctuations superimposed on this basic shape. The secondary fluctuations seen in peripheral arteries are a consequence of wave reflection in the upper and lower parts of the body [2]. With aging, there are characteristic changes in the flow pattern both in the ascending aorta and in peripheral arteries. In the ascending aorta, there is a reduction in flow acceleration with the consequent decline in slope of the upstroke of the flow-velocity profile. This is associated with a reduction in peak-flow velocity [157]. In more muscular arteries, there are also characteristic changes in the pattern of the secondary fluctuations [158]. Changes in flow-velocity profile occurring with hypertension also have been investigated recently by Japanese workers [159]. These investigators have recorded the flow-velocity profile in the ascending aorta and have interpreted changes in the downstroke of the flow-velocity wave as being due to alteration in timing and intensity of wave reflection secondary to increasing arterial stiffness of the peripheral vasculature.

Alteration of pressure within an artery also causes change in diameter. The contour of the diameter pulse is virtually identical to the pressure-pulse contour [2]. There are subtle differences between the pressure and diameter waves due to nonlinear elastic properties and to the viscosity of the arterial wall. As discussed previously, the larger, more elastic arteries have a greater diameter change for any given pressure change than do the less distensible peripheral arteries. While there is a similarity in contour of pressure and diameter waves, the absolute magnitude of the diameter pulsation is very small relative to the mean diameter of an artery; thus, measurement of arterial-diameter waves is less precise and more impractical than measurement of pressure or flow waves.

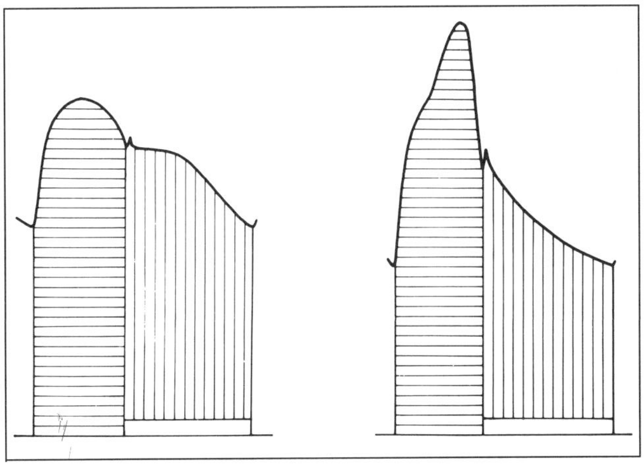

Fig. 6-8. Diagrammatic representation of the effects of arterial degeneration (right) on aortic systolic pressure time index (horizontally lined area) and aortic diastolic pressure time index (vertically lined area). Arterial degeneration results in increased systolic pressure load on the heart and decreased coronary perfusion pressure. (Reproduced with permission from MF O'Rourke. Arterial Function in Health and Disease. Edinburgh: Churchill-Livingstone, 1982.)

Ventricular-Vascular Interaction

The study of the effect of increasing arterial stiffness on ventricular function has been a difficult area, because adequate study of this topic requires appropriate definition and measurement of arterial compliance, of aortic load, and of left ventricular function. Further, there has been much debate as how best to measure indices of left ventricular function and aortic compliance, particularly with a view to obtaining parameters of ventricular and arterial function that can be used in the same plane to obtain a measure of ventriculo-arterial interaction [160].

Comparison of the patterns of left ventricular flow and aortic impedance in patients with compliant and stiffened vasculatures indicates that reduced arterial compliance would have a deleterious effect on left ventricular function. In youth, maximal flow output from the heart occurs at minimum impedance. With aging, impedance changes so that maximal flow output is opposed by high impedance (see Fig. 6-4) [161]. In addition, arterial stiffening produces a change in contour of the aortic pressure wave whereby systolic pressure and hence oxygen demand are increased at the same time as diastolic coronary perfusion pressure is reduced (Fig. 6-8). Although it has been widely accepted that reduced aortic compliance has adverse effects on cardiac contractile function and energetic efficiency, this hypothesis had remarkably little direct supporting data until recently.

For example, when isolated canine heart studies were performed to assess the utility of the end-systolic pressure-volume relation (derived from on-line measurement of left ventricular pressure-volume loops) as a load-independent index of ventricular contractile state, workers reported little change in the end-systolic pressure-volume relation despite twofold changes in total arterial compliance, characteristic impedance, and resistance [162]. These workers used a three-element Windkessel model of the arterial circulation that was computer generated and loaded on to an isolated canine heart. Myocardial efficiency, defined by the relation between total pressure-volume work (pressure-volume area) and oxygen consumption, also has been shown to be little affected by vascular load or type of ejection [163,164]. All these canine isolated heart models, however, have used lumped-parameter models of the circulation and have tended to neglect the indirect effects of reduced arterial compliance, namely, the distributed properties of the vascular tree and the timing and intensity of wave reflections. Various methods of stiffening the aorta have been used to measure the in situ effects of cardiac ejection into a stiff vasculature [165–168]. These studies focused largely on the effect of mechanical stiffening on vascular properties with little direct assessment of ventricular performance or energetics. Furthermore, none of these studies demonstrated increased myocardial oxygen consumption from ejection into a stiffened aorta.

More recently, an open-chest canine aortic bypass model has been developed in which the normally compliant canine aorta is bypassed by a stiff plastic conduit. The combined effect of the plastic tube and the apparatus used to secure it creates conditions of reduced aortic compliance and wave reflection such that haemodynamic features of human arterial degeneration are reproduced [70]. In adult humans, pressure-volume loops are characterized by a progressive rise in pressure throughout the period of systolic ejection. In the canine model, the increased pulsatile load that produced this late peaking loop produced a dramatic reduction in measured aortic compliance but produced only a very small change in mean peripheral resistance. In this canine model, cardiac efficiency, defined as the ratio of stroke work to oxygen consumption, was lowered by an average of 16 percent. More strikingly, for the heart to maintain the same systemic blood flow, myocardial oxygen consumption increased by between 30 percent and 50 percent when arterial load was associated with late peaking loops. These findings are consistent with the previous animal studies that showed that stiffening of the aorta increased pulsatile energy losses in the circulation and reduced load-dependent indices of contractile states. Stiffening of the aorta in this canine model also has been shown to prolong significantly the time constant of diastolic relaxation [169,170]. It should be noted that all these canine studies have, of course, assessed altered loading conditions on normal hearts. The question of whether left ventricular hypertrophy or concurrent myocardial ischemia amplifies the deleterious effects of aortic compliance on left ventricular function remains.

With the data from the Framingham Study showing left ventricular hypertrophy to be an independent predictor of future cardiovascular events [171], there has been renewed interest in the effects of arterial stiffness on left ventricular mass. While hypertension is the main cause of left ventricular hypertrophy, the correlation between standard sphygmomanometric blood-pressure level and left ventricular mass is not strong [148]. Improved correlation has been found by modifying blood-pressure-recording techniques, such as 24-hour recordings, peak systolic pressure during exercise, diastolic pressure during physical work, and long-term blood-pressure levels during longitudinal follow-up [171]. Both current and long-term follow-up show a better correlation between systolic pressure and left ventricular mass than diastolic pressure [171], again emphasizing the role of arterial stiffness as a determinant of cardiac hypertrophy. Indeed, there is evidence that reduced arterial compliance and enhanced wave reflection are related to left ventricular mass even at normotensive blood-pressure levels, as assessed by brachial measurements [172]. As previously discussed, brachial systolic pressure may be quite different from the central aortic pressure with which the heart directly interacts. Monitoring of central aortic pressure may thus be more relevant in assessing risk of ventricular hypertrophy or the ability to regress hypertrophy with specific antihypertensive medications, which is discussed next.

Therapeutic Strategies

The increased large-artery stiffness that occurs with age, hypertension, and cardiac failure has important implications with respect to treatment strategies. In hypertension, the relation between aortic stiffness and left ventricular hypertrophy has already been discussed. While many antihypertensive agents may be equally efficacious in reducing brachial sphygmomanometric pressure, not all drugs are equal in their ability to improve target-organ damage, such as left ventricular hypertrophy or end-stage renal failure.

Many studies have been reported on the differential effects of antihypertensive drugs on regression of left ventricular hypertrophy, although few have adequately compared agents in a double-blinded fashion with control of confounding variables. Meta-analysis of these many trials shows that calcium-channel blockers and angiotensin-converting enzyme inhibitors are most effective at reducing left ventricular hypertrophy [173]. These are the same classes of agents that improve indices of arterial stiffness in addition to lowering brachial sphygmomanometric pressure [82]. Attention now is being directed specifically at the effects of drugs on the stiffness of conduit and smaller muscular arteries and on left ventricular mass [174–178].

Similarly, in congestive cardiac failure, while it is known that many drugs are useful in improving a patient's symptomatic status, only the angiotensin-converting-enzyme (ACE) inhibitors and the nitrates have been shown to be effective in improving the patient's prognosis [179]. Several recent studies confirm the increased large-artery stiffness that occurs in dilated cardiomyopathy [22,69,91,140,180,181]. Those drugs that have been shown to improve mortality in heart failure are precisely those that have been shown to have ameliorative effects on large-artery function. The beneficial effects of ACE inhibitors on arterial stiffness have been alluded to in the preceeding discussion on antihypertensive treatment. Angiotensin itself produces an increase in arterial stiffness and wave reflection (Fig. 6-9) [182]. A large body of evidence documents the effect of nitroglycerin in reducing pulsatile load on the heart through improved arterial compliance and reduced wave reflection [88–90,149,150, 182,183]. Hence, an appreciation of arterial compliance is germane to the future development of treatment strategies in heart failure [22,184].

With improved prognosis from coronary artery disease and transplantation available for end-stage cardiac failure, together with an aging population, the hitherto neglected role of age-related changes in vascular function assume renewed importance. Consideration of the effects of drugs on the systemic vasculature rightly has moved away from a preoccupation with peripheral vascular resistance and arteriolar function to one that encompasses the effects of drugs on the systemic vasculature as a whole. Integral to this approach is the effect of drugs on large-artery function. In hypertension, our therapeutic approach would be improved if an antihypertensive drug not only reduced peripheral arteriolar resistance but also improved arterial compliance. Reference has already been made to the fact that studies thus far seem to show varying effects of the currently available anti-hypertensive drugs on the elastic properties of the larger, more central arteries, with the ACE inhibitors and calcium-channel blockers in particular improving compliance characteristics of conduit arteries. In addition, peripheral arteriolar dilatation will result in a reduction in mean distending pressure throughout the vascular system and hence shift the arteries in their stress-strain relationship to a position where they are more compliant. Finally, there is the important effect of drugs on the timing and intensity of wave reflection from the periphery. Drugs that dilate the small muscular arteries or arteriolar beds will reduce the intensity and delay the timing of wave reflection and so ameliorate ventricular-vascular coupling.

Monitoring

Assessment of the effects of arterial stiffness has now become germane to the treatment of cardiovascular dis-

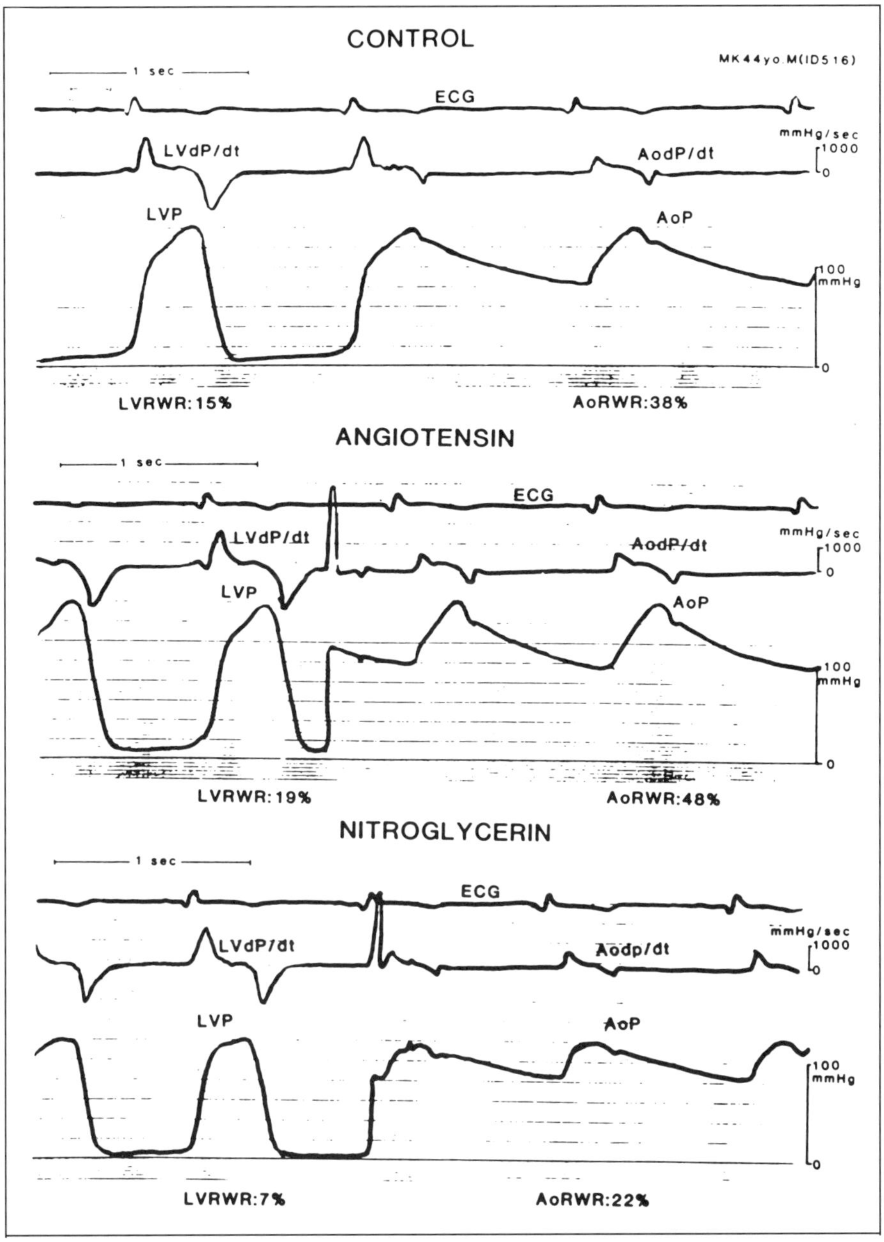

Fig. 6-9. Pressure recordings in the left ventricle and the ascending aorta of a 44-year-old man under normal conditions (top), after angiotensin infusion (center), and after sublingual administration of nitroglycerin (bottom). LV dP/dt = first derivative of left ventricular pressure; LVP = left ventricular pressure; AodP/dt = first derivative of aortic pressure; AoP = ascending aortic pressure. Reflected wave ratios are given below each panel for the left ventricle (LVRWR) and ascending aorta (AoRWR). (Reproduced with permission from K Takazawa. A clinical study of the second component of left ventricular systolic pressure. J Tokyo Med Coll 1987; 45(2):256–270.)

ease. Given that blood pressure is not the same in all arteries, there is a need to develop an approach that will detect changes in the aortic pressure with which the heart interacts when such changes are not readily detectable by standard sphygmomanometry. In disease states such as hypertension, sphygmomanometric pressure is now considered but one of many windows on a systemic process affecting the arterial vasculature at all levels [185].

As discussed, there are many ways of measuring arterial stiffness. Noninvasive measures may be applied to the bedside clinical situation to aid in diagnosis and therapy. Measurement of pulse-wave velocity has been used in the diagnosis of change in arterial properties in connective-tissue disorders and other degenerative disease states [132–135], although it has found its greatest use in the assessment of arterial compliance in large-scale epidemiologic studies [74,155]. Japanese workers have utilized the

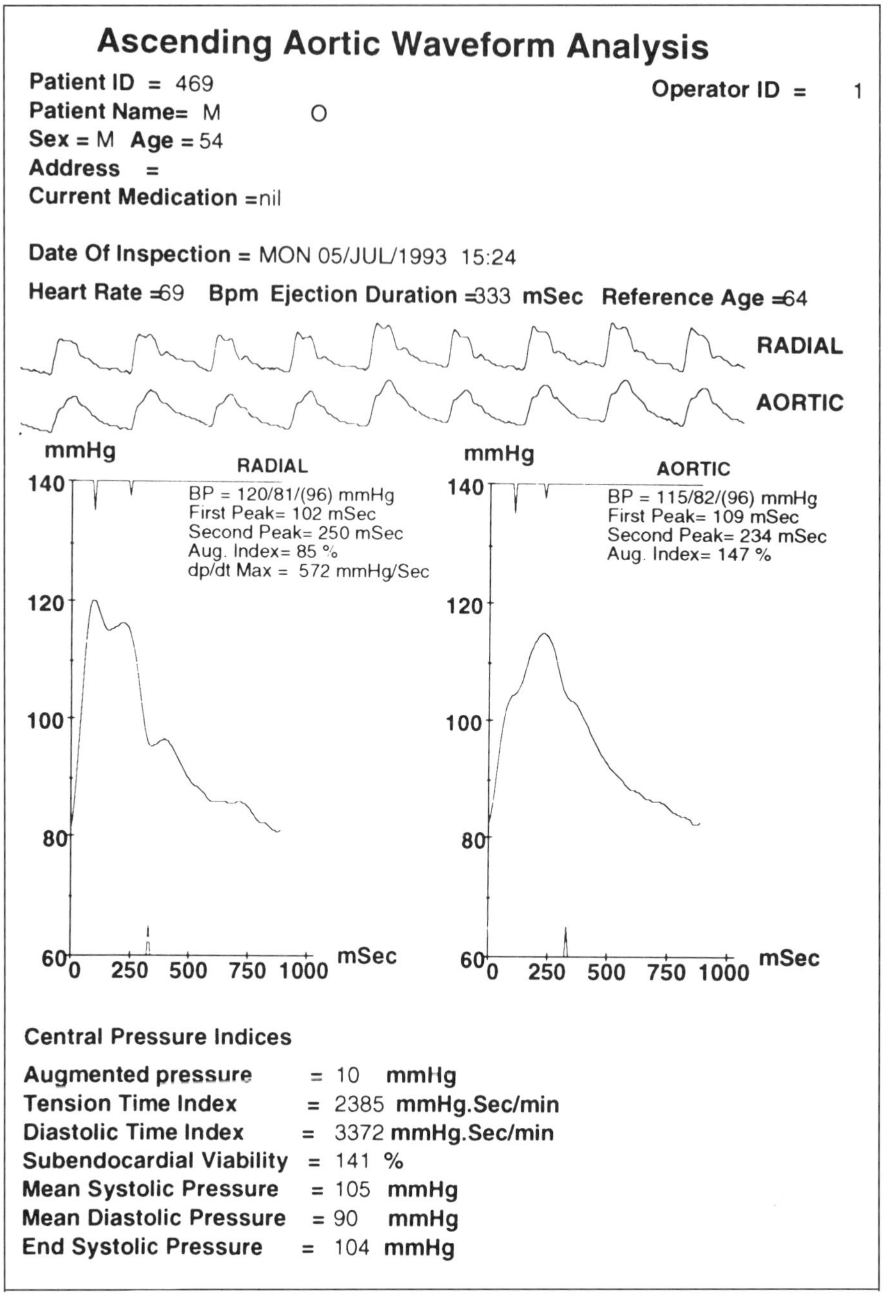

Fig. 6-10. A report on the pressure-wave analysis of a 54-year-old man. A series of radial-artery-pressure waves are recorded by applanation tonometry with systolic and diastolic pressure values calibrated by brachial syphymomanometry. A generalized upper-limb transfer function is applied to synthesize the ascending aortic pressure waves, which are displayed below the radial waves. On the enlarged illustrations, features of the radial-pressure waves (first and second systolic peak, or shoulder) and dicrotic notch are detected automatically by the algorithm, and corresponding points are placed on the derived ascending aortic pressure trace. Central-pressure indices calculated from such information include heart rate, ejection duration, reference age (from comparison of augmentation with an internal standard), mean pressure, time to first and second sytolic pressure peaks, pressure wave augmentation as percentage and in mm Hg, systolic tension-time index, diastolic pressure-time index, Buckberg's subendocardial viability ratio (ratio of diastolic index to systolic index), mean pressure during systole, mean pressure during diastole, and pressure at end-systole.

signal from a finger plethysmograph to assess arterial stiffness characteristics in individual subjects [186]. Plethysmography has been used to assess forearm arterial compliance characteristics [47]. Using ultrasound methods, Hoeks [187] has developed an arterial wall–tracking system that gives on-line arterial-diameter changes, allowing calculation of vessel distensibility in various conditions. Others have used conventional B-mode imaging of a vessel to obtain measures of arterial compliance by combining measured diameter changes with noninvasive pressure signal [55]. These plethysmographic and ultrasound techniques provide information on the distensibility of the local vascular bed but do not give a global measure of arterial function as do pulse-wave-velocity measurements.

Pulse-wave-contour analysis provides information on both direct and indirect effects of arterial stiffening [93]. While clinicians are used to feeling the pulse as part of clincial assessment, the interpretation of pulse-wave contour lags far behind the emphasis placed on interpretation of electrocardiographic electrical waves. A recently developed transcutaneous pulse recorder allows pressure waves to be recorded from traditional pulse points such as the radial and carotid sites using the principle of applanation tonometry as was originally developed for assessment of intra-ocular pressure [76,149].

One particular advance made in recent years is the combination of sphygmomanometric pressure measurement and tonometric pressure recording of the radial pulse to obtain a calibrated noninvasive recording. By use of a transfer function, the calibrated peripheral pulse can be used to synthesize a predicted central aortic pulse as part of the patient's routine bedside assessment [93]. In adults, a change in arterial stiffness produces a change in central aortic systolic pressure characterized by a decrease or an increase in the late systolic peak. While these changes in central pulse contour may not be accompanied by any change in brachial systolic or diastolic pressure, they are always associated with some change in the contour of the brachial or radial pulse. By using a transfer function, the peripheral-pulse-contour changes can be used to determine the central aortic pulse contour changes [188]. Such a system has been developed as a compact personal computer–based system which can be used in an office practice. Tonometric recordings of the radial pulse are taken, calibrated by sphygmomanometric measurements. An algorithm is applied to synthesize ascending aortic waves simultaneously. A series of waves, recorded over a respiratory cycle is ensemble-averaged and displayed (Fig. 6-10). Multiple physiologic parameters are derived, including central aortic systolic and diastolic pressures, augmentation index (the height of the late systolic peak), subendocardial perfusion estimates, and mean aortic systolic and diastolic pressures. Knowledge of such aortic-pressure parameters will allow day-to-day patient management to be based on information that hitherto could be obtained only by catheterization of the ascending aorta.

Summary

Arterial stiffness is an old concept but one that is assuming increased significance as advances are made in the study of the epidemiology, pathophysiology, and treatment of cardiovascular disease. There are many ways of defining and measuring stiffness, from the material elastic modulus of the wall to the capacitative or compliance property of the intact vessel. Studies have shown direct (reduced capacitance) and indirect (enhanced wave reflection) effects of increased arterial stiffness with aging and degenerative-disease states. The extent of arterial stiffening and the response to vasoactive drugs vary in different parts of the systemic vasculature, with clear differences evident between larger, elastic arteries and smaller, more muscular arteries. These changes in arterial function have important implications for efficient coupling between cardiac and systemic arterial function. Therapeutic strategies to ameliorate arterial stiffness and to optimize ventriculo-arterial coupling require adequate monitoring of large-artery function. New techniques have been developed and are now available, since standard sphygmomanometric measurements are inadequate in assessing overall arterial function or in measuring the central aortic pressure with which the heart interacts.

References

1. O'Rourke MF. Arterial Function in Health and Disease. Edinburgh: Churchill-Livingstone, 1982.
2. Nichols WW, O'Rourke MF. McDonald's Blood Flow in Arteries. London: Arnold, 1990.
3. O'Rourke M. Arterial stiffness, systolic blood pressure, and logical treatment of arterial hypertension. Hypertension 1990; 15(4):339–347.
4. Rutan GH, McDonald RH, Kuller LH. A historical perspective of elevated systolic vs diastolic blood pressure from an epidemiological and clinical trial viewpoint. J Clin Epidemiol 1989; 42:663–673.
5. Kannel WB, et al. Systolic blood pressure, arterial rigidity and risk of stroke: The Framingham Study. JAMA 1981; 245:1225–1229.
6. Amery A, et al. Efficacy of antihypertensive drug treatment according to age, sex, blood pressure and previous cardiovascular disease in patients over the age of 60. Lancet 1986; ii:589–592.
7. Franklin SS, Weber MA. Measuring hypertensive cardiovascular risk: the vascular overload concept. Am Heart J 1994; 128:793–803.
8. The Systolic Hypertension in Elderly Program Cooperative Research Group (SHEP): Implications of the systolic hypertension in the elderly program. Hypertension 1993; 21:335–343.
9. Fisher CM. The ascendancy of diastolic blood pressure over systolic. Lancet 1985; 1:1349–1350.
10. Mackenzie J. Principles of diagnosis and treatment of heart affections, 3rd ed. London: Frowde, 1917.
11. Young T. Hydraulic investigations, subservient to an intended Croonian Lecture on the Motion of the Blood. Philos Trans R Soc Lond 1908; 98:164–180.
12. Young T. On the functions of the heart and arteries (The Croonian Lecture). Philos Trans R Soc Lond 1909; 99:1–31.
13. Bright R. Reports of medical cases selected with a view of illustrating the symptoms and cure of diseases by a reference to morbid anatomy. London: Longmans, 1827.
14. Roy CS. The elastic properties of the arterial wall. J Physiol 1880; 3:125–159.
15. Bramwell JC, Hill AV. Velocity of transmission of the pulse wave and elasticity of arteries. Lancet 1922; 1:891–892.

16. O'Rourke M, Safar M, Dzau V. Arterial Vasodilation: Mechanisms and Therapy. London: Edward Arnold, 1993.
17. Boutouyrie P, et al. Opposing effects of ageing on distal and proximal large arteries in hypertensives. J Hypertens 1992; 10[Suppl 6]:S87–S91.
18. Feldman RL, Pepine CJ, Conti CR. Magnitude of dilation of large and small coronary arteries by nitroglycerine. Circulation 1981; 64:324–333.
19. Kutz MA, Lamping KG, J.N. B, et al. Mechanisms responsible for the heterogenous coronary microvascular response to nitroglycerine. Circ Res 1991; 68:847–855.
20. Laurent S, et al. Mechanism of nitrate-induced improvement on arterial compliance depends on vascular terrritory. J Cardiovasc Pharmacol 1992; 19:641–649.
21. O'Rourke MF, Kelly RP. Wave reflection in the systemic circulation and its implications in ventricular function. J Hypertens 1993; 11:327–667.
22. Laskey WK, Kussmaul WG. Arterial wave reflection in cardiac failure. Circulation 1987; 75:711–722.
23. McDonald DA. Blood Flow in Arteries, 2nd ed. London: Edward Arnold, 1974.
24. Krafka JJ. Comparative study of the histophysics of the aorta. Am J Physiol 1939; 125:1–14.
25. Learoyd BM, Taylor MG. Alterations with age in the viscoelastic properties of human arterial walls. Circ Res 1966; 18:278–292.
26. Peterson LH, Jensen RE, Parnell J. Mechanical properties of arteries in vivo. Circ Res 1960; 8:622–639.
27. Mulvany MJ. A reduced elastic modulus of vascular wall components in hypertension? Hypertension 1992; 20(1):7–9.
28. Fung YC. Biomechanics: Mechanical Properties of Living Tissues. New York: Springer, 1981.
29. Patel DJ, Vaishnav RN. The rheology of large blood vessels. In DE Bergel, ed. Cardiovascular Fluid Dynamics. New York: Academic, 1972.
30. Dobrin PB, Rovrick AA. Influence of vascular smooth muscle on contractile mechanics and elasticity of arteries. Am J Physiol 1969; 217(6):1644–1651.
31. Gow BS. Circulatory correlates: vascular impedance, resistance and capacity. In DF Bohr, AP Somlyo, HV Sparks, eds. Handbook of Physiology, Section 2: The Cardiovascular System. Bethesda: American Physiological Society. 1980. Pp. 353–408.
32. Roach M, Burton AC. Reason for the shape of the distensibility curves of arteries. Can J Biochem Physiol 1957; 35: 681–690.
33. Dobrin PB, Mrkvicka R. Estimating the elastic modulus of non-atherosclerotic elastic arteries. J Hypertens 1992; 10[Suppl 6]:S7–S10.
34. Bergel DH. The static elastic properties of the arterial wall. J Physiol 1961; 156:445–457.
35. Bramwell JC, Hill AV. The velocity of the pulse wave in man. Proc Soc Exp Biol Med 1922; 93:298–306.
36. Milnor WR. Haemodynamics, 2nd ed. Baltimore: Williams & Wilkins, 1989.
37. Gribbin A, Steptoe A, Sleight P. Pulse wave velocity as a measure of blood pressure change. Psychophysiology 1976; 13(1):86–90.
38. McDonald DA, Taylor MG. The hydrodynamics of the arterial circulation. Prog Biophys Mol Biol 1959; 9:107–173.
39. Avolio AP, et al. Effects of ageing on changing arterial compliance and left ventricular load in Northern Chinese urban community. Circulation 1983; 68:50–58.
40. Kawasaki T, et al. Non-invasive assessment of the age related changes in stiffness of major branches of human arteries. Cardiovasc Res 1987; 21:678–687.
41. Hirai T, et al. Stiffness of systemic arteries in patients with myocardial infarction. Circulation 1989; 80:78–86.
42. Dart AM, et al. Aortic distensibility in patients with isolated hypercholesterolaemia, coronary artery disease, or cardiac transplant. Lancet 1991; 338:270–273.
43. Hayashi K, et al. Biomechanical study of the constitutive laws of vascular walls. Exp Mechan 1974; 14:440–444.
44. Watt TB, Burrus CS. Arterial pressure contour analysis for estimating human vascular properties. J App Physiol 1976; 40(2):171–176.
45. Finkelstein SM, et al. Arterial vascular compliance in heart failure. IEEE Engineering Med and Biol Soc 1990; 12(2): 548–549.
46. Westling H, et al. Vasoactive drugs and elastic properties of human arteries in vivo, with special reference to the action of nitroglycerine. Eur Heart J 1984; 5:609–616.
47. Fitchett D, et al. Forearm arterial compliance: the validation of a plethysmographic technique for the measurement of arterial compliance. Clin Sci 1984; 67:69–72.
48. Emilio A, et al. Noninvasive characterization of peripheral vascular compliance with age. IEEE Engineering Med and Biol Soc 1990; 12(2):541–542.
49. Shimazu H, et al. Noninvasive measurement of beat to beat vascular viscoelastic properties in human fingers and forearms. Med Biol Eng Comput 1985; 23:43–47.
50. Starc V, et al. Peripheral compliance as seen by laser doppler. IEEE Engineering Med and Biol Soc 1990; 12(2):543–544.
51. Stefanadis C, et al. Aortic distensibility abnormalities in coronary artery disease. Am J Cardiol 1987; 59:1300–1304.
52. Mohhiaddin RH, et al. Regional aortic compliance studied by magnetic resonance imaging: the effects of age, training and coronary artery disease. Eur Heart J 1990; 11:990–996.
53. Levenson JA, et al. Plused doppler: Determination of diameter, blood flow velocity, and volumic flow of brachial artery in man. Cardiovasc Res 1981; 15:164–170.
54. Reneman RS, et al. Flow velocity patterns and distensibility of the carotid artery bulb in subjects of various ages. Circulation 1985; 71(3):500–509.
55. Roman MJ, et al. Parallel cardiac and vascular adaptation in hypertension. Circulation 1992; 86:1909–1918.
56. Hokanson DE, et al. A phase locked echo tracking system for recording arterial diameter changes in vivo. J Appl Physiol 1972; 32(5):728–733.
57. Tardy Y, et al. Assessment of the elastic behaviour of peripheral arteries from a non-invasive measurement of their diameter pressure curves. Clin Phys Physiol Meas 1991; 12:39–54.
58. Patel DJ, et al. Noninvasive determination of small vessel distensibility in man. J Biomech 1986; 8:607–611.
59. Fitchett DH. Forearm arterial compliance: a new measure of arterial compliance? Cardiovasc Res 1984; 18:651–656.
60. Hayoz D, et al. Conduit artery compliance and distensibility are not necessarily reduced in hypertension. Hypertension 1992; 20:1–6.
61. Lehmann ED, Gosling RG. Measuring aortic distensibility. Lancet 1991; 338:1075.
62. Lehmann ED, et al. Validation and reproducibility of pressure corrected aortic distensibility measurements using pluse-wave velocity doppler ultrasound. J Biomed Eng 1993; 15:221–228.
63. Chiu YC, et al. Determination of pulse wave velocities with computerised algorithms. Am Heart J 1991; 121(5):1460–1470.
64. Gosling RG. Extraction of physiological information from spectrum analysed doppler shifted continuous-wave ultrasound signals. In PW Hill, PW Watson, eds. IEE Modern Electronics Monographs. Stevenage: Peter Peregrinus, 1976.
65. Latham RD, et al. Regional wave travel and reflections along

the human aorta: a study with six simultaneous micromanometric pressures. Circulation 1985; 72:1257–1269.

66. Ting CT, et al. Regional pulse wave velocities in hypertensive and normotensive humans. Cardiovasc Res 1990; 24:865–872.
67. Merillon JP, et al. Evaluation of the elasticity and characteristic impedance of the ascending aorta in man. Cardiovasc Res 1978; 12:401–406.
68. Gundel W, et al. Aortic input impedance in man: acute response to vasodilator drugs. Circulation 1981; 63:1305–1314.
69. Laskey WK, et al. Characteristics of vascular hydraulic load in patients with heart failure. Circulation 1985; 72:61–71.
70. Kelly RP, Tunin R, Kass DA. Effect of reduced aortic compliance on cardiac efficiency and contractile function of in situ canine left ventricle. Circ Res 1992; 71:490–502.
71. Hayward CS, et al. Noninvasive determination of femoral vascular impedance using applanation tonometry and continuous wave doppler flowmetry. Proc Aust Physiol Pharmacol 1986; 17(2):212P.
72. Gribbin B, Pickering TG, Sleight P. Arterial distensibility in normal and hypertensive man. Clin Sci 1979; 56:413–417.
73. Smulyan H, et al. Effect of age on arterial distensibility in asymptomatic humans. Arteriosclerosis 1983; 3:199–205.
74. Avolio AP, et al. Effects of aging on arterial distensibility in populations with high and low prevalence of hypertension: comparison between urban and rural communities in China. Circulation 1985; 71(2):202–210.
75. Liu Z, Brin K, Yin FCP. Estimation of total arterial compliance: an improved method and evaluation of current methods. Am J Physiol 1983; 252:H588–H600.
76. Kelly R, et al. Noninvasive registration of the arterial pressure pulse waveform using high-fidelity applanation tonometry. J Vasc Med Biol 1989; 1(3):142–149.
77. Glagov S, Wolinsky H. Aortic wall as a "two-phase" material. Nature 1963; 199:606–608.
78. Wolinsky H, Glagov S. Structural basis for the static mechanical properties of the aortic media. Circ Res 1964; 14:400–413.
79. Clark JM, Glagov S. Transmural organization of the arterial media—The lamellar unit revisited. Arteriosclerosis 1985; 5:19–34.
80. Glagov S, et al. Microarchitecture and composition of arterial walls: relationships to location, diameter and distribution of medial stress. J Hypertens 1992; 10:S101–S104.
81. O'Rourke MF. Systolic blood pressure in an ageing population. J Clin Med 1992; 35(11):14–26.
82. Safar ME, et al. Peripheral large arteries and the response to antihypertensive treatment. Hypertension 1983; 5[Suppl 3]:63–68.
83. Simon A, et al. Action of vasodilating drugs on small and large arteries of hypertensive patients. J Cardiovasc Pharmacol 1983; 5:626–631.
84. Levenson J, Simon A. Heterogeneity of response of peripheral arteries to antihypertensive drugs in essential hypertension: basic effects and functional consequences. Drugs 1988; 35:34–39.
85. Simon AC, O'Rourke M, Levenson J. Arterial distensibility and its effect on wave reflection and cardiac loading in cardiovascular disease. Coronary Artery Disease 1991; 2:1111–1120.
86. O'Rourke MF, Avolio AP. Structural basis for increased distensibility of systemic muscular arteries with arterial vasodilator agents. J Mol Cell Cardiol 1985; 18[Suppl 2]:374.
87. Fitchett DH. Effects of vasodilator drugs on calibre and distensibility of small peripheral arteries. In M O'Rourke, M Safar, V Dzau, eds. Arterial Vasodilation: Mechanisms and Therapy. London: Edward Arnold, 1993. Pp. 190–199.
88. Yaginuma T, et al. Effect of glyceryl trinitrate on peripheral arteries alters left ventricular hydraulic load in man. Cardiovasc Res 1986; 20(2):153–160.
89. Fitchett DH, et al. Reflected pressure waves in the ascending aorta: Effect of glyceryl trinitrate. Cardiovas Res 1988; 22:494–500.
90. Latson TW, et al. Effect of nitroglycerine on aortic impedance, diameter, and pulse-wave velocity. Circ Res 1988; 62:884–890.
91. Carroll JD, et al. Arterial mechanical properties in dilated cardiomyopathy. J Clin Invest 1991; 87:1002–1009.
92. Slørdahl SA, et al. Segmental aortic wall stiffness from intravascular ultrasound at normal and subnormal aortic pressure in pigs. Acta Physiol Scand 1991; 143:227–232.
93. O'Rourke MF, Kelly R, Avolio A. The Arterial Pulse. Philadelphia: Lea & Febiger, 1992.
94. Kawarada A, et al. Non-invasive automatic measurement of arterial elasticity in human fingers and rabbit forelegs using photoelectric plethysmography. Med Biol Eng Comput 1986; 24:591–596.
95. Benetos A, et al. Alteration in the carotid artery wall properties with ageing and high blood pressure level. J Hypertens 1991; 9[Suppl 6]:S112–S113.
96. Benetos A, et al. Arterial alterations with aging and high blood pressure: A noninvasive study of carotid and femoral arteries. Arteriosclerosis and Thrombosis 1993; 13:90–97.
97. Safar M. Geometry and stiffness of the arterial wall in essential hypertension. In ME Safar, MF O'Rourke, eds. The Arterial System in Hypertension. Dordrecht: Kluwer, 1993. Pp. 135–153.
98. Lüscher TF, Tanner FC. Endothelial regulation of vascular tone and growth. Am J Hypertens 1993; 6:283S–293S.
99. Henrich WL. The endothelium—a key regulator of vascular tone. Am J Med Sci 1991; 302(5):319–328.
100. Stewart DJ, et al. Elevated endothelin-1 in heart failure and loss of normal response to postural change. Circulation 1992; 85:510–517.
101. Kostic MM, Schrader J. Role of nitric oxide in reactive hyperemia of the guinea pig heart. Circ Res 1992; 70:208–212.
102. Moncada S, Higgs A. The L-arginine-nitric oxide pathway. N Engl J Med 1993; 329:2002–2012.
103. Said SI. Nitric oxide and vasoactive intestinal peptide: Co-transmitters of smooth muscle relaxation. NIPS 1992; 7:181–183.
104. Vanhoutte PM. Is endothelin involved in the pathogenesis of hypertension? Hypertension 1993; 21:747–751.
105. Vallance P, Calver A, Collier J. The vascular endothelium in diabetes and hypertension. J Hypertens 1992; [Suppl 10](1):S25–S29.
106. Ho K. Effects of ageing on arterial distensibility and left ventricular load in an Australian population. [Thesis for Bsc(Med), University of New South Wales, 1982.]
107. Schimmler W. Untersuchungen zu Elastizitatsproblemen der Aorta. Archiv für Kreislaufforschung 1965; 47(3):189–233.
108. Mitchell JRA, Schwartz CJ. Arterial Diseases. Oxford: Blackwell, 1965.
109. O'Rourke MF. Effects of aging on aortic distensibility and on aortic function in man. In H Boudoulas, P Toutouzas, eds. 1st International Symposium on the Functional Abnormalities of the Aorta. Mount Kisco NY: Futura, 1994.
110. Gosling RG, et al. The area ratio of normal aortic junctions—aortic configuration and pulse-wave reflection. Br J Radiol 1971; 44:850–853.
111. Langewouters GJ. Viscoelasticity of the human aorta in vitro, in relation to pressure and age. [PhD Thesis. Free University of Amsterdam, 1982.]
112. O'Rourke MF, et al. Age-related changes of elastic lamellae in the human thoracic aorta. J Amer Coll Cardiol 1987; 9:53A.

113. Virmani R, et al. Effect of aging on aortic morphology in populations with high and low prevalence of hypertension and atherosclerosis. Am J Path 1991; 139(5):1119–1129.
114. Eagle KA, De Sanctis RW. Diseases of the aorta. In E Braunwald, ed. Heart Disease, 4th ed. Philadelphia: Saunders, 1992. Pp. 1528–1557.
115. Sandor B. Fundamental of cyclic stress and strain. Madison: University of Wisconsin, 1972.
116. Gent AN. Fracture of elastomers. In H Liebowitz, ed. Fracture. New York: Academic Press, 1972. P. 316.
117. Caldwell SM, et al. Dynamic fatigue life of rubber. Chemistry 1940; 12:19–23.
118. Lindley PB. Engineering design with natural rubber. Malayan Rubber Fund Board. The Natural Rubber Producers' Research Association Technical Bulletin, 4th ed. 1974; 8:17–19.
119. Kohn RR. Principles of Mammalian Aging, 2nd ed. Englewood Cliffs: Prentice-Hall, 1978.
120. Rucker RB, Tinker D. Structure and metabolism of arterial elastin. Int Rev Exp Pathol 1977; 17:1–47.
121. Broom ND. An "in vitro" study of mechanical fatigue in glutaraldehyde-treated porcine aortic valve tissue. Biomaterials 1980; 1:3–8.
122. Mahomed FA. The etiology of Bright's Disease and the prealbuminuric stage. Med Chir Trans 1874; 57:197–228.
123. O'Rourke MF. Pulsatile arterial haemodynamics in hypertension. Aust N Z J Med 1976; 6[Suppl 2]:40–48.
124. Merillon JP, et al. Aortic input impedance in heart failure: comparison with normal subjects and its changes during vasodilator therapy. Eur Heart J 1984; 5:447–455.
125. Ting CT, et al. Arterial hemodynamics in human hypertension. J Clin Invest 1986; 78:1462–1471.
126. Simon AC, et al. Estimation of forearm arterial compliance in normal and hypertensive men from simultaneous pressure and flow measurements in the brachial artery, using a pulsed Doppler device and a first-order arterial model during diastole. Cardiovasc Res 1983; 17:331–338.
127. van Merode T, et al. Carotid artery wall properties in normotensive and borderline hypertensive subjects of various ages. Ultrasound Med Biol 1988; 14(7):563–569.
128. Laurent S, et al. Isobaric compliance of the radial artery is increased in patients with essential hypertension. J Hypertens 1993; 11:89–98.
129. Nakashima T, Tanikawa J. A study of human distensibility with relation to atherosclerosis and aging. Angiology 1971; 27:477–490.
130. Lehmann ED. Elastic properties of the aorta. Lancet 1993; 342:1417.
131. Boudoulas H, Toutouzas P. 1st International Symposium on the Functional Abnormalities of the Aorta. Mount Kisco N.Y.: Futura, 1994.
132. Hirata K, et al. The Marfan Syndrome: Abnormal aortic elastic properties. J Am Coll Cardiol 1991; 18:57–63.
133. Yin FCP, et al. Arterial hemodynamic indexes in Marfan's syndrome. Circulation 1989; 79:854–862.
134. Francois B, et al. Pulse wave velocity recordings in a family with ecchymotic Ehlers-Danlos syndrome. Int Angiol 1986; 5:1–5.
135. Eliakim M, Sapoznikov D, Weinman J. Pulse wave velocity in healthy subjects and in patients with various disease states. Am Heart J 1971; 82(4):448–457.
136. Lax H, Feinberg AW. Abnormalities of the arterial pulse wave in young diabetic subjects. Circulation 1959; 20:1106–1110.
137. Woolam GL, et al. The pulse wave velocity as an early indicator of atherosclerosis in diabetic subjects. Circulation 1962; 25:533–539.
138. Avolio AP, et al. Change of arterial distensibility with age in subjects with familial hypercholesterolaemia. Aust N Z J Med 1985; 15:516.
139. Hayoz D, et al. Spontaneous diameter oscillations of the radial artery in humans. Am J Physiol 1993; 264:H2080–H2084.
140. Cohn JN, Finkelstein SM. Abnormalities of vascular compliance in hypertension, aging, and heart failure. J Hypertens 1992; 10[Suppl 6]:S61–S64.
141. O'Rourke MF, Avolio AP. Structural basis for increased distensibility of systemic muscular arteries with arterial vasodilator agents. J Mol Cell Cardiol 1986; 18[Suppl 2]:374.
142. Yaginuma T, O'Rourke MF. Modification of wave travel and reflection by vasodilator therapy. In MF O'Rourke, ME Safar, VJ Dzau, eds. Arterial Vasodilation: Mechanisms and Therapy. London: Edward Arnold, 1993. Pp. 50–61.
143. Kelly RP, et al. Arterial dilation and reduced wave reflection: Benefit of dilevalol in hypertension. Hypertension 1989; 14:14–21.
144. Asmar RG, et al. Comparison of effects of felodipine versus hydrochlorothiazide on arterial diameter and pulse-wave velocity in essential hypertension. Am J Cardiol 1993; 72:794–798.
145. Selke FW, et al. Influence of vessel size on the sensitivity of porcine coronary microvessels to nitroglycerin. Am J Physiol 1990; 258:H515–H520.
146. Levenson J, et al. Diuretics and arteriolar resistance and arterial compliance in human hypertension. Eur Heart J 1992; 13[Suppl G]:48–52.
147. Pannier BE, et al. Lisinopril versus Atenolol: Decrease in systolic versus diastolic blood pressure with converting enzyme inhibition. Cardiovasc Drugs Ther 1991; 5:775–782.
148. Frohlich ED, et al. The heart in hypertension. N Engl J Med 1992; 327:998–1008.
149. Kelly RP, et al. Nitroglycerin has more favourable effects on left ventricular afterload than apparent from measurement of pressure in a peripheral artery. Eur Heart J 1990; 11:138–144.
150. O'Rourke MF, et al. Effects of arterial dilator agents on central aortic systolic pressure and on left ventricular hydraulic load. Am J Cardiol 1989; 63:38 I–44 I.
151. Simkus GJ, Fitchett DH. Radial arterial pressure measurements may be a poor guide to the beneficial effects of nitroprusside on left ventricular systolic pressure in congestive heart failure. Am J Cardiol 1990; 66:323–326.
152. Takazawa K, et al. Underestimation of effect of vasodilator agents by peripheral blood pressure measurement: the cause and strategy. Circulation 1993; 88(4, part 2):I-263.
153. Remington JW, Wood EH. Formation of peripheral pulse contour in man. J Appl Physiol 1956; 9:433–442.
154. O'Rourke MF, Taylor MG. Vascular impedance of the femoral bed. Circ Res 1966; 18:126–139.
155. Avolio AP. Pulse wave velocity and hypertension. In ME Safar, et al. eds. The Cardiovascular System in Essential Hypertension. Paris: Martinus-Nijhoff, 1987.
156. Murgo JP, et al. Aortic input impedance in normal man: relationship to pressure wave shapes. Circulation 1980; 62:105–116.
157. Gardin JM, et al. The evaluation of blood flow velocity in the ascending aorta and main pulmonary artery of normal subjects by Doppler echocardiography. Am Heart J 1984; 107:310–319.
158. Mills CJ, et al. Pressure-flow relations and vascular impedance in man. Cardiovasc Res 1970; 4:405–417.
159. Miyashita H, et al. A Doppler index for evaluating the influence of aortic wave reflection on left ventricular ejection. Circulation 1993; 88:I-69.

160. Kass D, Kelly R. Ventriculo-vascular coupling: a review. Ann Biomed Eng 1992; 20:41–62.
161. O'Rourke MF, Avolio AP, Nichols WW. Left ventricular-systemic arterial coupling in humans and strategies to improve coupling in disease states. In FCP Yin, ed. Ventricular/Vascular Coupling: Clinical, Physiological, and Engineering Aspects. New York: Springer, 1987. Pp. 1–19.
162. Maughan WL, et al. Effect of arterial impedance changes on the end-systolic pressure-volume relation. Circ Res 1984; 54:595–610.
163. Suga H. Total mechanical energy of a ventricle model and cardiac oxygen consumption. Am J Physiol 1979; 236:H498–H505.
164. Suga H, et al. Constant mechanical efficiency of contractile machinery of canine left ventricle under different loading conditions. Jpn J Physiol 1984; 34:679–698.
165. Urschel CW, et al. Effects of decreased aortic compliance on performance of the left ventricle. Am J Physiol 1968; 214:298–304.
166. O'Rourke MF. Steady and pulsatile energy losses in the systemic circulation under normal conditions and in simulated arterial disease. Cardiovasc Res 1967; 1:313–326.
167. Salisbury PF, Cross CE, Rieben A. Ventricular perfomance modified by elastic properties of outflow system. Circ Res 1962; 11:319–328.
168. Randall OS, Van den Bos GC, Westerhof N. Systemic compliance: does it play a role in the genesis of essential hypertension? Cardiovasc Res 1984; 18:455–462.
169. Yabe R, et al. The influence of ascending aortic augmentation index (reflection coefficient) to left ventricular relaxation. Circulation 1991; 84:565.
170. Kelly R, Kass D. Effect of increased pulsatile load on diastolic function. Circulation 1992; 86:I-554.
171. Levy D, et al. Prognostic implications of echocardiographically determined left ventricular mass in the Framingham Heart Study. N Eng J Med 1990; 322:1561–1566.
172. Saba PS, et al. Relation of carotid pressure waveforms to left ventricular anatomy in normotensive subjects. Circulation 1992; 86:I-65.
173. Dahlöf B, Pennert K, Hansson L. Reversal of left ventricular hypertrophy in hypertensive patients. Am J Hypertens 1992; 5:95–110.
174. Safar ME, et al. Arterial dynamics, cardiac hypertrophy and anti-hypertensive treatment. Circulation 1987; 75[Suppl I]: I-156–I-161.
175. Asmar RE, et al. Reversion of cardiac hypertrophy and reduced arterial compliance after converting enzyme inhibition in essential hypertension. Circulation 1988; 78:941–950.
176. Zusman RM, et al. Nifedipine, but not propranolol, improves left ventricular systolic and diastolic function in patients with hypertension. Am J Cardiol 1989; 64:51F–61F.
177. Schulman SP, et al. The effects of antihypertensive therapy on left ventricular mass in elderly patients. N Engl J Med 1990; 322(19):1350–1356.
178. Pfeffer MA, Pfeffer JM. Reversing cardiac hypertrophy in hypertension. N Engl J Med 1990; 322(19):1388–1389.
179. Braunwald E. ACE inhibitors—a cornerstone of the treatment of heart failure. New Eng J Med 1991; 325:351–353.
180. Arnold JMO, et al. Large artery function in patients with chronic heart failure: Studies of brachial artery diameter and hemodynamics. Circulation 1991; 84:2418–2425.
181. Kelly R. Congestive heart failure and cardiac transplantation. In R Kelly, ed. Systemic Arterial Function in Health and Disease: Clinical Determinants and Measurement. [MD Thesis. University of New South Wales: Sydney, Australia, 1989.]
182. Takazawa K. A clinical study of the second component of left ventricular systolic pressure. J Tokyo Med Coll 1987; 45(2):256–270.
183. Yin FCP, et al. Effects of nitroprusside on hydraulic vascular loads on the right and left ventricle of patients with heart failure. Circulation 1983; 67:1330–1339.
184. Francis GS, Cohn JN. Mechanisms of cardiac and vascular dysfunction and the rationale for pharmacologic intervention. FASEB J 1990; 4:3068–3075.
185. Devereux RB, Alderman MH. Role of preclinical cardiovascular disease in the evolution from risk factor exposure to development of morbid events. Circulation 1993; 88(4):1444–1455.
186. Takazawa K, Ibukiyama C. Acceleration plethysmogram. Gendai Iryou 1988; 20:948–955.
187. Spek JJ, et al. Differences in vessel wall properties of large arteries in obese and lean subjects. J Hypertens 1994; 12:S210.
188. Karamanoglu M, et al. An analysis of the relationship between central aortic and peripheral upper limb pressure waves in man. Eur Heart J 1993; 14:160–167.

Normal Mechanisms of Hemostasis and Fibrinolysis

Douglas E. Vaughan
Andrew I. Schafer
Joseph Loscalzo

The hemostatic system evolved to arrest the flow of blood at sites of vascular injury, while its counterpart, the fibrinolytic system, evolved to ensure recanalization of vessels during the reparative process. These two systems act in concert with each other and in conjunction with vascular-wall products that modulate their activities to ensure blood flow. It is important to recognize that under both normal and pathologic conditions, the elements of hemostasis and fibrinolysis act simultaneously and are tightly coupled through important regulatory molecules that can influence both systems, such as thrombin and activated factor XII.

Hemostasis

Circulating platelets, plasma-coagulation proteins, and the vessel wall are the three major components of hemostasis. Their activities are closely integrated to ensure the maintenance of blood fluidity under normal circumstances. In response to vascular injury, they work in a carefully orchestrated manner to arrest bleeding and repair damage with dazzling precision and speed. Constantly poised in a delicate physiologic balance between its procoagulant and anticoagulant potentials, the hemostatic system can be disrupted by an extraordinary variety of pathologic events to cause either clinical bleeding or thrombosis. Thrombosis has been thought to result from inappropriate or unregulated hemostasis. Therefore, understanding the pathophysiology of thrombotic disorders requires a brief outline of the normal scheme of hemostasis.

The intact endothelial lining of the intimal surfaces of blood vessels—the only cells in the body to which circulating blood is normally exposed—is endowed with remarkable thromboresistant properties. In fact, the coagulation system probably is activated whenever blood comes into contact with any surface other than healthy endothelium, including components of damaged vessels, extravascular tissues, or artificial surfaces. Disruption of endothelial contiguity by various forms of injury attracts circulating platelets to attach initially in a monolayer to the damaged vessel wall. This process of platelet **adhesion** (platelet-vascular interaction) is provoked both by loss of endothelial thromboresistant activities (e.g., the potent antiplatelet and vasodilator autocoids, prostacyclin, and endothelium-derived relaxing factor) and by the exposure of platelet-activating subendothelial structures (e.g., collagen). Platelet adhesion is mediated primarily by the adhesive macromolecule, von Willebrand factor. The critical importance of this multimeric protein is illustrated by the serious bleeding problems that result from quantitative or qualitative plasma deficiencies of von Willebrand factor (vWF) (von Willebrand's disease, or vWD) or from loss of platelet receptors for vWF (Bernard-Soulier syndrome).

Following adhesion, activated platelets undergo the release reaction, during which prepackaged platelet granule constituents (including adenosine diphosphate or ADP, from dense granules and fibrinogen from alpha granules) are selectively discharged. This secretion process is partly dependent on the *de novo* formation of thromboxane A_2, an eicosanoid produced from platelet arachidonic acid that promotes hemostasis as a potent platelet activator and vasoconstrictor. Thromboxane A_2 directly antagonizes the actions of the major vascular arachidonic acid metabolite, prostacyclin. The importance of the release reaction in mediating subsequent platelet-plug formation is exemplified by bleeding disorders that can be caused by either the morphologic absence of specific platelet granules (storage-pool diseases) or the functional inhibition of thromboxane A_2 formation (with the use of aspirin or other nonsteroidal anti-inflammatory drugs).

The products of the platelet-release reaction promote further platelet activation, recruiting platelets to the site of vascular injury and stimulating the formation of an occlusive platelet plug. This process of platelet **aggregation** (platelet-platelet interaction) is mediated by other macromolecules that, like von Willebrand factor, are normal constituents of plasma as well as platelet alpha granules. They bind to platelet surface membrane glycoprotein determinants that are expressed only on activated platelets. Fibrinogen is probably the most important of these proteins under low shear conditions, while von Willebrand factor is the primary aggregating ligand in regions of the circulation where higher shear stress levels prevail. Fibronectin and thrombospondin also may be involved in the assembly of the platelet plug. Clinical disorders of fibrinogen (afibrinogenemia or dysfibrinogenemia) or loss of platelet receptors for fibrinogen (thrombasthenia) result in impaired platelet aggregation and a bleeding diathesis.

The relatively fragile platelet plug that is rapidly formed following vascular injury must be anchored by the insoluble protein meshwork of fibrin to achieve stable hemostasis. Fibrin is formed from its soluble plasma precursor fibrinogen by the action of the serine protease thrombin. This enzyme selectively cleaves polypeptides from the $A\alpha$ and $B\beta$ chains of fibrinogen (forming the by-product fibrinopeptides A and B, respectively) to convert fibrinogen to fibrin. Rapid polymerization of fibrin results in a growing fibrin clot. The fibrin polymers are finally covalently cross-linked through transamidination reactions catalyzed by thrombin-activated factor XIII (XIIIa). The formation of the pivotal coagulation enzyme thrombin is the culmination of a series of tightly linked proteolytic reactions (the coagulation cascade) in which plasma proteins normally devoid of biologic activity serve as enzyme precursors (zymogens) to be converted to their corresponding serine proteases, which then catalyze a subse-

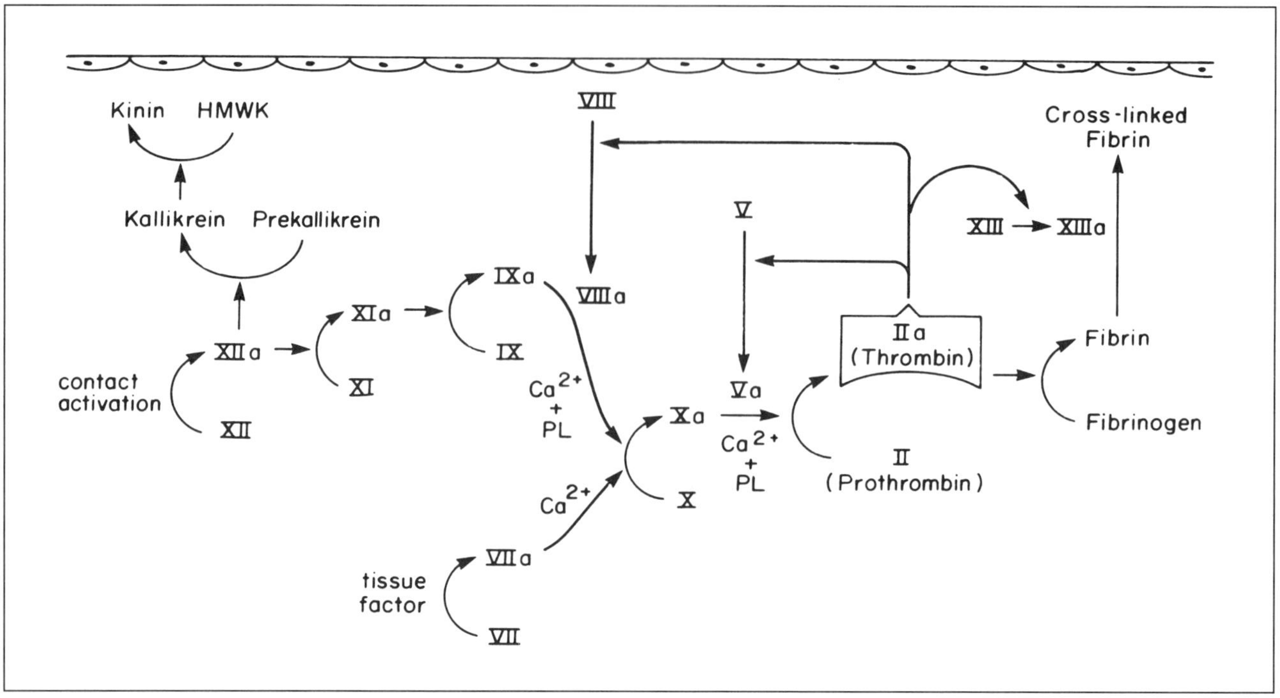

Fig. 7-1. Normal pathways of coagulation leading to intravascular fibrin generation.

quent zymogen-protease conversion [1–6]. In the activation of the coagulation system, zymogens are converted to proteases either through conformational changes (as in the initial steps of the cascade) or by specific proteolytic cleavages. The coagulation cascade thus acts as a self-amplifying scheme, in which a trivial stimulus may culminate explosively in the formation of large quantities of thrombin and the rapid generation of a fibrin clot (Fig. 7-1).

Thrombin is formed from its inactive zymogen precursor prothrombin by the action of activated factor X (Xa). Factor Xa cleaves specific sites in the prothrombin molecule to produce thrombin, in the process releasing by-product polypeptides F_1 and F_2, which can be measured in plasma as markers of thrombin generation, just as fibrinopeptides A and B can be measured as markers of fibrin formation. In addition to the substrate prothrombin and the enzyme Xa, the prothrombinase complex that yields thrombin also includes cofactors Va (the activated form of factor V), calcium, and an acidic phospholipid surface that can be efficiently provided by activated (but not quiescent) platelets. The Ca^{2+} in this reaction serves to form a bridge to bind gamma-carboxyglutamic-acid residues (Gla residues) on both Xa and prothrombin to negatively charged platelet membrane phospholipid surfaces, thus concentrating the prothrombinase complex to facilitate and localize thrombin generation. (The gamma-carboxylation of glutamic-acid residues on certain coagulation proteins is a vitamin K–dependent postsynthetic modification that is blocked by coumarin anticoagulants.) Thrombin is devoid of Gla residues following its cleavage from prothrombin by Xa and can thus be released from this Ca^{2+}-bound, cell surface–dependent complex. The reactions initiated by Xa leading to the formation of fibrin traditionally have been termed the **common pathway** of coagulation.

Activation of factor X to produce Xa can be achieved through either an **extrinsic pathway** or an **intrinsic pathway** of coagulation. Although traditionally conceptualized as separate and alternate pathways of factor-X activation, it is now recognized that important interactions occur between the extrinsic and intrinsic pathways. Furthermore, the absence of clinical bleeding complications in patients with hereditary deficiencies of any of the contact activation factors, such as factor XII, prekallikrein, and high-molecular-weight kininogen (HMWK), has challenged the physiologic relevance of the intrinsic pathway in initiating the coagulation cascade. In vivo coagulation is probably initiated by activation of the extrinsic (tissue factor) pathway.

The extrinsic pathway of coagulation leading to activation of factor X is triggered by the formation of the activated factor VII (VIIa)–tissue factor complex. Tissue factor [7] is an integral membrane-associated glycoprotein that is expressed on the surfaces of cells that are normally in contact with blood (e.g., endothelial cells, leukocytes) only in response to some perturbation of those cells, such as that caused by endotoxin, immune complexes, activated complement, or other inflammatory mediators. Tissue factor is also constitutively present on subendothelial tissues (e.g., fibroblasts, smooth muscle cells) that are exposed to blood as a result of vascular injury [8]. The mechanism whereby factor VII appears in the circulation in its activated form (factor VIIa) remains unclear. It is possible that trace amounts of factor VIIa are always present in blood. Alternatively, unlike the other coagulation-factor zymogens that are enzymatically inert, factor VII may actually possess endogenous proteolytic activity. Whatever the mechanism, factor VIIa is hemostatically ineffective until it is bound to its cofactor, tissue factor. This occurs when vascular injury exposes tissue factor to circulating factor VIIa. The trace amounts of factor VIIa–tissue factor complex thus generated induce the autocatalytic conversion of factor VII to VIIa, thereby amplifying the formation of the factor VIIa–tissue factor complex. The factor VIIa–tissue factor complex then activates factor X (or factor IX, as discussed later). Factor VIIa and its substrate factor X both contain Gla residues, through which calcium can form a bridge to phospholipid surfaces, permitting efficient and localized formation of factor Xa.

The intrinsic pathway is initiated by contact activation of factor XII on exposure of blood to negatively charged surfaces (e.g., glass, kaolin, celite) under experimental conditions in vitro and to subendothelial structures such as collagen or basement membrane at sites of vascular intimal damage under pathophysiologic conditions [9]. Activated factor XII not only initiates the intrinsic pathway of coagulation by activating factor XI (to XIa), it also triggers other proteolytic plasma systems that are involved in a complex fashion in the inflammatory response, complement activation, fibrinolysis, and the regulation of vascular tone [9–11]. Factor XIIa cleaves the zymogen prekallikrein to the serine protease kallikrein as well as XI to XIa; the generation of both kallikrein and XIa requires the complexing of their respective precursor zymogens to the cofactor HMWK. Kallikrein can cleave HMWK to form the nonapeptide bradykinin, which is an extremely potent vasodilator and enhancer of capillary permeability. Initial contact activation of factor XII involves limited proteolysis of factor XII to XII fragments (XIIf): XIIf retains the enzyme-active site of XIIa but loses its surface-binding site, thus allowing it to diffuse into plasma. The ability of kallikrein and XIa (as well as other proteases such as plasmin) to generate more activated factor XII from its zymogen precursor represents an autocatalytic circuit that serves to magnify the initial stimulus-activating factor XII [12].

Factor XIa can be formed by the action of XIIa or XIIf on factor XI. Physiologically, factor XIa is more likely to be generated by either autoactivation or by thrombin. It converts the zymogen factor IX to IXa. Factor IXa, in turn, activates factor X to Xa utilizing the cofactor VIIIa (the activated form of factor VIII), calcium, and a phospholipid surface provided by platelets. This so-called Xase (or tenase) complex, similar to the prothrombinase complex that is assembled to generate thrombin, is concentrated on cell surfaces for efficient and localized activation of factor X through calcium bridging of Gla residues on factors IXa and X to negatively charged cellular phospholipid surfaces. The cofactor in this reaction, factor VIII, also is known as the antihemophilic factor (AHF): it circulates in blood noncovalently associated with the distinct protein vWf. Deficiency of AHF causes classic hemophilia, a coagulation disorder, while deficiency of vWf causes vWD, a disorder of primary hemostasis characterized by defective platelet adhesion.

The convergent extrinsic and intrinsic pathways of coagulation are now recognized as not strictly alternate pathways for the activation of factor X. Complex interactions between these pathways are known to be operative [10,13]. Specifically, the factor VIIa–tissue factor complex can activate factor IX. Thus, this complex can activate factor X either directly or indirectly via factor-IX activation. Kinetic analysis has suggested that factor IX is the preferred substrate for the enzymatic action of the factor VIIa–tissue factor complex when both factors IX and X are simultaneously presented to it. It is also clear, however, that both the extrinsic and intrinsic pathways are required to provide completely normal hemostasis, since deficiency of either a strictly intrinsic-pathway coagulation factor (XI) or a strictly extrinsic-pathway coagulation factor VII can cause a systemic bleeding disorder. It is also of practical clinical utility to separate the intrinsic, extrinsic, and common pathways in the evaluation of patients with suspected coagulopathies: the activated partial thromboplastin time (aPTT) is a measure of the integrity of the intrinsic and common pathways of coagulation (HMWK; prekallikrein; factors XII, XI, IX, VIII, X, and V; prothrombin; and fibrinogen), whereas the prothrombin time (PT) is a measure of the integrity of the extrinsic and common pathways of coagulation (factors VII, X, and V; prothrombin; and fibrinogen). Neither the aPTT nor the PT detects a deficiency of factor XIII.

The events of primary hemostasis (platelet activation, platelet–vessel wall interactions) and secondary hemostasis (the coagulation cascade) do not operate independently or consecutively following injury. Complex interrelationships have been identified between the activation of platelets and coagulation factors. For example, the conversion of prothrombin to thrombin occurs on the surfaces of activated platelets much more efficiently than in fluid phase. The generation of thrombin on platelet surfaces then acts as a potent stimulus for further platelet activation. Thus, thrombin production and platelet activation can be seen as developing in a reciprocal and mutually amplifying manner to culminate in the rapid formation of a tightly localized hemostatic plug consisting of platelets and fibrin (Fig. 7-2).

The critical role of other blood and vascular cells in modulating the hemostatic system is also becoming recognized. Platelets as well as perturbed monocytes, macrophages, and endothelial cells also have procoagulant capabilities, possessing surface-expressed prothrombinase activity that can efficiently promote local thrombin generation. Furthermore, as noted above, monocytes, endothelial cells, and other vascular cells can also act in a procoagulant capacity by expressing tissue factor to activate factor VII. The relative importance of the procoagulant activities of those cells in the regulation of hemostasis is unknown, but it probably depends on complex factors such as the intravascular or extravascular site of thrombin generation, the local availability of coagulation factor substrates, and cell-specific stimuli. It is likely that the critical steps in hemostasis in vivo proceed predominantly on cell surfaces rather than in the fluid phase.

Endothelial cells, situated at the interface between blood and the vessel wall, play a pivotal role in regulating the homeostatic balance of hemostasis [14]. When perturbed

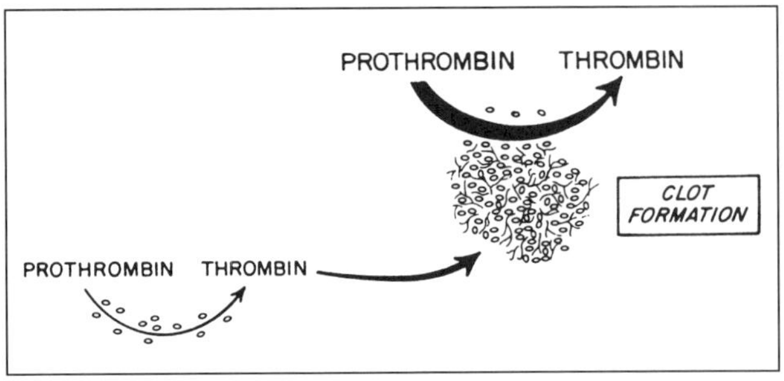

Fig. 7-2. Amplification and localization of formation of the hemostatic plug by interactions between platelets and thrombin. Activated platelet surfaces promote the markedly accelerated and localized conversion of prothrombin to thrombin. Thrombin then acts as a potent platelet agonist to activate platelets further and thus provide increased cell surface for further thrombin generation, leading to the rapid formation of a platelet-fibrin hemostatic plug.

(e.g., by injury or in response to inflammatory mediators), endothelial cells can promote coagulation by expressing procoagulant properties (tissue factor, prothrombinase activity), by releasing vWF and an inhibitor of fibrinolysis (plasminogen activator inhibitor type I), and by binding some coagulation factors. On the other hand, depending on the delicate balance of hemostatic modulators, endothelial cells also possess highly effective antithrombotic properties. These thromboresistant actions of endothelium are physiologically critical in maintaining blood fluidity and containing a thrombus to the confines of vascular damage.

Physiologic antithrombotic systems act in concert with the fibrinolytic system to prevent thrombus formation under normal circumstances and to focus the clot and localize it to the site of vascular damage in pathologic states. The major antithrombotic mechanisms are discussed in Chapter 10; fibrinolysis is discussed next.

Fibrinolysis

Several proteins have been identified as playing a direct role in physiologic clot dissolution (Fig. 7-3), and others have been shown to act as profibrinolytic cofactors or specific inhibitors of that system. Thus far, comparatively few specific deficiencies or abnormalities of the fibrinolytic system have been identified or described that lead to inadequate or excessive clot dissolution. It seems likely that abnormalities of the fibrinolytic system do contribute to the pathogenesis of thromboembolic disease; however, these abnormalities may be focal in nature and exceedingly difficult to detect clinically. Although the constituent proteins of the fibrinolytic system circulate in detectable quantities, their proteolytic activities are in many respects controlled by the clot itself. Systemic activation appears to occur only in the setting of the pharmacologic administration of a plasminogen activator or when the hemostatic system is grossly deranged, as in disseminated intravascular coagulation (DIC).

Several recurring themes are apparent in the physiology of the fibrinolytic system. Among these are the structural similarities of the primary constituent proteins and the enhancement of their activity as serine proteases by the presence of fibrin. An appreciation of this structural and functional homology is crucial to our current understanding of the fibrinolytic system (Table 7-1).

Plasminogen, tissue-type plasminogen activator (t-PA), and single-chain urokinase-type plasminogen activator (scu-PA) are released into the circulation as single-chain molecules that undergo one or more enzymatic cleavages during activation. In the aminoterminal portion of all three molecules, triple-looped disulfide-bonded structures, called kringles, can be identified. Kringles contain approximately 80 amino-acid residues and are held together by three disulfide bridges. Plasminogen contains five kringles, t-PA contains two, and scu-PA contains one [15–17]. There is marked homology in the sequence of these kringle structures, both within and between molecules, implying significant genetic conservation.

Both plasminogen and t-PA bind to fibrin, and it is that characteristic of those molecules that effectively localizes their activity to the clot [18,19]. The kringle structures appear to be the primary sites of fibrin binding, although other structural domains may be involved, including the finger region of t-PA (Table 7-2) [20–22]. With one kringle in its aminoterminus, scu-PA preferentially activates fi-

Fig. 7-3. Major molecules in plasminogen activation. Solid lines indicate activation; dashed lines indicate inhibition.

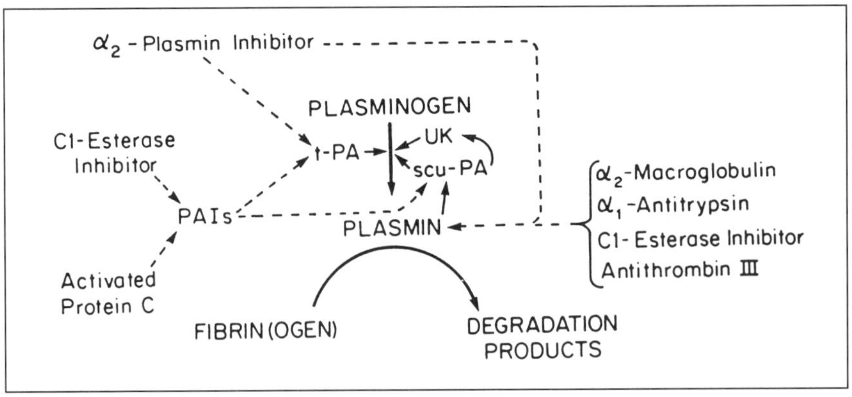

Table 7-1. Proteins of the human fibrinolytic system

Cellular product	Source	Active forms	Specific inhibitors
Glu-plasminogen	Liver	Glu-plasmin Lys-plasmin	α2-antiplasmin
sct-PA	Endothelium	sct-PA tct-PA	PAI-1, PAI-2, protease nexin
scu-PA	Endothelium	scu-PA tcu-PA LMW-UK	— PAI-1, PAI-2, protease nexin

brin-bound plasminogen, although it does not bind to fibrin.

Plasmin, t-PA, and scu-PA all belong to the generic class of enzymes called serine proteases [23]. The proteolytic locus of each of the molecules resides in their carboxyterminal regions and is specifically mediated through three amino acids: histidine, serine, and aspartic acid. The specificity of each enzyme for its particular substrate is a function of the three-dimensional structure of each individual molecule and the topology imparted to the active site by that structure.

Plasmin is ultimately responsible for the degradation of fibrin. It is generated by the sequential cleavage of plasminogen, which circulates as a single-chain protein with a molecular mass of 92,000 daltons (Fig. 7-4).

Plasminogen is synthesized primarily in the liver [24]. The native form of plasminogen, Glu-plasminogen, is a single-chain molecule containing 24 disulfide bridges and 790 amino acids [16]. Plasminogen is converted to plasmin by the cleavage of a single peptide bond, between residues Arg_{560} and Val_{561}, which converts the molecule to a two-chain entity [25]. The molecule may undergo additional cleavage of 76 amino-acid residues from the aminoterminus, either before or after the conversion of plasminogen to plasmin. Once amino acids 1 to 76 are removed from Glu-plasminogen, specific lysine-binding regions of the molecule are exposed that facilitate the physiologically important binding of the molecule (called Lys-plasminogen) to fibrin [26].

The kringle structures found on the A chain of plasminogen are particularly interesting and markedly homologous to the aminoterminal kringles found in prothrombin, t-PA, and scu-PA. Specific lysine-binding sites correspond to the fibrin-avid regions and are localized to kringles 1 and 4, with kringle 1 exhibiting the strongest binding properties [27].

The active site for plasmin is located in the B chain of the molecule and consists of three amino acid residues: His_{602}, Asp_{645}, and Ser_{740}. This site is remarkably similar to that of serine proteases found in other mammalian systems [28]. Although these amino acids are remote from each other in the primary sequence of the molecule, in the three-dimensional structure of the enzyme, they make up the active site.

Once plasmin is formed, it is capable of hydrolyzing proteins containing an accessible Arg-Lys bond [29]. Although the enzyme is relatively specific for fibrin, it will hydrolyze intact fibrinogen; convert Glu-plasminogen to the lysine form; and proteolyze coagulation factors V and VIII, serum complement components, and some hormones, including adrenocorticotropic hormone (ACTH) and growth hormone [30].

t-PA is functionally the most important endogenous protein that converts plasminogen to plasmin. It is synthesized in a number of different organs and tissues but predominantly by the vascular endothelium [31]. The human gene for t-PA is localized to chromosome 8 [32] and has been isolated, sequenced, and utilized through recombinant technology to produce pharmacologic quantities of the protein [33]. The protein structure of t-PA is similar to that of plasminogen in the broadest sense in that it contains kringles and a serine protease–active site near the carboxyterminus of the molecule.

t-PA contains additional structural domains that are very similar to those found in adhesive molecules and endothelial products. Near its aminoterminus, t-PA has two discrete regions: a finger region, analogous to the finger of fibronectin [25], and a growth factor domain [34], similar in structure and sequence to the well-characterized epidermal growth factor (EGF). The functions of these two regions are not completely clear at present, but it appears that the finger region may be responsible for the binding of t-PA to fibrin in the initial stages of fibrinolysis, whereas the major fibrin-binding site appears to reside in kringle 2 [24,35]. The EGF domain likely plays a role in the binding of t-PA to cell-surface receptors, which have been identified on endothelial cells [36], hepatocytes [37], and platelets [38]. Deletion of the EGF domain in recombinant mutant t-PA molecules prolongs the circulatory half-life of the protein, and it seems likely that the EGF domain is recognized by and binds to the receptors involved in the clearance of t-PA from plasma [39].

t-PA is produced by endothelial cells as a single-chain molecule with a molecular mass of approximately 72,000 daltons. The normal concentration of t-PA in plasma is approximately 5 ng/ml, but that concentration can be increased significantly through a number of provocative maneuvers, both pharmacologic and mechanical. Its circu-

Table 7-2. Fibrin-binding sites

Plasminogen	Kringles 1 and 4
t-PA	Finger region, Kringle 2

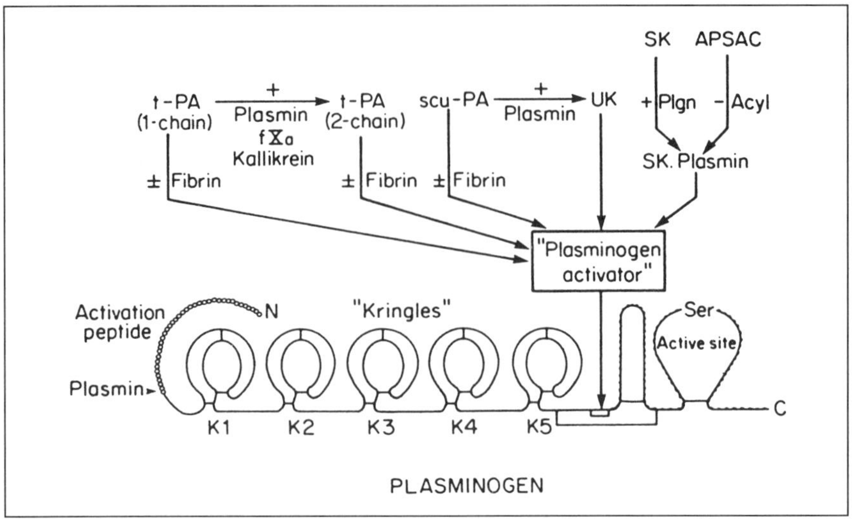

Fig. 7-4. Relationship of plasminogen to plasminogen activators.

lating half-life is approximately 4 minutes, and its primary clearance site is the liver.

t-PA acts to convert plasminogen to plasmin by cleaving the essential arginyl-valine bond that links the A (heavy) and B (light) chains of plasminogen. Plasmin, in a biologic example of reciprocity, converts single-chain, native t-PA to a two-chain form by cleaving the bond between Arg_{275} and Ile_{276}. This cleavage converts t-PA to a two-chain entity, with its aminoterminal end designated the A, or heavy, chain, and possessing the finger, EGF, and kringle regions. The fibrin avidity of t-PA appears to reside solely in the A chain [19]. The B, or light, chain of t-PA includes the remainder of the molecule and contains the catalytic, trypsinlike serine protease–active site, which in t-PA is composed of His_{325}, Asp_{374}, and Ser_{481} [40]. t-PA is relatively selective for its primary substrate (plasminogen), but it is capable of cleaving other circulating proteins, including prorenin [41], fibronectin [42], and fibrinogen itself [43]. The importance of these other proteolytic functions of t-PA has yet to be determined in vivo.

Both the single- and two-chain species of t-PA are capable of converting plasminogen to plasmin, but in the absence of fibrin, two-chain t-PA appears to be a more active molecule, having a greater catalytic efficiency than the single-chain form. Both single-chain and two-chain t-PA bind to fibrin, and that binding and the attendant conformational changes in the molecules [44] lower the K^m of single-chain t-PA for its substrate plasminogen from 65 μM to 0.16 μM [45]. The simplicity and biologic elegance of this system explains the mechanism of focality of action so critical to endogenous fibrinolysis. t-PA and its substrate plasminogen both bind to fibrin, a principal constituent of thrombi, and this binding itself enhances, catalyzes, and localizes the t-PA-mediated proteolysis of plasminogen to plasmin. The specificity of t-PA for fibrin-bound plasminogen is only relative and is much less apparent when administered in pharmacologic doses.

scu-PA is a glycoprotein containing 411 amino acids and, as its name implies, is released as a single-chain entity [17]. It has been isolated from urine and immortalized kidney cells in culture [46], but it is probably synthesized in vivo primarily by endothelial cells. scu-PA is the precursor of both HMW urokinase and low-molecular-weight (LMW) urokinase [47]. Plasmin and kallikrein convert scu-PA to the HMW two-chain form by cleavage of a single peptide bond (Lys_{158}-Ile_{159}). LMW urokinase is formed by additional plasmin-mediated proteolysis of the Lys_{135}-Lys_{136} bond, removing the sole kringle of scu-PA and HMW two-chain urokinase in the process. scu-PA circulates in plasma at levels similar to the basal levels of t-PA, that is, at approximately 8 to 10 ng/ml. The plasma half-life is approximately 10 minutes. Regulatory mechanisms in vivo for the synthesis and release of this protein have not been well characterized. scu-PA does not appear to convert plasminogen to plasmin to any significant degree in the absence of fibrin [48]. The fibrin selectivity of scu-PA has been attributed to its selective activation of fibrin-bound plasminogen [49].

Specific inhibitors of the active enzymes of the fibrinolytic system have been identified and well characterized. These inhibitors are members of the serine protease inhibitor, or serpin, class, and they circulate in plasma, rapidly neutralizing any fibrinolytic protease not bound to the clot surface. These fibrinolytic inhibitors thereby mediate a secondary system that effectively prohibits systemic fibrinolysis and confines fibrinolytic activity to the thrombus.

A number of specific and nonspecific inhibitors of plasmin have been identified, the most important of which is a single-chain glycoprotein with a molecular mass of 67 kDa, termed alpha$_2$-plasmin inhibitor (or alpha$_2$-antiplasmin). It is synthesized primarily in the liver and freely circulates in plasma with an average concentration of 6.9 mg/dl. Two characteristics of alpha$_2$-plasmin inhibitor deserve special emphasis. First, it rapidly neutralizes any circulating free plasmin in one of the fastest protein-protein interactions known. This binding is mediated through a lysine-binding region of alpha$_2$-plasmin inhibitor. Following this initial, reversible reaction, a slower, irreversible molecular interaction takes places that stabilizes the complex and renders the bound plasmin molecule permanently inactive [50]. Second, alpha$_2$-plasmin inhibitor can become covalently cross-linked to fibrin by factor XIII, as a result of which it may modulate plasmin activity within the clot, as well [51]. Alpha$_2$-plasmin inhibitor is the primary inhibitor of circulating plasmin, but other inhibitors are also present in plasma, including alpha$_2$-macroglobulin, alpha$_1$-antitrypsin, C_1-esterase inhibitor, and antithrombin III.

Several specific endogenous inhibitors of plasminogen activators also have been identified. At least four immunologically distinct groups of plasminogen activator inhibitors (PAI) exist [52]. These include PAI-1, derived from endothelial cells and platelets and the best-characterized thus far; PAI-2, derived from placental tissue and macrophages; PAI-3 isolated from human plasma and urine; and a fourth, nonspecific inhibitor called protease nexin-1.

PAI-1 appears to be the most important circulating inhibitor of t-PA [53]. Like antiplasmin and antithrombin III, PAI-1 belongs to the superfamily of serine protease inhibitors (serpins). It is produced in a number of different cells, including endothelial cells, liver cells, smooth muscle cells, and platelets [54,55]. PAI-1 appears to be the predominant protein in the subendothelial matrix, as determined by immunologic methods [56].

The normal PAI-1 level in plasma is approximately 20 ng/ml, although the range of concentration is wide [57]. Thrombin stimulates the release of PAI-1, from both platelets and endothelial cells [58,59]. Circulating plasma levels of PAI-1 also increase in the setting of inflammation, and this serpin can be categorized as an acute phase reactant. The PAI activity in normal, healthy individuals manifests a significant diurnal fluctuation [52]; approximately 60 percent of circulating PAI activity is due to PAI-1 [60].

PAI-1 has a plasma half-life of approximately 7 minutes and is apparently cleared by the liver [61]. It is capable of binding with and inactivating t-PA and two-chain and LMW urokinase, but not scu-PA [60].

PAI-2 is derived from human placental tissue and macrophages and, like PAI-1, can inhibit both t-PA and the urokinases. It was first described in 1968 [62] and has a molecular mass of 48 kDa. It appears to have a relatively greater affinity for scu-PA, HMW urokinase, and two-chain t-PA than for single-chain t-PA [63]. Normal levels of PAI-2 are similar to those of PAI-1 but can increase up to 20-fold in the third trimester of pregnancy, to concentrations as high as 100 ng/ml [52].

PAI-3 has been isolated from human urine and plasma [64], with concentrations in the latter of approximately 5 ng/ml. This 51-kDa protein inhibits single- and two-chain t-PA, HMW and LMW urokinase, and thrombin. Recent data suggest that PAI-3 and the inhibitor of activated protein C (APCI), also a serpin with arginine at its active center, are the same molecule [65], the physiologic role for which has yet to be identified.

Protease nexin is a 47-kDa glycoprotein synthesized by fibroblasts, renal epithelial cells, and cardiomyocytes [66,67]. It is a relatively promiscuous serine protease inhibitor, complexing to single- and two-chain t-PA, urokinase, plasmin, trypsin, factor Xa, and, in the presence of heparin, thrombin. Owing to this broad specificity, its undetectability in blood, and its relatively low binding affinity to these proteases, it is believed to act as a local modulator of serine protease activity [68].

In addition to the profibrinolytic proteases already discussed and their respective inhibitors, other circulating proteins can modulate the function of the fibrinolytic system in humans. In protein C, the link between coagulation and fibrinolysis becomes apparent, since this naturally occurring anticoagulant protein can inhibit PAI-1 [69]. PCI forms a one-to-one complex with PAI-1; thus, it now appears that protein C has dual roles in maintaining vascular patency: first, by inhibiting thrombus formation directly (because it inhibits coagulation factors V and VIII) and, second, by promoting fibrinolysis through the deactivation of PAI-1 [70].

Fibrinolytic activity is also regulated by the presence of receptors found on the endothelial surface that bind fibrinolytic proteins. Specific receptors have been identified and characterized that bind single- or two-chain u-PA [71,72], plasminogen [73], and t-PA [36,74]. These receptors enhance fibrinolytic activity by co-localizing plasminogen with plasminogen activators, which enhances plasminogen activation by up to 20-fold. Binding to these receptors also appears to provide some protection from circulating inhibitors [36,75]. On the platelet, assembly of t-PA and plasminogen bound to their respective receptors establishes an autocatalytic mechanism for cell-surface activation of plasminogen [76].

Intravascular clotting is by definition pathologic and is defined as **thrombosis**. In the arterial circuit, it has the propensity to occur at sites of atheromata. In the venous system, thrombosis most often occurs at sites of stasis (especially the lower extremities) and is not always initiated by an abnormal endothelial surface. Experimental studies have demonstrated the likely sequence of events in diseased vessel walls that leads to thrombus formation. The simple exposure of platelets to collagen induces their adherence to the vessel wall. Similarly, collagen can provoke the activation of factor VII and the generation of thrombin and, subsequently, fibrin through the intrinsic coagulation cascade. The exposure of factor XII to tissue factor in the vessel wall can likewise activate the extrinsic coagulation pathway.

The fibrinolytic system is poised to dismantle fibrin thrombi almost as quickly as they form. The physiologic stimuli for the induction of fibrinolysis are conveniently coupled to those that initiate thrombosis and are modulated by the direct effects of thrombus formation, as well. Thrombin is a key molecule in this regard (Fig. 7-5). Apart from its role in fibrin formation and amplification of clotting, thrombin directly stimulates the release of t-PA and PAI-1 from endothelial cells. Furthermore, in conjunction with its endothelial-derived cofactor, thrombomodulin, it activates protein C, which itself serves dual roles. APCI inhibits factors Va and VIIIa and thereby modulates coagulation. It also inactivates PAI-1 and indirectly promotes fibrinolysis. Many fibrinolytic proteins bind to and are activated by fibrin itself. Ischemia, brought on by throm-

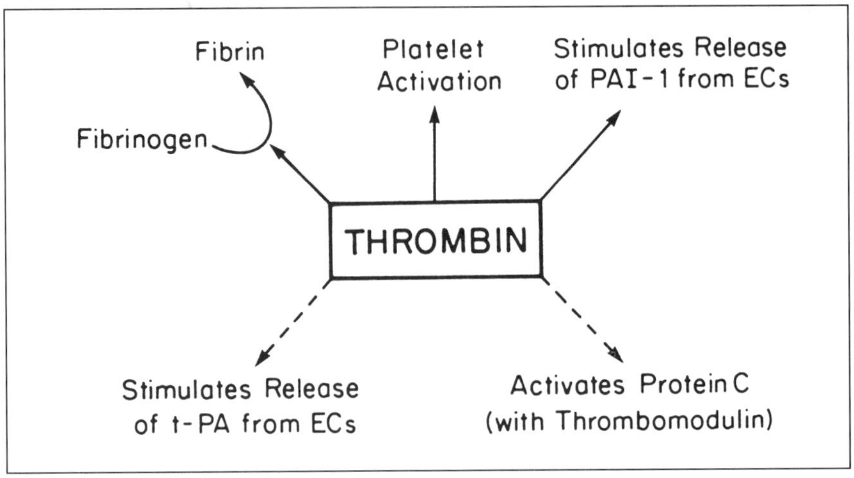

Fig. 7-5. Central role of thrombin in thrombosis and thrombolysis. Solid lines indicate prothrombotic events; dashed lines indicate antithrombotic or profibrinolytic events. (ECs = endothelial cells.)

botic vascular occlusion, also can stimulate the release of t-PA [77].

As described in Chapter 10, abnormalities in the fibrinolytic system have been implicated in the pathogenesis of thromboembolic disease. Abnormal plasminogen molecules with primary structural abnormalities (single amino-acid substitutions) have been isolated in several families with histories of recurrent deep venous thrombosis [78,79]. These individuals have normal antigenic levels of plasminogen, but the functional activity of the molecule is diminished. No human diseases have yet been identified to result from the primary, defective quantitative production of plasminogen activator molecules, either t-PA or scu-PA. The recent development of a murine model in which the genes for plasminogen activators are inactivated ("knocked out") [80] confirms the lack of important prothrombotic effect in individuals without t-PA and u-PA. Rates of fibrinolysis are attenuated yet proceed nevertheless. Recent observations on the role of macrophages and their aspartyl protease, cathepsin D, in promoting an alternative mechanism for fibrinolysis suggest that plasmin may not be the sole proteolytic enzyme responsible for the clearance of fibrin from the circulation [81,82]. Genetic polymorphisms also have not yet been identified. It recently has been reported that plasma t-PA levels can serve as an important predictor of risk for subsequent myocardial infarction or stroke in middle-aged healthy males [83,84]. The mechanism of this paradoxical relationship is uncertain, but it has been hypothesized that elevated levels of t-PA serve as a marker for preclinical atherosclerosis.

Increased levels of PAI-1 have been identified in youthful survivors of myocardial infarction [85] and are associated with increased risk of reinfarction [86]. Transgenic mice that are engineered to overexpress PAI-1 develop spontaneous thromboses [87], and tissue PAI-1 levels are markedly increased in atherosclerotic human arteries [88]. Defective release of t-PA has been described in several families with recurrent deep venous thrombosis [89,90], and one recent study measured a decreased fibrinolytic potential in one-third of patients diagnosed with deep venous thrombosis [91]. Conversely, recent reports have described patients with lifelong bleeding disorders apparently caused by deficiencies of PAI-1 [92–94]. Resistance to APCI recently has been reported to serve as a basis for venous thrombosis likely through the inability of factor Va to be degraded [95]; the role of APCI in inactivating PAI-1 has not been evaluated in this disorder.

References

1. Davie EW, Ratnoff OD. Waterfall sequence for intrinsic blood clotting. Science 1964; 145:1310–1312.
2. Macfarlane RG. An enzyme cascade in the blood clotting mechanism and its function as a biochemical amplifier. Nature 1964; 202:498–499.
3. Schafer AI. Coagulation cascade: an overview. In J. Loscalzo, AI Schafer, eds. Thrombosis and Hemorrhage. Boston: Blackwell, 1994.
4. Furie B, Furie BC. The molecular basis of blood coagulation. Cell 1988; 53:505–518.
5. Roberts HR, Lozier JN. New perspectives on the coagulation cascade. Hosp Pract 1992; 27:97–112.
6. Rapaport SI. Blood coagulation and its alterations in the hemorrhagic and thrombotic disorders. West J Med 1993; 158:156–161.
7. Spicer EK, et al. Isolation of cDNA s tissue factor: primary structure of the protein and cDNA. Proc Natl Acad Sci USA 1987; 84:5148–5152.
8. Wilcox JN, et al. Localization of tissue factor in the normal vessel wall and in the atherosclerotic plaque. Proc Natl Acad Sci USA 1989; 86:2839.
9. Colman RW. Surface-mediated defense reactions. The plasma contact activation system. J Clin Invest 1984; 73:1249–1253.
10. Lammle B, Griffin JH. Formation of the fibrin clot: the balance of procoagulant and inhibitory factors. Clin Haematol 14:281–342.
11. Cochrane CG, Griffin JH. The biochemistry and pathophysiology of the contact system of plasma. Adv Immunol 1982; 33:241–306.

12. Rosenberg RD. Hemorrhagic disorders. I: Protein interactions in the clotting mechanism. In WS Beck, ed. Hematology, 4th ed. Cambridge: MIT Press, 1985. Pp. 401–431.
13. Bauer KA, et al. Factor IX is activated in vivo by the tissue factor mechanism. Blood 1990; 76:731–736.
14. Nawroth P, Kisiel W, Stern D. The role of endothelium in the homeostatic balance of haemostasis. Clin Haematol 1985; 14:531–546.
15. Sottrup-Jensen L, et al. The primary structure of human plasminogen: isolation of two lysine-binding fragments and one "mini"-plasminogen by elastase-catalyzed-specific limited proteolysis. In JF Davidson, et al., eds. Progress in Chemical Fibrinolysis and Thrombosis, vol. 3. New York: Raven, 1978. Pp. 191–209.
16. Verstraete M, Collen D. Thrombolytic therapy in the eighties. Blood 1986; 76:1529–1541.
17. Guenzler WA, et al. The primary structure of high molecular mass urokinase from human urine. The complete amino acid sequence of the A chain. Hoppe-Seyler's Z Physiol Chem 1982; 363:1155–1165.
18. Thorsen S. Differences in the binding to fibrin of native plasminogen and plasminogen modified by proteolytic degradation. Influence of omega-aminocarboxylic acids. Biochim Biophys Acta 1975; 393:55–65.
19. Camiolo SM, Thorsen S, Astrup T. Fibrinogenolysis and fibrinolysis with tissue plasminogen activator, urokinase, streptokinase-activated human globulin, and plasmin. Proc Soc Exp Biol Med 1972; 28:65–74.
20. Lucas MA, Fretto LJ, McKee PA. The binding of human plasminogen to fibrin and fibrinogen. J Biol Chem 1983; 258:4249–4256.
21. van Zonneveld AJ, Veerman H, Pannekoek H. On the interaction of the finger and the kringle-2 domain of tissue-type plasminogen activator with fibrin. J Biol Chem 1986; 261:14214–14217.
22. Banyai L, Varadi A, Patthy L. Common evolutionary origin of the fibrin-binding structures of fibronectin and tissue-type plasminogen activator. FEBS Lett 1983; 163:37–41.
23. Jackson CM, Nemerson Y. Blood coagulation. Ann Rev Biochem 1980; 49:765–811.
24. Raum D, et al. Synthesis of human plasminogen by the liver. Science 1980; 208:1036–1037.
25. Robbins KC, et al. The peptide chains of plasmin. Mechanism of activation of human plasminogen to plasmin. J Biol Chem 1967; 242:2333–2342.
26. Banyai L, Patthy L. Importance of intramolecular interactions in the control of the fibrin affinity and activation of human plasminogen. J Biol Chem 1984; 259:6466–6471.
27. Vali Z, Patthy L. Location of the intermediate and high affinity epsilon-aminocarboxylic acid-binding sites in human plasminogen. J Biol Chem 1982; 257:2104–2110.
28. Hartley BS. Homologies in serine proteases. Philos Trans Royal Soc Lond (Biol) 1970; 257:277.
29. Weinstein MJ, Doolittle RF. Differential specificities of thrombin, plasmin, trypsin with regard to synthetic and natural substrates and inhibitors. Biochim Biophys Acta 1972; 258:577–590.
30. Sherry S, Alkjaersig N, Fletcher AP. Fibrinolysis and fibrinolytic activity in man. Physiol Rev 1959; 39:343–360.
31. Loskutoff DJ, Edgington DS. Synthesis of a fibrinolytic activator and inhibitor by endothelial cells. Proc Natl Acad Sci 1977; 74:3903–3907.
32. Raput B, et al. Chromosomal location of human tissue plasminogen activator and urokinase genes. Science 1985; 215:672–674.
33. Pennica D, et al. Cloning and expression of human tissue-type plasminogen activator cDNA in *E. coli*. Nature 1983; 301:214–221.
34. Ny T, Elgin F, Lund B. The structure of the human tissue-type plasminogen activator gene: correlation of intron and exon structures to functional and structural domains. Proc Natl Acad Sci 1984; 81:5355–5359.
35. Ichinose A, Takio K, Fujikawa K. Localization of the binding site of tissue-type plasminogen activator to fibrin. J Clin Invest 1986; 78:163–169.
36. Hajjar KA, et al. Binding of tissue plasminogen activator to cultured human endothelial cells. J Clin Invest 1987; 80:1712–1719.
37. Owensby DA, Sobel BE, Schwartz AL. Receptor-mediated endocytosis of tissue-type plasminogen activator by the human hepatoma cell line Hep G2. J Biol Chem 1988; 253:10587–10594.
38. Vaughan DE, et al. Characterization of the binding of human tissue-type plasminogen activator to platelets. J Biol Chem 1989; 264:15869–15874.
39. Browne MJ, et al. A tissue-type plasminogen activator mutant with prolonged clearance in vivo. Effect of removal of the growth factor domain. J Biol Chem 1988; 263:1599–1602.
40. Pohl GM, et al. Tissue plasminogen activator: peptide analyses confirm an indirectly derived amino acid sequence, identify the active serine residue, establish glycosylation sites, and localize variant differences. Biochemistry 1984; 23:3701–3707.
41. Tang SS, Loscalzo J, Dzau VJ. Tissue plasminogen activator activates the renin angiotensin system. Hypertension 1987; 10:355.
42. Quigley JP, et al. Limited cleavage of cellular fibronectin by plasminogen activator purified from transformed cells. Proc Natl Acad Sci 1987; 84:2776–2780.
43. Weitz JI, et al. Human tissue-type plasminogen activator (t-PA) releases fibrinopeptides A and B from fibrinogen. J Clin Invest 1988; 82:1700–1707.
44. Loscalzo J. Structural and kinetic comparison of single-chain and two-chain tissue plasminogen activator. J Clin Invest 1988; 82:1391–1397.
45. Hoylaerts M, et al. Kinetics of the activation of plasminogen by human tissue plasminogen activator. Role of fibrin. J Biol Chem 1982; 257:2912–2919.
46. Husain SS, Gurewich V, Lipinski V. Purification and partial characterization of a single-chain, high-molecular-weight form of urokinase from human urine. Arch Biochem Biophys 1983; 220:31–38.
47. Wun TC, Ossowski L, Reich E. A proenzyme form of urokinase. J Biol Chem 1982; 257:7262–7268.
48. Collen D, et al. Activation of plasminogen by pro-urokinase II. Kinetics. J Biol Chem 1986; 261:1259–1266.
49. Pannell R, Black J, Gurewich V. Complementary modes of action of tissue-type plasminogen activator and prourokinase by which their synergistic effect on clot lysis may be explained. J Clin Invest 1988; 81:853–859.
50. Wiman B, Collen D. On the kinetics of the reaction between human antiplasmin and plasmin. Eur J Biochem 1978; 84:573–578.
51. Sukata Y, Aoki N. Cross-linking of alpha-2 plasmin inhibitor to fibrin by fibrin-stabilizing factor. J Clin Invest 1980; 65:290–297.
52. Sprengers ED, Kluft C. Plasminogen activator inhibitors. Blood 1987; 69:381–387.
53. Kruithof EKO, Ransijn A, Bachmann F. Inhibition of tissue plasminogen activator by human plasma. In JF Davidson, F Bachmann, EKO Kruithof, eds. Progress in Fibrinolysis 6. Edinburgh: Churchill-Livingstone, 1983. Pp. 365–369.
54. Kruithof EKO, Tran-thang C, Bachmann F. Studies on the

release of plasminogen activator inhibitor by human platelets. Thromb Haemost 1986; 55:201–205.
55. van Mourik JA, Lawrence DA, Loskutoff DJ. Purification of an inhibitor of plasminogen activator (antiactivator) synthesized by endothelial cells. J Biol Chem 1984; 259:14914–14921.
56. Knudsen BS, Harpel PC, Nachman RL. Plasminogen activator inhibitor is associated with the extracellular matrix of cultured bovine smooth muscle cells. J Clin Invest 1987; 80:1082–1089.
57. Juhan-Vague I, et al. Plasma levels of a specific inhibitor of tissue-type plasminogen activator (and urokinase) in normal and pathologic conditions. Thromb Res 1984; 33:523–530.
58. Gelehrter TD, Szneyeer-Laszuk R. Thrombin induction of plasminogen activator inhibitor in cultured human endothelial cells. J Clin Invest 1986; 77:165–169.
59. Erickson LA, Ginsberg MH, Loskutoff DJ. Detection and partial characterization of an inhibitor of plasminogen activator in human platelets. J Clin Invest 1984; 74:1465–1472.
60. Sprengers ED. A sensitive assay, specific for endothelial cell type plasminogen activator inhibitor in blood plasma. Thromb Haemost 1986; 55:74–77.
61. Colucci M, Paramo JA, Collen D. Generation in plasma of a fast-acting inhibitor of plasminogen activator in response to endotoxin stimulation. J Clin Invest 1985; 75:818–824.
62. Kawano T, Morimoto K, Uemura Y. Urokinase inhibitor in human placenta. Nature 1968; 217:253–254.
63. Lecander I, Roblin R, Astedt B. Differential inhibition of two molecular forms of melanoma cell plasminogen activator by a placental inhibitor. Brit J Haematol 1984; 57:407–412.
64. Stump DC, Thienpont M, Collen D. Purification and characterization of a novel inhibitor of urokinase from human urine. J Biol Chem 1986; 261:12759–12766.
65. Heeb MJ, Espana F, Geiger M, et al. Immunological identity of heparin-dependent plasma urinary protein C inhibitor and plasminogen activator inhibitor-3. J Biol Chem 1987; 262:15813–15816.
66. Eaton DL, Baker JB. Evidence that a variety of cultured cells secrete protease nexin and produce a distinct cytoplasmic serine protease-binding factor. J Cell Physiol 1983; 117: 175–182.
67. Van Nostrandt W, Cunningham D. Purification of protease nexin II from human fibroblasts. J Biol Chem 1987; 262:8508–8514.
68. Mayer M. Biochemical and biological aspects of the plasminogen activator system. Clin Biochem 1990; 23:197–211.
69. van Hinsbergh VWM, et al. Activated protein C decreases plasminogen activator-inhibitor activity in endothelial cell-conditioned medium. Blood 1985; 65:444–451.
70. Sakata Y, et al. Mechanism of protein C-dependent clot lysis: role of plasminogen activator inhibitor. Blood 1986; 68:1218–1223.
71. Blasi F, Stoppelli MP, Cubellis MV. The receptor for urokinase-plasminogen activator. J Cell Biochem 1986; 32:179–186.
72. Roldan AL, et al. Cloning and expression of the receptor for human urokinase plasminogen activator, a central molecule in cell surface, plasmin dependent proteolysis. EMBO Journal 1990; 9:467–474.
73. Hajjar KA, et al. Binding of plasminogen to cultured human endothelial cells. J Biol Chem 1986; 261:11656–11662.
74. Hajjar KA. The endothelial cell tissue plasminogen activator receptor. J Biol Chem 1991; 266:21962–21970.
75. Miles LA, et al. Plasminogen receptors, urokinase receptors and their modulation on human endothelial cells. Blood 1988; 72:628–633.
76. Ouimet H, Freedman J, Loscalzo J. Kinetics and mechanism of platelet surface plasminogen activation by tissue-type plasminogen activation. Biochemistry 1994; 33:2970–2976.
77. Tappy L, Hauert J, Bachmann F. Effects of hypoxia and acidosis on vascular plasminogen activator release in the pig ear perfusion system. Thromb Res 1984; 33:117–124.
78. Aoki N, et al. Abnormal plasminogen: a hereditary molecular abnormality found in a patient with recurrent thrombosis. J Clin Invest 1978; 61:1186–1195.
79. Kazama M, et al. Abnormal plasminogen, a case of recurrent thrombosis. Thromb Res 1981; 21:517–522.
80. Carmeliet P, Schoonjans L, Kieckens, et al. Physiological consequences of loss of plasminogen activator gene function in mice. Nature 1994; 368:419–424.
81. Simon DI, Ezratty, Francis SA, et al. Fibrin(ogen) is internalized and degraded by activated human monocytoid cells via Mac-1 (CD11b/CD18): a non-plasmin fibrinolytic pathway. Blood 1993; 82:2414–2422.
82. Simon DI, Ezratty AM, Loscalzo J. The fibrin(ogen)olytic properties of cathepsin D. Biochemistry 1994; 33:6555–6563.
83. Ridker PM, et al. Endogenous tissue-type plasminogen activator and the risk of future myocardial infarction. Lancet 1993; 341:1165–1168.
84. Ridker PM, et al. A prospective study of tissue-type plasminogen activator and the risk of stroke. Lancet 1994; 343:940–943.
85. Hamsten A, et al. Increased plasma levels of a rapid inhibitor of tissue plasminogen activator in young survivors of myocardial infarction. N Engl J Med 1985; 313:1557–1563.
86. Hamsten A, et al. Plasminogen activator inhibitor in plasma. Risk factor for recurrent myocardial infarction. Lancet 1987; 2:3–7.
87. Erickson LA, et al. Development of venous occlusions in mice transgenic for the plasminogen activator inhibitor-1 gene. Nature 1990; 346:74–76.
88. Schneiderman J, et al. Increased type 1 plasminogen activator inhibitor gene expression in atherosclerotic human arteries. Proc Natl Acad Sci 1992; 89:6998–7002.
89. Nilsson IM, Ljunger H, Tengborn L. Two different mechanisms in patients with venous thrombosis and defective fibrinolysis: low concentration of plasminogen activator or increased concentration of plasminogen activator inhibitor. Brit Med J 1985; 290:1453–1456.
90. Wiman B, et al. The role of the fibrinolytic system in deep vein thrombosis. J Lab Clin Med 1985; 105:265–270.
91. Juhan-Vague I, et al. Deficient t-PA release and elevated PA inhibitor levels in patients with spontaneous or recurrent deep venous thrombosis. Thromb Haemost 1987; 57:67–72.
92. Schleef RR, et al. Bleeding diathesis due to decreased junctional activity of type 1 plasminogen activator inhibitor. J Clin Invest 1989; 83:1747–1752.
93. Dieval J, et al. A lifelong bleeding disorder associated with deficiency of plasminogen activator inhibitor type 1. Blood 1991; 77:528–532.
94. Fay WP, et al. Complete deficiency of plasminogen activator inhibitor type 1 due to a frame shift mutation. N Engl J Med 1992; 327:1729–1733.
95. Svensson PJ, Dahlback B. Resistance to activated protein C as a basis for venous thrombosis. N Engl J Med 1994; 330:517–522.

II

Pathophysiology of Vascular Disease

Vascular Injury

Stephen M. Schwartz

Twenty years ago, reviews of vascular biology treated the vessel wall as a pipe lined with a semipermeable membrane to control permeability faced with an antithrombotic anticoagulant surface to contain blood and supported by a mechanical-structural layer able to regulate lumen size [1–3]. Anticoagulant and antithrombotic properties were seen as physical attributes based on the absence or the presence of appropriate charge groups on the endothelial surface. The ability of the vessel wall to control transport was seen as depending on the physical structure of pores penetrating the vascular lining. The largest part of the vessel wall, the tunica media, comprised smooth muscle cells and was seen as a mechanical structure supporting the endothelial lining of the vessel and regulating blood flow by responding to the vasoactive substances and neural inputs. Most pathologists saw vascular diseases as alterations in mechanical function; increased contractility of muscle cells leading to excessive resistance; loss of the endothelial function as a semipermeable membrane leading to edema; accumulation of lipids in the vessel wall forming the atherosclerotic lesion; or endothelial denudation with exposure of thrombogenic subendothelial surface leading to thrombotic occlusion.

We now see the vessel as made up of living tissues with complex, biochemical functions [4–12]. Antithrombotic, anticoagulant, hemostatic functions, and even the permeability functions of the endothelial cells depend on specific structural proteins, receptors, endocrine factors, and enzymes synthesized by the endothelial cell. Smooth muscle cells not only provide a motor to control vessel-wall tone, they secrete proteins important to vessel-wall structure and synthesize molecules that may control their own growth.

Perhaps even more important than this focus on molecules produced by vessel-wall cells is the understanding that the vessel wall is a tissue comprising living cells and the realization that many vascular diseases involve disorders of cell growth. Smooth muscle hypertrophy and hyperplasia are central to current concepts of the morphologic changes underlying the major diseases involving obstruction of the vascular lumen: atherosclerotic vascular disease and hypertension [13,14]. This chapter will review the state of our knowledge about the common mechanisms underlying smooth muscle proliferation in these two common diseases.

Cells of the Vessel Wall

A modern view of vascular pathology must begin by reviewing how endothelial and smooth muscle cells come together to form blood vessels [7]. This two-cell structure means that blood vessels have a simpler structure than most other organs. Much of the pathology of blood vessels can be understood by analyzing the functions and dysfunctions of these two cells.

Embryonic Development of Blood Vessels

The earliest vascular primordia in the embryo are isolated cells that display endothelial and primitive hematopoietic immunologic markers [15]. These hemangioblasts coalesce to form **blood islands**, which consist of endothelium and primitive blood cells. The islands extend by sprouting and remodeling, forming a network (Fig. 8-1). The network eventually becomes connected with the heart to form the primitive circulation (Fig. 8-1c) [16–18]. These endothelial tubes become surrounded by locally derived, irregularly shaped mesenchymal cells which include the precursors of smooth muscle cells and adventitial fibroblasts (Fig. 8-1c) [19–22]. In the fourth fetal month, the three coats of the arterial wall become clearly evident. Cell layers delimited by elastic lamellae become more identifiable in large arteries, and the cells take on a more characteristic structural appearance [23]. At parturition, most arteries appear to have developed their adult number of layers of smooth muscle [24]. After this stage, the number of layers in the wall does not increase, and the medial thickening is due to the production of connective tissue, an increase of cell number, or an increase of cell mass [25,26]. Expression of the phenotype of smooth muscle cells is not seen until the third trimester [27].

The best evidence is that endothelial cells signal differentiation of smooth muscle cells from the surrounding embryonic milieu. This is supported by studies of isolated and cultured vessel-wall cells. Studies from this laboratory attempted to explore the ability of adult bovine endothelial cells to induce changes in the developing chick embryo. The bovine endothelial cells elicited a marked angiogenic response in the chicken system. Bovine fibroblasts and smooth muscle cells were not similarly angiogenic [28]. Endothelial cells also have been shown to produce fibroblast growth factor (FGF), a peptide that is angiogenic [29], as well as being mitogenic for smooth muscle cells and platelet-derived growth factor (PDGF), a peptide that is mitogenic and chemotactic for smooth muscle cells [30–35]. Perhaps one of these peptides is responsible for the recruitment of smooth muscle cells. More direct evidence for endothelial induction of a smooth muscle count comes from a recent study of vascular embryology. Using quail-chick hybrids, Ekblom et al. [4] showed that smooth muscle cells of the kidney vasculature are derived locally, while the endothelium is derived entirely from endothelial cells in the primitive vessels that vascularize the renal precursor.

Layers of the Arterial Wall

One of the simplest facts of vascular pathology is that the two most important lesions of vessels are localized to specific layers of the vessel wall. The major lesion of atherosclerosis is in the tunica intima, the innermost layer, which includes the endothelium and the connective tissue internal to the internal elastic lamina (IEL) (Fig. 8-2). While

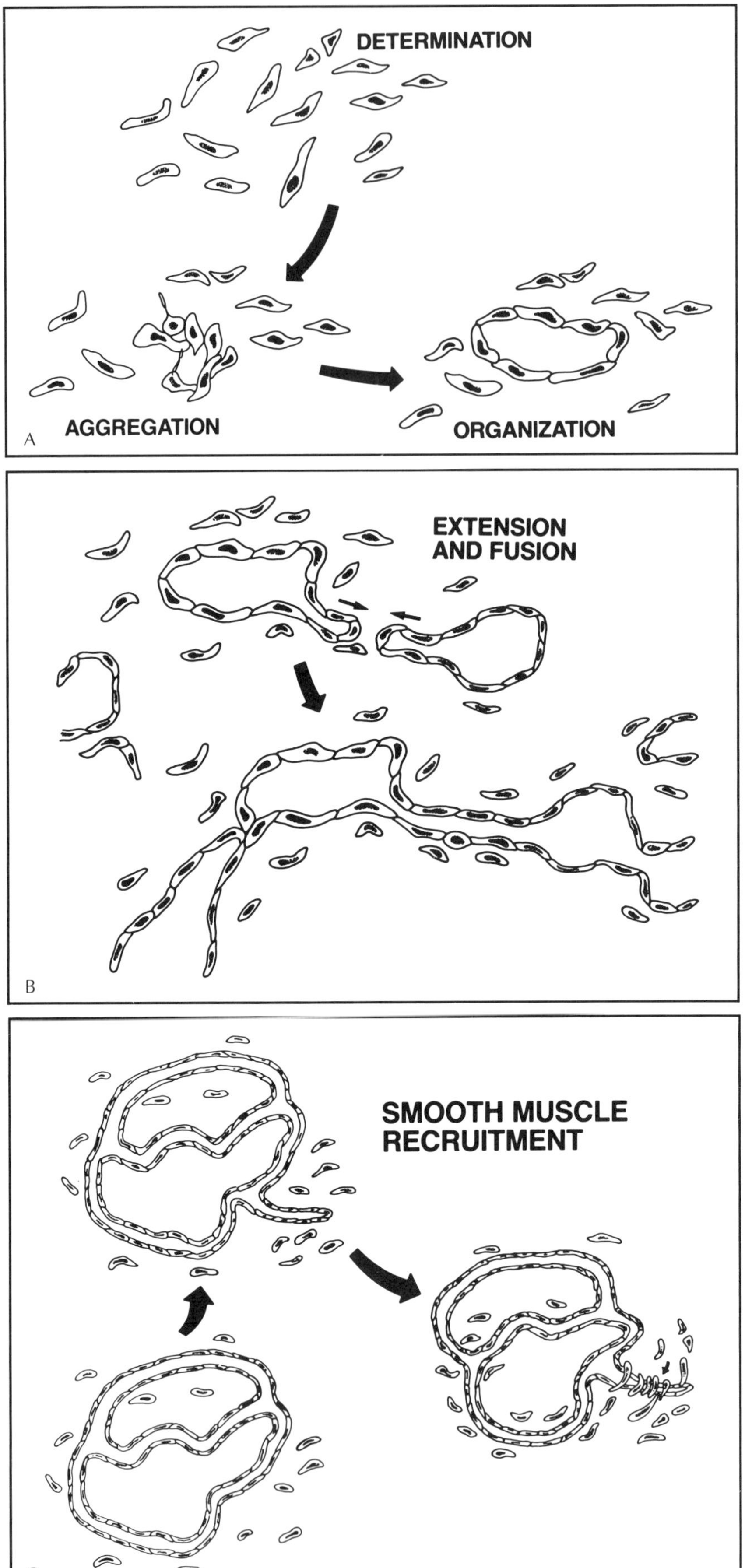
DETERMINATION
AGGREGATION
ORGANIZATION
A
EXTENSION
AND FUSION
B
SMOOTH MUSCLE
RECRUITMENT
C

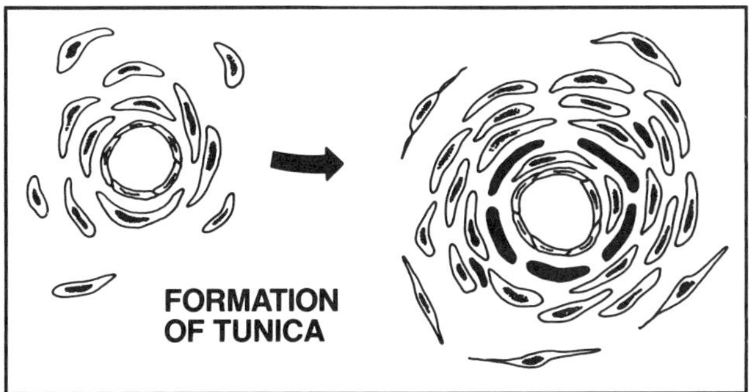

Fig. 8-2. Organization of the vessel wall into layers. The presumptive smooth muscle cells become separated from the endothelium by a layer of elastin (black), called the internal elastic lamella (IEL). The smooth muscle cells now make up the tunica media, the surrounding fibroblasts are called the tunica adventitia, and the part of the vessel wall within the IEL is called the tunica intima.

atherosclerosis afflicts both the elastic arteries, (i.e., major conduits like the aorta) and the larger muscular arteries [36], clinical atherosclerotic disease depends on occlusion of muscular arteries supplying an organ. Thus, atherosclerotic occlusion mainly represents the pathology of the tunica intima of larger muscular arteries. The major cell type between the endothelium and the IEL is the intimal smooth muscle cell. Other resident cells include lymphocytes, macrophages, and other inflammatory cells derived from the blood [37–39]. As the vascular tree branches, the thickness of the muscular arteries is decreased, and the tunica intima disappears. The tunica intima of small arteries is normally very thin, containing only the endothelium and some basal lamina. Even in large vessels, very little tunica intima is seen at birth, although the intima thickens as we age [40–42].

Hypertension affects all layers of the vessel, but the most important functional changes are due to pathology of the tunica media (Fig. 8-3). The tunica media is made up of the layers of smooth muscle cells that compose the bulk of the vessel wall. The structure of the tunica media is complicated by the invasion of autonomic nervous fibers, which control vascular contractility, and in thicker vessels by vasa vasorum, which are small branches of adventitial vessels that penetrate and nourish the media.

The tunica media of small muscular arteries regulates blood flow. The narrow lumen of these vessels produces an increased resistance that reduces blood pressure to levels appropriate for exchange across the thin-walled capillaries where exchange occurs. Thus, these vessels reduce pressure to maintain systemic capillary levels while increasing systemic pressure by regulation of total peripheral resistance. Pathologic change in the ratio of wall thickness to size of the lumen is central to elevation of blood pressure in hypertension [12].

Control of Smooth Muscle Proliferation

At least three mechanisms have been proposed for the control of smooth muscle proliferation: growth factors released from blood cells, inhibitors derived from the vessel wall, and growth stimulants produced by the cells of the vessel wall themselves.

The first, and predominant, hypothesis of proliferation suggests that cell growth is initiated by actions of growth factors derived from platelets or leukocytes. The factor uually discussed is PDGF [36]. The idea that a platelet factor controls smooth muscle replication grew out of the observation that smooth muscle cells would not replicate in serum prepared without platelet release [36], which led to the suggestion that PDGF was required for smooth muscle replication. This hypothesis was supported by the observation by Stemerman and others that denudation of arteries by a balloon embolectomy catheter produces intimal proliferation. Immediately after balloon catheterization, the denuded surface shows a prominent platelet carpet [43,44]. Antiplatelet serum inhibits the smooth muscle proliferative response [45].

The observation that whole blood serum (WBS) contains a platelet-derived mitogen led to the purification and cloning of PDGF [46]. Perhaps most startling, however, has been the more recent identification of the oncogene c-sis as the gene for one of the two PDGF peptide chains [47,48]. This oncogene is itself capable of transforming cells, raising the possibility that atherosclerosis is the result of secretion of an oncogenic peptide within the vessel wall. As will be discussed later, this observation is of considerable importance to the interesting possibility that smooth muscle replication may be controlled by factors intrinsic to the vessel wall. The second known requirement for cell-cycle progression is availability of somatomedin C, also known as insulin-like growth factor (IGF-1). IGF-1 is a cofactor that smooth muscle cells require for completion of the cell cycle following stimulation with PDGF [49–52]. IGF-1 itself can be synthesized by smooth muscle cells, and antibodies to IGF-1 inhibit cell-cycle progression [53]. These data suggest that PDGF is capable of stimulating production of its own progression factor.

It is important to point out that mitogenic substances other than PDGF also may be present at sites of vascular-wall injury. Platelets also contain a protein resembling epidermal growth factor (EGF) [54,55] and a factor able

Fig. 8-1. **A.** Origins of the vasculature: The earliest step is the commitment of some primitive mesenchymal cells to become endothelial cells. These cells aggregate and form small sacks, called blood islands. The endothelium of the blood islands is one cell thick. **B.** Organization into a network: Processes, usually called sprouts, extend from the blood islands, forming an interconnected network of endothelium-lined channels. **C.** Organization of channels into vessels: As the network becomes complete, the heart is connected and the endothelial channels acquire a coat of smooth muscle cells.

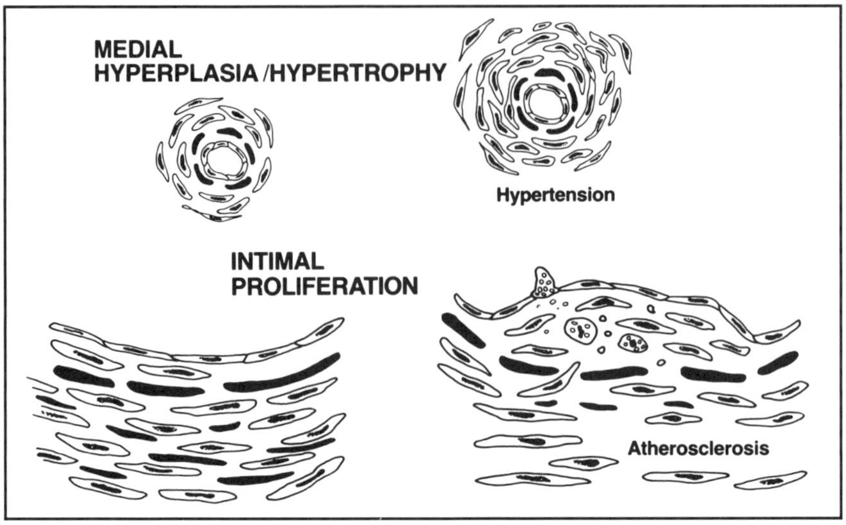

Fig. 8-3. Effects of vascular pathology on specific layers of the vessel wall. Hypertension is primarily a disease of the tunica media. This may take the form of increased contractile force or actual structural changes in vessel-wall mass. Atherosclerosis affects larger arteries and is specific for smooth muscle cells trapped in the tunica intima or those arteries.

to assist growth of cells in suspension called tumor growth factor β [56]. As already noted, FGF may be released from many cells as those cells are lysed [31]. Perhaps most relevant to atherosclerosis, the most obvious stimulus may be a growth factor derived from macrophages. Since these cells accumulate in the intima soon after commencement of a high-fat diet [57–59], these monocytes could be critical to smooth muscle proliferation. In vitro, monocytes or macrophages produce an as yet undefined polypeptide mitogen [60,61]. Recent evidence has shown that some of this mitogen is similar to or identical to PDGF [62].

Monocytes are likely to play a critical role in smooth muscle replication in atherosclerotic lesions forming in fat-fed animals. At least in animal models, we know that denudation does not appear until after initial events in the development of atherosclerotic lesions [58,59,63]. Recent studies on fat-fed animals, however, show a rapid initial monocytosis of the vessel wall with invasion and formation of intimal foam cell masses. At that point, endothelial continuity is still present [58,59,63]. Although there may be transient breaks as the lining of the vessel is penetrated by the monocytes, it is unlikely that any substantial platelet accumulation occurs at this early stage. Endothelial denudation occurs after monocyte accumulation [59]. What causes this endothelial disruption is unknown, but it is interesting to note that activated leukocytes can cause discontinuity of endothelial-cell monolayers, either by cell death [64] or by nonlethal mechanisms [65,66]. The relationship of this disruption to smooth muscle proliferation is an important unknown. Although two studies show that smooth muscle proliferation occurs prior to denudation [67,68], it is likely that the bulk of the proliferation in fat-fed animals occurs at later times [58].

There is also evidence that the vessel wall normally contains inhibitors of smooth muscle proliferation. The best studied of these are proteoglycans belonging to the heparan class. Clowes et al. discovered that exogenous heparin could inhibit proliferation in response to removal of the endothelium [69–71]. That effect may have mimicked the actions of materials present in the normal vessel wall and identified as crude extracts by previous studies. Nam et al. [72] showed that an aqueous extract of pig aorta injected intraperitoneally into eight-week-old living swine, in quantities as low as 500 g of protein, drastically reduced the rate of entry of arterial smooth muscle cells into mitosis, with no demonstrable effect on epidermal mitosis. Eisenstein et al. [73] reported two classes of molecules derived from bovine aortic extracts that are able to inhibit cell growth. One class, comprising structural polyanions, including heparans and proteoglycans, inhibited the growth of both smooth muscle and endothelial cells. Alcohol precipitates from aqueous extracts of the pig intima plus media were fractionated to produce both stimulators and inhibitors of synthetic-state smooth muscle in culture [74].

The most obvious question is the source of synthesis of such inhibitors. Possible cellular sources are suggested by studies showing that cultured vessel-wall cells, including both endothelium and smooth muscle, can synthesize heparan sulfates capable of inhibiting smooth muscle growth [75–78]. Smooth muscle cells themselves can synthesize a growth inhibitor for their own growth. Fritze et al., continuing the work of Castellot, have shown that smooth muscle cells also make a growth inhibitory heparan sulfate. This material is most prominent in quiescent cultures. By analogy to smooth muscle cells in vivo, the quiescent, untraumatized wall may be refractory to stimulation by PDGF [77]. It is conceivable that heparan sulfate released from quiescent endothelial cells could inhibit smooth muscle-cell proliferation as the region becomes covered with endothelium. Maintenance of the normal wall in a quiescent state could reflect heparan-sulfate synthesis by both endothelial cells and smooth muscle cells.

The role of endogenous heparan sulfates in controlling

cell proliferation after an arterial wound provides an alternative to the usual hypothesis that growth requires stimulation by release of a mitogen into the injured wall. One could imagine that balloon denudation results in a release of enzymes that digest the extracellular matrix, removing its inhibitory effect and thereby allowing the cells to replicate. Platelets contain a heparan sulfate–degrading endoglycosidase that could act in this way [79–81]. Incubation of endothelial cells with a crude platelet enzyme preparation or with a partially purified preparation of heparan sulfate–degrading endoglycosidase from the same source causes a marked release of cell-surface heparan sulfate, which appears in the incubation medium as oligosaccharides. Castellot et al. [82] proposed that following endothelial denudation or injury, platelets are deposited on the subendothelium, releasing heparitinase, platelet factor 4, and PDGF. The heparitinase cleaves heparinlike substances on the endothelium and smooth muscle into fragments that diffuse away, with additional inactivation of the substance by platelet factor 4 [83]. Thus, it is possible that balloon injury allows growth by initiating breakdown of heparan sulfate.

The hypothesis that growth is initiated by platelet-released factors at the site of denuding injury does not easily explain the continuation of proliferation lasting weeks after a balloon injury, while platelet release lasts only hours to days [84,85]. Several possibilities exist. The possibility that has just been discussed is that growth may depend on loss of inhibitors; nothing is known about how long a time would be required to restore endogenous inhibitory factors. Somewhat anecdotal evidence supports the possibility that mitogens might be released from cells within the plaque. Gajdusek and Schwartz reported that dead, cultured smooth muscle cells release a cytoplasmic mitogen distinct from PDGF [86]. More recent reports suggest that this material is FGF [31], a suggestion that seems consistent with evidence in vivo that FGF is a critical mitogen following angioplasty. Interestingly, Imai et al. [87] found a high correlation of evidence of cell death and stimulation of smooth muscle proliferation in fat-fed swine. They attributed this correlation to the extent of oxidation in cholesterol preparations used to feed the animals. Thus, cell death and platelet release in the plaque may be synergistic in the release of mitogens and hydrolysis of heparin-like molecules. FGF is very sticky [88,89] and could remain active in the wall for many days. Vlodavsky and his colleagues have suggested that FGF in vivo may be stored as a bound form localized in the extracellular matrix [90–92]; they found that residual PDGF on the culture dish could maintain smooth muscle-cell growth for days even in the presence of medium containing no PDGF. FGF, possibly released from dying cells, also is very sticky and might persist in areas of cell death for very long times. The sticky properties of growth factors may explain the claims of Savion et al. [93] that cells can grow on "extracellular matrices" prepared by detergent solubilization of cell cultures grown in the presence of growth factors.

The third possible mechanism for control of smooth muscle-cell replication depends on growth factors synthesized by the vessel-wall cells themselves. Cultured endothelial cells secrete soluble polypeptide mitogens that can stimulate smooth muscle replication. Part of this activity is due to a material that competes with the PDGF receptor and is neutralized by the PDGF antibody [94]. The identity of the non-PDGF mitogen remains unknown [95,96]. Although FGF is synthesized by endothelial cells, the protein either is not secreted or remains bound to the extracellular matrix [31,90]. The PDGF gene is expressed at high levels by cultured endothelial cells, while only low levels of expression of the PDGF gene are seen in endothelium in vivo [97]. At least in culture, production of PDGF by endothelium appears to be controlled by several factors, including the state of differentiation, exposure to thrombin, or exposure to lipoproteins. [30,32,98]. We do not know whether levels of PDGF-protein production can be altered in vivo. Two recent studies, however, suggest that endothelial cells in atherosclerotic plaques can synthesize message for PDGF. Barrett and Benditt [99] used Northern hybridization of human carotid-artery plaques to detect message in patterns of atherosclerotic plaques. They found mRNA for von Willebrand factor (an endothelial protein), *fms* (a leukocyte marker), smooth muscle actin, and both PDGF genes. Correlations between the concentrations of these messages suggested that macrophages were the major source of PDGF B-chain, but left open the possibility that endothelium could be involved. Wilcox and his collaborators [100] used in situ hybridization on the same tissue and found a high level of B-chain localization and some A-chain over small vessels penetrating the plaques. The large masses of macrophages were negative, suggesting that Barrett's Northern blot hybridizations may have been detecting *fms* in macrophage associated with these small vessels and suggesting that plaque endothelium is the major source of PDGF B-chain message. As noted below, however, plaque smooth muscle cells may also be an important source of these mRNAs. Libby and co-workers extended these studies by cell culture showing that plaque smooth muscle cells synthesize PDGF-A [101]. Ross and his colleagues used a monoclonal antibody and came to a somewhat different conclusion. Their data suggested that monocytes were the major source of PDGF-B. They did not study PDGF-A, so the data are not inconsistent with the earlier reports of Wilcox and Libby [13].

Perhaps more surprising is recent evidence that smooth muscle cells themselves may be able to stimulate their own growth by synthesis of both PDGF and IGF-1. Clemmons and his colleagues have found that PDGF is able to stimulate smooth muscle cells to produce IGF-1. This is particularly interesting because of evidence cited previously that IGF-1 is a cofactor that smooth muscle cells require for completion of the cell cycle following stimulation with PDGF [49–52]. The role of IGF-1 in growth responses of the vessel wall is unexplored. The discovery that cultured smooth muscle cells from fetal rats spontaneously produce PDGF-like material grew out of the observation that growth of smooth muscle cells derived from newborn-rat aortas cannot be arrested by putting cells in PDGF-deficient serum [102]. The culture medium from these fetal cells stimulates 3T3 cell and smooth muscle-cell replication. The mitogen responsible for this activity is inactivated by anti-PDGF antibody, and the conditioned medium competes for the PDGF receptor. Thus, it appears likely that fetal smooth muscle cells, at least in one species, can make this important mitogen [102]. There is also evidence that adult smooth muscle cells can be induced to produce similar material. Primary cultures of smooth muscle from aorta express A-chain message and synthesize a PDGF-like protein, and the A chain can also be detected in fresh aortic tissue [103,104]. With passage, however, cultured rat arterial smooth muscle cells produce low or absent levels of PDGF-like material unless those cells are derived from balloon injured vessels, these cells produced levels similar to the levels seen in cultured cells from immature aorta [68]. It is important to point out that since the observations of protein production can be made only on cells placed in culture, there is no direct evidence for comparable levels of production in vivo. Nonetheless, the appearance of activity in cells derived from the balloon injured vessel implies that some dramatic change has occurred in the capabilities of the smooth muscle cells making up the injured vessel wall. It is intriguing to consider the possibility that this change could be responsible for both the commitment to replication and the maintenance of replication during the days and weeks after injury [105]. As with observations of endothelial cell–derived mitogens, interpretation of these observations depends on whether the results reflect some property in vivo. As already noted, Wilcox and his colleagues began to address this question using in situ hybridization. These studies have shown localization of PDGF message in two cells in human carotid lesions. One cell type, already noted, is the endothelial lining of the capillaries found inside plaques; the other cell type is the intimal mesenchymal cells, presumably a dedifferentiated smooth muscle cell [100]. These results are somewhat surprising, given the high level of PDGF production by macrophages in vitro [36]. It will be important to ask whether protein, as well as message, is being produced in the plaques.

New Studies in Humans and Rats

Recent advances in animal models and data from human tissue have challenged the conventional wisdom not only about the role of growth factors but the role of proliferation itself. New markers of cell proliferation have failed to show smooth muscle proliferation in advanced [106] or even early [107] atherosclerotic lesions. Thus, we need to keep in mind that proliferation is not implied by growth factors in lesions.

The response to angioplasty may be more relevant to growth-factor biology. At least in the rat, several growth factors seem to play a role in the changes occurring after balloon injury. Critical molecules include angiotensin, PDGF, FGF, and transforming growth factor β (TGF-β). The balloon injury model begins with complete destruction of the endothelium as well as extensive death of medial smooth muscle cells [108]. The first response to balloon injury, called **first wave**, consists of medial smooth muscle-cell proliferation and begins about 24 hours after the injury. In elegant studies, Reidy and colleagues have shown that this wave of replication can be completely accounted for by release of basic FGF (bFGF) from dying smooth muscle cells [109,110]. Among other candidate molecules, studies with infused PDGF, as well as studies with anti-PDGF antibodies, have shown that this molecule does not play a significant role as a mitogen [111,112]. In addition, other molecules may be active, since more limited data suggest that alpha-adrenergic antagonists and angiotensin II (AII) can block medical replication [113–115].

The migration of smooth muscle cells across the internal elastic lamina to form the intima constitutes the **second wave**. Smooth muscle cells are readily observed on the luminal side of the internal elastic lamina four days after injury [108]. The duration of the second wave is not known. Several molecules can contribute to smooth muscle migration, including PDGF, TGF-β, bFGF, and AII. The relative contributions of these different molecules are not known, nor do we know whether other molecules are involved [110,115,116]. Interestingly, the effects of angiotensin-converting enzyme (ACE) inhibitors may result from the ability of these drugs to elevate bradykinin levels by preventing its degradation rather than the expected effect of these agents on lowering levels of AII. ACE inhibitors are not specific for the conversion of AI to AII [117–120]. Among other effects, these drugs inhibit degradation of bradykinin, and there is evidence from studies involving bradykinin antagonists that elevation of bradykinin can explain part of the effect of ACE inhibitors on neointimal formation [117,120]. The effect of PDGF is noteworthy, given the emphasis from in vitro studies that this molecule is a mitogen, despite the apparent lack of mitogenicity in vivo [111].

Once smooth muscle cells arrive in the intima, they may replicate for weeks to months [105]. This replication is the **third wave**. At the time of this writing, no specific molecular antagonist has been shown to inhibit this replication. Even antibodies to bFGF, which are so effective in inhibiting the first wave, are impotent against third-wave replication [110]. Therefore, although we cannot say that any specific molecule has been identified definitively as a third-wave mitogen, a few potential candidates appear to be present in the intima. For example, PDGF-A chain is overexpressed in the intima but will not stimulate replication if infused, nor do antibodies to PDGF suppress third-wave replication [111,122,123]. Other growth-control molecules that appear to be overexpressed in rat neointima include the AII receptor and TGF-β [116,124]. IGF-1 is also overexpressed following injury; however, it is overexpressed in the media [125]. While we cannot identify the critical molecules that sustain elevated replication in the third wave, we do know that the neointima can be stimulated to show a further increase of replication by infusion of other molecules. This increased responsiveness to mitogens can be called a **fourth wave**, and involves at least TGF-β, bFGF, or AII as agonists [109,113,116]. Again, PDGF does not appear to be mitogenic [111].

The role of the angiotensin system in neointimal formation is of particular relevance because of the failure of extensive clinical trials using ACE inhibitors to prevent restenosis [126]. With all the evidence from studies in the rat, why did the clinical studies fail? One explanation may lie in a misunderstanding of the pharmacology of converting enzyme inhibitors. Existing studies with ACE inhibitors are inconclusive in part because higher drug doses are needed to achieve significant suppression of intimal thickening (3–30 mg/kg/day) than to obtain a maximal (20%) reduction of blood pressure in the same strain of normotensive rats (3 mg/kg/day) [127]. This difference in dosage requirements may reflect the higher doses necessary to achieve inhibition of vascular-tissue ACE or to effectively block degradation of bradykinin at the site of injury [128]. The latter is of special interest because of evidence that bradykinin elevation as a result of inhibition of the normal catabolism by converting enzyme may act as an endogenous inhibitor of neointimal formation [117]. Finally, recent studies have identified a second enzyme able to produce active AII: chymase. Chymase is present in plaque and could be an important factor in the local production of angiotensin [129,130]. The best studied model for in vivo replication, neointimal formation, is the response of rat carotid artery to balloon angioplasty [44,108,131]. It is important to realize that this model is much simpler than the same response in larger, more complex human arteries that already have disease. First, rat carotid artery has only rare intimal cells [132]. Even normal arteries in larger animals have a pre-existing intima [133,134]. Second, unlike the response of arteries in larger animals, including rabbits, swine, and nonhuman primates, the response of rat arteries to most injuries involves platelets, but there is no deposition of fibrillar fibrin or adherence of leukocytes [135–144]. The simplicity of the rat model has made it possible to develop methods for detailed kinetic analyses of the processes leading to neointimal formation and to define four waves of response to injury with the molecules responsible for each of those waves [45,71,84,145–147].

In summary, the emerging picture of growth control in arterial smooth muscle is a complex balance of at least three kinds of forces. We simply do not know to what extent endogenous versus exogenous factors are active in vivo, nor do we understand the relative role of stimulating versus inhibitory growth factors.

Atherosclerotic Vascular Disease

As previously discussed, the cells of the tunica intima of arteries include smooth muscle cells and blood-derived white blood cells. This population is the ground in which smooth muscle cells proliferate to form the characteristic morphology of atherosclerosis.

Two different lesions have been proposed as the initial lesion of atherosclerosis [148,149]. The simplest is a local accumulation of fat in the vessel wall, resulting in a lesion sometimes referred to as a **fatty spot** or **fatty streak**. Alternatively, atherosclerosis may begin with focal accumulations of intimal smooth muscle cells called **intimal cell masses**.

Fatty streaks can be seen both in young humans and in experimental animals fed high-fat diets. Originally it was thought that the major fatty cell of the lesion was the macrophage. Interest in the macrophage decreased with the discovery in the early 1970s that many of the fat-filled cells were modified smooth muscle cells [148,150,151]. A balanced view today suggests that those cells with the greatest amount of lipid are indeed macrophages; however, smooth muscle cells also may contain fat. Fat-filled macrophages and fat-filled smooth muscle cells together are called **foam cells**.

There is reason to believe that the fatty spot is not the initial lesion. Children who die accidentally at a young age usually show large numbers of fatty spots in many parts of their arterial tree. The distribution of fatty infiltration in children, however, is somewhat unlike the distribution of more characteristic atherosclerotic lesions in adults. For example, fatty infiltration is common in the thoracic aorta, while atherosclerosis in adults is typical in the abdominal aorta. Nonetheless, many investigators believe that fatty infiltration represents the initial lesion of atherosclerosis with other factors controlling the distribution of the final, more clinically significant lesions [149,152].

The alternative candidate for the initial lesion is the intimal cell mass [7,153]. The intimal cell mass consists of accumulations of smooth muscle cells and associated connective tissue (see Fig. 8-3). Intimal cell masses near arterial-branch sites are called **cushions**. Intimal cell masses may be found in other locations within the intima [153,154]. Studies of fat-fed swine, as well as autopsy studies of human material, suggest that these focal accumulations of smooth muscle cells may have a predilection to the development of atherosclerotic lesions [40,152,153,155].

The presence of intimal cell masses in normal young people suggests that the initial stages of lesion development may occur early in the human life span. Accumulation of smooth muscle cells in the intima is, however, a normal part of the aging process. Arteries from older people show diffuse intimal thickening. Since this is part of the aging process and since it occurs diffusely throughout large arteries, many investigators would like to distinguish "normal" intimal thickening from the focal, pathologic events leading to atherosclerosis [149].

Despite these reservations, there is compelling evidence that smooth muscle proliferation is an essential part of atherosclerosis and intrinsic to its earliest phases. Morphologic studies of fat-fed animals, as well as later studies using tritiated thymidine autoradiography, demonstrate that smooth muscle proliferation is a major part of the response of animals to fat feeding [36,156]. Moreover, careful cell kinetic studies imply that the proliferative lesion in fat-fed pigs also begins in a pre-existing intimal cell mass [153].

While labeling studies have not been done in people, advanced atherosclerotic lesions have been labeled in vitro with ^{3}H-thymidine using tissue excised into organ culture. These studies suggest that smooth muscle replication at this stage of lesion development is, if anything, quite low [157,158]. These data are supported by more recent studies using cell cycle–specific markers to identify replicating cells in atherosclerotic plaques [106,107,159–161]. Evidence for proliferation in the early stages of human atherosclerotic lesions comes from a surprising direction. Many tumors can be shown to be the result of monoclonal proliferations because the presence of genetic markers specific for only a small number of the cells in the tissue of origin can be used to detect clonal growths. For example, we know that the leiomyoma of the uterus is monoclonal. This conclusion depends on the fact that a large proportion of black women are heterozygotic for glucose-6-phosphate dehydrogenase (G-6-PD). The gene for G-6-PD is located on the X chromosome. Each female cell turns off one or the other X chromosome early during differentiation. In a heterozygotic individual, each tissue consists of a mosaic of cells, some expressing one allele and other cells expressing the other allele of G-6-PD. The mixture of alleles in a cell mass, when compared with the random mixture in the underlying tissue, is a measure of the clonality of proliferation. Benditt utilized that fact to study the origins of human atherosclerotic lesions. He observed that a large proportion of atherosclerotic plaques of vessels in black females were monoclonal. The individual lesions showed a high preponderance of one or the other alleles, well beyond the chance distribution that might be expected from a random selection of large numbers of cells from underlying tissue [162].

This observation can be explained only by some form of smooth muscle-cell proliferation intrinsic to formation of atherosclerotic lesions. As hypothesized by Benditt, it seems likely that each lesion arises from one or, at most, a few smooth muscle cells. Moreover, these data are consistent with Thomas's studies in fat-fed swine [153] if we imagine that Thomas's intimal cell mass is a pre-existing monoclonal accumulation of intimal smooth muscle cells.

IS REPLICATION SLOW OR RARE IN ATHEROSCLEROSIS?

It is important to put this discussion in perspective. First, very few doublings would be required to convert the mass of the normal intima into the mass of an occlusive lesion. Such doublings might occur at rare intervals, intervals too rare to detect by the random samplings we now have. These doublings might even occur in bursts, consistent with angiographic studies that demonstrate rapid growth, or at least loss of lumen, at sites that are initially relatively normal [163]. Finally, we also need to consider proliferation of cells other than smooth muscle cells. A recent study from this laboratory shows focal levels of endothelial replication as high as 10 percent [161]. This may be evidence that angiogenesis is a very active and chronic process adding to plaque mass. Finally, while most studies have focused attention on the smooth muscle cell, Gordon et al. found more impressive evidence for macrophage replication than for smooth muscle replication [106].

We also need to consider the possible pathologic effects that might occur if the intima were to undergo hyperplasia. It is not obvious, for example, that the result would be a narrowed lumen. For example, Glagov et al. noted that human vessels can undergo massive accumulations of atherosclerotic mass without lumen narrowing [164]. The vessel wall compensates for the new mass by dilating to permit a normal level of blood flow until an adaptational limit is exceeded. This limit appears to occur when approximately 40 percent or more of the area bounded by the internal elastic lamina is occupied by intimal mass. The compensatory dilation is a structural change in the vessel wall and is usually called **remodeling**. Decreased lumen size probably does not occur until Glagov's limit is exceeded and may depend on pharmacologic mechanisms associated with the neointima or the plaque that cause a failure of normal remodeling events.

Remodeling is a normal response that allows the vessel to maintain normal levels of blood flow and wall stress and can be seen in small muscular arteries as well as in large elastic arteries [12,165]. Branching patterns of conduit vessels seem to be genetically determined [166]. Thus, the only way arteries can respond to a demand for an increase or a decrease in blood flow is by changing vessel caliber. These changes rely on rearrangement of existing vessel-wall components rather than synthesis of new mass or cell replication [167]. Until recently, the concept of vessel-wall remodeling as a part of the response to injury had been largely ignored in animal models of arterial injury and repair. The extent of remodeling versus loss of lumen due to intimal formation is illustrated by an important experiment by Jamal and co-workers. When Jamal and colleagues studied balloon-injured rabbit carotid artery, they found no narrowing of the lumen despite a 100-percent increase in wall thickness [165]. The same study, however, showed a significant (14%) narrowing in response to an experimental restriction of flow in the vicinity of the thyroid artery where endothelium had regenerated. This effect of the endothelium in an injured vessel is consistent with observations that structural adaptation to changes in flow requires an endothelium [165]. Since re-endothelialization generally correlates with a diminution of intimal thickening, these data may even imply a negative correlation of intimal mass with luminal narrowing [168]. The role of the endothelium in controlling lumen size may be especially important given the often neglected fact that plaques have a prominent microcirculation that comprises capillaries arising from the adventitia [169–171]. The role of these small vessels in regulating structural change or, for that matter, contractile properties of the atherosclerotic vessel remains unexplored.

If the correlation of intimal (or plaque) mass with lumen caliber is not a simple one, how do we account for angiographic changes seen after aggressive lipid-lowering therapy [172–174]? The actual degree of improvement of stenosis diameter in these studies is small (e.g., 0.7%–5.3%, or an increase of 0.003 to 0.117 mm in minimum absolute diameter). To put these results in perspective, one should note that six months after percutaneous coronary angioplasty, there is an average improvement of 16-percent diameter stenosis units and a 0.47-mm increase in minimum absolute diameter [175]. It is critical to realize that angiographic studies provide no insight into the mechanisms that may account for loss of lumen caliber. Thus, it is possible that apparent changes in mass reflect changes in adherent thrombotic material or state of vasospasm rather than in the extent of lumen narrowing due to accumulation of lipid and necrotic material in the atherosclerotic intima [176].

These angiographic regression studies showed only a modest change in lumen caliber compared to the beneficial change in clinical events [172,174]. This raises the intriguing possibility that lipid-lowering therapies may improve clinical outcome by stabilizing the lesion rather than by altering the lumen. Davies and others have suggested that the formation of fissures in plaques is the critical step leading to vascular occlusion [177–179]. They propose that fissuring results from a combination of biochemical events that weaken the fibrous cap over lesions and may include the expression of certain proteases [180]. Another group has added to this concept by proposing that accumulation of tumor necrosis factor α may lead to necrotic changes that result in plaque rupture [39]. While Arbustini and colleagues were unable to find a clear correlation of fissuring with acute ischemic heart disease, and Davies et al. found a high incidence of fissuring in atherosclerotic "control" arteries of patients dying of noncoronary events, the control patients may have had undetected myocardial infarctions and these fissures may simply represent sequelae of advanced atherosclerosis [39,178,181]. Davies's hypothesis would imply that we may be able to develop diagnostic tests, based on plaque composition as assessed by MRI, intravascular ultrasound (IVUS), or even gene expression patterns in atherectomy specimens, that might indicate lesion prognosis or the effectiveness of drugs targeted at stabilizing the lesion.

DOES REPLICATION OCCUR IN RESTENOSIS?

Restenosis seems like a simple problem: When 30 percent or more of angioplasties fail, most investigators assume that this is the result of a neointimal formation by hyperplasia, as discussed previously. This point of view is supported by morphologic studies that show proliferative smooth muscle cells in restenotic tissue. **Proliferation**, as used here, however, is a term describing only a morphologic change. Until recently, no one had asked whether the cells that make up restenotic tissue were actually replicating by objective criteria.

As discussed, we have used immunocytochemical labeling for the proliferating cell nuclear antigen (PCNA) to determine the proliferative profile of atherosclerotic lesions and found only very low levels of smooth muscle replication. We have used the same method to study 100 restenotic coronary atherectomy specimens [160]. To our surprise, the vast majority of the restenotic specimens (74%) showed no evidence of PCNA labeling. Moreover, in those specimens with proliferation, only a modest number of PCNA-positive cells were present per slide (typically < 50 cells per slide). PCNA labeling was detected over a wide time interval after the initial procedure (e.g., 1 day to 390 days) with no obvious proliferative peak. These were no differences in the proliferative profiles of restenotic specimens collected in the first three months, 4–6 months, 7–9 months, or more than 9 months after the initial interventional procedure (Spearman rank correlation coefficient $= 0.081$, $p = 0.43$). Furthermore, only 12 of 30 specimens obtained within 60 days of the initial coronary interventional procedure had one or more PCNA-positive nuclei per slide (including nine specimens collected within six days of the initial procedure, only three of which had immunolabeling of 1, 7, and 20 cells per slide). In support of these findings, a recent preliminary study using in vitro bromodeoxyuridine labeling also found low levels of proliferation in restenotic atherectomy specimens [182]. Similarly, Strauss et al. found no PCNA-positive cells in atherectomy specimens from seven restenotic stented coronary artery lesions [183].

These results and those of Strauss [183] contrast with a recent report by Pickering et al. [184]. In the latter study, both primary and restenotic coronary and peripheral arterial specimens had surprisingly high percentages of cells that were considered PCNA positive (e.g., mean $\pm$ SD: $15.2 \pm 13.6\%$ and $20.6 \pm 18.2\%$ by immunocytochemistry and in situ hybridization, respectively). However, only four of the 19 restenotic atherectomy specimens were obtained from coronary artery lesions, and none were obtained within one month of the initial interventional procedure (e.g., 1.6, 5.2, 6.1, and 7.9 months). Overall, the labeling indices reported by Pickering et al. seem exceptionally high (e.g., as high as 59% of cells being PCNA-positive) and resemble those of malignant neoplasms [185]. It is important, however, to realize that PCNA is not a direct measure of replication. Thus, the detection of differences in the frequency of PCNA-positive cells in the Pickering study should raise concerns that differences between primary and restenotic tissue in Pickering's study could reflect changes specific to peripheral arterial lesions, a tissue not included in our study.

These data return us to the discussion of remodeling. We cannot assume that an increase in intimal mass after angioplasty would narrow a vessel. Further, animal studies may be misleading, and we must reconsider the relevance of animal models to the human problem. Almost all animal studies, particularly those done in the rat, measure a decrease in lumen size from the initially normal situation. This can rightly be called **stenosis**. In contrast, the clinical problem is defined by the extent of dilatation that is lost after an atherosclerotic vessel has been dilated to achieve what the interventional cardiologist believes is an optimal diameter. The loss of this optimal diameter, rather than the pre-existing vessel caliber, is rightly called **restenosis** (e.g., a popular clinical definition of restenosis is $> 50\%$ loss of initial luminal diameter gain). By current angiographic criteria, even a return of the human vessel to its predilation diameter would be defined as restenosis, despite no change in intimal mass. To the best of our knowledge, angiographic studies in humans do not show that angioplasty produces stenoses similar to those seen in animal models. This would be difficult, of course, to demonstrate angiographically, because the initial lesion usually already has a critical stenosis. Furthermore, animal models, perhaps by design, require that all manipulated arteries show narrowing, that is, stenosis. There is no animal model in which 50 percent (or any significant percentage) of manipulated arteries remain dilated beyond their initial, unmanipulated caliber, yet this 50-percent rate (or higher) is the success rate seen when atherosclerotic human arteries are dilated with an angioplasty balloon. Perhaps, with more than 50 percent of human arteries remaining free of restenosis months after angioplasty, we may want to ask whether we have a sufficient animal model that allows us to explain why angioplasty is ever successful in the first place.

Finally, as noted in the discussion of atherosclerotic lesions, it is difficult to imagine that replication does not occur sometime during the formation of those lesions as well. It is important to remember that only a very few doublings, occurring episodically after angioplasty, would be enough to produce a large intimal mass by geometric progression. Detecting such a transient and rare event may be too difficult for current methods.

Theories of Atherosclerosis

At least three hypotheses have been offered to explain the origins of the characteristic atherosclerotic lesion. These hypotheses are not mutually exclusive; each hypothesis provides part of a sequence of discrete mechanisms that explain one or more of the accepted facts about the origins of the lesion.

THE INSUDATION HYPOTHESIS

The insudation hypothesis suggests that the lipid component of the plaque is derived from plasma lipoproteins. This hypothesis is substantiated, along with other evidence, by good analyses of plaque lipid showing that the lipid in the wall is derived from serum lipoproteins [186]. Of course, many questions remain unanswered. While we know that plaque lipid is derived from blood lipids, the mechanism of accumulation is unknown, and the role of lipid accumulation as the initial step in lesion formation remains to be demonstrated.

Satisfying as the insudation hypothesis is, any hypothesis based only on lipid accumulation is incomplete. No clinically significant atherosclerotic lesion is made up only of a lipid accumulation. Even if the lesion begins as a fatty accumulation, we do not know how the deposited cholesterol might induce the smooth muscle proliferation. Studies in cell culture have supported a role for lipoproteins in promoting smooth muscle growth [187–189]. Interpretation of these studies is problematic because the mitogenic concentrations of lipoproteins always are present in culture in amounts well below their concentrations in plasma. It is conceivable that fatty deposition injures cells, releasing growth factors that could stimulate cell proliferation.

THE PLATELET HYPOTHESIS

The idea that platelet accumulation is a critical part of plaque growth arose from the observation that atherosclerotic plaques contain recognizable platelet products as well as fibrin [2,190]. Proponents of this hypothesis proposed that material from the blood deposited on the inner surface of the arteries and degenerated. Plaque lipid was supposed to be derived from degenerated platelets. While we now know that the bulk of the fat in lesions is derived from plasma lipoproteins, the encrustation hypothesis also proposed that expansion of the plaques resulted from continued or repeated episodes of thrombosis and organization. The proliferative response to thrombosis is now accepted as part of the more general response-to-injury hypothesis of Ross.

The original encrustation hypothesis was missing a specific molecular basis for the stimulation of plaque growth, that is, "organization" in response to thrombosis. This was contributed by a set of ideas first proposed by Ross and colleagues as part of the general discussion of mechanisms of smooth muscle-growth control [36,46]. Their response-to-injury hypothesis proposed that smooth muscle proliferation depended on platelets accumulating at sites of endothelial denudation and on release from the platelets of polypeptide growth factors able to stimulate replication of smooth muscle cells in the vessel wall. Ross and Glomset discerned that smooth muscle cells become quiescent when they are put into serum prepared without platelet release (plasma-derived serum, or PDS), as opposed to the usual serum preparations (whole blood serum or WBS). This led to the purification, cloning, and identification of PDGF as a major cell mitogen.

The original response-to-injury hypothesis has undergone modifications over the years. We now know, for example, that smooth muscle replication can occur in fat-fed animals prior to endothelial denudation [191–193]. In fact, extensive intimal masses can occur as a result of accumulation of monocytes [56,58,194,195]. Since, as already noted, monocytes are also a source of growth factors, Ross has proposed that these cells may initiate smooth muscle growth [36]. Finally, the hypothesis also includes the possibilities that mitogens derived from vessel-wall cells themselves may initiate smooth muscle growth. This, however, leaves open the question of control of expression of autocrine growth factors by vessel-wall cells.

The response-to-injury hypothesis is complicated further by the recent observation that the atherosclerotic plaque also contains T-cells [37,38,196]. The expression of HLA-DR antigens on both endothelial cells and smooth muscle cells in plaques implies that these plaque lymphocytes have released lymphokines, presumably including gamma interferon and interleukin-1 (IL-1), into the plaque. It is intriguing to consider the possibility that the T-cells represent some kind of an autoimmune mechanism that could be important to the initiation and progression of lesions. Observations of T-cells so far is confined to the advanced human lesion. It is not known at what stage in lesion development T-cells first appear. Their presence, however, raises the possibility that lymphokines and monokines may play an as yet largely unstudied role in the propensity of vessel-wall cells to form lesions.

While a variety of pro- and antimitogenic factors likely to be present in the vessel wall have been reviewed, the original emphasis on the platelet remains likely to be valid as part of the picture of plaque growth over time, particularly in those periods when endothelium does break down and massive platelet release ensues. As will be discussed later, the response-to-injury hypothesis also may be important in the ontogeny of microvascular lesions in hypertension. Finally, while the response to injury hypothesis provides an attractive model of the complex factors promoting smooth muscle growth, this set of mechanisms sheds little light on the initial events leading to the observation that human atherosclerosis is a monoclonal proliferation.

THE MONOCLONAL "HYPOTHESIS"

This hypothesis proposes that atherosclerosis begins as a mutation or viral hit, transforming a single, isolated smooth muscle cell into the progenitor of a proliferative clone. The term *monoclonal hypothesis* is somewhat misleading. As already presented, we know from analysis of the G-6-PD allotypes that at least many human atherosclerotic plaques are derived from cells having a single allotype. The data for plaque monoclonality is as good as data for any neoplasm. Thus, monoclonality of plaques is more an observation than a hypothesis.

The term *monoclonal hypothesis*, however, has been used to identify Benditt's extension of his observation to the proposal that monoclonality is the result of neoplastic change [162]. Neoplastic transformation is one of several interpretations of a monoclonal G-6-PD allotype. The hypotheses that have been discussed include: (1) origin as single cells, as seen in neoplasms; (2) origin from very small numbers of cells; and (3) population giving rise to the proliferation itself consisting of only a single allotyped selection for a subset of cells bearing one or the other allotype.

Since sampling of normal wall does not support the third hypothesis, and since both allotypes are represented in individual lesions of each human, Benditt concluded that lesions must be either monoclonal or at most oligoclonal [162]. Because this pattern is known to occur only in neoplasia, Benditt further proposed that smooth muscle-cell replication depends on transformation to a benign neoplastic state. Pearson and his colleagues confirmed Benditt's observations in human plaques, comparing the plaque to the cutaneous scars [197]. Particularly interesting was their finding that monoclonality of atherosclerotic plaques at different stages of development was more definitive in advanced lesions, that is, in lesions with well-formed fibrous caps, than in fatty streaks [198]. This finding might have been expected, since the smooth muscle cells of the early fatty streak are diluted by large numbers of presumably polyclonal monocytes. In contrast to advanced plaques, cutaneous scars were polyclonal, that is, both allotypes of G-6-PD were represented equally. This would be expected if the response to a wound was a diffuse process involving stimulation of proliferation in many different cells, as proposed above.

Lee, Thomas, and their collaborators have offered a different interpretation of monoclonality [153,199–202]. This group has attempted to reconcile the data in humans with their own experimental work in animal models. Extensive cell kinetic analyses of fat-fed swine have been interpreted as showing that smooth muscle proliferation occurs by repetitive waves of replication and cell death. On the basis of a mathematical model, they argued that monoclonality might arise by a repeated resampling of a proliferative population in which several clones have become expanded. While this model might appear attractive mathematically, it is important to point out that the group has been unsuccessful in producing monoclonal lesions in fat-fed animals. This experiment was performed in hybrid hares bred between two species differing in the G-6-PD allotype. The failure to demonstrate monoclonality in the animal model must be seen as a serious reservation in our interpretation of smooth muscle-cell proliferation in animal model systems [198,203,204].

Benditt's hypothesis has much to recommend it. By definition, a benign neoplasm is a focal overgrowth of a single cell type. Benign neoplasms do not metastasize or invade. Thus, a nodule of smooth muscle cells growing in the uterus is called a **leiomyoma**. This may seem like semantics, but it is worth noting that if the plaque comprises a focal proliferation of smooth muscle cells, then the atherosclerotic plaque is, *by definition*, a benign neoplasm of smooth muscle cells.

The equation of plaques with leiomyomas leads to intriguing questions. For example, Benditt has proposed that the risk associated with smoking might be due to the accumulation of mutagens from cigarette smoke [162]. Interestingly, he observed that polycyclic aromatic hydrocarbons distribute in lipoproteins and that human vascular smooth muscle cells respond to chemical mutagens, as of course might be expected [205]. An additional avenue stimulated by the observation of monoclonality has been the search for possible oncogenic viruses. The Fabricants and their collaborators have reported that the incidence of fatty lesions in chickens is greatly increased by infection with Marek's disease virus, [206,207] which is a virus of the herpes group. In collaboration with McDougall, Benditt and Barrett showed that herpes virus genomes could be detected in atherosclerotic plaques by in situ hybridization [208]. This observation has been confirmed by Gyorkey et al. [209]. In addition, Melnik et al. reported the presence of cytomegalovirus antigen in human arterial smooth muscle cells and high levels of antibody in the serum of patients undergoing vascular surgery to treat atherosclerosis [210,211].

Benditt's neoplasm hypothesis needs to be considered in the context of current concepts of the control of normal and neoplastic growth. The last decade has seen the identification of a number of proteins, initially identified as mRNA species or as genomic DNA sequences specific for neoplasia. These mammalian genomic species were identified by their presence in transforming retroviruses. The discovery that these were originally derived from mammalian genomic sequences has turned out to be a powerful tool to understanding the normal replication of the cell. Alterations in activity of the protein products of these genes, including structural alterations in the protein so as to increase or decrease their activity as well as alterations in the gene so as to increase or decrease the amount of protein synthesis may cause severe imbalances that control cell replication and an overproliferation of cells [212].

Benditt's hypothesis that atherosclerosis is a benign neoplasm depends on identification of the gene responsible for loss of control of smooth muscle proliferation. Penn et al. [213] used DNA transfection to demonstrate that there are transforming sequences in human atherosclerotic tissue. This assay depends on the shearing of cellular DNA and the insertion of that DNA into target assay cells, usually the NIH 3T3 cell line. When that is done, there is always a small frequency of transformation [214]. An increased frequency of transformation may be seen either when the source DNA contains genomic species that are altered in some way so as to stimulate cell proliferation or when the source DNA is inserted into the recipient cells in such a way as to cause overexpression. Penn et al. [213] found an increased frequency of positive transformants. It is difficult to decide what that means. The sequence responsible for transformation is not known. Even if the sequence were known, the possibility exists that this sequence is a normal cellular gene, somehow made more available for transfection by the content of the plaque. Even that result, however, would illustrate an important point: By elucidating a smooth muscle–derived transforming gene, we might learn more about normal mechanisms of smooth muscle-growth control.

In summary, the monoclonal part of the monoclonal "hypothesis" is probably a fact. As with insudation, knowledge of that fact leaves several open questions, especially questions about the original stimulus to smooth muscle proliferation. In any case, clonal origin must be among the earliest events in ontogeny of the atherosclerotic plaque.

A Unifying Hypothesis for Atherosclerosis

We may be able to rationalize the various mechanisms proposed for atherosclerosis if we begin by listing the generally accepted facts about the lesion.

1. All clinically significant atherosclerotic lesions involve smooth muscle cells. While we do not know whether replication of smooth muscle cells is a result or a cause of the lesion, there is the suggestive evidence that focal accumulations of smooth muscle cells may precede the formation of atherosclerotic lesions.
2. Focal smooth muscle masses are found in the intima shortly after birth. These masses correlate with the location of lesions in later life. Fatty lesions also are seen early in life, but their distribution does not match that of adult lesions.
3. Nothing is known about the teleologic significance of the separation of the vessel wall into three layers. Atherosclerotic plaques are found only in the intima, suggesting something special about the intimal environment and about the subset of smooth muscle cells that become trapped in the intima.
4. The smooth muscle component of atherosclerotic lesion arises from one or, at most, a small number of cells. The mechanism of this "monoclonal" proliferation is not known.
5. Clinically significant atherosclerosis is greatly accelerated by a variety of forms of hyperlipemia. In populations where blood cholesterol is low, the incidence of clinically significant atherosclerotic disease is also low. It is likely, therefore, that lipid accumulation is necessary for progression to a clinically significant lesion.
6. The active atherosclerotic plaque contains a variety of cells known to give rise to growth-promoting factors in vitro. Based both on studies in vitro and on animal studies in vivo, it seems probable that these factors are active in the lesion-causing acceleration of progression of atherosclerosis.
7. Several other components of the lesions suggest that mechanisms similar to those involved in the response of any other tissue to injury may also occur in the vessel wall. This includes the presence of a prominent neovascular component as well as the presence of activated T-cells.

These facts cover a set of events in the ontogeny of the lesion beginning as early as birth, or before, and lead to a hypothesis based on concepts of how arteries develop. In this view, focal accumulation of smooth muscle cells, as in Benditt's observation of monoclonality or Thomas's observation of the intimal cell mass, is the first event. It is possible that the intimal cell mass suggests that intimal cell masses occur spontaneously during development as a result of the trapping of a few smooth muscle cells inside the developing internal elastic lamella. The complex geometry of maintaining structures while the vessel grows could explain the predilection for complicated structures, for example, branch sites, to develop both intimal cell masses and later atherosclerotic lesions. This "trapping" hypothesis could provide an alternative explanation of monoclonality [145]. A clone of intimal cells could result from one cell proliferating in response to a mutational or a viral change in a gene that controls growth. Alternatively, proliferation of the small number of cells trapped in the intima, like growth of sparsely plated cells in a culture dish, would produce the appearance of monoclonality, and that property would be intrinsic to the earliest stages of the plaque.

The trapping of smooth muscle cells in the intima might be complicated by migration of smooth muscle cells from the media into the intima. There is good evidence that arterial injury can elicit migration of smooth muscle cells into the intima after the vessel is formed. The most direct evidence for this comes from cell kinetic studies [84,215,216]. In the most detailed study, rats with balloon-denuded carotid arteries were labeled by continuous infusion with tritiated thymidine. All cells entering the cell cycle over 2 weeks were detected by autoradiography. During this interval, the increase in DNA of the media could be accounted for by about three cell doublings. About 90 percent of the cells in the intima were labeled and, therefore, must represent cells that moved into the intima and replicated on one or both sides of the internal elastic lamina. Since the average labeled cells must have divided three times, the 10 percent of the cells remaining unlabeled represent about 50 percent of the total migration into the intima (one cell with three divisions = eight labeled cells; one cell with migration alone = one unlabeled cell). Thus, substantial amounts of migration occur even without replication. Controls over migration have only begun to be explored, although a strong contender for that role is PDGF. This peptide not only is mitogenic for smooth muscle cells but is chemotactic as well [217]. In contrast, other mitogens are not chemotactic. Thus, PDGF by itself could account for several major features of atherosclerosis.

While the intimal cell mass may explain monoclonality and the localization of lesions to the intima, we still need to explain why cells in this site proliferate. Several ideas have been offered, and all might operate together:

1. Relatively sparse intimal smooth muscle cells might escape density-dependent inhibition by neighboring cells, perhaps due to a deficiency of endogenous heparan-sulfate glycosaminoglycans [218].
2. Cells in the intima could see higher concentrations of

mitogens released by platelets at the luminal surface or by entry of macrophages [36].
3. Intimal smooth muscle cells could have a proliferative advantage due to selection [200].
4. Intimal cells might be more subject to mutation by circulating polycyclic compounds bound to lipoproteins [219].

However the intimal cell mass begins, progression to an advanced, clinically significant lesion is likely to depend on problems of lipid accumulation. Properties of the smooth muscle cells and the types of connective tissue synthesized by cells in the intimal cell mass might make the sites prone to lipid accumulation. Alternatively, growth of the smooth muscle lesion might in some way injure the overlying endothelium, leading to increased permeability to lipids and further access to PDGF. Lipid insudation could lead to release of mitogens from the cytoplasm of injured cells with the accumulation of growth factors with the effects proposed in the response-to-injury hypothesis.

Initial Lesion of Hypertension

Whatever the mechanism of initiation of blood pressure, most studies agree that the maintenance of blood pressure depends on fixed structural changes sometimes called **chronic autoregulation** [12,220]. Folkow [12] has suggested that these changes themselves may be important for the maintenance of elevated blood pressure. An understanding of the mechanisms involved in modeling or remodeling of blood vessels very well may be important to our understanding of the pathologic consequences of this disease (see Fig. 8-1).

The possible significance of this smooth muscle pathology depends on an understanding of the central role played by **peripheral resistance** in control of blood pressure. The vasculature is a simple circuit, not unlike a high school science laboratory demonstration in which a transformer, some large wires, some resistors, and capacitors are connected together. The resistors in that circuit are the small arteries and arterioles. Vascular resistance is controlled either by restriction of lumen size, called arterial narrowing, or by a decrease in the number of vessels called rarefaction. In the former case, narrowing can be the result of increased wall thickness or active contraction. Most studies, however, show that increased wall thickness is a common feature of chronic hypertension regardless of the mechanism initiating elevation of pressure [221–223]. Morphometric studies have further shown that this increase includes all components of the vessel wall, that is, smooth muscle cell mass and connective tissue are both elevated [224,225]. Since the cell's own mass and the surrounding connective tissue are both synthesized by smooth muscle cells, hypertension is characterized by a fundamental, morphologic smooth muscle lesion. This review will concentrate on the evidence for an increased vascular mass and discuss possible mechanisms underlying that increase.

MORPHOLOGIC PATHOLOGY OF HYPERTENSION

It is important to realize that an increase in vascular smooth muscle mass occurs in resistance vessels in a wide variety of forms of hypertension, including forms in which we know the increase in mass is not itself the primary etiology. Forms of hypertension due to changes in blood volume may effectively increase resistance due to increased flow of blood through the microvascular bed. For example, Cowley and his colleagues made dogs hypertensive by resection of two-thirds of the renal mass followed by infusion of salt and water [220,226]. The initial response was an elevated cardiac output and blood volume. Peripheral resistance actually decreased. By 48 hours, however, cardiac output and blood volume were within normal limits and maintenance of pressure elevation was due to increased peripheral resistance [220]. While Cowley used this experiment to illustrate the central role of volume even when no elevation of volume is measurable, it is also apparent that the elevation of pressure depended on restriction of the lumen of the resistance vessels.

The lumen may be restricted by active contraction of the vessel wall, by increase in the structural mass of the vessel wall, or by both (see Fig. 8-3). The rapid drop in blood pressure when hypertensive animals or people are treated with smooth muscle relaxants implies that active constriction is important. Folkow [12], however, has pointed out that it is important to think of the increased mass not only in terms of its passive role in obstructing the vessel lumen but as amplifying the artery's response to extrinsic vasoactive stimuli. He has suggested that some component of elevation of blood pressure in humans and animals with hypertension must be attributed to a structural change.

If there are structural changes, we might expect to be able to measure a morphologic change in wall mass. Such changes have been analyzed by careful morphometric analysis of the vessel wall. It is important to point out that very small changes in radius should produce a massive increase in resistance. Since resistance is inversely proportional to the fourth power of the radius, a change of only 5 percent in the radius of a 100-micron resistance vessel would be expected to produce a 20-percent increase in blood pressure [12]. Against that background, it is likely that morphologic changes will be detectable only when there is significant elevation of pressure. Very surprising to note is that some authors have found evidence for an increase in vascular mass prior to changes in blood pressure [227,228].

The changes in wall mass seen in morphometric studies are subtle quantitative changes that are believable only when carefully analyzed on a population basis. It is not surprising, therefore, that most pathologists find that the morphology of hypertensive vascular thickening is not diagnostic of hypertension. Other changes have been claimed to be more diagnostic. Diffuse intimal thickening of elastic arteries and large muscular arteries, hyaline change, and reduplication of the internal elastic lamina in resistance arteries or arterioles are a normal part of the aging process. These changes are called **benign arteriosclerosis** and are said to appear at an accelerated rate in individuals with hypertensive atherosclerosis of large arteries and are also accelerated in individuals with chronic hypertension.

Severe elevations of blood pressure, for example, malignant hypertension, produce more dramatic changes at the microvascular level. The retinal vessels of hypertensive individuals are sufficiently abnormal to allow the diagnosis of hypertension on the basis of ophthalmoscopy alone. Arteries show segmental constriction and dilation, the arterioles are unable to resist the change in pressure, resulting in aneurysmal formation, hemorrhage, and scarring. These changes are typical of the pathology of other resistance vessels with severe rapid elevation of blood pressure, typically to diastolic blood pressures above 110 mm Hg. Smooth muscle cells in the vessel wall in dilated segments undergo necrosis, endothelial integrity is lost, and there are great increases in vascular permeability [229,230]. Studies of animals undergoing a rapid severe elevation of pressure show that the period of acute injury is reflected by endothelial denudation in the dilated segments followed by exudation of plasma proteins and deposition of platelets [231,232]. In humans and in animals, the result is necrosis, deposition of fibrin, and entry of plasma proteins into the vessel wall. This combination has been called **fibrinoid necrosis**. This breakdown of vascular integrity is followed by smooth muscle proliferation, with a dramatic increase in the numbers of layers of smooth muscle cells seen in hypertensive vessels, sometimes called **onion skinning**.

MECHANISM OF SMOOTH MUSCLE REPLICATION IN MALIGNANT HYPERTENSION

The proliferation of smooth muscle cells at sites of endothelial denudation and vascular dilation in small resistance vessels subjected to severe elevations in pressure [229–232] is not surprising given our knowledge of the response of larger arteries to mechanical denudation, described in the discussion of atherosclerosis. It is reasonable to propose that smooth muscle proliferation at these sites is the result of release of mitogens from platelets and necrotic vessel-wall cells at the site of injury.

The key observations began in the 1970s with autoradiographic studies by Crane and Dutta and later by Bevan showing that smooth muscle replication was markedly increased in response to acute elevation of blood pressure [233]. Bevan [234], using a coarctation model, demonstrated that DNA synthesis occurs in response to hypertension. Although the microvascular data were not quantitative, she showed a rough correlation of replication in small resistance vessels with the replication observed in large vessels. The latter showed an increase within 3 days of onset of hypertension with a gradual decrease over the following days and weeks [234].

The presence of endothelial denudation in small arterioles has been shown in several animal models for high blood pressure [229–232]. Furthermore, this microvascular change is specifically associated with focal areas of extreme dilation with high levels of permeability to plasma solutes [229,230,232] and endothelial denudation with thrombosis [229–231]. Indirect evidence supposes the proposition that a platelet-dependent mechanism may be operative. Crane and Dutta [233] published an interesting autoradiographic study. They found a diffusion gradient of replication at sites of hypertensive injury. Replication was prominent in the endothelium and smooth muscle cells of small renal arteries. Low levels were seen in the adjacent fibroblasts, and still lower but significant levels of replication were seen in adjacent epithelium of the collecting tubules. As they propose, these data suggest a role for a diffusible factor released at the site of injury [233]. The hypertensive microvessel may well be the best candidate for a vascular wall undergoing a proliferative response following release of platelet factors.

MECHANISM OF SMOOTH MUSCLE REPLICATION IN MODERATE HYPERTENSION

The mechanism eliciting smooth muscle replication in resistance vessels during moderate elevations in pressure may be less obvious. As just discussed, endothelial denudation is a prominent feature of acute hypertension induced by a variety of vasoactive agents. Thus, it is reasonable to attempt to explain smooth muscle replication in small arteries of Goldblatt hypertensive animals by the response to injury mechanism. As far as we know, however, mild hypertension, even the chronic elevation of pressure seen in a hypertensive rat, does not cause endothelial denudation. Even severe hypertension does not cause denudation in large arteries. There is also evidence that changes in vessel-wall mass occur in coarctation hypertension, even in protected vessels. This suggests the presence of a humoral trophic factor that might also affect DNA synthesis [235].

Unlike the acute changes in pressure seen in hypertensive models studied by Bevan [234] and by Crane and Dutta [233], the spontaneously hypertensive rat (SHR) shows only a slow increase in pressure. There are no reports of endothelial denudation or platelet deposition in either the microvessels or the large vessels of this rat strain. Before discarding denudation as an important component of hypertensive smooth muscle proliferation, it is interesting to note that Lee and colleagues found evidence of apparently necrotic endothelial cells in the microvasculature of the salt-fed Dahl hypertensive rat, another animal model where the rise in blood pressure is relatively small [236]. It is certainly possible that microvascular injury occurs episodically in the SHR. Nonetheless, it would be dangerous to conclude from the presence of hyperplasia in the microvasculature of chronically hypertensive animals that the mechanism of increase in smooth muscle cells is the same as that occurring in malignant hypertension or in the response of large vessels to the balloon catheter.

The sympathetic nervous system is an attractive alternative candidate for regulation of smooth muscle growth. Motor neurons can exert a trophic influence on skeletal muscle [237]. Similarly, sympathetic nerves exert a trophic influence on the structure and function of smooth muscle. Bevan and Tsuru [238] found that sympathectomy inhibited the increase in DNA mass of developing rabbit-ear artery. Similarly, extracts of sympathetic ganglia were shown to maintain cultured smooth muscle cells in a differentiated state [74]. Finally, Rorive et al. [239], among others, found that the ability of antihypertensive drugs to inhibit smooth muscle DNA replication depended on the presence or absence of effects on the sympathetic nervous system. (Table 8-1). We do know that hypertension

Table 8-1. Effects of pharmacologic intervention in hypertension on the cardiac and vascular hypertrophy associated with hypertension

Drug	Initiation/ termination	BP	Route	Body weight	Cardiac hyper- tension	Vascular hypertension	Model	Vessels	Refer- ence
ACE INHIBITORS									
Captopril prenatal	1, 14 wk	nr	oral		d	d csa aorta, renal, intra-renal	SHR	aorta, renal, intrarenal	[240]
	6, 20 wk	d	oral	ns	d	d aorta wt/length, mes w/l	SHR	aorta, mes	[241]
	8, 20 wk	d	water	sd	d	d csa, wt; nr ploidy	SHR	aorta	[242]
	25, 31 wk	d	oral			no effect w/l, lumen diameter, media t	SHR	mes, cer	[243]
	1 day, 6 wk	nr				i DNA, collagen content	1K1C	aorta	[239]
	1, 3 wk	d	water		nc	nc wt, DNA content	1K1C	aorta	[244]
	3, 5 wk	d	water		nc	nc wt, DNA content	1K1C	aorta	[244]
SYMPATHOLYTIC									
Reserpine	1 day, 6 wk	nr				d DNA, collagen content	1K1C	aorta	[239]
	0, 3 wk	d	sc			d coll s	DOCA	aorta, mes	[245]
Methyldopa	12, 15 wk	d	water			d aortic wt/body wt, coll s nc collagen content	SHR	aorta	[246]
	1, 3 wk	d	water		d	d wt, DNA content	1K1C	aorta	[244]
	3, 5 wk	d	water		nc	nc wt, DNA content	1K1C	aorta	[244]
6 hydroxydopamine	0, 3 wk	d	inj	sd	nc	d w/l WKY, nc SHR	SHR	mes	
Clonidine	1, 3 wk	d	water		d	d wt, DNA content	1K1C	aorta	[244]
	3, 5 wk	d	water		nc	nc wt, DNA content	1K1C	aorta	[244]
β-BLOCKERS									
Propranolol	0, 1 wk	no	oral		d	d aorta wt/body wt	NA	aorta	[247]
	1 day, 6 wk	no	water		nc	nc aorta wt/body wt, nr ploidy	DOCA	aorta	[248]
	7, 9 wk	no	oral		d	d protein, RNA	SPSHR	aorta	[247]
	8, 20 wk	no	water	sd	nc	nc csa, wt, ploidy	SHR	aorta	[242]
	1, 3 wk	no	water		nc	nc wt, DNA content	1K1C	aorta	[244]
	3, 5 wk	no	water		nc	nc wt, DNA content	1K1C	aorta	[244]
Atenolol	0, 1 wk	d	oral		d	d aorta wt	NA	aorta	[247]
α-BLOCKERS									
Phentolamine	0, 1 wk	nr	sc		d	d aorta wt	NA	aorta	[247]
Prazosin	6 wk	d	oral			nc diameter, wall t	SHR	mes, cer	[249]
CA ENTRY BLOCKERS									
Verapamil	0, 4 wk	d	sc		d	d media t	pul	lung arterioles	[250]
Nifedipine	0, 4 wk	d	sc		d	d media t	pul	lung arterioles	[250]
Felodipine	6, 12 wk	d			nc	nc w/l	SHR	mes	[251]
	6, 14 wk	d	water	ns	nc	nc media-to-lumen ratio	SHR	mes	[252]
VASODILATORS									
Hydralazine prenatal	21 wk	nr	water			nc	SHR	renal, mes	[227]
	4, 12 wk	nr			d	i media t, lumen diameter	SHR	mes	[251]
	4, 27 wk	nr	water	ns	d	i lumen d; d w/l	SHR	mes	[252]
	6, 20 wk	d	oral	ns	nc	d aorta wt/length	SHR	aorta, mes	[241]
	7, 9 wk	nr	oral		nc	nc	SPSHR	aorta, mes	[247]
	10, 12 wk	d	water	sd		d actomyosin content; nc aorta wt	SHR	aorta	[253]
	2, 5 mo	nr	water	ns	nc	d wt, ploidy; nc csa	SHR	aorta	[242]
	0, 4 wk	d	sc			nc media t	pul	lung arterioles	[250]
DIURETICS									
Hydrochlorothiazide	21, 27 wk	no			nc	d aorta area, nc renal w/l	SHR	aorta, renal	[254]
Furosemide	1, 3 wk	d	water		nc	nc wt, DNA content	1K1C	aorta	[244]
	3, 5 wk	no	water		nc	nc wt, DNA content	1K1C	aorta	[244]

Table 8-1 (continued)

Drug	Initiation/ termination	BP	Route	Body weight	Cardiac hyper-tension	Vascular hypertension	Model	Vessels	Refer-ence
COMBINATION TREATMENTS									
Hydralazine, reserpine, hydrochlorothiazide	25, 48 wk	d			d	d media t, smc content	SHR	mes	[255]
	4, 5 wk	d	water	ns		d wall csa, lg/sm arterioles	2K1C	cer arterioles	[256, 257]
	16, 18 wk	d	water	ns		d wall csa, sm arterioles	SHR	cer arterioles	[256, 257]
	7, 42 wk	d	water	ns		d aorta, intrarenal media t d w/l	SHR	aorta, intrarenal	[258]
	22, 42 wk	d	water	sd		d aorta, intrarenal media t d w/l			
	7, 22 wk	d	water	ns		no effect			
	3, 5 mo	d	water		d	d csa, smc V_V	SHR	aorta	[259]
	5, 7 mo	d	water		d	d csa, smc V_V			
Hydralazine, hydrochlorothiazide	21, 27 wk	d			d	d aorta area, t d renal w/l	SHR	aorta, renal	[260]
Captopril, hydrochlorothiazide	21, 27 wk	d			d	d aorta area, t d renal w/l	SHR	aorta, renal	[260]
Hydralazine, guanethidine	11, 36 wk	d				d media t	SHR	aorta	[261]
Anti-NGF, guanethidine	2, 28 days	nr	ip	sd		d csa lg mes	SHR	mes	[262]
Metoprol, felodipine	1,4 mo	d				d w/l	SHR	basal	[263]
	4, 6 mo	d				d w/l	SPSHR	cer	

cer = cerebral arteries
csa = cross-sectional area
d = decrease
DOCA = DOCA salt hypertension
i = increase
ip = intraperitoneal injection
mes = mesenteric arteries
NA = noradrenaline infusion
nc = no change
nr = no rise
ns = not significant
pul = pulmonary hypertension
sc = subcutaneous injection
sd = significant decrease
SHR = spontaneously hypertensive rat
smc = smooth muscle cell
SPSHR = stroke-prone SHR
t = thickness
w/l = wall-to-lumen ratio
wt = weight
V_V = partial volume
1K1C = 1 kidney, 1 clip
2K1C = 2 kidneys, 1 clip

increases the DNA content as well as the mass of large vessels.

SMOOTH MUSCLE MASS VERSUS SMOOTH MUSCLE-CELL NUMBER

Until this point, smooth muscle proliferation and wall thickening have been discussed as if they were one thing. By definition this need not be true—organ mass can increase by increasing cell number, hyperplasia by increasing cell mass, and hypertrophy or both may occur at the same time. For example, Owens and Schwartz [264,265] measured cell size in smooth muscle cells extracted from the aorta of spontaneously hypertensive or Goldblatt hypertensive rats. They found that individual cells of the hypertensive animals were bigger and the increase in cell size was adequate to account for the increase in wall mass. When, however, the DNA content of the isolated cells was corrected for cell number, there was more DNA than there should have been given the normal mammalian content of DNA per cell. A combination of image analysis and flow cytometric techniques were used to demonstrate that this increase in DNA was due to an increase in smooth muscle ploidy. In other words, there were no more smooth muscle cells, but there was more DNA. This work has been confirmed by others [248,266]. Polyploid cells account for most of the increased mass of the hypertensive rat vessel [264,267]. Thus, it appears that, at least in large vessels of the rat, DNA synthesis is important to the increase in mass.

Two reservations need to be expressed about these observations. First, the data have been obtained only from the rat. We have recently obtained limited data from humans [78]. In a study of about 200 autopsies at the University of Washington, we were able to examine ploidy in the aorta of seven hypertensive and seven control patients. Our postmortem diagnosis of hypertension was based on a combination of patient history and confirmed by the presence of a hypertrophied heart in these individuals. Clinical data were, however, very limited. There was no evidence in this study of an increase in ploidy and mean ploidy levels between the hypertensives and the controls. There was, however, a startling correlation between the frequency of elevated ploidy and the age of patients in the hypertensive but not the control population. That, at least, suggests that we may have been seeing a progressive change whose magnitude was limited by the use of antihypertensive therapy in this small number of patients.

The second reservation has to do with vessel size. While large vessels may be affected by hypertension, the possibility of an increase in total cell number is more important for microvessels. Obviously, the microvascular resistance vessels provide the major source of peripheral resistance and therefore the site of most interest in hypertension. As already noted, resistance vessels in humans and all other animals with hypertension show an increase in total mass. The available data suggest that these vessels show a true hyperplasia, that is, an increase in the number of diploid cells [268–270]. These studies, however, only estimated the number of cells by counting profiles in sections. There are not sufficient data in a two-dimensional image of a complex structure to permit anything more than a rough estimate of the number of cells from the number of profiles that can be seen in a single plane of section. Several attempts have been made to circumvent this problem.

Five different approaches have been used to estimate the number of cells in vessel walls. Todd [271] used three-dimensional reconstruction techniques to derive a model of all the smooth muscle cells located in the vessel wall. This arduous technique provided important and detailed data on the structure of the vessel wall and could, at least in theory, be used to count the number of cells in microvessels. The problem obviously is the limited number of vessels that could be studied in this way. As yet, Todd's method has not been applied to the problem of hypertensive small vessels. A more limited sampling approach has been employed by Thomas and colleagues to estimate the numbers of cells in the aorta of atherosclerotic swine. These investigators used serial sections to estimate the length of different cells [201]. They argued that differences in cell length were inversely proportional to differences in frequency of representation of cells in section. Estimates of cell length could be used to derive correction factors that could be applied to data gained in section. This relatively simple approach has not been applied to microvessels perhaps because of concerns that changes in the size or shape of cells in different conditions would invalidate the approximation.

A third technique grows out of the work on cell ploidy. If one knows the ploidy of cells in a vessel, it is possible to calculate the number of cells directly from the biochemical measurement of total DNA. The limitation of applying this method to microvessels is the difficulty in getting pure samples of microvascular smooth muscle cell free of endothelial cells and adventitial cells. A fourth approach has been applied to hypertensive vessels by Lee and his colleagues. These workers used the relationship of cell surface to cell volume as a means of estimating the probability of an increase in numbers of profiles of smooth muscle cells representing an increase in cell number or an increase in mass. They argued that increased numbers of objects, without a change in size or shape, should not change the ratio of surface area to volume. An increase in cell size should appear as a decrease in the surface-volume relationship. This method has been applied to the microvasculature, and the authors have interpreted their data as supporting an increase in cell number in the hypertensive microvasculature [225]. The fifth and most practical approach has come from the work of Mulvany et al. [272] on a technique called the **dissector**. The dissector depends on the assumption that the numbers of bottoms of nuclei seen in successive serial sections is proportional to the total number of cells.

Mulvany used the dissector to study mesenteric arteries of SHRs. These arteries contained an increased number of cells, consistent with the semiquantitative conclusions by others. The dissector, like most morphometric approaches, is arduous, and only small numbers of vessels were studied. This has led to some surprising findings. Mulvany, studying both animal and human microvessels, was unable to find a change in either cell number or total wall mass of hypertensive vessel walls. However, since physiologic studies tell us that these vessel walls must be thickened to account for the contractile properties of the hypertensive wall, Mulvany concludes that the primary wall change must be a rearrangement or remodeling of the existing vessel-wall mass, rather than an accretion of new mass [273,274].

Unfortunately, we have very few data on the mechanism underlying remodeling. Obviously, few clues can come from studies of smooth muscle replication after injury, and the distinction between hyperploid replication and true proliferation may not be critical to the most important implication of a proliferative response to hypertension. Nonetheless, maintenance of high blood pressure implies either chronic stimulation by a stimulus exogenous to the vessel wall or a chronic change in the responsiveness of the vessel wall.

On the other hand, the dissector is not necessarily conclusive. The method is arduous and might allow changes in cell number at a level that is biologically significant. One might imagine some sort of initial stimulus, an as yet undefined injury, that results in a chronic change we recognize as high blood pressure and is associated with an increase in cell number. This sort of "memory" might occur at many levels, ranging from resetting of renal or central physiologic mechanisms, positive feedback regulation of electrolyte levels, or direct changes in the effector system—the smooth muscles themselves. Change in DNA content of the vessel wall is a special alternative. If one imagines that the microvasculature replicates in response to episodes of acute hypertension, then the wall would retain an increased DNA content as a memory of the earlier event. In turn, this increased DNA could alter the ability of the vascular system to regulate synthesis and degradation of the contractile protein mass of arterial smooth muscle cells, possibly producing a fixed increase in peripheral vessel-wall mass. Such a mechanism might account for the well-established increase in structural resistance of the peripheral vasculature in humans and animals with hypertension [12,275].

Treatment studies may be important in the concept of a memory of vascular mass. The reversal of mass changes in SHR resistance vessels was accomplished by proportional reductions in cellular and extracellular material [255]. Is there a change in cell number with treatment? Warshaw et al. showed that the number of profiles of smooth muscle cells in vessel cross sections were reduced by 12 percent in treated SHRs. As discussed previously, this measure can give only a rough estimate of cell number. Carlier and Rorive [244] have shown that early treatment of renal hypertension by unclipping can reverse DNA content changes, but that after 3 weeks of hypertension these DNA changes were permanent. DNA synthesis, elevated in renal and genetic hypertension, is decreased with treatment in both these models [239,242,276]. It would be interesting to see if models of hypertension with different degrees of DNA change would react differently to subsequent episodes of hypertension. Freis et al. [277] have found that treatment of spontaneous hypertension can effectively reduce pressure, but when treatment is released, pressure rapidly rises to pretreatment levels and then proceeds to rise at the same rate as untreated controls. Limas et al. [258] studied effects of treatment release on aortic medial wall thickening in SHR and found that treatment prevented further wall thickening, but release resulted in a return to hypertensive levels after 20 weeks. This further suggests an internally coded memory of the appropriate response to hypertension, and indeed a programmed response may be resumed at the same stage present in this memory. Changes in ploidy of vascular smooth muscle are not reversed in SHR by treatment [259] or in desoxycorticosterone acetate (Doca) hypertension by a low-salt diet [278]. These results, as well as those of Carlier, imply that DNA changes could well be involved as irreversible events (memory) resulting from hypertension and resulting in structural hypertrophy.

Whether increases in arterial DNA are important in maintenance of elevated peripheral resistance depends on as yet unanswered questions: (1) Is the dissector sensitive enough to detect small changes in vessel wall cell number? (2) How does an increase in the number of cells, the amount of DNA per cell, or total DNA per vessel length affect the steady-state mass of the vessel wall? (3) If DNA content changes, how does an increase in DNA affect the response of the vessel wall to trophic stimuli from nerves or circulating factors? (4) How does an increased amount of DNA affect the response to subsequent hypertensive episodes?

RELATIONSHIP OF MASS CHANGES TO REPLICATION

The most obvious reason for being interested in this increase in DNA is the possibility that our available knowledge of the control of DNA synthesis might provide insights to the control of vascular mass in resistance vessels. The fact that most known changes in vascular mass are associated with increases in DNA content leads one to think that the two cellular changes may somehow be related.

Relatively little is known about the factors controlling vessel-wall mass. Two recent experiments, however, seem particularly relevant. The first, reported by Langille et al., studied the adaptation of the common carotid to decreased flow. This was accomplished by ligating the external carotid artery. Within 48 hours, the remaining carotid artery underwent active contraction, decreasing the effective lumen size. Within 2 weeks, this was followed by remodeling so that the vessel had an increased wall thickness and a decreased lumen diameter [279,280]. These changes that occurred in a large vessel are strikingly similar to changes described by Joshua et al. [281] in the cremasteric circulation of rats with 1 kidney–1 clip hypertension. Initially, they found an active constriction of the precapillary arterioles. By 2 weeks, this was converted to a structural change in the larger vessels, restricting flow in a fashion no longer relaxable with papaverine. With time, the structural component spread to smaller vessels. Joshua and his colleagues suggested that the structural changes in the larger vessels were in local response adapted to protecting the smaller vessels from damage by elevated pressure [281]. It is tempting to equate these hyperplastic changes to Cowley's findings of increased peripheral resistance due to autoregulation after a few days of high-volume hypertension due to excess salt intake [220].

Langille's experiment also provides possible clues as to the mechanisms controlling vascular mass independent of replication. Endothelial denudation of the common carotid prevented both the active contraction and the later remodeling change. Two known functions of the endothelium may be relevant. First, the endothelium is the source of endothelial-derived relaxing factor (EDRF) [282–284]. Whether EDRF somehow interacts with the underlying wall to maintain normal tone is not known, although it obviously is difficult to see how the presence of a source of a relaxing factor would encourage vasoconstriction. Second, and easier to consider, is the discovery, reviewed above, that endothelial cells are a potent source of polypeptide mitogens, including PDGF. While these peptide hormones traditionally have been thought of as growth factors, they also have been shown to be vasoactive [285,286]. It is possible that endothelial-derived PDGF, released in response to some flow-dependent stimulus, causes both an initial constriction response and a later trophic remodeling response.

Another possible clue comes from reports of the effects of various therapeutic regimes in cardiovascular mass. If there is a relationship between blood pressure and cardiovascular mass, then reversal or prevention of hypertension should prevent or reverse structural changes seen in hypertensive animals. As shown in Table 8-1, a substantial literature shows that antihypertensive agents can reverse or prevent cardiovascular hypertrophy. However, the efficacy of pharmacologic treatment is not universal and depends in part on the model and duration of hypertension, the form and duration of reversal, and the type of structural change of interest. For example, when blood pressures were controlled by captopril, aortic hypertrophy was prevented in SHR [241], but the DNA synthesis associated with renal hypertension was not [239]. Reserpine, however, was effective in preventing DNA synthesis in renal hypertension [239]. There is evidence that the reversal of SHR hypertension requires extended treatment [241,287], whereas in early stages of renal hypertension, treatment effects are relatively rapid [271]. Established renal hypertension is more difficult to reverse than developing renal hypertension [287,288]. A number of reports show that cardiac hypertrophy induced by hypertension can be prevented by captopril but not by hydralazine, although both treatments achieve normotension [241,254]. Hydralazine has an effect on the ratio of aortic weight to length after prolonged treatment but not in mesenteric vessels [241].

It is intriguing to consider the possibility that the link is control of vascular mass by the sympathetic nervous system. Probably the best evidence from treatment studies is the differential effects of vasodilators, which may reduce blood pressure but not affect cardiovascular mass, or sympathetic agents, calcium-channel blockers and angiotensin antagonists, which do prevent or reduce cardiovascular hypertrophy (see Table 8-1).

Hydralazine prevents hypertension but also stimulates sympathetic output, while captopril reduces sympathetic stimulation by reducing AII levels [241,254]. The effects of sympathetic agents are more direct, such as reserpine, which rapidly depletes catecholamines, providing a clearer view of the possible mechanism of sympathetic control over mass. It has already been noted that Bevan found unilateral sympathectomy of the ear of developing rabbits decreased growth in ear-artery DNA content. Wall-to-lumen ratio of Wistar-Kyoto mesenteric vessels also has been reduced by sympathectomy [252]. Sympathectomy can prevent hypertrophy [289,290] in hypertensive vessels, but it appears that the completeness and maintenance of sympathectomy are important issues in how effective this treatment is [252,260].

An alternative hypothesis has been proposed by Loeb et al., who found that calcium-channel blockers were effective in preventing hypertension-induced aortic DNA synthesis. They have argued that similar effects by captopril and hydralazine also were calcium mediated. This was further supported by ouabain treatment of normal animals that also stimulated DNA synthesis. The separation of hypertension from DNA synthesis and the lack of control over possible sympathetic stimulation by ouabain makes these results difficult to interpret. The effectiveness of calcium-channel blockers in reducing or preventing hypertrophy is also somewhat unpredictable (see Table 8-1), but this interesting hypothesis deserves further study.

In summary, the stimuli controlling smooth muscle replication in hypertension remain unknown. Growth factors released by platelets may play an important role in microvascular changes in malignant hypertension, but platelet-released factors are not likely to be involved in large vessels or in any vessel affected by milder and more chronic forms of high blood pressure. Wall tension and sympathetic activity are intriguing alternatives that need more exploration.

Summary

The emerging picture of growth control in arterial smooth muscle is a complex balance of forces. Denudation, thrombosis, and macrophage-derived growth factors almost certainly are critical to plaque progression in atherosclerosis. In addition to exogenous stimuli to cell growth, the vessel wall is capable of synthesis of endogenous growth inhibitors and growth stimulants.

This idea that intrinsic growth-factor production by vessel-wall cells themselves may be important is more consistent with our knowledge of smooth muscle replication in chronic hypertension where there is no evidence that endothelial denudation occurs. In atherosclerosis itself, the critical initial event may be developmental abnormality in smooth muscle proliferation. The best evidence for this is the fact that smooth muscle cells in plaques appear to be monoclonal. This could mean that the initial accumulation cells resulted from a rare proliferative event, for example, a mutation, as suggested by Benditt, or a developmental trapping, as proposed here. In any case, the initial event almost certainly is affected in its progression to a more advanced lesion by the presence of growth factors derived from platelets, monocytes, or possibly T-cells that interact with the damaged vessel wall.

In hypertension, the major question is probably not how smooth replication is controlled, but whether replication of smooth muscle cells matters to the progress of the disease. Most modern hypotheses of hypertension put elevated peripheral resistance at a central point. From a cell biologist's point of view, however, peripheral resistance is a poorly defined entity. Is it due to elevated protein synthesis, increase in cell number, or synthesis of increased extracellular mass? These are important distinctions because they imply quite different mechanisms of control at a biochemical level. This chapter suggests that DNA replication of smooth muscle cells in the vessel wall might constitute a kind of "memory," making the vessel more able to develop increased structural mass and, therefore, making the animal more prone to elevated peripheral resistance and hypertension.

References

1. Majno G. Ultrastructure of the vascular membrane. Am Physiol Soc 1965; 3:2293–2375.
2. French JE. Atherosclerosis in relation to the structure and function of the arterial intima, with special reference to the endothelium. Int Rev Exp Pathol 1966; 5:253–354.
3. Ryan GB, Majno G. Acute inflammation: a review. Am J Pathol 1977; 86:185–276.
4. Ekblom P, et al. The origin of the glomerular endothelium. Cell Differ 1982; 11:35–39.
5. Gabbiani G. The cytoskeleton of rat aortic smooth muscle cells. Normal conditions, experimental intimal thickening, and tissue culture. Ann NY Acad Sci 1986; 488:196–198.
6. Skalli O, Vandekerckhove J, Gabbiani G. Actin-isoform pattern as a marker of normal or pathological smooth muscle and fibroblastic tissues. Differentiation 1987; 33:232–238.
7. Schwartz SM, Campbell GR, Campbell JH. Replication of smooth muscle cells in vascular disease. Circ Res 1986; 58:427–444.
8. Gimbrone MA Jr, Buchanan MR. Interactions of platelets and leukocytes with vascular endothelium: in vitro studies. Ann NY Acad Sci 1982; 401:171–183.
9. Ryan JW, Ryan US. Endothelial surface enzymes and the dynamic processing of plasma substrates. Int Rev Exp Pathol 1984; 26:1–43.
10. Pober JS, et al. Interactions of T lymphocytes with human vascular endothelial cells: role of endothelial cells surface antigens. Immunobiology 1984; 168:483–494.
11. Ryan US. Metabolic activity of pulmonary endothelium: modulations of structure and function. Annu Rev Physiol 1986; 48:263–277.
12. Folkow B. Physiological aspects of primary hypertension. Physiol Rev 1982; 62:347–504.

13. Ross R. The pathogenesis of atherosclerosis—A perspective for the 1990's. Nature 1993; 362:801–809.
14. Schwartz SM, Heimark RL, Majesky MW. Developmental mechanisms underlying pathology of arteries. Physiol Rev 1990; 70:1177–1209.
15. Pardanaud L, et al. Vasculogenesis in the early quail blastodisc as studied with a monoclonal antibody recognizing endothelial cells. Development 1987; 100:339–349.
16. Le Douarin NM. Cell migrations in embryos. Cell 1984; 38:353–360.
17. Peault BM, Thiery JP, Le Douarin NM. A surface marker for the hemopoietic and endothelial cell lineages in the quail species defined by a monoclonal antibody. Proc Natl Acad Sci USA 1983; 80:2976–2980.
18. Noden DM. Origins and assembly of avian embryonic blood vessels. Ann NY Acad Sci 1990; 588:236–249.
19. Manasek FJ. The ultrastructure of embryonic myocardial blood vessels. Dev Biol 1971; 26:42–54.
20. De Simone-Santoro I, Renda T. Recherches ultrastructurales, histochimiques et histoenzymologiques sur la paroi aortique pendant sa morphogenese chez l'embryon de poulet. Annales d'Histochimie 1971; 16:171–181.
21. Blatt HJ. Uber die Entwicklung der Coronararterien bei der Ratte Licht- und elektronenmikroskopische Untersuchungen. Z Anat Entwicklungsgesch 1973; 142:53–64.
22. Gonzalez-Crussi F. Vasculogenesis in the chick embryo. An ultrastructural study. Am J Anat 1971; 130:441–460.
23. Karrer HE. An electron microscope study of the aorta in young and aging mice. J Ultrastruct Res 1961; 5:1–27.
24. Wolinsky H, Glagov S. A lamellar unit of aortic medial structure and function in mammals. Circ Res 1967; 20:99–101.
25. Looker T, Berry CL. The growth and development of the rat aorta. II. Changes in nucleic acid and scleroprotein content. J Anat 1972; 113:17–34.
26. Olivetti G, et al. Morphometric study of early postnatal development of the thoracic aorta in the rat. Circ Res 1980; 47:417–424.
27. Bochaton-Piallat ML, et al. Cultured aortic smooth muscle cells from newborn and adult rats show distinct cytoskeletal features. Differentiation 1992; 49:175–185.
28. Harris-Hooker SA, et al. Neovascular responses induced by cultured aortic endothelial cells. J Cell Physiol 1983; 114:302–310.
29. Montesano R, et al. Basic fibroblast growth factor induces angiogenesis in vitro. Proc Natl Acad Sci USA 1986; 83:7297–7301.
30. Gajdusek CM, et al. Activation of coagulation releases endothelial cell mitogens. J Cell Biol 1986; 103:419–428.
31. Schweigerer L, et al. Capillary endothelial cells express basic fibroblast growth factor, a mitogen that promotes their own growth. Nature 1987a; 325:257–259.
32. Fox PL, DiCorleto PE. Modified low density lipoproteins suppress production of a platelet-derived growth factor-like protein by cultured endothelial cells. Proc Natl Acad Sci USA 1986; 83:4774–4778.
33. Abraham JA, et al. Human fibroblast growth factor: nucleotide sequence and genomic organization. EMBO J 1986; 5:2523–2528.
34. Tong BD, et al. Isolation and sequencing of a cDNA clone homologous to the v-sis oncogene from human endothelial cells. Mol Cell Biol 1986; 6:3018–3022.
35. Burgess WH, et al. Structural evidence that endothelial cell growth factor-β is the precursor of both endothelial cell growth factor-α and acidic fibroblast growth factor. Proc Natl Acad Sci USA 1986; 83:7216–7220.
36. Ross R. The pathogenesis of atherosclerosis—An update. N Engl J Med 1986; 314:488–500.
37. Jonasson L, et al. Regional accumulations of T cells, macrophages, and smooth muscle cells in the human atherosclerotic plaque. Arteriosclerosis 1986; 6:131–138.
38. Gown AM, Tsukada T, Ross R. Human atherosclerosis. II. Immunocytochemical analysis of the cellular composition of human atherosclerotic lesions. Am J Pathol 1986; 125: 191–207.
39. Arbustini E, et al. Coronary atherosclerotic plaques with and without thrombus in ischemic heart syndromes: A morphologic, immunohistochemical, and biochemical study. Am J Cardiol 1991; 68:36B–50B.
40. Velican D, Velican C. Intimal thickening in developing coronary arteries and its relevance to atherosclerotic involvement. Atherosclerosis 1976; 23:345–355.
41. Stary HC, Strong JP. The fine structure of non-atherosclerotic intimal thickening of developing and of regressing atherosclerotic lesions at the bifurcation of the left coronary artery. Adv Exp Med Biol 1976; 67:89–108.
42. Sims FH, Gavin JB, Vanderwee MA. The intima of human coronary arteries. Am Heart J 1989; 118:32–38.
43. Stemerman MB, Ross R. Fibrous plaque formation in primates, an electron microscope study. J Exp Med 1972; 136: 769–789.
44. Schwartz SM, Stemerman MB, Benditt EP. The aortic intima. II. Repair of the aortic lining after mechanical denudation. Am J Pathol 1975; 81:15–42.
45. Friedman RJ, et al. The effect of thrombocytopenia on experimental atherosclerotic lesion formation in rabbits. Smooth muscle cell proliferation and re-endothelialization. J Clin Invest 1977; 60:1191–1201.
46. Ross R, Raines EW, Bowen-Pope DF. The biology of platelet-derived growth factor. Cell 1986; 46:155–169.
47. Doolittle RF, et al. Simian sarcoma virus onc gene, v-sis, is derived from the gene (or genes) encoding a platelet-derived growth factor. Science 1983; 221:275–277.
48. Waterfield MD, et al. Platelet-derived growth factor is structurally related to the putative transforming protein p28-sis of simian sarcoma virus. Nature 1983; 304:35–39.
49. O'Keefe EJ, Pledger WJ. A model of cell cycle control: sequential events regulated by growth factors. Mol Cell Endocrinol 1983; 31:167–186.
50. Singh JP, et al. Persistence of the mitogenic response to platelet-derived growth factor (competence) does not reflect a long-term interaction between the growth factor and the target cell. J Cell Biol 1983; 96:1497–1502.
51. Clemmons DR. Interaction of circulating cell-derived and plasma growth factors in stimulating cultured smooth muscle cell replication. J Cell Physiol 1984; 121:425–430.
52. Clemmons DR, Underwood LE, Chatelain PG, Van Wyk JJ. Liberation of immunoreactive somatomedin-C from its binding proteins by proteolytic enzymes and heparin. J Clin Endocrinol Metabol 1983; 56:384.
53. Russell WE, Van Wyk JJ, Pledger WJ. Inhibition of the mitogenic effects of plasma by a monoclonal antibody to somatomedin C. Proc Natl Acad Sci USA 1984; 81:2389–2392.
54. Oka Y, Orth DN. Human plasma epidermal growth factor/ β-urogastrone is associated with blood platelets. J Clin Invest 1983; 72:249–259.
55. Assoian RK, et al. Cellular transformation by coordinated action of three peptide growth factors from human platelets. Nature 1984; 309:804–806.
56. Tucker RF, et al. Growth inhibitor from BSC-1 cells closely related to platelet type-β transforming growth factor. Science 1984; 226:705–707.
57. Gerrity RG. The role of the monocyte in atherogenesis. I. Transition of blood-borne monocytes into foam cells in fatty lesions. Am J Pathol 1981; 103:181–190.

58. Faggiotto A, Ross R. Studies of hypercholesterolemia in the nonhuman primate. II. Fatty streak conversion to fibrous plaque. Arteriosclerosis 1984; 4:341–356.
59. Faggiotto A, Ross R, Harker L. Studies of hypercholesterolemia in the nonhuman primate. I. Changes that lead to fatty streak formation. Arteriosclerosis 1984; 4:323–340.
60. Leibovich SJ, Ross R. A macrophage-dependent factor that stimulates the proliferation of fibroblasts in vitro. Am J Pathol 1976; 84:501–513.
61. Curwen KD, Gimbrone MA Jr, Handin RI. In vitro studies of thrombo-resistance. The role of prostacyclin (PGI_2) in platelet adhesion to cultured normal and virally transformed human vascular endothelial cells. Lab Invest 1980; 42:366–374.
62. Shimokado K, Raines EW, Ross R. Activated macrophages secrete a PDGF-like molecule (abstract). J Cell Biochem 1985; [Suppl] 9A:137.
63. Goode TB, et al. Aortic endothelial cell morphology observed in situ by scanning electron microscopy during atherogenesis in rabbits. Atherosclerosis 1977; 27:235–251.
64. Boogaerts MA, et al. Enhancement of granulocyte-endothelial cell adherence and granulocyte-induced cytotoxicity by platelet release products. Proc Natl Acad Sci USA 1982; 79:7019–7023.
65. Harlan JM, et al. Neutrophil-mediated endothelial injury in vitro: mechanisms of cell detachment. J Clin Invest 1981; 68:1394–1403.
66. Territo M, Berliner JA, Fogelman AM. Effect of monocyte migration on low density lipoprotein transport across aortic endothelial cell monolayers. J Clin Invest 1984; 74:2279–2284.
67. Scott RF, et al. Distribution of intimal smooth muscle cell mass and their relationship to early atherosclerosis in the abdominal aortas of young swine. Atherosclerosis 1979; 34:291–301.
68. Walker LN, Bowen-Pope DF, Reidy MA. Secretion of platelet-derived growth factor (PDGF)-like activity by arterial smooth muscle cells is induced as a response to injury. J Cell Biol 1984; 99:416a.
69. Clowes AW, Karnovsky MJ. Suppression by heparin of smooth muscle cell proliferation in injured arteries. Nature 1977; 265:625–626.
70. Clowes AW, Clowes MM. Kinetics of cellular proliferation after arterial injury. IV. Heparin inhibits rat smooth muscle mitogenesis and migration. Circ Res 1986; 58:839–845.
71. Majesky MW, et al. Heparin regulates smooth muscle S phase entry in the injured rat carotid artery. Circ Res 1987; 61:296–300.
72. Nam SC, et al. Population dynamics of arterial smooth muscle cells. III. Inhibition by aortic tissue extracts of proliferative response to intimal injury in hypercholesterolemic swine. Exp Mol Pathol 1974; 21:259.
73. Eisenstein R, et al. Growth regulators in connective tissue. II. Evidence for the presence of several growth inhibitors in aortic extracts. Paroi Arterielle 1979; 5:163–169.
74. Chamley-Campbell JH, Campbell GR. Development of smooth muscle and autonomic nerves in culture. In Burnstock G, O'Brien R, Vrbova, G, eds. Somatic and Autonomic Nerve-Muscle Interactions. Amsterdam: Elsevier, 1983. Pp 35–56.
75. Castellot JJ Jr, et al. Cultured endothelial cells produce a heparin-like inhibitor of smooth muscle cell growth. J Cell Biol 1981; 90:372–379.
76. Campbell GR, Campbell JH. Smooth muscle phenotypic changes in arterial wall homeostasis: implications for the pathogenesis of atherosclerosis. Exp Mol Path 1985; 42:139–162.
77. Fritze LMS, Reilly CF, Rosenberg RD. An antiproliferative heparan sulfate species produced by postconfluent smooth muscle cells. J Cell Biol 1985; 100:1041–1049.
78. Reilly DF, Gordon D, Schwartz SM. Determination and comparison of the aortic polyploid smooth muscle content of human hypertensive subjects and normotensive controls. Acta Physiol Scand 1988; 133[Suppl 571]:181–188.
79. Wasteson A, Hook M, Westermark B. Demonstration of a platelet enzyme, degrading heparan sulphate. FEBS Letters 1976; 64:218–221.
80. Wasteson A, et al. Effect of a platelet endoglycosidase on cell surface associated heparan sulphate of human cultured endothelial and glial cells. Thrombosis Res 1977; 11:309–321.
81. Oosta GM, et al. Purification and properties of human platelet heparitinase. J Biol Chem 1982; 257:11249–11255.
82. Castellot JJ Jr, et al. Inhibition of vascular smooth muscle cell growth by endothelial cell-derived heparin. Possible role of a platelet endoglycosidase. J Biol Chem 1982; 257:11256–11260.
83. Handin RI, Cohen JH. Purification and binding properties of human platelet factor four. J Biol Chem 1976; 251:4273–4282.
84. Clowes AW, Schwartz SM. Significance of quiescent smooth muscle migration in the injured rat carotid artery. Circ Res 1985; 56:139–145.
85. Reidy MA, et al. Endothelial regeneration. VI. Chronic nondenuding injury in baboon vascular grafts. Am J Pathol 1986a; 123:432–439.
86. Gajdusek CM, Schwartz SM. Comparison of intracellular and extracellular mitogen activity. J Cell Physiol 1984; 121:316–322.
87. Imai H, et al. Angiotoxicity and arteriosclerosis due to contaminants of USP-grade cholesterol. Arch Pathol Lab Med 1976; 100:565–572.
88. Vlodavsky I, et al. Aortic endothelial cells synthesize basic fibroblast growth factor which remains cell associated and platelet-derived growth factor-like protein which is secreted. J Cell Physiol 1987a; 131:402–408.
89. Baird A, Ling N. Fibroblast growth factors are present in the extracellular matrix produced by endothelial cells in vitro: implications for a role of heparinase-like enzymes in the neovascular response. Biochem Biophys Res Commun 1987; 142:428–435.
90. Vlodavsky I, et al. Endothelial cell-derived basic fibroblast growth factor: synthesis and deposition into suendothelial extracellular matrix. Proc Natl Acad Sci USA 1987b; 84:2292–2296.
91. Bar-Ner M, et al. Inhibition of heparanase-mediated degradation of extracellular matrix heparan sulfate by non-anticoagulant heparin species. Blood 1987; 70:551–557.
92. Smith JC, et al. Growth factors adherent to cell substrate are mitogenically active in situ. Nature 1982; 296:154–156.
93. Savion N, et al. Synthesis and distribution of cytoskeletal elements in endothelial cells as a function of cell growth and organization. J Cell Physiol 1982; 110:129–141.
94. DiCorleto PE, Bowen-Pope DF. Cultured endothelial cells produce a platelet-derived growth factor-like protein. Proc Natl Acad Sci USA 1983; 80:1919–1923.
95. DiCorleto PE. Cultured endothelial cells produce multiple growth factors for connective tissue cells. Exp Cell Res 1984; 153:167–172.
96. Gajdusek CM. Release of endothelial cell-derived growth factor (ECDGF) by heparin. J Cell Physiol 1984; 121:13–21.
97. Barrett TB, et al. Polyploid nuclei in human artery wall smooth muscle cells. Proc Natl Acad Sci USA 1983; 80:882–885.
98. Jaye M, Maciag T. Modulation of the sis gene transcript during endothelial cell differentiation in vitro. Science 1985; 228:882–884.

99. Barrett TB, Benditt EP. Platelet-derived growth factor gene expression in human atherosclerotic plaques and normal artery wall. Proc Natl Acad Sci USA 1988; 85:2810–2814.
100. Wilcox JN, et al. Platelet-derived growth factor mRNA detection in human atherosclerotic plaques by in situ hybridization. J Clin Invest 1988; 82:1134–1143.
101. Libby P, et al. Production of platelet-derived growth factor-like mitogen by smooth muscle cells from human atheroma. N Engl J Med 1988; 318:1493–1498.
102. Seifert RA, Schwartz SM, Bowen-Pope DF. Developmentally regulated production of platelet-derived growth factor-like molecules. Nature 1984; 311:669–671.
103. Nilsson J, et al. Arterial smooth muscle cells in primary culture produce a platelet-derived growth factor-like protein. Proc Natl Acad Sci USA 1985; 82:4418–4422.
104. Majesky MW, Benditt EP, Schwartz SM. Expression and developmental control of platelet-derived growth factor A-chain and B-chain/sis genes in rat aortic smooth muscle cells. Proc Natl Acad Sci USA 1988; 85:1524–1528.
105. Clowes AW, Clowes MM, Reidy MA. Kinetics of cellular proliferation after arterial injury. III. Endothelial and smooth muscle growth in chronically denuded vessels. Lab Invest 1986; 54:295–303.
106. Gordon D, et al. Cell proliferation in human coronary arteries. Proc Natl Acad Sci USA 1990; 87:4600–4604.
107. Katsuda S, et al. Human atherosclerosis IV. Immunocytochemical analysis of cell activation and proliferation in lesions of young adults. Am J Pathol 1993; 142:1787–1793.
108. Clowes AW, Clowes MM, Reidy MA. Kinetics of cellular proliferation after arterial injury. I. Smooth muscle growth in the absence of endothelium. Lab Invest 1983; 49:327–333.
109. Lindner V, Reidy MA. Proliferation of smooth muscle cells after vascular injury is inhibited by an antibody against basic fibroblast growth factor. Proc Natl Acad Sci USA 1991; 88:3739–3743.
110. Olson NE, et al. Intimal smooth muscle cell proliferation after balloon catheter injury. The role of basic fibroblast growth factor. Am J Pathol 1992; 140:1017–1023.
111. Jawien A, et al. Platelet-derived growth factor promotes smooth muscle migration and intimal thickening in a rat model of balloon angioplasty. J Clin Invest 1992; 89:507–511.
112. Ferns GAA, et al. Inhibition of neointimal smooth muscle accumulation after angioplasty by an antibody to PDGF. Science 1991; 253:1129–1132.
113. Daemen MJAP, et al. Angiotensin II induces smooth muscle cell proliferation in the normal and injured arterial wall. Circ Res 1991; 68:450–456.
114. Van Kleef EM, et al. α-1-adrenoreceptor blockade reduces the angiotensin II-induced vascular smooth muscle cell DNA synthesis in the rat thoracic aorta and carotid artery. Circ Res 1992; 70:1122–1127.
115. Prescott M, Webb R, Reidy MA. ACE inhibitors vs. AII, AT1 receptor antagonist: Effects on smooth muscle cell migration and proliferation after balloon catheter injury. Am J Pathol 1991; 139:1291–1302.
116. Majesky MW, et al. Production of transforming growth factor β1 during repair of arterial injury. J Clin Invest 1991; 88:904–910.
117. Farhy RD, et al. Role of kinins and nitric oxide in the effects of angiotensin-converting enzyme inhibitors on neointima formation. Circ Res 1993; 72:1202–1210.
118. Kauffman RF, et al. Losartan, a nonpeptide AII receptor antagonist, inhibits neointima formation following balloon injury to rat carotid arteries. Life Sci 1991; 49:PL223–PL228.
119. Dzau VJ, Gibbons GH, Pratt RE. Molecular mechanisms of vascular renin-angiotensin system in myointimal hyperplasia. Hypertension 1991; 18[Suppl 4]:II100–II105.
120. Bunning P, Holmquist B, Riordan JF. Substrate specificity and kinetic characteristics of angiotensin-converting enzyme. Biochem 1983; 22:103–110.
121. deBlois D, Schwartz SM.
122. Majesky MW, et al. Platelet-derived growth factor (PDGF) ligand and receptor gene expression during repair of arterial injury. J Cell Biol 1990; 111:2149–2158.
123. Jackson CL, et al. Role of endogenous platelet-derived growth factor in arterial smooth muscle cell migration after balloon catheter injury. Arterioscler Thromb 1993; 13:1218–1226.
124. Viswanathan M, et al. Balloon angioplasty enhances the expression of angiotensin II AT1 receptors in neointima of rat aorta. J Clin Invest 1992; 90:1707–1712.
125. Cercek B, et al. Induction of insulin-like growth factor 1 messenger RNA in rat aorta after balloon denudation. Circ Res 1990; 66:1755–1760.
126. MERCATOR Study Group. Does the new angiotensin-converting enzyme inhibitor cilazapril prevent restenosis after percutaneous transluminal coronary angioplasty? Circulation 1992; 86:100–110.
127. Powell JS, et al. The proliferative response to vascular injury is suppressed by angiotensin-converting enzyme inhibition. J Cardiovasc Pharmacol 1990; 16[Suppl 4]:S42–S49.
128. Rakugi H, Dzau VJ, Pratt RE. Importance of tissue angiotensin-converting enzyme (ACE) in neointimal hyperplasia. Circulation 1992; 86[Suppl I]:I–169.
129. Kaartinen M, Penttila A, Kovanen PT. Mast cells of two types differing in neutral protease composition in the human aortic intima. Demonstration of tryptase- and tryptase/chymase-containing mast cells in normal intimas, fatty streaks, and the shoulder region of atheromas. Arterioscler Thromb 1994; 14:966–972.
130. Urata H, et al. Identification of a highly specific chymase as the major angiotensin II-forming enzyme in the human heart. J Biol Chem 1990; 265:22348–22357.
131. Baumgartner HR. Eine neue methode zur erzeugung der thromben durch gezielte uberdehnung der gefasswand. Z Ges Exp Med 1963; 137:227–234.
132. Salisbury BG, Hajjar DP, Minick CR. Altered glycosaminoglycan metabolism in injured arterial wall. Exp Molec Pathol 1985; 42:306–319.
133. Vesselinovitch D. Animal models and the study of atherosclerosis. Arch Pathol Lab Med 1988; 112:1011–1017.
134. Anderson PG. Animal models and morphometric techniques in studies of the vascular response to injury. Cardiovasc Pathol 1992; 1:263–278.
135. Schwartz SM, Haudenschild CC, Eddy EM. Endothelial regeneration. I. Quantitative analysis of initial stages of endothelial regeneration in rat aortic intima. Lab Invest 1978; 38:568–580.
136. Bjorkerud S. Reaction of the aortic wall of the rabbit after superficial, longitudinal, mechanical trauma. Virchows Arch 1969; 347:197–210.
137. Reidy MA, et al. Vascular injury: Quantification of experimental focal endothelial denudation in rats using indium-111-labeled platelets. Arteriosclerosis 1986b; 6:305–311.
138. Richardson M, et al. Wound healing in the media of the normolipemic rabbit carotid artery injured by air drying or by balloon catheter de-endothelialization. Am J Pathol 1990; 137:1453–1465.
139. Reddick RL, et al. Coronary atherosclerosis in the pig. Induced plaque injury and platelet response. Arteriosclerosis 1990; 10:541–550.
140. Weidinger FF, et al. Hypercholesterolemia enhances macrophage recruitment and dysfunction of regenerated endothe-

lium after balloon injury of the rabbit iliac artery. Circulation 1991; 84:755–767.
141. Scott RF, et al. Lining cell and intimal smooth muscle cell response and Evans blue staining in abdominal aortae of young swine after denudation by balloon catheter. Exp Molec Pathol 1980; 33:185–202.
142. Stadius ML, et al. Time course and cellular characteristics of the iliac artery response to acute balloon injury. An angiographic, morphometric, and immunocytochemical analysis in the cholesterol-fed New Zealand white rabbit. Arterioscler Thromb 1992; 12:1267–1273.
143. Groves HM, Kinlough-Rathbone RL, Richardson M. Platelet interaction with damaged rabbit aorta. Lab Invest 1979; 40:194–206.
144. Nichols TC, et al. Role of von Willebrand factor in arterial thrombosis. Studies in normal and von Willebrand disease pigs. Circulation 1991; 83[Suppl 6]:IV56–IV64.
145. Schwartz SM, Reidy MA, Clowes A. Kinetics of atherosclerosis, a stem cell model. Ann NY Acad Sci 1985; 454:292–304.
146. Miano JM, et al. Smooth muscle cell immediate-early gene and growth factor actin follows vascular injury. A putative in vivo mechanism for autocrine growth. Arterioscler Thromb 1993; 13:211–219.
147. Hanke H, et al. Time course of smooth muscle cell proliferation in the intima and media of arteries following experimental angioplasty. Circ Res 1990; 67:651–659.
148. Haust MD, More RH, Movat HZ. The role of smooth muscle cells in the fibrogenesis of arteriosclerosis. Am J Pathol 1960; 37:377–389.
149. McGill HC Jr. Persistent problems in the pathogenesis of atherosclerosis. Arteriosclerosis 1984; 4:443–451.
150. Geer JC. Fine structure of human aortic intimal thickening fatty streaks. Lab Invest 1965; 14:1764–1783.
151. Parker F, Odland GF. A correlative histochemical, biochemical and electron microscopic study of experimental atherosclerosis in the rabbit aorta with special reference to the myointimal cell. Am J Pathol 1966; 48:197–239.
152. Wissler RW, McCallister HA Jr, Vesselinovitch D. A histopathologic study of the fatty streak in aortas and coronary arteries of young American military personnel. Am J Pathol 1975; 78:64a.
153. Thomas WA, Lee KT, Kim DN. Cell population kinetics in atherogenesis. Cell births and losses in intimal cell mass-derived lesions in the abdominal aorta of swine. Ann NY Acad Sci 1985; 454:305–315.
154. Velican C, Velican D. Differences in the pattern of atherosclerotic involvement between non-branched regions and adjacent branching points of human coronary arteries. Atherosclerosis 1985; 54:333–342.
155. Velican C, Velican D. The precursors of coronary atherosclerotic plaques in subjects up to 40 years old. Atherosclerosis 1980; 37:33–46.
156. Stary HC, McMillan GC. Kinetics of cellular proliferation in experimental atherosclerosis. Arch Path 1970; 89:173–183.
157. Spagnoli LG, et al. Autoradiographic studies of the smooth muscle cells in human arteries. Paroi Arterielle 1981; 7:107–112.
158. Villaschi S, Spagnoli LG. Autoradiographic and ultrastructural studies on the human fibro-atheromatous plaque. Atherosclerosis 1983; 48:95–100.
159. Rekhter M, et al. Cell proliferation in human arteriovenous fistulas used for hemodialysis. Arterioscler Thromb 1993; 13:609–617.
160. O'Brien ER, et al. Proliferation in primary and restenotic coronary atherectomy tissue: Implications for antiproliferative therapy. Circ Res 1993; 73:223–231.
161. O'Brien ER, et al. Angiogenesis in human coronary atherosclerotic plaques. Am J Pathol 1994; 145:883–894.
162. Benditt EP, Gown AM. Atheroma: the artery wall and the environment. Int Rev Exp Path 1980; 21:55–118.
163. Waters D, et al. Effects of monotherapy with an HMG-CoA reductase inhibitor on the progression of coronary atherosclerosis as assessed by serial quantitative arteriography. Circulation 1994; 89:959–968.
164. Glagov S, et al. Compensatory enlargement of human atherosclerotic coronary arteries. N Engl J Med 1987; 316:1371–1375.
165. Jamal A, Bendeck M, Langille BL. Structural changes and recovery of function after arterial injury. Arterioscler Thromb 1992; 12:307–317.
166. Dilley RJ, Schwartz SM. Vascular remodeling in the growth hormone transgenic mouse. Circ Res 1989; 65:1233–1240.
167. Mulvany MJ. Determinants of vascular structure. J Cardiovasc Pharmacol 1992; 19[Suppl 5]:S1–S6.
168. Haudenschild CC, Schwartz SM. Endothelial regeneration. II. Restitution of endothelial continuity. Lab Invest 1979; 41:407–418.
169. Koester W. Endarteritis and arteritis. Berl Klin Wochenschr 1876; 13:454–455.
170. Geiringer E. Intimal vascularization and atherosclerosis. J Pathol Bacteriol 1951; 63:201–211.
171. Barger AC, et al. Vasa vasorum and neovascularization of human coronary arteries. N Engl J Med 1984; 310:175–177.
172. Brown BG, et al. Regression of coronary artery disease as a result of intensive lipid-lowering therapy in men with high levels of apolipoprotein B. N Engl J Med 1990; 323:1289–1298.
173. Blankenhorn DH, et al. Beneficial effects of colestipol niacin therapy on coronary atherosclerosis and coronary venous bypass grafts. JAMA 1987; 257:3233–3240.
174. Watts GF, et al. Effects on coronary artery disease of lipid-lowering diet, or diet plus cholestyramine, in the St. Thomas' Atherosclerosis Regression Study (STARS). Lancet 1992; 339:563–569.
175. Gould KL. Quantitative analysis of coronary artery restenosis after coronary angioplasty—Has the rose lost its bloom? J Am Coll Cardiol 1992; 19:946–947.
176. Kragel AH, Reddy SG, Wittes JT, Roberts WC. Morphometric analysis of the composition of atherosclerotic plaques in the four major epicardial coronary arteries in acute myocardial infarction and in sudden coronary death. Circulation 1989; 80:1747–1765.
177. Constantinides P. Plaque fissures in human coronary thrombosis. J Atheroscler Res 1966; 6:1–17.
178. Davies MJ, Thomas AC. Plaque fissuring—The cause of acute myocardial infarction, sudden ischemic death, and crescendo angina. Br Heart J 1985; 53:363–373.
179. Falk E. Morphologic features of unstable atherothrombotic plaques underlying acute coronary syndromes. Am J Cardiol 1989; 63:114E–120E.
180. Henney AM, et al. Localization of stromelysin gene expression in atherosclerotic plaques by in situ hybridization. Proc Natl Acad Sci USA 1991; 88:8154–8158.
181. Davies MJ. Anatomic features in victims of sudden coronary death. Coronary artery pathology. Circulation 1992; 85:[Suppl 1]I19–I24.
182. Leclerc G, et al. Assessment of cell kinetics in human restenotic lesions by in vitro bromodeoxyuridine labeling of excised atherectomy specimens (Abstract). Clin Res 1993; 41:343A.
183. Strauss BH, et al. Directional atherectomy for treatment of restenosis within coronary stents: Clinical, angiographic and histological results. J Am Coll Cardio 1992; 20:1465–1473.
184. Pickering JG, et al. Proliferative activity in peripheral and

coronary atherosclerotic plaque among patients undergoing percutaneous revascularization. J Clin Invest 1993; 91:1469–1480.

185. Garcia RL, Coltrera MD, Gown AM. Analysis of proliferative grade using anti-PCNA/cycin monoclonal antibodies in fixed, embedded tissues: Comparison with flow cytometric analysis. Am J Pathol 1989; 134:733–739.
186. Fry DL. Mass transport, atherogenesis, and risk. Arteriosclerosis 1987; 7:88–100.
187. Fischer-Dzoga K, et al. The role of hyperlipidemic serum on the proliferation and necrosis of aortic medial cells in vitro. Exp Mol Pathol 1977; 26:359–374.
188. Fless GM, et al. Serum low density lipoproteins with mitogenic effect on cultured aortic smooth muscle cells. Atherosclerosis 1982; 41:171–183.
189. Florentin RA, et al. Stimulation of DNA synthesis and cell division in vitro by serum from cholesterol-fed swine. J Cell Biol 1969; 41:641–645.
190. Packham MA, Mustard JF. The role of platelets in the development and complications of atherosclerosis. Semin Hematol 1986; 23:8–26.
191. Walker LN, Reidy MA, Bowyer DE. Morphology and kinetics of fatty streak lesion formation in the hypercholesterolemic rabbit. Am J Pathol 1986; 125:450–459.
192. Scott RF, et al. Intimal cell mass-derived atherosclerotic lesions in the abdominal aorta of hyperlipidemic swine. Part 2. Investigation of endothelial cell changes and leukocyte adherence associated with early smooth muscle cell proliferative activity. Atherosclerosis 1986b; 62:27–38.
193. Scott RF, et al. Atherosclerotic lesions in coronary arteries of hyperlipidemic swine. Part 2. Endothelial cell kinetics and leukocyte adherence associated with early lesions. Atherosclerosis 1986; 62:1–10.
194. Schaffner T, et al. Arterial foam cells with distinctive immunomorphologic and histochemical features of macrophages. Am J Pathol 1980; 100:57–74.
195. Rosenfeld ME, et al. Fatty streak expansion and maturation in Watanabe heritable hyperlipemic and comparably hypercholesterolemic fat-fed rabbits. Arterioslcerosis 1987; 7:24–34.
196. Tsukada T, et al. HHF35, a muscle-actin-specific monoclonal antibody: I. Immunochemical and biochemical characterization. Am J Pathol 1987; 126:51–60.
197. Pearson TA, et al. Clonal characteristics of cutaneous scars and implications for atherogenesis. Am J Pathol 1981; 102: 49–54.
198. Pearson TA, Dillman JM, Heptinstall RH. Clonal mapping of the human aorta. Relationship of monoclonal characteristics, lesion thickness, and age in normal intima and atherosclerotic lesions. Am J Pathol 1987; 126:33–39.
199. Lee KT, et al. Evidence for a polyclonal origin and proliferative heterogeneity of atherosclerotic lesions induced by dietary cholesterol in swine. Ann NY Acad Sci 1976; 275:336–347.
200. Thomas WA, et al. Alterations in population dynamics of arterial smooth muscle cell during atherogenesis. IV. Evidence for a polyclonal origin of hypercholesterolemia diet-induced atherosclerotic lesions in young swine. Exp Mol Pathol 1976; 24:244–260.
201. Thomas, WA, et al. Population dynamics of arterial cells during atherogenesis. VIII. Separation of the roles of injury and growth stimulation in early aortic atherogenesis in swine originating in pre-existing intimal smooth muscle cell masses. Exp Mol Pathol 1979a; 31:124–144.
202. Thomas WA, et al. Population dynamics of arterial cells during atherogenesis. X. Study of monotypism in atherosclerotic lesions of black women heterozygous for glucose-6-phosphate dehydrogenase (G-6-PD). Exp Mol Pathol 1979b; 31:367–386.
203. Lee KT, et al. Mosaicism in female hybrid hares heterozygous for glucose-6-phosphate dehydrogenase. VII. Evidence for selective advantage of one phenotype over the other in ditypic samples from aortas of hares fed cholesterol oxidation products. Exp Mol Pathol 1985; 42:71–77.
204. Pearson TA, et al. Cholesterol-induced atherosclerosis. Clonal characteristics of arterial lesions in the hybrid hare. Arteriosclerosis 1983; 3:574.
205. Bond JA, et al. Metabolism of benzo[a]pyrene and 7,12-dimethylbenz[a]anthracene in cultured human fetal aortic smooth muscle cells. Life Sci 1979; 25:425–430.
206. Minick CR, et al. Atheroarteriosclerosis induced by infection with a herpesvirus. Am J Pathol 1976; 96:673–706.
207. Fabricant CG, et al. Herpesvirus-induced atherosclerosis in chickens. Fed Proc 1983; 42:2476–2479.
208. Benditt EP, Barrett T, McDougall JK. Viruses in the etiology of atherosclerosis. Proc Natl Acad Sci USA 1983; 80:6386–6389.
209. Gyorkey F, et al. Herpesviridae in the endothelial and smooth muscle cells of the proximal aorta in arteriosclerotic patients. Exp Mol Pathol 1984; 40:328–339.
210. Melnick JL, et al. Cytomegalovirus antigen within human arterial smooth muscle cells. Lancet 1983; 2:644–647.
211. Adam E, et al. High levels of cytomegalovirus antibody in patients requiring vascular surgery for atherosclerosis. Lancet 1987; 2:291–293.
212. Stiles CD. The biological role of oncogenes—insights from platelet-derived growth factor. Cancer Res 1985; 45:5215–5218.
213. Penn A, et al. Transforming gene in human atherosclerotic plaque DNA. Proc Natl Acad Sci USA 1986; 83:7951–7955.
214. Weinberg RA. The action of oncogenes in the cytoplasm and nucleus. Science 1985; 230:770–776.
215. Hassler O. The origin of the cells constituting arterial intimal thickening. An experimental autoradiographic study. Lab Invest 1970; 22:286–295.
216. Webster WS, Bishop SP, Geer JC. Experimental aortic intimal thickening. I. Morphology and source of intimal cells. Am J Pathol 1974; 76:245–284.
217. Grotendorst GR. Alteration of the chemotactic response of NIH/3T3 cells to PDGF by growth factors, transformation, and tumor promoters. Cell 1984; 36:279–285.
218. Martin G, Ogburn C, Sprague C. Senescence and vascular disease. Adv Exp Med Biol 1975; 61:163–193.
219. Benditt EP, Gown AM. Immunohistochemistry: new vistas in biology and pathology. In Histochemistry: The Widening Horizons, Stoward PJ, Polak JM (eds). New York: John Wiley and Sons, 1981. Pp. 21–29.
220. Cowley AW. The concept of autoregulation of total blood flow and its role in hypertension. In Laragh JH, ed. Topics in Hypertension. New York: Yorke Medical Books. Pp 184–200.
221. Mulvany MJ, Hansen PK, Aalkjaer C. Direct evidence that the greater contractility of resistance vessels in spontaneously hypertensive rats is associated with a narrowed lumen, a thickened media, and an increased number of smooth muscle cell layers. Circ Res 1978; 43:854–863.
222. Aalkjaer C, Heagerty AM, Mulvany MJ. In vitro characteristics of vessels from patients with essential hypertension. J Clin Hypertens 1987; 3:317–322.
223. Wolinsky H. Response of the rat aortic media to hypertension. Morphological and chemical studies. Circ Res 1970; 26:507–522.
224. Pang SC, Scott TM. Stereological analysis of the tunica media of the aorta and renal artery during the development of

hypertension in the spontaneously hypertensive rat. J Anat 1981; 133:513–526.
225. Lee RM, et al. Ultrastructural changes in mesenteric arteries from spontaneously hypertensive rats. A morphometric study. Blood Vessels 1983; 20:72–91.
226. Cowley AW, Guyton AC. Baroreceptor reflex effects on transient and steady-state hemodynamics of salt-loading hypertension in dogs. Circ Res 1975; 36:536.
227. Lee RMKW. Vascular changes at the prehypertensive phase in the mesenteric arteries from spontaneously hypertensive rats. Blood Vessels 1985; 22:105–126.
228. Loeb AL, et al. Increased aortic DNA synthesis precedes renal hypertension in rats. An obligatory step? Hypertension 1986; 8:754–761.
229. Goldby FS, Beilin LJ. Relationship between arterial pressure and the permeability of arterioles to carbon particles in acute hypertension in the rat. Cardiovasc Res 1972a; 6:384–390.
230. Goldby FS, Beilin LJ. How an acute rise in arterial pressure damages arterioles. Cardiovasc Res 1972b; 6:569–584.
231. Reidy MA, Schwartz SM. A technique to investigate surface morphology and endothelial cell replication of small arteries. A study in acute angiotensin-induced hypertensive rats. Microvasc Res 1982; 24:158–167.
232. Giese J. Renin, angiotensin and hypertensive vascular damage: a review. Am J Med 1973; 55:315–331.
233. Crane WAJ, Dutta LP. The utilisation of tritiated thymidine for deoxyribonucleic acid synthesis by the lesions of experimental hypertension in rats. J Path Bact 1963; 86:83–97.
234. Bevan RD. An autoradiographic and pathological study of cellular proliferation in rabbit arteries correlated with an increase in arterial pressure. Blood Vessels 1976; 13:100–128.
235. Plunkett WC, Overbeck HW. Increased arteriolar wall-to-lumen ratio in a normotensive vascular bed in coarctation hypertension. Am J Physiol 1985; 249:H859–H866.
236. Lee RM, Triggle CR. Morphometric study of mesenteric arteries from genetically hypertensive Dahl strain rats. Blood Vessels 1986; 23:199–224.
237. Gutmann E. Neutrophic relations. Ann Rev Physiol 1976; 38:177–216.
238. Bevan RD, Tsuru H. Long-term denervation of vascular smooth muscle causes not only functional but structural damage. Blood Vessels 1979; 16:109–112.
239. Rorive GL, Carlier PJ, Foidart JM. Hyperplasia of rat arteries smooth muscle cells associated with development and reversal of renal hypertension. Clin Sci 1980; 59:335–338.
240. Henrichs KJ, et al. Is arterial media hypertrophy in spontaneously hypertensive rats a consequence of or a cause for hypertension? Clin Sci 1980; 59:331s–333s.
241. Freslon JJ, Giudicelli JF. Compared myocardial and vascular effects of captropil and dihydralazine during hypertension development in spontaneously hypertensive rats. Br J Pharmacol 1983; 80:533–543.
242. Owens GK. Influence of blood pressure on development of aortic medial smooth muscle hypertrophy in spontaneously hypertensive rats. Hypertension 1987; 9:178–187.
243. Marcoux FW, Mongeon SA, Halpern W. Mechanical and morphological properties of mesenteric (MES) and cerebral (CER) resistance arteries following chronic captopril (CAP) treatment of WKY and SHR rats (abstract). Fed Proc 1983; 42:645.
244. Carlier PG, Rorive GL. Pathogenesis and reversibility of the aortic changes in experimental hypertension. J Cardiovasc Pharmacol 1985; 7:S46–S51.
245. Ooshima A, et al. Increased collagen synthesis in blood vessels of hypertensive rats and its reversal by antihypertensive agents. Proc Natl Acad Sci USA 1974; 71:3019–3023.
246. Ehrhart LA, Ferrario CM. Collagen metabolism and reversal of aortic medial hypertrophy in spontaneously hypertensive rats treated with methyldopa. Hypertension 1981; 3:479–484.
247. Yamori Y, Tarazi RC, Ooshima A. Effect of β-receptor-blocking agents on cardiovascular structural changes in spontaneous and noradrenaline-induced hypertension in rats. Clin Sci 1980; 59:457s–460s.
248. Leitschuh M, Chobanian AV. Inhibition of nuclear polyploidy by propranolol in aortic smooth muscle cells of hypertensive rats. Hypertension 1987; 9:III-106–III-109.
249. Marcoux FW, Mongeon SA, Halpern W. Effects of chronic prazosin treatment on resistance arteries of WKY and SHR rats (abstract). Blood Vessels 1984; 21:194.
250. Stanbrook HS, Morris KG, McMurty IF. Prevention and reversal of hypoxic pulmonary hypertension by calcium antagonists. Am Rev Resp Dis 1984; 130:81–85.
251. Mulvany MJ, Korsgaard N, Nyborg N. Evidence that the increased calcium sensitivity of resistance vessels in spontaneously hypertensive rats is an intrinsic defect of their vascular smooth muscle. Clin Exp Hypertension 1981; 3:749–761.
252. Nyborg NCB, Mulvany MJ. Lack of effect of antihypertensive treatment with felodiprine on cardiovascular structure of young spontaneously hypertensive rats. Cardiovasc Res 1985; 19:528–536.
253. Seidel CL, Allen JC, Bowers RL. Mechanical and biochemical alterations of aorta induced by hydralazine hypotension. J Pharmacol Exp Ther 1980; 213:514–519.
254. Limas C, Westrum B, Limas CJ. Comparative effects of hydralazine and captopril on the cardiovascular changes in spontaneously hypertensive rats. Am J Pathol 1984; 117: 360–371.
255. Warshaw DM, Root PT, Halpern W. Effects of antihypertensive drug therapy on the morphology and mechanics of resistance arteries from spontaneously hypertensive rats. Blood Vessels 1980; 17:257–270.
256. Harper SL. Effects of antihypertensive treatment on the cerebral microvasculature of spontaneously hypertensive rats. Stroke 1987a; 18:450–456.
257. Harper SL. Antihypertensive drug therapy prevents cerebral microvascular abnormalities in hypertensive rats. Circ Res 1987b; 60:229–237.
258. Limas C, Westrum B, Limas CJ. Effect of antihypertensive therapy on the vascular changes of spontaneously hypertensive rats. Am J Pathol 1983; 111:380–393.
259. Owens GK. Differential effects of antihypertensive drug therapy on vascular smooth muscle cell hypertrophy, hyperploidy, and hyperplasia in the spontaneously hypertensive rat. Circ Res 1985; 56:525–536.
260. Lee RMKW, Smeda JS. Primary versus secondary structural changes of the blood vessels in hypertension. Can J Physiol Pharmacol 1985; 63:392–401.
261. Sapru HN, Wang SC. Modification of aortic baroceptor resulting in the spontaneously hypertensive rat. Am J Physiol 1976; 230:664–674.
262. Lee RMKW, et al. Structural and functional consequence of neonatal sympathectomy on the blood vessels of spontaneously hypertensive rats. Hypertension 1987; 10:328–338.
263. Nordborg C, Hardebo JE, Kahrstrom J. Does sympathectomy or antihypertensive treatment affect the morphology of basal cerebral arteries in spontaneously hypertensive rats? Acta Physiol Scand 1986; 552[Suppl]:62–65.
264. Owens GK, Schwartz SM. Alterations in vascular smooth muscle mass in the spontaneously hypertensive rat. Role in cellular hypertrophy, hyperploidy, and hyperplasia. Circ Res 1982; 51:280–289.
265. Owens GK, Schwartz SM. Vascular smooth muscle cell hypertrophy and hyperploidy in the Goldblatt hypertensive rat. Circ Res 1983; 53:491–501.

266. Lichtenstein AH, Brecher P, Chobanian AV. Effects of deoxycorticosterone-salt hypertension on cell ploidy in the rat aorta. Hypertension 1986; 8:II-50–II-54.
267. Goldberg ID, et al. Isolation and culture of a tetraploid subpopulation of smooth muscle cells from the normal rat aorta. Science 1984; 226:559–561.
268. Halpern W, Warshaw DM, Mulvany MJ. Mechanical and morphological properties of arterial resistance vessels in young and old spontaneously hypertensive rats. Circ Res 1979; 45:250–259.
269. Mulvany MJ. Blood pressure regulation and characteristics of small arteries in hypertension. Acta Med Scand 1982; 670[Suppl]:21–28.
270. Mulvany MJ. Determinants of vascular hemodynamic characteristics. Hypertension 1984; 6:III-13–III-18.
271. Todd ME, Laye CG, Osborne DN. The dimensional characteristics of smooth muscle in rat blood vessels: a computer-assisted analysis. Circ Res 1983; 53:319–331.
272. Mulvany MJ, Baandrup U, Gundersen HJG. Evidence for hyperplasia in mesenteric resistance vessels of spontaneously hypertensive rats using a three-dimensional dissector. Circ Res 1985; 57:794–800.
273. Mulvany MJ. Resistance vessel structure in hypertension: Growth or remodeling? J Cardiovasc Pharmacol 1993; 22[Suppl 5]:S44–S47.
274. Falloon BJ, et al. In vitro perfusion studies of resistance artery function in genetic hypertension. Hypertension 1993; 22:486–495.
275. Folkow B. Brief historical background and clinical implications of early structural changes. Hypertension 1984; 6:III-1–III-3.
276. Loeb AL, Bean BL. Antihypertensive drugs inhibit hypertension-associated aortic DNA synthesis in the rat. Hypertension 1986; 8:1135–1142.
277. Freis ED, et al. Alteration of the course of hypertension in the spontaneously hypertensive rat. Circ Res 1972; 31:1–7.
278. Chobanian AV, Lichtenstein AH, Schwartz JH, Hanspal J, Brecher P. Effects of deoxycorticosterone/salt hypertension on cell ploidy in rat aortic smooth muscle cells. Circulation 1987; 75:I-102–I-106.
279. Langille BL, Reidy MA, Kline RL. Injury and repair of endothelium at sites of flow disturbances near abdominal aortic coarctations in rabbits. Arteriosclerosis 1986; 6:146–154.
280. Langille BL, O'Donnell F. Reductions in arterial diameter produced by chronic decreases in blood flow are endothelium-dependent. Science 1986; 231:405–407.
281. Joshua IG, et al. Progressive microvascular alterations with the development of renovascular hypertension. Hypertension 1984; 6:61–67.
282. Radomski MW, Palmer RMJ, Moncada S. Comparative pharmacology of endothelium-derived relaxing factor, nitric oxide and prostacyclin in platelets. Br J Pharm 1987; 92:181–187.
283. Cocks TM, et al. Release and properties of endothelium-derived relaxing factor (EDRF) from endothelial cells in culture. J Cell Physiol 1985; 123:310–320.
284. Vanhoutte PM. Could the absence or malfunction of vascular endothelium precipitate the occurrence of vasospasm? J Mol Cell Cardiol 1986; 18:67–89.
285. Berk BC, et al. Early agonist-mediated ionic events in cultured vascular smooth muscle cells. Calcium mobilization is associated with intracellular acidification. J Biol Chem 1987; 262:5065–5072.
286. Berk BC, et al. Vasoconstriction: a new activity for platelet-derived growth factor. Science 1986; 232:87–90.
287. Lundgren Y. Adaptive changes of cardiovascular design in spontaneous and renal hypertension. Hemodynamic studies in rats. Acta Physiol Scand Suppl 1974; 408:1–62.
288. Carlier PG, Rorive GL. Evolution at aortic hyperplasia after reversal of renovascular hypertension in the rat. Arch Int Physiol Biochem 1983; 91:205–213.
289. Sadoshima S, et al. Effect of chronic sympathetic denervation on cerebrovascular hypertrophy during the development of hypertension in rats. Brain Res 1986; 379:205–209.
290. Hart MN, Heistad DD, Brody MJ. Effect of chronic hypertension and sympathetic denervation on wall/lumen ratio of cerebral vessels. Hypertension 1980; 2:419–423.

Other References

Barrett TB, et al. Expression of the sis gene by endothelial cells in culture and in vivo. Proc Natl Acad Sci USA 1984; 81:6772–6774.

Chamley-Campbell JH, Campbell GR, Ross R. Phenotype-dependent response of cultured aortic smooth muscle to serum mitogens. J Cell Biol 1981; 89:379–383.

Friedman RJ, et al. The effect of thrombocytopenia on experimental atherosclerotic lesion formation in rabbits. Smooth muscle cell proliferation and re-endothelialization. J Clin Invest 1970; 60:1191–1201.

Jespersen LT, et al. Cardiac mass and peripheral vascular structure in hydralazine-treated spontaneously hypertensive rats. Hypertension 1985; 7:734–741.

Nyborg NCB, Korsgaard N, Mulvany MJ. Neonatal sympathectomy of normotensive Wistar-Kyoto and spontaneously hypertensive rats with 6-hydroxydopamine: effect on resistance vessel structure and sensitivity to calcium. J Hypertension 1986; 4:455–461.

Reidy MA. Neointimal proliferation: The role of basic FGF on vascular smooth muscle cell proliferation. Thromb Haemost 1993; 70:172–176.

Schweigerer L, et al. Basic fibroblast growth factor in human rhabdomyosarcoma cells: implications for the proliferation and neovascularization of myoblast-derived tumors. Proc Natl Acad Sci USA 1987b; 84:842–846.

Endothelial Dysfunction in Vascular Disease

Joseph A. Vita
John F. Keaney, Jr.
Joseph Loscalzo

Located at the interface between blood and tissue, the endothelium regulates vascular function through synthesis and release of a number of products that act locally in the adjacent vessel wall or lumen. As discussed in detail in Chapter 1, the presence of normal endothelium maintains appropriate vasodilation, inhibits platelet activity, suppresses growth of intimal cells, and contributes to the maintenance of the balance between thrombosis and fibrinolysis. There is growing appreciation that disturbances of the metabolic and regulatory functions of the endothelium contribute to the pathophysiology of specific disease states. Clinical manifestations of such disturbances include vasospasm, intravascular thrombosis, plaque rupture, and intimal growth. Mendelsohn and Loscalzo coined the term **endotheliolopathy** to describe clinical entities in which endothelial pathology contributes to the clinical expression of disease [1]. A partial list of such diseases is presented in Table 9-1. Our growing understanding of the pathophysiologic importance of the endothelium in such conditions has naturally led to the development of new therapeutic strategies directed toward restoring its normal function.

In this chapter, we will focus on coronary atherosclerosis as a paradigm for endothelial dysfunction in vascular disease because of its prevalence in our society and because extensive research has provided critical insights into the pathophysiologic importance of endothelial-cell action in this disease. We will first review studies that emphasize the contribution of vascular dysfunction to the clinical expression of coronary artery disease. We will provide a brief review of normal endothelial control of blood flow and fluidity and then present studies of the pathophysiologic mechanisms of endothelial dysfunction in atherosclerosis. We will also briefly review mechanisms of endothelial dysfunction in related disease states, including diabetes mellitus and hypertension. The bulk of studies in this field have focused on endothelial control of vasomotion and, in particular, on the action of endothelium-derived relaxing factor (EDRF). However, recent studies have also emphasized that altered endothelial control of fibrinolysis and intimal growth influence the clinical expression of atherosclerosis. Finally, we will outline recent attempts to reverse abnormal coronary endothelial function and application of those measures to management of patients. We anticipate that an increased understanding of the pathophysiologic role of endothelial dysfunction may lead to new therapeutic approaches for other disease states, including those listed in Table 9-1.

Pathophysiology of Myocardial Ischemia in Coronary Artery Disease

It is clear that vascular dysfunction contributes to the pathophysiology of coronary atherosclerosis. Clinical management of patients with this disease traditionally has focused on the presence and the severity of fixed coronary arterial stenoses, and it is well established that the number of stenosed vessels is inversely related to survival [2]. However, the anatomic severity of atherosclerotic coronary stenoses, that is, the percent stenosis or minimal lumen diameter, does not necessarily relate to their potential for producing acute and chronic myocardial ischemia [3,4]. Instead, functional vascular abnormalities in atherosclerosis, which may lead to thrombus formation and vasospasm, appear to play more important roles in the pathogenesis of acute ischemic syndromes. Autopsy studies have revealed that fissuring or rupture of coronary atherosclerotic plaque with associated thrombus formation is an important feature of unstable angina and myocardial infarction [5]. These events also are associated with local platelet aggregation and release of vasoconstrictor substances, such as thrombin, serotonin, and thromboxane A_2, that may contribute to decreased coronary blood supply and to the production of ischemia and infarction [6–8]. Angiographic studies of patients following thrombolytic therapy for acute myocardial infarction demonstrate that, in the majority of patients, there is a relatively mild residual stenosis in the infarct-related artery (less than 60–70%), suggesting that thrombus formation, not progression of disease, accounts for those syndromes [9,10]. Similarly, in series of patients who underwent coronary angiography prior to presenting with a myocardial infarction or unstable angina, there was no correlation between the angiographic severity of a stenosis and its likelihood of causing clinical ischemia [11].

In stable angina, stenosis severity also correlates poorly with the expression of disease. In patients with single-vessel coronary disease enrolled in the Angioplasty versus Medical Therapy Study, stenosis severity failed to correlate with exercise capacity [4]. Computer-assisted quantitative angiography provided no advantage over visual estimation of stenosis severity, further arguing against the importance of the anatomic severity of the stenosis for the clinical expression of disease. A growing number of studies suggest that vascular dysfunction, particularly abnormal coronary vasomotion, contributes to the pathophysiology of myocardial ischemia in stable coronary disease. In a group of stable patients undergoing cardiac catheterization, Gage and colleagues observed that angiographically normal coronary arteries dilated during bicycle exercise, while atherosclerotic coronary arteries constricted in response to similar degrees of exertion [12]. Comparable constrictor responses of atherosclerotic vessels have been observed in response to other clinically relevant stimuli for ischemia, including the cold pressor test, emotional stress, and pacing [13–15]. In the setting of increased myocardial demand and some component

Table 9-1. Disease states characterized by endothelial dysfunction

Amyloidosis
Atherosclerosis
AIDS
Behçet's disease
Diabetes mellitus
Hemolytic uremic syndrome/thrombotic thrombocytopenic purpura
Hyperhomocyst(e)inemia
Hypercholesterolemia
Hyperhomocyst(e)inemia
Infectious hypertension
Endotoxemia
Rickettsial infection
Kawasaki disease
Primary pulmonary hypertension
Reperfusion injury
Toxemia
Transplantation endotheliopathy
Vsculitides
Systemic lupus erythematosus
Rheumatoid arthritis
von Willebrand disease

of fixed obstruction, such constrictor responses have the potential to decrease coronary blood supply significantly and contribute to the production of myocardial ischemia.

Endothelial Control of Vascular Tone and Platelet Activity

The vascular endothelium plays a central role in the control of vascular tone and thrombosis through the release of a number of substances that act locally in the vascular wall and adjacent vessel lumen. In 1980, Furchgott and Zawadzki demonstrated that exposure of isolated rabbit aorta to acetylcholine induces release of a vasodilator substance or substances, EDRF [16]. Since this initial report, extensive studies indicate that endothelial cells generate a variety of biochemical species that produce vasodilation and inhibit platelet deposition. EDRF has been identified as nitric oxide (NO) [17] or a closely related redox form of NO [18]. NO is a reactive free-radical species that is synthesized from L-arginine in endothelial cells by an NO synthase (*Nos 3*, previously termed eNos) [19]. Like exogenous nitrovasodilators, EDRF/NO relaxes vascular smooth muscle and inhibits platelet activity by activating soluble guanylyl cyclase and increasing intracellular cyclic 3′,5′-guanosine monophosphate (cGMP) concentration [20]. EDRF is synthesized constitutively and contributes to maintenance of basal vascular tone. In addition, EDRF release is stimulated by a variety of agents, including aggregating platelets, serotonin, thrombin, acetylcholine, substance P, alpha$_2$ adrenergic agonists, and bradykinin, all of which act through specific endothelial-cell membrane receptors [21]. EDRF release is also induced by shear stress resulting from increased blood flow through activation of a shear-sensitive calcium-dependent potassium channel [22–26].

The vascular endothelium produces other vasorelaxant substances, including the cyclooxygenase product prostacyclin [27] and the less well characterized endothelium-derived hyperpolarizing factor (EDHF) [28,29]. Prostacyclin relaxes vascular smooth muscle and inhibits platelet aggregation by activating adenylyl cyclase and increasing intracellular cyclic 3′,5′-adenosine monophosphate (cAMP). Many studies of EDRF action were performed in the presence of indomethacin or other cyclooxygenase inhibitor to exclude prostacyclin effects; however, there is evidence to suggest that the antiplatelet [30] and vasorelaxant [31] effects of prostacyclin and EDRF are synergistic, possibly through an effect of NO as an activator of cyclooxygenase [32]. By inhibiting platelet activation and adhesion, EDRF and prostacyclin release also limit indirectly the vasoconstrictor effects of platelet-derived thromboxane A_2. Endothelial cells also produce vasoconstrictor substances, including the polypeptide endothelin [33] and a prostanoid, endothelium-derived constricting factor (EDCF) [34,35]. All these substances act in concert with EDRF to mediate endothelial control of vascular tone and platelet activity.

ENDOTHELIAL DYSFUNCTION IN ATHEROSCLEROSIS AND RELATED VASCULAR DISEASE STATES

Endothelial control of arterial tone and blood flow is impaired in hypercholesterolemia and atherosclerosis. Arterial tissue obtained from patients with coronary disease demonstrates impaired endothelium-dependent relaxation with preserved relaxation to exogenous nitrates [36,37]. In cholesterol-fed animals, endothelium-dependent relaxation of conduit vessels is impaired in response to aggregating platelets, serotonin, thrombin, acetylcholine, substance P, and alpha$_2$-adrenergic agonists [36,38–41]. Atherosclerosis is also associated with impaired endothelial vasodilator function in resistance vessels in the coronary and peripheral circulation, and these abnormalities also have the potential to affect tissue perfusion adversely [41,42]. The degree of impairment varies with agonist and model, but in general, receptor-dependent vasorelaxation is lost before receptor-independent responses. In swine, EDRF release by receptors coupled to a pertussis toxin–sensitive G_i protein, such as serotonin and alpha$_2$-adrenergic agonists, is impaired early in the course of cholesterol feeding [43]. At this early stage, EDRF release via receptors linked to other signal-transduction systems (bradykinin, adenosine 5′-diphosphate) and receptor-independent release (calcium ionophore, A23187) are preserved [43,44]. In more advanced stages of cholesterol feeding and under conditions of endothelial regeneration following injury, loss of EDRF action appears to be more generalized [44].

The majority of studies suggest that relaxation to exogenous nitrovasodilators remains unimpaired in these models, arguing against a defect in the ability of vascular smooth muscle to relax. However, Creager and colleagues observed a defect in nitroprusside-mediated dilation in the brachial circulation of patients [45]. Recent work in atherosclerotic rabbits demonstrated an impairment in maximal guanylyl cyclase activity following exposure to nitrovasodilators [46]. This impairment of guanylyl cyclase activity has been related to an effect of oxidized low-density lipoprotein (LDL) [47].

Endothelial regulation of vascular tone also has been shown to be impaired in other related disease states. In models of hypertension, endothelium-dependent relaxation to acetylcholine and other receptor-dependent agonists is impaired in conduit [48] and resistance vessels [49,50]. Under certain experimental conditions, treatment of hypertension tends to restore endothelium-dependent relaxation [51], although such an effect was not observed in patients [52]. There is evidence that in addition to impaired EDRF action, release of prostanoid EDCF(s) also may contribute to abnormal regulation of vascular tone in hypertension [35,53].

Endothelium-dependent dilation is also impaired in animal models of diabetes mellitus. Exposure of vascular tissue to high glucose concentrations in vitro produces an impairment of endothelium-dependent relaxation to acetylcholine but not to A23187 or nitroprusside [54]. Similar observations were made in animals rendered diabetic by alloxan or streptozotocin treatment [55,56]. Abnormal endothelium-dependent relaxation is reversed by inhibitors of prostaglandin synthesis and specific antagonists of prostaglandin H_2/thromboxane A_2. Tesfamariam and colleagues also demonstrated increased production of vasoconstrictor prostaglandins in diabetic rabbits and isolated abdominal aortae exposed to high glucose concentrations [54]. Thus, a number of well-done studies currently support the view that endothelium-dependent vasodilator function is impaired in atherosclerosis and related disease states, including hypercholesterolemia, hypertension, and diabetes mellitus.

CLINICAL STUDIES OF IMPAIRED EDRF ACTION

In patients with atherosclerosis, endothelial vasomotor dysfunction has been demonstrated in coronary and peripheral arteries. In the coronary circulation, Ludmer and colleagues observed dilation of angiographically normal coronary arteries during acetylcholine infusion in a group of young patients with few coronary risk factors [57]. In patients with angiographic evidence of atherosclerosis, acetylcholine infusion produced "paradoxical" coronary constriction, an effect that likely reflected loss of EDRF release and unopposed direct effects of acetylcholine to constrict vascular smooth muscle. Vita and colleagues demonstrated constriction of angiographically normal coronary arteries during acetylcholine infusion in patients with coronary risk factors, including hypercholesterolemia, male gender, and total number of risk factors, suggesting that endothelial dysfunction precedes the development of angiographically apparent atherosclerosis (Fig. 9-1) [58]. Constrictor responses to acetylcholine have also been observed in angiographically normal arteries in patients with angiographic evidence of atherosclerosis in other coronary vessels [59]. In addition to its effects on epicardial coronary arteries, acetylcholine also dilates coronary resistance vessels, producing an increase in coronary blood flow; this response is impaired in the setting of hypercholesterolemia and angiographic evidence of atherosclerosis [60,61].

Support for the EDRF-dependent nature of the dilator response to acetylcholine in these studies was provided by the finding that N^G-monomethyl-L-arginine (L-NMMA), a specific inhibitor of NO synthase, blocked acetylcholine-mediated epicardial coronary dilation [62]. Interestingly, acetylcholine-mediated increases in coronary blood flow, reflecting dilation of resistance vessels, were not inhibited by L-NMMA, suggesting a non-EDRF-dependent mechanism for vasodilation in that vascular bed. Hemoglobin infusion, which scavenges NO, also prevented acetylcholine-induced epicardial coronary dilation [63]. Although, the constrictor response to acetylcholine in atherosclerosis likely reflects loss of EDRF action, the possibility remains that acetylcholine also stimulates release of endothelium-derived constrictor substances or that loss of other endothelium-dependent dilators contributes to the observed coronary constriction [35,64].

Dilation in response to other stimuli for EDRF release is also impaired in patients with coronary atherosclerosis, including serotonin [65], substance P [66], and increased blood flow [67]. Loss of acetylcholine-mediated dilation occurs relatively early in the course of coronary artery disease, while impaired flow-mediated dilation and vasoconstrictor responses to complex stimuli, such as the cold pressor test, are manifested later in the disease process [58,61,68]. The response to acetylcholine infusion may be impaired in patients even prior to the development of intimal proliferation detected by intracoronary ultrasound in patients with hyperlipidemia and other risk factors [69]. Impairment of endothelium-dependent dilation of epicardial and coronary resistance vessels to acetylcholine infusion also has been reported in patients with hypertension [70,71], diabetes mellitus [72], cigarette smoking [73], and advancing age [74,75].

A number of studies convincingly suggest that impaired coronary endothelial vasomotor function contributes to the pathogenesis of clinical ischemia. In patients with coronary atherosclerosis, loss of endothelium-dependent dilation to acetylcholine correlated with an abnormal coronary constrictor response to exercise, the cold pressor test, and mental stress [15,68,76]. These complex, clinically relevant stimuli are normally associated with increased coronary blood flow as well as activation of the sympathetic nervous system with an increase in circulating catecholamines. In atherosclerotic vessels, endothelial dysfunction impairs flow-mediated dilation [67] and is associated with increased vasoconstriction to alpha-agonists [77]. Thus, coronary-constrictor responses during exercise and other stimuli for ischemia may reflect, in part, loss of endothelial vasodilator function.

Regarding unstable coronary syndromes, endothelial dysfunction in atherosclerotic coronary arteries may lead to more severe constriction in response to locally produced thrombin, serotonin, aggregating platelets, and other vasoconstrictors [7,8,78], and there is evidence that serotonin is released into the coronary circulation of patients with unstable angina [7]. Under those conditions, the antiplatelet effects of EDRF also would be lost. Okumura and colleagues recently demonstrated that acetyl-

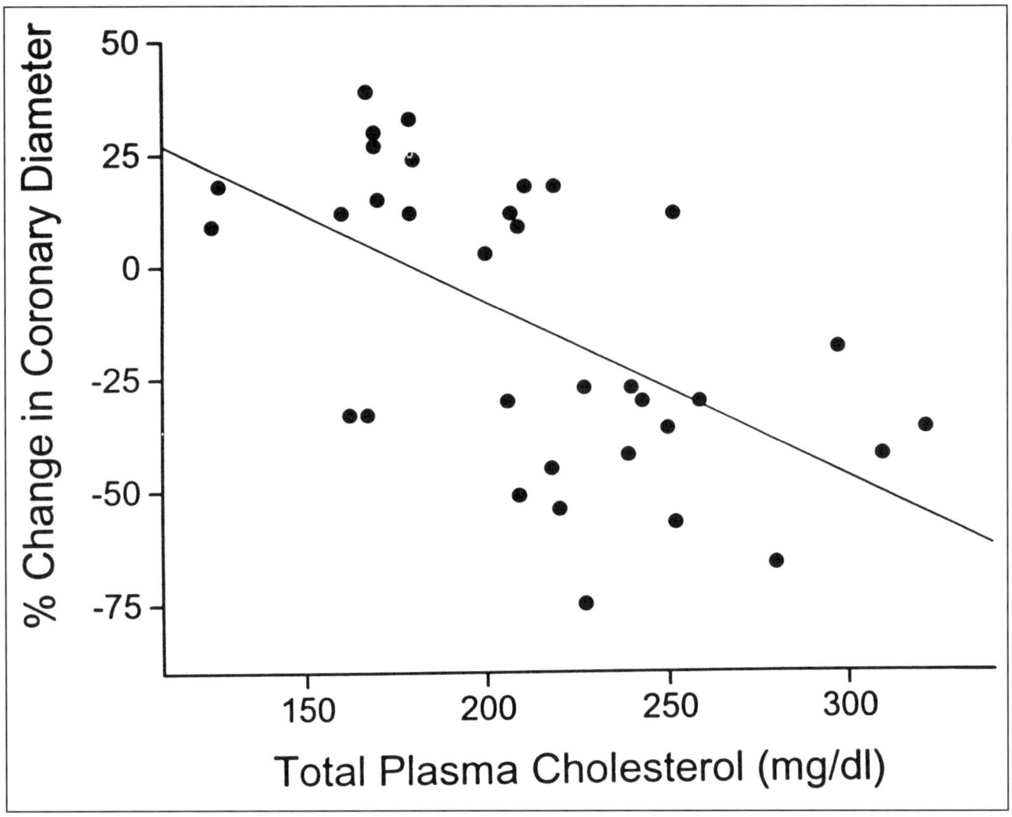

Fig. 9-1. Plasma cholesterol and coronary endothelial vasomotor function in humans. Displayed is a scatterplot of total plasma cholesterol and the vasomotor response to intracoronary acetylcholine infusion (final concentation 1 μM) expressed as percent change in coronary diameter from baseline in 34 subjects with angiographically normal coronary arteries. There is a highly significant relationship between total cholesterol and the acetylcholine response ($r = 0.58$, $p = 0.003$). (Adapted with permission from JA Vita et al. Coronary vasomotor response to acetylcholine relates to risk factors for coronary artery disease. Circulation 1990; 81:491–497.)

choline-induced constriction was significantly worse in infarct-related coronary arteries than in non-infarct-related arteries with equivalently severe stenoses [79]. Thus, impaired endothelial control of vasomotion appears to play important pathophysiologic roles in both stable and unstable coronary syndromes.

Although clinically relevant, the coronary circulation often is inaccessible for study in patients not requiring cardiac catheterization. For this reason, important information about the clinical expression of endothelial vasomotor dysfunction has been gained from examination of peripheral arteries. In the brachial circulation, intra-arterial methacholine or acetylcholine infusion produces dilation of resistance vessels and increased blood flow in normal patients. This response is impaired in patients with hypercholesterolemia [45] (Fig. 9-2), hypertension [80], and diabetes mellitus [81]. L-NMMA partially inhibited the forearm blood-flow response to acetylcholine, suggesting that EDRF synthesis contributes, at least in part to this response [82].

Recently, Creager and colleagues [83–85] and other investigators [86,87] developed a noninvasive method for assessment of flow-mediated dilation in the brachial artery using high-resolution duplex ultrasonography during hyperemic flow following cuff-occlusion of the limb (Fig. 9 3). Several investigators have recently confirmed that this response depends on NO synthesis using L-NMMA [88,89]. Using this methodology, impaired flow-mediated dilation has been demonstrated in patients with hypercholesterolemia, diabetes mellitus, and documented coronary atherosclerosisl [85,87,89,90]. In children with increased plasma LDL level as a result of heterozygous familial hypercholesterolemia and elevated lipoprotein(a), impaired dilation to flow in the femoral circulation was also demonstrated using this methodology [90]. A recent preliminary report suggests that noninvasive brachial responses correlate with the response of coronary arteries to acetylcholine infusion [84]. If that important finding is confirmed, this simple noninvasive technique may be useful for larger-scale screening of patients for evidence of coronary endothelial vasomotor dysfunction and for serial studies during interventions.

MECHANISMS OF IMPAIRED EDRF ACTION

A number of potential causes of endothelial dysfunction in atherosclerosis have been proposed, including inadequate EDRF production or release, excess degradation, altered end-organ sensitivity, or some combination of these effects. Recent studies suggest that a particularly important mechanism of impaired EDRF action in athero-

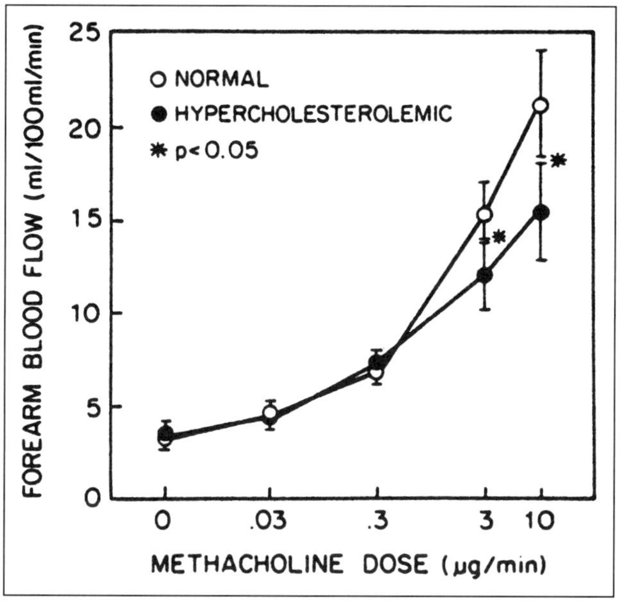

Fig. 9-2. Effect of hypercholesterolemia on forearm resistance vessel endoehtlial function. Dose response curves for forearm blood flow in response to methacholine infusion are displayed for a group of normal patients and a group of matched patients with hypercholesterolemia. Endothelium-dependent increases in blood flow are significantly impaired in patients with hypercholesterolemia. (Reproduced with permission from MA Creager et al. Impaired vasodilation of forearm resistance vessels in hypercholesterolemic humans. J Clin Invest 1990; 86:228–234.)

sclerosis is increased oxidative stress [91]. Increased production of reactive oxygen species and oxidative modification of LDL may lead to impaired EDRF action through several of these potential mechanisms.

A major source of oxidative stress in the vasculature is superoxide anion, which is produced by a number of enzymatic sources in vascular cells under physiological conditions [92]. Superoxide anion interferes with EDRF action by reacting with NO, thereby limiting its biologic activity [93–95]. In the setting of hypercholesterolemia, superoxide anion production in vascular tissue is markedly increased [96–99], and thus increased destruction of EDRF may be an important mechanism of endothelial vasodilator dysfunction in atherosclerosis. A recent study further demonstrated that dietary reduction of plasma cholesterol is associated with decreased superoxide anion production and improved endothelial function in cholesterol-fed rabbits [98]. In patients with coronary atherosclerosis, Levine and colleagues demonstrated that acute administration of ascorbic acid, a potent scavenger of superoxide anion, improves flow-mediated brachial dilation [100]. This finding supports the hypothesis that superoxide anion plays a pathophysiological role in impaired EDRF action in human atherosclerosis.

Superoxide anion and NO may react to form peroxynitrous acid, which may initiate lipid peroxidation [97] or serve as a source of cytotoxic hydroxyl radicals [102]. The potential importance of NO and superoxide anion interaction is further emphasized by observations that NO synthase is capable of superoxide generation when L-arginine concentration is limiting [103]. Superoxide anion may also undergo dismutation to H_2O_2, followed by reduction of H_2O_2 to the hydroxyl radical via the Fenton reaction. H_2O_2 may mediate endothelial cell injury [104] and impair EDRF production from cultured cells [105]. It also impairs relaxation to nitrovasodilators, including authentic NO, possibly through oxidation of intracellular thiols [105,106]. The hydroxyl radical may be involved in tissue damage resulting from reperfusion injury and inflammation [107] and may be present in atherosclerotic lesions [108]; however, the direct effects of hydroxyl radical in the action and metabolism of EDRF are relatively unknown.

According to the oxidative hypothesis of atherosclerosis, oxidative modification of LDL leads to foam-cell formation and is an important early event in atherogenesis [109]. In addition, the formation of oxidized LDL (ox-LDL) may interfere with EDRF action by a number of mechanisms. Ox-LDL leads to recruitment and retention of leukocytes in the vascular wall and subsequent release of reactive oxygen species that may degrade EDRF and further oxidize LDL [110–113]. In addition, ox-LDL has direct cytotoxic effects against endothelial cells [114]. Finally, ox-LDL impairs receptor-mediated release of EDRF [115] by a mechanism attributable to formation of lysophosphatidylcholine in the LDL particle [115–117]. Lysophosphatidylcholine appears to interfere with endothelial-cell-membrane signal transduction [118]. Such amphiphilic compounds are known to alter the activity of membrane enzymes, ligand-receptor coupling, transmembrane ion transport, and function of G proteins [44,119–121]. Recent studies suggest that lysophosphatidylcholine stimulates endothelial expression of the intercellular adhesion molecule-1 (ICAM-1) [122] and stimulates superoxide production [123], both via a mechanism dependent on activation of protein kinase C. The potential importance of lysophosphatidylcholine for endothelial dysfunction is further supported by the finding that its content is increased severalfold in atherosclerotic tissue [124].

Oxidative stress also appears to contribute to the mechanism of impaired EDRF action in other vascular disease states, including diabetes and hypertension. In isolated vessels exposed to elevated glucose and in vessels from animals rendered diabetic by exposure to alloxan, SOD and catalase restored endothelium-dependent relaxation to acetylcholine [125,126]. Deferoxamine, a chelator of iron and a hydroxyl-radical scavenger, and allopurinol, a xanthine oxidase inhibitor and free-radical scavenger, also prevented glucose-induced endothelial dysfunction [125]. In addition, vascular tissue isolated from animals consuming the lipid-soluble antioxidant probucol was resistant to the adverse effects of acute glucose exposure [125]. Endothelial dysfunction in diabetes is also prevented by cyclooxygenase inhibitors and the prostaglandin PGH_2 receptor blockade, and there is evidence that PGH_2 synthesis is coupled to superoxide production [127] and activation of protein kinase C [128,129]. Bucala and colleagues demonstrated that phospholipid and lipoprotein glycosylation promotes lipid peroxidation [130] and that gly-

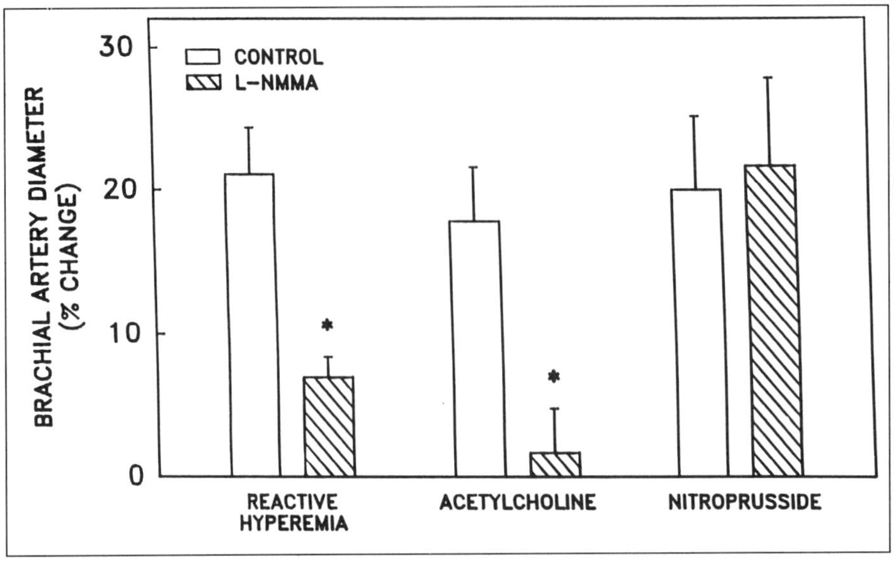

Fig. 9-3. Non-invasive assessment of endothelium-dependent vasodilation in the brachial artery. Using high resolution brachial ultrasound, brachial artery diameter was measured during reactive hyperemia, which induces NO release by increasing shear stress at the endothelial surface, during intra-arterial infusion of the endothelium-dependent vasodilator acetylcholine, and during infusion of the endothelium-independent vasodilator sodium nitroprusside. Vasodilator responses are expressed as percent change from baseline (± SEM). After infusion of the NO synthase antagonist, L-NMMA (hatched bars), the vasodilator response to hyperemia and acetylcholine was reduced, confirming the importance of NO synthesis in these responses. L-NMMA did not affect endothelium-independent vasodilation caused by nitroprusside. (Data provided by Mark A. Creager, M.D. and used with his permission.)

cosylation end-products impair endothelial vasomotor function [131]. In animal models of hypertension, superoxide production also has been implicated as a contributor to vascular dysfunction [132,133]. Thus, oxidative stress appears to contribute to the mechanisms of endothelial dysfunction in a number of clinically relevant vascular disease states.

Another proposed mechanism of endothelial dysfunction in atherosclerosis involves decreased availability of L-arginine, the substrate for EDRF synthesis. Studies in rabbits suggest that both acute and chronic administration of L-arginine improves endothelium-dependent dilation in cholesterol-fed animals [134,135]. In patients, acute intravenous administration of L-arginine improved the resistance-vessel vasodilator response to methacholine in the brachial circulation [136]. In the coronary circulation, intra-arterial L-arginine improved the resistance vessel but not the epicardial vasodilator responses to acetylcholine [60]. However, in a slightly older patient population, Casino and colleagues found that intra-arterial L-arginine had no effect on the impaired vasodilator effect of acetylcholine [137]. The mechanism of L-arginine's effect on endothelium-dependent vasodilation remains unclear. In both normal and hypercholesterolemic rabbits [134] and patients [136], plasma L-arginine concentrations exceed the K_m of endothelial NO synthase by approximately 30-fold [138], arguing against decreased substrate plasma availability as the primary defect in atherosclerosis.

Finally, increased production of vasoconstrictor substances may play a role in impaired vasodilator responses in atherosclerosis, diabetes, and hypertension. Circulating and coronary arterial tissue immunoreactive endothelin-1 was elevated in hypercholesterolemic swine, and, in addition, intracoronary acetylcholine infusion markedly increased systemic endothelin concentration, which correlated with the degree of coronary constriction [64]. Increased circulating endothelin concentration also has been demonstrated in the plasma of patients with advanced atherosclerosis [139]. Interestingly, ox-LDL stimulates endothelin release from cultured endothelial cells and intact swine aorta [140,141]. As already noted, diabetes mellitus is associated with increased release of endothelial-derived vasoconstrictor prostanoids [54,125]. Vasoconstrictor cyclooxygenase products also contribute to endothelial dysfunction in animal models of hypertension [35,53]. Thus, increased production of vasoconstrictor products coupled with decreased production or availability of vasodilator products may combine to promote vasoconstrictor responses in a number of clinically relevant disease states.

INTERVENTIONS TO IMPROVE ENDOTHELIAL VASOMOTOR FUNCTION

Lipid Lowering. It is now firmly established that cholesterol-lowering therapy reduces cardiovascular and total mortality in patients with coronary artery disease. A meta-analyses of 22 primary- and secondary-prevention trials indicated that for every 10-percent reduction in total plasma there was a 20-percent reduction in cardiovascular mortality [142]. Recently, a randomized, double-blind, placebo-controlled trial involving 4,444 patients with proven coronary disease demonstrated a 25-percent reduction in total plasma cholesterol and a 30-percent reduction in total mortality in patients with established coronary disease receiving simvastatin over a 5-year period [143]. Interestingly, the improvement in outcome was apparent after 1 to 2 years of therapy. Investigators have hypothesized that the beneficial effects of lipid-lowering therapy is the result of regression of atherosclerotic lesions, and a sizable number of angiographic regression trials have been completed to test this hypothesis [144]. Despite treatment with potent lipid-lowering agents and reductions of total and LDL cholesterol comparable to the mortality studies previously mentioned, serial angiography has demonstrated only modest effects on the angiographic severity of coronary lesions [144]. For example, in the Familial Atherosclerosis Treatment Study (FATS), treatment with lovastatin plus cholestyramine for 2.5 years reduced total cholesterol by 33.8 percent and reduced all cardiovascular events by 73 percent compared to placebo [145]. These effects were associated with only minimal changes in the average percent diameter stenosis of all atherosclerotic lesions: progression of lesion severity by 2.0 ± 3.7 percent for the control group and regression of lesion severity by 0.3 ± 5.0 percent in the lovastatin/cholestyramine group. These extremely modest effects on angiographic severity are unlikely to account for the profound reduction in event rate, particularly when one consideres that the coefficient of variation for percent stenosis in this study was 3.4 percent. In addition, the hypothesis that lesion regression explains the mortality benefits of lipid-lowering therapy is not supported by available data that fail to demonstrate a correlation between lesion severity and clinical ischemic syndromes [3,4].

Since lesion regression is an inadequate mechanistic explanation for the beneficial effects of lipid lowering, investigators have proposed a number of alternative explanations including reduced susceptibility to plaque rupture, and improved endothelial vasomotor function [144,146]. There is now strong evidence from animal and human studies that lipid-lowering therapy improves the vasodilator properties of the endothelium. In monkeys and rabbits rendered atherosclerotic by diet, reduction of dietary cholesterol is associated with improved endothelium-dependent relaxation [98,147]. In patients, Leung and colleagues demonstrated that a 28.7-percent reduction in total plasma cholesterol with cholestyramine was associated with marked improvement in epicardial endothelial vasomotor function over a six-month period as assessed by vasomotor responses to acetylcholine infusion (Fig. 9-4) [148]. Two recent, well-controlled trials have confirmed that lipid-lowering therapy with lovastatin for 6 to 12 months is associated with improved coronary endothelial function [149,150]. Restoration of the vasodilator and antithrombotic properties of the endothelium may explain, in part, the reduced event rate observed in patients on lipid-lowering therapy.

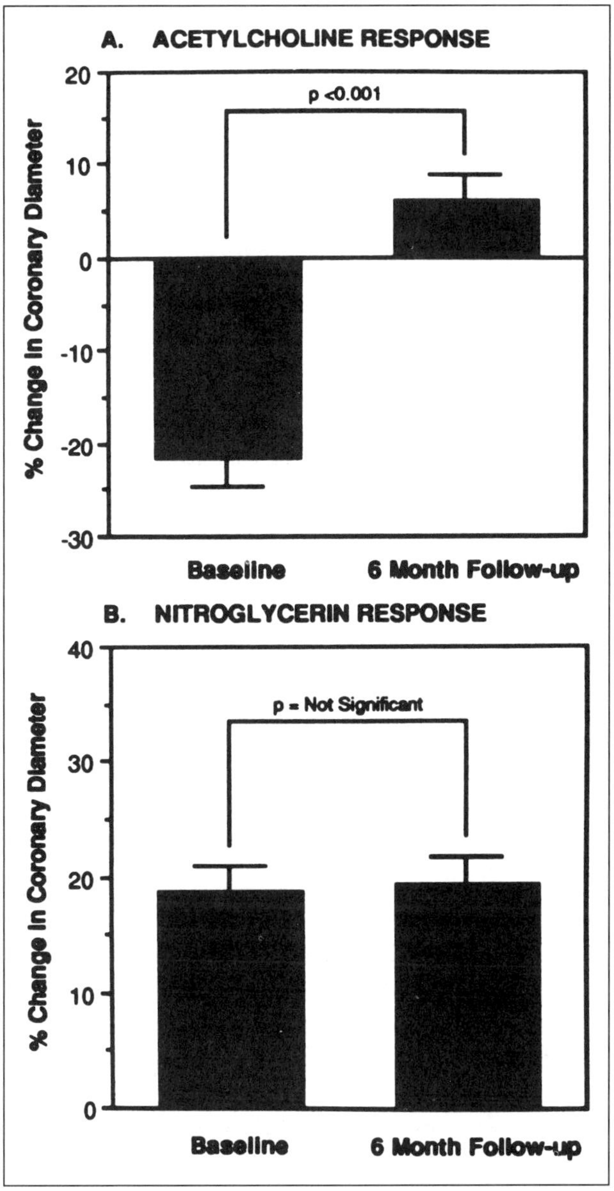

Fig. 9-4. Effect of cholesterol-lowering on coronary endothelial vasomotor function in patients. Plot demonstrating the coronary diameter response to intracoronary acetylcholine (A) and nitroglycerin (B) infusions before and after 6-month treatment with cholestyramine and cholesterol lowering diet in a group of patients with angiographically smooth coronary arteries. Reduction in total cholesterol (28.7%) was associated with a significant improvement in he vasomotor response to acetylcholine. (Reproduced with permission from WH Leung et al. Beneficial effect of cholesterol-lowering treatment on coronary endothelium-dependent relaxation in hypercholesterolemic patients. Lancet 1993; 341:1496–1500.)

Antioxidants. A similar argument may be made to explain the beneficial effects of antioxidants in coronary disease. There is considerable epidemiologic evidence that reducing oxidative stress with dietary lipid-soluble antioxidants reduces the clinical expression of coronary atherosclerosis. In the Health Professional Follow-up Study involving 39,910 men followed for four years, increasing dietary intake of vitamin E was independently associated with a lower risk of coronary artery disease (fatal coronary disease, nonfatal myocardial infarction, coronary bypass grafting, and coronary angioplasty) [151]. In that study, beta-carotene intake was inversely related to risk only in smokers, while higher vitamin-C intake was not associated with a reduced risk of coronary artery disease. Likewise, in the Nurses' Health study, the consumption of vitamin E supplements was associated with a 34-percent reduction in the risk of major coronary artery disease (fatal coronary disease or confirmed myocardial infarction) [152]. These dietary studies are supported by observations that plasma levels of vitamins A and E also inversely correlate with ischemic heart disease mortality [153].

In addition to primary prevention, there also is evidence that dietary lipid-soluble antioxidants may be beneficial for patients with established atherosclerosis. In a preliminary subgroup analysis of the Physicians' Health Study, Gaziano and colleagues reported that beta-carotene treatment reduced cardiovascular events by 51 percent in 333 male physicians with previously established coronary artery disease [154]. As was discussed previously for lipid-lowering therapy, investigators have also postulated that antioxidant therapy exerts its beneficial effects by limiting progression or inducing regression of established atherosclerotic lesions, but recent studies have failed to support this hypothesis. The Probucol Quantitative Regression Swedish Trial (PQRST) demonstrated that three years of probucol treatment had no effect on the severity of femoral atheroma [155]. Recently, Hodis and colleagues retrospectively examined the relationship between progression of coronary atherosclerosis nd antioxidant vitamin intake, assessed by dietary records, in patients enrolled in the Cholesterol Lowering Atherosclerosis Study (CLAS) [156]. They reported that average lesion severity progressed 2.0 percent in patients consuming less than 100 IU of vitamin E daily, but regressed 0.8 percent in patients with a higher vitamin E intake over the 2-year period of the randomized, lipid-lowering angiographic trial [156]. Although statistically significant, these modest effects on angiographic severity are unlikely to explain the mortality benefits in subjects with higher antioxidant intake.

The considerable evidence suggesting that increased oxidative stress may impair EDRF action naturally leads to the hypothesis that reducing vascular oxidative stress may improve endothelial function [91]. In animal models, dietary lipid-soluble antioxidants have markedly beneficial effects on endothelial vasomotor function. In rabbits, Keaney and colleagues demonstrated that consumption of a 1-percent cholesterol diet produced marked impairment of endothelium-dependent dilation, while supplementation of the 1-percent cholesterol diet with beta-carotene or alpha-tocopherol led to complete preservation of endothelium-dependent dilation in responses to acetylcholine and A23187 [157] (Fig. 9-5). In that model, preservation of endothelium-dependent dilation in atherosclerosis could not be explained by beneficial effects of antioxidants on the lipoprotein profile or the extent of atherosclerosis. Studies from that and other groups suggest that lipid-soluble antioxidants are concentrated in the vascular wall and limit LDL oxidation, limit superoxide production, and protect endothelial cells against the adverse effects of ox-LDL [99,158,159,160]. These effects of lipid-soluble antioxidants have the potential to restore the action of EDRF in the setting of atherosclerosis. Enhancement of the vasodilator and antiplatelet actions of EDRF may better explain the reduction in cardiovascular risk associated with increased intake of lipid-soluble antioxidants. Several large, randomized, placebo-controlled trials to prospectively test the effects of antioxidant therapy on cardiovascular events are currently ongoing.

Estrogen. Natural and replacement estrogens appear to have a protective effect against the development and clinical expression of atherosclerosis. Overall, women have a lower incidence of coronary artery disease than men; however, after natural or surgical menopause, atherosclerosis is accelerated [161]. Epidemiologic studies have demonstrated that estrogen replacement independently reduces the risk of cardiovascular events [162]. Replacement therapy also improves survival in women with established coronary atherosclerosis, suggesting that estrogens do more than limit atherogenesis [163]. In animal models, estrogens reduce the extent of atherosclerosis [164] and limit early steps in atherogenesis, including uptake of cholesteryl ester into the arterial wall [165]. Estrogen replacement raises plasma high-density lipoprotein (HDL) and lowers LDL [161]. However, multivariate analyses suggest that only 25 to 50 percent of the reduction in cardiovascular events in patients can be explained by these lipid effects [166]. Treatment of women with the partial estrogen antagonist tamoxifen also is associated with a reduction in cardiovascular events [167].

A number of studies suggest that estrogens influence regulation of vascular tone. In normocholesterolemic animals, 17β-estradiol enhances basal release of EDRF [168] and acetylcholine-mediated arterial relaxation [169]. Supraphysiologic 17β-estradiol concentrations attenuated the constrictor effects of endothelin and inhibited the constrictor responses to a direct calcium-channel agonist, suggesting an effect on calcium-channel function [170]. In pathologic states, estrogen also limits the development of endothelial dysfunction. In spontaneously hypertensive rats, estrogen lowered blood pressure and improved endothelium-dependent relaxation [171]. In atherosclerotic ovariectomized monkeys, Williams and colleagues demonstrated that chronic 17β-estradiol replacement abolished coronary artery constriction mediated by acetylcholine infusion, and there was an associated reduction in plasma cholesterol and coronary lesion extent [172]. In the same model, acute administration of 17β-estradiol also prevented acetylcholine-mediated coronary constriction [173]. Keaney and colleagues observed that estrogen replacement preserved endothelium-dependent relaxation in ovariectomized, cholesterol-fed miniature swine [174]. This protection of endothelial function was associated with protection of LDL against copper-mediated oxidation, suggesting that estrogens act, at least in part, through an antioxidant mechanism [174]. These findings are consistent with the known antioxidant properties of phenolic estrogens [175–177], including 17β-estradiol, and nonsteroidal estrogen analogues, such as tamoxifen [178].

In patients, estrogen status also appears to influence endothelial vasomotor function. Vita and colleagues demonstrated that female gender correlated with preservation of endothelium-dependent dilation to acetylcholine [58]. Lieberman and colleagues demonstrated that chronic es-

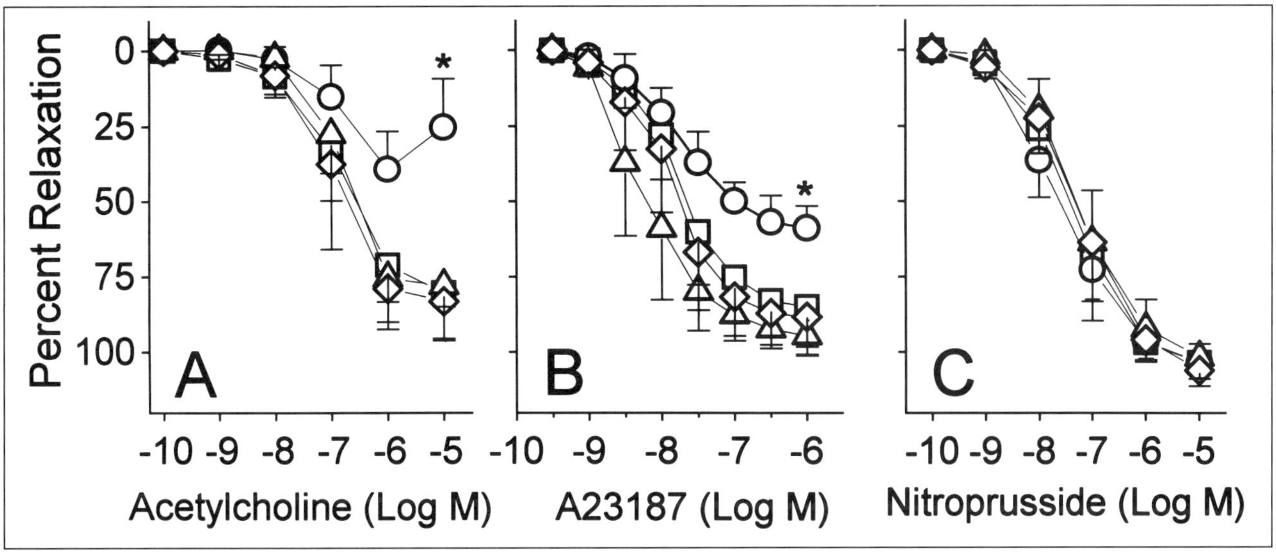

Fig. 9-5. Plot demonstrating the effect of dietary alpha-tocopherol and beta-carotene on endothelium-dependent arterial relaxation in cholesterol-fed rabbits. Aortic rings from rabbits fed chow (△), 1% cholesterol (○), 1% cholesterol with beta-carotene (□), and 1% cholesterol with alpha-tocopherol (◇) were exposed to increasing concentrations of acetylcholine (A), calcium ionophore A23187 (B), or sodium nitroprusside (C). These lipid-soluble antioxidants completely preserved endothelium-dependent dilation in the setting of hypercholesterolemia. (Reproduced with permission from JF Keaney Jr. et al. Dietary antioxidants preserve endothelium-dependent vessel relaxation in cholesterol-fed rabbits. Proc Natl Acad Sci USA 1993; 90:11880–11884.)

trogen administration in postmenopausal women improved flow-mediated dilation in the brachial artery [84]. In support of the hypothesis that estrogen exerts its protective effects on the endothelium through antioxidant mechanisms, Sack and colleagues recently demonstrated that LDL isolated from postmenopausal women receiving estrogen replacement was more resistant to copper-mediated oxidation than LDL isolated during a control period [179]. Relevant to the known effects of estrogens on the relaxation of vascular smooth muscle, acute administration of 17β-estradiol had direct vasodilator effects and blocked acetylcholine-mediated vasoconstriction in conduit and resistance vessels of postmenopausal women with endothelial dysfunction at baseline [180].

The observed improvement in endothelial vasomotor function with estrogen treatment provides a mechanistic explanation for the observed protective effects of intact ovarian function and estrogen replacement in postmenopausal women in regard to cardiovascular events. There are contradictory data regarding the effects of estrogen-containing oral contraceptives on cardiovascular mortality in both women and men [161]. Previously reported adverse effects of oral contraceptives may reflect, in part, the relatively high estrogen and the progestin content of older contraceptive preparations and also may reflect the interaction of other risk factors such as age and smoking history. Moreover, morbidity and mortality associated with oral-contraceptive use appears to be a consequence of thromboembolism rather than atherosclerosis or endothelial function per se [181].

Exercise. Although the cardiovascular adaptation to chronic exercise is multifactorial, one potentially important consequence of exercise training is improvement of endothelium-dependent arterial dilation. In chronically instrumented dogs, Wang and colleagues demonstrated improved endothelium-dependent epicardial coronary dilator responses to acetylcholine and increased blood flow following 7 days of daily treadmill exercise, an effect that was inhibited by L-NMMA [182]. Such an effect also has been demonstrated in coronary resistance vessels of normocholesterolemic swine after 16 to 20 weeks of treadmill exercise [183]. This effect has been postulated to result in part from chronic alterations in local blood flow. In addition to the acute effects of shear stress on release of EDRF described above [22,25,26], Miller and colleagues demonstrated enhanced endothelium-dependent dilation in vessels chronically exposed to increased blood flow in the setting of an arteriovenous anastomosis [184]. Recently, Sessa and colleagues demonstrated increased acetylcholine-stimulated nitrite production in coronary epicardial and resistance vessels in dogs after 10 days of regular treadmill exercise, reflecting increased NO synthesis [185]. In that model, exercise also was associated with enhanced aortic endothelial *Nos 3* gene expression [185]. The effect of exercise training on arterial endothelium-dependent has not been examined in patients, but such an effect could contribute to the beneficial effects of exercise on blood pressure and cardiovascular outcome [186].

Endothelial Control of Fibrinolysis and Thrombosis

In addition to regulating vascular tone, the endothelium participates in the regulation of fibrinolysis through the release of several factors, including tissue-type plasminogen activator (t-PA) and plasminogen activator inhibitor-1 (PAI-1). t-PA is a 72-kD serine protease that is synthesized and secreted basally by endothelial cells, which appear to be the only source of circulating t-PA [187]. Control of t-PA release is poorly understood, although in patients, circulating levels increase in response to venous occlusion [188], physical exercise [189], and infusion of 1-desamino-8-D-arginine (dDAVP) [190]. In tissue culture, thrombin [191], activated protein C [192], histamine [193], and shear stress [194] stimulate t-PA production. Forskolin, which induces an increase in cAMP, decreases synthesis of t-PA in endothelial cells [195]. Endothelial cells express t-PA receptors that serve to localize plasminogen activation to the endothelial surface and enhance local antithrombotic effects [196].

PAI-1, a 52-kD glycoprotein, is synthesized by endothelial cells [197] as well as by platelets [198] and placental tissue [199]. PAI-1 is the most important inhibitor of t-PA in plasma [200]. Its synthesis is regulated by a number of relevant factors, including endotoxin [201], interleukin-1 [202] and other inflammatory cytokines [203–205], phorbol esters [206], lipoproteins [207,208], thrombin [209], and angiotensin II [210].

The vascular endothelium also participates in control of thrombosis through the synthesis of von Willebrand factor (vWF), which is the polymeric glycoprotein that carries factor VIII in plasma. vWF mediates platelet adhesion to injured surfaces in vessels [211] and incorporation of platelets into evolving platelet-fibrin thrombi [212]. Additional, anticoagulant functions of endothelial cells include production of heparan sulfate proteoglycans [213] and acceleration of protein-C activation through the action of the endothelial-cell surface receptor thrombomodulin on thrombin's substrate specificity [214]. Finally, as described above, the vascular endothelium regulates platelet aggregation and activity through the action of EDRF, prostacyclin, or both. Like other nitrovasodilators, EDRF impairs platelet activity as assessed in vitro using aggregometry [215–217] and in the model of acute coronary ischemia developed by Folts [218]. Thus, factors that impair EDRF vasodilator activity may also lead to increased platelet activity; conversely, interventions that improve EDRF vasodilator action may also favorably affect platelet activity and have the potential to decrease myocardial ischemia in patients with coronary artery disease.

ENDOTHELIAL REGULATION OF FIBRINOLYSIS IN ATHEROSCLEROSIS

Endothelial control of fibrinolysis is altered in hypercholesterolemia and atherosclerosis, and this impairment may have an effect on the clinical expression of coronary artery disease. Increased circulating levels of t-PA antigen were strongly associated with increased risk for myocardial infarction [219] in apparently healthy males enrolled in the Physicians' Health Study (Fig. 9-6). In a smaller group of patients with angina and documented coronary artery disease, t-PA antigen also predicted cardiovascular events [220]. Plasma level of t-PA antigen has been shown to correlate with reduced HDL concentration and possibly with total cholesterol [219,221,222]. When other coronary risk factors, including decreased HDL, are taken into account, the predictive value of elevated t-PA antigen for coronary events was lost [221,223]. However, t-PA antigen was an independent predictor of stroke in the Physician's Health Study, even after controlling for lipoprotein profile and other coronary risk factors [223]. To explain the unexpected finding that an apparent increase in fibrinolytic capacity was associated with an increase in thrombotic events, Ridker and colleagues suggested that there is a generalized activation of the fibrinolytic system in the presence of atherosclerosis. They argued that progressive or active atherosclerosis "triggers a range of reactive mechanisms," including the fibrinolytic system, and that increased t-PA antigen is a "result rather than a cause" of active coronary disease [219]. Increased t-PA antigen previously has been reported to correlate with other acute-phase proteins, including fibrinogen and C-reactive protein, in patients with coronary disease [224].

More consistent with an increased tendency for intracoronary thrombosis in atherosclerosis is the finding that PAI level and activity are also increased in patients with coronary artery disease. In young survivors of myocardial infarction, Hamsten and colleagues found decreased t-PA activity at baseline and following the stress of venous occlusion, and they demonstrated that these findings were explained in large part by increased PAI-1 activity [225] (Fig. 9-7). In a subsequent report, these investigators demonstrated that increased plasma PAI was an independent risk factor for recurrent myocardial infarction [226]. Several other investigators have reported increased t-PA antigen level with decreased t-PA activity and increased PAI activity in patients with coronary artery disease [227–229] and diabetes [230]. Increased PAI-1 activity and decreased fibrinolytic activity of plasma also have been consistently shown to correlate with elevated plasma triglyceride levels [220,225,227,229] and with elevated plasma insulin concentrations [224]. However, the precise relationship among triglycerides, insulin, and PAI-1 release remains undefined. Cultured human endothelial cells exposed to LDL cholesterol demonstrate a prothrombotic phenotype with increased secretion of PAI-1 [207]. Relevant to the effects of ox-LDL on endothelial function, Weis and colleagues observed that ox-LDL increased human endothelial cell tissue-factor activity and reduced activation of protein C [230]. Kugiyama and colleagues demonstrated that ox-LDL and lysophosphatidylcholine also stimulated PAI-1 and inhibited t-PA release from endothelial cells [231]. Thus, hypercholesterolemia and atherosclerosis are associated with an alteration in the fibrinolytic and antithrombotic functions of the endothelium that could contribute to the clinical expression of coronary artery disease.

Recently, Vaughan and colleagues demonstrated that the vascular renin-angiotensin system influences endothelial control of fibrinolysis. Angiotensin II induces release of PAI-1 from cultured endothelial cells [210] and increases circulating levels of PAI-1 in patients [232]. Two clinical trials that examined the effects of angiotensin converting enzyme (ACE) inhibitors on outcome in patients with left ventricular dysfunction following myocardial infarction demonstrated that treatment with those agents

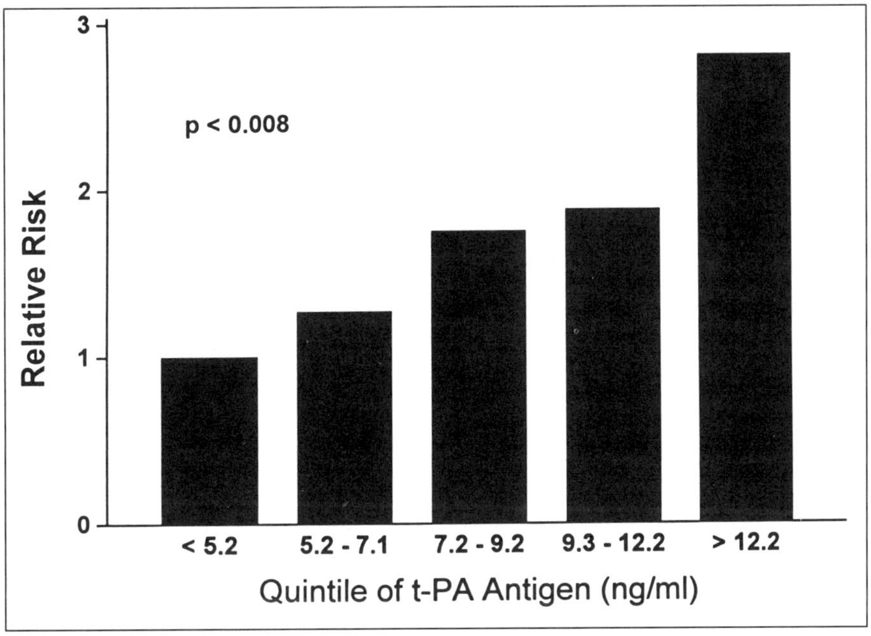

Fig. 9-6. Plot demonstrating the relative risk for myocardial infarction by quintile of t-PA antigen concentration in a cohort of patients enrolled in the Physician's Health Study. Increased t-PA antigen concentration was associated with a significant increase in risk for myocardial infarction. (Adapted with permission from PM Ridker, et al. Endogenous tissue-type plasminogen activator and risk of myocardial infarction. Lancet 1993; 341:1165–1168.)

also reduced recurrent myocardial infarction [233,234]. Vaughan and colleagues hypothesized that ACE inhibitors may reduce coronary thrombosis by reducing angiotensin II formation and, thus, reducing PAI-1 release [232]. Further support for that hypothesis is provided by the observation that hypertensive patients with increased plasma renin concentrations, and presumably increased angiotensin II concentrations, have an increased risk of myocardial infarction compared to hypertensive patients with normal or low plasma renin profile [235]. ACE inhibitors also inhibit bradykinin degradation [236], and by this mechanism, they have the potential to increase EDRF and prostacyclin release. Those effects could potentially reduce ischemic events through favorable effects on platelet activation and vasomotion in the coronary circulation.

Several studies indicate links between atherosclerosis and other endothelium-dependent regulators of thrombosis. In swine, deficiency of vWF is associated with a reduction in susceptibility to atherosclerosis [237,238]. However, a direct effect of atherosclerosis to alter endothelial control of thrombosis through vWF or heparan production has not been demonstrated. It is possible that decreased heparan production or a shift in total vWF production or multimer distribution could also contribute to an increased propensity for vascular thrombosis in atherosclerosis. Such an increase in vWF production has been demonstrated in the setting of diabetes [239]. In hyperhomocyst(e)inemia, a disorder characterized by endothelial damage, arterial thrombosis, and increased risk of coronary atherosclerosis, impaired endothelial thrombomodulin expression may contribute to the prothrombotic diathesis [240]. This disorder is also associated with impaired EDRF action, which could contribute to increased thrombosis through a loss of EDRF's antiplatelet and vasodilator effects [241].

Endothelial Control of Intimal Growth and Atherogenesis

The vascular endothelium is an important regulator of cell growth in the vascular wall, and a number of endothelial products may promote or inhibit proliferation of vascular smooth muscle cells. Mechanical removal of the endothelium is followed by proliferation of the intima [242,243]. The endothelial layer is regrown following denudation, but the regenerated endothelial layer demonstrates impaired EDRF action for weeks to months following injury [244,245]. Weidinger and colleagues demonstrated that the extent of intimal proliferation following femoral balloon injury in hypercholesterolemic rabbits correlates inversely with the degree of relaxation to acetylcholine, suggesting that the release of EDRF or other endothelium-dependent vasodilators could contribute to suppression of intimal growth [245]. NO-generating vasodilators and a prostacyclin analog inhibit smooth muscle-cell proliferation in culture [246,247]. Marks and colleagues recently demonstrated that local administration of a stable NO adduct, S-nitrosoalbumin, limited platelet adhesion and prevented smooth muscle proliferation in rabbit femoral arteries following endothelial denudation (Fig. 9-8) [248]. EDRF/NO may secondarily inhibit intimal growth by inhibiting platelet and leukocyte adhesion to the vascular wall and subsequent release of growth factors, including platelet-derived growth factor (PDGF) and epidermal growth factor [39,249].

In addition to release of EDRF/NO, the endothelium may also inhibit growth of vascular smooth muscle

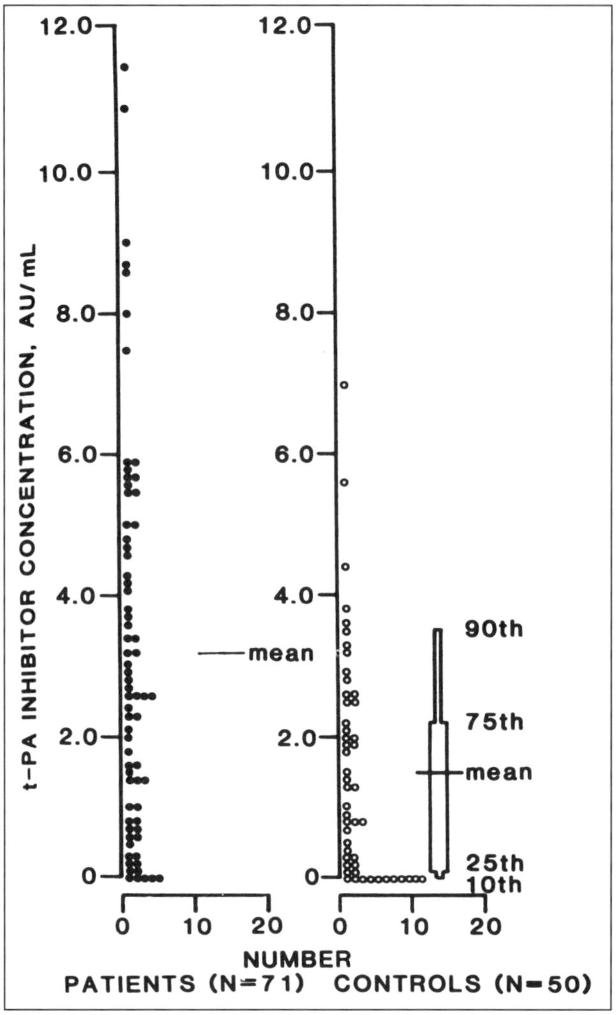

Fig. 9-7. Plot demonstrating the distribution of t-PA inhibitor (PAI) concentration in plasma from young survivors of myocardial infarction compared to matched controls. PAI concentrations were significantly higher in patients with myocardial infarction than in the controls. (Reproduced with permission from A Hamsten, et al. Increased plasma levels of a rapid inhibitor of tissue plasminogen activator in young survivors of myocardial infarction. N Engl J Med 1985; 313:1557–1563.)

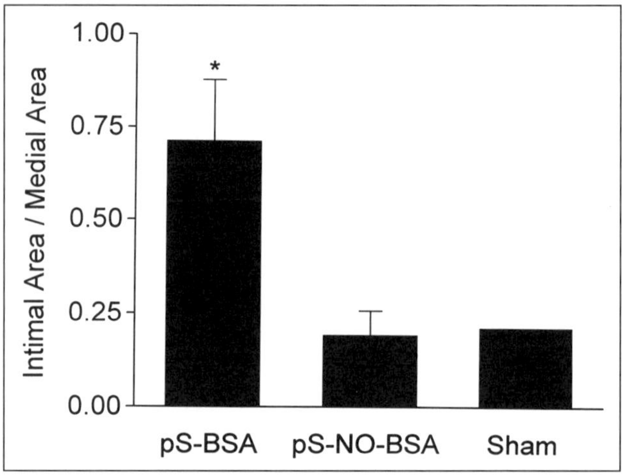

Fig. 9-8. Plot demonstrating femoral-artery intima to media ratio 2 weeks following balloon injury according to treatment with poly-S-nitroso-albumin or polythiolated albumin control. Treatment with this unique adduct of NO markedly inhibited smooth muscle proliferation following balloon injury. (Adapted with permission from DM Marks, et al. Complete inhibition of neointimal hyperplasia following vascular injury by a unique adduct of nitric oxide. J Clin Invest. In press.)

through expression of heparan sulfate proteoglycans [250]. Conversely, vasoconstrictor endothelial products, including endothelin and angiotensin II, may act to promote smooth muscle-cell growth [251]. The endothelium also elaborates a number of other growth-promoting factors, including PDGF, basic fibroblast growth factor (bFGF), insulinlike growth factor (IGF), and other cytokines [252–254]. Transforming growth factor beta (TGF-β), also released by endothelial cells, has antimitogenic properties [252–254]. One may speculate about other potential antiproliferative effects of NO, including (1) inhibition of ribonuclease reductase [255], (2) impairment of electron transport in mitochondria, (3) inhibition of anaerobic glycolysis through an effect on glyceraldehyde-3-phosphate dehydrogenase (GAPDH) ribosylation [256], and (4) apoptosis.

EDRF/NO elaboration appears to influence the development of spontaneous atherosclerotic lesions in the setting of cholesterol feeding. There is evidence that NO inhibits oxidative modification of LDL and subsequent foam-cell formation [257]. Cooke and colleagues demonstrated that chronic treatment of cholesterol-fed rabbits with the EDRF precursor L-arginine limited the development of endothelial vasomotor dysfunction and decreased the extent of atherosclerosis in the thoracic aorta and coronary arteries [258]. L-arginine treatment also inhibited in vitro endothelial binding of monocytes to aortae from cholesterol-fed rabbits, and L-NMMA increased monocyte binding in the same model [259]. Administration of another NO synthase inhibitor, nitro-L-arginine-methyl ester (L-NAME), at a dose that did not increase blood pressure, worsened lesion formation and inhibited endothelium-dependent relaxation in cholesterol-fed rabbits [260]. Thus, the action of EDRF inhibits key events in the atherogenic process,and loss of EDRF action promotes atherogenesis.

Under conditions of hypercholesterolemia, the endothelium also expresses leukocyte adhesion molecules that promote atherogenic process by contributing to the recruitment of monocytes into the vascular wall [111]. Lysophosphatidylcholine-stimulated expression of ICAM-1 in culture human and rabbit endothelial cells [261], and lysophosphatidylcholine- and ox-LDL-stimulated ICAM-1 expression, increased leukocyte adhesiveness and impaired endothelium-dependent relaxation in procine coronary arteries [122]. Expression of adhesion molecules in advanced atherosclerotic plaques leading to increased monocyte recruitement has also been proposed as a mechanism of increased vulnerability to plaque rupture and, thus, clinical expression of the disease [262]. Altered function of the endothelium, therefore, contributes to atherosclerosis by multiple mechanisms and in both eary and late stages of the disease process.

Summary

There is substantial evidence to support the idea that endothelial dysfunction is an important mechanism in the clinical expression of coronary artery disease and possibly the pathogenesis of atherosclerosis. Loss of EDRF action and the effects of other endothelium-derived vasodilators may contribute to the production of myocardial ischemia by promoting vasospasm and platelet activation in atherosclerotic coronary arteries. A shift in the production of t-PA and PAI-1 has the potential to promote coronary thrombosis and the development of myocardial infarction or unstable angina. The mechanisms of the effects of hypercholesterolemia and atherosclerosis on endothelial function remain controversial, but there is convincing evidence supporting the hypothesis that an increase in oxidative stress in the vasculature plays an important role. Increased production of reactive oxygen species, including superoxide anion, may inactive EDRF/NO or promote the formation of other reactive species. Oxidative modification of LDL may lead to impaired release of EDRF in part through the effects of lysophosphatidylcholine on endothelial membrane receptor and G-protein function. Ox-LDL also promotes the accumulation of leukocytes in the vascular wall and additional production of reactive oxygen species. Studies demonstrating the importance of vasoconstrictor endothelial products and L-arginine supplementation serve to emphasize the multifactorial nature of endothelial dysfunction in atherosclerosis.

Several modalities have the potential to improve endothelial vasomotor function in atherosclerosis, including lipid lowering, antioxidant supplementation, estrogen replacement in postmenopausal women, and exercise. In fact, the effects of some of these interventions on endothelial vasomotor and antithrombotic function may provide a better explanation for improved patient outcome than a simple slowing of lesion progression or reversal of stenosis severity. Similarly, endothelial effects, such as reduced PAI-1 expression and decreased bradykinin metabolism, may contribute to the beneficial effects of ACE inhibitors on cardiovascular events. There is a paucity of studies that examine different aspects of endothelial-cell function in parallel. Thus, it is unknown, for example, whether or not increased PAI-1 expression and impaired EDRF release occur independently in atherosclerosis. The finding that lysophosphatidylcholine-mediated impairment of EDRF release and promotion of PAI-1 expression may both depend on activation of protein kinase C suggests that those pathologic abnormalities of endothelial function may, in fact, be linked. Similarly, it remains unknown whether interventions that improve endothelial vasomotor function also favorably influence endothelial control of fibrinolysis or intimal growth.

Although coronary atherosclerosis is a well-studied example of the importance of endothelial dysfunction in vascular disease, it is also apparent that abnormalities of endothelial function contribute importantly to the pathophysiology of a number of other vascular disease states. We have touched on some common mechanisms in related conditions, including diabetes mellitus and hypertension. Investigation of the mechanism and means to reverse endothelial dysfunction in those and other conditions may prove a fruitful strategy for the development of new approaches to therapy and better patient management.

References

1. Mendelsohn ME, Loscalzo J. The Endotheliopathies. In J Loscalzo, MA Creager, VJ Dzau, eds. Vascular Medicine. Boston: Little, Brown,, 1992. Pp. 279–306.
2. Proudfit WJ, et al. Fifteen year survival study of patients with obstructive coronary artery disease. Circulation 1983; 68:986–997.
3. Ambrose JA, et al. Angiographic progression of coronary artery disease and the development of myocardial infarction. J Am Coll Cardiol 1988; 12:56–62.
4. Folland ED, et al. Relation between coronary artery stenosis assessed by visual, caliper, and computer methods and exercise capacity in patients with single vessel coronary artery disease. Circulation 1994; 89:2005–2014.
5. Richardson PD, Davies MJ, Born GV. Influence of plaque configuration and stress distribution on fissuring of coronary atherosclerotic plaques. Lancet 1989; 2:941–944.
6. Fuster V, et al. The pathogenesis of coronary artery disease and the acute coronary syndromes. N Engl J Med 1992; 326:310–318.
7. van den Berg E, et al. Transcardiac serotonin concentration is increased in selected patients with limiting angina and complex coronary lesion morphology. Circulation 1989; 79:116–124.
8. Willerson JT, et al. Specific platelet mediators and unstable coronary artery lesions. Experimental evidence and potential clinical implications. Circulation 1989; 80:198–205.
9. Brown GB, et al. Incomplete lysis of thrombus in the moderate underlying atherosclerotic lesion during intracoronary infusion of streptokinase for acute myocardial infarction: Quantitative angiographic observations. Circulation 1986; 73:653–661.
10. Jackett D, Davies G, Maseri A. Pre-existing coronary stenoses in patients with first myocardial infaction are not necessarily severe. Eur Heart J 1988; 8:1172–1181.
11. Ambrose JA, et al. Angiographic morphology and the pathogenesis of unstable angina pectoris. J Am Coll Cardiol 1985; 5:609–616.
12. Gage JE, et al. Vasoconstriction of stenotic coronary arteries during dynamic exercise in patients with classic angina pectoris: reversibility by nitroglycerin. Circulation 1986; 73:865–876.
13. Nabel EG, et al. Dilation of normal and constriction of atherosclerotic coronary arteries caused by the cold pressor test. Circulation 1988; 77:43–52.
14. Nabel EG, Selwyn AP, Ganz P. Paradoxical narrowing of atherosclerotic coronary arteries induced by increases in heart rate. Circulation 1990; 81:850–859.
15. Yeung AC, et al. The effect of atherosclerosis on the vasomotor response of coronary arteries to mental stress. N Engl J Med 1991; 325:1551–1556.
16. Furchgott RF, Zawadzki JV. The obligatory role of endothelial cells in the relaxation of arterial smooth muscle by acetylcholine. Nature 1980; 288:373–376.
17. Ignarro LJ, et al. Endothelium-derived relaxing factor produced and released from artery and vein is nitric oxide. Proc Natl Acad Sci USA 1987; 84:9265–9269.

18. Stamler JS, Singel DJ, Loscalzo J. Biochemistry of nitric oxide and its redox-activated forms. Science 1992; 258:1898–1902.
19. Palmer RM, Ashton DS, Moncada S. Vascular endothelial cells synthesize nitric oxide from L-arginine. Nature 1988; 333:664–666.
20. Ignarro LJ, et al. Association between cyclic GMP accumulation and acetylcholine-elicited relaxation of bovine intrapulmonary artery. J Pharmacol Exp Ther 1984; 228:682–690.
21. Furchgott R. Role of endothelium in responses of vascular smooth muscle. Circ Res 1983; 35:557–573.
22. Rubanyi GM, Romero JC, Vanhoutte PM. Flow-induced release of endothelium-derived relaxing factor. Am J Physiol 1986; 250:H1145–H1149.
23. Olesen SP, Clapham DE, Davies PF. Haemodynamic shear stress activates a K+ current in vascular endothelial cells. Nature 1988; 331:168–170.
24. Pohl U, Lamontagne D. Impaired tissue perfusion after inhibition of endothelium-derived nitric oxide. Basic Res Cardiol 1991; 86[Suppl 2]:97–105.
25. Cooke JP, et al. Flow stimulates endothelial cells to release nitrovasodilator that is potentiated by reduced thiol. Am J Physiol 1990; 259:H804–H812.
26. Cooke JP, et al. Flow activates an endothelial potassium channel to release endogenous nitrovasodilator. J Clin Invest 1991; 88:1663–1671.
27. Oates JA, et al. Clinical implications of prostaglandin and thromboxane A2 formation. N Engl J Med 1988; 319:689–698.
28. Chen G, Suzuki H, Weston AH. Acetylcholine releases endothelium-derived hyperpolarizing factor and EDRF from rat blood vessels. Br J Pharmacol 1988; 95:1165–1174.
29. Cowan CL, et al. Potassium channel-mediated relaxation to acetylcholine in rabbit arteries. J Pharmacol Exp Ther 1993; 266:1482–1489.
30. Radomski MW, Palmer RMH, Moncada S. The anti-aggregating properties of vascular endothelium: interactions between prostacylin and nitric oxide. Br J Pharmacol 1987; 92:639–646.
31. Shimokawa H, et al. Prostacyclin releases endothelium-derived relaxing factor and potentiates its action in coronary arteries of the pig. Br J Pharmacol 1988; 95:1197–1203.
32. Salvemini D, et al. Nitric oxide activates cyclooxygenase enzymes. Proc Natl Acad Sci USA 1993; 90:7240–7244.
33. Yanagisawa M, et al. A novel potent vasoconstrictor peptide produced by vascular endothelial cells. Nature 1988; 332:411–415.
34. Miller VM, Vanhoutte PM. Endothelium-dependent contractions to arachidonic acid are mediated by products of cyclooxygenase. Am J Physiol 1985; 248:H432–H437.
35. Luscher TF, Vanhoutte PM. Endothelium-dependent contractions to acetylcholine in the aorta of the spontaneously hypertensive rat. Hypertension 1986; 8:344–348.
36. Bossaller C, et al. Impaired muscarinic endothelium-dependent relaxation and cyclic guanosine 5′-monophosphate formation in atherosclerotic human coronary artery and rabbit aorta. J Clin Invest 1987; 79:170–174.
37. Forstermann U, et al. Selective attenuation of endothelium-mediated vasodilation in atherosclerotic human coronary arteries. Circ Res 1988; 62:185–190.
38. Cohen RA, et al. Loss of selective endothelial cell vasoactive functions caused by hypercholesterolemia in pig coronary arteries. Circ Res 1988; 63:903–910.
39. Shimokawa H, Vanhoutte PM. Impaired endothelium-dependent relaxation to aggregating platelets and related vasoactive substances in porcine coronary arteries in hypercholesterolemia and atherosclerosis. Circ Res 1989; 64:900–914.
40. Freiman PC, et al. Atherosclerosis impairs endothelium-dependent vascular relaxation to acetylcholine and thrombin in primates. Circ Res 1986; 58:783–790.
41. Heistad DD, et al. Augmented responses to vasoconstrictor stimuli in hypercholesterolemic and atherosclerotic monkeys. Circ Res 1984; 54:711–780.
42. Sellke FW, Armstrong ML, Harrison DG. Endothelium-dependent vascular relaxation is abnormal in the coronary microcirculation of atherosclerotic primates. Circulation 1990; 81:1586–1593.
43. Shimokawa H, Flavahan NA, Vanhoutte PM. Loss of endothelial pertussis toxin-sensitive G-protein function in atherosclerotic porcine coronary arteries. Circulation 1991; 83:652–660.
44. Flavahan NA. Atherosclerosis or lipoprotein-induced endothelial dysfunction: potential mechanisms underlying reduction in EDRF/nitric oxide activity. Circulation 1992; 85:1927–1938.
45. Creager MA, et al. Impaired vasodilation of forearm resistance vessels in hypercholesterolemic humans. J Clin Invest 1990; 86:228–234.
46. Schmidt K, Klatt P, Mayer B. Hypercholesterolemia is associated with a reduced response of smooth muscle guanylyl cyclase to nitrovasodilators. Arteriosclerosis and Thromb 1993; 13:1159–1163.
47. Schmidt K, et al. Activation of soluble guanylate cyclase by nitrovasodilators is inhibited by oxidized low-density lipoprotein. Biochem Biophys Res Commun 1990; 172: 614–619.
48. Luscher TF, Raij L, Vanhoutte PM. Endothelium-dependent vascular responses in normotensive and hypertensive Dahl rats. Hypertension 1987; 9:157–163.
49. Wright CE, Angus JA. Effects of hypertension and hypercholesterolemia on vasodilation in the rabbit. Hypertension 1986; 8:361–371.
50. Dohi Y, et al. Activation of endothelial L-arginine pathway in resistance arteries: Effects of age and hypertension. Hypertension 1990; 16:170–179.
51. Clozel M, Kuhn H, Hefti F. Effects of angiotensin converting enzyme inhibitors and of hydralazine on endothelial function in hypertensive rats. Hypertension 1990; 16:532–540.
52. Panza JA, et al. Effect of antihypertensive treatment on endothelium-dependent vascular relaxation in patients with essential hypertension. J Am Coll Cardiol 1993; 21:1145–1151.
53. Diederich D, et al. Impaired endothelium-dependent relaxations in hypertensive resistance arteries involve cyclooxygenase pathway. Am J Physiol 1990; 258:H445–H451.
54. Tesfamariam B, et al. Elevated glucose promotes generation of endothelium-derived vasoconstrictor prostanoids in rabbit aorta. J Clin Invest 1990; 85:929–932.
55. Tesfamariam B, Jakubowski JA, Cohen RA. Contraction of diabetic rabbit aorta due to endothelium-derived PGH2/TXA2. Am J Physiol 1989; 257:H1327–H1333.
56. Oyama Y, et al. Attenuation of endothelium-dependent relaxation in aorta from diabetic rats. Eur J Pharmacol 1986; 132:75–78.
57. Ludmer PL, et al. Paradoxical vasoconstriction induced by acetylcholine in atherosclerotic coronary arteries. N Engl J Med 1986; 315:1046–1051.
58. Vita JA, et al. Coronary vasomotor response to acetylcholine relates to risk factors for coronary artery disease. Circulation 1990; 81:491–497.
59. Werns SW, et al. Evidence of endothelial dysfunction in angiographically normal coronary arteries of patients with coronary artery disease. Circulation 1989; 79:287–291.
60. Drexler H, et al. Correction of endothelial dysfunction in coronary microcirculation of hypercholesterolemic patients by l-arginine. Lancet 1991; 338:1546–1550.

61. Egashira K, et al. Impaired coronary blood flow response to acetylcholine in patients with coronary risk factors and proximal atherosclerotic lesions. J Clin Invest 1993; 91:29–37.
62. Lefroy DC, et al. Effect of inhibition of nitric oxide synthesis on epicardial coronary artery caliber and coronary blood flow in humans. Circulation 1993; 88:43–54.
63. Collins P, et al. Hemoglobin inhibits endothelium-dependent relaxation to acetylcholine in human coronary arteries in vivo. Circulation 1993; 87:80–85.
64. Lerman A, et al. Circulating and tissue endothelin immunoreactivity in hypercholesterolemic pigs. Circulation 1993; 88:2923–2928.
65. Golino P, et al. Divergent effects of serotonin on coronary artery dimensions and blood flow in patients with coronary atherosclerosis and control patients. N Engl J Med 1991; 324:641–648.
66. Crossman DC, et al. Responses of atherosclerotic human coronary arteries in vivo to substance P. Circulation 1991; 84:2001–2010.
67. Cox DA, et al. Atherosclerosis impairs flow-mediated dilation of coronary arteries in humans. Circulation 1989; 80:458–465.
68. Zeiher AM, et al. Modulation of coronary vasomotor tone in humans. Progressive endothelial dysfunction with different early stages of coronary atherosclerosis. Circulation 1991; 83:391–401.
69. Reddy KG, et al. Evidence that selective endothelial dysfunction may occur in the absence of angiographic or ultrasound atherosclerosis in patients with risk factors for atherosclerosis. J Am Coll Cardiol 1994; 23:833–843.
70. Treasure CB, et al. Hypertension and left ventricular hypertrophy are associated with impaired endothelium-mediated relaxation in human coronary resistance vessels. Circulation 1993; 87:86–93.
71. Treasure CB, et al. Epicardial coronary artery responses to acetylcholine are impaired in hypertensive patients. Circ Res 1992; 71:776–781.
72. Nitenberg A, et al. Impairment of coronary vascular reserve in and ACH-induced coronary vasodilation in diabetic patients with angiographically normal coronary arteries and normal left ventricular systolic function. Diabetes 1993; 42:1017–1025.
73. Nitenberg A, Antony I, Foult JM. Acetylcholine-induced coronary vasoconstriction in young, heavy smokers with normal coronary arteriographic findings. Am J Med 1993; 95:71–77.
74. Zeiher AM, et al. Endothelium-mediated coronary blood flow modulation in humans. Effects of age, atherosclerosis, hypercholesterolemia, and hypertension. J Clin Invest 1993; 92:652–662.
75. Egashira K, et al. Effects of age on endothelium-dependent vasodilation of resistance coronary artery by acetylcholine in humans. Circulation 1993; 88:77–81.
76. Gordon JB, et al. Atherosclerosis influences the vasomotor response of epicardial coronary arteries to exercise. J Clin Invest 1989; 83:1946–1952.
77. Vita JA, et al. Patients with evidence of coronary endothelial dysfunction as assessed by acetylcholine infusion demonstrate marked increase in sensitivity to constrictor effects of catecholamines. Circulation 1992; 85:1390–1397.
78. Hirsh PD, et al. Release of prostaglandins and thromboxane into the coronary circulation in patients with ischemic heart disease. N Engl J Med 1981; 304(12):685–691.
79. Okumura K, et al. Effect of acetylcholine on the highly stenotic coronary artery: Difference between the constrictor response of the infarct-related coronary artery and that of the noninfarct-related artery. J Am Coll Cardiol 1992; 19: 752–758.
80. Panza JA, et al. Abnormal endothelium-dependent vascular relaxation in patients with essential hypertension. N Engl J Med 1990; 323:22–27.
81. Johnstone MT, et al. Impaired endothelium-dependent vasodilation in patients with insulin-dependent diabetes mellitus. Circulation 1993; 88:2510–2516.
82. Casino PR, et al. The role of nitric oxide in endothelium-dependent vasodilation of hypercholesterolemic patients. Circulation 1993; 88:2541–2547.
83. Uehata A, et al. Non-invasive assessment of flow-mediated vasodilation in brachial arteries: Diminished response in young males compared to females. Circulation 1992; 86:I-620.
84. Lieberman EH, et al. Estrogen improves flow-mediated dilation of the brachial artery in post-menopausal women. Ann Intern Med 1994; 121:936–941.
85. Uehata A, et al. Close relationship of endothelial dysfunction in coronary and brachial artery. Circulation 1993; 88:I-618.
86. Laurent S, et al. Flow-dependent vasodilation of brachial artery in essential hypertension. Am J Physiol 1990; 258:H1004–H1011.
87. Celermajer DS, et al. Non-invasive detection of endothelial dysfunction in children and adults at risk of atherosclerosis. Lancet 1992; 340:1111–1115.
88. Joannides R, et al. Nitric oxide is responsible for flow-dependent dilatation of human peripheral conduit arteries in vivo. Circulation 1995; 91:1314–1319.
89. Lieberman EH, et al. Flow-mediated vasodilation is impaired in the brachial artery of patients with coronary disease or diabetes mellitus. Clin Res 1993; 41:217A (Abstr).
90. Sorensen KE, et al. Impairment of endothelium-dependent dilation is an early event in children with familial hypercholesterolemia and is related to the lipoprotein (a) level. J Clin Invest 1994; 93:50–55.
91. Keaney JF, Jr., Vita JA. Atherosclerosis, oxidative stress and antioxidant protection in EDRF action. Prog Cardiovasc Dis 1995; 38:129–154.
92. Rosen GM, Freeman BA. Detection of superoxide generated by endothelial cells. Proc Natl Acad Sci USA 1984; 81:7269–7273.
93. Gryglewski RJ, Palmer RM, Moncada S. Superoxide anion is involved in the breakdown of endothelium-derived vascular relaxing factor. Nature 1986; 320:454–456.
94. Rubanyi GM, Vanhoutte PM. Superoxide anions and hyperoxia inactivate endothelium-derived relaxing factor. Am J Physiol 1986; 250:H822–H827.
95. Omar HA, et al. Inhibition of coronary artery superoxide dismutase attenuates endothelium-dependent and -independent nitrovasodilator relaxation. Circ Res 1991; 69:601–608.
96. Ohara Y, Peterson TE, Harrison DG. Hypercholesterolemia increases endothelial superoxide anion production. J Clin Invest 1993; 91:2546–2551.
97. White CR, et al. Superoxide and peroxynitrite in atherosclerosis. Proc Natl Acad Sci USA 1994; 91:1044–1048.
98. Ohara Y, et al. Dietary treatment of hypercholesterolemia normalizes endothelial superoxide production. Circulation 1993; 88:I-467(Abstr).
99. Keaney JF, et al. Dietary probucol preserves endothelial function in cholesterol-fed rabbits by limiting vascular oxidative stress and superoxide production. J Clin Invest 1995; 95:2520–2529.
100. Levine GN, et al. Ascorbic acid improves endothelial function in patients with coronary artery disease. Circulation 1996. In press.
101. Wei EP, et al. Superoxide generation and reversal of acetylcholine-induced cerebral arteriolar dilation after acute hypertension. Circ Res 1985; 57:781–787.
102. Beckman JS, et al. Apparent hydroxyl radical production by

peroxynitrite: implications for endothelial injury from nitric oxide and superoxide. Proc Natl Acad Sci USA 1990; 87:1620–1624.

103. Pou S, et al. Generation of superoxide by purified brain nitric oxide synthase. J Biol Chem 1992; 267:24173–24176.

104. Weiss SJ, et al. Role of hydrogen peroxide in neutrophil-mediated destruction of cultured endothelial cells. J Clin Invest 1981; 68:714–722.

105. Wei EP, Kantos HE. H_2O_2 and endothelium-dependent cerebral arteriolar dilation. Implications for the identity of endothelium-derived relaxing factor generated by acetylcholine. Hypertension 1990; 16:162–169.

106. Marczin N, Ryan US, Catravas JD. Effects of oxidant stress on endothelium-derived relaxing factor-induced and nitrovasodilator-induced cGMP accumulation in vascular cells in culture. Circ Res 1992; 70:326–340.

107. Fantone JD, Ward PA. Role of oxygen-derived free radicals and metabolites in leukocyte-dependent inflammatory reactions. Am J Pathol 1982; 107:397–403.

108. Smith C, et al. Stimulation of lipid peroxidation and hydroxyl radical generation by the contents of human atherosclerotic lesions. Biochem J 1992; 286:901–905.

109. Goldstein JL, et al. Binding site on macrophages that mediates uptake and degradation of acetylated low density lipoprotein, producing massive cholesterol deposition. Proc Natl Acad Sci USA 1979; 76:333–337.

110. Cushing SD, et al. Minimally modified low density lipoprotein induces monocyte chemotactic protein 1 in human endothelial cells and smooth muscle cells. Proc Natl Acad Sci USA 1990; 87:5134–5139.

111. Cybulsky MI, Gimbrone MA J. Endothelial expression of a mononuclear leukocyte adhesion molecule during atherogenesis. Science 1991; 251:788–791.

112. McNally AK, et al. Activated human monocytes oxidize low-density lipoprotein by a lipoxygenase-dependent pathway. J Immunol 1990; 145:254–259.

113. Hiramatsu K, et al. Superoxide initiates oxidation of low density lipoprotein by human monocytes. Arteriosclerosis 1986; 7:55–60.

114. Negre-Salvayre A, et al. Protective effect of 17beta estradiol against the cytotoxicity of minimally oxidized LDL to cultured bovine aortic endothelial cells. Atherosclerosis 1992; 99:207–217.

115. Kugiyama K, et al. Impairment of endothelium-dependent arterial relaxation by lysolecithin in modified low-density lipoproteins. Nature 1990; 344:160–162.

116. Parthasarathy S, Barnett J. Phospholipase A2 activity of low density lipoprotein: evidence for an intrinsic phospholipase A2 activity of apoprotein B-100. Proc Natl Acad Sci USA 1990; 87:9741–9745.

117. Yokoyama M, et al. Lysophosphatidylcholine: essential role in the inhibition of endothelium-dependent vasorelaxation by oxidized low density lipoprotein. Biochem Biophys Res Commun 1990; 168:301–307.

118. Inoue N, et al. Lysophosphatidylcholine inhibits bradykinin-induced phosphoinositide hydrolysis and calcium transients in cultured bovine aortic endothelial cells. Circ Res 1992; 71:1410–1421.

119. Scheir WT, et al. Regulation of guanylate and adenylate cyclase activities by lysolecithin. Proc Natl Acad Sci USA 1976; 73:1586–1590.

120. Briggs NN, Lefkowitz RJ. Parallel modulation of catecholamine activation of adenylate cyclase and formation of the high affinity agonist-receptor complex in turkey erythrocyte membranes by temperature and cis-vaccenic acid. Biochemistry 1980; 19:4461–4466.

121. Seldis SP, et al. Lysophosphatidylcholine potentiates Ca^{2+} accumulation in rat cardiac myocytes. Am J Physiol 1983; 244:H32–H38.

122. Sugiyama S, et al. Lysophosphatidylcholine in oxidized low-density lipoprotein increases endothelial susceptibility to polymorphonuclear leukocyte-induced endothelial dysfunction in porcine coronary arteries. Role of protein kinase C. Circ Res 1994; 74:565–575.

123. Ohara Y, et al. Lysophosphatidylcholine increases vascular superoxide anion production via protein kinase C activation. Arterioscler thromb 1994; 14:1007–1013.

124. Vidaver GA, Ting A, Lee JW. Evidence that lysolecithin is an important causal agent in atherosclerosis. J Theor Biol 1985; 115:27–41.

125. Tesfamariam B, Cohen RA. Free radicals mediate endothelial cell dysfunction caused by elevated glucose. Am J Physiol 1992; 263:H321–H326.

126. Pieper GM, Gross G. Oxygen-derived free radicals abolish endothelium-dependent relaxation in diabetic rat aorta. Am J Physiol 1988; 255:H825–H833.

127. Kukreja RC, et al. PGH synthase and lipoxygenase generate superoxide in the presence of NADH or NADPH. Circ Res 1986; 59:612–619.

128. Tesfamariam B, Brown ML, Cohen RA. Elevated glucose impairs endothelium-dependent relaxation by activating protein kinase C. J Clin Invest 1991; 87:1643–1648.

129. Lee T-S, et al. Activation of protein kinase C by elevation of glucose concentration: proposal for a mechanism in the development of diabetic vascular complications. Proc Natl Acad Sci USA 1989; 86:5141–5145.

130. Bucala R, et al. Lipid advanced glycosylation: pathway for lipid oxidation in vivo. Proc Natl Acad Sci USA 1993; 90:6434–6438.

131. Vlassara H, et al. Exogenous advanced glycosylation end products induce complex vascular dysfunction in normal animals: a model of diabetic and aging complications. Proc Natl Acad Sci USA 1992; 89:12043–12047.

132. Nakazono K, et al. Does superoxide underlie the pathogenesis of hypertension? Proc Natl Acad Sci USA 1991; 88:10045–10048.

133. Griendling KK, et al. Angiotensin II stimulates NADH and NADPH oxidase activity in cultured vascular smooth muscle cells. Circ Res 1994; 74:1141–1148.

134. Cooke JP, et al. Antiatherogenic effects of L-arginine in hypercholesterolemic rabbits. J Clin Invest 1992; 90:1168–1172.

135. Girerd XJ, et al. 1-Arginine augments endothelium-dependent vasodilation in cholesterol-fed rabbits. Circ Res 1990; 67:1301–1308.

136. Creager MA, et al. 1-Arginine improves endothelium-dependent vasodilation in hypercholesterolemic humans. J Clin Invest 1992; 90:1248–1253.

137. Casino PR, et al. Investigation of decreased availability of nitric oxide precursor as the mechanism responsible for impaired endothelium-dependent vasodilation in hypercholesterolemic patients. J Am Coll Cardiol 1994; 23:844–850.

138. Nathan C. Nitric oxide as a secretory product of mammalian cells. FASEB 1992; 6:3051–3064.

139. Lerman A, et al. Circulating and tissue endothelin immunoreactivity in advanced atherosclerosis. N Engl J Med 1991; 325(14):997–1001.

140. Boulanger CM, et al. Oxidized low density lipoproteins induce mRNA expression and release of endothelin from human and porcine endothelium. Circ Res 1992; 70(6): 1191–1197.

141. Horio T, et al. Stimulation of endothelin-1 release by low density and very low density lipoproteins in cultured human endothelial cells. Atherosclerosis 1993; 101(2):185–190.

142. Yusuf S, Wittes J, Friedman L. Overview of results of ran-

domized clinical trials in heart disease. II. Unstable angina, heart failure, primary prevention with aspirin, and risk factor modification. JAMA 1988; 260:2259–2263.

143. Scandinavian Simvastatin Survival Study Group. Randomized trial of cholesterol lowering in 444 patients with coronary heart disease: The Scandinavian Simvastatin Survival Study (4S). Lancet 1994; 344:1383–1389.
144. Levine GN, Keaney JF, Jr., Vita JA. Cholesterol reduction in cardiovascular disease: Clinical benefits and possible mechanisms. N Engl J Med 1995; 332:512–521.
145. Brown G, et al. Regression of coronary artery disease as a result of intensive lipid-lowering therapy in men with high levels of apolipoprotein B. N Engl J Med 1990; 323:1289–1298.
146. Loscalzo J. Regression of coronary atherosclerosis. N Engl J Med 1990; 323:1337.
147. Harrison DG, et al. Restoration of endothelium-dependent relaxation by dietary treatment of atherosclerosis. J Clin Invest 1987; 80:1808–1811.
148. Leung WH, Lau CP, Wong CK. Beneficial effect of cholesterol-lowering therapy on coronary endothelium-dependent relaxation in hypercholesterolemic patients. Lancet 1993; 341:1496–1500.
149. Treasure CB, et al. Beneficial effects of cholesterol-lowering therapy on the coronary endothelium in patients with coronary artery disease. N Engl J Med 1995; 332:481–487.
150. Anderson TJ, et al. The effect of cholesterol lowering and antioxidant therapy on endothelium-dependent coronary vasomotion. N Engl J Med 1995; 332:488–493.
151. Rimm EB, et al. Vitamin E consumption and the risk of coronary heart disease in men. N Engl J Med 1993; 328:1450–1456.
152. Stampfer MJ, et al. Vitamin E consumption and the risk of coronary heart disease in women. N Engl J Med 1993; 328:1444–1449.
153. Gey KF, Puska P. Plasma vitamins E and A inversely correlated to mortality in ischemic heart disease in cross-cultural epidemiology. Ann NY Acad Sci 1989; 570:268–282.
154. Gaziano JM, et al. Beta carotene therapy for chronic stable angina. Circulation 1990; 82:III–201(Abstr.)
155. Walldius G, et al. The effect of probucol on femoral atherosclerosis: the Probucol Quantitative Regression Swedish Trial (PQRST). Am J Cardiol 1994; 74:875–883.
156. Hodis HN, et al. Serial Coronary Angiographic Evidence that Antioxidant Vitamin Intake Reduces Progression of Coronary Artery Atherosclerosis. JAMA 1995; 273:1849–1854.
157. Keaney JF Jr, et al. Dietary antioxidants preserve endothelium-dependent vessel relaxation in cholesterol-fed rabbits. Proc Natl Acad Sci USA 1993; 90:11880–11884.
158. Cunningham DG, Vita JA, Keaney JR, Jr. Alpha-tocopherol prevents endothelial dysfunction due to oxidized LDL. Clin Res 1994; 42:175A (Abstr).
159. Simon BC, Haudenschild CC, Cohen RA. Preservation of endothelium-dependent relaxation in atherosclerotic rabbit aorta by probucol. J Cardiovasc Pharmacol 1993; 21:893–901.
160. Navab M, et al. Monocyte transmigration induced by modification of low density lipoprotein in cocultures of human aortic wall cells is due to induction of monocyte chemotactic protein 1 synthesis and is abolished by high density lipoprotein. J Clin Invest 1991; 88:2039–2046.
161. Barrett-Connor E, Bush TL. Estrogen and coronary heart disease in women. JAMA 1991; 265:1861–1867.
162. Colditz GA, et al. Menopause and the risk of coronary heart disease in women. N Engl J Med 1987; 316:1105–1110.
163. Sullivan JM, et al. Estrogen replacement and coronary artery disease. Effect on survival in post-menopausal women. Arch Intern Med 1990; 150:2557–2562.
164. Adams MR, et al. Inhibition of coronary artery atherosclerosis by 17-beta estradiol in ovariectomized monkeys. Lack of an effect of added progesterone. Arteriosclerosis 1990; 10:1051–1057.
165. Kushwaha RS, Hazzard WR. Exogenous estrogens attenuate dietary hypercholesterolemia and atherosclerosis in the rabbit. Metabolism 1981; 30:359–366.
166. Bush TL, et al. Cardiovascular mortality and noncontraceptive use of estrogen in women: results from the Lipid Research Clinics Program Follow-up Study. Circulation 1987; 75:1102–1109.
167. McDonald CC, Sewart HJ. Fatal myocardial infarction in the Scottish adjuvant tamoxifen trial. British Medical Journal 1991; 303:435–437.
168. Hayashi T, et al. Basal release of nitric oxide from aortic rings is greater in female rabbits than in male rabbits: implications for atherosclerosis. Proc Natl Acad Sci USA 1992; 89:11259–11263.
169. Miller VM, Vanhoutte PM. Progesterone and modulation of endothelium-dependent responses in canine coronary arteries. Am J Physiol 1991; 261:R1022–R1027.
170. Jiang C, et al. Acute effect of 17-beta estradiol on rabbit coronary artery contractile responses to endothelin-1. Am J Physiol 1992; 263:H271–H275.
171. Williams SP, et al. Endothelium-dependent relaxation in estrogen-treated spontaneously hypertensive rats. Eur J Pharmacol 1988; 145:205–207.
172. Williams JK, Adams MR, Klopfenstein HS. Estrogen modulates responses of atherosclerotic coronary arteries. Circulation 1990; 81:1680–1687.
173. Williams JK, et al. Short-term administration of estrogen and vascular responses of atherosclerotic coronary arteries. J Am Coll Cardiol 1992; 20:452–457.
174. Keaney JF Jr, et al. 17beta-estradiol preserves endothelial vasodilator function and limits LDL oxidation in hypercholesterolemic swine. Circulation 1994; 89:2251–2259.
175. Mazière C, et al. Estrogens inhibit copper and cell-mediated modification of low density lipoprotein. Arteriosclerosis 1991; 89:175–182.
176. Sugioka K, Shimosegawa Y, Nakano M. Estrogens as natural antioxidants of membrane phospholipid peroxidation. FEBS Lett 1987; 219:37–39.
177. Yagi K, Komura S. Inhibitory effect of female hormones on lipid peroxidation. Biochem Int 1986; 13:1051–1055.
178. Wiseman H, et al. Protective actions of tamoxifen and 4-hydroxytamoxifen against oxidative damage to human low-density lipoproteins: a mechanism accounting for the cardioprotective action of tamoxifen. Biochem J 1993; 292:635–638.
179. Sack MN, Rader DJ, Cannon RO 3rd. Oestrogen and inhibition of oxidation of low-density lipoproteins in postmenopausal women. Lancet 1994; 343:269–270.
180. Reis SE, et al. Ethinyl estradiol acutely attenuates abnormal coronary vasomotor responses to acetylcholine in postmenopausal women. Circulation 1994; 89:52–60.
181. Stadel BV. Oral contraceptives and cardiovascular disease. N Engl J Med 1981; 305:612–615.
182. Wang J, Wolin MS, Hintze TH. Chronic exercise enhances endothelium-mediated dilation of epicardial coronary artery in conscious dogs. Circ Res 1993; 73:829–838.
183. Muller JM, Myers PR, Laughlin H. Vasodilator responses of coronary resistance arteries of exercise-trained pigs. Circulation 1994; 89:2308–2314.
184. Miller VM, Vanhoutte PM. Enhanced release of endothelium-derived relaxing factor by chornic increases in blood flow. Am J Physiol 1988; 255:H446–H451.
185. Sessa WC, et al. Chronic exercise in dogs increases coronary vascular nitric oxide production and endothelial cell nitric oxide synthase gene expression. Circ Res 1994; 74:349–353.

186. Blair SN, et al. Statement on exercise. Circulation 1992; 86:340–344.
187. Hekman CM, Loskutoff DJ. Fibrinolytic pathways and the endothelium. Semin Thromb Hemost 1987; 13:514–527.
188. Holvoet P, Cleemput H, Collen D. Assay of human tissue-type plasminogen activator (t-PA) with an enzyme-linked immunosorbent assay (ELISA) based on three murine monoclonal antibodies to t-PA. Thromb Haemost 1985; 54:684–687.
189. Wiman B, Mellbring G, Ranby M. Plasminogen activator release during venous stasis and exercise as determined by a new specific assay. Clin Chim Acta 1983; 127:279–288.
190. Rijken DC et al. Measurement of human tissue-type plasminogen activator by two-site immunoradiometric assay. J Lab Clin Med 1983; 101:274.
191. Levin EG, et al. Thrombin stimulates tissue plasminogen activator release from cultured human endothelial cells. J Clin Invest 1984; 74:1988–1995.
192. Sakata Y, et al. Activated protein C stimulates the fibrinolytic activity of cultured endothelial cells and decreases antiactivator activity. Proc Natl Acad Sci USA 1985; 82:1121–1125.
193. Hanss M, Collen D. Secretion of tissue-type plasminogen activator and plasminogen activator inhibitor by cultured human endothelial cells: modulation by thrombin, endotoxin, and histamine. J Lab Clin Med 1987; 109:97–104.
194. Diamond SL, Eskin SG, McIntire LV. Fluid flow stimulates tissue plasminogen activator secretion by cultured human endothelial cells. Science 1989; 243:1483–1485.
195. Santell L, Levin EG. Cyclic AMP potentiates phorbol ester stimulation of tissue plasminogen activator release and inhibits secretion of plasminogen activator inhibitor-1 from human endothelial cells. J Biol Chem 1988; 263:16802–16808.
196. Hajjar KA, Hamel NM. Identification and characterization of human endothelial cell membrane binding sites for tissue plasminogen activator and urokinase. J Biol Chem 1990; 265:2908–2916.
197. Loskutoff D, Edgington T. Synthesis of a fibrinolytic activator and inhibitor by endothelial cells. Proc Natl Acad Sci USA 1977; 74:3903–3907.
198. Erickson LA, Hekman CM, Loskutoff DJ. The primary plasminogen-activator inhibitors in endothelial cells, platelets, serum, and plasma are immunologically related. Proc Natl Acad Sci USA 1985; 82:8710–8714.
199. Philips M, et al. Immunological relationship between the fast-acting plasminogen activator inhibitors from plasma, blood platelets and endothelial cells demonstrated with a monoclonal antibody against an inhibitor from placenta. Thromb Haemost 1986; 55:213–217.
200. Sprengers ED, Kluft C. Plasminogen activator inhibitors. Blood 1987; 69:381–387.
201. Suffredini AF, Harpel PC, Parrillo JE. Promotion and subsequent inhibition of plasminogen activation after administration of intravenous endotoxin to normal subjects. N Engl J Med 1989; 320:1165–1172.
202. Bevilacqua MP, et al. Regulation of the fibrinolytic system of cultured human vascular endothelium by interleukin 1. J Clin Invest 1986; 78:587–591.
203. Emeis JJ, Kooistra T. Interleukin 1 and lipopolysaccharide induce an inhibitor of tissue-type plasminogen activator in vivo and in cultured endothelial cells. J Exp Med 1986; 163:1260–1266.
204. Colucci M, Paramo JA, Collen D. Generation in plasma of a fast-acting inhibitor of plasminogen activator in response to endotoxin stimulation. J Clin Invest 1985; 75:818–824.
205. Saksela O, Moscatelli D, Rifkin DB. The opposing effects of basic fibroblast growth factor and transforming growth factor beta on the regulation of plasminogen activator activity of capillary endothelial cells. J Cell Biol 1987; 105:957–963.
206. Scarpati EM, Sadler JE. Regulation of endothelial cell coagulant properties. Modulation of tissue factor, plasminogen activator inhibitors, and thrombomodulin by phorbol 12-myristate 13-acetate and tumor necrosis factor. J Biol Chem 1989; 264:20705–20713.
207. Stiko-Rahm A, et al. Secretion of plasminogen activator inhibitor-1 from cultured umbilical vein endothelial cells is induced by very low density lipoprotein. Arteriosclerosis 1990; 10:1067–1073.
208. Etingin OR, et al. Lipoprotein (a) regulates plasminogen activator inhibitor-1 expression in endothelial cells. A potential mechanism in thrombogenesis. J Biol Chem 1991; 266:2459–2465.
209. Gelehrter TD, Sznycer-Laszuk R. Thrombin induction of plasminogen activator-inhibitor in cultured human endothelial cells. J Clin Invest 1986; 77:165–169.
210. Vaughan DE, Lazos SC. Angiotensin II induces plasminogen activator inhibitor (PAI-1) in vitro. Circulation 1992; 86[Suppl 1]:I-557.
211. Meyer D, Baumgartner HR. Role of von Willebrand factor in platelet adhesion to the subendothelium. Br J Haematol 1983; 54:1–9.
212. Turitto VT, Weiss HJ, Baumgartner HR. Platelet interaction with rabbit subendothelium in von Willebrand's disease: altered thrombus formation distinct from defective platelet adhesion. J Clin Invest 1984; 74:1730–1741.
213. Marcum JA, Rosenberg RD. Heparin-like molecules with anticoagulant activity are synthesized by cultured endothelial cells. Biochem Biophys Res Commun 1985; 126:365–372.
214. Esmon NL, Owen WG, Esmon CT. Isolation of a membrane bound cofactor for thrombin-catalyzed activation of protein C. J Biol Chem 1982; 257:859–864.
215. Azuma H, Ishikawa M, Sekizaki S. Endothelium-dependent inhibition of platelet aggregation. Br J Pharmacol 1986; 88:411–415.
216. Stamler JS, et al. N-acetylcysteine potentiates platelet inhibition by endothelium-derived relaxing factor. Circ Res 1989; 65:789–795.
217. Simon DI, et al. Antiplatelet properties of protein S-nitrosothiols derived from nitric oxide and endothelium-derived relaxing factor. Arteriosclerosis and Thromb 1993; 13:791–799.
218. Rovin JD, et al. Sodium nitroprusside, an endothelium-derived relaxing factor congener, increases platelet cyclic GMP levels and inhibits epinephrine-exacerbated in vivo platelet thrombus formation in stenosed canine coronary arteries. J Cardiovasc Pharmacol 1993; 22:626–631.
219. Ridker PM, et al. Endogenous tissue-type plasminogen activator and risk of myocardial infarction. Lancet 1993; 341:1165–1168.
220. Jansson JH, Nilsson TK, Olofsson BO. Tissue plaminogen activator and other risk factors as predictors of cardiovascular events in patients with severe angina pectoris. Eur Heart J 1991; 12:157–161.
221. Ridker PM, et al. A cross-section study of endogenous tissue plaminogen activator, total cholesterol, HDL cholesterol, and apolipoproteins A-1, A-II, and B-100. Arteriosclerosis and Thromb 1993; 13:1587–1592.
222. Crutchley DJ, et al. Levels of three hemostatic factors in relation to serum lipids. Monocyte procoagulant activity, tissue plasminogen activator, and type-1 plasminogen activator inhibitor. Arteriosclerosis 1989; 9:934–939.
223. Ridker PM, et al. Prospective study of endogenous tissue plasminogen activator and risk of stroke. Lancet 1994; 343:940–943.
224. Juhan-Vague I, et al. Plasma plasminogen activator inhibitor-1 in angina pectoris. Influence of plasma insulin and acute-phase response. Arteriosclerosis 1989; 9:362–367.

225. Hamsten A, et al. Increased plasma levels of a rapid inhibitor of tissue plasminogen activator in young survivors of myocardial infarction. N Engl J Med 1985; 313:1557–1563.
226. Hamsten A, et al. Plasminogen activator inhibitor in plasma: risk factor for recurrent myocardial infarction. Lancet 1987; 2:3–9.
227. Aznar J, et al. Plasminogen activator inhibitor activity and other fibrinolytic variables in patients with coronary artery disease. Br Heart J 1988; 59:535–541.
228. Paramo JA, et al. Plasminogen activator inhibitor in the blood of patients with coronary artery disease. British Medical Journal 1985; 291:573–574.
229. Nilsson TK, Johnson O. The extrinsic fibrinolytic system in survivors of myocardial infarction. Thromb Res 1987; 48:621–630.
230. Weis JR, et al. Oxidized low-density lipoprotein increases cultured human endothelial cell tissue factor activity and reduces protein C activation. FASEB 1991; 5:2459–2469.
231. Kugiyama K, et al. Transferable lipids in oxidized low-density lipoprotein stimulate plasminogen activator inhibitor-1 and inhibit tissue-type plasminogen activator release from endothelial cells. Circ Res 1993; 73:335–343.
232. Ridker PM, et al. Stimulation of plasminogen activator inhibitor in vivo by infusion of angiotensin II. Evidence of a potential interaction between the renin-angiotensin system and fibrinolytic function. Circulation 1993; 87:1969–1973.
233. Pfeffer MA, et al. Effect of captopril on mortality and morbidity in patients with left ventricular dysfunction after myocardial infarction. N Engl J Med 1992; 327:676–677.
234. The SOLVD investigators: Effect of enalapril on survival in patients with reduced left ventricular ejection fractions and congestive heart failure. N Engl J Med 1991; 325:293–302.
235. Alderman MH, et al. Association of the renin-sodium profile with the risk of myocardial infarction in patients with hypertension. N Engl J Med 1991; 324:1098–1104.
236. Williams GH, Hollenberg NK. Accentuated vascular and endocrine response to SQ20,881 in hypertension. N Engl J Med 1977; 297:194–201.
237. Griggs TR, et al. Susceptibility to atherosclerosis in aortas and coronary arteries of swine with von Willebrand's disease. Am J Pathol 1981; 102:137–145.
238. Bowie EJ, et al. The role of Willebrand factor in platelet–blood vessel interaction, including a discussion of resistance to atherosclerosis in pigs with von Willebrand's disease. Philosophical Transactions of the Royal Society of London 1991; 294:267–279.
239. Colwell JA, et al. New concepts about the pathogenesis of atherosclerosis in diabetes mellitus. Am J Med 1983; 30:67–80.
240. Lentz SR, Sadler JE. Inhibition of thrombomodulin surface expression and protein C activation by the thrombogenic agent homocysteine. J Clin Invest 1991; 88:1906.
241. Stamler JS, et al. Adverse vascular effects of homocysteine are modulated by endothelium-derived relaxing factor and related oxides of nitrogen. J Clin Invest 1993; 91:308–318.
242. Clowes AW, Reidy MA, Clowes MM. Kinetics of cellular proliferation after arterial injury. I. Smooth muscle growth in the absence of endothelium. Lab Invest 1983; 49:327–333.
243. Reidy MA. Biology of Disease. A reassessment of endothelial injury and arterial lesion formation. Lab Invest 1985; 53:513–520.
244. Shimokawa H, Vanhoutte PM. Impaired endothelium-dependent relaxation to aggregating platelets and related vasoactive substances in porcine coronary arteries in hypercholesterolemia and atherosclerosis. Circ Res 1989; 64:900–914.
245. Weidinger FF, et al. Persistent dysfunction of regenerated endothelium after balloon angioplasty of rabbit iliac artery. Circulation 1990; 81:1667–1679.
246. Garg UC, Hassid A. Nitric oxide-generating vasodilators and 8-bromo-cyclic guanosine monophosphate inhibit mitogenesis and proliferation of cultured rat vascular smooth muscle cells. J Clin Invest 1989; 83:1774–1777.
247. Koh E, et al. Effects of beraprost sodium, a stable analogue of prostacyclin, on hyperplasia, hypertrophy and glycosaminoglycan synthesis of rat aortic smooth muscle cells. Artery 1993; 20:242–252.
248. Marks DS, et al. Inhibition of Neointimal Proliferation in rabbits following vascular injury by a single treatment with a protein adduct of nitric oxide. J Clin Invest. In press.
249. Kubes P, Suzuki M, Granger DN. Nitric oxide: an endogenous modulator of leukocyte adhesion. Proc Natl Acad Sci USA 1991; 88:4651–4655.
250. Castellot JJ Jr, et al. Cultured endothelial cells produce a heparin-like inhibitor of smooth muscle cell growth. J Cell Biol 1981; 90:372–379.
251. Berk BC, Alexander RW. Commentary: Vasoactive effects of growth factors. Biochem Pharm 1989; 38:219–225.
252. Ross R. The pathogenesis of atherosclerosis: a perspective for the 1990s. Nature 1993; 362:801–809.
253. Schwartz SM, Heimark RL, Majesky MW. Developmental mechanisms underlying pathology of arteries. Physiol Rev 1990; 70:1177–1209.
254. Gibbons GH, Dzau VJ. The emerging concept of vascular remodeling. N Engl J Med 1994; 330:1431–1438.
255. Lepoivre M, Flaman J-M, Henry Y. Early loss of the tyrosyl radical of ribonucleotide reductase of adenocarcinoma cells producing nitric oxide. J Biol Chem 1992; 267:22994–23000.
256. Molina y Vedia L, et al. Nitric oxide-induced S-nitrosylation of glyceraldehyde-3-phosphate dehydrogenase inhibits enzymatic activity and increases endogenous ADP-ribosylation. J Biol Chem 1993; 267:24929–24932.
257. Jessup W, et al. The participation of nitric oxide in cell free- and its restriction of macrophage-mediated oxidation of low-density lipoprotein. Biochim Biophys Acta 1992; 1180:73–82.
258. Cooke JP, et al. Antiatherogenic effects of l-arginine in the hypercholesterolemic rabbit. J Clin Invest 1992; 90:1168–1172.
259. Tsao PS, et al. Enhanced endothelial adhesiveness in hypercholesterolemia is attenuated by l-arginine. Circulation 1994; 89:2176–2182.
260. Cayette AJ, et al. Chronic inhibition of nitric oxide production accelerates neointima formation and impairs endothelial function in hypercholesterolemic rabbits. Arteriosclerosis and Thromb 1994; 14:753–759.
261. Kume N, Cybulsky MI, Gimbrone MA Jr. Lysophosphatidylcholine, a component of atherogenic lipoproteins, induces mononuclear leukocyte adhesion molecules in cultured human and rabbit arterial endothelial cells. J Clin Invest 1992; 90:1138–1144.
262. O'Brien KD, et al. Vascular cell adhesion molecule-1 is expressed in human coronary atherosclerotic plaques. Implications for the mode of progression of advanced coronary atherosclerosis. J Clin Invest 1993; 92:945–951.

Pathophysiology of Thrombosis

Andrew I. Schafer

Although the coagulation system is constantly poised to respond to vascular injury and other thrombogenic stimuli by rapidly forming a platelet-fibrin clot, several important physiologic antithrombotic mechanisms operate to prevent thrombus formation under normal circumstances and to focus the clot and localize it precisely to the site where it is needed in pathologic states [1,2]. The major physiologic antithrombotic mechanisms currently recognized are prostacyclin, endothelium-derived relaxing factor (EDRF) or nitric oxide (NO), adenosine diphosphatase (ADPase), antithrombin, protein C and protein S, tissue factor pathway inhibitor (TFPI), and the fibrinolytic system (Table 10-1). Prostacyclin, EDRF/NO, and ADPase are potent inhibitors of platelets. Antithrombin, protein C, and TFPI are inhibitors of fibrin formation. The fibrinolytic system digests and clears the fibrin clot. These mechanisms probably do not act mutually exclusively on platelets or fibrin, however, and complex interactions occur among them. For example, the fibrinolytic protease plasmin not only digests fibrin but also affects platelet function [3,4] and acts synergistically with prostacyclin to inhibit platelet activation [5]. Most of these antithrombotic mechanisms require the presence of intact endothelium, and many are probably activated or at least locally amplified by the actual formation of a clot.

Prostacyclin (PGI_2), the major oxygenated metabolite of arachidonic acid in endothelial cells) promotes blood fluidity as a vasodilator and inhibitor of platelet aggregation [6,7]. It is a labile eicosanoid that probably exerts its antithrombotic effects locally in the immediate proximity of vascular injury rather than as a systemically circulating hormone. Prostacyclin synthesis by intact endothelium adjacent to a site of vascular injury may be focally amplified through the unidirectional transcellular transfer of common intermediates from activated platelets to the endothelial cells [8–10]; this has been thought to localize platelet plug formation efficiently by preventing further accrual of platelets to the hemostatic plug.

Impaired formation or release of prostacyclin from blood vessels would be expected to cause platelet hyperreactivity and a thrombotic tendency. Congenital deficiency of vascular cyclooxygenase has been reported, but the clinical consequences of decreased prostacyclin production in that case are apparently offset by the simultaneous deficiency of platelet cyclooxygenase, thus leading to decreased platelet thromboxane A_2 formation [11]. No specific thrombotic diathesis has yet been directly linked pathogenetically to defective formation or release of prostacyclin. However, diminished vascular prostacyclin formation has been found in thrombotic thrombocytopenic purpura [12], diabetes mellitus [13,14], and in patients with the lupus anticoagulant [15]—acquired clinical conditions that are associated with a thrombotic tendency.

EDRF, a major component of which is NO [16], has a biologic profile similar to that of prostacyclin, acting as a vasodilator and inhibitor of platelet activation [17], although they act through different cyclic nucleotide–dependent mechanisms: EDRF/NO via cyclic guanosine monophosphate (cGMP) and prostacyclin via cyclic adenosine monophosphate (cAMP). EDRF/NO and prostacyclin are synergistic inhibitors of platelet aggregation [18]. Loss of EDRF/NO has been associated with atherosclerotic cardiovascular disease, particularly coronary artery disease [19–29].

Endothelial cells also have ecto-ADPase activity that contributes to their platelet inhibitory properties [30]. The endothelial membrane ADPase acts as an apyrase by hydrolyzing and inactivating extracellular adenine nucleotides, including platelet-stimulatory adenosine diphosphate (ADP), which may be released from platelets themselves or other cells [31–33]. No clinical thrombotic or vascular disorders have as yet been linked to a specific deficiency of endothelial-cell ADPase activity.

Antithrombin III exerts its actions as a physiologic anticoagulant by binding to and neutralizing the activity of thrombin and some other serine proteases (XIIa, XIa, IXa, and Xa) in the coagulation cascade (Fig. 10-1) [34]. Heparin markedly potentiates the actions of antithrombin III by binding to lysyl residues on the antithrombin, thus inducing conformational changes in the molecule that facilitate its reaction with the active serine centers of thrombin and other coagulation proteases. Once the thrombin–antithrombin III complex has formed, it dissociates from heparin, permitting the free heparin to promote further thrombin–antithrombin III reactions [35]. Heparinlike substances actually occur naturally on the surfaces of blood vessels, tightly bound to endothelial cells [36]. The density of these endothelial proteoglycans varies throughout the vascular tree, the highest concentrations being found in the microvasculature. Thus, antithrombin III probably functions in vivo not predominantly in fluid phase but rather on endothelial surfaces, where such heparinlike proteoglycans normally are available to promote its neutralizing reactions with thrombin and other serine proteases of the coagulation cascade [37]. Another antithrombin (termed heparin cofactor II) that is antigenically distinguishable from antithrombin III may also participate as a similar physiologic anticoagulant [38]. Both quantitative deficiencies and functional defects of antithrombin III have been linked to a predisposition to thrombosis, presumably due to unchecked thrombin generation.

Protein C represents another critical physiologic anticoagulant system [39], the activation and actions of which are shown in Fig. 10-2. Thrombin converts the inactive zymogen protein C to activated protein C (protein Ca), a serine protease. The activation of protein C by thrombin is greatly accelerated on vascular intimal surfaces, which possess a receptor for thrombin termed **thrombomodulin** [40,41]. Once bound to endothelial-cell thrombomodulin, thrombin loses its ability to clot fibrinogen [42]. Thus,

Table 10-1. Endogenous antithrombic mechanisms

System	Actions
Prostacyclin (PGI_2)	Inhibits platelet activation; dilates blood vessels
Endothelium-derived relaxing factor (EDRF)/nitric oxide (NO)	Inhibits platelet activation; dilates blood vessels
Ecto-ADPase	Inhibits platelet activation
Antithrombin (AT)	Binds and neutralizes thrombin (accelerated by heparin binding to AT)
Protein C	Inactivates factors Va and VIIIa; may stimulate fibrinolysis (activated by thrombin binding to thrombomodulin; requires cofactor protein S)
Fibrinolysis	Digests fibrin

thrombomodulin serves as an endothelium-dependent physiologic anticoagulant system both by removing thrombin from the circulation and by providing a site for the activation of protein C. The anticoagulant action of protein Ca is due to its rapid inactivation of factors Va and VIIIa [43] and the stimulation of fibrinolysis [44–46], although the latter aspect of its activity has been disputed [47]. Thus, whereas thrombin activates factors V and VIII (to Va and VIIIa, respectively), thrombin-activated protein C (protein Ca) limits the action of thrombin by destroying Va and VIIIa. Protein S [48,49] serves as a cofactor for the expression of the anticoagulant activity of protein Ca. Both protein C and protein S are glycoproteins that require vitamin K–dependent postsynthetic γ-carboxylation of glutamic acid residues (to form Gla residues) for expression of their activities. Thus, unlike the other vitamin K–dependent clotting factors (X, IX, VII, and prothrombin) that act as procoagulants, these proteins are actually anticoagulants. Protein Ca and protein S form a complex on cellular phospholipid surfaces and can inactivate both free and platelet-bound factor Va [50]. As discussed below, quantitative and functional deficiencies of protein C or protein S cause a thrombotic tendency.

TFPI, formerly known as lipoprotein-associated coagulation inhibitor or extrinsic pathway inhibitor, has been identified recently as a major physiologic inhibitor of the tissue factor pathway of coagulation [51,52]. TFPI is associated with plasma lipoproteins and requires the presence of factor Xa to inhibit the factor VIIa–tissue factor complex reversibly. As yet, no abnormalities of TFPI have been found to be associated with a predisposition to thrombosis.

The fifth major physiologic antithrombotic mechanism is the fibrinolytic system [53–55]. In that system, the active fibrin-digesting enzyme plasmin is formed from its inactive plasma zymogen plasminogen by the action of plasminogen activators (Fig. 10-3). Plasminogen activators (PAs) have been found in a variety of tissues, but they can be classified into two immunologically distinct types: tissue-type PAs (t-PAs), which are primarily the vascular PAs, and urokinaselike PAs (u-PAs), which were originally isolated from urine. These two types of PAs have considerable structural homology but are produced by distinct genes that have been cloned and sequenced [56–58]. Both types of PAs are serine proteases that activate plasminogen by cleaving the same arginine-valine bond. u-PAs can activate plasminogen directly, whereas t-PAs must bind to fibrin as a cofactor to exert this activity. Thus, t-PAs generate plasmin primarily within the interstices of the fibrin clot. Although vascular endothelium produces t-PA, it also produces a fast-acting PA inhibitor [59–61]. This has led to the concept that net fibrinolytic activity is determined by a balance between endothelial release of PA and PA inhibitor into the circulation, so that agents or conditions that alter fibrinolytic activity can do so by changing either PA or PA inhibitor [62].

Fig. 10-1. Mechanisms of action of antithrombin III (AT). Heparinlike molecules on endothelial-cell surfaces bind AT, causing conformational changes in AT that markedly increase its ability to bind and thus neutralize thrombin and other serine proteases (activated coagulation factors), including XIIa, XIa, IXa, and Xa.

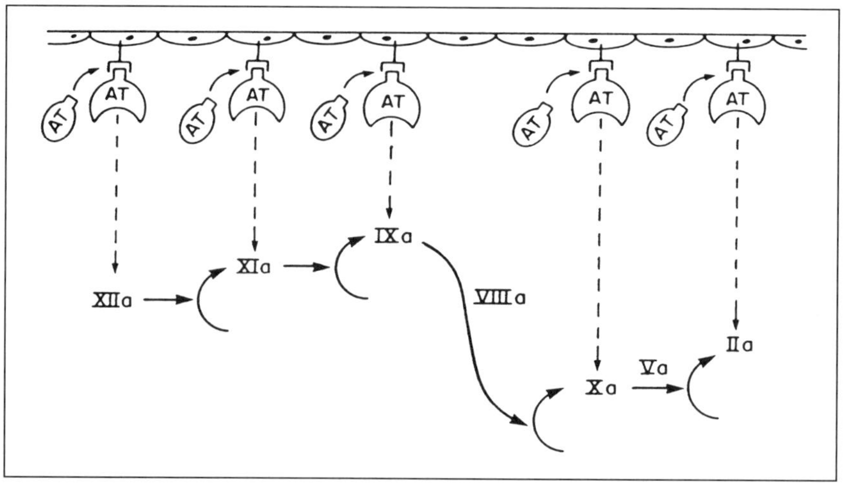

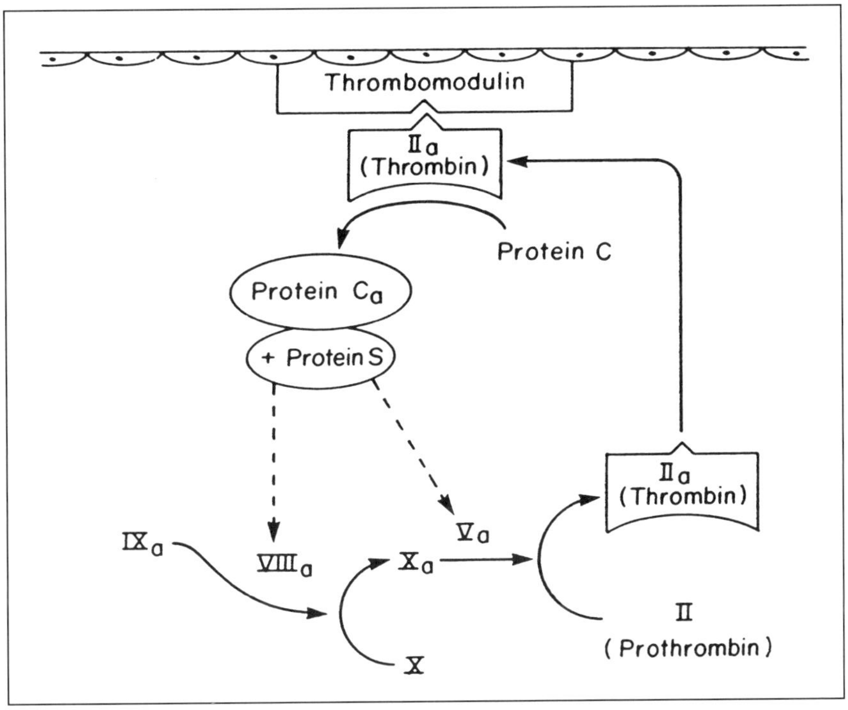

Fig. 10-2. Mechanisms of action of protein C. Thrombin (factor IIa) binds to endothelial-cell-surface sites termed thrombomodulin, on which protein C is activated to protein Ca. Protein Ca acts with its cofactor, protein S, to inactivate VIIIa and Va.

Plasmin cleaves fibrin(ogen) at a specific site that is distinct from that cleaved by thrombin, releasing the fragment Bβ-1-42, which can be measured in plasma by radioimmunoassay [63]. The remaining fragment X of fibrin(ogen) is subsequently degraded into smaller soluble cleavage products (fibrin-degradation products). The major physiologic plasma inhibitor of plasmin is α_2-antiplasmin: It forms a stable one-to-one stoichiometric complex with plasmin that is devoid of protease activity [64–66] in a manner that mirrors the neutralizing action of antithrombin on thrombin. When plasmin is formed in excess of plasma antiplasmin-binding capacity, circulating free plasmin produces a systemic thrombolytic state. At the level of the thrombus, plasmin bound to (and acting on)

Fig. 10-3. Mechanisms of action of the fibrinolytic system. Tissue-type plasminogen activator is released from endothelial cells by certain stimuli (e.g., thrombin), converting plasma plasminogen to plasmin and thus promoting fibrin digestion.

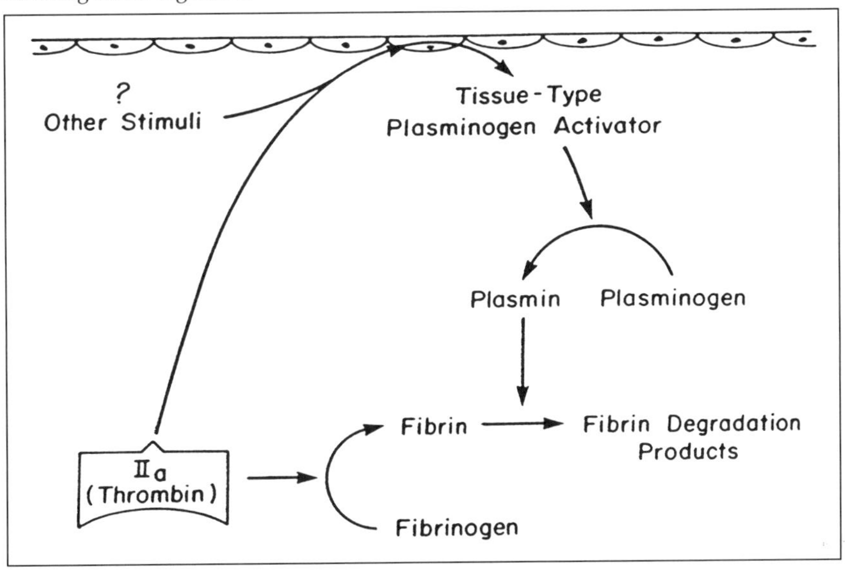

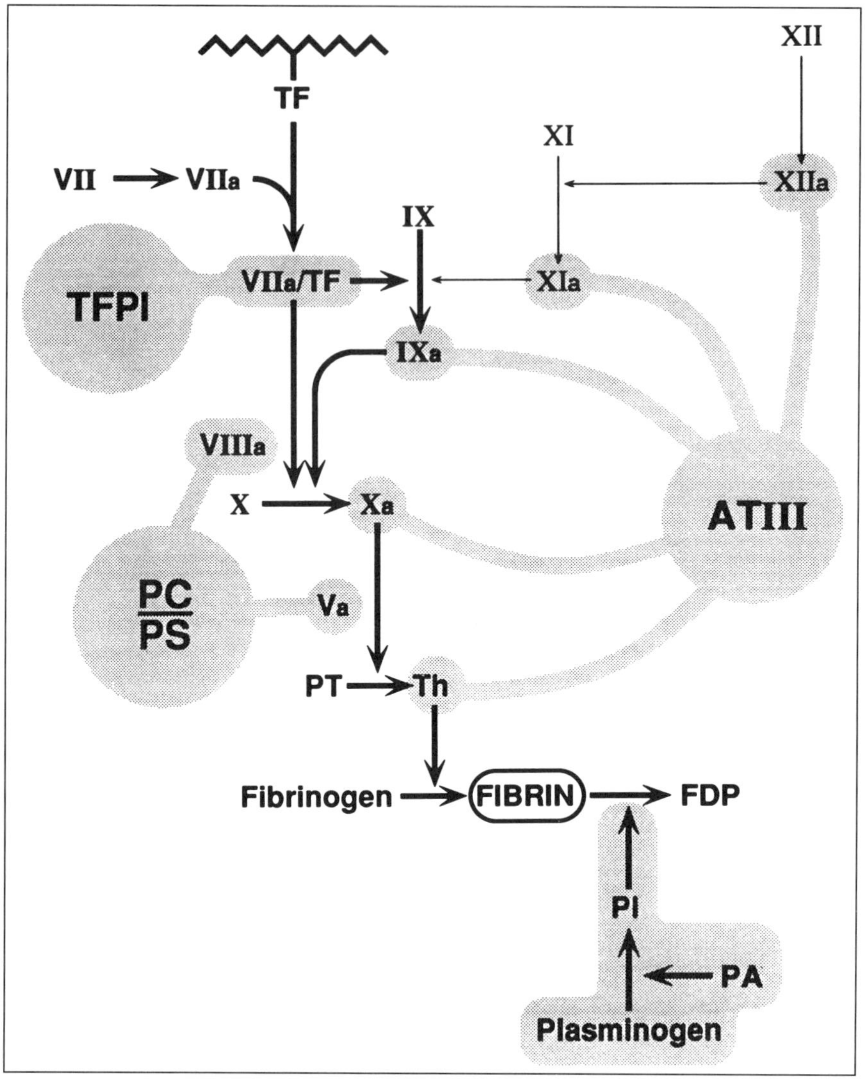

Fig. 10-4. Sites of action of the four major physiological antithrombotic pathways currently recognized: antithrombin III (ATIII); protein C/protein S (PC/PS); tissue factor pathway inhibitor (TFPI); the fibrinolytic system, consisting of plasminogen, plasminogen activator (PA), and plasmin (Pl). (Reproduced with permission from AI Schafer. Hypercoagulable states: molecular genetis to clinical practice. Lancet 1994; 344:1739–1742.)

fibrin is relatively protected from the actions of α_2-antiplasmin. A variety of abnormalities of the fibrinolytic system (e.g., those affecting plasminogen, PA, PA inhibitor) can cause a predisposition to thrombosis.

The major physiologic antithrombotic systems that regulate fibrin formation and removal are summarized in schematic form in Fig. 10-4.

The Hypercoagulable States

The **hypercoagulable state** is a poorly defined term that has been widely applied to the clinical problems of patients who are unusually predisposed to thromboembolism. In many cases, a specific abnormality of one of the previously described physiologic antithrombotic mechanisms causes a true prethrombotic state. Those disorders, which generally are inherited, are referred to as **primary hypercoagulable states** [67]. However, many other patients have a variety of acquired clinical conditions that are known to be associated with a high risk of thromboembolic complications. In those cases, referred to as **secondary hypercoagulable states,** the pathophysiologic basis for thrombosis is not currently well defined and appears to involve multifactorial or complex coagulopathies. An acquired secondary hypercoagulable state is frequently the stimulus that triggers a clinical thrombotic episode in a patient with a primary hypercoagulable state who has an inherited predisposition to thrombosis [68].

PRIMARY HYPERCOAGULABLE STATES

All the presently established primary hypercoagulable states (Table 10-2) involve defects in the proteins of the coagulation or fibrinolytic systems rather than platelet abnormalities. With rare exceptions, the primary hypercoagulable states are inherited disorders. Therefore, the specific coagulopathies in these patients generally are fixed and persistent throughout life [69], even though

Table 10-2. Primary hypercoagulable states

ANTITHROMBIN AND HEPARIN DISORDERS
Antithrombin III deficiency
Heparin cofactor II deficiency
PROTEIN C AND PROTEIN S DISORDERS
Protein C deficiency
Protein S deficiency
Activated protein C resistance
FIBRINOLYTIC DISORDERS
Hypoplasminogenemia
Dysplasminogenemia
Plasminogen activator deficiency
Decreased tissue plasminogen activator
Increased plasminogen activator inhibitor
Increased histidine-rich glycoprotein
Dysfibrinogenemia

the actual clinical thrombotic events occur episodically. Furthermore, some patients with primary hypercoagulable states are entirely asymptomatic and are diagnosed by laboratory findings in the course of family studies. The discrete thrombotic events in these patients are probably precipitated by clinical or subclinical acquired insults to an underlying abnormal coagulation system that is constantly poised for thrombosis but is chronically compensated by other antithrombotic mechanisms [67,70].

Several studies have estimated the prevalence of an underlying identifiable primary hypercoagulable state in younger patients (under age 45) presenting with an initial episode of venous thromboembolism to be about 20 percent [71]. One large series of consecutive patients with acute deep-vein thrombosis found an overall prevalence of deficiencies of antithrombin III, protein C, protein S, or plasminogen of only 8.3 percent [72]. This latter report suggests that the prevalence is too low to make screening all patients with deep-vein thrombosis cost effective at this time. However, as noted below, the recent reports of remarkably high prevalence of activated protein C resistance suggest that a primary hypercoagulable state should be identifiable in the majority of patients presenting with venous thromboembolism.

Certain generalizations can be made regarding the clinical manifestations of the various primary hypercoagulable states listed in Table 10-2. The most frequently encountered thrombotic complications in these patients are common venous thromboembolic problems, such as deep-vein thrombosis of the lower extremities and pulmonary embolism. Arterial thrombosis is a distinctly unusual manifestation of the primary hypercoagulable states, although a number of cases have been described, particularly with protein S deficiency [73]. Arterial thromboembolism may also originate from clinically occult venous thrombi in patients with patent foramen ovale [74]. Although the initial thrombotic episode may occur at any age, ranging from the neonatal period to old age, most of these patients first present with clinical symptoms in

Table 10-3. Assays of major types of inherited antithrombin III deficiency

		Activity	
Type	Antigen	Heparin cofactor	Progressive ATIII
I ("classic")	↓	↓	↓
II (active-site defect)	N	↓	↓
II (heparin-binding-site defect)	N	↓	N

ATIII = antithrombin III; N = normal.

early adulthood, in the second or third decade of life. Many patients with primary hypercoagulable states apparently are healthy and have no obvious predisposing risk factors for thrombosis. However, a specific precipitating event preceding the acute thromboembolism (e.g., pregnancy, use of oral contraceptives, surgery, trauma, infection) often can be identified with careful examination [75]. It is important for the clinician to recognize such additive risk factors that predispose patients with primary hypercoagulable states to thrombotic complications.

Antithrombin III Deficiency. Congenital deficiency of antithrombin III, the major physiologic antagonist of thrombin and other activated clotting factors, may be considered the prototype of the primary hypercoagulable states. The incidence of antithrombin III deficiency in the general population has been estimated to be 1 in 2,000 to 5,000 [76]. However, more recent studies using functional assays of heparin cofactor activity have determined the prevalence of antithrombin III deficiency in the general population to be 0.2 to 0.4 percent [77,78]. In typical cases, the biochemical defect is inherited in an autosomal dominant fashion [79,80]. Heterozygote patients have antithrombin III levels between 25 percent and 60 percent of normal. Because these levels sometimes overlap with the range of normal values, identification of affected persons can pose a diagnostic problem.

Inherited antithrombin III deficiency is now recognized as a heterogeneous disease [81]. Table 10-3 outlines the major types of antithrombin III deficiency. In the classic cases, deficiencies of similar proportions are found with both antigenic and functional assays of antithrombin III. These patients have a reduced synthesis of biologically normal antithrombin (type I antithrombin III deficiency). However, variants of antithrombin III deficiency have now been recognized in which normal immunologically determined levels of antithrombin are associated with a lowered functional level of the inhibitor. These patients (type II antithrombin III deficiency) have quantitatively normal production of a functionally defective molecule [82]. Patients with type II antithrombin III deficiency have a functional defect in either the heparin cofactor activity or both the heparin cofactor activity and the progressive protease inhibitor activity (in the absence of heparin) of the molecule. Clinical thrombosis is common in heterozygous subjects with type I disease or type II disease involving an active site defect, but it appears to be confined to homozygous subjects with type II disease who have only a heparin-binding site defect [71]. A more refined molecular classification of antithrombin III deficiencies also has been proposed [83]. A number of different mutant antithrombins have been isolated [84]. Molecular heterogeneity exists even among patients with phenotypically "classic" (type I) inherited antithrombin III deficiency; in some, deletion of a large segment of the gene is responsible for the disorder, whereas in others, small deletions, insertions, or single base substitutions have been found [85–90].

Since familial antithrombin III deficiency may be caused by functional or qualitative variants that do not lower the immunoreactive quantity of the protein in plasma, functional rather than immunologic assays should be used to screen for the deficiency state. Several complicating factors that may interfere with the clinical assay should be considered in the timing of the blood samples obtained for testing. In the acute phase of a massive thromboembolic event, plasma levels of antithrombin III (as well as other proteins involved in the physiologic anticoagulant systems, such as protein C) may be transiently lowered into the abnormal range in patients without congenital deficiency states. Therefore, although the finding of a normal functional level of antithrombin III during this acute period would exclude the diagnosis of antithrombin III deficiency, abnormally low levels cannot be considered diagnostic. Anticoagulation can also interfere with the assays for antithrombin III. Heparin may lower functional levels of the protein. Warfarin does not affect antithrombin III levels in most cases, but its use occasionally raises levels of antithrombin III into the normal range in congenitally deficient patients [91], thus potentially masking the diagnosis.

Acquired antithrombin III deficiency [92] may occur as a result of urinary excretion of the protein in patients with the nephrotic syndrome and may contribute to renal-vein thrombosis and other thromboembolic complications [93]. Decreased antithrombin III levels have also been noted in patients with advanced diseases of the liver (a major site of synthesis of the protein), in women using oral contraceptives [94], and in patients on L-asparaginase chemotherapy [95]. However, a causal relationship between acquired antithrombin III deficiency and thrombosis in these cases has not been clearly established.

Familial heparin cofactor II deficiency, inherited as an autosomal dominant trait, has been described in association with clinical thrombosis [96,97]. In the original cases reported, deficiency was due to decreased protein synthesis, with equivalent reductions in heparin cofactor II activities and antigenic concentrations.

Protein C and Protein S Deficiency. Inherited protein C deficiency [98,99,100] is transmitted as an autosomal trait. As is the case with antithrombin III deficiency, heterozygous patients may suffer from lifelong recurrent thrombosis. Homozygous protein C deficiency, characterized by complete or nearly complete absence of immunoreactive protein C in plasma, has been reported in association with massive and fatal neonatal thrombosis (purpura fulminans neonatalis) in infants born to consanguineous parents with heterozygous protein C deficiency [101,102]. Using a sensitive particle concentration fluorescence immunoassay, approximately 0.3 percent of a normal population screened has been found to be protein C deficient, although this report emphasized the difficulty in establishing clear quantitative criteria for the heterozygous deficiency state and the lack of predictability of thrombotic risk in deficient subjects [103]. While the vast majority of heterozygotes in the general population are asymptomatic [103], about 50 percent of heterozygotes belonging to families who do have a history of symptomatic thrombosis also can be expected to have thrombotic complications [104].

As with antithrombin III deficiency, functional variants of protein C deficiency have been reported. These patients have normal protein C antigen levels associated with subnormal protein C activity [105–108]. Patients with classic (type I) inherited protein C deficiency, who have quantitatively deficient synthesis of a qualitatively normal protein C molecule, most commonly have nonsense or missense point mutations in the protein C gene [109–112]. Specific mutations also have been reported in patients with functional defects of protein C (type II protein C deficiency) [113].

Acquired protein C deficiency has been found in patients with disseminated intravascular coagulation [114–116], as well as in other patients with a variety of acute illnesses [117]. As with acquired antithrombin III deficiency, in these clinical situations, transient depression of plasma levels of the protein presumably is due to rapid activation and clearance. Likewise, simultaneous depression of protein C and antithrombin III levels can occur due to the synthetic dysfunction of advanced liver disease [118]. One report has described a patient with an acquired inhibitor of protein C who died of purpura fulminans and disseminated intravascular coagulation [119].

Recent reports have shown that from 21 percent to 64 percent of patients with previously undiagnosed venous thrombophilia had a defect in the in vitro anticoagulant reponse to activated protein C [120–122]. In these patients, the impaired ability of activated protein C to prolong the activated partial thromboplastin time may reflect an inherited deficiency of an activated protein C cofactor [123], which has been recently isolated as an anticoagulant function of factor V [124].

Familial deficiency of protein S, the cofactor for protein Ca, also has been found to be associated with a hypercoagulable state [125,126] Testing of such patients [127] is complicated by the presence of two types of protein S in plasma: free protein S, which serves as the active cofactor for protein Ca, and protein S bound to the complement pathway inhibitor C4b-binding protein, which is inactive as an anticoagulant cofactor of protein Ca. Affected patients with protein S deficiency may have reduced levels of free protein S but normal levels of bound protein S [39,128].

Although heparin therapy does not generally interfere with clinical testing for protein C or protein S deficiency, the use of warfarin poses problems that are important to recognize. Since both protein C and protein S are vitamin K–dependent proteins, their plasma levels predictably are suppressed in nondeficient patients who are taking oral anticoagulants. To circumvent this problem, the simultaneous measurement of protein C or S and another vitamin K–dependent protein (e.g., prothrombin) should reveal a disproportionately low level of protein C or S in congenitally deficient patients [98].

Chronic warfarin therapy has been found to be clinically effective in preventing recurrent thrombosis in patients with protein C deficiency, even though use of this drug further suppresses congenitally low levels of the anticoagulant protein [98,99]. However, skin necrosis caused by cutaneous microvascular thrombosis may occasionally complicate the initiation of warfarin therapy in these patients [129,130]. The lesions, which initially tend to involve the lower extremities, abdominal wall, breast, or penis, can progress to fulminant hemorrhagic bullae and full-thickness skin infarctions [39]. Since protein C has a shorter half-life (about 6 hours) than most of the other vitamin K–dependent proteins, initiation of warfarin therapy may cause a temporary prothrombotic imbalance in congenitally protein C–deficient patients, leading to skin necrosis. In contrast, the long-term beneficial effects of warfarin in these patients are presumably due to the net antithrombotic effect of lowering levels of the vitamin K–dependent coagulation factors in spite of suppression of the protein C to below the congenitally deficient baseline level.

Fibrinolytic Disorders. A thrombotic tendency has been associated with several specific congenital and acquired abnormalities in the various components of the fibrinolytic system that lead to the impaired clearance of fibrin. Recurrent thrombosis caused by ineffective plasmin generation may be due to defective synthesis or release of plasminogen activator from the vasculature, presumably representing a primary dysfunction of endothelial cells [131], and quantitative [132] or qualitative [133] abnormalities of the plasminogen substrate for plasminogen activators. Molecular heterogeneity has been found among patients with functional plasminogen abnormalities predisposing to thrombosis [134]. Impaired plasminogen activation leading to thrombosis also can be due to the presence of circulating inhibitors of plasminogen activator [135] or pharmacologic inhibition with ε-aminocaproic acid or tranexamic acid [136].

Blunted fibrinolytic activity also has been a frequent finding in young survivors of myocardial infarction [137]. Subnormal t-PA activity measured in the blood of these patients following venous occlusion was found to be caused mainly by high levels of t-PA inhibitor and, to a lesser extent, by impaired t-PA release. The decreased fibrinolytic capacity in these cases correlated with elevations of serum triglycerides, a relationship that has been previously noted [138,139] but not clearly understood. Decreased fibrinolytic capacity caused by high plasma levels of t-PA inhibitor also has been found in patients with deep-vein thrombosis [140].

Dysfibrinogenemia. Although functional defects in fibrinogen activity are more frequently associated with a bleeding diathesis due to impaired fibrin formation, dysfibrinogenemias also have been found in occasional patients with a thrombotic tendency [141–146]. In some of these hypercoagulable states, the qualitatively defective fibrinogen molecule presumably forms fibrin gels that are abnormally rigid and resistant to the lytic effect of plasmin; in others, the mutant fibrinogen fails to bind thrombin normally, possibly leading to increased circulating thrombin.

Factor XII Deficiency. Patients with congenital deficiencies of the contact activation coagulation factors (factor XII, high-molecular-weight kininogen, and prekallikrein) characteristically have markedly prolonged partial thromboplastin times but a notable lack of apparent problems with hemostasis. The first patient described with factor XII (Hageman factor) deficiency actually died of pulmonary embolism [147]. Largely anecdotal and inconclusive evidence has now been reported that suggests that factor XII deficiency is, in fact, associated with a thrombotic rather than a bleeding tendency [148–151]. As noted, factor XII, high-molecular-weight kininogen, and prekallikrein are involved not only in the initiation of the intrinsic pathway of coagulation to promote hemostasis but also in the activation of the fibrinolytic system and the generation of vasodilator kinins, actions that promote blood fluidity. Therefore, depending on the balance of these conflicting actions, it is possible that congenital deficiency of a contact activation factor may cause a hypercoagulable state [152].

Treatment of the Primary Hypercoagulable States. The treatment and prophylactic management of thromboembolism with primary hypercoagulable states are controversial in some patients [153]. Asymptomatic individuals who are diagnosed in the course of family screening studies do not require chronic prophylactic oral anticoagulation. At the other end of the spectrum, patients with recurrent thromboembolic events should be committed to lifelong oral anticoagulant therapy. It has not been established whether the risks of recurrent thrombosis outweigh the risks of chronic anticoagulation in patients with primary hypercoagulable states who have suffered a single episode of thrombosis. Temporary prophylaxis should be considered in any patient with a primary hypercoagulable state, regardless of previous history of clinical thrombotic complications, who is exposed to a high-risk situation for thrombosis, for example, pregnancy, immobilization, or the postoperative setting. Treatment under those circumstances usually involves short-term prophylactic anticoagulation with warfarin or subcutaneous heparin. In patients with antithrombin III deficiency, replacement therapy with antithrombin III concentrate can be administered [154–157]. Purified protein C concentrate also has been used to treat homozygous protein C–deficient patients with neonatal purpura fulminans [158].

SECONDARY HYPERCOAGULABLE STATES

A wide variety of clinical conditions are known to be associated with an increased risk of thrombosis. In contrast to the primary hypercoagulable states, these second-

Table 10-4. Secondary hypercoagulable states

ABNORMALITIES OF COAGULATION AND FIBRINOLYSIS
Malignancy
Pregnancy
Use of oral contraceptives
Nephrotic syndrome
Lupus anticoagulant
ABNORMALITIES OF PLATELETS
Myeloproliferative disorders
Paroxysmal nocturnal hemoglobinuria (PNH)
Diabetes mellitus
Hyperlipidemia
Cushing's syndrome
Heparin-induced thrombocytopenia
ABNORMALITIES OF BLOOD VESSELS AND RHEOLOGY
Immobilization
"Effort" thrombosis
Postoperative state
Artificial surfaces
Vasculitis
Chronic obliterative arterial diseases
Homocystinuria
Hyperviscosity
Thrombotic thrombocytopenic purpura (TTP)

ary hypercoagulable states (Table 10-4) generally are acquired disorders with complex and incompletely defined pathophysiology [67]. Some acquired secondary hypercoagulable states may precipitate thrombotic complications when they develop in patients with preexisting congenital primary hypercoagulable states. The clinical importance of recognizing these associations lies in the possibility of eliminating or lowering the risk of thrombosis by treating the underlying systemic disorder.

Although the pathophysiologic basis of most secondary hypercoagulable states is complex and multifactorial, these conditions are categorized in Table 10-4 by currently recognized predominant mechanisms. In general, venous thrombosis develops more frequently in secondary hypercoagulable states caused predominantly by coagulation and fibrinolytic abnormalities, and arterial thrombosis develops more frequently in states caused by platelet or vascular abnormalities. However, both venous and arterial thromboembolic episodes may occur in any of these patients, and characteristic types of thrombosis may be associated with certain secondary hypercoagulable states.

Malignancy. The overall incidence of thrombosis in patients with malignancies is about 5 to 15 percent, but with some tumors, notably carcinoma of the pancreas, the incidence may be as high as 50 percent [159,160]. In addition to more commonly encountered deep-vein thrombosis of the lower extremities and pulmonary embolism, patients with malignancies may develop two characteristic types of thromboembolic complications. The syndrome of recurrent migratory superficial thrombophlebitis (Trousseau's syndrome) occurs typically in patients with pancreatic carcinoma and other mucin-secreting adenocarcinomas of the gastrointestinal tract [161] and may antedate by months or even years the clinical diagnosis of cancer. Unexplained migratory superficial thrombophlebitis should arouse suspicion of an underlying occult neoplastic disease. Nonbacterial thrombotic endocarditis (NBTE) occurs most commonly in patients with malignant tumors, particularly adenocarcinomas [162]. In patients with NBTE, arterial embolization from bland cardiac valve thrombi typically develops on damaged valves and leads to clinical manifestations of vascular insufficiency, ischemic necrosis of peripheral organs, and cerebral, coronary, splenic, or renal emboli.

In contrast to the established relation between known cancer and subsequent venous thromboembolism, the risk of occult malignancy in patients who present with venous thromboembolism has been unclear [163–167]. In a more recent prospective study of patients with idiopathic venous thrombosis (i.e., thrombosis not associated with another well-recognized risk factor), who were followed over a two-year period, a statistically significant association was found with the subsequent development of clinically overt cancer (cumulative incidence, 7.6%) [168]. The incidence of cancer in this latter study was particularly increased in patients with recurrent thrombosis. Nevertheless, the clinical implications of those findings remain unclear: it is not known if there is any benefit of early detection of cancer by extensive diagnostic testing in patients who present with venous thromboembolism [169].

Localized anatomic problems, such as tumor compression and venous stasis, may be important factors in precipitating thrombosis in cancer patients. However, complex systemic changes in the coagulation system also accompany malignancy in many cases [170,171]. A general activation of the clotting system characteristically develops, resulting in chronic disseminated intravascular coagulation (DIC) with secondary fibrinolysis [159,160,172–177]. The coagulopathies of patients with malignancies may range from the subclinical laboratory abnormalities of compensated or overcompensated DIC to intravascular coagulation with thrombosis to fulminant decompensated DIC with bleeding, depending on the delicate hemostatic balance between activation of coagulation, inhibition of coagulation, and clot lysis. Tumors may directly activate blood coagulation, as in certain human and animal tumors that elaborate a unique procoagulant cysteine protease to activate factor X directly [178], or acute promyelocytic leukemia, in which the leukemic cells release thromboplastic substances to activate the extrinsic pathway of coagulation [179,180]. Alternatively, tumor antigens may stimulate monocytes and macrophages to express procoagulant properties indirectly [160]. Certain chemotherapeutic agents used to treat cancer may actually contribute to the thrombotic tendency in these patients [181,182].

Pregnancy and Oral Contraceptives. The steep rise in the risk of thrombosis in the puerperium [183,184] increases with maternal age, parity, hypertension, eclampsia or preeclampsia, and cesarean section [185,186]. Venous compression and stasis caused by increased intra-abdominal pressure, hormonal relaxation of vascular smooth muscle, and altered blood rheologic properties are factors that may predispose to thromboembolism in pregnancy. Systemic coagulation changes develop progressively during the course of pregnancy and are characterized by increasing low-grade activation of intravascular coagulation [187]. Laboratory manifestations of this process include increasing plasma levels of factors VII, VIII, IX, X, and XII, particularly striking elevations of fibrinogen (approaching levels in late pregnancy that are double that of the non-pregnant state), and concomitant depletion of antithrombin III [188]. The hypercoagulability of pregnancy is further enhanced by a marked depression of fibrinolytic activity, which is promptly restored within an hour of delivery of the placenta [189], although more recent studies using specific assays of plasminogen activators and PA inhibitors suggest that alterations in the different components of the fibrinolytic system during pregnancy are more complex than originally thought [190]. This systemic activation of the coagulation system in pregnancy is probably initiated locally in the uteroplacental circulation and may occur as a physiologic mechanism for preparing the expectant mother for the hemostatic trauma of placental separation. However, the process also places the mother in a highly vulnerable position for thrombotic complications.

A significantly increased risk of mortality from cardiovascular disease has been established in women on oral contraceptives [185,191–193] Specific associations have been clearly shown between oral contraceptive use and increased risk of deep-vein thrombosis and pulmonary embolism [194–196], postoperative thrombosis [197], and cerebrovascular accidents, particularly thrombotic strokes in women with a history of migraine [198,199]. The relationship with coronary artery disease is not as clear [200], although it appears that oral contraceptives act synergistically with other cardiac risk factors [201,202]. The use of newer, low-dose estrogen combination pills reduces but does not eliminate the thrombotic risk [203], and progestogens also have been implicated in thrombogenesis [191]. Estrogens are likewise associated with an increased incidence of thromboembolism when they are used to prevent lactation [204] and to treat arterial disease [205] and prostate cancer in a dose-related manner [206]. The mechanism of estrogen-induced hypercoagulability is multifactorial, including alterations in blood flow, increased venous distensibility resulting in stasis [207], and increased blood viscosity [208] associated with impaired red-cell deformability [209]. Furthermore, estrogen dose- and time-dependent systemic activation of the coagulation system occurs as in late pregnancy [210–212], without the pregnancy-associated depression of the fibrinolytic response.

Nephrotic Syndrome. Patients with nephrotic syndrome are predisposed not only to renal-vein thrombosis but also to systemic thromboembolic complications [213,214]. No single cause of hypercoagulability in the nephrotic syndrome has been established. Urinary loss of antithrombin III may lead to acquired antithrombin III deficiency in some cases, but a causal relationship with thrombosis has been disputed [215,216]. Other possible pathophysiologic mechanisms include factor XII deficiency [217,218], high plasma levels of other coagulation factors, and abnormal fibrinolytic activity [216,219], platelet hyperreactivity [216,220], or other factors, such as the frequently accompanying hyperlipidemia. Hypoalbuminemia associated with hypertrophic gastropathy (Ménétrier's disease) is likewise complicated by thromboembolic problems [221].

Lupus Anticoagulant and Antiphospholipid Syndrome. The **lupus anticoagulant** is an immunoglobulin acquired by some patients with systemic lupus erythematosus, other autoimmune disorders, malignancies, and infections in response to certain drugs or spontaneously without apparent underlying disease. This antibody prolongs phospholipid-dependent coagulation reactions in vitro by binding to the phospholipid portion of the prothrombinase complex, thus causing prolongation of the activated partial thromboplastin time (aPTT) and sometimes also the prothrombin time (PT). Despite these abnormalities of coagulation tests, patients with the lupus anticoagulant rarely bleed excessively and may in fact be paradoxically at increased risk of thrombotic complications [222–227]

Other tests for antiphospholipid antibodies may be positive in patients with a lupus anticoagulant. These include anticardiolipin antibodies and a biologic false-positive test for syphilis utilizing the Venereal Disease Research Laboratories (VDRL) reagent. When any one or a combination of these antiphospholipid antibodies occurs in association with arterial or venous thrombosis, recurrent spontaneous abortions, or thrombocytopenia, the clinical disorder is referred to as the **antiphospholipid syndrome** [228]. The mechanism for the hypercoagulable state associated with the antiphospholipid syndrome is largely unknown. Possible mechanisms that have been proposed include decreased prostacyclin production [229], increased platelet activation and thromboxane A_2 synthesis [230], inhibition of the activation or function of protein C [231–235], and direct vascular immunoinjury [236,237]. None of these mechanisms, however, has been directly demonstrated to be pathogenetically linked to thrombosis in the antiphospholipid syndrome. An increased incidence of cardiac valvular lesions has been found in patients with antiphospholipid syndrome [238–243]. The valvular abnormalities include bland verrucous endocardial lesions (Libman-Sacks vegetations) that may be clinically asymptomatic or may cause valve dysfunction. These patients may be at increased risk of cerebral embolic events [244].

Although patients with antiphospholipid antibodies may develop a variety of thromboembolic problems, a striking association has been noted with recurrent first-trimester spontaneous abortions and second- or third-trimester fetal deaths [245–247]. In one series of 31 pregnancies in women with lupus anticoagulants, 30 resulted in spontaneous abortions or fetal deaths and only one in a live-born infant [246]. The placenta in these cases characteristically shows a decidual vasculopathy with extensive infarctions. Therapeutic modalities that have been attempted to improve the outcome of pregnancy, with varying degrees of success and morbidity, include aspirin [248,249], corticosteroids [248–250], subcutaneous heparin [249,251] and intravenous immune globulin [252].

Myeloproliferative Disorders and Paroxysmal Nocturnal Hemoglobinuria. Injury to the pluripotent hematopoietic stem cell of the bone marrow can lead to myeloproliferative disorders, including chronic myelogenous leukemia, polycythemia vera, myeloid metaplasia with or without myelofibrosis, and essential thrombocythemia. Paroxysmal nocturnal hemoglobinuria (PNH) is a related stem cell disorder. Although the clinical hematologic manifestations vary, all three bone marrow cell lines (leukocytes, erythrocytes, and platelets) are affected in these diseases. Major causes of morbidity and mortality in patients with these disorders are bleeding and, paradoxically, thrombosis [253–255]. Deep-vein thrombophlebitis and pulmonary embolism are commonly encountered thrombotic manifestations of these stem-cell diseases. However, three other specific syndromes of vascular occlusion are characteristically seen in patients with myeloproliferative disorders and PNH. These stem-cell diseases are the most frequently identified underlying conditions associated with hepatic-vein thrombosis (Budd-Chiari syndrome) [256]. In fact, it has been suggested that many patients with apparently idiopathic Budd-Chiari syndrome actually may have occult myeloproliferative disorders even in the absence of clinical hematologic manifestations [257]. The most characteristic clinical manifestation of small arterial vascular occlusion of the extremities in the myeloproliferative disorders is the syndrome of erythromelalgia [258,259], in which patients develop burning pain, redness, and warmth in one or more digits. Pulses in the large arteries remain easily palpable. Erythromelalgia results from inflammation, intimal proliferation, and platelet thrombosis of arterioles [260]. Digital ischemia syndromes caused by microvascular thrombosis sometimes progress to pregangrenous and gangrenous changes [261]. Thrombotic obstruction of the cerebral microcirculation may cause a variety of neurologic symptoms [262]. The arterial (digital and cerebrovascular) occlusive syndromes most frequently are seen in essential thrombocythemia, may be the initial manifestations of the myeloproliferative disorders, and are important to recognize since they may respond rapidly and dramatically to a lowering of the platelet count, treatment with aspirin, or both [253].

Several factors are involved in the pathogenesis of thrombosis in the myeloproliferative disorders and PNH. In patients with polycythemia vera, the increased whole-blood viscosity associated with erythrocytosis clearly is related to the thrombotic risk [263]. However, this cannot be the sole determinant of thrombosis, since only patients with extreme degrees of secondary polycythemia (e.g., in congenital cyanotic heart disease) are likewise at risk of thrombosis. The role of thrombocytosis in those disorders remains highly controversial [253]. In most cases, the level of the platelet count does not correlate with thromboembolic complications [264], and patients with secondary or reactive types of thrombocytosis generally are not considered to be prone to thrombosis. Qualitative defects in platelet function probably are more important than thrombocytosis in the development of hemostatic problems in these stem-cell diseases. A variety of morphologic and biochemical abnormalities of platelets have been described in the myeloproliferative disorders and PNH [253,265–275]. Functionally defective platelets in these patients presumably arise from megakaryocytes that share abnormalities with the bone marrow stem cell. However, none of the qualitative platelet defects has been specifically shown to cause a hypercoagulable state.

Diabetes Mellitus and Hyperlipidemia. Thrombosis has been considered to be a major component of the pathogensis of diabetic angiopathy [276]. The occlusive macrovascular and microvascular complications to which patients with **diabetes** are predisposed have been attributed in large part to platelet-vascular hyperreactivity. Multiple studies have demonstrated abnormal platelet function in diabetics [277]. Platelet aggregates characteristically are seen in microvascular thrombi [278,279], and laboratory evidence of in vivo platelet activation has been noted [280–282]. Platelet hyperaggregability in vitro is a frequent finding, which has been reported to be correlated with the degree of diabetic control [283–288]. Reduced platelet membrane fluidity [289] and altered cellular calcium and sodium transport [290] may be involved in the platelet hyperreactivity of diabetes. Unbalanced vascular prostacyclin-platelet thromboxane formation may contribute to these functional abnormalities, since diabetic vessels have been found to produce subnormal amounts of the antiplatelet vasodilator eicosanoid prostacyclin [13,14], and diabetic platelets produce increased amounts of the platelet-activating vasoconstrictor eicosanoid thromboxane A_2 (TXA_2) [291,292]. Nonenzymatic glycosylation of collagen in diabetic vessels, which increases platelet reactivity, may also contribute to these abnormalities [293]. A basic unresolved problem is whether the platelet-vascular hyperreactivity in diabetes mellitus is caused by a primary platelet or vascular defect. Furthermore, it is unclear if these abnormalities are directly related to glucose intolerance or other complicating problems, such as hyperlipidemia [288]. The hypercoagulable state of diabetes mellitus also may be associated with increased plasma levels of von Willebrand factor [294,295], impaired fibrinolysis [296–298], increased blood viscosity [299], and enhanced adhesion of red cells to vascular endothelium [300]. The pathogenesis of diabetic angiopathy is now recognized as involving complex interactions among abnormalities in hemostasis, red-blood-cell function, and lipoprotein metabolism [301].

Familial **type II hyperbetalipoproteinemia** is characterized by premature onset of atherosclerosis and increased morbidity and mortality from thrombosis. As in diabetes, in-vitro platelet hyperaggregability and increased production of TXA_2 have been found in this disorder [302–305]. This increased sensitivity of platelets to aggregating agents has been found to correlate with platelet membrane cholesterol content [305], and it can be reproduced by in-vitro cholesterol loading of normal platelets [304].

Patients with Cushing's syndrome or those receiving corticosteroid therapy have been found to have an increased risk of thromboembolic complications [306–308]. It is not clear if this is due directly to the hyperadrenocorticism or to associated problems such as diabetes and hypertension.

Heparin-Associated Thrombocytopenia and Thrombosis. Heparin can cause mild thrombocytopenia and affect platelet function directly by nonimmune mechanisms; however, this does not generally cause clinical problems. In contrast, antibody-mediated idiosyncratic heparin-associated thrombocytopenia apparently can be paradoxically associated with severe arterial or venous thromboembolic complications [309–313]. The reported frequency of heparin-associated thrombocytopenia varies considerably [310], and depends on a number of variables, including the clinical setting for administration of the anticoagulant and the preparation of the drug. The immune-mediated form of heparin-induced thrombocytopenia that may be associated with thrombosis is not dependent on the dose of heparin used: it can be initiated and sustained by small amounts of heparin used in prophylactic regimens, heparin flushes, or even heparin-coated central venous catheters.

The thrombotic complications associated with heparin therapy have been attributed primarily to intravascular platelet aggregation leading to the formation of microthrombi. More recently, sera from some patients with heparin-associated thrombocytopenia have been found to contain antibodies that react with heparin bound to vascular endothelial cells, suggesting that the seemingly paradoxical occurrence of thrombocytopenia and thrombosis in these cases may be due to concurrent immune injury to both platelets and endothelial cells [314].

Abnormalities of Blood Vessels and Rheology. **Prolonged immobilization** promotes the risk of thrombosis in a variety of clinical settings. A high incidence of thrombosis occurs in patients who are bedridden, immobilized before surgery, or paraplegic or hemiplegic, the last instance particularly involving the paralyzed leg [315–320]. Venous stasis in these situations may precipitate thrombosis by causing vascular endothelial damage through localized hypoxia [321] and by retarding the clearance of activated clotting factors from an area of vascular injury [322]. Vascular intimal damage has also been thought to be a contributory factor in the pathogenesis of axillary and subclavian venous thrombosis in otherwise healthy people who subject their upper extremities to repeated strenuous physical exertion (**''effort'' thrombosis**) [323–325]. The complication of **postoperative thromboembolism** depends on several factors, including underlying disease and independent individual risk factors, such as advanced age, heart disease, malignancy, obesity, pregnancy, use of oral contraceptives, previous history of thrombosis, and a coexisting primary hypercoagulable state. The type and duration of surgery is also an important variable: isotopically detected postoperative venous thrombosis occurs in approximately 70 percent of elderly patients with hip fractures, 50 percent of patients undergoing elective hip replacement, 30 percent of general-surgical patients, and 15 percent of gynecologic patients following hysterectomy for nonmalignant disease [326]. Although mechanical factors such as intraoperative tissue manipulation and immobilization probably contribute to the postoperative thrombotic tendency in those patients, reproducible systemic changes in coagulation have been difficult to demonstrate. Laboratory evidence of an imbalance between fibrin formation and fibrinolysis has been reported to antedate the development of clinical thrombosis in some patients undergoing neurosurgery [327].

Artificial materials exposed to circulating blood have a significant thrombogenic potential [328,329]. Platelet adhesion and aggregation invariably occur on exposure of blood to foreign surfaces, accompanied by activation of the coagulation system. The consequences are localized thrombosis and the risk of embolization of the fibrin-platelet masses when they are washed off by changes in the shear rate of blood. Localized and systemic thromboembolism may occur in various clinical settings, including hemodialysis, hemoperfusion, and cardiopulmonary bypass, and in patients with intra-aortic balloon-pumping devices, prosthetic heart valves, and vascular grafts and catheters [67].

In patients with cutaneous **vasculitis**, systemic lupus erythematosus, and scleroderma, an increased incidence of thrombosis has been attributed to inflammatory damage disrupting the normal antithrombotic properties of vascular endothelium: reduced fibrinolytic activity, impaired release of plasminogen activator, and systemic activation of the coagulation system have been reported in these disorders [330–334]. The hypercoagulable state in the subset of patients with antiphospholipid antibodies is discussed above. In patients with Kawasaki disease (mucocutaneous lymph node syndrome), acute vasculitis and perivasculitis of small blood vessels may progress to vascular fibrosis and thrombotic occlusions, leading to serious coronary, mesenteric, and digital vascular complications [335]. The most common thrombotic manifestations in patients with Behçet's disease are recurrent superficial and deep migratory thrombophlebitis. Phlebitis appearing at venipuncture sites may be characteristic. However, inferior and superior vena cava obstruction, Budd-Chiari syndrome, intracranial venous thrombosis, pulmonary artery thrombosis, and arterial thrombosis of the extremities also have been reported [336–341]. The predominant histopathologic lesion in Behçet's syndrome is vasculitis [342]. The hypercoagulable state of Behçet's disease is caused primarily by vascular endothelial dysfunction [343], and impaired fibrinolytic activity is found in many cases [343,344].

The **chronic obliterative arterial diseases** of the extremities include degenerative (atherosclerotic) and inflammatory (thromboangiitis obliterans, giant cell arteritis, Takayasu's disease) arteriopathies. These diseases are characterized by insidiously progressive symptoms of vascular insufficiency and occasional episodes of acute thromboembolism [345]. Thromboangiitis obliterans (Buerger's disease) is an inflammatory occlusive disease of the peripheral arteries and veins that typically affects young men who smoke heavily. Pathologically, segmental vasculitis combined with thrombosis results in vascular obliteration. Whether thrombosis or vasculitis is the primary process in this disease remains uncertain [346].

Predominantly arterial thrombosis (causing occlusive peripheral arterial, renovascular, cerebrovascular, and coronary artery disease), often occurring before or during the third decade of life, is a major cause of morbidity and mortality in patients with homozygous **homocystinuria** [347]. Furthermore, through use of a standardized methionine-loading test, heterozygous homocystinuria (which occurs in the normal population at a frequency of 1 in 70) also has been found to predispose to the development of premature occlusive arterial disease [348]. Heterozygosity for homocystinuria (hyperhomocysteinemia) has been considered to be an indepenent risk factor for vascular disease [349,350]. Young patients with homocystinuria may present with recurrent arterial thrombosis in the absence of any other clinical manifestations of the disease, such as mental retardation, ectopia lentis, or skeletal abnormalities [351]. Premature vascular occlusive disease has been thought to be initiated by sustained homocystine-induced vascular injury, which is characterized by patchy endothelial desquamation and intimal and medial fibrosis [352,353]. Vascular intimal damage and arterial thrombosis have been reproduced by homocystine infusion into experimental animals [353]. Increased platelet turnover, presumably due to damage or consumption of platelets in thrombi on the deendothelialized endarterial surfaces, has been shown in some [353] but not all [354] patients with homocystinuria. Homocysteine also may be atherogenic by promoting vascular smooth muscle cell–mediated auto-oxidation of low-density lipoprotein cholesterol [355], and thrombogenic by altering the thromboresistant properties of endothelial cells [356]. The intracellular transport of multiple endothelial-cell proteins may be altered in patients with homocystinuria [357]. Homocysteine also inhibits binding of t-PA to endothelial cells, thereby interfering with assembly of the fibrinolytic system on vascular surfaces and further promoting a prothrombotic state [358].

Hyperviscosity of blood can be caused by increased cell counts (as in polycythemia or leukemia), loss of blood-cell deformability, or increased concentrations of plasma proteins [359]. In certain situations, abnormal blood rheology can be directly implicated in the pathogenesis of thrombosis [360,361]. Uncontrolled polycythemia can cause thrombosis, particularly cerebrovascular accidents [362], and the elevated hematocrit correlates with reduced cerebral blood flow in patients with polycythemia vera [363] and secondary or relative polycythemia [364]. In some patients with polycythemia vera, coexisting abnormalities of platelet function undoubtedly contribute to the thrombotic risk. However, patients with extreme secondary polycythemia (e.g., congenital cyanotic heart disease) also are clearly at risk for thrombosis as a direct result of increased whole-blood viscosity [365]. The vaso-occlusive complications of sickle-cell disease are precipitated at least in part by abnormal rheology due to the sickled erythrocytes and their increased adhesiveness to vascular endothelium [366,367]. Unusually large von Willebrand factor multimers may preferentially mediate adhesion of sickle red cells to endothelial cells [368]. In some clinical situations, leukocytes also may be primarily involved in the thrombotic process. This occurs in some patients with acute or chronic leukemias, in whom microcirculatory occlusion can be caused by leukostasis, enhanced leukocyte-dependent procoagulant expression, and endothelial injury induced by activated leukocytes or by the hypoxia resulting from leukocyte oxygen consumption. Complement-stimulated granulocytes may cause pulmonary vascular leukostasis during hemodialysis using complement-activating dialyzer membranes [369] and in some forms of vasculitis [370].

Thrombotic Thrombocytopenic Purpura. Thrombotic thrombocytopenic purpura (TTP) is an acute or chronic relapsing disorder of probably diverse etiologies, which is characterized by thrombocytopenia and microangiopathic hemolytic anemia [371]. Neurologic, renal, and other systemic clinical manifestations are considered to be due to disseminated microvascular platelet thrombosis, typically not accompanied by activation of the coagulation system. A related thrombotic microangiopathy seen most commonly in children is the hemolytic uremic syndrome (HUS). Microthrombi-occluding arterioles and capillaries of different organs are characteristically found on pathologic examination. Based on experimental and clinical therapeutic information, the primary abnormality in TTP has been alternatively considered to reside in platelets, the blood vessel, or composition of plasma [372]. Evidence of endothelial damage includes the loss of fibrinolytic activity in diseased microvascular segments [373] and the finding of unusually large multimers of von Willebrand factor in the remission plasma of patients with chronic relapsing TTP [374,375]. Support for a plasma factor in the pathogenesis of TTP includes the frequent therapeutic response to plasma exchange [376], the experimental finding of loss of a plasma factor that stimulates vascular prostacyclin production [12], immune injury to endothelial cells [377,378], and the presence of a plasma platelet-agglutinating factor [379] in some cases.

Thrombotic microangiopathy resembling TTP has been described following chemotherapy with several antineoplastic agents, including mitomycin, cisplatin (in combination with bleomycin and vinca alkaloids), and combinations of asparaginase-vincristine-prednisone for childhood acute lymphoblastic leukemia and cytosine arabinoside-daunorubicin for acute myeloblastic leukemia. Patients may develop acute thrombosis or slowly progressive vascular occlusions. In many cases, this complication occurs in patients who are free of tumor, implicating the chemotherapeutic agents rather than the neoplasm itself in the pathogenesis of thrombosis [380–382].

Laboratory Tests of Hypercoagulability

The laboratory approach to the evaluation of hypercoagulability can be divided into two types of tests. First, a variety of markers of hemostatic activation have been developed that can detect ongoing subclinical thrombosis or hypercoagulability and provide some pathophysiologic clues by demonstrating which components of the hemostatic system have been involved. However, such tests cannot identify the specific cause of the hypercoagulable state. Second, laboratory tests can be directed at determining the specific nature of the thrombotic tendency by assessing the presence of one of the primary hypercoagulable states or an underlying systemic disorder that can cause a secondary hypercoagulable state. (A clinical approach to this type of laboratory evaluation is discussed in the next section.)

Traditionally, most clinical laboratory tests of hemostasis have been designed to evaluate bleeding, not thrombotic problems. It does not necessarily follow that, because a low platelet count, prolonged bleeding time, prolonged PT or aPTT often are associated with a hemorrhagic tendency, abnormalities in those tests in the opposite direction will be associated with hypercoagulability [383]. Furthermore, coagulation factors in their inert or zymogen form (as measured in the clinical laboratory) are present in normal plasma in great excess. Although severe deficiencies of coagulation factors may cause bleeding, higher-than-normal levels do not necessarily enhance coagulation. Several of the coagulation factors (e.g., factor VIII and fibrinogen) are acute-phase reactants, the levels of which increase in a variety of diseases. Therefore, elevations of plasma concentrations of these coagulation factors in patients with active thrombosis probably are secondary to the thrombosis or an underlying associated disease process (i.e., secondary hypercoagulable state). Nevertheless, it is interesting to note that increased plasma levels of fibrinogen [384,385], von Willebrand factor, and factor VIII:C [385] have been reported to be markers of risk for stroke and myocardial infarction, although a direct causal relationship with thrombogenesis in these situations remains entirely unclear.

A large array of tests that serve as markers of activation of various components of the hemostatic system (coagulation, fibrinolysis, and platelet and vascular reactivity) have been developed recently [386,387]. Although many of these assays are ingenious, most are flawed by a serious lack of sensitivity or specificity as well as potential sampling and technical artifacts. Despite their limitations, some of these tests are useful research tools to gain insight into basic pathophysiologic mechanisms of thrombosis in specific disorders. They also are of considerable clinical potential for the detection of hypercoagulable states in asymptomatic subjects and the monitoring of efficacy of antithrombotic therapy. Only some of the more widely used or more recently developed and promising assays are discussed here (Table 10-5).

When prothrombin interacts with factor Xa to generate thrombin, an inactive fragment called F_{1+2} is released. A sensitive and specific radioimmunoassay for F_{1+2} has been developed, the measurement of which in plasma quantitatively reflects the degree of systemic prothrombin activation [70]. The binding of antithrombin III to thrombin generated by this reaction results in the formation of circulating thrombin-antithrombin complexes (T-AT), which can also be measured by radioimmunoassay as an index of prothrombin activation [70]. The initial fibrin-generating action of free thrombin formed during activation of the coagulation system is to cleave fibrinopeptide A (FPA) from the aminoterminal end of the A-chain of fibrinogen. A commercially available radioimmunoassay for plasma FPA has been developed [388] that has proven to be a sensitive and specific marker for thrombin action and activation of the coagulation system [389]. Thrombin-induced activation of protein C results in the release of a specific activation peptide from the aminoterminus of the heavy chain. A radioimmunoassay for the protein C activation peptide (PCP) also has been developed [390]. Activated protein C can also be directly measured in blood by the use of immunoenzymatic methods [391,392].

Table 10-5. Laboratory markers of activation of hemostasis

ACTIVATION OF COAGULATION AND FIBRINOLYSIS
Fibrinopeptide A
F_{1+2} fragment
Thrombin-antithrombin complexes
Protein C activation peptide
Bβ related peptides
ACTIVATION OF PLATELETS
Platelet aggregation in vitro
Circulating platelet aggregates
Platelet-specific proteins
Platelet factor 4
β-thromboglobulin
Antibody binding to activated platelet membrane glycoproteins
In-vivo metabolites of TXA_2 and PGI_2

Measurements of F_{1+2}, T-AT, FPA, and PCP have been used to detect subclinical activation of the coagulation system in a variety of hypercoagulable states, and suppression of circulating levels of these markers of hemostatic activation provides sensitive assays for monitoring the efficacy of antithrombotic therapy. Furthermore, the finding of chronically elevated levels of F_{1+2} and FPA in asymptomatic patients with primary hypercoagulable states has provided evidence for a persistent state of hemostatic activation in these conditions [393]. In asymptomatic individuals with heterozygous protein C or protein S deficiency, the levels of F_{1+2} fragments are significantly increased in comparison to age-matched controls [394–396]. In subjects with heterozygous protein C deficiency, protein C activation (as measured by either PCP or the activated protein C assay) is reduced by about 50 percent [391,396]. The reduced indices of in-vivo protein C activation and the increased indices of in-vivo thrombin generation in protein C deficiency can be normalized by transfusion of protein C concentrate [397]. Similar studies in patients with antithrombin III deficiency have been more complicated to interpret. Initial observations of elevated F_{1+2} levels in asymptomatic heterozygotes with antithrombin III deficiency [398] were subsequently attributed to an in-vitro heparin anticoagulant effect [399]. Subsequent studies found either normal [394] or elevated plasmal levels of F_{1+2} [400] in antithrombin III–deficient individuals, although FPA levels were normal in those subjects [394,400].

The state of activation of the fibrinolytic system can be assessed by measurement of plasma levels of plasminogen, α_2-antiplasmin, and released t-PA and PAI, using both functional and immunologic assays. Plasmin formed during activation of the fibrinolytic system cleaves specific peptides from the B chains of fibrinogen or fibrin. The formation of these Bβ-related peptides of varying chain length (designated Bβ 1-42, Bβ 1-118, Bβ 15-42) can be detected by radioimmunoassays of plasma samples and represents a sensitive measure of subclinical activation of the fibrinolytic system [63,401]. By simultaneous assays of FPA and Bβ-related peptides, the relative contributions of coagulation and fibrinolysis can be determined in clinical situations involving complex hemostatic abnormalities.

Several methods have been developed to attempt to measure platelet activation in vivo. Each of these tests assesses a specific step in platelet activation (e.g., alterations in membrane glycoproteins, degranulation and release, prostanoid formation, aggregation), but no single general "marker" of in-vivo platelet activation is available. A relatively insensitive but widely used method is a test for the heightened reactivity of platelets to various agonists in vitro as an indication of in vivo platelet activation [402,403]. Different parameters of platelet-aggregation response have been applied to these studies, such as changes in the threshold concentration of agonists required to trigger aggregation. Another technique that has been used to measure in vivo platelet hyperreactivity is the detection of circulating platelet aggregates in paraformaldehyde-fixed specimens of peripheral blood [404]; blood-sampling techniques must be rigorously controlled for valid results to be obtained by this method [405–407].

The platelet-release reaction in vivo has been measured in blood samples by the use of radioimmunoassays of platelet factor 4 (PF4) and β-thromboglobulin (β-TG), two structurally closely related platelet-specific proteins that are secreted from granules [408–412]. Radioimmunoassays of PF4 and β-TG in plasma as indices of platelet activation in vivo are complicated by the possibility of artifactual in-vitro platelet release during venipuncture or processing of the blood specimen. Because PF4 is cleared from the circulation more rapidly than β-TG, possibly because of binding to vascular endothelial cells, it has been proposed that the finding of an increased ratio of plasma β-TG to PF4 in the same blood sample can distinguish in-vivo release from artifactual in-vitro release [409]. A more recent approach to detecting in-vivo platelet activation has used the binding of monoclonal antibodies to integral platelet-membrane proteins that become externally exposed only on activation and secretion of platelets [413,414]. Flow cytometry is used most often to detect activated platelets and platelet microparticles with this approach [415]. Although potentially less specific for platelets, the detection of alterations in platelet-surface glycoproteins directly with iodine-125-labeled monoclonal antibodies in fixed whole-blood samples can circumvent some problems of membrane alterations produced artifactually in vitro during platelet-isolation procedures [416,417]. With this method, different patterns of glycoprotein expression on intact platelet membranes and platelet-membrane microparticles have been found in different clinical platelet activation syndromes [417].

Radioimmunoassay of thromboxane B_2, the breakdown product of thromboxane A_2, has been used in blood samples as an index of in-vivo platelet activation associated with arachidonic-acid release and metabolism. Such measurements are susceptible to serious problems associated with invasive sampling, as are many of the previously noted markers of activation of coagulation and platelets. However, thromboxane biosynthesis can be assessed noninvasively by a specific and sensitive method of measurement of one of its major urinary enzymatic metabolites, 2,3-dinor-thromboxane B_2 [418,419], or its major plasma enzymatic metabolite, 11-dehydro-thromboxane B_2 [420]. Similarly, in-vivo prostacyclin formation can be determined by measurement of its urinary metabolite, 2,3-dinor-6-keto-prostaglandin F_1 [421]. Determinations of these in-vivo metabolites by gas chromatography–mass spectrometry have been applied to various clinical conditions associated with in-vivo platelet activation [422–425].

Pathogenesis of the Hypercoagulable States

Major advances in molecular genetics have begun to elucidate the relationship between the inherited predisposition to thrombosis and its clinical consequences [426]. The problem is well illustrated with inherited protein C deficiency [68]. The vast majority of individuals with heterozygous protein C deficiency, as well as the heterozygous parents of infants with homozygous protein C deficiency and neonatal purpura fulminans, are completely free of thrombotic complications. This suggests that protein C deficiency is an autosomal recessive disease. At the same time, a strong association has been found between heterozygous protein C deficiency and thrombosis among members of families with a clinical thrombotic diathesis. These observations would suggest that protein C deficiency is an autosomal dominant disease with high penetrance. The striking phenotypic variability of the primary hypercoagulable states strongly suggests that multigene interactions are operative. It has been proposed that an inherited predisposition to thrombosis results from combinations of prothrombotic mutations in two or more genes [426]. Thus, for example, heterozygous protein C deficiency by itself is considered only a risk factor for thrombosis; when it is combined with one or more additional prothrombotic mutations, however, it can have serious clinical consequences. In the future, direct sequencing strategies of a growing list of candidate genes for prothrombotic mutations should reveal how multigene interactions can generate a clinically significant hypercoagulable state.

An inherited predisposition to thrombosis, even when more than one mutation is involved, is probably insufficient to cause a clinical thrombotic event. As studies using markers of coagulation activation have suggested, patients with primary hypercoagulable states are at constant, lifelong risk of thrombosis. While patients with certain primary hypercoagulable states are thus continuously at risk for thrombosis throughout life, clinical thrombosis occurs episodically. This suggests that an acquired thrombogenic insult (e.g., one of the secondary hypercoagulable states) is the trigger that initiates a thrombotic event in a patient with a primary hypercoagulable state. In fact, clinical studies have suggested that predisposing events (e.g., pregnancy, surgery) can be identified in most cases of thrombosis in patients with primary hypercoagulable states [427]. Figure 10-5 depicts the concept that clinical thrombosis results from the unpropitious convergence of an inherited predisposition to thrombosis (hypercoagulability) [67,428,429] with an acquired thrombogenic stimulus.

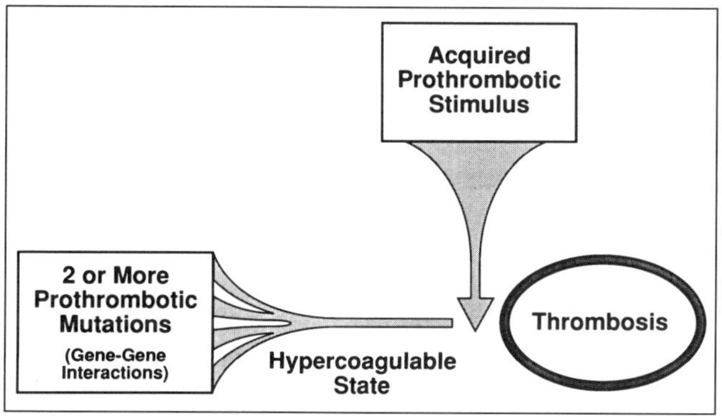

Fig. 10-5. A model of thrombogenesis. Multigene interactions involving prothrombotic mutations create an inherited predisposition to thrombosis (hypercoagulable state). In such patients, a thrombotic event is triggered by an acquired prothrombotic stimulus. (Reproduced with permission from AI Schafer. Hypercoagulable states: molecular genetics to clinical practice. Lancet 1994; 344:1739–1742.)

Clinical Approach to the Patient with a Hypercoagulable State

Although the laboratory tests discussed in the previous section may detect the presence of a hypercoagulable state, they cannot identify the specific cause of a thrombotic tendency. In the diagnostic approach to such patients, the various secondary and primary hypercoagulable states should be considered systematically.

The practical importance of identifying a systemic disorder causing a secondary hypercoagulable state lies in the possibility of improving the thrombotic tendency by treatment of the underlying disorder. Rather than indiscriminately exhaustive testing for each of the secondary hypercoagulable states listed in Table 10-4, individualized clinical judgment should direct the type and extent of such an evaluation. The clinical presentation of the patient may help to guide the search for an underlying disease. In general, patients with predominantly arterial thrombotic events are more likely to have platelet or vascular problems (e.g., myeloproliferative disorders, diabetes mellitus, hypercholesterolemia, homocystinuria), whereas in patients with primarily venous thrombosis a coagulation defect may be more likely. Furthermore, specific types of thrombotic events may provide important clues to the etiology. For example, a history of migratory superficial thrombophlebitis or NBTE suggests the presence of an occult malignancy. Patients presenting with the Budd-Chiari syndrome may be suspected of having a myeloproliferative disorder or paroxysmal nocturnal hemoglobinuria. Women with a history of habitual abortions should be evaluated for the lupus anticoagulant. Multiple arterial occlusions in a young person may indicate homocystinuria. Basic screening laboratory tests also can provide useful information. Thrombosis occurring in a patient with a prolonged aPTT would suggest the possibility of factor XII deficiency or a lupus anticoagulant. Thrombosis developing in the setting of a low platelet count may indicate TTP or heparin-induced thrombocytopenia.

After consideration of the secondary hypercoagulable states, clinical evaluation should focus on the possible diagnosis of a primary hypercoagulable state. It should be emphasized that identification of a secondary hypercoagulable state does not exclude the presence of a coexisting primary hypercoagulable state. In fact, as previously stressed, acquired disorders associated with secondary hypercoagulable states frequently supervene and precipitate thrombotic episodes in patients with underlying primary hypercoagulable states. Assays for many of the physiologic antithrombotic proteins, such as antithrombin III, protein C, and protein S, as well as activated protein C resistance, are becoming increasingly available in clinical coagulation laboratories. The timing of obtaining blood samples for these tests, the effect of concurrent use of anticoagulants, and the interpretation of the results should be critically considered. The decision to pursue the diagnosis of a primary hypercoagulable state through specialized research facilities is a matter of individual judgment. Several clinical features may indicate the presence of a primary hypercoagulable state. First, most of these patients develop venous rather than arterial thromboembolic complications. A strong family history of thrombosis is an important indicator of a congenital thrombotic tendency. Other clinical characteristics seen in patients with some primary hypercoagulable states include recurrent thrombosis without apparent precipitating factors, thrombosis occurring at unusual anatomic sites, thrombosis developing at an early age, and unusual resistance to conventional antithrombotic therapy. The practical importance of making the diagnosis of a specific primary hypercoagulable state includes the probable need for lifelong prophylactic anticoagulation in patients with previous recurrent thrombotic complications and the indication for family studies to identify asymptomatic affected relatives who should be vigilant for risk factors that might precipitate thrombosis.

References

1. Rosenberg RD, Rosenberg JS. Natural anticoagulant mechanisms. J Clin Invest 1984; 74:1–6.
2. Schafer AI. Focussing of the clot: normal and pathologic mechanisms. Ann Rev Med 1987; 38:211–220.
3. Schafer AI, Adelman B. Plasmin inhibition of platelet aggregation and of arachidonic acid metabolism. J Clin Invest 1985; 75:456–461.
4. Coller BS. Platelets and thrombolytic therapy. N Engl J Med 1990; 322:33–42.
5. Schafer AI, et al. Synergistic inhibition of platelet activation by plasmin and prostaglandin I_2. Blood 1987; 69:1504–1507.
6. Weksler BB. Prostacyclin. Prog Hemost Thromb 1982; 6:113–138.
7. Moncada S, Vane JR. Arachidonic acid metabolites and the interactions between platelets and blood-vessel walls. N Engl J Med 1979; 300:1142–1147.
8. Bunting S, et al. Arterial walls generate from prostaglandin endoperoxides a substance (prostaglandin X) which relaxes strips of mesenteric and coeliaca arteries and inhibits platelet aggregation. Prostaglandins 1976; 12:897–913.
9. Marcus AJ, et al. Synthesis of prostacyclin from platelet-derived endoperoxides by cultured human endothelial cells. J Clin Invest 1980; 66:979–986.
10. Schafer AI, Crawford DD, Gimbrone MA, Jr. Unidirectional transfer of prostaglandin endoperoxides between platelets and endothelial cells. J Clin Invest 1984; 73:1105–1112.

11. Pareti FI, et al. Congenital deficiency of thromboxane and prostacyclin. Lancet 1980; 1:898–900.
12. Remuzzi G, et al. Prostacyclin and thrombotic microangiopathy. Semin Thromb Hemost 1980; 6:391–394.
13. Silberbauer K, et al. Decreased vascular prostacyclin in juvenile-onset diabetes (Letter). N Engl J Med 1979; 300:366–367.
14. Harrison HE, Reece AH, Johnson M. Effect of insulin treatment on prostacyclin in experimental diabetes. Diabetologia 1980; 18:65–68.
15. Carreras LO, Vermylen JG. "Lupus" anticoagulant and thrombosis—possible role of inhibition of prostacyclin formation. Thromb Haemost 1982; 48:33–40.
16. Palmer RMJ, Ferrigo AG, Moncada S. Nitric oxide release accounts for the biological activity of endothelium-derived relaxing factor. Nature (London) 1987; 327:524–525.
17. Furchgott RF, Vanhoutte PM. Endothelium-derived relaxing and contracting factors. FASEB J 1989; 3:2007–2018.
18. Macdonald PS, Read MA, Dusting GJ. Synergistic inhibition of platelet aggregation by endothelium-derived relaxing factor and prostacyclin. Thromb Res 1988; 49:437–449.
19. Ludmer PL, et al. Paradoxical vasoconstriction induced by acetylcholine in atherosclerotic coronary arteries. N Engl J Med 1986; 315:1046–1051.
20. Harrison DG, et al. Restoration of endothelium-dependent relaxation by dietary treatment of atherosclerosis. J Clin Invest 1987; 80:1808–1811.
21. Bossaller C, et al. Impaired muscarinic endothelium-dependent relaxation and cyclic guanosine 5′-monophosphate formation in atherosclerotic human coronary artery and rabbit aorta. J Clin Invest 1987; 79:170–174.
22. Cohen RA, et al. Loss of selective endothelial cell vasoactive functions caused by hypercholesterolemia in pig coronary arteries. Circ Res 1988; 63:903–910.
23. Werns SW, et al. Evidence of endothelial dysfunction in angiographically normal coronary arteries of patients with coronary artery disease. Circulation 1989; 79:287–291.
24. Osborne J, et al. Cardiovascular effects of acute hypercholesterolemia in rabbits—reversal with lovastatin treatment. J Clin Invest 1990; 83:465–473.
25. Creager MA, et al. Impaired vasodilation of forearm resistance vessels in hypercholesterolemic humans. J Clin Invest 1990; 86:228–234.
26. Treasure CB, et al. Loss of the coronary microvascular response to acetylcholine in cardiac transplant patients. Circulation 1992; 86:1156–1164.
27. Treasure CB, et al. Hypertension and left ventricular hypertrophy are associated with impaired endothelium-dependent relaxation in the human coronary resistance vessels. Circulation 1993; 87:86–93.
28. Briner VA, Luscher TF. Role of vascular endothelial abnormalities in clinical medicine: atherosclerosis, hypertension, diabetes, and endotoxemia. Adv Intern Med 1994; 39:1–22.
29. Lowenstein CJ, Dinerman JL, Snyder SH. Nitric oxide: a physiologic messenger. Ann Intern Med 1994; 120:227–237.
30. Marcus AJ, et al. Inhibition of platelet function by an aspirin-insensitive endothelial cell ADPase. Thromboregulation by endothelial cells. J Clin Invest 1991; 88:1690–1696.
31. Slakey LL, Gordon EL, Pearson JD. A comparison of ecto-nucleotidase activities on vascular endothelial and smooth muscle cells. Ann NY Acad Sci 1990; 603:366–379.
32. Boeynaems JM, Pearson JD. P2 purinoceptors on vascular endothelial cells: physiological significance and transduction mechanisms. Trends Pharmacol Sci 1990; 11:34–37.
33. Yagi K, et al. ATP disphosphohydrolase is responsible for ecto-ATPase and ecto-ADPase activities in bovine aorta endothelial and smooth muscle cells. Biochem Biophys Res Commun 1991; 180:1200–1206.
34. Rosenberg RD, Damus PS. The purification and mechanism of action of human antithrombin-heparin cofactor. J Biol Chem 1973; 248:6490–6505.
35. Bjork I, Nordenman B. Acceleration of the reaction between thrombin and antithrombin III by non-stoichiometric amounts of heparin. Eur J Biochem 1976; 68:507–511.
36. Marcum JA, et al. Microvascular heparinlike species with anticoagulant activity. Am J Physiol 1983; 245:H725–733.
37. Marcum JA, McKenney JB, Rosenberg RD. Acceleration of thrombin-antithrombin complex formation in rat hindquarters via heparinlike molecules bound to the endothelium. J Clin Invest 1984; 74:341–350.
38. Tollefsen DM, Majerus PW, Blank MK. Heparin cofactor II. Purification of a heparin-dependent inhibitor of thrombin in human plasma. J Biol Chem 1982; 257:2162–2169.
39. Clouse LH, Comp PC. The regulation of hemostasis: the protein C system. N Engl J Med 1986; 314:1298–1304.
40. Esmon CT, Owen WG. Identification of an endothelial cell cofactor for thrombin-catalyzed activation of protein C. Proc Natl Acad Sci USA 1981; 78:2249–2252.
41. Esmon NL, Owen WG, Esmon CT. Isolation of a membrane-bound cofactor for thrombin-catalyzed activation of protein C. J Biol Chem 1982; 257:859–864.
42. Esmon CT, Esmon NL, Harris KW. Complex formation between thrombin and thrombomodulin inhibits both thrombin-catalyzed fibrin formation and factor V activation. J Biol Chem 1982; 257:7944–7947.
43. Marlar RA, Kleiss AJ, Griffin JH. Mechanism of action of human activated protein C, a thrombin-dependent anticoagulant enzyme. Blood 1982; 59:1067–1072.
44. Comp PC, Esmon CT. Generation of fibrinolytic activity by infusion of activated protein C into dogs. J Clin Invest 1981; 68:1221–1228.
45. van Hinsbergh VWM, et al. Activated protein C decreases plasminogen activator-inhibitor activity in endothelial cell-conditioned medium. Blood 1985; 65:444–451.
46. Sakata Y, et al. Mechanism of protein C-dependent clot lysis: role of plasminogen activator inhibitor. Blood 1986; 68:1218–1223.
47. Colucci M, Stassen JM, Collen D. Influence of protein C activation on blood coagulation and fibrinolysis in squirrel monkeys. J Clin Invest 1984; 74:200–204.
48. Di Scipio RG, et al. A comparison of human prothrombin, factor IX (Christmas factor), factor X (Stuart factor), and protein S. Biochemistry 1977; 16:698–706.
49. Walker FJ. Regulation of activated protein C by a new protein: a possible function for bovine protein S. J Biol Chem 1980; 255:5521–5524.
50. Walker FJ. Regulation of activated protein C by protein S: the role of phospholipid in factor Va inactivation. J Biol Chem 1981; 256:11128–11131.
51. Novotny WF, et al. Purification and characterization of the lipoprotein-associated coagulation inhibitor from human plasma. J Biol Chem 1989; 264:18832–18839.
52. Rapaport SI. Inhibition of factor VIIa / tissue factor-induced blood coagulation: with particular emphasis upon a factor Xa-dependent inhibitory mechanism. Blood 1989; 73:359.
53. Collen D. On the regulation and control of fibrinolysis. Thromb Haemost 1980; 43:77–89.
54. Aoki N, Harpel PC. Inhibitors of the fibrinolytic enzyme system. Semin Thromb Hemost 1984; 10:24–41.
55. Bachman F, Kruithof EKO. Tissue plasminogen activator: chemical and physiological aspects. Semin Thromb Hemost 1984; 10:6–17.
56. Edlund T, et al. Isolation of cDNA sequences coding for a part of human tissue plasminogen activator. Proc Natl Acad Sci USA 1983; 80:349–352.

57. Pennica D, et al. Cloning and expression of human tissue-type plasminogen activator cDNA in *E. coli.* Nature 1983; 301:214–221.
58. Verde P, et al. Identification and primary sequence of an unspliced human urokinase poly (A)+RNA. Proc Natl Acad Sci USA 1984; 81:4727–4731.
59. Dosne AM, Dupuy E, Bodevin E. Production of a fibrinolytic inhibitor by cultured endothelial cells derived from human umbilical vein. Thromb Res 1978; 12:377–387.
60. Levin EG. Latent tissue plasminogen activator produced by human endothelial cells in culture: evidence for an enzyme-inhibitor complex. Proc Natl Acad Sci USA 1983; 80:6804–6808.
61. Loskutoff DJ, et al. Detection of an unusually stable fibrinolytic inhibitor produced by bovine endothelial cells. Proc Natl Acad Sci USA 1983; 80:2956–2960.
62. Erickson LA, et al. The fibrinolytic system of the vascular wall. Clin Haematol 1985; 14:513–530.
63. Nossel HL. Reactive proteolysis of the fibrinogen B-β chain by thrombin and plasmin as a determinant of thrombosis. Nature 1981; 291:165.
64. Moroi M, Aoki N. Isolation and characterization of alpha 2-plasmin inhibitor from human plasma. A novel proteinase inhibitor which inhibits activated-induced clot lysis. J Biol Chem 1976; 251:5956–5965.
65. Mullertz S, Clemmensen I. The primary inhibitor of plasmin in human plasma. Biochem J 1976; 159:545–553.
66. Wiman B, Collen D. Purification and characterization of human antiplasmin, the fast-acting plasmin inhibitor in plasma. Eur J Biochem 1977; 78:19–26.
67. Schafer AI. The hypercoagulable states. Ann Intern Med 1985; 102:814–828.
68. Schafer AI. Hypercoagulable states: molecular genetics to clinical practice. Lancet 1994; 344:1739–1742.
69. Bauer KA. Elevated factor Xa activity in the blood of asymptomatic patients with congenital antithrombin deficiency. J Clin Invest 1985; 76:826–836.
70. Rosenberg RD, Bauer KA. New insights into hypercoagulable states. Hosp Pract 1986; 21:131–147.
71. Hirsh J. Congenital antithrombin III deficiency. Incidence and clinical features. Am J Med 1989; 87[Suppl 3B]:34S–38S.
72. Heijboer H, et al. Deficiencies of coagulation-inhibiting and fibrinolytic proteins in outpatients with deep-vein thrombosis. N Engl J Med 1990; 323:1512–1516.
73. Schafer AI, Kroll MH. Nonatheromatous arterial thrombosis. Annu Rev Med 1993; 44:155–170.
74. Lechat P, et al. Prevalence of patent foramen ovale in patients with stroke. N Engl J Med 1988; 318:1148–1152.
75. Winter JH, et al. Familial antithrombin III deficiency. Q J Med 1982; 51:373–395.
76. Rosenberg RD. Actions and interactions of antithrombin and heparin. N Engl J Med 1975; 292:146–151.
77. Meade TW, et al. Antithrombin III and procoagulant activity; sex differences and effects of the menopause. Br J Haematol 1990; 74:77–81.
78. Tait RC, et al. Antithrombin III activity in healthy blood donors: age and sex related changes and the prevalence of asymptomatic deficiency (Letter). Br J Haematol 1990; 75:141–142.
79. Egeberg O. Inherited antithrombin deficiency causing thrombophilia. Thromb Diath Haemorrh 1965; 13:516–530.
80. Thaler E, Lechner K. Antithrombin III deficiency and thromboembolism. Clin Haematol 1981; 10:369–390.
81. Lane DA, et al. Antithrombin III: a database of mutations. Thromb Haemost 1991; 66:657–661.
82. Sas G, et al. Abnormal antithrombin III (antithrombin III "Budapest") as a cause of a familial thrombophilia. Thromb Diath Haemorrh 1974; 32:105–115.
83. Prochownik EV. Molecular genetics of inherited antithrombin III deficiencies. Am J Med 1989; 87[Suppl 3B]:15S–18S.
84. Bauer KA, et al. Antithrombin "Chicago": a functionally abnormal molecule with increased heparin affinity causing familial thrombophilia. Blood 1983; 62:1242–1250.
85. Prochownik EV, et al. Molecular heterogeneity of inherited antithrombin III deficiency. N Engl J Med 1983; 308:1549–1552.
86. Bock SC, Prochownik EV. Molecular genetic survey of 16 kindreds with hereditary antithrombin III deficiency. Blood 1987; 70:1273–1278.
87. Olds RJ, et al. A frameshift mutation leading to type I antithrombin deficiency and thrombosis. Blood 1990; 76:2182–2186.
88. Gandrille S, et al. Molecular basis for hereditary antithrombin III quantitative deficiencies: a stop codon in exon IIIa and a frameshift in exon VI. Br J Haematol 1991; 78:414–420.
89. Grundy CB, et al. Recurrent deletion in the human antithrombin III gene. Blood 1991; 78:1027–1032.
90. Daly M, et al. Insertions/deletions in the antithrombin gene: 3 mutations associated with non-expression. Thromb Haemost 1992; 67:521–525.
91. Marciniak E, Farley CH, DeSimone PA. Familial thrombosis due to antithrombin III deficiency. Blood 1974; 43:219–231.
92. Hathaway WE. Clinical aspects of antithrombin III deficiency. Semin Hematol 1991; 28:19–23.
93. Lieberman E, et al. Thrombosis, nephrosis and corticosteroid therapy. J Pediatr 1968; 73:320–328.
94. Conard J, Samama M, Salomon Y. Antithrombin III and the estrogen content of combined estro-progestagen contraceptives. Lancet 1972; 2:1148–1149.
95. Conard J, et al. L-asparaginase, antithrombin III and thrombosis (Letter). Lancet 1980; 1:1091.
96. Tran TH, Marbet GA, Duckert F. Association of hereditary heparin co-factor II deficiency with thrombosis. Lancet 1985; 2:413–414.
97. Sie P, et al. Constitutional heparin co-factor II deficiency associated with recurrent thrombosis. Lancet 1985; 2: 414–416.
98. Griffin JH, et al. Deficiency of protein C in congenital thrombotic disease. J Clin Invest 1981; 68:1370–1373.
99. Broekmans AW, Veltkamp JJ, Bertina RM. Congenital protein C deficiency and venous thromboembolism: a study of three Dutch families. N Engl J Med 1983; 309:340–344.
100. Marciniak E, Wilson HD, Marlar RA. Neonatal purpura fulminans: a genetic disorder related to the absence of protein C in blood. Blood 1985; 65:15–20.
101. Branson HE, et al. Inherited protein C deficiency and coumarin-responsive chronic relapsing purpura fulminans in a newborn infant. Lancet 1983; 2:1165–1168.
102. Seligsohn U, et al. Homozygous protein C deficiency manifested by massive venous thrombosis in the newborn. N Engl J Med 1984; 310:559–562.
103. Miletich JP, Sherman L, Broze G, Jr. Absence of thrombosis in subjects with heterozygous protein C deficiency. N Engl J Med 1987; 317:991–996.
104. Allaart CF, et al. Increased risk of venous thrombosis in carriers of hereditary protein C deficiency defect. Lancet 1993; 341:134–138.
105. Comp PC, Nixon RR, Esmon CT. Determination of functional levels of protein C, an antithrombotic protein, using thrombin-thrombomodulin complex. Blood 1984; 63:15–21.
106. Barbui T, et al. Hereditary dysfunctional protein C (protein C Bergamo) and thrombosis. Lancet 1984; 2:819.
107. Bertina RM, et al. The use of a functional and immunologic

assay for plasm protein C in the study of the heterogeneity of congenital protein C deficiency. Thromb Haemost 1984; 51:1–5.
108. Miletich JP. Laboratory diagnosis of protein C deficiency. Semin Thromb Hemostas 1990; 16:169–176.
109. Reistma PH, et al. Protein C deficiency: a database of mutations. Thromb Haemost 1993; 69:77–84.
110. Romeo G, et al. Hereditary thrombophilia: identification of nonsense and missense mutations in the protein C gene. Proc Natl Acad Sci USA 1987; 84:2829–2832.
111. Grundy C, et al. Protein C deficiency and thromboembolism: recurrent mutation at Arg 306 in the protein C gene. Hum Genet 1992; 88:586–588.
112. Yamamoto K, et al. Impaired secretion of the elongated mutant of protein C (protein C-Nagoya). J Clin Invest 1992; 90:2439–2446.
113. Bovill E, et al. Protein $C_{Vermont}$: symptomatic type II protein C deficiency associated with two GLA domain mutations. Blood 1992; 79:1456–1465.
114. Griffin JH, et al. Protein C, an antithrombotic protein, is reduced in hospitalized patients with intravascular coagulation. Blood 1982; 60:261–264.
115. Mannucci PM, Vigano S. Deficiencies of protein C, an inhibitor of blood coagulation. Lancet 1982; 2:463–467.
116. Marlar RA, Endres-Brooks J, Miller C. Serial studies of protein C and its plasma inhibitor in patients with disseminated intravascular coagulation. Blood 1985; 66:59–63.
117. Sheth S, Cavalho A. Protein S and C alterations in acutely ill patients. Am J Hematol 1991; 36:14–19.
118. Rodeghiero F, et al. Liver dysfunction rather than intravascular coagulation as the main cause of low protein C and antithrombin III in acute leukemia. Blood 1984; 63:965–969.
119. Mitchell C, et al. A fatal thrombotic disorder associated with an acquired inhibitor of protein C. N Engl J Med 1987; 317:1638–1642.
120. Griffin JH, et al. Anticoagulant protein C pathway defective in majority of thrombophilic patients. Blood 1993; 82:1989–1993.
121. Koster T, et al. Venous thrombosis due to poor anticoagulant response to activated protein C: Leiden Thrombophilia Study. Lancet 1993; 342:1503–1506.
122. Svensson PJ, Dahlback B. Resistance to activated protein C as a basis for venous thrombosis. N Engl J Med 1994; 330:517–522.
123. Dahlback B, Carlsson M, Svensson PJ. Familial thrombophilia due to a previously unrecognized mechanism characterized by poor anticoagulant response to activated protein C: Prediction of a cofactor to activated protein C. Proc Natl Acad Sci USA 1993; 90:1004–1008.
124. Dahlback B, Hildebrand B. Inherited resistance to activated protein C is corrected by anticoagulant cofactor activity found to be a property of factor V. Proc Natl Acad Sci USA 1994; 91:1396–1400.
125. Comp PC, Esmon CT. Recurrent venous thromboembolism in patients with a partial deficiency of protein S. N Engl J Med 1984; 311:1525–1528.
126. Schwarz HP, et al. Plasma protein S deficiency in familial thrombotic disease. Blood 1984; 64:1297–1300.
127. Edson JR, Vogt JM, Huesman DA. Laboratory diagnosis of inherited protein S deficiency. Am J Clin Pathol 1990; 94:176–186.
128. Comp PC, et al. Familial protein S deficiency is associated with recurrent thrombosis. J Clin Invest 1984; 74:2082–2088.
129. Broekmans AW, et al. Protein C and the development of skin necrosis during anticoagulant therapy. Thromb Haemost 1983; 49:251.
130. McGehee WG, et al. Coumarin necrosis associated with hereditary protein C deficiency. Ann Intern Med 1984; 101:59–60.
131. Stead NW, et al. Venous thrombosis in a family with defective release of vascular plasminogen activator and elevated plasma factor VIII/von Willebrand's factor. Am J Med 1983; 74:33–39.
132. Lottenberg R, Dolly FE, Kitches CS. Recurring thromboembolic disease and pulmonary hypertension associated with severe hypoplasminogenemia. Am J Hematol 1985; 19:181–193.
133. Aoki N, et al. Abnormal plasminogen: a hereditary molecular abnormality found in a patient with recurrent thrombosis. J Clin Invest 1978; 61:1186–1195.
134. Ichinose A, et al. Two types of abnormal genes for plasminogen in families with a predisposition for thrombosis. Proc Natl Acad Sci USA 1991; 88:115–119.
135. Nilsson IM, et al. Severe thrombotic disease in a young man with bone marrow and skeletal changes and with a high content of an inhibitor in the fibrinolytic system. Acta Med Scand 1961; 169:323–337.
136. Naeye RL. Thrombotic state after a hemorrhagic diathesis, a possible complication of therapy with epsilon-aminocaproic acid. Blood 1962; 19:694–701.
137. Hamsten A, et al. Increased plasma levels of a rapid inhibitor of tissue plasminogen activator in young survivors of myocardial infarction. N Engl J Med 1985; 25:1557–1563.
138. Epstein SE, et al. Impaired fibrinolytic response to exercise in patients with type-IV hyperlipoproteinaemia. Lancet 1970; 2:631–634.
139. Simpson HCR, et al. Hypertriglyceridaemia and hypercoagulability. Lancet 1983; 1:786–789.
140. Wiman B, et al. The role of the fibrinolytic system in deep vein thrombosis. J Lab Clin Med 1985; 105:265–270.
141. Egeberg O. Inherited fibrinogen abnormality causing thrombophilia. Thromb Diath Haemorrh 1967; 17:176–187.
142. Al-Mondhiry HAB, Bilezikian SB, Nossel HL. Fibrinogen "New York"—an abnormal fibrinogen associated with thromboembolism: functional evaluation. Blood 1975; 45:607–619.
143. Carrell N, et al. Hereditary dysfibrinogenemia in a patient with thrombotic disease. Blood 1983; 62:439–447.
144. Engesser L, et al. Fibrinogen Nijmegeh: congenital dysfibrinogenemia associated with impaired t-PA mediated plasminogen activation and decreased binding of t-PA. Thromb Haemostas 1988; 60:113–120.
145. Koopman J, et al. The molecular basis of fibrinogen Naples associated with defective -thrombin binding and congenital thrombophilia: homozygous substitution of B 68 Ala-Thr. Thromb Haemost 1991; 65:809.
146. Koopman J, et al. Molecular basis for fibrinogen Dusart (A arg cys) and its association with abnormal fibrinogen polymerization and thrombophilia. J Clin Invest 1993; 1637–1643.
147. Ratnoff OD, Burse RJ, Sheon RP. The demise of John Hageman. N Engl J Med 1968; 279:760–761.
148. Aznar J, Fernandez Pavon A. Thromboembolic accidents in patients with congenital deficiency of factor XII. Thromb Diath Haemorrh 1974; 31:525–526.
149. Goodnough LT, Saito H, Ratnoff OD. Thrombosis or myocardial infarction in congenital clotting factor abnormalities and chronic thrombocytopenias: a report of 21 patients and a review of 50 previously reported cases. Medicine (Baltimore) 1983; 62:248–255.
150. Samlaska CP, James WD, Simel DL. Superficial migratory thrombophlebitis and factor XII deficiency. J Am Acad Dermatol 1990; 22:939.
151. Lammle B, et al. Thromboembolism and bleeding tendency

in congenital factor XII deficiency—a study of 74 subjects from 14 Swiss families. Thromb Haemost 1991; 65:117–121.
152. Hedner U, Nilsson IM. The role of fibrinolysis. Clin Haematol 1981; 10:327–342.
153. Bauer KA. Hypercoagulability—a new cofactor in the protein C anticoagulant pathway. N Engl J Med. 1994; 330: 566–567.
154. Menache D. Replacement therapy in patients with hereditary antithrombin III deficiency. Semin Hematol 1991; 28:31–38.
155. Owen J. Antithrombin III replacement therapy in pregnancy. Semin Hematol 1991; 28:46–52.
156. Francis CW, et al. Prophylaxis of venous thrombosis following total hip and total knee replacement using antithrombin III and heparin. Semin Hematol 1991; 28:39–45.
157. Menache D, et al. Evaluation of the safety, recovery, half-life and clinical efficacy of antithrombin III (human) in patients with hereditary antithrombin III deficiency. Blood 1990; 75:33–39.
158. Dreyfus M, et al. Treatment of homozygous protein C deficiency and neonatal purpura fulminans with a purified protein C concentrate. N Engl J Med 1991; 325:1565–1568.
159. Bick RL. Alterations of hemostasis associated with malignancy. Semin Thromb Hemost 1978; 5:1–26.
160. Rickles FR, Edwards RL. Activation of blood coagulation in cancer: Trousseau's syndrome revisited. Blood 1983; 62: 14–31.
161. Trousseau A. Phlegmasia alba dolens. Clin Med Hotel Dieu de Paris 1865; 3:94.
162. Deppisch LM, Fayemi AO. Non-bacterial thrombotic endocarditis: clinicopathologic correlations. Am Heart J 1976; 92:723–729.
163. Gore JM, et al. Occult cancer in patients with deep vein thrombosis. Ann Intern Med 1982; 96:556–560.
164. Goldberg RJ, et al. Occult malignant neoplasm in patients with deep venous thrombosis. Arch Intern Med 1987; 147:251–253.
165. Aderka D, et al. Idiopathic deep vein thrombosis in an apparently healthy patient as a premonitory sign of occult cancer. Cancer 1986; 57:1846–1849.
166. Griffin MR, et al. Deep venous thrombosis and pulmonary embolism: risk of subsequent malignant neoplasm. Arch Intern Med 1987; 147:1907–1911.
167. Monreal M, et al. Occult cancer in patients with venous thrombosis: a systematic approach. Cancer 1991; 67:541–545.
168. Prandoni P, et al. Deep-vein thrombosis and the incidence of subsequent symptomatic cancer. N Engl J Med 1992; 327:1128–1133.
169. Silverstein RL, Nachman RL. Cancer and clotting—Trousseau's warning (Editorial). N Engl J Med 1992; 327:1163–1164.
170. Luzzatto G, Schafer AI. The prethrombotic state in cancer. Semin Oncol 1990; 17:147–159.
171. Patterson WP, Ringenberg QS. The pathophysiology in cancer. Semin Oncol 1990; 17:140–146.
172. Sack GH, Jr, Levin J, Bell WR. Trousseau's syndrome and other manifestations of chronic disseminated coagulopathy in patients with neoplasms: clinical, pathophysiologic, and therapeutic features. Medicine (Baltimore) 1977; 56:1–37.
173. Sun NC, et al. Hemostatic abnormalities in malignancy, a prospective study of one hundred eight patients. Part I: Coagulation studies. Am J Clin Pathol 1979; 71:10–16.
174. Slichter SJ, Harker LA. Hemostasis in malignancy. Ann NY Acad Sci 1974; 230:252–261.
175. Weick JK. Intravascular coagulation in cancer. Semin Oncol 1978; 5:203–211.
176. Yoda Y, Abe T. Fibrinopeptide A (FPA) level and fibrinogen kinetics in patients with malignant disease. Thromb Haemost 1981; 46:706–709.
177. Colman RW, Rubin RN. Disseminated intravascular coagulation due to malignancy. Semin Oncol 1990; 17:172–186.
178. Gordon SG, Cross BA. A factor X-activating cysteine protease from malignant tissue. J Clin Invest 1981; 67:1665–1671.
179. Gralnick HR, Abrell E. Studies on the procoagulant and fibrinolytic activity of promyelocytes in acute promyelocytic leukaemia. Br J Haematol 1973; 24:89–99.
180. Gouault-Heilmann M, et al. The procoagulant factor of leukaemic promyelocytes: demonstration of immunologic cross reactivity with human brain tissue factor. Br J Haematol 1975; 30:151–158.
181. Levine MN, et al. The thrombogenic effect of anticancer drug therapy in women with stage II breast cancer. N Engl J Med 1988; 318:404–407.
182. Wall JG, et al. Arterial thrombosis associated with adjuvant chemotherapy for breast carcinoma: a Cancer and Leukemia Group B Study. Am J Med 1989; 87:501–504.
183. Siegel DG. Pregnancy, the puerperium and the steroid contraceptive. Milbank Mem Fund Q 1972; 50[Suppl 2]:15–23.
184. Sipes SL, Weiner CP. Venous thromboembolic disease in pregnancy. Semin Perinatol 1990; 14:109–118.
185. Tooke JE, McNicol GP. Thrombotic disorders associated with pregnancy and the pill. Clin Haematol 1981; 10:613–630.
186. Treffers PE, et al. Epidemiological observations of thromboembolic disease during pregnancy and in the puerperium, in 56,022 women. Int J Gynecol Obstet 1983; 21:327–331.
187. Bonnar J. Hemostatic function and coagulopathy during pregnancy. Obstet Gynecol Ann 1978; 7:195–217.
188. Biland L, Duckert F. Coagulation factors of the newborn and his mother. Thromb Diath Haemorrh 1973; 29:644–651.
189. Bonnar J, McNicol GP, Douglas AS. Fibrinolytic enzyme system and pregnancy. Br Med J 1969; 3:387–389.
190. Kruithof EKO, et al. Fibrinolysis in pregnancy: a study of plasminogen activator inhibitors. Blood 1987; 69:460–466.
191. Kaplan NM. Cardiovascular complications of oral contraceptives. Ann Rev Med 1978; 29:31–40.
192. Durant JL, Bressler R. Clinical pharmacology of the steroidal oral contraceptives. Adv Intern Med 1979; 24:97–126.
193. Stubblefield PG. Cardiovascular effects of oral contraceptives: a review. Int J Fertil 1989; 34[Suppl]:40–49.
194. Oral contraceptives and venous thromboembolic disease, surgically confirmed gallbladder disease, and breast tumours: report from the Boston Collaborative Drug Surveillance Programme. Lancet 1973; 1:1399–1404.
195. Sagar S, et al. Oral contraceptives, antithrombin-III activity, and postoperative deep-vein thrombosis. Lancet 1976; 1:509–511.
196. Vessey MP, Mann JI. Female sex hormones and thrombosis: epidemiological aspects. Br Med Bull 1978; 34:157–162.
197. Greene GR, Sartwell PE. Oral contraceptive use in patients with thromboembolism following surgery, trauma, or infection. Am J Public Health 1972; 62:680–685.
198. Collaborative Group for the Study of Stroke in Young Women. Oral contraception and increased risk of cerebral ischemia or thrombosis. N Engl J Med 1973; 288:871–878.
199. Collaborative Group for the Study of Stroke in Young Women. Oral contraceptives and stroke in young women: associated risk factors. JAMA 1975; 231:718–722.
200. Engel H-J, Engel E, Lichtlen PR. Coronary atherosclerosis and myocardial infarction in young women—role of oral contraceptives. Eur Heart J 1983; 4:1–6.
201. Shapiro S, et al. Oral-contraceptive use in relation to myocardial infarction. Lancet 1979; 1:743–746.
202. Jugdutt BI, et al. Myocardial infarction, oral contraception,

cigarette smoking, and coronary artery spasm in young women. Am Heart J 1983; 106:757–761.
203. Stolley PD, et al. Thrombosis with low-estrogen oral contraceptives. Am J Epidemiol 1975; 102:197–208.
204. Daniel DG, Campbell H, Turnbull AC. Puerperal thromboembolism and suppression of lactation. Lancet 1967; 2: 287–289.
205. Coronary Drug Project Research Group. The coronary drug project: initial findings leading to modifications of its research protocol. JAMA 1970; 214:1303–1313.
206. Blackard CE, et al. Incidence of cardiovascular disease and death in patients receiving diethylstilbestrol for carcinoma of the prostate. Cancer 1970; 26:249–256.
207. Goodrich SM, Wood JE. Peripheral venous distensibility and velocity of venous blood flow during pregnancy or during oral contraceptive therapy. Am J Obstet Gynecol 1964; 90:740–744.
208. Aronson HB, Magora F, Schenker JG. Effect of oral contraceptives on blood viscosity. Am J Obstet Gynecol 1971; 110:997–1001.
209. Oski FA, Lubin B, Buchert ED. Reduced red cell filterability with oral contraceptive agents. Ann Intern Med 1972; 77:417–419.
210. Poller L. Oral contraceptives, blood clotting and thrombosis. Br Med Bull 1978; 34:151–156.
211. Lindberg UB, et al. A comparison between effects of estradiol valerate and low dose ethinyl estradiol on haemostatic parameters. Thromb Haemost 1989; 61:65–69.
212. Bonnar J. Coagulation effects of oral contraception. Am J Obstet Gynecol 1987; 157:1042–1048.
213. Kendall AG, Lohmann RC, Dossetor JB. Nephrotic syndrome, a hypercoagulable state. Arch Intern Med 1971; 127:1021–1027.
214. Keusch G. Thrombotic complications in the nephrotic syndrome. Schweiz Med Wochenschr 1989; 119:1080–1085.
215. Kauffman RH, et al. Acquired antithrombin III deficiency and thrombosis in the nephrotic syndrome. Am J Med 1978; 65:607–613.
216. Panicucci F, et al. Comprehensive study of haemostasis in nephrotic syndrome. Nephron 1983; 33:9–13.
217. Thompson AR. Factor XII and other hemostatic protein abnormalities in nephrotic syndrome patients. Thromb Haemost 1982; 48:27–32.
218. Lange LG III, et al. Activation of Hageman factor in the nephrotic syndrome. Am J Med 1974; 56:565–569.
219. Vaziri ND. Nephrotic syndrome and coagulation and fibrinolytic abnormalities. Am J Nephrol 1983; 3:1–6.
220. Jackson CA, et al. Relationship between platelet aggregation, thromboxane synthesis and albumin concentration in nephrotic syndrome. Br J Haematol 1982; 69:77.
221. Searcy RM, Malagelada J-R. Ménétrier's disease and idiopathic hypertrophic gastropathy. Ann Intern Med 1984; 100:565–570.
222. Mueh JR, Herbst KD, Rapaport SI. Thrombosis in patients with the lupus anticoagulant. Ann Intern Med 1980; 92(2 pt 1):156–159.
223. Carreras LO, Vermylen JG. "Lupus" anticoagulant and thrombosis—possible role of inhibition of prostacyclin formation. Thromb Haemost 1982; 48:33–40.
224. Elias M, Eldor A. Thromboembolism in patients with the lupus-type circulating anticoagulant. Arch Intern Med 1984; 144:510–515.
225. Parke AL. Antiphospholipid antibody syndrome. Rheum Dis Clin N Am 1989; 15:275–286.
226. Harris EN, Asherton RA, Hughes GR. Antiphospholipid antibodies—autoantibodies with a difference. Ann Rev Med 1988; 39:261–271.
227. Love PE, Santoro SA. Antiphospholipid antibodies. Ann Intern Med 1990; 112:682–698.
228. Alving BM. Lupus anticogulants, anticardiolipin antibodies, and the antiphospholipid syndrome. In J Loscalzo, AI Schafer, eds. Thrombosis and Hemorrhage. Boston: Blackwell, 1994.
229. Watson KV, Schorer AE. Lupus anticoagulant inhibition of *in vitro* prostacyclin release is associated with a thrombosis-prone subset of patients. Am J Med 1991; 90:47–53.
230. Lellouche F, et al. Imbalance of thromboxane/prostacyclin biosynthesis in patients with lupus anticoagulant. Blood 1991; 78:2894–2899.
231. Freyssinet J-M, et al. An IgM lupus anticoagulant that neutralizes the enhancing effect of phospholipid on purified endothelial thrombomodulin activity—a mechanism for thrombosis. Thromb Haemost 1986; 55:309–313.
232. Cariou R, et al. Effect of lupus anticoagulant on antithrombogenic properties of endothelial cells—inhibition of thrombomodulin-dependent protein C activation. Thromb Haemost 1988; 60:54–58.
233. Marciniak E, Romond EH. Impaired catalytic function of activated protein C: a new in vitro manifestation of lupus anticaogulant. Blood 1989; 74:2426–2432.
234. Malia RG, et al. Inhibition of activated protein C and its cofactor protein S by antiphospholipid antibodies. Br J Haematol 1990; 76:101–107.
235. Lo SCL, et al. Studies of natural anticoagulant proteins and anticardiolipin antibodies in patients with the lupus anticoagulant. Br J Haematol 1990; 76:380–386.
236. Cines DB, et al. Presence of complement-fixing anti-endothelial cell antibodies in systemic lupus erythematosus. J Clin Invest 1984; 73:611–625.
237. Vismara A, et al. Relationship between anti-cardiolipin and anti-endothelial cell antibodies in systemic lupus erythematosus. Clin Exp Immunol 1988; 74:247–253.
238. Leung W-H, et al. Association between antiphospholipid antibodies and cardiac abnormalities in patients with systemic lupus erythematosus. Am J Med 1990; 89:411–419.
239. Nihoyannopoulos P, et al. Cardiac abnormalities in systemic lupus erythematosus. Association with raised anticardiolipin antibodies. Circulation 1990; 82:369–375.
240. Khamashta MA, et al. Association of antibodies against phospholipids with heart valve disease in systemic lupus erythematosus. Lancet 1990; 335:1541–1544.
241. Galve E, et al. Valvular heart disease in the primary antiphospholipid syndrome. Ann Intern Med 1992; 116:293–298.
242. Chartash EK, et al. Aortic insufficiency and mitral regurgitation in patients with systemic lupus erythematosus and the antiphospholipid syndrome. Am J Med 1989; 86:407–412.
243. Gleason CB, et al. A comparison of valvular involvement in the primary antiphospholipid syndrome versus anticardiolipin-negative systemic lupus erythematosus. Am Heart J 1993; 125:1123–1129.
244. Pope JM, Canny CLB, Bell DA. Cerebral ischemic events associated with endocarditis, retinal vascular disease, and lupus anticoagulant. Am J Med 1991; 90:299–309.
245. Lubbe WF, et al. Lupus anticoagulant in pregnancy. Br J Obstet Gynaecol 1984; 91:357–363.
246. Branch DW, et al. Obstetric complications associated with lupus anticoagulant. N Engl J Med 1985; 313:1322–1326.
247. Triplett DA. Antiphospholipid antibodies and recurrent pregnancy loss. Am J Reprod Immunol 1989; 20:52–67.
248. Ordi J, et al. Fetal loss treatment in patients with antiphospholipid antibodies. Ann Rheum Dis 1989; 48:798–802.
249. Cowchock FS, et al. Repeated fetal losses associated with antiphospholipid antibodies: a collaborative randomized

trial comparing prednisone with low-dose heparin treatment. Am J Obstet Gynecol 1992; 166:1318–1323.
250. Lockshin MD, Druzin ML, Qamar T. Prednisone does not prevent recurrent fetal death in women with antiphospholipid antibody. Am J Obstet Gynecol 1989; 160:439–443.
251. Rosove MH, et al. Heparin therapy for pregnant women with lupus anticoagulant or anticardiolipin antibodies. Obstet Gynecol 1990; 75:630–634.
252. Carreras LO, et al. Lupus anticoagulant and recurrent fetal loss: successful treatment with gammaglobulin. Lancet 1988; 2:393–394.
253. Schafer AI. Bleeding and thrombosis in the myeloproliferative disorders. Blood 1984; 64:1–12.
254. Mitus AJ, Schafer AI. Thrombocytosis and thrombocythemia. Hematol/Oncol Clin N Am 1990; 4:157–178.
255. Schafer AI. Essential thrombocythemia. Prog Hemostas Thromb 1991; 10:69–96.
256. Mitchell MC, et al. Budd-Chiari syndrome: etiology, diagnosis, and management. Medicine (Baltimore) 1982; 61:199–218.
257. Valla D, et al. Primary myeloproliferative disorder and hepatic vein thrombosis: a prospective study of erythroid colony formation in vitro in 20 patients with Budd-Chiari syndrome. Ann Intern Med 1985; 103:329–334.
258. Kurzrock R, Cohen PR. Erythromelalgia and myeloproliferative disorders. Arch Intern Med 1989; 149:105–109.
259. Drenth JPH, Michiels JJ. Three types of erythromelalgia. BMJ 1990; 301:454.
260. Michiels JJ, et al. Erythromelalgia caused by platelet-mediated arteriolar inflammation and thrombosis in thrombocythemia. Ann Intern Med 1985; 102:466–471.
261. Singh AK, Wetherley-Mein G. Microvascular occlusive lesions in primary thrombocythaemia. Br J Haematol 1977; 36:553–564.
262. Jabaily J, et al. Neurologic manifestations of essential thrombocythemia. Ann Intern Med 1983; 99:513–518.
263. Pearson TC, Wetherley-Mein G. Vascular occlusive episodes and venous haematocrit in primary proliferative polycythaemia. Lancet 1978; 2:1219–1221.
264. Kessler CM, Klein HG, Havlik RJ. Uncontrolled thrombocytosis in chronic myeloproliferative disorders. Br J Haematol 1982; 50:157–167.
265. Murphy S. Thrombocytosis and thrombocythaemia. Clin Haematol 1983; 12:89–106.
266. Maldonado JE, Pintado T, Pierre RV. Dysplastic platelets and circulating megakaryocytes in chronic myeloproliferative diseases. I: The platelets: ultrastructure and peroxidase reaction. Blood 1974; 43:797–809.
267. Gerrard JM, et al. Platelet storage pool deficiency and prostaglandin synthesis in chronic granulocytic leukaemia. Br J Haematol 1978; 40:597–607.
268. Bolin RB, Okumura T, Jamieson GA. Changes in distribution of platelet membrane glycoproteins in patients with myeloproliferative disorders. Am J Hematol 1977; 3:63–71.
269. Kaywin P, et al. Platelet function in essential thrombocythemia: decreased epinephrine responsiveness associated with a deficiency of platelet α-adrenergic receptors. N Engl J Med 1978; 299:505–509.
270. Cooper B, et al. Platelet resistance to prostaglandin D_2 in patients with myeloproliferative disorders. Blood 1978; 52:618–626.
271. Moore A, Nachman RL. Platelet F_c receptor: increased expression in myeloproliferative disease. J Clin Invest 1981; 67:1064–1071.
272. Jubelirer SJ, et al. Platelet arachidonic acid metabolism and platelet function in ten patients with chronic myelogenous leukemia. Blood 1980; 56:728–731.
273. Okuma M, Uchino H. Altered arachidonate metabolism by platelets in patients with myeloproliferative disorders. Blood 1979; 54:1258–1271.
274. Schafer AI. Deficiency of platelet lipoxygenase activity in myeloproliferative disorders. N Engl J Med 1982; 306: 381–386.
275. Dixon RH, Rosse WF. Mechanism of complement-mediated activation of human blood platelets in vitro: comparison of normal and paroxysmal noctural hemoglobinuria platelets. J Clin Invest 1977; 59:360–368.
276. Colwell JA. Vascular thrombosis in type II diabetes mellitus (Editorial). Diabetes 1993; 42:8–11.
277. Glassman AB. Platelet abnormalities in diabetes mellitus. Ann Clin Lab Sci 1993; 23:47–50.
278. Timperley WR, Preston FE, Ward JD. Cerebral intravascular coagulation in diabetic ketoacidosis. Lancet 1974; 1:952–956.
279. Timperley WR, et al. A reassessment of small vessel disease in diabetic neuropathy. Diabetologia 1975; 11:379–380.
280. Abrahamsen AF. Platelet survival studies in man (with special reference to thrombosis and atherosclerosis). Scand J Haematol 1968; Suppl 3:1–53.
281. Preston FE, et al. Elevated -thromboglobulin levels and circulating platelet aggregates in diabetic microangiopathy. Lancet 1978; 1:238–240.
282. Burrows AW, Chavin SI, Hockaday TDR. Plasma-thromboglobulin concentrations in diabetes mellitus. Lancet 1978; 1:235–237.
283. Colwell JA, Halushka PV. Platelet function in diabetes mellitus. Br J Haematol 1980; 44:521–526.
284. Heath H, et al. Platelet adhesiveness and aggregation in relation to diabetic retinopathy. Diabetologia 1971; 7: 308–315.
285. O'Malley BC, et al. Platelet abnormalities in diabetic peripheral neuropathy. Lancet 1975; 2:1274–1276.
286. Sagel J, et al. Increased platelet aggregation in early diabetes mellitus. Ann Intern Med 1975; 82:733–738.
287. Peterson CM, et al. Reversible hematologic sequelae of diabetes mellitus. Ann Intern Med 1977; 86:425–429.
288. Mustard JF, Packham MA. Platelets and diabetes mellitus (Editorial). N Engl J Med 1984; 311:665–667.
289. Winocour PD, et al. Reduced membrane fluidity in platelets from diabetic patients. Diabetes 1990; 39:241–244.
290. Mazzanti L, et al. Altered cellular Ca^{2+} and Na^{+} transport in diabetes mellitus. Diabetes 1990; 39:850–854.
291. Halushka PV, et al. Increased platelet thromboxane synthesis in diabetes mellitus. J Lab Clin Med 1981; 97:87–96.
292. Davi G, et al. Thromboxane biosynthesis and platelet function in type II diabetes mellitus. N Engl J Med 1990; 322:1769–1774.
293. Le Pape A, et al. Nonenzymatic glycosylation increases platelet aggregating potency of collagen from placenta of diabetic human beings. Biochem Biophys Res Commun 1983; 111: 602–610.
294. Coller BS, et al. Plasma cofactors of platelet function: correlation with diabetic retinopathy and hemoglobins $A_{1a\text{-}c}$. Ann Intern Med 1978; 88:311–316.
295. Borkenstein MH, Muntean WE. Elevated factor VIII activity and factor VIII-related antigen in diabetic children without vascular disease. Diabetes 1982; 31:1006–1009.
296. Fuller JH, et al. Haemostatic variables associated with diabetes and its complications. Br Med J 1979; 2:964–966.
297. Geiger M, Binder BR. Plasminogen activation in diabetes mellitus. J Biol Chem 1984; 259:2976–2981.
298. Juhan-Vague I, et al. Increased plasminogen activator inhibitor activity in noninsulin dependent diabetic patients—relationship with plasma insulin. Thromb Haemostas 1989; 61:370–373.

299. Prentice CRM, Lowe GDO. Blood viscosity and the complications of diabetes. Adv Exp Med Biol 1984; 164:99–103.
300. Wautier J-L, et al. Increased adhesion of erythrocytes to endothelial cells in diabetes mellitus and its relation to vascular complications. N Engl J Med 1981; 305:237–242.
301. Banga JD, Sixma JJ. Diabetes mellitus, vascular disease and thrombosis. Clin Haematol 1986; 15:465–492.
302. Carvalho ACA, Colman RW, Lees RS. Platelet function in hyperlipoproteinemia. N Engl J Med 1974; 290:434–438.
303. Tremoli E, et al. Platelet aggregation and malondialdehyde formation in type IIA hypercholesterolemic patients. Haemostasis 1979; 8:47–53.
304. Shattil SJ, et al. Platelet hypersensitivity induced by cholesterol incorporation. J Clin Invest 1975; 55:636–643.
305. Stuart MJ, Gerrard JM, White JG. Effect of cholesterol on production of thromboxane B_2 by platelets in vitro. N Engl J Med 1980; 302:6–10.
306. Cosgriff SW. Thromboembolic complications associated with A.C.T.H. and cortisone therapy. JAMA 1951; 147:924–926.
307. Sjöberg HE, Blombäck M, Granberg PO. Thromboembolic complications, heparin treatment and increase in coagulation factors in Cushing's syndrome. Acta Med Scand 1976; 199:95–98.
308. Patrassi GM, et al. Further studies on the hypercoagulable state of patients with Cushing's syndrome. Thromb Haemost 1985; 54:518–520.
309. Weismann RE, Tobin RW. Arterial embolism occurring during systemic heparin therapy. Arch Surg 1958; 76:219–227.
310. Kelton JG, Levine MN. Heparin-induced thrombocytopenia. Semin Thromb Hemost 1986; 12:59–62.
311. Warkentin TE, Kelton JG. Heparin-induced thrombocytopenia. Ann Rev Med 1989; 40:31–44.
312. Schmitt PB, Adelman B. Heparin-associated thrombocytopenia: a critical review and pooled analysis. Am J Med Sci 1993; 305:208–215.
313. Anderson GP. Insights in heparin-associated thrombocytopenia. Br J Haematol 1992; 80:504–508.
314. Cines DB, Tomaski A, Tannenbaum S. Immune endothelial-cell injury in heparin-associated thrombocytopenia. N Engl J Med 1987; 316:581–589.
315. Gallus AS. Venous thromboembolism: incidence and clinical risk factors. In JPL Madden, M Hume, eds. Venous Thromboembolism: Prevention and Treatment. New York: Appleton-Century-Crofts, 1976.
316. Hirsh J, Genton E, Hull R. Venous Thromboembolism. New York: Grune & Stratton, 1981. P. 13.
317. Gibbs NM. Venous thrombosis of the lower limbs with particular reference to bed-rest. Br J Surg 1957; 45:209–236.
318. Warlow C, Ogston D, Douglas AS. Venous thrombosis following strokes. Lancet 1972; 1:1305–1306.
319. Cope C, Reyes TM, Skversky NJ. Phlebographic analysis of the incidence of thrombosis in hemiplegia. Radiology 1973; 109:581–584.
320. Heatley RV, et al. Preoperative or postoperative deep-vein thrombosis? Lancet 1976; 1:437–439.
321. Hamer JD, Malone PC, Silver IA. The PO_2 in venous valve pockets: its possible bearing on thrombogenesis. Br J Surg 1981; 68:166–170.
322. Shattil SJ. Diagnosis and treatment of recurrent venous thromboembolism. Med Clin N Am 1984; 68:577–600.
323. Kleinsasser LJ. Effort thrombosis of the axillary and subclavian vein. Arch Surg 1949; 59:258–274.
324. Adams JT, DeWeese JA. "Effort" thrombosis of the axillary and subclavian veins. J Trauma 1971; 11:923–930.
325. Harley DP, et al. Pulmonary embolism secondary to venous thrombosis of the arm. Am J Surg 1984; 147:221–224.
326. Morris GK. Preoperative prediction of postoperative deep vein thrombosis. Thromb Haemost 1979; 41:27–32.
327. Owen J, et al. Thrombin and plasmin activity and platelet activation in the development of venous thrombosis. Blood 1983; 61:476–482.
328. Forbes CD. Thrombosis and artificial surfaces. Clin Haematol 1981; 10:653–668.
329. Hakim RM, Ault K, Himmelfarb J. Interaction of blood with artificial surfaces. In J Loscalzo, AI Schafer, eds. Thrombosis and Hemorrhage. Boston: Blackwell, 1994.
330. Cunliffe WJ, Menon IS. The association between cutaneous vasculitis and decreased blood fibrinolytic activity. Br J Dermatol 1971; 84:99–105.
331. Angles-Cano E, Sultan Y, Clauvel JP. Predisposing factors to thrombosis in systemic lupus erythematosus: possible relation to endothelial cell damage. J Lab Clin Med 1979; 94:312–323.
332. Cronlund M, et al. Fibrinopeptide A in plasma of normal subjects and patients with disseminated intravascular coagulation and systemic lupus erythematosus. J Clin Invest 1976; 58:142–151.
333. Furey NL, et al. Arterial thrombosis in scleroderma. Br J Dermatol 1975; 93:683–693.
334. Jordan JM, Allen NB, Pizzo SV. Defective release of tissue plasminogen activator in systemic and cutaneous vasculitis. Am J Med 1987; 82:397–400.
335. Mercer S. Kawasaki disease and its complications. Compr Ther 1981; 7:52–54.
336. Haim S, Barzilai D, Hazani E. Involvement of veins in Behçet's syndrome. Br J Dermatol 1971; 84:238–241.
337. Chamberlain MA. Behçet's syndrome in 32 patients in Yorkshire. Ann Rheum Dis 1977; 36:491–499.
338. Shimizu T, et al. Behçet's disease (Behçet's syndrome). Semin Arthritis Rheum 1979; 8:223–259.
339. Chajek T, Fainaru ML. Behçet's disease: report of 41 cases and a review of the literature. Medicine (Baltimore) 1975; 54:179–196.
340. O'Duffy JD, Carney JA, Deodhar S. Behçet's disease: report of 10 cases, 3 with new manifestations. Ann Intern Med 1971; 75:561–570.
341. Wilkey D, et al. Budd-Chiari syndrome and renal failure in Behçet's disease: report of a case and review of the literature. Am J Med 1983; 75:541–550.
342. Vermylen J, et al. Thrombosis and immune disorders. Clin Haematol 1986; 15:393–412.
343. Schmitz-Huebner U, Knop J. Evidence for an endothelial cell dysfunction in association with Behçet's disease. Thromb Res 1984; 34:277–285.
344. Chajek T, Aronowski E, Izak G. Decreased fibrinolysis in Behçet's disease. Thromb Diath Haemorrh 1973; 29:610–618.
345. Verstraete M, Vermylen J, Verhaeghe RH. Peripheral arterial diseases. Clin Haematol 1981; 10:669–689.
346. Williams G. Recent views on Buerger's disease. J Clin Pathol 1969; 22:573–578.
347. Wilcken DE, Dudman NP. Mechanisms of thrombogenesis and accelerated atherogenesis in homocysteinaemia. Haemostasis 1989; 19[Suppl 1]:14–23.
348. Boers GHJ, et al. Heterozygosity for homocystinuria in premature and peripheral and cerebral occlusive arterial disease. N Engl J Med 1985; 313:709–714.
349. Malinow MR. Hyperhomocyst(e)inemia. A common and easily reversible risk factor for occlusive atherosclerosis. Circulation 1990; 81:2004–2006.
350. Clarke R, et al. Hyperhomocysteinemia: an independent risk factor for vascular disease. N Engl J Med 1991; 324:1149–1155.

351. Newman G, Mitchell JRA. Homocystinuria presenting as multiple arterial occlusions. Q J Med 1984; 53:251–258.
352. McCully KS. Vascular pathology of homocysteinemia: implications for the pathogenesis of arteriosclerosis. Am J Pathol 1969; 56:111–128.
353. Harker LA, et al. Homocystinemia: vascular injury and arterial thrombosis. N Engl J Med 1974; 291:537–543.
354. Uhlemann ER, et al. Platelet survival and morphology in homocystinuria due to cystathionine synthetase deficiency. N Engl J Med 1976; 295:1283–1286.
355. Heinecke JW, et al. The role of sulfur-containing amino acids in superoxide production and modification of low density lipoprotein by arterial smooth muscle cells. J Biol Chem 1987; 262:10098–10103.
356. Rodgers GM, Conn MT. Homocysteine, an atherogenic stimulus, reduces protein C activation by arterial and venous endothelial cells. Blood 1990; 75:895–901.
357. Lentz SR, Sadler JE. Homocysteine inhibits von Willebrand factor processing and secretion by preventing transport from the endoplasmic reticulum. Blood 1993; 81:683–689.
358. Hajjar KA. Homocysteine-induced modulation of tissue plasminogen activator binding to its endothelial cell membrane receptor. J Clin Invest 1993; 91:2873–2879.
359. Bloch KJ, Maki DG. Hyperviscosity syndromes associated with immunoglobulin abnormalities. Semin Hematol 1973; 10:113–124.
360. Smith BD, La Celle PL. Blood viscosity and thrombosis: clinical considerations. Prog Hemost Thromb 1982; 6:170–201.
361. Goldsmith HL, Turitto VT. Rheological aspects of thrombosis and haemostasis: basic principles and applications. Thromb Haemostas 1986; 55:415–435.
362. Newton LK. Neurologic complications of polycythemia and their impact on therapy. Oncology 1990; 4:59–64.
363. Thomas DJ, et al. Cerebral blood-flow in polycythaemia. Lancet 1977; 2:161–163.
364. Humphrey PRD, et al. Cerebral blood-flow and viscosity in relative polycythaemia. Lancet 1979; 2:873–876.
365. Balcerzak SP, Bromberg PA. Secondary polycythemia. Semin Hematol 1975; 12:353–382.
366. Hoover R, et al. Adhesion of normal and sickle erythrocytes to endothelial monolayer cultures. Blood 1979; 54:872–876.
367. Hebbel RP, et al. Erythrocyte adherence to endothelium in sickle-cell anemia. N Engl J Med 1980; 302:992–995.
368. Wick TM, et al. Unusually large von Willebrand factor multimers preferentially promote young sickle and non-sickle erythrocyte adhesion to endothelial cells. Am J Hematol 1993; 42:284–292.
369. Craddock PR, et al. Complement and leukocyte-mediated pulmonary dysfunction in hemodialysis. N Engl J Med 1977; 296:769–774.
370. Craddock PR, et al. Granulocyte aggregation as a manifestation of membrane interactions with complement: possible role in leukocyte margination, microvascular occlusion, and endothelial damage. Semin Hematol 1979; 16:140–147.
371. Ruggenenti P, Remuzzi G. Thrombotic thrombocytopenic purpura and related disorders. Hematol Oncol Clin N Am 1990; 4:219–241.
372. Bukowski RM. Thrombotic thrombocytopenic purpura: a review. Prog Hemost Thromb 1982; 6:287–337.
373. Kwaan HC. Role of fibrinolysis in thrombotic thrombocytopenic purpura. Semin Thromb Hemost 1980; 6:395–400.
374. Moake JL, et al. Unusually large plasma factor VIII: von Willebrand factor multimers in chronic relapsing thrombotic thrombocytopenic purpura. N Engl J Med 1982; 307:1432–1435.
375. Moake JL, et al. Therapy of chronic relapsing thrombotic thrombocytopenic purpura with prednisone and azathioprine. Am J Hematol 1985; 20:73–79.
376. Rock GA, et al. Comparison of plasma exchange with plasma infusion in the treatment of thrombotic thrombocytopenic purpura. N Engl J Med 1991; 325:393–397.
377. Burns ER, Zucker-Franklin D. Pathologic effects of plasma from patients with thrombotic thrombocytopenic purpura on platelets and cultured vascular endothelial cells. Blood 1982; 60:1030–1037.
378. Wall RT, Harker LA. The endothelium and thrombosis. Ann Rev Med 1980; 31:361–371.
379. Lian EC-Y, et al. Presence of a platelet aggregating factor in the plasma of patients with thrombotic thrombocytopenic purpura (TTP) and its inhibition by normal plasma. Blood 1979; 53:333–338.
380. Fields SM, Lindley CM. Thrombotic microangiopathy associated with chemotherapy: case report and review of the literature. DICP 1989; 23:582–588.
381. Walker RW, et al. Carboplatin-associated thrombotic microangiopathic hemolytic anemia. Cancer 1989; 64:1017–1020.
382. Byrnes JJ, Moake JL. Thrombotic thrombocytopenic purpura and the haemolytic-uraemic syndrome: evolving concepts of pathogenesis and therapy. Clin Haematol 1986; 15:413–442.
383. Ratnoff OD. The role of haemostatic mechanisms. Clin Haematol 1981; 10:261–281.
384. Wilhelmsen L, et al. Fibrinogen as a risk factor for stroke and myocardial infarction. N Engl J Med 1984; 311:501–505.
385. Meade TW, et al. Haemostatic function and cardiovascular death: early results of a prospective study. Lancet 1980; 1:1050–1054.
386. Fareed J, et al. Molecular markers of hemostatic activation: future perspectives. Semin Thromb Hemost 1984; 10: 329–332.
387. Bauer KA. Inherited hypercoagulable states. In J Loscalzo, AI Schafer, eds. Thrombosis and Hemorrhage. Boston: Blackwell, 1994.
388. Nossel HL, et al. Radioimmunoassay of human fibrinopeptide A. Proc Natl Acad Sci USA 1974; 68:2350–2353.
389. Walenga JM, et al. Performance characteristics of a simple radioimmunoassay for fibrinopeptide A. Semin Thromb Hemost 1984; 10:219–227.
390. Bauer KA, et al. Detection of protein C activation in humans. J Clin Invest 1984; 74:2033–2041.
391. Gruber A, Griffin JH. Direct detection of activated protein C in blood from human subjects. Blood 1992; 79:2340–2348.
392. Orthner CL, Kolen B, Drohan WN. A sensitive and facile assay for the measurement of activated protein C activity levels *in vivo*. Thromb Haemost 1993; 69:441–447.
393. Bauer KA, et al. Elevated factor Xa activity in the blood of asymptomatic patients with congenital antithrombin deficiency. J Clin Invest 1985; 76:826–836.
394. Mannucci P, et al. Markers of procoagulant imbalance in patients with inherited thrombophilic syndromes. Thromb Haemost 1992; 67:200–202.
395. Leroy-Matheron C, Gouault-Heilmann M, Levent M. Prothrombin fragment 1 + 2 levels in patients with inherited deficiency in coagulation inhibitors. Thromb Haemost 1991; 65:1208.
396. Bauer KA, et al. Hemostatic enzyme generation in the blood of patients with hereditary protein C deficiency. Blood 1988; 71:1418–1426.
397. Conard J, et al. Normalization of markers of coagulation activation with a purified protein C concentrate in adults with homozygous PC deficiency. Blood 1993; 82:1159–1164.
398. Bauer KA, et al. Elevated factor Xa activity in the blood of

asymptomatic patients with congenital antithrombin deficiency. J Clin Invest 1985; 76:826–836.
399. Bauer KA, Barzegar S, Rosenberg RD. Influence of anticoagulants used for blood collection on plasma prothrombin fragment F_{1+2} measurements. Thromb Res 1991; 63:617–628.
400. Demers C, et al. Measurements of markers of activated coagulation in antithrombin III deficient subjects. Thromb Haemost 1992; 67:542–544.
401. Walenga JM, et al. Diagnostic efficacy of a simple radioimmunoassay test for fibrinogen/fibrin fragments containing the B-β 15–42 sequence. Semin Thromb Hemost 1984; 10: 252–263.
402. Born GVR. Aggregation of blood platelets by adenosine diphosphate and its reversal. Nature 1962; 194:927–929.
403. Thompson SG, Vickers MV. Methods in dose response platelet aggregometry. Thromb Hemost 1985; 53:216–218.
404. Wu KK, Hoak JC. A new method for the quantitative detection of platelet aggregates in patients with arterial insufficiency. Lancet 1974; 2:924–926.
405. Packham MA. Methods for detection of hypersensitive platelets. Thromb Haemost 1978; 40:175–195.
406. Weksler BB, Dougherty JH. Detecting of circulating platelet aggregates in cerebrovascular and coronary artery disease. In HJ Day, H Holmsen, MB Zucker, eds. Platelet Function Testing. Washington, D.C.: DHEW Publication NIH 78-1087, U.S. Government Printing Office, 1978. Pp. 410–415.
407. Packham MA, Mustard JF. Normal and abnormal platelet activity. In A Lasslo, ed. Blood Platelet Function and Medicinal Chemistry. New York: Elsevier, 1984. Pp. 61–128.
408. Handin RI, McDonough M, Lesch M. Elevation of platelet factor 4 in acute myocardial infarction: measurement by radioimmunoassay. J Lab Clin Med 1978; 91:340–349.
409. Kaplan KL, Owen J. Plasma levels of β-thromboglobulin and platelet factor 4 as indices of platelet activation in vivo. Blood 1981; 57:199–202.
410. Bolton AE, et al. Three approaches to the radioimmunoassay of β-thromboglobulin. Br J Haematol 1976; 33:233–238.
411. Bolton AE, et al. A radioimmunoassay for platelet factor 4. Thromb Res 1976; 8:51–58.
412. Kerry PJ, Curtis AD. Standardization of β-thromboglobulin (β-TG) and platelet factor 4 (PF4): a collaborative study to establish international standards for β-TG and PF4. Thromb Haemost 1985; 53:51–55.
413. McEver RP, Martin MN. A monoclonal antibody to a membrane glycoprotein binds only to activated platelets. J Biol Chem 1984; 259:9799–9804.
414. Berman CL, et al. A platelet alpha granule membrane protein that is associated with the plasma membrane after reactivation. J Clin Invest 1986; 78:130–137.
415. Abrams C, Shattil SJ. Immunological detection of activated platelets in clinical disorders. Thromb Haemost 1991; 65: 467–473.
416. Montgomery RR, et al. Diagnosis of Bernard-Soulier syndrome and Glanzmann's thrombasthenia with a monoclonal assay on whole blood. J Clin Invest 1983; 71:385–389.
417. George JN, et al. Platelet surface glycoproteins. Studies on resting and activated platelets and platelet membrane microparticles in normal subjects, and observations in patients during adult respiratory distress syndrome and cardiac surgery. J Clin Invest 1986; 78:340–348.
418. Lawson JA, et al. Measurement of urinary 2,3-dinor-thromboxane B_2 using bonded-phase phenylboronic acid columns and capillary gas chromatography-negative-ion chemical ionization mass spectrometry. Anal Biochem 1985; 150: 463–470.
419. Patrono C, et al. Estimated rate of thromboxane secretion into the circulation of normal humans. J Clin Invest 1986; 77:590–594.
420. Catella F, et al. 11-Dehydro-thromboxane B_2: a quantitative index of thromboxane A_2 biosynthesis in the human circulation. Proc Natl Acad Sci USA 1986; 83:5861–5865.
421. FitzGerald GA, et al. Estimated rate of prostacyclin secretion into the circulation in normal man. J Clin Invest 1981; 68:1272–1276.
422. FitzGerald GA, et al. Increased prostacyclin biosynthesis in patients with severe atherosclerosis and platelet activation. N Engl J Med 1984; 310:1065–1068.
423. Reilly IAG, et al. Increased thromboxane biosynthesis in a human preparation of platelet activation: biochemical and functional consequences of selective inhibition of thromboxane synthase. Circulation 1986; 73:1300–1309.
424. Reilly IAG, Roy L, FitzGerald GA. Biosynthesis of thromboxane in patients with systemic sclerosis and Raynaud's phenomenon. Br Med J 1986; 292:1037–1039.
425. Fitzgerald DJ, et al. Platelet activation in unstable coronary disease. N Engl J Med 1986; 315:983–989.
426. Miletich JP, et al. Inherited predisposition to thrombosis. Cell 1993; 72:477–480.
427. Demers C, et al. Thrombosis in antithrombin-III-deficient persons. Report of a large kindred and literature review. Ann Intern Med 1992; 116:754–761.
428. Nachman RL, Silverstein R. Hypercoagulable states. Ann Intern Med 1993; 119:819–827.
429. Alving BM. The hypercoagulable states. Hosp Pract 1993; 28:109–121.

Pathogenesis of Atherosclerosis: Cell Biology

Russell Ross

Prior to discussing the cellular changes and interactions that occur during the development of the lesions of atherosclerosis, it is necessary to review the cellular architecture of the normal muscular and elastic artery and the cellular constituents of the lesions themselves. This will set the stage for a review of the capacities and properties of each of the cells involved in atherogenesis and the significance of their interactions in this process.

The Normal Artery

All elastic (large) and muscular (small and medium) arteries contain three layers: the innermost layer, or intima; the middle layer, or media; and the outer layer, or adventitia [1].

THE INTIMA

The intima is bounded on the luminal surface by a continuous monolayer of endothelial cells and on its outer aspect by the internal elastic lamina, a highly fenestrated sheet of elastic fibers. During development, the endothelial cells turn over at varying rates. During adulthood, they are generally quiescent, although "hot spots" have been observed that consist of regions of increased endothelial turnover located at branches and bifurcations as well as other regions of the artery [2]. The endothelium is not a passive layer of cells; the endothelial cells not only line the blood container but create an important permeability barrier that determines which molecules enter the artery wall. Endothelial cells are joined together by both tight junctions and gap junctions. The tight junctions make the layer impermeable, while the gap junctions provide a means of interendothelial communication. The permeability of the endothelium is determined by vesicular transport and by junctional permeability. Active transport occurs via vesicles that are presumed to shuttle back and forth across the endothelial cells. The surface of the endothelium is nonthrombogenic due to a cell-surface coat that contains heparan sulfate (due to the formation of eicosanoids, such as prostacyclin) and enzymes (such as an endothelial ecto-adenosine diphosphatase [ecto-ADPase]), which prevent platelet adherence, aggregation, and thrombosis. Endothelial cells are also capable of forming relaxing factors and connective-tissue proteins, and when injured or appropriately stimulated, they form growth factors (or mitogens) that can induce connective-tissue cells, such as smooth muscle, to multiply. The endothelium rests on a collagen matrix called the basal lamina, which it is also responsible for forming. Endothelial cells can have both procoagulant and anticoagulant activities. As a consequence of all of these activities, the endothelium represents a dynamic layer of cells that is important in the pathogenesis of the lesions of atherosclerosis. (See Chapter 1 for a complete discussion of the endothelium).

THE MEDIA

The media of the artery is bounded on its inner aspect by the internal elastic lamina and on its outer aspect by another, less well developed, fenestrated sheet of elastic fibers, the external elastic lamina. The fenestrate of the elastic laminae are holes large enough for cells and cell processes to pass through. They also permit nutrients and other substances to traverse the artery wall. The normal media contains only a single cell type, the smooth muscle cell. During growth and development these smooth muscle cells can develop an extensive rough endoplasmic reticulum and Golgi apparatus and form large amounts of secretory protein, including collagen, elastin, and proteoglycans. During adulthood, they are relatively quiescent cells and contain few organelles other than mitochondria and bundles of contractile myofilaments. (See Chapter 2 for a complete discussion of smooth muscle.) The media of elastic arteries contains numerous lamellar units, each of which consists of a bundle of smooth muscle cells bounded on its inner and outer aspects by an elastic lamina. Muscular arteries contain a single inner and outer elastic lamina, whereas elastic arteries contain variable numbers of these laminae, depending on the size of the artery. It has been demonstrated that once an elastic artery contains more than 29 laminae, the capacity of the lumen of the artery to provide adequate nutrients for the outermost layers of the artery appears to be insufficient. When that occurs, vasa vasora penetrate from the outer aspect (adventitia) of the artery into the media to provide nutrition to the outermost layers of the artery wall [3].

THE ADVENTITIA

The outermost layer of the artery, the adventitia, is bounded on its inner aspect by the external elastic lamina and on its outer aspect by varying amounts of less compact connective tissue matrix, including collagen and proteoglycan together with small blood vessels and fatty tissue. The connective-tissue cells in the adventitia consist of a mixture of fibroblasts and smooth muscle.

The Lesions of Atherosclerosis

THE CELLS OF THE LESIONS AS IDENTIFIED WITH MONOCLONAL ANTIBODIES

Although the lesions of atherosclerosis have been recognized for many centuries and have been described by histologists and pathologists for many decades, there has been relatively little substantive advance in our understanding of the cellular constituents of the lesions until recently. Since hypercholesterolemia is the dominant risk factor associated with atherosclerosis in the United States and Western Europe, the foam-cell components in the lesions have been commonly observed and have been ascribed to both macrophages and smooth muscle cells. Once a cell has become so laden with lipid that it takes on the characteristics of a foam cell, determination of the cell of origin becomes particularly difficult. For that reason, the literature describing the lesions of atherosclerosis contains many potentially erroneous statements regarding cell composition.

Several monoclonal antibodies have been developed that permit identification of macrophages, smooth muscle cells, and lymphocytes. Monoclonal antibody HHF-35 was made against human myocardial actin [4]. This antibody recognizes alpha and gamma actin from skeletal, cardiac, and smooth muscle cells but not from fibroblasts or macrophages. It is, therefore, specific for smooth muscle cells when arterial tissue is examined. A second monoclonal antibody, HAM-56, was made against a cytoplasmic antigen derived from human alveolar macrophages [5]. The specific antigen recognized in the macrophage is not yet known. HAM-56 recognizes circulating blood monocytes and macrophages in every tissue known to contain resident macrophages or histiocytes but does not cross-react with any other cell except a particular type of capillary endothelial cell in some tissues, such as myocardium [5]. Monoclonal antibody T-200 is directed against T- and B-lymphocytes. The use of these three monoclonal antibodies and appropriately prepared tissues has made it possible to identify definitively the cellular constitution of lesions of atherosclerosis wherever they may occur and under whatever circumstances. These lesions and their composition are explained next.

THE FATTY STREAK

The fatty streak is a ubiquitous lesion of atherosclerosis, found at all ages in both sexes. It is seen frequently in infants and children and is widespread in young adults [6]. It occurs in the same anatomic sites in young individuals as in adults, as well as in other regions of the arterial tree that apparently are not prone to the development of advanced, complicated lesions of atherosclerosis. Using the monoclonal antibodies described above, it has been demonstrated that the fatty streak consists principally of one cell type, the lipid-laden macrophage. A few smooth muscle cells can be observed interspersed among the macrophages, and, as the fatty streak expands and grows, smooth muscle cells begin to accumulate beneath it. However, the fatty-streak lesion consists essentially of macrophages and varying numbers of T-lymphocytes (CD8+ and CD4+). Most of the macrophages are full of cholesteryl ester droplets, which give the cells the appearance of foam cells.

THE FIBROUS PLAQUE AND ADVANCED COMPLICATED LESION

The fibrous plaque is the lesion responsible for the principal clinical sequelae of atherosclerosis: myocardial infarction and cerebral infarction. It is usually found at branches, bifurcations, and bends in the arterial tree or at sites where the arterial tree is more fixed to adjacent structures than in straight parts of the artery. The fibrous plaque characteristically is covered by a dense band of connective tissue containing a special, modified, pancake-shaped form of smooth muscle cell; this region is called the fibrous cap [7]. This fibrous cap principally contains smooth muscle cells with some interspersed, nonlipid-containing macrophages. Beneath the fibrous cap is a highly cellular region consisting largely of macrophages, many of which are lipid laden, together with interspersed smooth muscle cells and a fair number of lymphocytes [5]. Below this is another very cellular region containing large numbers of smooth muscle cells, many of which contain lipid. The amount of lipid in a lesion reflects, in part, the level of lipid in the plasma of the affected individual. Given this cellular distribution, it appears that approximately 30 to 50 percent of the cells of the fibrous plaque are smooth muscle, approximately 30 to 50 percent are macrophages, and 5 to 15 percent are lymphocytes, principally T-cells [5,8].

The fibrous plaque can undergo a series of degenerative changes, including the development of ulcers and fissures. These changes appear to occur at sites in advanced lesions of atherosclerosis (fibrous plaques), which appear to be the weakest due to their relatively low content of fibrous connective tissue and relative enrichment in macrophages. When they are coupled with rheologic, stress-induced changes, due to alterations in flow patterns, such as occur at branches and bifurcations, these changes can lead to hemorrhage or thrombosis and may serve as a basis for thrombotic episodes that can lead to sudden death or to further lumenal narrowing of the affected artery.

THE CELLS OF THE BLOOD AND THE ARTERY WALL

The principal cells of the artery wall, the lining endothelium and smooth muscle cells, are affected during the process of atherogenesis. The endothelium may undergo a series of alterations, depending on the causative or injurious agent. In hypercholesterolemia, the surfaces of the endothelial cells are altered, as are the junctional complexes that help retain endothelial continuity. Eventually, "injury" to the endothelium may lead to a series of phenotypic changes and, in some anatomic sites, to increased endothelial turnover.

Hyperlipidemia and other risk factors appear to induce alterations in the lining endothelium associated with the onset of specialized types of inflammation. These alterations include the formation of a series of adhesive cell-surface proteins with specific affinities for ligands on circulating monocytes and T-lymphocytes. Proteins, such as vascular cell adhesion molecule-1 (VCAM-1), intercellular adhesion molecule-1 (ICAM-1), E-selectin, and P-selectin, may be formed on these endothelial cells, providing a basis for increased rolling and adhesion of monocytes, coupled with their transmigration between endothelial cells into the subendothelial space, leading to the first ubiquitous lesion of atherosclerosis, the fatty streak.

A significant effect of endothelial injury on the smooth muscle cell is an attraction to migrate from the media of the artery into the intima, where some of the cells proliferate and ultimately produce an intimal proliferative lesion, the fibrous plaque or complicated lesion, that causes clinical sequelae. The growth factors that are probably responsible for this intimal smooth muscle proliferation apparently derive in some cases from platelets [9], in many cases from injured endothelium [10], and, most important, from activated macrophages [11] that have accumulated during fatty-streak formation. In some instances, the growth factors derive from the proliferating smooth muscle cells themselves [12].

Smooth muscle cells from newborn rat aortas [13] and from neointimal proliferative lesions induced by balloon catheter de-endothelialization of rat carotid artery [12] have both been shown to be capable of secreting platelet-derived growth factor (PDGF). As a consequence, smooth muscle cells may be involved during embryogenesis and growth of the rat arterial system through an autocrine mechanism. This same effect may occur in induced intimal proliferative lesions. It is probable, however, that most of the growth-regulatory molecules and cytokines that play a role in the lesions are induced by an interacting network between smooth muscle, monocyte-derived macrophages, T-lymphocytes present in the lesions, and platelet thrombi (when platelets become associated with the lesions), as well as by the overlying endothelium. Growth factors, such as M-colony-stimulating factors (M-CSF) and GM-colony-stimulating factors (GM-CSF), are probably involved in macrophage replication, whereas PDGF, possibly heparin-binding epidermal growth factor–like growth factor (HB-EGF), and possibly fibroblast growth factor (FGF) may be involved in smooth muscle migration and proliferation. The cytokines, interleukin-1 (IL-1) and tumor necrosis factor alpha (TNF-α), as well as transforming growth factor beta (TGF-β), all can induce smooth muscle proliferation via a secondary induction of PDGF through their actions on endothelium to induce paracrine secretion of PDGF or on smooth muscle cells to induce autocrine secretion of PDGF-AA [14].

THE PLATELET

The platelet plays an integral role in atherogenesis at those anatomic sites where platelet interactions have been observed in experimental animals, such as nonhuman primates [15–18], swine [19], and rabbits [20,21], although it must be kept in mind that platelet interactions are not the common denominator in the formation of all lesions. They may occur at particular anatomic sites such as branches and bifurcations; however, lesions may form with no evidence of platelet interactions whatsoever. Where platelet interactions occur in the nonhuman primate, rapid formation of proliferative lesions occurs at similar sites. The presumption that the platelet provides the growth factors that initiate lesion formation under those circumstances is based on the fact that following adherence and aggregation induced by factors such as thrombin or by exposure to collagen, platelets contain and can secrete mitogens, including PDGF, epidermal growth factor (EGF) or transforming growth factor alpha (TGF-α), platelet-derived endothelial cell growth factor (PD-ECGF), and TGF-β [22]. In the artery wall, PDGF and TGF-β may be potent mitogens that could be chemotactic for smooth muscle cells and induce the cells that migrate into the intima to proliferate. Platelets also could play an important role in the organization of thrombi. Since large amounts of PDGF would be present in a thrombus, there would be migration and proliferation of smooth muscle cells during thrombus organization. It would be difficult, however, to explain lesion progression based solely on platelet-derived PDGF. The logical candidate responsible for lesion progression, and perhaps for the initiation of the majority of lesions, is the activated macrophage.

THE MONOCYTE/MACROPHAGE

Macrophages are capable of secreting growth factors for smooth muscle cells and fibroblasts [23]. Studies show that the activated macrophage, whether derived from the circulating monocyte, the lung, or the peritoneum, has the capacity to synthesize and secrete growth factors, including PDGF [24], FGF [25], EGF/TGF-α [26], IL-1 [27], and TGF-β [28]. When the monocyte is in the circulation, it does not express the genes for any of these growth factors except TGF-β, and none of these growth factors is secreted by nonactivated peripheral blood monocytes. Once activated to become macrophages, these cells are stimulated to express the genes for these various growth factors and can, with appropriate stimulation, synthesize and secrete each of them and possibly all or varying combinations of them. On that basis, it is assumed that macrophages, which are found in fatty streaks and as significant components of all advanced lesions of atherosclerosis, probably serve as the principal source of growth factors. Consequently, they probably bear the major responsibility for smooth muscle proliferation during the pathogenesis and progression of the lesions of atherosclerosis. Unlike platelets, which can release only prestored material, macrophages can be a continuing source of growth factors. In theory, these growth factors could chronically release mitogens based on their capacity to synthesize and secrete proteins.

Macrophages, as well as smooth muscle cells, play a key role in cell replication during atherogenesis. In many lesions, there is as much macrophage as smooth muscle replication. In numerous instances, the macrophage may be the dominant replicating cell. This case raises a host of questions on the role of macrophage replication and gene expression for growth-regulatory molecules and cytokines in determining the ultimate fate of the lesions of atherosclerosis. Macrophages not only can make these molecules but can be an active source of proteolytic enzymes, including enzymes that lyse extracellular matrix molecules. Excessive turnover of connective tissue induced by macrophages could lead to alterations in lesions that can result in lysis of areas of lesions and lesion weakness, possibly leading to aneurysmal change, as well as to weak spots that could be sites of fissures, cracking, and sudden thrombosis. Macrophages probably are the prime source of growth-regulatory and chemotactic molecules in the lesions and thus a key factor in lesion progression. Their interaction with T-lymphocytes is poorly understood. The T-lymphocytes may represent some form of immune response in the lesion and, if so, could serve to activate macrophages, and vice versa, in the process of atherogenesis.

Growth Factors

A number of mitogenic factors, termed growth factors, have been discovered after salivary glands were found to contain a source of growth factor activity for epithelial cells, EGF. Since that time, other mitogenic substances have been identified, isolated, purified, and characterized, and each of them appears to have a relative trophism for given cell types. These include the three different isoforms of PDGF (the AB, AA, and BB forms), PD-ECGF, FGF (both acidic and basic FGF), TGF-α, and TGF-β. Like EGF, TGF-α originally was found to be a mitogen principally for epithelial cells. TGF-α binds to the same receptor as EGF and was first thought to derive only from transformed or neoplastic cells but is now known to derive from diploid cells as well, including the activated macrophage [26]. The principal mitogens for connective-tissue–forming cells, such as fibroblasts and smooth muscle, are the different forms of PDGF and the acidic and basic forms of FGF. Unlike PDGF, however, FGF is also a mitogen for vascular endothelial cells, and thus it is a potent angiogenic agent. Most of the mitogens that have been discovered appear to have a relatively specific trophism for cells such as epithelium, endothelium, or mesodermally derived connective-tissue–forming cells such as fibroblasts and smooth muscle.

TGF-β probably should not be called a growth factor, since its principal activity appears to be inhibition of cell proliferation and induction of cell differentiation. In the presence of other growth factors such as EGF or PDGF, TGF-β has been shown to facilitate growth of particular types of cells in three-dimensional gel systems such as soft agar. TGF-β has a bimodal effect on connective-tissue cells such as smooth muscle. At low doses, TGF-β induces smooth muscle to express the gene for PDGF-A. It synthesizes and secretes PDGF-AA, stimulating proliferation. At higher doses, TGF-β continues to stimulate PDGF-AA but also downregulates the receptor required for PDGF-AA, thus inhibiting the autocrine response [29]. The field of growth-regulatory–molecule research is expanding rapidly, and our understanding of the roles of each of these substances in normal biology and in pathologic events is likewise increasing. Each molecule appears to exert its effects by binding to specific cell-surface, high-affinity receptors, which then stimulate intracellular signals that ultimately culminate in cell replication. In addition, they also induce numerous other cellular events, ranging from chemotaxis to increased RNA and protein synthesis and cell contraction.

THE CELLULAR INTERACTIONS THAT OCCUR DURING ATHEROGENESIS

With the knowledge of cellular constituents of the fatty streak and fibrous plaque and the physiologic properties of those cells, it becomes possible to appreciate the significance of the cellular interactions that lead to the development of each type of lesion and the factors that may be responsible for those interactions. The type and chronology of the cell interactions that occur during atherogenesis have been studied in a number of different animal species, including nonhuman primates [15–18], swine [19], rabbits [20,21], pigeons [30], and rats [31]. In each species, hypercholesterolemia has been induced by diet. In the case of the rabbit, the Watanabe heritable hyperlipidemic rabbit (WHHL) model of homozygous familial hypercholesterolemia (FH) was used. Atherosclerosis also has been studied in hypertensive animals, homocystinemic baboons, and diabetic animals. The cellular interactions that are best understood are those observed in the hypercholesterolemic nonhuman primate, swine, and rabbit.

Faggiotto and colleagues [15,16] and Masuda and colleagues [17,18] studied nonhuman primates made hypercholesterolemic by diet to levels equivalent to those found in human FH patients or in humans with common atherosclerosis. The levels of plasma cholesterol in those two studies ranged from 500 to 1200 mg/dl and 200 to 400 mg/dl, respectively. Under those conditions, the first changes that were observed involved adherence to endothelium of clusters of leukocytes, principally monocytes, together with small numbers of lymphocytes. These were attached in clusters located randomly throughout the arterial tree 7 to 12 days (at high levels of cholesterol) or several months (at lower levels) after inducing hypercholesterolemia.

The leukocytes adhere to each other, to other cell types, and to extracellular matrix via a series of cell-surface molecules that regulate their movement and interactions. These molecules include the immunoglobulin superfamily, including the ICAMs and the VCAMs; the integrin family, which includes a series of adhesion receptors, consisting of alpha and beta subunits, by which cells adhere to different forms of extracellular matrix; and the selectins, which are molecules with an N terminal lectin domain that play diverse roles in adhesion. In lesions of atherosclerosis, it appears that selectins may be involved in the rolling of leukocytes and that VCAM-1 and ICAM-1 may be two of the principal molecules involved in leukocyte adhesion to endothelium. Other molecules may be involved in the transmigration of these cells between the endothelium into the intima of the artery [32].

The monocytes move around on the surface, probe between junctions of the endothelial cells, and are chemotactically attracted into the space beneath the endothelial cells. As a consequence, they slide between the endothelial cells and localize in the intima. These monocytes then become converted rather rapidly to foam cells by taking up large quantities of extracellular lipoprotein, which they store largely in the form of cholesteryl ester. These collections of subendothelial, lipid-filled macrophages constitute the first and ubiquitous lesion of atherosclerosis, the fatty streak. The fatty streaks expand by continued chemotactic attraction of monocytes into the intima. Eventually, the intima contains one or two layers of large numbers of lipid-filled macrophages, and the overlying endothelium is stretched and thinned, providing a highly irregular surface containing domelike structures and deep crevices, as seen with the scanning electron microscope. The fatty streak also expands by the migration of some smooth muscle cells that are attracted from the media into the intima, where they also begin to accumulate lipid. Thus, the fatty streak becomes multilayered, with two or three layers of macrophages, each layer separated by small numbers of smooth muscle cells. Identical observations related to fatty-streak formation have been made in hypercholesterolemic swine [19] and in WHHL rabbits, as well as in rabbits with diet-induced hypercholesterolemia [20,21].

A second set of cellular interactions occurs in the hypercholesterolemic nonhuman primates after approximately

5 to 6 months of hypercholesterolemia (high levels of plasma cholesterol) or after 2 to 3 years (lower levels of plasma cholesterol). These occur at branches and bifurcations, first in the leg arteries and then, at subsequent monthly intervals, at the iliac bifurcation, followed by the abdominal aorta, the thoracic aorta, and ultimately the coronary arteries. The change consists of apparent dysjunction of endothelial cells and endothelial retraction over some areas of fatty streaks, particularly at branches and bifurcations, where the blood flow may contain eddy currents and back currents. This endothelial retraction exposes the underlying lipid-filled macrophages to the circulation, and some of them appear to migrate back into the lumen and are swept into the circulation. With this occurrence, platelets may adhere and thrombi form at sites of exposed connective tissue and, in most instances, on the exposed surface of the macrophages themselves. At the sites where these platelet interactions occur, massive proliferative smooth muscle lesions develop into fibrous plaques within two months. The fibrous plaque that forms contains a fibrous cap of dense connective tissue, made up of numerous flat smooth muscle cells, some of which contain lipid mixed with a few interspersed macrophages. This fibrous cap covers a mixture of smooth muscle cells and macrophages, both of which often contain numerous lipid droplets and appear as foam cells. In many instances, therefore, the fatty streak appears to be converted into a fibrous plaque either by platelet interactions, which often occur at branches and bifurcations where endothelial dysjunction and retraction occur, or possibly at other sites in the artery wall over a longer period of time, by attraction of smooth muscle cells from the media into the intima and induction of additional smooth muscle proliferation. This raises the interesting question as to what induces the proliferative response of the smooth muscle cells; it also gives rise to the need to understand factors responsible for the initial chemotactic attraction of the monocytes into the artery wall that leads them to develop into macrophages and foam cells.

In addition to smooth muscle cells, numerous macrophages have also been shown to proliferate actively within the lesions of atherosclerosis in hypercholesterolemic rabbits [33], in human lesions [34], and in monkeys [unpublished data]. Thus the multiplication of macrophages may be another critical factor in the process of atherogenesis. Macrophages also have been shown to contain PDGF-B protein within lesions of nonhuman primate and human atherosclerosis at all stages of development, indicating that macrophages are a source of PDGF-BB during lesion formation and progression [35].

The most probable explanation for these changes relates to the formation and secretion of growth factors by a number of cells, including platelets as they interact with the artery, activated macrophages, activated endothelial cells, and smooth muscle cells themselves. A number of growth factors may play a role in these phenomena, including PDGF, which can be secreted by platelets, activated macrophages, endothelial cells, and smooth muscle cells. In addition, FGF can be released from dying cells such as activated macrophages, and TGF-β, which modulates growth response, can be released by all the cells involved. The possible role of these growth-regulatory molecules and the other components associated with the development of the lesions of atherosclerosis are discussed next.

The Response-to-Injury Hypothesis of Atherosclerosis

The response-to-injury hypothesis was formulated based on many observations demonstrating that endothelial "injury" can lead to a sequence of cellular events in animals culminating in fibroproliferative lesions that appear very similar to those of atherosclerosis in humans.

The hypothesis suggests that some form of injury occurs to the lining endothelial cells as the initiating event. The injury may be very subtle, so that the endothelial cells remain phenotypically unchanged and morphologically intact, but endothelial function is altered. For example, the permeability characteristics of the endothelium may be altered, the endothelial cells may turn over at a greater rate, the endothelial cells may synthesize and secrete growth factors such as PDGF into the underlying artery wall, or the endothelial cells may be stimulated to synthesize vasoactive agents. Elements that could induce changes and injury to the endothelium could include substances derived from cigarette smoking, hypercholesterolemia, diabetes, hypertension, or viruses. It is postulated that appropriate endothelial injury could eventually lead to alterations in the surface characteristics of the endothelium and potentially in circulating monocytes, as well, leading them to become stickier and thus to interact with one another, inducing a chemotactic event in which monocytes first attach and then enter between the endothelial cells and lodge in the subendothelium. Support for this aspect of the hypothesis derives from the observations detailed previously and also from observations made in hypertensive animals [36]. Fatty streaks can thus develop in hypercholesterolemic or nonhypercholesterolemic conditions by localization in the intima of monocyte-derived macrophages. If such macrophages are properly activated, they could then become an important source of growth factors. Activated macrophages have the potential to secrete or release PDGF, FGF, EGF/TGF-α, TGF-β, colony-stimulating factor (CSF-1), and IL-1. Many of these growth factors, individually or in appropriate combinations, could have striking effects, including the capacity to attract smooth muscle cells chemotactically from the underlying media into the intima if the growth factors are secreted by the activated macrophages within the intimal space. According to this hypothesis, the fatty streak itself could become the principal source of growth factors over a prolonged period of time if the macrophages were properly activated. This would lead to conversion of the fatty streak into a fibroproliferative lesion, the fibrous plaque or complicated lesion of atherosclerosis (Fig. 11-1).

Furthermore, the response-to-injury hypothesis indicates that if the injury to the endothelium is sufficiently severe, endothelial dysjunction and retraction may occur. Further injury to the endothelium could come from the activated macrophages themselves, which could release toxic substances such as superoxide anion, oxidized lipoproteins, or other toxic substances that could lead to endo-

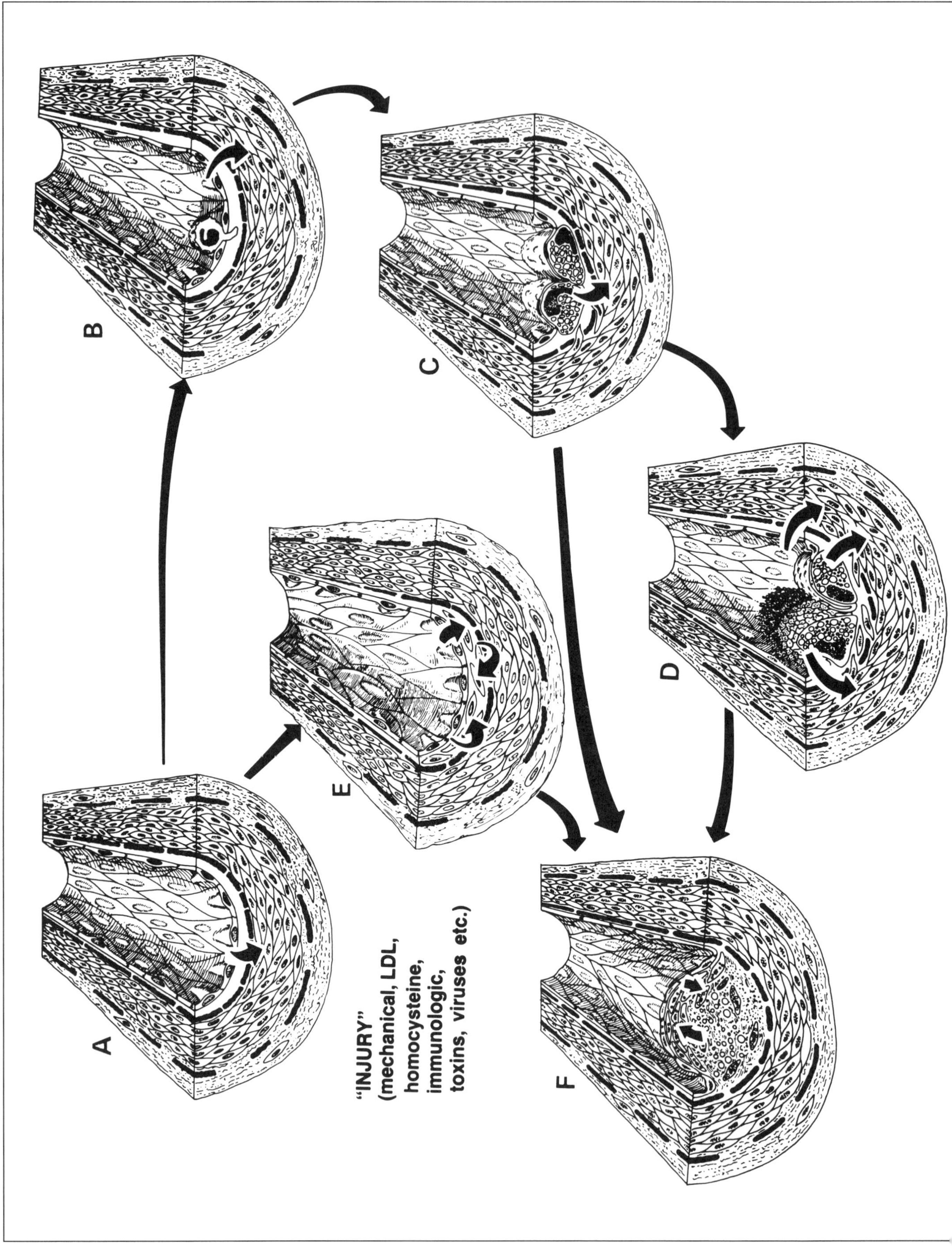
A
B
C
D
E
F
"INJURY"
(mechanical, LDL,
homocysteine,
immunologic,
toxins, viruses etc.)

thelial dysjunction. Endothelial dysjunction could result from the pressure of a constantly expanding fatty streak, caused by continued accumulation of subendothelial foam cells or by the local release of protease by foam cells, which can digest underlying connective tissue to which the endothelial cells are tethered. In either case, the endothelial retraction would then permit the interaction of a second blood cell, the platelet, with either or both the exposed macrophages and connective tissue. When that happens, platelet adherence and degranulation could occur, releasing all of the growth factors contained by the platelets, which also include PDGF, PDECGF, EGF/TGF-α, and TGF-β. Thus, the platelet, a potent source of growth factors, could accelerate the smooth muscle chemotactic and intimal proliferative response and play a role in the more rapidly progressing lesions of atherosclerosis [37].

The fatty streak is completely reversible in the nonhuman primate if a normal diet is restored. The fibrous plaque can also regress if hypercholesterolemia is aggressively approached using diet and lipid-lowering reagents in nonhuman primates and in humans. Thus, the understanding of how and where these molecules work provides numerous opportunities for intervention.

Plaque Regression

There is clear evidence that experimentally induced fatty streaks can completely regress when animals are taken off high-fat, high-cholesterol diets. Furthermore, there is evidence that some fibrous plaques can also regress in nonhuman primates in which atherosclerosis has been induced. Angiographic studies of human lesions have demonstrated that a certain percentage of advanced lesions can regress when patients are able to reduce their levels of plasma cholesterol for sufficient periods of time. Cell turnover is a key element of lesion regression. The fact that lesions susceptible to hypercholesterolemia can be induced to regress by alterations of diet suggests that this approach will be extremely important in reversing the injury that results from hypercholesterolemia, which leads to the formation of the fibrous plaque.

When a fibrous plaque progresses, it probably does so either by continuing alterations of injury to the endothelial cells, permitting continuing ingress of monocyte/macrophages, or perhaps in some cases by platelet interactions. Mural thrombosis on the surface of plaques may represent a major mode of plaque progression with increase in the size of the plaque and, thus, decrease in the effective lumen of the artery at such sites. The vasa vasorum in plaques may derive from endothelium at the luminal surface or from small vessels in the adventitia that serve to vascularize the lesion as the wall of the artery is thickened by lesion progression. The endothelial cells in the vasa vasorum, if they are appropriately activated, could potentially serve as sources of growth factors (PDGF in particular) and thus play a role in further progression of the lesions.

There is sufficient biochemical, cell and molecular biology, and in vivo data to suggest that the response-to-injury hypothesis has provided a basis for understanding how the lesions of atherosclerosis form and what steps may be taken to prevent lesion formation [37,38].

References

1. Ross R, Glomset JA. The pathogenesis of atherosclerosis. N Engl J Med 1976; 295:369–77, 420–5.
2. Schwartz SM, Benditt EP. Clustering of replicating cells in aortic endothelium. Acad Sci USA 1976; 73:651–53.
3. Glagov S. Hemodynamic risk factors; mechanical stress, mural architecture, medial nutrition and the vulnerability of arteries to atherosclerosis. In RW Wissler, JC Geer, eds. The Pathogenesis of Atherosclerosis. Baltimore: Williams & Wilkins, 1972. Pp. 164–99.
4. Tsukada T, et al. HHF35, a muscle-actin-specific monoclonal

Fig. 11-1. The response-to-injury hypothesis. Advanced intimal proliferative lesions of atherosclerosis may occur by at least two pathways. The pathway demonstrated by the long arrows has been observed in experimentally induced hypercholesterolemia. Injury to the endothelium **A.** may induce growth-factor secretion (short arrow), which may help induce monocytes to attach to endothelium **B.** Monocytes and endothelial cells may secrete growth factor (short arrow) into the subendothelium. Subendothelial migration of monocytes **C.** may lead to fatty streak formation and release of growth factors (short arrow) from the lipid-containing macrophages. Fatty streaks may be directly converted to fibrous plaques (long arrow from C to F) through release of growth factors from macrophages, endothelial cells, or both. Macrophages may also stimulate or injure the overlying endothelium. In some cases, macrophages may lose their endothelial cover, and platelet attachment may occur **D.**, providing three possible sources of growth factors: platelets, activated macrophages, and activated endothelium (short arrows). Some smooth muscle cells in the proliferative lesion **F.** may also form and secrete growth factors (short arrows).

Another pathway for development of advanced lesions of atherosclerosis is shown by the arrows from A to E to F. In this case, the endothelium may be injured but remain intact. Increased endothelial turnover and "injury" to the endothelium may result in growth-factor formation by endothelial cells **A.** This may stimulate migration of smooth muscle cells from the media into the intima, accompanied by endogenous production of PDGF by smooth muscle as well as growth-factor secretion from the injured endothelial cells **E.** These interactions could then lead to fibrous-plaque formation and further lesion progression **F.** (Reproduced with permission of New England Journal of Medicine from R. Ross. The pathogenesis of atherosclerosis—an update. N Engl J Med 1986; 314:488–500.)

antibody. I: Immunocytochemical and biochemical characterization. Am J Pathol 1987; 126:51–60.
5. Gown AM, Tsukada T, Ross R. Human atherosclerosis. II: Immunocytochemical analysis of the cellular composition of human atherosclerotic lesions. Am J Pathol 1986; 125:191–207.
6. McGill HC Jr, ed. The Geographic Pathology of Atherosclerosis. Baltimore: Williams & Wilkins, 1968. Pp. 1–193.
7. Ross R, et al. Human atherosclerosis. I: Cell constitution and characteristics of advanced lesions of the superficial femoral artery. Am J Pathol 1984; 114:79–93.
8. Jonasson L, et al. Regional accumulations of T cells, macrophages, and smooth muscle cells in the human atherosclerotic plaque. Arteriosclerosis 1986; 6:131–8.
9. Ross R, et al. A platelet-dependent serum factor that stimulates the proliferation of arterial smooth muscle cells in vitro. Proc Natl Acad Sci USA 1974; 71:1207–10.
10. Gajdusek C, et al. An endothelial cell–derived growth factor. J Cell Biol 1980; 85:467–72.
11. Glenn KC, Ross R. Human monocyte-derived growth factor(s) for mesenchymal cells: activation of secretion by endotoxin and Concanavalin A. Cell 1981; 25:603–15.
12. Walker LN, et al. Production of platelet-derived growth factor–like molecules by cultured arterial smooth muscle cells accompanies proliferation after arterial injury. Proc Natl Acad Sci USA 1986; 83:7311.
13. Seifert RA, Schwartz SM, Bowen-Pope DF. Developmentally regulated production of platelet-derived growth factor–like molecules. Nature 1984; 311:669–71.
14. Raines EW, Ross R. Platelet-derived growth factor in vivo. In Biology of Platelet-derived Growth Factor. Cytokines, B Westermark, C Sorg, eds. Basel: Karger, 1993. Vol 5. Pp. 74–114.
15. Faggiotto A, Ross R, Harker L. Studies of hypercholesterolemia in the nonhuman primate. I: Changes that lead to fatty streak formation. Arteriosclerosis 1984; 4:323–340.
16. Faggiotto A, Ross R. Studies of hypercholesterolemia in the nonhuman primate. II: Fatty streak conversion to fibrous plaque. Arteriosclerosis 1984; 4:341–356.
17. Masuda J, Ross R. Atherogenesis during low-level hypercholesterolemia in the nonhuman primate. I: Fatty streak formation. Arteriosclerosis 1990; 10:164–177.
18. Masuda J, Ross R. Atherogenesis during low-level hypercholesterolemia in the nonhuman primate. II: Fatty streak conversion to fibrous plaque. Arteriosclerosis 1990; 10:178–187.
19. Gerrity RG. The role of the monocyte in atherogenesis. I: Transition of blood-borne monocytes into foam cells in fatty lesions. Am J Pathol 1981; 103:181–190.
20. Rosenfeld ME, et al. Fatty streak initiation in Watanabe heritable hyperlipemic and comparably hypercholesterolemic fat-fed rabbits. Arteriosclerosis 1987; 7:9–23.
21. Rosenfeld ME, et al. Fatty streak expansion and maturation in Watanabe heritable hyperlipemic and comparably hypercholesterolemic fat-fed rabbits. Arteriosclerosis 1987; 7:24–34.
22. Ross R, Raines EW, Bowen-Pope DF. The biology of platelet-derived growth factor. Cell 1986; 46:155–69.
23. Leibovich SJ, Ross R. A macrophage-dependent factor that stimulates the proliferation of fibroblasts in vitro. Am J Pathol 1976; 84:501–513.
24. Shimokado K, et al. A significant part of macrophage-derived growth factor consists of at least two forms of PDGF. Cell 1985; 43:277–286.
25. Baird A, Mormede P, Bohlen P. Immunoreactive fibroblast growth factor in cells of peritoneal exudate suggests its identity with macrophage-derived growth factor. Biochem Biophys Res Commun 1985; 126:358–364.
26. Madtes DK, et al. Induction of transforming growth factor-alpha in activated human alveolar macrophages. Cell 1988; 53:285–293.
27. Dohlman JG, Payan DG, Goetzl EJ. Generation of a unique fibroblast-activating factor by human monocytes. Immunology 1984; 52:577–584.
28. Assoian RK, et al. Expression and secretion of type β transforming growth factor by activated human macrophages. Proc Natl Acad Sci USA 1987; 84:6020–6024.
29. Battegay EJ, et al. TGF-β induces bimodal proliferation of connective tissue cells via complex control of an autocrine PDGF loop. Cell 1990; 63:515–524.
30. Jerome WG, Lewis JC. Early atherogenesis in white Carneau pigeons. I: Leukocyte margination and endothelial alterations at the celiac bifurcation. Am J Pathol 1984; 116:56–68.
31. Joris I, et al. Studies on the pathogenesis of atherosclerosis. I: Adhesion and emigration of mononuclear cells in the aorta of hypercholesterolemic rats. Am J Pathol 1983; 113:341–358.
32. Springer TA. Adhesion receptors of the immune system. Nature 1990; 346:425–434.
33. Rosenfeld ME, Ross R. Macrophage and smooth muscle cell proliferation in atherosclerotic lesions of WHHL and comparably hypercholesterolemic fat-fed rabbits. Arteriosclerosis 1990; 10:680–687.
34. Gordon D, et al. Cell proliferation of human coronary arteries. Proc Natl Acad Sci USA 1990; 87:4600–4604.
35. Ross R, et al. Localization of PDGF-B protein in macrophages in all phases of atherogenesis. Science 1990; 248:1009–1012.
36. Chobanian AV, Brecher PI, Haudenshild CC, Effects of hypertension and of antihypertension therapy on atherosclerosis. State of the Art Lecture. Am Soc Proc[Suppl I] 1986; 8:15–21.
37. Ross R. The pathogenesis of atherosclerosis—an update. N Engl J Med 1986; 314:488–500.
38. Ross R. The pathogenesis of atherosclerosis: a perspective for the 1990s. Nature 1993; 362:801–809.

Pathogenesis of Atherosclerosis: Cellular Interactions

Peter Libby

Until the last dozen or so years, the prevailing concepts of the cellular events during atherogenesis considered primarily responses to soluble elements derived from blood or blood platelets. Attention was focused on blood-derived substances such as cholesterol-rich lipoproteins, for example, low-density lipoprotein (LDL), and mediators derived from platelet alpha granules, that is, platelet-derived growth factor (PDGF), as likely candidates for mediating atherogenesis. This view resembles in principle an **endocrine model**, in which local vascular cells respond to blood-borne stimuli. Current views have shifted to accord a more prominent role to signals exchanged at short distances among neighboring cells (a **paracrine model**). Cells can even generate signals to which they themselves respond, a model of information exchange known as **autocrine**. Hence, **cellular interactions** rather than simple responses to blood-borne substances currently assume a greater portion of our thinking regarding the pathogenesis of this complex disease.

This chapter will consider these cellular interactions in greater detail to illustrate current concepts of intercellular information exchange during atherogenesis. As an organizing principle, we will use the chronology of lesion development that has emerged from morphologic studies over the last decade. Notably, the cross-talk among cells of varying types during atherogenesis involves more than just the intrinsic cells of the arterial wall, the endothelium, and the vascular smooth muscle. Indeed, the mononuclear phagocyte probably also is an important contributor to atherogenesis. Thus, any discussion of cellular interactions during atherogenesis must consider the mononuclear phagocyte.

Monocyte-Endothelial Interactions

MONOCYTE ADHERENCE TO LESION-PRONE ENDOTHELIUM

Interactions between white blood cells and the endothelium figure prominently in many homeostatic and pathologic processes. For example, nascent leukocytes in the bone marrow must traverse the endothelium to gain access to the circulation. Leukopoeisis may even involve some signal exchanges between microvascular endothelial cells in the bone marrow and leukocytic precursors. The homeostasis of the normal cellular immune system involves constant lymphocyte recirculation from the lymph into the general circulation. This process clearly involves interaction of lymphocytes with various categories of endothelial cells (e.g., specialized venules in lymph nodes). During cellular immune responses, recruitment of lymphocytes to specific sites also probably involves selective interaction of lymphocytes with endothelial cells activated to their specific adhesion molecules [1].

This pattern of lymphocyte-endothelial interaction also pertains to acute and chronic inflammatory responses. For example, polymorphonuclear leukocytes accumulate in large numbers at sites of acute inflammation. This selective recruitment of granulocytes appears to involve the expression on the surface of activated endothelial cells of well-characterized adhesion molecules (E- and P-selectin) that interact selectively with cognate ligands expressed at high levels by polymorphonuclear leukocytes [2]. This type of lymphocyte-endothelial interaction constitutes the molecular mechanisms of pus formation at sites of acute bacterial infection or tissue injury.

In chronic inflammation, recruitment of mononuclear leukocytes predominates over recruitment of cells of the granulocytic series. A similar mechanism involving the expression of particular leukocyte adhesion molecules on the endothelial surface appears to be at work in this situation as well [3]. Mononuclear leukocytes, including lymphocytes and monocytes, can express surface molecules that interact selectively with receptors on the endothelium that are members of the immunoglobulin gene superfamily. These molecules are known as the vascular cell adhesion molecule-1 (VCAM), which interacts with the VLA-4 integrin molecule on the surface of mononuclear leukocytes, and the intercellular adhesion molecule-1 (ICAM), which interacts with LFA-1, a member of the CD-11/CD-18 subclass of the integrin superfamily [4,5]. Atherosclerosis, as a special case of chronic inflammation in arteries, may recapitulate this general model for endothelial-leukocyte interaction [6].

The initial phases of atherogenesis in humans probably occur in the first decades of life and seldom become accessible for pathologic analysis. Therefore, animal models of atherosclerosis, usually involving a diet enriched in cholesterol and saturated fats, provide insight into the early phases of the biology of the process. One of the first morphologically evident consequences of initiating an atherogenic diet is increased adhesive interactions of monocytes with the endothelium and subsequent local accumulation of mononuclear phagocytes within the intima of affected arteries. Poole and Florey clearly recognized this phenomenon in the 1950s in rabbits fed an atherogenic diet [7]. Subsequently, Gerrity and colleagues showed early monocyte-endothelial adhesive interaction in swine consuming an atherogenic diet [8]. Joris and colleagues described a similar sequence of events in rats fed a diet designed to induce atherosclerosis-like lesions [9]. Ross and co-workers defined a similar sequence of events in the nonhuman primate consuming an atherogenic diet and in mice bearing a genetically engineered mutation rendering them susceptible to diet-induced lesion formation [10–12]. Thus, in a range of diverse animal species with varying susceptibilities to atherosclerosis, increased monocyte-endothelial interaction constitutes an important early feature.

In 1958, Poole and Florey wrote, "It is clear that a patchy alteration in the endothelial surface takes place as manifested by lipoid accumulation and interaction with monocytes. Unfortunately, this cannot be pursued with profit [7]." In the 1980s, Gimbrone formulated the **endothelial-leukocyte adhesion molecule (E-LAM) hypothesis**. Gimbrone proposed that activated endothelial cells express on their surface more or less specific adhesion molecules that govern their adhesive interactions with various leukocyte classes [13]. As previously discussed, subsequent molecular characterization and functional studies on a variety of leukocyte adhesion molecules have verified the E-LAM hypothesis in its major aspects. In the context of atherogenesis, Cybulsky and Gimbrone proposed the existence of athero-E-LAMs that would mediate the selective monocyte-endothelial interaction established by the aforementioned experimental studies. These workers applied a monoclonal antibody strategy to identify a structure expressed selectively on the surfaces of endothelial cells overlying atherosclerotic lesions in rabbits that would have a monocyte-adhesive function. In 1991, Cybulsky and Gimbrone reported success with that strategy [14]. The molecule with athero-E-LAM function that they identified turned out to be the rabbit homologue of a recently described human endothelial-leukocyte adhesion molecule-1. This member of the immunoglobulin gene superfamily class of adhesion molecules binds to the VLA-4 integrin on mononuclear leukocytes. Those findings immediately suggested that VCAM-1 might participate in monocyte recruitment during early atherosclerotic-lesion development.

To test that possibility, we explored the early kinetics of VCAM expression by aortic endothelial cells in rabbits consuming an atherogenic diet [15]. In the normal rabbit aorta, few cells express VCAM-1. At four days following initiation of the atherogenic diet, even lesion-prone regions of the rabbit aorta displayed scant VCAM expression. However, seven days after commencement of the cholesterol-rich diet, most animals studied displayed focal VCAM-1 expression on the endothelial cells in lesion-prone regions of the aorta. At three weeks postinitiation of the diet, intimal monocyte-derived foam cells colocalized with VCAM-1 bearing endothelial cells were collected. This sequence of events supports the conjecture that VCAM-1 is one of the adhesion molecules that mediates monocyte adhesion to the endothelium in the early phases of atherogenesis.

Indeed, other adhesion molecules are also likely to be involved in this selective monocyte recruitment. For example, endothelial cells in developing atherosclerotic lesions may express higher levels of ICAM-1 as well [16,17]. At least two laboratories have employed monoclonal antibody strategies to identify athero-E-LAMs [18,19]. However, to date no molecular structures have emerged from those studies, although they remain an intriguing realm for future development in this area.

As noted, it is difficult to obtain appropriate specimens for studying the earliest phases of human atherosclerosis. Most observations on complicated human atheroma have not disclosed high levels of VCAM-1 expression on the overlying endothelium. However, the microvessels that form the neovascular plexi common in advanced atherosclerotic lesions do express VCAM-1 [20]. Taken together, the experimental observations on early atherogenesis and the study of advanced human lesions suggest the following overall scenario for monocyte recruitment during the life history of an atherosclerotic lesion. In the initial phases of fatty-streak formation, there are no intimal microvessels. Monocyte recruitment likely takes places via the macrovascular luminal endothelium. Later in the history of the lesion, when extensive plexi of microvessels have formed, they provide an enormous surface area for leukocyte trafficking. We know nothing of the kinetics of mononuclear phagocytes trafficking in atherosclerosis. However, the finding of VCAM-bearing microvessels in advanced human plaques suggests ongoing recruitment of mononuclear leukocytes through microvessels rather than the macrovascular endothelium.

LEUKOCYTE PENETRATION OF THE ENDOTHELIUM BY DIRECTED MIGRATION

Adhesion molecules can account for the initial phase of monocyte recruitment to nascent atherosclerotic lesions. However, their adhesive interaction is insufficient to account for their intimal accumulations of these phagocytes. It is likely that the directed migration of monocytes adherent to the activated endothelium requires chemoattractant molecules that provoke penetration into the intima [21]. Monocyte-chemoattractant protein-1 (MCP-1) constitutes a likely candidate for such a chemoattractant molecule [22]. Endothelial and smooth-muscle cells can elaborate MCP-1 when appropriately stimulated [23–25]. Human and experimental atherosclerotic lesions contain MCP-1 RNA transcripts or protein [26,27]. Again, MCP-1 is only one example, currently recognized, of a family of monocyte chemoattractants that may contribute to the accumulation of mononuclear phagocytes in the developing atheroma.

Before leaving the subject of monocyte-endothelial interaction, we must consider what stimuli account for the local expression of monocyte adhesion molecules and chemoattractants at particular sites of lesion predilection. One characteristic of lesion-prone areas of arteries is increased resonance time for lipoprotein particles. There is evidence for accumulation of oxidatively modified lipoproteins in atheroma. Therefore, induction of adhesion-molecule or chemoattractant expression by constituents of oxidized lipoproteins presents an intriguing link between dyslipidemia and early local changes in endothelial-monocyte interaction in the arterial wall. Kume and Gimbrone have shown that lysophosphatidyl choline can enhance VCAM-1 gene expression in endothelial cells [28,29]. This observation provides a potential molecular mechanism for this intriguing link between lipoproteins and VCAM expression.

Because it is the entire vasculature that experiences hypercholesterolemia, the mere existence of dyslipidemia does not explain the focal development of atherosclerotic lesions at predictable sites. Altered shear stress characterizes such lesion-prone areas [30]. Thus, local hydrodynamic forces constitute another likely candidate signaling focal adhesion-molecule expression on endothelial cells at sites of lesion formation. Indeed, shear stress does regulate the expression of the ICAM-1 gene [31]. However, there is no evidence that VCAM stress regulates the VCAM-1 gene. Resnick, working in Gimbrones' group, has identified a motif in the promoter region of certain shear stress–regulated genes that appears to confer that response to hydrodynamic forces [32]. This shear stress response element (SSRE), GAGACC, is not present in the promoter region of VCAM-1. Thus, no direct evidence supports shear stress as a regulator of endothelial VCAM expression during lesion formation. Interestingly, this transcriptional mechanism does mediate shear stress augmentation of ICAM-1 expression by endothelial cells. Furthermore, stress can induce MCP-1 expression by endothelial cells [33]. Our knowledge of this area is still rudimentary and based solely on in vitro models. It is likely that future research will continue to expand our understanding of the potential control of monocyte-adhesion recruitment by hydrodynamic forces.

Another potential signaling mechanism for focal adhesion-molecule and chemoattractant expression emerges from the consistent finding that cytokines—protein mediators of inflammation and immunity—may induce the expression of many adhesion molecules and chemoattractants. For example, in vitro and in organoid cultures of aortic tissue, cytokines such as tumor necrosis factor-α (TNF-α) or interleukin-1 (IL-1) can augment VCAM expression on endothelium [4,15,34–36]. Since oxidized lipoproteins can enhance the expression of certain cytokine genes in vascular cells, this pathway constitutes another potential link between deranged lipid metabolism and phagocyte accumulation during atherogenesis [37,38].

CONCLUSIONS REGARDING MONOCYTE-ENDOTHELIAL INTERACTIONS

In summary, work that has merged over the last few years provides a foundation for the understanding, in molecular terms, of the earliest phases of atherosclerotic lesion development at the level of endothelial-monocyte interaction. The concept of endothelial-leukocyte adhesion molecules as applied to atherogenesis now stands fully established. Our precise list of adhesion molecule and cognate ligands doubtless remains incomplete. The further concept of locally produced chemoattractants participating in monocyte recruitment, exemplified by MCP-1, does not exclude that other molecules, some as yet undiscovered, may also participate in this process. Finally, the signals that initiate endothelial activation at particular foci of lesion development remain conjectural. It is hard conceptually to exclude the involvement of sensors for the local hemodynamic environment, although the precise nature of such mechanisms in this context remains uncertain. Multiple coincident signals, requiring permissive hemodynamics, altered lipid metabolism, and other features likely coexist to explain focal endothelial activation during atherogenesis. Finally, we know too little of the economy of phagocyte trafficking during atherogenesis. It seems likely that leukocytes must be able to egress from lesions as well as to enter them. For example, fatty streaks, local accumulations of lipid-laden macrophages, are ubiquitous even in human populations that have low incidence of atherosclerosis. Fatty streaks commonly occur in children. Although they may mark sites of future lesion formation, in many cases they appear to regress. This observation suggests that we must keep a dynamic view of endothelial-monocyte interaction in mind. We must consider bidirectional trafficking to explain fatty-streak resorption. A mastering of these concepts undoubtedly will aid in our attempts to manipulate and promote regression of atherosclerotic lesions.

Macrophage–Smooth Muscle Cell Interactions

The foregoing section considered the adherence of monocytes to the endothelium and their entry into the intima by directed migration. Upon entry into the intima, macrophages gain access to smooth muscle cells already resident in the intima and have the opportunity for close contact with smooth muscle cells in the subjacent tunica media of the artery, which comprises multilayers of smooth muscle cells. Products of activated mononuclear phagocytes may indeed contribute to smooth muscle-cell replication in the intima and to recruitment of medial smooth muscle cells via migration. Macrophages are "professional" cytokine-secreting cells. By elaborating chemoattractants for smooth muscle cells such as PDGF, these cells may promote intimal smooth muscle-cell accumulation. Furthermore, cytokines such as IL-1 or TNF-α can activate many functions of smooth muscle cells, including their production of autocrine growth factors; the expression of adhesion molecules, which may promote macrophage retention in lesions; and the elaboration of lipid mediators such as prostaglandin E_2, which may alter local cholesterol metabolism.

On the other hand, smooth muscle cells may elaborate factors that influence macrophage functions. For example, as already mentioned, smooth muscle cells when activated elaborate the monocyte chemoattractants MCP-1 [25]. Also, smooth muscle cells can secrete macrophage-colony stimulating factor (M-CSF) [38]. M-CSF activates monocytes, and these phagocytic cells actually require M-CSF for their survival. Thus, smooth muscle cell–derived M-CSF may play a crucial role in maintaining viability of macrophages once they reside in evolving atherosclerotic lesions. The M-CSF secreted by smooth muscle cells can enhance functions of mononuclear phagocytes related to their transition from blood monocytes to the lipid-laden foam cells characteristic of atherosclerotic lesions. Specifically, M-CSF can augment the expression of the scavenger receptor for modified lipoproteins on the surface of human peripheral blood monocytes [38]. This receptor promotes the accumulation of altered lipoproteins, in contrast to the classical LDL receptor, in which high local concentrations of cholesterol do not suppress the expression of the scavenger receptor [39,40]. Transfection of cells with scavenger receptor confers on them the ability to accumulate the large amounts of cholesterol required for foam-cell formation. Thus, increased scavenger receptor expression induced by smooth muscle cell–derived M-CSF likely figures significantly in the transition from monocyte to foam cell observed during atherogenesis.

M-CSF also may regulate macrophage functions involved in reverse-cholesterol transport and, thus, lesion regression. We must view cholesterol economy in lesions as a dynamic process, much as that depicted for leukocytes. The net accumulation of cholesterol in lesions results from the balance between deposition and removal. Epidemiologic, cellular, and biochemical evidence suggests that high density lipoproteins (HDL) may contribute to cholesterol egress from lesions by a process known as **reverse cholesterol transport**. Macrophages stimulated with M-CSF express apolipoprotein E [38]. This locally produced apolipoprotein E can associate with HDL particles that have taken up cholesterol from lesions. The association of HDL particles with apolipoprotein-E bearing may promote their enhanced peripheral catabolism via the classic LDL receptor [41,42]. This LDL receptor actually has a higher affinity for apolipoprotein E than for the characteristic apolipoprotein of the LDL particle, apolipoprotein B. In that manner, smooth muscle cell–derived M-CSF may promote reverse cholesterol transport by inducing local macrophage apolipoprotein-E expression.

In vitro experiments have furnished much of the basis for these speculations regarding apolipoprotein-E expression and M-CSF. If these models pertain to human atherogenesis, one would predict increased expression of both M-CSF and apolipoprotein E in atherosclerotic lesions. Indeed, in a survey of gene expression in human atheroma, of a number of candidates tested, we found mRNA-encoding apolipoprotein E the most prominently elevated [43]. Plaque extracts contained manyfold greater concentrations of apolipoprotein-E mRNA than did control nonatherosclerotic arterial tissue. That study documented accumulation of apolipoprotein-E protein in association with macrophages and smooth muscle cells in advanced human atheroma. We have also found increased expression of M-CSF RNA and protein in human atherosclerotic lesions [38]. These observations support the models of smooth muscle cell–macrophage interactions proposed above. Studies in rabbits also disclose increased M-CSF and apolipoprotein-E expression in atherosclerotic lesions [44]. Mice deficient in apolipoprotein E show marked susceptibility to diet-induced atherosclerosis [45,46]. That finding is particularly noteworthy in light of the notorious resistance of rodents to atherosclerosis, even in the face of hypercholesterolemia. The availability of such mutant mice, in combination with mice bearing mutations that prevent expression of various mediators, such as M-CSF, should permit critical testing of the potential roles of factors such as M-CSF in cholesterol economy and the cellular events during atherosclerosis in vivo.

In summary, macrophages may influence smooth muscle function during atherogenesis, including the migration, proliferation, and production of locally active mediators [47]. On the other hand, smooth muscle cells can influence macrophage functions, enhancing their accumulation in the intima by chemoattractant production, expression of adhesion molecules, and M-CSF production. M-CSF may promote macrophage viability in lesions and may induce the expression of scavenger receptor, which promotes foam-cell formation. Finally, by augmenting macrophage apolipoprotein-E production, smooth muscle cell–derived M-CSF may promote reverse cholesterol transport, which is important in lesion progression. Once again, these models, which are based on current knowledge, merely provide examples of smooth muscle cell–mononuclear phagocyte interactions. Many more facets of this bidirectional cross-talk likely will emerge from future studies.

Endothelial Cell–Smooth Muscle Cell Interactions

The endothelium plays a crucial role in atherogenesis through its interactions with monocytes, as discussed above. In addition, endothelial cells are ideally situated for interacting with smooth muscle cells, particularly in the early phases of atherosclerotic-lesion development. During ontogeny, blood-vessel primordia consist of endothelial tubes that recruit their investment with smooth muscle cells from local mesenchyme. In human arteries, early in life, smooth muscle cells take up residence within the intima, where they may form the substrate for subsequent atheroma formation. Signals derived from the endothelium likely promote smooth muscle accumulation during blood-vessel ontogeny and during arterial intima formation. PDGF is one plausible candidate for an endothelial-derived smooth muscle chemoattractant and growth stimulator [48]. Two distinct genes encode the A and B isoforms of PDGF that must assemble into a dimer to attain biologic activity [49]. Although originally identified in platelets, many cells, including endothelial cells, can produce PDGF subunits. In particular, the endothelial cell appears to elaborate isoforms of PDGF that contain the B chain, although they can express the genes that encode both PDGF A and B chains [50–52]. Dimers of PDGF that contain the B chain potently stimulate smooth muscle migration and growth in vitro. After experimental arterial injury in rats, PDGF appears to act as a potent smooth muscle-cell chemoattractant [53–55].

The elaboration by endothelial cells of PDGF appears subject to tight regulation. For example, thrombin, likely to be generated at sites of arterial injury, augments PDGF gene expression by cultured endothelial cells [56]. Other products of coagulation, such as factor Xa, also enhance PDGF release from endothelial cells [57]. The gene that encodes the B chain of PDGF contains the hexanucleotide motif referred to above as the SSRE [32]. Thus, local hydrodynamics may influence PDGF expression by endothelial cells and thus promote smooth muscle-cell accumulation in the intima. This phenomenon might explain the finding of cushions of smooth muscle cells in the intima of lesion-prone areas of blood vessels, such as the proximal left-entry descending coronary artery in humans.

In addition to roles in smooth muscle-cell migration and growth control, the endothelium regulates another key function of vascular smooth muscle cells: their contractile response. In 1980, the seminal observations of Furchgott and colleagues established the obligatory role of the endothelium in determining the contractile response of vascular smooth muscle cells to a variety of vasodilators, notably the neurotransmitter acetylcholine [58]. Subsequent work reviewed elsewhere in this volume established the identity of the endothelial-derived relaxing factor (EDRF) as the nitric oxide (NO) radical or a closely related species [59]. Experimental work from a number of laboratories demonstrated that atherosclerotic levels exhibit impaired vasodilator responses to acetylcholine [60]. Observations in human coronary and peripheral arteries likewise demonstrated impaired vasodilator responses to exogenously supplied endothelial-dependent vasodilators such as acetylcholine [61].

These studies originally were interpreted as indicating dysfunction of the endothelium of atherosclerotic vessels manifested by impaired production of NO. Subsequent experiments by Harrison and his group demonstrated that the endothelium of atherosclerotic arteries actually elaborates increased amount of NO when stimulated by acetylcholine [62]. They further suggested that the impaired vasodilator response to acetylcholine actually results from increased inactivation of NO by locally produced superoxide anion [63]. Indeed, lesional macrophages may be a source for this oxygen radical, which annihilates the NO radical. Thus, it is not precisely correct to refer to impaired responses to acetylcholine in atherosclerotic vessels as "endothelial dysfunction." This phenomenon furnishes an example of trilateral cellular interactions in the atherosclerotic vessel among the endothelium (which appears to elaborate increased amounts of NO in response to acetylcholine), the macrophage (which appears to elaborate superoxide anion, which neutralizes the NO), and the smooth muscle cell (which ultimately receives less of the vasodilatory signal and exhibits impaired relaxation). The contractile apparatus of the smooth muscle cells in atherosclerotic vessels does appear to retain the capacity to relax. Administration of endothelial-independent vasodilators such as nitroprusside or the organic nitrates demonstrates the expected vasodilator response. In contrast, atherosclerotic arteries often display a paradoxical vasoconstriction when challenged with endothelial-dependent vasodilators such as acetylcholine [64].

Interactions among Smooth Muscle Cells

As noted at the beginning of this chapter, cells may elaborate mediators that act on themselves or on neighboring cells of the same type. Smooth muscle cells are an excellent example in the context of atherosclerosis for such an autocrine mode of information exchange. The preceding section provided examples of how PDGF isoforms can regulate functions of smooth muscle cells important during atherogenesis. As noted, endothelial cells particularly elaborate isoforms of PDGF that contain the B chain. Smooth muscle cells can also express PDGF genes. It has been known for many years that smooth muscle cells, particularly those from the aorta of neonatal rats or from the intimal cells of rat carotid arteries following an injury, elaborate a PDGF-like mitogen [65]. In vitro rat smooth muscle cells can elaborate PDGF-like mitogens and appear to express the B chain for PDGF. In contrast to these observations on rat smooth muscle cells, we have found that human smooth muscle cells, particularly those cultured from human atherosclerotic lesions, can express exclusively the A chain of PDGF [66]. That observation appears particularly interesting because the AA homodimer isoform of PDGF interacts only with the alpha isoform of the PDGF receptor and appears much less potent as a mitogen for vascular smooth muscle cells than B chain–containing isoforms [67]. Thus, the autocrine form of PDGF elaborated by human vascular smooth muscle cells probably acts less potently as a mitogen than endothelial- or platelet-derived isoforms. What function might this A chain homodimeric form of PDGF elaborated by arterial smooth muscle cells serve? Autocrine PDGF-A isoforms have been invokved as the proximate mediators of the growth-promoting effects of certain cytokines such as IL-1 or TNF-α [68,69]. However, it may be narrow minded to perseverate on the pro-proliferative effects of PDGF, particularly the AA isoform, which actually appears rather weakly mitogenic. One possibility is that PDGF-AA serves as a "survival" factor for smooth muscle cells. As noted previously, mononuclear phagocytes require M-CSF for survival. In the absence of this trophic factor, monocytes or macrophages will undergo programmed cell death, or apoptosis [70]. Perhaps PDGF-A isoforms serve a similar function for smooth muscle cells.

Other autocrine factors secreted by smooth muscle cells may include members of the heparin-binding growth factor family. For example, smooth muscle cells can express acidic fibroblast growth factor [71]; when stimulated by cytokines such as IL-1, they can express the gene encoding basic fibroblast growth factor, a competent smooth muscle mitogen [69]. Smooth muscle cells can produce heparin-binding epidermal growth factor (HB-EGF)–like molecule, another member of the heparin-binding growth factor family that may promote smooth muscle cell growth [72,73]. The in vivo role of HB-EGF remains unexplored, although both macrophages and smooth muscle cells appear capable of producing this potential mitogen.

T-Cell Interactions with Other Cell Types in Atherosclerotic Lesions

Hansson and colleagues and others demonstrated unequivocally the presence of substantial infiltrates of T-lymphocytes in human atherosclerotic lesions using monoclonal antibody-identification techniques [74,75]. These cells appear to be in a state of chronic activation [76]. A variety of lines of evidence suggest that complicated atherosclerotic plaques contain a polyclonal population of T-cells [77,78]. Although the stimuli for chronic activation of these T-cells remain unknown, these cells secrete lymphokines that may alter the function of neighboring cells in atherosclerotic lesions in significant ways [79]. T-cells can elaborate many of the same mediators produced by other cell types in the lesion. For example, activated T-cells can release TNF and the related molecule lymphotoxin. However, T-cells, unique among the cell types involved in atherosclerosis, can elaborate gamma-interferon. This lymphokine can induce a particular spectrum of functions of lesion-associated cells, as illustrated by the following examples.

Endothelial cells were the first recognized target for gamma interferon in the blood vessel. Under usual circumstances, human vascular endothelial cells express low levels of class II histocompatibility antigens. Yet when cocultured with activated lymphocytes or exposed to recombinant gamma interferon, endothelial cells readily display surface class II–histocompatibility molecules [80]. This property serves as a marker for activated endothelial cells in certain pathologic processes. Moreover, class II–histocompatibility antigens are absolutely required for initiation of the cellular immune response. In that manner, endothelial expression of class II–histocompatibility molecules, uniquely induced by gamma interferon, may contribute decisively to the pathogenesis of accelerated atherosclerosis in transplanted organs. Currently, such graft vascular disease constitutes the major limitation to long-term survival of solid-organ allografts [81]. Gamma interferon also can elicit the expression of various leukocyte-adhesion molecules on endothelial cells and thus contribute to leukocyte accumulation during atherogenesis, as described above.

Smooth muscle cells also response to gamma interferon by expression of functions that may prove pivotal in the evolution of atherosclerotic lesions. Hansson and colleagues first observed smooth muscle cells that expressed class II–histocompatibility antigens in regions of human atherosclerotic plaques containing T-cell infiltrates [82]. As in the case of endothelium, gamma interferon appears uniquely capable of inducing expression of class II–histocompatibility molecules in smooth muscle cells [83]. The expression by lesional smooth muscle cells of class II antigens has unknown functional consequences, although it provides strong evidence for the presence of gamma interferon in those lesions [83–85].

Gamma interferon also produces other important effects on smooth muscle cells. For example, it can inhibit the proliferation of rat and human smooth muscle cells [84,86]. In addition gamma interferon has a remarkable inhibitory effect on the expression of interstitial collagen genes by smooth muscle cells [87]. By elaborating procollagen molecules, smooth muscle cells provide the foundation for the vascular extracellular matrix. Complicated atherosclerotic lesions, as well as lesions that form following arterial injury such as percutaneous transluminal angioplasty, contain abundant extracellular matrix. In fact, the volume of such lesions occupied by matrix exceeds by far that occupied by cells in mature lesions. Thus, by inhibiting interstitial collagen gene expression, the T-cell product, gamma interferon, may contribute to the balance of vascular matrix accumulation. Regions of plaque rupture contain T-cells, macrophages, and smooth muscle cells bearing the footprints of gamma interferon action, that is, class II–histocompatibility molecule expression. We have speculated, therefore, that gamma interferon derived from T-cells in particular regions of human atheroma may inhibit collagen gene expression and contribute to the weakening of the fibrous cap of the atherosclerotic lesions [88]. This disruption of the integrity of the lesion's matrix might predispose to plaque rupture and promote the transition from chronic to acute phases of atherosclerosis.

The preceding section introduced the role of the macrophage scavenger receptor for modified lipoproteins in the formation of macrophage-derived foam cells. Later in the history of most atherosclerotic lesions, foam cells derived from smooth muscle cells also form. The smooth muscle cells can also express the scavenger receptor [89]. Gamma interferon can induce the expression of the scavenger receptor on smooth muscle cells cultured from rabbit aorta [90]. Although the expression by human smooth muscle cells of the scavenger receptor remains controversial, these observations provide yet another example of the interaction of smooth muscle cells with the T-cell–derived lymphokine gamma interferon.

T-cells also may influence macrophage functions by elaborating gamma interferon. In the case of the macrophage, gamma interferon appears to reduce scavenger receptor expression, which would tend to promote extracellular cholesterol accumulation within lesions [91]. Gamma interferon also potently activates mononuclear phagocytes. Many of the properties of macrophages associated with cytolytic effects and elaboration of various cytokines depend on gamma interferon [92]. Moreover, macrophages from rodents can express the inducible form of NO synthase, the enzyme that catalyzes the formation of NO radical, the potent vasodilatory molecule referred to in the context of endothelial-dependent vasorelaxation [93]. The ability of human macrophages and smooth muscle cells to express inducible NO synthase remains controversial. Cell culture experiments, however, consistently indicate that gamma interferon, usually in combination with another cytokine such as TNF-α, participates in the induction of this gene encoding the inducible isoform of NO synthase. In addition to its vasodilating effects, this molecule may alter platelet function [94], smooth muscle-growth control [95], and formation of cytotoxic derivatives such as peroxynitrite radical, among others.

These examples demonstrate how the T-cell–derived cytokine gamma interferon may affect endothelial cells, smooth muscle cells, and macrophages in atherosclerotic lesions. The functions induced in these various cell types by gamma interferon may profoundly influence aspects of lesion development. Gamma interferon often opposes the actions of other cytokines or growth factors, for example, by inhibiting smooth muscle-cell proliferation and collagen synthesis rather than promoting those processes. Thus, T-cell–derived cytokine gamma interferon may modify many potentially atherogenic functions of vascular wall cells.

Other Aspects of Cell-Cell Interaction during Atherogenesis

The discussion so far has focused on atherogenesis and cytokines as autocrine and paracrine mediators of intercellular communication during atherogenesis. In reality, much richer modes of communication probably interlink these cells. For example, lipid mediators such as prostaglandins constitute a long-recognized class of mediators of cell-cell communication in the context of atherosclerosis. Some of the apparent beneficial effects of certain unsaturated fatty acids on atherosclerosis may result from interfering with the usual pathways of prostanoid biosynthesis by vascular wall cells and lesional leukocytes. More recent work has brought to the fore other classes of lipid mediators that may be important in the pathogenesis of atherosclerosis [96]. The leukotrienes and lipoxins furnish examples of nonprostanoid lipid mediators that may mediate cell-cell communication during the formation of atherosclerotic lesions [97]. Transcellular metabolism of the lipid mediators such as the prostanoids furnishes a particularly apt illustration of the importance of cell-cell interaction in modulating the effects of various mediators. Furthermore, as alluded to briefly, prostanoids can alter the economy of cholesterol metabolism in smooth muscle cells, providing yet another link between cholesterol homeostasis and intercellular mediators of vascular functions.

Future Directions in the Study of Cell-Cell Interaction during Atherogenesis

Heretofore, most of the interest in atherosclerosis has focused on the intima, where the lesions form. Although logical, this focus on the intima to the exclusion of the other layers of the blood vessel may unduly limit our perspective of the true complexity of atherogenesis. Students of atherosclerosis usually regard the adventitia as "uninteresting." However, the adventitia furnishes the vasa vasorum from which many of the microvessels of the complicated atherosclerotic plaque arise. I have already considered the effect of these microvascular plexi as sites for leukocyte trafficking during lesion evolution. The microvessels derived from the adventitia also may furnish a source of endothelial mediators of smooth muscle function as considered. Finally, these microvessels, which may be as pliable as those that form in the diabetic retina, may readily hemorrhage, causing thrombin generation in situ and even contributing to acute lesion expansion by hematoma formation.

The adventitia also contains mast cells. Mast-cell granules contain heparan sulfate glycosaminoglycans, which may work in concert with angiogenic peptides to promote microvessel formation. The intimal and medial layers of arteries do not contain fibroblasts. However, fibroblasts may occur in the adventitia. As multipotent mesenchymal cells, the fibroblasts may respond in the adventitia in a manner similar to smooth muscle cells in the media and the intima. Thus, adventitial fibroblasts may contribute to the vessel remodeling that accompanies atherogenesis. Finally, the adventitia may constitute an important focus for inflammation in vascular diseases. After arterial injury, many investigators have focused on the intima and the media as sites of altered cellular function. The adventitia, however, exhibits many signs of inflammation and may contribute signals to the ongoing and sustained phases of the response to arterial injury [98]. In the case of atherosclerotic aortic aneurysms, the adventitia often contains exuberant collections of inflammatory cells. Thus, the ectasia of atherosclerotic vessels and aneurysm formation may depend in part on the cell-cell signaling that takes place in the adventitia of the vessel rather than in the more lumenal layers, which traditionally have been the focus of atherosclerosis researchers.

The neuron also has received scant attention as a cell type to consider in the context of atherogenesis. Yet control of vascular tone by vasomotor neurotransmitters is well established. Many substances first recognized in other contexts of vascular control have turned out to be neurotransmitters as well. For example, NO, endothelin, atrial natriuretic peptide, substance P, and a variety of other peptide mediators can derive from neurons. All our cell-culture studies of vascular cell function and most of the pharmacology performed on vessel strips have ignored the contribution of neurons. In our attempts to integrate fully current concepts of cell-cell interaction into the broad picture of atherogenesis, we must not neglect the neuron.

Summary

This chapter has summarized a wealth of work from many laboratories throughout the world that relates to the subject of cellular interactions during atherogenesis. The discussion is necessarily biased toward the interest of the author. Yet the principles put forth will likely prove generally applicable. Our current concepts of atherogenesis evoke a complex cast of characters as potential mediators of cell-cell interactions. This list is likely to evolve in opposing directions as we refine our knowledge. A few factors will doubtless emerge that may play pivotal roles in atherogenesis. Other factors, currently accorded crucial roles in this process, may be dethroned by experiments made possible by genetically modified animals that will permit critical testing of the roles of specific factors and aspects of atherosclerosis. The complexities of the signaling network and of the multilateral communication represent a challenge for understanding the pathogenesis of atherosclerosis and for developing effective preventive strategies and therapies aimed at lesion regression or stabilization.

References

1. Pober JS, Cotran RS. Cytokines and endothelial cell biology. Physiol Rev 1990; 70:427.
2. Bevilacqua MP, Nelson RM. Selectins. J Clin Invest 1993; 91:379–387.
3. Springer TA. Adhesion receptors of the immune system. Nature 1990; 346:425–434.
4. Osborn L, et al. Direct expression cloning of vascular cell adhesion molecule-1, a cytokine-induced endothelial protein that binds to lymphocytes. Cell 1989; 59:1203–1211.
5. Elices MJ, et al. VCAM-1 on activated endothelium interacts with the leukocyte integrin VLA-4 at a site distinct from the VLA 4/fibronectin binding site. Cell 1990; 60:577–584.
6. Munro JM, Cotran RS. The pathogenesis of atherosclerosis: atherogenesis and inflammation. Laboratory Investigation 1988; 58:249–261.
7. Poole JCF, Florey HW. Changes in the endothelium of the aorta and the behavior of macrophages in experimental atheroma of rabbits. J Path Bact 1958; 75:245–253.
8. Gerrity RG, et al. Dietary-induced atherogenesis in swine: Morphology of the intima in prelesion stages. Am J Pathol 1979; 95:775–786.
9. Joris T, et al. Studies on the pathogenesis of atherosclerosis. I. Adhesion and emigration of mononuclear cells in the aorta of hypercholesterolemic rats. Am J Pathol 1983; 113:341–358.
10. Faggiotto A, Ross R, Harker L. Studies of hypercholesterolemia in the nonhuman primate. I. Changes that lead to fatty streak formation. Arteriosclerosis 1984; 4:323–340.
11. Faggiotto A, Ross R. Studies of hypercholesterolemia in the nonhuman primate. II. Fatty streak conversion to fibrous plaque. Arteriosclerosis 1984; 4:341–356.
12. Nakashima Y, et al. ApoE-deficient mice develop lesions of all phases of atherosclerosis throughout the arterial tree. Arteriosclerosis & Thrombosis 1994; 14:133–140.

13. Gimbrone MAJ, Bevilacqua MP, Cybulsky MI. Endothelial-dependent mechanisms of leukocyte adhesion in inflammation and atherosclerosis. Ann NY Acad Sci 1990; 598:77–85.
14. Cybulsky MI, Gimbrone Jr, MA. Endothelial expression of a mononuclear leukocyte adhesion molecule during atherogenesis. Science 1991; 251:788–791.
15. Li H, et al. An atherogenic diet rapidly induces VCAM-1, a cytokine regulatable mononuclear leukocyte adhesion molecule, in rabbit endothelium. Arteriosclerosis & Thrombosis 1993; 13:197–204.
16. Printseva O, Peclo MM, Gown AM. Various cell types in human atherosclerotic lesions express ICAM-1. Further immunocytochemical and immunochemical studies employing monoclonal antibody 10F3. Am J Pathol 1992; 140:889–896.
17. Poston RN, et al. Expression of intercellular adhesion molecule-1 in atherosclerotic plaques. Am J Pathol 1992; 140:665–673.
18. Calderon TM, et al. An endothelial cell adhesion protein for monocytes recognized by monoclonal antibody IG9. Expression in vivo in inflamed human vessels and atherosclerotic human and Watanabe rabbit vessels. Laboratory Investigation 1994; 70:836–849.
19. Butcher EC, et al. Interactions between endothelial cells and leukocytes. J Cell Biochem 1986; 30:121–131.
20. O'Brien K, et al. Vascular cell adhesion molecule-1 is expressed in human coronary atherosclerotic plaques: Implications for the mode of progression of advanced coronary atherosclerosis. J Clin Invest 1993; 92:945–951.
21. Gerrity RG, Goss JA, Soby L. Control of monocyte recruitment by chemotactic factor(s) in lesion-prone areas of swine aorta. Arteriosclerosis 1985; 5:55–66.
22. Charo I. Monocyte-endothelial cell interactions. Current Opinion Lipodol 1992; 3:335–343.
23. Rollins BJ, et al. Cytokine-activated human endothelial cells synthesize and secrete a monocyte chemoattractant, MCP-1/JE. Am J Pathol 1990; 136:1229–1233.
24. Cushing SD, et al. Minimally modified low density lipoprotein induces monocytes chemotactic protein-1 in human endothelial cells and smooth muscle cells. Proc Natl Acad Sci USA 1990; 87:5134–5138.
25. Wang J, et al. Expression of monocyte chemotactic protein and interleukin-8 by cytokine-activated human vascular smooth muscle cells. Arteriosclerosis 1991; 11:1166–1174.
26. Nelken N, et al. Monocyte chemoattractant protein-1 in human atheromatous plaques. J Clin Invest 1991; 88:1121–1127.
27. Yla-Herttuala S, et al. Expression of monocyte chemoattractant protein-1 in macrophage-rich areas of human and rabbit atherosclerotic lesions. Proc Natl Acad Sci USA 1991; 88:5252–5256.
28. Kume N, Cybulsky MI, Gimbrone Jr, MA. Lysophosphatidylcholine, a component of atherogenic lipoproteins, induces mononuclear leukocyte adhesion molecules in cultured human and rabbit arterial endothelial cells. J Clin Invest 1992; 90:1138–1144.
29. Kume N, Gimbrone M, Jr. Lysophosphatidylcholine transcriptionally induces growth factor gene expression in cultured human endothelial cells. Journal of Clinical Investigation 1994; 93:907–911.
30. Nerem RM, et al. Hemodynamics and vascular endothelial biology. [Review]. Journal of Cardiovascular Pharmacology 1993; 21:S6–S10.
31. Nagel T, et al. Shear stress selectively upregulates intercellular adhesion molecule-1 expression in cultured human vascular endothelial cells. Journal of Clinical Investigation 1994; 94:885–891.
32. Resnick N, et al. Platelet-derived growth factor B chain promoter contains a cis-acting fluid shear-stress-responsive element [published erratum appears in Proc Natl Acad Sci USA 1993 Aug 15; 90(16);7908]. Proceedings of the National Academy of Sciences of the United States of America 1993; 90:4591–4595.
33. Shyy YJ, et al. Fluid shear stress induces a biphasic response of human monocyte chemotactic protein 1 gene expression in vascular endothelium. Proceedings of the National Academy of Sciences of the United States of America 1994; 91:4678–4682.
34. Carlos TM, et al. Vascular cell adhesion molecule-1 mediates lymphocyte adherence to cytokine-activated cultured human endothelial cells [published erratum appears in Blood 1990 Dec 1; 76(11):2420]. Blood 1990; 76:965–970.
35. Carlos T, et al. Human monocytes bind to two cytokine-induced adhesive ligands on cultured human endothelial cells: endothelial-leukocyte adhesion molecule-1 and vascular cell adhesion molecule-1. Blood 1991; 77:2266–2271.
36. Neish AS, et al. Functional analysis of the human vascular cell adhesion molecule-1 promoter. Journal of Experimental Medicine 1992; 176:1583–1593.
37. Rajavashisth TB, et al. Induction of endothelial cell expression of granulocyte and macrophage colony-stimulating factors by modified low-density lipoproteins. Nature 1990; 344:254–257.
38. Clinton S, et al. Macrophage-colony stimulating factor gene expression in vascular cells and in experimental and human atherosclerosis. Am J Path 1992; 140:301–316.
39. Kodama T, et al. Binding properties of a purified acetyl-LDL receptor. Circulation 1989; 80:II–333.
40. Krieger M, et al. Molecular flypaper, host defense, and atherosclerosis. Structure, binding properties, and functions of macrophage scavenger receptors. J Biol Chem 1993; 268: 4569–4572.
41. Brown MS, Goldstein JL. Lipoprotein metabolism in the macrophage: implications for cholesterol deposition in atherosclerosis. Ann Review Biochem 1983; 52:223–261.
42. Mahley RW. Apolipoprotein E: cholesterol transport protein with expanding role in cell biology. Science 1988; 240:622–630.
43. Salomon RN, et al. Increased apolipoprotein E and c-fms gene expression without elevated interleukin 1 or 6 levels indicate selective activation of macrophage functions in advanced human atheroma. Proc Natl Acad Sci USA 1992; 89:2814–2818.
44. Rosenfeld M, et al. Macrophage colony-stimulating factor mRNA and protein in atherosclerotic lesions of rabbits and humans. Am J Path 1992; 140:291–300.
45. Plump AS, et al. Severe hypercholesterolemia and atherosclerosis in apolipoprotein E-deficient mice created by homologous recombination in ES cells. Cell 1992; 71:343–353.
46. Piedrahita JA, et al. Generation of mice carrying a mutant apolipoprotein E gene inactivated by gene targeting in embryonic stem cells. Proc Natl Acad Sci USA 1992; 89:4471–4475.
47. Libby P, Clinton SK. The role of macrophages in atherogenesis. Current opinion in lipidology 1993; 4:355–363.
48. Ross R. The pathogenesis of atherosclerosis: a perspective for the 1990s. Nature 1993; 362:801–809.
49. Betsholtz C, et al. cDNA sequence and chromosomal localization of human platelet-derived growth factor A-chain and its expression in tumour cell lines. Nature 1986; 320:695–699.
50. Barrett TB, et al. Expression of the sis gene by endothelial cells in culture and in vivo. Proc Natl Acad Sci USA 1984; 81:6772–6774.
51. Collins T, et al. Cultured human endothelial cells express platelet-derived growth factor chain 2: cDNA cloning and structural analysis. Nature 1985; 316:748–750.
52. Collins T, et al. Cultured human endothelial cells express platelet-derived growth factor A chain. Am J Pathol 1987; 127:7–12.
53. Fingerle J, et al. Role of platelets in smooth muscle cell prolifer-

ation and migration after vascular injury in rat carotid artery. Proc Natl Acad Sci USA 1989; 86:8412–8416.

54. Jawien A, et al. Platelet-derived growth factor promotes smooth muscle migration and intimal thickening in a rat model of balloon angioplasty. J Clin Invest 1992; 89:507–511.
55. Ferns GA, Reidy MA, Ross R. Balloon catheter de-endothelialization of the nude rat carotid. Response to injury in the absence of functional T lymphocytes. Am J Pathol 1991; 138:1045–1057.
56. Daniel TO, et al. Thrombin stimulates c-sis gene expression in microvascular endothelial cells. J Cell Biol 1986; 261:9579–9582.
57. Gajdusek C, et al. Activation of coagulation releases endothelial cell mitogens. J Cell Biol 1986; 103:419–428.
58. Furchgott RF, Zawadzki JV. The obligatory role of endothelial cells in the relaxation of arterial smooth muscle by acetylcholine. Nature 1980; 288:373–376.
59. Palmer RM, Ferrige AG, Moncada S. Nitric oxide release accounts for the biological activity of endothelium-derived relaxing factor. Nature 1987; 327:524–526.
60. Shimokawa H, et al. Effects of dietary supplementation with cod-liver oil on endothelium-dependent responses in porcine coronary arteries. Circulation 1987; 76:898–905.
61. Liao JK, et al. Differential impairment of vasodilator responsiveness of peripheral resistance and conduit vessels in humans with atherosclerosis. Circulation Research 1991; 68:1027–1034.
62. Minor R, Jr, et al. Diet-induced atherosclerosis increases the release of nitrogen oxides from rabbit aorta. Journal of Clinical Investigation 1990; 86:2109–2116.
63. Ohara Y, Peterson TE, Harrison DG. Hypercholesterolemia increases endothelial superoxide anion production. Journal of Clinical Investigation 1993; 91:2546–2551.
64. Ludmer PL, et al. Paradoxical vasoconstriction induced by acetylcholine in atherosclerotic coronary arteries. N Engl J Med 1986; 315:1046–1051.
65. Walker LN, et al. Production of platelet-derived growth factor-like molecules by cultured arterial smooth muscle cells accompanies proliferation after arterial injury. Proceedings of the National Academy of Sciences of the United States of America 1986; 83:7311–7315.
66. Libby P, et al. Production of platelet-derived growth factor-like mitogen by smooth muscle cells from human atheromata. New Engl J Med 1988; 318:1493–1498.
67. Hart CE, et al. Two classes of PDGF receptor recognize different isoforms of PDGF. Science 1988; 240(4858):1529–1531.
68. Raines EW, Dower SK, Ross R. Interleukin-1 mitogenic activity for fibroblasts and smooth muscle cells is due to PDGF-AA. Science 1989; 243:393–396.
69. Gay CG, Winkles JA. Interleukin 1 regulates heparin-binding growth factor 2 gene expression in vascular smooth muscle cells. Proc Natl Acad Sci USA 1991; 88:296–300.
70. Libby P, Clinton SK. Cytokines as mediators of vascular pathology. Nouv Rev Fr Hematol 1992; 34:S47–S53.
71. Winkles JA, et al. Human vascular smooth muscle cells both express and respond to heparin-binding growth factor I (endothelial cell growth factor). Proc Natl Acad Sci USA 1987; 84:7124–7128.
72. Dluz SM, et al. Heparin-binding epidermal growth factor-like growth factor expression in cultured fetal human vascular smooth muscle cells. Induction of mRNA levels and secretion of active mitogen. Journal of Biological Chemistry 1993; 268:18330–18334.
73. Nakano T, et al. Glucocorticoid inhibits thrombin-induced expression of platelet-derived growth factor A-chain and heparin-binding epidermal growth factor-like growth factor in human aortic smooth muscle cells. Journal of Biological Chemistry 1993; 268:22941–22947.
74. Jonasson L, et al. Regional accumulations of T cells, macrophages, and smooth muscle cells in the human atherosclerotic plaque. Arteriosclerosis 1986; 6:131–138.
75. Tsukada T, et al. Immunocytochemical analysis of cellular components in lesions of atherosclerosis in the Watanabe and fat-fed rabbit using monoclonal antibodies. Arteriosclerosis 1986; 6:601–613.
76. Stemme S, Holm J, Hansson GK. T lymphocytes in human atherosclerotic plaques are memory cells expressing CD45RO and the integrin VLA-1. Arterioscler Thromb 1992; 12:206–211.
77. Stemme S, Rymo L, Hansson GK. Polyclonal origin of T lymphocytes in human atherosclerotic plaques. Lab Invest 1991; 65:654–660.
78. Swanson S, et al. Diversity of T-cell antigen receptor V beta gene utilization in advanced human atheroma. Arteriosclerosis 1994; 14:1210–1214.
79. Libby P, Hansson GK. Involvement of the immune system in human atherogenesis: Current knowledge and unanswered questions. Lab Invest 1991; 64:5–15.
80. Pober JS, et al. Ia expression by vascular endothelium is inducible by activated T cells and by human gamma interferon. Journal of Experimental Medicine 1983; 157:1339–1353.
81. Libby P, et al. Arteriosclerosis in transplanted hearts: too much and too soon. Can J Cardiol 1991; 7:XI–XII.
82. Jonasson L, et al. Expression of class II transplantation antigen on vascular smooth muscle cells in human atherosclerosis. J Clin Invest 1985; 76:125–131.
83. Warner SJC, Friedman GB, Libby P. Regulation of major histocompatibility gene expression in cultured human vascular smooth muscle cells. Arteriosclerosis 1989; 9:279–288.
84. Hansson GK, et al. Gamma interferon regulates vascular smooth muscle proliferation and Ia expression in vivo and in vitro. Circ Research 1988; 63:712–719.
85. Hansson GK, Holm J, Jonasson L. Detection of activated T lymphocytes in the human atherosclerotic plaque. Am J Pathol 1989; 135:169–175.
86. Warner SJC, Friedman GB, Libby P. Immune interferon inhibits proliferation and induces 2′-5′-oligoadenylate synthetase gene expression in human vascular smooth muscle cells. J Clin Invest 1989; 83:1174–1182.
87. Amento EP, et al. Cytokines positively and negatively regulate interstitial collagen gene expression in human vascular smooth muscle cells. Arteriosclerosis 1991; 11:1223–1230.
88. Galis Z, et al. Increased expression of matrix metalloproteinases and matrix degrading activity in vulnerable regions of human atherosclerotic plaques. J Clin Invest 1994; in press:
89. Pitas RE. Expression of the acetyl low density lipoprotein receptor by rabbit fibroblasts and smooth muscle cells. Upregulation by phorbol esters. J Biol Chem 1990; 265:12722–12727.
90. Li H, Freeman M, Libby P. Regulation of smooth muscle cell scavenger receptor expression in vivo by atherogenic diet and in vitro by cytokines. J Clin Invest 1995; 95:122–133.
91. Geng YJ, Hansson GK. Interferon-gamma inhibits scavenger receptor expression and foam cell formation in human monocyte-derived macrophages. J Clin Invest 1992; 89:1322–1330.
92. Nathan CF. Secretory products of macrophages. J Clin Invest 1987; 79:319–326.
93. Nathan C. Nitric oxide as a secretory product of mammalian cells. FASEB J 1992; 6:3051–3064.
94. Radomski MW, Palmer RM, Moncada S. Modulation of platelet aggregation by an L-arginine-nitric oxide pathway. Trends Pharmacol Sci 1991; 12:87–88.
95. Garg UC, Hassid A. Nitric oxide-generating vasodilators and

8-bromocyclic guanosine monophosphate inhibit mitogenesis and proliferation of cultured rat vascular smooth muscle cells. J Clin Invest 1989; 83:1774–1777.
96. Hajjar DP, Pomerantz KB. Signal transduction in atherosclerosis: integration of cytokines and the eicosanoid network. FASEB 1992; 6:2933–2941.
97. Serhan CN. Lipoxin biosynthesis and its impact in inflammatory and vascular events. [Review]. Biochimica at Biophysica Acta 1994; 212:1–25.
98. Tanaka H, et al. Sustained activation of vascular cells and leukocytes in the rabbit aorta after balloon injury. Circulation 1993; 88:1788–1803.

Pathogenesis of Atherosclerosis: Lipid Metabolism

David P. Via
John R. Guyton
Antonio M. Gotto, Jr.

The evidence for a major causative role of lipids in atherogenesis rests on three cornerstones: the high cholesterol content of atherosclerotic lesions, the production of atherosclerosis in animals fed high-fat diets, and clinical data linking plasma lipoprotein levels with atherosclerotic disease in human populations. Although the broad outlines of this evidence were established by the 1950s, a progression of new research techniques from ultracentrifugation to gene cloning has brought vastly improved understanding of lipid metabolism and atherogenesis. The prediction of atherosclerotic risk from lipoprotein analysis has undergone continuing refinement. The fraction of plasma cholesterol contained in high-density lipoproteins (HDL) is as powerful a negative predictor of coronary heart disease (CHD) as the total plasma cholesterol is a positive predictor [1]. Other factors that may be of comparable or greater predictive power include lipoprotein(a), or Lp(a); apoprotein, or apo, B; and apo A-I [2–5]. Thus, plasma lipids, lipoproteins, and apoproteins make a major contribution to cardiovascular risk. Moreover, interventions that reduce total cholesterol and low-density lipoprotein (LDL) cholesterol are effective in reducing risk for CHD. From the results of the Lipid Research Clinics Coronary Primary Prevention Trial and other studies, it appears that a 1-percent lowering of plasma cholesterol in a hypercholesterolemic person can lead to a 2-percent reduction in risk [6,7].

These facts emphasize the importance of an understanding of lipid and lipoprotein metabolism in devising strategies for the prevention or treatment of atherosclerotic disease, which remains the leading single cause of death in the industrialized world. Knowledge about factors affecting lipoprotein metabolism, although incomplete, has advanced to the point that hypercholesterolemic patients previously considered resistant to therapy can now be expected to respond to treatment. Despite this progress, the process of lipid deposition in the arterial wall, its role in lesion progression, and its relation to fibrocellular proliferation remain poorly understood.

Plasma Lipoproteins and Atherosclerosis

LIPIDS AND LIPOPROTEINS

The low aqueous solubility of lipids at physiologic pH, even polar lipids such as fatty acids and phospholipids, has important implications for their biologic behavior. The solubility of cholesterol is extremely low, about 10 nmol [8,9]. This lack of solubility and consequent self-association of lipid molecules make it possible for phospholipids and cholesterol to form the essential structure of cell membranes. Excessive accumulation of fatty acids or cholesterol, however, can have deleterious effects on cells. Toxicity may be due in part to the detergent properties of fatty-acid anions or to the decreased fluidity of cellular membranes with a very high cholesterol content [10]. On the other hand, the nonaqueous sequestration of lipid allows efficient transport in body fluids of esterified fatty acids and esterified cholesterol—which are completely insoluble in aqueous fluids—and their storage in cellular deposits. For circulatory transport, cholesterol, cholesteryl ester, triglyceride, and phospholipid are packaged together with apoproteins in micellar structures called **plasma lipoproteins** (Fig. 13-1) [11].

Plasma lipoproteins are separable by ultracentrifugation into fairly distinct classes on the basis of their equilibrium densities (Table 13-1). It is useful to think of lipoproteins as cholesterol rich, characterizing LDL; protein rich, characterizing HDL; or triglyceride rich, characterizing chylomicrons and their remnants, very low-density lipoprotein (VLDL) and intermediate-density lipoproteins (IDL). The flotation behavior of triglyceride-rich and protein-rich lipoproteins is comparable to the common observation that a fat person floats easily in a swimming pool, whereas a muscular person tends to sink. LDL, which is rich in cholesterol, has flotation properties between the extremes. An older nomenclature referred to lipoproteins on the basis of their electrophoretic mobilities, which are listed in Table 13-1.

APOPROTEINS

The apoproteins (Table 13-2) play essential roles in the determination of lipoprotein structure and the regulation of lipid transport. Apoproteins are designated by letters and numerals, such as apo A-I or apo C-III, which originally indicated members of families of apoproteins. Although the names persist, the basis of this nomenclature is no longer accepted. Every apoprotein sequenced thus far contains one or more alpha-helical regions, in which hydrophobic amino acids form one face of the helix and charged amino acids form the opposite face. The amphipathic character of these helical domains accounts for the binding of the protein to a lipid-water interface [11–14].

All lipoproteins of density less than 1.063 g/ml contain apo B. Two forms of apo B, apo B-48 and apo B-100, are associated with such lipoproteins derived from the intestine, but those derived from the liver have only apo B-100. A single apo B-100 molecule is contained in each VLDL particle in the liver and remains with the particle through its metabolism to IDL and LDL. The binding of apo B to lipoprotein particles is essentially permanent, lasting until cellular uptake and lysosomal hydrolysis of the particle occurs. This behavior is unique among the apoproteins and is probably explained by the presence of large hydrophobic domains in the amino-acid sequence of apo B [15].

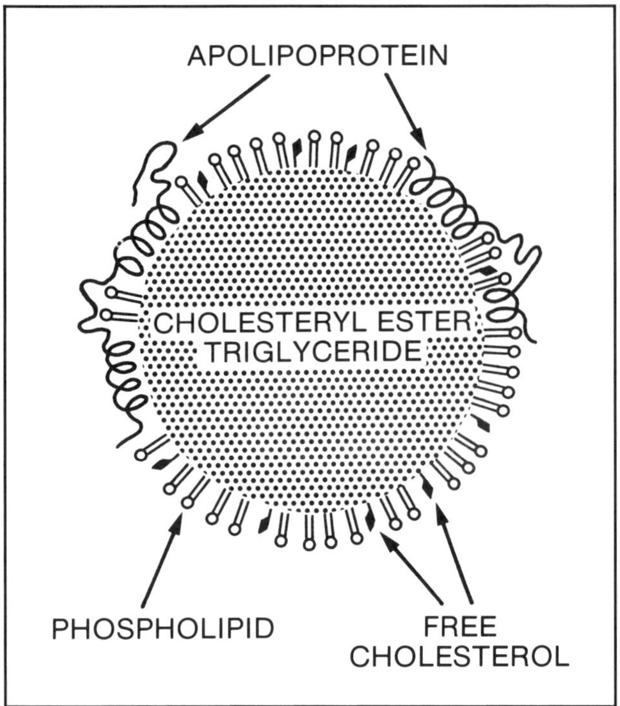

Fig. 13-1. Lipoprotein structure. Plasma lipoproteins are spherical particles containing a hydrophobic core composed predominantly of triglyceride, cholesteryl ester, or both and having a surface coat whose primary component is a phospholipid monolayer. Interspersed in the phospholipid coat are free cholesterol and apolipoproteins.

LIPOPROTEIN METABOLISM

Pathways for lipoprotein transport from the central organs, gut, and liver to peripheral tissues are shown in Fig. 13-2. Chylomicrons are synthesized in the gut and carry dietary, or exogenous, triglyceride and cholesterol; triglyceride is the major lipid constituent. VLDL, which is made in the liver, has as its primary function the transport of endogenously synthesized triglyceride to peripheral tissues. IDL represents an intermediate in the conversion of VLDL to LDL; this conversion depends on lipolytic enzymes located in the peripheral circulation and the liver. Lipoprotein lipase, the peripheral enzyme, participates in both the exogenous and endogenous pathways of triglyceride-rich lipoprotein metabolism. Absence of lipoprotein lipase or its apoprotein cofactor, apo C-II, leads to massive plasma triglyceride accumulation in chylomicrons (type I hyperlipoproteinemia) with resultant abdominal pain and pancreatitis; however, this condition is not associated with atherogenesis. Surface phospholipids and apoproteins liberated by lipoprotein lipase action on triglyceride-rich lipoproteins are transferred to HDL (Fig. 13-3); this metabolic link may help to explain the strong inverse relation between plasma levels of triglyceride and HDL.

Chylomicron remnants, IDL, and LDL are taken up by cells and digested in the lysosomes. To a large degree, cellular uptake is mediated by specific cell-surface receptors. Genetic defects in receptor-mediated lipoprotein uptake processes, shown in Fig. 13-2, can lead to atherogenic elevations of plasma lipids. Chylomicron remnants contain apo E, which mediates their binding and uptake by hepatocytes. Isomorphic forms of apo E that differ in their degree of positive charge exhibit varied affinities for receptor binding, with concomitant changes in the clearance of lipoprotein particles from the circulation. Dysbetalipoproteinemia (type III hyperlipoproteinemia), a rare disorder characterized by high plasma levels of chylomicron remnants and IDL, is associated with homozygosity for apo E_2, the isomorph with the weakest binding affinity, in combination with another metabolic alteration affecting plasma lipids [16,17]. Familial hypercholesterolemia, a rel-

Table 13-1. Plasma lipoproteins

					Mass composition				
					Surface			Core	
	Density (g/cm)	Diameter (nm)	Molecular weight (kDa)	Electrophoretic mobility	PROT	PL	C	CE	TG
Chylomicrons*	0.93	75–1200	~400,000	Origin	2	7	2	3	86
VLDL	0.93–1.0006	30–80	10,000–80,000	Pre-beta	8	18	7	12	55
IDL*	1.006–1.019	25–35	5,000–10,000	Slow pre-beta	19	19	9	29	23
LDL	1.091–1.063	18–25	~2300	Beta	22	22	8	42	6
Lp(a)*	1.050–1.125	24–26	3,000–5,000	Slow pre-beta	30	22	10	35	3
HDL_2	1.063–1.125	9–12	~360	Alpha	40	33	5	17	5
HDL_3	1.125–1.210	5–9	~175	Alpha	55	25	4	13	3

PROT = protein; PL = phospholipid; C = cholesterol; CE = cholesteryl ester; TG = triglycerides.
* These lipoproteins usually are not major components in fasting plasma. Chylomicrons normally circulate only postprandially. IDL is formed continuously from VLDL but is rapidly cleared or metabolized to LDL. Lp(a) is a minor lipoprotein in most individuals, but in some persons an inherited tendency leads to substantial Lp(a) plasma concentrations.
Sources: Data from RL Jackson, AM Gotto Jr. Hypothesis concerning membrane structure, cholesterol, and atherosclerosis. Atherosclerosis Reviews 1976; 1:1–21. AM Gotto Jr, HJ Pownall, RJ Havel. Introduction to the plasma lipoproteins. Methods Enzymol 1986; 128:1–41. LC Smith et al. Structure and dynamics of human plasma lipoproteins. In G Pifat, JN Herak, eds. Supramolecular Structure and Function. New York: Plenum, 1983. RJ Havel, JL Goldstein, MS Brown. Lipoproteins and lipid transport. In PK Bondy, LE Rosenberg, eds. Metabolic Control and Disease. Philadelphia: Saunders, 1980.

Table 13-2. Apoproteins

	Molecular weight (kDa)	Distribution	Function
A-I	28,000	HDL, chylomicrons	Activates lecithin-cholesterol acyltransferase
A-II	17,000	HDL, chylomicrons	Unknown
A-IV	46,000	HDL, chylomicrons	Unknown
B-48	264,000	Chylomicrons and remnants	Structural role in intestine-derived lipoproteins
B-100	550,000	LDL, IDL, VLDL, chylomicrons	Ligand for LDL receptor binding
C-I	5800	HDL, IDL, VLDL, chylomicrons	Activates lecithin-cholesterol acyltransferase
C-II	9100	VLDL, IDL, HDL, chylomicrons	Activates lipoprotein lipase
C-III	8750	VLDL, IDL, HDL, chylomicrons	Inhibits hepatic uptake of lipoproteins
D	22,000	HDL	Unknown, may participate in cholesteryl ester transfer
E	34,000	IDL, VLDL, chylomicrons, HDL	Ligand for binding to chylomicron remnant receptor and to LDL receptor
(a)	~500,000	Lp(a), chylomicrons	Unknown

Sources: Data from AM Gotto Jr, HJ Pownall, RJ Havel. Introduction to the plasma lipoproteins. Methods Enzymol 1986; 128:1–41. LC Smith et al. Structure and dynamics of human plasma lipoproteins. In G Pifat, JN Herak, eds. Supramolecular Structure and Function. New York: Plenum, 1983. RJ Havel, JL Goldstein, MS Brown. Lipoproteins and lipid transport. In PK Bondy, LE Rosenberg, eds. Metabolic Control and Disease. Philadelphia: Saunders, 1980.

Fig. 13-2. Lipoprotein pathways. In the exogenous lipid transport pathway, chylomicrons enter the circulation after being secreted into lymph by intestinal mucosal cells. Lipoprotein lipase, located on the luminal surface of capillary endothelium, hydrolyzes triglycerides and some phospholipids in the chylomicrons, allowing free fatty acids to diffuse into parenchymal tissue. Some surface components from the chylomicrons are transferred to HDL (see Fig. 13-3). The chylomicron remnants thus produced are rapidly taken up by hepatocytes. In the endogenous lipid transport pathway, VLDL is secreted by the liver and acted on by lipoprotein lipase in an analogous manner. IDL, which represents remnant particles from VLDL, may be taken up via hepatocyte LDL receptors or may be further metabolized with the help of hepatic lipase to form LDL. There are three possible fates for circulating LDL: (1) uptake via hepatic LDL receptors, (2) uptake by genetically identical LDL receptors located on peripheral cells, and (3) nonspecific uptake by peripheral ("scavenger") cells or by binding to extracellular tissue components.

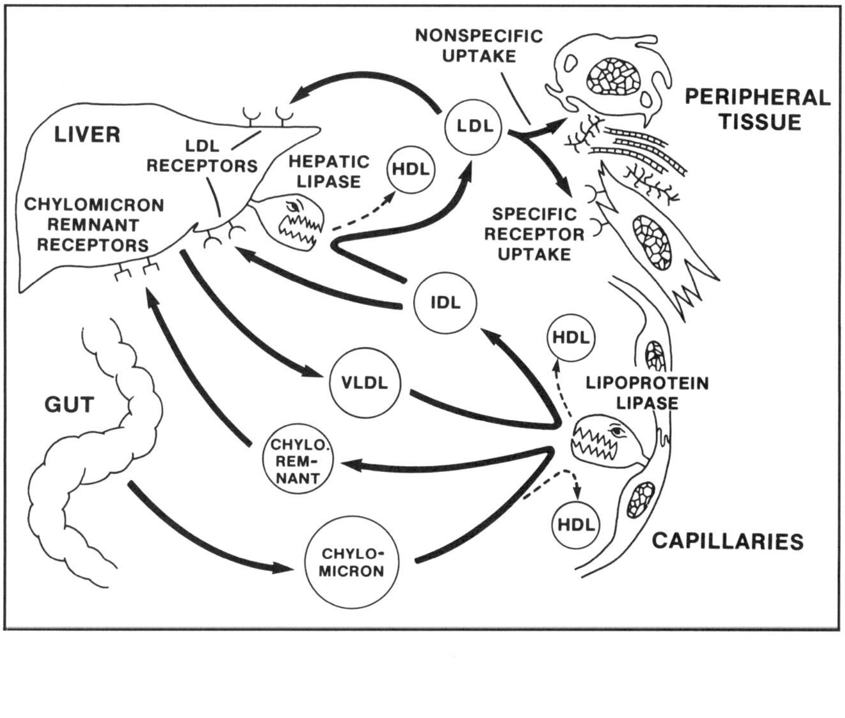

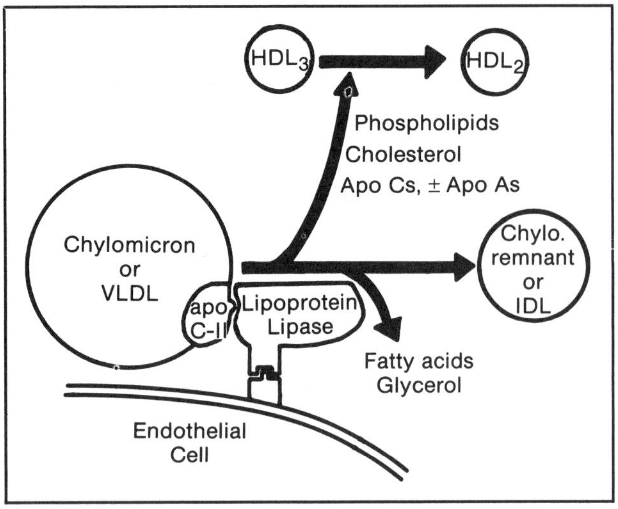

Fig. 13-3. Lipolysis of triglyceride-rich lipoproteins. Lipoprotein lipase is noncovalently bound to carbohydrate moieties on the surface of peripheral capillary endothelial cells, from which it can be released into the circulation by pharmacologically administered heparin. With aid of its cofactor, apo C-II, the enzyme hydrolyzes triglyceride from the lipoprotein core, producing free fatty acids and glycerol. As the lipoprotein core shrinks, surface components—phospholipids, cholesterol, and apo Cs—are transferred to HDL. This process causes conversion of HDL_3 to HDL_2. Chylomicrons, but not VLDL, contain apo A-I and apo A-II, which are transferred to HDL during lipolysis.

atively common atherogenic condition characterized by high plasma LDL levels, is caused by a genetic deficiency of or abnormality in LDL receptors.

Peripheral cells are limited in their capacity to deal with excess cholesterol. They can store excess cholesterol in esterified form but generally cannot further metabolize it or dispose of it. Therefore, cholesterol must be transported back to the liver for disposal and for regulation of body cholesterol content. Multiple interactive mechanisms for reverse cholesterol transport have been described (Fig. 13-4), but the relative quantitative importance of these diverse pathways is unknown [18–22]. Reverse cholesterol transport may account for the inverse epidemiologic relation between HDL and atherosclerotic disease. However, it has been impossible thus far to quantify reverse cholesterol transport directly. Genetic deficiency of lecithin:cholesterol acyltranferase (LCAT) (see Fig. 13-4) is associated with marked deficiency of cholesteryl ester in plasma lipoproteins and with early atherosclerosis [22]. Reverse cholesterol transport may be deficient in this syndrome.

LIPOPROTEIN ASSOCIATIONS WITH ATHEROGENESIS

Cholesterol-Rich Lipoproteins. LDL, which carries most of the plasma cholesterol, is the best-understood atherogenic lipoprotein. Analytic studies of LDL usually show a single, broad-based peak by ultracentrifugation, but some individuals show distinct subpopulations of particles. Increased atherogenicity has been associated with LDL that has an increased protein-to-cholesterol ratio and greater heterogeneity of particle size [23]. Clinically, this condition can be recognized as an elevation of apo B-100 concentration in LDL relative to LDL cholesterol [3]. This finding is most common in hypertriglyceridemic patients. It has been proposed that when VLDL is abundant, LDL becomes enriched in triglyceride and depleted in cholesteryl ester by a process of reciprocal transfer with VLDL. The resulting LDL particles are subject to lipolysis, which removes the triglyceride and leaves a smaller particle somewhat depleted of lipid [24]. The mechanism whereby small LDL might promote atherogenesis is unknown, although increased penetration of the arterial intima is a possibility.

Lp(a) consists of an LDL particle to which a large glycoprotein, apo (a), is joined by a disulfide linkage to the apo B-100 [2,25]. Lp(a) has a higher density than LDL; however, in the usual clinical methods for lipoprotein cholesterol determination, Lp(a) cholesterol is included in the LDL cholesterol fraction when the precipitation method is used or in the VLDL cholesterol fraction when the electrophoretic method is used. The physiologic role of Lp(a) remains enigmatic. It is synthesized primarily in the liver [26]. It is still unclear to what extent the LDL-receptor pathway is involved in Lp(a) catabolism, since evidence for and against its involvement has accumulated [27]. In terms of concentration, Lp(a) is usually a minor lipoprotein that carries about 5 mg/dl of cholesterol in the average person. However, Lp(a) levels can be much higher because of genetic factors, and levels above 13 mg/dl are strongly associated with early coronary disease [2]. Such high levels are found in approximately one fifth of individuals in white and Oriental populations. Blacks have higher levels of Lp(a) than whites, but the atherogenicity of this particle has not been proved in the black population. When considered on a per-particle basis, Lp(a) may be considerably more atherogenic than LDL. Preferential accumulation in the vascular wall of apo (a) compared with apo B has been demonstrated in humans [28]. Apo (a) shares a high degree of sequence homology with plasminogen, which suggests a possible link between Lp(a) levels and impaired fibrinolysis that could result in an enhanced tendency toward arterial thrombosis. Although competitive inhibition of fibrinolytic pathways by Lp(a) has been shown in vitro, the in-vivo significance of this connection remains hypothetical [29].

Protein-Rich Lipoproteins. In epidemiologic studies, the inverse relation between HDL cholesterol and CHD is usually as strong as the direct relation between total or LDL cholesterol and CHD. In the Framingham study, low HDL cholesterol was a much better predictor of CHD than high total or LDL cholesterol in men and women ages 49–82 years [1]. A heritable deficiency of apo A-I and apo C-III, which are gentically linked, is characterized by marked HDL deficiency and premature atherosclerotic disease. In another genetic syndrome, known as Tangier disease, apo A-I, apo A-II, and HDL all exhibit hypercatabolism. HDL is virtually absent, although LDL cholesterol is also reduced, and LDL is enriched in triglyceride. CHD may occur after age 40 in Tangier disease, but overwhelming atherosclerosis at an earlier age has not been described [30]. Elevated plasma HDL, or hyperalphalipoproteine-

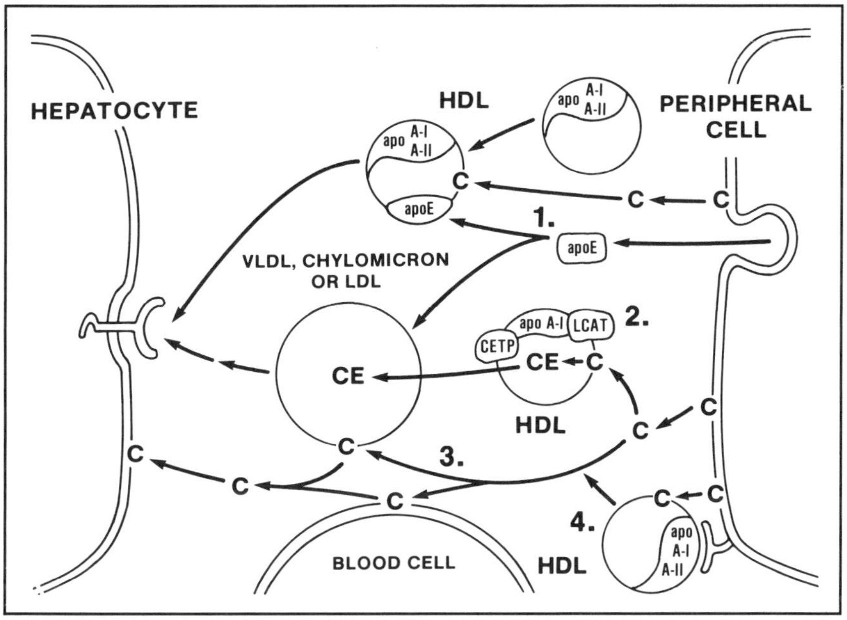

Fig. 13-4. Reverse cholesterol transport. Multiple interactive mechanisms for reverse cholesterol transport—from peripheral tissues back to the liver—have been described. (1) When their cholesterol content is high, certain peripheral cells, such as macrophages, begin to secrete apo E, which associates with nearby lipoprotein particles. Apo E facilitates receptor-mediated uptake of lipoproteins, especially HDL, by the liver. (2) HDL has a limited capacity for uptake of free cholesterol in its surface layer, but lecithin : cholesterol acyltransferase (LCAT) functions with its cofactor apo A-I to esterify cholesterol and move it into the oily interior of the lipoprotein particle. From there the cholesteryl ester can be distributed among all circulating lipoproteins via the activity of cholesteryl ester transfer protein (CETP). (3) Free cholesterol readily transfers via the aqueous phase from the plasma membrane of peripheral cells or from extracellular cholesterol deposits to the surface membranes of nearby lipoproteins or blood cells. In the hepatic microcirculation, a similar process can transfer free cholesterol to the hepatocyte plasma membrane. (4) Binding sites for HDL on the plasma membrane of peripheral cells may facilitate the exit of free cholesterol from the cell, either via the aqueous phase or by direct membrane-to-lipoprotein transfer.

mia, has been described as a familial syndrome associated with reduced rates of atherosclerotic disease and with longevity [31].

The two major HDL ultracentrifugal subfractions are HDL_2 and HDL_3. During lipolysis of triglyceride-rich lipoproteins by lipoprotein lipase, HDL_3, a smaller, heavier particle, is converted to HDL_2, a larger, lighter particle, by the transfer of phospholipid and other components from the triglyceride-rich lipoproteins (see Fig. 13-3). Fasting HDL_2 cholesterol levels vary interindividually, ranging from near 0 to greater than 50 mg/dl. Most of the clinical factors affecting HDL cholesterol levels, including gender, hormones, obesity, and exercise, primarily affect HDL_2. However, ethanol intake tends to raise both HDL_2 and HDL_3 levels. Apo A-I and apo A-II plasma levels are also elevated by ethanol [32].

Apo A-I is found in all HDL. Other apoproteins are variably present to form a diverse population of HDL particles. Apo A-II is found in most HDL_3 and some HDL_2. Apo E and other apoproteins are also found in some HDL [33].

An important question is whether HDL is directly antiatherogenic through its participation in reverse cholesterol transport or other mechanisms, or whether a depressed level of HDL merely correlates with an atherogenic condition. Injection of high levels of autologous HDL into cholesterol-fed rabbits decreases the severity of disease and promotes regression of established disease [34,35]; these results suggest some type of direct effect. Transgenic mice expressing human apo A-I (see "Animal Models," later in this chapter) also have been reported to be more atherosclerosis resistant than control mice. If oxidation of LDL is important in initiating the accumulation of lipid in the arterial wall (see "LDL Oxidation," later in this chapter), then the observations that HDL inhibits LDL oxidation [36] and acts as a major carrier of lipid hydroperoxides for hepatic removal [37] identify another mechanism for HDL-associated reduction in CHD risk. An inhibitor of the complement cascade, apo J, has also been identified as a component of HDL [38]. Complement binding to membranes enhances HDL binding, which, through interference with C9 polymerization, prevents formation of the pore-forming complex that disrupts the cell membrane [39]. Since complement deposition is an early event in experimental models of atherosclerosis, the protective effect of HDL may be of great significance in limiting damage to the arterial wall.

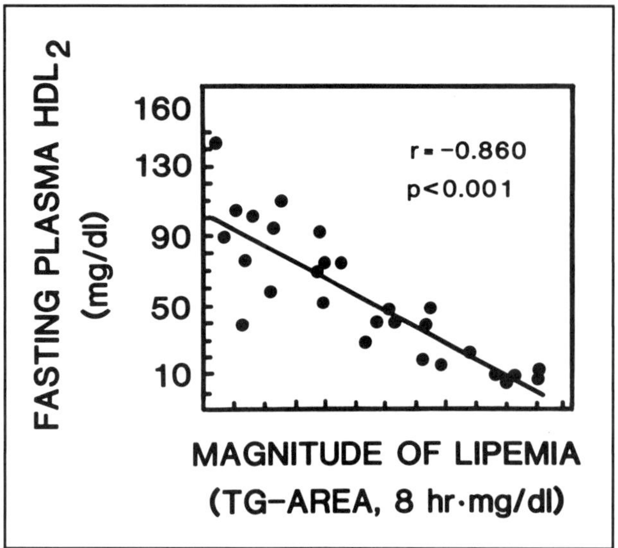

Fig. 13-5. Inverse relationship between fasting HDL_2 level and the integrated 8-hour response of plasma triglycerides to a fatty meal. (Reproduced with permission from JR Patsch et al. Inverse relationship between blood levels of high density lipoprotein subfraction 2 and magnitude of postprandial lipemia. Proc Nat Acad Sci USA 1983; 80:1449–1453.)

The precise contribution of these additional protective mechanisms versus the role of HDL in reverse cholesterol transport remains to be established. Although HDL cholesterol is a powerful predictor of CHD, it is unclear what clinical effects various physiologic and pharmacologic manipulations of HDL levels have.

Triglyceride-Rich Lipoproteins. A reasonable argument can be made that triglyceride-rich lipoproteins are directly atherogenic. Most epidemiologic studies have shown a positive relation between triglyceride levels and atherosclerotic disease. However, on multivariate analysis this association has not remained significant in men [40], although the Framingham Heart Study found elevated triglyceride levels to be a significant independent risk factor in women [41]. This may be attributable to the strong inverse relation between triglyceride and HDL cholesterol. Furthermore, fasting triglyceride levels, which were utilized in these epidemiologic analyses, may not be the best indicator of the atherogenicity of triglyceride-rich lipoproteins. For example, chylomicron remnants, which appear after a fatty meal, may have deleterious effects [42]. In type III hyperlipoproteinemia, which is commonly associated with atherosclerosis, these particles accumulate massively, even in fasting plasma. Additionally, in many individuals who are otherwise normal, plasma triglyceride levels rise excessively and remain elevated for 6 hours or more following a fatty meal. This phenomenon of triglyceride intolerance shows a remarkable inverse correlation with fasting HDL_2 levels (Fig. 13-5) [43]. Thus, the inverse correlation between HDL and atherosclerotic disease may be explained by high levels of triglyceride-rich lipoproteins during much of the day in subjects with low HDL_2 levels. Enrichment of HDL_2 particles with triglyceride transferred from postprandially accumulating chylomicrons may promote the conversion of HDL_2 to HDL_3 by hepatic lipase [44] and lead to low levels of circulating HDL_2. The abnormality underlying this atherogenic state may be a relative deficiency of peripheral lipoprotein lipase activity; this enzyme itself has exhibited an inverse correlation with CHD [45]. Cellular interactions of chylomicron remnants and other triglyceride-rich lipoproteins that may promote atherogenesis are described below. Modifications of VLDL that promote cellular receptor binding in hypertriglyceridemic patients apparently are due to proteolytic processing of apoproteins during the prolonged residence of VLDL particles in the circulation [46]. Those findings may provide models for other types of atherogenic modification of circulating lipoproteins.

Mechanisms of Arterial Lipid Accumulation

LIPOPROTEIN TRANSPORT IN THE NORMAL ARTERIAL WALL

Cholesterol in normal and atherosclerotic arteries derives mainly from plasma lipoproteins [47]. The thickened intima of large arteries bears a higher concentration of lipoproteins than any other tissue in the body, with the possible exception of blood plasma. The arterial intima normally contains no capillaries or lymphatics and is bounded on both inner and outer aspects by structures that represent major permeability barriers to macromolecular transport. Plasma constituents entering the intima first must cross the endothelium and then traverse a second barrier composed of multiple musculoelastic lamellae in the tunica media, before reaching lymphatic drainage in the outer media or adventitia. The net result may be accumulation and stagnation of lipoproteins in the arterial intima.

Lipoprotein Transport into the Arterial Wall. Transcytosis across the endothelial cell monolayer is the normal pathway for lipoprotein entry into the arterial wall (Fig. 13-6). Lipoproteins enter the pinocytic infoldings, or caveolae, of the endothelial plasma membrane; the caveolae detach from the cell surface to become free cytoplasmic vesicles, then reattach randomly to the endothelial surface [48]. This process of **transcytosis** utilizes uncoated pinocytic caveolae and vesicles. It should be distinguished from **endocytosis**, which is the uptake of lipoproteins in coated pits by a process that culminates in lysosomal digestion. In hypercholesterolemia and acute hypertension, arterial endothelial permeability apparently is increased [49,50], possibly because of increased rates of transcytosis, although further studies are needed.

Gaps in endothelial continuity may result from endothelial-cell death or the transendothelial migration of a blood leukocyte. Of particular interest are the large gaps in endothelial continuity that may form over the surface of intimal foam-cell lesions termed **fatty streaks**. The appearance of such gaps in a monkey model of dietary atherogenesis occurs just before the onset of intense lipid deposition and cellular proliferation in deeper intimal layers [51]. Greatly increased endothelial permeability to lipoproteins may be involved in this phenomenon, but

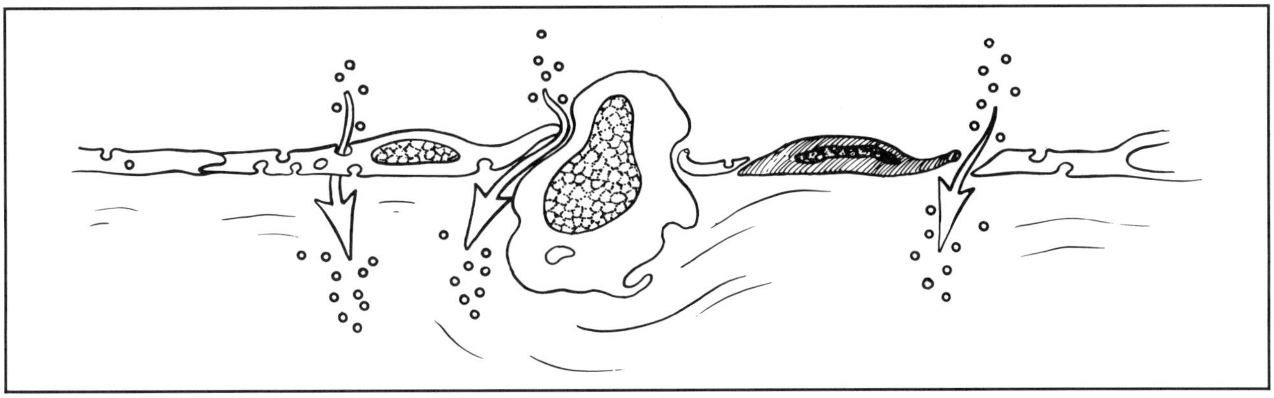

Fig. 13-6. Lipoprotein transport across arterial endothelium. Transcytosis is the major normal pathway. Passage of lipoproteins via the junctions between adjacent endothelial cells is thought to occur only when the junctions are opened due to leukocyte diapedesis or endothelial-cell death.

measurements of permeability have not yet been performed.

Lipoprotein transport in the arterial wall can be described using the principles of fluid mechanics. Lipoproteins may be carried through arterial tissue by fluid flow, which is also termed convection or solvent drag, or they may diffuse through the tissue independently of fluid flow (Fig. 13-7). In one analysis, convection and diffusion were estimated to be about equally important in LDL transport in rabbit aortic media [52]. If so, then lipoprotein diffusion would be expected to be the dominant transport process in the thickened intima of large human arteries, in which intima-media thickness is 3 to 10 times greater than that of rabbit aortic media (the greater thickness of these arteries diminishes convection, but not diffusion, in the inner layers. The third pathway in Fig. 13-7 illustrates the special importance of widely spaced but highly permeable gaps in the endothelial layer. Mathematical analysis suggests that such gaps may be remarkably effective in increasing the overall entry rate of lipoproteins into the arterial wall [53].

Lipoprotein Accumulation in Normal Arteries. LDL in human arterial intima has been detected immunohistochemically (Fig. 13-8) and quantified by electroimmunoassay. Saline-extractable LDL in normal intima contains on average 5–12 μg of apo B or 12–25 μg of cholesterol per milligram of dry defatted tissue weight [54,55]. Estimation of the volume of tissue containing these amounts of LDL indicates that the concentration of LDL in normal arterial intima, per unit volume, is nearly equal to or perhaps even greater than plasma LDL concentration [55,56]. Lp(a)

Fig. 13-7. Lipoprotein transport in the arterial wall. Convection is illustrated on the left, diffusion in the center, and the special conditions related to a highly permeable endothelial gap on the right. Represented at the bottom of the figure is the tunica media, which is relatively impermeable to lipoproteins in comparison with the tunica intima.

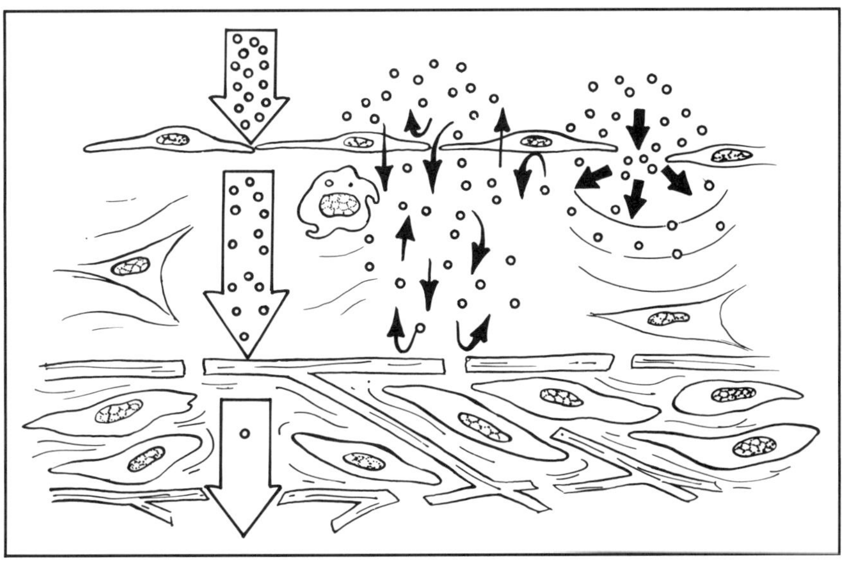

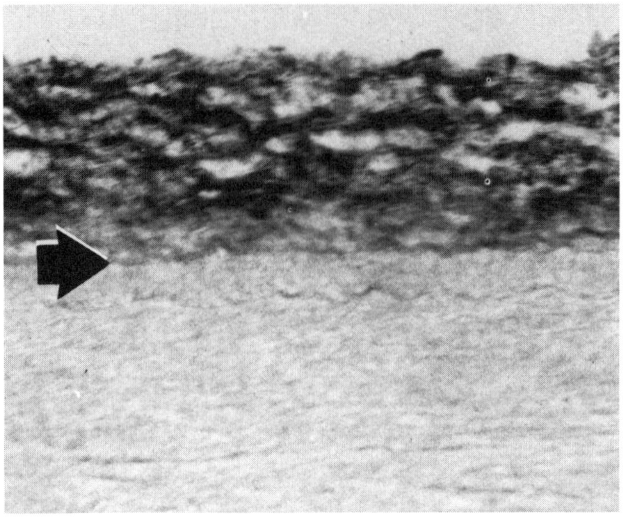

Fig. 13-8. Immunohistochemical staining for apo B in human arterial intima due to the presence of LDL. The tunica media shows no specific staining. Arrow shows location of internal elastic lamina. (Magnification × 137.)

accumulation in the intima is approximately fourfold in excess of plasma levels. The accumulation of LDL in normal arterial intima is age dependent and selective. By age 40, average apo B concentration in normal aortic intima may be five to six times higher than apo A-I concentration [57], despite the similar plasma concentrations of these two apoproteins.

Medial concentrations of lipoproteins are strikingly lower than intimal concentrations (see Fig. 13-8). Apo B and Apo A-I are undetectable in the tunica media by electroimmunoassay [56,58]. There are two possible explanations for the selective retention of LDL by the intima. One is that LDL may bind to various extracellular structural macromolecules within intimal tissue, which include proteoglycans, collagen, and elastin. The other possible explanation is that arterial medial tissue is relatively impermeable to particles as large as lipoproteins, to the extent that its resistance to lipoprotein transport is equal to or greater than that of the endothelium. A medial permeability barrier presumably would operate largely as a result of steric exclusion, which is likewise a function of extracellular tissue macromolecules [58].

Flux and Residence Time of Arterial Lipoproteins. The net flux of radioiodinated LDL into normal thoracic aortic wall in rabbits has been estimated in terms of the volume of plasma "cleared" by the aorta in one hour. This flux averages 70 nl plasma equivalent/cm^2 aortic surface area/hour [59], which is in reasonably good agreement with earlier work [60]. In another study, arterial LDL transport in humans was investigated by injecting radioiodinated LDL into comatose patients up to two weeks prior to death. Tissue radioactivity relative to plasma in the inner portion of the arterial wall eventually reached levels of 20 to 30 percent and did not seem to reach a plateau within the two-week period [61]. Since interstitial fluid accounts for only a fraction of total intimal volume, these data are consistent with the suggestion of high levels of LDL in the interstitial fluid of the arterial intima [56]. Moreover, the equilibration between plasma and intimal LDL may be relatively slow, on the order of weeks. Further data on LDL flux and concentration in the arterial intima are greatly needed; studies using animal models should examine regions of diffuse intimal thickening.

Lipid Accumulation in Normal Arteries. Beginning at about age 20, cholesteryl ester concentration in the normal arterial intima begins to rise linearly with age [55]. At age 60, cholesteryl ester may comprise 2 to 3 percent of the total wet weight of nonatherosclerotic intima. Only a small fraction of this lipid is contained in intact lipoproteins, as judged by the apo B measurements cited above. Another small portion of the cholesteryl ester in aortic intima is found within cells. Most of the lipid is found in extracellular perifibrous deposits in the deeper intimal layers. The evidence for a direct interaction between lipoproteins and extracellular matrix components, which may account for perifibrous lipid deposition, is summarized later in this chapter.

LIPOPROTEIN-CELL INTERACTION

Nonhepatic cells in vivo derive most of their required cholesterol from plasma lipoproteins. Some basic pathways of lipid and lipoprotein handling by cells are now well established (Fig. 13-9), but detailed knowledge about the critical factors in atherogenic lipid accumulation and foam-cell formation is still lacking.

As established by the work of Brown and Goldstein [62,63] and others, the level of unesterified cholesterol in a cell appears to be tightly regulated by three basic responses to excess cellular cholesterol or closely allied metabolites. The first response is inhibition of cholesterol

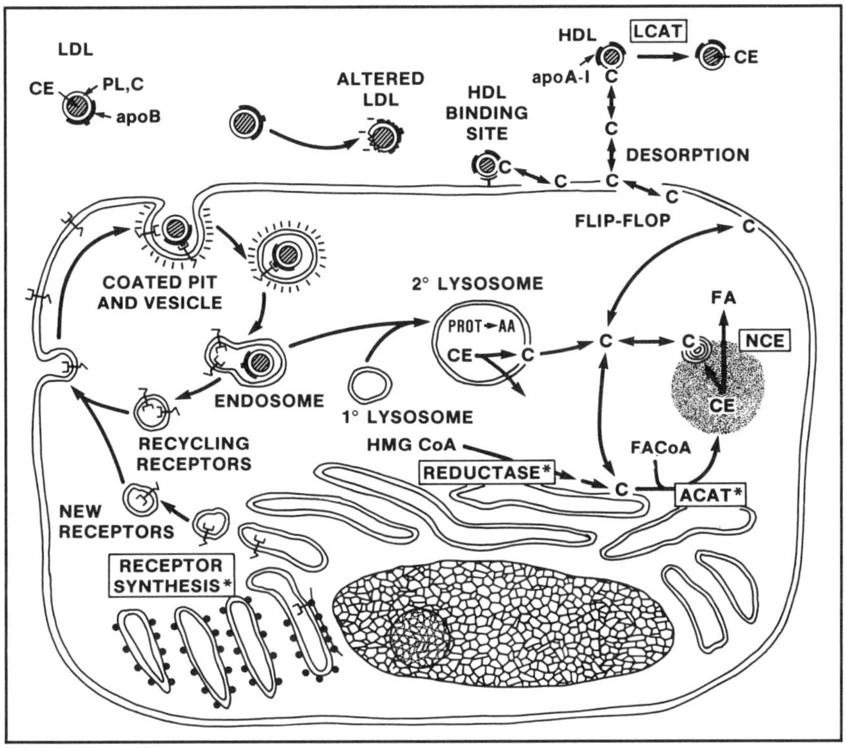

Fig. 13-9. Cellular cholesterol metabolism. Transmembrane LDL receptors are synthesized in the endoplasmic reticulum and transported via Golgi vesicles to the cell surface. The receptors diffuse laterally along the plasma membrane to localize in coated pits, where LDL is bound. Invagination produces a coated vesicle that rapidly loses its cytoplasmic coat and may coalesce with similar vesicles, forming the endosome. Acidification of the endosome interior causes dissociation of LDL and its receptor. A smaller vesicle containing the LDL receptors then buds off from the endosome and recycles the receptors to the cell surface. The other portion of the endosome fuses with a lysosome, within which LDL protein (PROT) and cholesteryl ester (CE) are hydrolyzed. Free cholesterol thus produced can diffuse through the aqueous phase to various cellular membranes (a process possibly accelerated by a cytoplasmic sterol carrier protein). Re-esterification of cholesterol is accomplished by a microsomal enzyme, acyl-CoA : cholesterol acyltransferase (ACAT), forming nonmembrane-bounded cytoplasmic droplets of cholesteryl ester. Three processes indicated by asterisks are responsive to the level of cellular free cholesterol or some closely allied metabolite. High cellular cholesterol suppresses LDL receptor synthesis, suppresses cellular cholesterol synthesis via HMG CoA reductase, and stimulates ACAT. Cytoplasmic cholesteryl ester can be hydrolyzed by a neutral-pH cholesteryl esterase (NCE), responsive to cyclic adenosine monophosphate (cAMP) levels. Cholesterol may exit the cell via aqueous transfer to the inner plasma membrane, transmembrane flip-flop, and aqueous desorption or direct transfer to HDL. Activity of lechithin : cholesterol acyltransferase (LCAT) can facilitate the uptake of unesterified cholesterol by HDL, by converting it to cholesteryl ester, which enters the lipoprotein core, leaving surface sites on HDL available for further cholesterol adsorption. A final important aspect of cellular lipoprotein metabolism is the oxidation of pericellular LDL, producing a more electronegative particle with partially hydrolyzed phospholipid and apo B.

synthesis via a decrease in the activity of the rate-limiting enzyme 3-hydroxy-3-methylglutaryl-coenzyme A (HMG-CoA) reductase. The product of this enzymatic reaction, mevalonic acid, is a precursor not only of cholesterol but also other important isoprenoid compounds—the isopentenyl group of transfer RNAs, ubiquinone, and dolichol [55]. HMG-CoA reductase activity is decreased by increased degradation of the enzyme and decreased mRNA production [62]. Lovastatin (formerly called mevinolin) and similar fungal metabolites are potent pharmacologic inhibitors of HMG-CoA reductase [64] and have shown promising results in clinical trials for the treatment of hypercholesterolemia. The second response is activation of acyl coenzyme A : cholesterol acyltransferase (ACAT), which catalyzes cholesterol esterification to cholesteryl oleate and thereby sequesters it in cytoplasmic droplets. This response protects the cell from the deleterious effects of unesterified cholesterol.

The third cellular response to excess cholesterol is downregulation of LDL receptors on the cell surface, caused by decreased mRNA for the receptors. This response limits the uptake of circulating cholesterol by the cell. The LDL receptor is a transmembrane glycoprotein localized in clathrin-coated pits on the surface of all mammalian cells. It binds LDL with high affinity ($K_D = 10^{-9}$ M). The process of LDL uptake in coated pits and vesicles and subsequent delivery to lysosomes is illustrated in Fig. 13-9.

Familial hypercholesterolemia is the monogenic disorder resulting from defective LDL receptor production or function. Mutant alleles may be divided into at least four classes based on functional characteristics. The most common type of mutation leads to a lack of synthesis of any immunoprecipitable receptor molecules. A second class of mutation specifies receptors that fail to undergo complete carbohydrate processing in the endoplasmic reticulum and Golgi apparatus and do not reach the cell surface. Variants of this mutation, which have been found in several human cases and in the Watanabe heritable hyperlipidemic rabbit, demonstrate slow intracellular processing of receptor protein. A small fraction of receptors is eventually expressed on the cell surface, but these do not bind LDL normally. A third class of mutant alleles in familial hypercholesterolemia produces receptors that reach the cell surface normally but cannot bind LDL. In a fourth class of mutant alleles, abnormal receptors are expressed on the cell surface and bind LDL normally but are unable to migrate to coated pits, where the LDL-receptor complex is internalized. Molecular defects in this class have been found in the cytoplasmic tail of the transmembrane receptor protein, indicating the importance of this region for localization in coated pits [57].

Patients with heterozygous familial hypercholesterolemia, whose cells exhibit only half the normal number of functional LDL receptors, commonly have plasma cholesterol levels of 300–500 mg/dl. Homozygous patients may have plasma cholesterol levels of 800 mg/dl or more and typically die with severe atherosclerosis in childhood or adolescence. A key metabolic feature of this disorder is the loss of normal lipoprotein uptake mediated by LDL receptors in the liver (see Fig. 13-2). This deficiency reduces the rate of plasma LDL catabolism and causes a loss of the normal feedback inhibition of hepatic cholesterol synthesis by plasma LDL cholesterol. Furthermore, since a substantial fraction of IDL is normally removed from plasma by hepatic LDL receptors, the lack of these receptors may allow more efficient conversion of IDL to LDL, thereby increasing LDL production.

The propensity for atherogenesis in familial hypercholesterolemia suggests that LDL receptors on arterial-wall cells may not be important in atherogenesis. Instead, one or more alternative receptor pathways, non-receptor-mediated cellular uptake of lipoproteins, and accumulation of lipid in association with extracellular tissue components may be the major mechanisms for arterial lipid deposition in these patients.

Alternative Lipoprotein Receptors. An attractive hypothesis to explain excessive lipid accumulation in the artery wall is that modified forms of lipoproteins are taken up into arterial cells after binding to alternative lipoprotein receptors. Goldstein et al. were able to demonstrate the presence of a receptor on macrophages that recognizes LDL made more electronegative by acetylation [65]. Uptake of those particles resulted in massive cholesteryl ester deposition in the cells, producing the in-vitro equivalent of the foam cells seen in atherosclerotic lesions. Unlike the LDL receptor, this receptor, termed the **scavenger receptor**, was not downregulated by cholesterol accumulation [66]. Subsequent studies conducted to define more physiologically relevant ligands for the macrophage scavenger receptor have demonstrated that LDL modified by exposure to malondialdehyde or aggregating platelets [67] or oxidized by cells [68–70] or metal ions such as copper [71,72] bind to this receptor and load cells with lipid. LDL isolated from inflammatory fluid [73] and, in some cases, extracted from the artery wall [74,75] also exhibit scavenger-receptor binding. Recently, peroxynitrate-modified LDL, which may form through the interaction of nitric oxide and superoxide with LDL, was reported to bind to the scavenger receptor [76]. The common feature of all these ligands is the net negative charge of the lipoprotein.

The macrophage scavenger receptor was identified in our laboratory as a 260,000-kD glycoprotein that can bind multiple types of charge-modified lipoproteins [77]. After molecular cloning, its structure has been deduced to be three monomeric subunits in triple-helical formation [78,79]. One region of the molecule has a high homology to collagen, and that region is the one responsible for binding various charge-modified lipoproteins [80,81]. The receptor is expressed at high levels in foam cells of atherosclerotic lesions [82]. This single receptor does not account for all scavenger-receptor activity on the macrophage [83,84]; expression cloning has indicated that the FcIIIb receptor also functions as a scavenger receptor for oxidized LDL (Ox-LDL) [85]. Thus, a family of scavenger receptors seems to exist.

Macrophages also exhibit poorly regulated uptake of variant VLDL particles, which leads to foam-cell formation. Cholesteryl ester–rich VLDL with beta electrophoretic mobility, or β-VLDL, is found in the plasma of cholesterol-fed animals and in the plasma of patients with dysbetalipoproteinemia (type III hyperlipoproteinemia). Uptake of β-VLDL by macrophages is mediated by binding to a modified form of the LDL receptor or to a macrophage receptor distinct from the acetyl-LDL, or scavenger, receptor [86]. β-VLDL causes cholesteryl ester loading of macrophages. VLDL from hypertriglyceridemic patients appears to bind to a distinct macrophage receptor because of partial proteolysis of apo B on the lipoprotein surface [87,88]. These VLDL particles cause triglyceride loading of the macrophage and, perhaps because of similar receptors on the endothelium, are toxic to the endothelium [88]. A 190-kD protein has been suggested as a candidate receptor for binding VLDL particles in hypertriglyceridemic patients [87].

In contrast to macrophages, smooth muscle cells in culture are quite resistant to cholesterol loading. Yet cholesteryl ester droplets have been observed in smooth muscle cells at lesion sites. One study attempting to resolve that paradox demonstrated ingestion by smooth muscle cells of preformed cholesteryl ester droplets released from macrophages [89]. More recently, scavenger receptor activity was demonstrated in rabbit smooth muscle cells after phorbol ester treatment, and lipid loading of the cells occurred after incubation with acetyl-LDL [90] or Ox-LDL

[91]. Scavenger-receptor activity in rabbit intimal smooth muscle cells isolated from the lesion site also has been demonstrated [92]. The scavenger receptor in the smooth muscle cells is structurally similar to that in the macrophages [93], and scavenger-receptor mRNA has been expressed in human smooth muscle cells treated with platelet-derived growth factor B or phorbol 12-myristate 13-acetate (PMA) [94]. These observations suggest that scavenger-receptor activity may be switched on in smooth muscle cells at some point during lesion formation and may eventually give rise to smooth muscle–derived foam cells.

While endothelial cells do not form foam cells, they too have scavenger-receptor activity [95]. The scavenger receptor on endothelial cells may provide a first line of defense against the accumulation of modified lipoproteins in the circulation. Modified lipoproteins such as acetyl-LDL injected intravenously into animals have a half-life of only 1.5 minutes before they are cleared from the circulation by scavenger receptors on liver sinusoidal endothelial cells [96,97]. This protective function also may be operational at the local level, since endothelial cells in the arterial wall aid in the removal of any modified lipoprotein as it is formed. It appears that one reason foam-cell formation does not occur in endothelial cells is that cholesterol re-esterification is very inefficient. Current studies in our laboratory [unpublished data] and elsewhere [93] suggest that the endothelial-cell scavenger receptor and the macrophage scavenger receptor, while functionally equivalent, may not be identical molecules. Hybridization with macrophage scavenger receptor–nucleic acid probes fails to detect a signal in endothelial cells, and Western blotting indicates that the endothelial-cell scavenger receptor protein is slightly smaller.

Lipid loading of macrophages can occur by other, non-receptor-mediated mechanisms. Phagocytic lipid loading of macrophages occurs when macrophages are presented with aggregated complexes, including cholesteryl ester-albumin [66], LDL-heparin-fibronectin-gelatin [98], and insoluble proteoglycan-LDL complexes [99]. Steinberg and colleagues [100] have demonstrated that LDL aggregates formed by vortexing are taken up into macrophages and result in lipid loading. This uptake does not occur through the scavenger receptor but appears to involve both phagocytosis and the LDL-receptor pathway. Aggregation may also play a role in loading cells with oxidized forms of LDL [101].

The Fate of Cholesterol Inside Cells. A relative deficiency of lysosomal hydrolysis of cholesteryl ester in proportion to the lipoprotein load presented to the lysosomes has been suggested to account for cellular cholesterol accumulation in atherosclerosis. Indeed, young patients with Wolman disease, who have a rare congenital deficiency of acid cholesteryl esterase, develop severe arterial lesions resembling atherosclerosis. However, Fowler and co-workers did not find a deficiency of lysosomal cholesteryl ester hydrolysis in experimental atherosclerosis in rabbits and monkeys. The accumulation of cellular lipid in comparable amounts in both lysosomes and cytoplasmic droplets, as shown by ultrastructural cytochemistry, implies that hydrolysis and re-esterification are occurring [102,103]. Much of the lysosomal lipid has been found to consist of free cholesterol, which also indicates hydrolysis. Acid cholesteryl esterase activity under optimal assay conditions was found to be three times higher in lipid-laden, atheromatous cells than in cells in normal arterial walls [104].

The activity of ACAT (see Fig. 13-9), which is responsible for forming cytoplasmic cholesteryl ester droplets, is greatly increased in arteries with lipid accumulation in foam cells. It has been suggested that ACAT might provide a biochemical trapping mechanism for cholesterol in the arterial wall. Specific ACAT inhibitors have been shown to retard arterial lipid deposition [105]. Now that the ACAT enzyme has been cloned [106], a greater understanding of the role of ACAT in the cholesterol-deposition process should be forthcoming.

A third major enzyme for intracellular cholesterol metabolism is a cytoplasmic cholesteryl esterase with optimal activity at neutral pH [107]. This enzyme is localized at the surface of cytoplasmic lipid droplets [108], and its activity is stimulated by cyclic adenosine monophosphate (cAMP). Further studies are needed to assess the role of this enzyme in foam-cell formation.

Cholesterol Removal. A deficiency or an overactivity of any single enzymatic step would not sufficiently explain the apparent accumulation of free and esterified cholesterol in both lysosomes and cytoplasmic droplets in foam cells. However, blocking the exit of cholesterol from the cell, especially if combined with abnormally high uptake of lipoproteins, might result in cholesterol accumulation, which occurred in the studies of Fowler and colleagues [102–104]. The mechanism of cholesterol removal from cells involves the desorption of unesterified cholesterol from the plasma membrane into the aqueous phase [109]. Because of the extremely low aqueous solubility of cholesterol, the removal of a significant quantity of cholesterol requires the nearby presence of cholesterol acceptors such as albumin, phospholipid, or HDL. Binding sites for HDL on the cell surface [110] may facilitate this process (see Fig. 13-4 and Fig. 13-9). Initial studies indicate the possible presence of specific HDL-binding sites on the surface of fibroblasts. Binding of HDL to those receptors, in contrast to other types of lipoprotein receptors, does not result in uptake and degradation of the lipoprotein. Subsequent work has identified a 110-kD protein in fibroblasts that is upregulated by cholesterol loading of cells [111]. It has been cloned recently and is not a previously known protein [112]. Whether it is the only HDL receptor remains to be established. In macrophages [113] and hepatocytes [114], HDL is bound to the surface of the cell, endocytosed, and then returned to the extracellular milieu intact through a process termed retroendocytosis. In lipid-loaded cells, HDL binding appears to cause mobilization of intracellular cholesterol pools that subsequently move to the cell surface. Protein kinase C inhibitors block the efflux [115], and cAMP has been reported to promote efflux [116]; therefore, two separate signal transduction pathways may be involved. In the arterial wall, cholesterol removal may be limited by the relatively slow diffusion of soluble cholesterol acceptors through interstitial fluid, causing saturation of available acceptor sites in the vicinity of the cells. This suggestion, however, is merely speculation at present.

LDL Oxidation. Oxidation of LDL was first demonstrated by overnight incubation of LDL with cultures of endothelial cells [117]. LDL treated in that way is more electronegative than normal LDL and bonds to macrophage scavenger receptors. Ox-LDL is characterized by a loss of cholesterol, hydrolysis of phosphatidylcholine at the 2 position, and breakdown of apo B. Macrophages [69], smooth muscle cells [70,118], fibroblasts, and lymphocytes [119] all can oxidize LDL under appropriate conditions. Cell-mediated oxidation of LDL can be mimicked in cell-free conditions in appropriate media or buffers containing sufficient levels of copper ions [71]. Less oxidized forms can be generated in the presence of iron ions [120].

Chemically, the oxidation process is complex [71,119]. It is thought that peroxidized lipid products formed in cells through the action of 15-lipoxygenase are transferred to the lipoprotein particles. A propagation phase mediated by copper ions ensues, during which additional lipoperoxides are formed. This propagation leads to breakdown of fatty acids and generation of reactive aldehydes that react with both apo B and phospholipid. Modification by these reactive groups of the critical lysine residues of apo B, which are required for interaction with the LDL receptor, leads to the loss of LDL-receptor specificity and the appearance of scavenger-receptor specificity.

Considerable evidence now supports the existence of Ox-LDL in vivo. Antibodies specific for oxidized forms of LDL react with material in the atherosclerotic lesion [121–123]. Human serum samples have been demonstrated to contain autoantibodies to forms of Ox-LDL [122], and in one study [124], the levels of autoantibodies were excellent predictors of subsequent progression of atherosclerosis. Lipoproteins extracted from the artery wall have been shown in some cases to have many of the properties of LDL oxidized in vitro, including scavenger-receptor uptake [125]. Immunoglobulin IgG extracted from lesion sites also demonstrates specificity for Ox-LDL [119]. While extensively oxidized LDL particles have never been found in circulation, presumably because of hepatic clearance by sinusoidal scavenger receptors, a small fraction of LDL with an altered charge reportedly has been isolated [126].

Specific antioxidants can have dramatic effects on experimental atherosclerosis in animal models. Probucol, probucol derivatives, and other antioxidants such as butylated hydroxytoulene (BHT) and phenylenediamine significantly reduce by up to 70 percent the size and number of atherosclerotic lesions in hypercholesterolemic rabbits [127–130]. This effect of probucol is independent of its lipid-lowering ability [127,129]. Whether all the antiatherosclerotic effects of probucol are due to its antioxidant effects, however, is currently an open question. Probucol also reduces the secretion from treated macrophage of interleukin-1β, a smooth muscle-cell mitogen [131]. In another study, probucol reduced the number of macrophages in the lesion site without altering the immunoreactivity of lesion tissue for an antibody specific for Ox-LDL [132].

Recent epidemiologic studies examining the effectiveness of common antioxidants have lent further credence to the association between Ox-LDL and atherosclerosis in humans. Prospective studies in which 40,000 men [133] and 80,000 women [134] were followed for up to eight years showed that high doses of vitamin E supplements significantly reduced the risk of CHD. Supplementation for two or more years was required to see significant benefit. The antioxidant beta-carotene was not effective in male nonsmokers but did reduce the risk in male smokers [133]. Female smokers and nonsmokers derived no benefit [134]. LDL from smokers has been shown to be more susceptible to oxidation than LDL from nonsmokers [135]. Conflicting results have been obtained with vitamin C. In those two prospective studies, no effect was seen in either men or women [133,134], but in another study, conducted in 11,000 men, an inverse correlation between CHD mortality and vitamin C intake was observed [136]. For now, the use of large supplements of vitamin antioxidants is not recommended, and a call has been made for a randomized, double-blind, long-term trial to ensure efficacy and safety of antioxidant use [137]. The Probucol Quantitative Regression Swedish Trial (PQRST) has provided evidence that probucol reduces susceptibility to oxidation of LDL isolated from treated subjects [138]. The results of analysis of the antioxidant contribution of probucol to changes in atherosclerosis versus probucol-mediated changes in lipid lowering in those subjects are being awaited.

There are multiple mechanisms through which Ox-LDL may affect lesion initiation and progression [139,140]. These mechanisms reflect the diversity of phenotypic changes these lipoprotein particles can induce in monocyte-macrophages, endothelial cells, smooth muscle cells, and activated T-cells at the lesion site. High levels of Ox-LDL particles are toxic to many cell types and thus can be a source of injury to the endothelium. These particles are directly chemotactic for monocytes because of their increased lysolecithin content and so may recruit monocytes to the artery wall. The Ox-LDL particles have scavenger-receptor specificity, and their uptake results in lipid loading of macrophages at the lesion site to form foam cells. Macrophages that have taken up Ox-LDL show decreased mobility; thus, the lipoprotein can maintain high levels of macrophages at the lesion site. Ox-LDL also induces tissue factor in macrophages and may influence the coagulation cascade at the lesion site. Interleukin-1-beta production in macrophages is switched on by treatment with Ox-LDL or the fatty acid oxidation product 9-hydroxyoctadecadienoic acid (free or cholesterol esterified). Endothelin production is elevated almost 10-fold after treatment of macrophages with Ox-LDL. In endothelial cells, mildly Ox-LDL stimulates the production of colony-stimulating factors that can enhance macrophage survival and smooth muscle-cell proliferation. The lysolecithin of Ox-LDL stimulates the binding of monocytes to the endothelium, which is the initial step in lesion formation, through upregulation of vascular adhesion molecule-1

(VCAM-1) on the endothelial cells. Lysolecithin also promotes the secretion of heparin-binding epidermal growth factor, a potent smooth muscle-cell mitogen, from the macrophage [141] and decreases the relaxation of vessels exposed to acetylcholine. The vascular tone of the artery, therefore, may be adversely affected. Monocyte chemotactic protein (MCP-1) production by the endothelial cells is increased after interaction with Ox-LDL. Macrophages lipid loaded by acetyl-LDL and Ox-LDL also have elevated levels of urokinase-type plasminogen activator and, through the generation of plasmin from plasminogen, cause the release of extracellular matrix-bound smooth muscle growth factors [142]. Smooth muscle cells respond to Ox-LDL by increasing production of platelet-derived growth factor A, a potent smooth muscle-cell mitogen. T-cells are activated by Ox-LDL, and the activated T-cells can produce a plethora of cytokines that affect each of the other cell types at the lesion site, causing, for example, the secretion of smooth muscle mitogen, and also participate in other immune-type reactions occurring at the site. Thus, it is clear that the presence of Ox-LDL at the lesion site can have extremely important consequences for lesion development.

Cytokine Control of Lipid Metabolism at the Lesion Site. As discussed by Ross in this book (see Chapter 11) and recently reviewed in detail [143], all the cell types at the lesion site are capable of secreting a myriad of cytokines that can have significant impact on the phenotypes of the surrounding cells. Evidence has been accumulating that suggests that some of those cytokines may directly affect the metabolism of charge-modified lipoproteins by macrophages at the lesion site. Colony-stimulating factor, which can be produced by macrophages and endothelial cells, stimulates the level of expression of the macrophage scavenger receptor [144]. Elevated levels of colony-stimulating factor and its receptor at the lesion site have been detected [145,146]. Long-term treatment of monocyte-derived macrophages with interferon-gamma (IFN-γ) produces a marked reduction in the expression of the macrophage scavenger receptor [147]. Studies in our laboratory suggest that the effects of IFN-γ depend on the stage of differentiation of the macrophage. Freshly isolated monocytes treated with IFN-γ show a stimulation of scavenger-receptor levels, while more fully differentiated cells treated with IFN-γ show a decline in receptor activity and mRNA levels. IFN-γ is a T-cell product, and both activated T-cells and IFN-γ have been demonstrated to be present at the lesion site [148,149]. Interestingly, injection of polynucleotide inducers of interferon or IFN-γ into cholesterol-fed rabbits reduces the severity of lesion formation [150,151]. Preliminary data from our laboratory suggest that interleukin-4, also a T-cell product, is a potent stimulator of macrophage scavenger receptors in fully differentiated macrophages. These data suggest that the composition of the cytokine milieu at the lesion site has an impact on the degree of uptake of modified lipoprotein such as Ox-LDL. Furthermore, these cytokine-mediated effects on lipid metabolism may differ depending on the residence time in the lesion of the target cells. A monocyte that has freshly migrated into the lesion area may not have the same response to a given cytokine as one that has been present in the lesion site for an extended period of time.

IFN-γ also decreases the secretion of apo E by macrophages and inhibits lipoprotein lipase secretion in human monocyte-derived macrophages [152]. Inhibition of apo E secretion may prevent apo E-mediated immunosuppression of lymphocytes and reduce foam-cell formation. Inhibition by IFN-γ of lipoprotein lipase secretion may also serve to limit foam-cell formation [153].

Smooth muscle-cell metabolism of lipoproteins also may be influenced by cytokines at the lesion site. Macrophage colony-stimulating factor has been noted to increase scavenger receptor activity in lesion-derived smooth muscle cells [32].

From the preceding discussion, it is clear that cytokines may be important factors in the regulation of lipoprotein metabolism at the lesion site. As detailed, modified lipoproteins such as Ox-LDL can have a significant impact on cytokine secretion by cells at the lesion site. Thus, both proatherogenic and antiatherogenic activities occur simultaneously at the lesion site. The relative strengths of cytokine effects on lipoprotein metabolism and of modified lipoprotein effects on cytokine secretion may have a direct influence on the degree of progression of the lesion.

PHYSICAL CHEMISTRY OF LIPID DEPOSITS

The most obvious forms of lipid deposition in mature fibrous-plaque atherosclerosis are solid crystals of cholesterol monohydrate and liquid or liquid-crystalline (mesophase) droplets composed predominantly of cholesteryl ester. Only the surface molecules of these deposits are available for heterogeneous chemical reactions or for transfer to other species such as lipoproteins, which can diffuse through the aqueous phase in and out of the arterial intima. The interior lipid molecules in these deposits are sequestered and resistant to removal processes. An understanding of the formation, growth, and regression of these large lipid deposits is essential to the understanding of atherogenesis. Small has advanced the theory that lipids in both normal and atherosclerotic arteries usually exist in a thermodynamically stable state and that the physical forms of the lipids are governed predominantly by lipid-lipid interactions [154,155]. The validity of this theory is demonstrated by the prediction of the observed physical phases of lipid in arterial tissue by a triangular phase diagram in which only the three major lipid components are considered (Fig. 13-10). Certain small and potentially transitional lesions, including **fibrolipid lesions** [156] and those termed **intermediate lesions** by Katz and co-workers [157], are exceptions to this rule and often appear to contain unesterified cholesterol in a supersaturated, thermodynamically unstable state.

In addition to cholesterol crystals and cholesteryl ester droplets, a phospholipid-rich phase of arterial lipid can be discerned. This phase takes the familiar form of bileaflet membranes, including cellular membranes. Unesterified cholesterol can be incorporated or "dissolved" in phospholipid membranes at molar ratios up to about 1 : 1, and cholesterol crystals are formed only when the molar ratio exceeds that level. Even in the absence of crystals, a high

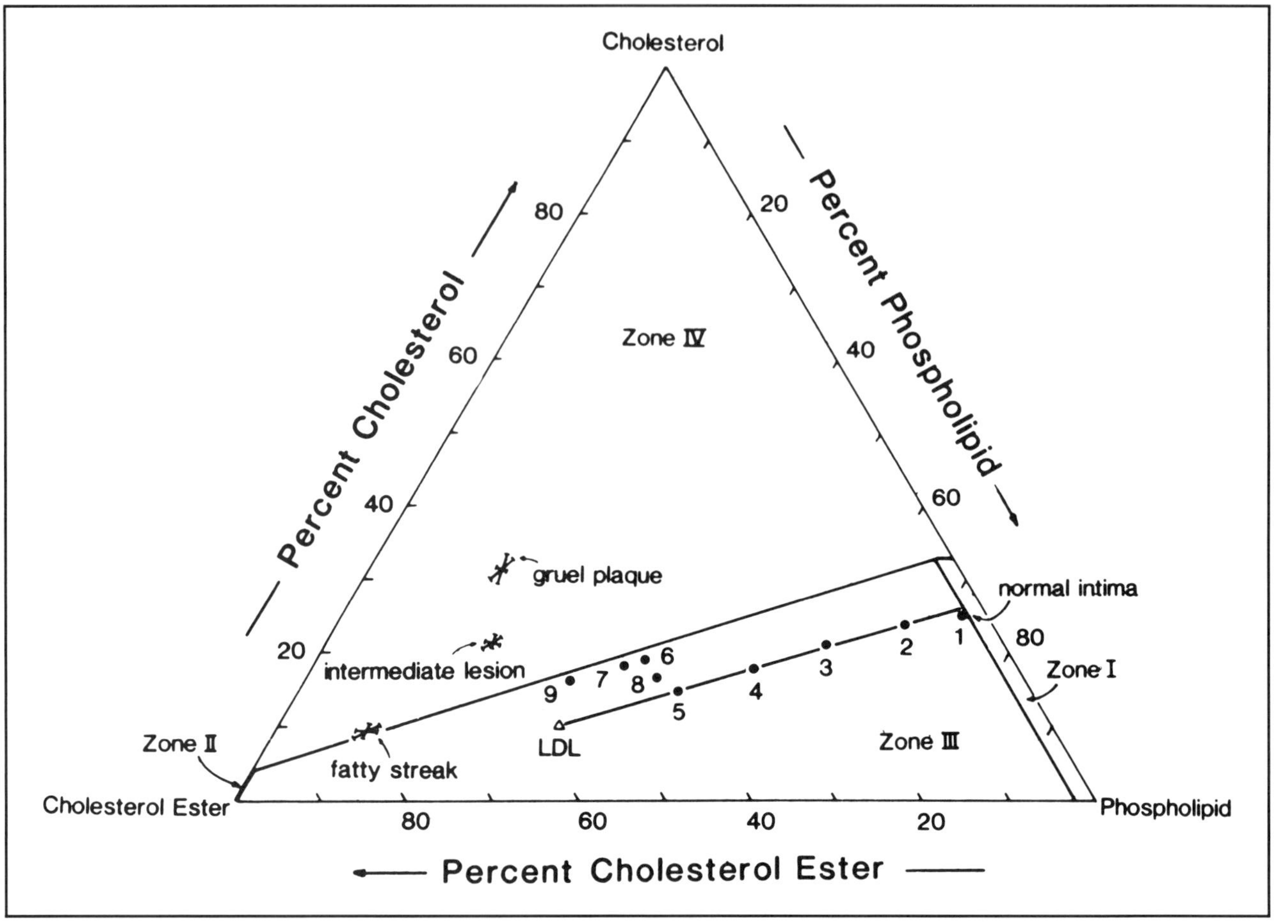

Fig. 13-10. Phase diagram of the major lipids of the arterial intima. Lipid mass composition is plotted on the triangular coordinates. Coordinate location determines the phases present. Zone I is a single phase made up of phospholipid bilayers containing up to 33% cholesterol and minimal cholesteryl ester. Zone II is a cholesteryl ester phase with minimal cholesterol and no phospholipid. Zone III is a two-phase region consisting of both of these phases. Zone IV is a three-phase region in which the third phase consists of cholesterol monohydrate crystals. Numbered points represent the average arterial lipid compositions of nonlesioned intima during decades of life; the line drawn through the first four decades suggests that lipid with the composition of LDL is being added to the intima. Mean lipid compositions of atherosclerotic lesions are plotted. Fatty streaks have two lipid phases (Zone III), gruel (fibrous) plaques have three (Zone IV), and intermediate lesions may have two or three. (Reproduced with copyright permission of the American Society of Clinical Investigation from DM Small et al. Physicochemical and histological changes in the arterial wall of nonhuman primates during progression and regression of atherosclerosis. J Clin Invest 1984; 73(6):1590–1605.)

concentration of cholesterol may decrease fluidity of cell membranes and thereby cause cellular toxicity. Recent evidence indicates that some extracellular lipid deposits take the form of membrane vesicles composed primarily of phospholipid and cholesterol [158]. Whether the vesicles originate from cellular debris or from de-novo extracellular assembly of component lipid molecules is uncertain. These vesicles probably account for the recently described, round, extracellular lipid particles that stain with filipin, a flourescent dye that specifically binds to unesterified cholesterol. Such particles have been found in a variety of human and animal atherosclerotic lesions [159].

Although the equilibrium-phase diagram describes the physical forms of lipid in the arterial wall (see Fig. 13-10), it does not explain net lipid accumulation. The driving forces for lipid accumulation remain unknown, although they may include some combination of lipoprotein-transport characteristics, interactions of lipoproteins and lipids with cells and with extracellular tissue, and lipid-lipid thermodynamics.

SUMMARY OF ARTERIAL LIPID DEPOSITION

Figure 13-11 represents diagrammatically several current theories of arterial lipid deposition. The complexity of the diagram is, unfortunately, a measure of the present state of ignorance. Nevertheless, a few generalizations can be made. A high load of cholesterol is presented to the arterial

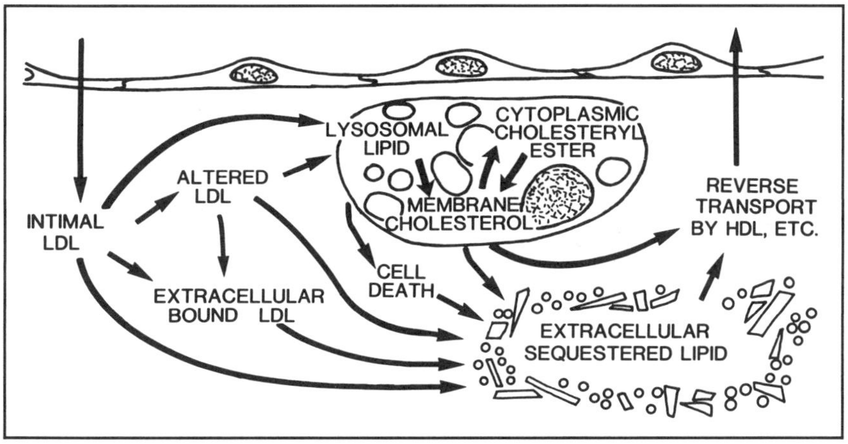

Fig. 13-11. Summary of pathways for lipid flux in arterial intima. LDL is considered the principal source of arterial cholesterol; HDL and other cholesterol acceptors are the means of removal. Intimal LDL may bind to extracellular sites, be taken up by cells, or become altered by oxidation or some other process. Extracellular sequestered lipid (cholesterol crystals and cholesteryl ester droplets) makes up the bulk of arterial lipid in fibrous plaques. This lipid could accumulate by at least five alternative routes. Individual lipid molecules could transfer from nearby normal or altered LDL. Alternatively, normal or altered LDL may bind in the form of intact particles to extracellular sites, then undergo loss of protein and phospholipid, leaving free and esterified cholesterol behind. Accumulation of lipid in cells may be an important preliminary step for part or even most of extracellular lipid accumulation. Cellular cholesterol could become extracellular by two major alternative processes: (1) the desorption of free cholesterol from the plasma membrane and subsequent deposition at extracellular sites and (2) cell necrosis, leaving behind cholesteryl ester droplets and some free cholesterol.

intima in the form of intimal LDL. The best current theories for foam-cell formation involve alteration or complexation of intimal LDL and cellular uptake via alternative lipoprotein receptors or phagocytosis. Death of foam cells is observed, but there are also instances of lipid deposits so intimately enmeshed in elastin or collagen fibers (see Fig. 13-12) that those deposits could not have resulted directly from foam-cell death. More information is needed about the binding of lipids or lipoproteins to the extracellular matrix. Even in the case of extracellular lipid deposition, the cellular role should not be minimized because synthesis of matrix constituents, cell-mediated alteration of lipoproteins, and desorption of excess cellular cholesterol from the plasma membrane are all potentially important mechanisms. The final step shown in Fig. 13-11 is the uptake of free cholesterol by diffusible particles, such as HDL, and subsequent diffusion or convection of those particles out of the intima. Very little is known about the details of the process; although it does seem to be a final common pathway for the removal of cholesterol from both cellular and extracellular sites, it may be relatively deficient since cholesterol accumulates at both sites.

Atherosclerosis-Lesion Development

HUMAN LESIONS

Fibrous Plaques. The fibrous plaque is the clinically important lesion of human atherosclerosis. It is the standard to which various experimental models, whether in animals or in vitro, must ultimately be compared. A fibrous plaque usually is considered synonymous with a raised, uncomplicated lesion, but plaques are sometimes subdivided according to their macroscopic surface appearance into categories of fibrous, fatty, and gelatinous. The constant feature of fibrous plaques is an accumulation of excessive intimal tissue due to proliferation and fibrogenesis of smooth muscle cells. An additional feature, which

Fig. 13-12. Electron micrograph of human aortic intima, showing cholesteryl ester deposition in the form of small droplets in an elastic fiber (top) and in two large droplets in a smooth muscle cell (bottom). (Magnification × 16,500.)

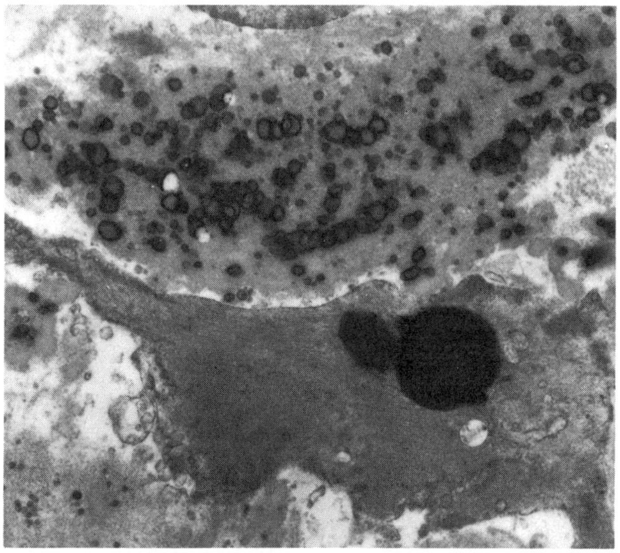

Table 13-3. Contrasting features of human atherosclerotic lesions

	Fatty streak	Gelatinous lesion	Fibrolipid lesion	Fibrous plaque
Contour	Flat	Raised	Minimally raised	Raised
Size	< 2 mm unless confluent	Variable, some > 1 cm	< 5 mm by definition	Any size
Sites of maximal involvement	Thoracic aorta, proximal coronaries	Abdominal aorta and elsewhere	Abdominal, then thoracic aorta; near ostia	Abdominal, then thoracic aorta; proximal coronaries
Chronology	Maximum in teenagers	Mostly age 20+	Age 20+	Age 20+
Epidemiology	Blacks = whites	Unknown	Unknown	Blacks < whites
Foam-cell infiltrates	Yes	No	Yes	Variable
Extracellular lipid	No	Perifibrous lipid	Deep-lying core region	Usually, in core region
Cholesterol crystals	No	No	In one-third of lesions	Usually, in core region
Unesterified/total cholesterol [47,105]	0.19	0.25	0.46	0.36
Fatty acyl groups in cholesterol ester [47]	50% 18:1 15% 18:2	Similar to fibrous plaque	Unknown	27% 18:1 42% 18:2

although common is not always found, is a core region of cellular necrosis and intense accumulation of extracellular lipid, principally free and esterified cholesterol. About three-fourths of fibrous plaques at an early stage of development contain a definable core region. Whether this fraction increases or decreases in larger, more mature plaques is unknown.

The fatty streak is a flat, lipid-containing intimal lesion of no immediate clinical consequence. Microscopically, the aortic fatty streak is characterized by collections of lipid-laden foam cells in a superficial location, almost always within 300 μm of the luminal surface [160]. Fatty streaks in the coronary arteries may have a different underlying histology than aortic fatty streaks, since they show abundant extracellular lipid and lipid contained within spindle-shaped cells, as well as scattered foam cells [161].

A continuing question about human atherogenesis is whether fatty streaks may progress to become fibrous plaques. A related question is whether cellular lipid accumulation is an early metabolic step leading to extracellular lipid deposition in the core region of the fibrous plaque. Data based on human atherosclerotic lesions are summarized in Table 13-3. The study of lesion topography and epidemiology has made it clear that many aortic fatty streaks are **not** progressive, particularly in populations that experience low rates of clinical cardiovascular disease [162]. Furthermore, if core-region lipid deposits of fibrous plaques have their origin in foam cells, then several chemical alterations of the lipid must take place during lesion progression. Most notable is an increase in the unesterified cholesterol content of the lesion. Smith and others have noted that fibrous-plaque cholesteryl esters have linoleate as their major fatty acyl group in a pattern very similar to that of plasma lipoproteins [55]. Fatty streaks, which contain predominantly intracellular cholesteryl ester, contain markedly more cholesteryl oleate and less cholesteryl linoleate, which appears to be due to the hydrolysis of cholesteryl ester from internalized lipoproteins and its subsequent re-esterification in the cell (see Fig. 13-9). The re-esterifying enzyme, ACAT, exhibits a specific preference for oleyl-CoA as substrate. These fatty acyl patterns led Smith to propose that much of the cholesteryl ester in the fibrous plaque is derived directly from plasma lipoproteins, bypassing the pathway of internalization, hydrolysis, and re-esterification in cells. Although a major role for cellular lipid accumulation in the fibrous plaque cannot be excluded, Smith's interpretation of the cholesteryl ester patterns has gained a great deal of acceptance. Within phospholipids accumulating in the fibrous-plaque core region, the ratio of sphingomyelin to lecithin rises to about five times higher than that found in either fatty streaks or plasma lipoproteins [55]. The processes responsible for those and other alterations in plaque lipids are not well understood, although differential exchange of various lipid classes is one possibility.

Gelatinous Lesions. Smith has proposed the gelatinous lesion as the precursor for most fibrous plaques [55,163]. Gelatinous lesions are best identified in fresh tissue by rather subjective criteria: translucent and edematous in appearance, slightly to frankly raised, and yielding to touch. Because of the difficulty of identification, lesions of this type often have been misclassified as normal intima or fibrous plaques. Microscopically, the gelatinous lesion is characterized by wide separation of connective tissue fibers, signifying edema. Tissue concentrations of LDL are increased, but an increase in nonlipoprotein lipid is found in only a minority of cases. Fibromuscular proliferation is a regular feature of larger gelatinous plaques. The study of gelatinous lesions has been hampered by the lack of standardized objective criteria for identification and by the lack of an animal model for these lesions.

Fibrolipid Lesions. Fibrolipid lesions are small, lipid-containing raised lesions that represent an early stage in fibrous-plaque development. Histologically, fibrolipid lesions show focal intimal thickening and a cholesterol-rich core region; by such features, the lesions can be classified as a subset of fibrous plaques. Fibrolipid lesions also resemble fatty streaks, however, because of the presence of numerous foam cells in the superficial intima [106]. The early formation of the atherosclerotic, lipid-rich core region of fibrolipid lesions has been described. Based on several lines of evidence—including the discrepant locations of the superficial foam cells and the deep early core region, the morphology of extracellular core-lipid droplets, and the association of these droplets with elastin and collagen—it is proposed that early core-lipid deposition proceeds through the extracellular assembly of droplets and vesicles. This hypothesis is in accordance with the data of Smith discussed above. Further studies are needed to clarify the contributions of cellular and extracellular lipid accumulation and metabolism at all stages of fibrous-plaque development.

Complicated Lesions. Complicated lesions are characterized by one or more of the following features: rupture or ulceration, thrombosis, intraplaque hemorrhage, and calcification. (See "Specific Features of Atherosclerotic Lesions," later in this chapter.)

ANIMAL MODELS

Animal experimentation provides an essential link between the understanding of the atherogenesis at the molecular and cellular level and the interpretation of human pathology and epidemiology. Animal models are used to examine the effects of new dietary interventions on atherosclerosis and to test other new interventional strategies ranging from new antilipidemic drugs to gene therapy. The major animal models currently in use in atherosclerosis research are rabbits, swine, primates, and transgenic mice. The ease of inducing atherosclerosis and the type of lesion produced seem to depend on three factors: the size of the animal, the average blood pressure, and the presence of a plasma component, allowing cholesteryl esters to be transferred among the various lipoprotein fractions. Cholesteryl ester–transfer activity is lacking in atherosclerosis-resistant species, such as the dog and the rat, but is significant in species more susceptible to atherosclerosis, such as rabbits, monkeys, and humans [164]. Induction of atherosclerosis in dogs and rats requires plasma cholesterol levels greater than 750 mg/dl, in combination with high levels of fat and antithyroid agents [165,166]. Diet-induced atherogenesis usually is achieved in susceptible species by feeding a diet containing 0.5–2.0 percent cholesterol. Cholesterol intake of 0.5 percent of total calories is approximately four times higher than that of the average American diet. Semipurified, high-fat diets with minimal cholesterol content can produce lesions in some species, including rabbits and monkeys. Highly saturated fats, such as lard, butterfat, other animal fats, and coconut oil, usually cause greater elevations of plasma cholesterol and are more atherogenic than unsaturated fats in animal studies.

The cholesterol-fed rabbit has been a convenient, readily accessible, economically feasible, and extensively used animal model. Supplementation of diet with cholesterol leads to very high plasma cholesterol (up to 2,000 mg/dl) in 2 to 4 weeks. Lesions produced are composed primarily of foam cells, and the complex lesions found in human atherosclerosis rarely are seen without special manipulations, such as intermittent feeding of a cholesterol-rich diet or injury to the arterial wall. Unlike in humans, in rabbits the lesions are distributed mainly in the thoracic aorta, and the major clinical manifestations of atherosclerosis in human (e.g., stroke, heart attack) are absent. In contrast, the Watanabe heritable hyperlipidemic (WHHL) rabbit strain is an excellent model for human familial hypercholesterolemia [123,124,126,132]. These rabbits exhibit spontaneous, complex atherosclerotic lesions and can have both heart attacks and strokes. Lesion development requires 6 to 9 months, which is longer than in the cholesterol-fed rabbit. The animals are not yet commercially available. The time required to establish a breeding colony, difficulty in breeding the animals, and the high mortality of newborn pups has restricted their use to a small number of laboratories.

The swine model of atherosclerosis has been used in a number of laboratories [105,167]. The choice of strain used can be crucial because some are quite resistant to lesion formation of any type. Lesions that form in appropiate strains fed high-fat, high-cholesterol diets have many of the same features seen in human atherosclerosis. Spontaneous atherosclerosis can occur in older animals fed a diet similar to a normal human diet. One noticeable difference in the pig model is the absence of sex difference in severity of disease. Of course, special facilities are required to maintain these animals.

Primates are excellent models for studies because the results are more readily extrapolated to humans [168,169]. These animals generally have a low level of spontaneous atherosclerosis. On the appropriate diet, however, they will develop the full spectrum of atherosclerotic lesions seen in humans, ranging from foam cell lesions to complex lesions, and exhibit the same types of clinical manifestations. The pattern of lesion distribution is quite similar to that in humans. As with the swine model, the sex differences seen in humans are not evident in primates. Primate experiments are expensive to conduct, and the supply of animals is limited. Although few institutions can afford to maintain a colony, regional facilities are available in several parts of the country for conducting research.

The transgenic mouse model has recently been applied to questions of importance in atherosclerosis, often with intriguing results. There are two categories of transgenic mice. Transgenic overproducers are formed by the incorporation of an additional gene, usually human, into the genomic DNA. This is accomplished by microinjection of a laboratory-derived DNA construct into fertilized murine eggs, which are then reimplanted into the female mouse. In transgenic knockout mice, an endogenous gene has been deleted by homologous recombination of a laboratory-derived DNA construct with DNA in embryonic stem cells. Selected stem-cell lines are then injected into blastocytes and reimplanted into the animal.

Transgenic overproducers have been derived for apo A-I, apo A-II, apo C-III, apo E, Lp(a), cholesteryl ester transfer protein (CETP), and the LDL receptor. Transgenic overproducers of apo A-I show elevated levels of HDL cholesterol [170,171]. They respond to high-fat diets by further increasing apo A-I and HDL cholesterol levels [172] and respond to probucol by decreasing HDL cholesterol and apo A-I levels, just as in human subjects [172,173]. In both instances, the mRNA levels and the fractional catabolic rate of apo A-I did not change, suggesting some type of post-transcriptional regulation not previously discovered. In overproducers of apo A-II, HDL cholesterol levels were not affected [174], suggesting that apo A-I is the prime controller of HDL levels. When introduced into C57BL/6 mice, which are susceptible to diet-induced atherosclerosis, the human apo A-I gene reduced aortic sinus foam-cell formation [175]. This result reinforces the idea that elevated apo A-I and HDL cholesterol levels have a protective effect against atherogenesis. Interestingly, if overproducers of apo A-I and apo A-II are crossed, the offspring are more susceptible to atherosclerosis than mice in which apo A-I alone is expressed. Therefore, apo A-I particles appear to be the more important in HDL-mediated protection against atherogenesis.

Surprisingly, transgenic overproducers of apo C-III were associated with hypertriglyceridemia [176] and so provide the first animal model of that disease. The plasma VLDL from these animals is enriched in apo C-III at the expense of apo E and is less avidly taken up by cells in vitro; consequently these particles may circulate longer in the blood. Genetic studies linking hypertriglyceridemia directly with alterations in apo C-III levels in humans have been initiated in several laboratories.

Overexpression of apo-E results in decreased plasma levels of LDL cholesterol and VLDL cholesterol and renders the mice resistant to diet-induced atherogenesis [177]. In contrast, overexpression of an apo E_3 mutant, which is associated with type III hyperlipoproteinemia, results in elevated basal levels of cholesterol and triglyceride in VLDL and LDL [178]. These animals respond to dietary cholesterol manipulation with additional increases in cholesterol and triglyceride and so provide a model for the study of type III hyperlipoproteinemia. Overexpression of the apo (a) molecule does not result in its incorporation into mouse lipoprotein particles [179]. However, expression in mice that are normally atherosclerosis resistant results in aortic sinus foam-cell formation with dietary challenge [180]. This finding suggests that the apo (a) protein is itself atherogenic and further supports the association between elevated apo (a) levels and increased risk for CHD.

Mice overexpressing the LDL receptor show increased hepatic clearance of injected LDL [181] and demonstrate resistance to a dietary challenge that significantly increased the LDL and VLDL levels in control mice [182]. Mice overexpressing the Type I bovine macrophage scavenger receptor were generated to give liver specific expression of the transgene (214). These mice had enhanced clearance of intravenously injected Ac-LDL as compared to the normal mice. In addition, on a high fat/cholesterol diet, the transgenic heterogygotes and homogygotes showed a marked (70%) suppressionof the rise in ApoB containing lipoprotein cholesterol compared to the normal mice. Compared to control mice, liver cholesteryl esters were reduced by 59% in the liver of transgenic animals. The livers of transgenic animals did not develop the fatty appearance of livers from the control animals on the high fat diet. These data strongly support a protective role for the scavenger receptor in the liver in prevention of atherosclerosis.

Transgenic knockout mice are available for apo E, apo A-I, and the LDL receptor. Homozygous apo E-knockout mice on low-fat, low-cholesterol diets have cholesterol levels of 500 mg/dl because of delayed plasma clearance of lipoproteins, and they show foam-cell formation within 10 weeks of birth [183,184]. These animals are remarkably sensitive to dietary challenge, and in one study that used a typical Western diet, had cholesterol levels of up to 3,000 mg/dl at 30 weeks. On a typical Western diet, the animals show lesion progression from foam-cell formation to complex lesion formation, as occurs in humans [185,186]. This is the first mouse model to show such typical lesion progression and will no doubt be used extensively. It is interesting to note that heterozygous apo E knockout mice have normal plasma clearance of lipoproteins. Crossbreeding apo E-deficient mice with apo A-I-overproducing mice has been reported to eliminate the susceptibility to atherosclerosis of the offspring. This finding strongly supports a direct protective role for HDL in the atherosclerosis process. Apo A-I-knockout mice have lowered plasma HDL cholesterol levels as expected [187], but no information is yet available on their susceptibility to atherosclerosis. Mice with the LDL receptor gene knocked out have been produced by Brown and Goldstein [188]. Those animals demonstrate elevated basal levels of serum cholesterol caused by increased levels of IDL and LDL and respond to a dietary cholesterol challenge by further increases in the cholesterol content of IDL and LDL compared with that in wild-type animals.

Several other animal models of atherosclerosis are used less frequently. The Carneau racing pigeon [189] has high blood pressure and develops a human-like fibrous plaque on cholesterol feeding. Genetically atherosclerosis-resistant lines are available for comparison with the more susceptible lines. A chicken model for atherosclerosis also is available. Chickens infected with the Marek's disease virus have an accelerated form of atherosclerosis in which smooth muscle foam cells predominate [190]. Hamsters have been used in a number of studies and respond well to dietary challenges [191].

SPECIFIC FEATURES OF ATHEROSCLEROTIC LESIONS

Lipid-Rich Core Region. The lipid-rich core region of the atherosclerotic lesion is an area of intense extracellular lipid deposition within most fibrous plaques and is usually centrally located. Such a core region may occupy most of the plaque volume of an advanced coronary lesion. The core region is usually acellular, but it may be hypocellular. **Atheronecrosis** is the term used to describe the loss of cells. The core region is distinguished by the presence of cholesterol crystals (or, if histologic preparation dissolves the crystals, clefts) and is usually more extensive than the area containing the cholesterol crystals. Early, small core regions may be devoid of cholesterol crystals.

The importance of the lipid-rich core region is underscored by the finding that more than 90 percent of transmural myocardial infarctions with early fatal outcomes are associated with thrombosis at a site of plaque rupture or ulceration [192]. Coronary angioscopy in patients with unstable angina has revealed either thrombus, which is probably associated with intimal ulceration, or frankly ragged, ulcerated intima as the underlying anatomic lesion [193]. Pathologic evidence indicates that the core region tends to expand or erode viable tissue toward the vessel lumen with time, undermining the fibrous cap of the lesion [130]. This process can result in plaque rupture, sudden exposure of flowing blood to the contents of the lipid-rich core, and catastrophic thrombosis or thromboembolism. Ulceration also may occur. In most cases of plaque rupture, blood enters the core region and partially mixes with its contents. This occurrence is the most common cause of plaque hemorrhage.

The developmental stages of the core region in a fibrous plaque are not entirely known. In one study, a distinct core region was already present in about three-fourths of the smallest detectable raised lesions in human aortic fibrolipid lesions. That finding suggests that a persistent focus of deep, extracellular lipid may serve as an inciting agent in fibrous-plaque development. It remains to be resolved whether lipid deposition occurs when cells are exposed to cytotoxic conditions or whether the lipid deposits themselves contain substances toxic to cells, such as oxidized sterols.

Capillary Formation. No capillaries are found in the arterial intima unless it is greatly thickened or has advanced atherosclerosis. Geiringer has suggested that the innermost 0.35 to 0.50 mm of arterial wall thickness is normally avascular, regardless of whether that critical depth is composed of intima, media, or a combination of the two [194]. The adventitia is always vascularized, and capillaries extend from the adventitia into the arterial wall to the critical depth. In advanced atherosclerosis, a marked proliferation of new vasa vasorum occurs in the adventitia of the vessel and penetrates from there into the media and the intima [195]. Intimal capillary ingrowth in the vicinity of the lipid-rich core region is associated with the presence of macrophages, macrophage-derived foam cells, and even giant cells, which may represent an attempt to resorb some of the lipid from the tissue [196].

A form of vascularization sometimes seen in advanced atherosclerosis is the presence of multiple luminal channels in an almost totally occluded vessel. This histologic appearance indicates the past occurrence of an occlusive thrombus that became recanalized at the same time that it was being organized and incorporated into arterial tissue. A similar process occurring in mural thrombi may explain the presence of giant capillaries in some plaques originating in the arterial lumen rather than the adventitia [194,197].

Calcium. The calcium content of the arterial wall rises steadily with age, even in the absence of atherosclerosis. Calcium is deposited in the form of apatite similar to that found in bone. In normal arteries, it is localized primarily near the surfaces of medial elastic fibers in association with the microfibrillar component [198,199]. With the onset of fibrous-plaque atherosclerosis, calcific nodules are associated with lipid deposits in the early core region [200]. Extensive calcification of lipid-rich areas occurs in many advanced fibrous plaques. Despite the dramatic pathologic presentation of calcified vessels, few clinical consequences have been ascribed thus far to the calcification itself or to the increased rigidity of the vessels.

A timely question is whether extracellular calcium deposition or cellular calcium metabolism plays an important role in the atherogenic process. Two human metabolic disorders associated with calcification of the arterial media—diabetes mellitus and chronic renal disease—are also strongly associated with atherosclerosis. In animals, hypervitaminosis D promotes atherogenesis, and the administration of agents that retard soft-tissue calcification, such as lanthanum and diphosphonates, inhibits atherogenesis [201]. It has been suggested that the administration of calcium channel–blocking agents also may inhibit atherogenesis in animals, and that hypothesis raises the question of a role for cellular calcium metabolism in atherogenesis [202,203]. It seems likely that more than one mechanism may be responsible for those diverse effects. Despite initial interest, the use of ethylenediaminetetraacetic-acid (EDTA) chelation therapy for the treatment of atherosclerosis has no scientific basis and does not belong in the ethical therapeutic armamentarium at this time.

Fibrocellular Proliferation. Lipid deposition and fibrocellular proliferation are easily recognized as the two major processes in atherosclerotic development, but, surprisingly, the relationship between those processes is difficult to explain. The answer may lie in the involvement of monocyte-macrophages in the lesion. By mechanisms as yet unclear, hypercholesterolemia leads to adherence and transmigration of large numbers of circulating monocytes through the arterial endothelium into the intima. In the intima, monocytes progress to become macrophages, many of which accumulate lipid to become foam cells [204,205]. Macrophages and perhaps macrophage-derived foam cells produce a potent polypeptide growth factor for smooth muscle cells [206,207]. Thus, the recruitment of monocyte-macrophages into an atherosclerotic lesion may explain the connection between hypercholesterolemia and smooth muscle-cell proliferation. Unexplained by that hypothesis, however, is why many foam-cell lesions, such as aortic fatty streaks, can remain stable, apparently without proliferation or progression, for decades. The trigger that may cause fatty streaks to progress to fibrous plaques or that may cause cellular proliferation in relatively normal intima is not known.

Stimulation of smooth muscle-cell proliferation by lipoproteins has been reported. In some studies, the availability of LDL was shown to be a limiting factor in cells otherwise stimulated to proliferate rapidly [208]. There is no evidence to suggest, however, that smooth muscle growth in the arterial intima is limited by LDL availability. In other studies, LDL from hypercholesterolemic humans and monkeys was shown to stimulate growth of primary monkey smooth muscle cultures, but LDL from normolipidemic subjects was ineffective even at high doses [209];

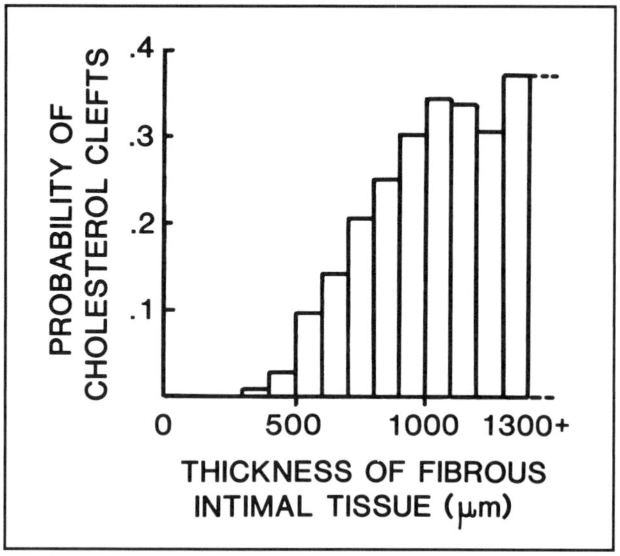

Fig. 13-13. Probability of finding cholesterol clefts in human aortic intima according to the thickness of fibrous intimal tissue. The lipid-rich core region does not develop when intimal thickness is less than 300 μmeters. (From data of RE Tracy et al. Atheronecrosis and its fibroproliferative base and cap in the thoracic aorta. Lab Invest 1979; 41(6):546–552.

LDL from hypercholesterolemic monkeys caused greater cholesterol accumulation in monkey smooth muscle cells than did LDL from normocholesterolemic monkeys, although the amount of cholesteryl ester increase was insufficient to create foam cells [210,211].

Another hypothesis is that fibrocellular proliferation in the intima may foster lipid deposition. After stimulation by growth factors, smooth muscle cells express additional LDL receptors, presumably to increase cellular cholesterol stores just prior to growth [212]. That mechanism, especially if not synchronized well with actual cell proliferation, could trap cholesterol in the intima. An obvious accompaniment of intimal growth is an increased distance to be crossed for diffusion of lipoproteins, oxygen, nutrients, and wastes, distance that is greatest for the deeper intimal layers. The deepest sublayer of the intima is the region where the smallest, presumably earliest, core accumulations of extracellular lipid are found. Tracy and coworkers have shown that cholesterol clefts occur in human aortic intima only when the total intimal depth exceeds a threshold of about 300 μm (Fig. 13-13) [213]. Thus, intimal growth—whether physiologic, in the case of diffuse intimal thickening, or pathologic, in the case of fibrous plaque development—appears to be a prerequisite for the massive extracellular lipid deposition associated with the core region.

Strategies for Intervention

An understanding of the role of lipid metabolism in atherogenesis will lead to improved plans for prevention and treatment. Modification of diet is the safest and most effective strategy that can be employed within an entire population. Such therapy eventually may include not only the avoidance of high-fat foods that raise plasma cholesterol levels but also the ingestion of certain plant fibers and gums, if the suggested lowering of plasma cholesterol by those dietary components is confirmed. Effective pharmacologic treatment of hypercholesterolemia is also available, but the combination of hypertriglyceridemia and reduced levels of HDL cholesterol remains a difficult clinical problem. Drugs capable of raising HDL levels are available, and more are under development, but it is not yet clear that their use will reduce the incidence of atherosclerotic disease.

Further progress in understanding the atherosclerotic process will lead to new clinical strategies. For example, clinical trials with antioxidants may lead to recommendations for dietary supplementation to decrease the risk of formation of oxidized forms of LDL. New drugs such as ACAT inhibitors and cholesterol-biosynthesis inhibitors (the statins) provide additional possibilities for limiting the atherosclerotic process. Gene-therapy approaches [106] are a new and exciting direction that holds great promise for interventional strategies. Finally, the role of the lipid-rich core region in causing intimal rupture and catastrophic thrombosis suggests another possible therapeutic strategy: If core expansion and spreading necrosis can be inhibited to allow a sturdy, endothelialized fibrous cap to develop over the lesion, then it may not always be necessary to achieve total regression of the atherosclerotic plaque.

References

1. Gordon T, et al. High density lipoprotein as a protective factor against coronary heart disease. The Framingham Study. Am J Med 1977; 62(5):707–714.
2. Dahlen GH, et al. Association of levels of lipoprotein Lp[a], plasma lipids, and other lipoproteins with coronary artery disease diagnosed by angiography. Circulation 1986; 74(4): 758–765.
3. Sniderman A, et al. Association of coronary atherosclerosis with hyper*apo*betalipoproteinemia [increased protein but normal cholesterol levels in human plasma low density (β) lipoproteins]. Proc Natl Acad Sci USA 1980; 77(1):604–608.
4. Kottke BA, et al. Apolipoproteins and coronary artery disease. Mayo Clin Proc 1986; 61(5):313–320.
5. Miller NE, et al. Relation of angiographically defined coronary artery disease to plasma lipoprotein subfractions and apolipoproteins. BMJ 1981; 282(6278):1741–1744.
6. Lipid Research Clinics Program: The Lipid Research Clinics Coronary Primary Prevention Trial results. I. Reduction in incidence of coronary heart disease. JAMA 1984; 251(3): 351–364.
7. Lipid Research Clinics Program: The Lipid Research Clinics Coronary Primary Prevention Trial results. II. The relationship of reduction in incidence of coronary heart disease to cholesterol lowering. JAMA 1984; 251(3):365–374.
8. Small DM. The Physical Chemistry of Lipids: from Alkanes to Phospholipids. New York: Plenum, 1986.
9. Renshaw PF, Janoff AS, Miller KW. On the nature of dilute aqueous cholesterol suspensions. J Lipid Res 1983; 24(1): 47–51.
10. Jackson RL, Gotto AM Jr. Hypothesis concerning membrane structure, cholesterol, and atherosclerosis. Atherosclerosis Reviews 1976; 1:1–21.
11. Gotto AM Jr, Pownall HJ, Havel RJ. Introduction to the plasma lipoproteins. Methods Enzymol 1986; 128:1–41.

12. Smith LC, et al. Structure and dynamics of human plasma lipoproteins. In G Pifat, JN Herak, eds. Supramolecular Structure and Function. New York: Plenum, 1983.
13. Havel RJ, Goldstein JL, Brown MS. Lipoproteins and lipid transport. In PK Bondy, LE Rosenberg, eds. Metabolic Control and Disease. Philadelphia: Saunders, 1980.
14. Segrest JP, et al. A molecular theory of lipid–protein interactions in the plasma lipoproteins. FEBS Lett 1974; 38(3): 247–253.
15. Yang C-Y, et al. Sequence, structure, receptor-binding domains and internal repeats of human apolipoprotein B-100. Nature 1986; 323(6090):738–742.
16. Breslow JL, et al. Studies of familial type III hyperlipoproteinemia using as a genetic marker the apoE phenotype E2/2. J Lipid Res 1982; 23(8):1224–1235.
17. Weisgraber KH, Innerarity TL, Mahley RW. Abnormal lipoprotein receptor-binding activity of the human E apoprotein due to cysteine–arginine interchange at a single site. J Biol Chem 1982; 257(5):2518–2521.
18. Glomset JA. The plasma lecithin: cholesterol acyltransferase reaction. J Lipid Res 1968; 9(2):155–167.
19. Norum KR, et al. Transport of cholesterol. Physiol Rev 1983; 63(4):1343–1419.
20. Fielding CJ, Fielding PE. Cholesterol transport between cells and body fluids: role of plasma lipoproteins and the plasma cholesterol esterification system. Med Clin North Am 1982; 66(2):363–373.
21. Fielding CJ. The origin and properties of free cholesterol potential gradients in plasma, and their relation to atherogenesis. J Lipid Res 1984; 25(13):1624–1628.
22. Glomset JA, Norum KR, Gjone E. Familial lecithin: cholesterol acyltransferase deficiency. In Stanbury JB, et al, eds. The Metabolic Basis of Inherited Disease. New York: McGraw–Hill, 1983.
23. Fisher WR. Heterogeneity of plasma low density lipoproteins: manifestations of the physiologic phenomenon in man. Metabolism 1983; 32(3):283–291.
24. Eisenberg S, et al. Abnormalities in very low, low, and high density lipoproteins in hypertriglyceridemia: reversal toward normal with bezafibrate treatment. J Clin Invest 1984; 74(2):470–482.
25. Gaubatz JW, et al. Human plasma lipoprotein [a]: structural properties. J Biol Chem 1983; 258(8):4582–4589.
26. Tomlinson JE, McLean JW, Lawn RM. Rhesus monkey apolipoprotein(a). Sequence, evolution, and sites of synthesis. J Biol Chem 1989; 264(10):5957–5965.
27. Howard GC, Pizzo SV. Lipoprotein(a) and its role in atherothrombotic disease. Lab Invest 1993; 69(4):373.
28. Cushing GL, et al. Quantitation and localization of apolipoproteins[a] and B in coronary artery bypass vein grafts resected at re-operation. Arteriosclerosis 1989; 9(5): 593–603.
29. Gotto AM Jr, Morrissett JD, eds. Second International Conference on Lipoprotein[a]. Chem Phys Lipids 1994; 67/68:1.
30. Schaefer EJ. Clinical, biochemical, and genetic features in familial disorders of high density lipoprotein deficiency. Arteriosclerosis 1984; 4(4):303–422.
31. Glueck CJ, et al. Familial hyper-alpha-lipoproteinemia: studies in eighteen kindreds. Metabolism 1975; 24(11):1243–1265.
32. Camargo CA Jr, et al. The effect of moderate alcohol intake on serum apolipoproteins A-I and A-II. A controlled study. JAMA 1985; 253(19):2854–2857.
33. Weisgraber KH, Mahley RW. Subfractionation of human high density lipoproteins by heparin–Sepharose affinity chromatography. J Lipid Res 1980; 21(3):316–325.
34. Badimon JJ, et al. High density lipoprotein plasma fractions inhibit aortic fatty streaks in cholesterol-fed rabbits. Lab Invest 1989; 60(3):455–461.
35. Badimon JJ, Badimon L, Fuster V. Regression of atherosclerotic lesions by high density lipoprotein plasma fraction in the cholesterol-fed rabbit. J Clin Invest 1990; 85(4):1234–1241.
36. Parthasarathy S, Barnett J, Fong LG. High-density lipoprotein inhibits the oxidative modification of low-density lipoprotein. Biochim Biophys Acta 1990; 1044(2):275–283.
37. Bowry VW, Stanley KK, Stocker R. High density lipoprotein is the major carrier of lipid hydroperoxides in human blood plasma from fasting donors. Proc Natl Acad Sci USA 1992; 89(21):10316–10320.
38. Jenne DE, et al. Clusterin (complement lysis inhibitor) forms a high density lipoprotein complex with apolipoprotein A-I in human plasma. J Biol Chem 1991; 266(17):11030–11036.
39. Hamilton KK, Zhao J, Sims PJ. Interaction between apolipoproteins A-I and A-II and the membrane attack complex of complement. Affinity of the apoproteins for polymeric C9. J Biol Chem 1993; 268(5):3632–3638.
40. Hulley SB, et al. Epidemiology as a guide to clinical decisions. The association between triglyceride and coronary heart disease. N Engl J Med 1980; 302(25):1383–1389.
41. Castelli WP. The triglyceride issue: a view from Framingham. Am Heart J 1986; 112(2):432–437.
42. Zilversmit DB. Atherogenesis: a postprandial phenomenon. Circulation 1979; 60(3):473–485.
43. Patsch JR, et al. Inverse relationship between blood levels of high density lipoprotein subfraction 2 and magnitude of postprandial lipemia. Proc Natl Acad Sci USA 1983; 80(5): 1449–1453.
44. Patsch J, et al. High density lipoprotein$_2$: relationship of the plasma levels of this lipoprotein species to its composition, to the magnitude of postprandial lipemia, and to the activities of lipoprotein lipase and hepatic lipase. J Clin Invest 1987; 80(2):341–347.
45. Breier C, et al. Essential role of post-heparin lipoprotein lipase activity and of plasma testosterone in coronary artery disease. Lancet 1985; 1(8440):1242–1244.
46. Bradley WB, et al. Apolipoprotein-E degradation in human very low density lipoproteins by plasma protease(s): chemical and biological consequences. Biochem Biophys Res Commun 1982; 109(4):1360–1367.
47. Newman HAI, Zilversmit DB. Quantitative aspects of cholesterol flux in rabbit atheromatous lesions. J Biol Chem 1962; 237(7):2078–2084.
48. Vasile E, Simionescu M, Simionescu N. Visualization of the binding, endocytosis, and transcytosis in low-density lipoprotein in the arterial endothelium in situ. J Cell Biol 1983; 96(6):1677–1689.
49. Stefanovich V, Gore I. Cholesterol diet and permeability of rabbit aorta. Exp Mol Pathol 1971; 14(1):20–29.
50. Hüttner I, Moore RH, Rona G. Fine structural evidence of specific mechanism for increased endothelial permeability in experimental hypertension. Am J Pathol 1970; 61(3):395–412.
51. Faggiotto A, Ross R. Studies of hypercholesterolemia in the nonhuman primate. II: Fatty streak conversion to fibrous plaque. Arteriosclerosis 1984; 4(4):341–356.
52. Bratzler RL, Colton CK, Smith KA. Theoretical models for transport of low-density lipoproteins in the arterial wall. In GW Manning, MD Haust, eds. Atherosclerosis: Metabolic, Morphologic, and Clinical Aspects. New York: Plenum, 1977.
53. Pfeffer R, et al. Diffusion of macromolecules across the arterial wall in the presence of multiple endothelial injuries. J Biomech Eng 1981; 103(3):197–203.
54. Hoff HF, et al. Quantification of apolipoprotein B in grossly normal human aorta. Circ Res 1977; 40(1):56–64.

55. Smith EB. The relationship between plasma and tissue lipids in human atherosclerosis. Adv Lipid Res 1974; 12: 1–49.
56. Smith EB, Ashall C. Low-density lipoprotein concentration in interstitial fluid from human atherosclerotic lesions. Relation to theories of endothelial damage and lipoprotein binding. Biochim Biophys Acta 1983; 754(3):249–257.
57. Heideman CL, Hoff HF. Lipoproteins containing apolipoprotein A-I extracted from human aortas. Biochem Biophys Acta 1982; 711(3):431–444.
58. Comper WD, Laurent TC. Physiological function of connective tissue polysaccharides. Physiol Rev 1978; 58(1):255–315.
59. Carew TE, et al. Measurement in vivo of irreversible degradation of low density lipoprotein in the rabbit aorta. Predominance of intimal degradation. Arteriosclerosis 1984; 4(3): 214–224.
60. Bratzler RL, et al. The distribution of labeled low-density lipoproteins across the rabbit thoracic aorta in vivo. Atherosclerosis 1977; 28(3):289–307.
61. Scott PJ, Hurley PJ. The distribution of radio-iodinated serum albumin and low-density lipoprotein in tissues and the arterial wall. Atherosclerosis 1970; 11(1):77–103.
62. Brown MS, Goldstein JL. A receptor-mediated pathway for cholesterol homeostasis. Science 1986; 232(4746):34–47.
63. Goldstein JL, et al. Receptor-mediated endocytosis: concepts emerging from the LDL receptor system. Annu Rev Cell Biol 1985; 1:1–39.
64. Alberts AW, et al. Mevinolin: a highly potent competitive inhibitor of hydroxymethylglutaryl-coenzyme A reductase and a cholesterol-lowering agent. Proc Natl Acad Sci USA 1980; 77(7):3957–3961.
65. Goldstein JL, et al. Binding site on macrophages that mediates uptake and degradation of acetylated low density lipoprotein, producing massive cholesterol deposition. Proc Natl Acad Sci USA 1979; 76(1):333–337.
66. Brown MS, Goldstein JL. Lipoprotein metabolism in the macrophage: implications for cholesterol deposition in atherosclerosis. Annu Rev Biochem 1983; 52:223–261.
67. Fogelman AM, et al. Malondialdehyde alteration of low density lipoproteins leads to cholesteryl ester accumulation in human monocyte-macrophages. Proc Natl Acad Sci USA 1980; 77(4):2214–2218.
68. Steinbrecher UP, et al. Modification of low density lipoprotein by endothelial cells involves lipid peroxidation and degradation of low density lipoprotein phospholipids. Proc Natl Acad Sci USA 1984; 81(12):3883–3887.
69. Parthasarathy S, et al. Macrophage oxidation of low density lipoprotein generates a modified form recognized by the scavenger receptor. Arteriosclerosis 1986; 6(5):505–510.
70. Morel DW, DiCorleto PE, Chisolm GM. Endothelial and smooth muscle cells alter low density lipoprotein in vitro by free radical oxidation. Arteriosclerosis 1984; 4:357–364.
71. Esterbauer H, et al. Biochemical, structural, and functional properties of oxidized low-density lipoprotein. Chem Res Toxicol 1990; 3(2):77–92.
72. Lenz ML, et al. Lipid hydroperoxy and hydroxy derivatives in copper-catalyzed oxidation of low density lipoprotein. J Lipid Res 1990; 31(6):1043–1050.
73. Raymond TL, Reynolds SA, Swanson JA. Lipoproteins of the extravascular space: enhanced macrophage degradation of low density lipoproteins from interstitial inflammatory fluid. J Lipid Res 1985; 26(11):1356–1362.
74. Goldstein JL, et al. Stimulation of cholesteryl ester synthesis in macrophages by extracts of atherosclerotic human aortas and complexes of albumin/cholesteryl esters. Arteriosclerosis 1981; 1(3):210–226.
75. Hoff HF, O'Neil J. Lesion-derived low density lipoprotein and oxidized low density lipoprotein share a lability for aggregation, leading to enhanced macrophage degradation. Arterioscler Thromb 1991; 11(5):1209–1222.
76. Graham A, et al. Peroxynitrite modification of low-density lipoprotein leads to recognition by the macrophage scavenger receptor. FEBS Lett 1993; 330(2):181–185.
77. Via DP, et al. Murine macrophage tumors are a source of 260,000-Dalton acetyl-low density lipoprotein receptor. J Biol Chem 1985; 260(12):7379–7386.
78. Kodama T, et al. Type I macrophage scavenger receptor contains α-helical and collagen-like coiled coils. Nature 1990; 343(6258):531–535.
79. Matsumoto A, et al. Human macrophage scavenger receptors: primary structure, expression and localization in atherosclerotic lesions. Proc Natl Acad Sci USA 1990; 87(23): 9133–9137.
80. Doi T, et al. Charged collagen structure mediates the recognition of negatively charged macromolecules by macrophage scavenger receptors. J Biol Chem 1993; 268(3):2126–2133.
81. Acton S, et al. The collagenous domains of macrophage scavenger receptors and complement component C1q mediate their similar, but not identical, binding specificities for polyanionic ligands. J Biol Chem 1993; 268(5):3530–3537.
82. Yla-Herttuala S, et al. Gene expression in macrophage-rich human atherosclerotic lesions. 15-lipoxygenase and acetyl low density lipoprotein receptor messenger RNA colocalize with oxidation specific lipid–protein adducts. J Clin Invest 1991; 87(4):1146–1152.
83. Sparrow CP, Parthasarathy S, Steinberg D. A macrophage receptor that recognizes oxidized low density lipoprotein but not acetylated low density lipoprotein. J Biol Chem 1989; 264(5):2599–2604.
84. Arai H, et al. Multiple receptors for modified low density lipoproteins in mouse peritoneal macrophages: different uptake mechanisms for acetylated and oxidized low density lipoprotein. Biochem Biophys Res Commun 1989; 159(3): 1375–1382.
85. Stanton LW, et al. A macrophage Fc receptor for IgG is also a receptor for oxidized low density lipoprotein. J Biol Chem 1992; 267(31):22446–22451.
86. Koo C, Wernette-Hammond ME, Innerarity TL. Uptake of canine β-very low density lipoproteins by mouse peritoneal macrophages is mediated by a low density lipoprotein receptor. J Biol Chem 1986; 261(24):11194–11201.
87. Gianturco SH, et al. The β-VLDL receptor pathway of murine P388D$_1$ macrophages. J Lipid Res 1986; 27(4):412–420.
88. Gianturco SH, Gotto AM Jr, Bradley WA. Hypertriglyceridemia: lipoprotein receptors and atherosclerosis. In D Kritchevsky, WL Holmes, R Paoletti, eds. Drugs Affecting Lipid Metabolism VIII. New York: Plenum, 1985.
89. Wolfbauer G, et al. Development of the smooth muscle foam cell: uptake of macrophage lipid inclusions. Proc Natl Acad Sci USA 1986; 83(20):7760–7764.
90. Pitas RE. Expression of the acetyl low density lipoprotein receptor by rabbit fibroblasts and smooth muscle cells. Upregulation by phorbol esters. J Biol Chem 1990; 265(21):12722–12727.
91. Dejager S, Mietus-Snyder M, Pitas RE. Oxidized low density lipoproteins bind to the scavenger receptor expressed by rabbit smooth muscle cells and macrophages. Arterioscler Thromb 1993; 13(3):371–378.
92. Inaba T, et al. Expression of M-CSF receptor encoded by *c-fms* on smooth muscle cells derived from arteriosclerotic lesion. J Biol Chem 1992; 267(8):5693–5699.
93. Bickel PE, Freeman MW. Rabbit aortic smooth muscle cells express inducible macrophage scavenger receptor messen-

ger RNA that is absent from endothelial cells. J Clin Invest 1992; 90(40):1450–1457.
94. Inaba T, et al. Platelet-derived growth factor induces c-*fms* and scavenger receptor genes in vascular smooth muscle cells. J Biol Chem 1992; 267(18):13107–13112.
95. Stein O, Stein Y. Bovine aortic endothelial cells display macrophage-like properties toward acetylated ^{125}I-labelled low density lipoprotein. Biochim Biophys Acta 1980; 620(3): 631–635.
96. Nagelkerke JF, Barto KP, van Berkel TJC. In vivo and in vitro uptake and degradation of acetylated low density lipoprotein by rat liver endothelial, Kupffer, and parenchymal cells. J Biol Chem 1983; 258(20):12221–12227.
97. van Berkel TJC, De Rijke YB, Kruijt JK. Different fate in vivo of oxidatively modified low density lipoprotein and acetylated low density lipoprotein in rats. Recognition by various scavenger receptors on Kupffer and endothelial liver cells. J Biol Chem 1991; 266(4):2282–2289.
98. Falcone DJ, et al. Lipoprotein–heparin–fibronectin-denatured collagen complexes enhance cholesteryl ester accumulation in macrophages. J Cell Biol 1984; 99:1266–1274.
99. Salisbury BGJ, Falcone DJ, Minick CR. Insoluble low-density lipoprotein–proteoglycan complexes enhance cholesteryl ester accumulation in macrophages. Am J Pathol 1985; 120(1):6–11.
100. Khoo JC, et al. Enhanced macrophage uptake of low density lipoprotein after self-aggregation. Arteriosclerosis 1988; 8(4):348–358.
101. Hoff HF, et al. Aggregation as well as chemical modification of LDL during oxidation is responsible for poor processing in macrophages. J Lipid Res 1993; 34(11):1919–1929.
102. Shio H, Haley NJ, Fowler S. Characterization of lipid-laden aortic cells from cholesterol-fed rabbits. II: Morphometric analysis of lipid-filled lysosomes and lipid droplets in aortic cell populations. Lab Invest 1978; 39(4):390–397.
103. Fowler S, et al. Characterization of cell populations isolated from aortas of rhesus monkeys with experimental atherosclerosis. Circ Res 1980; 46(4):520–530.
104. Haley NJ, Fowler S, deDuve C. Lysosomal acid cholesteryl esterase activity in normal and lipid-laden aortic cells. J Lipid Res 1980; 21(8):961–969.
105. Bocan TM, et al. Inhibition of acyl-CoA cholesterol O-acyltransferase reduces the cholesteryl ester enrichment of atherosclerotic lesions in the Yucatan micropig. Atherosclerosis 1993; 99(2):175–186.
106. Chang CCY, et al. Molecular cloning and functional expression of human acyl-coenzyme A: cholesterol acyltransferase cDNA in mutant Chinese hamster ovary cells. J Biol Chem 1993; 268(28):20747–20755.
107. Hajjar DP, Minick CR, Fowler S. Arterial neutral cholesteryl esterase. A hormone-sensitive enzyme distinct from lysosomal cholesteryl esterase. J Biol Chem 1983; 258(1): 192–198.
108. McGookey DJ, Anderson RGW. Morphological characterization of the cholesteryl ester cycle in cultured mouse macrophage foam cells. J Cell Biol 1983; 97(4):1156–1168.
109. Rothblat GH, Phillips MC. Mechanism of cholesterol efflux from cells. Effects of acceptor structure and concentration. J Biol Chem 1982; 257(8):4775–4782.
110. Biesbroeck R, et al. Specific high-affinity binding of high density lipoproteins to cultured human skin fibroblasts and arterial smooth muscle cells. J Clin Invest 1983; 71(3): 525–539.
111. Graham DL, Oram JF. Identification and characterization of a high density lipoprotein-binding protein in cell membranes by ligand blotting. J Biol Chem 1987; 262(16): 7439–7442.
112. McKnight GL, et al. Cloning and expression of a cellular high density lipoprotein-binding protein that is up-regulated by cholesterol loading of cells. J Biol Chem 1992; 267(17): 12131–12141.
113. Schmitz G, et al. Interaction of high density lipoproteins with cholesteryl ester-laden macrophages: Biochemical and morphological characterization of cell surface receptor binding, endocytosis and resecretion of high density lipoproteins by macrophages. EMBO J 1985; 4(3):613–622.
114. DeLamatre JG, et al. Metabolism of apoE-free high density lipoproteins in rat hepatoma cells. Evidence for a retroendocytic pathway. J Lipid Res 1990; 31(2):191–202.
115. Mendez AJ, Oram JF, Bierman EL. Protein kinase C as a mediator of high density lipoprotein receptor-dependent efflux of intracellular cholesterol. J Biol Chem 1991; 266(16): 10104–10111.
116. Bernard DW, et al. cAMP stimulates cholesteryl ester clearance to high density lipoproteins in J7774 macrophages. J Biol Chem 1991; 266(2):710–716.
117. Henriksen T, Mahoney EM, Steinberg D. Enhanced macrophage degradation of low density lipoprotein previously incubated with cultured endothelial cells: recognition by receptors for acetylated low density lipoproteins. Proc Natl Acad Sci USA 1981; 78(10):6499–6503.
118. Peng S-K, et al. Effect of auto-oxidation products from cholesterol on aortic smooth muscle cells. An in vitro study. Arch Pathol Lab Med 1978; 102(2):57–61.
119. Witztum JL. Role of oxidised low density lipoprotein in atherogenesis. Br Heart J 1993; 69[1 suppl]:S12–S18.
120. Heinecke JW, Rosen H, Chait A. Iron and copper promote modification of low density lipoprotein by human arterial smooth muscle cells in culture. J Clin Invest 1984; 74(5):1890–1894.
121. Haberland ME, Fong D, Cheng L. Malondialdehyde-altered protein occurs in atheroma of Watanabe heritable hyperlipidemic rabbits. Science 1988; 241(4862):215–218.
122. Palinski W, et al. Low density lipoprotein undergoes oxidative modification in vivo. Proc Natl Acad Sci USA 1989; 86(4):1372–1376.
123. Boyd HC, et al. Direct evidence for a protein recognized by a monoclonal antibody against oxidatively modified LDL in atherosclerotic lesions from a Watanabe heritable hyperlipidemic rabbit. Am J Pathol 1989; 135(5):815–825.
124. Salonen JT, et al. Autoantibody against oxidised LDL and progression of carotid atherosclerosis. Lancet 1992; 339(8798):883–887.
125. Yla-Herttuala S, et al. Evidence for the presence of oxidatively modified low density lipoprotein in atherosclerotic lesions of rabbit and man. J Clin Invest 1989; 84(4):1086–1095.
126. Avogaro P, Bittolo Bon G, Cazzolato G. Presence of a modified low density lipoprotein in humans. Arteriosclerosis 1988; 8(1):79–87.
127. Carew TE, Schwenke DC, Steinberg D. Antiatherogenic effect of probucol unrelated to its hypocholesterolemic effect: evidence that antioxidants in vivo can selectively inhibit low density lipoprotein degradation in macrophage-rich fatty streaks slowing the progression of atherosclerosis in the Watanabe heritable hyperlipidemic rabbit. Proc Natl Acad Sci USA 1987; 84(21):7725–7729.
128. Bjorkhem I, et al. The antioxidant butylated hydroxytoluene protects against atherosclerosis. Arterioscler Thromb 1991; 11(1):15–22.
129. Mao SJT, et al. Attenuation of atherosclerosis in a modified strain of hypercholesterolemic Watanabe rabbits with use of a probucol analogue (MDL 29,311) that does not lower serum cholesterol. Arterioscler Thromb 1991; 11:1266–1285.
130. Sparrow CP, et al. Low density lipoprotein is protected

from oxidation and the progression of atherosclerosis is slowed in cholesterol-fed rabbits by the antioxidant N,N′-diphenyl-phenylenediamine. J Clin Invest 1992; 89(6):1885–1891.
131. Akeson AL, et al. Inhibition of IL-1β expression in THP-1 cells by probucol and tocopherol. Atherosclerosis 1991; 86(2–3):261–270.
132. O'Brien K, et al. Probucol treatment affects the cellular composition but not anti-oxidized low density lipoprotein immunoreactivity of plaques from Watanabe heritable hyperlipidemic rabbits. Arterioscler Thromb 1991; 11(3): 751–759.
133. Rimm EB, et al. Vitamin E consumption and the risk of coronary artery disease in men. N Engl J Med 1993; 328(20):1450–1456.
134. Stampfer MJ, et al. Vitamin E consumption and the risk of coronary artery disease in women. N Engl J Med 1993; 328(20):1444–1449.
135. Scheffler E, et al. Smoking influences the atherogenic potential of low-density lipoprotein. Clin Investig 1992; 70:263.
136. Enstrom JE, Kanim LE, Klein MA. Vitamin C intake and mortality among a sample of the United States population. Epidemiology 1992; 3(3):194–202.
137. Steinberg D. Antioxidant vitamins and coronary heart disease (Editorial). N Engl J Med 1993; 328(20):1487–1489.
138. Walldius G, et al. The role of lipids and antioxidive factors for development of atherosclerosis. The Probucol Quantitative Regression Swedish Trial (PQRST). Am J Cardiol 1993; 71(6):15B–19B.
139. Berliner JA, Haberland ME. The role of oxidized low-density lipoprotein in atherogenesis. Current Opinion in Lipidology 1993; 4(5):373–381.
140. Witztum JL, Steinberg D. Role of oxidized low density lipoprotein in atherogenesis. J Clin Invest 1991; 88(6): 1785–1792.
141. Nakano T, et al. Lysophosphatidylcholine upregulates the level of heparin-binding epidermal growth factor-like growth factor mRNA in human monocytes. Proc Natl Acad Sci USA 1994; 91(3):1069–1073.
142. Falcone DJ, et al. Macrophage and foam cell release of matrix-bound growth factors. Role of plasminogen activation. J Biol Chem 1993; 268(16):11951–11958.
143. Ross R. The pathogenesis of atherosclerosis: a perspective for the 1990s. Nature 1993; 362(6423):801–809.
144. Ishibashi S, et al. Monocyte colony-stimulating factor enhances uptake and degradation of acetylated low density lipoproteins and cholesterol esterification in human monocyte-derived macrophages. J Biol Chem 1990; 265(24):14109–14117.
145. Clinton SK, et al. Macrophage colony-stimulating factor gene expression in vascular cells and in experimental and human atherosclerosis. Am J Pathol 1992; 140(2):301–316.
146. Rosenfeld ME, et al. Macrophage colony-stimulating factor mRNA and protein in atherosclerotic lesions of rabbits and humans. Am J Pathol 1992; 140(2):291–300.
147. Geng YJ, Hansson GK. Interferon-gamma inhibits scavenger receptor expression and foam cell formation in human monocyte-derived macrophages. J Clin Invest 1992; 89(4):1322–1330.
148. Hansson GK, Holm J, Jonasson L. Detection of activated T lymphocytes in the human atherosclerotic plaque. Am J Pathol 1989; 135(1):169–175.
149. Hansson GK, et al. Localization of T lymphocytes and macrophages in fibrous and complicated human atherosclerotic plaques. Atherosclerosis 1988; 72(2–3):135–141.
150. Kuo PT, et al. Suppression of experimental atherosclerosis in rabbits by interferon-inducing agents. J Am Coll Cardiol 1984; 3(1):129–134.
151. Wilson AC, et al. Suppression of aortic atherosclerosis in cholesterol-fed rabbits by purified rabbit interferon. Arteriosclerosis 1990; 10(2):208–214.
152. Brand K, Mackman N, Curtiss LK. Interferon-gamma inhibits macrophage apolipoprotein E production by post-translational mechanisms. J Clin Invest 1993; 91(5):2031–2039.
153. Jonasson L, et al. Interferon-gamma inhibits lipoprotein lipase in human monocyte-derived macrophages. Biochim Biophys Acta 1990; 1053(1):43–48.
154. Small DM. Cellular mechanisms for lipid deposition in atherosclerosis. N Engl J Med 1977; 297(16):873–877, 297(17): 924–929.
155. Small DM, et al. Physicochemical and histological changes in the arterial wall of nonhuman primates during progression and regression of atherosclerosis. J Clin Invest 1984; 73(6):1590–1605.
156. Bocan TMA, Guyton JR. Human aortic fibrolipid lesions. Progenitor lesions for fibrous plaques, exhibiting early formation of the cholesterol-rich core. Am J Pathol 1985; 120(2):193–206.
157. Katz SS, Shipley GG, Small DM. Physical chemistry of the lipids of human atherosclerotic lesions. Demonstration of a lesion intermediate between fatty streaks and advanced plaques. J Clin Invest 1976; 58(1):200–211.
158. Guyton JR, Klemp KF. The lipid-rich core region of human atherosclerotic fibrous plaques: prevalence of small lipid droplets and vesicles by electron microscopy. Am J Pathol 1989; 134(3):705–717.
159. Kruth HS. Localization of unesterified cholesterol in human atherosclerotic lesions. Demonstration of filipin-positive, oil-red-O-negative particles. Am J Pathol 1984; 114(2): 201–208.
160. Tracy RE, et al. Spatial dispersion of foam cells in the human thoracic aorta. Lab Invest 1983; 49(6):693–701.
161. Robertson WB, et al. The fate of the fatty streak. Exp Mol Pathol 1963; 2[Supp 1]:28–39.
162. McGill HC Jr. Fatty streaks in the coronary arteries and aorta. Lab Invest 1968; 18(5):560–564.
163. Smith B. Identification of the gelatinous lesion. In FG Schettler, et al., eds. Atherosclerosis VI: Proceedings of the Sixth International Symposium. Berlin: Springer, 1983.
164. Tall AR. Plasma lipid transfer proteins. J Lipid Res 1986; 27(4):361–367.
165. Still WJS, O'Neal RM. Electron microscopic study of experimental atherosclerosis in the rat. Am J Pathol 1962; 40(1): 21–35.
166. Mahley RW, et al. Canine hyperlipoproteinemia and atherosclerosis. Accumulation of lipid by aortic medial cells in vivo and in vitro. Am J Pathol 1977; 87(1):205–226.
167. Sassen LM, et al. Development and regression of atherosclerosis in pigs. Effects of n-3 fatty acids, their incorporation into plasma and aortic plaque lipids, and granulocyte function. Arterioscler Thromb 1993; 13:651–660.
168. Wissler RW, et al. Arterial lesions and blood lipids in rhesus monkeys fed human diets. Exp Mol Pathol 1983; 38(1): 117–136.
169. Wolfe MS, et al. Childhood consumption of dietary polyunsaturated fat lowers risk for coronary artery atherosclerosis in African green monkeys. Arterioscler Thromb 1993; 13(6):863–875.
170. Walsh A, et al. Intestinal expression of the human apoA-I gene in transgenic mice is controlled by a DNA region 3′ to the gene in the promoter of the adjacent convergently transcribed apoC-III gene. J Lipid Res 1993; 34(4):617–623.

171. Rubin EM, et al. Expression of human apolipoprotein A-I in transgenic mice results in reduced plasma levels of murine apolipoprotein A-I and the appearance of two new high density lipoprotein size subclasses. Proc Natl Acad Sci USA 1991; 88(2):434–438.
172. Hayek T, et al. Dietary fat increases high density lipoprotein (HDL) levels both by increasing the transport rates and decreasing the fractional catabolic rates of HDL cholesteryl ester and apolipoprotein (apo) A-I: presentation of a new animal model and mechanistic studies in human apo A-I transgenic and control mice. J Clin Invest 1993; 91(4):1665–1699.
173. Hayek T, et al. Probucol decreases apolipoprotein A-I transport rate and increases HDL cholesteryl ester fractional catabolic rate in control and human apo A-I transgenic mice. Arteriosclerosis Thrombosis 1991; 11(5):1295–1302.
174. Schultz JR, et al. Expression of human apolipoprotein A-II and its effect on high density lipoproteins in transgenic mice. J Biol Chem 1992; 267(30):21630–21636.
175. Rubin EM, et al. Inhibition of early atherogenesis in transgenic mice by human apolipoprotein AI. Nature 1992; 353(6341):265–267.
176. Aalto-Setää K, et al. Mechanism of hypertriglyceridemia in human apolipoprotein (apo) CIII transgenic mice: diminished very low density lipoprotein fractional catabolic rate associated with increased apo CIII and reduced apo E on the particles. J Clin Invest 1992; 90(5):1889–1900.
177. Shimano H, et al. Plasma lipoprotein metabolism in transgenic mice overexpressing apolipoprotein E. Accelerated clearance of lipoproteins containing apolipoprotein B. J Clin Invest 1992; 90(5):2084–2091.
178. van der Maagdenberg AMJM, et al. Transgenic mice carrying the apolipoprotein E3-Leiden gene exhibit hyperlipoproteinemia. J Biol Chem 1993; 268(14):10540–10545.
179. Chiesa G, et al. Reconstitution of lipoprotein(a) by infusion of human low density lipoprotein into transgenic mice expressing human apolipoprotein(a). J Biol Chem 1992; 267(34):24369–24374.
180. Lawn RM, et al. Atherogenesis in transgenic mice expressing human apolipoprotein(a). Nature 1992; 360(6405):670–672.
181. Hoffman SL, et al. Overexpression of low density lipoprotein (LDL) receptor eliminates LDL from plasma in transgenic mice. Science 1988; 239(4845):1277–1281.
182. Yokode M, et al. Diet-induced hypercholesterolemia in mice: prevention by overexpression of LDL receptors. Science 1990; 250(4985):1273–1275.
183. Piedrahita JA, et al. Generation of mice carrying a mutant apolipoprotein E gene inactivated by gene targeting in embryonic stem cells. Proc Natl Acad Sci USA 1992; 89(10):4471–4475.
184. Plump AS, et al. Severe hypercholesterolemia and atherosclerosis in apolipoprotein E-deficient mice created by homologous recombination in ES cells. Cell 1992; 71(2): 343–353.
185. Nakashima Y, et al. ApoE-deficient mice develop lesions of all phases of atherosclerosis throughout the arterial tree. Arterioscler Thromb 1994; 14(1):133–140.
186. Reddick RL, Zhang SH, Maeda N. Atherosclerosis in mice lacking apo E. Evaluation of lesional development and progression. Arterioscler Thromb 1994; 14(1):141–147.
187. Williamson R, et al. Marked reduction of high density lipoprotein cholesterol in mice genetically modified to lack apolipoprotein A-I. Proc Natl Acad Sci USA 1992; 89(15): 7134–7138.
188. Ishibashi S, et al. Hypercholesterolemia in low density lipoprotein receptor knockout mice and its reversal by adenovirus-mediated gene delivery. J Clin Invest 1993; 92(2): 883–893.
189. Schwenke DC, St Clair RW. Influx, efflux, and accumulation of LDL in normal arterial areas and atherosclerotic lesions of white Carneau pigeons with naturally occurring and cholesterol-aggravated aortic atherosclerosis. Arterioscler Thromb 1993; 13(9):1368–1381.
190. Capron L. Viruses and atherosclerosis. Rev Prat 1990; 40(24):2227–2233.
191. Quinet EM, et al. Adipose tissue cholesteryl ester transfer protein mRNA in response to probucol treatment: cholesterol and species dependence. J Lipid Res 1993; 34(5): 845–852.
192. Ridolfi RL, Hutchins GM. The relationship between coronary artery lesions and myocardial infarcts: ulceration of atherosclerotic plaques precipitating coronary thrombosis. Am Heart J 1977; 93(4):468–486.
193. Sherman CT, et al. Coronary angioscopy in patients with unstable angina pectoris. N Engl J Med 1986; 315(15): 913–919.
194. Geiringer E. Intimal vascularisation and atherosclerosis. J Pathol Bacteriol 1951; 63(2):201–211.
195. Barger AC, et al. Hypothesis: vasa vasorum and neovascularization of human coronary arteries. A possible role in the pathophysiology of atherosclerosis. N Engl J Med 1984; 310(3):175–177.
196. Bayliss High OB, Adams CWM. The role of macrophages and giant cells in advanced human atherosclerosis. Atherosclerosis 1980; 36(3):441–447.
197. Roberts WC. Does thrombosis play a major role in the development of symptom-producing atherosclerotic plaques? (Editorial) Circulation 1973; 48(6):1161–1166.
198. Gardner MB, Blankenhorn DH. Aortic medical calcification. An ultrastructural study. Arch Pathol 1968; 85(4):397–403.
199. Haust MD, Geer JC. Mechanism of calcification in spontaneous aortic arteriosclerotic lesions of the rabbit. An electron microscopic study. Am J Pathol 1970; 60:329–346.
200. Tanimura A, McGregor DH, Anderson HC. Calcification in atherosclerosis. I: Human studies. J Exp Pathol 1986; 2(4): 261–273.
201. Kramsch DM, Aspen AJ, Apstein CS. Suppression of experimental atherosclerosis by the Ca^{++}-antagonist lanthanum. J Clin Invest 1980; 65(5):967–981.
202. Henry PD, Bentley KI. Suppression of atherogenesis in cholesterol-fed rabbit treated with nifedipine. J Clin Invest 1981; 68(5):1366–1369.
203. Sugano M, et al. Suppression of atherosclerosis in cholesterol-fed rabbits by diltiazem injection. Arteriosclerosis 1986; 6(2):237–241.
204. Gerrity RG. The role of the monocyte in atherogenesis. I: Transition of blood-borne monocytes into foam cells in fatty lesions. Am J Pathol 1981; 103(2):181–190.
205. Gown AM, Tsukada T, Ross R. Human atherosclerosis. II: Immunocytochemical analysis of the cellular composition of human atherosclerotic lesions. Am J Pathol 1986; 125(1): 191–207.
206. Glenn KC, Ross R. Human monocyte-derived growth factor(s) for mesenchymal cells: activation of secretion by endotoxin and concanavalin A. Cell 1981; 25(3):603–615.
207. Martin BM, et al. Stimulation of nonlymphoid mesenchymal cell proliferation by a macrophage-derived growth factor. J Immunol 1981; 126(4):1510–1515.
208. Brown BG, Mahley R, Assman G. Swine aortic smooth muscle in tissue culture. Some effects of purified swine lipoproteins on cell growth and morphology. Circ Res 1976; 39(3):415–424.
209. Fischer-Dzoga K, Kuo Y-F, Wissler RW. The proliferative

effect of platelets and hyperlipidemic serum on stationary primary cultures. Atherosclerosis 1983; 47(1):35–45.
210. Eisele B, Bates SR, Wissler RW. Interaction of low density lipoproteins from normal and hyperlipemic rhesus monkeys with arterial smooth muscle cells in culture. Atherosclerosis 1980; 36(1):9–24.
211. St Clair RW, Greenspan P, Leight M. Enhanced cholesterol delivery to cells in culture by low density lipoproteins from hypercholesterolemic monkeys. Correlation of cellular cholesterol accumulation with low density lipoprotein molecular weight. Arteriosclerosis 1983; 3(1):77–86.
212. Chait A, et al. Platelet-derived growth factor stimulates activity of low density lipoprotein receptors. Proc Natl Acad Sci USA 1980; 77(7):4084–4088.
213. Tracy RE, et al. Atheronecrosis and its fibroproliferative base and cap in the thoracic aorta. Lab Invest 1979; 41(6):546–552.

Pathophysiology of Ischemic Syndromes

Antonio Fernandez-Ortiz
Valentin Fuster

The vasculature supplies oxygen and nutrients to the tissues and removes metabolites resulting from biologic reactions. Normally, oxygen supply is closely matched to metabolic oxygen demands, and tissue demands are generally unable to exceed the normal oxygen-supply capacity. Oxygen supply is determined by blood perfusion and the oxygen-carrying capacity of the blood. Ischemia occurs when there is an imbalance between tissue oxygen demands and oxygen supply as a consequence of reduced blood perfusion. Ischemia should be distinguished from hypoxia, which is a condition of reduced oxygen supply to tissue despite adequate perfusion, and anoxia, which is an absence of oxygen supply despite adequate perfusion.

The most common underlying condition of reduced oxygen supply in ischemic syndromes is atherosclerotic disease, which either causes direct luminal arterial narrowing (**stable lesion**) or produces an acute arterial obstruction by inducing thrombus formation (**unstable lesion**). Atherosclerotic disease in the coronary artery system may manifest in the form of stable or unstable angina, acute myocardial infarction, or sudden cardiac death. Atherosclerotic disease in the cerebral arterial system (including the intracranial and extracranial arteries) may manifest in the form of transient ischemic attack or cerebral ischemic infarction. And atherosclerotic disease in the peripheral arterial system may manifest in the form of intermittent claudication or acute ischemia of the extremities (Fig. 14-1).

More than 70 million Americans—more than one in four—have some form of cardiovascular disease [1]. Cardiovascular diseases cause almost as many deaths as accidents, cancer, infections, and all other diseases combined. In 1991, 43 percent of all deaths in the U.S. population were due to cardiovascular disorders. Atherosclerosis was the underlying disease in 72 percent of those deaths [2]. Overall, coronary atherosclerosis and subsequent ischemic heart disease are the most lethal cardiovascular events in both sexes, exacting a large toll in disability and quality of life, mainly in the elderly. The prevalence of coronary artery disease estimated by the National Heart Interview Survey was 2.9 percent of the population in 1989 (6.9 million), and there were 498,000 coronary deaths that year, accounting for more than one-fourth of the deaths in persons over age 35 [3]. For cerebral ischemia, in 1989 the prevalence was 1 percent of the population (2.6 million) (that prevalence, however, rose to 7.8 percent for men aged 75 and over), and deaths due to cerebrovascular disease were 147,000 [3]. For peripheral arterial disease, epidemiology has been much less well defined because standards of diagnosis have varied widely. Much of the available information is confined to the incidence and prevalence of intermittent claudication, which appears to result in a dramatic underestimation of the true prevalence of peripheral atherosclerosis. Intermittent claudication has been reported in 1 to 2 percent of the general population in the United States [4,5], with rates up to two times higher in men than in women [6,7]. Every year, 55,000 men and 44,000 women have a first-listed diagnosis of chronic peripheral arterial disease, and 229,000 men and 184,000 women have chronic peripheral arterial disease noted at discharge. Comorbid coronary disease in patients with peripheral arterial disease may exceed 50 percent, and there is an excess prevalence of cerebrovascular occlusive disease as well [8]. Such comorbidity is to be expected, given the similarity of risk factors for atherosclerosis in the various arterial beds [9].

The Framingham Heart Study [10] has provided reliable data for 36 years of follow-up in a population sample of 5,209 men and women aged 35 to 94. Average annual rates of major cardiovascular events rose from 5 percent at ages 35–44 to 59 percent at ages 85–94. In people under age 75, coronary artery disease is the predominant ischemic disorder; in those older than 75, the proportion of cerebrovascular events is higher than that of coronary events. Recently, efforts have been made to link the natural history of the various ischemic syndromes with the biology and the evolution of atherosclerotic lesions [11,12]. Many investigators are intrigued by the cellular mechanisms responsible for the transformation of stable atherosclerotic plaques into unstable lesions in which rupture and thrombosis develop. This chapter will provide pathophysiologic explanation for the broad spectrum of ischemic syndromes based on our current understanding of atherosclerosis, thrombosis, and vasospasm.

Determinants of Blood Flow and Ischemia

The amount of oxygen used by the tissues is directly related to blood flow, the oxygen content of arterial blood, and the amount of oxygen extracted from the blood by the tissue. Of these considerations, blood flow has the most practical importance since the oxygen-carrying capacity of the blood cannot be significantly increased unless considerable hypoxemia is present. Furthermore, organs like the heart and the skeletal muscles extract a high and relatively fixed amount of oxygen from the circulation. Even during rest, 70 to 80 percent of the oxygen in the blood perfusing the coronaries is extracted by the myocardium [13]. Therefore, augmentation of flow is the only practical mechanism by which increased metabolic demands can be met (Fig. 14-2). Blood flow depends on the perfusion pressure and the resistance offered by the vascular bed. The perfusion, or driving pressure, is the gradient between the pressure in supplying tissue arteries and the pressure in draining veins. Abnormalities of arteries or arteriolae, such as those caused by atherosclerotic disease, may reduce driving pressure and consequently flow to nutrient capillary beds, resulting in ischemia. Certain factors determine blood flow and the pathophysiol-

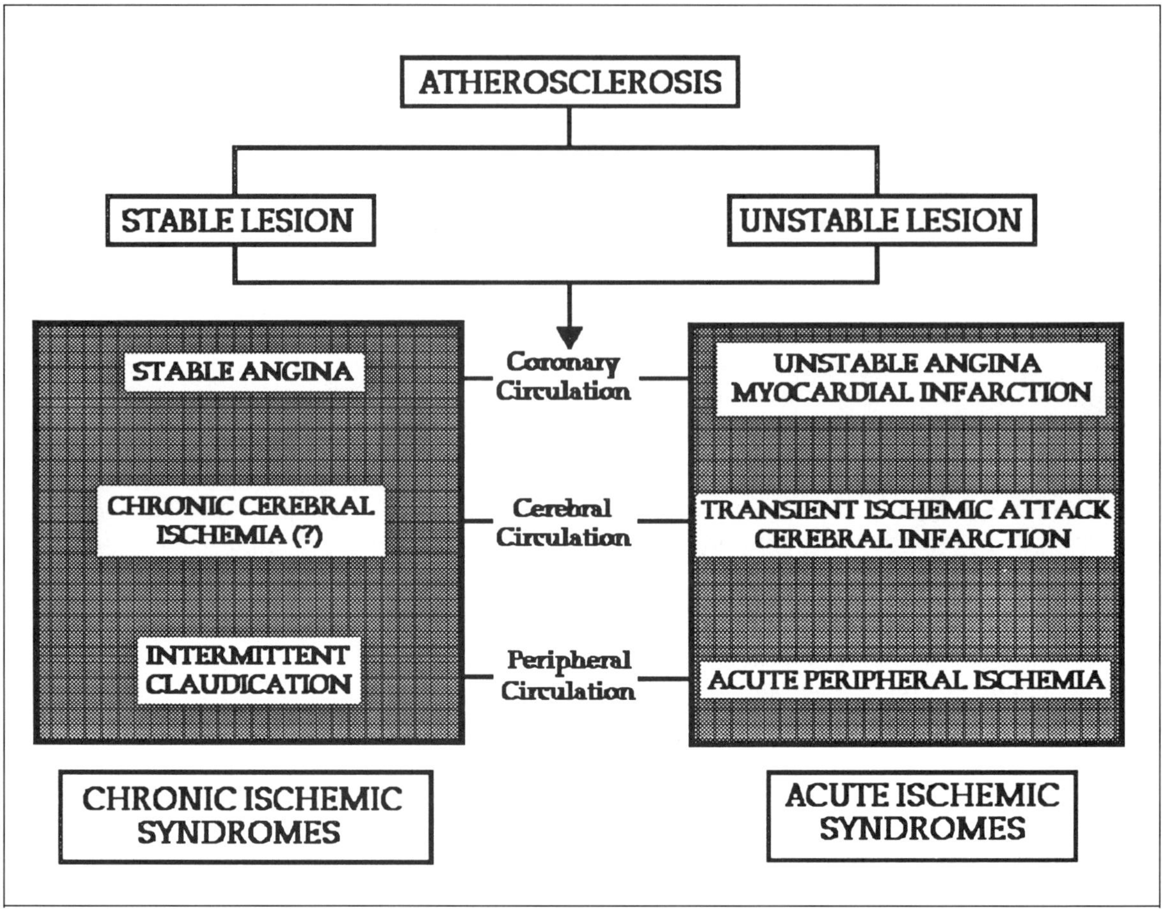

Fig. 14-1. Atherosclerosis is the most common recognized underlying condition in ischemic syndromes. Stable lesions, by direct luminal arterial narrowing in the coronary, cerebral, or peripheral circulation, may cause stable angina, chronic cerebral ischemia, or intermittent claudication, respectively. Unstable lesions, by inducing acute thrombus formation in the coronary, cerebral, or peripheral circulation, may cause unstable angina and myocardial infarction, transient ischemic attacks and cerebral infarction, or acute peripheral ischemia, respectively.

ogy of ischemia in the heart, the brain, and the lower extremities.

CORONARY CIRCULATION

The coronary circulation differs from other circulations in that the resistance offered by the vascular bed is strongly influenced by phasic systolic compression of the coronary vessels. Effective perfusion pressure is not constant throughout the cardiac cycle. The intramyocardial vascular tree is compressed during systole, and systolic flow through intramyocardial vessels is substantially reduced, making aortic dyastolic pressure a major determinant in coronary blood flow. In addition, because coronary vessels are also exposed to intramyocardial pressure during diastole, the net driving force responsible for maintaining coronary flow during diastole must be the difference between aortic diastolic pressure and intramyocardial diastolic pressure. The latter is related to left ventricular diastolic pressure, which when elevated, as may occur during episodes of angina pectoris, may significantly reduce myocardial blood flow. At the other side of the balance, oxygen demands by the myocardium may vary greatly depending on heart rate; tension developed in the left ventricular wall, which is a function of systolic blood pressure and cardiac size; and the contractile state of the myocardium.

Abundant evidence suggests that the coronary arteries are not just passive conduits for blood but exhibit active vasomotion under a variety of stimuli. When an atherosclerotic plaque causes coronary-artery narrowing, pressure distal to the obstruction is reduced, and ischemia is avoided by a compensatory decrease in vascular resistance at the distal arteriolar bed [14]. This coronary autoregulation has been suggested to be mediated by metabolites accumulated in the myocardium when flow is insufficient. For example, adenosine, a powerful coronary vasodilator, may be a major factor responsible in restoring the balance between oxygen supply and demand by decreasing the resistance of coronary vessels [15]. It is likely, however, that different control mechanisms account for normal *versus* diseased vessels and that numerous other mediators of vascular tone, such as those derived from

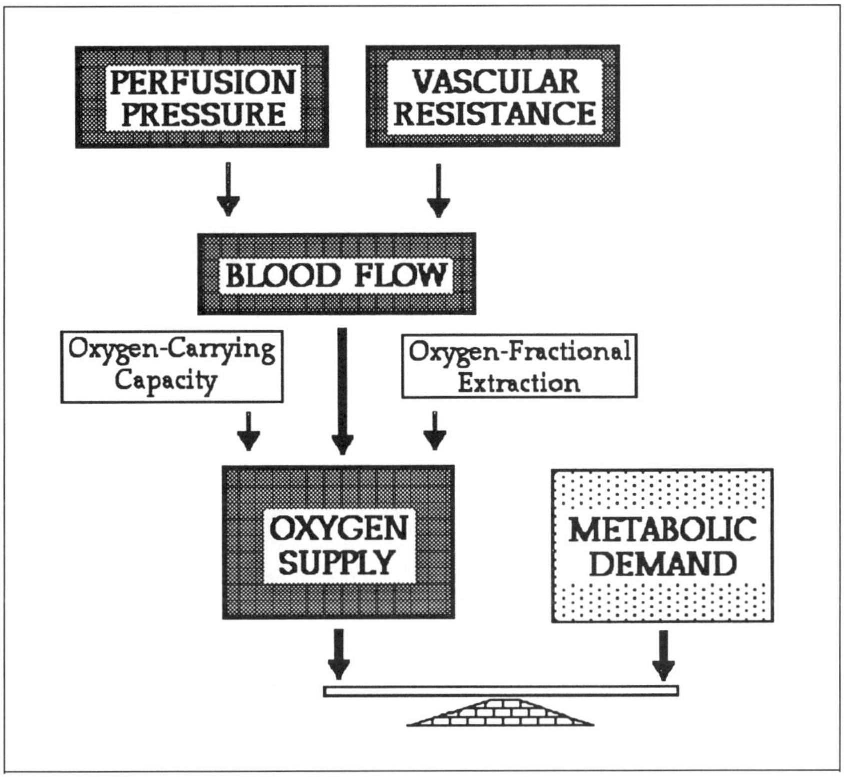

Fig. 14-2. Factors influencing oxygen supply. Increase in blood flow, by means of decrease in vascular resistances or increase in perfusion pressure, is the most important mechanism by which oxygen supply can be matched to metabolic oxygen demands.

the endothelium, adrenergic receptors, prostaglandins, serotonin, platelets, and probably even cholesterol, may be involved in determining coronary blood flow [16–19].

CEREBRAL CIRCULATION

Characteristically, cerebral tissue is much less influenced by the physical determinants of oxygen demands. When cerebral perfusion pressure is normal, blood flow is regulated primarily by changes in arteriolar size [20], and there is a direct correlation between cerebral blood flow and intravascular cerebral blood volume. Cerebral blood flow is also closely matched to the metabolic demands of the tissue. As a result, there is a uniform value throughout the brain for the fractional extraction of oxygen from the blood. This cerebral oxygen-extraction fraction is approximately one-third in normal resting humans [21]. As perfusion pressure falls, the first compensatory response is arterial vasodilatation. Flow is then maintained by a decrease in vascular resistance. Both blood volume and the volume-flow ratio will increase, but oxygen extraction will remain normal. As perfusion pressure falls further, the capacity for compensatory vasodilatation will be overwhelmed, and blood flow will begin to fall. At that stage, cerebral oxygen metabolism is maintained by an increase in oxygen extraction. If cerebral perfusion pressure falls further, the compensatory mechanisms of the brain will be exhausted, and cerebral ischemia may occur [22]. These complex compensatory mechanisms, together with an extensive network of collaterals, may explain why atherosclerosis in the cerebrovascular system remains largely asymptomatic until an acute arterial occlusion develops.

PERIPHERAL CIRCULATION

In studying the peripheral circulation, one must consider separately the physiology of muscle and cutaneous blood flow. Blood flow to resting muscle is quite low. In fact, at rest, blood flow is normal or nearly normal in most people with peripheral vascular disease [23]. During exercise, local ischemia may induce vasodilatation, which, combined with an increase in cardiac output, may increase blood flow to leg muscles 5- to 10-fold. However, although skin requirements to maintain nutrition and integrity also are low, the arteriolar network of the skin is under strong autonomic control and is subject to marked extremes of vasoconstriction and vasodilatation.

Since the foot is composed mostly of skin and subcutaneous tissue, significant ischemia may not occur until arterial insufficiency is quite advanced. Muscle may have adequate blood flow in the resting state even when the foot has become gangrenous. However, during exercise, even with maximal dilation, arteries supplying the muscle cannot afford the enormous increase in blood flow that is necessary for walking. It is not surprising, then, that intermittent claudication is usually the first symptom of arterial insufficiency in active individuals. On the other hand, if arterial occlusion is confined predominantly to the distal tibial arteries, beyond the branching of most of the muscle blood supply, rest pain in the foot may be the first symptom of peripheral atherosclerosis.

Pathophysiology of Chronic Ischemic Syndromes

As pointed out, the most frequently recognized cause of ischemia is atherosclerotic disease, which either causes direct luminal arterial narrowing (**stable plaques**) or produces acute obstruction by inducing thrombus formation (**unstable plaques**). Vasoconstriction occuring at the site of an atherosclerotic plaque may significantly increase obstruction to blood flow, and the presence of adequate collateral circulation may finally determine the clinical outcome of the ischemic insult.

UNDERLYING PROCESS: STABLE ATHEROSCLEROTIC LESION

Plaque Initiation. Formation of atherosclerotic lesions is initiated by endothelial dysfunction at certain lesion-prone sites characterized by areas of low shear stress [24]. The combination of increased uptake of low-density lipoproteins and enhanced monocyte recruitment are pivotal initiating events for atherosclerosis [25,26]. The morphologic studies by Stary have provided many answers about plaque initiation and evolution [27,28]. Initial atherosclerotic lesions (types I and II), consisting of isolated groups of macrophages filled with lipid droplets (fatty streaks), were found in areas of adaptive eccentric intimal thickening in the coronary arteries of 45 percent of infants in the first 8 months of life [28]. Progression beyond the fatty-streak stage is associated with the accumulation of extracellular lipid, which replaces the intercellular matrix proteoglycans and fibers, driving smooth muscle cells apart (type III). Multiple scattered pools of extracellular lipid may progress to a massive, confluent accumulation of lipids, or **lipid core** (type IV). Simultaneously or soon thereafter, smooth muscle cells migrate into and proliferate in the plaque, forming a layer, or cap, over the lumina side of the lipid core [27,29]. More and more collagen is produced, and plaque size increases. The process culminates in what is known as a **raised fibrolipid** or **advanced plaque** (type V) (Fig. 14-3).

Mechanisms of Atherosclerotic Plaque Growth. Arteries may show all stages of plaque development, implying that new lesions are generated throughout life. Even in the same individual, there are major plaque-to-plaque variations in the relative proportions of extracellular lipid and collagen that are present [30–32]. The work by Stary indicates that a plaque can take from 10 to 15 years to fully develop. In the first three decades of life, the composition of the lesions is predominantly lipidic and relatively predictable. From the fourth decade on, however, the composition of advanced lesions becomes unpredictable because some lesions continue to increase by mechanisms other than lipid deposition [11,28]. Angiographic studies have shown that the progression of early atherosclerotic lesions to clinically manifest, enlarging atherosclerotic plaques, such as those that cause blood-flow impairment, is neither linear nor predictable [33]. New high-grade lesions often appear in segments of arteries that were normal at previous angiographic examination. This unpredictable and episodic progression can be explained by plaque rupture with subsequent mural thrombosis leading to intermittent plaque growth (Fig. 14-4).

Small plaque fissures may allow blood to enter and expand the plaque. Plaque expansion produces acute changes in plaque geometry with subsequent alterations in local rheology that may further stimulate lesion progression [24]. Analyses of the coronary tree in patients who died of ischemic heart disease have shown a morphologic appearance consistent with previously healed fissues at different stages of thrombosis and thrombus organization [34]. Furthermore, studies using monoclonal antibodies to identify fibrin, fibrinogen, and their degradation products also have supported the evidence for thrombosis and thrombus incorporation as part of plaque progression [35]. Additionally, the healing organization process of intraplaque thrombi also may contribute to subclinical progression of the lesions through interactions between thrombotic elements and vascular cells. Several studies have demonstrated that, besides platelets [25,36], thrombin is a potent mitogen for mesenchymal-derived cells and is chemotactic for monocytes [37,38] and that fibrin(ogen) and its degradation products, by their ability to stimulate vascular-cell proliferation, may also contribute to lesion progression [39]. In earlier phases of the disease, fibrinogen accumulation in atherosclerotic plaques also has been related to increased endothelial permeability rather than incorporation of mural thrombus to the plaque [40], and fibrinogen has been attributed a critical role in the extracellular retention of lipoproteins into the lesion [41–44].

Although rupture-mediated progression is clinically silent in most cases, it has an important prognostic value. In a recent study, clinically silent coronary atherosclerotic progression, assessed by angiography, was shown to be a strong and independent predictor of future coronary events, particularly cardiac death [45]. Interestingly, this atherosclerotic progression is often more rapid in persons with coronary risk factors and in lesions with certain topographic characteristics [11,46]. In the Coronary Artery Surgery Study (CASS) [46], diabetes, proximal or midvessel coronary lesion location, elevated cholesterol, interval from myocardial infarction, and complex lesion morphology were identified as predictors of angiographic progression. Clinical studies also support the hypothesis that thrombogenic factors are important contributors to the progression of atherosclerosis. Results of a 5-year trial of platelet-inhibitor therapy [47] indicate that antiplatelet agents are helpful in preventing the angiographic progression of coronary disease. Also, heparin recently has been reported to improve the exercise tolerance and reduce ischemic symptoms in patients with stable angina pectoris [48].

Alternative to plaque rupture and thrombus-mediated growth, atherosclerotic lesions may grow by means of smooth muscle-cell proliferation and collagen-rich matrix synthesis giving rise to an advance sclerotic plaque. Such lesions, consisting entirely or almost entirely of scar collagen, are found more often in arteries of lower extremities.

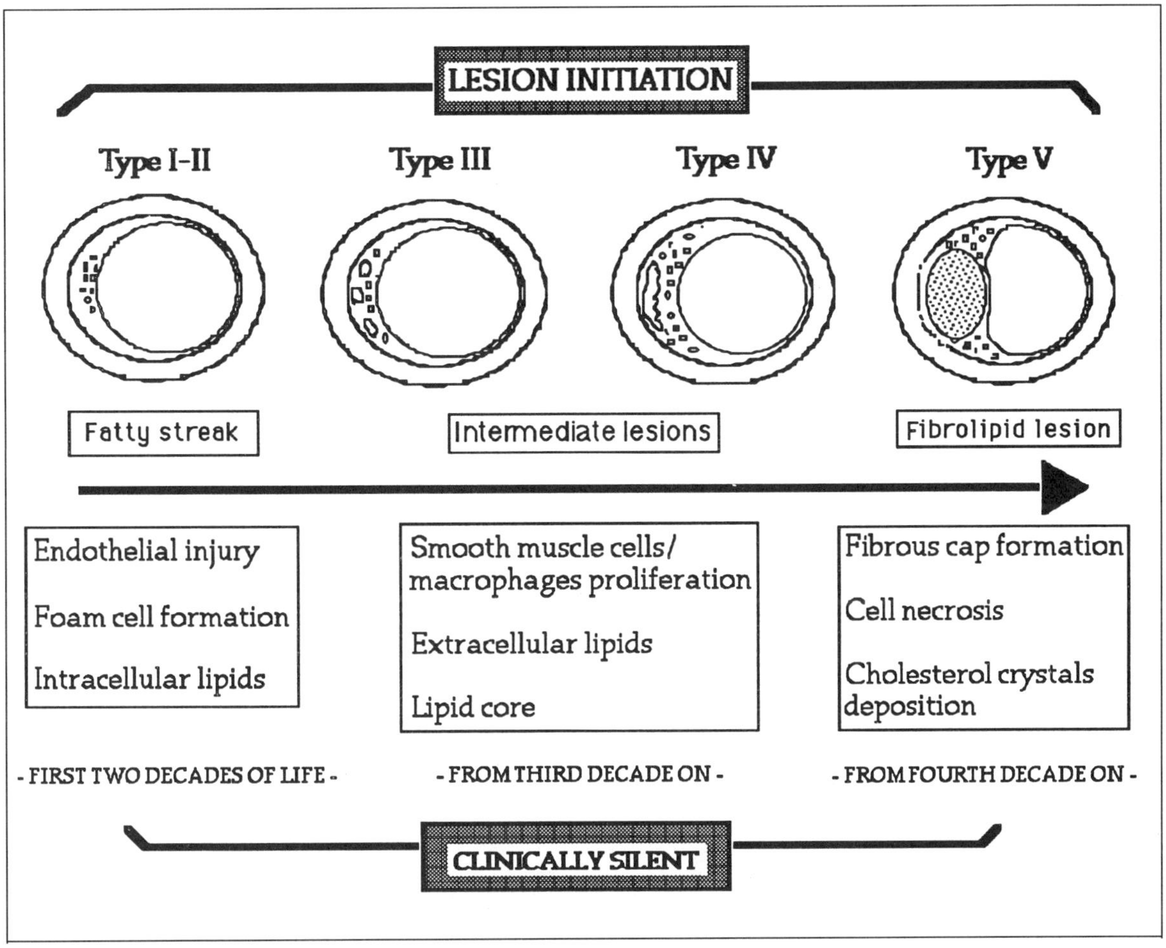

Fig. 14-3. Diagrammatic representation of the process of atherosclerotic-plaque initiation. In the first three decades of life, lesions grow slowly by means of intracellular and extracellular lipid accumulation. In the fourth decade, mature fibrolipid lesions are formed, but at this stage lesions may still be clinically silent.

Lipid may have regressed, or it may never have been in the lesion [28] (see Fig. 14-4).

CLINICAL SYNDROMES

Stable Angina. In patients with stable coronary artery disease, angina commonly results from increases in myocardial oxygen demand that outstrip the ability of stenosed coronary arteries to increase oxygen delivery. Stable angina pectoris is angina that has not changed in frequency, severity, or duration in the last 6 to 8 weeks. The pain characteristically occurs with exertion, emotional stress, or other stimuli that increase myocardial oxygen consumption. The threshold for pain is usually fixed but may be somewhat variable; that is, a stimulus that causes angina on one occasion may not on another, although a consistent pattern usually can be determined. Furthermore, when assessed by ambulatory Holter monitoring, ischemia may be noted to occur at different heart rates [49]. This inconsistency in anginal threshold in daily life likely is due to alterations in blood-flow delivery, probably as a result of changes in vasomotor tone rather than to unperceived changes in oxygen demands.

Pathologic studies have found that in patients with stable angina severe atherosclerotic lesions (> 75% cross-sectional area luminal narrowing, equivalent to 50% diameter reduction) consist of either advanced fibrolipid plaques (60%) or predominantly pure fibrotic lesions (40%) [30]. There is usually no plaque ulceration or thrombosis; however, intraplaque hemorrhage and rests from thrombus organization may be observed. Generally, the pattern of angina does not correlate with extent or severity of the atherosclerotic disease. Mild or infrequent angina does not imply mild or insignificant disease. It appears that prognosis in stable angina is most accurately predicted by the number and the severity of individual obstructions of the three major coronary arteries and by left ventricular function [50]. All this information is obtained by cardiac catheterization with coronary arteriography and left ventriculography.

Chronic Cerebrovascular Ischemia. Stable atherosclerotic disease in the cerebrovascular system is usually asymptomatic. Complex compensatory mechanisms and extensive collateral circulation protect the brain against the hemody-

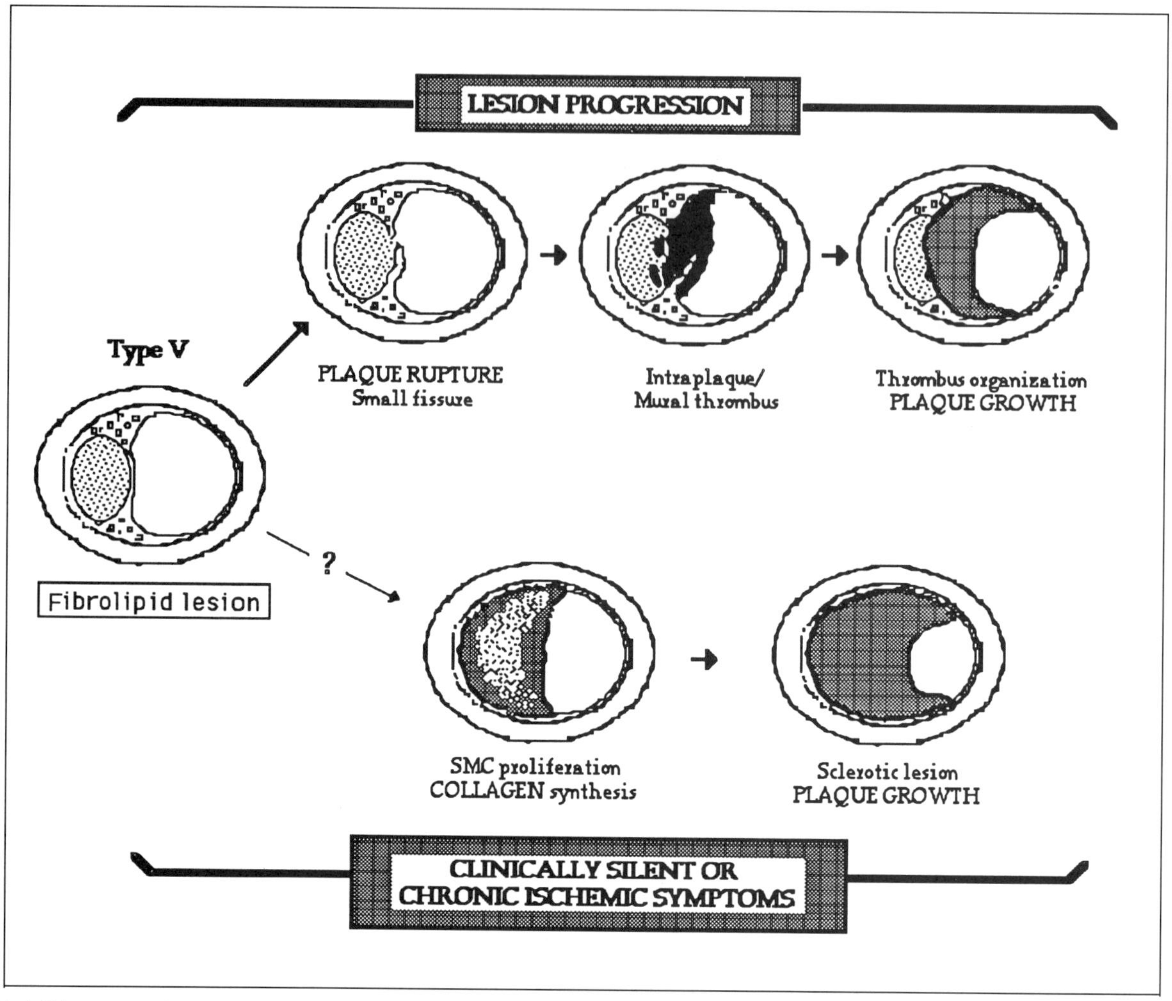

Fig. 14-4. Diagrammatic representation of the mechanisms involved in plaque growth and atherosclerotic progression. Mature fibrolipid lesions may undergo plaque rupture and subsequent resealing by small thrombus formation, contributing to plaque growth. Alternatively, the continuous process of smooth muscle cell (SMC) proliferation and collagen-rich matrix synthesis enlarges plaque volume, giving rise to a mature sclerotic lesion. These stable lesions are clinically silent until a hemodynamically significant stenosis develops and stable ischemic symptoms appear.

namic effects of fixed, stable atherosclerotic lesions. Although the great majority of patients with carotid artery lesions are asymptomatic, often a systolic bruit over the carotid artery in the midneck just behind and below the angle of the mandible is audible. A bruit is most likely to be heard when the stenosis approaches 50 percent of the lumen and often is not present over stenoses greater than 80 percent. The prevalence of asymptomatic carotid bruits has been found to be between 3 and 12 percent in the population over 45 years of age [51–54].

Occasionally, transient ischemic attacks may be very brief and are often manifested by rather mild symptoms such as momentary clumsiness, occasional dropping of objects, fleeting scotomas, or transient loss of memory or speech. Patients may not always recall these episodes or attribute any importance to them. Evidence that these transient attacks result from progressive luminal narrowing leading to precarious hemodynamic insufficiency or from transient thromboembolism into cerebral arteries is controversial. Certainly, poor collateral circulation to the ischemic areas may play a prominent role, but factors such as blood viscosity, vessel-wall compliance, and other unknown factors are needed to explain why blood-flow reduction and ischemia are transient.

Another pathogenic mechanism for chronic cerebral ischemia may be intimal thickening and fibrosis of small intracranial arteries and arteriolae. Such changes have been correlated with the occurrence of microinfarctions, often called lacunae, throughout the internal capsule, cerebellar white matter, brain stem, and basal ganglia [55]. Clinical signs and symptoms secondary to lacunar infarcts generally do not occur before the seventh or eighth decades in normotensive individuals but may appear earlier in hypertensive ones. Patients with lacunar disease may have a variety of neurological findings from ataxia, dysarthria, or hemiplegia to a demential process.

Intermittent Claudication. A peripheral vascular obstruction (stenosis or occlusion) that diminishes arterial blood flow sufficiently to alter function may be manifested as exercise-induced limb claudication (intermittent claudication) or ischemic tissue injury (i.e., ulcers or nonhealing wounds). Intermittent claudication is a clinical condition characterized by symptoms, mostly pain, in the muscles of the lower extremities during exercise. This usually occurs first in the gastrocnemius muscle, because of its high oxygen requirement during ambulation. Thus, intermittent claudication represents the skeletal-muscle counterpart to stable angina pectoris.

Chronic lower-extremity ischemia has a broad spectrum of severity. The most widely used classification is that developed by Fontaine, which encompasses four stages of severity based on signs and symptoms [56]. Stages I and II include ischemia only with exercise, while stages III and IV include ischemia at rest. As the severity of the disease progresses, physical findings of ischemia develop before the onset of symptoms at rest; these findings include atrophy of the skin, loss of hair, ridging of the toenails, and slow or poor healing of breaks in the skin. Ulceration and gangrene are manifestations of far-advanced arterial insufficiency (stage IV). Worsening of symptoms in a patient with stable claudication usually is caused by occlusion of previously stenotic axial vessels or one of the major collaterals that circumvent an obstruction. Two-thirds to three-fourths of patients with peripheral arterial disease who survive for several years after diagnosis will have stable symptoms, while the remaining one-third to one-fourth will show deterioration or progression. One to 5 percent eventually will require amputation [8]. Patients with ischemia at exercise have a favorable prognosis and traditionally are not considered for surgery until the symptoms become truly incapacitating. However, current availability of percutaneous revascularization techniques make these patients candidates for treatment earlier in the course of the disease than would conventional surgical procedures [56].

Pathophysiology of Unstable Ischemic Syndromes

Thrombosis occurs only in arteries containing atherosclerosis. Rupture of the surface of an atherosclerotic plaque has been confirmed to initiate thrombosis by numerous clinical and autopsy studies [57–60]. Extension of thrombus following plaque rupture is believed to be the major determinant of clinical outcome in acute ischemic syndromes.

UNDERLYING PROCESS: UNSTABLE ATHEROSCLEROTIC LESION

Plaque Rupture. In an advanced fibrolipid lesion, the atheromatous gruel is separated from the vascular lumen by a fibrous cap, which is often thinnest and macrophage-richest where it joints the adjacent, more normal intima [29]. Rupture occurs when the strain within the fibrous cap exceeds the deformability of its component material [61]. In the coronary tree, marked oscillations in shear stress, acute changes in coronary pressure or tone, and bending and twisting of an artery during each heart contraction could contribute to plaque rupture. However, determinants of plaque rupture in the cerebrovascular and peripheral circulation are poorly defined. Interestingly, plaque rupture may not always occur at the regions of highest stress, suggesting that local variations in plaque-material properties also contribute to plaque rupture [62]. Compared with intact caps, ruptured ones contain less collagen, and their tensile strength is reduced [63]. Recently, by use of cell-specific monoclonal antibodies, it was shown that the site of ruptured atherosclerotic plaques is invariably associated with large numbers of macrophages and T-cells and lack of smooth muscle cells, suggesting that a localized inflammatory process contributes to rupture and instability [64]. Macrophages within the cap are capable of degrading extracellular matrix by phagocytosis or by secreting proteolytic enzymes such as plasminogen activators and metalloproteinases [29,65]. Macrophages, therefore, may weaken the fibrous cap, predisposing it to rupture. Recent pathoanatomic studies also have indicated that atheromatous core size, cap thickness, and cap macrophage density are major determinants of plaque vulnerability to rupture [66].

Thrombotic Response. As discussed earlier, thrombi resulting from plaque rupture may be small and clinically silent and may become organized, contributing to the growth of the atherosclerotic lesion. When thrombi are large, however, they can contribute to acute ischemic syndromes such as unstable angina or non-Q-wave myocardial infarction by intermittent occlusion of blood flow, Q-wave myocardial infarction by permanent occlusion of blood flow, and cerebral infarction or acute peripheral ischemia by distal thrombus embolization [67–69] (Fig. 14-5). Most ruptured plaques probably are resealed by a small mural thrombus, and only sometimes a major luminal thrombus evolves. It is likely that many variables determine whether an unstable plaque proceeds rapidly to an occlusive thrombus with the potential for acute ischemic events or persists at an intermediate stage as a mural nonocclusive thrombus. Local factors such as quantity (fissure size) and quality of thrombogenic substrate exposed after plaque rupture (plaque composition), as well as rheology of blood flow at the site of rupture, are the major local determinants of thrombotic response after plaque rupture [70]. Systemic factors such as the fibrinolytic system, catecholamines, and lipoprotein(a) also modulate thrombosis, but it is unknown if they are less or more influential than substrate thrombogenicity and rheology in determining the outcome of plaque rupture [11,12].

Not only are atheromatous plaques containing lipid-rich "gruel" the most vulnerable plaques to rupture, the lipid core of such plaques, when exposed to flowing blood after rupture, is also the most thrombogenic component of the plaque, being about sixfold more thrombogenic than the collagen-rich sclerotic component [71] (Fig. 14-6). The atheromatous gruel is thought to be derived from retained lipids, necrotic and disintegrated cells (preferentially macrophage-foam cells), and degraded extracellular matrix. It contains cholesterol crystals, cholesteryl esters (soft lipid), lipoprotein(a), phospholipids, cellular debris, and collagen-degradation products. The component(s) responsible for the high thrombogenicity found in the gruel

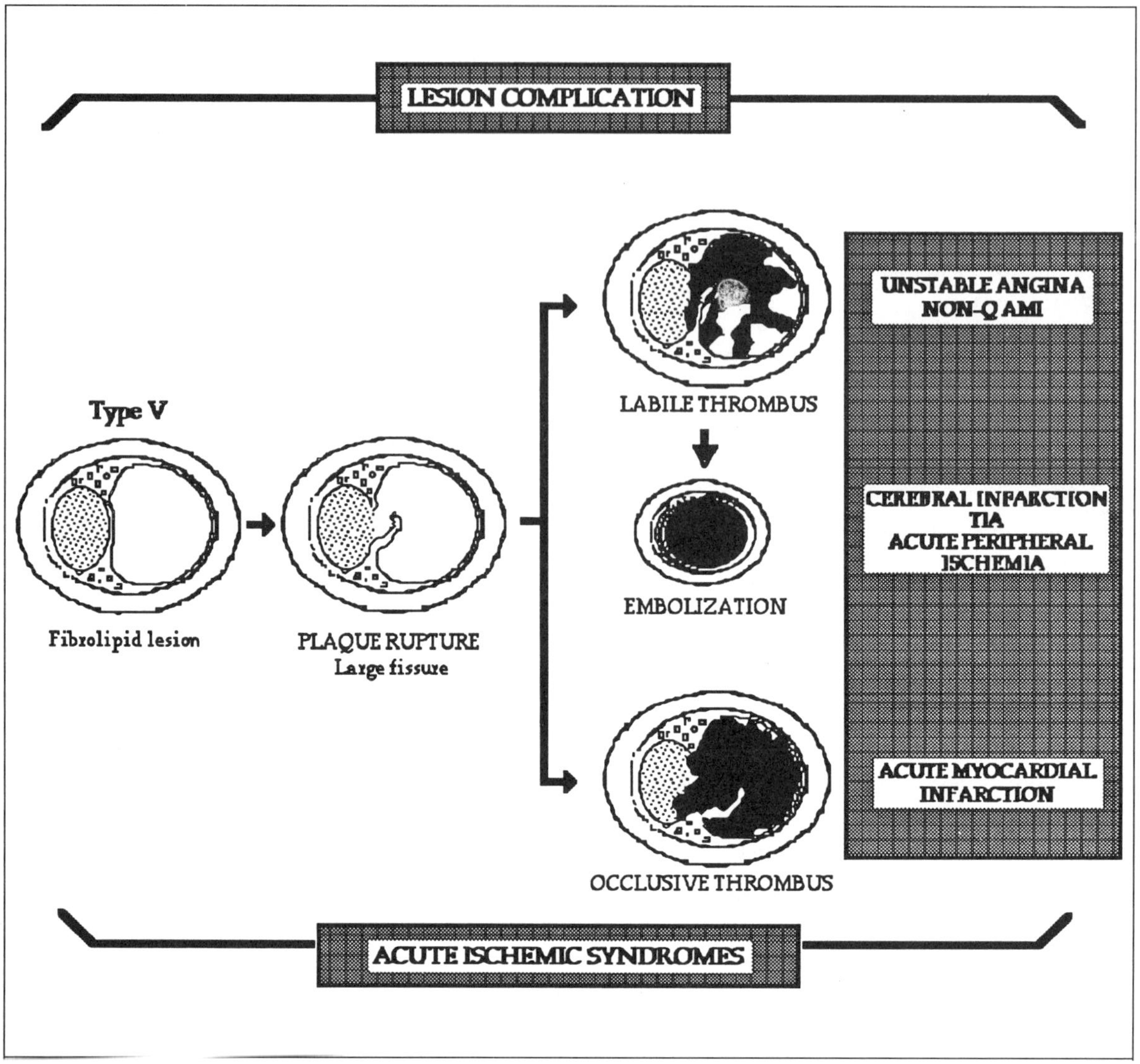

Fig. 14-5. Diagrammatic representation of the mechanisms underlying acute ischemic syndromes. Mature fibrolipid lesions may undergo plaque rupture. Local factors (thrombogenic substrate and rheology) and systemic factors determine thrombotic response after plaque rupture. Labile thrombus, by intermittent occlusion of blood flow, may cause unstable angina or non-Q-wave acute myocardial infarction (AMI). Distal embolization of thrombus formed at the site of plaque rupture may cause cerebral infarction, transient ischemic attacks (TIA), or acute peripheral ischemia. Finally, fixed, occlusive thrombus may cause acute transmural myocardial infarction.

is unknown. Tissue factor protein (derived from disintegrated macrophages?) has been identified immunohistochemically in a scattered pattern within the atheromatous core of human carotid plaques [72], but its role in activating the coagulation cascade after plaque rupture has not been established. It is likely that other components of the gruel, such as lipids, also might induce platelet aggregation and activation of the coagulation system [73].

Besides the nature of the exposed thrombogenic material, local rheologic conditions following plaque rupture are of paramount importance for the thrombotic outcome (mural versus occlusive thrombus). Platelet thrombus may indeed form and grow within a severe stenosis, predominantly at the apex where the blood velocity and shear forces are highest [74]. Therefore, if the rupture site includes the apex of the plaque, platelet deposition will be enhanced. In addition to local flow disturbances caused by degree of stenosis and the presence of flaps, as well as dissections and fissures at the site of plaque rupture, recent data derived from ex-vivo perfusion studies on human aortic atherosclerotic plaques have shown that the roughness of the exposed surface also influences thrombogenicity [71]. As roughness increases, thrombogenicity increases probably due to the effect of local flow disturbances on the surface irregularities.

Besides local factors, clinical and experimental evidence has suggested that systemic factors can influence the outcome of ischemic syndromes. Four systemic factors during plaque rupture may enhance thrombogenicity: (1) serum epinephrine levels (e.g., stress, smoking, early morning)

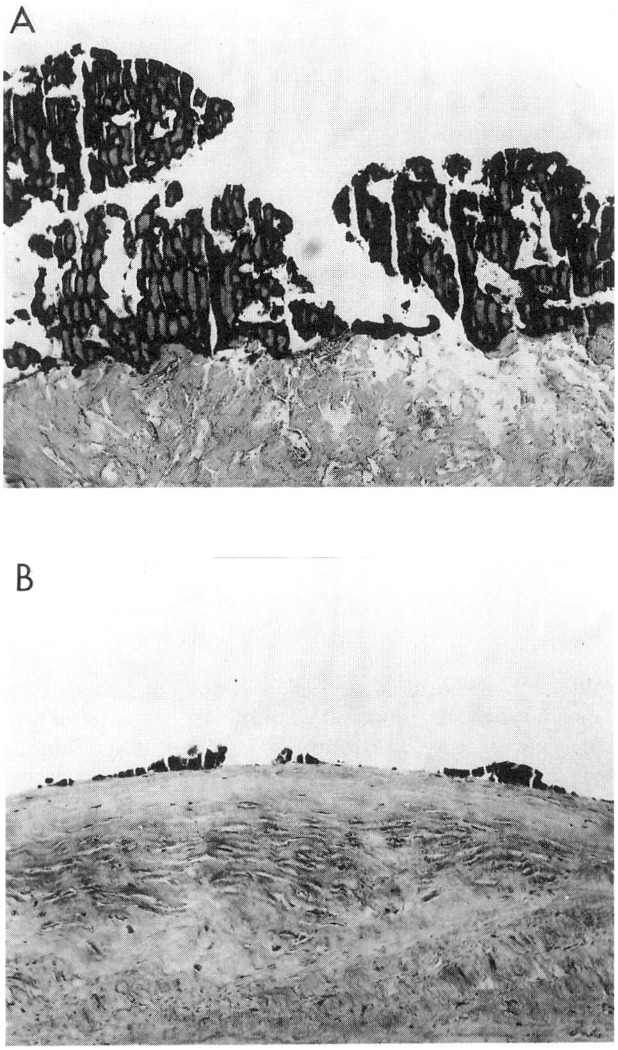

Fig. 14-6. The lipid-rich gruel from atheromatous human aortic lesions is more thrombogenic than the collagen-rich matrix from sclerotic lesions. Exposure of the lipid-rich core with abundant cholesterol crystals **A.** to flowing blood, in an ex-vivo perfusion system, resulted in higher thrombus formation than exposure of collagen-rich matrix **B.** (Original magnification × 75.)

[75]; (2) serum cholesterol levels [76]; (3) impaired fibrinolysis (e.g., high serum lipoprotein(a) levels, plasminogen activator inhibitor) [77]; and (4) hypercoagulability states marked with high levels of fibrinogen, $fragments_{1,2}$, and fibrinopeptide A [78–80].

CLINICAL SYNDROMES

Acute Coronary Syndromes. About 75 percent of thrombi responsible for acute coronary syndromes (unstable angina, acute myocardial infarction, and sudden death) are precipitated by plaque rupture whereby thrombogenic material is exposed to the flowing blood [81]. Minor and superficial intimal irregularities, but not frank rupture, are found beneath the rest of the thrombi, usually in combination with a severe atherosclerotic stenosis.

In unstable angina, a relatively small fissuring or disruption of an atherosclerotic plaque may lead to an acute change in plaque structure and a reduction in coronary blood flow, resulting in exacerbation of angina. Transient episodes of thrombotic vessel occlusion at the site of plaque injury may occur, leading to angina at rest [82,83]. This thrombus is usually labile and results in temporary vascular occlusion, perhaps lasting only 10–20 minutes [67]. In addition, secondary to release of vasoactive substances by platelets, vasoconstriction may contribute to a reduction in coronary flow. These alterations in perfusion and myocardial oxygen supply probably account for two-thirds of episodes of unstable angina; the rest may be caused by transient increases in myocardial oxygen demands [83].

In non-Q-wave infarction, more severe plaque damage would result in more persistent thrombotic occlusion, perhaps lasting up to 1 hour. About one-fourth of patients with non-Q-wave infarction may have an infarct-related vessel occluded for more than 1 hour, but the distal myocardial territory usually is supplied by collaterals [84]. ST segment elevation in the electrocardiogram, an early peak in plasma creatine kinase concentration, and a high rate of angiographic patency of the involved vessel in early angiograms support those speculations. Resolution of vasospasm also may be pathogenically important in non-Q-wave infarction [85,86]. Therefore, spontaneous thrombolysis, spasm resolution, or presence of collateral circulation is important in preventing the formation of Q-wave infarction by limiting the duration of myocardial ischemia.

In Q-wave infarction, larger plaque fissures may result in the formation of a fixed and persistent thrombus. That leads to an abrupt cessation of myocardial perfusion for more than 1 hour, resulting in transmural necrosis of the involved myocardium. The coronary lesion responsible for the infarction frequently is only mildly to moderately stenotic, which suggests that plaque rupture with superimposed thrombus rather than the severity of the underlying lesion is the primary determinant of acute occlusion [87,88]. It is conceivable that in patients with severe coronary stenosis, well-developed collaterals prevent or reduce the extent of infarction [67]. In perhaps one-fourth of patients, coronary thrombosis results from superficial intimal injury or blood stasis in areas of high-grade stenosis [59]. Additionally, myocardial infarction may be promoted by alterations in hemostasis, such as increased activation of the coagulation system (increased epinephrine, fibrinogen, or cholesterol levels), or impairment of the fibrinolytic system (increased lipoprotein(a) or plasminogen-activator inhibitor levels).

Sudden coronary death probably involves a rapidly progressive coronary lesion in which plaque rupture and resultant thrombosis lead to ischemia and fatal ventricular arrhythmias [59,60]. Absence of collateral flow to the myocardium distal to the occlusion or platelet microemboli [89] perhaps contribute to the development of sudden ischemic death.

In summary, the natural history of acute coronary syndromes probably mirrors that of the underlying ruptured plaque. Stabilization would correspond to resealing of a rupture, accentuation of symptoms to development of mural thrombosis, non-Q-wave infarction to development of transient occlusion, and transmural Q-wave infarction to establishment of a persistent occlusive thrombus. Furthermore, this natural history may be modified by vascular tone and presence of collateral circulation.

Acute Cerebral Ischemia. Clinical manifestations of atherosclerotic disease in the cerebral circulation (intracranial and extracranial arteries) results in a spectrum of acute cerebral ischemic syndromes ranging from transient ischemic attacks to full-blown cerebral infarction. Transient ischemic attacks are brief episodes of focal loss of brain function with a rapid onset and usually lasting minutes. Arbitrarily, episodes lasting less than 24 hours are classified as transient ischemic attacks, although the longer the episode, the greater the likelihood of a cerebral infarction to develop. As in acute coronary syndromes, duration of thrombotic occlusion and presence of collateral circulation are key elements in determining the outcome of the ischemic cerebrovascular syndromes. Although thrombosis over a disrupted atherosclerotic plaque probably plays a key pathogenic role in a great majority of patients suffering from cerebrovascular events, in contrast to acute coronary syndromes, other pathogenic mechanisms such as arterial embolism, cardiogenic embolism, intracranial hemorrhage, and subarachnoid hemorrhage also play a role in a substantial proportion of these patients.

The exact mechanism by which carotid atherosclerotic lesions lead to cerebrovascular ischemic syndromes remains speculative. Recently, as in coronary syndromes, plaque fissuring and exposure of plaque content to flowing blood has been suggested as being necessary for thrombus formation in the carotid system [90]. Mural thrombi can either contribute to obstruction and progression of the lesion or, more important, give rise to emboli. It has been assumed that fragments of mural thrombi of extracranial atheromatous plaques break down and cause cerebral ischemia by impacting within distal intracranial arteries [91,92]. However, other sources of emboli, such as the cardiac chambers, may be important contributors to the pathogenic mechanism of cerebral ischemia. Clinical data indicate that at least 25 percent of all cerebral ischemic events are associated with atrial fibrillation [93], and about one in three patients with atrial fibrillation will experience a cerebral ischemic event during his or her lifetime.

As in coronary lesions, plaque composition in carotid lesions might be a key factor in determining the likelihood of rupture and thrombotic response. Carotid ultrasound studies have shown that complex, echolucent plaques and those with stenosis greater than 75 percent are most likely to develop cerebrovascular symptoms [94]. Examination of endarterectomy specimens removed from patients with and without ischemic neurologic symptoms have found that plaques associated with symptoms have large atheromatous cores, focally disrupted fibrous caps, and juxtaposed regions of highly different composition. In such lesions, focal concentrations of circumferential stress may occur that might well lead to plaque fissuring [62]. At least one small series has clearly suggested plaque rupture and thrombosis as the pathogenic mechanism of cerebral ischemia in carotid artery disease [90], and results from the North American Symptomatic Carotid Endarterectomy Trial (NASCET) have recently shown that angiographically defined carotid ulceration is associated with an increased risk of stroke in patients with severe carotid stenosis [95]. The ongoing multi-institutional cooperative study NASCET-ACAS (Asymptomatic Carotid Atherosclerotic Study) Plaque Project [96] is likely to be helpful for comparing the pathophysiology of cerebral and coronary ischemic syndromes.

Acute Peripheral Ischemia. Acute peripheral ischemia is characterized by abrupt onset of excruciating pain and coldness in the distal portion of an extremity. The pain may be knifelike or have a burning, paresthetic quality. Up to a certain point, increasing ischemia creates more pain, but when ischemia is very marked, there actually may be less pain. When peripheral nerves become very ischemic, axonal degeneration occurs and the extremity becomes numb.

Major causes of acute peripheral occlusion include embolism, acute arterial thrombosis, intense vasospasm, and aortic dissection. Embolism is by far the most common cause of acute arterial occlusion of the extremities [97]. The source of thromboembolism may be the arterial system itself (mainly by rupture and thrombosis in atherosclerotic plaques located in the abdominal aorta) or the heart (valvular disease, arrhythmias, or cardiomyopathies). Embolism in a previously nonstenotic artery is more likely when symptoms occur suddenly in a patient without prior claudication and with risk factors for thromboembolism (such as atrial fibrillation, left ventricular failure, prosthetic heart valves, or aortic aneurysm). When that occurs, advanced ischemia is common, owing to inadequate time for development of collateral circulation. In such cases, limb acute ischemia may be a prelude to even more disastrous emboli in vital areas such as the cerebral, mesenteric, and renal arteries.

The second major category of acute arterial obstruction involves in-situ thrombosis. Most patients with acute arterial thrombosis in an extremity have had symptoms or signs of peripheral arterial disease before the acute event. In some cases, the vessel is so close to total obstruction before the acute event and collateral circulation so well established, that the patient notices only an increase in severity of the previous claudication. When in-situ thrombosis complicates an existing lesion, the presumed mechanism in many cases is also plaque rupture, as previously described, but stasis of blood flow in a severely stenotic lesion also may be important. The clinical outcome in such cases depends mostly on the adequacy of collateral circulation.

Role of Vasospasm

Disordered control of vasomotor tone with tendencies toward vasoconstriction is an important pathophysiologic mechanism involved across the spectrum of the various ischemic syndromes. Vasospasm causing ischemia was first demonstrated directly by angiography by Maseri and his colleagues in 1978 [98]. They showed spontaneous occlusive coronary vasospasm in patients with unstable angina pectoris.

The endothelium can profoundly affect vascular tone by releasing relaxing factors such as prostacyclin [99] and endothelium-derived relaxing factor. The latter, identified as nitric oxide, can also prevent platelet deposition [100]. Endothelium also releases contracting factors such as endothelin-1 [101]. Under physiologic conditions, endothelium-derived relaxing factor seems to predominate. However, under pathologic conditions, such as those of atherosclerosis, endothelium generates more mediators that enhance constriction and fewer mediators that enhance dilation. Mechanisms that may account for a decreased activity in endothelium-mediated vasodilatation include: (1) decreased production of nitric oxide [102,103]; (2) normal or even increased production of nitric oxide but increased degradation to inactive metabolites by the abnormal redox environment of the diseased artery with increased production of oxygen radicals [104–106]; (3) enhanced direct contractile sensitivity of vascular smooth muscle cells in diseased arteries; and (4) increased local concentration of vasoconstriction agents. Indeed, local secretion of endothelium-derived relaxing factor seems to be diminished in atherosclerotic human coronary arteries [107]. For example, a paradoxical vasoconstrictor response to acetylcholine has been demonstrated in atherosclerotic coronary arteries in humans [75,108], a response that has been attributed to endothelial dysfunction. Exercise [109] and cold pressor testing [110] dilated normal coronary arteries but constricted both minimally and advanced stenotic lesions. A recent coronary arteriographic study in humans suggested that there is a progressive impairment of endothelial vasoactive function, beginning with a selective endothelial dysfunction in angiographically normal arteries in patients with hypercholesterolemia and progressing to vasoconstriction in response to several agonists in atherosclerotic coronary arteries [111]. Furthermore, endothelial-dependent relaxation becomes defective with increasing risk factors, such as smoking and a family history for coronary artery disease, even before disease is angiographically apparent [112]. High-resolution ultrasound performed in femoral and brachial arteries of symptom-free children and young adults with risk factors for atherosclerosis also have demonstrated impairment in endothelium-dependent vasodilatation even before anatomic evidence of plaque formation [113]. Thus, endothelial-dependent dilation, probably the single most important intrinsic vasodilator system, is defective in atherosclerosis and undoubtedly contributes to the increased vasoconstriction and disordered vasomotor control in the disease.

Vasospasm also plays an important role in unstable ischemic syndromes. The constrictor predominance present in atherosclerotic disease may be enhanced further in the unstable state by increasing sensitivity to vasoconstrictors. Furthermore, when the endothelium has been injured or removed, such as occurs in plaque rupture, platelet-dependent vasoconstriction mediated by serotonin and thromboxane A_2 [114,115] and thrombin-dependent vasoconstriction may occur, suggesting a direct interaction of these substances with smooth muscle cells. This information, along with recent data obtained in humans after percutaneous angioplasty [116,117], supports the angiographic observation that transient vasoconstriction accompanies plaque disruption and thrombosis in the acute coronary syndromes [118].

In summary, in chronic ischemic syndromes, stable atherosclerotic disease is associated with abnormal vasodilatation or an exaggerated vasoconstriction response, due to dysfunction in endothelial-dependent dilation mechanisms. Similarly, the presence of atherogenic risk factors, such as hypercholesterolemia, may increase the likelihood of vasoconstriction, whereas in acute ischemic syndromes, there is a predisposition for platelet-dependent and thrombin-dependent transient vasoconstriction to occur at the site of plaque disruption and thrombosis.

Role of Collateral Circulation

An important anatomical factor that may modify the hemodynamic effects of an atherosclerotic obstruction is the presence of collateral circulation. Collaterals are anastomotic connections without an intervening capillary bed between portions of the same artery or between different arteries.

In human hearts, the distribution and the extent of collateral vessels are quite variable. Under physiologic conditions, collateral vessels generally are less than 40 μm in diameter and appear to have little or no function. However, when myocardial perfusion is compromised by obstructions affecting major vessels, collateral vessels enlarge, and blood flow through them increases [119]. Collaterals become angiographically visible only when coronary occlusion is complete or virtually so. Collaterals may equal perfusion through a vessel with 90 percent stenosis of the luminal diameter [120], providing perfusion just sufficient to maintain myocardial viability and prevent myocardial infarction. There is very little information regarding the ways in which coronary collateral circulation can be stimulated. Exercise [121,122] and gradual rather than abrupt coronary occlusion [120] appear to enhance the development of collaterals. New technologies aimed at the full understanding of collateral recruitment and angiogenesis and the therapeutic impact of growth factors are being investigated in several animal models.

Positron-emission tomography studies have shown that neither the presence nor the severity of unilateral carotid disease is a reliable indicator of the hemodynamic status distal to a stenosis in the ipsilateral cerebral hemisphere [20]. However, there exists a significant relation between the cerebral hemodynamic status and the pattern of collateral circulation as determined by carotid angiography. Arterial supply to the middle cerebral artery territory ipsilateral to a severe carotid lesion can be determined by flow through the carotid itself, through the anterior circle of Willis from the opposite carotid circulation, through the ipsilateral opthalmic artery from the external carotid artery, or through meningeal anastomotic channels across the surface of the brain from the anterior cerebral circulation [20]. Because of this extensive network of collaterals in the cerebrovascular system, little rationale exists for using the degree of stenosis to assume hemodynamic consequences and risk for stroke in carotid artery disease. Indeed, studies investigating the relation between the severity of carotid stenosis and the subsequent risk for stroke in patients with asymptomatic carotid artery disease have produced conflicting results. Some have shown an increased risk for stroke with increasing stenosis [123,124], whereas others have not [125,126]. As discussed earlier, patients with severe carotid artery disease may be at increased risk for subsequent stroke due to nonhemodynamic factors, such as atherosclerotic plaque instability, particularly plaque rupture and thromboembolism. Further, plaque composition rather than hemodynamic consequences of the stenosis may be more important in determining the prognosis of carotid artery disease.

In the lower extremities, atherosclerosis tends to be slowly progressive and, because extensive collateral circulation develops, to remain asymptomatic for long periods of time. Only about one-third of patients with definitive arterial occlusions will report intermittent claudication [127,128]. When an arterial occlusion develops, the severity of the insult depends to a large extent on the patient's ability to summon immediate collateral circulation. The speed of opening of collateral vessels is quite variable and is governed by several factors. The length of the occluded arterial segment, the prior status of the peripheral circulation, and the location of the occlusion affect the outcome [97]. A more proximally located occlusion allows more capacity for collateral flow than distal obstruction. Thus, an aortoiliac occlusion is less likely to threaten limb survival than a popliteal artery occlusion. Even when an artery is abruptly occluded, some collateral vessels may open immediately. A femoral arteriogram taken 24 hours after a traumatic occlusion of the popliteal artery often shows numerous collateral branches from the profunda femoral clustered around the hip; however, these vessels are not delivering much blood to vessels beyond the obstruction. In contrast, a femoral arteriogram of a patient with chronic femoropopliteal disease usually shows a wide profunda femoral artery extending halfway down the thigh with ramifications that meet elongated geniculate arteries or collaterals from the tibial arteries. In such cases, extensive blood flow through those alternate channels effectively nourishes the limb.

References

1. Shepherd JT, et al. Report of the task force on vascular medicine. Circulation 1994; 89:532–535.
2. National Heart, Lung and Blood Institute: NHLBI Fact Book, Fiscal Year 1992. Washington, D.C.: US Dept of Health and Human Services, National Institutes of Health, 1993.
3. Kannel WB, Thom TJ. Incidence, prevalence and mortality of cardiovascular diseases. In W Hurst, The Heart, 8th ed., RC Schlant, RW Alexander, eds. New York: McGraw-Hill, 1994.
4. Hughson WG, Mann JI, Garrod A. Intermittent claudication: prevalence and risk factors. Br Med J 1978; 1:1379–1381.
5. Kannel WB, et al. Intermittent claudication: incidence in the Framingham Study. Circulation 1970; 41:875–883.
6. Reunanen A, Takkunen H, Aromaa A. Prevalence of intermittent claudication and its effect on mortality. Acta Med Scand 1982; 211:249–256.
7. Fowkes FG, et al. Edinburgh Artery Study: prevalence of asymptomatic and symptomatic peripheral arterial disease in the general population. Int J Epidemiol 1991; 20:384–392.
8. Dormandy J, et al. Fate of the patient with chronic leg ischaemia. J Cardiovasc Surg 1989; 30:50–57.
9. Criqui MH, et al. Peripheral arterial disease in large vessels is epidemiologically distinct from small vessel disease: an analysis of risk factors. Am J Epidemiol 1989; 129:1110–1129.
10. Gordon T, Kannel WB. Premature mortality from coronary heart disease: The Framingham Study. JAMA 1971; 215: 1617–1625.
11. Fuster V, et al. The pathogenesis of coronary artery disease and the acute coronary syndromes. N Eng J Med 1992; 326: 242–250, 310–318.
12. Fuster V. Lewis A. Connor Memorial Lecture: Mechanisms leading to acute myocardial infarction: Insights from studies in vascular biology. Circulation 1993; 88:I-A–I-B.
13. Berne RM, Rubio R. Coronary circulation. In RM Berne, S Sperelakis, SR Geiger, eds. Handbook of Physiology, Sec 2: The Cardiovascular System, Vol 1: The Heart. Bethesda, MD: American Physiological Society 1979. Pp. 873–952.
14. Gould KL, Lipscomb K, Calvert C. Compensatory changes of the distal coronary vascular bed during progressive constriction. Circulation 1975; 51:1085–1094.
15. Berne RM. The role of adenosine in the regulation of coronary blood flow. Cir Res 1980; 47:807–813.
16. Feigl EO. Coronary Physiology. Physiol Rev 1983; 63:54–96.
17. Furchgott RF. Role of endothelium in responses of vascular smooth muscle. Cir Res 1983; 53:557–573.
18. Moncada S, Vane JR. Pharmacology and endogenous roles of prostaglandin endoperoxides, thromboxabe A_2 and prostacyclin. Pharmacol Rev 1978; 30:293–331.
19. Heistad DD, et al. Augmented responses to vasoconstrictor stimuli in hypercholesterolemic and atherosclerotic monkeys. Cir Res 1984; 54:711–718.
20. Powers WJ, et al. The effect of hemodynamically significant carotid artery disease on the hemodynamic status of the cerebral circulation. Ann Inter Med 1987; 106:27–35.
21. Powers WJ, et al. Cerebral blood flow and cerebral metabolic rate of oxygen requirements for cerebral function and viability in humans. J Cereb Blood Flow Metab 1985; 5:600–608.
22. Powers WJ, Raichle ME. Positron emission tomography and its application to the study of cerebrovascular disease in man. Stroke 1985; 16:361–76.
23. Friedman SA. Arteriosclerosis obliterans of the lower extremities. In SA Friedman, ed. Vascular Diseases: a Concise Guide to Diagnosis, Management, Pathogenesis and Prevention. Boston: 1982. Pp. 1–30.
24. Gibson CM, et al. Relation of vessel wall shear stress to atherosclerosis progression in human coronary arteries. Atherosclerosis and Thrombosis 1993; 13:310–315.
25. Ross R. The pathogenesis of atherosclerosis: a perspective for the 1990s. Nature 1993; 362:801–809.
26. van der Wal AC, et al. Adhesion molecules on the endothelium and mononuclear cells in human atherosclerotic lesions. Am J Pathol 1992; 141:1427–1433.
27. Stary HC. Evolution and progression of atherosclerotic lesions on coronary arteries of children and young adults. Arteriosclerosis 1989; 9:I19–I32.
28. Stary HC. Composition and classification of human atherosclerotic lesions. Virchows Archiv A Pathol Anat 1992; 421:277–290.
29. Falk E. Why do plaques rupture? Circulation 1992; 86:III30–III42.
30. Davies MJ. A macro and micro view of coronary vascular insult in ischemic heart disease. Circulation 1990; 82[Suppl II]:II38–II46.
31. Bouch DC, Montgomery GL. Cardiac lesions in fatal cases of recent myocardial ischaemia from a coronary care unit. Br Heart J 1970; 32:795–803.

32. Hangartner JRW, et al. Morphological characteristics of clinically significant coronary artery stenosis in stable angina. Br Heart J 1986; 56:501–508.
33. Bruschke A, et al. The anatomic evaluation of coronary artery disease demonstrated by coronary angiography in 256 non-operated patients. Circulation 1981; 63:527–540.
34. Davies MJ, Thomas AC. Plaque fissuring: The cause of acute myocardial infarction, sudden ischemic death and crescendo angina. Br Heart J 1985; 53:363–373.
35. Bini A, et al. Identification and distribution of fibrinogen, fibrin and fibrin(ogen) degradation products in atherosclerosis: Use of monoclonal antibodies. Arteriosclerosis 1989; 9:109–121.
36. Ferns GAA, et al. Inhibition of neointimal smooth muscle accumulation after angioplasty by an antibody to PDGF. Science 1991; 253:1129–1132.
37. Berk BC, et al. Thrombin stimulated events in cultured vascular smooth muscle cells. Biochem J 1991; 265:17334–17340.
38. Jones A, Geczy CL. Thrombin and factor Xa enhance the production of interleukin-1. Immunology 1990; 71236–71241.
39. Naito M, et al. Effects of fibrinogen and fibrin on the migration of vascular smooth muscle cells in vitro. Atherosclerosis 1990; 83:9–14.
40. Zhang Y, et al. Plasma protein insudation as an index of early coronary atherogenesis. Am J Patho 1993; 143:496–506.
41. Smith EB, Keen GA, Grant A. Factors influencing the accumulation in fibrous plaques of lipid derived from low-density lipoprotein. I. Relation between fibrin and immobilization of apo B-containing lipoprotein. Atherosclerosis 1990; 84:165–171.
42. Smith EB, Cochran S. Factors influencing the accumulation in fibrous plaques of lipid derived from low-density lipoprotein. II. Preferential immobilization of lipoprotein[a] (lp[a]). Atherosclerosis 1990; 84:173–181.
43. Niendorf A, et al. Morphological detection and quantitation of lipoprotein(a) deposition in atheromatous lesions of human aorta and coronary arteries. Virchows Arch A Pathol Anat 1990; 417:105–111.
44. Beisiegel U, et al. Lipoprotein(a) in the arterial wall. Eur Heart J 1990; 11(E):174–183.
45. Waters D, Craven TE, Lespérance J. Prognostic significance of progression of coronary atherosclerosis. Circulation 1993; 87:1067–1075.
46. Alderman EL, et al. Five-year angiographic follow-up of factors associated with progression of coronary artery disease in the Coronary Artery Surgery Study (CASS). J Am Coll Cardiol 1993; 22:1141–1154.
47. Chesebro J, et al. Antiplatelet therapy in coronary artery disease progression: reduced infarction and new lesion formation (Abstr). Circulation 1989; 80:II266.
48. Melandri G, et al. Benefit of adding low molecular weight heparin to the conventional treatment of stable angina pectoris. A double-bind, randomized, placebo-controlled trial. Circulation 1993; 88:2517–2523.
49. Deedwania PC. Increased myocardial oxygen demand and ischemia during daily life: Resurrection of an age-old concept. J Am Coll Cardiol 1992; 20:1099–1100.
50. Ringqvist I, et al. Prognostic value of angiographic indices of coronary artery disease from the coronary artery surgery study (CASS). J Clin Invest 1983; 71:1854.
51. Wolf PA, et al. Asymptomatic carotid bruit and risk of stroke—The Framingham Study. JAMA 1981; 245:1442–1445.
52. Heyman A, et al. Risk of stroke in asymptomatic persons with cervical arterial bruits. N Eng J Med 1980; 302:838–841.
53. Cutjer JL. Cerebrovascular disease in an elderly population. Circulation 1967; 36:394–399.
54. Sandock BA, et al. Carotid artery bruits-Prevalence survey and differential diagnosis. Mayo Clin Proc 1982; 57:227–230.
55. Friedman SA. Ischemic disease of the brain. In SA Friedman, ed. Vascular Diseases: a Concise Guide to Diagnosis, Management, Pathogenesis and Prevention. Boston. Pp. 279–305; 1982.
56. Pentecost MJ, et al. Guidelines for peripheral percutaneous transluminal angioplasty of the abdominal aorta and lower extremity vessels. A statement for health professionals from a special writing group of the Councils on Cardiovascular Radiology, Arteriosclerosis, Cardio-Thoracic and Vascular Surgery, Clinical Cardiology, and Epidemiology and Prevention, the American Heart Association. Circulation 1994; 89:511–531.
57. Richardson PD, Davies MJ, Born GVR. Influence of plaque configuration and stress distribution on fissuring of coronary atherosclerotic plaques. Lancet 1989; 2:941–944.
58. Falk E. Unstable angina with fatal outcome: dynamic coronary thrombosis leading to infarction and/or sudden death: autopsy evidence of recurrent mural thrombosis with peripheral embolization culminating in total vascular occlusion. Circulation 1985; 71:699–708.
59. Davies MJ, et al. Factors influencing the presence or absence of acute coronary thrombi in sudden ischemic death. Eur Heart J 1989; 10:203–208.
60. Davies MJ, Thomas A. Thrombosis and acute coronary artery lesions in sudden cardiac ischemic death. N Eng J Med 1984; 310:1137–1140.
61. McIsaac AI, Thomas JD, Topol EJ. Toward the quiescent coronary plaque. J Am Coll Cardiol 1993; 22:1228–1241.
62. Cheng GC, et al. Distribution of circumferential stress in ruptured and stable atherosclerotic lesions. A structural analysis with histopathological correlation. Circulation 1993; 87:1179–1187.
63. Kragel AH, et al. Morphometric analysis of the composition of atherosclerotic plaques in the four major epicardial coronaries in acute myocardial infarction and sudden coronary death. Circulation 1989; 80:1747–1756.
64. van der Wall AC, et al. Site of intimal rupture or erosion of thrombosed coronary atherosclerotic plaques is characterized by an inflammatory process irrespective of the dominant plaque morphology. Circulation 1994; 89:36–44.
65. Shah PK, et al. Human monocyte-derived macrophages express collagenase and induce collagen breakdown in atherosclerotic fibrous caps: implications for plaque rupture. Circulation 1995; 92:1565.
66. Davies MJ, et al. Risk of thrombosis in human atherosclerotic plaques: role of extracellular lipid, macrophages, and smooth muscle cell content. Br Heart J 1993; 69:377–381.
67. Fuster V, et al. Insights into the pathogenesis of acute ischemic syndromes. Circulation 1988; 77:1213–1220.
68. Constantinides P. Pathogenesis of cerebral artery thrombosis in man. Arch Pathol 1967; 83:422–428.
69. Sherman DG, Hart RG. Stroke and transient ischemic attack: Thromboembolism and antithrombotic therapy. In Thrombosis in Cardiovascular Disorders. V Fuster, ed. Philadelphia: Saunders, 1992. Pp. 409–422.
70. Chesebro JH, et al. Antithrombotic therapy and progression of coronary artery disease: Antiplatelets versus antithrombins. Circulation 1992; 86[Suppl III]:III100–III111.
71. Fernandez-Ortiz A, et al. Characterization of the relative thrombogenicity of atherosclerotic plaque components: Implications for consequences of plaque rupture. J Am Coll Cardiol 1994. In press.
72. Wilcox JN, et al. Localization of tissue factor in the normal vessel wall and in the atherosclerotic plaque. Proc Natl Acad Sci USA 1989; 86:2839–2843.

73. Lyford CL, et al. The coagulant and thrombogenic properties of human atheroma. Circulation 1967; 35:284–293.
74. Badimon L, Badimon JJ. Mechanism of arterial thrombosis in nonparallel streamlines: Platelet thrombi grow on the apex of stenotic severely injured vessel wall. J Clin Invest 1989; 84:1134–1144.
75. Yeung AC, et al. The effect of atherosclerosis in the vasomotor response of coronary arteries to mental stress. N Engl J Med 1991; 325:1551–1556.
76. Badimon JJ, et al. Platelet deposition at high shear rates is enhanced by high plasma cholesterol levels: in vivo study in the rabbit model. Arterioscler Thromb 1991; 11:395–402.
77. Moliterno DJ, et al. Relation of plasma lipoprotein(a) to infarct artery patency in survivors of myocardial infarction. Circulation 1993; 88:935–940.
78. Woodhouse PR, et al. Seasonal variations of plasma fibrinogen and factor VII activity in the elderly: winter infections and death from cardiovascular disease. Lancet 1994; 343:435–439.
49. Rapold HJ, et al. Plasma fibrinopeptide A levels in patients with acute myocardial infarction treated with alteplase. Correlation with concomitant heparin, coronary artery patency, and recurrent ischemia. Circulation 1992; 85:928–934.
80. Fon EA, et al. Hemostatic markers in acute transient ischemic attacks. Stroke 1994; 25:282–286.
81. Falk E. Coronary thrombosis: Pathogenesis and clinical manifestations. Am J Cardiol 1991; 68:28B–35B.
82. Sherman CT, Litvak F, Grundfest W. Coronary angioscopy in patients with unstable angina. N Eng J Med 1986; 315:913–919.
83. Gotoh H, et al. The role of intracoronary thrombus in unstable angina: Angiographic assessment and thrombolytic therapy during ongoing anginal attacks. Circulation 1988; 77:526–534.
84. DeWood MA, et al. Coronary arteriographic findings soon after non-Q-wave myocardial infarction. N Eng J Med 1986; 315:417–423.
85. Gibson RS, et al. The prevalence and clinical significance of residual myocardial ischemia 2 weeks after uncomplicated non-Q-wave infarction: A prospective natural history study. Circulation 1986; 73:1186–1198.
86. Timmis AD, et al. The effects of early coronary patency on the evolution of myocardial infarction: A prospective angiographic study. Br Heart J 1987; 58:345–351.
87. Ambrose J, et al. Angiographic progression of coronary artery disease and the development of myocardial infarction. J Am Coll Cardiol 1988; 12:56–62.
88. Little WC, et al. Can coronary angiography predict the site of a subsequent myocardial infarction in patients with mild-to-moderate coronary artery disease? Circulation 1988; 78:1157–1166.
89. Fuster V, et al. Atherosclerosis plaque rupture and thrombosis: Evolving concepts. Circulation 1990; 82:II47–II49.
90. Ogata J, et al. Rupture of atheromatous plaque as a cause of thrombotic occlusion of stenotic internal carotid artery. Stroke 1990; 21:1740–1745.
91. Bogousslavsky J, Van Melle G, Regli F. Middle cerebral arterial pial territory infarcts: a study of the Lausanne stroke registry. Ann Neurol 1989; 25:555–560.
92. Fieschi C, et al. Clinical and instrumental evaluation of patients with ischemic stroke within the first six hours. J Neurol Sci 1989; 91:311–312.
93. Halperin J, Hart R. Atrial fibrillation and stroke. New ideas and persisting dilemmas. Stroke 1988; 19:937–947.
94. Langsfeld M, Gray-weale AC, Lusby RJ. The role of plaque morphology and diameter reduction in the development of new symptoms in asymptomatic carotid arteries. J Vasc Surg 1989; 9:548–557.
95. Eliasziw M, et al. Significance of plaque ulceration in symptomatic patients with high-grade carotid stenosis. Stroke 1994; 25:304–308.
96. Fisher M, et al. The NASCET-ACAS Plaque Project. Stroke 1993; 24[Suppl I]:I-24–I-25.
97. Friedman SA. Acute arterial obstruction. In SA Friedman, ed. Vascular Diseases: a Concise Guide to Diagnosis, Management, Pathogenesis and Prevention. Boston: 1982. Pp. 31–62.
98. Maseri A, et al. Coronary vasospasm as a possible cause of myocardial infarction. A conclusion derived from the study of "preinfarction" angina. N Eng J Med 1978; 299:1271–1277.
99. Moncada S, et al. An enzyme isolated from arteries transforms prostaglandin endoperoxides to an unstable substance that inhibits platelet aggregation. Nature 1976; 263:663–665.
100. Palmer RMJ, Ashton DS, Moncada S. Vascular endothelial cells synthesize nitric oxide from L-arginine. Nature 1988; 333:664–666.
101. Yanagisawa M, et al. A novel potent vasoconstrictor peptide produced by vascular endothelial cells. Nature 1988; 332:411–415.
102. Cooke JP, et al. Antiatherogenic effects of L-arginine in the hypercholesterolemic rabbit. J Clin Invest 1992; 90:1168–1172.
103. Rossitch E Jr, et al. L-arginine normalizes endothelial function in cerebral vessels from hypercholesterolemic rabbits. J Clin Invest 1991; 87:1295–1299.
104. Minor RL Jr, et al. Diet-induced atherosclerosis increases the release of nitrogen oxides from rabbit aorta. J Clin Invest 1991; 86:2109–2116.
105. Ohara Y, Peterson TE, Harrison DG. Hypercholesterolemia increases endothelial superoxide anion production. J Clin Invest 1993; 91:2546–2551.
106. Mugge A, et al. Chronic treatment with polyethylene-glycolated superoxide dismutase partially restores endothelium-dependent vascular relaxations in cholesterol-fed rabbits. Circ Res 1991; 69:1293–1300.
107. Chester AH, et al. Low basal and stimulated release of nitric oxide in atherosclerotic epicardial coronary arteries. Lancet 1990; 336:897–900.
108. McLenachan JM, et al. Early evidence of endothelial vasodilator dysfunction of coronary branch points. Circulation 1990; 82:1169–1173.
109. Gordon JB, et al. Atherosclerosis influences the vasomotor response of epicardial coronary arteries to exercise. J Clin Invest 1989; 83:1946–1952.
110. Nabel EG, et al. Dilatation of normal and constriction of atherosclerotic coronary arteries caused by the cold pressor test. Circulation 1988; 77:43–52.
111. Zeiher AM, et al. Modulation of coronary vasomotor tone in humans: progressive endothelial dysfunction with different early stages of coronary atherosclerosis. Circulation 1991; 83:391–401.
112. Vita JA, et al. Coronary vasomotor response to acetylcholine relates to risk factors for coronary artery disease. Circulation 1990; 81:491–497.
113. Celermajer D, et al. Non-invasive detection of endothelial dysfunction in children and adults at risk of atherosclerosis. Lancet 1992; 340:1111–1115.
114. Willerson JT, et al. Specific platelets mediators and unstable coronary artery lesions: experimental evidence and potential clinical implications. Circulation 1989; 80:198–205.
115. Lam JYT, et al. Is vasospasm related to platelet deposition? Relationship in a porcine preparation of arterial injury in vivo. Circulation 1987; 75:243–248.

116. Fishell TA, et al. Coronary artery vasoconstriction routinely occurs after percutaneous transluminal coronary angioplasty. Circulation 1988; 78:1323–1324.
117. el-Tamimi H, et al. Abnormal vasomotor changes early after coronary angioplasty. Circulation 1991; 84:1198–1202.
118. Hackett D, et al. Intermittent coronary occlusion in acute myocardial infarction: value of combined thrombolytic and vasodilatory therapy. N Eng J Med 1987; 317:1055–1059.
119. Habib GB, et al. Influence of coronary collateral vessels on myocardial infarct size in humans: Results of Phase I Thrombolysis in Myocardial Infarction (TIMI) Trial. Circulation 1991; 83:739–746.
120. Patterson RE, et al. Differences in collateral myocardial blood flow following gradual vs abrupt coronary occlusion. Cardiovasc Res 1983; 17:207–213.
121. Cohen MV, Yipintsoi T, Scheuer J. Coronary collateral stimulation by exercise in dogs with stenotic coronary arteries. J Appl Physiol 1982; 52:664–671.
122. Bloor CM, White FC, Sanders M. Effect of exercise on collateral development in myocardial ischemia in pigs. J Appl Physiol 1984; 56:656–665.
123. Roederer GO, et al. The natural history of carotid arterial disease in asymptomatic patients with cervical bruits. Stroke 1984; 15:605–613.
124. Durward QJ, Ferguson GG, Barr HWK. The natural history of asymptomatic carotid bifurcations plaques. Stroke 1982; 13:459–464.
125. Grotta JC, et al. The significance of carotid stenosis or ulceration. Neurology 1984; 34:437–442.
126. Roederer GO, et al. Natural history of carotid artery disease on the side contralateral to endarterectomy. J Vasc Surg 1984; 1:62–72.
127. Fiedman SA, Pandya M, Greif E. Peripheral arterial occlusion in patients with acute coronary heart disease. Am Heart J 1973; 86:415–419.
128. Marinelli MR, et al. Noninvasive testing versus clinical evaluation of arterial disease. JAMA 1979; 241:2031–2039.

Pathogenesis of Essential Hypertension

Jeffrey C. Webber
Allen J. Naftilan

Essential hypertension is undoubtedly the consequence of a variety of diseases; therefore, a single cause probably never will be identified. Many of the physiologic changes seen in hypertensive patients and often hypothesized to be a possible cause are actually the result of compensatory mechanisms rather than truly etiologic. Although hypertension has been demonstrated to cluster in families, environmental factors also contribute to the final blood pressure, rendering the search for genetic causes difficult. Further complicating the picture is the fact that a definitive normal for blood pressure is not available, and people are arbitrarily called hypertensive if their blood pressure deviates from the norm of a unimodal distribution curve. Despite those difficulties, many factors have been implicated as potentially causative. With the advances in molecular biology and genetics, a number of investigators have begun to dissect the individual genes that may be responsible for some forms of human hypertension. It would not be possible to discuss all the possible etiologies of hypertension, so this chapter will be limited to four major topics: the genetics of hypertension and the role of the central nervous system, the role of the kidney, and the possible role of abnormal vasculature as possible etiologies of hypertension.

Genetics

As early as 1761, when Morgagni [1] observed that the father of a patient who died of cerebral apoplexy died from the same cause, it has been noted that high blood pressure clusters in families. Based on the early studies of Weitz [2] and Platt [3], who both found an increased incidence of hypertension in adult siblings of hypertensive probands and evidence for transmission over three generations, it initially was felt that hypertension was inherited as a dominant trait. Those studies were later refuted by the classic St. Mary's Hospital studies [4–6], which concluded that hypertension was inherited as a continuously distributed characteristic rather than a discrete Mendelian trait. In those studies, the blood pressures of 2,031 individuals from the general population were ascertained to determine the distribution of blood pressures in the general population. The blood pressures of first-degree relatives of hypertensive patients were then measured. After adjustment for age and sex, the investigators determined an overall correlation between siblings of 0.24 for systolic blood pressure and 0.22 for diastolic blood pressure. More recent studies from Tecumseh, Michigan, and Framingham, Massachusetts [7,8], have attempted to correct for the added effects of environmental factors. Although their correlations are slightly lower, both studies still support the same conclusions as the St. Mary's Hospital studies. A number of the Framingham sibling pairs were followed for 16 years; despite their living in different households, the correlation coefficients remained unchanged [9].

Many researchers believe that hypertension in an individual is determined by higher genetic susceptibility to environmental factors. To separate those factors, studies of both adoptees and twins have been used. The most extensive studies of adopted children have been performed on a series of families from Montreal, Canada [10], where blood pressure comparisons between 756 adopted children and 445 natural children and 1,176 parents involving 606 households were made. After correcting for a number of known factors that can influence blood pressure, a much greater correlation was observed between natural parents and their children and between siblings than between adoptive parents and children. From that observation, researchers concluded that genetic factors account for 34 percent of the variability in systolic blood pressure and 30 percent of the variability in diastolic blood pressure. A number of twin studies have also supported a strong genetic influence on blood pressure [11,12]. Correlations for monozygotic twins have ranged around 0.80 and for dizygotic twins around 0.40. These numbers must be viewed with caution, however, because it appears that twins exhibit excessive sharing of sociocultural environments, which would tend to exaggerate the effects of genetics. A study of Utah twins [12] suggested that adjustment for weight and other life-style factors may be much more important in twin studies compared to other genetic studies.

A variety of other methods have been used to determine the genetic influence on blood pressure. Schull et al. [13] used the family-set approach to study a black population in Detroit. In that method, the correlation between an individual and two biologic relatives (a sibling and a cousin) is compared to that between two unrelated individuals (the spouse and a cousin). The design takes into account the influence of immediate family environment, neighborhood environment, and genetic factors. Initially, analysis of the data suggested that genetic factors were relatively unimportant, but reanalysis of the data utilizing path analysis [14,15] concluded that approximately 30 percent of the blood-pressure distribution could be explained by genetic factors. Path analysis is based on the concept that every observed correlation can be defined in terms of the underlying factors thought to influence familial resemblance. Relationships are specified as partial regression coefficients of blood pressure and underlying factors, and the squares of those coefficients specify the relative contribution of the factor.

A difficult aspect of studying the genetics of hypertension is that, rather than being a distinct phenotype, hypertension represents a continuum of blood pressure above a normal distribution. The final phenotype is the consequence of a number of physiologic abnormalities that interact with environmental influences. Those physiologic

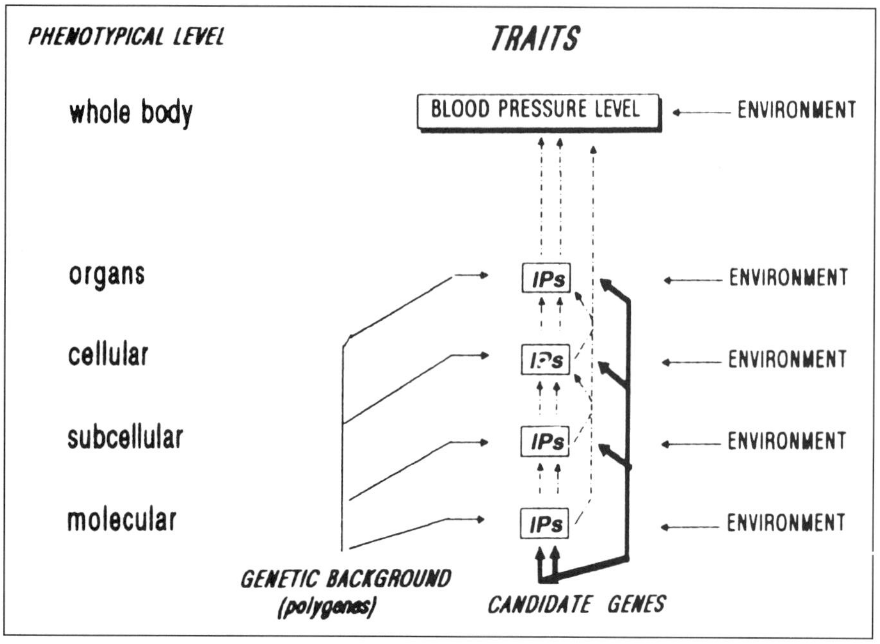

Fig. 15-1. Dissection of a complex trait at different levels of biological organization. IPs = intermediate phenotypes. (Reproduced with permission from A Camussi, G Bianchi. From the unimodal-bimodal controversy to molecular technology. Hypertension 1988; 12:620–628.)

factors have been termed intermediate phenotypes, and there have been numerous attempts to identify the multitude of intermediate phenotypes that contribute to the final blood pressure. Once an intermediate phenotype is defined, the responsible alleles can be identified and mapped. An illustration of how all these factors may interact has been proposed by Camussi and Bianchi [16] and is shown in Fig. 15-1. Once an intermediate phenotype has been identified by the use of molecular techniques, mutagenic alleles can be identified and the interaction of the multiple phenotypes studied.

One possible intermediate phenotype that has been extensively studied because of the potential importance of intracellular sodium in hypertension is transport systems that move sodium across the cell membrane. The best studied of these systems is red blood cell Na^+-Li^+ countertransport. Numerous studies in both hypertensive patients and experimental animals have demonstrated a 1.5- to 2-fold increase in countertransport in hypertensives [17–25]. A likely candidate gene responsible for Na^+-Li^+ countertransport is the gene that encodes for the Na^+-H^+ antiporter [26]. Lifton and colleagues have tested this hypothesis in a series of elegant studies [27,28]. They first localized the Na^+-H^+ antiporter gene to chromosome 1 near the Rh gene and then genotyped 200 individuals in 14 Utah pedigrees for the antiporter gene and 2 flanking markers. They reported a logarithm of the odds (LOD) score of −5.9, excluding linkage of the antiporter gene with Na^+-Li^+ countertransport. To test for linkage of the antiporter gene to hypertension, 93 hypertensive sibling pairs were genotyped. Because the number of shared antiporter genes between hypertensive siblings (0.93) was not greater than expected (1.0), linkage to hypertension was excluded.

Several other intermediate phenotypes have been studied. A number of investigators [29,30] have reported that 40 to 50 percent of patients with essential hypertension are **nonmodulators**, that is, they do not increase their renal plasma flow in response to a high-sodium diet. In addition, they demonstrate a blunted response to infused angiotensin II with respect both to changes in renal blood flow and to stimulation in aldosterone secretion. This trait demonstrates familial aggregation in that a high percentage of patients with a family history of hypertension also are nonmodulators [31], suggesting that this would be a useful trait to map genetically. Although no data have been generated that link this trait to a specific locus, studies are ongoing and may soon provide a clue as to a genetic cause for hypertension.

Two general methods are used to dissect further the genetic cause of a disease: reverse genetics, or positional cloning, and the candidate-gene approach. Linkage studies are performed utilizing random genetic markers, suspected loci are identified, and eventually the responsible gene is identified. This approach has been used successfully for a variety of single-gene diseases, the most publicized of which is cystic fibrosis [32]. Linkage studies are difficult and can be quite time consuming. This is especially true for a polygenic disease such as hypertension, so a candidate-gene approach also has been employed. In the latter method, a gene is identified that may contribute to the hypertensive phenotype, polymorphisms in that gene are identified, and then either a formal linkage analysis is performed in a large family or affected relative-pairs, such as siblings, are studied. In relative-pair analysis, cosegregation of the marker and the disease is evaluated by seeking an excess sharing of the suspected genotype between the two affected siblings. The approach has the advantage of enabling the use of a large number of families, each of a small size, and one does not need to make assumptions concerning the dominance of the locus. The method is limited, however, by its lack of power for finding a formal linkage, which requires the use of a large number of families.

Because of their potential importance in blood pressure regulation, components of the renin-angiotensin system have been studied for genetic abnormalities that may contribute to the genetic phenotype. Since the rate-limiting step in the generation of angiotensin II is the generation of angiotensin I by renin, it was reasonable to assume that a genetic alteration in the renin gene could contribute to the hypertensive phenotype. An initial study demonstrated the lack of any linkage of a renin-gene polymorphism to either hypertension or plasma-renin activity (PRA) in a large Utah family [33]. That study has been reconfirmed in two independent studies. The first report demonstrated no association of a renin-gene polymorphism and essential hypertension [34], while the second performed a sibling-pair analysis in 133 subjects from 57 families and found no linkage of renin genotype to hypertension [35]. The gene for angiotensin-converting enzyme (ACE) also has been studied for potential linkage to human hypertension. Cambien et al [36] first reported that there was a familial resemblance of plasma ACE levels suggesting that there was segregation of a major gene. Since the converting-enzyme gene had been recently demonstrated to be a candidate gene for hypertension in a rat model, Jeunemaitre et al. [37] used the highly polymorphic marker at the human growth hormone locus on chromosome 17, which maps close to the converting-enzyme gene, to perform a sibling-pair linkage study. This analysis was performed on 132 controls and 149 hypertensive subjects in Utah and failed to demonstrate any linkage between the ACE gene and hypertension.

One component of the renin-angiotensin system has been linked to human essential hypertension. In a recent report, Jeunemaitre et al [38] studied linkage of the angiotensinogen gene to hypertension in a sibling-pair analysis. Angiotensinogen is the specific substrate for renin, and the reaction generates angiotensin I. This is the rate-limiting step in the formation of angiotensin II, and since an earlier study had demonstrated a significant correlation between plasma-angiotensinogen concentration and blood pressure [39], the angiotensinogen gene appeared to be an important gene to study. A total of 215 siblingships were studied, 132 from Utah identified in the general population and 83 from Paris accessed from a hypertension clinic. Linkage did not reach significance in the Utah population but did in the group from Paris. When both populations were pooled, significance also was achieved. A more significant linkage was observed when the analysis was restricted to patients with more severe hypertension. It was felt that the lack of significance seen in the Utah population alone was due to the fact that siblingship was ascertained from the general population, and they tended to have less severe hypertension than the Paris population, which was ascertained from a referral hypertension clinic. An alternative explanation could be the more narrowly defined population base in the Utah patients. This hypothesis was supported by the higher level of significance achieved in the patients with severe hypertension. It is also important to note that higher plasma-angiotensinogen levels were noted in carriers of the genotype most commonly associated with hypertension. Certainly these data support the hypothesis that an abnormality in the angiotensinogen gene may contribute to the hypertensive phenotype in the populations studied. Currently, a number of groups are repeating similar studies in different populations, and a definitive answer on the role angiotensinogen plays in essential hypertension awaits the results of these studies.

Another approach to identifying the genetic cause of hypertension is to perform linkage studies in animal models, identify potential genes of interest, and then test the identified gene in human linkage studies. Genetic studies in laboratory animals have the advantage that selective breeding can be conducted to manipulate the phenotype and cross-breeding performed to fix the genetic composition of the strain. Through selective breeding for blood pressure extremes, a number of hypertensive mouse and rat strains have been developed (Table 15-1). Most of these models are in rats, since mice are difficult to perform physiologic studies on due to their small size. The most widely studied of these are the spontaneously hypertensive rat (SHR) strain developed by Okamato et al. [42] and the salt-sensitive and resistant strains developed by Dahl et al. [41] (Dahl-R and Dahl-S, respectively). A set of four criteria have been proposed by Rapp [47] that must be met for a biochemical or physiologic trait to be accepted as causing a genetic difference in blood pressure:

1. A difference in the trait must be demonstrated between the two strains.
2. The trait must follow Mendelian inheritance.
3. The genes identified must cosegregate with an increment in blood pressure that is greater than zero.
4. There must be some logical link between the trait and blood pressure.

Both the candidate-gene approach and positional cloning have been used to identify possible genes involved in blood pressure control in these animal strains. One of the first descriptions of an abnormal genotype possibly contributing to hypertension is the report by Rapp and his colleagues [48,49] that a polymorphism in the renin gene segregated with the salt-sensitive allele in an F1 and F2 population of a Dahl-S and Dahl-R cross. By examining the blood pressure of the F2 population as a function of genotype, they were able to estimate that the polymorphism in the renin allele in the S-rat accounted for approximately a difference of 10 mm Hg in blood pressure. It is important to note, however, that these data do not prove that an alteration in the renin gene contributes to hypertension in the Dahl rat, since an abnormality in an unknown gene closely linked to the renin gene on the same chromosome would give the same results. More recently, Deng and Rapp [49a] have documented highly significant cosegregation of the inducible nitric oxide synthase locus (*Nos 2*) with blood pressure in the Dahl-S rat. A similar study in the SHR has been reported by Kurtz et al [50].

Table 15-1. Rodent strains selectively bred for blood pressure

Strain	Lines[a]	Original stock	Generations[b]	Systolic BP[c]	Year first reported, reference
RATS					
New Zealand (Dunedin): genetically hypertensive (GH) rats	H, C	Wistar-derived	25	180	Smirk et al. [40]
USA (Brookhaven): salt-sensitive (S) and salt-resistant (R) rats	H, L	Sprague-Dawley	7	170	Dahl et al. [41]
Japan (Kyoto): spontaneously hypertensive rats (SHR)	H	Wistar-derived	4	200	Okamoto et al. [42]
Israel (Jerusalem): Doca-salt-sensitive (SBH) and -resistant (SBN) rats	H, L	Not given	6	185	Ben-Ishay et al. [43]
France: Lyon hypertensive (LH), Lyon normotensive (LN), and Lyon low blood pressure (LL) rats	H, C, L	Sprague-Dawley	5	180	Dupont et al. [44]
Italy: Milan hypertensive strain (MHS) and Milan normotensive (MNS) rats	H, C	Wistar	5	175	Bianchi et al. [45]
MOUSE					
USA: BP 1	H, C, L	8-way cross of inbred lines	17	150	Schlager [46]

[a] H = line selected for high blood pressure; C = control line, unselected, random bred; L = line selected for low blood pressure.
[b] Number of generations to achieve maximum response in the hypertensive line.
[c] Systolic blood pressure (mm Hg) of the hypertensive line at plateau of selection response.

They found that a polymorphism that marked the SHR renin gene in a F2 population generated by a cross with the Lewis rat segregated with an increased blood pressure. Again, further studies will be needed to clearly define if an abnormal renin gene really contributes to the elevated blood pressure seen in these rats or if a closely linked gene is responsible for the differences in blood pressure.

A further advantage of studying genetics in animals is the ease with which one can perform positional cloning since multiple crosses can be easily examined. This kind of study was performed by two groups independently [51,52] on a cross between the Wistar-Kyoto (WKY) rat and the spontaneously hypertensive stroke-prone rat, a substrain of the original SHR. This cross had been performed and phenotypically analyzed previously [53], and the DNA from the F2 population was available for analysis. Both groups found linkage (LODs > 5) to rat chromosome 10 (corresponding to human chromosome 17). This region is closely linked to the ACE gene in both rats and humans, raising the possibility that the ACE gene is a candidate gene in essential hypertension. At the time, the one human study that looked for linkage of the ACE gene with hypertension in a large patient population was negative [37]. Also, even though linkage to a region near the ACE gene in rats has been demonstrated, that by no means demonstrates that an abnormality in the gene product is responsible for hypertension.

In an effort to find new candidate genes that contribute to hypertension, Iwai and Inagami [54] performed differential screening for messenger RNA species expressed in SHR and WKY rat kidneys. One of these genes, called SA, was expressed at least at 10-fold higher levels in the SHR compared to the WKY rat. This gene was mapped to chromosome 1, and evidence for cosegregation of SA or closely linked markers and hypertension has been described in a number of SHR and WKY-rat crosses [55,56]. Recently, Iwai et al. [57] found an association between a polymorphism in the human SA gene and essential hypertension in a small Japanese population, providing preliminary evidence that SA may be a candidate gene worthy of further study. The function of the SA gene is at present unknown, but elucidation of its function could provide new insight into the pathophysiology of essential hypertension. Of course, its elevation in the kidney of the SHR could be just a consequence of the hypertension, but further studies should help answer that question.

In summary, it is clear that a number of genes contribute to the hypertensive phenotype. Although a number of candidates in both humans and animal models have been found, no genetic abnormality that definitively elevates blood pressure has been identified. Further research using both animal models and improved gene-mapping techniques in patients should provide new data soon.

The Role of The Kidney

The kidneys exert a powerful influence on blood pressure regulation and act as the primary organ system through which multiple, complex regulatory pathways maintain blood volume and pressure homeostasis. An important function of the kidney is to monitor and normalize blood volume, chiefly by controlling the rate and the extent of sodium excretion. Sodium is the principal extracellular ion in vertebrates, and perturbations in net sodium excretion may adversely modulate total body volume, cardiac output, and arterial blood pressure through multiple mechanisms.

The kidney is also the primary organ involved in the renin-angiotensin-aldosterone system (RAS). The juxta-

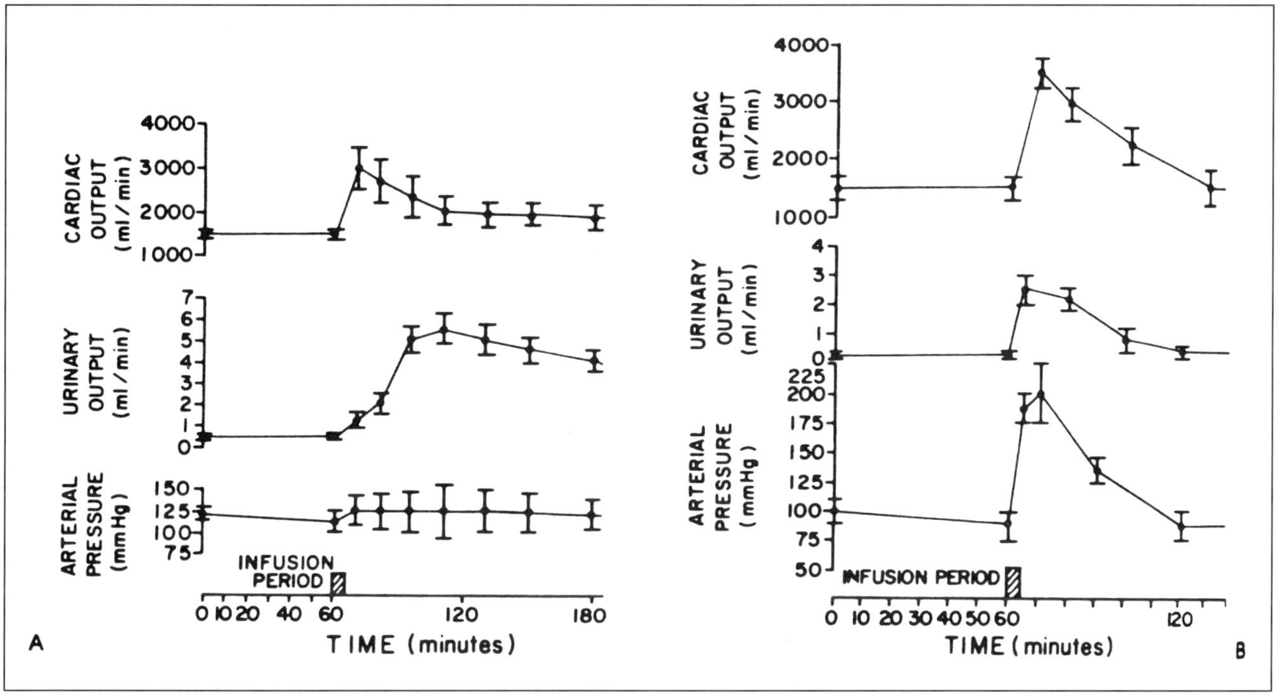

Fig. 15-2. Effect of transfusing a volume of blood into dogs equal to approximately 40 percent of the animal's own blood volume over a period of 4 minutes with either (**A**) intact cardiovascular neural reflexes or (**B**) after destruction of the nervous system to block all cardiovascular neural reflexes. (Reproduced with permission from WA Dobbs, JW Prather, AC Guyton. Relative importance of nervous control of cardiac output and arterial pressure. Am J Cardiol 1971; 27:507–512.)

glomerular cells located in each individual nephron unit produce renin, the enzyme responsible for the conversion of angiotensinogen (produced mainly in the liver) to angiotensin I, which eventually is converted by ACE in the lungs to angiotensin II, a potent vasoconstrictor and mediator of aldosterone secretion. This chain of events beginning in the kidney results in further sodium retention by virtue of aldosterone's effects on the distal renal tubule, as well as angiotensin II's effect on glomerular afferent arteriolar tone and, perhaps to a lesser extent, by the vasoconstrictive effects of angiotensin II on peripheral vascular resistance. The contribution of the RAS to renovascular hypertension in patients exhibiting significant renal artery stenosis is well known. However, data also suggest that dysfunction of this system might play an important role in patients with essential (as opposed to renovascular) hypertension, as well. Experimental-animal data demonstrate different temporal determinants of blood pressure regulation. Short-term (minutes to a few hours) regulators of blood pressure control exert their influences primarily via the nervous system. Baroreceptor, chemoreceptor, and central nervous system ischemic mechanisms provide rapid, transient modulating influences on arterial blood pressure control and tend to obscure the other, more chronic (several hours to days) determinants, including the RAS and the influences of fluid-volume homeostasis.

The temporal distinction between short-term and long-term determinants is well demonstrated in a study performed in dogs during the early 1970s [58]. Guyton et al. performed blood transfusions equaling 40 percent of the anesthetized dogs' total blood volume in a 4-minute period (Fig. 15-2). In the first set of dogs (whose cardiovascular reflexes remained intact), the arterial pressure rose very little in spite of marked increases in cardiac and urinary output. However, a second set of dogs, whose cardiovascular nervous system reflexes had been intentionally destroyed prior to study, exhibited marked increases in arterial pressure as well as cardiac and urinary output. These data demonstrate the importance of short-term modulators of blood pressure control and show that these modulators are neurally mediated. Without their influence, large, rapid fluid shifts can have a profound impact on arterial blood pressure.

The important relationship between arterial blood pressure and volume status in normotensive individuals is depicted by the so-called renal-function curve shown in Fig. 15-3 [59]. In that curve, the equilibrium point represents the blood pressure at which volume homeostasis is achieved. Any other given arterial pressure will lead to a decrease or an increase in blood volume, depending on whether it lies above or below, respectively, the horizontal line transecting the equilibrium point. That point represents the net fluid volume that must be excreted by the kidneys after accounting for all other fluid eliminated via extrarenal pathways (insensible losses, etc.).

From the renal-function curve, it becomes clear that as arterial blood pressure increases returning back to the equilibrium point requires the excretion of body fluid. This is achieved via pressure natriuresis and diuresis,

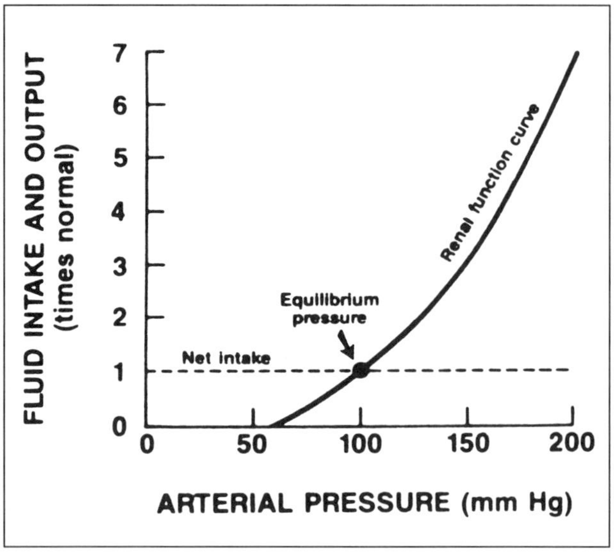

Fig. 15-3. Renal-function curve demonstrating the relationship between arterial pressure and fluid intake and output. This renal volume mechanism allows for long term regulation of blood pressure. (Reproduced with permission from AC Guyton. Textbook of Medical Physiology. Philadelphia: Saunders, 1976. P. 282.)

whereby sodium and water excretion facilitate a return to the prehypertensive state depicted by the equilibrium point. The relative steepness of the curve illustrates the concept that, in individuals with normal renal function, dietary sodium intake may vary substantially with relatively little arterial blood pressure change. If intervening processes were to prevent the requisite natriuresis from restoring volume homeostasis, or if new events were to change the slope of the renal-function curve, one could conceive of how a new equilibrium setpoint might be achieved through which a net positive fluid-volume status would be associated with sustained hypertension. In other words, altered natriuretic responses would contribute to a sustained hypertensive state. Four general mechanisms have been proposed whereby impaired renal function might lead to inadequate natriuretic responses and, thus, hypertension: nephron loss (loss of renal mass), heterogeneity of nephrons, increased renal-sympathetic-nerve activity, and alterations in nephron-cell-membrane ion transport.

Research performed in animal models reveals the development of an abnormal renal-function curve and the propensity toward hypertension in subjects sustaining a reduction in renal mass. Guyton and colleagues, for example, surgically reduced the renal mass of anesthetized dogs by approximately 70 percent and documented the preservation of relatively normal arterial pressures when the dogs were fed a low-sodium diet [60]. However, dramatic increases in blood pressure were observed in the dogs when they were switched to a high-sodium diet. In the setting of reduced renal mass, the renal-function curve generated from these dogs was flatter and shifted to the right, confirming that in that setting mild changes in sodium intake are associated with substantial changes in arterial pressure.

Koletsky and Goodlett confirmed the progressive increase in salt sensitivity with reduced renal mass by exploring the incidence of hypertension in rats exhibiting various decrements in renal mass [61]. Sixty-six percent of control rats (having normal renal mass) fed a high-sodium diet for 8 months became hypertensive. However, when similar rats underwent uninephrectomy (50% nephrectomy) and were then subjected to a high-sodium diet, 94 percent became hypertensive by 4 months. When 75-percent nephrectomies were subsequently performed on a similar set of rats, 100 percent became hypertensive within 2 weeks.

Epidemiologic data gathered from humans with various congenital kidney diseases lend further credence to the purported connection between reduced nephron numbers or loss of renal mass and hypertension. Patients born with a solitary kidney exhibit a higher incidence of hypertension [62], as do patients with oligomeganephronia, a rare congenital disease consisting of bilateral renal hypoplasia [63,64]. Brenner and colleagues hypothesize that the number of nephrons with which people are born is variable and that some people enter this world with deficient glomerular filtration surface areas (FSA) [65]. The reduced FSA forces the remaining glomeruli to filter excessive volumes of plasma, thereby predisposing them to glomerular sclerosis; that in turn reduces the FSA further and perpetuates a cycle of progressive loss of FSA.

A quantitative reduction in nephrons, therefore, seems like a plausible contributor to hypertension. Histologic studies, however, by Sommers et al. [66] of renal-biopsy specimens performed in patients with uncomplicated essential hypertension revealed that only 8 percent of the glomeruli were obsolescent. Instead, focal spasm of afferent renal arterioles, vascular smooth muscle cell hypertrophy with widening of the internal elastic lamina with hyaline leading to focal luminal narrowing, and hyperplasia of juxtaglomerular cells were noted. These observations led Laragh and colleagues to propose the heterogeneity-of-nephrons hypothesis [67,68]. According to that hypothesis, patients with essential hypertension are born with two qualitatively different populations of nephrons. One subset of nephrons is chronically ischemic due to afferent arteriolar vasoconstriction or intrinsic luminal narrowing. They theorize that those nephrons exhibit impaired sodium excretion and, due to local ischemic conditions, secrete high levels of renin. The second subset of nephrons is not ischemic and, therefore, produces normal levels of renin and is capable of normal (or even hyper-) natriuresis.

Laragh's group speculates that the high renin levels produced by the ischemic nephrons circulate and eventually impair sodium excretion in both nephron populations by [68] (1) increasing tubular reabsorption in the hyperfunctioning nephrons; (2) increasing tissue growth factor–mediated afferent arteriolar vasoconstriction in hyperfunctioning nephrons; or (3) providing inadequate renin levels to support efferent arteriolar tone in the hypoperfused nephrons due to the mixing of high renin levels from the ischemic subset with the relatively normal renin levels from the majority hyperfunctioning subset. The net result is that all nephrons are exposed to inappropriate levels of angiotensin II, which in turn leads to sodium retention and subsequent hypertension owing to the pressure-volume relationship discussed previously.

Although the existence of two discrete subpopulations of nephrons is a difficult task to prove, circumstantial evidence does exist in support of this intriguing theory. For example, Laragh [68] reminds us of the wide splay in renin levels seen in patients with essential hypertension, and that ACE inhibitors often exhibit a significant blood pressure effect even in patients with normal renin levels. According to this theory, those observations also indicate that, in patients with hypertension, "normal" renin levels are inappropriately high for their hypertensive condition. Moreover, patients with essential hypertension fail to suppress completely aldosterone secretion on a high-sodium diet or to stimulate aldosterone secretion maximally while on a low-sodium diet [69] or during diuretic therapy [70]. Again, such abnormal hormonal responses might well be due to the presence of inappropriately high circulating levels of renin.

Laragh and colleagues also remind us that patients with essential hypertension demonstrate a hypernatriuretic response when administered intravenous saline, the degree and immediacy of which are intermediate between that noted in normotensive subjects [71–73] and patients with primary hyperalderosteronism [74]. Patients with primary hyperaldosteronism exhibit complete suppression of renin secretion and, hence, a dramatic natriuretic response to saline infusion [74]. According to Laragh's group, essential hypertensives exhibit a lesser natriuretic response to saline infusion because of the production of renin by the subset of ischemic nephrons. On the other hand, their natriuretic response exceeds that of normotensive subjects because of a large subset of adapting hypernatriuretic nephrons. The heterogeneity-of-nephrons theory, therefore, unifies several important features noted in essential hypertension: a morphogenetic basis (two functionally different subsets of nephrons at birth), stereotypic natriuretic responses (hypernatriuresis with saline infusion challenge), and a coherent contributory role of the RAS.

The role of the renal sympathetic nervous system in modulating arterial hypertension has been the focus of intense research for the past quarter century. Urinary sodium and water excretion are known to be regulated in part by the renal sympathetic nerves, which exert their influence by altering renal hemodynamics via changes in renal vascular resistance; modulating renin release from cells of the juxtaglomerular apparatus, leading to changes in angiotensin II production; and innervating renal tubular cells and thereby altering cellular sodium transport directly.

In 1977, Katholi et al. [75] published an important animal study providing a possible link between renal sympathetic input and chronic hypertension. Using a crossover treatment schema, the hemodynamic responses, PRA, and plasma aldosterone levels of conscious, uninephrectomized dogs receiving chronic intrarenal infusions of norepinephrine were compared with those of similar animals receiving chronic infusions of norepinephrine via the inferior vena cava. They noted the development of sustained hypertension associated with transient increases in PRA and plasma aldosterone levels, yet a positive sodium balance in those dogs subjected to chronic intrarenal infusion of norepinephrine (Fig. 15-4). The hemodynamic responses were abolished by the infusion of phentolamine (a selective alpha-1 adrenoreceptor inhibitor), but not by the angiotensin II antagonist Sar^1, Ala^8 angiotensin II (saralasin), implicating the sympathetic nervous system, and not the RAS, and its direct effects on sodium handling as the mediator of this sustained hypertensive response. On the other hand, those dogs treated with norepinephrine infused via the inferior vena cava exhibited only transient elevations in blood pressure coinciding with brief elevations of PRA and plasma aldosterone secretion and an early net natriuresis. These data provide further evidence that increased renal sympathetic nerve activity might play a significant role in the development or maintenance of

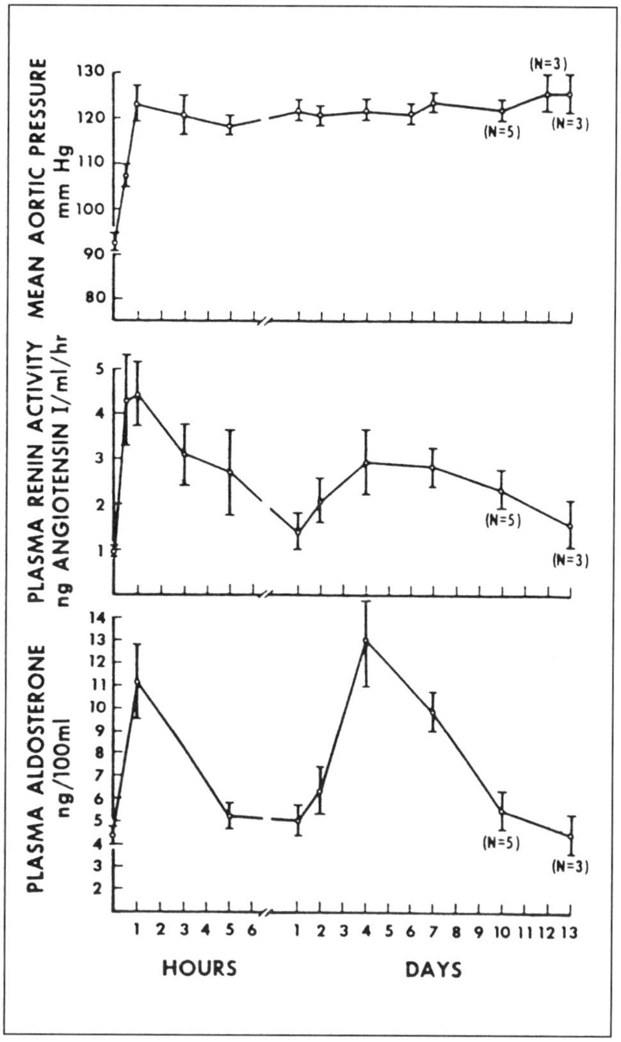

Fig. 15-4. Response to intrarenal norepinephrine infusions of mean arterial pressure (top panel), plasma renin activity (middle panel), and plasma aldosterone level (bottom panel) in dogs. It is important to note the sustained hypertension in this model and the lack of a pressure natriuresis. (Reproduced with permission from RE Katholi et al. Production of sustained hypertension by chronic intrarenal infusion in conscious dogs. Circulation 1977; 40[Suppl I]:I118–I126.)

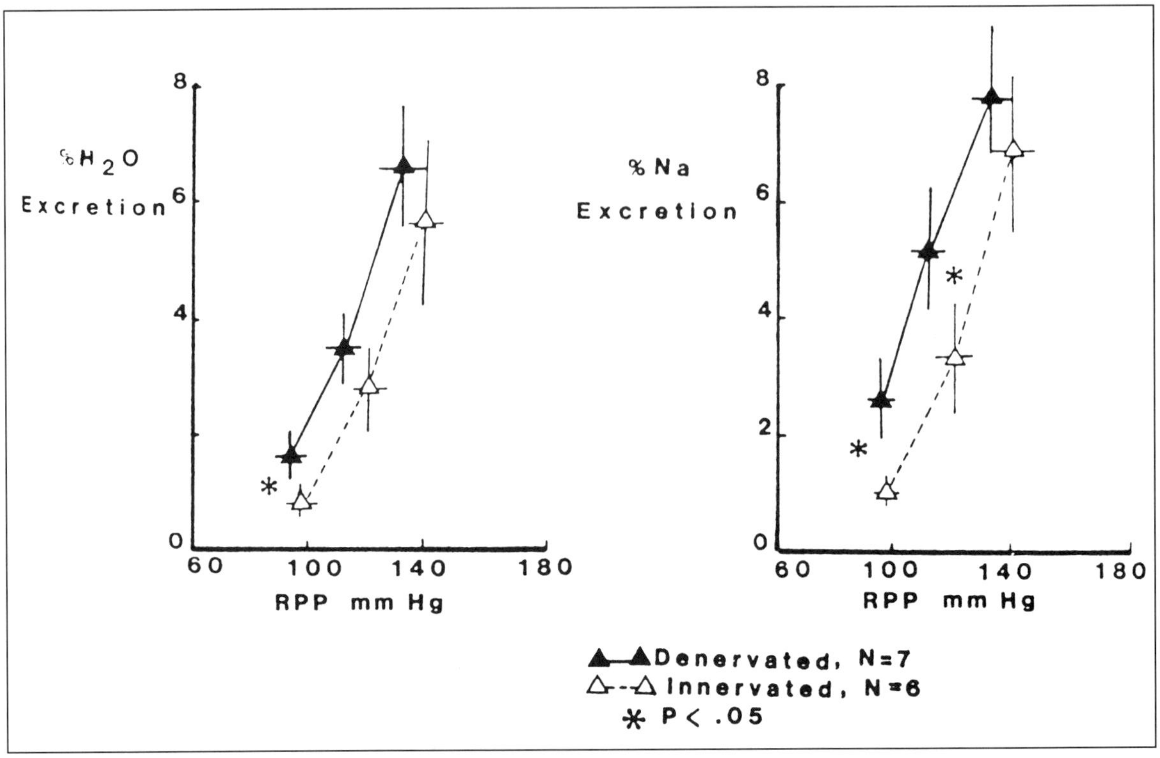

Fig. 15-5. The influence of the renal nerves on the relationship of water (left) and sodium (right) excretion to renal perfusion pressure (RPP). (Reproduced with permission from RJ Roman, AW Cowley Jr. Characterization of a new model for the study of pressure-natriuresis in the rat. Am J Physiol 1985; 248:F190–F198.)

essential hypertension, perhaps due to abnormalities in the compensatory mechanism of pressure natriuresis.

The concept that renal sympathetic tone directly influences renal sodium excretion was further explored by Roman and Cowley, who evaluated the effects of renal denervation in Sprague-Dawley rats by varying renal perfusion pressures (regulated via specially designed aortic clamps) [76]. Renal denervated, adrenalectomized, uninephrectomized rats (i.e., rats whose neural and humoral influences were controlled) exhibited greater urinary sodium excretion and hence urine flow at any given renal perfusion pressure when compared with innervated controls (Fig. 15-5). The steep slope of that relationship, as depicted in Fig. 15-5, indicates that small changes in renal perfusion pressure are capable of effecting large increases in sodium excretion. These data suggest that the important interrelationship between natriuresis, diuresis, and renal perfusion pressure is modified by renal sympathetic tone.

Innervation of the kidneys involves essentially two types of nerve fibers: efferent renal sympathetic and afferent sympathetic nerves. The efferent nerve fibers modulate the tubular transport of sodium and water into the proximal and distal tubules as well as the loop of Henle [77]. In addition, efferent nerves modify the rate and the extent of renin secretion from the juxtaglomerular cells. Afferent renal sympathetic nerves, on the other hand, act as mechanoreceptors and chemoreceptors that transmit data concerning tubular stretch and sodium content in the plasma filtrate. Although much speculation has arisen regarding the role of afferent renal innervation in initiating or perpetuating essential hypertension, solid evidence linking the two remains elusive. On the other hand, evidence for a supporting role of the efferent renal sympathetic nervous system in the pathogenesis of essential hypertension is much more compelling. Several rat models of hypertension provide important insights into the role of the sympathetic renal nervous system in hypertension. Rather than enumerate all of the models, we will focus on studies involving three: the SHR, the desoxycorticosterone acetate–sodium chloride (Doca-NaCl) hypertensive rat, and the borderline hypertensive rat (BHR).

The SHR shares many characteristics with humans suffering from essential hypertension. These rats develop progressive increases in blood pressure with increasing age. Overall sympathetic activity is increased and correlates well with the development of hypertension when compared to normotensive WKY rats. As in humans, the hypertension noted in these animals appears to be associated with altered renal function, and a subset of SHR tends to be salt sensitive, exhibiting worsening hypertension when dietary sodium intake is increased. Several studies have explored the role of the renal sympathetic nervous system in the development of hypertension in the SHR, a special strain of rat (also known as the Okamoto strain) that is acquired through repeated inbreeding of those WKY rats that tended toward the hypertensive state. Winternitz et al. [78] showed that bilateral renal denervation in the SHR delays the onset and development of hypertension compared to sham-operated rats and that those events were accompanied by significant increases in urinary sodium excretion. The effects of renal sympathetic denervation were time dependent in that none of the rats older than 17 weeks at the time of denervation went on to develop hypertension or increased natriuresis. It therefore appears that the renal sympathetic nervous system plays a role in the development of hypertension in this particular rat model by somehow altering renal sodium excretion at a young age. Oparil and colleagues performed dorsal rhizotomies (selective renal afferent nerve denervation) in SHR and showed no significant increases in blood pressure or sodium excretion compared with control animals [79]. This is in striking contrast to SHR undergoing total renal denervation (destruction of both afferent and efferent limbs) with phenol, in which large reductions in blood pressure and sodium excretion occurred. These data indicate that, at least in the SHR model, the efferent but not the afferent sympathetic system is the primary renal neural modulator of hypertension.

Another rat model of essential hypertension, the DOCA-NaCl hypertensive rat, exhibits renal nerve function characteristics similar to those seen in the SHR. These rats are uninephrectomized Sprague-Dawley rats that develop sustained hypertension after the dietary administration of Doca and 1 percent NaCl. Katholi et al. [80] found that renal denervation performed before the initiation of Doca-NaCl treatment in these rats delayed and blunted the hypertensive response, much like the response noted in SHR. Moreover, they found in this study that those effects could not be reproduced in similar rats undergoing renal denervation several weeks after treatment with Doca-NaCl had been initiated. Therefore, the development and the severity of hypertension secondary to neurally mediated sodium retention can be slowed and blunted, respectively, in young Doca-NaCl rats undergoing renal denervation.

The BHR is another interesting animal model that suggests a renal neural contribution to the development of hypertension. This model comprises the first filial offspring of SHR and the WKY rat and therefore contains genetic contributions from both hypertensive and normotensive parents. It has been examined as a genetic model of environmentally induced hypertension. Researchers have noted that the BHR can become permanently hypertensive when subjected to limited periods of environmental stress [81] or a high-salt diet [82]. Lawler et al. [83] found that renal denervation performed early (but not late) prevents the development of hypertension in BHR subjected to behavioral stress. In that study, "unstressed" rats were compared to rats undergoing 5 weeks of daily 2-hour sessions of cutaneous tail shock. Each group was further subdivided into sham-operated and operated subjects, in which the operated subjects underwent bilateral renal denervation. "Early" operations (performed after 5 weeks of stress, rat age = 18 weeks) were compared with "late" operations (performed after 11 weeks of stress, rat age = 24 weeks). They discovered that the BHR developed significant increases in arterial blood pressure in response to stress and that those increases could be eliminated by early but not late bilateral renal denervation [84]. Therefore, stress-induced hypertensive responses in BHR can be blunted successfully if bilateral renal denervation is performed at an early stage. These findings parallel those results, discussed earlier, noted in SHR and Doca-NaCl-sensitive rats subjected to high-salt diets, namely that a critical period exists in these animal models in which sympathetic neural renal input determines the future blood pressure state of the rat.

DiBona and colleagues have evaluated the effects of high-salt diet and environmental stress on the development of hypertension, exaggeration of natriuretic responses to isotonic saline loading, and augmentation of blood pressure responses to acute environmental stress [85]. They compared the blood pressure responses, urinary sodium excretion, and efferent renal sympathetic nerve activity (ERSNA) of BHR, SHR, and control WKY rats in the presence of normal (1% NaCl) and high-salt (8% NaCl) diets. They demonstrated that BHR fed a high-salt diet manifested an increase in arterial pressure associated with an exaggerated natriuretic response to isotonic saline loading. This exaggerated natriuretic response correlates with an abrupt withdrawal of ERSNA and is blunted by prior renal denervation. Moreover, BHR fed a high-salt diet exhibited greater rises in blood pressure and ERSNA and a decrease in urinary sodium excretion when stressed with air jet. All these abnormal responses mimicked those seen in SHR. On the other hand, BHR fed a 1-percent NaCl diet exhibited responses more nearly similar to control WKY rats. This study highlights the important impact of environmental influences on hypertension and shows that those effects are at least partially mediated through ERSNA.

While many animal models of essential hypertension have provided evidence for a principal role of the sympathetic renal nervous system in the development of essential hypertension, similar data in human studies have been much more elusive. For one, our ability to quantitate sympathetic neural influences on renal function have been hindered by inaccessibility of those nerves to microneurographic analysis. In addition, tremendous technical difficulties have been encountered in determining isolated renal norepinephrine synthesis and turnover rates [86]. Nonetheless, a small number of studies have demonstrated increased renal norepinephrine spillover in patients with essential hypertension [87], particularly those who are young adults [88–90]. This measure of sympathetic activity (which evaluates the rate at which the neurotransmitter norepinephrine is released into the plasma) was accompanied by normal renal extraction of radiolabeled norepinephrine, suggesting that the increased spillover of norepinephrine in these subjects was due to increased renal sympathetic nerve activity and not due to defective neuronal reuptake of norepinephrine. In summary, the process of natriuresis assumes a critical, prominent role in the maintenance of blood pressure control. The multifactorial means by which the kidneys succeed or fail to carry out that role determine in large part the boundary between normotensive and hypertensive states. The difficulty in this discussion is that currently it is difficult to differentiate between cause and effect. Further studies should help decide if the changes in renal sympathetic nerve activity are a cause or just an effect of the elevation in blood pressure.

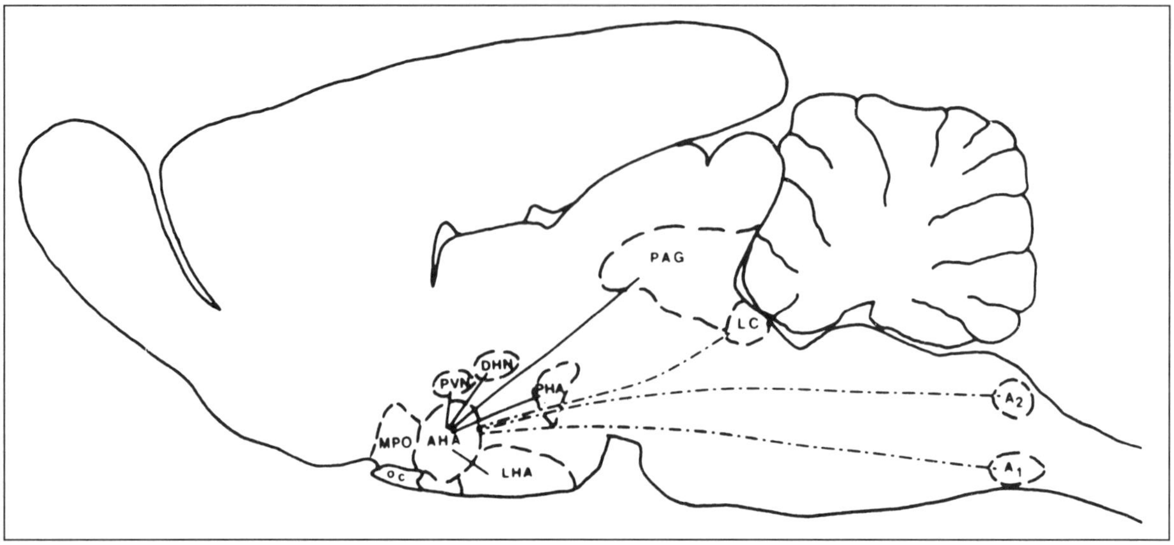

Fig. 15-6. Parasagittal reconstruction of rat brain to demonstrate the major afferent projections (solid lines) to the anterior hypothalamic area (AHA), as well as the efferent projections (dashed lines) from the AHA to the pressor nuclei in the hypothalamus. A_1, A_2 = brain-stem noradrenergic nuclei; PAG = periaqueductal gray; PHA = posterior hypothalamic area; PVN = paraventricular nucleus; MPO = median preoptic nucleus; OC = optic chiasm; LHA = lateral hypothalamic area; DHN = dorsal hypothalamic nuclei. (Reproduced with permission from JM Wyss, S Oparil, YF Chen. The role of the central nervous system in hypertension. In JH Laragh, BM Brenner, eds. Hypertension: Pathophysiology, Diagnosis, and Management. New York: Raven, 1990. P. 687.)

Role of the Central Nervous System

The sympathetic nervous system is called on to maintain blood pressure control via local influences on the kidney, as described above. But equally important are the global influences of blood pressure homeostasis that the sympathetic nervous system imparts via the central nervous system (CNS). To understand better the role of the CNS in the pathogenesis of hypertension, the methodology used by scientists to analyze the association between neuroanatomy and pathophysiology must be understood. Research involving animal models of hypertension has shed considerable light on the CNS mechanisms of blood pressure modulation. Several of these studies have depended on the formation of site-specific lesions in the CNS of animals to prevent, slow, or in some cases trigger the development of hypertension. Lesions involving the brain stem include those in the nucleus tractus solitarius (NTS). The NTS integrates sensory input from ascending afferent fibers such as those from carotid and aortic baroreceptors, modulates efferent sympathetic activity responsible for controlling cardiorespiratory functions, and influences vasopressin release [91]. Bilateral lesions involving the NTS result in loss of arterial baroreceptor reflexes [92] and alterations in normal systemic levels of renin and aldosterone levels, leading to hypertensive crises in rats while precipitating a more indolent form of hypertension in other animal species [93,94].

Other sites in the medulla known to be associated with blood pressure control include the C-1 neurons in the ventrolateral medulla, the A-1 neurons located in the caudal ventrolateral medulla, and the A-2 group of neurons located in the dorsal medulla (Fig. 15-6). The C-1 neurons innervate the sympathetic autonomic nuclei located in the spinal cord and provide tonic vasomotor control. Lesions involving those neurons lead to reductions in blood pressure similar to those observed following spinal cord transsection [95]. The A-1 neurons provide inhibitory control over sympathetic discharge and thus tend to lower blood pressure. Their influence is exerted indirectly on sympathetic nerves in the spinal cord via their interaction with the C-1 neurons. Therefore, lesions involving the A-1 group of neurons lead to hypertension due to disinhibition of sympathetic nervous activity [96]. The A-2 group of neurons represents adrenergic neurons that supply the NTS; lesions involving these neurons result in hypertension as well [97], suggesting that both the A-1 and A-2 groups of neurons modulate blood pressure control by providing inhibitory feedback on the sympathoadrenomedullary axis.

Lesions involving specific sites in the hypothalamus also can alter blood pressure responses in various animal models. For example, stimulation of paraventricular and supraoptic nuclei in the hypothalamus result in arterial blood pressure increases [97]. Lesions involving the anteroventral portion of the third ventricle in the anterior hypothalamus (AV3V) reverse or prevent the development of hypertension in Doca-salt- and Dahl salt-sensitive rats [98] but not SHR [99].

While studies such as these have concentrated on focal CNS injury, other animal studies have examined the relationship among hypertension, peripheral sympathetic nerve stimulation, and CNS input. For example, Doca-NaCl rats exhibit decreased storage of norepinephrine in peripheral adrenergic nerve endings consistent with increased turnover of peripheral norepinephrine [99]. DeChamplain and colleagues determined that this increased peripheral catecholamine turnover is related to increased peripheral sympathetic nerve activation, which occurs following a decrease in central noradrenergic activity [100]. Spinal-cord sectioning at the C-6,7 level resulted in a rapid decline in blood pressure but did not appreciably affect the norepinephrine content in hypothalamic adrenergic neurons. That indicates that the low levels of norepinephrine found in the brain stem were not secondarily caused by systemic hypertension but likely represented a primary event.

Oparil and colleagues noted similar findings in the SHR. They discovered that young SHR fed a high-salt diet develop hypertension accompanied by increased peripheral sympathetic nerve activity and altered norepinephrine content in the hypothalamic nuclei [101]. They evaluated the level of hypothalamic noradrenergic input in SHR by treating salt-sensitive SHR (SHR-S) and salt-resistant SHR (SHR-R) with both 8-percent and 1-percent-salt diets. They subsequently noted the onset of hypertension, diminished release of norepinephrine in nerve terminals in the anterior hypothalamus, decreased input of depressor neurons innervating the anterior hypothalamus, and resultant increased sympathetic activity peripherally in SHR-S subjects fed the 8-percent-salt diet [101]. These changes were less dramatic, yet still present, in SHR-S subjects fed a 1-percent-salt diet, and no such pressor response was noted in WKY control or SHR-R animals. That observation suggests that the development of hypertension in those particular animal models is mediated by decreased central depressor adrenergic nerve activity brought on by high-salt feeding at a susceptible age.

Evidence supporting a contributory role of the CNS to the development of hypertension in humans has been to date primarily circumstantial and anecdotal. Clinical observations have demonstrated associations between certain disease states or surgical manipulations involving the CNS and the subsequent development of hypertension. For example, hypertension is a well-known entity in certain stroke syndromes and represents one of the components of the Cushing reflex, which frequently accompanies massive cerebrovascular accidents [102,103]. Episodes of labile hypertension also have been reported in patients undergoing carotid endarterectomy, a phenomenon presumably mediated through disruption of nerve fibers innervating carotid sinus baroreceptors [104]. Occasionally, patients suffering the Guillain-Barré syndrome, with its attendant neurologic deficits, have developed refractory hypertension [105], but since this is a peripheral neuropathy, it is difficult to implicate the CNS.

Earlier this century, patients with severe hypertension were not infrequently treated with thoracodorsal sympathectomy [106]; disruption of the sympathetic ganglia in this region provided dramatic, albeit temporary, decreases in blood pressure. Pharmacologic therapy gradually replaced surgical intervention in most forms of hypertension, with many of the early antihypertensive agents mediating blood pressure control via well-described effects on the CNS. Clonidine and alpha-methyldopa are two examples of such agents, whose primary antihypertensive effects appear to emanate from their activity as alpha$_2$ adrenergic agonists, which results in stimulation of brain-stem and hypothalamic nuclei [107].

Several centrally acting agents are well known for their propensity to precipitate hypertensive responses when withdrawn too rapidly in humans. Aside from the well-known response to clonidine withdrawal [108], rapid withdrawal of opiates and alcohol, for example, likewise can result in large rises in blood pressure [109,110]. Data both from animal models and from humans support the concept that the CNS imparts a powerful influence on systemic blood pressure control and that the means by which it exerts its influence depends on complex feedback loops as well as diverse neurotransmitter-receptor interactions. The observations described here raise more questions than they answer, yet they do provide a stimulating framework for future inquiry into the mechanisms by which the CNS contributes to essential hypertension.

Vascular Growth

An increase in peripheral vascular resistance is one of the hallmarks of hypertension. Folkow [111,112] was the first to appreciate fully the significance of vascular smooth muscle cell proliferation in the pathogenesis of hypertension. He found that the resistance vessels from hypertensive animals exhibited increased vascular resistance compared to controls, even when they were maximally dilated (Fig. 15-7). When those vessels were vasoconstricted, they also exhibited a steeper slope in the resistance curve than controls. The responses could be mathematically modeled by assuming that there was a 30-percent increase in arterial-wall thickness, resulting in a decrease in the wall-to-lumen ratio. That increase in wall thickness is at least partially an adaptive response to the elevated blood pressure in that it reduces wall stress, but it also results in an increase in peripheral vascular resistance at any level of vasoconstriction. The increase in resistance will both accentuate and perpetuate the hypertension. There is even accumulating data [113,114] that smooth muscle cells from genetically hypertensive rats grow abnormally fast, suggesting that an abnormality in the vascular smooth muscle cell itself may be one participating factor in hypertension. The increased thickness of the smooth muscle layer of resistance vessels, whether a cause or a consequence of the increased blood pressure, in turn can act as a vascular amplifier, further raising arterial pressure.

There has been a great deal of research concerning the pathology of the smooth muscle changes seen in hypertension. Early work by Owens and Schwartz demonstrated a 50-percent increase in smooth muscle mass in the thoracic aorta, with a 50-percent increase in cellular protein in both the SHR [115] and the Goldblatt hypertensive rat [116]. Interestingly, there was no increase in cell number, with only a modest increase in DNA content, which could be attributed to an increase in cell ploidy, with as many as 50 percent of the cells exhibiting tetraploid or greater DNA content. This increase in ploidy also has been seen in aorta from aging humans [117]. These results indicate that the increase in smooth muscle cell mass seen in thoracic aortae is due to cellular hypertrophy rather than hyperplasia.

Although the smooth muscle changes observed in the thoracic aorta are due to hypertrophy, that does not ap-

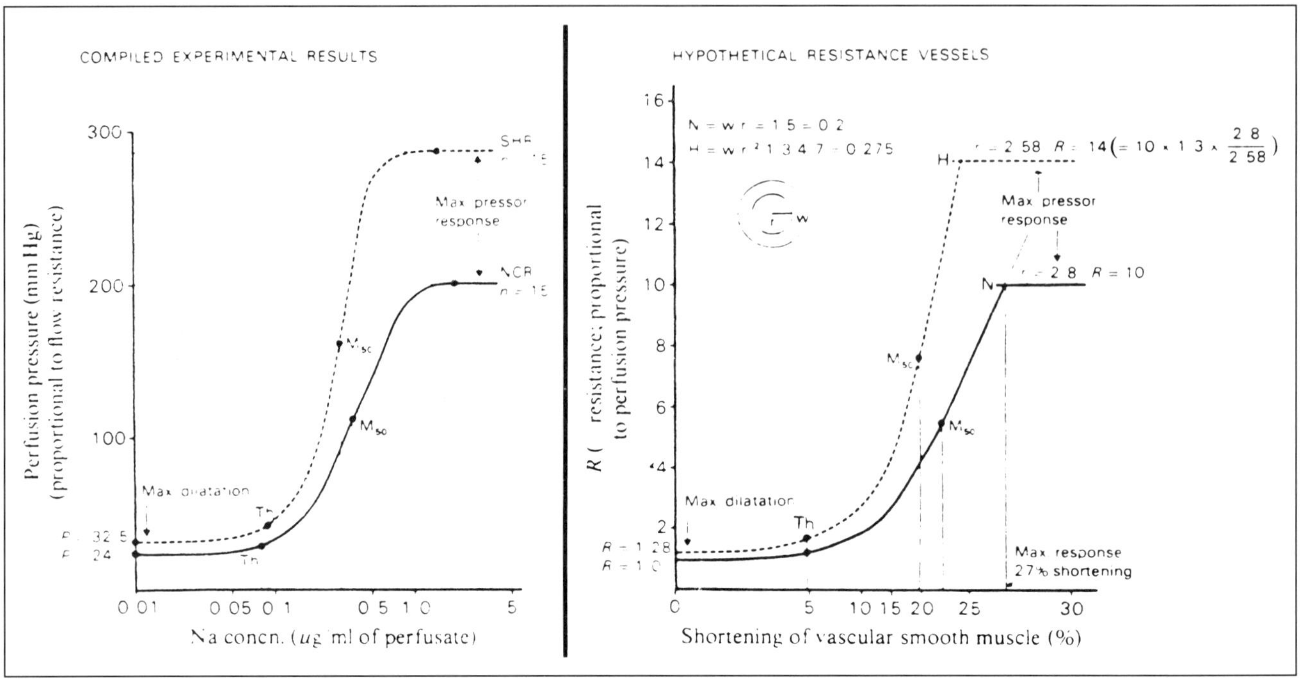

Fig. 15-7. (Left): Average resistance curves for SHR and normotensive Wistar control rat (NCR) perfused hindquarter vascular beds. Graded vasoconstriction responses were induced by intra-arterial norepinephrine at concentrations up to supramaximal levels. (Right): Mathematically deduced resistance curves for two hypothetical resistance vessels, H and N, where H differs from N only by a 30-percent increase of media thickness encroaching on the lumen already at maximal smooth muscle relaxation. Note the striking similarities between the two sets of resistance curves, especially with respect to resistance at maximal relaxation threshold (Th); steepness of the curves; 50 percent of the maximal pressor (resistance) response (M_{50}); and maximal pressor (resistance) response. (Reproduced with permission from B Folkow. Cardiovascular structural adaptation: its role in the initiation and maintenance of primary hypertension. Clin Sci 1978; 55:3s–22s.)

pear to be true in the smaller resistance vessels. Using a three-dimensional dissector, Mulvany et al. [118] demonstrated an increase in the number of cells per unit length in the mesenteric resistance vessels of the SHR compared to the WKY rat. They found no concomitant increase in smooth muscle cell volume, indicating that in those vessels the increase in smooth muscle mass was due primarily to hyperplasia and not hypertrophy, as seen in the thoracic aorta. These results have been confirmed by Owens et al. [119], using the same careful morphometric methods they had used for the thoracic aorta. It thus appears that different vascular beds can respond to an elevation in blood pressure in at least two different ways. A third mechanism by which hypertension leads to decreased intravascular luminal area is remodeling, where the smooth muscle cells rearrange themselves into increased layers, resulting in an increase in wall thickness and decreasing luminal diameter. This is especially true in the cerebral vasculature, where Baumbach and Heistad [120] have reported that remodeling is the key element responsible for decreasing the luminal diameter in the SHR. These authors hypothesize that an increase in vascular wall thickness is protective of the microcirculation in that it restores wall stress to normal. Similar remodeling changes have been reported in subcutaneous arteries from patients with essential hypertension [121,122], indicating that that mechanism may be very important.

The triggers that cause the increase in smooth muscle mass are not clear. Owens provided the first clue when he treated SHR with various antihypertensive medications and evaluated the effect on blood pressure and thoracic aorta smooth muscle mass [123,124]. Treatment with the ACE inhibitor captopril resulted in a significantly greater reduction in smooth muscle mass than did hydralazine, despite equal reductions in blood pressure. In those studies, captopril also significantly reduced smooth muscle mass in the control WKY rats. These data suggest that a non-pressor-related factor, such as angiotensin II, may have an important role in smooth muscle cell growth. Similar data have been reported by Wang and Pruitt [125] who found that ACE inhibitors prevented smooth muscle cell growth in the one kidney–one clip Goldblatt rat. This is a non-renin-dependent model of hypertension, and ACE inhibitors had no effect on blood pressure, yet a significant decrease in medial smooth muscle mass was observed in both the thoracic aorta and the mesenteric resistance vessels. Numerous other investigators have reported similar results with a variety of ACE inhibitors in the renal, coronary, cerebral, mesenteric, and limb vasculature [126–128]. Infusion of angiotensin II also has been reported to increase smooth muscle growth directly [129] and increase both aortic and cardiac fibrosis and fibronectin expression [130,131]. Further evidence of the importance of angiotensin II comes from the work of Griffin et al. [132], who infused angiotensin II into rats at doses that increased systolic blood pressure to 200 mm Hg and found increases in medial smooth muscle mass in the mesenteric vasculature. When those animals were treated with hydralazine to normalize the blood pressure, the increase in medial smooth muscle mass still was observed. It is also possible that the antiproliferative effects of ACE inhibitors are due to an increase in bradykinin. Bradykinin can inhibit smooth muscle cell mitogenesis presumably via induction of nitric oxide production [133]. In support of this hypothesis are the reports that a bradykinin antagonist blocked the antiproliferative effects of an ACE inhibitor following rat carotid injury [134,135]. Those studies, while not definitive, certainly warrant further investigation.

The growth promoting effects of angiotensin II also can be appreciated in cultured vascular smooth muscle cells. When angiotensin II is added to quiescent cultures of rat thoracic smooth muscle cells, there is a 20- to 50-percent increase in cellular protein content with no increase in cell number and only a small increase in cellular DNA content [136,137]. This is associated with a rapid induction of a number of the early-growth-response genes [138–140] and a delayed induction of the genes for the platelet-derived growth factor (PDGF) A-chain and transforming growth factor beta (TGF-β) [141–143]. This property of angiotensin II may be related to its ability to contract smooth muscle cells, since mechanical stretch has been demonstrated to stimulate growth of rabbit aortic smooth muscle cells grown on elastic membrane [144], and both serotonin and arginine vasopressin stimulate smooth muscle cell growth in vitro [145,146]. In vivo, phenylephrine infused into a rat has been demonstrated to increase c-*fos*, c-*jun* and PDGF expression in the aorta [147]. Taken together, these data suggest that agents that stimulate smooth muscle contraction act to increase smooth muscle cell growth, perhaps via an autocrine stimulation of growth factors such as PDGF or TGF-β.

There is also evidence that there may be a genetic abnormality in the smooth muscle cells isolated from hypertensive animals. These cells exhibit enhanced responsiveness to angiotensin II, PDGF, and epidermal growth factor [113,114]. It also has been reported that TGF-β may be mitogenic to smooth muscle cells isolated from SHR yet growth inhibitory to cells isolated from Sprague-Dawley rats [142,143]. If there is a genetic predisposition for an abnormal smooth muscle response to a variety of growth factors, the trigger that stimulates the release of those factors is unknown. It is important to note that in the intact vessel the smooth muscle cell is not an isolated entity. The endothelial cell layer overlying the smooth muscle cells could obviously play an important role since it can secrete a wide variety of growth factors and cytokines. As discussed elsewhere in this text, endothelial dysfunction has been described in hypertension; how that affects vascular resistance is an unanswered question. The extracellular matrix is also a rich source of smooth muscle mitogens, including heparin, thrombospondin and fibroblast growth factor. To elucidate the mechanisms of enhanced smooth muscle growth in hypertension, it is necessary to understand the interactions of the various growth factors and cell types and how they affect smooth muscle cells, which may be phenotypically abnormal.

Diet

SODIUM

Epidemiologic studies concerning the role of dietary salt remain controversial. Early studies demonstrated a positive correlation between dietary sodium intake and the prevalence of hypertension in various populations [148–151]. Generally, as seen in Fig. 15-8, there is a higher prevalence of hypertension in populations with a high-sodium excretion [152]. These studies are difficult to interpret, however, because they are not controlled for genetic or other environmental factors. In contrast to those general population studies, however, within-population studies have not showed this clear relationship in unselected subjects [153,154]. To clarify this issue, Weinberger et al. [155] studied both hypertensive and normotensive patients and their response to rapid volume expansion and contraction. They classified 51 percent as salt sensitive, meaning that they exhibited an increase of at least 10 mm Hg in blood pressure in response to a sodium load. That finding has been reported by others as well [156,157] and most investigators find approximately 50 percent of patients to be salt sensitive, perhaps being slightly higher among African-American patients [158].

The cause for this salt sensitivity is not clear, but a number of groups have suggested that it is an inherited trait [159–162]. That view is substantiated by work in laboratory animals. In the early 1960s, Dahl and coworkers [163,164] inbred Sprague-Dawley rats for their sensitivity to NaCl intake. They were able to develop both the Dahl resistant and Dahl sensitive strains of rats. On a normal sodium diet, the blood pressures of the two strains are equal; after placement on an 8-percent NaCl diet, however, the sensitive strain exhibits an increase in blood pressure of 60 to 80 mm Hg. A similar salt-sensitive strain of rats has been reported by Oparil and her colleagues [165,166], who found that SHR from the Taconic Farms breeding colony demonstrated a significant rise of 20 mm Hg in systolic blood pressure when placed on an 8-percent NaCl diet. In contrast, SHR from other sources, such as Charles River Breeding laboratories, were resistant to sodium loading. Numerous mechanisms have been proposed to account for the salt sensitivity, including impaired renal sodium handling, alterations in membrane pumps, increases in sensitivity to contractile agonists, and increased sympathetic nerve activity, and have been extensively reviewed [167]. The role of abnormal renal sodium handling is this model has been discussed elsewhere in this chapter.

Evidence for an abnormal response of the sympathetic nervous system to a sodium load is extensive. Salt-sensitive patients and animals have inappropriately high plasma norepinephrine levels during sodium loading [168–170], and a selective reduction in norepinephrine stores in the anterior hypothalamus of salt-sensitive SHR following sodium loading has been described [171]. An exaggerated pressor response to circulating norepinephrine and angiotensin II also has been reported [172–176] and may well contribute to the hypertensive response.

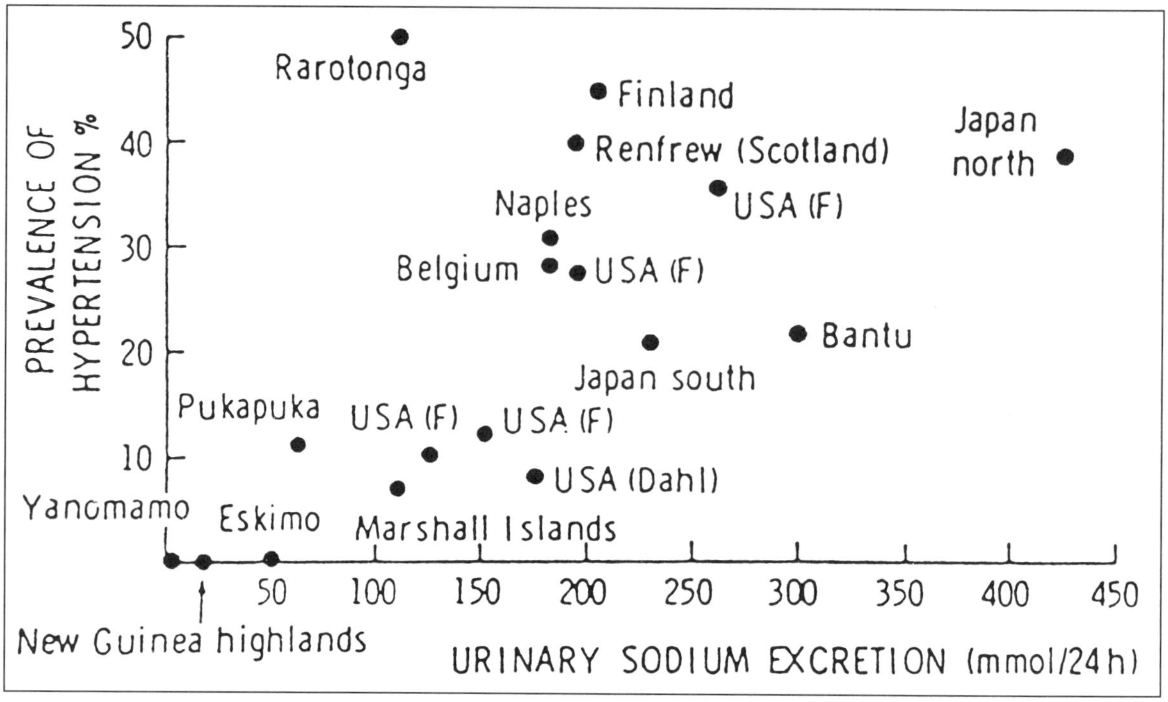

Fig. 15-8. Prevalence of hypertension based on urinary sodium excretion from different geographical distributions. Hypertension is defined as a diastolic pressure of 90 mm Hg or systolic pressure of 40 mm Hg. (Reproduced with permission from GA MacGregor. Sodium is more important than calcium in essential hypertension. Hypertension 1985; 7:628–637.)

Abnormalities in several cellular transport mechanisms also have been reported in patients with salt sensitivity, including the Na^+ pump [177–181], the Na^+-K^+-Cl^- cotransport [182–184], and the Na^+-H^+ antiporter [185,186]. Despite intensive research, it is not clear whether any of these abnormalities are a consequence or a cause of hypertension. Obviously, all these possible causes of salt sensitivity in humans and laboratory animals may interact, and much more research is needed before we can clearly define each of their individual roles. Recently, the INTERSALT trial investigated the interaction between salt and blood pressure in over 10,000 men and women aged 20 to 59 in 52 centers [187]. The major conclusion was that although there was a relationship between blood pressure and dietary salt intake, it was weaker than the relationship between blood pressure and body mass index. Despite this conclusion, a reduction in salt intake would significantly reduce the incidence of hypertension seen in the 30- to 59-year-old age group.

CALCIUM

The evidence for a role of dietary calcium in hypertension comes from early observations that the incidence of hypertension was lower in populations that had water with a high calcium content [188]. More recent evidence has supported that finding [189,190], and the National Health and Nutrition Examination Survey (NHANES-1) concluded that calcium intake was the best single dietary predictor of blood pressure [189,190]. Actually more than 20 epidemiologic studies have found an inverse relationship between dietary calcium and blood pressure (see 191 for review). A decrease in calcium intake results in a slight increase in parathyroid hormone (PTH), reduced serum phosphorus, and an increase in urinary calcium excretion. Similar findings on the effects of calcium have been observed in experimental animals. In SHR, a decrease in plasma ionized calcium compared to WKY controls has been found, and large increases in calcium intake can blunt the development of hypertension in the SHR [192–197].

In patients, a number of well-controlled trials have found a significant reduction in blood pressure with supplementation of 1 g of calcium a day [189,190,198]. These groups have been classified into responders and nonresponders, and in one trial 43 percent of hypertensives and 13 percent of normotensives responded to calcium with a decrease in blood pressure of at least 10 mm Hg. Proposed mechanisms accounting for this effect of calcium are numerous. Many parameters change as dietary calcium changes, including PTH, calcitrol, calcitonin gene-related peptide (CGRP), the renin-angiotensin system, and the sympathetic nervous system. Many of these factors have vasoactive properties and could certainly affect blood pressure. It also has been proposed that dietary calcium may alter blood pressure by altering the metabolism of other electrolytes, particularly sodium. None of these mechanisms have been conclusively proven at this time and continue to remain the subject of intensive research [191].

POTASSIUM

Epidemiologic data suggest that there is an inverse relationship between dietary potassium intake and systemic blood pressure. Early surveys, perhaps due to methodologic problems, at first failed to demonstrate any relationship between urinary potassium excretion and blood pressure [199–202]. In contrast, population studies in both the United States and Japan suggested that blood pressure was higher in those populations ingesting a low-potassium diet [203,204]. More recent data analyzing the National Health and Nutrition Evaluation (NHANES I) have found a significant association between potassium intake and blood pressure [205,206], with blood pressure correlating inversely with potassium. When the data are analyzed by defining people as either hypertensive or not, a potassium intake of less than 900 mg/day is associated with a 12- to 14-percent risk of hypertension [206,207]. A more comprehensive study was the INTERSALT study [188,208], in which 52 study groups from 32 countries investigated the effects of dietary potassium on the incidence of high blood pressure. A total of 10,000 individuals were enrolled, and dietary consumption was assessed by 24-hour urine excretion of sodium and potassium. After correction for age, sex, body mass, and other variables, a significant negative correlation between potassium and blood pressure was found. Animal studies have supported that finding: potassium dietary supplementation attenuates the hypertension and dramatically reduces the mortality in the spontaneously hypertensive stroke-prone rat [204,209,210]. It also has been demonstrated to prevent the development of renal lesions in the Dahl rat model [211,212].

The mechanism by which potassium affects systemic blood pressure is probably multifactorial. Potassium loading has been shown to induce a natriuresis in both dogs [213] and rats [214,215]. In humans, potassium loading has been demonstrated to increase 24-hour urinary sodium excretion [216,217], but it is difficult to document that that is responsible for the decreases seen in blood pressure. Another factor that also may be altered by potassium is the renin-angiotensin system, but the effects are not clear. Stimulation of renin activity is not always seen following potassium loading in patients [216,218,219], and numerous investigators have found that potassium directly suppresses renin release [216,220–222]. In addition to effects on renin release, vascular reactivity to angiotensin II has been reported to be depressed by potassium [223].

Potassium also may have direct effects on smooth muscle cells. When smooth muscle is exposed to potassium, vascular resistance drops in hypertensive rats [224,225] and infusion of potassium decreases forearm vascular resistance when infused into the brachial artery [226,227]. Despite this, no change in total vascular resistance has been noted in humans on a potassium-supplemented diet [228], making it difficult to implicate this mechanism. Other mechanisms that have been proposed include effects on eicosanoid metabolism [229,230], as well as an increase in production of renal kallikrein [231]. None of these mechanisms has been clearly established; thus, the mechanism by which potassium may influence blood pressure remains unclear.

It should be obvious from this discussion that the pathogenesis of essential hypertension still is not clear. It also should be apparent that the causes of this disease are multifactorial and involve a number of the mechanisms discussed here. With the rapid advances in molecular and cellular biology in the next few years, new, important insights into the genetics and pathogenesis of hypertension should be achieved.

References

1. Morgagni JB. De Sedibus et Causus Morboreum per Anatomen Indagatis, Vol. 1. Venice: Ramondiana, 1761.
2. Weitz, W. Zur aetiologie der genuinen oder vascularen hypertension. Z Klin Med 1923; 96:151.
3. Platt R. Heredity in hypertension. Q J Med 1947; 16:111.
4. Hamilton M, et al. The etiology of essential hypertension. 1. The arterial pressure in the general population. Clin Sci 1954; 13:11–35.
5. Hamilton M, et al. The etiology of essential hypertension. 2. Scores for arterial blood pressure adjusted for differences in age and sex. Clin Sci 1954; 13:37–49.
6. Hamilton M, et al. The etiology of essential hypertension. 4. The role of inheritance. Clin Sci 1954; 13:273–304.
7. Havlik RJ, et al. Blood pressure aggregation in families. Am J Epidemiol 1979; 110:304–312.
8. Johnson BC, Epstein FH, Kuelsberg MO. Distributions and familial studies of blood pressure and serum cholesterol in a total community—Tecumseh, Michigan. J Chronic Dis 1965; 18:147–160.
9. Kannel WB. Host and environmental determinants of hypertension. In H Hesteloot, JV Joosens, eds. Epidemiology of Arterial Blood Pressure. The Hague: Martinus Nijhoff, 1976. Pp. 265–295.
10. Biron P, Mongeau J-G. Familial aggregation of blood pressure and its components. Pediatr Clin 1978; 25:29–33.
11. Schwartz JT, Wagner JO. The NHLBI twin study of cardiovascular disease risk factors: Methodology and summary of results. Am J Epidemiol 1977; 106:284–295.
12. Slatery ML, et al. Lifestyle and blood pressure levels in male twins in Utah. Genet Epidemiol 1988; 5:277–287.
13. Schull WJ, et al. A family set method for estimating heredity and stress. II. Preliminary results of the genetic methodology in a pilot survey of Negro blood pressure. J Chronic Dis 1970; 23:83–92.
14. Moll PP, et al. Heredity, stress and blood pressure, a family set approach: The Detroit project revisited. J Chronic Dis 1983; 36:317–328.
15. Keller JB. Environmental and genetic sources of familial aggregation of blood pressure in Tecumseh, Michigan. Am J Epidemiol 1984; 120:131–144.
16. Camussi A, Bianchi G. From the unimodal-bimodal controversy to molecular technology. Hypertension 1988; 12: 620–628.
17. Canessa ML, et al. Increased sodium-lithium countertransport in red cells of patients with essential hypertension. N Engl J Med 1980; 302:772–776.
18. Adragna NC, et al. Red cell lithium–sodium countertransport and sodium–potassium cotransport in patients with essential hypertension. Hypertension 1982; 4:795–804.
19. Canali M, et al. Increased erythrocyte lithium–sodium countertransport in essential hypertension: its relationship to family history of hypertension. Clin Sci 1980; 61:13s–15s.
20. Boerwinkle E, et al. Analysis of the distribution of erythrocyte sodium–lithium countertransport in a sample representative of the general population. Genet Epidemiol 1986; 3:365–378.
21. Woods JW, et al. Increased red-cell sodium–lithium countertransport in normotensive sons of hypertensive parents. N Engl J Med 1982; 306:593–595.
22. Weder AB, Torretti BA, and Julius S. Racial differences

in erythrocyte cation transport. Hypertension 1984; 6:115–123.
23. Trevisan M, et al. Abnormal red blood cell ion transport and hypertension. Hypertension 1983; 5:363–367.
24. Wiley JS, et al. Erythrocyte cation cotransport and countertransport in essential hypertension. Hypertension 1984; 6:360–368.
25. Hasstedt SJ, et al. Hypertension and sodium–lithium countertransport in Utah pedigrees: Evidence for major-locus inheritance. Am J Human Genet 1988; 43:14–22.
26. Seifter JL, Aronson PS. Properties and physiologic roles of the plasma membrane sodium–hydrogen exchanger. J Clin Invest 1986; 78:859–864.
27. Lifton RP, et al. Cloning of the human genomic amiloride-sensitive Na^+/H^+ antiporter gene, identification of genetic polymorphisms, and localization on the genetic map of chromosome 1p. Genomics 1990; 7:131–135.
28. Lifton RP, et al. Exclusion of the Na^+-H^+ antiporter as a candidate gene in human essential hypertension. Hypertension 1991; 17:8–14.
29. Lifton RP, et al. Evidence for heritability of non-modulating essential hypertension. Hypertension 1989; 13:884–889.
30. Brown NJ, Ryder D, Nadeau J. Caffeine attenuates the renal vascular response to angiotensin II infusion. Hypertension 1993; 22:847–852.
31. Williams GH, et al. Non-modulation as an intermediate phenotype in essential hypertension. Hypertension 1992; 20:788–796.
32. Riordan JR, et al. Identification of the cystic fibrosis gene: cloning and characterization of complementary DNA. Science 1989; 245:1066–1080.
33. Naftilan AJ, et al. A lack of genetic linkage of renin gene restriction fragment length polymorphisms with human hypertension. Hypertension 1989; 14:614–618.
34. Soubrier F, et al. Similar frequencies of renin gene restriction fragment length polymorphisms in hypertensive and normotensive subjects. Hypertension 1990; 16:712–717.
35. Jeunemaitre X, et al. Sib pair linkage analysis of renin gene haplotypes in human essential hypertension. Hum Genet 1992; 88:301–306.
36. Cambien F, et al. Familial resemblance of plasma angiotensin-converting enzyme level: The Nancy study. Am J Hum Genet 1988; 43:774–780.
37. Jeunemaitre X, et al. Absence of linkage between the angiotensin converting enzyme locus and human essential hypertension. Nature Genetics 1992; 1:72–75.
38. Jeunemaitre X, et al. Molecular basis of human hypertension: Role of angiotensinogen. Cell 1992; 71:169–180.
39. Walker WG, et al. Relationship between blood pressure and renin, renin substrate, angiotensin II, aldosterone and urinary sodium and potassium in 574 ambulatory subjects. Hypertension 1979; 1:287; 291.
40. Smirk FH, Hall WH. Inherited hypertension in rats. Nature 1958; 182:727–728.
41. Dahl LK, Heine M, Tassinari L. Role of genetic factors in susceptibility to experimental hypertension due to chronic excess salt ingestion. Nature 1962; 194:480.
42. Okamoto K, Aoki K. Development of a strain of spontaneously hypertensive rats. Jpn Circ J 1963; 27:282–293.
43. Ben-Ishay D, Saliternik R, Welner A. Separation of two strains of rats with inbred dissimilar sensitivity to Doca-salt hypertension. Experientia 1972; 28:1321–1322.
44. Dupont J, et al. Selection of three strains with spontaneously different levels of blood pressure. Biomedicine 1973; 19: 36–41.
45. Bianchi G, Fox U, Imbasciati E. The development of a new strain of spontaneously hypertensive rats. Life Sci 1974; 14:339–347.
46. Schlager G. Selection for blood pressure levels in mice. Genetics 1974; 76:537–549.
47. Rapp JP. A paradigm for identification of primary genetic causes of hypertension in rats. Hypertension 1983; 5[Supp I]:I-198–I-203.
48. Rapp JP, Wang SM, Dene H. A genetic polymorphism in the renin gene of Dahl rats cosegregate with blood pressure. Science 1989; 243:542–544.
49. Wang SM, Rapp JP. Structural differences in the renin gene of Dahl salt-sensitive and salt-resistant rats. Mol Endocrinol 1989; 3:288–294.
49a. Deng AY, Rapp JP. Locus for the inducible, but not a constitutive, nitric oxide synthase congregates with blood pressure in the Dahl salt-sensitive rat. J Clin Invest 1995; 95:2170–2177.
50. Kurtz TW, et al. Cosegregation of the renin allele of the spontaneously hypertensive rat with an increase in blood pressure. J Clin Invest 1990; 85:1328–1332.
51. Hilbert P, et al. Chromosomal mapping of two genetic loci associated with blood-pressure regulation in hereditary hypertensive rats. Nature 1991; 353:521–529.
52. Jacob HJ, et al. Genetic mapping of a gene causing hypertension in the stroke-prone spontaneously hypertensive rat. Cell 1991; 67:213–224.
53. Lindpaintner K, Takahashi S, Ganten D. Structural alterations of the renin gene in stroke-prone spontaneously hypertensive rats: examination of genotype-phenotype correlations. J Hypertens 1990; 8:763–773.
54. Iwai N, Inagami T. Isolation of preferentially expressed genes in the kidneys of hypertensive rats. Hypertension 1991; 17:161–169.
55. Lindpaintner K, et al. Molecular genetics of the SA gene: Cosegregation with hypertension and mapping to rat chromosome 1. J Hypertens 1993; 11:83–88.
56. Samani NJ, et al. A gene differentially expressed in the kidney of the spontaneously hypertensive rat cosegregates with increased blood pressure. J Clin Invest 1993; 92:1099–1103.
57. Iwai N, et al. Human SA gene locus as a candidate locus for essential hypertension. Hypertension 1994; 23:375–380.
58. Dobbs WA, Prather JW, Guyton AC. Relative importance of nervous control of cardiac output and arterial pressure. Am J Cardiol 1971; 27:507–512.
59. Guyton AC, et al. The dominant role of the kidneys in the long-term regulation of arterial pressure in normal and hypertensive states. In JH Laragh, BM Grenner, eds. Hypertension: Pathophysiology, Diagnosis, and Management. New York: Raven, 1990. P. 1030.
60. Guyton AC. Arterial Pressure and Hypertension. Philadelphia: Saunders,1980.
61. Koletsky S, Goodsitt AM. Natural history and pathogenesis of hypertension. Arch Pathol 1960; 69:654–662.
62. Maschio G, et al. Clinical features of patients with solitary kidneys. Nephron 1986; 43:10–15.
63. Fetterman GH, Habib R. Congenital bilateral oligonephronic renal hypoplasia with hypertrophy of nephrons (oligomeganephronie). Am J Clin Pathol 1969; 52:199–207.
64. Lieberman E. Essential hypertension in children and youth: a pediatric perspective. J Pediatr 1974; 85:1–11.
65. Brenner BM, Garcia DL, Anderson S. The renal abnormality in hypertension. In JH Laragh, BM Brenner, eds. Hypertension: Pathology, Diagnosis, and Management, New York: Raven, 1995. Pp. 1151–1152.
66. Sommers SC, Relman AS, Smithwick RH. Histologic studies of kidney biopsy specimens from patients with hypertension. Am J Pathol 1958; 34:685–715.

67. Sealey JE, et al. On the renal basis of essential hypertension: nephron heterogeneity with discordant renin secretion and sodium excretion causing a hypertensive vasoconstrictor-volume relationship. Journal of Hypertension 1988; 6:763–777.
68. Laragh JH. Nephron heterogeneticity: clue to the pathogenesis of essential hypertension and effectiveness of angiotensin-converting enzyme inhibitor treatment. Am J Hypertension 1989; 87(61S):2S–14S.
69. Collins RD, et al. Abnormally sustained aldosterone secretion during salt loading in patients with various forms of benign hypertension: relation to plasma renin activity. J Clin Invest 1970; 49:1415–1526.
70. Weber MA, et al. Disparate patterns of aldosterone response during diuretic treatment of hypertension. Ann Intern Med 1977; 87:558–563.
71. Farnsworth EB. Renal reabsorption of chloride and phosphate in normal subjects and in patients with essential arterial hypertension. J Clin Invest 1946; 25:897–905.
72. Cottier PT, Weller JM, Hooblerr SW. Effect of an intravenous sodium chloride load on renal hemodynamics and electrolyte excretion in essential hypertension. Circulation 1958; 17:750–760.
73. Papper S, Belsky JL, Bleifer KH. The response to the administration of an isotonic sodium chloride-lactate solution in patients with essential hypertension. J Clin Invest 1960; 39:876–884.
74. Laragh JH, Cannon PJ, Ames RP. Aldosterone secretion and various forms of hypertensive vascular disease. Ann Intern Med 1963; 59:117–120.
75. Katholi RE, et al. Production of sustained hypertension by chronic intrarenal norepinephrine infusion in conscious dogs. Circulation 1977; 40[Suppl I]:I118–I126.
76. Roman RJ, Cowley AW Jr. Characterization of a new model for the study of pressure-natriuresis in the rat. Am J Physiol 1985; 248:F190–F198.
77. Wyss JM, Oparil S, Sripairojthikoon W. Neuronal control of the kidney: contribution to hypertension. Can J Pharmacol Physiol 1992; 70:760.
78. Winternitz SR, Katholi RE, Oparil S. Role of the renal sympathetic nerves in the development and maintenance of hypertension in the spontaneously hypertensive rat. J Clin Invest 1980; 66:971–978.
79. Oparil S, Sripairojthikoon W, Wyss JM. The renal afferent nerves in the pathogenesis of hypertension. Can J Pharmacol Physiol 1987; 65:1548–1558.
80. Katholi RE, Naftilan AJ, Oparil S. Importance of renal sympathetic tone in the development of DOCA-salt hypertension in the rat. Hypertension 1980; 2:266–273.
81. Lawler JE, et al. Effects of stress on blood pressure and cardiac pathology in rats with borderline hypertension. Hypertension 1981; 3:496–505.
82. Lawler JE, et al. Hypertension produced by a high sodium diet in the borderline hypertensive rat. Clin Exp Hypertens 1987; (A) 9:1713–1731.
83. Lawler JE, et al. Bilateral renal denervation can prevent the development of stress-induced hypertension in the borderline hypertensive rat. Clin and Exper Hyper-Theory and Practice 1989; A11(8):1549–1563.
84. Sanders BJ, Lawler JE. The borderline hypertensive rat (BHR) as a model for environmentally-induced hypertension: a review and update. Neuroscience and Behavioral Reviews 1992; 16:207–217.
85. DiBona GF, Jones SY. Renal manifestations of NaCl sensitivity in borderline hypertensive rats. Hypertension 1991; 17:44–53.
86. Esler M, et al. Assessment of human sympathetic nervous system from measurements of norepinephrine turnover. Hypertension 1988; 11(1):3–20.
87. Esler M, et al. Mechanism of elevated plasma noradrenaline in the course of essential hypertension. J Cardiovasc Pharmacol 1986; 8[Suppl 5]:S39–S43.
88. Esler M, et al. Mild high-renin essential hypertension: a neurogenic human hypertension? N Engl J Med 1977; 296:405–411.
89. London GM, et al. Renal and systemic hemodynamics in sustained essential hypertension. Hypertension 1984; 6: 743–754.
90. Hollenberg NK, Williams GH, Adams DF. Essential hypertension: abnormal renal vascular and endocrine responses to a mild psychological stimulus. Hypertension 1981; 3:11–17.
91. Abboud FM. The sympathetic nervous system in hypertension. Clin and Exper Hyper-Theory and Practice 1984; A6(1&2):43–60.
92. Doba N, Reis DJ. Hypertension produced by brainstem lesions in rat. Circulation Research 1973; 34:293–301.
93. Nathan MA, Reis DJ. Chronic labile hypertension produced by lesions of the nucleus tractus solitarii in the cat. Circulation Research 1977; 40:72–80.
94. Carey MR, et al. Production of sustained hypertension by lesion in the nucleus tractus solitarii of the American Foxhound. Hypertension 1979; 1:246–254.
95. Ross CA, et al. Tonic vasomotor control by the rostral ventrolateral medulla: Effect of electrical or chemical stimulation of the area containing C1 adrenaline neurons on arterial pressure, heart rate, and plasma catecholamines and vasopressin. J Neurosci 1984; 4(2):474–494.
96. Oparil S, et al. Pathogenesis of Hypertension. In HA Fozzard et al, eds. The Heart and Cardiovascular System. New York: Raven, 1992. Pp 295–331.
97. Ciriello J, Calaresu FR. Role of paraventricular and supraoptic nuclei in central cardiovascular regulation in the cat. Am J Physiol 1980; 239:R137–R142.
98. Knuepfer MM, et al. Effects of afferent renal nerve (ARN) stimulation and baroreceptor activation on unit activity (UA) in the anteroventral third ventricle (AV3V) region. Fed Proc 1984; 39:837–845.
99. deChamplain J, Krakoff LR, Axelrod J. Relationship between sodium intake and norepinephrine storage during the development of experimental hypertension. Circ Res 1968; 23:479–491.
100. van Ameringen M, deChamplain J, Imbeault S: Participation of central noradrenergic neurons in experimental hypertension. Can J Physiol Pharmacol 1976; 55:1246–1251.
101. Chen Y-F, et al. High NaCl diet reduces hypothalamic norepinephrine turnover in hypertensive rats. Hypertension 1988; 11:55–62.
102. Emmanuele MA, et al. Basilar artery aneurysm simulating phaechromocytoma. Neurology 1981; 31:1560–1561.
103. Ito A, Omae T, Katsuki S. Acute changes in blood pressure following vascular diseases in the brainstem. Stroke 1973; 4:80–84.
104. Towne JB, Bernhard VM. The relationship of postoperative hypertension to complications following carotid endarterectomy. Surgery 1980; 88:575–580.
105. Ventura HO, Messerli FH, Barron RE. Norepinephrine induced hypertension in Guillain-Barré syndrome. Hypertension 1986; 4:265–267.
106. Guyton AC. Hypertension: A neural disease? Arch Neurol 1988; 45:178–182.
107. Rudd P, Blaschke TF. Antihypertensive agents and the drug therapy of hypertension. In: AG Goodman et al., eds. The Pharmacological Basis of Therapeutics. Pp 788–792.
108. Reid JL, et al. Clonidine withdrawal in hypertension.

Changes in blood pressure and plasma and urinary noradrenaline. Lancet 1977; 36:1171–1174.
109. Gold MS, Kleber HD. Clinical utility of clonidine in opiate withdrawal: a study of 100 patients. In: Psychopharmacology of Clonidine, H Lal, S Fielding, eds. Pp 299–306.
110. Beevers D, eds. et al. Alcohol and hypertension. Contrib Nephrol 1982; 30:92–97.
111. Folkow B. Cardiovascular structural adaptation: its role in the initiation and maintenance of primary hypertension. Clin Sci 1978; 55:3s–22s.
112. Folkow B. Physiological aspects of primary hypertension. Physiol Rev 1982; 62:347–504.
113. Hadrava V, Tremblay J, Hamet P. Abnormalities in growth characteristics of aortic smooth muscle cells in spontaneously hypertensive rats. Hypertension 1989; 13:589–597.
114. Haudenschild CC, Grunwald J, Chobanian AV. Effects of hypertension of migration and proliferation of smooth muscle in culture. Hypertension 1985; 7[Suppl I]:I-101–I-104.
115. Owens G, Schwartz S. Alterations in vascular smooth muscle mass in the spontaneously hypertensive rat. Role of cellular hypertrophy, hyperploidy, and hyperplasia. Circ Res 1982; 51:280–289.
116. Owens G, Schwartz S. Vascular smooth muscle cell hypertrophy and hyperploidy in the Goldblatt hypertensive rat. Circ Res 1983; 534:491–501.
117. Barrett T, et al. Polyploid nuclei in human artery wall smooth muscle cells. Proc Natl Acad Sci 1983; 80:882–885.
118. Mulvany M, Baandrup U, Gundersen H. Evidence for hyperplasia in mesenteric resistance vessels of spontaneously hypertensive rats using a three-dimensional disector. Circ Res 1985; 57:794–800.
119. Owens GK, Schwartz SM, McCanna M. Evaluation of medial hypertrophy in resistance vessels of spontaneously hypertensive rats. Hypertension 1988; 11:198–207.
120. Baumbach GL, Heistad DD. Remodeling of cerebral arterioles in chronic hypertension. Hypertension 1989; 13:968–972.
121. Korsgaard N, et al. Cellular basis of the increased vascular pressor response in essential hypertension (Abstract). J Hypertension 1990; 8[Suppl 3]:S118.
122. Short D. Morphology of the intestinal arterioles in chronic human hypertension. Br Heart J 1966; 28:184–188.
123. Owens G. Differential effects of antihypertensive therapy on vascular smooth muscle cell hypertrophy, hyperploidy, and hyperplasia in the spontaneously hypertensive rat. Circ Res 1985; 56:525–536.
124. Owens GK. Influence of blood pressure on development of aortic medial smooth muscle hypertrophy in spontaneously hypertensive rats. Hypertension 1987; 9:178–187.
125. Wang D-H, Prewitt RL. Captopril reduces aortic and microvascular growth in hypertensive and normotensive rats. Hypertension 1990; 15:68–77.
126. Clozel JP, Kuhn H, Hefti F. Vascular protection with cilazapril in hypertension. J Cardiovasc Pharmacol 1992; 19[Suppl 5]: S28–S33.
127. Levy BI, Safar ME. Remodeling of the vascular system in response to hypertension and drug therapy. Clin Exp Pharmacol Physiol 1992; 19[Suppl 19]:33–37.
128. Novo S, et al. Regression of structural vascular changes in hypertensives after captopril treatment. Eur Heart J 1992; 13:1135–1137.
129. Daemen MJAP, et al. Angiotensin II induces smooth muscle proliferation in the normal and injured rat arterial wall. Circ Res 1991; 68:450–456.
130. Himeno IT, et al. Angiotensin II alters aortic fibronectin independently of hypertension. Hypertension 1994; 23:823–826.
131. Crawford DC, Chobanian AV, Brecher P. Angiotensin II induces fibronectin expression associated with cardiac fibrosis in the rat. Circ Res 1994; 74:727–739.
132. Griffin SA, et al. Angiotensin II causes vascular hypertrophy in part by a non-pressor mechanism. Hypertension 1991; 17:626–635.
133. Gary VC, Hassid A. Nitric Oxide generating vasodilators and 8-bromo-cyclic guanosine monophosphate inhibit mitogenesis and proliferation of cultured rat smooth muscle cells. J Clin Invest 1989; 83:1774–1777.
134. Fahry RD, et al. Kinins mediate the antiproliferative effect of ramapril in rat carotid artery. Biochem Biophys Res Comm 1992; 182:283–288.
135. Lenz W, Wiemer G, Scholkens BA. Contribution of bradykinin to the cardiovascular effects of ramapril. J Cardiovasc Pharmacol 1993; 22[Suppl 9]:51–58.
136. Geisterfer AA, Peach MJ, Owens GK. Angiotensin II induces hypertrophy, not hyperplasia, of cultured rat aortic smooth muscle cells. Circ Res 1988; 62:749–756.
137. Berk BC, et al. Angiotensin II-stimulated protein synthesis in cultured rat aortic smooth muscle cells. Hypertension 1989; 13:305–314.
138. Naftilan AJ, et al. Angiotensin II induces c-fox expression in smooth muscle via transcriptional control. Hypertension 1989; 13:706–711.
139. Naftilan AJ, et al. Induction of the proto-oncogene c-jun by angiotensin II. Mol Cell Biol 1990; 10:5536–5540.
140. Taubman MB, et al. Angiotensin II induces c-fox mRNA in aortic smooth muscle. J Biol Chem 1989; 264:526–530.
141. Naftilan AJ, Pratt RE, Dzau VJ. Induction of platelet-derived growth factor a-chain and c-myc gene expressions by angiotensin II in cultured rat vascular smooth muscle cells. J Clin Invest 1989; 83:1419–1424.
142. Gibbons GH, Pratt RE, Dzau VJ. Vascular smooth muscle cell hypertrophy vs. hyperplasia. Autocrine transforming growth factor -1 expression determines growth response to angiotensin II. J Clin Invest 1992; 90:456–461.
143. Stouffer GA, Owens GK. Angiotensin II-induced mitogenesis of spontaneously hypertensive rat-derived cultured smooth muscle cells is dependent on autocrine production of transforming growth factor. Circ Res 1992; 70:820–828.
144. Leung D, Glagov S, Mathews M. A new in vitro method for studying cell responses to mechanical stimulation: Different effects of cyclic stretching and agitation on smooth muscle cell biosynthesis. Exp Cell Res 1977; 109:285–298.
145. Geisterfer A, Peach MM, Owens GK. Angiotensin II induces hypertrophy, not hyperplasia, of cultured rat aortic smooth muscle cells. Circ Res 1988; 62:749–756.
146. Nemecek GM, et al. Stimulation of aortic smooth muscle cell mitogenesis by serotonin. Proc Natl Acad Sci USA 1980; 83:674–678.
147. Majesky MW, et al. $_1$-Adrenergic stimulation of platelet-derived growth factor A-chain gene expression rat aorta. J Biol Chem 1990; 265:1082–1088.
148. Gleibermann L. Blood pressure and dietary salt in human populations. Ecol Food Nutr 1973; 2:143–156.
149. McCarron DA, Henry HJ, Morris CD. Human nutrition and blood pressure regulation: an integrated approach. Hypertension 1982; 4[Suppl III]:III-2–III-3.
150. Dahl LK. Evidence for an increase intake of sodium in hypertension based on urinary excretion of sodium. Proc Soc Exp Biol Med 1957; 94:23.
151. Stamler J, et al. Dietary and hormonal factors in experimental atherogenesis and blood pressure regulation. In G Pincus, ed. Recent Progress in Hormone Research. New York: Academic, 1955. Pp 401–452.
152. MacGregor GA. Sodium is more important than calcium in essential hypertension. Hypertension 1985; 7:628–637.

153. Kawasaki T, et al. The effect of high-sodium and low-sodium intake on blood pressure and other related variables in human subjects with idiopathic hypertension. Am J Med 1978; 64:193.
154. Watt GCM. Does salt sensitivity exist? Klin Wochenschr 1981; 69[Suppl 25]:30–35.
155. Weinberger MH, et al. Definitions and characteristics of sodium sensitivity and blood pressure resistance. Hypertension 1986; 8[Suppl II]:II-127–II-134.
156. Sullivan JM, Retts JF. Sodium sensitivity in human subjects: hemodynamic and hormonal correlates. Hypertension 1988; 11:717–723.
157. Campese VM, et al. Abnormal relationship between Na^+ intake and sympathetic nervous system activity in salt-sensitive patients with essential hypertension. Kidney Int 1982; 21:371–378.
158. Falkner B, et al. Sodium sensitivity, growth and family history of hypertension in young blacks. J Hypertension 1986; 4[Suppl 5]:5381–5383.
159. Campese VM, et al. Abnormal renal hemodynamics in black salt-sensitive patients with hypertension. Hypertension 1991; 18:805–812.
160. Blaustein MP, Hamlyn JM. Pathogenesis of essential hypertension: a link between dietary salt and high blood pressure. Hypertension 1991; 18[Suppl III]:III-184–III-195.
161. Dahl LK, Leitt G, Heine M. Influence of dietary potassium and sodium potassium molar ratios on the development of salt hypertension. J Exp Med 1972; 136:318.
162. Kurtz TW, Al-Bander HA, Morris RC Jr. 'Salt-sensitive' essential hypertension in men. N Engl J Med 1987; 317:1043–1048.
163. Dahl LK, Heine M. Primary role of renal homografts in setting blood pressure levels in rats. Circ Res 1975; 36:692.
164. Dahl LK, Knudsen KD, Iwai J. Genetic influence of the kidney in hypertension-prone rats. Circ Res 1970; 26/27[Suppl II]:II-277–II-289.
165. Oparil S, et al. The neural basis of salt sensitivity in the rat: Altered hypothalamic function. Am J Med Sci 1988; 295(4): 360–369.
166. Oparil S, et al. The neuronal basis of salt sensitivity. In R Rettig, D Ganten, FC Luft, eds., Salt and Hypertension. Berlin: Springer, 1989. Pp. 83–96.
167. Campese VM. Salt sensitivity in hypertension. Renal and cardiovascular complications. Hypertension 1994; 23:531–550.
168. Campese VM, et al. Abnormal relationship between sodium intake and sympathetic nervous system activity in salt-sensitive patients with essential hypertension. Kidney Int 1982; 21:371.
169. Koolen MI, Van Brummelen P. Adrenergic activity and peripheral hemodynamics in relation to sodium sensitivity in patients with essential hypertension. Hypertension 1984; 6:820.
170. Koepke JP, Jones S, DiBona GF. High sodium intake increases sensitivity of central alpha-2 adrenoceptors in spontaneously hypertensive rats. Hypertension 1988; 11:326–333.
171. Chen Y-F, et al. High NaCl diet reduces hypothalamic norepinephrine turnover in hypertensive rats. Hypertension 1988; 11:55–62.
172. Mendlowitz M, et al. Vascular responsiveness in hypertensive and hypotensive rats. Geriatrics 1965; 20:797–807.
173. Vlachakis N. Blood pressure response to noradenaline infusion in relationship to plasma catecholamines and renin activity in man. J Clin Pharmacol 1979; 19:654–661.
174. Iimura O, Kikuchi K, Sato S. Plasma noradenaline concentration and pressor response to infused noradenaline in patients with borderline hypertension, and mild or moderate essential hypertension. Jpn Circ J 1984; 48:159–167.
175. Bianchetti MG, et al. Correction of cardiovascular hypertensivity to norepinephrine by potassium supplementations in normotensive members of hypertensive families and patients with essential hypertension. J Hypertens 1984; 2[Suppl 3]:445–448.
176. Campese VM, et al. Pressor reactivity to norepinephrine and angiotensin in salt-sensitive hypertensive patients. Hypertension 1993; 21:301–307.
177. Weder AB. Membrane sodium transport and salt sensitivity of blood pressure. Hypertension 1991; 17[Suppl I]:I-74–I-80.
178. Rygielski D, et al. Erythrocyte ghost Na^+-K^+-ATPase and blood pressure. Hypertension 1987; 10:259–266.
179. Garay RP, et al. Inherited defect in a Na^+K^+ cotransport system in erythrocytes from essential hypertension. Nature 1980; 284:281–283.
180. Tuck ML, et al. Kinetic analysis of erythrocyte Na^+K^+ pump and cotransport in essential hypertension. Hypertension 1987; 10:204–211.
181. Canessa M, et al. Does sodium intake modify red cell Na transport in normal and hypertensive subjects? Am J Hypertens 1989; 2:513–523.
182. Canessa M, et al. Na-K-Cl cotransport and Na pump in red cells of young blacks and blood pressure response to salt loading. J Clin Hypertens 1986; 2:101–108.
183. Rosskopf D, Dusing R, Siffert W. Membrane sodium–proton exchange and primary hypertension. Hypertension 1993; 21:607–617.
184. Aviv A, Livne A. The Na^+/H^+ antiport, cytosolic free Ca^{2+}, and essential hypertension: a hypothesis. Am J Hypertens 1988; 1:410–413.
185. Berk BC, et al. Spontaneously hypertensive rat vascular smooth muscle cells in culture exhibit increased growth and Na^+/H^+ exchange. J Clin Invest 1989; 83:822–829.
186. Livne A, et al. Increased platelet Na^+-H^+ exchange rates in essential hypertension: application of a novel test. Lancet 1987; 1:533–536.
187. INTERSALT Cooperative Research Group. Intersalt: an international study of electrolyte excretion and blood pressure. Results for 24 hour urinary sodium and potassium excretion. Br Med J 1988; 297:319–328.
188. Schroeder HA. Relation between mortality from cardiovascular disease and treated water supplies: Variations in states and 163 largest municipalities of the United States. JAMA 1960; 172:1902.
189. Harlan WR, Harlan LC. Calcium intake and blood pressure: An epidemiologic perspective. In H Langford, B Levine, LE Bogen, eds. Nutritional Factors in Hypertension. New York: Alan R. Liss, 1990. Pp. 175–197.
190. McCarron DA. Calcium metabolism in health and chronic diseases: An overview. In H Langford, B Levine, LE Bogen, eds., Nutritional Factors in Hypertension. New York: Alan R. Liss, 1990. Pp. 99–106.
191. Hatton DC, McCarron DA. Dietary calcium and blood pressure in experimental models of hypertension: A review. Hypertension 1994; 23(4):513–530.
192. Wright GL, Rankin GO. Concentrations of ionic and total calcium in plasma of our models of hypertension. Am J Physiol 1982; 243:H365–H370.
193. Bindels RJM, et al. Increased plasma calcitonin levels in young spontaneously hypertensive rats: role in disturbed phosphate homeostasis. Pflugers Arch 1987; 408:395–400.
194. Stern N, et al. Effects of high calcium intake on blood pressure and calcium metabolism in young SHR. Hypertension 1984; 6:639–646.
195. McCarron DA, et al. Disturbances of calcium metabolism

in the spontaneously hypertensive rat. Hypertension 1981; 3[Suppl I]:I-162–I-173.

196. Hano T, et al. Antihypertensive effects of oral calcium supplementation in spontaneously hypertensive rats. Contrib Nephrol 1991; 90:36–41.
197. Hatton DC, et al. Blood pressure development and serum calcium in suckling spontaneously hypertensive rat pups: effects of maternal dietary calcium. J Hypertens 1986; 4[Suppl 3]:S465–S467.
198. McCarron DA, et al. Blood pressure and nutrient intake in the United States. Science 1984; 224:1392–1398.
199. Luft FC, et al. Effects of volume expansion and contraction on potassium homeostasis in normal and hypertensive humans. J Am Coll Nutr 1986; 5:357–369.
200. Tuomilehto J, et al. Sodium and potassium excretion in a sample of normotensive and hypertensive persons in eastern Finland. J Epidemiol Community Health 1980; 34:174–178.
201. Doyle AE, Chua KG, Duffy S. Urinary sodium, potassium and creatinine excretion in hypertensive and normotensive Australians. Med J Aust 1976; 2:898–900.
202. Grim CE, et al. Racial differences in blood pressure in Evans County, Georgia: relationship to sodium and potassium intake and plasma renin activity. J Chronic Dis 1980; 33:87–94.
203. Langford HG. Dietary potassium and hypertension: Epidemiologic data. Ann Intern Med 1983; 98(5 pt. 2):770–772.
204. Tobian L. Potassium and hypertension. Nutr Rev 1988; 46(8):273–283.
205. Frisancho AR, Leonard WR, Bollettino LA. Blood pressure in blacks and whites and its relationship to dietary sodium and potassium intake. J Chronic Dis 1984; 37(7):515–519.
206. McCarron DA, et al. Blood pressure and nutrient intake in the United States. Science 1984; 224:1392–1398.
207. Harlan WR, et al. Dietary intake and cardiovascular risk factors, part I. Blood pressure correlates: US, 1971–75. DHHS 1983; publication no. (PHS)83–1676.
208. INTERSALT Study. An international co-operative study on the relation of blood pressure to electrolyte excretion in populations. I. Design and methods. J Hypertens 1986; 4:781–787.
209. Dietz R, et al. Partial replacement of sodium by potassium in the diet restores impaired noradrenaline inactivation and lowers blood pressure in stroke-prone spontaneously hypertensive rats. Clin Sci 1981; 61:69S–71S.
210. Sugden AL, Bean BL, Straw JA. Na^+, K^+ and water balance in young spontaneously hypertensive rats: relationship to blood pressure after high K^+ treatment. Clin Sci 1987; 72:321–327.
211. Tobian L, et al. Potassium protection against lesions of the renal tubules, arteries, and glomeruli and nephron loss in salt-loaded hypertensive Dahl S rats. Hypertension 1984; 62(2 pt. 2):I170–176.
212. Dahl LK, Leitl G, Heine M. Influence of dietary potassium and sodium potassium molar ratios on the development of salt hypertension. J Exp Med 1972; 136:318–330.
213. Kahn M, Bohrer NK. Effect of potassium-induced diuresis on renal concentration and dilution. Am J Physiol 1967; 212:1365–1375.
214. Wright FS, et al. Potassium secretion by distal tubule after potassium adaptation. Am J Physiol 1971; 221(2):437–448.
215. Brandis M, Keyes J, Windhager EE. Potassium-induced inhibition of proximal tubular fluid reabsorption in rats. Am J Physiol 1972; 222(2):421–427.
216. Brunner HR, et al. The influence of potassium administration and of potassium derivation on plasma renin in normal and hypertensive subjects. J Clin Invest 1970; 49:2128–2138.
217. Smith SJ, et al. Does potassium lower blood pressure by increasing sodium excretion? A metabolic study in patients with mild to moderate essential hypertension. J Hypertens 1983; 1[Suppl 2]:27–30.
218. Tabuchi Y, et al. Hypotensive mechanism of potassium supplementation in salt-loaded patients with essential hypertension. J Clin Hypertens 1985; 2:145–152.
219. Iimura O, et al. Studies on the hypotensive effect of high potassium intake in patients with essential hypertension. Clin Sci 1981; 61:77s–80s.
220. Vander AJ. Direct effects of potassium on renin secretion and renal function. Am J Physiol 1970; 219(2):455–459.
221. Sealey JE, et al. Potassium balance and the control of renin secretion. J Clin Invest 1970; 49:2119–2127.
222. Nasjletti A, et al. High potassium intake selectively increases urinary PGF_2 excretion in the rat. Am J Physiol 1985; 17:F382–F388.
223. Campbell WB, Schmitz JM. Effect of alterations in dietary potassium on the pressure and steroidogenic effects of angiotensins II and III. Endocrinology 1978; 103:2098–2104.
224. Overbeck HW, Clark DWJ. Vasodilator responses to K^+ in genetic hypertensive and in renal hypertensive rats. J Lab Clin Med 1975; 86(6):973–983.
225. Webb RC, Bohr DF. Potassium relaxation of vascular smooth muscle from spontaneously hypertensive rats. Blood Vessels 1979; 16:71–79.
226. Lowe RD, Thompson JW. The effect of intra-arterial potassium chloride infusion upon forearm blood flow in man. J Physiol 1962; 162:69P–70P.
227. Overbeck HW, et al. Attenuated vasodilator responses to K^+ in essential hypertensive men. J Clin Invest 1974; 53:678–686.
228. Fujita T, Ando K. Hemodynamic and endocrine changes associated with potassium supplementation in sodium loaded hypertensives. Hypertension 1984; 6:184–192.
229. Zusman RM, Keiser HR. Regulation of prostaglandin E_2 synthesis by angiotensin II, potassium, osmolality, and dexamethasone. Kidney Int 1980; 17:277–283.
230. Klotman PE, et al. Captopril enhances aminoglycoside nephrotoxicity in potassium-depleted rats. Kidney Int 1985; 28:118–127.
231. Horwitz D, Margolius HS, Keiser HR. Effects of dietary potassium and race on urinary excretion of kallikrein and aldosterone in man. J Clin Endocrinol Metab 1978; 47:296–299.

OTHER REFERENCES

Canessa M, et al. Increased sodium–lithium countertransport in red cells of patients with essential hypertension. N Engl J Med 1980; 302:772–776.

DeChamplain J, Krakoff LR, Axelrod J. Interrelationships of sodium intake, hypertension, and norepinephrine storage in the rat. Circ Res 1969; 24[Suppl I]:75–92.

Genain CP, et al. Failure of salt loading to inhibit tissue norepinephrine turnover in prehypertensive Dahl sensitive rats. Hypertension 1988; 12:568–573.

Gordon FJ, et al. Effect of anteroventral third ventricle (AV3V) lesions on the development of hypertension in spontaneously hypertensive rats. Jpn Heart J 1979; 20:116–118.

Miura M, Reis DJ. The role of the solitary and paramedian reticular nuclei in mediating cardiovascular reflex response from carotid baro- and chemoreceptors. J Physiol 1972; 239:525–548.

Winternitz SR, Oparil S. Sodium-neural interactions in the development of spontaneous hypertension. Clin Exp Hypertens 1982; 4:751–760.

Pathophysiology of Vasospasm

John P. Cooke
Victor J. Dzau

Vasospasm may be defined as excessive constriction of a vessel resulting in ischemia of the tissue that it subserves (Fig. 16-1A). **Venospasm** may be similarly defined as excessive constriction of a vein inducing a pathologic impedance to venous outflow from the tissue it drains. In general, vasospasm is due to a disruption of the normal balance of vasoconstrictor and vasodilator influences. Thus, in the absence of a fixed narrowing in the vessel wall, excessive vasoconstriction (vasospasm) can create pathophysiologic reductions in blood flow.

The definition of vasospasm becomes more difficult in the presence of a fixed lesion, such as an atherosclerotic plaque. In that case, tissue ischemia might result from normal vasomotion superimposed on a hemodynamically significant lesion (Fig. 16-1B). The symptoms and signs related to that event may be indistinguishable from true vasospasm. Indeed, changes in blood fluidity may induce symptoms mimicking those of vasospasm in the absence of vasomotion, as in the case of platelets transiently aggregating at the site of a highly stenotic lesion (Fig. 16-1C). The astute clinician and investigator, however, are cognizant of the different pathophysiologic processes that may present as vasospasm and are careful to differentiate, for example, primary from secondary Raynaud's phenomenon and true coronary vasospasm from normal vasomotion superimposed on a highly stenotic lesion.

The term *vasospasm* is frequently misused. Four decades ago, Pickering gently chided his colleagues for invoking vasospasm uncritically as the cause of transient ischemia in a variety of situations:

> . . . many of the manifestations of disease that have been ascribed to abnormal contraction of a single artery, or group of arteries, are in fact due to other circumstances, of which the chief is organic arterial occlusion or obstruction. These phenomena can be interpreted in terms of known pathologic or physiologic processes, without assuming that arteries behave like whimsical children and react violently to a perfectly ordinary stimulus or to none at all [1].

His words remain a useful caveat today, since the term *vasospasm* is used often but not often used well. Conscious of Pickering's caution, Prinzmetal eschewed the term *vasospasm* in his landmark article describing variant angina, postulating instead that attacks were precipitated by "a normal increase in tonus of the vessel wall" superimposed on an atherosclerotic lesion [2]. Despite Prinzmetal's thoughtful analysis, *coronary vasospasm* is most frequently incriminated in the disorder that bears his name. One may argue that it is an issue of semantics to distinguish between true vasospasm and other causes of dynamic fluctuation in luminal diameter, particularly given the clinical observation that these all respond to vasodilator therapy. However, the development of improved and specific therapies for these different pathophysiologic processes will be facilitated by the distinction [3].

Similarly, vasospasm of the digital arteries should not be reflexively indicted in Raynaud's phenomenon, particularly when associated with conditions, such as scleroderma, that make normal fluctuations in tone superimposed on a fixed lesion the more likely mechanism [4]. Cerebral vasospasm occurs after a subarachnoid hemorrhage, but in later stages of the process the narrowed lumen is due primarily to structural changes in the vessel wall [5]. Less appropriate is the use of vasospasm to describe the phenomenon in severely hypertensive patients in which segments of the retinal vessels assume a narrow caliber in comparison to adjacent segments. In truth, it is the narrow segments that are responding with normal vasomotion to an increased systemic pressure, whereas the dilated segments have lost their capacity to autoregulate [6].

The pathogenesis of vasospasm is not yet completely understood, but it is likely that multiple determinants are responsible and that these vary in importance depending on the circulatory bed involved and the associated disease states. An understanding of the mechanisms of vasospasm requires a fundamental knowledge of the physiology of vasomotion.

Physiology of Vasomotion

Vasomotor tone is finely regulated by both systemic and local forces. A variety of vasoconstrictor and vasodilator influences form a complex system of checks and balances that allows the vessel to respond to changes in systemic hemodynamics or local tissue demands. A disturbance of the balance between vasoconstrictor and vasodilator influence may lead to vasospasm. Therefore, a discussion of vasospasm best begins with a review of the determinants of vasomotion.

NEUROGENIC CONTROL

Blood vessels are innervated to varying degrees by sympathetic nerve fibers, ranging from no innervation at all, as in the umbilical vessels, to dense sympathetic innervation, as in the digital arteries. The sympathetic nerve fibers course through the vessel in the adventitia and external one-third of the media forming a network of slender processes (about 0.1 μm in diameter). At regular intervals along these fibers, localized swellings can be seen. These varicosities are closely apposed to the vascular smooth muscle; they contain granular vesicles in which the neurotransmitter substances are stored.

Norepinephrine released from the sympathetic nerve ending stimulates postjunctional alpha adrenoceptors on the smooth muscle to initiate vasoconstriction. In most vessels, these alpha-adrenergic receptors are of the $alpha_1$ subtype, although in a few vascular beds, postjunctional

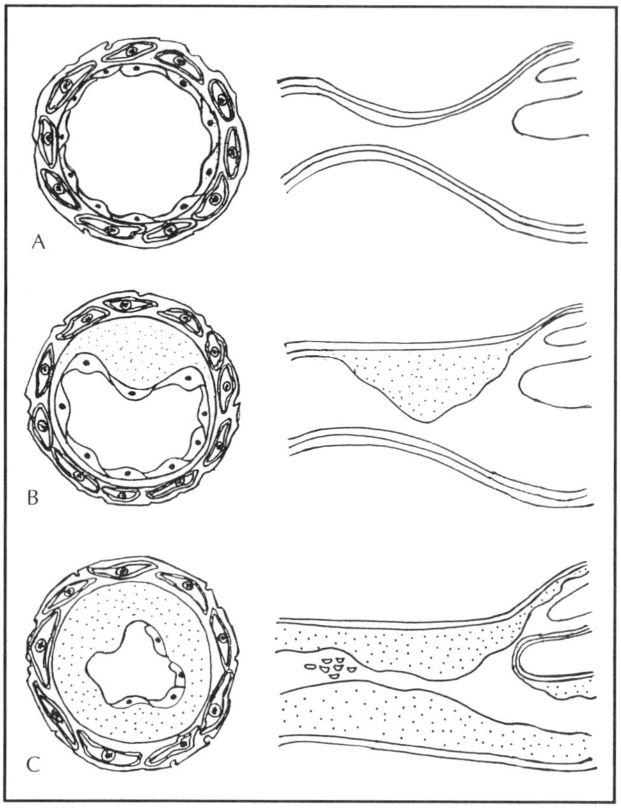

Fig. 16-1. Transient regional ischemia in the absence of increased oxygen demand may be secondary to **A.** excessive vascoconstriction, **B.** normal vasomotion superimposed on reduced perfusion pressure or a fixed structural change in the vessel wall, or **C.** transient rheologic changes (e.g., platelet aggregation, precipitation of cold agglutinins) often superimposed on fixed or dynamic changes (or both) in the vessel wall.

$alpha_2$ adrenoceptors contribute to the contractile response [7–9]. In the coronary artery, beta-adrenergic receptors predominate over alpha adrenoceptors on the postjunctional smooth muscle [10]. In that tissue, release of norepinephrine from adrenergic nerves thereby induces vasodilation of the epicardial coronary arteries mediated by the beta adrenoceptors.

Prejunctional receptors (on the nerve ending) modulate the release of norepinephrine. Some of these receptors are facilitatory and, when stimulated, augment the release of neurotransmitter. Such receptors include those for angiotensin II and epinephrine. Other receptors, when stimulated, inhibit neurotransmission, including those for acetycholine, 5-hydroxytryptamine, and histamine [11].

Vascular smooth muscle is also innervated by cholinergic fibers. Release of acetylcholine from these nerve endings generally induces vasodilation, presumably via stimulation of prejunctional muscarinic receptors on the sympathetic nerve ending. As previously mentioned, stimulation of those receptors by acetylcholine reduces release of norepinephrine from the adrenergic nerve ending. Acetylcholine released from cholinergic fibers also may stimulate the endothelium to release endothelium-derived relaxing factor (EDRF). That effect of neuronally released acetylcholine has not been established, however, and seems unlikely to occur in the conduit vessels in which acetylcholine likely would be metabolized before it could diffuse through the media to the endothelium.

Disturbances in adrenergic or cholinergic neurotransmission likely play a role in vasospasm in some vascular beds. Other neurotransmitters that may modulate smooth muscle tone to a lesser degree include dopamine, adenosine triphosphate (ATP), and the neuropeptides substance P, neuropeptide Y, and vasoactive intestinal peptide. There is no evidence yet that these substances play a major role in vasospastic disorders.

CIRCULATING VASOACTIVE SUBSTANCES

Vasoconstrictors. The primary vasoconstrictor hormones are norepinephrine, angiotensin II, and arginine vasopressin (AVP). Circulating norepinephrine is released from adrenergic nerve endings and secreted by the adrenal medulla. Its effect on vascular tone is potentiated by angiotensin II. In addition to its direct effect to induce vasoconstriction, angiotensin II stimulates neurons in the central nervous system to increase sympathetic nerve activity. In the periphery, angiotensin II facilitates the release of norepinephrine from adrenergic nerve endings by virtue of its excitatory presynaptic effects. It also inhibits neuronal uptake of norepinephrine to increase the half-life of norepinephrine released at the neuromuscular junction. Furthermore, by augmenting aldosterone release, angiotensin II increases intracellular sodium concentration within the vessel wall. That leads to an increase in intracellular calcium (via sodium-calcium exchange) and thus to a more reactive vessel. Angiotensin II traditionally is viewed as a hormonal product involving the participation of the liver, kidney, and endothelium. More recently it has become apparent that a local renin-angiotensin system exists in the vessel wall by virtue of its intrinsic synthesis of angiotensinogen, renin, and converting enzyme [12]. There is good evidence that a disturbance of the vascular renin-angiotensin system may participate in hypertension, but no role has been defined for it in vasospasm.

The neurohypophyseal peptide AVP promotes water reabsorption by the kidney and causes constriction in most peripheral vascular beds. In cerebral vessels, however, this hormone induces endothelium-dependent vasodilation [13]. AVP also induces vasodilation of the forearm musculature [14]. This vasoactive hormone is released in response to shock or hemorrhage and probably acts to redistribute blood flow to cerebral and skeletal-muscle circulations. The combined actions may serve to maintain blood pressure and redistribute blood flow to sustain critical tissue function during hypotensive states.

Circulating endogenous inhibitors of the sodium-potassium ATPase pump are putative hormones thought to play a role in natriuresis and vasoconstriction [15]. These agents have yet to be characterized fully, but evidence for circulating ouabainlike substances has been obtained in a number of mammalian species, including humans. Like the cardiac glycosides, these agents inhibit the sodium-potassium ATPase pump to depolarize vascular smooth muscle and thereby increase sodium-calcium exchange across the cell membrane. These actions increase intracellular calcium concentration, augment the contractile state of vascular smooth muscle, and increase neuronal release of norepinephrine. The importance of these substances in hypertensive states is under investigation.

Vasodilators. Epinephrine has greater affinity for beta-adrenergic receptors than alpha-adrenergic receptors on the vascular smooth muscle and generally induces vasodilation. In certain vascular beds in which alpha adrenoceptors predominate, however, epinephrine acts as a vasoconstrictor. Furthermore, in the presence of beta-adrenoceptor blockade, epinephrine may induce unopposed alpha-adrenergic vasoconstriction. Epinephrine is also a strongly positive inotropic agent; because it increases cardiac output and heart rate, mean arterial pressure is maintained despite the drop in systemic resistance mediated by beta-adrenergic vasodilation.

Atrial natriuretic peptide (ANP) also acts as a vasodilator [16]. The vasodilation elicited by ANP is mediated by cyclic guanosine monophosphate (cGMP), which is generated by activation of particulate guanylate cyclase. This is in contradistinction to the action of nitrovasodilators, which induce a rise in tissue GMP via soluble guanylate cyclase. The vasodilation induced by ANP subsequently reduces venous return and mean arterial pressure, thereby reducing the atrial distention that is the stimulus for its release.

The primary role of insulin and glucagon is to maintain normoglycemia, but those hormones also have direct effects on the vasculature. Glucagon induces vasodilation by a cyclic adenosine monophosphate (cAMP)–dependent mechanism [17]. Insulin also acts as a vasodilator independently of its effects on plasma glucose. Infusion of insulin into the brachial artery increases blood flow in the human forearm [18]. That effect is antagonized by propranolol and is thus likely mediated by beta-adrenergic receptors.

THE ENDOTHELIUM

The endothelium is much more than a sheet of nucleated cellophane, to echo the words of Lord Florey, the experimental pathologist and Nobel laureate [19]. It is, rather, a metabolic factory that actively participates in the hemostatic process, regulates vasomotion, and influences vascular structure by synthesizing and secreting a wide variety of substances (Fig. 16-2). Those substances include factors that modulate the interaction of circulating blood elements with the vessel wall, coagulation factors, inhibitors and activators of fibrinolysis, growth factors, and regulators of vascular smooth muscle tone [20–25]. Prostacyclin is a vasodilator of major importance. An endothelial product derived from arachidonic acid by the action of cyclo-oxygenase, prostacyclin acts as a potent inhibitor of vascular reactivity and platelet aggregation [24,25]. Its importance as a modulator of vessel tone is highlighted by the in vitro observation that inhibitors of cyclooxygenase cause vascular rings to contract [26].

Yet another potent vasodilator is EDRF [27]. EDRF is now known to be nitric oxide, derived from the metabolism of L-arginine [28–30]. It acts as a nitrovasodilator in that its effect is mediated by increases in vascular levels of cGMP and is antagonized by inhibitors of soluble guanylate cyclase. Its importance in regulating vasomotion is underscored by its demonstration throughout the vascular tree in a wide range of species, from lower vertebrates to humans [31,32]. EDRF modulates a multitude of stimuli impinging on the vessel wall. Aggregating platelets induce endothelium-dependent vasodilation in the presence of intact endothelium but vasoconstriction after endothelial injury [33,34]. The direct vasoconstrictor actions of serotonin, norepinephrine, and vasopressin are opposed by simultaneous stimulation of their specific receptors on the endothelium and subsequent release of EDRF [13,34,35]. In addition, the endothelium actively metabolizes norepinephrine and serotonin to attenuate their effects [36].

Flowing blood induces endothelium-dependent vasodilation that is largely due to the action of EDRF, although prostacyclin may play a lesser role [37–41]. Endothelial shear stress imposed by flow also opens potassium channels to hyperpolarize the cell [42]. That wave of hyperpolarization may spread via gap junctions to underlying vascular smooth muscle to contribute to flow-mediated vasodilation. In addition to EDRF, the endothelium also releases a hyperpolarizing factor (EDHF) to induce vasodilation [43].

The endothelium also secretes substances that may participate in states of hypertonus. In addition to angiotensin II, endothelial cells synthesize histamine, as do mast cells in the perivascular tissue. Endothelin is yet another product of the endothelium [44]. Endothelin is a peptide that evokes an intense and prolonged vasoconstriction that is slow in onset. Synthesis of endothelin is known to be triggered by epinephrine or thrombin and by a reduction in endothelial shear stress (as in a low-flow state). In addition to being the most potent peptide vasoconstrictor known, endothelin also stimulates proliferation of vascular smooth muscle [45].

BLOOD ELEMENTS

In the presence of an intact endothelium, aggregating platelets induce vasodilation, which is predominantly mediated by adenosine diphosphate released from the platelets [34]. In addition, epinephrine and 5-hydroxytryptamine (serotonin) released from aggregating platelets may contribute to endothelium-dependent relaxation [33,35]. When the endothelium is injured, those same substances may trigger vasoconstriction via the activation of alpha-adrenergic and serotonergic receptors, respectively, on the vascular smooth muscle. Thromboxane A_2 also contributes to the vasoconstriction induced by platelets aggregating in an area of intimal injury.

Other blood elements modulate vasomotion. Under certain circumstances, neutrophils may release a vasodilator that resembles EDRF in its action [46]. Conversely, activated neutrophils release the vasoconstrictor superoxide anion that inactivates EDRF and precipitates lipid peroxidation and endothelial injury [47,48]. White blood cells also release vasoconstrictor leukotrienes in addition to thromboxane A_2. The vasoconstrictor leukotrienes (LTC_4, LTD_4, and LTE_4) are potent coronary constrictors in the

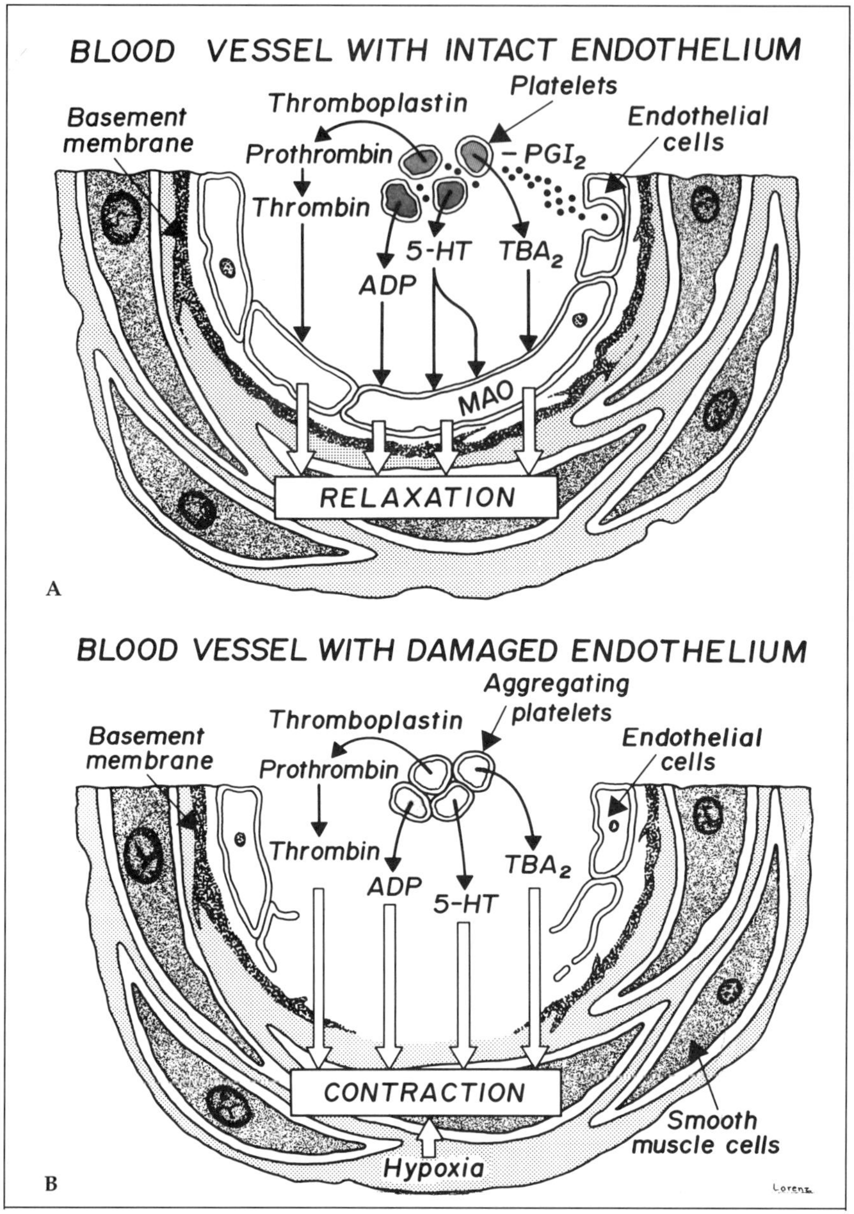

Fig. 16-2. Role of the endothelium in modulating vasoreactivity. **A.** An intact endothelium favors vasodilation. Prostacyclin (PGI_2) released from the endothelium inhibits platelet and vascular reactivity. EDRF has similar activity and is released in response to substances derived from aggregating platelets and circulating vasoconstrictors. The endothelial cell also degrades many vasoactive substances. **B.** The injured or dysfunctional endothelium favors vasoconstriction. Platelets aggregate in the absence of prostacyclin and EDRF and release vasoactive substances, which now induce excessive vasoconstriction without the buffering influence of the endothelium. Hypoxic endothelium releases vasoconstrictor prostanoids and perhaps increased amounts of endothelin. 5-HT = serotonin; ADP = adenosine diphosphate. (Reproduced with permission from JT Shepherd, PM Vanhoutte. Spasm of the coronary arteries; causes and consequences [the scientist's viewpoint]. Mayo Clin Proc 1985; 60:33–46.)

feline circulation but preferentially constrict the resistance vessels in the atherosclerotic miniature swine; in the latter model of epicardial coronary artery spasm, leukotrienes do not appear to play a major role [49,50].

Free hemoglobin augments vessel tone by virtue of its ability to scavenge EDRF and inactivate soluble guanylate cyclase (the enzyme required for the intracellular synthesis of the vasodilator cGMP) [51]. Hemoglobin also releases norepinephrine from sympathetic nerve endings. Furthermore, the oxidation of oxyhemoglobin to methemoglobin liberates superoxide anion, a reaction that occurs slowly in vivo [52].

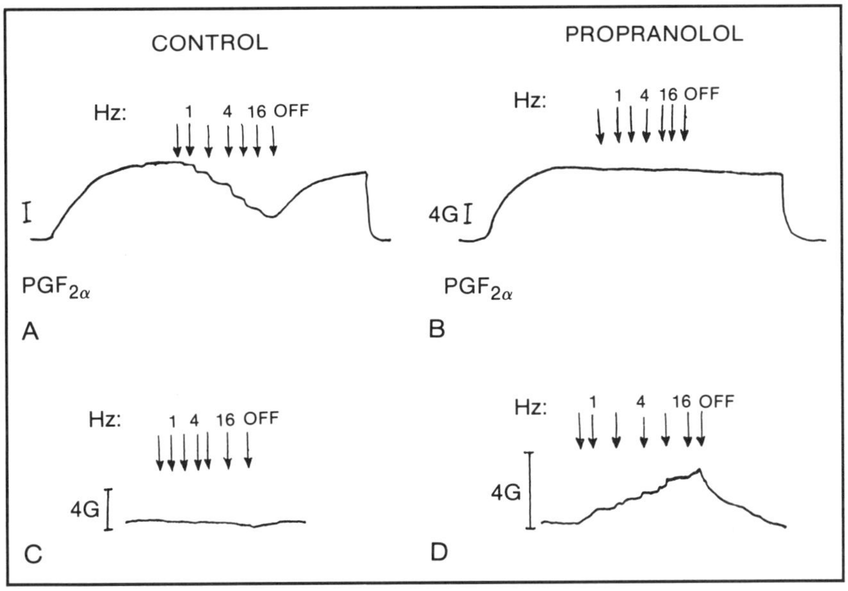

Fig. 16-3. The beta-adrenergic antagonist propranolol unmasks alpha-adrenergic contraction to nerve-released norepinephrine. **A.** In vitro, a vascular ring taken from canine left circumflex coronary artery contracts with the administration of prostaglandin F_2 alpha ($PGF_{2\alpha}$) and then relaxes to increasing frequency of electrical stimulation (measured in Hz). The relaxation is due to activation of beta-adrenergic receptors in the vascular smooth muscle by norepinephrine released from the electrically stimulated nerve endings. **B.** After administration of propranolol, the relaxation to nerve-released norephinephrine is blocked. **C.** When the ring is not contracted, electrical stimulation has no effect on basal tension. **D.** After administration of propranolol, the ring contracts to nerve-released norepinephrine, due to unopposed activation of alpha adrenoceptors. (Modified from PM Vanhoutte. Automonic nerves, aggregating platelets and contraction of coronary arterial smooth muscle. In FL Abel, WH Newman, eds. Functional Aspects of the Normal, Hypertrophied and Failing Heart. Boston: Martinus Nijhoff, 1984. Pp. 135–148.)

EXOGENOUS INFLUENCES

Normally, a delicate interplay between endogenous vasoconstrictor and vasodilator influences serves to regulate vasomotion in response to changes in systemic hemodynamics or local tissue demand. A number of exogenous influences (e.g., drugs) can disturb that balance to induce vasospasm.

Cocaine potentiates adrenergic neurotransmission to elicit vasoconstriction. This agent blocks neuronal uptake of norepinephrine, thereby increasing the concentration of nerve-released norepinephrine at the neuromuscular junction. Recreational use of cocaine may result in paroxysmal vasoconstriction of coronary arteries with ischemic injury and occasionally a fatal outcome even in subjects with apparently normal epicardial coronary vessels [53,54].

In some circumstances, the beta-adrenergic antagonists are known to precipitate vasospasm in the coronary, cerebral, and digital circulations, probably by altering the balance between alpha- and beta-adrenergic response. When beta-adrenoceptors are antagonized by propranolol, alpha-adrenergic vasoconstriction is unmasked in the canine coronary artery (Fig. 16-3) [10]. Similarly, paralysis of the sodium-potassium ATPase pump by cardiac glycosides inactivates the beta adrenoceptors, leaving the alpha receptor unopposed [55]. Those findings may explain the observation that symptoms may be aggravated by propranolol or digoxin in some patients with ischemic syndromes [56–58].

Likewise, ergot drugs and methysergide can exacerbate symptoms in patients with significant coronary artery disease or vasospasm. These drugs likely stimulate serotonergic and alpha-adrenergic receptors to activate vascular smooth muscle and have been reported to aggravate ischemic syndromes. Inhalation of tobacco smoke also exacerbates ischemic syndromes. In addition to accelerating atherosclerosis, smoking increases sympathetic outflow from the central nervous system to increase coronary tone [59]. Coronary- and digital-artery vasospasm also may occur in munitions workers chronically exposed to industrial nitroglycerin, typically on weekends [60]. The latter phenomenon is thought to be due to the sudden withdrawal of nitrate action.

The oncologic agents 5-fluorouracil, vinblastine, and bleomycin may precipitate coronary vasospasm and Raynaud's phenomenon [61,62]. The pathophysiologic mechanism is not understood. Industrial exposure to vinyl chloride polymerization processes also may induce Raynaud's phenomenon (as well as acro-osteolysis of the distal phalanges) in a small percentage of workers [63].

In addition to drugs, physical influences may precipitate spasm. Coronary catheters induce focal spasm in a small percentage of patients undergoing angiography, but this phenomenon is clinically unrelated to variant angina.

At least 5 percent of angioplasty procedures are attended by vasospasm, which may be due to endothelial injury [64]. After angioplasty, coronary vasoconstriction is also seen as a response to the restoration of normal perfusion pressure in the segment of vessel distal to the stenosis [65].

In stenotic arteries, passive changes in vessel diameter may precipitate symptoms that mimic those of vasospasm. Physical forces that may cause passive changes in the diameter of the coronary lumen include blood flow and perfusion pressure. Increases in blood-flow velocity normally evoke endothelium-dependent vasodilation, but in the presence of a significant atherosclerotic lesion, increased velocity may reduce luminal diameter [66]. That is due to the fact that increases in velocity cause a larger drop in transluminal pressure across a stenosis. By that mechanism, angina may be aggravated by vasodilators that preferentially act on resistance vessels to increase blood-flow velocity (such as dipyridamole). Blood-vessel diameter also is dependent on perfusion pressure. In a certain physiologic range, changes in vessel diameter with changes in perfusion pressure are minor due to the phenomenon of autoregulation. However, major reductions in systemic pressure passively reduce the luminal diameter.

Pathophysiology of Vasospasm

VASOSPASM OF THE CORONARY ARTERIES

Coronary vasospasm is manifested by anginal pain not related to exertion and classically is associated with the electrocardiographic finding of ST segment elevation [2,67]. It is confirmed by the angiographic demonstration of dynamic narrowing of a coronary artery, occurring spontaneously or provoked by intravenous administration of ergonovine maleate and inducing a total or subtotal (> 75%) occlusion (Fig. 16-4) [67–70]. Episodes usually are relieved by nitroglycerin. Prolonged paroxysms may induce arrhythmias, myocardial necrosis, or both [71].

It is probably useful to distinguish coronary vasospasm occurring in an angiographically normal (or minimally diseased) vessel from vasoconstriction superimposed on a significant fixed coronary stenosis. As outlined next, the pathophysiologic mechanisms and the progression of disease appear to be different in these two cases.

In the cardiac catheterization laboratory, the diagnosis of coronary vasospasm can be made using intravenous ergonovine maleate [72]. This provocative test has a sensitivity and specificity exceeding 90 percent and is superior to the cold pressor and exercise tests [73,74]. Initially, it was thought that the action of ergonovine was mediated by alpha-adrenergic receptors, but it is now apparent that a serotonergic mechanism predominates [75,76]. In normal coronary arteries, ergonovine elicits a mild diffuse vasoconstriction; in patients with variant angina, this agent precipitates intense focal or diffuse vasoconstriction of the culprit arteries. The vasospasm is usually associated with anginal pain and ST segment elevation. In normal subjects, it seems likely that ergonovine simultaneously stimulates serotonergic receptors on the vascular smooth muscle (to induce vasoconstriction) and endothelium (to release EDRF) with a resultant mild vasoconstriction. In patients with atherosclerotic coronary artery disease, the buffering influence of the endothelium is lost in such a way that a more marked vasoconstriction obtains.

Endothelial dysfunction probably plays a major role in coronary vasoconstriction, causing transient myocardial ischemia in patients with atherosclerotic coronary artery disease. Its role in precipitating true vasospasm in patients with minimal atherosclerosis is less secure. Nevertheless, injury to the endothelium permits vasoconstrictor influences to predominate. After balloon-catheter denudation of the endothelium followed by a high-cholesterol diet, the coronary artery in miniature swine becomes hyperresponsive to vasoconstrictors [77]. Ergonovine maleate, serotonin, and histamine trigger vasospasm in the injured segments of the coronary artery. Although endothelium regenerates to resurface an injured area, this new tissue is morphologically and functionally abnormal [78,79]. The endothelial cells are cuboidal and not aligned in the direction of flow, and endothelium-dependent vasodilation in vitro is attenuated or absent [79].

Similarly, vessels from hypercholesterolemic swine, monkeys, and rabbits are hyperresponsive to vasoconstrictor agents, largely because of attenuated endothelium-dependent relaxation, although a direct action of cholesterol on the smooth muscle membrane to facilitate calcium entry or to alter signal transduction may play a role [80–83]. In humans, intracoronary administration of acetylcholine induces vasoconstriction of atherosclerotic vessels but vasodilation of angiographically normal vessels [84]. The paradoxical response to acetylcholine chloride likely is due to an imbalance between its direct vasoconstrictor action and its indirect action to release EDRF. Likewise, the increase in forearm blood flow with intra-arterial administration of methacholine chloride is attenuated in hypercholesterolemic subjects [85]. The abnormality in both circulations is due to a diminished activity of EDRF and can be corrected by infusion of the EDRF precursor, L-arginine [86,87].

Hypoxic injury to the endothelium can incite spasm. In dogs, ischemia followed by reperfusion of a coronary artery disrupts the ultrastructure of the endothelium and abrogates its vasodilator influence [88,89]. Oxygen free radicals released during reperfusion damage the cell membrane and quench EDRF [47,48]. Under those pathologic conditions, the endothelium also generates vasoconstrictor substances [90]. Together, these processes may be responsible for the increased frequency of coronary vasospasm following myocardial infarction [77]. They also may contribute to the frustrating clinical scenario of early reocclusion after successful reperfusion of the coronary artery using thrombolytic agents.

Additional evidence that endothelial dysfunction plays a role in alterations in coronary tone comes from the observation that flow-mediated vasoconstriction, rather than vasodilation, may occur in patients with coronary disease. In normal subjects, exercise elicits vasodilation of the epicardial coronary arteries that is proportional to increases in coronary artery flow. In patients with coronary disease, angina may be precipitated by exercise, which appears to be due to a paradoxical vasoconstriction with augmented flow [91]. In animal models, flow-mediated vasodilation is lost after endothelial injury [37,40].

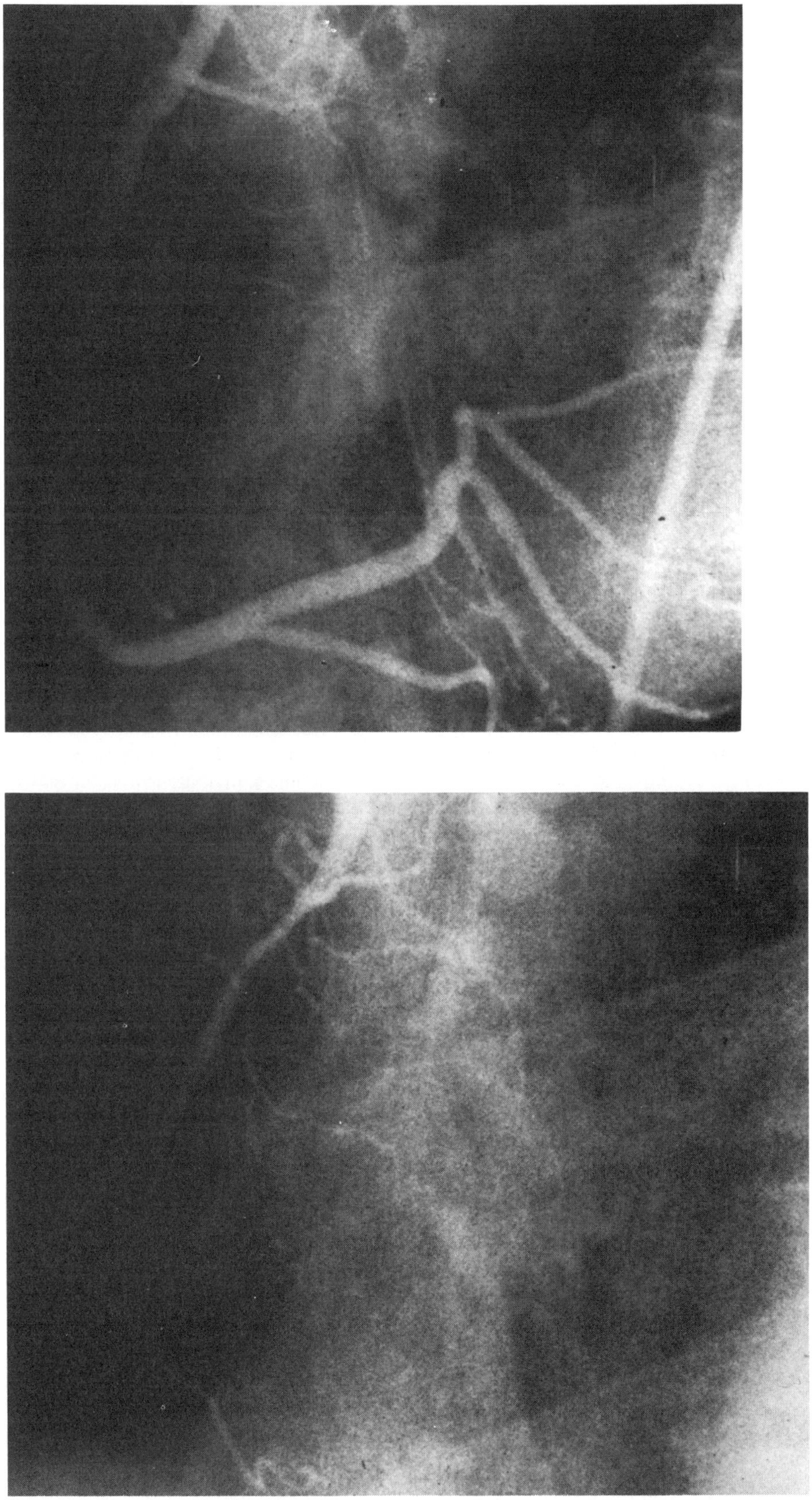

A

B

Fig. 16-4.

Damage to the endothelium reduces release of prostacyclin as well as of EDRF. The importance of this vasodilator is highlighted by observations using the cyclooxygenase inhibitor indomethacin, which abrogates synthesis of prostacyclin. Indomethacin provokes vasoconstriction in the canine coronary artery, demonstrated in vivo by angiography [92]. In humans, indomethacin increases coronary vascular resistance and may exacerbate anginal symptoms [93]. Even in the absence of antagonists, production of prostacyclin is reduced in segments of the vessel wall harboring atherosclerotic plaque [94]. That may explain in part the tendency for vasospasm to occur in the vicinity of atherosclerotic lesions.

Although an endothelial vasodilator dysfunction almost certainly contributes to transient myocardial ischemia in patients with atherosclerotic coronary stenoses, it is not clear whether vasospasm occurring in angiographically normal coronary arteries has the same pathophysiologic mechanism. Indeed, the endothelium-dependent vasodilation to substance P and to low doses of intracoronary acetylcholine is preserved in patients with coronary vasospasm and normal baseline coronary arteriograms [95].

It is also possible that vasodilator influences of the endothelium may be eclipsed by its vasoconstrictor properties under certain circumstances. That possibility was put forward by Osler, who postulated that a "perverted internal secretion" was responsible for coronary vasospasm [96]. A possible candidate substance is histamine [97]. In the human coronary artery, histamine acts as a vasoconstrictor, and its effect is intensified in atherosclerotic vessels [98,99]. Furthermore, the levels of endogenous histamine are elevated in those tissues [99]. Those findings may explain the observation that histamine provokes spasm in some patients with variant angina [100]. In the miniature-swine model of coronary vasospasm, histamine is as effective as ergonovine in provoking spasm [77]. In that model, there is a close spatial correlation between the site of spasm and the atherosclerotic portion of the coronary artery. The increased response of the vascular smooth muscle is specific for histamine, since the smooth muscle response to other agonists is not affected. Endothelium-dependent vasodilation to histamine and serotonin also is attenuated in those atherosclerotic pigs. Endothelin also may play a role in coronary hypertonus. Levels of that vasoconstrictor peptide are increased in the vessel wall and in plasma of hypercholesterolemic swine and patients with atherosclerosis [101,102]. Specific endothelin antagonists under clinical investigation will provide information regarding the contribution of the vasoconstrictor in pathophysiologic states.

In addition to endothelial vasodilator dysfunction, an aberration of adrenergic response may contribute to vasospasm in some cases. Subcutaneous administration of epinephrine has been reported to precipitate episodes [103], whereas phentolamine alleviates symptoms of coronary vasospasm in some patients [104]. The cold pressor test augments sympathetic outflow to the heart and may also trigger attacks [105]. In subjects with atherosclerosis, the cold pressor test increases coronary vascular resistance, suggesting that atherosclerosis may alter the balance between alpha- and beta-adrenergic response [106]. That is supported by the in-vitro finding that atherosclerotic human coronary arteries are hyperresponsive to norepinephrine (as well as to histamine and serotonin) [99]. Another explanation is that in those patients, there is an endothelial vasodilator dysfunction and a reduction in the release of endothelial vasodilators that normally act as a countervailing force to sympathetic activation [107, 108].

In most cases of variant angina, alpha-adrenergic response does not play a major role. Since beta adrenoceptors predominate in the coronary smooth muscle, local release of endogenous norepinephrine normally produces vasodilation. Furthermore, prior to a true vasospastic attack, it is unusual to observe signs of increased sympathetic activity to the heart (manifested by an increase in heart rate or prolongation of the Q–T interval) [109]. Only in a minority of patients is spasm precipitated by the cold pressor test or by administration of adrenergic agonists [74,109]. Adrenergic antagonists are not effective therapy for the majority of patients with variant angina, and the response to surgical denervation is inconsistent [109–111]. Furthermore, vasospasm has been reported following cardiac transplantation, a setting in which the coronary arteries are divorced from direct nervous control [112].

Platelets contribute in a major way to abnormal vasomotion in the coronary circulation. Infusion of serotonin into the coronary arteries of normal individuals causes mild vasodilation at lower doses and only mild constriction at higher doses [113]. By contrast, in patients with stable angina, serotonin causes only vasoconstriction, and at higher doses patients develop angina and electrocardiographic changes. Patients with variant angina have a more pronounced vasoconstriction to serotonin, with coronary occlusion at the higher doses [113]. In patients with variant angina and in those with unstable angina, there is biochemical evidence of platelet activation during attacks manifested by elevated levels of thromboxane metabolites or of platelet factor 4 [114,115]. In patients with unstable angina or rest pain, fresh thrombus in association with a disrupted atherosclerotic plaque is observed by arteriography or angioscopy [116,117]. In those syndromes, vasodilators and antiplatelet agents often are of therapeutic benefit since aggregating platelets release a variety of potent vasoconstrictors [33,34,118]. In addition, serotonin released from aggregating platelets may be taken up by adrenergic nerve endings in vessels with endothelium. Later, the serotonin is coreleased with norepinephrine to stimulate excitatory serotonergic receptors, thereby blunting beta-adrenergic vasodilation [119].

Fig. 16-4. **A.** A coronary angiogram demonstrating minimal irregularities of the right coronary artery in a patient with symptoms suggestive of coronary artery vasospasm. **B.** The coronary angiogram is repeated after an intravenous bolus of ergonovine to reveal marked vasospasm of the right coronary artery with occlusion in its midportion.

Transient episodes of angina not related to exertion are usually ascribed to vasospasm, but it is possible that in some patients with high-grade stenosis, luminal obstruction by platelet aggregates in the absence of vasoconstriction may be responsible. Folts and colleagues have found cyclic flow reductions due to platelet aggregates in dogs with experimental stenosis of the coronary artery [120]. Antiplatelet agents were more effective than vasodilators in preventing those cyclic flow reductions.

Despite the contribution of platelets to coronary vasomotion in the setting of a high-grade stenosis, antagonists of platelet-derived vasoconstrictors have not been effective in variant angina. The thromboxane synthase inhibitor dazoxiben as well as the serotonin antagonist ketanserin have failed to provide therapeutic benefit in most cases [121,122]. However, the doses of ketanserin used may not have been great enough to block the high concentrations of serotonin that are known to exist at the surface of the vessel [123]. Furthermore, it may be necessary to antagonize thromboxane and serotonin simultaneously to have an effect. In one study of six patients with variant angina, however, aspirin reduced thromboxane B_2 levels to less than 3 percent of control values but did not alter episodes of ischemia [124]. Those studies indicate that the mechanism of coronary vasospasm is different from that of unstable angina.

The question has been raised whether coronary vasospasm is linked to the progression of disease. Experimental data have suggested that vasospasm may induce alterations in endothelial cytostructure and the integrity of the endothelial surface, possibly due to local hemodynamic disturbances [125]. Coronary vasospasm also has been implicated in rapid expansion of lesions by rupturing intralesional capillaries and causing intramural hemorrhage [126]. Moreover, endothelial vasodilator dysfunction may promote processes that accelerate the progression of atherosclerosis. Specifically, endothelium-derived nitric oxide and prostacyclin are both potent inhibitors of platelet aggregation, vascular smooth muscle proliferation, and leukocyte–vessel wall interaction [127,128]. The first observable event in atherogenesis, the adherence of monocytes to the endothelium, is inhibited by endothelium-derived nitric oxide. Therefore, it is conceivable that a loss of endothelial vasodilator dysfunction could promote atherogenesis. Indeed, all the known risk factors for atherosclerosis (hypercholesterolemia, hypertension, diabetes mellitus, lipoprotein(a), tobacco use, age, homocystinemia) are associated with reduced endothelium-dependent vasodilation, even prior to the development of clinically apparent atherosclerosis [129–133]. Moreover, when the elaboration of endothelium-derived nitric oxide is restored, atherogenesis is markedly inhibited in hypercholesterolemic animals [134]. By contrast, inhibition of nitric oxide synthase accelerates atherogenesis in animal models [135,136].This acceleration of atherosclerosis by endothelial vasodilator dysfunction may occur in humans. Indeed, in 239 patients with ischemic heart disease followed for up to 10 years, a positive ergonovine test was predictive of progression and subsequent myocardial infarction [137].

Although endothelial vasodilator dysfunction exists in ischemic heart disease and may play a role in progression, its role in true coronary vasospasm is not clear. As previously mentioned, endothelium-dependent vasodilation appears to be preserved in true coronary vasospasm [96]. In addition, progression of atherosclerosis at the site of vasospasm does not occur at a faster rate than nonspastic segments in individuals with typical Prinzmetal's angina [138].

The initiators of coronary vasospasm likely are multifactorial, and among patients different factors may predominate. Moreover, different pathophysiologic mechanisms may be operative in different ethnic groups. For example, in the United States and in Europe, up to 24 percent of patients with coronary vasospasm have completely normal arteriograms (prior to provoking the spasm), whereas over 50 percent of patients in Japan have no fixed lesions by arteriography [139–145].

VASOSPASM OF DIGITAL ARTERIES

Raynaud's phenomenon is classically manifested by triphasic color changes of the hands and feet, accompanied by paresthesia and pain. On exposure to cold or with emotional stress, the affected part becomes pale (due to reduced blood flow), then, somewhat later, cyanotic (due to desaturation of oxyhemoglobin), and finally red (due to reactive hyperemia as the blood vessels finally relax). When Raynaud's phenomenon occurs in the absence of organic arterial disease, it is thought to be due to digital artery vasospasm, an entity known as Raynaud's disease [146,147].

Acrocyanosis and primary livedo reticularis may be variants of Raynaud's disease, since these conditions are associated with reduced skin blood flow intensified by cold or emotional upset [146,147]. Acrocyanosis is manifested clinically by a persistent cyanotic hue of the skin of the digits. Livedo reticularis presents as a reddish blue mottling of the skin in a reticulated pattern. Both conditions are thought to be due to vasospasm of small cutaneous arteries or arterioles leading to a reduction in blood flow with desaturation of oxyhemoglobin. That at least some cases of Raynaud's disease may have a mechanism common to that of coronary vasospasm is underscored by the observation that patients with variant angina have a higher incidence of Raynaud's disease [148]. Therefore, the preceding discussion of the pathogenesis of coronary vasospasm applies in part to digital vasoreactivity.

There are differences, however, between coronary and digital arteries in the determinants of vasomotion. Unlike the coronary arteries, alpha-adrenergic contraction predominates over beta-adrenergic relaxation in limb arteries. The limb vessels are richly innervated by sympathetic fibers and are highly responsive to changes in sympathetic tone. Both $alpha_1$ and $alpha_2$ adrenergic subtypes are present on the postjunctional smooth muscle and initiate contraction when stimulated [8]. Conversely, stimulation of the presynaptic $alpha_2$ adrenergic receptors results in a negative feedback inhibition of norepinephrine release from sympathetic nerves.

The importance of the adrenergic system in digital vasomotion is highlighted by the clinical improvement in patients with Raynaud's disease following sympathectomy

[146,147]. Cohen and Coffman found that arteriovenous shunt flow was normal but that nutritional flow was reduced in the digits of patients [149]. They also implicated the sympathetic nervous system, since the decreased capillary flow during body cooling was partially reversed with body warming. Those observations would support Raynaud's contention that overactivity of the sympathetic nerves is responsible for the disorder [150].

Reflex sympathetic dystrophy is likely a genuine form of sympathetic overactivity inducing Raynaud's phenomenon. In that disorder, often two phases may be observed. In the first phase, sympathetic tone appears to be reduced, and the limb is dry, edematous, and noticeably warmer than the contralateral extremity. This first stage may be variably followed by a vasospastic phase in which the limb becomes persistently cold, hyperhydrotic, edematous, cyanotic or pale, and atrophic. The limb is unusually sensitive to cold exposure and to physical stimulation. In some cases, chemical or surgical sympathectomy may afford relief [146].

Although sympathetic overactivity plays a major role in the vasospasm of reflex sympathetic dystrophy, in the usual case of Raynaud's disease, normal fluctuations in sympathetic tone superimposed on a **local fault** in the vessel likely is responsible for the signs and symptoms observed. The concept that a local fault of the digital arteries predisposes to vasospasm was first suggested by Lewis, who noted that attacks could be precipitated after anesthesia of the sympathetic nerves or after sympathectomy [151,152]. Furthermore, he observed that local cooling could induce an attack and that local warming could abort an episode in one finger without influencing the other digits.

Although hand blood flow is reduced in patients with Raynaud's disease, after sympathetic release induced by body warming, hand blood flow rises to normal levels [153,154], leading Peacock to conclude that there were no structural arterial lesions in patients with Raynaud's disease. That theory was supported by the observations of Lewis, who found that in arterial biopsies of three patients with mild cases of vasospasm, the vessels appeared normal [155]. Therefore, the local fault in the digital arteries remains an enigma. Some investigators have proposed that a functional disorder of the postjunctional $alpha_2$ adrenergic receptors may be responsible [9,156]. That hypothesis is based on the finding that in canine cutaneous vessels changes in responsiveness of the postjunctional $alpha_2$ adrenoceptor mediate the vasodilation to warming and the vasoconstriction to cooling [156–158]. In normal volunteers, vasoconstriction triggered by ambient or local cooling is antagonized by intra-arterial or iontophoretic administration of $alpha_2$- but not $alpha_1$-adrenergic antagonists [159,160]. Finally, in patients with Raynaud's disease, there is an increased density of $alpha_2$ adrenoceptors on the platelet membrane [161]; if the same phenomenon occurs in the vascular smooth muscle of patients with Raynaud's disease, that might be responsible for the heightened vasoconstriction to cold.

Raynaud's disease occurs five times more frequently among women than men [162]. That may be due to the observation that women have a lower hand blood flow than men under standard environmental conditions, which likely is due to increased sympathetic outflow to the limbs [163]. Increased sympathetic outflow to the limbs may cause a downregulation of adrenergic receptors, which would explain the observation that intra-arterial administration of adrenergic agonists has less effect on finger blood flow in women than in men [164].

Other endogenous vasoconstrictors may contribute to digital vasoconstriction. ATP is a known cotransmitter with norepinephrine in adrenergic nerve endings. It is released with norepinephrine from sympathetic nerves to contribute to the vasoconstriction with cooling in canine cutaneous vessels [165].

Serotonin also is a vasoconstrictor in the finger circulation. Intra-arterial infusions of serotonin reduce finger capillary and arteriovenous shunt flow [166]. Aggregating platelets contract human digital arteries in vitro by releasing serotonin and thromboxane A_2 [167]. Each of these vasoconstrictors makes approximately equal contributions to the vasoconstriction induced by platelet aggregation in the digital vessels. Serotonin may contribute to the vasoconstriction induced by environmental cooling, since the latter is partly reversed with blockade of serotonergic receptors [166]. Ergot drugs stimulate alpha-adrenergic and serotonergic receptors in the digital circulation. An overdose of ergot preparation may precipitate severe vasospasm in the limbs (Fig. 16-5).

Raynaud's phenomenon may be secondary to normal increases in tone superimposed on intraluminal obstructions. Raynaud's phenomenon secondary to that mechanism occurs in approximately 80 percent of patients with systemic scleroderma and 30 percent of patients with systemic lupus erythematosus, and it has been reported in a wide range of disorders that induce occlusive arterial disease (Table 16-1) [146,147]. Unlike Raynaud's disease, which is due to increased vasomotion, Raynaud's phenomenon associated with occlusive arterial disease is due to normal fluctuations in vessel tone superimposed on fixed lesions. Furthermore, as the occlusive arterial disease progresses, severe tissue ischemia and necrosis may occur, a stage that is exceedingly rare in true Raynaud's disease and that is only superficial when it does occur. Raynaud's disease usually can be distinguished from secondary cases of Raynaud's phenomenon, although the latter is often mistaken for "vasospasm." The confusion dates back to Raynaud's original thesis, in which he grouped together patients with transient ischemia of the digits and those with gangrene (Fig. 16-6).

Raynaud's phenomenon sometimes develops in workers using vibrating pneumatic tools and in certain other workers whose occupations involve repeated trauma to the hands (e.g., pianists, typists, mechanics, and farmers) [146]. Occupational arterial occlusive disease is the likely mechanism; arteriograms often reveal arterial occlusions in the radial, ulnar, palmar arch, or digital arteries [168]. Biopsies of these vessels may reveal medial muscular hypertrophy or subintimal fibrosis, although there are reports of normal arterial biopsies in some cases [169,170].

Prolonged changes in environmental temperature may alter thermosensitivity of the cutaneous vasculature in humans. After 10 or more years of daily exposure to iced

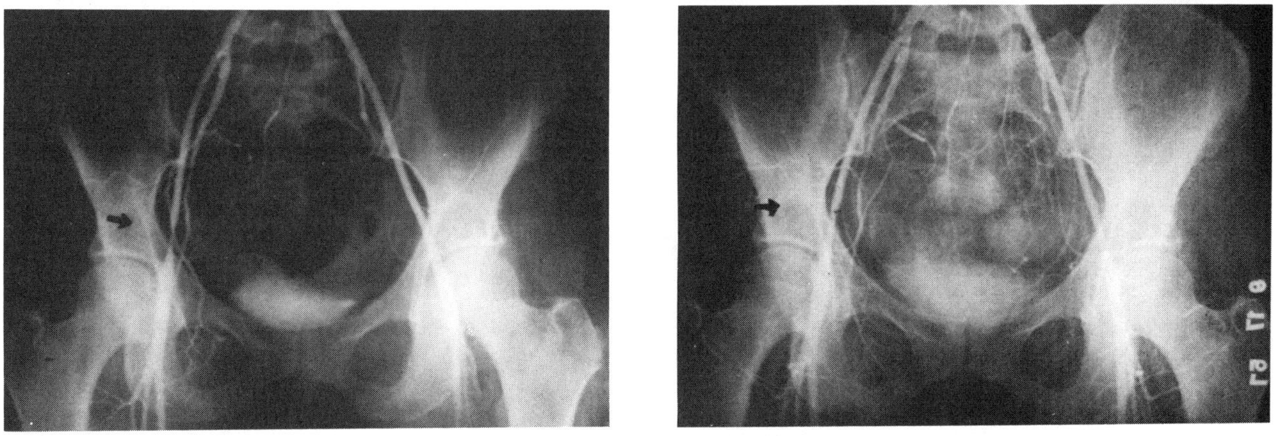

A B

Fig. 16-5. Photographs of abdominal aortic angiograms performed in a 41-year-old woman complaining of intermittent hip and thigh claudication occurring at variable distances. This patient had a history of frequent use of an ergotamine suppository for migraine headaches. **A.** Initial angiogram reveals vasospasm of left external iliac artery (arrow) and tapered narrowing of multiple intrainguinal vessels. **B.** Angiogram 5 days later (off ergots) reveals resolution of vasospasm (arrow). (Courtesy of John Joyce, M.D., Mayo Clinic, Rochester, Minn.)

fish, 90 percent of frozen-fish filleters develop Raynaud's phenomenon [171]. The symptoms of Raynaud's disease may be ameliorated by conditioning the hands using short periods of exposure to warm water during environmental cooling [172].

Raynaud's phenomenon also may be secondary to changes in rheologic properties of blood. Cold agglutinins, cryoproteins, or hyperviscosity due to other disorders of serum proteins may induce intermittent ischemia of the digits in the absence of vasospasm.

VASOSPASM OF THE CEREBRAL ARTERIES

Migraine Syndrome. Migraine headaches are thought to be a manifestation of vasomotor instability. That hypothesis is strengthened by the observation that other vasospastic disorders occur in association with migraines [173,174]. The eighteenth-century British physician Robert Whytt may have been the first to propose a vasospastic etiology for migraine headaches, but surely the more memorable argument in favor of that hypothesis was made a century later by the Berlin professor DuBois-Reymond [175,176]. The eminent physiologist was struck by the vasomotor manifestations of his own migraine headaches and described them in vivid detail. He concluded his account by stating, "I maintain that in my Migraine a Tetanus takes place in the muscular coats of the vessels of the affected half of the head; in other words, a Tetanus in the territory of the cervical portion of the right sympathetic" [176]. Indeed, vasospasm in the retinal or cerebral vessels (or both) is thought to be responsible for the subjective visual disturbances and other cortical symptoms at the onset of an attack, whereas subsequent vasodilation may be responsible for the headache, facial flushing, congestion of the conjunctiva and nasal mucosa, and tenderness of the temporal artery on the side of the headache. The beneficial effect of ergotamine tartrate on the headache may be to counteract this vasodilation.

Table 16-1. Arterial occlusive diseases associated with Raynaud's phenomenon

Arteriosclerosis
Thromboangiitis obliterans
Collagen vascular disease
Necrotizing vasculitides
Occupational occlusive disease
Cold injury
Coagulopathy (paraneoplastic syndrome; deficiencies of protein C, protein S, or antithrombin III)
Hyperviscosity (macroglobulinemia, cold agglutinins, cryoglobulins)
Embolism (originating from a diseased proximal vessel, or cardiac chamber, or vein in the presence of a right-to-left shunt)

Electroencephalographic changes consistent with cortical ischemia (indicating vascular obstruction) have been observed during an episode; so too has transient occlusion of the retinal arteries [177,178]. Prompt abolition of the visual or neurologic symptoms may be obtained by administration of nitrates [179].

The trigger for cycles of vasoconstriction and vasodilation with migraine headaches is not known. Humoral factors, substances released from aggregating platelets, or both may play a role. In some patients, attacks are followed by increased excretion of the metabolites of norepinephrine, epinephrine, and serotonin [180]. Furthermore, the serotonin antagonist methysergide prevents attacks

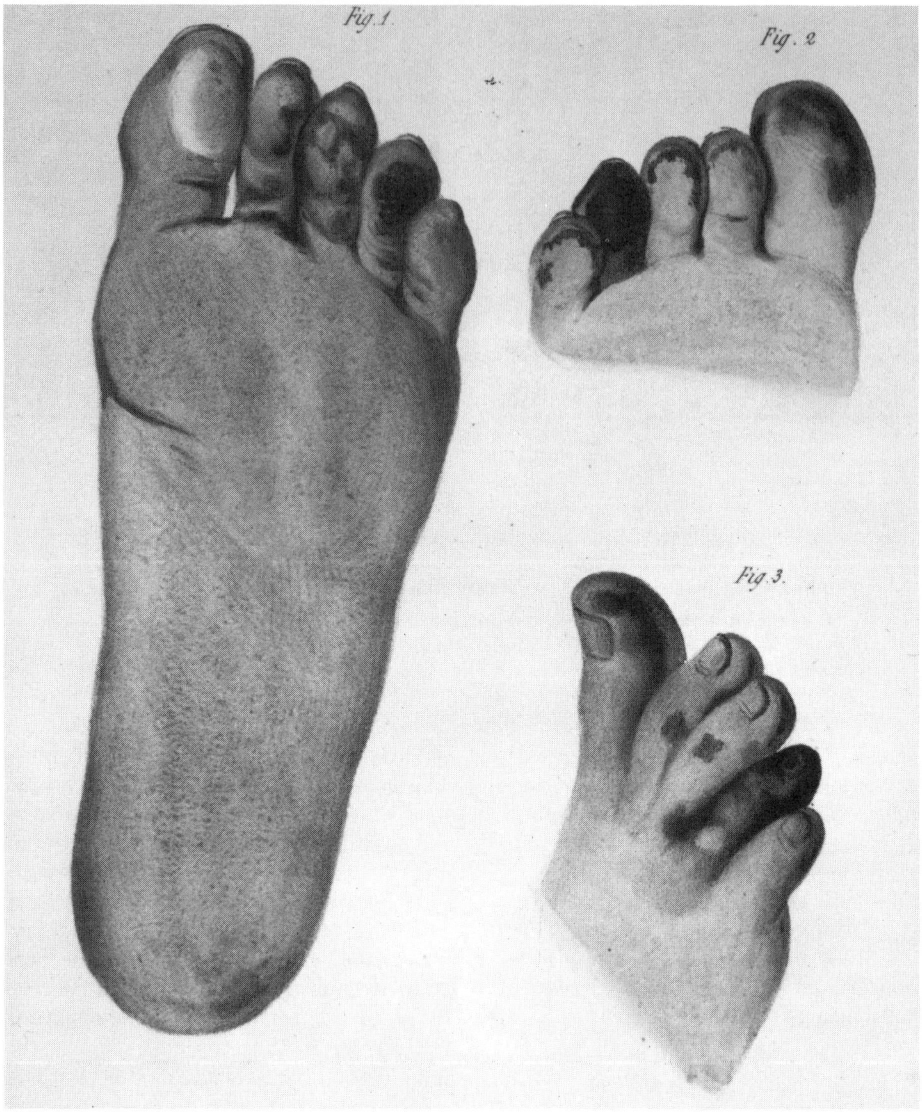

Fig. 16-6. Reproduction from Raynaud's original thesis. Originally Raynaud included patients with gangrene (as shown here) in his description of the syndrome that now bears his name. Later he was to correctly distinguish between intermittent, transient ischemia of the digits (Raynaud's phenomenon) and gangrene. (Reproduced from M. Raynaud. Local aphyxia and symmetrical gangrene of the extremities. New Sydenham Society, 1862. Courtesy of Boston Medical Library in the Francis A. Countway Library of Medicine.)

in some individuals. The increase in platelet aggregability in migraine patients is further support for a role of serotonin [181]. Some individuals link their attacks to certain foods, such as chocolate, cheese, and wine. Phenylethylamine is a constituent of those substances and has been shown to precipitate headaches, possibly because it is a precursor for a wide variety of sympathomimetic agents [181,182].

Cerebral Vasospasm after Subarachnoid Hemorrhage. Although there is much inferential evidence that migraine headaches are precipitated by vasospasm, angiographic confirmation is rarely obtained. Conversely, there is angiographic support for cerebral vasospasm in patients following subarachnoid hemorrhage. There are approximately 30,000 cases annually of aneurysmal subarachnoid hemorrhage in North America; one-third of those patients die or are permanently disabled. Narrowing of the cerebral arteries occurs in approximately 20 percent of patients surviving the initial hemorrhage, and in half of these patients it leads to stroke or death [183]. The likelihood of vasospasm appears to be related to the amount of hemorrhage [184]. The cerebral conduit vessels are nourished by cerebrospinal fluid in the subarachnoid space, a process that may be physically interrupted by the presence of thrombus. Thrombus may obstruct nutrient and oxygen delivery to the vessels; the resulting hypoxia is known to release a nonprostanoid vasoconstrictor from the endothelium that has yet to be characterized [185]. Hypoxic damage to the vascular smooth muscle incites an inflammatory response [186]. White blood cells infiltrate the media and release vasoconstrictor leukotrienes as well as superoxide anion; the latter may contribute to endothelial injury as well as to direct chemical inactivation of EDRF [48,186–190]. Superoxide anion is also released by the thrombus surrounding the vessel due to the oxidation of free hemoglobin to methemoglobin. Subsequent lipid peroxidation injures the media and endothelium, precipitating endothelial desquamation and platelet adherence [189].

In the canine basilar artery, endothelial injury reverses relaxation by AVP to a contraction [185]. In experimental models of cerebral vasospasm, endothelium-dependent relaxations to thrombin, AVP, and ATP are reduced [188,189]. Besides causing endothelial injury or dysfunction, hemoglobin released by a subarachnoid hemorrhage may quench EDRF [51]. Endothelium-dependent relaxations in the canine basilar artery are reduced in vitro by hemoglobin or by cerebrospinal fluid from patients with subarachnoid hemorrhages [190]. Damage to the endothelium may be responsible for the observation that vascular prostacyclin is reduced after subarachnoid hemorrhage [191–193]. Loss of the buffering influence of the endothelium after experimental subarachnoid hemorrhage likely is responsible for the augmented contractile response to 5-hydroxytryptamine and vasoconstrictor prostanoids in vitro [189].

In addition to dynamic changes in vessel tone, structural changes in the vessel wall contribute to the disorder. As early as 30 minutes after subarachnoid hemorrhage, endothelial convolutions can be seen along with subendothelial fluid accumulation due to increased endothelial-cell permeability [194]. Myonecrosis and the resulting inflammatory response cause additional swelling of the vessel wall. In later stages, fibromuscular hyperplasia further narrows the lumen [5,195]. The structural changes in the vessel wall contribute in a major way to the luminal narrowing and likely are responsible for the poor response of symptoms to vasodilators. Whereas the luminal narrowing that may occur immediately after subarachnoid hemorrhage likely is due to true vasospasm, the more common cause occurring later in its course is luminal narrowing due to alterations in vascular structure.

Autoregulation is disturbed following a subarachnoid hemorrhage, which also may be secondary to endothelial injury. In-vitro studies indicate that a vasoconstrictor prostanoid released from endothelial cells may play a role in autoregulation [196]. In those investigations, it was found that the canine basilar artery responds to a sudden stretch with further contraction if the endothelium is present. That contraction is abolished by removal of the endothelium or by administration of indomethacin.

VENOSPASM

Venospasm occasionally occurs in response to venous catheterization, usually with large-bore catheters or with vigorous manipulation. Its cause is not known, but venospasm usually responds to direct injection into the vein of lidocaine, papaverine, or contrast agent. This entity represents a more serious problem when it occurs in the setting of bypass surgery using a venous graft. Often vasodilators are of benefit, but occasionally the venospasm leads to acute thrombosis and failure of the graft.

The cutaneous veins are densely innervated by sympathetic nerves and respond strongly to release of endogenous norepinephrine or to exogenous alpha-adrenergic agonists [9,197]. Cooling causes further contraction of the vessels, probably due to an augmentation of the receptor-agonist interaction [156–158].

Conversely, the deeper veins dilate in response to cold and vasoconstrict with warming [198]. The differential response to temperature of the cutaneous and deep veins likely serves a homeostatic purpose [11]. During environmental cooling, the superficial veins constrict, and venous blood is shunted to the deep veins. Cooled blood from the periphery dilates the deep veins, allowing them to accept the increased flow. That serves the purpose of conserving body heat. Conversely, when the body core temperature increases, deep veins constrict, while the superficial veins dilate to accept increased venous flow and to radiate heat to the environment. In that way, heat is lost to the environment to reduce the core temperature. Therefore, changes in local venous tone in response to temperature contribute to thermoregulation.

Besides alpha-adrenergic receptors, the venous smooth muscle also has receptors for serotonin [199]. These receptors likely mediate the contraction to dihydroergotamine tartrate, a venoconstrictor occasionally given to reduce venous pooling in patients at risk for venous thrombosis [200,201].

In contrast to arteries, only a few substances induce endothelium-dependent relaxation of veins, and generally they are not very potent. For example, endothelium-dependent contraction occurs in the veins in response to arachidonic acid, in contrast to the vasodilation seen in arteries [202].

Summary

There is a great heterogeneity in the determinants of smooth muscle tone from one vascular bed to another. Consequently, the provocateurs of spasm in the coronary, cerebral, and digital circulations are not identical. Furthermore, symptoms of transient ischemia, in the absence of increased tissue demand for oxygen, may not always represent hypertonus or "vasospasm." Indeed, in many cases, these ischemic syndromes are due to normal fluctuations in tone superimposed on a fixed stenosis of the lumen. Indeed, the symptoms of so-called vasospasm may even be due to rheologic changes induced by platelet aggregates or aberrant serum proteins rather than changes in vasomotor tone. As our knowledge of vasomotion expands, the classification of the vasospastic disorders will be clarified and more enlightened therapeutic strategies implemented.

References

1. Pickering GW. Vascular spasm. Lancet 1951; 2:845–850.
2. Prinzmetal M, et al. Angina pectoris I: a variant form of angina pectoris. Am J Med 1959; 27:375–388.

3. Maseri A, et al. Coronary artery spasm and vasoconstriction: The case for a distinction. Circulation 1990; 81:1983–1991.
4. Dabich L, et al. Digital arteries in patients with scleroderma. Arch Int Med 1972; 130:708–719.
5. Conway LW, McDonald LW. Structural changes of the intradural arteries following subarachnoid hemorrhage. J Neurosurg 1972; 37:715–723.
6. Jampol LE. Ocular manifestations of selected systemic diseases. In GA Peyman, DR Sanders, MF Goldberg, eds. Principles and Practices of Ophthalmology. Philadelphia: Saunders, 1980. P. 1639.
7. Flavahan NA, et al. Characterization of postjunctional alpha-1 and alpha-2 adrenoceptors activated by exogenous or nerve-released norepinephrine in the canine saphenous vein. J Pharmacol Exp Ther 1984; 230:699–705.
8. Flavahan NA, et al. Human postjunctional alpha-1 and alpha-2 adrenoceptors: differential distribution in arteries of the limbs. J Pharm Exp Ther 1986; 241:361–365.
9. Cooke JP. Alpha-adrenergic receptors in vascular smooth muscle: Characterization of subtypes and modulation of response by alterations in temperature and calcium availability (Thesis). Rochester, MN: Mayo Graduate School of Medicine, 1985.
10. Cohen RA, Shepherd JT, Vanhoutte PM. Prejunctional and postjunctional actions of endogenous norepinephrine at the sympathetic neuroeffector junction in canine coronary arteries. Circ Res 1983; 52:16–25.
11. Shepherd JT, Vanhoutte PM. Neurohormonal Regulation in the Human Cardiovascular System: Facts and Concepts. JT Shepherd, PM Vanhoutte, eds. New York: Raven, 1980.
12. Kifor I, Dzau VJ. Endothelial renin-angiotensin pathway: Evidence for intracellular synthesis and secretion of angiotensins. Circ Res 1987; 60:422–428.
13. Katusic ZS, Shepherd JT, Vanhoutte PM. Vasopressin causes endothelium-dependent relaxations of the canine basilar artery. Circ Res 1984; 55:575–579.
14. Hirsch AT, et al. Vasopressin-mediated forearm vasodilation in normal humans. Evidence for a vascular vasopressin V2 receptor. J Clin Invest 1989; 84:418–426.
15. De Wardener HE, MacGregor GA. The relation of a circulating sodium transport inhibitor (the natriuretic hormone?) to hypertension. Medicine 1983; 62:310–326.
16. Winquist RJ. Pharmacologic effects of atrial natriuretic peptide. Endocrinol Metab Clin N Amer 1987; 16:163–182.
17. Gagnon G, Regoli D, Rioux F. A new bioassay for glucagon. Br J Pharmacol 1978; 64:99–108.
18. Creager MA, Liang CS, Coffman JD. Beta adrenergic-mediated vasodilator response to insulin in the human forearm. J Pharmacol Exp Therap 1985; 235:709–714.
19. Florey L. The endothelial cell. Br Med J 1966; 2:487–490.
20. See Chapter 9, The Endothelial Dysfunction in Vascular Disease, in this volume.
21. Jaffe EA. Endothelial cells and the biology of factor VIII. N Engl J Med 1977; 296:377–383.
22. Cooke JP, Tsap P. Cytoprotective effects of nitric oxide. Circulation 1993; 88:2451–2454.
23. Dzau VJ, et al. Vascular biology and medicine in the 1990s: Scope, concepts, potentials, and perspectives. Circulation 1993; 87:705–719.
24. Moncada S, et al. Differential formation of prostacyclin (PGX or PGI_2) by layers of the arterial wall. An explanation for the anti-thrombotic properties of vascular endothelium. Thromb Res 1977; 11:323–344.
25. Moncada S. Prostacyclin and arterial wall biology. Arteriosclerosis 1982; 2:193–207.
26. Kalsner S. Endogenous prostaglandin release contributes directly to coronary tone. Can J Physiol Pharmacol 1975; 53:560–565.
27. Furchgott RF, Zawadzki JV. The obligatory role of endothelial cells in the relaxation of arterial smooth muscle by acetylcholine. Nature 1980; 288:373–376.
28. Ignarro LJ, et al. Endothelium-derived relaxing factor from pulmonary artery and vein possesses pharmacologic and chemical properties identical to those of nitric oxide radical. Circ Res 1987; 61:866–879.
29. Palmer RMJ, Ferrige AG, Moncada S. Nitric oxide release accounts for the biological activity of endothelium-derived relaxing factor. Nature 1987; 327:524–526.
30. Palmer RMJ, Ashton DS, Moncada S. Vascular endothelial cells synthesize nitric oxide from L-arginine. Nature 1988; 333:664–666.
31. Miller VM, Vanhoutte PM. Endothelium-dependent responses in isolated blood vessels of lower vertebrates. Blood Vessels 1986; 23:225–235.
32. Luscher TF, et al. Endothelium dependent relaxations in human arteries. Mayo Clin Proc 1987; 62:601–606.
33. Cohen RA, Shepherd JT, Vanhoutte PM. Inhibitory role of the endothelium in the response of isolated coronary arteries to platelets. Science 1983; 221:273–274.
34. Houston DS, Shepherd JT, Vanhoutte PM. Adenine nucleotides, serotonin and endothelium-dependent relaxations to platelets. Am J Physiol 1985; H389-H395.
35. Cocks TM, Angus JA. Endothelium-dependent relaxation of coronary arteries by noradrenaline and serotonin. Nature 1983; 305:627–630.
36. Vanhoutte PM, Shepherd JT. Components of the cardiovascular system: how structure is geared to function. In PM Vanhoutte, JT Shepherd, eds. The Human Cardiovascular System: Facts and Concepts. New York: Raven, 1980. Pp. 21–22.
37. Holtz J, et al. Flow-dependent, endothelium-mediated dilation of epicardial coronary arteries in conscious dogs: Effects of cyclooxygenase inhibition. J Cardiovasc Pharmacol 1984; 6:1161–1169.
38. Cooke JP, et al. Flow stimulates endothelial cells to release a nitrovasodilator that is potentiated by reduced thiol. Am J Physiol 1990; 28:H804-H812.
39. Frangos JA, et al. Flow effects on prostacyclin production by cultured human endothelial cells. Science 1985; 227:1477–1479.
40. Cooke JP, et al. Flow activates an endothelial potassium channel to release an endogenous nitrovasodilator. J Clin Invest 1991; 88:1663–1671.
41. Ohno M, et al. Shear stress elevates endothelial cGMP: Role of a potassium channel and G protein coupling. Circulation 1993; 88:193–197.
42. Olesen SP, Clapham DE, Davies PF. Haemodynamic shear stress activates a K^+ current in vascular endothelial cells. Nature 1988; 331:1168–1170.
43. Komori K, Lorenz RR, Vanhoutte PM. Nitric oxide, ACh and electrical and mechanical properties of canine arterial smooth muscle. Am J Physiol 1988; 255:H207–H212.
44. Yanagisawa M, et al. A novel potent vasoconstrictor peptide produced by vascular endothelial cells. Nature 1988; 332:411–415.
45. Dubin D, et al. Endothelin, a potent vasoconstrictor, is a vascular smooth muscle mitogen. J Vasc Med Biol 1989; 1:150–154.
46. Rimele TJ, et al. Interaction of neutrophils with vascular smooth muscle: identification of a neutrophil-derived relaxing factor. J Pharm Exp Therap 1988; 245:102–111.
47. Fridovich I. The biology of oxygen radicals. Science 1978; 201:875–880.

48. Rubanyi GM, Vanhoutte PM. Superoxide anions and hyperoxia inactivate endothelium-derived relaxing factor. Am J Physiol (Heart Circ Physiol 19) 1986; 250:H822–H827.
49. Roth DM, Lefer AM. Studies on the mechanism of leukotriene induced coronary artery constriction. Prostaglandins 1983; 26:573–581.
50. Tomoike H, et al. Leukotriene C_4- and D_4-induced diffuse peripheral constriction of swine coronary artery accompanied by ST elevation on the electrocardiogram: Angiographic analysis. Circulation 1987; 76:480–487.
51. Martin W, et al. Selective blockade of endothelium dependent and glyceryl trinitrate-induced relaxation by haemoglobin and by methylene blue in the rabbit aorta. J Pharmacol Exp Ther 1985; 232:708–716.
52. Sano K. Cerebral vasospasm is a deficiency syndrome. In RH Wilkinson, ed. Cerebral Vasospasm. New York: Raven, 1988. Pp. 285–295.
53. Isner JM, et al. Acute cardiac events temporally related to cocaine abuse. N Engl J Med 1986; 315:1438–1443.
54. Ascher EK, Stauffer JCE, Gaasch WH. Coronary artery spasm, cardiac arrest, transient electrocardiographic Q waves and stunned myocardium in cocaine-associated acute myocardial infarction. Am J Cardiol 1988; 61:939–941.
55. Cooke JP, Shepherd JT, Vanhoutte PM. Vasoconstriction induced by ouabain in the canine coronary artery: contribution of adrenergic and nonadrenergic responses. Cardiovasc Drugs Therapy 1988; 2:255–263.
56. Robertson RM, et al. Exacerbation of vasotonic angina pectoris by propranolol. Circulation 1982; 65:281–285.
57. Balcon R, Hoy J, Sowton E. Haemodynamic effect of rapid digitalization following acute myocardial infarction. Br Heart J 1968; 30:373–376.
58. Crawford MH, et al. Combined propranolol and digoxin therapy in angina pectoris. Ann Intern Med 1975; 83:449–455.
59. Coffman JD. The attenuation of reserpine or guanethidine of the cutaneous vasoconstriction caused by tobacco smoking. Am Heart J 1967; 74:229.
60. Lange RL, et al. Nonatheromatous ischemic heart disease following withdrawal from chronic industrial nitroglycerin exposure. Circulation 1972; 46:666–678.
61. Kleiman NS, et al. Prinzmetal's angina during 5-fluorouracil chemotherapy. Am J Med 1987; 82:566–568.
62. Vogelzang NJ, et al. Raynaud's phenomenon: A common toxicity after combination chemotherapy for testicular cancer. Ann Intern Med 1981; 95:288–292.
63. Wilson RH, et al. Occupational acro-osteolysis: report of 31 cases. JAMA 1967; 201:577.
64. Cowley MS, et al. Acute coronary events associated with percutaneous transluminal coronary angioplasty. Am J Cardiol 1984; 53:12C–16C.
65. Fischell TA, Bausback KN, McDonald TV. Evidence for altered epicardial coronary artery autoregulation as a cause of distal coronary vasoconstriction after successful percutaneous transluminal coronary angioplasty. J Clin Invest 1990; 86:575–584.
66. Santamore WP, et al. Synergistic effects of pressure, distal resistance, and vasoconstriction on stenosis. Am J Physiol 1982; 243:H236–H242.
67. Maseri A, et al. Variant angina: one aspect of a continuous spectrum of vasospastic myocardial ischemia. Am J Cardiol 1978; 42:1019–1035.
68. Dhurandhar RW, et al. Prinzmetal variant form of angina with arteriographic evidence of coronary arterial spasm. Am J Cardiol 1972; 30:902–905.
69. Oliva PB, Potts DE, Pluss RA. Coronary arterial spasm in Prinzmetal angina: documentation by coronary arteriography. N Engl J Med 1973; 288:745–751.
70. Schroeder JS, et al. Provocation of coronary spasm with ergonovine maleate: new test with results in 57 patients undergoing coronary arteriography. Am J Cardiol 1977; 40:487–491.
71. Myerburg RJ, et al. Life-threatening ventricular arrhythmias in patients with silent myocardial ischemia due to coronary artery spasm. N Engl J Med 1992; 326:1451–1455.
72. Curry RC Jr, et al. Effects of ergonovine in patients with and without coronary artery disease. Circulation 1977; 56:803–809.
73. Bertrand ME, et al. Frequency of provoked coronary arterial spasm in 1089 consecutive patients undergoing coronary arteriography. Circulation 1982; 65:1299–1306.
74. Waters DD, et al. Comparative sensitivity of exercise, cold pressor and ergonovine testing in provoking attacks of variant angina in patients with active disease. Circulation 1983; 67:310–315.
75. Brazenor RM, Angus JA. Ergometrine contracts isolated canine coronary arteries by a serotonergic mechanism: No role for alpha adrenoceptors. J Pharmacol Exp Therap 1981; 218:530–536.
76. Henry PD, Yokoyama M. Supersensitivity of atherosclerotic rabbit aorta to ergonovine. Mediation by a serotonergic mechanism. J Clin Invest 1980; 66:306–313.
77. Yamamoto Y, et al. Attenuation of endothelium-related relaxation and enhanced responsiveness of vascular smooth muscle to histamine in spastic coronary arterial segments from miniature pigs. Circ Res 1987; 61:772–778.
78. Shimokawa H, Lawrence LA, Vanhoutte PM. Porcine coronary arteries with regenerated endothelium have a reduced endothelium-dependent responsiveness to aggregating platelets and serotonin. Circ Res 1987; 61:256–269.
79. Weidinger F, et al. Persistent dysfunction of regenerated endothelium after balloon angioplasty of rabbit iliac artery. Circulation 1990; 81:1667–1679.
80. Shimokawa H, Kim P, Vanhoutte PM. Endothelium-dependent relaxation to aggregating platelets in isolated basilar arteries of control and hypercholesterolemic pigs. Circ Res 1988; 63:604–612.
81. Verbeuren TJ, et al. Effect of hypercholesterolemia on vascular reactivity in the rabbit. Circ Res 1986; 58:552–564.
82. Yokoyama M, Henry PD. Sensitization of isolated canine coronary arteries to calcium ions after exposure to cholesterol. Circ Res 1979; 45:479–486.
83. Galle J, Bassenge E, Busse R. Oxidized low density lipoproteins potentiate vasoconstrictions to various agonists by direct interaction with vascular smooth muscle. Circ Res 1990; 66:1287–1293.
84. Ludmer PL, et al. Paradoxical vasoconstriction induced by acetylcholine in atherosclerotic coronary arteries. N Engl J Med 1986; 315:1046–1051.
85. Creager MA, et al. Impaired vasodilation of forearm resistance vessels in hypercholesterolemic humans. J Clin Invet 1990; 86:228–234.
86. Creager MA, et al. L-arginine normalizes endothelial response in the forearm circulation of hypercholesterolemic humans. J Clin Invest 1992; 90:1248–1253.
87. Drexler H, et al. Correction of endothelial dysfunction in the coronary microcirculation of hypercholesterolemic patients by L-arginine. Lancet 1991; 338:1546–1550.
88. VanBenthuysen KM, McMurtry IF, Horwitz LD. Reperfusion after acute coronary occlusion in dogs impairs endothelium-dependent relaxation to acetylcholine and augments contractile reactivity in vitro. J Clin Invest 1987; 79:265–274.
89. Ku DD. Coronary vascular reactivity after acute myocardial ischemia. Science 1982; 218:576–578.
90. Rubanyi GM, Vanhoutte PM. Hypoxia releases a vasocon-

strictor substance from the canine vascular endothelium. J Physiol 1985; 364:45–56.
91. Gage JE, et al. Vasoconstriction of stenotic coronary arteries during dynamic exercise in patients with classic angina pectoris: reversibility by nitroglycerin. Circulation 1986; 73: 865–876.
92. Lane GE, Bove AA. The effect of cyclooxygenase inhibition on vasomotion of proximal coronary arteries with endothelial damage. Lab Invest 1985; 72:389–396.
93. Friedman PL, et al. Coronary vasoconstrictor effect of indomethacin in patients with coronary artery disease. N Engl J Med 1981; 305:1171–1175.
94. D'Angelo, Mysliwiec M, Donati MB. Defective fibrinolytic and prostacyclin-like activity in human atheromatous plaques. Thromb Haemostas 1978; 39:535–536.
95. Egashira K, et al. Preserved endothelium-dependent vasodilation at the vasospastic site in patients with variant angina. J Clin Invest 1992; 89:1047–1052.
96. Osler W. The Lumleian lectures on angina pectoris. Lancet 1910; March 26:839–844.
97. Hollis TM, Rosen LA. Histidine decarboxylase activities of bovine aortic endothelium and intima-media. Proc Soc Exp Biol Med 1972; 141:978–987.
98. Ginsburg R, et al. Quantitative pharmacologic responses of normal and atherosclerotic isolated human epicardial coronary arteries. Circulation 1984; 69:430–440.
99. Kalsner S, Richards R. Coronary arteries of cardiac patients are hyperreactive and contain stores of amines: A mechanism for coronary spasm. Science 1984; 223:1435–1437.
100. Ginsburg R, et al. Histamine provocation of clinical coronary artery spasm: implications concerning pathogenesis of variant angina pectoris. Am Heart J 1981; 102:819–822.
101. Lerman A, et al. Circulating and tissue endothelin immunoreactivity in hypercholesterolemic pigs. Circulation 1993; 88:2923–2928.
102. Lerman A, et al. Circulating and tissue endothelin immunoreactivity in advanced atherosclerosis. N Engl J Med 1991; 325:997–1001.
103. Yasue H, et al. Prinzmetal's variant form of angina as a manifestation of alpha-adrenergic receptor-mediated coronary artery spasm: Documentation of coronary arteriography. Am Heart J 1976; 91:148–155.
104. Ricci DR, et al. Altered adrenergic activity in coronary arterial spasm: insight into mechanism based on study of coronary hemodynamics and the electrocardiogram. Am J Cardiol 1979; 43:1073–1079.
105. Raizner AE, et al. Provocation of coronary artery spasm by the cold pressor test. Hemodynamic, arteriographic and quantitative angiographic observations. Circulation 1980; 62:925–932.
106. Mudge GH Jr, et al. Reflex increase in coronary vascular resistance in patients with ischemic heart disease. N Engl J Med 1976; 295:1333–1337.
107. Vita JA, et al. Patients with evidence of coronary endothelial dysfunction as assessed by acetylcholine infusin demonstrate marked increase in sensitivity to constrictor effects of catecholamines. Circulation 1992; 85:1390–1397.
108. Drexler H, Zeiher AM. Progression of coronary endothelial dysfunction in man and its potential clinical significance. Basic Res Cardiol 1991; 86[Suppl 2]:223–232.
109. Chierchia S, et al. Alpha-adrenergic receptors and coronary spasm: An elusive link. Circulation 1984; 69:8–14.
110. Winniford MD, Filipschuck N, Hillis D. Alpha-adrenergic blockade of variant angina: a long-term, double blind randomized trial. Circulation 1983; 67:1185.
111. Clark DA, et al. Coronary artery spasm: medical management, surgical denervation, and autotransplantation. J Thorac Cardiovasc Surg 1977; 73:332–339.
112. Buda AJ, et al. Coronary artery spasm in the denervated transplanted human heart. Am J Med 1981; 70:1144–1148.
113. McFadden EP, et al. Effect of intracoronary serotonin on coronary vessels in patients with stable angina and patients with variant angina. N Engl J Med 1991; 324:648–654.
114. Sobel M, et al. Circulating platelet products in unstable angina pectoris. Circulation 1981; 63:300–306.
115. Fitzgerald DJ, et al. Platelet activation in unstable coronary disease. N Engl J Med 1986; 315:983–989.
116. Sherman CT, et al. Coronary angioscopy in patients with unstable angina pectoris. N Engl J Med 1986; 315:913–919.
117. Bresnahan DR, et al. Angiographic occurrence and clinical correlates of intraluminal coronary artery thrombus: role of unstable angina. J Am Coll Cardiol 1985; 6:285–289.
118. Ellis EF, et al. Coronary arterial smooth muscle contraction by a substance released from platelets: evidence that it is thromboxane A_2. Science 1976; 193:1135–1137.
119. Cohen RA, Zitney KM, Weisbrod RM. Accumulation of 5-hydroxytryptamine leads to dysfunction of adrenergic nerves in canine coronary artery following intimal damage in vivo. Circ Res 1987; 61:829–833.
120. Folts JD, Gallagher K, Rowe GG. Blood flow reductions in stenosed canine coronary arteries: vasospasm or platelet aggregation? Circulation 1982; 65:248–255.
121. Yui Y, et al. Selective thromboxane A2 synthetase inhibition in vasospastic angina pectoris. J Am Coll Cardiol 1986; 7:25–29.
122. DeCaterina R, Carpeggiani C, L'Abbate A. A double-blind, placebo-controlled study of ketanserin in patients with Prinzmetal's angina: Evidence against the role of serotonin in the genesis of coronary vasospasm. Circulation 1984; 69:889.
123. Benedict CR, et al. Correlation of plasma serotonin changes with platelet aggregation in an in vivo dog model of spontaneous occlusive thrombus formation. Circ Res 1986; 58: 58–67.
124. Chierchia S, et al. Failure of thromboxane A_2 blockade to prevent attacks of vasospastic angina. Circulation 1982; 66:702–705.
125. Gertz SD, et al. Endothelial cell damage and thrombus formation after partial arterial constriction: Relevance to the role of coronary artery spasm in the pathogenesis of myocardial infarction. Circulation 1981; 63:476–486.
126. Kuga T, et al. Role of coronary artery spasm in progression of organic coronary stenosis and acute myocardial infarction in a swine model. Circulation 1993; 87:573–582.
127. Moncada S, Higgs A. Mechanisms of disease: The L-arginine-nitric oxide pathway. N Engl J Med 1993; 329:2002–2012.
128. Cooke JP, Tsao PS. Is NO an endogenous antiatherogenic molecule? Arterioscler Thromb 1994; 14:653–655.
129. Celermajer DS, et al. Aging is associated with endothelial dysfunction in healthy men years before the age-related decline in women. J Am Coll Cardiol 1994; 24:471–476.
130. Sorensen KE, et al. Impairment of endothelium-dependent dilation is an early event in children with familial hypercholesterolemia and is related to the lipoprotein(a) level. J Clin Invest 1994; 93:50–55.
131. Celermajer DS, et al. Cigarette smoking is associated with dose-related and potentially reversible impairment of endothelium-dependent dilation in healthy young adults. Circulation 1993; 88:2149–2155.
132. Celermajer DS, et al. Non-invasive detection of endothelial dysfunction in children and adults at risk of atherosclerosis. Lancet 1992; 340(8828):1111–1115.
133. Panza JA, et al. Abnormal endothelium-dependent vascular

relaxation in patients with essential hypertension. N Engl J Med 1990; 323:22–27.
134. Cooke JP, et al. Anti-atherogenic effects of L-arginine in the hypercholesterolemic rabbit. J Clin Invest 1992; 90:1168–1172.
135. Naruse K, et al. Prostaglandin H2 does not contribute to impaired endothelium-dependent relaxation and long-term inhibition of nitric oxide synthesis promotes atherosclerosis in hypercholesterolemic rabbit thoracic aorta. Arterioscler Thromb 1994; 14:746–752.
136. Cayatte AJ, et al. Chronic inhibition of nitric oxide production accelerates neointima formation and impairs endothelial function in hypercholesterolemic rabbits. Arterioscler Thromb 1994; 14:753–759.
137. Nobuyoshi M, et al. Progression of coronary atherosclerosis: Is coronary spasm related to progression? J Am Coll Cardiol 1991; 18:904–910.
138. Kaski JC, et al. Variant angina pectoris: Role of coronary spasm in the development of fixed coronary obstruction. Circulation 1992; 85:619–626.
139. Maseri A, Chierchia S. Coronary artery spasm: Demonstration, definition, diagnosis and consequences. Prog Cardiovasc Dis 1982; 25:169–192.
140. MacAlpin RN. Relation of coronary arterial spasm to sites of organic stenosis. Am J Cardiol 1980; 46:143–153.
141. Maseri A, et al. "Variant" angina: One aspect of a continuous spectrum of vasospastic myocardial ischemia. Am J Cardiol 1978; 42:1019–1035.
142. Severi S, et al. Long-term prognosis of "variant" angina with medical treatment. Am J Cardiol 1980; 46:226–232.
143. Wiener L, et al. Spectrum of coronary arterial spasm: Clinical, angiographic, and myocardial metabolic experience in 29 cases. Am J Cardiol 1976; 38:945–955.
144. Kimura E, Kishida H. Treatment of variant angina with drugs: A survey of 11 cardiology institutes in Japan. Circulation 1981; 63:844–848.
145. Nakamura M, Takeshita A, Nose Y. Clinical characteristics associated with myocardial infarction, arrhythmias, and sudden death in patients with vasospastic angina. Circulation 1987; 75:1110–1116.
146. Coffman JD, Davies WT. Vasospastic diseases: a review. Prog Cardiovasc Dis 1975; 18:123–146.
147. Creager MA. Vasospastic diseases of the extremity. In J Loscalzo, MA Creager, VJ Dzau, eds. Vascular Medicine. Boston: Little, Brown, 1992.
148. Robertson D, Oates JA. Variant angina and Raynaud's phenomenon. Lancet 1978; 1:452.
149. Coffman JD, Cohen AS. Total and capillary fingertip blood flow in Raynaud's phenomenon. N Engl J Med 1971; 285:259.
150. Raynaud M. On local asphyxia and symmetrical gangrene of the extremities [1862]. New researches on the nature and treatment of local asphyxia of the extremities [1874]. T Barlow, trans. In Selected Monographs. London: The New Sydenham Society, 1988.
151. Lewis T. Experiments relating to peripheral mechanisms involved in spasmodic arrest of circulation in fingers, variety of Raynaud's disease. Heart 1929; 15:7.
152. Lewis T, Pickering GW. Observations upon maladies in which the blood supply to the digits cease intermittently or permanently, and upon bilateral gangrene of digits; observations relevant to so-called Raynaud's disease. Clin Sci 1934; 1:327.
153. Peacock JH. A comparative study of the digital cutaneous temperatures and hand blood flows in the normal hand, primary Raynaud's disease and primary acrocyanosis. Clin Sci 1959; 18:25.
154. Peacock JH. Vasodilation in the human hand. Observations on primary Raynaud's disease and acrocyanosis of the upper extremities. Clin Sci 1957; 17:575.
155. Lewis T. The pathological change in the arteries supplying the fingers in warm handed people and in cases of so-called Raynaud's disease. Clin Sci 1938; 3:287.
156. Vanhoutte PM, et al. Modulation of postjunctional alpha-adrenergic responsiveness by local changes in temperature. Clin Sci 68:121s–123s.
157. Cooke JP, Shepherd JT, Vanhoutte PM. The effect of warming on adrenergic neurotransmission in canine cutaneous vein. Circ Res 1984; 54:547–553.
158. Flavahan NA, et al. Cooling and alpha 1- and alpha 2-adrenergic responses in cutaneous veins: role of receptor reserve. Am J Physiol 1985; 249(5 Pt 2):H950–H955.
159. Ekenvall L, et al. Alpha-adrenoceptors and cold-induced vasoconstriction in human finger skin. Am J Physiol 1988; 255(5 Pt 2):H1000–H1003.
160. Coffman JD, Cohen RA. Role of alpha-adrenoceptor subtypes mediating sympathetic vasoconstriction in human digits. Eur J Clin Invest 1988; 18:309–313.
161. Edwards JM, et al. Alpha 2-adrenergic receptor levels in obstructive and spastic Raynaud's syndrome. J Vasc Surg 1987; 5:38–45.
162. Hines EA, Christensen NA. Raynaud's disease among men. JAMA 1945; 129:1.
163. Cooke JP, et al. Sex differences in sympathetic control of hand blood flow. Circulation 1990; 82:1607–1615.
164. Freedman RR, Savharwal SC, Desai N. Sex differences in peripheral vascular adrenergic receptors. Circ Res 1987; 61:581–585.
165. Flavahan NA, Vanhoutte PM. Sympathetic purinergic vasoconstriction and thermosensitivity in a canine cutaneous vein. J Pharmacol Exp Therap 1986; 239:874.
166. Coffman JD, Cohen RA. Serotonergic vasoconstriction in human fingers during reflex sympathetic responses to cooling. Am J Physiol (Heart Circ Physiol 23) 1988; 254:H889–H893.
167. Moulds RFW, Iwanov V, Medcalf RL. The effects of platelet-derived contractile agents on human digital arteries. Clin Sci 1984; 66:443–451.
168. Shatz IJ. Occlusive arterial disease in the hands due to occupational trauma. N Engl J Med 1963; 268:281.
169. Gurdjian ES, Walker LW. Traumatic vasospastic disease of the hand (white fingers). JAMA 1945; 129:668.
170. Ash WF, Cook WT, Old JW. Raynaud's phenomenon of occupational origin. Arch Environ Health 1962; 5:333.
171. Mackeiwicz Z, Piskorz A. Raynaud's phenomenon following long-term repeated application of great difference in temperature. J Cardiovasc Surg 1977; 18:151.
172. Jobe JB, et al. Induced vasodilation as treatment of Raynaud's disease. Ann Intern Med 1982; 97:706–709.
173. Zahavi I, et al. Prevalence of Raynaud's phenomenon in patients with migraine. Arch Intern Med 1984; 144:742–744.
174. Miller D, et al. Is variant angina the coronary manifestation of a generalized vasospastic disorder? N Engl J Med 1981; 304:763–768.
175. Whytt R. The Works of Robert Whytt, M.D. Edinburgh: 1768. P. 621.
176. DuBois-Reymond E. Zur kentniss der hemikrania. In Archiv fur Anatomie Physiologie und Wissenschaftliche Medizin. Leipzig: 1860. Pp. 461–468.
177. Engel GL, Ferris EB Jr, Romano J. Focal encephalographic changes during episodes of migraine. Am J Med Sci 1945; 209:650.
178. Graveson GS. Retinal artery occlusion in migraine. Br Med J 1949; 2:838.

179. Schumacker GA, Wolff HG. Experimental studies in headache. Arch Neural Psychiat (Ohio) 1941; 45:199.
180. Adams RD. Headache. In KL Isselbacher, et al. eds. Harrison's Principles of Internal Medicine, 9th ed. New York: McGraw-Hill, 1980.
181. Couch JR, Hassaneim RS. Platelet aggregability in migraine. Neurology 1977; 27:843.
182. Innes IR, Nickerson M. Norepinephrine, epinephrine and the sympathomimetic amines. In LS Goodman, A Gilman, eds. The Pharmacological Basis of Therapeutics, 5th ed. New York: Macmillan, 1975.
183. Kassel N, Drake C. Timing of aneurysm surgery. Neurosurgery 1982; 10:514–519.
184. Fisher CM, Kistler JP, David JM. Relation of cerebral vasospasm to subarachnoid hemorrhage visualized by computerized tomographic scanning. Neurosurgery 1980; 6:1–9.
185. Katusic CS, Vanhoutte PM. Anoxic contractions in isolated canine cerebral arteries. J Cardiovasc Pharmacol 1986; 8:S97–S101.
186. Liszcak TM, et al. Cerebral arterial constriction after experimental subarachnoid hemorrhage is associated with blood components within the arterial wall. J Neurosurg 1983; 58:18–26.
187. Yokota M, et al. Leukotrienes in experimental cerebral vasospasm. In RH Wilkinson, ed. Cerebral Vasospasm. New York: Raven, 1988. Pp. 275–284.
188. Kim P, Sund TM, Vanhoutte PM. Alterations in endothelium-dependent responsiveness of the canine vascular artery after subarachnoid hemorrhage. J Neurosurg 1988; 69:239–246.
189. Nakagomi T, et al. Endothelial damage and cerebral vasospasm. In RH Wilkinson, ed. Cerebral Vasospasm. New York: Raven, 1988. Pp. 137–143.
190. Kanamaru K, et al. Inhibition of endothelium-dependent relaxation by hemoglobin and cerebrospinal fluid from patients with aneurysmal subarachnoid hemorrhage: a possible mechanism in relation to cerebral vasospasm. In RH Wilkinson, ed. Cerebral Vasospasm. New York: Raven, 1988. Pp. 163–168.
191. Boullin DJ, et al. Responses of human and baboon arteries to prostaglandin endoperoxides in biologically generated and synthetic prostacyclin: Their relevance to cerebral arterial spasm in man. Br J Clin Pharmacol 1979; 7:139–147.
192. Seifert B, et al. Arachidonic acid metabolism following aneurysm rupture: Evaluation of cerebrospinal fluid and serum concentration of 6-keto prostaglandin F_1 alpha and thromboxane B_2 in patients with subarachnoid hemorrhage. Surg Neurol 1987; 24:243–252.
193. Walker B, et al. Effects of subarachnoid haemorrhage on intracranial prostaglandins. J Neurol Surg Psych 1983; 46:119–125.
194. Mayberg MR, et al. Acute structural changes in feline cerebral arteries after subarachnoid hemorrhage. In RH Wilkinson, ed. Cerebral Vasospasm. New York: Raven, 1988. Pp. 231–246.
195. Smith RR, et al. The constrictive angiopathy of subarachnoid hemorrhage: an immunopathological approach. In RH Wilkinson, ed. Cerebral Vasospasm. New York: Raven, 1988. Pp. 247–252.
196. Katusic Z, Shepherd JT, Vanhoutte PM. Endothelium-dependent contraction to stretch in canine basilar arteries. Am J Physiol (Heart Circ Physiol) 1987; 21:H671-H673.
197. Flavahan NA, et al. Characterization of postjunctional alpha-1 and alpha-2 adrenoceptors activated by exogenous or nerve-released norepinephrine in the canine saphenous vein. J Pharmacol Exp Ther 1984; 230:699–705.
198. Vanhoutte PM, Lorenz RR. Effect of temperature on reactivity on saphenous, mesenteric and femoral veins of the dog. Am J Physiol 1970; 218:1746–1750.
199. Rowley DA. Venous constriction is the cause of increased vasopermeability produced by 5-hydroxytryptamine, histamine, bradykinin and 48/80 in the rat. Br J Exp Pathol 1964; 45:56–67.
200. Multicenter Trial Committee. Dihydroergotamine-heparin prophylaxis of postoperative deep vein thrombosis: A multicenter trial. JAMA 251:2960–2966.
201. Kakkar VV, et al. Prophylaxis for postoperative deep vein thrombosis: synergistic effect of heparin and dihydroergotamine. JAMA 1979; 241:39–42.
202. Vanhoutte PM, Miller VN. Heterogeneity of endothelium-dependent responses in mammalian blood vessels. J Cardiovasc Pharmacol 1985; 7[Suppl 3]:S12–S23.

Pathophysiology of Vasculitis

Kenneth M. Pariser
Sheldon M. Wolff

The pathophysiologic basis of most vasculitides is presumed to be hypersensitivity. **Hypersensitivity** is an exorbitant response to or overexposure to an antigen that results in excessive degree of tissue damage. It is historically divided into four types, which are listed in Table 17-1. In animal models of vasculitis and in human disease, the most thoroughly studied immunologic mechanism that produces the hypersensitivity response is immune complex deposition. Immune complex–mediated hypersensitivity, or Type III hypersensitivity, most commonly results from the persistent exposure to excessive amounts of antigen. The fusion of antigens with antibody(ies) produces complexes—immune complexes—which may deposit in tissues, giving rise to an acute inflammatory response and tissue damage.

Cell-mediated hypersensitivity, or Type IV delayed-type hypersensitivity, is mediated by T lymphocytes. It results from an exaggerated response by previously primed memory T lymphocytes, which release lymphokines into the region that attract and stimulate macrophages and other T cells. Those cells in turn are capable of causing significant tissue damage. Although delayed-type hypersensitivity is potentially of great importance in the generation of the granulomatous vasculitides, until recently it has received less attention than Type III hypersensitivity. Similarly, little is known about antibodies directed at vascular antigens, or Type II hypersensitivity. In that mechanism, autoantibodies directed at antigens on the vessel surface or in the vessel wall may induce an acute inflammatory response resulting in damage to the wall. Type II hypersensitivity may play a role in some vasculitides.

Three models of the role of immune complexes in the production of a vasculitic lesion have been particularly valuable: the Arthus reaction, experimentally induced serum sickness, and passively administered immune complexes [1]. The **Arthus reaction** is induced by the intradermal injection of soluble antigen into a previously immunized animal. The injected antigens are bound to antibody-forming precipitated immune complexes. These complexes induce an intense local inflammatory reaction via complement activation, mast-cell degranulation, and acute infiltration of polymorphonuclear cells. Human serum sickness results from the injection of large doses of nonhuman immunoglobulin. The foreign proteins provoke the formation of antibodies, which bind to the circulating foreign immunoglobulin, creating soluble immune complexes. If there is significant antigen excess, as will exist early in the antibody response, some of the soluble antigen-antibody complexes (immune complexes) will deposit in the vessel wall, producing a clinical condition called **serum sickness**. Fever, lymphadenopathy, rash, arthritis, and hematuria frequently are noted in this syndrome. In human vasculitides, including cryoglobulinemia, hepatitis B–related vasculitis, Henoch-Schönlein purpura, and many cases of polyarteritis nodosa, soluble immune complexes appear to play a similar significant pathogenetic role [2–6].

Immune Complexes in Vasculitis

In the normal immune response, antibodies attach to and immobilize foreign antigens, forming immune complexes that usually allow for the ultimate degradation of the antigen without significant host injury. This process of formation of immune complexes is influenced by factors in the host as well as properties of the antigen. The size, type, ratio of antibody to antigen, affinity of antibody to antigen, and rate of clearance of immune complexes have significant bearing on the potential of these complexes to induce disease (Table 17-2).

The size of immune complexes partially determines their fate. Animal models of serum sickness suggest that intermediate-sized, slightly greater than 19 Svedberg units, soluble complexes are deposited in vessel walls [7]. This size complex is frequently found when antigen exists in molar excess to antibody and can produce a hypersensitivity response. Significantly larger complexes, formed in antibody excess, rapidly fix complement and are phagocytosed by mononuclear cells in the liver and the spleen, where they usually are destroyed. Smaller complexes remain in the circulation and are less likely to deposit in vessels and induce inflammation [8]. The size of the complex is influenced by (1) the molar ratio of antigen to antibody, (2) the number of epitopes of the antigen, (3) the immunoglobulin class and subclass of the antibodies, and (4) the affinity of the antibody for the antigen [8]. For example, a large antigen with many epitopes likely will result in larger complexes, which are readily taken up by phagocytic cells.

The ability of immune complexes to fix complement, a function of the number, affinity, and class of antibodies, also plays a key role in the ultimate fate of the immune complexes. The name **complement** is given to a series of proteins capable of producing an amplified effect from a triggering stimulus. The pathway that is capable of being activated by the polysaccharides found on micro-organisms alone or by immunoglobulin A (IgA) bound to antigen is called the **alternative complement pathway**. The **classic complement pathway** is activated by interaction with immunoglobulin G (IgG) or immunoglobulin M (IgM), which is bound to antigen. The activation of complement, in particular C3, opsonize the complexes, that is, it facilitates their phagocytosis by cells of the reticuloendothelial system. Complement activation also stimulates phagocytes, triggers release of mediators from mast cells and basophils, induces chemotaxis of neutrophils, and vasodilates capillaries and increases their permeability. Through both the classic and the alternative complement

Table 17-1. Hypersensitivity reactions

Type	Name	Mechanism
I	Anaphylactic hypersensitivity	Cross-linkage of IgE molecules bound to mast cells.
II	Antibody (non-IgE)–mediated hypersensitivity	Ig-coated target is damaged by inflammatory reaction.
III	Immune complex–mediated hypersensitivity	Immune complexes deposit on tissues and induce an inflammatory reaction.
IV	Cell-mediated (delayed type) hypersensitivity	Activated T lymphocytes induce effector cells to produce tissue damage.

pathways C3b, a cleavage fragment of C3 binds to the immune complexes, preventing immune precipitation and bringing about the formation of a immune complexes that can bind to the C3b receptor, CR1 [9].

CR1 exists on erythrocytes, neutrophils, monocytes, some T- and B-lymphocytes, and glomerular podocytes. Up to 90 percent of the CR1 receptors in the human circulation are on erythrocytes [10]. Immune complexes injected into primates bind to CR1 on erythrocytes, which transport the soluble complexes to the Kupffer cells in the liver. Besides providing immune-complex transport, CR1 inhibits full activation of the complement cascade [11]. Thus, CR1 functions as a mechanism to protect against the deposition of immune complexes in the blood vessels and tissues (where activation of complement could lead to tissue destruction) by transporting those complexes to the fixed macrophages in the liver and the spleen, where they can be disposed of safely.

Failure to clear immune complexes can result in their deposition in vessel walls. A number of processes can create that situation. A deficiency in the early classic complement components (inherited deficiencies of C1q, C1r, C1s, C4, or C2) may lead to decreased complement activation and less C3b available for binding to CR1. In fact, patients with inherited deficiencies of early complement components are more likely to develop vasculitis [12]. Immune complexes composed of antibodies (e.g., IgA) that do not activate the classic complement components also may bind poorly to CR1. Those complexes are not as rapidly cleared by the liver and may deposit in tissue such as that of the kidney and the lung [13]. Depletion or deficiency of CR1 or dysfunction of the fixed macrophages also may result in slowed clearance of circulating immune complexes and increased deposits in the vasculature [14].

Table 17-2. Factors that determine the fate of immune complexes

Immunoglobulin class of the antibody
Molar ratio of antibody to antigen
Ability of the antibody to fix complement
Affinity of the antigen-binding site on the antibody
Surface charge of the antigen
Valence of the antigen (number of antibody-binding sites)
State of the CR1 receptors

Other factors may contribute to the deposition of immune complexes in vessels. The electrical charge of the antigen and antibody will influence deposition [15,16]. For example, in animal models the cationic, not the anionic, immune complexes deposit and localize in the glomerular basement membrane [16]. Vasodilatation of the vessels brought about by mediators released by endothelial cells—prostacyclin, nitric oxide, endothelial derived growth factor, and platelet-activating factor—play an important role by increasing vessel permeability and neutrophil migration [17]. Histamine and serotonin released by platelets, basophils, or mast cells after binding to immune complexes, as well as bradykinin, C3a, C5a, and platelet-activating factor, also are capable of producing vasodilatation and increased vascular permeability, resulting in greater immune-complex deposition [1,18]. Prostacyclin and leukotrienes enhance that effect, and their production by endothelial cells is increased by interleukin-1 and tumor necrosis factor [17]. Mechanical factors such as turbulence (at branching points), hypertension, and hydrostatic pressure also increase deposition of immune complexes in vessel walls [19].

Once deposited in the vessel wall, immune complexes are capable of further activating the complement cascade, releasing anaphylatoxins (C4a, C3a, and C5a) and chemoattractants (C3b and C5a). The anaphylatoxins increase vascular permeability. Chemoattractants and endothelial-cell adhesion molecules direct neutrophil migration to the sites of the immune complexes. Activated neutrophils bind to vascular cell adhesion molecule-1 (VCAM-1) and intercellular adhesion molecule-1 (ICAM-1), which are leukocyte adhesion molecules on the endothelial cells and whose expression is markedly increased in patients with vasculitis such as Wegener's granulomatosis [20]. Those molecules also recruit unstimulated neutrophils and activate them so they participate in the inflammatory process [21].

Subsequently, the neutrophils phagocytose the immune complexes utilizing their Fc, CR1, and CR3 receptors. Although those surface receptors are helpful in clearing the immune complexes, the neutrophils also release their lysosomal contents, which can damage local tissues and activate kinins. The inflammation results in further activation of the complement membrane attack complex (C5b-C9) and release of leukotrienes, creating more tissue damage [1,22] (Fig. 17-1).

The result of this inflammatory onslaught is the loss of the integrity of the blood vessels and local tissue ischemia and destruction, that is, **vasculitis**. Control of this inflammatory cascade is less well understood. Phagocytosis and degradation of the immune complexes is one way in which the inflammatory process is contained. Transport of the complexes to the fixed macrophage system in the liver and the spleen is a second mechanism [14]. Prostaglandins may modulate this process by suppression of the response of inflammatory cells [23]. Inhibitors of the complement pathway, kinin inhibitors, and protease inhibitors also are important modulators. Sporadic reports

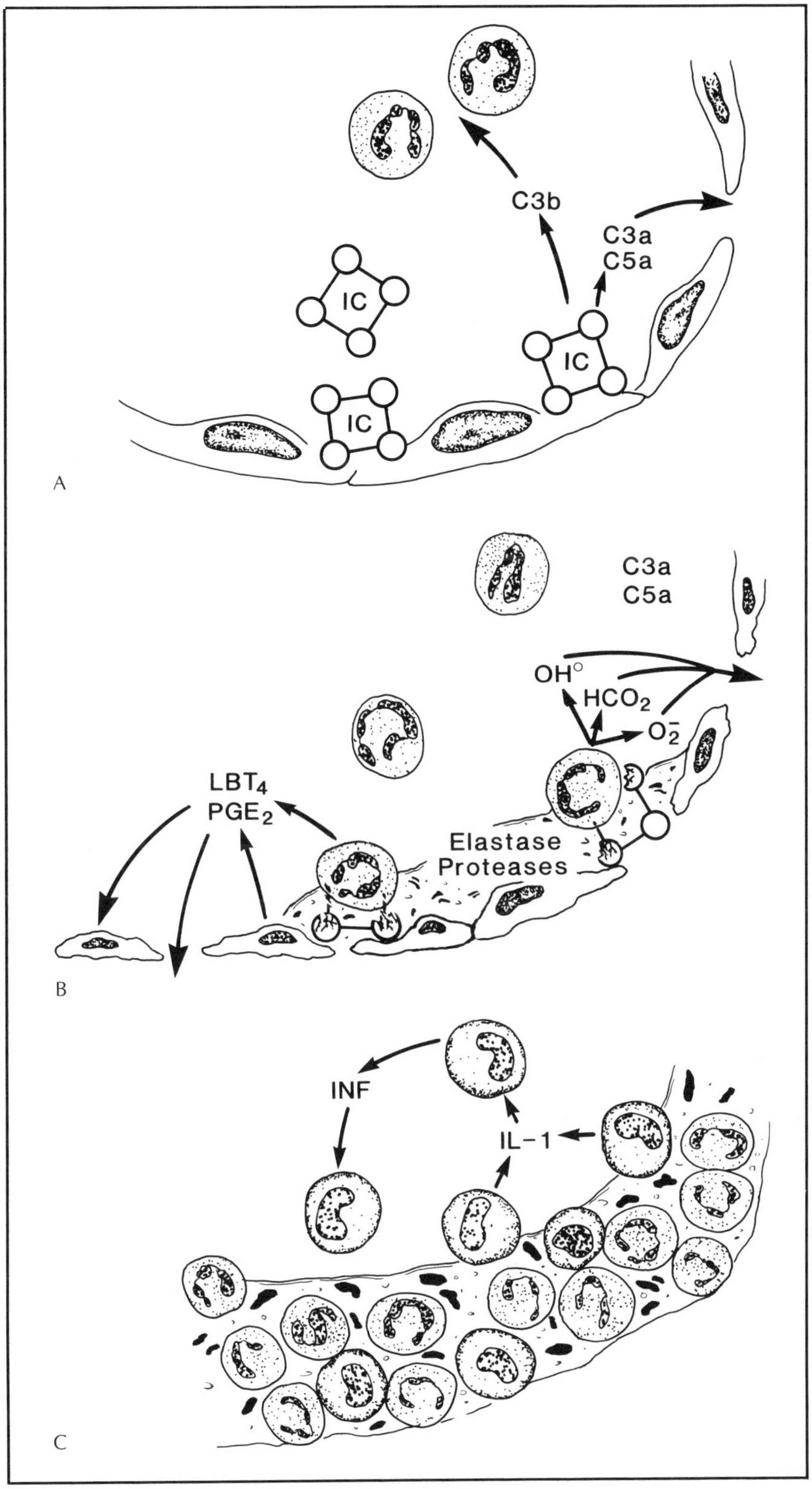

Fig. 17-1. Immune complexes in vasculitis. **A.** Immune complexes deposited on vessel walls, releasing anaphylatoxinc (C3a, C5a) and chemoattractants (C3b), producing endothelial cell retraction and attracting and activating neutrophils. **B.** Neutrophils responding to C3b and other factors phagocytose the immune complexes and release lysosomal enzymes, superoxide anions, leukotrienes, and prostaglandins, all of which damage the vessel wall and attract additional leukocytes. **C.** The release of interleukins and interferons activates the local inflammatory cells to greater metabolic activity and creates systemic effects such as fever, leukocytosis, and the production of acute phase reactants.

of cutaneous and systemic vasculitis associated with alpha$_1$-antitrypsin deficiency suggest that those control mechanisms play a significant role that deserves further investigation [24,25].

Immune Complexes in Human Disease

Although serum sickness is the classic human disease in which circulating immune complexes have been demonstrated to have a major pathophysiologic role, other vasculitides have been associated with circulating immune complexes [3,6]. Hepatitis B surface antigen has been shown to be a part of immune complexes that deposit in vasculitic lesions in some patients with systemic necrotizing vasculitis (polyarteritis) [5,26–28]. Henoch-Schönlein purpura has been associated with IgA immune complexes in both children and adults [4,29]. Cryoglobulinemia with vasculitis is immune complex mediated. The antigen in the complex may be either hepatitis C antibody or viral antigen [30]. Both hepatitis C antibody and hepatitis C RNA have been detected in concentrated amounts along with the cryoglobulin in the cryoprecipitate [31]. Necrotizing vasculitis of the skin also has been shown to be immune complex mediated [32]. The role of immune complexes in the granulomatous vasculitides, such as Wegener's granulomatosis, giant cell arteritis, and Churg-Strauss syndrome, is less well accepted [33].

Hypersensitivity induced vessel damage also can result from autoantibodies directed at the constituents of the vessel wall. The direct attack on the integrity of the vessel by antibody has the potential to induce an inflammatory reaction by a mechanism similar to that induced by immune-complex deposition. Complement activation, chemotaxis and adherence of polymorphonuclear cells, and release of lysosomal contents producing tissue destruction can be generated in that model. In human disease, circulating autoantibodies directed at vessel walls have been identified [34,35]. Detection at the site of vessel damage in human disease is not reported.

Cellular Immune-Mediated Vasculitis

In contrast to immune complex deposition, the role of direct lymphocyte-mediated vessel wall damage is less well studied. This mechanism has particular relevance to those vasculitides characterized histologically by lymphocyte and macrophage infiltration and the formation of granulomata such as giant-cell arteritis.

At least two potential pathways exist for direct lymphocyte-mediated vasculitis. Through a type IV immune reaction, sensitized T lymphocytes may bind to antigens and release cytokines [36]. The cytokines discharged by those cells, some of which are listed in Table 17-3, enlist other cells, particularly macrophages and lymphocytes, for amplification of the inflammatory response. Activated macrophages may phagocytose antigen or immune complexes and then release lysosomal enzymes, producing damage similar to what the polymorphonuclear cells induce when reacting to immune complexes [36]. Continued stimulation of the T lymphocytes by persistent antigen results in a localized collection of activated macrophages, some of which may be transformed into epithelioid cells and multinucleated giant cells. This may produce a classic granuloma, as seen in the granulomatous vasculitides [37].

Table 17-3. Selected cytokines

Interleukin-1	Activates resting T cells; stimulates production of other cytokines; activates macrophages and endothelial cells
Interleukin-2	Activates natural killer cells; is a growth factor for activated T cells and cytotoxic T cells
Interleukin-4	T cell growth factor; increases immunoglobulin production and suppresses cytokines production by macrophages; released by TH-2 lymphocytes
Interleukin-6	Growth factors for activated B cells; promotes differentiation of B cells to plasma cells
Interleukin-8	Secreted by endothelial cells; attracts and activates neutrophils
Interferon gamma	Activates macrophages and endothelial cells; augments B cell stimulating lymphokines and natural-killer-cell activity
Tumor necrosis factor alpha	Secreted by monocytes, macrophages, and T lymphocytes, synergy with other cytokines to induce inflammation
Tumor necrosis factor beta	Stimulates production of lymphokines; activates macrophages and endothelial cells

In giant cell arteritis, immunohistochemical studies show that CD4+ T-lymphocytes and macrophages are the dominant cell types. CD8+ T cells and B-lymphocytes are rarely found [38]. Analysis of the CD4+ T lymphocytes (T helper cells) indicates that these are a selected subpopulation, TH1 helper cells [39]. This local aggregation of TH1 helper cells suggests that there is local recognition of antigen. In the same study, identification of interleukin-2 mRNA and interferon-gamma in the biopsies of patients with giant cell arteritis supports the notion of local antigen processing with the release of cytokines, amplifying the vasculitic lesion [39]. Shared clonal types of T cells in the vascular lesions of patients with giant cell arteritis also suggest the possibility of local antigenically stimulated T cells [40]. Selective expansion and stimulation of T cells expressing restricted T cell receptors in giant cell arteritis and Kawasaki disease suggest that certain populations of T cells are selected by their recognition of disease-related antigens [41,42].

A second pathway is direct delayed-type hypersensitivity reaction to vascular antigens. Smooth muscle cells, endothelial cells, and the internal elastic lamina have been proposed as the target antigens for cellular immune-mediated damage in giant cell arteritis. In fact, activated cytotoxic lymphocytes have been found circulating in some patients with systemic vasculitides [43]. Animal models of experimental autoimmune delayed-type hypersensitivity vasculitis exist [44,45]. Those models employ vascular smooth muscle or endothelial cells as the antigen for T lymphocytes. Histologically, these animals develop a vasculitis with mononuclear cells invading the media and

Table 17-4. HLA associations with vasculitis

Disease	HLA antigen	Percent with antigen	Relative risk	Reference
Behçet's syndrome	B51	63	18.2	[55]
Giant cell arteritis	Cw3	57	5.65	[56]
Giant cell arteritis	DRB1*0401	62	—	[57]
Kawasaki disease	A2, B44, Cw5	25	8.9	[58]
Kawasaki disease	Bw51	30	14.8	[59]
Wegener's granulomatosis	DR2	65	—	[60]
Wegener's granulomatosis	B8	39	—	[61]
Takayasu arteritis	Bw52	46	—	[62]

adventitia of arterioles and venules in most organs. Some animals developed a granulomatous vasculitis in the pulmonary arterioles [46].

Vascular endothelial cells express relatively unique antigens as well as major histocompatibility complex (MHC) class II antigens [47,48]. Endothelial cells also appear to have the ability to substitute for macrophages as antigen-presenting cells [49]. This could either induce or aggravate an ongoing autoimmune process, resulting in an intense inflammatory response in the vessel wall. MHC class II molecules on endothelial cells have been identified in polyarteritis nodosa along with CD4+ T lymphocytes and activated macrophages, suggesting that endothelial cells may play such a role in human vasculitides [50]. A similar finding has been reported in the coronary arteries of patients with Kawasaki disease [51]. Dendritic cells are also present in vasculitic lesions, especially in early lesions [50]. Dendritic cells are critical in initiating an immune reaction, because they function as antigen-presenting cells. As lesions age, dendritic cells disappear, leaving macrophages and endothelial cells as the likely antigen-presenting cells.

Immunogenetic Factors in the Pathogenesis of Vasculitis

Each of the mechanisms for vasculitis proposed so far implicates an altered or abnormal immune response. In mice, immune-response genes are linked to the histocompatibility system. In humans, a similar finding, although more difficult to demonstrate, appears to exist between the immune-response genes and the class II MHC antigens. A statistical association has been found between immune responsiveness to ragweed, streptococcus, influenza A, vaccinia, tetanus, and human leukocyte antigens (HLA) [52]. Those connections and studies demonstrating linkage between HLA antigens and autoantibodies, as well as diseases with abnormal immune reactivity, suggest that certain vasculitides may be associated with HLA antigens (Table 17-4) [53,54]. The mechanism through which MHC antigens predispose individuals to those diseases is unclear. The relatively weak relationships seen in most of the reported series and the differences seen in separate ethnic groups indicate that the genetic mechanisms are complex and may be controlled from several chromosomal loci.

ANTINEUTROPHIL CYTOPLASMIC AUTOANTIBODIES

Antineutrophil cytoplasmic autoantibodies (ANCAs) were first described in 1982 in patients with segmental necrotizing glomerulonephritis with few immune deposits in the glomerulus and clinical features suggestive of vasculitis [63]. Eight patients complained of myalgias and arthralgias, and four had dyspnea and hemoptysis in addition to their glomerulonephritis. The lack of immunoglobulin deposition in their glomeruli distinguished their condition from Goodpasteur's syndrome or systemic lupus erythematosus. The report was confirmed two years later [64]. Subsequently, ANCAs were found in a majority of patients with Wegener's granulomatosis and primary crescentic pauci-immune glomerulonephritis as well as in some patients with microscopic polyarteritis nodosa, Churg-Strauss syndrome, and polyangiitis overlap syndrome [65–67]. Studies of ANCAs in vitro have demonstrated that they can enhance the activity of polymorphonuclear cells. In the presence of cytokines, such as interferon-gamma, neutrophils express proteinase-3 and myeloperoxidase on their membranes. Since these are the primary antigens for ANCA, their expression by activated neutrophils on their membranes makes them targets for this ANCA [68]. This may enhance neutrophil damage to local tissues and induce both local and systemic inflammation, which overwhelms the normal controlling mechanisms of inflammation [69].

ANCA immunofluorescence staining in a coarse cytoplasmic pattern with central accentuation (C-ANCA) correlates with antibody to proteinase-3 and has a nearly 90-percent specificity for Wegener's granulomatosis [68]. Perinuclear staining, P-ANCA, has a high correlation with antibody to elastase and myeloperoxidase detected by enzyme-linked immunosorbent assays (ELISA) [70,71]. While P-ANCA staining can be detected in patients with Wegener's granulomatosis, microscopic polyarteritis, and pauci-immune crescentic glomerulonephritis, the interpretation of the pattern is more complicated because of other disease associations, including inflammatory bowel disease, Felty's syndrome, autoimmune hepatitis, and other rheumatic conditions [69]. It is uncertain whether ANCAs are pathogenic or merely a marker for disease [72].

Other Pathogenetic Mechanisms

In addition to the immunopathogenesis, Behçet's syndrome, thromboangiitis obliterans, and occasionally other systemic vasculitides demonstrate an increased tendency to thrombosis both in clinical features and pathologic specimens [73–74]. Studies of localized and systemic vasculitides have shown a variety of abnormalities in fibrinolysis. Defective release of tissue plasminogen-activator antigen has been found in rheumatoid vasculitis, Behçet's syndrome, and cutaneous necrotizing venulitis [75–77]. Elevated levels of plasminogen-activator inhibitor also have been found in livedoid vasculitis [78]. These decreased levels of fibrinolytic activity appear to be due to reduced release of plasminogen activator from the endothelial cells of the venules [77], which may result in increased fibrin deposits intravascularly as well as in the vessel wall. The deposits potentially can augment the ischemic process initiated by the immune-complex deposits in the vessel wall. Whether the decreased fibrinolytic activity represents a reaction to the inflammation around the endothelial cell and the vessel wall or actually contributes to the pathogenesis of these disorders is unclear.

Direct viral deposition and growth in the vessel wall also has been demonstrated to induce a vasculitis in animals [79]. Rubella has, on rare occasion, induced a similar lesion in humans [80]. Herpes zoster virus induces an arteritis with direct local replication of the virus in the cerebral vessels [81]. Human immunodeficiency virus (HIV) has been associated with a necrotizing and nonnecrotizing arteritis affecting medium-sized vessels. Hypersensitivity vasculitis with small-vessel involvement is also seen. HIV antigens and HIV RNA have been detected in both large- and small-vessel lesions [82].

Direct invasion of the blood vessel with abnormal or malignant cells, as seen in angiocentric immunoproliferative lesion, is another potential mechanism. In angiocentric immunoproliferative lesion, atypical lymphocytoid and plasmacytoid cells are seen in conjunction with granulomatous inflammation in an angiocentric and angiodestructive pattern [83]. Toxic injury to vessels, as postulated in Buerger's disease with tobacco smoke and as reported in Spain with consumption of adulterated rapeseed oil, demonstrates that mechanisms other than immune-mediated destruction may induce a vasculitis [73,84].

Summary

Currently, the best-studied pathogenetic mechanism for human vasculitis is immune-complex deposition. With few exceptions (e.g., hepatitis B surface antigen), the antigens remain unknown that induce an immune response needed to create the soluble circulating immune complexes of the right size, charge, and constituents to deposit in vessel walls rather than to be transported to the fixed-macrophage system for proper disposal. Similarly, the host factors that contribute to that dysfunctional immune and inflammatory response, although outlined in broad terms, are not well understood.

The role of delayed-hypersensitivity cell-mediated immune response in the induction of the vasculitides is even less well understood. The techniques necessary to begin to assess the function of those cells are only now available. Work in nonimmune pathogenetic areas that may contribute to these processes are clearly in their infancy.

References

1. Cochrane CG, Weigle WO. The cutaneous reaction to soluble antigen-antibody complexes. A comparison with the Arthus reaction. J Exp Med 1958; 108:591.
2. Barrett J, et al. Circulating immune complexes in cutaneous and systemic vasculitis: clinicopathological correlations. Ann Rheum Dis 1982; 41:25–29.
3. Agnello V, Chung RT, Kaplan LM. A role for hepatitis C virus infection in type II cryoglobulinemia. N Engl J Med 1992; 327:1490–1495.
4. Levinsky RJ, Barratt TM. IgA immune complexes in Henoch-Schönlein purpura. Lancet 1979; 2:1100–1103.
5. Marcellin P, et al. Latent hepatitis B virus (HBV) infection is systemic necrotizing vasculitis. Clin Exp Rheumatol 1991; 9:23–28.
6. Lawley TJ, et al. A prospective clinical and immunologic analysis of patients with serum sickness. N Engl J Med 1984; 311:1407–1413.
7. Cochrane CG, Hawkins D. Studies on circulating immune complexes. III: Factors governing the ability of circulating complexes to localize in blood vessels. J Exp Med 1968; 127:137.
8. Mannik M. Physiochemical and functional relationships of immune complexes. J Invest Dermatol 1980; 74:333–338.
9. Schifferli JA, Peters DK. Complement mediated inhibition of immune precipitation. II: Analysis by sucrose density gradient ultracentrifugation. Clin Exp Immunol 1982; 47:563–569.
10. Siegel I, Liu TL, Gleicher N: The red-cell immune system. Lancet 1981; 2:556–559.
11. Yeh CG, et al. Recombinant soluble human complement receptor type 1 inhibits inflammation in the reversed passive arthus reaction in rats. J Immunol 1991; 146:250–256.
12. Agnello V: Complement deficiency states. Medicine 1978; 57:1–23.
13. Waxman FJ, et al. Differential binding of immunoglobulin A and immunoglobulin G1 immune complexes to primate erythrocytes in vivo: immunoglobulin A immune complexes bind less well to erythrocytes and are preferentially deposited in glomeruli. J Clin Invest 1986; 77:82–89.
14. Schifferli JA, Ng YC, Peters DK. The role of complement and its receptor in the elimination of immune complexes. N Engl J Med 1986; 315:488–495.
15. Gauthier VJ, Striker GE, Mannik M. Glomerular localization of preformed immune complexes prepared with anionic antibodies or with cationic antigens. Lab Invest 1984; 50:634–644.
16. Joselow SA, Mannik M. Localization of preformed, circulating immune complexes in murine skin. J Invest Dermatol 1984; 82:335–340.
17. Zavoico GB, et al. Interleukin-1 and related cytokines enhance thrombin-stimulated PGI2 production in cultured endothelial cells without affecting thrombin-stimulated von Willebrand factor secretion or platelet activating factor biosynthesis. J Immunol 1989; 142:3993–3999.
18. Cochrane CG. Studies on the localization of circulating antigen–antibody complexes and other macromolecules in vessels. I: Structural studies. J Exp Med 1963; 118:489–502.
19. Kniker WT, Cochrane CG. The localization of circulating immune complexes in experimental serum sickness. The role of vasoactive amines and hydrodynamic forces. J Exp Med 1968; 127:119.
20. Stegeman CA, et al. Serum levels of soluble adhesion molecules intercellular adhesion melecule 1, vascular cell adhesion molecule 1, and E-selectin in patients with Wegener's granulomatosis, Arthritis Rheum 1994; 37:1228–1235.
21. Pober JS, Coltran RS. The role of endothelial cells in inflammation. Transplantation 1990; 50:537–44.

22. Mayer MM. Membrane damage by complement. Johns Hopkins Med J 1981; 148:243–258.
23. Scales WE, et al. Regulation of monokine gene expression: Prostaglandin E_2 suppresses tumor necrosis factor but not interleukin-1 alpha or beta mRNA and cell-associated activity. J Leukoc Biol 1989; 45:416–421.
24. Fortin PR, et al. Alpha-1-antitrypsin deficiency and systemic necrotizing vasculitis. J Rheumatol 1991; 18:1613–1619.
25. Lewis M, et al. Severe alpha-1-antitrypsin deficiency associated with cutaneous vasculitis, rapidly progressive glomerulonephritis, and colitis. Am J Med 1985; 79:489–494.
26. Fye KH, et al. Immune complexes in hepatitis B antigen-associated periarteritis nodosa: detection by antibody-dependent cell mediated cytotoxicity and the Raji cell assay. Am J Med 1977; 62:783.
27. Gocke DJ, et al. Vasculitis in association with Australian antigen. J Exp Med 1971; 134:330s.
28. Marcellin P, et al. Latent hepatitis B virus (HBV) infection in systemic necrotizing vasculitis. Clin Exp Rheumatol 1991; 9:23–28.
29. Baart de la Faille-Kuyper EH, et al. IgA deposits in cutaneous blood vessel walls and mesangium in Henoch-Schönlein syndrome. Lancet 1973; 1:892–893.
30. Chad D, et al. The pathogenesis of cryoglobulinemic neuropathy. Neurology 1982; 32:725–729.
31. Agnello V, Chung RT, Kaplan LM. A role for hepatitis C virus infection in type II cryoglobulinemia. N Engl J Med 1992; 327:1490–1495.
32. Soter NA. Clinical presentations and mechanisms of necrotizing angiitis of the skin. J Invest Dermatol 1976; 67:354–359.
33. Ronco P, et al. Immunopathological studies of polyarteritis nodosa and Wegener's granulomatosis: a report of 43 patients with 51 renal biopsies. Quart J Med 1983; 206:212–223.
34. Tizard EJ, et al. Antiendothelial cell antibodies detected by a cellular based ELISA in Kawasaki disease. Arch Dis Child 1987; 79:468–472.
35. Dhingra R, et al. An enzyme linked immunosorbent assay for detection of anti-aorta antibodies in Takayasu arteritis patients. Int J Cardiol 1993; 40:237–242.
36. Akai KI, et al. Cytokines: coordinators of immune and inflammatory response. Annu Rev Biochem 1990; 59:783–836.
37. Lie JT, American College of Rheumatology Subcommittee on Classification of Vasculitis. Illustrated histopathologic classification criteria for selected vasculitis syndromes. Arthritis Rheum 1990; 33:1074–1087.
38. Cid MC, et al. Immunohistochemical analysis of lymphoid and macrophage subsets and their immunologic activation markers in temporal arteritis. Arthritis Rheum 1989; 32:884–893.
39. Weyland CM, et al. Tissue cytokine patterns in patients with polymyalgia rheumatica and giant cell arteritis. Ann Int Med 1994; 121:484–491.
40. Weyland CM, et al. Distinct vascular lesions in giant cell arteritis share identical T cell clonotypes. J Exp Med 1994; 179:951–960.
41. Abe J, et al. Characterization of T cell repertoire changes in Kawasaki disease. J Exp Med 1993; 177:791–796.
42. Grunewald J, et al. CD4+ and CD8+ cell expansions using selected TCR V and J gene segments at the onset of giant cell arteritis. Arthritis Rheum 1994; 37:1221–1227.
43. Bland AD, Scott DGI. Activated cytotoxic lymphocytes in systemic vasculitis. Rheumatol Int 1991; 11:69–72.
44. Hart MN, et al. Experimental autoimmune type of vasculitis resulting from activation of mouse lymphocytes to cultured endothelium. Lab Invest 1983; 48:419–427.
45. Moyer CF, Reinisch CL. The role of vascular smooth muscle cells in experimental autoimmune vasculitis. Am J Pathol 1984; 117:380–390.
46. Hart MN, et al. Autoimmune vasculitis resulting from in vitro immunization of lymphocytes to smooth muscle. Am J Pathol 1985; 119:448–455.
47. Cui YC, et al. A vascular endothelial cell antigen with restricted distribution in human foetal, adult and malignant tissues. Immunol 1983; 49:183–189.
48. Rosa F, Fellows M. The effect of gamma-interferon on MHC antigens. Immunol Today 1984; 5:261–262.
49. Hirschberg H, Bergh OJ, Thorsby E. Antigen-presenting properties of human vascular endothelial cells. J Exp Med 1980; 152:249–255.
50. Cid MC, et al. Immunohistochemical characteristics of inflammatory cells and immunologic markers in muscle and nerve biopsy specimens from patients with systemic polyarteritis nodosa. Arthritis Rheum 1994; 37:1055–1061.
51. Terai M, et al. Class II histocompatibility antigen expression on coronary artery endothelium in a patient with Kawasaki disease. Hum Pathol 1990; 21:231–234.
52. Koopman WJ. Genetic control of immune responses. In WN Kelley ed. Textbook of Rheumatology. Philadelphia: Saunders, 1985. P. 58.
53. Scherak O, Smolen JS, Mayr WR. HLA-DRw3 and systemic lupus erythematosus. Arthr Rheum 1980; 23:954.
54. Stastny P, et al. The human immune response region (HLA-D) and disease susceptibility. Immunol Rev 1983; 70:113–153.
55. Arber N, et al. Close association of HLA-B51 and B52 in Israeli patients with Behçet's syndrome. Ann Rheum Dis 1991; 50:351–353.
56. Hansen JA, Healey LA, Wilske KR. Association between giant cell (temporal) arteritis and HLA-Cw3. Hum Immunol 1985; 13:193–198.
57. Weyland CM, et al. HLA-DRB1 alleles in polymyalgia rheumatica, giant cell arteritis and rheumatoid arthritis. Arthritis Rheum 1994; 37:514–520.
58. Kaslow RA, et al. Association of epidemic Kawasaki syndrome with the HLA-A2, B44, Cw5 antigen combination. Arth Rheum 1985; 28:938–940.
59. Krensky AM, et al. HLA antigens in mucocutaneous lymph node syndrome in New England. Pediat 1981; 67:741–743.
60. Elkon KB, et al. HLA antigen frequencies in systemic vasculitis: increase in HLA-DR2 in Wegener's granulomatosis. Arth Rheum 1983; 26:102–105.
61. Katz P, et al. Association of Wegener's granulomatosis with HLA-B8. Clin Immun Immunopath 1979; 14:268–270.
62. Yajima M, Moriwaki R, Numano F, Park YB, Cho YD. Comparative studies between Japanese and Korean patients: comparison of the findings of angiography, HLA-Bw52, and clinical manifestations. Heart-Vessels 1992; [Suppl 7]: 102–105.
63. Davies DJ, et al. Segmental necrotising glomerulonephritis with antineutrophil antibody: possible arbovirus aetiology? BMJ 1982; 2:606.
64. Hall JB, et al. Vasculitis and glomerulonephritis: a subgroup with an antineutrophil cytoplasmic antibody. Aust NZ J Med 1984; 14:277–278.
65. Hoffman GS, et al. Wegener's granulomatosus: an analysis of 158 patients. Ann Intern Med 1992; 116:488–489.
66. Falk RJ, Jennette JC. Anti-neutrophil cytoplasmic autoantibodies with specificity for myeloperoxidase in patients with systemic vasculitis and idiopathic necrotising and crescentic glomerulonephritis. N Eng J Med 1988; 318:1651–1657.
67. Cohen Tervaert JW, et al. Detection of autoantibodies against myeloid lysosomal enzymes: a useful adjunct to classification of patients with biopsy proven necrotizing arteritis. Am J Med 1991; 91:59–66.

68. Hagen EC, et al. Fundamental and clinical aspects of antineutrophil eytoplasmic antibodies. Autoimmunity 1992; 11:199–207.
69. Kallenberg CGM, et al. Anti-neutrophil cytoplasmic antibodies: current diagnostic and pathophysiologic potential. Kidney Int 1994; 46:1–15.
70. Charles LA, et al. Antibodies against granule proteins activate neutrophils in vitro. J Leukoc Biol 1991; 50:539–546.
71. Gross WL, Csernok E, Schmitt, LOH. Antineutrophil cytoplasmic autoantibodies: Immunologic aspects. Klin Wochenscher 1991; 69:558–566.
72. Jennette JC. Pathogenic potential of anti-neutrophil cytoplasmic autoantibodies (Editorial). Lab Invest 1994; 70:135–137.
73. McKusick VA, et al. Buerger's disease: a distinct clinical and pathologic entity. JAMA 1962; 181:5–12.
74. Koc Y, et al. Vascular involvement in Behçet's disease. J Rheumatol 1992; 19:402–410.
75. Toki N, Yamura T. Studies on the blood fibrinolytic involvement in Behçet's disease. J Rheumatol 1992; 19:402–410.
76. Lau CS, et al. Abnormal plasma fibrinolysis in patients with rheumatoid arthritis and impaired endothelial fibrinolytic response in those complicated by vascultis. Ann Rheum Dis 1993; 52:643–649.
77. Lotti T, et al. Mesoglycan treatment restores defective fibrinolytic potential in cutaneous necrotizing venulitis. Int J Dermatol 1993; 32:368–371.
78. Klein KL, Pittelkow MR. Tissue plasminogen activator for treatment of livedoid vasculitis. Mayo Clin Proc 1992; 67:923–938.
79. Estes PC, Cheville NF. The ultrastructure of vascular lesions in equine viral arteritis. Am J Pathol 1970; 58:235.
80. Fortain NJ, Morrow AG, Roberts WC. Late vascular manifestations of the rubella syndrome: a roentgenographic-pathologic study. Am J Med 1971; 51:134.
81. Martin JR, Mitchell WJ, Henken CK. Neurotropic herpesviruses, neural mechanisms and arteritis. Brain Pathol 1990; 1:6–10.
82. Gherardi R, et al. The spectrum of vasculitis in human immunodeficiency virus infected patients. Arthritis Rheum 1993; 36:1164–1174.
83. Liebow AA, Carrington CRB, Friedman PJ. Lymphomatoid granulomatosis. Hum Pathol 1972; 3:457–558.
84. Martinez-Tello FJ, et al. Pathology of a new toxic syndrome caused by ingestion of adulterated oil in Spain. Virchows Arch (Pathol Anat) 1982; 397:261–285.

III

Diagnostic Methods in Vascular Disease

Examination of the Patient with Vascular Disease

John W. Joyce

The essence of clinical diagnosis is circumscribed by history, examination, and knowledge of the behavior of the process under assessment. Laboratory testing then accomplishes confirmation, quantitation, and, in some instances, clarification of uncertainties. Competent historic and physical examination skills are the prime tools of the clinician. They endure throughout a career, whereas testing and therapeutic modalities continue to evolve and change. A logical, efficient plan of investigation and treatment has as its soundest foundation a well-performed clinical assessment.

The cardiovascular system is a particularly rich field for this logic, because its multiple structural and hydraulic disorders cause clearly defined symptoms and findings so often accessible to the eye, ear, and hand. A broad array of testing modalities is well developed. This chapter presents an approach to the historic and physical examination of diseases of the arterial, venous, and lymphatic systems. Full discussion of the natural history of specific entities and the testing useful in their evaluation is developed in subsequent chapters. It is hoped that, by utilizing these parallel resources, the reader will be assisted in the prime responsibility of accurate diagnosis and that the opening thesis will then become diagnosis by directed history, sensitized examination, and selective testing.

It is axiomatic that appreciation of the whole patient is intrinsic to any vascular examination. This may have been accomplished by another physician or it may be the primary responsibility of the examiner. The following examples are self-apparent: the comorbidity of atherosclerosis in the coronary, carotid, renal, and visceral arteries; the heart as a source of dyspnea, edema, and emboli; the importance of impaired cardiac, renal, and pulmonary function and of associated hematologic, metabolic, and systemic disease in therapeutic decisions; the settings of trauma, bedrest, infections, and prior procedures that predispose to arterial and venous problems; the importance of risk factors such as tobacco smoking, diabetes mellitus, hypertension, and lipid disorders in long-term management of atherosclerosis; the value of body habitus and skin findings as markers of unusual diseases. The converse is an equally valid corollary: The vascular system can offer clues, just as do the eyes, skin, and nails, to diseases of other organ systems [1]. A systematic recording of historic and examination data is essential for later comparisons in both acute and chronic vascular diseases and for providing information useful to therapy and prognosis. The use of objective tests, including photography, where appropriate, often substantiates the patient's account or the physician's notations on subsequent review. The examining physician can rapidly acquire a comfortable degree of confidence in the diagnosis of vascular disorders when the findings of sound, well-directed examinations are confirmed by the clinical course or laboratory findings.

The Arterial System

HISTORIC EXAMINATION

An effective medical history has two components: the patient's account and directed questions from an interested and informed examiner. Gentle instruction or redirection may be necessary with the circumlocutory patient. Observations of others often are essential in extracting sound information from an impaired or forgetful patient. The patient's primary concern and all other significant observations are pursued by interrogation prompted by the differential diagnosis of that symptom or disease process. The best questions are informed but not leading, brief, and in language that is clearly understood by those interviewed. Five additional avenues of information are often fruitful: essential negatives that eliminate other diagnoses; knowledge of circumstances that aggravate or alleviate the problem; time relationships of the symptom to other medical events and whether the complaint is intermittent or constant; the tempo of the process in terms of seconds, minutes, hours, days, or longer; and a listing of drugs or prior events, such as arterial punctures, surgery, or radiation, that can have a significant relationship to the process being evaluated. These general observations apply to all medical interviews.

Many patients will be seen with a diagnosis already assigned. Proper consultation requires a review of the history, examination, and data supporting the diagnosis. A fresh reconstruction may clarify or extend the original conclusions and identify underappreciated etiologic factors or systemic problems.

CHRONIC OCCLUSIVE ARTERIAL DISEASE

The symptoms produced by stenosis or occlusion of major arteries are governed by the location of the lesion, its severity, and the status of the collateral flow of that system. Most patients present with lesions partly compensated by collateral circulation and complain initially of claudication in muscle groups deprived of full blood supply. Progressive limitation is usual, and the tempo, depending on risk factors and etiology, may be measured in weeks, months, or years. When the occlusive process is extensive, when local trauma or infection are superimposed, or when collateral flow is lost, inadequate tissue perfusion can cause rest pain, neuropathic distress, tissue infarction, or ulceration.

Claudication. Claudication is a stereotyped, reproducible distress in a muscle group, induced by exercise and relieved by rest. A patient may describe the distress as pain, cramping, tightness, weakness, heaviness, fatigue, or "giving out." With progression of the occlusive process, the symptom may change character, location, or intensity, and local muscle tenderness can persist for a while during recovery. Common muscular cramps differ from claudication in that most occur at rest, and those occurring with exercise are random and accompanied by the muscle contraction characteristic of all cramps.

Sustained exercise, most commonly walking for the legs and hair grooming or tool use for the arms, is required to induce claudication. Many patients walk significant cumulative distances at work without symptoms because their efforts are intermittent, only to experience claudication on the more prolonged effort of walking home, to their transportation, or during recreation. Because claudication results from a disparity between supply and demand of blood flow, symptoms occur more quickly with an accelerated pace, when carrying a burden, walking uphill, or on difficult terrain. Many patients alertly question why they are able to cycle or use various exercise devices for much longer periods, compared to their usual walking time, before claudication occurs: When leg exercise is done in the sitting position, the work load is less because the effect of gravity is reduced.

Symptom relief begins when exercise is stopped and commonly requires 2 to 5 minutes, occasionally longer. More rapid recovery is observed by some when weight is shifted from the symptomatic leg or after sitting. It is essential to establish that muscle groups are the primary site of the discomfort and whether relief is complete and timely with rest. When those criteria are not clearly met, and when the symptoms also occur in the standing, sitting, or supine position without exercise, musculoskeletal, neurologic, and mechanical problems should be pursued as the cause of the distress. It is critical to question each patient suspected of having claudication for these prime observations. Should the answer be unclear or should there be other sources of distress to compound or confuse the history, the presence or absence of occlusive disease can be clarified by observing the symptoms produced and the distal blood pressure response with exercise testing.

Claudication, as defined and detailed, is a most specific and reliable symptom. Quantitation, however, is quite variable by history alone, owing to differences in pace, estimates of distance, and variations in work load. Often, patients consider their claudication stable when, in fact, they have accommodated to progressive limitation by changes in pace and life-style. When quantitation is desired for longitudinal observation of claudication, whether treated medically or surgically, objective testing is essential. Proof of diagnosis and simple, reliable measurements are provided by periodic ankle-brachial pressure indices taken both at rest and after standardized treadmill exercise testing. It is of singular importance to determine what impact the claudication has on the patient's life-style. Decisions regarding the advisability of surgical or interventional therapy are based in part on whether the claudication significantly impairs the patient's productivity or, in some instances, recreation.

The site of claudication suggests the approximate location of the occlusive process when a single focal lesion is present. Isolated pedal claudication results from foot or low-calf vessel disease. This condition is common in thromboangiitis obliterans but rare in atherosclerosis. Foot claudication is usually accompanied by low-calf distress and caused by lesions of the tibial-peroneal vessels. Popliteal occlusive disease localizes claudication to the lower third of the calf and lesions of the superficial femoral artery to the upper two-thirds or all of the calf. Common femoral lesions induce claudication of the calf, thigh, or both, depending on the patient's gait. Aortoiliac disease yields bilateral calf, thigh, buttock, and occasionally back distress. The order of appearance of the symptoms is usually from distal to cephalad, but this may be reversed, and symptoms may be limited to the calf or to the buttocks and thighs. Again, this may depend on the patient's gait, but in some instances the differences are governed by associated occlusive problems in the internal iliac or profunda femoris arteries. When the occlusive process is at multiple levels, the initial site of claudication usually reflects the most distal significant lesion or the area with the poorest collateral flow. It is not uncommon for patients to experience a different quality or distribution of their usual distress when performing treadmill exercise testing. This is most logically explained by the requirement of different muscle activity to handle the incline of the machine. Occlusive arterial disease is often bilateral, yet the patient may report only unilateral symptoms. This occurs because a hemodynamically significant lesion in the symptomatic limb causes the patient to stop before the level of exercise critical for claudication is reached in the contralateral leg with lesser disease.

Questions regarding the onset, distribution, and tempo of claudication are a fundamental requirement of a competent history. This information can confirm the behavior expected of arteriosclerosis obliterans, the most common cause of claudication, whereas deviations from the usual patterns can suggest other or even specific disease mechanisms. Claudication caused by atherosclerosis may first be experienced with random extremes of activity, such as hunting, hiking, or running. This is often established retrospectively by careful questioning when the patients present a year or two later with symptoms now part of their daily life. The limitation and the extent of involvement progress slowly over several years, and many patients report stability of their symptoms for five or more years [2]. A more rapid progression usually indicates operative risk factors such as diabetes mellitus, cigarette smoking, or inadequately controlled hypertension. Abrupt decreases in claudication distance are explained by thrombosis in situ of occlusive or aneurysmal disease and, on occasion, by embolism from those sources or the heart. Such events can be silent or overlooked by the patient and may occur during hospitalization for other illnesses. Patients may report further limitation on resuming usual walking patterns after a period of reduced activity (such as weather or illness might induce) but then gradually improve to their usual performance level. This is explained by deconditioning.

Several specific problems underscore the value of establishing during the interview the mode of onset and the tempo of claudication. Abrupt branch-vessel deficit is a hallmark of acute dissection, which is manifest by pulse deficits, claudication, and, often, varying degrees of ischemia when limb vessels are involved. Dissection occurs primarily in the thoracic aorta and rarely in the abdominal aorta or limb vessels, and it may be induced by arterial instrumentation. Thoracic dissection is usually diagnosed

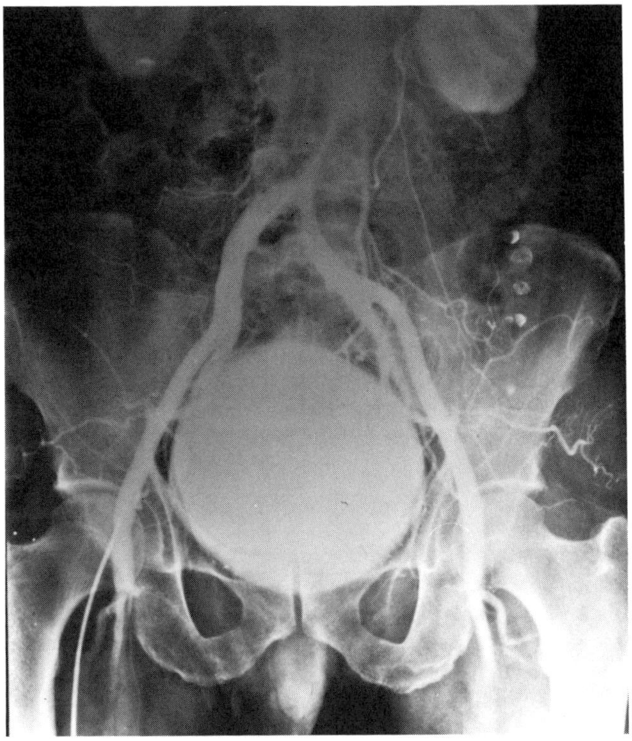

A

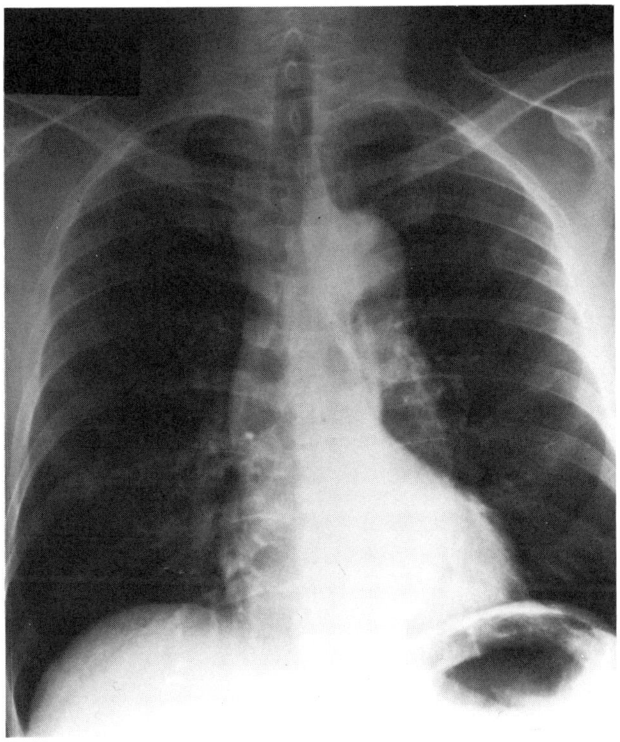

B

Fig. 18-1. **A.** Translumbar arteriogram of 54-year-old male with buttock, thigh, and calf claudication, found after recovery from a major episode of chest pain three months earlier, diagnosed as pericarditis. Note compression of distal aorta by false lumen of dissection of descending aorta. **B.** Chest x-ray taken when patient was assessed for claudication. Note aneurysmal descending thoracic aorta at aortic knob.

readily by its catastrophic clinical and radiologic features, but on occasion claudication is the first clue when the process has been obscured by unconsciousness, overlooked (Fig. 18-1), or silent. The overuse of ergot, usually by rectal suppository for migraine, can induce arterial insufficiency in any or all limbs. Of note, the syndrome evolves over only a few hours or days. Depending on the dose, the episodes manifest as claudication, which may be progressive in its severity and distribution, or even ischemia and gangrene. On occasion, attacks of claudication or ischemia are intermittent and relate to the periodicity of the migraine attack and its treatment [3]. Thromboangiitis obliterans (Buerger's disease), second only to atherosclerosis as a cause of claudication in youthful patients, characteristically begins distally in the feet or hands. Its tempo is an additional useful diagnostic feature. Both the cephalad progression of involvement and the severity of the claudication and ischemia evolve over only a few years [4]. Limiting claudication and pulse deficits may develop within a 6- to 12-week period in both temporal and Takayasu's arteritis. Tissue ischemia is rare. Arm vessels are involved more frequently than those of the legs, and bilaterality is common. Indeed, development of simultaneous bilateral arm or leg claudication (and on occasion of all four limbs) over a few weeks' time is pathognomonic of temporal arteritis in patients beyond age 50. Significant anemia can unmask asymptomatic, underlying occlusive disease and cause transient periods of claudication (and angina pectoris) that clears as the anemia is corrected.

A broad array of diseases and mechanisms can cause claudication (Table 18-1). The clinical profiles are detailed in subsequent chapters. Both acute arterial occlusion and atherosclerotic occlusive disease are frequent in active medical and surgical practice. Knowledge of their usual behavior and variations is the best preparation for recognizing less common or rare disorders. The value of the general principles of interrogation outlined above is apparent on a brief review of Table 18-1. Many of the diagnoses are suggested by historic events, such as acute arterial occlusion, radiation therapy, instrumentation, or ergot use. Some are suggested by age (thromboangiitis obliterans, temporal and Takayasu's arteritis, popliteal-artery entrapment) or by the disease tempo. Ancillary physical findings establish the diagnosis of a few (coarctation of the aorta, pseudoxanthoma elasticum, neurofibromatosis), and some diagnoses are defined only by laboratory testing (retroperitoneal fibrosis, primary arterial tumor, anemia).

Variants of Claudication. Two well-defined entities may generate a quandary for the physician assessing the pa-

Table 18-1. Processes that cause claudication

Acute arterial occlusion
Thrombosis
Embolism
Trauma
Limb-vessel dissection
Atherosclerosis (arteriosclerosis obliterans)
Thromboangiitis obliterans
Arterial fibrodysplasia
Occluded limb aneurysms
Thoracic outlet syndrome
Radiation fibrosis
Retroperitoneal fibrosis
Popliteal-artery entrapment
Adventitial cystic disease (popliteal or femoral)
Aortic coarctation
Thoracic
Abdominal
Temporal arteritis
Takayasu's arteritis
Pseudoxanthoma elasticum
Primary arterial tumor
Ergot toxicity
Iliac endofibrosis of athletes

tient with leg distress induced by exertion. In the first entity, often called **vasospastic claudication,** the patient provides a history for claudication from aortoiliac or femoropopliteal occlusive disease, yet on examination, all vessels are fully pulsatile and no bruits are present. Such a patient should ascend the examining table step repetitively until the symptoms are reproduced (usually fewer than 50 ascents are required) and then be promptly reexamined. Pedal pulses are now absent, bruits are present over the stenotic arteries, and the feet often are pale. Both the symptoms and the findings clear with a few minutes of rest. The syndrome is even better defined by observing the symptoms during treadmill testing; resting pressures and indices are normal, drop with exercise, and then recover. This perplexing phenomenon was originally ascribed to vasospasm [5], but it is the result of fixed occlusive disease, which angiography confirms. In explanation, the stenosis is subcritical at rest, but with exercise, increased blood flow to dilated muscular beds just distal to the stenosis deprives downstream vessels of pressure and flow [6]. Atherosclerosis is the usual etiology. Popliteal entrapment syndrome, in which the artery passes through the medial head of the gastrocnemius muscle or is compressed by other anomalous muscles or ligaments, can also yield a negative examination in the face of a positive history in its early phase. Disappearance of pedal pulses with passive dorsiflexion or active plantar flexion of the foot against resistance is a useful screening test. Treadmill testing confirms the reduction of pressure with exercise, and angiography defines the diagnosis [7]. (For the sake of clarity, it should be noted that the spasm induced by ergot toxicity causes a fixed lesion, demonstrable on arteriography, that clears over days as the drug is eliminated from the body.)

Pseudoclaudication is the second problematic variant of claudication. It may be of neurogenic or muscular origin. In neurogenic claudication, the history is positive and the arterial exam negative. Neurologic clues may be absent or subtle at rest. The patient focuses on leg distress, usually bilateral, that is induced by exercise and clears with rest. Several historic details, however, define neurogenic pseudoclaudication. Almost always, the distress also occurs with prolonged standing or in given, fixed positions. Second, rest relief may be slow or require a specific posture. Third, the distress often has a dysthetic, numb quality in addition to pain, and the patient can complain of becoming clumsy or weak as walking progresses. A history of current or prior back distress is common. Often these historic details are not fully expressed by the patient and must be elicited. Such questions are part of the essential negatives in assessing all claudicants. Pseudoclaudication is caused by compression of the distal spinal cord or cauda equina by hypertrophic spinal stenosis and, on occasion, by protruded disk fragments or tumor [8,9]. The absence of occlusive arterial disease can be confirmed by exercise testing. When both arterial and neurogenic disease are present, observing the symptomatology and measuring arterial indices with exercise testing can help identify the dominant lesion.

Amyotrophic lateral sclerosis, the muscular dystrophies, and McArdle syndrome can produce muscular distress relieved by exercise. Examination defines these myogenic pseudoclaudicators, and the absence of arterial disease can be established by exercise testing.

Three additional entities causing limb distress with exercise warrant attention. Each has characteristic historic features differing from arterial claudication as defined and normal pulses at rest and after effort. Some patients with extensive iliocaval venous obstruction experience a congestive distress of the legs, often described as "bursting," with exercise that is relieved slowly by standing but more rapidly by lying with the legs elevated. Signs of venous obstruction or incompetence are apparent on examination, and the syndrome is called **venous claudication.**

Chronic compartment syndromes occur recurrently in some young athletes after sustained, high-impact leg use. They report muscle pain, tenderness, and sometimes swelling localized to one of the four calf-muscle compartments, on occasion accompanied by local or pedal dysesthesias. Recovery is slow, often taking hours after each episode. The diagnosis is confirmed by documenting elevated compartment pressures after exercise by manometry [10].

The author has documented a patient who demonstrated spinal cord ischemia induced by walking. The patient reported ascending numbness and became progressively weaker in both legs to the point of falling after 100 feet. Absent calf and thigh strength and the disappearance of reflexes were present on examination at this point. Repair of a high-grade left common iliac stenosis eliminated the symptoms, and it is postulated that the left internal iliac artery was a critical collateral for spinal cord perfusion.

Persistent Pain. Persistent pain in the presence of occlusive arterial disease indicates chronic tissue ischemia and is of two types: rest pain and ischemic neuropathy. Pulse deficits are noted proximally when large-vessel occlusive disease is responsible, but distal pulses may be present when the ischemic process is in the acral and digital vessels or in the microcirculation, as occurs with thromboangiitis obliterans, collagen-vascular disease, various thrombosing disorders, and microembolization.

REST PAIN. With advanced perfusion deficits, the patient experiences a constant, deep, agonizing pain that usually is confined to the digits and the forefoot when the skin is intact. It may be more localized when chronic ischemia is complicated by local infarctions, ulceration, or infection, even with lesions of just a few millimeters in size. Such lesions may result from microembolization or local thrombosis, but more often they represent trauma that is superimposed on an area of borderline perfusion. A history of direct injury, a switch to new shoes, activity with increased foot use, an ingrown nail, or recent trimming of callus or toe nails often can be elicited.

Initially the pain may be present only at night, interrupting or even preventing sleep. It is characteristically ameliorated by hanging the limb dependently from the bed, sleeping in a chair, or by walking about for several minutes. The pain extends into the day with progression, although the night remains the worst time. The involved areas are very tender and sensitive to the slightest pressure of clothing, bed sheets, or touch. Examination must be accomplished with great gentleness and patience. Contractures of ankle, knee, or hip joints can ensue over a few weeks as the patient protects the limb by immobility and fixed postures. Standard dosages of anodynes often are inadequate; the pain may suppress appetite and weight; and the patient can be demoralized, if not frankly depressed.

ISCHEMIC NEUROPATHY. This distress occurs when larger areas of a limb suffer chronic ischemia, and it is less localized than rest pain. The patient describes a constant aching that may shift about, pulling or tearing sensations, and often a throbbing or burning quality of distress that involves large areas below the knee or elbow. Random jabs of severe, lancinating pain shooting up the limb often are superimposed on the chronic distress. Vasomotor phenomena of cyanosis or rubor may occur when the chronic pain exacerbates in paroxysms of several hours' duration. Like rest pain, ischemic neuropathy is more severe during the night.

ACUTE ARTERIAL OCCLUSION

Acute arterial occlusion is an abrupt event evolving over moments or a few hours and manifested by pulse deficits with varying degrees of distal ischemia. Skin and muscle changes produce the most important findings, but in advanced, prolonged ischemia, nerves, arteries, and veins in the zone of damage contribute. The triad of trauma, thrombosis in situ, and embolism, each with important subdivisions, constitutes a time-honored logic of differential diagnosis. To that should be added three exceptions: dissection of the aorta or limb arteries, severe ergot toxicity, and the low-output state. It is quite apparent from this differential diagnosis that both the limb and the overall clinical setting must be assessed to ensure proper management: both life and limb may be in jeopardy.

The historic and physical events caused by acute occlusion of a limb artery may yield a spectrum of events, depending on the site and the extent of the occlusion, the integrity of collateral flow, and the preexisting status of that vascular bed. Presentations range from a dramatic episode to simple shortening of claudication distance on a given day or perhaps just the silent loss of a pulse when a paired artery compensates for the loss of its mate, as can occur in the forearm. The patient with a major limb occlusion can complain of sudden and severe pain, abnormal or absent sensation, weakness, claudication, and pallor. Examination confirms absent pulses and, distal to that, varying degrees of coolness and pallor of the skin, tenderness and even hardening of the muscles, and reduced or absent motor and sensory power. These phenomena are often simplified into a traditional teaching aphorism: the five Ps of acute arterial occlusion—pain, pallor, paralysis, paresthesias, and pulselessness.

Further comments are pertinent to an appreciation of the scope of acute limb-vessel occlusion. At onset, the pain may be severe enough to stop the patient or even induce a fall. It may continue to intensify or ameliorate over hours as collateral flow comes into play, clots lyse, or fragmentation with distal migration occurs. The phenomenon of fragmentation also can explain the late lowering of the occlusion level sometimes seen. Conversely, clot propagation may extend the initial severity and location over a few hours or days, either gradually or in episodes. The initial pain may be modest and can disappear in hours. A significant number of patients experience only dysesthesias rather than pain at the onset; claudication is then noted on subsequent efforts. As mentioned, a change in claudication distance alone marks some events. The abruptness of onset does **not** distinguish embolic from thrombotic occlusion. With each type of occlusion, about half of patients have equally instantaneous onset; in the other half, symptom complex evolves over 3 or 4 hours [11]. Reduction in motor and sensory power reflects advanced degrees of severity and muscle tenderness, and, later, induration indicates severe ischemia. An additional, uncommon sign of advanced ischemia is superficial phlebitis in the zone of damage and, on occasion, deep venous thrombosis. The latter, of course, may also reflect prolonged bedrest or concomitant local mechanical or clotting problems.

Two findings are helpful in localizing the site of acute occlusion. First, the site is always distal to the lowest palpable pulse. Second, the level of skin pallor and, particularly, coolness gives an approximate location of the site when collateral flow is intact. The transition of skin temperature occurs in the ankle for tibioperoneal lesions, the low calf for popliteal obstruction, the high calf for superficial femoral occlusion, the midthigh for common femoral blockage, and bilaterally at the groin or lower abdomen for aortoiliac obstruction. When thrombosis in situ occurs in a limb already without limb pulses from chronic occlusive disease, the level of skin coolness becomes most useful in localizing the acute changes. It is intact collateral flow that locates the clinical findings several inches below the site of obstruction. Significantly, then, the level of coolness becomes almost identical to the site of occlusion when collateral flow also is impaired. An illustration is acute thrombosis of a popliteal aneurysm extending to the adductor hiatus that also obliterates the geniculate collateral, producing coolness at or above the patellar, rather than in the upper third of the calf, as would be expected. Another example of the importance of collateral circulation occurs in saddle embolism that occludes both superficial femoral arteries: The temperature transition (and overall ischemia) is at a higher level on one side if the profunda femoris artery also lodges some clot.

Physical Examination. The presence or absence of pulses, aneurysms, and bruits and their quantitation are the essentials of the arterial examination. Four extensions of these three basics can be required by specific clinical problems: the Allen test, exercise testing, evaluation of tissue perfusion, and the thoracic outlet maneuvers. It is a fundamental corollary, often unspoken, that the skin and general habitus of the patient are noted and the ocular fundus examined when indicated. The three basic observations should be an integral part of all general examinations, and they add less than a minute to the screening of a normal patient. These techniques are mandatory when any complaint potentially of cardiac or vascular origin is the focus of consultation, because of the comorbidity and interrelationships of the cardiac, arterial, and venous systems. A physician's confidence in these skills grows quickly when repetitive examinations are confirmed by the subsequent course or objective testing.

PULSES. The author routinely examines the following pulses: radial, ulnar, brachial, subclavian, carotid, aortic, common femoral, popliteal, posterior tibial, and dorsalis pedal. When a pulse is abnormal or absent, its course is tracked as far as local muscle or bony anatomy allows. Additional pulses, given below, are examined when indicated.

The following techniques are recommended:

1. Both patient and examiner should be in a relaxed posture.
2. Use the surface area of three or four fingers whenever possible.
3. Control and relax the nearby joint with the other hand.
4. Begin with light pressure. Increase and vary pressure for difficult examinations.
5. Avoid use of the thumb, as the examiner's own pulse is sometimes transmitted. If transmission is suspected, having an associate count out the patient's pulse at another site can clarify the problem if there is a significant difference between the examiner's rate and the patient's rate.

The most challenging pulse is the absent pulse. Often the history and ancillary findings support that it is occluded. When in doubt, Doppler signals and pressures should be assessed to establish whether the pulse is absent or just obscured.

Individual pulses are palpated as the arms, neck, trunk, and legs are sequentially examined. Bilateral vessels are compared. The **radial artery** is quite accessible, particularly when the examiner uses a second hand to relax the flexor tendons by cupping the patient's wrist or uses the handshake position to induce partial flexion. The **ulnar artery** often is obscured by a well-developed wrist, requiring good wrist relaxation by these techniques. The Allen test is frequently needed to decide if a nonpalpable ulnar artery is absent or merely obscured. The **brachial artery** is easily found in the antecubital fossa when the elbow is partially flexed and muscle groups relaxed by supporting the forearm. It can be traced cephalad to the axilla along the medial, inferior border of the biceps muscle in lean patients, when clinically useful. The **subclavian pulse** is best felt with the patient in the sitting position and by cupping three or four fingertips into the supraclavicular fossa with slowly increasing pressure. The **carotid artery** is palpated along the anterior margin of the sternocleidomastoid muscle, using three or four fingers on two overlapping areas from the clavicle to the mandibular angle to cover its length. It is prudent to examine the carotid with the patient semirecumbent when there is a history of syncope or ischemic cerebral events.

For examination of the **abdominal aorta,** the patient should be supine on a firm surface, with knees flexed and arms at sides, and encouraged to breathe to obtain good relaxation. The examiner should be standing. Begin with gentle pressure of eight fingers across the epigastrium, then gradually bring two or three fingers of each hand slowly deeper on either side of the aorta until its pulsation and dimensions are defined throughout its palpable length. Coaching the patient to relax and breathe, warning the patient that modest discomfort may be felt, and penetrating a bit further with each expiration are useful maneuvers in a difficult examination. The **common femoral artery** is palpated just below the inguinal ligament medial to the quadriceps muscle. A few centimeters of the **external iliac artery** can be felt above the inguinal ligament in lean patients. The legs should be uncrossed to avoid interference by tense muscles. When obesity obscures landmarks, these additional techniques are useful: rotate the leg laterally, move any overhanging panniculus cephalad with one hand, and, using three or four fingers, palpate in the area of the medial third or fourth of the limb mass closest to the groin with gradually increasing pressure.

The **popliteal artery** can be most challenging because of poor relaxation or obscuring obesity and musculoskeletal structures. With the patient preferably supine, the author cradles the patient's knee in both hands, inviting relaxation, and then uses eight fingers in the popliteal crevice, varying pressure according to resistance. When a pulse is not found, palpating lower for the artery, between the heads of the gastrocnemius muscle, can be helpful. The popliteal examination must be completed by palpation to the adductor hiatus by compressing the adductor muscles between two hands in search for occult aneurysmal disease (Fig. 18-2).

The **posterior tibial artery** normally is easy to identify. The examiner controls and relaxes the patient's ankle with one hand and curls three or four fingers of the other

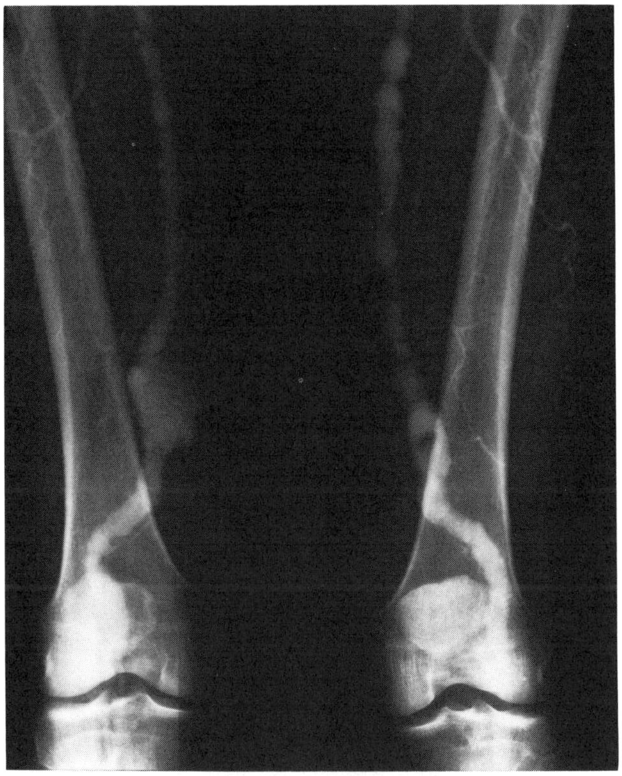

Fig. 18-2. Bilateral popliteal aneurysms discovered by palpation of the adductor muscle mass. This 61-year-old male sought opinion regarding operation for an abdominal aortic aneurysm. The popliteal lesions were overlooked in two prior vascular consultations for the abdominal aneurysm. Note the dilated, irregular superficial femoral arteries, typical of arteriomegaly.

hand about the posterior-inferior surface of the medial malleolus. The **dorsalis pedal pulse** is commonly between the tendons of the first and second toe and is best felt 2 to 3 inches below the joint crevice. It may be located more laterally, however, and is congenitally absent in 8 to 10 percent of patients [12].

ADDITIONAL PULSES. The **temporal** and **occipital arteries** warrant examination when temporal arteritis is part of the differential diagnosis. These vessels may be visibly enlarged, inflamed and tender, reduced, or absent. Rarely, the temporal artery may be involved by periarteritis nodosa or Buerger's disease [13]. Significant coarctation of the thoracic aorta induces collateral flow of such magnitude that pulsations may be felt about the **scapulae** and also along the **lower margins of ribs 3 through 9.** Similarly, complete occlusion of the juxtarenal abdominal aorta can generate collateral flow through the lower **intercostal** and the **superficial hypogastric** and **inferior epigastric arteries** that may be palpable and even visible (Fig. 18-3). On occasion, both **medial** and **lateral geniculate arteries** become palpable collaterals with long-standing popliteal artery occlusion.

Aneurysms. Arterial aneurysms are a significant cause of death and disability. Because their natural history is reasonably well defined and repair is effective, the detection of aneurysmal disease stands as a primary clinical goal and the vascular examination as a primary tool. Aneurysms of the thoracic aorta and the visceral and iliac arteries are most often diagnosed incidental to surgery or imaging. The three most common lesions, however, those of the abdominal aorta and popliteal and femoral arteries, are usually accessible to sound clinical examination. Aneurysms tend to be multiple, and additional lesions can be found during the initial assessment or later in the patient's life. Up to half of femoral and popliteal aneurysms are bilateral. Aneurysmal disease should be sought in the presence of ectasia or aneurysm of any other artery or when arteriomegaly is found, and it is intrinsic to the differential diagnosis of acute arterial occlusion, microembolism, and secondary livedo reticularis (Fig. 18-4). It should be considered when there is a long history of significant cigarette smoking or hypertension or a family history of aneurysmal disease.

Arterial size and the vigor of pulsation vary with patient stature and conditioning. For a given patient, all pulses are quite similar in magnitude, with the exception of the dorsalis pedal and ulnar arteries, which can be less prominent. When a pulse is slightly larger or more forceful than others in an individual patient, ectasia is suspected. An arbitrary definition of an aneurysm is a focal enlargement one-and-a-half or more times larger than the usual diameter of that artery. Tortuosity, particularly of the right common carotid, abdominal aorta, or radial artery, may mimic aneurysms. Careful palpation may define the difference, but ultrasound or arteriographic studies may be required for clarification. Diagnosis of an aneurysm is made with confidence when a palpable and often visible pulsation is transmitted to the fingers on either side of an enlarged vessel. Seroma surrounding an arterial graft creates a mass that violates that rule; the tense fluid may transmit bilateral pulsation from a normal prosthesis coursing through it. If pulsation is consistently found on only one side of a mass, the findings represent a mass plus a transmitted pulse. Lesions near the abdominal aorta that can produce this phenomenon include horseshoe kidney, mesenteric and pancreatic cysts, and retroperitoneal tumor. Primary arterial tumors such as hemangioendothelioma or sarcoma also may be pulsatile. The firm and often irregular surface of such lesions helps distinguish them from a true aneurysm. Thyroid cancer and hypernephroma can produce pulsatile metastases that suggest aneurysm. Their location in soft tissue or bone is a useful differential feature.

The examination techniques described in earlier paragraphs identify 70 to 80 percent of operated **abdominal aortic aneurysms.** The lesion may be noted at the umbilicus, below the xiphoid, and often fills the entire area. Most abdominal aortic aneurysms center to the left of the midline, but aortic tortuosity on occasion swings the mass right of midline. Pulsation below the normal position of the umbilicus may represent overlap of a large aneurysm but more often suggests extension of the process into the common iliac arteries. Palpation should always begin gently, but rather firm pressure may be needed to define

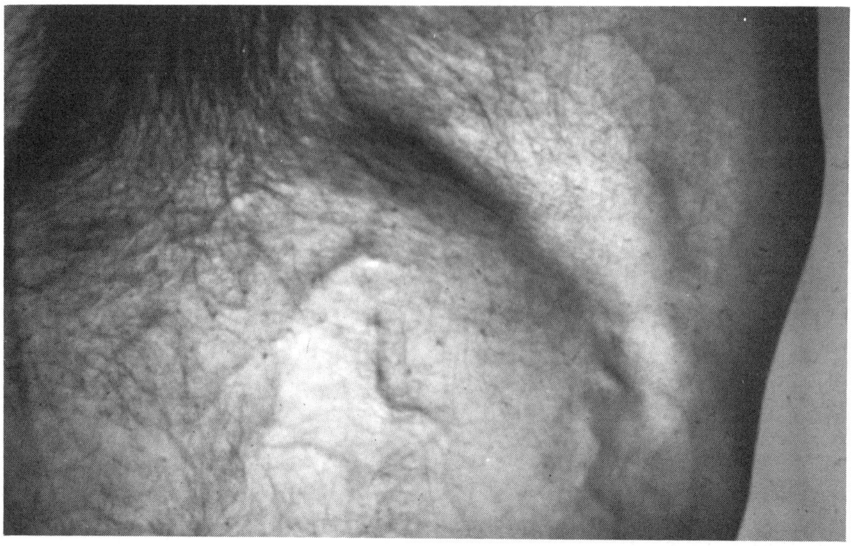

A

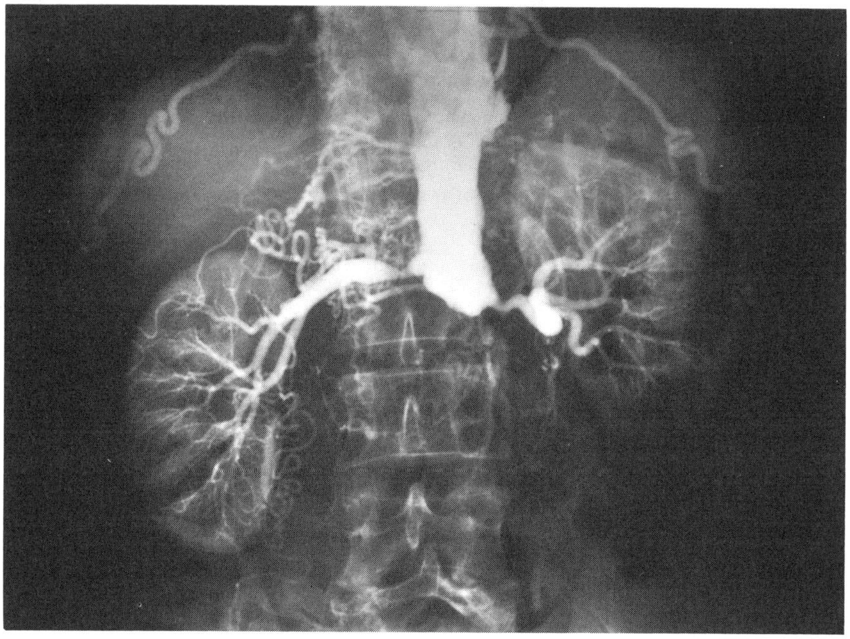

B

Fig. 18-3. **A.** Pulsatile superficial epigastric artery right lower quadrant. This 42-year-old male, seen in consultation for hypertension, presented to gastrointestinal service with abdominal pain; these vessels were initially viewed as venous collaterals. Final diagnoses: renovascular hypertension, abdominal angina, and claudication. **B.** Retrograde brachial arteriogram. Note juxtarenal aortic occlusion, absence of all mesenteric vessels, bilateral renal artery stenosis, and enlarged lower intercostal arteries that contribute to collateral circulation to the legs.

the lateral margins. When the abdominal aorta is routinely examined on all patients, the examiner can develop an appreciation of aneurysmal size and identify lesions as small as 3 or 4 cm in diameter in lean patients. Slight patient discomfort is not uncommon, but significant tenderness should suggest recent expansion, contained rupture, or an inflammatory aneurysm. In answer to a common question, the author is unaware of rupture during examination of any of several thousand abdominal aortic aneurysms seen in over four decades in his institution. Of note, a solitary instance of rupture of an isolated iliac aneurysm during digital examination of the rectum has been experienced. The patient survived repair.

Femoral and **popliteal aneurysms** yield readily to the examination methods described. Patients are often first to note a femoral aneurysm while bathing. In contrast,

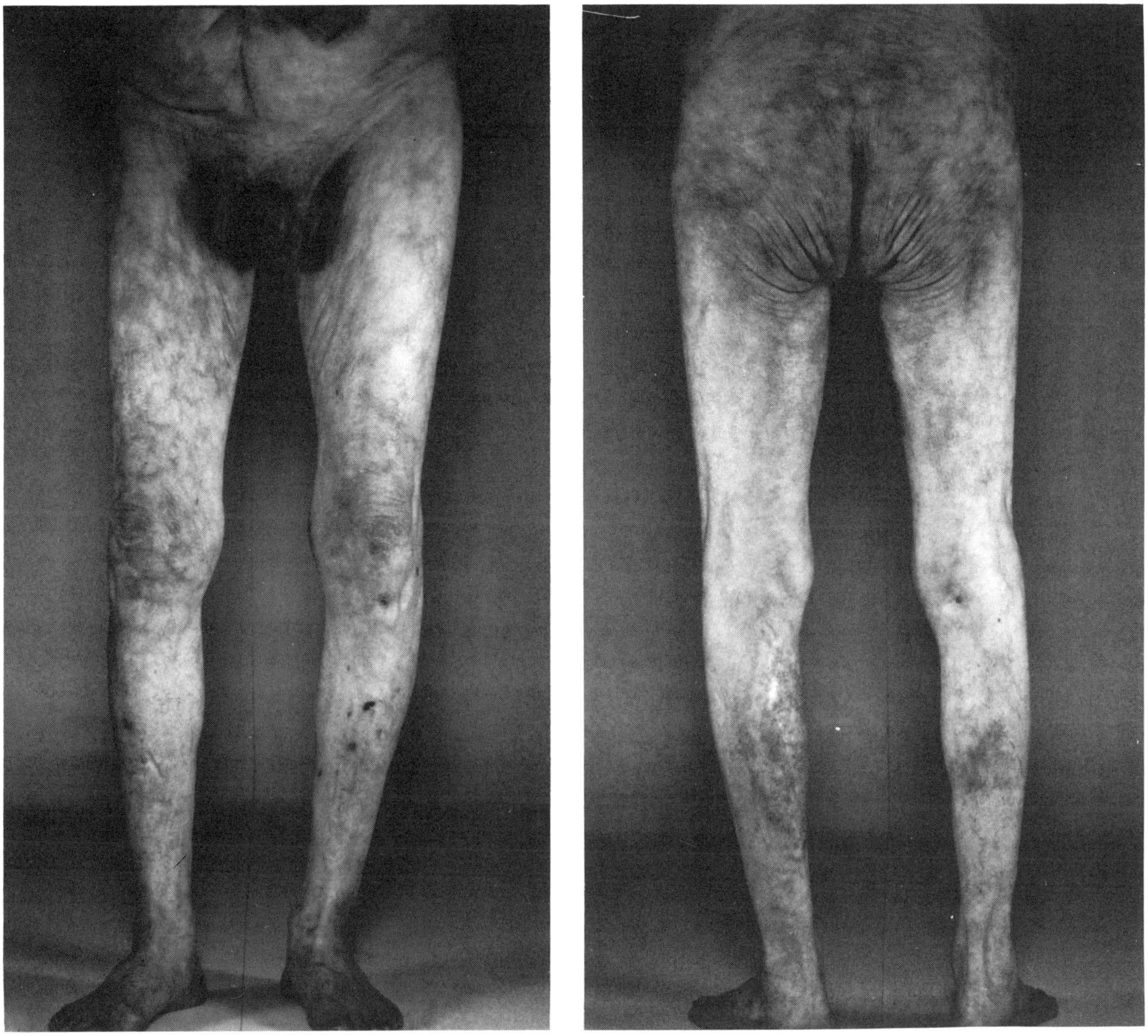

A B

Fig. 18-4. **A.** This 63-year-old male presented with ischemic rest pain of all toes. Note cyanotic forefeet and secondary livedo reticularis to level of waist. An abdominal aortic aneurysm was found by palpation. **B.** Posterior view. The aneurysm was resected, the toes healed slowly, and patient survived an additional 21 years.

popliteal aneurysms are easily overlooked by the patient and indeed by the physician when the latter accepts full pedal pulses as indirect proof of popliteal patency. The popliteal artery must be deliberately examined to avoid that error, both at the joint crevice and in its course cephalad to the adductor hiatus, where the medial muscle mass can obscure a significant aneurysm, as previously emphasized (see Fig. 18-2). Popliteal and femoral aneurysms embolize, producing additional findings. Macroemboli can occlude distal pulses and produce ischemic changes. Microembolization may also occur and is manifest by cyanotic or infarcted digits and forefoot skin and scattered punctate cutaneous lesions (Fig. 18-5). Further, both aneurysms often compress the adjacent vein, causing distal edema and increased venous pattern. Secondary venous thrombosis may occur. Larger aneurysms may also cause femoral or popliteal neuropathy by compression. Rupture of those aneurysms is rare but is most apparent from the painful hematoma, which often has overlying ecchymosis that can gravitate distally over subsequent days [14,15].

The majority of **thoracic aortic aneurysms** are discovered by imaging. When such studies are not common for a given patient or population, signs and symptoms introduce the diagnosis. The lesions can cause pain from expansion or rupture and cough, dysphagia, hemoptysis, and dysphonia by compression of nearby mediastinal

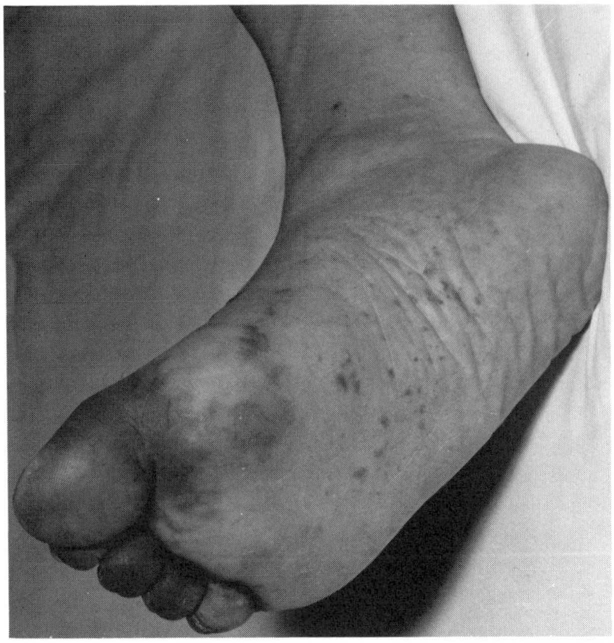

Fig. 18-5. Cyanotic forefoot and scattered cutaneous infarcts caused by embolic shower from a popliteal aneurysm. Amputation was required. Contralateral popliteal aneurysm repaired with saphenous vein bypass graft.

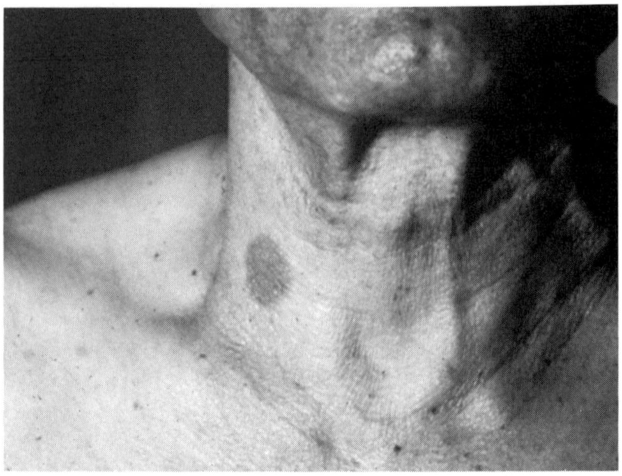

Fig. 18-6. Unilateral jugular venous distention. This is caused most often by osseous deformity or postural changes in the elderly. Other causes include primary and secondary mediastinal and thoracic tumors. This 67-year-old male had an asymptomatic aneurysm of the high descending thoracic aorta, which was resected.

structures. Physical findings divide into three groups: dysfunction of the aortic valve, effects of the aneurysmal mass, and effects of rupture. Aortic-valve stenosis can cause significant poststenotic aneurysm formation. Aortic valve incompetence, with its multiple signs and symptoms, occurs when cystic medial disease or healed dissection of the ascending aorta dilates the aortic ring. Early signs of compression include cough, hemoptysis, dysphonia, and elevation of the jugular venous pressure. Right, left, or bilateral jugular venous distention can correlate with ascending, arch, or high descending thoracic aneurysm (Fig. 18-6). Particularly large aneurysms may produce a palpable or even visible precordial heave, and massive lesions can erode the sternum and be dramatically visible under the skin. Rupture of the ascending aorta within the pericardial sac causes the ominous findings of pericardial tamponade. The features of hemothorax, either unilateral or bilateral, can occur with leakage or rupture of any thoracic aneurysm.

Extension of an abdominal aortic aneurysm into the **iliac arteries** occurs in one-third or more of instances. Isolated aneurysms of the common, the external, and, rarely, the internal iliac arteries are usually diagnosed incidental to imaging procedures, during unrelated surgery, or at the time of laparotomy for intra-abdominal hemorrhage. Fewer than one-fifth are detected by examination of the lower abdomen or are suggested from pulsatility noted during digital examination of the rectum or pelvis. It is fortunate that this occult aneurysm is uncommon, because rupture is its most common complication [16].

Aneurysms of the **carotid, subclavian,** and **axillary arteries** are easily appreciated when those areas are palpated during the examination routine. Atherosclerosis and trauma are the usual causes. Type IV Ehlers-Danlos syndrome should be remembered when multiple, often bilateral, and bizarre aneurysms involve these vessels. Thoracic outlet syndromes, chiefly those associated with skeletal deformities or cervical ribs, commonly have dilation found in the supraclavicular space or just below the clavicle. Complications of large-vessel or digital embolization already may be present when the lesion is detected. Aneurysms of the muscular portions of the **limbs, scalp, hands,** and **feet** are random events, and almost all are the result of trauma, procedures, or infected emboli. On rare occasions, periarteritis nodosa produces small aneurysms of the **limb, skin,** or **temporal arteries.** Large arteriovenous fistulas can cause aneurysmal dilation of either or both the involved artery and vein.

Bruits. The term **bruit** (from the French *braire,* to bray, to roar) is used in the United States to label sounds heard from blood vessels, which are usually silent. By convention, the term **murmur** is confined to prolonged, abnormal sounds produced by the heart. Bruits are caused by turbulent flow in arteries or veins and can be induced by stenosis or extrinsic compression, aneurysms, and hyperdynamic flow. In most instances, a bruit heard over an aneurysm represents stenosis in that or a nearby artery. The proximal limit of a bruit closely localizes the lesion. The sound usually transmits for an additional 4 to 6 cm downstream from its origin and often as much as 15 or 20 cm in vessels with high flow, such as the abdominal aorta and the common carotid artery. The turbulence that causes some bruits is such that it may be palpable as a thrill over the site of origin.

Both the pitch and the duration of a bruit are useful and warrant description. Coarse, low-pitched bruits are common to larger vessels such as the aorta and the carotid and proximal limb arteries. Bruits of higher pitch are generated by smaller vessels, such as renal or mesenteric arteries, or by a high-grade stenosis of any vessel. Both the duration and the pitch of a bruit increase as a stenosis progresses but may disappear when the lesion becomes critically narrow. These observations are most useful when following a lesion over time. An early stenosis may be silent, only to generate a bruit when flow is increased by exercise, emotion, or pharmacologic stimuli. That explains disparities noted at different times or by other examiners [17].

A bruit that rises and falls throughout all of systole and diastole and begins again, without pause, with the next cardiac cycle is called a **continuous bruit.** It is pathognomonic for arteriovenous fistula at the site of its greatest intensity. Continuous bruits heard over the parenchyma of the lung or liver usually indicate a congenital fistula, including those seen with Rendu-Osler-Weber disease. Continuous bruits may occur spontaneously in necrotic tumors and at biopsy or interventional sites. Patients may report hearing constant or continuous bruits. These come from arteriovenous fistulas of the scalp, dura, or intracranial vessels and often can be documented by auscultation of the head or ocular globe.

The examiner should be aware of three innocent bruits: jugular venous hum and supraclavicular and epigastric bruits. The venous hum is heard at the base of the neck in the supraclavicular fossa from childhood through the mid-30s in certain patients. The sound is continuous and may be rumbling, swishing, coarse, or whistling. It is most often noted with the patient sitting, can disappear or intensify with rotation or tilt of the head, and commonly disappears with the Valsalva maneuver or when the patient is supine. It is best diagnosed by occluding the cephalad jugular vein with gentle pressure, which completely eliminates the sound and proves its benign, venous origin [17]. The innocent supraclavicular bruit is heard in the same age range. It is typically midsystolic and of low, coarse pitch, and its functional nature is demonstrated by hyperextending the shoulders backward, causing the sound to disappear [17]. Most epigastric bruits represent occlusive disease. Some are caused by compression of the celiac axis by the crus of the diaphragm. In the absence of hypertension, renal insufficiency, or intestinal symptoms, the epigastric bruit can be observed [18].

Extensions of the Arterial Examination. To perform the **Allen test,** the examiner occludes the patient's radial or ulnar artery with firm pressure by one or two fingers and instructs the patient to exsanguinate the hand by making a fist and then to relax both the hand and wrist. When the noncompressed artery is patent, the hand flushes to normal color in less than 3 seconds. When refilling is delayed, stenosis or occlusion of the noncompressed vessel is diagnosed. The maneuver is then repeated on the opposite vessel. When only part of the palm or certain digits fail to flush, occlusive disease of the palmar arch or digital vessels is confirmed. It is critical that the wrist be relaxed. Many patients hyperextend the wrist on release, and a normal artery can be compressed by tense ligamentous structures, giving a false positive test. To avoid this, the author controls the wrist with his nonexamining hand and repeats the maneuver until satisfied that the test is valid. The Allen test is quite accurate in assessing occlusive disease of the radial, ulnar, palmar, and digital arteries [19].

The **exercise test** has already been described for the patient giving a positive history but having a negative examination (vasospastic claudication). It is equally useful for the patient with a positive examination but negative history, creating the work load necessary to bring out symptoms of claudication, which some patients do not attain in their daily activities. A third application of the exercise test is to clarify and separate out observations from the patient who has several different pains or who gives an unclear history. Having the patient ascend the examining table step accomplishes a greater work load in less time than toe stands or corridor walking and avoids the delay of undressing, which the latter usually requires.

Elevation-dependency testing traditionally has been used at the bedside to assess distal perfusion of the legs. With the patient supine, both feet are elevated to 60 degrees for a minute. Pallor with the leg still supine indicates severe ischemia, and pallor before 15 seconds suggests inadequate perfusion for healing ischemic ulcers or infarction. Slow healing can be expected when pallor occurs between 30 and 45 seconds. The patient then is assisted to the upright position, and refilling of the pedal veins is timed. Normal patients fill in less than 15 seconds. Venous filling between 30 and 45 seconds supports slow healing, and values of 60 seconds or longer indicate severe ischemia. Currently, reconstructive surgery is offered when the stage of ulceration is reached. It may not be technically feasible in some instances, however, and these guidelines can be useful in deciding if conservative care is worth trying. It should be noted that venous filling times are invalidated by deep or superficial venous incompetency, and the test is not practical in edematous or obese limbs.

Compression of the neurovascular bundle at the thoracic outlet may cause distinctive clinical syndromes. A single component usually is involved, and neurogenic pain is the most frequent presentation, while arterial and venous problems each comprise fewer than 5 percent of events. Involvement of two systems, and rarely all three, may occur. Neurogenic or venous compression is caused predominantly by fibrous bands or muscles and rarely by bone. In contrast, most arterial compression results from cervical ribs or deformities of the clavicle and upper ribs.

Venous occlusion may cause intermittent episodes of edema but most often presents as an acute axillosubclavian-vein thrombosis with edema and suffusion of the arm and hands, congestive distress, and venous collaterals visible on the upper arm and pectoral area. Pulmonary embolism may occur [20]. Arterial compression is initially noted as claudication with the arms used above the shoulders. Later, stenosis, but more often a subtle aneurysm forms at the site of chronic compression: reduced distal pulses, enlargement of the axillosubclavian artery inferior

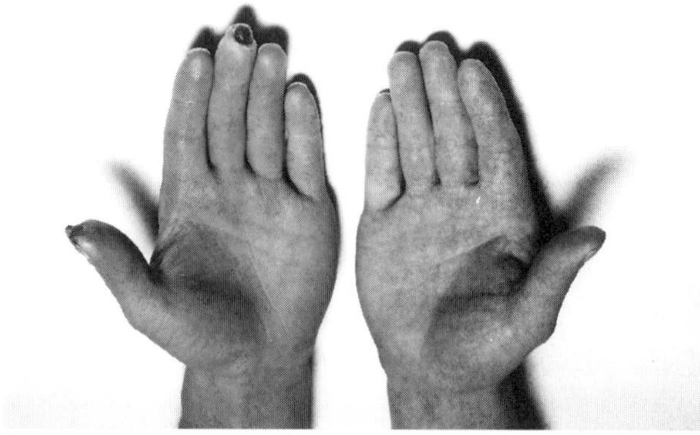

A

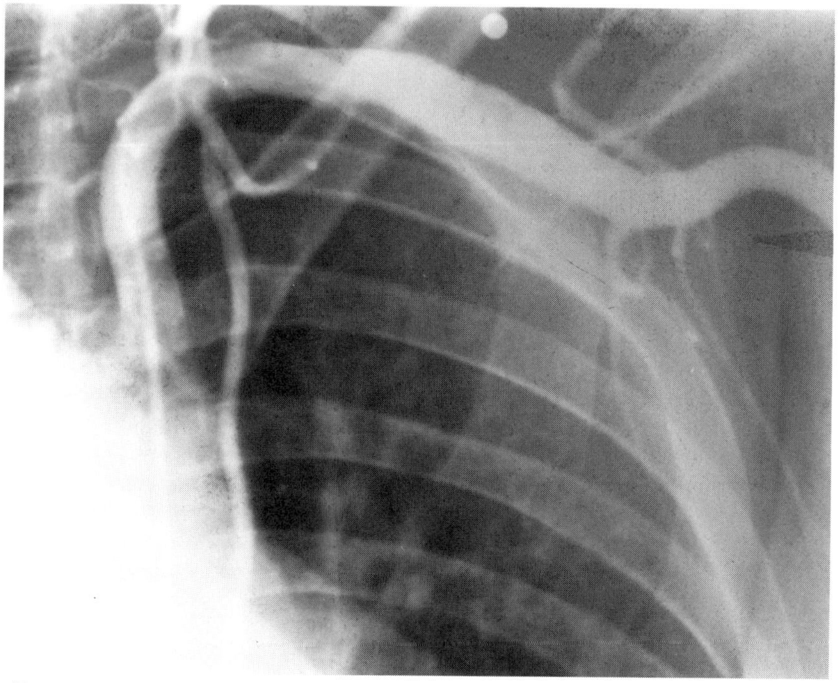

B

Fig. 18-7. **A.** A Infarcted pads digits 1 and 3, left hand, with normal right hand. Patient experienced Raynaud's phenomenon on left fingers 2 to 5 on cold exposure for 4 years, and the finger ulcers developed following minor trauma just prior to examination. **B.** Arch aortogram of the same patient. Dilation of axillary artery distal to the clavicle with a small area of clot just visible on the upper border of the aneurysm. This area was a small ulceration with thrombus formation when seen at surgery.

to the clavicle, and a cervical rib may be appreciated by palpation. Acute occlusions are late events, often first bringing the patient to care. This may be thrombosis at the site of compression, macroembolization to the brachial and distal vessels, or microembolization to the digits and skin, manifest as pallor, cyanosis, infarction, nail bed splinters, or Raynaud's phenomenon [21] (Fig. 18-7). Neurogenic compression produces pain syndromes most commonly in the ulnar distribution, but compression of upper plexus nerves can cause shoulder, neck, and head pain. The differential of these syndromes is broad, electromyography usually is negative and useful predominantly in excluding other disorders, and careful clinical correlation is required to establish the diagnosis [22].

Three outlet maneuvers traditionally are described; with each, the radial pulse is monitored by palpation or continuous-wave Doppler sounds and pulse traces. Disappearance of the radial pulse is abnormal and a positive test. In the **hyperabduction maneuver,** the arm is raised from the side, in the plane of the shoulder, through an arch approaching 180 degrees and pulse disappearance recorded at the level it occurs. **Costoclavicular maneuvers** thrust both shoulders backward and downward maximally, as in a military bracing posture; this maneuver is done both actively by the patient and repeated passively by the examiner. The **Adson maneuver** asks the patient to rotate the head maximally both backward and upward, as though looking for a star over his or her shoulder, first to the right and then to the left. Each of these tests can obliterate the radial pulse in normal patients and have diagnostic significance only if symptoms are reproduced.

The **elevated arm stress test** (EAST) is the most reliable maneuver for neurogenic outlet compression. The patient elevates both elbows to 90 degrees and braces them back behind the plane of the shoulders (as if facing a hold-up), then makes fists repetitively for 3 minutes. The test correlates well with surgical relief if the patient's symptoms are reproduced. The involved hand often becomes pallid with a positive test [22].

The Skin. The skin is highly vascular because of its function as a heat exchanger. Occlusive arterial disease can alter skin temperature, color, and nutrition, and it is chiefly the skin that is damaged by occlusive digital and microcirculatory disease. Both acute and chronic occlusive disease reduce skin temperature in the zone of poor perfusion. Temperature changes are felt better by the back of the hand rather than the calloused palm, and differences as small as 1°C or 2°C can be appreciated. Comparison to the contralateral limb or more proximal skin should be made. The value of a change in temperature for localizing an acute occlusion has been discussed. Profound coolness indicates severe ischemia. Generalized coolness of all limbs may reflect poor cardiac output, hemorrhage, or shock. Chronically cool hands and feet, a common office complaint, usually reflects the patient's basic vasomotor tone. Such patients also respond more dramatically to environmental cooling or emotional stimuli, and some also demonstrate primary livedo reticularis, Raynaud's phenomenon, or acrocyanosis. Limbs damaged by neurologic disease such as polio, stroke, or paraparesis of any cause often are cooler than normal. Coolness is also common to disuse syndromes and reflex sympathetic dystrophy. Edema often accompanies those states and obscures pulses. Doppler systolic pressures establish whether the changes are secondary to vasomotor activity or occlusive disease. The color of skin varies with blood flow and, therefore, with temperature, physical activity, and emotional stimuli. Pallor is usual with marked acute ischemia or on elevation with chronic ischemia. A cyanotic hue is more common with digital and microcirculatory or vasospastic vascular disease. A red or violet coloration is characteristic of long-standing ischemia of the forefoot with rest pain. It is felt to represent chronic dilation of the arterioles in response to inadequate flow [23].

Microcirculatory and digital ischemic events may be acute or chronic. They are manifest by nailbed splinter hemorrhages, cyanosis, infarction, gangrene, and ulcer. Secondary livedo reticularis and Raynaud's phenomenon may accompany those changes. Cyanosis that blanches with pressure is to be distinguished from that which does not: the first can usually heal, the latter goes on to local tissue loss. Areas of ischemia may be single or multiple. Lesions may measure only 1 to 2 mm and be confined to a phalynx or digit, or they may involve all digits and large proximal zones of skin. These diseases can be classified into three groups: local trauma superimposed on chronic ischemia from large-vessel disease, atherothrombotic microembolism, and disease caused by systemic or hematologic disease. Atherothrombotic microemboli come almost exclusively from proximal stenotic or aneurysmal disease, rarely from the heart. The shower can be small and focal (Fig. 18-8), regional (see Fig. 18-2), or extensive (see Fig. 18-4), depending on the source and the magnitude of the lesion shedding debris. In major showers, muscle may be damaged, and parenchymal organs such as the gut and kidney may sustain lethal insult. Episodes tend to be recurrent but random and the damage cumulative.

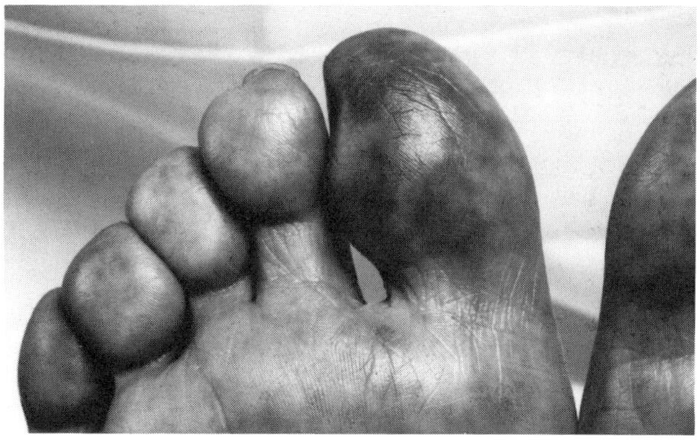

Fig. 18-8. Multiple microembolic lesions on both feet. Distal aortic stenosis repaired by endarterectomy of aortoiliac segment. The lesion was highly ulcerated. The toes had minimal sensitivity and no spontaneous pain. The right great toe healed after minor surface sloughing.

The various necrotizing vasculitides are the usual systemic diseases causing microcirculatory deficits. Some are cutaneous only, although a small number later become systemic. Hematologic causes include polycythemia vera, primary thrombocytosis, diffuse intravascular coagulopathy, cold agglutinens, heparin-induced thrombocytopenia, and cryoproteins. All digits of two or more limbs and often nearby skin commonly are damaged when a hematologic mechanism is operative.

Skin chronically deprived of blood may become thin, translucent, shiny, and red and may develop thicker callus and nails. These findings are also the result of age and various dermatologic disorders, however, and a circulatory deficit should be established by physical or laboratory examination before presuming a causal role.

The Venous System

The assessment of venous disorders often is less precise than that of arterial ones. The findings can be more subtle, owing to lower pressure, and many of the cardinal manifestations can be produced by other disease processes. Objective tests often are required; tests have varying degrees of specificity and sensitivity and must be carefully chosen to match the question being asked. In contrast to arteriography, false-positive or false-negative venograms are common, owing to the low pressures, the large quantities of contrast sometimes required, and the diluting effect of tributary veins.

Table 18-2. Possible causes of the swollen, painful calf

Deep venous thrombosis
Deep venous incompetence
Orthostatic edema
Postvascular surgery or postorthopedic surgery
Lymphedema
Acute cellulitis
Muscle or tendon tears
Ruptured Baker's cyst
Bone or soft-tissue tumor
Hematoma
Trauma
Blood dyscrasia
Popliteal space mass
Cyst
Aneurysm
Tumor

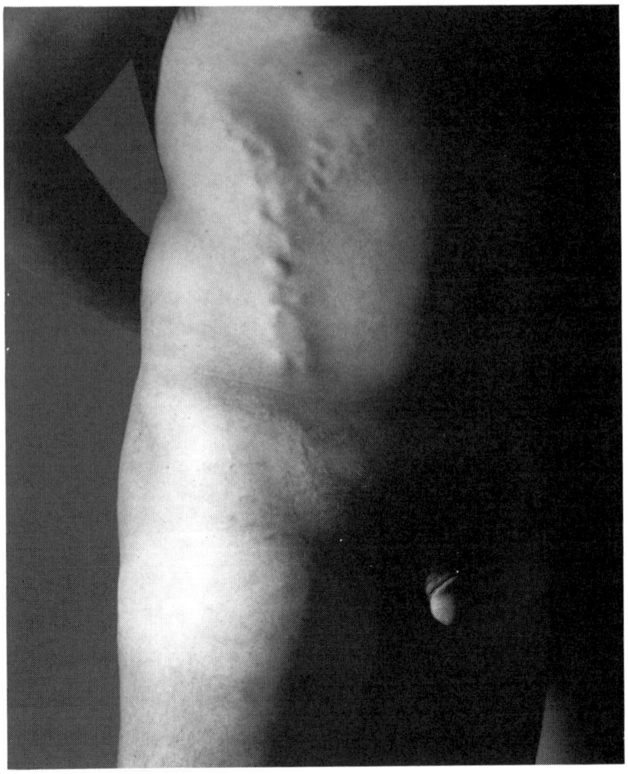

Fig. 18-9. Collateral venous flow through the superficial hypogastric-epigastric system. Inferior caval occlusion had occurred 8 years earlier as an extension of iliofemoral thrombosis following leg fracture and casting.

VARICOSE VEINS

A varicosity starts as a slight bulge in a vein at the site of an incompetent valve. Patients may be predisposed by heredity or because they use the muscle pump of their calves minimally in their daily life, with much orthostatic pressure. As the segment enlarges further, distal valves become progressively incompetent, the vein stretches further and elongates, and tortuosity occurs. Stasis changes with ulceration are a late sequela. Varicose veins may be locally tender and may itch, burn, or ache. Some very extensive varicosities are asymptomatic. Complications include stasis dermatitis, ulceration, thrombosis in situ, superficial phlebitis, and subcutaneous or, on occasion, external rupture, either spontaneous or after local trauma. Death by exsanguination is rare, occurring when the patient cannot apply the gentle pressure needed to stop bleeding because of injury, disability, or toxicity.

Varicose veins are classified as primary when there is no component of deep or perforator incompetence. Varicosities can be secondary to arteriovenous fistula, proximal compression, right heart disease, and most frequently to deep and perforator vein incompetence. The **Trendelenburg test** can be used at the bedside to differentiate deep and superficial venous incompetence. With the patient supine, the leg is elevated and the veins are emptied. A tourniquet or blood pressure cuff inflated to 60 or more mm Hg is placed around the thigh, and the patient then stands. If the varicosities begin to fill within 30 seconds, deep and perforator disease is present. If the veins do not fill, the tourniquet is released. If the veins then fill downward from above, superficial disease alone is suspected. The test is imprecise in heavy legs. Various techniques such as Doppler auscultation, duplex imaging, and exercise plethysmography are more precise in defining the problem.

SUPERFICIAL PHLEBITIS

Inflammation, induration, erythema, and tenderness along the anatomic course of a superficial vein make this diagnosis self-apparent in most instances. On occasion, a long red streak in the medial thigh must be differentiated from acute lymphangitis. The absence of systemic signs, such as fever, chills, and nausea, and of inguinal nodes suggests phlebitis as the diagnosis. Indeterminate problems can be solved using the Doppler or ultrasound scanning. On occasion, superficial phlebitis presents in the form of a round nodule. This may occur with Buerger's disease and cutaneous vasculitis, or it may be idiopathic and recurrent. A biopsy is often prudent to confirm the diagnosis. The common causes of superficial thrombophlebitis are thrombosis in a varix and an indwelling apparatus. Recurrent episodes lasting 2 to 3 weeks may occur in Buerger's disease and Behçet's disease, often as the initial manifestation, and also with vasculitis or in an idiopathic form. Superficial phlebitis can occur in the zone of ischemia with severe acute arterial occlusion. Superficial phlebitis with malignancy and primary idiopathic migrating thrombophlebitis are rare.

DEEP VENOUS THROMBOSIS

The cardinal manifestations of deep venous thrombosis of the limbs are venous hypertension, edema, and increased muscle turgidity and tenderness. All may be absent in major proximal vein thrombosis, particularly when the patient is at bedrest. In turn, many other mechanisms can cause each or all of these signs. Finally, venous compression by an adjacent mass such as aneurysm, bone tumor,

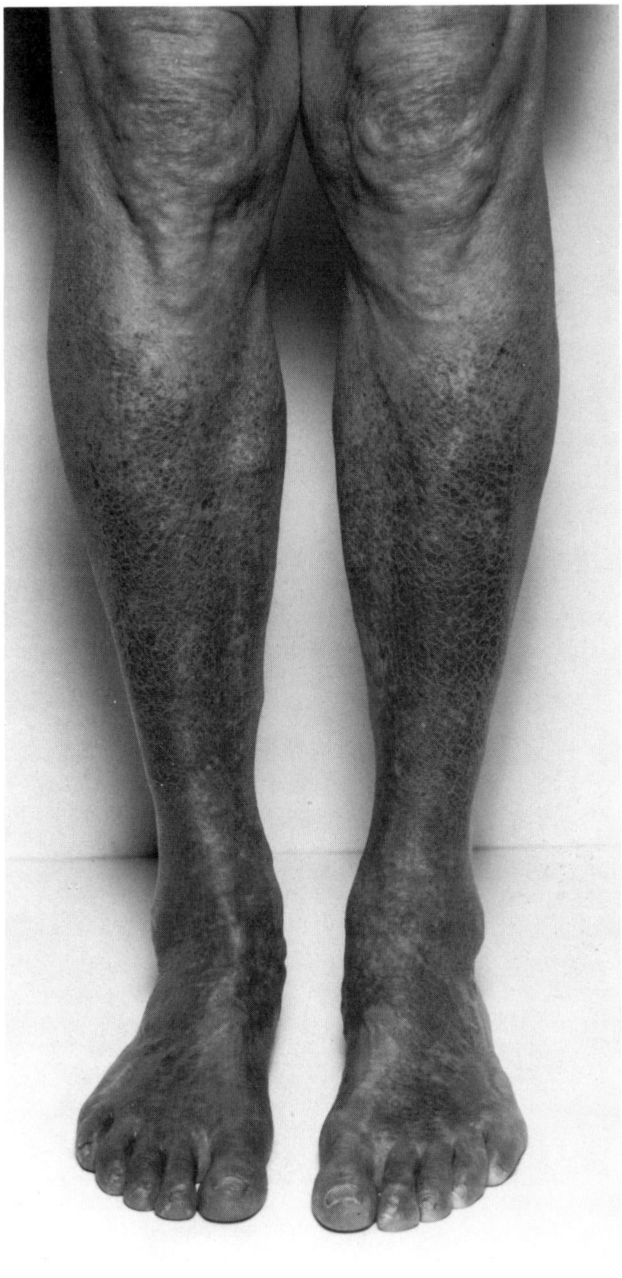

Fig. 18-10. Purpura simplex caused by 15 years of anticoagulant therapy for a cardiac prosthesis. Note pedal involvement.

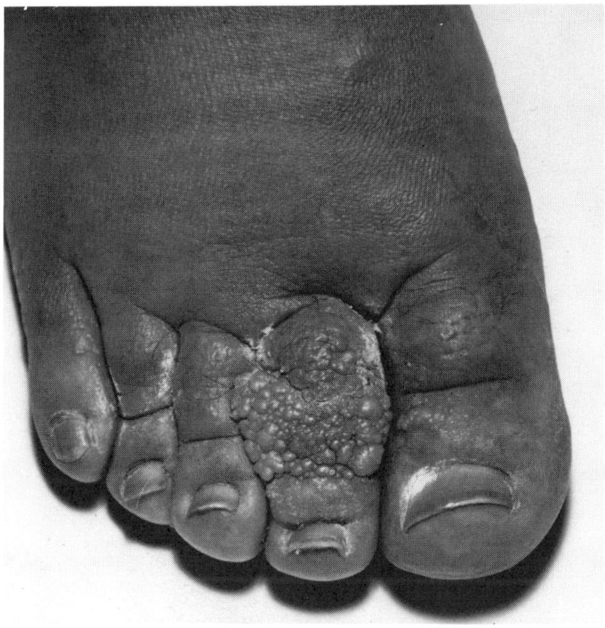

Fig. 18-11. Verucca formation on toes in patient with chronic lymphedema praecox.

or joint cyst can produce those findings without true thrombosis being present. Up to half of all patients referred to a vascular laboratory with probable deep venous thrombosis do not have the disease [24].

The examination can be enhanced in several ways. First, the leg examination should always be done with the patient standing. Lighting should be indirect, neither too bright nor too dim. Subtle degrees of edema can be appreciated with the calf and thigh contours just touching each other for comparison, and by inspecting the malleolar hollows from behind. Increased venous pattern is best appreciated with the patient standing, and then often only over bony prominences such as the tibial plateau, the knee, or the iliac crest. Both anterior-posterior and lateral compression of the involved muscle mass are preferred to the Homans' sign. This allows a more precise appreciation of pain and induration as the process is followed through to resolution. Examination of the popliteal space and the groin is necessary to localize possible compressing masses. Axillosubclavian thrombosis assessment requires bilateral thoracic outlet maneuvers and palpation of the supraclavicular space and axilla for masses. Objective testing is mandatory when there is any doubt about the diagnosis, or when the question must be settled definitively because of the risk of therapy or ancillary disease. The author uses objective tests routinely. Lesions that can create a difficult differential diagnosis are listed in Table 18-2. Clinical clues for each of those lesions yield to a careful history or examination.

CAVAL OCCLUSIVE SYNDROMES

Occlusion of the superior vena cava can be caused by gradual compression, acute thrombosis, or both. The onset may, therefore, be gradual, with increased venous pattern over the chest and neck and modest edema of the neck and face. With abrupt occlusion—a syndrome of extensive neck, face, and eye edema—protruding eye globes, distorted vision, severe headache and mental confusion, and lethargy may result. Occlusion of the inferior vena cava also can be abrupt or gradual, and the distal edema modest or massive, sometimes involving the penis and the scrotum. Collateral flow on the abdominal wall can be very subtle and apparent only in the standing position (Fig. 18-9). Portal vein occlusion develops these same collaterals, and direction of flow can help differentiate the

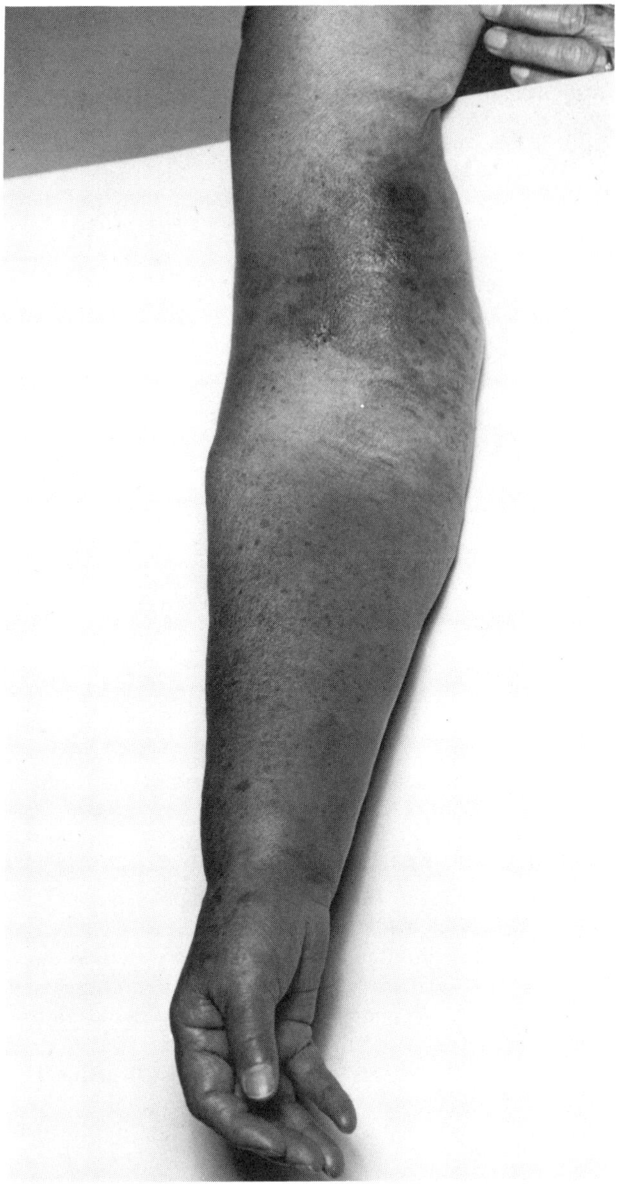

Fig. 18-12. Postmastectomy lymphedema. The upper-arm lesion is bluish red and somewhat warm. It was treated for several weeks with antibiotics as cellulitis. Biopsy confirmed an infiltrating lymphangiosarcoma.

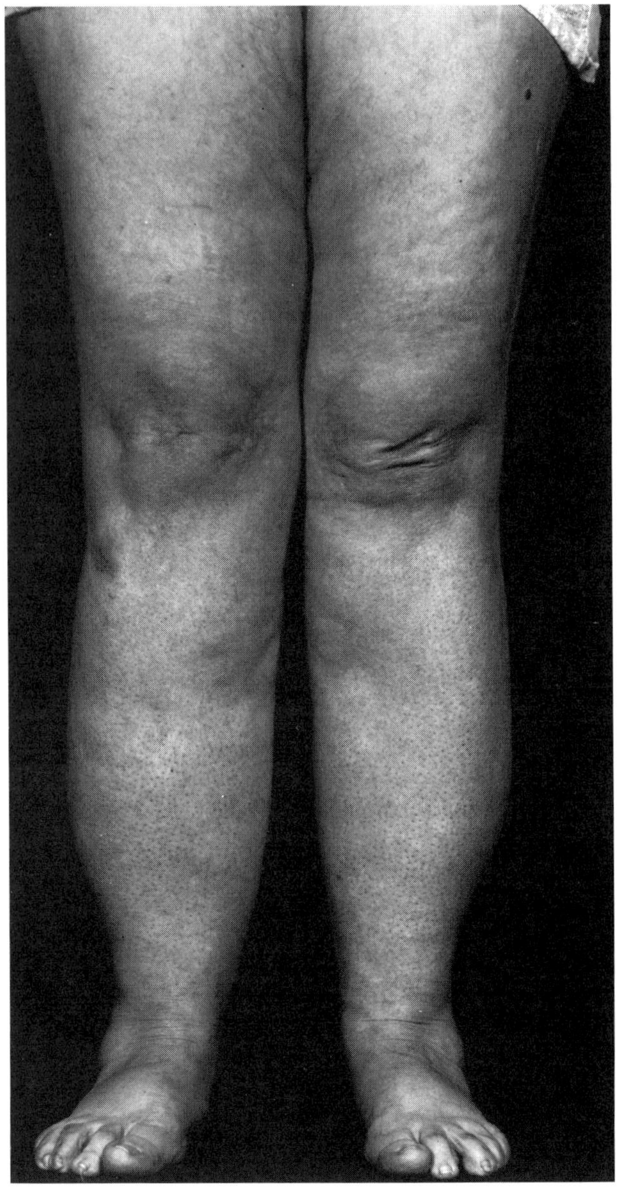

Fig. 18-13. Moderate lipedema. Note modest orthostatic edema of dorsum of foot.

two lesions: flow is caudad in portal obstruction and cephalad with inferior caval occlusion. Over 80 percent of superior caval occlusions are associated with primary or secondary malignancy of the thorax and neck. Benign causes include fibrosing mediastinitis, indwelling devices, and clotting disorders. Approximately half of inferior caval obstructions are of nonmalignant origin. Many are an extension of lower leg venous disease, and compressing aneurysms and clotting disorders are recognized etiologic mechanisms.

VENOUS INSUFFICIENCY

The physical findings of venous insufficiency are caused by an increased orthostatic column secondary to incompetent valves and, to a lesser degree, proximal obstruction, or a combination of both. This yields three major findings: venous hypertension, edema, and hemosiderin deposition in the skin. The latter two, in turn, can induce any of a varying combination of reactions, including fibrosis, sterile cellulitis, pruritus, lichenification, and, eventually, ulceration. Approximately 20 percent of venous insufficiency is secondary to primary varicose veins and the majority to disease of the deep and perforating veins. Edema tends to be less prominent in patients with superficial incompetence and the venous pattern less noticeable in patients with deep incompetence. Combinations of both diseases can exist in a given patient and alter those findings. The differential between deep venous disease with obstruction and incompetence is most accurately performed by utilizing Doppler or ultrasound imaging of the venous system. Several conditions that resemble deep venous insufficiency but that are mimics are arteriovenous shunts, disease of the right heart and tricuspid valve, purpura simplex (Fig. 18-10 on p. 411), and the early stage of Kaposi's sarcoma, which may begin as a deposition of elevated hemosiderin in the skin of the feet and ankles.

Lymphatic Disease

Diseases that affect the circulatory function of the lymphatic system of the limbs include lymphedema and acute lymphangitis and cellulitis. Acute lymphangitis and cellulitis can be classically manifested by a prodromal period of chills and fever followed by nausea and malaise, with the subsequent eruption of erythematous patches on the involved extremity 6 to 8 hours later. In some, the cutaneous findings occur without systemic symptoms. A lymphangitic streak and regional lymph nodes are seen in a small proportion of cases. The fever may reach levels as high as 104°F. Often there is a portal of entry, which is usually trichophytosis of the toe webs and feet, less commonly an extremity injury, and on occasion an upper respiratory infection. Lymphedema of the extremities is characterized by two features: increased thickness of the dermis and involvement of the hand or foot and digits in the process. Those features easily differentiate lymphedema from chronic venous edema. In the acute phase, however, venous edema can involve the foot.

Lymphedema is a bedside diagnosis and can be confirmed by lymphoscintigraphy when needed. Complications include progression, acute lymphangitis and cellulitis, verucca formation of the toes (Fig. 18-11 on p. 411), and, on rare occasion, lymphangiosarcoma (Fig. 18-12). **Lipedema** is a commonly seen, inherited tendency for abnormal fat deposition of the calves, thighs, or buttocks, and it occurs predominantly in women after puberty. No circulatory or cellular cause has been identified for this abnormal distribution of adipose tissue. It is differentiated from lymphedema and venous edema by its history and by its very symmetric distribution. A component of orthostatic edema frequently is present, with the foot involvement and improvement of the limb overnight that is typical of orthostatic edema (Fig. 18-13). Pitting edema is more common in lipedema and venous disease, but it can occur in lymphedema; therefore, it is not a criterion of diagnosis.

References

1. Joyce JW. The vascular examination: clues and correlations of various diseases. In JA Spittell, ed. Clinical Medicine, vol. 6. New York: Harper & Row, 1981.
2. Juergens JL, Barker NW, Hines EA Jr. Arteriosclerosis obliterans: review of 520 cases with special reference to pathogenic and prognostic factors. Circulation 1960; 21:188–195.
3. Maples M, et al. Arterial complications of ergotism. Amer Surgeon 1981; 5:224–227.
4. Shionoya S. Buerger's disease (thromboangiitis obliterans). In RB Rutherford, ed. Vascular Surgery. Philadelphia: Saunders, 1995. Pp. 235–244.
5. Leary WV, Allen EV. Intermittent claudication as a result of arterial spasm induced by walking. Am Heart J 1941; 22:719–725.
6. DeWeese JA. Pedal pulses disappearing with exercise. N Engl J Med 1960; 262:1214–1217.
7. Whelan TJ. Popliteal artery entrapment. In RB Rutherford, ed. Vascular Surgery. Philadelphia: Saunders, 1989. Pp. 783–791.
8. Goodreau JJ, et al. Rational approach to the differentiation of vascular and neurogenic claudication. Surgery 1978; 84: 749–757.
9. Hall S, et al. Lumbar spinal stenosis: clinical features, diagnostic procedures and results of surgical treatment in 68 patients. Ann Intern Med 1985; 103:271–275.
10. Turnipseed WD, Detmer DE, Girdley F. Chronic compartment syndrome: an unusual cause of claudication. Ann Surg 1989; 219:557–563.
11. Jacobs AL. Arterial embolism in the limbs. Edinburgh: Livingstone, 1959.
12. Barnhorst DA, Barner HB. Prevalence of congenitally absent pedal pulses. N Engl J Med 1968; 278:264–265.
13. Lie JT. Diagnostic histopathology of major systemic and pulmonary vasculitic syndromes. Rheum Dis Clin North Am 1990; 16:269–292.
14. Pappas G, et al. Femoral aneurysms: review of surgical management. JAMA 1964; 190:489–493.
15. Wychulis AR, Spittell JA Jr, Wallace RB. Popliteal aneurysms. Surgery 1970; 68:942–951.
16. McCready RA, et al. Isolated iliac artery aneurysms. Surgery 1983; 93:688–693.
17. Perloff JK. Physical Examination of the Heart and Circulation. Philadelphia: Saunders, 1982. P. 171.
18. McLoughlin MJ, Colapinto RF, Hobbs BB. Abdominal bruits: clinical and angiographic correlation. JAMA 1975; 232:1238–1242.
19. Kamienski RW, Barnes RW. Critique of the Allen test for continuity of the palmar arch assessed by Doppler ultrasound. Surg Gynec Obstet 1976; 142:861–864.
20. Machleder HI. Axillary-subclavian vein thrombosis. In RB Rutherford, ed. Vascular Surgery, Fourth Edition. Philadelphia: WB Saunders, 1995. Pp. 999–1007.
21. Kieffer E, Ruotolo C. Arterial complications of thoracic outlet compression. In RB Rutherford, ed. Vascular Surgery, Fourth Edition. Philadelphia: WB Saunders, 1995. Pp. 992–998.
22. Roos DB. Thoracic outlet nerve compression. In RB Rutherford, ed. Vascular Surgery, Third Edition. Philadelphia: WB Saunders, 1989. Pp. 858–874.
23. Strandness DE, Sumner DS. Hemodynamics for Surgeons. New York: Grune & Stratton, 1975. Pp. 278–279.
24. Barnes RW, Wu K, Hoak J. Fallibility of the clinical diagnosis of venous thrombosis. JAMA 1975; 234:605–607.

Noninvasive Vascular Testing

Mark A. Creager
Daniel H. O'Leary
Peter M. Doubilet

In patients with peripheral vascular disorders, diagnostic and therapeutic decisions are guided primarily by a careful history and physical examination. The noninvasive vascular laboratory has become an important adjunct in the evaluation of a variety of vascular diseases. Advances in technology have enabled a more thorough assessment of blood-flow disturbances and better visual resolution of diseased vessels.

This chapter reviews the principles of noninvasive vascular testing and discusses the utility of the noninvasive vascular laboratory in the diagnosis of specific vascular disorders. The techniques and application of ultrasound to detect changes in blood flow and abnormalities in vascular structure are stressed. Discussion also focuses on the various plethysmographic and blood pressure–measuring techniques used to evaluate arterial and venous occlusive disorders. The role of radionuclide tests, magnetic resonance imaging, and computed tomography as diagnostic tools for vascular disease is reviewed in subsequent chapters.

Methods of Noninvasive Vascular Testing

DOPPLER ULTRASONOGRAPHY

Ultrasonic transducers are constructed of piezoelectric materials that are capable of emitting and receiving an echo signal. When an electrical stimulus is applied, the material transmits an ultrasonic signal of a fixed frequency. When deformed by a reflected ultrasonic pressure wave, the transducer generates a voltage.

Alterations in the frequency of the reflected signal can be used to measure blood velocity. When the target is stationary relative to the scan head, the frequency of the emitted signal and that of the returning signal are identical. When a sound wave of a fixed frequency strikes a moving particle, however, the reflected signal frequency is shifted by an amount proportional to the velocity of the target. The change in the perceived frequency of an energy wave, when either the source or the receiver is moving relative to the other, is termed the **Doppler shift.** Christian Doppler first elucidated this principle in a paper titled "On the Colored Light of the Double Stars and Certain Other Stars of the Heavens," which he presented to the Royal Bohemian Society of Sciences in Prague in 1843 [1]. The Doppler principle is given by the following classic equation:

$$Df = 2VF \cos \theta / c$$

where Df is the frequency shift, V is the velocity of the target, F is the frequency of the transmitted sound, θ is the angle between the transmitted sound beam and the velocity vector, and c is the velocity of sound in tissue. The first practical proof of the validity of Doppler's theory came in 1845, when Buys Ballot, a Dutch mathematician and physicist, placed several horn players in chairs on a flat car attached to a locomotive [2]. The musicians played a constant note on their instruments, and stationary listeners noted that the pitch of the note appeared higher as the train approached and diminished as the train moved away. Doppler's theory is universal to all energy waveforms, although it was not until the twentieth century that its applicability to light as well as to sound could be validated by scientific experiment.

Review of the Doppler equation shows that it is subject to a number of variables. There is a direct relationship between the frequency of the transmitted signal and the perceived frequency shift. Increasing one increases the other. There is also a linear relationship between the velocity of the target along its axis and the perceived frequency shift. The higher the velocity, the greater the change in frequency. The Doppler shift is affected in an inverse fashion by the angle at which the ultrasound beam intersects the axis of the target. The maximum change is observed at 0 and 180 degrees to the axis of motion. As the angle of interrogation changes from 0 or 180 degrees toward the perpendicular, the detected Doppler shift decreases until, at 90 degrees, no Doppler shift should be observed. Three variables have practical importance in the choice of equipment used and on the interpretation of test results: (1) the frequency of the emitted ultrasound signal, (2) the velocity of the moving target, and (3) the angle of the intersecting ultrasound beam relative to the moving target. Altering the angle of interrogation, the frequency of the emitted signal, or the velocity of the target affects the significance of the Doppler shift detected.

Doppler instruments can be of two basic types, **continuous wave** and **pulse wave** [3,4]. Continuous-wave systems transmit constantly and require two crystals in the transducer head, one to generate an outgoing signal and one to receive the returning signal. By detecting positive or negative shifts in the returning signal, the system can determine whether the target is moving toward or away from the transducer source [5]. Systems that have this capability are termed **bidirectional.** Continuous-wave systems cannot relate the emitted signal to a phase-shifted returning signal and thus lack spatial resolution. Therefore, they cannot assign the frequency shift to a specific depth. Pulse-wave systems, conversely, transmit only brief bursts of energy [6]. Following transmission, they close down for a predetermined length of time, then open, or "gate," the ultrasound receiver. The same crystal is used to transmit and receive. It can be utilized for only one of those two functions at a time. By varying the moment when the crystal is activated to receive the returning signals, pulse-wave systems are able to sample the reflected waves from specific depths and thus offer spatial

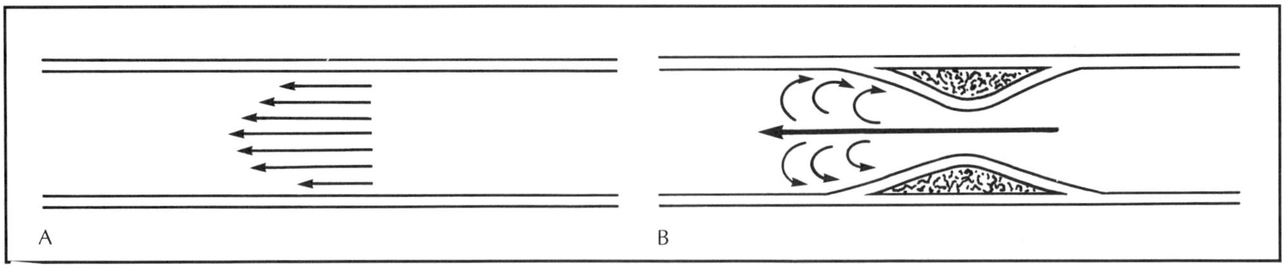

Fig. 19-1. **A.** Laminar flow in a normal vessel. The red cells moving at the center of the artery have the highest velocity, whereas those at the periphery have the lowest velocity. **B.** Turbulent flow in a stenosed vessel. Also, the velocity of the red cells increases at the point of maximum narrowing.

information when flow disturbances are present. By varying the length of time the system is gated, the size of the sample volume can be altered.

Pulsing the emitted signal does impose a limit on the maximum frequency shift that can be unambiguously identified. The Doppler shift can be sampled only once during each complete pulse cycle. Thus, the sampling frequency of the Doppler system, known as the pulse repetition frequency (PRF), defines the upper limits of detectable flow disturbance. If the sampling limit, called the Nyquist limit, is exceeded by the frequency of the returning signal, those higher-frequency signals will not be adequately sampled and will be displayed as low-frequency shifts. This phenomenon, known as **aliasing,** occurs only with pulse-wave Doppler systems and only when frequency shifts of greater than one-half the PRF are present.

DOPPLER ANALYSIS

The Doppler frequency shift is caused by numerous red cells moving at varying speeds. Accordingly, the reflected signal is made up of many single-frequency signals. Typically, emitted Doppler frequencies are in the range of 1 MHz (million cycles per second) to 10 MHz. The perceived frequency shift is between 1 kHz (thousand cycles per second) and 20 kHz and is thus within the audible range. Although experienced operators are able to obtain a great deal of useful information simply by listening to the Doppler-shifted signal, the complexity of blood flow, particularly in diseased states, requires further processing of the signal. The most widely used method of signal processing is spectrum analysis. Spectrum analysis identifies the frequencies that make up a sound and determine the intensity or power of each frequency present during the interval measured. The spectrum analyzer takes a signal and employs a mathematic calculation called a fast Fourier transform to separate the composite signal into its basic frequency components. From that, numerous clinically useful parameters can be calculated, including maximum velocity, mean velocity, end-diastolic velocity, and spectral broadening.

In normal vessels, flow is laminar [7]. The red cells moving at the center of the artery have the highest velocity, and those at the periphery have the lowest velocity. There is little difference between the speed of the fastest-moving cell and the slowest (Fig. 19-1A). The velocity of the cells varies during the cardiac cycle; the highest velocities occur at peak systole. With stenosis, two changes are apparent: The velocity of the red cells increases at the point of maximum narrowing, and turbulence is generated downstream from the point of maximal stenosis [8] (Fig. 19-1B). Spectral waveform analysis of the peak systolic frequency or velocity at the point of maximal narrowing and of the range of frequencies or velocities that occur distal to the stenosis (spectral broadening) provide a means of determining the amount of disease present (Fig. 19-2).

COLOR DOPPLER

Technologic developments now permit instantaneous color coding of Doppler-shift information within the entire field sampled by the ultrasound beam, permitting it to be superimposed on the gray-scale image [9,10]. With standard pulse-echo techniques, the examiner places the range-gated sample volume at any site in the visualized vessel to provide image and flow information simultaneously; thus, only one region can be sampled in a vessel at a time. Multiple sites must be interrogated in this fashion to ensure that the site of maximal disease is sampled.

With color Doppler, the phase or frequency-shift information contained in the returning ultrasound signal is processed in real time to form a velocity display in the direction of sampling over the entire imaging field. Doppler frequency-shift data is available for every point imaged. The information is then superimposed on the gray-scale image to provide a composite real-time display of both anatomy and flow (Plates 1 and 2). When motion is detected, it is assigned a color, typically red or blue, determined by whether the frequency shift is toward or away from the probe. Color assignment is arbitrary and can be altered, but most users assign the color red to arteries and blue to veins. With increasing Doppler frequency shifts, the hue and the intensity of the color display changes, with a progressive desaturation of the color and a shift toward white at the highest detectable velocities.

When stenosis is present, the velocity of blood flowing across a narrowed lumen is increased. That point is easily identifiable if the operator has preset the color scale with respect to an arbitrary maximum. If flow exceeds that level, either color desaturation or actual color aliasing is perceived immediately (Plate 3). Aliasing, as described earlier, refers to the artifactual folding over of a Doppler

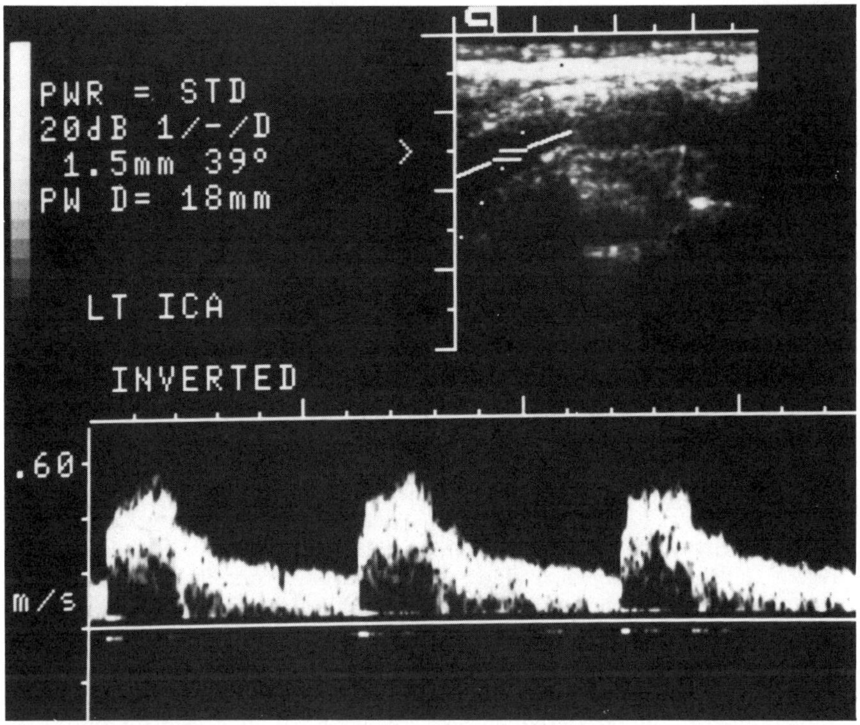

A

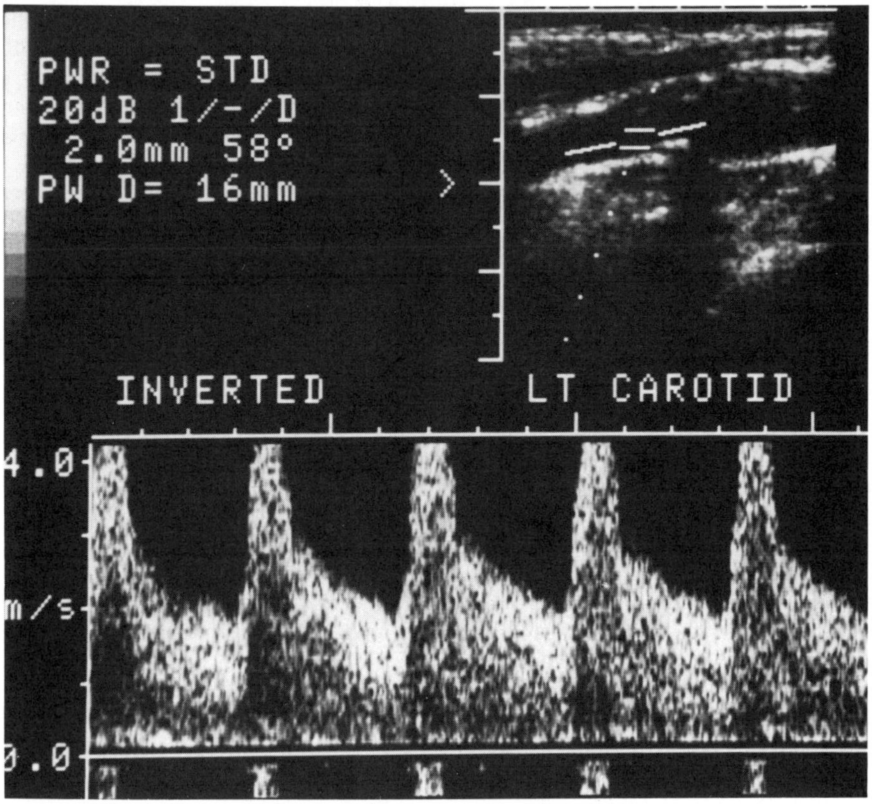

B

Fig. 19-2. **A.** Doppler velocity waveform with spectral analysis derived from a normal vessel. There is a narrow velocity envelope, since most red cells travel at a similar speed. The velocity of the cells varies during the cardiac cycle; the highest velocities occur at peak systole. **B.** Doppler velocity waveform with spectral analysis from a stenosed vessel. The peak velocity is higher than that found in a normal vessel. Turbulence creates a wide range of red-cell velocities, causing spectral broadening.

signal because of inadequate sampling rates; therefore, the color display may falsely suggest low-frequency shifts [11,12]. The perturbed blood flow can extend quite distal to the site of maximal stenosis, and it varies with the degree of stenosis. With mild stenoses, the zone of perturbation manifests itself as zones of swirling or reversed flow immediately distal to the stenosis [13]. As the severity of the narrowing increases, the zone of mildly perturbed flow progresses into a more chaotic and turbulent pattern (see Plate 3). Thus, even when an area of significant stenosis goes unrecognized, possibly because of shadowing from plaque mineralization, the presence of this pattern of chaotic flow and flow reversal downstream suggests the need for more careful study. Normal flow patterns visualized beyond zones of calcification imply absence of a significant stenosis.

There is a reasonably linear relationship between the degree of disease present and the velocity or frequency shift detected once the cross-sectional vessels are narrowed by 50 to 60 percent [14]. Color systems alias at quite low frequencies. Because color systems sample the entire field of view, they are limited in their pulse-repetition frequency and thus limited in the peak frequencies they can identify. Therefore, once the area of maximal stenosis is identified, the degree of narrowing cannot be extrapolated from the data presented in the color format. Furthermore, since color Doppler information is extracted from a large number of sample volumes, the time spent interrogating any single one of those is limited. Color Doppler systems compute the mean, rather than the maximum, velocity in each sample volume. When a zone of high mean flow is identified, however, the probability that it represents the site of maximum flow disturbance is high. Once an area of flow abnormality is identified, the color component may be turned off and the site of maximal flow disturbance interrogated using conventional range-gated Doppler techniques.

ULTRASONOGRAPHIC IMAGING

High-frequency sound waves, typically in the range of 2 to 10 MHz, are used to construct an image of the anatomy that underlies the ultrasound transducer [15]. The transducer, which generates the image, houses a piezoelectric crystal that transmits pulses of sound into the body and receives reflected sound waves. The image can be constructed because of fluctuations in the acoustic properties of tissues that the beam encounters as it travels through the body. When the beam of sound waves encounters an interface between tissues that differ in acoustic impedance or velocity or both, part of the beam is reflected back to the transducer. Each reflected sound wave corresponds to an interface at a single point in the body. Sound travels at a relatively constant velocity in soft tissues. Therefore, the site of the reflector can be determined from the direction of the wave as it left the transducer and the time elapsed between the sound beam leaving and returning to the transducer. Each returning echo is displayed as a gray dot on a video screen using a brightness mode (B-mode), in which the brightness of the dot depends on the strength of the reflected wave.

A two-dimensional image is created by sequentially transmitting waves in multiple directions in a single plane and combining the reflected echoes into a single display. The beam, directed by an internal motor or electronic circuitry, sweeps through the region of interest rapidly, yielding images at the rate of 10 to 60 per second. To the human eye, this produces a continuously changing image. Internal movements are thereby observed at the rate at which they are actually occurring, leading to the term **real-time scanning.** Real-time scanning has two features that are critical for vascular imaging. First, it allows the operator to examine multiple planes quickly, permitting a more rapid selection of the plane that optimally depicts the structure of interest. That is very helpful, for example, in obtaining a long-axis view of a blood vessel that travels obliquely through the body. Second, it allows the user to make diagnoses that depend on seeing a particular kind of internal movement. The vessel walls reflect the ultrasound beam and are easily imaged, whereas the lumen or normal vessels that contain only flowing blood appears black, or anechoic, because the blood cells are too small to generate strong reflections. Visualizing a pulsating structure may enable the examiner to distinguish a vascular structure, such as an aneurysm (or pseudoaneurysm) from a cyst or a hematoma. In view of these advantages, the older, static (non-real-time) scanners have become obsolete for vascular (and other) imaging applications.

Most real-time scanners utilize either a linear or a sector-image format. This categorization refers to the shape of the image and the direction of the individual sound waves with respect to the body. A linear-array transducer produces a rectangular image made up of a series of sound waves that emanate perpendicular to the transducer face (Fig. 19-3A). A sector scanner produces images in a "pie-slice" shape, made up of waves that emanate radially from a smaller transducer face (Fig. 19-3B). The most evident difference between the two types of scanners relates to the width of the image close to the transducer (i.e., close to the skin surface) and far from the transducer (i.e., deep into the body). A linear format gives a wider field of view in the near field than does a sector scanner, making the former generally preferable for imaging superficial structures (e.g., carotid artery, superficial femoral vein). A linear format typically (but not always) has a more restricted field of view in the far field than does a sector format. That, together with the ease of imaging between ribs with the smaller-headed sector transducer, makes sector scanning generally preferable for abdominal applications.

These general rules have important exceptions. By inserting a gap (filled with water or other homogeneous medium) between the ultrasound probe and the patient, the near field of a sector scanner can be widened considerably. A sector scanner with a water-filled gap (or water gap) can be used to image superficial structures. Other developments, such as the introduction of curved linear arrays, which are a hybrid between linear and sector scanners, further blur the distinctions between the two scanner types and their range of applications.

There are several types of sector scanners, including mechanical, electronic (phased array), and annular array [15]. A mechanical sector scanner steers the sound wave by moving the piezoelectric crystal in a rotating or oscillat-

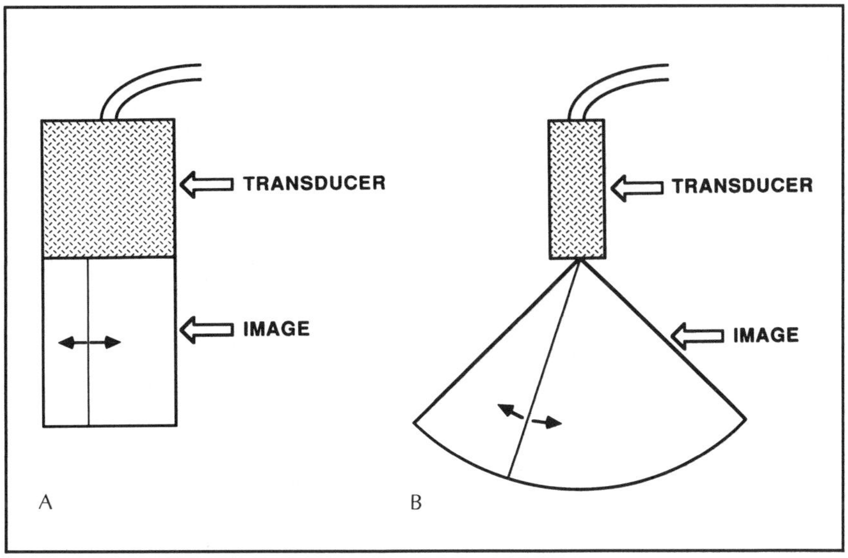

Fig. 19-3. Real-time scanning formats. **A.** In a linear array, sound waves emanate in a beam perpendicular to the broad-based linear-array transducer. Sweeping of the beam from side to side (solid arrows) generates a rectangular image. **B.** In a sector scanner, sound waves emanate radially from the transducer. Motion of the beam (solid arrows), accomplished mechanically or electronically, generates a sector-shaped image.

ing motion or via an oscillating mirror. The movement, produced by an electric motor, occurs in the housing of the transducer. A phased array produces a sector-shaped image electronically, without moving parts. The transducer contains several piezoelectric crystals arranged side by side, and the beam is steered in different directions by exciting the various crystals at slightly different times. The timing pattern determines the beam direction and allows the beam to be focused at variable depth in the scan plane. An annular-array transducer has both mechanical and electronic features. It has several ring-shaped crystals arranged concentrically, which, when fired at different times, can focus the beam in two planes, both in and perpendicular to the image plane. The beam is steered mechanically to produce a sector-shaped image. Any of these sector-scanning methods can be used to assess the abdominal vasculature. With a water gap and sufficiently high emission frequency (see "Sound Wave Frequency"), they also can be used to examine superficial vessels, such as the carotid arteries.

SOUND WAVE FREQUENCY

Every piezoelectric crystal emits sound waves at a characteristic frequency. For ultrasonographic imaging, the desired emission frequency is related to two key features of any ultrasound transducer: (1) resolution, or ability to distinguish between two closely spaced structures, and (2) penetrance, or ability to image structures deep in the body. The higher the frequency emitted by a transducer, the greater its resolution and the worse its penetrance. This trade-off between resolution and penetrance limits the diagnostically useful frequency range to 2 to 10 MHz when scanning from the skin surface. Frequencies below 2 MHz have insufficient resolution, and those above 10 MHz have inadequate penetrance. Endoluminal transducers, which can be used to scan from within blood vessels, use frequencies of 20 MHz or higher. As a general rule, it is important to use the highest-frequency transducer that can penetrate to the structure of interest. Scanning a deep structure, such as the abdominal aorta, requires a low-frequency transducer in the 2- to 5-MHz range (typically, 3.5 MHz). High-frequency transducers (5–10 MHz), on the other hand, are appropriate for superficial structures, such as the carotid artery.

PLETHYSMOGRAPHY

Plethysmographic techniques in vascular diseases are designed to measure changes in limb volume. *Plethysmos* derives from the Greek word meaning "to enlarge." By detecting changes in limb volume, these techniques can be used to measure limb blood flow as well as limb venous capacitance; therefore, they are useful in the assessment of arterial and venous disorders [16].

The fundamentals of plethysmography are best exemplified by the water plethysmograph. With this technique, the part of the limb to be examined is encased in a water-filled container. Increases or decreases in limb volume displace or are replaced by an equal amount of water. Changes in the water level can be detected by a transducer placed at the top of the water column. Thus, the change in limb volume that occurs with each pulse can be recorded and subsequently analyzed.

In 1953, Whitney introduced the **strain-gauge** plethysmograph [17]. The mercury-in-rubber strain gauge used by Whitney has been modified to a mercury-in-silastic strain gauge. This mercury-filled silicone tube is closed at both ends with copper contacts, ensuring electrical continuity with the mercury column. As the length of the strain gauge varies, the resistance of the mercury column also changes. Variation in the voltage drop across the gauge can be detected by a Wheatstone bridge, amplified, and subsequently recorded. By knowing the length of the strain gauge, one can determine limb volume (V) by the equation $V = r^2l$, where r is the radius of the limb under the strain gauge and l is the length of forearm covered by the strain gauge. Because the length remains constant, change in volume can be detected by determining the change in radius. Because $r = C/2\pi$, where C is the circumference of the limb, changes in volume can be determined by measuring changes in circumference [18]. Changes in circumference are reflected by changes in the length and therefore the resistance of the strain gauge.

Air plethysmography is based on the principle that volume change is related to pressure change in a closed system. The limb segment of interest is encased in an airtight chamber. Increases in the volume of the limb segment decrease the surrounding air volume and thereby increase the pressure in the system. The changes can be detected by a pressure transducer and graphically illustrated. Typically, the chambers are constructed of plastic. An adaptation of this technique utilizes a pneumatic cuff that is placed around the limb segment [19]. The cuff is inflated to a modest level of pressure. As the limb volume increases or decreases, the pressure inside the cuff changes accordingly. The pressure change can be transduced and graphically recorded.

Impedance plethysmography utilizes principles that relate blood volume in the limb to electrical impedance [6]. The conduction of electricity in a biologic segment is related to the volume of blood in that segment. Electrical impedance expresses the resistance to conduction and is, therefore, inversely proportional to blood volume. Resistance can be determined by applying a known current across a biologic segment while measuring the change in voltage across that segment according to Ohm's law, which states that voltage equals current times resistance. Accordingly, the impedance plethysmograph utilizes a series of electrodes placed circumferentially around the limb. A small current is passed between the electrodes, and the subsequent voltage changes are recorded. Measurement of the voltage change enables an indirect assessment of limb volume. Although this technique has been used to measure blood flow and assess pulse volume, its principal application in the noninvasive vascular lab is to test for deep-vein thrombosis.

Venous-occlusion plethysmography can be used to quantitate the rate of blood flow into most parts of the limb, including forearm, hand, finger, calf, foot, and toe (Fig. 19-4). Typically, a pneumatic cuff is placed on the limb proximal to the area of interest. The cuff is rapidly inflated to a pressure sufficient to prevent venous efflux yet allow blood flow into the limb. Changes in limb volume detected by a plethysmograph are recorded over a series of several cardiac cycles (Fig. 19-5). The cuff is then deflated, and the limb volume returns to its baseline level. Calibration of the plethysmograph enables precise definition of the volume change in the limb over a time period and thereby the quantitation of blood flow. When forearm or calf blood flow is being measured, a pneumatic cuff is placed on the wrist or ankle and inflated to suprasystolic pressure to eliminate the contribution of hand or foot blood flow to the measurements. Although water plethysmography is a very accurate method for assessing pulse volume and quantitating limb blood flow, the apparatus is bulky and somewhat difficult to use efficiently. Therefore, it is not typically used in modern noninvasive vascular labs. It has been replaced by other, more efficient techniques, such as strain-gauge or air plethysmography.

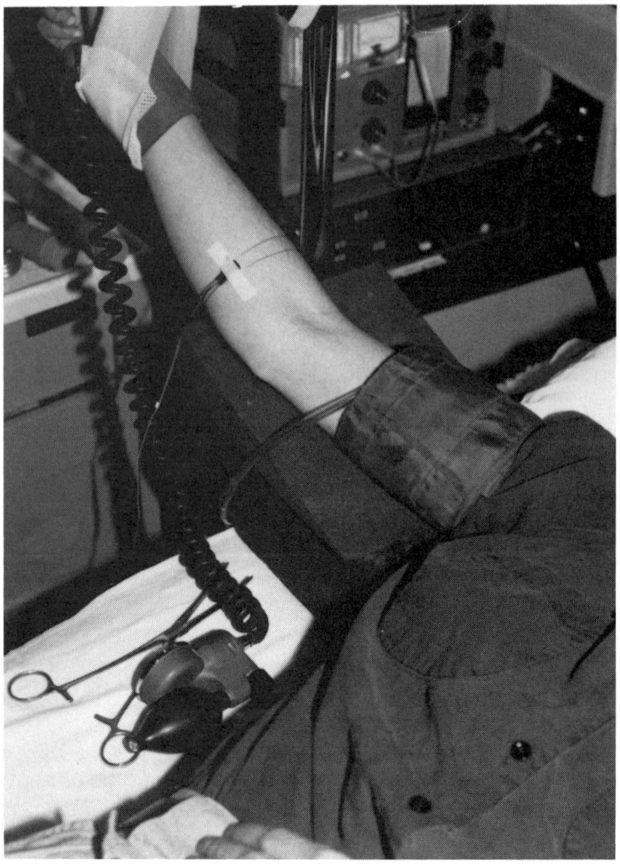

Fig. 19-4. Venous-occlusion plethysmography. The extremity is elevated above the level of the heart. A strain gauge is applied to the area of interest (in this case, the forearm). A venous-occlusion cuff is placed on the upper arm. The cuff on the wrist is inflated to suprasystolic pressure to exclude hand blood flow.

Photoplethysmography is a technique that qualitatively assesses pulse volume. The photoplethysmograph employs a light source and photosensor. The light source usually consists of incandescent lamps or light-emitting diodes that emit red or near-infrared light to reduce interference by hemoglobin. A variety of photosensors are available, including silicon solar cells, cadmium sulfide, and cadmium selenide photoresistors and phototransistors. Blood reflects and scatters light emitted from the source. As blood volume increases, there is greater dispersion of light and, therefore, less reflected light is received by the sensor. Electrical signals from the photosensor can be amplified and displayed graphically. The appearance

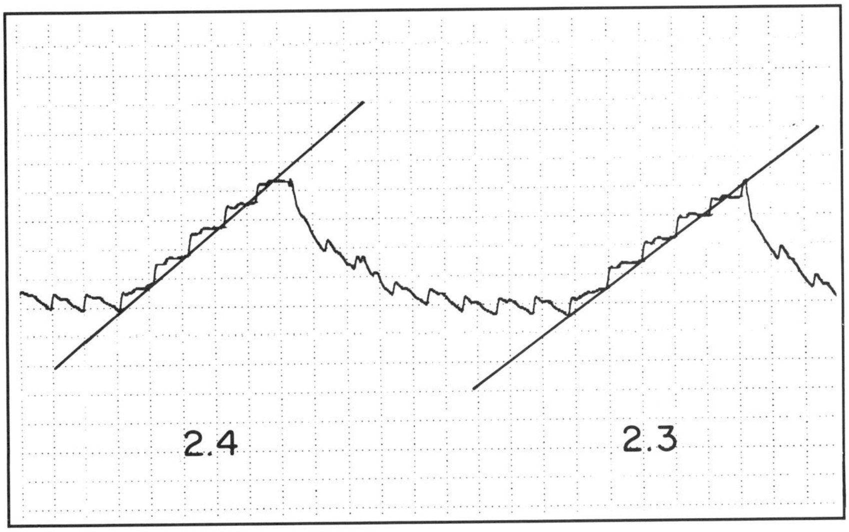

Fig. 19-5. Graphic recording obtained during venous-occlusion plethysmography. With each upper-arm cuff inflation, the forearm volume increases proportional to the rate of blood flow. Since the strain gauge is calibrated, forearm blood flow can be calculated.

of the pulse volume obtained with photoplethysmographic techniques is similar to that obtained with other plethysmographic techniques [20].

LASER DOPPLER

Another technique for assessing limb perfusion is the laser Doppler flowmeter. This instrument combines laser physics and the Doppler principle to measure the velocity of red cells in cutaneous tissues [21]. Low-powered laser light is emitted from a probe to an area of interest. When encountering blood cells, the light undergoes a shift in wave frequency not unlike that which occurs with Doppler ultrasonography. The reflected light is detected by optical fibers on the probe. The instrument is capable of calculating the red-cell velocity according to the equation

$$V = F \times \lambda$$

where V is velocity, F is the frequency shift of the light wave, and λ is the emitted wave length. As with duplex ultrasonography, laser Doppler flowmeters are capable of assessing red-cell velocity, but they are limited in their ability to quantitate volumetric flow. Furthermore, their utility is limited primarily to the skin.

DETERMINATION OF BLOOD PRESSURE

The kinetic energy for blood pressure is created by a cardiac contraction and maintained by the structural properties of the conductance and resistance vessels. Pressure energy is lost throughout the smaller vessels, arterioles, capillaries, and, ultimately, the venous system as a result of frictional forces [22]. In the larger vessels, frictional forces play a lesser role. Thus, blood pressure is maintained throughout the large and medium-size vessels. In fact, as a result of reflection of blood pressure waves, systolic pressure in the more distal vessels is higher than systolic pressure in the aorta and proximal vessels [22].

In the presence of an arterial stenosis, there is loss of pressure energy secondary to frictional forces created by the stenosis and the development of turbulence in the poststenotic area. Thus, one of the most useful tests to assess the severity of an arterial stenosis is the measurement of blood pressure proximal and distal to the lesion. An important determinant of a pressure gradient is the cross-sectional area of the stenosis. This is apparent by an examination of Poiseuille's law, which states the following:

$$Q = \frac{\pi \Delta P r^4}{8 \eta l}$$

where Q is the volume flow, ΔP is the pressure gradient, r is the vessel radius, η is viscosity, and l is the length of the vessel. Although the length of the stenosis also contributes to the pressure drop, that component has less effect on determining the pressure gradient [23]. From the equation, it is apparent that the magnitude of the pressure gradient also is proportional to the rate of blood flow in the vessel. In states of higher blood flow, there is a greater fall in blood pressure across a given stenosis. Thus, in states of high flow, such as during exercise, the pressure fall across a stenosis is likely to be higher than it was when measured under resting conditions [24]. It is also for that reason that multiple stenoses along the course of a vessel do not result in a blood pressure gradient that is simply additive from that caused by each single stenosis. As flow progressively falls subsequent to each stenosis, the pressure gradient across successive stenoses is proportionately less [25].

When measured under resting conditions, a pressure gradient usually does not develop until the cross-sectional area of the stenosed segment is at least 60 percent of the unobstructed vessel [26]. When flow is increased, as during exercise or reactive hyperemia, a pressure gradient can be detected in a stenotic lesion whose area is even less than 60 percent of the unobstructed vessel. As the cross-sectional area of the stenosis decreases further, there is a rather precipitous fall in blood pressure. With total occlusions, the pressure gradient depends on the resistance in the collateral vessels around the occlusion [27].

TECHNIQUES TO MEASURE LIMB BLOOD PRESSURE

There are multiple noninvasive techniques to measure blood pressure. These techniques include the auscultatory method, palpation, Doppler ultrasonography, plethysmography, and isotope clearance techniques. Each method utilizes blood pressure cuffs and manometers. The blood pressure cuffs are applied over the areas of interest. In the absence of an arterial stenosis in the upper extremities, the brachial artery pressure can be used as a frame of reference. Pressure cuffs placed along the legs can therefore be utilized to detect the presence of stenotic lesions sufficient to create a pressure gradient.

Since the size of the limbs varies from location to location and from individual to individual, selection of cuff size is important. The American Heart Association has recommended that the cuff size be based on limb circumference [28]. The width of the cuff bladder should be at least 40 percent of the limb circumference. The length of the cuff bladder should be enough to encircle at least 80 percent of the arm in adults. Commercially manufactured blood pressure cuffs are available for use on the upper and the lower arm, thigh, calf, and ankle. Either a mercury gravity manometer or an aneroid manometer can be aligned through tubing and control valves to the blood pressure cuffs.

The noninvasive measurement of systolic blood pressure was initiated with the development of the manometric cuff by Riva-Rocci in 1896 [29]. An occluding cuff is inflated to suprasystolic pressures. The examiner palpates a pulse distal to the occluding cuff during gradual deflation of the cuff. The pressure indicated on the manometer when the first pulse is detected is interpreted as the systolic blood pressure. Unfortunately, the utility of this rather simple technique is limited in patients with peripheral arterial occlusive disease. In those patients, pulses distal to a significant stenosis often are not palpable.

In 1905, Korotkoff described the auscultatory method for measuring systolic and diastolic blood pressure [30]. With this method, a stethoscope is placed over an artery distal to an occluding cuff. The cuff is inflated to suprasystolic pressures. As the cuff is deflated, a series of sounds are created, beginning at systolic pressure and terminating at the diastolic pressure. The first Korotkoff cuff sounds are characterized by a loud snapping. The initial appearance of these sounds denotes systole. The sounds in the second phase are softer in intensity, sounds in the third phase increase in intensity, and in the fourth phase, sounds decrease in intensity. The fifth phase is the disappearance of sounds, and it usually correlates with diastole. In patients in whom sounds are detected down to 0 mm Hg, the fourth phase of Korotkoff sounds correlates best with diastole. Although the auscultatory method is useful in measuring systolic and diastolic blood pressure over the brachial artery, its utility in detecting lower-extremity blood pressure is limited because it is frequently difficult to hear those sounds over the popliteal fossa or over the pedal arteries.

The most useful technique to measure limb systolic blood pressure involves the detection of blood velocity with Doppler instruments. (The principles of Doppler-shift flow detection are described in "Doppler Ultrasonography," earlier in this chapter.) A Doppler flow probe is placed over the blood vessel of interest distal to the occluding cuff. The cuff is inflated to suprasystolic pressure. As the cuff is deflated, systolic blood pressure is signaled by the onset of blood flow detected either acoustically or via a graphic recorder aligned to the flow probe. Since even minimal amounts of flow can be detected by a Doppler instrument, this method is particularly useful in patients with peripheral arterial occlusive disease.

As described earlier, a variety of plethysmographic techniques can be used to determine blood flow in the extremity. Water plethysmography is too tedious a technique for routine use in a clinical noninvasive vascular laboratory even though the technique has been successfully employed in the research laboratory. Strain gauges, air displacement transducers, and photoplethysmographs are devices that can be placed along the extremity to detect the appearance of pulses. As with the other techniques, an occluding cuff is inflated to suprasystolic pressures. As the cuff is deflated, flow is detected by the appearance of pulses detected by the plethysmograph and displayed on a graphic recorder. These techniques are particularly useful over the digital vessels, where it is often difficult to detect blood flow using Doppler instruments.

Noninvasive Vascular Testing for Specific Disease States

CEREBROVASCULAR DISEASE

Examination of the carotid arteries is performed using instruments that combine real-time B-mode imaging, color Doppler, and Doppler ultrasound with spectral waveform analysis. Although each modality could be interpreted independently, it is advantageous to combine independent information to improve the sensitivity, specificity, and predictability of disease severity.

Imaging devices using 7- to 10-MHz imaging transducers are currently employed to visualize the carotid artery because it lies within 3 cm of the surface of the neck. The operator images the common, internal, and external carotid arteries by moving the probe along the course of the vessels (Fig. 19-6). The common carotid artery lies parallel to the surface of the skin and ascends in the neck from a point just above the clavicle to an area slightly below the angle of the mandible, where it bifurcates into internal and external branches. Proximal to the bifurcation, a slight dilatation of the common carotid artery, representing the carotid bulb, can be seen. The upper limit of the carotid bulb is defined by the inferior tip of the flow divider, which marks the point where the external and internal carotid arteries originate. The external carotid artery usually lies anterior and slightly medial to the internal carotid artery. The external carotid is the smaller of the two, and it gives rise to branches in the neck that supply the neck and face. The internal carotid artery has

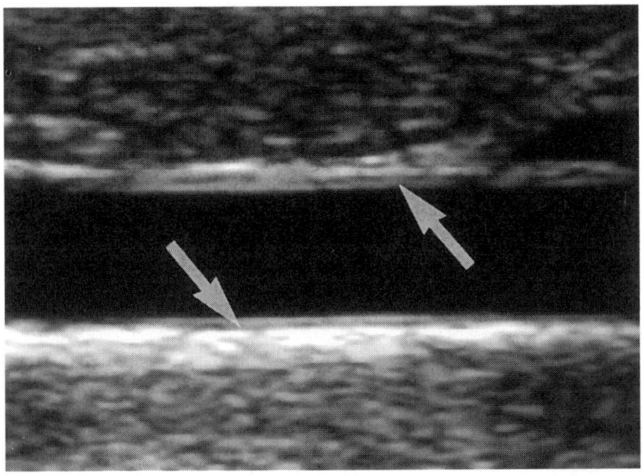

Fig. 19-6. B-mode image of normal common carotid artery. The near- and far-wall intima and adventitia boundaries appear as two parallel echogenic lines separated by a hypoechoic space (arrows).

no branches in the neck and ascends into the calvarium to supply the brain.

In practice, it can be difficult to distinguish between the internal and the external carotid artery simply by viewing the gray-scale image. Since incorrect identification of lesion location has significant clinical implications, gated-pulse Doppler ultrasound should be employed routinely to distinguish the two vessels. The internal carotid artery is a low-resistance system; the external carotid artery is a high-resistance one. Because the Doppler waveforms from each are usually quite different, Doppler ultrasound is an effective way to identify each artery. The tracing on the monitor should be observed and the auditory signal carefully examined. If the Doppler gate is in the internal carotid artery, the flow pattern is that of a low-resistance bed. The signal has a rapid upstroke and a quasi-steady flow through systole and diastole. The graphic display indicates antegrade flow above a zero baseline. It should not fall to baseline or reverse during diastole. The characteristics of the Doppler signal from the external carotid artery include forward flow with a sharp upstroke during early systole, a rapid deceleration with reversed flow in early diastole, and a return to baseline in late diastole.

The internal and external carotid arteries also can be distinguished from each other by color Doppler. The unique characteristics of the color Doppler signal from the external carotid artery consist of a rapid acceleration of flow in early systole, followed by either absence or reversal of flow during diastole. In the internal carotid artery, there is a more uniform antegrade flow pattern. Color Doppler can detect branch arteries arising from the external carotid artery, whereas the internal carotid artery has no branches in the neck.

High-resolution B-scan imaging can identify the boundaries between the different layers of the arterial wall in normal individuals. With longitudinal views of the carotid arteries, the layers appear as two parallel echogenic lines separated by a hypoechoic space (see Fig. 19-6). They usually are best observed in the common carotid artery where the vessel courses parallel to the skin surface and thus presents a target at right angles to the ultrasound beam. The first echo along the far wall is derived from the lumen-intima interface, and the second, usually brighter echo along the far wall originates from the media-adventitia interface. Between those interfaces lies the media, which appears as an anechoic zone between the lumen-intima interface and the media-adventitia interface. The adventitia is highlighted along its inner margin by the media. The periadventitia, depending on location, is composed of loose areolar tissue and, in most instances, is echolucent. The same interfaces also can be seen along the near wall. When near- and far-wall interfaces are not at right angles to the ultrasound beam, they become a more difficult target to visualize. It often is difficult to demonstrate interfaces in vessel segments that are curvilinear. In the carotid bulb, where the walls flare, only short segments of wall may be seen on any single frame. That same phenomenon may be observed in the proximal portion of the internal carotid artery, where the walls may not be parallel and, hence, suboptimally visualized. Other reasons for loss of wall interfaces are not related to scanning technique and include the presence of plaque or, possibly, the presence of fat in the arterial wall.

The earliest changes of atherosclerosis as detected by ultrasound imaging consist of wall thickening and disruption of normal wall interfaces [31–34]. Intima-media thickness increases with age and is greater in hypercholesterolemic than in normocholesterolemic individuals [34–36]. As disease progresses, focal plaque can be identified (Fig. 19-7). Progression or regression of plaque or of intima-media thickness as documented by ultrasound currently is being used as a surrogate end point in a number of studies.

Epidemiologic studies have shown that high-grade stenoses are rare in the general population but that wall thickening is not. Using that measure permits much broader characterization of risk for individuals or populations. What is not known convincingly as yet is whether the presence of increases in wall thickness beyond those predicted by age and gender may identify individuals at higher risk for coronary disease and stroke.

Attempts have been made to relate the different echo patterns of plaques with specific histologic findings and then to predict clinical outcome [37–43]. Even in the absence of significant lumen narrowing, certain categories of plaque might be responsible for a large proportion of neurologic events [44,45]. These "active" lesions are defined in terms of **plaque morphology** and **surface characteristics.** Plaques that demonstrate a uniform echogenicity across lesion width are termed homogeneous; those that do not are designated heterogeneous. Calcified plaque on the vessel wall leads to very strong reflections at the blood-mineral interface and so-called acoustic shadowing beneath the plaque, resulting from the inability of the ultrasound beam to penetrate the calcium. Plaque surface can be described as smooth, irregular, or ulcerated. It has not been determined whether such char-

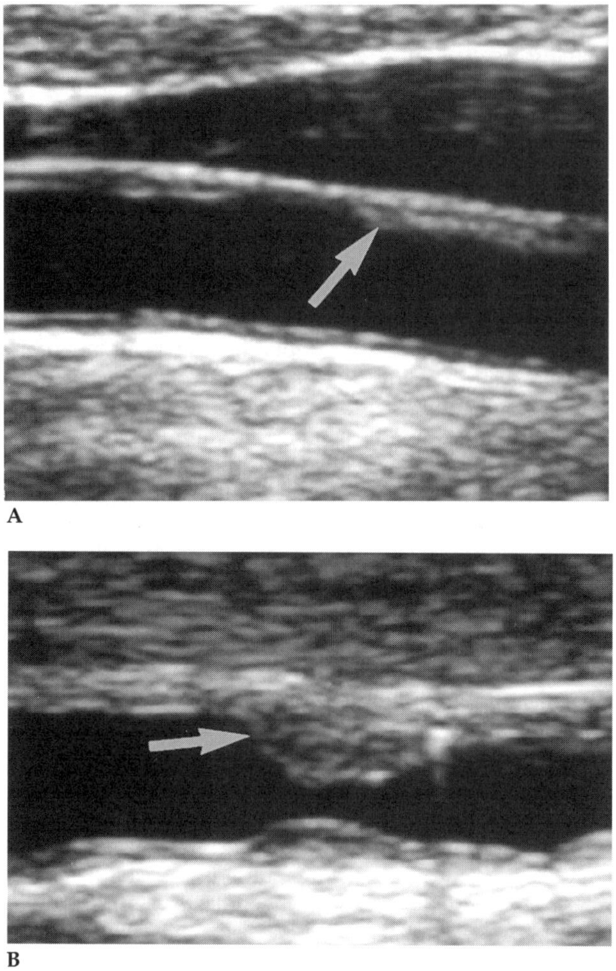

Fig. 19-7. **A.** B-mode image of a carotid artery showing mild intimal-medial thickening (arrow). **B.** B-mode image of a carotid artery showing severe intimal medial thickening (arrow).

acterizations based on ultrasound study will prove clinically useful.

Ultrasound imaging techniques are capable of delineating mild to moderate atherosclerotic plaque, whereas Doppler techniques are necessary to assess the severity of more advanced stenoses. The early atherosclerotic lesion consists of focal intimal thickening. At that stage, the Doppler velocity waveform is normal because significant hemodynamic abnormalities have not occurred. With increasing severity of disease and encroachment on the vascular lumen, laminar flow is disrupted [8], and a broader range of frequencies is encountered in the Doppler velocity waveform. Spectral broadening becomes more pronounced, although peak velocity shifts are not significantly altered until there is at least a 50-percent reduction in lumen diameter [14]. When an increase in velocity is detected, stenoses are considered hemodynamically significant. Velocity or frequency shifts increase as the severity of stenosis increases, reflecting progressive acceleration of red cells through the site of maximal narrowing (see Fig. 19-2 and Plate 2). A direct relationship exists between the amount of disease present and the Doppler shift encountered. Peak internal carotid velocities of less than 125 cm/second are considered normal in patients with normal cardiac function and stroke volume. Although atherosclerotic plaque may be present and obvious on gray-scale images, narrowing of the lumen of more than 50 percent is not likely to be present if the velocity is less than 125 cm/second. Velocities of 125 to 250 cm/second correspond to stenosis of 50 to 80 percent, and velocities exceeding 250 cm/second are found with diameter stenosis of greater than 80 percent. When flow in the carotid arteries is reduced because of diminished cardiac output, ratios of internal carotid artery to common carotid artery velocity can be used. An internal carotid artery to common carotid artery peak-velocity ratio of 2:1 would suggest a greater than 50-percent stenosis. A ratio of 3:1 would suggest narrowing of 75 percent or greater.

If an artery is occluded, no Doppler signal is obtained. It is cautioned, however, that absence of a Doppler-shift signal may be related to other phenomena, including poor placement of the sample volume, misregistration of the sample gate, or simply failure to push the correct button. In that situation, color Doppler ultrasound is quite useful in identifying total occlusion of the internal carotid artery because flow can be visually demonstrated in the external carotid artery but not in the internal carotid artery.

Carotid ultrasound has some limitations. It requires 6 to 12 months to become skilled in the technique. Most errors can be traced to lack of operator skills rather than equipment failure. The position of the internal and external carotid arteries may be reversed, causing misinterpretation of the location of the lesion. The presence of calcium may cause shadowing as well as poor vessel and lesion definition. Total occlusions may be mistaken for normal vessels and normal vessels for occlusions because thrombus can have the same echogenic properties as flowing blood. It may be impossible to distinguish pseudo-occlusion from occlusion, even when using meticulous technique. Soft plaque may be overlooked, and reverberation artifact may be mistaken for disease.

Color Doppler ultrasound avoids some of those pitfalls and also is helpful in avoiding the misdiagnosis of occlusion. Vessel tortuosity, shadowing caused by plaque mineralization, poor scanning technique, weak returning Doppler signals distal to a point of extreme stenosis—each can lead to the false-positive diagnosis of occlusion. Alternatively, with occlusion of the internal carotid artery, branching of the external carotid artery can be mistaken for the normal carotid bifurcation (see Plate 3). The last error can be reinforced if the main stem of the external carotid artery has become a significant source of collateral flow. When occlusion is not present, color Doppler ultrasound permits rapid identification of the bifurcation (see Plate 1). Once two vessels have been identified, the color image facilitates sampling of the velocity profile of vessels. In addition, the internal carotid artery can be identified higher in the neck, well away from the bifurcation. Also, color Doppler ultrasound may detect deeply placed vessels that otherwise might be overlooked. Those vessels can then be traced backward to their origin. Flow may abruptly reverse and then cease at an origin of the occluded internal carotid artery. Absence of a color Doppler flow signal in a visualized vessel can be quite striking. When occlusion is suspected, it is helpful to rotate the transducer into the short axis and advance the probe through the bifurcation with the color option activated. It may be necessary to angle the probe head slightly to obtain a good color Doppler signal. When the internal carotid artery is not occluded, the appearance of flow splitting into the internal and external carotid artery is obvious to the examiner. If the internal carotid artery is occluded, no color Doppler signal is detected in that vessel even though flow would be present in the adjacent patent external carotid artery.

TRANSCRANIAL DOPPLER

Doppler also can be used to obtain flow information from intracranial cerebral arteries. The transcranial Doppler technique was first described by Aaslid and his co-workers in 1982 to record flow velocity in basal cerebral arteries [46]. Since the thickness of the skull prevents the propagation of high-frequency ultrasound waves, lower-frequency probes, having a transmission frequency of 1–2 MHz, are employed to gain access to intracranial vessels. The most commonly utilized cranial "window" is the temporal bone. A pulse Doppler probe is placed against the skull just above the zygomatic arch, where the bone is thin. By adjusting the depth of the beam and the angle of insonation, a skilled examiner is able to identify signals from the anterior, middle, and posterior cerebral arteries. The upper portion of the vertebral arteries and basilar artery are studied by the suboccipital route. Normal systolic, diastolic, and mean velocities in the middle cerebral artery approximate 90, 45, and 60–75 cm / second, respectively [47,48]. In the posterior cerebral artery, normal mean velocity approximates 30 cm / second [47]. Mean velocities greater than 80 cm / second suggest significant stenosis in the middle cerebral artery; mean velocities greater than 70 cm / second are consistent with significant stenosis in the posterior cerebral and basilar arteries [49].

The clinical utility of transcranial Doppler in adults has been to monitor intracranial vasospasm after subarachnoid bleed, detection of middle cerebral-artery disease, the study of collateral circulation in patients with carotid-artery disease, determination of brain death, and evaluation of arteriovenous malformations of the brain [47–50]. In infants, performing an examination through the patent anterior fontanel permits direct visualization of the vessels under study. Whether transcranial Doppler will become a widely used clinical tool is uncertain.

Diseases of the Abdominal Aorta and Its Major Branches

GENERAL CONSIDERATIONS AND SCANNING TECHNIQUES

Real-time ultrasound is useful for the evaluation of the abdominal aorta and its major branches. These vessels appear as anechoic structures because they are fluid filled. They stand out distinctly in the midst of the surrounding soft tissues. The flexibility in choosing scanning planes enables the examiner to follow vessels and display them longitudinally and transversely. The dynamic nature of real-time ultrasonography facilitates visualization of arterial pulsations and, thus, differentiation of arteries from other anechoic structures. Duplex ultrasonography provides a two-dimensional image as well as information on the direction and the velocity of flow in a wide variety of abdominal vessels. Color Doppler sonography can assist in identifying and following blood vessels, since both arteries and veins stand out as colored structures superimposed on a gray-scale background.

The examination of the abdominal arterial system, from the upper abdominal aorta to the common iliac arteries, usually is performed with the patient in a supine position. Patient preparation consists of fasting for 8 hours to minimize the presence of bowel gas. The abdominal aorta should be examined both longitudinally and transversely. At each level, the transducer is oriented so that the maximal length of the segment is visualized (Fig. 19-8A). The transducer is then rotated 90 degrees to achieve a transverse view (Fig. 19-8B). This procedure requires particular care in patients with a tortuous aorta. Anteroposterior and transverse diameters of the normal abdominal aorta gradually taper from 3 cm in the upper abdomen to approximately 1.5 cm near the aortic bifurcation (Fig. 19-8C). If bowel gas is a problem, application of downward pressure on the anterior abdominal wall may displace the gas toward both flanks, thus permitting an unobstructed view of the aorta. Alternatively, the aorta can be visualized in a coronal plane through either flank, with or without placing the patient in a decubitus position [51].

The celiac artery can be identified superiorly in the abdomen at its anterior origin from the aorta. A transverse view of the aorta at the origin of the celiac artery demonstrates the celiac artery as it branches into the common hepatic and splenic arteries (Fig. 19-8D); the left gastric artery also can be seen in some patients. The superior mesenteric artery is visualized at its origin on the anterior surface of the aorta, just caudad to the celiac axis (see Fig. 19-8A). It usually can be followed for several centimeters, running almost parallel on a longitudinal view, and appears as an anechoic round area surrounded by an echogenic rim anterior to the aorta on a transverse view. The renal arteries often can be seen exiting laterally from the aorta. They are identified via a transverse view of the aorta (Fig. 19-8E) or when visualized through the kidneys by placing the transducer over the patient's flanks. The right renal artery also can be seen passing under the inferior vena cava on a longitudinal scan of the latter vessel. The aortic bifurcation and the common iliac arteries can be examined in several planes. Transverse views of the aorta as it bifurcates into the common iliac arteries can be obtained by sliding the transducer caudally. The transducer can then be rotated along the long and short axes of each of the two arteries. The aortic bifurcation can also be visualized via a coronal plane through either flank.

AORTIC ANEURYSMS

An aneurysm, or abnormal dilation, of the abdominal aorta is diagnosed when the luminal diameter exceeds 3 cm or when there is a focal bulge. At least 90 percent of aortic aneurysms are associated with atherosclerosis. Other etiologies include syphilitic or mycotic aneurysms

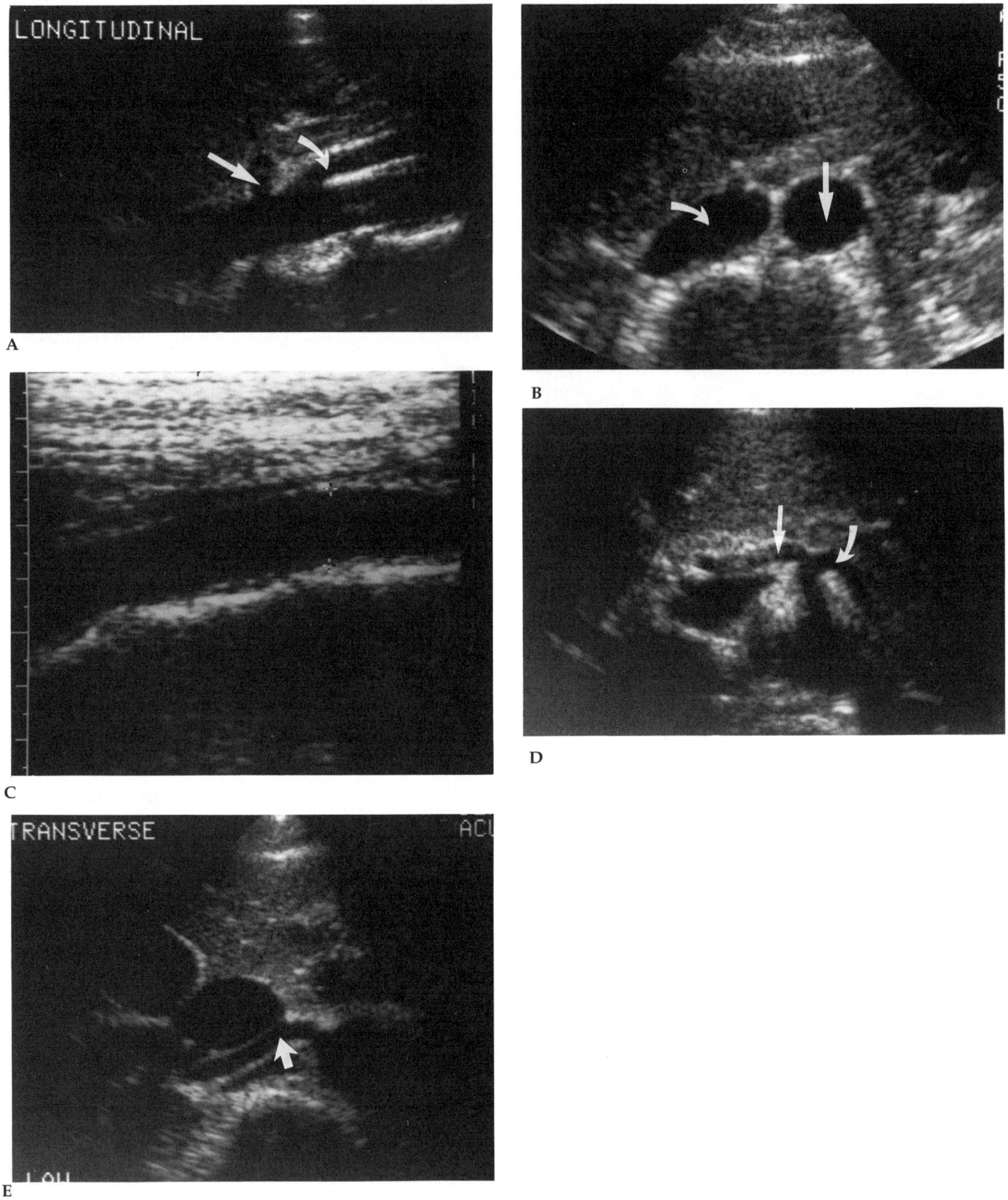

Fig. 19-8. Abdominal aorta and its major branches: normal sonographic anatomy. **A.** Longitudinal view of upper abdominal aorta, demonstrating takeoff of celiac (straight arrow) and superior mesenteric (curved arrow) arteries. **B.** Transverse view of abdominal aorta (straight arrow) and inferior vena cava (curved arrow). **C.** Longitudinal view of lower abdominal aorta: caliber is smaller than that of upper abdominal aorta. **D.** Celiac artery emerging from aorta, branching into common hepatic (straight arrow) and splenic (curved arrow) arteries. **E.** Right renal artery (arrow) emerging from the aorta and traveling under the inferior vena cava.

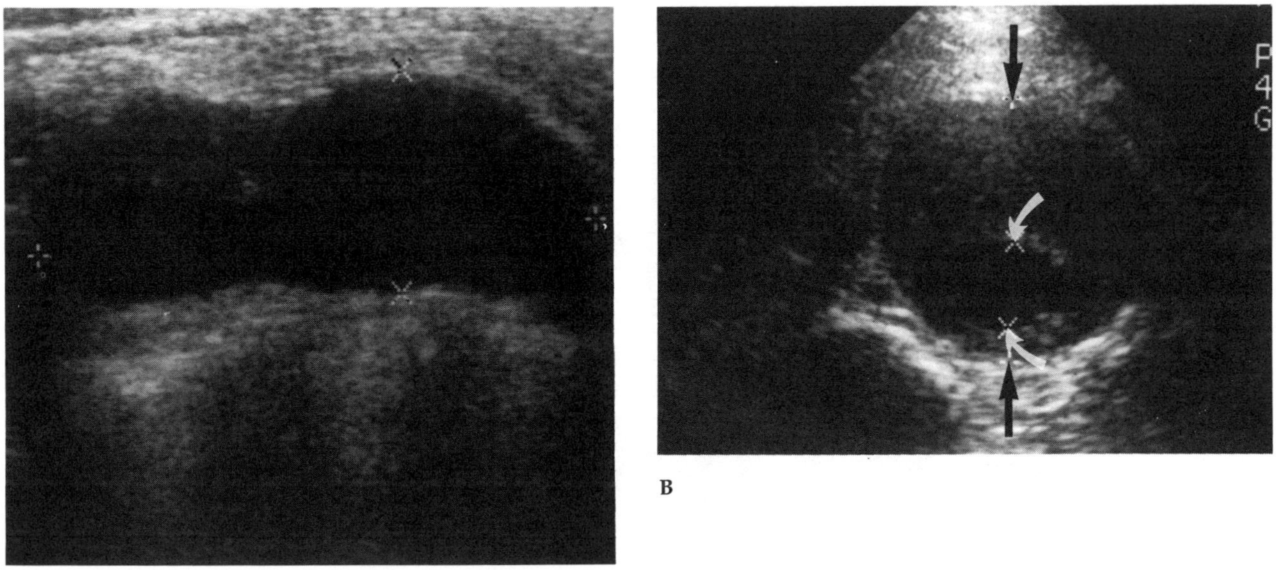

B

A

Fig. 19-9. Abdominal aortic aneurysm. **A.** Longitudinal view of mid-to-lower abdominal aorta. Anteroposterior diameter (between "×" cursors) is 4.5 cm, and length (between "+" cursors) is 10.3 cm. **B.** Transverse view demonstrates aneurysm with central anechoic lumen (surrounded by straight arrows) is 4.5 cm, and luminal diameter (between curved arrows) is 1.5 cm.

(e.g., due to salmonella or staphylococcus). Most occur below the renal arteries, often extending caudally to involve the common iliac arteries [52]. When aneurysm is suspected clinically, on the basis of a pulsatile abdominal mass or other signs or symptoms, ultrasonography provides an accurate means of diagnosis [53]. If present, ultrasound can provide information on the size and location of an aneurysm; this technique also assesses the relationship of an aortic aneurysm to major arterial branches, including the renal and common iliac arteries. Such relationships, however, can be examined in greater detail by computed tomography, magnetic resonance imaging, and angiography [54,55].

Sonographic findings of aortic aneurysm include a diameter greater than 3 cm in the anteroposterior diameter, when measured from outside wall to outside wall on a transverse view, and focal dilation (Fig. 19-9). Thrombus is commonly seen in the lumen, and calcifications often are present in or adjacent to the vessel wall. Thrombus appears as hypoechoic or heterogenous material surrounding part or all of the anechoic central lumen. Careful scanning technique and optimal machine settings may be necessary to distinguish hypoechoic thrombus from anechoic lumen [56,57]. The ultrasonographic assessment of an abdominal aortic aneurysm also should include a determination of its cephalocaudal length and, if possible, define its relationship to major branches of the aorta.

Rupture is the most feared consequence of an abdominal aortic aneurysm. Once it occurs, the untreated mortality approaches 100 percent, and mortality is high even if surgery is performed. If the patient presents in shock secondary to acute aneurysm rupture, the emergent nature of the problem may preclude ultrasonographic evaluation. With less severe ruptures or chronic leaks that do not cause cardiovascular collapse, ultrasound may aid in the diagnosis by detecting a retroperitoneal hematoma [58]. A hematoma appears as a soft-tissue mass, typically hypoechoic, surrounding the aorta and silhouetting the psoas muscles. The kidneys may be displaced laterally by the hematoma. Computed tomography is superior for displaying the size and the extent of the hematoma, because of the potential for obscuration of ultrasound images by bowel gas.

Another complication of abdominal aortic aneursym is the development of periaortic fibrosis, an entity called inflammatory aortic aneurysm. The periaortic inflammatory mass is associated with increased surgical morbidity and mortality rates. The involved area may include ureters, the inferior vena cava, and renal veins. The ultrasonographic appearance includes an echogenic aortic wall surrounded by a hypoechoic inflammatory mantle [59]. When this appearance is encountered, a computed tomography examination may be performed to determine the full extent of the inflammatory process.

AORTIC DISSECTION

Aortic dissection refers to a hematoma in the media of the aorta, associated with an intimal tear. When dissection extends to the abdominal aorta, the diagnosis can be made ultrasonographically by visualization of the intimal flap [60–62]. This appears as a linear collection of echoes that undulates with the cardiac cycle during real-time observation (Fig. 19-10). The finding is easy to recognize in most cases, but care must be taken to distinguish it from lique-

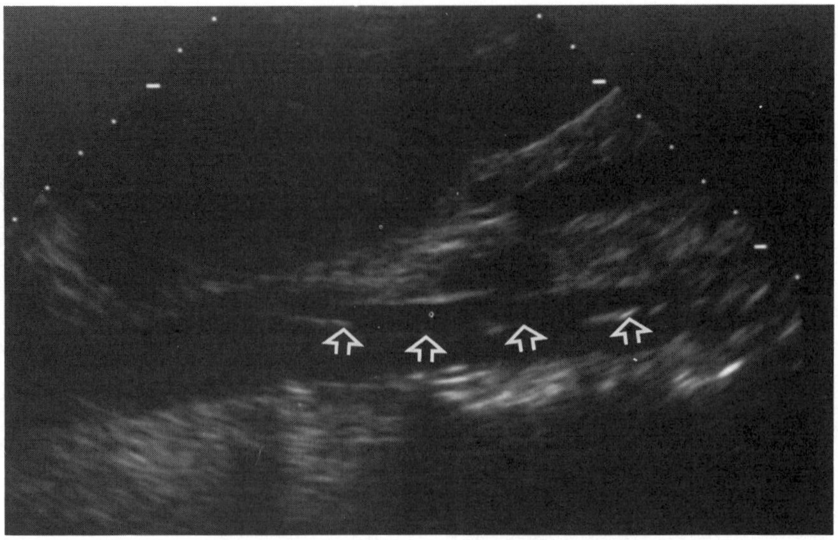

Fig. 19-10. Aortic dissection. Longitudinal view of upper abdominal aorta demonstrates intimal flap (arrows) that was seen to undulate with the cardiac cycle during real-time observation.

faction that may occur around a solid thrombus (Fig. 19-11) [63]. When dissection is suspected or diagnosed by ultrasound examination, computed tomography or angiography should be performed to define more precisely the full extent of the lesion.

ANEURYSMS OF OTHER ABDOMINAL ARTERIES

Aneurysms occur in a variety of intra-abdominal arteries. They have been diagnosed sonographically in the celiac, common hepatic, left and right hepatic, splenic, superior mesenteric, and renal arteries [64–69]. The two-dimensional image may be insufficient as an isolated test to make the diagnosis because an aneurysm in these vessels is often difficult to distinguish from a cyst, pseudocyst, or abscess. Aneurysms of branches of the renal arteries, for example, can be confused with simple renal cysts, and common hepatic, celiac, and superior mesenteric artery aneurysms may be diagnosed incorrectly as pancreatic pseudocysts. The diagnosis of aneurysm is facilitated by observing the lesion to be pulsatile during real-time scan-

Fig. 19-11. Transverse view of abdominal aortic aneurysm, with liquefaction (straight arrows) surrounding the more echogenic thrombus (curved arrows).

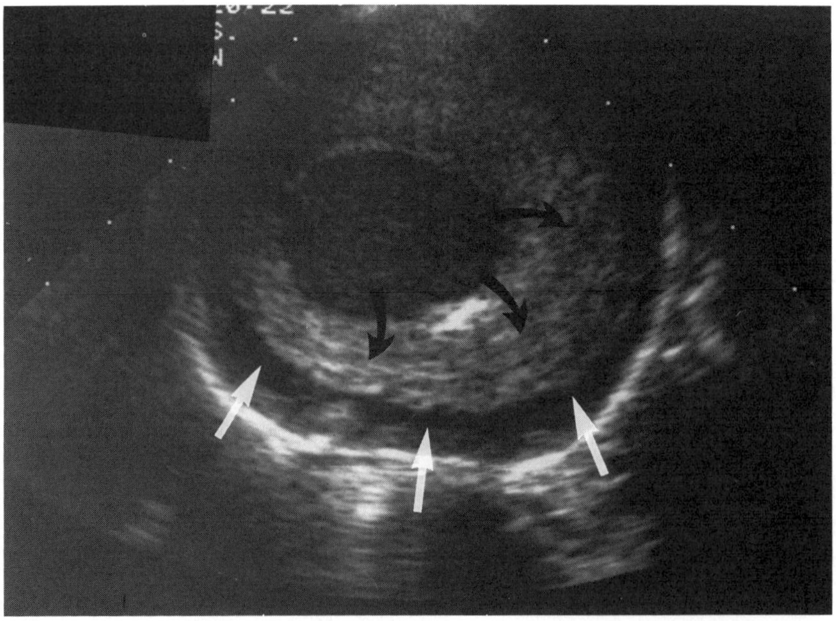

ning or, more reliably, by documenting blood flow in the lesion via pulse-wave or color Doppler examination.

ILIAC ARTERY ANEURYSMS

Iliac artery aneurysms can occur either as an extension of abdominal aortic aneurysms or as isolated lesions. The cause of the majority of these aneurysms is atherosclerosis. Other etiologies include trauma and infection. The ultrasonographic evaluation of an aortic aneurysm should always include examination of the iliac arteries. Sonography of the iliac arteries is useful to evaluate the patient with a pulsatile mass or other findings that suggest the presence of an iliac aneurysm.

The normal diameter of the common iliac arteries is less than 1 cm [70]. Aneurysms are diagnosed by identifying focal or diffuse enlargement of the vessel [70–72]. They can occasionally be very large. Ultrasound is useful not only for detecting and measuring the aneurysm but for diagnosing related complications such as perforation or ureteral obstruction.

PSEUDOANEURYSMS

Pseudoaneurysms are contained arterial ruptures or perforations, often comprising a hematoma that is connected via a patent channel to an adjacent artery. A pseudoaneurysm may result from trauma, needle puncture, or vascular surgery. It is a potential complication of angiographic procedures at the site of the arterial perforation [73]. Pseudoaneurysms have been reported to occur in the hepatic, superior mesenteric, splenic, and celiac arteries secondary to chronic pancreatitis [74,75].

The sonographic diagnosis is established via duplex ultrasonography or color Doppler examination. The lesion appears as an anechoic mass adjacent to an artery. The demonstration of the pulsatile blood flow via the Doppler study [73,74] distinguishes the lesion from a simple hematoma (Fig. 19-12). The track connecting the artery and the pseudoaneurysm can be visualized, in some cases, by color Doppler.

Renal Artery Stenosis. The high prevalence of hypertension in the population and the fact that renovascular hypertension is a potentially treatable form of blood pressure elevation have led numerous investigators to examine whether Doppler ultrasound might be a useful noninvasive test for renal artery stenosis. Attempts to diagnose renal artery stenosis have employed Doppler measurements of either the main renal artery or the intrarenal arteries.

The Doppler criteria proposed to diagnose renal artery stenosis are analogous to those that have been proved accurate for diagnosing carotid stenosis. Those derived from Doppler interrogation of the main renal artery include peak systolic velocity above 125 cm/second; ratio of peak systolic velocity in the renal artery to that in the abdominal aorta of greater than 3.5; and spectral broadening. The renal-to-aorta peak systolic velocity ratio is reported to have a sensitivity of 84–98 percent and specificity of 95–97 percent [76–79]. Locating the main renal artery and obtaining a reliable Doppler waveform is time consuming and cannot be accomplished in many patients because of obesity or overlying bowel gas. Also, some studies have suggested that the criteria used for evaluating the main renal artery are insensitive [80,81]. Reasons for inaccuracy include inability to angle-correct when the course of the renal artery cannot be determined or, in many cases, to interrogate the main renal artery at an angle of less than 60 degrees, as well as failure to detect accessory renal arteries [82].

Fig. 19-12. Right femoral artery pseudoaneurysm. Fluid-filled structure in the right groin 2 days following a femoral artery puncture. Doppler signal from within the lesion demonstrates pulsatile arterial flow.

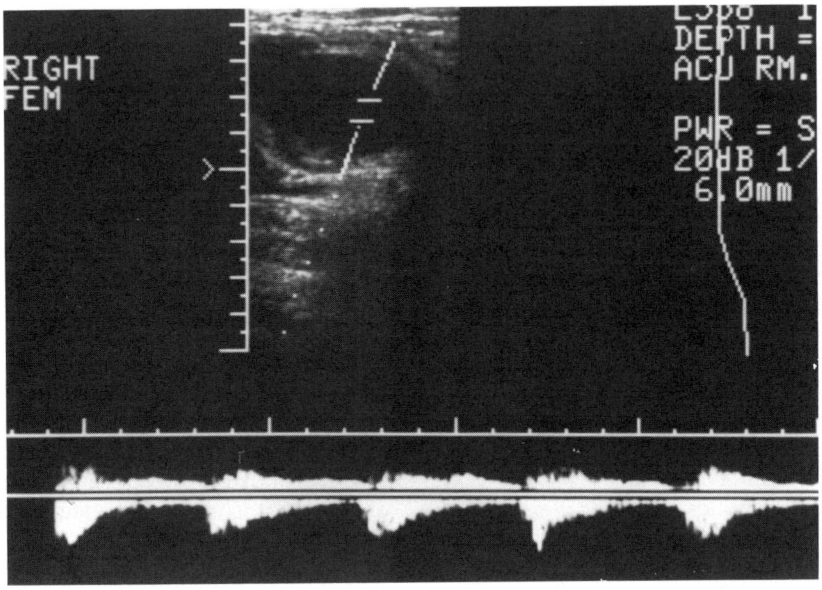

Table 19-1. Noninvasive tests to diagnose arterial occlusive disease of the extremities

Doppler ultrasonography
Pulse volume recording
Extremity segmental pressure measurements
Exercise testing
Reactive hyperemia
Oximetry
Ultrasound imaging

In view of these problems and limitations, some investigators have used Doppler to interrogate the intrarenal arteries as a means to diagnose renal artery stenosis [83–86]. These vessels are closer to the skin surface than is the main renal artery, so that Doppler signals can be obtained more easily. The rationale for interrogating these vessels is that, in the presence of a stenotic lesion in the main renal artery, the downstream intrarenal vessels will display a **pulsus tardus-parvus** pattern: slow systolic upstroke and diminished peak systolic velocity. Proposed criteria for renal artery stenosis using Doppler measurements of the intrarenal arteries include prolonged systolic acceleration time (≥ 0.07 seconds), diminished systolic acceleration index (< 3 m/second), and abnormal configuration of the early systolic peak. Some studies have suggested that these criteria are sensitive (78–95%) and specific (83–97%) for renal artery stenosis [85,86]. At least one investigation, however, has failed to replicate those results, finding no significant difference between stenotic (>50% diameter narrowing) and nonstenotic vessels for any of the tardus-parvus parameters [87]. In view of these conflicting results, further studies will be needed to clarify what role, if any, Doppler ultrasound has in screening hypertensive patients for renal artery stenosis.

Mesenteric Artery Stenosis. The potential role of Doppler in diagnosing superior mesenteric artery stenosis also has been examined, using measurements of the peak systolic and end-diastolic velocities. To minimize intraobserver variability when obtaining Doppler velocity measurements from this artery, Doppler interrogation should be performed using an insonation angle of at most 60 degrees and with the patient in a fasting state [88–90]. In one study comparing duplex Doppler ultrasonography with angiography, the Doppler criteria found to be useful for diagnosing superior mesenteric artery stenosis (≥50% diameter reduction) included peak systolic velocity greater than 300 cm/second (sensitivity of 63%, specificity of 100%) and end-diastolic velocity greater than 45 cm/second (sensitivity of 100%, specificity of 92%) [91].

Arterial Occlusive Disease of the Extremities

This section describes in detail the techniques used in the noninvasive vascular laboratory to evaluate patients with arterial disease in the extremities. Many of the noninvasive tests discussed earlier in this chapter are utilized in patients with arterial disease of the extremities (Table 19-1). These tests are useful when following the patient's clinical course, whether the condition is treated conservatively or with surgical intervention. The tests used most frequently in the noninvasive vascular laboratory include Doppler ultrasonography, pulse volume analysis, extremity blood pressure measurements, exercise testing, postocclusive reactive hyperemic blood flow measurements, transcutaneous oximetry, and ultrasound imaging.

DOPPLER ULTRASOUND

Doppler ultrasonography is a useful qualitative technique to identify vessels with significant stenotic lesions. Blood flow through a vessel can be detected and evaluated by an auditory assessment of the Doppler signal. In addition, conversion of Doppler signals to an analogue output enables a graphic display of the pulse-wave velocity. The typical Doppler operating frequency is 8 to 10 MHz for superficial arteries and 5 MHz for deeper blood vessels, such as the iliac arteries.

The Doppler probe is usually positioned at a 60-degree angle over the common femoral, superficial femoral, popliteal, dorsalis pedal, and posterior tibial arteries. With the exception of the popliteal artery, the patient can remain in a supine position. Analysis of the popliteal artery may be facilitated by placing the patient in the prone position. The Doppler probe can be used to evaluate arterial disease in the upper extremity by placing it over the subclavian artery in the supraclavicular fossa, over the brachial artery near the axilla as well as in the antecubital fossa, and over the radial and ulnar arteries on the volar aspect of the wrist. In addition, the Doppler probe is useful for evaluating the presence of blood flow in the palmar arch, as well as along the digital arteries.

It should be recalled that the Doppler frequency shift is proportional to the velocity of blood flow. Normally, the pulse-velocity waveform has three components: a rapid forward-flow component during systole, a transient flow reversal during early diastole, and a slower forward-flow component during late diastole (see Fig. 19-13A). If the probe is placed distal to an arterial stenosis, the normal triphasic waveform is altered. The appearance of the waveform depends on the severity of the stenosis (Fig. 19-13B and C). In the presence of a severe stenosis or occlusion, the waveform usually is dampened, the systolic peak is lower, and the rate of rise is delayed. At the peak of the systolic upstroke, flutter may be detected. The reverse-flow component disappears, and the final descending portion becomes very shallow. In the presence of severe ischemia, no flow whatsoever may be detected. If the probe is positioned directly over a stenosis, the signal may become high pitched and turbulent. By placing a probe over multiple areas of the extremity's vessels, the examiner can assess the location of stenotic lesions. For example, if the Doppler waveform is abnormal over the common femoral artery, the patient may have significant aortoiliac occlusive disease. If the waveform over the common femoral artery has a normal triphasic appearance, however, but the waveform over the popliteal artery is abnormal, it is likely that a significant stenosis is present between the two locations. Further dampening of the pulse-velocity waveform over the dorsalis pedal pulse would imply additional distal stenoses.

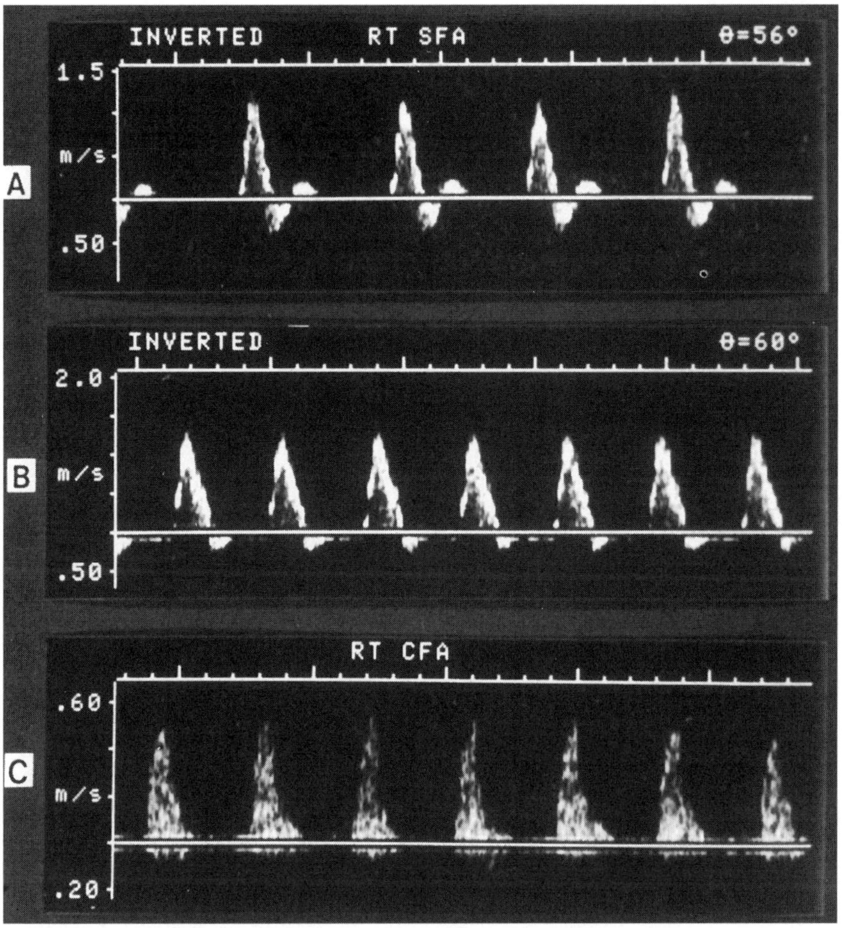

Fig. 19-13. **A.** Normal Doppler pulse-velocity waveform. There is a rapid forward-flow component during systole, a transient flow reversal during early diastole, and a slower forward-flow component during late diastole. **B.** Doppler velocity waveform recorded distal to a mild stenosis. The wave form becomes biphasic, losing the forward-flow component during late diastole. **C.** Doppler velocity waveform recorded distal to a severe stenosis. The waveform is dampened, the systolic peak is lower, and the rate of rise is delayed.

Most commercially available Doppler devices convert the signals to an analogue waveform by using a zero crossing detector. The analogue waveform signal can be used to detect and assess the severity of an arterial stenosis. The waveform becomes abnormal distal to a stenosis. Frequently, it is difficult to analyze the analogue waveform signal if the signal-to-noise ratio is low or when venous flow is also present. The use of frequency analysis by Fourier transformation provides a more sophisticated method for processing Doppler signals. Frequency analysis enables graphic display of all Doppler-shift frequencies that are detected by the Doppler probe.

PULSE VOLUME RECORDING

The pulse volume recording is another useful noninvasive test for the detection of peripheral arterial occlusive disease. This technique utilizes the principles of plethysmography to evaluate changes in leg volume with each pulse.

The normal pulse volume recording resembles a blood pressure waveform [92]. It is composed of a systolic upstroke with a sharp systolic peak and a downslope that is concave toward the baseline and that includes a prominent dicrotic wave. The waveform becomes progressively more abnormal with increasing severity of the arterial stenosis. One can qualitatively analyze the waveform as being mildly abnormal, moderately abnormal, or severely abnormal [93–101] (Fig. 19-14). A mildly abnormal waveform has a sharp systolic peak, but the dicrotic wave is absent, and the downslope is convex in relation to the baseline. A moderately abnormal waveform has a flat systolic peak. In addition, the upslope and downslope time are approximately equal, and the dicrotic wave is invariably absent. A severely abnormal waveform is characterized by a very low amplitude. Occasionally, in the presence of very severe ischemia, the waveform is entirely absent. It should be noted, however, that the dicrotic wave may be absent, even in normal vessels. That occurs particularly when resistance in the vessels is low, as might occur after exercise [93,94]. The presence of the dicrotic wave indicates a normal vessel. There may be wide variation

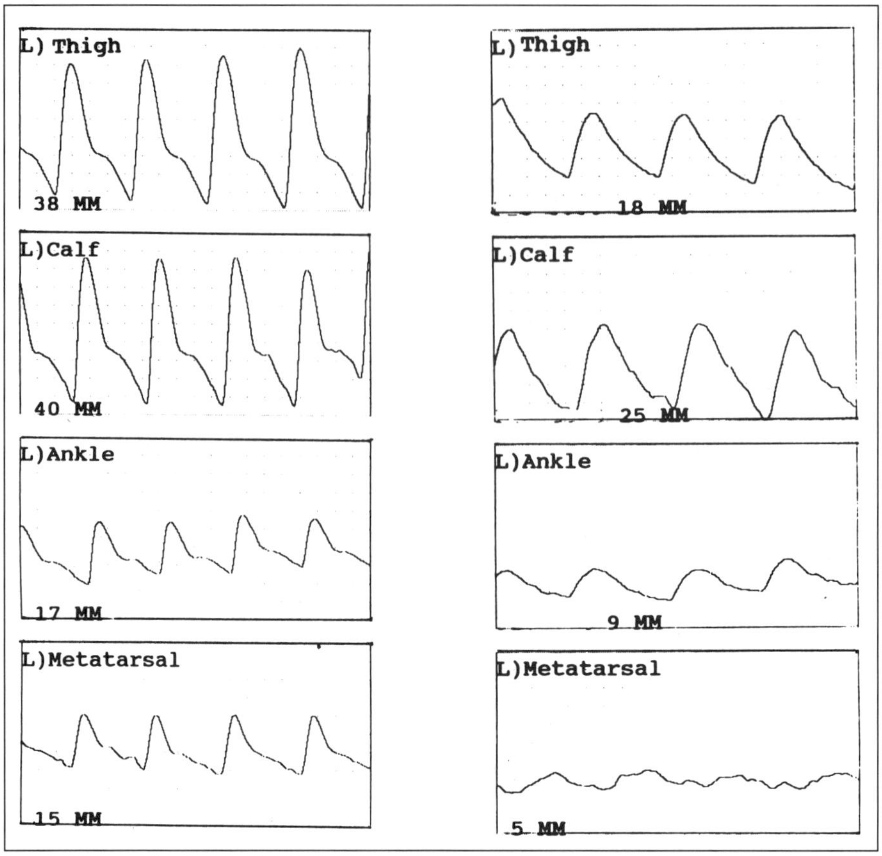

Fig. 19-14. (Left) Normal pulse volume recording. Tracings derived from the thigh, upper calf, and ankle and metatarsal segments. The pulse volume contour displays a normal upstroke, dicrotic notch, and downstroke at each level. (Right) Pulse volume recording from a patient with arterial occlusive disease. The amplitude of the pulse volume is diminished, the upstroke is delayed, and there is no dicrotic notch.

in the amplitude of the waveform, even in normal limbs. The amplitude may be affected by stroke volume, blood pressure, or vascular tone as well as the patency of the vessel. A unilateral amplitude reduction suggests underlying arterial stenosis.

A moderately or severely abnormal pulse volume recording may identify hemodynamically significant lesions in 95 percent of extremities [95]. This test is useful in following the natural course of disease, because the amplitude of the pulse volume recording is usually reproducible in the same patient over time. A reduction in pulse volume amplitude frequently correlates with the progression of underlying peripheral arterial occlusive disease [95]. The pulse volume recording is particularly useful when calcified vessels preclude accurate interpretation of leg pressure measurements. It also is useful to assess digital blood flow. An abnormal pulse volume recording may reflect impaired blood supply to the digits. It is often difficult, however, to distinguish decreased digital blood flow secondary to vasospasm from that secondary to occlusive disease. The pulse volume recording is used in the evaluation of thoracic outlet syndrome, popliteal artery entrapment, and graft patency.

The technique for pulse volume recording employs the placement of pneumatic cuffs or strain gauges at multiple levels of the limb, including the upper and lower thigh, the upper and lower calf, and along the digits. As with Doppler ultrasonography, an abnormal pulse volume recording usually reflects disease proximal to the location of the sensor cuff or strain gauge. The principal limitation of pulse volume recordings is that the cuffs or strain gauge cannot be placed high enough on the thigh to distinguish superficial femoral-artery stenoses from lesions in more proximal vessels. Thus, an abnormal pulse volume recording in the upper thigh may be secondary to proximal superficial femoral, common femoral, iliac artery, or aortic stenoses. In that situation, Doppler ultrasonography is more useful because the probe can be placed along the iliac arteries as well as over the common femoral artery.

EXTREMITY PRESSURE MEASUREMENT

Noninvasive assessment of systolic blood pressure in the extremities is probably the most frequently used noninvasive test to detect the presence of hemodynamically significant arterial stenosis. Pneumatic cuffs typically are positioned on the leg over the upper thigh, above the knee, below the knee, and just above the ankle. During assessment of the upper extremity, the cuffs can be placed on the upper arm, on the forearm just below the elbow, and at the wrist. Each cuff is inflated to a suprasystolic pressure. The pressure at which blood flow resumes during deflation of the cuff is the systolic blood pressure. The onset of flow is usually detected with a Doppler ultrasound flow detector. In the lower extremities, the probe can be placed over the posterior tibial, dorsalis pedal, and peroneal arteries. To measure blood pressure in the thigh, the probe can be placed over the popliteal artery. In the upper extremities, Doppler probes can be placed over the radial or ulnar arteries and occasionally over the brachial arteries in the antecubital fossa. Other methods used to detect the onset of flow include strain-gauge plethysmography, photoplethysmography, and isotope-clearance techniques.

Normally, the systolic blood pressure in the thigh approximates that determined from the brachial artery [97,98]. The amplitude of the pressure wave increases as the wave travels distally because of increased stiffness of the arterial walls in the more peripheral vessels and the presence of reflective waves [99]. In the aorta, approximately 90 percent of the cross-sectional area must be narrowed before there is a change in distal pressure or blood flow, whereas in the carotid, iliac, and femoral arteries, a stenosis of 70 to 90 percent is sufficient to cause a fall in blood pressure [24,101]. An ankle-to-brachial systolic blood pressure ratio less than 0.97 is considered abnormal. Patients with leg claudication frequently have ankle-brachial indices of 0.5 to 0.8 [101–103]. In patients with significant ischemia at rest, the ankle-brachial index often is less than 0.5 [97–99]. In the lower extremity, a gradient in excess of 20 mm Hg between successive cuffs suggests significant interval disease [104]. In the upper extremity, a gradient greater than 10 mm Hg between sequential cuffs suggests significant stenosis. It should be noted that the systolic blood pressure in the fingers and the toes may normally approximate 60 percent of the systolic pressure in the wrist and the ankle, respectively [105]. A toe-to-brachial pressure index less than 0.6 is considered abnormal. An absolute systolic blood pressure less than 50 mm Hg in the toes is abnormal [104].

Systolic pressure measurements are used to complement the history and the physical examination. These measurements are helpful in locating and quantifying the severity of stenotic lesions and in the differential diagnosis of patients with claudication. For example, patients with pseudoclaudication secondary to spinal stenosis, arthritis, or muscular disorders have normal systolic pressure measurements. Leg pressure measurements are useful to follow the natural course of disease in an individual patient. Furthermore, these tests can be used to follow the outcome of revascularization procedures, allowing early detection of graft stenosis. Systolic pressure measurements also are used to determine prognoses in patients with ischemia and skin lesions and to determine sites of amputation as well as to predict the success of those procedures. For example, healing is usually poor if the ankle pressure is less than 55 mm Hg or the toe pressure is less than 30 mm Hg [106]. Leg pressure measurements are an objective means of following the responses to medical therapy, including the use of investigational drugs, smoking cessation, and exercise programs.

Transcutaneous Oximetry. The measurement of transcutaneous oxygen tension is used to assess the severity of skin ischemia in patients with peripheral arterial occlusive disease. Oxygen-sensing electrodes are placed on the legs, including the dorsum of each foot, and on the chest wall. Measurements are made with the patient in the supine position. In normal individuals, the resting foot transcutaneous oxygen tension approximates 60 mm Hg [107], and the ratio of foot-to-chest transcutaneous oxygen tension, called the **regional perfusion index,** approximates 0.90 [108]. These values decrease in relative proportion to the severity of ischemia. Patients with claudication, but without ischemia at rest, may have values that overlap with normal subjects. In many patients, however, the values are decreased, often ranging from 40 to 60 mm Hg, corresponding to a regional perfusion index of approximately 0.80. In patients with resting ischemia, or impending tissue loss, foot transcutaneous oxygen tension often is less than 40 mm Hg, corresponding to a regional perfusion index of less than 0.5 [108]. Tissue transcutaneous oxygen tension can be used to predict the likelihood of healing following amputation. Healing usually occurs if the tissue oxygen tension is greater than 40 mm Hg, whereas wound healing is unlikely to occur if transcutaneous oxygen tension is less than 20 mm Hg [109,110]. Provocative maneuvers such as leg elevation or exercise may improve the sensitivity of transcutaneous oximetry to assess the severity of peripheral arterial occlusive disease. Following exercise, foot transcutaneous oxygen tension falls in patients with peripheral arterial occlusive disease but not in normal individuals [107,111]. Foot transcutaneous oxygen tension is lower in diabetics than in nondiabetics [108,112]. As such, it may be a useful test to assess the severity of arterial occlusive disease, particularly in those individuals in whom calcification precludes accurate measurements of ankle pressures [108].

EXERCISE TESTING

Under basal conditions a lesion that narrows a peripheral artery to less than 70 percent of its cross-sectional area may not cause a decrease in distal systolic pressure. As flow through the lesion increases, however, there is further loss of energy and a subsequent fall in blood pressure. This is reflected in Poiseuille's law, which relates changes in flow to changes in blood pressure across a stenosis. Treadmill exercise is an intervention that increases blood flow to the lower extremities. Thus, it is a sensitive way to determine whether an arterial stenosis is present. During exercise, vascular resistance in the exercising muscle falls [113]. As a result, blood flow to that extremity increases. Under those conditions, an arterial stenosis creates a pressure gradient. Also, the contracting muscles increase the tissue pressure extrinsic to the vessel [114]. If the extravascular pressure exceeds the intravascular perfusion pressure, the vessel can collapse. Therefore, it is possible to create a fall in the ankle-to-brachial index during exercise, even with lesions that are less than 70 percent of the cross-sectional area of the artery [115–117].

Treadmill exercise testing has become a useful way to evaluate peripheral arterial occlusive disease, particularly in patients with borderline lesions. A variety of exercise protocols can be used to study the effects of exercise on leg blood flow or leg blood pressure. These protocols usually employ a motorized treadmill that uses fixed or progressive speeds and angles of incline. The fixed or constant-load treadmill test utilizes speeds of 1.5 to 2.0 miles per hour and a single grade ranging from 0 to 12 percent. Progressive- or graded-treadmill protocols vary the speed or the grade (or both) of the treadmill. Traditional protocols used to assess cardiac disease, such as the Bruce or Naughton protocols, gradually increase both speed and treadmill grade [118,119]. For the evaluation of peripheral arterial disease, some progressive protocols maintain a constant speed of 2 miles per hour and gradually increases the grade from 0 to 17.5 percent [120,121]. Alternatively, the protocol may keep the grade constant at 12 percent and maintain a speed of 1.5 to 2 miles per hour.

Brachial and ankle systolic blood pressures are determined at rest, immediately following exercise, and repeatedly until they return to basal values. In normal individuals, blood pressure typically increases during exercise. The increase in blood pressure occurs in both the upper and the lower extremities. Therefore, the ankle-to-brachial index remains constant whether measured at rest or following exercise. In patients with peripheral arterial occlusive lesions, the change in blood pressure is disproportionate. The increase in blood pressure in the upper extremity is not matched by a comparable increase in blood pressure in the lower extremity. Indeed, there may be a fall in blood pressure in the lower extremity. Thus, the ankle-to-brachial index decreases. The fall in the ankle-to-brachial pressure index following exercise is proportional to the severity of the stenosis. Furthermore, it takes longer for the ankle-to-brachial pressure index to return to baseline values following exercise. This is because the exercise-induced vasodilation persists longer in patients with more severe ischemia. The objective end points in patients with peripheral arterial occlusive disease who are undergoing treadmill exercise tests include the exercise time, the ankle-to-brachial pressure index immediately following exercise, and the time required for return of the ankle-to-brachial index to basal value.

The treadmill exercise test is not only a sensitive method for evaluating arterial stenoses, it also provides additional information. It is frequently difficult to evaluate a patient's exercise limitations based on historic information alone. By objectively measuring exercise capacity in patients limited by claudication, the examiner gains a much clearer understanding of a patient's limitations. Many patients with atherosclerosis of the extremities also have coronary artery disease. With the implementation of cardiac monitoring, treadmill exercise testing may be useful in detecting underlying myocardial ischemia. If patients are significantly limited by claudication, they may not achieve an adequate work load to sufficiently stress their heart and provoke myocardial ischemia. However, the presence of electrocardiographic changes during low levels of exercise may indicate the presence of severe coronary artery disease [122]. This test may be particularly useful, therefore, in patients undergoing evaluation of their peripheral vascular status, particularly if they are potential candidates for surgery. The treadmill exercise test also is useful in following the natural course of patients with peripheral arterial occlusive disease and in monitoring responses to conservative therapy, investigational drugs, and exercise programs. Furthermore, this test is useful in following the outcome of patients after revascularization procedures.

REACTIVE HYPEREMIA

The vasodilation that accompanies recovery from an ischemic stimulus is called **reactive hyperemia.** Ischemia can be produced by inflation of a pneumatic cuff to suprasystolic pressure. Vasodilation occurs as a consequence of autoregulatory phenomena. Inflation of a pneumatic cuff about the thigh to suprasystolic pressures for at least 5 minutes usually is adequate to cause sufficient ischemia. Release of the pneumatic cuff allows a surge of blood flow into the dilated resistance vessels of the lower extremity. Normally, because of the vasodilation, there is a slight fall in leg pressure compared to upper-extremity pressure [123,124]. Nonetheless, the ankle-to-brachial pressure index usually is greater than 0.9 during the first minute following release of the pneumatic cuff. Blood pressure distal to a stenotic lesion decreases further during periods of increased flow. Thus, an ankle-to-brachial index less than 0.8 following release of an ischemic stimulus is abnormal and indicative of arterial occlusive disease [125,126].

The strain-gauge plethysmograph or the photoplethysmograph can be used to detect pulses following the release of an ischemic stimulus [127]. Normally, following the release of an ischemia, there is a return of the pulse volume to at least 50 percent of its basal value within 3.5 seconds [127]. In the presence of stenotic lesions, the pulse reappearance time may be considerably prolonged, sometimes exceeding 60 seconds. Plethysmographic techniques also are available to assess changes in blood flow during reactive hyperemia. They are particularly useful in the research laboratory but have found limited application in the clinical setting. Blood flow may be quantitated using venous occlusion water or strain-gauge plethysmography [128]. Basal blood flow may be comparable in normal subjects and in patients with moderate arterial occlusive disease, but the blood-flow response is diminished during reactive hyperemia in patients with diseased vessels [128].

Thus, the measurement of blood pressure or pulse reappearance time during reactive hyperemia can be a sensitive method of predicting the presence of an arterial stenosis. This intervention has some advantages over treadmill exercise. First, it requires much less equipment: Only blood pressure cuffs and a Doppler ultrasound detector are needed to create the ischemic stimulus and to evaluate the arm and leg blood pressure during reactive hyperemia. Second, this test can be used to evaluate patients who are unable to walk on the treadmill. Its limitation is that it does not allow objective assessment of exercise capacity. Also, the inflation of a pneumatic cuff for 5 minutes to induce ischemia is frequently uncomfortable and not well tolerated by many patients.

COLOR-ASSISTED DUPLEX ULTRASONOGRAPHY

Duplex ultrasonography has not yet achieved widespread acceptance for evaluating infrainguinal arteries, but it is being employed in some laboratories as a preoperative screening test or to assess the results of percutaneous transluminal angioplasty. The location of the vessel is first assessed by placing the transducer in a transverse position over the common femoral artery. Thereafter, the transducer is oriented longitudinally to image the common femoral artery, the femoral artery bifurcation, the superficial femoral artery, and the popliteal artery. The posterior tibial and peroneal arteries are best imaged when the transducer is placed along the medial aspect of the calf, and the anterior tibial arteries are imaged best from the lateral approach. Gray-scale imaging is useful to identify areas of intimal thickening, plaque formation, and calcification. Color Doppler imaging will detect abnormal flow jets caused by arterial stenoses. The abrupt loss of color and the absence of a Doppler waveform is indicative of occlusion. Criteria for defining a stenosis vary among laboratories. Most suggest that a peak systolic velocity greater than 160 cm / second or a twofold increase in peak systolic velocity is consistent with a stenosis of at least 50 percent [129–131]. The sensitivity of this technique for detecting significant stenoses in the femoral or popliteal arteries ranges from 78 to 85 percent and for detecting occlusions 90 to 100 percent, whereas the specificity for stenoses approximates 90 to 100 percent and for occlusions also 90 to 100 percent [129–136]. This technique is also useful to assess patency in the tibial and peroneal arteries, but it is less reliable for evaluating the severity of stenoses in those vessels [135–137].

The patency of infrainguinal bypass grafts can be assessed by color-assisted duplex ultrasound. Approximately 20 to 30 percent of these grafts fail over a 5-year period [138,139]. Early graft failure usually is attributed to technical problems such as retained valve leaflets, intimal flaps, valvulotone injury, kinks, and perianastomotic stenoses [140,141]. Graft failure occurring between 6 months and 2 years is often a consequence of intimal hyperplasia, primarily occurring in anastomotic regions. Late failures occur when progression of atherosclerosis in native vessels compromises flow either into or exiting the graft. Ultrasound surveillance of infrainguinal bypass grafts has been used to identify sites of stenosis that might presage graft failure. Once identified, these local problems can be corrected readily by surgical intervention, thereby precluding graft failure.

The proximal anastomosis is identified and examined by placing the transducer parallel to the graft. The conduit of the graft is scanned by moving the longitudinally oriented transducer down the graft, adjusting the color window as required by the course of the graft. As in native arteries, color Doppler imaging will detect abnormal flow jets in areas of stenosis. Pulse Doppler interrogation is performed at anastomotic sites, approximately every 5 to 10 cm along the graft conduit, in contiguous native arteries, and at sites of abnormal flow detected by color Doppler. Normal velocity varies among grafts but usually ranges between 50 and 120 cm / second. A peak systolic velocity below 45 cm / second identifies a graft that has an increased likelihood of incipient failure [142–147]. A twofold increase in peak systolic velocity is indicative of stenosis of at least 50 percent, whereas a threefold increase in peak systolic velocity or an end diastolic velocity higher than 20 cm / second is suggestive of stenosis greater than 75 percent [148–153]. Infrainguinal bypass graft ultrasonography has been used to identify technical problems intraoperatively, enabling appropriate corrections before the patient leaves the operating room [147–151]. A number of laboratories have used the technique in surveillance protocols to monitor grafts postoperatively and have noted that significant stenoses often are identified even before there is significant change in the ankle-brachial index [142,144,152–154]. Protocols to survey grafts postoperatively vary among the laboratories. Based on the incidence of graft failures, a reasonable protocol is to survey grafts at 1 month, 3 months, 6 months, 12 months, and annually thereafter following bypass graft surgery.

RAYNAUD'S PHENOMENON

Raynaud's phenomenon is characterized as episodic digital vasospasm. The diagnosis of Raynaud's phenomenon usually is made by a history that includes the occurrence of digital pallor, cyanosis, and erythema provoked by exposure to cold or by emotional stress. A variety of serologic tests are employed to distinguish primary from secondary Raynaud's phenomenon. Few noninvasive vascular tests, however, are clinically useful to distinguish patients with Raynaud's phenomenon from other individuals with digital ischemia, acrocyanosis, or simply cold extremities. Tests that have been used in some laboratories include digital pulse volume recordings, measurements of digital blood flow, and digital systolic pressure [155–158].

The digital pulse volume contour can be measured during local warming and after systemic or local cooling. Air, strain-gauge, or photoelectric plethysmographic techniques can be used to record the pulse volume waveform. (Features of normal and abnormal pulse wave contours were described earlier in this chapter.) Exposing the digits to local heating should produce a normal pulse waveform if no obstructive lesions are present in proximal vessels or in the digital arteries [159]. Thus, patients with digital ischemia secondary to atherosclerosis, thromboangiitis obliterans, or digital vascular pathology would be most likely to have an abnormal pulse waveform contour during local heating [160]. Patients with primary Raynaud's phenomenon should have a normal pulse waveform during local heating because obstructive lesions are not present. Cooling can be produced systemically by lowering the room temperature or by applying cooling blankets. Systemic cooling, particularly if supplemented with local digital cooling, often produces an abnormal pulse waveform in patients with Raynaud's phenomenon. The difficulty in using pulse volume recordings to evaluate patients with Raynaud's phenomenon is underscored by the fact that there is considerable overlap in the responses of normal individuals, patients with Raynaud's phenomenon, and patients with digital ischemia secondary to obstructive lesions [160]. Therefore, the predictive value of this technique is not high.

The determination of digital systolic pressure has been used by some laboratories to diagnose patients with Raynaud's phenomenon [158]. A sphygmomanometric cuff is placed on the proximal aspect of the digit and inflated to suprasystolic pressures. During deflation of the cuff, systolic digital blood pressure is determined by the appearance of digital blood flow as detected by plethysmographic or isotope-clearance techniques. Usually, the digital systolic pressure is approximately 25 mm Hg less than the brachial artery pressure [161]. Several studies have suggested that digital systolic pressure is lower in patients with Raynaud's phenomenon than in age- and sex-matched normal individuals [162,163]. As noted with pulse volume recordings, however, there is considerable overlap between those two groups such that the measurement of digital systolic pressure alone is insufficient to make the diagnosis of Raynaud's phenomenon. It has been shown, however, that systemic and local cold exposure causes digital systolic pressure to fall dramatically in patients with Raynaud's phenomenon but not in normal individuals or those with acrocyanosis [164–168]. During this maneuver, the systolic pressure in patients with primary Raynaud's phenomenon may fall to zero.

Quantitation of digital blood flow using plethysmographic or radioisotope-clearance techniques has been evaluated as a potential means to diagnose patients with Raynaud's phenomenon [169]. Although many patients with Raynaud's phenomenon have an abnormally low digital blood flow, there remains considerable overlap between them and normal individuals, thereby obviating the diagnostic utility of this measurement in patients with Raynaud's phenomenon.

Venous Diseases

The noninvasive vascular laboratory is particularly useful in evaluating diseases of the veins. Its principal utility has been in the diagnosis of deep-vein thrombosis. Many noninvasive vascular laboratories are also employing tests to evaluate chronic venous insufficiency and venous varicosities.

A variety of noninvasive tests have been used to evaluate patients for deep-vein thrombosis, including Doppler ultrasonography, impedance plethysmography (IPG), iodine-125 fibrinogen scanning, and venous ultrasound imaging. As techniques have improved and technology has progressed, the noninvasive vascular laboratory has evolved from a preliminary testing area that often preceded venography to a highly reliable unit capable of diagnosing deep-vein thrombosis with high degrees of accuracy. The venous ultrasound imaging examination has been the principal diagnostic test that has catapulted the noninvasive vascular laboratory into a prominent role in the diagnosis of deep-vein thrombosis. The relative ease and safety of these examinations have supplanted the need for venography in many centers. Descriptions of some of the other noninvasive tests are provided here, not only for historic purposes, but because these tests often are useful as adjunct studies.

DOPPLER ULTRASONOGRAPHY

Doppler ultrasonography was one of the first noninvasive tests used to evaluate patients suspected of having deep-vein thrombosis [170–173]. A continuous-wave Doppler probe of approximately 7.5 MHz is applied over selected sites of the venous system of the lower extremities. These sites usually include the common femoral, superficial femoral, popliteal, and posterior tibial veins. The examiner listens for the presence of venous flow, which typically varies with respiration. Flow in the veins of the lower extremities increases during expiration and decreases during inspiration. This respiratory-variation flow probably is caused by changes in extrinsic pressure applied on the inferior vena cava by the diaphragm. If a thrombus is present in a vein proximal to the location of the ultrasound probe, the respiratory variation is not present in venous flow. Another aspect of the test involves manual compression of the foot or calf. During this maneuver, flow accelerates in the veins. The increased flow can be detected by the ultrasound probe. If thrombus is present between the area of compression and the location of the probe, no flow acceleration occurs. In the absence of a deep-vein thrombosis, release of manual compression causes accelerated flow in distal veins. An abnormal response is characterized by no increase in flow in the distal vein. For example, the probe can be placed on the posterior tibial vein as the calf is sequentially compressed and released. A normal response is an acceleration of flow in the posterior tibial vein and selected calf veins such as the posterior tibial vein. Release of proximal compression can be used to examine common femoral, superficial femoral, and popliteal veins. The technique of Doppler ultrasonography for the diagnosis of deep-vein thrombosis is limited by its subjectivity. In experienced hands, however, this test's sensitivity and specificity in patients with venographically confirmed proximal deep-vein thrombosis are approximately 85 and 90 percent, respectively [170]. Sensitivity is less than 50 percent in patients with calf-vein thrombosis [170].

IMPEDANCE PLETHYSMOGRAPHY

With impedance plethysmography, small amounts of electric current are transmitted to electrodes placed on the leg, the change in voltage across two electrodes is measured, and impedance is determined. Graphic display of impedance allows qualitative evaluation of changes in leg volume. With this technique, a sphygmomanometric cuff is placed on the thigh and inflated to a pressure sufficient to impair venous efflux. This maneuver increases the volume in the calf, which is recorded as an upward deflection on the impedance plethysmograph. The cuff is suddenly deflated, and calf volume decreases as blood exits through a patent venous system. The decrease is recorded as a rapid downward deflection on the graphic recorder. The presence of a proximal deep-vein thrombosis results in a basal increase in calf volume. Thus, thigh-cuff inflation causes only a modest increase in calf volume. Furthermore, with abrupt thigh-cuff deflation, the impedance plethysmograph records only a gradual decrease in calf volume. Normal rates of rise during cuff inflation and falls during cuff deflation have been established [170,174–176]. Deviation from the normal values is very suggestive of the presence of a deep-vein thrombosis in proximal veins such as the iliac, common femoral, superficial femoral, or popliteal veins. Deep-vein thrombosis of a calf vein usually is insufficient to affect the volume responses to thigh-cuff inflation and deflation, and therefore it usually is not detected by this technique. For proximal deep-vein thrombosis, both the sensitivity and the specificity of impedance plethysmography have been estimated at approximately 90 percent [170].

IODINE-125 FIBRINOGEN SCANNING

Iodine-125 fibrinogen scanning is included in this section because of its special role in diagnosing deep-vein thrombosis. The basis for this test is the fact that fibrinogen is incorporated into a propagating thrombus. Thus, if fibrinogen is marked with a radioisotope, its incorporation into a thrombus can be detected by a nuclear scanning device.

With this technique, 100 microcuries (μCi) of iodine-125 fibrinogen is administered to patients suspected of having deep-vein thrombosis. Prior to the administration of iodine-125 fibrinogen, patients receive a potassium iodide solution (100 mg) orally to block thyroidal uptake of the radioisotope. Potassium iodide should be given daily for 2 weeks. The legs are divided into 7- to 10-cm sections and marked accordingly. Scanning is performed and isotope counts are recorded over the heart and each of the marked areas. Scanning is repeated on a daily basis for several days. The radiolabeled fibrinogen is incorporated into a propagating thrombus, usually within 24 to 72 hours following isotope administration. At that time, the scanning device detects an increase in count over the involved area. Typically, a 20-percent increase in isotope counts, compared to the corresponding site on the other leg, is required to make the diagnosis of deep-vein thrombosis.

In contrast to the other noninvasive tests used to evaluate venous disease, iodine-125 fibrinogen scanning has been particularly useful in diagnosing calf-vein thrombosis. The sensitivity and the specificity of this technique in patients with calf-vein thrombosis approximate 80 and 75 percent, respectively [170,177–179]. The test has been less useful in very proximal deep-vein thrombosis because the large blood volume in the proximal part of the thigh may give falsely high counts. False-positive tests may be caused by inflammation, hematoma, superficial-vein thrombosis, or venous varicosities. Some centers use iodine-125 fibrinogen scanning as a complement to another technique, such as impedance plethysmography, to examine the entire leg for proximal and distal deep-vein thrombosis.

Iodine-125 fibrinogen scanning has several limitations. First, it may take several days before the test becomes positive, which means that anticoagulant treatment must be withheld for that period of time. Anticoagulant therapy would prevent thrombus propagation and thereby limit incorporation of the radiolabeled fibrinogen into a venous thrombus. Second, it is a somewhat tedious technique to perform. Third, it requires familiarity with radiopharmaceuticals. Finally, its only advantage over other noninvasive tests is that it is more sensitive for diagnosing calf-vein thrombosis. Although the issue remains controversial, many physicians elect to withhold anticoagulant therapy in patients with isolated calf-vein thrombosis because the incidence of pulmonary embolism from that site is low. Those physicians prefer to follow the patients with serial examination until evidence of proximal deep-vein thrombosis develops or until sufficient time passes to assure them that proximal propagation has not occurred. For those reasons, the majority of noninvasive vascular laboratories do not use iodine-125 fibrinogen scanning as a routine noninvasive test to diagnose deep-vein thrombosis.

VENOUS ULTRASOUND

Venous ultrasound studies employ duplex ultrasonographic equipment. Because the veins of the lower extremity can be quite deep, a 5-MHz probe is used to permit deeper penetration. Venous ultrasound has been shown to be very sensitive and specific in diagnosing proximal deep-vein thrombosis [180–186]. In most series, sensitivity and specificity range from 90 to 100%.

The principal criteria for the diagnosis of deep-vein thromboses by ultrasound include (1) failure of the vein to collapse on direct compression, (2) visualization of thrombus within the lumen (Plate 4), and (3) an absent or abnormal Doppler shift signal from the vein. Of the three, noncompressibility of a vein when the examiner applies direct pressure with the probe has proved to be the most reliable finding for identifying deep venous thromboses [187,188] (Fig. 19-15).

The study of the lower extremities begins at the level of the groin crease. Proximal veins lie deep in the pelvis and cannot be reliably studied with high-resolution ultrasound. Scanning is done in the short-axis projection. Deep veins and arteries lie together in the leg. Usually, each leg has only a single common femoral, deep femoral, superficial femoral, and popliteal vein. The calf veins are paired. Two veins travel with each of the three major arteries present in the calf. In addition, a superficial venous network and numerous penetrating veins connect the superficial and deep systems. The normal vein appears as an echo-free channel. It usually is larger than the accompanying artery and has typical venous pulsations. These pulsations may be obvious on inspection alone; if not, the Doppler sample volume can be placed in the visualized vessel and the flow pattern studied to determine whether the vessel is an artery or a vein. The probe is held lightly on the skin and advanced along the course of the vein. Every few centimeters, pressure is applied by compressing the transducer head against the skin. If no thrombus is present, the vein appears to collapse. The diagnosis of deep-vein thrombosis is suggested if the vein fails to collapse [188]. The vein must collapse completely; partial or nearly complete collapse may occur when very early or nonocclusive thrombus is present. If the examiner is uncertain as to whether sufficient pressure is being applied, two additional tests are helpful. First, if the pressure required to collapse the vein results in distortion of the accompanying artery, the study is probably abnormal and consistent with deep-vein thrombosis. Second, the opposite leg can be used as a control, since deep-vein thrombosis is seldom a bilateral process. In acute deep-vein thrombosis, the size of the involved vein increases markedly. The opposite side can be used for comparison. Identification of thrombus in a vein is diagnostic of deep-vein thrombosis [183], but that finding is rare. Thrombus, par-

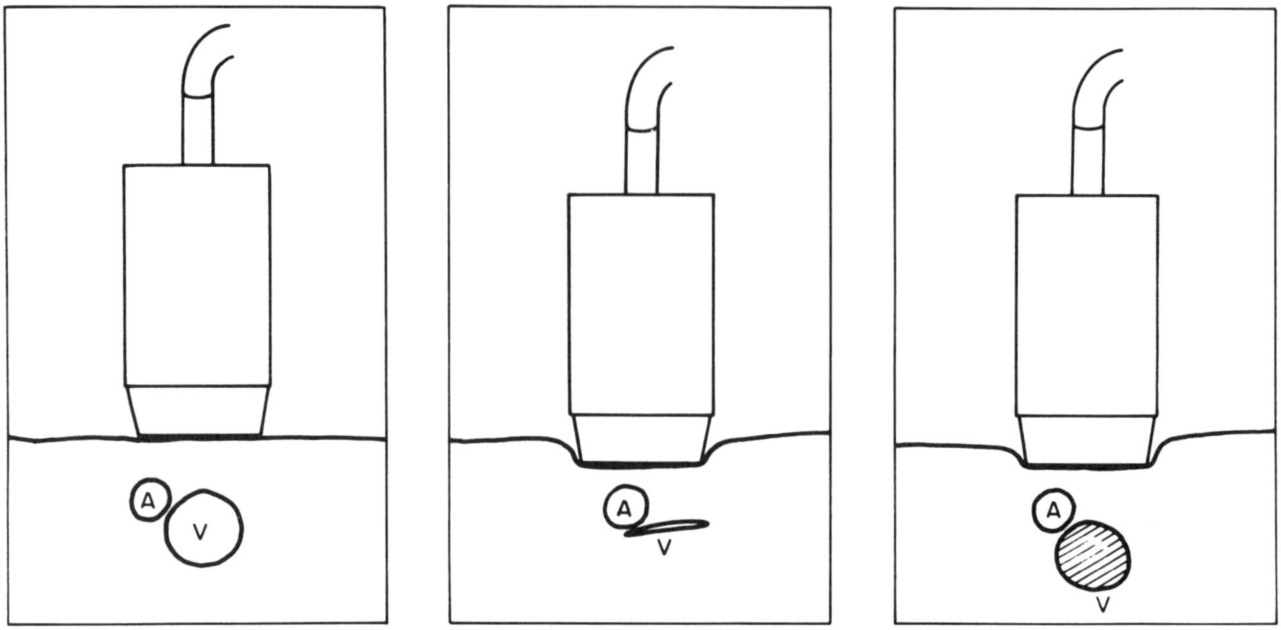

Fig. 19-15. B-mode ultrasound illustrating a normal vein prior to direct compression (left) and after direct compression (center). The vein collapses readily with compression. A thrombosed vein does not collapse during the compression maneuver (right).

ticularly fresh thrombus, often is isoechoic to flowing blood and thus cannot be distinguished from it. Nonocclusive thrombus adjacent to flowing blood is easier to visualize than is total occlusive thrombus, where the echo pattern is uniform across the entire vessel (see Plate 4). The absence of a Doppler signal from a vessel supports the presence of thrombus. Color Doppler examination is helpful in that regard, because flow is not visualized in the thrombosed vein.

Duplex ultrasonography, though extremely sensitive and specific for proximal deep-vein thrombosis, is not as predictive for calf-vein thrombosis [189]. Color Doppler testing, however, has aided in extending the examination to the calf level [190,191]. The vessels there are small and difficult to distinguish from other structures. The color Doppler examination permits rapid identification of the anterior and posterior tibial arteries and the peroneal artery. The veins then can be located because they lie in close proximity. Even when veins are not visualized, their patency can be assessed using augmentation maneuvers, such as calf compression, to increase venous flow that can be visualized by the color Doppler.

Venous ultrasonography may enable discrimination between acute and chronic deep-vein thrombosis. With chronic deep-vein thrombosis, the walls of the vein may be thickened and the transverse diameter of the involved segment may be small; there also may be a pattern of increased echoes within the lumen. With chronic deep-vein thrombosis, extensive collateral channels develop, which can be misinterpreted as normal deep veins. That error can be avoided by remembering that the major veins run parallel to the arteries. If no accompanying artery is found, the likelihood that the vessel is a collateral vein is increased. A collateral channel tends to be tortuous and irregular in its course. When a collateral is suspected, the artery at that level of the leg should be identified and a search undertaken for an accompanying thrombosed vein.

Venous ultrasound has proved to be a highly accurate method of identifying deep-vein thrombosis from the level of the common femoral vein at the groin crease to the popliteal vein. Improved resolution of imaging devices and color Doppler is expanding the utility of this technique to study calf veins. Venous ultrasound also can be employed to study the venous system of the upper extremities and the neck. It also can be used for other studies of the venous system, including venous mapping prior to grafting and assessment of venous competence. Because the technique is relatively easy to learn, and because it complements existing physiologic tests, venous ultrasound has become the most widely used test in the noninvasive vascular laboratory to diagnose deep-vein thrombosis.

CHRONIC VENOUS DISORDERS

Chronic venous insufficiency may occur as a consequence of deep-vein thrombosis or incompetence of venous valves. Following an episode of deep-vein thrombosis, the valve leaflets become thickened and shortened, and the vein wall becomes somewhat rigid. Those changes impair the vein's ability to prevent retrograde flow of blood. Furthermore, although many veins recanalize after an episode of thrombosis, large proximal veins may remain occluded. Several noninvasive tests are used to determine the underlying cause of chronic venous insufficiency. Duplex ultrasonography can be used to diagnose chronic venous occlusion as well as valvular incompetence. The thickened vein wall can be visualized by high-resolution B-mode imaging. Venous collaterals also can be visualized by this technique. Furthermore, the use of color Doppler ultrasound is useful in assessing the direction of blood flow in the veins during selected maneuvers. For example, a Valsalva maneuver or manual compression of the extremity should not result in retrograde venous flow if the valves are intact and functioning normally. In the presence of deep-vein valvular incompetence, retrograde venous flow occurs during those maneuvers. The precise location of the abnormal valves can be detected if each maneuver is repeated as the venous system is mapped with the ultrasound probe. If an imaging system is not available, a reasonable assessment of valvular incompetence can be made with continuous-wave Doppler ultrasound. The probe is placed over the common femoral, superficial femoral, or popliteal vein. Valsalva and proximal compression maneuvers are repeated, and the presence of regurgitant flow is assessed either audibly or by a graphic recorder.

Doppler ultrasound and plethysmographic techniques can be used to detect incompetence in the perforating veins [192–197], which are communicating veins that connect the superficial and deep venous systems. Ultrasound can detect the direction of blood flow in the perforating veins during selected maneuvers, such as proximal compression. Plethysmographic techniques also have been used to map the presence and extent of incompetent perforating veins.

Both strain-gauge plethysmography and photoplethysmography have been used to assess the presence and the severity of chronic venous insufficiency [193–195]. The strain-gauge or photoelectric probe is placed near the ankle. The patient is then requested to exercise by, for example, plantar-flexing the foot repeatedly. Following cessation of exercise, restoration of venous volume occurs sooner in patients with venous insufficiency than in normal individuals. To identify the specific location of incompetent perforating veins, this test can be repeated as a tourniquet is applied along sequential sites of the leg. The tourniquet prevents the superficial venous system from contributing to an abnormal response, enabling the examiner to identify the level of incompetent perforating veins.

Varicose veins are classified as primary or secondary. Primary varicose veins originate in the superficial system; secondary varicose veins may occur either as a consequence of deep venous insufficiency and incompetent perforating veins or from chronic deep venous occlusion. The noninvasive tests described here may be helpful in distinguishing primary from secondary varicose veins [192–194]. Deep venous insufficiency caused by valvular incompetence as well as chronic deep venous occlusive disease can be assessed by those techniques. The presence of incompetent perforating veins may be determined by Doppler ultrasound or plethysmographic techniques. Thus, noninvasive tests can exclude disorders of the deep venous system. In addition, the superficial veins can be studied by using ultrasound techniques in a manner similar to that described for the deep system. The direction of flow in the superficial venous system can be determined with maneuvers such as Valsalva and proximal compression [192,196]. Retrograde flow suggests superficial venous valvular incompetence. Furthermore, improved resolution with B-mode imaging devices makes possible the mapping of the presence and the extent of superficial venous varicosities.

References

1. Doppler C. Über das farbige Licht der Doppelsterne und einiger anderer Gestirne des Himmels. Prague: Abhandlinger der königlichen böhmischer Gesellschaft der Wissenschafter, 1843. Pp. 465–482.
2. Buys Ballot CHD. Akustische Versuche auf der Niederländischen Eisenbahn nebst gelegentlichen Bemerkungen zur Theorie des Hrn. Prof. Doppler. Pogg Ann 1845; 66:321.
3. Greene ER, Eldridge MW, Voyles WF. Quantitative evaluation of atherosclerosis using Doppler ultrasound. In MG Bond, et al. eds. Clinical Diagnosis of Atherosclerosis. New York: Springer, 1983. Pp. 139–168.
4. Strandness DE, Bell JW. Peripheral vascular disease: diagnosis and objective evaluation using a strain-gauge. Ann Surg[Suppl] 1965; 161:1.
5. McLeod FD Jr. A directional Doppler flowmeter. In Digest of the Seventh International Conference of Medical and Biological Engineering. Uppsala: Almquist & Wiksell, 1967. P. 213.
6. Wells PNT. Basic principles and Doppler physics. In KJW Taylor, PN Burns, PNT Wells, eds. Clinical Applications of Doppler Ultrasound. New York: Raven, 1988. Pp. 1–25.
7. Satormura S. Study of the flow patterns in peripheral arteries by ultrasonics. J Acoust Soc Japan 1959; 15:151.
8. Blackshear WM, et al. Carotid artery velocity patterns in normal and stenotic vessels. Stroke 1980; 11:67–71.
9. Merritt CRB. Doppler color flow imaging. J Clin Ultrasound 1987; 15:591–597.
10. Zierler RE, et al. Noninvasive assessment of normal carotid bifurcation hemodynamics with color-flow ultrasound imaging. Ultrasound Med Biol 1987; 13:471–476.
11. Baker D. Applications of pulsed Doppler techniques. Radiol Clin N Am 1980; 18:79–103.
12. Waag RC, Gramick R. Ultrasound basics. In R Gramick, RC Waag, eds. Cardiac Ultrasound. St Louis: Mosby, 1975. Pp. 1–18.
13. Middleton WD, Foley WD, Lawson TL. Color-flow Doppler imaging of carotid artery abnormalities. AJR 1988; 150: 419–425.
14. Zwiebel WJ, et al. Correlation of peak Doppler frequency with lumen narrowing in carotid stenosis. Stroke 1982; 13:386–391.
15. Kremkau FW. Diagnostic Ultrasound: Principles and Instruments, 4th ed. Philadelphia: Saunders, 1993.
16. Hyman C, Winsor T. History of plethysmography. J Cardiovasc Surg 1961; 2:506.
17. Whitney RJ. Measurement of volume changes in human limbs. J Physiol (Lond) 1953; 121:1.
18. Hokanson DE, Sumner DS, Strandness DE Jr. An electrically calibrated plethysmograph for direct measurement of blood flow. IEEE Trans Biomed Eng 1975; 22:25.
19. Cranley JJ. Phleborheography. R I Med J 1975; 58:111–120.
20. Barendsen GJ. Plethysmography. In MD Verstraete, ed. Methods in Angiology. The Hague: Martinus Nijhoff Publishers, 1980. Pp. 38–92.
21. Schabauer AMA, Rooke TW. Cutaneous laser Doppler flowmetry: Applications and findings. Mayo Clin Proc 1994; 69:564–575.
22. Kroeker EJ, Wood EH. Beat-to-beat alterations in relationship of simultaneously recorded central and peripheral arterial

pressure pulses during Valsalva maneuver and prolonged expiration in man. J Appl Physiol 1956; 8:483.
23. Young DF, Cholvin NR, Roth AC. Pressure drop across artificially induced stenoses in the femoral artery of dogs. Circ Res 1975; 36:735–743.
24. Schultz RD, Hokanson DE, Strandness DE Jr. Pressure-flow and stress-strain measurements of normal and diseased aortoiliac segments. Surg Gynecol Obstet 1967; 124:1267–1276.
25. Flanigan DP, et al. Multiple subcritical stenoses. Ann Surg 1977; 186:663–668.
26. Newman DL, Walesby RK, Bowden NLR. Hemodynamic effects of acute experimental aortic coarctation in the dog. Circ Res 1975; 36:165–172.
27. Thulesius O. Principles of pressure measurement. In EF Bernstein, ed. Noninvasive Diagnostic Techniques in Vascular Disease. St. Louis: Mosby, 1985. Pp. 79–82.
28. Perloff D, et al. Human blood pressure determination by sphygmomanometry. Circulation 1993; 88:2460–2467.
29. Riva-Rocci S. Un nuovo sfigmomanometro. Gaz Med Torino 1896; 47:981.
30. Korotkoff NS. On the subject of methods of measuring blood pressure. Bull Imp Mil Med Acad 1905; 11:365.
31. Glagov S, Zarins CK. Quantitating atherosclerosis: problems of definition. In MG Bond, et al., eds. Clinical Diagnosis of Atherosclerosis. New York: Springer, 1983. Pp. 11–35.
32. Pignoli P, et al. Intimal plus medial thickness of the arterial wall: a direct measurement with ultrasound imaging. Circulation 1986; 74:1399–1406.
33. Wolverson MK, et al. Carotid atherosclerosis: high resolution real-time sonography correlated with angiography. AJR 1983; 40:355–361.
34. Poli A, et al. Ultrasonographic measurement of the common carotid artery wall thickness in hypercholesterolemic patients. A new model for the quantitation and follow-up of preclinical atherosclerosis in living human beings. Atherosclerosis 1988; 70:253–261.
35. O'Leary DH, et al. Use of sonography to evaluate carotid atherosclerosis in the elderly: The Cardiovascular Health Study. Stroke 1991; 22:1155–1163.
36. Salonen R, et al. Prevalence of carotid atherosclerosis and serum cholesterol levels in Eastern Finland. Arteriosclerosis 1988; 8:788–792.
37. Edwards JH, et al. Atherosclerotic subintimal hematoma of the carotid artery. Radiology 1979; 133:123–129.
38. Imparato AM, Riles TS, Gorstein F. The carotid bifurcation plaque: pathologic findings associated with cerebral ischemia. Stroke 1979; 10:238–245.
39. Lusby RJ, et al. Carotid plaque hemorrhage: its role in production of cerebral ischemia. Arch Surg 1982; 117:1479–1488.
40. Reilly LM, et al. Carotid plaque histology using real-time ultrasonography: clinical and therapeutic implications. Am J Surg 1983; 146:188–193.
41. O'Donnell TF Jr, et al. Correlation of B-mode ultrasound imaging and arteriography with pathologic findings at carotid endarterectomy. Arch Surg 1985; 120:443–449.
42. Bluth EI, et al. Sonographic characterization of carotid plaque: detection of hemorrhage. AJR 1986; 146:1061–1065.
43. O'Leary DH, et al. Carotid bifurcation disease: prediction of ulceration with B-mode ultrasound. Radiology 1987; 162: 523–525.
44. Leahy AL, et al. Duplex ultrasonography and the selection of patients for carotid endarterectomy: plaque morphology or luminal narrowing? J Vasc Surg 1988; 8:558–562.
45. Bassiouny HS, et al. Critical carotid stenosis: morphologic and chemical similarity between symptomatic and asymptomatic plaques. J Vasc Surg 1989; 9:202–212.
46. Aaslid R, Markwalder TM, Nornes H. Noninvasive transcranial Doppler ultrasound recording of flow velocity in basal cerebral arteries. J Neurosurg 1982; 57:769–774.
47. Aaslid R. Transcranial Doppler sonography. New York, Springer, 1986. P. 57.
48. Martin PJ, Evans DH, Naylor AR. Transcranial color-induced sonography of the basal cerebral circulation. Reference data from 115 volunteers. Stroke 1994; 25:390–396.
49. Rorick MB, Nichols PT, Adams RJ. Transcranial Doppler correlates with angiography in detection of intracranial stenosis. Stroke 1994; 25:1931–1934.
50. Seiler RW, et al. Cerebral vasospasm evaluated by transcranial ultrasound correlated with clinical grade and CT-visualized subarachnoid hemorrhage. J Neurosurg 1986; 64:594–600.
51. Steiner E, et al. Sonographic examination of the abdominal aorta through the left flank: a prospective study. J Ultrasound Med 1986; 5:499–502.
52. Gomes MN. Clinical and surgical aspects of abdominal aortic aneurysms. Sem Ultrasound 1982; 3:156.
53. Yucel EK, et al. Sonographic measurement of abdominal aortic diameter: Interobserver variability. J Ultrasound Med 1991; 10:681–683.
54. Amparo EG, et al. Comparison of magnetic resonance imaging and ultrasonography in the evaluation of abdominal aortic aneurysms. Radiology 1985; 154:451–456.
55. Eriksson I, Hemmingsson A, Lindgren PG. Diagnosis of abdominal aortic aneurysms by aortography, computer tomography, and ultrasound. Acta Radiol Diagn 1980; 21:209–214.
56. Harter LP, et al. Ultrasonographic evaluation of abdominal aortic thrombus. J Ultrasound Med 1982; 1:315–318.
57. Anderson JC, Baltaxe HA, Wolf GL. Inability to show clot: one limitation of ultrasound of the abdominal aorta. Radiology 1979; 132:693–696.
58. Clayton MJ, Walsh JW, Brewer WH. Contained rupture of abdominal aortic aneurysms: sonographic and CT diagnosis. AJR 1982; 138:154–156.
59. Cullenward MJ, et al. Inflammatory aortic aneurysm (periaortic fibrosis): radiologic imaging. Radiology 1986; 159:75–82.
60. Gooding GAW. Aneurysms of the abdominal aorta, iliac, and femoral arteries. Sem Ultrasound 1982; 3:170.
61. Conrad MR, et al. Real-time ultrasound in diagnosis of acute dissecting aneurysm of the abdominal aorta. AJR 1979; 132:115–116.
62. Dee P, Granato JE, Gibson RS. The CT and ultrasound diagnosis of aortic aneurysm. Sem US, CT, MR 1985; 6:146.
63. King PS, Cooperberg PL, Madigan SM. The anechoic crescent in abdominal aortic aneurysms: not a sign of dissection. AJR 1986; 146:345–348.
64. Herzler GM, et al. Celiac artery aneurysm: ultrasonic diagnosis. J Clin Ultrasound 1981; 9:141–143.
65. Athey PA, et al. Sonography in the diagnosis of hepatic artery aneurysms. AJR 1986; 147:725–727.
66. Warshauer DM, Keefe B, Mauro MA. Intrahepatic hepatic artery aneurysm: computed tomography and color-flow Doppler ultrasound findings. Gastrointest Radiol 1991; 16:175–177.
67. Derchi LE, et al. Aneurysms of the splenic artery: noninvasive diagnosis by pulsed Doppler sonography. J Ultrasound Med 1984; 3:41–44.
68. Mourad K, Guggiana P, Minasian H. Superior mesenteric artery aneurysm diagnosed by ultrasound. Br J Radiol 1987; 60:287–288.
69. Verma BS, et al. Superior mesenteric artery branch aneurysm diagnosed by ultrasound. Br J Radiol 1991; 64:169–171.
70. Neiman HL, Yao JST, Silver TM. Grey-scale ultrasound diag-

nosis of peripheral arterial aneurysms. Radiology 1979; 130:413–416.

71. Marcus R, Edell SL. Sonographic evaluation of iliac artery aneurysms. Am J Surg 1980; 140:666–670.
72. Baron RL, Banner MP, Pollack HM. Isolated internal iliac artery aneurysms presenting as giant pelvic masses. AJR 1983; 140:784–786.
73. Mitchell DG, et al. Femoral artery pseudoaneurysm: diagnosis with conventional duplex and color Doppler ultrasound. Radiology 1987; 165:687–690.
74. Falkoff GE, Taylor KJ, Morse S. Hepatic artery pseudoaneurysm: diagnosis with real-time and pulsed Doppler ultrasound. Radiology 1986; 158:55–56.
75. Gooding GA. Ultrasound of a superior mesenteric artery aneurysm secondary to pancreatitis: a plea for real-time ultrasound of sonolucent masses in pancreatitis. J Clin Ultrasound 1981; 9:255–256.
76. Olin JW, et al. The utility of duplex ultrasound scanning of the renal arteries for diagnosing significant renal artery stenosis. Ann Int Med 1995; 122:833–838.
77. Greene ER, Avasthi PS, Hodges JW. Noninvasive Doppler assessment of renal artery stenosis and hemodynamics. J Clin Ultrasound 1987; 15:653–659.
78. Taylor DC, et al. Duplex ultrasound scanning in the diagnosis of renal artery stenosis: A prospective evaluation. J Vasc Surg 1988; 7:363–369.
79. Strandness DE. Duplex scanning in diagnosis of renovascular hypertension. Surg Clin North Am 1990; 70:109–117.
80. Berland LL, et al. Renal artery stenosis: prospective evaluation of diagnosis with color duplex as compared with angiography. Radiology 1990; 174:421–423.
81. Desberg AL, et al. Renal artery stenosis: evaluation with color Doppler flow imaging. Radiology 1990; 177:749–753.
82. Middleton WD. Doppler US evaluation of renal artery stenosis: past, present, and future. Radiology 1992; 184:307–308.
83. Lafortune M, et al. Renal arterial stenosis: slowed systole in the downstream circulation—experimental study in dogs. Radiology 1992; 184:475–478.
84. Patriquin HB, et al. Stenosis of the renal artery: assessment of slowed systole in the downstream circulation with Doppler sonography. Radiology 1992; 184:479–485.
85. Stavros AT, et al. Segmental stenosis of the renal artery: pattern recognition of tardus and parvus abnormalities with duplex sonography. Radiology 1992; 184:487–492.
86. Schwerk WB, et al. Renal artery stenosis: grading with image-directed Doppler US evaluation of renal resistive index. Radiology 1994; 190:785–790.
87. Kliewer MA, et al. Renal artery stenosis: analysis of Doppler waveform parameters and tardus-parvus pattern. Radiology 1993; 189:779–787.
88. Moneta GL, et al. Duplex ultrasound measurement of postprandial intestinal blood flow: effect of meal composition. Gastroenterology 1988; 95:1294–1301.
89. Rizzo RJ, et al. Mesenteric flow velocity variations as a function of angle of insonation. J Vasc Surg 1990; 11:688–694.
90. Perko MJ, Sven J. Duplex ultrasonography of superior mesenteric artery: interobserver variability. J Ultrasound Med 1993; 5:259–263.
91. Bowersox JC, et al. Duplex ultrasonography in the diagnosis of celiac and mesenteric artery occlusive disease. J Vasc Surg 1991; 14:780–788.
92. Raines JK. The pulse volume recorder in peripheral arterial disease. In EF Bernstein, ed. Noninvasive Diagnostic Techniques in Vascular Disease. St. Louis: Mosby, 1985. Pp. 563–574.
93. Raines JK, et al. Vascular laboratory criteria for the management of peripheral vascular disease of the lower extremities. Surgery 1976; 79:21–29.
94. Kempczinski RF, Rutherford RB. Current status of the vascular diagnostic laboratory. Adv Surg 1978; 12:1–52.
95. Kempczinski, RF. Segmental volume plethysmography in the diagnosis of lower extremity arterial occlusive disease. J Cardiovasc Surg (Torino) 1982; 23:125–129.
96. Carter SA. Clinical measurement of systolic pressures in limbs with arterial occlusive disease. JAMA 1969; 207:1869–1874.
97. Thulesius O, Gjores JE. Use of Doppler shift detection for determining peripheral arterial blood pressure. Angiology 1971; 22:594–603.
98. Yao ST, Hobbs JT, Irvine WT. Ankle systolic pressure measurements in arterial disease affecting the lower extremities. Br J Surg 1969; 56:676–679.
99. Taylor MG. Wave travel in arteries and the design of the cardiovascular system. In EO Attinger, ed. Pulsatile Blood Flow. New York: McGraw-Hill, 1964.
100. May AG, et al. Critical arterial stenosis. Surgery 1963; 54:250.
101. Yao ST. Haemodynamic studies in peripheral arterial disease. Br J Surg 1970; 57:761–766.
102. Cutajar CL, Marston A, Newcombe JF. Value of cuff occlusion pressures in assessment of peripheral vascular disease. Br Med J 1973; 2:392–395.
103. Lennihan R Jr, Mackereth MA. Ankle blood pressures as a practical aid in vascular practice. Angiology 1975; 26:211–224.
104. Strandness DE Jr, Bell JW. Peripheral vascular disease: diagnosis and objective evaluation using a mercury strain gauge. Ann Surg 1965; 161[Suppl 4]:1.
105. Carter SA, Lezack JD. Digital systolic pressures in the lower limb in arterial disease. Circulation 1971; 43:905–914.
106. Carter SA. The relationship of distal systolic pressures to healing of skin lesions in limbs with arterial occlusive disease, with special reference to diabetes mellitus. Scand J Clin Lab Invest 1973; 31[Suppl 128]:239–243.
107. Byrne P, et al. The use of transcutaneous oxygen tension measurements in the diagnosis of peripheral vascular insufficiency. Ann Surg 1984; 200:159–165.
108. Rooke TW, Osmundson PJ. The influence of age, sex, smoking, and diabetes on lower limb transcutaneous oxygen tension in patients with arterial occlusive disease. Arch Intern Med 1990; 150:129–132.
109. Bacharach JM, et al. Predictive value of transcutaneous oxygen pressure and amputation success by use of supine and elevation measurements. J Vasc Surg 1992; 15:558–563.
110. Christensen KS, Klarke M. Transcutaneous oxygen measurement in peripheral occlusive disease. An indicator of wound healing in leg amputation. J Bone Joint Surg 1986; 68:423–426.
111. Hauser CJ, Shoemaker WC. Use of transcutaneous PO_2 regional perfusion index to quantify tissue perfusion in peripheral vascular disease. Ann Surg 1983; 197:337–343.
112. Hauser CJ, et al. Superiority of transcutaneous oximetry in noninvasive vascular diagnosis in patients with diabetes. Arch Surg 1984; 119:690–694.
113. Jorfeldt L, Wahren J. Leg blood flow during exercise in man. Clin Sci 1971; 41:459–473.
114. Coffman JD. Intermittent claudication and rest pain: physiologic concepts and therapeutic approaches. Prog Cardiovasc Dis 1979; 22:53–72.
115. Cappelen C Jr, Hall KV. The effect of obstructive arterial disease on the peripheral arterial blood pressure. Surgery 1960; 48:888.
116. King LT, Strandness DE Jr, Bell JW. The hemodynamic response of the lower extremities to exercise. J Surg Res 1965; 5:167.

117. Strandness DE Jr, Bell JW. An evaluation of the hemodynamic response of the claudicating extremity to exercise. Surg Gynecol Obstet 1964; 119:1237.
118. Bruce RA, Kusumi F, Hosmer D. Maximal oxygen intake and nomographic assessment of functional aerobic impairment in cardiovascular disease. Am Heart J 1973; 85:546–562.
119. Patterson JA, et al. Treadmill exercise in assessment of the functional capacity of patients with cardiac disease. Am J Cardiol 1972; 30:757–762.
120. Hiatt WR, et al. The evaluation of exercise performance in patients with peripheral vascular disease. J Cardiopulmonary Rehabil 1988; 12:525–532.
121. Gardner AW, et al. Progressive vs single-stage treadmill tests for evaluation of claudication. Med Sci Sports Exerc 1991; 23:402–408.
122. Goldschlager N, Selzer A, Cohn K. Treadmill stress tests as indication of presence and severity of coronary artery disease. Ann Intern Med 1976; 85:277–286.
123. Dornhorst AC, Sharpey-Schafer EP. Collateral resistance in limbs with arterial obstruction: spontaneous changes and effects of sympathectomy. Clin Sci 1951; 10:371.
124. Johnson WC. Doppler ankle pressure and reactive hyperemia in the diagnosis of arterial insufficiency. J Surg Res 1975; 18:177–180.
125. Keagy BA, et al. Comparison of reactive hyperemia and treadmill tests in the evaluation of peripheral vascular disease. Am J Surg 1981; 142:158–161.
126. Coffman JD, Davies WT. Vasospastic diseases: a review. Prog Cardiovasc Dis 1975; 18:123–146.
127. Fronek A, Coel M, Bernstein EF. The pulse-reappearance time: an index of overall blood flow impairment in the ischemic extremity. Surgery 1977; 81:376–381.
128. Sumner DS. Volume plethysmography in vascular disease: an overview. In EF Bernstein, ed. Noninvasive Diagnostic Techniques in Vascular Disease. St. Louis: Mosby, 1985. Pp. 97–118.
129. Zeuchner J, et al. Angiography and colour flow duplex ultrasonography in the evaluation of peripheral ischaemic occlusive arterial disease. Acta Radiol 1994; 35:270–274.
130. Sacks D, et al. Evaluation of the peripheral arteries with duplex US after angioplasty. Radiology 1990; 176:39 44.
131. Sacks D, et al. Peripheral arterial Doppler ultrasonography: diagnostic criteria. J Ultrasound Med 992; 11:95–103.
132. Vashisht R, et al. Colour-coded duplex ultrasonography in the selection of patients with endovascular surgery. Br J Surg 1992; 79:1030–1031.
133. Mewissen MW, et al. The role of duplex scanning versus angiography in predicting outcome after balloon angioplasty in the femoropopliteal artery. J Vasc Surg 1992; 15:860–866.
134. Moneta GL, et al. Noninvasive localization of arterial occlusive disease: a comparison of segmental Doppler pressures and arterial duplex mapping. J Vasc Surg 1993; 17:578–582.
135. Hatsukami TS, et al. Color Doppler imaging of infrainguinal arterial occlusive disease. J Vasc Surg 1992; 16:527–533.
136. Kohler TR, et al. Duplex scanning for diagnosis of aortoiliac and femoropopliteal disease: a prospective study. Circulation 1987; 76:1074–1080.
137. Cossman DV, et al. Comparison of contrast arteriography to arterial mapping with color-flow duplex imaging in the lower extremities. J Vasc Surg 1989; 10:522–599.
138. Taylor LM, Edward JM, Porter JM. Present status of reversed vein bypass grafting: five-year results of a modern series. J Vasc Surg 1990; 11:193–206.
139. Donaldson MC, Mannick JA, Whittemore AD. Femoro-distal bypass with in situ greater saphenous vein: long-term results using the Mills valvatome. Ann Surg 1991; 213:457–465.
140. Bergamini TM, et al. Experience with in situ saphenous vein bypasses during 1981 to 1989: determinant factors of long-term patency. J Vasc Surg 1991; 13:137–149.
141. Donaldson MC, Mannick JA, Whittemore AD. Causes of primary graft failure after in situ saphenous vein bypass grafting. J Vasc Surg 1992; 15:113–120.
142. Mills JL, et al. The importance of routine surveillance of distal bypass grafts with duplex scanning: a study of 379 reversed vein grafts. J Vasc Surg 1990; 12:379–389.
143. Laborde AL, et al. A prospective comparison of ankle/brachial indices and color duplex imaging in surveillance of the in situ saphenous vein bypass. J Cardiovasc Surg 1992; 33:420–425.
144. Bandyk DF, Cato RF, Towne JB. A low flow velocity predicts failure of femoropopliteal and femorotibial bypass grafts. Surgery 1985; 98:799–809.
145. Polak JF, et al. Determination of the extent of lower-extremity peripheral arterial disease with color-assisted duplex sonography: comparison with angiography. AJR 1990; 155:1085–1089.
146. Robison JG, Elliott BM. Does postoperative surveillance with duplex scanning identify the failing distal bypass? Ann Vasc Surg 1991; 5:182–185.
147. Schmitt DD, et al. Early patency of in situ saphenous vein bypasses as determined by intraoperative velocity waveform analysis. Ann Vasc Surg 1990; 4:270–275.
148. Bandyk DF, et al. Hemodynamics of vein graft stenosis. J Vasc Surg 1988; 8:688–695.
149. Polak JF, et al. Early detection of saphenous vein arterial bypass stenosis by color-assisted duplex sonography: a prospective study. AJR 1990; 154:857–861.
150. Bandyk DF. Essentials of graft surveillance. Semin Vasc Surg 1993; 6:92–102.
151. Bandyk DF, Jorgensen RA, Towne JB. Intraoperative assessment of in situ saphenous vein arterial grafts using pulsed Doppler spectral analysis. Arch Surg 1986; 121:292–299.
152. Bandyk DF, et al. Monitoring functional patency of in situ saphenous vein bypasses: the impact of a surveillance protocol and elective revision. J Vasc Surg 1989; 9:286–296.
153. Buth J, et al. Color-flow duplex criteria for grading stenosis in infrainguinal vein grafts. J Vasc Surg 1992; 14:716–728.
154. Gooding GAW, et al. Lower-extremity vascular grafts placed for peripheral vascular disease: Prospective evaluation with duplex Doppler sonography. Radiology 1991; 180:379–386.
155. Lau CS, et al. Digital blood flow response to body warming, cooling, and rewarming in patients with Raynaud's phenomenon. Angiology 1995; 46:1–10.
156. Thulesius O, Borgnis F, Dvorak T. Analysis of photoplethysmographic pulse curves with electronic derivation. Scand J Clin Lab Invest 1973; 31[Suppl 128]:159–162.
157. Bollinger A, Schlumpf M. Finger blood flow in healthy subjects of different age and sex and in patients with primary Raynaud's disease. Acta Chir Scand[Suppl] 1976; 465:42–47.
158. Hirai M, Nielsen SL, Lassen NA. Blood pressure measurements of all five fingers by strain-gauge plethysmography. Scand J Clin Lab Invest 1976; 36:627–632.
159. Sumner DS. Digital plethysmography. In RB Rutherford, ed. Vascular Surgery, 2nd ed. Philadelphia: Saunders, 1984.
160. Thulesius O. Methods for the evaluation of peripheral vascular function in the upper extremities. Acta Chir Scand[Suppl] 1976; 465:53–54.
161. Hirai M. Arterial insufficiency of the hand evaluated by digital blood pressure and arteriographic findings. Circulation 1978; 58:902–908.
162. Cohen RA, Coffman JD. Reduced fingertip arterial pressures in Raynaud's disease. J Vasc Med Biol 1989; 1:21–26.

163. Cohen RA, Coffman JD. Digital vasospasm: the pathophysiology of Raynaud's phenomenon. Intl Angiol 1984; 3:47.
164. Krahenbuhl B, Nielsen SL, Lassen NA. Closure of digital arteries in high vascular tone states as demonstrated by measurement of systolic blood pressure in the fingers. Scand J Clin Lab Invest 1977; 37:71–76.
165. Nielsen SL, Lassen NA. Measurement of digital blood pressure after local cooling. J Appl Physiol: 1977; 43:907–910.
166. Hoare M, et al. The effect of local cooling on digital systolic pressure in patients with Raynaud's syndrome. Br J Surg 1982; 69[Suppl]:S27–S28.
167. Corbin DOC, Wood DA, Housley E. An evaluation of finger systolic-pressure response to local cooling in the diagnosis of primary Raynaud's phenomenon. Clin Physiol 1985; 5:383–392.
168. Carter SA, Dean E, Kroeger EA. Apparent finger systolic pressures during cooling in patients with Raynaud's syndrome. Circulation 1988; 77:988–996.
169. Coffman JD, Cohen AS. Total and capillary fingertip blood flow in Raynaud's phenomenon. N Engl J Med 1971; 285:259–263.
170. Hirsh J, Genten E, Hull R. Venous Thromboembolism. New York: Grune & Stratton, 1981. Pp. 234–318.
171. Evans DS. The early diagnosis of deep-vein thrombosis by ultrasound. Br J Surg 1970; 57:726–728.
172. Barnes RW, et al. Accuracy of Doppler ultrasound in clinically suspected venous thrombosis of the calf. Surg Gynecol Obstet 1976; 143:425–428.
173. Lindqvist R. Ultrasound as a complementary diagnostic method in deep vein thrombosis of the leg. Acta Med Scand 1977; 201:435–438.
174. Hull R, et al. Impedance plethysmography using the occlusive cuff technique in the diagnosis of venous thrombosis. Circulation 1976; 53:696–700.
175. Hull R, et al. Impedance plethysmography: the relationship between venous filling and sensitivity and specificity for proximal vein thrombosis. Circulation 1978; 58:898–902.
176. Wheeler HB, et al. Occlusive impedance phlebography: a diagnostic procedure for venous thrombosis and pulmonary embolism. Prog Cardiovasc Dis 1974; 17:199–205.
177. Browse NL, et al. Diagnosis of established deep vein thrombosis with the ^{125}I-fibrinogen uptake test. Br Med J 1971; 4:325–328.
178. Kakkar VV, Nicolaides AN, Renney JTG. ^{125}I-labelled fibrinogen test adapted for routine screening for deep vein thrombosis. Lancet 1970; 1:540–542.
179. Hirsh J, Gallus AS. ^{125}I-labelled fibrinogen scanning: use in the diagnosis of venous thrombosis. JAMA 1975; 233:970–973.
180. Polak JF. Peripheral Vascular Sonography: A Practical Guide. Baltimore: Williams & Wilkins, 1992. Pp. 155–214.
181. O'Leary DH, Kane RA, Chase BA. A prospective study of the efficacy of B-scan sonography in the detection of deep venous thrombosis in the lower extremities. J Clin Ultrasound 1988; 16:1–8.
182. Lensing AW, et al. Detection of deep-vein thrombosis by real-time B-mode ultrasonography. N Engl J Med 1989; 320:342–345.
183. Sullivan ED, Peter DJ, Cranley JJ. Real-time B-mode venous ultrasound. J Vasc Surg 1984; 1:465–471.
184. White RH, et al. Diagnosis of deep-vein thrombosis using duplex ultrasound. Ann Int Med 1989; 111:297–304.
185. Heijboer H, et al. A comparison of real-time compression ultrasonography with impedance plethysmography for the diagnosis of deep-vein thrombosis in symptomatic outpatients. N Engl J Med 1993; 329:1365–1369.
186. Rose SC, et al. Symptomatic lower extremity deep venous thrombosis: accuracy, limitations, and role of color duplex flow imaging in diagnosis. Radiology 1990; 175:639–644.
187. Dauzat MM, et al. Real-time B-mode ultrasonography for better specificity in the noninvasive diagnosis of deep venous thrombosis. J Ultrasound Med 1986; 5:625–631.
188. Raghavendra BN, et al. Deep venous thrombosis: detection by probe compression of veins. J Ultrasound Med 1986; 5:89–95.
189. Cronan JJ, Dorfman GS, Grusmark J. Lower extremity deep venous thrombosis: further experience with and refinements of ultrasound assessment. Radiology 1988; 168:101–107.
190. Polak JF, Cutler SS, O'Leary DH. Deep veins of the calf: assessment with color Doppler flow imaging. Radiology 1989; 171:481–486.
191. Simons GR, et al. Utility of leg ultrasonography in suspected symptomatic isolated calf deep venous thrombosis. Am J Med 1995; 99:43–47.
192. van Bemmelen PS, et al. Quantitative segmental evaluation of venous valvular reflux with duplex ultrasound scanning. J Vasc Surg 1989; 10:425–431.
193. Folse R, Alexander RH. Directional flow detection for localizing venous valvular incompetency. Surgery 1970; 67:114–121.
194. Abramowitz HB, et al. The use of photoplethysmography in the assessment of venous insufficiency: a comparison to venous pressure measurements. Surgery 1979; 86:434–441.
195. Barnes RW, et al. Noninvasive quantitation of venous reflux in the postphlebitic syndrome. Surg Gynecol Obstet 1973; 136:769–773.
196. Barnes RW, Ross EA, Strandness DE. Differentiation of primary from secondary varicose veins by Doppler ultrasound and strain gauge plethysmography. Surg Gynecol Obstet 1975; 141:207–211.
197. Tibbs DJ, Fletcher EWL. Direction of flow in superficial veins as a guide to venous disorders in lower limbs. Surgery 1983; 93:758–767.

Magnetic Resonance Imaging of Vascular Disease

Joseph F. Polak
Mary K. Adamis
Mahesh R. Patel

The use of magnetic fields for the evaluation of blood flow is not a new concept. First introduced in the mid 1950s, electromagnetic flowmeters are still in use today. These devices measure the induced current caused by blood moving perpendicular to an applied magnetic field. The magnitude of the induced current is proportional to the flow rate of blood through a vessel [1].

Today, magnetic fields are used quite differently for the noninvasive evaluation of the vascular tree. Magnetic resonance imaging was born in 1973, when Lauterbur showed that two-dimensional imaging could be performed on a living object placed in a highly homogeneous magnetic field. That technique, referred to as zeumatography, uses appropriately superimposed magnetic field gradients [2] to create an image and has led to a plethora of imaging algorithms that are still evolving and increasing in complexity and numbers. Magnetic resonance imaging can provide anatomic detail of the major and medium-sized vessels. It also can be used to depict blood flow in various arteries and veins.

Magnetic resonance also can be used to detect the effects of vascular disease on the metabolism of end organs by phosphorus-31 (P-31) spectroscopy. Evolving from early in-vitro work in the late 1970s, this technique is being investigated with a view to achieving true in-vivo mapping of P-31 and its metabolites [3]. Magnetic resonance spectroscopy can detect and grade energy-source depletion in end organs secondary to a decreased delivery of nutrients and sequentially monitor end-organ function during therapy. The technique remains investigational, however, and is not part of routine clinical practice. This chapter will concentrate mainly on vascular imaging by proton nuclear magnetic resonance (NMR) techniques. P-31 spectroscopy will be discussed only briefly.

Principles of Instrumentation

NONIMAGING

The electromagnetic flowmeter uses magnetic fields to monitor blood flow [1], which is of historic interest since the principle used to measure flowing blood is quite different from that used in magnetic resonance imaging. The electromagnetic flowmeter measures the current induced by blood flowing between the poles of a magnet (Fig. 20-1). The motion of the blood in the field causes a change in current or voltage, which is subsequently measured with electrodes. The measurement is invasive, requiring exposure of the vessel being imaged. In magnetic resonance imaging or spectroscopy, it is not an induced electric current that is detected but rather the radio frequency (RF) waves emitted subsequent to the excitation of nuclei (protons) placed in a highly homogeneous magnetic field. The technique, therefore, is inherently noninvasive.

A brief review of the electromagnetic spectrum quickly situates the energy range of the RF waves used in magnetic resonance with respect to the frequencies used for vision and for radiographic examinations in general. The wavelengths involved are quite large (Fig. 20-2). For example, a frequency of 64 MHz, which is currently used for body imaging at 1.5 tesla, corresponds to a wavelength of a few meters, which is in sharp contrast to the submicron wavelengths used in standard radiography. The difference in wavelengths, in part, distinguishes magnetic resonance techniques from other radiologic imaging approaches. In general, radiography and radionuclide-emission scanning rely on protons either emitted or attenuated by tissues in the body. The major physical parameter being measured is electron density, as related to atomic number and tissue density. The transmitted (radiography) or emitted (radionuclide scanning) protons are collimated and either captured on film or detected by a gamma camera. In the case of NMR, RF waves permeate the object, and the actual frequency of the wave holds information as to the location of a group of photons placed in a magnetic field. These RF waves cannot be collimated and, as such, cannot be mapped on a RF–sensitive emulsion. Their location must be decoded using more sophisticated mathematic techniques. The magnetic spin properties of the nuclei of interest are responsible for the signals being detected.

A basic understanding of the principles behind magnetic resonance imaging can be achieved using either the classic or the quantum mechanic approach. When a patient is placed in a magnetic field, a very small number of the nuclei in the tissues—in essence, hydrogen protons—line up with the magnetic field. The protons try to attain a minimal energy configuration, with some aligning parallel, others antiparallel, to the applied field (Fig. 20-3). This quantum mechanic explanation can be extended to explain the NMR effect by the following: When an RF wave is matched to the difference in energy levels of the aligned protons, a transition can occur. In essence, a small number of those protons increase their energy level and are then capable of reemitting the energy they have absorbed. This reemitted energy is detected and permits magnetic resonance imaging.

The classic model of nuclear magnetic resonance imaging allows an intuitive understanding of the physical principles involved. The nuclei themselves can be viewed as spinning tops. The influence of the magnetic field on the nucleus is similar to the influence of gravity on a spinning top. The nuclei precess, or turn about, the main magnetic field. The frequency of their precession defines the RF that is necessary to excite them. If two distant nuclei under the influence of a magnetic gradient are at slightly different precession frequencies, the RF necessary to modify the motion of either spinning top is also slightly

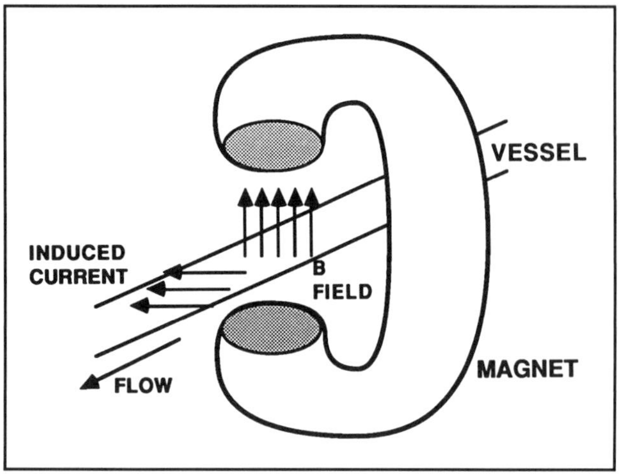

Fig. 20-1. How an electromagnetic flowmeter works. The two magnet poles are positioned on both sides of the vessel to be studied. The flowing blood is a conductor; as it crosses the magnetic lines, an electric current proportional to blood flow is induced. Once calibrated, the device can measure changes in blood flow with an accuracy of 5 to 10 percent.

different (Fig. 20-4). The relationship between the rate at which a nucleus spins and the applied (external) magnetic field is called the **gyromagnetic ratio**. For a given nucleus, it relates the frequency of precession (Larmor frequency) to the magnetic field strength.

What happens when an RF wave is used to excite nuclei (protons) in the magnetic field? If an RF wave of the appropriate value is turned on for a short amount of time, the protons start changing their relative angle of precession with respect to the main magnetic field. As long as this RF is turned on, the angle of the spinning top or proton continues to change with respect to the main magnetic field. For example, if the RF is turned on for an amount of time, T_A, the protons will change their orientation relative to the main field by a corresponding angle, α. The rate of precession is not affected. If the length of the radio-frequency exposure is doubled, then twice as much angular displacement results (Fig. 20-5). Similarly, multiples of T_A will result in multiples of angular displacement. In the true physical sense, this is an ideal situation since dissipative processes make the actual linear correspondence between length of RF excitation and actual angular displacement inaccurate for longer-duration RF excitations (longer RF-pulse duration).

In NMR imaging, many factors are responsible for the signal strengths originating from tissues. First and most important, the amplitude of detected signals depend on the relative amount of protons. The tissue concentration of hydrogen is approximately 80 M, whereas the concentration of phosphorus-31 is, at most, in the millimolar range. Second, the rate at which protons excited by an RF pulse return to their equilibrium position is variable. Two mechanisms are responsible for this effect. The first, commonly referred to as T_1, or spin lattice relaxation, causes

Fig. 20-2. One of the fundamental differences between magnetic resonance and other diagnostic imaging techniques can be appreciated in this diagram of the electromagnetic spectrum. Because the wavelengths in magnetic resonance are so large, they cannot be effectively collimated and used to directly map the density or other equivalent characteristics of body tissues. The location of radiofrequency signals must be ascertained by a completely different mechanism, that is, by encoding the spatial characteristics of the resonant protons by local magnetic field changes.

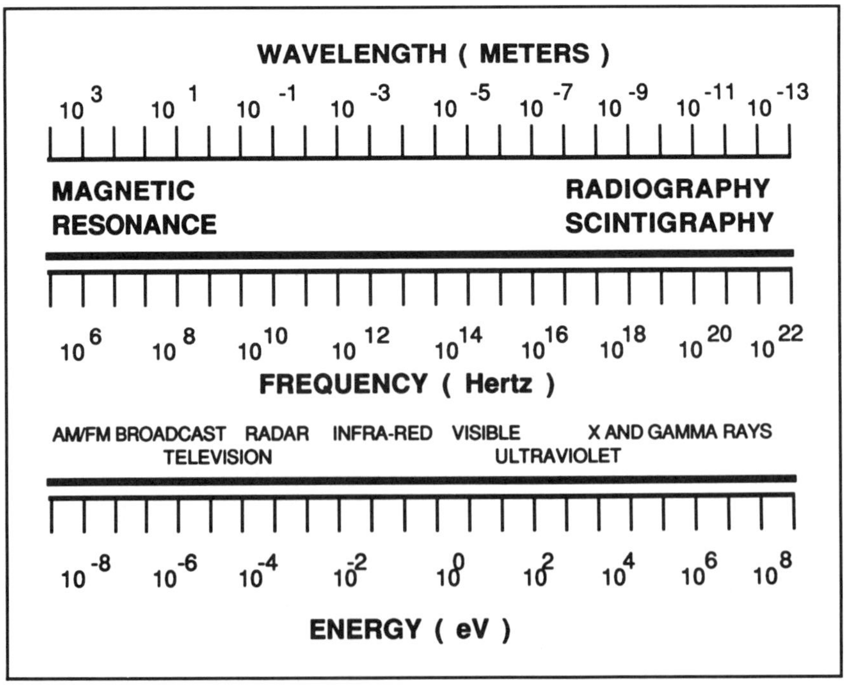

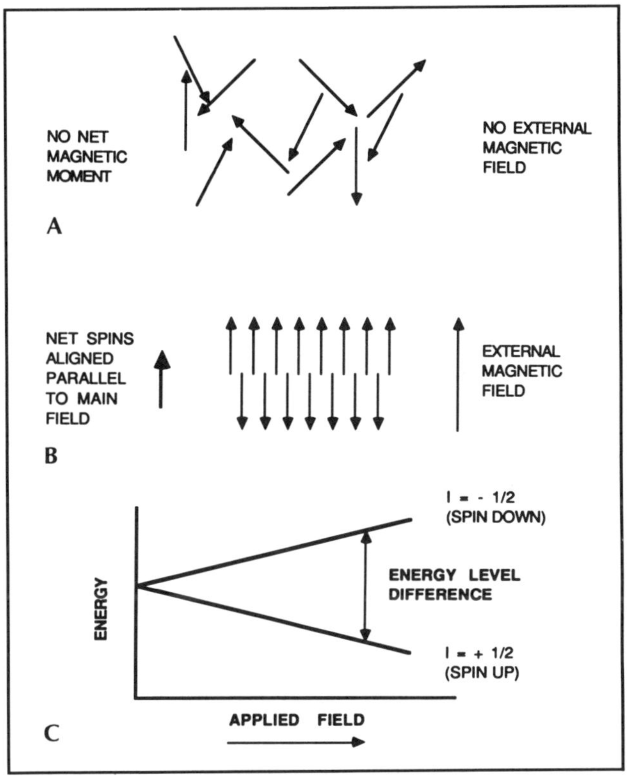

Fig. 20-3. Quantum mechanical explanation for the origin of the proton (H-1) signals used in NMR imaging. **A**. With no magnetic field turned on, the magnetic dipoles of hydrogen nuclei have no preferential alignment. **B**. The effect of an externally applied magnetic field. A slightly larger number of nuclei are aligned with the field, typically 1.00007 of those aligned against. **C**. The energy or radio frequency that can be used to excite the nuclei is greater as the field strength increases. Currently, only those nuclei with unitary spin quantum number (+½, −½ spin values) are used for imaging.

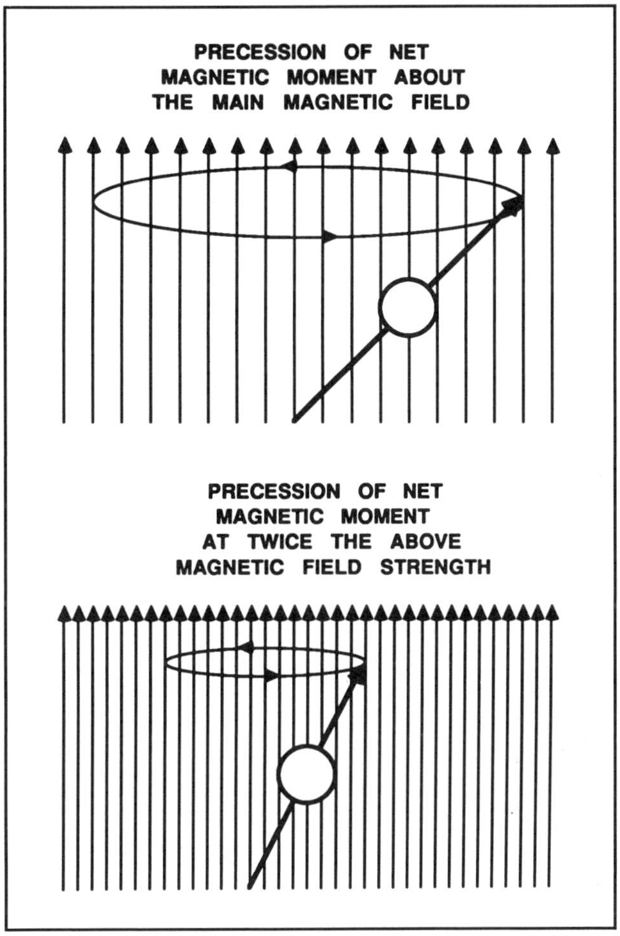

Fig. 20-4. A summary of the classic explanation of the NMR experiment. The net (total) magnetization in a given volume is thought to precess about the main magnetic field. As the field increases, the frequency of precession increases. The relationship between field strength and frequency is defined by the Larmor constant. This constant is different for each nucleus.

the protons to give back energy into the surrounding lattice as they "relax" back to their equilibrium position with respect to the main field. T_1 is defined as the time needed to regain 63.2 percent of this equilibrium magnetization. It typically measures in the range of hundreds to thousands of milliseconds for water protons in tissues. The underlying mechanism for this effect is proton-proton dipole interaction. Its principal determinant is the tumbling motion of water molecules, both rotational and translational.

Another process that accounts for signal loss is that of T_2, or spin-spin relaxation. In addition to dipole-dipole interactions, small local fluctuations of the magnetic field contribute an additional dephasing or scrambling of the spins. For example, the pulse lengths needed to align protons in the plane perpendicular to the static field (the transverse plane) of the magnet is 90 degrees. Additional values can achieve that result if their length is prolonged by adding 180-degree pulse length increments, that is, 270 degrees, 450 degrees, and so on (Fig. 20-6). Loss of signal intensity in the transverse plane following this excitation is referred to as the **free induction decay**, or FID, signal. FID is a function of local magnetic field inhomogeneities, and its decay constant is referred to as T_2^*. Many of these superimposed inhomogeneities can be eliminated by the use of a simple pulse sequence that refocuses the signal as an echo (Fig. 20-7). What is achieved is a signal that is dependent on the inherent T_2 relaxation characteristics of the tissues and that is less than T_2^*. T_2 is, in all cases, shorter than T_1.

Signal intensity on an image depends on proton intensity, T_1, T_2^*, T_2, and flow. The effect of blood flow is more subtle. Flow can either replenish or remove excited protons within a vessel and therefore affect signal intensity differently (Fig. 20-8). The RF signal reemitted by the hydrogen nuclei within tissues following a 90-degree RF pulse depends on additional factors. A hydrogen proton in water precesses at a given frequency defined by the magnetic field: the gyromagnetic ratio. The same proton, if it is part of a hydroxyl group in fat, precesses at a slightly different frequency corresponding to approximately a 3-parts-per-million change in the local magnetic

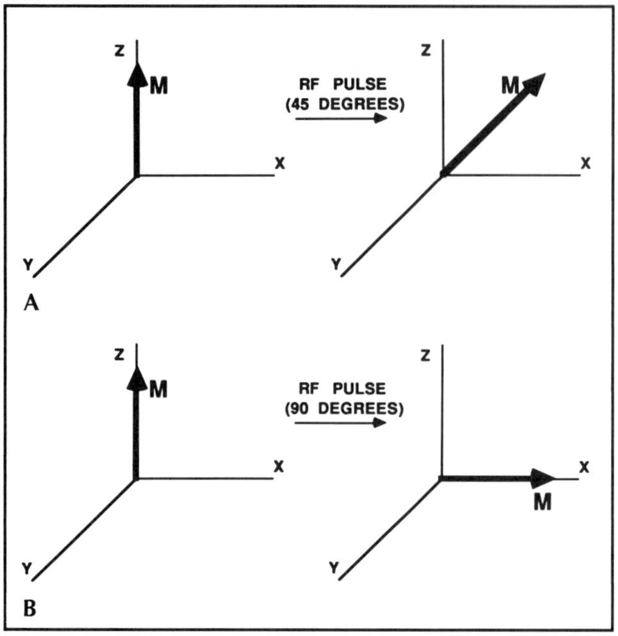

Fig. 20-5. **A**. A 45-degree RF pulse has been applied. The effect of this pulse is to "tilt" the net magnetization of a sample volume by 45 degrees with respect to the main magnetic field. The signal can be sensed only along the x-y plane and is therefore proportional to M × sin (45 degrees). **B**. A 90-degree pulse now tilts the magnetization vector onto the x-y plane. The detected signal is maximum and proportional to M. This effect can be achieved either by increasing the duration of the RF pulse or by increasing its energy over the same time interval.

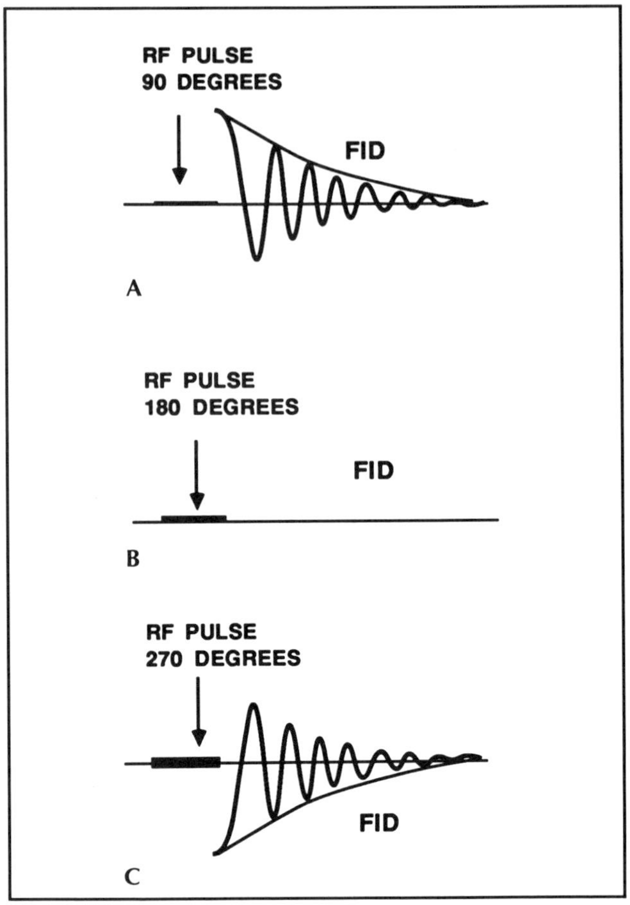

Fig. 20-6. How a signal is detected by an RF coil. **A**. A 90-degree pulse causes a maximal response in the signal. The detected signal is called an FID (free induction decay). The time constant for the loss of the signal is a combination of two effects: the T_2 characteristic of the tissue and the local magnetic field inhomogeneities (T_2*). **B**. A 180-degree pulse causes no detectable signal because the magnetization vector is again perpendicular to the x-y plane. **C**. A 270-degree RF pulse again causes a maximal signal to be detected, but the signal issues from the negative part of the x-y plane. The phase of this FID is shifted with respect to the one shown in (A).

field. This different precession frequency is due to local shielding of the magnetic field by the neighboring carbon atoms. Similarly, the phosphorus-31 protons of adenosine triphosphate (ATP) have different resonant frequencies depending on their proximity to other phosphorus hydroxyl groups. If a homogeneous sample of water and fat or a suspension of ATP and adenosine diphosphate (ADP) is excited, the relative number of protons in the mixture can be determined by measuring the signal intensity at the corresponding resonant frequency, which is in the concept of a spectrum (Fig. 20-9). The example of two groups of similar nuclei having slightly different precession frequencies due to the presence of a gradient also can be analyzed by such a technique. Nuclei in an object placed at a given location along the gradient can be plotted out as a function of their Larmor frequency (Fig. 20-10). If two separate objects are placed in the gradient, the RF detector would detect both signals superimposed as one. The signals are processed with the aid of a mathematic process called a Fourier transformation. Two peaks are readily identified on the resultant spectrum: Their positions on the spectrum correspond to the physical locations of the objects (Fig. 20-11). The most clinically useful protons are hydrogen and P-31. Although other protons can be used, such as fluorine-19 and sodium-24, the relatively low concentration of those compounds in the human body make their routine clinical use impractical.

The spectra of organs might be expected to be well defined and sharp since they are well-defined mixtures of water and fat or of P-31 metabolites. These nuclei are actually subjected to more complex magnetic environments, which widen their spectral waveform. Such is the situation in vivo for P-31: There is such an admixture of small local magnetic microenvironments that there is broadening over a large bandwidth of the frequency spectrum, which makes high-resolution decomposition of the spectrum impossible [4]. The in-vitro approach often must be utilized for correct characterization of metabolites. In fact, removal of water and suspension in nonaqueous inert solutions is necessary for high-resolution spectroscopy [5].

IMAGE CREATION

The presence of a magnetic field gradient superimposed on a large steady magnetic field leads to slight differences

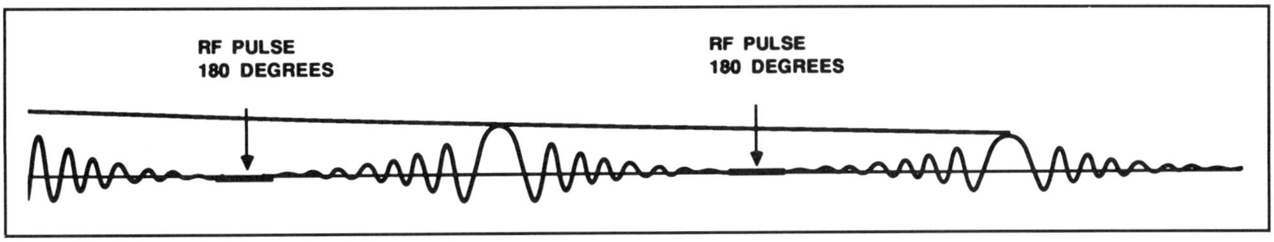

Fig. 20-7. The differences between FID and T_2 decay. The decay component due to T_2^* causes the rapid decay of FID. T_2 itself can be recovered if the signal is refocused by applying 180-degree pulses at regularly spaced intervals, which is represented by the upper line showing a longer exponential decay of the serial FID peak signals.

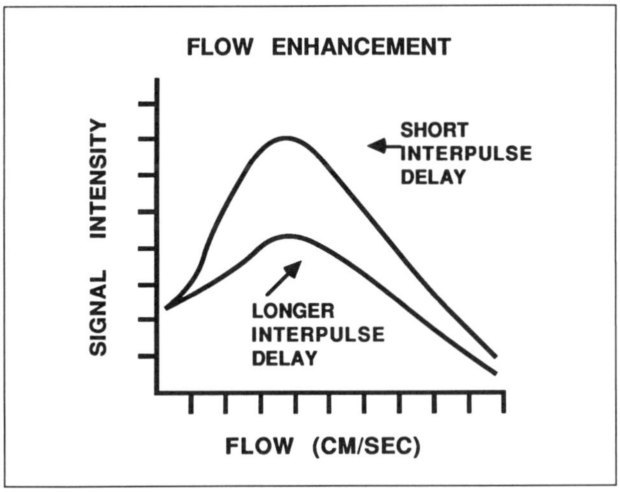

Fig. 20-8. The flow-enhancement effect is seen in an image plane perpendicular to the direction of flow. At low enough flow velocities, new protons enter the slice of interest and produce more signal. As velocity increases, the protons leave the imaging plane in the time between the RF pulses and therefore do not contribute to the signal.

in the RF at which protons situated along a gradient resonate (see Fig. 20-10). That is why the frequency of the detected RF signal changes as a function of position in the magnetic field. A judicious combination of these gradients can be used to selectively interrogate different portions of a three-dimensional object. This approach originally was used to pick a specific tissue volume in a body, excite that volume, and, finally, detect the amount of resonant protons present in it [6]. The location of the volume being interrogated was then shifted by varying the gradient in two directions. By continuing the process, it is possible to interrogate every portion of an object and to reconstruct an actual proton-density map of the object. This approach is, however, quite time consuming. Subsequent improvements have permitted whole lines through the Fourier transform space of an object to be excited and then interrogated [7,8].

More complex approaches permit rapid two-dimensional image reconstructions [2,7] and were first described by Lauterbur in 1973 [2]. There are two approaches to spatially encoding the RF signals from an object to obtain

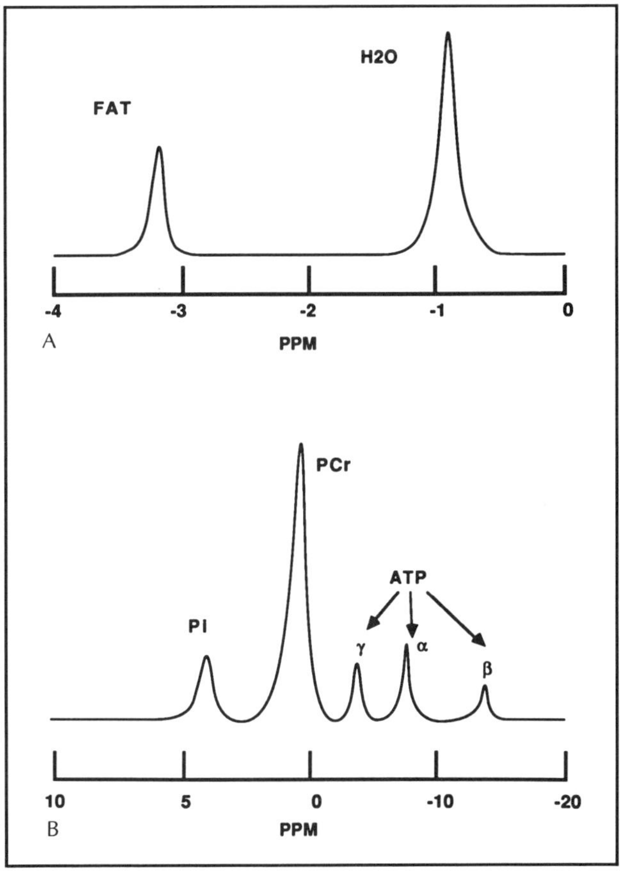

Fig. 20-9. **A.** A typical example of a spectrum (moderate to high resolution) of a mixture of water and fat in a homogeneous magnetic field. Two peaks are clearly defined. The areas underneath both peaks correspond to the relative amount of water and fat in the mixture. **B.** The P-31 peaks of ATP and its precursors are more complex. There is an admixture of inorganic and organic phosphate signals. Again, the sample is kept in a highly homogeneous field. In both cases, the separation of the resonance frequency of the different constituent peaks is a reflection of local magnetic field shielding effects caused by adjacent nuclei, that is, carbon proximity to hydrogen in fat versus oxygen and hydrogen in water.

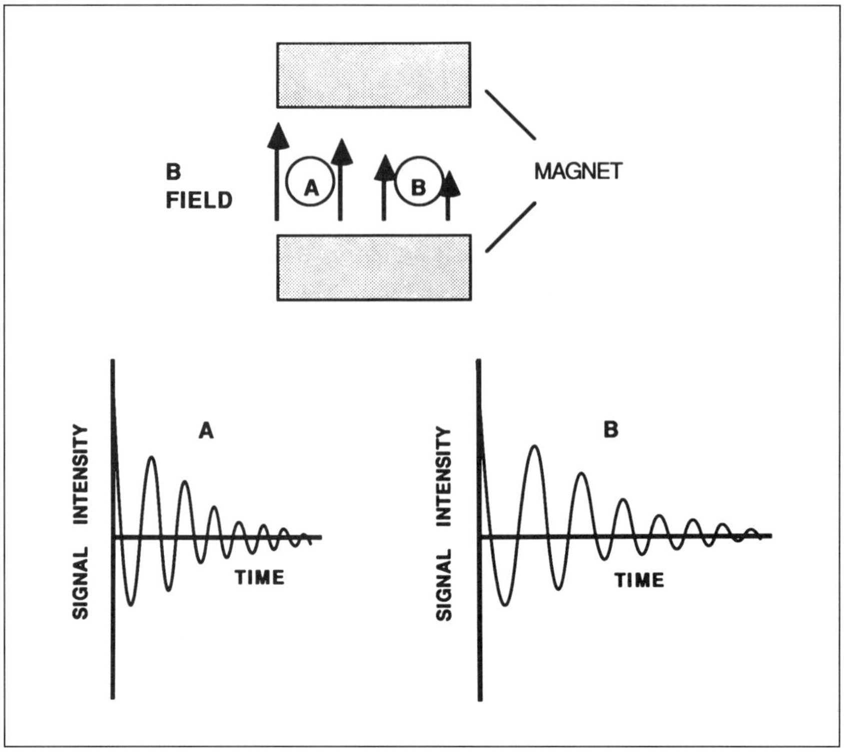

Fig. 20-10. The effect of a magnetic field gradient superimposed on the main magnetic field. Objects A and B are composed of the same homogeneous material. A is in a zone of higher magnetic field and therefore resonates at a higher frequency. B is at a slightly lower field and resonates at a lower frequency.

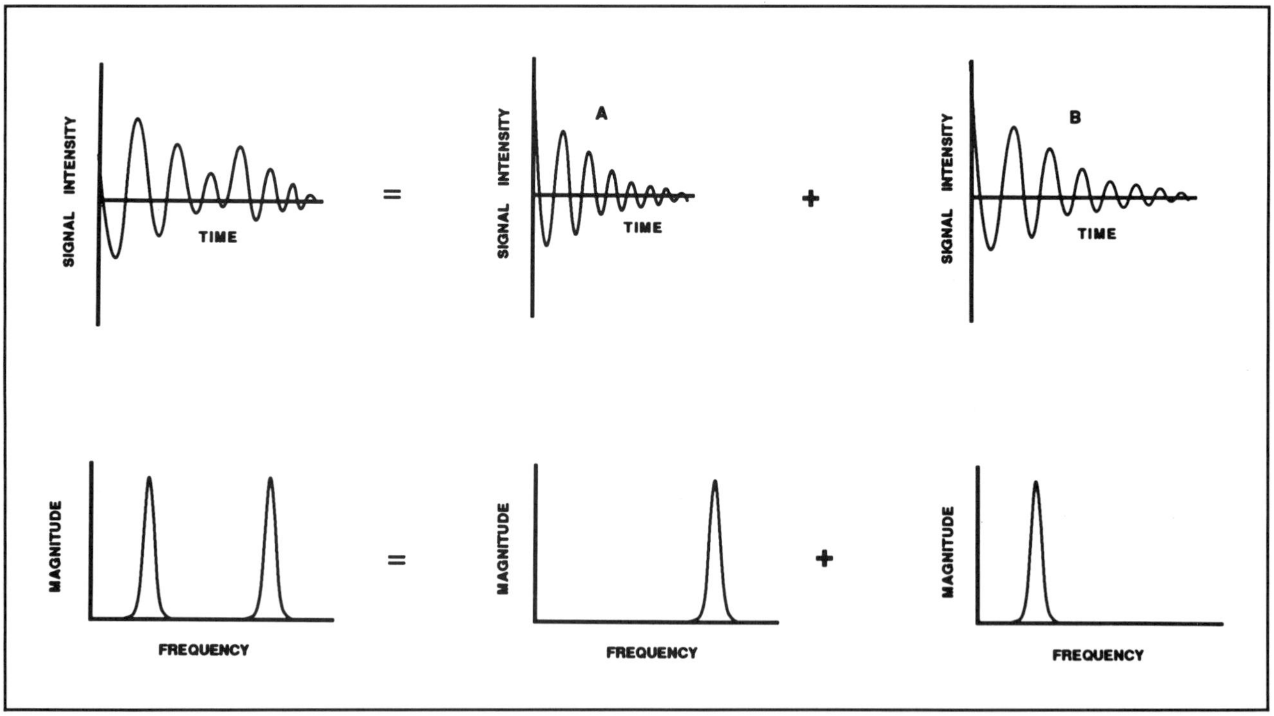

Fig. 20-11. The effect of detecting signals from objects A and B in Fig. 20-10. (Top) The combined detected RF signal is due to the superimposition of the respective RF signals, which occur if only object A or object B is in the magnet. (Bottom) The corresponding Fourier transforms (or spectra) are shown. One of the characteristics of Fourier transformation is that the superimposed waveforms can be decomposed and resolved.

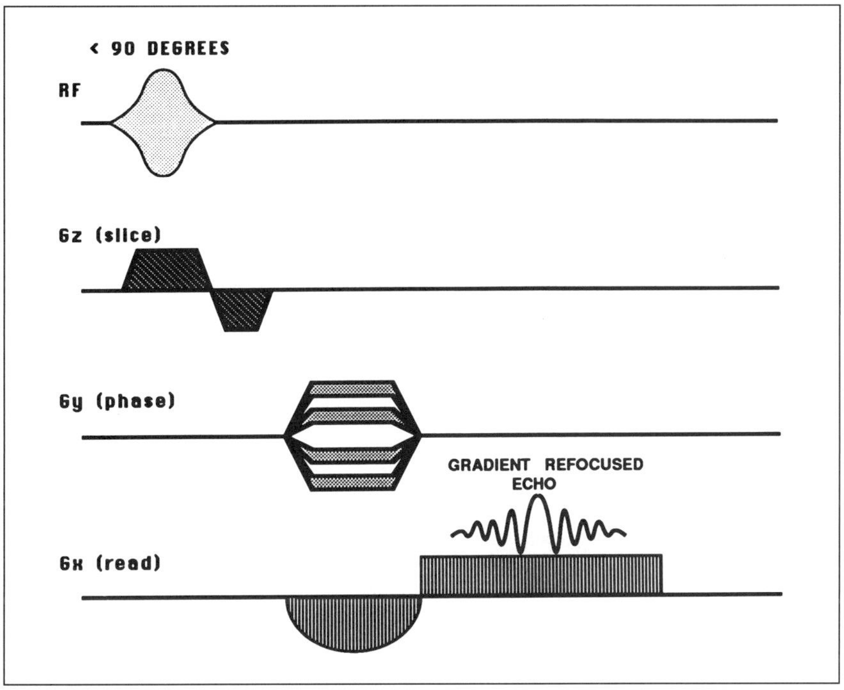

Fig. 20-12. A typical gradient-refocused pulse sequence consists of repetitive RF pulses (<90 degrees), typically between 15 and 40 degrees and of a gradient used to refocus the echo (Gx read). The Gz slice select gradient is used to select a slice of interest. The Gy phase gradient is used to encode spatial information along the axis perpendicular to the read (x) axis. Many variations exist in the way this pulse sequence is implemented, each with a proprietary abbreviation: FLASH, FISP, GRASS. All are variants of sequences referred to as steady-state free precession, since the interval between successive RF pulses (TR) is typically 20 to 40 milliseconds, which causes a steady state in the magnetization vector once the sequence starts running.

a tomographic picture. The first, called back-projection, is now rarely used. With it, magnetic field gradients of different values are simultaneously applied in two directions perpendicular to each other. An RF excitation pulse is then sent into the object. The value of the two perpendicular gradients is varied, and the acquired signals are used to reconstruct an image. This technique is akin to that used in single photon emission computed tomography (SPECT).

The second approach relies on two-dimensional Fourier transform techniques [8]. An image projection is defined by using a constant applied magnetic gradient in one direction: the read direction. Signals acquired as a gradient perpendicular to this read gradient—the phase encode direction—are varied in amplitude or duration. Varying the second gradient creates a synthetic set of frequencies along this direction. In the decoding of those frequencies, an image is reconstructed. The relative signal intensities of tissues or blood within the tomographic image are influenced by T_1 and T_2 as well as by blood flow and motion. Contrast differences between tissues and blood also can be emphasized by the use of specially designed pulse sequences.

Imaging time and the relative contrast between blood, moving blood, and surrounding soft tissues depend on the pulse sequences used. The sequence used to increase signal strength of moving blood is called **gradient recall imaging** [8]. Protons in a given slice are subjected to a selective RF pulse matched to the magnetic field gradient. By reapplication of the magnetic field gradient in the opposite direction, the dephasing effect can be reversed and a signal detected (Fig. 20-12). This signal, called a **gradient echo**, can have increased signal strength when it comes from moving blood. In the spin-echo technique, unlike in the gradient-echo techniques, the refocusing is achieved by a 180-degree RF pulse [8], which compensates for the effect of static magnetic field inhomogeneities present in the magnet (Fig. 20-13). Another technique currently being used is a variant of spin-echo imaging that decreases imaging times by using multiple 180-degree pulses and echoes for each RF pulse [9].

In a simple imaging experiment, such as the spin-echo imaging sequence, a selective 90-degree pulse is applied while a magnetic field gradient is turned on to select a given slice in an object (Fig. 20-13). After an interval commonly referred to as one-half the echo-time, or TE/2, that pulse is followed by another pulse, this time 180 degrees, which forces the spins to rephase. The rephasing causes a signal at an interval of TE/2 from the 180-degree pulse and therefore TE from the original 90-degree pulse: This is an echo of the original signal. For maximal signal intensity, the pulse sequence should be repeated at an interval long enough to permit full T_1 relaxation of the protons in the slice being imaged. This repetition interval,

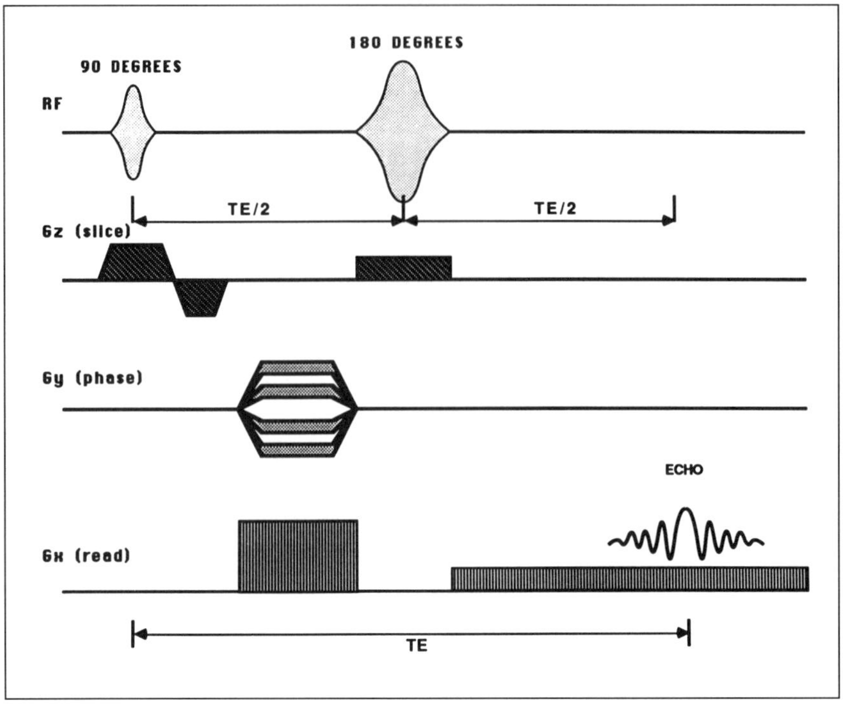

Fig. 20-13. Compared to Fig. 20-12, the spin-echo sequence depicted here uses a 180-degree RF pulse to refocus the spins. The time at which this occurs is the TE interval. An extra gradient is turned on during this selective 180-degree pulse to refocus only the spins in the slice, which makes the sequence more sensitive to flow. A nonselective 180-degree pulse might refocus moving spins from outside the slice of interest and cause an in-slice flow-related artifact.

which is the interpulse delay time, also commonly referred to as TR, should be longer than five times the T_1 of the constituent protons in the slice. If the TR is shorter, protons have not had sufficient time to completely relax, and there is a corresponding loss in signal intensity. If the TR is longer than four to five times the T_1 of the tissues in the image, the resultant image is a proton-density image. If the TR is shorter, the image is T_1 weighted. The length of the echo-time TE also affects the image. With a short TE, say, in the range of 10 to 15 milliseconds, the difference between the different T_2 values of the tissues in the image may not be distinguished. If the echo-time is increased to longer values, then tissues with longer T_2 values will have more signal than those with short T_2. Signal from flowing blood also is lost. Interestingly, the signal lost because of fluctuations in the local magnetic fields and slow blood flow can be partially recovered by a second echo obtained following the application of a second 180-degree pulse. This refocusing of some of the static inhomogeneities present in the image is commonly referred to as even-echo rephasing. Spin-echo imaging sequences can be made more efficient if multiple echoes are acquired during a given TR interval. This rapid acquisition with relaxation enhancement (RARE) keeps some of the T_2 imaging characteristics of tissues [9].

Long acquisition times are needed to minimize the saturation effects and partial relaxation seen with short TR values. More rapid imaging sequences are possible. Currently, gradient-refocused imaging sequences are utilized (see Fig. 20-12). Here, instead of using the 180-degree echo to refocus the spins, gradients are used to refocus the signal more quickly. However, because excitation is occurring at very short TR intervals, signals can easily saturate. RF energy deposition is also large if the duration of the RF pulses is kept at 90 degrees. Reducing the angle of excitation to values less than 90 degrees, for example, 30 degrees, not only decreases the deposition of energy in the patient but also improves contrast between moving blood and stationary tissues. There are multiple variants of these gradient-refocused methods, each having slightly different effects on image contrast and sensitivity to blood flow. These imaging sequences are frequently used in flow imaging and magnetic resonance angiography.

FLOW IMAGING

The first magnetic resonance images clearly showed that moving fluids had either absent signal or less signal than stationary objects [10]. When imaging is performed at a given plane, the motion of protons—that is, blood flow—out of that plane between the 90-degree and 180-degree pulses of a spin-echo sequence can almost eliminate the protons available to the refocusing 180-degree pulse. The loss of signal due to blood flow is commonly referred to as the **flow void effect** or **time-of-flight loss** [11]. The loss of signal is due to the actual elimination of protons from the slice of interest (Fig. 20-14). Increased signal in the vessel can be achieved by exciting the slice proximal to the imaging slice of interest with a 90-degree slice selective pulse and then applying a 180-degree pulse downstream from that point. The image shows that blood

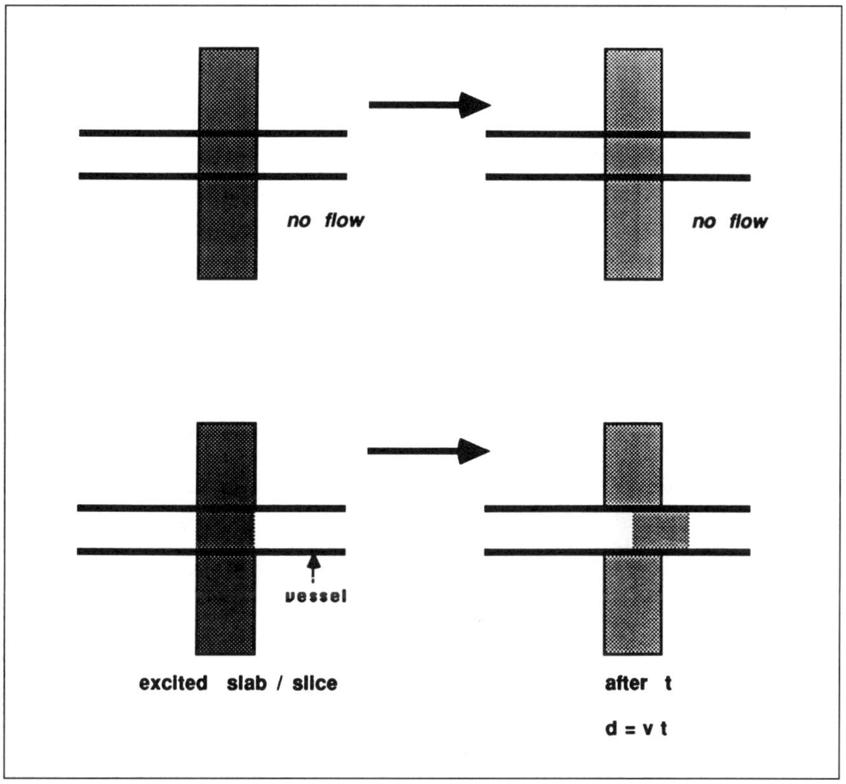

Fig. 20-14. The mechanism responsible for the flow-void effect. (Top) With absent flow, signal loss between two RF pulses is due to T_2 and T_1 effects. (Bottom) Signal from flowing blood is lost not only due to T_1 and T_2 effects but also because of physical displacement outside the imaging slice.

entering the imaging volume has high signal intensity [11]. The signal is clearly seen in normal vessels, while turbulence cancels out any signals and a flow void will develop in the artery or vein being imaged [12]. The flow-void and spin-label effects can be achieved by the use of selected imaging sequences. This approach is complicated and time consuming because of the number of imaging acquisitions and the inherent slowness of the imaging sequences [13–15].

Flow imaging has been achieved with spin-echo phase-sensitive [16–18] and gradient-refocused imaging sequences [19,20]. With the phase-sensitive spin-echo approach, motion causes dephasing of protons in the direction of the applied magnetic field gradient. The magnitude of the resultant signal is proportional to the intensity of the magnetic field and the length of time that the protons are submitted to the dephasing effect. The image sequence is gated with an electrocardiogram to early systole and to early diastole. The images are subtracted, and the resultant image shows the protons that have moved (Fig. 20-15). This approach can give excellent images of the peripheral vasculature [18]. It is limited by a preferential flow sensitivity along a selected axis, most often the read gradient. Obtaining blood flow information along another axis requires that the direction of the read gradient be changed and that an additional set of images be acquired. Both images are then added to give a more accurate representation of blood flow distribution.

The signal lost by protons moving in a magnetic field gradient can be recovered, in part, by applying a reverse magnetic field gradient in the opposite direction. If a unipolar magnetic field dephases all static protons by a fixed amount, a reversed magnetic gradient of the same strength can refocus the nonmoving protons. Protons with a constant velocity accumulate a larger phase shift (Fig. 20-16). If bipolar gradients are used, then all constant-velocity terms can be canceled (Fig. 20-17). Similarly, a more complex gradient can be used to correct for constant acceleration [21].

Magnetic resonance angiography does not, in general, rely on spin-echo sequences. The rapid gradient echo-imaging sequences are used almost exclusively. The short repetition time of these imaging sequences permits entry of fresh protons in the imaging plane. Inflowing blood shows up as a region of high signal intensity [20,22]. There are, however, two conditions to the efficient use of these sequences: (1) Imaging is best done in the plane perpendicular to the direction of moving blood, and (2) the length of the RF pulse must be kept short. The phenomenon responsible for the increased signal intensity of fresh blood entering the imaging plane is called **flow replenishment**. As shown in Fig. 20-18, the signals from the nonmoving tissues around the vessel are partly saturated due to the rapid repetition time of the sequence. Blood flowing into the slice has not been previously saturated and can therefore give a strong signal. The RF pulse is less than 90 degrees. Contrast between blood and surrounding nonmoving tissues is increased if the pulse length is be-

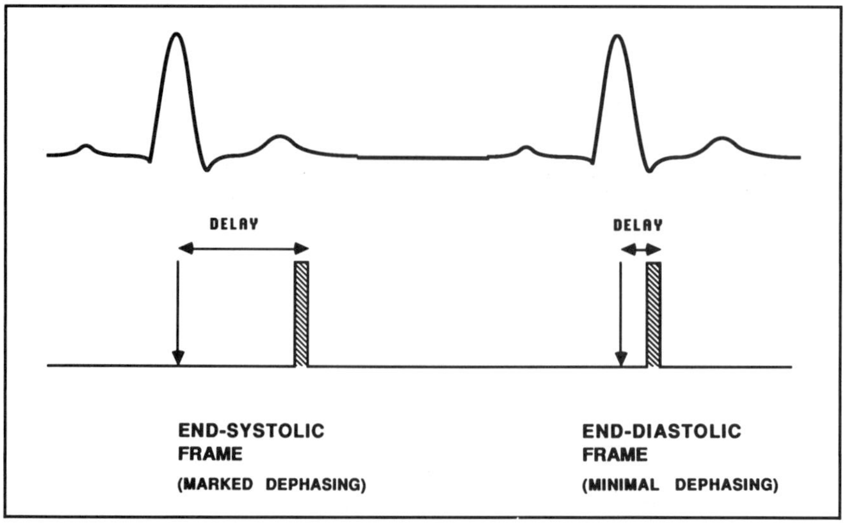

Fig. 20-15. For subtraction of the vessels using electrocardiographic gating, signal must be detected within a vessel. This is more likely to occur for more slowly flowing blood near end-diastole. Signal void is expected on the image taken near end-systole. By subtracting the end-systolic image from the end-diastolic, an image of the vessel lumen can be obtained.

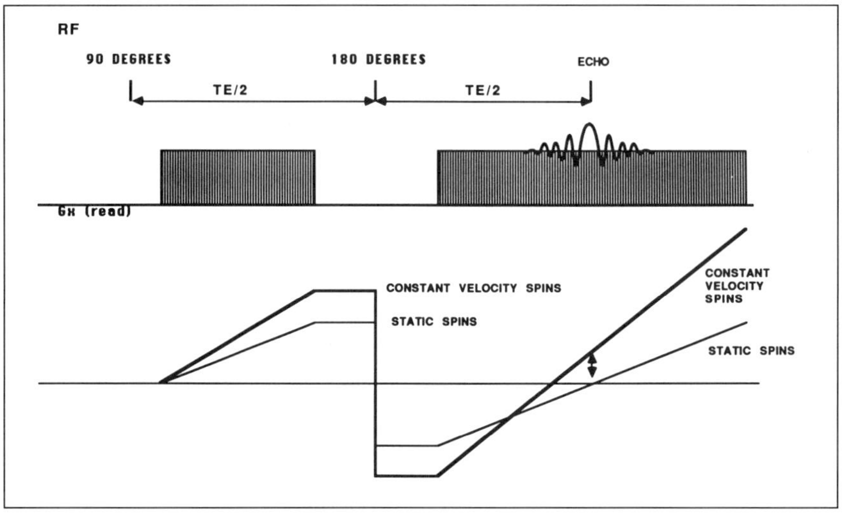

Fig. 20-16. The effect of the magnetic field gradient used to encode in the read direction. Because moving spins (here at a constant velocity) accumulate a different amount of phase than static spins, the two signals do not refocus at the same point, which causes additional signal loss and artifact on the image.

tween 15 degrees and 40 degrees. The decreased pulse length limits the deposition of RF energy (manifested as heating and an increase in patient temperature) to acceptable levels. High flow velocities, turbulence, and eddy effects will cause a loss in signal intensity. The gradient-refocused techniques are also very sensitive to magnetic field inhomogeneities, and signal loss can occur wherever metallic objects are present or at the interface between tissues of differing magnetic susceptibilities, for example, the interface of soft tissue with calcium. Despite these problems, the gradient-refocused sequences are used extensively for vascular imaging. They can be applied to a volume of tissue and used to obtain sets of two- or three-dimensional images. The three-dimensional approaches are limited by the fact that they are more sensitive to motion artifacts. The two major types of magnetic resonance angiograms are generated with the help of gradient-refocused sequences in one of two ways: the time-of-flight approach and the phase-sensitive approach [10].

Areas of high signal intensities on time-of-flight images are created when fresh protons—that is, blood within a vessel—enter into the imaging plane due to flow-related enhancement (see Fig. 20-18). The vessel of interest generally lies perpendicular to the imaging plane. A final image of the vessel is created after the sequentially acquired images are processed. Acquiring multiple two-dimen-

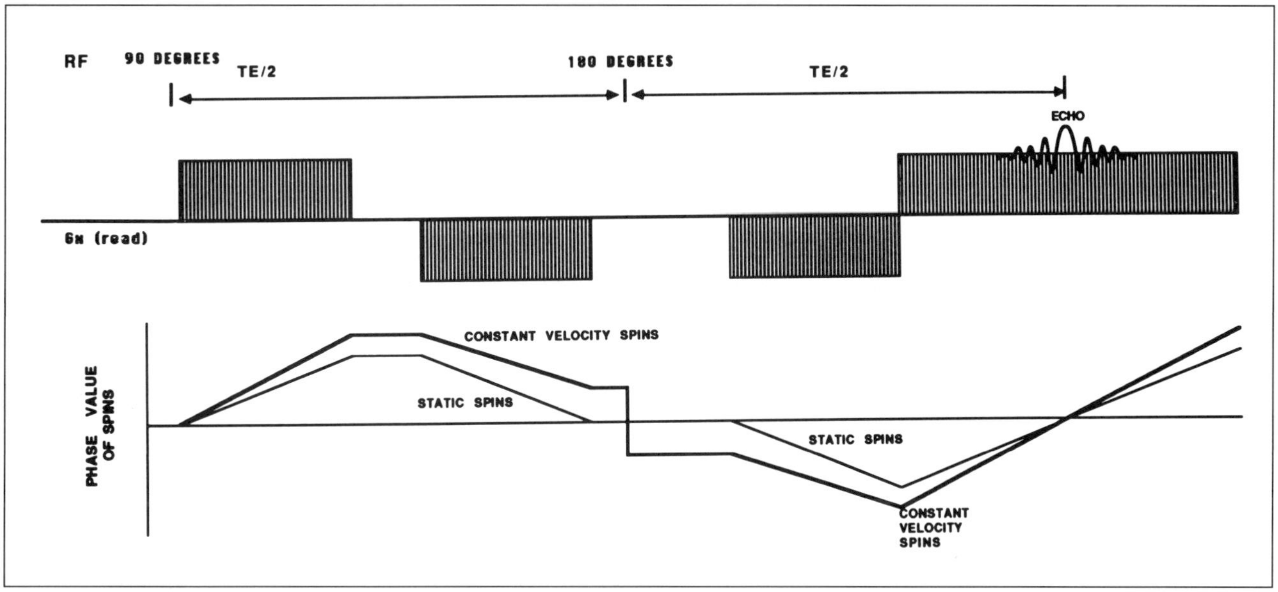

Fig. 20-17. Bipolar gradients (gradient moment nulling) can be used to refocus the moving spins at the same point as the static spins. This combination can be used to cancel the effect of spins moving at a constant velocity. More complex gradients are needed to cancel the effects of acceleration. Variants of these sequences are used to encode information on the velocity of moving blood, which is accomplished by combining a pair of pulse sequences, one sensitive to motion and one not sensitive. Subtracting one from the other gives an image containing flow-velocity information.

sional images and then stacking them to form a volume improves contrast, and each image can be done while the patient holds his or her breath, allowing motionless imaging of blood vessels. Images obtained by two- or three-dimensional techniques usually are reconstructed using a maximum intensity projection (MIP) algorithm. An MIP algorithm projects only the brightest pixel along a ray (usually the blood vessels in a bright-blood-technique image). Images can be rotated to display the area or the vessel of interest at the optimum obliquity. The phase-sensitive methods rely on the acquisition of paired images, each with a different sensitivity to flowing blood [23]. These images are acquired in either two or three directions and amalgamated into a final three-dimensional image. They are more sensitive to motion than the time-of-flight images. Although capable of displaying quantitative velocity values for moving blood, the phase-sensitive method requires some a priori knowledge of the velocity distribution of the blood velocities in the vessel of interest. This imaging technique sets a window over which it can measure blood-flow velocity. If the window is set too high, information is lost; if it is set too low, rapidly moving blood is misregistered as more slowly moving blood. Display of this information also is achieved by the MIP algorithm.

METABOLISM

P-31 spectroscopy has been used principally for in-vitro systems. A series of coils are positioned around different organs, which are perfused ex vivo. Shifts in the ATP peaks are measured, and perturbations in metabolism can then be documented [4,5,24].

The use of surface coils to detect the signals from deeper structures in the body is technically demanding. The intervening tissues give off signals, which are superimposed on the signals from the organs of interest. Different schemes have been adopted to compensate for this effect. One scheme is the use of concentric surface coils so that only a small area of interest is excited by the inner coil while the outer surface coil detects the signal [25]. Another approach is the use of judiciously designed RF pulses to excite a specific volume of interest at a given depth [26]. Extrinsic gradients also can be used to create a coarse image [27]. In-vivo measurements have been made on muscles of the lower extremities [28], as well as the more anterior portions of the myocardial wall [29]. More selective depth resolution has not yet been achieved for reasonable imaging acquisition time intervals except in the case of the brain. The low concentration of phosphorus metabolites restricts this approach to large volumes and long imaging times. Changes in different metabolites, such as lactate, also can be measured in vivo using proton spectroscopy [30]. The problems in detecting this peak include those already mentioned, as well as the need to suppress signals from neighboring component nuclei of water and fat [31].

Magnetic resonance spectroscopy can be used to quantify the metabolic changes due to alterations in oxygen delivery. Although in-vivo measurements are now possible, spectroscopic methods are not in widespread clinical use at this time. The major constraint is the low concentrations of these metabolites; measurements must be made over large volumes and take large amounts of time. Increased acquisition time and number of signal averages

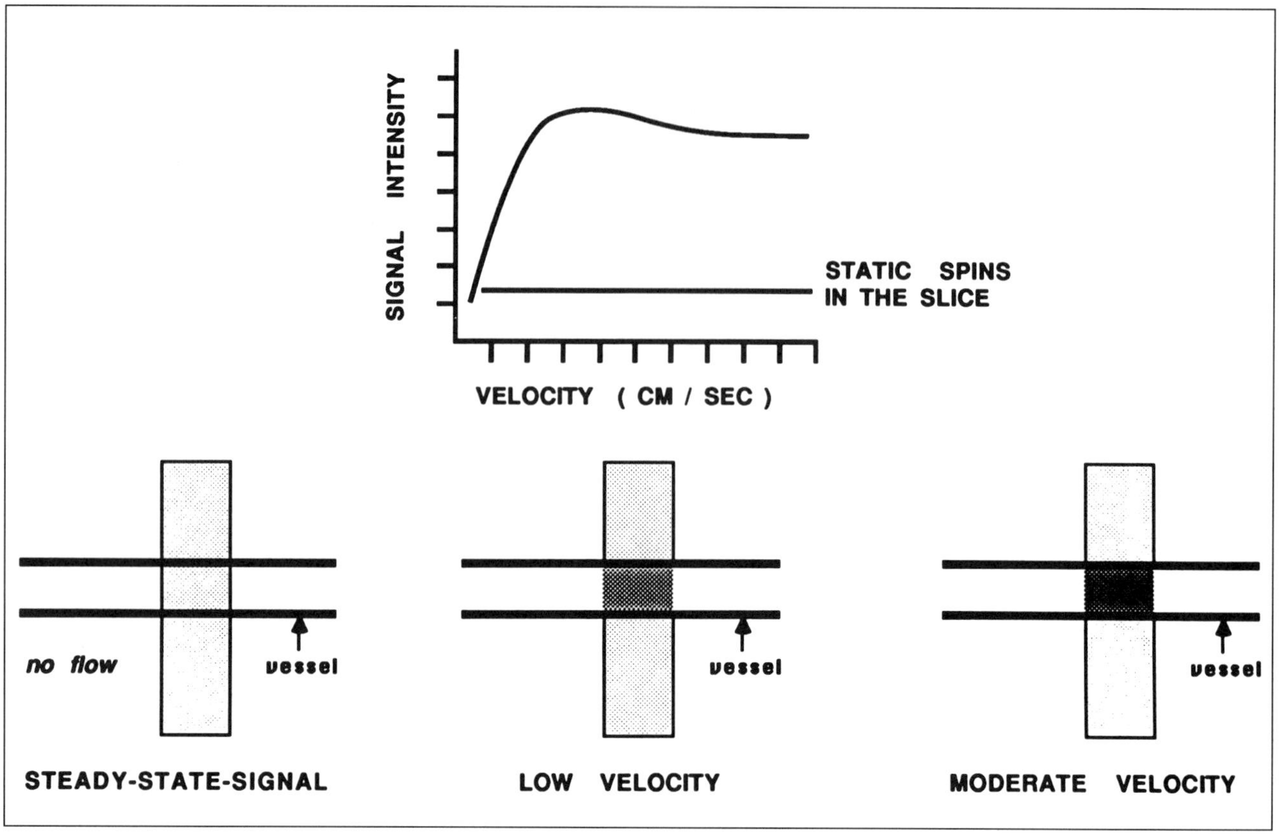

Fig. 20-18. The gradient-refocused pulse sequences cause an increase in the signal originating from spins entering the slice. These sequences are, therefore, sensitive to flow perpendicular to the slice of interest. They can be used to confirm that a vessel is patent. They also are used for cardiac imaging since the blood pool has a high signal intensity. Stenotic, regurgitant lesions, or any lesions that cause turbulence, are seen as well-defined zones of signal void.

increases signal-to-noise ratio. Increased sample volume decreases imaging time but compromises spatial localization (typical ranges are 1 to 10 cc). If needed, the ATP–inorganic phosphate balance can be studied in large volumes, such as the muscles of the leg or the anterior wall of the left ventricle.

A novel approach to the problem is to increase the number of nuclei that are participating in a metabolic pathway. An example is the injection of C-13–enriched glycogen. The subsequently obtained spectra reflect the balance between aerobic and anaerobic metabolism [32].

PARAMAGNETIC COMPOUNDS

Paramagnetic compounds consist of paramagnetic nuclei that are often linked to a carrier such as diethylene triamine pentacetic acid (DTPA). A typical example is that of gadolinium coupled to DTPA. Gadolinium serves as the active paramagnetic center [33], while DTPA stabilizes it and gives it the pharmacokinetics of a compound that is distributed in the extracellular space. Early on, this complex was used in the evaluation of myocardial ischemia or infarction [34]. Following injection, the compound is rapidly distributed to well-perfused tissues, such as normal muscle. The interaction with water in the extracellular space causes an increase in the signal intensity on T_1-weighted images detected from the tissue due to shortening of the T_1 relaxation time. Severely ischemic or infarcted tissues are not affected. In time, the ischemic tissues have a relatively larger concentration of contrast material than the surrounding tissues, and the signal intensity reverses [35]. These compounds also can be used to increase the contrast between tissue and blood vessels and enhance signal intensity in rapidly moving blood [36]. Rapid imaging techniques also offer the possibility of dynamically following a bolus of a paramagnetic complex and thereby assessing regional perfusion [37].

Compounds such as manganese chloride [38] and the nitroxide free radicals [39] have come into disfavor because of possible toxicity effects. Iron complexes have been used to image the gastrointestinal tract but do not offer any advantages in the vascular tree. Complexes of chromium and dysprosium also have been investigated [40].

Applications in Arterial Diseases

CEREBROVASCULAR DISEASES

One of the first uses of magnetic resonance imaging has been the diagnosis of central nervous system disorders. Standard spin-echo magnetic resonance imaging can be used to detect cerebral infarcts because signal changes are

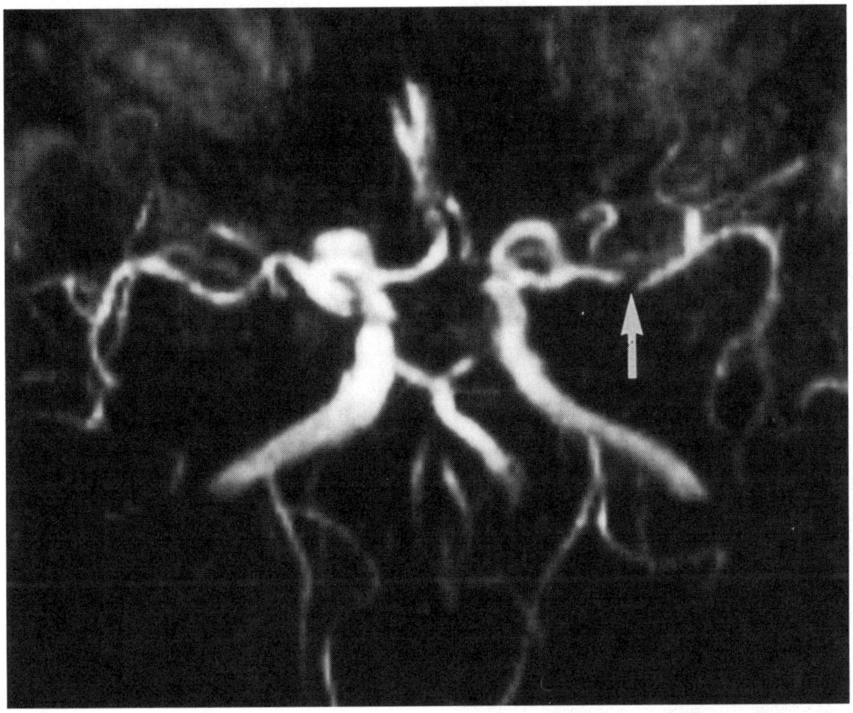

Fig. 20-19. An MR angiogram showing the major intracranial arteries. A zone of signal loss in the left middle cerebral artery (arrow) is due to a focal intracranial stenosis.

caused by the extent of local edema, damage to the blood-brain barrier, and the presence of hemorrhage.

The sensitivity of magnetic resonance imaging is better than that of computed tomography in early (acute) infarcts [41]. Magnetic resonance imaging is very sensitive for detecting early edema and blood-brain barrier damage, but it cannot detect early parenchymal or subarachnoid hemorrhage that occurs in the first 48 hours following a stroke [42,43]. With time, hemorrhage becomes visible due to the paramagnetic effects caused by the local accumulation of methemoglobin as well as other red blood cell–breakdown products [42,43].

Magnetic resonance can detect intracranial vascular malformations and aneurysms. In arteriovenous malformations, feeding vessels can be seen on standard spin-echo images as heterogeneous zones of flow void [44]. Zones of previous hemorrhage may show up as local areas of signal loss [45]. Arteriovenous malformations leading to thrombosis of the cavernous sinus can be quite elegantly diagnosed by magnetic resonance [46]. In the broad category of occult cerebrovascular malformations (including capillary telangiectasia, cavernous angioma, and small thrombosed arteriovenous malformations), magnetic resonance offers the possibility of making a specific diagnosis. Finally, venous angiomas can be clearly shown by magnetic resonance [47].

By combining spin-echo with gradient-refocused imaging, flowing blood can be clearly delineated. On spin-echo images, the signal intensity in the vessel or vascular structure often is decreased. With gradient-refocused imaging, signal intensity of flowing blood is increased. When both sequences are combined, the diagnosis of intra-arterial aneurysms can be made for aneurysms of 5 mm or greater [20,48,49]. However, they tend to miss the most important sign of a ruptured aneurysm, that is, subarachnoid blood.

Time-of-flight or phase-contrast magnetic resonance angiograms of the intracranial vessels also can be used to detect focal intracranial stenoses (Fig. 20-19).

P-31 spectroscopy has been used to document evidence of cerebral ischemia, which has been best described in premature infants [50]. The potential for monitoring developmental changes has yet to be exploited.

EXTRACRANIAL AND INTRACRANIAL VESSELS

The flow sensitivity of the two pulse sequences used for magnetic resonance angiography varies markedly. Three-dimensional phase-contrast imaging can be used to map out the intracranial vascular tree [23], since the intracranial vessels are less likely to move during image acquisition than the extracranial branches. Time-of-flight imaging is more easily applied to the extracranial carotid system [51,52]. Specialized RF coils are placed over the neck to improve signal-to-noise ratio of the magnetic resonance angiograms. Finally, the whole extent of the vascular tree can be imaged over a relatively small volume and short time, making it possible to reconstruct the vessels in three dimensions. With gradient-refocused imaging, a window showing flowing blood within a velocity range of 1 cm/second to 1–2 m/second can be visualized. Unfortunately, the turbulence and stasis that arise in the carotid artery distal to a stenosis cause signal-intensity loss. Therefore, it

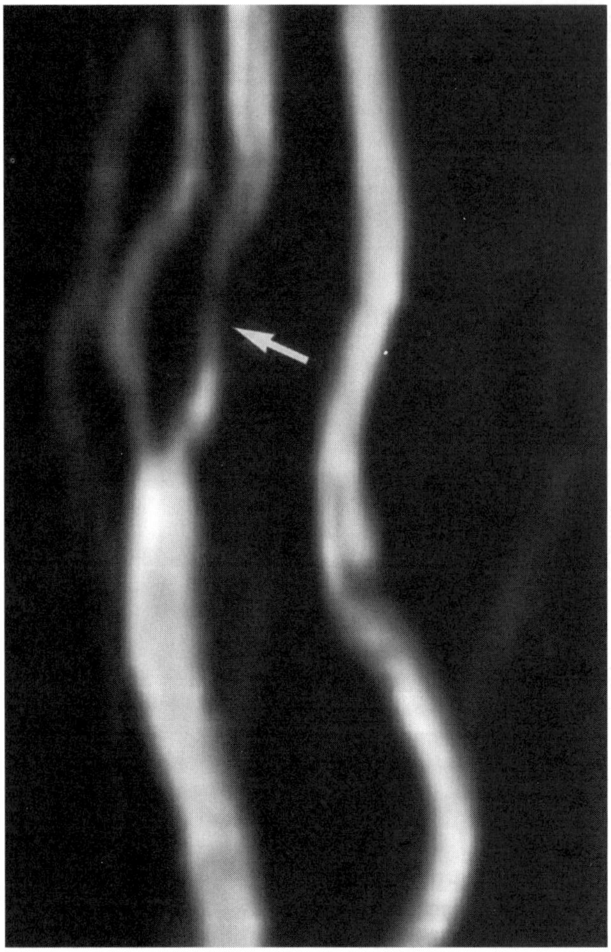

Fig. 20-20. This two-dimensional time-of-flight magnetic resonance angiogram shows a 50-percent narrowing (arrow) distal to the origin of the internal carotid artery.

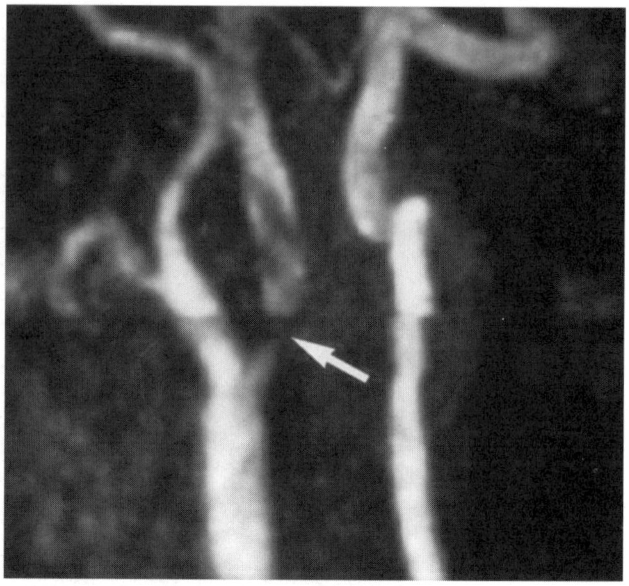

Fig. 20-21. A projection angiogram showing a zone of signal loss in the proximal internal carotid artery (arrow), which corresponds to a 90-percent-diameter stenosis on a contrast arteriogram.

is not possible to accurately measure blood-flow-velocity changes in the higher ranges normally seen with moderately severe stenoses.

The two-dimensional gradient-focused images are acquired as a series of stacked images of 0.8- to 1.5-cm thickness over distances of 8 to 10 cm. A projection angiogram is then created and the images used to estimate stenosis severity [53]. Magnetic resonance angiography has a diagnostic accuracy sufficiently high to be considered an effective screening test for detecting the presence of significant carotid lesions [51,54,55]. The projection angiogram of the carotid bifurcation resembles that of the traditional arteriogram (Fig. 20-20). The limited spatial resolution may make it difficult to adopt this examination as a full substitute for arteriography. Instead, in the two-dimensional time-of-flight images, the appearance of a zone of signal loss, or flow gap (Fig. 20-21), can be used to infer the presence of a significant (>70%) stenosis. The three-dimensional time-of-flight sequences are less sensitive to the artifacts generated by flowing blood and can depict a high-grade stenosis as an area of focal narrowing. These images are, however, more susceptible to artifacts generated by patient motion [52]. If magnetic resonance angiography alone is used to evaluate the carotid bifurcations, the source images as well as the projection angiogram must be inspected carefully before a diagnosis is made [56].

The aortic arch is accessible to this technique. It requires a separate imaging coil than the smaller one used for imaging the neck, thereby adding to the length of the examination. Magnetic resonance angiography can therefore be used to image the arch and exclude high-grade lesions at the origin of the carotid arteries.

CORONARY ARTERY DISEASE

Cardiac imaging offers the possibility of obtaining noninvasive measurements of myocardial mass [57], ventricular volumes [58], wall motion [59], and valvular function [60]. In all cases, some form of gating or electrocardiographic synchronization must first be available. Respiratory gating, once thought to be a prerequisite for cardiac imaging, is not essential.

The standard gated cardiac exam will trigger a signal acquisition within a fixed interval of time following the R-wave of the electrocardiogram. If triggered immediately following the R-wave (typically 4–10 milliseconds), a first echo image can be acquired 20–40 milliseconds later, close enough to be called an end-diastolic image. If close to the T-wave (200–300 milliseconds later), then an end-systolic image can be taken. In essence, for a single slice, which can be taken either in the transverse plane used in computed tomography or along the axis used for echocardiography or angiography, a minimum of 128 to 256 heartbeats is needed. The signal intensity of the myocardium is then a function of the R-R interval, which then becomes the

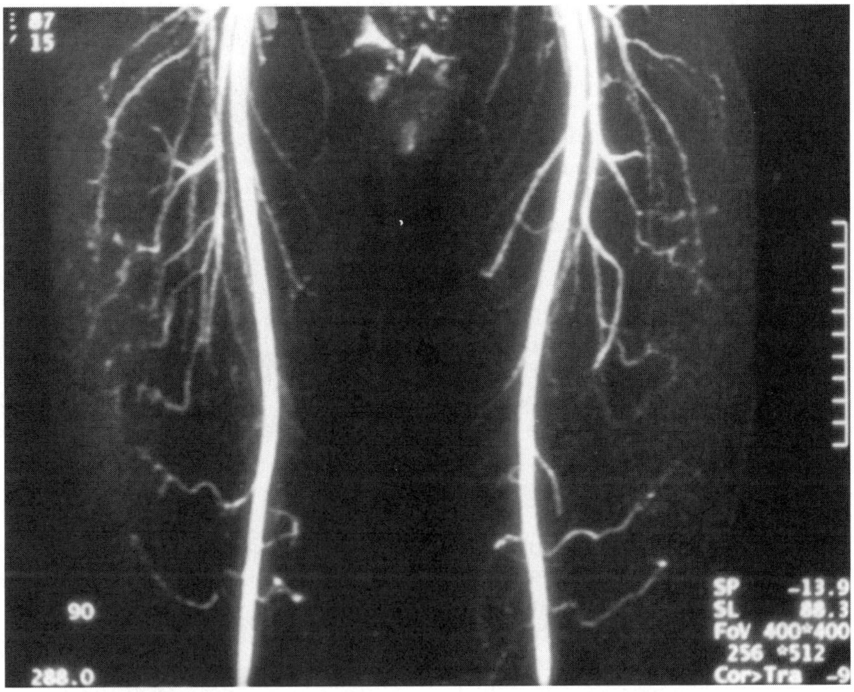

Fig. 20-22. Coronal, contrast-enhanced, two-dimensional, gradient-echo magnetic resonance angiogram of the legs from the femoral arteries to below the knees shows normal arterial anatomy.

TR (repetition interval). The image can be oriented along any axis with respect to the heart (long-axis view, short-axis view) by electronically adjusting the magnetic gradients used to encode the image. Although 128 heartbeats are the minimum required for each image of the heart frozen in a specific portion of the cardiac cycle, it is possible to acquire slices parallel to that image, each in a different portion of the cardiac cycle.

If the same slice is imaged more than once during a given R-R interval, the signal from the myocardium is then weighted by a shorter effective TR. Changes in wall thickness between diastole and systole can then be determined. More slices can be taken by interleaving them irregularly during the cardiac cycle. Such a strategy shortens acquisition time but weights the signal intensities in each image differently. Measurements of ventricular volumes, mass, and wall motion still can be performed, but the T_1 and T_2 characteristics of the myocardium are lost. In fact, this strategy is now used for cine magnetic resonance, which uses gradient-refocused images where the blood pool has a strong signal. Images are synchronized to the cardiac cycle. From 16 to 32 frames are acquired in a given projection. When played back, the images recreate a dynamic cinematic display, or movie, of the heart as it contracts and relaxes. On the images, high-intensity signals correspond to the blood in the cardiac chambers. The presence of jets due to mitral stenosis or regurgitation causes zones of signal void proportional to the severity of valvular dysfunction [60]. Myocardial wall motion abnormalities also can be seen from a dynamic movie playback.

Aorto-saphenous coronary graft patency can be documented, either by signal void on a spin-echo image or by signal presence on gradient-refocused imaging [61]. In the first approach, it is difficult to locate the patent graft. For the second, image artifacts limited to the nature of gradient-refocused imaging are aggregated by the presence of surgical appliances (clips). Magnetic resonance angiography also can be used for evaluating the coronary arteries [62], which requires very rapid acquisition during a voluntary breath hold [63]. In addition, it is better suited for the proximal coronary arteries and may give inconsistent results for the distal segments of the posterior descending and the anterior descending coronary arteries.

The major contribution to cardiac imaging has been the anatomic detail possible with patients who have congenital abnormalities or pericardial diseases [64–68]. Applications to the study of myocardial ischemia and function have not developed rapidly. Myocardial ischemia or infarction can be detected, confirming the presence of ventricular wall–motion abnormalities. The signal intensity of damaged (infarcted) myocardium shows serial changes, which can then be used to measure the extent of the infarcts. Early on, the T_1 and T_2 of the infarcted tissue increase in parallel with edema and increased water content. Later, as scarring develops, these effects reverse [69].

The detection of ischemic myocardium can be investigated by the injection of a paramagnetic compound, such as gadolinium-DTPA, that distributes to viable myocardium in proportion to its blood supply. Gadolinium-DTPA can also detect myocardial infarcts by virtue of a late phase of signal enhancement when it enters damaged tissues [63]. Whether such approaches will gain widespread use remains to be seen.

EXTREMITIES

In general, the signal from flowing blood is lost during standard spin-echo imaging. This effect is more marked when the direction of flow is perpendicular to the image. Another effect can be documented when blood flow is parallel to the slice. The signal loss is then due to two processes. The first process is caused by the gradients used for imaging and the second by the distribution of flowing blood in the vessel of interest. This dephasing can be used to image the vessels as follows: An image obtained at systole is subtracted from diastole, thereby showing a map of flowing blood in the extremity. This scheme relies on the relative dephasing of moving blood during systole and the relative signal coherence of stagnant blood during end-diastole [17]. This approach is time consuming and is not in routine clinical use.

Variants of the phase-contrast magnetic resonance angiogram also have been been used. The advantage is that the subtracted image need not be gated [70]. This imaging approach has been almost completely replaced by time-of-flight techniques. Early clinical results have shown that it is possible to map out the extent of femoral and popliteal artery stenosis with accuracies approaching 90 percent [71]. Magnetic resonance angiography can evaluate patients with severe peripheral arterial disease and may, in those patients, be superior to arteriography for evaluating the distal runoff arteries of the calf and foot [72]. The accuracy of the technique is decreased in the presence of artifacts generated by surgical clips [73,74], which can cause false-positive findings for the presence of a stenosis. Nevertheless, magnetic resonance angiography may become a substitute for traditional arteriography [75] (Fig. 20-22).

RENOVASCULAR

Spin-echo images are poorly suited to the evaluation of the renal arteries, a reflection of those arteries' varied orientations and number of accessory branches. In addition to showing the renal-artery origins, spin-echo images also give information on the renal parenchyma. The relationship of the main renal arteries to other renal branches and to pathologic processes such as aneurysms can often be shown.

Gradient-refocused sequences can generate images useful for the confirmation of the volume of blood flow in the renal arteries [76]. Early results also suggest that magnetic resonance angiography may be an accurate means of detecting the presence of proximal renal artery stenosis [77,78], and there is possible utility in patients with renal insufficiency [79] (Fig. 20-23). The major limitation to this approach is the consistent weakness of magnetic resonance angiography in identifying accessory renal artery branches [78,80].

Rapid imaging of the kidney following the injection of a paramagnetic substance can show the transit of the material into and out of the kidney, which reflects on global as well as regional perfusion [81]. This method, albeit indirect, may prove useful in confirming the presence of significant arterial stenosis. The differences in transit time caused by a stenosis would change the arrival of the agent and affect the appearance of the kidney (Fig. 20-24).

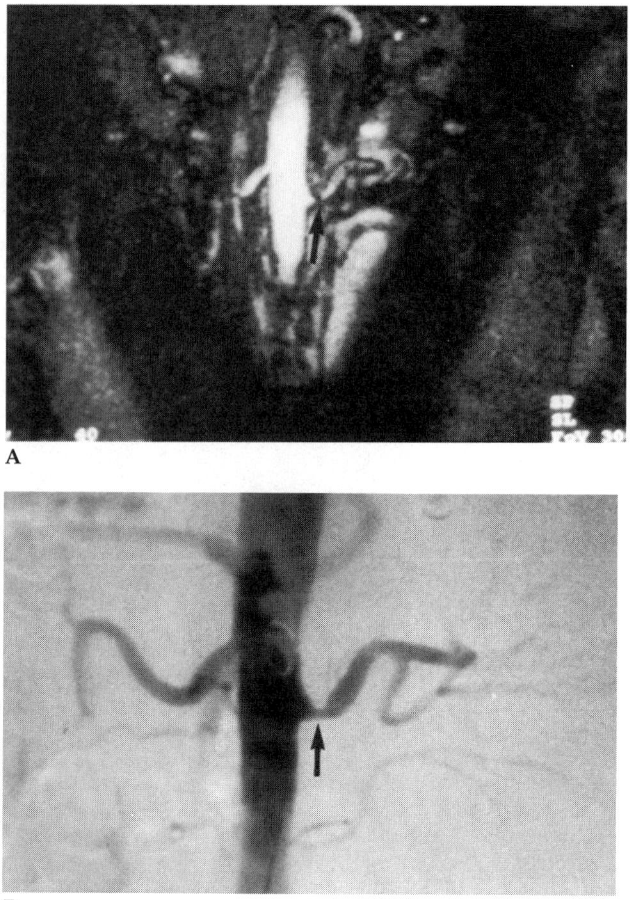

A

B

Fig. 20-23. **A**. Coronal, two-dimensional time-of-flight, bright-blood, magnetic resonance angiographic image of the proximal renal arteries shows a severe stenosis of the left renal artery just beyond the ostium (arrow). Dark oblique lines over the kidneys represent saturation bands to eliminate signal from the renal veins and the inferior vena cava. **B**. Conventional angiogram shows an approximately 70-percent stenosis of the left renal artery (arrow). Magnetic resonance angiograms tend to overestimate the degree of stenosis, as in this case.

MESENTERIC VESSELS

Clinical studies evaluating the utility of magnetic resonance for assessing the mesenteric arteries are few [80]. Experimental studies suggest that changes in signal intensity in mesenteric fat may be used to document mesenteric infarction [82], but that has yet to be proved clinically.

AORTIC DISEASES

Magnetic resonance contributes significantly to the evaluation of diseases that affect the aorta (Fig. 20-25). The lack of signals in the vessel lumen aids in making the differential diagnosis of aneurysm versus dissection

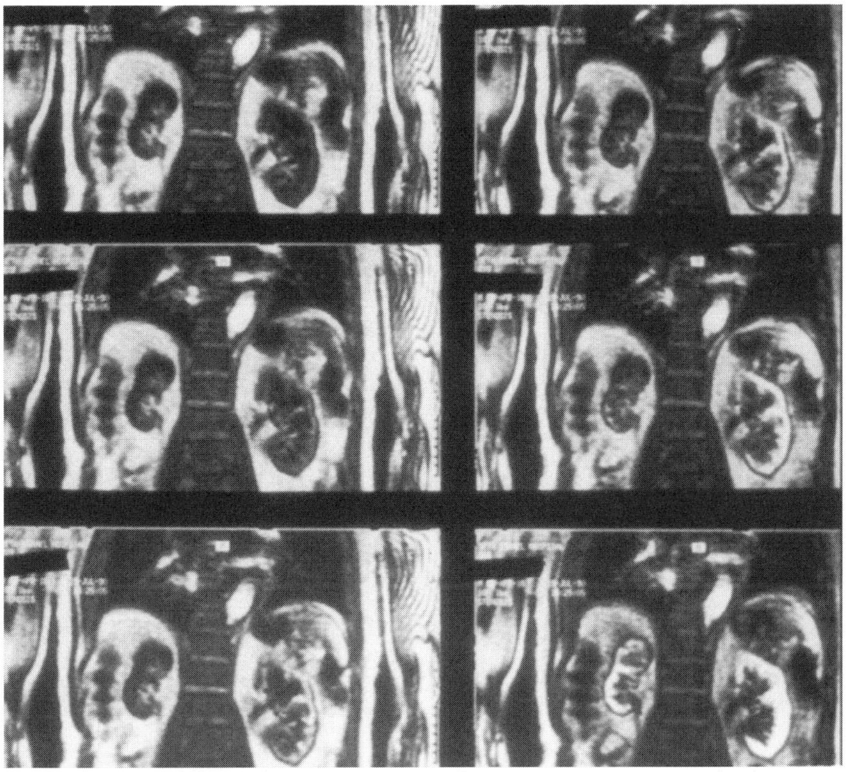

Fig. 20-24. Rapid, coronal, T_1-weighted, turbo-FLASH magnetic resonance images of the kidneys during a bolus of gadolinium-DTPA shows a small right kidney with delayed perfusion. The right kidney was affected with a severe renal artery stenosis.

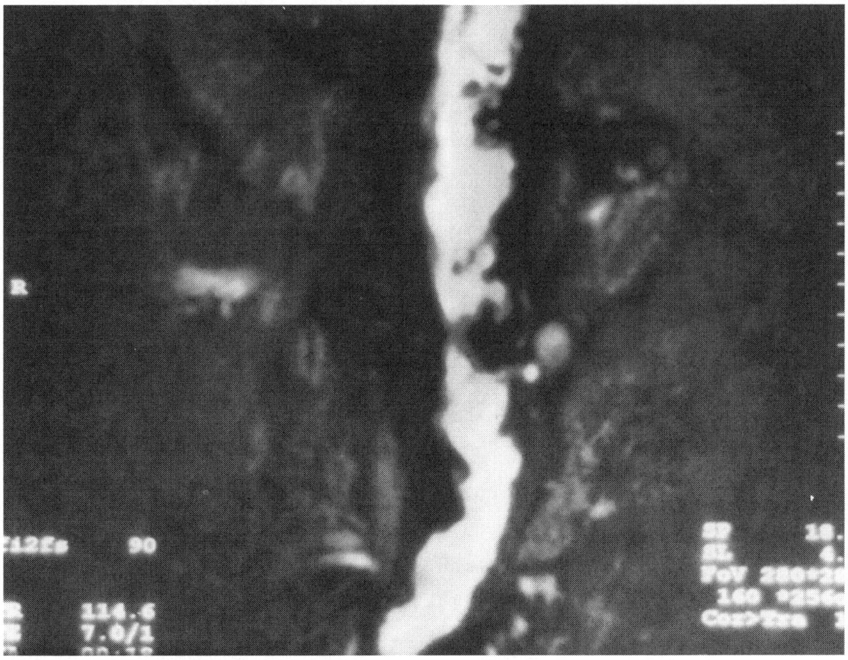

Fig. 20-25. Coronal, T_1-weighted, contrast-enhanced, gradient-echo magnetic resonance image of the abdominal aorta demonstrates diffuse atherosclerotic disease with extensive mural irregularity.

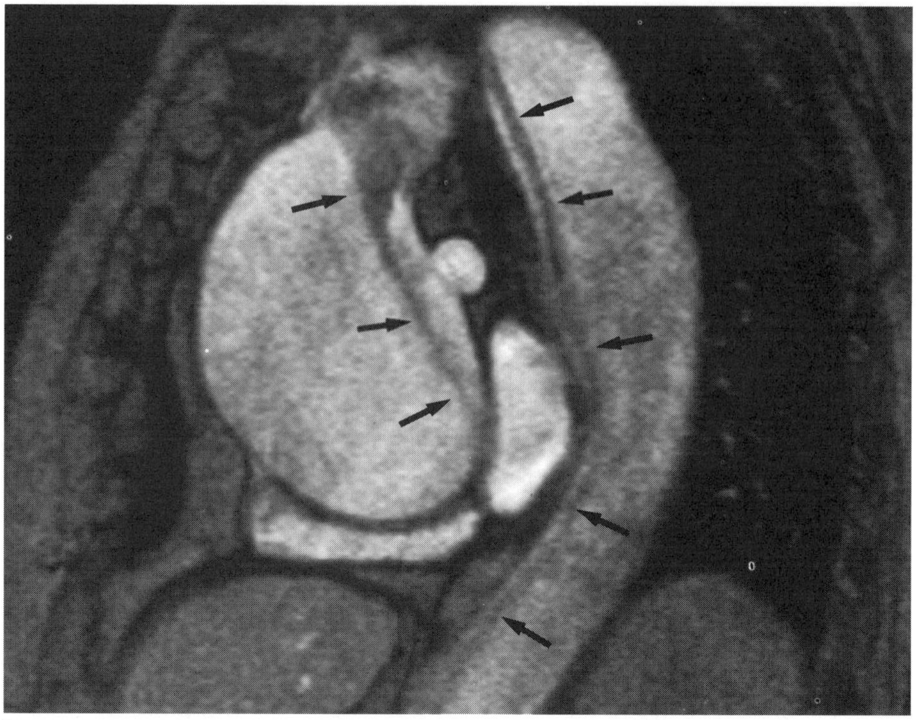

A

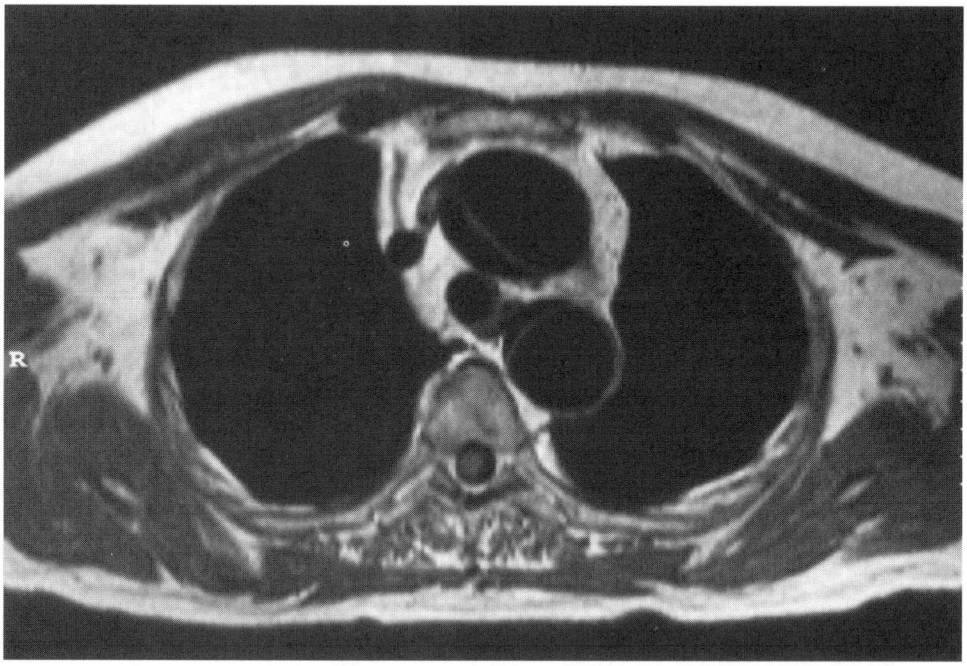

B

Fig. 20-26. **A**. Sagittal-oblique, bright-blood, segmented turbo-FLASH magnetic resonance angiographic image of the thoracic aorta demonstrates a type I aortic dissection with the dissection flap extending from the ascending aorta throughout the visualized descending aorta (arrows). The ascending aorta is also dilated. **B**. T_1-weighted, EKG-gated axial magnetic resonance image just beyond the aortic arch shows the dissection flap to involve both the ascending and descending aorta.

[83,84]. In the former, the full extent of the abnormality and associated thrombus can be clearly mapped out. In the latter, the intimal flap can be clearly delineated. The added advantages of magnetic resonance over computed tomography are the ability to directly image the aortic arch in the coronal plane and the possibility of assessing aortic valve incompetence in patients with type I dissection. The full extent of a dissection also can be easily mapped out down to the abdominal aorta (Fig. 20-26). Gradient-refocused imaging can help in assessing the extent of aortic aneurysm thrombus and in locating the origins of the major branches [84] (Fig. 20-27). Thus, the magnetic resonance techniques are superior to computed tomography for the evaluation of aortic dissections and aneurysms [85].

DEEP-VEIN THROMBOSIS

Magnetic resonance angiography (venography) can be used to detect deep-vein thrombosis in the lower extremities and pelvis (Fig. 20-28). Patent veins show up with increased signals due to flowing blood. Thrombus has lower signal intensities [86,87]. Although the widespread use of this modality is limited by the large expense, it is nevertheless very accurate for the detection of deep-vein thrombosis [88]. Sensitivity and specificity are reported to be greater than 90 percent in the femoral and popliteal veins [89].

Assessment of suspected inferior vena cava and superior vena cava thrombosis [22,90] is reliably performed with magnetic resonance imaging [91]. Normally patent veins show normal signal enhancement. Thrombus shows lack of signal. Extension of renal-vein thrombus from renal-cell carcinoma into the inferior vena cava can be mapped accurately. Appropriate decisions can then be made if surgical intervention has been deemed necessary.

PULMONARY EMBOLISM

Early data showed that thrombus could be visualized on gated spin-echo imaging [92]. This, unfortunately, is practical only for cases of large central pulmonary emboli. Gradient-refocused imaging during a breath hold can show blood vessel signal beyond the segmental branches of the pulmonary arteries [93]. Although this imaging sequence performs well in normal subjects, it is difficult to implement in patients who are short of breath.

An indirect way of determining the presence of thrombosis is persistent parenchymal signal during the cardiac cycle. Attempts to pursue this strategy have not been consistently successful [94].

PULMONARY HYPERTENSION

Pulmonary arterial hypertension can be diagnosed by virtue of a morphologic enlargement of the main pulmonary arteries [95]. Functional evaluation of blood-flow velocity has yet to be studied with magnetic resonance angiography, although the presence of tricuspid regurgitation can be seen in all cases of pulmonary hypertension when rapid imaging sequences are used [96].

SUMMARY

Magnetic resonance has become a valuable approach in the evaluation of vascular diseases. Rapid imaging sequences and two-dimensional rendering of three-dimensional flow information are combined to create magnetic resonance angiograms of the neck and leg arteries. These angiograms can compete in accuracy with traditional arteriography.

Imaging of the coronary arteries is now feasible. The presence of coronary artery disease also can be inferred from magnetic resonance imaging of changes in myocardial signal intensity seen in myocardial scarring and ischemia.

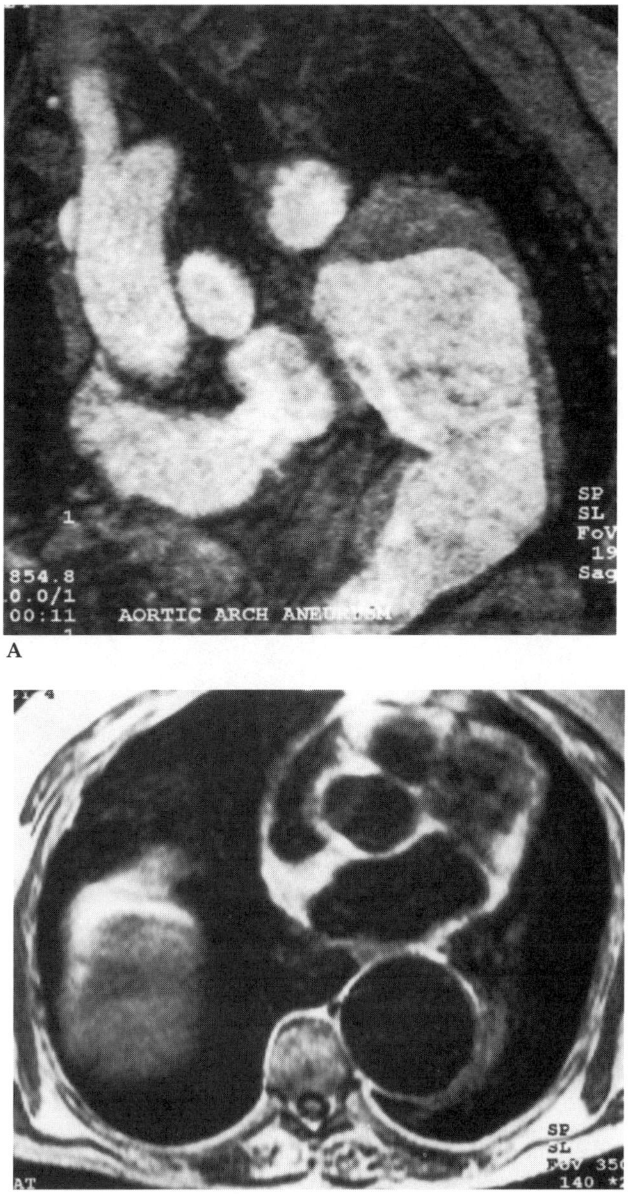

A

B

Fig. 20-27. **A**. Sagittal-oblique, bright-blood, segmented turbo-FLASH magnetic resonance angiographic image of the thoracic aorta shows a large descending aortic aneurysm with plaque formation posteriorly. **B**. T_1-weighted, EKG-gated axial magnetic resonance image through the descending aorta demonstrates the aneurysm, with posterior plaque, and no dissection flap.

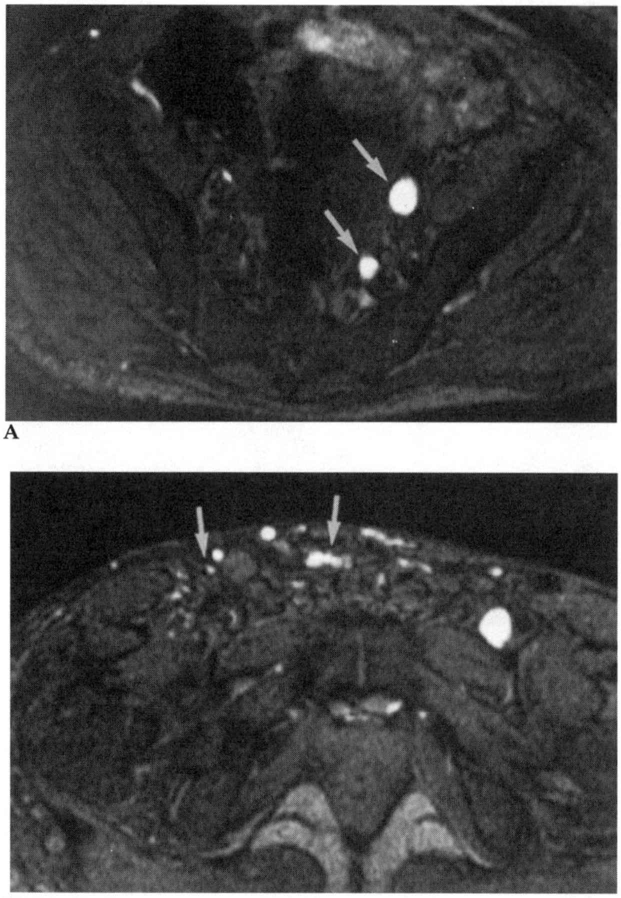

Fig. 20-28. **A**. Axial, bright-blood, two-dimensional time-of-flight magnetic resonance image of the pelvis shows normal venous flow in the left external and internal iliac veins (arrows) and no flow signal in the contralateral veins. **B**. More inferiorly, normal flow is present in the left common femoral vein. No flow signal is identified in the right common femoral vein, with collateral vessels anteriorly (arrows). The appearance is consistent with chronic deep venous thrombosis of the right pelvic and femoral veins. A saturation band was placed over the aorta to eliminate arterial flow.

Although spectroscopy might emerge for wider clinical uses in the next few years, the cost effectiveness of that approach remains to be seen.

References

1. Kolin A. Improved apparatus and technique for electromagnetic determination of blood flow. Rev Sci Instr 1952; 23:236.
2. Lauterbur PC. Image formation of induced local interactions: examples employing NMR. Nature 1973; 242:190–191.
3. Hoult DI, et al. Observation of tissue metabolites using ^{31}P nuclear magnetic resonance. Nature 1974; 252:285–287.
4. Chance B, et al. Detection of ^{31}P nuclear magnetic resonance signals in brain by in-vivo and freeze-trapped assays. Proc Natl Acad Sci USA 1978; 75:4925–4929.
5. Gyulai L, et al. Phosphorylethanolamine: the major constituent of the phosphomonoester peak observed by ^{31}P-NMR on developing dog brain. FEBS Lett 1984; 178:137–142.
6. Hinshaw WS. Spin mapping: the application of moving gradients to NMR. Phys Lett 1974; 48A:87.
7. Maudsley AA. Multiple line scanning spin density imaging. J Magn Res 1980; 41:1120.
8. Bottomley PA. NMR imaging techniques and applications: a review. Rev Sci Instr 1982; 53:1319–1330.
9. Melki PM, et al. Comparison of the Faise method with conventional dual-echo sequences. J Magn Reson Imag 1991; 1: 319–324.
10. Axel L. Blood flow effects in magnetic resonance imaging. AJR 1984; 143:1157–1166.
11. Bradley WG, et al. Blood flow: magnetic resonance imaging. Radiology 1985; 154:443–450.
12. Bradley WG, et al. The appearance of rapidly flowing blood on magnetic resonance images. AJR 1984; 143:1167–1174.
13. Wherli FW, et al. Approaches to in-plane and out-of-plane flow imaging. Noninvasive Med Imaging 1984; 1:127–136.
14. Axel L, et al. A time-of-flight method of measuring flow velocity by magnetic resonance imaging. Magn Reson Imaging 1986; 4:190–205.
15. Stahlberg F, et al. Quantitative study of flow dependence in NMR images at low flow velocities. Comput Assist Tomogr 1986; 10:1006–1015.
16. Bryant DJ, et al. Measurement of flow with NMR imaging using a gradient pulse and phase difference technique. J Comput Assist Tomogr 1984; 8:588–593.
17. Wedeen VJ, et al. Projective MRI angiography and quantitative flow-volume densitometry. Magn Reson Med 1986; 3: 226–241.
18. Meuli RA, et al. MR gated subtraction angiography: evaluation of lower extremities. Radiology 1986; 159:411–418.
19. Frahm J, et al. NMR imaging of dynamic processes using the FLASH technique. Magn Reson Med 1986; 3:321–327.
20. Atlas SW, et al. Vascular intracranial lesions: applications of gradient-echo MR imaging. Radiology 1988; 169:455–461.
21. Lenz GW, et al. In-plane vascular imaging: pulse sequence design and strategy. Radiology 1988; 166:875–882.
22. Unger EC, et al. Single breath-holding scans of the abdomen using FISP and FLASH at 1.5 T. J Comput Assist Tomogr 1988; 12:575–583.
23. Dumoulin CL, et al. Three-dimensional phase contrast angiography. Magn Reson Med 1989; 9:139–149.
24. Nunnally RL, et al. Assessment of pharmacological treatment of myocardial infarction by phosphorus-31 NMR with surface coils. Science 1981; 211:177–180.
25. Styles P, et al. A concentric surface-coil probe for the production of homogeneous B1 fields. J Magn Res 1985; 62:397.
26. Bendall MR, et al. Theoretical description of depth pulse sequences on and off resonance including improvements and extensions thereof. Magn Reson Med 1985; 2:91–113.
27. Bottomley PA, et al. In-vivo solvent-suppressed localized hydrogen nuclear magnetic resonance spectroscopy: a window on metabolism? Proc Natl Acad Sci USA 1985; 82:2148–2152.
28. Wilson JR, et al. Evaluation of energy metabolism in skeletal muscle of patients with heart failure with gated phosphorus-31 nuclear magnetic resonance. Circulation 1985; 71:57–62.
29. Bottomley PA, et al. The fate of inorganic phosphate and pH in regional myocardial ischemia and infarction: a noninvasive ^{31}P NMR study. Magn Reson Med 1987; 5:129–142.
30. Kameda K, et al. Localized proton spectroscopy of focal brain pathology in humans: significant effects of edema on spin-spin relaxation time. Magn Reson Med 1994; 31:537–540.
31. Bottomley PA, et al. Noninvasive detection and monitoring of regional myocardial ischemia in situ using depth-resolved 31P NMR spectroscopy. Proc Natl Acad Sci USA 1985; 82: 8747–8751.
32. Sillerud LO, et al. Structure and metabolism of mammalian

liver glycogen monitored by carbon-13 nuclear magnetic resonance. Biochemistry 1983; 22:1087–1094.
33. Carr DH, et al. Intravenous chelated gadolinium as a contrast agent in NMR imaging of cerebral tumours. Lancet 1984; 1:484–486.
34. Wesby GE, et al. Effect of gadolinium-DPTA on the relaxation times of normal and infarcted myocardium. Radiology 1984; 153:165–169.
35. Saeed M, et al. Reversible and irreversible injury in the reperfused myocardium: differentiation with contrast material-enhanced MR imaging. Radiology 1990; 175:633–637.
36. Lin W, et al. Gadolinium-enhanced high-resolution MR angiography with adaptive vessel tracking: preliminary results in the intracranial circulation. J Magn Reson Imag 1992; 2: 277–284.
37. Atkinson DJ, et al. First-pass cardiac perfusion: evaluation with ultrafast MR imaging. Radiology 1990; 174:641–643.
38. Wolf GL, et al. Cardiovascular toxicity and tissue proton T_1 response to manganese injection in the dog and rabbit. AJR 1983; 141:193–197.
39. Couet WR, et al. Factors affecting nitroxide reduction in ascorbate solution and tissue homogenates. Magn Reson Imaging 1985; 3:83–88.
40. Runge VM, et al. Work in progress: potential oral and intravenous paramagnetic NMR contrast agents. Radiology 1983; 147:789–791.
41. Bradley WG, et al. Comparison of CT and MR in 400 patients with suspected disease of the brain and cervical spinal cord. Radiology 1984; 152:695–702.
42. Bradley WG, et al. Effect of methemoglobin formation on the MR appearance of subarachnoid hemorrhage. Radiology 1985; 156:99–103.
43. DeLaPaz RL, et al. NMR imaging of intracranial hemorrhage. J Comput Assist Tomogr 1983; 8:599–607.
44. Lee BC, et al. MR imaging of cerebral vascular malformations. AJNR 1985; 6:863–870.
45. Gomori JM, et al. Occult cerebral vascular malformations: high-field MR imaging. Radiology 1986; 158:707–713.
46. Savino PJ, et al. High-field magnetic resonance imaging in the diagnosis of cavernous sinus thrombosis. Arch Neurol 1986; 43:1081–1082.
47. Scott JA, et al. Magnetic resonance imaging of a venous angioma. AJNR 1985; 6:284–286.
48. Ross JS, et al. Intracranial aneurysms: evaluation by MR angiography. AJR 1990; 155:159–165.
49. Huston III J, et al. Blinded prospective evaluation of sensitivity of MR angiography to known intracranial aneurysms: Importance of aneurysm size. AJNR 1994; 15:1607–1614.
50. Hope PL, et al. Cerebral energy metabolism studied with phosphorus NMR spectroscopy in normal and birth-asphyxiated infants. Lancet 1984; 2:366–370.
51. Polak JF, et al. Detection of internal carotid artery stenosis: comparison of MR angiography, color Doppler sonography, and arteriography. Radiology 1992; 182:35–40.
52. Masaryk AM, et al. 3DFT MR angiography of the carotid bifurcation: potential and limitations as a screening examination. Radiology 1991; 179:797–804.
53. Litt AW, et al. Diagnosis of carotid artery stenosis: comparison of 2DFT time-of-flight MR angiography with contrast angiography in 50 patients. AJR 1991; 156:611–616.
54. Riles TS, et al. Comparison of magnetic resonance angiography, conventional angiography, and duplex scanning. Stroke 1992; 23:341–346.
55. Huston J, et al. Carotid artery: prospective blinded comparison of two-dimensional time-of-flight MR angiography with conventional angiography and duplex US. Radiology 1993; 186:339–344.
56. Wilkerson DK, et al. The comparative evaluation of three-dimensional magnetic resonance for carotid artery disease. J Vasc Surg 1991; 14:803–811.
57. Katz J, et al. Estimation of human myocardial mass with MR imaging. Radiology 1988; 169:495–498.
58. Sechtem V, et al. Measurement of right and left ventricular volumes in healthy individuals with cine MR imaging. Radiology 1987; 163:697–702.
59. Edelman RR, et al. Cardiac function: evaluation with fast-echo MR imaging. Radiology 1987; 162:611–615.
60. Utz JA, et al. Valvular regurgitation: dynamic MR imaging. Radiology 1988; 168:91–94.
61. Gomes AS, et al. Coronary artery bypass grafts: visualization with MR imaging. Radiology 1987; 162:175–179.
62. Manning WJ, et al. A preliminary report comparing magnetic resonance coronary angiography with conventional angiography. N Engl J Med 1993; 328:828–832.
63. Atkinson DJ, et al. Cineangiography of the heart in a single breath hold with a segmented turbo-FLASH sequence. Radiology 1991; 178:357–360.
64. Soulen RL, et al. Advances in noninvasive evaluation of congenital anomalies of the thoracic aorta. Radiol Clin N Am 1985; 23:727–736.
65. Didier D, et al. Congenital heart disease: gated MR imaging in 72 patients. Radiology 1986; 158:227–235.
66. Soulen RL, et al. Postoperative evaluation of complex congenital heart diseases by magnetic resonance imaging. Radiographics 1987; 7:975–1000.
67. Sechtem V, et al. MRI of the abdominal pericardium. AJR 1986; 147:245–252.
68. Kersting-Sommerhoff BA, et al. Magnetic resonance imaging of congenital heart disease: sensitivity and specificity using receiver operating characteristic curve analysis. Am Heart J 1989; 118:155–162.
69. Canby RC, et al. Proton nuclear magnetic resonance relaxation times in severe myocardial ischemia. J Am Coll Cardiol 1987; 10:412–420.
70. Gullberg GT, et al. MR vascular imaging with a fast gradient refocusing pulse sequence and reformated images from transaxial sections. Radiology 1987; 165:241–246.
71. Mulligan SA, et al. Peripheral arterial occlusive disease: prospective comparison of MR angiography and color duplex US with conventional angiography. Radiology 1991; 178:695–700.
72. Owen RS, et al. Magnetic resonance imaging of angiographically occult runoff vessels in peripheral arterial occlusive disease. N Engl J Med 1992; 326:1577–1581.
73. Owen RS, et al. Symptomatic peripheral vascular disease: selection of imaging parameters and clinical evaluation with MR angiography. Radiology 1993; 187:627–635.
74. Yucel EK, et al. Atherosclerotic occlusive disease of the lower extremity: prospective evaluation with two-dimensional time-of-flight MR angiography. Radiology 1993; 187:637–641.
75. Cambria RP, et al. The potential for lower extremity revascularization without contrast arteriography: Experience with magnetic resonance angiography. J Vasc Surg 1993; 17:1050–1057.
76. Wolf RL, et al. Measurement of normal renal artery blood flow: cine phase-contrast MR imaging vs clearance of p-Aminohippurate. AJR 1993; 161:995–1002.
77. Kent CD, et al. Magnetic resonance imaging: a reliable test for the evaluation of proximal atherosclerotic renal arterial stenosis. J Vasc Surg 1991; 13:311–318.
78. Debatin JF, et al. Imaging of the renal arteries: value of MR angiography. AJR 1991; 157:981–990.
79. Yucel EK, et al. Time of flight renal MR angiography in patients with renal insufficiency. Magn Reson Imaging 1993; 11:925–930.

80. Kaufman JA, et al. MR imaging (including MR angiography) of abdominal aortic aneurysms: comparison with conventional angiography. AJR 1994; 163:203–210.
81. Mitchell DG, et al. Induced renal artery stenosis in rabbit magnetic resonance imaging angiography, and radionuclide determination of blood volume and blood flow. Magn Reson Imaging 1988; 6:113–124.
82. Cohen JR, et al. Superior mesenteric artery balloon occlusion: a nonoperative model of small bowel ischemia in dogs. Invest Radiol 1987; 22:871–874.
83. Kersting-Sommerhoff BA, et al. Aortic dissection: sensitivity and specificity of MR imaging. Radiology 1988; 166:651–655.
84. Dinsmore RE, et al. Magnetic resonance imaging of thoracic aortic aneurysms: comparison with other imaging methods. AJR 1986; 146:309–314.
85. Cigarroa JE, et al. Diagnostic imaging in the evaluation of suspected aortic dissection: old standards and new directions. N Engl J Med 1993; 328:35–43.
86. Spritzer CE, et al. Deep venous thrombosis evaluation with limited-flip-angle, gradient-refocused MR imaging: preliminary experience. Radiology 1988; 166:371–375.
87. Rapoport S, et al. Venous clots: evaluation with MR imaging. Radiology 1987; 162:527–530.
88. Evans AJ, et al. Detection of deep venous thrombosis: prospective comparison of MR imaging with contrast venography. AJR 1993; 161:131–139.
89. Erdman W, et al. Deep venous thrombosis of extremities: role of MR imaging in the diagnosis. Radiology 1990; 174:425–431.
90. McMurdo K, et al. Normal and occluded mediastinal veins. Radiology 1986; 159:33–38.
91. Hansen M, et al. Assessing the patency of mediastinal and thoracic inlet veins: value of MR imaging. AJR 1991; 155:1177–1182.
92. White RD, et al. MR imaging of pulmonary arterial hypertension and pulmonary emboli. AJR 1987; 149:15–21.
93. Wielopolski PA, et al. Three-dimensional MR imaging of the pulmonary vasculature: preliminary experience. Radiology 1992; 183:465–472.
94. Ovensfors CO, et al. Diagnosis of peripheral pulmonary emboli by MR imaging: an experimental study in dogs. Magn Reson Imaging 1988; 6:487.
95. Didier D, et al. Estimation of pulmonary vascular resistance by MRI in patients with congenital cardiovascular shunt lesions. AJR 1986; 146:919–924.
96. Frank H, et al. Detection and quantification of pulmonary artery hypertension with MR imaging: results in 23 patients. AJR 1993; 161:27–31.

Vascular Nuclear Medicine

Finn Mannting
Joseph F. Polak

In 1927, Blumgart first used an intravenous injection of radium to determine the mean circulation time in humans [1]. In the following years, cumbersome external detectors often were used to measure cardiac output, organ transit times, and shunt lesions [2–4]. With the introduction of external imaging devices in the 1950s and 1960s [5,6], it became possible to map the distribution of radioisotopes in different vascular beds. Since then, the use of computers and the development of newer radiopharmaceuticals have expanded the diagnostic possibilities of nuclear medicine.

Despite these improvements, the limitations in intrinsic resolution of the radionuclide technique make it impossible to image vascular anatomy accurately. What is possible, and therefore the purpose of nuclear medicine vascular studies, is the assessment of functional abnormalities in a given vascular bed or organ secondary to abnormalities in the feeding or draining vessels. Two examples of this approach are myocardial perfusion imaging using thallium-201 (Tl-201) and the detection of functional renal-artery stenosis using radiolabeled tracers excreted by the kidneys. This chapter reviews the principles and the current status of radionuclides applied in vascular diseases.

Radionuclides

The administration of radioactive materials to humans raises immediate concerns about radiation exposure and potential carcinogenic effects. Once administered, the ideal radiopharmaceutical should reach the organ of interest instantly and reside in it for just enough time to permit imaging. It then should be rapidly eliminated. The isotope should ideally emit radiation of only gamma energy, and that energy should be matched to the imaging device. Unfortunately, this scenario is physically impossible. This chapter's discussion of the basic principles of radionuclide imaging will reveal its utility and its limitations.

There are three forms of radioactive decay: gamma emission, beta emission, and alpha decay. The term **x-ray** refers to gamma rays (photons) produced by the impact of electrons on a metal target. The mode of production of these photons is different in the case of an administered radionuclide [7,8]. These photons are, in essence, the product of a transition in the energy state of a nucleus (nuclear isomerism). A typical example is that of technetium-99m (Tc-99m) (Fig. 21-1). Here, the decay of molybdenum-99 (Mo-99) obtained as a fission product leads to Tc-99m, which has a half-life of 6.03 hours. Transitions in nuclear energy levels yield three photon energies—γ_1, γ_2, and γ_3—only one of which, γ_2, is suitable for imaging. Of the remaining two, γ_3 is emitted too infrequently, and γ_1 is emitted with too low an energy to be of any use for imaging. Any nucleus that has a gamma decay also has the finite probability that a portion of the energy destined to become a gamma ray is, instead, transferred to conversion electrons. Unfortunately, those electrons, in turn, transfer their energy to the surrounding tissues and therefore can account for a significant proportion of the radiation dose during isotope decay. This process is referred to as **internal conversion**. The lower the internal conversion fraction, the smaller the dose that is absorbed.

In the second mode of decay, beta emission, the transformation of one nucleus into another is associated with the emission (or absorption) of a particle. This process can take place in one of three ways. The first way, beta decay, consists of the emission of an electron as a neutron transforms into a proton. The electrons emitted with a range of energies in this way interact with surrounding tissues, bleeding off their energy locally. They cannot be used to image (Fig. 21-2). In the second way, positron decay, a proton transforms into a neutron, and a positive particle is emitted. That particle has an energy greater than 1.022 MeV (megaelectron volts). In contrast to the emission of an electron, however, energy is not completely given up to surrounding tissues. A positron can combine with an electron in the surrounding tissues, thereby liberating a pair of photons of 511 keV (kiloelectron volts) emitted at 180 degrees to each other (Fig. 21-3). The distance covered by the positron before the emission of the photons is typically 1 to 5 mm. Since the photons are emitted in opposite directions, they can be detected and used in positron tomography. Finally, a process called electron capture consists of the absorption by the nucleus of one of the electrons of the atomic shell. Again, a proton is transformed into a neutron. The vacancy created in the electronic shell is then reshuffled as electrons redistribute themselves. As this occurs, photons of characteristic energy are emitted (Fig. 21-4). These photons are called characteristic x-rays because their origin is similar to that of photons generated in x-ray tubes. Electron capture and positron emission can occur in the same nucleus if the energy level difference between the nuclei is greater than 1.022 MeV.

The final form of decay, alpha decay, consists of the liberation of a helium nucleus from a very heavy, large nucleus (Fig. 21-5). This process results in large amounts of energy deposition in tissues and is not used for imaging.

Gamma decay and beta decay are commonly encountered in imaging applications. Ideally, photons emitted between 80 and 300 keV can be used for imaging with optimal results at roughly the energy of Tc-99m (140 keV). The use of varied forms of isotopic compounds has to do with their biodistribution (i.e., Tl–201 in the myocardium), their ease of chemical preparation (i.e., I-125 fibrinogen), or their incorporation in metabolic pathways (i.e., carbon-11 (C-11) palmitate). Compounds having similar biologic behaviors are preferable if they can be labeled with iso-

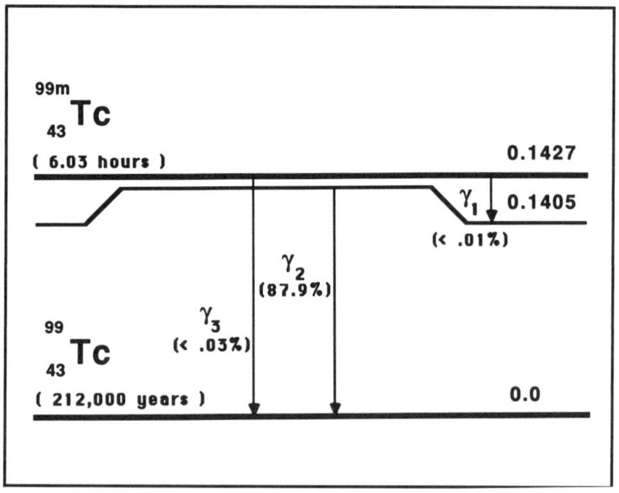

Fig. 21-1. Decay scheme of Tc-99m. The gamma ray with 140-keV energy transition (γ_2) is the one used for imaging. Nuclear isomerism entails that the energy level of the nucleus changes without any change in the number of protons or neutrons.

topes having decay characteristics resembling those of Tc-99m.

Instrumentation

PRINCIPLES

Scintillation detectors such as sodium iodide (NaI) (thallium-activated) have long been the instruments used to map the distribution of radiocompounds in the body. In its simplest form, a detector consists of a NaI crystal, in which an incident photon interacts. This interaction takes place in a somewhat complex manner in that three physical processes are involved: Compton scattering, photoelectric effect, and pair production. The end point is the production of a flash of light, the intensity of which is proportional to the incident photon energy. This flash is processed by a photomultiplier tube into a voltage pulse, which is also proportional to the gamma photon energy (Fig. 21-6). It is therefore possible to tune in to a specific energy range of emitted photons, within limitations.

The first of these limitations is that the processes responsible for dispersing energy in the detector crystal are also at work in the patient. After injection, an isotope loses significant amounts of the total gamma rays emitted. This attenuation of the number of photons is a function of the depth of the target organ or vessel in the body. The energy lost by the photons is reemitted at lower energies, contributing to a background of scattered photons that makes unreliable the quantitative evaluation of the number of photons or radioactivity in a target organ. The other limitation or restriction is that higher-energy photons may not be detected accurately since they might not deposit all their energy in the imaging crystal. That is the case when photons bounce back from the crystal or take a grazing trajectory sideways toward the crystal casing. At sufficiently high energies, the photons may literally traverse the crystal while depositing only a fraction of their energy. A final restriction of this process is that low-energy photons may not exit the patient from deeper organs or, if they do, may be very difficult to detect due to scattering from higher-energy photons in both patient and crystal (Fig. 21-7).

Ideally, although crystals can function from 30 to 40 keV up to 1,000 keV, operating ranges of 100 keV are apt to yield the best results. The limitation of using a single crystal to detect radioactivity in a patient is that spatial localization is poor. With the probe over the lungs, the transit of a radioactive bolus injected intravenously can be followed. Differences between flow to upper and lower lobes can be measured with two appropriately positioned probes. Carrying out this process leads to mapping isotopic distribution by moving a probe over the body while encoding the spatial location. Although this process is well suited to steady-state uptake and prolonged retention of a radiopharmaceutical, it does not permit simultaneous dynamic imaging over large portions of the body.

Fig. 21-2. **A.** Beta emission. The transition of P-32 to S-32 is associated with the transformation of a neutron into a proton and an electron. That accounts for the atomic number increase from 15 to 16. **B.** The electrons are emitted as a spectrum or "distribution" of energies. The mean energy of the electrons is one-third the E_{max} value (maximum energy).

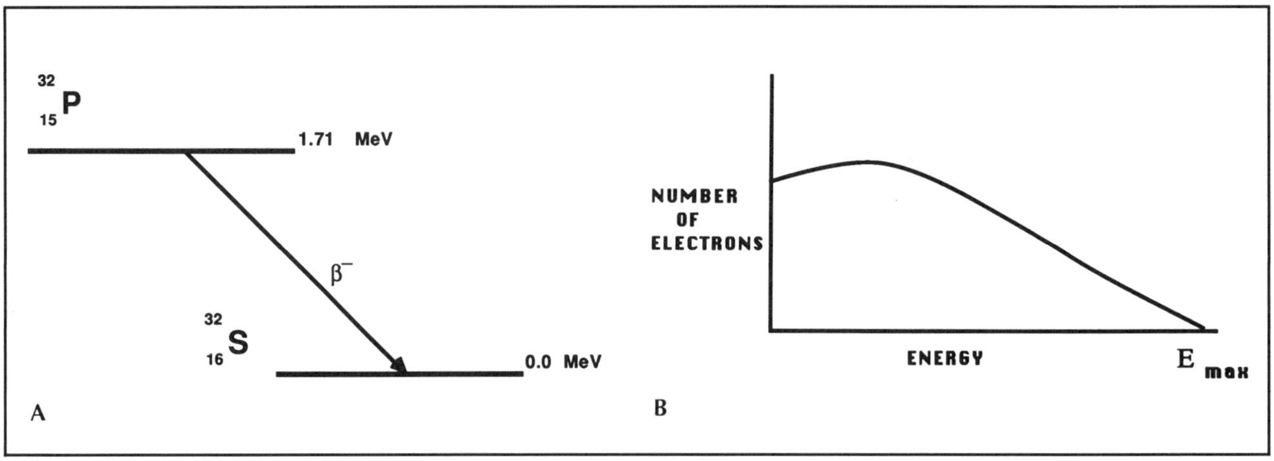

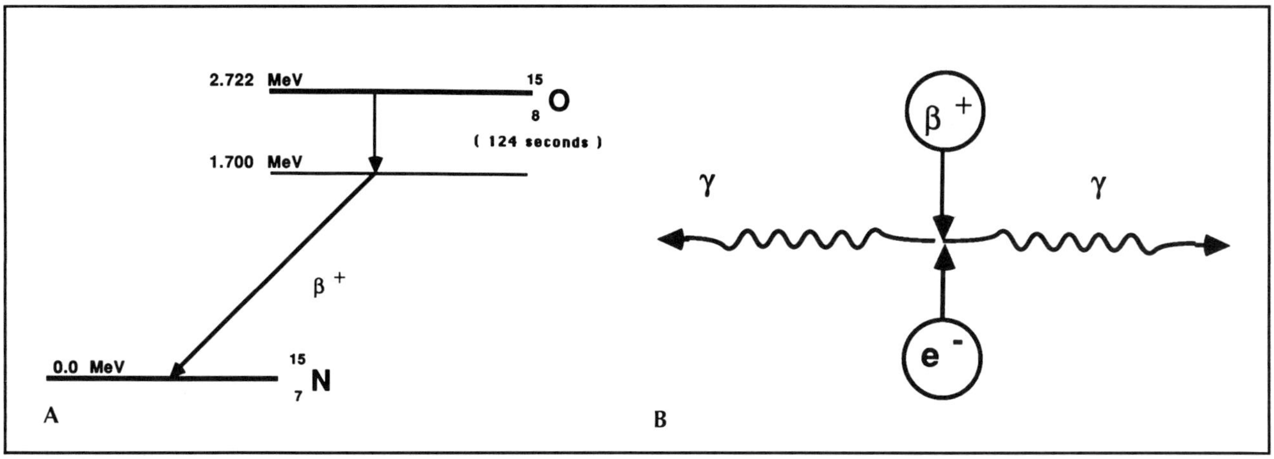

Fig. 21-3. **A.** Positron emission. The transition of O-15 to N-15 is also associated with the transformation of a proton into a neutron and a positron. That accounts for a decrease in the atomic number from 8 to 7. At least a 1.022-MeV energy level difference is required for this to occur. The positron emitted has a supplemental energy above the rest mass of 511 keV, which is distributed in a fashion similar to beta emission (Fig. 21-2B). The greater this excess energy, the greater the distance covered before combining with an electron. The distance can vary from 1 to 5 mm. **B.** When a resting positron (511-keV rest mass) combines with a resting electron (511-keV rest mass), two 511-keV photons are emitted at 180 degrees to each other.

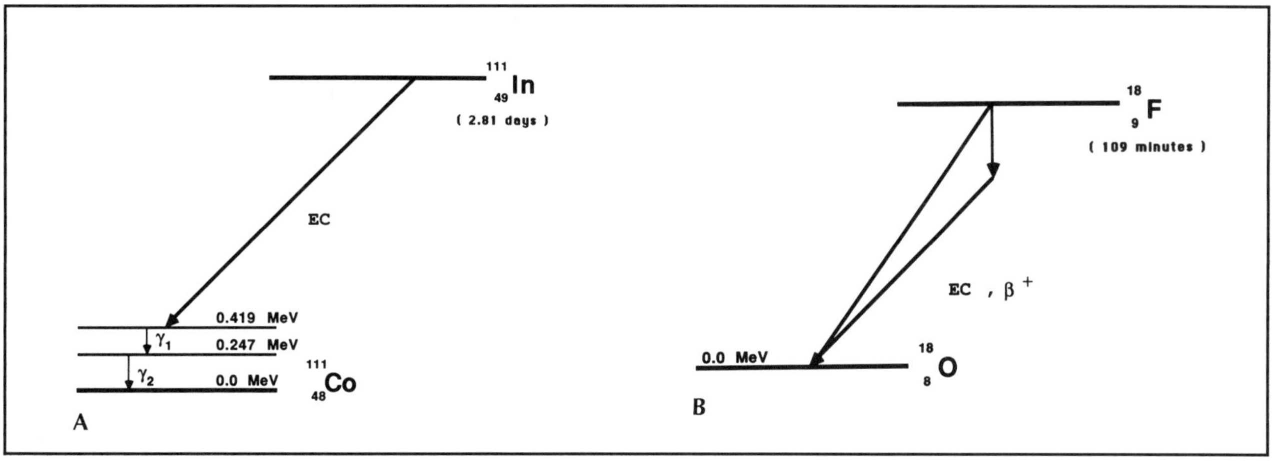

Fig. 21-4. **A.** Electron capture. Electron capture tends to occur when the energy-level differences are not sufficient to induce the emission of a positron. The atomic number decreases since a proton is lost as it combines with an electron. **B.** Positron emission and electron capture. If the energy-level difference is high enough (> 1.022 MeV), electron capture competes with positron emission. Positron emission tends to predominate, however.

PLANAR IMAGING

A gamma camera consists of a large NaI crystal and a series of photomultiplier tubes (Fig. 21-8). This arrangement mimics an array of single crystals, each encoding the position of a gamma ray originating from a patient. There are two critical differences, however. First, a collimator is needed to ensure proper spatial encoding. Because of this design feature, there is a 1,000-fold loss in sensitivity, that is, only one of 1,000 emitted photons reaches the crystal. Second, to improve resolution or the ability to distinguish organ boundaries or small focal areas of pharmaceutical uptake, the crystal thickness is kept to a minimum, which reduces sensitivity further. Typically, for Tc-99m, a 0.25-inch crystal has only 82 percent of the efficiency of a 1-inch crystal.

It is obvious, therefore, that efficiency, or the ability to image smaller amounts of radioactivity, is jeopardized when higher resolution is sought. The major advantage of the current generation of gamma cameras is the possibility of acquiring serial images over an organ of interest. In general, rates of two frames per second can be used to perform dynamic imaging over most organs. With a higher temporal resolution of milliseconds, it becomes possible to acquire studies such as the gated radionuclide

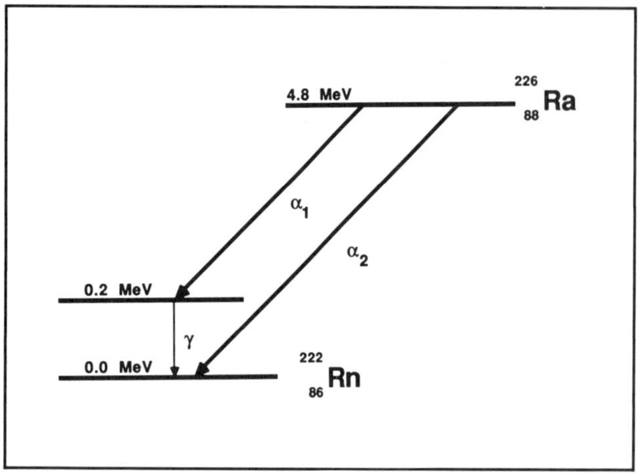

Fig. 21-5. Alpha decay. The alpha decay process cannot be used for imaging. A helium nucleus is emitted, which accounts for a large amount of deposited energy in the tissues.

ventriculogram. Here, the output of the gamma camera consists of an x-y coordinate pair on the crystal surface encoded as to the occurrence of emission during the cardiac cycle. Typically, a series of frames or time windows of 25 to 50 milliseconds spanning the cardiac cycle is acquired and summed for each of 100 to 300 cardiac cycles. What is acquired and subsequently used to determine ejection fraction is the fluctuation of blood volume in the cardiac chambers during the cardiac cycle (Fig. 21-9). A variant of the gated radionuclide study, first-pass radionuclide ventriculography, requires not only similar temporal resolution but also the capability of acquiring large numbers of photons over small time increments (Fig. 21-10). When a full dose of a radiopharmaceutical is viewed by the camera during its transit through right heart, lungs, and then left heart, it becomes possible to saturate the electronic capabilities of the camera (see Fig. 21-9). Obviously, this consideration limits the amount of radioactivity that can be injected. Were it not for this limitation, short half-life tracers, such as tantalum-178 (Ta-178) and iridium-191m (Ir-191m), could be used in large quantities and still offer the advantage of low deposited radiation doses.

Since the 1980s, hybrid cameras equipped with microprocessors have been capable of yet higher counting rates or high spatial resolution. The devices responsible for transforming the signals into digital data have grown more rapid. For yet more rapid imaging, designs have focused on subsegmenting the photomultiplier tubes into groups or smaller segments, each having a better throughput rate than its predecessor. Yet the truly digital gamma cameras remain somewhat specialized, design compromises still being made in favor of rapid acquisition rates in exchange for slightly decreased resolution.

By the use of ionization detectors containing gases such as xenon under high pressure, it is possible to achieve both high resolution and rapid rates of acquisition. These gas chambers encode position with the aid of small wire electrodes, hence the name multiwire proportional chambers. The limiting factor to their wide distribution and manufacture is the restricted energy range over which they are efficient. This range is typically below 80 keV, an energy above which most imaging is performed. Nevertheless, special applications such as first-pass radionuclide angiocardiograms can be performed with an isotope such as Ta-178.

The devices discussed thus far are, in essence, capable of planar imaging and thereby give only one projection of the isotopic distribution in a vessel or organ. With tomography, it is possible to reconstruct the three-dimensional distribution of an isotope.

TOMOGRAPHY

The mathematic principle underlying tomography is that to re-create a section from data acquired from multiple projections, it must be reprojected (back-projected) after compensating for the summation effects due to the superposition of counts originating from the tissues. For example, consider imaging by acquiring data from multiple projections of a simple point of radioactivity. The data from, say, 64 projections are stored in a computer. By reconstructing the point and projecting the acquired data onto a slice, the computer automatically localizes the point within the section. However, this reprojection, by itself, ends up giving a picture that features maximal radioactivity in the expected location of the original point source but that includes added activity around the point.

Fig. 21-6. In this schematic of a detector, a photomultiplier processes the flash of light originating in a NaI crystal following the interaction of a gamma ray. This flash of light is picked up by a photodetector and transformed into a stream of electrons, which are accelerated by sequentially placed dynodes. The amplified stream of electrons hits an anode, leading to a voltage pulse.

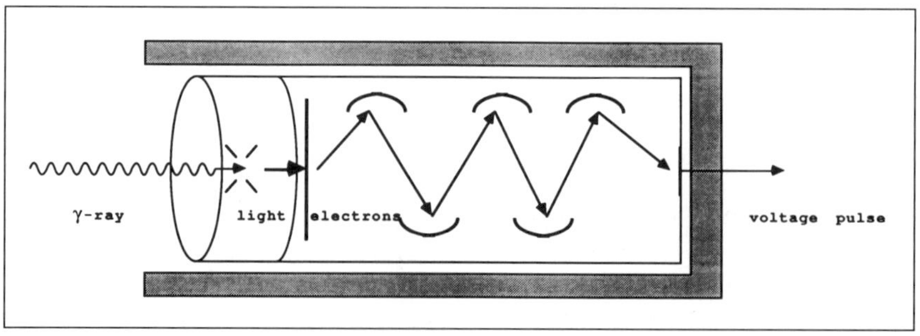

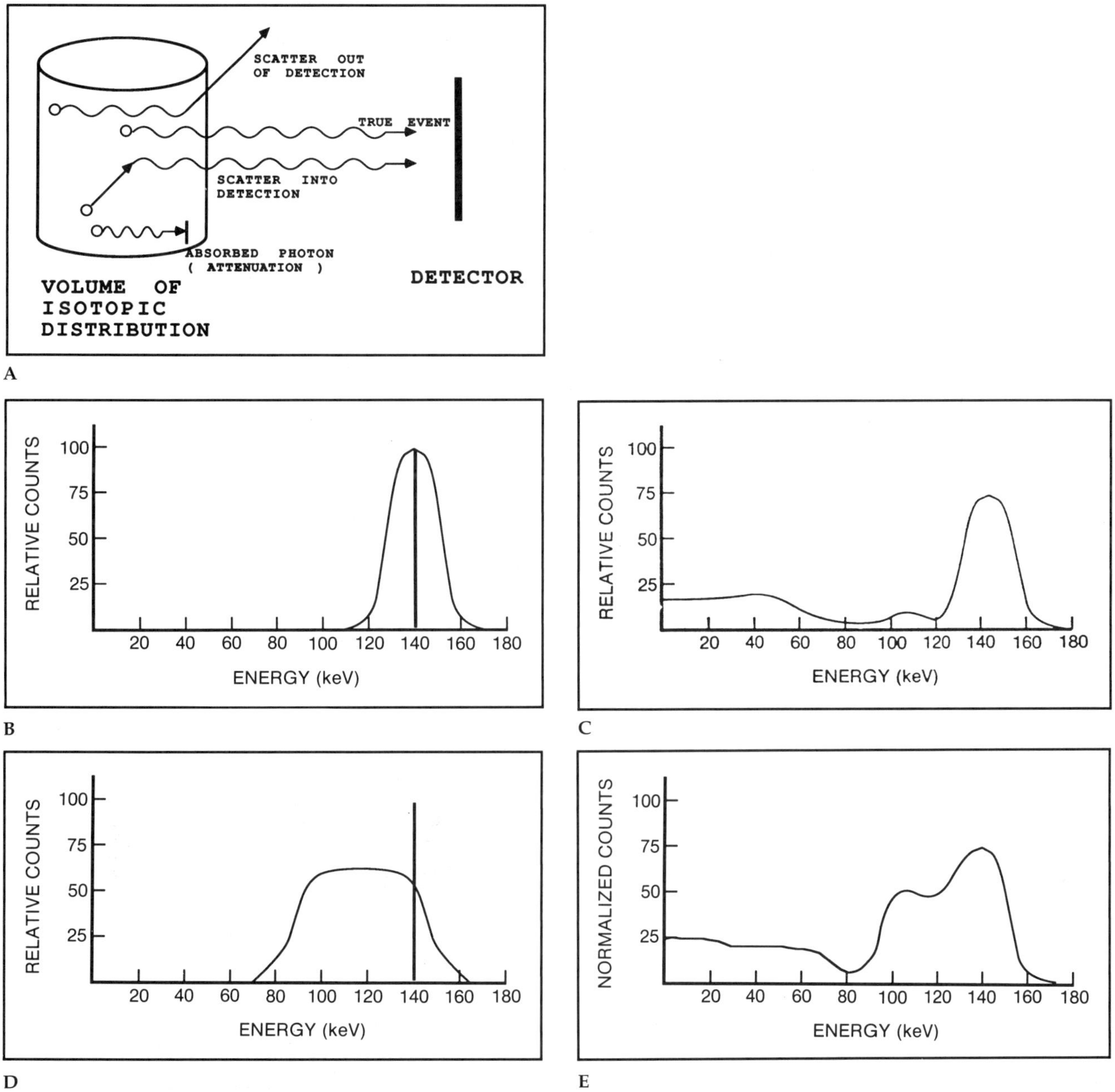

Fig. 21-7. **A.** Summary of the tissue interactions that can occur to a gamma ray within the body. The photon may be emitted as is or lose all its energy within the tissue. Photons of lower energy emitted due to scattering may be detected or may scatter out of the field of view. **B.** The ideal detector response to a 140-keV photon (dark bar) is a broad gaussian curve originating from stochastic process occurring during the detection process (i.e., instrument noise). **C.** The processes responsible for the detection of the photons in the NaI crystal detector add lower energies to the spectrum. This is due to Compton-scattering events or to interactions in the crystal housing. **D.** The energy emitted from an isotopic source depicted in (A) is much broader, with a larger number of photons in the lower energies. **E.** Combining (D) with (C) yields the typical spectrum detected outside the body for Tc-99m (140 keV).

This is more information than the original data set contained! A mathematic operator called a kernel—in essence, a digital filter—is used to compensate and correct for this effect.

Three-dimensional reconstruction is possible after reconstructing a series of these stacked sections and selecting planes of interest. For example, it is possible to acquire first a series of transverse scans through the myocardium. After reconstruction, the isotopic distribution can be displayed in either the short axis or the long axis of the left

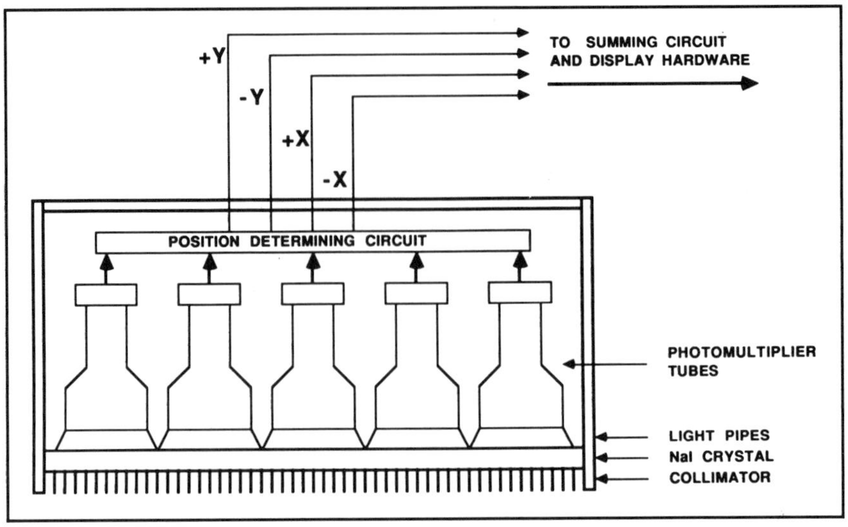

Fig. 21-8. Components of the gamma camera used for most nuclear medicine imaging procedures. A collimator made from either cast lead or lead foil ensures the detection of parallel rays. The sodium iodide (NaI) crystal absorbs the incident photons, transforming their energy into light photons. These are then detected by a bank of photomultiplier tubes that interface with the NaI crystal via light pipes. The resultant voltage pulses are proportional not only to the photon energy but also to the relative position of the detected event. This voltage information is further decoded and sent electronically to the display component of the gamma camera.

ventricle after reprocessing the stacked data along the selected planes.

The first clinical applications, which emerged in the 1970s, used dedicated arrays of single-NaI (or other scintillation) detectors able to scan one section of 1- to 3-cm thickness [9]. Changes in blood volume in the brain were studied early on [10]. The limitations of single-photon-emission computed tomography (SPECT) were those discussed earlier in this chapter: the intrinsic limits of resolution of NaI crystals and the loss of photon signals with depth within the body. For the former, limits of 1 cm and 1.5 to 2.0 cm are the norm for the head and the body, respectively. In the body, this attenuation effect is more significant at lower energies, but, for a point lying in the middle of the abdomen or the heart, up to 85 percent of the signal can be lost. Attenuation compensation schemes have evolved over the last few years. These algorithms are still inherently limited, and only semiquantitative estimates can be made of the true distribution of an isotope such as Tc-99m. SPECT is currently available and widely used with rotation gamma cameras that acquire multiple sections simultaneously. Quality control is much more difficult for these devices than for planar imaging since the slightest change in the uniformity of the detector response can irretrievably corrupt the reconstructed images. Such technical requirements have only been met by the more recent generations of gamma cameras.

With positron-emission tomography (PET), the information from simultaneously ejected photons (180 degrees from each other) is used to encode spatial information. The reconstruction process is similar to that for SPECT, but the attenuation correction process is simpler because of the higher photon energy (511 keV). Coincidence detection of the two ejected photons also helps to improve resolution (7–10 mm in the brain) at the cost of decreased

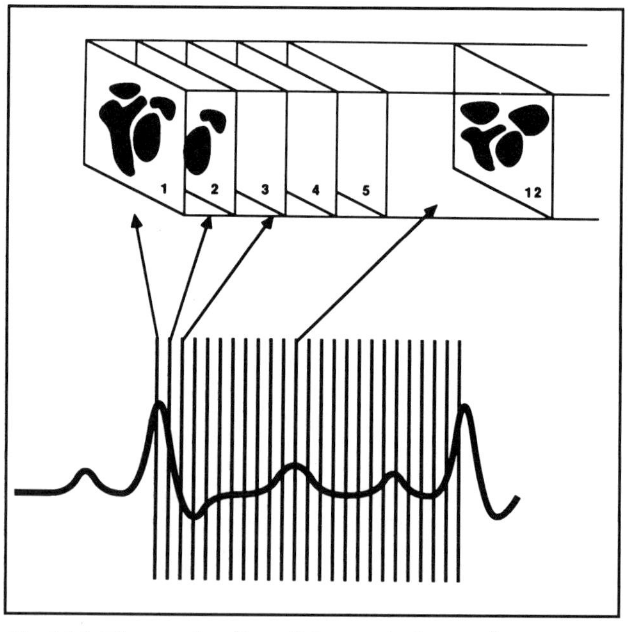

Fig. 21-9. The gated radionuclide ventriculogram is synchronized to the electrocardiogram. The first image is taken during the first 25 msec following the R wave and is formed by all photons detected during that time interval. The second image correspond to the time interval between 25 and 50 msec from the R wave. The pattern repeats for many cardiac cycles, so that each image is the summation of all events during the corresponding time interval with respect to the R wave. Typically, 300 cardiac cycles are needed for such a study.

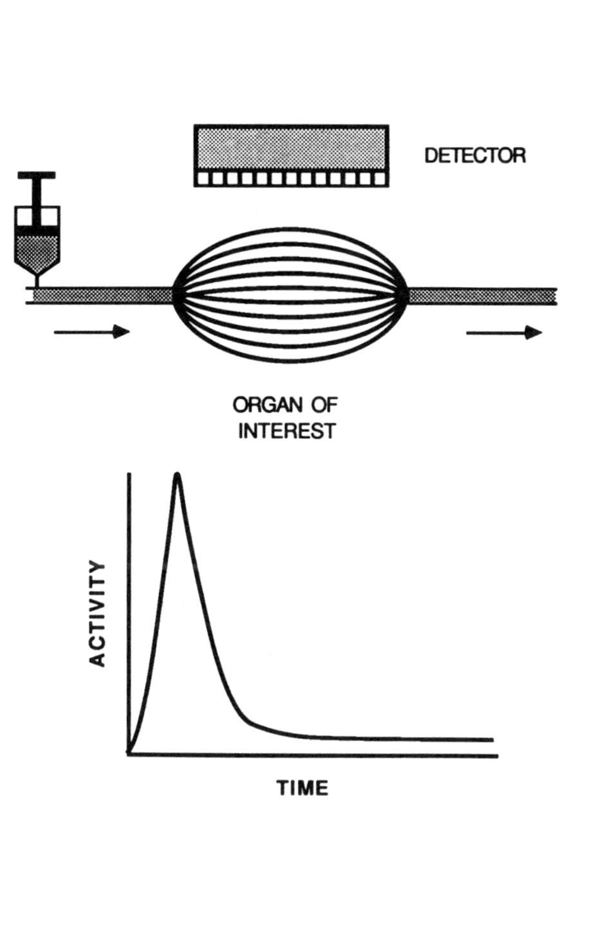

Fig. 21-10. (**top**) Intravascular tracers such as Tc-99m–labeled red blood cells reach a steady state or equilibrium within a few minutes of their injection. (**Bottom**) The early portion of the time-activity curve is the first-pass effect through the organ of interest. The shape of this curve reflects blood flow and size of the intravascular compartment. The latter portion of the curve is the steady-state or equilibrium phase of the isotope, which corresponds to a given amount of activity per cubic centimeter.

efficiency. Because of the short half-lives involved, it is possible to administer larger doses initially. To cope with the higher ensuing counting rates, cesium fluoride (CsF) detectors are used, since these can achieve higher counting rates. Most positron emitters have short half-lives measurable in minutes (Table 21-1), which necessitate the use of specialized chemistry facilities to complex the isotopes quickly to a targeting pharmaceutical. Luckily, C-11 can be incorporated into compounds such as palmitate, and fluorine-18 (F-18) to glucose. For perfusion imaging, oxygen-15 (O-15) extraction can be measured, whereas C-11 carbon monoxide can be used as a blood-volume tracer.

Although gamma cameras and PET ring detectors are currently available, the versatility of the various nuclear-medicine approaches to vascular imaging is primarily due to the wide range of radiopharmaceuticals that can be injected.

Radiopharmaceuticals

Radionuclides used for imaging are administered intravenously either in their pure ionic form, for example, Tl-201 and gallium-67 (Ga-67), or more commonly bound to specific carriers with known biochemical and physiologic behavior, for example, iodohippuran-123, and microspheres labeled with Tc-99m) (Table 21-2). The trend in recent years has been toward tracers of the latter type. More and more substances with well-known biologic properties are being labeled with appropriate radioactive tracers. The tracers simply serve as indicators of where the carrier travels and how it is handled in the organ. Information and data extracted from nuclear-medicine studies are thus functional and physiologic information rather than anatomic images.

Blood-volume tracers can be used either to determine intravascular transit times or to perform static imaging of the body's blood pool (see Fig. 21-10). The first complex used in vascular imaging was I-131–labeled albumin [11]. This tracer is imaged within a few minutes of its injection, since the early biodistribution is that of the intravascular space. Thereafter, the labeled isotope builds up slowly in the interstitium and lymphatic channels. Over long time intervals, it is degraded in the liver. Another complex utilized is chromium-15 (Cr-51)–labeled red blood cells [12]. The radioisotope is complexed to hemoglobin in the cell; its subsequent injection fully parallels the blood-volume distribution. Damaged red cells tend to be cleared by functioning splenic tissue. Cr-51 has a high radiation burden per millicurie of injected dose and a poor imaging energy of 320 keV. Both Tc-99m labeled to human serum albumin (HSA) and indium-113m (In-113m) transferrin complex have been used as blood-pool-imaging agents [13]. Currently, the ideal blood-pool tracer is Tc-99m–labeled red blood cells. The principle is that a reducing agent, tin (stannous ion), first enters the red blood cell. If Tc-99m is then administered in its normally available form as pertechnetate (Tc-99m O_4), it enters the pretreated red cells and binds to the heme moiety of hemoglobin. This preparation is quite stable in vivo.

There are two major variants to the Tc-99m approach. The first, called **in-vivo labeling**, [14], is performed by injecting a compound containing 200 to 400 μg of stannous ion, in this case, the contents of a pyrophosphate kit. After 20 minutes, the injection of 20 mCi of Tc-99m O_4 is sufficient to label red blood cells with an efficiency of 80 to 90 percent. The remaining free pertechnetate distributes into the interstitial spaces, showing preferential thyroid, stomach, and choroid plexus uptake as well. The free isotope is also excreted into the bowel and urinary tract. The second approach, **in-vitro labeling** [15,16], involves taking a sample of blood (10–20 ml) from the patient and incubating it sequentially with pyrophosphate (stannous ion) and Tc-99m O_4. After washing in saline to remove the nonbound pertechnetate, the labeled cells are reinjected into the patient. In this approach, because of the volume involved, a sharp bolus cannot be injected. First-pass radionuclide ventriculogram or first-pass shunt studies are then more difficult to perform. With time, typically within 10 minutes, the tracer is at equilibrium with the body's blood pool. Changes in the blood volume of a

Table 21-1. Isotopes (positron emitters) used for cardiovascular imaging

Isotope	Half-life	Form	Use
Carbon-11	20.3 minutes	Carbon monoxide Labeled palmitate Labeled glucose, pyruvate Labeled amino acids	Cerebral blood volume Cardiac fatty acid metabolism Cardiac glucose metabolism Amino acid metabolism
Nitrogen-13	10.0 minutes	Ammonia Labeled amino acids	Myocardial perfusion Amino acid metabolism
Oxygen-15	124 seconds	Oxygen Labeled water or labeled hemoglobin Labeled carbon monoxide	Oxygen utilization Organ perfusion (brain, heart) Blood-pool imaging
Fluorine-18	108 minutes	Fluoro-2-deoxyglucose	Carbohydrate metabolism
Rubidium-82	75.0 seconds	Dissolved in saline	Myocardial perfusion
Gallium-68	68.3 minutes	Ethylenediaminetetraacetic acid (EDTA) complex	Blood volume Transit-time measurement

cardiac chamber can then be followed as a function of the cardiac cycle [17,18]. Similarly, changes in blood volume of an extremity can be monitored and then measured as a function of exercise or body position [19]. Lack of venous compliance in peripheral vessels can be documented in patients with heart failure. Changes in splenic volume have been measured in humans before, during, and following exercise [20]. Not only can the abnormal vascular spaces of hemangiomas be detected [21,22], but changes in brain blood volume as a function of systemic carbon dioxide partial pressure (pCO_2) can be monitored [23]. Detecting either acute or intermittent gastrointestinal hemorrhage over 24 hours also is possible [24,25].

Many tracers not only distribute in the intravascular spaces but also in the extracellular spaces of tissues. A simple injection of Tc-99m O_4 mimics distribution in the extracellular space but in an imperfect fashion: This compound also has affinity for proteins in plasma and other specific tissue binding sites (choroid plexus, thyroid cells, goblet cells of the stomach). A true extravascular tracer such as labeled inulin remains the gold-standard substance in this category of isotopes [26]. Although studies

Table 21-2. Isotopes (nonpositron emitters) used for cardiovascular imaging

Isotope	Half-life	Form	Use
Technetium-99m	6.03 hours	Varied complexes (pertechnetate, diethylene triamine pentacetic acid [DTPA]) Blood pool (labeled red cells) Brain specific (PAO complex) Myocardial specific (isonitril complex) Aggregated albumin (capillary blockade) Infarct specific (phosphate complex)	Transit-time measurements Early uptake for perfusion Left-to-right shunt lesions Ventricular function Venous patency Bleeding sites Hemangioma Active uptake, to measure perfusion Lung scintigraphy Right-to-left shunt lesions Organ perfusion by intraarterial injection Myocardial infarct
Thallium-201	73 hours	Thallous chloride (potassium analogue)	Myocardial/muscle perfusion Damaged blood-brain barrier
Xenon-133	5.24 days	Gas, dissolved (injected intraarterial) gas (inhaled)	Organ perfusion Lung ventilation Organ perfusion
Iodine-131	8.04 days	Renal specific (iodohippuran) Infarct specific (antimyosin antibody)	Renal perfusion and function Myocardial infarct imaging
Iodine-123 (substitute for I-131)	13.3 hours	Iodofatty acids	Myocardial metabolism/ischemia
Iodine-125	60 days	Thrombus binding (fibrinogen)	Calf vein thrombosis
Indium-111	67 hours	Thrombus binding (labeled platelets) Infarct binding (DTPA, antimyosin)	Arterial or venous thrombosis Myocardial infarct imaging
Gallium-67	78 hours	Infection site (gallium citrate)	Abscess detection

were conducted to measure distribution of these spaces in humans with either I-125 inulin or cobalt (Co-58) bound to vitamin B12, the small quantities of material used to minimize patient dose have relegated such approaches to nonimaging applications. Total body extracellular fluid spaces were measured, and estimates of the interstitial space were made by subtracting the intravascular volume space, derived by either a direct measurement or an estimate made from the blood volume, from the total counts. With newer radioisotopic complexes, such as Tc-99m diethylene triamine pentacetic acid (DTPA) or In-111 DTPA, compounds that distribute in the extracellular spaces are readily available. Although imaging is clearly possible, these compounds are unstable in vivo, and true steady-state measurements are less reliable than with inulin or Co-58 ethylenediaminetetraacetic acid (EDTA). These tracers are used mostly to estimate transit times in either the lung or the kidney. In the lung, shunt studies or estimates of pulmonary transit times as part of double-indicator dilution methods are possible [27,28]. In the kidney, estimates of renal perfusion or transit curves can be used to screen for renal hypertension or to monitor incipient rejection or vascular injury to renal transplants [29,30]. An advantage (or disadvantage) of all true extracellular fluid tracers is their typical renal excretion, which, barring protein binding or active transport in the renal tubules, tends to be proportional of glomerular filtration rate (GFR). Differential estimates of renal function can then be assessed during imaging [31].

In the two approaches discussed above—in-vivo and in-vitro labeling—the isotope complex is injected and fully distributed throughout the body. This is not true with capillary blockade, in which a labeling isotope is complexed to small particulate aggregates (albumin microspheres) and injected proximal to a capillary bed (Fig. 21-11). Such an approach can be used to measure the proportion of blood flow to different parts of the organs [32,33]. In experimental situations, microspheres made of carbon are tagged with different isotopes, injected, and counted in organs of interest after sacrificing the animal. In patients, degradable human albumin microspheres with diameters of roughly 28 μm, or macroaggregated albumin with a size range between 20 and 100 μm, normally are injected intravenously to perform lung-perfusion imaging (or lung scanning). These complexes degrade slowly in vivo. The lung arterioles normally trap all the injected particles, which typically number 200,000 to 1,000,000. The proportion of obstructed arterioles is low (0.01 percent) and unlikely to cause ill effects. The only exceptions are patients with severe pulmonary hypertension. In such cases, the arteriolar bed is restricted in that the injection of a particle with a 30-μm diameter obstructs a more proximal arteriole, which typically has a small diameter (due to myointimal hyperplasia) and therefore compromises a larger portion of the lung. Also, in most cases of chronic obstructive disease, there is frank lung destruction and a reduced vascular bed. For both those reasons, the microemboli caused during lung scanning may acutely jeopardize right-heart function in a manner similar to the pathophysiology of pulmonary embolism if the number and the size of particles are not appropriately reduced

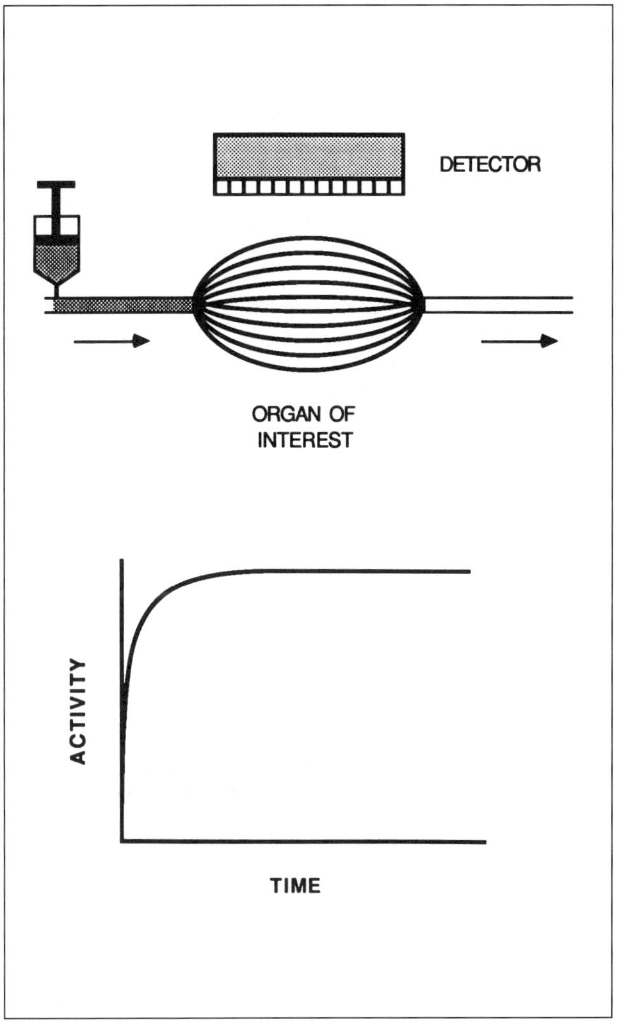

Fig. 21-11. Full extraction and trapping. The injection of appropriately sized labeled particles in an artery feeding a capillary bed can result in trapping of those particles and of the radioactivity they contain. This is the principle behind lung-perfusion scintigraphy. Over a given organ, regional differences in radioactivity reflect regional blood flow. Similar approaches have been used to measure perfusion in arterial beds such as those of the heart or the muscles of the lower extremities.

[34]. Labeled microspheres can be injected into varied arterial beds and used to measure the effects of vascular disease. Selective injections into the coronaries can map out perfusion patterns to different territories and used to quantify the significance of stenoses [35,36]. In the periphery, labeled isotopes have been used to assess impaired muscle perfusion from atherosclerosis, both at rest and following exercise or the administration of vasodilators [37,38]. Finally, capillary blockade can be used to detect vascular shunts or arteriovenous malformations. For example, a right-to-left cardiac shunt is documented by the presence of cerebral and renal activity following a lung-perfusion scan [39]. Using a similar approach, Rhodes and colleagues were able to disprove the existence of small arterial shunts in patients with Paget's disease [40].

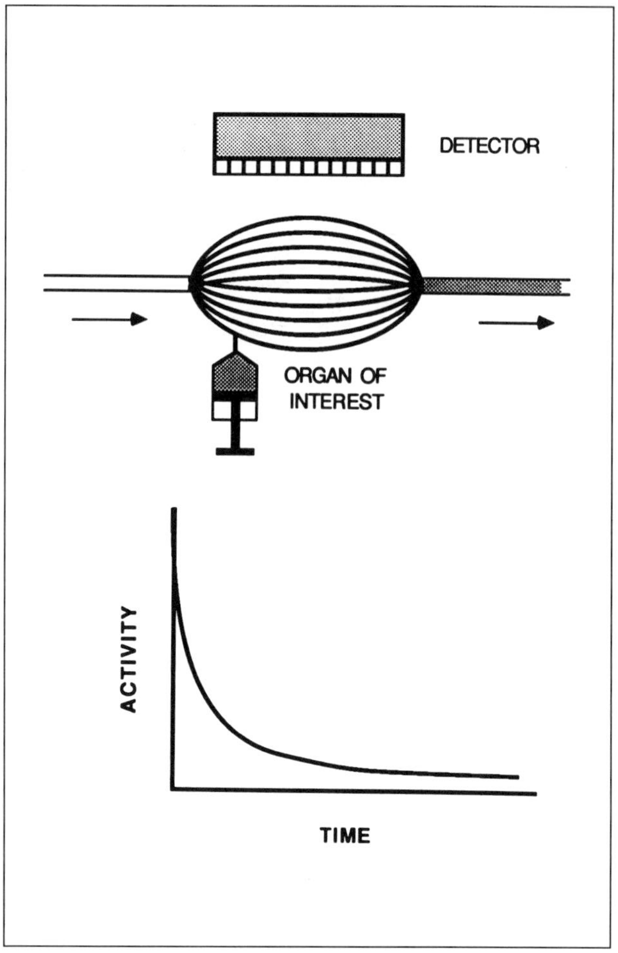

Fig. 21-12. Diffusible tracers. (**Top**) A diffusible tracer, most commonly the radioactive isotope of an inert gas, is injected either directly into a tissue of interest or into the feeding artery. The subsequent clearance rate of the isotope reflects tissue perfusion. (**Bottom**) By measuring the slope of the logarithm of the time-activity curve and knowing the tissue, the partition coefficient of the gas in the tissue perfusion can be estimated directly in cubic centimeters per second.

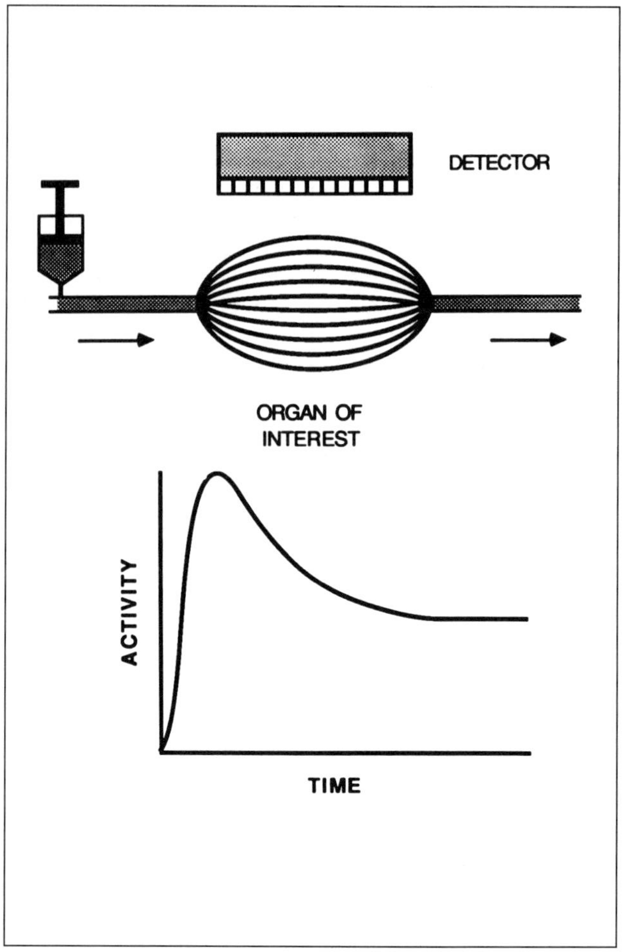

Fig. 21-13. Cellular trapping and extraction. Radiopharmaceuticals that show preferential organ uptake normally show two distinct temporal effects.The first is uptake proportional to blood flow, a reflection of isotope delivery. That, in combination with the extraction efficiency of the organ or its constituents, accounts for the proportion of isotope that remains in the organ soon after the injection. The second effect is a slow equilibrium of the isotope, which reflects trapping by the cell or by receptors in the organ.

When capillary blockade is used to estimate organ perfusion, these measurements can be transformed to cubic centimeters per minutes if the true cardiac output is estimated by other, independent means. Using inert diffusible gases such as xenon-133 (Xe-133) or krypton-85 (Kr-85), it is possible to measure absolute organ perfusion in cubic centimeters per second directly. Those gases, when delivered to an arterial bed as a sharp bolus, tend to leave the organ as a function of their retention in the tissue compartments (Fig. 21-12). Therefore, knowing what is called the partition coefficient, it is possible to determine absolute organ blood flow by ensuring radioisotope egress from the organ [41,42]. Such an approach has been used to determine renal hemodynamics in various disease states [43], to measure peripheral limb blood flow as a predictor of limb salvage or ulcer healing [44], and to document changes in coronary hemodynamics following various interventions [45,46]. This approach is best used as an adjunct to arteriography. It is, however, possible to measure organ perfusion, for example, to the brain, if a combined measurement of isotope uptake in the vascular tree is made during breathing of the isotope [47]. This requires complex data acquisition and analysis, and it cannot offer the same accuracy as the direct intra-arterial approach.

Finally, a broad family of isotopes and radiopharmaceuticals manifest preferential organ or compartment uptake during imaging (Fig. 21-13). An example of physiologic uptake by an isotope is that of potassium. Soon after the injection of potassium or of analogues such as rubidium or Tl-201, distribution in muscle, including myocardium, is proportional to blood flow [3,48]. Subsequently, with time, myocardial or muscle mass can be estimated [49,50]. Overall, Tl-201 is the best analogue currently available, despite the low energies of the mercury-201 (Hg-201) x-rays that make up its decay scheme.

Most metabolic precursors available for imaging are

complexed to positron emitters, for which there are two principal reasons. First, carbon, oxygen, and nitrogen isotopes have low atomic numbers and therefore tend to decay by positron emission. Second, carbon, hydrogen, oxygen, and nitrogen naturally make up most of the metabolic precursors that can be used safely. The inherent drawback to using these isotopic complexes is the need for sophisticated and rapid chemistry as well as a specialized production facility consisting of an on-site cyclotron and a PET scanner. These radiopharmaceuticals can be used to determine perfusion indirectly by monitoring changes in the energetics (i.e., the uptake of C-11 palmitate or N-13 ammonium) of the ischemic myocardium [51,52]. In the brain, precursors such as F-18 fluorodeoxyglucose can monitor overall metabolic activity and delineate zones of decreased perfusion [53].

Another behavior of radiopharmaceuticals comes under the broad category of binding or incorporation. Under specific circumstances, binding to a product released due to cell death, such as myosin labeled to antimyosin antibody, is an indirect indicator of severely reduced perfusion in the zone of a myocardial infarction [54]. Similarly, the lack of binding newer Tc-99m isonitrile complexes to myocardium is an indirect indicator of absent perfusion since radiopharmaceutical delivery depends on blood flow [55]. Active binding of I-125 fibrinogen or Ir-111–labeled platelets to a forming thrombus are examples of the use of direct labels binding to an active component of the clotting mechanism [56,57]. The limitations imposed on the use of those complexes for imaging are inherent to their biologic behavior. For example, there is nonspecific binding of fibrinogen at sites of active inflammation, leading to false-positive exams [58]. Conversely, heparin interferes with labeled platelet binding to thrombus, leading to false-negative exams [59].

Principles of Measurement

Before selecting a radioisotope for vascular imaging, one must determine what form of physiologic information is desired. Blood flow can be measured by the use of indicator dilution methods, inert gas washout, capillary blockade, or relative changes in local distribution of a bound radiopharmaceutical. Regional changes in metabolic activity also reflect local changes in blood flow. Finally, active binding of a complex can be used to image focal areas of thrombosis or infarction directly.

INDICATOR DILUTION

The indicator dilution method can be used to determine cardiac output or organ perfusion. Its application requires a tracer having a volume of distribution restricted either to the intravascular or the extracellular fluid space. This method, in principle, permits full mixing of the injected compound in the compartment to be measured. For example, if labeled red cells were injected into a peripheral vein and a peripheral artery were then sampled, a curve could be built of radioactivity per milliliter of blood over time. This curve represents the transit time of the various labeled red cells through the circulation [60]. It is assumed that all the radioactivity is injected as a very short bolus, reaching the heart almost instantaneously. It has been shown that a mathematical function called a gamma variate best describes the curve's shape [61,62]:

$$tm = \frac{C(t)t\,dt}{C(t)\,dt}$$

where tm is the transit time, and $C(t)$ is the radioactivity/ml. A single pass through the system is assumed.

To measure the total amount of radioactivity injected into the patient, the cardiac output (CO) is calculated as

$$CO = \frac{\textit{injected radioactivity}}{C(t)\,dt}$$

This expression describes a total cardiac output measurement similar to the indocyanine green method. A gamma camera can be used in a similar fashion to determine mean organ transit time from outside the patient.

The same approach can be used to quantify left-to-right cardiac shunts [63]. For example, with the use of an extracellular tracer such as Tc-99m DTPA, a time-activity curve can be constructed for radioactive counts detected by a gamma camera. After correcting for gamma camera dead time, the time-activity curve can be used to measure mean lung transit time. Again, it is assumed that a small bolus is delivered intravenously. It has been shown that recirculation and shunt lesions create a second visible peak in the lung time-activity curve (Fig. 21-14). It is as-

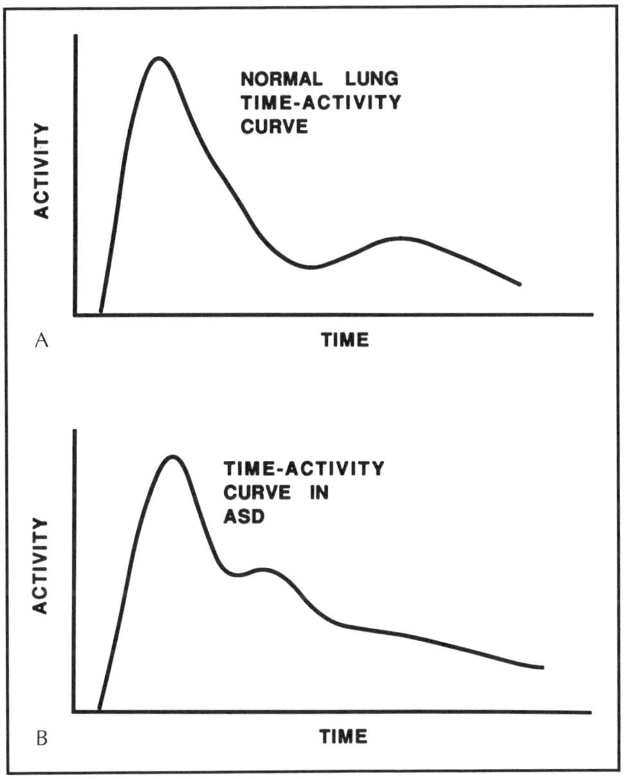

Fig. 21-14. The normal lung time-activity curve does not show a significantly early second peak. **A.** The second peak reflects passage through the systemic circulation. **B.** This curve exemplifies the early recirculation peak seen with a shunt lesion. The relative amplitude of this peak can be used to quantify the size of the shunt. (ASD = atrial septal defect.)

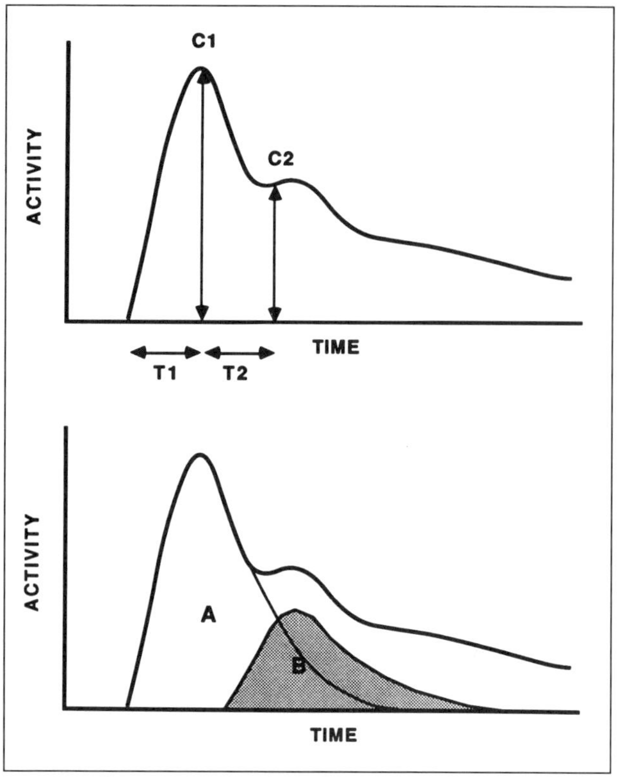

Fig. 21-15. Two commonly used methods of quantifying shunt lesions from the time-activity curve measured over a lung. These are first corrected for gamma camera dead time. **A.** The time-activity curve is shown at a time (T2) equal to the time between the arrival of the isotope and peak activity (T1). If the Ratio C2:C1 is greater than 0.35, a shunt is most likely present. This ratio can be used to quantify the shunt lesion. **B.** A more sophisticated mathematic fit is made to the gamma variate function. The curve with surface A measures pulmonary blood flow, which combines systemic and shunt flow. The curve with area B is proportional to shunt flow proper. A − B is, therefore, systemic blood flow. The pulmonary-to-systemic shunt ratio is, therefore, A/(A − B).

sumed that both curves are typical of gamma variate function. The early portion of the curve is first fitted to a gamma variate, that is, it represents the true forward output of the right heart chamber. After subtracting the first curve fitted to a gamma variable function, the resultant curve is again fitted to a gamma variate. This second curve represents radioactivity returning to the pulmonary circulation via left-to-right shunts (Fig. 21-15). Thus, the first fitted curve (A) is total pulmonary blood flow, and the second (B) represents shunt flow. The QP:QS, or pulmonary-to-systemic shunt ratio, is then A/(A − B). This value is typically 1 to 1.2 in normals. The value greater than unity is thought to represent flow via the bronchial arteries, which technically behave as small shunt lesions.

In case of prolonged delivery of isotope, a mathematic adjustment is made for the actual shape of the prolonged bolus. This process, called **deconvolution**, can help in more accurate quantitation of transit times [64]. Besides pulmonary transit times, there have been few clinical applications of the transit time estimate in other organs. Analysis of the transit times has been proposed for diagnosing renal transplant rejection, for example, or hepatic cirrhosis, but this method has not been implemented.

If an isotope of a short half-life is used, the activity curves must be adjusted for continuing radioactive decay. In fact, for short enough half-lives, no significant activity reaches the left heart. It is then possible to isolate and measure right-heart function with an isotope such Ir-191 ($t^{1/2}$ = 5 seconds) [65].

DIFFUSIBLE TRACERS

Regional blood flow can be determined directly by the use of diffusible tracers instead of nondiffusible tracers [43,46,66,67]. Isotopes such as Xe-133, Xe-127, Kr-85, and Kr-81m are typical of freely diffusible gases: They are not metabolized, and they do not, for practical purposes, recirculate. Assuming instantaneous delivery via an arterial catheter, the externally detected activity decreases as a monoexponential function of time [41,42].

Knowing $-K$, the slope of the log of the time-activity curve in the organ of interest, and λ, the partition coefficient for the gas in the organ (typically, 0.72 for myocardium), blood flow is measured from the following equation:

$$\frac{-F}{w} = \frac{\lambda \times K}{\delta \times 100}$$

where w is the organ weight, F is the flow in milliliters per minute, K is the slope, and δ is the density in grams per milliliter. The major objection to this approach is that homogeneity of the partition coefficient is assumed for the whole organ irrespective of pathologic processes that may involve the organ.

CAPILLARY BLOCKADE

Capillary blockade remains a powerful means of determining regional blood flow. First, the amount of injected radioactivity is measured. The relative uptake of the isotope is then determined from planar images taken in anteroposterior and posteroanterior projections. The geometric average is then used to estimate the amount of radioactivity in specific regions. The relative blood flow to a target organ is the fraction measured over that organ. For example, consider a right-to-left shunt lesion. Following the injection, there is radioactivity in brain, kidneys, and other portions of the body [39]. A good approximation of the shunt is the ratio of total counts minus counts in the lung to total counts in the body.

ORGAN UPTAKE

Early uptake of pharmaceuticals, in general, reflects delivery and, therefore, blood flow (Fig. 21-16). During the ensuing minutes to hours, the agents redistribute as a function of physiologic uptake by a target tissue or by specific attachment to either specific or nonspecific binding sites.

Potassium and its analogues are prime examples of physiologic uptake by a target tissue. For example, Tl-201, a potassium analogue, normally is not present, as is potassium, in muscle cells. Due to similarities in handling

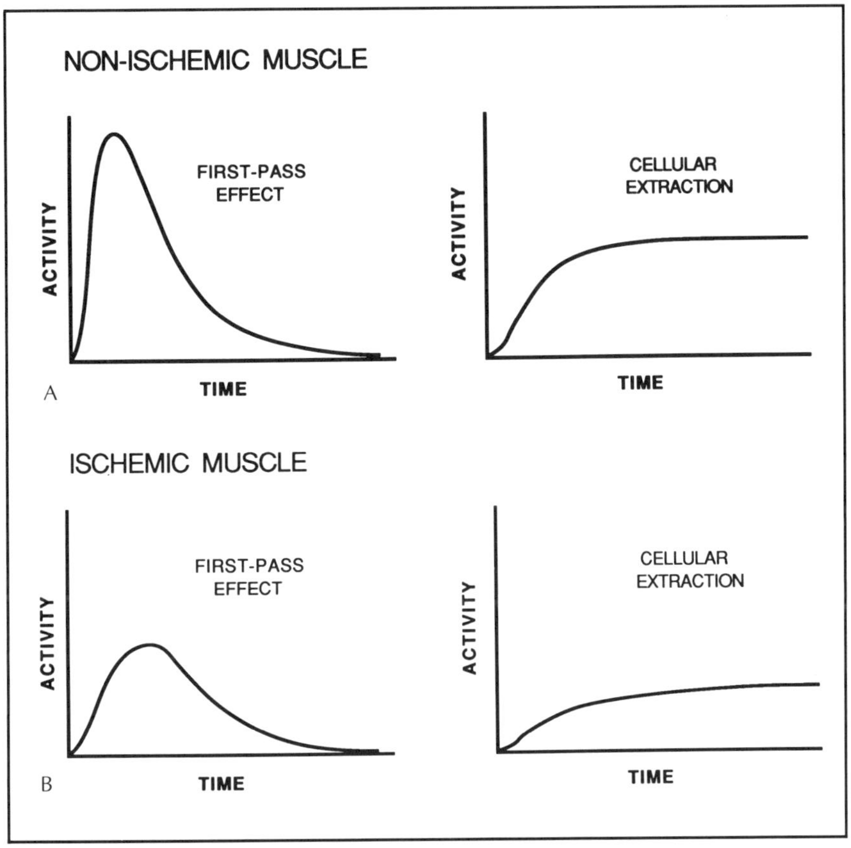

Fig. 21-16. **A.** In nonischemic muscle, the early uptake of an isotope such as Tl-201 reflects local blood flow and extraction efficiency. The first curve is the variable to be measured. The second curve is assumed to hold constant over a wide physiologic range. **B.** In ischemic muscle, the early transit of the isotope is blunted. Although extraction efficiency remains quite high (> 80%), the decreased delivery of the isotope due to a proximal stenosis decreases the isotope that is trapped early.

by the cells, however, the final uptake of the isotope reflects the passive potassium "pool." It is therefore possible to image such a pool and to quantify the amount of actively metabolizing, or "live," muscle cells. This pool, by itself, does not contain much information on perfusion. However, the early uptake following injection (most commonly as part of a stress test) reflects perfusion (Fig. 21-17). The extent of live yet ischemic muscle cells can then be inferred if the perfusion image is subtracted from an image of the passive potassium pool [50,67,68].

Binding of pharmaceuticals can be either specific or nonspecific. The former is exemplified by antigen-antibody (Ag-Ab) reactions, where blood flow is not directly related to the uptake of the labeled pharmaceutical. The use of antimyosin-labeled antibodies is a prime example of such an approach. Lack of perfusion can be inferred only by the presence of dead cells, as documented by uptake of the labeled pharmaceutical. Direct muscle injury, such as occurs in electric shock, also can cause uptake of the pharmaceutical.

Nonspecific binding of a compound also can reflect regional blood flow. Uptake of the radiopharmaceutical is then a function of regional perfusion. In bone, the uptake of Tc-99m–labeled phosphates and phosphonates is directly linked to blood flow. Cardiac uptake of the newer isonitrile Tc-99m complexes (teboroxime, sestamibi) reflects myocardial blood flow. Similarly, cerebral perfusion can be measured by the uptake of iodoamphetamines (IMP) and, more recently, by the Tc-99m–labeled propyleneamine oxide (PAO) analogues [69,70,71].

METABOLISM

Radiopharmaceuticals used to estimate metabolic activity also can be used to measure regional perfusion. Again, the estimates are made indirectly, since early uptake of a labeled precursor depends on blood flow. This approach is limited, because uptake is influenced by additional metabolic factors, and dissociation of perfusion and local metabolism is seen following strokes. For example, F-18–labeled deoxyglucose uptake generally is proportional to blood flow. Another exception is the avid uptake by brain tumors [72,73]. In the heart, fatty-acid analogues, such as C-11 palmitate or I-123–labeled fatty acids, can be used to determine the volume and distribution of actively metabolizing cells [74,75]. A dissociation between their uptake and regional perfusion has been shown to occur. The reverse phenomenon—increased perfusion in a region of lowered oxygen utilization—has been seen in the brain; it is referred to as **luxury perfusion** [76].

Another facet of local perfusion is the function of a

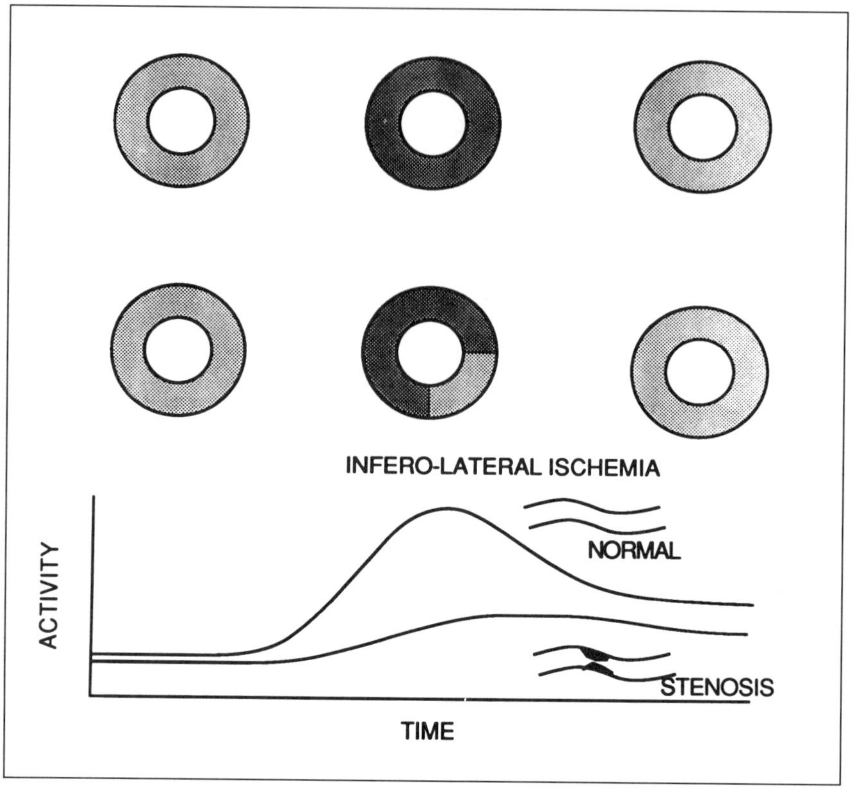

Fig. 21-17. The early distribution of Tl-201 (or analogues) peaks early in normal myocardium. The zone of ischemia in the inferolateral wall on this representation of a short-axis view is characterized by the decreased isotope uptake. Thus, the early perfusion image (middle column) of the short-axis myocardial images reflects a difference of isotope concentration. With time, the isotope equilibrates evenly into the myocyte, creating an image of myocardial mass (right column). The previously ischemic myocardium then looks similar to the nonischemic muscle.

target organ. The heart's function can be measured with radionuclide ventriculography and the determination of regional contraction [77]. For the kidney, uptake and excretion of iodohippurate or DTPA are indirect indicators of preserved organ vascularity [78,79].

A special situation arises with the detection of acute venous thrombosis. The presence of thrombosis in the major draining veins of the lower or upper extremities reflects abnormal patterns of blood flow during radionuclide venography [80,81]. In addition, a compound such as Tc-99m–labeled sulfur colloid often "sticks" to an acute thrombosis [82]. Similarly, labeled fibrinogen binds to thrombus in formation, as do In-111–labeled platelets, with which heparin interferes. A simpler, but less sensitive, method of visualizing deep venous thrombosis can be implemented by imaging the blood pool of the lower extremities. The deep veins show absence of blood-pool activity when an acute thrombus has replaced blood in the lumen of the involved vein [83].

Radionuclide Imaging of Vascular Disorders

CEREBROVASCULAR DISEASE

Radionuclide angiography, with bolus injection of the tracer and dynamic imaging (2 to 4 images per second), is used occasionally to evaluate patients with cerebrovascular disease. When such a sequence of dynamic images is played back as an endless cine loop, information on the flow to the brain, asymmetry in the flow, or lack of flow is demonstrated. This technique is especially useful when performed with one of the newer cerebral-perfusion agents, which are trapped in brain tissue according to flow. In addition to dynamic images of the flow, static images of regional uptake in the brain (if any) are possible (84). The combined information—flow in the major arteries and cortical perfusion (uptake)—are important in establishing the diagnosis of brain death [85].

The newer brain-perfusion agents introduced in the mid 1980s have completely replaced the older brain-imaging agents (Tc-pertechnetate, DTPA, glucoheptonate) of the extracellular distribution type. The older agents did not cross the blood-brain barrier but did provide a radionuclide angiogram. Cerebral uptake was a sign of an interrupted barrier. Xe-133 inhalation and registration of the isotope by a single gamma camera or by multiple detectors placed over the cortex offers certain advantages [86,87], but that technique is not used routinely. Iodoamphetamine (IMP) (labeled with I-123) crosses the blood-brain barrier. It has very effective cortical uptake proportional to flow; redistribution occurs over hours. This agent was widely used in the late 1980s and early 1990s but is no longer available. The most widely used new agent, hexamethyl propyleneamine oxide (HMPAO) labeled with Tc-99m, is lipid soluble, crosses the blood-brain barrier, and is extracted by brain tissue in proportion to regional perfusion [88]. Once trapped, it is contained for hours, thus enabling imaging procedures of long duration and at selected times after the administration. HMPAO Tc-99m works like microspheres and is very suitable for SPECT studies. HMPAO studies provide detailed information concerning differences in regional perfusion [89]. Also, perfusion to the cortex as well as to deep structures can be demonstrated. HMPAO has been used successfully to study regional cerebral perfusion during and after interventions. Evaluation of the functional significance of obstructions in the major cerebral arteries is performed by HMPAO Tc-99m imaging after administration of acetazolamide (Diamox) [90,91] or carbon dioxide [92,93] inhalation (Plate 5) [94].

Cerebral perfusion during seizures and between seizures has been used to identify epileptic foci (high flow and reduced flow) [95,96]. Evaluation of cortical perfusion with mapping of functional centers is done during visual or auditory stimuli [97]. HMPAO is prepared and labeled with Tc-99m shortly before injection. The shelf-life after preparation is only 30 minutes, a limitation of its usefulness. A competing new agent, Tc-99m labeled with ethyl cysteinate dimer (ECD), works according to the same principles [98,99] but has a longer shelf life after preparation.

Cerebral perfusion expressed in milliliters per gram of tissue and metabolic activity reflecting regional cerebral function of a group of neurons can be studied with positron-emitting tracers and dedicated scanners [100]. These tracers and equipment supply unique biologic information but at a price often difficult to justify in the clinical context. As a research tool, however, the technique is invaluable. Radionuclides, decaying by positron emission with creation of two opposite directed 511-keV photons, are short-lived tracers and must be created on location using cyclotrons. Dedicated tomographic detectors, PET scanners, are used to register this type of radiation. Oxygen-15 ($t\frac{1}{2}$ = 124 seconds) as carbon monoxide or O-15 water is used as a perfusion tracer and for the mapping of metabolic activity thereafter [101,102]. F-18 ($t\frac{1}{2}$ = 108 minutes) labeled deoxyglucose (FDG) is the classic metabolic tracer-complex, widely used for studies of regional cerebral metabolic activity [103], reflecting neuronal activity and regional blood flow. Deoxyglucose and its radioactive marker are taken up by neurons like glucose, using the same membrane transport system. Like glucose, deoxyglucose undergoes enzymatic phosphorylation, yielding FDG-6-phosphate (FDG-6-P), which is not metabolized further and is trapped in proportion to metabolic activity (glucose uptake). The short half-life of the positron emitters allows for higher administered doses, leading to high counts. That, in combination with the high photon energy, sophisticated scanners, and attenuation methods, ensures images with high anatomical resolution and reliable quantitative data. The cost of the hardware and the staff of physicists, chemists, and engineers required to produce the radionuclides and operate the equipment makes PET scanning an expensive diagnostic tool.

Recently, conventional gamma cameras have been modified to work at the energy level (511 keV) of positron emitters. The preliminary results with those systems are promising, and commercial systems are now available, makine metabolic imaging available and realistic in clinical settings.

CORONARY ARTERY DISEASE

Perfusion Imaging. Tl-201 is the agent classically used for myocardial perfusion imaging [104] and has been available since the mid-1970s [105]. The hydrated thallium ion, Tl^+, has approximately the same atom radius as potassium and is biologically handled like a potassium ion, K^+. After intravenous injection, thallium is extracted from the circulation of all tissues and accumulates intracellularly, like potassium, and becomes part of the same cation pool. The early uptake in the tissues is linearly related to flow over a wide range. Less than 5 percent of the injected dose accumulates in the myocardium, reflecting the coronary flow fraction of the cardiac output. The remaining thallium is taken up in tissues and organs according to flow at the moment of injection and tissue-extraction coefficients. For example, when injected into a patient intravenously during peak stress on a treadmill, about 5 percent of the tracer will accumulate in the myocardium, but a considerable portion will go to the leg muscles performing the work. This is easily demonstrated by whole-body imaging. Such images even show which muscle groups are responsible for performing the work on the treadmill, a pattern that differs from exercise performed on a bicycle. The difference in muscular uptake relative to flow to muscles or part of the muscle group also is seen in the myocardial muscle and is the general principle for myocardial perfusion imaging. Regions (or vascular territories) with high flow at the moment of injection will show high tracer uptake, whereas regions (vascular territories) with low flow will show less tracer uptake (ischemia). Regions (vascular territories) with no flow will show no uptake (obstruction or scar).

The components of an exercise test with thallium imaging include stressing the patient to achieve a sufficient cardiac workload, injection of the tracer at peak stress, imaging of differences in regional uptake, determining relative hypoperfusion (which almost always represents ischemia), and relating regional hypoperfusion to vascular territory. The initial thallium content observed shortly after administration changes over time (so-called **wash-out**). The rate of wash-out varies in different pools even within the same organ. Over time, wash-out takes place in some tissues and wash-in in other tissues, ending with a redistribution state in which only minor changes in regional content occur.

In the classical thallium myocardial perfusion imaging protocol [106], thallium was injected during peak stress, and redistribution imaging was performed 3 to 4 hours later, on the presumption that redistribution had taken place during that period of time [107]. Regional-uptake differences in the stress images that disappeared in the redistribution images were considered ischemia, while areas with reduced uptake in stress images that did not change significantly in the redistribution images were considered fixed, representing scar. This rationale was undisputed for many years but later was shown [108,109] to be misleading in up to 40 percent of patients. Thallium redistribution is a variable phenomenon. In some cases, it occurs fast (within 30 minutes to 4 hours), but in many cases it takes much longer. With the use of imaging 24 hours after stress injection, it has been shown that many "fixed defects" in the traditional redistribution images filled in, that is, they were false-positive fixed defects [110]. Delayed imaging, therefore, is preferable for distinguishing reversible from fixed perfusion defect, but it is a cumbersome strategy. Injection of an additional thallium dose (half the stress dose), so-called **reinjection**, 3 to 4 hours after the stress dose, has been shown to accomplish the same as the 24-hour delayed imaging [107], namely, discrimination between true fixed defects and defects with prolonged redistribution. The reinjection image is basically a rest image superimposed on the residual stress image, and in most cases it is close to a true rest image [107]. The reinjection protocol is more practical than 24-hour delayed imaging. It also has the advantage of better image quality. A further refinement of the reinjection protocol includes imaging 3 to 4 hours after the reinjection, thereby detecting very late redistribution. These new thallium imaging protocols can detect stress-induced ischemia (stress versus reinjection images) [108] and distinguish viable but hibernating myocardium (delayed images) [109]. To determine the extent of myocardial viability, injection with early (10–20 minutes) and delayed imaging (3–6 hours) is the protocol of choice. Hibernating myocardium is defined as noncontractile myocardium with no or low flow [107]. Such myocardium has preserved cellular integrity and metabolism, contrasting with true fixed defects, which represent scar. In hibernating myocardium, the chronically ischemic cells have down-regulated metabolism to a minimum and utilize glucose. Such cells potentially can regain contractile function and left ventricular function may improve.

The gold standard for the detection of hibernating myocardium is a PET study of perfusion and metabolism. Typically, hypoperfusion is demonstrated with N-13 ammonia [111] or rubidium-82 (Rb-82) [112] and glucose metabolism (not fatty-acid metabolism, which is the normal substrate for myocytes) with F-18 deoxyglucose (FDG) [113]. Several studies have shown that myocardium with these characteristics may regain contractile function in about 80 percent of the cases after revascularization, in spite of akinesis preoperatively [111]. Assessment of myocardial viability with PET scanning and thallium protocols using reinjection and delayed imaging have been compared. It has been consistently shown that the thallium reinjection methods detect 80 to 90 percent of the areas with viable myocardium that are detected by PET [109]. The difference in cost between thallium and PET studies and the limited availability of PET justify the thallium technique, except for very difficult cases.

Recently, several Tc-99m–based tracers have been developed as alternatives to Tl-201 [114]. One of these, 2-methoxyisobutylisonitrile (sestamibi) has been compared to and found equivalent to thallium for the detection of myocardial ischemia [114,115]. Sestamibi is the only widespread accepted and clinically used Tc-based perfusion agent. This tracer complex is based on a large molecule in the isonitrile family and is supplied as a kit for labeling with Tc-99m locally. The tracer complex has many advantages over Tl-201, including a shorter half-time (6 hours versus 72 hours), allowing for higher doses, which lead to better image quality; photon energy better suited for the gamma camera (140 keV versus 80 keV); and being supplied as a kit for labeling locally. For sestamibi, regional myocardial uptake is a function of flow within a wide range. The mechanism of uptake for sestamibi differs from that of thallium. The driving force in sestamibi uptake is the negative membrane potential, and in cells sestamibi accumulates in the mitochondria, where the membrane potential is even more negative [116]. Sestamibi uptake requires the presence of membrane potential, whereas thallium uptake requires functioning sodium-potassium pumps. Thus, both uptake mechanisms rely on metabolically active cells. Once it is intracellular, sestamibi remains constant for hours without significant redistribution. Imaging can, therefore, be performed several hours after injection yet still serve as a fingerprint of perfusion at the moment of injection. This is another advantage over thallium, where redistribution is unpredictable and varies, requiring imaging as soon as possible after injection. Many comparative studies have confirmed the high concordance (about 90%) between the results of myocardial perfusion imaging with thallium and with sestamibi [114]. However, for assessment of myocardial viability and hibernating myocardium, protocols using thallium have been better validated than those with sestamibi.

Two injections are used to detect and assess ischemia, the first at rest with imaging 1 hour later, followed by a three-times higher dose at peak exercise, with imaging after 30 minutes to 1 hour (Plate 6). The opposite order of injection also can be used [117]. Pharmacologic stress testing is an alternative to physical stress testing, if physical stress is considered difficult or contraindicated or if the patient is unable to perform predictably on the treadmill. Dipyridamole-induced coronary vasodilation [118] by intravenous infusion of standard dose [56 mg/kg/min for 4 minutes] followed by tracer injection 4 to 6 minutes after infusion, is well established and considered by many to be as effective as physical stress (Plate 7). An alternative protocol uses adenosine [119,120], an effective vasodilator that has a very short half-life and that is soon to be approved for this indication. Dobutamine infusion [119,121] in standardized incremental doses is a new and attractive alternative. It allows titration of doses to achieve increases in heart rate and blood pressure at a desired level. The tracer (thallium or sestamibi) is injected at peak infusion, with imaging stipulated by the tracer used. The dobutamine protocol resembles a physical stress test by increasing heart rate and blood pressure. The side effects and complications of the pharmacologic tests are comparable and few [120,122].

Digital images and tomographic (SPECT) imaging have replaced analog and planar imaging in most institutions. Tomographic technique improves the anatomical resolution considerably, leading to better assessment of perfusion abnormalities but with surprisingly little improvement in overall sensitivity and specificity for detection of coronary artery disease (from 80% to 90%). Sophisticated computer techniques are in use for reconstruction of the data to standardized short- and long-axis cuts according to the individual true cardiac axis. It is crucial that these reconstructed stress and rest slices be aligned carefully, ensuring that the same portions of the myocardium are compared in the two studies. High-resolution monitors and color coding are used to enhance the images. Thus, processed and arranged images may be read visually. To minimize intra- and interobserver variability and to improve accuracy, quantification of regional-tracer-uptake perfusion has been developed. These methods compare actual data with a database of normals, identifying abnormal areas and calculating the extent and severity of perfusion abnormalities, which are expressed in arbitrary units. Such quantitative data are displayed graphically as images in which the large amount of data from SPECT studies are compressed into one functional image [123]. The bulls-eye configuration (Plate 8) is a commonly used method to display a large amount of data in one easy-to-view image.

Myocardial Function. Left and right ventricular function can be assessed by radionuclide angiography. Two types of radionuclide angiography are in clinical use: first-pass and equilibrium radionuclide angiography.

First-pass radionuclide angiography [124] is performed by injection of Tc-99m pertechnetate as a bolus. A gamma camera registers the tracer passage through the right ventricle, the lungs, and the left ventricle. Curves demonstrating changes in tracer content in the ventricles during the cardiac cycle are generated (Fig. 21-18). Ejection fractions for each ventricle are calculated according to the formula (*end-diastolic counts − end-systolic counts*)/*end-diastolic*) × 100%. This method provides a reliable right ventricular ejection fraction but is a less accurate measurement of left ventricular ejection fraction since the tracer is diluted when it reaches the left side. The first-pass technique is rapid and can be used during exercise or intervention. The method is affected by the bolus injection and by arrhythmias. Furthermore, the standard gamma camera is not really suitable for the high count rates achieved with this method. A dedicated first-pass camera built for high count rates is commercially available but not widely used. Left-to-right cardiac shunts can be assessed accurately with the first-pass technique (see Fig. 21-14 and Fig. 21-15) [125].

Equilibrium radionuclide angiography is also referred to as **multiple-gated acquisition** (MUGA), **radionuclide angiography** (RNA), **radionuclide ventriculography** (RVG), **gated blood pool** (GBP), and **equilibrium radionuclide angiography** (ERNA). It is the most commonly used radionuclide method for assessment of left and right ventricular function [126]. Red blood cells are pretreated with tin (stannous chloride) and labeled with Tc-99m.

Fig. 21-18. Summary of the difference between gated-equilibrium and first-pass radionuclide ventriculography. (**Top**) The first-pass study is acquired with high court rates over a short time interval (range indicated by arrows). Determination of ventricular volumes and ejection fraction is made over 3 to 5 cardiac cycles, as a bolus injected into a vein transverses the lung and heart. (**Bottom**) The gated-equilibrium study is performed when a steady amount of radioactivity is present in the blood pool, that is, the counts per milliliter of blood are constant (at equilibrium).

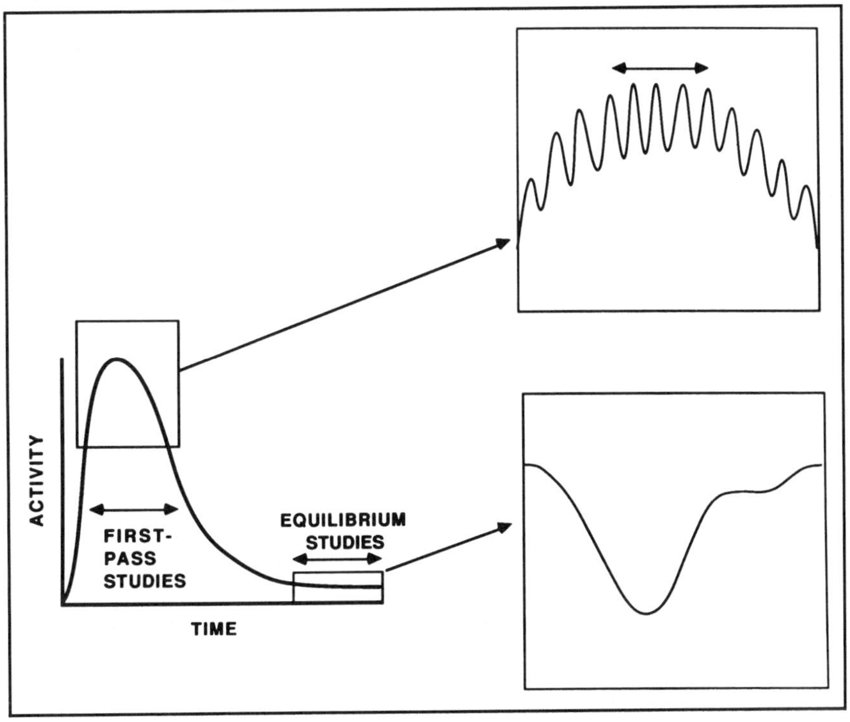

Stannous chloride accumulates in the erythrocytes and binds to hemoglobin. When the Tc-99m molecules are added and enter the red blood cell, they are reduced from oxygenated state VII to IV, as the stannous chloride is oxygenated. Tc-99m in the reduced state (IV) binds firmly to the hemoglobin molecule and leaves the red blood cell gradually over hours. The labeling procedure can be performed in vivo, in vitro, or partially in vitro [127]. The semi-in-vitro technique is practical and commonly used, yielding labeling efficiency of about 90 percent—midway between the in-vivo (75%) and the in-vitro (> 95%) technique. The labeled cells are allowed time (10–15 minutes) to equilibrate in the total blood volume. Any organ or structure with significant volume of blood can be imaged with a standard gamma camera. The relatively large volumes of blood in the ventricle and the spleen, the lesser volumes in larger arteries and veins, and also the small volumes in hemangiomas are visualized with this technique. The erythrocyte labeling (blood-volume labeling) is stable; thus, imaging can be performed for hours.

Imaging is typically done in the "best septal" left anterior oblique projection, that is, the projection where the septum best separates the left ventricular and right ventricular cavities. The imaging procedure utilizes the patient's electrocardiogram as a trigger. An interfaced computer is programmed to detect the R wave and define that time point as the start of the cardiac cycle. Information is collected in bins of 25–40 milliseconds during the cardiac cycle for a predefined time or amount of detected photons (see Fig. 21-9). Typically, 24 to 32 frames per cardiac cycle and an acquisition time of 5–6 minutes or 300–400 cycles are used. The acquired data are displayed as an endless loop cine for assessment of wall-motion abnormalities. Advanced edge-detection algorithms are used to define the end-diastolic and end-systolic left ventricular delineation and generate time-activity curves. These curves describe average changes in tracer content in the left ventricular cavity. From the volume curve ejection fraction, ejection and filling rates are computed, and regional ejection fractions are generated for assessment of regional function [126]. The advantages of the radionuclide method for assessment of left ventricular function are high reproducibility, independence of volume estimations, observer independence, applicability to stress situations and interventions, and limited influence by minor arrhythmias. Major arrhythmias may be a problem, and atrial fibrillation is a relative contraindication. Radionuclide angiography is not as popular as it was in the 1980s, because two-dimensional echocardiography can give the requested information with sufficient accuracy. Currently, the principal indications for radionuclide angiography are situations where quality echocardiography cannot be obtained and situations where changes in function occurring over time are important (e.g., during cardiotoxic chemotherapy [128] or when following patients with aortic valve regurgitation). Assessment of left ventricular function during physical, pharmacologic, or mental stress are reliable and reproducible with radionuclide angiography [129,130]. Also, this method is useful for cardiac-risk stratification to follow ventricular function after events or interventions [131]. A recent promising development is tomographic (SPECT) radionuclide angiography, with three-dimensional computer display of the beating left ventricle. This technique assesses regional function with high anatomical resolution and renders accurate volume calculations.

Myocardial Infarction. Radionuclide methods for imaging myocardial infarction have been used since the 1970s. Tc-99m–labeled pyrophosphate agents are relatively successful if administered 1½ to 3 days after the acute event. The pyrophosphate carrier accumulates in areas with recent cellular necrosis in which there is release of calcium. These infarct-avid (hot-spot) images are difficult to interpret because a myocardial infarction can have all possible forms and sizes and because there are few anatomical references in the images. However, the pyrophosphate scan has not supplanted more conventional biochemical and electrocardiographic methods to diagnose myocardial infarction. Recently, monoclonal antibodies against myosin labeled with In-111 were introduced [132] (in use in Europe but not yet approved in the United States). This technique is more specific but is subject to the same limitations for clinical use as the pyrophosphate scans. A possible niche is in the diagnosis of acute myocarditis [133]. Information pertaining to the extent and the degree of uptake in the myocardium may have prognostic implications.

Myocardial Autonomic Innervation. Imaging of myocardial sympathetic innervation is accomplished by metaiodobenzylguanidine (MIBG) labeled with I-123 or I-133 [134]. MIBG is a norepinephrine analogue that, after intravenous injection, accumulates in the sympathetic nerve endings. Imaging (planar or SPECT) has been applied to clinical situations where the state of the sympathetic innervation has been considered important for diagnosis or treatment. In terminal congestive heart failure, secondary to ischemic heart disease or dilated idiopathic cardiomyopathy, the method has demonstrated sympathetic neural abnormalities [135]. In postinfarction patients, this type of imaging has shown that the myocardial volume associated with deinnervation is much larger than the infarction itself [136].

Myocardial Metabolism. The myocyte's primary metabolic substrate is free-fatty acids and, to a much lesser degree, glucose (80% and 20%, respectively). During acute or chronic ischemia, myocardial metabolism switches to anaerobic glucolysis. Fatty-acid metabolism has been studied with I-123–labeled beta-methyl-branched fatty-acid analogues like beta-methyl-pentadecanoic acid using a gamma camera SPECT technique [137]. These labeled fatty-acid analogues have initial myocardial uptake like ordinary fatty acids. Due to a modification in C2 (beta) position, they are not metabolized further in the beta oxidation chain, that is, trapped according to regional metabolic rate; thus, they serve as quantitative markers of fatty-acid metabolism. Ischemic myocardium appears in these studies as uptake-deficient zones (cold spots). Myocardium with predominant glucose metabolism, that is, ischemic myocardium (acute or chronic), has been studied extensively with FDG and PET scanning [138]. As for the modified fatty acids described above, the modified and labeled glucose molecules are trapped in accordance with the regional glucose metabolic rate. Ischemic myocardium appears as zones with high uptake (hot spots). FDG studies have been useful in detecting hibernating myocardium [139], that is, myocardium with low or no flow, no contractile function, but detectable metabolism. Such myocardium, if revascularized, is potentially able to regain function.

EXTREMITIES

The arterial and venous systems in the extremities can be imaged by means of tracer bolus injection or by red blood cell labeling after equilibrium [140]. In practice, those methods have found little use. The only exception is the upper-extremity venous system when obstruction is suspected [141]. Following injection of a bolus dose of Tc-99m pertechnetate, dynamic images (two to four frames per second) are obtained and stored in the computer. Playback of the images as an endless-loop cine demonstrates the flow from the site of injection, often an antecubital vein, through the extremity's venous system, superior vena cava, and right atrium and ventricle. The method is useful for demonstration of spontaneous venous thrombus, external obstruction (mass) of venous inflow, obstructions associated with intravenous catheters, and malfunction of implanted intravenous dosing devices. Injection of tracer bolus on the contralateral site is very useful for comparison of vascular anatomy and flow pattern between the suspected site and the normal site.

RENAL VASCULAR DISEASE

Radionuclides have been widely utilized in recent years in the diagnosis of renal vascular disease. Historically, radionuclide angiography was used to visualize renal-artery flow after bolus injection of the tracer. Later, computer-generated curves of the tracer flowing through the renal arteries were used to assess renal-artery stenosis. It is now clear that such attempts at direct assessment of the flow in the arteries have little or no diagnostic value, except for the fact that flow per se can be documented. In transplant patients, serial assessment of a perfusion index, calculated as kidneys–arterial flow (Hilson index), may be helpful to follow the early posttransplantation phase [142].

With the use of filtration agents like Tc-99m DTPA [143] or tubular secreted agents like Iodohippuran-123 [144] or Tc-99m–mercapto acetyltriglycine (MAG-3) [145], reliable information on renal perfusion and transit can be obtained. The accumulation of these agents early (1–3 minutes) after injection, that is, the rising phase of the computer-generated renogram, is related to kidney perfusion. Decreased upslope, prolonged time to peak, and delayed transit time are quantitative evidence of decreased perfusion. These measurements have been applied extensively to diagnose renal artery stenosis, yielding sensitivity and specificity approximating 70–80 percent [143,145].

Marked improvement in the accuracy of this diagnostic procedure is achieved by means of angiotensin converting enzyme (ACE) inhibitor challenge [142–146]. The presumption is that a hemodynamically significant renal-artery stenosis leads to a decrease in glomerular pressure. That decrease triggers the juxtamedullary system to produce renin, which converts angiotensinogen to angiotensin. Angiotensin II is a potent vasoconstrictor that increases systemic blood pressure. Locally, angiotensin II causes efferent arteriolar constriction, which reestablishes the filtration pressure. Thus, kidney function is preserved at the expense of systemic hypertension. A widely accepted, standardized renogram protocol using the ACE inhibitor captopril is as follows:

1. No ACE inhibitors 2–3 days before the test;
2. Captopril per os (25–50 mg) given crushed 1 hour before the test or enalapril intravenously (40 μg/kg) 10 minutes prior to the test;
3. Hydration (10 ml/kg) 30 minutes to 1 hour before the test;
4. A filtration agent (Tc-99m DPTA) or tubular agent (MAG-3) given intravenously and images obtained every 15–30 seconds for 20–30 minutes.

Computer-generated background subtracted renograms for each kidney are created from these images (Fig. 21–19), and specific measurements of tracer uptake, transit, and retention are computed for each kidney. If the captopril renogram is abnormal, a baseline study is performed, and the specific variables are compared for each kidney. Using standardized preparation protocols, imaging, and measurements, the diagnostic accuracy of the captopril renogram includes sensitivity and specificity approximating 90 percent for diagnosis of renovascular hypertension [143,144,145]. Follow-up studies and positive and negative predictive values of more than 90 percent have documented the method's potential to predict cure or improvement in hypertension after successful intervention [145]. Even bilateral renal-artery stenosis can be diagnosed with this technique, since each kidney is compared with itself with and without ACE inhibition, that is, the test is not based on asymmetric function between the kidneys. In patients with a single kidney, the method applies as well and for the same reasons. The method has been widely applied in patients with kidney failure, and the tubular agents seem best suited for those patients. The prevalence of renovascular hypertension in the general population is less than 5 percent. If the prevalence of renovascular hypertension in the population investigated can be increased to 40–50 percent by selection of clinical moderate-to-high probability cases (abdominal bruit, abrupt onset or worsening of hypertension, severe or difficult-to-control hypertension, signs of kidney failure), then captopril renography will serve as a cost-effective screening method for renovascular hypertension [147].

MESENTERIC VASCULAR DISEASE

Radionuclide techniques generally are not applicable to diagnosing mesenteric vascular disease, but they can be used to localize gastrointestinal bleeding [148], in which case, Tc-99m–labeled red blood cells are used. After an intravenous injection of the labeled red blood cells, images are obtained in bins of 5 minutes, usually for 1 hour or shorter if bleeding is obvious. Playback of the images as

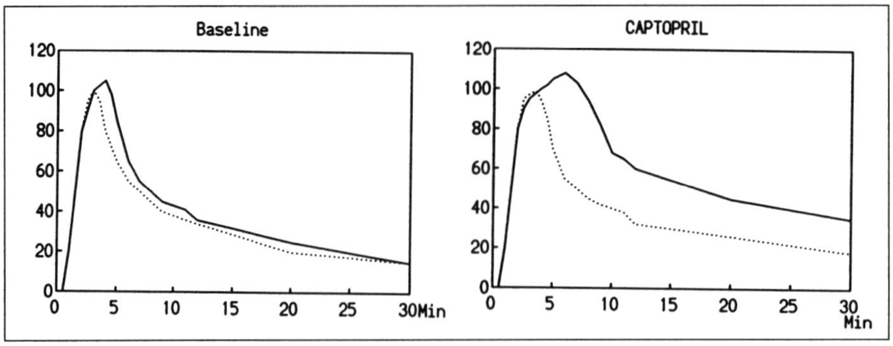

Fig. 21-19. Baseline and captopril renograms in a patient with hypertension. At baseline, both the left kidney (stippled) and the right kidney (solid line) renograms appear normal (time to peak < 5 minutes and residual cortical activity at 20 minutes < 20%). During captopril challenge, no significant change is detected in the left kidney renogram, while the right kidney shows an increase in time to maximum (4 minutes to 6.5 minutes) and higher retention (from 24% to 42%). This is consistent with functionally significant renal artery stenosis; therefore, renovascular hypertension is likely (>90% probability).

an endless-loop cine improves the diagnostic accuracy of the study. The first intraluminal occurrence of labeled red blood cells is taken as the bleeding site. The intraluminal movement of tracer assists in interpretation of the images; however, the fact that bowel content does not necessarily move distally but occasionally moves upstream is a pitfall. Bleeding as low as a few milliliters per minute has been detected with this technique.

AORTIC DISEASES

Except in rare situations like aortitis or aortic root abscess, which can be imaged with Ga-67– or In-111–labeled white blood cells [149], nuclear medicine has little to contribute in the diagnosis of aortic diseases.

Radionuclide Imaging of Venous Disease

ACUTE DEEP VENOUS THROMBOSIS

The injection and subsequent incorporation of I-125 fibrinogen into a propagating thrombus have been used to diagnose venous thrombosis (see Chap. 19). Radionuclide venography, while potentially useful, is rarely used to diagnose deep venous thrombosis. Imaging of deep-vein thrombosis using labeled thrombocytes or antifibrin has been available since the mid-1980s but has found little clinical use. Recent progress in labeling efficiency and carriers may change that situation.

PULMONARY EMBOLISM

Imaging of pulmonary perfusion is accomplished with Tc-99m–labeled particles [150]. Macroaggregated albumin (MAA) or albumin microspheres (AM) are used and are supplied commercially as kits, which contain particles sized 5–50 μm and 20–40 μm, respectively. The lungs contain about 350 million capillaries with diameters that approximate 10 μm. About 300,000 particles labeled with Tc-99m are injected slowly with the patient sitting and respiring normally; 80 percent of the particles are trapped in the pulmonary capillaries. The tracer distribution in the lungs reflects perfusion distribution during the injection. Less than 0.1 percent of the capillaries are blocked by the particles, which dissolve gradually over hours. Except for rare cases of severe pulmonary hypertension, in which there is a reduced amount of functioning capillaries, the method is safe. Lung-perfusion abnormalities, which are relatively nonspecific, are seen in many situations, including infections, atelectases, tumors, primary vascular diseases, pulmonary hypertension, and other respiratory disorders.

A perfusion scan is used in combination with a ventilation scan, most often X-133, to diagnose pulmonary embolism. Tc-99m aerosols and krypton are also used. The ventilation scan is obtained in the projection where the perfusion abnormalities are best seen. Ventilation scans are performed by having the patient inhale the radioactive gas as a single deep breath, followed by steady-state ventilation in a closed system, and ending with a wash-out phase after the patient is disconnected from the gas-delivery system. A perfusion abnormality of the segmental type combined with normal ventilation, that is, perfusion-ventilation (V/Q) mismatch, is the classic sign of pulmonary embolism (Fig. 21-20). Because of the documented high degree of variability in the pattern of perfusion and ventilation abnormalities in pulmonary embolism, several sets of criteria for diagnosis of pulmonary embolism have been suggested. The Prospective Investigation of Pulmonary Embolism Diagnosis (PIOPED) study [150,151] is the largest and most ambitious prospective study ever of pulmonary embolism with angiographic and clinical follow-up and included more than 800 patients. The study (PIOPED I) [150] and a revision (PIOPED II) [151] provided clinically useful diagnostic criteria and probabilities for diagnosing pulmonary embolism (Table 21-3). If a perfusion-ventilation scan is performed, the scintigraphic probability of pulmonary embolism should be expressed as low, intermediate, or high. In the lung, perfusion defects can be seen for months or years following an acute episode of pulmonary embolism.

CHRONIC VENOUS DISORDERS

The contribution of radiopharmaceuticals to the diagnosis of chronic venous disorders is somewhat limited. In the realm of direct venous imaging, the filling of superficial

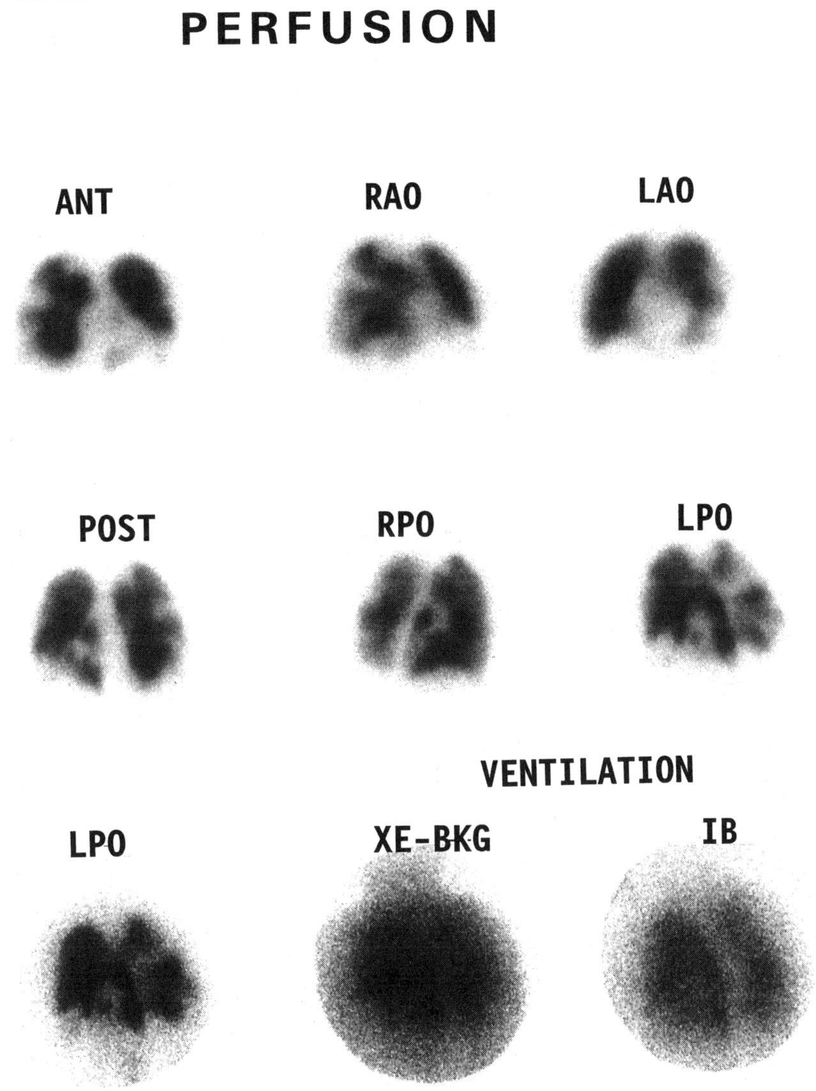

Fig. 21-20. Perfusion and ventilation scans in a patient with high clinical suspicion of acute pulmonary embolism shortly after coronary artery bypass surgery. (**Top and middle rows**) Perfusion scan in anterior (ANT), right anterior oblique (RAO), left anterior oblique (LAO), posterior (POST), right posterior oblique (RPO), and left posterior oblique (LPO) projections. (**Bottom row**) LPO images of perfusion, xenon background (Xe-BKG), and first-breath xenon ventilation. There are multiple segmental and subsegmental perfusion defects in both lungs but with near normal ventilation, that is, V/Q mismatch. The combination of a high clinical probability and a high V/Q scan probability of pulmonary embolism indicates a very high likelihood of pulmonary embolism.

venous structures can be seen after the application of tourniquets when venography is performed. When blood-pool imaging is performed, chronic absence of a blood pool in the deep veins of the thigh and knee can sometimes be seen [19].

Radionuclide Imaging of Other Disorders

CONGENITAL DISORDERS

Cavernous hemangiomas can be detected with Tc-99m–labeled red blood cells in the equilibrium phase. The increased blood volume in the hemangiomas are detected as hot spots [152], that is, areas hotter (more blood volume per gram of tissue) than the organ itself. SPECT imaging increases the sensitivity of the method significantly, which has found widespread use in the evaluation of benign CT abnormalities in the liver (adenoma versus focal nodular hyperplasia versus cavernous hemangioma) [153]. Cavernous hemangiomas in the brain have recently been detected with high-resolution cameras and combined perfusion–blood volume imaging. Myocardial perfusion abnormalities secondary to coronary artery anomalies can be demonstrated with the standard myocardial perfu-

Table 21-3. Criteria for diagnosis of pulmonary embolism (PIOPED)*

Probability of pulmonary embolism	Ventilation/perfusion pattern
High	1. Three or more large ventilation/perfusion mismatches, or 2. One large and two moderate ventilation/perfusion mismatches, or 3. Four moderate ventilation/perfusion mismatches
Intermediate	1. One moderate to two large ventilation/perfusion mismatches, or 2. One moderate matched ventilation/perfusion abnormality with clear chest x-ray
Low	1. Extensive matched ventilation/perfusion abnormality with clear chest x-ray, or 2. Any perfusion defect with substantially larger abnormality on chest x-ray (ventilation irrelevant), or 3. Small perfusion defect (any number) with clear chest x-ray (ventilation irrelevant), or 4. Nonsegmental perfusion defect and abnormal chext x-ray as follows: a. Cardiomegaly, enlarged aorta or hila, elevated diaphragm b. Pleural effusion c. Linear opacity or subsegmental atelectasis

Large perfusion abnormality, >75% of segment; moderate perfusion abnormality, 25–75% of segment; small perfusion abnormality, <25% of segment.

When compared to angiography, the positive predictive value of a high probability scan approximates 90%. The negative predictive value of a low probability scan is 90%.

*Criteria for diagnosis of Pulmonary Embolism based on the PIOPED study. A recent chest X-ray is required. Perfusion (Q) imaging with labeled particles, ventilation (V) imaging (single breath) with gas or aerosol. Perfusion and ventilation defects are scored as segment/nonsegmental, and as small/moderate/large. Perfusion and ventilation defects may be matched or mismatched [150,151].

sion–imaging methods [154] and has been applied even in children.

INFLAMMATORY AND IMMUNOLOGIC DISORDERS

Vasculitis secondary to rheumatic and immunologic diseases are in principle imaged in the same manner as other vascular diseases in the organ of interest. For example, scleroderma with involvement of the coronary or pulmonary arteries is imaged by myocardial-perfusion imaging [155] and lung-perfusion imaging.

HYPERTENSION

Nuclear medicine studies have gained an essential role in evaluation of secondary hypertension. Renovascular hypertension is diagnosed using filtration or tubular radionuclides after challenge with an ACE inhibitor, as discussed previously. Pheochromocytomas and other neuroendocrine tumors associated with hypertension can be detected with I-123–labeled MIBG (a norepinephrine analogue) or the recently approved somatostatin analogue octreotide labeled with In-111 [156]. The success rate for detection of these tumors with octreotide scanning approximated 80 percent in a large recent study involving more than 1,000 patients [156].

INFECTIOUS DISORDERS

Specific diagnosis of infectious vasculitis [149], infected prosthetic grafts [157,158], and infected valves or abscesses can be made using Ga-67, white blood cells labeled with In-111, or labeled with HMPAO Tc-99m. Ga-67 is very nonspecific and accumulates in infections, inflammations, and tumors. It takes 2–3 days after injection before Ga has diminished in the circulation and accumulated sufficiently in the target, for imaging to be performed. Labeled white blood cells clear the circulation and accumulate faster and more specifically in foci of infection. Imaging with HMPAO–Tc-99m–labeled white blood cells is performed within hours, whereas imaging with In-111–labeled white blood cells is usually done after 24 hours. In-111–labeled white blood cells have some advantages over other tracers for imaging vascular infections or infections close to vascular structures because of higher specificity and a longer half-life. That allows for more complete clearance of the blood pool while the tracer accumulates in infectious foci. Newly developed carriers with higher specificity are in clinical testing [159].

References

1. Blumgart HL, Weiss S. Studies on the velocity of blood flow. II: The velocity of blood flow in normal resting individuals, and a critique of the method used. J Clin Invest 1927; 4:15–31.
2. Veall N, Vetter H. Radioisotope Techniques in Clinical Research and Diagnosis. London: Butterworth, 1958. Pp. 350–361.
3. Sapirstein LA. Regional blood flow by fractional distribution of indicators. Am J Physiol 1958; 193:161–168.
4. Folse R, Braunwald E. Pulmonary vascular dilution curves recorded by external detection in the diagnosis of left-to-right shunts. Br Heart J 1962; 24:166–172.
5. Kuhl DE, et al. A high-contrast photographic recorder for scintillation counter scanning. Radiology 1956; 66:730–739.
6. Anger HO. Scintillation camera. Rev Sci Instrum 1958; 29:27–33.
7. Dillman LT. Radionuclide decay schemes and nuclear parameters for use in radiation-dose estimation. MIRD Pamphlet 4. J Nucl Med 1969; 10[Suppl 2]:1–32.
8. Dillman LT, Van der Lage FC. Radionuclide decay schemes and nuclear parameters for use in radiation-dose estimation. MIRD Pamphlet 10. J Nucl Med 1975; 16[Suppl 7]:1–125.
9. Kuhl DE, Edwards RQ. The Mark III scanner: a compact device for multiple-view and section scanning of the brain. Radiology 1970; 96:563–570.
10. Kuhl DE, et al. Local cerebral blood volume determined by three-dimensional reconstruction of radionuclide scan data. Circ Res 1975; 36:610–619.
11. Reli AM, MacIntyre WJ, Friedell HL. A radioisotope method of visualization of blood pools. AJR 1958; 79:129–137.
12. Gray SJ, Frank H. The simultaneous determination of red cell mass and plasma volume in man with radioactive sodium chromate and chromic chloride. J Clin Invest 1953; 32:1000–1004.
13. Bonte FJ, Curry TS III. Blood-pool scanning with technetium-99m human serum albumin. Radiology 1965; 85:1120–1122.

14. Pavel DG, Zimmer AM, Patterson VN. In vivo labeling of red blood cells with ^{99m}Tc: a new approach to blood pool visualization. J Nucl Med 1977; 18:305–308.
15. Hegge FN, et al. Cardiac chamber imaging: a comparison of red blood cells labeled with Tc-99m in vitro and in vivo. J Nucl Med 1978; 19:129–134.
16. Callahan RJ, et al. A modified method for the in vivo labeling of red blood cells with Tc-99m: concise communication. J Nucl Med 1982; 23:315–318.
17. Zaret BL, et al. A noninvasive scintiphotographic method for detecting regional ventricular dysfunction in man. N Engl J Med 1971; 284:1165–1170.
18. Burow RD, et al. Analysis of left ventricular function from multiple gated acquisition cardiac blood pool imaging. Comparison to contrast angiography. Circulation 1977; 56:1024–1028.
19. Clements IP, et al. Radionuclide evaluation of peripheral circulatory dynamics: new clinical application of blood pool scintigraphy for measuring limb venous volume, capacity, and blood flow. Am Heart J 1981; 102:980–983.
20. Konstam MA, et al. Effect of exercise on erythrocyte count and blood activity concentration after technetium-99m in vivo red blood cell labeling. Circulation 1982; 66:638–642.
21. Engel MA, et al. Differentiation of focal intrahepatic lesions with ^{99m}Tc-red blood cell imaging. Radiology 1983; 146:777–782.
22. Brodsky RI, et al. Hepatic cavernous hemangioma: diagnosis with ^{99m}Tc labeled red cells and single-photon emission CT. AJR 1987; 148:125–129.
23. Kuhl DE, et al. Local cerebral blood volume in head-injured patients. Determination by emission computed tomography of 99m Tc-labeled red cells. J Neurosurg 1980; 52:309–320.
24. Alavi A, et al. Scintigraphic detection of acute gastrointestinal bleeding. Radiology 1977; 124:753–756.
25. Winzelberg GG, et al. Evaluation of gastrointestinal bleeding by red blood cells labeled in vivo with technetium-99m. J Nucl Med 1979; 20:1080–1086.
26. Cotlove E. Mechanism and extent of distribution of inulin and sucrose in chloride space of tissues. Am J Physiol 1954; 176:396–410.
27. Spach MS, et al. Radioisotope-dilution curves as an adjunct to cardiac catheterization. I: Left to right shunts. Am J Cardiol 1965; 16:165–175.
28. Weissler AM, McCraw BH, Warren JV. Pulmonary blood volume determined by a radioactivity tracer technique. J Appl Physiol 1959; 14:531–534.
29. Hilson AJ, et al. Dynamic renal transplant imaging with Tc-99m DTPA (Sn) supplemented by a transplant perfusion index in the management of renal transplants. J Nucl Med 1978; 19:994–1000.
30. Arlart I, et al. Predictive value of radionuclide methods in the diagnosis of unilateral renovascular hypertension. Cardiovasc Radiol 1979; 2:115–125.
31. Gates GF. Glomerular filtration rate: estimation from fractional renal accumulation of ^{99m}Tc-DTPA (stannous). AJR 1982; 138:565–570.
32. Ashburn WL, et al. Myocardial perfusion imaging with radioactive-labeled particles injected directly into the coronary circulation of patients with coronary artery disease. Circulation 1971; 44:851–865.
33. Taplin GV, MacDonald NS. Radiochemistry of macroaggregated albumin and newer lung scanning agents. Semin Nucl Med 1971; 1:132–152.
34. Vincent WR, Goldberg SJ, Desilets D. Fatality immediately following rapid infusion of macroaggregates of ^{99m}Tc albumin (MAA) for lung scan. Radiology 1968; 91:1181–1184.
35. Quinn JL III, Serratto M, Kezdi P. Coronary artery bed photoscanning using radioiodine albumin macroaggregates (RAMA). J Nucl Med 1966; 7:107–113.
36. Kirk GA, et al. Particulate myocardial perfusion scintigraphy: its clinical usefulness in evaluation of coronary artery disease. Semin Nucl Med 1977; 7:67–84.
37. Jones EL, Wagner HN Jr, Zuidema GD. New method for studying peripheral circulation in man. Arch Surg 1965; 91:725–734.
38. Rhodes BA, et al. The distribution of radioactive microspheres after intraarterial injection in the legs of patients with peripheral vascular disease. AJR 1973; 118:820–826.
39. Gates GF, Orme HW, Dore EK. Measurement of cardiac shunting with technetium-labeled albumin aggregates. J Nucl Med 1971; 12:746–749.
40. Rhodes BA, et al. Absence of anatomic arteriovenous shunts in Paget's disease of bone. N Engl J Med 1972; 287:686–689.
41. Kety SS. I: Blood-tissue exchange methods: theory of blood-tissue exchange and its application to measurement of blood flow. Meth Med Res 1960; 8:223–227.
42. Zierler KL. Equations for measuring blood flow by external monitoring of radioisotopes. Circ Res 1965; 16:309–321.
43. Hollenberg NK. Renal blood flow in hypertension and in renal disease. Prog Nucl Med 1972; 2:200–234.
44. Silberstein EB, et al. Predictive value of intracutaneous xenon clearance for healing of amputation and cutaneous ulcer sites. Radiology 1983; 147:227–229.
45. Maseri A, et al. Possibilities, limitations, and technique for the study of regional myocardial perfusion in man by xenon-133. Cardiovasc Res 1977; 11:277–290.
46. Cannon PJ, Weiss MB, Sciacca RR. Myocardial blood flow in coronary artery disease: studies at rest and during stress with inert gas washout techniques. Prog Cardiovasc Dis 1977; 20:95–120.
47. Obrist WD, et al. Determination of regional cerebral blood flow by inhalation of 133-xenon. Circ Res 1967; 20:124–135.
48. Love WD, et al. Differences in the relationships between coronary blood flow and myocardial clearance of isotopes of potassium, rubidium, and cesium. Am Heart J 1968; 76:353–355.
49. Wackers FJ, et al. Noninvasive visualization of acute myocardial infarction in man with thallium-201. Br Heart J 1975; 37:741–744.
50. Pohost GM, et al. Differentiation of transiently ischemic from infarcted myocardium by serial imaging after a single dose of thallium-201. Circulation 1977; 55:294–302.
51. Schelbert HR, et al. C-11 palmitate for the noninvasive evaluation of regional myocardial fatty acid metabolism with positron computed tomography. III: In vivo demonstration of the effects of substrate availability on myocardial metabolism. Am Heart J 1983; 105:492–504.
52. Schelbert HR, et al. Regional myocardial perfusion assessed with N-13 labeled ammonia and positron emission computerized axial tomography. Am J Cardiol 1979; 43:209–218.
53. Reivich M, et al. The [18F] fluorodeoxyglucose method for the measurement of local cerebral glucose utilization in man. Circ Res 1979; 44:127–137.
54. Khaw BA, et al. Scintigraphic quantification of myocardial necrosis in patients after intravenous injection of myosin-specific antibody. Circulation 1986; 74:501–508.
55. Holman BL, et al. Myocardial imaging with technetium-99m CPI: initial experience in the human. J Nucl Med 1987; 28:13–18.
56. Kakkar V. The diagnosis of deep vein thrombosis using the 125I fibrinogen test. Arch Surg 1972; 104:152–159.
57. Grimley RP, et al. Imaging of 111In-labelled platelets—a new method for the diagnosis of deep vein thrombosis. Br J Surg 1981; 68:714–716.

58. Hirsh J, Gallus AS. 125-I-labeled fibrinogen scanning. Use in the diagnosis of venous thrombosis. JAMA 1975; 233:970–973.
59. Fedullo PF, et al. Indium-111-labeled platelets: effect of heparin on uptake by venous thrombi and relationship to the activated partial thromboplastin time. Circulation 1982; 66:632–637.
60. Bassingthwaighte JB. Circulatory transport and the convolution integral. Mayo Clin Proc 1967; 42:137–154.
61. Starmer CF, Clark DO. Computer computations of cardiac output using the gamma function. J Appl Physiol 1970; 28:219–220.
62. Gamel J, et al. Pitfalls in digital computation of the impulse response of vascular beds from indicator-dilution curves. Circ Res 1973; 32:516–523.
63. Maltz DL, Treves S. Quantitative radionuclide angiocardiography: determination of Qp:Qs in children. Circulation 1973; 47:1049–1056.
64. Alderson PO, et al. Deconvolution analysis in radionuclide quantitation of left-to-right cardiac shunts. J Nucl Med 1979; 20:502–506.
65. Treves S, et al. Iridium-191 angiocardiography for the detection and quantitation of left-to-right shunting. J Nucl Med 1980; 21:1151–1157.
66. Marcus ML, Bischof CJ, Heistad DD. Comparison of microsphere and xenon-133 clearance method in measuring skeletal muscle and cerebral blood flow. Circ Res 1981; 48:748–761.
67. Okada RD, et al. Improved diagnostic accuracy of thallium-201 stress test using multiple observers and criteria derived from interobserver analysis of variance. Am J Cardiol 1980; 46:619–624.
68. Strauss HW, et al. Thallium-201 for myocardial imaging. Relation of thallium-201 to regional myocardial perfusion. Circulation 1975; 51:641–645.
69. Winchell HS, Baldwin RM, Lin TH. Development of I-123-labeled amines for brain studies: localization of I-123-iodophenylalkyl amines in rat brain. J Nucl Med 1980; 21:940–946.
70. Hill TC, et al. Initial experience with SPECT (single-photon computerized tomography) of the brain using N-isopropyl I-123 p-iodoamphetamine: concise communication. J Nucl Med 1982; 23:191–195.
71. Volkert WA, et al. ^{99m}Tc-propyleneamine oxime (^{99m}Tc-PnAO); a potential brain radiopharmaceutical. Eur J Nucl Med 1984; 9:511–516.
72. Dichiro G, et al. 18F-2-fluoro-2-deoxyglucose positron emission tomography of human cerebral gliomas. J Cereb Blood Flow Metab 1981; [Suppl 1]:S11–12.
73. Kuhl DE, et al. Effects of stroke on local cerebral metabolism and perfusion: mapping by emission computed tomography of 18FDG and 3NH3. Ann Neurol 1980; 8:47–60.
74. Lerch R, et al. Localization of viable, ischemic myocardium by positron-emission tomography with 11C-palmitate. Circulation 1981; 64:689–699.
75. Feinendegen LE, et al. Noninvasive analysis of metabolic reactions in body tissues, the case of myocardial fatty acids. Eur J Nucl Med 1981; 6:191–200.
76. Lenzi GL, Frackowiak RSK, Jones T. Cerebral oxygen metabolism and blood flow in human cerebral ischemic infarction. J Cerebral Blood Flow Metab 1982; 2:321–335.
77. Burow RD, et al. Analysis of left ventricular function from multiple gated acquisition cardiac blood pool imaging. Comparison to contrast angiography. Circulation 1977; 56:1024–1028.
78. Keim HJ, et al. Computer-assisted static/dynamic renal imaging: a screening test for renovascular hypertension. J Nucl Med 1979; 20:11–17.
79. Keane JM, Schlegel JU. The use of a scintillation camera system for screening of hypertensive patients. J Urol 1972; 108:12–14.
80. Sy WM, Lao RS. Collateral pathways in superior vena caval obstruction as seen on gamma images. Br J Radiol 1982; 55:294–300.
81. Hayt DB, et al. Radionuclide venography of the lower extremities and inferior vena cava by continuous injection and moving bed gamma camera technique. Radiology 1976; 121:748–750.
82. Verma RC, et al. Radionuclide venography and the role of radionuclides in the detection of venous disease. Vasc Surg 1977; 11:227–240.
83. Lisbona R, et al. Tc-99m red blood cell venography in deep venous thrombosis of the lower limb. Clin Nucl Med 1985; 10:208–224.
84. de la Riva A, et al. Diagnosis of brain death: superiority of perfusion studies with 99Tcm HMPAO over conventional radionuclide cerebral angiography. Br J Radiol 1992; 65:289–294.
85. Schlake HP, et al. Determination of cerebral perfusion by means of planar brain scintigraphy and 99Tcm-HMPAO in brain death, persistent vegetative states, and severe coma. Intensive Care Med 1992; 18:76–81.
86. Lassen NA, Rommer P. Cerebral blood flow tomography by single photon emission computed tomography using 133-Xe in cerebrovascular disease. Monogr Atheroscler 1986; 14:71–82.
87. Sackeim HA, et al. Regional cerebral blood flow in mood disorders. II. Comparison of major depression and Alzheimer's disease. J Nucl Med 1993; 34:1090–1101.
88. Neirinckx R, et al. Technetium-99m d.l-HM-PAO: a new radiopharmaceutical for SPECT imaging of regional cerebral blood perfusion. J Nucl Med 1987; 28:191–202.
89. Andersen AC, et al. Quantitative measurements of cerebral flow using SPECT and (99m-Tc) d.l-HM-PAO compared to Xe-133. J Cereb Blood Flow Metab 1988; 8:S69-S81.
90. Lassen NA, et al. Effect of acetazolamide on cerebral blood flow and brain tissue oxygenation. Postgrad Med J. 1987; 63:185–187.
91. Knop J, et al. Tc-99m HMPAO SPECT with acetazolamide challenge to detect hemodynamic compromise in occlusive cerebrovascular disease. Stroke 1992; 23:1733–1742.
92. Ringelstein EB, Eyck SV, Mertens I. Evaluation of cerebral vascular vasomotor reactivity by various vasodilatation stimuli: comparison of CO2 and acetazolamide. J Cereb Blood Flow Metab 1992; 12:162–168.
93. Oku N, et al. Carbon dioxide reactivity by consecutive Tc-99m-HMPAO SPECT in patients with chronically obstructed major cerebral artery. J Nucl Med 1994; 35:32–40.
94. Machac J, Vallagholosula A. Cerebral versus myocardial stress perfusion imaging: role of pharmacological intervention in diagnostic assessment of flow reserve. (Editorial) J Nucl Med 1994; 35:41–43.
95. Rowe CC, et al. Visual and quantitative analysis of interictal SPECT with Tc-99m-HMPAO in temporal lobe epilepsy. J Nucl Med 1991; 32:1688–1694.
96. Bauer SH, Feistel H. Regional cerebral flow during focal seizures of temporal and frontocortical onset. Ann Neurol 1990; 27:162–166.
97. Crosson B, et al. A technique to localize activation in the human brain with technetium-99m-HMPAO SPECT: A validation study using visual stimulation. J Nucl Med 1994; 35:755–763.
98. Holman BL, et al. Biodistribution, dosimetry, and clinical evaluation of Tc-99m-ethyl cysteinate dimer in normal sub-

jects and in patients with chronic cerebral infarction. J Nucl Med 1989; 30:1018–1024.
99. Leville J, Demoneau G, Walovitch RC. Intersubject comparison between Tc-99m ECD and Tc-99m-HMPAO in healthy human subjects. J Nucl Med 1992; 33:480–484.
100. Albert NM, Erickson L, Chang JY. Strategy for measurement of regional cerebral blood flow using short-lived tracers and emission tomography. J Cereb Blood Flow Metab 1984; 4:28–34.
101. Lammertsma AA, Jones T. Correction for presence of intravascular oxygen-15 in the steady-state technique for measuring regional oxygen extraction ratio in the brain. J Cereb Blood Flow Metab 1983; 3:416–424.
102. Mejia MA, et al. Simplified nonlinear correction of oxygen-15-water regional cerebral blood flow images without blood sampling. J Nucl Med 1994; 35:1870–1977.
103. Phelps ME, et al. Tomographic measurement of local cerebral glucose metabolic rate in humans with (F18)2-fluoro-2 deoxy-D -glucose: validation of the method. Ann Neurol 1979; 6:371–388.
104. Dahlberg ST, Leppo JA. Myocardial kinetics of radiolabelled perfusion agents: Basis for perfusion imaging. J Nucl Cardiol 1994; 1:189–197.
105. Wackers F Th, et al. Noninvasive visualization of acute myocardial infarction in man with thallium-201. Br Heart J 1975; 37:741–744.
106. Pohost GM, et al. differentiation of transiently ischemic from infarcted myocardium by serial imaging after a single dose of thallium-201. Circulation 1977; 55:294–302.
107. Zaret BI, Wackers F Th. Nuclear Cardiology Review part one. N Eng J Med 1993; 329:775–783.
108. Dilsizian V, et al. Enhanced detection of ischemic but viable myocardium by the reinjection of thallium after stress-redistribution imaging. N Eng J Med 1990; 323:141–146.
109. Bonow RO, et al. Identification of viable myocardium in patients with chronic coronary artery disease and left ventricular dysfunction. Comparision of thallium scintigraphy with reinjection and PET imaging with F-18-deoxyglycose. Circulation 1991; 83:26–37.
110. Kiat H, et al. Late reversibility of tomographic myocardial thallium-201 defects. An accurate marker of myocardial viability. J Am Coll Cardiol 1988; 12:1456–1463.
111. Tamaki N, et al. Value of rest-stress myocardial positron tomography using N-13 ammonia for preoperative prediction of reversible asynergy. J Nucl Med 1989; 30:1302–1310.
112. Gould KL, et al. Myocardial metabolism of flourodeoxyglucose compared to cell membrane integrity for the potassium analogue Rubidium-82 for assessment of infarct size in man by PET. J Nucl Med 1991; 32:1–9.
113. Schweiger M, Hicks R. The clinical role of metabolic imaging of the heart by positron emission tomography. J Nucl Med 1991; 32:565–578.
114. Wackers F Th, et al. Technetium 99m hexakis 2 methylisobutyl isonitrile: Human biodistribution, dosimetry, safety and preliminary comparison with thallium 201 for myocardial perfusion imaging. J Nucl Med 1989; 30:301–311.
115. Taillifer R, et al. Technetium-99m-sestamibi myocardial perfusion imaging in detection of coronary artery disease: comparison between initial (1-hour) and delayed (3-hour) postexercise images. J Nucl Med 1991; 32:1961–1965.
116. Piwnica-Worms D, et al. Effect of metabolic inhibition on technetium-99m-MIBI kinetics in cultured chicken myocardial cells. J Nucl Med 1990; 31:464–472.
117. Taillefer R, et al. Same day injection of Tc-99m methoxy isobutyl isonitrile (hexamibi) for myocardial tomographic imaging: Comparison between rest-stress and stress-rest injection sequence Eur J Nucl Med 1989; 15:113–117.
118. Gould KL. Non-invasive assessment of coronary stenosis by myocardial perfusion imaging during pharmacologic coronary vasodilatation: I Physiologic basic and experimental validation. Am J Cardiol 1978; 41:267–278.
119. Iskandrian AS, Verani MS, Heo J. Pharmacologic stress testing: Mechanism of action, hemodynamic responses, and results in detection of coronary artery disease. J Nucl Cardiol 1994; 1:94–111.
120. Cerqueira MD, et al. Safety profile of adenosine stress perfusion imaging: results from the Adenoscan Multicenter trial registry. J Am Coll Cardiol 1994; 23:384–389.
121. Verani MS. Dobutamine myocardial perfusion imaging. J Nucl Med 1994; 35:737–739.
122. Mertes H, et al. Symptoms, adverse effects, and complications associated with Dobutamine stress echocardiography. Experience in 1118 patients. Circulation 1993; 88:15–19.
123. Garcia EV. Quantitative myocardial perfusion single-photon emission computed tomography imaging: Quo vadis? (Where do we go from here ?). J Nucl Cardiol 1994; 1:83–94.
124. Jones RH. Radionuclide angiocardiography in patients with coronary artery disease. In BL Zaret, GA Beller, eds. Nuclear Cardiology: State of the Art and Future Directions. St Louis: Mosby, 1993. Pp. 111–122.
125. Maltz Dl, Treves S. Quantitative radionuclide angiocardiography: determination of Qp:Qs in children. Circulation 1973; 47:1049–1056.
126. Zaret Bl, Wackers F Th. Nuclear Cardiology Review part two. N Eng J Med 1993; 329:855–863.
127. Callahan RJ, et al. A modified method for in vivo labelling of red blood cells with Tc-99m: concise communication. J Nucl Med 182; 23:315–318.
128. Schwartz RG, et al. Congestive heart failure and left ventricular dysfunction complicating doxyrubicin therapy: Seven year experience using serial radionuclide angiography. Am J Med 1987; 82:1109–1118.
129. Setaro JF, et al. Long term outcome in patients with congestive heart failure and intact systolic left ventricular performance. Am J Card 1992; 69:1212–1216.
130. Bonow RO, et al. Exercise induced ischemia in mildly symptomatic patients with coronary artery disease and preserved left ventricular function: identification of subgroups at risk of death during medical therapy. N Eng J Med 1984; 311:1339–1345.
131. Zaret BL, Wackers F Th, Terrin ML. Assessment of global and regional left ventricular function at rest and during exercise after thrombolytic therapy for acute myocardial infarction: results of the Thrombolysis in Myocardial Infarction (TIMI) II study. Am J Cardiology 1992; 69:1–9.
132. Khaw BA. Myocardial damage delineated by indium-111 antimyosin FAB and technetium-99m pyrophosphate. J Nucl Med 1987; 28:76–83.
133. Carrio I, et al. Indium-111 antimyosin scintigraphy to assess myocardial damage in patients with suspected myocarditis and cardiac rejection. J Nucl Med 1993; 29:1893–1899.
134. Sisson J, et al. Metaiodobenzylguanidine to map scintigraphically the adrenergic nervous system in man. J Nucl Med 1987; 28:1625–1632.
135. Schofer J, et al. Iodine-123 meta-iodobenzylguanidine scintigraphy: a noninvasive method to demonstrate myocardial adrenergic nervous system disintegrety in patients with idiopathic dilated cardiomyopathy. J Am Coll Cardiol 1988; 12:1252–1258.
136. McGhie AI, et al. Regional cardiac adrenergic function using I-123 meta-iodobenzylguanidine tomographic imaging after myocardial infarction. Am J Cardiol 1991; 67:236–242.
137. Reske SN. Experimental and clinical experience with iodine

123-labeled iodophentylpentadecanoic acid in cardiology. J Nucl Cardiol 1994; 1:S58–S64.
138. Gropler RJ. Methodology governing the assessment of myocardial glucose metabolism by positron emission tomography and fluorine 18-labelled flourodeoxyglucose J Nucl Cardiol 1994; 1:S4–14.
139. Tamaki N. Current status of viability assessment with positron tomography. J Nucl Card 1994; 1:S40–47.
140. Dhenke RD, Moore WH, Long SE. Radionuclide venography in iliac and inferior vena caval obstruction. Radiology 1982; 144:597–602.
141. Hartshorne MF, et al. Chest radionuclide angiography in the evaluation of pulmonary masses. J Clin Nucl Med 1984; 16:756–1763.
142. Hilson AJ, et al. Dynamic renal imaging with Tc-99m DTPA (sn) supplemented by a transplant perfusion index in the management of renal transplants. J Nucl Med 1978; 9:994–1000.
143. Setaro JF, et al. Simplified captopril renography in diagnosis and treatment of renal artery stenosis. Hypertension 1991; 18:289–298.
144. Erbsloh-Moller B, et al. Furosemide-133-I-Hippuran renography after angiotensin-converting enzyme inhibitor for the diagnosis of renovascular hypertension. Am J Medicine 1991; 90(1):23–29.
145. Dondi M, et al. Prognostic value of captopril renal scintigraphy in renovascular hypertension. J Nucl Med 1992; 33:22040–2044.
146. Nally JV Jr, Black HRS. State-of-the-art review: Captopril renography—Pathophysiological considerations and clinical observations. Seminars in Nuclear Medicine 1992; 22:85–97.
147. Davidson R, Wilcox CS. Diagnostic usefulness of renal scanning after angiotensin converting enzyme inhibitors. Hypertension 1991; 18:299–303.
148. Hattner RS, Engelstad BL. An advance in identification and localization of gastrointestinal hemorrhage. Gastroenterology 1983; 83:484–485.
149. Moosa HH, et al. Inflammatory aneurysms of the abdominal aorta. Arch Surg 1989; 124:673–675.
150. PIOPED. Value of the ventilation/perfusion scan in acute pulmonary embolism. JAMA 1990; 263:2753–2759.
151. Gottschalk A, et al. Ventilation perfusion scintigraphy in the PIOPED study. Part II. Evaluation of the scintigraphic criterias and interpretations. J Nucl Med 1993; 34:1119–1126.
152. Front D, et al. Evaluation of hemangiomas with technetium-99m-labeled RBC's: Perfusion–blood pool mismatch. JAMA 1983; 249:1488–1490.
153. Rubin EA, Lichtenstein G R, Alavi A. Hepatic scintigraphy of solitary liver masses. J Nucl Med 1993; 34:697–705.
154. Katsuragi M, et al. Thallium-201 myocardial SPECT in Bland-White-Garland syndrome: Two adult patients with inferior posterior defects. J Nucl Med 1993; 34:2182–2184.
155. Gustafsson R, et al. Cold-induced myocardial reversible ischemia in systemic sclerosis. Lancet 1989; 2:475–479.
156. Krenning EP, et al. Somatostatin receptor scintigraphy with (111-In-DTPA-d-Phe) and (123-I-Thyr3) -OCTREOTIDE: The Rotterdam experience with more than 1000 patients. Eur J Nucl Med 1993; 20:716–731.
157. LaMuaglia G, et al. Utility of the In-111-labeled human immunoglobulin G scan for detection of focal vascular graft infection. J Vasc Surg 1989; 10:20–27.
158. Vorne M, et al. 99m-Tc leucocyte scintigraphy in prosthetic vascular graft infections. Nucl Med 1989; 28:95–98.
159. Seabold JE, Rosenbrough SF. Will a radiolabelled antibody replace In-111-platelets to detect active thrombus? J Nucl Med 1994; 1738–1740.

Principles of Angiography

Michael A. Bettmann
Michael F. Meyerovitz

History

Angiography has played a central role in both the diagnosis and, more recently, the therapy of peripheral vascular disease. Improved understanding and treatment of this common disease has paralleled developments in cardiovascular radiologic techniques. The potential value of imaging the blood vessels was noted shortly after the discovery of x-rays by Roentgen in Germany in late 1895. By January 1896, a study was published concerning the evaluation of amputated extremities [1]. Later that year, a volume was published suggesting the use of x-rays for evaluation of blood vessels in surgery and in autopsies [2]. Interest in the visualization of vessels by the use of x-rays continued over the next 25 years, limited largely by the lack of an appropriate contrast material, one that would allow visualization of the vessels in vivo without causing significant damage. In the early 1920s, Sicard and Forestier began to use an iodized oil formation, initially in animals and subsequently in patients, for venous and right-heart studies [3]. In 1923, Berberich and Hirsch performed arterial and venous studies in patients utilizing strontium bromide [4]. Although film quality was good, the contrast agent was toxic and therefore of limited practical utility. Subsequently, Brooks utilized sodium iodide for arteriography, again with good visualization of arterial anatomy but marked discomfort during injection [5]. Coincident with the developments in contrast agents, selective angiography was undertaken, with a catheter placed by a surgical cutdown. In 1928, Moniz and colleagues described the utility of carotid angiography [6], and Forssmann, a German, inserted a catheter into his antecubital vein and advanced it into the right atrium [7]. In 1929, dos Santos and colleagues described probably the first transcutaneous approach, the technique of translumbar aortography, for visualization of the abdominal aorta and its branches [8].

Also in 1929, Swick, an American urologist working in Germany, described the use of the first organic iodide compound [9]. Iodine was an effective radiopaque agent, but it was impractical in its inorganic form because of toxicity. The discovery that organic iodide formulations were generally fairly well tolerated for arteriography, urography, and cardiac studies led to the increased utilization of angiography. In the 1930s, several different kinds of contrast agents were synthesized and utilized clinically. During that decade, both translumbar aortography and brachial and femoral angiography, utilizing catheters placed via cutdown, were fairly widely used. A significant limitation at the time, however, was the relatively poor quality of fluoroscopic images as well as the difficulty of obtaining multiple x-ray exposures over short periods of time. Farinas, in 1941, was the first to report on retrograde aortography utilizing the femoral approach [10].

In the 1940s, marked improvements in fluoroscopy were achieved by the use of image amplification, through the work of Chamberlain [11], Coltman [12], and Sturm and Morgan, who essentially developed the modern image intensifier [13]. Those developments led to both improved images and decreased radiographic doses. Coincident with improvements in image production, various workers developed methods of imaging abdominal and peripheral vascularity with multiple, rapid exposures. These and related developments have been extensively reviewed by Abrams [14].

Perhaps the most important development in the 1950s was Seldinger's development of a method that allowed percutaneous arterial catheterization, eliminating the need for a cutdown [15]. Although the cutdown approach for coronary arteriography was developed further and is still fairly widely used, the percutaneous, or Seldinger, technique was perhaps the single most important technical advance in the history of angiography.

Also in the 1950s, the use of tri-iodinated, fully substituted benzene rings as clinical contrast agents began. With minor changes, these particular contrast agents remain in wide clinical use. Grainger has reviewed the evolution of contrast agents [16]. Similarly, the image-amplification system perfected by Sturm and Morgan in the late 1940s fostered the development of the current generation of high-resolution, large-field image intensifiers. Film changers also have evolved, with extremely reliable rapid film changers becoming available in the last 10 years. These changers consist of feeding and receiving magazines that allow four to six exposures per second of large-size films. Exquisite detail can be achieved using short exposure times, which has proved extremely helpful for definition of disease and surgical reconstruction.

Equipment

Angiography currently depends on several types of equipment: contrast agents, catheters and guidewires, image production and amplification chains, and x-ray tubes and tables. Improvements in all these areas have led to angiography's prominent role in the diagnosis of vascular disease and, increasingly, to angiography's role in the treatment of many types of vascular disease.

IMAGING EQUIPMENT

Imaging equipment in current use is extremely complex as well as extremely expensive. The price of an angiography suite currently ranges from $500,000 to $2 million. Each suite has several key components. The size of the equipment, as well as the near-surgical approach to angiographic procedures, requires a large, well-circumscribed, lead-lined room. X-ray tables for use in angiography generally consist of a tabletop that can be easily moved in all directions and to which there is ready access for both angiographic procedures and, when necessary, resuscitation. In the past, x-ray tubes for use in angiographic rooms were ceiling mounted. If angulated views of a particular area were necessary, patients had to be moved. In the 1970s, movable x-ray tubes mounted on C-shaped or U-shaped arms were developed. The x-ray tubes are mounted in conjunction with an image intensifier and a film-changer system, with one component above and the other below the patient. This allows not only oblique views but also cranial or caudal angulation [17], maneuvers that have proven particularly important in selective coronary angiography. Further developments include the availability of tube-film changer combinations that can be rotated 360 degrees. Additionally, longer imaging arms have been developed, which have two advantages: first, even tall patients can be imaged from head to toe without being turned on the table, and second, patients can be easily and rapidly moved onto and off the table.

An important consideration in room design is the availability of a long-field film changer or a stepping table. The former, generally consisting of a ceiling-mounted tube and a 3- to 4-foot-long film holder, allows imaging of the entire lower extremities without patient movement. A stepping table allows precise movement of the patient with continued exposure during a single injection of contrast. In such an arrangement, the film and tube remain stationary and the patient moves, in conjunction with contrast injection, to three or four preprogrammed positions. As with a long-field film holder, the entire arterial system of the lower extremities can be visualized during a single injection of contrast material. The advantages of the more common stepping table are that the tube need not be a separate, ceiling-mounted one and that it allows greater latitude in obtaining good arterial visualization, since multiple exposures can be made at each station. A fixed field is satisfactory for imaging abdominal, cerebral, and upper-extremity vasculature. Because of continuous movement by the heart, cardiac angiography is best accomplished with 35-mm cine film rather than cut film. This is essentially a movie, at a frame rate adjustable from 30 to 60 frames per second.

An x-ray generator, generally positioned outside the room, controls the production of x-rays by the tube in the room. A high-energy charge causes the production of electrons from a coil, which are directed toward a target. When the electrons strike the target, which generally is a tungsten alloy, x-rays are produced. The x-rays are then directed through a window in the tube housing to penetrate the designated area of interest. X-rays penetrate patients as a function of several variables, perhaps most important the differences in density of different structures, and are received on the image-intensifier screen. The image-intensifier system, which both decreases exposure and increases the clarity of the image, was largely the work of Morgan and Sturm in the 1940s [13]. An image intensifier, as the name implies, enhances the energies of the x-rays that penetrate the target, or body part, and reach the imaging receiver. The resultant images are projected onto a television screen or directly onto film or are transformed into digital format, which can be manipulated to produce images. Intensifiers have become more sensitive, allowing lower x-ray exposures to obtain the same information. They have also become larger. The increased size allows the visualization of larger areas more rapidly but necessitates an increase in patient and operator exposure to produce sufficient x-ray photons (and consequently scatter) to cover the screen.

Digital imaging has played a major role in the recent expansion of angiography. The basic concept, an old one, is that images are obtained before contrast is injected. Following the injection of contrast, the initial image is subtracted from the contrast-containing image to leave a picture of the contrast-filled vessels alone. Background structures that may detract from the image, such as bones, are subtracted. Direct film subtraction has long been utilized, particularly in neuroradiologic procedures, to improve contrast sensitivity. Levin and co-workers have thoroughly discussed digital subtraction imaging [18]. The basic principle is that an initial image obtained during fluoroscopy, prior to contrast injection, is used as a mask image. Subsequently, images accumulate during contrast injection at rates ranging from one every 2 seconds to as many as 64 per second. The images are initially formed on the image intensifier and then picked up by a TV camera. The images are then digitized, and the masked image is subtracted from the contrast-containing images. Digital-subtraction imaging has several theoretical advantages: First, lower exposure levels are necessary to gather the information on image-intensifier screens, so lower radiation doses are expected than with normal cut-film imaging. This has not yet proven to be true, due to inefficiency in image gathering and the need for the accumulation of multiple images to form one satisfactory subtracted image. Second, digital-subtraction imaging was initially heralded as usable for intravenous injections of contrast, possibly obviating the need for intra-arterial injections in many diagnostic situations. This also has not proven feasible, primarily due to difficulties in maintaining and timing the contrast bolus and preventing patient movement (and, therefore, loss of superimposibility of mask and subsequent images). A major practical advantage of arterial digital subtraction, however, has been that lower doses of contrast material can be injected due to the high-contrast sensitivity of digital-subtraction imaging. This has cost advantages, but, more important, it increases patient comfort. Further, the images are immediately available, so multiple angiographic runs can be accomplished in relatively short periods of time, without the delay of removal and development of cut films. The use of large-field image intensifiers, as large as 16 inches in diameter rather than standard ones 9 in. in diameter, also has broadened the applicability of this approach.

In most systems currently utilized, an initial analogue image is digitized from the TV camera for image manipulation and display. To obtain hard copies, however, reconversion to an analogue image is performed, and that image is then photographed. This process leads to some inherent loss of resolution. Laser printers now are available that, with appropriate software connections, allow direct copies to be made from the digitized images. Efforts are being made to modify the imaging chain, primarily the image intensifier and TV camera, so that images are directly digitized rather than converted from the output tube of the TV camera. These developments will help to lower the radiation dose and to improve the quality of images. Although the contrast resolution of digital-subtraction angiography (DSA) is inherently superior to that of film-screen angiography, its spatial resolution is inferior. This is not a problem with large vessels, but it can be important in attempting to visualize smaller ones. Further optimization of digital imaging also depends on computer software development. As the quality of the image depends in part on the number of pixels per field, increasing pixels increases resolution, but it also increases the computer storage space needed. Most current systems have 512 × 512 and 1024 × 1024 image matrices. Whether the increased computer space and the increased exposure needed are worth the extra information remains to be determined. The digital approach, then, is an extremely promising one for angiography, because of improved speed, perhaps improved patient safety, and theoretical advantages of image storage and manipulation.

CONTRAST AGENTS

The contrast agents utilized for angiography have evolved significantly over the last 10 years. Although the fully substituted ionic organic iodine compounds initially developed in the 1950s are still the contrast agents most widely used, several new compounds have been developed since the early 1970s [16]. A major problem with radiographic contrast agents, perhaps the single most important factor in explaining the relatively unusual severe adverse reactions, is the marked hyperosmolality of all these agents to blood. Utilizing two different approaches, several new agents have been developed that are still hyperosmolar to blood but far less so than previously. These agents are currently far more expensive than the conventional agents. They are far more comfortable for patients during peripheral arteriography—a significant consideration, since conventional agents often cause feelings of relatively intense pain and heat on injection into certain arteries, such as the distal abdominal aorta or pelvic or lower-extremity arteries. These new agents also appear to decrease the incidence of nausea, vomiting, and other minor reactions to contrast use. Whether these new agents decrease the incidence of more severe adverse reactions, such as bronchospasm or cardiovascular arrest, remains open to question [19]. Because conventional contrast agents remain, in general, extremely safe, and because discomfort related to these agents is markedly reduced with digital imaging, the role of the new agents is still evolving. As experience with them increases, and as newer, lower-cost agents become available [20], the use of these low-osmolality agents is likely to increase.

The low-osmolality agents are currently used most often in selected patients who are particularly likely to benefit from their use [21]. These patients include those with prior documented reactions, such as severe urticaria or laryngeal edema, not merely feelings of heat, pain, or even nausea, which most likely are related primarily to hyperosmolality. Patients with a very strong allergic diathesis also may benefit from their use. In the past, it was felt that patients with shellfish allergies are particularly susceptible to contrast reactions, but this has not been borne out by more recent studies. Additionally, patients with significant cardiovascular disease or instability are likely to benefit from the use of low-osmolality agents, because those agents cause less alteration in cardiac function than do high-osmolality agents, that is, less fall in blood pressure and tachycardia on injection [20,22]. Patients with marked anxiety, severe trauma, or severe CNS disease may also benefit, since motion induced by discomfort as well as vagally mediated adverse events secondary to discomfort may be detrimental to such patients. Perhaps most important, the low-osmolality contrast media are beneficial in patients undergoing painful procedures. In peripheral arteriography, for example, the pain and heat experienced with the injection of conventional high-osmolality agents is often significant. With low-osmolality agents, these symptoms, although sometimes still considerable, are generally markedly reduced. It is also apparent that agents differ in ways other than osmolality [23]. Appropriate prior discussion with the patient combined with good premedication, such as midazolam and fentanyl, is effective in lessening discomfort [24]. As noted, DSA generally is performed with dilute contrast material. The dilution serves to lower the osmolality, and DSA is, therefore, generally free of discomfort, even with conventional high-osmolality contrast agents.

CATHETERS AND GUIDEWIRES

In contrast to the initial use of relatively simple plastic tubes as catheters, the catheters and guidewires currently used offer tremendous variety, latitude, and safety. The catheters used through the 1960s generally were handmade from various types of plastic tubing. Using hot water or steam, individual angiographers converted straight shapes to various curves, as deemed necessary. The technology of catheters has since advanced as impressively as the technology of other areas of angiography. Polyethylene, polyurethane, and nylon are now most commonly used for catheters, and catheters are available preformed in a wide variety of shapes and sizes. For diagnostic angiography, catheters most commonly range from 5 to 7 F (1.7 to 2.3 mm in outer diameter). An important consideration in catheters is torque control, that is, the balance between stiffness and maneuverability that allows a catheter to be selectively placed. Torque control is often achieved by utilizing a thin metal mesh in two layers of plastic. Another alternative has been to use an inner layer made up of a material with high tensile strength, such as nylon, and an outer layer of a softer, smoother material, such as a polyethylene.

In addition to torqueability, the ease of insertion, ease of advancement, and thrombogenicity are major concerns in catheter design. Catheters should be smooth enough to be inserted easily and advanced easily, even through tortuous vessels. They also must be soft enough to be advanced selectively into vessels, as well as stiff enough to be directed. This inherent contradiction is partially dealt with through the use of various catheter shapes and guidewires. The thrombogenicity of catheters has been a major consideration. Many of the complications of angiography relate to thrombus formation on the catheter, both at the tip and at the entry site. These problems have been dealt with in various ways, primarily by modification of catheter materials and by improved smoothness of the catheter walls [25].

There also has been a tendency toward the use of smaller catheters; 4- and 5-F catheters (1.33 and 1.67 mm in diameter) are now available for routine diagnostic use. Previously, 7- and 8-F (2.3 and 2.7 mm) catheters were routinely used. It is generally felt that the smaller the catheter, the less likely it is to damage the arterial wall, particularly at the catheter-entry site. Smaller catheters have smaller internal diameters, however, which decrease the possible flow rate, but there are various ways to compensate. To achieve rates of flow of contrast sufficient to replace blood in the aorta, a pigtail catheter is usually used. This catheter has a circular shape over the distal few centimeters, with multiple side holes. Rapid injection of contrast material (e.g., 20–40 ml per second) is possible because of outflow through the side holes. The shape and the side holes tend to balance the catheter in the middle of the aorta, even at high flow rates, avoiding damage to the wall. Conversely, if a straight catheter with a single end hole is used, the end of the catheter may recoil vigorously during a high-volume injection and lead to wall damage and even a dissection. When smaller vessels, such as the popliteal, are evaluated, a lower flow rate is possible, and a single-end-hole catheter with a shape advantageous for selective catheterization of a specific vessel is safe and effective. Various commonly utilized catheter shapes are shown in Fig. 22-1.

An additional key piece of angiographic equipment is the guidewire (Fig. 22-2). Guidewires generally fit inside the catheter; are available in various lengths, sizes, and materials; and are essential for initial placement of the catheter as well as selective catheterization. A guidewire generally consists of a stainless steel core wrapped with a smaller wire. The core is welded to the wrapping near the distal end, and it ends short of the tip, leaving the tip soft and atraumatic. Tips with various shapes are available, such as straight or J-shaped with a 1.5-, 3.0-, or 15-mm radius of curvature, as are wires ranging in stiffness from very soft to very firm and in diameter from 0.012 in. to 0.045 in. The most commonly used guidewires are those with a 3- or 15-mm J-shaped tip, a core that ends 5 cm from the end, and a diameter of 0.038 in. The combination of such a wire with various catheters has been shown to allow relatively easy and very safe access to the arterial system.

Angiographic Approaches and Anatomy

The major contribution of angiography in vascular disease is precise, high-resolution definition of anatomy. Any angiographic examination must be tailored to the questions to be answered in the specific patient. The vast bulk of arteriograms in patients with peripheral vascular disease are undertaken to define the nature and the extent of vascular obstruction. With the availability of noninvasive tests for peripheral vascular disease coupled with patient history and physical examination, it is unusual to use arteriography to diagnose peripheral disease. The same pertains to most other types of angiography. The specific access used, then, depends on the location and the extent of disease, the purpose of the study (diagnostic or therapeutic), and the patient's condition. If a patient has a threatened right leg with an asymptomatic left, for example, many angiographers would approach the study from the right femoral artery, with the thought that the normal limb should be left undisturbed. Others would feel that using the right, with the attendant need to shave and sterilize the area, might predispose to infection should the patient have surgery soon after angiography. In general, the percutaneous femoral approach is used, and there are no data to support utilizing the affected or the unaffected side preferentially. Alternative approaches to the femoral are the translumbar, the percutaneous axillary or high brachial, and the antecubital brachial. These approaches are relatively safe, although the incidence of complications, particularly since the femoral approach is used so much more often than others, is higher [26]. The translumbar approach has been widely used and has a low incidence of complications, but it has two problems. First, the translumbar approach is contraindicated in patients with hypertension or severe abdominal aortic disease, since compression of the puncture site is impossible. Second, the ability to maneuver the catheter that has been inserted or to exchange it is very limited, which eliminates this approach for subselective catheterization or interventional procedures. The percutaneous axillary approach is similarly limited, because control of the puncture site is often more difficult than with the femoral artery. Also, the high brachial and axillary artery segments are smaller, and the consequences of arterial damage or leak are more significant than with the femoral artery. These problems have led to a preference for the femoral approach for interventional procedures. The brachial cutdown approach at the level of the antecubital fossa is often used for coronary angiography [27], in large part for historic reasons. The percutaneous approach to the brachial artery in the antecubital fossa has replaced the cutdown in many institutions.

SELECTIVE ANGIOGRAPHY

The Aorta. In younger patients, the aorta must be visualized angiographically to exclude traumatic damage. Following automobile trauma with seatbelts or "deceleration" injuries, as in a fall from a height, the most common site of pathology is in the region of the ductus ligament, in the high descending thoracic aorta. In older patients, the thoracic aorta is studied most commonly to exclude a spontaneous dissection. The abdominal aorta is evaluated in elderly patients most often for assessment of aneurysms and arterial occlusive disease. There is ongoing debate about which imaging modality is most useful for each particular abnormality. For thoracic aortic pathology, some authors feel that contrast-enhanced CT is as accurate as angiography and is clearly less invasive. Others maintain that there are false negatives with CT that limit its utility. MRI has been shown to be capable of imaging the thoracic aorta with accuracy, but its role in the trauma patient remains unclear. That is because of limitations imposed by the relatively long imaging time needed, impeded access to a patient while undergoing the exam, and lack of data concerning accuracy. Angiography has the

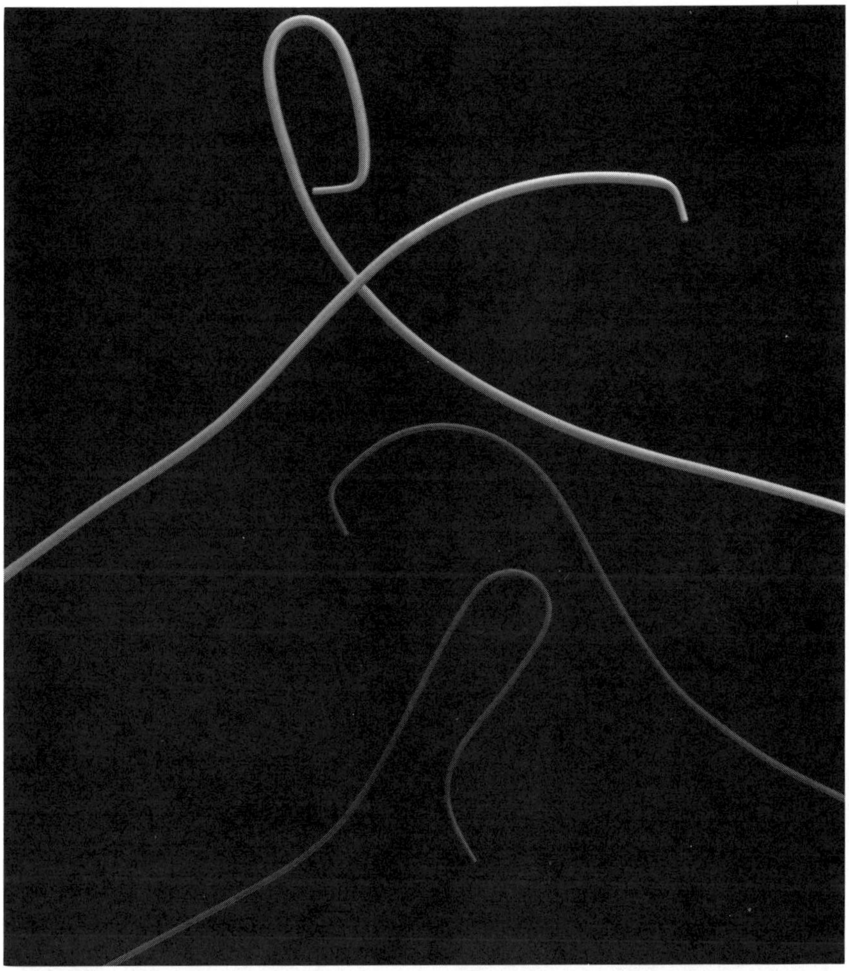

Fig. 22-1. Commonly used selective catheters. From top to bottom, left Judkins catheter (for left coronary artery), right Judkins catheter (for right coronary artery), Cobra catheter (for selective visceral angiography), Simmons catheter (also for selective visceral arterial catheterization).

limitations of being an invasive procedure and not being universally available. Its accuracy, also, is probably not complete, yet it is clearly at least as accurate overall as any of the other modalities and is generally accepted as the gold standard for thoracic aortic pathology [28].

The question as to when angiography should be undertaken in patients with chest trauma is also a difficult one. Classically, angiography is performed on an emergency basis in patients with a widened mediastinum on a good-quality chest radiograph. Because angiography is an invasive procedure, with a finite morbidity in any situation, it is important to utilize it only when it is appropriately indicated. In such trauma cases, the chest film obtained is often a portable one taken in the anteroposterior position, with resultant magnification of the more anterior structures of the mediastinum. Although the consequences of missing an aortic tear clearly are greater than the risks of angiography, care still must be taken to avoid unnecessary examinations. Some investigators feel that aortography is indicated on an emergency basis in patients with mechanism-of-injury situations, that is, in individuals who have had deceleration trauma, even in the presence of a normal chest radiograph. Although it is conceivable that significant aortic trauma may occur in that setting, it has not been shown to occur more than very rarely. At most, elective aortography is indicated, and screening with CT is probably a better choice in that situation. Two additional points must be kept in mind in regard to arch aortography in aortic trauma. The mortality from arch rupture is greatest within the first hour of the incident, so most patients who die from that process die before reaching an angiographic laboratory. Second, in most cases in which the mediastinum is truly widened, the cause is venous bleeding. This is virtually always self-limited and cannot be visualized by angiography.

High-quality angiography requires two projections, which generally are obtained simultaneously in a unit with biplane filming capability or by using first a left anterior oblique projection (to open the aortic arch) followed by an anteroposterior or, preferably, right anterior oblique projection. Findings range from obvious to subtle. A true aortic transection is rarely seen, because such pa-

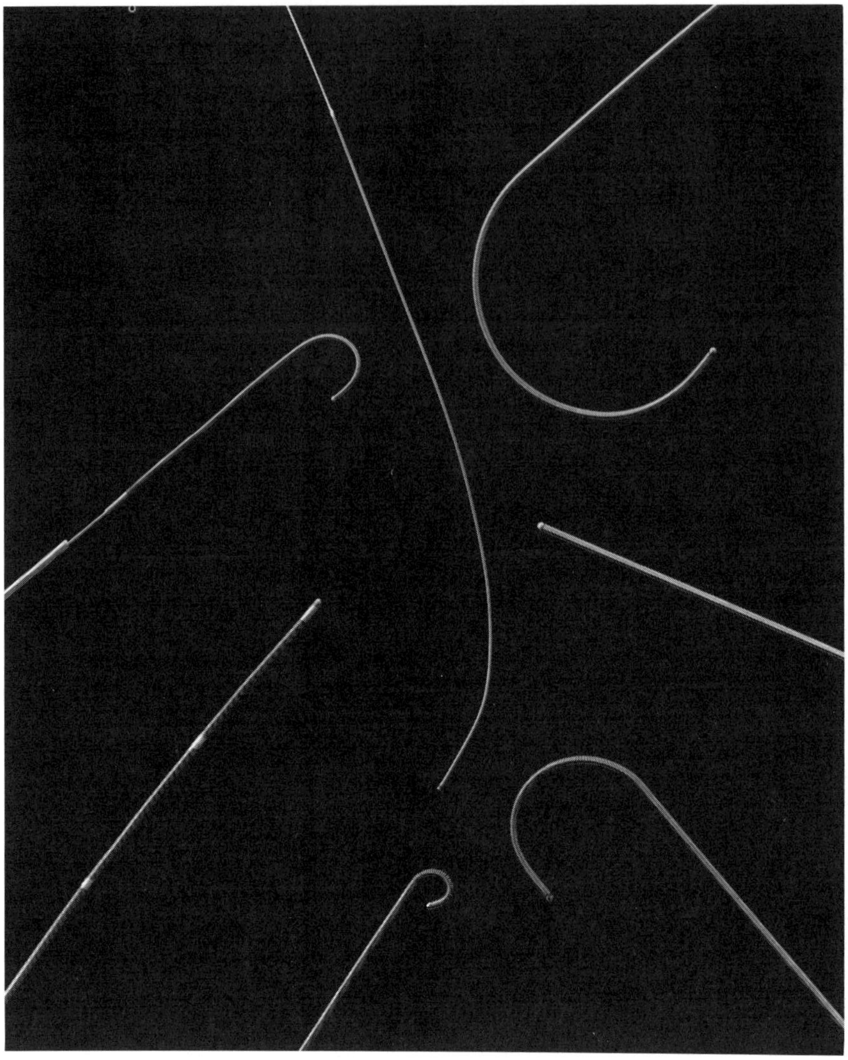

Fig. 22-2. Commonly used guidewires, with straight, 1.5-mm J-shape, 3.0-mm J, 10-mm J, and 15-mm J tips.

tients generally are, at best, too critical to allow angiography. A pseudoaneurysm, indicative of focal disruption of the aortic wall, may be seen, particularly at the level of the ductus diverticulum or ductus ligament in the high descending portion of the thoracic aorta. A minor wall tear, generally thought to require immediate surgical repair, may be manifest by visualization of a small area of extraluminal contrast seen in only one view.

Spontaneous aortic dissection, generally heralded by classic symptoms of tearing chest pain or high back pain, is another indication for emergency angiography. CT and MRI are thought by some to be as accurate as angiography in diagnosis of the presence or absence of a dissection. CT is not as reliable, however, in defining the origin of a dissection. This is particularly true in defining the reentry point of a dissection that begins in the aortic root and in determining if a dissection involves the origins of the great vessels. Both mortality and treatment depend on the extent and the origin of the dissection. The operative approach to such patients clearly depends on accurate assessment, and one reasonable approach is to utilize CT initially, followed by angiography if any doubt exists. That is, if contrast-enhanced CT is equivocal or suggests a dissection, angiography can be used to definitively confirm or exclude one. If a dissection is present, angiography can define the entry and exit points of the false channel.

Dissections are seen primarily in two settings. In the elderly, they are generally related to atherosclerosis and hypertension. That type of dissection most often begins in the descending thoracic aorta, distal to the left subclavian artery. Such dissections can lead to aortic rupture, but most often they are self-limited if blood pressure is controlled. Dissections associated with cystic medial necrosis, with or without Marfan's syndrome, can involve any part of the aorta or all of it. Classically, patients with this underlying aortic pathology have teardrop-shaped aortic-valve sinuses, and the dissection begins in the aortic root. Surgical repair often involves placement of a conduit in the ascending thoracic aorta, with or without an attached aortic valve prosthesis, depending on the degree of aortic regurgitation present. In these patients, presumably because of the underlying aortic disease, partial detachment of the conduit is not uncommon, with formation of a new false channel. That condition also can be defined either by angiography or by dynamic contrast-enhanced CT. MRI may also prove useful in this situation, since patients usually are stable with an enlarging mediastinum on chest radiograph. MRI is extremely sensitive to flow patterns, and cardiac gating is easily accomplished [29].

The abdominal aorta is often studied angiographically to define aneurysms, which generally are diagnosed on physical examination; their size can be accurately determined by ultrasound. Angiography is often performed preoperatively to define the relationship of the aneurysm to the renal arteries and to determine whether the aneurysm extends into the iliac arteries. Those factors dictate the surgical approach and the type of graft placed. Currently, angiography is used only for such anatomic determinations. It is possible that in the future MRI will replace angiography for this indication. The findings of abdominal aortic aneurysms are generally those of an ectatic segment of aorta. Usually, the abnormal segment begins just inferior to the renal arteries and ends proximal to the aortic bifurcation (Fig. 22-3). Also, a large part of the aneurysm may be filled with thrombus, giving a misleading image of a straight border and normal or mildly enlarged aortic diameter. The true size of the aneurysm usually is definable either by a calcified rim or by displacement of adjacent vessels, particularly the superior mesenteric artery. The inferior mesenteric artery is occluded in most patients with aortic aneurysms.

Peripheral Arterial Occlusive Disease. The anatomy imaged in peripheral arterial occlusive disease is fairly simple. In imaging of the lower extremities, the abdominal aorta is visualized both for general information and for the nature and extent of disease. That is, the presence, appearance, and location of the celiac axis, superior mesenteric artery, renal arteries, and inferior mesenteric artery are evaluated (Fig. 22-4). The pelvic vessels are visualized, primarily the distal abdominal aorta and its bifurcation, the common iliac arteries, and the internal (hypogastric) and external iliac arteries (Figs. 22-5 and 22-6; see also Fig. 22-4). Below the inguinal ligament, the common femoral arteries, profunda femoris, and superficial femoral arteries are evaluated (Fig. 22-7). Frontal as well as oblique views of the iliac and femoral bifurcations are helpful to ensure that eccentric lesions are not missed. The superficial femoral artery passes laterally into the adductor canal in the distal thigh to become the popliteal. Generally, the popliteal gives off the anterior tibial artery high in the calf, which traverses the interosseous membrane and then proceeds distally on that structure to the lateral malleolus (see Fig. 22-5C). Just distal to the anterior tibial origin, the common posterior tibial-peroneal trunk divides into the more lateral peroneal artery, which ends at the ankle, and the medially positioned posterior tibial. The anterior and posterior tibial arteries then traverse the foot to supply the dorsalis pedis and the distal posterior tibial arteries, respectively.

The most common findings, those of atherosclerosis, cover a wide spectrum. The abdominal aorta in patients with peripheral vascular disease is often involved by fairly extensive atherosclerosis of varying degrees of severity. Mild wall irregularity almost invariably is present. As with all angiography, it is important to keep in mind that only the lumen of the vessel is visualized, not the entire wall thickness (see Fig. 22-3). Marked diffuse wall thickening, with resultant luminal narrowing, may not be evident as anything other than mild irregularity and focal narrowing. Occlusion of the distal abdominal aorta generally is heralded by a typical picture of a smoking history and severe bilateral claudication. Occasionally, however, femoral pulses may be preserved in such patients due to good collateral inflow (Figs. 22-8 and 22-9).

In the pelvis and lower extremities, the findings of peripheral vascular disease are both common and fairly similar for all vessels. Aneurysms and ectatic changes are rare; wall irregularity, stenoses, and occlusions of varying length are common. Iliac-artery stenoses may involve any portion of the common or external iliac arteries (Fig. 22-10; see also Figs. 22-6, 22-8, and 22-9). Internal iliac disease is not infrequent, but it is rarely felt to be related to significant symptoms. Impotence, although often associated with distal aortic, common, or internal iliac disease, is usually related to diffuse disease or to focal small-vessel disease. When related to major-vessel occlusion, impotence almost invariably occurs only with occlusion of both internal iliac arteries. If one is patent, cross-pelvic collaterals generally are sufficient to maintain function. Occlusions in the iliac system, as elsewhere, are most commonly related to a more distal lesion, with back thrombosis to the first major branch point (see Figs. 22-8 and 22-10). Interventional therapy often is helpful not only in alleviating symptoms but in defining the underlying lesions that precipitated the occlusion.

Common femoral and profunda femoris artery disease is, empirically, less common than disease in the superficial femoral artery (Fig. 22-11). Two types of occlusive involvement of the superficial femoral artery are relatively frequent. The first is diffuse proximal disease just beyond the origin; the second is focal disease at the entrance to the adductor canal. The second type is presumably related to long-term recurrent extrinsic vessel-wall trauma. Occlusion of the entire superficial femoral artery, from its origin to the origin of the popliteal artery, is also a fairly common finding. The profunda femoris is generally patent in such cases and provides collateral flow to the superior geniculate branches of the popliteal artery (Fig. 22-12). It is fairly common, then, to be able to visualize well the popliteal artery and distal vessels in the presence of superficial femoral artery occlusion (Figs. 22-13, 22-14, and 22-15).

In the popliteal artery and beyond, attention is directed at defining the extent of disease. That is, it is important in contemplating surgical bypass of a femoral artery occlusion to know whether the popliteal artery is sufficiently intact above the knee joint to allow above-knee placement of the distal end of a graft. If not, the graft must be placed across the knee joint (see Fig. 22-15F). Similarly, it is useful

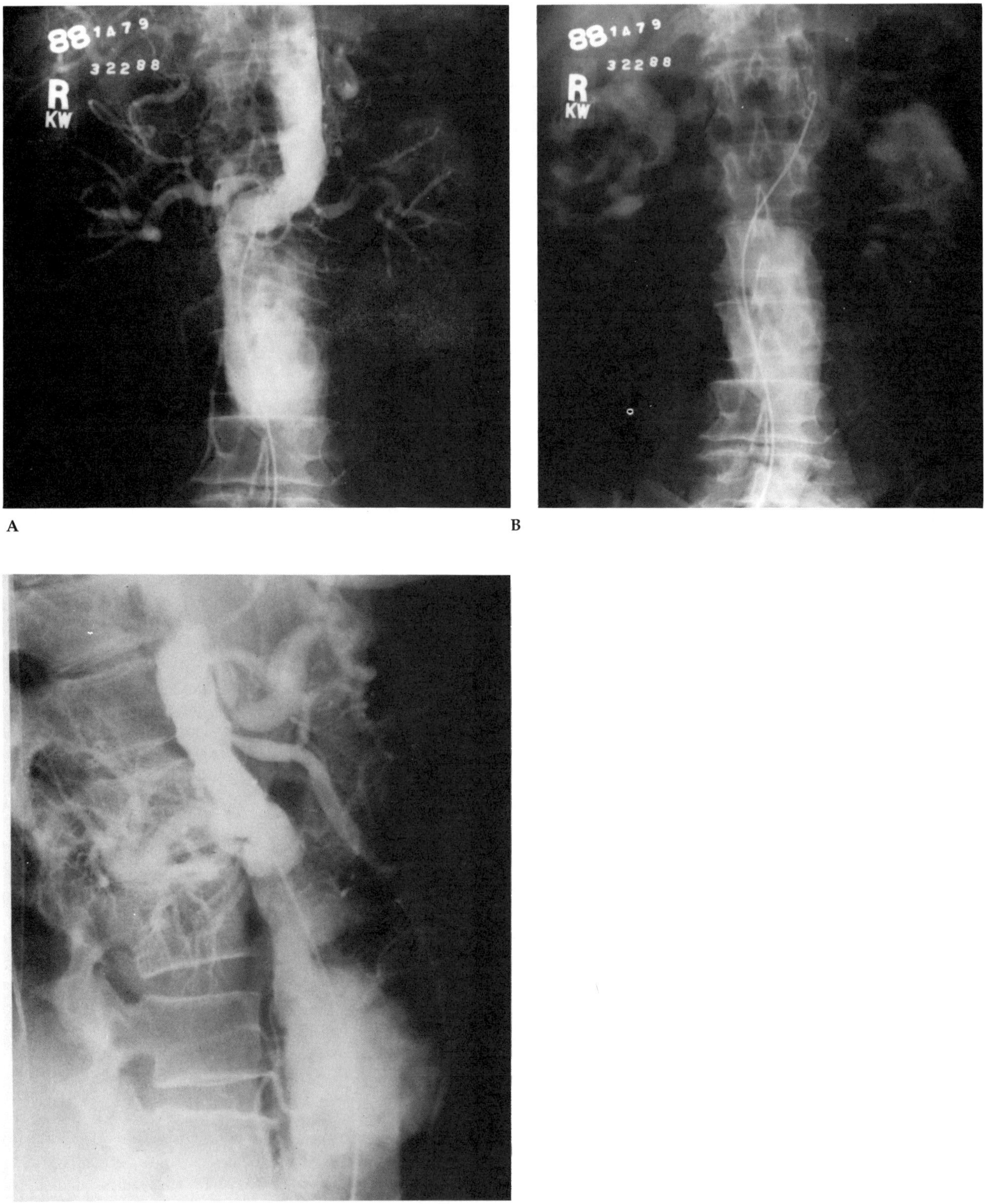

A B

C

Fig. 22-3. Abdominal aortic aneurysm. **A.** Frontal view early in injection. **B.** Late film from frontal view. **C.** Lateral view, early. Note marked tortuosity and origin of aneurysm just inferior to stenosed left renal artery. Also note calcification to left of spine, well lateral to the portion of the lumen that fills with contrast; this is the thrombosed portion of the lumen of the aneurysm. Also note anterior displacement of superior mesenteric artery over the aneurysm in the lateral view. Ectatic segment of aorta extended into the iliac arteries.

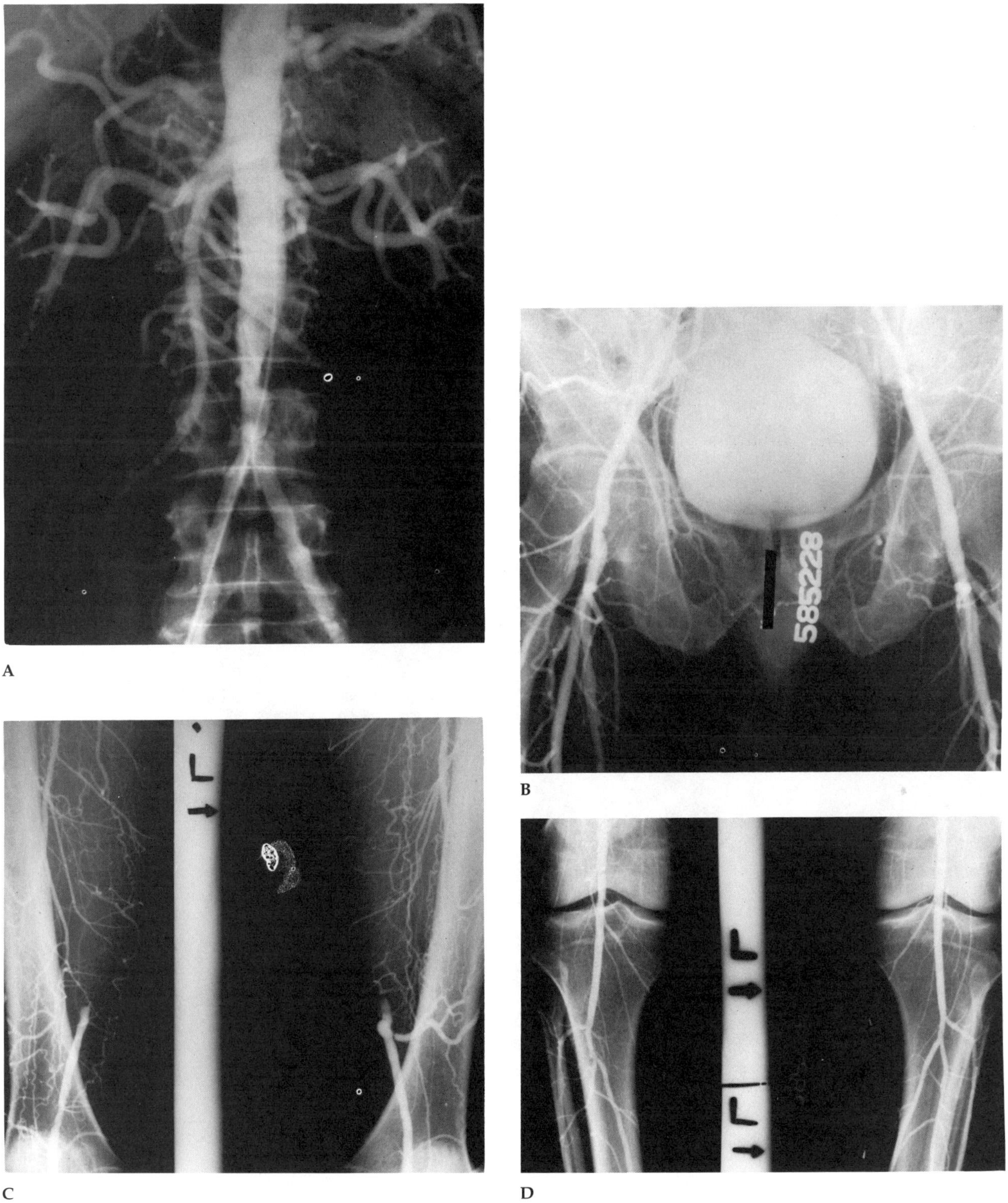

Fig. 22-4. A 58-year-old man with severe claudication, right worse than left. **A.** Severely atherosclerotic abdominal aorta, with normal visceral vessels. **B.** Patent iliac arteries and common femoral arteries. **C.** Bilateral superficial femoral-artery occlusions with good collateral reconstitution of popliteal arteries above the knee bilaterally. **D.** Good distal-vessel runoff bilaterally.

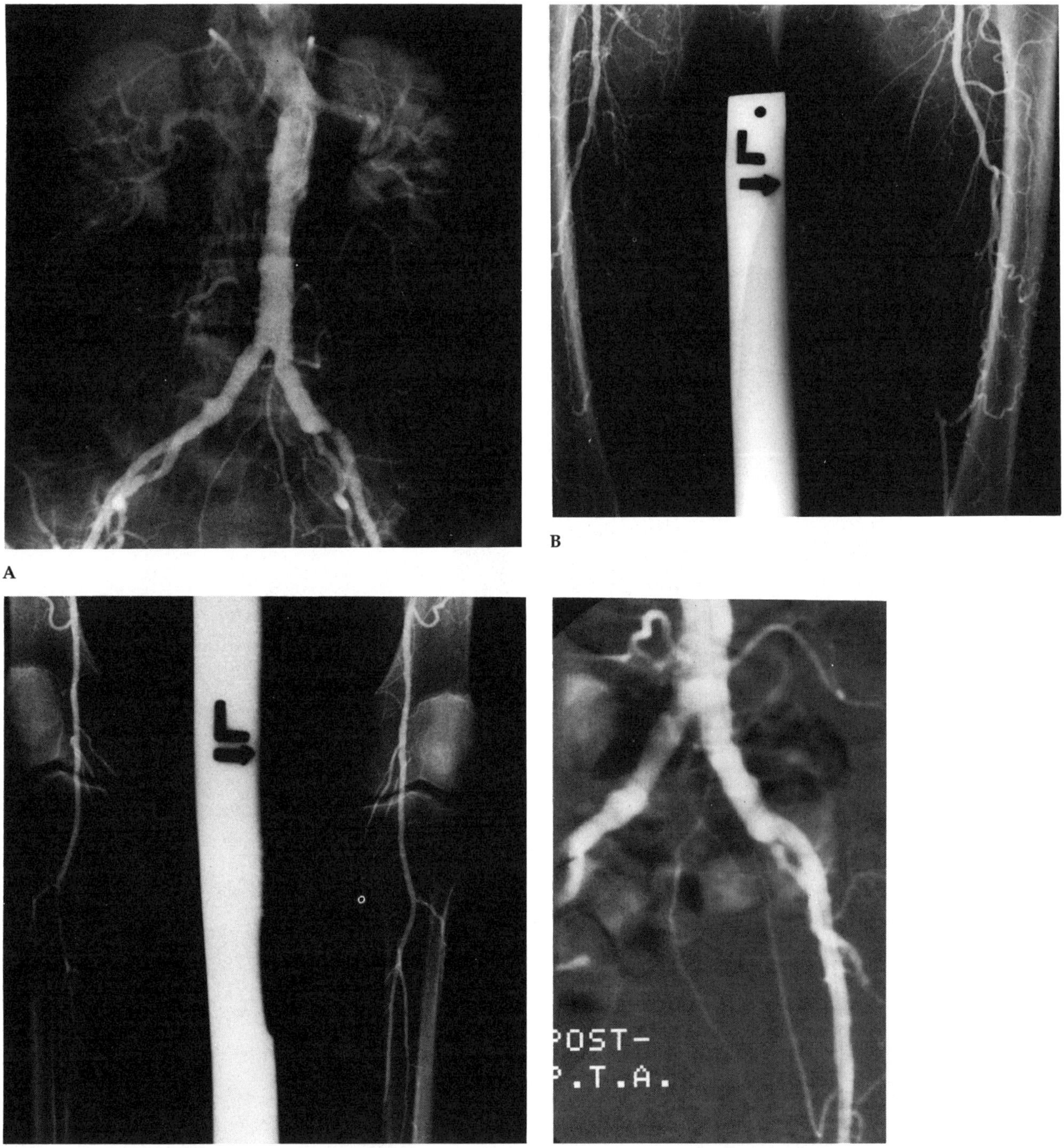

A B C D

Fig. 22-5. A 72-year-old female with mild aortic atherosclerosis, severe left common iliac stenosis, bilateral superficial femoral-artery occlusions, and good distal runoff. **A.** Mildly tortuous abdominal aorta with normal renal arteries. Note tight left external iliac artery stenosis. **B.** View of the upper legs demonstrates bilateral superficial femoral-artery occlusion, with good reconstitution of the left popliteal artery via collaterals. **C.** Good popliteal arteries bilaterally with bilateral runoff via anterior tibial (lateral), posterior tibial (medial), and peroneal (middle) arteries. **D.** Digital-subtraction image of left external iliac artery, showing excellent result from percutaneous transluminal angioplasty.

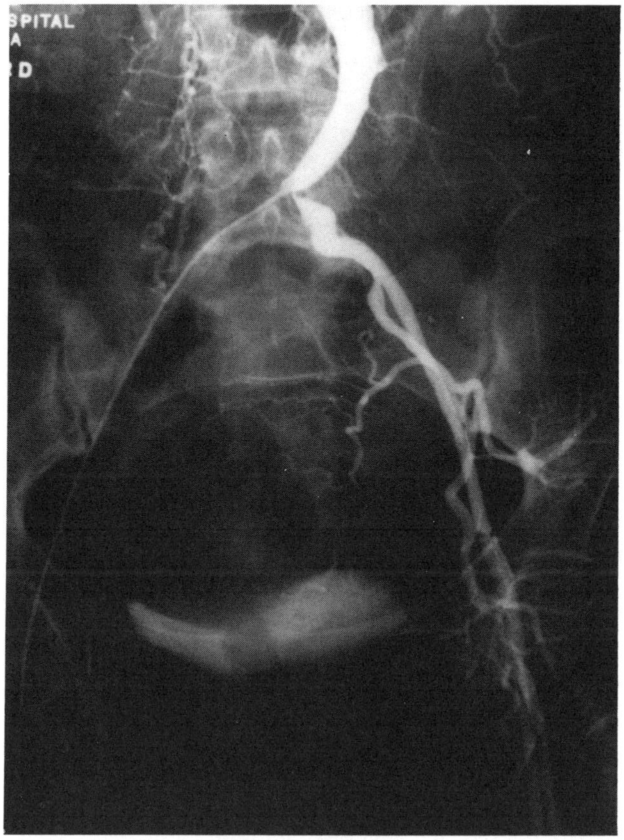

Fig. 22-6. A 50-year-old male with severe claudication. Note marked narrowing of distal aorta and obvious stenosis of origin of left common iliac artery. Right iliac origin is so narrowed that the catheter introduced through it occludes antegrade flow.

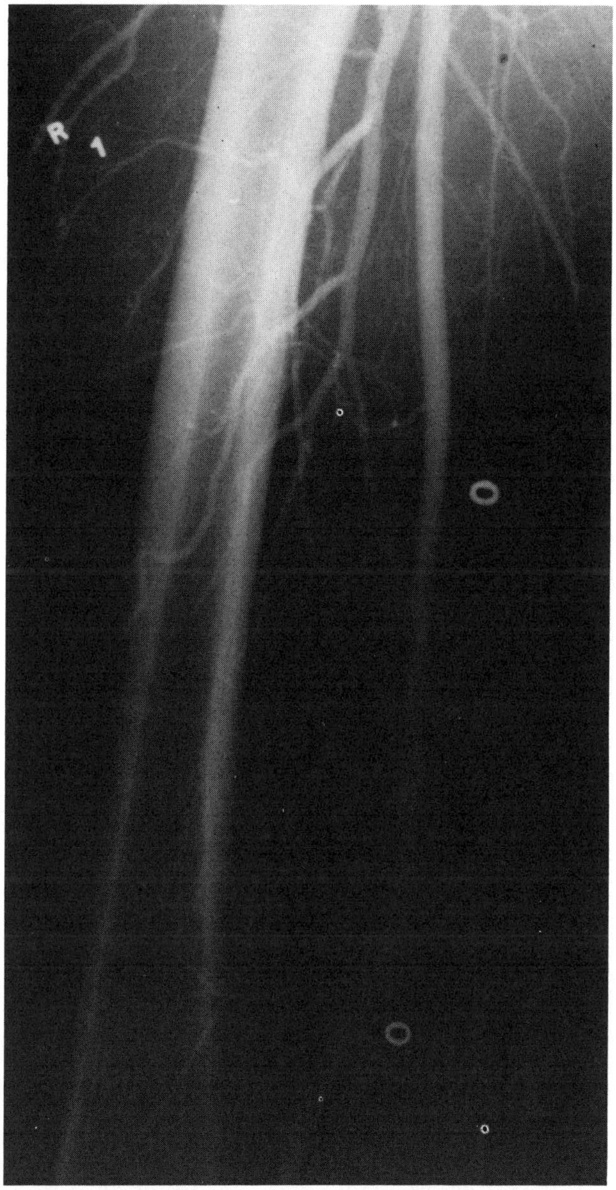

Fig. 22-7. Normal right profunda femoris artery (lateral) and superficial femoral artery (medial). The latter becomes the popliteal as it enters the adductor canal, just proximal to where it crosses the cortex of the distal femur.

to visualize the more distant runoff vessels—a function that currently only angiography can perform in a practical fashion (Fig. 22-16; see also Fig. 22-15). Both surgically and percutaneously, treatment of below-knee vascular disease is becoming more widely available as well as more effective. It is often advantageous to use a combination of cut-film and digital imaging, with the higher spatial resolution of the former and superior contrast resolution of the latter (see Figs. 22-16A and 22-16C).

Another important function of angiography is the definition of vascular grafts and their associated native vessels (see Figs. 22-15C, 22-15D, and 22-15F). Both artificial and natural (i.e., autologous vein) grafts can be safely punctured for angiographic procedures (Fig. 22-17). Interventional procedures such as thrombolysis and angioplasty have come to play a large role in the treatment of stenosed or occluded grafts. Diagnosis of abnormalities of grafts, of their anastomoses, or of progression of disease proximal or distal to grafts is an increasingly important function of angiography. In such studies, a therapeutic intervention such as thrombolysis is important not only to resolve symptoms but also to define reasons for recurrence of such symptoms, that is, the etiology of graft failure. In evaluating grafts, it is generally accepted that if failure occurs in 1 month or less, a technical problem is responsible. If failure occurs in 1 to 6 months, fibromuscular proliferation at or near the anastomosis is the most likely cause. Subsequent failure is generally related to progressive atherosclerosis (Fig. 22-18).

Trauma is another important reason for performing angiography. Following acute trauma, angiography may be useful to define the precise abnormality if distal pulses are clearly diminished or absent, to rule out major arterial abnormalities (as opposed to venous or small-arterial-branch pathology) in the presence of a falling hematocrit or an expanding hematoma, or to exclude arterial damage

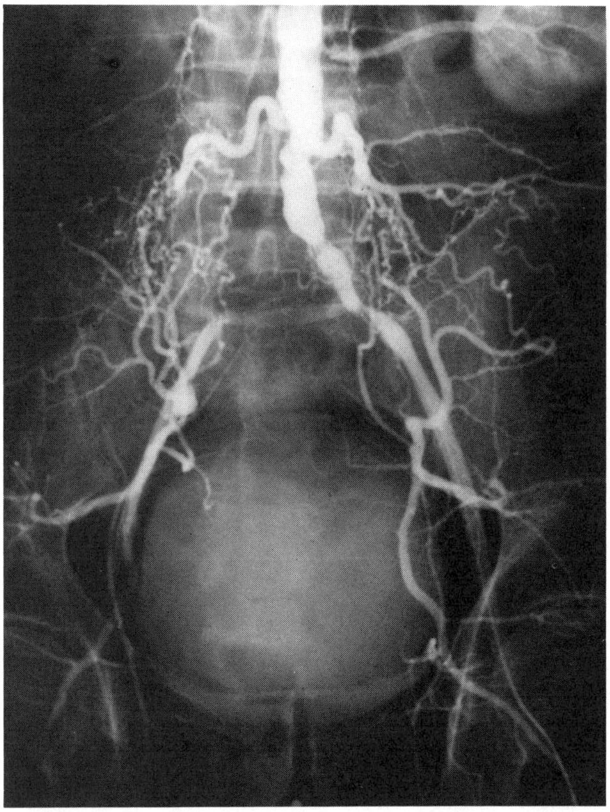

Fig. 22-8. Marked distal aortic disease extending into iliac arteries in a 65-year-old male with bilateral claudication. There are two focal stenoses of the left common iliac artery and a focal occlusion of the right common iliac artery. Two markedly enlarged distal lumbar arteries provide good collateral filling bilaterally. Note stenosis of origin of accessory left lower-pole renal artery.

in the presence of injury in proximity to an artery (Fig. 22-19). The role of emergency angiography, particularly in the absence of altered distal pulses, has been debated. The best evidence currently suggests that the yield is extremely low from arteriography for extremity trauma in the absence of altered pulses or an expanding hematoma [30]. In such situations, angiography should be performed on an elective basis or not at all. Patients can be watched judiciously and further evaluation performed as clinically warranted. This view has been supported not only by the low yield of arteriography in the absence of specific signs of arterial damage but also by the benign nature of abnormalities noted on elective angiography.

Iatrogenic trauma leads to arterial abnormalities that are often subacute or chronic in presentation. Most such arterial injury is related to surgery or to prior angiography [31,32]. Probably the most common injury is a pseudoaneurysm at a graft site. This injury can present at any time following placement of a vascular graft, usually as a gradually expanding pulsatile mass. Often, physical diagnosis confirmed by ultrasound examination is sufficient to allow optimal surgical repair. Angiography may be helpful in defining the relationship of the mass to the graft-native vessel anastomosis and thus may facilitate preservation of the graft. It may also prove useful in confirming that the mass actually communicates with the native vessel and does not represent a seroma or abscess surrounding the artery. A pseudoaneurysm also may occur following inadvertent vessel-wall damage during surgery on adjacent tissues, for example, femoral-artery damage during a total hip replacement. Pseudoaneurysms, particularly subacute ones, are probably most common following angiographic procedures performed with percutaneous placement of large catheters in a femoral artery. Pseudoaneurysms may be seen following percutaneous intra-aortic counter-pulsation balloon placement, due to both the 10-F or larger arterial sheath and the need for concurrent anticoagulation and, for similar reasons, after percutaneous transluminal coronary angioplasty. It is generally felt that pseudoaneurysms have a high likelihood of life-threatening rupture and should be repaired as soon as possible after diagnosis.

Another peripheral arterial condition is vessel rupture related to surgical embolectomy or to percutaneous angioplasty. Both generally present with sudden onset of hemodynamic instability, often accompanied by flank or groin pain if the iliac system is the site of rupture, as is most often the case. A small leak, related to the arterial puncture, can also occur and lead to significant blood loss. This is most often related to a high arterial puncture, of the external iliac artery above the inguinal ligament rather than of the common femoral artery below. Persistent bleeding from the puncture site is thought to occur because the external iliac artery lies retroperitoneally, and it is difficult to compress the arterial entry site successfully. In contrast, the common femoral artery can be successfully compressed against adjacent musculature below the inguinal ligament.

Pathology other than trauma or atherosclerosis is rarely encountered on lower-extremity angiography. Involvement of major lower-extremity vessels by a vasculitis is rare, far less common than involvement of visceral arteries or those of the upper extremity (Fig. 22-20). Congenital anomalies are also unusual. Although there are well-described variations in the distribution of the branches of the popliteal artery, they are usually of no clinical significance. An exception is the popliteal entrapment syndrome, in which there is anomalous insertion of portions of the gastrocnemius muscle with lateral displacement of the popliteal artery [33]. This may predispose to aneurysm formation or to obstruction at the level of the joint. Abnormalities of the midpopliteal artery are rare in the absence of such anatomic variants. The etiology is thought to be recurrent extrinsic trauma, an explanation similar to that commonly given for the frequent occlusion of the distal superficial femoral artery as it enters Hunter's canal in the low thigh (see Figs. 22-13A and 22-15C). Various other abnormalities of the lower-extremity arteries occur infrequently. These include other congenital abnormalities (almost invariably asymptomatic), developmental abnormalities (e.g., unilateral hypoplasia of the femoral-artery system secondary to cardiac catheterization in infancy), arteriovenous malformations, and vascular infections (rare and most frequently associated with prosthetic grafts).

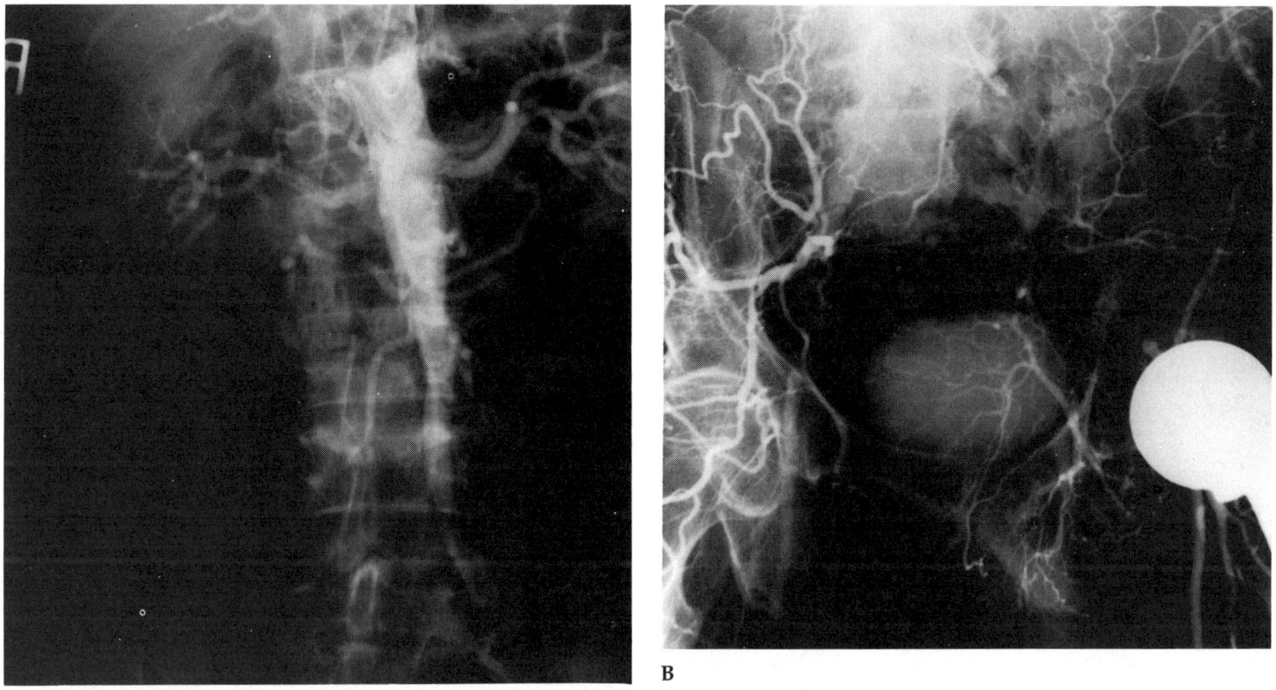

A B

Fig. 22-9. A 58-year-old male with trace femoral pulses bilaterally. **A.** Distal aortic narrowing with occlusion of right common iliac artery at its origin and on the left distally. **B.** Good collateral reconstitution of common and superficial femoral arteries bilaterally.

Upper-Extremity Angiography. The technique for evaluation of upper-extremity arteries is similar to that for any selective arterial study. A catheter of a shape suited to placement in the major artery supplying the area in question is advanced from the arterial entry site, in combination with a guidewire. For the arm, this generally means use of the retrograde femoral approach for catheterization of the subclavian artery, directly on the left or by traversing the innominate trunk on the right. In such selective maneuvers, many factors must be considered, including care in catheterization to avoid damage to the vessel wall as well as attention to underlying abnormalities such as an anomalous origin (e.g., the left subclavian origin proximal to the innominate). Also, contrast injection must be limited, to prevent inadvertent blood-brain-barrier damage due to excessive amounts injected into the carotid circulation, and care must be taken to avoid selective catheterization of the vertebral artery or costocervical trunk, which may provide blood supply to the anterior cervical-thoracic spine. Like lower-extremity angiography, upper-extremity angiography may be painful, particularly if high-osmolality, high-iodine-content contrast agents are utilized, which may lead to patient motion and resultant loss of detail. By diluting the contrast material (to lower osmolality) and using digital-subtraction imaging, this problem can be largely obviated (see Figs. 22-20A and 22-20B).

The major indication for upper-extremity angiography is trauma, either extrinsic (e.g., knife wound or gunshot; see Fig. 22-19) or iatrogenic. As in the lower extremity, sharp or blunt trauma with alteration of distal pulses or an expanding hematoma are indications for emergency arteriography. Although most such examinations do not show acute arterial damage of large vessels, it is important to exclude occlusion of a major branch or wall abnormalities, such as an intimal flap, which may progress to occlusion. In patients with similar trauma but no pulse change or expanding hematoma, elective arteriography may be performed, again with the intention of excluding wall damage, if the trauma is felt to have occurred in proximity to a major artery. Again, most such studies are negative, but they are still justifiable in the appropriate clinical setting. Iatrogenic trauma relates mainly to the use of the brachial artery for cardiac catheterization, either percutaneously or, more often, via cutdown. In experienced hands, the cutdown approach has an incidence of complications as low as the percutaneous femoral one. As a function of decreasing experience, however, the incidence of complications increases [34]. Complications usually manifest as loss of pulse, but acute ischemia or hand claudication may occur. Both require surgical intervention, with thrombectomy and repair if symptoms occur soon after an occlusion or with placement of a graft for remote injury [35]. Particularly when the injury is more than 24 to 48 hours old, angiography is helpful in defining the extent of the occlusion.

Upper-extremity angiography is useful in some patients with manifestations of Raynaud's phenomenon or digital

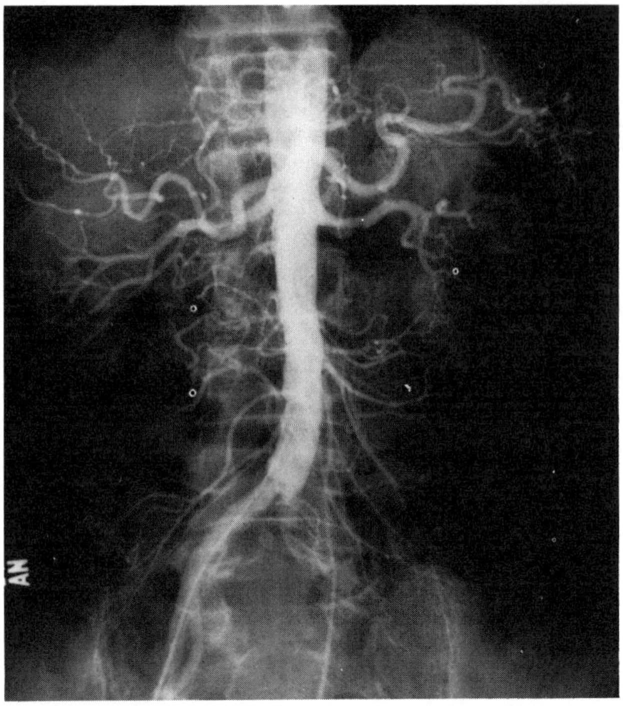

A

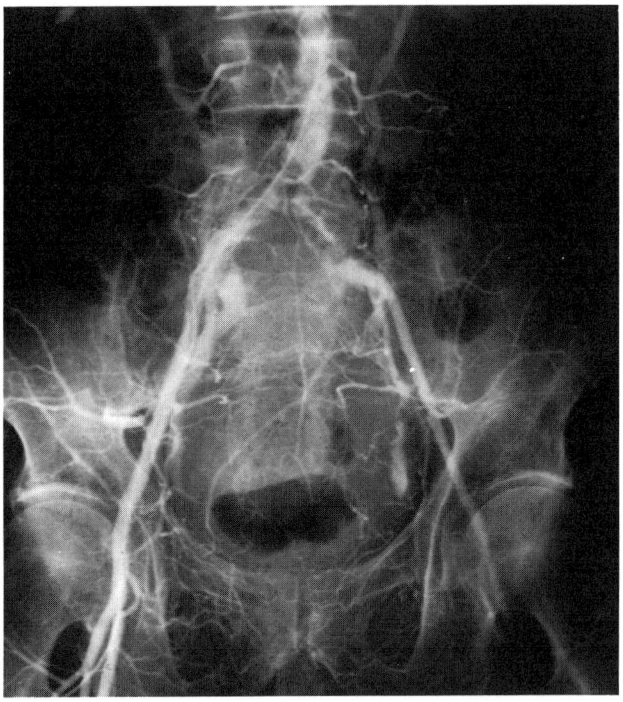

B

Fig. 22-10. A 62-year-old male with normal abdominal aorta **(A)** and short left common iliac artery occlusion **(B)** with good collateralization, resulting in reconstitution at the iliac bifurcation.

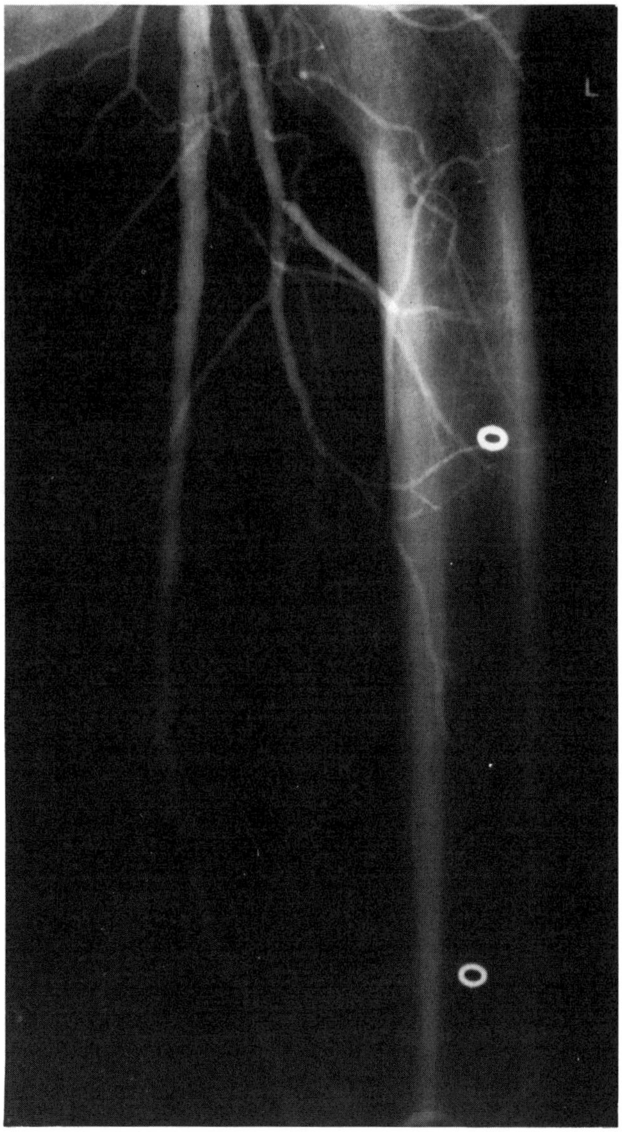

Fig. 22-11. Patent superficial femoral and profunda femoris arteries, with minor atherosclerotic changes, which are more marked in the former.

ischemia (see Fig. 22-20). Distal vessels in the hand are often occluded in patients with necrotizing vasculitis. Occlusion of larger hand vessels and even of the distal radial or ulnar arteries may occur in some connective tissue diseases, such as scleroderma or systemic lupus erythematosus. In patients with digital ischemia, angiography may be helpful in defining the underlying disease and planning appropriate therapy.

Renal Angiography. Renal angiography is most often indicated as part of the workup for severe hypertension, donation of a kidney, evaluation of renal trauma, or preoperative mapping prior to planned partial nephrectomy. It is rarely necessary as part of the workup for renal

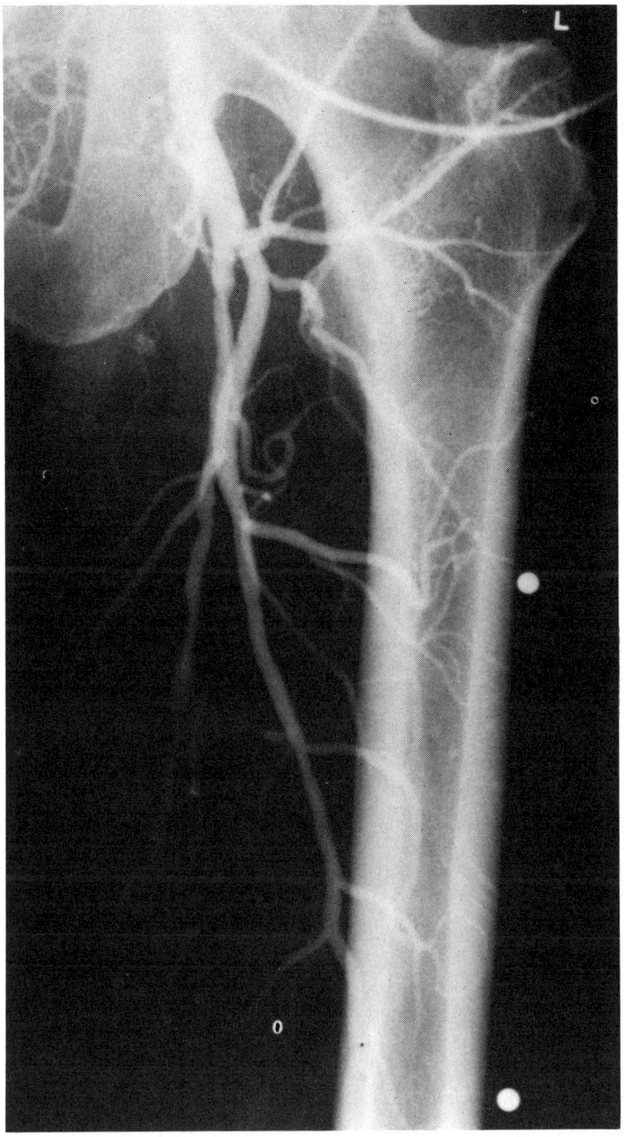

Fig. 22-12. A 49-year-old man with left-leg claudication. There is occlusion of the mid and distal superficial femoral artery. The profunda femoris artery is patent.

masses, due to the accuracy of CT and ultrasound. In the investigation of hypertension, aortography is usually sufficient for assessment of renal artery stenosis (see Fig. 22-8). In equivocal cases, selective renal angiography is performed. Measurement of arterial pressure proximal and distal to stenoses may help define hemodynamic significance in such cases. The true utility of selective renal-vein renin assays in determining the significance of stenoses remains controversial [36]. In the workup of renal donors, angiography is used to determine the number of renal arteries. The presence of an unrecognized polar renal artery, as seen in Fig. 22-8, may lead to complications for both the donor and the recipient at the time of surgery. Also, angiography can rule out small vascular abnormalities, such as fibromuscular dysplasia or an arteriovenous

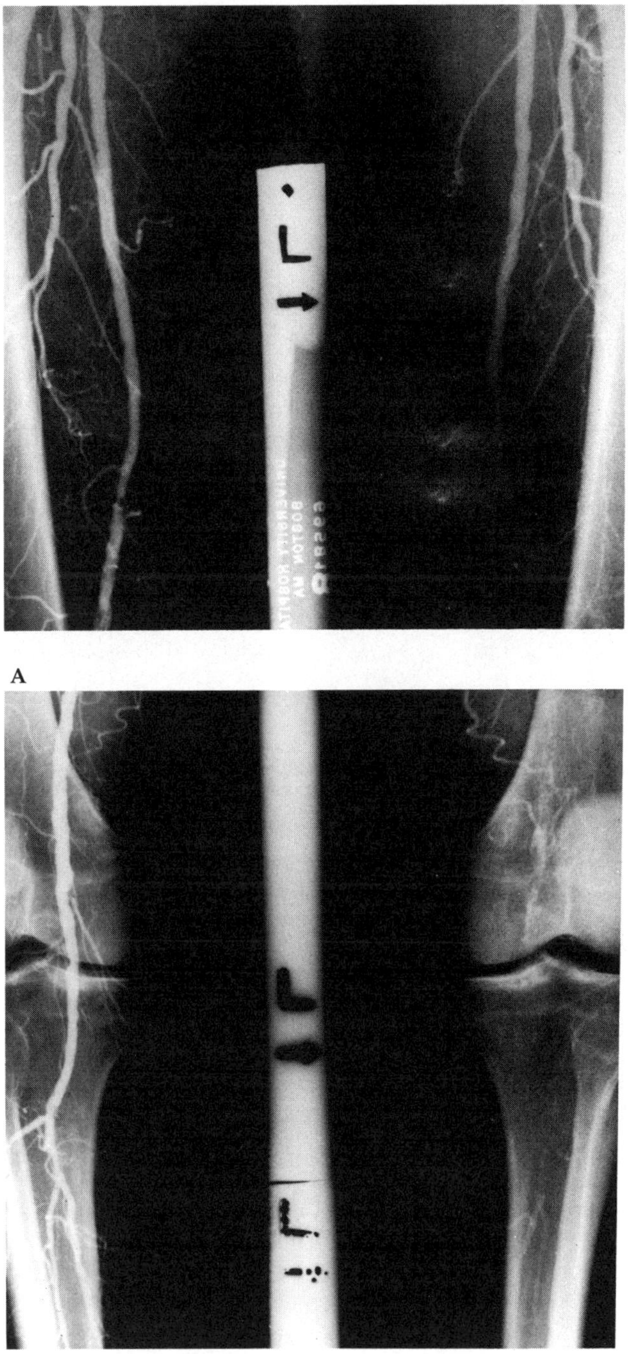

A

B

Fig. 22-13. A 55-year-old male with tight stenosis of right superficial femoral artery at the adductor canal, with occlusion of the left superficial femoral artery at the same level **(A)**, moderate right popliteal disease with good runoff, and minimal left popliteal reconstitution **(B)**. Note fair collateral reconstitution of left posterior tibial and peroneal arteries.

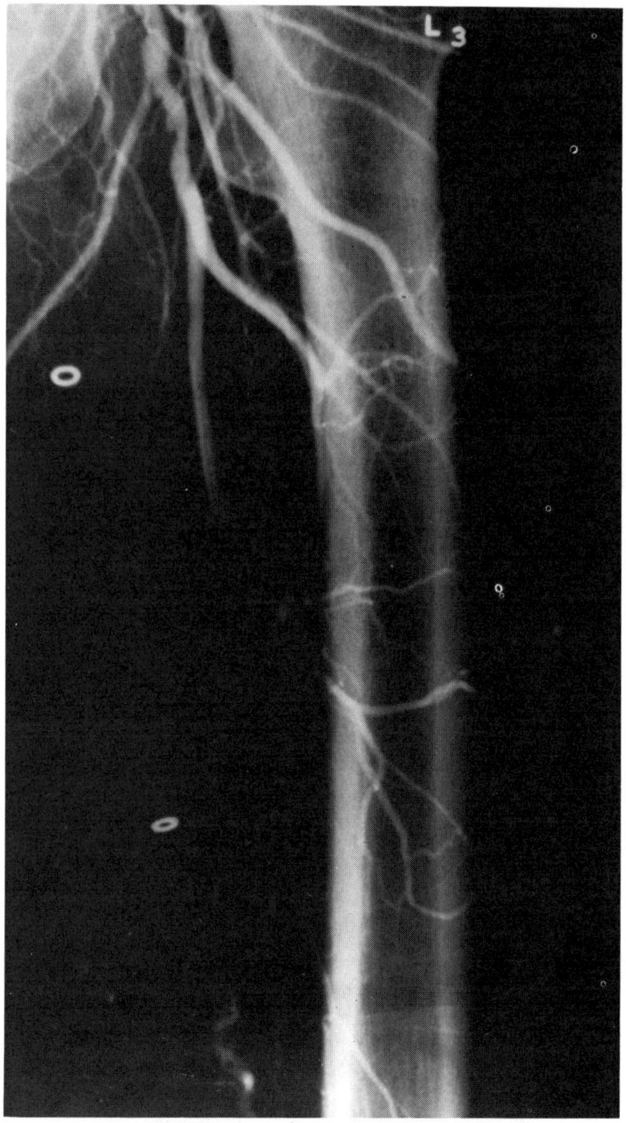

Fig. 22-14. Occlusion of left superficial femoral artery at its origin, with fairly good reconstitution of the popliteal artery above the knee via collaterals from the profunda femoris artery.

ties, such as fibromuscular dysplasia or an arteriovenous malformation, that may contraindicate donation. When partial nephrectomy is planned, either as bench surgery or in situ, angiography is helpful in defining the precise vascular anatomy and the relationship of the mass to the major arteries. Preoperative embolization of tumors has been utilized either immediately or several days to several weeks preoperatively, to shrink tumor mass, limit blood loss, and facilitate surgery.

Visceral Angiography. As with renal angiography, the role of visceral-artery angiography has changed over the past decade due to the efficacy of ultrasound, CT, and, to a lesser extent, radionuclide imaging. Currently, angiography is useful chiefly in defining vascular anatomy prior to surgery and in confirming and treating enteric bleeding. The use of angiography purely for diagnosis of vascular disease is unusual. In that regard, it is necessary to confirm the diagnosis of intestinal angina, which is characterized by occlusion of two or three major visceral arteries and stenosis of the third (i.e., the celiac axis, superior mesenteric artery, and inferior mesenteric artery). Occasionally, intestinal angina can be treated by angioplasty. Angiography is also imperative when a diagnosis of nonocclusive or occlusive mesenteric ischemia is entertained. In the former, early diagnosis and selective intra-arterial infusion of papaverine is thought to be the most effective treatment. In the past, angiography was used to make the diagnosis of gastrointestinal bleeding, but now radionuclide studies offer a significant advantage. Even marked active gastrointestinal bleeding may not correlate well with symptoms in the sense that symptoms may not occur until bleeding has slowed or stopped. Further, most bleeds are intermittent. Angiography in this setting provides a very accurate anatomic definition, but only of a discrete point in time. Using the 99m-labeled erythrocyte technique, dynamic scanning can be carried out over time, even up to 24 hours after injection. Patients can then be followed, and intermittent bleeding documented. Also, blood-pool scanning in this fashion can help to localize the bleeding site in general terms. This makes angiography far more effective by avoiding studies in patients who are not actively bleeding, as well as by performing studies tailored to when and where the bleed is occurring. Angiography, then, can be used for selective localization and treatment of a bleeding source.

In patients with chronic intermittent intestinal bleeds, angiography is used to exclude angiodysplasia. Classically, angiodysplasias occur in the submucosa of the ileocecal region, but they have been found throughout the large and small bowels. They often present with chronic intermittent blood loss and are said not to be visible on endoscopy unless actively bleeding. Angiographically, they are diagnosed by the presence of an early draining vein (caused by arteriovenous shunting), early arterial filling, and a small caput of abnormal vessels. The treatment of choice is focal surgical excision.

Angiography for other vascular diseases in the visceral and hepatic circulation is less frequent. Celiac-axis and superior-mesenteric-artery injections often are performed to demonstrate splenic- and portal-vein patency prior to shunt surgery for portal hypertension. Occasionally, angiography is useful for definition of hepatic arterial anatomy prior to partial hepatic resection of metastatic deposits (e.g., colon carcinoma) or hepatoma. Trauma to the liver may require angiography, both for definition of anatomy and for treatment to control bleeding. This is true more for iatrogenic trauma, such as bleeding following percutaneous liver biopsy or placement of a transhepatic drainage tube, than for other types of trauma that tend to lead to major-vessel injury and hemodynamic collapse necessitating emergency surgery. Angiography occasionally is undertaken for patients with vasculitis, particularly Takayasu's arteritis, or peculiar abdominal symptoms, to exclude major vascular pathology. In general, visceral angiography is currently less useful than in the era prior to

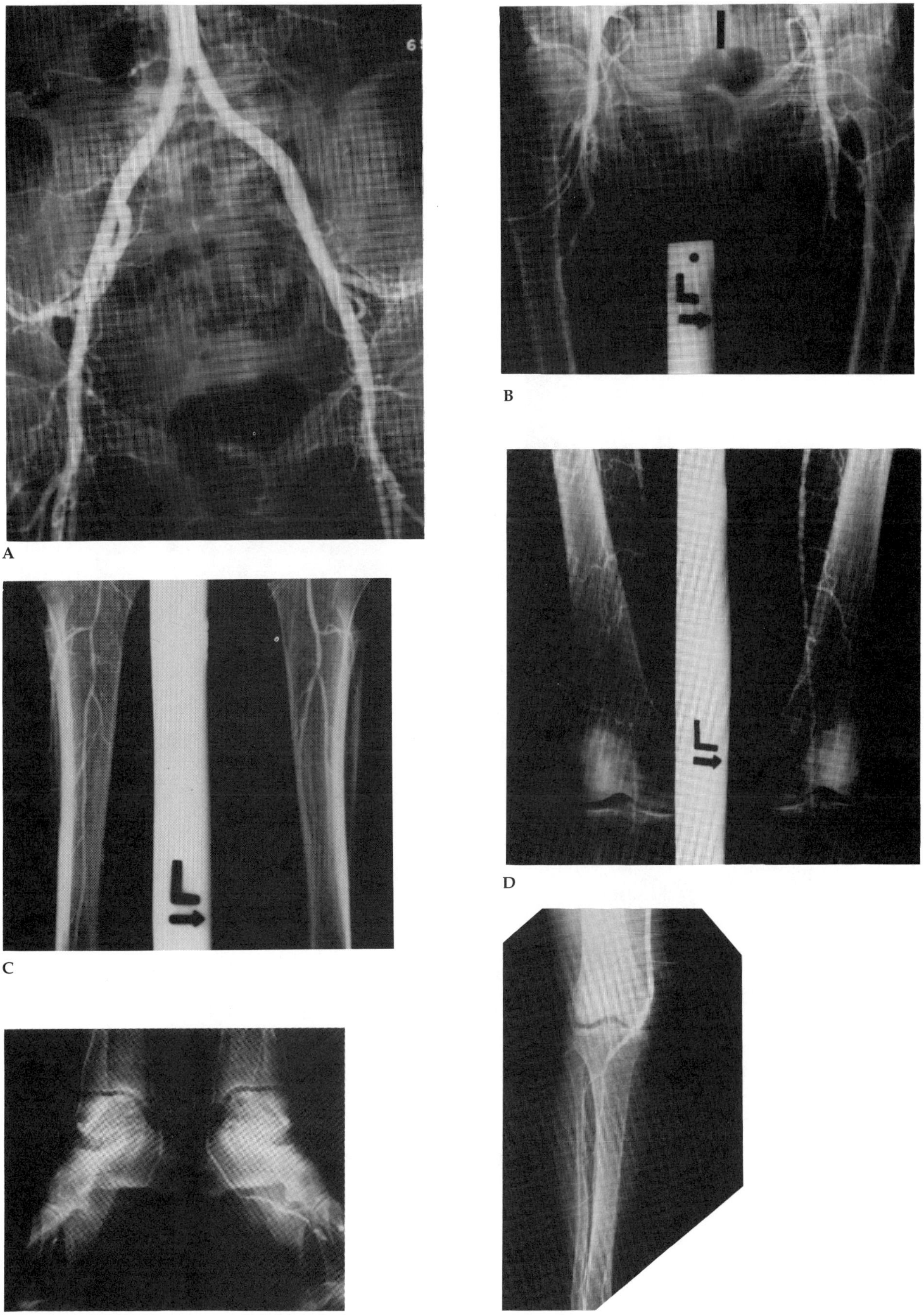

Fig. 22-15. An 81-year-old female with right-leg claudication. **A., B.** Aorta, iliac arteries, and common femoral arteries are essentially normal in appearance. **C.** The right superficial femoral artery is occluded, with good collateral reconstitution of the popliteal artery. The left is diffusely diseased but patent. **D.** Runoff on the right is via a diffusely diseased anterior tibial artery and the peroneal artery. The posterior tibial artery is occluded. On the left there is runoff via the posterior tibial (medially) and the peroneal, with an occluded anterior tibial artery. **E.** In the right foot, the dorsalis pedis artery fills faintly, going to the dorsum, and the posterior tibial artery is reconstituted. In the left foot, the peroneal artery is seen ending normally just above the ankle, and the posterior tibial artery is widely patent into the metatarsal region. **F.** Distal portion of a below-knee femoral-popliteal graft on the right. Note collateral filling of posterior tibial artery.

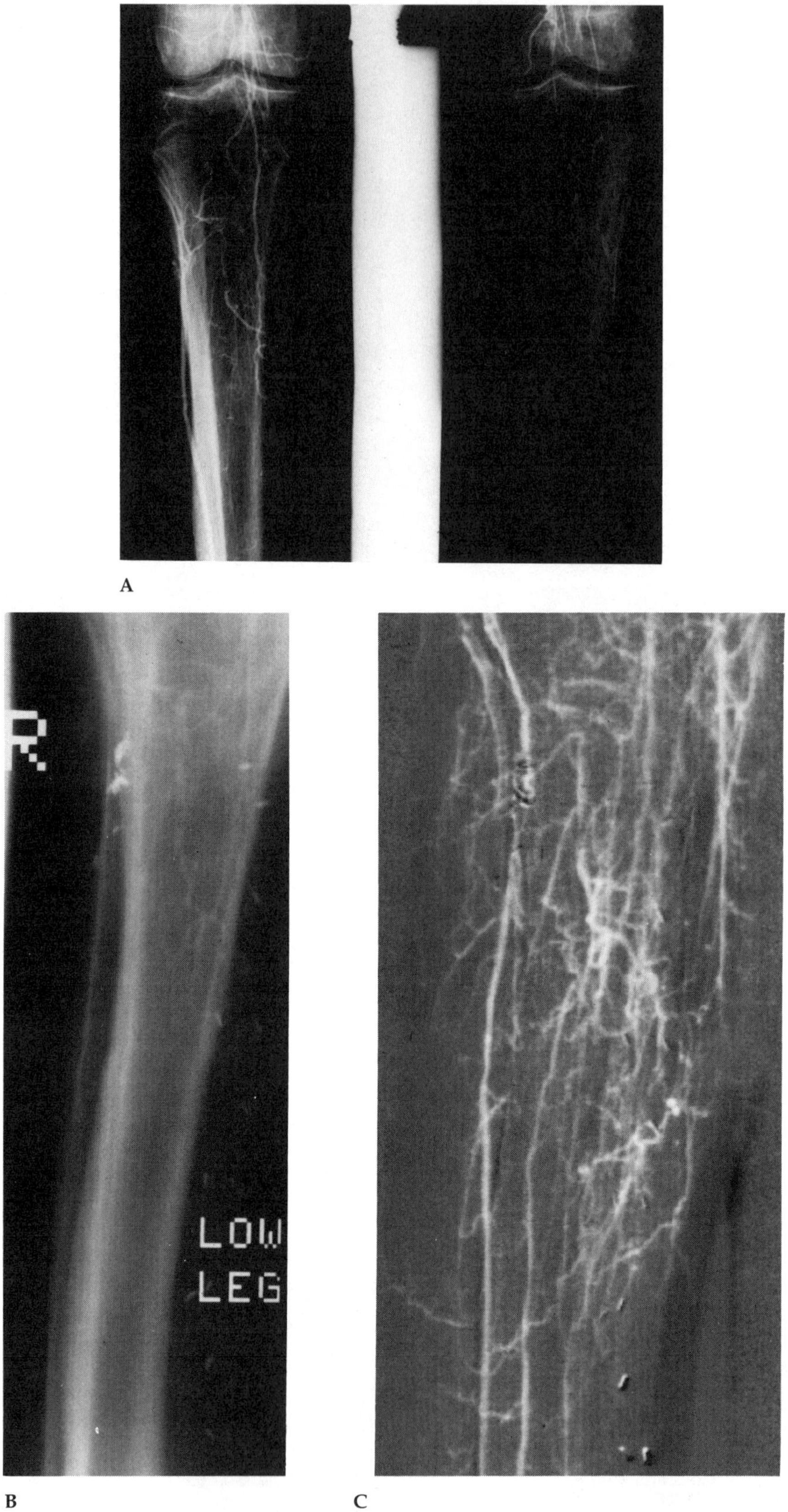

Fig. 22-16. A 70-year-old male with severe distal disease. **A.** Note left below-knee amputation and poor visualization of distal vessels on the right, distal to an occluded popliteal artery. **B.** Digital-subtraction view of right lower leg superimposed on mask. **C.** DSA view of right lower leg showing collateral reconstitution of the anterior tibial and peroneal arteries, both of which appear suitable for a graft. Note superior contrast resolution on digital subtraction image.

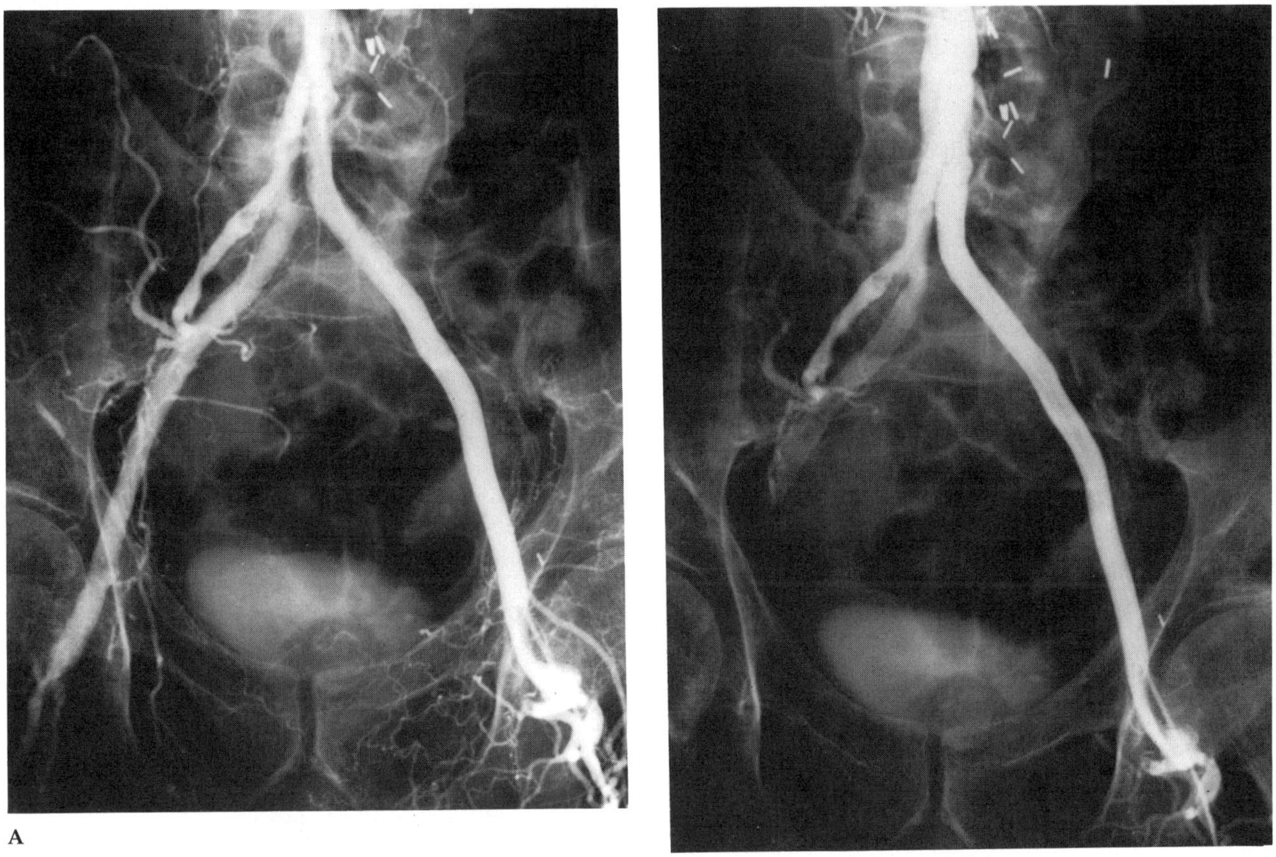

A B

Fig. 22-17. Aortobifemoral graft, with access via puncture of the femoral component on the left. The right native common and internal iliac arteries are patent. **A.** Early arterial filling. **B.** Later arterial phase.

pool radionuclide scanning. It remains useful for diagnosis in certain specific situations. As in other vascular beds, its utility for therapy continues to evolve.

Cerebral Angiography. Evaluation of the extracranial carotid arteries is most often performed with duplex ultrasound, in conjunction with other noninvasive modalities. Angiography generally is reserved for patients with equivocal noninvasive findings, as preoperative evaluation, and for patients with questionable intracerebral vascular disease. The aim of angiography is to define the severity of carotid artery disease. Noninvasive studies may not be able to distinguish between very tight stenosis and occlusion, and the treatment of the two differs markedly. It may also be important to study the intracerebral vasculature to ensure that repair of extracranial disease is likely to be beneficial. Other than in the investigation of atherosclerosis, angiography is occasionally used for vascular mapping prior to tumor therapy. It is also important in the assessment of aneurysms to define their location and relationship to major arteries. As in other body areas, cerebral angiography as a diagnostic modality is less useful than it was prior to the availability of CT and MRI. As with peripheral vascular disease, however, angiographic treatment is increasing in importance, in the form of angioplasty of subclavian arteries and transcatheter ablation of aneurysms and vascular malformations.

Cardiac Angiography. Coronary artery definition, in terms of clinical utility, currently is feasible only with angiography. Fast CT and MRI both have shown promise, but neither is yet clinically useful for this purpose [37]. Conversely, angiography for definition of cardiac function and clarification of congenital heart disease has been replaced to a large extent by ultrasound and radionuclide studies. A comprehensive discussion of coronary angiography is beyond the scope of this chapter, but the technique is used primarily in atherosclerosis to define the nature and extent of coronary lesions. It also plays a role in excluding coronary artery disease in patients in whom other, noninvasive studies are equivocal, and similarly in assessing coronary anatomy in patients with other lesions that may cause chest pain. Such conditions are hypertrophic cardiomyopathies and aortic-valve stenosis or regurgitation. Coronary angiography also may be of interest in patients with dilated cardiomyopathies, to distinguish those with an ischemic cause.

Advances in cardiac angiography over the last decade

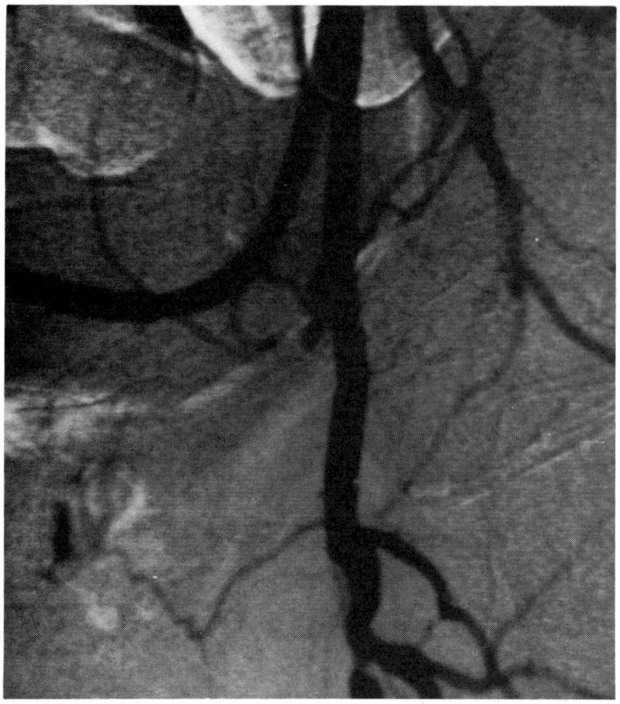

Fig. 22-18. Digital-subtraction angiogram of left inguinal region in patient with patent left-to-right femoral-femoral graft and occluded 5-year-old left femoral-popliteal graft. Note patent profunda femoris artery with branch stenosis and nubbin of graft from common femoral artery.

have been mainly technical [38]. Except for minor alterations, catheterization technique and catheters have changed little. Because of the constant, complex movement of the heart, digital-subtraction imaging has not yet proven practical, although digital imaging per se offers the possibility of more accurate quantification of lesions. The development of x-ray stands with a C-arm or U-arm configuration has allowed routine use of complex angles for imaging the coronary arteries. This development is extremely helpful because of the overlap of vessels that occurs in any single projection, particularly on selective injection of the left main coronary artery. By using multiple views with altered craniocaudal and side-to-side angulation, any given segment can be defined. There has been an accompanying improvement in the generators that produce the x-rays and in the film used to record images, so that improved images are attained with equal or decreased radiation. As with angiography of other parts of the vascular system, percutaneous interventional procedures are becoming increasingly important. It is likely that noninvasive modalities such as ultrasound or MRI will be refined to such a degree that they can largely obviate diagnostic coronary angiography. Therapy using angiographic equipment and technique, however, is likely to increase in importance.

Venography. Almost all the veins in the body can be visualized using one of several imaging radiologic techniques: duplex ultrasound, CT, MRI, or conventional angiography. The lower-extremity venous system is most commonly imaged using duplex ultrasound to evaluate for deep venous thrombosis; this modality can also be used to detect incompetent venous valves and for preoperative venous mapping to evaluate possible venous conduits for arterial bypass procedures. Lower-extremity venography usually is reserved for the evaluation of infrapopliteal venous thrombosis (where duplex ultrasound is less sensitive and when the venous ultrasound examination is unable to visualize proximal veins) and for the evaluation of incompetent perforating veins in patients with varicose veins and the postphlebitic syndrome. The inferior vena cava is best evaluated noninvasively with MRI, but it can be easily visualized with conventional angiographic

Fig. 22-19. Subclavian angiogram in 19-year-old male with stab wound to right shoulder, intact pulses distally, and an expanding supraclavicular hematoma. A pseudoaneurysm is present, with a small focal arterial injury and clear arterial leak. This was repaired by oversewing.

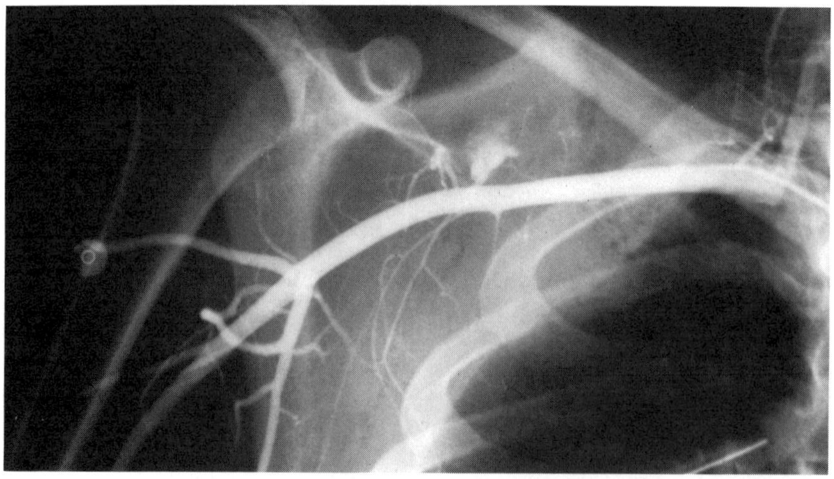

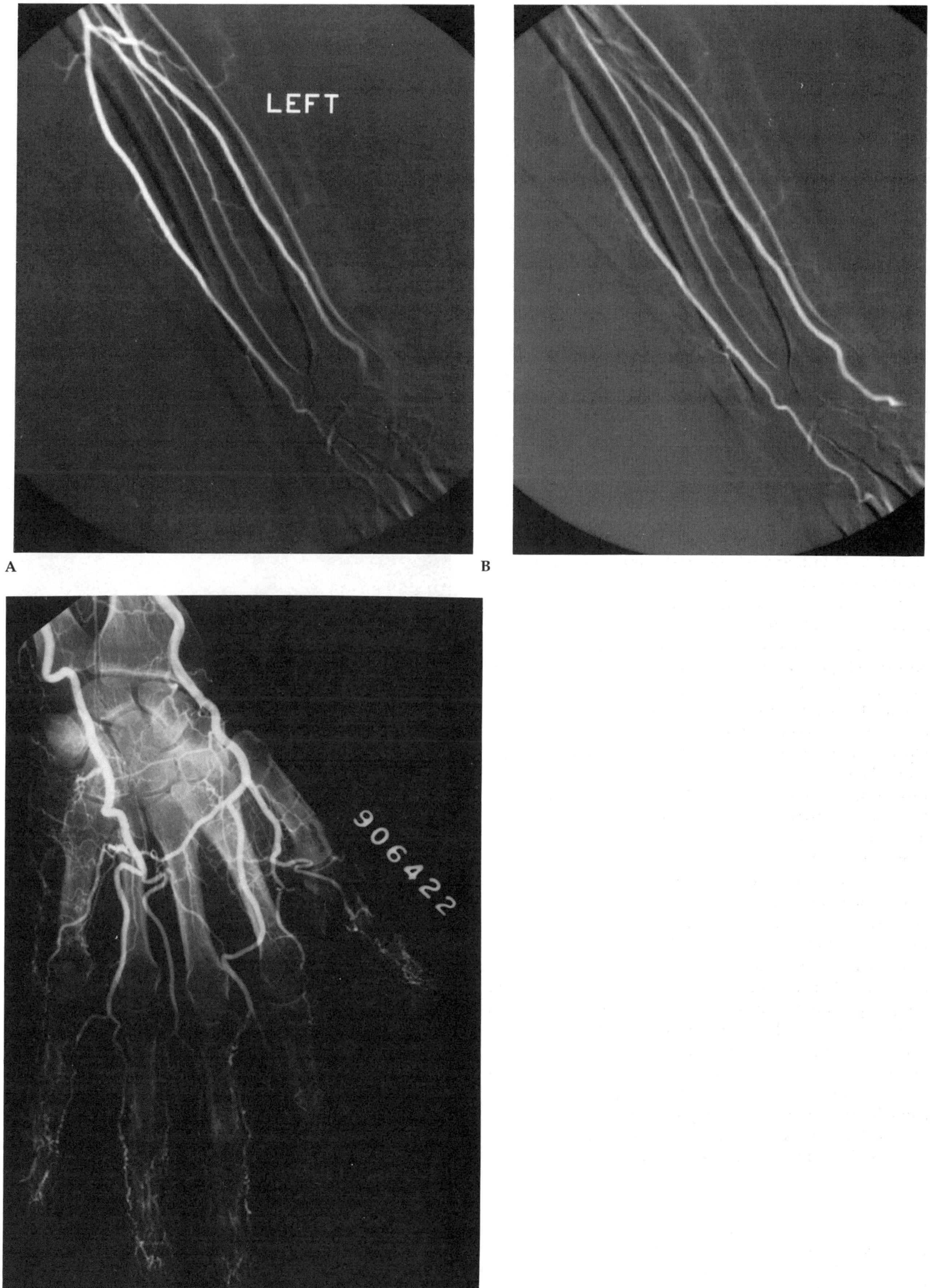

A B C

Fig. 22-20.

techniques utilizing the percutaneous approach, usually via the femoral vein. The most common indication for the latter procedure is prior to deployment of an inferior vena caval filter, to check caval patency and the location of renal veins. The upper-extremity venous system can be evaluated with conventional venography, duplex ultrasound, or MRI. Conventional venography is quick and easy, requiring only an intravenous line in the affected limb for contrast-medium injection, and allows for examination of all the veins draining the upper extremity.

Conventional angiographic evaluation of veins involves similar principles to the angiographic evaluation of arteries. Contrast medium is injected into the particular vein or venous system under study, and serial digital or cut-film radiographs are obtained. Direct venography of veins such as the renal veins requires selective catheterization utilizing a percutaneous-catheter approach. In the case of renal veins, the approach is usually via the common femoral vein. Direct venography of the portal venous system requires either a percutaneous transhepatic approach or a transjugular approach.

Lower-extremity venography is performed using the technique described by Rabinov and Paulin [39]. A pedal vein on the dorsum of the foot is cannulated with a No. 23 or No. 21 butterfly needle, and contrast medium (in a concentration of approximately 43%) is slowly injected under fluoroscopic guidance with the patient tilted in a reverse Trendelenberg position. If there is inadequate opacification of the deep venous system, tourniquets can be applied above the ankle and knee joint. When the deep venous system is adequately opacified, radiographs are obtained, usually in several obliquities below the knee and in a single posteroanterior projection above the knee. Opacification of the iliac and common femoral vein requires laying the table flat, releasing the tourniquets, and proper timing of the radiograph. The diagnostic criterion for venous thrombosis is the demonstration of an intraluminal filling defect outlined by contrast medium. Although nonfilling of particular deep veins may be due to thrombosis, this diagnosis cannot be made with certainty unless the filling defect is demonstrated, since veins occasionally may not fill with contrast medium because of preferential flow patterns (Fig. 22-21).

Venography to demonstrate the existence and locations of incompetent perforating veins in varicose veins and the postphlebitic syndrome requires the application of a tourniquet above the ankle and early radiographs with contrast-medium injection. The incompetent perforating veins are demonstrated by the retrograde flow of contrast medium from the deep veins to the superficial veins. Occasionally, descending venography may be performed to demonstrate incompetent valves. Here, contrast medium is injected into the common femoral vein with the patient in the semi-erect position. If the valves are competent, contrast medium will flow retrogradely from the leg.

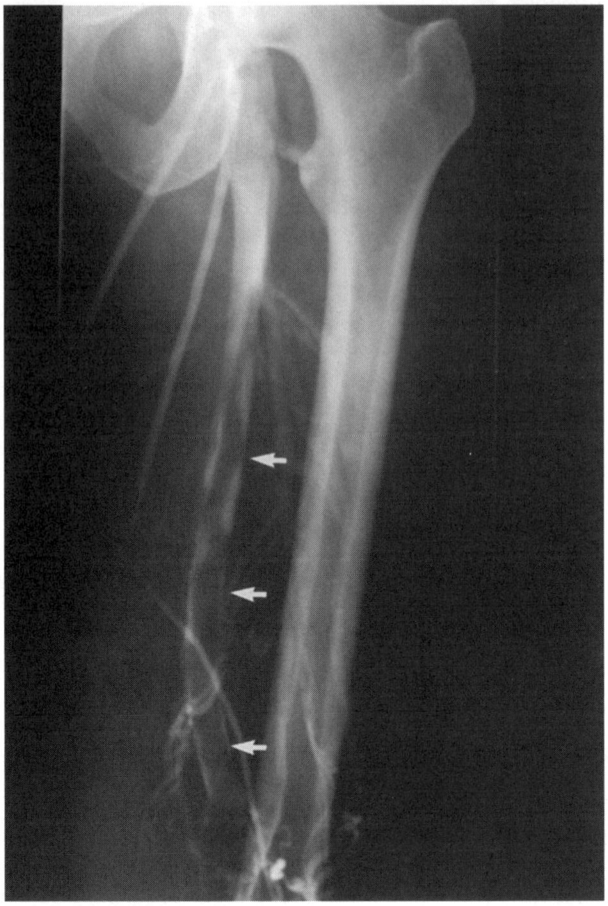

Fig. 22-21. Left-lower-extremity venogram reveals thrombus in superficial femoral vein (arrows).

Pulmonary Angiography. The most common indication for pulmonary angiography is suspected acute pulmonary embolism. Other indications include pulmonary hypertension due to suspected chronic pulmonary hypertension, pulmonary arteriovenous malformations, hemoptysis due to a suspected pulmonary vascular abnormality, and preoperative planning for partial pulmonary resection or lung transplantation.

As with all angiographic procedures, the patient is evaluated by the angiographer prior to the procedure, and informed consent is obtained. Particular notice must be taken of electrocardiographic evidence of left bundle branch block, since that will necessitate having a pacing

Fig. 22-20. A 56-year-old female with Raynaud's syndrome. **A., B.** DSA views of the right forearm show slow filling of radial, ulnar, and interosseous arteries to the wrist and into the hand. **C.** Magnification cut-film angiogram shows occlusion of the distal paired digital arteries of the thumb and index finger and of the medial aspect of the middle finger. This pattern of multiple tapering distal occlusions is typical of vasculitis but otherwise nonspecific.

catheter in the right ventricle (or at least readily at hand for rapid insertion) during the procedure, in case complete heart block should develop from catheter manipulation. If the patient is heparinized, heparin should be discontinued prior to the procedure.

In the angiographic suite, electrocardiographic monitoring is established for the duration of the procedure. Pulmonary angiography is most commonly performed from a transfemoral approach. Before advancing the catheter through the iliac vein or inferior vena cava, it is wise to check the patency of those vessels by hand injections of contrast medium under fluoroscopy. It is important to obtain right-heart pressure measurements through the arteriographic catheter, and in patients with clinical evidence of left ventricular failure, pulmonary capillary wedge pressure recordings with a Swan-Ganz catheter should be obtained. A 7-F pigtail catheter (maximum flow rate 35 ml/second), together with a tip deflector wire, or a pulmonary artery–seeking pigtail catheter is used [40,41]. If a double lumen Swan-Ganz catheter is utilized initially to measure the pulmonary capillary wedge pressure, an exchange wire can be used to place the pigtail catheter in the pulmonary artery. If the transfemoral route is contraindicated, pulmonary arteriography can be performed either through an antecubital vein or by using a transjugular approach. With either approach, a polyethylene pigtail catheter and deflector wire system or a closed-end multiple-sidehole catheter such as an NIH or Eppendorf catheter may be used. The pigtail catheter system is preferred since there is less likelihood of cardiac perforation [42]. Selective left and right pulmonary arteriography are performed using low osmolar contrast medium injected at a rate of 20-25 ml/second for 2 seconds. If there is elevation of the pulmonary artery pressure, lower injection rates should be used.

Difficulties in the diagnosis of pulmonary embolism may arise because of overlapping vessels or overlying pulmonary radiolucencies. Multiple projections with oblique views usually overcome those problems [43–45]. There is no consensus among authors as to which view is the best initial projection for pulmonary angiography. Most emboli tend to lodge in the lower lobes, and the ipsilateral posterior oblique view shows the lower-lobe arteries to best advantage (particularly in patients with lower-lobe atelectasis). To visualize the right main pulmonary artery, the anteroposterior projection is best, while to visualize the left main pulmonary artery, the right posterior oblique projection is best. The radionuclide perfusion lung scan should be used to direct the pulmonary arteriogram. If there are bilateral abnormalities on the lung scan, at least two angiographic views of each lung are essential to exclude pulmonary emboli. If the lung-scan abnormality is unilateral, at least two views of the ipsilateral lung and a single view of the contralateral lung usually are adequate to exclude embolism. In questionable areas, magnification views may be of great help in defining the abnormality and demonstrating the embolus. If overlapping vessels remain a problem, a superselective injection into the involved segment may be useful [46]. Rarely, a balloon-occlusion pulmonary arteriogram may be necessary to define the abnormality with a high degree of certainty. This is performed with a balloon-occlusion catheter such as a Swan-Ganz catheter and a gentle hand injection of 5–10 ml of contrast medium [47].

In the majority of angiographic laboratories, cut film has been the radiographic recording medium of preference for pulmonary angiography and has been widely regarded as the gold standard. Another angiographic approach to pulmonary embolism is the use of biplane cine angiography where it is available [48]. The patient is instructed to continue breathing during the cine angiogram—this leads to scissoring of the vessels with each breath so that during at least some portion of the filming sequence, vascular superimposition is maximized. Scissoring may also aid in ascertaining the nature of radiolucent filling defects, which may be caused by a nonvascular structure such as rib margins and bronchi on end. Cine angiography also helps in defining spurious filling defects caused by streaming of contrast medium in a vessel because of the 30 frames-per-second cine rate. One of the most striking findings on many of the cine studies in patients with emboli is a to-and-fro motion of the clot with each cardiac contraction, which increases the visibility of emboli. On the late phase of the cine run, the pattern of left ventricular contraction can be observed. Recently, with the advent of high-quality digital acquisition of angiographic images using a 1024 $\times$ 1024 matrix and rapid filming (seven frames per second or faster), digital pulmonary angiography is becoming widely used. The latter method has the advantage of rapid image display and the ability to use digital-subtraction techniques, but there has been no formal comparison with cut-film pulmonary angiography.

Pulmonary angiography is an invasive procedure; possible complications include contrast-medium reaction, cardiac perforation, cardiac arrhythmias, cardiac arrest, and death. The mortality rate in patients with pulmonary angiography is reported as 0.2 percent, with deaths occurring in patients with pulmonary hypertension who did not tolerate injection of contrast medium [42]. To avoid this, pulmonary angiography should be performed with caution in patients with a right ventricular end diastolic pressure (RVEDP) of 20 mm Hg or greater. This degree of elevation in the RVEDP indicates a severely compromised right ventricle that probably cannot tolerate any further rise in pulmonary artery pressure. With severe elevation of the RVEDP, the use of low-osmolar contrast medium is essential, and subselective angiography should be considered. Cardiac perforation is usually the result of use of an NIH or Eppendorf catheter; this complication is exceedingly unlikely with the use of a pigtail catheter.

The only truly definitive diagnostic signs of embolism on pulmonary angiography are intraluminal filling defects and abrupt arterial cutoff with the trailing edge of the embolus outlined by contrast medium (Fig. 22-22). The secondary angiographic signs, which are not in themselves diagnostic, are peripheral perfusion defects and increased transit time of contrast medium. Arterial cutoff without the visualized intraluminal tail of the embolus outlined by contrast medium can be caused by conditions other than pulmonary embolism, such as extrinsic compression or tumor invasion.

Although pulmonary angiography has been generally

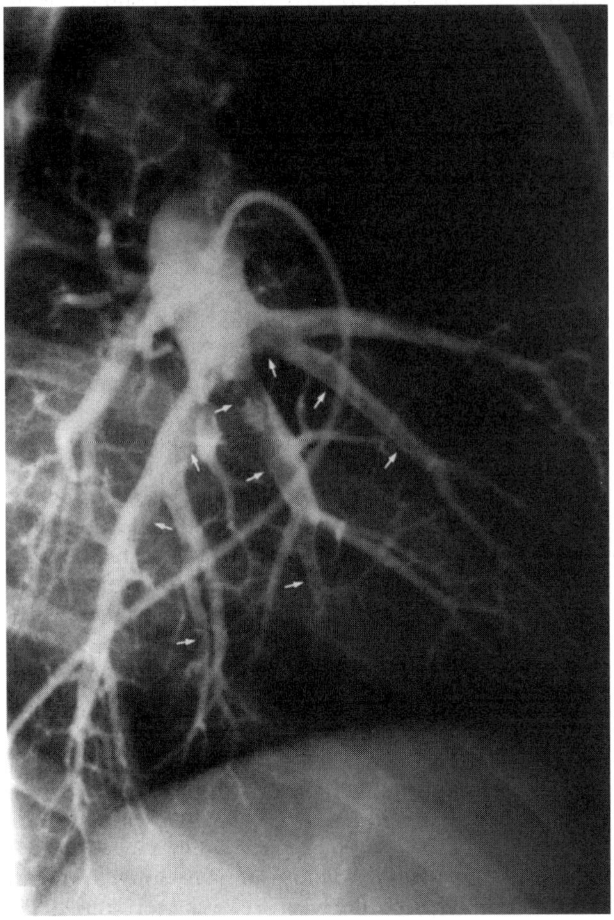

Fig. 22-22. Left pulmonary arteriogram reveals emboli in lingula and lower-lobe branches (arrows).

accepted as the gold standard for the diagnosis of pulmonary embolism, the true diagnostic accuracy of angiography is difficult to define since there is no other test (including postmortem findings) with a higher degree of diagnostic accuracy. Novelline et al. [49] studied the clinical course of patients with suspected pulmonary embolism and a negative pulmonary arteriogram to determine whether there was any clinical significance from emboli that may have been missed on the arteriogram; none of the untreated patients died as a result of thromboembolic disease, and none of the patients suffered recurrent embolism during follow-up. They concluded, therefore, that high-quality pulmonary angiography performed within 24 to 48 hours of the onset of symptoms can effectively rule out clinically significant pulmonary thromboembolism. For that reason, pulmonary angiography remains the gold standard.

Summary

Angiography remains a complex, expanding field. This chapter is intended to give an overview of the field, not be a comprehensive guide to it. Angiography began almost as soon as x-rays were discovered. Coincident with the emergence of other, less invasive imaging modalities, angiography has become increasingly important as a therapeutic subspecialty. It is likely to become even more central to medical practice, particularly in regard to therapy, with continued evolution of equipment. The major areas of advancement over the next decade, as over the last two decades, probably will be in decreased radiation, improved quantitative imaging, and improved therapeutic tools.

References

1. Haschek E, Lindenthal OT. A contribution to the practical use of the photography according to Roentgen. Wien Klin Wochenschr 1896; 9:63.
2. Morton WG, Hammer EW. The x-ray, or, photography of the invisible and its value in surgery. New York: American Technical Book Company, 1896.
3. Sicard JA, Forestier G. Injections intravasculaires d'huile iodée sous controle radiologique. CR Soc Biol (Paris) 1923; 88:1200.
4. Berberich J, Hirsch S. Die roentgenographische Darstellung der Arterien and Venen am Lebenden. München Klin Wochenschr 1923; 49:2226.
5. Brooks B. Intraarterial injection of sodium iodide. JAMA 1924; 82:1016.
6. Moniz E, Diaz A, Lima A. La radioarteriographie et la topographie cranioencephalique. J Radiol Electrol Med Nucl 1928; 12:72.
7. Forssmann W. Ueber Kontrastdarstellung der Hoehlen des levenden rechten Herzens und der Lungenschlagader. Munchen Med Wochenschr 1931; 78:489.
8. dos Santos R, Lamas AC, Peirera-Caldas J. L'arteriographie des membres de l'aorte et de ses branches abdominales. Bull Mem Soc Natl Chir 1929; 55:587.
9. Swick M. Darstellung der Niere and Harnwege in Roentgenbild durch intravenoese Einbingung eines neuen Kontraststoffes, des Uroselectans. Klin Wochenschr 1929; 8:2087.
10. Farinas PL. A new technique for the arteriographic examination of the abdominal aorta and its branches. Am J Roentgen 1941; 46:641.
11. Chamberlain WE. Fluoroscopes and fluoroscopy; Carman lecture. Radiology 1942; 38:383.
12. Coltman JW. Fluoroscopic image brightening by electronic means. Radiology 1948; 51:359.
13. Sturm RE, Morgan RH. Screen intensification systems and their limitations. Am J Roentgen 1949; 62:617.
14. Abrams HL. Introduction and Historical Notes. In HL Abrams, ed. Angiography. Boston: Little, Brown, 1982. Pp. 3–13.
15. Seldinger SI. Catheter replacement of needle in percutaneous arteriography: new technique. Acta Radiol (Stockholm) 1953; 39:368.
16. Grainger RG. Intravascular contrast media—the past, the present and the future. Brit J Radiol 1982; 55:1–15.
17. Harrington DP, et al. Compound angulation for the angiographic evaluation of renal artery stenosis. Radiology 1983; 146:829–831.
18. Levin DC, et al. Digital subtraction angiography: principles and pitfalls of improvement techniques. Am J Roentgen 1984; 143:447–454.
19. Powe NR, et al. Contrast medium-induced adverse reactions: economic outcome. Radiology 1988; 169:163–168.
20. Regan K, et al. Double-blind study of a new nonionic contrast agent for cardiac angiography. Radiology 1988; 167:409–413.
21. Bettmann MA. Guidelines for the use of low osmolality contrast agents. Radiology 1989; 172:901–903.
22. Feldman RL, et al. Contrast media-related complications during cardiac catheterization using Hexabrix or Renografin in high-risk patients. Am J Cardiol 1988; 61:1334–1337.

23. Smith DC, et al. Three new low-osmolality contrast agents: a comparative study of patient discomfort. Am J Neuroradiol 1988; 9:1376.
24. Lind LJ, Mushlin PS. Sedation, analgesia and anasthesia for radiologic procedures. Cardiovasc Intervent Radiol 1987; 10:247–253.
25. Kido DP, et al. Thrombogenicity of heparin and non-heparin-coated catheters: clinical trial. Am J Neuroradiol 1982; 3:535–539.
26. Hessel SJ, Adams DF, Abrams HL. Complications of angiography. Radiology 1981; 138:273–281.
27. Sones FM Jr, Shirey EK. Cine coronary arteriography. Mod Concepts Cardiovasc Dis 1962; 31:732–738.
28. Rose SC, Moore EE. Emergency trauma angiography: accuracy, safety and pitfalls. Am J Roentgenol 1987; 165:643–649.
29. Guthaner DF. Cardiovascular magnetic resonance imaging—state of the art 1988: summary of a symposium. Cardiovasc Intervent Radiol 1989; 12:213–225.
30. McCort JJ. President's address: caring for the major trauma victim: role for radiology. Radiology 1987; 163:1–12.
31. Formanek G, Frech RS, Amplatz K. Arterial thrombus formation during clinical percutaneous catheterization. Circulation 1970; 41:833–839.
32. Siegelman SS, Caplan LH, Annes GP. Complications of catheter angiography: Study with oscillometry and "pullout" angiograms. Radiology 1968; 91:251–253.
33. Collins PS, McDonald PT, Lim RC. Popliteal artery entrapment: an evolving syndrome. J Vasc Surg 1989; 10:484–489.
34. Davis K, et al. Complications of coronary arteriography from the collaborative study of coronary artery surgery (CASS). Circulation 1979; 59:1105–1112.
35. Brenner J, Couch NP. Peripheral arterial complications of left heart catheterization and their management. Am J Surg 1973; 125:521–526.
36. Martin LG, Cork RD. Renal vein renin analysis in patients treated with renal angioplasty (Abstr). Radiology 1989; 173(p):74.
37. Aurigemma GP, et al. Noninvasive determination of coronary artery bypass graft patency by cine magnetic resonance imaging. Circulation 1989; 80:1595–1602.
38. Levin DC, Dunham LR, Stueve R. Causes of cine image quality deterioration in cardiac catheterization laboratories. Am J Cardiol 1983; 52:881–886.
39. Rabinov K, Paulin S. Roentgen diagnosis of venous thrombosis in the leg. Arch Surg 1972; 104:134–144.
40. Courey WR, deVillasante JM, Waltman AC. A quick, simple method of percutaneous transfemoral pulmonary arteriography. Radiology 1974; 113:475–477.
41. Grooman JH, Renner JW. Transfemoral pulmonary angiography: update on technique. AJR 1981; 136:624–626.
42. Mills SR, et al. The incidence, etiologies, and avoidance of complications of pulmonary angiography in a large series. Radiology 1980; 136:295–299.
43. Johnson BA, James AE Jr, White RI Jr. Oblique and selective pulmonary angiography in the diagnosis of pulmonary embolism. AJR 1973; 118:801–808.
44. Gomes AS, Grollman JH Jr, Mink J. Pulmonary angiography for pulmonary emboli: rational selection of oblique views. AJR 1977; 129:1019–1025.
45. Bossart PJ, et al. Pulmonary angiography: the importance of multiple projections. Cardiovasc Intervent Radiol 1982; 5:105–107.
46. Bookstein JJ. Segmental pulmonary arteriography in pulmonary embolism. Radiology 1969; 93:1007–1012.
47. Wilson JE, Bynum LJ. An improved pulmonary angiographic technique using a balloon-tipped catheter. Am Rev Respir Dis 1976; 114:1137–1144.
48. Meyerovitz MF, et al. Evaluation of optimized biplane cine pulmonary angiography. Invest Rad 1985; 20:945–949.
49. Novelline RA, et al. The clinical course of patients with suspected pulmonary embolism and a negative pulmonary arteriogram. Radiology 1978; 126:561–567.

Computed Tomography in Vascular Disorders

Sabah S. Tumeh
Steven E. Seltzer
Ay-Ming Wang

Computed tomography (CT) first captured the scientific limelight in 1979, when the Nobel Prize in medicine was awarded to Godfrey Hounsfield and Alan Cormack for their contributions toward the development of the imaging device [1,2]. Considering the progress that has been made with CT, it is astonishing to realize that this tool has been in existence for only little more than a decade. In the past 15 years, the exposure time required to produce a CT image has dropped by a factor of 5,000. Whereas 4 to 5 minutes were necessary in the early days, some ultrafast scanners currently make images with exposures as short as 50 milliseconds. Advances in x-ray hardware, computer software, and display technology have permitted CT scanning to play a prominent role in the diagnosis of vascular disorders.

This chapter is divided into three sections. The first section reviews the mechanical principles of CT scanners. The intent is to inform the practitioner about the strengths, weaknesses, and limitations of the device. The second section explores the role of this new technology and illustrates its usefulness in the diagnosis of extracranial vascular disease. The third section examines the CT appearance of the normal anatomy and pathology of intracranial vessels. Abnormalities of arteries and veins and the sequelae of abnormal brain perfusion are presented. It is hoped that this chapter will give the practitioner an understanding of how CT scanners work, a sense of their role in vascular medicine, and a familiarity with the appearance of vascular disorders on CT images.

Principles of CT Scanner Operation

FORMATION OF THE CT IMAGE

CT images are produced in three basic steps [3,4]. First, multiple x-ray exposures or images of an object are produced. Second, the image is reconstructed with the aid of a computer. Third, the image is displayed in various shades of gray.

Step 1: Multiple X-Ray Exposures. At least five different approaches to the task of obtaining multiple x-ray exposures have been used by CT scanner manufacturers. Each approach uses a new generation of scanner design (Fig. 23-1). Scanners of the **first generation** employ one x-ray tube with a tightly collimated, pencil-shaped CT beam and one x-ray detector. The tube and the detector move across the patient in a coordinated motion (termed a translation) and then rotate 1 degree on their axes and repeat the process (translate-rotate geometry). After 365 degrees of rotation, a full, cross-sectional set of exposures has been made. Exposure times as long as 4 to 5 minutes are required to obtain one complete data set. First-generation scanners were used almost exclusively for brain imaging.

Second-generation scanners replace the pencil-shaped x-ray beam and the single x-ray detector of the original devices with a fan-shaped beam and a bank that contains as many as 30 x-ray detectors. The tube and the detectors still move in a translate-rotate fashion, but by rotating through a greater arc (up to 30 degrees), they have shortened imaging times to between 10 and 90 seconds. These second-generation scanners were the first to perform extracranial, nonneurologic CT imaging.

Third-generation scanners employ a much wider, fan-shaped x-ray beam and an arc of up to 700 detectors. The x-ray tube and the detector array rotate opposite each other through a complete 360-degree motion (rotate-rotate geometry). There are no translational movements. Scan times can be as short as a single second.

In **fourth-generation** scanners, a ring of x-ray detectors completely surrounds the patient. Only the x-ray tube moves, exposing the stationary detectors that fall in the path of the fan-shaped beam (rotate-stationary geometry). Exposure times with this type of scanner are again as short as 1 second.

Third- and fourth-generation scanners are considered state-of-the-art instruments, and thousands are in clinical use today. They have the ability to image all parts of the body, although images of moving structures (such as the heart) are still degraded somewhat by artifacts.

RECENT ADVANCES. An important technological breakthrough that has made enormous contributions to vascular imaging has been the development of **spiral** or helical CT imaging systems. Both third- and fourth-generation scanners are capable of spiral CT. Prior to 1990, the x-ray tube and the detectors of all CT systems were connected to their gantry by electrical cables. The wires conducted power from the generator to the tube and data from the detectors to the host computer. Because of the presence of the cables, the tube-detector array could rotate only about 360 degrees in one direction before it would have to stop and reverse, to avoid winding the cable into a knot. After 1990, it became possible on commercially available systems to replace the cables with electro-optical slip rings. These products of the fiberoptic revolution allowed the tube-detector complex to rotate continuously in the same direction, obviating the need to stop and rewind. This breakthrough permitted the execution of prolonged, continuous x-ray exposures coupled with movement of the patient couch. The geometry of the resulting exposure is a spiral. From the spiral CT exposure is collected a volumetric dataset that spans the region of interest in the body. From that dataset, slices are reconstructed at arbitrary table positions.

The advent of spiral CT led to several critical advances in CT angiographic techniques. First, the ability to cover

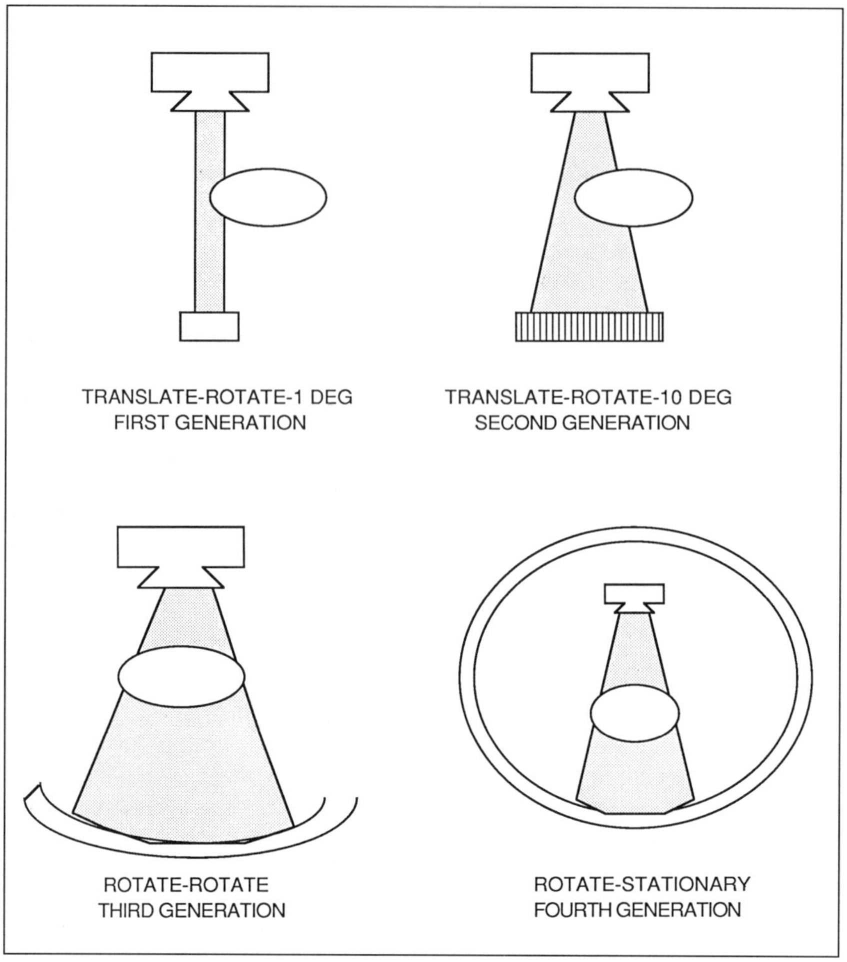

Fig. 23-1. Four generations of CT scanners. In each drawing, the CT apparatus is represented in schematic form, viewed from the foot of the patient couch. The patient is represented as an oval in the center. The course of the radiation beam is represented by the shaded area.

the entire region of interest (say, the abdominal aorta from the diaphragm to the iliac bifurcation) in one 30- to 40-second exposure allowed all the CT scan data to be collected during the first pass of an intravenously administered bolus of contrast agent through the arterial tree. That allows imaging at the time of peak arterial opacification. Second, the ability to reconstruct large numbers of finely spaced slices from one CT scan exposure allowed the production of high-quality three-dimensional reconstructions of the arteries of interest. The resulting three-dimensional angiograms have found widespread clinical applications in virtually all large vascular beds [5].

Despite the tremendous advances allowed by spiral CT, even the most modern systems are not capable of the extremely short exposure times required to produce stop-action views of the heart and vascular structures. Because of those limitations, efforts to develop a CT unit with an ultrafast exposure have centered on redesigning the basic apparatus. In 1983, Boyd and Lipton introduced a scanner capable of producing images in 50 milliseconds [6]. In this so-called **fifth-generation** scanner, the x-ray tube itself has been redesigned and actually takes the form of a circle that surrounds the patient. As indicated in Fig. 23-2, a beam of electrons is aimed at target rings composed of tungsten. Collimated x-rays produced by this bombardment are collected by a ring of detectors that also surround the patient. There are no moving mechanical parts. Magnets sweep the electron beam around the exposure circle. A tube designed in this way is able to store large amounts of heat, permitting exposures with reasonable photon statistics to be made in a short period of time. These so-called **electron-beam** or ultrafast CT systems have made clinical contributions to the diagnosis of both vascular and cardiac disorders [7,8].

Step 2: Computer-Aided Reconstruction. Sensitive x-ray detectors measure the flux of x-ray photons during the CT exposure. Aided by a powerful array processor, a computer solves millions of simultaneous equations to calculate the linear x-ray attenuation coefficient of the tissue exposed to the CT beam. First tabulating the flow of x-rays through the patient from every point around the circle, the computer uses mathematic algorithms (such as filtered-back projection) to reconstruct a cross-sectional im-

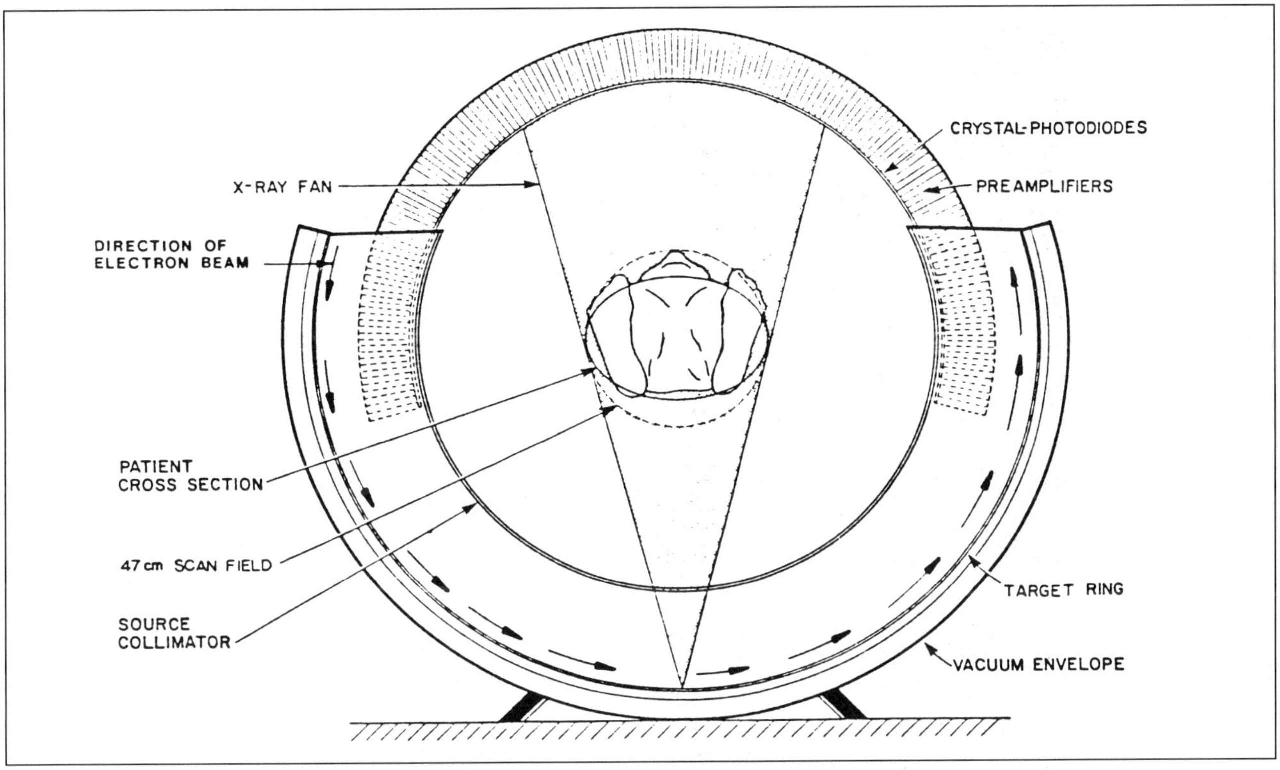

Fig. 23-2. Fifth-generation cine-CT scanner. (Courtesy of Imatron, Inc., South San Francisco, Calif.)

age of the patient and store it in the computer memory. The mathematic principles of such reconstructions have been known for decades, but because they require making millions of calculations in seconds, this kind of image was impractical before the advent of modern computer equipment.

RECENT ADVANCES. Improvements in computer hardware and software and dramatic advances in the capabilities of array processors have shortened image-reconstruction times to the point where CT examinations can be monitored virtually as they take place. Usually, each image is reconstructed and viewed before the next is obtained. New algorithms have been written so that images emphasizing edge enhancement, high degrees of spatial resolution, or low noise can be created from the same set of scanning data.

Advances in information-storage technology have opened up new ways to store and retrieve the tremendous amount of data associated with CT images. An image reconstructed on a 512×512 format requires 2^{18} (262,144) pieces of information. Sophisticated recording media will permit easier access to and longer, safer storage of CT images. For vascular imaging, it is vital to have enough computer memory and storage to acquire a large number of detailed images rapidly.

Step 3: Image Display. After the CT computer calculates the linear x-ray attenuation coefficient for each portion of the CT image, the coefficients are translated onto a scale that is easier to understand and interpret. Generally, the coefficients are normalized to a reference material (water) and magnified to a whole number. These numbers, known as CT values, generally range from −1,000 Hounsfield units (HU) for air, to 0 HU for water, up to over 1,000 HU for dense bone.

The CT values that the image comprises are then translated into shades of gray for display on a television monitor and subsequent recording onto conventional x-ray film. From the broad range of CT numbers in the image, a narrow segment is selected to be displayed in shades of gray, while the numbers above and below that range are shown as all white or all black, respectively. The CT value selected to be at the center of the displayed gray scale and the width of the range of CT values displayed as shades of gray can be manipulated by the viewer.

By appropriately manipulating the center and the width of the gray scale, small density differences between objects often can be discerned. It is possible to determine and display with great precision the actual CT values from an area of interest in an image. For example, the change in the CT values before and after the administration of contrast material can demonstrate blood flow parameters and be an important indicator of the perfusion of a tissue.

RECENT ADVANCES. Modern CT scanners have 256 levels of gray for image display. The revolution in mini- and microcomputers has allowed the development of low-cost, independent, operator-controlled workstations that interface directly with the CT computer and do not interfere with scanning. These increasingly powerful review consoles permit the diagnostician to evaluate images, edit

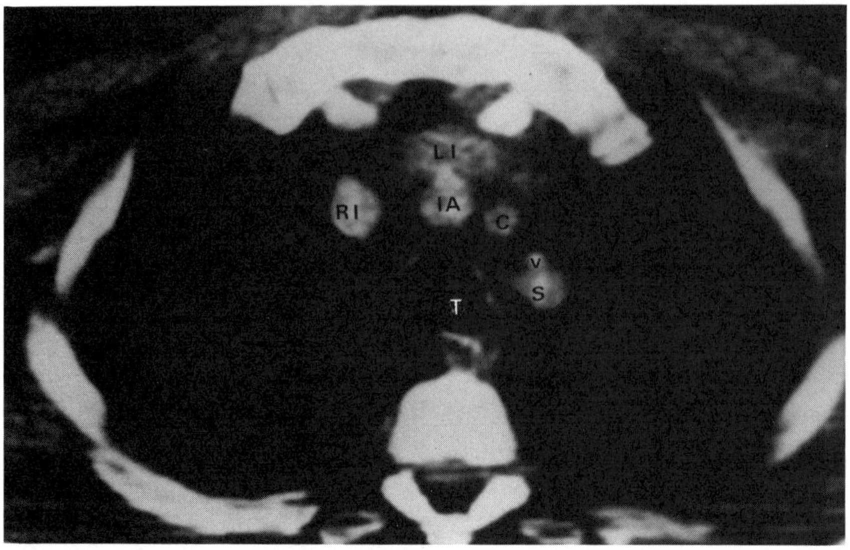

A

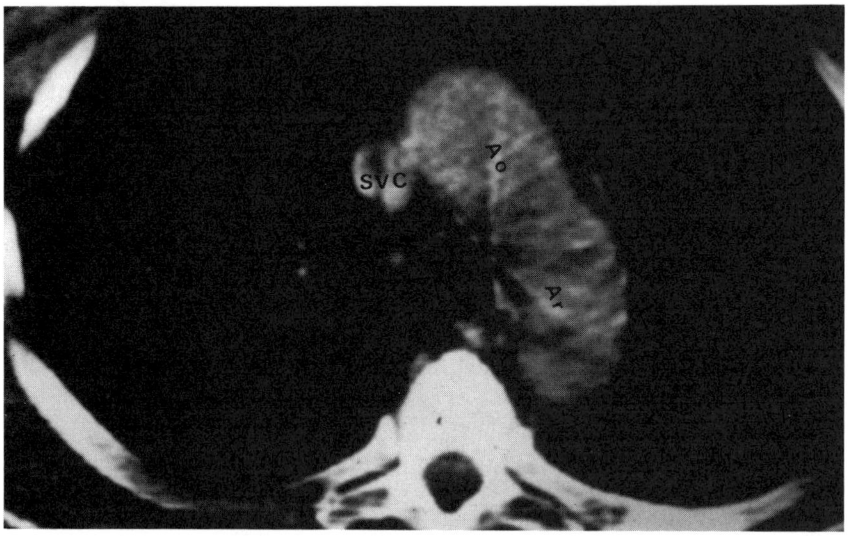

B

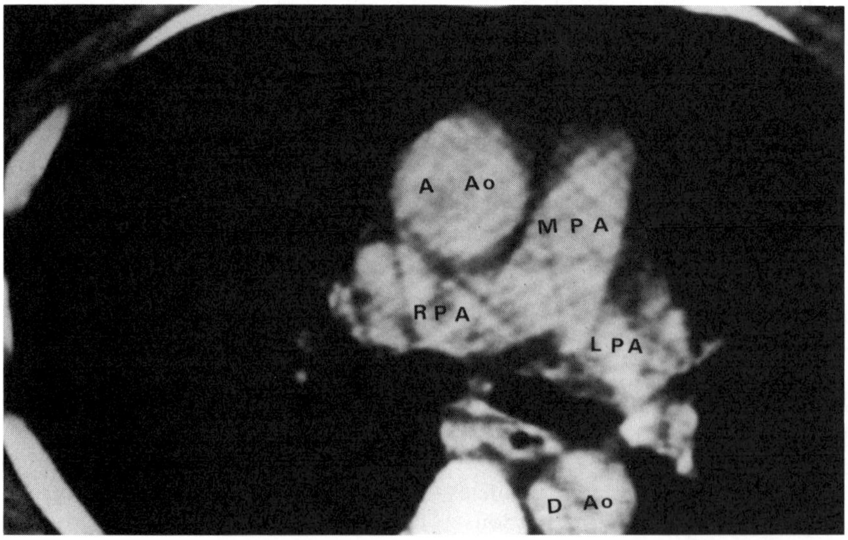

C

them, and create three-dimensional and other advanced displays to highlight characteristics of a particular tissue.

Advances also have been made in recording media. Previously, most CT images viewed by the radiologist were made by photographing the face of a cathode-ray tube. This analogue process suffered from distortion and a loss of the digital nature of the CT information. Now, laser printers similar to those used with word processors are more widely available for use with CT. These devices take digital information directly from the CT computer's memory and translate the stored values into film density. The CT values determine the laser's intensity as it blackens the film. Laser-produced images are very sharp, and they convey the digital CT data with great fidelity.

Tremendous advances in image processing have produced tools useful for the rendering and display of CT angiographic images. The three-dimensional images produced from spiral CT datasets can be portrayed either as shaded-surface displays, which highlight vessel surfaces and contours, or as maximum-intensity projection displays, which portray vessels as bright, translucent structures [9]. Either type of display can be viewed from any angle or rotated in space to allow the viewer to extract as much information as possible about the vascular anatomy.

Characteristics of CT Scanning in Diagnosis of Vascular Disorders

IMAGE CHARACTERISTICS

CT images have some special characteristics that make them particularly valuable in the diagnosis of vascular disorders. Because they are cross-sectional in nature, they can show blood vessels and other tissues without the confusion from overlapping structures that often limits conventional radiographs. CT images combine excellent contrast resolution with good spatial resolution. They depict soft tissues with far better clarity than do conventional radiographs. The quantitative nature of both the image and the display is valuable in measuring precisely the x-ray densities of various tissues and the density changes produced by contrast media.

CONTRAST ENHANCEMENT

Intravenous contrast agents are commonly used in the evaluation of vascular structures by CT. These iodinated agents are the same ones used in conventional radiography (for urography and angiography). They are often administered as a compact intravenous bolus, after which multiple scans are obtained to document the transit of contrast through a vessel or a tissue. The lumina of vessels can actually be seen, and regions of flowing blood can be differentiated from thrombus-filled areas.

It is also possible to use xenon gas as a contrast agent for cerebrovascular perfusion measurements. While patients inhale nonanesthetic amounts of xenon, CT scans are performed rapidly. Analysis of time-density curves from various regions of the brain give quantitative information about local blood flow.

DYNAMIC (RAPID) SCANNING

As described previously, conventional CT scanners have exposure duration times as short as 1 second and interscan delay times as short as 3 seconds. In the spiral scanning mode, continuous data acquisition for up to 40 to 50 seconds is now possible. The more experimental electron-beam scanners have exposure times as short as 50 milliseconds and virtually no interscan delay. The ability to perform dynamic (rapid) scans with short interscan delay permits measurement of the transit of contrast-laden blood through vessels and assessment of relative tissue perfusion. These scanners are able to take virtual stop-action views of the heart in various portions of the cardiac cycle to assess regional wall motion.

WEAKNESSES OF CT SCANNING

The weaknesses of CT for the diagnosis of vascular disorders derive largely from the physical limitation of the technique. Although CT's spatial resolution is good, it does not match that of conventional radiographs. Vessels smaller than 2 mm in diameter are unlikely to be visible on CT scans. Cross-sectional display has advantages for showing soft-tissue structures, but it cannot easily be used to trace long, tubular structures like blood vessels through their entire course. The availability of three-dimensional reconstructions have largely overcome this problem. Although exposure times and interscan delay times have shortened dramatically, images from most scanners are degraded by motion artifact when a moving object like the heart is in the field.

In addition, CT angiography requires the use of iodinated contrast agents, with their attendant risks and complications. Recent developments in magnetic resonance angiography, which requires no contrast agents, have made that technique exciting for a variety of clinical vascular imaging applications, especially in the brain. Magnetic resonance angiography and vascular ultrasound should be considered the noninvasive vascular imaging proce-

Fig. 23-3. Normal anatomy of thoracic vessels. **A.** CT section above the level of the aortic arch demonstrating the following vessels: RI = right innominate vein; LI = left innominate vein; IA = innominate artery; C = left common carotid; V = left vertebral artery; S = left subclavian artery; T = trachea. Notice that the left innominate vein crosses behind the manubrium, anterior to the major arteries, to join the right innominate vein. **B.** CT scan at the level of the aortic arch demonstrates the arch (Ao Ar) and superior vena cava (SVC). **C.** CT scan below the level of the aortic arch, at the level of the pulmonary arteries. A Ao = ascending aorta; D Ao = descending aorta; MPA = main pulmonary artery; RPA = right pulmonary artery; LPA = left pulmonary artery.

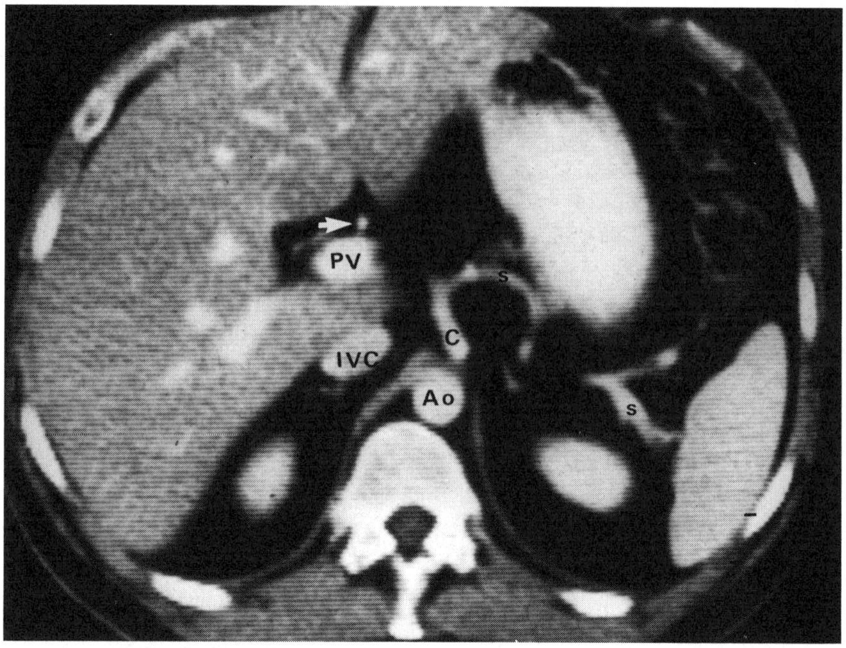

A

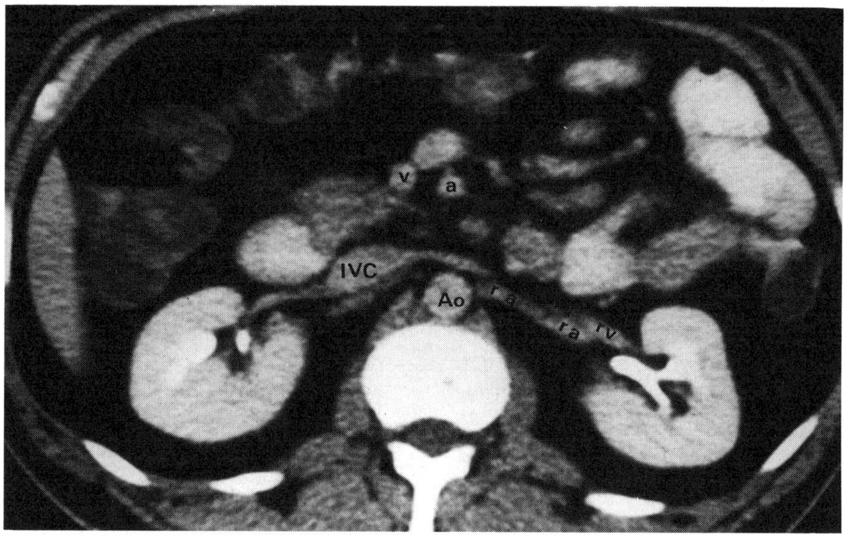

B

Fig. 23-4. Normal anatomy of abdominal vessels. **A**. Ao = aorta; IVC = inferior vena cava; C = celiac axis; S = splenic artery; PV = portal vein. **B**. CT scan at the level of the renal vessels. Ao = aorta; a = superior mesenteric artery; IVC = inferior vena cava; ra = renal artery; rv = renal vein; v = superior mesenteric vein.

dures of choice in patients with contraindications to iodinated contrast agents.

Dosimetry: Complications and Precautions

The radiation dose from a CT scan slice varies with different scanners, but it averages 3 rems to the skin surface [10,11]. Because the tightly collimated CT beam gives off only a small amount of scattered radiation, there is little additive dose from performing sequential, contiguous slices through an area of interest. If scans through the same anatomic area are repeated, however, the dose from the second examination is added to that of the first.

The radiation dose from CT is from 20 to 50 times greater than that of low-dose examinations such as conventional chest radiographs but is on a par with that of urography or contrast studies of the gastrointestinal tract.

Complications of intravenous contrast use are well known to most physicians [12]. Major reactions include anaphylaxis and respiratory or cardiac compromise; minor ones include skin rashes and urticaria. Nausea and vomiting are common but are not thought to be allergic in nature. Contrast agents are also known to be implicated in acute renal failure, which is often a risk in patients with vascular disorders or diabetes mellitus. The dose of

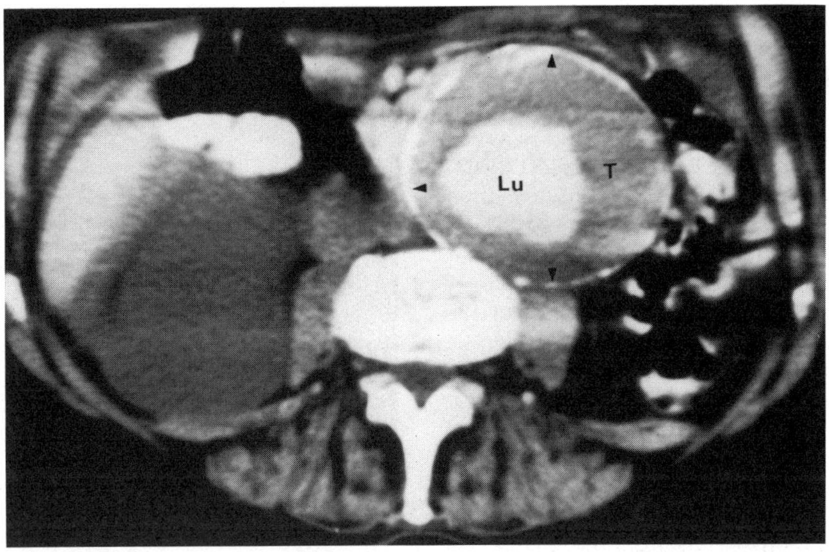

Fig. 23-5. Atherosclerotic aneurysm of the abdominal aorta. CT scan of the lower abdomen reveals a large atherosclerotic aneurysm of the abdominal aorta. Notice the thin circumferential calcifications in the wall (arrowheads). There is a large thrombus (T) completely surrounding the patent lumen (Lu), which is enhanced by intravenous contrast medium.

contrast agent employed is often up to 29 g of iodine, a value similar to that used in urography and less than that used in detailed angiographic examinations. Hence, it is important in patients who are scheduled for CT examinations to document a history of prior allergic reactions to contrast materials or other drugs. Similarly, it is important to know about the patient's renal function and the presence of medical conditions (such as diabetes or dehydration) that might increase the risk of contrast-induced renal failure. Female patients should be asked whether they might be pregnant. With spiral CT, the amount of intravenous contrast medium used could be reduced substantially, almost by 50 percent, without compromising the quality of the examination [13].

Clinical Use of CT in Diagnosis of Extracranial Vascular Disorders

CT has revolutionized noninvasive imaging of the aorta and the venae cavae and their major branches and tributaries, as well as of the main pulmonary arteries and veins. Direct visualization by CT of normal and pathologic conditions of those structures in the head, neck, chest, and abdomen is now routine clinical practice.

THE AORTA AND GREAT ARTERIES

Normal Appearance. Because of the transaxial nature of CT, most large vessels appear as circular soft-tissue densities, with the exception of the aortic arch, which runs transaxially in the chest and therefore appears tubular. The left subclavian, left common carotid, and innominate arteries are visualized as three circular densities at a level above the aortic arch. The descending thoracic and abdominal aorta each appear as a circular soft-tissue density lying in front of the vertebral column (Fig. 23-3). The caliber of the abdominal aorta decreases as it approaches the bifurcation at about the level of L4. The major branches that can be depicted by CT are the celiac axis and its main branches, the superior mesenteric artery, and the renal and iliac arteries (Fig. 23-4). The inferior mesenteric artery can be seen in some cases.

If the wall of the aorta is not calcified, it cannot be differentiated from nonenhanced intraluminal blood, which measures about 50 to 70 HU. If the density of intraluminal blood is low, as in anemia, or high, as with contrast enhancement, then differentiation of the aortic wall is possible.

Congenital Anomalies. CT with contrast enhancement is reasonably accurate in the evaluation of congenital anomalies of the great vessels in adults. Most of these patients are asymptomatic, and CT is usually done either to confirm chest radiographic findings or to investigate more subtle conditions such as bronchiectasis or small tumors. CT should be confined to cases such as these and not be used to investigate complicated problems, particularly those associated with congenital heart disease. Disorders that have been studied with CT include aberrant subclavian arteries, right-sided aortic arch, double aortic arch, and coarctation of the aorta.

In the presence of aberrant right subclavian artery—a commonly studied anomaly—CT shows a higher than normal aortic arch that has an anteroposterior orientation [14]. The aberrant vessel arises from the most posterior part of the aortic arch or descending aorta. The origin of that artery may be dilated and, in severe cases, is called a diverticulum, which may be confused with an aortic aneurysm if it is not recognized [9].

An aberrant subclavian artery is less common on the left than on the right. Ten percent of these patients have congenital heart disease. The CT findings are similar to those of aberrant right subclavian artery.

In aortic arch anomalies (coarctation, double- and right-sided arch), CT findings have been described in a few cases of each condition [14–16]. In those cases, CT has shown the congenital lesions accurately.

Atherosclerotic Disease and Its Complications. Atherosclerotic changes are readily depicted by CT and include tortuosity, mural calcifications, dilatation, and aneurysm formation (Fig. 23-5).

The normal aorta is seen anterior and slightly to the left of the vertebrae. A tortuous, atherosclerotic aorta deviates from that course and may be seen to the right of the vertebral column. The true aortic wall in atherosclerotic disease is thin and consists almost entirely of avascular connective tissue; the wall may also have some calcifications [17], which are responsible for the thin peripheral curvilinear calcifications seen on CT. Mural calcifications may be very dense, however. Atherosclerotic calcification may be seen in the lumen of the aorta as well [18]. These central calcifications should alert the examiner to the possibility of aortic dissection or leaking [18], although calcifications in an intraluminal thrombus or atheroma may have a similar appearance.

Aortic Aneurysm. Atherosclerosis is the most common cause of aortic aneurysm in the United States. Other causes are dissecting hematoma, infection, and inflammatory conditions. Most aortic aneurysms are fusiform. Abdominal aortic aneurysms commonly arise below the renal arteries and extend to involve the iliac arteries. CT is able both to diagnose and to size these lesions accurately [19]. The largest diameter of an aneurysm can be precisely measured, the length determined from serial scans, and the relationship to major branches such as the renal arteries accurately demonstrated. If contrast enhancement is used, intraluminal atheromatous plaques or thrombi can be readily seen as low-attenuation areas adjacent to the wall (see Fig. 23-5). Up to 100 percent of all intraluminal thrombi are visible on CT [20] and are most commonly seen as a complex ring surrounding the aortic lumen [20] (see Fig. 23-5). They may have lenticular shapes, however.

Rupture is the most serious complication of an abdominal aortic aneurysm. If the triad of pain, pulsating abdominal mass, and hypotension is noted, the diagnosis is made clinically [21], and emergency surgery should be performed without any imaging interventions. However, the CT findings of a leaking aneurysm include the aneurysm itself, a high-density fluid collection (fresh blood) in the retroperitoneum displacing the kidneys, and an indistinct margin of the aorta [22] (Fig. 23-6). Rarely, an abdominal aortic aneurysm may rupture into the vena cava (aortocaval fistula). The acute form is characterized by severe low-back pain, abdominal mass, a murmur, and signs and symptoms of venous hypertension in the pelvis and lower extremities [23]. In addition to showing the aneurysm and the blood around the aorta, CT may also show the actual communication [24], which most commonly involves the right posterolateral wall of the aorta and the distal inferior vena cava.

Dissecting Hematoma. Aortic dissection is due to a tear in the vessel wall and an ensuing flow of blood between its inner third and outer two-thirds. The newly created channel is called the **false channel** or **lumen**. Factors predisposing to aortic dissection include weakness of the media (as in Marfan syndrome), cystic medial necrosis, Ehlers-Danlos syndrome, or, less frequently, atherosclerosis or syphilis.

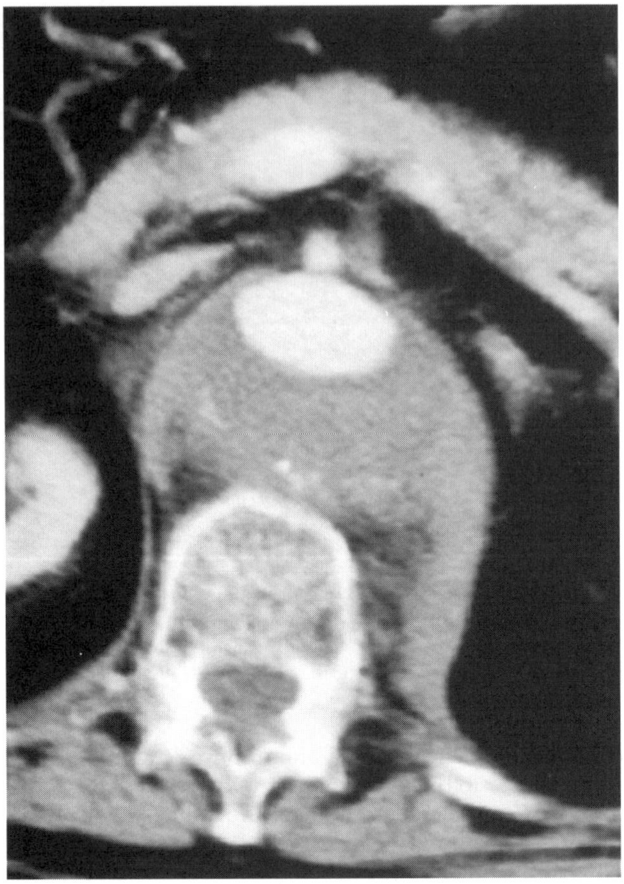

Fig. 23-6. Ruptured aortic aneurysm. CT image with contrast enhancement shows a large aortic aneurysm. The lumen is opacified. The posterior wall of the aneurysm is just anterior to the vertebra (notice the calcifications). The high-density material dissecting behind the left diaphragmatic crus represent acute leak.

CT is very accurate in making the diagnosis of aortic dissection (Fig. 23-7), showing its extent with a sensitivity and a specificity of 88.5 and 100 percent, respectively [25]. Without intravenous contrast enhancement, a CT scan may show enlarged aortic diameter (greater than 5 cm in most cases), centrally displaced intimal calcifications, and a difference in density between the two lumina. These findings are not specific, however, and may represent other entities, such as an atherosclerotic aneurysm with a calcified intraluminal thrombus. Diagnosis can be made with greater confidence when contrast enhancement is used. The most reliable clue is the demonstration of two channels that, because of the slower flow in the false lumen, opacify at different rates [25]. The demonstration

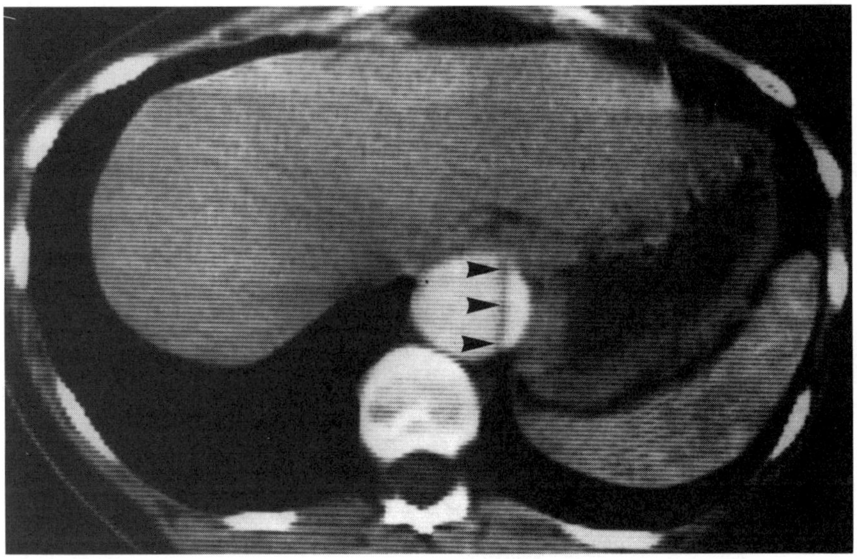

Fig. 23-7. Aortic dissection. A CT scan of the upper abdomen shows dissection of the descending aorta. Notice the intimal flap that runs in an anteroposterior direction (arrowheads).

of an intimal flap also is a very reliable diagnostic sign [26]. Care should be exercised if streak artifacts are present on the image because they may mimic the flap [27].

Apart from acute dissection, CT also has proved useful in the follow-up of patients with chronic dissection and after surgery. The majority of patients with chronic dissection are treated medically, and CT can be used to confirm the diagnosis, determine extent, and look for complications (rupture, extension, and pseudoaneurysm formation). Following surgical treatment, there is a high incidence of persistent patency of the false lumen [28,29] (Fig. 23-8). Prosthetic implants that are inserted at the site of the proximal tear also may be detected on nonenhanced CT scans. Dacron implants have a higher density than nonopacified blood and surrounding soft tissues (130–149 HU) [30] (see Fig. 23-8). These prostheses can be seen in

Fig. 23-8. Postoperative appearance of aortic dissection. CT scan of the chest at the level of the pulmonary artery shows a Dacron implant in the ascending aorta (large arrowhead). These implants usually have higher density than surrounding tissue and appear opaque. Notice the persistence of the intimal flap (small arrowheads) and the false lumen in the descending aorta.

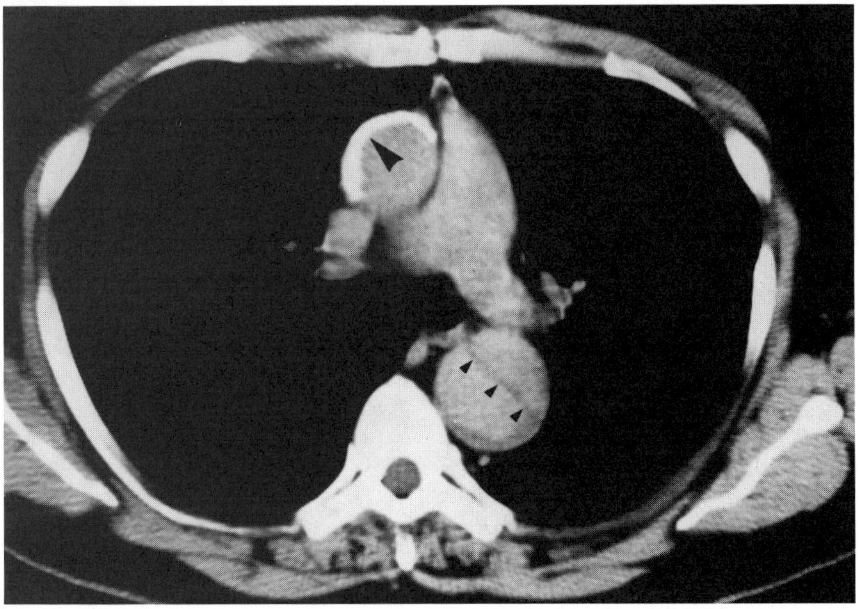

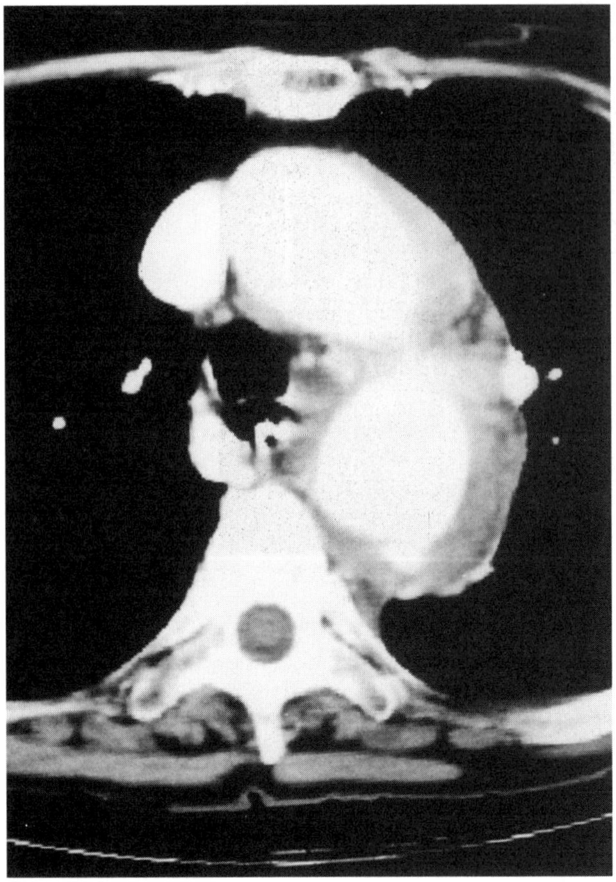

Fig. 23-9. Penetrating atherosclerotic ulcer (PAU). CT image just below the aortic arch done with intravenous contrast enhancement. There is an out-pocketing of contrast medium arising from the posterior wall of the descending aorta representing a penetrating ulcer. Notice the blood surrounding the aorta, most probably from the PAU.

82 percent [28] to 96 percent [30] of cases. Teflon prostheses have lower density and may be seen in some cases. If grafts stay in place long enough, they may calcify and become easier to visualize on CT.

Penetrating Atherosclerotic Ulcers. Penetrating atherosclerotic ulcer (PAU) is a poorly understood, potentially catastrophic complication of atherosclerotic disease that predominantly affects the middle or distal parts of the descending aorta. It is thought to develop as a small ulcer in an atheromatous plaque that penetrates the internal elastic lamina, allowing a hematoma to develop in the media. The ulcer and associated dissection may be localized due to the presence of medial fibrosis related to the atherosclerotic disease. Typically, the patient is an elderly hypertensive who presents with chest or back pain; commonly, the picture is confused with aortic dissection. The management of this potentially fatal acute condition is controversial. While some authors advocate immediate surgery and antihypertensive treatment [31,32], others believe that conservative treatment may be effective unless the patient becomes hemodynamically unstable or symptoms persist or recur despite medical treatment [33,34]. The diagnosis of PAU is possible by CT. In one series of patients, a focal ulcer was seen in about 93 percent, displaced intimal calcifications in 80 percent, pleural and extrapleural fluid collections in 43 percent, and mediastinal fluid in 25 percent [34]. A thick or enhancing aortic wall could be seen in about a third of the patients (Fig. 23-9).

Inflammatory Aortic Aneurysm (Periaortic Fibrosis). Inflammatory aneurysm of the abdominal aorta is a distinct entity and accounts for 5 to 23 percent of all abdominal aortic aneurysms [35], with a male-to-female ratio of 25 : 1. Pathologically, it is characterized by a dense inflammatory mass surrounding a thickened aortic wall. The mass is hypervascular and goes beyond the adventitia of the aorta; it may be large enough to be confused with para-aortic lymphadenopathy. Of the adjacent organs, the ureters are most commonly involved [36]. The inferior vena cava, renal veins, and duodenum also may be enmeshed, and obstruction of those structures may produce the presenting symptoms. The obstruction may present in an acute condition difficult to differentiate from aortic rupture or dissection. CT may differentiate those conditions.

Fig. 23-10. Inflammatory aneurysm of the abdominal aorta. CT image through the abdominal aorta just above the level of the renal hila reveals infiltration of the periaortic tissues by low-density material (unlike fresh blood, which has high density) and obliteration of the fat planes. These findings should suggest the inflammatory nature of the process.

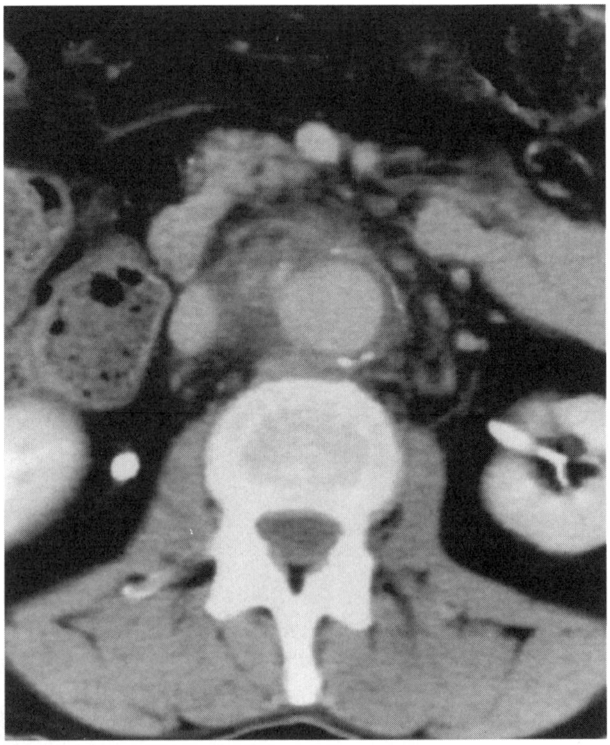

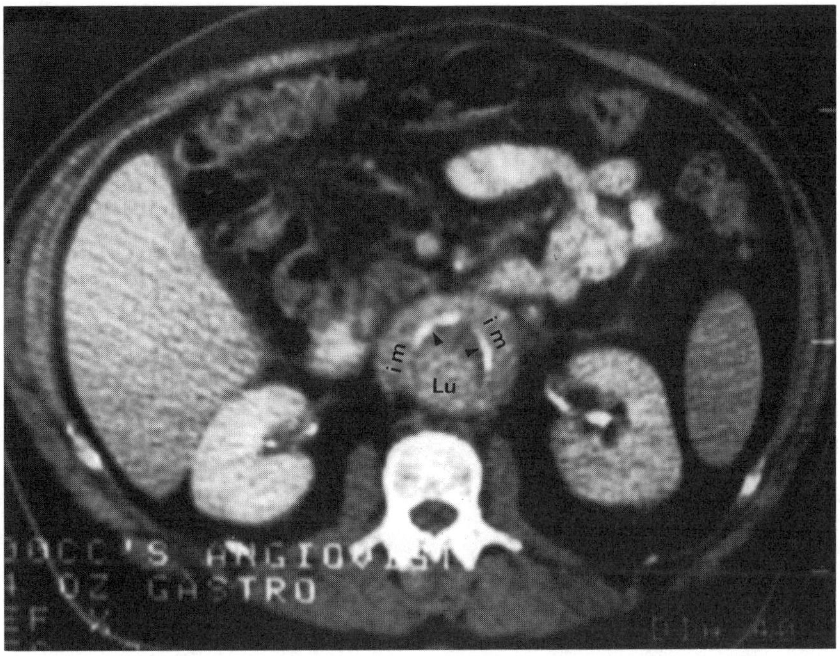

Fig. 23-11. Inflammatory aneurysm of the abdominal aorta. CT scan at the level of the renal hila shows an inflammatory aneurysm of the abdominal aorta. Notice the inflammatory mass (im) that surrounds the aorta anteriorly and laterally with relative sparing of the posterior wall. This inflammatory mass enhances with intravenous contrast injection (compare density to that of the back muscles). Calcifications are also seen in the aortic wall (arrowheads). Patent aortic lumen (Lu).

In inflammatory aneurysm, CT will show atherosclerotic changes in the aorta. The surrounding tissues will be infiltrated by the inflammatory fluid, which has a similar or lower density to that of the aortic lumen (Fig. 23-10), while extravasated blood from the aortic rupture has a higher density (Fig. 23-6). Inflammatory aneurysms are less likely to rupture than noninflammatory aneurysms (15% versus 40%).

Preoperative evaluation of these lesions is very important, to measure the extent of disease and to determine

Fig. 23-12. Mycotic aneurysm of the abdominal aorta. There is a large mass (Ma) displacing the abdominal aorta (Ao) to the right. Notice the high density and irregular borders of the mass.

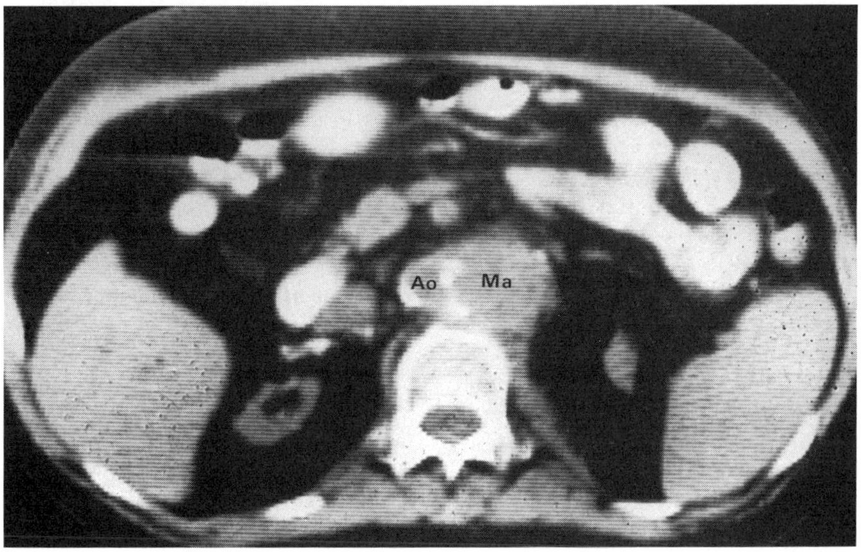

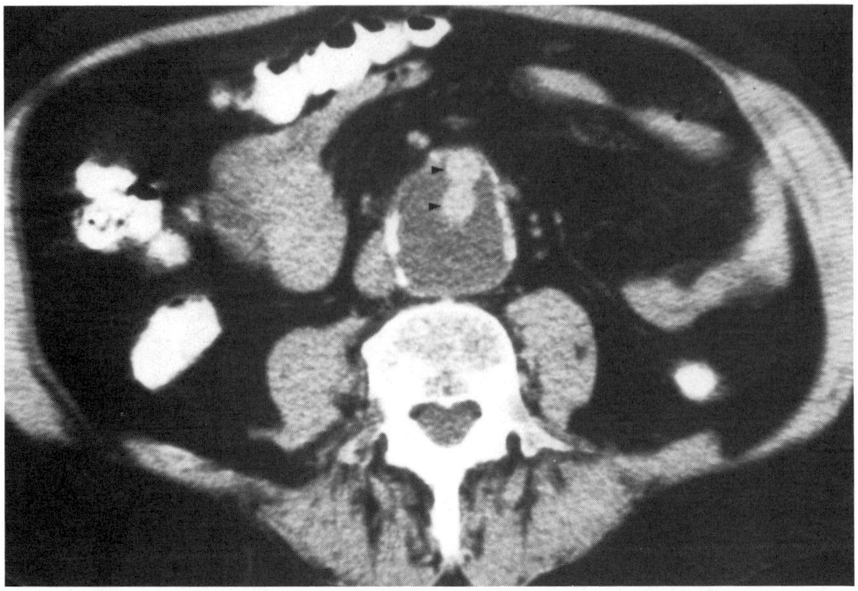

Fig. 23-13. Postoperative appearance of the abdominal aorta. This is a patient who has had aortobifemoral bypass. Notice the two concentric circles (arrowheads), which represent the grafts. They have a higher density than the surrounding hematoma within the native aortic shell, indicating patency. Notice the presence of calcifications in the native aortic shell.

adjacent-organ involvement (such as hydronephrosis secondary to ureteral occlusion). CT can be useful for such purposes. In the presence of an inflammatory aneurysm, CT shows a thickened, sometimes calcified aortic wall surrounded by a low-density soft-tissue mass that often spares the posterior wall [37] (Fig. 23-11). The mass is enhanced if intravenous contrast medium is used (see Fig. 23-11). Dynamic CT shows rapid enhancement of the aortic lumen followed by slow enhancement of the inflammatory mass [37]. Separation of the lumen from the inflammatory mass may be seen in patients with very thick aortic walls due to long-standing disease. CT also has been utilized to demonstrate shrinkage of the inflammatory mass following corticosteroid therapy [37].

Mycotic Aneurysms. Mycotic aortic aneurysms are uncommon, accounting for only 2.6 percent of cases [38]. (This figure dates to 1955 and may not reflect the current true prevalence.) Although some factors, such as diabetes mellitus, immune compromise, sepsis, and prior arterial trauma, may predispose to the development of mycotic aneurysms [39], bacterial endocarditis remains the most likely cause. The infection may spread to the aorta by embolization of the vasa vasorum or by direct extension from inside or outside the vessel. The most common site of involvement is the ascending aorta, but disease of the descending aorta also has been reported [39,40]. Although the presentation could be catastrophic, featured by aortic rupture, sepsis, or massive gastrointestinal bleed due to aortic-enteric fistula, it is more common to be insidious, allowing time for diagnosis. However, since the mortality rate is as high as 50 percent, early diagnosis is extremely important. Although no diagnostic CT features have been reported, the presence of an aneurysm that does not possess characteristic findings of atherosclerotic disease should arouse suspicion. The presence of infiltration of the periaortic tissues by low-density material should suggest the diagnosis (Fig. 23-12). Irregular luminal shape and adjacent soft-tissue mass (see Fig. 23-12), with or without gas, suggest that an aneurysm is mycotic in nature. If the infectious process extends to bone, destruction of an adjacent vertebral body may be seen.

The Postoperative Abdominal Aorta. The CT appearance of the postoperative aorta depends on the type of procedure done. After endoaneurysmorrhaphy, where the native aortic shell is loosely wrapped and sutured around the graft, two concentric circles are seen (Fig. 23-13). The outer circle represents the aortic aneurysmal shell and the inner one, the graft. After aortobifemoral bypass, two nonconcentric circles may be seen (Fig. 23-14). If resection is complete, only one lumen is seen.

The CT appearance of the postoperative abdominal aorta depends on the presence or absence of complications, which include hemorrhage, pseudoaneurysm formation, infection, occlusion, aortoduodenal fistula, and pancreatitis [41]. Thrombosis of the graft is readily apparent when the lumen fails to enhance following intravenous contrast injection. Distal anastomotic pseudoaneurysms can be demonstrated as fluid collections around the distal anastomotic site [41]. The only suggestion of infection may be the presence of gas bubbles in a fluid collection next to the aorta (Fig. 23-15). Otherwise, infected and sterile fluid collections are difficult to tell apart.

Pseudoaneurysm. Pseudoaneurysms of the aorta are either

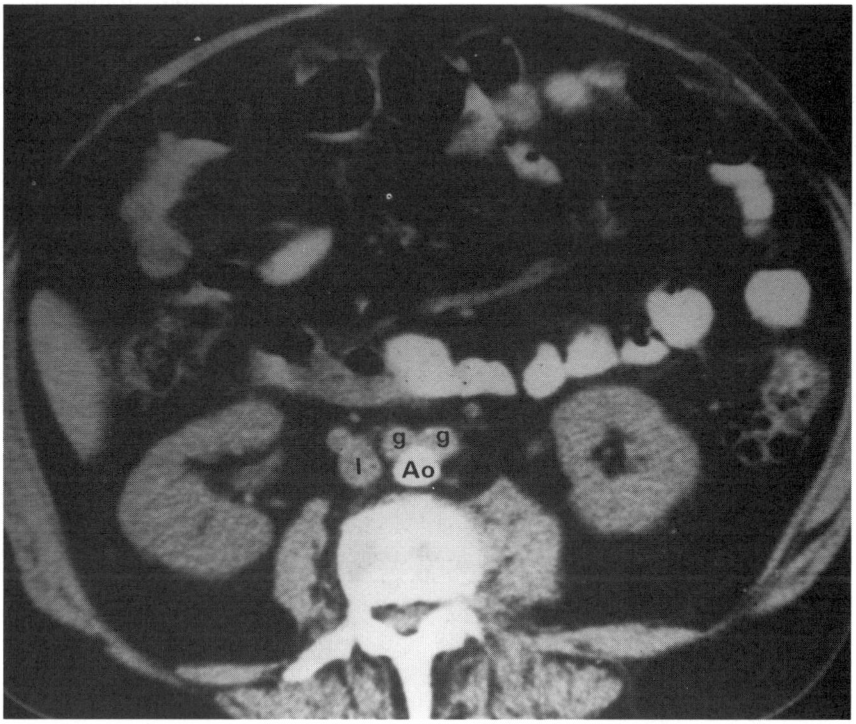

Fig. 23-14. Aortobifemoral bypass. Notice the two round structures (g) in front of the aorta (Ao), representing the bypass grafts.

traumatic (Fig. 23-16) or postsurgical (Fig. 23-17). CT plays an important role in the evaluation of traumatic injury to the aorta. It also has an important role in excluding mediastinal hematoma as a cause of mediastinal widening on chest radiographs, without reducing sensitivity. In a large series of 326 patients, no false-negative CT was found [42]. On the other hand, CT depicted mediastinal hematoma in 7.5 percent of patients with normal chest radiographs. CT showed improvement in specificity, accuracy, and positive predictive value. When used in conjunction with chest radiography, CT reduced the need for angiography by 56 percent [42] in those patients. The role of CT in the diagnosis of traumatic pseudoaneurysms remains controversial. Although CT is noninvasive and very accurate in detecting associated mediastinal hematoma, it may not show the aortic laceration. Angiography remains the procedure of choice in evaluating patients suspected of having suffered aortic trauma [43].

PULMONARY ARTERIES

The anatomy of the pulmonary arteries and veins has been well studied by CT (see Fig. 23-3). The arteries are posterior and lateral to the bronchi; the veins are usually inferior and anterior to the arteries. The vessels are seen as round or tubular densities, but they are very hard to visualize beyond the first division.

Although CT is useful in studying some congenital anomalies (such as anomalous pulmonary venous return and arterial slings) and some acquired lesions (such as arteriovenous malformation or aneurysms of the pulmonary arteries) [44], angiography is more accurate in evaluating these lesions and the complex cardiac defects that may coexist. In cases of hilar enlargement, CT remains the procedure of choice in identifying either dilated pulmonary vessels or hilar mass as the cause. Contrast-medium injection is extremely helpful in that setting and would be readily seen to fill dilated vessels; hilar masses never enhance to the same degree.

CT also has been used to evaluate pulmonary hypertension. O'Callaghan measured the diameter of the intrapericardial division of the right pulmonary artery and correlated it with pulmonary hypertension [45]. The mean diameter of the normal artery was 13.3 mm $\pm$ 1.5 mm (one standard deviation). The upper limit of normal was 16.6 mm, and hypertensive patients had a mean right pulmonary artery diameter of 22.4 mm. O'Callaghan noted, however, that CT cannot quantitate the severity of the hypertension.

MAJOR ABDOMINAL ARTERIES

CT is very useful in visualizing abnormalities (especially aneurysms) of hepatic, splenic, celiac, superior mesenteric, and renal arteries. Wall calcifications, if present, usually have a circumferential pattern (Fig. 23-18). When contrast medium is injected intravenously, the aneurysms themselves enhance in a similar fashion to that of adjacent arteries or the abdominal aorta (Fig. 23-19). Recognition of this enhancement pattern is important, because it differentiates aneurysms from soft-tissue masses, particularly when the former arise within an organ (see Fig. 23-19).

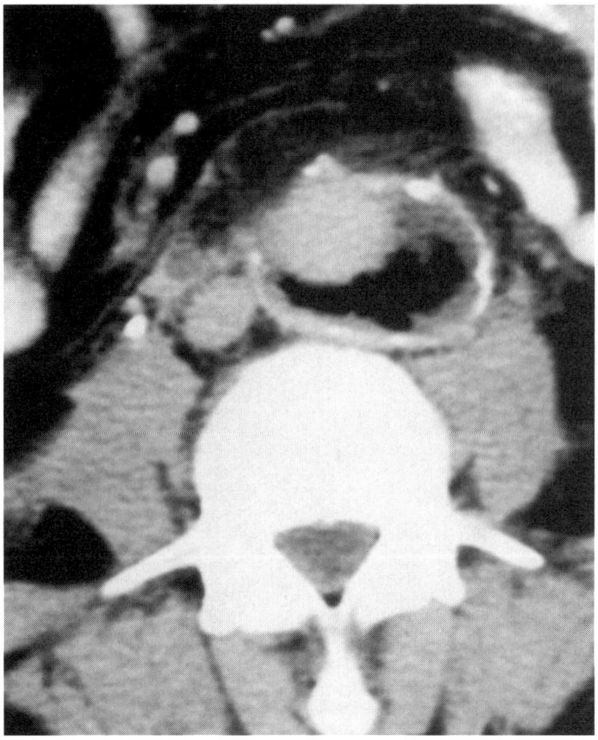

Fig. 23-15. Infected aortic graft. CT image obtained with contrast enhancement shows air within the native shell. Although the presence of air in the immediate postoperative period is expected without infection, it is very suggestive of an infection later on.

Although CT is able to detect these lesions with high sensitivity, it is not etiology specific. For example, CT cannot differentiate mycotic from other types of aneurysm in the absence of air.

Spiral CT three-dimensional angiography has found widespread applications in the abdomen. The abdominal aorta is easily visualized in multiple projections, as are its major branches (Fig. 23-20). Using thin slices, spiral CT angiography images have been shown capable of depicting renal-artery diameter in sufficient detail that several authors have suggested it to be a potential screening tool for the detection of renal-artery stenosis [46,47].

CORONARY ARTERIES

Until now, CT has not played a significant role in the evaluation of coronary artery disease. The major drawbacks in this situation are image degradation by cardiac motion and the transverse cross-sectional nature of CT images. The cross-sectional character poses a real problem because of the need to visualize the entire tree of a coronary artery at one time if localized stenoses are to be identified with certainty. To that end, orthographic reprojections of CT images have been prepared, but some stenotic lesions were obscured because of the superimposition inherent in the technique. Recently, however, electron-beam CT systems have shown greater promise in their ability to detect coronary artery calcifications. Studies have shown sensitivities ranging from 88 to 100 percent, but specificities have been lower. The accuracy of the technique appears to depend on the age group studied and on criteria for diagnosing coronary disease [8].

CT has been evaluated in the study of coronary bypass-graft patency. In one series, its sensitivity and specificity in that regard were 93 and 95 percent, respectively [48]. Other series showed a lower sensitivity for CT, depending on the anatomic location of the graft and ranging from 77.5 percent (for left anterior and right coronary arteries) to 40 percent (for the circumflex and obtuse marginal) [49]. CT images of a patent graft may be misleading, since they provide no information about the state of myocardial perfusion distally.

Carotid Arteries. Spiral CT angiography has shown promise as a means to evaluate the carotid artery in the region of its bifurcation (Fig. 23-21). Studies addressing the relative accuracy of spiral CT angiography, magnetic resonance angiography, and conventional angiography have shown mixed results [50,51,52]. Further refinements in CT scans as well as in image editing and rendering-method techniques may be necessary for CT angiography of carotid stenoses to reach its full potential.

Tissue Infarction. Before the advent of CT, the diagnosis of infarction of abdominal organs was difficult to make. Renal infarction (Fig. 23-22), for example, was difficult to diagnose clinically because the symptoms of abdominal or flank pain, nausea, vomiting, and leukocytosis are nonspecific and may be seen in other diseases [53]. In most cases, angiography was needed to establish the diagnosis. After bolus administration of contrast, large segmental or global infarcts, which commonly are due to trauma, show as sharply marginated areas of no enhancement surrounded by a high-attenuation cortical rim on CT. Small scattered areas of low attenuation may be seen in associa-

Fig. 23-16. Aortic transection in a patient who had a motor vehicle accident. **A**. Supine film of the chest reveals widening of the mediastinum with loss of definition of the aortic knob and the presence of a left apical cap (arrowheads). These findings are extremely suggestive of injury to the thoracic aorta. **B**. CT scan of the same patient obtained following intravenous contrast enhancement reveals a small hematoma (H) lateral to the aorta (Ao). The presence of the mediastinal hematoma was the only sign of aortic injury on CT. No definite pseudoaneurysm was seen. **C**. An aortogram reveals aortic transection just beyond the left subclavian artery with a pseudoaneurysm formation (Ps An). This case demonstrates the superiority of aortography over CT in the evaluation of traumatic injury to the thoracic aorta.

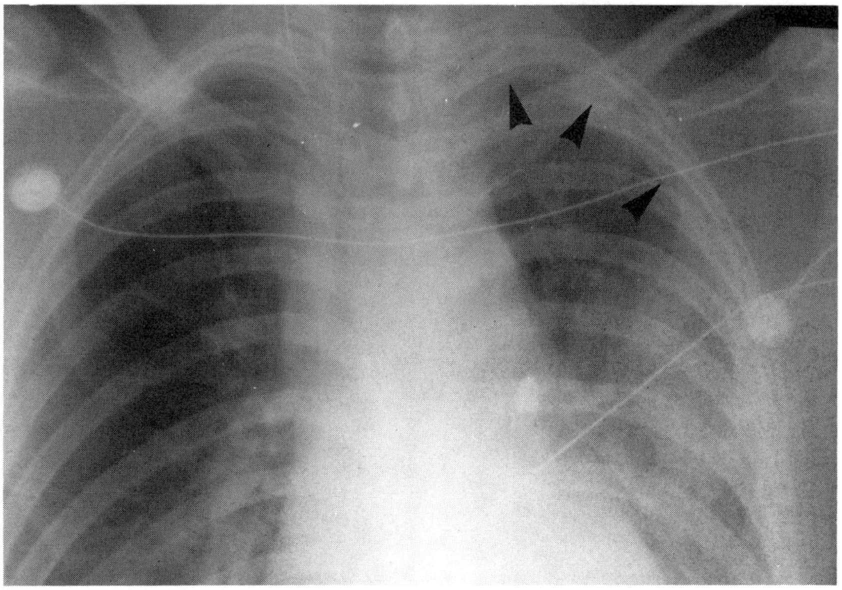

A

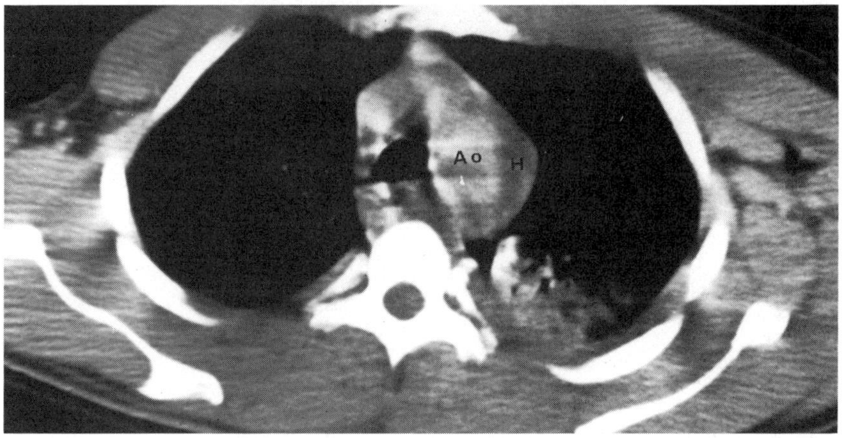

B

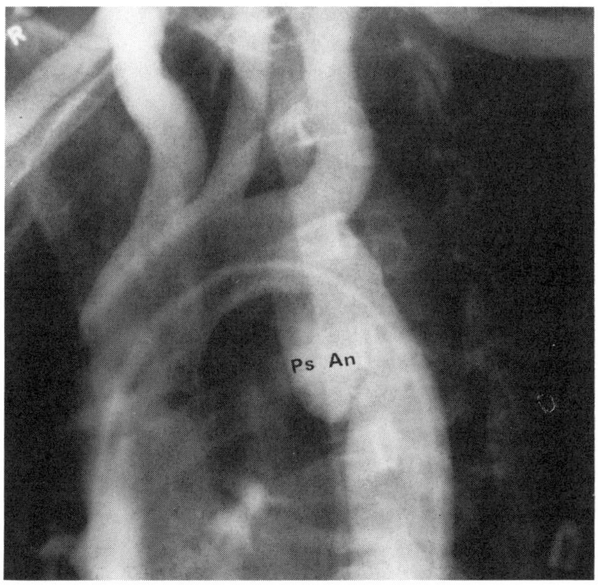

C

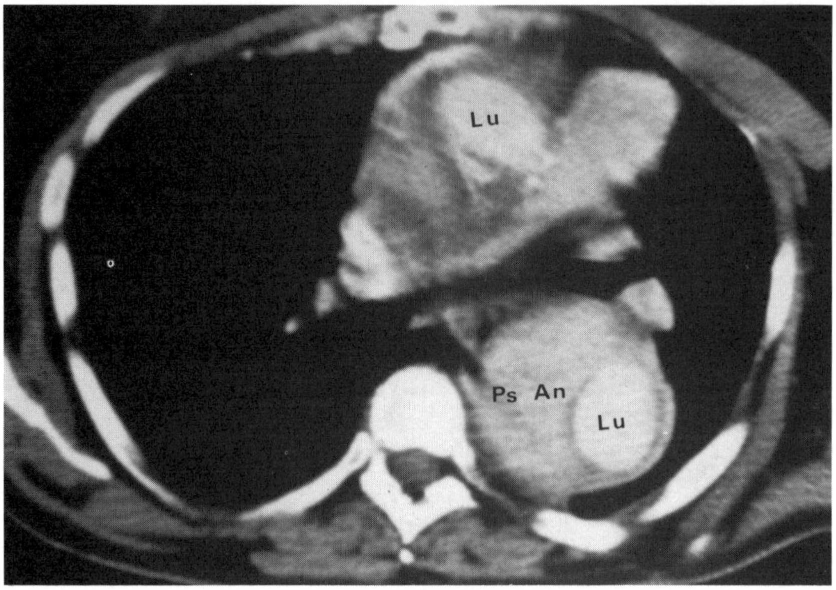

A

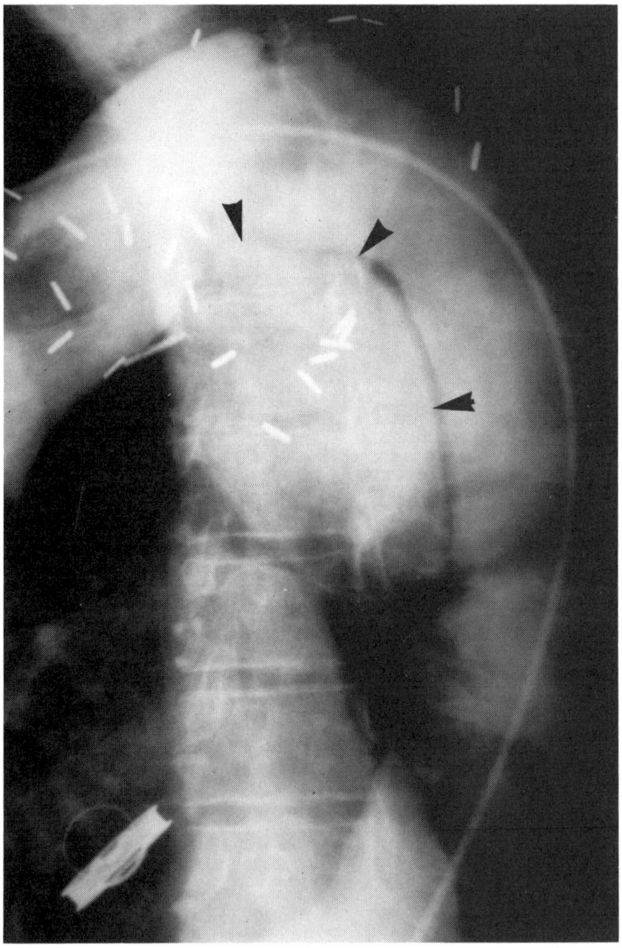

B

Fig. 23-17. Postsurgical pseudoaneurysm. This patient had an aortic valve replacement and aortic surgery for dissection. **A**. CT scan done at the level of the main pulmonary artery following intravenous injection of contrast medium reveals patent aortic lumen (Lu). There is a large enhancing space surrounding the ascending as well as the descending aorta, suggestive of a large pseudoaneurysm (Ps An). **B**. Aortogram reveals a large pseudoaneurysm located within the aortic arch (arrowheads). Notice the displaced aortic valve.

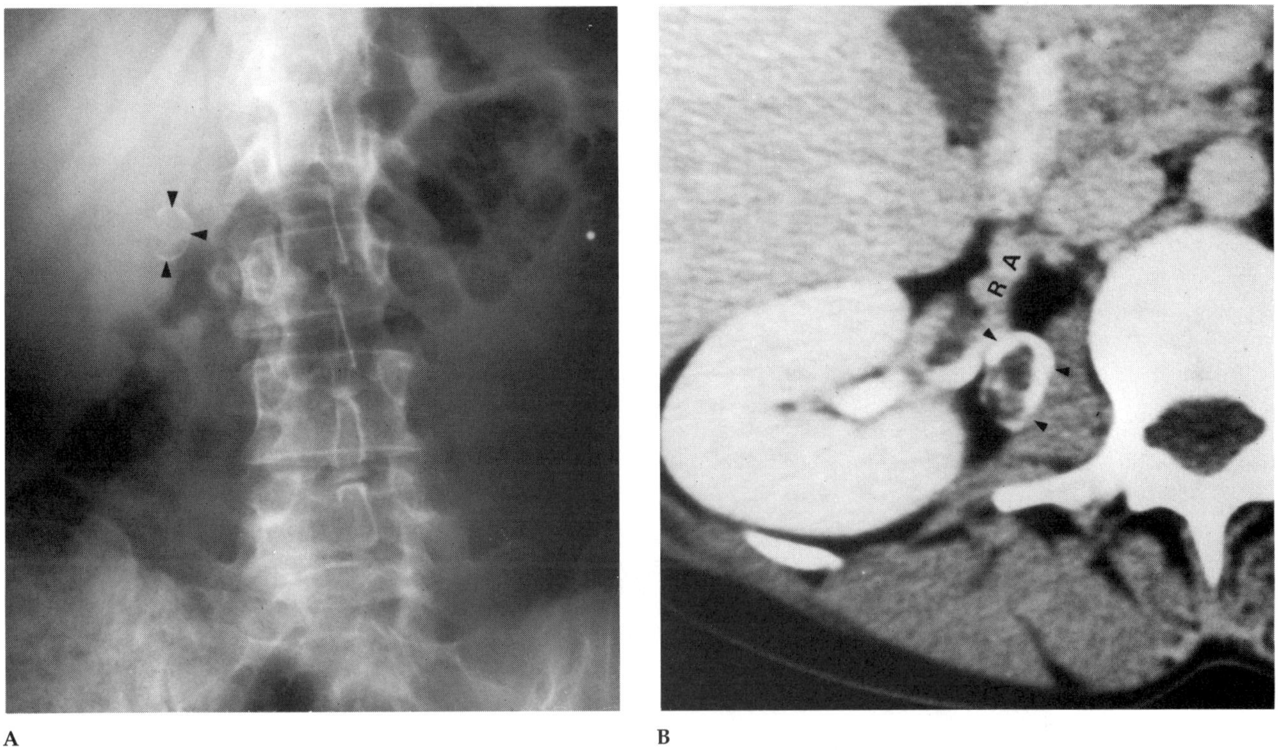

Fig. 23-18. Renal artery aneurysm. **A.** Supine film of the abdomen reveals a calcified pseudoaneurysm of the right renal artery (arrowheads). Notice the circular distribution of calcifications in the wall of the aneurysm. **B.** CT scan of the same patient reveals the aneurysm of the right renal artery. Notice the circular shape of the calcifications. Also, notice that the lumen of the aneurysm has a lower density than the adjacent renal artery (RA), indicating at least partial thrombosis of the aneurysm.

tion with small embolic infarcts. CT scans performed without use of intravenous contrast medium may fail to demonstrate any abnormality [54].

Splenic infarcts are well examined by CT. The presence of a wedge-shaped defect, with its apex toward the hilum and its base near the capsule, is very characteristic of an infarct. Small infarcts, however, may present as small foci of low density, which is not specific for this entity (Fig. 23-23). Chronic infarcts may calcify and appear as high-density areas on CT. This is particularly true in patients with sickle-cell disease, in which condition the spleen is very small, and high-density areas, representing calcium and iron deposition, may be seen.

Liver infarction is uncommon because of the dual blood supply to that organ [55]. Although anemic infarction was reported following thrombosis of the hepatic veins and main extrahepatic portal vein with complete patency of the hepatic artery [56], most of the reported cases are due to occlusion of the hepatic artery. This lesion has been reported as a complication of a variety of clinical situations, such as abdominal neoplasia, bacterial endocarditis, sickle-cell disease, cholesterol emboli, catheter-placement progressive systemic sclerosis, and toxemia of pregnancy. Periarteritis nodosa remains the leading cause of hepatic infarction [57]. CT shows a triangular area of low density that would not enhance, with its base next to the capsule and its apex close to the hilum (Fig. 23-24). CT can also play an important role in the follow-up of those patients (see Fig. 23-24).

Infarcts of the gastrointestinal tract vary in presentation, from a severe catastrophic event to a very mild episode of abdominal pain. Angiography remains the procedure of choice in examining the major mesenteric arteries and their branches. CT can be used to study the superior mesenteric artery, which should be seen in all patients. Thrombosis of this vessel may be demonstrated on CT [58]. CT also can show the effect of ischemia on bowel by demonstrating wall thickening and edema (Fig. 23-25). CT can be utilized in the follow-up of those conditions.

THE VENAE CAVAE AND THEIR TRIBUTARIES

Computed tomography may be the first examination to disclose a congenital anomaly or a pathologic state of the venae cavae and their tributaries. Differentiation of these anomalies from other processes, such as enlarged retroperitoneal lymph node or masses, is important and can be made by demonstrating their continuity with other veins and aided by the fact that they enhance with contrast.

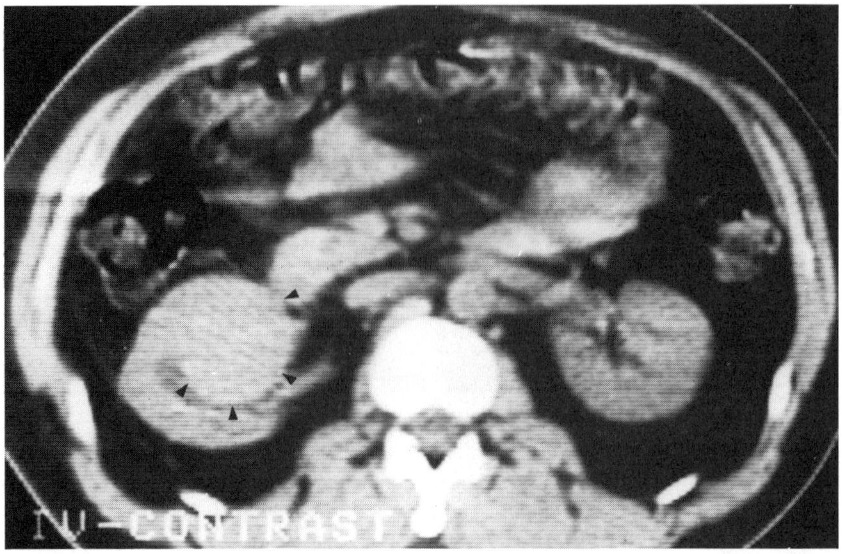

A

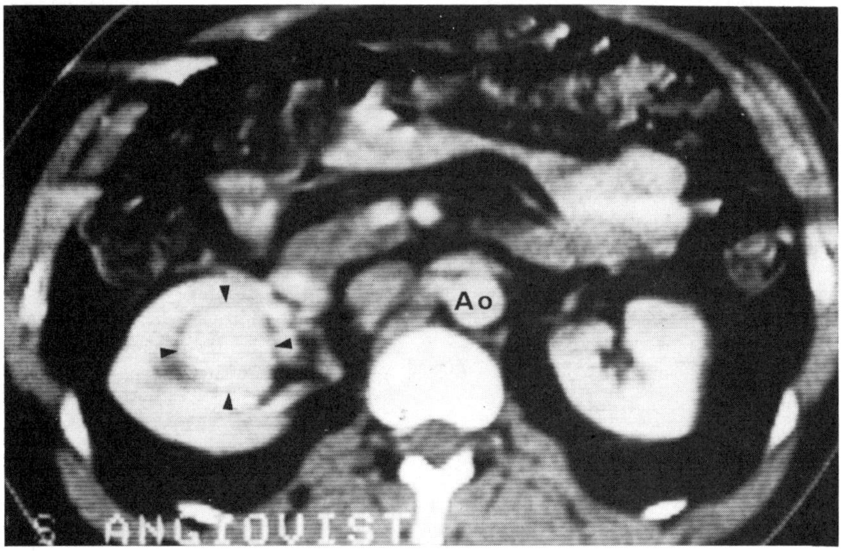

B

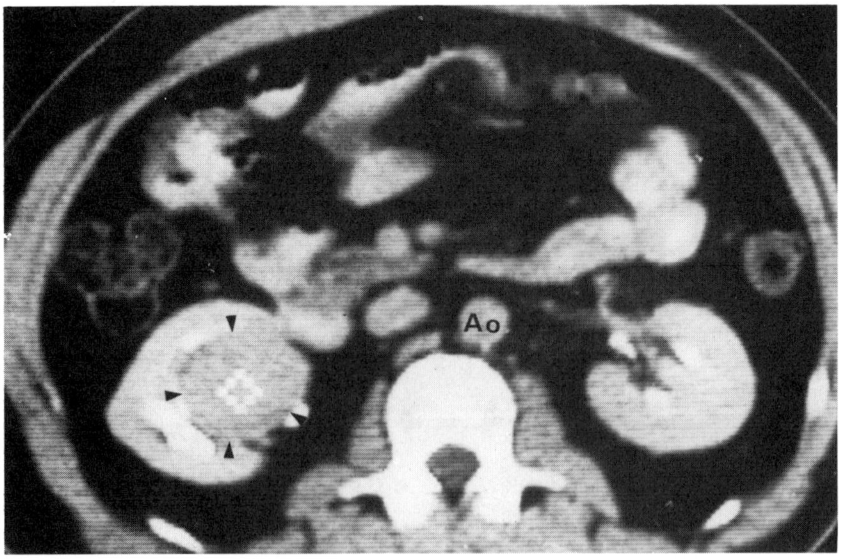

C

The Inferior Vena Cava. The inferior vena cava (IVC) is formed by the common iliac veins at the level of L5. It ascends in front of the vertebral bodies and to the right of the abdominal aorta. Moving cephalad, it becomes more anterior until it joins the right atrium.

CONGENITAL ANOMALIES. Many congenital anomalies may involve the inferior vena cava with or without involving other organs. When the vessel is interrupted with azygous or hemiazygous continuation, the suprarenal segment of the cava fails to connect with the hepatic veins. Blood returns to the heart via the azygous, hemiazygous, or accessory hemiazygous veins. Although this lesion may be isolated, it is sometimes associated with asplenia or polysplenia. In that case, CT would demonstrate a normal cava from the junction of the iliac veins to just above the renal veins, where the cava fails to continue cephalad and join the hepatic veins. The azygous or hemiazygous veins would be dilated [59].

One anomaly, a **duplicated left-sided IVC**, starts at the level of the iliac veins and travels on the left side of the aorta to the level of the renal veins, where it empties into the right cava via a vessel that crosses in front of or behind the aorta. Although this vessel causes no clinical problems, it may cause some confusion on CT. First, this anomaly may be mistaken for enlarged lymph nodes—a problem easily resolved by using intravenous contrast enhancement to follow the course of the vein. Second, it may be mistaken for an enlarged gonadal vein on that side. Following the vein caudally usually resolves that issue; the duplicated vena cava ends at the level of the iliac veins, whereas the gonadal vein courses more caudally to the level of the inguinal canal [60].

Anomalies of the renal veins can be detected readily on CT. A retroaortic left renal vein is seen to course behind the aorta either at the same level of a normal vein or a little more caudad. It represents persistence of the retroaortic supracardinal vein, with regression of the anterior subcardinal vein. If both veins persist, a circumaortic left renal vein results. In this condition, the veins form a vascular ring in front of and behind the aorta. The retroaortic vein is usually about two vertebrae caudad to the anterior vein, which follows a normal course.

THROMBOSIS. Thrombosis of major abdominal veins is always due to a clot, either with or without tumor. CT offers an invaluable tool not only to document the presence of thrombosis but also to differentiate the two entities.

A number of characteristic changes are seen on CT in most cases of venous thrombosis. The involved vessel is usually enlarged [61], and in the majority of cases, the thrombus fills the vascular lumen completely (Fig. 23-26). In some cases, however, it may be incomplete and appear as a semilunar filling defect with blood flowing around it. The clot density depends on its age. Hyperdense clots have been seen in the very acute situation [62]. As the clot organizes it becomes isodense with blood and therefore difficult to detect. Later on, it becomes less dense than surrounding blood. Caution should be exercised when evaluating a filling defect in the vena cava following intravenous contrast administration. Flow defects secondary to streaming of unopacified blood may mimic an intraluminal thrombus [63]. The involved vessel wall is sharply defined and enhances with intravenous contrast administration [61,64]. This enhancement reflects increased blood flow through the vasa vasorum. An indirect but frequently seen sign is the presence of venous collaterals, which appear as tortuous tubular structures, enhancing after intravenous contrast administration. They are more commonly proximal than distal to the area of obstruction.

Differentiation of tumor from nontumor thrombus is possible by CT, since the former is usually denser (Fig. 23-27) and may demonstrate similar morphologic features to the primary tumor [47]. Tumor thrombi may be isodense with blood initially and show enhancement following intravenous contrast injection, reflecting their hypervascularity. Direct invasion from an adjacent primary may be seen. Rarely, a metastatic focus, especially in the liver, may invade adjacent veins.

CT has proved very helpful in the diagnosis of hepatic vein occlusion (Budd-Chiari syndrome), the clinical diagnosis of which is difficult. CT demonstrates multifocal hypodense parenchymal lesions along with patchy enhancement following intravenous contrast injection [65]. Failure to visualize normal hepatic veins, particularly after contrast enhancement on CT, is diagnostic of this entity (Fig. 23-28).

Superior Vena Cava and Its Tributaries

CONGENITAL ANOMALIES. CT detection of developmental anomalies of the great thoracic veins has been well documented [66]. Injection of contrast medium is necessary to identify these anomalous structures and their relationship to adjacent vessels. Usually the anomalies are picked up as incidental findings on CT done for other reasons or done to clarify abnormal shadows seen on plain chest radiographs. In addition, 4.4 percent of patients with congenital heart disease have persistent left superior vena cava.

THE SUPERIOR VENA CAVA SYNDROME. Development of the superior vena cava (SVC) syndrome is an ominous sign, since it is usually due to malignancy: bronchogenic carcinoma, lymphoma, or metastatic disease [67]. Benign eti-

Fig. 23-19. Intrarenal renal artery aneurysm. **A**. Precontrast CT scan reveals a large mass within the right renal sinus (arrowheads). The density of the mass is similar to that of the surrounding renal parenchyma, indicating that it is not a simple cyst. **B**. CT scan immediately following the intravenous administration of contrast medium shows the same space-occupying lesion (arrowheads). Notice that the density of this mass is similar to that of the abdominal aorta (Ao). **C**. A delayed scan through the same area again shows the same lesion (arrowheads). Notice again that the density of that lesion is similar to that of the abdominal aorta.

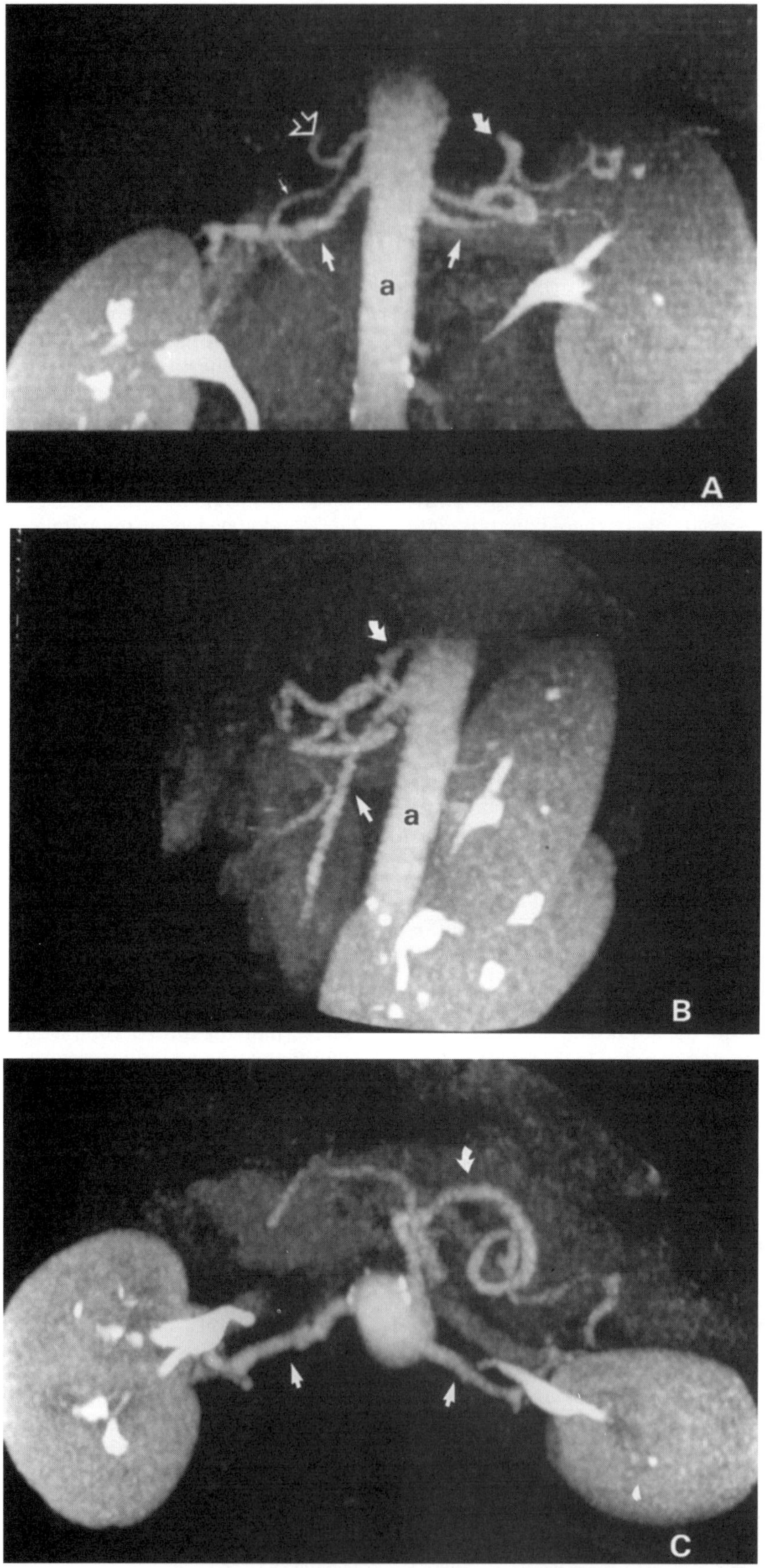
a
A
a
B
C

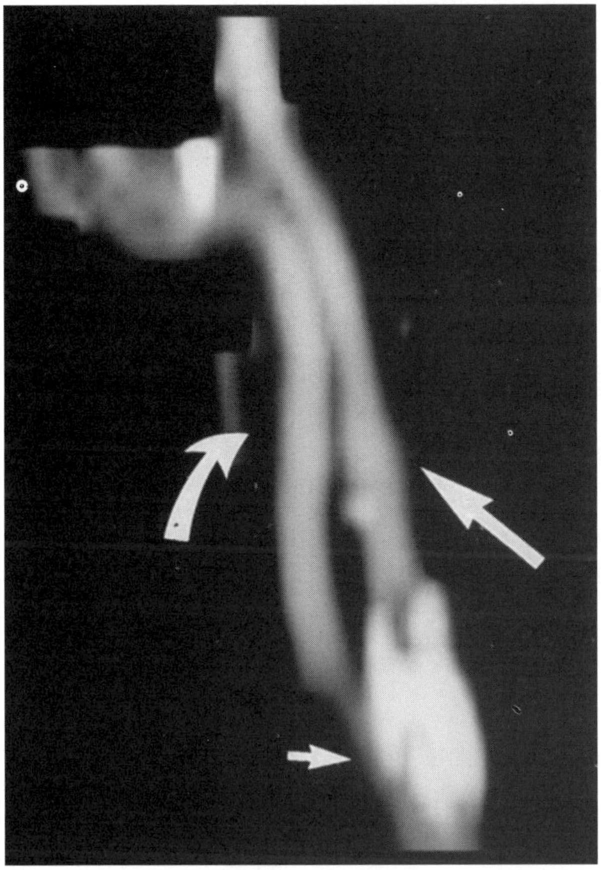

Fig. 23-21. Lateral projection of a three-dimensional spiral CT angiogram of the carotid artery at and above its bifurcation. The internal carotid (curved arrow) and external carotid (straight arrow) are both well seen. A large calcified plaque (short arrow) is seen at the bifurcation. The vessels can be rotated into any oblique position desired to maximize the view of the bifurcation. (Courtesy Richard B. Schwartz, M.D., Brigham and Women's Hospital, Boston, Mass.)

ologies include fibrosing mediastinitis [68]. Indwelling intravenous devices, such as subclavian venous catheters [68], pacemakers [69], and LeVeen shunts also have been incriminated. In the setting of the SVC syndrome, CT provides detailed information about the site and extent of an obstructing thrombus or an invading mediastinal lesion. It also provides guidance for percutaneous biopsy of an unsuspected lesion and aids in planning surgery and radiation therapy.

Extracranial Tissue Perfusion. The blood flow to extracranial tissues can be assessed by means of dynamic CT coupled with bolus administration of contrast. Because contrast media mix thoroughly in the blood pool, the flow of iodine can be tracked through an organ and iodine transit used as a reflection of tissue blood flow. Usually, a time-tissue density curve is constructed and the rate of density-curve upswing (a measure of tissue blood flow), peak curve height, and the area under the curve (a measure of tissue distribution volume) are determined [70]. In analyzing renal blood flow, the appearance time of contrast media in the renal artery, cortex, medulla, and pelvis can be tabulated [71]. Patterns and contrast enhancement can reveal global or regional perfusion abnormalities.

INTRACRANIAL VESSELS

CT often can depict normal intracranial vessels and delineate the regions or territories supplied by major arterial trunks (Figs. 23-29 and 23-30).

Aneurysm. Intracranial aneurysms are classified as saccular or berry (most common), atherosclerotic, mycotic, tumor induced, traumatic, or dissecting [72].

Saccular or berry aneurysms result from a congenital defect in the arterial wall. Most of them arise at or near the circle of Willis. The common sites are at the anterior communicating artery (Fig. 23-31A, B), the origin of the posterior communicating from the internal carotid artery, and the middle cerebral artery bifurcation (Fig. 23-31C, D). Ninety percent of these aneurysms arise from the internal carotid system and its branches; the few that have their origin in the vertebral-basilar arterial system are most commonly found at the tip of the basilar artery, with a few in the posterior inferior cerebellar artery.

Five percent of the population may harbor saccular aneurysms [72], whereas 20 to 25 percent have multiple intracranial aneurysms [73–75]. Congenital aneurysms sometimes may be familial [74]. There is an increase of incidence of aneurysms of the feeding artery or arteries of an arteriovenous malformation [75]. Aneurysms have been associated with several diseases, including coarctation of the aorta, polycystic disease of the kidneys, fibromuscular hyperplasia of the carotid arteries, Marfan syndrome, pseudoxanthoma elasticum, Ehlers-Danlos syndrome, and moyamoya disease [72]. Patients with subacute bacterial endocarditis may be found to harbor mycotic aneurysms, as may those with congenital heart disease with right-to-left shunt and those who use drugs intravenously [76]. Such lesions tend to be peripheral in location. Aneurysms are more common in women after the age of 40 [77], which suggests that there may be an

Fig. 23-20. Three-dimensional spiral CT angiogram of the midabdominal aorta and its branches. The kidneys are opacified and are excreting contrast material. **A.** Frontal projection showing the aorta (a), both renal arteries (straight arrows), the splenic artery (curved arrow), the hepatic artery (open arrow), and the gastroduodenal artery (small arrow). **B.** Lateral projection showing the celiac artery (curved arrow) and the superior mesenteric artery (straight arrow) originating from the ventral aspect of the aorta (a). **C.** Axial projection showing the renal arteries (straight arrows) and the splenic artery (curved arrow) to advantage.

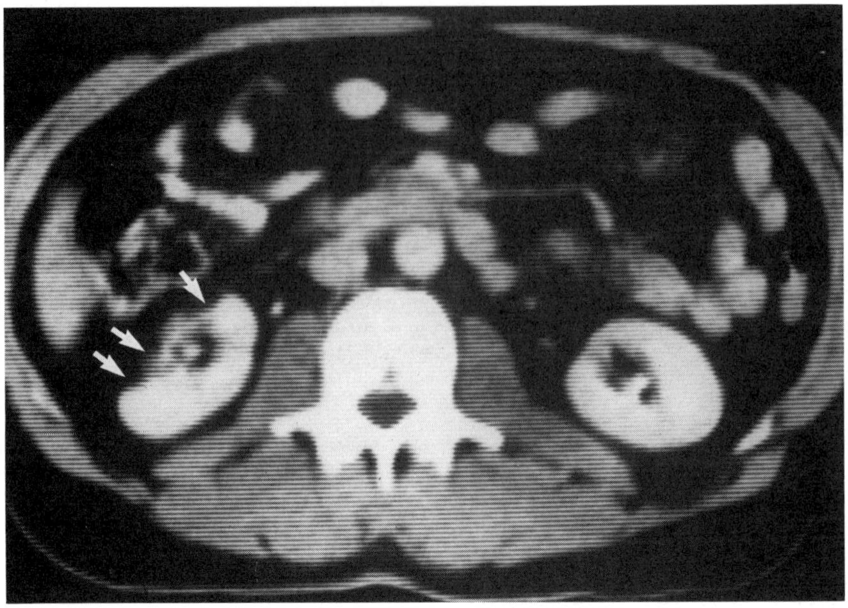

Fig. 23-22. Renal infarct. CT of the midabdomen reveals marked and irregular loss of renal parenchyma on the right (arrows). This finding is very suggestive of renal infarct.

inherited feature of female blood vessels that makes them susceptible to aneurysm formation. Complications from ruptured aneurysm can be serious and include subarachnoid, ventricular, and parenchymal hemorrhage. (For further detail, see "Nontraumatic Intracranial Hemorrhage," later in this chapter.)

CT FINDINGS IN PATIENTS WITH ANEURYSM. On contrast-enhanced CT scans, small aneurysms (less than 5 mm in diameter) are usually not visible because their size is not much larger than that of the parent artery [78]. Giant aneurysms (larger than 2.5 cm) are easily identified, but they can be confused with other pathologic mass lesions. Calcium may outline part or all of the wall. What appears on CT as a partly thrombosed, broad-necked, giant aneurysm may have the angiographic appearance of a small aneurysm with a distinct neck. CT is more reliable than angiography to evaluate size. If the aneurysm is partially or entirely clotted, contrast enhancement is valuable. A mural thrombus may be seen as a crescentic zone of nonenhancement on CT, but an almost completely throm-

Fig. 23-23. Splenic infarct in a patient with atrial fibrillation. Notice the low-attenuation area in the anterior tip of the spleen, suggestive of splenic infarct.

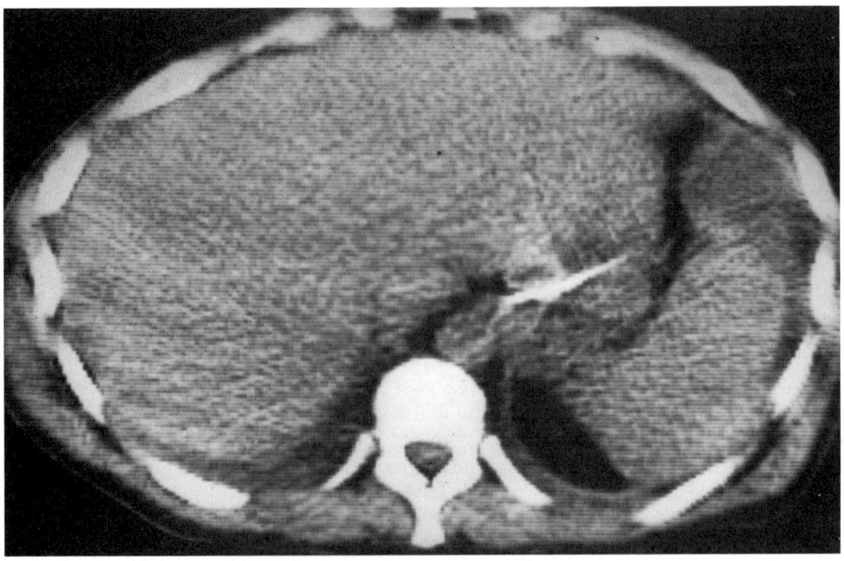

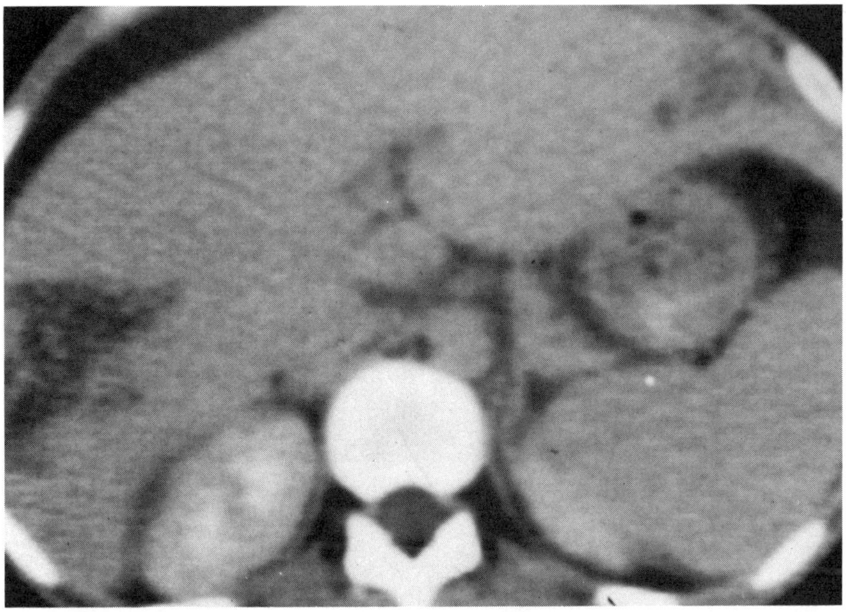

A

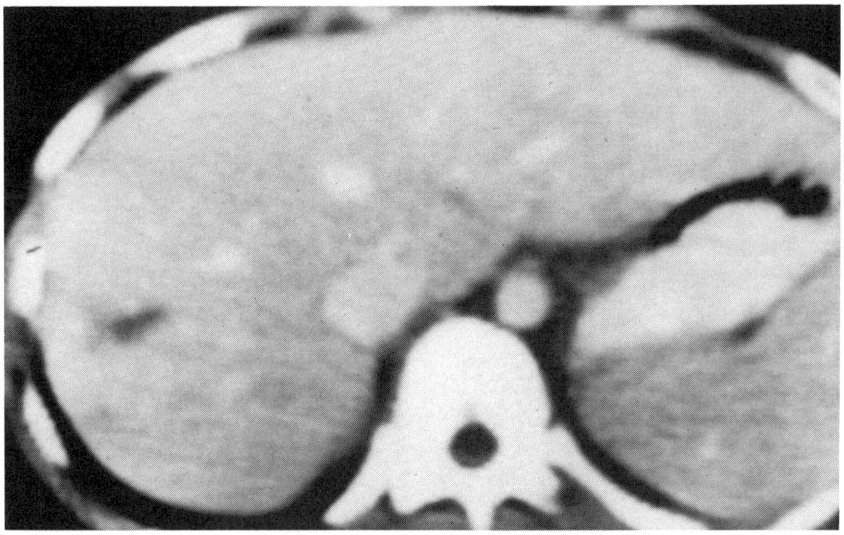

B

Fig. 23-24. Liver infarct. **A**. CT scan of the upper abdomen in a patient with toxemia of pregnancy and disseminated intravascular coagulopathy (DIC) and elevated liver function tests. Notice the wedge-shaped area of decreased attenuation in the right lobe of the liver, with its base in the subcapsular area and the head pointing toward the hilum. These findings suggest a liver infarct. **B**. Follow-up CT of the liver in the same patient reveals marked resolution of the previous infarct. Notice the residual attenuation area in the right lobe.

bosed aneurysm may resemble a target or bull's eye, with the persisting lumen at the center (Fig. 23-32). Occasionally, only the wall of the thrombosed aneurysm will enhance due to the presence of vaso vasorum. Because a brain tumor may mimic a giant aneurysm, angiography is the procedure of choice for diagnosis (Fig. 23-33). Rapid dynamic scanning immediately after contrast injection may differentiate aneurysm from neoplasm [79].

Vascular Malformation. Arteriovenous malformation (AVM) results from failure of a capillary bed to develop between an artery (or arteries) and a vein (or veins) [75]. The dura, the pia, or the ventricular ependymal surface may be the site of AVM, which is considered congenital and may either enlarge over time [80] or disappear spontaneously [81]. Parenchymal, ventricular, and subarachnoid hemorrhage (or all three) may be seen on the nonenhanced

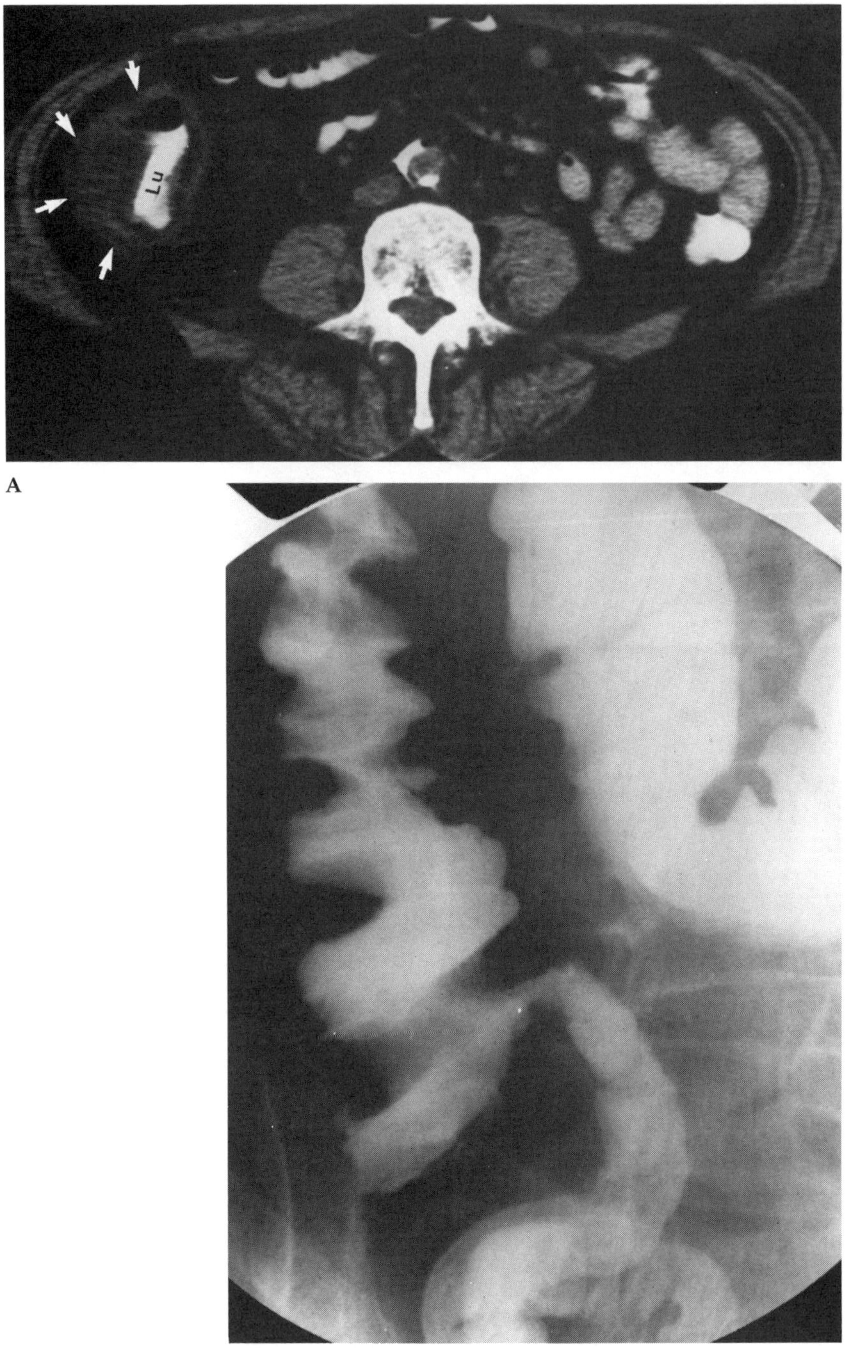

Fig. 23-25. Ischemic bowel disease. **A**. CT scan of the lower abdomen reveals marked thickening of the wall of the cecum resulting in a mass effect (arrows). Notice the compression of the bowel lumen (Lu), which is filled with contrast medium. **B**. A barium enema done in the same patient reveals marked thickening of the wall of the ascending colon with thumbprinting, very suggestive of ischemia.

CT scan when an AVM bleeds. (For further detail, see "Nontraumatic Intracranial Hemorrhage," later in this chapter.) The brain surrounding an AVM may be dysplastic or atrophic due to diversion of blood away from normal brain. The adjacent ventricles may be either reduced from the mass effect or enlarged by atrophic change; prominent vessels also may characterize the CT scan (Fig. 23-34). Angiography demonstrates the feeding arteries and draining veins.

Cerebral cavernous hemangioma is a rare vascular

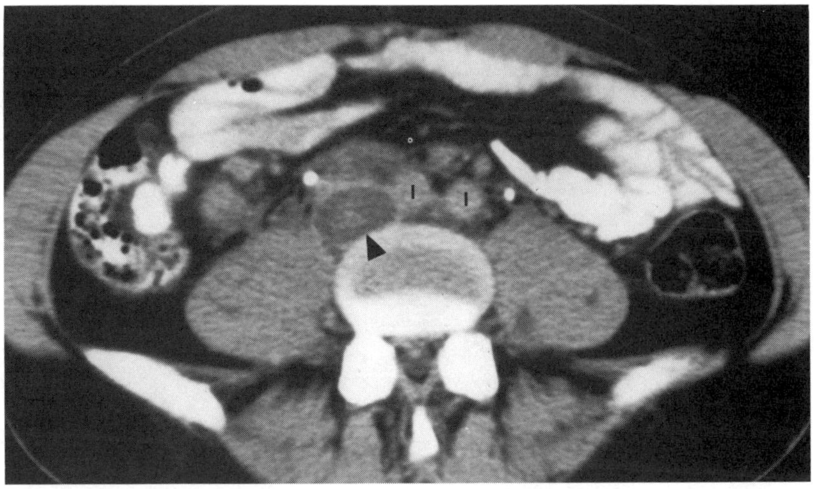

A

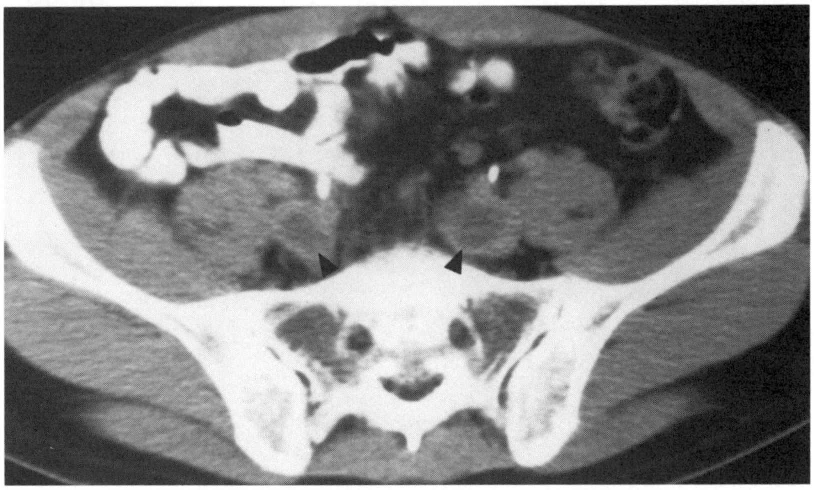

B

Fig. 23-26. Thrombosis of inferior vena cava. **A**. CT scan at the level of the aortic bifurcation (I = common iliac artery). Notice the enlargement of the inferior vena cava (arrowhead). Notice the low-density center of the cava compared to that of the iliac arteries; this is a large thrombus occupying the entire IVC lumen. **B**. CT scan done at the level of the upper pelvis in the same patient reveals extension of the thrombosis into the common iliac veins (arrowheads). Notice enlargement of the iliac veins, which are completely occupied by a large thrombus that has a low attenuation value.

malformation that is surgically curable. It is not easily detected by angiography. A well-demarcated, heterogeneously dense area with mild or no mass effect may be found on nonenhanced CT scan (Fig. 23-35). The enhanced CT scan shows only mild enhancement. Cavernous hemangioma of the middle fossa may mimic a meningioma on CT [82]. It may bleed and can be detected on the nonenhanced scan.

Carotid-Cavernous Fistula. Internal carotid-artery-to-cavernous-sinus fistula may result either from rupture of an intracavernous carotid aneurysm or from traumatic laceration of the internal carotid artery within the cavernous sinus. Contrast-enhanced CT scan (Fig. 23-36) may demonstrate an enlarged cavernous sinus and an enlarged superior ophthalmic vein [83]. Proptosis (enlargement of the extraocular muscles) also may be seen on CT, particularly when the condition is acute. Associated abnormalities such as fracture or adjacent postoperative defect may be seen. The findings of enlarged cavernous sinus and superior ophthalmic vein, ptosis, and enlarged extraocular muscles may disappear completely or regress following spontaneous resolution or therapeutic obliteration of the fistula.

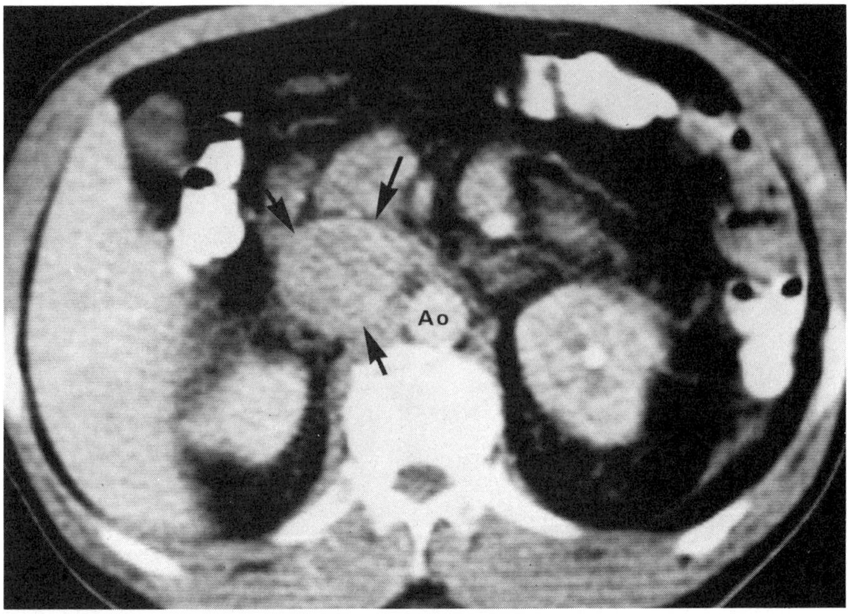

A

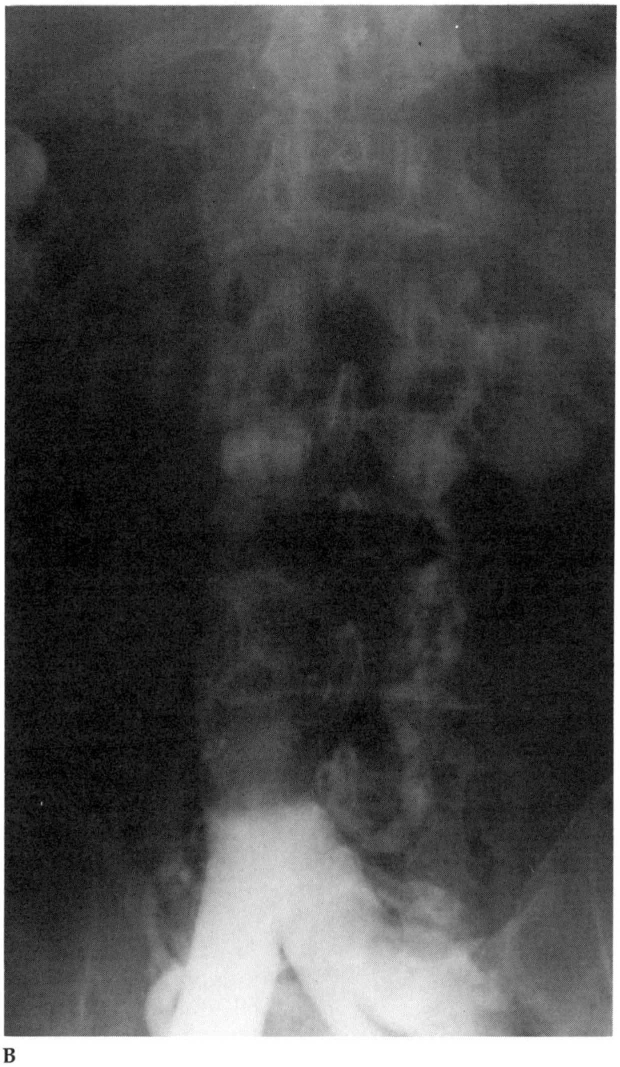

B

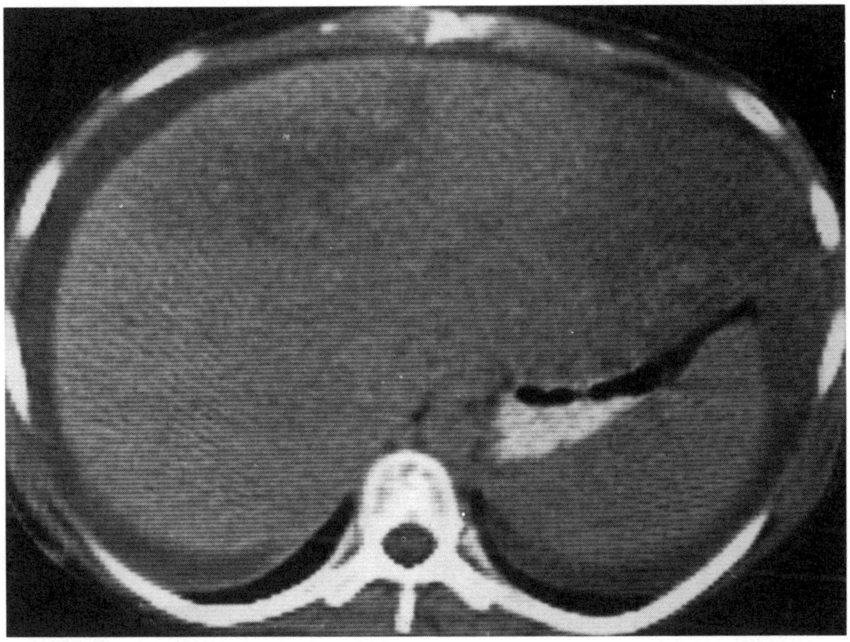

Fig. 23-28. Budd-Chiari syndrome. A CT scan of the upper abdomen in a patient with suspected hepatic vein thrombosis reveals an ill-defined area of low attenuation in the liver anteriorly. Notice that the hepatic veins cannot be identified. Such findings are very suggestive of Budd-Chiari syndrome. There is also some ascitic fluid in the peritoneal cavity.

Ischemic Cerebrovascular Syndromes. Cerebral ischemia is a prevalent disease that affects 500,000 Americans annually. Thrombosis and embolization of the cerebral arterial systems are its most important causes. The severity of the neurologic defects depends on how well collateral circulation is established. If a collateral blood supply is available and the patient's vascular compromise is slight, the patient might not have symptoms; however, if the collaterals are absent or inadequate, symptoms of ischemia result. If the neurologic defects resolve within 24 hours, the incident is termed a transient ischemic attack (TIA); the longer they persist, however, the more likely they are to evolve into complete stroke. Venous thrombosis may produce venous infarction (see "Cerebral Venous Occlusive Disease," later in this chapter). CT plays a critical role in the evaluation of stroke because of its ability to differentiate ischemic infarct from hemorrhage. Hemorrhage appears as a focus of high density on the nonenhanced CT scan, and ischemic infarct appears as either isodense or low-density lesions in the brain parenchyma. CT has minimal value in distinguishing between TIA and reversible ischemic neurologic deficits.

CT scans provide additional information about density values of the lesion, the presence or absence of mass effect, and the pattern of contrast enhancement. This information permits more complete evaluation of ischemic infarcts. For example, within 12 hours after ictus (seizure), no changes in infarct density can be detected (Fig. 23-37). Between 12 and 24 hours after ictus, a poorly circumscribed, hypodense area may be seen, which is the earliest evidence of bland infarct. Beyond 24 hours, sharply delineated hypodensity of the infarcted brain conforming to a vascular distribution is a constant finding (see Fig. 23-37B, C). After 7 to 10 days, when more than three-fourths of all infarcts are discernible, the attenuation values increase as the edema is subsiding. Some infarcts revert to normal density temporarily (foggy effect) or permanently, but many necrotic infarcts become cysts with low-attenuation value similar to that of cerebrospinal fluid (CSF). Focal dilatation of the adjacent CSF spaces also may occur.

Although mass effect is always present in an ischemic infarct, due to increased intracellular or extracellular fluid, only 23 to 47 percent of cases can be demonstrated by CT [84]. The mass effect is usually maximal by the fifth day and tends to subside thereafter. By the twenty-fifth day,

Fig. 23-27. Tumor thrombosis of the inferior vena cava in a patient with renal-cell carcinoma. **A**. CT scan of the midabdomen shows marked enlargement of the inferior vena cava (arrows) compared to the aorta (Ao). Notice the high density in the inferior vena cava compared to the previous case (see Fig. 23-20). This high attenuation value reflects vascularity of that tumor thrombus. **B**. Inferior vena cavogram in the same patient reveals complete obstruction just distal to the common iliac vein. Notice the enlarged lumbar collaterals.

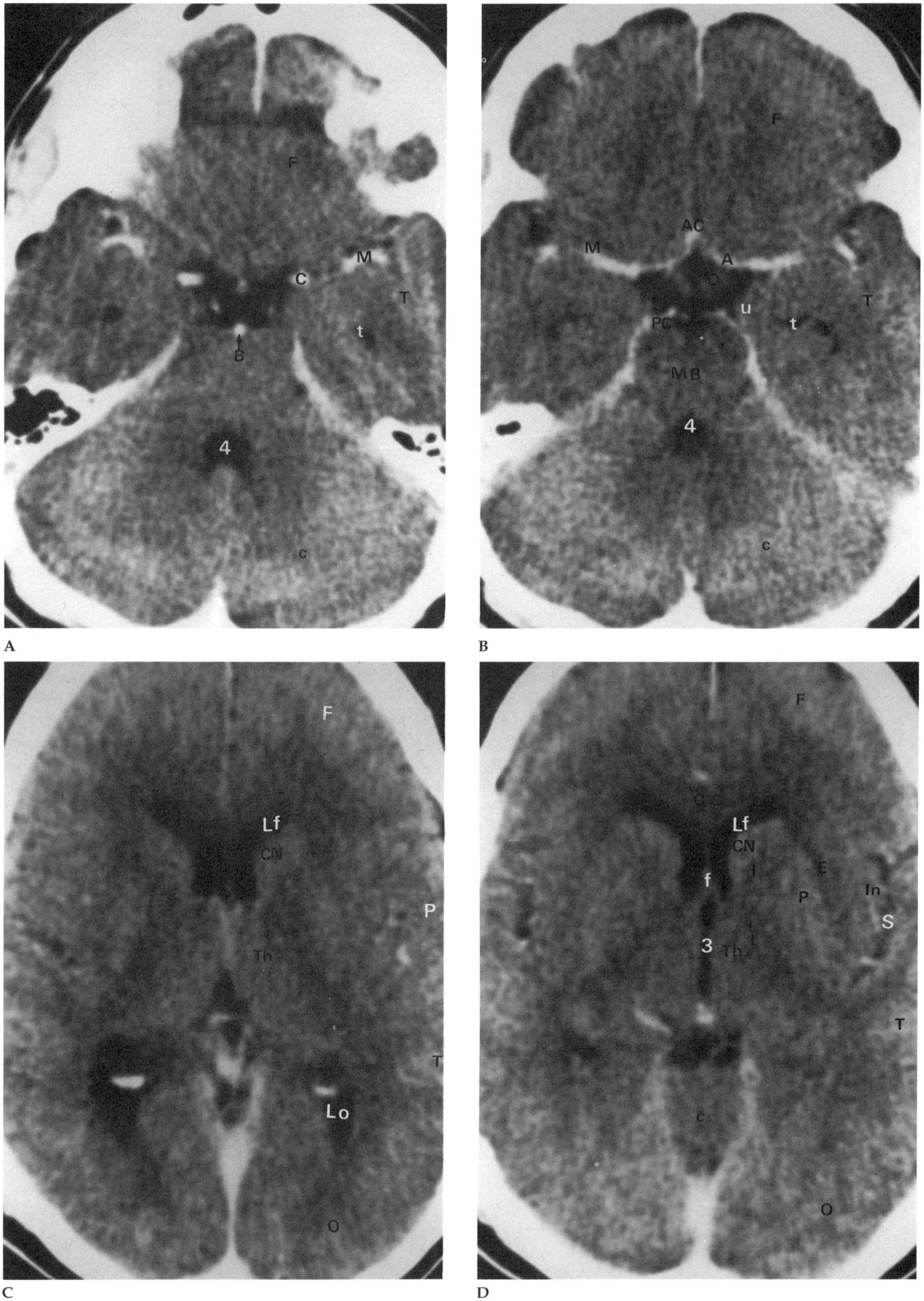
F
M
C
T
t
B
4
c
A
F
AC
M
A
C
u
T
PC
t
MB
4
c
B
F
Lf
CN
P
Th
T
Lo
O
C
F
CC
Lf
CN
f
I
E
P
In
S
3
Th
I
T
c
O
D

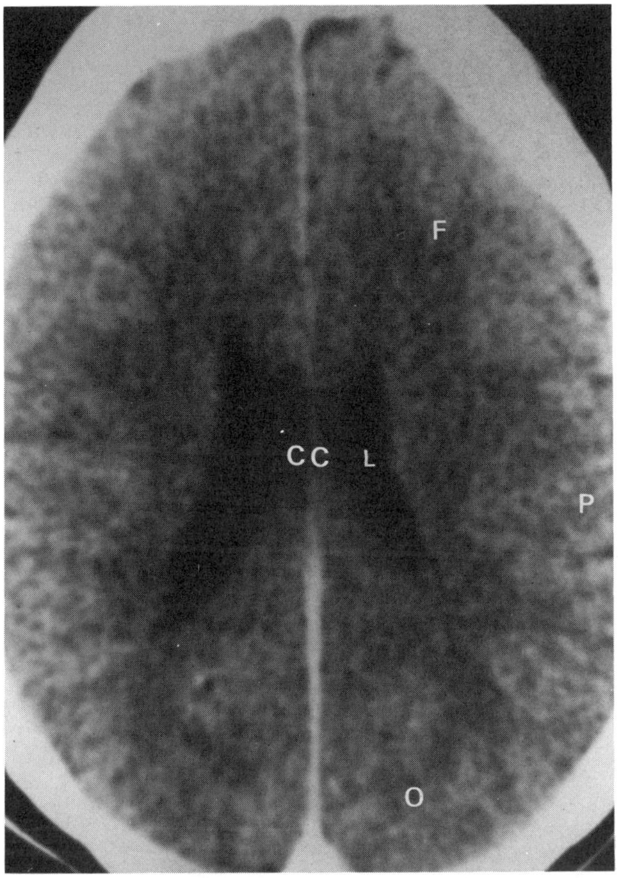

E

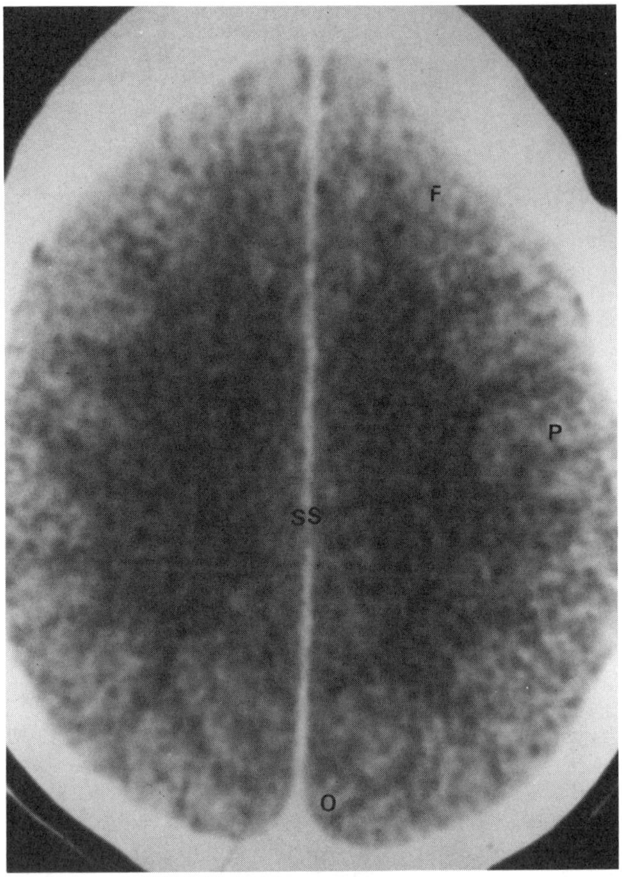

F

Fig. 23-29. Normal axial contrast-enhanced cranial CT scans at the levels of fourth ventricle **(A)**, midbrain **(B)**, third ventricle **(C)**, occipital horn of the lateral ventricles **(D)**, body of the lateral ventricles **(E)**, high convexity **(F)**. A = anterior cerebral artery; AC = anterior communicating artery; B = basilar artery; C = internal carotid artery; c = cerebellum; CC = corpus callosum; CN = caudate nucleus; E = external capsule; F = frontal lobe; f = fornix; I = internal capsule; In = insula; L = body of lateral ventricle; Lf = frontal horn of lateral ventricle; Lo = occipital horn of lateral ventricle; M = middle cerebral artery; MB = midbrain; O = optic chiasm; P = parietal lobe; s = sylvian fissure; SS = superior sagittal sinus; T = temporal lobe; t = temporal horn of lateral ventricle; Th = thalamus; u = uncus; 3 = third ventricle; 4 = fourth ventricle.

it is usually absent. If there is any residual mass beyond day 25, brain tumor should be suspected.

Following contrast administration, a lack or paucity of enhancement in the affected cortical region suggests an infarct. Abnormal enhancement seldom occurs before the third day of ictus; its presence becomes rapidly more likely during the third week but is unusual during or after the second month. Gyral (Fig. 23-38A) or basal ganglia enhancement (Fig. 23-38B) may be seen in infarct enhancement patterns. The patterns of enhancement are nonspecific, and contrast medium may be neurotoxic and vasotoxic in patients with acute cerebral infarct if the iodine dosage exceeds 42 g [84].

Nontraumatic Intracranial Hemorrhage. CT is very sensitive for the detection of intracranial hemorrhage. It can be used to determine the cause of bleeding as well as to monitor the progression or resolution of the bleeding. This section reviews CT findings in intracranial hemorrhage from a variety of causes. Rupture of an intracranial aneurysm can produce subarachnoid, ventricular, or parenchymal hemorrhage (or all three) and occasionally subdural hematoma. Nonenhanced CT can show blood in the subarachnoid space (Fig. 23-39), the ventricular system, the brain parenchyma, and the subdural space; it can also demonstrate complications from aneurysmal rupture, such as communicating hydrocephalus and dila-

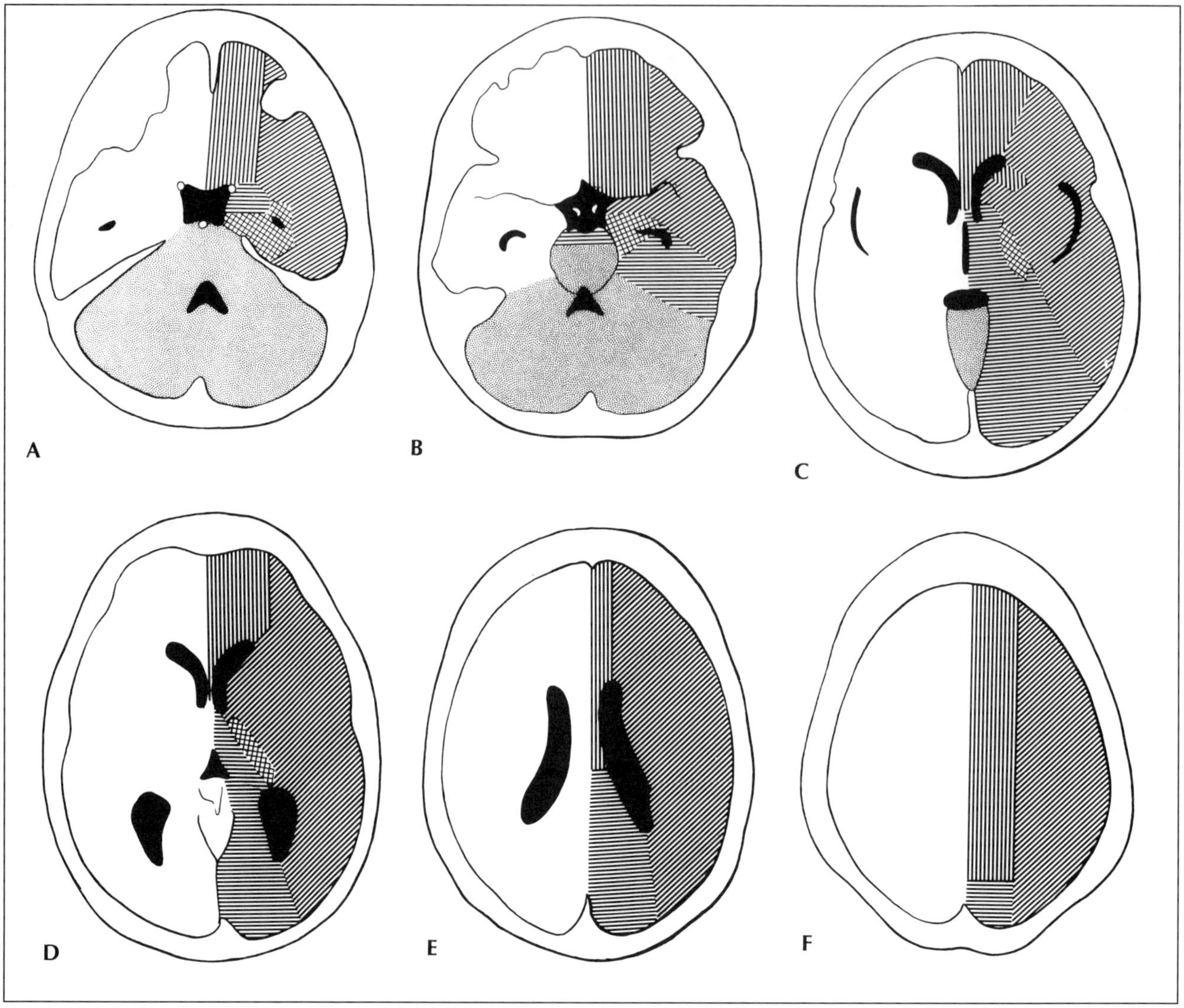

Fig. 23-30. Axial views corresponding to Fig. 23-29, at the levels of the fourth ventricle **(A)**, midbrain **(B)**, third ventricle **(C)**, occipital horn of lateral ventricle **(D)**, body of lateral ventricle **(E)**, and high convexity **(F)**. Vertical shading = anterior cerebral artery; diagonal shading = middle cerebral artery; horizontal shading = posterior cerebral artery; cross-hatching = anterior choroid artery; dotted areas = basilar artery and its branches.

tation of the ventricles, infarction due to vascular spasm, mass effect, and edema. If a patient is suspected of having a ruptured aneurysm, a baseline nonenhanced cranial CT scan should be obtained as soon as possible. This usually locates the rupture and confirms the diagnosis by demonstrating high-density subarachnoid blood. If CT shows a subarachnoid hemorrhage, then a lumbar puncture is not necessary; if it shows hydrocephalus and mass effect from intracerebral hematoma, lumbar puncture should be avoided. The detection of blood in the subarachnoid space depends on the volume and the duration of hemorrhage and the patient's hemoglobin value [85]. Despite CT's sensitivity for detection of blood, 25 percent of subarachnoid hemorrhages detected by lumbar puncture from ruptured aneurysm are not detectable on CT scan.

The location of the bulk of the subarachnoid hemorrhage and associated intracerebral hematoma or intraventricular hemorrhage may suggest the site of the broken aneurysm [86]. It helps the selection of the artery to catheterize first during an arteriogram. Rupture of a posterior fossa aneurysm seldom produces visible blood in the suprasellar and sylvian fissure cisterns. For example, rupture of supratentorial aneurysm results in a widespread distribution of blood in the subarachnoid spaces [87].

If a pial or pial-dural AVM bleeds, the parenchymal hemorrhage must be peripheral. Contrast-enhanced CT scan may show prominent vessels (draining vein and feeding artery) (Fig. 23-40). The AVM may appear as an enhancing mass that mimics a tumor. A cryptic AVM may bleed into the parenchyma and may have no abnormal enhancement and a normal cerebral angiogram. If the AVM is ependymal, the hemorrhage may be confined to

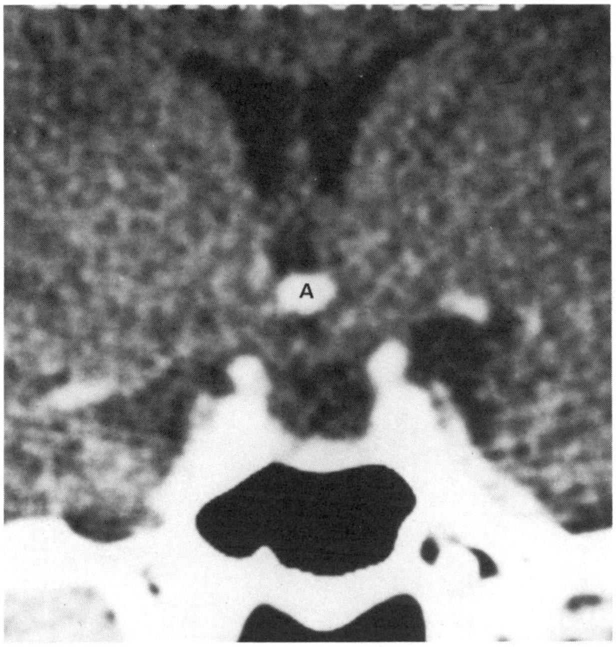

A

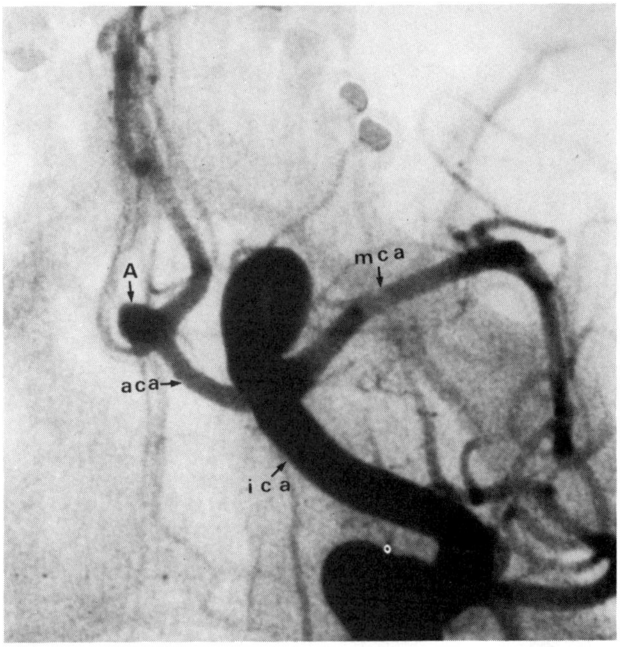

B

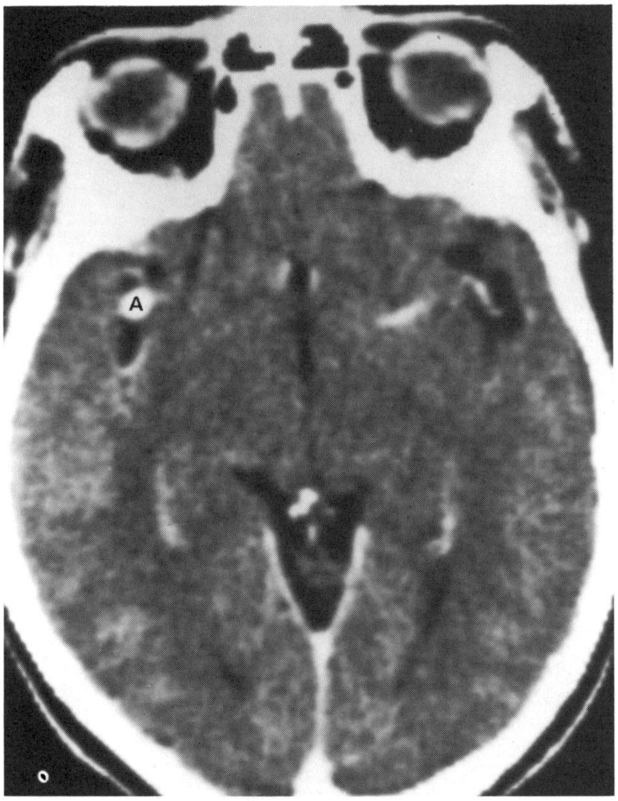

C

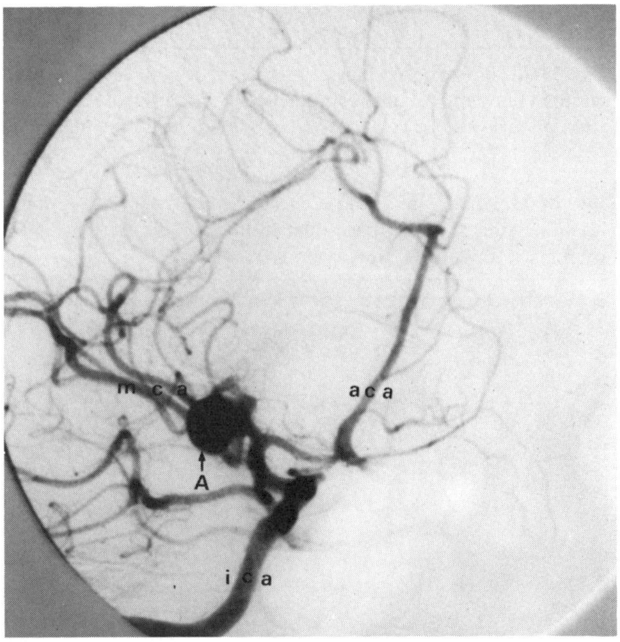

D

Fig. 23-31. Aneurysms of anterior communicating and middle cerebral arteries. **A**. Direct contrast-enhanced coronal cranial CT demonstrating a 5-mm-diameter anterior communicating artery aneurysm (A). **B**. Basal view of left internal carotid arteriogram demonstrating an anterior communicating artery aneurysm (A), which was seen on CT scan. (ACA = anterior cerebral artery; MCA = middle cerebral artery; ICA = internal carotid artery.) **C**. Axial contrast-enhanced cranial CT demonstrating an 8-mm aneurysm at the right middle cerebral artery trifurcation (A). **D**. Frontal projection of the right internal carotid arteriogram confirmed the right middle cerebral artery (MCA) trifurcation aneurysm (A).

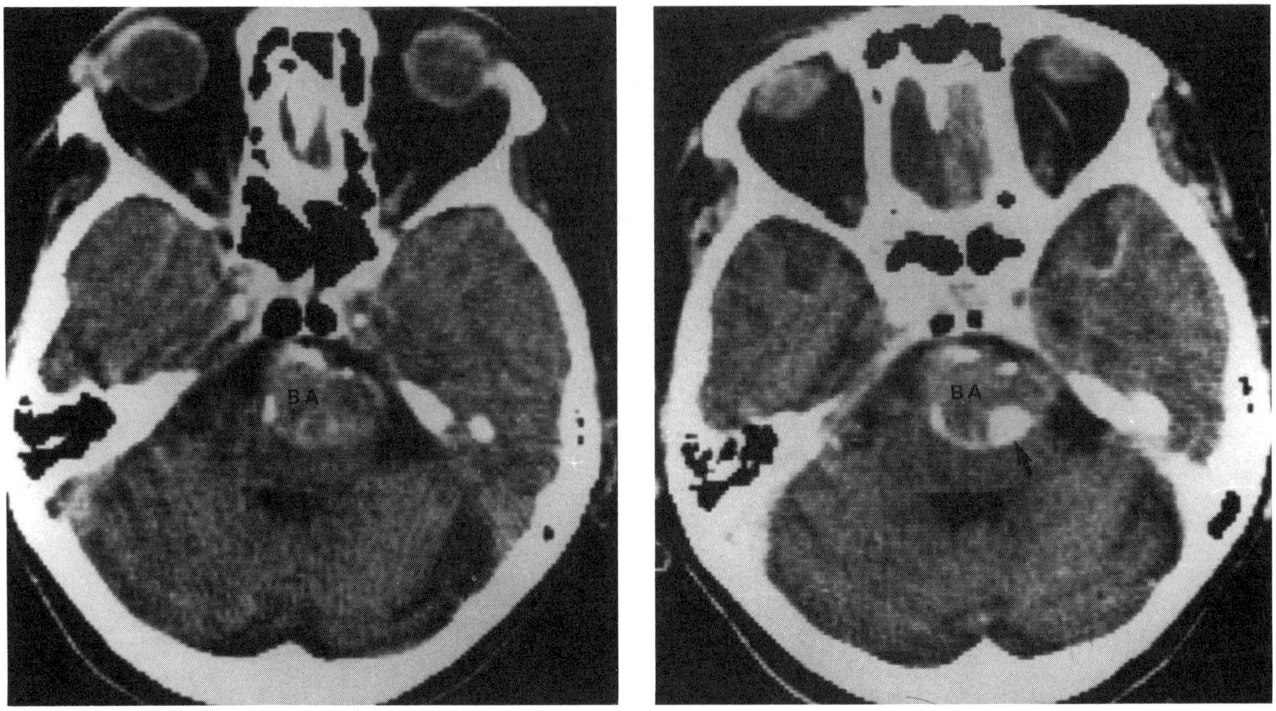

A B

Fig. 23-32. Thrombosed basilar artery aneurysm. Axial cranial CT scan without **A**. and with **B**. IV contrast showing a bull's-eye persistent lumen (arrow) in a calcified thrombosed basilar artery (BA) aneurysm.

Fig. 23-33. Aneurysm of the internal carotid artery. **A**. Axial contrast-enhanced cranial CT showing an enhancing mass (A) parasellar in location on the right. **B**. Right internal carotid angiogram demonstrating a large aneurysm (A).

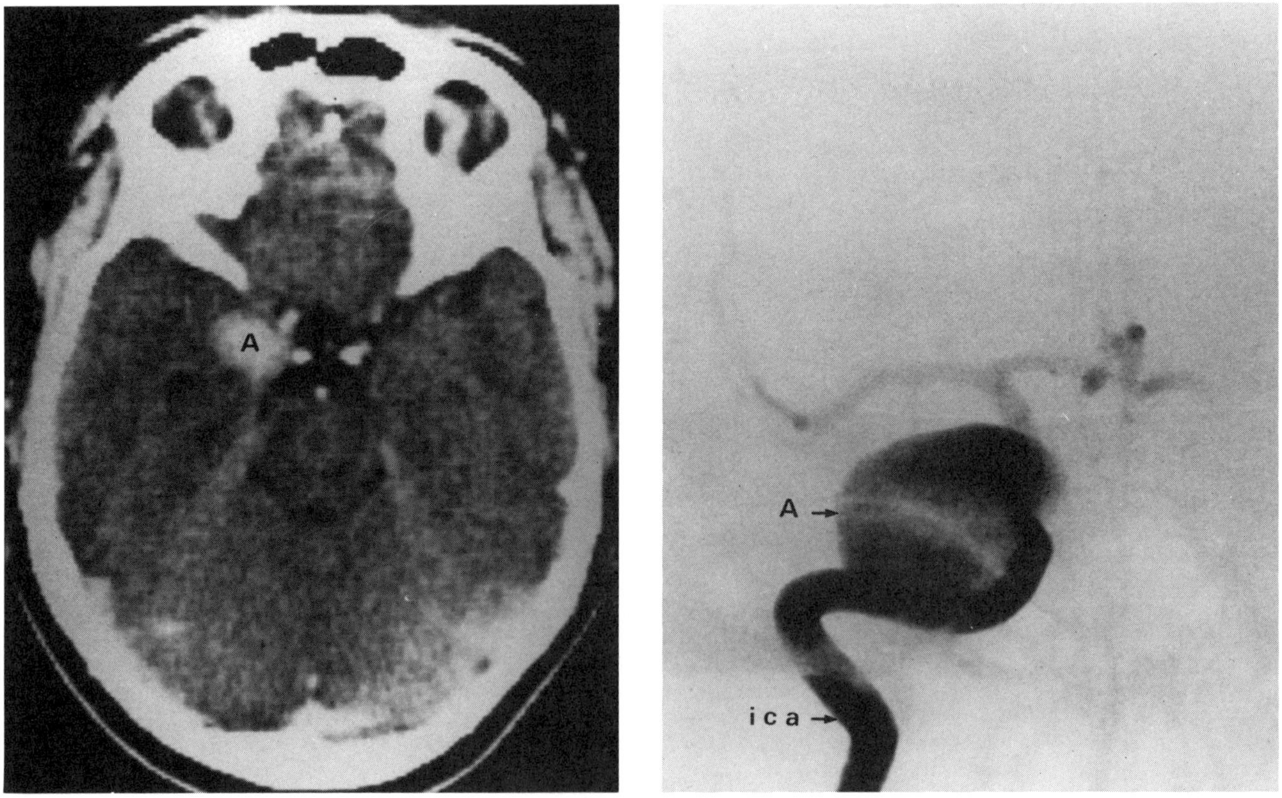

A B

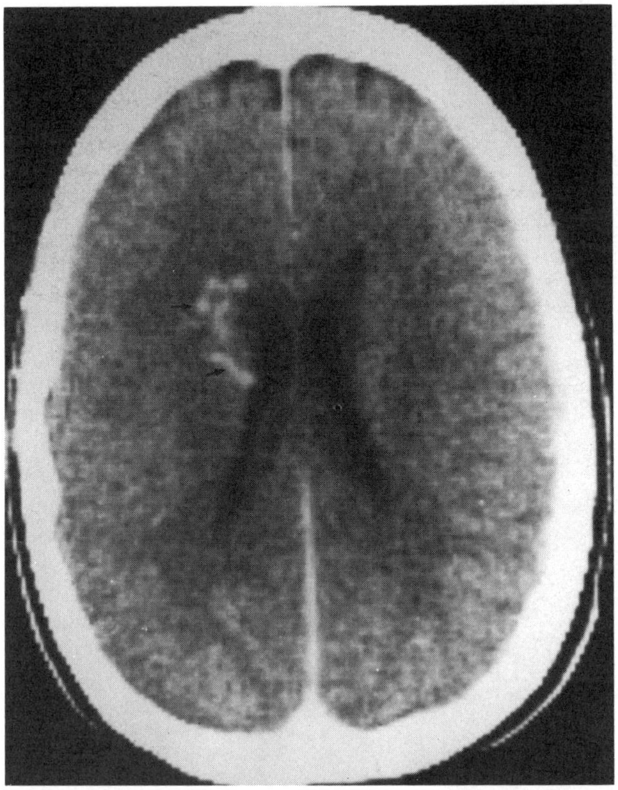

A

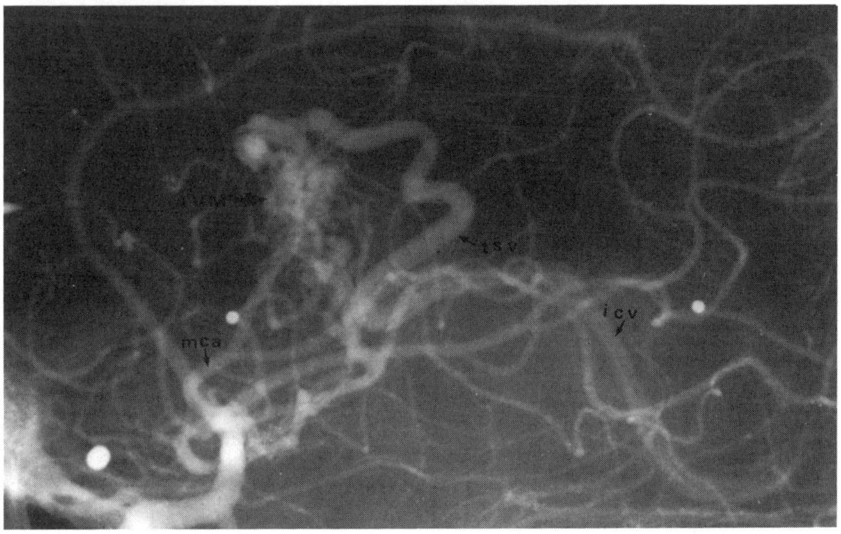

B

Fig. 23-34. Arteriovenous malformation (AVM). **A**. Contrast-enhanced CT shows AVM presented as prominent vessels in the right deep frontal region and medial basal ganglia (arrows). **B**. Right internal carotid angiogram shows the AVM fed by the middle cerebral artery (MCA) and drained into thalamostriate (TSV) and internal cerebral veins (ICV).

the ventricular system or extend into the adjacent parenchyma. Venous angiomas and cavernous hemangiomas may also occasionally bleed.

Hypertensive cerebral hemorrhage is a catastrophic event; it is usually massive and commonly involves the basal ganglia and thalamus. Intraventricular extension is common. Another common site is the dentate nucleus of the cerebellum [88]. When CT is performed immediately after ictus, the high-density area can be readily demonstrated (Fig. 23-41).

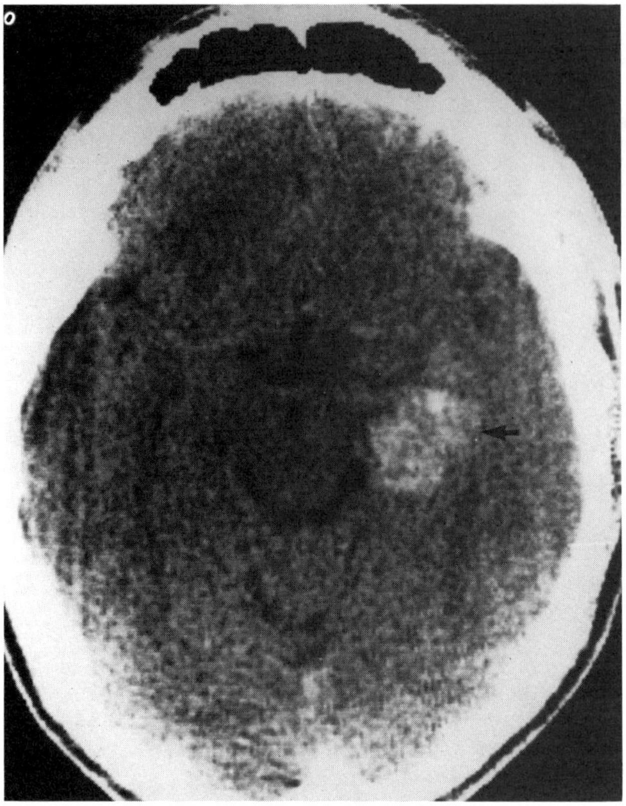

Fig. 23-35. Contrast-enhancing CT scan showing a high-density mass in the right medial temporal lobe with mild enhancement. The angiogram was normal. At surgery, a cavernous hemangioma was found (arrow).

Low-birth-weight newborns have a high incidence of germinal matrix hemorrhage [89], which has been divided into four categories. Grade 1 hemorrhage is limited to the germinal matrix (subependymal hemorrhage); grade 2 extends into the ventricles; grade 3 extends into ventricles with ventricular dilatation. Grade 4 implies germinal matrix and diffuse cerebral parenchymal hemorrhage. The prognosis is related to the grade of hemorrhage. CT scan can demonstrate blood in the germinal matrix, ventricles, or cerebral parenchyma; evaluate the size of the ventricle; and monitor response to therapy.

Primary brain tumors as well as metastases (especially melanoma and carcinoma of the lung) may bleed. The hemorrhage is detectable on noncontrast-enhanced CT, and enhanced scans may show tumor enhancement surrounding the parenchymal hemorrhage.

Six percent of patients with clinically diagnosed cerebral infarcts may have **hemorrhagic** infarcts, which appear to be formed by coalescence areas of petechial bleeding. The shape of this hemorrhage may mirror that of specific cerebral arteries. The combination of hyperdensity to the cerebral cortex with hypodensity localized in the adjacent white matter may be reasonably specific for hemorrhagic infarct (Fig. 23-42A). Parenchymal hemorrhage in the territory of ischemic infarct (Fig. 23-42B) or subdural hematoma (Fig. 23-42C, D) may be seen in patients undergoing anticoagulant treatment.

Cerebral amyloidosis, toxemia, coagulopathies caused by disease or chemotherapy, decreased platelets (Fig. 23-43), and intravenous drug abuse may be associated with intracranial hemorrhage.

INTRACRANIAL VEINS

Cerebral Venous Angiomas. Cerebral venous angiomas represent a rare intracranial vascular malformation in which a collection of abnormal vessels lacks normal quantities of smooth muscle or elastic tissue. Their walls are composed of fibrous connective tissue with a flat endothelium. Their feeding arteries are not increased in number or size. The characteristic angiographic findings are those of a radiating collection of medullary veins deep within the brain parenchyma, draining centrally into one or several large veins and terminating in a superficial cortical vein or dural sinus (Fig. 23-44). It is possible to recognize bleeding from a cerebral venous angioma on a plain CT scan. Contrast-enhanced scans often show a focal round or linear density corresponding to the angioma (see Fig. 23-44). Other CT signs may include an increase in brain parenchymal density (common) secondary to intravascular blood in the myriad of medullary veins or a large draining vein in the sylvian fissure [90].

Aneurysm of Galen's Vein. Aneurysm of Galen's vein is actually a misnomer describing a large arteriovenous fistula involving Galen's vein. CT scan may show obstructive hydrocephalus and a large, high-density midline mass with dense enhancement in the vicinity of Galen's vein.

Cerebral Venous Occlusive Disease. Venous occlusion can have a wide variety of causes, including trauma, infection, tumors (primary or metastatic), pregnancy and puerperium, oral contraceptive use, severe dehydration, acute right-heart failure, and some hematologic disorders (such as disseminated intravascular coagulation, sickle-cell disease, and leukemia) [91,92].

CT findings for cerebral venous occlusion include the following [93]:

1. Visualization of the thrombosed cortical vein ("cord sign") (Fig. 23-45A); this vein may show enhancement because of perivenous, localized blood-brain barrier breakdown or intramural inflammation of the vein wall.
2. Superior sagittal sinus thrombosis presented as "empty triangle," or "delta sign" (Fig. 23-45B). A low density in the sinus is seen, attributable to the thrombosed sinus surrounded by the collateral circulation of the parasagittal dural venous plexus.
3. Multiple bilateral parasagittal hemorrhagic foci or solitary parenchymal hematoma.
4. Intense tentorial enhancement, gyral enhancement, or both.
5. Severe brain edema.
6. Normal CT scan.

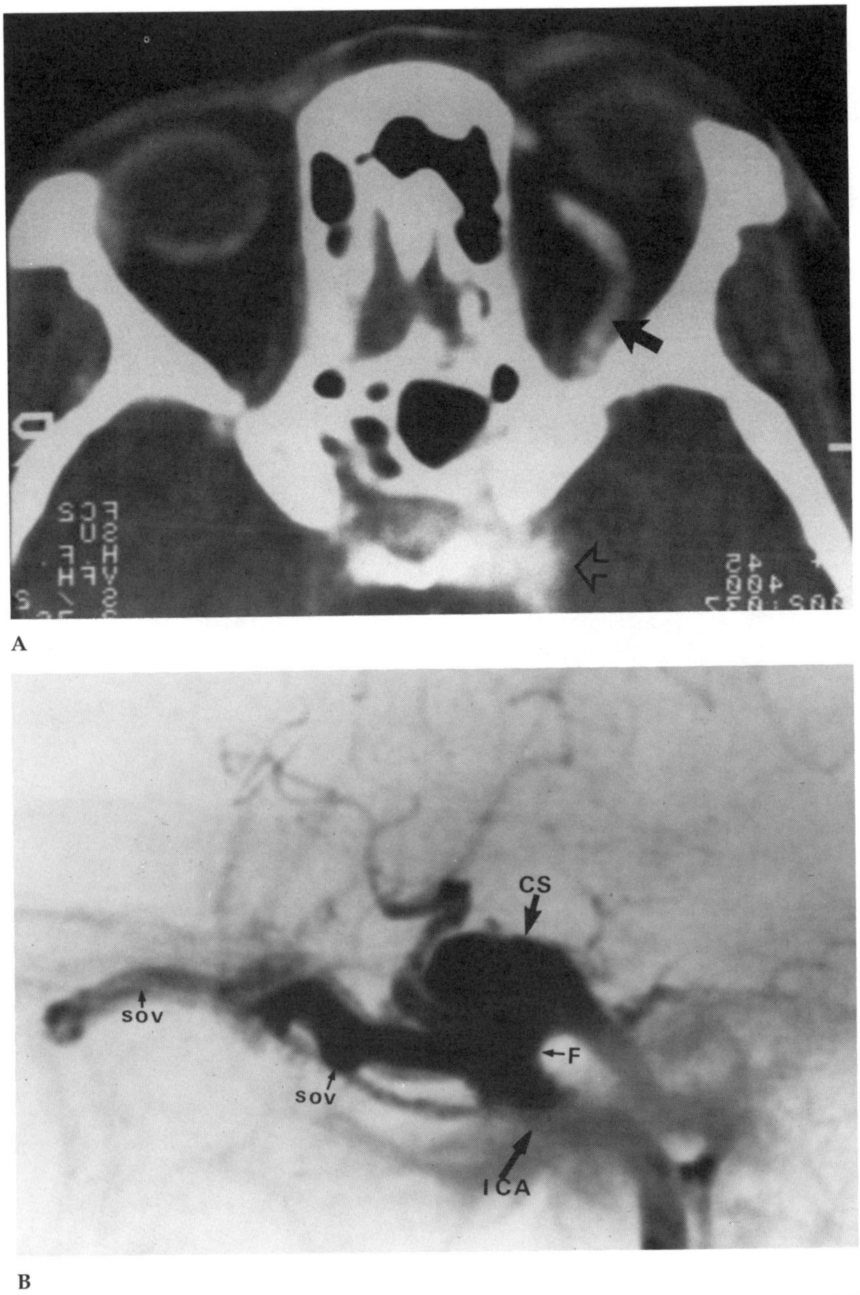

Fig. 23-36. Carotid cavernous fistula. **A**. Contrast-enhanced CT scan demonstrating enlarged left cavernous sinus (open arrow) and superior ophthalmic vein (arrow). **B**. Lateral view of the left internal carotid (ICA) arteriogram demonstrating carotid cavernous sinus (CS) fistula (F) and the enlarged superior ophthalmic vein (SOV).

Internal jugular vein thrombosis may be seen in patients with septic thrombophlebitis. It may also result from central venous catheterization, compression of the internal jugular vein by abscess or tumor of the head and neck, or oral contraceptive use following intravenous drug injection directly into the internal jugular vein [94]. The characteristic CT finding is enlargement of the thrombosed internal jugular vein, which is seen to have a low-density lumen and sharply enhanced wall (Fig. 23-46).

INTRACRANIAL PERFUSION

Rapid-sequence dynamic CT is performed by state-of-the-art CT scanners. Contrast medium is injected as a compact bolus through an 18-gauge catheter in a large antecubital vein; multiple images of the same preselected levels are

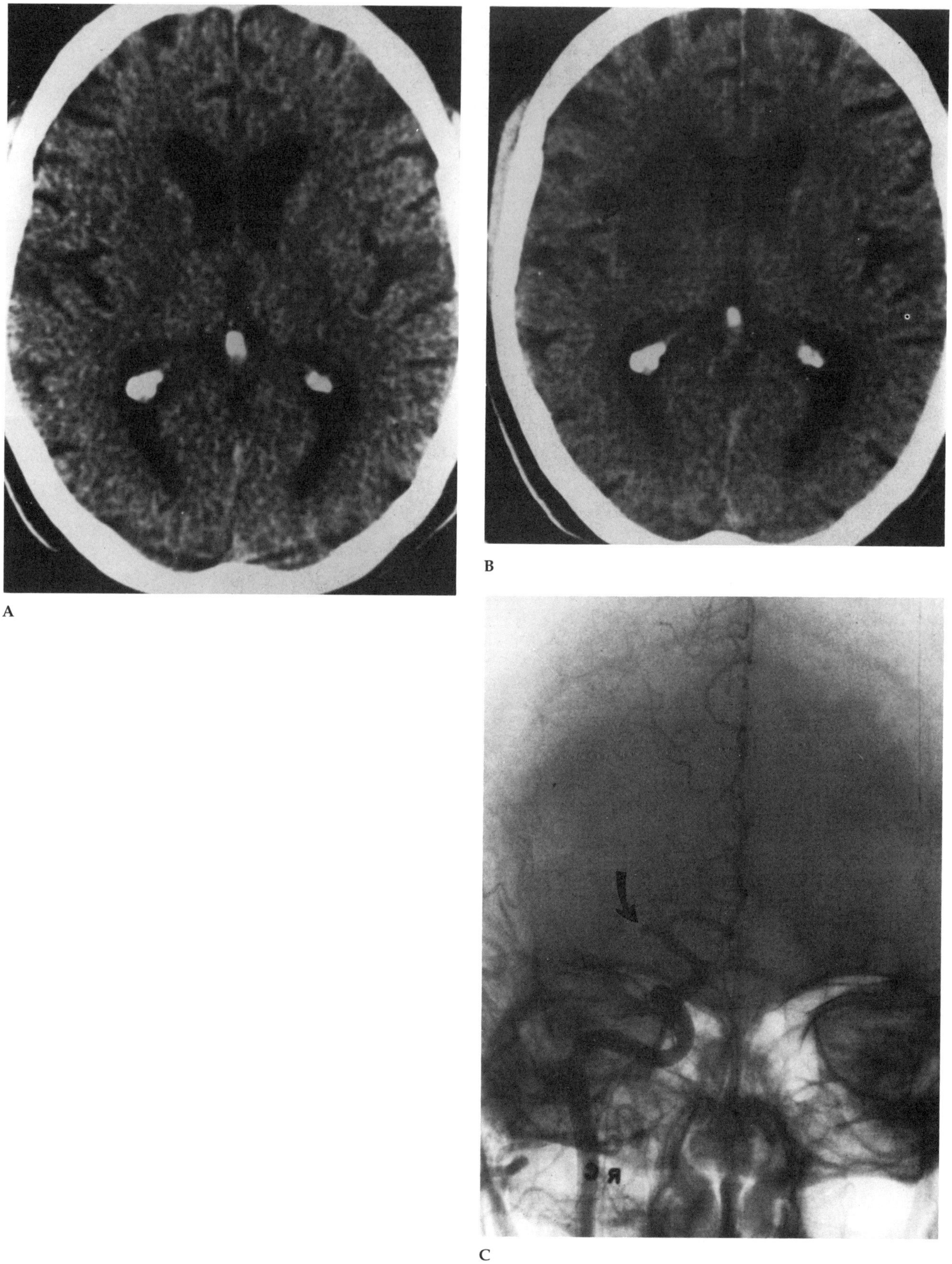

A

B

C

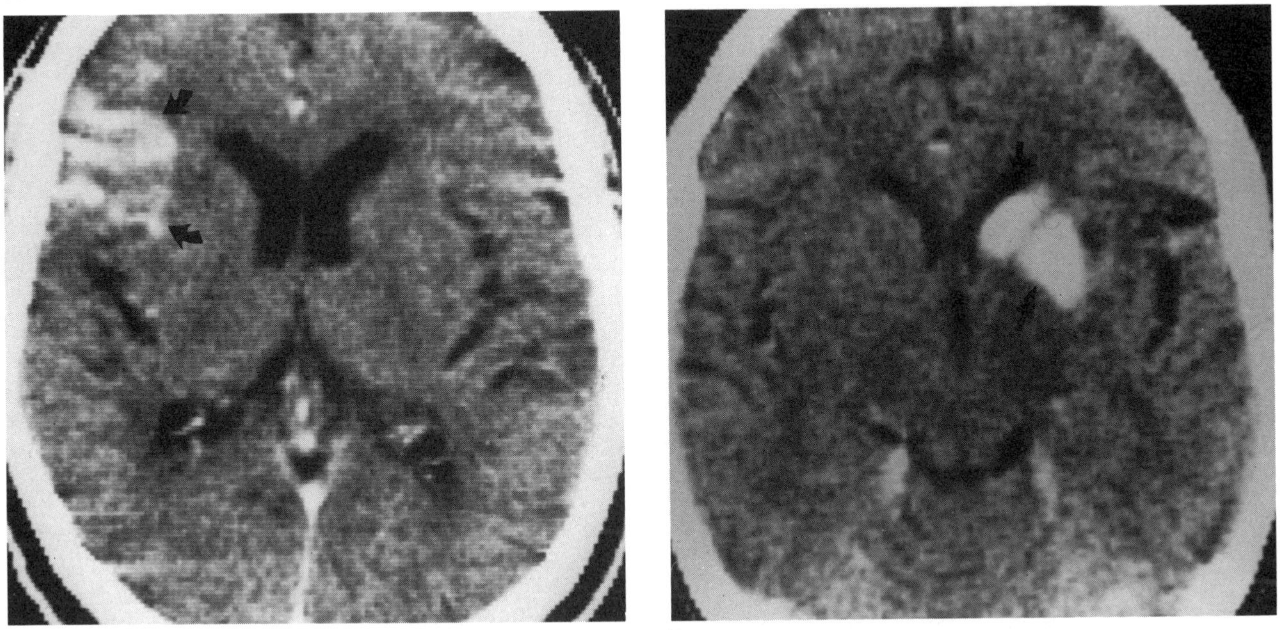

A B

Fig. 23-38. Ischemic stroke-enhancing pattern. **A.** Contrast-enhanced CT showing gyri enhancement in the right frontal ischemic infarct at 20 days after the ictus. **B.** Contrast-enhanced CT demonstrating an enhancement (arrows) in the left caudate nucleus and putamen, caused by an ischemic infarct sparing the internal capsule, at 16 days after the ictus.

then obtained with minimum interscan delay (1.5 to 6.5 seconds). The transit pattern of contrast media in a vascular structure is displayed as a contrast density-time flow graph, consisting of rapid wash-in, peak, and wash-out phases [95,96]. Dynamic CT may predict the patency of the cervical internal carotid artery, differentiate an intracranial giant aneurysm from intracranial tumor, differentiate a parasellar aneurysm from a pituitary tumor, and demonstrate anatomic details (encasement of vessels or the location of vascular structures on the edges of the lesions).

However, since the tight junction of the endothelial cells in the cerebral capillaries restricts passage of many materials through the blood-brain barrier, most of the clinically available contrast media do not freely cross this barrier. This means that although rapid-sequence CT scanning using intravenous iodinated contrast medium can be used to determine total cerebral blood flow, flow through regions of the brain parenchyma cannot be determined quantitatively. Cerebral perfusion and metabolism can be quantitatively studied either by single-photon-emission computed tomography (SPECT) or by positron-emission tomography (PET).

Stable Xenon-Enhanced CT. The stable xenon-enhanced (Xe-enhanced) CT study is based on the time-dependent changes in density of brain tissue on CT that occur while the patient breathes and then stops breathing a mixture of nonradioactive xenon gas and oxygen or a mixture of xenon and air. A baseline cranial scan is obtained at each selected level, and then four to six Xe-enhanced cranial CT scans are obtained during a 4- to 6-minute inhalation period. The baseline CT images are subtracted from the Xe-enhanced CT images. The buildup and wash-out of xenon in the brain can be appreciated as a function of the measured enhancement of the CT images. Two- or three-dimensional cerebral blood-flow mapping can be obtained [97]. This technique may be useful clinically for study and diagnosis of ischemic cerebral vascular disease, head trauma, brain death, seizure disorders, and degenerative CNS disease. The high-resolution flow maps from an anatomic cross-section can be displayed beside the routine CT image for direct comparison.

Summary

CT has come a long way since its advent a little more than 20 years ago. Technically, it has evolved from first-

Fig. 23-37. Acute middle cerebral artery stroke CT scans at 4 hours **A.** and 26 hours **B.** **A.** Normal CT scan. **B.** Low-density infarct involving the right basal ganglia with mass effect on the frontal horn of the right lateral ventricle. **C.** Right internal carotid arteriogram demonstrates occlusion of the proximal portion of M1 segment of the right middle cerebral artery (curved arrow).

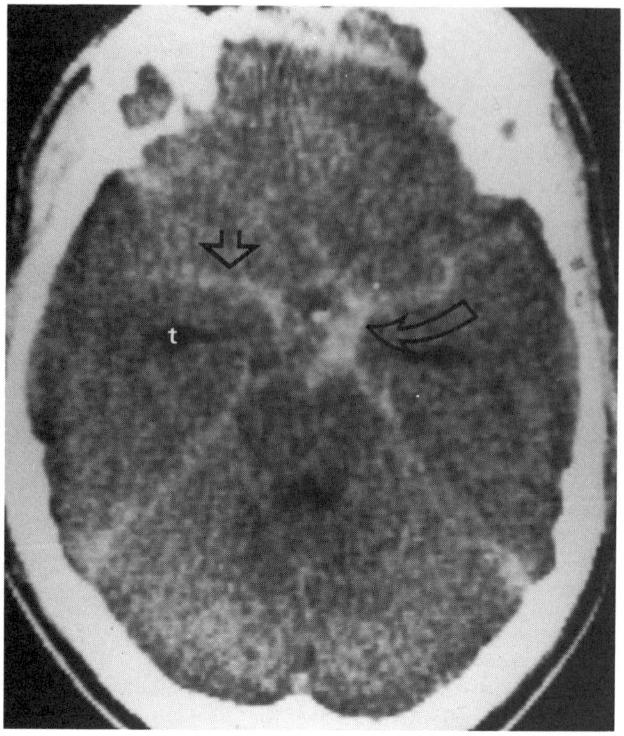

A

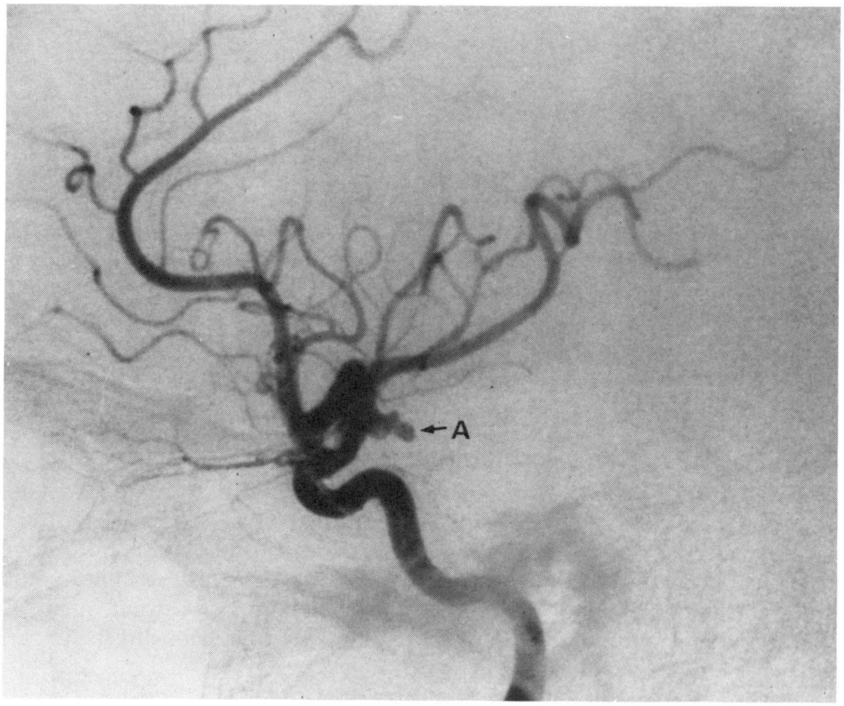

B

Fig. 23-39. Ruptured aneurysm. **A**. Nonenhanced cranial CT scan demonstrates high attenuation, representing blood in the suprasellar cistern (curved arrow) and the sylvian fissure cistern (open arrow) and dilatation of the temporal horns (t). **B**. Arteriogram of the left internal carotid demonstrating an aneurysm (A) originating from the origin of the posterior communicating artery with irregular contour, suggesting rupture.

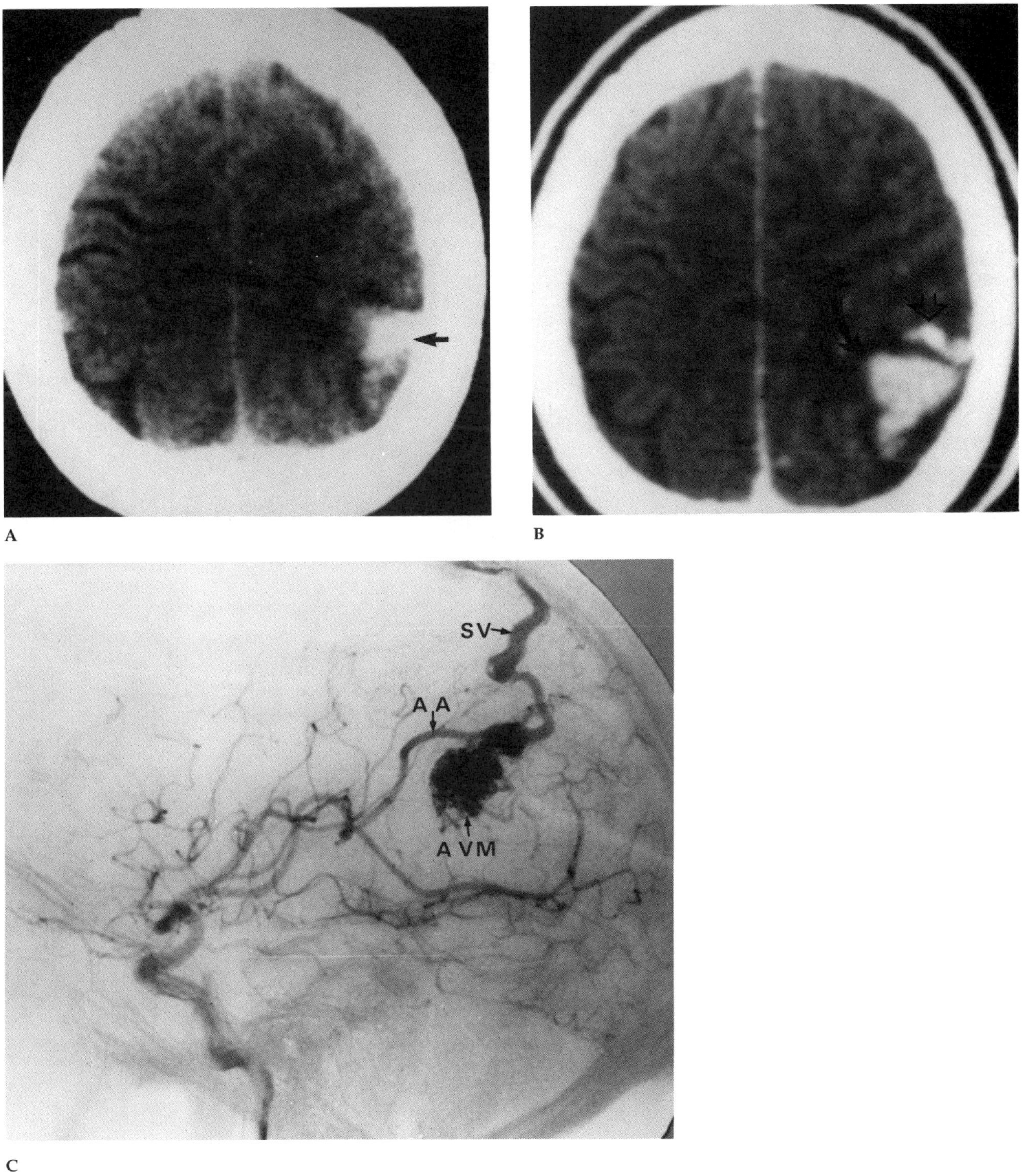

Fig. 23-40. Arteriovenous malformation presenting with cerebral hemorrhage. **A**. Nonenhanced CT demonstrates cerebral hematoma (arrow) in the angular gyrus of the left parietal lobe. **B**. Contrast-enhanced CT scan demonstrates linear enhancement (open arrow) anterior to the hematoma (curved arrow), representing dilated vein. **C**. Lateral view of the left internal carotid arteriogram demonstrates AVM fed by the dilated angular artery (AA) and draining to a superficial cortical vein (SV) entering superior sagittal sinus.

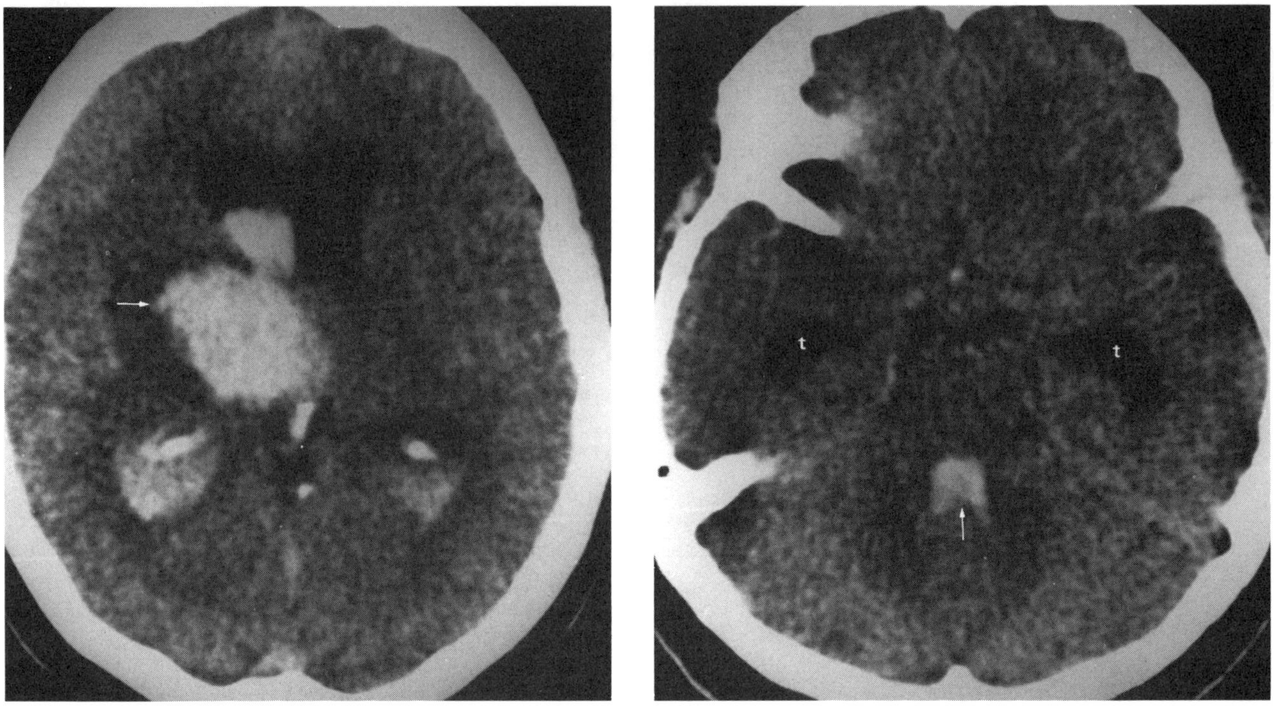

A B

Fig. 23-41. Hypertensive hemorrhage. **A**. CT scans of a hypertensive patient with sudden onset of headache and progressive unresponsiveness. An extensive hemorrhage in right basal ganglia (arrow) with severe mass effect on the right lateral ventricle and the third ventricle, with midline shift to the left. Hemorrhage extending to third ventricle and in the lateral ventricle. **B**. Blood clot in the fourth ventricle (arrow) and marked dilatation of the temporal horn of the lateral ventricles (t).

generation scanners that required 4- to 5-minute exposure times to subsecond electron-beam systems and spiral CT. CT has had a significant impact on medical practice in many areas, such as the CNS and the mediastinum. Diseases of the vascular system are studied well by CT. In some situations, CT has replaced other imaging modalities. On the other hand, CT's role in the evaluation of conditions such as aortic rupture remains controversial. Furthermore, because of technical factors, CT has failed to play a significant role in the evaluation of coronary artery disease. Tissue perfusion is another area where CT has played only a limited role. Although rapid-sequence enhanced CT can be utilized to study changes in contrast density that should reflect perfusion in specific tissues, technical factors have prevented wide use of CT in that field.

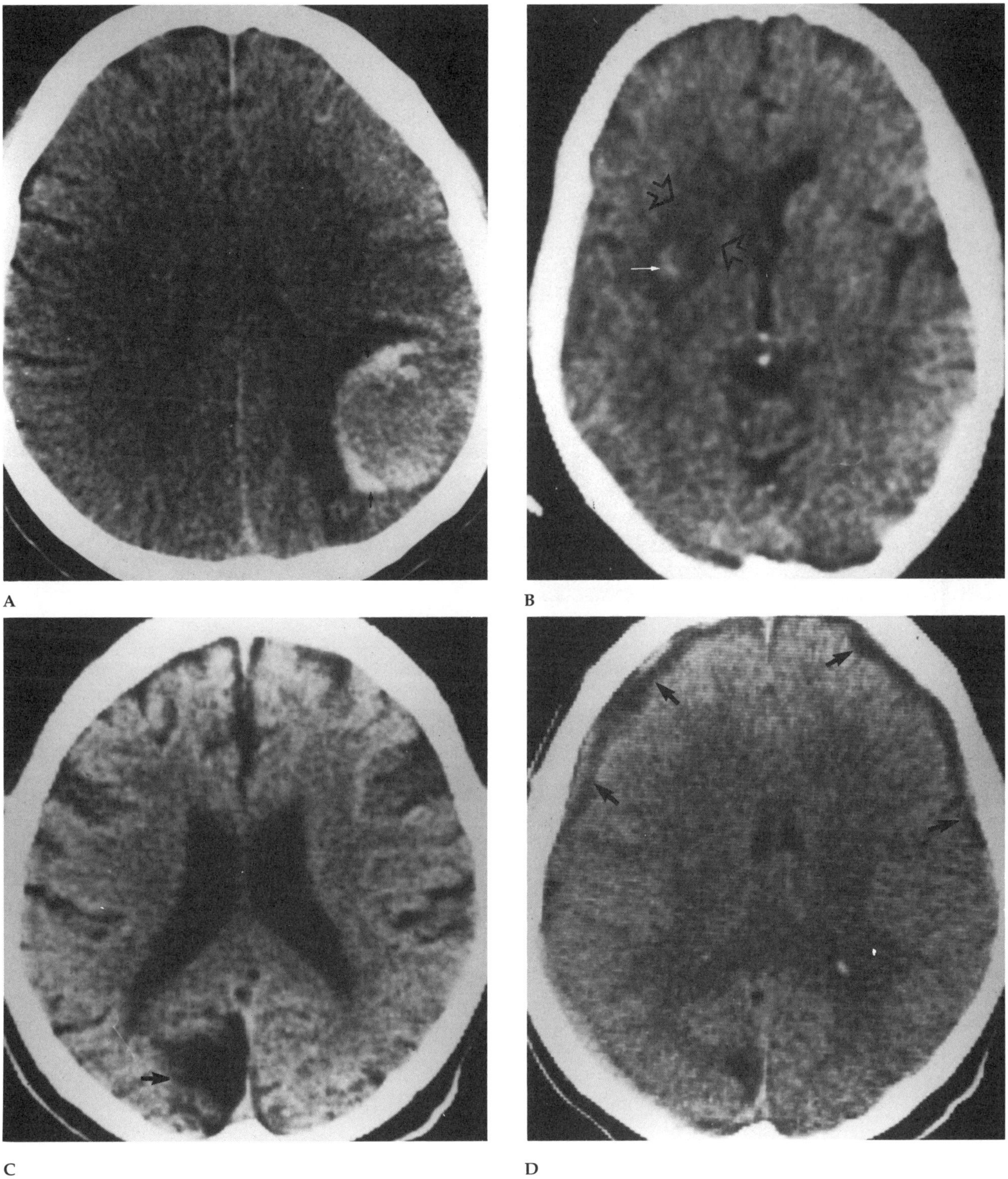

Fig. 23-42. Cerebral hemorrhage. **A**. CT scan showing hemorrhagic infarct (arrows) in the left parieto-occipital lobe. **B**. CT scan showing hemorrhage (arrow) in the patient with ischemic infarct (open arrows) in the right basal ganglia after patient treated with heparin. **C**. In the patient with right occipital lobe ischemic infarct (arrow) treated with coumadin. **D**. CT scan showing subdural hematoma (arrows).

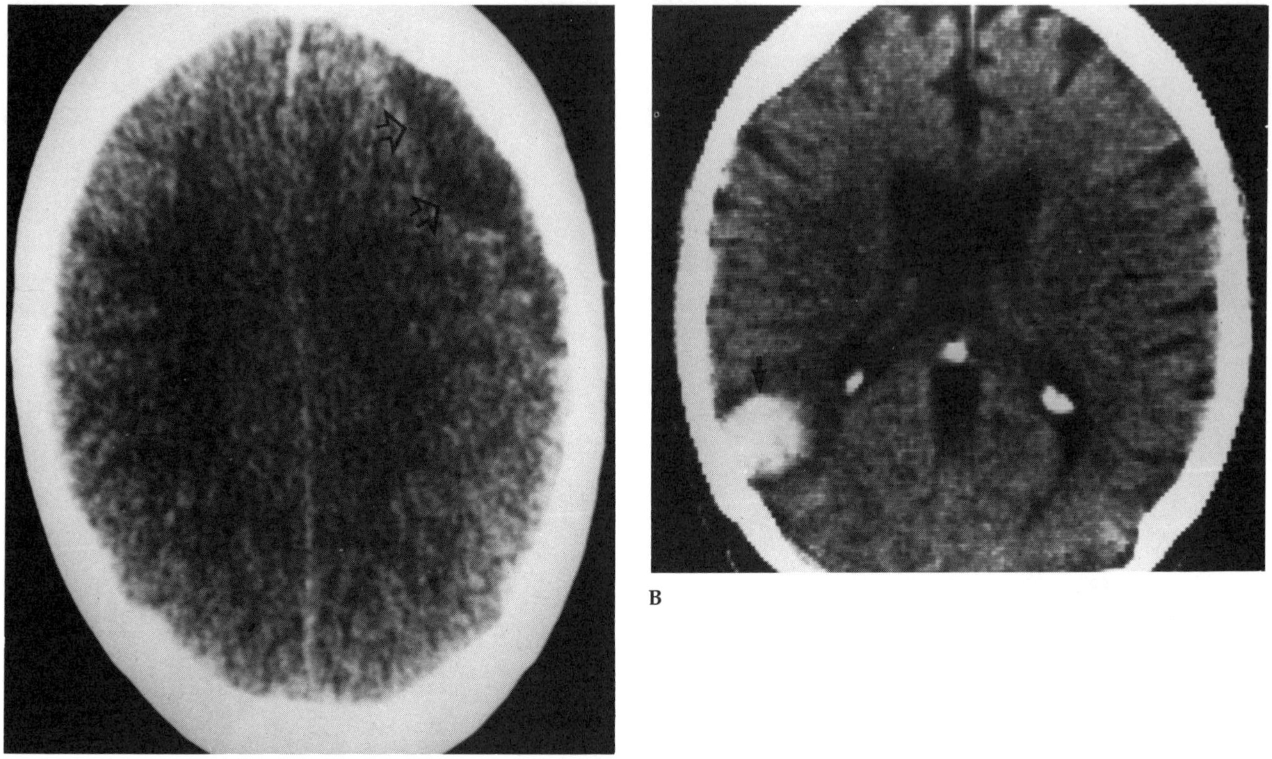

A

B

Fig. 23-43. Subdural and cerebral hemorrhage complicating chemotherapy. Patients with acute myelogenous leukemia received chemotherapy with significant decrease of platelets producing **A**. left frontal SDH (open arrows), **B**. parenchymal hemorrhage (arrow) in the right parieto-occipital region.

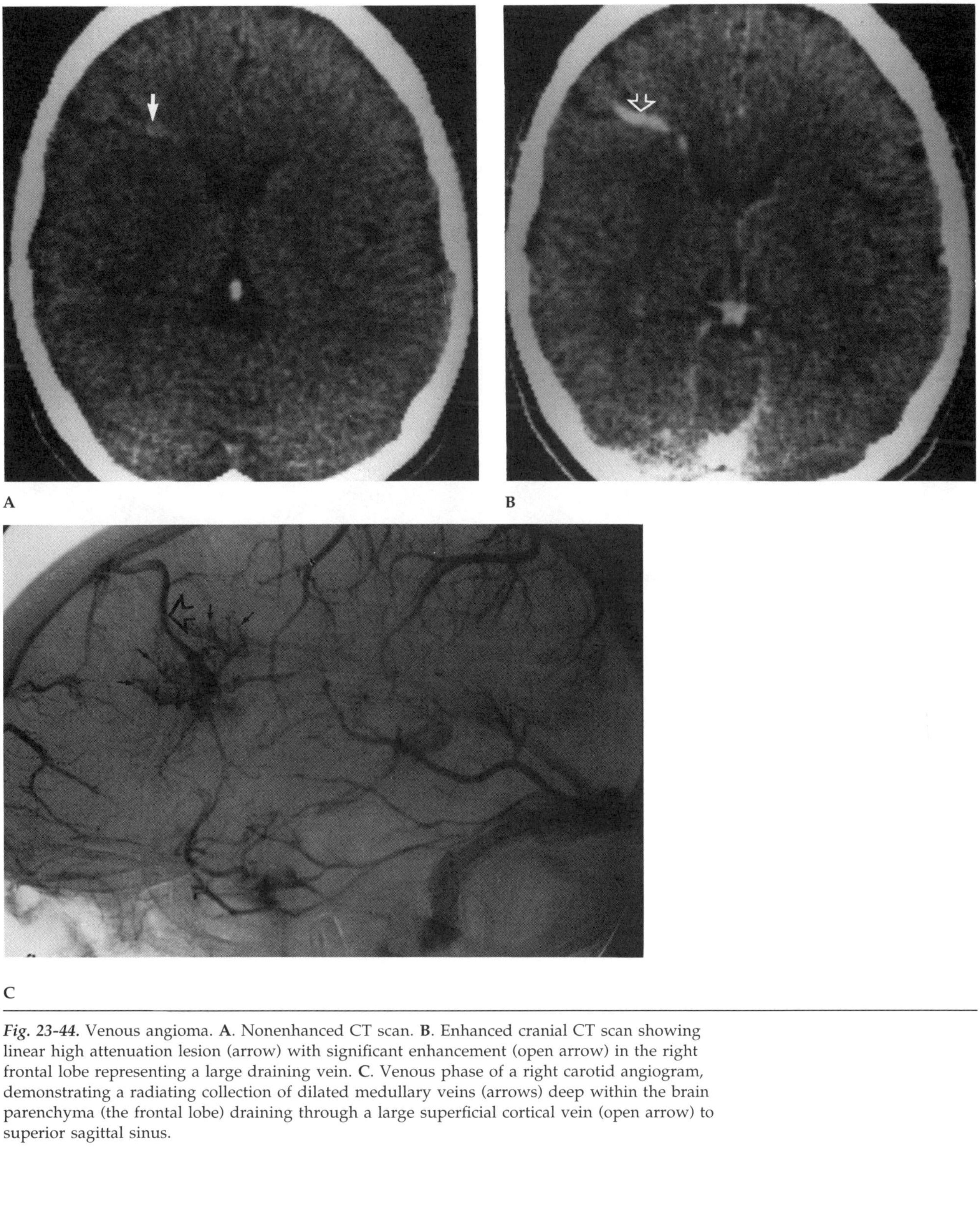

Fig. 23-44. Venous angioma. **A**. Nonenhanced CT scan. **B**. Enhanced cranial CT scan showing linear high attenuation lesion (arrow) with significant enhancement (open arrow) in the right frontal lobe representing a large draining vein. **C**. Venous phase of a right carotid angiogram, demonstrating a radiating collection of dilated medullary veins (arrows) deep within the brain parenchyma (the frontal lobe) draining through a large superficial cortical vein (open arrow) to superior sagittal sinus.

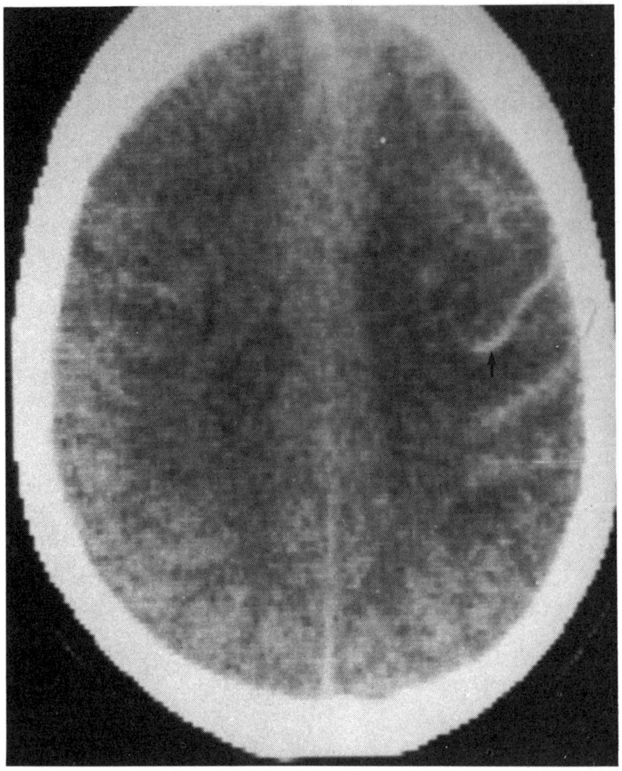

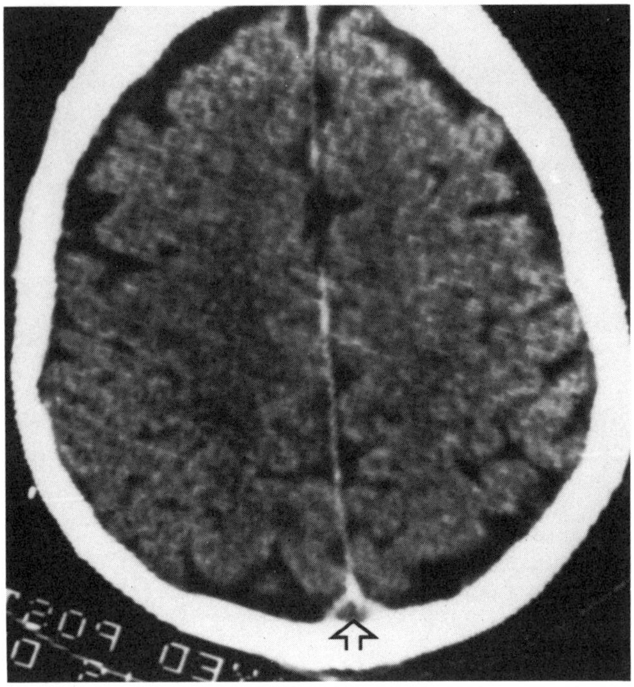

B

A

Fig. 23-45. Venous thrombosis. **A**. Nonenhanced CT scan demonstrating thrombosed cortical vein (arrow), and diffuse severe brain edema. **B**. Contrast-enhanced CT scan demonstrating an empty triangle sign (open arrow) in the posterior superior sagittal sinus, which was confirmed by cerebral angiogram as a thrombosed superior sagittal sinus.

Fig. 23-46. Jugular vein thrombosis. **A**. Nonenhanced axial CT of neck demonstrates enlarged internal jugular vein (arrow). **B**. Contrast-enhanced axial CT of neck demonstrates dilated internal jugular vein with sharply enhanced wall (arrows) and low density within the lumen (thrombosis). **C**. Coronal computer reformatted image demonstrates the whole length of the thrombosed internal jugular vein (arrows).

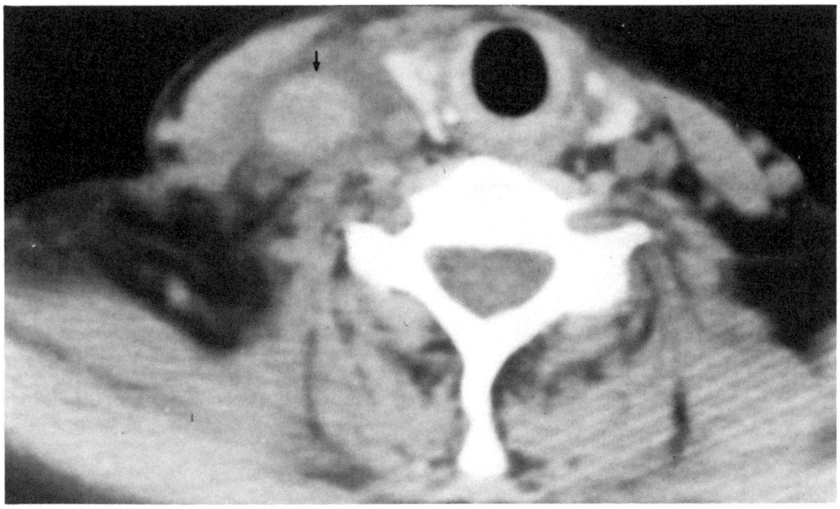

A

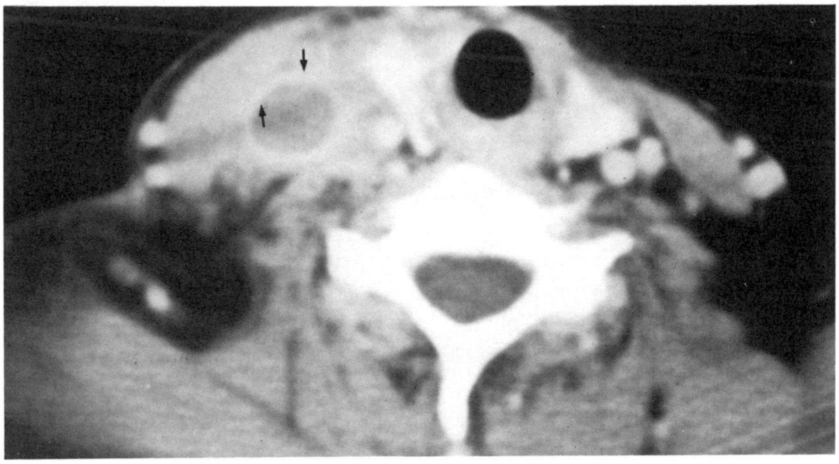

B

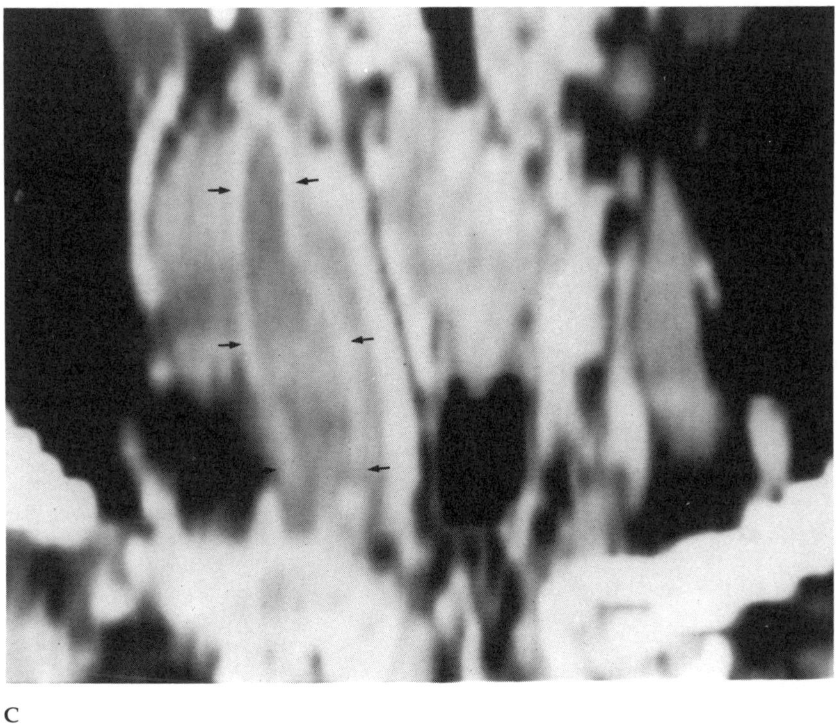

C

References

1. Hounsfield GN. Computed medical imaging. Nobel lecture, December 8, 1979. J Comput Assist Tomogr 1980; 4:665-674.
2. Cormack AM. Early two-dimensional reconstruction (CT scanning) and recent topics stemming from it. Nobel lecture, December 8, 1979. J Comput Assist Tomogr 1980; 4:658–664.
3. Curry TS, Dowdey JE, Murry RC. Christinsen's Introduction to the Physics of Diagnostic Radiology. Philadelphia: Lea & Febiger, 1984. Pp. 320–350.
4. McCullough EW. Factors affecting the use of quantitative information from a CT scanner. Radiology 1977; 124:99–107.
5. Dillon DH, et al. Spiral CT angiography. AJR 1993a; 160:1273–1278.
6. Boyd DP, Lipton MJ. Cardiac computed tomography. Proc IEEE 1983; 71:298-307.
7. Tannenbaum SR, et al. Detection of calcific deposits in coronary arteries by ultrafast computed tomography and correlation with angiography. Am J Cardiol 1989; 63:870–872.
8. Kaufman RB, et al. Detection of heart calcification with electron beam CT: interobserver and intraobserver reliability for scoring quantification. Radiology 1994; 190:347–352.
9. Rubin GD, et al. Three-dimensional spiral CT angiography of the abdomen: initial clinical experience. Radiology 1993; 186:147–152.
10. Brasch RC, Boyd DP, Gooding CA. Computed tomography scanning in children: comparison of radiation dose and resolving power of commercial CT scanners. AJR 1978; 131:95–101.
11. Brasch RC, Cann CE. Computed tomographic scanning in children II: An updated comparison of radiation dose and resolving power of commercial scanners. AJR 1982; 138:127–133.
12. Shehadi WH, Toniolo G. Adverse reactions to contrast media. Radiology 1980; 137:299–302.
13. Costello P, et al. Spiral CT of the thorax with reduced volume of contrast material: A Comparative Study. Radiology 1992; 183:663–666.
14. Webb WR, et al. CT demonstration of mediastinal aortic arch anomalies. J Comput Assist Tomogr 1982; 6:445.
15. Godwin JD, et al. Evaluation of coarctation of the aorta by computed tomography. J Comput Assist Tomogr 1981; 5:153.
16. McLoughlin MJ, et al. Computed tomography in congenital anomalies of the aortic arch and great vessels. Radiology 1981; 138:399.
17. Haust MD. Atherosclerosis—lesions and sequelae. In M Silver, ed. Cardiovascular Pathology, Vol. 1. New York: Churchill-Livingstone, 1983. P. 277.
18. Heiberg E, et al. CT characteristics of aortic atherosclerotic aneurysm versus aortic dissections. J Comput Assist Tomogr 1985; 9:78–83.
19. Gomes NM, Hufnagel CA. CT scanning: a new method for the diagnosis of abdominal aortic aneurysms. J Cardiovasc Surg 1979; 20:511–515.
20. Machinda K, Tasaka A. CT patterns of mural thrombus in aortic aneurysms. J Comput Assist Tomogr 1980; 4:840.
21. Schwartz S, ed. Principles of Surgery, 2d ed. New York: McGraw-Hill, 1974. Pp. 887–894.
22. Rosen A, et al. CT diagnosis of ruptured abdominal aortic aneurysm. AJR 1984; 143:265–268.
23. Reckless JPD, McCall I, Taylor GW. Aorto-caval fistulae: an uncommon complication of abdominal aortic aneurysm. Br J Surg 1972; 59:461.
24. Ginaldi S, Long WD. Concurrent dissection and intracaval rupture of an abdominal aortic aneurysm: CT findings. J Comput Assist Tomogr 1985; 9:369–371.
25. Vasile N, et al. Computed tomography of thoracic aortic dissection: accuracy and pitfalls. J Comput Assist Tomogr 1986; 10:211–215.
26. Oudkerk M, Overbosch E, Dee P. CT recognition of acute aortic dissection. AJR 1983; 141:671–676.
27. Gallagher S, Dixon AK. Streak artifacts of the thoracic aorta, pseudodissection. J Comput Assist Tomogr 1984; 8:688–693.
28. Mathieu D, et al. Postoperative CT follow-up of aortic dissection. J Comput Assist Tomogr 1986; 10:216–218.
29. Turley K, et al. Repair of thoracic aortic dissection: evaluation of false lumen utilizing computed tomography. J Thorac Cardiovasc Surg 1981; 81:61.
30. Jacobs NM, et al. Evaluation of the grafted ascending aorta with computed tomography. Radiology 1982; 145:749–753.
31. Stanson AW, et al. Penetrating atherosclerotic ulcer of the thoracic aorta: Natural history and clinicopathological correlation. Ann Vasc Surg 1986; 1:15–23.
32. Cooke JP, Kazmier FJ, Orszuhak TA. Penetrating atherosclerotic ulcer: pathologic manifestations, diagnosis and management. Mayo Clinic 1933; 63:718–725.
33. Hussain S, et al. Penetrating atherosclerotic ulcers of the thoracic aorta. J. Vasc Surg 1989; 9:710–717.
34. Kazerooni EA, Bree RL, Williams DM. Penetrating atherosclerotic ulcers of the descending thoracic aorta: Evaluation with CT and distinction from aortic dissection.
35. Crawford JL, et al. Inflammatory aneurysms of the aorta. J Vasc Surg 1985; 2:113–124.
36. Bainbridge ET, Woodward DAK. Inflammatory aneurysms of the abdominal aorta with associated mesenteric obstruction or medial deviation. J Cardiovasc Surg 1982; 23:365–370.
37. Cullenward MJ, et al. Inflammatory aortic aneurysm (periaortic fibrosis) radiology imaging. Radiology 1986; 159:75–82.
38. Parkhurst GF, Decker JP. Bacterial aortitis and mycotic aneurysm of the aorta: report of 12 cases. Am J Pathol 1955; 31:821–835.
39. Johansen K, Devin J. Mycotic aortic aneurysms: a reappraisal. Arch Surg 1983; 118:583-588.
40. Atlas SW, et al. CT diagnosis of a mycotic aneurysm of the thoracoabdominal aorta. J Comput Assist Tomogr 1984; 8(6):1211–1212.
41. Hilton S, et al. Computed tomography of the postoperative abdominal aorta. Radiology 1982; 145:403–407.
42. Raptopoulas V, et al. Traumatic aortic tear: Screening with chest CT. Radiology 1992; 182:667–673.
43. Egan TJ. Computed tomography in the diagnosis of aortic aneurysm, dissection or traumatic injury. Radiology 1980; 136:141–146.
44. Daykin EL, Irwin GAL, Harrison DA. CT demonstration of a traumatic aneurysm of the pulmonary artery. J Comput Assist Tomogr 1986; 10:323–324.
45. O'Callaghan JP. CT evaluation of pulmonary artery size. J Comput Assist Tomogr 1982; 6:101–104.
46. Rubin GD, et al. Spiral CT of renal artery stenosis: comparison of three-dimensional rendering techniques. Radiology 1994; 190:181–189.
47. Galanski M, et al. Renal artery stenoses: spiral CT angiography. Radiology 1993; 189:185–192.
48. Brundage BH. Detection of patent coronary artery bypass grafts by computed tomography: a preliminary report. Circulation 1980; 61:826–831.
49. Guthauer DF. The use of computed tomography in the diagnosis of coronary artery bypass graft patency. Intervent Radiol 1980; 3:3–8.
50. Castillo M. Diagnosis of disease of the common carotid artery bifurcation: CT angiography vs catheter angiography. AJR 1993; 161:395–398.
51. Dillon EH, et al. CT angiography: application to the evaluation of carotid artery stenosis. Radiology 1993b; 189:211–219.

52. Schwartz RB, et al. Common carotid artery bifurcation: evaluation with spiral CT—work in progress. Radiology 1992; 185:513–519.
53. Kassirer JP. Thrombosis and embolism of the renal vessels. In LE Early, CW Gottschalk, eds. Strauss and Welt's Diseases of the Kidney, 3d ed. Boston: Little, Brown, 1979. Pp. 1385–1393.
54. Hilton S, et al. CT findings in acute infarction. Urol Radiol 1984; 6:158-163.
55. Michaels NA. Newer anatomy of the liver-variant blood supply and collateral circulation. JAMA 1960; 172:125–132.
56. Ghaudur-Mnaymneh L. Anemic infarction of the liver resulting from hepatic and portal vein thrombosis. Johns Hopkins Med J 1976; 139:78–81.
57. Carroll R. Infarction of the human liver. J Clin Pathol 1963; 16:133–136.
58. Nichols DM. Computed tomography in acute mesenteric vein thrombosis. J Comput Assist Tomogr 1984; 8:171–172.
59. Breckingridge JW, Kinlaw WB. Azygous continuation of the inferior vena cava: CT appearance. J Comput Assist Tomogr 1980; 4:392–397.
60. Royal SA, Callen PW. CT evaluation of anomalies of the inferior vena cava and left renal vein. AJR 1979; 132:759–763.
61. Zerhouni EA, Barth KH, Siegelman SS. Demonstration of venous thrombosis by computed tomography. AJR 1980; 134:753–758.
62. Castillo M, Munez D, Morillo G. Review of computed tomography findings in thrombosis of the major abdominal venous pathways. J Comput Assist Tomogr 1986; 10:205–214.
63. Barnes PA, Bernardino ME, Thomas JL. Flow phenomenon mimicking thrombus: a possible pitfall of the pedal infusion technique. J Comput Assist Tomogr 1982; 6:304–306.
64. Vigo M, et al. CT demonstration of portal and superior mesenteric vein thrombosis in hepatocellular carcinoma. J Comput Assist Tomogr 1980; 5:627–629.
65. Becker CD, Scheidegger J, Marincek. Hepatic vein occlusion: morphologic features on CT and ultrasonography. Gastrointest Radiol 1986; 11:305–311.
66. Webb WR, et al. Computed tomographic demonstration of mediastinal venous anomalies. AJR 1982; 139:157–161.
67. Lochridge SK, Knibbe WP, Doty DB. Obstruction of the superior vena cava. Surgery 1979; 85:14–24.
68. Mahajan V, et al. Benign superior vena cava syndrome. Chest 1975; 68:32–35.
69. Chamorrow H, Rao G, Wholey MH. Superior vena cava syndrome: a complication for transvenous pacemaker implantation. Radiology 1978; 126:377–378.
70. Axel L, et al. Functional imaging of the liver. New information from dynamic CT. Invest Radiol 1984; 19:23–29.
71. Ishikawa I, et al. Renal cortex visualization and analysis of dynamic CT curves kidney. J Comput Assist Tomogr 1981; 5:695–701.
72. Sekhar LN, Hervas RC. Origin, growth and rupture of saccular aneurysms (a review). Neurosurgery 1981; 8:248–260.
73. Zack DJ. Multiple intracranial aneurysms. AJR 1978; 130: 180–182.
74. Fox JL, Ko JP. Familial intracranial aneurysms: six cases among 13 siblings. J Neurosurg 1980; 52:501–503.
75. Newton TH, Troost BT. Arteriovenous malformations and fistulae. In TH Newton, DG Potts, eds. Radiology of the Skull and Brain, Vol. 2. St. Louis: Mosby, 1984.
76. Caplain LR, Hier DB, Banks G. Current concepts of cerebrovascular disease: stroke and drug abuse. Stroke 1982; 13: 869–872.
77. Andrews RJ, Spiegel PK. Intracranial aneurysms: age, sex, blood pressure and multiplicity in an unselected series of patients. J Neurosurg 1979; 51:27–32.
78. David KR, et al. A neuroradiologic approach to the patient with a diagnosis of subarachnoid hemorrhage. Radiol Clin N Am 1982; 20:87–94.
79. Cohen WH, Pinto RS, Kricheff II. The value of dynamic scanning. Radiol Clin N Am 1982; 20:23–25.
80. Peeters FLM. Angiographically demonstrated large vascular malformation in a patient with a normal angiogram 23 years before. Neuroradiology 1982; 23:113–114.
81. Conforti P. Spontaneous disappearance of cerebral arteriovenous angioma. Case report. J Neurosurg 1971; 34:432–434.
82. Ishikawa M, et al. Computed tomography of cerebral cavernous hemangiomas. J Comput Assist Tomogr 1980; 4:587–591.
83. Weisberg LA. Computed tomographic findings in carotid-cavernous fistula. Comput Tomogr 1981; 5:31–36.
84. Houser OW, et al. Radiologic evaluation of ischemic cerebrovascular syndromes with emphasis on computed tomography. Radiol Clin N Am 1982; 20:123–142.
85. Davis JM, et al. Cranial computed tomography in subarachnoid hemorrhage: relationship between blood detected by CT and lumbar puncture. J Comput Assist Tomogr 1980; 4:794–796.
86. Bell BA, Kendall BE, Symon L. Computed tomography in aneurysmal subarachnoid hemorrhage. J Neurol Neurosurg Psychiatry 1980; 43:522.
87. Lilequist B, Lindquist M, Valdimarsson E. Computed tomography and subarachnoid hemorrhage. Neuroradiology 1977; 14:21–26.
88. Wiggins WS, et al. Clinical and computerized tomographic study of hypertensive intracerebral hemorrhage. Arch Neurol 1978; 35:832–833.
89. Popile LA, et al. Incidence and evolution of subepedymal and intraventricular hemorrhage. A study of infants with birth weights less than 1500 gm. J Pediatr 1978; 92:529–534.
90. Olson E, Gilmor RL, Richmond B. Cerebral venous angiomas. Radiology 1984; 151:97–104.
91. Vines FS, Davis DO. Radiological correlation in cerebral venous occlusive disease. Radiology 1971; 98:9–22.
92. Zilkha A, Diaz AS. Computed tomography in the diagnosis of superior sagittal sinus thrombosis. J Comput Assist Tomogr 1980; 4:124–126.
93. Buonanno FS, et al. Computed cranial tomographic findings in cerebral sinovenous occlusion. J Comput Assist Tomogr 1978; 2:281–290.
94. Patel S, Brennan J. Diagnosis of internal jugular vein thrombosis by computed tomography. J Comput Assist Tomogr 1981; 5:197–200.
95. Dobben GD, et al. Evaluation of brain circulation by rapid rotational computed tomography. Radiology 1979; 133: 105–111.
96. Traupe H, et al. Perfusion patterns in CT transit studies. Neuroradiology 1980; 19:181–191.
97. Yonas H, et al. Mapping cerebral blood flow by xenon-enhanced computed tomography: clinical experience. Radiology 1984; 152:435–442.

IV

General Principles of Therapy

Epidemiology of Risk-Factor Reduction

J. Michael Gaziano

Cardiovascular disease (CVD) remains the number one cause of death in the United States, accounting for nearly half of all deaths among both men and women. Age-adjusted death rates from CVD increased during the first half of the twentieth century, but there have been substantial reductions in both stroke and coronary heart disease (CHD) mortality rates over the last three decades (Fig 24-1). These reductions have occurred among both whites and blacks, men and women, and in all age groups. Advances in treatment, particularly of coronary heart disease, including the establishment of emergency medical systems and coronary care units, life-saving therapies such as revascularization and thrombolytic therapy, and the increased use of beta blockers, aspirin, and ACE inhibitors, have clearly contributed to reduced mortality rates. However, the major decline in CVD mortality rates can be attributed to the preventive measures that have been encouraged throughout the population [1].

The process of disease prevention involves several steps, including understanding disease mechanisms, identifying risk factors, establishing intervention strategies that will reduce risk, weighing the benefits of any given intervention against the risks and costs, establishing guidelines for health providers and the general public, and, finally, implementing those guidelines. Basic and animal research data, while important in establishing a causal link between any one factor and disease, are discussed elsewhere in this text. This chapter reviews the principles used in the development of preventive strategies, followed by a summary of the evidence on the role of the major modifiable risk factors in the development of atherosclerotic disease.

Three risk factors for which the strength and consistency of their association with atherosclerotic disease indicate a causal relationship and for which the benefits of intervention are well documented include cigarette smoking, elevated serum cholesterol, and hypertension. There is little doubt that diabetes mellitus, physical inactivity, and menopause increase the risk of CHD, but the precise reduction in risk attributable to intervention in these risk-factor areas has been difficult to document. Other potential factors include obesity, moderate alcohol consumption, hemostatic factors, psychological factors, prophylactic aspirin, and antioxidant intake. For each risk factor, the available data on the strength of its association with CHD from both observational studies and randomized trials will be summarized. The estimates from observational data may not always agree with those from randomized trials, and the possible reasons for those discrepancies also will be examined. Finally, intervention strategies and their costs will be discussed briefly for those factors where data are available.

The Role of Epidemiology in Risk Reduction

The complex nature of atherogenesis as a multifactorial process makes it difficult to define clearly the risk attributable to any one factor. Potential risk factors for atherosclerotic disease include unmodifiable factors such as age, sex, and race; behavioral characteristics such as smoking and exercise; and biochemical markers such as serum cholesterol level. The correlations and complex interactions among factors can lead to difficulties in the establishment of associated risk. The situation is further complicated by imprecision in the definition of some potential risk factors. Techniques in multivariate analysis allow epidemiologists to consider simultaneously a multiplicity of factors in very large databases.

A risk factor that is causally linked to a particular disease should be strongly and consistently associated with that disease. However, the apparent strength of the association may depend on whether or not analysts control for other related factors. Inadequate control for related factors could result in underestimation or overestimation of the true relationship of any factor with disease. Control for factors in the causal pathway would tend to underestimate the true association. For example, obesity is clearly associated with increased risk of CHD, but the association appears to be mediated, at least in part, by lipoprotein abnormalities, hypertension, and diabetes mellitus. The apparent strength of the association of obesity with CHD depends on whether those other factors are in the model, and much is left to the discretion of the investigator in this regard.

The role of epidemiology in the development of preventive strategies involves a number of complementary methodologies [2]. These include descriptive studies, observational analytic studies (case-control studies and prospective cohort studies), randomized trials, meta-analyses, and cost- and risk-benefit analyses (Table 24-1).

Descriptive studies include case reports, case series, cross-sectional surveys, cross-cultural studies, and studies of population-based temporal trends. Case reports and case series describe characteristics associated with a particular disease usually at the time of presentation. In cross-sectional surveys, the prevalence of both disease and exposure variables are assessed at the same time among a group of individuals. Cross-cultural studies describe differences between populations in disease rates and the prevalence of potential risk factors, while population-based temporal trends describe changes in disease rates and potential risk factors within a population over time. The value of these studies is in the generation of hypotheses that can be tested in more analytic epidemiologic studies, such as case-control and prospective cohort studies as well as randomized trials.

The major contribution of descriptive studies, particularly cross-cultural studies and studies of temporal trends, has been the strong suggestion that environmental factors play an important role in the development of atherosclerotic disease. The relatively high rates of heart disease in northern Europe compared to southern Europe, the differences in CVD rates between industrialized and less

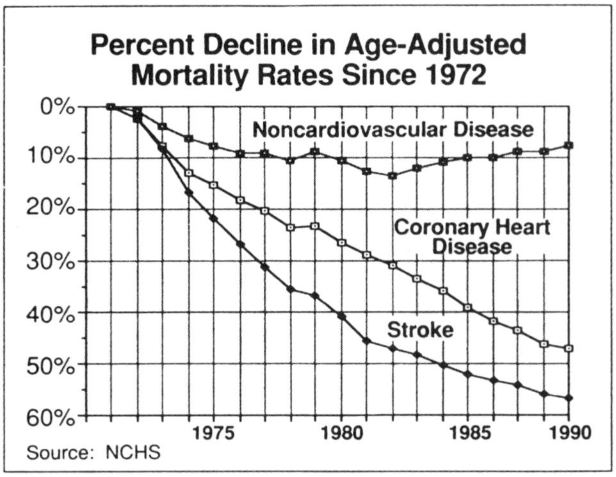

Priority Area Lead Agency:
National Institutes of Health
Bernadine P. Healy, M.D.
Director

Collaborating Agencies:
Food and Drug Administration
Centers for Disease Control
Health Resources and Services Administration
Agency for Health Care Policy and Research
Health Care Financing Administration

Healthy People 2000 Coordinator:
Office of Disease Prevention and
Health Promotion
J. Michael McGinnis, M.D.
Director

Fig. 24-1. Percent decline in age-adjusted mortality rates since 1972. (Source: National Center for Health Statistics.)

developed nations, and changing heart disease rates over the past three decades in the United States and other industrialized nations strongly suggest an important environmental component in the pathogenesis of atherosclerotic disease. Migration studies such as the Ni-Hon-San study, which showed increasing heart disease rates as Japanese men migrated from Japan to Honolulu and San Francisco, indicated that genetic factors do not explain a large portion of the cross-cultural differences in heart disease rates [3].

The weakness of descriptive studies derives from the inability to control adequately for potential factors that may confound any apparent association, thus making it difficult to link any single factor causally with disease. Potential confounders include genetics and life-style characteristics, as well as differences in the availability of health care resources. For example, worldwide heart disease rates are correlated with the number of television sets per capita, but that does not imply a causal relationship. The number of television sets per capita is merely

Table 24-1. Methodologies used in developing preventive strategies

Descriptive studies
Case reports
Case series
Cross-sectional surveys
Cross-cultural studies
Studies of temporal trends
Observational analytic studies
Case-control studies
Prospective cohort studies
Randomized trials
Meta-analysis
Cost- and risk-benefit analyses

a marker for other risk factors that confound the relationship. Because of their weaknesses, descriptive studies generally do not allow for the establishment of causal relationships; therefore, the following discussion of evidence supporting an association of a given factor with CVD will be confined largely to more analytic studies.

In contrast to descriptive studies, observational analytic studies (case-control and prospective cohort studies) enable researchers to attempt to control for potential confounders. Case-control studies are designed to identify cases of a particular disease and appropriately matched controls and to compare exposure status of potential risk factors obtained at the time disease status is established. Although case-control studies are more efficient and less costly than prospective cohort studies, selection and recall bias may affect risk estimates, since exposure status is ascertained after disease occurrence. Selection of both cases and matched controls may introduce bias, since selected cases or controls may not adequately represent the intended source populations. Cases may recall information regarding exposure status in a systematically different way than do controls.

In prospective cohort studies, researchers ascertain exposure status at the beginning of the study and follow individuals for subsequent events. Like case-control studies, prospective studies are less subject to the biases of descriptive studies because the outcome, as well as the exposure data, is available for each individual in the study population, thus allowing control for many potential confounders. Furthermore, in contrast to case-control studies, in prospective cohort studies, exposure is measured prior to the development of clinically apparent disease, thus minimizing the impact of recall and selection bias.

Case-control and prospective cohort studies are quite useful in establishing risk attributable to a single factor, particularly when the effect of a given risk factor is large. When the effect size is large, it often is not necessary or feasible to conduct randomized trials. The observational data on cigarette smoking and increased risk of lung cancer were so overwhelming that it would have been unethical to randomize individuals to cigarette smoking. On the other hand, when searching for small to moderate effects, the amount of uncontrolled confounding in observational studies may be as large as the likely risk reduction itself.

In that case, randomized trials may be helpful in confirming an association and quantitating its magnitude. In addition, when there are competing risks and benefits, randomized trials may be useful in determining the net effect of any given intervention. Estrogen replacement therapy, for example, appears to confer a protective effect in terms of CHD, but those benefits must be weighed against the potential risks of uterine and possibly breast cancer. In randomized trials, investigators allocate subjects to various treatment groups and observe for subsequent effects of each treatment. Randomized trials of adequate size overcome some of the limitations of observational epidemiologic studies by equally distributing the known as well as the unknown confounders among treatment groups.

In some instances, data from individual observational studies or randomized trials are not sufficient to establish a clear risk or benefit of a factor or intervention. Therefore, it may be helpful to pool data from several studies in an overview, or meta-analysis. Pooling data from either observational studies or randomized trials may be difficult if there are major differences in study design, interventional strategies, or definitions of exposure variables or outcome measures. Meta-analyses must be interpreted cautiously because the results may depend on the underlying assumptions that dictate which studies to include in any analysis or how the data are summarized.

Once reasonable estimates of risk and benefit for a particular risk factor or intervention have been established, cost- and risk-benefit analyses can be helpful in establishing guidelines for intervention. Similar to estimates derived from meta-analyses, those from cost- and risk-benefit analyses often are quite dependent on the underlying assumptions for a given analysis, and thus must be interpreted cautiously.

Modifiable Risk Factors of Cardiovascular Disease

CIGARETTE SMOKING

Prevalence. In the United States per capita cigarette consumption rose dramatically in the first half of this century (Fig. 24-2). Over 65 percent of men born between 1911 and 1920 were smoking by 1945 [4]. Cigarette-smoking rates have declined from the peak of 41 percent of the adult population in 1965 to 26 percent in 1991 [5,6]. The rate of decline among men has been different from that among women. Among men, smoking rates have been cut by almost one-half, from a peak of over 50 percent of the adult male population in the early 1960s to 28 percent in 1991, while among women, rates have dropped by about one-third (34% in 1965 to 24% in 1992). The slower rate of decline among women has been attributed to increased rates among women under 30 years of age. Smoking rates tend to be higher among blacks, those with lower socioeconomic status, and those with only a high school education or less.

Smoking and Risk of CHD. By the middle of this century, seminal studies linking smoking and heart disease were published by English et al. [7], Doll and Hill [8], and Hammond and Horn [9]. The Surgeon General's report in 1964 reaffirmed the epidemiologic relationship [10], and by 1983 the Surgeon General firmly established cigarette smoking as a leading avoidable cause of CVD [11]. The Surgeon General's report in 1989 presented definitive data from observational case-control and cohort studies, largely among men, that demonstrate that smoking increases CHD mortality by 50 percent and doubles the incidence of CHD [12]. Willett et al. [13] and Rosenberg et al. [14] have demonstrated a similar increase in relative risk for fatal and nonfatal CHD among women. The risk of a CHD event increases with age, and there is a clear dose-response relationship for cigarette consumption [15] with relative risks as high as 5.5 for fatal CHD among heavy smokers compared to nonsmokers [13]. The strength, consistency, and dose-responsive character of the relationship in observational epidemiology make any explanation other than a causal one extremely unlikely.

Reduction in Risk Associated with Smoking Cessation. There are virtually no large-scale randomized trial data on reduction in risk associated with smoking cessation as an isolated intervention. The Multiple Risk Factor Intervention Study tested a multifaceted risk-modification program among men at high risk for CHD. After 10.5 years, the intervention group had a 24-percent lower death rate from myocardial infarction (MI) and a 10.6-percent reduction in total CHD mortality, which was associated with a 29-percent reduction in the prevalence of smoking [16]. However, because smoking cessation was only one of several risk-factor modifications, it is impossible to determine the magnitude of the smoking effect.

Most data on the efficacy of smoking cessation have been generated by prospective cohort studies [17]. The risk of MI declines more rapidly than that of CHD death. The greatest proportion of risk reduction of MI occurs in the first several months after cessation. The risk of MI is just slightly above that of nonsmokers by 2 years. The decline in risk of CHD death also is greatest in the first several months after cessation, but even after 10 years, the risk is slightly greater than for nonsmokers. These reductions in risk occur regardless of the duration or level of daily consumption. The risk of CHD is reduced even among those with established coronary disease [18]. The rapid early decline followed by a gradual late decline in risk suggests that more than one mechanism may be involved. It has been postulated that the early risk reduction may be due to rapid reversal of thrombogenic tendencies [19–21], while the late risk reduction may be due to slowing of atherosclerotic progression mediated by changes in traditional risk factors [22,23].

Interventional Strategies. The vast majority of those who give up smoking do not use an organized cessation program. The efficacy of smoking intervention programs range from a 6-percent 1-year success rate for physician counseling to 18 percent for self-help programs and 20–26 percent for pharmacologic interventions with nicotine gum or patch [24,25]. Data on the role of other pharmacologic interventions such as clonidine in smoking cessation are not consistent. Since smoking cessation programs gen-

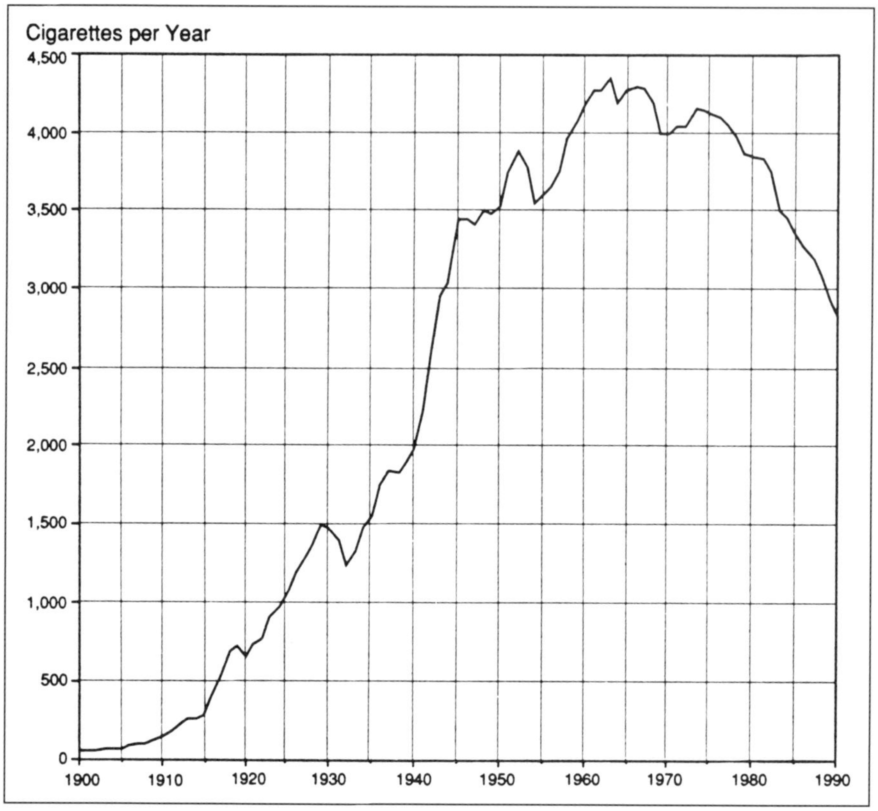

Fig. 24-2. U.S. per capita cigarette consumption for adults aged 18 and older (1900 to 1990). (Source: U.S. DHHS, 1991.)

erally cost less than continued smoking, there is little doubt of the cost-effectiveness of this intervention.

SERUM CHOLESTEROL

Prevalence of Elevated Serum Cholesterol. In 1991, one-half of all American adults ages 20 through 74 years of age had cholesterol levels greater than 200 mg/dl, and 20 percent of American adults had cholesterol levels of 240 mg or greater [26]. Almost 30 percent of American adults meet the National Cholesterol Education Program (NCEP) guidelines for dietary intervention for hypercholesteremia, and 7 percent meet the guidelines for management by medication [27]. Based on data from several national surveys, mean age-adjusted cholesterol levels have shown a modest decline in the United States since the early 1960s [28,29].

Risk Associated with Elevated Serum Cholesterol. A number of case-control and prospective cohort studies have documented an increased risk of CHD with elevated serum cholesterol. There appears to be a linear relationship with an increase in 1 percent of serum cholesterol associated with an increased risk of CHD of about 2 percent [30]. This effect occurs at any level of cholesterol; a recent study analyzing the relationship between total cholesterol levels and heart disease among those with serum cholesterol between 160 and 190 mg/dl indicated that a 10-percent increase in baseline cholesterol was associated with a 21-percent increase in risk from CHD [31]. These relationships are apparent in men and women, blacks and whites. Furthermore, there appears to be an even higher risk with increases in serum cholesterol at earlier age. Specifically, in a recent meta-analysis of 10 observational studies that included follow-up data from over 500,000 subjects, a 10-percent increase in serum cholesterol was found to increase the incidence of ischemic heart disease by 54 percent at age 40, 39 percent at age 50, 27 percent at age 60, and 20 percent at age 70 [32].

These estimates from prospective data may underestimate the true risk associated with lipoprotein abnormalities, because the relationship generally is based on a single measure of serum total cholesterol [33,34]. The basis of this underestimation rests on two forms of bias: (1) regression-dilution bias, which is the bias that results from random fluctuation of cholesterol levels over time in any subject and from inaccuracies in the assays, and (2) surrogate-dilution bias, which results from less than perfect correlation in low density lipoprotein (LDL) cholesterol with total cholesterol levels. In a prospective cohort among over 21,500 men, 5,700 of whom were tested repeatedly for total and LDL cholesterol, the observed increased risk associated with a 10-percent increase in serum cholesterol was 17 percent, which increased to 27 percent after adjustment for the two forms of bias [34].

In addition to total and LDL cholesterol, other lipoprotein abnormalities also may be independent predictors of CHD. High density lipoprotein (HDL) cholesterol has emerged as an important independent predictor of CHD.

Researchers with the Framingham Heart Study found that for every 1-mg/dl decrease in HDL cholesterol, there is a 3- to 4-percent increase in coronary artery disease [35–37]. An emerging body of evidence now indicates that the ratio of total or LDL cholesterol to HDL cholesterol may be an important predictor of the risk of CHD. Data from the Physicians' Health Study suggest that a one-unit decrease in this ratio decreases the risk of myocardial infarction by 53 percent [38]. Elevated triglycerides clearly are associated with CHD, particularly in the setting of low HDL cholesterol levels and among women, but whether they represent an independent factor after control for other factors remains unclear.

Reduction in Risk Associated with Treatment of Serum Cholesterol. Randomized trial data clearly demonstrate a reduction in risk of CHD with treatment to lower serum cholesterol. Meta-analyses of randomized trials generally have shown a reduction in risk of both fatal and nonfatal CHD in both primary and secondary prevention trials [39–42]. Those results were confirmed in a recent overview of 28 trials, which summarized data from primary and secondary trials of cholesterol reduction based on 4,000 CHD events among 46,000 participants [43]. Law et al. [43] reported a reduction in ischemic heart disease mortality of 10 percent (95% confidence interval, or CI = 3%–16%; $p < 0.004$) and a reduction in ischemic heart disease events of 18 percent (95% CI = 13%–22%; $p < 0.001$) for a 10-percent reduction in serum cholesterol. The effect is greatest with increasing duration of treatment. A 10-percent reduction in cholesterol was associated with a 7-percent (95% CI = 0%–14%) reduction in CHD events among those treated for less than 2 years, 22 percent (95% CI = 15%–28%) among those treated from 2.1 to 5 years, and 25 percent (95% CI = 15%–36%) among those treated for more than 5 years. The estimate for those treated for the longest duration is consistent with estimates from observational studies. In the Scandinavian Simvastatin Survival Study (4S), the first of the large-scale trials of HMG CoA reductase inhibitors, total and LDL cholesterol reductions were greater than previous trials [44]. In this placebo-controlled, double-blind trial 4,444 subjects with known CHD and elevated serum cholesterol about 5.5 mmol/L mean changes in total, LDL, and HDL cholesterol were −25 percent, −35 percent, and +8 percent, respectively. During a median follow-up of 5.4 years, among those assigned to simvastatin compared with those randomized to placebo, the risk of a cardiovascular event, coronary death, and death from any cause were significantly lower (relative risk of 0.66 [$P < 0.001$], 0.58 [$P < 0.001$] and 0.70 [$P < 0.001$], respectively).

The totality of evidence from basic research, observational epidemiologic studies, and randomized trials provides strong support for the judgment that lowering serum cholesterol decreases the risk of CHD [45]. Furthermore, the observational data are consistent with the randomized trial data when duration of treatment is 5 years or more. The strength and consistency of the association as well as the apparent dose-response relation argue strongly for a causal link.

Table 24-2. Risk of non-CHD death among those with low compared to those with high cholesterol by study type

Cause of death	Employment-based cohorts	Community-based cohorts
Non-CHD vascular	0.92 (0.80–1.05)	1.12 (0.98–1.28)
Cancer	1.00 (0.91–1.10)	1.23 (1.17–1.30)
Trauma	0.95 (0.70–1.30)	1.29 (1.13–1.47)
Other	1.08 (0.97–1.21)	1.62 (1.47–1.78)
Total	1.00 (0.94–1.06)	1.20 (1.15–1.24)

Source: Adapted from Law MR, Thompson SG, Wald NJ. Assessing possible hazards of reducing serum cholesterol. Br Med J 1994; 308:373–379.

Nonvascular Mortality. While there is little doubt that cholesterol reduction results in reduced risks of CHD, questions regarding the increased risk of nonvascular causes have been raised [46]. An interesting and consistently held finding from observational studies is that individuals with very low (less than 160 mg/dL) cholesterol levels have higher rates of noncardiovascular mortality [30]. It is unclear, however, if low cholesterol is just an marker for or a cause of nonvascular disease. In a recent review by Law et al. [43], the association of increased non-CHD mortality from prospective cohort studies varied depending on whether the populations studied were employment- or community-based (see Table 24-2). In employment-based cohorts, there was no evidence of increased non-CHD mortality among those with low cholesterol, which was defined as less than 5 mmol/liter (193 mg/dl) (relative risk = 1.00; 95% CI = 0.94–1.06). In addition to the point estimate indicating a null result, the upper bound of the confidence interval (1.06) excludes any substantial risk. In contrast, there was an apparent increased risk of non-CHD deaths among those in community-based cohorts (relative risk [RR] = 1.20; 95% CI = 1.15–1.24). If we assume a causal link between low cholesterol and non-CHD mortality, these discrepant results are difficult to explain. An alternative explanation for the inverse relationship in the less healthy community-based populations may be the higher prevalence of premorbid disease, such as cancer, liver disease, and depression, all of which are associated with low cholesterol. This explanation is also supported by the attenuation of the inverse association if deaths in the first 5 years were excluded [30], providing additional evidence that the association is unlikely to be causal.

Data from individual randomized trials have been insufficient to address the issue of nonvascular mortality. The lack of a statistically significant benefit in overall mortality has led some to speculate that this is evidence of an offsetting of the reduction in risk by an increase in nonvascular mortality [46]. In the two most comprehensive overviews, the observed reduction in total mortality from all randomized trials was 4 percent, which is quite consistent with the expected 6-percent decline anticipated by the overall 10-percent decline in CHD death if there were no excess risk of nonvascular death [43,47]. There was no evidence that cholesterol reduction increases mortality from any single cause. It should be noted that mean cholesterol reduction in these early trials was relatively modest (6–10 mg/dl). In the Scandinavian Simvastatin Survival Study (4S) where drug therapy resulted in a 25 percent reduction in total cholesterol there was no increase in nonvascular deaths (49 in placebo versus 46 in the treatment group) [44]. Ongoing randomized trials with the statins (HMG CoA reductase inhibitor), which will result in greater cholesterol reduction (25–30%), will have increased power to detect an effect on nonvascular mortality.

Interventional Strategies. Recent estimates suggest that 30 percent of the adult U.S. population would be eligible for nonpharmacologic intervention [27]. Reduction in fat intake results in reduction in serum cholesterol [48,49], and dietary interventions have been shown to reduce the risk of CHD events [50] and delay the progression of coronary artery disease [51]. While most cholesterol-reduction diets stress reduction in saturated fats, replacement of those fats with carbohydrates or monounsaturated or polyunsaturated fats remains controversial. Replacement of saturated fats with carbohydrates reduces not only LDL cholesterol but also HDL cholesterol, while replacement with monounsaturated fats reduces LDL and may maintain HDL levels [52]. Recent data suggest that transfatty acids found in hydrogenated vegetable oils may increase LDL cholesterol and reduce HDL cholesterol, thereby potentially increasing the risk of CHD [53]. Foods high in these transfatty acids include margarine, vegetable shortening, and processed foods such as cookies, crackers, and candies. Exercise, obesity, smoking, hormone replacement therapy, and alcohol consumption also can have an impact on lipoprotein profile. Intensive life-style modification comes without the potential risks associated with drug therapy and tends to be less costly than drug intervention.

Drug therapy has focused on those at higher risk and is based on LDL targets. Approximately 7 percent of the adult population meet NCEP Adult Treatment Panel (ATP) II guidelines for pharmacologic intervention. Lipid-lowering therapy should be considered as an adjunct to life-style modification. Combinations of various agents at lower doses (which may reduce toxicities) are currently under investigation. Despite the increased risk of CHD among those with low HDL in the setting of a desirable LDL cholesterol, research on the efficacy of drug therapy in this group is scant. For that reason, the revised NCEP guidelines do not recommend drug therapy for isolated low HDL. A stronger emphasis is being placed on the choice of LDL cholesterol–lowering drugs, depending on the level of HDL. Many cholesterol-lowering drugs increase HDL to some degree, although niacin and gemfibrozil are particularly effective at raising HDL levels. While the role of triglycerides in the development of atherosclerotic disease is unclear, the NCEP guidelines recommend consideration of triglyceride levels when choosing cholesterol-lowering drugs. Niacin and gemfibrozil have a favorable affect on triglyceride levels. The cost effectiveness of pharmacologic cholesterol reduction depends on the risk of CHD for each individual. Pharmacologic interventions are generally considered cost effective for those with existing coronary disease and those with multiple coronary risk factors.

HYPERTENSION

Prevalence. The Fifth Report of the Joint National Committee on Detection, Evaluation, and treatment of High Blood Pressure (JNC V) defines optimal blood pressure as a systolic blood pressure (SBP) less than 120 mm Hg and a diastolic blood pressure (DBP) less than 80 mm Hg; high-normal blood pressure as an SBP of 130–139 mm Hg and a DBP of 85–89 mm Hg; and hypertension as SBP above 140 mm Hg or DBP above 90 mm Hg [54]. Data from two national surveys suggest that 30 percent of American adults are hypertensive and that the prevalence of hypertension is greater among blacks than whites and among men than women; there is a clear increase in prevalence with older age, increasing from 9 percent among those aged 19–24 to 75 percent of those over 75 years of age [55,56].

Risk Associated with High Blood Pressure. Elevation of systolic or diastolic blood pressure has consistently been associated with an increased risk of CHD. In a recent meta-analysis, MacMahon et al. [33] examined the relationship of DBP and SBP to CHD from nine, large prospective observational studies among over 400,000 participants who accrued over 4,850 CHD events during follow-up and found a strong, positive relationship of both DBP and SBP with CHD. The relationship was linear with no threshold effect (Fig. 24-3); risk was increased even in the ranges of mild-to-moderate hypertension. In addition, there was no increase in risk associated with low blood pressure. An increase of 7 mm Hg in DBP from any baseline blood pressure was associated with a 27-percent increase in CHD risk and a 42-percent increase in stroke risk. Using data from the screenees for the Multiple Risk Factor Intervention Trial (MRFIT), Stamler et al. [57] also found a similar strong linear relationship between relative risk and SBP. Further, compared to those with SBPs less than 110 mm Hg, 32 percent of the excess risk of CHD associated with hypertension occurred in those with optimal to high-normal blood pressures (SBPs of 110 to 139 mm Hg).

Reduction in Risk with Treatment of Hypertension. For patients with malignant hypertension (defined as diastolic blood pressure greater than 115 mm Hg), the benefits of pharmacologic intervention are clear and uncontroversial. Beginning in the late 1960s, a number of randomized trials have confirmed the protective effect of treatment of mild-to-moderate hypertension, and these early trial data led to the establishment of treatment guidelines in the 1970s [58,59]. The most precise estimates of risk reduction have come from several recent meta-analyses. Collins et al. [60] summed data from 14 randomized trials that included 37,000 subjects treated for 3 to 5 years. A blood pressure

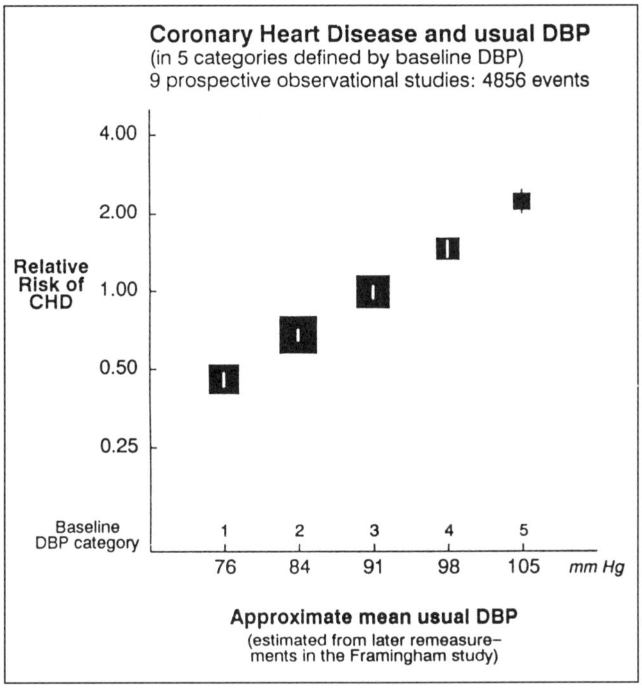

Fig. 24-3. Relative risk of CHD by level of diastolic blood pressure. (Source: MacMahon et al., Blood pressure stroke and coronary heart disease I: prolonged differences in blood pressure; prospective observational studies corrected for regression dilution bias. Lancet 1990; 335:765–774.)

decrease of 5 to 6 mm Hg resulted in a 42-percent reduction in risk of stroke and a 14-percent reduction in risk of CHD events. These results are supported by a subsequent meta-analysis by Hebert et al., which includes an additional three trials [61]. Hebert estimated a 16-percent reduction in risk of CHD events. While the reductions in stroke are consistent with what would have been anticipated by the observational data, that is not the case for CHD. The observed reduction in risk of CHD of 14–16 percent is about half of what was anticipated by observational data. This blunted effect may have been due to the short duration of treatment in randomized trials, assuming that risk of CHD declines more slowly than stroke risk. Alternatively, some investigators have speculated that the discrepancy could be explained by atherogenic side effects (including effects on lipids and glucose) of some of the antihypertensive agents used in the trials [62,63].

Interventional Strategies. The JNC V report recommends nonpharmacologic modifications in life-style alone for mild hypertensives and as an adjunct to pharmacologic intervention in moderate-to-severe hypertensives [54]. The optimal strategy to reduce SBP to below 140 and DBP to below 90 mm Hg will depend on the other risk factors present. Nonpharmacologic therapies that have been shown to be effective in the management of hypertension and that are recommended in the JNC V report include weight loss, limitation of alcohol intake to no more than 1 oz. of ethanol per day, aerobic exercise, and reduction of sodium intake [54]. Inexpensive nonpharmacologic interventions may be advisable in those with high-normal blood pressure, and a substantial percentage of those with mild-to-moderate hypertension can control blood pressure with diet (reduced caloric, sodium, and alcohol intake) and exercise alone. The Dietary Intervention Study in Hypertension found that blood pressure could be successfully lowered through weight loss in overweight patients and sodium reduction in normal-weight patients [64]. The efficacy of pharmacologic therapy has been well documented, and the cost appears to be approximately $24,000 per life year saved for those with moderate hypertension [65].

DIABETES MELLITUS

In the United States, approximately 14 million people carry the diagnosis of diabetes. Approximately 90 percent of those are non-insulin-dependent diabetics. Over the last decade, the prevalence of both non-insulin-dependent diabetes mellitus (NIDDM) and insulin-dependent diabetes mellitus (IDDM) appear to be increasing, which may be a reflection of increasing body-mass index (BMI) [66] and continuously improved survival in the reproductive years. Major determinants of NIDDM are diet, weight, and family history.

CHD is a major complication of both NIDDM and IDDM. There is little doubt that diabetes increases the risk of atherosclerotic disease. By age 40, CHD is the number one cause of death in both diabetic males and females with IDDM [67]. Among those with IDDM, the onset of clinically apparent CHD occurs at an early age with markedly increased risks by the third decade of life. The risk is related to the duration of diabetes and not the age of onset [68]. In the Danish Steno Hospital Study, mortality from MI alone was 12.5 percent after 35 years of diabetes, regardless of the age of onset [69]. Age-adjusted rates for CHD are two to three times higher among diabetic men and three to seven times higher among diabetic women with NIDDM than among nondiabetics [70,71].

The precise risk attributable to asymptomatic hyperglycemia remains unclear. In recent reports from the Framingham Heart Study and the East Boston Elderly Cohort, glycosylated hemoglobin was independently associated with risk of CHD among nondiabetics [72].

Data on the reduction of risk of CHD associated with tight glycemic control of diabetics are scant. While recent trial data support a benefit of tight control in reducing microvascular and renal complications of diabetes [73], there are no large-scale randomized trial data suggesting a benefit in terms of CHD reduction. In the Diabetes Control and Complications Trial (DCCT), there was an apparent reduction in CHD events among those with IDDM that did not achieve statistical significance likely because of the small numbers of events in this relatively young cohort. In a recent trial among non-insulin-dependent diabetics, those randomized to tight control with insulin were at increased risk of suffering a CHD event during a mean follow-up period of 27 months [74].

In stark contrast to well-controlled IDDM, those with NIDDM are much more likely to have multiple cardiovascular risk factors, including dyslipidemia, hypertension, and obesity, than are the general population [67,75,76].

The overall prevalence of hypertension among diabetics in the National Health and Nutrition Examination Survey II was 63–70 percent, compared with 40 percent among nondiabetics [77]. Diabetics are much more likely to have low HDL and high triglycerides [78]. In the DCCT, there were significant improvements in lipoprotein profile with a statistically significant reduction in LDL cholesterol in patients who were treated with tight control.

Diet and exercise are an integral component of the treatment strategy for any diabetic. In many obese, non-insulin-dependent diabetics, glycemic control can be achieved with a modest-weight-loss diet [79]. While oral hypoglycemic agents and insulin can improve glycemic control, their role in the reduction of risk from macrovascular complications of NIDDM remains unclear. Treatment of NIDDM with insulin often results in weight gain. Reduction of risk from CHD in diabetics also should include intensive modification of the other traditional risk factors.

PHYSICAL INACTIVITY

Despite widespread interest in exercise in the United States, data on the level of activity of the nation are limited. Data from the National Health Interview Survey estimated that 40 percent of the adult population exercise regularly (43% of males, 38% of female, and 23% of those over 65), but only 4–8% of adults engage in vigorous exercise for 20 minutes or more three or more times per week [80,81]. The number of adults considered sedentary declined from over 40 percent in the early 1970s to 27 percent by 1985.

Epidemiologic study of the role of exercise in heart disease is particularly problematic, in that the true quantity of physical activity is, unlike smoking behavior, cholesterol levels, and hypertension, a difficult variable to quantify and monitor. Also, an individual's interest in physical activity may co-vary with other aspects of a healthy life-style. Physical activity is generally assessed by report. Formal exercise testing has been used to quantitate physical fitness, but few epidemiologic studies have examined the relationship of physical fitness and risk of CHD. Since Morris et al. [82] first reported in the mid-1950s that CHD rates were lower among bus conductors and mail carriers compared to sedentary coworkers (bus drivers and postal supervisors, respectively), a number of observational studies have reported a similar inverse association between activity level and CHD [83]. In the early reports, physically active occupations tended to be associated with reduced risks of CHD; however, interpretation of the early occupational studies was limited owing to the potential for confounding effects (perhaps those who chose active occupations were healthier than those who chose sedentary jobs) and by an inability to include leisure activity.

Morris et al. [84] developed questionnaires to incorporate estimates of leisure-time activity in their analyses. In this study among civil servants with sedentary jobs, those who engaged in vigorous sports were half as likely to suffer MI as those who did not. This relationship between activity of any kind and lower risk of CHD has been confirmed in a number of studies. Paffenberger et al. [85] found that, among Harvard graduates, vigorously active alumni (defined as expending more than 2,000 kcal per week in physical activity) experienced a 39-percent lower rate of CHD than less active alumni (expending less than 2,000 kcal per week). Subjects who were physically active as students but who had not continued an active life-style as adults experienced the same risk as subjects who were never physically active as students or in their adult years [86]. Researchers in the MRFIT found that subjects in the highest tertile of activity experienced a lower risk of CHD compared to the lowest tertile [87]. In addition, poor baseline-exercise treadmill performance was a predictor of subsequent CHD mortality in that study. In a recent meta-analysis of 27 observational cohort studies of leisure-time and occupational activity, the risk of CHD event was almost twice that compared to inactive individuals after controlling for other coronary risk factors [83].

While regular activity appears to reduce the risk of CHD, sporadic, intense physical exertion has been associated with an increased risk of MI and sudden death, particularly among individuals who do not regularly engage in physical activity [88–90].

No large-scale, randomized trials have been conducted to determine the benefit of exercise intervention. Cessation of activity appears to result in increased risk of CHD. There are clear benefits of physical activity in terms of other cardiovascular risk factors. A physically active life-style increases the level of HDL, reduces the level of LDL and triglycerides, increases insulin sensitivity, and reduces resting blood pressure [36,91,92]. However, the efficacy of exercise counseling has not been clearly established. The physician's office appears to be an important location for the promotion of physical activity, but physician counseling is only moderately effective [93].

POSTMENOPAUSAL ESTROGEN THERAPY

In the United States, CHD is the number one cause of death among men after the age of 40 years. However, it is the number one killer among women by age 60 [94]. At every age, men exhibit a higher incidence of and mortality rates from CHD. After menopause, the gap narrows substantially [95]. The risk of CHD rises rapidly among women after both natural menopause and following oophorectomy [96–98]. Women presenting with first MI tend to be older and mortality is higher; however, after adjustment for age and other indicators of severity and comorbidity, theses differences are greatly attenuated [99,100].

A wide range of factors may explain the postmenopausal increased risk in CHD, including the adverse changes in lipid and glucose metabolism following menopause, which result in an increase in LDL cholesterol, a decrease in HDL cholesterol, and an increase in glucose intolerance, as well as changes in hemostatic factors and vascular function. Endogenous estrogens appear to play a major role in reducing the risk of CHD in women. There is substantial improvement in lipoprotein profile with a reduction in LDL and an increase in HDL following hormone replacement therapy [101–103]. In addition, there appears to be a protective effect on vascular function, and estrogens can protect LDL from oxidation [104]. Estrogens also may have a role in maintaining normal hemostasis and improving glucose tolerance.

The effects of postmenopausal hormone therapy on the risk of CHD have been widely studied in a number of case-control and prospective cohort studies. Recent overviews suggest that treatment with estrogen replacement therapy reduces the risk of CHD by 44 percent [105,106]. In the Nurses' Health Study (NHS), the largest prospective cohort study to address this question, current users had about half the risk of CHD (RR = 0.51; 95% CI = 0.37–0.70) as nonusers [107]. There appears to be an even stronger effect among those with known CHD [108]. Those data, however, are limited by their observational nature. It is quite possible that those who self-select for estrogen therapy engage in other protective behaviors that confound this relationship. The strength and the consistency of the epidemiologic data would strongly argue for an overall protective effect.

The apparent benefits in terms of CVD must be weighed against the known or potential risks of hormone replacement therapy. Estrogen replacement therapy increases the risk of endometrial cancer, which can be attenuated by the addition of progestin. In addition, some data suggest that hormone replacement therapy may increase the risk of breast cancer. An additional benefit of estrogen replacement is reduced risk of osteoporosis-related fractures. There also may be differential effects of oral and transdermal estrogen: Transdermal estrogens, which do not have a first-pass effect on the liver, appear to have less of an effect on lipoprotein levels.

Large-scale, randomized trial data are not yet adequate to assess fully the risks and benefits of postmenopausal hormone replacement. The ongoing Women's Health Initiative will address the risks and benefits of treatment of postmenopausal women with estrogen alone, as well as the use of estrogen and progestin in combination, compared to placebo. Currently available observational data suggest that the benefits of hormone replacement therapy outweigh the risks.

OBESITY

Over 20 percent of the U.S. population is obese, which is defined as being 20 percent over the desirable weight level [109]; the problem seems to be more prevalent among women than men. Despite growing awareness of the ill health effects of obesity, the proportion of the U.S. population that is overweight has increased steadily over the past two decades among both men and women [110,111].

While few data would dispute the association of obesity with CHD, there remains controversy on the independent status of this risk factor. The difficulty in assessing the independent status of obesity stems from two factors. First, there are multiple ways to measure obesity. Weight can be standardized to a desirable level or compared in relative terms. BMI is a widely used measure of weight distribution. It also can be assessed and quantified by various anthropomorphic measures, such as the thickness of skin folds or waist-hip ratio. It appears that distribution of body fat may play an important role in predicting risk, with central or abdominal adiposity imparting greater risk than peripheral or diffuse adiposity [112,113]. In addition to waist-hip ratio, visceral adiposity can be estimated by computerized tomography or magnetic resonance imaging.

The presence of confounding determinants in the analysis is a second issue that complicates assessment of the relationship of obesity with CHD. Smoking and chronic disease tend to reduce body weight. Lack of control for those factors may underestimate the impact of obesity as a risk factor. Other risk factors such as hypertension, lipid abnormalities, and insulin resistance are associated with increased weight [109,114,115]. Data from the Framingham Heart Study suggests that change in weight is associated with a corresponding change in those risk factors [116]. Some have argued that to determine the independent risk of obesity, one must control for those risk factors, while others suggest that control for those factors, which are in the causal pathway, would underestimate the true impact of obesity on CHD.

As a result of these methodologic concerns, reports on the association of obesity with CHD have been understandably conflicting. After control for coronary risk factors, several studies among both men and women tended to show no association of obesity with risk of CHD [117–119]. This lack of effect stands in contrast to a report by Hubert [115], which summarized the prospective data largely among men and found an independent effect of obesity after controlling for other risk factors. In the NHS [120], where lipoprotein abnormalities, hypertension, and diabetes were not included in the multivariate model, there was a greater than threefold increased risk of fatal and nonfatal CHD among those with the highest BMI (greater than or equal to 29) as well as an 80-percent increase in the moderately obese (BMI of 25 to 29). Obesity clearly is associated with CHD. Whether there is residual increased risk associated with obesity after controlling for hypertension, serum lipoprotein levels, and diabetes remains unclear at this time.

The effect of weight reduction on the risk of CHD remains uncertain. Data from prospective studies are limited, because of the small numbers of individuals who have managed to lose weight and keep the weight off for long periods of time. There are no large-scale trials of weight reduction as an isolated intervention on which to estimate the benefits of this intervention. However, given the improvements in glucose tolerance, blood pressure, and lipoprotein profile, which have been clearly documented, the consensus is that weight reduction should be part of an overall prevention program [121,114]. It should be pointed out that dieting to lose weight, particularly with the reduction in fat intake, will result in a reduction in LDL cholesterol and also in HDL. For that reason, many advocate an increase in exercise as part of a weight reduction program to maintain HDL levels. Manson et al. [122] have estimated that maintenance of ideal body weight could reduce the risk of CHD by 35–50 percent compared to being obese, based largely on prospective studies.

There is little consensus on the ideal approach to weight reduction. Promoting life-style changes to encourage weight reduction or maintenance of ideal body weight has been universally disappointing. While 30–40 percent of the American population report attempts at weight reduction, failure rates are exceedingly high [123]. Effective treatment strategies generally involve a multifaceted approach, including dietary counseling, behavioral modification, and increased physical activity, as well as psychosocial support [123,124]. Without precise estimates of the benefit and with variability in the intervention strategy, it is impossible to estimate the cost-benefit ratio of this intervention.

MODERATE ALCOHOL CONSUMPTION

The effects of alcohol consumption on CVD are complex. Epidemiologic data are derived almost entirely from observational studies. While heavy alcohol intake increases total [125,126] and CVD mortality [127,128], moderate intake appears to exert a protective effect on CHD compared to no alcohol intake [129–131]. The evidence from both observational and experimental studies suggests that alcohol raises total HDL and that approximately 50 percent of the risk reduction attributable to alcohol consumption is explained by changes in total HDL as well as HDL_2 and HDL_3, both of which are beneficial in reducing the risk of CHD [132,133]. Thus, moderate alcohol consumption appears to reduce the risk of CHD by raising HDL cholesterol levels. In most case-control and cohort studies, benefit is derived from beer, wine, and distilled beverage consumption, which suggests that it is the alcohol that is the major factor responsible for the protective association. Some have suggested, largely on the basis of ecologic data, that there might be an additional benefit to red wine consumption. While some observational data suggest that the risk reduction is greater for wine drinkers compared to drinkers of beer and other alcoholic beverages, this may be due to other confounding factors, since wine drinkers tend to be more educated and have higher incomes. In addition, wine tends to be consumed with meals, which, some have speculated, has metabolic advantages.

With respect to total mortality, there seems to be a J-shaped association, with a significant increased hazard among heavy drinkers. However, in a recent meta-analysis, Maclure [134] suggests an L-shaped threshold effect for CHD, with reduced risks beginning at three drinks per week and no additional benefit for more than one drink per day. From a public policy standpoint, whether the benefits for CHD persist at heavy drinking levels or are attenuated is moot, since clear harm in terms of overall mortality outweighs any benefits in the reduction of heart disease.

While the association of alcohol and CHD is likely to be causal, any individual or public health recommendations must consider the complexity of alcohol's metabolic, physiologic, and psychological effects. With alcohol, the differences between daily intake of small-to-moderate and large quantities may be the difference between preventing and causing disease. A discussion of alcohol intake should be a part of routine preventive counseling. One or two drinks per day may be safe, in general. However, counseling must be individualized; other medical problems, including other coronary risk factors (particularly hypertension and diabetes), liver disease, tendency toward excess, family history of alcoholism, and possibly breast and colon cancer, should be taken into account when discussing alcohol consumption.

PSYCHOLOGICAL FACTORS

It has been postulated by many investigators that psychological factors may play a role in disease. Extensive research efforts have been directed at the role psychological factors may play in the development of CHD. There is mounting evidence for an association between CHD and several psychological factors, with the strongest evidence for stress, type-A personality, anger, lack of social support, and depression [135–139]. The associations have been more consistent in case-control studies than in prospective studies.

While associations of various psychological factors with CHD have been strong, many difficulties in establishing a casual link exist. As has been the case for obesity and physical activity, there is no single, well-defined measure of psychological wellness that can be universally applied in epidemiologic research. While it may be difficult to establish independent risk factor status for the various psychological factors associated with CHD, there may be a psychological component to many of the traditional behavioral risk factors. There appears to be an impact of psychological factors on various behaviors such as smoking, diet, and physical activity. Mental stress may be linked to lipids [140], vascular function [141], and various hemostatic factors, which may explain the association of stressful situations with ischemia [142,143] and MI [144].

Few studies have independently assessed the impact of psychological interventions alone. The nature of the interventions preclude the use of blinded, randomized trial designed to address this question. Most interventional studies have been conducted among those with existing coronary artery disease. Several studies have shown a benefit of a life-style modification program that contained a psychological component. Benefits have been apparent in terms of regression of coronary stenoses among those with documented coronary artery disease [145,146] and reduced infarction rate in those following infarction [147]. It is not yet possible to tease out the independent effects of the psychological or other interventions.

It remains possible that counseling, emphasizing entire life-style change, may have led to increased compliance with other risk factor–modification efforts or medical therapies in these studies. There does, however, appear to be a benefit of programs with a behavioral component that stress modification of multiple factors. This is a fertile area for future research. Blinded, randomized trials of pharmacologic treatment for depression after MI are in the design phase and could add valuable information to our understanding of the independent impact of psychological factors on the risk of CHD.

HEMOSTATIC RISK FACTORS

Lipoprotein(a)—Lp(a)—appears to be associated with risk of atherosclerotic disease [148]. While case-control data suggest a strong association [148,149], prospective cohort data are not all consistent with that view. The largest prospective cohort study to evaluate the association of Lp(a) with subsequent CHD is the Lipid Research Clinics Coronary Prevention Trial [150]. In that study, Lp(a) levels were significantly associated with the risk of CHD. A second, smaller prospective study reported similar results [151]. Data from the Framingham Heart Study suggest that Lp(a) is a predictor of heart disease in women but not in men, and data from the Physicians' Health Study (PHS) reported no association with subsequent risk of MI in men [152]. It should be noted that the PHS represents a relatively healthy population and the range of Lp(a) levels was narrow, which may make it difficult to detect the apparent modest risk reported in other studies.

A number of hemostatic variables, including fibrinogen, von Willebrand factor, and factor VII, have been associated with other traditional cardiovascular risk factors [153–157]. All three factors have been associated with increased risks of CHD, but the association for fibrinogen is the strongest and most consistent. Case-control and prospective cohort studies have consistently demonstrated a positive association between fibrinogen levels and CHD [155–157] and stroke [158]. In a recent meta-analysis [159], fibrinogen was shown to confer an increased risk of CHD independent of other risk factors. Both increased platelet count and aggregability have been associated with risk of subsequent CHD event [160,161]. In addition, antiplatelet agents have been demonstrated to reduce the risk of CHD and stroke, particularly among those individuals with underlying atherosclerotic disease [162].

Several case-control studies suggest tissue-type plasminogen activator (t-PA) and plasminogen activator inhibitor levels are elevated among patients with coronary heart disease. Those findings have been supported by recent, prospective cohort data from the PHS, in which premorbid levels of endogenous t-PA antigen were increased among those who went on to develop MI or stroke during a follow-up period of 5 years [163,164]. While increased levels of t-PA antigen appear to be associated with CHD and stroke risk, there seems to be an inverse association of t-PA activity with risk of CHD [165].

Whether each of these hemostatic risk factors represents an independent risk factor for atherosclerotic disease or is in the causal pathway for other risk factors is not entirely clear. Other risk factors, such as cigarette smoking, affect the levels of various hemostatic risk factors [166] and may enhance platelet aggregability. Lipoprotein abnormalities and moderate alcohol consumption are associated with t-PA levels. Additional observational data as well as interventional trials aimed at altering hemostatic factors will provide valuable information on the role of those factors in the treatment and prevention of atherosclerotic disease.

PROPHYLACTIC LOW-DOSE ASPIRIN

Reduction of risk during or immediately following MI has been demonstrated for beta blockers, thrombolytic agents, and aspirin, and in the secondary prevention of subsequent events for beta blockers, aspirin, and angiotensin converting enzyme (ACE) inhibitors (among those with low ejection fraction); however, the use of any of these agents, with the exception of aspirin, in the primary prevention of CHD events is precluded because of potential side effects and cost.

Two large-scale studies in men assessed the benefits of prophylactic low-dose aspirin in the prevention of CVD [167,168]. There was a significant reduction of 44 percent in the risk of first MI among those randomly assigned to aspirin compared to placebo in the PHS ($p = 0.001$) [167]. That outcome is in contrast with the results of the British Doctors' Study, where no risk reduction was observed [168]. This contrasting outcome may have been due, in part, to noncompliance in both treatment arms of the unblinded British trial [168]. Combining data from these two trials reveals a 33-percent reduction in risk of MI. The benefit in the PHS was confined to those individuals older than 50 years of age. There was an apparent, though not statistically significant, increased risk of stroke in this study cohort. There are observational data in women [169] but no available randomized trial data as yet. The ongoing Women's Health Study will address the risk-to-benefit ratio of treatment with aspirin in women.

DIETARY ANTIOXIDANTS

Mounting evidence from basic and animal research suggests a role for oxidative damage in the development of atherosclerosis [170], raising the possibility that natural antioxidants may prevent or impede its progression [171]. Although antioxidants can inhibit in-vitro LDL oxidation [172], preserve endothelial function [173], inhibit platelet aggregability [174], and reduce atherosclerotic progression in animals [175–177], whether dietary supplementation with antioxidants will reduce the risk of atherosclerotic disease in humans remains unclear.

Descriptive data suggest that consumption of fruits and vegetables is associated with reduced risk of CHD. Two recent prospective cohort studies suggest that supplementation with vitamin E, in particular, is associated with a reduced risk of atherosclerotic disease [178,179]. The evidence from observational dietary intake and some blood-based studies is somewhat stronger for the lipid-soluble antioxidants alpha-tocopherol and beta-carotene than for the water-soluble antioxidant vitamin C. This difference may be due to the relatively low rates of vitamin C deficiency in the populations studied, or it could be due to mechanistic differences.

Randomized trial data on the effects of supplementation are limited. In a subgroup of 333 subjects with angina pectoris, treatment with beta-carotene appeared to be associated with a reduced risk of CHD [180]. A recent, large-scale randomized trial of vitamins in the prevention of cancer among a poorly nourished population in Linxian, China, reported a reduction in overall mortality among those consuming a mixture of beta-carotene (15 mg daily), alpha-tocopherol (30 mg daily), and selenium (50 μg daily) that was largely due to a reduction in stomach cancer mortality [181]. While mortality from ischemic heart disease was less than 9 percent of the total, cerebrovascular mortality accounted for 26 percent of the total. There was an apparent, though nonsignificant, reduction in the risk of CVD mortality (relative risk = 0.90; 95% CI = 0.76–1.07). In that population, the majority of strokes is likely to be hemorrhagic rather than thromboembolic.

While the latter type are generally due to atherosclerotic disease, that is not the case for the former. Therefore, the relevance of these findings in terms of atherosclerotic disease prevention is not yet clear.

The Alpha-Tocopherol Beta-Carotene Cancer Prevention Trial (ATBC Trial) is the first large-scale, randomized trial of antioxidant vitamins in a well-nourished population [182]. This 2 × 2 factorial trial tested the effect of alpha-tocopherol (50 mg daily) and beta-carotene (20 mg daily) in the prevention of lung cancer among 29,133 Finnish male smokers [182]. After adjustment for testing multiple hypotheses, there were no increases or decreases in risk that could not be explained plausibly by chance. Nevertheless, some findings were unexpected. For alpha-tocopherol, there was no clear reduction in risk of ischemic heart disease or ischemic stroke mortality (658 total ischemic deaths among those assigned alpha-tocopherol compared to 704 among those assigned placebo). The apparent benefits in those who took vitamin E in the NHS and the Health Professional Follow-up Study were largely confined to those who used a dose of 100 IU or more per day, which is higher than the 50 mg used in this trial. There was a possible increase in the risk of hemorrhagic stroke in the alpha-tocopherol treatment group compared to those assigned to placebo (66 versus 44), a finding not compatible with the lower stroke rates among those assigned antioxidant vitamins in the Linxian, China, trial. Hemorrhagic stroke was not a prespecified endpoint, and while this finding is compatible with an antiplatelet effect of vitamin E, it remains plausible that it could be the result of chance. With respect to beta-carotene, there also was no apparent protective effect of supplementation with respect to deaths from ischemic heart disease and stroke; in fact, there were more ischemic heart disease deaths in the treated group (653 versus 586). The ATBC Trial results do not disprove the value of antioxidant vitamins, nor do they incriminate those vitamins as harmful. They do, however, raise the possibility that some of the previously reported benefits may have been overestimated and that there may be some adverse effects. The available randomized trial data are not yet sufficient to assess fully the risk-to-benefit ratios for antioxidants. Additional randomized trial data should be forthcoming in the near future that will further define the role of antioxidants in the primary and secondary prevention of atherosclerotic disease.

Free iron, as well as other transition metals, can catalyze free-radical formation. For that reason, iron and copper are tightly bound to transport and storage proteins to prevent their involvement in free-radical formation. It has been hypothesized that increased iron intake or iron stores may promote atherogenesis by increasing oxidative stress. While one early report from a prospective study among Finnish males reported a positive association of ferritin levels with CHD [183], subsequent reports have been conflicting. In a recent prospective study (the National Epidemiologic Survey and Follow-up Study), increased transferritin saturation was not associated with increased risk of CHD; in fact, there was a trend in the opposite direction [184]. Iron-intake studies also have been conflicting. One recent prospective study reported no association for iron intake in general but an increased risk associated with intake of heme iron derived largely from red meat [185]. In a recent retrospective autopsy study, there was no evidence of increased atherosclerotic disease among those with significant iron overload (hemochromatosis or multiorgan hemosiderosis) [186]. In fact, advanced or severe coronary atheroscleroses was present in 12 percent of iron-overload cases compared with 38 percent of age-, sex-, and race-matched controls ($p = 0.01$). Some investigators have suggested that the conflicting results arise from the difficulty in assessing iron stores using plasma markers or intake. At this point, it is unclear whether iron status or intake represents a risk factor for CHD.

Summary

Current epidemiologic data strongly support a role for risk-factor modification in the prevention of CHD. The strength of evidence for an association with CVD for each risk factor is summarized in Table 24-3. Smoking cessation, cholesterol reduction, and control of hypertension all appear to have a clear benefit on reducing the risk of CHD in a cost-effective manner. Public policy measures as well as individual counseling are clearly warranted for all three modifications. While open debate should continue on who should be aggressively treated with lipid-lowering drugs, there is little debate over those at highest risk, particularly those with existing disease. Existing data support nonpharmacologic public health measures to lower the serum cholesterol of the population.

While it is clear that diabetes substantially increases the risk of CHD, data on interventions to maintain normoglycemia among diabetics are insufficient to provide estimates on risk reduction of CHD. Tight control appears to reduce renal and microvascular disease risk, but data on glycemic control and risk of CHD are conflicting. Some data even suggest increased risk associated with insulin use among non-insulin-dependent diabetics. Aggressive management of other cardiovascular risk factors are clearly warranted among diabetics.

With regard to physical inactivity and obesity, there is little doubt that these factors are associated with substantial increases in the risk of CHD. There are few trial data suggesting a benefit of exercise or weight reduction in lowering the risk of CHD, and it is unlikely that such randomized trial data will be available in the near future. It is clear that regular exercise and maintenance of ideal body weight improve other cardiovascular risk factors and, therefore, justify their importance as part of a preventive program. In clinical practice, efforts at reducing prevalence of physical inactivity and obesity, however, have been disappointing.

Recent evidence also suggests that hormone replacement therapy in postmenopausal women may substantially reduce the risk of CHD. Randomized trial data, such as those obtained from the Women's Health Initiative, will provide valuable information with regard to the competing risks and benefits of estrogen therapy alone, as well as estrogen therapy with progestin. Currently available observational data suggest that the benefits of treatment outweigh the risks.

The independent impact of psychological factors, such as depression, stress, and personality type on the risk

Table 24-3. Summary of the strength of evidence on the association of risk factors with CVD and the efficacy of intervention

Risk factor	Strength of evidence of association with CVD from observational data	Strength of evidence of association from randomized trials	Efficacy of intervention to modify risk factor
Cigarette smoking	+++	NA	++
Serum cholesterol	+++	+++	+++
Hypertension	+++	+++	+++
Diabetes mellitus	++	NA	++
Physical inactivity	++	NA	+/−
Obesity	++	NA	+/−
Menopause	+++	+	NA
Moderate alcohol consumption	++	NA	NA
Psychological factors	+	NA	NA
Hemostatic factors	+	NA	NA
Prophylactic aspirin	++	++	NA
Antioxidants	++	+/−	NA

NA: sufficient data not available.

of CHD remains unclear; further data will be needed to confirm or refute the relationship and to establish the efficacy of interventional strategies. Multifaceted therapeutic interventions with a psychological component can lower subsequent risk of CHD; however, the independent contribution of the psychological component remains unclear.

The totality of evidence suggests an inverse association between moderate alcohol consumption and MI, which is mediated, in large part, by changes in HDL levels. Hemostatic risk factors represent a promising area for future research. At this point, recommendations specifically targeted at modifying these factors are premature. While mounting basic and human data suggest a role for oxidation in the development of atherosclerotic disease, the efficacy as well as the risk of supplementation with antioxidants remain unclear. Randomized trial data will become available from ongoing trials on which rational decisions can be based.

In summary, primary and secondary prevention have contributed substantially to the reduction in CHD and stroke morality rates over the last several decades. In addition to development of a better understanding of mechanistic and epidemiologic determinants of atherosclerotic disease, considerably more attention must be given to effective strategies for implementation of existing guidelines for risk-factor modification. Further research on the cost- and risk-benefit ratios will enable better targeting of interventions for maximal individual and societal benefit. More widespread use of multifaceted self-help and health professional–directed prevention programs should help sustain the decline in CVD mortality rates in the United States.

References

1. Goldman L, Cook EF. The decline in ischemic heart disease mortality rates. An analysis of the comparative effects of medical interventions and changes in lifestyle. Ann Intern Med 1984; 101:825–836.
2. Hennekens CH, Buring JE. Epidemiology in Medicine. Boston: Little, Brown, 1987.
3. Worth RM, et al. Epidemiologic studies of coronary heart disease and stroke in Japanese men living in Japan Hawaii and California: mortality. Am J Epidemiol 1975; 102:481–490.
4. U.S. Department of Health and Human Services Public Health Service National Institutes of Health National Cancer Institute. Smoking and Tobacco Control Monographs 1: Strategies to Control Tobacco Use in the United States: a Blueprint for Public Health action in the 1990's. Washington, D.C.: U.S. Department of Health and Human Services, 1991. NIH Publ No. 92-3316.
5. McGinnis JM, Shopland D, Brown C. Tobacco and health: trends in smoking and smokeless tobacco consumption in the United States. Ann Rev Publ Health 1987; 8:441–467.
6. Centers for Disease Control and Prevention. Cigarette smoking among adults: United States 1991. Morbidity and Mortality Weekly Report 1993; 42:230–233.
7. English JP, Willius FA, Berksan J. Tobacco and coronary disease. JAMA 1940; 115:1327–1329.
8. Doll R, Hill AB. Lung cancer and other causes of death in relation to smoking. A second report on the mortality of British doctors. Br Med J 1956; 2:1071–1081.
9. Hammond EC, Horn D. Smoking and death rates: report on forty-four months of follow-up of 187,783 men. II. Death rates by cause. JAMA 1958; 166:1294–1308.
10. U.S. Public Health Service: Smoking and Health. Report of the advisory committee to the Surgeon General of the Public Health Service. Washington D.C.: 1964; Government Printing Office PHS Publ No 1103.
11. U.S. Department of Health and Human Services. The health consequences of smoking: cardiovascular disease. A report of the Surgeon General. Washington D.C.: 1983; Government Printing Office. DHHS Publication No. (PHS) 84-50204.
12. U.S. Department of Health and Human Services. Reducing the health consequences of smoking: 25 years of progress. A report of the Surgeon General. Washington D.C.: 1989; Government Printing Office, DHSS Publication No. (CDC)89-8411.
13. Willett WC, et al. Relative and absolute excess risks of coronary heart disease among women who smoke cigarettes. N Eng J Med 1987; 317:1303–1309.

14. Rosenberg L, Palmer JR, Shapiro S. Decline in the risk of myocardial infarction among women who stop smoking. N Engl J Med 1990; 322:213–217.
15. Doll R, Peto R. Mortality in relation to smoking: 20 years' observation on male British doctors. Br Med J 1976; 2:1525–1536.
16. Multiple Risk Factor Intervention Trial Research Group. Relationship between baseline risk and coronary heart disease and total mortality in the Multiple Risk Factor Intervention Trial. Prev Med 1986; 15:254–273.
17. U.S. Department of Health and Human Services. The Health Benefits of Smoking Cessation. A Report of the Surgeon General. Washington D.C.: Government Printing Office, 1990.
18. Omen GS, et al. The temporal pattern of reduction of mortality risk after smoking cessation. J Prev Med 1990; 6:251–257.
19. O'Connor NTJ, et al. Hypercoagulability and coronary artery disease. Br Heart J 1984; 52:614–616.
20. Fitzgerald GA, Oates JA, Nowak J. Cigarette smoking and hemostatic function. Am Heart J 1988; 115:267–271.
21. Murray JJ, et al. Platelet-vessel wall interactions in individuals who smoke cigarettes. Adv Experiment Med Biol 1990; 273:189–198.
22. Mjos OD. Lipid effects of smoking. Am Heart J 1988; 115:272–275.
23. Robertson D, Tseng CJ, Appalsamy M. Smoking and mechanisms of cardiovascular control. Am Heart J 1988; 115: 258–263.
24. Schwartz JL. Review and evaluation of smoking cessation methods: the United States and Canada 1978–1985. Washington D.C.: Government Printing Office, 1987. NIH Publication No. 87-2940.
25. Transdermal Nicotine Study Group. Transdermal nicotine for smoking cessation: six month results from two multicenter controlled clinical trials. JAMA 1991; 266:3133–3138.
26. Sempos CT, et al. Prevalence of high blood cholesterol among U.S. adults. An update based on guidelines from the Second Report of the National Cholesterol Education Program Adult Treatment Panel. JAMA 1993; 269:3009–3014.
27. Expert Panel on Detection Evaluation and Treatment of High Blood Cholesterol in Adults. Summary of the second report of the National Cholesterol Education Program (NCEP) expert panel on detection evaluation and treatment of high blood cholesterol in adults (Adult Treatment Panel II). JAMA 1993; 269:3015–3023.
28. National Center for Health Statistics—National Heart Lung and Blood Institute Collaborative Lipid Group: Trends in serum cholesterol levels among US. adults aged 20 to 74 years: data from the National Health and Nutrition Examination Surveys 1960 to 1980. JAMA 1987; 257(7):937–942.
29. Schucker B, et al. Change in cholesterol awareness and action: results from national physician and public surveys. Arch Intern Med 1991; 151:666–673.
30. LaRosa JC, et al. The cholesterol facts: a summary of the evidence relating dietary fats serum cholesterol and coronary heart disease: a joint statement by the American Heart Association and the National Heart Lung and Blood Institute. AHA Medical/Scientific Statement 1990; 1721–1733.
31. Chen Z, et al. Serum cholesterol concentration and coronary heart disease in population with low cholesterol concentrations. Br Med J 1991; 303:276–282.
32. Law MR, Wald NJ, Thompson SG. By how much and how quickly does reduction in serum cholesterol concentration lower risk of ischemic heart disease. Br Med J 1994; 308:367–372.
33. MacMahon S, et al. Blood pressure stroke and coronary heart disease I: prolonged differences in blood pressure; prospective observational studies corrected for regression dilution bias. Lancet 1990; 335:765–774.
34. Law MR, et al. Systematic underestimation of association between serum cholesterol concentration and ischemic heart disease in observational studies: data from the BUPA study. Br Med J 1994; 308:363–366.
35. Gordon DJ, et al. High-density lipoprotein cholesterol and cardiovascular disease: Four prospective American studies. Circulation 1989; 79:8–15.
36. Gordon DJ, Rifkind BM. High-density lipoprotein—the clinical implications of recent studies. N Engl J Med 1989; 321:1311–1316.
37. Jacobs DR Jr, et al. High density lipoprotein cholesterol as a predictor of cardiovascular disease mortality in men and women: the follow-up study of the Lipid Research Clinics Prevalence Study. Am J Epid 1990; 131:32–47.
38. Stampfer MJ, et al. A prospective study of cholesterol apolipoproteins and the risk of myocardial infarction. N Engl J Med 1991; 325:373–381.
39. Rossouw JE, Lewis B, Rifkind BM. The value of lowering cholesterol after myocardial infarction. N Engl J Med 1990; 323:1112–1119.
40. Holme I. An analysis of randomized trials evaluating the effects of cholesterol reduction on total mortality and coronary heart disease incidence. Circulation 1990; 82: 1916–1924.
41. Muldoon MF, Manuck SB, Matthew KA. Lowering cholesterol concentrations and mortality: a quantitative review of primary prevention trials. Br Med J 1990; 301:309–314.
42. Ravnskov U. Cholesterol lowering trials in coronary heart disease: frequency of citation and outcome. Br Med J 1992; 305:15–19.
43. Law MR, Thompson SG, Wald NJ. Assessing possible hazards of reducing serum cholesterol. Br Med J 1994; 308:373–379.
44. Scandinavian Simvastatin Survival Study Group. Randomized trial of cholesterol lowering in 4444 patients with coronary heart disease: the Scandinavian Simvastatin Survival Study (4S). Lancet 1994; 344:1383–1389.
45. Consensus Conference. Lowering blood cholesterol to prevent heart disease. JAMA 1985; 253:2080–2086.
46. Oliver MF. Might treatment of hypercholesterolemia increase non-cardiac mortality? Lancet 1991; 337:1529–1531.
47. Peto R. Personnel communication.
48. Keys A. Serum cholesterol response to dietary cholesterol. Am J Clin Nutr 1984; 40:351–359.
49. Hegsted DM. Dietary fat and serum lipids: an evaluation of the experimental data. Am J Clin Nutr 1993; 57:875–883.
50. Dayton S, et al. A controlled clinical trial of a diet high in unsaturated fat in preventing complications of atherosclerosis. Circulation 1969; [39/40 Suppl] II:II1–II63.
51. Watts GF, et al. Effects on coronary artery disease of lipid lowering diet plus cholestyramine in the St. Thomas Atherosclerosis Regression Study (STARS). Lancet 1992; 339: 563–569.
52. Mensink RP, Katan MB. Effect of dietary fats on serum lipids and lipoproteins. Arteriosclerosis and Thrombosis 1992; 12:911–919.
53. Ascherio A, et al. Trans fatty acids intake and risk of myocardial infarction. Circulation 1994; 89:94–101.
54. Joint National Committee on Detection, Evaluation, and Treatment of High Blood Pressure. The Fifth Report of the Joint National Committee on the Detection, Evaluation, and Treatment of High Blood Pressure (JNC V). Arch Intern Med 1993; 153:154–183.
55. Subcommittee on Definition and Prevalence of the Joint National Committee on Detection, Evaluation, and Treatment

of High Blood Pressure, 1984. Hypertension prevalence and the status of awareness, treatment, and control in the United States. Hypertension 1985; 7(3):457–468.

56. Working Group on Primary Prevention of Hypertension: Report of the National High Blood Pressure Education Program Working Group on Primary Prevention of Hypertension. Arch Intern Med 1993; 153:186–208.
57. Stamler J, Stamler R, Neaton JD. Blood pressure, systolic and diastolic, and cardiovascular risks: U.S. population data. Arch Intern Med 1993; 153:598–615.
58. National Conference on High Blood Pressure Education. Report on Proceedings. Bethesda, MD: U.S. Department of Health, Education and Welfare, Public Health Service, National Institutes of Health, 1973. USDHEW Publ No. (NIH) 73-486.
59. Report of the Joint National Committee on Detection, Evaluation and Treatment of High Blood Pressure: A cooperative study. JAMA 1977; 237:255–261.
60. Collins R, et al. Blood pressure, stroke, and coronary heart disease, II: short-term reductions in blood pressure: overview of randomized drug trials in their epidemiological context. Lancet 1990; 335:827–838.
61. Hebert PR, et al. Recent evidence on drug therapy of mild to moderate hypertension and decreased risk of coronary heart disease. Arch of Int Med 1993; 53(5):578–581.
62. Pollare T, Lithell H, Berne C. A comparison of the effects of hydrochlorothiazide and captopril on glucose and lipid metabolism in patients with hypertension. N Engl J Med 1989; 321:868–873.
63. Weinberger MH. Antihypertensive therapy and lipids: evidence, mechanisms, and implications Arch Intern Med 1985; 145:1102–1105.
64. Langford JG, et al. Dietary therapy slows the return of hypertension after stopping prolonged medication. JAMA 1985; 253:657–664.
65. Edelson JT, Weinstein MC, Tosteson ANA. The long term cost-effectiveness of various initial monotherapies for mild to moderate hypertension. JAMA 1990; 263:408–413.
66. Prevalence and Incidence of Diabetes—United States, 1980–1987. Morbidity and Mortality Weekly Report 1990; 39:809–821.
67. Kleinman JC, et al. Mortality among diabetics in a national sample. Am J Epidemiol 1988; 128:389–401.
68. Krolewski AS, Warram JH, Christleib, AR. Onset, course, complications, and prognosis of diabetes mellitus. In. A Marble et al, eds. Joslin's Diabetes Mellitus. Philadelphia: Lea & Febiger, 1985.
69. Kannel WB, McGee DL. Diabetes and glucose intolerance as risk factors for cardiovascular disease: the Framingham Study. Diabetes Care 1979; 2:120–126.
70. Krolewski AS, et al. Magnitude and determinants of coronary artery disease in juvenile-onset, insulin-dependent diabetes mellitus. Am J Cardiol 1987; 59:750–755.
71. Deckert T, Poulsen JE, Larsen M. Prognosis of diabetics with diabetes onset before age thirty-one. I. Survival, causes of death, and complications Diabetologia 1978; 14:363–370.
72. Fields TS, et al. Glycosylated hemoglobin A_{1c} and increased mortality from cardiovascular disease in elderly women. Circulation 1994; (Abstr) 89:941.
73. The Diabetes Control and Complications Trial Research Group. The effect of intensive treatment of diabetes on the development and progression of long-term complications in insulin-dependent diabetes mellitus. N Engl J Med 1993; 329:977–986.
74. VA Cooperative Study on Glycemic Control and Complications in Type II Diabetes, 1994.
75. Ruderman NB, Haudenschild C. Diabetes as an atherogenic factor. Progr Cardiovas Dis 1984; 26:373–412.
76. Kannel WB. Lipid, diabetes, and coronary heart disease: insights from the Framingham Study. Am Heart J 1985; 110:1100–1107.
77. Harris MI. Non-insulin dependent diabetes mellitus in black and white Americans. Diabetes/Metabolism Rev 1990; 6:71–90.
78. DeFronzo RA, et al. New concepts in the pathogenesis and treatment of noninsulin-dependent diabetes mellitus Am J Med 1983; 74:52–81.
79. Henry RR, Gumbiner B. Benefits and limitations of very-low-calorie diet therapy in obese NIDDM. Diabetes Care 1991; 14:802–823.
80. U.S. Department of Health and Human Services. Health Promotion and Disease Prevention United States, 1985. Data from the National Health Interview Survey. Hattysville, MD: National Center for Health Statistics, 1988. Series 10, #163. USDHHS Publ No. 88–1591.
81. Powell KE, et al. The status of the 1990 objectives for physical fitness and exercise. Public Health Reports 1986; 101:15–20.
82. Morris JN, et al. Coronary heart disease and physical activity of work. Lancet 1953; 2:1053–1057; 1111–1120.
83. Berlin JA, Colditz GA. A meta-analysis of physical activity in the prevention of coronary heart disease. Am J Epidemiol 1990; 132:612–628.
84. Morris JN, et al. Vigorous exercise in leisure time and the incidence of coronary heart disease Lancet 1973; 1:333–339.
85. Paffenbarger RS, Wing AL, Hyde RT. Physical activity as an index of heart attack risk in college alumni. Am J Epidemiol 1978; 108:161–175.
86. Lee IM, Paffenbarger RS, Hsieh CC. Time trends in physical activity among college alumni, 1962–1988. Am J Epidemiol 1992; 135:915–925.
87. Leon AS, et al. Leisure-time physical activity levels and risk of coronary heart disease and death: the Multiple Risk Factor Intervention Trial. JAMA 1987; 258:2388–2395.
88. Mittelman MA, et al. Triggering of acute myocardial infarction by heavy physical exertion-protection against triggering by regular exertion. N Engl J Med 1993; 329: 1677–1683.
89. Thompson PD, et al. Incidence of death during jogging in Rhode Island from 1975 through 1980. JAMA 1982; 247:2535–2538.
90. Willich SN, et al. Physical exertion as a trigger of acute myocardial infarction. N Engl J Med 1993; 329:1684–1690.
91. Haskell B. Exercise-induced changes in plasma lipids and lipoproteins. Prev Med 1984; 13:23–36.
92. Rauramaa R. Relationship of physical activity, glucose tolerance, and weight management. Prev Med 1984; 13: 37–46.
93. U.S. Preventive Services Task Force. Guide to Clinical Preventive Services: an Assessment of the Effectiveness of 169 Interventions. Baltimore: Williams and Wilkins, 1989.
94. U.S. Department of Health and Human Services. Morbidity and Mortality Chart Book on Cardiovascular, Lung, and Blood Diseases, 1990. Bethesda, MD: National Institutes of Health: National Heart, Lung, and Blood Institute, 1990.
95. Eaker ED, Castelli WP. Coronary heart disease and risk factors among women in the Framingham Study. In ED Eaker, et al, eds. Coronary Heart Disease in Women: Proceedings of an NIH Workshop. New York: Haymarket Doyma, 1987.
96. Bush TL. The epidemiology of cardiovascular disease in postmenopausal women. Ann NY Acad Sci 1990; 592:263–271.

97. Eaker ED, et al. Cardiovascular disease in women. Circulation 1993; 88:1999–2009.
98. Palmer JR, et al. Reproductive factors and risk of myocardial infarction. Am J Epidemiol 1992; 136:408–416.
99. Robinson K, et al. Risk factors and in-hospital course of first episode of myocardial infarction or acute coronary insufficiency in women. J Am Coll Cardio 1988; 11:932–936.
100. Fiebach NH, Viscoli CM, Horwitz RI. Differences between women and men in survival after myocardial infarction. Biology or methodology? JAMA 1990; 263:1091–1096.
101. Bush TL, Miller VT. Effects of pharmacologic agents used during menopause: impact on lipids and lipoproteins. In DR Mischell Jr, ed. Menopause: Physiology and Pharmacology. Chicago: Year Book Medical Publishers, 1987.
102. Henderson BE, et al. Estrogen use and cardiovascular disease. Am J Obstet Gynecol 1986; 154:1181–1186.
103. Lobo RA. Estrogen and cardiovascular disease. Ann NY Acad Sci 1990; 592:286–294.
104. Keaney JF Jr, et al. 17 beta-estradiol preserves endothelial vasodilator function and limits low-density lipoprotein oxidation in hypercholesterolemic swine. Circ 1994; 898:2251–2259.
105. Stampfer MJ, Colditz GA. Estrogen replacement therapy and coronary heart disease: a quantitative assessment of the epidemiologic evidence. Prev Med 1991; 20:47–63.
106. Barrett-Connor E. Postmenopausal estrogen and prevention bias. Ann Int Med 1991; 115:455–456.
107. Stampfer MJ, et al. Postmenopausal estrogen therapy and cardiovascular disease: ten-year follow-up from the Nurses' Health Study. N Engl J Med 1991; 325:756–762.
108. Bush TL, et al. Cardiovascular mortality and noncontraceptive use of estrogen in women: results from the Lipid Research Clinics Program Follow-up Study. Circulation 1987; 75:1102–1109.
109. National Institutes of Health Consensus Development Panel on the Health Implications of Obesity. Health implications of obesity; National Institutes of Health Consensus Development conference statement. Ann Intern Med 1985; 103:1073–1077.
109. Harlan WR, et al. Secular trends in body mass in the United States, 1960–1980. Am J Epidemiol 1988; 128:1065–1074.
111. National Center for Health Statistics. Plan and operation of the Second National Health and Nutrition Examination Survey, 1976–1980. Vital and health statistics. Series 1, No. 15. Washington, D.C.: Government Printing Office, 1981. DMMS Publ No. (PHS) 81-1317.
112. Folsom AR, et al: Body fat distribution and 5-year risk of death in older women. J Amer Med Assoc 1993; 269:483–487.
113. Lapidus L, et al. Distribution of adipose tissue and risk of cardiovascular disease and death: A 12-year follow-up of participants in the population study of women in Gothenberg, Sweden. Br Med J 1984; 289:1257–1261.
114. Mann GV. The influence of obesity on health. N Engl J Med 1974; 291:178–185; 226–232.
115. Hubert HB. The importance of obesity in the development of coronary risk factors and disease: the epidemiologic evidence. Ann Rev Public Health 1986; 7:493–502.
116. Ashley FW, Kannel WB. Relation of weight change to changes in atherogenic traits: the Framingham Study. J Chron Dis 1974; 27:103–114.
117. Pooling Project Research Group. Relationship of blood pressure, serum cholesterol, smoking habit, relative weight, and ECG abnormalities to incidence of major coronary events: final report of the Pooling Project. J Chron Dis 1978; 31:201–306.
118. Noppa H, et al. Obesity in relation to morbidity and mortality from cardiovascular disease. Am J Epidemiol 1980; 111:682–692.
119. Tuomilehto J, et al. Body weight and risk of myocardial infarction and death in the adult population of eastern Finland. Br Med J 1987; 295:623–627.
120. Manson JE, et al. A prospective study of obesity and risk of coronary heart disease in women. N Engl J Med 1990; 322:882–889.
121. Bierman EL, Hirsch J. Obesity. In RH Williams, ed. Textbook of Endocrinology. Sixth Ed. Vol 1. Philadelphia: Saunders, 1981.
122. Manson JE, Tosteson H, Ridker PM. The primary prevention of myocardial infarction. N Engl J Med 1992; 326: 1406–1416.
123. Committee on Diet and Health. Diet and health: implications for reducing chronic disease risk. Washington, D.C.: National Academy Press, 1989.
124. Dwyer JT. Treatment of obesity: conventional programs and fad diets. In P Bjorntorp, BN Brodoff, eds. Obesity. Philadelphia: Lippincott, 1992.
125. Klatsky AL, Friedman GD, Siegelaub AB. Alcohol and mortality. A ten-year Kaiser-Permanente experience. Ann Intern Med 1981; 95(2):139–145.
126. Pell S, D'Alzono CA. A five year mortality study of alcoholics. J Occup Med 1973; 15:120–125.
127. Fraser GE, Upsdell M. Alcohol and other discriminants between cases of sudden death and myocardial infarction. Am J Epidemiol 1981; 114(4):462–476.
128. Duetscher S, Rockette HE, Krishnswami V. Evaluation of habitual excessive alcohol consumption on myocardial infarction risk in coronary disease patients. Am Heart J 1984; 108(4):988–995.
129. Moore RD, Pearson TA. Moderate alcohol consumption and coronary artery disease: a review. Medicine 1986; 65:242–267.
130. Gordon T, Kannel WB. Drinking habits and cardiovascular disease: The Framingham Study. Am Heart J 1983; 105: 667–673.
131. Stampfer MJ, et al. A prospective study of moderate alcohol consumption and the risk of coronary disease and stroke in women. N Engl J Med 1988; 319(5):267–273.
132. Criqui MH, et al. Lipoproteins as mediators for the effects of alcohol consumption and cigarette smoking on cardiovascular mortality: results from the lipid research clinics follow-up study. Am J Epidemiol 1987; 126(4):629–637.
133. Gaziano JM, et al. Moderate alcohol intake, increased levels of high-density lipoprotein and its subfractions, and risk of myocardial infarction. N Engl J Med 1993; 329:1829–1834.
134. Maclure M. Demonstration of deductive meta-analysis: ethanol intake and risk of myocardial infarction. Epidemiol (Rev) 1993; 15:328–351.
135. Haynes SG, Feinleib M, Kennel WB. The relationship of psychological factors to coronary heart disease in the Framingham Heart Study. II. Eight year incidence of coronary heart disease. Am J Epidemiol 1980; 111:37–58.
136. Krantz DS, et al. Environmental stress and biobehavioral antecedents of coronary heart disease. J Consult Clin Psych 1988; 56:333–341.
137. Booth-Kewley S, Friedman HS. Psychological predictors of heart disease: a quantitative review. Psych Bull 1987; 101:343–362.
138. Smith TW, Barefoot JC. The assessment of hostility: implications for research and practice. Paper presented at the annual meeting of the American Psychosomatic Society. Charleston, SC: 1993.
139. Broadhead WE, et al. The epidemiologic evidence from a

relationship between social support and health. Am J Epidemiol 1983; 117:320–325.
140. Niaura R, Stoney CM, Herbert N. Lipids in psychological research: the last decade. Biological Psychology 1992; 34:1–43.
141. Yeung AC, et al. The effect of atherosclerosis on the vasomotor response of coronary arteries to mental stress. N Engl J Med 1991; 325:1551–1556.
142. Rozanski A, et al. Mental stress and the induction of silent myocardial ischemia in patients with coronary artery disease. New Engl J Med 1988; 318:1005–1012.
143. Burg MW, et al. Role of behavioral and psychological factors in mental stress-induced silent left ventricular dysfunction in coronary artery disease. J Am Coll Cardiol 1993; 22:440–448.
144. Tofler GH, et al. Analysis of possible triggers of acute myocardial infarction (The MILIS Study). Am J Cardiol 1990; 66:22–27.
145. Ornish D, et al. Can lifestyle changes reverse coronary heart disease? Lancet 1990; 336:129–133.
146. Shuler G, et al. Myocardial perfusion and regression of coronary artery disease in patients on a regimen of intensive physical exercise and low fat diet. J Am Coll Cardiol 1992; 19:34–42.
147. Friedman M, et al. Alteration of type-A behavior and its effect on cardiac recurrences in post myocardial infarction patients: summary results of the recurrent coronary prevention project. Am Heart J 1986; 112:653–665.
148. Loscalzo J. Lipoprotein(a): a unique risk factor for atherothrombotic disease Arteriosclerosis 1990; 10:671–679.
149. Scanu AM. Lipoprotein(a): a genetic risk factor for premature coronary heart disease. JAMA 1992; 267:3326–3329.
150. Schaeffer EJ, et al. Elevated lipoprotein(a) levels predict CHD incidence in the prospective Lipid Research Clinics Coronary Primary Prevention Trial (LRC-CPPT). Circulation 1992; 86:3231(A).
151. Rosengren A, et al. Lipoprotein(a) and coronary heart disease: a prospective case-control study in a general population of middle aged men. Br Med J 1990; 301:1248–1251.
152. Ridker PM, Hennekens CH, Stampfer MJ. A prospective study of lipoprotein(a) and the risk of myocardial infarction JAMA 1993; 270:2195–2199.
153. Yang XL, et al. Relation of hemostatic factors to other risk factors for CHD and to sex hormones in men. Arteriosclerosis Thromb 1993; 13:467–471.
154. Green D, et al. Hemostatic factors in the Coronary Artery Risk Development in Young Adults (CARDIA) Study. Arteriosclerosis Thromb 1994; 14:686–693.
155. Rainer C, et al. Changes in blood rheology in patients with stable angina pectoris as a result of coronary artery disease. Circulation 1987; 76:15–20.
156. Meade TW, et al. Hemostatic function and ischemic heart disease. Principle results of the Nortwick Park Heart Study. Lancet 1986; 2:533–537.
157. Yarnell JWG, et al. Fibrinogen, viscosity, and white blood cell count are major risk factors for ischemic heart disease. The Caerphilly and Speedwell Collaborative Heart Disease Studies. Circulation 1991; 83:836–844.
158. Wilhemsen L, et al. Fibrinogen as a risk factor for stroke and myocardial infarction. NEJM 1984; 311:501–505.
159. Ernst E, Resch KL. Fibrinogen as a cardiovascular risk factor. A meta-analysis and review of the literature. Ann Int Med 1993; 118:956–963.
160. Trip MD, et al. Platelet hyperreactivity and prognosis in survivors of myocardial infarction. NEJM 1990; 322:1549–1554.
161. Thaulow E, et al. Blood platelet count and function are related to total cardiovascular death in apparently healthy men Circulation 1991; 84:613–617.
162. Antiplatelet Trialist Collaboration: Secondary prevention of vascular disease by prolonged antiplatelet treatment. Br Med J 1988; 296:320–331.
163. Ridker PM, et al. Endogenous tissue-type plasminogen activator and risk of myocardial infarction. Lancet 1993; 341:1165–1168.
164. Ridker PM, et al. A prospective study of endogenous tissue-type plasminogen activator and risk of stroke. Lancet 1994; 343:940–943. (In press 1994)
165. Meade TW, et al: Fibrinolytic activity, clotting factors, and long term incidence of ischemic disease in the Northwick Park Heart Study. Lancet 1993; 342:1076–1079.
166. Stratton JR, et al. Effects of physical conditioning on fibrinolytic variables and fibrinogen in young and old healthy adults. Circulation 1991; 83:565–569.
167. Steering Committee of the Physician's Health Study Research Group. Final report on the aspirin component of the ongoing Physicians' Health Study. N Engl J Med 1989; 321:129–135.
168. Peto R, et al. A randomized trial of the effects of prophylactic daily aspirin among male British doctors. Br Med J 1988; 296:313–316.
169. Manson JE, et al. A prosecutive study of aspirin use and primary prevention of cardiovascular disease in women. JAMA 1991; 266:521–527.
170. Steinberg D, et al. Beyond cholesterol: modifications of low density lipoprotein that increase its atherogenicity. N Engl J Med 1989; 320:915–924.
171. Gaziano JM, et al. Dietary antioxidants in cardiovascular disease. Ann of NY Acad of Sci 1992; 249–259.
172. Esterbauer H, et al. The role of lipid peroxidation and antioxidants in oxidative modification of LDL. Free Radic Biol & Med 1992; 13:341–390.
173. Keaney JF Jr, et al. Dietary antioxidants preserve endothelium-dependent vessel relaxation in rabbits. Proc Natl Acad Sci 1993; 90:11880–11884.
174. Oda T, et al. Alpha-tocopherol inhibits platelet and neutrophil activation during cyclic flow variations in dogs with coronary stenosis and endothelial injury. Circulation 1993; 88[Suppl]:1–35 Abstr 0173.
175. Smith TL, Kummerow FA. Effect of dietary vitamin E on plasma lipids and atherogenesis in restricted ovulatory chickens. Atherosclerosis 1989; 75:105–109.
176. Carew T, et al. Antiatherogenic effect of probucol unrelated to its hypocholesterolemic effect: evidence that antioxidants in vivo can selectively inhibit low density lipoprotein degradation in macrophage-rich fatty streaks and slow the progression of atherosclerosis in the Watanabe heritable hyperlipidemic rabbit. Proc Natl Acad Sci USA 1987; 84:7725–7729.
177. Verlangieri AJ, et al. Effects of d-alpha-tocopherol supplementation on experimentally induced primate atherosclerosis J Am Coll Nutr 1992; 11:131–138.
178. Stampfer MJ, et al. A prospective study of vitamin E consumption and risk of coronary disease in women. New Engl J Med 1993; 328:1444–1449.
179. Rimm EB, et al. Dietary intake and risk of coronary heart disease among men. NEJM 1993; 328:1450–1456.
180. Gaziano JM, et al. Beta carotene therapy for chronic stable angina. Circulation 1990; 82[Suppl III]:202.
181. Blot WJ, et al. Nutritional intervention trials in Linxian, China: Supplementation with specific vitamin / mineral combinations, cancer incidence, and disease specific mortality in the general population. J Natl Cancer Inst 1993; 85:1483–1492.

182. The Alpha-Tocopherol, Beta-Carotene Cancer Prevention Study Group. The effect of vitamin E and beta carotene on the incidence of lung cancer and other cancers in male smokers. New Engl J Med 1994; 330:1029–1035.
183. Salonen JT, et al. High stores iron levels are associated with excess risk of myocardial infarction in Eastern Finnish men. Circulation 1992; 86:803–811.
184. Sempos CT, et al. Body iron stores and the risk of CHD. N Engl J Med 1994; 330:1119–1124.
185. Ascherio A, et al. Dietary iron intake and risk of coronary disease among men. Circulation 1994; 89:969–974.
186. Miller M, Grover M, Hutchins MD. Hemochromatosis, multiorgan hemosiderosis, and coronary artery disease. JAMA 1994; 272:231–233.

The Atherogenic Dyslipoproteinemias

Allan D. Sniderman
Katherine Cianflone

In this chapter, we will review the common atherogenic dyslipoproteinemias, which substantially increase the risk of premature vascular disease. Usually the rarer causes receive the most attention and the commonest the least. That approach will not be our practice here. However common or rare, significant dyslipoproteinemias are not present in all patients with premature vascular disease. Even so, we consider that arteriosclerosis is almost always the result of a complex interaction between two principal determinants: the atherogenic plasma lipoproteins and elements of the arterial wall itself. In this model, the classical nonlipoprotein risk factors for vascular disease such as smoking, diabetes, and hypertension act wholly or in part by altering the properties of the lipoproteins or by changing critical properties of the arterial wall. Smoking, for example, causes the number of atherogenic particles in plasma to increase [1,2] and also causes interendothelial junctions to widen [3,4], thereby facilitating entry of lipoproteins into the subintimal space. Diabetes mellitus, on the other hand, results in glycation of lipoprotein particles [5,6] and components of the arterial wall [7–10], the net effect of which is to multiply the atherogenic risk attributable to low-density lipoprotein (LDL) by increasing the likelihood that such particles are trapped or oxidized in the vessel. Hypertension has obvious and important effects on the arterial wall, with thickening of the subintimal space likely to contribute to trapping of LDL particles within it [11]. To the extent, therefore, that these nonlipoprotein risk factors operate through their effects on lipoproteins, lowering the levels of the atherogenic plasma lipoproteins in such patients becomes even more of a priority than it would be otherwise.

This leads to the second introductory point we would like to make, namely, the importance of elements of the vascular wall in the development of the disease process. Atherogenesis is much more than just the accumulation of cholesterol in the arterial wall. Indeed, too much attention has been paid for too long to the plasma lipoproteins and too little to the roles that the elements of the wall itself play in this intricate and prolonged process of injury and response to injury. Each component that enters into the formation of a lesion almost certainly can vary so as to increase or decrease the risk of vascular disease. At the moment, unfortunately, almost nothing is known of these factors.

Our point of view, therefore, is that in some patients abnormalities in the plasma lipoproteins are sufficiently pronounced as to be causal, and these are the dyslipoproteinemias we will review. In many other patients, even though the plasma lipoprotein levels are less extreme, other risk factors or metabolic defects in the vascular wall are acting synergistically to multiply their adverse biologic effects. Thus, we believe that in most cases of vascular disease the plasma lipoproteins play a necessary role in the development and evolution of the arterial disease process. If so, lowering the level of the atherogenic lipoproteins is likely to produce clinical benefit in both groups of patients.

The Flow of Fatty Acids and Cholesterol

Lipoproteins transport cholesterol and triglycerides (three fatty acids bound to a glycerol backbone) in the circulation from one site to another. Most emphasis has focused on understanding the transport of cholesterol and very little on understanding the transport of fatty acids. This narrow focus is unfortunate because dietary and endogenously synthesized fatty acids represent the major fuel for cardiac and skeletal muscle. Thus, understanding the flow of fatty acids in the organism is critical to understanding how energy can be mobilized when needed. The concept is also critical to understanding the pathogenesis of some of the most common dyslipoproteinemias associated with premature coronary artery disease.

The fatty-acid cycle can be summarized as follows: dietary fatty acids enter the circulation as triglycerides formed in the intestine, which are then packaged in the interior of chylomicrons, the very large triglyceride-rich lipoprotein particles secreted by enterocytes. As illustrated in Fig. 25-1A, chylomicrons transport the fatty acids principally to adipocytes but also to myocytes. In adipocytes, they are re-formed into triglycerides, and during that process the energy they contain is stored for future use. In the myocyte, fatty acids are oxidized almost immediately, and the energy generated is used to support contraction. Once most of the triglyceride has been removed, the chylomicron particles, with their store of cholesterol intact, are now called **chylomicron remnants**, which are rapidly taken up by the liver. The chylomicron, therefore, has disposed of the major dietary lipids in different sites: fatty acids to adipocytes and myocytes; cholesterol to the liver.

Given the limited store of glycogen in muscle, an alternative and, preferably inexhaustible, source of energy is essential to meet any substantial energy requirement, such as that in the fasting state. That source is fatty acids, which are released from adipocytes when triglyceride molecules in them are hydrolyzed by the enzyme hormone-sensitive lipase (Fig. 25-1B). This enzyme, as its name implies, is activated when a wide variety of hormones, particularly catecholamines, interact with their receptors at the adipocyte membrane surface. The fatty acids released from adipocytes can be taken up and oxidized by muscle as required, but the numbers released are not carefully calibrated against need. Rather, an excess is liberated to ensure that myocytes do not even transiently fall short of their energy requirements.

Because fatty acids in excess are cytotoxic and because there are no barriers to their entry into cells, plasma con-

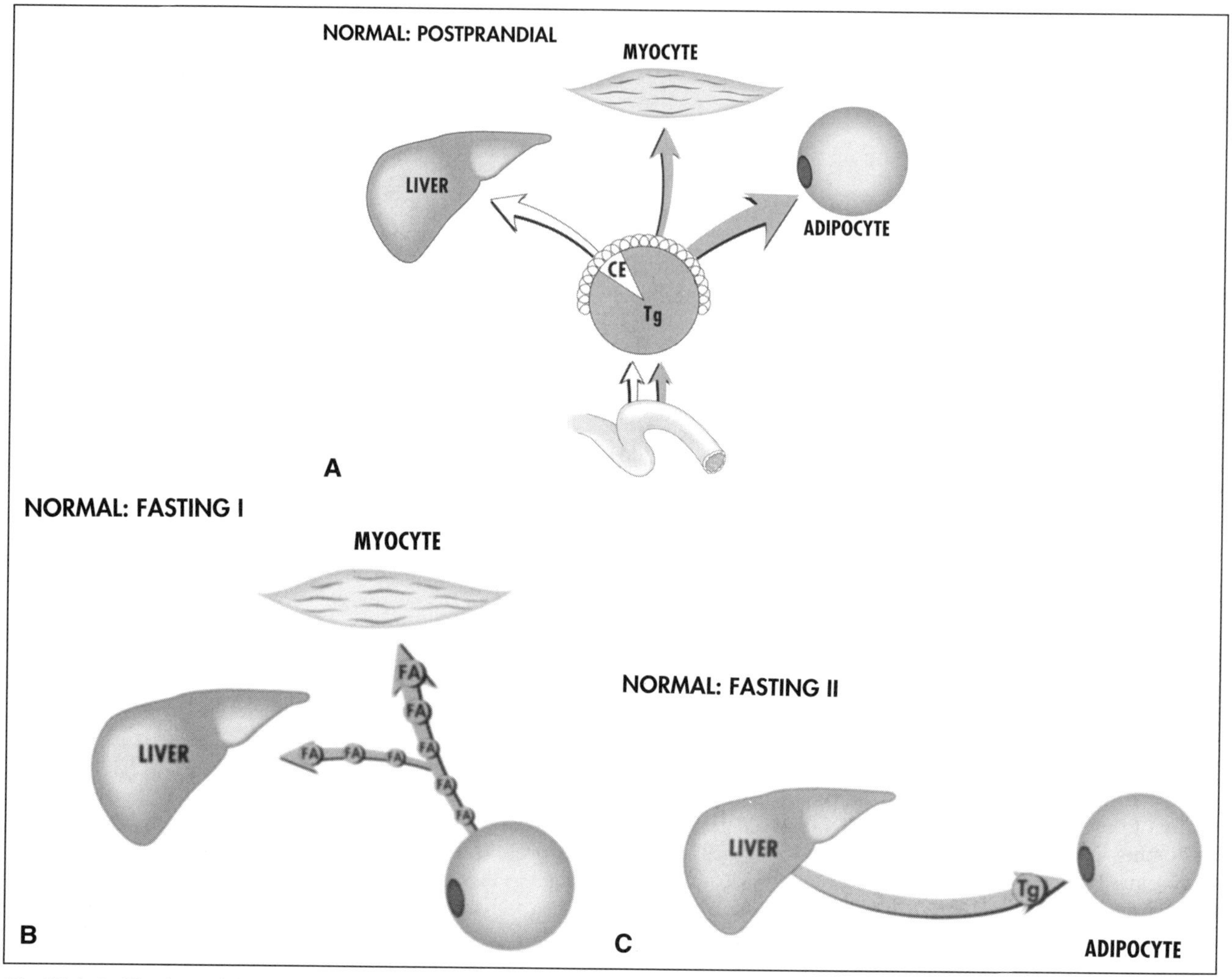

Fig. 25-1. **A.** The fate of the triglyceride and cholesteryl ester in a chylomicron particle. Chylomicrons are very large triglyceride-rich particles. They are spherical with an outer coat consisting of a phospholipid monolayer and several apoproteins, only one of which, B48 (the coil partially encircling the particle), is illustrated. In their interior are triglyceride (Tg)—the predominant lipid—and cholesteryl ester (CE). Chylomicrons are formed in the enterocytes and enter the circulation through the thoracic duct. In the microcirculation, they bind to the enzyme lipoprotein lipase, which, in the presence of its cofactor, apoCII, hydrolyzes the triglyceride in them. The fatty acids released are taken up principally by adipocytes but also, to a certain degree, by myocytes. The remnant particle, which contains little of the original triglyceride but most of the cholesterol, is then rapidly cleared by the liver. **B.** Fatty-acid release during fasting. To meet the energy requirements of the heart and skeletal muscle, triglyceride in the adipocyte is hydrolyzed by the enzyme hormone-sensitive lipase. The fatty acids released from the cell bind to albumin and are rapidly dispersed throughout the circulation. Those required are taken up by the tissues that need them but only to the degree necessary for energy at that moment, since only adipocytes can store energy in any quantity for later use. Those fatty acids not required are removed from the circulation by the liver, thus preventing the level of fatty acids in plasma from increasing significantly. **C.** In the liver, the fatty acids that have been removed from the circulation are almost all resynthesized into triglycerides and released from the liver in VLDL. The triglyceride in the VLDL particle undergoes the same fate as that in the chylomicron, that is, hydrolysis by lipoprotein lipase and either oxidation by monocytes or smooth muscle cells or storage in adipocytes.

centrations must be carefully regulated to avoid cell injury. Short-term protection against excessive levels occurs by virtue of hepatic uptake, a process that is concentration dependent and virtually unsaturable [12]. The liver has a limited capacity to store or oxidize these fatty acids; thus, the majority are reformed into triglycerides and secreted as very low density lipoprotein (VLDL) particles [13]. The triglyceride from these particles is hydrolyzed much as that in chylomicrons; as a result, many of the fatty acids in VLDL are restored to adipocytes (Fig. 25-1C). However, unlike chylomicrons, most of the VLDL remnant particles in humans are not immediately removed from plasma but instead are transformed into cholesterol-rich atherogenic LDL particles, which have a long plasma half-life compared to VLDL.

The Plasma Lipoproteins

CHYLOMICRONS

Not all plasma lipoproteins pose significant atherogenic risk. Chylomicron particles appear to be too large to enter the arterial wall; thus, the metabolic errors that produce marked elevation of plasma triglycerides, such as the absence of lipoprotein lipase [14] or its essential cofactor, apoCII [15,16], increase the risk of pancreatitis but not of premature coronary disease. Chylomicrons are thought to be metabolized in two successive steps: triglycerides are first extracted, and the cholesterol-rich remnant particles are then rapidly removed by the liver [17]. Rarely, as in type III hyperlipoproteinemia, large numbers of these remnant particles accumulate in plasma, and atherogenic risk is thereby markedly increased [18]. Whether chylomicron remnants contribute importantly to risk in other clinical settings in which they are present in far less but still elevated concentrations is unclear. Certainly, impaired clearance of chylomicron remnants is a common finding in patients with coronary disease [19,20]. However, as we will discuss, other abnormalities are often also present in those patients, making it difficult to identify with certainty the specific metabolic importance of remnants in producing atheromatous disease.

THE HEPATIC APOB100 LIPOPROTEINS

The classical model of the members of the hepatic poB100 lipoprotein family and their metabolic relationships are illustrated in Fig. 25-2. There are three generations of lipoprotein particle, each one denser than its predecessor. In VLDL and LDL classes, as we will discuss, there is also important variation in particle composition. In humans all lipoprotein particles of hepatic origin contain one molecule of apoB100, whereas all those of intestinal origin have a single molecule of a smaller homologue of apoB100, apoB48. Thus, apoB100 content identifies a lipoprotein of hepatic origin, while apoB48 content indicates intestinal origin. Since all hepatic lipoproteins have one molecule of apoB100 per particle, the total mass of apoB100 in plasma correlates with the exact number of hepatic lipoprotein particles.

The hepatic lipoproteins are spherical particles that comprise a coat and a core. VLDL is the largest and the most buoyant of the group and contains, in addition to its single molecule of apoB100, several other apoproteins

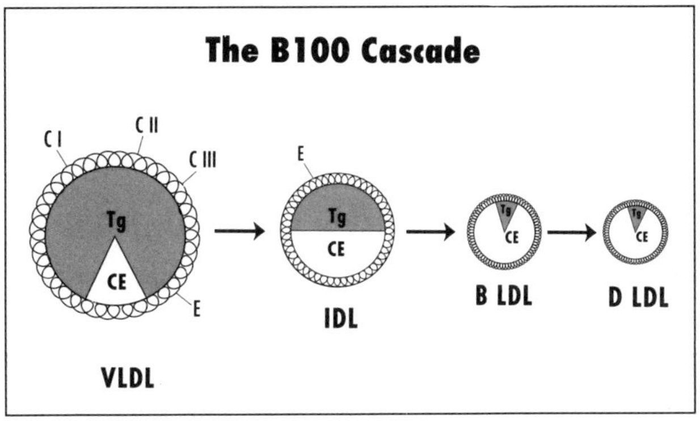

Fig. 25-2. The classic view of the apoB100 cascade. On the left is a VLDL particle secreted by the liver. Like the chylomicron, it is spherical. In its coat, however, is a molecule of apoB100 rather than apoB48 (represented by the coil completely encircling the particle). The apoB100 molecule is twice as large as apoB48 and contains the region that binds to the LDL receptor in the additional protein section. Additional apoproteins are present—apoE, CI, CII, and CIII—all of which may influence the metabolic fate of the particle. As the triglyceride (Tg) in VLDL is being hydrolyzed, the particle becomes smaller because it is losing core mass and most of the apoproteins on its surface except apoB100. Each VLDL particle contains one molecule of apoB100, and that molecule stays with the particle throughout its natural life. An intermediate particle—IDL—is represented next. In contrast to VLDL, the atherogenicity of which remains in doubt, this particle is certainly small enough to promote atherosclerosis. Once more of the triglyceride and all the apoproteins except the single molecule of apoB100 have been removed, a cholesterol-rich remnant, LDL, is produced. These particles are heterogeneous in composition, with some larger and more buoyant (B LDL) and others smaller and denser (D LDL). The larger ones contain more cholesteryl ester (CE) in their cores and are likely the precursors of the smaller ones, which contain less.

(apoE, apoCI, CII, and CIII) in its coat [22]. The coat itself comprises a monolayer of phospholipid molecules with some free cholesterol intercalated in it, while the core consists of the most hydrophobic lipids, which are principally triglycerides, and cholesteryl ester. As the triglyceride in VLDL is hydrolyzed and thus extracted from the particle, apoproteins other than apoB100 dissociate from the particle surface, and the particle becomes smaller, denser, and relatively enriched in cholesterol. When its density exceeds 1.006 g/ml, it is defined as an intermediate density lipoprotein (IDL). Further removal of triglyceride and apoproteins yields a still denser cholesterol-rich LDL particle (LDL d 1.019–1.063 g/ml), the only protein within which is apoB100.

In normals, for every three VLDL particles secreted by the liver, two become LDL, the third having been irreversibly removed from the plasma compartment during metabolism [21]. This metabolic processing should result in more VLDL than LDL particles in plasma. This is not the case, however, since the plasma half-life of an LDL particle is approximately 10 times that of a VLDL particle [21]. IDL, LDL, and lipoprotein(a) [Lp(a)] each contain one molecule of B100, and all are atherogenic.

Thus, measurement of plasma apoB provides a clinically precise estimate of the atherogenic risk posed by the cumulative pool of apoB-containing particles. Since approximately 90 percent of total apoB-containing particles are LDL [23,24], total plasma apoB, for clinical purposes, is equivalent to LDL apoB.

HIGH DENSITY LIPOPROTEIN (HDL)

High density lipoprotein (HDL) is a complex family of particles, the smallest and densest of the major lipoprotein classes. Cholesterol is the major lipid component of HDL, and apoA1 and apoAII are the two major apoproteins in these particles. The smaller, denser HDL particles are called HDL3, and the larger, more buoyant ones HDL2. HDL particles can be characterized in other ways, as well, such as by their apoprotein composition, in which case they are divided into AI-only and AI-AII particles [25]. The classic physiologic role of HDL is as the key lipoprotein particle involved in reverse cholesterol transport [26].

The metabolic path a cholesterol molecule takes as it ultimately enters the liver for excretion in the bile acid pool is convoluted. First, free cholesterol in the cell membrane is transferred to a small, dense HDL fraction. Once in the phospholipid monolayer of this particle, a fatty acyl group from the phospholipid pool is transferred to the cholesterol by the enzyme lecithin-cholesterol acyltransferase (LCAT) to form a molecule of cholesteryl ester, which then partitions in the interior of the particle [27]. The cholesteryl ester may then be returned through its HDL-carrier particle directly to the liver, but more often it is transferred to VLDL in exchange for triglyceride; this exchange is mediated by a plasma protein, cholesteryl ester transfer protein (CETP) [28]. In humans, most of the cholesterol present in VLDL is derived by CETP action, after which it is returned to the liver through receptor-mediated uptake of VLDL or its products, IDL or LDL.

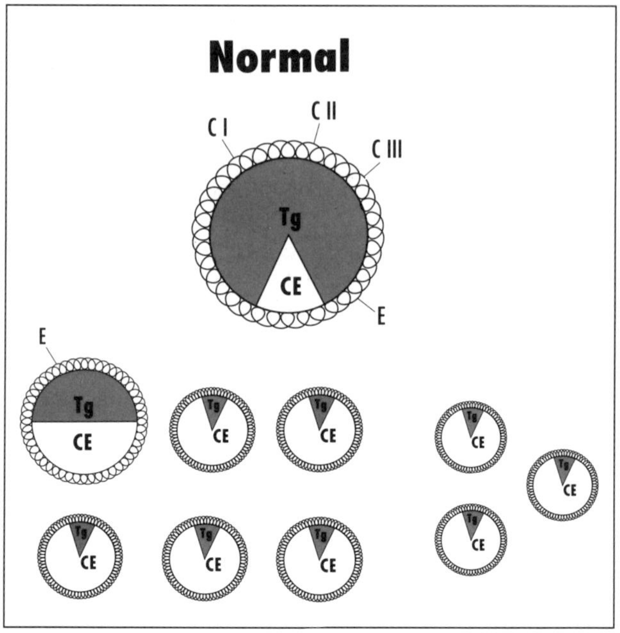

Fig. 25-3. ApoB100 lipoprotein distribution in a normal individual. Even though VLDL is the precursor of IDL and LDL, the much longer half-life of LDL results in its representing more of the product than the parent particle. An IDL particle is also illustrated, containing more triglyceride with additional apoproteins. The LDL particles as shown differ somewhat in size, composition, and density. The identity of the lipoprotein particles is the same as in Figure 2, with VLDL, IDL, B LDL and D LDL ranging from largest to smallest, respectively.

VLDL and LDL Heterogeneity

VLDL and LDL each comprise a class of lipoprotein particles within which there is considerable variation in size and density. As noted previously, since there is always only one molecule of apoB100 per particle, the number of particles in each class can be determined by measuring the concentration of apoB100 within that class. The mean size of particles in each class can also be derived from the ratio of the dominant core lipid to the concentration of apoB100 in each particle class.

Increased numbers of small, dense LDL particles are common findings in coronary disease [29–32]. Because their association with premature disease has been shown to be so powerful, it is important to understand their origin. Even in normals, not all LDL particles are identical in composition [33,34] (Fig. 25-3). Rather, they are heterogeneous, with some larger and more buoyant, and others smaller and denser.

As to the mechanisms responsible for this heterogeneity, exchange of core lipid is the principal determinant. The plasma protein, CETP, facilitates transfer of cholesteryl ester and triglycerides among the plasma lipoprotein fractions [28] (Fig. 25-4). Exchange is stoichiometric, that is, cholesteryl ester can be transferred from HDL or LDL to, for example VLDL, in return for which either a cholesteryl ester or triglyceride molecule will be transferred from VLDL to HDL. When LDL and HDL are involved, since cholesteryl ester is the dominant core lipid of both, there is little net change in the composition of either. By contrast, when VLDL and LDL are involved in exchange, major changes in particle composition result. Since the principal core lipid in VLDL is triglyceride and in LDL is cholesteryl ester, cholesteryl ester will move from LDL to VLDL in return for which triglyceride will move from VLDL to LDL. The resulting LDL particle now contains more triglyceride but is about the same size and density because cholesteryl ester and triglyceride differ little in these properties.

Subsequent steps modify particle size and density. If the triglyceride in the core of the LDL particle is hydrolyzed, the amount of core lipid is reduced and the particle is consequently smaller. Given that proteins are considerably denser than lipids, the particle is denser, as well, because the lipid-to-protein ratio decreases. Since there is less cholesteryl ester and since most of the cholesterol in LDL is present in the esterified form, the ratio of cholesterol to apoB100 is less in small, dense LDL particles than in larger, more buoyant LDL particles. The pattern-B phenotype described by Austin and Krauss, which is associated with increased risk of vascular disease [31], refers to patients in whom the majority of LDL particles are of the small, dense distribution. It is important to note that

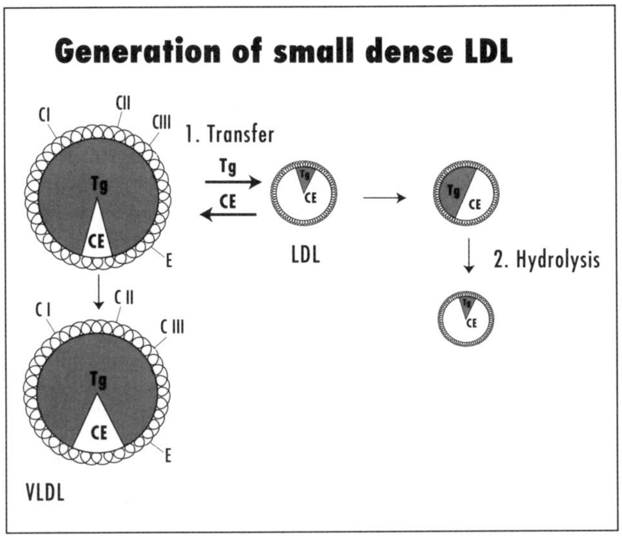

Fig. 25-4. The processes responsible for the heterogeneity of LDL particles. Two steps are involved: First, there is transfer of the core lipids between the particles (1. Transfer). The transfer and exchange are mediated by a plasma protein, cholesteryl ester transfer protein (CETP). Since the density of cholesteryl ester (CE) and triglyceride (Tg) differ little, the composition of the particle, but not its size or density, has been changed by the first step. However, once the triglyceride that has entered the LDL particle is hydrolyzed (2. Hydrolysis), the particle is now smaller and denser. Note that the conformation of the apoB100 molecule changes as the particle gets smaller; these changes may well affect its metabolic fate. The same steps can occur when HDL particles encounter triglyceride-rich lipoproteins, which would result in a lower HDL cholesterol.

exactly the same metabolic sequence can occur among HDL particles and the triglyceride-rich lipoproteins. The end result of that metabolic sequence is a lower HDL cholesterol, which is likely the most common course for the low-HDL cholesterol measured so frequently in patients with vascular disease.

The Atherogenicity of Small, Dense LDL

LDL is not atherogenic simply because it delivers and deposits cholesterol in the vessel wall. LDL binding to the endothelial surface results in expression of adhesion molecules [35], which facilitate monocyte recruitment into the arterial wall from the plasma compartment [36]. LDL also profoundly impairs the normal vasoactive responses of the arterial wall [37–41], and there is now evidence that LDL composition and particle number relate more precisely to those adverse consequences than do plasma or LDL cholesterol levels. Dyce and colleagues have recently shown that impaired coronary vasodilation relates most powerfully to small dense LDL and to an increase in LDL particle number rather than to total or LDL cholesterol [42]. Small, dense LDL increases thromboxane secretion more than does larger LDL [43]. Moreover, owing to its smaller size, small, dense LDL penetrates the arterial wall more easily [44], and once there, is more likely to oxidize [45–47] and to adhere to glycosaminoglycans than larger LDL [48]. Small, dense LDL causes intracellular calcium to increase in vascular smooth muscle cells more than does contact with larger LDL, a difference that may contribute to altered second-messenger responses [49]. In summary, it is now obvious that LDL particles are more than passive vehicles that deliver cholesterol to the arterial walls; thus, measurement of LDL cholesterol only imperfectly describes the atherogenic risk it poses.

Limitations of the Lipoprotein Phenotyping System

The system currently used to categorize patients clinically, the lipoprotein-phenotyping system introduced by Fredrickson and colleagues [50], is demonstrably inadequate for that purpose. Indeed, it was realized to be inadequate even as it was introduced, principally because it incompletely addresses lipoprotein physiology [51].

Classic lipoprotein phenotyping has, in our view, four major flaws. The first is that it treats dyslipoproteinemias as if they altered only one, or at most two, lipoproteins at a given time. Type I represents elevation of chylomicrons; type II, LDL; type III, remnants; type IV, increased VLDL; and type V, the simple sum of types I and IV. Clearly, this view is an oversimplification of the facts. For example, the most common dyslipoproteinemia associated with premature coronary artery disease, hyperapoB100 [52], involves abnormal chylomicron metabolism [53,54], increased VLDL production [55–57] with often elevated levels of VLDL [58], usually elevated levels of IDL, and very frequently lower levels of HDL cholesterol, as well [59,60]. All these abnormalities are present in most affected individuals, and several may play important roles in atherogenesis in addition to that attributable to the feature that is the hallmark of the disorder, the elevated LDL particle number itself [28,52].

Second, the classification implies that within each type there are no important phenotypic differences and that one genetic error should not produce multiple phenotypes. Again, in the case of hyperapoB100, that is clearly not the case. Affected individuals may have any of a number of lipid phenotypes and may change their lipid phenotype quite frequently, including during periods in which they may be normolipidemic.

Third, not only is the neat but artificial packaging of this long-established system physiologically incorrect, parameters of great contemporary interest, such as HDL cholesterol and Lp(a), are not included. And finally, as we have just reviewed, if all we measure are lipoprotein lipids, then the number and composition of the plasma lipoprotein particles remain obscure, and, as we will demonstrate in the discussion of the dyslipoproteinemias, clinical distinctions of importance cannot be made. A more contemporary classification of the primary dyslipoproteinemias is presented in Table 25-1, while Table 25-2 lists the plasma levels of apoB100 for the various Fredrickson lipoprotein phenotypes. Note particularly that measurement of apoB may establish that normolipidemic individuals are by no means normal and that approximately one-third of the patients with type IV hyperlipoproteinemia have an elevated LDL particle number.

Table 25-1. Plasma profiles of primary dyslipoproteinemias

	Plasma profile					
Dyslipoproteinemia	apoB	TC	Tg	LDL cholesterol	HDL cholesterol	Lp(a)
HyperapoB	↑ or ↑ ↑	N or ↑	N or ↑	N or ↑	N or ↓	
Familial hypertriglyceridemia (FHTG)	N	N	↑	N	~↓	
HDL deficiency	N or ↑	N	N or ↑		↓	
Familial hypercholesterolemia (FH) and familial defective B100	↑ ↑	↑ ↑	N	↑ ↑	N	N or ↑
Type III	N	↑	↑	N	N or ↓	
Lp(a)						↑

Abbreviations: apoB = plasma apolipoprotein B100; TC = plasma total cholesterol; Tg = plasma triglycerides; Lp(a) = lipoprotein Lp(a). Arrows indicate major (↑ ↑) or moderate (↑) increases and moderate (↓) or slight decreases (~ ↓); N = normal.

THE ATHEROGENIC DYSLIPOPROTEINEMIAS

HyperapoB100 (Familial Combined Hyperlipidemia)

HyperapoB100 is that atherogenic dyslipoproteinemia characterized by an increased LDL particle number due to increased secretion of apoB100 lipoprotein particles by the liver [52,55]. The increased secretion of VLDL particles from the liver increases their number in plasma and frequently results in hypertriglyceridemia. More important, at least so far as atherogenesis is concerned, the increased secretion rate of VLDL lipoprotein particles leads to increased numbers of IDL and LDL particles, both of which are small enough to enter the arterial wall readily. VLDL, by contrast, is much larger and, accordingly, much less likely to penetrate between endothelial junctions [61]. As well, even in hypertriglyceridemic patients, there are many fewer VLDL particles than LDL particles [23,24]; thus, independent of size, far more of the latter will enter an artery than the former. It must be emphasized that in hyperapoB100 there is no error in the LDL degradation pathway—the process by which LDL is removed from plasma—as there is in familial hypercholesterolemia (FH) or the familial defective apoB100 syndrome [54]. Rather, owing to the limited capacity of the normal LDL pathway to remove LDL particles from plasma, the number of plasma LDL particles will rise when the rate at which they are produced is high enough that the capacity to clear them is exceeded.

The terms *hyperapoB100* and *familial combined hyperlipidemia* (FCH), arose at different times, but for all practical purposes they are interchangeable. FCH was first described in 1973 by Goldstein and colleagues [62] and defined as the presence of hypertriglyceridemia and hypercholesterolemia in different family members. In 1980, hyperapoB100 was described as a dyslipoproteinemia characterized by an elevated level of LDL apoB100 in the face of a normal or near-normal LDL cholesterol [52]. Studies have now shown that the major pathophysiologic features of FCH and hyperapoB100—the overproduction of VLDL [55–57], the increased plasma apoB100 level [52,63], and the increased numbers of smaller, denser LDL particles [28,63]—are the same.

Notwithstanding that they describe the same metabolic error [64], important practical distinctions can be made between hyperapoB100 and FCH. The diagnosis of FCH cannot be made unless the family can be studied. For the practicing physician who must deal with a given patient,

Table 25-2. Fredrickson-Levy-Lees lipoprotein phenotying system

Lipoprotein phenotype	Lipoprotein class affected	Tg	TC	LDL cholesterol	apo B
Normolpidemic	None	N	N	N	N or ↑
I	Chylomicrons	↑ ↑	↑	N	N
II A	LDL	N	↑ or ↑ ↑	↑ or ↑ ↑	↑ or ↑ ↑
II B	LDL/VDL	↑	↑ or ↑ ↑	↑ or ↑ ↑	↑ or ↑ ↑
III	Chylomicron} VLDL	↑ ↑	↑ ↑	N	N
IV	VLDL	↑	N	N	⅔ N, ⅓ ↑ or ↑ ↑
V	↑ Chylomicrons ↑ VLDL	↑ ↑	↑	N	Usually N, rarely ↑

Abbreviations: apoB = plasma apolipoprotein B100; Tg = plasma triglycerides; TC = plasma total cholesterol. Arrows indicate major (↑ ↑) or moderate (↑) increases; N = normal.

this often is not feasible; thus, the diagnosis cannot be made. If FCH is not diagnosed and if all the physician has available are the lipoprotein lipids, the patient who is hypertriglyceridemic and at increased risk cannot be distinguished from the patient is also hypertriglyceridemic but who is not at increased risk of vascular disease [58,65–68]. Equally unfortunately, a normolipidemic individual with increased LDL particle number will be dismissed as normal. By contrast, hyperapoB100 is a diagnosis made in an individual patient in whom the key feature is an elevated apoB100 and, therefore, an increased IDL and LDL particle number. Making this diagnosis, then, directs the physician to therapy aimed to reduce IDL and LDL particle number, whatever the lipoprotein phenotype.

PATHOPHYSIOLOGY OF HYPERAPOB100

The physiologic raison d'être of the hepatic apoB lipoproteins is to maintain the balance of lipid in the liver, thus preventing the accumulation in hepatocytes of undue amounts of either triglyceride or cholesteryl ester. At the moment, all the recognized causes of the increased secretion of VLDL involve an increased supply of fatty acids to the liver [69], although, undoubtedly, differences in the intracellular metabolism of sterols in the hepatocyte will soon be recognized as causes, as well. By contrast, there is little evidence supporting changes in the structure or composition of apoB100 as a cause of its overproduction [70–73].

The rate of secretion of apoB100 particles depends not only on the rate of synthesis of the apoB100 molecules but also on the concurrent rates of synthesis of core lipids in the hepatocytes [74–76]. More apoB100 molecules are synthesized than are incorporated into lipoprotein particles because an important proportion are hydrolyzed soon after they have been synthesized in the rough endoplasmic reticulum. Most important, it is also now clear that a major mechanism responsible for the increased secretion of apoB100 particles in hyperapoB100 is delivery of excess fatty acids to the liver, which results in secretion of increased numbers of VLDL particles that are near normal in composition [77,78]. In that instance, increased synthesis of core lipids results in a greater proportion of the apoB100 molecules actually being used for the purpose for which they were intended, namely, to export excess lipid from the hepatocyte.

The reason for the increased flux of fatty acids to the liver appears to lie in failure of adipocytes to take up fatty acids at a normal rate in these patients [79]. How does this occur? Adipocytes are the only cells in the body with the capacity to store energy in any important amounts. For example, a healthy, nonobese, 70-kg male has 15 kg of adipose tissue, representing an energy source of 140,000 kcal. By contrast, his muscle mass contains only 225 mg glycogen, which will yield only 900 kcal. To store fatty acids, the triglycerides in the chylomicrons and VLDL must be hydrolyzed by the enzyme lipoprotein lipase, and the fatty acids that are released enter the adipocytes and are reincorporated in triglycerides. It has been assumed that the rate at which this process occurs is controlled by the activity of lipoprotein lipase and that the adipocyte has an unlimited capacity to take up fatty acids and convert them into triglyceride. That assumption is incorrect: The correlation between the rate at which triglycerides are cleared from plasma and the amount of lipoprotein lipase present on the endothelium is, in fact, quite poor [80]. Moreover, the rate at which triglycerides are synthesized in adipocytes is now known to be regulated by the adipsin–acylation-stimulating protein (ASP) pathway.

The adipsin-ASP pathway has only recently been described [81,82] and appears to be the major mechanism that regulates the rate of triglyceride synthesis in adipose tissue. Human adipocytes can secrete the three proteins of the alternate complement pathway: factor B, factor D (or adipsin), and the third component of complement (C3). These molecules interact to produce ASP, which is identical to C3adesarg, a small fragment of C3. ASP interacts with the cell to increase specific membrane transport of glucose [83]. By contrast, ASP does not appear to affect membrane transport of fatty acids [83]; rather, uptake of fatty acids increases secondarily to their increased incorporation into triglyceride molecules owing to stimulation of the activity of the last enzyme involved in this process, diacylglycerol acyltransferase [84].

It is now established that patients with hyperapoB100 have impaired clearance of triglyceride-rich lipoproteins and elevated plasma free-fatty-acid levels [53,54,85,86]. In normals, plasma ASP levels rise after an oral fat load, and the degree to which they do correlates with the rate at which triglycerides are cleared from plasma [87]. In a substantial number of patients with hyperapoB100, this pathway is defective owing to decreased response of cells to ASP [88,89]. If it is defective, the rate at which triglycerides can be synthesized in adipocytes is limited, and, as a result, fatty acids accumulate in the capillary space causing lipoprotein lipase to dissociate from the endothelium and, thus, inhibiting triglyceride hydrolysis [90]. The fatty acids are transported to the liver, but equally important, so are the partially hydrolyzed chylomicron and VLDL particles. These particles are not meant to be taken up by the liver until virtually all their triglyceride has been removed (see Fig. 25-1). However, once the process of hydrolysis has begun, even if it is incomplete, any remnant particles that arrive at the liver will be rapidly taken up [91], and since they contain fatty acids in the form of triglycerides, they constitute a second mechanism by which excess fatty acids are delivered to the liver.

The consequences of impaired removal of fatty acids extend beyond these abnormal metabolic events. LDL-receptor activity, and therefore LDL clearance, decreases as fatty-acid delivery to the liver increases [92], an effect that would tend to elevate plasma LDL. Insulin clearance also decreases [93] and hepatic gluconeogenesis increases [94], thus producing the key elements of syndrome X, hyperinsulinemia and a tendency to hyperglycemia. The results of several studies make it obvious that an increased number of small, dense LDL particles and insulin resistance are often coincident [95–97]. Indeed, we now conceive of a triangle de risque in such patients: the insulin-glucose abnormalities; the hyperapoB100 dyslipoproteinemia (hypertriglyceridemia, low HDL cholesterol, and

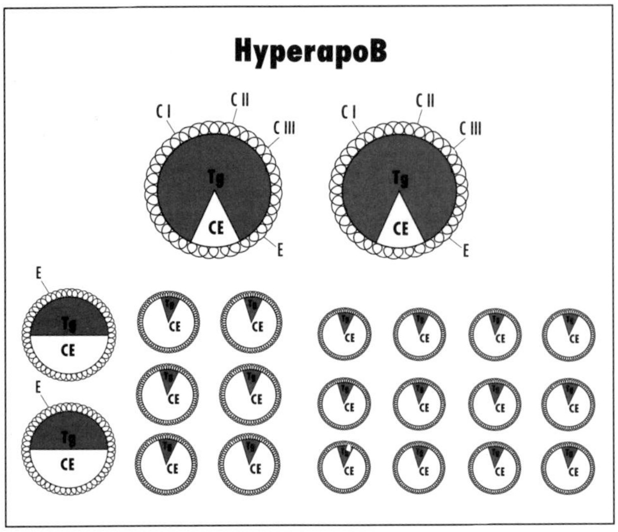

Fig. 25-5. The number and composition of the B100 lipoproteins in a typical patient with hyperapoB100, which can be contrasted with the findings in a normal individual (see Fig. 25-3). Owing to overproduction, the number of VLDL and IDL particles is increased. Because they account for few of the apoB100 particles, the most impressive changes, insofar as particle number is concerned, are in the LDL range, where the number is markedly increased. Note that the LDL particles are heterogeneous in composition, but many are smaller with less cholesteryl ester (CE) in their core than was seen in the normal case (see Fig. 25-3). Note also that the composition of the VLDL particles differs little from normal. The identity of the lipoprotein particles is the same as in Fig. 25-2, with VLDL, IDL, B LDL, and D LDL ranging from largest to smallest, respectively.

increased numbers of small, dense LDL particles); and the third component, a procoagulant state. Both VLDL and LDL stimulate the secretion of plasminogen activator inhibitor type 1 (PAI-1) by endothelial cells [98,99]. The elevated VLDL and LDL particle number in patients with hyperapoB100 may, then, explain why the same investigators find both elevated apoB and elevated PAI-1 [100–102] in patients with premature coronary disease.

CLINICAL AND LABORATORY PROFILES IN HYPERAPOB

The clinical manifestations of this biochemical chaos are restricted to the vascular tree. Tuberous and eruptive xanthomas are not seen in hyperapoB100, and while hyperapoB100 is frequently found in patients with xanthelasmata [103], xanthelasmata are not a good diagnostic marker for either hyperapoB100 or coronary artery disease. The hallmark of the disorder is an elevated apoB100 level in plasma (Fig. 25-5). Plasma apoB100 is also elevated in disorders that impair LDL clearance, but in hyperapoB100, the LDL cholesterol-to-apoB100 ratio is normal or reduced. The pattern of the lipoprotein lipids in hyperapoB100 is quite variable (see Table 25-1). Some patients are normolipidemic, others hyperlipidemic. The latter may manifest type IV or type II hyperlipoproteinemia, usually type IIB but not infrequently type IIA; rarely, a type V pattern may be present. HDL cholesterol is often reduced [104,105] for the reasons noted above. Most important, the lipid phenotype of an individual patient may be quite variable, with elevated apoB100 the only constant. It is also important to note that the measurement of apoB100 has now been standardized [106], which is not the case for lipoprotein lipids.

Therapy for all the dyslipidemias will be discussed later, but the major principle of therapy in hyperapoB100 is to reduce LDL particle number by reducing the rate at which particles are produced as well as increasing the rate at which they are cleared from plasma. Of all the drugs now at our disposal, HMGCoA reductase inhibitors are the first choice in therapy. LDL particle number is markedly reduced and chylomicron remnant clearance improved, as well, with these agents [54,107]. The first and most important effect, the lowering of apoB100, is achieved in part by improving clearance [108] but to an equal or perhaps even greater extent by decreasing production of LDL particles [109–112].

Familial Hypertriglyceridemia

Familial hypertriglyceridemia (FHTG) was originally defined as a monogeneic pattern of hypertriglyceridemia, that is, type IV hyperlipoproteinemia, within a family. Initially, patients with FHTG were thought to be at increased risk of vascular disease [62]. Later, however, that view was felt to be incorrect [67], and the contradiction has never been resolved. The contradiction is not an arcane or academic issue: Should affected patients be treated to reduce their risk of vascular disease? If so, how should they be treated? Further, how can some patients with type IV hyperlipoproteinemia be at increased risk and others not? We suspect the contradiction and attendant confusion stem from case selection and incomplete characterization of the lipoprotein profile. In the original study [62], the index cases all had coronary disease, whereas in the later study none did [67]. In the later publication, although all patients studied had type IV hyperlipoproteinemia, none had elevated apoB100. ApoB100 levels were not measured in the original study, but we suspect they would have been elevated. This issue should be resolved soon, since the controversy is now under thorough investigation.

In any case, the findings in the more recent and more complete analysis of the lipoprotein profile in FHTG reveals a picture (Fig. 25-6) much the same as seen in carbohydrate-induced hypertriglyceridemia. Both conditions are characterized by triglyceride-enriched VLDL particles that are secreted [113–117] at a normal rate. LDL particle number is not elevated, and plasma apoB100 is on the lower side of normal since fewer of the triglyceride-rich VLDL are converted to LDL than usual [118]. An increase in bile-acid synthesis has been reported in some patients with FHTG, but how this observation affects pathogenesis has not yet been elucidated. Because VLDL are large lipoproteins, they tend not to enter the arterial wall easily [61]. In FHTG, they are even larger and so even less likely to gain entry inside the vessel wall. It is the normal LDL particle number in FHTG that we believe explains why atherogenic risk in these patients is not increased. By contrast, atherogenic risk is increased in hypertriglyceridemic patients with hyperapoB100 because their LDL particle number is elevated [58,65–68]. However, severely

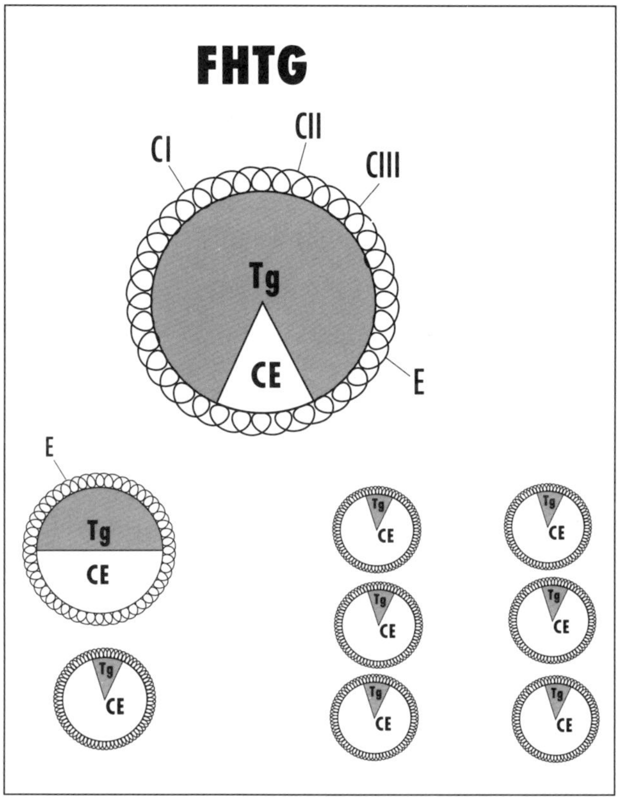

Fig. 25-6. The findings in a patient with familial hypertriglyceridemia (FHTG). The number of VLDL particles is normal, but the particles are much larger than normal with much more triglyceride (Tg) in their cores. The number of LDL particles often is slightly less than normal because fewer of these triglyceride-enriched VLDL particles tend to be converted into LDL particles. The identity of the lipoprotein particles is the same as in Fig. 25-2, with VLDL, IDL, B LDL, and D LDL ranging from largest to smallest, respectively.

hypertriglyceridemic patients are at risk for pancreatitis, and prevention of that complication is an indication in some for pharmacologic therapy, usually with a fibric-acid derivative.

LABORATORY PROFILE

We earlier criticized the traditional lipoprotein-phenotyping system and indicated the value of measuring apoB100. Type IV hyperlipoproteinemia is one of the clearest examples of the value of apoB100, because without it being measured there is no way to distinguish between hypertriglyceridemic patients who are at increased risk and patients with an identical lipoprotein profile who are not at substantially increased risk of atherosclerosis.

HDL Deficiency (Hypoalphalipoproteinemia)

That low levels of HDL are associated with an increased risk of coronary disease is incontrovertible. What remains unknown is by what mechanism or mechanisms that increased risk is expressed. Do lower plasma HDL levels, as is often thought, reflect reduced return of cholesterol from peripheral tissues to the liver, and does that lead to excessive accumulation of cholesterol in the arterial wall? Or is the low HDL cholesterol simply a marker of another, more important atherogenic abnormality? Perhaps surprisingly, given the force of conventional wisdom, the latter and not the former now seems much more commonly the problem.

The causes of hypoalphalipoproteinemia can be divided into primary and secondary ones. The primary causes are rare and produce marked reduction in HDL cholesterol (generally <10 mg/dl). They include Tangier disease [118], the apoA-1 deficiency states [119–123], apoA-1 variants [124], lecithin-cholesterol acyltranferase (LCAT) deficiency [125], and fish eye disease [126]. The A1 deficiency states are due to deletions, rearrangements, or point mutations in the apoA1-CIII-AIV gene complex. Depending on the specific cause, such errors result in a lack of expression of any or all three of these apoproteins. In such disorders, A1 synthesis is reduced, whereas with Tangier disease and LCAT deficiency, A1 clearance is increased.

Much more commonly, however, low HDL cholesterol is less pronounced and due to or associated with another metabolic disorder. The exchange of cholesteryl ester and triglyceride between lipoprotein particles (see Fig. 25-4) is largely responsible for the well-known inverse relation between plasma triglycerides and HDL cholesterol (higher values of the former leading to lower values of the latter). This relationship is crucial to appreciate, because in most instances a low HDL cholesterol is likely secondary to a high plasma triglyceride or an increased secretion rate of apoB100-containing lipoproteins, even in the absence of frank hypertriglyceridemia [127]. Of particular importance is the recent report by Genest and colleagues [128] of an increase in apoB100 in familial hypoalphalipoproteinemia. The index cases all had coronary disease, again demonstrating the relation between elevated apoB100 levels and vascular risk.

LABORATORY PROFILE

By definition, in primary hypoalphalipoproteinemia, HDL cholesterol levels are low. Other lipid values should be normal. But as just noted, this represents yet another instance of the limited information available to the clinician if only plasma lipoprotein lipids are measured. If apoB100 is elevated in such patients, the therapeutic dilemma is defined as whether to attempt to raise the HDL cholesterol or to lower the plasma apoB100 and triglycerides. The evidence from (1) the series of angiographic trials that the progression of disease can be diminished by any of a series of therapies that markedly lower the level of LDL in plasma [129–143]) and (2) the finding from meta-analysis that clinical events are also substantially reduced [144] suggests that the prime objective of therapy should be to lower LDL particle number in this group of patients, as well. The issue, however, is far from resolved. Measurement of HDL cholesterol seems likely to prove a more sensitive index of cardiac risk than will measurement of its major apoprotein, A1.

Familial Hypercholesterolemia and Familial Defective apoB100 Syndrome

The pathophysiology of the increased levels of LDL in both familial hypercholesterolemia (FH) and familial defective apoB100 syndrome is the same as is the clinical picture of the heterozygous form of both disorders; thus, the two will be considered together. In both dyslipoproteinemias, the normal process by which LDL is removed from plasma is defective. The pathway by which that occurs was described by Brown and Goldstein [145], who were awarded the Nobel prize for this achievement. In brief, a region of the apoB100 molecule on the LDL particle binds to a specific receptor sited in coated pits on the cell membrane surface. The bound particle is internalized, the receptor dissociates from the complex and returns to the cell surface, the apoB100 is hydrolyzed in the lysosome, and the cholesterol released in the cell causes both cholesterol and receptor synthesis to decrease. In other words, the cell makes all the appropriate adaptations to prevent excess accumulation of cholesterol.

In FH, more than 30 molecular defects have been reported that interfere with the synthesis of the receptor or with its siting on the cell membrane surface [146]. In the familial defective B100 syndrome, the LDL pathway itself is normal, but the ligand, the apoB100 molecule, has been altered by a single critical amino acid substitution at position 3500 so as to render it unable to bind to its receptor, the first essential step in the pathway [147–149]. Thus, FH is due to a defect of the receptor, whereas familial defective B100 represents the other side of this metabolic coin of failure, a defect of the ligand.

These are the primary reasons for impaired function of the LDL pathway. Other influences, however, require consideration. Insufficient levels of thyroid hormone, for example, also result in impaired function of this pathway, which is the mechanism for the increased levels of LDL that occur so often in hypothyroid patients [150]. Diet also influences the level of their expression, with higher intakes of cholesterol and fatty acids leading to lower levels of LDL receptors in hepatocyte membranes, thus reducing the rate of LDL clearance from plasma.

The composition of LDL particles in plasma is altered in FH such that they become larger and cholesterol enriched (Fig. 25-7) [28]. This particle modification likely relates both to failure of clearance of some of the larger IDL particles and to increased opportunity for transfer of cholesterol from HDL to LDL because of the prolonged half-life in plasma of these LDL particles. In the heterozygote, the normal pathway is available but reduced in effectiveness, whereas in the homozygote, it is not present at all. Because the central pathway represents the high-affinity removal route, if it does not operate normally, more LDL particles than usual are removed by processes that are less specific and less effective, causing the LDL particle number in plasma to rise substantially. For many, if not all, of these other routes to operate, the LDL particle first must be altered by some event such as oxidation. Once that occurs, if entry of the altered LDL then occurs by a so-called scavenger pathway, its entry is unrestricted, and cells such as macrophages are converted into foam cells. This pathway is present in all of us but operates at a much lower level than in persons with FH and, which is important, is not feedback regulated, in contrast to the normal LDL receptor pathway. In FH patients, its enhanced importance as a removal mechanism is evidenced

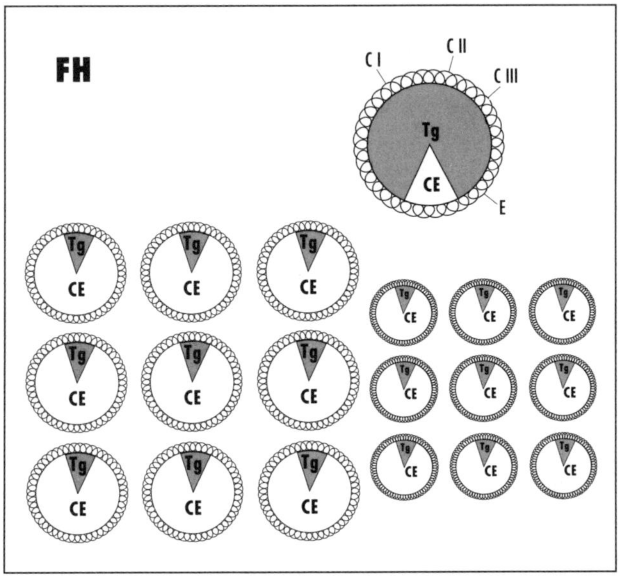

Fig. 25-7. Findings in a typical patient with familial hypercholesterolemia (FH). The number of LDL particles is markedly increased, and many are larger and cholesterol-enriched compared to normal. The identity of the lipoprotein particles is the same as in Fig. 25-2, with VLDL, IDL, B LDL, and D LDL ranging from largest to smallest, respectively.

by atheroma generation and by extravascular foam cell formation, such as tendon xanthomas.

CLINICAL AND LABORATORY FEATURES

The frequency of FH has been estimated to be 1 in 500, and that of familial defective B100 syndrome to be approximately the same, although more recent estimates suggest that the former is less common than previously thought [149]. Homozygotes for either are exceedingly rare. In work performed 20 years ago, FH was thought to account for approximately 10 percent of premature coronary disease, but its prevalence is much less in more modern surveys [151]. The clinical picture is worth description because, in contrast to hyperapoB100, the diagnosis involves characteristic clinical as well as laboratory findings. Tendon xanthomas are the key to clinical diagnosis appearing in the heterozygote after age 20 and the homozygote in early childhood. These lesions are hard, not soft, and they are deep but not attached to the skin. The most common sites are the extensor tendons of the hand and the Achilles tendons, although other sites are often involved, such as the triceps tendon. Two other quite rare disorders can cause tendon xanthoma, betasitosterolemia [152] and cerebrotendinous xanthomatosis [153]. In neither disorder is marked hypercholesterolemia present; by contrast, both have been associated with hyperapoB100 type dyslipoproteinemias [154,155].

Although occasionally expression is not as clear-cut, characteristically, both FH and familial defective B100 syndrome produce marked elevations of total cholesterol, LDL cholesterol, and apoB100. Thus, the average serum cholesterol in adult heterozygotes is approximately 350 mg/dl and in homozygotes greater than 600 mg/dl. With values less than 350 mg/dl, the majority of patients will have some other reason for elevated LDL, such as hyperapoB. In FH, LDL cholesterol and apoB levels obviously are markedly increased, and the LDL cholesterol-to-apoB100 ratio is high, as well [29]. Of interest and of potential clinical significance, the level of Lp(a) is higher than would be expected by chance alone in such patients [156].

The atherosclerotic burden of this metabolic disorder is high but not distributed evenly between the sexes. Men are at substantially higher risk than women, with about half of male heterozygotes dying before 60 as opposed to only one-sixth of affected women [157]. The coronary arteries clearly are susceptible, but the relative rarity of vascular disease in other territories is noteworthy and not observed in the other dyslipoproteinemias we will review. By contrast, in homozygotes the accumulation of cholesterol in the proximal aorta and the aortic cusps can be so excessive as to cause hemodynamically severe aortic stenosis [158]. Some evidence of this tendency can also be seen in some heterozygotes.

The principle of therapy is straightforward: Lower LDL by all possible means. Appropriate dietary advice rarely produces substantial change but should not be ignored. A variety of pharmacologic approaches have been developed and include HMGCoA reductase inhibitors, bile-acid sequestrants, and nicotinic acid, with the first two often used in combination. Effective pharmacologic therapy has been shown to reduce the rate of coronary artery disease progression. In homozygotes, these approaches rarely work, and far more aggressive measures such as LDL apheresis [159] and liver transplantation [160] may be required.

Type III Hyperlipoproteinemia

Type III hyperlipoproteinemia is characterized by the accumulation in plasma of chylomicron and VLDL remnants (Fig. 25-8). Clinically, it is associated with premature coronary and peripheral vascular disease, markedly increased plasma cholesterol and triglyceride, and characteristic tuberous and palmar xanthomas [161,162]. The xanthomas were, in fact, the features that led to the first description of the syndrome in 1851 by Addison and Gull [163]. They produce a yellow-orange discoloration of the palmar skin creases, and occasionally, are also present in the palmar creases of the fingers and wrists. The other common lesions are tuberous xanthomas that are found most often on the surfaces of the elbows and knees but also over the Achilles tendons, where they must be distinguished from the tendon xanthoma of FH and familial defective B100 syndrome. Clinical expression is unusual before the third decade in men and tends to occur even later in women.

A number of conditions are often found concomitantly in patients with this disorder, some of which may be critical in its pathogenesis in individual patients. Obesity and glucose intolerance are common, the two perhaps being interrelated. Hypothyroidism can produce type III hyperlipoproteinemia, and thyroid function should always be assessed in these patients [164]. Estrogen status often plays a role in that in females type III is much more common after than before menopause, and estrogen

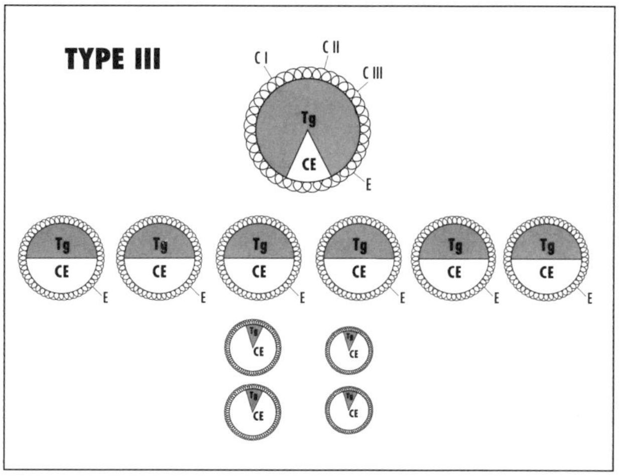

Fig. 25-8. Findings in a patient with type III hyperlipoproteinemia. The major abnormality is an increase in remnant particles, which are of two kinds: those of hepatic origin, containing apoB100 (shown here), and those of intestinal origin, containing apoB48 (not illustrated). The number of LDL particles is normal; that accounts for the high plasma apoE-to-B ratio, which can be seen in this disorder. The identity of the lipoprotein particles is the same as in Fig. 25-2, with VLDL, IDL, B LDL, and D LDL ranging from largest to smallest, respectively.

therapy can produce marked amelioration of the dyslipidemia in many affected females [165,166].

Our understanding of the pathogenesis of type III hyperlipoproteinemia remains frustratingly incomplete [167]. Its hallmark is elevation of chylomicron and VLDL remnants, which occurs because their clearance from plasma is impaired. But the pathways that remove these lipoprotein particles from plasma have not been precisely defined. One molecular defect in type III that has been clearly identified is genetic alteration of apoE, which obviously must play some crucial role in the removal process. Several alleles code for this protein with three isoforms and, therefore, six phenotypes present in the population. The most frequent isoform is E3 and the other two represent variants thereof. Position 112 of E3 is cysteine and 158 is arginine. By contrast, E4 has arginine rather than cysteine at positions 112 and 158, whereas E2 has cysteine at both. E2/E2 remnant particles bind poorly to cells, E4/E4 bind best, and E3/E3 particles are intermediate in this respect. Interestingly, in general, lower levels of cholesterol are associated with the E2 allele and higher ones with E4.

Abnormalities in apoE obviously are key to the pathogenesis of type III, with most patients manifesting an E2/E2 phenotype. Rarely, other errors have been described, with complete absence of apoE also having been reported [167,168]. But abnormalities in apoE are not the whole story because only a very small proportion of individuals who are homozygous for E2 develop type III. Because of that clinical observation, it generally is agreed that the clinical disorder represents a double metabolic disorder—abnormal apoE plus some other genetic or acquired metabolic disorder. Our hypothesis is that many of these patients will be shown to have abnormalities in peripheral triglyceride clearance and may therefore represent compound mosaics of an abnormal apoE and an abnormal adipsin-ASP pathway.

LABORATORY PROFILE

The usual laboratory features of type III are as follows. Both cholesterol and triglyceride are substantially elevated, and if expressed in mg/L, they are often comparable in magnitude. Although rarely used now, either paper or agarose gel electrophoresis demonstrates a broad beta band. Most helpful is the demonstration of a cholesterol-to-triglyceride ratio less than 0.30 in VLDL isolated by ultracentrifugation. The basis for this abnormality is that the delayed clearance of these particles leads to increased cholesteryl ester–triglyceride exchange, producing the cholesterol-enriched remnant particle. An increased number of remnants is also evident by a high apoE-to-apoB100 ratio [169]. If the technology is available, the demonstration of a characteristic abnormality in apoE phenotype—usually homozygosity for the E2 allele—completes the diagnostic work-up.

Although rare, the diagnosis is an important one to make clinically because therapy is surprisingly simple. A wide range of approaches has been shown to work, from diet to pharmacologic therapy with either fibrates or HMGCoA reductase inhibitors.

Lipoprotein (a) and Coronary Artery Disease

In the past several years, much effort has been spent attempting to define the pathophysiologic basis for the relation between the lipoprotein (a), or Lp(a), class and premature vascular disease. Lp(a) is a class of lipoprotein particles [170] characterized by one molecule of apoB100 linked by a disulfide bridge to a molecule of apo(a) [171]. The apoB100 molecule, as always, is associated with a mass of lipid. This lipid is usually predominantly cholesteryl ester; in this case, the particles have a density similar to that of LDL, although they are larger in size. A small proportion of Lp(a) particles are enriched in triglyceride, in which case they more closely resemble VLDL.

Apo(a) itself is a glycoprotein with a polypeptide chain that varies between 300 and 800 kDa. Its structural similarity to plasminogen is considerable [172], although kringles 1–3 of plasminogen are not found in apo(a). Rather, there is a single copy of kringle 5 and between 13 to 37 copies of kringle 4. In plasminogen, by contrast, a single copy of each kringle is present. The variable number of repeats of kringle 4 in apo(a) produces isoforms of very different size, one consequence of which is that measurement of mass by immunoassay does not translate automatically, as it does in the case of apoB, into measurement of particle number. In general, the smaller isoforms produce higher plasma concentrations [173].

A considerable number of studies have shown that increased levels of Lp(a) are associated with increased risk of premature vascular disease. Of interest, Lawn and colleagues have recently shown that mice transgenic for apolipoprotein(a) when fed a high-cholesterol, high-fat diet manifest much greater aortic lesions than do controls [174]. The interpretation of those results is complicated by the fact that in mice, in contrast to humans, the apolipoprotein(a) is not associated with lipid or apoB100, the inference being that apo(a) itself is directly atherogenic. The distribution of Lp(a) levels in Caucasians is skewed with almost a 1,000-fold range in concentration [175]. About 20 percent of the population have a level above 30 mg/dl total Lp(a), the value above which vascular risk appears significantly elevated. The distribution in black Americans, however, is different, with much higher levels in this group overall and with values present as a normal distribution [175].

Apo(a) is made in the liver, and it is not yet clear whether association with the apoB100-lipid complex occurs in the hepatocyte or following secretion from the cell. Similarly, what physiologic role, if any, this lipoprotein plays also remains unknown. As to the mechanisms by which it increases atherogenic risk, hypothesis outruns evidence by far. What is clear is that Lp(a) can infiltrate arterial and saphenous-vein bypass grafts, since substantial amounts of antigen are evident in and around atheromatous lesions in such vessels [176,177]. Whether entry into the subintimal space is a simple function of the plasma concentration of Lp(a) is not yet certain. The similarity in structure to plasminogen plus the fact that apo(a) cannot be converted into an active fibrinolytic enzyme owing to an arginine-cysteine substitution at the activation site suggest the lipoprotein may act to inhibit fibrinolysis at the endothelial surface. Although much work of interest has been done in vitro, there still is no evidence such a mechanism is operative in vivo.

One of the more important recent concepts is that whatever the precise mechanism(s) by which it promotes atherogenesis, Lp(a) is an important determinant of atherogenesis only in the presence of elevated levels of LDL. This concept is based principally on evidence from cross-sectional studies in FH [178,179]. Indeed, given the present limitation in our ability to lower levels of Lp(a) by dietary or pharmacologic therapy (modest to moderate reductions are possible with moderate- or high-dose nicotinic acid) [180], this relation might be critical clinically since levels of LDL are now relatively easy to control. The factors that control plasma levels of Lp(a) remain largely unknown, but for most individuals the level tends to be quite constant. Some interesting clinical observations may turn out to shed some light on regulation of plasma levels of Lp(a): A number of reports have appeared documenting higher levels in diabetics, particularly those with nephropathy [181–183]. Similarly, Lp(a) levels appear to be systematically higher in both hemodialysis and peritoneal dialysis patients [184,185]. The physiologic mechanisms responsible for those associations have yet to be elucidated, and their role in atherogenic risk in those unique patient populations have yet to be defined.

Secondary Hyperlipidemias

DIABETES MELLITUS

The importance of vascular disease in determining the clinical outcome in patients with diabetes mellitus cannot be overstated. Indeed, the natural history of the disease is very much the rate at which the vascular complications, both microvascular and macrovascular, occur. The microvascular pathologies—retinopathy, neuropathy, and nephropathy—may well relate to the level of glycemic control. The macrovascular pathologies, particularly coronary disease, relate much more closely, we believe, to the dyslipoproteinemias present in such patients than many consider to be the case. Certainly, the very large differences in risk of vascular disease in diabetics from different regions of the world argue strongly against hyperglycemia being the only, or perhaps even the preeminent, mechanism of macrovascular injury [186].

The lipid profiles of patients with insulin-dependent diabetes mellitus (IDDM) and those with non–insulin-dependent diabetes mellitus (NIDDM) share important similarities as well as differences. In neither group is total or LDL cholesterol frequently markedly elevated. Triglycerides often are high [187], whereas, at least in IDD patients, HDL cholesterol levels are often not as low as might be anticipated. These similarities are to be contrasted with important differences that may shed new light on pathogenesis of the disorders themselves. In IDDM, apoB100 and, therefore, LDL particle number, tend to be normal with triglyceride-enriched remnantlike particles often present [188]. By contrast, in at least a subset of NIDDM, the picture resembles more that in hyperapoB100, with increased numbers of small, dense LDL particles present [189]. In such patients, we suspect that abnormalities in fatty-acid metabolism may be responsible not just for the lipid abnormalities but for the elevated blood glucose and insulin levels, as well. Some [190], but not all [191], studies have reported increased Lp(a) in patients with NIDDM. In IDDM, some correlation between glycemic control and levels of Lp(a) has been noted, which has not been observed in NIDDM [192]. The most consistent changes in Lp(a) have been the increases noted with the onset of nephropathy. If pharmacologic therapy is chosen, the objective might be either to reduce triglycerides with fibric acid derivatives or to reduce LDL particle number with HMGCoA reductase inhibitors.

HYPOTHYROIDISM

The usual consequences of hypothyroidism are elevated cholesterol and apoB100 levels due to reduced activity of the LDL pathway [150]. Hepatic cholesterol synthesis also increases, which tends to increase apoB100 secretion [193,194]. Less commonly, triglyceride levels are increased, probably due to reduced lipoprotein lipase activity with increased numbers of triglyceride-and apoE-rich remnant particles being the consequence. When hypothyroidism is the cause, thyroid hormone replacement is the only therapy necessary.

DEEP ABDOMINAL OBESITY

Obesity per se is not associated with increased cardiovascular risk, whereas male-type omental obesity is. The increased risk in the latter is likely the consequence of the associated metabolic complications: insulin resistance and hyperapoB100 [195–197]. Both may relate to abnormalities in fatty-acid metabolism. Omental adipocytes clear chylomicron triglycerides less well than their subcutaneous counterparts [198]. The consequences of incomplete hydrolysis and premature release of triglyceride-rich remnant particles have been detailed above and apply to omental obesity as they do to hyperapoB100 due to defective or deficient ASP response. Stimulated lipolysis also appears to be more pronounced in omental adipocytes, which could also tend to increase portal-vein fatty-acid levels excessively [199–201]. Elevated plasma fatty acids, particularly in the portal circulation, lead to increased apoB production [74] plus reduced insulin [93] clearance and increased gluconeogenesis [94] by the liver. The objective of therapy in these patients should be reduction in their mass of omental adipose tissue.

RENAL DISEASE

In patients with chronic renal failure and those with end-stage renal disease treated with hemodialysis, HDL cholesterol levels are low, triglycerides high, but apoB100 and total cholesterol normal or low. This pattern contrasts with patients being treated with peritoneal dialysis in whom HDL cholesterol levels are low, triglycerides and cholesterol somewhat higher, and apoB100 often frankly elevated [202,203]. In dialysis patients of either type and in diabetics with nephropathy, Lp(a) levels have been reported to be substantially increased [204].

The nephrotic syndrome, of course, produces the most abnormal of the secondary dyslipoproteinemias [205]. In those patients, LDL levels characteristically are profoundly elevated, sometimes to the same degree as in homozygous familial hypercholesterolemia. The LDL particles are also enriched in cholesterol, although only modest reductions at most in LDL clearance have been documented in this disorder [206]. Less commonly, but by no means infrequently, plasma VLDL levels are increased, as well. In our view, HMGCoA reductase inhibitors are the preferred therapeutic approach in such patients.

MEDICATIONS

A wide range of medications produce a wide range of adverse effects on lipoprotein metabolism, effects that have generated considerable interest and concern. In most instances, however, the effects, while clear in the aggregate, are not pronounced in the individual. The exception is steroids, which produce a hyperapoB100-type dyslipidemia with variable lipid phenotype [207–209]. Their impact is obvious in transplant patients, although other immunosuppressive drugs may contribute to dyslipoproteinemia. HDL cholesterol levels may be markedly increased, but such patients do not seem spared vascular disease, although more follow-up is required [210,211]. Thiazide diuretics raise triglycerides and lower HDL cholesterol [212]. The effects of beta blockers are complex in that their use leads to somewhat higher triglyceride and lower HDL cholesterol levels. In that case, apoB100 and LDL levels also rise [213,214]. The most pronounced lipid changes in this class appear to be related to agents such as propranolol, which are no longer commonly used. Also, their impact on serum lipids diminishes over time. All in all, their effects are rarely so substantial as to justify any hesitancy in their clinical use.

THERAPY

Rationale and Clinical Evidence of Benefit

The emphasis throughout this chapter has been on IDL and LDL as being the two classes of lipoproteins that are clearly atherogenic. By contrast, low levels of HDL or high levels of plasma triglycerides due to increased amounts of VLDL alter the statistical probability of disease, but the mechanisms by which they might produce disease remain obscure. More important, in our view, there is now strong clinical evidence that lowering the number of atherogenic apoB100 particles in plasma is beneficial [144,215,216], whereas this evidence is much weaker to nonexistent with regard to lowering plasma triglyceride or raising HDL cholesterol. This point, plus the fact that modern pharmacologic therapy makes therapeutic alteration of plasma apoB100 levels achievable in most patients, should, we believe, govern our management decisions. Full review of this body of evidence would require extensive discussion. For present purposes, only our major conclusions will be outlined. We would emphasize that, while strong, the evidence still is incomplete, and the therapeutic approaches we suggest are presented with full awareness that the decisive clinical trials are still underway and that their findings could alter these recommendations. On the other hand, the evidence is incontrovertible that without therapeutic intervention, atherosclerosis is a progressive disease in the vast majority of patients [217,218], that anatomic progression is associated with subsequent clinical events [218], and that the risk of progression and clinical events both are related to the plasma levels of LDL [219].

The evidence of benefit with therapy comes from a variety of sources. We noted earlier that increased levels of LDL, particularly small, dense LDL, resulted in impaired flow-mediated vasodilation [42], raising the hope that reduction of LDL particle number would produce improved myocardial oxygen supply-demand imbalance. There is now evidence that this view is correct. Leung and coworkers [220] were the first to show that reduction of serum cholesterol resulted in improved response to acetylcholine challenge and, thus, more normal flow-mediated vasodilatation responses. Recently Gould and colleagues [221], using positron emission tomography, have confirmed and extended this finding by documenting decreases in size and severity of dipyridamole-induced perfusion abnormalities after marked lowering of LDL.

Clinical trials can be divided into trials of primary and secondary prevention with interventions that range from a number of dietary approaches to a series of pharmacologic therapies. The trials of primary prevention were the first completed, and while suggestive of benefit, the results are not definitive [222]. The evidence has become much stronger with the recent series of angiographic trials of prevention of progression [129–143]. The principal goal of these trials was to determine if marked lowering of plasma LDL in patients with documented coronary or carotid disease would reduce the rate of progression of disease. While the interventions in the coronary trials varied widely from dietary and lifestyle alteration to administration of a series of pharmacologic agents to partial ileal bypass, all produced at least a 20-percent lowering of plasma LDL. Only preliminary reports are available from a number of these trials. Nevertheless, all except one [142] demonstrated that progression of disease as assessed angiographically was significantly reduced and several—in general, those with greater reduction in serum LDL—demonstrated regression in a significant number of lesions.

Such anatomic findings are suggestive but, of course, far from clinical proof. A meta-analysis we recently performed, however, indicated significant reduction in clinical events in these trials [144]. Death and nonfatal myocardial infarction both were reduced by 30 percent, with an even greater reduction in the percentage of interventions such as bypass surgery and angioplasty in the treated compared to the control group. Conclusions based on meta-analysis should, of course, always be regarded as provisional; that is particularly true in this case, given that one trial, the Program on Surgical Control of the Hyperlipidemias (POSCH) trial [132], was so much larger and lasted so much longer than the other trials included in the analysis. On the other hand, there are now five separate coronary angiographic trials [132,136,137,139,143] and two carotid trials [223,224], all showing independent evidence for significant clinical benefit. Given the minimal risk of therapy for lowering LDL markedly, the risk-benefit ratio, in our opinion, strongly favors therapy in patients with vascular disease, and such therapy should include pharmacologic as well as dietary interventions.

As to the objectives of therapy, marked rather than moderate reduction in LDL particle number seems the most reasonable goal in patients with established vascular disease. Two further studies should be noted in this regard. First, post-facto analysis of the data in the FATS trial [225] indicated that the group of patients whose cholesterol was not markedly elevated had less angiographic evidence of progression and more angiographic evidence of regression than the group with the higher levels of cholesterol. Even more important, evidence of clinical benefit was clear in this group, while only a trend to benefit was present in the group with the high cholesterol levels. In both groups, LDL particle number was elevated at the onset because all patients in the trial had increased apoB100. Even though the percent reduction in LDL cholesterol and apoB100 was about the same in both groups, only in the first group was the LDL particle number reduced to normal. In the second, while it decreased significantly, the mean value merely entered the upper limit of the normal range. These results suggest to us that, for the moment, the key to angiographic and clinical success is maximal reduction in LDL particle number; simply achieving an LDL cholesterol within midpoint of the normal range is not sufficient.

Pharmacologic Therapy

Although dietary therapy should never be ignored, it is rarely sufficient either in patients with vascular disease or in patients with clear-cut dyslipidemias in whom the objective of therapy is to reduce the risk of vascular disease. Pharmacologic therapy is called for in almost all these patients. The reader is referred to the appropriate sources for detailed instructions as to the use of such

Table 25-3. Effect of pharmacologic agents on plasma lipid and lipoprotein profiles

Pharmacologic agent	Plasma profile apoB	TC	Tg	LDL cholesterol	HDL cholesterol	Lp(a)
HMGCoA reductase inhibitors	↓↓	↓↓	~↓	↓↓	~↑	NC
Bile-acid sequestrants	↓	↑	↓	↓		NC
Nicotinic acid	↓↓	↓↓	↓↓	↓↓	↑	~↓
Fibrates	~↓	~↓	↓↓	~↓	↑	NC

Abbreviations: apoB = plasma lipoprotein B; TC = plasma total cholesterol; Tg = plasma triglycerides; Lp(a) = lipoprotein Lp(a). Arrows indicate major (↓↓), moderate (↓), or slight decreases (~↓) and moderate (↑) or slight increases (~↑); NC = no change.

agents presented in Table 25-3. Here we will only indicate our personal preference for the order in which they should be used.

In our opinion, the class of first choice to reduce IDL and LDL particle number in plasma is the HMGCoA reductase inhibitor group [226]. These agents are effective, and the side effects are well defined and relatively infrequent. Their major effects are on the concentration of LDL, but there are often additional though quantitatively less important beneficial effects on plasma VLDL and HDL levels. The principal effect—that of lowering LDL levels—occurs by virtue of improvement in clearance and decrease in production, both almost certainly relating to their effect on hepatic cholesterol synthesis. With the exception of homozygous FH, HMGCoA reductase inhibitors are effective in all situations characterized by increased levels of LDL and IDL [227–230]. Side effects are relatively infrequent, with hepatotoxicity and myocytolysis the two of particular importance. The latter may rarely be sufficiently severe as to impair renal function and, thus, be life threatening. However, this side effect virtually occurs only if these agents have been used in combination with erythromycin, cyclosporin, nicotinic acid, or fibrates [230]. HMGCoA reductase inhibitors should not be given to patients with cholestasis. Their principal drawback in usual practice, however, is cost, a problem that, unfortunately, applies to some other hypolipidemic agents, as well.

The exception to this last point is nicotinic acid, which is both effective and affordable. It lowers VLDL and LDL and raises HDL [231]. The drawbacks in this case are the length of time to achieve a therapeutically adequate dose and side effects. These are of two kinds: those of immediate discomfort to the patients but not of clinical significance, such as flushing and pruritus, and those with clinical consequence, such as gout, diabetes, and duodenal ulcer. Nicotinic acid likely acts by multiple mechanisms, which include reduction in fatty-acid release from adipose tissue and inhibition of secretion of VLDL by the liver. Doses of between 3–6 g/day must be achieved to have significant clinical benefit. The drug is contraindicated in patients with gouty arthritis or significant hyperuricemia, active liver disease, a history of peptic ulcer disease, or, some authorities suggest, type II diabetes.

Bile-acid sequestrants now represent second-line agents, which we use most often to supplement the effect of the HMGCoA reductase inhibitors. They lower LDL levels by depleting the hepatic bile-acid pool and, thus, the hepatic cholesterol pool. Consequently, LDL clearance increases, and plasma LDL levels fall [232,233]. Maximal doses are rarely justified, because the dose-response curve is not linear. Gastrointestinal side effects are common, and these agents may interfere with the absorption of several medications, including digoxin, thyroxin, thiazides, and beta blockers. Absorption of folate and fat-soluble vitamins can also be impaired. In patients who are already hypertriglyceridemic, bile-acid sequestrants should be used cautiously or not at all, because plasma triglycerides may rise substantially.

The last class of agents we will consider are fibrates, agents that will consistently lower plasma triglycerides and raise HDL cholesterol. These agents also produce LDL profile shifts from the smaller, more atherogenic particles to the larger, possibly less dangerous variety [234]. Their impact on LDL particle number varies, but it is rarely pronounced; thus, we do not regard them as preferred agents for this purpose. By contrast, an agent of this group was associated with a positive clinical outcome in the Helsinki heart trial [235], and, therefore, the use of these agents to reduce the likelihood of ischemic events cannot be dismissed. The mechanisms by which triglycerides are reduced are likely multiple and include activation of lipoprotein lipase, reduction of fatty-acid release from adipose tissue, and increase in triglyceride synthesis in adipocytes. Cholesterol secretion into bile increases; therefore, fibrates have the potential to increase the risk of cholelithiasis [236]. At least two of the agents in this class, clofibrate and bezafibrate, may potentiate the action of warfarin anticoagulants.

Combination therapy often is used either in individuals with markedly elevated LDL levels or when maximal reduction is chosen as the therapeutic approach. Certain combinations, such as HMGCoA reductase inhibitors and bile-acid sequestrants, are relatively easy to use. In carefully selected patients, fibrates or nicotinic acid have been used in combination with HMGCoA reductase inhibitors. With such an approach, there is a small but significant risk of important myocytolic damage with its attendant complications; thus, it would seem prudent to restrict such usage to those with considerable experience and interest in that area.

References

1. Hostmark AT, et al. Coronary risk factors in middle-aged men as related to smoking, coffee intake and physical activity. Scand J Soc Med 1992; 20(4):196–203.
2. Jarvik GP, et al. Host and environmental effects on plasma apolipoprotein B. Intern J Clin Lab Res 1993; 23:215–220.
3. Allen DR, Browse NL, Rutt DL. Effects of cigarette smoke, carbon monoxide and nicotine on the uptake of fibrinogen by the canine arterial wall. Atherosclerosis 1989; 77:83.
4. Pittilo RM, et al. Effects of cigarette smoking on the ultrastructure of rat thoracic aorta and its ability to produce prostacyclin. Thromb Haemost 1982; 48:173.
5. Curtis LK, Witztum JL. Plasma apolipoproteins AI, AII, B, C1 and E are glycosylated in hyperglycaemic diabetic subjects. Diabetes 1985; 34:452–461.
6. Witzum JL, et al. Non-enzymatic glycosylation of human low density lipoprotein alters its biologic activity. Diabetes 1982; 31:283–291.
7. Brownlee M, Vlassara H, Cerami A. Nonenzymatic glycosylation products in collagen covalently trap low-density lipoprotein. Diabetes 1985; 34:938–941.
8. Schinder SL, Kohn RR. Effects of age and diabetes mellitus on the solubility and nonenzymatic glycosylation of human skin collagen. J Clin Invest 1981; 67:1630–1635.
9. Tarsio JF, Reger LA, Furcht LT. Molecular mechanisms in basement membrane complications of diabetes. Diabetes 1988; 37:5332–5340.
10. Brownlee M. Advanced products of nonenzymatic glycosylation and the pathogenesis of diabetic complications. In H Rifkin, D Porte, eds. Diabetes Mellitus—Theory and Practice. New York: Elsevier, 1990. Pp. 279–291.
11. Demer LL. Mechanical factors in artery wall function and atherogenesis. In AJ Lasis, JJ Rotter, RS Sparkes, eds. Molecular Genetics of Coronary Artery Disease. Candidate Genes and Processes in Atherosclerosis. Monogr Hum Genet., vol 14. Basel: Karger, 1992. Pp. 82–97.
12. Heimberg M, Weinstein I, Kohout M. The effects of glucagon, dibutyryl cyclic adenosine 3′5′ monophosphate and concentration of free fatty acid on hepatic lipid metabolism. J Biol Chem 1969; 244:5131–5139.
13. Fukuda N, Ontko J. Interactions between fatty acid synthesis, oxidation, and esterification in the production of triglyceride-rich lipoproteins by the liver. J Lipid Res 1984; 25:831-842.
14. Schaefer EJ, Levy RI. The pathogenesis and management of lipoprotein disorders. N Engl J Med 1985; 312:1300–1310.
15. Breckinridge WC, et al. Hypertriglyceridemia associated with a deficiency of apolipoprotein C-II. N Engl J Med 1978; 198:1265–1273.
16. Baggio G, et al. Apolipoprotein C-II deficiency syndrome. Clinical features, apoprotein characterization, lipase activity, and correction of hypertriglyceridemia after apolipoprotein C-II administration in two affected patients. J Clin Invest 1986; 77:520–527.
17. Redgrave TG. Formation of cholesteryl ester-rich particulate lipid during metabolism of chylomicrons. J Clin Invest 1970; 49:465–471.
18. Brewer HB Jr, et al. Type III hyperlipoproteinemia diagnosis, molecular defect, pathology, and treatment. Ann Intern Med 1983; 98:623–640.
19. Groot PHE, et al. Postprandial lipoprotein metabolism in normolipidemic men with and without coronary artery disease. Arterio & Thromb 1991; 11:653.
20. Simons LA, et al. Chylomicrons and chylomicron remnants in coronary artery disease: A case-control study. Atherosclerosis 1987; 65:181.
21. Havel RJ. The formation of LDL: Mechanisms and regulation. J Lipid Res 1984; 25:1570–1576.
22. Elovson J, et al. Plasma VLDL contain a single molecule of apolipoprotein B. J Lipid Res 1988; 29:1461–1473.
23. Durrington PN, Bolton CH, Hartog M. Serum and lipoprotein apolipoprotein B levels in normal subjects and patients with hyperlipoproteinemia. Clin Chim Acta 1978; 82:151–160.
24. Sniderman AD, Vu H, Cianflone K. The effect of moderate hypertriglyceridemia on the relation of plasma total and LDL apoB levels. Atherosclerosis 1991; 89(2–3):109–116.
25. Cheung MC, Albers JJ. Characterization of lipoprotein particles isolated by immunoaffinity chromatography: Particles containing A-I and A-II and particles containing A-1 but no A-II. J Biol Chem 1984; 259:12201.
26. Swenson, TL. Transfer proteins in reverse cholesterol transport. Curr Opin Lipid 1992; 3:67–74.
27. Kostner GM, et al. The role of LCAT and cholesteryl ester transfer proteins for the HDL and LDL structure and metabolism. Adv Exp Med Biol 1987; 210:79.
28. Tall AR. Plasma cholesteryl ester transfer protein. J Lipid Res 1993; 34:1255–1274.
29. Teng B, et al. Composition and distribution of low-density lipoprotein fractions in hyperapobetalipoproteinemia, normolipidemia and familial hypercholesterolemia. Proc Natl Acad Sci USA 1983; 80(21):6662–6666.
30. Crouse JR, et al. Studies of low density lipoprotein molecular weight in human beings with coronary artery disease. J Lipid Res 1985; 26:566–574.
31. Austin MA, et al. Low-density lipoprotein subclass phenotypes and the risk of myocardial infarction. JAMA 1988; 13:1917–1921.
32. Campos H, et al. Low density lipoprotein particle size and coronary artery disease. Arterio & Thromb 1992; 12:187–195.
33. Shen MMS, et al. Heterogeneity of serum low density lipoproteins in normal subjects. J Lipid Res 1981; 22:236–244.
34. Krauss RM, Burke JD. Identification of multiple subclasses of plasma low density lipoproteins in normal humans. J Lipid Res 1982; 23:97–104.
35. Cilbulsky M, Gimbrone M. Endothelial expression of mononuclear leukocyte adhesion molecule during atherogenesis. Science 1991; 251:778–791.
36. Yla-Herttaala S, et al. Expression of monocyte chemoattractant protein atherosclerotic lesions. Proc Natl Acad USA 1991; 88:5252–5256.
37. Vita JA, et al. The coronary vasomotor response to acetylcholine related to risk factors for coronary artery disease. Circulation 1990; 81:491–497.
38. Chin J, Azhar S, Hoffman BB. Inactivation of endothelial derived relaxing factor by oxidized lipoproteins. J Clin Invest 1992; 89:10–18.
39. Mitchell JA, et al. Native LDL inhibits the release of endothelial derived relaxing factor by reducing the activity of endothelial nitric oxide synthase. Circ Res 1990; 66:18–27.
40. Vita JA, et al. Endothelial dysfunction leads to increased coronary constriction to catecholamines in patients with early atherosclerosis. J Am Coll Cardiol 1990; 15:158.
41. Shimokawa H, Vanhoutte PM. Impaired endothelium-dependent relaxation of aggregating platelets and related vasoactive substances in porcine coronary arteries in hypercholesterolemia and atherosclerosis. Circ Res 1989; 64:900–914.
42. Dyce MC, et al. Indices of LDL particle size closely relate to endothelial dysfunction (Abstr). Circ 1993; I-466.
43. Weisser B, et al. Low density lipoprotein subfractions in-

crease thromboxane formation in endothelial cells. BBRC 1993; 192:1245–1250.
44. Zilversmit DB, Nordestguard BG. Comparison of arterial intimal clearances of LDL from diabetic and non-diabetic cholesterol-fed rabbits. Arteriosclerosis 1989; 9:176–183.
45. DeGraaf J, et al. Enhanced susceptibility to in vitro oxidation of the dense low density lipoprotein subfraction in healthy subjects. Arteriosclerosis 1991; 11:298–306.
46. Dejager S, Bruckert E, Chapman JM. Dense low density lipoprotein subspecies with diminished oxidative resistance predominate in combined hyperlipidemia. J Lipid Res 1993; 34:295–308.
47. DeGraaf J, et al. Identification of multiple dense LDL subfractions with enhanced susceptibility to in vitro oxidation among hypertriglyceridemic subjects. Arterio & Thromb 1993; 13:712–719.
48. Hurt-Camejo E, et al. Differential uptake of proteoglycan-selected subfractions of low density lipoprotein by human macrophages. J Lipid Res 1990; 31:1387–1398.
49. Weisser B, Locher R, deGraaf J. Low density lipoprotein subfractions and [Ca^{2+}] in vascular smooth muscle cells. Circ Res 1993; 73:118–124.
50. Fredrickson DS, Levy RI, Lees RS. Fat transport in lipoproteins—an integrated approach to mechanisms and disorders. N Engl J Med 1967; 267:34–44, 94–103, 148–156, 215–225, 273–281.
51. Fredrickson DS. Phenotyping on reaching Base Camp (1950–1975). Circulation 1993; 87:III1–15.
52. Sniderman AD, et al. Association of coronary atherosclerosis with hyperapobetalipoproteinemia [increased protein but normal cholesterol levels in human plasma low-density (B) lipoproteins]. Proc Natl Acad Sci USA 1980; 77(1):604–608.
53. Genest J, et al. Hyperapobetalipoproteinemia: Plasma lipoprotein responses to oral fat load. Arteriosclerosis 1986; 6(3):297–304.
54. Cabezas MC, et al. Simvastatin improves chylomicron remnant removal in familial combined hyperlipidemia without changing chylomicron conversion. Metabolism 1993; 42:497–503.
55. Teng B, et al. Metabolic basis of hyperapobetalipoproteinemia: Turnover of apolipoprotein B in low-density lipoprotein and its precursors and subfractions compared with normal and familial hypercholesterolemia. J Clin Invest 1986; 77(3):663–672.
56. Kissebah AH, Alfarsi A, Adams PW. Integrated regulation of very low density lipoprotein triglyceride and apolipoprotein B kinetics in man: Normolipidemic subjects, familial combined hyperlipidemia. Metabolism 1981; 30:856–868.
57. Venkatesan S, et al. Stable isotopes show a direct relation between VLDL apoB production and serum triglyceride levels and indicate a metabolically and biochemically coherent basis for familial combined hyperlipidemia. Arterio & Thromb 1993; 13:1110–1118.
58. Sniderman AD, et al. Association of hyperapobetalipoproteinemia with endogenous hypertriglyceridemia and atherosclerosis. Ann Intern Med 1982; 97(6):833–839.
59. Brunzell JD, et al. Apoprotein B and A1 and coronary artery disease in humans. Arterio & Thromb 1984; 4:79–83.
60. Kwiterovich PO Jr. HyperapoB: A plerotropic phenotype characterized by dense low density lipoproteins and associated with coronary artery disease. Clin Chem 1988; 34[Suppl B1–B135]:B71–B83.
61. Shaik M, et al. Quantitative studies of transfer in vivo of low density, Sf12–60, and Sf60–400 lipoproteins between plasma and arterial intima. Arterio & Thromb 1991; 11:569–577.
62. Goldstein JL, et al. Hyperlipidemia in coronary heart disease. II: Genetic analysis of lipid levels in 176 families and delineation of a new inherited disorder, combined hyperlipidemia. J Clin Invest 1973; 52:1544–1577.
63. Brunzell JD, et al. Plasma lipoproteins in familial combined hyperlipidemia and monogenic familial hypertriglyceridemia. J Lipid Res 1983; 24:147–155.
64. Grundy SM, Chait A, Brunzell JD. Familial Combined Hyperlipidemia Workshop. Arterioscler 1987; 7:203–207.
65. Kukita H, et al. Clinical significance of measurement of serum apolipoproteins AI, AII and B in hypertriglyceridaemic male patients with and without coronary artery disease. Atherosclerosis 1985; 55:143–149.
66. Barbir M, et al. High prevalence of hypertriglyceridemia and apolipoprotein abnormalities in coronary artery disease. Br Heart J 1988; 60:397–403.
67. Brunzell JD, et al. Myocardial infarction in the familial forms of hypertriglyceridemia. Metabolism 1976; 25:313–320.
68. Durrington PN, et al. Serum apolipoproteins AI and B and lipoproteins in middle aged men with and without previous myocardial infarction. Br Heart J 1986; 56:206–212.
69. Sniderman AD, Cianflone K. Metabolic disruptions in the adipocyte-hepatocyte fatty acid axis as causes of hyperapoB. Symposium Proceeding. Intl J Obesity 1995; 19:527–533.
70. Young SG. Recent progress in understanding apolipoprotein B. Circulation 1989; 82:1574–1594.
71. Raugh G, et al. Genetic evidence from 7 families that apolipoprotein B gene is not involved in familial combined hyperlipidemia. Atherosclerosis 1990; 83:81–87.
72. Houlston R, Lewis B, Humphries SE. Polymorphisms of the apolipoprotein B and E genes and their possible roles in familial and non-familial combined hyperlipaemia. Disease Markers 1991; 9:319–325.
73. Deeb SS, et al. Association of apolipoprotein-B gene variants with plasma apo-B and low-density-lipoprotein (LDL) cholesterol levels. Hum Genet 1992; 88(4):463–470.
74. Gibbons GF. Assembly and secretion of hepatic very-low-density lipoprotein. Biochem J 1990; 268:1–13.
75. Dixon JL, Ginsberg HN. Regulation of hepatic secretion of apolipoprotein B containing lipoproteins: Information obtained from cultured liver cells. J Lipid Res 1993; 34:167–179.
76. Sniderman A, Cianflone K. Substrate delivery as a determinant of hepatic apoB secretion. Arterio & Thromb 1993; 13(5):629–636.
77. Cianflone K, et al. Regulation of apoB secretion from HepG2 cells: Evidence for a critical role for cholesterol ester synthesis in the response to a fatty acid challenge. J Lipid Res 1990; 31(11):2045–2055.
78. Cianflone K, et al. Pathogenesis of carbohydrate induced hypertriglyceridemia using HepG2 cells as a model system. Arterio & Thromb 1992; 12:271– 277.
79. Sniderman AD, et al. From familial combined hyperlipidemia to hyperapoB: Unravelling overproduction of hepatic apoB lipoproteins. Curr. Opin. Lipid 1992; 3(2):137–142.
80. Olivecrona T, Bengtsson-Olivecrona G. Lipoprotein lipase and hepatic lipase. Curr Opin Lipid 1990; 1:222–230.
81. Baldo A, et al. The adipsin-acylation stimulating protein system and regulation of intracellular triglyceride synthesis. J Clin Invest 1993; 92:1543–1558.
82. Sniderman AD, Baldo A, Cianflone K. The potential role of acylation stimulating protein as a determinant of plasma triglyceride clearance and intracellular triglyceride synthesis. Curr. Opin. Lipid 1992; 3(3):202–207.
83. Germinario R, et al. Coordinate regulation of triacylglycerol

synthesis and glucose transport by acylation stimulating protein. Metabolism 1993; 40(5):574–580.
84. Yasruel Z, et al. Effect of acylation stimulating protein on the triacylglycerol synthetic pathway of human adipose tissue. Lipids 1991; 26(7):495–499.
85. Sniderman AD, Kwiterovich PO Jr. Hyperapobetalipoproteinemia and LDL and HDL_2 heterogeneity. NIH meeting proceedings. U.S. Department of Health and Human Services. Proceedings of Workshop on Lipoproteins Heterogeneity. Washington, D.C.: NIH Publication No. 87-2646, 1987.
86. Castro Cabezas M, et al. Impaired fatty acid metabolism in familial combined hyperlipidemia: A mechanism associating hepatic apolipoprotein B overproduction and insulin resistance. J Clin Invest 1993; 92(1):160–168.
87. Cianflone K, et al. The metabolic response of ASP to an oral fat load. J Lipid Res 1989; 30(11):1727–1733.
88. Cianflone K, Maslowska M, Sniderman AD. Impaired response of fibroblasts in patients with hyperapobetalipoproteinemia to Acylation Stimulating Proteins. J Clin Invest 1990; 85:722–730.
89. Kwiterovich PO Jr, Motevalli M, Miller M. The effect of three serum basic proteins on the mass of lipids in normal and HyperapoB fibroblasts. Arterio & Thromb 1994; 14:1–7.
90. Saxena U, Witte LD, Goldberg IJ. Release of endothelial cell lipoprotein lipase by plasma lipoproteins and free fatty acids. J Biol Chem 1989; 264:4349–4355.
91. Evans AJ, et al. Lipolysis is a prerequisite for lipid accumulation in HepG2 cells induced by large hypertriglyceridemic very low density lipoproteins. J Biol Chem 1992; 267:1–9.
92. Horton JD, Cuthbert JA, Spady DK. Dietary fatty acids regulate hepatic low density lipoprotein (LDL) transport by altering LDL receptor protein and mRNA levels. J Clin Invest 1993; 92:743–749.
93. Svedberg J, et al. Fatty acids in the portal vein of the rate regulate hepatic insulin clearance. J Clin Invest 1991; 88:2054–2058.
94. Golay A, et al. Relationships between plasma free fatty acid concentration, endogenous glucose production, and fasting hyperglycemia in normal and non-insulin dependent diabetic individuals. Metabolism 1987; 36:692–696.
95. Reaven GM, et al. Insulin resistance and hyperinsulinemia in individuals with small, dense, low density lipoprotein particles. J Clin Invest 1993; 92:141–146.
96. Hunt SC, et al. Apoprotein, low density apoprotein subfraction, and insulin associations with familial combined hyperlipidemia: Study of Utah patients with familial dyslipidemic hypertension. Arterio & Thromb 1989; 9:335–344.
97. Selby JV, et al. LDL subclass phenotypes and the insulin resistance syndrome in women. Circulation 1993; 88:381–387.
98. Stiko-Rahm A, et al. Secretion of plasminogen activator inhibitor-1 from cultured human umbilical vein endothelial cells is induced by very low density lipoprotein. Arteriosclerosis 1990; 10:1067–1073.
99. Hamsten A. Coagulation factors and hyperlipidemia. Curr Opin Lipid 1991; 2:226–271.
100. Hamsten A, et al. Increased plasma levels of rapid inhibitor of tissue plasminogen activator in young survivors of myocardial infarction. N Engl J Med 1985; 313:1557–1563.
101. Tornvall P, et al. Relation of plasma levels and composition of apolipoprotein B-containing lipoproteins to angiographically defined coronary artery disease in young patients with myocardial infarction. Circulation 1993; 88(Part 1):2180–2189.
102. Glueck CJ, et al. Relationships between Lp(a) lipids, apolipoproteins basal and stimulated fibrolytic regulations and D-dimer. Metabolism 1993; 42:236–246.
103. Douste-Blazy P, et al. Increased frequency of apoE-ND phenotype and hyperapobetalipoproteinemia in normolipidemic subjects and xanthelasmas of the eyelids. Ann Intern Med 1982; 96:164–169.
104. Brunzell JD, et al. Apoprotein B and A-1 and coronary artery disease in humans. Arterio & Thromb 1984; 4:79–83.
105. Kwiterovich PO Jr. HyperapoB: a pleiotropic phenotype characterized by dense low density lipoproteins and associated with coronary artery disease. Clin Chem 1988; 34[Suppl B-1–B-135]:B71–B83.
106. Marcovina SM, et al. Hannon International Federation of Clinical Chemistry Standardization Project for Measurements of Apolipoprotein A-1 and B: Comparability of apolipoprotein B values by use of international reference material. Clin Chem 1994; 40:586–592.
107. Cianflone K, et al. Modulation of chylomicron remnant metabolism by an HMG CoA reductase inhibitor. Metabolism 1990; 39(3):274–280.
108. Bilheimer DW, et al. Mevinolin and colestipol stimulate receptor-mediated clearance of low density lipoprotein from plasma in familial hypercholesterolemia heterozygotes. Proc Natl Acad Sci USA 1983; 80:4124–4128.
109. Vega GL, Krauss RM, Grundy SM. Pravastatin therapy in primary moderate hypercholesterolemia: Changes in metabolism of apolipoprotein B-containing lipoproteins. J Intern Med 1990; 227:81–94.
110. Arad Y, Ramakrishnan R, Ginsberg HN. Lovastatin therapy reduces low density lipoprotein apoB levels in subjects with combined hyperlipidemia by reducing the production of apoB-containing lipoproteins: Implications for the pathophysiology of apoB production. J Lipid Res 1990; 30:567–582.
111. Arad Y, Ramakrishnan R, Ginsberg HN. Effects of lovastatin therapy on very-low-density lipoprotein triglyceride metabolism in subjects with combined hyperlipidemia: Evidence for reduced assembly and secretion on triglyceride-rich lipoproteins. Metabolism 1992; 41:487–493.
112. Cortner J, et al. The effect of lovastatin in very low-density lipoprotein apolipoprotein B production by the liver in familial combined hyperlipidemia. J Inherit Metab Dis 1993; 16:127–134.
113. Melish J, et al. Dissociation of apoprotein B and triglyceride production in very-low-density lipoproteins. Am J Physiol 1980; 239:E354–E362.
114. Abbott WGH, et al. Effect of a high carbohydrate, low saturated-fat diet on apolipoprotein B and triglyceride metabolism in Pima Indians. J Clin Invest 1990; 86:642–650.
115. Cianflone K, et al. Pathogenesis of carbohydrate induced hypertriglyceridemia using HepG2 cells as a model system. Arterio & Thromb 1992; 12:271–277.
116. Ruderman NB, et al. A biochemical and morphologic study of very low density lipoproteins in carbohydrate-induced hypertriglyceridemia. J Clin Invest 1971; 50:1355–1368.
117. Packard CJ, et al. Metabolism of apolipoproteinB in large triglyceride-rich very low density lipoproteins in hypertriglyceridemic subjects. J Clin Invest 1986; 77:663–672.
118. Fredrickson DS, Altrocchi PH, Avioli LC. Tangier disease: Combined clinical staff conference at the National Institutes of Health. Ann Intern Med 1961; 55:1016–1031.
119. Deeb SS, et al. A mutation in human apolipoprotein A-I gene. Dominant effect on the level and characteristics of plasma high density lipoproteins. J Biol Chem 1991; 277:13654–13660.
120. Matsunaga T, et al. Apolipoprotein A-I deficiency due to a codon 84 nonsense mutation of the apolipoprotein A-I gene. Proc Natl Acad Sci USA 1991; 88:2793–2797.

121. Schaefer EJ, et al. Familial apolipoprotein A-I and C-III deficiency, variant II. J Lipid Res 1985; 26:1089–1101.
122. Karathanasis SK, Ferris E, Haddad IA. DNA inversion within the apolipoproteins AI/CIII/AIV encoding gene cluster of certain patients with premature atherosclerosis. Proc Natl Acad Sci USA 1987; 84:7198–7202.
123. Ordovas JM, et al. Familial apolipoprotein A-I, C-III and A-IV deficiency and premature atherosclerosis due to deletion of a gene complex on chromosome 11. J Biol Chem 1989; 264:16339–16342.
124. Weisgraber KH, et al. A-I Milano apoprotein: Isolation and characterization of a cysteine-containing variant of the A-I apoprotein from human high density lipoproteins. J Clin Invest 1980; 66:901–909.
125. Glomset JA, Norum KR, Gjone E. Familial lecithin: cholesterol acyltransferase deficiency. In JB Stanbury, JB Wyngaarden, DS Fredrickson, eds. The Metabolic Basis of Inherited Disease. New York: McGraw-Hill, 1983. Pp. 643–654.
126. Carlson LA. Fish-eye disease: A new familial conditions with massive corneal opacities and dyslipoproteinemia. Eur J Clin Invest 1982; 12:41–53.
127. Ginsberg HN, et al. Increased production rates of LDL are common in individuals with low plasma levels of HDL cholesterol, independent of plasma triglyceride concentrations. Arterio & Thromb 1993; 13:842–851.
128. Genest J Jr, et al. Familial hypoalphalipoproteinemia in premature coronary artery disease. Arterio & Thromb 1993; 13:1728–1737.
129. Brensike JF, et al. Effects of therapy with cholestyramine on progression of coronary atherosclerosis: Results of the NHLBI Type II Coronary Intervention Study. Circulation 1984; 69:313–324.
130. Blankenhorn DH, et al. Beneficial effects of combined colestipol niacin therapy on coronary atherosclerosis and coronary venous bypass grafts. JAMA 1987; 257:3233–3240.
131. Cashin-Hemphill L, et al. Beneficial effects of colestipol-niacin on coronary atherosclerosis. A four year follow-up. JAMA 1990; 264:3013–3017.
132. Buchwald H, et al. Effect of partial ileal bypass surgery on mortality and morbidity from coronary heart disease in patients with hypercholesterolemia: Report of the program on surgical control of the hyperlipidemias (POSCH). N Engl J Med 1990; 323:946–955.
133. Ornish D, et al. Can lifestyle changes reverse coronary heart disease? Lancet 1990; 336:129–133.
134. Kane JP, et al. Regression of coronary atherosclerosis during treatment of familial hypercholesterolemia with combined drug regimens. JAMA 1990; 264:3007–3012.
135. Tatami R, et al. for the LARS Investigators. Regression of coronary atherosclerosis by combined LDL-apheresis and lipid-lowering drug therapy in patients with familial hypercholesterolemia: A multicenter study. Atherosclerosis 1992; 95:1–13.
136. Watts GF, et al. Effects on coronary artery disease of lipid-lowering diet or diet plus cholestyramine in the St. Thomas' Atherosclerosis Regression Study (STARS). Lancet 1992; 339:563–569.
137. Haskell WL, et al. Effects of intensive multiple risk factor reduction on coronary atherosclerosis and clinical cardiac events in men and women with coronary artery disease: The Stanford Coronary Risk Intervention Project (SCRIP). Circulation 1994; 89(3):975–990.
138. Schuler G, et al. Myocardial perfusion and regression of coronary artery disease in patients on a regimen of intensive physical exercise and low fat diet. J Am Coll Cardiol 1992; 19:34–42.
139. Brown BG, et al. Regression of coronary artery disease as a result of intensive lipid-lowering therapy in men with high levels of apolipoproteinB. N Engl J Med 1990; 323:1289–1298.
140. Blankenhorn DH, et al. Coronary angiographic changes with lovastatin therapy. The monitored Atherosclerosis Regression Study (MARS). The MARS Research Group. Ann Intern Med 1993; 119(10):969–976.
141. Waters D, et al. Effects of monotherapy with an HMG-CoA reductase inhibitor in the progression of coronary atherosclerosis as assessed by serial quantitative arteriography: The Canadian Coronary Atherosclerosis Intervention Trial. Circulation 1994; 89:959–968.
142. Sacks FM, et al. The effect on coronary artery stenosis if intensive pharmacologic step therapy to improve LDL and HDL in patients with normal plasma lipid levels. Circulation 1992; 86:1–743.
143. Pitt B, et al. Pravastatin limitation of atherosclerosis in the coronary arteries (PLACI). J Am Coll Cardiol 1994; 131A:1A–484A.
144. Sniderman AD, Ghezzo R. A meta-analysis of the clinical outcomes of the recent quantitative angiographic trials to lower plasma LDL in patients with coronary artery disease. Can J Cardiol 1994 In press.
145. Brown MS, Kovanen PT, Goldstein JL. Evolution of the LDL receptor concept—from cultured cells to intact animals. Ann NY Acad Sci 1980; 348:48–68.
146. Russell DW, Esser V, Hobbs HH. Molecular basis of familial hypercholesterolemia. Arteriosclerosis 1989; 9:1–8.
147. Innerarity TL, et al. Familial defective apoB-100: Low density lipoproteins with abnormal receptor binding. Prac Natl Acad Sci USA 1987; 84:6919–6923.
148. Innerarity TL, et al. Familial defective apolipoprotein B-100 a mutation of apolipoprotein B that causes hypercholesterolemia. J Lipid Res 1990; 31:1337–1349.
149. Myant NB. Familial defective apolipoprotein B-100: A review, including some comparisons with familial hypercholesterolemia. Atherosclerosis 1993; 104:1–18.
150. Thompson GR, et al. Defects of the receptor-mediated low density lipoprotein catabolism in homozygous familial hypercholesterolemia and hypothyroidism in vivo. Proc Natl Acad Sci USA 1981; 78:2591–2595.
151. Genest JJ, et al. Prevalence of familial lipoprotein disorders in patients with premature coronary artery disease. Circulation 1992; 85:2025–2033.
152. Bhattacharyya AK, Conner WE. β-sitosterolaemia and xanthomatosis. J Clin Invest 1974; 53:1033–1043.
153. Salen G, Shefer S, Berginer VM. Familial diseases with storage of sterols other than cholesterol: cerebrotendinous xanthomatosis and sitosterolaemia with xanthomatosis. In JB Stanbury, et al., eds. The Metabolic Basis of Inherited Disease. 5th Edition. New York: McGraw-Hill, 1983. Pp. 713–730.
154. Beathy TH, et al. Genetic analysis of plasma sitosterol, apoprotein B and lipoproteins in a large Amish pedigree with sitosterolemia. Am J Hum Genet 1986; 38(4):492–504.
155. Lussier-Cacan S, et al. Tendon xanthomas associated with cholestonolosis and hyperapobetalipoproteinemia. Clin Invest Med 1986; 9(2):94–99.
156. Seed M, et al. Relation of serum lipoprotein(a) concentration and apolipoprotein (a) phenotype to coronary heart disease in patients with familial hypercholesterolemia. N Engl J Med 1990; 322:1494–1499.
157. Slack J. Risks of ischaemic heart-disease in familial hyperlipoproteinaemia states. Lancet 1969; 2:1380–1382.
158. Allen JM, et al. Cardiovascular complications of homozy-

gous familial hypercholesterolemia. Br Heart J 1980; 44:361–368.
159. Thompson GR, Lowenthal R, Myant NB. Plasma exchange and the management of homozygous familial hypercholesterolemia. Lancet 1978; 1:1208–1210.
160. Bilheimer DW, et al. Liver transplantation to provide low-density lipoprotein receptors and lower plasma cholesterol in a child with homozygous familial hypercholesterolemia. N Engl J Med 1984; 311:1658–1664.
161. Morganroth J, Levy RI, Fredrickson DS. The biochemical, clinical and genetic features of type III hyperlipoproteinaemia. Ann Intern Med 1975; 82:158–174.
162. Brewer HB, et al. Type III hyperlipoproteinaemia. Diagnosis, molecular defects, pathology and treatment. Ann Intern Med 1983; 98:623–640.
163. Addison T, Gull W. On a certain affection of the skin. Guy's Hospital Res Ser II 1851; 7:265–270.
164. Hazzard WR, Bierman EL. Aggravation of broad-beta disease (type 3 hyperlipoproteinaemia) by hypothyroidism. Arch Intern Med 1972; 130:822–828.
165. Kushwaha RS, et al. Type III hyperlipoproteinaemia: paradoxical hypolipidaemic response to estrogen. Ann Intern Med 1977; 87:517–525.
166. Falko JM, et al. Effect of estrogen therapy on apolipoprotein E in type III hyperlipoproteinaemia. Metabolism 1979; 28:1171–1177.
167. Mahley RW, Rall SC Jr. Type III hyperlipoproteinemia. In Scriver CR, Beaudet AL, Sly WS, et al eds. The Metabolic Basis of Inherited Disease. 6th Edition. New York: McGraw-Hill, 1989. Pp. 1195–1250.
167a. Ordovas J, et al. Apolipoprotein E isoform phenotyping methodology and population frequency with identification of apoE1 and apoE5 isoforms. J Lipid Res 1987; 28:371–380.
168. Ghiselli G, et al. Type III hyperlipoproteinaemia associated with apolipoprotein E deficiency. Science 1981; 214:1239–1241.
169. Marz W, et al. Apolipoprotein E to B ratios: A marker for type III hyperlipoproteinemia. Eur J Clin Chem Clin Biochem 1993; 31:743–747.
170. Berg K. A new serum type system in man—the Lp system. Acta Pathol Microbiol Scand 1963; 59:369–382.
171. Fless GM, Rolih CA, Scanu AM. Heterogeneity of human plasma lipoprotein(a): Isolation and characterization of the lipoprotein subspecies and their apoproteins. J Biol Chem 1984; 259:11470–11478.
172. McLean JW, et al. cDNA sequence of human apolipoprotein(a) is homologous to plasminogen. Nature 1987; 330:132–137.
173. Utermann G, et al. Genetics of the quantitative Lp(a) lipoprotein trait. I. Relation of Lp(a) glycoprotein phenotypes to Lp(a) lipoprotein concentrations in plasma. Hum Genet 1988; 78:41–46.
174. Lawn RL, et al. Atherogenesis in transgenic mice expressing human apolipoprotein(a). Nature 1992; 360(17):670–672.
175. Scanu AM, Scandiani L. Lipoprotein(a): Structure, biology, and clinical relevance. In GH Stollerman, et al. eds. Advances in Internal Medicine. St. Louis: Mosby Year Book, 1991. Pp. 249–270.
176. Smith EB, Cochran S. Factors influencing the accumulation in fibrous plaques of lipid derived from low density lipoprotein II. Preferential immobilization of lipoprotein(a) (Lp(a)). Atherosclerosis 1990; 84:173–181.
177. Cushing GL, et al. Quantitation and localization of apolipoproteins(a) and B in coronary artery bypass vein grafts resected at a reoperation. Arteriosclerosis 1989; 9:593–603.
178. Seed M, et al. Relation of serum lipoprotein(a) concentration and apolipoprotein(a) phenotype to coronary heart disease in patients with familial hypercholesterolemia. N Engl J Med 1990; 322:1494–1499.
179. Wiklund O, et al. Apolipoprotein(a) and ischaemic heart disease in familial hypercholesterolemia. Lancet 1990; i:1360–1363.
180. Carlson LA, Hamsten A, Asplund A. Pronounced lowering of serum levels of lipoprotein (a) in hyperlipidaemic subjects treated with nicotinic acid. J Intern Med 1989; 226:271–276.
181. Jenkins AJ, et al. Increased plasma apolipoprotein(a) levels in IDDM patients with microalbuminuria. Diabetes 1991; 40:787–790.
182. Takegoshi T, et al. Alterations of lipoprotein(a) in patients with diabetic nephropathy. Atherosclerosis 1990; 83:99–100.
183. Kapelrud H, et al. Serum Lp(a) lipoprotein concentrations in insulin dependent diabetic patients with microalbuminuria. Br Med J 1991; 303:675–678.
184. Parra MJ, et al. Lp(a) lipoprotein in patients with chronic renal failure treated by hemodialysis. Clin Chem 1987; 33:721–724.
185. Thillet J, et al. Lipoprotein (a) in patients treated by continuous ambulatory peritoneal dialysis. Am J Kid Dis 1993; 22(1):226–232.
186. Sniderman AD, Michel C, Racine N. Heart disease in patients with diabetes mellitus. J. Clin Epidemiol 1992; 45(12):1357–1370.
187. Nikkila EA. Triglyceride metabolism in diabetes mellitus. Progr Biochem Pharmacol 1973; 8:271–299.
188. Winocour PH, et al. Lipoprotein abnormalities in insulin-dependent diabetes mellitus. Lancet 1986; i:1176–1178.
189. Schonfeld G, et al. Apolipoprotein B levels and altered lipoprotein composition in diabetes. Diabetes 1974; 23:927–934.
190. Joven J, Vilella E. Serum levels of lipoprotein (a) in patients with well controlled noninsulin dependent diabetes mellitus. JAMA 1991; 265:1113–1114.
191. Haffner SM, et al. Lp(a) concentrations in NIDDM. Diabetes 1992; 41:1267–1272.
192. Arauz C, Lackner C, Ramirez LC. Lipoprotein (a) levels in diabetic patients and correlations with the metabolic control. Diabetes 1990; 39[Suppl 1]:64A.
193. Abrams JJ, Grundy SM. Cholesterol metabolism in hypothyroidism and hyperthyroidism in man. J Lipid Res 1981; 22:323–338.
194. Kosykh VA, et al. Cholesterol can stimulate secretion of apolipoprotein B by cultured human hepatocytes. Biochim Biophys Acta 1985; 836:385–389.
195. Desprès JP, et al. Regional differences of body fat, plasma lipoproteins and cardiovascular disease. Arteriosclerosis 1990; 10:497–511.
196. Anderson AJ, et al. Body fat distribution, plasma lipids, and lipoproteins. Arteriosclerosis 1988; 8:88–94.
197. Karhapaa P, et al. Obese men with type IIB hyperlipidemia are insulin resistant. Arterio & Thromb 1993; 13:1469–1475.
198. Maslowska MH, et al. Regional differences in triacylglycerol synthesis in adipose tissue. J Lipid Res 1993; 34:219–228.
199. Rebuffé-Scrive M, et al. Metabolism of adipose tissue in intraabdominal depots of nonobese men and women. Metabolism 1989; 38:453–458.
200. Ostman J, et al. Regional differences in the control of lipolysis in human adipose tissue. Metabolism 1979; 28:1198–1205.
201. Bolinder J, et al. Differences at the receptor and post-receptor levels between human omental and subcutaneous adi-

pose tissue in the action of insulin and lipolysis. Diabetes 1983; 32:117–123.
202. Sniderman AD, et al. Hyperapobetalipoproteinemia: The major dyslipoproteinemia in patients with chronic renal failure treated with chronic ambulatory peritoneal dialysis. Athero 1987; 65(3):257–264.
203. Steel J, et al. Lipids, lipoproteins and apolipoproteins tissues in continuous ambulatory peritoneal dialysis. Atherosclerosis 1989; 79:47–50.
204. Murphy BG, et al. Increased serum apolipoprotein (a) in patients with chronic renal failure treated with continuous ambulatory peritoneal dialysis. Atherosclerosis 1992; 93:53–57.
205. Newmark SR, et al. Lipoprotein profiles in adult nephrotics. Mayo Clin Proc 1975; 50:354–364.
206. Vega GL, Grundy SM. Lovastatin therapy in nephrotic hyperlipidemia: Effects on lipoprotein metabolism. Kidney Intl 1988; 33:1160–1168.
207. Ettinger WH, et al. Dyslipoproteinemia in systemic lupus erythematosus. Effect of corticosteroids. Am J Med 1987; 83:503–508.
208. Ettinger WH, Hazzard WH. Prednisone increases VLDL and HDL in healthy men. Metabolism 1988; 37:1055–1058.
209. Ettinger WH Jr, Hazzard WR. Elevated apolipoprotein-B levels in corticosteroid-treated patients with systemic lupus erythematosus. J Clin Endocrinol Metab 1988; 67:425–428.
210. Lowry RP, et al. Type II hyperlipoproteinemia, hyperapobetalipoproteinemia and hyperalphalipoproteinemia following renal transplantation: Prevalence and precipitating factors. Transplant Proc 1987; 19(1 Pt. 3):2229–2232.
211. Bilodeau M, et al. Dyslipoproteinemia following heart and heart-lung cardiac transplantation. Potential relation to accelerated graft arteriosclerosis. J Heart Transplant 1989; 8(6):454–459.
212. Moser M. Lipid abnormalities and diuretics. Am Fam Phys 1989; 40:213–220.
213. Miller NE. Effects of adrenoreceptor-blocking drugs on plasma lipoprotein concentrations. Am J Cardiol 1987; 60:17E–23E.
214. Genest JJ, et al. Lipoprotein cholesterol, apolipoprotein A-I, B and Lp(a) abnormalities in men with premature coronary disease. J Am Coll Cardiol 1992; 19:792–802.
215. Law MR, Wald NG, Thompson SG. By how much and how quickly does reduction in serum cholesterol lower risk of ischemic heart disease. Br Med J 1994; 308:367–372.
216. Brown BG, et al. Lipid lowering and plague regression: New insights into prevention of plaque disruption and clinical events in coronary disease. Circ 1993; 87:1781–1791.
217. Campeau L, et al. The relationship of risk factors to the development of atherosclerosis in saphenous-vein bypass grafts and progression of disease in the native circulation. A study 10 years after aortocoronary bypass surgery. N Engl J Med 1984; 311(21):1329–1332.
218. Waters D, Craven T, Lespérance J. Prognostic significance of progression of coronary artery atherosclerosis. Circ 1993; 87:1067–1075.
219. Rossouw JE. The effects of lowering serum cholesterol on coronary heart disease risk. Medical Clinics of North America 1994; 78(1):181–195.
220. Leung WH, Lau CP, Wong CK. Beneficial effect of cholesterol-lowering therapy on coronary endothelium-dependent relaxation in hypercholesterolaemic patients. Lancet 1993; 341:1496–1500.
221. Gould KL, et al. Short-term cholesterol lowering decreases size and severity of perfusion abnormalities by positron emission tomography after dipyridamole in patients with coronary artery disease. Circulation 1994; 89:1530–1538.
222. Robinson JG, Leon AS. The prevention of cardiovascular disease: Emphasis on secondary prevention. In D.B. Hunninghake, eds. Lipid Disorders. The Medical Clinics of North America 1994; 78(1):69–98.
223. Blyington RP, et al. Plac-2: Effects of pravastatin on progression of carotid atherosclerosis and clinical events. (Abstr) J Am Coll Cardiol 1993; 21(2):71A.
224. Furberg C, Blyington R. ACAPS: Effects of lovastatin on progression of carotid atherosclerosis and clinical events. Circ 1993; 88:1–386.
225. Stewart BF, et al. The benefits of lipid-lowering therapy in men with elevated apolipoprotein B are not confined to those with high LDLc. J Am Coll Cardiol 1994; 23(4):899–906.
226. Maher VM, Thompson GR. HMG CoA reductase inhibitors as lipid-lowering agents: Five years experience with lovastatin and an appraisal of simvastatin and pravastatin. Q J Med 1990; 74:165.
227. Betteridge DJ, et al. Treatment of familial hypercholesterolemia—United Kingdom Lipid Clinics Study of pravastatin and cholestyramine. Br Med J 1992; 304:1355.
228. Illingworth DR, Bacon SP, Larsen KK. Long term experience with HMG CoA reductase inhibitors in the therapy of hypercholesterolemia. Atheroscler Rev 1988; 18:161.
229. Mol MJTM, Stalenhoef AFH. HMG CoA reductase inhibitors. Curr Opin Lipidol 1993; 4:41.
230. Tobert JA. Efficacy and long-term adverse effect pattern of lovastatin. Am J Cardiol 1988; 62:28J.
231. Drood JM, Zimetbaum PJ, Frishman WH. Nicotinic acid for treatment of hyperlipoproteinemia. J Clin Pharmacol 1991; 31:641.
232. Hunninghake DB. Resin therapy. Adverse effects and their management. In J Fears, ed. Pharmacological Control of Hyperlipidemia. Barcelona: Prous Science Publishers, 1986. P 67.
233. Shepherd J, et al. Cholestyramine promotes receptor mediated low density lipoprotein catabolism. N Engl J Med 1980; 302:1219.
234. Tsai Y, Yuan J, Hunninghake DB. Effect of gemfibrozil on composition of lipoproteins and distribution of LDL subspecies. Athero 1992; 95:35.
235. Frick MH, et al. Helsinki Heart Study: Primary-prevention trial with gemfibrozil in middle-aged men with dyslipidemia. Safety of treatment, changes in risk factors, and incidence of coronary heart disease. N Engl J Med 1987; 317:1237.
236. Palmer RH. Effects of fibric acid derivatives on biliary lipid composition. Am J Med 1987; 83:37.

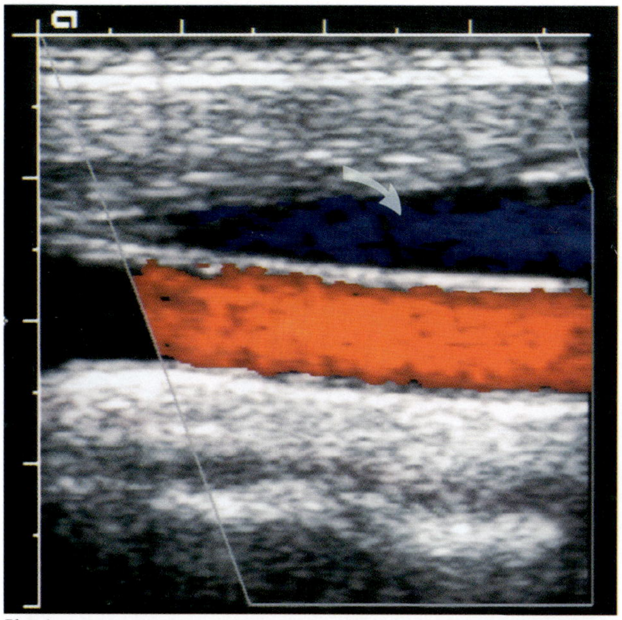

Plate 1

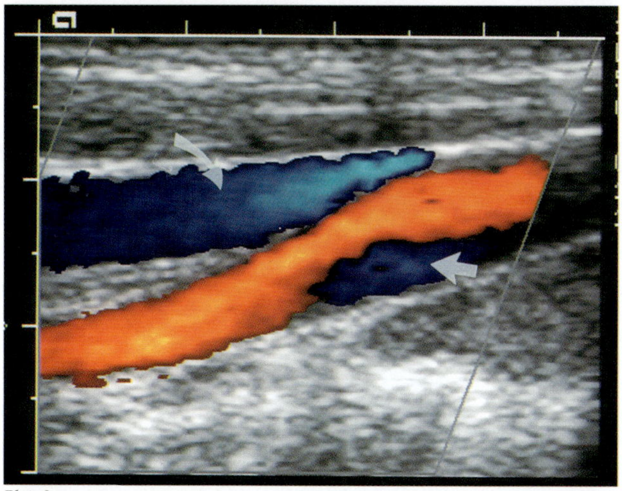

Plate 2

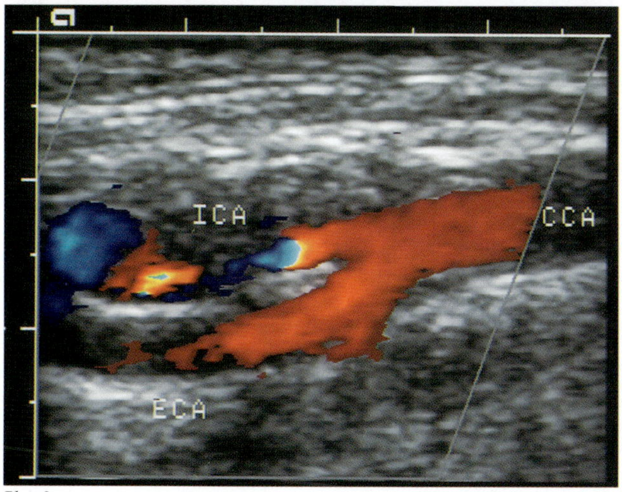

Plate 3

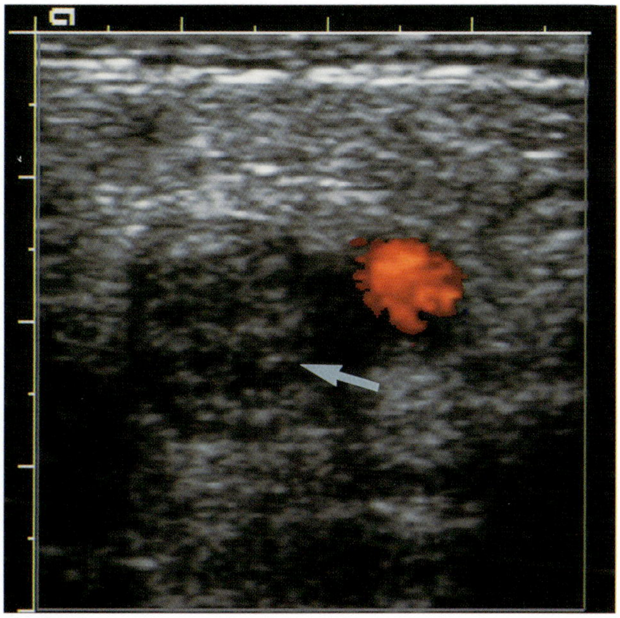

Plate 4

Plate 1. Color Doppler image of a normal common carotid artery. When red blood cell motion is detected, it is assigned a color, determined by its direction and frequency. In this example, normal laminar blood flow in the common carotid artery is depicted in red. The vessel in blue, anterior to the common carotid artery, is the internal jugular vein.
(See Chap. 19.)

Plate 2. Color Doppler image of a normal internal carotid artery just distal to the carotid-artery bifurcation. The antegrade flow in the internal carotid artery is depicted in red. At its proximal portion is an area of flow reversal, depicted in blue (arrow), which results from red cells separating at the flow divider between the internal and external carotid artery. The internal jugular vein is anterior to the internal carotid artery (curved arrow).
(See Chap. 19.)

Plate 3. Color Doppler image of a stenosed internal carotid artery. There is acceleration and turbulence of blood flow in the area of the stenosis, which is depicted as color desaturation (red to orange to yellow) and reversal of flow (blue). Key: ECA = external carotid artery, ICA = internal carotid artery, CCA = common carotid artery.
(See Chap. 19.)

Plate 4. Color Doppler image illustrating a cross-sectional image of a large thrombus (arrow) in the common femoral vein. There is no blood flow detected in this vessel. The femoral artery (red) lies alongside the common femoral vein.
(See Chap. 19.)

Plate 5. Patient with recent cerebrovascular accident secondary to middle-cerebral-artery stenosis. **Top row**. Transverse MRI images. Note lesion in left posterofrontal and temporal regions. **Middle row**. Baseline transverse perfusion images (Tc-99m labeled HMPAO). The size of the perfusion defect corresponds to pathoanatomy found with MRI. **Bottom row**. Transverse perfusion images with tracer injection during Diamox provocation. The perfusion defect is much larger than at baseline.
(See Chap. 21.)

Plate 6. Patient with atypical chest pain and severe peripheral arterial disease who was unable to perform standard exercise test. Preoperative risk evaluation with intravenous dipyridamole. **Rows 1 and 3**. Baseline (rest) transverse myocardial perfusion images (Tc-99m sestamibi) revealed no perfusion abnormalities. Therefore, there is no evidence of prior MI. **Rows 2 and 4**. Transverse perfusion images with tracer administration during pharmacologic stress. Hypoperfusion (ischemia) is evident in the lateral wall extending from base to apex, typical of left circumflex (LCX) coronary-artery territory. A significant volume of myocardium involved (approximately 20% of total).
(See Chap. 21.)

Plate 7. Patient with typical chest pain and ST-segment depression during treadmill exercise. Coronary angiography demonstrated a 75-percent left anterior descending (LAD) coronary-artery stenosis, and 60-percent left circumflex (LCX) coronary-artery stenosis. **Top row**. Resting coronal perfusion images (oriented like a short-axis ECHO). A mild perfusion defect is present in the apical portion of the anterior wall, consistent with a small nontransmural myocardial infarction (left anterior descending [LAD] coronary-artery territory). **Second row**. Coronal perfusion images after the tracer administration during stress. There is moderate to severe ischemia in the anterior wall, septum, and apex, that is, LAD coronary-artery territory. No ischemia is found in the lateral wall (left circumflex [LCX] coronary-artery territory). **Third and fourth rows**. Transverse rest and stress images, respectively. Ischemia is evident in the septum and apex, while the lateral wall is unaffected.
(See Chap. 21.)

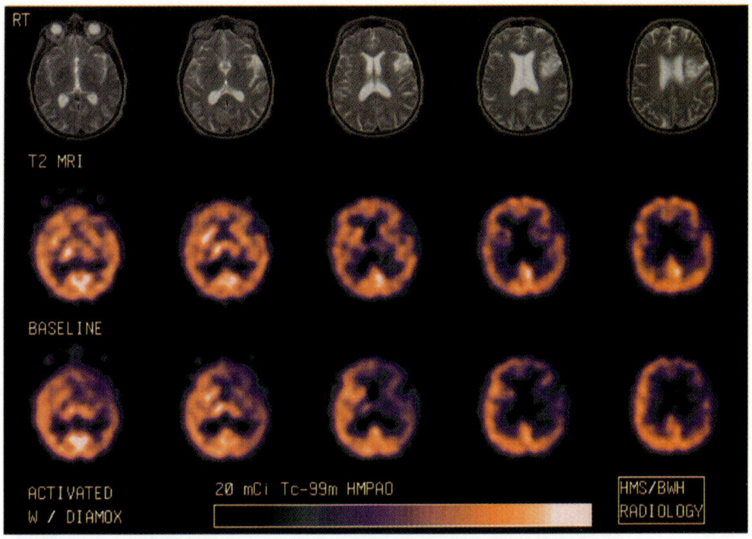

Plate 5

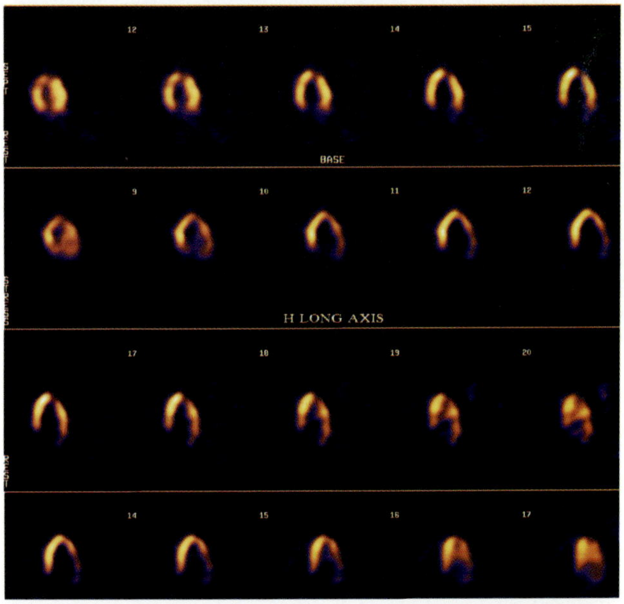

Plate 6

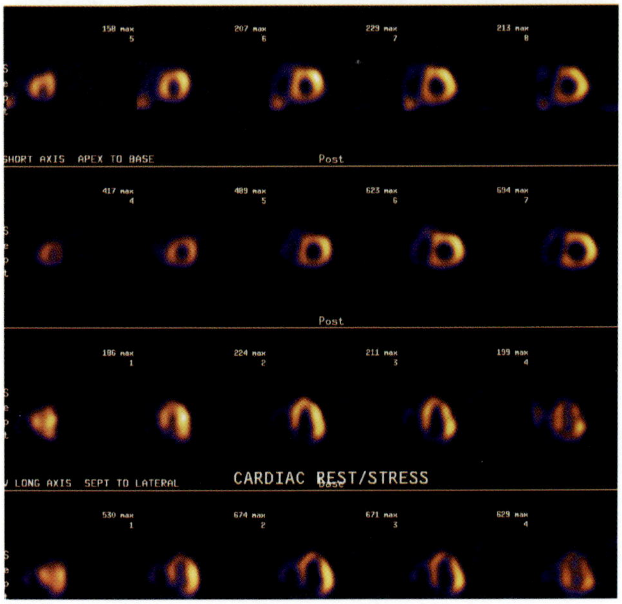

Plate 7

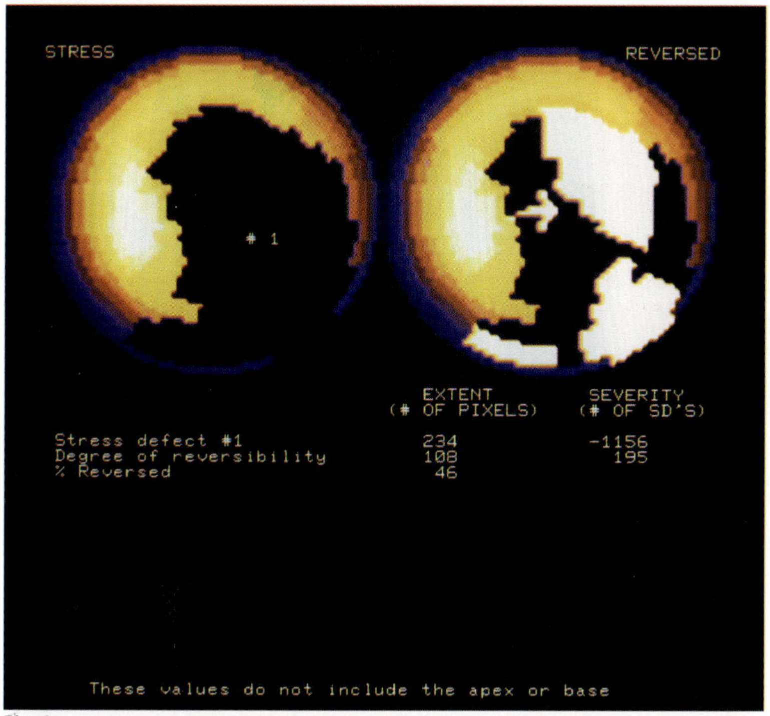
STRESS
REVERSED
1
EXTENT
(# OF PIXELS)
SEVERITY
(# OF SD'S)
Stress defect #1
Degree of reversibility
% Reversed
234
108
46
-1156
195
These values do not include the apex or base

Plate 8

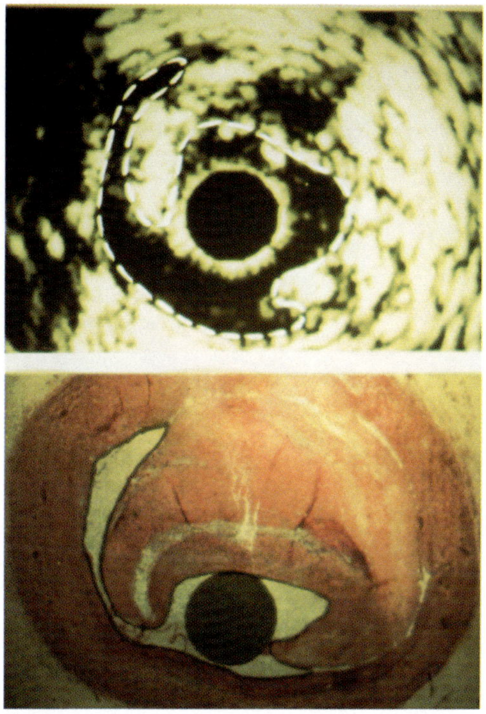

Plate 9

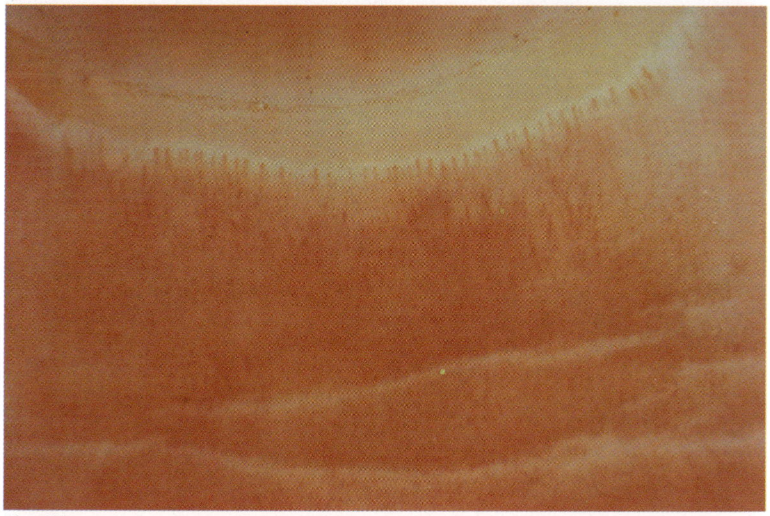

Plate 10A

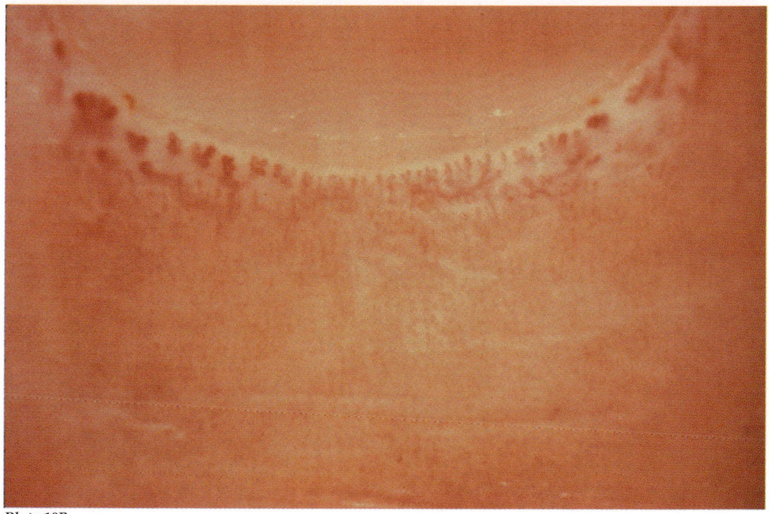

Plate 10B

Plate 8. Bull's-eye display of quantified SPECT data. In the coronal images, the myocardium is divided into sectors (5 degrees), and tracer uptake is calculated. The results from all sectors and coronal slices are normalized to the segment with highest uptake, and the relative data are displayed as a bull's-eye: the observer looks directly at the apex, that is, the center of the image. The base is in the distance; the anterior wall is up; the lateral wall is right; the inferior wall is down; the septum is to the left. The right ventricle is not seen. The black area on the stress image is an area with abnormally low uptake. White on top of black in the rest image depicts an area with reversible changes, defined as more than a 12-percent change from stress to rest. The extent and the severity of abnormalities are computed.
(See Chap. 21.)

Plate 9. Correlation between intravascular ultrasound (IVUS) and histology. **Top**. IVUS image obtained of angioplasty (PTA) site in iliac artery, demonstrating extensive plaque fracture. Patient expired 24 hours later from unrelated cause. **Bottom**. Histologic section corresponding to PTA site, depicting nearly identical morphologic features as those seen by IVUS.
(See Chap. 31.)

Plate 10A. Nailfold capillary microscopic examination of a healthy subject. The superficial capillaries are regularly spaced hairpin loops.
(See Chap. 42.)

Plate 10B. Nailfold capillary microscopic examination of a patient with scleroderma. Avascular areas and enlarged and deformed capillary loops are characteristic of this connective tissue disorder. (Courtesy of Dr. Hildegard Maricq.)
(See Chap. 42.)

Plate 11. Acrocyanosis is characterized by persistent violaceous discoloration of the digits and hands. (Courtesy of Dr. Karen McCoy, reproduced with permission.)
(See Chap. 42.)

Plate 12. This patient has chronic pernio, with characteristic pigmented lesions affecting the toes. (Courtesy of Dr. Jeffrey Olin, reproduced with permission.)
(See Chap. 42.)

Plate 13. Erythromelalgia. Characteristic erythema affecting the feet of a woman with polycythemia vera. She had chronic, intense burning pain in both feet, causing her to soak her feet in water throughout the day. This patient is the same one illustrated in Fig. 42-14.
(See Chap. 42.)

Plate 14. Plantar ulcer in an ischemic foot, complicated by a lack of protective sensation on the foot and repeated trauma from weight bearing and walking. Motor neuoropathy has accelerated loss of the arch and normal weight distribution. The foot has been recently revascularized.
(See Chap. 51.)

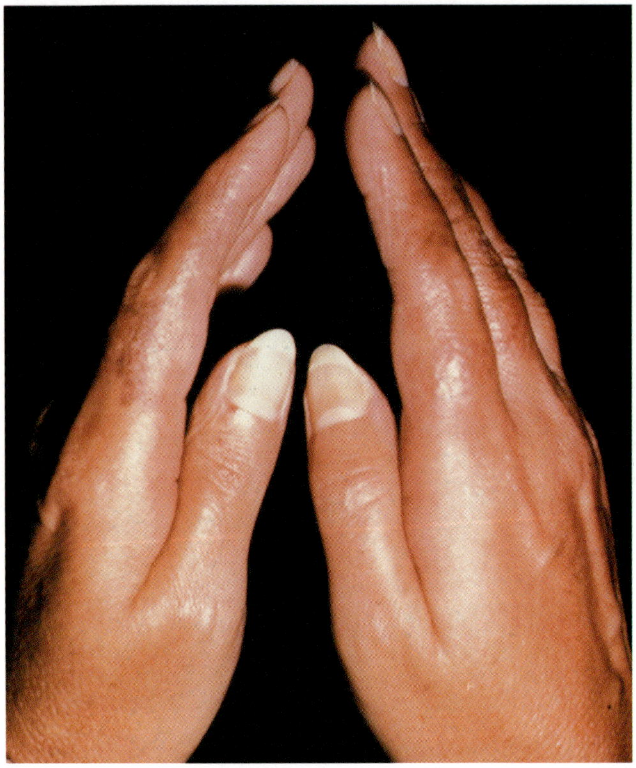

Plate 11

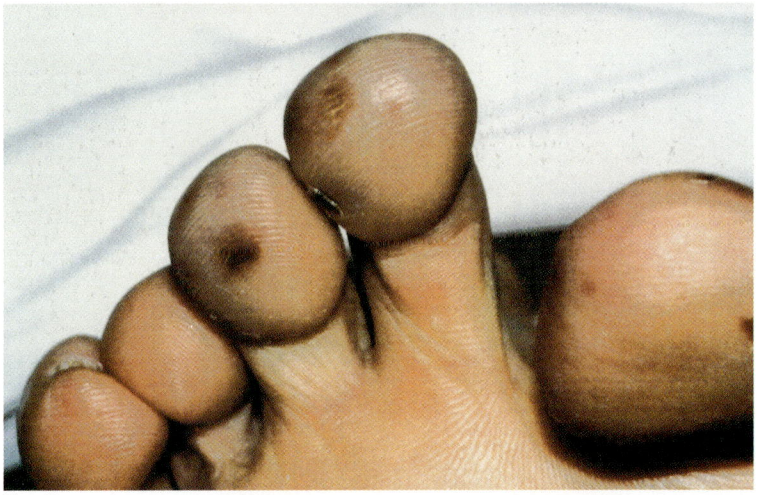

Plate 12

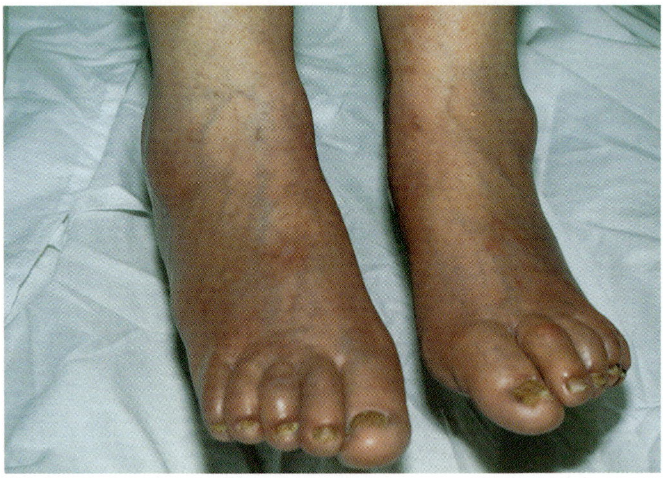

Plate 13

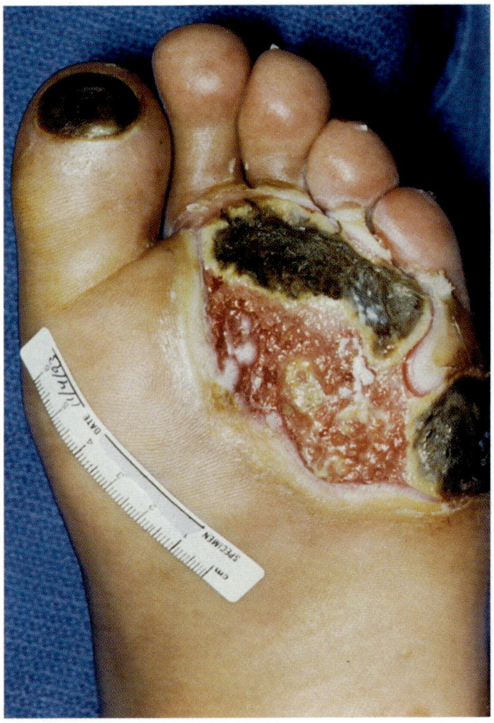

Plate 14

Hypertension: Evaluation and Management

Peter Rudd
Victor J. Dzau

Hypertension is one of the major cardiovascular risk factors contributing to myocardial infarction, cerebrovascular accidents, congestive heart failure, peripheral vascular insufficiency, and premature mortality. It is the most common reason for office visits to internists and the most common indication for the use of prescription medication in the United States [1,2]. In 1988, stroke alone cost Americans about $23.3 billion a year in direct and indirect costs. Much of the cost is attributable to uncontrolled hypertension [3]. The health care costs attributable to coronary heart disease are even greater. In 1992, the total annual direct costs of antihypertensive medications alone were estimated at $7 billion [4]. The overall cost-effectiveness of interventions to control hypertension depend on careful diagnosis, optimized adherence, treatment minimization, parsimonious selection of tests and treatments, and practice efficiency [5].

ESTABLISHING THE DIAGNOSIS AND RISK PROFILE

Definition

Classic definitions of hypertension have used indirect sphygmomanometric levels of 140 mm Hg systolic or 90 mm Hg diastolic to delimit the lower bounds of abnormality [6].

The epidemiologic reality is more complex. Blood pressure (BP), like most physiologic variables, exhibits a bell-shaped distribution with no simple cut-off to demarcate "safe" from "dangerous" levels of blood pressure elevation. There is also marked variability from day to day and by method of measurement [7]. Actuarial data have long confirmed that even moderate elevations carry incremental risk over those at average risk (~128/82 mm Hg). Consensus groups have generally selected higher levels to define hypertension, usually in the range 140/90 to 160/100 mm Hg, arguing that lower levels would burden medical care systems excessively for any important, demonstrable benefit [8]. Epidemiologic data have consistently shown a continuous, positive, linear relationship between systolic and diastolic blood pressure and the incidence of stroke and heart attack. No single threshold level distinguishes those who will have a cardiovascular event from those who will not [9].

Risk Factor versus Disease

Hypertension mediates most of its adverse effects via acceleration of atherosclerosis and vascular remodeling, especially in large to medium-sized blood vessels. As such, hypertension most properly fits as a risk factor, among many others, rather than as a disease in itself. Analogies with hypercholesterolemia are apt, since the principal mainfestations of disease come from the consequences of the elevations rather than from the elevations themselves. In 1981, hypertension accounted for the loss of about two million years of life and 500,000 years of productive life in the United States [2].

Hypertension often keeps close company with a multitude of other cardiovascular risk factors, including diabetes mellitus, dyslipidemia, hyperinsulinemia, and exogenous obesity [9,10]. In the National Health and Nutrition Examination Survey (NHANES) II, the prevalence of hypertension (BP $\geq$ 160/95) was 2.9 times higher among those who were overweight compared to those who were not. The obese were also 2.9 times more likely to have diabetes mellitus and 1.5 times more likely to have hypercholesterolemia. A number of intriguing hypotheses have emerged to explain the clustering, whether mediated through relative insulin resistance [11] or changes in cytosolic calcium [12]. Although the precise mechanism is unconfirmed, high levels of renin relative to sodium excretion may confer up to a sevenfold increased risk compared to those with normal renin profiles, even among individuals who lack other cardiovascular risk factors [13]. The preeminent nonendogenous factor remains cigarette smoking, which directly and indirectly leads to endothelial damage and accelerated atherosclerosis.

Most of the individual factors, like hypercholesterolemia and obesity, exhibit a curvilinear relation to subsequent rates of adverse outcomes, rising disproportionately as risk factors increase. Not surprisingly, in combination, these risk factors are multiplicative rather than simply additive. In most patients, the adverse consequences play out over years and decades rather than over weeks or months. Once hypertension develops, it tends to be self-perpetuating via amplifying mechanisms mediated by secondary structural changes in the blood vessels, heart, and kidney. These adaptive structural changes magnify and perpetuate hypertension by increasing systemic vascular resistance, enhancing cardiac output, or impairing renal sodium and water excretion. The long-term sequelae of hypertensive structural changes in those end organs are complications of atherosclerotic vascular disease, cardiac hypertrophy and failure, stroke, and renal dysfunction [14].

Prevalence

By single BP determinations, nearly one in every four, or 50 million, adult Americans have hypertension, when defined as being on antihypertensive medication or having systolic blood pressure (SBP) greater than 140 or diastolic blood pressure (DBP) greater than 90 mm Hg [15]. Using the somewhat more stringent criteria of intercurrent antihypertensive drug therapy or more than two occasions with sustained BP elevations, the prevalence falls to 30–40 million Americans. The prevalence rises progressively with advancing age from less than 5 percent among

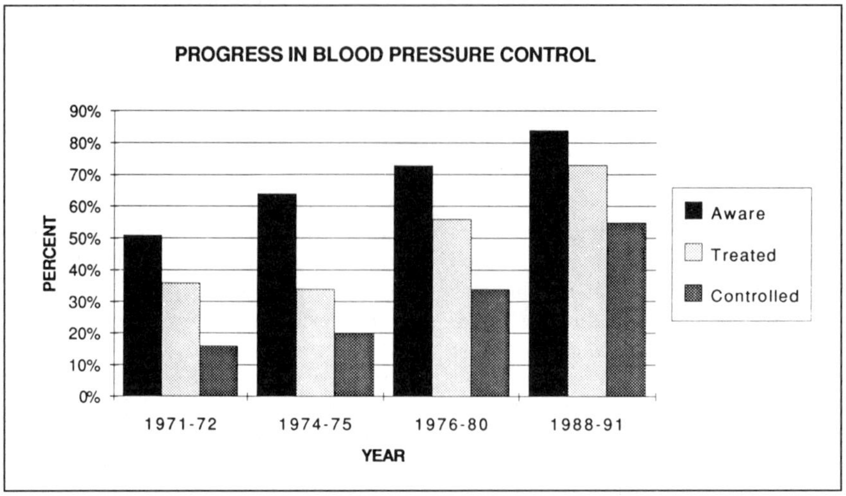

Fig. 26-1. Changing prevalence of hypertensive patients in the United States, 1971–1991, by blood pressure ≥ 160/95 mm Hg and status of awareness of the diagnosis, receiving treatment for the condition, and achieving BP control. Data from NHANES I, II, and III for BP ≥ 160/95 mm Hg as cited in Joint National Committee on Detection, Evaluation, and Treatment of High Blood Pressure. The fifth report of the Joint National Committee on Detection, Evaluation, and Treatment of High Blood Pressure (JNC V). Arch Intern Med 1993; 153:154–183.

individuals under age 29 to more than 50 percent among those over age 60 [16]. Other important associations for having hypertension include black race and male gender during middle age. On average, black women develop hypertension 10 years before white women do. As the population ages and women tend to outlive men, the number of hypertensive women continues to predominate, with higher attributable risk over that of men, even though men and women develop hypertension at comparable rates [2].

The risks of cardiovascular morbidity and mortality increase curvilinearly with increasing BP, both for systolic and diastolic pressure. The historical disinterest in systolic pressure has passed. Primary prevention trials from the United States [17], Sweden [18], and the United Kingdom [19] have each confirmed the net benefit of diagnosing and treating isolated systolic hypertension, which occurs predominantly among the elderly. Each year, approximately two million new hypertensive patients are added to the pool of Americans who may benefit from antihypertensive intervention [20].

Estimates from the 1988–1991 NHANES III survey indicate substantial improvement in our national efforts to detect, evaluate, and treat hypertension over the past two decades (Fig. 26-1). By the criteria of 160/95 mm Hg, 84 percent of those with elevated BP at a single determination appear aware of their hypertension. Fully 73 percent of those with hypertension (defined as BP ≥ 160/95 mm Hg or on antihypertensive medications) are receiving antihypertensive therapy, and 55 percent of those treated have BP ≤ 160/95 mm Hg. By the more stringent criteria of ≤ 140/90, the rates are only 65, 49, and 21 percent, respectively [16]. Rate-limiting hurdles curtail success at every step. Even when started on antihypertensive therapy, individuals with elevated BP may experience adverse drug reactions or otherwise fail to take their medications as prescribed. Table 26-1 summarizes the prevalences of selected cardiovascular risk factors by age group.

Risk Factors

OBESITY

Both cross-sectional and prospective observational studies confirm a strong association between body weight and BP [21,22]. The association includes stepwise increases in BP with higher body weight and higher prevalence of hypertension among those with greater weight. Obesity yields a two- to sixfold increase in the risk of developing hypertension and may account for 20–30 percent of the attributable exposure [23]. By NHANES II criteria (body mass index = weight in kg/[height in meters]^2 > 27.8 for men and > 27.3 for women), the prevalence of obesity among American adults varies from less than 20 percent among younger white males to more than 60 percent among older black females [24]. Upper-body or android fat patterns are more dangerous cardiovascularly than lower body or gynoid patterns, in both men and women. The patterns may be most objectively measured by calculating the ratio of minimum waist circumference to maximum hip circumference, yielding a more reliable predictor of subsequent cardiovascular disease than total weight or body mass index [25].

Obesity interacts with other risk factors to compound its adverse effects. Obese individuals display lower normalized left ventricular (LV) peak filling rates than do lean subjects as well as greater LV end-diastolic and systolic dimensions, LV wall thickness, and LV mass—a constellation of findings that predispose the obese hypertensive to cardiac enlargement and impaired LV filling [26]. Obesity also predisposes to glucose intolerance, type II diabetes mellitus, hyperinsulinemia, and insulin resistance. The common link among these results may be the development of deranged cellular calcium homeostasis within

Table 26-1. Prevalence (%) of selected cardiovascular risk factors

Age (years)	Inactivity[a]	Obesity[b]	Hypertension[c]	Smoking[d]	Diabetes[e]	Hypercholesterolemia[f]	LVH by ECG[g]
MEN							
35–44	12.1	12.5	13.5	48.6	1.1	20.2	2.9
45–54	16.9	14.7	18.3	43.1	1.1	25.7	4.8
55–64	21.0	12.5	22.3	37.4	3.3	23.5	10.1
65–74	27.1	12.7	27.1	22.8	3.2	21.6	7.1
WOMEN							
35–44	13.3	20.1	8.5	38.8	0.8	12.9	0.9
45–54	19.3	24.2	18.2	36.1	2.9	28.0	3.6
55–64	30.8	30.9	31.2	24.2	3.2	49.7	4.1
65–74	39.0	27.2	47.6	10.2	6.1	51.0	9.6

[a]Average oxygen consumption < 0.30 l/minute (1954–1958).
[b]Weight ≥ 20% above median (1960–1962).
[c]BP ≥ 160/90 (1960–1962).
[d]Current habit of cigarette smoking (1970).
[e]Diabetes mellitus requiring medication treatment (1960–1962).
[f]Serum cholesterol ≥ 260 mg/dl (1960–1962).
[g]Electrocardiographic pattern of left ventricular hypertrophy (1948–1953).
Source: Adapted from Kaplan NM. Coronary heart disease risk factors and antihypertensive drug selection. J Cardiovasc Pharmacol 1982; 4[Suppl 2]:S187–S189.

vascular smooth muscle. Whereas insulin physiologically attenuates vascular smooth muscle's contractile responses to vasoactive factors, increased cellular calcium from insulin resistance can lead to increased vascular tone and peripheral resistance [27].

PHYSICAL INACTIVITY

Recent studies have focused attention more on leisure-time activity or exercise capacity than on work-related physical exercise. They confirm a significant inverse relationship between activity classification and BP in both sexes, in all races, and at all ages, independent of weight [28].

DYSLIPIDEMIA

Hypertension and dyslipidemia also coexist more commonly than would be predicted by chance, especially for hypertriglyceridemia and lowered levels of high density lipoprotein (HDL) cholesterol. One study observed a 47-percent prevalence of lipid abnormalities among individuals with onset of hypertension before age 60 and their siblings, including 20–40 percent concordance for specific dyslipidemic patterns [29]. More recent work indicates that hypercholesterolemia, even in the absence of atherosclerosis, may diminish the arterial wall's responsiveness to direct vasodilator influences [30]. Elevated serum lipids lead to vessel-wall responses, including endothelial dysfunction, smooth-muscle-cell proliferation, lipid accumulation, foam-cell formation, and, eventually, necrosis and plaque development. Hypertension may induce shear-related injury to the vessel. Endothelial injury (caused by hypertension) and vascular cell proliferation (induced by increased pressure or vasoactive substances) are effects that amplify the atherosclerotic process [31].

EXCESS SODIUM INTAKE

Our hunter-gatherer ancestors probably consumed only 200–500 mg/day of sodium. Most modern societies consume approximately 10 times as much: 2.5–5 g/day sodium (6–12 g/day, or 100–200 mmol/day, salt), far in excess of any physiologic need [32]. Analysis of 47,000 individuals in 24 communities indicates that differences in sodium intake of 100 mmol/day can produce SBP differences of 5–10 mm Hg, especially at older age ranges [33].

The cause-and-effect relationship is complicated by measurement difficulties, wide biologic variability, and marked variation in sodium consumption [34]. Stratified analysis in the INTERSALT study investigated 10,079 patients at 52 centers in 32 countries and concluded that the average prevalence of hypertension was highest among centers with a high sodium intake, whether or not body-mass index or alcohol consumption was low [35].

ALCOHOL CONSUMPTION

Most of the more than 30 published cross-sectional studies on alcohol as risk factor indicate that its use is associated with higher BP [36]. Consuming three or more alcoholic drinks a day (~ 40 g ethanol per day) increases BP, even when controlling for body mass index, cigarette smoking, and age [32]. As much as 5–7 percent of the overall prevalence of hypertension can be attributed to alcohol intake of three or more drinks a day, which appears to be a threshold. Consumption substantially higher than this level may cause less optimal outcomes [38].

SMOKING

Smoking emerges as a principal, independent risk factor for cardiovascular disease, but it also covaries significantly with hypertension. In many primary prevention trials, the prevalence of smoking among hypertensive subjects approaches 35 percent, and an additional 30 percent may be exsmokers [39]. Epidemiologically, smoking is negatively associated with BP, relative body weight, and physical activity during leisure. In contrast, smoking is positively associated with total cholesterol, psychological stress, and alcohol abuse [40]. Although it might be predicted that smoking cessation should lead to weight gain and BP elevation, the Multiple Risk Factor Intervention Trial observed no increase in BP after smoking cessation, after controlling for weight [41]. Acutely, for about 15 minutes, smoking one to two cigarettes may produce a rise in BP of 8–10 mm Hg among habitual smokers who abstain from smoking overnight [42].

STRESS

Stressful stimuli can elevate SBP and DBP, increase circulating levels of catecholamines, cortisol, vasopressin, endorphins, and aldosterone, and reduce urinary sodium excretion [16]. By cross-sectional, case-control, and prospective trials, the emerging data are consistent with stress serving as an important component in the development and maintenance of hypertension [43,44]. The observational studies confirm the association between stress and hypertension, even when controlling for age, race, body-mass index, type A behavior, alcohol consumption, family history of hypertension, urinary sodium excretion, and physical activity.

Some have argued that the critical ingredient in stress is the absence of feasible means to reduce the stress, whether at the worksite or in other settings [45]. This constellation of factors might arise most commonly among minority populations and those with limited education or economic prospects [46].

HIGH RENIN PROFILE

One of the most intriguing but incomplete stories related to hypertension pathogenesis surrounds the renin-angiotensin system and the precise role of renin-sodium profiling [13]. To make sense of the heterogeneity of pathophysiologic features and clinical sequelae of hypertension, some investigators have focused on prognostic categorization of patients by level of renin, corrected for urinary sodium excretion. Early retrospective studies showed inconsistent results, either useful [47] or not useful [48] for predicting subsequent myocardial infarction (MI). Renin-sodium profiles, obtained by plotting plasma-renin activity against the urinary excretion of sodium, permit classification of patients into high, normal, and low groupings.

In one prospective study, patients with high renin-sodium profiles followed for an average of 8.3 years displayed more than a fivefold increase in MI per 1,000 person-years compared to those with low profiles, when adjusted for age, sex, and race. Cox proportional-hazards analysis confirmed the relationship for MI but not for stroke or noncardiovascular event after adjustment for race, sex, age at entry, serum cholesterol, smoking status, LV hypertrophy by electrocardiography, blood glucose, body-mass index, history of cardiovascular disease or treatment, blood pressure, and use of beta blockers [13]. This promising report of association carries methodologic cautions, since more than 20 percent of the initial subjects had to be excluded for questionable urinary sodium collections, and plasma renin activity determinations occurred only once for each patient.

Previous work by the same investigators has established an inverse relation between plasma-renin activity and sodium balance, measured by 24-hour urinary sodium excretion. Thus, individuals with high profiles generate augmented plasma-renin activity for their state of sodium balance. Replication of the findings has been confounded by the need for standardization of renin-sampling procedures and renin assay [49]. Pathophysiologically, the renin excess may be a marker for increased angiotensin, which in turn may stimulate vascular smooth-cell migration and growth [50].

Level of BP for Concern

Two dissimilar thresholds affect operationalizing hypertension definitions. The first deals with the **diagnosis of hypertension,** whether for epidemiologic studies, insurance risk classification, or casual warnings to individuals with mild elevations too insignificant to start active treatment. Most frequently, this threshold appears around 135–140/85–90 mm Hg. The other threshold relates to the **initiation of antihypertensive treatment** on the basis of BP level alone, usually in excess of 160/100 mm Hg [8]. Between those two threshold levels, a variety of other considerations govern therapeutic decisions, including the presence of one or more major cardiovascular risk factors (e.g., dyslipidemia or smoking); the existence of relevant comorbidity (e.g., diabetes mellitus or renal dysfunction), which increases the likelihood of subsequent target-organ damage; or the discovery of preexisting target-organ damage (e.g., LV hypertrophy, peripheral arterial insufficiency, or angina). Of these considerations, preexistence of target-organ damage carries the greatest degree of absolute risk for subsequent morbidity and mortality.

As described, the thresholds refer to therapeutic decisions for individuals. Some have argued that this approach alone will not prevent all the BP-related cardiovascular and renal disease in the community, since the BP-risk relationship is continuous, curvilinear, and progressive [16]. One alternative set of strategies focuses on larger groups, either in the general population or in high-risk subgroups. Targeted subgroups might include African-Americans, persons with borderline high BP, those with a positive family history for hypertension and atherosclerotic complications, and those with potentially dangerous lifestyle patterns. Overall, the benefits of screening asymptomatic adults for hypertension outweigh the risks and costs involved, especially for older adults and men more than women [51]. The cost effectiveness of screening is highly sensitive to the cost of therapy for mild hypertension and the efficacy of therapy to prevent premature deaths [52,53]. The costs of therapy include initial drug acquisition, supplemental drug acquisition, laboratory monitoring, clinic visits, and treatment of side effects [54].

RISKS VERSUS BENEFITS FROM TREATMENT

Epidemiologic data have long confirmed a continuum of risk for hypertension [55]. Since hypertension is a heterogeneous condition and BP level alone does not fully predict subsequent events, controversy has surrounded the optimal degree of BP lowering to maximize benefit and minimize risk. No one argues about the merits of treating severe or malignant hypertension. As the BP level falls, however, the likelihood of unambiguous benefit falls, and the number of individuals needed to treat to demonstrate clear benefit rises [56].

Some of the difficulty reflects problems in study design and analysis. Not all the primary prevention trials have paid sufficient attention to issues of using the instudy blood pressure rather than the beginning and ending BP levels. The studies have not always corrected for risk profile at entry, performed other than linear analysis, allowed sufficient follow-up time, provided consistent intensity of antihypertensive therapy, or supplied complete characterization of subgroups [57]. Even when methodologically pure, primary prevention trials may yield mixed results, especially with mild hypertension and when comparing different monotherapies among subgroups with dissimilar risk profiles [58].

In recent years, consistent support has emerged for antihypertensive drug therapy as producing net benefit, even among the elderly with isolated systolic hypertension [17,19,59] without compromising their quality of life [60]. The benefit is especially marked among those with higher pretreatment blood pressures [61] and those with multiple risk factors, rather than those with just hypertension [62].

J-CURVE PHENOMENON

In addition to these cautions, a number of investigators have reported a J-shaped relationship between decrease of cardiovascular events and degree of BP reduction [57,63,64]. A subgroup of individuals presenting with hypertension may be especially vulnerable to increased rates of cardiovascular events when more than modest BP reduction occurs. The most consistent data cluster on the dangers of marked falls in diastolic blood pressure associated with increased rates of coronary ischemia and MI. Less convincing data are available for stroke and for SBP [57]. The specific medications used for antihypertensive therapy are less critical than the magnitude of BP decline [65].

Implications for diagnosis include the importance of watching carefully for any evidence of ischemia, whether directly for the coronary circulation or indirectly such as from LV hypertrophy. Therapeutically, the desired goal for DBP should be no less than 80–85 mm Hg [66]. Since excessive lowering of the BP alone may be dangerous, clinicians should emphasize reducing all cardiovascular risk factors rather than just hypertension. Finally, the concomitant use of antiplatelet therapy may be beneficial to minimize thromboembolic complications.

MORBIDITY AND MORTALITY AMONG MILD HYPERTENSIVES

While persons with the highest blood pressures are at the greatest risk and may be the most satisfying to treat on an individual basis, they contribute only a small proportion to the overall impact from high blood pressure. In 1980, approximately 410,000 deaths occurred in American males and females of at least age 45 related to SBP elevations. The corresponding number of stroke deaths was 175,000. The majority of such cardiovascular complications occur among individuals who have only a slight increase in attributable risk. Because 70–75 percent of individuals with hypertension have only mild BP elevations, almost 60 percent of the cardiovascular complications from elevated SBP result from levels less than 160 mm Hg. Similar patterns emerge for DBP less than 90 mm Hg [67]. Fully 57 percent of all heart attacks and almost half of all strokes in the Framingham study occurred in persons with normal blood pressure [9]. As the population shifts to longer survival, the frequency and the distribution of cardiovascular disease related to BP will show a growing proportion of complications among those without major BP elevations.

On the flip side, BP elevations alone do not guarantee prompt, bad outcomes. During 15 years of follow-up in the Framingham study, less than one-third of those with SBP 195 mm Hg or higher as their only risk factor had a stroke or heart attack [62]. Interactions among cardiovascular risk factors exert critical influence. For example, only minor net benefit may come from treating nonsmoking women with sustained SBP 195 mm Hg and higher in contrast to dramatic reductions in cardiovascular morbidity and mortality for women with comparable BPs who smoke [63]. By Markov cohort modeling, the average remaining life expectancy of two patients of identical age and level of diastolic pressure may vary by 10–24 years, depending on the presence of other risk factors. In some hypertensive men, the benefits of smoking cessation were three to eight times greater than the expected benefits from antihypertensive therapy [70]. The key conclusion is that antihypertensive treatment strategy should be driven by analysis of overall risk benefit rather than by a mechanical focus on BP threshold alone [9].

VARIABILITY OF BP

Indirect versus Direct. Compared to direct assessment of BP by intra-arterial measurement, most indirect methods tend to underestimate SBP and overestimate DBP, presumably in part because of limitations in detecting bloodflow and auscultatory sounds through soft tissue. For obvious logistic and patient acceptance reasons, interarterial assessment usually is reserved for research settings or rare situations in which validation of BP is essential [71].

Office versus Basal. The optimal technique to determine BP remains controversial. The common standard has long been mercury sphygmomanometers applied to patients' arms, while generally in the sitting position, and via a single determination. An extensive literature confirms the relevance of several confounding influences [72].

The major pitfalls involve setting, equipment, examiner, and technique. The **setting** of the clinician's office, even when protected from distractions, interruptions, and irritations, often yields higher BP levels than when determinations occur in less stressed environments, such as home. On the one side, office recordings remain the basis for most epidemiologic correlations with subsequent cardiovascular morbidity and mortality. On the other side, office BP values correlate less well with target-organ damage rates than do basal rates obtained from home determinations or ambulatory monitoring: for eye [73], heart [74], arteries [75], and kidney [76]. Home or ambulatory monitoring provides the benefit of additional data, especially over a variety of physiologic conditions, compared to the relatively brief times spent in clinicians' offices [77]. Home determinations may reduce the need or frequency of physician visits with improved BP control and reduced costs [78]. Important cautions about using home BP determinations include thorough instruction in proper BP-taking technique and validation that the specific BP-measuring device is accurate [33]. Important deviations and miscalibrations may be frequent [33]. Finally, home determinations may serve to facilitate medication compliance by offering feedback about treatment effectiveness or by helping to involve reinforcing family members [79].

Equipment issues usually revolve around manometer calibration and the selection of the appropriate cuff size. All manometers, especially aneroid units, may lose accuracy over time. Periodic recalibration offers reassurance against some diagnostic errors. In one study of physicians' office practices, 8 percent of mercury sphygmomanometers were out of calibration by 4 or more mm Hg and 30 percent of aneroid sphygmomanometers deviated by 10 or more mm Hg [80]. In the same study, only 3 percent of the physicians used the appropriate cuff size on all patients. Several recent reviews point out trade-offs among available models [81–83].

Characteristics of the **examiner** may play an additional role. Artifactually higher BP readings may result when the examiner is male rather than female and the examiner was wearing a white coat rather than dressed in casual clothing [72].

Many problems arise as artifacts of the measurement **techniques** themselves. Perhaps the most critical factors are selection of optimal cuff size for the patient's arm [84], sufficient initial elevation of cuff pressure with confirmation by palpation to avoid auscultatory gaps [85], and proper preparation of the patient. The last factor includes avoiding full-bladder or -bowel conditions; uncomfortable ambient temperature, especially cold; and caffeine compounds, smoking, or physical exertion within 30 minutes of measurement [86]. Table 26-2 summarizes the fifth report of the Joint National Committee on Detection, Evaluation, and Treatment of High Blood Pressure (JNC V) classification of BP for adults [6].

Table 26-2. BP classification

Category[a]	Systolic (mm Hg)	Diastolic (mm Hg)
Normal	< 130	< 85
High normal	130–139	85–89
Hypertensive[b]		
Stage 1 (mild)	140–159	90–99
Stage 2 (moderate)	160–179	100–109
Stage 3 (severe)	180–209	110–119
Stage 4 (very severe)	≥ 210	≥ 120

[a]Adults age 18 and older, not taking antihypertensive drugs, and not acutely ill.
[b]Determined by the average of two or more measurements taken during two or more visits.
Source: Adapted from Joint National Committee on Detection, Evaluation, and Treatment of High Blood Pressure. The fifth report of the Joint National Committee on Detection, Evaluation, and Treatment of High Blood Pressure (JNC V). Arch Intern Med 1993; 153:154–183.

Home BP Monitoring. The inherent variability in BP confounds simple diagnosis and predisposes to both under- and overdiagnosis. An obvious alternative to high-technology solutions is to have patients measure their own BPs over a variety of conditions in the midst of usual activities. Efforts at self-measurement may be limited by inaccuracy of available equipment and the need for training [72]. While mercury manometers are the most accurate and unlikely to have faulty calibration, they are relatively expensive and inconvenient to transport. Electrical devices may be less accurate and more difficult to calibrate, but they are generally easier to use than manual aneroid models.

Home monitoring carries the advantages of simple instructions, relatively low cost, and possible improvement in subsequent compliance with treatment. Unfortunately, concomitant disadvantages include possible inaccuracies of measurement, need for regular calibration of equipment, times of BP measurement selected by the patient, small likelihood of recording short-lived events, patient inconvenience, and adequate patient levels of hearing, visiion, and dexterity [87].

Ambulatory BP Monitoring. In contrast, ambulatory BP monitoring (ABPM) may readily produce multiple BP measurements at specified, frequent intervals, both at home and in work settings, as well as during sleep. Such measurements permit evaluation of circadian rhythm, short-lived events, and BP changes that may not be signaled by symptoms. Equipment failure, equipment misapplication, disturbance of patient's work or sleep, local reactions to the cuff, limited normative data, and cost all limit the usefulness of the technology [88].

The typical, fully automated device for ABPM is battery driven. It consists of an arm cuff inflated by air compressor or gas cylinder. The two most common techniques for ABPM involve auscultatory or oscillometric methods. The **auscultatory technique** employs a modified microphone to detect Korotkoff sounds with internal signal checking, error assessment, and sometimes R-wave gating on the electrocardiographic signal to screen out ambient noise. The method requires great care in placing the microphone to optimize signals and to minimize artifact. The **oscillometric method** detects SBP and mean BP and uses algorithms to calculate DBP, a procedure that may not be appropriate for all subjects. Vibrations and muscle artifacts may generate distortions by the oscillometric technique.

None of the devices is accurate when cardiac rate is irregular. Careful calibration on device application is essential. The ideal time to perform ABPM is a typical day, reflecting the full array of events and stressors. The concomitant use of a patient diary for activities, positions, medications, emotions, and other potential influences maximizes the yield of the recording.

Table 26-3. Indications for ambulatory BP monitoring

Borderline hypertension
Labile or episodic hypertension
Possible disparity between office and other BP readings
Rule out "white-coat hypertension"
Target-organ damage despite normal office BP
Monitoring of antihypertensive drug efficacy
Duration of effect
Dosage ranging
Resistant or refractory hypertension
Other research purposes

Source: Adapted from Zachariah PK, Sheps SG, Smith RL. Clinical use of home and ambulatory blood pressure monitoring. Mayo Clin Proc 1989; 64(11):1436–1446.

Table 26-4. Initial history of hypertensive patient

SOCIODEMOGRAPHICS. Age, sex, race, occupation, education, psychosocial constraints

HYPERTENSION HISTORY. Duration, monitoring intervals, past evaluations, response to past therapy, recent weight changes

SYMPTOMS OF HYPERTENSION COMPLICATIONS. Transient ischemic attack, cerebrovascular attack (CVA), angina, congestive heart failure, peripheral vascular disease, claudication

SYMPTOMS OF SECONDARY HYPERTENSION. Episodic headaches, palpitations, sweating, weight loss (pheochromocytoma), muscular weakness, cramps, paresthesia, and polyuria (primary hyperaldosteronism), weight gain, acne, bruising, hirsuitism (Cushing's syndrome), and lower-extremity claudication (coarctation of aorta)

CARDIOVASCULAR RISK FACTORS. Dyslipidemia, diabetes mellitus, smoking, high salt intake, saturated fat intake, stress, low activity level, alcohol use, gout; family history of hypertension, coronary artery disease (especially if < age 60), CVA, diabetes mellitus dyslipidemia

COMPLICATING COMORBIDITY. Renal or hepatic dysfunction, chronic obstructive pulmonary disease or asthma, obesity, gout

MEDICATIONS. All, including pressors (amphetamines, cocaine, appetite suppressants, diet and cold capsules, nasal sprays), fluid retainers (birth control pill, adrenal steroids, nonsteroidal anti-inflammatory drugs), and other (cyclosporine, monoamine oxidase inhibitors, erythropoietin, licorice, thyroid hormones)

Most individuals interpreting the ABPM data examine the record for BP patterns, mean values and variation, and correlation with potentially explanatory factors. No consensus currently exists about the optimal analysis for ABPM data, although the concept of BP load has gained special prominence. **BP load** refers to the percentage of readings during which the systolic or diastolic pressure exceeds predefined limits, such as 140/90 mm Hg while awake and 120/80 mm Hg during sleep. In one study, when the BP load exceeded 40 percent, the probability of increased LV mass index or decreased LV filling rate was 61 percent versus only 17 percent when the load was less than 40 percent [89]. Alternative strategies include interpretations based on Fourier analysis and smoothing techniques in search of chronobiologic patterns. Under those conditions, BPs tend to be highest at work, lower at home, and lowest during sleep in most individuals [90].

There remains considerable controversy about the optimal place of the technology [72,88,91]. Possible indications for noninvasive ABPM are listed in Table 26-3. Several investigators have confirmed the existence of **white-coat hypertension,** a syndrome in which BP in medical settings remains substantially higher than those in other settings [92–94]. Most clinical use of ABPM appears consistent with national guidelines and yields modest changes in diagnosis, evaluation, and therapy [95]. The overall cost effectiveness of ABPM would be warranted for selected subgroups, such as low-risk patients with borderline hypertension seeking to avoid drug therapy [72].

EVALUATION OF THE HYPERTENSIVE PATIENT

General Assessment

The goals of the general assessment consist of (1) confirming the diagnosis, (2) considering the possibility of secondary hypertension, (3) evaluating evidence for target-organ damage, and (4) seeking clues for optimal future management. Each component rests on a foundation of a thoughtful history and physical examination as well as selective use of laboratory, radiologic, and other tests.

Establishing the diagnosis of hypertension draws data from both the history and the physical examination. The principal components are outlined in Table 26-4. Of special importance in the history is the presence or absence and the degree of other cardiovascular risk factors as well as the duration and the extent of BP elevations. Commonly, hypertension may present in a transient or borderline fashion, only to become more sustained in later years. The age of onset and the clinical context, such as pregnancy, may be important considerations. The assessment is complicated by two distinct kinds of vascular problems from hypertension: (1) hypertensive complications of small arteries and arterioles (lacunar infarction, intracerebral hemorrhage, nephrosclerosis, and medial dissection of the aorta) and (2) atherosclerotic disease of the large and medium-sized arteries (thromboembolic stroke, coronary insufficiency, intermittent claudication, aortic aneurysm, and renal-artery stenosis).

Physical Examination

The principal components of the focused physical examination are summarized in Table 26-5. Most critical are attention to optimal techniques of BP determination, including proper sized cuff, preparation of the patient, and multiple determinations [96]. During the initial visit, the examiner should obtain BP in both the supine and upright positions and compare blood pressures in the two arms, noting discrepancies of 10 mm Hg or more and taking future BP determinations in the higher arm. The cuff bladder should encircle at least 80 percent of the arm circumference and its width should be 15 cm or more in the average adult. A cuff that is too narrow can falsely elevate

Table 26-5. Initial physical examination of hypertensive patient

Vital signs, including two or more BP determinations (averaged) both supine or sitting and standing, separated by at least 2 minutes; notation and selection of "higher" arm if asymmetrical BPs; ankle-brachial index or arm and leg BP
Weight, height, calculation of body-mass index (weight in kg/[height in meters]^2)
Fundoscopic exam for retinopathy
Neck exam for carotid artery, jugular venous distention, thyromegaly
Cardiac and chest exam for heart size, murmurs, gallops, arrhythmias, rales
Abdominal exam for masses, bruits, abnormal aortic pulsations
Extremity exam for peripheral vascular pulses, bruits, edema
Neurologic exam
Check for stigmata of gout, dyslipidemia, thyroid dysfunction, Cushing's syndrome, neurofibromatosis

the readings [97]. Rolled sleeves constricting the arm may distort BP values, but thinly sleeved arms display no significant effect [97]. To avoid underestimating SBP in an auscultatory gap, the examiner should palpate the radial or brachial pulse during inflation and begin auscultation only after the pulse disappears. The systolic pressure is the point at which the Korotkoff sounds first become audible with each heart beat. Most commonly, diastolic pressure is recorded when heart sounds disappear, except in unusual circumstances in which disappearance (phase V) extends close to zero. In such circumstances, using phase IV (muffling) will reasonably approximate DBP. When obtaining two or more BP determinations, the second reading is almost always lower than the first, sometimes by 5–10 mm Hg. Little subsequent change in BP is generally obtained after the second determination [98]. Table 26-6 lists potential errors in BP measurement.

The remainder of the physical examination should search for target-organ damage and evidence of atherosclerotic disease, concentrating on evidence for cardiomegaly, vascular insufficiency, and bruits as well as possible stigmata of secondary hypertension or comorbidities, such as hepatic or renal dysfunction, which complicate therapy.

Baseline Tests

The selection of additional tests should properly reflect the need for baseline assessments, likely cardiovascular risk factors, and sometimes consideration of secondary hypertension. Current status and changes in renal function may be particularly important, since they affect selection of drug therapy and may worsen despite good BP control [99]. Routine chest radiographs and electrocardiograms have only limited usefulness in the workup of most hypertensives and are therefore not essential [100]. Recommended tests for routine evaluation of all hypertensive patients are listed in Table 26-7.

Table 26-6. Potential errors in BP measurement

EQUIPMENT
Inaccurate or uncalibrated manometer
Improper sphygomamanometer bladder size
PATIENT PREPARATION
Not resting for ≥5 minutes in quiet, comfortable environment
Drinking caffeine-containing beverage or smoking within 30 minutes
OBSERVER TECHNIQUE
Not supporting arm or torso to decrease muscle artifact
Not keeping arm position at heart level
Not centering cuff bladder on brachial artery
Not estimating SBP by palpating radial pulse before auscultation
Not keeping eyes at level of mercury manometer
Not consistently using Korotkoff phase IV or phase V sounds for DBP
Inflating bladder too slowly or deflating it too fast
Not measuring in both arms at first to establish symmetry
Not completely deflating cuff and waiting 1–2 minutes before remeasurement
GENERAL CAVEATS
Misinterpreting any auscultatory gap
Not integrating distortion from any cardiac arrhythmias
Ignoring observer bias, digit preference

Table 26-7. Initial tests for hypertensive patient

	Purpose	Specific tests
Initial	Establish baseline levels; search for cardiovascular risk factors	Serum potassium, creatinine, blood glucose (preferably fasting), total and HDL cholesterol, urinalysis
Desirable but not essential	Establish baseline levels; search for cardiovascular risk factors	Complete blood count, uric acid, triglycerides, electrocardiogram
Sometimes useful	Establish baseline levels; search for cardiovascular risk factors	Plasma renin–urinary sodium ratio, echocardiogram, home or ambulatory blood pressure monitoring

Evaluation for Secondary Forms of Hypertension

PREVALENCE

Additional tests, especially those for possible secondary hypertension, generally offer limited yield because curable secondary hypertension is rare, especially in unselected, primary care settings. Most important, there is little justification for aggressive evaluation of every hypertensive patient at the first visit in the absence of important

Table 26-8. Prevalence of primary and secondary hypertension

Type of patients	Referred series			Unselected series				
Reference number	[101]	[102]	[103]	[104]	[105]	[106]	[107]	[108]
Author(s)	Gifford	Ferguson	Bech and Hilden	Iimura (Men only)	Berglund et al. (Men only, age 47–54)	Rudnick et al.	Greminger et al.	Lewin et al.
Country	USA	USA	Denmark	Japan	Sweden	Canada	Switzerland	USA
Study year	1969	1975	1975	1973	1976	1977	1977	1985
Number of patients	4,392	246	482	448	689	665	854	5,485
Diagnoses (percent)								
Primary hypertension	88.9	89.4	79.4	87.3	94.3	94.3	92.9	97.2
Renal parenchymal disease	5.2	2.4	12.9	5.7	4.5	4.7	5.0	2.6
Renovascular hypertension	4.4	2.9	5.0	—	0.6	0.2	0.8	0.1
Operated	1.0	1.6	1.0	—	0.3	0.2	—	—
Cured	NA	NA	NA	—	—	—	—	—
Coarctation of aorta	0.6	—	—	—	0.1	0.2	0.6	—
Primary aldosteronism	0.4	0.8	0.4	0.9	0.1	—	0.2	0.1
Cushing syndrome	0.3	—	—	—	—	0.2	—	—
Pheochromocytoma	0.2	—	0.2	0.2	—	—	—	—
Primary hyperparathyroidism	—	—	—	—	0.3	—	—	—
Oral contraceptive induced	—	4.5	1.5	—	—	0.2	0.5	0.1
Other or unspecified	—	—	—	5.9	0.1	0.2	—	—

NA = Not available.

clues, and the diagnostic process may resume if patients later exhibit new clues or refractoriness to treatment. Table 26-8 summarizes the prevalence distribution of primary versus secondary hypertension among referred and unselected populations. There is remarkable uniformity among unselected series: primary hypertension is the ultimate etiology in 93–94 percent of cases, renal parenchymal disease is an additional 5–6 percent (rarely reversible), and all other causes of presumably reversible secondary hypertension account for 1–2 percent of the total. The full differential for secondary hypertension appears in Table 26-9. Several important clues from history, physical examination, or baseline testing may indicate a higher than usual likelihood of secondary hypertension. Those clues are summarized in Table 26-10.

RENAL PARENCHYMAL DISEASE

Renal parenchymal disease constitutes the single largest cause of secondary hypertension, although most of the conditions may not be reversible.

Presentation. A large array of different clinical situations may converge with hypertension in the presence of renal parenchymal disease. **Acute renal failure** may result from acute glomerulonephritis (especially postinfectious crescentic or focal segmental changes), vasculitis (especially systemic lupus erythematosus, scleroderma, or polyarteri-

Table 26-9. Differential diagnosis of secondary hypertension

RENAL PARENCHYMAL DISEASE
Anephric: volume dependency
Chronic dialysis: volume dependency; autonomic dysfunction
Posttransplantation
Chronic renal failure
Acute renal failure
Other
VASCULAR HYPERTENSION
Renovascular
Coarctation of the aorta
ENDOCRINOLOGIC HYPERTENSION
Glucocorticoid excess
Mineralocorticoid excess
Catecholamine-secreting tumors
Hyperthyroidism
Hyperparathyroidism
PHARMACOLOGIC HYPERTENSION
Vasoconstrictors
Volume expanders
Cyclosporine

Table 26-10. Secondary hypertension: an overview

	Clues from		
Condition	History	Physical	Early lab
RENAL PARENCHYMAL DISEASE	Renal disease, urinary-tract infections, diabetes mellitus, chronic analgesics	Flank or abdominal mass	Active urinary sediment, elevated creatinine, glycosuria, proteinuria, anemia
RENOVASCULAR HYPERTENSION	Age < 30, especially female; age > 60, especially male; new onset, rapid course; cardiovascular risk factors; family history of vascular anomalies	Flank bruit; peripheral vascular insufficiency	Proteinuria
COARCTATION OF THE AORTA		Asymmetrical pulses and BP, pulse delay arm-leg, systolic murmur or bruit	Ankle-brachial index; chest radiograph $\pm$ notching of ribs
CUSHING'S SYNDROME	Weight gain, acne, fluid retention, bruising	Abdominal mass; moon facies; truncal obsesity; striae, plethora, hirsuitism, weakness	Hyperglycemia
PRIMARY HYPERALDOSTERONISM	Weakness, paresthesia, polyuria, tetany		Hypokalemia, especially after potassium-wasting diuretics; [diagnosis excluded by potassium ≥ 4 mEq/l]
PHEOCHROMOCYTOMA	Paroxysmal hypertension; palpitations, headache, sweating, fainting, weight loss; procedure leading to attacks; family history of multiple endocrine neoplasm or neurofibromata	Orthostasis, tremor, perspiration; cardiomyopathy	Hyperglycemia; posterior mediastinal mass on chest radiography
HYPERTHYROIDISM	Nervousness, palpitations, dysphagia, weight loss	Tremor, goiter, wide pulse pressure, bruit, exophthalmos	
DRUG RESPONSE	Vasoconstrictors, fluid retainers, nephrotoxins		

*Bracketed words describe one example of a more comprehensive list.

tis), or acute obstruction. When the renal dysfunction is more insidious, **chronic renal failure** occurs, usually associated with loss of 80 percent or more of the nephrons. The most common causes are vasculitis, glomerular disease (especially diabetic nephropathy, crescentic and focal segmental glomerulitis) and polycystic renal disease [109]. Most of these patients have a volume-dependent form of hypertension, indicative of chronic glomerulonephritis and usually relatively easy to control. A less common subset of patients have nephrosclerosis, dependent on renin rather than volume and often more difficult to control. Most of the patients requiring **chronic dialysis** display both a volume dependency and variable degrees of autonomic dysfunction, while those with no functional kidneys, or **postbilateral nephrectomy,** usually are volume dependent.

Other, less common causes of hypertension associated with chronic renal disease include pyelonephritis, membranous and membranoproliferative glomerulonephritis, immunoglobulin A (IgA) nephropathy, renin-secreting tumors, or drug-induced renal dysfunction, such as that following phenacetin-containing analgesics [110]. Once **renal transplantation** has occurred, the hypertension may result from continuation of prior hypertension, excess renin from the native kidney, posttransplant renal-artery stenosis, immunosuppressive therapy (both corticosteroids and cyclosporine), chronic rejection, recurrent intrinsic renal disease, or volume overload.

Diagnosis and Management. Although the above conditions may present in a variety of ways, screening tests usually reveal azotemia, microalbuminuria or proteinuria, or abnormal urinary sediment. The most important management decisions usually revolve around the desirability and timing of dialysis or transplantation as well as the optimal management of the volume component of the hypertension. The volume component usually responds to diuretics or to dialysis, while the renin component may require beta blockers, angiotensin converting enzyme (ACE) inhibitors, or minoxidil. Several standard antihypertensive agents may need dose adjustments in chronic renal failure [110].

VASCULAR HYPERTENSION

Hypertension may result from physiologically significant stenosis of the renal arteries, the aorta, and a variety of other vascular structures.

Table 26-10 (continued)

Diagnostic tests			
Screening	Definitive	Comments	Therapy
24-hour urinary protein, creatinine clearance	Renal biopsy	False reassurance with "normal" serum creatinine in the elderly	Treat underlying condition; r/o transplant stenosis, immunosuppressive therapy, rejection, volume overload
Captopril renal scan, [MRI]*	Renal arteriography	Split-vein renins no longer required for diagnosis	Renal angioplasty, renal artery reconstruction
Echocardiogram	Aortography		Surgical repair
Overnight dexamethasone suppression test (1 mg) 24-hour urinary free cortisol	4–8 mg dexamethasone suppression test; CT or MRI scan CRH stimulation test		Surgical excision vs. drug suppression
24-hour urinary aldosterone; orthostatic test; stimulated plasma-renin activity	Abdominal CT or MRI; adrenal-vein sampling; response to glucocorticoids		Excision for adenoma after spironolactone trial; anti-aldosterone drugs for hyperplasia; [glucocorticoids]
Spot urinary metanephrine 24-hour urinary metanephrine, total catecholamines, VMA; clonidine-suppression test	CT or MRI scan; 131I-MIBG scan meta-iodobenzylguanidine [radiocholesterol scan]	Provocative tests no longer recommended; tumor palpation in operating room	Excision after pretreatment with alpha blockers, fluid; [phenoxybenzamine, labetalol]
Free thyroxine; thyroid-stimulating hormone	Thyroid uptake/scan; antithyroid antibodies		131-I vs. surgery vs. antithyroid meds

Renovascular

PATHOPHYSIOLOGY. Compromise of arterial flow to either or both kidneys may produce hypertension from activation of the renin-angiotensin-aldosterone system. Depending on the status and the participation of the contralateral kidney, the ischemic stimulus may elevate renin, promote fluid retention, or both.

CLINICAL SUBGROUPS. Two clinical subgroups comprise the majority of patients with the conditions of renovascular hypertension: fibromuscular dysplasia and atherosclerotic disease. **Fibromuscular dysplasia** of the renal arteries accounts for about 25 percent of all renovascular hypertension and occurs almost exclusively in younger patients, especially females. Although five pathologic subtypes are described, 70 percent of affected individuals display medial fibroplasia, and an additional 20 percent show perimedial fibroplasia. Both these subtypes exhibit classical beaded appearance on angiography [111]. Although the precise pathogenesis is uncertain, the natural history usually consists of slow progression of stenosis without frank occlusion.

Atherosclerotic disease, which makes up nearly 70 percent of the total, usually involves the proximal third of the renal artery with or without encroachment of the ostium itself. Lesions generally arise bilaterally, although one or the other side may predominate. Renal artery stenosis sometimes precedes and sometimes follows stenoses in other critical circulations. In fact, atherosclerotic disease may extend for years without signaling its presence with hypertension or even elevated serum creatinine. Left untreated, most lesions progress, including complete occlusion and renal failure [112]. If stenosis exceeds 75 percent, the probability of progression to full occlusion approaches 40 percent over 1 year [113]. Some estimate that 5–15 percent of individuals entering dialysis programs have previously undetected renovascular hypertension [112].

Other, less common causes of renovascular hypertension include Takayasu's arteritis, polyarteritis nodosa, aneurysms, radiation fibrosis, thromboemboli (including cholesterol emboli), and extrinsic compression of the renal arteries by tumor.

PRESENTATION. Given the most common clinical clusters, two scenarios are most likely to herald renovascular hypertension: (1) recent-onset hypertension in a young white woman with no family history of hypertension or (2) late onset or exacerbation of hypertension in an older man with strong evidence of coronary, cerebrovascular, or peripheral vascular insufficiency. Although abdominal bruits modestly increase the odds of significant stenosis, the presence or absence of bruits holds limited predictive value. Other potential clues include marked hypertensive retinopathy, worsening of renal function after ACE-inhibitor therapy, progressive worsening of azotemia despite adequate BP control, history of unilateral small kidney from incidental studies, history of smoking, and history of pulmonary edema [114].

DIAGNOSIS. Clues from the history and the physical examination alert the clinician to renovascular hypertension as a possibility. Baseline testing may demonstrate mild azotemia, proteinuria, or hypokalemia in fewer than 20 percent of individuals with the condition, modestly higher rates than among others with essential hypertension. No perfect screening test exists. Proponents exist for elevated peripheral plasma-renin activity with or without captopril stimulation [115], renal scans, renal digital subtraction angiography [116], intravenous pyelography, and prompt progression to arteriography [117]. Such arteriography remains the gold standard, although it is an invasive test. In recent years, the marginal utility of obtaining renal-vein renins to confirm unilateral versus bilateral disease has been questioned, given poor positive and negative predictive value [118]. One interesting alternative to direct angiography is the use of captopril scintigraphy, which combines radionuclide scanning of the kidney (especially with mercaptoacetyltriglycine) with captopril stimulation to enhance differences in renal blood flow [119]. In that context, the ACE inhibitor produces a fall in glomerular filtration rate more than a reduction in renal blood flow on the affected side. A positive scan correlates with successful angioplasty or surgical intervention in 90 percent or more of cases but may be less definitive in the presence of renal dysfunction [120]. Both doppler ultrasound and magnetic resonance technologies offer promising results but are not yet cost-effective alternatives [121].

MANAGEMENT. Extreme surgical maneuvers like nephrectomy rarely are necessary these days. Preserving renal function preferentially involves endarterectomy, aortorenal bypass with saphenous vein or hypogastric artery, or partial nephrectomy when multiple distal stenoses occur. While BP reductions occur in 50–60 percent of all patients undergoing such procedures, the rates of improvement are superior among those with fibromuscular dysplasia compared with those with atherosclerosis [122]. The latter carry a worse prognosis because of progression of the arteriosclerotic process. Similar differential improvements occur for angioplasty along with the advantage that the procedure may take place at the same time as diagnostic angiography [123].

The trade-offs for medical management are especially acute for atherosclerotic disease. Progression of the arteriosclerosis with occlusion and renal failure may occur even with adequate BP control. There have been no randomized, controlled trials directly comparing the two treatment strategies [112]. Useful drug classes have included ACE inhibitors (with cautions about hypotension, dose adjustment with renal dysfunction, and actual deterioration in renal function), beta blockers, and dihydropyridine calcium channel blockers.

AORTIC COARCTATION. A variety of congenital and acquired malformations of the aorta may produce hypertension. Although the majority present during childhood, an important minority may pass into adulthood before definitive diagnosis. The variations include a left, right, or double aortic arch, which produces tracheal, bronchial, and esophageal compression. The variations can be recognized on chest radiographs or esophagrams and confirmed by ultrasound, angiography, CT scan, or MRI. Other congenital lesions of the aortic arch are characterized by aortic obstruction and include supravalvular aortic stenosis, aortic-arch interruption or atresia, and coarctation [124].

Angioplasty and surgery remain the treatments of choice, although complications of the procedures include functional impairment, aneurysmal formation, and restenosis [125]. Useful, noninvasive ways to confirm the diagnosis and monitor for complications include Doppler ultrasound with exercise for arm-leg differences [126], transesophageal echocardiography [127], and MRI [125].

ENDOCRINOLOGIC HYPERTENSION

Cushing's Syndrome. Spontaneous Cushing's syndrome may be classified as (1) **corticotropin dependent** (Cushing's disease, ectopic corticotropin syndrome, and very rare ectopic corticotropin-releasing hormone syndrome) and (2) **corticotropin independent** (unilateral cortisol-producing adenomas and carcinomas). Rarely, bilateral adrenal hyperplasia, especially with functioning nodules, may yield the same clinical constellation of hypercortisolism, including hypertension. Even these distinctions have become blurred as the spectrum of ectopic adrenocorticotropic hormone (ACTH) hypersecretion has filled in and expanded [128]. Fully 70–90 percent of patients with ACTH-dependent hypercortisolism have a pituitary tumor, but sophisticated special testing and endocrinologic consultation still may be necessary once the syndrome has been confirmed.

In most patients, the physical stigmata are striking: truncal obesity, moon facies, buffalo hump, striae, and ecchymoses are coupled with osteoporosis, hyperglycemia, and hypertension. Up to 70 percent of individuals with the syndrome display hypertension, regardless of the subtype and independent of salt intake. Increased pressor responsiveness has been reported, probably due to local postsynaptic effector mechanisms in the resistance vessels, and circadian BP variations have been decreased, absent, or even reversed [129]. Initial screening for the diagnosis is best performed by a 1-mg overnight dexamethasone-suppression test and/or a 24-hour urinary free cortisol 2-mg dexamethasone-suppression test. Further distinctions require repeated plasma ACTH measurements by radioimmune assay along with the 8-mg dexamethasone suppression test [130] or a corticotropin releasing hormone (CRH) stimulation test with inferior petrosal sinus sampling [131]. Further localization may require CT, MRI, or ^{131}I-6 beta-iodomethyl-19-norcholesterol (NP-59) scanning, a marker of adrenocortical cholesterol uptake, accurately localizing adrenal cortex dysfunction [132].

The majority of individuals with Cushing's disease undergo transsphenoidal exploration, with remission rates of about 80 percent, especially for noninvasive, relatively small tumors [133]. Postoperative courses, particularly for those undergoing adrenalectomy, may be stormy, in part because of cardiac complications associated with LV hypertrophy [134]. Recently described medical options include metyrapone, bromocriptine, and ketoconazole [135].

Primary Aldosteronism

CLINICAL SUBGROUPS. While Cushing's syndrome reflects glucocorticoid excess, a variety of other conditions exhibit mineralocorticoid excess, including primary hyperaldosteronism (adenoma, carcinoma, or bilateral hyperplasia), enzymatic deficiencies (11-OH-hydroxylase deficiency, 17-OH-hydroxylase deficiency, and 11-OH-dehydrogenase deficiency syndromes), or chronic licorice ingestion. Although all these conditions are relatively rare, the most common (60–90% of the total) is benign, unilateral adenoma of the adrenal (aldosterone-producing adenoma, or APA), secreting inappropriately large and autonomous secretion of aldosterone with predictable metabolic and pathophysiologic consequences. Less common variants include idiopathic hyperaldosteronism (IHA) (bilateral hyperplasia), nodular adrenocortical hyperplasia, aldosterone-producing renin-responsive adenoma, and glucocorticoid-suppressible hyperaldosteronism [136].

PATHOPHYSIOLOGY. The autonomous secretion of aldosterone occurs in distinction to the usual diurnal variation in plasma aldosterone, linked to plasma cortisol concentrations in normal subjects. Nonhormonal factors like increased serum potassium or decreased serum sodium can stimulate aldosterone synthesis directly. Once secreted, aldosterone increases distal tubular sodium resorption and potassium secretion, increases intravascular volume, and suppresses renin secretion. When secreted in excess, aldosterone produces a volume-dependent hypertension, although there is physiologic escape from incessant sodium retention before frank edema develops.

PRESENTATION. Patients with primary hyperaldosteronism have no distinguishing symptoms from others with hypertension, although they may display nonspecific weakness, fatigue, polyuria, or cramps, presumably reflecting hypokalemia. APA is more common in women than in men, generally presenting in the third to sixth decade [137]. Most commonly, an excessive loss of potassium or refractoriness to treatment may prompt further investigation. Hypokalemia may reach panic values ($\leq$ 2.8 mEq/liter), especially after diuretic therapy, but may be in the low normal range ($\leq$ 4.0 mEq/liter) without provocation or after salt restriction in up to 38 percent of patients [138].

DIAGNOSIS. The diagnostic process for primary hyperaldosteronism consists of three components: confirmation of inappropriately high aldosterone secretion, distinction between excisable tumor and nonsurgical glandular hyperplasia, and exclusion of rare variants suitable for medical therapy other than aldosterone antagonists. Because of many other causes of hypokalemia and low-renin hypertension, the single best screening test for the condition is a 24-hour urinary collection for aldosterone [139]. The collection should occur after withdrawal of all diuretics and ACE inhibitors for 2 weeks or more and all aldosterone antagonists for 6 weeks or more and repletion of fluid status, sodium, and potassium to normal levels, if necessary with 3–5 days of salt loading to ensure 24-hour urinary sodium of 200 or more mEq/liter [137]. These steps are essential to avoid stimulation of aldosterone secretion by hyperkalemia or its inhibition by hypokalemia. Noninterfering antihypertensive drugs include $alpha_1$ blockers and ganglionic antagonists like guanadrel. Alternatively, a logistically simpler screening test may be the plasma aldosterone (PA) to plasma-renin activity (PRA) ratio, if patients can be withdrawn safely from antihypertensive medications for 2 or more weeks. A PA-PRA ratio greater than 30 and a PA greater than 20 ng/ml may yield a sensitivity of 90 percent, a specificity of 91 percent, a positive predictive value of 69 percent, and a negative predictive value of 98 percent. Some investigators have reported both consistent differentiation from essential hypertension and separation between APA and IHA, the two most common forms of primary hyperaldosteronism [140].

Once the triad of hypertension, high aldosterone, and low renin has been confirmed, the clinician can shift attention to detecting adenomata for which surgical excision is the treatment of choice and curative in 70 percent of cases [137]. The hypertension, hypokalemia, and hyperaldosteronism are generally higher in APA than in IHA, but the distinctions usually are too small to be clinically useful. Imaging studies like CT scans can detect adenomata of 0.7 cm or greater, but up to 8 percent of the normal population may have nonfunctioning, incidental adrenal adenomata, and MRI scanning offers no clear advantage. Dexamethasone and Lugol's solution pretreatment and NP-59 scanning may highlight a functioning mass while suppressing surrounding adrenal tissue and protecting the thyroid. Unfortunately, scanning must proceed over 2–5 days and carries only a 72-percent accuracy, which is highly dependent on the tumor's size [137].

Indirect confirmation of the pathophysiologic significance of such masses may come from orthostatic tests or selective venous sampling. Orthostatic tests for APA versus IHA are based on two complementary features: (1) APA usually displays autonomous aldosterone secretion, unaffected by physiologic stimuli, such as standing, but exquisitely sensitive to the diurnal variation in cortisol secretion; and (2) IHA exhibits no particular diurnal variation but is markedly responsive to renin-based stimuli like standing. Most critically, the change in plasma aldosterone from 8 a.m. to noon after overnight recumbency must be interpreted in the context of the concomitant changes in PRA and plasma cortisol. An increase in plasma cortisol during the procedure invalidates the test. Some investigators have reported both sensitivities of 85 percent with the criterion of less than 30 percent orthostatic increase in plasma aldosterone and an important subset of renin-responsive aldosterone producing adenoma [141].

Venous sampling of the adrenals may be justified despite the expense and risks if the CT scan is normal despite unsuppressible plasma aldosterone. Worrisome complications of the procedure include adrenal infarction. Technically difficult, the catheterization may fail to cannulate the right adrenal vein in up to 25 percent of cases, but, if successful, it permits direct measurement of aldosterone-cortisol ratios with lateralization ratios greater than 10 : 1. Concomitant infusion of ACTH or cosyntropin minimizes stress-related changes in plasma aldosterone.

MANAGEMENT. For the common subset of patients with APA, unilateral total adrenalectomy is the treatment of choice, if the patient is an acceptable surgical candidate. Preoperative management with high-dose spironolactone (200–600 mg / day in divided doses) for 2–6 weeks offers a good prediction of the surgical result with correction of hypertension and hypokalemia [142]. Despite careful workups and uncomplicated perioperative courses, long-term cure rates average less than 70 percent, even though most patients display improved BP control with simplified regimens. The BP may require 3–6 months postoperatively to fall to normal values [137].

For the remaining patients, no cure is available. Treatment usually consists of a low-sodium diet (≤ 80 mEq/ day), maintenance of near-optimal body weight, and aldosterone-antagonist therapy. Spironolactone is the drug of first choice as 200–600 mg / day in divided doses. Correction of hypokalemia occurs within days, while normalization of BP may require 1–2 months. Common side effects include painful gynecomastia, impotence, decreased libido, menstrual irregularities, and gastrointestinal discomfort. Alternative therapies include amiloride (10–40 mg / day), dihydropyridines (e.g., nifedipine 30–180 mg / day), and ACE inhibitors. In patients with the rare syndrome of glucocorticoid-suppressible aldosteronism, spironolactone therapy may be as effective and better tolerated than dexamethasone 2 mg daily [137].

Pheochromocytoma

CLINICAL SUBGROUPS. Pheochromocytomas and other catecholamine-secreting tumors (paragangliomas when arising outside the adrenal) may prompt some of the most dramatic moments in hypertension. The clinical spectrum is wide, ranging from previously unsuspected tumors that first gain recognition from hypertensive crisis after a procedure like anesthesia to incidentally discovered, slow-growing, metabolically almost inactive masses. On rare occasions, patients may present with fever, encephalopathy, and multiple-organ-system failure. Nearly 80 percent of the tumors are limited to the adrenal glands, usually unilaterally, although more likely to be bilateral or multiple in pediatric presentations or in familial forms such as neurofibromatosis, von Hippel-Lindau disease, and multiple endocrine neoplasia type 2a or 2b. An additional 10–20 percent arise in other intra-abdominal sites, fewer than 5 percent from intrathoracic sites along the neurosecretory crest or bladder, and a small number from intracranial sites. Up to 20 percent of tumors will be multiple. Fewer than 10 percent of all catecholamine-secreting tumors are malignant, although their presentation may be difficult to distinguish from their more benign equivalents. Prompt diagnosis and definitive treatment are essential to avoid cardiomyopathy, congestive failure, or other potentially lethal outcomes [143].

PATHOPHYSIOLOGY AND PRESENTATION. Disease manifestations reflect the direct and indirect effects of catecholamines, either hypersecreted at random intervals for variable durations or tonically released. The classic triad of episodic headache, palpitations with or without tachycardia, and inappropriate perspiration accompanying the hypertension may suggest the condition, but the full textbook description occurs less than half the time. Other findings that may indicate pheochromocytoma include nervousness and anxiety, tremor, nausea, abdominal or chest pain, orthostatic drops in BP, glucose intolerance, weight loss, pallor, and fatigue [143]. Usually the most spectacular symptoms accompany the most dramatic BP elevations. Although less likely without one or more of the classic symptoms, the diagnosis of pheochromocytoma should be considered in those unresponsive to appropriate triple-drug therapy, those with paroxysmal hypertension associated with clinical procedures, or those with hypertension developing after phenothiazine, tyramine, or tricyclic antidepressant therapy. Pregnancy may unmask the disease, as the growing uterus applies pressure on the adrenal, or following micturition for rare presentations of bladder wall–based tumors. Tumors that are metabolically nearly silent may grow to large size before detection, while metabolically active lesions generate enough symptoms to remain small when first discovered.

DIAGNOSIS. Under most circumstances, the diagnosis of catecholamine-secreting tumor receives first confirmation by elevated urinary levels of one or more of the vasoactive hormones. Most tumors secrete both norepinephrine and epinephrine, although the former usually predominates. Since any single hormone may or may not be elevated, most published guidelines call for collecting an array, usually consisting of metanephrine, total catecholamines, vanillylmandelic acid, norepinephrine, and epinephrine. Some have argued that a negative assay for a single catecholamine has a 98-percent predictive value for ruling out the disease in a primary care population [144]. Optimally, the diagnostic procedure consists of a 24-hour collection that includes both catecholamine and creatinine to monitor sufficiency of urine collection. Shorter timed intervals (e.g., 4–8 hours) may be useful, if full-day collections are impractical or if episodic symptoms are short-lived and potentially diluted by longer collections. Using a ratio of micrograms of catecholamine per milligram of creatinine, the clinician may extrapolate to a full day's collection. Urine collections should occur at times of sustained hypertension. Plasma catecholamines may be equally diagnostic, as long as collection procedures are assiduously followed to minimize false positives and false negatives [143]. Newer biochemical techniques usually obviate the need for dietary or drug restrictions [145].

The majority of patients with pheochromocytoma have dramatic elevations of catecholamines, at least twice the normal level. If the clinical suspicion is high but the urinary concentration is only equivocally elevated, the use of an oral clonidine-suppression test (plasma-catecholamine levels before and after clonidine 0.3 mg orally) [146] or an overnight clonidine-suppression test (clonidine 0.3 mg orally at 9 p.m. with overnight urine collections) [147] to minimize hypotensive reactions may assist in distinguishing clonidine-suppressible versus irrepressible secretion. Clonidine serves to reduce central sympathetic outflow among those with essential hypertension but leaves autonomous secretion unaffected. The provocative tests commonly recommended in prior decades are now relegated to use in the small number of individuals with ambiguously mild elevations but strong clinical suspicion.

Definitive diagnosis and full localization usually require both biochemical tests for catecholamines and scanning of potential sites by CT or MRI. On occasion, these scans may fail to localize the tumor. Scanning by [^{131}I] meta-iodobenzylguanidine (MIBG) uses a guanethidine analog with affinity for chromaffin tissue to search the entire body rather than a more focal study to detect an anatomic lesion, which generally must exceed 1 cm in diameter for identification. A number of antihypertensive medications, including labetalol, nifedipine, reserpine, diltiazem, verapamil, and tricyclic antidepressants, may interfere with the test [148].

MANAGEMENT. In most situations, patients with catecholamine-secreting tumors undergo curative resection as definitive therapy. Perioperative management usually includes several weeks of alpha-blocker therapy, especially phenoxybenzamine, and rehydration to avoid abrupt hypotension from withdrawal of the elevated catecholamines once the tumor pedicle has been clamped. Often the degree of alpha blockade, using phentolamine or nitroprusside, is only partial to assist the surgeon in localizing the tumor by direct palpation during the exploration and to ensure that BP falls with complete excision. Persistent BP elevations may indicate additional catecholamine-secreting tumors. Beta blockade can control arrhythmias during the perioperative period but should be administered only in conjunction with alpha blockers to avoid unopposed alpha-agonist effect. Up to 25 percent of those with benign, resected tumors remain hypertensive postoperatively, related perhaps to primary hypertension or hypertensive nephropathy [145].

Other Endocrinologic Causes of Hypertension. A variety of other conditions may cause hypertension, including hyperthyroidism and hyperparathyroidism. Usually the hypertension is not the most prominent manifestation of the hormonal derangement and responds over 1–2 months with correction of the underlying disease. Screening tests for hyperthyroidism consist of free-thyroxine concentration supplemented by a free-T3 assay only if the hormonal excess is suspected despite normal screening values. An ionized calcium and parathormone assay by immunoradiometric assay constitute the best screening tests for hyperparathyroidism.

PHARMACOLOGIC HYPERTENSION

A wide variety of medications can produce drug-mediated hypertension, correctable once the condition is recognized and the offending agent withdrawn. The drugs logically cluster into several groupings: (1) **vasoconstrictors** (phenylephrine, pseudoephedrine, phenylpropranolamine, beta-agonist bronchodilators, and other sympathetic amines, as well as stimulant abuse, antiadrenergic agent withdrawal, and monoamine oxidase inhibitor cotreatment with tyramine), (2) **volume expanders** (glucocorticoids; estrogens, especially at high doses as in oral contraceptives; nonsteroidal anti-inflammatory agents that inhibit protaglandins and thromboxane A_2 via cyclo-oxygenase) [149], and (3) *miscellaneous* other agents, like psychotropic drugs, that interfere with sympatholytic antihypertensive agents or those with poorly specified mechanisms such as cyclosporine or erythropoietin [150].

Cyclosporine-related hypertension has assumed special importance, both because of the critical utility of cyclosporine in many posttransplantation settings and because the incidence of hypertension in such a context can exceed 50 percent. Possible mechanisms of producing elevated BP include (1) direct nephrotoxicity, (2) renal vasoconstriction by either imbalanced production of renal vasoconstrictor eicosanoids or by failure of vasodilatory prostaglandin synthesis, (3) altered renin-angiotensin-aldosterone system status, (4) interference with physiologic mediators like endothelial-derived relaxation factor, and (5) increased renal-sympathetic-nerve activity with resultant vasoconstriction [151]. Perhaps as a consequence of cyclosporine's binding to cyclophilin, an intracellular calcium-binding protein, hypertensive patients treated with cyclosporine may be particularly sensitive to treatment by dihydropyridine therapy [152], while ACE-inhibitor therapy may worsen renal function and diuretic therapy may exacerbate hypomagnesemia. In the presence of worsening renal function or hyperkalemia, the clinician should reduce cyclosporine doses [151].

MANAGEMENT OF THE HYPERTENSIVE PATIENT

Goal of Antihypertensive Therapy

The overall goal of antihypertensive therapy is the prevention of cardiovascular and cerebrovascular morbidity and mortality. Important intervening variables include the level of BP achieved, the quality of life for treated patients, and their compliance with therapy, but these issues are not sufficient ends in themselves [153]. Management generally combines nonpharmacologic and drug therapy to optimize BP control. Table 26-11 summarizes recommendations for nondrug therapy.

Nonpharmacologic Treatment

WEIGHT REDUCTION

Loss of excess weight reduces both SBP and DBP. The Trials of Hypertension Prevention [154] produced an average weight loss of 3.8 kg at 18 months, reduction of SBP and DBP by 2.9 and 2.3 mm Hg, respectively, and a 51-percent reduction in hypertension incidence among individuals with high normal BP by using caloric restriction and modest physical activity. Similar results have been reported by two other randomized controlled trials of nondrug therapy [155,156]. None of the three trials reported adverse effects from weight loss. Other benefits of weight loss generally include improvement in lipid profile [157] and reduced rates of developing diabetes mellitus, breast cancer, and gout [16].

Most trials confirm that BP reduction is directly related to the weight loss achieved, although less than optimal weight loss may still reduce BP to levels below the need for supplemental treatment. Hypertension may return if

Table 26-11. Recommendations for nondrug therapy

	Normotensive individuals	Hypertensive patients	Health care professionals
Alcohol	≤ 2 drinks/day (8 oz. wine, 2 oz. liquor, 24 oz. beer)	≤ 2 drinks/day (8 oz. wine, 2 oz. liquor, 24 oz. beer); abstinence if BP still uncontrolled	Advise on effects of excess consumption, encourage reduction, refer as appropriate
Obesity	Goal body weight = BMI 20–27 kg/m^2	Reduce to acceptable BMI by diet and exercise	Inform patient, use proper BP cuff, refer as appropriate
Saturated fat	Total fat < 30% total calories; saturated fat < 10% of total calories; cholesterol < 100 mg/day	Total fat < 30% total calories; saturated fat < 10% total calories; cholesterol < 100 mg/day	Provide information on fat content of foods; counsel on methods to reduce fat and cholesterol intake over time
Sodium/salt	Avoid high-salt foods, minimize salt addition; reduce intake to < 100 mmol (< 2.3 g sodium, < 6 g salt)/day	Avoid high-salt foods, minimize salt addition; reduce intake to < 100 mmol (< 2.3 g sodium, < 6 g salt)/day	Provide information on salt content of foods; counsel on methods to reduce salt intake over time
Smoking	Stop smoking	Stop smoking	Advise on effects of smoking; encourage reduction, then abstinence; refer as appropriate
Exercise	Regular exercise as beneficial for weight regulation and reducing cardiovascular mortality	Regular, progressive exercise as beneficial for weight regulation and reducing cardiovascular mortality; avoid isometric exercise	Encourage regular, appropriate physical activity; refer as appropriate to community resources
Potassium	Eat potassium-rich diet (high in vegetables, fruits, low-fat dairy products)	Eat potassium-rich diet (high in vegetables, fruits, low-fat dairy products, especially if on potassium-losing diuretics)	Provide information on potassium-rich diet and optimal preparation (steaming better than boiling)
Other Calcium Magnesium Stress management	Data at present not sufficient to recommend inclusion	Data at present not sufficient to recommend inclusion	Data at present not sufficient to recommend inclusion

Sources: Adapted from Laidlaw JC, Chockalingam A. Canadian consensus conference on nonpharmacological approaches to the management of high blood pressure: Recommendations. J Cardiovasc Pharmacol. 1990; 16[Suppl 8]:S48–S50. Cressman MD. Management of hypercholesterolemia in the hypertensive patient. Cleve Clin J Med 1989; 56(4):351–358. Joint National Committee on Detection, Evaluation, and Treatment of High Blood Pressure. The fifth report of the Joint National Committee on Detection, Evaluation, and Treatment of High Blood Pressure (JNC V). Arch Intern Med 1993; 153:154–183.

weight gain recurs, but most trials suggest that the regain is only partial and that long-term benefits of BP reduction persist [154,156]. The critical component appears to be the weight loss itself rather than the substitution or avoidance of "high-energy" foods [158]. Weight loss carries the extra benefit of reducing all-cause mortality, especially when analyses correct for intercurrent smoking or antecedent disease [159].

EXERCISE

Adding more physical activity to a weight-loss program accelerates the weight loss and facilitates BP reduction. The precise mechanism likely involves decreases in cardiac output and peripheral resistance as well as modifications in serum norepinephrine levels, insulin sensitivity, electrolyte balance, neural and baroreflex mechanisms, and vascular structure [160].

Many of the published data reflect some methodological compromises. Yet they offer consistent evidence in support of exercise as beneficial. Following increased physical activity, BP falls up to 6–7 mm Hg for both SBP and DBP, independent of any weight changes [16]. All types of increased activity appear effective. Augmentation of daily activity level has been shown to be superior to concentrating workouts three times a week, and moderate-intensity endurance exercise (40–60% of maximum oxygen consumption) proves as effective as higher-intensity exercise for reducing BP [161]. In particular, frequent regular exercise appears to be partially protective against the potential trigger effect of strenuous physical exercise for acute MI [162]. Recent summaries of energy expenditures for representative activities and lists of contraindications may be helpful in planning exercise programs [163].

SODIUM RESTRICTION

Over 70 published studies have addressed the impact of reducing sodium intake on BP [164]. Despite crossover and parallel group comparisons in both normotensive and hypertensive trial populations, most trials have been too small to assess definitively the sodium hypothesis of hypertension causation. Pooled estimates suggest that BP reductions are most impressive among older individuals, those with higher baseline levels of BP, and particularly those who are "salt sensitive" [164,165]. Following reductions in dietary intake from the American average of 10 g/day of salt to about half that quantity, reductions in SBP and DBP average 5 and 3 mm Hg, respectively, among hypertensive subjects.

Not all hypertensives show sensitivity to sodium intake or to natriuresis for BP reduction [34]. Depending on the patient mix, the prevalence of such salt sensitivity equals 20–60 percent of the tested group, while the remainder of the population will exhibit negligible responses in BP to the same interventions [166]. Elderly and African-American patients may be especially susceptible to salt restriction. One possible mechanism for a special susceptibility may be the observation that subjects with a pulse rate 78 beats or more per minute have an exaggerated pressor effect from increased salt intake in contrast to those with heart rates less than 68 [167]. Most important, sodium restriction often allows reduction or even elimination of the need for antihypertensive medications, whether or not in combination with weight loss [168].

ALCOHOL RESTRICTION

Restricting habitual consumption to fewer than three alcoholic drinks/day can reduce BP in both normotensive and hypertensive individuals and may help prevent hypertension [16]. The use of low-alcohol beer for six weeks reduced SBP and DBP by 5 and 3 mm Hg, respectively, independent of weight change for systolic levels [169].

STRESS REDUCTION AND RELAXATION TRAINING

In light of consistent evidence that stress may elevate BP, many investigators have assessed stress-management interventions to prevent or reduce hypertension. Some benefit of relaxation, meditation, or biofeedback has been reported from both workplace and clinical settings [170,171]. One review of 25 published, randomized controlled trials enumerated 823 subjects on active treatment but many methodologic limitations: small sample sizes (17 of 25 studies had fewer than 40 subjects), short duration (average duration 3 months), and small effects [172]. Only two of five studies with more than 15 subjects per treatment arm and 12 months or more of treatment duration exhibited significant BP reductions. The one randomized controlled trial testing the value of stress management to prevent the development of hypertension could not demonstrate a clear benefit [154]. Current evidence, therefore, is lacking for strong endorsement of stress reduction as a principal treatment modality for hypertension.

OTHER DIETARY CHANGES

Potassium supplementation may carry a direct natriuretic effect, suppression of the renin-angiotensin system, and direct arterial vasodilatation. Most of the published trials have been small, short, and limited to normotensives or those with mild BP elevations. Even when the trials were larger, longer, or pooled for data analysis, the net effect of potassium supplementation was modest: 3–5 mm Hg net reduction in BP [16].

Several other conditions, especially osteoporosis, may be modified by sufficient intake of **calcium** (recommended daily allowance 800–1200 mg). The data in support of calcium's beneficial effect for hypertension are scant. Although 25 randomized controlled trials of calcium supplementation have been reported, most show small or inconsistent results. Even when pooling results from 23 of the trials, the average net reduction in BP was 0.5–1.0 mm Hg. Many of the published studies were observational and might have been confounded by sodium intake, which was often poorly measured [16].

Similarly disappointing results have emerged about **magnesium** supplementation. Of the nine published clinical trials, many are confounded by intercurrent use of antihypertensive medications [16]. In the one trial using 340 mg (15 mmol) or less of elemental magnesium, the net BP reduction was only 0.1–0.2 mm Hg [154]. Magnesium supplementation, moreover, frequently brought on indigestion, diarrhea, or other gastrointestinal complaints.

In the Multiple Risk Factor Intervention Trial, **saturated fat** percentage, dietary **cholesterol,** and **starch** independently showed high correlation with SBP. No association for BP was demonstrable for total dietary fat [172]. Replacing saturated fats with mono- or polyunsaturated fats produced no significant change in BP, although it still was beneficial for reducing overall cardiovascular risk. Reductions in dietary **protein** or increases in dietary **fiber** similarly show no net effect on BP. **Fish-oil** supplements of 3 g/day or more (at least two 100-g servings of fish or 6–10 fish-oil capsules) produced net reductions of 3–5 mm Hg among hypertensives, although accompanied by flatulence and a taste and smell found disagreeable by many patients and their families [174].

Drug Therapy

If 3–6 months of hygienic, nondrug therapy fail to reduce BP to acceptable levels for patients with mild-to-moderate hypertension, the clinician should consider antihypertensive medications. Direct comparison of nondrug and drug therapies suggests superior blood-pressure control with pharmacologic agents [175]. More than 60 distinct drugs exist for this purpose [176], and selection should reflect thoughtful evaluation of the patient's status and preferences.

Regardless of the agent chosen, the medication should achieve as many of the following objectives as possible [177]:

- Display efficacy as monotherapy in more than 50 percent of all patients.
- Provide 24-hour BP control during all activities.
- Offer once-daily dosing.
- Reduce vascular resistance.
- Improve arterial compliance.
- Preserve cardiac output.

- Maintain perfusion to critical organs.
- Avoid tolerance or pseudotolerance.
- Avoid reflex volume retention or stimulating neurohumoral mechanisms.
- Display favorable biochemical and metabolic effects.
- Reverse the pathologic structural changes (e.g., cardiac hypertrophy).
- Reduce ventricular ectopy if present.
- Minimize target-organ damage.
- Maintain normal hemodynamic response to exercise.
- Offer few side effects and good quality of life.
- Facilitate optimal compliance with drug regimen.
- Display favorable profiles in concomitant diseases or problems.

ALTERNATIVE APPROACHES

No single strategy for selecting antihypertensive-drug therapy is relevant and helpful for all patients. Four principal approaches have emerged as useful: stepped care, demographic analysis, renin profiling, and individualization.

Stepped Care. Over the past two decades, the concept of progressive, stepped care has evolved from a narrow set of incremental options to a broader set of guidelines in JNC V [6]:

Step 1. Prescribe life-style modifications, including weight reduction, moderated alcohol intake, regular physical exercise, reduced sodium intake, and smoking cessation.

Step 2. If response is inadequate, continue the life-style modification and add monotherapy for mild to moderate (stages 1 and 2) hypertension with thiazide diuretics or beta blockers, unless there is a contraindication. Other agents, like ACE inhibitors, calcium antagonists, $alpha_1$-blockers, and alpha-beta blockers, are satisfactory substitutes for patients with contraindications, although the drugs' long-term net benefits are not established.

Step 3. If response to initial treatment is inadequate, increase the drug dosage, substitute another antihypertensive drug, or add a second agent from a different drug class.

Step 4. If response still is inadequate, add a second or third agent of a different drug class (including an appropriate diuretic, if not already administered).

The major advantages of the stepped-care consist of simplicity of understanding and implementation, emphasis on administration of complementary drug classes for synergism, and titration to minimize toxicities. While the JNC V recommendations acknowledge that hypertensives are heterogeneous in their risk profiles, hemodynamics, and susceptibility to drug therapy, the committee's selection of thiazide diuretics and beta blockers as principal monotherapies remains controversial [178]. More important to some, the JNC V offers limited sensitivity to three issues: hemodynamic diversity among hypertensives, negative metabolic effects of thiazides and beta blockers, and the need for direct testing of stepped care versus alternative approaches. Several recent studies suggest either that all drug classes offer comparable short-term net benefits [179] or that some alternative antihypertensive agents may be superior to those recommended by JNC V in terms of antihypertensive efficacy after 1 year of therapy [180]. Reducing doses to the minimum level with acceptable antihypertensive efficacy yields the best results in costs and side effects [181].

Demographic Analysis. In discovering heterogeneity in hypertension, many authors have propounded useful if simplistic heuristics, summarizing relative responsiveness of demographic subgroups to different antihypertensive drug classes. Although the guidelines are helpful as generalizations, they reflect relative, not absolute, effectiveness.

In this context, **age** may predict the preponderance of elevated cardiac output (CO) versus increased systemic vascular resistance (SVR) by subgroup. Younger patients may exhibit high or normal CO, often associated with a sympathetically activated, hyperkinetic circulation, potentially responsive to antiadrenergic agents like beta blockers or to ACE inhibitors. Older patients more commonly display low or normal plasma-renin activity, volume expansion, and increased SVR. Such patterns often respond to diuretic or calcium-antagonist therapy.

In much the same way, analysis by **race** suggests useful subgroup differences. A majority of black hypertensive patients show volume-dependent, low-renin patterns, compared to about 10 percent among white hypertensives [182]. While diuretic therapy may be especially effective, other drug classes like beta blockers, calcium antagonists, and ACE inhibitors may also control BP among black hypertensives [183]. These and other demographic and hemodynamic differences offer modest support for the principles summarized in Table 26-12.

Renin-Profile Analysis. Classification of hypertensive patients into three renin-sodium strata may carry prognostic and therapeutic implications [13,49]. The process requires both assessment of PRA and 24-hour urinary sodium excretion of a stable diet. By such evaluation, hypertensive populations have been categorized into low renin (20–30% of group), normal renin (55–60%), and high renin (10–15%) subtypes. Recent reports of prospective studies indicate that pretreatment renin-sodium profiles predict differential rates of subsequent MI among high (14.7/1,000 person-years), normal (5.6), and low (2.8) renin-sodium profile subjects [13]. These differences occur despite comparable success in BP control in all three groups. No significant differences were observed over more than 8 years of follow-up for stroke or noncardiovascular events.

Therapeutically, high-renin hypertensives reportedly respond better to ACE inhibitors, central $alpha_2$ agonists, peripheral $alpha_1$ blockers, beta blockers, and nondihydropyridine calcium antagonists. In contrast, those with low-renin profiles display differential responsiveness to dihydropyridine calcium antagonists and diuretics. Despite the conceptual attractiveness and prognostic implications, renin profiling has not achieved wide acceptance as a method for selecting drug therapy [184]. Practical obstacles to its use include cost, inaccuracies and logistics

Table 26-12. Demographic/hemodynamic clustering of relative responsiveness to monotherapy by antihypertensive drug class

Factor	Diuretics	Beta blockers	Alpha$_1$ blockers	Ace inhibitors	Calcium antagonists
Older age (vs. younger)	+++	+	++	++	+++
Black race (vs. white)	+++	+	++	++	+++
Volume dependent (vs. not)	+++	+	++	+	++
High renin (vs. low)	+	+++	+	+++	+
↑ Sympathetic activity (vs. ↓)	+	+++	+++	++	++

Key: + = less effective; ++ = effective; +++ = more effective than comparison group.
Source: Modified from Dzau VJ. Evolution of the clinical management of hypertension: Emerging role of "specific" vasodilators as initial therapy. Am J Med 1987; 82[Suppl 1A]:36–43.

of 24-hour urinary collections, and suboptimal predictive characteristics. The PRA must be adjusted for technique, diet, age, race, sex, and posture, among other factors, further limiting its utility. Most clinicians find therapeutic trials of particular medications more feasible and less expensive.

Individualized Approach. The individualized approach is perhaps the most comprehensive strategy for selecting antihypertensive therapy. It factors in a patient's profile of hemodynamics and pathophysiology, cardiovascular risk analysis, concurrent medical conditions and therapies, demographics, quality-of-life analysis, and cost. Although the most complex, this approach most personalizes the drug selection to the particular patient [177].

The strategy consists of six components:

1. Responding to projected **pathophysiology and hemodynamics,** the clinician chooses medications to reverse the underlying circulatory dysregulation, adjusted for the patient's age, race, weight, and symptoms, lowering the vascular resistance if elevated while preserving cardiac output and maintaining perfusion to critical target organs, both at rest and with exercise, over the entire 24 hours.
2. Reflecting **cardiovascular risk-profile analysis,** the clinician avoids medications that worsen the known risk profile, such as rejecting thiazides in a patient with elevated low density lipoprotein (LDL) cholesterol [185]. In addition, the clinician prospectively monitors those regimen-affected factors that affect risk and continuously adjusts the regimen to minimize overall risk, whether related to atherosclerosis, major arrhythmias, congestive failure, or sudden death [184].
3. Aware of **concurrent medical conditions and therapies,** the clinician prescribes the fewest antihypertensive drugs to treat the greatest number of concomitant conditions, such as using beta blockers when both angina and hypertension are present in the absence of heart failure, peripheral vascular insufficiency, or bronchospasm [186]. Such therapeutic parsimony facilitates medication adherence by simplifying the overall regimen and minimizes adverse drug reactions and drug-drug interactions.
4. This approach uses the **demographic** patterns previously described but integrates the options related to age and race with the other factors as well.
5. To optimize adherence to the regimen, the clinician seeks to optimize the patient's **quality of life,** considering physical, mental, social, emotional, and sexual functions [179,180,187].
6. Finally, the strategy considers **cost:** the sum of drug-acquisition cost, required concomitant treatment (e.g., potassium supplementation for thiazide diuretics) and tests (e.g., monitoring serum potassium and renal function), clinician visits, hospitalizations and emergency evaluations, missed work from disease or side effects, and direct and indirect costs of long-term morbidity and mortality as well as lost wages and productivity [188].

HEMODYNAMICS OF ESSENTIAL HYPERTENSION AND DRUG EFFECTS

Physiology. Arterial blood pressure is the product of CO and SVR. SVR, in turn, reflects both peripheral vascular resistance and renal vascular resistance in both capacitance and resistance vessels. Among hypertensive patients, elevations in SVR constitute the primary hemodynamic abnormality as a function of blood viscosity and arteriolar vasoconstriction [189].

Some hemodynamic changes occur with aging [190]. The slight increases in CO observed among young hypertensives often result from augmented sympathetic nervous system activity and generate tachycardia and increased total body oxygen consumption at rest. With exercise, their CO and SVR both fall, but SVR levels remain higher than among normotensive controls. As hypertensive patients age, their CO gradually falls and their SVR progressively rises beyond levels associated with normal aging and accompanied by increased resistance in skeletal muscle and in the splanchnic and pulmonary circulations. Table 26-13 summarizes the effects of antihypertensive drug therapy on concomitant medical conditions and metabolic disorders, and Table 26-14 lists common drug interactions for antihypertensive therapy. Table 26-15 summarizes the dosing guidelines and the relative advantages and disadvantages of antihypertensive drugs.

Drug Clustering by Hemodynamic Effect. The optimal hemodynamic approach to antihypertensive drug treatment is

Table 26-13. Effects of antihypertensive drug therapy on concomitant medical conditions and metabolic disorders

	Conditions and disorders				
	Diuretics	Beta blockers	$Alpha_1$ blockers	Ace inhibitors	Calcium antagonists
Dyslipidemia	–	–	++	0	0
Diabetes mellitus	–	–	0	0	0
Hypokalemia	–	0	0	±	0
Hypercalcemia	–	0	0	0	0
Angina	0	++	0	±	++
Congestive failure	++	–	0	++	–
Arrhythmias	–	++	0	0	++
Bronchospasm	0	–	0	0	±

Key: – = adverse effect; ++ = beneficial effect; ± = may be beneficial or adverse; 0 = no effect.
Source: Modified from Dzau VJ. Evolution of the clinical management of hypertension: Emerging role of "specific" vasodilators as initial therapy. Am J Med 1987; 82[Suppl 1A]:36–43.

Table 26-14. Common drug interactions in antihypertensive therapy

Drug class	Antihypertensive drug	Interaction
Sympathomimetics Phenylephrine Phenylpropanolamine Ephedrine Cocaine Beta agonists for asthma	Sympatholytics: $alpha_2$ agonists (methyldopa, clonidine), guanethidine	↓ Antihypertensive effect
Tricyclic antidepressants	Sympatholytics: $alpha_2$ agonists (methyldopa, clonidine), guanethidine, guanadrel, reserpine	↓ Antihypertensive effect
Phenothiazines	Sympatholytics: $alpha_2$ agonists (methyldopa, clonidine), guanethidine, guanadrel, reserpine	↓ Antihypertensive effect ± Paradoxical hypertension
Monoamine oxidase inhibitors	Sympatholytics: $alpha_2$ agonists (methyldopa, clonidine), guanethidine, guanadrel, reserpine	↓ Antihypertensive effect ± Paradoxical hypertension
Lithium	Thiazide or loop diuretics	↓ Decreased lithium clearance
Volume expanders NSAIDs Oral contraceptives Corticosteroids	All agents, especially diuretics	↓ Antihypertensive effect
Potassium augmentors Potassium supplements Spironolactone Amiloride triamterene	ACE inhibitors (all); potassium-sparing diuretics (spironolactone, amiloride, triamterene)	Hyperkalemia, especially in context of renal dysfunction
Beta blockers (all)	Verapamil	Produce high grade A-V block, precipitate congestive failure
Miscellaneous Digitalis Warfarin Pyridoxine L-dopa Oral hypoglycemics	 Potassium-losing diuretics Thiazide diuretics Hydralazine Methyldopa Thiazide diuretics	 Hypokalemia ↑ Prothrombin time ↓ Pyridoxine effect ↓ Anti-Parkinsonian effect ↓ Hypoglycemic effect

to reduce SVR while preserving CO and perfusion of critical target organs, such as brain, heart, and kidney. Available medications for lowering BP conveniently fall into three subgroups by hemodynamic alterations:

The first group **reduces SVR while preserving CO and organ perfusion.** This group includes blockers (prazosin, terazosin, doxazosin, trimazosin), $alpha_2$ central agonists (clonidine, guanabenz, guanfacine, methyldopa), thiazide diuretics, ACE inhibitors (captopril, enalapril, lisinopril, ramipril, benazepril, quinopril, et al.), dihydropyridine calcium antagonists (nifedipine, nicardipine, nitrendipine, nimodipine, isradipine, felodipine, et al.), and direct vasodilators (hydralazine, minoxidil, pinacidil). Most of these agents may be administered as initial monotherapy with little compensatory neurohumoral response, except for the direct vasodilators, which induce reflex tachycardia, fluid retention, and increased myocardial work. Diuretics initially produce modest contraction of intravascular volume, but antihypertensive effect may be delayed for weeks or even months, as SVR falls and CO returns to near-normal levels. The precise mechanism of these changes is uncertain, but it may reflect calcium-mediated vascular tone. Although calcium antagonists share a common name, the subgroup of dihydropyridipines distinctively produces vasodilatation, decreased SVR, and reflex sympathetic stimulation with possible tachycardia, fluid retention, and vasodilatory headache.

The second group **elevates SVR and reduces CO.** Such medications are beta blockers both with (pindolol, acebutolol, carteolol, et al.) and without (propranolol, metoprolol, timolol, atenolol, nadolol, betaxolol, penbutolol, et al.) intrinsic sympathomimetic activity (ISA), although CO tends to be reduced less with those agents that possess ISA. Early reports suggested that beta blockers with ISA could lower BP with minimal reductions in SVR and CO while preserving heart rate and glomerular filtration. More recent studies indicate that all beta blockers share an unfavorable hemodynamic response to exercise and may compromise perfusion to skeletal muscle, liver, and kidneys. Distinctions between selective and nonselective beta blockers are dose dependent and tend to converge on nonselective features as administered dosage increases [177].

The third group both **reduces SVR and reduces CO;** it includes reserpine, guanethidine, guanadrel, combined alpha-beta agents (labetalol, carvedilol, et al.), and nondihydropyridine calcium antagonists (diltiazem, verapamil). While unpleasant side effects generally limit the utility of guanethidine and guanadrel, reserpine has received some renewed attention because of low cost, long duration of action to compensate for partial compliance, and demonstrable long-term efficacy, especially in combination with diuretic therapy [191]. Combined alpha-beta agents offer the convenience of reduced SVR from $alpha_1$ blockade and controlled heart rate from beta blockade [192]. Finally, the nondihydropyridine calcium antagonists promote both vasodilatation and negative inotropic and chronotropic cardiac effects.

Special Situations

HYPERTENSIVE CRISES

True hypertensive emergencies are unusual. Many reflect mismanagement, sometimes from patient nonadherence, sometimes from medical-system failures, sometimes from both factors [193]. The clinical priority should be the safe, prompt, and gradual lowering of BP without major side effects or complications rather than a search for secondary causes. Dangers exist from both undertreatment and overtreatment. Diuretic therapy usually is not needed, unless applied in the presence of frank fluid overload or with diazoxide or minoxidil therapy. Antiadrenergic agents carry the possibility of sedation, confounding the interpretation of altered mental status in hypertensive crisis, and therefore should best be avoided in favor of nonsedating alternatives. The principal drug classes useful in hypertensive crises reduce peripheral resistance. The clinician selects among them by assessing the need for prompt (e.g., diazoxide) versus less prompt (e.g., minoxidil) treatment, precisely controlled (e.g., nitroprusside) versus less controlled (e.g., nifedipine), and equipment-intensive (e.g., nitroprusside) versus uncomplicated (e.g., diazoxide) procedures. Most drug-induced complications can be minimized by anticipating which organs will receive pharmacologic effects, both short and long term.

Definitions. The clinician should define the crisis as urgent (no target-organ damage) or emergent on the basis of clinical decompensation rather than by BP level alone. Although systolic pressures often exceed 180–200 and diastolics 110–120 mm Hg, the absolute level is less important than the rate of rise and the absolute difference in BP between the patient's usual level and those observed during crisis. The typical patient in hypertensive crisis is middle-aged, male, and lacking consistent access to medical care, although all sociodemographic groups are at risk.

Clinical Features. Early pathophysiologic changes reflect arteriolar spasm, while later decompensation results from fibrinoid necrosis, release of vasoactive substances, further vasoconstriction, and myointimal proliferation. Target-organ damage may affect brain, eye, kidney, heart, and gut, among other tissues. Most patients offer few specific symptoms. Sometimes cardiovascular decompensation produces palpitations, angina, or congestive failure; neurologic manifestations may include headache, nausea, seizures, or obtundation. Clinical exam may demonstrate retinopathy, congestive heart failure, arrhythmias, or neurologic deficits, including focal findings. The usual screening tests include hematocrit, electrolytes, creatinine, urinalysis, electrocardiogram, and chest radiograph. Most screening laboratory tests are normal or nonspecific, such as mild azotemia, proteinuria, and hypokalemia.

Several patterns of clinical presentations deserve emphasis. The new onset of hypertension in the absence of prior BP elevations is most consistent with acute drug reactions (e.g., cocaine, amphetamines, phencyclidine, monoamine oxidase (MAO) inhibitor–tyramine reactions) or acute glomerulonephritis. In contrast, sudden, dramatic worsening of BP in a chronic hypertensive patient usually represents accelerated primary hypertension, renal parenchymal disease, or vasculitis. If BP elevation rather than improvement occurs after diuretic therapy, the clinician should consider extra stimulation of the renin-angiotensin-aldosterone system in the midst of vasoconstriction as causative.

Specific Clinical Situations. There is no single recipe for a hypertensive crisis. Each situation should be assessed individually for critical organ involvement, desired time frame for lowering BP (minutes, hours, or days), and

Table 26-15. Antihypertensive drug therapy summary

Class	Example(s)	Mechanism(s)	Initial dose	Usual dose	Maximal dose
DIURETICS					
Thiazides	Hydrochlorothiazide	Natriuresis	12.5–25 mg/d	25–50 mg/d	100 mg/d
	Chlorothiazide	Vasodilatation	125–250 mg/d	250–500 mg/d	1000 mg/d
	Bendroflumethiazide		2.5 mg/d	2.5–5 mg/d	10 mg/d
	Trichlorothiazide		1–2 mg/d	1–2 mg/d	4 mg/d
	etc.				
Thiazide-like	Chlorthalidone	Natriuresis	12.5–25 mg/d	25–50 mg/d	50 mg/d
	Indapamide	Vasodilatation	2.5 mg/d	2.5–5 mg/d	5 mg/d
	Metolazone		0.5–2.5 mg/d	0.5–5 mg/d	5 mg/d
K_+-sparing	Spironolactone	Natriuresis	25 mg/d	25–50 mg/d	100 mg/d
	Triamterene		25–50 mg/d	25–50 mg/d	75 mg/d
	Amiloride		5 mg/d	5–10 mg/d	10 mg/d
Loop	Furosemide	Natriuresis	10–20 mg/d	10–40 mg/d	120 mg/d
	Bumetanide		0.5 mg/d	0.5–1.0 mg/d	5 mg/d
	Ethacrynic acid		25 mg/d	25–50 mg/d	100 mg/d
ANTI-ADRENERGICS					
Beta-blockers					
Lipophilic	Propranolol	Peripheral beta	20–40 mg/d	40–160 mg/d	320 mg/d
	Timolol	blockers	10–20 mg/d	20–40 mg/d	80 mg/d
	Pindolol (ISA)	Anti-renin effect	5–10 mg/d	10–20 mg/d	60 mg/d
	Metoprolol		25–50 mg/d	50–100 mg/d	200 mg/d
	Labetalol	[a1 + b]	100 mg/d	100–200 mg/d	1200 mg/d
Hydrophilic	Nadolol	Decrease cardiac	20–40 mg/d	40–120 mg/d	320 mg/d
	Atenolol	output	25–50 mg/d	50–100 mg/d	200 mg/d
	Acebutolol (ISA)		200 mg/d	200–400 mg/d	1200 mg/d
	Betaxolol		5 mg/d	5–10 mg/d	20 mg/d
	etc.				
$Alpha_2$ agonists	Methyldopa	Decrease peripheral	125–250 mg/d	250–500 mg/d	2000 mg/d
	Clonidine	catecholamines	0.1–0.2 mg/d	0.1–0.6 mg/d	1.2 mg/d
	Clonidine patch	Decrease HR, CO	0.1 mg/d	0.1–0.3 mg/d	0.3 mg/d
	Guanabenz		2–4 mg/d	2–8 mg/d	64 mg/d
	Guanfacine		1 mg/d	1–2 mg/d	3 mg/d
$Alpha_1$ blockers	Prazosin	Peripheral postgan-	1 mg/d	1–2 mg/d	10 mg/d
	Terazosin	glionic blocker	1 mg/d	1–2 mg/d	10 mg/d
	Doxazosin	Vasodilatation	1 mg/d	1–2 mg/d	8 mg/d
Peripheral antagonists	Reserpine	Peripheral gangli-	0.1 mg/d	0.1–0.25 mg/d	0.25 mg/d
	Guanethidine	onic blocker	10 mg/d	10–50 mg/d	150 mg/d
	Guanadrel		10 mg/d	10–50 mg/d	100 mg/d
ACE INHIBITORS					
	Captopril	Decrease A-II, aldo	12.5 mg/d	25–75 mg/d	150 mg/d
	Enalapril	Decrease afterload	2.5–5 mg/d	10–20 mg/d	40 mg/d
	Lisinopril		5 mg/d	10–20 mg/d	40 mg/d
	Benazepril				
	etc.				
CALCIUM ANTAGONISTS					
Dihydropyridines	Nifedipine	Vasodilatation	30 mg/d	30–90 mg/d	180 mg/d
	Nicardipine	Reflex sympathetic	30 mg/d	30–90 mg/d	180 mg/d
	Nitrendipine	stimulation	5 mg/d	10–20 mg/d	40 mg/d
	Isradipine	Decrease afterload	5 mg/d	5–15 mg/d	15 mg/d
	Amlodipine		5 mg/d	5–15 mg/d	15 mg/d
	etc.				
Negative inotropic	Verapamil	Decrease HR, CO	80–120 mg/d	120–240 mg/d	480 mg/d
	Diltiazem		60 mg/d	90–240 mg/d	360 mg/d
VASODILATORS					
	Hydralazine	Peripheral vasodila-	25–50 mg/d	50–200 mg/d	300 mg/d
	Minoxidil	tation	2.5–10 mg/d	10–20 mg/d	40 mg/d

LVH = left ventricular hypertrophy; K_+ = potassium; 1o hyperaldo = primary hyperaldosteronism; TG = triglycerides; MI = myocardial infarction; CAD = coronary artery disease; HDL = high density lipoprotein cholesterol; ISA = intrinsic sympathomimetic activity; CHF = congestive heart failure; HR = heart rate; CO = cardiac output; LDL = low density lipoprotein cholesterol; AII = angiotensin II; aldo = aldosterone.

Table 26-15 (continued)

Usual doses/day	Advantages	Disadvantages	Comments
DIURETICS			
1	Potentiates other antihypertensives Low cost Proven end-organ efficacy	Hypokalemia Hyperuricemia Hypercholesterolemia Hyperglycemia	Especially effective among blacks, obese, elderly May increase LVH Mediated via low K_+
1	Lasts 24–48 hrs. Works even if GFR < 50 Works even if GFR < 50	Hypokalemia Hyperuricemia Hypercholesterolemia	Especially effective among blacks, obese, elderly May increase LVH
1–2	Spares K_+ No effect on glucose, uric acid, lipid	Gynecomastia Little hypotensive effect on its own	Higher doses in 1o hyperaldo Caution in renal dysfunction
1–2	More potent diuresis	Hypokalemia Hyperuricemia Hypercholesterolemia Hyperglycemia	Less effective antihypertensive effects despite greater diuresis
ANTI-ADRENERGICS			
1–2	Effective for secondary prevention of MIs Useful when CAD comorbidity is present May assist for coexistent agitation or tremor	Decrease exercise tolerance May cause bronchospasm Increase TG, decrease HDL except with ISA Predispose to CHF May cause sedation, nightmares, indigestion, vascular insufficiency	All beta blockers are equally effective antihypertensives Main differences are convenience of dosing and side-effect profile Those with ISA may be less cardioprotective
1–2	Decrease CO when contraindication to beta blockers May assist for coexistent agitation or tremor	May cause excess sedation, dry mouth, orthostasis, dermatitis from patch	Slow upward titration may minimize unpleasant side effects
1–2	Lowers LDL Raises HDL	"First-dose" phenomenon	Potentiated by diuretics
1–2	Long half-life (wks)	May cause depression, orthostasis, sedation, peptic exacerbations	[Reserpine] Little used but found effective and safe in low doses
ACE INHIBITORS			
2–3 1–2 1 1	Fewer side effects Useful for diabetic glomerulopathy	May cause proteinuria, dysgeusia, cough, rash May precipitate renal failure, especially with stenosis	Useful in context of congestive heart failure, LVH Use caution in context of renal dysfunction
CALCIUM ANTAGONISTS			
1–2	Effective in wide array of patients May help natriuresis	May cause headache, edema, flushing, weakness, tachycardia May predispose to CHF	May be useful in context of peripheral insufficiency, angina
1–2	Useful in context of CAD, arrhythmia	Constipation May precipitate CHF	Avoid cotreatment with beta blockers
VASODILATORS			
1–2	Useful step-3 agents	May cause angina, edema, pericarditis, lupus-like syndrome	Must control HR and fluid retention for good BP control

Table 26-16. Antihypertensive therapy of choice for hypertensive emergencies

Clinical situation	Agents of choice	Alternatives	Avoid or use cautiously
Malignant hypertension, no associated disease	Diazoxide Nitroprusside Minoxidil Nifedipine Nicardipine	Hydralazine Trimethaphan Clonidine Labetalol Captopril	
Intracerebral or subarachnoid hemorrhage	Nitroprusside	Trimethaphan Labetalol	Diazoxide Hydralazine Methyldopa Reserpine Clonidine
Ischemic heart disease	Nitrates Nitroprusside Labetalol	Morphine Trimethaphan Calcium antagonists	Diazoxide Hydralazine Minoxidil
Pulmonary edema	Furosemide Morphine, O_2	Other diuretics Nitrates Nitroprusside	Beta blockers Verapamil Diltiazem
Pregnancy, toxemia, trimethaphan	Nifedipine Hydralazine Methyldopa	Nitroprusside Diazoxide Labetalol	Nitrates Thiazides
Dissecting aortic aneurysm	Nitroprusside + beta blocker	Trimethaphan + beta blocker Labetalol	Diazoxide Hydralazine Minoxidil Diuretics
Renal failure or trimethaphan, acute nephritis	Diazoxide Nitroprusside Calcium antagonists	Hydralazine Methyldopa Minoxidil	Beta blockers
Pheochromocytoma	Phentolamine or phenoxybenzamine *plus* propranolol	Nitroprusside Prazosin Labetalol Hydralazine Diazoxide	Methyldopa Beta blockers alone
Postoperative trimethaphan, hypertension	Nitroprusside Diazoxide Esmolol	Hydralazine Methyldopa	

available options, including personnel and equipment. A summary of preferred treatments for hypertensive emergencies appears in Table 26-16.

Accelerated hypertension without major target-organ damage is the most common situation. It usually occurs in the context of inadequately treated primary hypertension but may also reflect renal parenchymal disease, withdrawal from antiadrenergic agents, vasculitis, or renovascular disease. In the absence of significant retinopathic, cardiovascular, or neurologic abnormality, the clinician may elect brief observation after initial response to therapy with close follow-up rather than automatic hospitalization [194].

More ominous are **CNS catastrophes,** which can result from hypertensive encephalopathy with failure of the cerebral blood flow's autoregulation, with or without focal neurologic findings. Less commonly, any cerebral insult, such as cerebrovascular accident (thrombotic, embolic, or hemorrhagic), trauma, subdural hematoma, neoplasia, encephalitis, vasculitis, and drug withdrawl, can produce transient hypertension. While autoregulation generally maintains cerebral blood flow (CBF) within narrow limits over a wide range of blood pressures, chronic BP elevations shift the curve to higher settings, and abrupt changes in BP carry risks of dangerous rises or falls in CBF [195]. Therapeutically, the clinician seeks a 10–20-percent reduction in BP over the first hour rather than full normalization, since more aggressive treatment may impair CBF [196].

Hypertension carries extra hazards for **ischemic heart disease.** While angina, like other acute pain, may briefly elevate BP, MI usually lowers cardiac output and subsequent BP. If persistent, hypertension may increase peri-infarction morbidity and mortality. Thoughtful selection of therapy can reduce pressure without augmenting myocardial work.

In the setting of **pulmonary edema** or **congestive heart failure,** the priority is to ameliorate the LV failure first, anticipating that BP reduction will naturally follow, rather than to focus exclusively on the hypertension. Diuretic therapy plays an important role in such situations of fluid overload, even though most other hypertensive crises offer little place for diuresis.

Aortic aneurysms that affect the proximal ascending

Table 26-17. Differential diagnosis of refractory hypertension

Specific identifiable disorder (secondary hypertension)	10%
Exogenous substances	15%
Agents that raise blood pressure in susceptible persons	
Agents that interfere with antihypertensive drug action	
Complicating biologic factors	5%
Inappropriate or inadequate drug regimen	45%
Noncompliance or partial compliance with regimen	25%

Source: Adapted from Setaro JF, Black HR. Refractory hypertension. N Engl J Med 1992; 327(8):543–547.

aorta are surgical emergencies and carry poor prognoses. Medical management in that context serves mainly to stabilize as much as possible before transfer to the operating room, if surgery is feasible. When localized distal to the left subclavian artery, such aneurysms may be triaged to surgery (good risk) or medical (poor risk) therapy. Drug therapy seeks to decrease the rate of pulse-wave propagation to limit aneurysmal extension as well as to lower BP overall.

During **pregnancy,** hypertension usually presents among primiparas after the twentieth week. Up to 40 percent of gestational hypertensives will have sustained hypertension within the subsequent two decades. Pregnancy may unmask previously unrecognized chronic renal disease, renovascular hypertension, and other secondary causes of hypertension. While delivery is the ultimate treatment of choice, interim therapy may include bedrest, hydralazine, methyldopa, or atenolol, avoiding ACE inhibitors.

In the **perioperative period,** hypertension constitutes a relative contraindication to elective surgery. The occurrence of abrupt hypertension during induction may suggest an occult pheochromocytoma. Sudden cessation of beta blockers, methyldopa, or clonidine in the immediate preoperative period may precipitate hypertensive crises [197].

REFRACTORY HYPERTENSION

Definition. Resistant, or refractory, hypertension, defined as failure to lower BP to less than 140/90 mm Hg despite a regimen of three or more antihypertensive agents, may occur from factors related to the prescribing clinician, the patient, the disease, or combinations of the three [198]. Such a definition assumes that careful and appropriate measurement of BP has occurred on several occasions, including adequate patient preparation, elimination of interfering substances, and use of proper instruments and techniques.

Differential. The differential diagnosis of refractory hypertension depends heavily on selective factors of primary care versus referral practice. While partial compliance with prescribed regimens may figure prominently in primary care, the most common cause of resistant hypertension usually is inappropriate or inadequate drug regimens in a referral practice [150]. Other causes of refractory hypertension are summarized in Table 26-17. Even in the context of refractory hypertension, specific, identifiable, secondary causes of hypertension comprise only approximately 10 percent of the total. Although not common, correctable secondary forms of hypertension may first appear more likely after treatment has started. Clues such as an increase in BP after starting ACE-inhibitor therapy may suggest occult conditions, such as renovascular hypertension.

Regimen Problems. Once the diagnosis of resistant disease has been confirmed, the clinician should review the regimen to confirm its sufficiency. The dosage of prescribed medications may be submaximal and may be reasonably increased as long as adverse drug reactions do not occur. In addition, most antihypertensive medications, especially when prescribed as monotherapy, prompt physiologic compensation. These compensatory reactions usually include reflex tachycardia, fluid retention, or other stimulation of the renin-angiotensin-aldosterone system. Perhaps the most common difficulty is to recognize "pseudoresistance," which results from subclinical fluid retention, especially following the use of vasodilators or antiadrenergic agents. BP control usually follows quickly after (re)institution of adequate diuretic therapy to blunt fluid retention, commensurate with the level of renal function. Most thiazide diuretics lose antihypertensive potency as creatinine clearance falls below 40 ml/minute.

Inappropriate antihypertensive combinations also may occur. Using more than one drug of the same drug class or creating adverse drug-drug interactions, as summarized in Table 26-14, may blunt BP control.

Partial Compliance. In recent years, the failure of patients to adhere to prescribed regimens has received greater emphasis. Sometimes such partial compliance or adherence reflects suboptimal knowledge of the regimen or of the importance of consistent medication taking. When queried nonconfrontationally, many patients acknowledge that a variety of "hassle" factors interfere, such as complex regimens, disruption of daily schedules, side effects, and cost [199]. Other concerns for some patients may include unsupportive health beliefs, especially about the significance of the hypertension diagnosis or the effectiveness of the prescribed treatment [200].

Better measures of medication-taking behavior have demonstrated several important epidemiologic patterns. While 50–60 percent of individuals appear to take their regimens consistently and accurately, 5–10 percent demonstrate poor adherence with negligible compliance and early dropout from treatment. In addition, an intermediate group of partial compliers, comprising 30–40 percent of the total, demonstrate highly variable medication-taking behavior. They appear to accept the principle of antihypertensive therapy but have difficulty with consistent adherence. On occasion, they demonstrate important gaps in medication taking, lasting for days, which predispose to withdrawal, rebound, or other side effects as well as submaximal benefit [201].

In parallel, patients may have difficulty adhering to both pill taking and life-style changes such as weight loss, regular exercise, salt restriction, and reducing smoking,

Table 26-18. Guidelines for antihypertensive management

A. INITIAL MONOTHERAPY
1. Project likely pathophysiologic cluster.
2. Consider important comorbidities and cardiovascular risk factors.
3. Integrate data from past treatments, side effects, fears, or reactions.
4. Select low initial dose.
5. Instruct about likely side effects, time course of response, therapeutic goal.
6. Schedule return visit consistent with drug action to reinforce regimen.
B. ADDING A SECOND DRUG
1. Consider noncompliance or partial compliance; inquire nonconfrontationally.
2. Consider pseudoresistance (is the diuretic component satisfactory?).
3. Consider the optimal dose in light of pathophysiologic cluster, past responses.
4. Consider drug-drug interactions.
5. Consider secondary hypertension.
6. Select complementary antihypertensive agent.
7. Repeat steps A2–6.
C. THIRD DRUGS VERSUS OTHER OPTIONS
1. Repeat steps B1–7.
2. Consider ambulatory BP monitoring, inpatient observation, electronic medication monitoring.

alcohol consumption, or other substance abuse. Recognition of the problem often is confounded by physicians' disinterest in noncompliance as well as by the insensitivity of patient self-report, clinician opinion, and prescription refill rates [202].

Management. Confronted with a patient who demonstrates refractory hypertension, the clinician should review the regimen, the goal BP, and past patterns of BP control. Subsequent steps include ruling out confounding conditions such as drug-related side effects, excess salt intake, drug-drug interactions, and secondary hypertension. Inquiring about toxicities should be nonconfrontational and assess potentially embarrassing symptoms like altered libido, impotence, or incontinence. When relevant, the clinician should consider a change in regimen, especially the inclusion of an appropriate diuretic, commensurate with the level of renal function. Adjusting the regimen should permit simplification, tailoring the regimen details to the patient's daily life-style, and minimizing side effects. On occasion, powerful additional antihypertension agents such as minoxidil may be necessary. Table 26-18 summarizes guidelines for antihypertensive management.

References

1. Baum D, et al. Prescription drug use in 1984 and changes over time. Med Care 1988; 26:105–114.
2. Anastos K, et al. Hypertension in women: what is really known? The Women's Caucus, Working Group on Women's Health of the Society of General Internal Medicine. Ann Intern Med 1991; 115(4):287–293.
3. Roccella EJ, Lenfant C. Considerations regarding the cost and effectiveness of public and patient education programmes. J Hum Hypertens 1992; 6(6):463–467.
4. Manolio TA, et al. Trends in pharmacologic management of hypertension in the United States. Arch Intern Med 1995; 155(8):829–837.
5. Stason W. Opportunities for improving the cost-effectiveness of antihypertensive treatment. 1986; 81[Suppl 6C]:45–51.
6. Joint National Committee on Detection, Evaluation, and Treatment of High Blood Pressure. The fifth report of the Joint National Committee on Detection, Evaluation, and Treatment of High Blood Pressure (JNC V). Arch Intern Med 1993; 153:154–183.
7. Pickering G. Normotension and hypertension: The mysterious viability of the false. Am J Med 1978; 65:561–563.
8. Alderman MH, et al. International roundtable discussion of national guidelines for the detection, evaluation, and treatment of hypertension. Am J Hypertension 1993; 6:974–981.
9. Alderman MH. Blood pressure management: individualized treatment based on absolute risk and the potential for benefit. Ann Intern Med 1993; 119(4):329–335.
10. Haffner SM, et al. Clustering of cardiovascular risk factors in confirmed prehypertensive individuals. Hypertension 1992; 20(1):38–45.
11. Tuck M. Glucose, insulin, and insulin resistance as biochemical predictors of hypertension. Am J Hypertens 1991; 4(11):638S–641S.
12. Resnick LM. Cellular calcium and magnesium metabolism in the pathophysiology and treatment of hypertension and related metabolic disorders. Am J Med 1992; 93(2A):11S–20S.
13. Alderman MH, et al. Association of the renin-sodium profile with the risk of myocardial infarction in patients with hypertension. N Engl J Med 1991; 324:1098–1104.
14. Krieger JE, Dzau VJ. Molecular biology of hypertension. Hypertension 1991; 18[3 Suppl]:13–17.
15. Centers for Disease Control, National Center for Health Statistics, as cited in National High Blood Pressure Education Program Working Group Report on Primary Prevention of Hypertension. Arch Intern Med 1993; 153:187.
16. National High Blood Pressure Education Program Working Group. National High Blood Pressure Education Program Working Group Report on Primary Prevention of Hypertension. Arch Intern Med 1993; 153:186–208.
17. SHEP Cooperative Research Group. Prevention of stroke by antihypertensive drug treatment in older persons with isolated systolic hypertension. Final results of the Systolic Hypertension in the Elderly Program (SHEP). JAMA 1991; 265(24):3255–3264.
18. Dahlof B, et al. Morbidity and mortality in the Swedish Trial in Old Patients with Hypertension (STOP-Hypertension). Lancet 1991; 338:1281–1285.
19. MRC Working Party. Medical Research Council trial of treatment of hypertension in older adults: Principal results. Br Med J 1992; 304:405–412.
20. Coroni-Huntley J, LaCroix A, Havlik RJ. Race and sex differentials in the impact of hypertension in the United States: the National Heath and Nutrition Examination Survey. 1 Epidemiologic follow-up study. Arch Intern Med 1989; 149:780–788.
21. MacMahon S, et al. Obesity and hypertension: Epidemiological and clinical issues. Eur Heart J 1987; 8:57–70.
22. Stamler J. Epidemiologic findings on body mass and blood pressure in adults. Ann Epidemiol 1991; 1:347–362.
23. Van Itallie TB. Health implications of overweight and obesity in the United States. Ann Intern Med 1985; 103:983–988.
24. Beilin LJ. Epitaph to essential hypertension—a preventable disorder of known aetiology? J Hypertens 1988; 6:85–94.
25. Kaplan NM. The deadly quartet: Upper-body obesity, glu-

cose intolerance, hypertriglyceridemia, and hypertension. JAMA 1989; 149:1514–1520.
26. Grossman E, Oren S, Messerli FH. Left ventricular filling in the systemic hypertension of obesity. Am J Cardiol 1991; 68:57–60.
27. Sowers JR, et al. Mechanisms of hypertension in diabetes. Am J Hypertension 1991; 4:177–182.
28. Arroll B, Beaglehole R. Does physical activity lower blood pressure: A critical review of the clinical trials. J Clin Epidemiol 1992; 45:439–447.
29. Williams RR, Hunt SC, Hopkins PN. Familial dyslipidemic hypertension: Evidence from 58 Utah families for a syndrome present in approximately 12% of patients with essential hypertension. JAMA 1988; 259:3579–3586.
30. Creager MA, et al. Impaired vasodilation of forearm resistance vessels in hypercholesterolemic humans. J Clin Invest 1990; 86(1):228–234.
31. Dzau VJ. Atherosclerosis and hypertension: mechanisms and interrelationships. J Cardiovasc Pharmacol 1990; 15(5): S59–S64.
32. Intersalt Cooperative Research Group. INTERSALT: An international study of electrolyte excretion and blood pressure: Results for 24 hour urinary sodium and potassium excretion. Br Med J 1988; 297:319–328.
33. Mejia A, Julius S. Practical utility of blood pressure readings obtained by self-determination. J Hypertens Suppl 1989; 7(3):S53–S57.
34. Houston MC. Sodium and hypertension; A review. Arch Intern Med 1986; 146(1):179–185.
35. Stamler R. Implications of the INTERSALT study. Hypertension 1991; 17[Suppl 1]:I16–I20.
36. MacMahon S. Alcohol consumption and hypertension. Hypertension 1987; 9:111–121.
37. Criqui MH, et al. Multivariate correlates of adult blood pressures in nine North American populations: the Lipid Research Clinics Prevalence Study. Prev Med 1982; 11:391–402.
38. Fortmann SP, et al. The association of blood pressure and dietary alcohol: Differences by age, sex, and estrogen use. Am J Epidemiol 1983; 118:497–507.
39. Mancia G. Opening remarks: The need to manage risk factors of coronary heart disease. Am Heart J 1988; 115:240–241.
40. Wilhelmsen L. Coronary heart disease: Epidemiology of smoking and intervention studies of smoking. Am Heart J 1988; 115:242–249.
41. Schoenenberger JC. Smoking change in relation to changes in blood pressure, weight, and cholesterol. Prev Med 1982; 11:441–453.
42. Freestone S, Ramsay LE. Effect of coffee and cigarette smoking on the blood pressure of untreated and diuretic-treated hypertensive patients. Am J Med 1982; 73:348–353.
43. Pieper C, LaCroix AZ, Karasek RA. The relation of psychosocial dimensions of work with coronary heart disease risk factors: A meta-analysis of five United States data bases. Am J Epidemiol 1989; 129:483–494.
44. Schnall PL, et al. The relationship between "job strain," workplace diastolic blood pressure, and left ventricular mass. JAMA 1990; 263:1929–1935.
45. Johnson JV, Hall EM. Job strain, workplace social support, and cardiovascular disease: A cross-sectional study of a random sample of the Swedish working population. Am J Publ Health 1988; 78:1336–1342.
46. James SA. Psychosocial precursors of hypertension: A review of the epidemiologic evidence. Circulation 1987; 76[Suppl 1]:I60–I66.
47. Brunner HR, et al. Essential hypertension: Renin and aldosterone, heart attack and stroke. N Engl J Med 1972; 286: 441–449.
48. Kaplan NM. The prognostic implications of plasma renin in essential hypertension. JAMA 1975; 231:167–170.
49. Dzau VJ. Renin and myocardial infarction in hypertension. N Engl J Med 1991; 324:1128–1130.
50. Daemen MJAP, et al. Angiotensin II induces smooth muscle cell proliferation in the normal and injured rat arterial wall. Circ Res 1991; 68:450–456.
51. Bulpitt CJ, Fletcher AE. Cost-effectiveness of the treatment of hypertension. Clin Exp Hypertens 1993; 15(6):1131–1146.
52. Edelson JT, et al. Long-term cost-effectiveness of various initial monotherapies for mild to moderate hypertension. JAMA 1990; 263(3):407–413.
53. Littenberg B. A practice guideline revisited: screening for hypertension. Ann Intern Med 1995; 122(12):937–939.
54. Hilleman DE, et al. Cost-minimization analysis of initial antihypertensive therapy in patients with mild-to-moderate essential diastolic hypertension. Clin Ther 1994; 16(1):88–102.
55. Lew EA. High blood pressure, other risk factors and longevity: The insurance viewpoint. Am J Med 1973; 55:281–294.
56. Hansson L. What are we really achieving with long-term drug therapy? Am J Hypertens 1988; 1:414–420.
57. Berglund G. Goals of antihypertensive therapy: Is there a point beyond which pressure reduction is dangerous? Am J Hypertens 1989; 2:586–598.
58. Medical Research Council Working Party. Stroke and coronary heart disease in mild hypertension: Risk factors and the value of treatment. Br Med J 1988; 296:1565–1570.
59. Dahlof B, et al. Swedish Trial in Old Patients with Hypertension (STOP-Hypertension) analyses performed up to 1992. Clin Exp Hypertens 1993; 15(6):925–939.
60. Applegate WB, et al. Impact of the treatment of isolated systolic hypertension on behavioral variables. Results from the Systolic Hypertension in the Elderly Program. Arch Intern Med 1994; 154(19): 2154–2160.
61. Kawachi I, Malcolm LA. The cost-effectiveness of treating mild-to-moderate hypertension: a reappraisal. J Hypertens 1991; 9(3):199–208.
62. Kannel WB. An epidemiological perspective in hypertension problem solving. Cardiology 1994; 1:71–77.
63. Cruickshank JM. Coronary flow reserve and the J curve relation between diastolic blood pressure and myocardial infarction. Br Med J 1988; 297:1227–1230.
64. Farnett L, et al. The J-curve phenomenon and the treatment of hypertension; Is there a point beyond which pressure reduction is dangerous. JAMA 1991; 265:489–495.
65. Alderman MH, et al. Treatment-induced blood pressure reduction and the risk of myocardial infarction. JAMA 1989; 262:920–924.
66. Samuelsson OG, et al. The J-shaped relationship between coronary heart disease and achieved blood pressure level in treated hypertension: further analyses of 12 years of follow-up of treated hypertensives in the Primary Prevention Trial in Gothenburg, Sweden. J Hypertension 1990; 8:547–555.
67. Whelton PK, Klag MJ. Epidemiological considerations in the treatment of hypertension. Drugs 1986; 31[Suppl 4]:8–22.
68. Madhavan S, Alderman MH. The potential effect of blood pressure reduction on cardiovascular disease. A cautionary note. Arch Intern Med 1981; 141:1583–1586.
69. Australian National Blood Pressure Management Committee. The Australian therapeutic trial in mild hypertension. Lancet 1980; 1:1261–1267.
70. Kawachi I, Purdie G. Should treatment of mild to moderate hypertension be targeted? Results from a Markov cohort model incorporating multiple risk factors. J Hum Hypertens 1990; 4(6):651–658.
71. Mejia AD, et al. Artifacts in measurement of blood pressure and lack of target organ involvement in the assessment of

patients with treatment-resistant hypertension. Ann Intern Med 1990; 112(4):270–277.
72. Appel LJ, Stason WB. Ambulatory blood pressure monitoring and blood pressure self-measurement in the diagnosis and management of hypertension. Ann Intern Med 1993; 118(11):867–882.
73. Sokolow M, Perloff D, Cowan R. Contribution of ambulatory blood pressure to the assessment of patients with mild to moderate office blood pressure. Cardiovasc Rev Rep 1980; 1:295–303.
74. Pickering TG, et al. What is the role of ambulatory blood pressure monitoring in the management of hypertensive patients? Hypertension 1985; 7:171–177.
75. Asmar RG, et al. Arterial distensibility and ambulatory blood pressure monitoring in essential hypertension. Am J Cardiol 1988; 61:1066–1070.
76. Giaconi S, et al. Microalbuminuria and casual and ambulatory blood pressure monitoring in normotensives and in patients with borderline and mild essential hypertension. Am J Hypertension 1989; 2:259–261.
77. Julius S. Home blood pressure monitoring: advantages and limitations. J Hypertens Suppl 1991; 9(3):S41–S46.
78. Soghikian K, et al. Home blood pressure monitoring. Effect on use of medical services and medical care costs. Med Care 1992; 30(9):855–865.
79. Stahl SM, et al. Effects of home blood pressure measurement on long-term BP control. Am J Publ Health 1984; 74(7):704–709.
80. McKay DW, et al. Clinical assessment of blood pressure. J Hum Hypertens 1990; 4(6):639–645.
81. Evans CE, et al. Home blood pressure-measuring devices: a comparative study of accuracy. J Hypertens 1989; 7(2):133–142.
82. O'Brien E, et al. Inaccuracy of seven popular sphygmomanometers for home measurement of blood pressure. J Hypertens 1990; 8(7):621–634.
83. Mann S. Inaccuracy of electronic sphygmomanometers. J Occup Med 1992; 34(7):304–306.
84. Sprafka JM, et al. The effect of cuff size on blood pressure measurement in adults. Epidemiology 1991; 2(3):214–217.
85. Askey JM. The auscultatory gap in sphygmomanometry. Ann Intern Med 1974; 80:94–97.
86. Campbell NR, et al. Accurate, reproducible measurement of blood pressure. Can Med Assoc J 1990; 143(1):19–24.
87. Zachariah PK, Sheps SG, Smith RL. Clinical use of home and ambulatory blood pressure monitoring. Mayo Clin Proc 1989; 64(11):1436–1446.
88. National High Blood Pressure Education Program Working Group. National High Blood Pressure Education Program Working Group report on ambulatory blood pressure monitoring. Arch Intern Med 1990; 150(11):2270–2280.
89. White WB, Dey HM, Schulman P. Assessment of the daily blood pressure load as a determinant of cardiac function in patients with mild-to-moderate hypertension. Am Heart J 1989; 118(4):782–795.
90. Staessen J, et al. The diurnal blood pressure profile; A population study. Am J Hypertension 1992; 5:386–392.
91. Audet AM, et al. Automated ambulatory blood pressure and self-measured blood pressure monitoring devices: Their role in the diagnosis and management of hypertension. Ann Intern Med 1993; 118:889–892.
92. Hall CL, Higgs CM, Notarianni L. Home blood pressure recording in mild hypertension: value of distinguishing sustained from clinic hypertension and effect on diagnosis and treatment. Bath Health District Hypertension Study Group. J Hum Hypertens 1990; 4(5):501–507.
93. Julius S, et al. "White coat" versus "sustained" borderline hypertension in Tecumseh, Michigan. Hypertension 1990; 16(6):617–623.
94. Julius S, et al. White coat hypertension: a follow-up. Clin Exp Hypertens [a] 1992; 14(1–2):45–53.
95. Grin JM, McCabe EJ, White WB. Management of hypertension after ambulatory blood pressure monitoring. Ann Intern Med 1993; 118(11):833–837.
96. American Society of Hypertension. Recommendations for routine blood pressure measurement by indirect cuff sphygmomanometry. Am J Hypertension 1992; 5:207–209.
97. Hollerman DR, Westman EC, McCrory DC. The effect of sleeved arms on oscillometric blood pressure measurement. J Gen Intern Med 1993; 8:325–326.
98. Mathieu G, et al. Blood pressure determinations during medical examinations: How many? Canad J Publ Health 1974; 65:447–450.
99. Rosansky SJ, et al. The association of blood pressure levels and change in renal function in hypertensive and nonhypertensive subjects. Arch Intern Med 1990; 150:2073–2076.
100. Bartha GW, Nugent CA. Routine chest roentgenograms and electrocardiograms; Usefulness in the hypertensive workup. Arch Intern Med 1978; 138:1211–1213.
101. Gifford RW. Evaluation of the hypertensive patient with emphasis on detecting curable causes. Milb Mem Fund Q 1969; 47:170–186.
102. Ferguson RK. Cost and yield of the hypertensive evaluation: Experience of a community-based referral clinic. Ann Intern Med 1975; 82:761–765.
103. Bech K, Hilden T. The frequency of secondary hypertension. Acta Med Scand 1975; 197(1–2):65–69.
104. Iimura O. Actual incidence of secondary hypertension. Jpn Circ J 1973; 37(9):1040–1044.
105. Berglund G, Andersson O, Wilhelmsen L. Prevalence of primary and secondary hypertension: Studies in a random population sample. Br Med J 1976; 2:554–556.
106. Rudnick KV, et al. Hypertension in a family practice. Canad Med Assoc J 1977; 117:492–497.
107. Greminger P, et al. Primary and secondary hypertension in polyclinical patients. Schweiz Med Wochenschr 1977; 107(17):605–609.
108. Lewin A, et al. Apparent prevalence of curable hypertension in the Hypertension Detection and Follow-up Program. Arch Intern Med 1985; 145(3):424–427.
109. Gabow PA. Autosomal dominant polycystic kidney disease. N Engl J Med 1993; 329:332–342.
110. Heyka RJ, Vidt DG. Control of hypertension in patients with chronic renal failure. Cleve Clin J Med 1989; 56:65–76.
111. Harrison EG, McCormack LJ. Pathologic classification of renal arterial disease in renovascular hypertension. Mayo Clin Proc 1971; 46:161–167.
112. Rimmer JM, Gennari FJ. Atherosclerotic renovascular disease and progressive renal failure. Ann Intern Med 1993; 118:712–719.
113. Schreiber MJ, Pohl MA, Novick AC. The natural history of atherosclerotic and fibrous renal artery disease. Urol Clin N Amer 1984; 11:383–392.
114. Pickering TG, et al. Recurrent pulmonary oedema in hypertension due to bilateral renal artery stenosis: Treatment by renal angioplasty or surgical revascularization. Lancet 1988; 2:551–552.
115. Muller FB, et al. The captopril test for identifying renovascular disease in hypertensive patients. Am J Med 1986; 80:633–644.
116. Havey RJ, et al. Screening for renovascular hypertension; Is renal digital-subtraction angiography the preferred noninvasive test? JAMA 1985; 254:388–393.

117. Kumar R, Schreiber MH. The changing indications for excretory urography. JAMA 1985; 254:403–405.
118. Sellars L, Shore AC, Wilkinson R. Renal vein renin studies in renovascular hypertension—do they really help? J Hypertension 1985; 3:177–181.
119. Black HR, et al. The role of captopril scintigraphy in the diagnosis and management of renovascular hypertension: A consensus conference. Am J Hypertension 1991; 4(12 Part 2):661S–725S.
120. Mann SJ, Pickering TG. Detection of renovascular hypertension; State of the art: 1992. Ann Intern Med 1992; 117:845–853.
121. Strotzer M, et al. Noninvasive assessment of renal artery stenosis. A comparison of MR angiography, color Doppler sonography, and intraarterial angiography. Acta Radiol 1995; 36(3):243–247.
122. Novick AC, et al. Trends in surgical revascularization for renal artery disease. Ten years' experience. JAMA 1987; 257:498–501.
123. Kuhlmann U, et al. Long-term experience in percutaneous transluminal dilatation of renal artery stenosis. Am J Med 1985; 79:692–698.
124. Jaffe RB. Radiographic manifestations of congenital anomalies of the aortic arch. Radiol Clin North Am 1991; 29(2):319–334.
125. Kaemmerer H, et al. Follow-up using magnetic resonance imaging in adult patients after surgery for aortic coarctation. Thorac Cardiovasc Surg 1993; 41(2):107–111.
126. Teien D, et al. Estimation of Doppler gradients at rest and during exercise in patients with recoarctation of the aorta. Br Heart J 1991; 65(3):155–157.
127. Marelli AJ, Child JS, Perloff JK. Transesophageal echocardiography in congenital heart disease in the adult. Cardiol Clin 1993; 11(3):505–520.
128. Findling JW. The Cushing syndromes; An enlarging clinical spectrum. N Engl J Med 1989; 321(24):1677–1678.
129. Mantero F, Bascaro M. Glucocorticoid-dependent hypertension. J Steroid Biochem Mol Biol 1992; 43(5):409–413.
130. Tyrrell JB, et al. An overnight high-dose dexamethasone suppression test for rapid differential diagnosis of Cushing's syndrome. Ann Int Med 1986; 104(2):180–186.
131. Kaye TB, Crapo L. The Cushing syndrome: an update on diagnostic tests. Ann Intern Med 1990; 112(3):434–444.
132. Gross MD, Shapiro B. Scintigraphic studies in adrenal hypertension. Semin Nucl Med 1989; 19(2):122–143.
133. Carpenter PC. Cushing's syndrome: update of diagnosis and management. Mayo Clin Proc 1986; 61(1):49–58.
134. Sugihara N, et al. Cardiac characteristics and postoperative courses in Cushing's syndrome. Am J Cardiol 1992; 69(17):1475–1480.
135. Miller JW, Crapo L. The medical treatment of Cushing's syndrome. Endocr Rev 1993; 14(4):443–458.
136. Irony I, et al. Correctable subsets of primary aldosteronism. Primary adrenal hyperplasia and renin responsive adenoma. Am J Hypertens 1990; 3(7):576–582.
137. Young WF, Klee GC. Primary aldosteronism; Diagnostic evaluation. Endocr Metab Clin N Amer 1988; 17(2):367–395.
138. Young WF, et al. Primary aldosteronism: diagnosis and treatment. Mayo Clin Proc 1990; 65(1):96–110.
139. Bravo EL, et al. The changing clinical spectrum of primary aldosteronism. Am J Med 1983; 74(4):641–651.
140. Weinberger MH, Fineberg NS. The diagnosis of primary aldosteronism and separation of two major subtypes. Arch Intern Med 1993; 153:2125–2129.
141. Fontes RG, et al. Reassessment of the predictive value of the postural stimulation test in primary aldosteronism. Am J Hypertens 1991; 4(9):786–791.
142. Novick AC. Surgery for primary hyperaldosteronism. Urol Clin North Am 1989; 16(3):535–545.
143. Bravo EL, Gifford RW. Pheochromocytoma: diagnosis, localization and management. New Engl J Med 1984; 311(20)(11):1298–1303.
144. Young MJ, et al. Biochemical tests for pheochromocytoma: Strategies in hypertensive patients. J Gen Intern Med 1989; 4:273–276.
145. Falterman CJ, Kreisberg R. Pheochromocytoma: clinical diagnosis and management. Southern Med J 1982; 75(3): 321–328.
146. Bravo EL, et al. Clonidine-suppression test; a useful aid in the diagnosis of pheochromocytoma. Med Intelligence 1981; 305(11)(9):623–626.
147. MacDougall IC, et al. Overnight clonidine suppression test in the diagnosis and exclusion of pheochromocytoma. Am J Med 1988; 84:993–1000.
148. Khafagi FA, et al. Labetalol reduces iodine-131 MIBG uptake by pheochromocytoma and normal tissues. J Nucl Med 1989; 30(4):481–489.
149. Radack K, Deck C. Do nonsteroidal anti-inflammatory drugs interfere with blood pressure control in hypertensive patients? J Gen Intern Med 1987; 2:108–112.
150. Setaro JF, Black HR. Refractory hypertension. N Engl J Med 1992; 327(8):543–547.
151. Porter GA, et al. Cyclosporine-associated hypertension. Arch Intern Med 1990; 150:280–283.
152. Bellett M, et al. Systemic hypertension after cardiac transplantation: Effects of cyclosporine on renin-angiotensin-aldosterone system. Am J Cardiol 1985; 56:927–931.
153. Kawachi I, Wilson N. The evolution of antihypertensive therapy. Soc Sci Med 1990; 31(11):1239–1243.
154. The Trials of Hypertension Prevention Collaborative Research Group. The effects of nonpharmacologic interventions on blood pressure of persons with high normal levels: Results of the Trials of Hypertension Prevention, Phase I. JAMA 1992; 267:1213–1220.
155. Stamler R, et al. Primary prevention of hypertension by nutritional-hygienic means: Final report of a randomized, controlled trial. JAMA 1989; 262:1801–1807.
156. Hypertension Prevention Trial Research Group. The Hypertension Prevention Trial: Three-year effects of dietary changes on blood pressure. Arch Intern Med 1990; 150:153–162.
157. Fagerberg B, et al. Weight reduction versus antihypertensive drug therapy in obese men with high blood pressure: effects upon plasma insulin levels and association with changes in blood pressure and serum lipids. J Hypertens 1992; 10(9):1053–1061.
158. Weinsier RL, et al. Obesity-related hypertension: Evaluation of the separate effects of energy restriction and weight reduction on hemodynamic and neuroendocrine status. Am J Med 1991; 90:460–468.
159. Lee IM, et al. Body weight and mortality; A 27-year follow-up of middle-aged men. JAMA 1993; 270:2823–2828.
160. Franklin BA, Gordon S, Timmis GC. Exercise prescription for hypertensive patients. Ann Medicine 1991; 23:279–287.
161. Hagberg JM, et al. Effect of exercise training in 60- to 69-year-old persons with essential hypertension. Am J Cardiol 1989; 64:348–353.
162. Willich SN, et al. Physical exertion as a trigger of acute myocardial infarction. N Engl J Med 1993; 329:1684–1690.
163. Peterson DM. Exercise and physical activity in the adult population; A general internist's perspective. J Gen Intern Med 1993; 8:149–159.
164. Law MR, Frost CD, Wald NJ. By how much does dietary

salt reduction lower blood pressure? III. Analysis of data from trials of salt reduction. Br Med J 1991; 302:819–824.
165. Cutler JA, et al. An overview of randomized trials of sodium reduction and blood pressure. Hypertension 1991; 17[Suppl 1]:I27–I33.
166. Muntzel M, Drüeke T. A comprehensive review of the salt and blood pressure relationship. Am J Hypertension 1992; 5:1S–42S.
167. Staessen J, et al. Pulse rate and sodium intake interact to determine blood pressure. A population study. Am J Hypertension 1991; 4:107–112.
168. Little P, et al. A controlled trial of a low sodium, low fat, high fibre diet in treated hypertensive patients: effect on antihypertensive drug requirement in clinical practice. J Hum Hypertens 1991; 5(3):175–181.
169. Puddey IB, Beilin LJ, Vandongen R. Regular alcohol use raises blood pressure in treated hypertensive subjects. Lancet 1987; 1:647–651.
170. Patel C, et al. Trial of relaxation in reducing coronary risk: Four-year follow-up. Br Med J 1985; 290:1103–1106.
171. Agras WS, et al. Relaxation training for essential hypertension at the worksite. II. The poorly controlled hypertensive. Psychosom Med 1987; 49:264–273.
172. Johnson DW. The behavioral control of high blood pressure. Curr Psychol Res Rev 1987; 6:99–114.
173. Ascherio A, et al. A prospective study of nutritional factors and hypertension among US men. Circulation 1992; 86:1475–1484.
174. Appel LJ, et al. Does supplementation of diet with "fish oil" reduce blood pressure? A meta-analysis of controlled clinical trials. Arch Intern Med 1993; 153:1429–1438.
175. Cutler JA. Combinations of lifestyle modification and drug treatment in management of mild-moderate hypertension: a review of randomized clinical trials. Clin Exp Hypertens 1993; 15(6):1193–1204.
176. Drugs for hypertension. Med Letter 1995; 37(949):45–50.
177. Houston MC. Hypertension strategies for therapeutic intervention and prevention of end-organ damage. Prim Care 1991; 18(3):713–753.
178. Weber MA, Laragh JH. Hypertension: steps forward and steps backward. The Joint National Committee fifth report. Arch Intern Med 1993; 153(2):149–152.
179. Neaton JD, et al. Treatment of Mild Hypertension Study. Final results. JAMA 1993; 270(6):713–724.
180. Materson BJ, et al. Single-drug therapy for hypertension in men. A comparison of six antihypertensive agents with placebo. The Department of Veterans Affairs Cooperative Study Group on Antihypertensive Agents. N Engl J Med 1993; 328(13):914–921.
181. Maling TJ, Kawachi I. Minimum effective dosage in the drug treatment of hypertension: a cost effective strategy for prescribers. N Z Med J 1990; 103(890):231–233.
182. Mitas JA, et al. Racial analysis of the volume-renin relationship in human hypertension. Arch Intern Med 1979; 139(2):157–160.
183. Saunders E, et al. A comparison of the efficacy and safety of a beta-blocker, a calcium channel blocker, and a converting enzyme inhibitor in hypertensive blacks. Arch Intern Med 1990; 150(8):1707–1713.
184. Materson BJ, Preston RA. Newer principles of patient profiling for antihypertensive therapy. Circulation 1989; 80[6 Suppl]:IV128–135.
185. Kasiske BL, et al. Effects of antihypertensive therapy on serum lipids. Ann Intern Med 1995; 122:133–141.
186. Kannel WB. The clinical heterogeneity of hypertension. Am J Hypertension 1991; 4:283–287.
187. Beto JA, Bansal VK. Quality of life in treatment of hypertension. A meta-analysis of clinical trials. Am J Hypertens 1992; 5(3):125–133.
188. Stason W. Opportunities for improving the cost-effectiveness of antihypertensive treatment. 1986; 81[Suppl 6C]:45–51.
189. O'Rourke MF. What is blood pressure? Am J Hypertens 1990; 3:803–810.
190. Fagard R, Thijs L, Amery A. Age and the hemodynamic response to posture and to exercise. Am J Geriat Cardiol 1993; (March/April):23–40.
191. Magarian GJ. Reserpine: a relic from the past or a neglected drug of the present for achieving cost containment in treating hypertension? J Gen Intern Med 1991; 6(6):561–572.
192. van Zwieten PA. An overview of the pharmacodynamic properties and therapeutic potential of combined alpha- and beta-adrenoceptor antagonists. Drugs 1993; 45(4):509–517.
193. Shea S, et al. Predisposing factors for severe, uncontrolled hypertension in an inner-city minority population. N Engl J Med 1992; 327(11):776–781.
194. Reuler JB, Magarian GJ. Hypertensive emergencies and urgencies; Definition, recognition, and management. J Gen Intern Med 1988; 3:64–74.
195. Strandgaard S, Paulson OB. Cerebral blood flow and its pathophysiology in hypertension. Am J Hypertension 1989; 2:486–492.
196. Calhoun DA, Oparil S. Treatment of hypertensive crisis. N Engl J Med 1990; 323(17):1177–1183.
197. Martin DE, Kammerer WS. The hypertensive surgical patient; Controversies in management. Surg Clin N Amer 1983; 63(5):1017–1033.
198. Schiff RL, Cohen MH, Balson A. What do you do when the blood pressure is up? An approach to the known hypertensive who has an elevated blood pressure. J Gen Intern Med 1991; 6(1):71–76.
199. Rudd P, Marshall G. Antihypertensive medication-taking behavior: Outpatient patterns and implications. In J Rosenfeld, ed. Hypertension Control in the Community. London: John Libbey, 1985:232–236.
200. Huertin-Roberts S, Reisen E. The relation of culturally influenced lay models of hypertension to compliance with treatment. Am J Hypertension 1992; 5:787–792.
201. Rudd P, et al. Gaps in cardiovascular medication taking: The tip of the iceberg. J Gen Intern Med 1993; 8:659–666.
202. Rudd P. Maximizing compliance with antihypertensive therapy. Drug Ther 1992; 22(12):25–32.

Anticoagulants, Antiplatelet Agents, and Fibrinolytics

Joseph Loscalzo
Andrew I. Schafer

Treatment of thrombotic disorders involves the use of agents that interfere with hemostasis or activate fibrinolysis. Among the first group, antiplatelet drugs and anticoagulants are the two primary classes, and plasminogen activators are used to induce fibrinolysis. Although agents in each class have been available for clinical use for a number of years, interest in antithrombotic therapies has surged recently, largely because of the outcomes of several large clinical trials such as the Physicians' Health Study and the development of novel endogenous agents for pharmacologic use, such as tissue-type plasminogen activator.

Anticoagulants

MECHANISMS OF ACTION

Two primary anticoagulants are available for clinical use: heparin and its low-molecular-weight derivatives and warfarin and its derivatives. Both classes of drugs act to inhibit fibrin formation, but they do so by very different mechanisms.

Heparin is a sulfated glycosaminoglycan polymer derived from porcine intestinal mucosa or beef lung. It has a weight-average molecular weight of 15,000, but typical commercial preparations range quite widely in size distributions and specific activities. Only about 20 percent of the molecules in commercial preparations have anticoagulant activity.

Heparin acts by catalyzing the association between antithrombin III and thrombin, as well as activated factors IX, X, XI, and XII (Fig. 27-1) [1]. Once the serine protease inhibitor (serpin)–enzyme complex forms, heparin dissociates and becomes available for catalyzing the formation of additional inhibited complexes. The antithrombin III–activating function of heparin depends on a critical pentasaccharide sequence within the glycosaminoglycan polymer [2]. Low-molecular-weight heparin preparations are produced from unfractionated heparin by enzymatic or chemical depolymerization. The critical pentasaccharide sequence, which is present in both conventional and low-molecular-weight preparations, is sufficient to accelerte antithrombin III–mediated inactivation of factor Xa. However, an additional 13 saccharide units are required to coordinate the binding of heparin to both antithrombin III and thrombin. Therefore, low-molecular weight heparins that contain fewer than 18 saccharide units cannot bind to and inactivate thrombin [3]. These relationships are schematized in Fig. 27-2.

Other anticoagulant functions of heparin that have recently been defined include the specific inhibition of thrombin mediated by heparin cofactor II, an effect that occurs only at relatively high concentrations of heparin [4]; inhibition of prothrombin activation by activated factor X in the absence of antithrombin III [5]; and inhibition of platelet aggregation [6]. Heparin also can induce thrombocytopenia in 3 to 10 percent of patients, primarily as a result of the induction of platelet aggregation mediated through immune mechanisms involving platelet-associated IgG [7]. This idiosyncractic phenomenon is said to be more common with bovine than porcine preparations of heparin [8], and it can be accompanied by thrombotic complications, which occurs with both unfractionated and low-molecular-weight preparations.

Warfarin and its congeners are oral anticoagulants of low molecular weight that have chemical structures similar to vitamin K. These agents block the conversion of vitamin K epoxide to vitamin K by vitamin K epoxide reductase (Fig. 27-3) [9]. Vitamin K epoxide is produced from vitamin K during the gamma-carboxylation of glutamic acid residues in the vitamin K–dependent procoagulant proteins: factors II, VII, IX, and X. Gamma-carboxylation is essential for the binding of these proenzymes to phospholipid groups through calcium bridges, a process that is necessary for full expression of their procoagulant action [10,11].

Two other vitamin K–dependent proteins that have been identified are protein C and protein S. These molecules function as natural anticoagulants in that activation of protein C in the presence of protein S and thrombomodulin by thrombin is associated with proteolytic inactivation of factors Va and VIIIa, thereby attenuating fibrin production. Given this important function of these vitamin K–dependent proteins, vitamin K antagonists have the theoretical potential for inducing thrombosis by suppressing protein C activity; such potential may be realized in those rare individuals who experience warfarin-induced skin necrosis. In those patients, microvascular thrombosis develops probably as a result of protein C inactivation in the setting of partial protein C deficiency. Newer direct thrombin inhibitors are currently under active investigation, including hirudin, hirulog, and argatroban.

CLINICAL USE: GENERAL PRINCIPLES

The use of anticoagulants to treat thromboembolic disease has been widely accepted since the original study of Barritt and Jordan showed their efficacy in patients with pulmonary embolism [12]. Anticoagulation has been shown to be of benefit in the prevention of thrombus extension in patients with deep venous thrombosis; the prevention of recurrence of pulmonary embolism; the prevention of recurrence of arterial embolism in patients with an intracardiac source of thrombus associated with valvular heart disease, atrial fibrillation, cardiomyopathy, or myocardial infarction; and prophylaxis against the formation of deep venous thrombus in postoperative or immobile states.

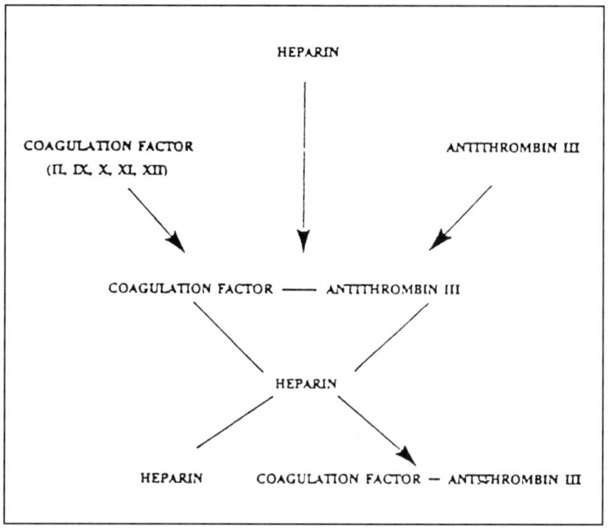

Fig. 27-1. Heparin catalyzes the inhibition of coagulation factors II, IX, X, XI, and XII by antithrombin III. Once the complex between the coagulation factor and antithrombin III has been formed, heparin dissociates from the ternary complex to be used again as a catalyst for additional complex information.

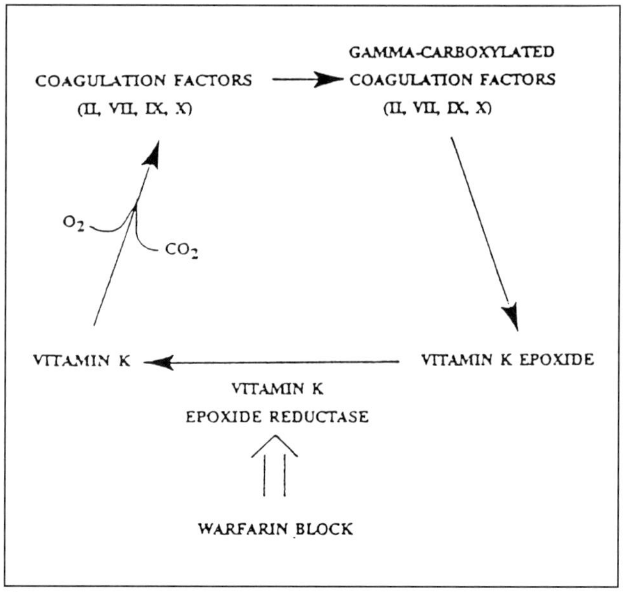

Fig. 27-3. Warfarin inhibits the conversion of vitamin K epoxide back to active vitamin K, a cofactor required for the gamma-carboxylation of glutamate residues in factors II, VII, IX, and X.

Heparin therapy [13] commonly is used in one of three regimens: (1) low-dosage subcutaneous administration for prophylaxis against venous thrombosis, (2) standard-dosage subcutaneous administration, or (3) continuous intravenous infusion. The second and third regimens are to prevent recurrence or propagation of clinically established thrombotic events.

Low-dosage prophylactic regimens usually involve the administration of a fixed dosage of 5,000 U of heparin 2 hours postoperatively, followed by 5,000 U every 8 or 12 hours [14]. In patients at high risk (e.g., those undergoing major orthopedic surgery or with a previous history of venous thrombosis), adjusted low-dose prophylactic heparin therapy (adjusted to the upper normal range of the activated partial thromboplastin time) should be considered.

Subcutaneous, dose-adjusted, full-dose regimens have been used for many years for full therapeutic anticoagulation. These regimens involve administering heparin at dosages averaging approximately 5,000 U every 4 to 6 hours, aiming to maintain the activated partial thromboplastin time (aPTT) at 1.5 times the control aPTT prior to instituting heparin therapy. The problem with subcutaneous administration is that wide swings in plasma levels of heparin are associated with the regimen, which can lead to periods during which the patient is more likely to

Fig. 27-2. **A.** Inactivation of thrombin. To inactivate thrombin, heparins must bind antithrombin III (ATIII) through the high-affinity pentasaccharide and to thrombin through an additional 13 saccharide units. Low-molecular-weight (LMW) heparins that contain fewer than 18 saccharide units cannot bind to thrombin and, therefore, are unable to inactivate thrombin. **B.** Inactivation of factor Xa. To inactivate factor Xa, heparins must bind to ATIII through the high-affinity pentasaccharide but do not need to bind to factor Xa. Therefore, both standard heparins and LMW heparins are able to inactivate factor Xa. (Reproduced with permission from Hirsh J, Levine MN. Low molecular weight heparin. Blood 1992; 79:1–17.)

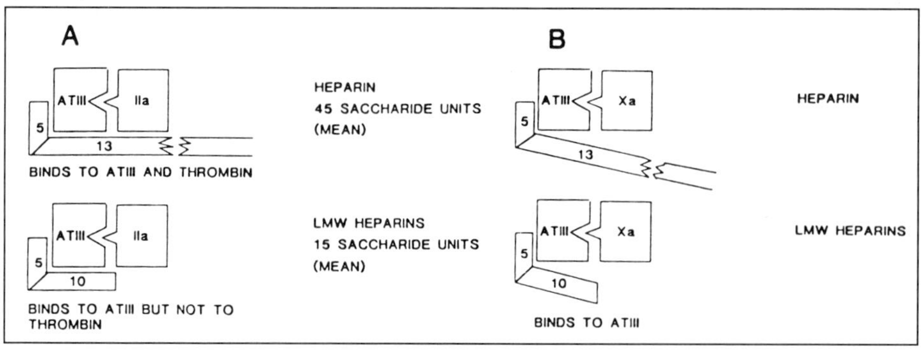

bleed alternating with periods during which thrombosis is likely. For those theoretical reasons, continuous infusion is the preferred method of administration for full anticoagulation. The continuous-infusion method involves the administration of a 5,000- to 20,000-U loading dose given as an intravenous bolus, followed by 1,000 to 2,000 U/hour as a continuous infusion. This method of administration is felt to provide safer anticoagulation with lower rates of hemorrhage, but it does so probably not because of elimination of the swings in plasma levels noted with subcutaneous administration but because of reduced total dosage for each 24-hour period [15]. In fact, no relationship has been found between the risk of bleeding while on heparin and the degree of prolongation of the aPTT, either with intermittent subcutaneous regimens [16] or continuous-infusion regimens [17]. Initial dosing may also be administered on a unit-per-weight basis. Standard regimens include an initial loading dose of 80 U/kg followed by 18 U/kg/hr as a continuous infusion or as indicated by a standard titration program [18].

Low-molecular-weight heparins have a longer plasma half-life, and their anticoagulant response to weight-adjusted doses is less variable than standard unfractionated heparin. Those properties permit low-molecular-weight heparins to be adminstered once daily and without laboratory monitoring [3]. Low-molecular-weight heparins have been shown to be efficacious in prophylaxis against deep veinous thrombosis in post-operation or immobile states and in the treatment of confined deep veinous thrombosis.

Warfarin is the most widely used vitamin K antagonist, primarily owing to its excellent bioavailability [19]. The average half-life of a single dose of warfarin is 35 hours, its absorption is influenced by diet and drugs, and its metabolism is affected by clinical disorders and drugs. Although 90 percent of warfarin sodium is bound to albumin, only the free fraction is therapeutically active.

The anticoagulant effects of warfarin derivatives are usually monitored by the one-stage prothrombin time (PT). The optimal range for prolongation of the PT has been a matter of considerable controversy over the years, primarily because of the nature of the thromboplastin reagent used in standard assays. In 1959, Sevitt and Gallagher showed that oral anticoagulants prevent venous thrombosis in patients with fractured hips [20]. They suggested that this effect was best achieved by prolongation of the PT to 2 to 2.5 times control. Based on that original observation, most physicians have followed these guidelines whenever warfarin is used for anticoagulation. Many physicians were not aware, however, that the thromboplastin reagent used in this landmark study was derived from human brain; in North America, thromboplastins are commonly derived from rabbit brain. Human-brain thromboplastin is a more sensitive reagent in assessing prolongation of the PT than is rabbit-brain thromboplastin. Prolongation of the PT by 2 to 2.5 times control using human-brain thromboplastin is equivalent to a 1.3- to 1.5-fold prolongation of the PT using rabbit-brain thromboplastin.

Poller and Taberner indicated in 1972 that most British physicians consider the therapeutically effective range of prolongation of the PT to be 1.8 to 2.1 times the normal control using human-brain thromboplastin [21]. That degree of prolongation is equivalent to 1.3 to 1.4 times the normal control using rabbit-brain thromboplastin. Hull and colleagues demonstrated convincingly that that so-called low-dosage (by North American standards) warfarin therapy is equally efficacious at preventing complications of deep venous thrombosis as full-dose therapy, with significantly fewer hemorrhagic side effects [22].

To minimize variability among laboratories and thromboplastin reagents used to measure the PT, most laboratories now report PT results as the international normalized ratio (INR). Thromboplastin reagents are standardized for activity against a World Health Organization reference preparation. Each thromboplastin lot is assigned an international sensitivity index (ISI) that correlates activity with the standard. Prothrombin times are converted to INRs by the following equation:

$$INR = (observed\ PT/control\ PT)^{ISI}$$

Anticoagulation has been shown to be beneficial in a variety of clinical disorders. Prophylactic regimens of both low-dosage heparin [14] (5,000 U subcutaneously 2 hours preoperatively and then every 8 or 12 hours thereafter) and low-dosage warfarin [23] (maintaining the PT at 1.3 times control using rabbit-brain thromboplastin at the time of surgery, then increasing it to 1.5 times control postoperatively) lower the incidence of postoperative deep venous thrombosis significantly without hemorrhagic complications. The latter regimen was studied in orthopedic patients undergoing hip or knee surgery for whom heparin prophylaxis was felt to be ineffective but for whom it has been convincingly shown by meta-analysis that even standard heparin therapy affords protection [24].

CLINICAL USE: SPECIFIC DISORDERS

Anticoagulation has been most commonly used in medical practice to treat deep venous thrombosis and pulmonary embolism. The evidence that heparin is effective in the treatment of pulmonary embolism stems primarily from a single study, that of Barritt and Jordon, who showed that the 25-percent mortality rate from pulmonary embolism was dramatically reduced by the administration of heparin and subsequent oral anticoagulants [12]. Convincing evidence that anticoagulation is useful in patients with deep venous thrombosis also exists. Before the introduction of anticoagulant therapy, Zilliacus showed that up to 27 percent of patients with clinical evidence of deep venous thrombosis developed symptoms and signs compatible with pulmonary embolism, and that in up to 22 percent of these patients, the embolic event was fatal [25]. The importance of long-term anticoagulant therapy in patients with deep venous thrombosis was studied by Hull and colleagues, who showed that treatment with oral anticoagulants after an initial course of standard heparin therapy prevented recurrent deep venous thrombosis in all patients studied, whereas low-dosage heparin treatment (5,000 U every 12 hours) failed to do so [22]. In patients treated with the heparin regimen, there was a

47-percent incidence of recurrence at 3 months, as documented by venography, but those treated with warfarin manifested no recurrences.

The other major area in which anticoagulants have been shown to be beneficial is among patients with atrial fibrillation with or without coexistent valvular heart disease. The problem of recurrent embolism secondary to chronic rheumatic heart disease complicated by atrial fibrillation was first defined by Cosgriff [26] and Askey and Cherry [27]. Subsequently, it has been shown that atrial fibrillation is present in 2 to 5 percent of the general population over the age of 60 years [28], that more than one-third of untreated patients with atrial fibrillation have evidence of systemic arterial embolism at autopsy [29,30], and that 35 percent of patients with atrial fibrillation who are not adequately anticoagulated sustain clinically significant embolic events premorbidly over a 4-year period [31] with a risk of stroke more than six times that of the general population [32]. Conversely, approximately 10 percent of patients with stroke have atrial fibrillation [33]. In addition to the increases in morbidity associated with atrial fibrillation, mortality rates also are significantly increased: the mortality rate among patients with chronic atrial fibrillation and mitral stenosis is increased 17.4-fold compared with control populations, whereas that among patients with chronic atrial fibrillation and coronary artery disease is increased 7.0-fold [34].

For those reasons, the use of chronic anticoagulation has been advocated in patients with atrial fibrillation for many years, but a controlled, prospective trial was not performed to quantitate carefully the expected benefit [26,35–38] until recently [39]. The results of uncontrolled trials were quite dramatic, showing up to a 90-percent decrease in the incidence of systemic emboli [38], thereby lessening enthusiasm for a controlled trial. The first truly prospective, controlled trials clearly show a benefit for anticoagulation in patients with nonrheumatic atrial fibrillation, both in terms of thromboembolic complications and vascular deaths [39–44]. Thus, anticoagulation with warfarin derivatives is recommended for all patients with chronic atrial fibrillation who cannot be successfully cardioverted or maintained in normal sinus rhythm. Among those with paroxysmal atrial fibrillation, anticoagulation is also recommended long-term unless paroxysms can be controlled with antiarrhythmic therapy. The reason for that approach stems from the observation by the Framingham group that stroke is a risk factor for the development of chronic atrial fibrillation [28], implying that patients with embolic stroke probably experience paroxysms of atrial fibrillation in association with the embolic event and that those paroxysms eventually evolve into persistent atrial fibrillation.

The use of anticoagulants in patients about to undergo cardioversion is also an area of some controversy. In that setting, the problems that arise include establishing the duration of atrial fibrillation prior to presentation, the duration of anticoagulation needed prior to cardioversion, and the duration of anticoagulation necessary after successful cardioversion. First, it is important to recognize that electrical and chemical cardioversion are equally risky from the standpoint of embolism. Second, emboli tend not to occur immediately on cardioversion but often 24 to 72 hours later, when auricular contraction becomes more organized. Finally, as with most disorders in which their use has been proved to be of benefit, anticoagulants do not eliminate the risk of embolization, they simply reduce it. As with the use of anticoagulants in patients with chronic atrial fibrillation, their use in patients about to undergo cardioversion is based more on usual clinical practice rather than the results of carefully designed, controlled clinical trials.

Most authorities recommend that patients in atrial fibrillation for more than 2 days receive anticoagulation for 2–3 weeks prior to attempted cardioversion. The recommended period is based on the estimated time for the endogenous fibrinolytic system to dissolve thrombi, the ongoing extension of which is prevented by the use of warfarin derivatives. The largest trial (nonrandomized) conducted thus far is that of Bjerkelund and Orning, who showed that 5.3 percent of unanticoagulated patients embolized, whereas only 0.8 percent of anticoagulated patients did so following a similar treatment regime [45]. A recent nonrandomized trial confirmed that benefit [46]. In the future, the use of transesophageal echocardiography may prove useful as a means to exclude the presence of left atrial thrombi and, thereby, limit the use of prophylactic anticoagulation in patients requiring cardioversion [47]. Once cardioversion has been successfully accomplished, anticoagulation should continue for 3 weeks, during which time the persistence of normal sinus rhythm should be documented by Holter monitoring.

Among the other areas in which anticoagulation has been considered include acute myocardial infarction, angina pectoris, transient ischemic attack, valvular heart disease, and prosthetic valve replacement. Among the more than 30 studies on the use of anticoagulants in acute myocardial infarction, only three have been of adequate size and statistical design for consideration here [48–50]. Of those three, only one showed a significant mortality benefit for short-term anticoagulation with heparin followed by phenindione, with a 30-percent reduction compared with the placebo group [50]. The proposed benefits of short-term anticoagulation in patients with acute infarction stem from preventing extension of coronary thrombosis, attenuating growth of or preventing development of mural thrombi, and preventing development of deep venous thrombosis and accompanying pulmonary embolism. The potential benefits of long-term anticoagulation in acute myocardial infarction also have been addressed in three well-designed trials of sufficient size to detect benefit in mortality or recurrent infarction [51–53]. Of those, two showed a mortality benefit of 30 and 4.3 percent [52,53]. The same two trials also showed a significant reduction in recurrent infarction of 50 and 25 percent. The soundest support for the use of anticoagulants after myocardial infarction comes from the Warfarin Reinfarction Study (WARIS), [54] in which patients were treated for 3 years with warfarin or placebo following an acute myocardial infarction. In that trial, warfarin use was shown to reduce mortality by 24 percent, nonfatal reinfarction by 49 percent, and cerebrovascular events by 55 percent. In patients with unstable angina pectoris,

Telford and Wilson originally showed in an appropriately designed trial that the combination of atenolol and heparin markedly reduced both the mortality rate and the infarction rate [55]. In that trial, however, almost half the patients enrolled subsequently were removed from the study, so the overall results must be viewed as inconclusive. More recently, a study conducted at the Montreal Heart Institute showed that heparin, aspirin, or both significantly improved the probability of an event-free outcome in patients with unstable angina [56,57].

Anticoagulants have not been shown to improve the outcome of patients with completed strokes [58]. Patients with progressive strokes [58] or those with transient ischemic attacks (TIAs) [58] may benefit acutely from anticoagulation [60]. In patients with a cardiac source of emboli, however, reduction in recurrent cerebral embolism has been demonstrated convincingly by several groups [48–50].

Finally, patients with valvular heart disease, particularly mitral stenosis with atrial fibrillation, and patients with prosthetic heart valves, particularly bioprostheses in the mitral position or mechanical prostheses in any position, require anticoagulation to prevent valve thrombosis and embolism. Patients with cardiomyopathy and patients with significant pulmonary hypertension also are generally considered candidates for lifelong anticoagulation.

COMPLICATIONS OF ANTICOAGULANT USE

The major complication of anticoagulation is, of course, bleeding. Hemorrhagic risk varies with the underlying disorder for which the individual is being anticoagulated and with the duration and intensity of the anticoagulant. For short-term anticoagulation with heparin (in patients with venous thromboembolism), the four best studies show a 1.3-percent total bleeding rate over a 6-month period; warfarin treatment over the same period is associated with a 19.9-percent total bleeding rate [22,61–63]. The use of low-dose warfarin, as described previously, is associated with significantly lower bleeding rates in the same time period with equal therapeutic efficacy [22]. Bleeding rates in studies using long-term anticoagulation with warfarin derivatives are substantial. In patients with ischemic cerebrovascular disease, total bleeding ranged from 10 to 68 events per 100 patient years, of which 2 to 9 events were fatal [64–66]; in patients with prosthetic heart valves, bleeding rates ranged from 1.8 to 6.4 events per 100 patient years, of which 0.2 to 0.8 were fatal [67–69]; and among patients treated with anticoagulation for myocardial infarction, total bleeding events ranged from 6.4 to 14.6 per 100 patient years, of which 0 to 1.0 were fatal [70–74]. It is important to recognize that major bleeding in patients treated for venous thromboembolism and cerebrovascular disease was almost always associated with an underlying risk factor. Cancer or recent surgery was common among patients with venous thromboembolism, whereas hypertension was common among patients with cerebrovascular disease [75]. Although less intense warfarin regimens have clearly been shown to be associated with lower bleeding rates [22], no quantitative correlation has yet been documented between the degree of prolongation of the PT or the aPTT and the risk of bleeding.

Nonhemorrhagic complications of heparin therapy include heparin-induced thrombocytopenia and thrombosis [76] and heparin-induced osteoporosis [77], the latter complication occurring in patients treated for prolonged periods. Warfarin use has been associated with skin necrosis thought to occur from microvascular thrombosis in patients with partial deficiency of protein C [78]. Given the short half-life of protein C, anticoagulation with warfarin derivatives without heparin treatment in those patients can be associated with a transient decrease in functional protein C at a time during which the longer-lived vitamin K–dependent procoagulants have not been sufficiently depleted. Warfarin embryopathy (in the first trimester) and central nervous system malformation (throughout pregnancy) also have been associated with warfarin use in pregnancy [79,80].

Antiplatelet Agents

OVERVIEW OF PLATELET ACTIVATION AND AGGREGATION

Most of the currently used and newer investigational antiplatelet agents exert their actions by interrupting specific pathways of platelet activation, modulating physiologic platelet inhibitory mechanisms, or both. Furthermore, several drugs used principally for other purposes (such as calcium channel blockers and beta blockers) may likewise interfere with normal platelet function. To understand the mechanisms of action of antiplatelet agents, therefore, a brief outline of the regulation of platelet activation is presented here.

Circulating platelets are activated whenever they come into contact with surfaces other than healthy vascular intimal endothelial cells. Clinical examples of this situation occur in patients with intravascular prosthetic devices (artificial cardiac valves, intra-aortic balloons, vascular grafts and shunts) and in patients undergoing extracorporeal circulation, such as open-heart surgery or hemodialysis. Vascular injury likewise disrupts endothelial contiguity and exposes circulating platelets to thrombogenic subendothelial structures, including collagen. Platelets respond to vascular damage by undergoing the process of adhesion, during which a monolayer of platelets is formed to cover the area of vessel intima denuded of endothelium. The platelet-vascular interaction is mediated by von Willebrand factor, which binds to specific platelet surface receptors localized to membrane glycoprotein Ib/IX (GPIb/IX). Adhesion is followed by the platelet release reaction, during which platelets degranulate and synthesize thromboxane A_2. Products released in the process recruit platelets from the circulation and activate them to form a hemostatic platelet plug. Platelet aggregation is mediated primarily by fibrinogen, which promotes platelet-platelet interactions after binding to specific receptors formed on activated platelet surfaces by the heterodimeric complex of the integrins, membrane glycoproteins IIb and IIIa (GPIIb/IIIa). Under pathologically elevated shear stress conditions (e.g., stenosed coronary arteries), von Willebrand factor substitutes for fibrinogen as the aggregating ligand.

The state of activation of platelets is dictated by the

balance of diverse physiologic signals, both positive and negative, that bind to specific surface receptors. These extracellular signals transmit information through the membrane and into the platelet by means of a family of G proteins, so called because they are activated by guanosine triphosphate (GTP). The G proteins then activate "amplifier" enzymes on the inner membrane surface, which convert precursor molecules into intracellular second messengers. Many positive extracellular stimuli (agonists) follow the general scheme of signal-response coupling by activating phospholipase C, which converts phosphatidylinositol bisphosphate (PIP_2) into two separate intracellular second messengers: diacylglycerol (DG), which activates protein kinase C (PKC), and inositol trisphosphate (IP_3), which mobilizes free ionized calcium from intracellular organelles. The synergistic actions of these two branching pathways of PIP_2 breakdown produce the full physiologic response of platelet release and aggregation. Free cytosolic ionized calcium, which also can be directly translocated from the extracellular medium by ionophores, not only initiates the contractile response of platelets but also activates phospholipase A_2. Phospholipase A_2 cleaves arachidonic acid (AA) from the carbon-2 position of membrane phospholipids to liberate free AA, a polyunsaturated fatty acid composed of 20 carbons and 4 double bonds (designated C20:4). Free AA is converted by cyclo-oxygenase (prostaglandin G/H synthase) to cyclic endoperoxides (PGG_2, PGH_2), which are then metabolized to thromboxane A_2 (TXA_2) by thromboxane synthase (TxS). The endoperoxides and TXA_2 are highly labile eicosanoids with potent hemostasis-promoting properties: they cause both vasoconstriction and platelet aggregation. Their platelet-activating actions are mediated by PGH_2-TXA_2 receptors that also are linked to G-protein-mediated phospholipase C activation, thus completing a positive feedback loop. Some physiologic platelet agonists (so-called "strong" agonists, such as thrombin) directly activate phospholipase C, but others (so-called "weak" agonists, such as epinephrine and adenosine diphosphate, or ADP) exert this effect indirectly through the generation of PGH_2 and TXA_2.

The major negative intracellular signals of platelets are cyclic adenosine monophosphate (cAMP) and cyclic guanosine monophosphate (cGMP). Increases in intracellular cAMP or cGMP inhibit or reverse platelet activation by blocking PIP_2 breakdown, calcium mobilization, and AA release by phospholipase A_2. The generation of cAMP follows the general scheme of signal-response coupling outlined above. Negative or inhibitory extracellular signals, such as prostaglandin I_2 (PGI_2, prostacyclin), bind to specific surface receptors linked to G proteins that stimulate adenylyl cyclase (AC): AC-stimulatory G proteins are designated G_s. The activated amplifier enzyme AC then converts adenosine triphosphate (ATP) to cAMP. The platelet inhibitory actions of cAMP are terminated by its breakdown to AMP by a phosphodiesterase (PD). Many platelet-stimulatory agonists bind to receptors that are linked not only to a phospholipase C–activating G protein but also to an AC-inhibitory G protein, designated G_i, that inhibits cAMP formation.

The major physiologic stimulus to raise platelet cAMP and thereby inhibit platelet function is PGI_2. PGI_2 is an eicosanoid synthesized by vascular endothelial cells following the release of free AA through the sequential actions of cyclo-oxygenase (as in platelets) and prostacyclin synthetase (PS); the latter enzyme operates in endothelial cells in place of the TxS of platelets. Endoperoxides that serve as substrates for both TxS in platelets and PS in endothelial cells can be shunted from activated platelets to endothelial cells to promote increased PGI_2 formation by the endothelial cells. This "endoperoxide steal" may occur adjacent to areas of vascular damage and platelet activation to enhance the generation of PGI_2 in an attempt to keep the platelet plug localized. The major physiologic stimulus to raise platelet intracellular cGMP is endothelium-derived relaxing factor (EDRF) or nitric oxide (NO). EDRF/NO binds to the heme-activator site of soluble guanylyl cyclase, inducing an increase in cGMP in the platelet and thereby inhibiting platelet function.

ASPIRIN: PHARMACOLOGY

Aspirin (acetylsalicylic acid) is absorbed readily from the stomach and the upper small intestine. It is partly hydrolyzed by esterases in the gut wall, representing an important form of presystemic metabolism. Further metabolism of aspirin occurs via esterases present in plasma, red cells, liver, and lungs [81]. The hydrolysis of aspirin results in the liberation of free-acetyl groups, which are then covalently bound to acetylate diverse proteins, such as albumin, hemoglobin, and cell-membrane constituents [82–84]. Acetyl groups released by aspirin hydrolysis selectively acetylate the hydroxyl groups of serine residues at position 529 of cyclo-oxygenase, causing the irreversible inhibition of its enzyme activity [85–88]. As shown in Fig. 27-4, acetylation of cyclo-oxygenase blocks its ability to convert AA to PGG_2 and PGH_2, thereby preventing the formation of TXA_2 in platelets (and prostacyclin in endothelial cells). Salicylic acid (salicylate), the other product of aspirin hydrolysis, lacks antiplatelet activity and may, in fact, block the effects of aspirin by inhibiting cyclo-oxygenase acetylation. Salicylate is further metabolized to glucuronic acid and glycine conjugates (Fig. 27-5). The in vivo plasma half-life of aspirin is 15 to 20 minutes, whereas that of salicylate is 2 to 3 hours [89,90].

Following the ingestion of 325 mg aspirin, the template bleeding times of normal subjects become moderately prolonged, typically reaching about twice baseline values at 12 hours and returning to normal within 24 to 48 hours. Bleeding times following aspirin administration tend to be more prolonged in men than in women [91], possibly accounting for the increased antithrombotic effects of aspirin in males in some clinical studies [92,93] and experimental models of thrombosis [94]. The consumption of alcohol, which by itself does not cause significant prolongation of the bleeding time, has been shown to potentiate aspirin-induced prolongation of the bleeding time [95]. Occasionally, aspirin use results in an exaggerated prolongation of the bleeding time. That effect has been thought to occur in patients with underlying mild functional platelet disorders or von Willebrand's disease, in whom the inges-

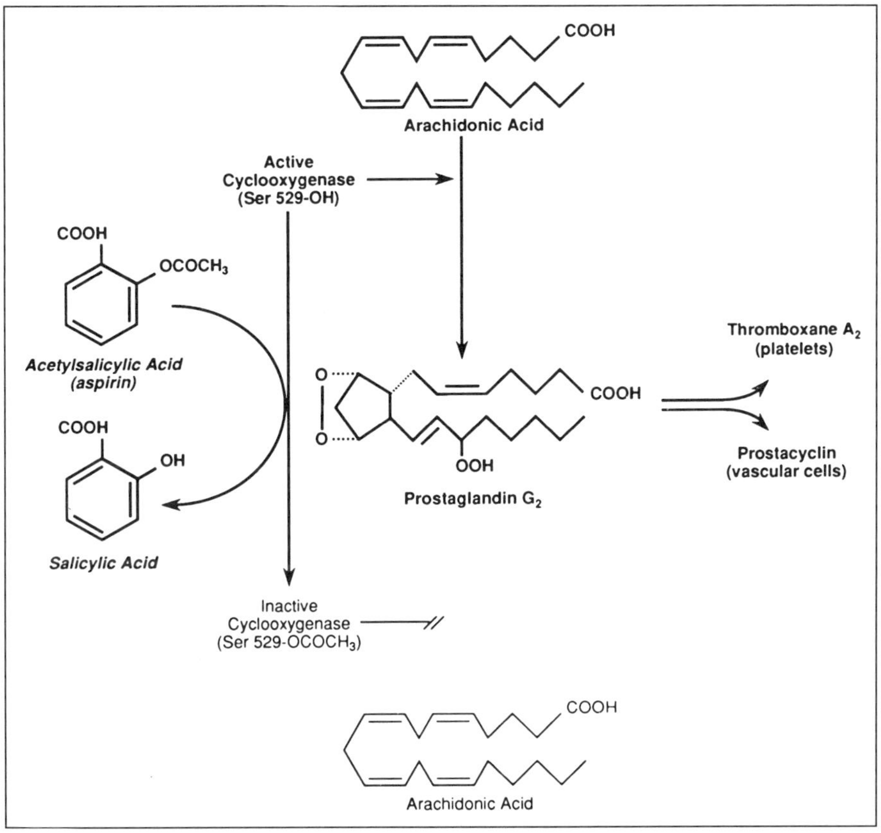

Fig. 27-4. Mechanism of action of aspirin. Cyclo-oxygenase (prostaglandin G/H synthase) oxygenates free arachidonic acid to the labile prostaglandin endoperoxides PGG_2 (and PGH_2). Endoperoxides and the metabolic intermediates in the synthesis of TXA_2 by thromboxane synthase (in platelets) or prostacyclin (PGI_2) by prostacyclin synthase (in vascular cells). Aspirin (acetylsalicylic acid) acetylates a serine residue at position 529 (Ser529) of cyclo-oxygenase, rendering the enzyme functionally inactive. Irreversible inactivation of cyclo-oxygenese by aspirin (or reversible inactivation by other NSAIDs) blocks the formation of TXA_2 and PGI_2 by platelets and vascular cells, respectively.

tion of aspirin presumably unmasks a subclinical hemostatic defect [96].

Aspirin does not significantly impair the process of platelet adhesion, as measured in vitro by platelet retention on glass-bead filters or adhesion of subendothelial structures of vessel walls. Aspirin does, however, inhibit platelet aggregation and release. Measurement of platelet aggregation in vitro by the turbidometric method characteristically shows that aspirin administration completely blocks aggregation in response to arachidonate, abolishes the second wave of irreversible aggregation in response to epinephrine and low concentrations of ADP, and partially inhibits collagen-induced aggregation. Those effects persist for 4 to 7 days after a single oral dose, when blood salicylate levels are no longer detectable [97], which corresponds to the life span of platelets and indicates the irreversibility of the inhibitory action of aspirin on platelets. The earlier normalization of the bleeding time reflects the emergence of a sufficient cohort of uninhibited platelets from the bone marrow following the decay of blood salicylate levels to achieve normal in-vivo primary hemostasis. The inhibitory effects of aspirin on aggregation are accompanied by inhibition of degranulation and secretion of ATP, ADP, serotonin, and other platelet-granule constituents.

Aspirin irreversibly inhibits cyclo-oxygenase by acetylating the enzyme [85–88]. Therefore, the capacity of a cell to recover from that inhibitory effect depends on *de-novo* synthesis of nonacetylated cyclo-oxygenase. Since platelets essentially are incapable of new protein synthesis, the formation of TXA_2 following the administration of aspirin is blocked for the remaining lifetime of exposed platelets. The inhibitory effect of aspirin on vascular cyclo-oxygenase that leads to PGI_2 production tends to neutralize its antiplatelet effect in inhibiting platelet cyclo-oxygenase and TXA_2 production, thus creating an "aspirin dilemma." That problem has prompted attempts to find a low, platelet-selective dose of aspirin that spares vascular endothelial cyclo-oxygenase. The issue of a differential sensitivity of platelet and vascular cyclo-oxygenase to aspirin remains unsettled [81,98–100]. It has been found that a single low dose of aspirin (40–80 mg) can almost completely inhibit platelet aggregation and TXA_2 synthesis while largely sparing endothelial PGI_2-forming capacity [100–103]. Repeated administration of very low doses of aspirin causes cumulative inhibition of platelet cyclo-

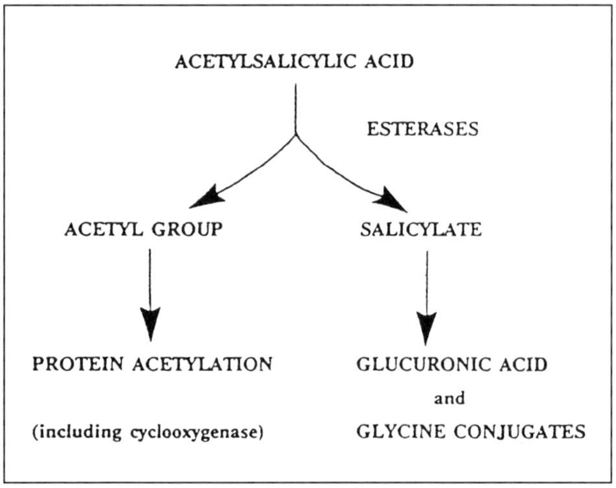

Fig. 27-5. Acetylsalicylic acid (aspirin) undergoes hydrolysis by esterases in the stomach and in peripheral tissues and is converted to acetyl groups and salicylate in the process. Acetyl groups acetylate a variety of proteins, the most important of which is cyclo-oxygenase in platelets and endothelial cells. Salicylate is inactive, although some evidence supports the view that this metabolic product of aspirin may inhibit acetylation of cyclo-oxygenase.

oxygenase. Steady-state inhibition of less than 90 to 95 percent of platelet TXA_2 formation is achieved with aspirin dosages of 20–40 mg/day in normal subjects and in patients with coronary artery disease [104–107]. However, long-term administration of conventially formulated aspirin at low dosages also partially suppresses vascular PGI_2 formation [108,109]. Therefore, biochemical selectivity of that regimen for platelets is relative, at best, and not absolute.

The relative selectivity of low-dosage aspirin in blocking the generation of platelet TXA_2, with less inhibition of endothelial PGI_2, may not be due simply to differences in the sensitivity of the cyclo-oxygenases of the two cell types to aspirin. An alternative explanation for apparent aspirin selectivity involves the previously noted presystemic metabolism of aspirin. Low-dosage aspirin administration sufficiently raises blood aspirin levels in the portal system to acetylate all platelets during presystemic recirculation. Because aspirin is extensively hydrolyzed in the liver and lungs, insufficient concentrations of aspirin are released into the systemic circulation to inhibit endothelial cyclo-oxygenase throughout the vascular tree [110]. Furthermore, the salicylate that accumulates in the systemic circulation after the presystemic metabolism of aspirin actually inhibits the acetylation of vascular cyclo-oxygenase by any residual circulating aspirin [111,112]. Low dosages of enteric-coated aspirin preparations may be particularly effective in that regard, since little or no aspirin escapes the portal circulation to reach the systemic circulation following their oral administration [113–116]. At the same time, such aspirin preparations prolong bleeding time, inhibit platelet aggregation, and inhibit more than 99 percent of TXA_2 production at a dosage of 325 mg every other day [117].

The question of dosage-selective inhibition of platelet cyclo-oxygenase remains unsettled, but platelets and endothelial cells clearly differ in their abilities to synthesize new uninhibited enzyme. Endothelial-cell PGI_2 production can rapidly recover from inhibition by aspirin because new, nonacetylated cyclo-oxygenase is synthesized with the decay of blood aspirin levels. In contrast, the anucleate platelet is virtually incapable of new-protein synthesis. Regardless of the dosage, however, there is overwhelming clinical evidence that aspirin's antithrombotic effects through TXA_2 inhibition, and possibly other mechanisms, predominate [118,119].

CLINICAL USE OF ASPIRIN

Aspirin has been clearly demonstrated to have beneficial effects in a variety of vascular and thrombotic disorders. In 1953, Dr. Lawrence L. Craven described his personal 7-year clinical experience of administering "one aspirin a day" to 1,465 healthy male subjects "who were overweight and known to lead a sedentary life"; he reported that "not one of them developed coronary occlusion or coronary insufficiency" [120]. Aspirin appears to be clinically effective in patients with unstable angina, myocardial infarction, aortocoronary bypass grafts, and transient cerebrovascular ischemic attacks. In some situations, other drugs administered concurrently appear to exert additive or synergistic beneficial actions. The optimal dosage and duration of aspirin therapy in these clinical situations remain controversial.

The Antiplatelet Trialists' Collaboration has recently published the results of meta-analyses combining patient data across all methodologically sound trials of prophylactic antiplatelet therapy available for review before March 1990 [120–123]. The most widely tested regimen was aspirin, 75 to 325 mg daily, although trials of other antiplatelet drugs also were included. The studies concluded that antiplatelet agents given to a wide range of patients at increased risk for occlusive vascular disease reduced all-cause mortality, vascular mortality, vascular events (including nonfatal myocardial infarction, nonfatal stroke, and vascular death), and nonfatal myocardial infarction. Benefit was observed among patients with unstable angina, suspected acute myocardial infarction, past history of myocardial infarction, nonfatal stroke, TIA, peripheral vascular disease, and those having vascular procedures. Low-risk patients receiving antiplatelet agents had reduced nonfatal myocardial infarction only.

The Physicians' Health Study reported the premature termination of a randomized, double-blind, placebo-controlled trial of aspirin in the primary prevention of mortality from cardiovascular disease [124]. In that trial of 22,000 male U.S. physicians 40 to 84 years of age, randomized to 325 mg of aspirin on alternate days or placebo, a significant 44-percent reduction in the risk of myocardial infarction was found in the aspirin group after an average follow-up of 5 years. Significant benefits of aspirin were found on both nonfatal and fatal myocardial infarction. Simultaneously, a study of a smaller number of British physicians on a different aspirin regimen (500 mg daily) for 6 years failed to demonstrate a significant beneficial effect of the drug on the incidence of first myocardial infarction, stroke, and total cardiovascular mortality [125].

Both the American and the British studies noted an increased risk of hemorrhagic strokes (statistically significant in the American study) among those in the aspirin group. Nevertheless, when all nonfatal myocardial infarctions, strokes, and vascular deaths from all causes were combined in the U.S. study, those receiving aspirin still showed a significant reduction in risk [126]. A number of additional randomized, placebo-controlled trials of the efficacy of aspirin in primary prevention are underway. These studies will be required to resolve whether the beneficial effects of aspirin outweigh its hazards, particularly intracranial hemorrhage, in primary prevention of myocardial infarction in both healthy and high-risk subjects. Information is notably deficient regarding the role of aspirin in primary prevention in women, a problem that is being currently addressed by the Nurses' Health Study of 40,000 nurses over 50 years of age with no previous history of cardiovascular disease [127].

A subgroup of the Physician's Health Study with chronic stable angina was found to benefit from aspirin in reducing the risk of first myocardial infarction to at least the same degree as the asymptomatic men in the trial [128]. The Swedish Angina Pectoris Aspirin Trial randomized patients with chronic stable angina (and without a history of prior myocardial infarction) to aspirin, 75 mg daily, or placebo: aspirin reduced the incidence of myocardial infarction and sudden death by 34 percent [129].

The value of aspirin in patients with unstable angina has been clearly established. Death and myocardial infarction, the principal end-points, were halved after 12 weeks in men with unstable angina given a daily dose of 325 mg buffered aspirin, compared with matching placebo [130]. The beneficial effects continued for up to 1 year after completion of the formal 12-week trial, and the concurrent use of beta blockers was found to have an additive effect. In another trial, men and women with unstable angina derived equal benefit from the use of aspirin, 325 mg four times daily [131]. In that study also, the incidence of cardiac death or nonfatal myocardial infarction was halved by aspirin. Sulfinpyrazone, either alone or in addition to aspirin, provided no benefit. Similar findings were reported by the Research Group on Instability in Coronary Artery Disease in Southeast Sweden (RISC—Risk of Myocardial Infarction or Death), in which an aspirin dose of 75 mg daily significantly reduced the risk of myocardial infarction and death in patients with unstable angina or non-Q-wave myocardial infarction after 3 months and after 1 year of study [132,133]. The RISC study noted a beneficial effect of aspirin in patients with both symptomatic and silent ischemia, as detected by predischarge exercise testing [134]. The study also found that its aspirin regimen reduced the risk of myocardial infarction and death after treatment for 5 days but had no effect during the first two days of treatment [132]. In another study, however, the risk of nonfatal and fatal myocardial infarction was markedly reduced in the early phase of unstable angina in patients receiving aspirin, 325 mg twice daily [135,136].

A number of well-conducted trials of aspirin (in daily dosages ranging from 300 mg to 2,000 mg) have evaluated the efficacy of aspirin in secondary prevention after myocardial infarction [137–145]. In most of those studies, a trend toward reduced mortality was found in patients treated with aspirin. When data from six of the trials were combined, using accepted statistical methods, the overall reduction in total mortality was estimated to be between 8 and 15 percent [137]. Subsequently, the second International Study of Infarct Survival (ISIS-2) in over 17,000 patients found that aspirin, 162.5 mg daily, started within 24 hours of acute myocardial infarction, with or without streptokinase, reduced the occurrence of cardiovascular mortality at 5 weeks. The combination of aspirin and streptokinase was significantly more effective than either drug alone [146]. More recently, aspirin, 50 mg daily, started 8 days after first myocardial infarction, was reported to decrease significantly the incidence of reinfarction when used in combination with either dipyridamole or ticlopidine in comparison with no antiplatelet therapy [147].

When aspirin (100 mg daily) was started 24 hours after aortocoronary bypass surgery, graft patency was significantly improved at 4 months from 68 to 90 percent in a placebo-controlled, prospective, double-blind trial [148]. Other trials have confirmed the efficacy of antiplatelet drugs, specifically aspirin, in that setting provided treatment is started before surgery or within 36 hours after the operation [148]. Antiplatelet prophylaxis started more than 48 hours after surgery has shown no benefit [138]. (The results of trials using dipyridamole in conjunction with aspirin to prevent bypass graft occlusion are reviewed later in this section.)

Aspirin has been found to be effective in preventing stroke or death in patients with TIAs and appears to be superior to oral anticoagulants in that setting [136,137]. Several large-scale trials have documented the efficacy of aspirin [92,150–152] and the lack of efficacy of dipyridamole or sulfinpyrazone in preventing these end-points in patients with TIAs. Following signal TIAs, the Swedish Aspirin Low-dose Trial (SALT) reported an 18-percent reduction in stroke or death in patients who began to take aspirin compared with placebo within 4 months of initial symptoms [153]. A coincidental finding in some of the trials of secondary prevention after myocardial infarction was a definite trend toward reduction in strokes by aspirin [49,55], confirming the benefit of aspirin in cerebrovascular ischemic syndromes. Although aspirin appears to decrease the risk of stroke or death in patients with TIAs, evidence for its effect in reducing the frequency of further TIAs is less convincing. Two trials have failed to confirm a reduction in TIA, stroke, or death by aspirin in patients with TIAs [154,155]. A study of the dose-effect of aspirin in patients with TIAs showed no difference in vascular outcomes over 2.6 years in patients treated with 30 mg/day or 283 mg/day aspirin [156]. A recent analysis suggests that higher-dosage aspirin may be more beneficial in these patients [157], but studies indicating improved efficacy of higher dosages used combinations of other antiplatelet drugs. Although there has been controversy concerning the efficacy of aspirin in stroke prevention in women, aggregate meta-analysis of the large antiplatelet trials do not indicate a differential effect of aspirin according to gender [158].

The reported efficacy of aspirin in a variety of other thrombotic and vascular disorders will require confirmation. Aspirin (900 mg/day) has been shown to retard the progression of atherosclerotic peripheral vascular diseases in one double-blind, placebo-controlled randomized trial [159]; the addition of dipyridamole (225 mg/day) enhanced the beneficial effect of aspirin. Other trials have demonstrated salutary effects of aspirin in some patients with peripheral vascular disease [121,160]. Although oral anticoagulants and heparin are the preferred therapy for the prophylaxis of venous thromboembolism, one study has demonstrated the effectiveness of aspirin in patients with fractured hips and those undergoing hip replacement [85], situations in which prophylaxis with anticoagulants is known to be more difficult. Another trial found the combination of aspirin and sulfinpyrazone to be effective in the prophylaxis of deep-vein thrombosis in patients undergoing total hip replacement [161]. The Antiplatelet Trialists' Collaboration analyzed 62 trials in 9,000 patients and concluded that antiplatelet therapy may reduce the incidence of deep-vein thrombosis and pulmonary embolism in a variety of surgical and medical settings [123]. Aspirin may be superior to warfarin in preventing recurrent stenoses after transluminal coronary angioplasty, especially in patients with longer histories of angina [162]. Aspirin also has been shown to limit reocclusion following successful thrombolysis [163]. Earlier studies suggested that antiplatelet therapy with a combination of aspirin and dipyridamole may be effective when given early in pregnancy to patients at high risk of preeclampsia, fetal-growth retardation, or both [164]. However, recently completed trials fail to support the routine use of aspirin in pregnant women at increased risk of preeclampsia or intrauterine growth retardation [165]. There is anecdotal evidence that aspirin, administered in conjunction with corticosteroids, may reduce the risk of spontaneous abortion in patients with lupus anticoagulants [166]. Aspirin (160 mg daily) has been found to be effective in preventing shunt thrombosis in patients undergoing chronic hemodialysis [167].

Despite improvements in valve design, thromboembolic complications remain a serious problem after cardiac valve replacement. Although lifelong high-intensity prophylactic anticoagulation with warfarin is used routinely in patients with mechanical valves and in patients with tissue valves complicated by atrial fibrillation or previous embolism, major systemic embolism still occurs at a rate of 2 to 3 percent per year [168]. To reduce that residual risk, the addition of an antiplatelet agent is recommended. The possible efficacy of dipyridamole is discussed below. Earlier studies found that the addition of aspirin at dosages of up to 1,200 mg daily significantly reduced embolic complications but caused an increased risk of serious bleeding [169,170]. More recently, a randomized, double-blind, placebo-controlled trial tested the efficacy and safety of adding aspirin (100 mg daily) to warfarin (target INR 3.0 to 4.5) in 370 patients with mechanical heart valves or with high-risk tissue valves. The addition of aspirin reduced mortality, particularly from vascular causes, together with major systemic embolism. Although there was some increase in bleeding, the risk of the combined treatment was more than offset by the considerable benefit [171].

As noted in the discussion of anticoagulants, warfarin has been the established prophylactic therapy to prevent systemic embolism in patients with nonrheumatic atrial fibrillation. However, the recently published Stroke Prevention in Atrial Fibrillation (SPAF) II trial [44], which compared warfarin (adjusted to an INR of 2.0–4.5) to aspirin (325 mg daily) in 1,100 patients with atrial fibrillation, found that although warfarin appeared to be more effective than aspirin for the prevention of ischemic strokes, it was associated with more hemorrhagic strokes. The study suggested that aspirin can be recommended for many younger, low-risk patients; in higher-risk groups (e.g., patients with previous TIAs or strokes and those with cardiac abnormalities), in whom the risk of thromboembolism during aspirin treatment was almost twice as high as for those taking warfarin, warfarin remains clearly indicated [172].

Despite an impressive volume of data that has accumulated in the literature to demonstrate the efficacy of aspirin in the primary and secondary prevention of a wide variety of vascular and thrombotic disorders, the shortcomings of aspirin as an antithrombotic agent must be considered. It is only partially effective in most clinical situations and completely ineffective in some others. Experimental studies have suggested that the antiplatelet effects of aspirin may be lost in settings where catecholamine surges and pathologically elevated shear stress are encountered [173].

OTHER NONSTEROIDAL ANTI-INFLAMMATORY DRUGS (NSAIDs)

Since the establishment of aspirin as a widely used antiplatelet drug, a number of newer agents have been introduced that also act primarily by inhibiting the formation or action of endoperoxides and TXA_2 or by shifting the balance of vascular PGI_2/platelet TXA_2 production to favor antiplatelet activity. These agents include other nonsteroidal anti-inflammatory drugs (NSAIDs), fish oils (omega-3 fatty acids), thromboxane synthase inhibitors, endoperoxide-TXA_2 receptor antagonists, and PGI_2 and its synthetic analogues. These predominantly investigational therapeutic modalities are briefly reviewed here.

Other NSAIDs, such as indomethacin, phenylbutazone, piroxicam, naproxen, diclofenac, meclofenamic acid, ibuprofen, and sulindac, interfere with platelet function through a mechanism similar to that of aspirin [174–176]. However, these drugs are reversible rather than irreversible inhibitors of cyclo-oxygenase. Therefore, their antiplatelet actions are short-lived, generally lasting no longer than 6 hours, depending on the half-life of the drug [177].

OMEGA-3 FATTY ACIDS

Epidemiologic studies of Greenland Eskimos in comparison with mainland Danes have suggested that a reduced incidence of coronary atherosclerosis, myocardial infarction, and occlusive vascular disease might be attributed to their distinctive diet, which is rich in marine lipids [178,179]. Subsequently, it has been found that the consumption of fish by a cohort of middle-aged Dutch men followed for 20 years lowered the mortality from coronary heart disease by more than 50 percent [180]. The Western

Electric Study likewise demonstrated an inverse correlation between fish ingestion and mortality from coronary artery disease [181]. This protective effect was observed with an average daily intake of as little as 30 g fish (equivalent to one or two fish dishes per week). More recently, striking pathologic evidence of retardation of the development and progression of coronary atherosclerosis has been reported in hyperlipidemic swine that were fed an atherogenic diet supplemented with cod liver oil [182]. There have been several randomized trials of fish-oil supplementation to prevent restenosis after coronary angioplasty. Review of those studies [183], which utilized up to 6 g/day of omega-3 fatty acids, have shown mixed results.

A number of factors may contribute to the protective effect of fish oils on atherosclerotic cardiovascular disease [184–186]. Omega-3 polyunsaturated fatty acid contained in fish oils have hypolipidemic effects, lowering serum cholesterol and low density lipoprotein (LDL) cholesterol and triglyceride levels without affecting high density lipoprotein (HDL) cholesterol [187,188], although other studies have reported elevations in LDL cholesterol concentrations in some cases [189]. The antithrombotic effects of fish oils also may be partly attributed to favorable alterations in blood rheology, cell-membrane fluidity [190], and anti-inflammatory effects [191]. Another significant antiatherogenic action of fish oils is thought to be mediated by their antiplatelet effects; individuals ingesting diets rich in these marine lipids have a mild clinical bleeding tendency, prolonged bleeding times, mild thrombocytopenia, and abnormalities in platelet aggregation in vitro.

The predominant polyunsaturated fatty acids in the Eskimo diet belong to the family of omega-3 (or N-3) fatty acids, so designated because the first double bond is always located on the third carbon atom from the methyl (omega) terminus [192]. The major omega-3 fatty acids in fish oils are eicosapentaenoic acid (EPA) and docosahexanoic acid (DHA). EPA is a 20-carbon polyunsaturated fatty acid with 5 double bonds and is therefore abbreviated C20 : 5, omega-3. DHA is a 22-carbon fatty acid with 6 double bonds, abbreviated C22 : 6, omega-3. In contrast, AA (C20 : 4) belongs to the omega-6 family of fatty acids. Cold-water fish contain the largest amounts of EPA and DHA.

The antithrombotic alterations in platelet-vascular interactions promoted by fish oils have been thought to be due, at least in part, to competition between EPA and AA for cyclo-oxygenase. TXA_2 formed from the action of cyclo-oxygenase on AA substrate in platelets is a potent activator of platelets and vasoconstrictor; however, TXA_3, which is produced from EPA, has virtually no biologic activity. In contrast, both PGI_2 (derived from AA) and PGI_3 (derived from EPA) produced by vascular endothelial cells have comparable actions as vasodilators and platelet inhibitors [193–197]. Thus, diets rich in omega-3 fatty acids promote the formation of TXA_3 and PGI_3 over TXA_2 and PGI_2 by platelets and blood vessels, respectively, favorably shifting the balance of those eicosanoids toward an antithrombotic effect. The relationships are shown in Fig. 27-6. It has been emphasized that rather large and potentially unpalatable doses of medicinal fish-oil supplements may be required to alter cell-membrane fatty-acid contents (ratios of EPA to AA in platelet membranes approximating unity) that simulate those attained with Eskimo diets [195].

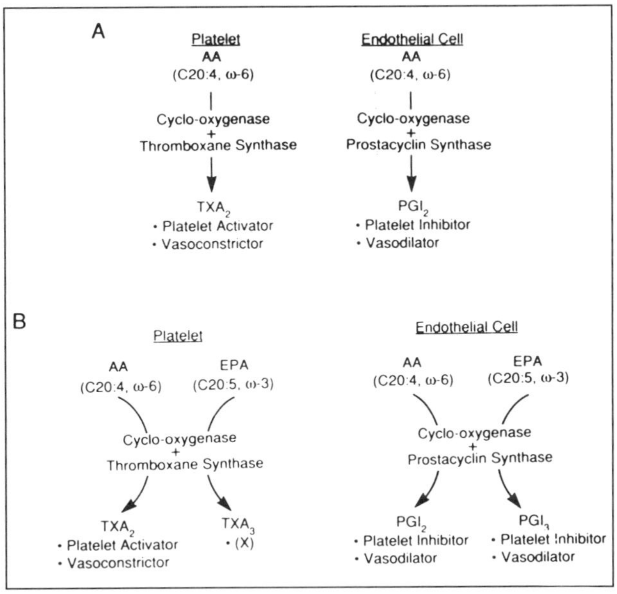

Fig. 27-6. Effects of omega-3 (ω-3) fatty acids on platelet–vessel wall interactions. **A.** The predominant substrate for cyclo-oxygenase in platelets and vascular endothelial cells of subjects ingesting a Western diet is arachidonic acid (AA), an ω-6 fatty acid. AA oxygenation in platelets leads to the formation of the potent platelet aggregator and vasoconstrictor TXA_2; the biologic actions of platelet TXA_2 tend to be offset by the production of the platelet inhibitor and vasodilator PGI_2 by oxygenation of AA in endothelial cells. **B.** In subjects ingesting an Eskimo diet or in those supplementing their diets with medicinal fish oil, eicosapentaenoic acid (EPA), an ω-3 fatty acid, competes with AA for cyclo-oxygenase in both platelets and endothelial cells. In platelets, EPA is converted to the biologically inactive TXA_3; in endothelial cells, it is converted to PGI_3, which retains the antithrombotic properties of PGI_2. (Reprinted with permission from Schafer AI. The platelet life cycle: normal function and qualitative disorders. In RI Handin, SE Lux, TP Stossel, eds., Blood. Principles and Practice of Hematology. Philadelphia; Lippincott, 1995. Pp. 1095–1127.)

THROMBOXANE-SYNTHASE INHIBITORS AND THROMBOXANE-RECEPTOR ANTAGONISTS

The failure of aspirin and other cyclo-oxygenase inhibitors to block completely platelet TXA_2 production without affecting vascular PGI_2 production could be circumvented by the use of platelet TxS inhibitors. Theoretically, such agents would offer the additional advantage of redirecting platelet-derived endoperoxides to neighboring endothelial cells to provide substrates for enhanced PGI_2 synthesis [198,199]. Imidazole compounds are known to act as TxS inhibitors, and dazoxiben has emerged from a series of substituted imidazoles as a potentially useful orally administered drug [200–204]. Administration of dazoxiben to human subjects leads, as expected, to marked suppression of TXA_2 formation [205]. However, in-vitro platelet aggregation is not consistently inhibited by TxS inhibitors [206–208]. That finding may be due to the direct agonist effects of endoperoxides, which accumulate with TxS inhibition and which themselves occupy and activate the platelet TXA_2 receptor. This explanation is supported by the finding of the additive inhibitory effects on platelet aggregation with the use of endoperoxide-thromboxane receptor antagonists [209].

Clinical experience with the use of TxS inhibitors has been generally disappointing to date. In addition to the possible agonist actions of accumulated endoperoxides during TxS inhibition noted above, these reversible TxS inhibitors have short plasma half-lives and provide only incomplete suppression of TXA_2 production during long-term dosing [208]. Dazoxiben has failed to produce improvement in the objective parameters of Raynaud's phenomenon in various trials [210–212]. Another imidazole analogue has been found to be ineffective in improving renal or liver function in the hepatorenal syndrome [213]. Short-term dosing studies with dazoxiben have failed to influence the time to exercise-induced angina [214,215], and beneficial effects of the drug on the hemodynamic response to atrial pacing in patients with chronic stable angina have been, at best, marginal [216,217].

Antagonists of thromboxane-endoperoxide receptors represent a potentially valuable antiplatelet therapeutic approach [218]. Several such drugs have been developed for clinical use, some of which relatively selectively block platelet TXA_2 receptors, while others also act on TXA_2 receptors in other tissues, such as vascular cells [219]. Thromboxane-receptor antagonists have the advantage over TxS inhibitors in that they block the effects of both TXA_2 and the endoperoxide PGH_2, whereas TxS inhibitors, as previously noted, do not prevent the agonist effects of endoperoxides if they accumulate. The possibility of the combined use of a TxS inhibitor and a thromboxane-receptor antagonist has particular appeal as clinical antiplatelet therapy: by blocking thromboxane receptors, the proaggregatory actions of the endoperoxides should be prevented, while endoperoxide diversion to endothelial cells is permitted and, hence, so is augmented vascular PGI_2 production [220].

Ridogrel, a dual thromboxane synthase inhibitor and thromboxane-endoperoxide receptor blocker, has been found to possess more potent antiplatelet effects than aspirin in human volunteers [221]. However, in a trial of 907 patients with myocardial infarction receiving streptokinase thrombolytic therapy, adjunctive ridogrel was not found to be superior to aspirin in potentiating fibrinolysis and preventing rethrombosis [222]. Those results, which show comparably suboptimal responses to aspirin and ridogrel, may be attributed to the relatively modest thromboxane-receptor antagonism of ridogrel or the possibility that pathways of platelet activation or stimuli to thrombosis-rethrombosis that are not affected by aspirin or ridogrel may be operative in this clinical setting.

STIMULI OF PLATELET cAMP AND cGMP

Agents that inhibit TXA_2 formation (such as aspirin) can block platelet aggregation and release in response to weak agonists, but they have little or no effect on aggregation and release in response to strong agonists and no effect on platelet adhesion, the initial event in the process of primary hemostasis. In contrast, drugs that increase platelet cAMP or cGMP, of which prostanoids (and their analogues) and NO donors are the most potent, can also prevent platelet aggregation induced by strong agonists, as well as platelet adhesion to varying degrees.

PGI_2, which raises platelet cAMP, is the most potent naturally occurring platelet inhibitor currently identified. Its clinical use, however, has been limited by its extreme lability at physiologic pH and its potent vasoactive effects. The possibility of in-vivo desensitization of platelet responsiveness with prolonged infusions of PGI_2 might also limit its therapeutic potential [223,224].

The clinical use of PGI_2 is currently largely restricted to extracorporeal circuits, such as cardiopulmonary bypass, charcoal hemoperfusion, and hemodialysis. In those settings, the regional administration of PGI_2 prevents extracorporeal platelet consumption and reduces the risk of platelet embolization and bleeding [225]. The intravenous infusion of PGI_2 has resulted in transient beneficial effects in coronary artery disease [226,227], peripheral obliterative arterial and vasospastic disorders [228,229], and thrombotic thrombocytopenic purpura [230].

Problems with the chemical instability, short in-vivo half-life and adverse hemodynamic actions of PGI_2 have prompted considerable research to synthesize stable analogues of the prostanoids. Carbacyclin analogues possess comparable antiplatelet and hemodynamic effects and offer the advantage of increased chemical stability. Like PGI_2, however, these compounds are rapidly metabolized and inactivated after infusion, leading to short-lived biologic activity in vivo [231]. Iloprost is a chemically stable synthetic PGI_2 analogue that is a more potent inhibitor of platelet aggregation than is PGI_2 or PGE_1 [232], has less pronounced vasoactive properties than the natural prostanoid [233], and can be administered orally. Infusions of iloprost (0.5–2.0 ng/kg/ml) have been reported to exert long-lasting beneficial clinical effects in patients with ischemia of the extremities [234]. However, hypercoagulability and enhanced platelet reactivity have been observed during and sometimes after iloprost infusion [235]. The development of a well-tolerated, orally effective analogue of long duration of activity and high selectivity for antiplatelet actions is still awaited [231].

Organic nitrates have platelet-inhibitory properties, acting through an increase in platelet cGMP [236,237]. NO donors inhibit both platelet adhesion and platelet thrombus formation in vivo [238], as well as having vasodilatory properties. Preliminary results of human trials that compare continuous infusion of the NO donor linsidomine (SIN-1) to isosorbide nitrate in unstable angina and NO donors to diltiazem with percutaneous transluminal coronary angioplasty have failed to demonstrate superior clinical benefit of the NO donors [239].

DIPYRIDAMOLE

Dipyridamole, unlike aspirin, does not prolong bleeding time [240]. Dipyridamole has been found to inhibit platelet adhesion in some but not all studies [241–244]. It inhibits platelet aggregation in vitro only at concentrations that are considerably higher than those attained in blood with clinical use [175,245,246]. Dipyridamole prolongs platelet survival in various thrombotic and vascular disorders that are characterized by rapid platelet turnover, such as arterial and venous thrombosis, prosthetic heart valves, prosthetic grafts, and possibly coronary artery disease [247–249]. The effects of dipyridamole contrast with those of aspirin, the use of which is associated with prolongation of bleeding time and impaired platelet aggregation but no changes in platelet survival.

The precise mechanism of antithrombotic action of dipyridamole remains unclear and may be multifactorial [136,249]. Some studies have suggested that the drug acts by directly stimulating the synthesis of PGI_2 by vascular endothelium [250,251], although that has been disputed [253,254]; potentiating the effects of PGI_2 [255] and inhibiting platelet TXA_2 formation [256]; inhibiting phosphodiesterase, thereby raising platelet cAMP levels [257,258]; and blocking the uptake of adenosine into endothelial cells, red cells, and leukocytes, resulting in the local accumulation of this platelet-inhibitory and vasodilating compound in the thrombotic microenvironment [250, 259–261]. Several of those effects may not occur at concentrations of dipyridamole that are attained in plasma during therapy.

In general, controlled clinical studies have failed to demonstrate any antithrombotic efficacy by dipyridamole when it is used alone [250]. In fact, dipyridamole has not been found to add to the beneficial effects of aspirin in the secondary prevention of myocardial infarction [139,140], maintaining coronary bypass graft patency [262], or reducing the incidence of stroke in patients with prior TIAs or stroke [150,263]. However, dipyridamole may exert additive or synergistic effects when used in combination with aspirin or warfarin in certain selected situations. Specifically, dipyridamole may be effective in the prevention of angiographically documented progression of peripheral occlusive arterial disease after 2 years when combined with aspirin [159]. The addition of dipyridamole to warfarin has been found to reduce significantly the incidence of major systemic embolism in patients with mechanical heart valves [264–266]. Data are not available on direct benefit and risk comparisons between aspirin [171] and dipyridamole as additions to oral anticoagulants in patients with high-risk cardiac valve prostheses.

SULFINPYRAZONE

Sulfinpyrazone is a uricosuric drug that has structural similarity to phenylbutazone [81,267]. Its antiplatelet effects were suggested when it was found to restore the shortened platelet survival of some patients with gout [268]. After gastrointestinal absorption, sulfinpyrazone is slowly metabolized from its sulfoxide form to a sulfide [269–271], possibly by bacterial degradation following biliary excretion of the parent drug [272]. In vitro, the sulfide metabolite has been found to be considerably more active than the parent compound in its antiplatelet actions [268,273]. The formation of a slowly formed active metabolite may account for the finding that the effects of sulfinpyrazone on platelets take several days to appear and disappear [154].

Similar to dipyridamole and unlike aspirin, sulfinpyrazone normalizes the shortened platelet survival in various clinical situations [268,274,275]. There is equivocal evidence that sulfinpyrazone also inhibits platelet adhesion in vitro [276,277]. Sulfinpyrazone acts as an incomplete and reversible inhibitor of platelet cyclo-oxygenase [278,279], but this effect is unlikely to account entirely for the antiplatelet actions of the drug [280].

The clinical efficacy of sulfinpyrazone in the secondary prevention of myocardial infarction has been the subject of considerable controversy [281–286]. Interpretation of study results has been complicated by the possible antiarrhythmic effects of the drug and the beneficial effects of the concomitant use of beta blockers. Sulfinpyrazone, used either alone or in combination with aspirin, has been found to have no beneficial effects in patients with TIAs [92] or unstable angina [131]. As has been reported with aspirin, sulfinpyrazone appears to prevent arteriovenous shunt thrombosis [287].

TICLOPIDINE

Ticlopidine and its analog, clopidogrel, are thienopyridine derivatives that cause potent inhibition of ADP-induced platelet aggregation. They also cause lesser degrees of inhibition of aggregation in response to other stimuli that act in part by releasing endogenous ADP from platelet-dense granules [288,289]. These drugs exert their antiplatelet action primarily by inhibiting the binding of ADP to its specific platelet receptors that are coupled to inhibition of platelet adenylyl cyclase [290,291]. Earlier studies demonstrating inhibition by ticlopidine of fibrinogen binding to its platelet membrane glycoprotein (GP) IIb/IIIa receptor [292] probably reflected a downstream event following ADP-receptor blockade. Unlike aspirin, ticlopidine also inhibits shear stress–induced platelet aggregation, which is partially mediated by released ADP [293].

Full antiplatelet activity is obtained only 3 to 5 days after ticlopidine administration, and the bleeding time is not maximally prolonged until 5 to 6 days after starting ticlopidine [294]. The effects of ticlopidine persist for 4 to 8 days after drug discontinuation, suggesting an irreversible antiplatelet effect. Maximal platelet antiaggregatory action is found only after oral administration and cannot be reproduced in vitro at pharmacologic concentrations of the drug; that suggests that biologic activity is mediated by a metabolite of ticlopidine [288].

The most established clinical indication for the use of ticlopidine is in the prevention of stroke. The Ticlopidine versus Aspirin Stroke Study (TASS) [295] compared aspirin (650 mg twice daily) and ticlopidine (250 mg twice daily) in over 3,000 randomized patients with a history of TIA or minor ischemic stroke. Ticlopidine was found to be superior to aspirin for preventing stroke, with significant relative risk reductions for the primary end-points of nonfatal stroke or death from any cause (12%) as well as fatal and nonfatal stroke (21%) at 3 years. Subgroup analysis also showed that ticlopidine is more effective than aspirin for the prevention of recurrent TIAs during a 5-year follow-up period [296]. However, many patients enrolled in TASS were "aspirin failures" at the time of their qualifying events; therefore, the relative efficacy of ticlopidine versus aspirin for preventing stroke or TIA in patients not previously treated with aspirin remains uncertain [297]. In the Canadian-American Ticlopidine study, ticlopidine was found to be superior to placebo in the secondary prevention of stroke [298], but ticlopidine and aspirin have not yet been directly compared for this indication.

Although ticlopidine appears to be more effective than aspirin in certain clinical settings of cerebrovascular ischemia, its advantage may be at least partially offset by its considerably higher expense and the complication of infrequent (< 1%) but severe neutropenia. At this time, ticlopidine is generally considered to be indicated (at a recommended dosage of 250 mg twice daily) for patients with TIA or stroke who have aspirin intolerance or who fail with aspirin treatment.

Ticlopidine also has been shown to be effective in placebo-controlled clinical trials to prevent coronary artery bypass graft reocclusion [299] and to prevent death or myocardial infarction in patients with unstable angina [300], intermittent claudication [301], and nonproliferative diabetic retinopathy [302].

PLATELET MEMBRANE GLYCOPROTEIN IIb/IIIa ANTAGONISTS

The limited clinical efficacy of many of the antiplatelet drugs described so far has been attributed in part to their targeting of only specific, single platelet receptors or platelet metabolic pathways. It has been proposed that broad inhibition of platelet function should provide greater antithrombotic efficacy. To that end, a number of agents have been developed recently to interrupt the final common pathway of platelet aggregation, the binding of fibrinogen to its platelet membrane GPIIb/IIIa receptor. Platelet activation by any stimulus leads to the transition of the GPIIb/IIIa receptor to a high-affinity ligand-binding state. The multivalent adhesive glycoproteins fibrinogen (at sites of lower shear stress) and von Willebrand factor (at sites of high shear stress) can then bind to two platelets simultaneously, forming bridges between platelets in a process of platelet cohesion or aggregation [303–305]. The peptide recognition sequence arginine-glycine-aspartic acid (abbreviated as RGD), which is present in these adhesive molecules, mediates their binding to the GPIIb/IIIa receptor. Two general strategies to develop inhibitors of fibrinogen-GPIIb/IIIa interactions have utilized (1) monoclonal antibodies to GPIIb/IIIa and (2) small-molecule RGD analogues that compete with fibrinogen (or von Willebrand factor) for binding to platelet GPIIb/IIIa.

Monoclonal antibodies that block the GPIIb/IIIa receptor are potent inhibitors of platelet aggregation, both in vitro and in vivo. The monoclonal antibody known as 7E3, originally developed by Coller [306], has been extensively investigated in animal and human antithrombotic trials. Those studies have used either the Fab fragment of the mouse antibody or the Fab fragment of a chimeric antibody containing the variable regions of the mouse antibody and the constant regions of a human antibody [303,307].

The Evaluation of 7E3 for the Prevention of Ischemic Complications (EPIC) Investigators have recently reported that a chimeric monoclonal-antibody Fab fragment of 7E3 (c7E3 Fab), administered as a bolus and infusion to over 2,000 patients undergoing high-risk coronary angioplasty or atherectomy, resulted in a 35-percent reduction in the composite-event rate, primarily in the rate of nonfatal myocardial infarction and the need for emergency repeat angioplasty or bypass surgery [308]. Substantial blood loss was observed in the trial, however, resulting in a significant increase in the use of blood products. Serious bleeding complications were particularly noted at sites of femoral puncture. A pilot trial by the European Cooperative Study Group randomized 60 patients with unstable angina to bolus and infusion of either c7E3 Fab or placebo [309]. All patients were concomitantly treated with aspirin, intravenous nitroglycerin, and heparin. Results showed a trend to reduced rates of ischemia, reduced major events (deaths, infarcts, urgent interventions) during hospital stay, and angiographically demonstrated improvement in Thrombolysis in Myocardial Infarction (TIMI) flow and quantitative improvement of the lesions with c7E3 Fab–treated patients. No excess bleeding complications were observed, although the doses of 7E3 used were the same as in the EPIC trial. Another study has reported improved coronary artery patency and a trend for fewer ischemic events when 7E3 was used (in conjunction with heparin and aspirin) following thrombolytic therapy for acute myocardial infarction [310]. Administration of the antibody (a nonchimeric murine 7E3 Fab, used in bolus injections) was not associated with a higher bleeding risk.

Potential problems of monoclonal antibodies are their lack of reversibility and immunogenicity, although the latter may, to some extent, be circumvented by the use of "humanized" chimeric antibodies. Peptides containing RGD or an analogous amino acid sequence have been developed that compete with fibrinogen (or von Willebrand factor) and thus reversibly prevent platelet aggregation in response to any stimulus. A number of these RGD-containing peptides (disintegrins) are derived from snake venoms and leeches [311–315]. Remarkably, nuclear magnetic resonance has determined that the structure of ornatin and decorsin, two RGD-containing GPIIb/IIIa inhibitors from leeches, possess the same protein scaffold but different binding epitopes as two other leech-derived antithrombotic proteins that affect hemostasis by very different mechanisms, namely hirudin, a thrombin inhibitor, and antistasin, a factor Xa inhibitor [316]. To increase the metabolic stability, potency, and selectivity of the disintegrins, a number of cyclic peptides, peptidomimetic, and nonpeptide RGD mimetics have been synthesized [317–324]. Integrelin, which has been shown to improve thrombolysis when administered with hirudin in a canine model of coronary thrombosis [325], is currently in human clinical trials.

Several general problems with the clinical use of any platelet GPIIb/IIIa antagonist must be considered. All GPIIb/IIIa inhibitors currently available require intravenous administration, which limits their use to acute situations of thrombosis and reocclusion. Orally active compounds will be needed for use as long-term preventive therapy. Early clinical experience with these drugs already has emphasized the need for careful assessment of the risk of bleeding, particularly when treatment is combined with invasive procedures. Pharmacologic blockade of platelet GPIIb/IIIa would mimic to a great extent the inherited bleeding disorder Glanzmann's thrombasthenia [326]. The limitation of bleeding risk, which applies to potent antiplatelet drugs in general, is due to the inability of any known antithrombotic agent to discriminate between a pathologic thrombus and a protective hemostatic plug in its target of action.

OTHER ANTIPLATELET AGENTS

A number of other promising antiplatelet strategies await assessment of clinical efficacy and bleeding risk. While platelet-membrane GPIIb/IIIa antagonists interfere with the **final** common pathway of platelet aggregation, agents that block the interaction of von Willebrand factor with its platelet receptor on GPIb/IX should produce a global antiplatelet defect by interfering with the **initial** event of platelet activation, the process of platelet adhesion to the damaged vessel wall. Such a therapeutic strategy offers the additional theoretical advantage of inhibiting the entire cascade of platelet-activating events that follows adhesion, including not only platelet aggregation but also the preceding secretory reaction, which releases mitogens from platelet granules into the vessel wall. Agents that interfere with the interaction of von Willebrand factor with platelet GPIb/IX include monoclonal antibodies against von Willebrand factor, monoclonal antibodies against GPIb/IX, recombinant von Willebrand factor fragments (which bind to GPIb/IX and inhibit the binding of von Willebrand factor multimers to the receptor), and aurin tricarboxylic acid (which binds to von Willebrand factor multimers and prevents their interaction with the receptor) [327,328].

The most potent platelet stimulus is thrombin. Therefore, direct antithrombins (e.g., hirudin) would not only interrupt the formation of fibrin but also concurrently inhibit platelet aggregation [303,304]. Unlike heparin, hirudin does not need to complex with antithrombin III to inhibit thrombin; therefore, it can more effectively inhibit fibrin-bound thrombin. Direct antithrombins are considerably more potent than heparin in reducing platelet-thrombus formation in animal models of thrombosis [329,330]. It is not yet known, however, whether the optimal antiplatelet regimen will also be the optimal anticoagulant regimen of direct thrombin inhibitors [303].

FIBRINOLYTIC AGENTS

Plasminogen activators of both exogenous and endogenous origin have been used to convert plasminogen to plasmin (Fig. 27-7) and thereby dissolve fibrin thrombi. Streptokinase (SK) is a 47,000-Da protein derived from beta-hemolytic streptococci. SK does not convert plasminogen to plasmin enzymatically but binds to plasminogen in a stoichiometric manner. The SK-plasminogen complex that forms expresses plasmin activity [331]. SK has a plasma half-life of approximately 23 minutes. Because of its bacterial origin, allergic reactions do occur with standard use.

Derivatives of SK have been synthesized that become activated in vivo. Anisoylated plasminogen-SK activator

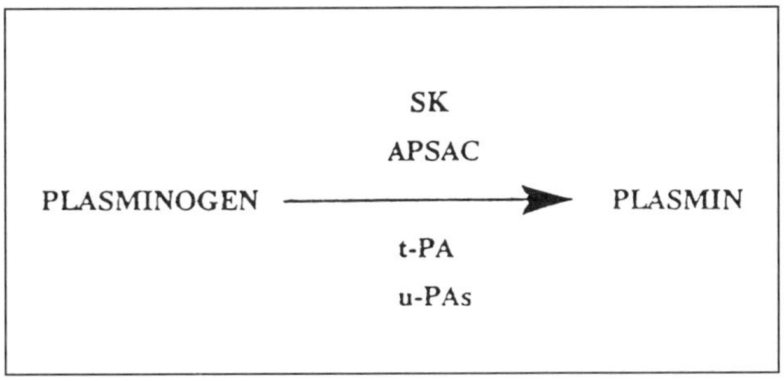

Fig. 27-7. Plasminogen activators convert plasminogen into plasmin. Streptokinase (SK) does so nonenzymatically, serving to induce an enzymatically active conformation in plasminogen on binding; the SK-derivative anisoylated plasminogen-streptokinase activator complex (APSAC) undergoes activation in plasma by the hydrolysis of the anisoyl group at the active site of plasminogen. Tissue-type plasminogen activators (t-PAs) and the urokinase-type plasminogen activator (u-PA), both endogenous activator classes, activate plasminogen enzymatically.

complex (APSAC) is one such agent in which the active site of plasminogen is acylated, then complexed to SK. Spontaneous deacylation occurs in vivo, which causes enzymatic activity to manifest. APSAC has a longer half-life than SK (90 minutes) and is not inhibited by endogenous plasmin inhibitors [332].

Urokinase (UK) is an endothelial-cell enzyme that converts plasminogen to plasmin directly. It is synthesized in a proenzymatic form known as single-chain urokinase-type plasminogen activator (scuPA) or prourokinase (PUK) [333]. This proenzyme has a molecular mass of 54 kDa and is converted to the enzymatically active form, high-molecular-weight two-chain urokinase (HMWtcUK) by proteolysis at the Lys 158-Ile 159 bond. The conversion occurs on exposure to plasmin; further proteolytic cleavage leads to the generation of a smaller molecule, conventional urokinase (low-molecular-weight two-chain urokinase, or LMWtcUK), which contains the active site but has lost the fibrin-binding domain (kringle region). scuPA is one of two important endogenous plasminogen activators that are fibrin specific by virtue of predominant activation of fibrin-bound plasminogen over ambient plasma plasminogen. scuPA itself may have slight intrinsic enzymatic activity that is attenuated by an endogenous plasma inhibitor [334]; alternatively, its selectivity may occur as a result of enhanced catalytic efficiency toward plasminogen bound to internal lysine-rich fibrin sequences [335]. scuPA and its derivatives have plasma half-lives ranging from 5 to 10 minutes.

Tissue-type plasminogen activator (t-PA) is the other major endogenous plasminogen activator [336]. It is a 67-kDa enzyme synthesized in a single-chain form by endothelial cells [337] that is converted to a two-chain form by the action of plasmin, factor Xa, or kallikrein [338]. It, too, is relatively fibrin selective, binding to fibrin and having greater catalytic efficiency toward plasminogen bound to fibrin than toward ambient plasma plasminogen [339]. The fibronectin "finger" domain and the second of two kringle domains confer fibrin-binding properties on the molecule [340]. The single-chain form of t-PA has an initial plasma half-life of 4 minutes and a terminal half-life of 46 minutes; the two-chain form has an initial half-life of approximately 5 minutes and a terminal half-life of approximately 46 minutes.

Thrombolytic agents have been used to lyse thrombi in virtually every vascular bed. Their use in deep venous thrombosis and pulmonary embolism was best characterized first in the Urokinase and Urokinase-Streptokinase Pulmonary Embolism Trials (UPET and USPET) [341,342]. In those trials, patients treated with UK with heparin or SK with heparin achieved more rapid pulmonary vascular reperfusion and reduction in pulmonary artery pressures than did patients treated with heparin alone. More recently, similar benefit has been demonstrated for t-PA [343]. Among the many trials of thrombolytic therapy in deep venous thrombosis, approximately one-half of patients manifest rapid lysis of 75 percent or more of thrombus in the proximal deep veins with thrombolytic treatment; that rate compares favorably with that observed with heparin alone (6%) [344]. Although these results for pulmonary embolism and deep venous thrombosis are encouraging, actual benefit to patients in terms of well-defined end-points, such as death and (recurrent) pulmonary embolism, have not been documented. Part of the problem in that regard stems from the relatively small patient sample sizes in the studies. Nevertheless, most authorities strongly recommend the use of lytic agents in patients with right ventricular dysfunction by echocardiography or massive pulmonary embolism to prevent acute cor pulmonale and sudden death [345] and in patients with extensive deep venous thrombosis to reduce the incidence of the postphlebitic syndrome [346–348]. Other venous disorders that are reportedly responsive to thrombolytic therapy include upper-extremity venous thrombosis [349], central retinal vein occlusion [350], Budd-Chiari syndrome [351], and right intracardiac thrombi [352].

Arterial thrombi also are susceptible to lysis by thrombolytic agents. In particular, in a variety of studies, intravenous SK and t-PA have been shown to be useful in acute coronary thrombosis associated with acute myocardial infarction. DeWood and colleagues showed in 1980 that coronary thrombus is present in at least 80 percent of patients who present within 6 hours of the onset of an acute Q-wave infarction [353]. Early attempts at treating evolving infarcts with thrombolytic agents were made over 25 years ago, but those trials involved prolonged infusions of SK or UK and were complicated by severe hemorrhagic complications [354]. Since the prospect of myocardial salvage depends critically on the rapidity of establishing reperfusion, later study designs have included relatively rapid administration of lytic agents to patients who present within 6 hours of the onset of pain. These studies [355–369] have demonstrated successful reperfusion using SK, t-PA, APSAC, UK, and scuPA, all of which involve brief (i.e., no more than 3 hours) infusions that minimize the incidence of hemorrhagic complications. The end-points of these studies differ significantly, but in general they illustrate the following points:

1. The earlier lytic therapy is begun, the better the outcome, as measured by improvements in ventricular function or mortality.
2. Functional benefit from reperfusion may extend beyond 6 hours after the onset of pain; however, the risk of myocardial rupture increases, especially between 12 and 24 hours.
3. Intravenous therapy is as efficacious as intracoronary therapy, is less costly, and, since it does not require cardiac catheterization, is associated with fewer hemorrhagic complications.
4. The clot-selective agents, t-PA and scuPA, are only relatively fibrinogen sparing at pharmacologically effective doses and appear not to be associated with a significantly lower incidence of hemorrhagic complications.
5. Thrombolytic therapy is, in general, a temporizing measure that should be followed at some later time with definitive mechanical therapy, such as angioplasty or bypass surgery.

Other arterial disorders in which thrombolytic therapy may be useful include peripheral arterial occlusion from emboli or atherothrombi [370,371] and selected patients with cerebrovascular occlusion [372,373]. As in patients with coronary atherothrombi, definitive correction of the residual stenosis after clot lysis remains an important issue.

The major complications of thrombolytic therapy that lessen enthusiasm for its use in patients with occlusive vascular disorders include hemorrhage and reocclusion. The incidence of hemorrhagic complications has been reduced by a variety of factors prevalent in the current therapeutic regimes, including the use of brief infusions of agent, minimizing of invasive vascular procedures, and excluding patients with hypertension or a history of stroke. Even with stringent adherence to those guidelines, however, hemorrhage remains a significant complication of therapy, with major hemorrhagic complications occurring in up to 15 percent of patients. Fibrin-selective agents were designed with the theoretical expectation that hemorrhagic complications would be reduced; unfortunately, despite the generation of a less lytic state with t-PA treatment than with, for example, SK, the incidence of bleeding is identical between the two patient groups. The reason for the apparent discrepancy is that even a relatively clot-selective thrombolytic agent cannot discriminate between an occlusive thrombus and a protective hemostatic plug [374]. Hence, measures that minimize exposure of patients with known or suspected hemostatic plugs in, for example, sites of arterial puncture, prior stroke, or prior gastrointestinal hemorrhage can be quite effective in minimizing hemorrhagic risk.

Reocclusion remains an additional vexing problem that appears to be more pronounced with SK (19%) [369,375] and t-PA (24%) [369,376] than with UK (4%) [377] in myocardial infarction. The pathophysiology of reocclusive phenomena has not been entirely explained, but it probably depends on the exposure of subendothelial matrix, which provides a surface rich in procoagulant activity and stimulatory to platelets. Thus far, heparin and aspirin therapy have not attenuated the incidence of reocclusion appreciably, although aspirin used with SK does provide additional mortality benefit compared with SK alone [163,360]. Interestingly, the thrombolytic agent that produces the greatest systemic lytic state, UK, is associated with the lowest incidence of reocclusion. For that reason, some authors have argued that a systemic lytic state is desirable and important for optimal outcome [376].

Among future developments in thrombolysis that may affect clinical practice are the use of combinations of agents (including adjunctive antiplatelet and antithrombin agents) to minimize cost and, possibly, hemorrhagic complications [335,377]. Other possibilities are identifying patients who are most likely to bleed and developing therapeutic strategies that optimize rates and times of reperfusion while minimizing the incidence of hemorrhage and reocclusion.

References

1. Rosenberg RD, Damus PS. The purification and mechanism of action of human antithrombin-heparin cofactor. J Biol Chem 1973; 248:6490–6505.
2. Rosenberg RD, Armand G, Lam L. Structure function relationships of heparin species. Proc Natl Acad Sci 1981; 75:3065–3068.
3. Hirsh J, Levine MN. Low molecular weight heparin. Blood 1992; 79:1–17.
4. Tollefsen DM, Majerus PW, Blank MK. Heparin cofactor II. J Biol Chem 1981; 257:2162–2169.
5. Walker FJ, Esmon CT. Interactions between heparin and factor Xa. Inhibition of prothrombin activation. Biochim Biophys Acta 1979; 585:405–415.
6. Kelton JG, Hirsh J. Bleeding associated with antithrombotic therapy. Sem Hematol 1980; 17:375–379.
7. Kelton JB, Levine MN. Heparin-induced thrombocytopenia. Semin Thromb Hemost 1986; 12:599–662.
8. King DJ, Kelton JG. Heparin-associated thrombocytopenia. Ann Int Med 1984; 100:535–540.
9. Whitlon DS, Sadowski JA, Suttie JW. Mechanism of coumarin action: significance of vitamin K epoxide reductase inhibition. Biochemistry 1978; 17:1371–1377.
10. Esmon CT, Sadowski MA, Suttie JW. A new carboxylation reaction. J Biol Chem 1975; 250:4744–4748.
11. Esmon CT, Suttie JW, Jackson CM. The functional significance of vitamin K action. Differences in phospholipid between normal and abnormal prothrombin. J Biol Chem 1975; 250:4095–4099.
12. Barritt DW, Jordan SC. Anticoagulant drugs in the treatment of pulmonary embolism. Lancet 1960; 1:1309–1311.
13. Hirsh J. Heparin. N Engl J Med 1991; 324:1565–1574.
14. Kakkar VV, Corrigan T, Spindler J. Efficacy of low doses of heparin in prevention of deep-vein thrombosis after major surgery. A double-blind randomized trial. Lancet 1972; 2:101–106.
15. Hirsh J, Genton E, Hull R. Treatment of venous thromboembolism. In J Hirsch, E Genton, R Hill, eds., Venous Thromboembolism. New York: Grune & Stratton, 1981. Pp. 122–144.
16. Salzman EW, et al. Management of heparin therapy. N Engl J Med 1975; 292:1046–1050.
17. Basu D, et al. A prospective study of the value of monitoring heparin treatment with the activated partial thromboplastin time. N Engl J Med 1972; 287:324–327.
18. Raschke RA, et al. The weight-adjusted heparin monogram compared with a standard monogram: a randomized controlled trial. Ann Int Med 1995; 119:874–881.
19. Hirsh J. Oral anticoagulant drugs. N Engl J Med 1991; 324:1865–1875.
20. Sevitt S, Gallagher NG. Prevention of venous thrombosis and pulmonary embolism in injured patients. Lancet 1959; 2:987–989.
21. Poller L, Taberner DA. Dosage and control of oral anticoagulants: an international collaborative survey. Brit J Haematol 1982; 1:479–485.
22. Hull R, et al. Different intensities of anticoagulation in the long-term treatment of proximal venous thrombosis. N Engl J Med 1982; 307:1676–1681.
23. Francis CW, et al. Two-step warfarin therapy. JAMA 1983; 249:374–378.
24. Collins R, et al. Reduction in fatal pulmonary embolism and venous thrombosis by perioperative administration of subcutaneous heparin. N Engl J Med 1988; 318:1162–1172.
25. Zilliacus H. On the specific treatment of thrombosis and pulmonary embolism with anticoagulants with particular reference to the post thrombotic sequelae. Acta Med Scand [Suppl] 1946; 171:1.
26. Cosgriff SW. Prophylaxis of recurrent embolism of intracardiac origin; protracted anticoagulant therapy on an ambulatory basis. JAMA 1950; 143:870–872.
27. Askey JM, Cherry CB. Thromboembolism associated with auricular fibrillation; continuous anticoagulant therapy. JAMA 1950; 144:97–100.
28. Kannel WB, et al. Epidemiologic features of clinical atrial fibrillation. N Engl J Med 1982; 306:1018–1022.
29. Hinton RC, et al. Influence of etiology of atrial fibrillation on incidence of system embolus. Am J Cardiol 1977; 40:509–513.
30. Aberg H. Atrial fibrillation: a study of atrial thrombosis and systemic embolism in necropsy material. Acta Med Scand 1969; 188:373–379.
31. Fisher CM. Reducing risks of cerebral embolism. Geriatrics 1979; 34:53–61, 65–66.
32. Wolf PA, et al. Epidemiologic assessment of chronic atrial fibrillation and risk of stroke: the Framingham study. Neurology 1978; 28:973–977.
33. Friedman GD, Loveland DB, Ehrlich SP. Relationship of stroke to other CV disorders. Circulation 1968; 38:533–541.
34. Gajewski J, Singer RB. Mortality in an insured population with atrial fibrillation. JAMA 1981; 245:1540–1544.
35. Wood JC, Conn HL Jr. Prevention of systemic atrial embolism in chronic rheumatic heart disease by means of protracted anticoagulant therapy. Circulation 1954; 10:177–523.
36. Szekely P. Systemic embolism and anticoagulant prophylaxis in rheumatic heart disease. Brit Med J 1964; 1:1209–1212.
37. Baker RN. Anticoagulation in treatment of cerebral infarction—report of a cooperative study. Neurology 1962; 2:823–830.
38. Owren W. Results of anticoagulation treatment in Norway. Arch Int Med 1963; 111:240–244.
39. Petersen B, et al. Placebo-controlled, randomized trial of warfarin and aspirin for the prevention of thromboembolic complications in chronic atrial fibrillation. Lancet 1989; 1:175–179.
40. Stroke prevention in Atrial Fibrillation Study Group Investigators. Preliminary report of the Stroke Prevention in Atrial Fibrillation Study. N Engl J Med 1990; 322:863–868.
41. Boston Area Anticoagulation Trial in Atrial Fibrillation Investigators. The effect of low-dose warfarin on the risk of stroke in patients with nonrheumatic atrial fibrillation. N Engl J Med 1990; 323:1505–1511.
42. Connolly SS, et al. Canadian atrial fibrillation anticoagulation (CAFA) Study. J Am Coll Cardiol 1991; 18:349–355.
43. Ezekowitz MD, et al. Warfarin in the prevention of stroke

associated with nonrheumatic atrial fibrillation. N Engl J Med 1992; 327:1406–1412.
44. SPAF-II Investigators. Warfarin versus aspirin for prevention of thromboembolism in atrial fibrillation: Stroke Prevention in Atrial Fibrillation II Study. Lancet 1994; 343:687–691.
45. Bjerkelund C, Orning OM. The efficacy of anticoagulant therapy in preventing embolism related to DC electrical conversion of atrial fibrillation. Am J Cardiol 1969; 23:200–216.
46. Arnold AZ, et al. Role of prophylactic anticoagulation for direct cardioversion in patients wtih atrial fibrillation or atrial flutter. J Am Coll Cardiol 1992; 19:856–857.
47. Manning WJ, et al. Cardioversion from atrial fibrillation without prophylactic anticoagulation with use of transesophageal echocardiography to exclude the presence of atrial thrombi. N Engl J Med 1993; 329:1577–1584.
48. Anticoagulants in acute myocardial infarction: results of a cooperative clinical trial. JAMA 1973; 225:724–729.
49. Assessment of short term anticoagulant administration after cardiac infarction: report of the Working Party on Anticoagulant Therapy in Coronary Thrombosis to the Medical Research Council. Brit Med J 1969; 1:335–342.
50. Drapkin A, Merskey C. Anticoagulant therapy after acute myocardial infarction: relation of therapeutic benefit to patients' age, sex and severity of infarction. JAMA 1972; 288:541–548.
51. Bredden D, et al. The German-Austrian Aspirin Trial: a comparison of acetylsalicylic acid, placebo and phenprocoumon in secondary prevention of myocardial infarction. Circulation 1980; 62[Suppl V]:63–72.
52. Second report of the Working Party on Anticoagulant Therapy in Coronary Thrombosis to the Medical Research Council. An assessment of long-term anticoagulant administration after cardiac infarction. Brit Med J 1964; 2:837–843.
53. United States Veterans Administration. Long-term anticoagulant therapy after myocardial infarction. 1965; JAMA 193:929–934.
54. Smith P, Arnesen H, Holme I. The effect of warfarin on mortality and reinfarction after myocardial infarction. N Engl J Med 1990; 323:147–152.
55. Telford AM, Wilson C. Trials of heparin vs. atenolol in prevention of myocardial infarction in intermediate coronary syndrome. Lancet 1981; 1:1225–1228.
56. Theroux P, et al. Aspirin, heparin, or both to treat acute unstable angina. N Engl J Med 1988; 319:1105–1111.
57. Theroux P, et al. Aspirin vs. heparin to prevent myocardial infarction during the acute phase of unstable angina. Circulation 1993; 88:2045–2048.
58. Kistler JP, Ropper AH, Heros RC. Therapy of ischemic cerebrovascular disease due to atherosclerosis. N Engl J Med 1984; 311:100–105.
59. Olsson JE, et al. Anticoagulant vs. antiplatelet therapy as prophylaxis against myocardial infarction in transient ischemic attacks. Stroke 1980; 11:4–9.
60. Estol CJ, Pessin MS. Anticoagulation: is there still a role in atherothrombotic stroke? Stroke 1990; 21:820–824.
61. Bynum LJ, Wilson JE. Low dose heparin therapy in the long-term management of venous thromboembolism. Am J Med 1979; 67:553–556.
62. Hull R, et al. Warfarin sodium versus low dose heparin in the long-term treatment of venous thromboembolism. N Engl J Med 1979; 301:855–858.
63. Hull R, et al. Adjusted SQ heparin versus warfarin in the long-term treatment of venous thrombosis. N Engl J Med 1982; 306:189–194.
64. Enger E, Boyesen S. Long-term aspirin therapy in patients with myocardial infarction. Acta Med Scand 1965; 178[Suppl]:7–55.
65. McDowell F, McDevitt E, Wright IS. Anticoagulant therapy: five years' experience with the patient with an established cerebrovascular accident. Arch Neurol 1963; 8:209–214.
66. Baker RN. An evaluation of anticoagulant therapy in the treatment of cerebrovascular disease: report of the Veterans Administration Cooperative Study of Atherosclerosis. Neurology 1961; 11:132–138.
67. Altman R, et al. Aspirin and prophylaxis of thromboembolic complications in patients with substitute heart valves. J Thorac Cardiovasc Surg 1976; 72:127–129.
68. Chesebro JH, et al. Trial of combined warfarin plus dipyridamole or aspirin therapy in prosthetic heart valve replacement: danger of aspirin compared with dipyridamole. Am J Cardiol 1983; 51:1537–1541.
69. Forfar JC. A 7-year analysis of hemorrhage in patients on long-term anticoagulant therapy. Brit Heart J 1979; 42:128–132.
70. Sixty-plus Reinfarction Study Research group. A double-blind trial to assess long-term anticoagulant therapy in elderly patients after myocardial infarction. Lancet 1982; 1:64–68.
71. Meuwissen O, et al. Double blind trial of long-term anticoagulant therapy after myocardial infarction. Acta Med Scand 1969; 186:361–368.
72. Loeliger EA, et al. A double-blind trial of long-term anticoagulant therapy after myocardial infarction. Acta Med Scand 1967; 182:549–566.
73. Bjerkelund CJ. Therapeutic level in long-term anticoagulant therapy after myocardial infarction: its relation to recent infarction and sudden death. Am J Cardiovasc 1963; 1:158–163.
74. Harvald B, Hilden T, Lund E. Long-term anticoagulant therapy after myocardial infarction. Lancet 1962; 2:626–630.
75. Levine MN, Raskob G, Hirsh J. Hemorrhagic complications of long-term anticoagulant therapy. Chest 1986; 89[Suppl 2]:165–255.
76. King DJ, Kelton JC. Heparin-induced thrombocytopenia. Ann Int Med 1984; 100:535–540.
77. Avioli LV. Heparin-induced osteoporosis: an appraisal. Adv Exp Med Biol 1975; 52:375–387.
78. McGehee WJ, et al. Coumarin necrosis associated with hereditary protein C deficiency. Ann Int Med 1984; 100:55–60.
79. Hall JG, Pacili RM, Wilson KM. Maternal and fetal sequelae of anticoagulant during pregnancy. Am J Med 1980; 68:122–140.
80. Iturbe-Alessio I, et al. Risks of anticoagulant therapy in pregnant women with artificial heart valves. N Engl J Med 1986; 315:1390–1393.
81. Pedersen AK, FitzGerald GA. The human pharmacology of platelet inhibition: pharmacokinetics relevant to drug action. Circulation 1985; 112:1164–1176.
82. Hawkins D, et al. Structural changes in human serum albumin induced by ingestion of acetylsalicylic acid. J Clin Invest 1969, 48:536–542.
83. Bridges KR, et al. The acetylation of hemoglobin by aspirin. J Clin Invest 1975; 56:201–207.
84. Green FA, Jung CY. Acetylation of erythrocyte membrane peptides by aspirin. Transfusion 1981; 21:55–58.
85. Roth GJ, Majerus PW. The mechanism of the effect of aspirin on human platelets. I: Acetylation of a particulate fraction protein. J Clin Invest 1975; 56:624–632.
86. Patrono C. Aspirin as an antiplatelet drug. N Engl J Med 1994; 330:1287–1294.
87. DeWitt DL, Smith WL. Primary structure of prostaglandin G/H synthase from sheep vesicular gland determined from the complementary DNA sequence. Proc Natl Acad Sci USA

1988; 85:1412–1416. [Erratum: Proc Natl Acad Sci USA 1988; 85:5056.]
88. Funk CD, et al. Human platelet-erythroleukemia cell prostaglandin G/H synthase: cDNA cloning, expression, mutagenesis and gene chromosomal assignment. FASEB J 1991; 5:2304–2312.
89. Rowland M, Riegelman S. Pharmacokinetics of acetylsalicylic acid and salicylic acid after intravenous administration in man. J Pharmacol Sci 1968; 57:1313.
90. Levy G. Clinical pharmacology salicylates: a reassessment. Brit J Clin Pharmacol 1980; 10[S-1]:285.
91. Young VP, et al. Sex differences in bleeding time and blood loss in normal subjects following aspirin ingestion. Thromb Res 1980; 20:705.
92. Canadian Cooperative Study Group. A randomized trial of aspirin and sulfinpyrazone in threatened stroke. N Engl J Med 1978; 299:53–59.
93. Harris WH, et al. Aspirin prophylaxis of venous thromboembolism after total hip replacement. N Engl J Med 1977; 297:1246.
94. Kelton JG, et al. Sex differences in the antithrombotic effects of aspirin. Blood 1978; 52:1073.
95. Deykin D, Janson P, McMahon L. Ethanol potentiation of aspirin-induced prolongation of the bleeding time. N Engl J Med 1982; 306:852–854.
96. Czapek EE, et al. Intermediate syndrome of platelet dysfunction. Blood 1978; 52:103–113.
97. Weiss HJ, Aledort LM, Kochwa S. The effect of salicylates on the hemostatic properties of platelets in man. J Clin Invest 1968; 47:2169.
98. Baenziger NL, Dillenden MJ, Majerus PW. Cultured human skin fibroblasts and arterial cells produce a labile platelet inhibiting prostaglandin. Biochem Biophys Res Commun 1977; 78:294.
99. Jaffe EA, Weksler BB. Recovery of endothelial cell prostacyclin production after low doses of aspirin. J Clin Invest 1979; 63:532.
100. Preston FE, et al. Inhibition of prostacyclin and platelet thromboxane A_2 after low-dose aspirin. N Engl J Med 1981; 304:76.
101. Hanley SP, et al. Differential inhibition by low-dose aspirin of human venous prostacyclin synthesis and platelet thromboxane synthesis. Lancet 1981; 1:969.
102. Masotti G, et al. Differential inhibition of prostacyclin production and platelet aggregation by aspirin. Lancet 1979; 2:1213.
103. Weksler BB, et al. Differential inhibition by aspirin of vascular and platelet prostaglandin synthesis in atherosclerotic patients. N Engl J Med 1983; 308:800.
104. FitzGerald GA, et al. Endogenous biosynthesis of prostacyclin by treatment of endothelium with aspirin. J Clin Invest 1979; 63:1089.
105. Villa S, Livio M, de Gaetano G. The inhibitory effect of aspirin on platelet and vascular prostaglandins in rats cannot be completely dissociated. Brit J Haematol 1979; 42:425.
106. Catalano PM, Smith JB, Murphy S. Platelet recovery from aspirin inhibition in vivo: differing patterns under various assay conditions. Blood 1981; 57:88.
107. de Caterina R, Patrono C. Selective inhibition of thromboxane-related platelet function by low-dose aspirin in patients after myocardial infarction. Am J Cardiol 1985; 55:589.
108. Ciabattoni G, et al. Radioimmunoassay measurement of 2,3-dinor metabolites of prostacyclin and thromboxane in human urine. Adv Prostaglandin Thromboxane Leukot Res 1987; 598–602.
109. Braden GA, Knapp HR, FitzGerald GA. Suppression of eicosanoid biosynthesis during coronary angioplasty by fish oil and aspirin. Circulation 1991; 84:679–685.
110. Pederson AK, FitzGerald GA. Dose-related kinetics of aspirin: presystemic acetylation of platelet cyclooxygenase. N Engl J Med 1984; 311:1206.
111. Cerletti C, Livio M, de Gaetano G. Nonsteroidal antiinflammatory drugs react with two sites on platelet cyclooxygenase. Biochim Biophys Acta 1982; 714:122.
112. de Gaetano G, et al. Pharmacology of platelet inhibition in humans; implication of the salicylate-aspirin interaction. Circulation 1985; 72:1185–1193.
113. Ali M, et al. Plasma acetylsalicylate and salicylate and platelet cyclooxygenase activity following plain and enteric coated aspirin. Stroke 1980; 11:9–13.
114. Ross-Lee LM, et al. Plasma levels of aspirin following effervescent and enteric coated tablets, and their effect on platelet function. Eur J Clin Pharmacol 1982; 23:545–551.
115. Siebert DJ, et al. Aspirin kinetics and platelet aggregation in man. Clin Pharmacol Ther 1983; 33:367–374.
116. Clarke RJ, et al. Suppression of thromboxane A_2 but not of systemic prostacyclin by controlled-release aspirin. N Engl J Med 1991; 325:1137–1141.
117. Stampfer MJ, et al. Effect of alternate-day regular and enteric-coated aspirin on platelet aggregation, bleeding time, and thromboxane A_2 levels in bleeding-time blood. Am J Med 1986; 81:400–404.
118. Hirsh J, et al. Aspirin and other platelet-active drugs: The relationship between dose, effectiveness, and side effects. Chest 1992; 102[Suppl]:327S–336S.
119. Fuster V, et al. Aspirin as a therapeutic agent in cardiovascular disease. Circulation 1993; 87:659–675.
120. Craven LL. Experiences with aspirin (acetylsalicyclic acid) in the non-specific prophylaxis of coronary thrombosis. Mis Valley Med J 1953; 75:38–44.
121. Antiplatelet Trialists' Collaboration. Collaborative overview of randomised trials of antiplatelet therapy—I: prevention of death, myocardial infarction, and stroke by prolonged antiplatelet therapy in various categories of patients. Br Med J 1994; 308:81–106.
122. Antiplatelet Trialists' Collaboration. Collaborative overview of randomised trials of antiplatelet therapy—II: maintenance of vascular graft or arterial patency by antiplatelet therapy. Br Med J 1994; 308:159–168.
123. Antiplatelet Trialists' Collaboration. Collaborative overview of randomised trials of antiplatelet therapy—III: reduction in venous thrombosis and pulmonary embolism by antiplatelet prophylaxis among surgical and medical patients. Br Med J 1994; 308:235–246.
124. Steering Committee of the Physicians' Health Study Research Group. Final report on the aspirin component of the ongoing Physicians' Health Study. N Engl J Med 1989; 321:129–135.
125. Peto R, et al. Randomized trial of prophylactic daily aspirin in British male doctors. Br Med J 1988; 296:313–316.
126. Relman AS. Aspirin for the primary prevention of myocardial infarction. N Engl J Med 1988; 318:245–246.
127. Manson JE, et al. A prospective study of aspirin use and primary prevention of cardiovascular disease in women. JAMA 1991; 266:521–527.
128. Ridker PM, et al. Low-dose aspirin therapy for chronic stable angina: a randomized, placebo-controlled clinical trial. Ann Intern Med 1991; 114:835–839.
129. Juul-Möller S, et al. Double-blind trial of aspirin in primary prevention of myocardial infarction in patients with stable chronic angina pectoris. Lancet 1992; 340:1421–1425.
130. Lewis HD, et al. Protective effects of aspirin against acute myocardial infarction and death in men with unstable an-

gina: results of a Veterans Administration Cooperative Study. N Engl J Med 1983; 309:396–403.
131. Cairns JA, et al. Aspirin, sulfinpyrazone, or both in unstable angina. N Engl J Med 1985; 313:1369–1375.
132. The RISC Group. Risk of myocardial infarction and death during treatment with low dose aspirin and intravenous heparin in men with unstable coronary artery disease. Lancet 1990; 336:827–830.
133. Wallentin LC, Research Group on Instability in Coronary Artery Disease in Southeast Sweden. Aspirin (75 mg/day) after an episode of unstable coronary artery disease: long-term effects on the risk for myocardial infarction, occurrence of severe angina and the need for revascularization. J Am Coll Cardiol 1991; 18:1587–1593.
134. Nyman I, Larsson H, Wallentin L. Research Group on Instability in Coronary Artery Disease in Southeast Sweden. Prevention of serious cardiac events by low-dose aspirin in patients with silent myocardial ischemia. Lancet 1992; 340:497–501.
135. Théroux P, et al. Aspirin, heparin, or both to treat acute unstable angina. N Engl J Med 1988; 319:1105–1111.
136. Théroux P, et al. Reactivation of unstable angina after the discontinuation of heparin. N Engl J Med 1992; 327:141–145.
137. Webster J, Douglas AS. Aspirin and other antiplatelet drugs in the prophylaxis of thrombosis. Blood Reviews 1987; 1:9–20.
138. Gallus AS. The use of antithrombotic drugs in artery disease. Clin Hematol 1986; 15:509–559.
139. Persantine-Aspirin Reinfarction Study Research Group. Persantine and aspirin in coronary heart disease. Circulation 1980; 621:449–461.
140. Klimt CR, et al. Persantine-aspirin reinfarction study. II: Secondary coronary prevention with Persantine and aspirin. J Am Coll Cardiol 1986; 7:251–269.
141. Elwood PC, et al. A randomized controlled trial of acetyl salicylic acid in the secondary prevention of mortality from myocardial infarction. Brit Med J 1974; 1:436–440.
142. Coronary Drug Project. Aspirin in coronary heart disease. J Chr Dis 1976; 29:625–642.
143. Breddin K, et al. Secondary prevention of myocardial infarction. Comparison of acetylsalicylic acid, phenprocomoun and placebo. A multicenter two-year prospective study. Thromb Haemost 1979; 41:225–236.
144. Elwood PC, Sweetman PM. Aspirin and secondary mortality after myocardial infarction. Lancet 1979; 2:1313–1315.
145. Aspirin Myocardial Infarction Study (AMIS) Research Group. A randomized controlled trial of aspirin in persons recovered from myocardial infarction. JAMA 1980; 243:661–669.
146. ISIS-2 (Second International Study of Infarct Survival) Collaborative Group. Randomised trial of intravenous streptokinase, oral aspirin, both, or neither among 17,187 cases of suspected acute myocardial infarction: ISIS-2. Lancet 1988; 2:349–360.
147. Ishikawa K, Kanamasa K, Ogawa I. Aspirin 50 mg per day combined with either dipyridamole or ticlopidine is effective to prevent recurrent myocardial infarction. Circulation 1992; 86:[Suppl]1:643.
148. Lorenz RL, et al. Improved aortocoronary bypass patency by low-dose aspirin (100 mg daily). Lancet 1984; 1:1261–1264.
149. Sanz G, et al. Prevention of early aortocoronary bypass occlusion by low-dose aspirin and dipyridamole. Circulation 1990; 82:765–773.
150. American-Canadian Cooperative Study Group. Persantine aspirin trial in cerebral ischemia. II: Endpoint results. Stroke 1985; 16:406–415.
151. Fields WS, et al. Controlled trial of aspirin in cerebral ischaemia. Stroke 1977; 8:301–305.
152. Fields WS, et al. Controlled trial of aspirin in cerebral ischaemia. Part II: Surgical Group. 1978; 9:309–319.
153. The SALT Collaborative Group. Swedish Aspirin Low-Dose Trial of 75 mg aspirin as secondary prophylaxis after cerebrovascular ischemic events. Lancet 1991; 338:L345–L349.
154. Sorensen PS, et al. Acetylsalicylic acid in the prevention of stroke in patients with reversible cerebral ischemic attacks. A Danish Cooperative Study. Stroke 1983; 14:15–22.
155. Guirand-Chaumeil B, et al. Prevention des recidives des accidents vasculaires cerebraux ischemiques par les antiagregants plaquettaires. Neurology (Paris) 1982; 138:368–385.
156. The Dutch TIA Trial Study Group. A comparison of two doses of aspirin in patients after a transient ischemic attack or minor ischemic stroke. N Engl J Med 1991; 325:1261–1266.
157. Dyken ML, et al. Low-dose aspirin and stroke: "it ain't necessarily so". Stroke 1992; 23:1395–1399.
158. Sivenius J, et al. The European Stroke Prevention Study: Results according to sex. Neurology 1991; 41:1189–1192.
159. Hess H, Mietaschk A, Deichsel G. Drug-induced inhibition of platelet function delays progression of peripheral occlusive arterial disease: a prospective double-blind angiographically controlled trial. Lancet 1985; 1:415–419.
160. Clagett GP, Graor RA, Salzman EW. Antithrombotic therapy in peripheral arterial occlusive disease. Chest 1992; 102[Suppl]:516S–528S.
161. Sautter RD, et al. Aspirin-sulfinpyrazone in prophylaxis of deep venous thrombosis in total hip replacement. JAMA 1983; 250:2649–2654.
162. Thornton MA, et al. Coumadin and aspirin in prevention of recurrence after transluminal coronary angioplasty: a randomized study. Circulation 1984; 69:721–727.
163. Roux S, Christeller S, Ludin E. Effects of aspirin on coronary reocclusion and recurrent ischemia after thrombolysis: a meta-analysis. J Am Coll Cardiol 1992; 19:678–680.
164. Beaufils M, et al. Prevention of pre-eclampsia by early antiplatelet therapy. Lancet 1985; 1:840–842.
165. CLASP (Collaborative Low-dose Aspirin Study in Pregnancy) Collaborative Group. CLASP: a randomised trial of low-dose aspirin for the prevention and treatment of pre-eclampsia among 9364 pregnant women. Lancet 1994; 343:619–629.
166. Ware Branch D, et al. Obstetric complications associated with the lupus anticoagulant. N Engl J Med 1985; 313:1322–1326.
167. Harter HR, et al. Prevention of thrombosis in patients on hemodialysis by low-dose aspirin. N Engl J Med 1979; 301:577–579.
168. Bloomfield P, et al. Twelve-year comparison of a Bjork-Shiley mechanical heart valve with porcine bioprostheses. N Engl J Med 1991; 324:573–579.
169. Dale J, et al. Prevention of arterial thromboembolism with acetylsalicylic acid: a controlled clinical study in patients with aortic ball valves. Am Heart J 1977; 94:101–111.
170. Altman R, et al. Aspirin and prophylaxis of thromboembolic complications in patients with substitute heart valves. J Thorac Cardiovasc Surg 1976; 72:127–129.
171. Turpie AGG, et al. A comparison of aspirin with placebo in patients treated with warfarin after heart-valve replacement. N Engl J Med 1993; 329:524–529.
172. White HD. Aspirin or warfarin for non-rheumatic atrial fibrillation? Lancet 1994; 343:683–684.
173. Folts JD, et al. Shortcomings of aspirin as an antithrombotic agent. Submitted for publication.
174. Simon LS, Mills JA. Nonsteroidal anti-inflammatory drugs. N Engl J Med 1980; 302:1179.

175. Weiss HJ. Platelets. In Pathophysiology and Antiplatelet Drug Therapy. New York: Alan R. Liss, 1982.
176. Patrono C, et al. Clinical pharmacology of platelet cyclooxygenase inhibition. Circulation 1985; 72:1177–1184.
177. Schafer AI. Effects of nonsteroidal anti-inflammatory drugs on platelet function and systemic hemostasis. J Clin Pharmacol 1995; 35:209–219.
178. Bang HO, Dyerberg J, Nielsen AB. Plasma lipid and lipoprotein pattern in Greenlandic West-Coast Eskimos. Lancet 1971; 1:1143–1145.
179. Bang HO, Dyerberg J. The bleeding tendency in Greenland Eskimos. Dan Med Bull 1980; 27:202–205.
180. Kromhout D, Bosscheiter EB, de Lezenne Coulander C. The inverse relation between fish consumption and 20-year mortality from coronary heart disease. N Engl J Med 1985; 312:1205–1209.
181. Shekelle RB, et al. Fish consumption and mortality from coronary heart disease. N Engl J Med 1985; 313:820.
182. Weiner BH, et al. Inhibition of atherosclerosis by cod-liver oil in a hyperlipidemic swine model. N Engl J Med 1986; 315:841–846.
183. Franklin SM, Faxon DP. Pharmacologic prevention of restenosis after coronary angioplasty: review of the randomized clinical trials. Coronary Artery Disease 1993; 4:232–242.
184. Fish oil for the heart. Med Lett 1987; 29:7–9.
185. Kantha SS. Dietary effects of fish oils on human health: a review of recent studies. Yale J Biol Med 1987; 60:37–44.
186. Israel DH, Gorlin R. Fish oils in the prevention of atherosclerosis. J Am Coll Cardiol 1992; 19:174–185.
187. Harris WS, Connor WE, McMurry MP. The comparative reductions of the plasma lipids and lipoproteins by dietary polyunsaturated fats: salmon oil vs. vegetable oils. Metabolism 1983; 32:179–184.
188. Phillipson BE, et al. Reduction of plasma lipids, lipoproteins, and apoproteins by dietary fish oil in patients with hypertriglyceridemia. N Engl J Med 1985; 312:1210–1216.
189. Sullivan DR, et al. Paradoxical elevation of LDL apoprotein B levels in hypertriglyceridaemic patients and normal subjects ingesting fish oil. Atherosclerosis 1986; 61:129–134.
190. Spector AA, Yorek MA. Membrane lipid composition and cellular function. J Lipid Res 1985; 26:1015–1035.
191. Lee TH, et al. Effects of dietary enrichment with eicosapentaenoic and docosahexaenoic acids on in vitro neutrophil and monocyte leukotriene generation and neutrophil function. N Engl J Med 1985; 312:1217–1224.
192. Leaf A, Weber PC. Cardiovascular effects of n-3 fatty acids. N Engl J Med 1988; 318:549–557.
193. Hamberg M, Svensson J, Samuelsson B. Thromboxanes: a new group of biologically active compounds derived from prostaglandin endoperoxides. Proc Natl Acad Sci USA 1975; 72:2994–2998.
194. Needleman P, et al. Triene prostaglandins: prostacyclin and thromboxane biosynthesis and unique biological properties. Proc Natl Acad Sci USA 1979; 176:944–948.
195. Knapp HR, et al. In vivo indexes of platelet and vascular function during fish-oil administration in patients with atherosclerosis. N Engl J Med 1986; 314:937–942.
196. Fischer S, Weber PC. Prostaglandin I_2 is formed in vivo in man after dietary eicosapentaenoic acid. Nature 1984; 307:165–168.
197. von Schacky C, Fischer S, Weber PC. Long-term effects of dietary marine omega-3 fatty acids upon plasma and cellular lipids, platelet function, and eicosanoid formation in humans. J Clin Invest 1985; 76:1626–1631.
198. Deckmyn H, et al. Manipulation of the local thromboxane and prostacyclin balance in vivo by the antithrombotic compounds dazoxiben, acetylsalicyclic acid and nafazatrom. Biochem Pharmacol 1983; 32:2757–2762.
199. FitzGerald GA, Oates JA. Selective and nonselective inhibition of thromboxane formation. Clin Pharmacol Ther 1984; 35:633.
200. Verstraete M, Kienast J. Pharmacology of the interaction between platelets and vessel wall. Clin Haematol 1986; 15:493–508.
201. Bunting S, Moncada S, Vane JR. The prostacyclin-thromboxane A_2 balance: pathophysiological and therapeutic implications. Brit Med Bull 1983; 39:271–276.
202. Randall MJ, et al. UK-37248, a novel, selective thromboxane synthetase inhibitor with platelet anti-aggregatory and antithrombotic activity. Thromb Res 1981; 83:145–162.
203. Tyler HM, Saxton CAPD, Parry MJ. Administration to man of UK-37,248-01, a selective inhibitor of thromboxane synthetase. Lancet 1981; 1:629–632.
204. Smith JB. Pharmacology thromboxane synthetase inhibitors. Fed Proc 1987; 46:139–143.
205. Vermylen J, et al. Thromboxane synthetase inhibition as antithrombotic strategy. Lancet 1981; 1:1073–1075.
206. Heptinstall S, et al. Effects of a selective inhibitor of thromboxane synthetase on human blood platelet behavior. Thromb Res 1980; 20:219–230.
207. Bertele V, et al. Inhibition of thromboxane synthetase does not necessarily prevent platelet aggregation. Lancet 1981; 1:1057–1058.
208. Gresele P, et al. Serum albumin enhances the impairment of platelet aggregation with thromboxane synthase inhibition by increasing the formation of prostaglandin D_2. Biochem Pharmacol 1984; 33:2083–2088.
209. FitzGerald GA, Reilly IAG, Pedersen AK. The biochemical pharmacology of thromboxane synthase inhibition in man. Circulation 1985; 72:1194–1201.
210. Belch JJF, et al. Dazoxiben, a thromboxane synthetase inhibitor, in the treatment of Raynaud's syndrome: a double blind trial. Brit J Clin Pharmacol 1983; 15:1135.
211. Luderer JR, et al. Dazoxiben, a thromboxane synthetase inhibitor in Raynaud's phenomenon. Clin Pharmacol Ther 1984; 36:105.
212. Ettinger WH, et al. Controlled double-blind trial of dazoxiben and nifedipine in the treatment of Raynaud's phenomenon. Am J Med 1984; 77:451.
213. Zipser RD, et al. Therapeutic trial of thromboxane synthesis inhibition in the hepatorenal syndrome. Gastroenterology 1984; 87:1228.
214. McGibney D, et al. Effects of UK 37,248, a thromboxane synthetase inhibitor, on platelet behavior in patients with coronary heart disease undergoing exercise to angina. Clin Sci 1983; 12:138.
215. Reuben SR, et al. Effects of dazoxiben and exercise performance in chronic stable angina. Brit J Clin Pharmacol 1983; 15:835.
216. Kiff PS, et al. Hemodynamic and metabolic effects of dazoxiben at rest and during atrial pacing. Brit J Clin Pharmacol 1983; 15:738.
217. Thaulow E, Dale J, Myhre E. Effects of a selective thromboxane synthetase inhibitor, dazoxiben, and acetyl salicylic acid on myocardial ischemia in patients with coronary heart disease. Am J Cardiol 1984; 53:1255.
218. Lefer AM, Darius H. A pharmacological approach to thromboxane receptor antagonism. Fed Proc 1987; 46:144–148.
219. Brittain RT, et al. AH23848: a thromboxane receptor-blocking drug that can clarify the pathophysiologic role of thromboxane A_2. Circulation 1985; 72:1208–1218.
220. Ritter JM, Dollery CT. Therapeutic opportunities in vasoocclusive disease. Circulation 1986; 73:240–243.

221. Hoet B, et al. R68070, a combined thromboxane/endoperoxide receptor antagonist and thromboxane synthase inhibitor, inhibits human platelet activation in vitro and in vivo: a comparison with aspirin. Blood 1990; 75:646–653.
222. The RAPT Investigators. Randomized trial of ridogrel, a combined thromboxane A_2 synthase inhibitor and thromboxane A_2/prostaglandin endoperoxide receptor antagonist, versus aspirin as adjunct to thrombolysis in patients with acute myocardial infarction. Circulation 1994; 89:588–595.
223. Bertele V, et al. Refractoriness of platelets to prostaglandins after prolonged infusion in rabbits. J Lab Clin Med 1985; 106:551–561.
224. MacDermot J. Desensitization of prostacyclin responsiveness in platelets. Biochem Pharmacol 1986; 35:2645–2649.
225. Lewis PJ, Dollery CT. Clinical pharmacology and potential of prostacyclin. Brit Med Bull 1983; 39:281–284.
226. Bergmann G, et al. Prostacyclin: haemodynamic and metabolic effects in patients with coronary artery disease. Lancet 1981; 1:569–572.
227. Henriksson P, Edhag O, Wennmalm A. Prostacyclin infusion in patients with acute myocardial infarction. Brit Heart J 1985; 53:173–179.
228. Szczeklik A, Skawinski A, Gluszko P. Successful therapy of advanced arteriosclerosis obliterans with prostacyclin. Lancet 1979; 1:1111–1114.
229. Belch JJF, et al. Epoprostenol (prostacyclin) and severe arterial disease. Lancet 1983; 1:315–317.
230. FitzGerald GA, et al. Intravenous prostacyclin in thrombotic thrombocytopenic purpura. Ann Int Med 1981; 95:319–322.
231. Whittle BJR, Moncada S. Platelet actions of stable carbocyclic analogues of prostacyclin. Circulation 1985; 72:1219–1225.
232. Fisher CA, et al. Comparison of equimolar concentrations of iloprost, prostacyclin, and prostaglandin E_1 on human platelet function. J Lab Clin Med 1987; 109:184–190.
233. Schor K, et al. The antiplatelet and cardiovascular actions of a new carbacyclin derivative (ZK 36 374)—equipotent to PGI_2 in vitro. Naunyn Schmiedebergs Arch Pharmacol 1981; 316:252–255.
234. Fiessinger JN, Schafer M. Trial of iloprost versus aspirin treatment for critical limb ischemia of thromboangiitis obliterans. Lancet 1990; 1:555–557.
235. Kovacs IB, Mayo SC, Kirby JD. Infusion of a stable prostacyclin analogue, iloprost, to patients with peripheral vascular disease: lack of antiplatelet effect but risk of thromboembolism. Am J Med 1991; 90:41–46.
236. Schafer AI, Alexander RW, Handin RI. Inhibition of platelet function by organic nitrate vasodilators. Blood 1980; 55: 649–654.
237. Stamler J, Loscalzo J. The antiplatelet effects of organic nitrates and nitroso-derivatives and their importance in cardiovascular disorders. J Am Coll Cardiol 1991; 18:1529–1536.
238. Groves PH, et al. SIN-1 reduces platelet adhesion and platelet thrombus formation in a porcine model of balloon angioplasty. Circulation 1993; 87:590–597.
239. Ferguson JJ. Meeting highlights: nitric oxide donors. Circulation 1994; 90:4.
240. Dale J, Myhre E, Rostwelt K. Effects of dipyridamole and acetylsalicylic acid on platelet functions in patients with aortic ball-valve prosthesis. Am Heart J 1975; 89:613–618.
241. Sullivan JM, Kagnoff MF, Gorlin R. Reduction of platelet-adhesiveness in patients with coronary artery disease. Am J Med Sci 1968; 255:292.
242. Rajah SM, et al. The effects of dipyridamole on platelet function: correlation with blood levels in man. Brit J Clin Pharmacol 1979; 4:129–133.
243. Weiss HJ, et al. Effect of aspirin and dipyridamole on the interaction of human platelets with subendothelium: studies using citrated and native blood. Thromb Haemost 1981; 45:136–141.
244. Graves HM, et al. Effect of dipyridamole and prostacyclin on rabbit platelet adherence in vitro and in vivo. J Lab Clin Med 1982; 99:548–558.
245. Emmons PR, et al. Effect of dipyridamole on human platelet behaviour. Lancet 1965; 2:603–606.
246. Mills DCB, Smith JB. The influence on platelet aggregation of drugs that affect the accumulation of adenosine 3′: 5′-cyclic monophosphate in platelets. Biochem J 1971; 121: 185–196.
247. Ritchie JL, Harker LA. Platelet and fibrinogen survival in coronary atherosclerosis: response to medial and surgical therapy. Am J Cardiol 1977; 39:595.
248. Harker LA, Slichter SJ. Platelet and fibrinogen consumption in man. N Engl J Med 1972; 287:999.
249. Genton E, Ellis J, Steele P. Comparative effects of platelet suppressant drugs on platelet survival time. Thromb Diath 1975; 34:522.
250. FitzGerald GA. Dipyridamole. N Engl J Med 1987; 316:1247–1257.
251. Masotti G, et al. Stimulation of prostacyclin by dipyridamole. Lancet 1979; 1:1412.
252. Van de Velde VJS, et al. Dipyridamole stimulates prostacyclin production in isolated rat aortic tissue. Arch Int Pharmacodyn Ther 1982; 256:327–328.
253. Boeynaems JM, Van Coevorden A, Demolle D. Dipyridamole and vascular prostacyclin production. Biochem Pharmacol 1986; 35:2897–2902.
254. Ciabattoni G, Boss AH, Patrignani P. Endogenous biosynthesis of thromboxane and prostacyclin and platelet function during chronic dosing with low dose aspirin and dipyridamole. Adv Prostaglandin Thromboxane Leukot Res. In press.
255. Moncada S, Korbut R. Dipyridamole and other phosphodiesterase inhibitors act as anti-thrombotic agents by potentiating endogenous prostacyclin. Lancet 1978; 1:1286–1289.
256. Best LC, et al. Mode of action of dipyridamole on human platelets. Thromb Res 1979; 16:367–379.
257. Tsien W-H, Sheppard H. The lack of correlation between inhibition of platelet aggregation of cAMP levels. Fed Proc 1981; 40:809.
258. Lam SC-T, et al. Effect of cAMP phosphodiesterase inhibitors on ADP-induced shape change, cAMP and nucleoside diphosphokinase activity of rabbit platelets. Thromb Haemost 1982; 47:90–95.
259. Gresele P, et al. Mechanism of the antiplatelet action of dipyridamole in whole blood: modulation of adenosine concentration and activity. Thromb Haemostas 1986; 55:12–18.
260. Born GVR, Mills DCB. Potentiation of the inhibitory effect of adenosine on platelet aggregation by drugs that prevent its uptake. Proc Physiol Soc 1969; 41P–42P.
261. Crutchley DJ, Ryan US, Ryan JW. Effects of aspirin and dipyridamole on the degradation of adenosine diphosphate by cultured cells derived from bovine pulmonary artery. J Clin Invest 1980; 66:29–35.
262. Brown BG, et al. Improved graft patency in patients treated with platelet-inhibiting therapy after coronary bypass surgery. Circulation 1985; 72:138–146.
263. Bousser MG, Eschwege E, Haguenau M. "AICLA" controlled trial of aspirin and dipyridamole in the secondary prevention of athero-thrombotic cerebral ischemia. Stroke 1983; 14:5–14.
264. Sullivan JM, Harken DE, Gorlin R. Pharmacologic control of thromboembolic complications of cardiac-valve replacement. N Engl J Med 1971; 284:1391–1394.
265. Chesebro JH, et al. Trial of combined warfarin plus dipyridamole or aspirin therapy in prosthetic heart valve replace-

ment: danger of aspirin compared with dipyridamole. Am J Cardiol 1983; 1:1537–1541.
266. Stein PD, Kantrowitz A. Antithrombotic therapy in mechanical and biological prosthetic heart valves and saphenous vein bypass grafts. Chest 1989; 95:[Suppl]107S–117S.
267. Margulies EH, White AM, Sherry S. Sulfinpyrazone: a review of its pharmacological properties and therapeutic use. Drugs 1980; 20:179.
268. Smythe HA, et al. The effect of sulfinpyrazone on platelet economy in man. Canad Med Assoc J 1965; 92:818.
269. Kirstein Pederson A, Jackobsen P. Sulphinpyrazone metabolism during long-term therapy. Brit J Clin Pharmacol 1981; 11:597.
270. Lecaillon JB, et al. Sulfinpyrazone kinetics after intravenous and oral administration. Clin Pharmacol Ther 1979; 26:611.
271. Jakobsen P, Pedersen AK. Two metabolites of sulfinpyrazone and their identification and determination by mass spectrometry. J Pharm Pharmacol 1981; 33:89.
272. Renwick AG, et al. The role of gut flora in the reduction of sulfinpyrazone in the rat. Biochem Pharmacol 1982; 31:2649.
273. Wallis RB. Mechanisms of actions of sulfinpyrazone. Thromb Res 1983; S-IV:31.
274. Steele P, et al. Effect of sulfinpyrazone on platelet survival time in patients with transient cerebral ischemic attacks. Stroke 1977; 8:396–398.
275. Steele P, et al. Platelet survival in patients with rheumatic disease. N Engl J Med 1974; 290:537.
276. Baumgartner HR. Effects of acetylsalicylic acid, sulfinpyrazone and dipyridamole on platelet adhesion and aggregation in flowing native and anticoagulated blood. Haemostasis 1979; 8:340.
277. Essien EM, Mustard JF. Inhibition of platelet adhesion to rabbit aorta by sulphinpyrazone and acetylsalicylic acid. Atherosclerosis 1977; 27:89.
278. Ali M, McDonald JWD. Effects of sulphinpyrazone on platelet prostaglandin synthesis and platelet release of serotonin. J Lab Clin Med 1977; 89:868–875.
279. FitzGerald GA, et al. Endogenous biosynthesis of prostacyclin and thromboxane and platelet function during chronic administration of aspirin in man. J Clin Invest 1983; 71:676.
280. Packham MA, et al. Alteration of the response of platelets to surface stimuli by pyrazole compounds. J Exp Med 1967; 126:171.
281. Hood WB. More on sulfinpyrazone after myocardial infarction. N Engl J Med 1982; 306:988–989.
282. The Anturane Reinfarction Trial Research Group. Sulfinpyrazone in the prevention of cardiac death after myocardial infarction: the Anturane Reinfarction Trial. N Engl J Med 1978; 298:289–295.
283. The Anturane Reinfarction Trial Research Group. Sulfinpyrazone in the prevention of sudden death after myocardial infarction. N Engl J Med 1980; 302:250–256.
284. Temple R, Pledger GW. The FDA's critique of the Anturane Reinfarction Trial. N Engl J Med 1980; 303:1488–1492.
285. The Anturane Reinfarction Trial Policy Committee. The Anturane Reinfarction Trial: reevaluation of outcome. N Engl J Med 1982; 306:1005–1008.
286. Sulphinpyrazone in post-myocardial infarction: report from the Anturane Reinfarction Italian Study. Lancet 1982; 1:237–242.
287. Kaegi A, et al. Arteriovenous shunt thrombosis. Prevention by sulfinpyrazone. N Engl J Med 1974; 290:304–306.
288. Murray JC, Kelly MA, Gorelick PB. Ticlopidine: a new antiplatelet agent for the secondary prevention of stroke. Clin Neuropharmacol 1994; 17:23–31.
289. Sattiel E, Ward A. Ticlopidine: a review of its pharmacodynamic and pharmacokinetic properties, and therapeutic efficacy in platelet-dependent disease states. Drugs 1987; 34:222–262.
290. Defreyn G, et al. Ticlopidine and clopidogrel (SR 25990C) selectively neutralize ADP inhibition of PGE_1-activated platelet adenylate cyclase in rats and rabbits. Thromb Haemostas 1991; 65:186–190.
291. Mills DCB, et al. Clopidogrel inhibits the binding of ADP analogues to the receptor mediating inhibition of platelet adenylate cyclase. Arteriosclerosis and Thromb 1992; 12:430–436.
292. Di Minno G, Cerbone AM, Mattioli PL. Functionally thrombasthenic state in normal platelets following the administration of ticlopidine. J Clin Invest 1985; 75:328–338.
293. Cattaneo M, et al. Shear-induced platelet aggregation is potentiated by desmopressin and inhibited by ticlopidine. Arteriosclerosis and Thromb 1993; 13:393–397.
294. Defreyn G, et al. Pharmacology of ticlopidine: a review. Semin Thromb Hemost 1989; 15:159–166.
295. Hass WK, et al. Ticlopidine Aspirin Stroke Study group—A randomized trial comparing ticlopidine hydrochloride with aspirin for the prevention of stroke in high-risk patients. N Engl J Med 1989; 321:501–507.
296. Bellavance A, for the Ticlopidine Aspirin Stroke Study Group. Efficacy of ticlopidine and aspirin for prevention of reversible cerebrovascular ischemic events. Stroke 1993; 24:1452–1457.
297. Rothrock JF, Hart RG. Ticlopidine hydrochloride use and threatened stroke. West J Med 1994; 160:43–47.
298. Gent M, et al., and the CATS Group. The Canadian-American Ticlopidin Study (CATS) in thromboembolic stroke. Lancet 1989; 1:1215–1220.
299. Limet R, et al. Prevention of aortocoronary bypass graft occlusion—Beneficial effect of ticlopidine on early and late patency rates of venous coronary bypass grafts: A double-blind study. J Thorac Cardiovasc Surg 1987; 94:773–783.
300. Balsano F, et al. and the STA I Group. Antiplatelet treatment with ticlopidine in unstable angina, a controlled multicenter trial. Circulation 1990; 82:17–24.
301. Balsano F, et al. Ticlopidine in the treatment of intermittent claudication: A 21-month double-blind trial. J Lab Clin Med 1989; 114:84–91.
302. TIMAD Study Group. Ticlopidine treatment reduces the progression of non-proliferative diabetic retinopathy. Arch Opthalmol 1990; 108:1577–1583.
303. Coller BS. Antiplatelet agents in the prevention and therapy of thrombosis. Annu Rev Med 1992; 43:171–180.
304. Harker LA. Platelets and vascular thrombosis. N Engl J Med 1994; 330:1006–1007.
305. Phillips DR, Charo IF, Scarborough RM. GP IIb-IIIa: the responsive integrin. Cell 1991; 65:359–362.
306. Coller BS. A new murine monoclonal antibody reports an activation-dependent change in the conformation and/or microenvironment of the platelet glycoprotein IIb/IIIa complex. J Clin Invest 1985; 76:101–108.
307. Coller BS, et al. Monoclonal antibodies to platelet GP IIb/IIIa as antithrombotic agents. Ann NY Acad Sci 1991; 614:193–213.
308. The EPIC Investigators. Use of a monoclonal antibody directed against the platelet glycoprotein IIb/IIIa receptor in high-risk coronary angioplasty. N Engl J Med 1994; 330:956–961.
309. Simoons ML, et al., and the European Cooperative Study Group. Randomized Trial of a GP IIb/IIIa platelet receptor blocker in refractory unstable angina. Circulation 1994; 89:596–603.
310. Dennis MS, et al. Platelet GP IIb/IIIa protein antagonists

from snake venoms: evidence for a family of platelet aggregation inhibitors. Proc Natl Acad Sci USA 1990; 87:2471–2475.

311. Huang TF, et al. Trigramin: a low molecular weight peptide inhibiting fibrinogen interaction with platelet receptors expressed on glycoprotein IIb/IIIa complex. J Biol Chem 1987; 262:16157–16163.
312. Gan ZR, et al. Echistatin: a potent platelet aggregation inhibitor from the venom of the Viper Echis Carinatus. J Biol Chem 1988; 262:19827–19832.
313. Gould RJ, et al. Distintegrins: a family of integrin inhibitory proteins from viper venoms. Proc Soc Exp Biol Med 1990; 195:168–171.
314. Kleiman NS, et al. Profound inhibition of platelet aggregation with monoclonal antibody 7E3 Fab following thrombolytic therapy: results of the TAMI 8 pilot study. J Am Coll Cardiol 1993; 22:381–389.
315. Mazur P, et al. Ornatins: potent glycoprotein IIb/IIIa antagonists and platelet aggregation inhibitors from the leech *Placobdella ornata*. Eur J Biochem 1991; 202:1073–1082.
316. Krezel AM, et al. Structure of the RGD protein decorsin: conserved motif and distinct function in leech proteins that affect blood clotting. Science 1994; 264:1944–1947.
317. Ruggeri ZM, et al. Inhibition of platelet function with synthetic peptide designed to be high affinity antagonists of fibrinogen binding to platelets. Proc Natl Acad Sci USA 1986; 83:5708–5712.
318. Nicholson NS, et al. In vitro and in vivo effects of a peptide mimetic (SC-47643) of RGD as an antiplatelet and antithrombotic agent. Thromb Res 1991; 62:567–578.
319. Nichols AJ, et al. Development of GP IIb/IIIa antagonists as antithrombotic drugs. Trends Pharmacol Sci 1992; 13:413–417.
320. Hartman GD, et al. Non-peptide fibrinogen receptor antagonists: I discovery and design of exosite inhibitors. J Med Chem 1992; 36:4640–4642.
321. Roux SP, et al. Effects of heparin, aspirin, and a synthetic platelet glycoprotein IIb-IIIa receptor antagonist (Ro 43-5054) on coronary artery reperfusion and reocclusion after thrombolysis with tissue-type plasminogen activator in the dog. J Pharmacol Exp Ther 1992; 264:501–508.
322. Kouns WC, et al. Reversible conformational changes in glycoprotein IIb-IIIa by a potent and selective peptidomimetic inhibitor. Blood 1991; 80:2539–2547.
323. Peerlinck K, et al. MK-383 (L-700,462), a selective nonpeptide platelet glycoprotein IIb/IIIa antagonist is active in man. Circulation 1993; 88:1512–1517.
324. Mousa SA, et al. Antiplatelet and antithrombotic efficacy of DMP 728, a novel platelet GP IIb/IIIa receptor antagonist. Circulation 1994; 89:3–12.
325. Nicolini FA, et al. Combination of platelet fibrinogen receptor antagonist and direct thrombin inhibitor at low doses markedly improves thrombolysis. Circulation 1994; 89:1802–1809.
326. Mousa SA, De Grado WF, Reilly TM. Platelet GP IIb/IIIa antagonists: how safe is this antithrombotic approach? Am J Med 1994; 96:300.
327. Alevriadou BR, et al. Real-time analysis of shear-dependent thrombus formation and its blockade by inhibitors of von Willebrand factor binding to platelets. Blood 1993; 81:1263–1276.
328. Ikeda Y, et al. The role of von Willebrand factor and fibrinogen in platelet aggregation under varying shear stress. J Clin Invest 1991; 87:1234–1240.
329. Chesebro JH, Fuster V. Dynamic thrombosis and thrombolysis: role of antithrombins. Circulation 1991; 83:1815–1817.
330. Lumsden AB, et al. Lasting safe interruption of endarterectomy thrombosis by transiently infused antithrombin peptide D-Phe-Pro-ArgCH_2Cl in baboons. Blood 1993; 81:1762–1770.
331. Kosow DP. Kinetic mechanism of the activation of human plasminogen by streptokinase. Biochemistry 1975; 14:4459–4460.
332. Monk JP, Heel RC. Anisoylated plasminogen streptokinase activation complex (ABAC): a review of its mechanism of action, clinical pharmacology and therapeutic use in acute myocardial infarction. Drugs 1987; 34:25–49.
333. Hussain SS, Gurewich V, Lipinski B. Purification and partial characterization of single-chain high-molecular-weight form of urokinase from human urine. Arch Biol Biophys 1983; 280:31–38.
334. Lijnen HR, et al. Activation of plasminogen by prourokinase. J Biol Chem 1986; 261:1253–1258.
335. Pannell R, Black J, Gurewich V. Complementary modes of action of tissue-type plasminogen activation and prourokinase by which their synergistic effect on clot lysis may be explained. J Clin Invest 1988; 81:853–859.
336. Rijken DC, Collen D. Purification and characterization of the plasminogen activation secreted by human melanoma cells in culture. J Biol Chem 1981; 256:7035–7041.
337. Levin EG. Latent tissue plasminogen activation produced by human endothelial cells in cultures: evidence for an enzyme inhibitor complex. Proc Natl Acad Sci 1983; 80:6804–6808.
338. Ichinose A, Kisiel W, Fujikawa K. Protection from activation of tissue plasminogen activator by plasmin and tissue enzymes. Fed Eur Biochem Soc Letts 1984; 175:412–418.
339. Rijken DC, Hoylaerts M, Collen D. Fibrinolytic properties of one-chain and two-chain human extrinsic (tissue-type) plasminogen activator. J Biol Chem 1982; 257:2920–2925.
340. von Zonnenveld A-J, Veerman H, Pannekoek A. On the interaction of the finger and kringle-2 domains of tissue-type plasminogen activator with fibrin. J Biol Chem 1986; 261:14214–14218.
341. The Urokinase Pulmonary Embolism Trial: a National Cooperative Study. Circulation 1973; 47[Suppl II]:1–108.
342. Urokinase-Streptokinase Embolism Trial: phase 2 results: a comparative study. JAMA 1974; 229:1606–1613.
343. Goldhaber SZ, et al. Acute pulmonary embolism treated with tissue plasminogen activator. Lancet 1986; 2:886–889.
344. Immelman EV, Jeffery PC. The postphlebitic syndrome; pathophysiology, prevention and management. Clin Chest Med 1984; 5:537–550.
345. Wolfe MW, Skibol K, Goldhaber SZ. Pulmonary embolic disease: diagnosis, pathophysiologic aspects, and treatment with thrombolytic therapy. Curr Prob Cardiol 1993; 18:587–663.
346. Johansson L, et al. Comparison of SK with heparin: late results in the treatment of deep vein thrombosis. Brit Med J 1969; 1:810–811.
347. Kakkar VV, et al. Late results of treatment of deep vein thrombosis. Brit Med J 1969; 1:810–811.
348. Kakkar VV, Lawrence D. Hemodynamics and clinical assessment of the therapy for acute deep vein thrombosis: a prospective study. Am J Surg 1985; 150:54–63.
349. Druy EM, et al. Lytic therapy with treatment of axillary and subclavian vein thrombosis. J Vasc Surg 1985; 2:821–827.
350. Kohner EM, et al. Streptokinase in central retinal vein occlusion: a controlled clinical trial. Brit Med J 1976; 1:550–553.
351. Greenwood LH, et al. Urokinase in the treatment of Budd-Chiari syndrome. Am J Roentgen 1983; 141:1057–1059.
352. Shenoy MM, et al. Streptokinase lysis of intraventrical thrombus and pulmonary embolism with resolution of acquired intracerebral shunt. Ann Int Med 1985; 103:65–66.
353. DeWood MA, et al. Prevalence of total coronary occlusion

during the early hours of transient myocardial infarction. N Engl J Med 1980; 303:897–902.

354. Yusef S, et al. Intravenous and intracoronary fibrinolytic therapy in acute myocardial infarction: review of results on mortality, reinfarction, and side-effects from 33 randomized controlled trials. Euro Heart J 1985; 6:556–585.
355. Gruppo Italiano per lo studio della streptochinasi nell' infarto miocardico (GISSI). Effectiveness of intravenous thrombolytic treatment in acute myocardial infarction. Lancet 1986; 1:397–402.
356. Gruppo Italiano per lo studio della streptochinasi nell' infarto miocardico (GISSI-2). A factorial randomized trial of alteplase versus streptokinase and heparin versus no heparin among 12,490 patients with acute myocardial infarction. Lancet 1990; 336:65–71.
357. Third International Study of Infarct Survival (ISIS-3). Presented at the annual meeting of the American College of Cardiology, Atlanta, Georgia (USA), March 1991.
358. The ISAM Study Group. A prospective trial of intravenous streptokinase in acute myocardial infarction (I.S.A.M.). Mortality, morbidity, and infarct size at 21 days. N Engl J Med 1986; 314:1465–1471.
359. Kennedy JW, et al. Western Washington randomized trial of intracoronary streptokinase in acute myocardial infarction. N Engl J Med 1983; 309:1477–1482.
360. ISIS-2 (Second International Study of Infarct Survival) Collaborative Group. Randomized trial of intravenous streptokinase, oral aspirin, both, or neither among 17,187 cases of suspected acute myocardial infarction: ISIS-2. Lancet 1988; 2:349.
361. White HD, et al. Effect of intravenous streptokinase on left ventricular function and early survival after acute myocardial infarction. N Engl J Med 1987; 317:850–856.
362. Chesebro JH, et al. Thrombolysis in myocardial infarction (TIMI) trial phase I: a comparison between intravenous tissue plasminogen activation and intravenous streptokinase. Circulation 1987; 76:142–154.
363. Verstraete M, et al. Randomized trial of intravenous recombinant tissue type plasminogen activator versus intravenous streptokinase in acute myocardial infarction. Report for the European Cooperative Study Group for Recombinant Tissue-type Plasminogen Activator. Lancet 1985; 1:842–847.
364. Wilcox RG, et al. Trial of tissue plasminogen activator for mortality reduction in acute myocardial infarction—Anglo-Scandinavian Study of Early Thrombosis (ASSET). Lancet 1988; 2:525–530.
365. Anderson JL, et al. Multicenter reperfusion trial of intravenous anisoylated plasminogen streptokinase activator complex (APSAC) in acute myocardial infarction: controlled comparison with intracoronary streptokinase. J Am Coll Cardiol, 1989; 13:988–997.
366. AIMS Trial Study Group. Long-term effect of intravenous anistreplase in acute myocardial infarction. Final Report of the AIMS Study. Lancet 1990; 2:422–431.
367. Mathey DG, et al. Intravenous urokinase in acute myocardial infarction. Am J Cardiol 1985; 55:878–882.
368. Muller J. From the Prourokinase-Myocardial Infarction Study Group. Clot-selective coronary thrombolysis with prourokinase. Circulation 1987; 76:121a.
369. The GUSTO Investigators. An international randomized trial comparing four thrombolytic strategies for acute myocardial infarction. N Engl J Med 1993; 329:673–682.
370. Avery A, et al. Outcome of recent thromboembolic occlusions of limb arteries treated with streptokinase. Brit Med J 1970; 4:639–644.
371. Belkin M, et al. Intra-arterial fibrinolytic therapy: efficacy of streptokinase vs. urokinase. Arch Surg 1986; 121:769–773.
372. Del Zoppo GJ, Zeumer H, Hortier A. Thrombolytic therapy in stroke: possibilities and hazards. Stroke 1986; 17:595–607.
373. Del Zoppo GJ. Antithrombotic therapy in cerebrovascular disease. In J Loscalzo, AI Schafer, eds. Thrombosis and Hemorrhage. Boston: Blackwell. Pp 1225–1252.
374. Marder VJ, Sherry S. Thrombolytic therapy: current status. N Engl J Med 1988; 318:1512–1520, 1585–1595.
375. Sherry S. Appraisal of various thrombolytic agents in the treatment of acute myocardial infarction. Am J Med 1987; 83[Suppl 27]:31–46.
376. Burket MW, et al. Relation of effectiveness of intracoronary thrombolysis in acute myocardial infarct to systemic thrombolytic state. Am J Cardiol 1985; 56: 441–444.
377. Collen D, et al. Synergism of thrombolytic agents in vivo. Circulation 1986; 74:838–842.

Future Molecular Approaches to the Treatment of Cardiovascular Disease: Gene Therapy

Heiko E. von der Leyen
Victor J. Dzau

As Paul Berg states, "There is no doubt that the development and application of recombinant DNA technology has put us at the threshold of new forms of medicine" [1].

The application of molecular biologic technology in cardiovascular research is widening so rapidly that traditional concepts of physiology and pharmacology have been revolutionized by the concept of cellular and molecular regulation in cardiovascular disease (the third paradigm, according to Katz [2]). We have witnessed a major evolution in thinking from the view that the heart and blood vessels are mechanical organs that respond to nerves and hormones to the recognition that the cardiovascular tissues are biologic, active organs capable of synthesizing active molecules that participate in the regulation of cardiac and vascular function [3].

At the beginning of this century, the work of the heart was understood mechanically as a beat-to-beat response to altered hemodynamics [4], and the vasculature was described as a passive conduit that transports blood to and from vital organs, as it was shown by William Harvey in 1628. Resulting therapeutic approaches according to these paradigms aimed at reducing heart work by, for example, bed rest or reducing the blood volume by more or less physical methods. As biophysical and biochemical methods became available in the middle of this century, new paradigms evolved in cardiovascular medicine, and it became clear that vascular function was regulated by humoral factors [5] and that, for example, calcium plays a pivotal role in controling cardiac contractility [6]. Subsequently, numerous therapeutic drugs were introduced that interact with the calcium metabolism and that influence myocardial contractility as well as vascular activity. It is now clear that the cardiovascular system is a complex organ capable of sensing its environment, transducing signals to cells in the cardiovascular tissue or to the surrounding tissue, and synthesizing local mediators that participate in the regulation of cardiac and vascular function [2,3,7]. Thus, a third paradigm is emerging in that cardiovascular function is regulated by altered gene expression in the cardiovascular system. This has led to the identification of genes involved in cardiovascular disease and created the concept of gene therapy as a potential approach to treat cardiovacsular disease. The molecular approach to cardiovascular disease consists of (1) the elucidation of pathobiologic processes, especially at the cellular and molecular levels using Northern blot, reverse transcriptase-polymerase chain reaction (RT-PCR), in-situ hybridization, and other techniques; (2) in-vivo gene manipulation and the development of animal models of diseases using gene transfer, antisense oligonucleotide application, and transgenic animals; and (3) the development of novel therapeutic strategies like gene replacement, gene correction, and gene augmentation (Table 28-1). In the 1970s, the molecular revolution transformed biology; now, in the 1990s, the molecular revolution is transforming medicine.

Several pivotal events in molecular biology and biochemistry as well as in medicine have led to the new concept of **in-vivo gene transfer** and **gene therapy** [8]. By the mid- to late 1960s, it was discovered that, in the course of transforming a cell from the normal to the neoplastic phenotype, the papovaviruses SV40 and polyoma integrated their genetic information or specific transforming regions covalently, stably, and heritably into the genomes of target cells [9]. Those experiments showed, for the first time, that an efficient genetic transformation of a cell by exogenous genetic information must be possible [10], and it was suggested that SV40 could be developed as a transducing vector to introduce exogenous DNA into mammalian cells [11]. Before the beginning of the recombinant-DNA era, the use of viruses to transfer therapeutic genes into cells and even into human patients (with no effect at the time) took place [12]. Stimulated by the advent of recombinant-DNA techniques [1] Friedmann and Roblin [13] first suggested, in 1972, that tumor viruses can be modified to carry recombinant genetic information to complement genetic defects and correct disease phenotypes. That concept was supported by Berg and colleagues [14], who prepared a recombinant SV40 vector that indeed was able to transfer foreign DNA sequences efficiently into mammalian cells. In 1979, the same group showed that even total cellular DNA could be introduced into mammalian cells efficiently and functionally [15]. It was clear that two tools were necessary for gene therapy: efficient methods of gene transfer (i.e., viral vectors) and specific genes in cloned form (i.e., recombinant-DNA technology).

The recent development of efficient gene-transfection procedures, together with the arsenal of recombinant-DNA technology, has led to a widespread application of transient or stable expressions of genes to study disease processes and the potential use of gene therapy. Over 200 patients worldwide have now received exogenous functional genetic material with therapeutic intent [16,17]. The results of these pioneering experiments cannot be expected to be startling—the systems used are relatively crude, and there are many problems still to be solved. However, the pace of research is fast, and it transcends the traditional boundaries of contemporary high-technology medicine in the development of transfection vectors and for the targeting and control of gene expression. This chapter focuses on attempts to aim gene modification at cardiovascular disorders, particularly diseases of the vas-

Table 28-1. A molecular approach to cardiovascular disease

1. Defination of pathobiological mediators
   - mRNA analysis/PCR, Northern blotting
   - In situ hybridization
2. Simulation of pathological conditions
   - Gene transfer of putative mediators
   - Antisense inhibition of putative mediators
   - Transgenic animals
3. Novel therapies
   - Gene augmentation
   - Antisense or decoy strategies
   - Gene replacement

culature. Table 28-2 summarizes the potential application of gene therapy in cardiovascular disease.

Gene-Transfer Techniques for the Cardiovascular System

To improve the efficiency of gene transfer, a number of alternatives to the classic precipitation techniques—calcium phosphate or diethylaminoethyl (DEAE)–dextran polymer [18]—have recently been developed (Table 28-3). The encapsulation of the DNA of interest in artificial lipid membranes (liposomes) resulted in a higher efficiency of gene transfer in certain cell types [19]. Microinjection has been used successfully to introduce purified recombinant proteins, neutralizing antibodies, and competitor oligonucleotides into cells, allowing a critical examination of the role of specific gene products in the acquisition of a variety of defined phenotypic features that can be assayed at the single-cell level [20,21]. The intramuscular injection of plasmid DNA into skeletal muscle showed transient expression of a foreign gene in different skeletal myotubes [22]. By extending direct gene injection to the heart muscle, the expression of a reporter gene was demonstrated for up to 4 weeks after the initial injection [23]. Furthermore, expression of injected genes can be targeted at specific cell types in vivo (e.g., cardiac muscle cells) and modulated by the hormonal status of the animal [24]. Another approach for gene delivery consists of viral vectors that recently have been used in growing numbers to express exogenous genes in vivo [25,26]. Effective therapy by in-vivo delivery of DNA requires efficient delivery, long-term maintenance of the DNA that is delivered, and physiologic levels of expression of the therapeutic gene. Full levels of physiologically controlled expression can be obtained after transfer of intact genes or fragments of DNA hundreds of kilobases in size, as has been demonstrated by the transfer of yeast artificial chromosomes into transgenic mice [27,28]. Long-term maintenance of input DNA could be achieved if the DNA carried replication origins, a centromere, and telomeres to allow maintenance and segregation in mammalian cells [29]. Those features could be combined as a mammalian artificial chromosome that would confer full levels of controlled expression as well as being maintained in any cell into which it was introduced [30].

Table 28-2. Gene therapy for cardiovascular disease

Gene therapy	Example of target gene
SYSTEMIC GENE THERAPY	
Familial hypercholesterolemia	Low-density lipoprotein receptor
Atherosclerosis	High-density lipoprotein
Hypercoagulable states	Tissue-plasminogen activator
Refractory diabetes mellitus	Insulin
LOCAL GENE THERAPY	
Restenosis after angioplasty	Cell-cycle regulatory gene
Transplant rejection	Leucocyte adhesion molecule
Transplant vasculopathy	Cytokine
Myocardial infarction	
Cardiac remodeling	Transforming growth factor-β
Angiogenesis	Fibroblast growth factor
Myocarditis	Cytokine
Congenital heart disease	Myocyte differentiation factors
Thrombosis	Tissue-plasminogen activator
Glomerular disease	Cytokine; cell-cycle regulatory gene
Aortic aneurysms	Protease inhibitor

Table 28-3. Experimental methods of gene transfer

- Viral-mediated
  - Retrovirus
  - Adenovirus
    - Replication deficient
    - Adenoviral coat/transferrin-polylysine
- Lipid-mediated
  - Liposomes
  - Cationic liposomes (Lipofectin®)
- Fusigenic liposome-mediated
  - Sendai virus–liposome complex
- Other methods
  - Microinjection
  - Microparticle bombardment
  - Implantation (myoblast)

Although calcium phosphate, DEAE dextran, cationic liposome, and electroporation have been widely employed in vitro to transfect foreign genes into various cells, those methods are usually characterized by low in-vivo transfection efficiency [31]. Currently, in-vivo gene-transfer techniques for cardiovascular applications include (1) viral gene transfer such as retrovirus or adenovirus, (2) liposomal gene transfer with cationic liposomes (Lipofectin ®), (3) fusigenic liposomes using Sendai virus (hemagglutinating virus of Japan, or HVJ) complexed with liposomes, and (4) direct (micro)injection, including myoblast implantation (Table 28-3). As outlined next, the in-vivo gene-transfer techniques have different advantages and disadvantages.

VIRAL MEDIATED GENE TRANSFER

Retroviral Mediated Gene Transfer. Retroviral expression vectors are constructed by incorporating the exogenous gene into the viral genome [32]. The recombinant viral vector can deliver the inserted gene into the cell with high efficiency [33]. A retroviral vector is constructed by several steps [34]. First, to render the vector nonreplicating, the structural genes required for viral replication are deleted from the retrovirus using appropriate restriction enzymes (although the packaging signals are left intact). Next, the exogenous gene of interest is inserted into the viral backbone by ligation. The recombinant retrovirus now contains the exogenous gene, regulatory sequences, and packaging signals, but it lacks the actual structural genes required to produce a complete virion. It requires a helper cell to produce infectious viral particles. The defective retroviral vector DNA is introduced into a packaging helper cell line that contains a second plasmid encoding the structural genes. When a retroviral vector, in which the structural genes are removed but the packaging signal remains intact, is introduced in such a packaging cell line, the packaging signal is recognized by the structural proteins provided by the second plasmid, and a complete infectious virion is produced. The defective retroviral vector then infects a host organism. The genome from the retroviral vector becomes incorporated in the host genome, and the host cell can express the gene of interest. In case of the **single-gene vector**, the structural genes of the retrovirus are replaced by a single gene that is then transcribed under the control of the viral regulatory sequences contained in the long terminal repeat (LTR) [33–35]. Such a recombinant virus can be used as a vector to transfer either a selectable marker or a nonselectable cellular gene. Nabel et al. [25,36] first demonstrated the feasibility of transfecting blood vessels with foreign DNA in vivo. Using a double-balloon catheter and direct infection with a murine amphotropic retroviral vector containing a recombinant beta-galactosidase gene, those authors showed in pig iliofemoral arteries that several cell types in the vessel wall were transduced, including endothelial and vascular smooth muscle cells. The reporter gene was expressed for at least 5 months. With a similar retroviral vector containing the beta-galactosidase gene, Wilson et al. [37] reported that prosthetic vascular grafts seeded with genetically modified endothelial cells expressed beta-galactosidase activity and protein up to 5 weeks, as detected by enzymatic assay and in-situ cytohistochemistry. Though it has a substantial transfection efficiency, the retroviral method does seem to have several disadvantages: (1) there is a limitation to the insert size because foreign genes must be inserted into the retrovirus; (2) stable transfection is related to cell replication, and no transfection efficiency can be achieved in terminally differentiated cells; (3) there is the possibility of developing deleterious side effects, such as viral infection and activation of oncogenes; (4) there is the potential of developing an autoimmune response against the intrinsic retroviral antigens; and (5) because the retroviral method results in stable transformation of target cells, the random integration could potentiate mutagenesis [31]. The retrovirus-mediated gene-transfer method may present higher risks to humans than other gene-transfer methods [38]. Indeed, monkeys have been reported to develop malignant T-cell lymphomas after undergoing bone marrow transplantation with a gene-transfer protocol in which a helper virus contaminated the retroviral vector preparation [39].

Adenovirus-Mediated Gene Transfer. Adenovirus vectors also have been shown to be useful vehicles for cardiovascular gene transfer. Like the herpes virus (a neurotropic virus that can transfect neuronal cells with high efficiency [40]), adenoviruses are DNA viruses that can transfect nondividing cells and generally do not integrate into the host genome. Two different methods using adenoviral gene transfer are currently under investigation: (1) a replication-deficient adenoviral vector similar to the retroviral approach and (2) coupling of adenoviral coat to transferrin-polylysine/DNA complexes. The first approach consists in insertion of the foreign genes into deleted regions of the adenovirus genome similar to the retroviral approach [41,42]. Replication-deficient recombinant adenoviral vectors can be manipulated to encode for recombinant-gene products limited to 7.5 kilobases. The recombinant virus can be propagated in certain mammalian cell lines that serve to complement the growth of replication-deficient adenovirus. Aortic smooth muscle cells [42] and cardiac myocytes [43] were successfully transfected using replication-defective adenovirus carrying the beta-galactosidase and chloramphenicol acetyltransferase reporter gene, respectively. Effective in-vivo transfection by direct infusion into vessels was demonstrated in vascular tissue with expression of the transgene for at least 2 weeks [42,44–46] and in myocardial tissue by direct injection into the myocardium [43,47]. Although adenoviral vectors represent a highly efficient gene-transfection method, they have the potential disadvantages of viral infection and viral antigen-induced immunity [48], which may limit the use of those vectors in humans. Adenovirus-mediated gene transfer into the lungs of baboons was associated with the development of alveolar inflammation at high doses of virus required to induce detectable gene expression [49].

The second adenoviral-mediated gene-transfer approach is reported by coupling adenovirus to DNA-polylysine complexes, resulting in a high transfection efficiency in tissue-culture cell lines [50]. Replication-deficient or chemically inactivated adenovirus is coupled to polylysine, either enzymatically through the action of transglutaminase or biochemically by biotinylating adenovirus and streptavidinylating the ploylysine moiety. Combination complexes containing DNA, adenovirus-polylysine, and transferrin-polylysine have the capacity to transfer the reporter gene into adenovirus-receptor- and transferrin-receptor-rich cells. The adenovirus and transferrin complexes are colocalized in endosomes. The virus, because of its endosomolytic properties, is thought to destroy the integrity of the endosomal membrane and to effect exit of the colocalized DNA into the cytoplasm and eventually to the nucleus [51]. This approach has many advantages similar to the HVJ method. For some tissues, such as the lung, the adenoviral gene transfer method is particularly attractive and efficacious. Recently, Willard et al. [52] reported the successful gene transfer into the blood vessels using that approach. An interesting extension of the adenoviral vector system was reported recently in abstract form [53]. A recombinant virus was constructed in which the firefly luciferase gene (serving as a reporter gene) was driven by a thyroid hormone–retinoic acid response element linked to the herpes simplex virus thymidine kinase promoter. Using that construct in vivo, reporter-gene activity was stimulated by injection of triiodo-thyronine (T3), which showed the potential to endogenously regulate the expression of genes transferred for the purpose of therapy.

LIPID-MEDIATED GENE TRANSFER

The liposomal method is safe and easy to use. The cationic lipid-mediated method (DNA mixed with a liposome suspension comprising cationic lipid) was first reported in 1987 [19]. The possible mechanism of this gene-transfer approach is that the negatively charged phosphate groups on DNA bind to the positively charged surface of the liposome and that the residual positive charge then presumably mediates binding to negatively charged sialic-acid residues on the cell surfaces. The cationic lipid-mediated method seems to be efficient for in-vitro transfer of DNA. In-vivo application of the method showed transfection of DNA into intact coronary and peripheral arteries [54]; however, the transfection efficiency was low, and the incubation time needed was long. The expression of liposome-mediated arterial gene transfer may be augmented in the presence of ongoing cellular proliferation (e.g., intimal proliferation after balloon injury) [55]. Using a single intravenous injection of expression plasmid-liposome complexes in adult mice, expression of the transgene could be targeted at specific tissues and cell types, depending on the promoter element used [56].

FUSIGENIC-LIPOSOME MEDIATED GENE TRANSFER

Sendai Virus (HVJ)/Liposome Technique. This method represents a combination of fusigenic proteins of the Sendai virus (HVJ) in conjunction with liposomes. It appears to possess several advantages for in-vivo gene transfer such as (1) efficiency independent of cell differentiation or replication, (2) safety (since the virus is inactivated before transfection, only the viral coat is used for delivery of the transgene), (3) simplicity of preparation, (4) brevity of incubation time (in vitro, 40 minutes; in vivo, 10–15 minutes), and (5) no limitation of inserted DNA size. Figure 28-1 illustrates the steps for preparation of Sendai virus–complexed liposomes for gene transfer. The DNA to be transfected is mixed with a nuclear protein (high-mobility group-1, or HMG-1). The nuclear protein can bind DNA and delivers the DNA to nuclei, thereby enhancing the integration of the transfected DNA into the nucleus [57,58]. Next, Sendai virus–liposome complexes are prepared by mixing dried lipids (containing phosphatidylserine, phosphatidylcholine, and cholesterol) with the DNA–HMG-1 solution and subsequently with UV-light–inactivated HVJ (purified Z strain). After purification by a sucrose density gradient centrifugation to remove unincorporated virus particles, the HVJ-liposome complex is ready for use in transfection experiments [59]. An interesting feature of the Sendai virus–liposome-mediated gene-transfer method is the fact that after fusion of the liposome complex with the cell membrane the DNA is released directly into the cytosol without endocytosis, thereby enhancing the nuclear uptake and reducing lysosomal destruction of the DNA construct [60]. The Sendai virus–liposome method was compared in vitro with the cationic liposome method using an angiotensin converting enzyme (ACE) gene construct [61]. Cellular ACE activity was significantly higher with the Sendai virus method (35-minute incubation time for transfection) than cationic liposome method (24-hour incubation time). In addition, human ACE cDNA transfected into the rat carotid artery in organ culture yielded high ACE expression in the tunica media at 3 days after transfection [61]. In-vivo experiments in rat carotid arteries using an SV40 large-T-antigen cDNA expression vector showed that the Sendai virus–liposome transfection method was efficient (up to 30% of the vessel wall showed SV40 T-antigen expression) without apparent toxicity [62]. One week after transfection, immunohistochemical staining revealed expression of the transgene in the tunica media of both injured and uninjured arteries.

The HVJ method has been employed successfully for gene transfer in vivo to many tissues, including liver [58],

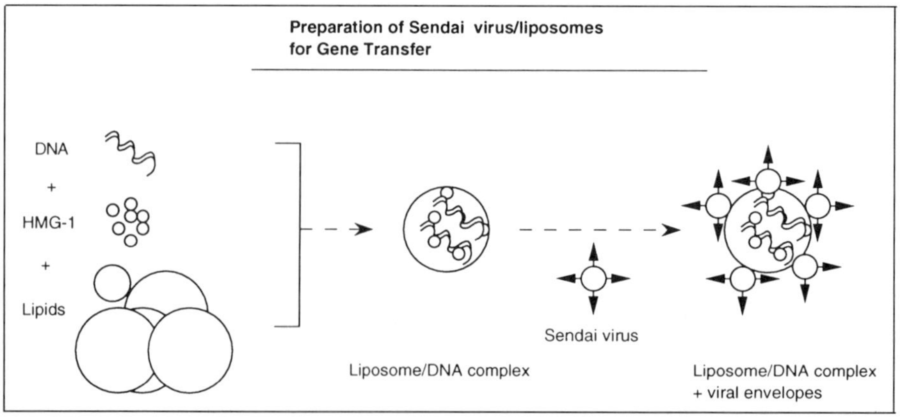

Fig. 28-1. Preparation of Sendai virus–liposome complex for gene transfer. HMG-1 = high mobility group-1.

kidney [63,64], and the vascular wall [26]. Due to the hemagglutinating activity of the Sendai virus, a nonspecific binding for red blood cells may be disadvantegeous. To avoid that side effect, a vessel segment has to be flushed with physiologic saline solution before introduction of the HVJ-liposome transfection solution. The Sendai virus–liposome method is also suitable for transfer of antisense oligonucleotides. It can result in a significant increase in the stability and the effectiveness of antisense oligonucleotides [65]. In-vivo transfer of fluorescein isothiocyanate (FITC)–labeled phosphothioate oligonucleotides into injured rat carotid arteries using the Sendai virus–liposome method resulted in widespread distribution of fluorescence in medial vascular cells at 10 minutes after transfection. The fluorescence was localized primarily in cell nuclei and persisted up to 2 weeks after transfection [26]. So far, in experiments using the Sendai virus–liposome transfection system, no evidence of side effects has been reported. Given the above-mentioned advantageous facts of the inactivated Sendai-virus vector, the Sendai virus–liposome methods seems to represent a very attractive gene-transfer method for the cardiovascular system.

OTHER GENE-TRANSFER METHODS

The potential use of genetically modified endothelial cells has been investigated. Wilson et al. [37] implanted vascular grafts that were genetically modified by retrovirus-mediated gene transfer, and Nabel et al. transferred genetically modified endothelial cells into the vessel wall in vivo [36]. Lynch et al. [66] reported the seeding of adenosine deaminase gene-transfected smooth muscle cells into endothelium-denuded blood vessels. Dichek and colleagues focused on the development of a stent coated with genetically modified endothelial cells for the prevention of restenosis [67]. They were able to detect small quantities of tissue-type plasminogen activator (t-PA) from stents seeded with genetically modified endothelial cells containing recombinant t-PA [68]. Another approach to deliver gene products is given by the implantation of genetically modified myoblasts or fibroblasts to muscular tissue providing systemic delivery of hormones [69]. The implanation of myoblasts transfected with human factor IX using a retrovirus vector resulted in secretion of the protein into the circulation for up to 1 month [70].

Application of Gene Transfer in Cardiovascular Therapy

Potential applications of gene transfer in cardiovascular gene therapy (see Table 28-2) include the treatment of vascular disorders (restenosis, atherosclerosis), cardiac diseases (myocardial infarction, cardiac remodeling, cardiomyopathy), metabolic disorders (diabetes mellitus, hypercholesterolemia, hypertension), and autoimmune diseases (glomerulonephritis).

The local delivery of genetically modified material to the vasculature includes a direct deposition of therapeutic agents into the vessel wall through an intravascular delivery system or administration of fusion toxins that have specific affinities to the vessel wall [71,72]. The development of catheter-based drug-delivery systems compatible with incubation times necessary for efficient gene transfer yet capable of maintaining tissue perfusion will be neccessary to elucidate the full potential of in-vivo gene transfer. Using a double-balloon catheter, Nabel et al. [73] reported the introduction, by direct gene transfer into porcine arteries, of a eukaryotic expression vector encoding a secreted form of fibroblast growth factor-1 (FGF-1) thereby inducing intimal thickening of the transfected vessels together with neocapillary formation. In the same model, the overexpression of transforming growth factor-β_1 (TGF-β_1) in normal arteries resulted in substantial extracellular matrix production accompanied by intimal and medial hyperplasia [74]. Those findings showed that TGF-β_1 differentially modulates extracellular matrix production and cellular proliferation in the arterial wall and could play a reparative role in response to arterial injury. Although the application of gene transfer is very helpful for evaluating the pathobiologic function of a specific gene (with the prospect of subsequent development of therapeutic agents), the main advantage of gene therapy is the application of recombinant DNA to directly treat cardiovascular diseases. We recently reported [75] the construction of an expression vector containing the endothelial cell–nitric oxide synthase (ec-NOS) cDNA driven by a beta-actin promoter and CMV enhancer. In-vivo transfection of that construct in balloon-injured rat carotid arteries not only restored nitric oxide production in the vessel wall but also significantly increased the vascular reactivity of the vessel. Furthermore, ec-NOS transgene expression resulted in a 70-percent inhibition of neointima formation after balloon injury (Fig. 28-2). Thus, using in-vivo gene-transfer techniques, it was shown that the loss of endothelial-derived nitric oxide may play a fundamental role in the pathogenesis of vascular diseases such as atherosclerosis [75]. This study documented for the first time therapeutic effects utilizing direct in-vivo gene transfer of a cDNA encoding a functional enzyme, and it was speculated that ec-NOS gene transfer may be useful for gene therapy of neointimal hyperplasia and associated local vasospasm. Another therapeutic approach was reported recently that used an adenoviral vector encoding the herpesvirus thymidine kinase (*tk*) [76]. After introduction of the vector in injured porcine arteries and vascular smooth muscle cells, the *tk* gene rendered the smooth muscle cells sensitive to the nucleoside analog ganciclovir given immediately after balloon injury. After one course of ganciclovir treatment, intimal hyperplasia decreased by about 50–70 percent. Also, by using an adenovirus-mediated gene transfer, Zoldhelyi et al. report that they were able to prevent balloon angioplasty–induced thrombotic complications in a pig model by transfer of prostaglandin H synthase-1 cDNA [77].

Intracellular targeting to inhibit factors necessary for cell proliferation and migration could be achieved by molecular-based approaches using the transfer of specific oligonucleotides [78]. This strategy theoretically provides a simple means to inhibit the expression of a specific gene [79,80]. mRNA contains sequences of nucleotides that encode for specific amino acids; this is the "sense" message that results in the translation of a protein product. The antisense oligonucleotide represents a 15- to 20-oligomer sequence of nucleotides complementary to the target

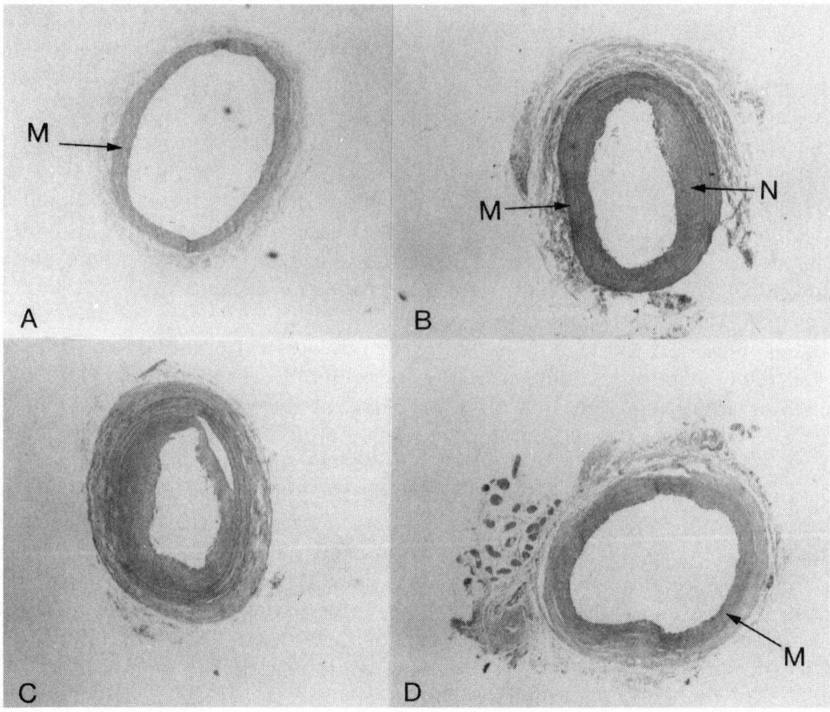

Fig. 28-2. Inhibition of neointimal hyperplasia by in-vivo gene transfer of endothelial cell-nitric oxide synthase construct. **A.** Normal artery; **B.** injured artery, untransfected; **C.** injured artery, control vector transfected; **D.** injured artery, NOS transfected. M = media, N = neointima. (Reproduced with permission from von der Leyen et al. Gene therapy inhibiting neointimal vascular lesion: in vivo gene transfer of endothelial-cell nitric oxide synthase gene. Proc Natl Acad Sci USA 1995; 92:1137–1141.)

mRNA that hybridizes with it. The effect of the antisense message is that it fails to encode a message that can be translated into a protein. In the case of a disease-related protein, the antisense strategy theoretically prevents expression of a given protein that caused the specific disease. Several groups have investigated the effects of antisense oligonucleotides on intimal hyperplasia after balloon injury. The administration of antisense oligonucleotides against c-myb (exceeding a concentration of 150 μM) using a pluronic gel applied to the adventitial layer of rat carotid arteries inhibited the development of neointimal hyperplasia in response to balloon injury [81]. Unfortunately, this periadventitial polymer delivery system is not a practical approach for the prevention of restenosis after percutaneous transluminal angioplasty in humans. The Sendai virus–liposome gene-transfer approach provides an intraluminal molecular delivery system that has several advantages over the periadventitial polymer delivery approach. The Sendai virus–liposome method seems to substantially increase the efficiency of uptake of oligonucleotides and appears to increase the stability of the oligonucleotides in intracellular compartments. We anticipate that the modification of antisense oligonucleotide pharmacokinetics by use of the HVJ-liposome complex may facilitate the potential clinical utility of the agents by (1) allowing for an abbreviated intraluminal incubation time to preserve organ perfusion, (2) prolonging the duration of biological action, and (3) enhancing efficacy such that the nonspecific effects of high doses (i.e., > 100 μM) of oligonucleotides can be avoided. Our recent data revealed that a single administration of antisense oligonucleotides against proliferating cell nuclear antigen (PCNA) and cdc2 kinase genes (15 μM) inhibited neointimal formation after balloon injury at least up to 8 weeks after transfection [82] (Fig. 28-3). The combination of antisense cdc2 and cdk2 oligonucleotides also resulted in nearly complete inhibition of neointima formation [26]. Given that the virus is inactivated by ultraviolet light, there is little potential for biologic hazard by the use of this method compared to retroviral mediated gene-transfer approaches. Using a retroviral vector, Bennett et al. [83] showed an inhibition of vascular smooth muscle cell proliferation by administration of c-myc antisense oligonucleotides to injured rat carotid arteries. Recently, two additional studies reported inhibition of neointima formation after antisense application. Delivery of antisense PCNA oligonucleotides by a Pluronic gel (in a rat carotid model) and of antisense c-myc oligonucleotides by direct application through a porous ballon (in a porcine coronary artery model) resulted in significant inhibition of neointimal hyperplasia [84,85]. We speculate that continuing development in the use of antisense oligonucleotide

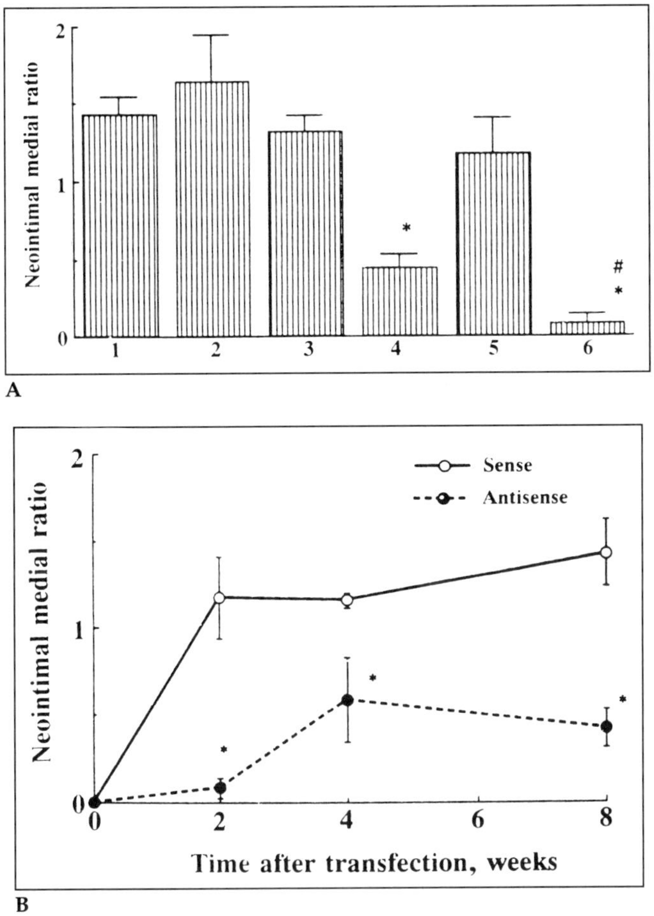

Fig. 28-3. **A.** Dose effect of cdc2 kinase and PCNA antisense and sense ODNs on intimal-medial area ratio. Bars: 1, injured vessels without any treatment; 2, injured vessels treated with HVJ–liposomes without ODN; 3, injured vessels treated with 3 μM sense HVJ–ODN; 4, injured vessels treated with 3 μM antisense HVJ–ODN; 5, injured vessels treated with 15 μM sense HVJ–ODN; 6, injured vessels treated with 15 μM antisense HVJ–ODN. *, $P < 0.01$ vs. sense treatment; #, $P < 0.01$ vs. 3 μM antisense ODN treatment. ODN = oligonucleotide. **B.** Long-term efficiency of cdc2 kinase and PCNA antisense and sense ODNs on intimal/medial area ratio. **, $P < 0.01$ vs. sense treatment. Morishita R, et al. Single intraluminal delivery of antisense cdc2 kinase and proliferating-cell nuclear antigen oligonucleotides results in chronic inhibition of neointimal hyperplasia. Proc Natl Acad Sci USA. 1993; 90:8474–8478.

technology will further characterize the biologic role of gene products activated in response to vascular injury as well as provide new therapeutic agents for use in humans.

The efficacy of aorto-coronary vein grafting is limited by early graft thrombosis and accelerated graft atherosclerosis. Recombinant adenovirus-mediated gene transfer of soluble cell adhesion molecules to porcine interposition vein grafts resulted in a high level of gene expression in vivo [86]. Therapeutic effects of this approach have not yet been reported. Our group recently demonstrated that the intraoperative transfer of antisense oligonucleotides direct against cell cycle regulatory genes (PCNA/cdc2 kinase) resulted in blockade of medial smooth muscle cell proliferation and prevented accelerated atherosclerosis responsible for graft failure [90]. The selective blockade of cell-cycle regulatory genes in rabbit jugular veins grafted into carotid arteries influenced the vascular remodeling process after grafting by directing remodeling away from neointimal hyperplasia toward medial hypertrophy, yielding conduits that more closely resembled normal arteries. More important, these grafts were resistant to diet-induced atherosclerosis.

Chronic heart failure also may represent a target for gene therapy. Lefkowitz and colleagues showed enhanced myocardial function in transgenic mice overexpressing the β_2-adrenergic receptor [87]. Because chronic heart failure in humans is accompanied by a reduction in the number of myocardial beta-adrenergic receptors and in inotropic responsiveness, these results suggest a potential gene-therapy approach to this disease. Grafted cardiomyocytes carrying a fusion gene of the alpha-cardiac myosin heavy-chain promoter might also provide a useful approach for myocardial repair, provided that the grafted cells can contribute to myocardial function [88]. Successful transfection after fluoroscopic-guided direct percutaneous delivery of a transgene expressing a reporter gene into cardiac muscle suggests that it might be feasible to deliver genetic material into the myocardium of patients [89]. Especially in ischemic cardiovascular diseases, the direct in-vivo gene transfer of FGF-1 or related genes could provide a method to stimulate angiogenesis and neovascularization to enhance collateral blood flow to ischemic myocardial tissue [73].

Now that gene therapy for cardiovascular disease appears to be not far from reality, it is time to address practical issues that eventually will determine the clinical potential of gene therapy in cardiovascular disease. Current problems in gene therapy are summarized in Table 28-4. In particular, the following questions must be addressed:

Table 28-4. Current problems in gene therapy

Low efficiency
Delivery system
Inactivation, or silencing, of transgene
Toxicity
Identification of appropriate targets
Human applications

1. **Safety**, which includes methodologic and ethical issues. Methodologically, we must develop safer and more efficient gene-transfer systems as well as an easy and noninvasive gene-delivery system.
2. **Persistence of gene expression and duration of treatment**.
3. **Regulation**. Ideal gene therapy should be regulated by intrinsic hormonal conditions, to avoid overexpression. However, hormone-regulated promoters are not ideal

for the strong expression necessary for the treatment of certain inherited disorders. In the future, we must find ideal and suitable promoters that can be regulated but express sufficient amounts of the product (e.g., a cut-off system) for effective gene therapy.

Although there still are many unresolved issues, human gene therapy for cardiovascular disease is now a reality. The application of new molecular technologies will bring considerable benefits to the diagonsis and treatment of many diseases, some extremely rare, such as inherited metabolic disorders, and others more common, such as cancer and cardiovascular disease.

References

1. Berg P. Dissections and reconstructions of genes and chromosomes. Science 1981; 213:296–303.
2. Katz AM. Molecular biology in cardiology, a paradigmatic shift. J Mol Cell Cardiol 1988; 20:355–366.
3. Dzau VJ., Re N. Tissue angiotensin system in cardiovascular medicine. A paradigm shift? Circulation 1994; 89:493–498.
4. Starling EH. On the circulatory changes associated with exercise. J Roy Army Med Corps 1920; 34:258–272.
5. Furchgott RF. The pharmacology of vascular smooth muscle. Pharmacol Rev 1955; 7:183–210.
6. Katz AM. Cyclic AMP effects on the myocardium: A man who blows hot and cold with one breath. J Am Coll Cardiol 1983; 2:143–149.
7. Dzau VJ, et al. Vascular biology and medicine in the 1990s: Scope, concepts, potentials, and perspectives. Circulation 1993; 87:705–719.
8. Friedmann T. A brief history of gene therapy. Nature Genetics 1992; 2:93–98.
9. Sambrook J, et al. The integrated state of viral DNA in SV40-transformed cells. Proc Natl Acad Sci USA 1968; 59:1288–1293.
10. Rogers S, Pfuderer P. Use of viruses as carriers of added genetic information. Nature 1968; 219:749–751.
11. Subramani S, Southern PJ. Analysis of gene expression using Simian virus 40 vectors. Anal Biochem 1983; 135:1–15.
12. Rogers S, et al. Induction of arginase activity with the Shope papilloma virus in tissue culture cells from an argininemic patient. J Exp Med 1973; 137:1091–1096.
13. Friedmann T, Roblin R. Gene therapy for human genetic disease? Science 1972; 178:648–649.
14. Jackson DA, Symons RH, Berg P. Biochemical method for inserting new genetic information into DNA of simian virus 40: Circular SV40 DNA molecules containing lambda phage genes and the galactose operon of Escherichia coli. Proc Natl Acad Sci USA 1972; 69:2904–2909.
15. Mulligan RC, Howard BH, Berg P. Synthesis of rabbit beta-globin in cultured monkey kidney cells following infection with a SV40 beta-globin recombinant genome. Nature 1979; 277:108–114.
16. Anderson WA. Human gene therapy. Science 1992; 256: 808–813.
17. Thompson L. At age 2, gene therapy enters a growth phase. Science 1992; 258:744–746.
18. Sambrook J, Fritsch EF, Maniatis T. Molecular Cloning, 2nd Edition. Cold Spring Harbor: Cold Spring Harbor Laboratory Press, 1989; Pp. 16.1–16.81.
19. Felgner PL, et al. Lipofectin: A highly efficient, lipid mediated DNA-transfection procedure. Proc Natl Acad Sci USA 1987; 84:7413–7417.
20. Capecchi M. High efficiency transformation by direct microinjection of DNA into mammalian cells. Cell 1980; 22:479–488.
21. Adams BA, et al. Intramembrane charged movement restored in dysgenic skeletal muscle by injection of dihydropyridine receptor cDNAs. Nature 1990; 345:569–572.
22. Wolff JA, et al. Direct gene transfer into mouse muscle in vivo. Science 1990; 247:1465–1468.
23. Lin H, et al. Expression of recombinant gene in myocardium in vivo after direct injection of DNA. Circulation 1990; 82:2217–2221.
24. Kitsis RN, et al. Hormonal modulation of a gene injected into rat heart in vivo. Proc Natl Acad Sci USA 1991; 88:4138–4142.
25. Nabel EG, Plautz G, Nabel GJ. Site-specific gene expression in vivo by direct gene transfer into the arterial wall. Science 1990; 249:1285–1288.
26. Morishita R, et al. Intimal hyperplasia after vascular injury is inhibited by antisense cdk 2 kinase oligonucleotides. J Clin Invest 1994; 93:1458–1464.
27. Peterson KR, et al. Transgenic mice containing a 210 kb human β locus YAC display proper developmental control of human globin genes. Proc Natl Acad Sci USA 1993; 90:7593–7597.
28. Schedl A, et al. A yeast artificial chromosome covering the tyrosinase gene confers copy-number-dependent expression in transgenic mice. Nature 1993; 362:258–261.
29. Brown WRA. Mammalian artificial chromosomes. Curr Opin Gene Dev 1992; 2:479–486.
30. Huxley C. Mammalian artificial chromosoms: a new tool for gene therapy. Gene Ther 1994; 1:7–12.
31. Flegner PL, Rhodes G. Gene therapeutics. Nature 1991; 349:351–352.
32. Varmus H. Retroviruses. Science 1988; 240:1427–1435.
33. Cone RD, Mulligan RC. High-efficiency gene transfer into mammalian cells: Generation of helper-free recombinant retrovirus with broad mammalian host range. Proc Natl Acad Sci USA 1984; 81:6349–6353.
34. Danos O, Mulligan RC. Expression of retroviral trans-acting functions from complementary crippled genomes: A system for helper free packaging of retroviral vectors. J Cell Biochem 1988; 12:172–178.
35. Cepko CL, Roberts BE, Mulligan RC. Construction and applications of a highly transmissible murine retrovirus shuttle vector. Cell 1984; 37:1053–1062.
36. Nabel EG, et al. Recombinant gene expression in vivo within endothelial cells of the arterial wall. Science 1989; 244:1342–1344.
37. Wilson JM, et al. Implantation of vascular grafts lined with genetically modified endothelial cells. Science 1989; 244:1344–1346.
38. Morgan RA, Anderson WF. Human gene therapy. Ann Rev Biochem 1993; 62:191–217.
39. Donahue RE, et al. Helper virus induced T cell lymphoma in nonhuman primates after retroviral mediated gene transfer. J Exp Med 1992; 176:1125–1135.
40. Breakefield XO, DeLuca NA. N Biol 1991; 3:203–218.
41. Berkner KL. Expression of heterologous sequences in adenoviral vectors. Curr Top Microbiol Immunol 1992; 158:39–66.
42. Guzman RJ, et al. Efficient and selective adenovirus-mediated gene transfer into vascular neointima. Circulation 1993; 88:2838–2848.
43. Kass-Eisler A, et al. Quantitative determination of adenovirus-mediated gene delivery to rat cardiac myocytes in vitro and in vivo. Proc Natl Acad Sci USA 1993; 90:11498–11502.
44. Barr J, et al. Efficient catheter-mediated gene transfer into the heart using replication-defective adenovirus. Gene Ther 1994; 1:51–58.
45. Lemarchand P, et al. In vivo gene transfer and expression in normal uninjured blood vessels using replication-deficient

recombinant adenovirus vectors. Circ Res 1993; 72:1132–1138.
46. Losordo DW, et al. Use of the rabbit ear artery to serially assess foreign secretion after site-specific arterial gene transfer in vivo. Circulation 1994; 89:785–792.
47. Guzman PJ, et al. Efficient gene transfer into myocardium by direct injection of adenovirus vectors. Circ Res 1993; 73:1202–1207.
48. Quantin B, et al. Adenovirus as an expression vector in muscle cells in vivo. Proc Natl Acad Sci USA 1992; 89:2581–2584.
49. Simon RH, et al. Adenovirus-mediated gene transfer of CFTR gene to lung of nonhuman primates: toxicity study. Human Gene Ther 1993; 4:771–780.
50. Wagner E, et al. Coupling of adenovirus to transferrin-polylysine/DNA complexes greatly enhances receptor-mediated gene delivery and expression of transfected genes. Proc Natl Acad Sci USA 1992; 89:6099–6103.
51. Curiel DT, et al. Adenovirus enhancement of transferrin-polylysine-mediated gene delivery. Proc Natl Acad Sci USA 1991; 88:8850–8854.
52. Willard JE, et al. Genetic modification of the vessel wall. Comparison of surgical and catheter-based techniques for delivery of recombinant adenovirus. Circulation 1994; 89(5):2190–2197.
53. Hayashi Y, et al. Expression of a thyroid hormone-responsive recombinant gene introduced into adult mice livers by replication-defective adenovirus can be regulated by endogenous thyroid hormone receptor. Journal of Biological Chemistry, 1994; 269(39):23872–23875.
54. Lim CS, et al. Direct in vivo gene transfer into the coronary artery and peripheral vasculatures in the intact dog. Circulation 1991; 83:2007–2011.
55. Takeshita S, et al. Increased gene expression after liposome-mediated arterial gene transfer associated with intimal smooth muscle cell proliferation. J Clin Invest 1994; 93:652–661.
56. Zhu N, et al. Systemic gene expression after intavenous DNA delivery into adult mice. Science 1993; 261:209–211.
57. Kaneda Y, Iwai K, Uchida T. Introduction and expression of the human insulin gene in adult rat liver. J Biol Chem 1989; 264:12126–12129.
58. Kaneda Y, Iwai K, Uchida T. Increased expression of DNA cointroduced with nuclear protein in adult rat liver. Science 1989; 243:375–378.
59. Morishita R, et al. Novel and effective gene transfer technique for study of vascular renin angiotensin system. J Clin Invest 1993; 91:2580–2585.
60. Okada Y, et al. Modification of cell membranes with viral envelopes during fusion of cells with HVJ (Sendai virus). Exp Cell Res 1975; 93:368–378.
61. Morishita R, et al. Novel in vitro gene transfer method for study of local modulators in vascular smooth muscle cells. Hypertension 1993; 21:894–899.
62. Morishita R, et al. In vivo gene transfer into intact blood vessels: a novel and efficient method (Abstr). Circulation 1992; 86[Suppl I]:I-227.
63. Tomita N, et al. Direct in vivo gene introduction into rat kidney. Biochem Biophys Res Comm 1992; 186:129–134.
64. Isaka Y, et al. Glomerulosclerosis induced by in vivo transfection of transforming growth factor-β or platelet-derived growth factor gene into the rat kidney. J Clin Invest 1993; 92:2597–2601.
65. Morishita R, et al. Pharmacokinetics of antisense oligodeoxyribonucleotides (cyclin B_1 and CDC 2 kinase) in the vessel wall in vivo: enhanced therapeutic utility for restenosis by HVJ-liposome delivery. Gene 1994; 149:13–19.
66. Lynch CM, et al. Long-term expression of human adenosine deaminase in vascular smooth muscle cells of rats: a model for gene therapy. Proc Natl Acad Sci USA 1992; 89:1138–1142.
67. Dichek DA, et al. Seeding of intravascular stents with genetically engineered endothelial cells. Circulation 1989; 80:1347–1353.
68. Dichek DA, et al. Enhancement of the fibrinolytic activity of sheep endothelial cells by retroviral vector-mediated gene transfer. Blood 1991; 77:533–541.
69. Barr E, Leiden JM. Systemic delivery of recombinant proteins by genetically modified myoblasts. Science 1991; 254:1507–1509.
70. Yao SN, Kurachi K. Expression of human factor IX in mice after injection of genetically modified myoblasts. Proc Natl Acad Sci USA 1992; 89:3357–3361.
71. Wilensky RL, et al. Methods and devices for local drug delivery in coronary and peripheral arteries. Trends Cardiovasc Med 1993; 5:163–170.
72. Riessen R, Issner JM. Prospects for site-specific delivery of pharmacologic and molecular therapies. J Am Coll Cardiol 1994; 23:1234–1244.
73. Nabel EG, et al. Recombinant fibroblast growth factor-1 promotes intimal hyperplasia and angiogenesis in arteries in vivo. Nature 1993; 362:844–846.
74. Nabel EG, et al. Direct transfer of transforming growth factor β1 gene into arteries stimulates fibrocellular hyperplasia. Proc Natl Acad Sci USA 1993; 90:10579–10763.
75. von der Leyen HE, et al. Gene therapy inhibiting neointimal vascular lesion: in vivo gene transfer of endothelial-cell nitric oxide synthase gene. Proc Natl Acad Sci USA 1995; 92:1137–1141.
76. Ohno T, et al. Gene therapy for vascular smooth muscle cell proliferation after arterial injury. Science 1994; 265:781–784.
77. Zoldhelyi P, et al. Prevention of balloon angioplasty-induced thrombotic complications in a pig model by adenovirus-mediated transfer of prostaglandin H synthase-1 cDNA (Abstr). Clin Res 1994; 42:237A.
78. Epstein SE, et al. The basis of molecular strategies for treating coronary restenosis after angioplasty. J Am Coll Cardiol 1994; 23:1278–1288.
79. Stein CA, Cohen JS. Oligonucleotides as inhibitors of gene expression: a review. Cancer Res 1988; 48:2659–2668.
80. Stein CA, Cheng YC. Antisense oligonucleotides as therapeutic agents—is the bullet really magical? Science 1993; 261:1004–1012.
81. Simons M, et al. Antisense c-myb oligonucleotides inhibit intimal arterial smooth muscle cell accumulation in vivo. Nature 1992; 359:67–70.
82. Morishita R, et al. Single intraluminal delivery of antisense cdc2 kinase and proliferating-cell nuclear antigen oligonucleotides results in chronic inhibition of neointimal hyperplasia. Proc Natl Acad Sci USA 1993; 90:8474–8478.
83. Bennett MR, et al. Inhibition of vascular smooth muscle cell proliferation in vitro and in vivo by C-myc antisense oligonucleotides. J Clin Invest 1994; 93:820–828.
84. Simons M, Edelman ER, Rosenberg RD. Antisense proliferating cell nuclear antigen oligonucleotides inhibit intimal hyperplasia in a rat carotid artery injury model. J Clin Invest 1994; 93:2351–2356.
85. Shi Y, et al. Transcatheter delivery of c-myc antisense oligomers reduces neointimal formation in a porcine model of coronary artery balloon injury. Circulation 1994; 90:944–951.
86. Chen S, Wilson JM, Muller DWM. Adenovirus-mediated gene transfer of soluble vascular cell adhesion molecule to porcine interposition vein grafts. Circulation 1994; 89:1922–1928.
87. Milano CA, et al. Enhanced myocardial function in transgenic

mice overexpressing the β_2-adrenergic receptor. Science 1994; 264:582–586.
88. Soonpaa MH, et al. Formation of nascent intercalated disks between grafted fetal cardiomyocytes and host myocardium. Science 1994; 264:98–101.
89. Gal D, et al. Direct myocardial transfection in two animal models. Evaluation of parameters affecting gene expression and percutaneous gene delivery. Lab. Invest. 1993; 68:18–25.
90. Mann MJ, et al. Genetic engineering of vein grafts resistant to atherosclerosis. Proc Natl Acad Sci USA 1995; 92:4502–4506.

Principles of Vascular Surgery

Anthony D. Whittemore
John A. Mannick

Surgical intervention for peripheral vascular disease that is either occlusive or aneurysmal in nature embraces an increasingly complex array of techniques and procedures, the advantages and disadvantages of each requiring careful consideration for the individual patient. In recognition of the growing complexity of the subspecialty, in 1983, the American Board of Surgery created special criteria for certification of vascular surgeons. Each year, new textbooks and journals have been added to the extensive existing literature on the subject, testifying to the growth of fundamental knowledge as well as legitimate controversy. From this rapid growth and ongoing controversy, certain principles emerge that guide our everyday management of patients with peripheral vascular disease. To delve deeply into each controversial area with an exhaustive review of individual current references is clearly beyond the scope of this chapter. Rather, it is our intent to distinguish between established principles and controversial treatments in an effort to provide an understanding of the surgical decision-making process.

Peripheral Vascular Occlusive Disease

EXTRACRANIAL CEREBROVASCULAR DISEASE

Appropriate candidates for surgical management of extracranial vascular disease are those patients with significant pathologic lesions resulting primarily from atherosclerosis and, less often, from fibrous intimal hyperplasia, tortuous vessels, arteritis, or dissection. The hemodynamic significance of the lesion usually is documented by noninvasive evaluation with a duplex scan combining Doppler and real-time B-mode imaging. Modern imaging techniques are sufficiently sensitive and specific as to preclude the necessity for routine cerebral contrast angiography. Risks associated with cerebral angiography are minimal but not negligible if the study produces rather than prevents a catastrophic neurologic event [1,2]. Magnetic resonance angiography provides images of variable quality and requires further evolution of both hardware and software for more precise and reproducible anatomical resolution.

While most atherosclerotic lesions involving the bifurcation of the common carotid artery are to some extent both stenotic and ulcerated, both characteristics usually are considered separately. A lesion stenotic to the point of hemodynamic significance, however, usually is associated with some degree of ulceration (Fig. 29-1), and it is the ulcer that represents the real threat. Conversely, an ulcerated plaque is not necessarily significantly stenotic. From a radiologic point of view, a stenotic lesion becomes hemodynamically significant when the internal diameter is diminished by 50 percent, resulting in a 75-percent reduction of the cross-sectional area [3]. Although this conclusion is based on the inverse relationship of the pressure drop to the fourth power of the radius, the actual velocity of flow measured distal to such a stenotic lesion depends on a number of variables, including the viscous properties of blood, surface characteristics of the lumen, and the length of stenotic segment. The neurologic risk and sequelae attributed to such hemodynamically significant lesions, however, remain controversial. Since neurologic deficits most often result from embolization of thrombus or atherosclerotic debris rather than from hypoperfusion, the pathologic sequelae of a hemodynamically significant lesion relate more to the morphologic complexity of associated ulceration rather than to the degree of stenosis [4]. Hemodynamically insignificant plaques that are nonetheless ulcerated may be classified by the degree of complexity. The simplest class A plaque represents a smooth, broad-based, shallow ulceration (Fig. 29-2), whereas the more complex class C plaque is multiulcerated with an irregular surface perhaps resulting from plaque rupture or dissection (Fig. 29-3). Some studies suggest that the risk of ipsilateral neurologic events correlates with the degree of plaque complexity [5].

Patients with stenotic or ulcerated lesions may be categorized into four clinical groups on the basis of symptoms: transient ischemic attacks (TIAs), asymptomatic lesions, fixed deficits, and stroke in evolution. The final decision regarding the advisability of endarterectomy is determined by the symptomatic status associated with the specific pathologic lesion.

The management of patients with transient ischemic attacks is currently the least controversial of the four groups [6–10]. Since publication of results from the North American Symptomatic Carotid Endarterectomy Trial (NASCET) and the European Carotid Surgery Trial (ECST), it is generally accepted that the risk of ipsilateral stroke associated with stenotic lesions in excess of 70 percent is significantly reduced with endarterectomy. The NASCET demonstrated a 26-percent incidence of stroke within 2 years of the onset of symptoms with optimal medical therapy, significantly higher than the 9-percent incidence following endarterectomy, an absolute risk reduction of 17 percent [9]. Similarly, in the ECST, 3 percent of surgical patients versus 17 percent of control patients sustained ipsilateral stroke, a sixfold reduction in risk [10]. Provided the incidence of perioperative stroke is less than 2 or 3 percent, as is the case for most well-trained vascular surgeons, endarterectomy remains the most appropriate alternative [11–14].

It is not clear yet whether carotid endarterectomy is beneficial for patients with symptoms and stenotic lesions less than 70 percent. Such patients, as well as those with simple class A plaques, should receive an initial trial of antiplatelet therapy with surgery reserved for persistent

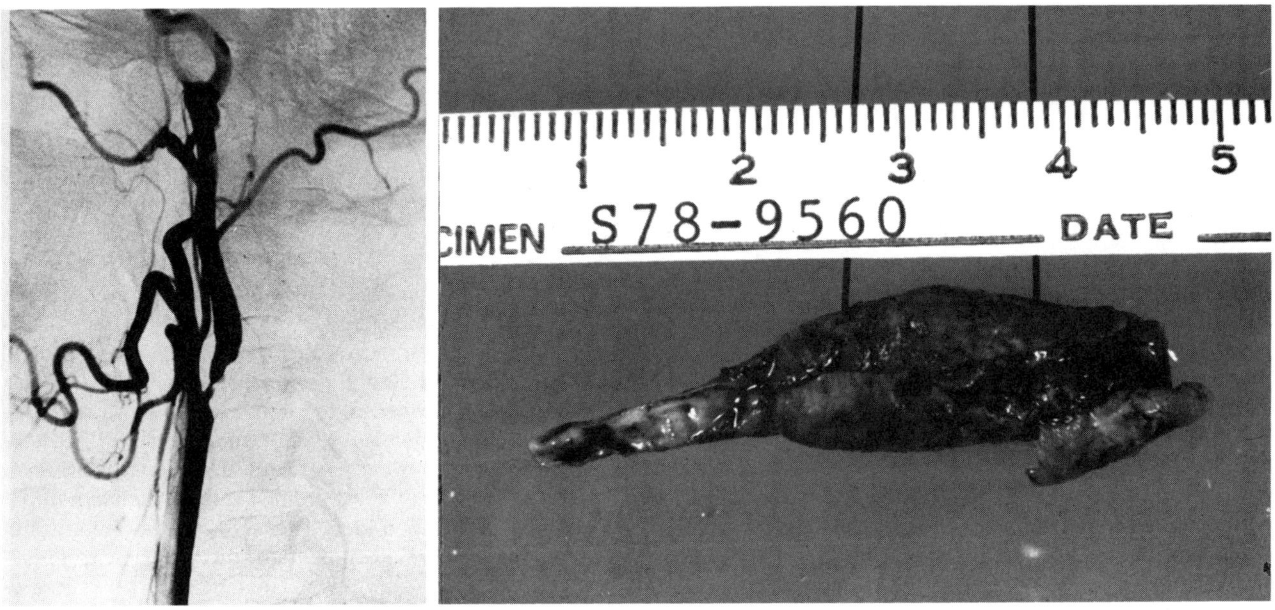

A B

Fig. 29-1. **A**. Intra-arterial digital subtraction demonstrating a high-grade stenotic atheroma at the origin of the internal carotid artery, resulting in a reduction of the luminal diameter by approximately 90 percent. **B**. Endarterectomized specimen demonstrates characteristic atheromatous plaque extending cephalad from the point of maximal stenosis, proximal to which is shown friable intraluminal atheromatous debris.

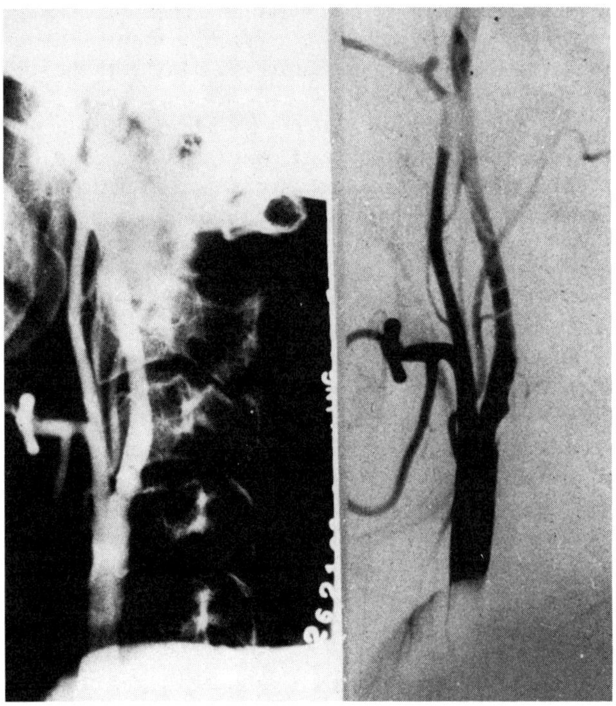

Fig. 29-2. Conventional arteriogram with subtracted film demonstrating a minimal atheroma at the origin of the internal carotid artery containing a shallow central ulceration.

or recurrent TIAs [4–10]. For symptomatic patients with hemodynamically significant stenoses or more complex plaque formation, however, initial endarterectomy clearly is indicated [15].

Asymptomatic patients with significant stenotic lesions constitute a far more controversial group. The controversy is fueled by an incomplete understanding of the disease's natural history, an understanding that may become more complete pending the outcome of the multicenter Asymptomatic Carotid Artery Stenosis (ACAS) study. It has been claimed that the majority of patients who eventually sustain a fixed stroke from extracranial vascular disease will demonstrate prodromal TIAs, thus allowing time for surgical intervention prior to an irreversible catastrophic event [16]. More recent evidence suggests that that may not pertain to patients whose lesions have progressed beyond 80-percent stenosis [17]. The patients may sustain a risk of significant neurologic events approaching 50 percent within 2 years, and nearly half of those that ultimately develop a fixed cerebrovascular accident (CVA) demonstrate no warning symptoms whatsoever [6]. Some 21 percent of asymptomatic patients with 80 percent or greater lesions demonstrate evidence of clinically silent cerebral infarctions on CT scan [18]. Evidence from the recently concluded multicenter Veterans Administration trial for asymptomatic carotid-artery lesions in excess of 50-percent stenosis was not conclusive [19]. The incidence of all ipsilateral neurologic events (TIA and stroke) was significantly lower after 4 years among surgical patients (8%) compared with medical management (21%). If one

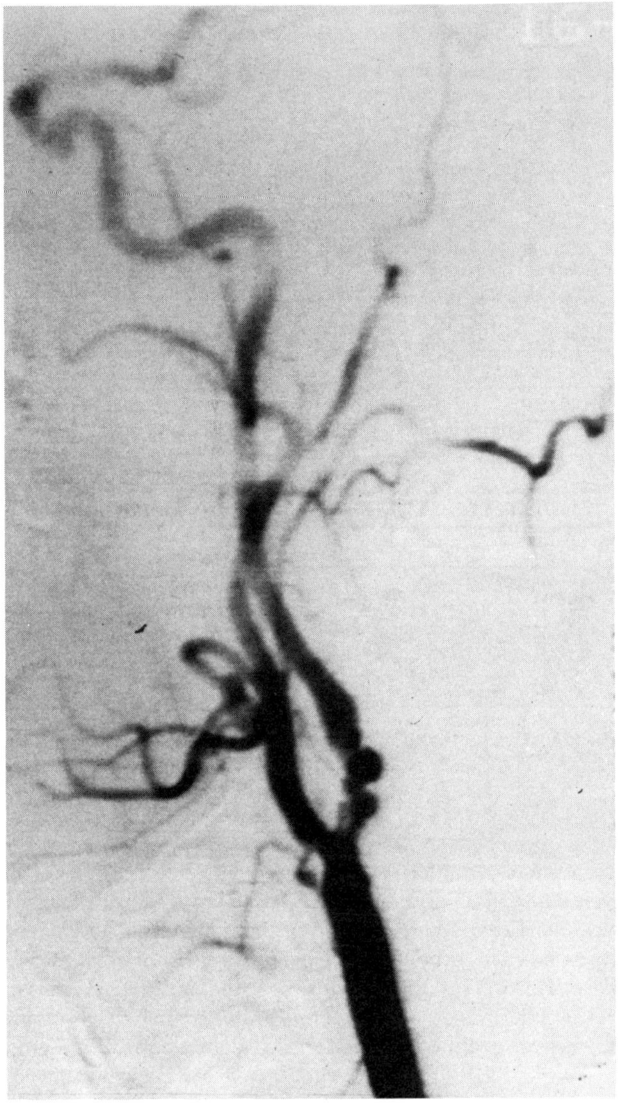

Fig. 29-3. Intra-arterial digital subtraction arteriogram demonstrating an exceptionally irregular luminal surface characterized by the presence of at least two deep ulcerations.

excludes TIAs, however, the difference in the incidence of stroke and death was not significant. On the other hand, the difference observed with respect to ipsilateral stroke among surgical (5%) and medical (10%) patients failed to achieve statistical significance by only the slimmest of margins ($p = 0.056$). The study also was somewhat flawed by the mandatory assignment to the surgical group of three strokes resulting from angiography, which produced a 30-day combined operative stroke and death rate of nearly 5 percent. Most vascular surgeons, then, recommend endarterectomy for asymptomatic lesions greater than 80-percent stenosis in otherwise appropriate candidates but reserve final judgment pending the outcome of the current ACAS trial.

Fixed neurologic deficits in patients with appropriate lesions represent a second, highly controversial indication for endarterectomy. The controversy stems from disastrous attempts at intervention during the 1960s [20,21]. Because accurate diagnosis was not possible, endarterectomy was inappropriately undertaken in patients with limited and massive cerebral infarcts. Those strokes resulted from hypertensive and hemorrhagic events as well as atheroembolic disease. The dismal experience led to the classic teaching that surgical intervention for patients with fixed neurologic deficits should be delayed for a 4- to 6-week period of "stabilization." With the use of angiographic evaluation earlier in the management of patients with cerebral vascular accidents, however, a subgroup of individuals with highly stenotic, preocclusive lesions emerged [2,22]. The patients in that subgroup remain at considerable risk for extension of their stroke or reinfarction within a 4- to 6-week period of time, which thus becomes anything but stabilizing [23–25]. More recent experience with endarterectomy for individuals with limited fixed deficits and, therefore, residual carotid territory at risk has not resulted in a perioperative stroke rate significantly different from that of elective endarterectomy [25–28]. From that initial experience, an approach has evolved that may allow more appropriate management of highly selected individuals with neurologic deficits, as illustrated in Fig. 29-4 [29]. Fewer surgeons continue to advocate a 6-week period of stabilization [30].

Once a decision has been reached to proceed with endarterectomy, several principles govern the conduct of the operation. Surgery may be undertaken comfortably with either local, regional, or general anesthesia. Local anesthesia usually consists of the superficial infiltration of a solution of lidocaine [31]. Regional anesthesia involves the deeper intrascalene deposition of a longer-acting local agent around the C3-C5 nerve roots [32]. General anesthesia, of course, requires endotracheal intubation for the administration of inhalational agents [33]. In experienced hands, all three methods have provided equally favorable results. The primary advantage of local and regional anesthesia lies in their provision of the most accurate monitor of cerebral function—an awake patient. Should clamping of the internal carotid result in deterioration of cerebral function, an indwelling shunt can be inserted and its subsequent function continuously and directly assessed. Although regional technique may produce less physiologic stress and obviate the known sequelae of a formal general anesthetic, it probably is inappropriate for an excessively anxious patient, particularly in the presence of a myocardium sensitive to catecholamines. A second disadvantage of the regional anesthetic is that it may become inadequate, particularly if cardiovascular complications ensue such that general anesthesia with endotracheal intubation becomes mandatory, an unpleasant situation for all concerned. Most surgeons and patients, therefore, prefer a general anesthetic, which has become increasingly safer with the advent of intraoperative EEG monitoring [33]. With such monitoring, the adequacy of cerebral perfusion can be assessed continuously and the selective use of a shunt governed by the occurrence of appropriate EEG changes [33–35]. While most perioperative strokes are caused by embolization rather than by hypoperfusion, it seems prudent to maintain ipsilateral cerebral perfusion as near to normal as possible. A common approach em-

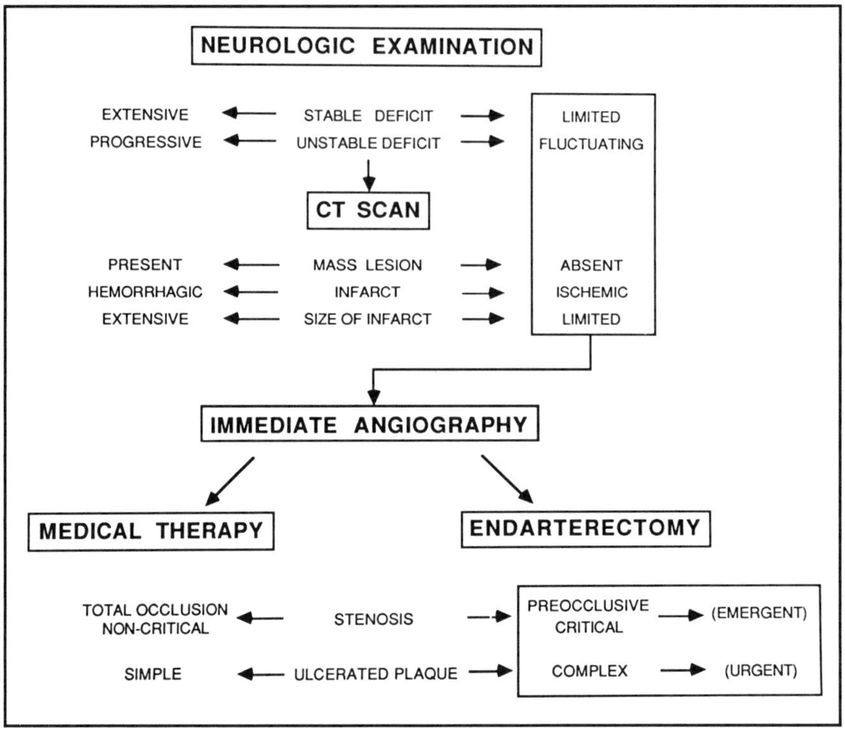

Fig. 29-4. Algorithm demonstrating the parameters utilized in the management of patients admitted to the hospital with a recent stroke.

ploys a general anesthetic with sophisticated, multichannel EEG monitoring.

The utilization of an intravascular shunt to provide continued cerebral perfusion during endarterectomy continues to evoke intense debate. Some surgeons advocate the routine use of a shunt, whereas others utilize it selectively based on intraoperative EEG changes or stump pressure measurements [33–35]. Still others do not use a shunt under any circumstances whatsoever [36–39]. Proponents of each method have produced excellent results, and the superiority of one method over another cannot be established. This controversy remains unsettled in large part because most intraoperative strokes result from embolization rather than hypoperfusion. Nevertheless, when an awake patient loses consciousness or an EEG tracing demonstrates profound global ischemia, those events should be reversed as quickly as possible. With the selective use of a shunt based on EEG monitoring, 16 percent of patients develop changes that require intravascular shunting for reversal [33]. It is important to note that this shunt requirement increases to 27 percent in patients who have a contralateral high-grade stenosis, to 40 percent in those with contralateral occlusion, and to 67 percent in patients with a fixed neurologic deficit and bilateral disease. The progression testifies to the increased risk of endarterectomy in such patients when operated on without cerebral protection [30].

The actual surgical procedure is initiated with an incision along the anterior border of the sternocleidomastoid muscle, with subsequent dissection of the distal segment of common carotid artery (Fig. 29-5). The dissection is continued cephalad with division of one or more facial veins and isolation of the internal and external carotid vessels. The distal dissection of the internal carotid artery must be carried beyond the extent of grossly evident disease. This may require elevation of the hypoglossal nerve, retraction of the marginal mandibular branch of the cervical nerve, and mobilization of the distal vagus. Following systemic anticoagulation, the vessels are occluded proximally and distally with atraumatic vascular clamps. A longitudinal arteriotomy is initiated in the distal common carotid artery and is extended through the atheromatous plaque into the internal carotid artery well beyond grossly evident disease. The arteriotomy must be carried sufficiently distal to ensure that all atheroma is removed and to allow expeditious insertion of an indwelling shunt if necessitated by concurrent EEG changes. These intraarterial shunts consist of flexible tubing of appropriate caliber and, if required, are usually inserted into the distal internal carotid artery first, allowed to backbleed, and inserted into the common carotid artery proximally. The shunt is secured in place with catheter tourniquets proximal and distal to the arteriotomy. Cerebral perfusion is thus restored and endarterectomy undertaken around the indwelling luminal shunt. The atheroma is separated from the underlying residual media with a spatula and removed. It is critical to ensure a clean distal intimal margin, which, if loosely adherent to the media, may occasionally require some fine tacking sutures. The orifice of the external carotid artery also is endarterectomized as thoroughly as possible to protect this important potential collateral.

Following removal of all atheromatous debris and inti-

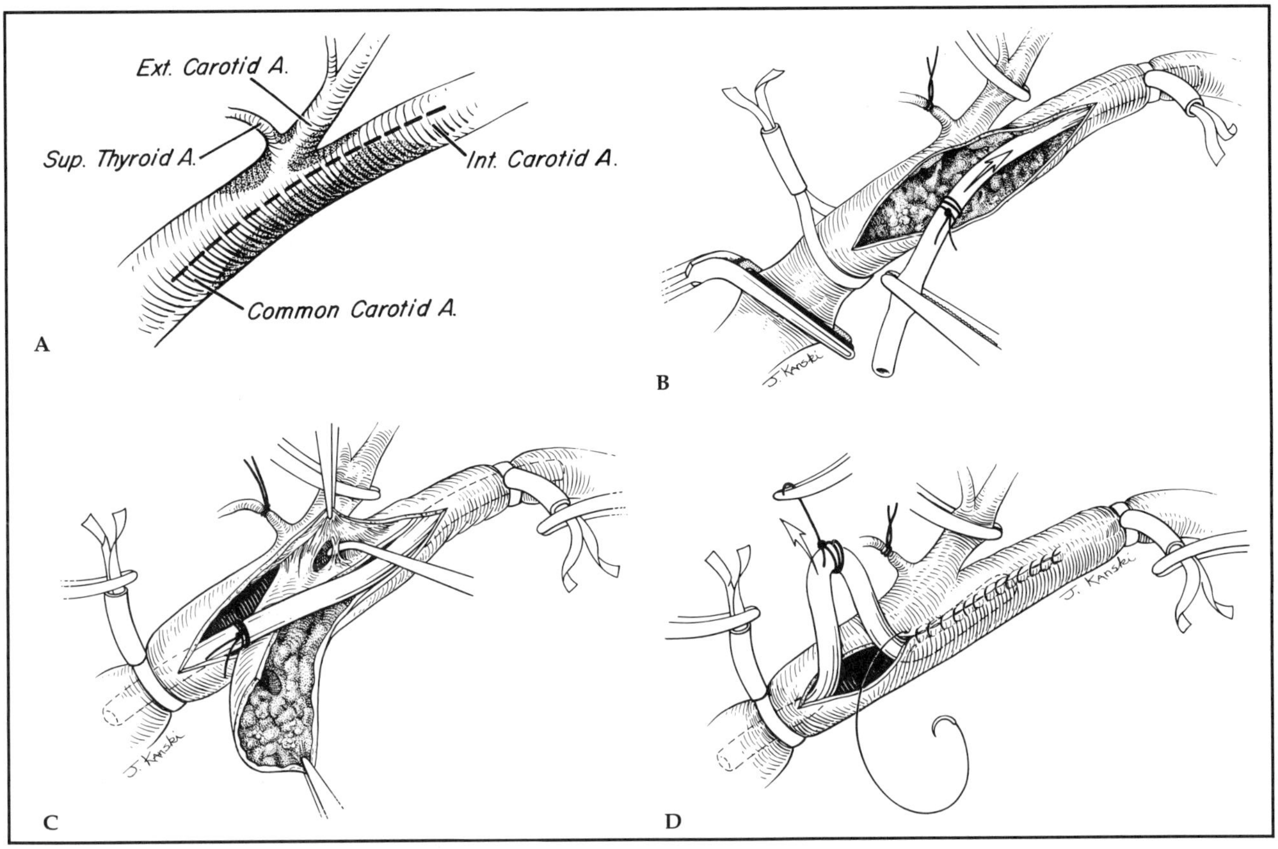

Fig. 29-5. Following a longitudinal arteriotomy through the origin of the internal carotid **(A)**, deterioration of baseline EEG tracing necessitated the insertion of an indwelling shunt **(B)**. With cerebral perfusion reestablished **(C)**, endarterectomy is carried out and the shunt removed **(D)** just prior to completion of the closure.

mal fragments, the arteriotomy is closed. Many surgeons prefer to close the arteriotomy with an elliptical patch of vein or prosthetic material to effect an angioplasty and diminish the likelihood of recurrent stenosis, but most have not found this necessary and prefer to close the arteriotomy primarily with fine polypropylene suture [40,41]. Just prior to completion of the angioplasty or closure, the shunt is removed and the vessels flushed. The occluding clamps then are removed in sequential fashion to ensure that any residual thrombus or atheromatous debris is carried into the external rather than the internal carotid artery. Anticoagulation may be reversed with protamine sulfate in an effort to reduce the incidence of postoperative cervical hematoma, or it may be continued to minimize postoperative thrombotic complications. Cervical drains generally are not used except in patients with diffuse incisional bleeding associated with the use of preoperative antiplatelet agents or persistent intraoperative anticoagulation. Prior to wound closure, however, intraoperative cerebral arteriography or duplex imaging should be routinely obtained [42]. A single hand injection of approximately 15 cc of contrast is administered through a needle inserted retrograde in the common carotid artery proximal to the endarterectomized segment. Should the film demonstrate an intraluminal filling defect or stenotic segment, appropriate corrective action is taken. Although this practice has not altered perioperative mortality or morbidity, it may reduce the likelihood of recurrent stenosis.

Patients are closely monitored either in a recovery area or in an intensive care unit with particular regard to blood pressure and neurologic status. Since fluctuations in blood pressure occur in approximately 30 percent of patients following carotid endarterectomy, prevention of extremes frequently is required. Within a few hours, however, hypertension usually resolves, and patients may be transferred to a regular floor prior to discharge, usually on the second postoperative day. This early discharge is predicated on the observation that most postoperative complications become apparent within the first 24 hours following surgery. Although most perioperative cerebral events are embolic in nature, an occasional patient develops acute thrombosis of the entire endarterectomized site. A patient developing a progressive neurologic deficit in the recovery room, therefore, should be returned immediately to the operating room and explored as expeditiously as possible.

Mortality and neurologic morbidity figures associated with carotid endarterectomy are listed in Table 29-1 and are representative of most series in the recent literature. It is important to understand that peripheral neurologic morbidity related to cranial nerves occurs in as many

Table 29-1. Operative mortality associated with carotid endarterectomy

Number	Deaths	CNS deficits: Fixed	CNS deficits: Transient
127 cases of general anesthesia, routine shunt	1 (0.8%)	2 (1.6%)	3 (2.4%)
110 cases of regional anesthesia, routine shunt	1 (0.9%)	1 (0.9%)	2 (1.8%)
219 cases of general anesthesia, EEG monitoring			
150 CEA[a] alone	1 (0.7%)	1 (0.7%)	1 (0.7%)
51 CEA = CABG[b] (elective)	1 (2.0%)	1 (2.0%)	2 (4.0%)

[a]Carotid endarterectomy
[b]Coronary artery bypass grafting

as 5 to 10 percent of patients and, although temporarily annoying, it is rarely of sustained significance. With mobilization of the hypoglossal nerve, some degree of tongue deviation and numbness may be apparent and usually resolves within a few days. Similarly, temporary dysfunction of the marginal mandibular branch of the cervical nerve results in paresis of the ipsilateral inferior orbicularis oris muscle, which should not be confused with a central facial deficit. Voice change is most frequently associated with cord edema resulting from endotracheal intubation, but it also may result from irritation of the vagus or superior laryngeal nerves. Difficulty swallowing frequently accompanies cervical edema but occasionally reflects dysfunction of the pharyngeal constrictors from trauma to the glossopharyngeal nerve. The spinal accessory nerve generally is protected by the sternocleidomastoid muscle and rarely becomes paretic. Most cranial nerve dysfunctions resolve in a matter of a few days, and virtually all resolve within 3 months.

Patients with bilateral carotid lesions deserve special consideration. The disease is generally symmetric to some extent, and the usual patient undergoes initial endarterectomy for a symptomatic lesion. If the contralateral lesion proves remotely symptomatic or hemodynamically significant, staged endarterectomy is advised [43].

The postoperative follow-up should include noninvasive evaluation at regular intervals, probably every 3 months during the first year. This schedule is recommended since the healing process of the endarterectomized site includes smooth-muscle proliferation and ultimate reendothelialization. The extent of the smooth muscle proliferative response may determine the degree of restenosis, which becomes clinically manifest in 2–5 percent of patients following initial surgery. While noninvasive evaluation has demonstrated a much higher occurrence of lesser degrees of asymptomatic restenosis, this is not surprising, nor does it carry the same significance as the original atherosclerotic stenosis since the pathology is quite different [40,41]. The early restenotic lesion often consists of fibromuscular hyperplasia, which produces a smooth, nonulcerated surface and probably poses less of a threat as a nidus for thrombus formation and subsequent embolization. Nevertheless, when a stenosis progresses beyond the 80-percent level or is associated with appropriate symptoms, reoperation generally is recommended. Such a procedure usually does not entail endarterectomy since no discrete plane can be conveniently developed and, therefore, it consists of a patch angioplasty using autogenous vein or prosthetic material.

OCCLUSIVE DISEASE OF THE UPPER EXTREMITIES

Occlusive disease of the upper extremities most frequently occurs in the innominate or proximal subclavian arteries. These lesions often are asymptomatic owing to their proximal location and availability of abundant collateral circulation. Significant disease is therefore suggested by the presence of an appropriate bruit or a discrepancy in blood pressure determinations between the upper extremities. Symptoms referable to significant disease include arm claudication, subclavian steal, and, rarely, peripheral embolization.

Patients with significant symptoms are candidates for revascularization, which can be accomplished with several approaches. Direct endarterectomy of the involved arterial segment, although conceptually attractive, often proves challenging for two major reasons. First, exposure of the innominate or proximal left subclavian artery requires median sternotomy, a more involved exposure than the alternative supraclavicular approach. Second, atherosclerotic brachiocephalic vessels frequently are friable and attenuated, making direct repair technically difficult. For those two reasons, a supraclavicular extra-anatomic approach, such as a carotid-subclavian bypass, is preferred [44].

Carotid-subclavian bypass is undertaken through a limited incision superior and parallel to the clavicle through which the distal subclavian and proximal common carotid arteries are exposed. With EEG monitoring, the proximal common carotid artery is occluded and a graft anastomosed end-to-side to a carotid arteriotomy. The necessity for an indwelling shunt is predicated on observed EEG changes. The graft is then delivered deep to the jugular vein for end-to-side anastomosis to the distal subclavian artery. The bypass then provides antegrade flow to the appropriate arm as well as retrograde subclavian flow to restore vertebral circulation. Prosthetic material or autogenous vein may be utilized with equally satisfactory results. The improved performance of prosthetic material

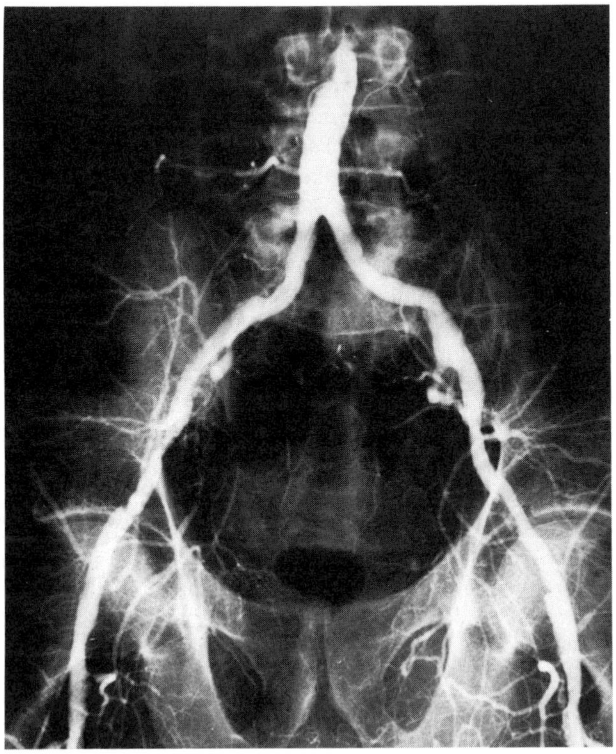

Fig. 29-6. Angiogram demonstrating diffuse aortoiliac atherosclerotic occlusive disease that resulted in significant disabling claudication.

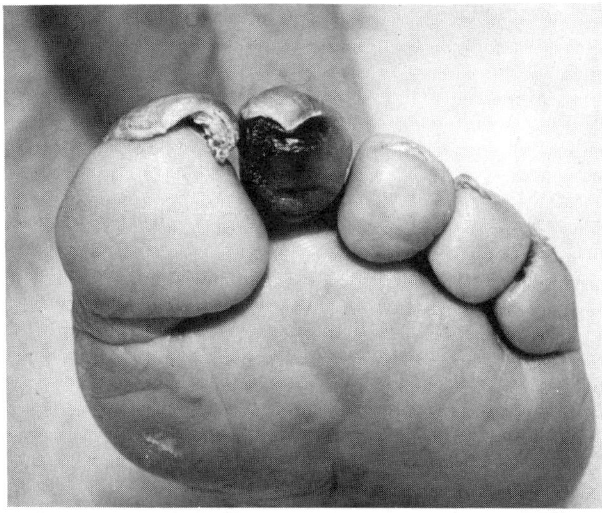

Fig. 29-7. Blue-toe syndrome, resulting from peripheral embolization of thrombus or atheromatous debris from proximal occlusive disease.

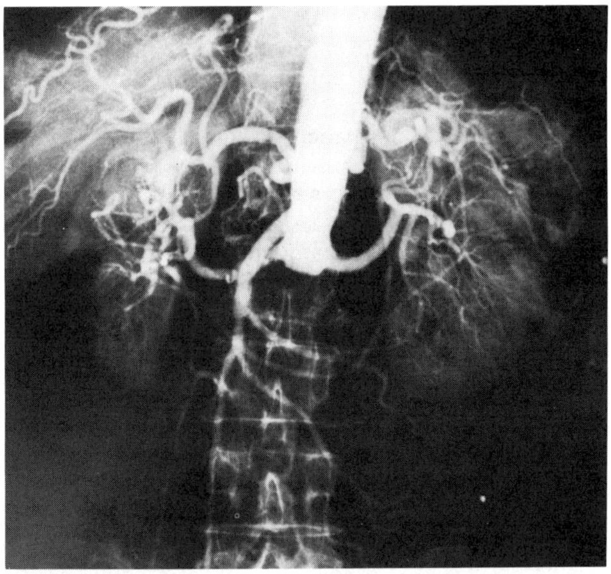

Fig. 29-8. Transaxillary ateriogram demonstrating total occlusion of the infrarenal abdominal aorta with propagation of thrombus to the level of the renal arteries.

in this location reflects the relatively high flow through the short length of graft required. Using this supraclavicular approach, a 5-year patency rate approaching 85 percent can be expected to provide significant relief of symptoms in the vast majority of patients [44].

AORTOILIAC OCCLUSIVE DISEASE

Aortoiliac occlusive disease most commonly becomes apparent with the onset of intermittent claudication (Fig. 29-6) [45]. Since adequate oxygen delivery to the hypogastric and deep femoral distribution also is diminished, the symptoms involve the musculature of the thigh and the buttocks as well as the calves. Although the triad of intermittent claudication, impotence, and diminished femoral pulses is relatively common, global atrophy of both lower extremities, as originally described by Leriche and Morrell, is not striking because patients are now referred earlier in their course [46]. Chronic ischemic rest pain occurs in these patients when aortoiliac disease is combined with tandem infrainguinal superficial femoral or tibioperoneal lesions. Occasionally, proximal occlusive disease becomes evident with the so-called blue-toe syndrome (Fig. 29-7), reflecting distal embolization of thrombus or atheromatous debris originating from the proximal diseased aortoiliac segment [47,48]. Finally, acute infrarenal aortic occlusion with inadequate aortoiliac collaterals may result in life- and limb-threatening distal ischemia (Fig. 29-8). Chronic aortic occlusion provides a setting for proximal propagation of thrombus that threatens patency of the visceral vessels in approximately 15 percent of such patients [49].

The presence of rest pain or total aortic occlusion, either chronic or acute, mandates angiographic evaluation and revascularization. Patients with symptoms limited to intermittent claudication, however, require careful consideration before surgical intervention is recommended. The majority of such patients (80%) remain stable or may improve following the onset of symptoms [50]. Furthermore,

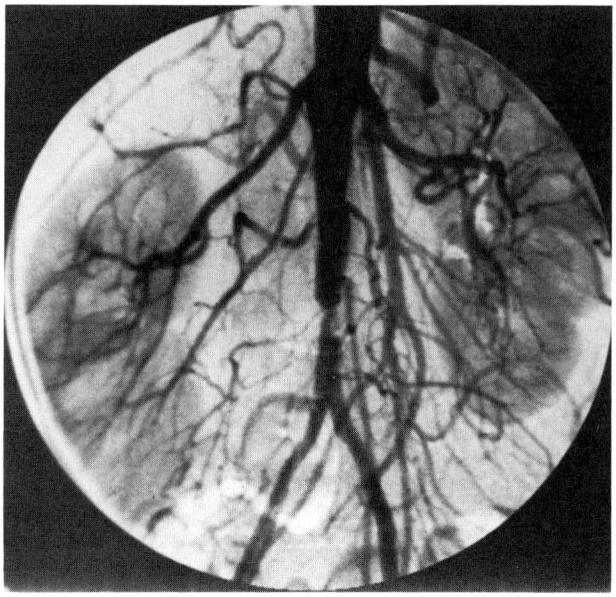

Fig. 29-9. Localized stenosis of the distal aorta, resulting in disabling claudication, amenable to endarterectomy.

the risk of amputation in patients with intermittent claudication is limited to 5 percent during their lifetime (slightly higher for diabetics) [50–52]. Thus, revascularization should be reserved for patients whose claudication progresses and remains severely disabling.

Once the need for intervention has been established, the operative procedure selected becomes a function of the anatomic pathology as delineated angiographically in the context of the patient's overall physiologic status. Aortoiliac endarterectomy generally is reserved for individuals with relatively short-segment, well-localized disease that does not extend into the external iliac system. This procedure is most appropriate for short-segment disease of the distal infrarenal aorta, commonly encountered in young female heavy smokers (Fig. 29-9). More extensive aortoiliac endarterectomy, however, involves substantial disruption of the autonomic plexus, which may result in impairment of sexual function [53].

The best candidates for iliac endarterectomy are those perhaps more appropriately treated at present with percutaneous transluminal angioplasty (PTA) (Fig. 29-10) [54]. The overall results achieved with proximal iliac PTA, however, may not be as favorable as initially reported. Earlier series suggested that the 5-year patency rate associated with iliac PTA approached 80 percent and was therefore comparable to surgical results with either short-segment endarterectomy or aortofemoral bypass [55–57]. Initial success rates approach 90 percent, but longer-term follow-up suggests a 5-year patency rate of 60 percent for common iliac PTA, 50 percent for external iliac PTA, and 40 percent for femoropopliteal PTA [58].

The most efficacious method of aortoiliac reconstruction for the majority of patients consists of the aortobifemoral bypass graft [59–62]. The aortobifemoral bypass consists of a bifurcated prosthesis that extends from the infrarenal aorta to both common femoral arteries in the groin (Fig. 29-11). This procedure negates the impact of progressive atherosclerosis in the distal iliac system and obviates the necessity for extensive dissection about the aortic bifurcation that results in damage to the autonomic plexus. Aortoiliac, in contrast to aortobifemoral, bypass is occasionally required, however, to provide antegrade

Fig. 29-10. **A.** Retrograde femoral arteriogram demonstrating relatively localized disease involving the right external iliac artery. **B.** This localized lesion was subsequently successfully dilated using percutaneous transluminal angioplasty.

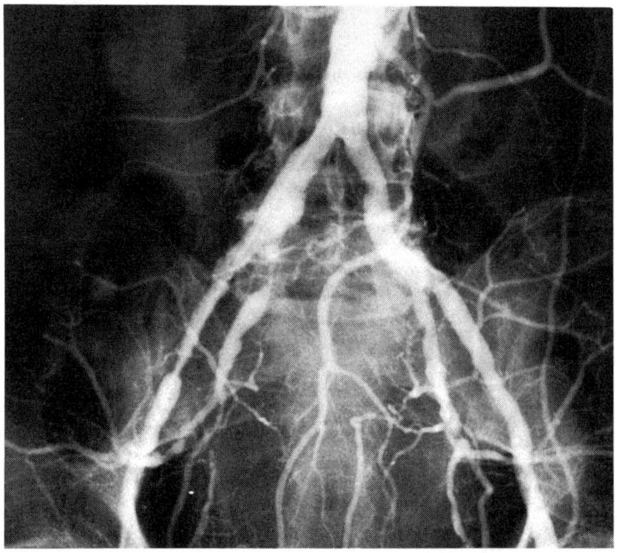

A

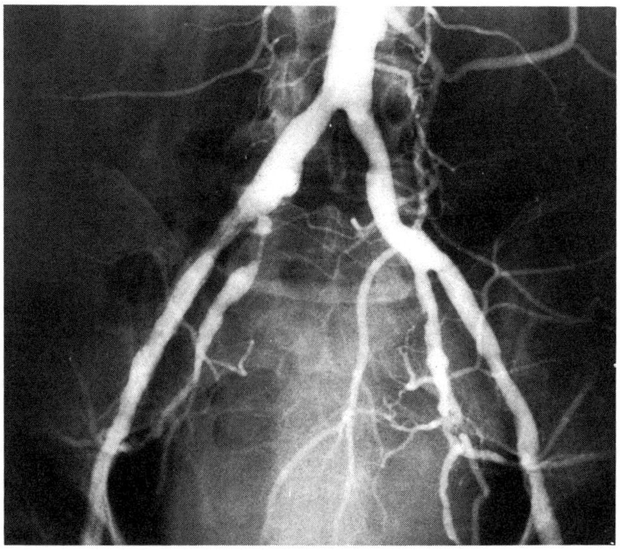

B

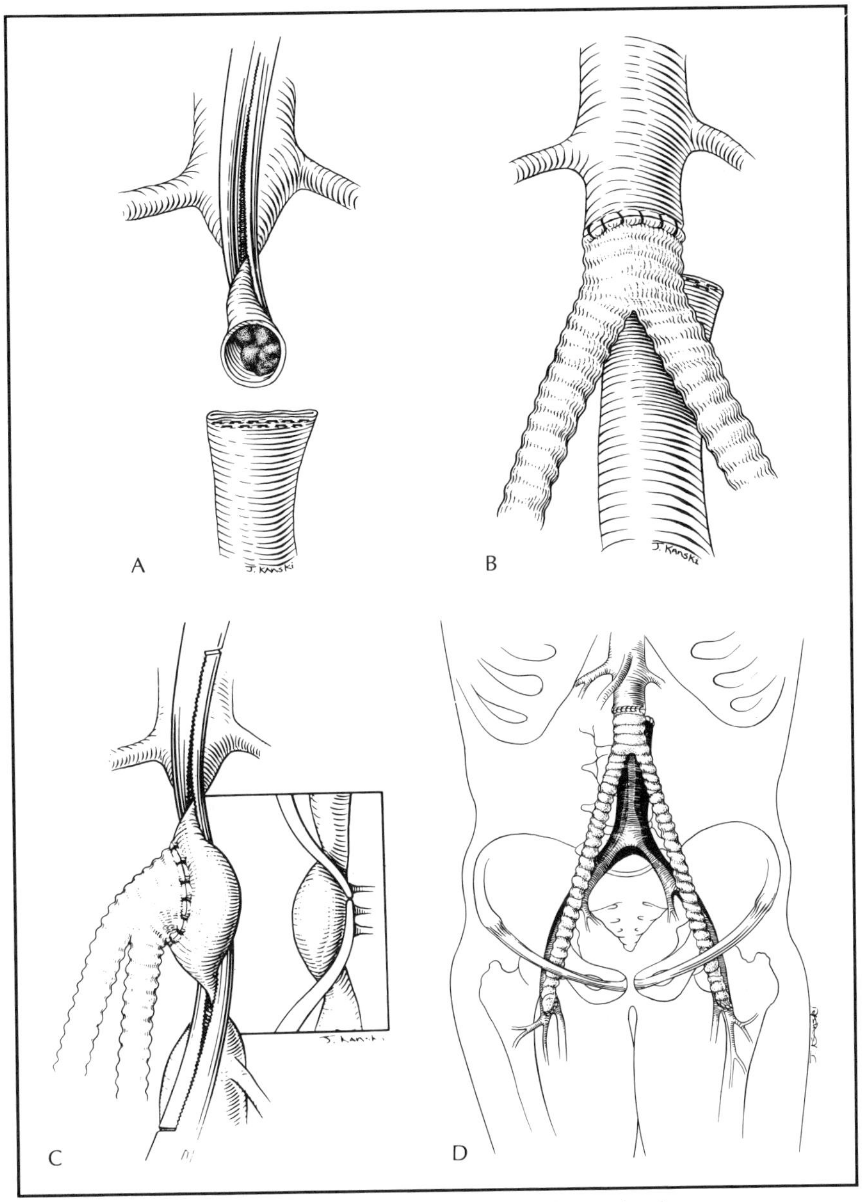

Fig. 29-11. **A**. During the course of aortobifemoral bypass graft, the infrarenal aorta has been transected proximal to a stapled closure following placement of a proximal occluding clamp. **B**. The thrombus in the proximal cuff is then endarterectomized prior to end-to-end anastomosis of a bifurcated prosthesis. **C**. In cases where retrograde perfusion of at least one pelvic vessel cannot be ensured, an end-to-side proximal anastomosis is advisable to preserve perfusion of at least one internal iliac vessel. **D**. The distal limbs are then delivered through retroperitoneal tunnels and anastomosed to the common deep femoral arteries bilaterally.

flow into at least one hypogastric artery. This is desirable in situations where retrograde perfusion of the native external iliac system from a distal femoral anastomosis is insecure. Pelvic perfusion thus is ensured by antegrade supply to the dominant hypogastric vessel. The proximal anastomosis can be constructed either end to side or, more commonly, end to end. Although no definitive proof exists to date, most surgeons feel the end-to-end technique provides improved hemodynamic flow across the anastomosis, resulting in fewer proximal suture-line complications such as false aneurysm or aortoduodenal fistula. End-to-end anastomosis also avoids potential distal embolic complications by excluding the infrarenal aortoiliac system. End-to-side anastomosis, however, may be necessary for patients who require continued antegrade perfusion of the distal infrarenal aorta or iliac vessels. This procedure is important to consider if an important visceral vessel requires continued antegrade perfusion, or if retrograde perfusion of at least one internal iliac artery is precluded by extensive external iliac disease.

Conventional aortobifemoral bypass is carried out under general anesthesia with cardiopulmonary monitoring appropriate to the particular patient. The peritoneal cavity is usually entered through a long midline incision and retroperitoneal exposure secured. The retroperitoneum is incised to the level at which the left renal vein crosses the aorta, and the tissues surrounding the aorta are dissected free just sufficient to allow the insertion of a cross-clamp. More extensive dissection results in a proportionate increase in third-space sequestration postoperatively and augments the potential for hemorrhage from posterior lumbar vessels. Retroperitoneal tunnels are bluntly created to join two short vertical groin incisions through which the distal common femoral arteries are exposed. The patient is then heparinized and the aorta cross-clamped proximally just below the origin of the renal artery. A second clamp or stapling device is placed 2 or 3 cm distally, just above the origin of the inferior mesenteric artery. The aorta is then transected and the distal stump secured with either the stapler or continuous suture. The proximal aortic cuff is endarterectomized as necessary and trimmed appropriately. Most surgeons prefer a knitted rather than a woven prosthesis for aortobifemoral bypass in the belief that the knitted graft is perhaps more rapidly and completely incorporated into the surrounding tissue, thereby reducing the chances for infection. The knitted graft, due to its higher porosity, requires preclotting with the patient's blood prior to systemic heparinization. More recently developed grafts are rendered impervious with a variety of coatings, including collagen, which precludes the necessity for preclotting even knitted grafts. The preclotted graft is then anastomosed end to end to the proximal aortic cuff, and the limbs of the prosthesis are subsequently delivered through the previously created retroperitoneal tunnels to both groin incisions. The distal anastomoses are then completed, most commonly using an arteriotomy that is introduced into the distal common femoral artery and then carried through the origin of the deep femoral vessel. The hood of the distal anastomosis, therefore, provides a patch angioplasty of the origin of the deep femoral artery, ensuring sustained outflow from the bypass in the event of progressive distal superficial femoral occlusive disease [58,63]. The latter consideration has undoubtedly improved the overall patency rates for aortobifemoral grafts to the current anticipated level of 85 to 90 percent at 5 years [58–62]. This patency rate is achieved at the expense of a 2-percent operative mortality accompanied by a 10-percent incidence of perioperative morbidity. Even in patients with claudication associated with both proximal aortoiliac disease and bilateral superficial femoral disease, the restoration of normal inflow to the groin level provided by the proximal bypass procedure is sufficient to result in satisfactory palliation in 85 percent of such individuals [62,63]. Thus, only 15 percent of patients ultimately require distal femoropopliteal revascularization. Rarely, patients operated on for ischemic rest pain and tandem disease require simultaneous proximal and distal arterial bypass.

In some instances, conventional aortobifemoral bypass graft may not be appropriate, and an alternative approach may be required. Since the results provided by these alternative methods are inferior to those associated with aortobifemoral bypass, they are reserved for poor-risk patients with limb-threatening ischemia or, in some instances, life-threatening infections. These extra-anatomic aortoiliac reconstructions embrace three major categories of procedures, depending on the donor vessel employed. The first approach consists of the femorofemoral technique, introduced by Vetto in 1962, which has provided excellent results for patients with unilateral iliac lesions (Fig. 29-12) [64]. An 8- to 10-mm graft is anastomosed end to side to a donor femoral artery, delivered through a suprapubic tunnel to the contralateral symptomatic lower extremity, and the second end-to-side femoral anastomosis is constructed. The procedure is minimally stressful since surgical dissection is limited and is carried out under regional anesthesia. The long-term patency rates are slightly inferior to those achieved with aortobifemoral bypass and range from 70 to 85 percent at 5 years [65–68]. The femorofemoral bypass also has proved useful in salvaging extremities threatened by a life-sustaining intra-aortic balloon pump [69].

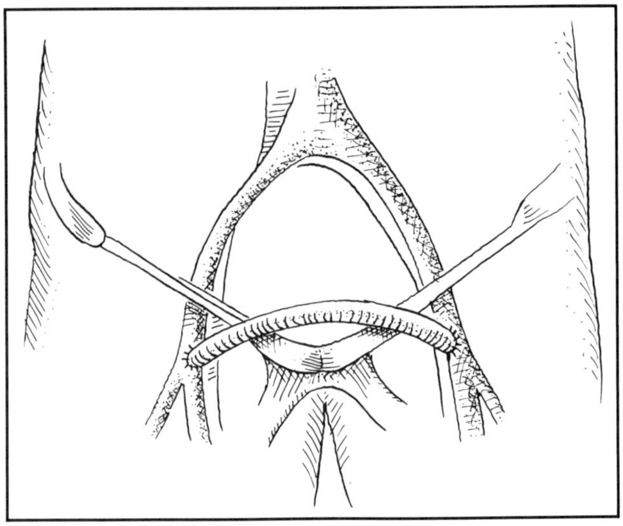

Fig. 29-12. The femorofemoral bypass offers a durable solution to unilateral aortoiliac disease.

The axillary artery also can be utilized as a donor vessel for the axillobifemoral graft, a second alternative to conventional aortofemoral reconstruction and introduced by Blaisdell and co-workers in 1960 [70]. Appropriate candidates include individuals felt to be at high physiologic risk for serious morbidity or mortality from conventional transabdominal reconstruction. More often, however, axillofemoral reconstruction is indicated for patients with intra-abdominal pathology consisting of sepsis, malignancy, or extensive prior surgery or radiation. Intra-abdominal sepsis from an infected previous vascular graft requires resection of the graft with extra-anatomic reconstruction. Axillofemoral bypass usually is carried out under light general anesthesia for construction of the transthoracic subcutaneous tunnel. In exceptionally high-risk individuals, however, regional anesthesia can be supplemented with local anesthesia for the infraclavicular incision.

The operative technique is initiated with exposure of

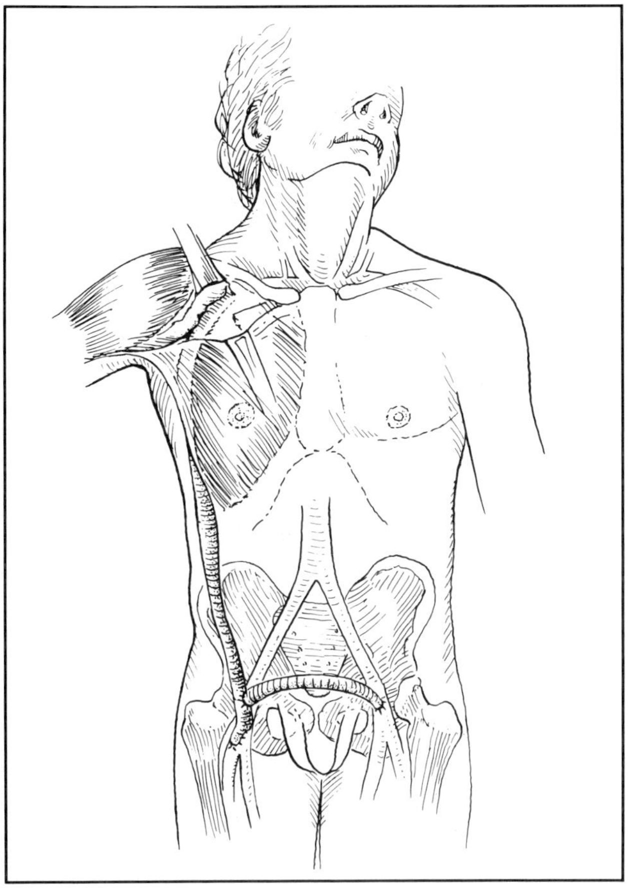

Fig. 29-13. For patients with bilateral aortoiliac occlusive disease and intra-abdominal pathology, sepsis, or radiation or who are at high physiologic risk for general anesthetic, the axillobifemoral graft is an alternative means of aortoiliac reconstruction.

the femoral vessels through bilateral short vertical groin incisions and exposure of the proximal axillary artery through an infraclavicular incision (Fig. 29-13). A long subcutaneous tunnel is constructed deep to the pectoral muscles in the midaxillary line to the iliac crest, where the tunnel extends anteriorly into the appropriate groin incision. A suprapubic tunnel similar to the femorofemoral tunnel then is created to the contralateral groin. An 8- to 10-mm graft, preclotted if necessary, is delivered through the axillary tunnel and, following systemic anticoagulation, an end-to-side anastomosis is constructed to the proximal axillary artery. The crossover limb is then anastomosed to the descending axillary limb in the ipsilateral groin incision. The graft is trimmed appropriately and sutured end to side to an ipsilateral common femoral arteriotomy extending across the origin of the deep femoral artery to ensure continued outflow in the event of progressive superficial femoral disease. The crossover limb is similarly anastomosed to the common and deep femoral arteries in the contralateral groin. Axillobifemoral bypass grafts thus constructed are associated with a 5-year patency rate approximating 70 percent [70–74]. Although the mortality rate is frequently higher (6%) than that associated with aortobifemoral bypass (2%), extra-anatomic reconstruction is carried out in patients preselected on the basis of more advanced systemic atherosclerosis, concomitant disease, or infection of a previous aortofemoral graft. Conversely, one of the major factors in the lower morbidity associated with conventional aortofemoral reconstruction is that patients with more advanced disease have been selected out for extra-anatomic bypass.

Unilateral axillofemoral bypass should be avoided but is occasionally necessary when removing an infected aortic prosthesis. Graft patency after 5 years is clearly inferior (50%) to bilateral reconstruction (70%) and reflects the significant reduction of flow through the descending unilateral axillary limb [72,74]. If outflow from a unilateral axillary graft is restricted to the deep femoral artery alone, 5-year patency rates are further diminished to 40 percent. When both deep and superficial femoral vessels are patent, however, increased flow through the long descending limb provides an improved 5-year patency rate of approximately 60 percent. Thus, a patient warranting revascularization primarily on the basis of resting ischemia in one lower extremity still requires bilateral reconstruction to sustain optimal 5-year patency.

The third major donor vessel consists of a patent common or external iliac artery that, when utilized in appropriate individuals, preserves the reduced operative morbidity and mortality characteristic of extra-anatomic reconstruction yet provides an improved 5-year patency [75]. The enhanced patency rate probably reflects the shorter donor prosthetic limb (Fig. 29-14). Iliofemoral reconstruction is carried out with retroperitoneal exposure of the appropriate donor iliac vessel through a short, transverse incision in the lower abdominal quadrant. Regional anesthetic technique usually is employed, and the morbidity and mortality inherent in the transabdominal approach are minimized. A prosthetic graft is anastomosed end to side to the distal common iliac or proximal external iliac artery and is carried through a retroperitoneal tunnel to the ipsilateral femoral vessels. A crossover limb may then be anastomosed to the prosthesis in the retroperitoneum or in the groin and delivered across to the contralateral common femoral artery. Patency rates associated with iliobifemoral reconstructions are comparable to those achieved with aortofemoral bypass, as might be expected, and therefore approach 90 percent at 5 years. Perioperative mortality is exceedingly rare, and the morbidity rate of approximately 3 percent compares favorably with that of alternative methods [75].

INFRAINGUINAL OCCLUSIVE DISEASE

Until recently, surgical intervention for infrainguinal occlusive disease has not been as satisfactory as proximal aortoiliac reconstruction. Surgeons therefore have been reluctant to recommend femoropopliteal bypass for patients with claudication as the only indication of peripheral ischemia. Infrainguinal reconstruction has been reserved primarily for those with advanced ischemic rest pain or with tissue necrosis evidenced by nonhealing ulceration or gangrene where surgery is warranted for limb salvage. More recently, however, increasingly favorable

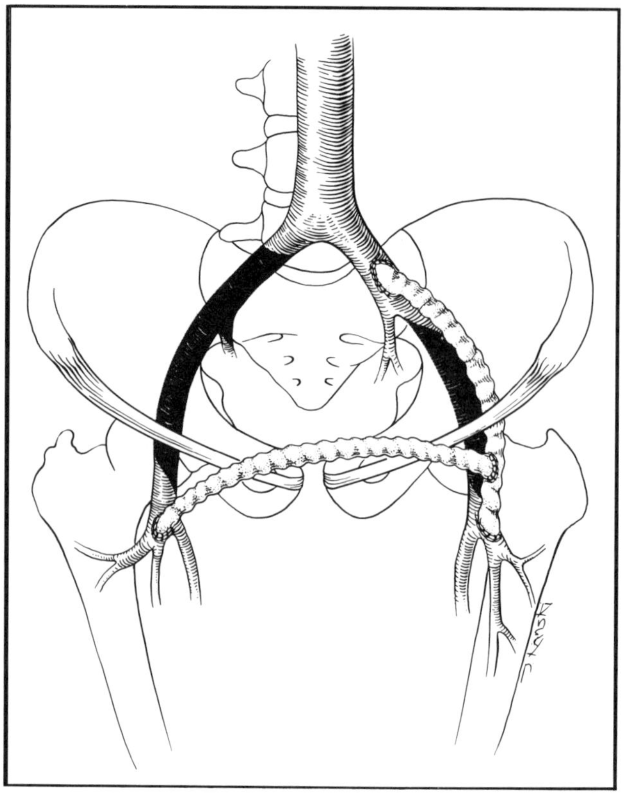

Fig. 29-14. In patients with a patent donor common iliac artery, the iliobifemoral bypass graft can be constructed with considerably less intraoperative stress than conventional aortofemoral bypass.

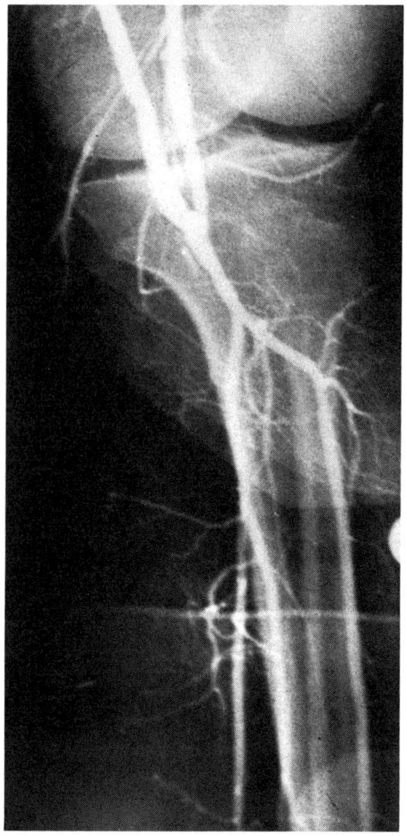

Fig. 29-15. Intraoperative completion arteriogram demonstrating satisfactory femoropopliteal bypass below the knee.

results with reconstruction utilizing autogenous vein have been documented, and therefore the controversy surrounding claudication as the sole indication for reconstruction has resurfaced. Since intermittent claudication in the vast majority of patients results from superficial femoral occlusion, and since, as mentioned previously, this symptom may remain stable or improve over the course of several years [50], claudication must result in significant disability before operative intervention can be recommended.

Femoropopliteal bypass with reversed autogenous saphenous vein was initially popularized in 1948 by Kunlin, whose basic technique established a standard approach to infrainguinal reconstruction that remained virtually unchanged until the early 1980s [76]. Preoperative arteriography demonstrates the distal anatomy and provides the basis for determining the most appropriate position for the distal anastomosis. Although some surgeons prefer general anesthesia, infrainguinal reconstruction frequently is carried out with regional anesthesia and is associated with a perioperative 30-day operative mortality rate of less than 3 percent [77–81].

The operative approach requires initial exposure of the femoral vessels through a vertical groin incision and, if possible, simultaneous exposure of the appropriate site for distal anastomosis. It is not uncommon to choose an anastomosis distal to that originally planned because intraoperative inspection of a vessel may reveal the presence of more disease than was initially visualized arteriographically. The saphenous vein is then exposed throughout its entire length or through multiple interrupted interval incisions. To produce satisfactory patency, the vein should be at least 3.5 mm in caliber at its distal end. The vein graft is removed from its native position after all tributaries are divided; it is then gently dilated and its proximal end reversed to align the valves in the direction of flow. The distal anastomosis is then constructed using fine monofilament suture. Following completion of the distal anastomosis, the graft is delivered through a tunnel extending proximally between the heads of the gastrocnemius through a subsartorial plane to the groin incision. The vein graft is then appropriately trimmed, bevelled, and sutured end to side to the common femoral artery or, as with a distal anastomosis of a proximal reconstruction, to an arteriotomy that extends across the origin of the deep femoral vessel to effect a patch angioplasty. Following completion of the bypass and release of all occluding clamps, arteriography is required to assess the adequacy of the reconstruction (Fig. 29-15). Completion angiography has minimized the number of technical failures by allowing immediate identification and repair of narrowed anastomoses, kinked grafts, stenotic segments, residual distal thrombus, and intimal flaps (Fig. 29-16).

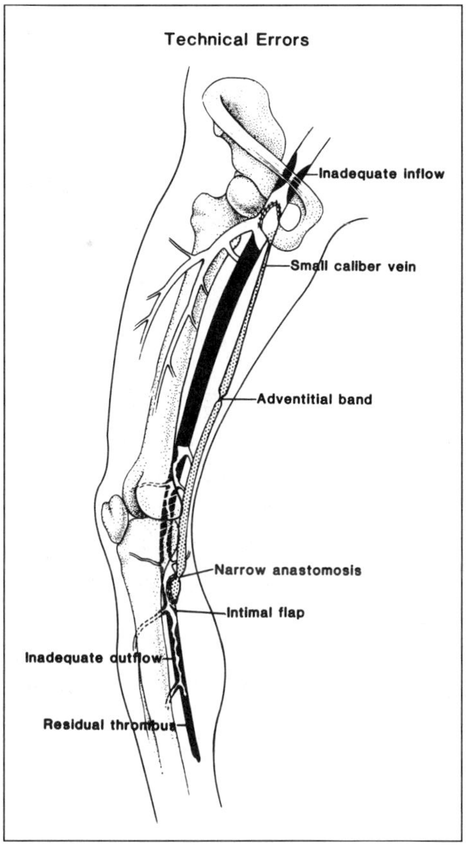

Fig. 29-16. Schematic representation of a reversed femoropopliteal bypass vein graft illustrating potential sources of early technical problems that may be identified with intraoperative completion arteriography.

Results associated with reversed autogenous saphenous vein bypass grafts to various distal vessels are tabulated in Table 29-2. The most favorable results with reversed grafts are those where the distal anastomosis is located above the knee [77–82]. The primary patency rates after 5 years then diminish as the distal anastomosis becomes located progressively more distally. The desire to place the distal anastomosis as proximally as possible, however, must be weighed against the presence of or potential for disease in the outflow segment just distal to that anastomosis. Most frequently, therefore, a patent but diseased midpopliteal artery requires a below-knee distal anastomosis. Occasionally, with more advanced infrainguinal atherosclerosis, runoff into the tibioperoneal system may be discontinuous, leaving an isolated popliteal segment. Such a segment remains useful as a site for distal anastomoses and results in a 65-percent 5-year graft patency rate [80]. Until recently, this isolated popliteal segment was the preferred site for reversed autogenous vein grafts in that situation because long vein grafts to the distal tibioperoneal system resulted in inferior patency rates [78]. This preference may no longer hold, since results with vein grafts to the tibioperoneal system have improved [83], and when an in-situ vein graft can be utilized, the distal tibioperoneal anastomosis is preferred.

VEIN GRAFT FAILURE

It is apparent from Table 29-2 that a substantial number of reversed infrainguinal vein grafts fail during the first 5 years. Although the underlying cause for occlusion remains obscure in approximately one-third of such failures, the responsible mechanisms can be determined in the majority [79,84,85]. A consistent group of failures occurs within the 30 days following initial bypass, resulting from technical errors or misjudgments during surgery or from systemic complications associated with myocardial infarction, hypotension, or hypercoagulable states. More commonly, however, fibrous intimal lesions within the vein graft develop within 6 months, with failure resulting from stenosis at the proximal anastomosis within the narrowest portion of the reversed vein graft or just proximal to the distal anastomosis (Fig. 29-17) [79]. Fibrous intimal hyperplasia also may occur in the midportion of the vein graft, perhaps at the site of a fibrotic valve (Fig. 29-18). A third major group of grafts fail after the first or second year due to progressive atherosclerosis in the native vasculature. A minority of graft thromboses are associated with embolic or septic events. There is no evidence to suggest a statistically significant correlation between known risk factors and ultimate graft failure, yet a distinct tendency for failure has been repeatedly observed in those patients who persist in smoking.

Secondary Reconstruction. Failing or thrombosed vein grafts can be successfully restored to secondary patency with a variety of reconstructive techniques. Prior to the advent of thrombolytic therapy, most patients were taken to the operating room with a totally occluded graft that necessitated initial catheter thrombectomy. Following restoration of flow, intraoperative arteriography was obtained to determine the causative lesion. This lesion frequently consisted of a short-segment stenosis near an anastomosis or within the graft itself and was amenable to simple vein-patch angioplasty, as illustrated in Fig. 29-19. Patch angioplasty following thrombectomy of an

Table 29-2. Results of infrainguinal arterial reconstruction

Material	Number of grafts	5-year cumulative patency (%)			
		Femoropopliteal bypass		Infrapopliteal bypass	
		Primary	Secondary	Primary	Secondary
Autogenous saphenous	440	78	86	66	78
Polytetrafluoroethylene	300	37	39	12	0

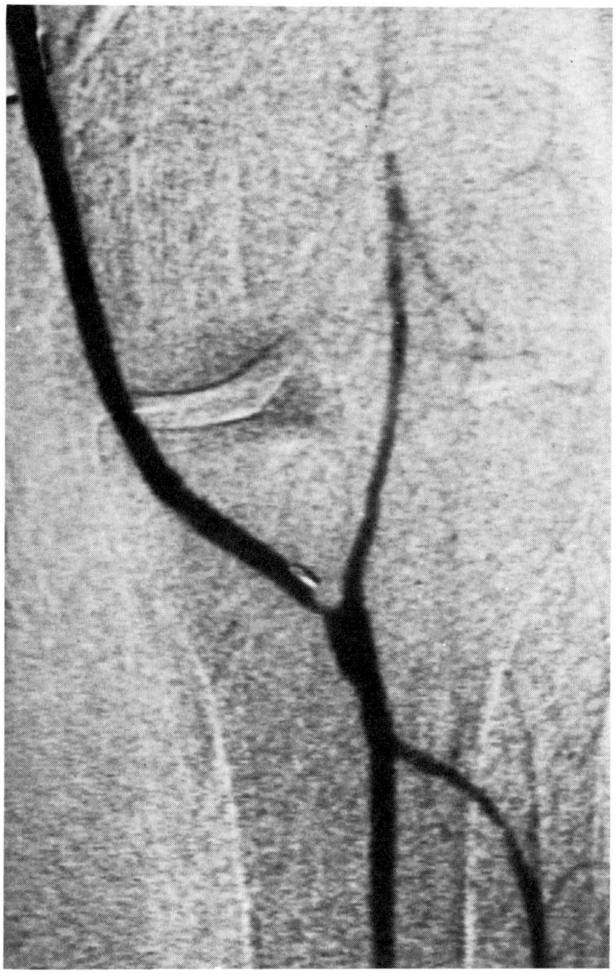

Fig. 29-17. Digital subtraction angiography demonstrating distal juxta-anastomotic stenosis that most likely is secondary to fibrous intimal hyperplasia.

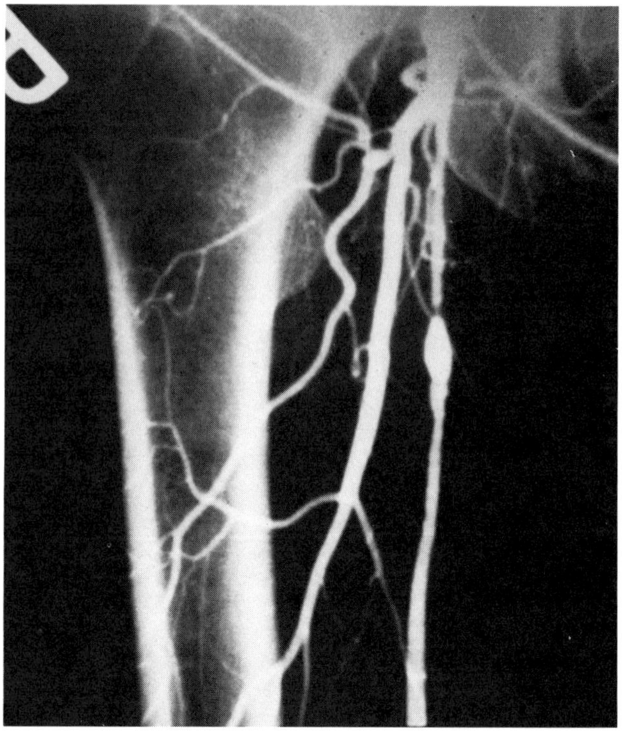

Fig. 29-18. Proximal stenosis occurring in a reversed vein graft with mild poststenotic dilatation.

occluded graft provides limited (28%) cumulative 5-year patency [86]. If, however, failure is noted prior to total occlusion such that secondary reconstruction does not require initial thrombectomy, the same patch-angioplasty technique yields an 82-percent 5-year patency rate. More extensive lesions involving a longer length of vein graft or of the adjacent native vessel may require a secondary vein graft. These secondary grafts may consist of either arm vein, greater or lesser saphenous, or a usable portion of the original vein graft (Fig. 29-20), with the expectation of a 50-percent 5-year patency rate [87].

From this experience, several broad concepts emerge. First, secondary revascularization, although associated with lower patency rates than primary bypass, provides a 5-year limb salvage rate in excess of 70 percent, such that over 90 percent of threatened limbs may be salvaged with one or more subsequent procedures. The operative mortality rate of secondary reconstruction, like that of primary bypass, remains less than 1 percent [87]. The operative mortality and secondary patency rates do not diminish with multiple reconstructive procedures. Second, the necessity for following patients frequently with duplex scans after primary bypass cannot be overemphasized since every effort must be made to intervene with secondary reconstruction **prior to** actual graft thrombosis. Early detection and subsequent repair of the underlying stenotic lesion results in dramatically improved patency and salvage rates. Whether this discrepancy reflects endothelial damage resulting from the initial thrombectomy catheter or merely the presence of adherent thrombus remains to be determined.

With the advent of thrombolytic therapy, it was hypothesized that initial thrombolysis of occluded grafts might in fact make catheter thrombectomy unnecessary and thereby improve the long-term patency associated with secondary reconstruction of totally occluded grafts [88]. Provided irreversible ischemic damage is not imminent, such patients currently are taken to the angiography suite for an initial trial of thrombolytic therapy. Using the intraarterial infusion of urokinase delivered within the occluding thrombus itself, initial thrombolysis is successful in the majority of patients (80%), and it allows the subsequent definition of a causative lesion, obviating the trauma inherent in catheter thrombectomy [88–91]. Preliminary results with secondary reconstruction following thrombolytic therapy are more successful than when initial catheter thrombectomy is required; however, they remain suboptimal compared to those achieved with secondary reconstruction prior to actual graft occlusion [88]. Thus, it remains critical to identify grafts prior to failure to ensure long-term secondary patency of infrainguinal re-

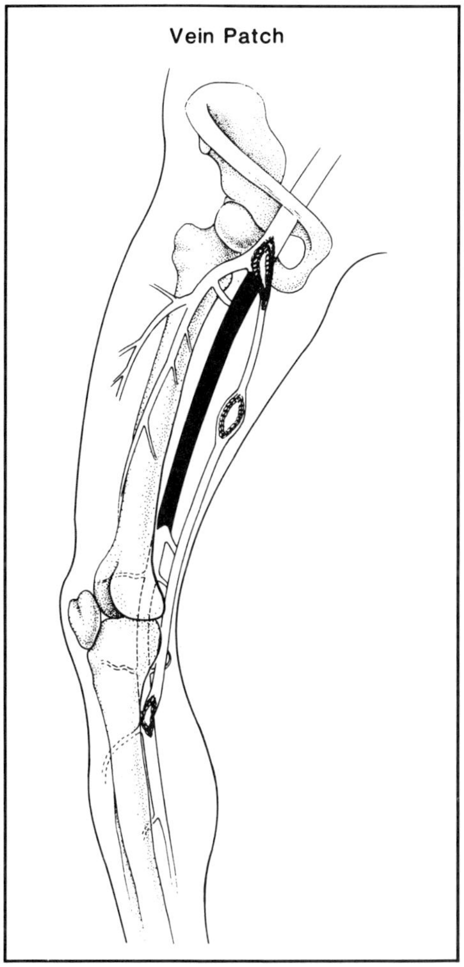

Fig. 29-19. Well-localized stenotic segments of patent vein grafts can be managed with simple vein-patch angioplasties.

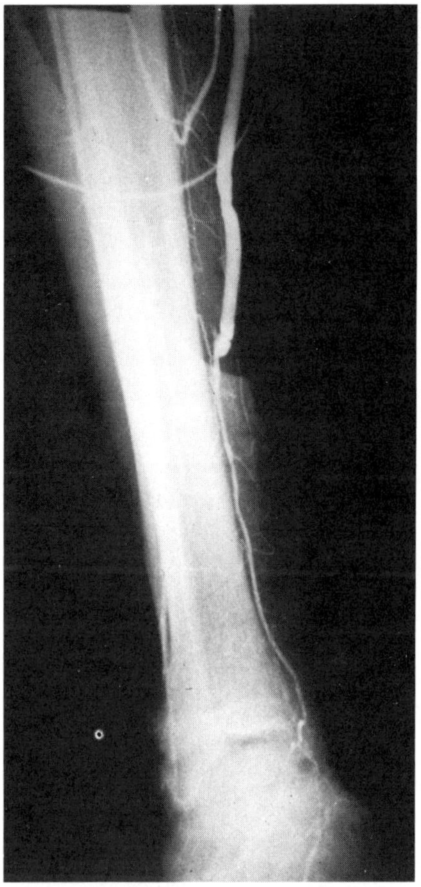

Fig. 29-20. A previous vein graft that has become diffusely stenotic throughout its distal portion can be successfully bypassed using a short segment of vein originating from the proximal portion of the original vein graft. This patient has had such an extension vein graft to the midposterior tibial artery utilizing cephalic vein.

constructions. It is currently recommended that such individuals be followed every 3 to 4 months with noninvasive evaluation during the first year after initial bypass. The first indication of a significant decrease in Doppler ankle pressures, recurrent ischemic symptoms, or significant alterations in flow velocity on Doppler scan should prompt angiographic evaluation.

The In-Situ Saphenous Vein Graft. Although the reversed autogenous vein graft has remained the standard approach to infrainguinal reconstruction since its introduction in 1948, the concept of an in-situ saphenous vein graft has been explored during several periods [92]. Recent improvements in instrumentation have allowed further refinement of the in-situ technique [93,94]. Rather than harvesting and inverting the saphenous vein graft, the vein is left in its natural bed (in situ) and, following adequate visualization, the valves are rendered incompetent with a valvulotome that incises the vein valve cusps (Fig. 29-21). Following exposure of the appropriate vessels, the patient is heparinized and the saphenofemoral junction transected. The proximal common femoral venotomy is oversewn and the first saphenous vein valve excised under direct vision. The proximal end of the vein graft is then anastomosed to the common femoral artery and the occluding clamps removed, allowing antegrade arterial flow through the saphenous vein. With arterial pressure apposing the vein valve cusps proximally, the cusps are progressively incised until all valves are incompetent and brisk arterial flow is observed distally. The saphenous vein is transected distally and anastomosed end to side to the distal anastomotic site. Residual arteriovenous fistulae resulting from patent saphenous-vein tributaries are ligated and completion arteriography undertaken as described previously.

This method provides several theoretic advantages over the reversed method, including preservation of the vasovasorum, preservation of more functional endothelium, improved size match at the anastomoses, and increased vein utilization, since smaller-caliber vein may be used for anastomoses to the very distal tibioperoneal vessels at the level of the malleolus. While many of these theoretic advantages remain controversial, the in-situ method is more expeditious and undoubtedly allows increased vein

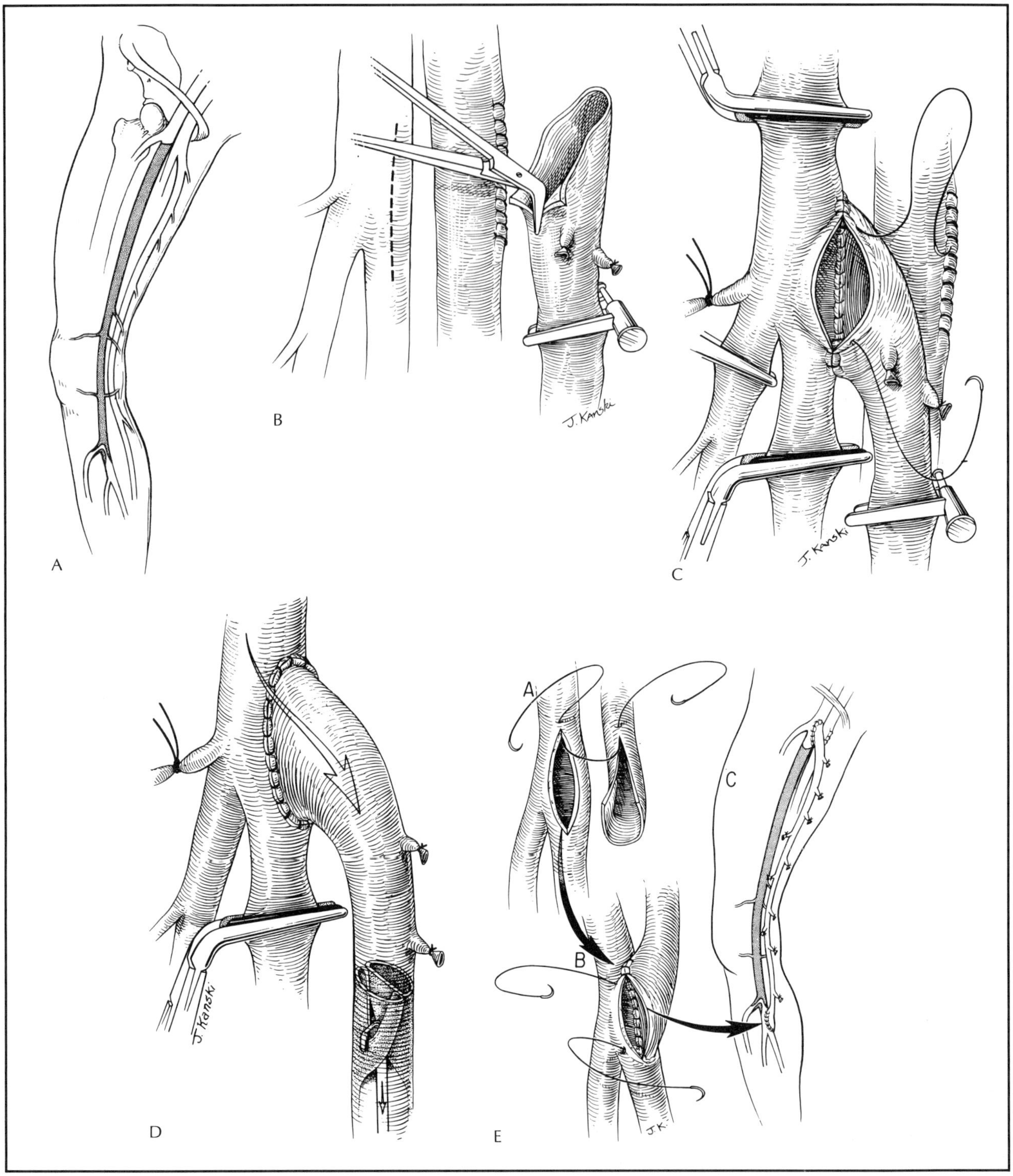

Fig. 29-21. The occluded superficial femoral and popliteal arteries (stippled vessels) can be reconstructed with an in-situ saphenous vein graft carried from the common femoral artery to the distal tibioperoneal trunk below the knee **(A)**. The saphenofemoral junction is transected in the groin, the venotomy in the femoral vein oversewn, and the proximal end of the saphenous vein prepared for anastomosis **(B)**. The vein graft is then anastomosed end to side to the femoral artery **(C)**. Following completion of the anastomosis, flow is restored through the vein graft and the valvulotome inserted through side branches at appropriate intervals to lyse the valve cusps **(D)**. Finally, the distal anastomosis is completed, in this case at the level of the distal tibioperoneal vessel **(E)**.

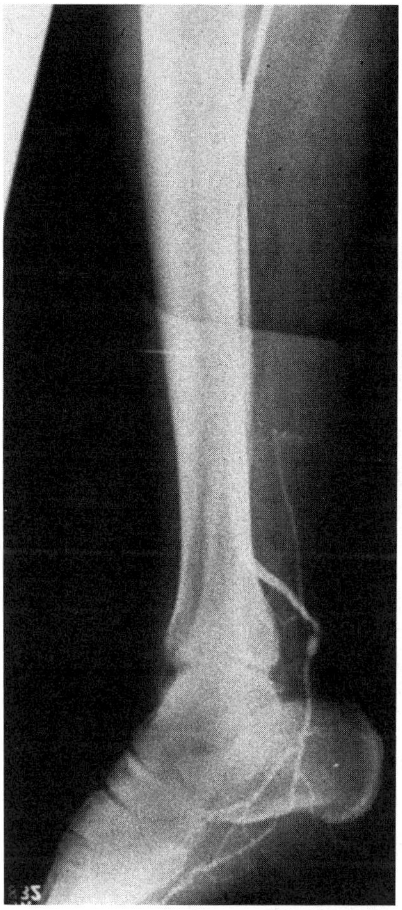

Fig. 29-22. Intraoperative completion arteriogram demonstrating an in-situ bypass from the common femoral artery to the distal posterior tibial artery at the level of the medial malleolus.

utilization, so that more patients of advanced age with advanced disease become appropriate candidates for reconstruction. The in-situ technique has resulted in 5-year patency rates of 85 percent in both femoropopliteal and femorotibial positions [81]. These vastly improved results in the femorotibial group contrast starkly with the lower patency (56%) associated with reversed grafts, a contrast augmented by the fact that as many as 25 percent of patients undergoing in-situ grafting would not have been candidates for the reversed technique due to the small caliber of vein or distal artery at the malleolar level (Fig. 29-22). A significant difference in patency rates between diabetics and nondiabetics has not been observed.

A variety of prosthetic materials have been utilized for small-caliber arterial bypass, but none has provided results comparable to those achieved with autogenous vein [95–99]. Disappointing experience with small-diameter Dacron prostheses in the 1960s prompted several trials utilizing alternatives such as bovine carotid artery and human umbilical vein grafts, both of which required tanning with either dialdehyde starch or glutaraldehyde. Both of these biologic grafts proved cumbersome and, although reinforced with an external synthetic mesh, demonstrated an increased tendency for delayed aneurysmal dilatation. Dissatisfaction with these biologic substitutes resulted in increased use of expanded polytetrafluoroethylene (PTFE) grafts, which possessed more desirable handling characteristics and held the promise of a more biocompatible nonthrombogenic luminal surface. Extensive clinical experience during the past decade, however, clearly has relegated PTFE to a position inferior to autogenous vein (see Table 29-2). The overall 5-year patency rates associated with infrainguinal PTFE grafts approximates 35 percent, higher for claudicators (57%) than when used for limb salvage (24%) [99]. When PTFE is utilized in the above-knee position, the patency is more acceptable (50–60%), whereas below-knee femoropopliteal reconstruction provides a reduced 30-percent patency rate. The results achieved with femorotibial PTFE grafts are generally so unsatisfactory (12% 5-year patency) that such reconstruction even for limb salvage is of questionable benefit. Given these discouraging results with prosthetic material, every effort is made to exhaust all possible sources of autogenous tissue, including lesser saphenous or arm vein [100].

Visceral Vessel Occlusive Disease

RENOVASCULAR RECONSTRUCTION

Patients with refractory hypertension or impaired renal function may be appropriate candidates for renal revascularization using one of several methods available. Percutaneous transluminal angioplasty has been shown to be most appropriate for patients with unilateral, nonostial atherosclerosis or for those with fibromuscular disease (Fig. 29-23) [101]. Patients failing percutaneous dilatation, however, and those with ostial lesions indicative of contiguous aortic plaque are more appropriately managed surgically (Fig. 29-24). Operative intervention includes endarterectomy, aortorenal bypass, or extra-anatomic reconstruction using either the common hepatic or splenic artery as a donor vessel. The most appropriate method of reconstruction is determined by individual anatomy, as defined by preoperative arteriography and by the surgeon's experience and preference. Patients with focal ostial lesions may be expeditiously revascularized with transaortic endarterectomy [102]. Through an abdominal incision, retroperitoneal aortic exposure is achieved as previously described and extended to allow mobilization of the left renal vein. The suprarenal aorta is dissected to the level of the origin of the superior mesenteric artery. Following systemic anticoagulation, the aorta is occluded proximal and distal to the renal arteries and a transverse incision made across the aorta and extended through the origin of both renal arteries. Plaque is then endarterectomized with a spatula and the distal intimal surfaces thoroughly inspected under direct vision. The aortic incision may be closed primarily or with a patch of either vein or prosthetic material to effect bilateral renal-artery angioplasties. That decision is governed by the caliber of the native vessels.

Alternatively, patients with more diffuse disease involving a longer length of the proximal renal artery are more appropriately treated with a bypass technique. The

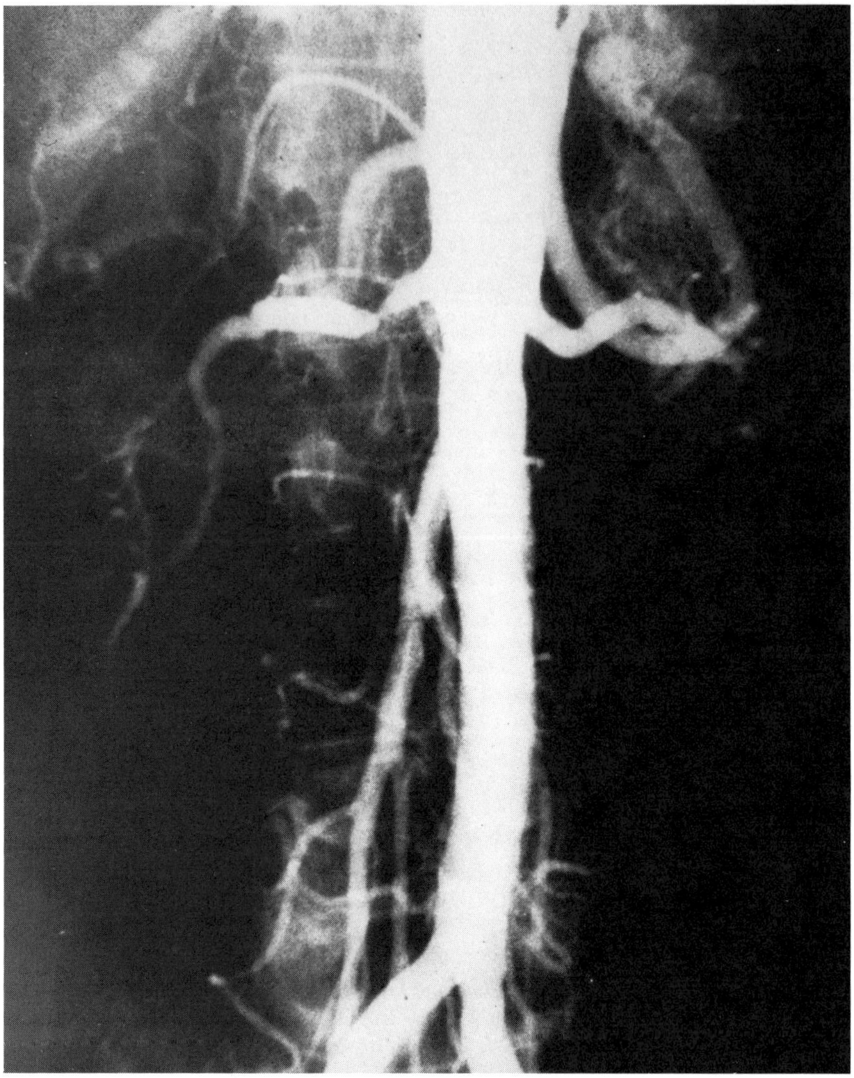

Fig. 29-23. Arteriogram demonstrating nonostial localized stenosis of the right renal artery, a very favorable lesion for percutaneous transluminal angioplasty.

best results are obtained with aortorenal bypass when the infrarenal aorta is relatively free of disease [103,104]. A severely diseased infrarenal aorta provides an insecure proximal anastomosis, which may compromise long-term patency. Aortorenal bypass can be effected using either autogenous or prosthetic material; the preference in most centers is saphenous vein (Fig. 29-25). After exposure of the retroperitoneal aorta, the renal arteries must be dissected and mobilized more completely. Following systemic anticoagulation, the distal renal artery at the anastomotic site is occluded with atraumatic clamps, and a 2-cm longitudinal arteriotomy is incised. The appropriate graft is bevelled and sutured end to side to the renal artery. Following completion of the initial distal anastomosis, the aorta is occluded and the proximal anastomosis constructed to a 2-cm aortotomy. To provide a satisfactory proximal anastomosis, a severely diseased infrarenal aorta may require replacement with a prosthetic graft or the use of an alternative donor site. The iliac artery and either the hepatic or splenic vessels provide appropriate alternatives [105–109]. When such patients require infrarenal aortic reconstruction for concomitant aortoiliac or aneurysmal disease, the choice clearly is the aortorenal bypass, using the prosthetic graft for the proximal anastomosis.

If indications for simultaneous infrarenal aortic reconstruction are absent, more appropriate reconstruction may be secured using the celiac axis as the donor vessel [108,109]. In the case of left-renal artery lesions, revascularization can be obtained using the splenic artery. The splenic artery is dissected free along the superior border of the pancreas, ligated distally near the hilum of the spleen, and passed through the retropancreatic plane to be anastomosed to the left renal artery. Revascularization of the right renal artery requires the use of an autogenous vein graft anastomosed distally end to side or end to

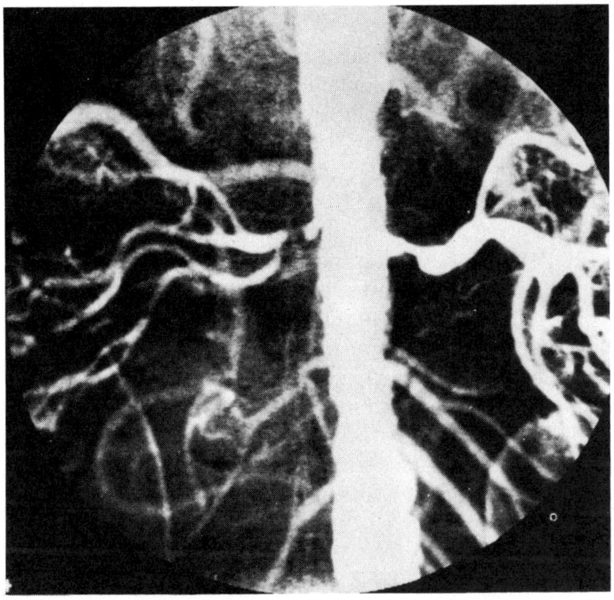

Fig. 29-24. Arteriogram demonstrating bilateral renal artery stenoses with contiguous aortic disease.

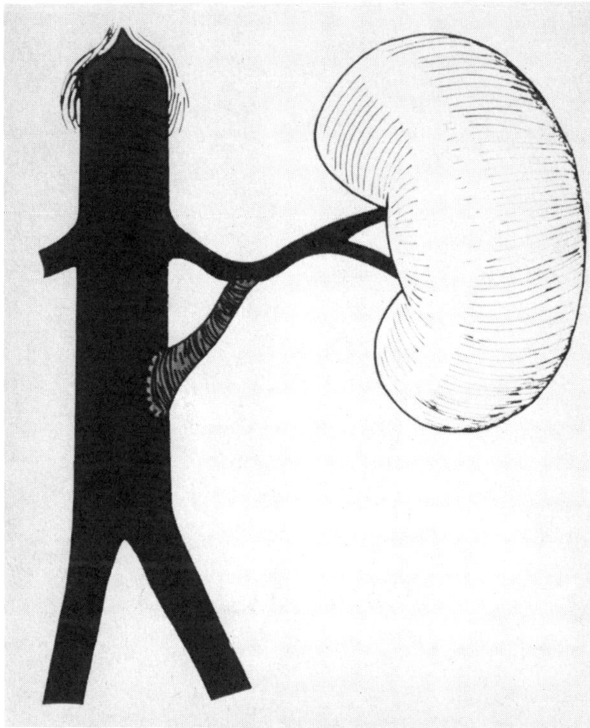

Fig. 29-25. The technique of aortorenal bypass using autogenous saphenous vein.

end to the renal artery and proximally end to side to the common hepatic artery. Both methods provide favorable long-term patencies, with cure or improvement in the majority of patients.

MESENTERIC REVASCULARIZATION

Mesenteric insufficiency results from the occlusion or severe stenosis of two of the three major mesenteric vessels, and affected patients often are referred only after several years of diffuse abdominal pain that may or may not be related to meals and accompanied by significant weight loss [110–113]. These patients represent a challenge to the vascular surgeon since mesenteric revascularization often is technically demanding [111]. It is not surprising that such patients are rare, given the extensive collateral network available to the splanchnic bed. Even with two of three vessels entirely occluded, available collateral vessels emanating from the third may suffice, as exemplified by the angiogram in Fig. 29-26, which was obtained from a patient without mesenteric symptoms. The most appropriate reconstruction remains controversial and must be tailored to individual anatomy. Nevertheless, when revascularization is indicated, many surgeons prefer to rearterialize at least two of the three visceral vessels [112], but others have had excellent results with celiac revascularization alone [111]. The more frequently revascularized vessels consist of the celiac axis and the superior mesenteric artery; the best results have been obtained with either endarterectomy of appropriate limited ostial lesions or with bypass grafting using autogenous tissue. Results with prosthetic material have been inferior, which, to some extent, is a reflection of the tortuous course such grafts must follow.

Endarterectomy is best undertaken through a retroperitoneal approach to the left lateral aspect of the suprarenal aorta, which is subsequently occluded proximally and distally [111]. The left lateral aorta is then incised, exposing the ostia of the celiac and superior mesenteric vessels, which subsequently are endarterectomized. In patients with more diffuse proximal disease, endarterectomy may be inappropriate and bypass necessary [112,113]. Infrarenal aortic or proximal common iliac origins of the bypass grafts are acceptable in patients with relatively disease-free aortoiliac vessels, but in patients with more advanced disease of the infrarenal aortoiliac system, a supraceliac origin may be required.

Arterial Aneurysm

Surgical management of aortic aneurysms originally consisted of aortic ligation proximal to the aneurysmal sac [114]. Results were predictably devastating due to inadequate collateral supply and subsequent peripheral ischemia. It was then theorized that controlled, progressive thrombosis might allow sufficient time for collateral to develop, and delayed occlusion was achieved with the introduction of wire into the aneurysm sac [115]. Although this approach certainly resulted in long-term survivors and has been reported effective as recently as the 1970s [116], far superior results are now achieved with direct repair. Early attempts at wrapping the aneurysm with cellophane or skin grafts also proved unsuccessful [117].

Modern aneurysm repair was introduced in 1951 by DeBost and colleagues, who successfully replaced a syphi-

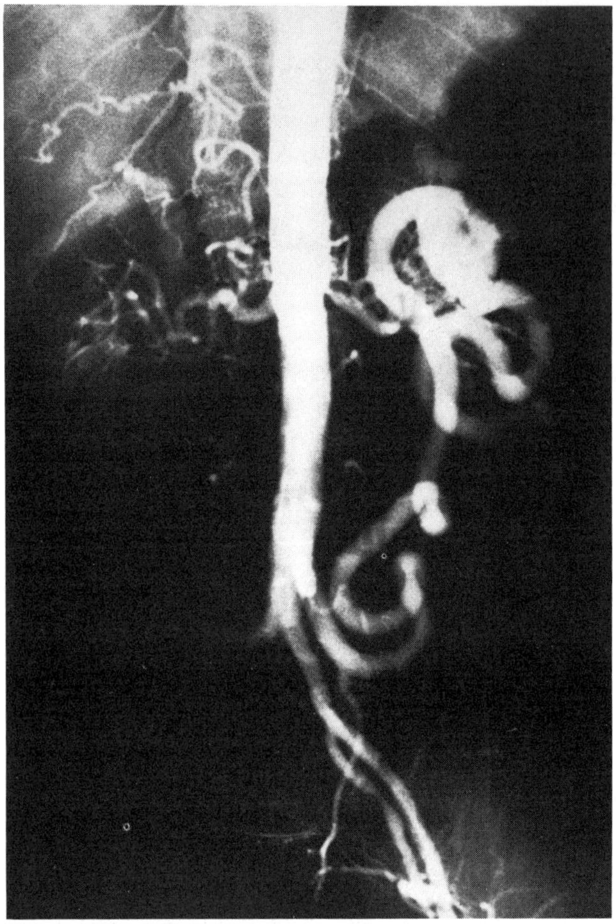

Fig. 29-26. Aortoiliac occlusive disease with complete occlusion of the right common iliac artery associated with occlusion of the celiac and superior mesenteric arteries and stenosis of the left renal artery. A large meandering mesenteric vessel originating from the inferior mesenteric artery supplies the entire gut. Aortoiliac reconstruction requires simultaneous proximal mesenteric endarterectomy, bypass, or reimplantation of the large mesenteric vessel or an end-to-side proximal anastomosis to preserve mesenteric flow.

litic aneurysm of the infrarenal aorta with an aortic homograft [118]. With the advent of prosthetic material, direct repair became the standard approach [119]. The mortality figures for operative repair, however, remained extraordinarily high during the early 1960s and approached 20 percent in some series [120–123]. A dramatic reduction in mortality has evolved during the intervening years from a multitude of factors, including concurrent improvements in anesthetic management, which reduced operative mortality to the 10-percent level by the end of the 1960s. More recent advances further reduced mortality figures, which currently range from zero to 5 percent [124–127]. First, Creech assimilated Matas's technique of endoaneurysmorrhaphy [128] in the context of observations made by Javid and colleagues [129] and began to advocate a nonexcisional approach to aneurysms [130]. Instead of removing the entire aneurysm, a maneuver that may require substantial operative time and extensive retroperitoneal dissection with resultant blood loss and postoperative third-space sequestration, the aorta was merely clamped proximal and distal to the aneurysm, the sac opened longitudinally, and a prosthetic graft inserted inside the aneurysm sac.

A second major factor contributing to the reduced operative mortality stemmed from the realization that successful operative management required knowing that most such patients have significant coronary artery disease, which may or may not be clinically evident [131–134]. Appreciation of the systemic manifestations of atherosclerotic disease thus became an important factor influencing the outcome of repair. A significant reduction in the operative mortality evolved from the observation that adequately hydrated patients demonstrated more stable intraoperative hemodynamics [135]. As afterload is increased during aortic cross-clamping, systemic resistance is simultaneously reduced with pharmacologic agents, which are terminated on removing the clamp. Such preoperative hydration is well tolerated in the vast majority of patients, but approximately 10 percent of individuals with a compromised myocardium do not tolerate increased left ventricular filling pressures. It therefore became necessary to monitor preoperative hydration and subsequent cardiac performance with the pulmonary artery thermistor-tipped catheter, whereby individual myocardial performance could be optimized at a given pulmonary artery wedge pressure [126]. While it is no longer feasible to admit patients undergoing aortic aneurysm repair to an intensive care unit during the evening preoperatively, pulmonary-artery and radial-artery catheters usually are inserted prior to induction of anesthesia and during volume loading. The wedge pressure is elevated in increments and the cardiac index measured to allow the determination of individual left ventricular performance. Wedge pressures subsequently are maintained perioperatively at a level that ensures optimal left ventricular performance for the individual patient.

Since the currently anticipated operative mortality rate approaches 2 percent, the decision regarding the advisability of aneurysm repair becomes relatively straightforward. Abdominal aortic aneurysms represent one of the few disease entities for which the natural history has been reasonably well documented [136–138]. Both Estes in 1950 and Szilagyi in 1966 and again in 1972 documented the mortality associated with large abdominal aortic aneurysms at approximately 50 percent after 2 years and 80 percent after 5 years following diagnosis. The majority of these deaths resulted from rupture of the aneurysm. In those series, a large aneurysm was defined as greater than 6 cm in transverse diameter. Smaller aneurysms have a reduced but finite tendency to rupture; therefore, most surgeons recommend repair of all aneurysms reaching the size of 5 cm in diameter. Recent evidence indicates that aneurysms that expand at a rate exceeding 0.5 cm during a 3- to 6-month interval also represent a sufficiently increased risk of rupture that repair should be undertaken even though the absolute diameter may not yet have reached 5 cm [138]. Routine abdominal ultrasonography therefore should be utilized at 3- to 6-month intervals

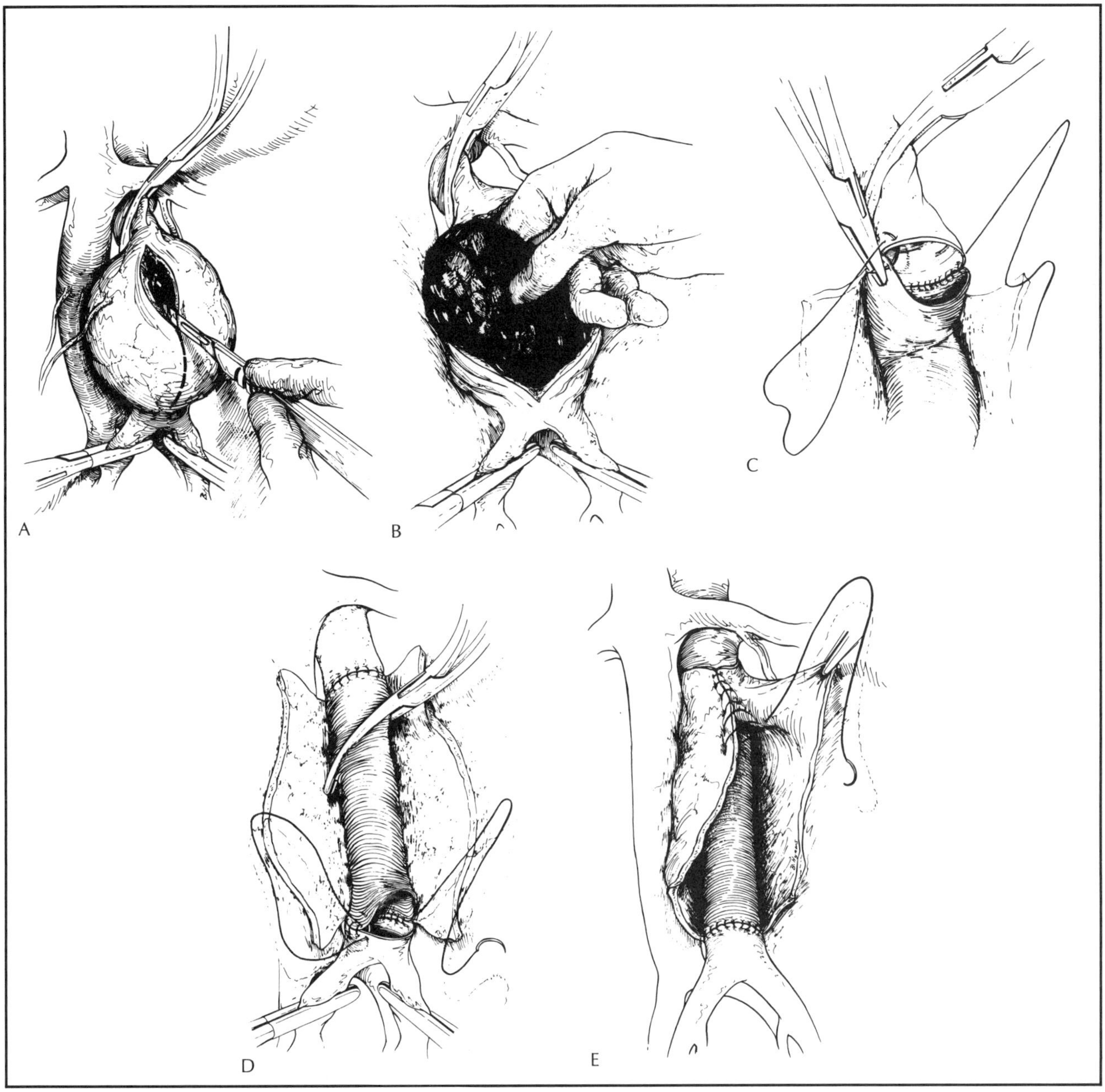

Fig. 29-27. **A**. Following retroperitoneal exposure, an infrarenal abdominal aortic aneurysm has been isolated between occluding clamps, and the sac is opened longitudinally. **B**. Extensive laminated intraluminal thrombus is evacuated, and any backbleeding lumbar vessels are oversewn. **C**. The proximal anastomosis of the repair is constructed by suturing the graft to the neck of the aneurysm end to end using a continuous monofilament suture. **D**. The distal anastomosis to the terminal aortic bifurcation is then completed with similar technique. **E**. After restoration of flow through the graft, the aneurysm sac is reapproximated over the graft to provide protection to the overlying viscera. (Modified with permission from RM Greenhalgh. Vascular Surgical Techniques: An Atlas. Philadelphia: Saunders, 1989.)

to monitor accurately the transverse diameter of aortic aneurysms [139].

Preoperative arteriography, although not absolutely mandatory [140], is helpful for determining the relationship of the visceral vessels to the neck of the aneurysm; it also may reveal aberrant renal vessels and provide some assessment of the iliac vessels. The majority of aneurysms can be repaired with a simple tube graft, ignoring ectatic or minimally aneurysmal iliac vessels [141]. Where the common iliac arteries are aneurysmal as well, however, repair is best effected with aortobifemoral reconstruction.

The operative approach for most patients consists of a long midline abdominal incision and, following retroperitoneal exposure, the retroperitoneum overlying the aneu-

Table 29-3. Operative morbidity associated with repair of abdominal aortic aneurysms

Year	Authors	Number of patients	30-day operative mortality rate (%)
1980	Whittemore et al. [126]	110	0
1981	Crawford et al. [125]	140	1.4
1989	Johnston et al. [124]	666	4.8
1990	Golden et al. [127]	500	1.6

rysm is incised cephalad to the level of the left renal vein (Fig. 29-27). The periaortic tissues are dissected free of the neck of the aneurysm laterally just sufficient to allow the insertion of a cross-clamp. In the case of a tube graft, the common iliac arteries are dissected distally to allow the insertion of temporary occluding clamps. If aortofemoral reconstruction is required, retroperitoneal tunnels are created to bilateral short vertical groin incisions through which the distal femoral vessels are isolated. Following systemic anticoagulation, the aorta proximal to the neck of the aneurysm is occluded, as are the distal iliac vessels. The aneurysm sac is opened longitudinally and evacuated of laminar thrombus. Backbleeding lumbar vessels are secured with figure-of-eight sutures. A straight prosthesis, usually woven, because this material is less porous than knitted grafts, is sutured proximally to the neck of the aneurysm using Creech technique with running prolene suture. The distal anastomosis is similarly constructed to the terminal aortic bifurcation or to both iliac and femoral vessels. Before completing the distal anastomoses, the aortic graft is thoroughly flushed of residual thrombus and atheromatous debris, and all occluding clamps are removed on completion. The aneurysm sac is irrigated and closed over the prosthesis to provide the first layer of autogenous tissue between the prosthetic graft and the overlying bowel. The retroperitoneum is similarly apposed to effect at least a two-layer retroperitoneal closure in an effort to reduce the incidence of aortoduodenal fistula. Intraoperative transfusion is necessary in only 50 percent of our patients at present, because shed blood can be processed and returned with a cell-saver apparatus. Using that approach, the perioperative 30-day mortality

Fig. 29-28. The graft inclusion method of repairing thoracoabdominal aneurysms, demonstrating techniques of anastomosing intercostal and visceral vessels. (Reproduced with permission from ES Crawford et al. Progress in treatment of thoracoabdominal and abdominal aortic aneurysms involving celiac, superior mesenteric, and renal arteries. Ann Surg 1978; 188:404).

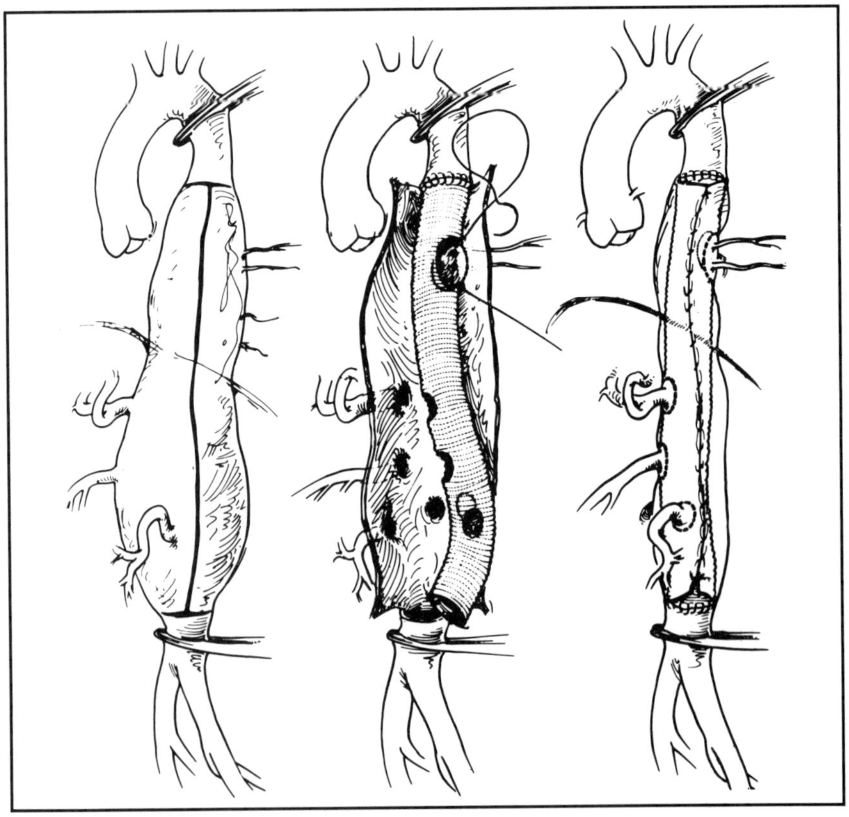

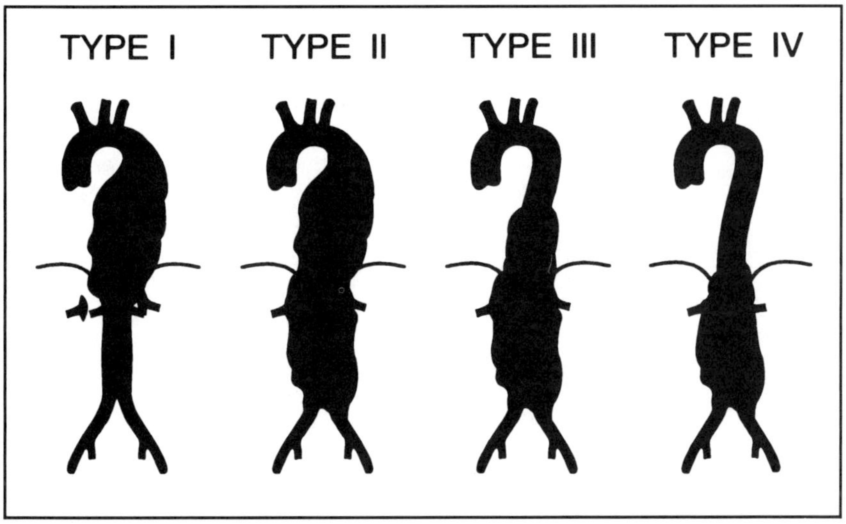

Fig. 29-29. Classification of thoracoabdominal aneurysms into the four major groups. The type II aneurysm requiring replacement of the entire aorta is associated with the highest risk (20%) of spinal cord injury. (Reproduced with permission from R Cambria et al. Recent experience with thoracoabdominal aneurysm repair. Arch Surg 1989; 124:620. Copyright 1989, American Medical Association.)

rate associated with elective aneurysm repair approximates 2 percent in most current series (Table 29-3). The incidence of postoperative cardiac events has been reduced substantially, and myocardial infarction currently occurs in fewer than 3 percent of patients [127].

Patients with a ruptured aneurysm who survive until they reach the hospital remain subject to inordinately high operative mortality. A major contributing factor to this excessive mortality is a persistent delay in initial diagnosis and the tendency to obtain multiple laboratory tests. The diagnosis of an intra-abdominal hemorrhagic catastrophe is, however, usually reasonably obvious, and immediate exploration is clearly indicated. Arteriography is seldom required for diagnostic purposes, and patients should be taken to the operating room expeditiously. The anticipated operative mortality is less than 20 percent for patients who arrive in the operating room normotensive but as high as 70 percent for patients who remain in shock [142–144]. Operative repair is similar to that described for intact aneurysms, except that anticoagulation is contraindicated since it only adds to the already high incidence of hemorrhagic diatheses. The best defense against ruptured aneurysm is, therefore, the elective repair of aneurysms greater than 5 cm in diameter or of smaller aneurysms demonstrating rapid expansion. Although nonresective therapy, such as axillobifemoral bypass after aortic ligation, is advocated by some [145,146], the vast majority of patients may be appropriately managed with direct repair despite marked cardiopulmonary compromise.

Thoracoabdominal Aneurysms

The surgical management of thoracoabdominal aneurysms has been improved dramatically during the past decade, in large part due to Dr. Stanley Crawford's monumental efforts with nearly 1,000 such patients [147,148]. His large personal experience has achieved a reduction in the overall operative mortality for patients with nondissecting thoracoabdominal aneurysms to 10 percent and the incidence of its most dreaded complication, paraplegia. Although the procedure produces enormous perioperative physiologic stress in patients with extensive associated cardiovascular disease, repair can now be recommended with acceptable risks, given the much higher risk characteristic of the natural history.

Repair requires a thoracoabdominal incision, clamping of the thoracic aorta, and replacement of varying lengths of aorta, depending on the pathologic anatomy involved. Replacement is carried out with incision of the left lateral aspect of the aorta and insertion of a graft from within the aneurysm sac, incorporating intercostal and visceral arterial ostia (Fig. 29-28). As with infrarenal aortic repair, the increased afterload associated with aortic clamping is reduced pharmacologically, and the renal arteries often are perfused with a chilled balanced salt solution.

Thoracoabdominal aneurysms can be divided into four types, according to the anatomic extent of aneurysmal disease (Fig. 29-29). Type I consists of patients with aneurysms confined primarily to the thoracic segment, whereas type II aneurysms involve the entire thoracic and abdominal aorta. Type III includes aneurysms involving the entire abdominal aorta and most of the descending distal thoracic segment, and type IV aneurysms are similar to those in type III but involve only the most distal thoracic aorta.

Paraplegia occurs in only 1 to 4 percent of patients with type I, III, or IV aneurysms but far more commonly (11%) in type II patients, presumably because repair excludes a longer segment of aorta and more arterial supply to the spinal cord. Although reimplantation of large intercostals

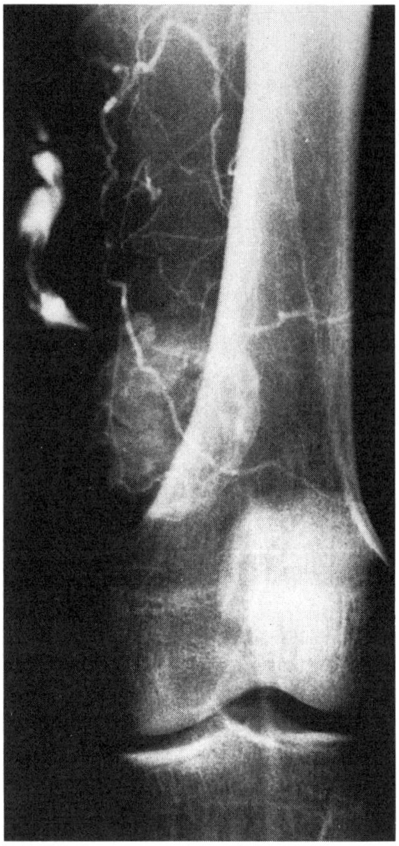

Fig. 29-30. Popliteal aneurysm demonstrated in the proximal popliteal artery just distal to the adductor hiatus.

seems to have reduced that complication, its etiology and prevention remain poorly understood. The incidence of spinal cord ischemia does not necessarily correlate with preoperative angiographic anatomy, intraoperative hypotension, hypothermia, length of cross-clamp time, or the use of shunts or extracorporeal bypass. Enthusiasm to repair extensive type II aneurysms must be tempered by a realistic expectation of a 10-percent incidence of paraplegia and a similar incidence of paraparesis. The decision to proceed with surgery, therefore, is highly individualized. Repair of all other types of thoracoabdominal aneurysm, however, should be undertaken without undue delay. When technically feasible, separate thoracic and abdominal aneurysms probably should be repaired during separate, staged procedures.

Peripheral Arterial Aneurysms

The most common peripheral arterial aneurysms are located in the popliteal artery and are bilateral in at least half of patients (Fig. 29-30). Elective repair is mandated on diagnosis since popliteal-artery aneurysms are associated with an inordinately high incidence of subsequent limb loss due to thrombotic occlusion or embolization [150,151]. The operative approach to such patients consists of excluding the aneurysm with a femoropopliteal bypass. Such reconstruction is carried out with autogenous tissue and requires ligation of the native popliteal artery proximal and distal to the aneurysm. Excision of the aneurysm usually is unnecessary, since subsequent thrombosis ensues with gradual reduction in size of the mass. Occasionally, exceptionally large popliteal aneurysms require excision to achieve adequate decompression of the popliteal fossa and, more specifically, the popliteal veins. Results with current methods of repair are excellent, with limb salvage rates approaching 90 percent at 5 years [151,152].

Femoral artery aneurysms are encountered less frequently and usually are bilateral [153]. The vast majority are associated with aortoiliac aneurysms, and 50 percent are associated with popliteal aneurysms. Repair is indicated when the aneurysm becomes greater than 3 cm in diameter. Common femoral-artery aneurysms are approached through a groin incision, and a short length of 8- or 10-mm prosthetic graft is interposed between the normal-caliber distal iliac artery and the bifurcation of the common femoral vessel. The femoral aneurysm sac may then be closed over the graft, as described for aortic aneurysm repair.

Visceral Arterial Aneurysms

The most common visceral arterial aneurysm involves the splenic artery and is said to occur in 1 percent of the population [154,155]. The majority are small, asymptomatic aneurysms less than 2 cm in diameter and are circumferentially calcified, a finding that once was thought to protect against rupture. Neither calcification nor normotension, however, are factors that can be relied on to rule out the possibility of rupture. The actual risk of rupture is unknown but seems highest when the aneurysm becomes greater than 2 cm in diameter or is associated with pregnancy. Therefore, large or expanding splenic aneurysms or those occurring in women of childbearing age should be addressed. The aneurysm may be excluded with proximal and distal ligature or excised. The splenic artery does not need to be reconstructed, nor is splenectomy necessary, because continued arterial supply to the spleen derives from the short gastric vessels [155].

Hepatic-artery aneurysms represent the next most common visceral-artery aneurysm, accounting for approximately 20 percent. Whereas the risk of rupture remains undetermined, it does occur as the presenting problem in nearly half of all patients with such aneurysms. The operative management of a hepatic arterial aneurysm depends on its location along the vessel [156]. Aneurysms of the common hepatic artery proximal to the origin of the gastroduodenal artery can be excluded with proximal and distal ligation without reconstruction, since blood supply from the superior mesenteric artery via the pancreaticoduodenal arcade generally is adequate. Aneurysms distal to the gastroduodenal branch involving the proper hepatic artery require reconstruction, most commonly carried out with autogenous saphenous vein. Intraparenchymal hepatic-artery aneurysms may require more extensive hepatic resection.

Isolated aneurysms of the proximal celiac trunk are extremely rare [157], but aneurysms involving the superior mesenteric artery trunk have been reported more often [158]. The majority of those aneurysms are mycotic;

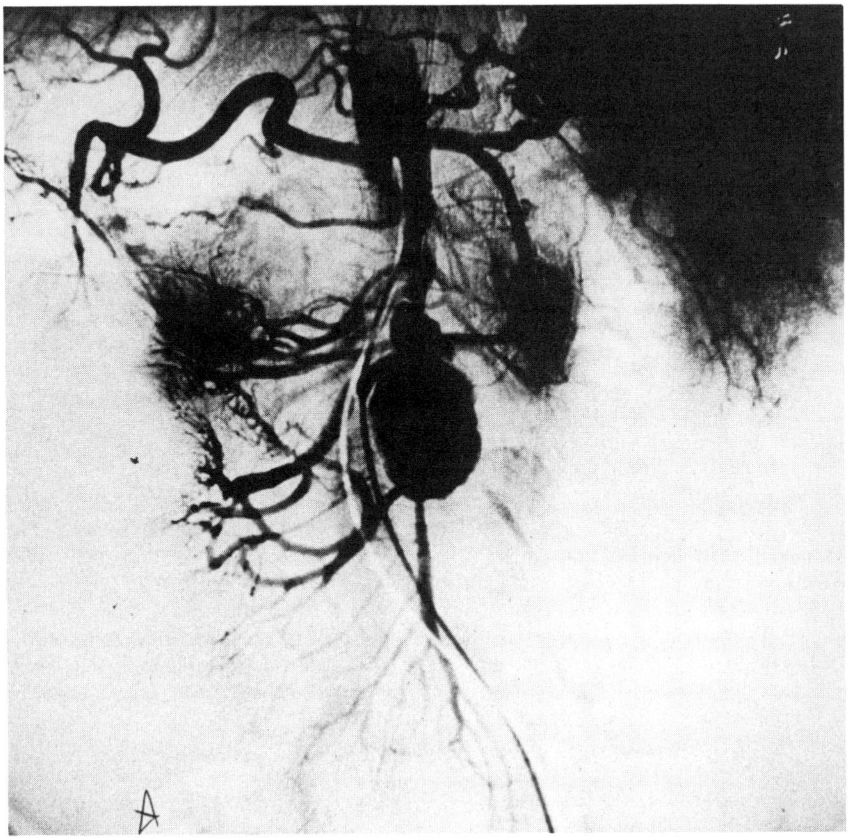

Fig. 29-31. Mycotic aneurysm of the superior mesenteric artery required excision and intestinal revascularization using autogenous saphenous vein grafts.

therefore, their repair requires resection and subsequent reconstruction using autogenous tissue (Fig. 29-31). Although primary ligation with excision has been advocated in the past, the incidence of distal intestinal ischemia is high; therefore, reconstruction is indicated [159].

Renal artery aneurysms are sometimes encountered and tend to be of more varied etiology [160,161]. The most common aneurysm is a true saccular lesion that tends to occur near the proximal bifurcations, a location that lends credence to the speculation that the aneurysms result from medial necrosis. The vast majority are asymptomatic and are found incidentally on arteriography for other indications. Such aneurysms should be repaired in women of childbearing age and in patients with renovascular hypertension or clinical symptoms.

References

1. Faught E, Trader SD, Hanna GR. Cerebral complications of angiography for transient ischemia and stroke: prediction of risk. Neurology (Minn) 1979; 29:4–15.
2. Eisenbert RL, Bank WO, Hedgcock MW. Neurologic complication of angiography in patients with critical stenosis of the carotid artery. Neurology (NY) 1980; 30:895.
3. Barnes RW. Hemodynamics for the vascular surgeon. Arch Surg 1980; 115:216.
4. Kistler JP, Ropper AH, Heros RC. Therapy of ischemic cerebral vascular disease due to atherothrombosis. N Engl J Med 1984; 311:27–34,100.
5. Dixon S, et al. Natural history of non-stenotic, asymptomatic ulcerative lesions of the carotid artery: a further analysis. Arch Surg 1982; 117:1493.
6. Fields WS, et al. Controlled trial of aspirin in cerebral ischemia. Stroke 1977; 8:301.
7. Fields WS, et al. Controlled trial of aspirin in cerebral ischemia. Part II: Surgical group. Stroke 1978; 9:309.
8. The Canadian Cooperative Study Group. A randomized trial of aspirin and sulfinpyrazone in threatened stroke. N Engl J Med 1978; 299:53.
9. North American Symptomatic Carotid Endarterectomy Trial Collaborators. Beneficial effect of carotid endarterectomy in symptomatic patients with high-grade carotid stenosis. N Engl J Med 1991;325:445–453.
10. European Carotid Surgery Trialists Collaborative Group. MRC European carotid surgery trial: interim results for symptomatic patients with severe (70–99%) or with mild (0–29%) carotid stenosis. Lancet 1991;337:1235–1243.
11. Fields WS, et al. Joint study of extracranial arterial occlusion. V: Progress report of prognosis following surgery or nonsurgical treatment for transient cerebral ischemic attacks and cervical carotid artery lesions. JAMA 1970; 211:1993–2003.
12. Rubin JR, et al. Carotid endarterectomy in a metropolitan community: the early results after 8535 operations. J Vasc Surg 1988; 7:256–260.

13. Moore WS. Carotid endarterectomy—is it safe in the community? J Vasc Surg 1986; 4:313.
14. Whittemore AD, et al. Routine electroencephalographic (EEG) monitoring during carotid endarterectomy. Ann Surg 1983; 197:707.
15. Moore WS, et al. Carotid endarterectomy: practice guidelines. Report of the ad hoc committee to the Joint Council of the Society for Vascular Surgery and the North American Chapter of the International Society for Cardiovascular Surgery. J Vasc Surg 1992;15:469–479.
16. Mohr JP, et al. The Harvard Cooperative Stroke Registry: a prospective registry. Neurology 1978; 28:754.
17. Roederer GO, et al. The natural history of carotid arterial disease in asymptomatic patients with cervical bruits. Stroke 1984; 15:605.
18. Ricotta JJ, et al. Use of computerized cerebral tomography in selection of patients for elective and urgent carotid endarterectomy. Ann Surg 1985;202:783–787.
19. Hobson RW, et al. Efficacy of carotid endarterectomy for asymptomatic carotid stenosis. N Engl J Med 1993; 328: 221–227.
20. Wylie EJ, Hein MF, Adams JE. Intracranial hemorrhage following surgical revascularization for treatment of acute strokes. J Neurosurg 1964;21:212.
21. Thompson JE, Austin DJ, Patman RD. Endarterectomy of the totally occluded carotid artery for stroke. Arch Surg 1967; 95:791–801.
22. Buonanno F, Toole JF. Management of patients with established ("completed") cerebral infarction. Stroke 1981; 12: 7–16.
23. Meyer FB, et al. Emergency carotid endarterectomy for patients with acute carotid occlusion and profound neurological deficits. Ann Surg 1985; 203:82.
24. Dosick SM, et al. Carotid endarterectomy in the stroke patient: computerized axial tomography to determine timing. J Vas Surg 1985; 2:214.
25. Goldstone J, Moore WS. Emergency carotid artery surgery in neurologically unstable patients. Arch Surg 1976; 111:1284.
26. Goldstone J, Moore WS. A new look at emergency carotid artery operations for the treatment of cerebrovascular insufficiency. Current concepts of cerebrovascular disease. Stroke 1978; 9:599.
27. Mentzer RM Jr, et al. Emergency carotid endarterectomy for fluctuating neurologic deficits. Surgery 1981; 89:60.
28. Whittemore AD, et al. Early carotid endarterectomy in patients with small, fixed neurologic deficits. J Vasc Surg 1984; 1:795.
29. Whittemore AD, Mannick JA. Surgical treatment of carotid disease in patients with neurologic deficits. J Vasc Surg 1987; 5:910.
30. Giordano JM, et al. Timing of carotid artery endarterectomy after stroke. J Vasc Surg 1985; 2:250.
31. Hafner CD, Evans WE. Carotid endarterectomy with local anaesthesia: results and advantages. J Vasc Surg 1988; 7:232-239.
32. Whittemore AD. Carotid endarterectomy—an alternative approach. Arch Surg 1980; 115:940.
33. Whittemore AD, et al. Routine electroencephalographic monitoring during carotid endarterectomy. Ann Surg 1983; 197:707.
34. Sundt TM, et al. Correlation of cerebral blood flow and electroencephalographic changes during carotid endarterectomy. Mayo Clin Proc 1981; 56(9):533.
35. Baker JD, et al. An evaluation of encephalographic monitoring for carotid study. Surgery 1975; 78(6):787.
36. Prioleau WH, Aiken AF, Hairston P. Carotid endarterectomy: neurologic complications as related to surgical techniques. Ann Surg 1977; 185(6):678–683.
37. Whitney DG, et al. Carotid artery surgery without a temporary indwelling shunt. Arch Surg 1980; 115(11):1393.
38. Baker WH, Dorner DB, Barnes RW. Carotid endarterectomy: is an indwelling shunt necessary? Surgery 1977; 82:321.
39. Imparato AM, et al. Cerebral protection in carotid surgery. Arch Surg 1982; 117:1073.
40. Curley S, Edwards WS, Jacob TP. Recurrent carotid stenosis after autologous tissue patching. J Vasc Surg 1987; 6:350.
41. Eikelboom BC, et al. Benefits of carotid patching: a randomized study. J Vasc Surg 1988; 7:240.
42 Dilley RB, Bernstein EF. A comparison of B-mode real-time imaging and arteriography in the intraoperative assessment of carotid endarterectomy. J Vasc Surg 1986; 4:457.
43. Bock RW, et al. The natural history of asymptomatic carotid artery disease. J Vasc Surg 1993; 17:160–171.
44. Vogt DP, et al. Brachiocephalic arterial reconstruction. Ann Surg 1982; 195:541.
45. Charcot JM. Sur la claudication intermittente observée dans un cas d'obliteration complete de l'une des artères iliaques primitives. Mem Soc Biol 1:225, 1858.
46. Leriche R, Morell A. The syndrome of thrombotic obliteration of the aortic bifurcation. Ann Surg 1948; 127:193.
47. Crane C. Atheroembolic embolism of lower extremities in arteriosclerosis. Arch Surg 1967; 94:96–101.
48. Karmody AM, et al. Blue toe syndrome. Arch Surg 1976; 111:1263.
49. Tapper SS, et al. Suprarenal aortic occlusion. J Vasc Surg 1993; 18:372–80.
50. Boyd AM. The natural course of arteriosclerosis of the lower extremities. Proc R Soc Med 1962; 55:591.
51. Imparato AM, et al. Intermittent claudication: its natural course. Surgery 1975; 78:795.
52. McAllister FF. The fate of patients with intermittent claudication managed non-operatively. Am J Surg 1976; 132:593.
53. Weinstein MH, Machleder HI. Sexual function after aortoiliac surgery. Ann Surg 1975; 181:787.
54. Gruntzig A. Die perkutane transluminale Rekanalisation chronischer Arterienverschlusse mit einer neuen Dilatationstechnik. Baden-Baden: G. Witzstrock Verlag, 1977.
55. van Andel GJ. Transluminal iliac angioplasty: long term results. Radiology 1980; 135:607.
56. Dotter CT. Transluminal angioplasty: a long view. Radiology 1980; 135:561.
57. Colapinto RF, Hannies-Jones EP, Johnston KW. Percutaneous transluminal dilatation and recanalization in the treatment of peripheral vascular disease. Radiology 1980; 135:583.
58. Johnston KW, et al. 5-year results of prospective study of percutaneous transluminal angioplasty. Ann Surg 1987; 206:403.
59. Brewster DC, Darling RC. Optimal methods of aortoiliac reconstruction. Surgery 1978; 84:739.
60. Szilagyi DE, et al. A thirty-year survey of reconstructive surgical treatment of aortoiliac occlusive disease. J Vasc Surg 1986; 3:421.
61. Crawford ES, et al. Aortoiliac occlusive disease: factors influencing survival and function following reconstructive operations over a twenty-five year period. Surgery 1981; 90:1055.
62. Malone JM, Moore WS, Goldstone J. The natural history of bilateral aortofemoral bypass grafts for ischemia of the lower extremities. Arch Surg 1975; 110:1300.
63. Morris GC Jr, et al. Surgical importance of profunda femoris artery. Arch Surg 1961; 82:32.
64. Vetto RM. The treatment of unilateral iliac artery obstruction

with a transabdominal, subcutaneous, femorofemoral graft. Surgery 1962; 52:342.

65. Plecha FR, Plecha FM. Femorofemoral bypass grafts: ten-year experience. J Vasc Surg 1984; 1:555.
66. Flanigan DP, et al. Hemodynamic and angiographic guidelines in selection of patients for femorofemoral bypass. Arch Surg 1978; 113:1257.
67. Mannick JA, Maini BS. Femoro-femoral grafting. Indications and late results. Am J Surg 1978; 136:190.
68. Dick LS, et al. A 12-year experience with femorofemoral crossover grafts. Arch Surg 1980; 115:1359.
69. Gold JP, et al. Femorofemoral bypass to relieve acute leg ischemia during intraaortic balloon pump cardiac support. J Vasc Surg 1986; 3:351.
70. Blaisdell FW, et al. Aorto-iliac substitution utilizing subcutaneous grafts. Ann Surg 1970; 172:775.
71. Mannick JA, Williams LE, Nabseth, DC. The late results of axillofemoral grafts. Surgery 1970; 68:1038.
72. LoGerfo FW, et al. A comparison of the late patency rates of axillobilateral femoral and axillounilateral femoral grafts. Surgery 1977; 81:33–40.
73. Eugene J, Goldstone J, Moore WS. Fifteen year experience with subcutaneous bypass grafts for lower extremity ischemia. Ann Surg 1977; 186:177.
74. Ray LI, et al. Axillofemoral bypass: a critical reappraisal of its role in the management of aortoiliac occlusive disease. Am J Surg 1979; 138:117.
75. Couch NP, et al. The iliac-origin arterial graft: a useful alternative for iliac occlusive disease. Surgery 1985; 97:83.
76. Kunlin J. Le traitement de l'arterite obliterante par la greffe veineuse. Arch Mal Coeur 1949; 42:371.
77. Maini BS, Mannick JA. Effect of arterial reconstruction on limb salvage. Arch Surg 1978; 113:1297–1304.
78. Kacoyanis GP, et al. Femoro-tibial and femoro-peroneal bypass vein grafts: a 15-year experience. Arch Surg 1981; 116:1529.
79. Whittemore AD, et al. Secondary femoro-popliteal reconstruction. Ann Surg 1981; 193:35–42.
80. Kaufman JL, et al. The fate of grafts to an isolated popliteal artery segment. Surgery 1982; 92:1027.
81. Fogle MA, et al. A comparison of in situ and reversed saphenous vein grafts for infrainguinal reconstruction. J Vasc Surg 1987; 5:46–52.
82. DeWeese JA, Rob CG. Autogenous venous grafts ten years later. Surgery 1977; 82:775.
83. Taylor Jr LM, Phinney ES, Porter JM. Present status of reversed vein bypass for lower extremity revascularization. J Vasc Surg 1986; 3:288.
84. Szilagyi DE, et al. Biologic fate of autogenous vein implants as arterial substitutes. Am Surg 1973; 178:232–246.
85. Brewster DC, et al. Factors affecting patency of femoropopliteal bypass grafts. Surg Gynecol Obstet 1983; 157:437.
86. Cohen JR, et al. Recognition and management of impending vein-graft failure. Arch Surg 1986; 121:758.
87. Belkin M, et al. Preferred strategies for secondary infrainguinal bypass surgery: lessons learned from 300 consecutive reoperations. Annual Meeting of the Society for Vascular Surgery, 1994.
88. Gardiner GA Jr, et al. Thrombolysis of occluded femoropopliteal grafts. AJR 1986; 147:621.
89. McNamara TO, Bomberger RA. Factors affecting initial and 6-month patency rates after intraarterial thrombolysis with high dose urokinase. Am J Surg 1986; 152:709.
90. Van Breda A, Katzen BT, Deutsch AS. Urokinase versus streptokinase in local thrombolysis. Radiology 1987; 165:109.
91. Graor RA, et al. Thrombolysis of peripheral arterial bypass grafts: surgical thrombectomy compared with thrombolysis. A preliminary report. J Vasc Surg 1988; 7:347–355.
92. Hall KV. The greater saphenous vein used in situ as an arterial shunt after extirpation of the vein valves. Surgery 1962; 51:492.
93. Leather RP, Powers SR, Karmody AM. A reappraisal of the in situ saphenous vein arterial bypass: its use in limb salvage. Surgery 1979; 86:453.
94. Leather RP, et al. Instrumental evolution of the valve incision method of in situ saphenous vein bypass. J Vasc Surg 1984; 1:113.
95. Campbell CD, Brooks DM, Bahnson HT. The use of expanded microporous polytetrafluoroethylene for limb salvage. A preliminary report. Surgery 1976; 79:485.
96. McAuley CE, Steed DL, Webster HW. Seven-year follow-up of expanded polytetrafluoroethylene (PTFE) femoropopliteal bypass grafts. Ann Surg 1984; 199:57–60.
97. Charlesworth PM, et al. The fate of polytetrafluoroethylene grafts in lower limb bypass surgery: a six-year follow-up. Br J Surg 1985; 72:896–899.
98. Veith FJ, et al. Six-year prospective multicenter randomized comparison of autologous saphenous vein and expanded polytetrafluoroethylene grafts in infrainguinal arterial reconstructions. J Vasc Surg 1986; 3:104.
99. Whittemore AD, et al. What is the proper role of polytetrafluoroethylene (PTFE) grafts in infrainguinal reconstruction? J Vasc Surg 1989; 10:299.
100. Kent KC, Whittemore AD, Mannick JA. Short-term and midterm results of an all autogenous tissue policy for infrainguinal reconstruction. J Vasc Surg 1989; 9:107.
101. Sos TA, et al. Percutaneous transluminal angioplasty in renovascular hypertension due to atheroma or fibromuscular hyperplasia. N Engl J Med 1983; 309:274.
102. Wylie EJ, Perloff DL, Stoney RJ. Autogenous tissue revascularization techniques in surgery for renovascular hypertension. Ann Surg 1969; 170:416.
103. Morris GC, et al. Late results of surgical treatment for renovascular hypertension. Surg Gynecol Obstet 1966; 122:1255.
104. Dean RM. Operative management of renovascular hypertension. In JJ Bergan, JST Yao, eds. Surgery of the Aorta and its Body Branches. New York: Grune & Stratton, 1979. Pp. 377–407.
105. Brewster DC, et al. Combined aortic and renal artery reconstruction. Am J Surg 1976; 131:457–463.
106. Dean RM, et al. Aortic and renal disease. Factors affecting the value of combined procedures. Ann Surg 1984; 200:336.
107. Stoney RJ, et al. Juxtarenal aortic atherosclerosis. Ann Surg 1984; 200:345–354.
108. Novick AC, et al. Splenorenal bypass in the treatment of stenosis of the renal artery. Surg Gynecol Obstet 1977; 144:891–898.
109. Moncure AC, et al. Use of the splenic and hepatic arteries for renal revascularization. J Vasc Surg 1986; 3:196–203.
110. Stoney RJ, Wylie EJ. Recognition and surgical management of visceral ischemic syndromes. Ann Surg 1966; 164:714–722.
111. Rapp JM, et al. Durability of endarterectomy and antegrade grafts in the treatment of chronic visceral ischemia. J Vasc Surg 1986; 3:799–806.
112. Hollier LH, et al. Surgical management of chronic intestinal ischemia: a reappraisal. Surgery 1981; 90:940.
113. Zelenock GB, et al. Splanchnic arteriosclerotic disease and intestinal angina. Arch Surg 1980; 115:497–501.
114. Matas R. Aneurysm of the abdominal aorta at its bifurcation into the common iliac arteries. Ann Surg 1940; 112:909.
115. Blakemore AM, King B. Electrothermic coagulation of aortic aneurysms. JAMA 1938; 111:1821.

116. Hicks GL, Rob C. Abdominal aortic aneurysm wiring: an alternative method. Am J Surg 1976; 131:664.
117. Lowenberg EL. Aneurysm of the abdominal aorta--report of two cases treated by "cutis grafting." Angiology 1950; 1:396–404.
118. DeBost C, Allary M, Oeconomos N. A propos de traitement des aneurysmes de l'aorte; ablation de l'aneurysme: retablissement de la continuite par graffe d'aorte conserve. Mem Acad Chir 1951; 77:381.
119. Voorhees AB, Jaretzky A, Blakemore AH. The use of tubes constructed from Vinyon-N cloth in bridging arterial deficits. Ann Surg 1952; 135:332.
120. DeBakey ME, et al. Aneurysm of the abdominal aorta; analysis of results of graft replacement therapy one to eleven years after operation. Ann Surg 1964; 160:622.
121. Voorhees AB Jr, McAllister FF. Long term results following resection of arteriosclerotic abdominal aortic aneurysms. Surg Gynecol Obstet 1963; 117:355.
122. Szilagyi DE, et al. Contribution of abdominal aortic aneurysmectomy to prolongation of life. Ann Surg 1966; 164:678.
123. May AG, et al. Surgical treatment of abdominal aortic aneurysms. Surgery 1968; 63: 711.
124. Johnston KW. Multicenter prospective study of nonruptured abdominal aortic aneurysm. Part II. Variables predicting morbidity and mortality. J Vasc Surg 1989; 9:437.
125. Crawford ES, et al. Aortic aneurysm: current status of surgical treatment. Surg Clin North Am 1979; 59:597–636.
126. Whittemore AD, et al. Aortic aneurysm repair: reduced operative mortality associated with maintenance of optimal cardiac performance. Ann Surg 1980; 192:414–421.
127. Golden MA, et al. Selective evaluation and management of coronary artery disease in patients undergoing repair of abdominal aortic aneurysm. Ann Surg 1990; 212:415–423.
128. Matas, R. Personal experience in vascular surgery. Ann Surg 1940; 112:802.
129. Javid M, et al. Complication of aortic aneurysm. Arch Surg 1962; 85:9650.
130. Creech O Jr. Endo-aneurysmorrhaphy and treatment of aortic aneurysms. Ann Surg 1966; 164:935.
131. Hertzer NR, et al. Routine coronary angiography prior to elective aortic reconstruction: results of selective myocardial revascularization in patients with peripheral vascular disease. Arch Surg 1979; 114:1336.
132. Brown OW, et al. Abdominal aortic aneurysm and coronary artery disease: a reassessment. Arch Surg 1981; 116:1484.
133. Hertzer NR, et al. Coronary artery disease in peripheral vascular patients. Ann Surg 1984; 199:223.
134. Crawford ES, et al. Infrarenal abdominal aortic aneurysms: factors influencing survival after operation performed over a 25-year period. Ann Surg 1981; 193:699–709.
135. Grindlinger GA, et al. Volume loading and vasodilators in abdominal aortic aneurysmectomy. Am J Surg 1980; 139:480.
136. Estes JE Jr. Abdominal aortic aneurysm: a study of one hundred and two cases. Circulation 1950; 2:258.
137. Szilagyi DE, Elliott JP, Smith RF. Clinical fate of the patient with asymptomatic abdominal aortic aneurysm and unfit for surgical treatment. Arch Surg 1972; 104:600.
138. Bernstein EF, Chan EL. Abdominal aortic aneurysm in high-risk patients. Ann Surg 1984; 200:255.
139. Hertzer NJ, Beven E. Ultrasound aortic measurement and elective aneurysmectomy. JAMA 1978; 240:1966.
140. Brewster DC, et al. Angiography in the management of aneurysms of the abdominal aorta. N Engl J Med 1975; 292:822.
141. Glickman MH, et al. Aortic aneurysm: to tube or not to tube. Surg 1982; 91:603.
142. Hiatt JCG, et al. Determinants of failure in the treatment of ruptured abdominal aortic aneurysm. Arch Surg 1984; 119:1264.
143. Shackleton CR, et al. Preoperative predictors of mortality risk in ruptured abdominal aortic aneurysm. J Vasc Surg 1987; 6:583.
144. Lowrie GM. Progress in the treatment of ruptured abdominal aortic aneurysm. World J Surg 1980; 4:653.
145. Karmody AM, et al. The current position of nonresective treatment of abdominal aortic aneurysm. Surgery 1983; 94:591.
146. Inahara T, et al. The contrary position to the non-resective treatment for abdominal aortic aneurysm. J Vasc Surg 1985; 2:42.
147. Crawford ES, et al. Progress in treatment of thoracoabdominal and abdominal aortic aneurysms involving celiac, superior mesenteric, and renal arteries. Ann Surg 1978; 188:404.
148. Crawford ES, et al. Thoracoabdominal aortic aneurysms: preoperative and intraoperative factors determining immediate and long-term results of operations in 605 patients. J Vasc Surg 1986; 3:389–404.
149. Cambria R et al. Recent experience with thoracoabdominal aneurysm repair. Arch Surg 1989; 124:620.
150. Szilagyi DE, Schwartz RL, Reddy DJ. Popliteal arterial aneurysms: the natural history and management. Arch Surg 1981; 116:724.
151. Anton GE, et al. Surgical management of popliteal aneurysms: trends in presentation, treatment, and results from 1952 to 1984. J Vasc Surg 1986; 3:125.
152. Reilly MK, Abbott WM, Darling RC. Aggressive surgical management of popliteal artery aneurysms. Am J Surg 1983; 145:498–502.
153. Graham LM, et al. Clinical significance of arteriosclerotic femoral artery aneurysms. Arch Surg 1980; 115:502.
154. Trastek VF, et al. Splenic artery aneurysms. Surgery 1982; 91:694.
155. Trastek VF, Pairolero PC, Bernatz PE. Splenic artery aneurysms. World J Surg 1985; 9:378.
156. Mathisen DJ, Athanasouhs CA, Malt RA. Preservation of arterial flow to the liver: goal in treatment of extrahepatic and post-traumatic intrahepatic aneurysms of the hepatic artery. Ann Surg 1982; 196:400.
157. Graham LM, et al. Celiac artery aneurysms: historic (1745–1949) versus contemporary (1950–1984) differences in etiology and clinical importance. J Vasc Surg 1985; 2:757.
158. Stanley JC, Thompson NW, Fry WJ. Splanchnic artery aneurysms. Arch Surg 1970; 101:689.
159. Graham JM, McCollum CH, DeBakey ME. Aneurysms of the splanchnic arteries. Am J Surg 1980; 140:797–801.
160. Stanley JC, et al. Renal artery aneurysms. Arch Surg 1975; 110:1327-1333.
161. Tham G, et al. Renal artery aneurysms. Ann Surg 1983; 197:348.

Assessment and Reduction of Cardiac Risk in Peripheral Vascular Surgery

Khether E. Raby

Surgery of carotid, aortic, and infrainguinal arteries is unique from other noncardiac surgery with respect to cardiac risk. The same disease process that accounts for peripheral arterial disease, atherosclerosis, also accounts for a high prevalence of coronary artery disease [1–4]. Patients with peripheral arterial disease also have a disproportionate prevalence of comorbidities such as older age, smoking, diabetes, and renal failure, which together conspire to make perioperative morbidity and mortality especially high [3]. As much as 50 percent of that morbidity and mortality is thought to be related to coronary artery disease and more specifically myocardial ischemia [1–5]. Patients with peripheral arterial disease frequently are sedentary due to claudication, prior stroke, associated lung or joint disease and hence do not manifest symptoms of myocardial ischemia that suggest higher risk. In fact, peripheral arterial surgery often represents their first and most comprehensive "stress test." Finally, factors such as pain perception, increased basal catecholamine levels, blood loss, or a hyperthrombotic state also may contribute to the unmasking of myocardial ischemia for the first time in the perioperative period [6–9].

For those same reasons, the long-term cardiac risk in patients with peripheral arterial disease is probably underevaluated when compared with other patients with coronary artery disease. Since the long-term cardiac risk of patients with peripheral arterial disease is also known to be high, preoperative risk assessment is especially important to identify patients whose short- and long-term prognoses may benefit from further interventions [1,5].

Despite the high cardiac risk involved, perioperative risk of peripheral arterial surgery appears to be decreasing [1–4,10–13]. Numerous modern trials tracking perioperative mortality and morbidity have shown a striking decrease in risk when compared with trials of a decade ago (Fig. 30-1) [1–4,10–13]. This pattern is particularly notable in patients undergoing abdominal aortic aneurysm repair, which not long ago was considered the highest-risk peripheral vascular procedure [10,12]. Reasons for this trend most likely include the routine use of perioperative risk assessment for patient selection, the proliferation of noninvasive cardiac testing, improved surgical and anesthesia techniques, treatment of myocardial ischemia, and better monitoring strategies in the perioperative period. While no definitive studies have been performed that validate a unified and multidisciplinary risk-reduction approach, it is clear that in the current era higher-risk patients are undergoing peripheral arterial surgery safely [10–12]. This chapter summarizes the many lessons learned in perioperative risk assessment and examines the treatment strategies available for the reduction of risk in patients undergoing peripheral arterial surgery.

Preoperative Clinical Evaluation

It has been said that the majority of all diagnoses can be made by history alone [14,15]—patients with peripheral arterial disease are no exception. Numerous retrospective and prospective trials have identified the following clinical markers from the history and the physical examination that are independent predictors of risk in peripheral arterial surgery.

1. **Age.** Since the 1960s, aging has been recognized as an independent risk factor for perioperative morbidity [16–19]. In particular, multiple studies have documented that age, independent of associated risk factors such as the prevalence of coronary artery disease, hypertension, and diabetes, predicts adverse perioperative cardiac events [16,19]. Some studies have found that patients age 65 and greater have more than a 20-fold increase in perioperative death when compared to younger counterparts [18].
2. **Diabetes.** Several features of diabetes mellitus make this systemic illness a strong risk factor of perioperative cardiac morbidity, including poor healing, the risk of perioperative infection, and the high prevalence of diffuse atherosclerosis and asymptomatic myocardial ischemia [20,21]. Several investigators have established the association of diabetes with adverse cardiac events in vascular surgery patients [19,22]. One well-supported strategy is that **all** diabetics with peripheral vascular disease who are about to undergo surgery, even in the absence of overt manifestations of coronary artery disease, should undergo noninvasive testing prior to clearance before surgery [19].
3. **Type of surgery.** Peripheral vascular surgery has always been viewed as high-risk surgery compared with other general surgery [2,16,19,23,24]. In particular, surgery involving the peritoneal space, including all aortic reconstructive surgery, has long been recognized as the highest risk of vascular surgery procedures [2,24]. Paradoxically, there is evidence in the literature that abdominal aortic aneurysm repair in particular is becoming a lower-risk procedure [10,12]. This phenomenon can be attributed in part to the recognition of risk associated with aortic surgery and the appropriate measures routinely taken to minimize such risk, including meticulous preoperative assessment, longer intensive-care stays, careful monitoring of cardiac hemodynamics, and sophisticated postoperative analgesia regimens [10]. The strategy of risk management in patients undergoing aortic surgery has proved so efficient, it can now be argued that infrainguinal surgery is associated with a higher cardiac risk.
4. **History of coronary artery disease.** In the landmark series from the Cleveland Clinic, Hertzer and colleagues

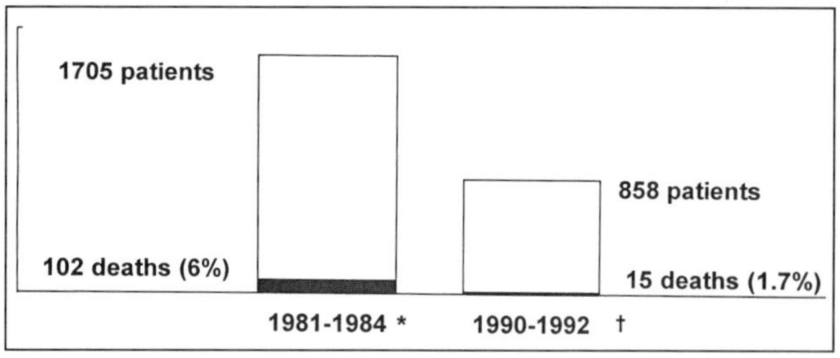

Fig. 30-1. Pooled cardiac mortality rates after vascular surgery comparing representative studies published 1981–1984 with representative studies 1991–1992. (1981–1984 studies include Jamieson, Circulation 1982; Hertzer, Surgery 1981; Hollier, J Vasc Surg 1984. 1990–1992 studies include Golden, Ann Surg 1990; Donaldson, Surgery 1991; Buul, J Vasc Surg 1992.)

Table 30-1. Cardiac risk index

Variable	Points
Coronary artery disease (angina/MI)	5–10
Congestive heart failure	10–20
Valvular heart disease (aortic stenosis)	20
Arrhythmia	5
Poor general condition	5
Age > 70 years	5
Emergency surgery	10

Source: Modified from AS Detsky et al. Predicting cardiac complications in patients undergoing cardiac surgery. J Gen Intern Med 1986; 141:1631–1634.

found that close to 40 percent of patients with peripheral arterial disease have anatomically significant coronary artery disease, and the vast majority of postoperative cardiac events occurred in this patient subgroup [25]. Not surprisingly, a recent history of myocardial infarction, angina pectoris, congestive heart failure, or ventricular arrhythmias has been shown to independently predict risk of perioperative cardiac morbidity [19,22,24,26–28]. In the 1970s, myocardial infarction occurring within 6 months of elective surgery was viewed as a significant enough risk factor to cause postponement of elective surgery [24]. More recently, patients who have had myocardial infarctions within 2–3 months of elective vascular surgery have been safely taken through surgery, again reflecting the impact of cardiac risk assessment and management in a well-identified subgroup [27]. Likewise, the history of symptomatic ischemic heart disease, particularly New York Heart Association class III or IV angina pectoris or heart failure, has also been shown to predict perioperative cardiac risk [26]. It should be noted, however, that the absence of such symptoms in sedentary vascular surgery patients (e.g., those who cannot walk more than one or two city blocks) is not adequate in ruling out the presence of significant myocardial ischemia [29]. Finally, while ventricular ectopy remains a controversial management issue in all patients with coronary artery disease, at least two independent studies have shown that the presence of ventricular ectopy on baseline 12 lead electrocardiograms were independent predictors of cardiac risk in vascular surgery patients [19,24].

5. **Valvular heart disease.** Significant aortic stenosis long has been recognized as an important risk factor for perioperative morbidity in all noncardiac surgery [24]. Less definitive data are available for aortic insufficiency, mitral valve disease, and right-sided valvular lesions. Because most significant valvular heart diseases cause symptoms of chest pain or congestive heart failure, their contribution to risk likely is reflected in the severity of symptoms and should be approached in the same way as symptomatic coronary artery disease.
6. **Hypertension and left ventricular hypertrophy.** Well-established evidence links hypertension and the resultant cardiac end-organ damage (left ventricular hypertrophy) with long-term cardiac risk [30]. The case for perioperative cardiac risk in vascular surgery patients is less well established. One recent study linked the presence of left ventricular hypertrophy on electrocardiograms with a high prevalence of postoperative myocardial ischemia but not directly with adverse postoperative cardiac events [22].

Since each of the markers is a significant predictor of risk, it should follow that the more markers an individual patient has, the higher the perioperative cardiac risk. That logic is best represented by the multiple attempts to quantify the predictive ability of a clinical evaluation via the development of risk indices [16,24,26,31]. The most well known of these indices is the time-honored cardiac risk index developed by Goldman and colleagues in the 1970s, which identified many of the factors listed here as well as other noncardiac issues that were then validated by multivariate analysis as important cumulative predictors of cardiac risk. The risk index developed a scoring system that weighted individual risk factors by significance, and a total score was used to create four distinct risk categories for general-surgery patients [16,24]. The cardiac risk index has been repeatedly validated and modified to be applicable to a population with a higher prevalence of coronary artery disease, such as patients undergoing peripheral arterial surgery (Table 30-1) [26]. Cardiac risk indices are important in confirming the effectiveness of a history, a physical examination, and a baseline electrocardiogram in identifying risk in a vast majority of patients, including those undergoing peripheral arterial surgery. However, risk indices tend to assume that cardiac symptoms are an accurate reflection of the activity of coronary artery disease. Unfortunately, in patients with disabling symptoms from claudication or prior stroke, the absence of symptomatic angina or congestive heart failure is not reassuring [29,31]. Moreover, while several reports underscored that cardiac risk indices (and by inference the clinical evaluation) are extremely useful in identifying high-risk patients, those identified at intermediate and low risk by clinical criteria alone may, in fact, still be at significant risk for perioperative cardiac morbidity [31,32].

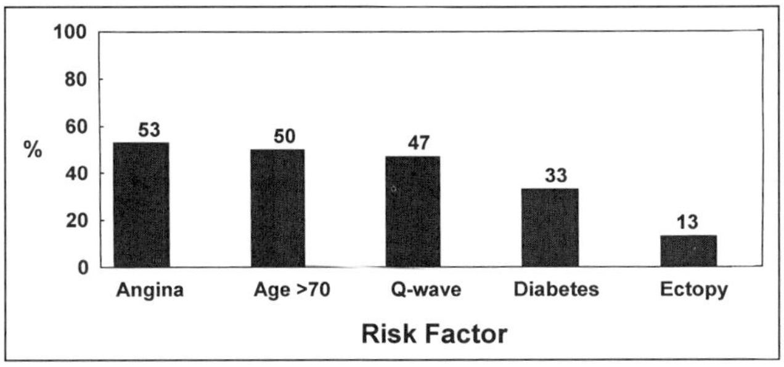

Fig. 30-2. Independent risk factors for postoperative myocardial ischemic events as identified by Eagle and colleagues. These risk factors serve as an excellent summary of the usefulness of clinical evaluation and are widely employed as a good starting point for cardiac risk assessment. (From KA Eagle et al. Combining clinical and thallium data optimizes preoperative assessment of cardiac risk from major vascular surgery. Ann Intern Med 1989; 110:859–866.)

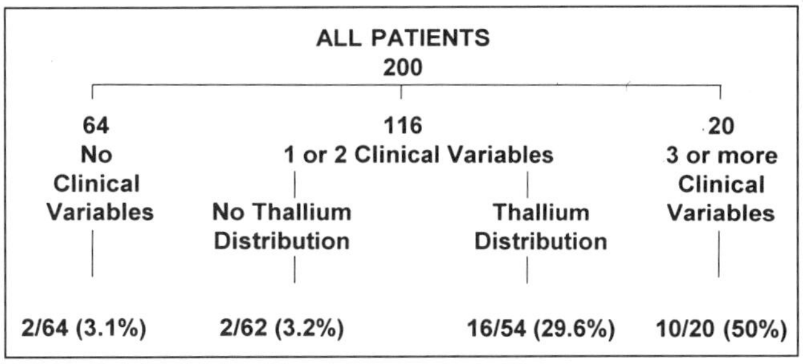

Fig. 30-3. A flow diagram summarizing the predictive value of dipyridamole thallium imaging for assessing risk of cardiac events after vascular surgery. Two hundred patients referred for dipyridamole thallium imaging. The 64 patients with no clinical variables identified in Fig. 30-2 had the lowest event rate. Twenty patients with three or more variables had the highest event rate. Those patients with one or two clinical variables had a median event rate and were most likely to benefit from the presence of abnormal thallium redistribution study. (Adapted from KA Eagle et al. Combining clinical and thallium data optimizes preoperative assessment of cardiac risk from major vascular surgery. Ann Intern Med 1989; 110:859–866.)

Eagle and colleagues have persuasively used the insights of these observations to propose a role for noninvasive cardiac testing as an adjunct to a clinical evaluation. The group identified five risk factors: advanced age, diabetes, myocardial infarction, ventricular ectopy on electrocardiography, and a history of angina pectoris or congestive heart failure as initial stratifiers of risk in patients undergoing peripheral arterial surgery (Fig. 30-2). Patients with none of these risk factors are at extremely low cardiac risk, and further noninvasive testing, even if abnormal, would not substantially affect risk assessment. Furthermore, patients who have three or more of the clinical markers are at such high risk a priori, that a normal noninvasive cardiac test would not substantially reduce the risk predicted. Finally, patients who are identified at intermediate risk (one or two markers) are most likely to benefit from further noninvasive cardiac testing (Fig. 30-3). Hence, the majority of patients have their risk correctly identified by clinical evaluation alone, and a substantial minority is then effectively identified for further testing and risk stratification [19]. Eagle's clinical markers were strikingly similar to those identified by risk indices in the 1970s and early 1980s (Table 30-1) [16,24,26], and the approach of noncardiac testing after clinical evaluation has been validated by an independent set of consecutive vascular surgery patients undergoing Holter monitoring for asymptomatic myocardial ischemia detection [33].

For practical purposes, Eagle's criteria have been widely recognized as an excellent starting point for the evaluation of preoperative risk among vascular surgery patients [19,29,33]. Since a substantial number of patients fall into the category of intermediate risk, extensive research has gone into identifying optimal noninvasive cardiac tests that might be effective in further estimating cardiac risk.

Noninvasive Cardiac Testing

EXERCISE TESTING

Treadmill exercise testing has long been established as an important method of assessing long-term risk in patients with coronary artery disease [34,35]. As a general rule, noninvasive cardiac tests that predict long-term risks also are useful for perioperative risk assessment. In the early 1980s, Cutler and colleagues showed that treadmill exercise testing was a useful technique in assessing preoperative risk in patients undergoing vascular surgery. While a positive exercise test predicted risk, a discrete measure of work load (in this case inability to reach 75% of maximal predicted heart rate), was also a predictor of perioperative risk [36]. Those observations have been confirmed independently by Gerson *et al.* in the mid-1980s [37] and more recently in an exclusive series of vascular surgery patients by McPhail and colleagues [38]. In all three studies, the theme of work load as a powerful predictor of risk was confirmed. McPhail found that the inability to reach 85% of maximal predicted heart rate was the strongest predictor of perioperative risk (Fig. 30-4) [38].

Investigators with extensive experience with treadmill exercise testing support the argument that peripheral arterial disease is not a contraindication to exercise testing. In a consecutive series of 176 patients who had peripheral vascular disease at Brigham and Women's Hospital in the late 1980s, almost 50 percent of all patients were judged able to exercise [33]. Patients with carotid stenosis or abdominal aortic aneurysms who do not have coincidental claudication often are able to exercise adequately. There is a relative contraindication to exercise in patients with large abdominal aortic aneurysms, because the hypertensive response that accompanies exercise may increase the risk of aneurysm rupture, although reports of that complication are extremely rare [39]. Even patients with lower-extremity disease that present for elective revascularization surgery sometimes can perform treadmill exercise testing. Some centers have developed modified protocols that employ more gradual and more frequent changes in treadmill speed and elevation, thereby maximizing the exercise capacity of disabled patients [40]. In addition, arm ergometry exercise has been successfully used in pre-

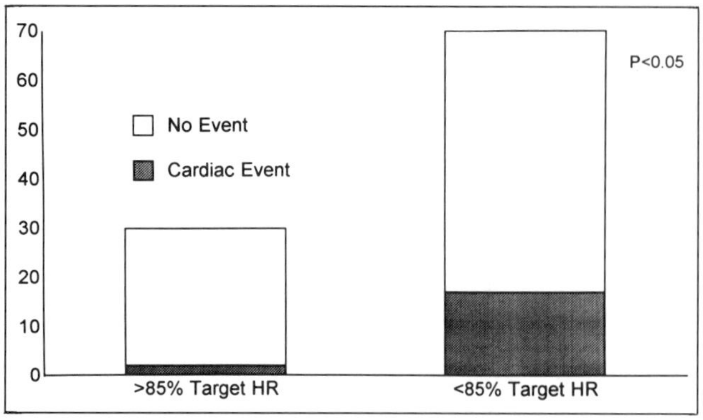

Fig. 30-4. Summary of the usefulness of treadmill exercise testing to predict risk of vascular surgery. Patients who achieved greater than 85 percent of target rate had a very low cardiac event rate. By contrast, patients who achieved less than 85 percent of target heart rate had a higher cardiac event rate. This study illustrates the importance of work load as a superior predictor of cardiac risk to ischemia on exercise testing (Adapted from N McPhail et al. The use of preoperative exercise testing to predict cardiac complications after arterial reconstruction. J Vasc Surg 1988; 7:60–68.)

operative risk assessment in vascular-surgery patients. The latter option, however, often is less standardized and less widely used than treadmill exercise testing [41,42].

All these observations suggest that exercise testing is underutilized in vascular-surgery patients. Since convincing evidence exists that exercise capacity is a good predictor of perioperative and long-term outcome, exercise testing should be the first option considered for preoperative cardiac risk assessment in those patients requiring noninvasive testing. That being said, a disadvantage of exercise testing is that a significant portion of vascular surgery patients are unable to reach 70–85 percent of their target heart rates because of claudication and not because of cardiac limitations. In those patients, exercise testing probably is not a useful option. In addition, many patients with peripheral vascular disease have baseline electrocardiographic abnormalities or are on digoxin, making exercise-induced electrocardiographic changes difficult to interpret with certainty and decreasing the positive predictive value of the test [43]. The addition of radionuclide imaging agents such as thallium or sestamibi circumvents that problem but adds to the complexity and expense of the test [44].

DIPYRIDAMOLE THALLIUM IMAGING FOR ISCHEMIA

This technique was developed in the mid-1980s in response to the need for a definitive preoperative noninvasive cardiac test in vascular-surgery patients who are unable to exercise. Intravenous dipyridamole causes significant vasodilation in normal coronary vessels and, to a lesser extent, in atherosclerotic vessels. This results in preferentially increased flow in vascular beds with normal arteries, and a relative steal syndrome in vascular beds with coronary stenoses. Hence, dipyridamole mimics the effect of exercise on both normal and stenotic coronary arteries. Simultaneous myocardial imaging with thallium or sestamibi (most recently modified by single photon emission computed tomography, or SPECT) demonstrates a lack of radionuclide distribution in regions supplied by stenotic coronary arteries, or defect. This defect is unchanged (fixed) on subsequent rest images if the underlying myocardium has undergone infarction. If, on the other hand, the myocardium is ischemic, the defect reperfuses or disappears on rest images. Dipyridamole radionuclide imaging can be analyzed for the number and size of fixed or reperfused defects, which correspond to coronary anatomy and inducible ischemia [45,46].

Table 30-2. Use of dipyridamole-thallium to predict cardiac events: study summaries

	# Points	Prevalence of defects	Relative risk
Eagle et al. [19]	200	41%	7
Leppo et al. [48]	89	47%	16
Lane et al. [54]	101	70%	4
Mangano et al. [55]	60	37%	1
Baron et al. [18]	457	35%	1

Most studies of dipyridamole thallium imaging have found that redistribution defects are associated with perioperative cardiac risk in vascular-surgery patients [47–50]. Others have found that the combination of fixed and reperfused defects were more predictive than reperfused defects alone, both for perioperative and long-term risk (Table 30-2) [49,50,51]. Recently, advances in the quantitation of dipyridamole thallium imaging has been shown to improve the predicted accuracy of the technique, although this quantitative analysis is not yet widely available [51,52].

One feature of all early dipyridamole thallium data is that patients studied were often referred for the specific purpose of preoperative risk assessment and therefore preselected for higher risk [47–53]. Most studies provided the results of the test to the managing clinicians, who were therefore unblinded [47–54]. In two recent series using dipyridamole thallium imaging for preoperative risk assessment, only consecutive nonselected patients were enrolled, and dipyridamole thallium imaging was found **not** to be a useful predictor of risk in that setting (see Table 30-2) [18,55]. The discrepancy underscores that no noninvasive cardiac test, including dipyridamole thallium imaging, is useful when used as a screening test for **all** patients undergoing vascular surgery, but testing may be very useful when targeted at only those patients whose clinical risk assessment requires further information.

Among the disadvantages of dipyridamole thallium imaging is expense and technical complexity. Dipyridamole is contraindicated in patients with severe bronchospasm and those on theophylline and caffeine preparations [45,46]. Hypotension induced by intravenous dipyridamole may be hazardous in patients with critical carotid stenoses. Some centers have replaced dipyridamole with adenosine or dobutamine as the vasodilator agent [56,57], with promising preliminary results. Despite disadvantages, a large volume of data supports the selective use of dipyridamole thallium imaging to predict preoperative and long-term cardiac risk in patients who cannot exercise and whose risk is not clearly identified by clinical evaluation alone [19,29].

ASSESSMENT OF LEFT-VENTRICULAR EJECTION FRACTION

The ejection fraction is an important prognostic predictor of long-term cardiac risk in patients with coronary artery disease [58], but its role in the perioperative assessment of risk in vascular-surgery patients remains controversial. Ejection fraction was thought to be an especially important factor in patients undergoing aortic reconstruction surgery. Specifically, Pasternack and colleagues found that the combination of low ejection fraction and aortic cross-clamping was more likely to cause significant cardiac morbidity postoperatively. By contrast, patients with preserved ejection fraction (≥55%) suffered little change through aortic surgery [59]. More recent studies, however, have refuted the predictive accuracy of ejection fraction in the perioperative setting. Newer data show that even patients with ejection fractions in the 30-percent range can safely undergo aortic reconstructive surgery [60,61]. The controversy may be explained in part by the proliferation of perioperative pulmonary-artery monitoring and sophisticated anesthesia techniques that have made surgery in patients with reduced ejection fraction safer. Comparative studies of ejection-fraction assessment and dipyridamole thallium imaging have demonstrated that dipyridamole thallium is superior in selected vascular-surgery patients, suggesting that the presence of myocardial ischemia is a more important predictor of risk in baseline ventricular function [62,63].

Nevertheless, the assessment of ejection fraction still may have a role in the perioperative assessment of risk. For example, patients who have myocardial ischemia documented by treadmill testing, dipyridamole thallium, or other techniques and who have normal left-ventricular ejection fractions may well be patients whose risk is manageable with medical therapy in the perioperative setting. By contrast, patients with documented myocardial ischemia and depressed ejection fraction not only have higher perioperative risk but represent a subgroup of patients with coronary artery disease whose risk can better be addressed with coronary revascularization therapy *a priori*. This was an important finding of the Coronary Artery Surgery Study (CASS) and appears to apply regardless of symptoms [64]. Some patients with especially low ejection fractions, with or without myocardial ischemia, have a poor long-term prognosis anyway and hence are not candidates for elective vascular surgery.

STRESS ECHOCARDIOGRAPHIC IMAGING

Studies that examine the value of ejection fraction in predicting perioperative risk have relied largely on radionuclide imaging of the left ventricle [59–63]. Few data are available on the value of transthoracic echocardiography, an excellent method for assessing ejection fraction in many settings. One promising advance has been the combined assessment of myocardial ischemia and ventricular function via the use of echocardiography in the setting of a stress agent. Dipyridamole has been used in conjunction with echocardiography for predicting cardiac risk in vascular-surgery patients, and preliminary data are promising [65]. More extensive data are available on dobutamine stress echocardiography. In one study, 136 patients who were unable to exercise underwent dobutamine stress echocardiography. The data were not available for clinical decision making, hence, clinicians who manage the patients were blinded. The only complication was one episode of reversible ventricular fibrillation induced by dobutamine. One hundred thirty-one patients had studies that were acceptable for analysis, and 35 had new or worsening wall-motion abnormalities under stress. All 15 cardiac events occurred in the patients who had wall-motion abnormalities induced. Most important, the absence of inducible wall-motion abnormalities provided an excellent negative predictive value (Table 30-3) [66]. Dobutamine stress echocardiography combines the advantages of tests that induce myocardial ischemia, such as treadmill exercise and dipyridamole thallium, with an assessment of ejection fraction. The expense of the study, the need for extensive expertise to interpret stress images, and the risk of potentially lethal arrhythmias have limited its use thus far [66–68].

Table 30-3. Cardiac risk assessment using dobutamine stress test

	Odds ratio
> 70 years	2.3
History of angina	5.1
History of infarction	4.0
Diabetes	3.5
WMA at rest	2.9
NWMA during test	72

Source: From D. Poldermans et al. Dobutamine stress echocardiography for assessment of cardiac risk before noncardiac surgery. Am J Cardiol 1991; 68:976–977.

HOLTER MONITORING FOR ASYMPTOMATIC ISCHEMIA

Ambulatory electrocardiographic (Holter) monitoring for asymptomatic myocardial ischemia is another modality for measuring the activity of coronary artery disease. ST depression on continuous ECG recording is reliable, reproducible, and a strong marker of myocardial ischemia [69–71] and predicts cardiac risk in a variety of settings [33,72–74]. Prior studies on silent myocardial ischemia have suggested that such episodes occur at heart rates far below those encountered during stress testing, thus suggesting that the technique may be useful in patients who are unable to undergo exercise to high work loads [71]. Several independent groups have shown that preoperative Holter monitoring for myocardial ischemia was predictive of perioperative cardiac risk in vascular-surgery patients (Table 30-4) [33,75–77]. In particular, the absence of ischemia carried a strong negative predictive value (Table 30-5) [33]. A recent report from the study of the Perioperative Ischemia Research Group (see Table 30-4 [78]) found preoperative ischemia detected by Holter

Table 30-4. Preoperative ischemia predicts cardiac events: study summaries

	Number points	Prevalence of ischemia (%)	Relative risk
Raby et al. [33]	176	18	32
Mangano et al. [78]	474	18	2
Fleisher et al. [76]	56	21	6
Pasternack et al. [75]	200	40	18

Table 30-5. Preoperative ischemia: correlation with postoperative cardiac events

	Ischemia n = 32 (18%)	No ischemia n = 144 (82%)
Cardiac event	38	1
No event	63	99

Source: KE Raby et al. Correlation between preoperative ischemia and major cardiac events after peripheral vascular surgery. N Engl J Med 1989; 321:1296–1300.

monitoring was a less useful risk predictor than postoperative ischemia [78]. Few data comparing Holter monitoring and other noninvasive tests are available. Small studies comparing Holter monitoring with dipyridamole echocardiography and dipyridamole thallium imaging have shown comparable risk prediction [79–81]. Since stress-radionuclide imaging and Holter monitoring have low positive predictive values, the combination of the two tests may increase the predictive value sufficiently to make for better risk assessment [81].

Holter monitoring for asymptomatic ischemia is the least expensive of the noninvasive tests and is technically simple to apply. However, it has similar disadvantages to exercise testing. Abnormal baseline EKGs, including left-bundle-branch block, left ventricular hypertrophy with strain pattern, and other ST-T changes (including those associated with digoxin), decrease the positive predictive value [43].

Treatment Options for High Risk Patients

It is clear that clinical evaluation and judicious use of noninvasive cardiac testing preoperatively correctly identify the risk in the vast majority of patients undergoing vascular surgery. For the most part, cardiac risk appears related to the prevalence of myocardial ischemia. Preoperative assessment of risk as outlined here is ultimately justified **only** if it triggers treatment strategies that decrease myocardial ischemia and reduces perioperative cardiac events.

CORONARY REVASCULARIZATION

For many years, investigators have argued that coronary revascularization therapy is the only viable alternative to decreasing cardiac risk in the vascular-surgery patient population [82–85]. Hertzer and colleagues showed that vascular-surgery patients who had undergone coronary artery bypass grafting had an extremely low risk after vascular surgery, whereas patients with coronary artery disease who had not undergone revascularization had a substantially higher risk after vascular surgery [2,5,24,82]. Those and other data were used to argue that coronary angiography and revascularization should be a uniform strategy in patients undergoing peripheral vascular surgery [82–85]. That strategy has proved impractical, since it exposes a majority of patients with peripheral vascular disease to the substantial risk of coronary angiography and coronary revascularization when it is clear that the overall preoperative risk is low. Since better clinical evaluation and noninvasive cardiac testing have made it easier to identify patients at highest risk from myocardial ischemia, some now advocate that patients undergoing vascular surgery who have "positive" preoperative noninvasive cardiac tests should undergo coronary angiography and revascularization [82–85]. Stated differently, peripheral vascular surgery and a positive noninvasive cardiac test are in and of themselves an indication for **prophylactic coronary revascularization therapy.** This line of thinking is supported by several uncontrolled trials that reported a low overall cardiac mortality after vascular surgery in patients who have had prior coronary revascularization [82–85]. Perhaps the most comprehensive of those trials was reported by Foster and colleagues, whose data are derived from 1,600 patients in the CASS registry who underwent noncardiac surgery. The investigators identified three groups of patients: (1) those without significant coronary disease, (2) those with coronary disease who had coronary bypass grafting prior to noncardiac surgery, and (3) those with coronary artery disease that was anatomically significant but who did not undergo bypass grafting prior to noncardiac surgery. The study showed that patients in group 3 experienced a higher mortality (2.4%) after noncardiac surgery than patients in groups 1 or 2 (Table 30-6) [83]. Modern data reported on smaller groups of vascular-surgery patients who had undergone prior coronary artery bypass grafting show mortality rates comparable to patients undergoing vascular surgery who have no evidence of coronary artery disease, while patients without prior coronary artery bypass grafting have post-vascular-surgery mortality rates ranging from 2–5 percent [84,85].

All the studies that address this issue, however, suffer from fundamental bias. Each trial cited identified patients who underwent coronary artery bypass grafting for well-established indications, such as symptomatic disease uncontrolled by medical therapy and persistent ischemia with compromised left-ventricular function. No large trial to date has identified patients undergoing vascular surgery who had **prophylactic revascularization therapy,** as is being advocated [82–85]. Widening the indication for coronary revascularization therapy to include planned peripheral vascular surgery may introduce a population of patients whose risk of coronary revascularization may be substantially worse [86–88]. More important, few of the large trials cited include the morbidity and mortality inherent to coronary revascularization therapy in the ultimate interpretation of their data and conclusions [86–88]. Some trials cited identified patients after they survived

Table 30-6. Cardiac risk after noncardiac surgery: CASS registry

Variable	No CAD	CAD/CABG	CAD/no CABG	P-value
Death	0.5%	0.9%	2.4%	<0.03
MI	0%	0.7%	1.1%	NS
Chest pain	4.5%	5.1%	8.7%	<0.01

Key: CAD = coronary artery disease; CABG = coronary artery bypass graft.
Source: ED Foster. Risk of non-cardiac operations in patients with defined coronary disease: the Coronary Artery Surgery (CASS) Registry experience. Ann Thorac Surg 1986; 41:42–48.

coronary artery bypass grafting without major sequelae. Hence, the process selected out candidates for vascular surgery who died or suffered significant morbidity in the course of coronary revascularization, thereby eliminating the highest-risk vascular-surgery patients [86–88]. Data available on the risk of coronary artery bypass grafting in patients with peripheral vascular disease suggest that that patient population is at especially high risk for morbidity and mortality from coronary revascularization [86–88]. Estimates of mortality from coronary bypass grafting in patients with peripheral vascular disease range from 5 to 17 percent, depending on the trial and the age of the patients [86–88]. Hence, in 1994, a patient with an abdominal aortic aneurysm who had no indication for coronary bypass grafting other than impending vascular surgery and an abnormal noninvasive cardiac test, if subjected to prophylactic coronary bypass surgery, would be exposed to about a 5-percent mortality risk prior to vascular surgery. Undergoing subsequent vascular surgery would then make the cumulative mortality risk about 6

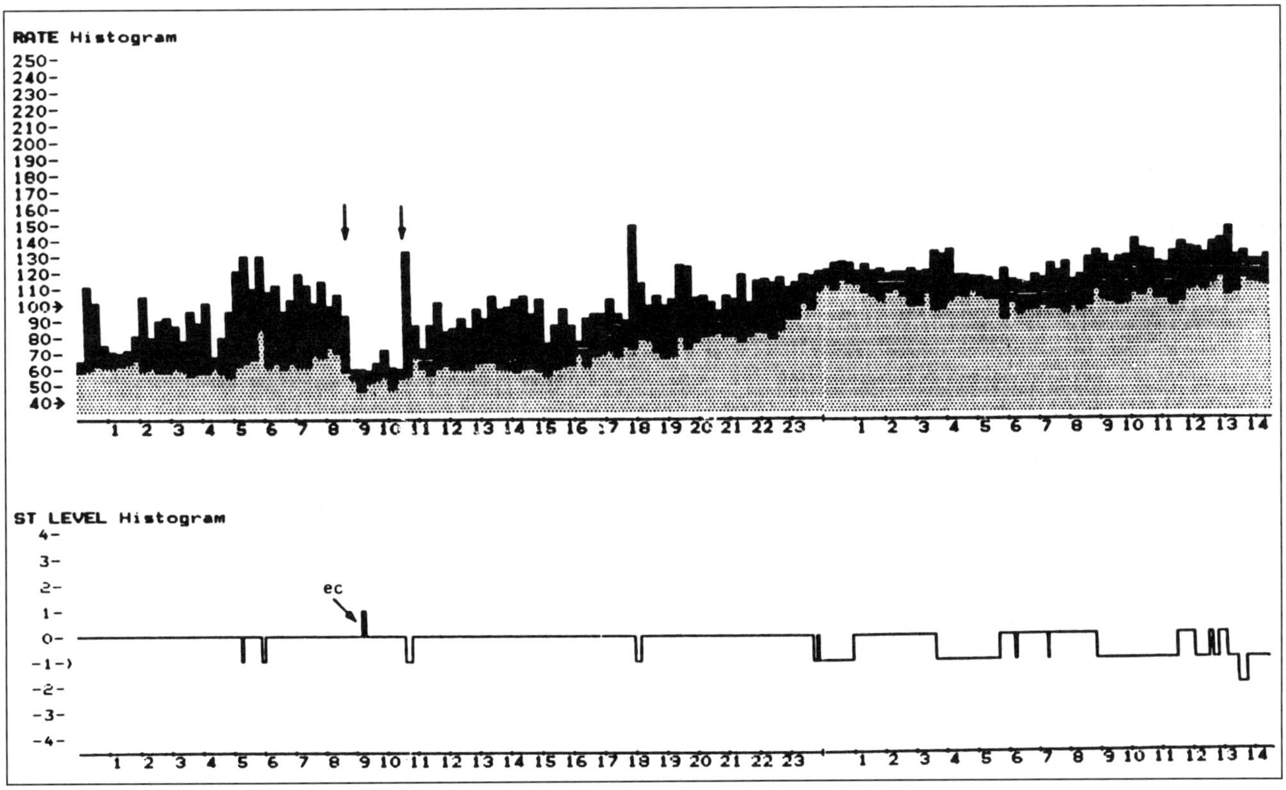

Fig. 30-5. Heart-rate and ST-level histogram from a patient undergoing general anesthesia. The record begins at midnight on the day of surgery and ends at 2 p.m. on postoperative day 1. Duration of anesthesia is indicated by the *arrows.* The *black bars* indicate maximum and minimum heart rates for each 15-minute time interval. The *stippled area* is the area under the minimum heart rate for computer integration purposes. EC-spurious ST elevation caused by electrocautery interference. Note that the heart rate is strictly controlled intraoperatively but rises gradually in the postoperative period and is accompanied by a higher prevalence of ischemia. (Adapted from RL McCann, FN Clements. Silent myocardial ischemia in patients undergoing peripheral vascular surgery. Incidence and association with cardiac morbidity and mortality. J Vasc Surg 1989; 9:583–587.)

to 7 percent. That figure is substantially higher than the worst modern mortality rates reported for high-risk patients undergoing aortic reconstructive surgery without the benefit of coronary artery bypass grafting (see Fig. 30-1). Until more definitive prospective control data are available, the use of prophylactic coronary artery bypass grafting for risk reduction prior to vascular surgery is not justified.

Fewer data are available for coronary angioplasty. Two studies exist that are anecdotal and suffer from the same flaws as data on coronary bypass grafting. Patients who survive coronary angioplasty appear to have a modest risk reduction after vascular surgery. If commonly accepted rates of angioplasty failure and associated morbidity and mortality are taken into account, that modest risk reduction does not justify prophylactic angioplasty [89,90].

The benefit of coronary revascularization may become substantial in long-term risk reduction [1,5,64]. However, while long-term cardiac risk among vascular-disease patients is high, it is not clear that prophylactic coronary artery bypass grafting or coronary angioplasty decreases mortality or reduces the risk of future myocardial infarction, save for a few small, well-identified subgroups [64]. Moreover, data that documented high morbidity and mortality from coronary artery disease in vascular-surgery patients were compiled largely in the late 1970s and early 1980s, a time when medical therapy for coronary artery disease risk was in its infancy. Now that the use of a beta blocker and antiplatelet therapy as well as aggressive risk-factor intervention have been shown to lower cardiac risk [91–93], the argument for prophylactic coronary revascularization to address long-term risk in vascular surgery patients remains, at best, unsettled.

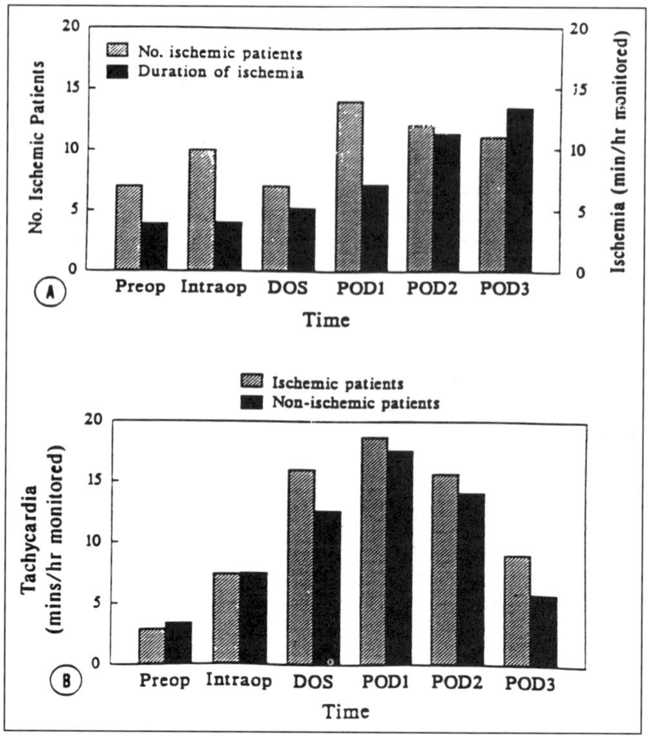

Fig. 30-6. Prevalence of myocardial ischemia **(A.)** and tachycardia **(B.)** in relation to time of surgery. The prevalence of ischemia is highest in postoperative days 1 and 2, a time when the incidence of tachycardia is highest. (Adapted from RL McCann, FN Clements. Silent myocardial ischemia in patients undergoing peripheral vascular surgery. Incidence and association with cardiac morbidity and mortality. J Vasc Surg 1989; 9:583–587.)

MEDICAL THERAPY

Intraoperative and postoperative Holter monitoring for asymptomatic ischemia has proved invaluable in the understanding of the mechanisms of developing myocardial ischemia in the perioperative setting [77,78,94–98]. While some controversy persists about the value of preoperative Holter monitoring in identifying risk in this patient population, there is wide consensus on the importance of intraoperative and postoperative Holter monitoring in identifying myocardial ischemia and risk during and after vascular surgery [77,78,94–98]. Multiple studies have shown that in vascular-surgery patients intraoperative myocardial ischemia is uncommon and not predictive of postoperative cardiac events [77,97,98]. The lower prevalence of intraoperative ischemia can be attributed in part to the strict control of heart rate, blood pressure, and pain perception that is routinely exercised in the operating room (Fig. 30-5) [77]. By contrast, the period beginning with waking from anesthesia and lasting up to 72 hours postoperatively is marked by the highest prevalence of ischemia among patients undergoing vascular surgery (Fig. 30-6) [77]. Postoperative ischemia is prevalent in 30 to 40 percent of high-risk vascular-surgery patients [77,78,97]. While the episodes of ischemia are not directly the result of discrete periods of increased heart rates, the overall time window is associated with a gradual increase in heart rate and pain perception (see Fig. 30-6) [77]. Even more important, asymptomatic ischemia precedes major cardiac events by a time window lasting up to several hours in the majority of cases where such an event ensues (Fig. 30-7) [97,99].

Several insights emerge from these observations. First, the intraoperatively strategy of strict control of blood pressure, heart rate, and pain perception achieves the greatest control of myocardial ischemia in high-risk patients. Once the effects of anesthesia begin to wane, pain perception returns, and less vigilant control of blood pressure and heart rate occurs, the prevalence of postoperative ischemia is at its highest (see Fig. 30-5). Since postoperative ischemia is highly predictive of perioperative cardiac risk [78,97], it follows that future strategies should aim to duplicate the hemodynamic and pain-perception control achieved in the operating room during the period of highest risk. Most cardiac events in vascular-surgery patients occur within the first 72 hours after surgery [94,97]. In addition, there is preliminary evidence to suggest that the postoperative period is a period of relatively high thrombogenesis, possibly as a result of catecholamine surges and the effect of anesthesia [100]. Hence, emerging medical strategies to control myocardial ischemia should include reducing myocardial oxygen demand (heart rate

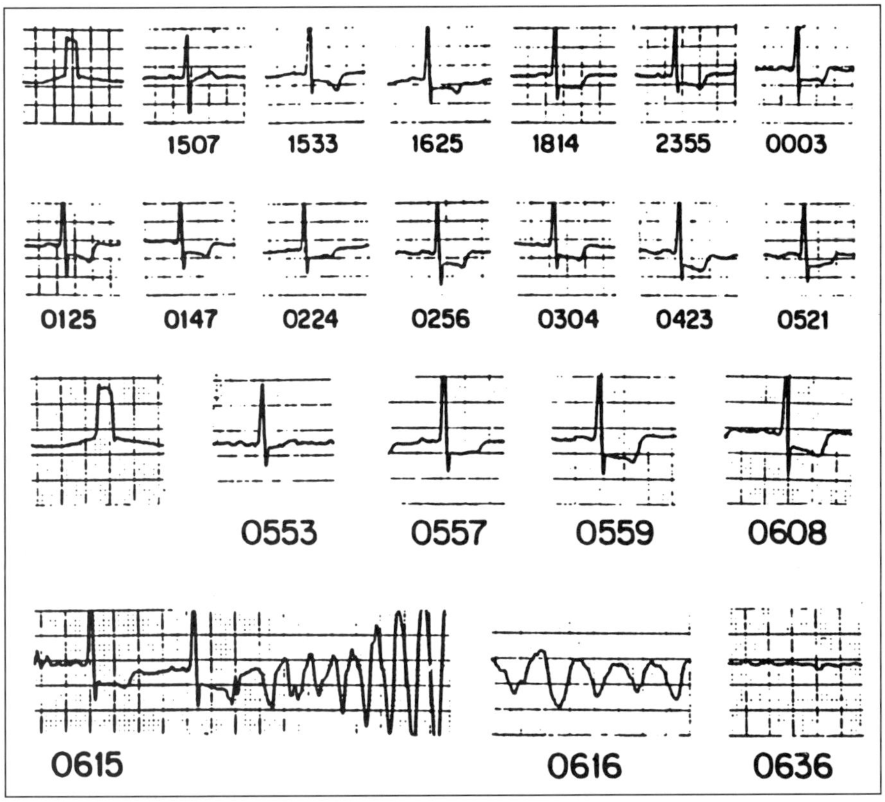

Fig. 30-7. Holter monitor tracing of the period after carotid endarterectomy of a patient with coronary artery disease. Holter monitoring during postoperative day 2. The unlabeled tracing is a standardization signal; the complex labeled 1507 (i.e., 3:07 p.m.) is the patient's baseline. The other 12 tracings represent discrete episodes of silent ischemia. At 5:53 a.m., the patient was at his baseline. Silent ischemia began at 5:57 a.m. and progressed during the visit of the surgical house staff. At 6:15 a.m., 3.5 mm of ST segment depression gave rise to polymorphic ventricular tachycardia, which degenerated quickly into ventricular fibrillation. (Adapted from L Ganz et al. Silent ischemia preceding sudden cardiac death in patients after vascular surgery. Am Heart J 1994; 127:1652–1654.)

and blood pressure) and reducing thrombogenesis (antiplatelet therapy).

Beta blockers reduce cardiac risk in patients with coronary artery disease over long-term follow-up [101]. Controlled trials examining the effect of beta-blocker therapy on ambulatory and perioperative myocardial ischemia have found a clear reduction in the number of episodes and total duration of ischemia as measured by Holter monitoring [102–104]. In one study, clinicians who were informed that their vascular-surgery patients had preoperative ischemia on Holter monitoring employed more aggressive medical therapy, including more extensive use of beta blockers, and significantly reduced ischemia and cardiac events in the first 48 hours postoperatively when compared to a cohort of historic controls whose preoperative ischemia was not revealed to the managing clinicians (Fig. 30-8) [105]. No randomized controlled trial as yet has demonstrated that beta-blocker therapy reduces both ischemia and cardiac events, but these preliminary data strongly suggest that beta blockers have a special role in risk management in the postoperative setting. Moreover, while it has long been thought that beta blockers are contraindicated in the long-term risk reduction of patients with claudication, a recent pooled analysis has refuted that [106]. Studies are underway to determine the effect of beta blockers on perioperative and long-term risk in a prospective controlled manner. In the mean time, vascular-surgery patients seem undertreated for cardiac risk when compared to counterparts with coronary artery disease. In one recent survey that examined the treatment of vascular-surgery patients who had coronary artery disease and preoperative ischemia, a surprising 50 percent were not receiving aspirin, and 60 percent were not receiving beta-blocker therapy despite no obvious contraindications [105]. Since the risks of aspirin and beta blockers are relatively low, maximizing medical therapy that has been proved effective seems prudent.

Some preliminary studies also have suggested that nitrate therapy reduces myocardial ischemia in the first 48 hours postoperatively [107]. Recent anesthesia data suggest that the type of anesthesia also may play a special role. More specifically, several trials have suggested that in vascular-surgery patients the use of regional or spinal anesthesia demonstrably reduces the incidence of thrombotic events, including cardiac thrombotic events, in the perioperative period when compared to general anesthe-

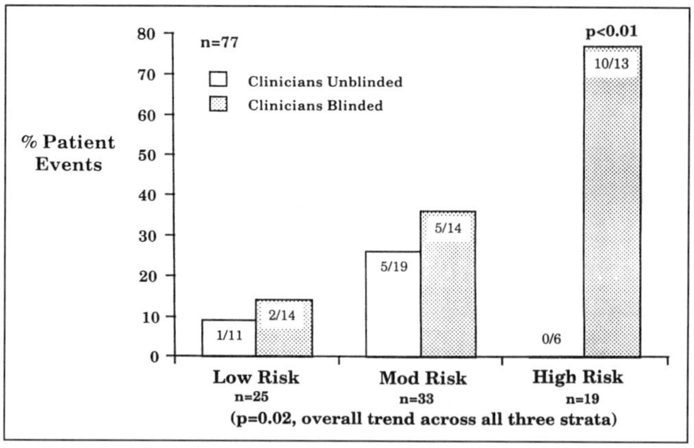

Fig. 30-8. Adverse cardiac event rates among 41 patients with preoperative ischemia on Holter monitoring whose clinicians were blinded to the Holter results versus 36 patients whose clinicians were unblinded to the results and who therefore received more intensive medical therapy. All patients were divided into terciles of risk based on a multivariate score derived from clinical characteristics, coronary artery disease severity, and type of vascular surgery. Intensive medical therapy in response to unblinding of the Holter result was most likely to reduce cardiac risk in the highest-risk subgroup. (Adapted from TC Andrews et al. Identification and treatment of perioperative myocardial ischemia in patients undergoing peripheral vascular surgery. J Vasc Med Biol 1994; vols: 8–15.)

sia [9,100,108]. The mechanism of that observation is thought to be that general anesthetics exert a hyperthrombotic effect, particularly in the high-risk perioperative period. Even in the absence of a prospective controlled trial, many centers have made spinal or epidural anesthesia the routine protocol in vascular-surgery patients. The spinal-anesthesia approach also has the added convenience of prolonging analgesia over the 48-hour high-risk postoperative period with analgesic agents administered via the epidural route. One preliminary report shows that increased perioperative pain control translates into a lower prevalence of postoperative myocardial ischemia [109]. Finally, prospective controlled data suggest that the use of pulmonary-artery monitoring and the optimization of cardiac output and filling pressures in high-risk vascular-surgery patients result in lower perioperative cardiac morbidity rates, as well as other thrombotic events when compared to a strategy of no monitoring [110,111]. While the number of patients included in these trials was low, the trials have been extremely influential in clinical practice, since pulmonary-artery monitoring is increasingly common, particularly in the management of aortic-surgery patients (Table 30-7) [111].

Summary

While the issues surrounding the evaluation of cardiac risk in vascular-surgery patients remain complex, it is clear that the perioperative risk of vascular-surgery patients is trending downward despite the inclusion of higher-risk patients. Causes of that trend include a higher prevalence of patients who have had their coronary artery disease previously treated, with either coronary revascularization or a medical therapy, improved risk assessment with widespread practice of routine preoperative clinical evaluation and the use of a variety of noninvasive cardiac tests, and significant improvement in surgical, anesthesia, and hemodynamic monitoring techniques. Whether this reduction in risk will translate into lower long-term cardiac risk is not yet clear. At least two investigators have shown that the long-term cardiac risk among vascular-surgery patients is in great part related to the perioperative cardiac events that these patients suffer [22,112], which gives reason to hope that advances in perioperative management also will yield long-term dividends. Nevertheless, patients with peripheral vascular disease and concomitant coronary artery disease are relatively underidentified and undertreated with medical or coronary revascularization therapy when compared to all other patients with coronary artery disease [105]. Because presentation for elective surgery is an excellent opportunity to identify and correct unrecognized cardiac risk, preoperative evaluation should remain a routine part of patient management.

The principal controversy is what to do with the high-risk vascular-surgery patient. The most prudent approach is that advocated by Wong and Detsky in a recent review [29] and summarized in Fig. 30-9. The authors carefully examined all available preoperative evaluation modalities and potential treatment options to arrive at a coherent

Table 30-7. Effect of pulmonary artery monitoring on adverse events among patients undergoing vascular surgery

Adverse event	Group 1[a] (n = 45)	Group 2[b] (n = 23)	Group 3[c] (n = 21)
Intraoperative arrhythmia tachycardia or hypotension	30[d]	15[d]	22
Postoperative cardiac morbidity	3[d]	2[d]	5
Early graft thrombosis	1[d]	1[d]	4
Death	1 (2.2%)	0	2 (9.5%)

[a]Group 1 = PA line 12 hours prior to surgery.
[b]Group 2 = PA line 3 hours prior to surgery.
[c]Group 3 = No PA line.
[d]$p < 0.05$ compared to group 3.
Source: Adapted from JF Berlauk et al. Preoperative optimization of cardiovascular hemodynamics improves outcome in peripheral vascular surgery. Ann Surg 1991; 214:289–297.

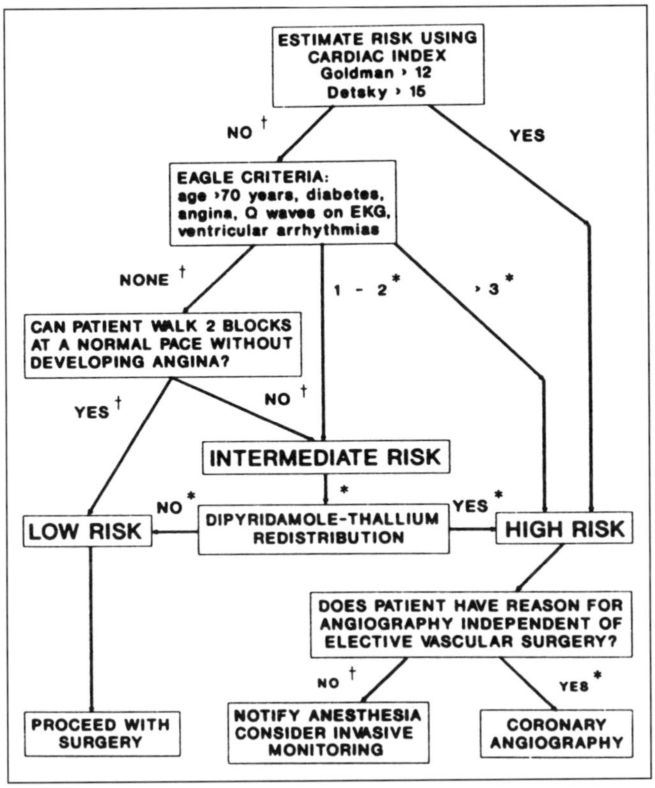

Fig. 30-9. Approach to cardiac risk stratification for patients having peripheral vascular surgery. (From T Wong, AS Detsky. Preoperative cardiac risk assessment in patients having peripheral vascular surgery. Ann Int Med 1992; 116:743–753.)

universal approach. Briefly, their approach is that high-risk vascular-surgery patients include those identified by a thorough history, physical, and basic laboratory data (e.g., those who have at least three of the clinical markers identified by Eagle and co-workers [19]) **and** patients who have only intermediate clinical risk but also an abnormal preoperative noninvasive cardiac test. Low-risk patients include those patients who are not felt to be high risk by an evaluating clinician (e.g., they have none of the clinical markers proposed by Eagle and colleagues) and those patients at intermediate clinical risk who also have a normal preoperative noninvasive cardiac test. Using that strategy, low-risk patients can proceed to surgery without further evaluation or precaution. It should be emphasized that the vast majority of these patients need not even receive a preoperative noninvasive cardiac test. High-risk patients who have an indication for angiography and coronary revascularization **other** than elective vascular surgery (e.g., patients with class III or IV angina, ischemia, or ventricular dysfunction) should undergo coronary angiography and subsequent elective preoperative coronary revascularization when anatomically feasible, since such patients would get that therapy even if they did not need vascular surgery. For high-risk patients with no such indication, prophylactic coronary revascularization cannot be justified for perioperative risk reduction alone. Such patients can undergo vascular surgery safely, particularly with modern anesthesia techniques, careful intraoperative or postoperative monitoring, and special attention to analgesia, blood pressure, and heart-rate control intraoperatively and in the first 72 hours postoperatively [77,94–98].

Which noninvasive cardiac tests should be used for preoperative assessment? Most experts have recommended dipyridamole thallium imaging, principally because it is the most widely used study for that purpose [29,113]. However, recent trials with dipyridamole thallium imaging enrolled consecutive patients and found no role in predicting perioperative risk [18,55]. Of the other options, Holter monitoring has been the only study shown to be effective in a consecutive series of patients whose clinicians were blinded to the test result [33]. Yet Holter monitoring is not widely used and has several disadvantages, as already mentioned. Dobutamine echocardiography also has been shown to be an effective test when clinicians were blinded to its results. It has the advantage of being less expensive than dipyridamole thallium imaging, and it provides information about baseline ejection fraction. This test, too, is not yet widely used [66–68].

Suffice it to say that none of the available tests is perfect. The best current recommendation is that no test should be used for blanket screening purposes. Clinical evaluation in the manner described is the best initial screening procedure. Those patients whose risk cannot be fully determined by clinical evaluation alone should receive the noninvasive cardiac test that the local clinician feels most expert at performing and interpreting [114]. Such an approach is likely to make peripheral vascular surgery a low-risk procedure despite the inherent high risk among most of its patients. Moreover, this approach likely will identify those patients at highest long-term risk and appropriately expose them to well-established medical and surgical interventions, thereby finally addressing the most significant remaining problem in this patient population.

References

1. Jamieson WR, et al. Influence of ischemic heart disease on early and late mortality after surgery for peripheral occlusive vascular disease. Circulation 1982; 66:I-92–I-97.
2. Hertzer NR. Myocardial ischemia. Surgery 1983; 93:97–101.
3. Cooperman M, et al. Cardiovascular risk factors in patients with peripheral vascular disease. Surgery 1978; 84:505–509.
4. Hollier LH, et al. Late survival after abdominal aortic aneurysm repair: influence of coronary artery disease. J Vasc Surg 1984; 1:290–299.
5. Hertzer NR. The natural history of peripheral vascular disease. Circulation 1991; 83:I-12–I-19.
6. Kim YD, et al. Changes in peripheral vascular and cardiac sympathetic activity before and after coronary artery bypass surgery: interrelationships with hemodynamic alterations. Am Heart J 1981; 102:972–979.
7. Scheinin B, et al. Sympatho-adrenal and pituitary hormone responses during and immediately after thoracic surgery—modulation by four different pain treatments. Acta Anesthsiol Scand 1987; 31:762–767.
8. Pathak KS, Anton AH, Sutheimer CA. Effects of low-dose morphine and fentanyl infusions on urinary and plasma catecholamine concentrations during scoliosis surgery. Anesth Analg 1985; 64:509–514.
9. Truman KJ, et al. Effects of epidural anesthesia and analgesia on coagulation and outcome after major vascular surgery. Anesth Analg 1991; 73:696–704.

10. Golden MA, et al. Selective evaluation and management of coronary artery disease in patients undergoing repair of abdominal aortic aneurysm. Ann Surg 1990; 212:415–423.
11. Donaldson MC, Mannick JA, Whittemore AD. Femoral-distal bypass with in situ greater saphenous vein. Long-term results using the Mills valvulotome. Ann Surg 1991; 213:457–465.
12. Bunt TJ. The role of a defined protocol of cardiac risk assessment in decreasing perioperative myocardial infarction in vascular surgery. J Vasc Surg 1992; 15:626–634.
13. Taylor LM Jr, et al. The incidence of perioperative myocardial infarction in general vascular surgery. J Vasc Surg 1991; 15:52–61.
14. Sandler G. The importance of the history in the medical clinic and the cost of unnecessary tests. Am Heart J 1980; 100:928–931.
15. Braunwald EB. Examination of the patient: the history. In EB Braunwald, Heart Disease, A Textbook of Cardiovascular Medicine. Philadelphia: Saunders, 1988. Pp. 1–12.
16. Goldman L. Multifactorial index of cardiac risk in non-cardiac surgery: ten year status report. J Cardiothorac Anesth 1987; 1:237–244.
17. Logue RB, Kaplan JA. The cardiac patient and non-cardiac surgery. Curr Probl Cardiol 1982; 7:1–49.
18. Baron JF, et al. Dipyridamole-thallium scintigraphy and gaited radionuclide angiography to assess cardiac risk for abdominal aortic surgery. N Engl J Med 1994; 330:663–669.
19. Eagle KA, et al. Combining clinical and thallium data optimizes preoperative assessment of cardiac risk from major vascular surgery. Ann Intern Med 1989; 110:859–866.
20. Rennart G, Slatz-Rennart H, Wanderman K. Size of acute myocardial infarction in patients with diabetes mellitus. Am J Cardiol 1985; 55:1629–1630.
21. Anderson RJ, et al. Infectious risk factors in the immunosuppressed host. Am J Med 1973; 54:453–460.
22. Hollenberg M, et al., for the Study of Perioperative Ischemia Research Group. Predictors of postoperative myocardial ischemia in patients undergoing non-cardiac surgery. JAMA 1992; 268:205–209.
23. Debakey ME, Lawrie GM. Combined coronary artery and peripheral vascular disease: recognition and treatment. J Vasc Surg 1984; 1:605–607.
24. Goldman L, et al. Multifactorial index of cardiac risk in non-cardiac surgical procedures. N Engl J Med 1977; 297:845–850.
25. Hertzer NR, et al. Coronary artery disease in peripheral vascular patients: classification of 1000 coronary angiograms and results of surgical management. Ann Surg 1984; 199:223–233.
26. Detsky AS, et al. Predicting cardiac complications in patients undergoing cardiac surgery. J Gen Intern Med 1986; 141:1631–1634.
27. Rao TL, Jacobs KH, El-Etr AA. Reinfarction following anesthesia in patients with myocardial infarction. Anesthesiology 1983; 59:499–505.
28. Von Knorring J. Postoperative myocardial infarction: a prospective study in a high risk group of surgical patients. Surgery 1981; 90:55–60.
29. Wong T, Detsky AS. Preoperative cardiac risk assessment for patients having peripheral vascular surgery. Ann Intern Med 1992; 116:743–753.
30. Cannel WB, McGee DL, Gordon T. A general cardiovascular risk profile: the Framingham Study. Am J Cardiol 1976; 38:46–51.
31. Lette J, et al. Multivariate clinical models and quantitative dipyridamole thallium imaging to predict cardiac morbidity and death after vascular reconstruction. J Vasc Surg 1991; 14:160–169.
32. Takase B, et al. Comparative prognostic value of clinical risk indices resting two-dimensional echocardiography and dipyridamole stress thallium 201 myocardial imaging for perioperative cardiac events in major non-vascular surgery patients. Am Heart J 1993; 126:1099–1106.
33. Raby KE, et al. Correlation between preoperative ischemia and major cardiac events after peripheral vascular surgery. N Engl J Med 1989; 321:1296–1300.
34. Bruce RA, et al. Enhanced risk assessment for primary coronary heart disease events by maximal exercise testing: ten years of experience at the Seattle Heart Watch study. J Am Coll Cardiol 1983; 2:569–573.
35. Giagnoni E, et al. Prognostic value of exercise EKG testing in asymptomatic, normotensive subjects: a prospective matched study. N Engl J Med 1983; 309:1085–1089.
36. Cutler BS, et al. Applicability and interpretation of electrocardiographic stress testing in patients with peripheral vascular disease. Am J Surg 1981; 141:501–506.
37. Gerson MC, et al. Cardiac prognosis in non-cardiac geriatric surgery. Ann Intern Med 1985; 103:832–837.
38. McPhail N, et al. The use of preoperative exercise testing to predict cardiac complications after arterial reconstruction. J Vasc Surg 1988; 7:60–68.
39. Puls A, Thadani U. Rupture of abdominal aortic aneurysm during exercise. Gated blood pool studies. Am J Med 1986; 81:887–889.
40. Panza JA, Quyyumi AA, Diodata JG. Prediction of the frequency and duration of ambulatory myocardial ischemia in patients with stable coronary artery disease by determination of the ischemic threshold from exercise testing: importance of the exercise protocol. J Am Coll Cardiol 1991; 17:657–663.
41. Goldman S, et al. Arm exercise testing with myocardial scintigraphy in asymptomatic patients with peripheral vascular disease. Chest 1989; 95:740–746.
42. Balady GI, et al. Value of arm exercise testing in detecting coronary artery disease. Am J Cardiol 1985; 55:37–39.
43. Kawai C, Hultgren HN. The effect of digitalis upon the exercise electrocardiogram. Am Heart J 1964; 68:409–411.
44. McCarthy DM, et al. Single dose myocardial perfusion imaging with thallium-201: Application in patients with nondiagnostic electrocardiographic stress tests. Am J Cardiol 1979; 43:899–903.
45. Leppo J, et al. Serial thallium-201 imaging after dipyridamole infusion: diagnostic utility in detecting coronary stenoses and relationship to regional wall motion. Circulation 1982; 66:649–657.
46. Francisco DA, et al. Tomographic thallium-201 myocardial perfusion scintigrams at the maximal vasodilation with intravenous dipyridamole. Circulation 1982; 66:370–379.
47. Boucher CA, et al. Determination of cardiac risk by dipyridamole-thallium imaging before peripheral vascular surgery. N Engl J Med 1985; 312:389–394.
48. Leppo J, et al. Noninvasive evaluation of cardiac risk before elective vascular surgery. J Am Coll Cardiol 1987; 9:269–276.
49. Younis LT, et al. Prognostic importance of silent myocardial ischemia detected by intravenous dipyridamole thallium myocardial imaging in asymptomatic patients with coronary artery disease. J Am Coll Cardiol 1989; 14:1635–1641.
50. McFalls EO, et al. Angina and persistent exercise thallium defects: independent risk factors in elective vascular surgery. J Am Coll Cardiol 1993; 21:1347–1352.
51. Lette J, et al. Preoperative and long-term cardiac risk assessment. Ann Surg 1992; 216:192–204.
52. Lette J, et al. Preoperative coronary artery disease risk stratification based on dipyridamole imaging and a simple three step, three segment model for patients undergoing non-car-

diac vascular surgery or major general surgery. Am J Cardiol 1992; 69:1553–1558.
53. Levinson JR, et al. Usefulness of semiquantitative analysis of dipyridamole-thallium-201 redistribution for improving risk stratification before vascular surgery. Am J Cardiol 1990; 66:406–410.
54. Lane SE, et al. Predictive value of quantitative dipyridamole-thallium scintigraphy in assessing cardiovascular risk after vascular surgery in diabetes mellitus. Am J Cardiol 1989; 64:1275–1279.
55. Mangano DT, et al. Dipyridamole-thallium-201 scintigraphy as a preoperative screening test: a re-examination of its predictive potential. Circulation 1991; 84:493–502.
56. Shaw L, et al. Determination of perioperative cardiac risk by adenosine thallium-201 myocardial imaging. Am Heart J 1992; 124:861–869.
57. Elliott BM, et al. Dobutamine-201 thallium imaging: assessing cardiac risk associated with vascular surgery. Circulation 1991; 84(III):54–60.
58. Morris KG, et al. Value of radionuclide angiography for predicting specific cardiac events after acute myocardial infarction. Am J Cardiol 1985; 55:318–322.
59. Pasternak PF, et al. The value of radionuclide angiogram in the prediction of perioperative myocardial infarction in patients undergoing lower extremity revascularization procedures. Circulation 1985; 72(II):13–17.
60. McCann RL, Wolfe WG. Resection of abdominal aortic aneurysms in patients with low ejection fractions. J Vasc Surg 1989; 10:240–244.
61. Kasmers A, Cerqueria MD, Gierler RE. Perioperative and late outcome in patients with left ventricular ejection fraction of 35% or less who require major vascular surgery. J Vasc Surg 1988; 8:307–315.
62. Takase B, et al. Comparative prognostic value of clinical risk indices resting 2-dimensional echocardiography and dipyridamole stress thallium-201 myocardial imaging for perioperative cardiac events in major non-vascular surgery patient. Am Heart J 123; 126:1099–1106.
63. McEnroe GS, et al. Comparison of ejection fraction in Goldman risk factor analysis to dipyridamole-thallium-201 studies in the evaluation of cardiac morbidity after aortic aneurysm surgery. J Vasc Surg 1990; 11:497–504.
64. Weiner DA, et al. The role of exercise testing in identifying patients with improved survival after coronary artery bypass surgery. J Am Coll Cardiol 1986; 8:741–748.
65. Tischler MD, et al. Prediction of major cardiac events after peripheral vascular surgery using dipyridamole echocardiography. Am J Cardiol 1991; 68:593–597.
66. Poldermans D, et al. Dobutamine stress echocardiography for assessment of cardiac risk in patients undergoing major vascular surgery. Circulation 1993; 87:1506–1512.
67. Lane RT, et al. Dobutamine stress echocardiography for assessment of cardiac risk before noncardiac surgery. Am J Cardiol 1991; 68:976–977.
68. Langan EM, et al. Dobutamine stress echocardiography for cardiac risk assessment before aortic surgery. J Vasc Surg 1993; 18:905–913.
69. Selwyn AP, et al. Myocardial ischemia in patients with frequent angina pectoris. Br Med J 1978; 2:1594–1596.
70. Selwyn AP, et al. Different physiology of painful and silent myocardial ischemia. Circulation 1986; 74(II):57.
71. Deanfield JE, et al. Transient ST-segment depression as a marker of myocardial ischemia during daily life. Am J Cardiol 1984; 54:1195–1200.
72. Gottlieb SO, et al. Silent ischemia as a marker of early unfavorable outcome in patients with unstable angina. N Engl J Med 1986; 314:1214–1219.
73. Tzivoni D, et al. Prognostic significance of ischemic episodes in patients with previous myocardial infarction. Am J Cardiol 1988; 62:661–664.
74. Hedblad B, et al. Increased mortality in men with ST segment depression during 24-hour ambulatory monitoring long-term EKG monitoring. Eur Heart J 1989; 10:149–158.
75. Pasternack PF, et al. Silent myocardial ischemia monitoring predicts late as well as perioperative cardiac events in patients undergoing vascular surgery. J Vasc Surg 1992; 16:171–180.
76. Fleisher LA, et al. Predictive value of preoperative ischemia for postoperative ischemic cardiac events in vascular and non-vascular surgery patients. Am Heart J 1991; 122:980–985.
77. McCann RL, Clements FN. Silent myocardial ischemia in patients undergoing peripheral vascular surgery. Incidence and association with cardiac morbidity and mortality. J Vasc Surg 1989; 9:583–587.
78. Mangano DT, et al. Association of perioperative myocardial ischemia with cardiac morbidity and mortality in men undergoing non-cardiac surgery. N Engl J Med 1990; 323:1781–1788.
79. Tischler MD, et al. Dipyridamole echocardiography versus ambulatory ischemia monitoring in the assessment of perioperative risk. J Am Coll Cardiol 1991; 17:264a.
80. Fleisher LE, et al. Preoperative dipyridamole-thallium imaging and Holter monitoring as a predictor of preoperative cardiac events and long-term outcome. J Am Coll Cardiol 1994; 23:158a.
81. Ruddy TD, et al. Cardiac risk stratification using dipyridanole myocardial perfusion imaging and ambulatory ECG monitoring prior to vascular surgery. Eur J Vasc Surg 1993; 7:151–155.
82. Hertzer NR, et al. Routine coronary angiography prior to elective aortic reconstruction. Arch Surg 1979; 114:1336–1344.
83. Foster ED, et al. Risk of non-cardiac operations in patients with defined coronary disease: the Coronary Artery Surgery (CASS) Registry experience. Ann Thorac Surg 1986; 41:42–48.
84. Nielsen JL, et al. Risk of major elective operation after myocardial revascularization. Am J Surg 1992; 164:423–424.
85. Reul TJ, et al. The effect of coronary bypass on the outcome of peripheral vascular operations in 1093 patients. J Vasc Surg 1986; 3:788–798.
86. O'Connor GT, et al. Prediction of in-hospital mortality associated with coronary artery bypass surgery. Circulation 1992; 85:2110–2118.
87. Mullaney CJ, et al. Early and late results after isolated coronary artery bypass surgery in 159 patients aged 80 years and older. Circulation 1990; 82(IV):229–236.
88. Gersh BJ, et al. Coronary arteriography and coronary artery bypass surgery: morbidity and mortality in patients ages 65 or older. A report from the Coronary Artery Surgery Study. Circulation 1983; 67:483–491.
89. Allen JR, Helling TS, Hartzler GO. Operative procedures not involving the heart after percutaneous transluminal coronary angioplasty. Surg Gyn Obstet 1991; 173:285–288.
90. Huber KC, et al. Outcome of non-cardiac operations in patients with severe coronary artery disease successfully treated preoperatively with coronary angioplasty. Mayo Clin Proc 1992; 67:15–21.
91. Pedersen TR. Six year follow-up of the Norwegian Multicenter Study on Timolol after acute myocardial infarction. N Engl J Med 1984; 313:1055–1058.
92. Hennekens CH, et al. Aspirin and other antiplatelet agents in the secondary and primary prevention of cardiovascular disease. Circulation 1988; 80:749–756.
93. Lipid Research Clinics Program. The Lipid Research Clinics

Coronary Primary Prevention Trial I: Reduction and incidence of coronary heart disease. JAMA 1984; 251:351–364.
94. Mangano DT, et al. Perioperative myocardial ischemia in patients undergoing non-cardiac surgery I. Incidence and severity during the four-day perioperative period. J Am Coll Cardiol 1991; 17:843–850.
95. Mangano DT, et al. Perioperative myocardial ischemia in patients undergoing non-cardiac surgery II. Incidence and severity during the first week after surgery. J Am Coll Cardiol 1991; 17:851–857.
96. Ouyang P, et al. Frequency and significance of early postoperative silent myocardial ischemia in patients having peripheral vascular surgery. Am J Cardiol 1989; 64:1113–1116.
97. Raby KE, et al. Detection and significance of intraoperative and postoperative myocardial ischemia in peripheral vascular surgery. JAMA 1992; 268:222–227.
98. Landesberg G, et al. Importance of long-delays in postoperative ST segment depression and cardiac morbidity after vascular surgery. Lancet 1993; 341:715–719.
99. Ganz L, et al. Silent ischemia preceding sudden cardiac death in a patient after vascular surgery. Am Heart J 1994; 127:1652–1654.
100. Rosenfeld BA, et al. The effects of different anesthetic regimens on fibrinolysis and the development of postoperative arterial thrombosis. Anesthesiology 1993; 79:435–443.
101. Yusuf S, et al. Beta-blockade during and after myocardial infarction: an overview of the randomized trial. Prog Cardiovasc Dis 1985; 27:335–371.
102. Frishman WH, Teicher M. Antianginal drug therapy for silent myocardial ischemia. Am Heart J 1987; 114:140–147.
103. Imperi GA, et al. Effects of titrated beta-blockade on silent myocardial ischemia in ambulatory patients with coronary artery disease. Am J Cardiol 1987; 60:519–524.
104. Pasternack PF, et al. The hemodynamics of beta-blockade in patients undergoing abdominal aortic aneurysm repair. Circulation 1987; 76(III):1–7.
105. Andrews TC, et al. Identification and treatment of perioperative myocardial ischemia in patients undergoing peripheral vascular surgery. J Vasc Med Biol 1994; 5:8–15.
106. Radack K, Deck C. Beta-adrenergic blocker therapy does not worsen intermittent claudication in subjects with peripheral arterial disease. Arch Intern Med 1991; 151:1769–1776.
107. Dodds TM, et al. Impact of prophylactic nitroglycerin infusion on the incidence of myocardial ischemia during noncardiac surgery. Society of Cardiovascular Anesthesiology, 1992 meetings (Abstr).
108. Gelman S. General versus regional anesthesia for peripheral vascular surgery. Anesthesiology 1993; 79:415–418.
109. Siliciano D, et al. Use of continuous versus intermittent narcotic after CABG surgery: effects on myocardial ischemia. Anesth Analg 1990; 70:S1–S450.
110. Whittemore AD, et al. Aortic aneurysm repair. Reduced operative mortality associated with maintenance of optimal cardiac performance. Ann Surg 1980; 192:414–420.
111. Berlauk JF, et al. Preoperative optimization of cardiovascular hemodynamics improves outcome in peripheral vascular surgery. Ann Surg 1991; 214:289–297.
112. Raby KE, et al. Long-term prognostic significance of myocardial ischemia detected by Holter Monitoring in patients with peripheral vascular disease. Am J Cardiol 1990; 66:1309–1313.
113. Fleisher LA, Beattie C. Current practice in the preoperative evaluation of patients undergoing major vascular surgery: a survey of cardiovascular anesthesiologists. J Cardiothorac Vasc Anesth 1993; 7:650–654.
114. Goldman L. Assessment of perioperative cardiac risk. N Engl J Med 1994; 330:707–709.

Percutaneous Revascularization in Peripheral Arterial Disease

Kenneth Rosenfield
Robert Schainfeld
Jeffrey M. Isner

The pioneering work of Dotter, Judkins, Gruentzig, and others opened the door for percutaneous, potentially less invasive strategies to treat peripheral artery disease (PAD) [1–3]. In the two to three decades since this seminal work, the results of the percutaneous approach have been overwhelmingly positive; consequently, its growth has been steady, although constrained by acknowledged limitations, most notably those of restenosis and the difficulty of treating diffusely diseased and occluded vessels. In the early years of percutaneous transluminal angioplasty (PTA), the availability of only large-profile balloons and stiff, nonyielding guide wires, coupled with the inherent difficulties of interpreting images provided by early generations of x-ray equipment (which dictated the need for large volumes of contrast), sometimes meant that the hazards of percutaneous therapy were comparable to that of surgical revascularization. Recent innovations, however, have resolved many of those early limitations associated with percutaneous techniques, and, while restenosis remains a vexing and tenacious problem, even that may be ameliorated by certain novel strategies.

Several factors have made percutaneous revascularization increasingly popular as the first line of therapy for PAD. First, technological improvements, by enabling safer and more effective angioplasty, are exerting a positive impact. Catheter profiles have been reduced considerably, limiting complications related to vascular access. The use of novel materials for balloon and guide-wire construction has facilitated passage through occluded vessels and permitted routine access to more remote vascular sites with less risk and greater efficacy. Directional and rotational atherectomy now enable "debulking" of atheroma and thereby facilitate angioplasty of lesions that are eccentric and heavily calcified, which had responded poorly to balloon dilation alone. Endovascular stents have been demonstrated to improve both short-term and long-term outcomes of aortoiliac, renal, and coronary PTA [4–6].

Second, improvements in imaging techniques have led to a better appreciation of the acute results of catheter-based intervention. Foremost among those improvements has been the introduction of intravascular ultrasound (IVUS), which provides a cross-sectional view of the vessel similar to a histologic section [7]. The improvement in on-line imaging using IVUS, along with digital enhancement of conventional contrast images, has led to better comprehension of the mechanisms responsible for successful and unsuccessful angioplasty. Concomitantly, the volume of contrast required during a given intervention has been reduced.

Third, an increased emphasis on health care costs has motivated providers, insurers, and patients themselves to reassess treatment modalities available for various conditions. PTA, which can be performed as a same-day or overnight-stay procedure, at a cost significantly less than that of surgical revascularization, is thus currently being viewed favorably as a cost-saving approach for treating symptomatic vascular disease. To the extent that the choice of revascularization strategy is patient driven, the percutaneous approach often is preferred by patients, who are increasingly aware of their treatment options. Many patients favor the reduced-morbidity potential of less invasive techniques, even if the symptomatic improvement in certain circumstances may not be as durable or the degree of revascularization not as complete. A lower-risk partial revascularization may suffice to treat symptoms and indeed be preferable to a higher-risk attempt at complete revascularization. Nowhere has the wisdom of this philosophy become more evident than in the treatment of infrapopliteal disease in high-risk patients with limb-threatening ischemic ulceration. Recognition that even short-term restoration of antegrade flow by PTA can result in ulcer healing and—barring any trauma to the limb—long-term limb salvage, has provided a viable alternative to surgery in those patients [8].

Last, as the population in the United States ages, the prevalence of PAD is increasing, thus compelling health care providers to optimize treatment strategies. People over 65 years of age, the stage when vascular disease achieves its peak prevalence, now constitute 12 percent of the population, a figure expected to double in the next 35 years. As pointed out in a recent U.S. Public Health Service document, ". . . improving the functional independence, not just the length, of later life is an important element in promoting the health of this age group" [9]. Judicious treatment of patients disabled by PAD may enable them to experience the well-documented benefits of exercise and physical activity. The availability of efficacious percutaneous options for revascularization in this group of patients with a high-risk profile due to comorbid conditions and associated vascular disease in other vital organs represents an attractive first line of therapy. Furthermore, the increasing awareness among physicians and patients that effective, less invasive therapy is available for disabling or lifestyle-limiting PAD has led to a reevaluation of the threshold for intervention. A patient whose claudication is not severe enough to warrant major surgical bypass may nonetheless be appropriate for PTA. Recognition that the threshold for PTA should not be equivalent to that for major surgical bypass has prompted a change in strategy for those patients. In certain patients with lifestyle-limiting claudication, it is reasonable to obtain a diagnostic angiogram and then to proceed with PTA if the lesion is suitable, but treat conservatively (non-surgically) if amelioration of symptoms would require high-risk PTA or surgery.

The increasing popularity of percutaneous therapy for PAD underscores the importance for vascular specialists and interventionalists to have a comprehensive understanding of the mechanisms of angioplasty, the indications for intervention, the expected short- and long-term outcome for a given revascularization procedure, and the potential complications.

Mechanisms of Successful Percutaneous Angioplasty

The mechanisms by which balloon dilation enhance lumen area have remained controversial since the procedure was introduced. The chief liability of the majority of studies examining this issue is that their conclusions are based on data obtained from assessment of either postmortem or in-vitro specimens. While pathologic evaluation of dilated vessels typically discloses plaque fractures and stretching of the arterial wall, the exact contribution of these factors versus plaque compression and other elements remains enigmatic. Most in-vivo attempts to identify the mechanisms responsible for successful or unsuccessful PTA have been limited by the lack of ability, using standard angiographic imaging methods, to adequately assess the morphology and geometry of a lesion before and after treatment and at the time of restenosis. Conventional contrast angiography has been the time-honored approach for lesion characterization and assessment. Angiography, however, remains limited by several factors, which have been well described [10–17]. Those limitations relate principally to the fact that contrast angiography depicts the vessel lumen only; plaque and vessel wall are viewed as a negative imprint on the contrast-filled lumen. While that view allows for characterization of lumen topography, irregularities in the vascular lumen vessel wall can only be inferred from the negative imprint. Angiography does not enable visualization or characterization of tissue elements below the intimal surface. This limitation becomes particularly problematic in a vessel with diffuse disease, in which case the vessel may appear angiographically normal due to the ubiquitous distribution of atherosclerotic plaque. Furthermore, contrast angiography is limited to a single planar view per injection; as such, information regarding the circumferential nature of the plaque cannot be directly recorded. Visualization of the vessel from alternative angles is possible, but only at the expense of additional injections of contrast material.

INTRAVASCULAR ULTRASOUND (IVUS)

IVUS has become a potent adjunct imaging technique to contrast angiography, addressing many of the limitations of the latter. IVUS is unequivocally superior to contrast angiography in its ability to demonstrate detailed characteristics at the interface of the lumen and vessel wall. IVUS also depicts structures below that interface, within the plaque and vessel wall. The expanding library of clinical experience with image interpretation has enabled us to glean several lessons from IVUS regarding lesion characteristics, mechanisms of balloon angioplasty, and effects of various novel interventional therapies.

Lesion Characterization by IVUS. To the extent that certain characteristics of a given lesion affect its response to intervention, it is critical to be able to assess accurately those characteristics. Because of the intraluminal location of the IVUS probe and the ability of ultrasound energy to penetrate tissues, IVUS provides information regarding the arterial wall that was previously unavailable in vivo but rather provided only by pathologic examination. Experimental and clinical experience to date indicates that IVUS images correlate remarkably well with histologic examination (Plate 9). IVUS is exquisitely sensitive in detecting plaque and other details that are angiographically silent [18–21]. Indeed, IVUS detects the presence of plaque not seen by angiography in virtually all patients undergoing interventional procedures [7]. Angiographically normal sites adjacent to target lesions almost always demonstrate significant disease when imaged by IVUS, a fact that has obvious implications regarding the selection of balloon or device size and in assessment of relative luminal narrowing.

Not uncommonly, an angiographically normal-appearing vessel is found by IVUS to have diffuse, ubiquitous distribution of plaque throughout, indicating a much more advanced stage of atherosclerosis than would have been presumed otherwise. The response to balloon dilation in such a diffusely diseased vessel might be expected to differ from that in a normal vessel with focal plaque. Inasmuch as the distinction between the two types of lesions is facilitated by IVUS, this modality may be instrumental in guiding the interventional strategy and defining the mechanism of lumen enlargement.

IVUS also has expanded our knowledge regarding plaque morphology. Calcified plaque, characterized by acoustic shadowing, is detected by IVUS in the majority of vessels undergoing angioplasty. This feature is underappreciated by angiography Honye et al., for example, identified calcific deposits by IVUS in 83 percent of patients undergoing angioplasty, whereas angiography identified calcium in only 14 percent of the same cohort [22]. Since calcium in the vessel wall undoubtedly affects the response to dilation (Figs. 31-1 and 31-2), identification of calcium is potentially important.

In occasional cases, IVUS may be uniquely informative with regard to details of plaque and wall pathology. The images shown in Fig. 31-3, for example, were recorded from a patient with recent onset of disabling claudication; hypoechoic foci suggested that plaque rupture and hemorrhage were responsible for the patient's accelerated symptoms. Tissue obtained by directional atherectomy documented findings of plaque fissure and hemorrhage, confirming the suspicion raised by IVUS that plaque rupture was the mechanism for the patient's acute onset of symptoms [23].

IVUS and Mechanisms of Angioplasty. Plaque fracture, plaque compression, and stretching of arterial wall components—all likely play a role in enhancing luminal dimensions, yet the relative contribution of each remains controversial. Furthermore, although certain angiographic parameters, such as a lesion on a bend or a long, irregular stenosis, are associated with an untoward angioplasty

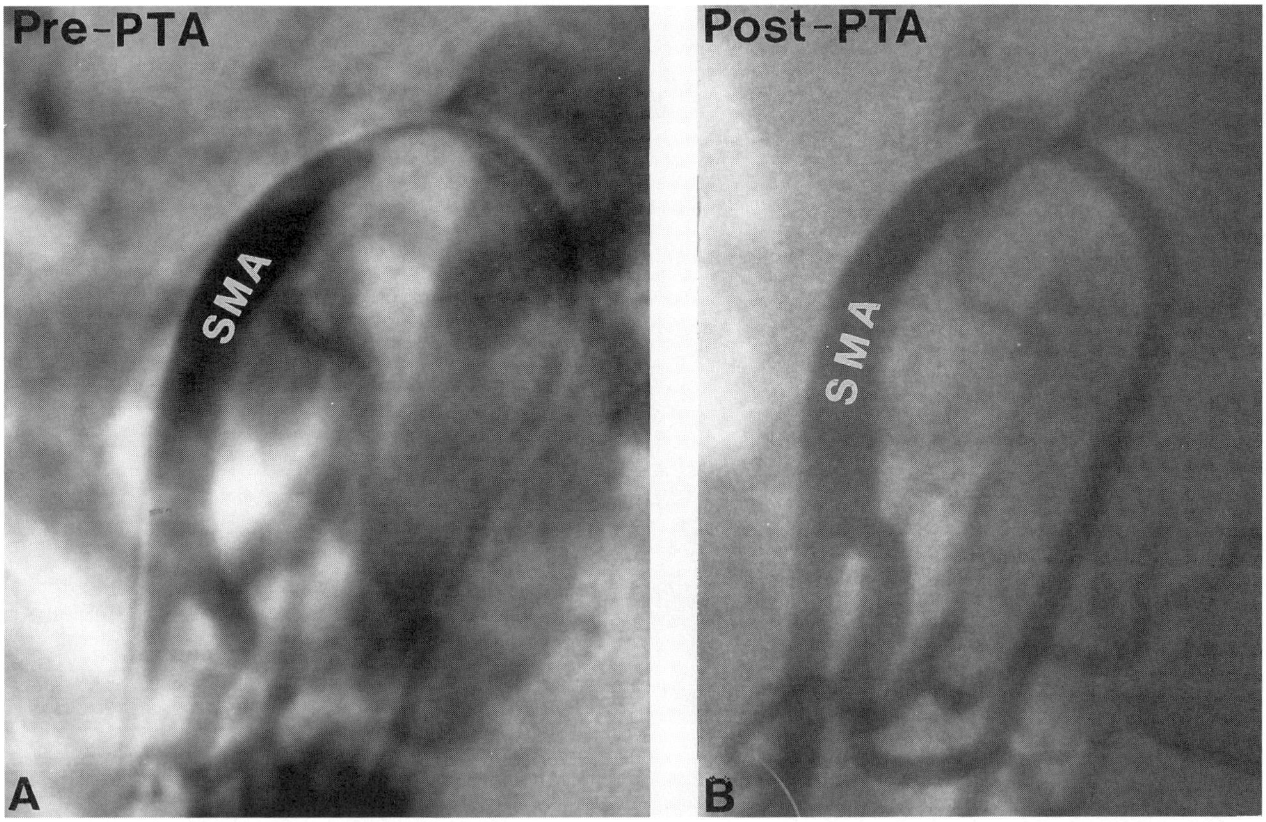

Fig. 31-1. Balloon angioplasty (PTA) of superior mesenteric artery (SMA) in elderly woman with severe intestinal angina. **A.** Selective angiography before PTA demonstrates critical ostial stenosis. Angiogram depicted was obtained only after test injections in multiple other, less optimal angles. **B.** Post-PTA plaque fracture is evident. Presence and distribution of calcium is difficult to discern by angiography and fluoroscopy.

outcome, it is impossible to predict how a given vessel will react to balloon dilation. IVUS, because it consistently demonstrates exquisite detail regarding morphologic alterations in the arterial wall and subjacent plaque, has provided new insight into the effects of angioplasty [24–27]. The fact that IVUS routinely depicts tomographic full-thickness images of the arterial wall, allows, in vivo, a perspective similar to that achieved by histologic examination. Furthermore, the ability to perform serial examinations in vivo enables documentation regarding pathologic alterations attributable to the specific instrumentation employed. These unique features of IVUS have been used to good advantage to study the mechanisms by which balloon angioplasty improves luminal patency.

Observations from IVUS suggest that plaque fracture or dissection is associated with balloon dilation in the majority of angiographically and hemodynamically successful procedures [21]. Indeed, recent data suggest that at least some degree of plaque fracture must be seen by IVUS for a successful long-term result following balloon angioplasty; vessels that display no such fractures may be more prone to recoil or restenosis [28,29]. Moreover, investigations using IVUS suggested that plaque fractures constitute the dominant contribution to the overall increase in luminal dimensions following balloon angioplasty. Losordo et al. [30], for example, evaluated IVUS images obtained before and after PTA in 40 patients and quantified the relative contributions of plaque fracture, plaque compression, and arterial stretch to the enhanced overall luminal area. Total luminal cross-sectional area more than doubled after PTA. The neolumen created by balloon-induced plaque fractures accounted for the majority (72%) of the total increase in luminal area. Compression of plaque made an important, but quantitatively less significant, contribution to postangioplasty increase in luminal area. Arterial stretching was demonstrated in only 25 percent of patients, and, even in that group, its contribution to increased area was minimal. Those IVUS data confirm previous observations from pathologic studies suggesting that plaque fracture constitutes the principal mechanism responsible for increased luminal patency after balloon angioplasty and contradict conclusions based on other studies [31–33] that have implicated stretching of the vessel wall as a major factor.

The presence and the location of calcific deposits also may influence angioplasty outcome. Waller et al. [34] have suggested, based on histologic studies, that tears and fractures typically occur along the border between calcific

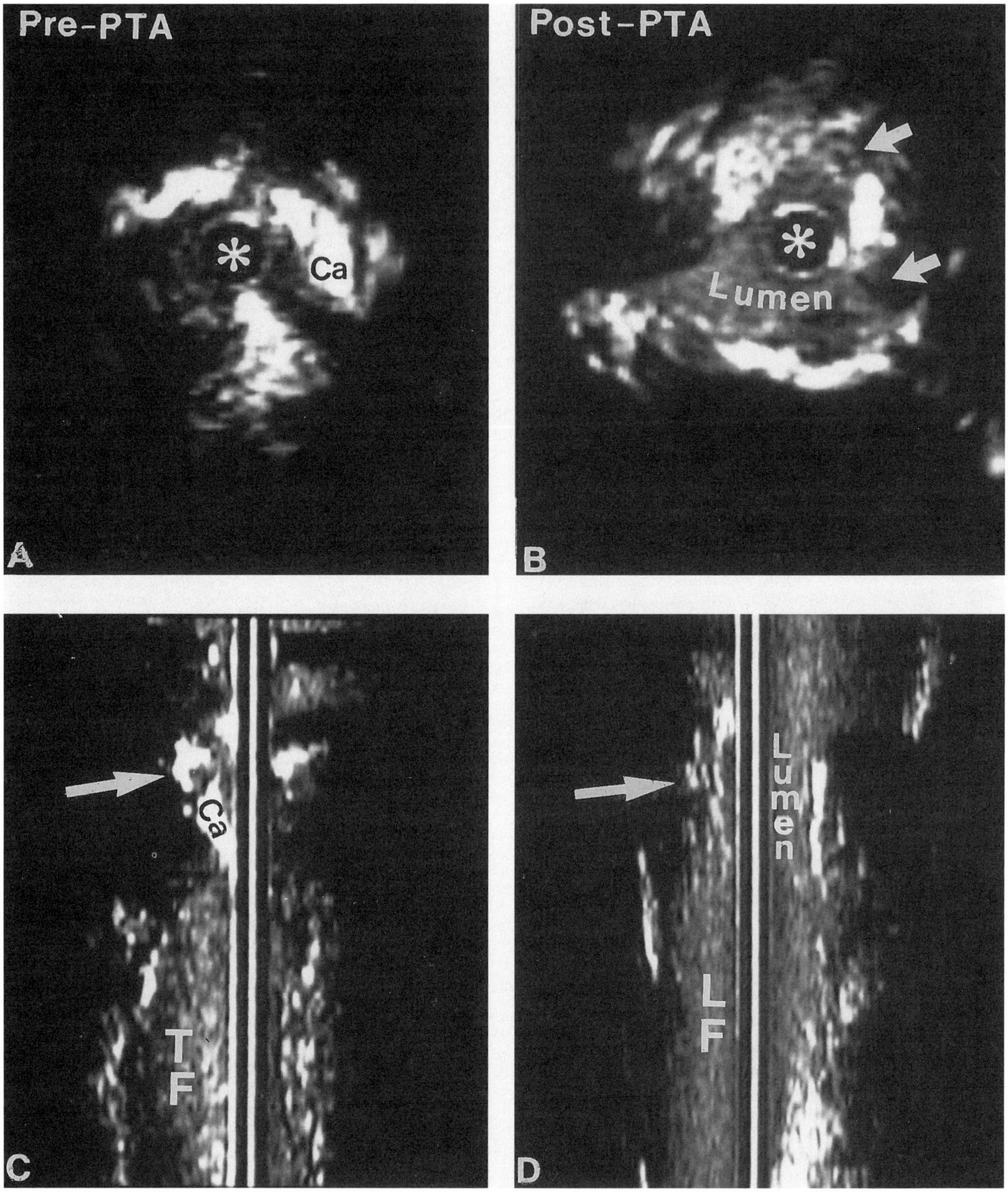

Fig. 31-2. IVUS and sagittal three-dimensional reconstruction during PTA of superior mesenteric artery from Fig. 31-1. **A.** IVUS before PTA demonstrates heavily calcified (Ca) plaque surrounding probe (*asterisk*), not appreciated by angiography (see Fig. 31-1). **B.** IVUS after PTA shows enlargement of lumen due to increased separation or fracture (*arrows*) between calcific deposits. **C.** Sagittal image from serial IVUS frames reconstructs vessel longitudinally, similar in orientation to angiogram, and shows calcific plaque (*arrow*) encroaching on lumen, which has normal dimensions more distally. Coarse echoes in distal lumen indicate turbulent flow (TF) through stenosis. **D.** Sagittal view following PTA. Proximal lumen is partially enlarged at lesion site (*arrow*), and echo signals corresponding to blood flow are now more uniform, indicating more laminar flow (LF).

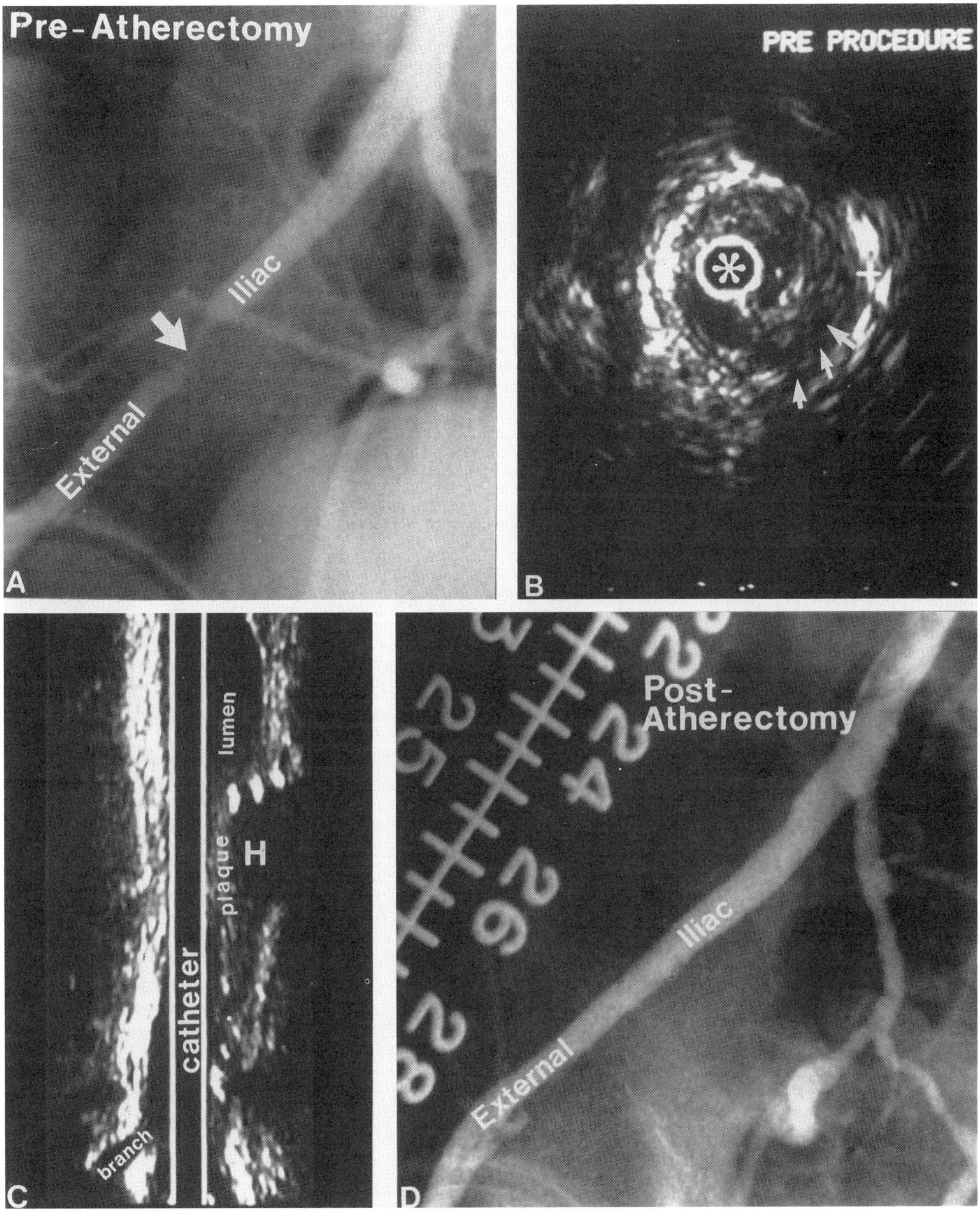

Fig. 31-3. Angiographic and IVUS findings in a patient with crescendo claudication. **A.** Diagnostic arteriogram showing irregular, high-grade stenosis (*arrow*) in right external iliac artery. **B.** Two-dimensional intravascular ultrasound (asterisk indicates the ultrasound transducer) obtained before atherectomy shows heterogeneous plaque with hypoechoic foci that are consistent with plaque hemorrhage (*arrows*), suggesting plaque rupture as possible mechanism for patient's recent onset of symptoms. **C.** Three-dimensional reconstruction of serial IVUS images showing right external iliac artery narrowed by segmental stenosis that abuts ultrasound catheter, encroaching on lumen; hypoechoic foci of plaque hemorrhage (H) now seen in longitudinal disposition. **D.** Angiogram obtained after atherectomy demonstrates successful revascularization.

plaque and softer tissue. Based on that assumption, the increased sensitivity of IVUS in detecting calcific deposits may be clinically relevant. Indeed, Fitzgerald et al. [35] observed that in their angioplasty patients with plaque fractures depicted by IVUS the location of the fracture was virtually always adjacent to a calcific deposit (see Fig. 31-2). Furthermore, the extent of dissection was greater in the patients with calcified vessels than in those with noncalcified vessels, suggesting that the presence of calcium may predict the location and the extent of plaque fracture. To the extent that large dissections may portend a poor angioplasty outcome, the detection and localization of calcium may become a relevant and practical application of IVUS. Further studies are necessary, however, to discriminate the characteristic pattern of those calcific deposits that represent a harbinger of a poor percutaneous transluminal coronary angioplasty (PTCA) result.

Preliminary evidence from in-vivo IVUS studies also has provided insight regarding the mechanisms by which directional atherectomy, stent deployment, and laser angioplasty enhance luminal area. In contrast to vessels undergoing balloon angioplasty, vessels in which directional atherectomy is performed demonstrate less prominent plaque-arterial wall disruption; instead, the perimeter of the neolumen is typically smooth and uninterrupted. In our initial series of patients [36], no plaque cracks were observed on postatherectomy IVUS examination. Instead, discrete "bites," corresponding to individual passes of the cutting blade and consistent with tissue removal, often were observed. Signs of arterial-wall trauma are most completely effaced on IVUS images recorded following delivery of an endovascular stent (Fig. 31-4): The fact that extensive trauma is observed at these same sites postballoon (prestent) suggests that stent implantation acutely ameliorates arterial-wall pathology [37,38].

Regions of Interest

As already mentioned, one of the most compelling justifications for redefining the indications for percutaneous revascularization is the evolution in techniques and technology that has occurred over the past two decades. These developments have not only permitted improved procedural results (e.g., routine treatment of infrapopliteal arteries) but, in some cases, have already documented improved long-term patency (e.g., iliac stents) [4]. Technical features, likelihood of success, and chances for clinical improvement vary in degree according to the region of interest in the peripheral circulation. Weighted consideration of these individual issues is required to determine, for any given combination of lesions, the appropriateness of nonsurgical revascularization. Accordingly, the purpose of this following section is to review briefly what may be anticipated following percutaneous revascularization applied to specific regions of interest in the peripheral vasculature, in terms of both acute and longer-term clinical results.

AORTOILIAC DISEASE

PTA remains the treatment of choice for aortoiliac stenoses (Fig. 31-5). Alternative devices, such as directional and rotational atherectomy, have not been widely employed for these lesions (except for diagnostic purposes [39]) for two reasons. First, the relatively large dimensions of devices typically required for all but the smallest iliac arteries create problems for noninflatable devices. Second, the application of endovascular prostheses (stents) to aortoiliac lesions has dramatically changed the short-term (Figs. 31-4, 31-6) as well as long-term results. Palmaz [40], Gunther [41], Rees [42], and Becker [43] have documented the extent to which stents may be used to rescue flow-limiting complications of iliac PTA. Preliminary findings reported by Richter and colleagues [4,44] have suggested that significant improvements in long-term patency may be achieved in patients randomized to PTA and stent versus PTA alone: the **angiographic** patency (93%) in patients studied at 5-year follow-up rivals the best **clinical** patency reported at a similar time interval in patients undergoing operative revascularization. Those excellent procedural and long-term results of percutaneous revascularization in patients with iliac lesions thus make the physical finding of a diminished femoral pulse a useful sign for identifying patients who are likely to benefit from percutaneous revascularization.

The extent to which lytic therapy may further optimize the treatment of iliac occlusions remains to be defined. There are two specific considerations in this regard. The first is the ability to traverse the segment of occluded artery. That issue already has been addressed by the use of hydrophilic guide wires [45] and novel technical approaches [46–48], the combination of which has yielded an extremely high procedural success rate (Figs. 31-6, 31-7). The second issue concerns distal embolization: it has been suggested that the larger mass required to occlude a large-diameter artery, such as the iliac, might increase the likelihood of embolic complications [49,50]. In patients with an ipsilateral occlusion of the superficial femoral artery (SFA) or single-vessel infrapopliteal runoff, embolic occlusion of the profunda or the tibial and peroneal arteries, respectively, may in fact lead to acute limb-threatening ischemia. Prophylactic administration of lytic therapy, therefore, may be of benefit to such patients.

While the specter of acute limb-threatening ischemia resulting from embolization to a single runoff vessel may serve as a deterrent to direct (nonlytic) recanalization of occluded iliac arteries, the current incidence of embolization in that setting is exceedingly low. Such is particularly the case if one employs a strategy of initial underdilation followed by stent deployment; the stent provides a scaffold that, in theory, affixes the thrombus or plaque to the vessel wall, thus reducing the likelihood of distal embolization. Given the low incidence of embolization with this strategy, primary recanalization and stenting—without lytic therapy—at least for patients with more than a single runoff vessel, provides excellent results and avoids the potential hazards of thrombolytic therapy (see Fig. 31-7).

Clearly, the most common indication for iliac angioplasty is claudication. In some patients with claudication and in rare patients with limb ischemia, the iliac lesion typically coexists with more distal disease involving the SFA or infrapopliteal vessels [51]; in such cases, initial treatment of the iliac obstruction is based on the premise that improving inflow will secondarily improve outflow,

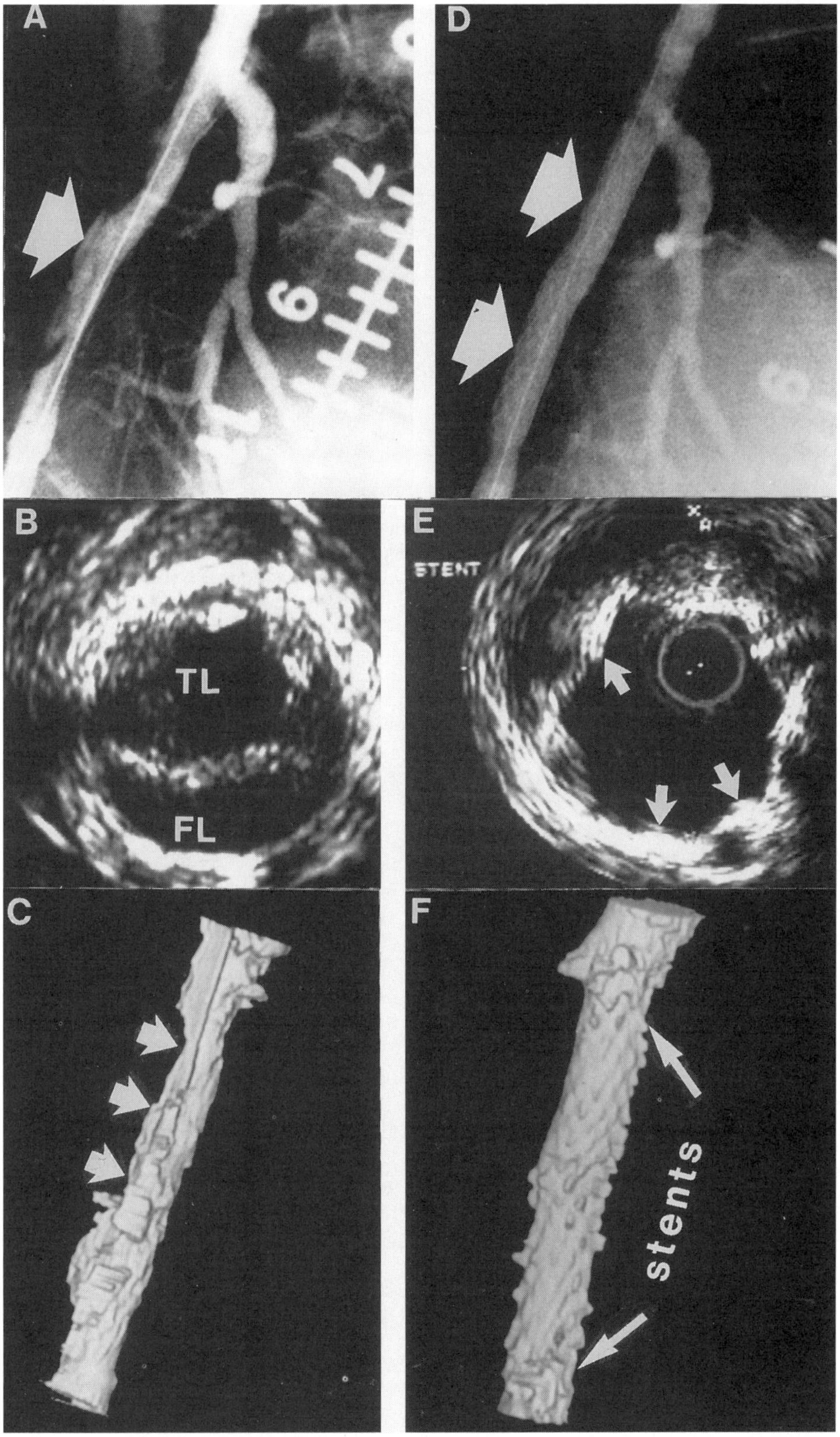

Fig. 31-4.

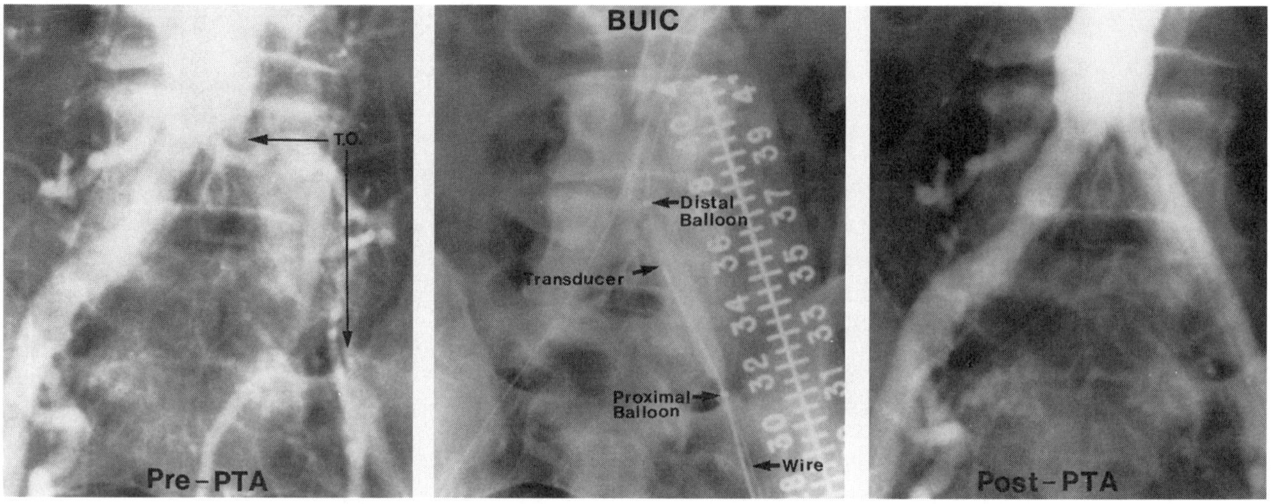

A B C

Fig. 31-5. Angiographic findings pre- and post-PTA of totally occluded left iliac artery using balloon-ultrasound-inflation catheter (BUIC) [29]. This 63-year-old man had been advised 8 years earlier that his symptoms did not warrant operative revascularization. For the subsequent 8 years, his symptoms had remained unchanged. With frequent stops to rest, he could manage several blocks of walking but had been forced to abandon leisure activities such as golfing. **A.** Left iliac totally occluded. **B.** "Pull-through" approach [155] was used to advance guide wire from introducer sheath in right common femoral artery, over aortic bifurcation, antegrade through occlusion, and distally into and through introducer sheath placed in left common femoral artery. Traction placed on externalized guide wire was used to advance BUIC across occluded segment. **C.** Final result. The patient returned to playing golf regularly and has remained asymptomatic during 5 years of follow-up examinations.

either via the profunda in the case of an occluded SFA (Fig. 31-8) or by increasing the head of perfusion pressure to that segment of the infrapopliteal circulation that remains patent. Implicit in this strategy is the lesser degree of technical difficulty, high incidence of procedural success, and low rate of restenosis associated with iliac PTA. Moreover, PTA avoids the complication of iatrogenic postoperative impotence, reported to complicate 10–25 percent of aortoiliac operations [52,53].

A similar strategy underlies the preparatory role of iliac angioplasty in patients undergoing surgical revascularization for treatment of distal disease [51,54,55]. Percutaneous revascularization of an iliac lesion may be required to facilitate patency of a downstream femoral-popliteal conduit designed to bypass an occluded SFA. Alternatively, nonsurgical revascularization of an iliac site may be employed in conjunction with surgery to lower the anastomotic site and thereby reduce the risk of operative revascularization in patients judged to be high risk due to coronary heart disease or other illnesses. For example, in the patient with a lengthy unilateral occlusion of one iliac artery and less extensive obstruction of the contralateral side, higher-risk aortofemoral bypass surgery may be obviated by percutaneous treatment of the less diseased iliac artery, followed by a cross-femoral graft to the contralateral femoral artery (Fig. 31-9).

Occasionally, even when the need for cross-femoral grafting is anticipated, treatment of the contralateral artery may enable better collateralization and unexpectedly obviate the need for surgery altogether. Such was the case

Fig. 31-4. Amelioration of post-PTA dissection of external iliac artery using stents. **A.** Post-PTA angiogram demonstrates extensive dissection (*arrow*) in external iliac artery. **B.** Representative IVUS frame shows extent of arterial wall trauma, with large dissection flap interposed between true lumen (TL) and false lumen (FL). **C.** Three-dimensional reconstruction of serial IVUS images creates a "cast" of the vascular lumen, narrowed by dissection and encroaching false lumen (*arrows*). **D.** Angiogram following deployment of two Palmaz stents (*arrows*) shows improved patency, but interface between stent and vessel wall not delineated. **E.** IVUS image from stent site demonstrates amelioration of arterial-wall pathology with effacement of dissection by expanded stent. Struts identified by arrows. **F.** Three-dimensional cast of stented iliac artery now depicts uniform dimensions throughout length of vessel, with resolution of luminal narrowing. Cobblestoned appearance of struts is evident.

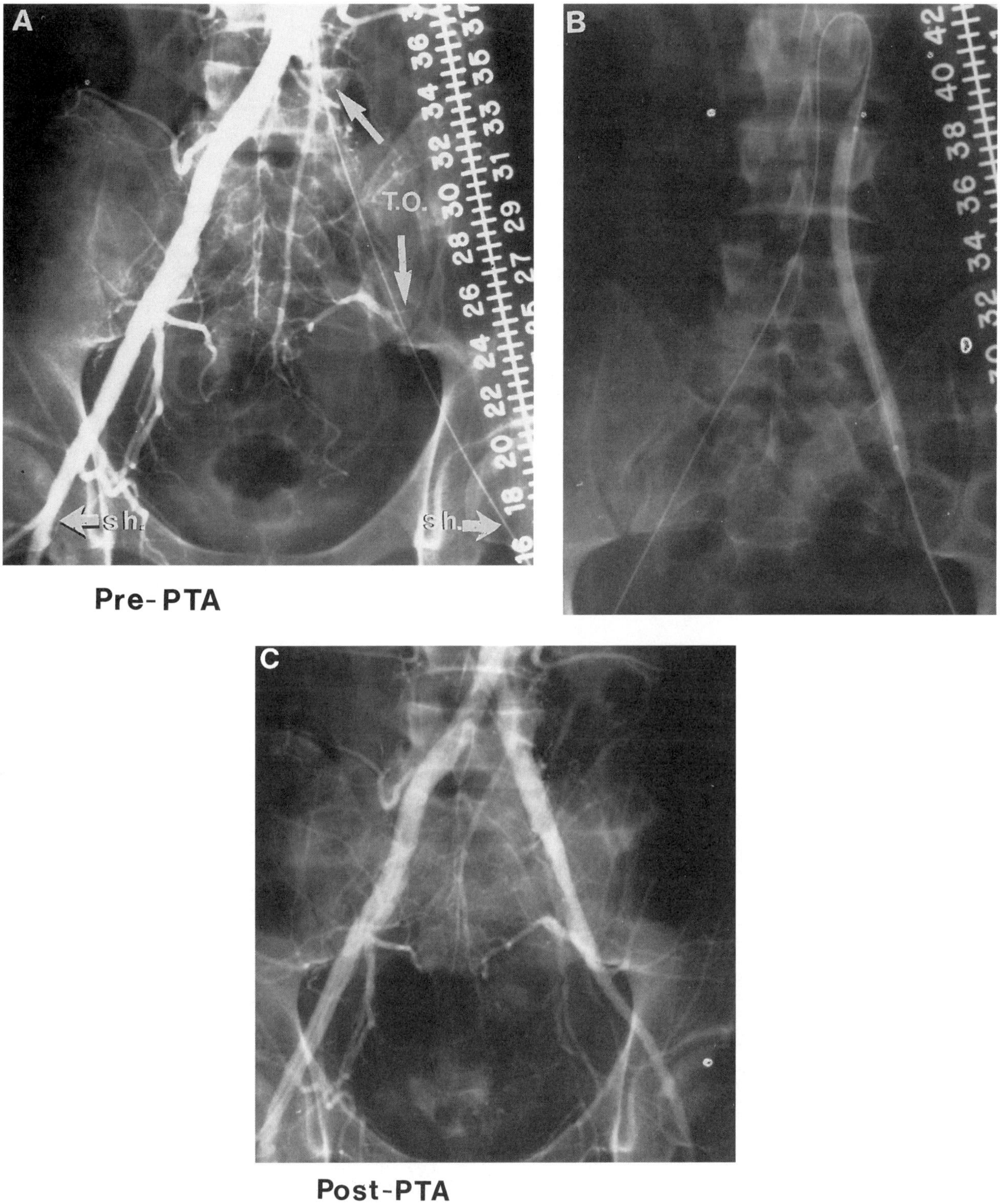

Fig. 31-6. Recanalization of 10 cm long common iliac occlusion using hydrophilic guide wire. This 39-year-old man complained of a 2-year history of left leg claudication at 1½ blocks, severely limiting his lifestyle. **A.** 10-cm occlusion was transversed with a hydrophilic guide wire (Glidewire, Terumo) antegrade from the contralateral (right) side, after unsuccessful attempts at retrograde recanalization. The guide wire was fed into the left femoral sheath, such that both ends of the same wire were outside the body ("pull-through" technique). **B.** The balloon was then advanced retrograde from the left, maintaining traction on the wire from the right to help pull through the resistant occlusion. **C.** Following PTA, left common iliac artery is patent. The patient was rendered asymptomatic, which he remains 4 years post-PTA.

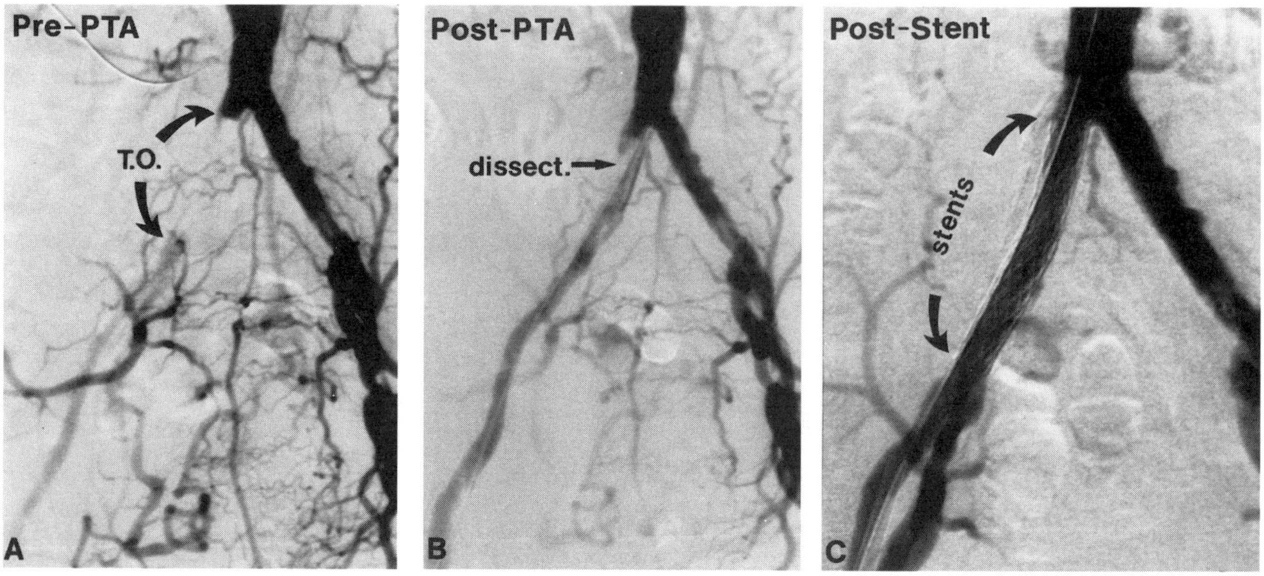

Fig. 31-7. PTA and stent deployment in chronically occluded right common iliac artery. **A.** Baseline angiogram demonstrates 5-cm total occlusion (T.O.) of right common iliac artery with reconstitution of external and internal iliac arteries. Occlusion was crossed using combination of angled and straight Glidewire, buttressed by a 4F catheter. **B.** Post-PTA angiogram demonstrating patent common iliac artery with extensive dissection. **C.** Final angiogram following deployment of two Palmaz stents. Common iliac artery is widely patent. Baseline mean gradient of 37 mm Hg was reduced to 1 mm Hg.

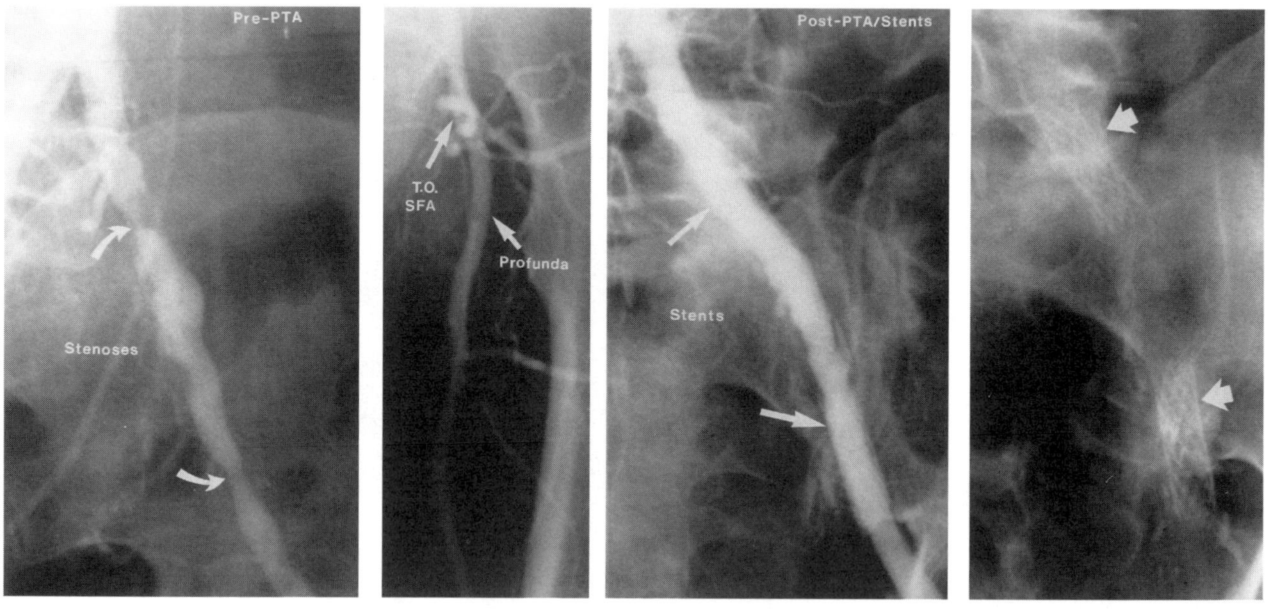

Fig. 31-8. PTA and stent used for serial stenoses in left iliac artery **A.** associated with flush total occlusion (T.O.) of left superficial femoral artery (SFA) **B.** Strategy in this case is designed to perform what is a technically more straightforward and durable percutaneous procedure—iliac PTA-stent **C.** versus recanalization of SFA T.O.—and utilize improved inflow from iliac to augment outflow via profunda. **D.** Radiograph of stents (*arrows*). Patient, formerly Rutherford class 3, remains asymptomatic 4 years postrevascularization.

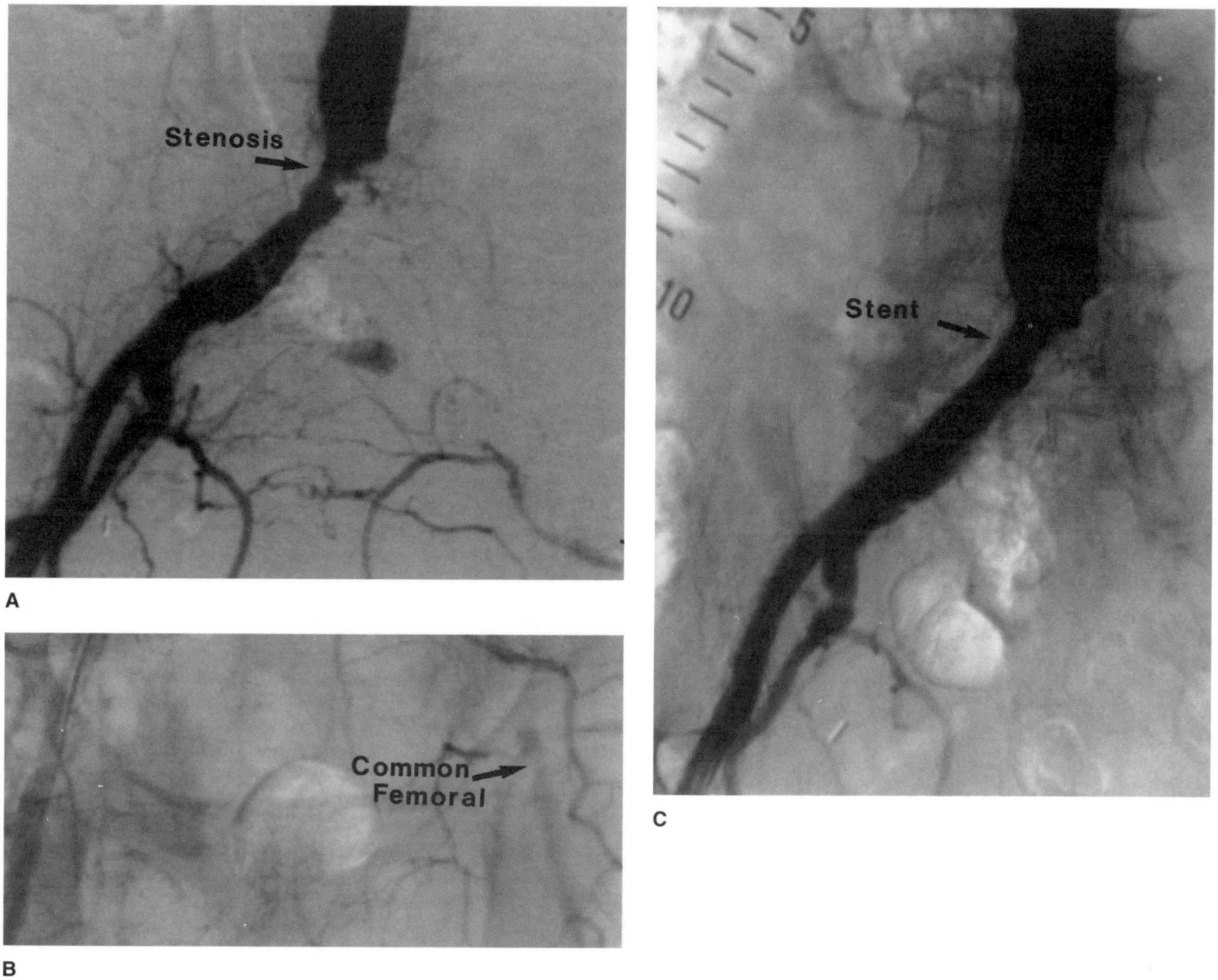

Fig. 31-9. Preparatory role of iliac PTA in patient undergoing surgical revascularization for distal disease. Patient had chronic lymphoma with extensive retroperitoneal and inguinal adenopathy and was a poor candidate for major (aortofemoral) reconstructive surgery. Surgical risk was reduced by PTA-stent therapy of right common iliac artery in preparation for cross-femoral grafting from right to left common femoral artery. **A.** Stenosis pre-PTA. **B.** Reconstitution of left common femoral artery. **C.** After stent deployment, normal flow and pressure were restored to right iliac artery, which subsequently served as the donor artery for cross-femoral grafting.

in the patient whose angiograms are demonstrated in Fig. 31-10. This 62-year-old woman with severe coronary artery disease and rest pain in the right leg underwent dilation of aortic and left common femoral artery stenoses, in preparation for left-to-right cross-femoral grafting. However, following the percutaneous procedure, symptoms in the right leg unexpectedly resolved, presumably the result of increased perfusion pressure to collateral vessels arising from the left internal iliac artery. Surgery was cancelled, and the patient remains asymptomatic 3 years later.

Two additional issues regarding percutaneous treatment of aortoiliac disease deserve specific comment. The first concerns the role of percutaneous revascularization in modifying the treatment of patients with cardiac disease undergoing vascular surgery [56]. Nowhere is this issue more relevant than in patients with coronary heart disease and aortoiliac occlusive disease, such as the patient just described, in whom abdominal surgery is associated with a marked increase in cardiac morbidity and mortality [57–60]. Recent work from several groups [61,62] has demonstrated the feasibility of intraluminal insertion of a graft-stent prosthesis for the treatment of abdominal aortic aneurysms. Although much less common than aneurysmal dilation, stenoses of the aorta are treated routinely and effectively by PTA [63–65] (Figs. 31-11 and 31-12; also see Fig. 31-10). Quite common is the situation described previously, in which percutaneous treatment of the aortoiliac lesion permits surgical revascularization to be adjusted one level caudal, obviating the risk associated with aortic-level surgery (see Fig. 31-9).

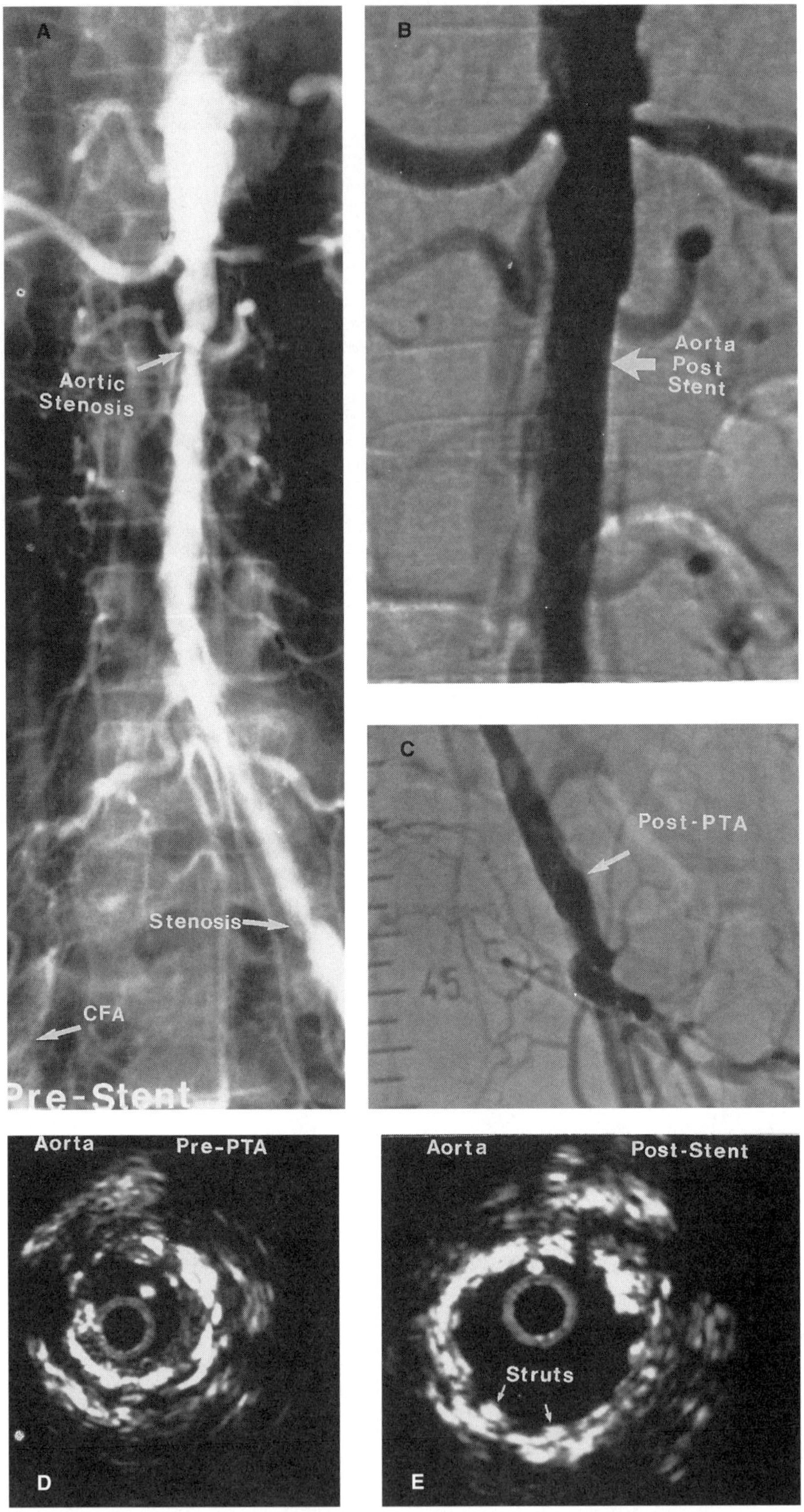

Fig. 31-10. PTA of aorta and common iliac artery in nonischemic (left) side in preparation for cross-femoral graft leads to unexpected resolution of ischemic pain. Patient is a 62-year-old woman, a poor surgical candidate, with rest pain and severe claudication in right leg **(A)**. Occlusion of right common iliac artery and stenoses in infrarenal aorta and left common iliac artery pre-PTA. Initial strategy was to dilate the stenotic sites, then graft from left to right common femoral artery (CFA). Following PTA-stent of aorta **(B)** and PTA alone of iliac artery **(C)** patient's right (contralateral) leg symptoms disappeared, presumably due to increased left-to-right collateral flow via internal iliac-artery tributaries. The planned cross-femoral bypass surgery was cancelled; patient remains asymptomatic 3 years post-PTA. PTA was guided by IVUS, which demonstrates marked improvement in lumen cross-sectional area of aortic lesion from pre-PTA **(D)** to post-stent **(E)**. Asterisk denotes IVUS catheter.

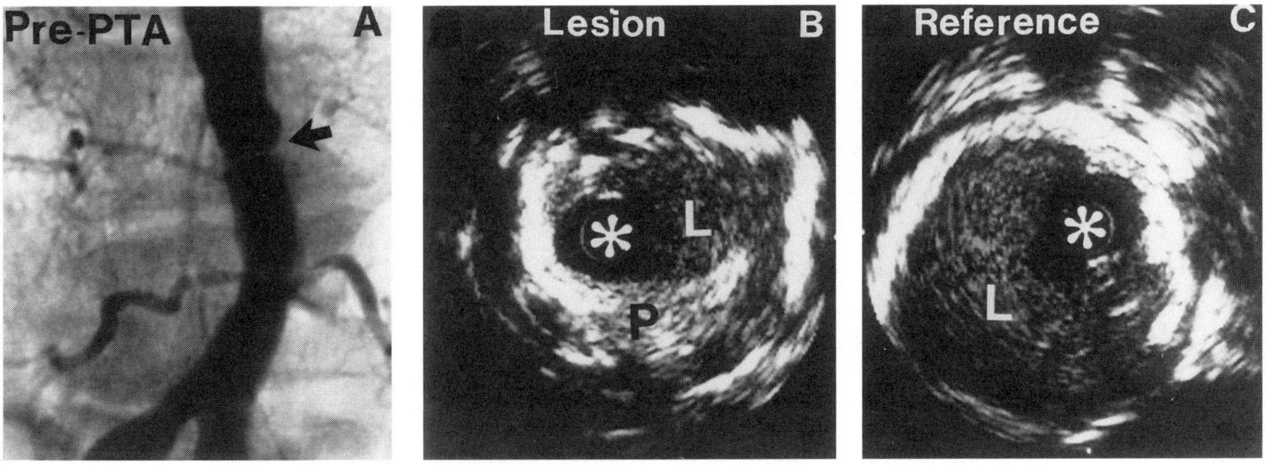

Fig. 31-11. Superior imaging of eccentric aortic lesion by IVUS compared to angiography. This 63-year-old woman presented with accelerated bilateral buttocks claudication, occurring at 1–2 blocks. **A.** Conventional anteroposterior angiography failed to disclose any significant stenosis; mild irregularity (*arrow*) was seen within the distal aorta. After discovering a large pressure gradient (see Fig. 31-13), IVUS exam was performed. **B.** IVUS image depicting focal, eccentric plaque (P) narrowing the lumen (L) in distal aorta. **C.** IVUS from reference site distal to stenosis depicts normal lumen dimensions. Asterisk indicates the IVUS catheter.

The second issue involves angiographic assessment of aortic and iliac stenoses. Clinical experience with IVUS has documented the extent to which conventional diagnostic angiography may underestimate hemodynamically significant luminal narrowing in tortuous common and external iliac arteries [66–70]. In particular, the ostium of the common iliac, as well as the common iliac bifurcation, may be problematic in this regard. Eccentric lesions in the distal aorta may pose the same problem (see Figs. 31-11 and 31-12). IVUS permits direct planimetry of luminal cross-sectional narrowing at these sites, obviating the multiple, angulated angiographic views required to unwind or eliminate sites of vessel overlap, which may obscure important luminal obstruction. The improved anatomic definition afforded by ultrasound examination can then be used in conjunction with physiologic indices, including intra-arterial measurement of translesion pressure gradient (Fig. 31-13) and intra-arterial Doppler-measurement of flow velocity [65], to identify those lesions appropriate for revascularization.

The importance of using multiple modalities—IVUS and pressure gradients—in addition to angiography is underscored in complex cases of percutaneous revascularization. This is particularly so in the aorta, where, due to its deep location, the difficulty in obtaining angulated views and the presence of multiple important side branches, the effect of dilation may be angiographically ambiguous. Delineation of the effects of intervention and subsequent guidance by IVUS may greatly facilitate the execution of percutaneous procedures at the aortic level, enabling safer and more effective treatment (Fig. 31-14).

FEMORAL AND POPLITEAL ARTERIES

Previous experience has failed to document any significant differences in either acute or long-term results for percutaneous revascularization of the SFA versus the popliteal arteries; accordingly, both will be considered here together under the heading of SFA. The acute procedural success for percutaneous revascularization of **nonocclusive**, that is, stenotic, lesions in the SFA using conventional guide wires and standard PTA currently approaches 100 percent. That rate contrasts with the results of earlier reports [71–75] that described acute success rates as low as 72 percent. It must be recognized, however, that the less optimal results described in the earlier reports reflect two issues. First, many of these reports combined analyses of total occlusions together with stenoses. Second, many of the patients described in those reports (including one as recent as 1985 [72]) included patients treated with nonballoon (coaxial 8-French/12-French Dotter catheters or tapered Teflon dilating) catheters. Routine use first of the double-lumen, polyvinylchloride-balloon dilating catheter introduced by Gruentzig in 1976 [3] and subsequently of catheters with lower-profile (5-French) shafts and polyethylene balloons accounts in large part for the consistently favorable acute results typical of current practice.

Stenoses of the SFA and Popliteal Artery. The acute procedural success that can be achieved in SFA stenoses is similar to that reported for iliac stenoses. Long-term patency in the SFA, however, is clearly inferior to that expected in iliac stenoses. Five-year patency rates varying from 47 percent to 70 percent [72–76] have been reported for SFA revascularization; the variability in long-term follow-up results is due, in part, to the multiple lengths and morphologies of SFA lesions selected for treatment, as well as the aforementioned mixture of stenoses with occlusions and nonballoon- with balloon-dilated cases. Those factors, however, pale by comparison to the variable manner in which vessel patency has been defined or evaluated,

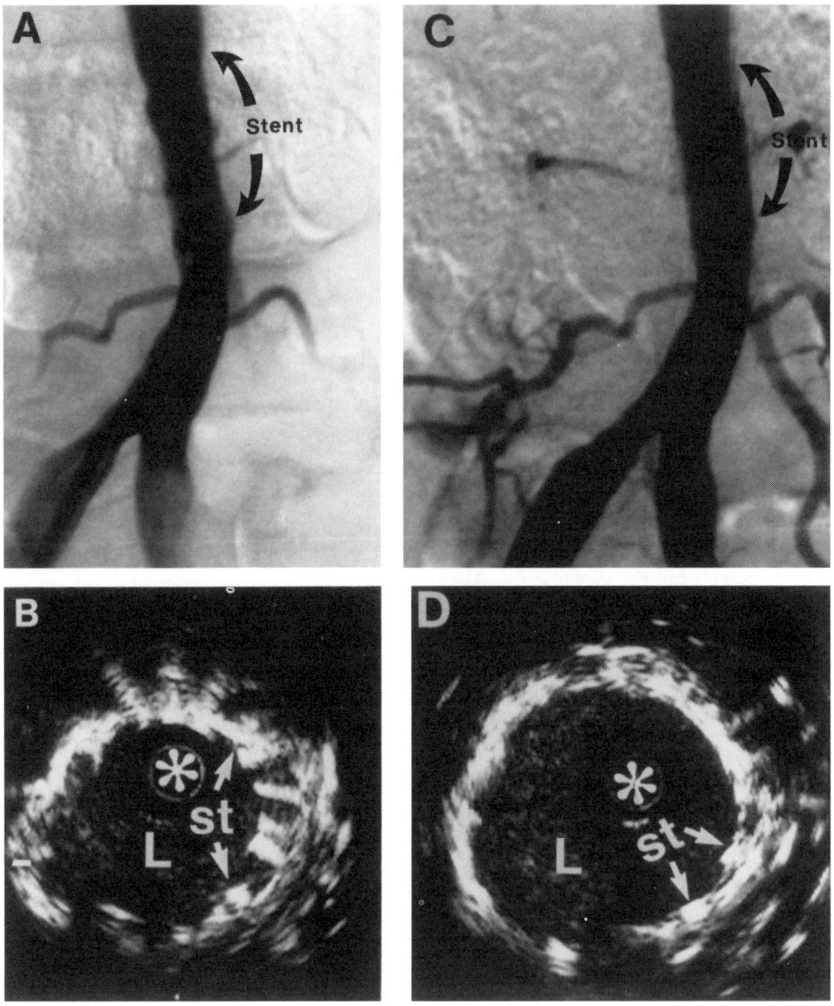

Fig. 31-12. Stent underexpansion detected by IVUS. PTA and stent deployment in eccentric aortic lesion from Fig. 31-11. **A.** Angiogram after deployment of Palmaz stent with 9-mm balloon depicts ostensibly good result, without obvious compromise in lumen or stent. **B.** Although lumen (L) is now enlarged compared to pre-PTA (Fig. 31-11), IVUS after 9-mm PTA-stent demonstrates stent underexpansion, with all struts (st) between 2 and 5 o'clock not in apposition to arterial wall. **C.** Angiogram following 12-mm PTA shows slight decrease in luminal irregularity where stent has been redilated (*arrows*). **D.** IVUS after 12-mm PTA demonstrates complete expansion of stent, with all struts (st) now completely apposed to arterial wall and overall lumen (L) area further increased.

whether initial failures are or are not excluded from long-term analyses, and the statistical measures employed to analyze long-term follow-up [77]. In a recently published prospective analysis of PTA of 208 lesions in 140 limbs (106 claudicants), Matsi and associates reported an overall technical (angiographic) success rate of 88 percent and a successful clinical outcome in 91 percent of SFA lesions [78]. Evaluation by Doppler waveforms 1 day post-PTA demonstrated hemodynamic success in 99 percent of stenoses and 80 percent of occlusions. Systematic, prospective long-term follow-up of all study patients using ankle-brachial indices and clinical symptoms revealed primary patency rates of 47 percent, 44 percent, and 43 percent in patients evaluated at the 1-, 2-, and 3-year marks, respectively. Secondary patency was 63 percent at 1 year and 59 percent at both 2 and 3 years. Predictors of long-term patency included fewer stenoses, shorter lesion length, better runoff, and concentric morphology.

A variety of novel technologies have been investigated as potential means of improving long-term patency and reducing restenosis following SFA revascularization. It must be emphasized that all these techniques, including directional atherectomy, laser angioplasty, rotational atherectomy, and endovascular stents, have in common the fact that they are wire guided and therefore limited to the treatment of stenoses or otherwise successfully recanalized occlusions. Among these new devices, directional atherectomy has been employed most widely. The fact that atherosclerotic plaque resected by directional atherectomy is preserved intact and in a form suitable for a

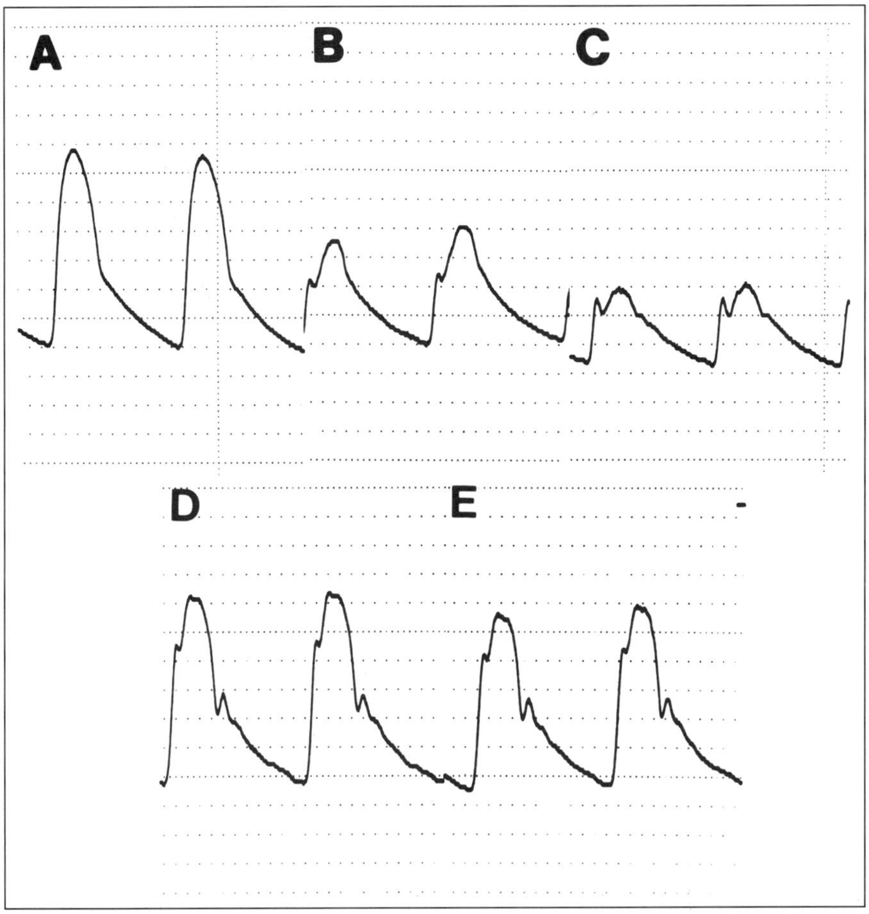

Fig. 31-13. Intra-arterial transstenotic pressure gradient pre- and post-PTA in patient from Figs. 31-11 and 31-12. **A.** Baseline BP from aorta proximal to lesion. **B.** BP obtained simultaneously from aorta distal to lesion demonstrates peak gradient of 30 mm Hg, which becomes exacerbated after administration of intra-arterial nitroglycerin **(C).** Proximal **(D)** and distal **(E)** aortic pressures post-PTA-stent are nearly identical, indicating hemodynamic improvement.

variety of laboratory analyses confers to that modality a unique diagnostic function. Studies of atherectomy specimens performed using conventional light microscopy [79,80] as well as more contemporary molecular biologic techniques [81–84] suggest that it may play a critical role in providing human tissues to develop novel biopharmaceutical agents for the treatment of restenosis. Moreover, recent attempts to exploit the biopsy capabilities unique to directional atherectomy have raised the intriguing possibility that application of molecular techniques to the analysis of atherectomy tissue might prospectively identify those patients likely to develop restenosis [85].

The superiority of directional atherectomy from a therapeutic standpoint remains less clear. In patients with short, eccentric lesions, directional atherectomy (with or without adjunctive PTA) appears to offer acute procedural results similar to those reported for PTA [80,86–90]. The impact of directional atherectomy on subsequent restenosis, however, remains controversial; unlike the recently completed Coronary Angioplasty Versus Excisional Atherectomy Trial (CAVEAT) [91], no randomized trial of PTA versus directional atherectomy has yet to be reported. Most nonrandomized studies [80,88,90] thus far have been unable to demonstrate, even for selected groups, significant reduction in restenosis among patients treated by directional atherectomy. These preliminary findings may be explained in part by the unpredictable extent to which augmented patency results from the catheter-versus-balloon-versus-cutter effects of the atherectomy device (Fig. 31-15).

Rotational atherectomy [92,93] has not yet been demonstrated to have an advantage for SFA revascularization, save for those rare patients in whom the extent of calcific deposits renders the lesions refractory to alternative techniques. Furthermore, the disproportionately large introducer sheath required to accommodate appropriately sized devices represents a potential disadvantage for SFA rotational atherectomy. In the smaller popliteal artery, it is possible that the debulking effect of rotational atherectomy ultimately may prove to offer some benefit over balloon angioplasty alone (Fig. 31-16).

The role of laser angioplasty in SFA revascularization remains investigational. A variety of laser sources have been investigated for this application, including thermal ("hot-tip") systems [94–99], continuous wave (CW) lasers such as Nd:YAG [100], and pulsed-laser systems using

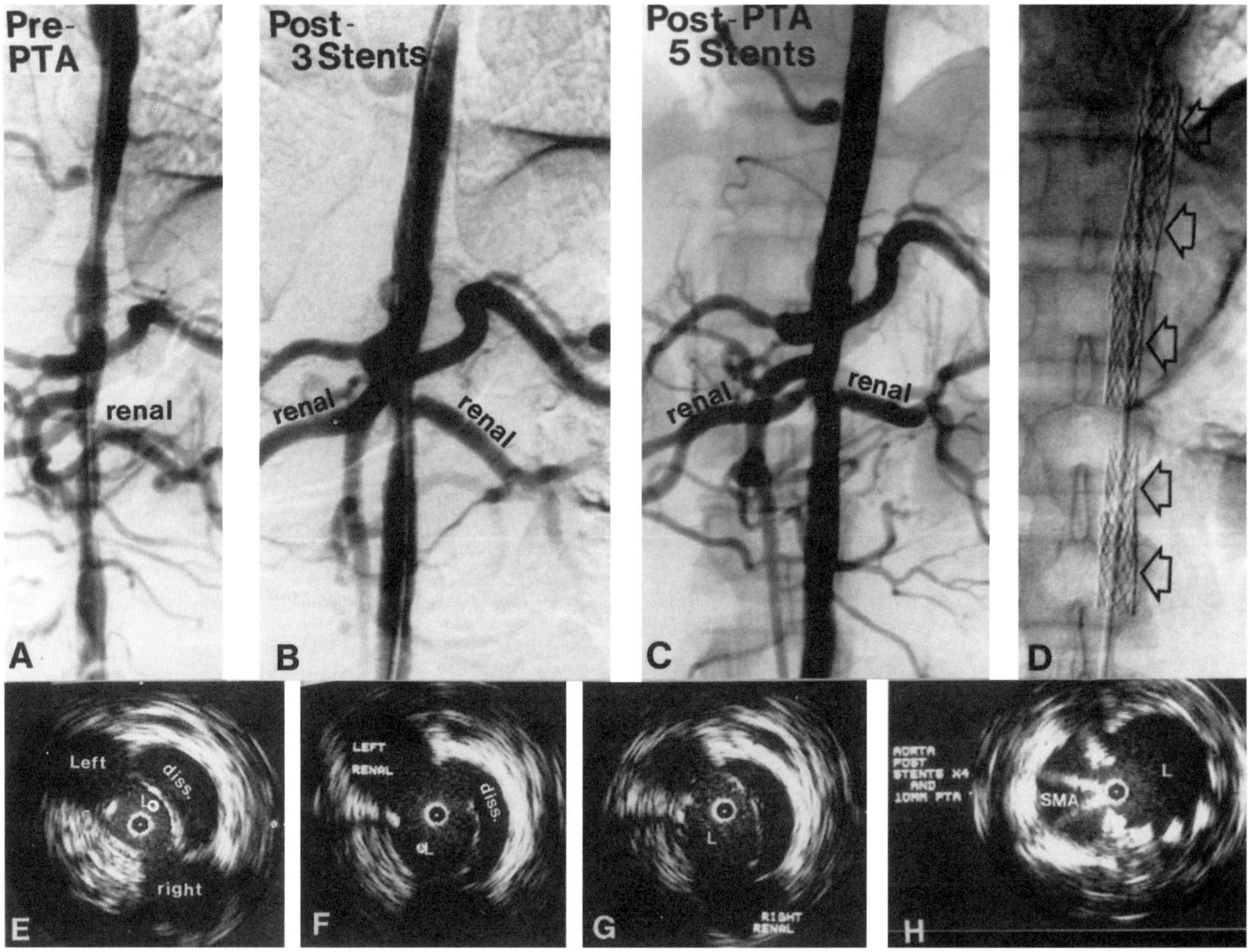

Fig. 31-14. Revascularization of abdominal aortic stenosis with PTA–multiple stents under IVUS guidance. This 30-year-old woman presented with malignant hypertension and nonpalpable femoral pulses due to abdominal aortic coarctation, thought to be secondary to Takayasu's disease, now apparently quiescent. **A.** Angiogram pre-PTA demonstrates extensive disease in the aorta, both above and below the renal arteries. **B.** Following PTA above and below the renal arteries and placement of three stents, result appears reasonable by angiography, although moderate stenosis remains below and at level of renal arteries. IVUS image **(E)** at take-off of renals (left, right) demonstrates large dissection (diss.) extending from proximal PTA site, encroaching on renal-artery ostia and narrowing aortic lumen (L). **C.** Redilated aorta, with two additional stents, shows no encroachment at level of renal arteries. IVUS frames **(F)** and **(G)** confirm persistence of dissection (diss.), but concurrent enlargement of aortic lumen (L) and elimination of obstruction leading into renal arteries (left renal, right renal). **D.** Stents (*arrows*) in aorta. **H.** IVUS of stent in mid-aorta depicts struts overlying origin of superior mesenteric artery (SMA); struts cast shadows into SMA but do not compromise blood flow **(C)**.

either visible (flash-lamp-pumped dye) [101–103], infrared (holmium) [104], or ultraviolet (excimer) [105] wavelengths. Thermal systems are now a dead issue: experience with the hot tip systems demonstrated in dramatic fashion the multiple unfavorable consequences of heat applied to the vasculature [106–109]. The lesser degree of heating resulting from pulsed-laser systems [110] is essential for vascular applications. While all three pulsed wavelengths continue to be investigated for SFA revascularization, our own clinical experience with the excimer (Figs. 31-17 and 31-18) has been more favorable than with the alternative wavelengths. In occasional cases, the excimer laser clearly has facilitated completion of revascularization that was refractory to conventional techniques (Fig. 31-19). While there is preliminary evidence [111] to suggest that the thrombolytic properties of excimer-laser radiation may be exploited to reduce the need for thrombolytic therapy in selected patients (Fig. 31-20), that application requires further confirmation. Evidence that excimer-laser angioplasty can reduce restenosis remains the subject of ongoing study [102,112].

In contrast to the documented reduction in restenosis

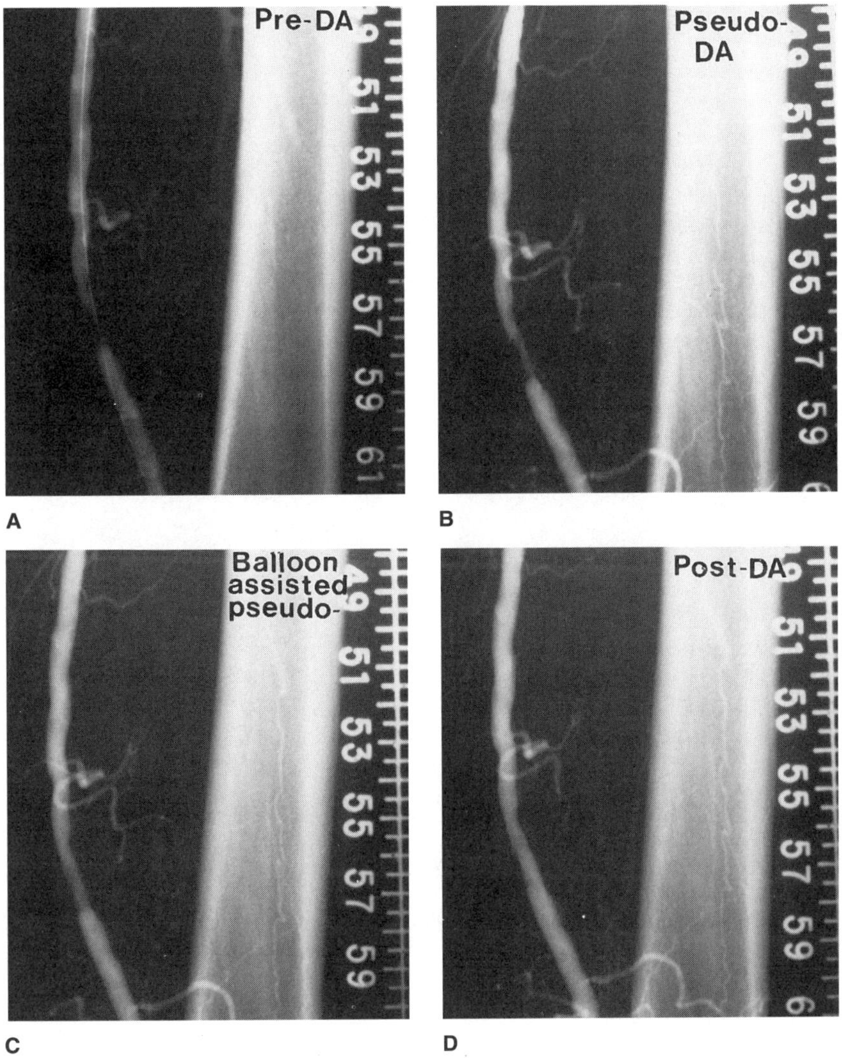

Fig. 31-15. Incremental luminal patency resulting from individual components of directional atherectomy (DA). **A.** Angiogram shows high-grade stenosis in superficial femoral artery (SFA), pre-DA. **B.** Angiogram shows improved luminal patency resulting from Dotter effect of advancing DA catheter through lesion (no balloon inflation, no atherectomy). **C.** Angiogram shows further improvement in luminal patency resulting from balloon inflation (2 atm) without activating cutter. **D.** Angiogram shows final result accomplished by activating cutter.

achieved by the use of endovascular stents for iliac PTA, early experience with endovascular stents in the SFA has been less favorable. Preliminary results with a variety of stent designs [41,113,114] have failed to demonstrate a significant reduction in restenosis following SFA revascularization. In further contrast to results reported for iliac applications, the use of stents in the SFA has been complicated by an unpredictable incidence of subacute thrombosis and, thus, uncertainty regarding the need for short-term and possibly even long-term anticoagulation [114]. Full analysis of these early results may ultimately identify certain anatomic factors—for example, lesion length and distal runoff—that may discriminate among optimal versus suboptimal candidates for SFA stents. It is likely, however, that the use of stents in the SFA will be governed principally by the size of the artery itself; in the coronary circulation, for example, current data suggest that the larger the dimensions of the native artery, the greater the likelihood of favorable short- and long-term outcome [5]. It remains to be seen whether stents in the SFA will further improve long-term patency, as has been the case for the iliac vessels. The issue is currently being addressed in the Femoral Artery Stent Trial (FAST), in which patients with SFA lesions 10 cm or shorter are randomized to receive either balloon angioplasty alone or Palmaz stents (Figs. 31-21 and 31-22).

Occlusion of the SFA and Popliteal Artery. In contrast to the coronary vasculature, in which stenotic lesions are the rule and occlusions the exception, the distribution of lesions in the SFA is the reverse: among patients studied angiographically for consideration of revascularization, occlu-

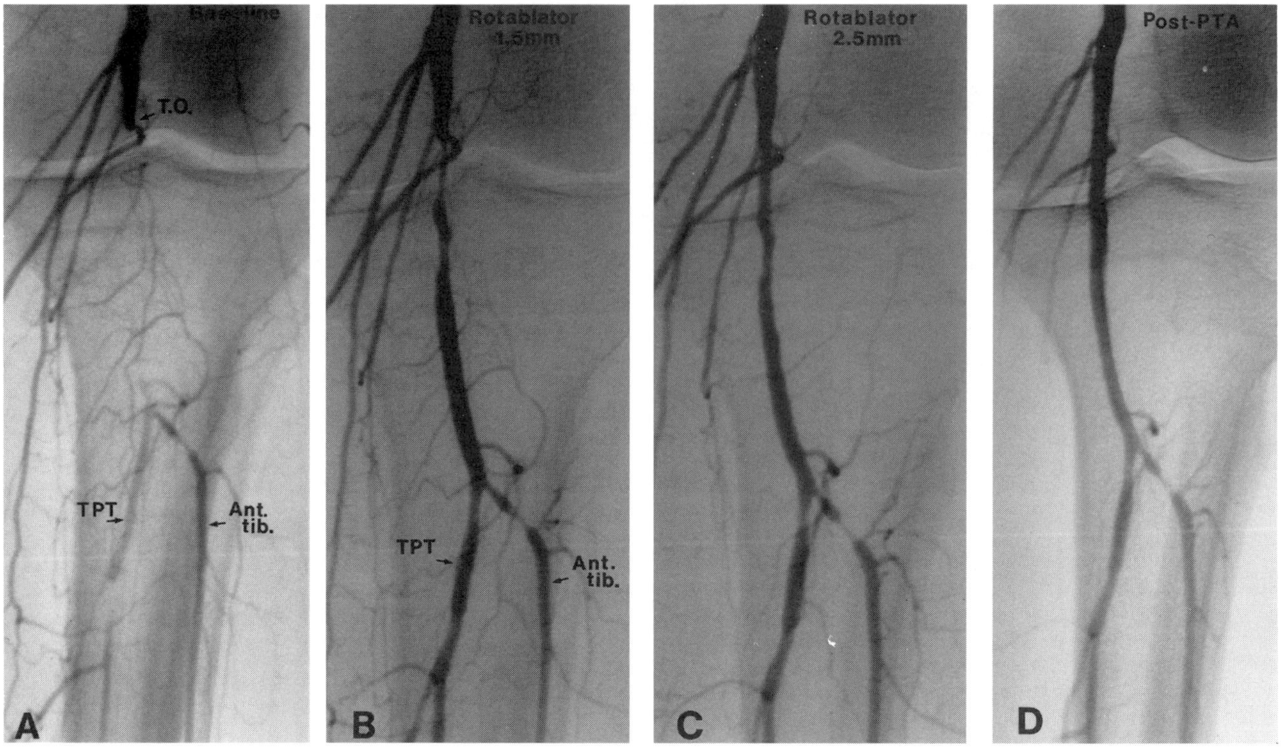

Fig. 31-16. Rotational atherectomy recanalization of occluded popliteal artery in a 74-year-old man with rest pain in the left ankle and foot. **A.** Baseline angiogram shows total occlusion of popliteal artery, with reconstitution of anterior tibial artery (Ant. tib.) and tibioperoneal trunk (TPT). Progressive enlargement of neolumen occurs after treatment with 1.5 mm **(B)** and 2.5 mm **(C)** rotational atherectomy burrs. **D.** Following angioplasty (5-mm balloon), popliteal artery restored to normal caliber without gross evidence of plaque fracture.

sions are more prevalent than stenoses. And while the long-term implications for revascularization of SFA and coronary occlusions are similar—both are associated with a high likelihood of recurrence [71–74,115,116]—the likelihood of achieving short-term patency, that is, acute procedural success, is higher for SFA occlusions. This is the case even for long (>10 cm) SFA occlusions (see Figs. 31-17 and 31-18) and is due largely to two technical modifications.

The first modification is the use of hydrophilic wires, for example, the Glidewire™*. Among 109 consecutive patients at our institution in whom the Glidewire was used to attempt percutaneous revascularization of SFA total occlusions, the Glidewire was successfully advanced across the occluded segment in 107 patients (98%); balloon angioplasty alone or in combination with directional atherectomy or laser angioplasty was then used to complete percutaneous revascularization in all 107 patients in whom Glidewire recanalization was successful [45]. Ankle-brachial index improved from 0.48 ± 0.02 prerevascularization to 0.82 ± 0.02 postrevascularization. Improvement in Rutherford class by one or more grades was observed in 96 (94%) of 102 patients seen at 1-month follow-up. This experience was noteworthy because, unlike most previous reports, which have excluded occlusions more than 10 cm long, patients in this series were not excluded on the basis of lesion length. Among the 107 SFA occlusions, 50 measured 5–10 cm in length, and 21 were more than 20 cm long; consequently, mean occlusion length (9.8 cm) exceeded that reported in most previous series.

The improved acute procedural success, described previously, achieved with the Glidewire has two important implications. First, the demonstrated efficacy of the Glidewire in a variety of anatomically complex, including lengthy, arterial occlusions clearly extends the spectrum of patients who may be candidates for percutaneous revascularization. Second, the high success rate achieved with the Glidewire constitutes a new standard against which novel instruments [94–97,104,117–120] developed for treatment of occluded peripheral arteries and grafts should be judged.

The second factor that has contributed to improved procedural success in crossing SFA occlusions is the increasingly aggressive use of thrombolytic therapy. Lytic therapy has, in fact, been advocated and proved effective even for *chronic* total occlusions. That is because occlusion of the lower-extremity arteries typically is characterized

* Glidewire is a registered trademark of the Terumo Corporation, Tokyo, Japan.

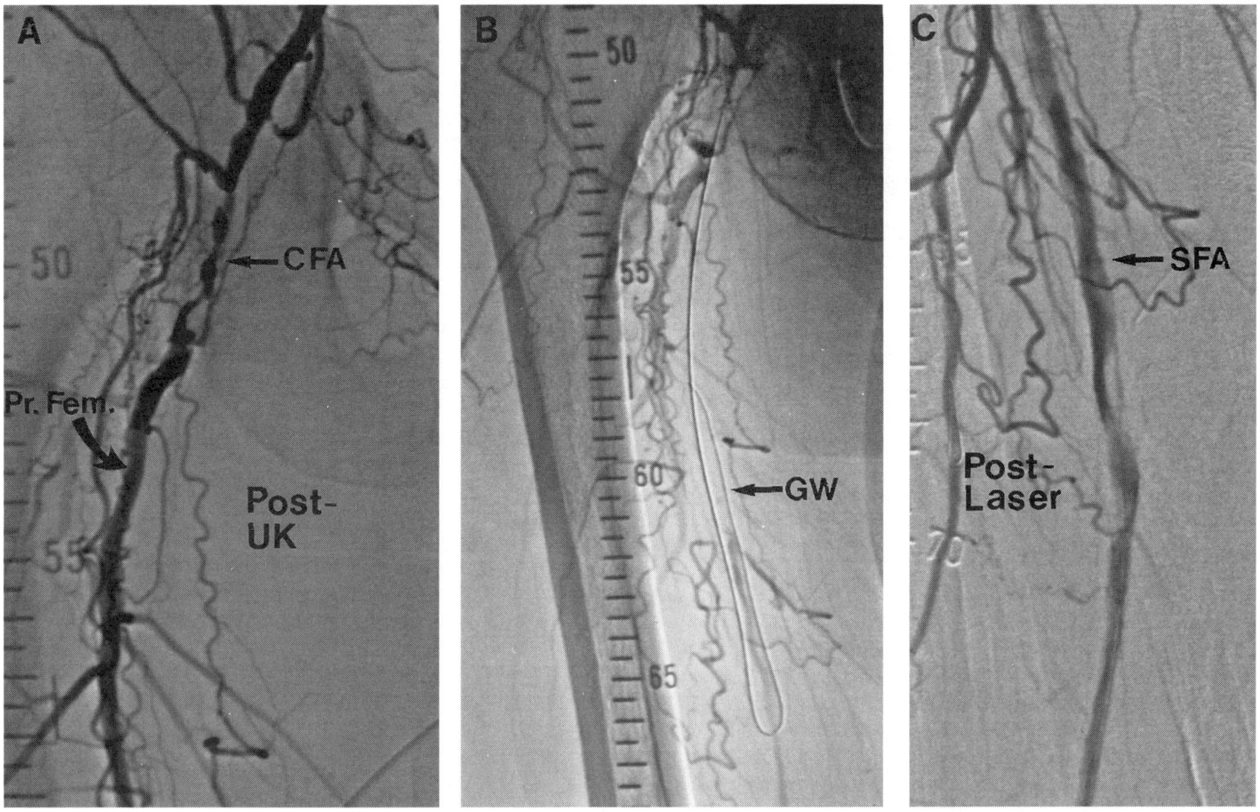

Fig. 31-17. Recanalization of occluded SFA using Glidewire and excimer laser. **A.** Angiogram demonstrating common femoral artery (CFA), with multiple high-grade stenoses, and SFA occlusion. Profunda femoris (Pr. Fem.) is seen below CFA. **B.** Glidewire (GW), configured with a loop at its leading edge, is advanced through entire length of SFA occlusion, following which occluded segment was treated with excimer-laser angioplasty. **C.** Post-laser angiogram demonstrates patent SFA with foci of residual haziness.

by a lengthy, metastable, submaximally organized, gelatin-like thrombus propagating retrograde from and superimposed on a less lengthy, high-grade atherosclerotic lesion. In such cases, lytic therapy can be effective in converting a long occlusion to one that is either shorter or no longer occlusive and thereby more amenable to mechanical revascularization. The efficacy of this approach recently underwent systematic, multicenter investigation in patients with lower-extremity occlusions who were randomized to lytic versus operative therapy in the Surgery and Thrombolysis for Ischemia of the Lower Extremity (STILE) Trial [121]. Preliminary data from the STILE Trial suggest that successful recanalization of *chronic* SFA occlusions using thrombolytic agents (tissue plasminogen activator [tPA] or urokinase) is technically feasible and, in many instances, associated with an excellent outcome. However, reestablishing patency by that approach is less reliable for lengthy or "flush" total occlusions than surgical bypass; for those lesions, the outcomes of surgery are more durable. The use of thrombolytic therapy for *acute* occlusions ($\leq$ 14 days' duration) appears to be more favorable, whether in the SFA or elsewhere (Fig. 31-23). Both the STILE Trial and a similar randomized investigation executed by Ouriel and associates [122] demonstrated that, for acute or subacute occlusions, thrombolysis and surgery were equivalent in terms of restoration of patency and limb salvage. An unexpected finding in Ouriel's study, with a similar trend in the STILE Trial, was a significant reduction in the frequency of both in-hospital complications and 12-month mortality in patients receiving thrombolysis versus those treated surgically. Thus, there is compelling evidence to support a strategy of primary thrombolysis for acute occlusions of the SFA.

All attempts to optimize acute procedural results in patients with lengthy total occlusions of the SFA must be tempered by the high frequency of restenosis following percutaneous revascularization of such lesions [71–74,116]. The basis for the higher incidence of restenosis associated with occluded, as opposed to stenotic, peripheral arteries has been clarified in part by in-vitro and in-vivo analyses. Tobis et al. [123] performed in-vitro studies to determine the mechanism of argon laser–mediated thermal-probe recanalization of SFA occlusions 0.5 to 26.0 cm in length. They observed that regardless of whether or not the laser was activated, the probe seldom penetrated the central (luminal) portion of a fibrous atheroma; instead, recanalization typically proceeded along an intramural course. We have used IVUS to address this

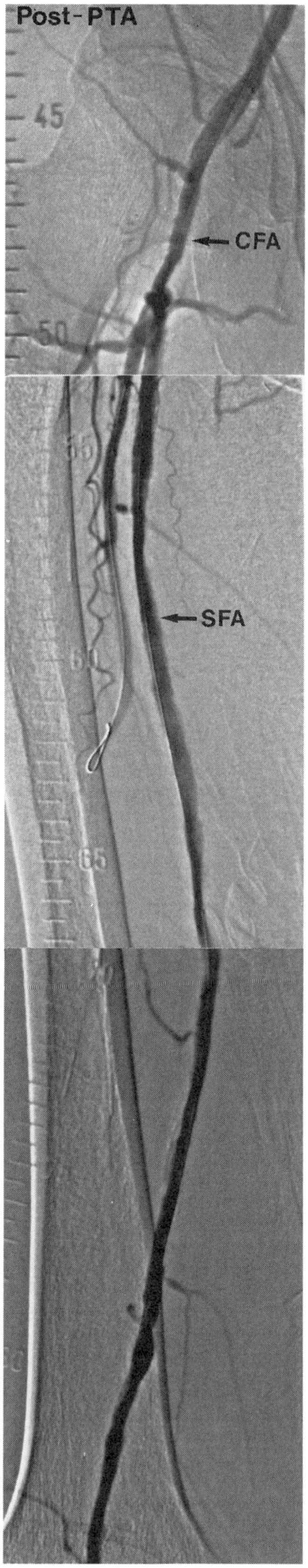

same issue in vivo. Three-dimensional reconstruction of ultrasound images from totally occluded peripheral arteries postrevascularization confirmed that, in many cases, clinically successful revascularization of totally occluded peripheral arteries does in fact include a significant intramural course [66,124,125] (Fig. 31-24).

Accordingly, the extent to which favorable acute procedural results in patients with chronic total occlusion will ultimately extend the role of percutaneous revascularization remains to be defined. Certainly for patients with nonhealing lesions or threatened limb loss in whom the risks of surgery are considered prohibitive or in whom veins are unavailable for distal bypass procedures, percutaneous revascularization of lengthy, occluded segments may facilitate healing. In similar types of patients with rest pain, PTA may be employed to achieve pain relief at a lower risk than conventional surgical reconstruction. For patients with less severe symptoms, improved ability to revascularize a chronically occluded artery does not in and of itself constitute a sufficient basis for routine invasive therapy.

Three anatomic issues concerning femoral arterial revascularization deserve additional, specific comment. The first issue involves clinical presentation of embolic complications apparently related to ulcerated or thrombotic lesions of the SFA, the so-called **blue-toe syndrome**. Emboli in such patients initially were inferred to result from friable plaque morphology that posed an unacceptable risk for percutaneous revascularization. It is now clear that such patients can be effectively treated by either PTA or directional atherectomy with both a high degree of procedural success and an acceptably low risk of further embolic complications [126–128]. The second issue involves stenotic and occlusive lesions of the common femoral artery. Such lesions certainly may be accessed without great difficulty from the contralateral limb (see Figs. 31-17 and 31-18). The acute results of common femoral PTA, however, are presumed to be less predictable. The concern that PTA-induced plaque fractures could propagate into the common femoral bifurcation, leading to potential compromise of both the SFA and the profunda, implicitly suggests that PTA of the common femoral artery must be undertaken with considerable caution. The third anatomic consideration is the combination of a stenotic profunda with a proximal occlusion of the SFA. Technically satisfactory results of profunda PTA have been described previously [129] and in this particular situation might well be more easily accomplished than revascularization of a coexisting, proximal, long SFA occlusion. Should revascularization of the profunda, a site not currently favored for stent deployment, be complicated by acute occlusion, however, complete interruption of antegrade flow via both femoral arteries may result in an acutely ischemic limb. For that reason, we advocate partic-

Fig. 31-18. Post-PTA angiography of vessels shown in Fig. 31-17. Common femoral artery (CFA) and native superficial femoral artery (SFA) are widely patent following excimer-laser angioplasty and PTA.

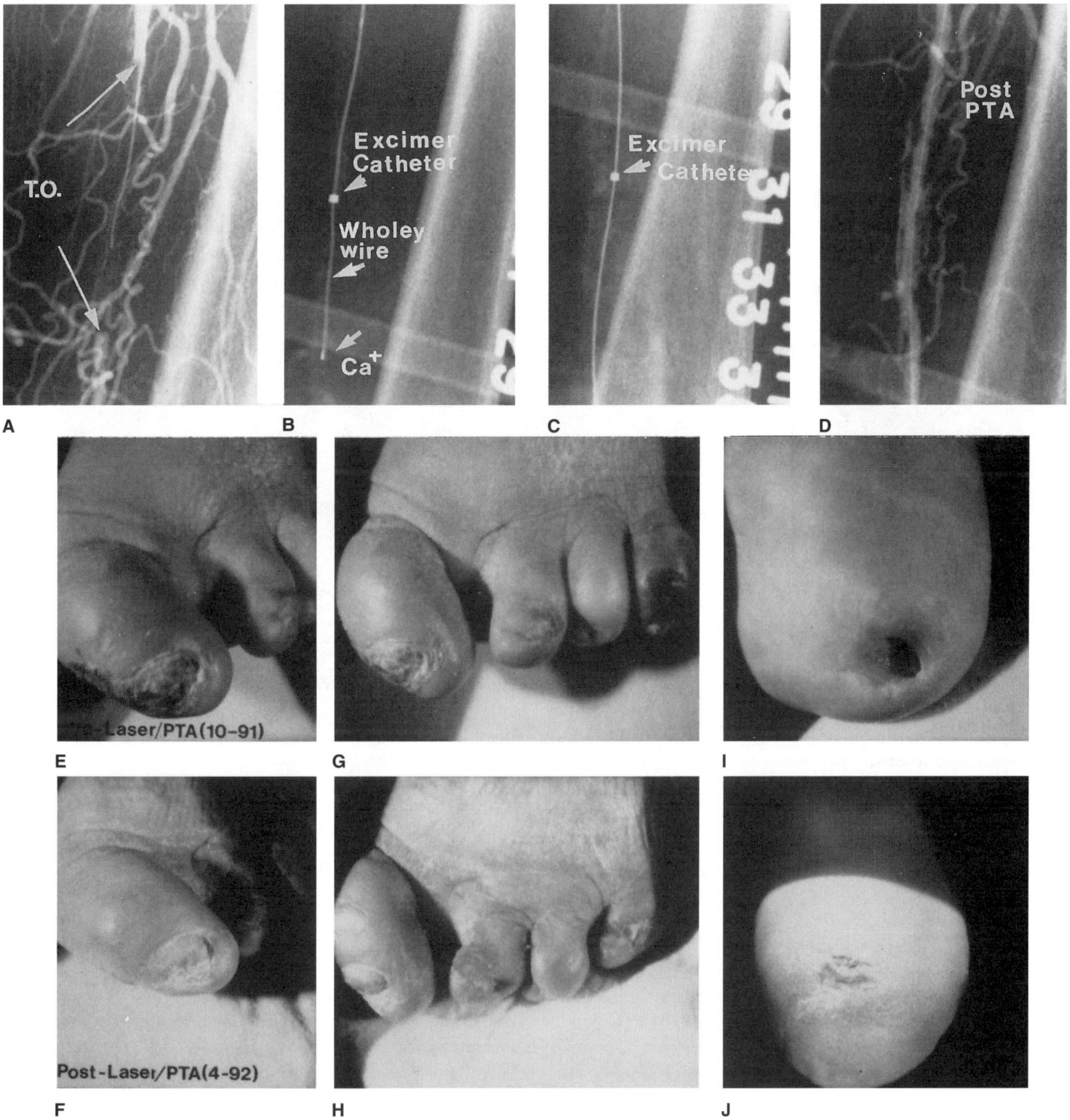

Fig. 31-19. Excimer laser–facilitated revascularization of totally occluded left superficial femoral artery in 86-year-old woman with nonhealing lesions of the first toe, fifth toe, and heel. **A.** Total occlusion (T.O.) of left SFA. **B.** Neither a hydrophilic Glidewire nor a Wholey wire, shown here, could be advanced beyond a nodular calcific deposit (Ca) in the distal left SFA. An excimer-laser catheter was therefore advanced over the Wholey wire and used to irradiate the proximal portion of the occlusion. **C.** Following excimer-laser irradiation of the nodular calcific deposit in the distal SFA, Wholey wire could then be advanced into the distal SFA. **D.** Final angiographic result following adjunctive PTA. (*Below*) Photographs of left foot taken pre- and postrevascularization demonstrate healing of lesions involving the first toe (**E, F**), fifth toe (**G, H**), and heel (**I, J**).

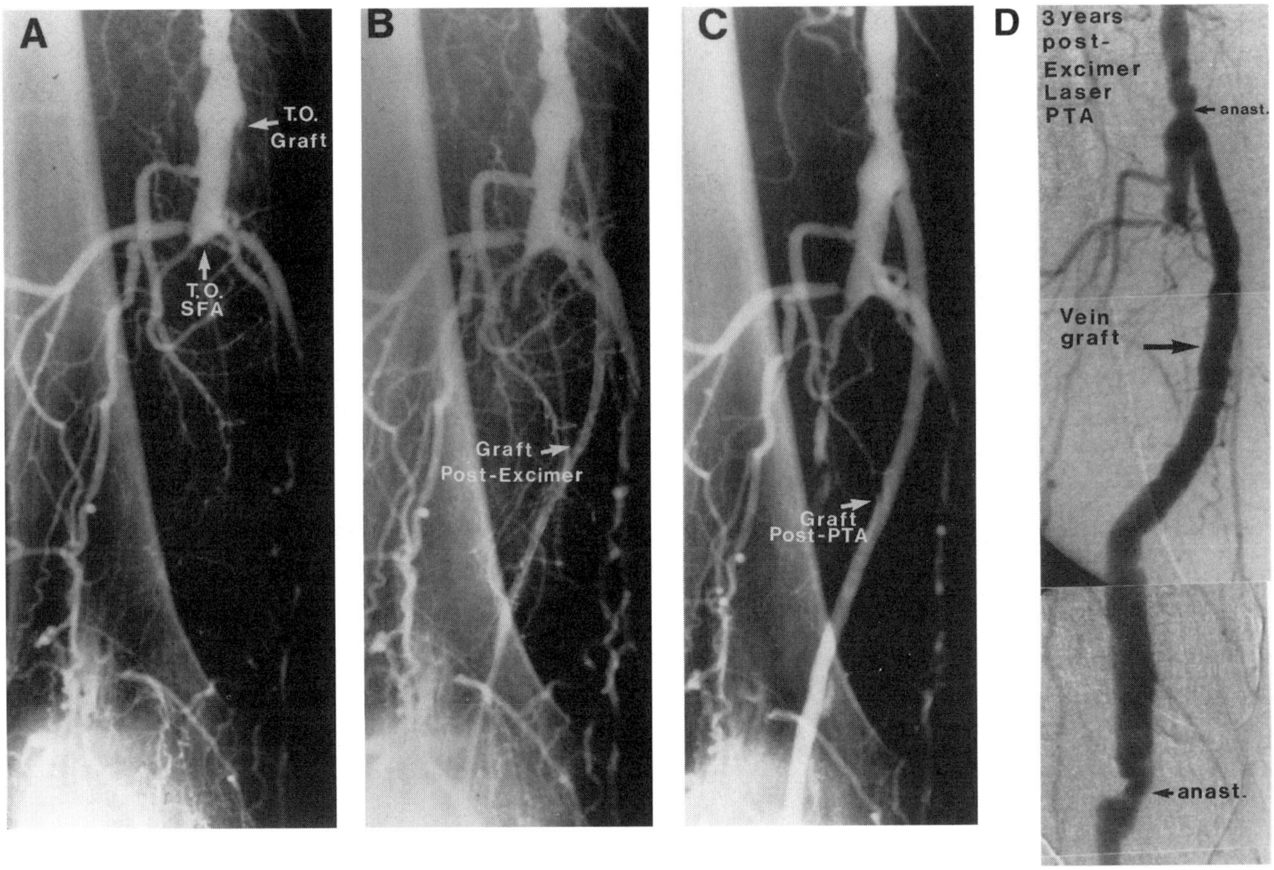

Fig. 31-20. Laser-assisted thrombolysis of occluded femoral-popliteal bypass graft. This 55-year-old man presented with clinical evidence of graft occlusion 3 months post–reverse saphenous vein bypass graft surgery. **A.** Following 24 hours of intra-arterial urokinase, there was no improvement in graft patency. **B.** Following wire-guided excimer-laser revascularization, antegrade flow through the graft is restored. **C.** Final result following adjunctive PTA. **D.** Follow-up angiography at 3 years postrevascularization demonstrates excellent graft patency. Both proximal and distal anastomoses (anast.) are patent. The patient remains free of symptoms.

ular caution when a percutaneous approach to this latter combination of lesions is being considered.

INFRAPOPLITEAL ARTERIES

Published clinical experience involving percutaneous revascularization of the anterior tibial, tibioperoneal trunk, posterior tibial, and peroneal arteries, while dating to the time of Dotter's original work [2], has been far more limited than that described here for aortoiliac and SFA sites. This is related to several issues, including the facts that claudication rarely is due to isolated disease of the infrapopliteal arteries; that knee-to-foot patency of one of the three major branches generally is regarded as sufficient to prevent critical lower-limb ischemia; that restenosis rates in these vessels typically have been the highest of any of the lower-extremity sites; and that obstructive disease in these arteries often is occlusive, severely diffuse, and complicated by heavy calcific deposits.

There is little question that application of techniques employed for coronary arterial revascularization, development of catheters having design features similar to those used for coronary interventions, and improvements in radiographic imaging equipment all have resulted in more widespread application of percutaneous revascularization for infrapopliteal disease. Prior to the use of coronary-type dilating equipment, for example, nonballoon, tapered angiographic or even nonangiographic catheters often were employed for infrapopliteal "angioplasty" [130]. Several reports [131–134] have now documented that with application of contemporary angioplasty equipment, stenotic and even short (< 2 cm) occlusions of one or more infrapopliteal arteries can be revascularized percutaneously with a very high degree of efficacy and at extraordinarily low risk.

Even lengthy total occlusions (Fig. 31-25), previously resistant to conventional techniques [135], often can be revascularized satisfactorily by combined use of hydrophilic guide wires, excimer-laser angioplasty, and rotational atherectomy. Among 20 consecutive patients with occlusion of one or more infrapopliteal arteries in whom percutaneous revascularization was performed in our institution, percutaneous revascularization was successfully

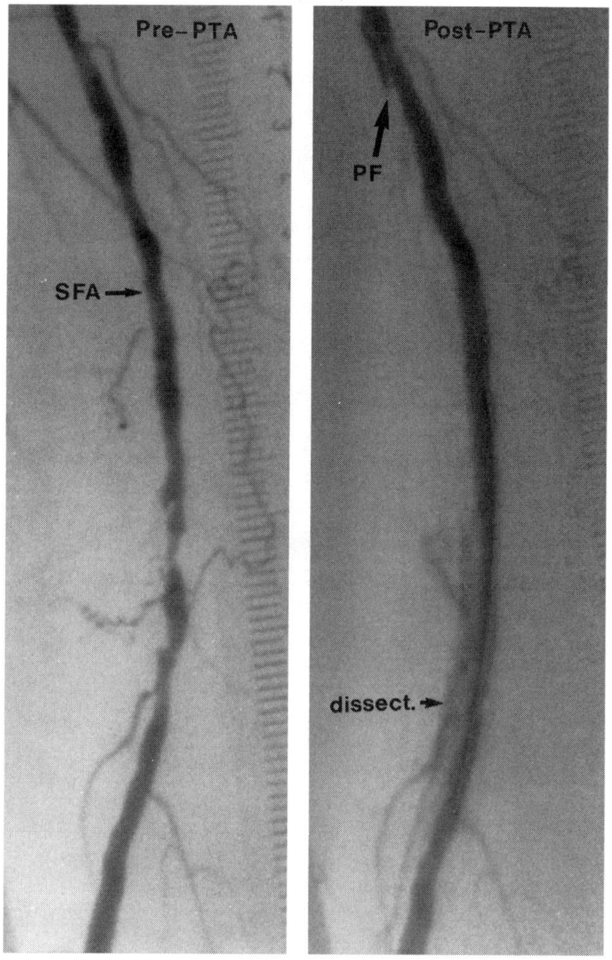

Fig. 31-21. PTA versus stenting in the SFA. Patient entered into the Femoral Artery Stenting Trial (FAST) was randomized to receive balloon angioplasty. Dilation of high-grade stenosis seen pre-PTA (left) leads to typical hazy dissection (right) and plaque fracture (PF) in proximal vessel. Despite these, the patient has had a good short-term clinical result. Clinical, noninvasive, and 6-month angiographic follow-up are planned as part of the trial.

completed in 19 (95%), including 11 occlusions 1–4 cm in length, and 9 measuring 5–10 cm long [45]. Postprocedural luminal-diameter narrowing was at all sites along the length of original occlusion less than 30 percent in 15, less than 40 percent in 17, and less than 50 percent in 19. Ankle-brachial index improved from 0.41 ± 0.06 prerevascularization to 0.77 ± 0.10 postrevascularization. Improvement in Rutherford class by one or more grades was observed at 1-month follow-up in 18 (94%) of 19 patients. Among 17 patients classified as Rutherford class 5 or 6, successful limb salvage was achieved in 15 (88%) of 17 patients.

Given this documented technical success, several factors combine to make nonsurgical revascularization particularly attractive for patients with infrapopliteal disease. The first factor is the well-documented, short-lived patency of prosthetic materials used as conduits for lower-extremity distal bypass surgery [136,137]. Consequently, use of the native vein—either as a reversed autologous graft or, more frequently, as an in-situ graft—has become the standard for surgical treatment in such patients. While the use of native vein and improved surgical techniques have led to improvements in short-term success and long-term patency, certain liabilities of this approach persist. Long-term patency still is inferior to that reported for suprapopliteal disease [138]. In-situ bypass surgery appears to have a higher risk of infectious complications than most other lower-extremity vascular procedures [139]. Finally, and most important, use of the saphenous vein for lower-extremity surgery precludes its future use, both as a conduit for coronary bypass surgery in a population of patients with a nearly universal incidence of coronary artery disease, as well as for subsequent lower-extremity vascular disease, including graft occlusive disease. If the latter is refractory to percutaneous or operative reconstruction, the patient often is left with limited options, including conservative therapy or eventual amputation.

Understandably, most vascular surgeons thus have advocated distal lower-extremity bypass surgery only for those patients with an advanced (4–6) Rutherford classification. For those groups, percutaneous therapy consequently becomes a very useful and appropriate alternative to reconstructive surgery. Even in patients with Rutherford class 4 (rest pain) or 5 (minor tissue loss), a percutaneous approach, if technically feasible, may have several advantages. First, it may defer definitive surgical therapy, thus preserving native veins. Second, it may accelerate healing of an ulcerative lesion or obviate superimposed infections. Third, in more advanced cases, it may lower the anatomic level of proposed amputation and thereby preserve patient mobility by helping to heal a more limited (e.g., transmetatarsal) amputation site [140].

It must be emphasized that the goals of infrapopliteal revascularization often differ from those of above-the-knee therapy. Because claudication rarely is the result of infrapopliteal obstruction alone, percutaneous treatment of those sites typically is performed in conjunction with SFA-popliteal revascularization. Even when present as an associated lesion or lesions, the requirement for angioplasty is not automatic: Uninterrupted patency of at least one of the three major infrapopliteal arteries generally is sufficient to obviate claudication or heal a distal ischemic lesion. In patients in whom infrapopliteal disease coexists with SFA-popliteal disease and in whom at least one of three vessels has no flow-limiting obstruction, it has been our practice to limit *associated* treatment of the infrapopliteal arteries to short (< 2 cm) stenoses and occlusions, if we choose to treat them at all.

More often, however, consideration of infrapopliteal angioplasty is necessary not for symptoms of lower-extremity ischemia but for signs of critical limb ischemia, such as nonhealing, ulcerated lesions with or without superimposed infection. In such patients, uninterrupted patency of at least one of the three infrapopliteal arteries may be anticipated to expedite healing of a distal lesion (Fig. 31-26) or a residual stump in patients requiring amputation. In the group of patients for whom the benefits of successful revascularization far outweigh the risks of

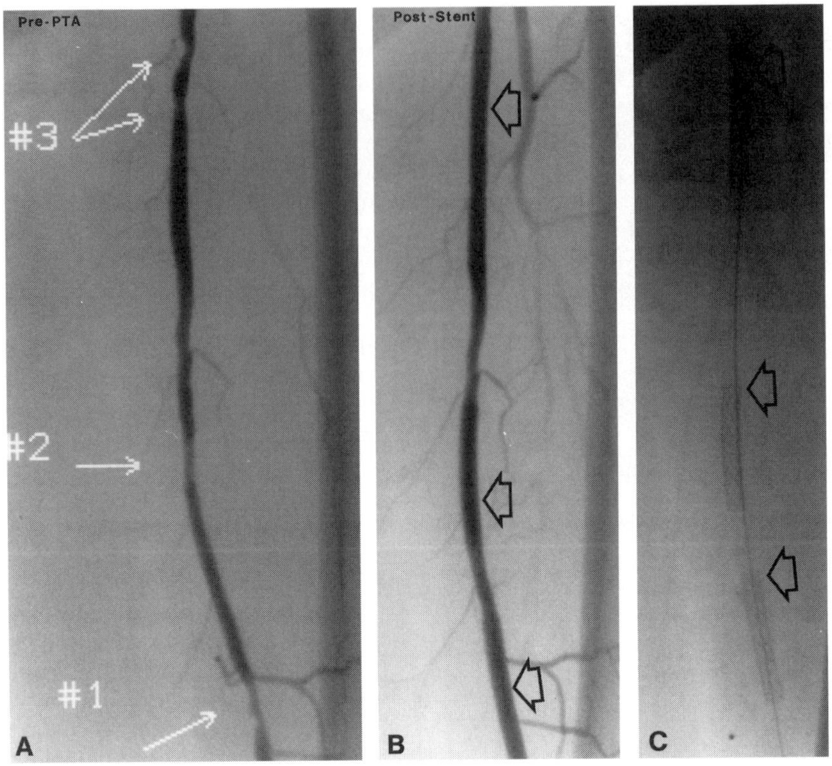

Fig. 31-22. Participant in the Femoral Artery Stenting Trial (FAST) randomized to receive stents. **A.** Moderate, proximal, and high-grade distal stenoses seen pre-PTA. **B.** Post-stent deployment. **C.** Stented sites (*arrows*) are uniform and widely patent. Sites between the stents, previously judged not to be significantly diseased, now paradoxically appear narrow relative to the stented areas.

a failed procedure, aggressive application of percutaneous revascularization may be expected to achieve extremely gratifying results, even in patients with calcified or lengthy total occlusions (Fig. 31-27).

Two points concerning percutaneous infrapopliteal revascularization require special emphasis. First, results previously achieved with conventional wires and balloon catheters do not represent what currently can be accomplished using more contemporary techniques [45,92]. There is little doubt that excimer-laser angioplasty (see Fig. 31-26) has facilitated percutaneous revascularization of long, total occlusions. Likewise, rotational atherectomy (see Fig. 31-16) may play an important role in the treatment of heavily calcified infrapopliteal arteries. Even in the presence of lengthy, multivessel occlusions, demonstrated reconstitution of one or more arteries suggests that percutaneous revascularization of at least one major artery should be possible. Consequently, recommendations based solely on previous experience with standard angioplasty equipment [135] should be reconsidered.

Second, the incidence of restenosis, which remains high in these patients irrespective of the technique employed, should not be a factor in the decision to employ a percutaneous approach for what is, in most of these patients, a short-term problem. If uninterrupted patency of even one vessel can be achieved, the improvement in antegrade nutrient flow typically is adequate to facilitate limb salvage. Once healed, most patients will do satisfactorily, even in the face of documented restenosis, if they can avoid subsequent foot trauma. This strategy is further supported by the fact that both the short-term and the long-term outcomes of distal surgical reconstruction for infrapopliteal disease are likewise imperfect.

BYPASS GRAFTS

Percutaneous revascularization represents an alternative to operative reconstruction for achieving so-called secondary patency [77] of failing or failed native or prosthetic conduits. Nonsurgical revascularization has several obvious advantages: It saves the patient the morbidity and additional hospitalization associated with a repeat surgical procedure; it does not require the availability or utilization of additional native veins; and, in certain cases, it may obviate the need to employ prosthetic materials for distal reconstruction, an application for which such materials have been shown to confer low patency rates [136,137].

The published experience with stenotic (i.e., compromised but nonoccluded) lower-extremity bypass grafts is extremely limited and, therefore, not surprisingly, variable. Cohen et al. [141] used PTA to treat 7 of 29 patients with "impending vein graft failure" and reported a 5-year cumulative patency rate of 43 percent for the group, versus a 5-year cumulative patency of 83 percent in the

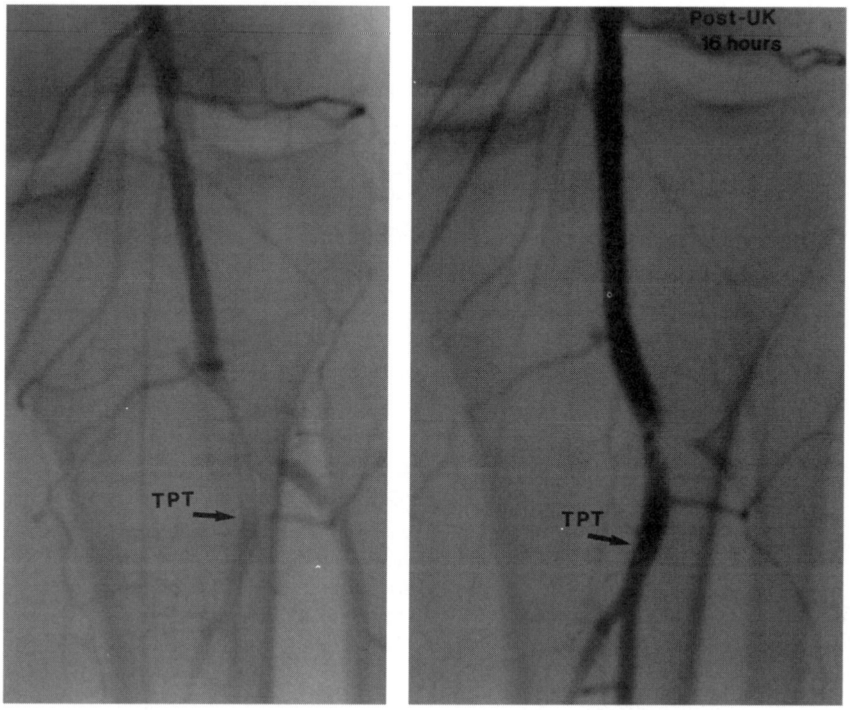

Fig. 31-23. Acute embolic occlusion in elderly woman with chronic atrial fibrillation. Rest pain resolved promptly after administration of urokinase. Patency was restored to tibioperoneal trunk (TPT). Patient remains asymptomatic 2½ years later.

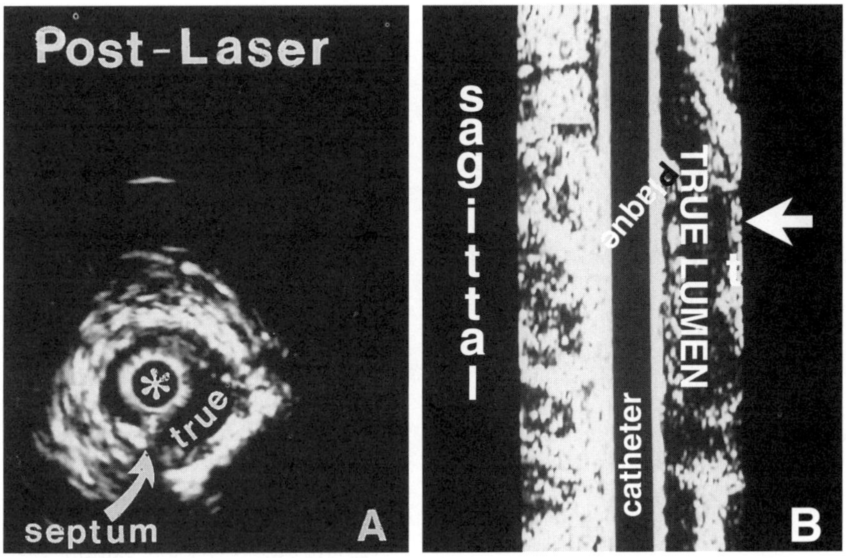

Fig. 31-24. Subintimal channel created during recanalization of 8-cm occlusion in SFA using guide wire (Terumo) followed by excimer laser angioplasty. **A.** Inspection by conventional two-dimensional reconstruction IVUS demonstrates "double-barrel" lumen. IVUS probe (*asterisk*) in subintimal channel separated by septum from second ("true") lumen. **B.** Sagittal image rendered by on-line three-dimensional reconstruction depicts subintimal pathway of ultrasound catheter as it enters atherosclerotic plaque, which separates catheter from true lumen at right. Arrow depicts level of ultrasound frame shown in (**A**).

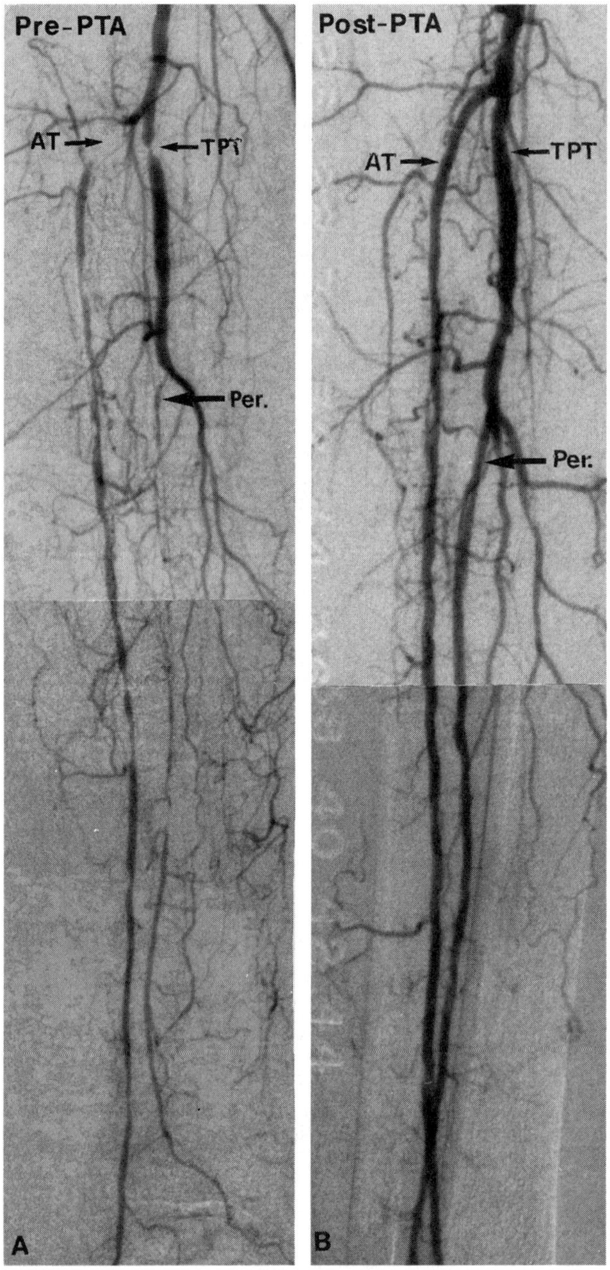

Fig. 31-25. PTA of occluded anterior tibial artery, tibioperoneal trunk, and peroneal artery in elderly patient with foot ulceration and threatened limb loss. **A.** Baseline angiogram demonstrates 2-cm occlusion of anterior tibial artery (AT), high-grade stenosis of tibioperoneal trunk (TPT), and lengthy occlusion of peroneal artery (Per.). All three segments were recanalized with Glidewire, followed by excimer-laser angioplasty and PTA. **B.** Final angiogram post-PTA demonstrates widely patent anterior tibial, tibioperoneal trunk, and peroneal artery.

remaining 22 patients treated by reconstruction with patch angioplasty. Perler et al. [142] described a 7-year experience during which a total of 19 grafts were treated by PTA: Primary and secondary patency rates at 36-month follow-up were 22 percent and 27 percent, respectively. Again, because a primary 5-year patency rate of 62 percent was achieved in nine vein graft stenoses revised surgically during the same time period, the authors concluded that surgical reconstruction was preferable to PTA for vein graft stenosis. Bandyk et al. [143] used PTA to perform 18 of 103 secondary procedures intended to correct primary or recurrent graft stenoses. Their case selection (13 involved an "adjacent artery stenosis," 3 a venous conduit, and 2 an anastomosis) reflected their bias that "PTA be reserved for management of atherosclerotic lesions that develop in arteries proximal or distal to graft anastomotic sites." Recurrent stenosis was observed in three cases early (< 3 months) and in five cases late post-PTA.

Whittemore et al. reviewed their institutional experience with balloon angioplasty applied to 54 stenotic lesions in 30 patients [144]. In none of the patients was PTA associated with a serious complication. While the overall 4-year patency rate was only 18 percent, the case mix demonstrated an important bimodal distribution: Vein grafts requiring only a single PTA had a patency rate of 59 percent at 3 years, as opposed to those requiring repetitive dilation in which 3-year patency was 6 percent. Neither anatomic nor clinical factors predicted protracted patency. While the authors are no doubt correct in concluding that PTA has "significant limitations in providing sustained secondary patency," their data also may be interpreted to argue for at least one PTA in those cases where it is technically feasible, given that up to two-thirds of impending graft failures may be obviated by a single percutaneous intervention.

In fact, among two more recently described, larger groups of patients with vein graft stenoses, the long-term outcome associated with PTA of vein graft stenoses appeared substantially improved. Berkowitz et al. [145] used PTA alone to treat 44 (61%) of 72 graft stenoses. The 5-year life table–assisted primary patency after correction of the stenotic lesion was 61 percent. In contrast to the above-reported experience, lesion location was a principal determinant of graft patency: Lesions in the proximal (including anastomosis) and distal graft had significantly better patency than mid-graft and distal anastomotic lesions.

Similarly, Sanchez et al. [146] reported encouraging results with PTA in the treatment of 156 (55%) of 285 lesions involving failing or threatened vein and polytetrafluoroethylene bypass grafts. For inflow or outflow lesions less than 5 cm in length, 5-year secondary patency was 58 percent. For graft stenoses less than 1.5 cm in length within vein grafts greater than 3 mm in diameter, the 24-month extended patency rate was 93 percent.

Our own approach to stenotic grafts (Figs. 31-28, 31-29, and 31-30), regardless of the dimensions or locations of the stenoses, is to make at least one attempt at percutaneous revascularization. This approach derives from consideration of several issues. First, percutaneous revascularization of stenotic grafts most often is technically straightforward. Second, the risk of serious complications is low. Third, the contribution of adjunctive diagnostic and therapeutic techniques, including IVUS, directional atherectomy (Fig. 31-31), excimer-laser angioplasty, and endovascular stents, to preservation of graft

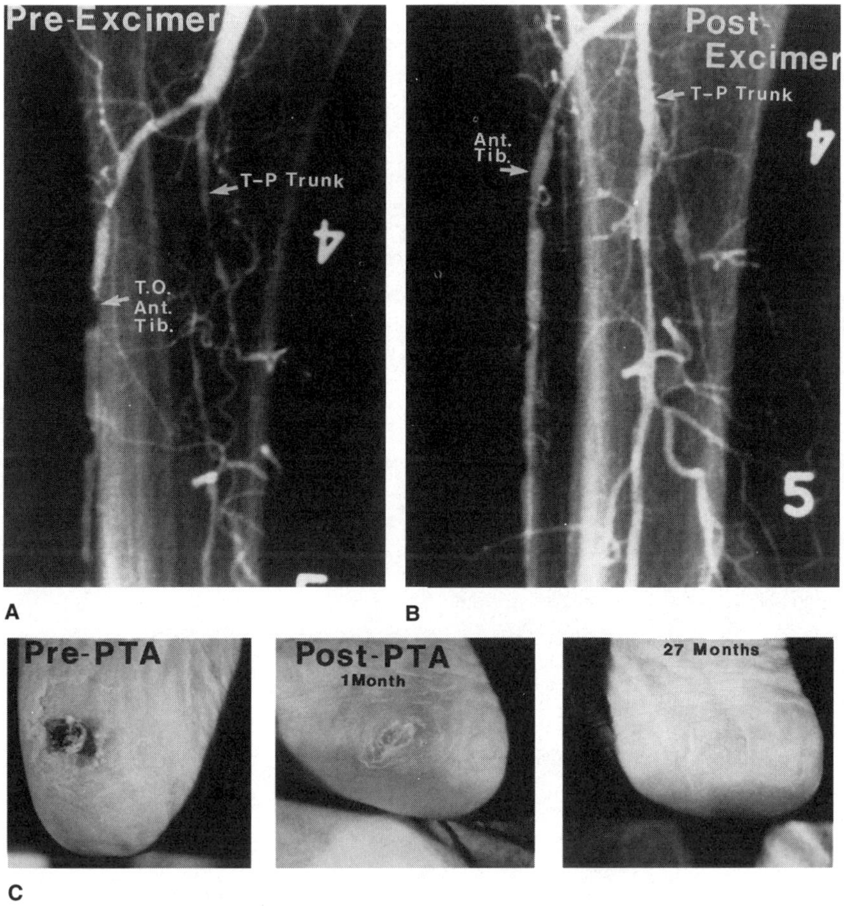

Fig. 31-26. Excimer-laser angioplasty of totally occluded (T.O.) anterior tibial (Ant. Tib.) and tibioperoneal (T-P) trunk in a 67-year-old woman with nonhealing lesion of the left heel. **A.** Baseline angiogram. **B.** Final angiogram following sole therapy with wire-guided excimer laser irradiation. **C.** Progressive healing of left heel lesion at 1 month (*middle*) and 27 months (*right*) postrevascularization. Patient remains asymptomatic 2 years later.

patency remains essentially untested; preliminary data, for example, suggest that stents in particular may reduce the incidence of restenosis in stenotic coronary artery bypass grafts [147,148]. Fourth, surgical revision itself is complicated by imperfect long-term patency [51,136,149–152]. Thus, given the uncertain long-term results of any form of revascularization in this setting, combined with the prospect of salvaging some unknown but nevertheless important percentage of bypass grafts at relatively low cost and low risk, it is likely that percutaneous revascularization of stenotic bypass conduits will continue, for the near future, to be expanded.

Limited published data [153–158] are available regarding comprehensive series of patients in whom *occluded* bypass conduits have been percutaneously revascularized without preemptive administration of thrombolytic therapy. In most of those reports, unspecified numbers of patients were excluded from consideration if the occlusion could not be crossed with a guide wire; lytic therapy was delivered primarily to the origin—as opposed to the "body"—of the thrombus; or PTA was performed following lytic therapy only in selected patients. Although not subclassified in terms of graft versus native arterial sites, McNamara and Fischer [153] observed that the ability to completely traverse the occluded site with the guide wire constituted the best single test for predicting the likelihood of recanalizing a given occlusion and obtaining complete clot lysis: In every case in which the guide wire was advanced completely through the occlusion, the ensuing infusion produced complete clot lysis.

Among 14 consecutive patients from our own institution in whom a bypass graft was successfully crossed with the Glidewire, revascularization was completed successfully in 12 (85%) [45]. The length of the occluded segment measured 3 cm in one patient, and was greater than 10 cm in the remaining 11. Residual luminal-diameter narrowing was less than 30 percent in all 12 patients. Postprocedural ankle-brachial indices improved from 0.37 ± 0.08 to 0.82 ± 0.08. Rutherford class, too, increased by one or more grades in all 12 patients, including 4 who were classified as class 5 or 6 preprocedure.

Our current approach to percutaneous revascularization of occluded grafts exploits not only the ability of the Glidewire to more readily traverse lengthy graft occlu-

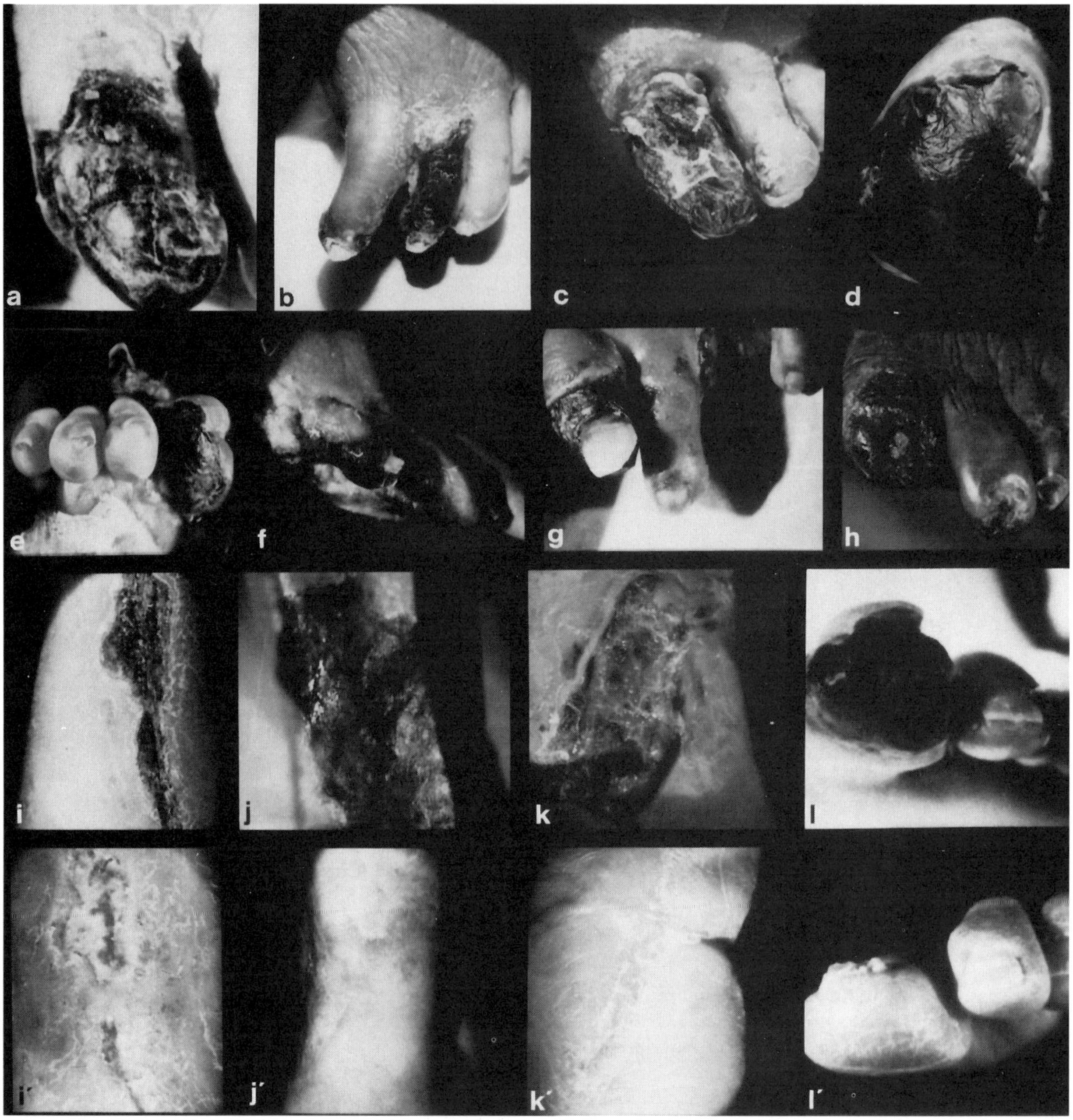

Fig. 31-27. Composite figure showing the extent of severely ischemic alterations that typically develop before patients or their doctors seek medical consultation regarding the basis for the findings and possible treatment options. In most of these cases, amputation ultimately was required. In the last four panels, the appearance of the foot is shown after percutaneous revascularization of the patients whose limbs were photographed at the time of initial presentation shown in the third row. These patients illustrate one of the most difficult groups of patients seen by specialists in vascular medicine. Earlier diagnosis and institution of therapy clearly are required to prevent the development of such extensive disease, if the risk of amputation is to be reduced. It should be recognized, however, that when the extent of disease has reached even this degree, amputation and bypass surgery are not the only available treatment options. Percutaneous revascularization often may be successful in rescuing limbs of these patients; regardless of the subsequent incidence of restenosis, in the absence of recurrent foot, ankle, or lower-leg trauma, such lesions often will remain clinically silent after satisfactory healing.

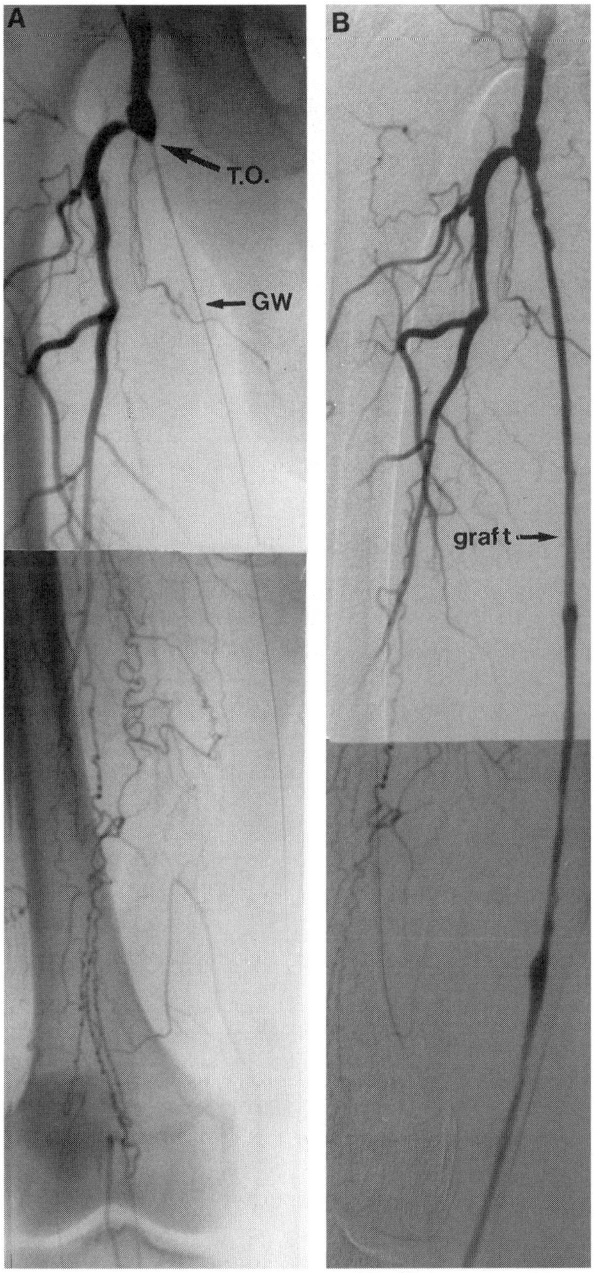

Fig. 31-28. Revascularization of occluded in-situ vein bypass graft in patient with continuous rest pain. **A.** Angiogram obtained after Glidewire (GW) is advanced through entire length of occluded femoral-anterior tibial in-situ vein bypass graft. **B.** Angiogram following Glidewire recanalization, thrombolytic therapy with urokinase, and balloon angioplasty demonstrates widely patent graft.

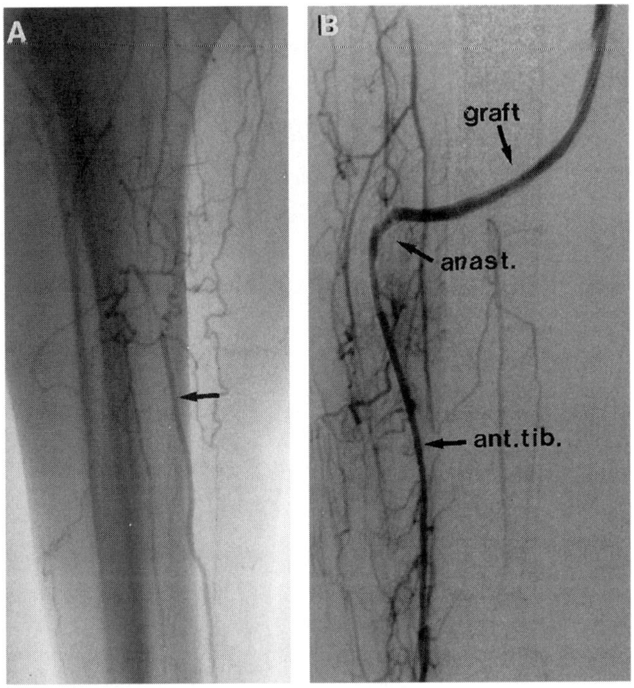

Fig. 31-29. Recanalization of distal graft and anastomosis in patient from Fig. 31-11. **A.** Baseline angiogram demonstrates absence of graft but filling of distal runoff vessels (*arrow*) via collaterals. **B.** Following thrombolysis and balloon angioplasty, distal graft and anastomosis (anast.) with anterior tibial (ant. tib.) artery now widely patent. Flow restored to ankle level, with restoration of palpable pulse and resolution of rest pain.

sions but, in addition, profits from the advent of low-profile catheter-wire perfusion systems that permit protracted delivery of lytic therapy directly into the occluding thrombus via side holes in the perfusion instrument. The extent to which these procedural factors were directly responsible for successful revascularization in the above-described cases will require further assessment in a larger patient cohort. It is noteworthy, however, that, similar to the experience of McNamara and Fischer [153], the one occluded graft in our own series that could not be successfully crossed with the Glidewire could not be salvaged with lytic therapy. The capability to nontraumatically salvage these conduits constitutes a potentially valuable treatment strategy in a group of patients who often have no remaining veins for repeat surgery and in whom use of prosthetic grafts to distal sites may be undesirable.

There are limited published data regarding the application of novel-device technology to the treatment of occluded bypass grafts. Consequently, the potential efficacy of novel mechanical approaches, including endovascular stents, cited above for reducing graft restenosis, remains undetermined. It is likely that efforts similar to those that have been proposed in the past to augment graft patency through genetic engineering [159] may, in the future, be applied percutaneously [160] to prevent restenosis following successful revascularization.

SUBCLAVIAN AND INNOMINATE ARTERIES

Angioplasty of the subclavian and innominate arteries has been performed since 1980 [161], with favorable outcomes and few complications. Both short- and long-term results with PTA appear to be comparable to those in aortoiliac vessels, which are of similar size. The results also compare favorably to surgical alternatives, including common-ca-

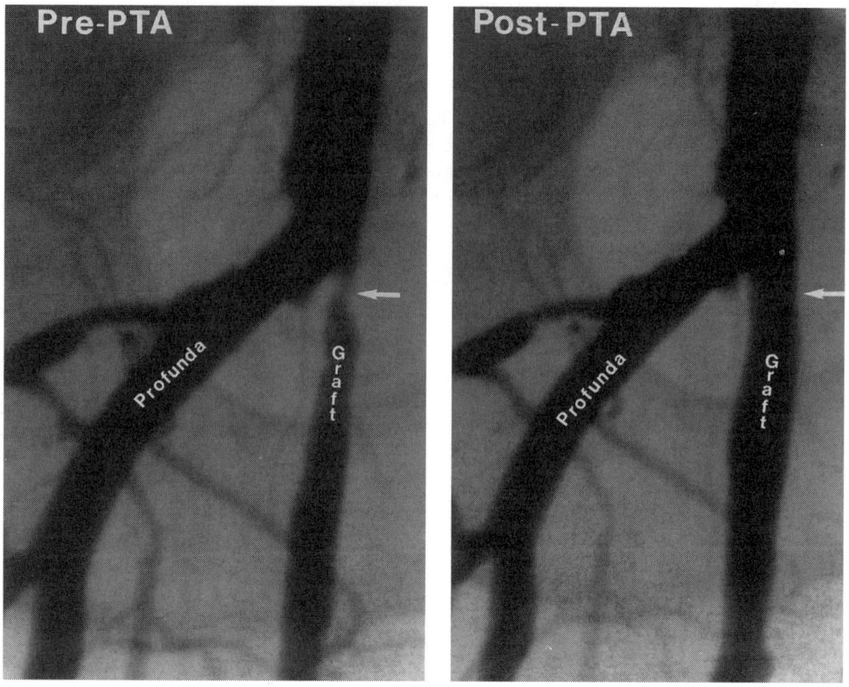

Fig. 31-30. Balloon angioplasty of proximal anastomosis in femoropopliteal vein graft 1 year postsurgery. Pre-PTA, focal stenosis (*arrow*) is evident. Post-PTA, after dilating with a 7-mm balloon, the stenosis has been relieved. At 1 year post-PTA, the patient has no symptoms, and duplex scan confirms patency of the dilated site.

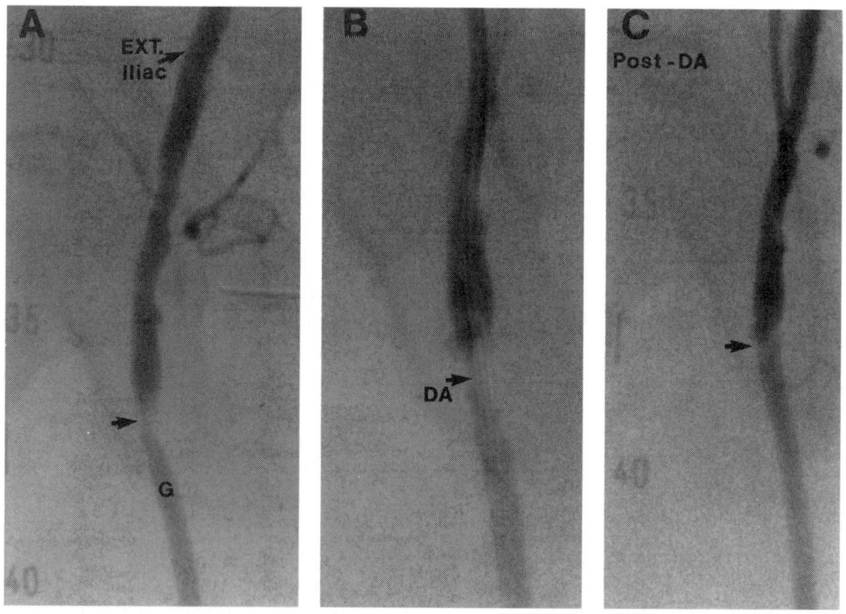

Fig. 31-31. Directional atherectomy of lesion (*arrow*) in proximal anastomosis of femoropopliteal Gore-tex® graft (G). **A.** Angiography shows focal stenosis. **B.** Directional atherecomy catheter (DA) advanced antegrade via ipsilateral common femoral artery. **C.** Final result is satisfactory. Patient is asymptomatic and graft widely patent by Doppler at 18 months.

rotid-to-subclavian bypass. However, the overall number of such patients included in published reports in whom revascularization was limited to PTA is well under 1,000. No randomized trials comparing surgery and PTA have been performed. Nonetheless, for proximal, focal subclavian stenoses, PTA is now considered first-line therapy. Occlusive disease is more controversial because of the difficulty occasionally experienced in crossing such lesions, and the potential for thrombus or atheroma to be dislodged into the intracerebral circulation. PTA has advantages over surgery, namely, obviating the need for general anesthesia and a prolonged hospital stay with significant morbidity. Not infrequently, the common carotid itself is stenotic and, therefore, unsuitable as a donor artery. Thus, while percutaneous recanalization of subclavian occlusions is technically feasible [162], the safety and efficacy of PTA versus surgery remain to be determined.

As indicated, most series of subclavian PTA reported in the literature are limited to small numbers of patients. In one of the largest individual series described to date, Millaire and colleagues recently presented the outcomes in 50 consecutive patients over 7 years (1984–1991) [163]. Confounding their results are the facts that there is a learning curve associated with the procedure and that equipment used in earlier years was less advanced. PTA was performed for symptomatic ischemia of the posterior fossa (N = 14), upper extremity (N = 13), or both (N = 7) in 34 (68%) of their patients. The remaining 16 (32%) were treated for preservation of flow, where further thrombosis would have devastating consequences. Subclavian steal syndrome (see Fig. 31-28) was frequently present (60%), as was concomitant involvement of other brachiocephalic vessels (52%).

Millaire achieved technical success (defined as < 30% residual stenosis and < 10 mm residual mean gradient) in 90 percent of cases. Failure usually was due to the inability to dilate a tightly narrowed or occluded vessel. Complications (10%) were related mainly to vascular access, although one stroke occurred, with subsequent partial resolution. Access-related complications were quite frequent when the axillary approach was used, occurring in three of nine patients. Long-term follow-up was available in 98 percent of the patients and indicated a persistent hemodynamic benefit in 84 percent at an average of 40 months postprocedure. Even in the seven patients with long-term hemodynamic failure, only one was chronically symptomatic. The results are similar to those reported in other, smaller series [164–170], and confirm the favorable results of PTA in the subclavian artery.

From a technical standpoint, subclavian PTA may be approached either from the femoral artery or from the ipsilateral arm. The latter may be more difficult in the case where brachial blood pressure is attenuated due to high-grade obstruction. We favor the femoral approach, which seems to be associated with fewer vascular complications and less risk of compromise to the upper-extremity vasculature. The availability of endovascular stents, while not yet examined systematically for subclavian arteries, may further optimize the acute and long-term outcome in selected patients undergoing subclavian or innominate PTA (Figs. 31-32 and 31-33).

RENAL ARTERIES

The primary goals of renal-artery revascularization are to preserve or restore renal function, improve control of hypertension, and eliminate congestive heart failure (CHF). Associated secondary benefits can include reduction in antihypertensive medications; the potential to retard progression of vascular disease; and, occasionally, elimination of the need for dialysis. For patients with chronic CHF or cardiomyopathy, correction of renal-artery stenosis (RAS) may enable safe institution of angiotensin converting enzyme (ACE) inhibitor therapy. Percutaneous techniques offer an attractive alternative to surgical bypass or endarterectomy, which are more invasive and associated with higher morbidity.

Prevalence and Indications for Therapy. The prevalence of RAS remains unknown, since currently available non-invasive diagnostic and screening techniques have poor predictive value. Previous population-based estimates suggested that at least 2 million to 4 million of approximately the 70 million people with hypertension in the United States have RAS [171]. Two recent studies, however, in which patients underwent routine screening angiography for renovascular disease, suggest that the prevalence is significantly higher than previous estimates. Vetrovec and colleagues systematically performed diagnostic renal angiography on patients undergoing cardiac catheterization [172]. Of their patients with a history of either hypertension or renal insufficiency, fully 23 percent of patients had significant RAS, defined as diameter narrowing of 50 percent or more. Another 7 percent had detectable RAS of a less severe nature (< 50% narrowed diameter). Significant RAS was present in a remarkable 64 percent of patients with renal insufficiency (creatinine > 1.5 in males, > 1.2 in females), whereas 18 percent of patients with hypertension alone had significant RAS. Additionally, Vetrovec demonstrated that, among patients with coronary artery disease, 29 percent had some degree of renal-artery narrowing. In a similar study, Harding and colleagues performed screening renal arteriograms in 1,651 consecutive patients undergoing routine coronary arteriography [173]. Fifteen percent had significant (≥ 50%) RAS. For those patients with a creatinine of 2.0 mg/dl or more, the incidence increased to nearly 40 percent. Surprisingly, almost one-half of the patients with documented renovascular disease did not exhibit hypertension. Thus, limiting screening to hypertensive patients excludes many with significant RAS, at risk for progressive azotemia. From those studies and similar ones, it would appear that the prevalence of RAS is significantly higher than that predicted from crude population-based studies of hypertensive patients. Such a finding would not be surprising, since most of the population-based studies were performed 15 or more years ago, when average life expectancy was shorter, the population younger, and the prevalence of vascular disease less. Indeed, among patients with generalized vascular disease in the older age group, whose legions are increasing yearly, RAS is likely to be common [174]. Additionally, there is now good evidence that the percentage of patients developing end-stage renal disease on the basis of renovascular insuffi-

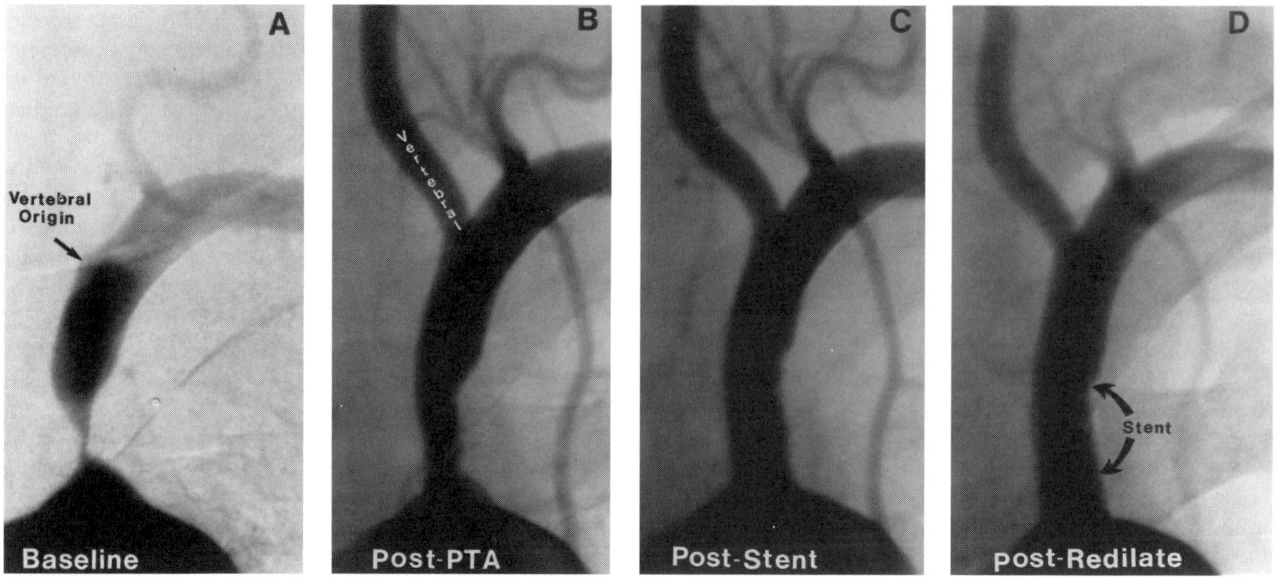

Fig. 31-32. PTA-stenting of subclavian artery stenosis with associated subclavian steal syndrome. **A.** Baseline angiogram depicts critical stenosis at origin of left subclavian artery. Vertebral artery is not visualized, because it has retrograde flow. Distal to origin of vertebral artery, mixing of blood from retrograde vertebral flow causes dilution of contrast material and, consequently, less density. **B.** Post-PTA, 7-mm balloon. Antegrade flow now restored in the vertebral artery, but significant recoil is present at the lesion site. **C.** Palmaz stent deployed with an 8-mm balloon, lumen enlarged; minor irregularities seen along border of stent. **D.** Postredilation with 9-mm balloon.

ciency, as opposed to nonvascular etiologies, is increasing. In a recent analysis of their dialysis patients, Mailloux and colleagues found that the percentage of patients with renal failure from RAS increased from approximately 8 percent between 1970 and 1982 to 16.5 percent between 1982 and 1985 [175]. Given the high prevalence of RAS in patients with baseline azotemia (64% in Vetrovec's study), Mailloux's findings are not surprising. Perhaps of even more concern are the consequences of developing renal failure from RAS. Mailloux found that patients in that category have a particularly poor prognosis once on dialysis, with a median survival of only 27 months and a 5-year survival of less than 10 percent. While the presence of associated cardiovascular disease is undoubtedly responsible for much of the increased mortality, renovascular patients also are typically more difficult to manage on dialysis, owing to persistence of hypertension, fluid retention, and intolerance of the stress of dialysis. Furthermore, dialysis itself, for unclear reasons, seems to be associated with an acceleration of the atherosclerotic process,

Fig. 31-33. IVUS during subclavian PTA-stenting. **A.** IVUS after 7-mm balloon dilation. Maximum diameter measures 4.8 mm, indicating significant recoil. **B.** Following stent deployment with 8-mm balloon, struts (*arrows*) still protrude slightly into lumen. **C.** Post-PTA 9 mm, struts (*arrows*) now well apposed to arterial wall. Asterisks indicate IVUS catheter.

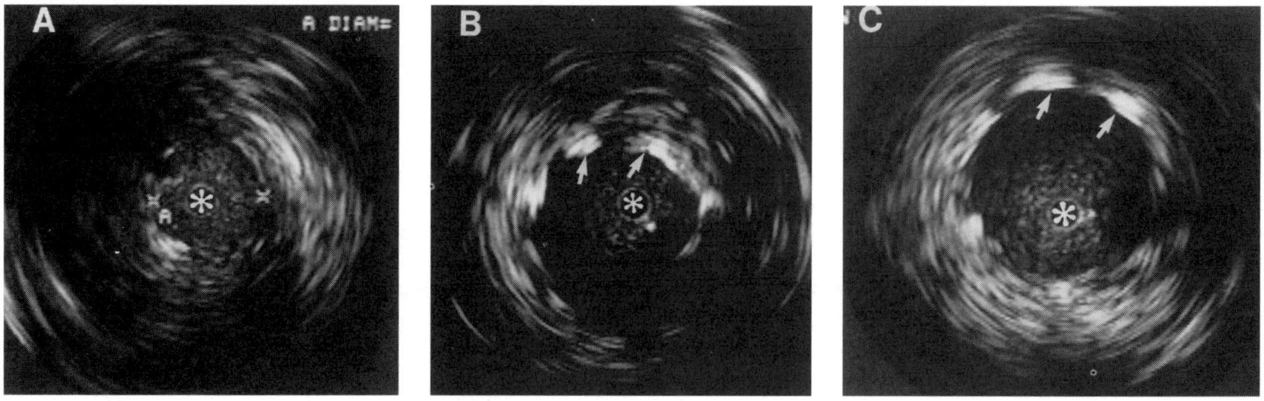

hastening the progression of coronary and cerebrovascular lesions.

For the patient not yet in renal failure, the combination of renovascular hypertension and renal insufficiency can have serious implications. It can be anticipated that the hypertension will exacerbate the progression of atherosclerosis, including coronary, renal, and cerebral. In the case of unilateral RAS, persistent hypertension can exert a negative effect on the contralateral kidney, which is not "protected" by lower perfusion pressure, inducing further intrinsic kidney damage and potentially exacerbating underlying azotemia. Beyond the vascular and intrarenal effects of hypertension, there are potentially deleterious hemodynamic consequences associated with hyperreninemia, including fluid retention and CHF [171].

Effective treatment of the offending stenotic renal-artery lesion(s) offers the prospect of preventing or delaying the consequences of persistent hypertension and progressive renal ischemia, improving morbidity and mortality, and reducing cost to the patient and the health care system. The latter should not be underestimated, since the yearly cost of maintaining a patient on hemodialysis exceeded $37,000 in 1991 and may be twice that amount now. In their recent review, Rimmer and Gennari point out that, despite our improved ability over the past 10 years to treat hypertension with medications, the same period of time has seen a sixfold increase in the occurrence of end-stage renal disease attributed to hypertensive nephrosclerosis [174]. Since only a small percentage of these patients were likely to have undergone diagnostic arteriography, there remains a significant possibility that many developed renal failure from progressive RAS. Rimmer and Gennari estimate conservatively that renovascular disease is the primary cause for more than 2,000 cases per year of new end-stage renal disease, requiring initiation of dialysis. Thus, they suggest that RAS could be responsible for in excess of $75 million per year for dialysis expenditures alone (using 1991 figures), excluding the costs related to increased patient comorbidity, lost wages, and disability. Early intervention with revascularization potentially could reduce this economic burden. There is good evidence, albeit preliminary, to suggest that preemptive renal-artery revascularization may not only eliminate or delay the need for dialysis but may improve long-term prognosis as well [174]. The reason for that improvement likely would be the reduction in comorbid conditions associated with renal failure and dialysis, including accelerated cardiovascular disease, myocardial infarction, CHF, and stroke.

Revascularization for RAS. Since Gruntzig first demonstrated successful use of balloon catheters for renal artery revascularization [176], controversy has persisted regarding which lesions to treat by PTA versus surgery and at what threshold revascularization should be recommended. The paucity of randomized controlled trials comparing medical therapy, surgery, and PTA or even of standardized definitions among reports as to what constitutes a successful therapeutic outcome precludes formulation of conclusions regarding the relative benefits and indications of each strategy.

Notwithstanding the lack of standardized data and randomized trials, the results of percutaneous renal angioplasty (PTRA) have generally been favorable, and some consensus has evolved regarding its application. Certain lesions are now deemed appropriate for percutaneous treatment; others, which respond less favorably, may be more definitively treated by surgical means or are best treated medically. The distinction between the anatomical substrates is based on lesion etiology (fibromuscular versus atherosclerotic) and lesion location (ostial, midvessel, or branch). Additional considerations include the condition of the adjacent aorta and the presence of comorbid conditions, such as coronary artery disease.

Fibromuscular Disease. Results of surgical revascularization for severe hypertension due to fibromuscular disease (FMD) can be exemplary in the hands of surgeons with extensive experience. For example, of 104 FMD patients operated on by Novick and colleagues, complete resolution of hypertension was seen in 66 (63%), improved BP control in 31 (30%), and failure in 7 (7%) [177]. Notably, however, the surgical population changed before 1980 and after 1980: Patients operated on before 1980 included predominantly those with main renal artery involvement (72%); in contrast, only 30 percent after 1980 had main renal involvement, and the majority were treated for branch disease. The declining role of surgery for FMD of the main renal artery is a reflection of the fact that that entity is treated quite effectively with PTRA (Fig. 31-34).

PTRA is now indeed the preferred treatment for FMD involving the main renal artery. The work of Klinge and colleagues [178] is fairly representative of most series regarding PTRA in FMD. Of 52 patients in their series undergoing PTRA for FMD, initial technical success exceeded 90 percent. Initial clinical success (elimination of or significant reduction in hypertension at 6 months) occurred in 87 percent. During 5 years of follow-up, only three patients (6%) with initially successful outcomes experienced a recurrence. Klinge's results mirror those of several other investigators [179–182], who demonstrated initial success rates between 82 percent and 100 percent.

While PTRA for main renal artery FMD is less invasive and less costly than surgery and equally effective, experience with PTRA for branch stenosis due to FMD is limited. The approach advocated thus far for such lesions has been surgical; however, Cluzel et al. recently reported successful technical and clinical outcomes in 21 of 25 (84%) renal branch arteries dilated for treatment of hypertension [183]. Those preliminary data suggest that PTRA may offer an effective alternative treatment for FMD in renal-artery branches, with reduced risk and morbidity compared to surgery.

Atherosclerotic RAS. Percutaneous treatment of atherosclerotic RAS has been less predictably gratifying than that of FMD. In a pooled analysis of multiple studies, Rimmer and Gennari demonstrate improvement in renal function in 43 percent of patients, stabilization in 35 percent, and continued worsening (e.g., no beneficial effect of PTRA) in 22 percent [174]. In a separate pooled analysis looking

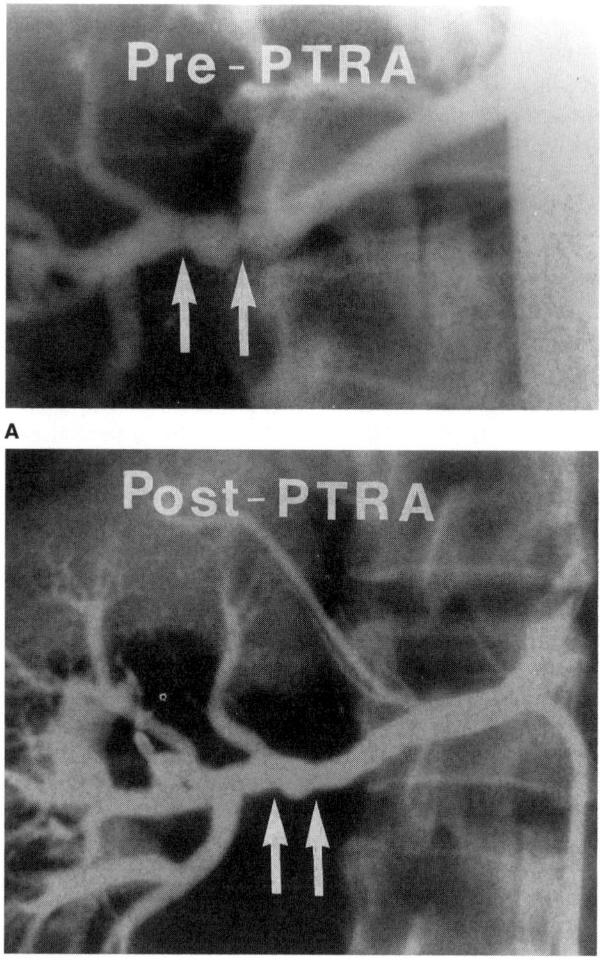

Fig. 31-34. Balloon angioplasty for FMD of right renal artery in a 28-year-old female with severe hypertension and prior left nephrectomy. **A.** Focal ring-like stenoses (*arrows*), typical of FMD, are evident in main renal artery. **B.** After balloon dilation, stenoses (*arrows*) are relieved. Patient's BP normalized, and medications were discontinued. BP and renal function remain normal at 5-year follow-up.

at initial technical and clinical outcomes of PTRA, 73 percent of patients with atherosclerotic RAS achieved a "favorable" outcome, compared to 89 percent of patients with FMD [178]. In one of the larger individual series with long-term follow-up, Klinge and colleagues analyzed the effect of PTRA on hypertension in their 115 patients with atherosclerotic RAS. At six months, 11 percent had achieved a "cure," and 78 percent were improved; at follow-up out to 8 years, only 13 percent of the patients with favorable outcomes had experienced recurrence of hypertension.

Interpretation of the results of PTRA in atherosclerotic RAS has been complicated by a lack of consistency regarding definitions of success and failure. Most investigators distinguish between technical results and clinical outcome. Whereas the criteria for a successful technical result tend to be relatively standardized (e.g., $< 50\%$ residual diameter stenosis), the criteria for clinical response have been far from uniform. Some investigators measure outcome in terms of renal function and others in terms of blood pressure. Additionally, standards defining "improvement," "stabilization," and "worsening" of hypertension and renal function vary from study to study, as do the time course and method (angiographic versus clinical) of follow-up. Alterations in antihypertensive medical regimen postintervention often are not specified. Assessment of the results of PTRA is further confounded by differences in technique; for example, some investigators recommend overdilation by as much as 150 percent [179], while others suggest more conventional balloon sizing [178]. Moreover, most reports make no distinction between results of PTRA early on, when the procedure and its technology were in their infancy, and later, after refinements in equipment and technique may have enabled superior outcomes.

Despite those caveats, balloon angioplasty appears to offer a safe and effective modality for renal revascularization, with a favorable risk-benefit ratio. The mortality rate in most series is less than 1 percent; contrast-related and atheroembolic events are surprisingly infrequent; and the majority of reported complications are related to vascular access. Renal-artery rupture occurs occasionally but appears to be predominantly associated with balloon oversizing. Surgical revascularization in appropriately selected cases also has been shown to be quite effective, both with regard to restoring or preserving renal function and reducing hypertension [174,184]. Nonetheless, while effective in restoring normal arterial flow and pressure to the ischemic kidney, the morbidity and mortality of surgical revascularization can be significant. Reported mortality has been between 2 and 17 percent, depending on patient age and etiology of the RAS [174,185–190]. Older patients with atherosclerotic disease demonstrate higher mortality and morbidity, although Novick reported that avoidance of the diseased aorta and use of alternative "donor" arteries may reduce risk of death in those patients to 2 percent or less [177,191]. As noted by Novick and colleagues, surgical experience and technique have progressed over the past 20 years of published reports, as have the indications for surgical revascularization and the patient population [177]. The same considerations hold true for balloon angioplasty, rendering analysis of the results of PTRA itself and a comparison between PTRA and surgery virtually impossible.

A balanced assessment regarding the role of PTRA versus surgery has recently been provided by Weibull and colleagues [192], who carried out one of the only randomized prospective trials comparing PTRA to surgical reconstruction in atherosclerotic RAS. Their study was limited to patients aged 70 years or less with unilateral, aorto-ostial (within 1 cm of the aorta) disease. Among the 58 patients randomized to PTRA or surgery, there was no statistically significant difference in acute outcome. At 24 months, the primary patency in the PTRA group was 62 percent, but secondary patency (90%), achieved by repeat PTRA or surgery, was comparable to that of patients initially randomized to surgery (97%). Results with regard to cure or improvement in hypertension were also similar,

90 percent for PTRA and 86 percent for surgery, at the end of all treatments (primary and secondary). Likewise, glomerular filtration rate did not differ significantly between groups. The frequency of complications also was reported as being similar. The conclusion of Weibull and associates was that a strategy of initial treatment with PTRA is indicated for RAS, with close clinical follow-up and additional PTRA or surgical revascularization, if indicated, for cases of initial failure or restenosis. Based on their data and employing that strategy, it can be expected that approximately 60 percent of patients will not require additional treatment after initial PTRA; of those with recurrent symptoms, one-half will require repeat PTRA, the other one-half surgery. Interestingly, over the 2-year study period, 14 percent of patients developed a new stenosis in the contralateral, nonrandomized renal artery, necessitating additional treatment, which may make the case for less invasive initial therapy even more compelling.

The factor that is most predictive of initial failure or recurrence following PTRA is lesion location (Fig. 31-35): Stenoses located at the ostium generally are associated with an acute success rate of 50 percent or less and exceedingly high restenosis rates [179,180,193]. While modifications in angioplasty technique, such as use of guiding catheters [194], and enhancement in imaging using IVUS [195] may facilitate PTRA, it is likely that the major limitation to successful dilation of ostial lesions will continue to be the elastic recoil of plaque, which is partially aortic in origin. Recent experiences using stents during PTRA to augment lumen size and reduce recoil, particularly for ostial stenoses, have been quite encouraging (Fig. 31-36). Several investigators have clearly demonstrated more complete initial amelioration of the stenosis and transstenotic gradient following stent deployment, compared to balloon angioplasty alone [6,196,197]. Dorros et al. showed a reduction in percent stenosis in 21 patients from 82 percent to 29 percent using balloon dilation alone, with a further reduction to 3 percent after stent placement [198]. Likewise, the transstenotic gradient was reduced from 94 to 23 mm Hg with PTA and to less than 1 mm Hg after stent deployment.

Restenosis, while not eliminated, may be reduced with stents (Fig. 31-37). Lewis and colleagues noted restenosis ($\geq$ 50% diameter stenosis) at 6-month angiography in 6 out of 16 (38%) patients in whom stents were used for ostial RAS [199]. In an unpublished series of 39 stented renal arteries from our institution, initial technical success was achieved in 100 percent of cases, and only 4 of 25 (16%) with 6-month angiograms have demonstrated restenosis (Fig. 31-38; also see Fig. 31-37). Those data compare favorably with data from balloon angioplasty alone for lesions at the renal ostium. Preliminary results support the use of stents for renal ostial stenoses, particularly if the residual stenosis after balloon angioplasty is 25 percent or greater or there remains a significant transstenotic gradient. Whether the application of stents in the treatment of atherosclerotic RAS will render percutaneous therapy superior to surgical revascularization remains to be determined.

Current Recommendations for the Treatment of RAS. Patients with progressive renovascular disease, as indicated by steady decline in renal function, hypertension that is accelerated or difficult to control, or recurrent CHF in the face of normal systolic cardiac function, generally will benefit from renal revascularization. Not uncommonly, patients who recently have developed end-stage renal disease, partly or wholly due to RAS, also may benefit from revascularization [187,190,200]; PTRA may enable such patients to discontinue or avoid imminent dialysis (Figs. 31-39 and 31-40). Occasionally, renal artery revascularization may be used prophylactically to reduce risk and prevent progression of disease in patients undergoing high-risk procedures, for example, the patient with renal insufficiency and labile hypertension undergoing coronary artery bypass surgery, in whom pretreatment of the offending RAS may facilitate postoperative management (see Fig. 31-37).

The favorable risk-benefit profile of PTRA, compared with the morbidity, mortality, and cost of surgical revascularization, justifies the use of the percutaneous approach as the first line of therapy. This is unarguably the case with FMD and atherosclerotic disease in the body of the main renal artery. For atherosclerotic ostial lesions, where short-term success and long-term outcome are relatively unfavorable using balloon angioplasty alone, decisions regarding therapy must be individualized based on the patient's ability to withstand surgery, the severity of the hypertension and the degree to which it can be controlled, and finally the degree of the renal dysfunction and its deleterious effects on hemodynamic status (CHF). If those factors indicate that the offending stenosis is clinically significant, then an initial attempt at percutaneous revascularization seems warranted. The chance of achieving a successful outcome with minimal risk is still reasonable and does not preclude subsequent surgical revascularization, if necessary. Finally, the availability of stents for PTRA may improve both acute and long-term results for ostial lesions.

HEMODIALYSIS CONDUITS

Patients dependent on hemodialysis because of end-stage renal disease number in excess of 120,000. Recent evidence shows that number to be increasing at a rate of 10 percent per year [201]. As the population of patients on dialysis expands and life expectancy on dialysis increases, preservation of vascular access sites has become increasingly important. The ideal dialysis access conduit has yet to be developed. Repeated large-gauge needle punctures three times per week, increased shear forces and intraluminal pressure during dialysis, and postdialysis compression of puncture sites are all factors that may contribute to the high incidence of stenosis and thrombosis that occur in dialysis conduits, be they arteriovenous (AV) fistulas or GORE-TEX®* grafts. Infections, subcutaneous hematomas, and hypercoagulable states also may contribute. AV fistulas tend to develop stricture-like stenoses at, and proximal to, sites of repeated puncture. GORE-TEX grafts develop stenoses principally localized to the venous anas-

* GORE-TEX is a registered trademark of W. L. Gore and Assoc., Inc., Flagstaff, Arizona.

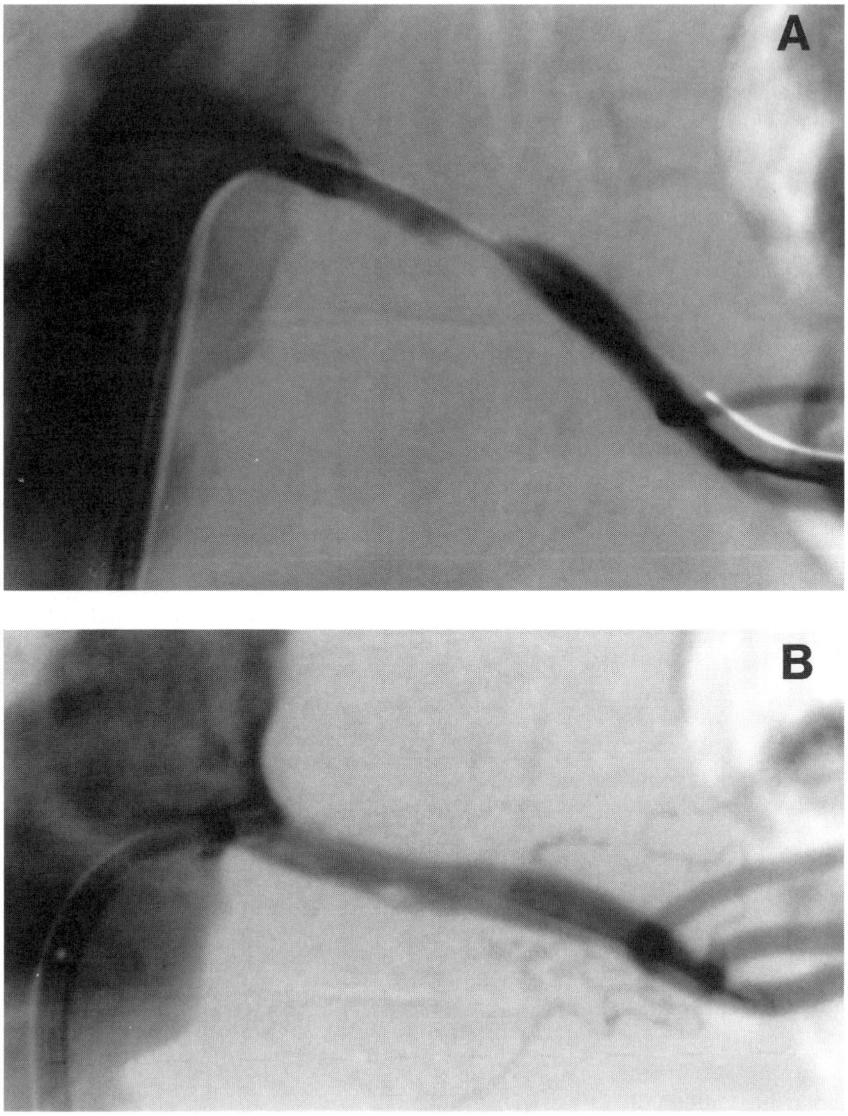

Fig. 31-35. Percutaneous balloon angioplasty of atherosclerotic stenosis of the left renal artery. Patient is elderly man with accelerated hypertension. Contralateral renal artery is occluded, and right kidney is nonfunctional. **A.** Angiogram depicts lesion in midportion of left renal artery. **B.** Post-PTA angiogram shows excellent result, typical for stenoses in midvessel. Patient's hypertension was easily controlled post-PTA and remains in control 2½ years postprocedure.

tomosis, although arterial anastomotic lesions also occur; accumulation of pseudointima in the body of the graft also may predispose to inadequate function and graft failure or thrombosis. Surgical revision, previously considered to be the standard approach for treating failed dialysis access sites, typically requires several days of hospitalization and placement of temporary access while the primary access site heals. The surgical approach is, therefore, expensive and inconvenient for the patient. A more important consequence of surgical revision, however, is the use of proximal native vein, which may limit options for future surgical management.

PTA has played an increasingly important role in maintaining the functional status of hemodialysis access conduits. The goals of percutaneous revascularization are to restore the normal hemodynamic function of the fistula or graft and to increase the longevity of the access. In that respect, the use of PTA for dialysis conduits requires a different perspective from PTA in general: Restenosis is tolerated at a higher frequency than nearly all other circumstances. That is because the patency of dialysis conduits is problematic, regardless of whether surgery or other approaches are utilized.

Percutaneous treatment of stenotic or occluded grafts or fistulae usually is technically straightforward. Acute successful rates of 70–95 percent have been reported [201–206]. However, restenosis rates are higher than for PTA in most other vascular beds, presumably because of the same factors that predispose to primary failure. Turmel-Rodrigues and colleagues reported primary patency of 44

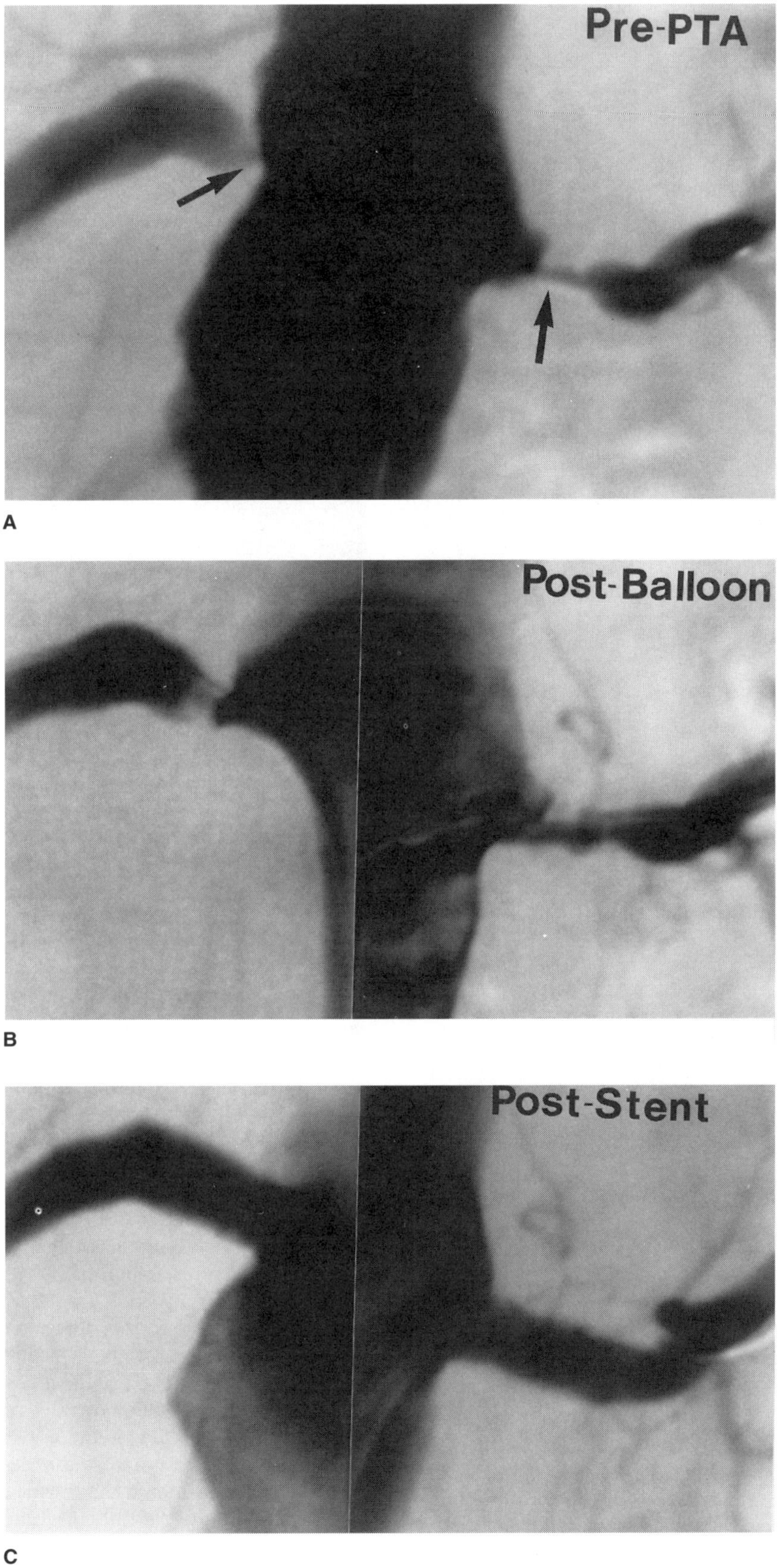

Fig. 31-36. Bilateral renal artery PTA and stenting for ostial stenoses. **A.** Bilateral renal ostial lesions (*arrows*) in 59-year-old woman with coronary artery disease, renal insufficiency (creatinine = 2.0), and accelerated hypertension (BP > 200 mm Hg on multiple medications). **B.** Typical suboptimal response to balloon dilation in renal ostial lesions. **C.** Complete effacement of plaque and normalization of lumen diameter after stent deployment and high-pressure balloon inflation.

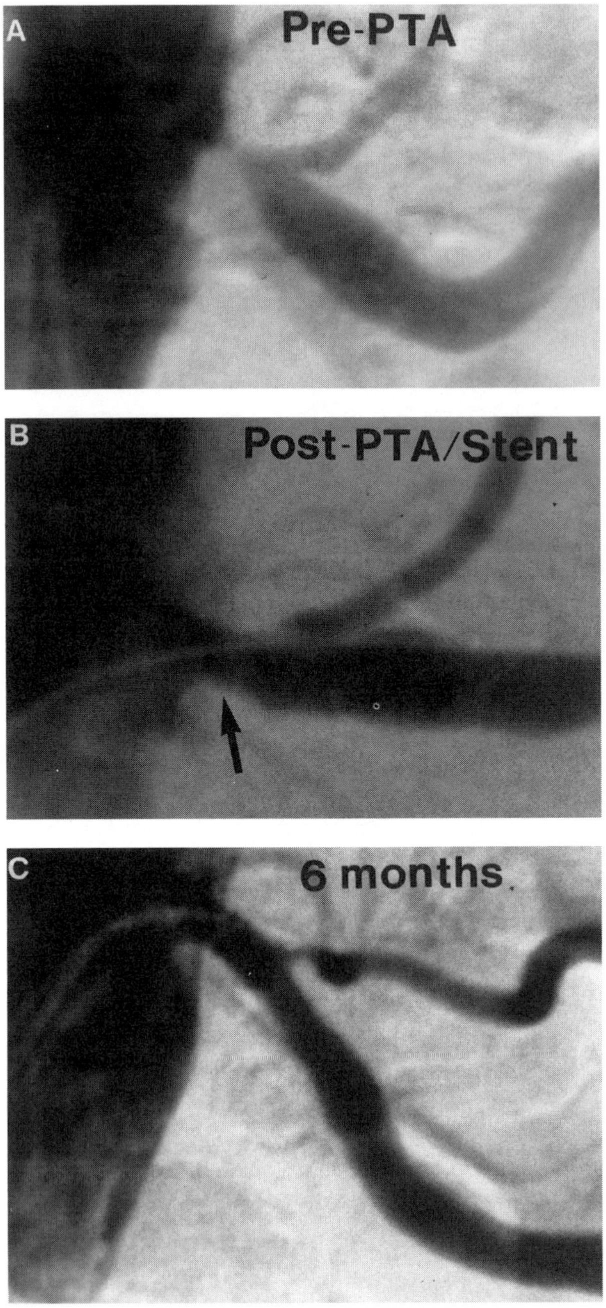

Fig. 31-37. Prophylactic renal-artery revascularization prior to coronary artery bypass surgery (CABG). Patient with highly unstable angina and three-vessel coronary disease requiring semiurgent CABG. Hypertension had recently accelerated (SBP > 200), and renal function had deteriorated; surgeon was concerned about possibility of labile hypertension and further renal compromise postoperatively. **A.** Baseline renal angiogram performed at same time as cardiac catheterization demonstrated occlusion of right renal artery and 99 percent stenosis in left renal artery. **B.** Angiogram immediately following PTA-stent (*arrow*) deployment shows restoration of lumen. BP normalized, and patient subsequently had uneventful CABG. **C.** Renal angiogram 6 months post-PTA demonstrates widely patent stent site.

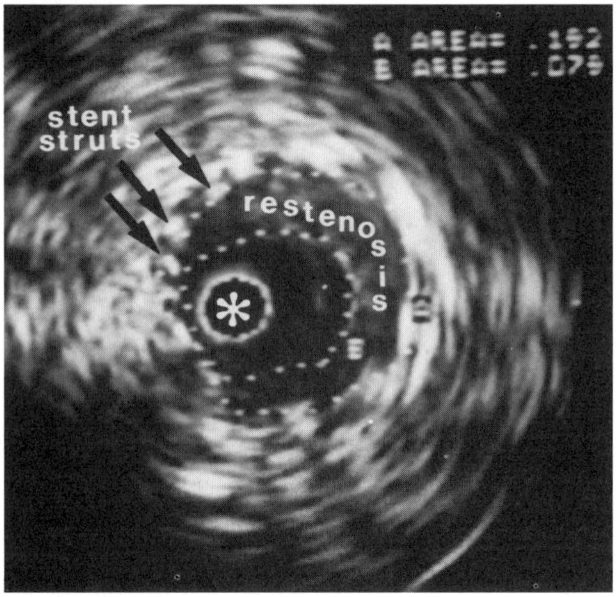

Fig. 31-38. IVUS of restenosis within stent in renal artery. Stent configuration remains circular and fully expanded, but crescent of neointimal tissue growth (restenosis) narrows the lumen cross-sectional area by approximately 50 percent. Asterisk indicates IVUS catheter.

percent at 1 year and 30 percent at 2 years in their 59 patients [203]. Similarly, Glantz and colleagues documented an initial success of 82 percent in 141 procedures performed over 7 years. Primary patency was 45 percent at 1 year and 24 percent at 2 years [206]. Complications of PTA, including graft thrombosis, perforation, and pseudoaneurysm at the PTA site, are uncommon and easily managed. Despite the unfavorable restenosis rate, secondary patency has been quite acceptable in series where the investigators closely monitored graft function and performed early graft angiography and repeat PTA in cases of recurrent stenosis. For example, in Turmel-Rodrigues' series, secondary patency was 82 percent at 1 year, 79 percent at 2 years, and 71 percent at 3 years [203]. Therefore, while the average graft may remain functional for 4 to 6 months after a single PTA, as opposed to 14 to 18 months after surgical revision [201], close monitoring of graft function and appropriately timed intervention can enhance the results of the percutaneous approach and delay the need for graft revision.

Failure of access sites typically presents in one of two ways: ineffective dialysis due to a flow-limiting stenosis or inability to obtain access due to graft thrombosis. In the case of the former, a diagnostic angiogram should be performed and appropriate treatment rendered based on the findings. Acute graft thrombosis traditionally has been managed with direct surgical thrombectomy. Nonetheless, recent successes with catheter-directed thrombolysis using urokinase suggest that percutaneous treatment is a viable alternative to surgery. As summarized by Kumpe et al., success rate in restoring patency with locally administered thrombolytic therapy is between 65 percent and

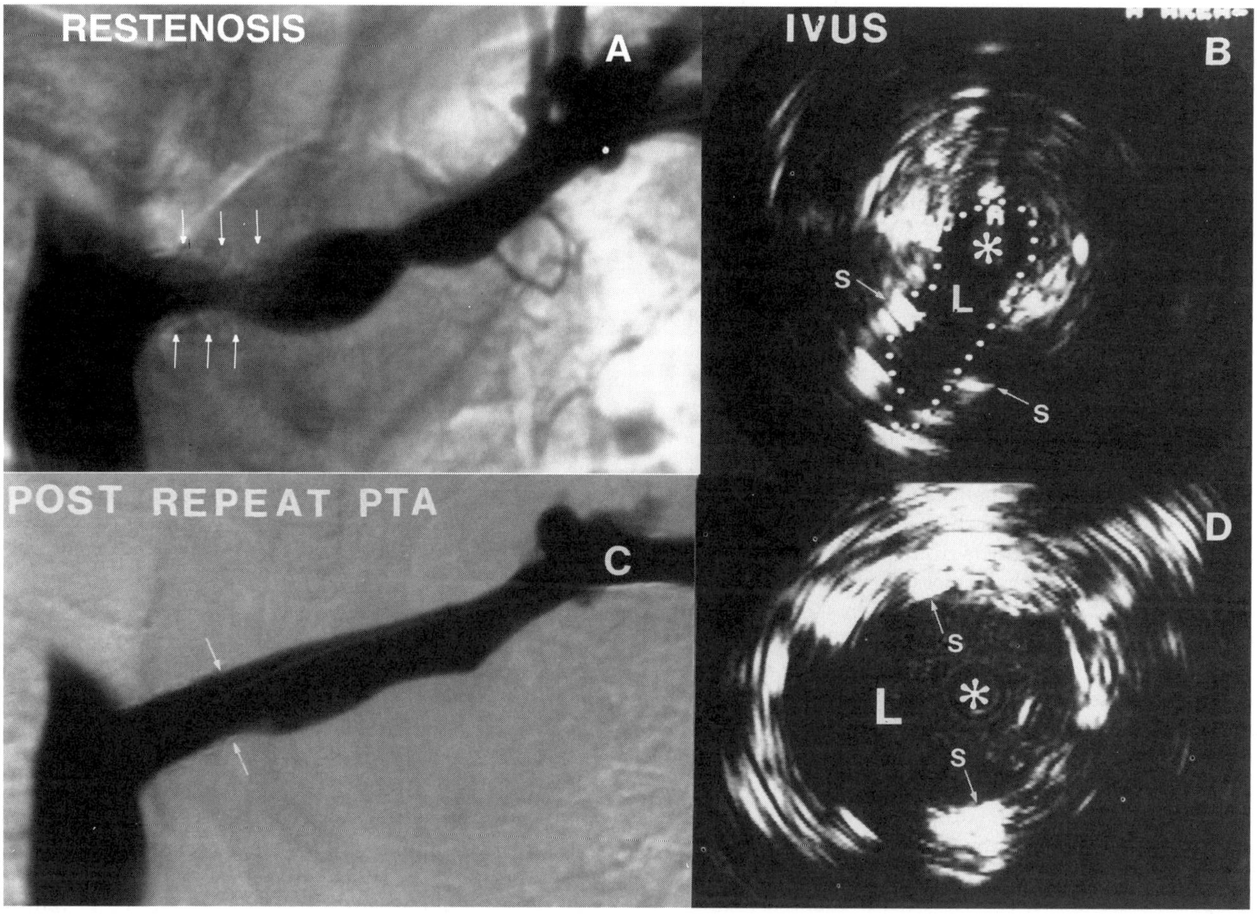

Fig. 31-41. Restenosis due to eccentric stent collapse. **A.** Angiogram of subclavian vein proximal to a dialysis graft 4 months postangioplasty and Palmaz stent deployment. Narrowed contrast column within stent, whose edges (*arrows*) show full expansion, suggests classic restenosis due to neointimal proliferation. **B.** IVUS image from restenotic site depicts absence of neointimal growth within stent but confirms eccentric collapse of the stent. Approximation of opposing struts (*arrows*) confers a narrowed, slit-like configuration to the stented lumen. **C.** Angiogram after repeat PTA depicts restoration of lumen. Contrast column now approaches stent borders (*arrows*). **D.** IVUS demonstrates reexpansion of stent to circular configuration and enlargement of lumen (L) area.

cerebrovascular disease, to restrict surgery to patients with altogether disabling claudication or threatened limb loss.

Currently, intervention at an earlier stage of symptomatic disability is possible due to the lower risks and lower costs of nonsurgical revascularization. As pointed out by Kumpe and Rutherford [53], "[T]he advantages to the patient able to undergo angioplasty rather than surgery . . . are lower initial morbidity and mortality, no need for general anesthesia, shorter hospital stay, (and) less trauma." That is true, even when the morbidity of PTA is added to that of diagnostic angiography. In a multicenter trial of 118,591 arteriographic procedures reported by Hessel et al. [208], for example, the incidence of complications with axillary, translumbar, and femoral approaches were 3.29 percent, 2.89 percent, and 1.73 percent, respectively; overall mortality was 0.025 percent. Complications of PTA are, for the most part, minor and typically do not require surgical treatment [209]. In contrast to PTCA, access-related events account for most complications (2% to 8% in most series [53,209–211]) and range from the less serious and more common (e.g., groin hematoma) to the serious but rare (e.g., retroperitoneal hematoma) [212]. The incidence of complications at the angioplasty site, 1 to 7 percent in most series [53,209–211], is similar to PTCA and consists principally of acute occlusion; as with PTCA, many complications can be managed with lytic or adjunctive mechanical therapy, including stents, so the need for emergent surgery due to a jeopardized limb is rare. Distal embolization has been reported in up to 5 percent of cases [210]; most, however, are clinically silent [209], and even those that might be potentially problematic often can be obviated pre-PTA or treated successfully post-PTA by judicious use of lytic therapy.

The conclusion that PTA is cost efficient is supported by several published analyses [213–216] that demonstrated that the initial costs of PTA are 18 to 34 percent those of surgical intervention, principally as a result of reduced length of hospitalization. The classic paper by Doubilet and Abrams [213], published in 1984, demonstrated the extent to which the cost of treating PAD would be progressively diminished by increased application of PTA. They estimated that in 1980 PTA was being utilized in lieu of surgery in approximately 6.7 percent of patients who required therapeutic intervention; the projected cost savings at that level was estimated to be $16.6 million. According to their analysis, if PTA were employed as the initial procedure in 40 percent of patients, the anticipated savings would approach $100 million. A subsequent analysis [214] suggested that the original estimates of Doubilet and Abrams might be conservative and that the estimated savings could exceed $180 million per year for femoral lesions and $117 million for iliac lesions.

More recently, Tunis et al. [217] called into question those projections. To assess the extent to which PTA was used and the associated changes in surgical management of lower-extremity vascular disease, Tunis and colleagues reviewed discharge abstracts from a database maintained by the Maryland Health Services Cost Review Commission. The patient cohort included patients 25 years of age or older who were discharged between January 1979 and December 1989 with a procedure code listed for lower-extremity bypass surgery, major lower-extremity amputation, or "other vessel repairs," the code used for PTA of lower-extremity arteries. The authors estimated that over that 10-year period, the annual rate of PTA rose from 1 to 24 per 100,000 residents; despite the apparent increase in the use of PTA, the annual rate of peripheral bypass surgery was estimated to have increased as well (from 32 to 65 per 100,000 residents), while the annual rate of lower-extremity amputation was estimated to remain unchanged. The suggestion that PTA and bypass surgery were being employed with increased frequency (and cost) without improved efficacy (as judged from the constant estimate in the rate of lower-extremity amputations) was widely interpreted as evidence contradicting the utility of peripheral revascularization in general and PTA in particular.

Certain aspects of the design and execution of that analysis have raised questions regarding the validity of its conclusions [218]. First, the procedural code employed to identify PTA ("other vessel repairs") was by no means specific for either percutaneous or lower-extremity procedures. The same code was used to code operative profundoplasty; percutaneous central-vein, visceral, and brachiocephalic PTA; and operative as well as percutaneous revision of dialysis fistulae. The importance of misclassifying the last group is underscored by 1984 data suggesting that up to 400 patients in the state of Maryland were candidates for dialysis-access PTA, compared to 245 patients who underwent PTA in that year. Second, the code employed to identify amputations did not differentiate the level of lower-extremity amputation. Such coding could therefore not identify those patients in whom PTA had been used effectively to lower the level of amputation required, a practice that has been well documented to preserve patients' mobility and psyche, particularly when amputation can be limited to a transmetatarsal procedure [140].

Apart from limitations inherent in the procedural codes employed, the study design obviated any opportunity to examine the likely possibility that PTA was employed with increasing frequency from 1979–1989 to treat patients with claudication, as opposed to limb-threatening ischemia. As the authors acknowledged [217], "The increased number of angioplasty and bypass procedures performed . . . may have reduced patients' discomfort and improved their functional status—*outcomes that we could not detect with the HSCRC data base*." The authors later reiterated that point in defense of their original paper, stating [219]:

> Concern about the accuracy of the Maryland hospital discharge abstract data is justified. . . . (Admittedly) . . . our analysis did not provide any direct evidence regarding . . . the clinical circumstances in which PTA . . . is either most effective or clinically indicated. . . . We thus do not think it is appropriate to draw conclusions regarding the circumstances in which PTA . . . is indicated from our data.

It is nevertheless true that both the risks and the cost of percutaneous revascularization increase with the complexity and the extent of anatomic involvement. The decision to revascularize the patient with claudication in 1995, therefore, must take into account two principal considerations. The first is the patient's symptoms. Reduction in pulse amplitude or inability to palpate one or more pulses on physical examination altogether supports a vascular basis for the patient's complaints. While noninvasive testing [147,220–226] continues to represent an indispensible and necessary initial step in the evaluation of PAD, failure to document an abnormal ankle-brachial index at rest does not exclude the presence of severe obstruction, particularly in diabetic or other patients with calcified, noncompressible arteries. Even in the absence of extensive vascular calcification, exercise or alternative stress testing may be required to elicit hemodynamic evidence of symptomatic vascular obstructions. Duplex [220], including color-flow [223], examinations may help to clarify such discrepancies. Angiographic examination, however, still is required to define the second consideration, namely, the full extent and complexity of the anatomic basis for symptomatic disability.

Once having clarified the anatomic basis for claudication, the recommendation to advise percutaneous revascularization is then individualized according to the two considerations described above. Two patients, for example, may be similarly limited, and in both, the degree of limitation may be inadequate to justify the risks of vascular surgical reconstruction. Diagnostic angiography may suggest that percutaneous revascularization has a high likelihood of technical success in one patient who may thus be a suitable candidate for percutaneous revascularization. In the second patient, certain risks and a complex of anatomical factors suggesting a low likelihood of acute or long-term success may dictate that only surgical revascularization would constitute effective therapy, in which case it may be appropriate to defer the risk of surgery until the patient is more critically disabled. Angiography thus may critically raise or lower the threshold for recommending that an intervention be performed. In earlier days, when higher-risk and higher-cost surgery represented the sole option to medical and exercise therapy, it reasonably could be argued that the decision to proceed with angiography came down to consideration of symptomatic disability only. The option of performing lower-risk and lower-cost PTA, however, implies that the threshold for responding to a given level of symptomatic disability may be raised or lowered, depending on the extent and the complexity of anatomic findings.

Should the patient treated by percutaneous revascularization return with clinical evidence of restenosis, repeat percutaneous intervention probably is indicated for the same reasons that led to the recommendation for the original procedure. A certain proportion of those patients, as has been clearly documented in certain patients undergoing one or more repeat coronary angioplasty procedures [227,228], will achieve a satisfactory long-term result following the second intervention. In those who fail repeated percutaneous attempts to achieve long-term patency, the decision to undergo surgical revascularization may involve a reassessment of the patient's anatomy and clinical status.

To adopt that approach with maximum concern for safety and efficacy clearly requires coordinated input from enlightened experts in vascular medicine, cardiology, radiology, and vascular surgery. The cost of underutilizing such enlightened and coordinated input will be reflected in loss of both dollars and patient years, which might have been otherwise fulfilling and useful.

References

1. Gruentzig AR. Transluminal dilatation of coronary artery stenosis (Letter to editor). Lancet 1978; 1:263.
2. Dotter CT, Judkins MP. Transluminal treatment of arteriosclerotic obstruction. Description of a new technic and a preliminary report of its application. Circulation 1964; 30: 654–670.
3. Gruentzig A. Die perkatane rekanalisation chronischer arterieller verschlusse (Dotter-Prinzip) mit einem neuem doppellumigen dilatationskatheter. Fortschr Geb Reontgenstr Nuklearmed 1976; 124:80–86.
4. Richter GM, et al. Prospective randomized trial: iliac stenting versus PTA (Abstract). Angiol 1992; 43:268.
5. Carrozza JP Jr., et al. Angiographic and clinical outcome of intracoronary stenting: immediate and long-term results for a large single-center experience. J Am Coll Cardiol 1992; 20:328–337.
6. Rees CR, et al. Palmaz stent in atherosclerotic stenoses involving the ostia of the renal arteries: preliminary report of a multicenter study. Radiology 1991; 181:507–514.
7. Rosenfield K, Isner JM. Intravascular ultrasound in patients undergoing coronary and peripheral arterial revascularization. In EJ Topol, ed. Textbook of Interventional Cardiology. 2nd ed. Philadelphia: Saunders, 1994. Pp. 1153–1185.
8. Isner JM, Pieczek A, Rosenfield K. Untreated gangrene in patients with peripheral artery disease. Circ 1994; 89: 482–483.
9. Public Health Service. Health People 2000. Department of Health and Human Services 1990; 91:327–328.
10. Vlodaver Z, et al. Correlations of the ante-mortem arteriogram and the post-mortem specimen. Circ 1973; 47: 162–169.
11. Grondin CM, et al. Discrepancies between cineangiographic and post-mortem findings in patients with coronary artery disease and recent myocardial revascularization. Circ 1974; 49:703–708.
12. Pepine CJ, Feldman RL, Nichols WW. Coronary arteriography: potentially serious sources of error in interpretation. Cardiovasc Med 1977; 2:747–752.
13. Arnett EN, et al. Coronary artery narrowing in coronary heart disease: comparison of cineangiographic and necropsy findings. Ann Intern Med 1979; 91:350–356.
14. Isner JM, et al. Accuracy of angiographic determination of left main coronary arterial narrowing: angiographic-histologic correlative analysis in 28 patients. Circ 1981; 63:1056–1064.
15. White CW, Wright CB, Doty DB. Does visual interpretation of the coronary arteriogram predict the physiologic importance of a coronary stenosis? N Engl J Med 1984; 310:819–824.
16. Isner JM, Donaldson RF. Coronary angiographic and morphologic correlation. Cardiol Clin 1984; 2:571–592.
17. Marcus ML, et al. Visual estimates of percent diameter coronary stenosis: "a battered gold standard". J Am Coll Cardiol 1988; 11:882–885.
18. Nissen SE, et al. Intravascular ultrasound assessment of lumen size and wall morphology in normal subjects and patients with coronary artery disease. Circ 1991; 84:1087–1099.
19. Gussenhoven WJ, et al. Intravascular echographic assessment of vessel wall characteristics: a correlation with histology. Int J Card Imaging 1989; 4:105–116.
20. Davidson CJ, et al. Intravascular ultrasonography versus digital subtraction angiography: a human in vivo comparison of vessel size and morphology. J Am Coll Cardiol 1990; 16:633–636.
21. Isner JM, et al. Percutaneous intravascular ultrasound examination as an adjunct to catheter-based interventions: preliminary experience in patients with peripheral vascular disease. Radiol 1990; 175:61–70.
22. Honye J, et al. Enhanced diagnostic ability of intravascular ultrasound imaging compared with angiography (Abstract). Circ 1992; 86:I-324–I-330.
23. Mecley M, et al. Atherosclerotic plaque hemorrhage and rupture associated with crescendo claudication. Ann Intern Med 1992; 117:663–666.
24. Tobis JM, et al. Intravascular ultrasound cross-sectional arterial imaging before and after balloon angioplasty in vitro. Circ 1989; 80:873–882.
25. Isner JM, et al. Clinical experience with intravascular ultrasound as adjunct to percutaneous recanalization in 101 consecutive patients (Abstract). J Am Coll Cardiol 1991; 17: 125A.
26. Nishimura RA, et al. Intravascular ultrasound imaging: in vitro validation and pathologic correlation. J Am Coll Cardiol 1990; 16:145–154.
27. Rosenfield K, et al. Qualitative assessment of peripheral vessels by intravascular ultrasound before and after interventions (Abstract). J Am Coll Cardiol 1990; 15:107A.
28. Honye J, et al. Morphological effects of coronary balloon angioplasty in vivo assessed by intravascular ultrasound imaging. Circ 1992; 85:1012–1025.
29. Isner JM, et al. Combination balloon-ultrasound imaging catheter for percutaneous transluminal angioplasty. Circ 1991; 84:739–754.
30. Losordo DW, et al. How Does Angioplasty Work? Serial analysis of human iliac arteries using intravascular ultrasound. Circ 1992; 86:1845–1858.
31. Farb A, et al. Plaque morphology and pathologic changes in arteries from patients dying after coronary balloon angioplasty. J Am Coll Cardiol 1990; 16:1421–1429.

32. Castaneda-Zuniga WR, Formanek A, Tadavarthy M. The mechanism of balloon angioplasty. Radiol 1980; 135:565–571.
33. The SHK, et al. Effect of balloon angioplasty on femoral artery evaluated with intravascular ultrasound imaging. Circ 1992; 86:483–493.
34. Waller BF, et al. Atherosclerotic plaque calcific deposits: an important factor in success or failure of transluminal coronary angioplasty (Abstract). Circ 1988; 78:II-376–II-380.
35. Fitzgerald PJ, Ports TA, Yock PG. Contribution of localized calcium deposits to dissection after angioplasty. An observational study using intravascular ultrasound. Circ 1992; 86:64–70.
36. Isner JM, et al. Percutaneous intravascular ultrasound for assessment of interventional techniques: initial findings in patients undergoing balloon angioplasty, atherectomy, and endovascular stent implants (Abstract). Circ 1989; 80: II-579.
37. Nakamura S, et al. Intracoronary ultrasound observations during stent implantation. Circulation 1994; 89:2026–2034.
38. Rosenfield K, et al. Three-dimensional reconstruction of human coronary and peripheral arteries from images recorded during two-dimensional intravascular ultrasound examination. Circ 1991; 84:1938–1956.
39. Mecley M, et al. Atherosclerotic plaque hemorrhage and rupture associated with crescendo claudication. Ann Int Med 1992; 117:663–666.
40. Palmaz JC, Richter GM, Noeldge G. Intraluminal stents in atherosclerotic iliac artery stenosis: preliminary report of multicenter study. Radiology 1988; 168:727–731.
41. Gunther RW, et al. Iliac and femoral artery stenoses and occlusions: treatment with intravascular stents. Radiology 1989; 172:725–730.
42. Rees CR, et al. Angioplasty and stenting of completely occluded iliac arteries. Radiology 1989; 172:953–959.
43. Becker GJ, Palmaz JC, Rees CR. Angioplasty-induced dissections in human iliac arteries: management with Palmaz balloon-expandable intraluminal stents. Radiology 1990; 176:31–38.
44. Richter GM, Roeren T, Brado M. Further update of the randomized trial: Iliac stent placement versus PTA-morphology, clinical success rates, and failure analysis. JVIR 1993; 4:30.
45. Pieczek AM, et al. Successful percutaneous revascularization of 180/190 (95%) consecutive peripheral arterial total occlusions using hydrophilic ("Glide") wire (Abstract). Circulation 1992; 86:I-704.
46. Ginsburg R, et al. Pull-through approach to percutaneous angioplasty of totally occluded common iliac arteries. Radiology 1989; 172:111–113.
47. Gains PA, Cumberland DC. Wire-loop technique for angioplasty of total iliac artery occlusions. Radiology 1988; 168:275–276.
48. Loose HW, Ryall CJ. Common iliac artery occlusion: treatment with pull-through angioplasty. Radiology 1988; 168: 273–274.
49. Ring E, et al. Percutaneous recanalization of common iliac artery occlusions: an unacceptable complication rate? AJR 1982; 139:587–589.
50. Auster M, Kadir S, Mitchell S. Iliac artery occlusion: management with intrathrombus streptokinase infusion and angioplasty. Radiology 1984; 153:385–388.
51. Veith FJ, et al. Changing arteriosclerotic disease patterns and management strategies in lower-limb-threatening ischemia. Ann Surg 1990; 212:402–414.
52. Health and Public Policy Committee, American College of Physicians. Percutaneous transluminal angioplasty. Ann Int Med 1983; 99:864–869.
53. Kumpe DA, Rutherford RB. Percutaneous transluminal angioplasty for lower extremity ischemia. In RB Rutherford, ed. Vascular Surgery, Third Edition. Philadelphia: Saunders, 1992. Pp. 759–761.
54. Kadir S, et al. Percutaneous transluminal angioplasty as an adjunct to the surgical management of peripheral vascular disease. Ann Surg 1982; 195:786–795.
55. Brewster DC, et al. Long-term results of combined iliac balloon angioplasty and distal surgical revascularization. Ann Surg 1989; 210:324–331.
56. Isner JM, Rosenfield K. Reducing the cardiac risk associated with vascular surgical procedures: balloons as prophylactics. Mayo Clinic Proc 1992; 67:95–98.
57. Eagle KA, et al. Combining clinical and thallium data optimizes preoperative assessment of cardiac risk before major vascular surgery. Ann Int Med 1989; 110:859–866.
58. Goldman L, Caldera DL, Nussbaum SR. Multifactorial index of cardiac risk in noncardiac surgical procedures. New Engl J Med 1977; 297:845–850.
59. Boucher CA, et al. Determination of cardiac risk by dipyridamole-thallium imaging before peripheral vascular surgery. New Engl J Med 1985; 312:389–394.
60. Lalka SG, et al. Dobutamine stress echocardiography as a predictor of cardiac events associated with aortic surgery. J Vasc Surg 1992; 15:831–842.
61. Mirich D, et al. Percutaneously placed endovascular grafts for aortic aneurysms: feasibility study. Radiology 1989; 170: 1033–1037.
62. Laborde JC, et al. Intraluminal bypass of abdominal aortic aneurysm: feasibility study. Radiology 1992; 184:185–190.
63. Velasquez G, et al. Nonsurgical aortoplasty in Leriche syndrome. Radiology 1980; 134:359–360.
64. Tegtmeyer CJ, et al. Percutaneous transluminal angioplasty in the region of aortic bifurcation: the two-balloon technique with results and long-term follow-up study. Radiology 1985; 157:661–665.
65. Isner JM, et al. Combined physiologic and anatomic assessment of percutaneous revascularization using a Doppler guidewire and ultrasound catheter. Am J Card 1993; 71: 700–860.
66. Rosenfield K, et al. Three-dimensional reconstruction of human coronary and peripheral arteries from images recorded during two-dimensional intravascular ultrasound examination. Circulation 1991; 84:1938–1956.
67. Isner JM, et al. Percutaneous intravascular ultrasound examination as an adjunct to catheter-based interventions: preliminary experience in patients with peripheral vascular disease. Radiology 1990; 175:61–70.
68. Isner JM, et al. Combination balloon-ultrasound imaging catheter for percutaneous transluminal angioplasty: validation of imaging, analysis of recoil, and identification of plaque fracture. Circulation 1991; 84:739–754.
69. Losordo DW, et al. How does angioplasty work? Serial in vivo morphometric analysis of mechanisms of angioplasty in humans using intravascular ultrasound. Circulation 1992; 86:1845–1858.
70. Isner JM, Rosenfield K. Enough with the fantastic voyage: will IVUS pay in Peoria? Cath Cardiov Diag 1992; 26: 192–199.
71. Zeitler E, et al. Results of percutaneous transluminal angioplasty. Radiology 1983; 146:57–60.
72. Krepel VM, et al. Percutaneous transluminal angioplasty of the femoropopliteal artery: initial and long-term results. Radiology 1985; 165:325–328.
73. Hewes RC, White RI, Murray RR. Long-term results of superficial femoral artery angioplasty. AJR 1986; 146:1025–1029.
74. Johnston KW, Rae M, Hogg-Johnston SA. Five year results

of a prospective study of percutaneous transluminal angioplasty. Ann Surg 1987; 206:403–413.

75. Gallino A, et al. Percutaneous transluminal angioplasty of the arteries of the lower limbs: a 5-year follow-up. Circulation 1984; 70:619–623.
76. Johnston KW. Femoral and popliteal arteries: reanalysis of results of balloon angioplasty. Radiology 1992; 183:767–771.
77. Rutherford RB, Becker GJ. Standards for evaluating and reporting the results of surgical and percutaneous therapy for peripheral arterial disease. Radiology 1991; 181:277–281.
78. Matsi PJ, et al. Femoropopliteal angioplasty in patients with claudication: primary and secondary patency in 140 limbs with 1–2-year follow-up. Radiology 1994; 191:727–733.
79. Johnson DE, et al. Primary peripheral arterial stenoses and restenoses excised by transluminal atherectomy: a histopathologic study. J Am Coll Cardiol 1990; 15:419–425.
80. vonPolnitz A, et al. Percutaneous peripheral atherectomy: angiographic and follow-up of 60 patients. J Am Coll Cardiol 1990; 15:682–688.
81. Leclerc G, et al. Evidence implicating nonmuscle myosin in restenosis: use of in situ hybridization to analyze human vascular lesions obtained by directional atherectomy. Circulation 1992; 85:543–553.
82. Nikol S, et al. Expression of transforming growth factor-β1 is increased in human vascular restenosis lesions. J Clin Invest 1992; 90:1582–1592.
83. Pickering JG, et al. Proliferative activity in peripheral and coronary atherosclerotic plaque among patients undergoing percutaneous revascularization. J Clin Invest 1993; 91:1469–1480.
84. Weir L, et al. Differential expression of nonmuscle myosin IIB mRNA in atherosclerosis: use of quantitative PCR to analyze gene expression in specimens obtained by directional atherectomy (Abstract). J Am Coll Cardiol 1993; 21:187A.
85. Simons M, et al. Relation between activated smooth muscle cells in coronary artery lesions and restenosis after atherectomy. New Engl J Med 1993; 328:608–613.
86. Simpson JB, et al. Transluminal atherectomy for occlusive peripheral vascular disease. Am J Cardiol 1988; 61:96G–101G.
87. Hofling B, et al. Percutaneous removal of atheromatous plaques in peripheral arteries. Lancet 1988; 384–386.
88. Dorros G, et al. Angiographic follow-up and clinical outcome of 126 patients after percutaneous directional atherectomy (Simpson AtheroCath™) for occlusive peripheral vascular disease. Cath Cardiov Diag 1991; 22:79–84.
89. Graor RA, Whitlow PL. Transluminal atherectomy for occlusive peripheral vascular disease. J Am Coll Cardiol 1990; 15:1551–1558.
90. Kim D, et al. Peripheral directional atherectomy: 4-year experience. Radiology 1992; 183:773–778.
91. Topol EJ, et al. For the CAVEAT Study Group: A comparison of directional atherectomy with coronary angioplasty in patients with coronary artery disease. New Eng J Med 1993; 329:221–227.
92. Dorros G, et al. Acute angiographic and clinical outcome of high speed percutaneous rotational atherectomy (Rotablator). Cath Cardiov Diag 1991; 22:157–166.
93. Zacca NM, Raizner AE, Noon GP. Treatment of symptomatic peripheral atherosclerotic disease with a rotational atherectomy device. Am J Cardiol 1989; 63:77–80.
94. Seeger JM, et al. Initial results of laser recanalization in lower extremity arterial reconstruction. J Vasc Surg 1989; 9:10–17.
95. Belli AM, et al. Total peripheral artery occlusions: conventional versus laser thermal recanalization with a hybrid probe in percutaneous angioplasty—results of a randomized trial. Radiology 1991; 181:57–60.
96. Odink HF, de Vaois HC, Eikelboom BC. Femoropopliteal arterial occlusions: laser-assisted versus conventional percutaneous transluminal angioplasty. Radiology 1991; 181: 61–66.
97. Berengolz-Zlochin SN, Westerhof PW, Mali WPTM. Nd: YAG laser-assisted angioplasty in femoropopliteal artery occlusions: "hot" versus "cold" recanalization with transparent contact probe. Radiology 1992; 182:409–414.
98. Sanborn TA, Cumerland DC, Greenfield AJ. Percutaneous laser thermal angioplasty: mitral results and 1-year follow-up in 129 femoropopliteal lesions. Radiology 1988; 168: 121–125.
99. Sanborn TA, et al. Infrapopliteal and below-knee popliteal lesions: treatment with sole laser thermal angioplasty. Radiology 1989; 172:89–93.
100. Lammer J, Karnel F. Percutaneous transluminal laser angioplasty with contact probes. Radiology 1988; 168:733–737.
101. Murray A, et al. Peripheral laser angioplasty with pulsed dye laser and ball-tipped optical fibers. Lancet 1989; 1471–1474.
102. Huppert PE, et al. Comparison of pulsed laser-assisted angioplasty and balloon angioplasty in femoropopliteal artery occlusions. Radiology 1992; 184:363–367.
103. Leon MB, Almagor Y, Bartorelli AL. Fluorescence-guided laser assisted balloon angioplasty in patients with femoropopliteal occlusions. Circulation 1990; 81:143–155.
104. White CJ, et al. Recanalization of arterial occlusions with a lensed fiber and a holmium:YAG laser. Lasers Surg Med 1991; 11:250–256.
105. Isner JM, et al. The excimer laser: gross, light microscopic, and ultrastructural analysis of potential advantages for use in laser therapy of cardiovascular disease. J Am Coll Cardiol 1985; 6:1102–1109.
106. Isner JM, et al. In vivo assessment of tissue pathology resulting from laser irradiation: analysis of 23 patients studied by directional atherectomy immediately following laser angioplasty. Circulation 1992; 85:2185–2196.
107. Steg PG, et al. Effect of argon laser irradiation on rabbit aortic smooth muscle: evidence for endothelium-independent contraction and relaxation. Cardiovasc Res 1988; 22:747–753.
108. Diethrich EB. Laser angioplasty: development, current status and future. Angiol 1990; 41:757–767.
109. White RA, White GH. Laser angioplasty: development, current status, and future perspectives. Sem Vasc Surg 1989; 2:123–142.
110. Clarke RH, et al. Gas chromotomic-light microscopic correlative analysis of excimer laser photoablation of cardiovascular tissues. Evidence for a thermal mechanism. Circ Res 1987; 60:429–439.
111. Rosenfield K, et al. Excimer laser thrombolysis for rapid clot dissolution in lesions at high risk for embolization: a potentially useful new application for excimer laser (Abstract). J Am Coll Cardiol 1992; 19:104A.
112. Litvack F, et al. Percutaneous excimer-laser and excimer-laser-assisted angioplasty of the lower extremities: results of initial clinical trial. Radiology 1989; 172:331–335.
113. Rousseau HP, et al. Treatment of femoropopliteal stenoses by means of self-expandable endoprostheses: midterm results. Radiology 1989; 172:961–964.
114. Sapoval MR, et al. Femoropopliteal stent placement: long-term results. Radiology 1992; 184:833–839.
115. Safian RD, et al. Initial success and long-term follow-up of percutaneous transluminal coronary angioplasty in chronic total occlusions versus conventional stenoses. Am J Cardiol 1988; 61:23G–28G.

116. Morgenstern BR, et al. Total occlusions of the femoropopliteal artery: high technical success rate of conventional balloon angioplasty. Radiology 1989; 172:937–940.
117. Sanborn TA, Cumberland DC, Greenfield AJ. Peripheral laser-assisted balloon angioplasty. Arch Surg 1989; 124:1099–1103.
118. Tobis JM, Conroy R, Deutsch LS. Laser-assisted versus mechanical recanalization of femoral arterial occlusions. Am J Cardiol 1991; 68:1079–1086.
119. Siegel RJ, et al. Percutaneous ultrasonic angioplasty: initial clinical experience. Lancet 1989; 2:272–274.
120. Rosenschein U, et al. Ultrasonic angioplasty in totally occluded peripheral arteries. Initial clinical histological, and angiographic results. Circulation 1991; 83:1976–1986.
121. Comerota AJ, et al. Surgery versus thrombolysis for occluded lower extremity bypass grafts: Results of a prospective randomized trial. Ann Surg 1994; 220:251–268.
122. Ouriel K, et al. A comparison of thrombolytic therapy with operative revascularization in the initial treatment of acute peripheral arterial ischemia. J Vasc Surg 1994; 19:1021–1030.
123. Tobis J, Smolin M, Mallery J. Laser-assisted thermal angioplasty in human peripheral artery occlusions: mechanism of recanalization. J Am Coll Cardiol 1989; 13:1547–1554.
124. Rosenfield K, et al. Three-dimensional reconstruction of intravascular ultrasound images recorded in 68 consecutive patients following percutaneous revascularization of totally occluded arteries: in vivo evidence that the neolumen frequently includes subintimal component (Abstract). Circulation 1991; 84:II-686.
125. Rosenfield K, et al. Human coronary and peripheral arteries: on-line three-dimensional reconstruction from two-dimensional intravascular US scans. Radiology 1992; 184:823–832.
126. Dolmatch B, et al. Blue toe syndrome: treatment with percutaneous atherectomy. Radiology 1989; 172:799–804.
127. Brewer ML, et al. Blue toe syndrome: treatment with anticoagulants and delayed percutaneous transluminal angioplasty. Radiology 1988; 166:31–36.
128. Kumpe DA, Zwerdinger S, Griffin K. Blue digit syndrome: treatment with percutaneous transluminal angioplasty. Radiology 1988; 166:37–44.
129. Motarjeme A, Keifer J, Ziska A. A percutaneous transluminal angioplasty case selection. Radiology 1980; 135:573–581.
130. Bakal CW, et al. Percutaneous transluminal angioplasty of the infrapopliteal arteries: results in 53 patients. AJR 1990; 154:171–174.
131. Schwarten DE, Cutclif WB. Arterial occlusive disease below the knee: treatment with percutaneous transluminal angioplasty performed with low-profile catheters and steerable guide wires. Radiology 1988; 169:71–74.
132. Dorros G, et al. Below-the-knee angioplasty: tibioperoneal vessels, the acute outcome. Cath Cardiov Diag 1990; 19: 170–178.
133. Horvath WH, Oertl M, Haidinger D. Percutaneous transluminal angioplasty of crural arteries. Radiology 1990; 177: 565–569.
134. Brown KT, et al. Percutaneous transluminal angioplasty of infrapopliteal vessels: preliminary results and technical considerations. Radiology 1988; 169:75–78.
135. Spies JB, et al. Guidelines of percutaneous transluminal angioplasty. J Vasc Interven Radiol 1990; 1:5–15.
136. Hallet JW Jr., Brewster DC, Darling RC. The limitation of polytetrafluoroethylene in the reconstruction of femoropopliteal and tibial arteries. Surg Gynecol Obstet 1981; 152:819–821.
137. Veith FJ, et al. Six-year prospective multicenter randomized comparison of autologous saphenous vein and expanded polytetra fluoroethylene grafts in infrainguinal arterial reconstructions. J Vasc Surg 1986; 3:104–114.
138. Leather RP, Shah DM. In situ saphenous vein arterial bypass. In RB Rutherford, ed. Vascular Surgery, Third Edition. Philadelphia: Saunders, 1992. Pp. 422–423.
139. Reifsnyder T, et al. Wound complications of the in situ saphenous vein bypass technique. J Vasc Surg 1992; 15:843–850.
140. Miller N, et al. Transmetatarsal amputation: the role of adjunctive revascularization. J Vasc Surg 1991; 13:705–711.
141. Cohen JR, et al. Recognition and management of impending vein-graft failure. Importance of long-term patency. Arch Surg 1986; 121:758–759.
142. Perler BA, et al. Balloon dilatation versus surgical revision of infra-inguinal autogenous vein graft stenoses: long-term follow-up. J Cardiovasc Surg 1990; 31:656–661.
143. Bandyk DF, et al. Durability of vein graft revision: the outcome of secondary procedures. J Vasc Surg 1991; 13:200–210.
144. Whittemore AD, et al. Limitations of balloon angioplasty for vein graft stenosis. J Vasc Surg 1991; 14:340–345.
145. Berkowitz HD, Fox AD, Deaton DH. Reversed vein graft stenosis: early diagnosis and management. J Vasc Surg 1992; 15:130–142.
146. Sanchez LA, et al. A ten-year experience with one hundred fifty failing or threatened vein and polytetrafluoroethylene arterial bypass grafts. J Vasc Surg 1991; 14:729–738.
147. Steward J, et al. Stenotic disease of saphenous vein coronary artery bypass grafts treated by self-expanding stents (Abstract). J Am Coll Cardiol 1992; 19:49A.
148. Leon MB, et al. Comparison of stent implantation in native coronaries and saphenous vein grafts (Abstract). J Am Coll Cardiol 1992; 19:263A.
149. Brewster DC, LaSalle AJ, Robison JG. Factors directing patency of femoropopliteal bypass grafts. Surg Gynecol Obstet 1983; 157:437–442.
150. Whittemore AD, Clowes AW, Couch NP. Secondary femoropopliteal reconstruction. Ann Surg 1981; 193:35–42.
151. Szilagyi ED, Elliott JP, Hageman JG. Biologic fate of autogenous vein implants as arterial substitutes. Ann Surg 1973; 178:232–251.
152. Barnes RW, et al. Serial noninvasive studies do not herald postoperative failure of femoropopliteal or femorotibial bypass grafts. Ann Surg 1989; 210:486–494.
153. McNamara TO, Fischer JR. Thrombolysis of peripheral arterial and graft occlusions: improved results using high-dose urokinase. AJR 1985; 144:769–775.
154. Durham JD, Geller SC, Abbott WM. Regional infusion of urokinase into occluded lower-extremity bypass grafts: long-term clinical results. Radiology 1989; 172:83–87.
155. Gardiner GA Jr., et al. Salvage of occluded arterial bypass grafts by means of thrombolysis. J Vasc Surg 1989; 9:426–431.
156. Meyerovitz MF, et al. Recombinant tissue-type plasminogen activator versus urokinase in peripheral arterial and graft occlusions: a randomized trial. Radiology 1990; 175:75–78.
157. Belkin M, Donaldson MC, Whittemore AD. Observations in the use of thrombolytic agents for thrombotic occlusion of infrainguinal vein grafts. J Vasc Surg 1990; 22:286–296.
158. Cragg AH, Smith TP, Corson JC. Two urokinase dose regimens in native arterial and graft occlusions: initial results of a prospective, randomized clinical trial. Radiology 1991; 171:681–686.
159. Wilson JM, et al. Implantation of vascular grafts lined with genetically modified endothelial cells. Science 1989; 244: 1344–1346.
160. Leclerc G, et al. Percutaneous arterial gene transfer in a rabbit model efficiency in normal and balloon-dilated atherosclerotic arteries. J Clin Invest 1992; 90:936–944.

161. Bachman DM, Kim RM. Transluminal dilatation for subclavian steal syndrome. AJR 1980; 135:995–996.
162. Burke DR, et al. Percutaneous transluminal angioplasty of subclavian arteries. Radiology 1987; 164:699–704.
163. Millaire A, et al. Subclavian angioplasty: immediate and late results in 50 patients. Cath Cardiov Diag 1993; 29:8–17.
164. Duber C, et al. Angioplastie der arteria subclavia. Technik, früh und spätergebnisse. Dtsch Med Wochenschr' 1989; 114:496–502.
165. Motarjeme A, et al. Percutaneous transluminal angioplasty for treatment of subclavian steal. Radiology 1985; 155: 611–613.
166. Hebrang A, Maskovic J, Tomac B. Percutaneous transluminal angioplasty of the subclavian arteries: long-term results in 52 patients. AJR 1991; 156:1091–1096.
167. Fraina C, et al. Percutaneous transluminal angioplasty versus surgery for subclavian artery occlusive disease. Am J Surg 1989; 158:511–514.
168. Wilms G, et al. Percutaneous transluminal angioplasty of the subclavian artery: early and late results. Cardiovasc Intervent Radiolo 1987; 10:123–128.
169. Dorros G, et al. Peripheral transluminal angioplasty of the subclavian and innominate arteries utilizing the brachial approach: acute outcome and follow-up. Cath Cardiov Diag 1990; 19:71–76.
170. Erbstein RA, Wholey MH, Smoot S. Subclavian artery steal syndrome: treatment by percutaneous transluminal angioplasty. AJR 1988; 151:291–294.
171. Pickering TG. Diagnosis and evaluation of renovascular hypertension. Indications for therapy. Circ 1991; 83:I-147–I-154.
172. Vetrovec GW, Landwehr DM, Edwards VL. Incidence of renal artery stenosis in hypertensive patients undergoing coronary angiography. J Interven Cardiol 1989; 2:69–76.
173. Harding MB, et al. Renal artery stenosis: prevalence and associated risk factors in patients undergoing routine cardiac catheterization. J Am Soc Nephrol 1992; 2:1608–1616.
174. Rimmer JM, Gennari FJ. Atherosclerotic renovascular disease and progressive renal failure. Ann Intern Med 1993; 118:712–719.
175. Mailloux LU, et al. Predictors of survival in patients undergoing dialysis. Am J Med 1988; 84:855–862.
176. Gruntzig A, et al. Treatment of renovascular hypertension with percutaneous transluminal dilation of a renal-artery stenosis. Lancet 1978; 1:801–802.
177. Novick AC, et al. Trends in surgical revascularization for renal artery disease: Ten years' experience. JAMA 1987; 257:498–501.
178. Klinge J, et al. Percutaneous transluminal renal angioplasty: initial and long-term results. Radiology 1989; 171:501–506.
179. Sos TA, Pickering TG, Phil D. Percutaneous transluminal renal angioplasty in renovascular hypertension due to atheroma or fibromuscular dysplasia. N Engl J Med 1983; 309: 274–279.
180. Tegtmeyer CJ, et al. Percutaneous transluminal dilatation of the renal arteries. Radiology 1980; 135:589–599.
181. Lohr E, et al. Percutaneous transluminal angioplasty of renal arteries: a therapeutic principle—case report of 128 patients with renovascular hypertension. In CT Dotter, et al., eds. Percutaneous Transluminal Angioplasty. Berlin: Springer, 1983. Pp. 281–285.
182. Schwarten DE, et al. Clinical experience with percutaneous transluminal angioplasty of stenotic renal arteries. Radiology 1980; 135:601–604.
183. Cluzel P, et al. Stenoses of renal branch arteries in fibromuscluar dysplasia: results of percutaneous transluminal angioplasty. Radiology 1994; 193:227–232.
184. Libertino JA, et al. Changing concepts in surgical management of renovascular hypertension. Arch Intern Med 1988; 148:357–359.
185. Franklin SS, et al. Operative morbidity and mortality in renovascular disease. JAMA 1975; 231:1148–1153.
186. Hansen KJ, et al. Management of renovascular hypertension in the elderly population. J Vasc Surg 1989; 10:266–273.
187. Jamieson GG, et al. Reconstructive renal vascular surgery for chronic renal failure. Br J Surg 1984; 71:338–340.
188. Messina LM, et al. Renal revascularization for recurrent pulmonary edema in patients with poorly controlled hypertension and renal insufficiency. J Vasc Surg 1992; 15:73–82.
189. Luft FC, Grim CE, Weinberger MH. Intervention in patients with renovascular hypertension and renal insufficiency. J Urol 1983; 130:654–656.
190. Libertino JA, et al. Renal revascularization to preserve and restore renal function. J Urol 1992; 147:1485–1487.
191. Novick AC, et al. Diminished operative morbidity and mortality in renal revascularization. JAMA 1981; 246:749–753.
192. Weibull H, et al. Percutaneous transluminal renal angioplasty versus surgical reconstruction of atherosclerotic renal artery stenosis: a prospective randomized study. J Vasc Surg 1993; 18:841–852.
193. Sos TA. Angioplasty for the treatment of azotemia and renovascular hypertension in atherosclerotic renal artery disease. Circ 1991; 83[Suppl I]:I-162–I-166.
194. White CJ, et al. Guiding catheter-assisted renal artery angioplasty. Cathet Cardiovasc Diagn 1991; 23:10–13.
195. Rosenfield K, et al. Intravascular ultrasound of renal arteries in patients undergoing percutaneous transluminal angioplasty: Feasibility, safety, and initial findings, including 3-dimensional reconstruction of renal arteries (Abstract). J Am Coll Cardiol 1991; 17:204A.
196. Dorros G, Prince C, Mathiak L. Stenting of a renal artery stenosis achieves better relief of the obstructive lesion than balloon angioplasty. Cathet Cardiovasc Diagn 1993; 29:191–198.
197. Hennequin LM, et al. Renal artery stent placement: long-term results with the Wallstent endoprosthesis. Radiology 1994; 191:713–719.
198. Dorros G, Prince C, Mathiak L. Stenting of a renal artery stenosis achieves better relief of the obstructive lesion than balloon angioplasty. Cath Cardiov Diag 1993; 29:191–198.
199. Lewis BE, et al. Improved hemodynamic, angiographic, and functional results after renal artery stenting. J Invas Cardiol 1994; 6:136–140.
200. Morris GC, DeBakey ME, Cooley DA. Surgical treatment of renal failure of renovascular origin. JAMA 1962; 182:609–612.
201. Gaylord GM, Taber TE. Long-term hemodialysis access salvage: problems and challenges for nephrologists and interventional radiologists. JVIR 1993; 4:103–107.
202. Kumpe DA, Cohen MA, Durham JD. Treatment of failing and failed hemodialysis access sites: comparison of surgical treatment with thrombolysis/angioplasty. Sem Vasc Surg 1992; 5:118–127.
203. Turmel-Rodrigues L, et al. Insufficient dialysis shunts: improved long-term patency rates with close hemodynamic monitoring, repeated percutaneous balloon angioplasty, and stent placement. Radiology 1993; 187:273–278.
204. Glanz S, Gordon DH, Butt KMH, Hong J, Lipkowitz GS. The role of percutaneous angioplasty in the management of chronic hemodialysis fistulas. Ann Surg 1987; 206:777–781.
205. Schwab SJ, Raymond JR, Saeed M. Prevention of hemodialysis fistula thrombosis. Early detection of venous stenoses. Kidney Int 1989; 36:707–711.
206. Glantz S, et al. Axillary and subclavian vein stenosis: percutaneous angioplasty. Radiology 1988; 168:371–373.

207. Sullivan KL, et al. Hemodynamics of failing dialysis grafts. Radiology 1993; 186:867–872.
208. Hessel SJ, Adams DF, Abrams HL. Complications of angiography. Radiology 1981; 138:273–278.
209. O'Keeffe ST, Woods BO, Beckmann CF. Percutaneous transluminal angioplasty of the peripheral arteries. In DJ Breslin, ed. Cardiology Clinics. Peripheral Vascular Disease in the Elderly. Philadelphia: Saunders, 1991. Pp. 519–521.
210. Gardiner Jr, GA, et al. Complications of transluminal angioplasty. Radiology 1986; 159:201–208.
211. Orron DE, Kim DS. Percutaneous transluminal angioplasty. In DS Kim, DE Orron, eds. Peripheral Vascular Imaging and Intervention. Philadelphia: Saunders, 1990. Pp. 393–408.
212. Trerotola SO, Kuhlman JE, Fishman EK. Bleeding complications of femoral catheterization: CT evaluation. Radiology 1990; 174:37–40.
213. Doubilet P, Abrams HL. The cost of underutilization: Percutaneous transluminal angioplasty for peripheral vascular disease. New Engl J Med 1984; 310:95–102.
214. Freiman DB, et al. Economic impact of transluminal angioplasty. Angiol 1985; 36:772–777.
215. Jeans WD, et al. A comparison of the costs of vascular surgery and balloon dilatation in lower limb ischaemic disease. Brit J Radiol 1986; 59:453–456.
216. Kinnison ML, et al. Cost incentives for peripheral angioplasty. AJR 1985; 145:1241–1244.
217. Tunis SR, Bass EB, Steinberg EP. The use of angioplasty, bypass surgery, and amputation in the management of peripheral vascular disease. New Engl J Med 1991; 325:556–562.
218. Becker GJ, et al. Angioplasty, bypass surgery and amputation for lower extremity peripheral arterial disease in Maryland: A closer look. Radiology 1993; 186:635–638.
219. Steinberg EP, Bass EB, Tunis SR. Interventional management of peripheral vascular disease: what did we learn in Maryland and where do we go from here? Radiology 1993; 186:639–642.
220. Kohler TR, et al. Duplex scanning for diagnosis of aortoiliac and femoropopliteal disease: a prospective study. Circulation 1987; 76:1074–1080.
221. Johnston KW, Hosang MY, Andrews DF. Reproducibility of noninvasive vascular laboratory measurements of the peripheral circulation. J Vasc Surg 1987; 6:147–152.
222. Prineas RJ, et al. Recommendations for use of non-invasive methods to detect atherosclerotic peripheral arterial disease—in population studies. AHA Council on Epidemiology. Circulation 1982; 65:1561A–1566A.
223. Rosenfield K, et al. Non-invasive assessment of peripheral vascular disease by color flow Doppler/two-dimensional ultrasound. Am J Cardiol 1989; 64:247–251.
224. Yao JST. Hemodynamic studies in peripheral artery disease. Br J Surg 1970; 57:761–766.
225. Bandyk DF. Postoperative surveillance of infrainguinal bypass. Surg Clin North Am 1990; 70:71–85.
226. Marinelli MR, Beach KW, Glass MJ. Noninvasive testing vs. clinical evaluation of arterial disease: a prospective study. JAMA 1979; 241:2031–2034.
227. Teirstein PS, et al. Repeat restenosis: efficacy of the third and fourth coronary angioplasty (Abstract). J Am Coll Cardiol 1987; 9:63A.
228. Quigley PJ, et al. Repeat percutaneous transluminal coronary angioplasty and predictors of recurrent restenosis. J Am Coll Cardiol 1989; 63:409–413.

Selective Intra-arterial Thrombolytic Therapy in Peripheral Arterial Disease

Krishna Kandarpa

The purpose of selective or local intra-arterial thrombolytic therapy (IATT) is to restore blood flow to the ischemic limb rapidly by dissolving the occlusive thrombus and to identify underlying lesions for treatment by surgical or percutaneous procedures. Although treatment of peripheral arterial occlusions by intravenous infusion of exogenous plasminogen activators, specifically streptokinase (SK), was attempted about three decades ago, this approach was limited by its low success and high complication rates [1,2]. Intra-arterial catheter delivery of concentrated lytic agent directly into the thrombus reduces the systemic concentration and the total dose of drug required for therapy while providing ready access for percutaneous revascularization procedures. In spite of those theoretical advantages, early studies by Dotter et al. [3,4] showed no significant improvement in results over intravenous delivery. Nonetheless, the improved results of later larger series utilizing more optimal treatment regimens [5–7] and the advent of percutaneous balloon angioplasty revived and consolidated the place of this therapeutic modality in the armamentarium of the vascular interventionalist.

The recognized limitations of balloon thromboembolectomy also have increased interest in regional thrombolytic therapy for peripheral arterial occlusions (PAO) [8]. Thromboembolectomy has been associated with a high incidence of residual thrombus, inability to clear thrombus in smaller peripheral branches, and endothelial disruption that results in subsequent intimal hyperplasia and diffuse luminal narrowing [9]. Consequently, local thrombolysis increasingly is being accepted as an alternative form of therapy as its role in the treatment of PAO is clarified with respect to patient selection by clinical and arteriographic criteria [7,10–12] and the sites and types of conduits suitable for treatment, for example, native arteries and bypass grafts of the extremities and dialysis access grafts [13–19]. Most important, an initial trial of selective thrombolytic therapy seldom compromises subsequent surgical procedures [10], and the extent of required surgery may be decreased with improvement in the outcome of the majority of successfully lysed patients [10,20].

Patient Selection

Regional thrombolytic therapy is indicated in patients who have new-onset claudication or limb-threatening ischemia as a result of thrombotic or embolic arterial occlusions [7,13,14,21,22]. Both acute and chronic thrombi can be successfully dissolved [10,11,15]. A few absolute contraindications to this therapy have been formulated to avoid the adverse consequences, albeit relatively rare, of the three general risks associated with it: severe internal bleeding, embolization from a remote source (e.g., left ventricle), and rapid reperfusion of a severely ischemic limb. The first two risks, in the absence of direct vascular injury, depend to a large degree on the systemic effects of the lytic agent.

Severe internal bleeding and its sequelae can be minimized by adhering to accepted absolute contraindications (Table 32-1) [7,13,14,21]: active internal bleeding; recent cerebrovascular accident (within 6 to 12 months, including transient ischemic attack within 2 months); and known intracranial neoplasm or recent (within 2 months) craniotomy. The bleeding complication rates reported vary with the specific plasminogen activator used and its ability to produce a systemic lytic state, the rate and duration of infusion, and the degree of concomitant anticoagulation [23–25].

Most relative contraindications (see Table 32-1) to local thrombolytic therapy also stem from the risk of bleeding and include recent (10–14 days) major (abdominal or thoracic) surgery, organ biopsy, trauma, gastrointestinal bleeding, pregnancy or postpartum status, and uncontrolled hypertension or diabetic hemorrhagic retinopathy. In such patients, thrombolytic therapy should not be contemplated unless the benefits far outweigh its risks. For example, elderly patients (age greater than 70 years) with hypertension (BP greater than 150/95 mm Hg), especially hypertension that is not controlled prior to fibrinolytic therapy, when treated with intravenous thrombolytic infusion for acute myocardial infarction (AMI) have been shown to have a significantly greater risk for intracerebral hemorrhage [26]. Although those results cannot be extrapolated directly to the peripheral system, it is prudent to screen and monitor such patients carefully when they are being considered for regional thrombolysis, especially if prolonged infusion is anticipated.

Special consideration should be given to patients who have undergone recent vascular surgery. The traditional waiting period before initiating thrombolytic therapy has been 1 week to 10 days to allow for wound healing. However, sealing of certain grafts (e.g., Dacron) by fibrin deposition within the interstices of the material and by the formation of a fibrin tunnel around the graft may take as long as 3 months [27]. Occasionally, an operative complication or a technical problem may force a request for thrombolytic therapy almost immediately after surgery. We have on rare occasion initiated infusions within a few days after peripheral arterial surgery limited to the limb, especially when signs of bleeding from the wound would be evident on visual inspection. However, the extent of the problem and the potential risks should be carefully analyzed and the decision to proceed with a brief trial of infusion should be based on a clear therapeutic goal. The surgeon and the interventional radiologist should agree to stop infusion or intervene surgically if problems arise.

Table 32-1. Contraindications for local thrombolytic therapy

ABSOLUTE
Active internal bleeding
Irreversible limb ischemia (severe sensory deficits, muscle rigor)
Recent stroke (arbitrary guidelines: TIA within 2 months or CVA within 6–12 months)
Intracranial neoplasm or recent (2 months) craniotomy
Protruding mobile left-heart thrombus
RELATIVE
History of gastrointestinal bleeding
Recent (10–14 days) major surgery, including biopsy
Recent trauma
Recent CPR
Severe uncontrolled high BP (DBP > 125 mm Hg)
Emboli from cardiac source (obtain echocardiogram if suspected)
Subacute bacterial endocarditis
Coagulopathy
Pregnancy and postpartum period (< 10 days)
Severe cerebrovascular disease
Diabetic hemorrhagic retinopathy

Sources: Compiled from [7,8,12–17,20–25].

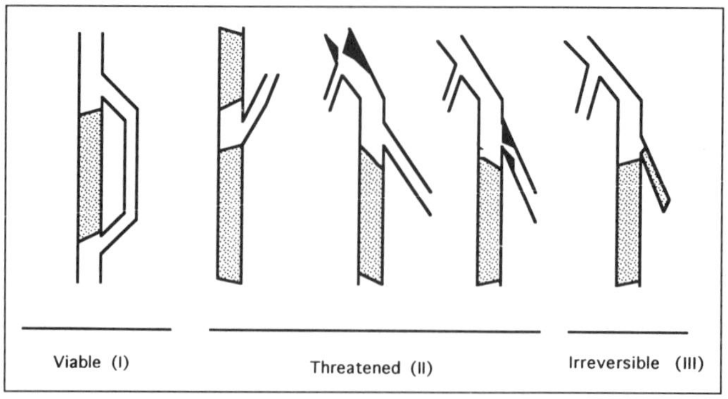

Fig. 32-1. Angiographic patterns typically corresponding to clinical acute ischemia categories. Viable limbs often show a single segmental occlusion with patent collaterals and reconstitution of calf runoff vessels. Threatened limbs can have tandem lesions in series or parallel with patent collaterals and reconstitution of calf runoff vessels. Irreversible ischemic limbs have extensive parallel thrombotic occlusions, occluded collaterals, and no distal reconstitution of runoff vessels. (Reprinted with permission from Kandarpa K and Aruny JE, Handbook of Interventional Radiologic Procedures (2nd ed.). Boston: Little, Brown, 1996.)

Thrombolysis is best avoided if a recently (<3 months) placed intra-abdominal or intrapelvic graft is present, since internal bleeding is more difficult to detect early in its course.

Patients with intracardiac thrombi have a greater risk of repeat embolization during lytic therapy [28]. Thus, if the heart is the suspected source of embolism, an echocardiogram should be obtained prior to the initiation of thrombolytic therapy. Demonstration of protrusion and mobility of the thrombus on echocardiography is predictive of a higher risk for embolization [29]; such patients should be absolutely excluded from consideration for thrombolysis. When these findings are absent, the rate of embolic stroke from thrombolysis is reportedly much less than 1 percent [30]. Although post–myocardial infarction, left ventricular laminar, adherent mural thrombi have been safely dissolved by intravenous urokinase (UK) administration [31], at least one case of death from recurrent massive embolization from the left ventricle during regional thrombolysis for PAO has been reported [28]. Elsewhere, the potential risk of distal embolization from thrombosed popliteal aneurysms also poses a relative contraindication to local lytic therapy. However, thrombolysis may be considered if all runoff vessels are occluded and there is a need to demonstrate a distal vessel prior to surgical bypass [32,33]. Other potential sources for peripheral embolization, such as in the aorta, also should be carefully evaluated prior to initiating thrombolytic therapy.

The consequences of rapid restoration of blood flow to a severely ischemic limb, referred to as **reperfusion syndrome**, have been recognized and described extensively in the surgical literature [34–36]. The larger the amount of jeopardized muscle mass (i.e., more proximal occlusion) and the more profound the ischemia, the greater is the risk of complication from reperfusing necrotic tissue. Although the reported incidence of this complication during thrombolytic therapy is under 1 percent, its seriousness demands emphasis. The most serious, and potentially fatal, consequences are cardiac dysfunction resulting from systemic acidemia and hyperkalemia, caused by the washout of metabolites from necrotic tissue, and renal failure, resulting from capillary entrapment of myoglobin released from necrotic muscle. Thrombolytic therapy is, therefore, best avoided in patients with irreversibly ischemic limbs, especially when a large amount of muscle mass is jeopardized. Physical examination of those limbs reveals the absence of distal pulses and capillary return (marbling of the skin), muscle paralysis (rigor), and severe sensory deficits (anesthesia). Both arterial and venous Doppler signals are absent on noninvasive ultrasound evaluation. On arteriography, all major branches and their collaterals are typically thrombosed, and there is no reconstitution of the calf runoff vessels [10] (Fig. 32-1). The unacceptably high risk of attempting to treat irreversibly ischemic limbs with regional thrombolysis was emphasized in an early study that utilized SK intra-arterially [37]. More recently, McNamara and Bomberger [10] reported a high rate of amputation (25%) and their only death (from reperfusion syndrome) in patients who had Society for Vascular Surgery/International Society for Cardiovascular Surgery (SVS/ISCVS) category III (irreversible) acute limb ischemia. In the same study no patients with viable (SVS/ISCVS category I) or threatened (SVS/ISCVS category II) limbs died, and the amputation rates for those patient categories were 0 percent and 8 percent, respectively. Thus, these patients generally are good candidates for regional thrombolytic therapy, barring other contraindications.

Procedural Considerations

PREPARATION

High-quality x-ray fluoroscopy and arteriography are absolute prerequisites for performing IATT. An initial diagnostic arteriogram of the limb will, in general, corroborate the clinical assessment of the status of the limb (see Fig. 32-1) and should serve as a baseline roadmap for judging the progress of thrombolytic therapy. Preparation for angiography should include informed consent from the patient or guardian, who should be told of the potential risks and alternative modes of treatment. Patients are asked to abstain from eating solid foods prior to angiography and during treatment. This is a precautionary measure in case the patient needs emergency surgery. Oral hydration is encouraged, and intravenous fluids are given in preparation for the administration of iodinated radiographic contrast media.

Initial laboratory evaluation consists of ensuring that baseline hemoglobin, hematocrit, platelet count, blood urea nitrogen, and creatinine are within acceptable limits. Assessment of systemic lytic (fibrinogen, fibrin degradation products [FDP], plasminogen levels, etc.) and coagulation (e.g., partial thromboplastin time [aPTT], activated clotting time [ACT] levels) status is of little use in the prediction of successful outcome or of hemorrhagic complications [24,25,30,38,39]. However, baseline assessment of coagulation parameters and fibrinogen levels and periodic (every 6–12 hours) reassessment may, when the parameters are extremely abnormal, be useful for management. For example, a decrease in fibrinogen level to under 100 mg/dl or a drop from the baseline level by 50 percent should alert the physician to the increased potential for bleeding. Obviously, an unexplained drop in the hematocrit should suggest the possibility of occult bleeding.

TECHNIQUE

A baseline arteriogram is performed to document the extent of thrombus and other luminal disease. Previous angiograms and noninvasive vascular studies should be reviewed before planning the access site. The selected puncture site should provide the most direct route possible to the thrombus to facilitate catheter manipulation and potential angioplasty or atherectomy (Figs. 32-2, 32-3, and 32-4). That strategy also will ensure that minimal catheter surface (which is thrombogenic) is exposed to the bloodstream. The use of an intra-arterial (IA) sheath is recommended because it facilitates catheter exchanges and minimizes trauma at the puncture site. When necessary, careful direct puncture of a graft may be attempted. Axillary-artery puncture should be avoided when thrombolysis is planned, since an axillary hematoma could result in brachial plexus compression. When an upper-extremity puncture cannot be avoided, a high brachial-, rather than an axillary-, artery puncture is recommended (see Fig. 32-4).

Following selective catheterization of the occluded vessel, an attempt is made to cross the entire length of thrombus with a straight, flexible-tipped guide wire, a hydrophilic-polymer-coated guidewire, or equivalent (see Fig. 32-2). A thrombus that is resistant to guide-wire passage (failure of **guide-wire traversal test**) probably is chronic and may be more difficult to lyse [10]. However, chronic thrombi per se should not discourage an attempt at thrombolysis [11]. If the guide wire fails to enter or cross the thrombus, a short trial of infusion with the catheter just proximal to the thrombus still is appropriate. After a few hours of treatment, many thrombi will "soften" proximally, and the guide wire and catheter can then be advanced into them. If the thrombus is crossed successfully, it can be macerated gently with a J-shape wire. Care must be taken to avoid excessive intimal damage, which can result in acute rethrombosis and possibly long-term intimal thickening.

Following successful guide-wire traversal, an infusion catheter is advanced into the thrombus. Placement of the catheter should be such that the entire thrombus is optimally bathed with the plasminogen activator. In addition, the catheter itself should not be occlusive to blood flow.

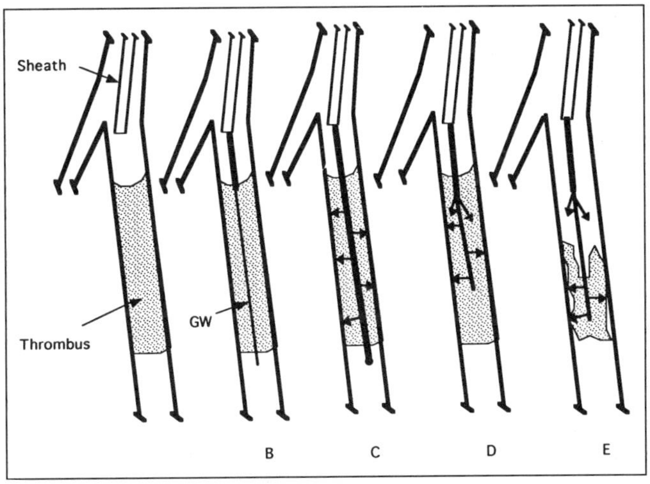

Fig. 32-2. Stages of regional thrombolysis. (A) An occluded segment of vessel is demonstrated angiographically. (B) A coaxial catheter is introduced through the intra-arterial sheath and advanced into the proximal thrombus, and a guide wire is then advanced to the distal end of the thrombus (guide-wire traversal test). (C) A tip-occluded multi-side-orifice catheter is advanced into the entire thrombus, which is saturated with a bolus dose of lytic agent deposited by rapid pulse-spray infusion. (Alternatively, an end-hole catheter or a catheter with fewer distal side holes is advanced distally and retracted proximally while depositing small doses of lytic agent at each station.) (D) Continuous infusion is administered with an end-hole catheter with its tip in the proximal thrombus and a smaller side-hole catheter, which is advanced much further into the clot. (A distal untreated segment of thrombus is shown here, but a tip-occluded side-hole catheter may be advanced so as to bathe the thrombus with lytic agent throughout its length.) (E) As thrombolysis progresses, both catheters may be advanced, but with this configuration the inner catheter alone may be advanced into the receding thrombus front. This is continued until the entire thrombus is dissolved and an underlying obstructing lesion is uncovered for treatment by angioplasty or surgery. (Reprinted with permission from Kandarpa K and Aruny JE, Handbook of Interventional Radiologic Procedures (2nd ed.). Boston: Little, Brown, 1996.)

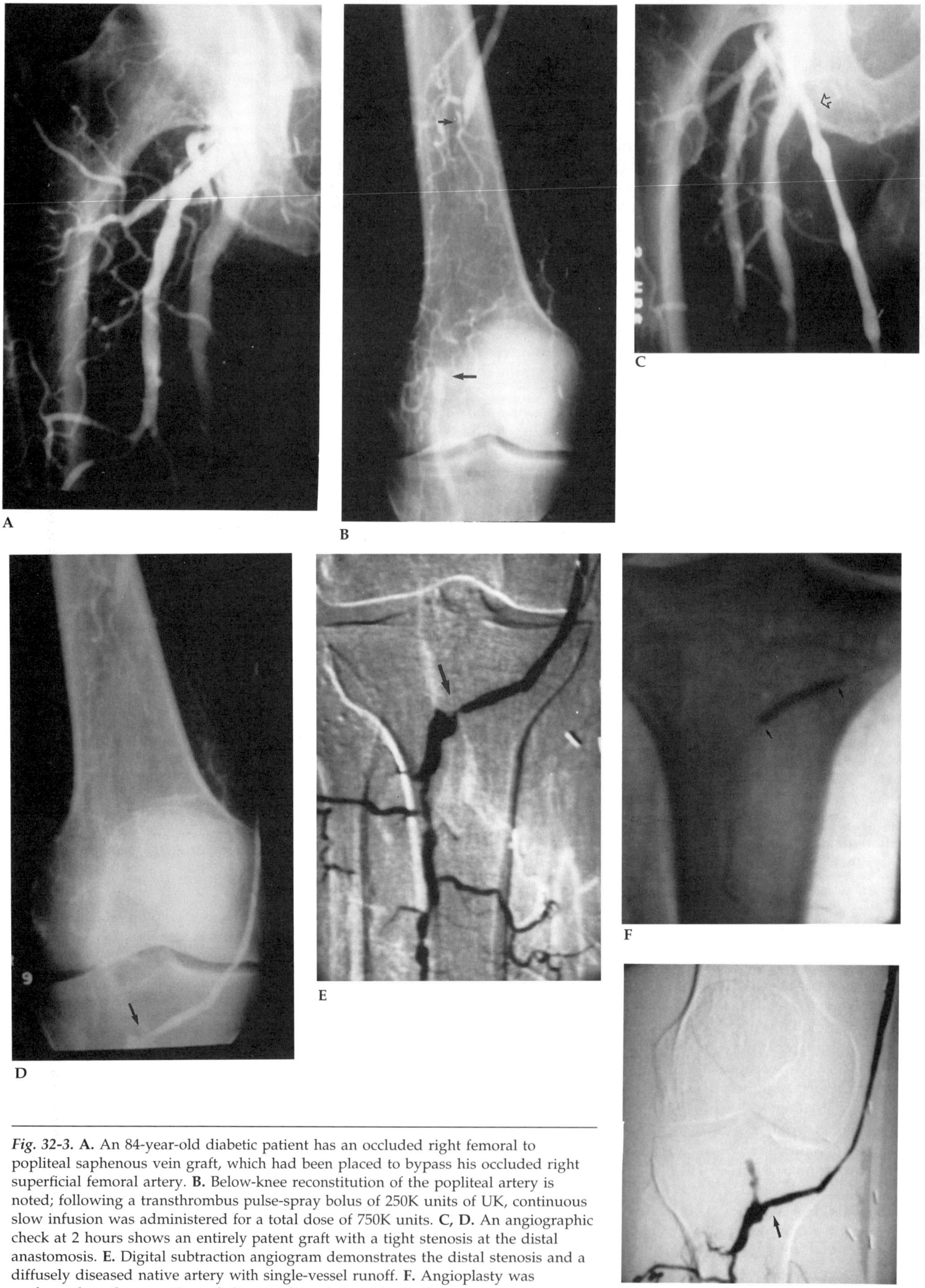

A

B

C

D

E

F

G

Fig. 32-3. **A.** An 84-year-old diabetic patient has an occluded right femoral to popliteal saphenous vein graft, which had been placed to bypass his occluded right superficial femoral artery. **B.** Below-knee reconstitution of the popliteal artery is noted; following a transthrombus pulse-spray bolus of 250K units of UK, continuous slow infusion was administered for a total dose of 750K units. **C, D.** An angiographic check at 2 hours shows an entirely patent graft with a tight stenosis at the distal anastomosis. **E.** Digital subtraction angiogram demonstrates the distal stenosis and a diffusely diseased native artery with single-vessel runoff. **F.** Angioplasty was performed on the stenosis, and **G.** a good result was obtained.

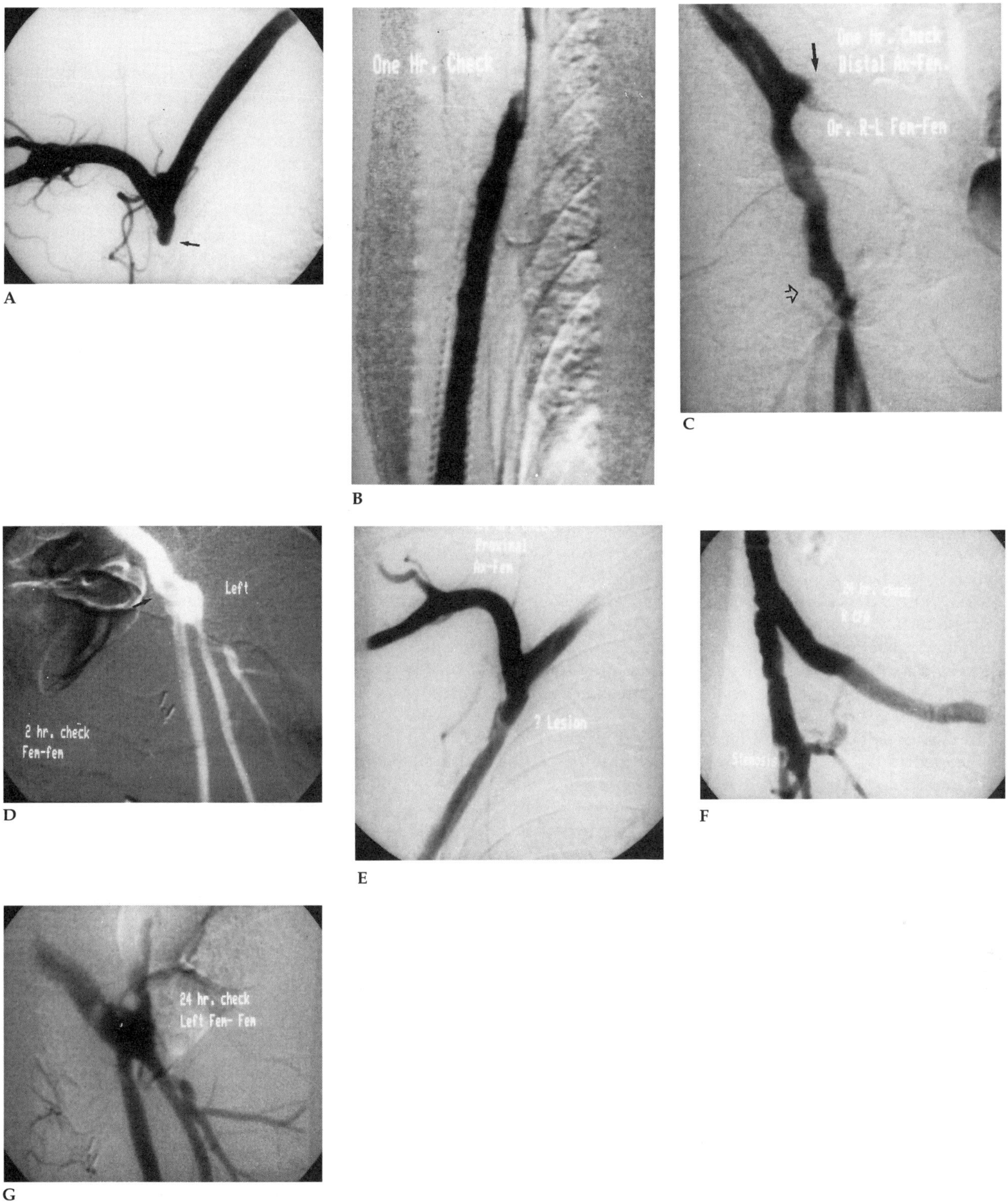

Fig. 32-4. **A.** An elderly male patient has a right axillary to right femoral and right-to-left cross-femoral graft for extensive aortoiliac occlusive disease. His limbs were acutely ischemic but viable. A high right brachial puncture was used, and the graft was entered via the proximal anastomosis, avoiding a perilous axillary puncture. **B, C.** 1 hour following intrathrombic pulse-spray bolusing of 300K units of UK, the right axillary-to-femoral portion of the graft is patent, but there is extensive thrombus in the right-femoral and cross-femoral limbs of the graft, with slow flow to the left site. **D.** At 2 hours, the cross-femoral limb is patent, but thrombus is present at the distal anastomosis without significant resolution of thrombus in the right femoral limb (not shown). **E.–G.** At 24 hours, nearly all of the thrombus is dissolved, and there is good flow into both lower extremities. A kink in the proximal graft was suspected of being a culprit lesion, but it was not. A patch-plasty was required at the right common femoral-artery anastomosis.

To avoid that, a larger catheter, for example, 5 French (5F), can be placed proximally and a smaller catheter, for example, 3F, introduced coaxially with its tip advanced into the thrombus.

When the catheter has been successfully advanced beyond the distal extent of the thrombus, a transthrombus deposition of the lytic agent is recommended to saturate the thrombus with the drug [40,41]. Sullivan et al. [40] suggested that high-dose "transthrombus bolusing" significantly decreases the time for completion of lysis and the total dose of agent. That is consistent with our own experience [41]. Bolusing is accomplished by depositing approximately 10K–25K IU of concentrated UK (10K–25K IU/ml) per 10 cm of thrombus, preferably using a catheter with multiple side orifices and pulsed-spray (forced-infusion) technique [41–43]. The bolusing should start distally, and the catheter should be retracted proximally. Some workers [43] advocate leaving a distal plug of thrombus in place to avoid possible embolization caused by forced infusion (pulse spray). That has not been a problem in our experience, and we bolus the entire thrombus to reestablish flow quickly. Small distal emboli of thrombus usually dissolve with continued infusion of the lytic agent [41,43] but also can often be removed by percutaneous suction thrombectomy.

Following initial intrathrombic bolusing, a continuous, slow infusion is started. Conventionally, continuous infusion is administered with a volumetric infusion pump and with a coaxial 3F end-hole catheter imbedded as distally into the thrombus as possible and an outer 5F catheter imbedded in the proximal portion of the thrombus [7]. The catheters are advanced distally as lysis progresses. The selected dose of lytic agent may be divided between the proximal and distal catheters, as desired. Currently, many commercially available side-hole infusion systems allow a variety of options for bathing the thrombus with lytic agents. By selecting the proper system, the entire thrombus or any segment(s) of it can be infused with lytic agent, while catheter manipulations are minimized. Unfortunately, the catheters can obstruct flow, and their surfaces are thrombogenic. Since blood flow to the ischemic limb must be restored as quickly as possible, the selected catheter(s) should be nonobstructively positioned. Residual thrombus, too, can serve as a nidus for further thrombus formation [44]. To minimize the problem of concurrent rethrombosis during therapy, intravenous anticoagulation with heparin is recommended. We favor an aggressive approach to anticoagulation: an intravenous bolus of heparin at 70 units/kg and continuous infusion at 600–1,200 units/hour [7,13,14]. This therapy can be initiated as soon as the thrombus has been negotiated with a wire. Heparin should be adjusted to maintain either aPTT or ACT [45] at a therapeutic range, as described below. Recent studies, however, suggest that a smaller dose (100 U/hour) through the ipsilateral intra-arterial sheath may be sufficient to prevent pericatheter thrombus formation because of the higher locally delivered concentration [46].

Our urokinase-infusion protocol is modified from McNamara's original high-dose regimen [7]. UK is mixed at a concentration of 3,000 IU/ml with sterile saline. A transthrombus bolus of 150K–250K IU is laced by either the end-hole or the side-hole pulse-spray technique. Then continuous infusion is administered as follows: 4,000 IU/minute for 2 hours, followed by 2,000 IU/minute for 2 hours, and finally 1,000 IU/minute for the duration of the treatment. On the occasions when recombinant tissue plasminogen activator (rt-PA) is employed, a transthrombus bolus of 5–10 mg is given. A continuous infusion of 0.5–3.0 mg/hour is then infused for the duration of the treatment. All patients are fully heparinized systemically.

Many of the available infusion systems can be used for both conventional (drip) slow-infusion and the newer (forced) pulsed-spray infusion method. Most of these catheters have side orifices distributed over different lengths to match the thrombus length. A new pulse-spray catheter (from AngioDynamics, Glens Falls, N.Y.) has pressure-responsive side-slit orifices, and is available in 4F and 5F sizes. The end hole is occluded by a 0.035-in. tip-occluding wire during pulse-spray infusion but is removed for slow continuous infusion; it is the only system designed for high-pressure infusion. The EDM multilumen multi-side-hole catheter (4.7F) (from Peripheral Systems Group, Mountain View, Calif.) is designed for uniform distribution of the infusate, but forceful infusion is hindered by the high resistance of the small inner luminae. The McNamara coaxial catheter infusion set (from Cook, Inc., Indianapolis) allows the infusion length to be varied (via the inner 3F catheter) as thrombolysis progresses without having to exchange the outer (5.5F) catheter. The Cook multi-side-port catheter (5F) infusion set has a ball-tip-occluding wire that can be used during side-port infusion. The Mewissen multi-side-hole, over-the-wire infusion catheter (5F) can be used either alone or in combination with a coaxially placed 0.035-in. Katzen infusion wire (both from Medi-Tech/Boston Scientific, Watertown, Mass.), thereby emulating the advantages of the McNamara catheter. These catheters can be used individually or in combination for pulse-spray infusion. In addition to the Katzen infusion wire, there are at least three other 3F end-hole catheters: Sos infusion wire (from Bard, Billerica, Mass.) and a 3F teflon catheter and the Cragg Convertible Wire (both by Medi-Tech), which can be used coaxially through an outer catheter (having a 0.038-in. inner diameter) for distal infusion when larger catheters may be occlusive to flow.

MONITORING AND TERMINATION OF INFUSION

Following satisfactory positioning of catheters and initiation of the infusions, a pressure bandage is placed over the arterial access site. If the intra-arterial sheath or the outer coaxial catheter is not being used for infusing the lytic agent, they should be slowly infused (keep vein open [KVO] rate) with dilute heparinized saline (1,500 U heparin in 500 ml NS). The patient is transferred to an intensive care unit, where the clinical status and vital signs are monitored frequently. In addition, pulses in the treated extremity (and the extremity used for access, if different) are checked by palpation or Doppler signals every 4 hours or more frequently if clinically indicated. The puncture site itself should be examined initially every 30 minutes for 4 hours, and then every 2 hours during infusion.

Laboratory evaluation is used primarily to ensure adequate anticoagulation and to detect occult hemorrhage. For the former, it is desirable to have a partial thromboplastin time (PTT) value approximately 2.0–2.5 times control level (with a control level of 35 seconds, target PTT would be 70–90 seconds). Alternatively, since the response to heparin is highly variable among individual patients [45,47,48], we prefer to monitor the ACT, which is maintained around 300 seconds. PTT and ACT levels are obtained every 2 hours, up to 4 hours, after the initiation of heparin infusion, and adjustments in infusion rates are made as necessary. Beyond that point, those values should be obtained on a daily basis, unless otherwise indicated. Similarly, daily hematocrit, BUN, serum creatinine, and fluid intake and output (a Foley catheter is suggested) are monitored with a view toward detecting occult bleeding or acute renal failure. We have not routinely obtained fibrinogen levels and do not find the practice to affect patient management significantly. However, if fibrinogen levels are being followed during prolonged infusions, follow-up measurements can be made at 6 hours, 12 hours, and then at every 12 hours. Again, this parameter is of use in alerting the physician to a higher potential for bleeding only when it is extremely abnormal. Precautions should be taken to avoid intramuscular injections and excessive manipulation of the patient during lytic therapy. In case of fever, acetaminophen is suggested, although there is no absolute contraindication to limited concomitant use of acetylsalicylic acid (aspirin).

A repeat angiogram is obtained at 4–12 hours after initiation of treatment to check for progress of thrombolysis, unless clinically indicated earlier. For logistical reasons, especially in patients whose infusions begin late in the day, the repeat study may be delayed until the next morning. During infusion it is not unusual for clot fragments to embolize distally and cause a temporary worsening of symptoms. In fact, that is to be expected, and the patient and the referring physician should be made aware of the possibility. Frequently, only clinical evaluation and reassurance are necessary, since most such emboli will resolve with continued lytic therapy, often without prolonging the treatment duration. On occasion, if symptoms fail to abate and a persistent deterioration in the limb is noted, an angiogram may be indicated to evaluate the severity of the problem. If distal embolization has occurred or a previously patent branch is now occluded, a small catheter can be advanced into the region and a concentrated bolus of lytic agent deposited in the immediate vicinity of the embolus, if not directly into it. Alternatively, suction thrombectomy can be employed.

On evidence of successful recanalization (clinical improvement, return of Doppler signals, and angiographic resolution of thrombus), infusion is terminated. Infusion also is terminated if treatment has failed or if a serious complication has occurred. The lytic agent and heparin are discontinued simultaneously. The inner catheter is removed, and the outer catheter is pulled back, leaving only a short segment of it in the artery. If an arterial sheath was employed, it is left in place, and both infusion catheters are removed from the patient. Dilute heparinized saline is infused through the outer catheter or IA sheath to keep them patent until they are removed when the patient's lytic and coagulation status have normalized (usually in 4–6 hours, but the lytic state may persevere longer in patients who have had prolonged infusions). Following successful thrombolysis, underlying stenoses are treated by percutaneous angioplasty or atherectomy (see Fig. 32-3) or, if the disease is more severe, by surgical revascularization [10,13,14]. If a delay in such definitive treatment is anticipated, the patient should remain adequately heparinized. Systemic anticoagulation may be restarted 4–6 hours after removal of the sheath and (uncomplicated) groin compression.

INFUSION TECHNIQUES FOR ACCELERATING THROMBOLYSIS: SHORTENING THE DURATION OF THERAPY

A current drawback of regional thrombolytic therapy is the prolonged infusion time needed to complete treatment. Duration of infusion increases morbidity [40] and costs. Besides using more rapidly acting plasminogen activators, several new infusion techniques have been developed for accelerating thrombolysis. Modifications of infusion protocols include initial transthrombus bolusing, pulse-spray (forced-intermittent) infusion, and a variety of new catheter systems that bathe the thrombus more effectively with the lytic agent. In a retrospective comparison of high-dose with low-dose transthrombus bolusing, but with similar continuous infusion rates, Sullivan et al. [40] reported that the high dose significantly shortened treatment times. However, a prospective trial comparing similar high-dose to low-dose bolus and continuous infusion rates by Cragg et al. showed no such difference [63]. In-vivo studies in animal models [64,65] showed that forceful infusion of the lytic agent into the thrombus accelerates thrombolysis. Recently, our group completed a randomized prospective clinical trial comparing conventional, slow infusion with forced intrathrombic infusion for treatment of PAO [41]. Initially both groups of patients received forced intrathrombus spray-bolusing of UK through a tip-occluded multi-side-slit (pressure-responsive orifice) catheter (from AngioDynamics, Glens Falls, N.Y.). Following that therapy, one group of 13 patients received slow, continuous-infusion (with an infusion pump from IMED, San Diego, Calif.), while the other group of 12 patients continued to receive spray-infusion (with a prototype PS Injector from AngioDynamics) for the 4-hour duration of the protocol. We were able to achieve antegrade flow and significant lysis ($\geq$ 95%) of the thrombus in the majority of patients in both groups in under 4 hours. However, the difference in total treatment time (to achieve 100% lysis of thrombus with clinical improvement) between the two groups was not statistically significant. Interestingly, our total treatment time was longer by a factor of 10 compared with the total treatment time (< 2 hours) reported by Bookstein and coworkers in their several, uncontrolled, retrospective studies [43,66]. Notably, when the two groups in our study were combined and the results of total treatment times were compared to our own recently documented historic record of treatment duration [56], we found that a significantly greater number of the study patients (78%) were completing their treatment within 24 hours than our pa-

Table 32-2. Results of peripheral arterial thrombolysis (%)

	UK[a]	rt-PA[b]	SK[c]
Clinical success	~90	~90	~60
Amputation[d]	8–11	15–20	16
Death	0–1.6	2–10	2–4

[a]Compiled from [7,8,10,16,22–25].
[b]Compiled from [23–25].
[c]Compiled from [5–7,16,23–25].
[d]As a consequence of the preexisting severity of ischemia.

Table 32-3. Overall incidence of complications of peripheral arterial thrombolysis

Complication	Incidence (%)
Major bleeding	6.6
Intracranial hemorrhage	0.5
Retroperitoneal hemorrhage	0.3
Minor bleeding	6.3
Limb-related complications	
Distal embolization	5.2
Amputation	
Due to distal embolization	0.8
Due to preexisting severe ischemia	8.0
Reperfusion syndrome	0.7
Compartment syndrome	2.0
Concurrent rethrombosis	3.0
Local arterial dissection	0.6
Systemic complications	
Acute renal failure	0.3
Acute myocardial infarction	0.2
Other	
Nonhemorrhagic stroke	≪1.0
Death	0.8

Sources: Compiled from [38] (n = 1,787 cases) and [30] (n = 1,000 cases).

tients previously had (fewer than 50%). We attributed this shortening to the aggressive initial spray bolusing, which both groups in our study received.

The early restoration of brisk, antegrade flow may reduce the effectiveness of continued pulse-spray infusion, perhaps accounting for the lack of a significant difference in total treatment time between the two groups. Pulse-spray infusion in our study, however, was as safe as conventional infusion. Based on those findings, we would recommend early and aggressive pulse-spray bolusing of the thrombus to achieve maximum infiltration of the thrombus by the lytic agent. When necessary, we favor continuing infusion overnight to eliminate all thrombus [67], based on evidence, primarily in studies on thrombolysis for AMI, that residual thrombus is itself highly thrombogenic [44,68] and that thrombolysis itself is associated with in-vivo activation of the coagulation system [69–71]. It should be noted that pulse-spray thrombolysis has been more effective in reducing treatment time of thrombosed dialysis access grafts than of occluded lower-extremity arteries. The treatment of dialysis grafts is completed in about 1 hour [18,19,43]. This is due in part to the fact that dialysis access occlusions are detected promptly and consist of freshly formed thrombi in contrast to the chronically organized thrombi of the extremities.

Results

INITIAL RESULTS

The published series [22,49,50] on thrombolysis with UK for acutely ischemic limbs suggest that a positive thrombolytic outcome can be expected in about 85–95 percent of cases (Table 32-2). The mean duration of infusion is approximately 24 hours. A rapid, early (< 2 hours) response to thrombolysis is associated with improved initial success [7]. Durations of infusion generally are reported to be shorter with rt-PA [50,51] and much longer with SK [7,13,49] but may vary with the doses and rates of infusion used. The most important positive influence on outcome is the presence of at least one runoff vessel below the knee [52].

Currently, UK is preferred over SK for peripheral arterial thrombolysis because it achieves a higher initial clinical success rate (see Table 32-2: 90% for UK vs. 60% for SK) with a lower incidence of complications (Table 32-3). McNamara [7] has reported a significantly shorter mean duration of treatment with UK (18 hours) compared with SK (42 hours); that experience has been confirmed by others [13,14,40]. Some of the differences in the success and complication rates are attributable to the pharmacokinetics of the drugs [24]. For example, SK has to form a complex with a molecule of plasminogen before it can convert a second molecule of plasminogen to plasmin, the enzyme that lyses fibrin. SK also causes a more rapid and profound depletion in fibrinogen compared to UK or rt-PA. The decrease in circulating fibrinogen hinders the ability to form new clots in response to vascular injury and may result in bleeding.

SK is a bacterial protein, which has two important consequences. First, patients who have had prior streptococcal infections may have antibodies that may cause hypersensitivity reactions during SK infusion or, if present in high levels, may reduce the bioavailability and efficacy of the agent [53]. Second, patients previously treated with SK can develop antibodies to it, and subsequent retreatment with SK may need to be delayed up to 6 months [54]. Several recent studies have compared the risks and benefits of IATT with UK and SK and have concluded that treatment of PAO with UK is more efficacious, safer, and, consequently, more cost effective than treatment with SK [16,21,49,50,53,55].

At the present time, UK also is preferred over rt-PA for peripheral arterial thrombolysis because UK has a lower reported incidence of complications, although initial clinical success rates are similar (see Tables 32-2 and 32-3). Tissue-type plasminogen activator has a greater catalytic efficiency when fibrin bound [24,54] than when free in the circulation. This property was believed to endow rt-PA with a rapid, "clot-specific" lytic effect with minimal systemic effects. Unfortunately, that view has not held up in practice. In an early study using rt-PA for thrombolysis in peripheral artery and bypass graft occlusions (mean duration < 6.5 days), Graor et al. [51] reported a 92-percent success rate (lysis and clinical improvement with a mean lysis time of 3.9 hours) and no major complications. However, a later prospective randomized comparison [56] of rt-PA with UK for treatment of peripheral arterial and graft occlusions (mean duration < 12 days) showed that, although lysis initially progressed more rapidly with rt-PA, there was no statistically significant difference between the two groups either in the number of patients achieving complete lysis at 24 hours or in the clinical outcome at 30 days. There were a significantly greater suppression of fibrinogen levels and more major bleeding complications with rt-PA, but the difference in the latter was not statistically significant. The rt-PA dosing in the two studies was similar. However, preliminary trans-thrombus bolusing and concomitant IV heparin anticoagulation were employed in all patients only in the randomized trial [56].

Recently, a study that specifically compared the relative risk of stroke with different lytic agents in patients being treated for AMI found that, although the incidence of stroke was not increased with thrombolysis per se, rt-PA had a significant excess of strokes in comparison with SK [57]. Unfortunately, none of the presently used agents is able to differentiate occlusive pathologic from protective physiologic thrombus.

Graor et al. [50] have reported the results of a retrospective analysis that compared the efficacy and safety of local intra-arterial infusion of SK (n = 200), UK (n = 200), and rt-PA (n = 65) for peripheral arterial occlusions. Complete thrombolysis with clinical improvement was achieved in 60 percent, 91 percent, and 95 percent of patients treated with SK, rt-PA, and UK, respectively. The highest incidence of major complications (bleeding, intracranial hemorrhage, death) occurred with SK and the lowest with UK, with rt-PA intermediate thereto. The incidences of major hemorrhage with SK, rt-PA, and UK were 28 percent, 12 percent, and 6 percent, respectively. There was a 2-percent incidence of intracranial hemorrhage with SK and rt-PA, and nil (no incidents) with UK. The incidence of death was 4 percent for SK, 2 percent for rt-PA, and nil for UK. The conclusion from that study was that UK was the safest and most efficacious of the three drugs. Cost-effectiveness studies comparing UK to rt-PA are awaited.

LONG-TERM RESULTS

Long-term patency is improved if the underlying lesions are treated promptly by percutaneous or surgical techniques [10,14,22,58]. Often, if thrombolysis fails, simple thrombectomy and graft revision also tend to fair poorly [13,58]. Long-term patency of successfully treated suprainguinal conduits generally is higher than for infrainguinal conduits [10,58], as it is for vein grafts in comparison to synthetic grafts [14]. However, the long-term patency of successfully lysed suprainguinal grafts may be slightly inferior to surgically achieved patency [58]. Early studies of Hess et al. [6] suggested that superior long-term patencies could be achieved with embolic as opposed to thrombotic arterial occlusions. The best long-term patencies are reported by Sullivan et al. [14], whose results suggest that grafts that have been successfully recanalized by thrombolysis followed by a definitive revascularization procedure (percutaneous transluminal angioplasty [PTA] or surgery) have two-year patencies of approximately 85 percent, comparable to patency rates of failing (stenosing) grafts that have been successfully repaired surgically (patch-plasty) prior to in-situ thrombotic occlusion [59] and superior to outright graft replacement. Lammer et al. [60] previously reported a 2-year cumulative patency rate of 81 percent following intra-arterial thrombolysis. Durham and Rutherford [58] have reported limb-salvage rates of 75 percent at 1 year and 55 percent at 2 years. However, the benefit of thrombolytic therapy on long-term vascular patency is questioned by some [61,62] and remains a controversial topic.

Complications

INCIDENCE

Selective (local) thrombolytic therapy does pose some risks to the patient. The reported total complication rates associated with this treatment may range as high as 50 percent [30,38]. Fortunately, the vast majority of those complications do not have significant clinical consequences. The overall major-complication rate (e.g., for stroke, AMI, amputation as a result of distal embolization during treatment, and death) is under 1 percent [30,38]. Serious complications may result from judgment errors involving inappropriate patient selection, failure to recognize bleeding or mismanagement of it, and failure to adhere to a well-tested infusion protocol [72]. Sullivan et al. [40] have determined that the probability of a major complication associated with lower-extremity thrombolysis increases with the duration of infusion from 4 percent at 8 hours to 34 percent at 40 hours. The risks of intra-arterial thrombolytic therapy can, therefore, be decreased by selecting patients who meet the clinical criteria associated with successful and safe outcome, by understanding the risk-benefit profiles of the available plasminogen activators, and by employing techniques that expedite treatment.

Undetected, remote, internal bleeding can have disastrous consequences. Fortunately, the overall risk of intracranial hemorrhage at approximately 0.5 percent is reasonably low [38]. This rate is influenced by the plasminogen activator used and the dosage administered [23–25,56]. Retroperitoneal hematoma occurs in about 0.3 percent of patients [30] and, if massive, will result in hypotension and may cause MI and possibly death. Nonetheless, the overall risk of MI associated with regional thrombolysis is only about 0.2 percent [38]. Retroperitoneal hematomas are more likely to occur when arterial punctures are made above the inguinal ligament. Blood can dissect from those sites into the pelvic and retroperitoneal spaces without manifesting superficial signs of bleeding. Complaints of persistent nausea and back pain, worsening of vital signs, or an unexplained drop in hematocrit should provide early clues to the possibility of retroperitoneal bleeding, which, if suspected, can be definitively diagnosed by computed tomography of the abdomen. Surgical intervention may be needed unless the bleeding stops spontaneously with the discontinuation of lytic and anticoagulant therapy or with other measures to reverse the hemorrhagic state.

Puncture-site hematomas and local oozing, usually managed by local arterial compression, constitute the majority of minor bleeding complications of 6 percent associated with selective thrombolytic therapy [38]. Occasionally, the caliber of the intra-arterial catheter or sheath may need to be increased to tamponade the puncture site. If it is determined that bleeding is occurring as a result of excessive anticoagulation, the intravenous heparin infusion rate needs to be decreased. Care must be taken, however, to make the adjustment appropriately so that it does not result in subtherapeutic anticoagulation and rethrombosis around the infusion catheter. Catheter-related trauma resulting in mural dissection or a puncture-site pseudoaneurysm occurs in fewer than 1 percent of cases, which may on occasion need surgical intervention [7,30,38,73].

Extravasation of blood can occur through a prosthetic graft (e.g., Dacron and Gore-Tex) of any age [74]. The site of extravasation usually is at the anastomosis, but seepage also can occur through the body of the graft. Often, infusion simply may be discontinued with no further consequence. Clearly, if the extravasation is superficial and confined to the limb, it is more easily detected and corrected than when it is deep within the abdomen. It would be imprudent, therefore, to subject a patient with a recently placed aortoiliac graft to thrombolytic therapy.

Distal migration (embolization) of thrombus fragments during treatment occurs overall in about 5 percent of cases [38]. Clinically, such embolization is manifested by a sudden onset of pain or loss of a distal pulse during infusion. Fortunately, most of these emboli resolve without significant clinical consequences with continued lytic therapy. On occasion, a small (3F) coaxial catheter might have to be advanced distally to infuse concentrated lytic agent directly into the embolized vessel or thrombus. Rarely, in under 1 percent of cases, limited amputation may be required as a direct result of such clot migration [38]. The risk of distal embolization can be decreased by avoiding excessive clot fragmentation and premature balloon angioplasty [30]. In general, amputation is more likely to be needed because of the preexisting severity of limb ischemia rather than as a result of a complication of lytic therapy [10,30]. The risk of reembolization from a remote (e.g., cardiac) source is small when the patients are properly screened with echocardiography [30].

Concurrent rethrombosis occurs in about 3 percent of cases undergoing regional thrombolytic therapy [7,38] but is more likely to occur if concomitant intravenous heparin is not administered [75]. Rethrombosis following successful recanalization is attributable to a low, local blood flow rate or the presence of an infusion catheter, which both can be occlusive to flow and serve as a thrombogenic surface [75]. Fibrin-bound thrombin contributes to thrombogenicity of residual thrombus [44]. Thrombolytic agents themselves may create a procoagulant state during infusion [68–71]. Careful maintenance of therapeutic anticoagulation during lytic therapy serves to avoid rethrombosis and unnecessary prolongation of the infusion.

The consequences of rapid reperfusion of a nonviable limb with a large burden of necrotic muscle have already been discussed. **Compartment syndrome,** another complication of rapid reperfusion noted in about 2 percent [30] of patients, is clinically manifested by pain, a tenseness over the muscle compartment, and progressive loss of muscle (loss of ability to dorsiflex the foot) and nerve function as a consequence of the elevated intracompartmental pressure from fluid retention and muscle edema. When indicated, fasciotomy successfully relieves the high pressure causing this symptom complex.

Rare complications of intra-arterial thrombolytic therapy, occurring in under 0.5 percent of cases, include acute renal failure related to the use of iodinated radiographic contrast agents (adequate hydration and use of digital subtraction angiography with diluted contrast media can decrease this risk) [76]; allergic reactions to the lytic agents, primarily to streptokinase; and sepsis [30,38,73]. In one study of PAO that retrospectively compared three lytic agents, the incidence of a major allergic reaction with SK or rt-PA was under 0.5 percent; with UK, it was nil [23]. Extremely rare occurrences of spontaneous splenic rupture and hemorrhage have been reported [77].

Death from local thrombolytic therapy is rare, under 1 percent, and is usually the result of remote bleeding (e.g, intracranial, retroperitoneal) or systemic complications from reperfusion of an irreversibly ischemic limb [23,25,30,38]. In the study by Graor et al. [23] there was a 4-percent death rate associated with regional thrombolysis with SK or rt-PA, but no deaths were associated with UK.

MANAGEMENT OF COMPLICATIONS

When severe bleeding occurs during thrombolytic therapy, both the thrombolytic agent and heparin should be discontinued immediately. If the bleeding continues in spite of these measures, fresh frozen plasma should be administered. If the bleeding results in an unacceptable drop in the hematocrit not attributable to hemodilution, transfusion of whole fresh blood or packed red blood cells may be indicated. For severe, continuing hemorrhage, epsilon aminocaproic acid (Amicar) should be considered. The most important intervention, however, is to find the source of internal bleeding and to take definite corrective action.

Distal embolization of thrombus usually resolves with continued lytic therapy or application of suction thrombectomy. Surgical embolectomy is needed on rare occasion. Allergic reactions are rare with UK and are more frequently associated with SK and rt-PA. Occasional episodes of mild bronchospasm, skin rash, and transient fever are reported with all three agents. Recently, there have been reports of chills and rigors following rapid infusion of large boluses (e.g., given during treatment of dialysis fistulae) of UK (Abbokinase, Abbott Labs, Chicago). This is thought to be related to cytokine production from the aging cell lines currently used for manufacturing this agent [personal communication with AA Sasahara, Abbott Labs]. These symptoms may be blocked by oral prophylaxis with 1 g acetaminophen and 50 mg diphenhydramine hydrochloride (Benadryl), given 30–60 minutes prior to UK infusion. If these symptoms occur during treatment, 50 mg meperidine hydrochloride (Demerol) may be given intravenously. Alternatively, histamine-2 blockers, such as 300 mg cimetidine or 50 mg ranitidine, may be given.

Summary

The accrued experience over the last decade has led to the increasing acceptance of selective IATT for PAO as an adjunct to definitive recanalization procedures. In addition to quickly restoring perfusion to an ischemic limb, this treatment serves to uncover underlying culprit obstructive lesions. In a minority of patients, it is the only treatment needed. Most focal stenoses can be treated with PTA, which may be the only adjunctive procedure necessary in certain patients. When diffuse occlusive disease is present, surgical revascularization can be performed almost immediately without adverse effects from the preceding thrombolytic therapy. Additionally, emergent surgery may be avoided, and more limited elective procedures are often possible. The latter can be of special benefit to patients with limited options for grafting material. Thrombolytic therapy is especially useful for those patients who have thrombosed runoff vessels, which not only must be demonstrated prior to surgery but whose presence also positively influences the long-term patency of any revascularization procedure [52].

The duration of infusion, which increases morbidity and cost, continues to limit the ready acceptance of selective thrombolysis. Newer infusion techniques have significantly decreased the treatment times, which nevertheless remain around 24 hours for lower-extremity occlusions in the experience of most workers. However, dialysis access grafts are lysed within an hour using pulse-spray infusion techniques. Work continues on the optimization of infusion methods [78,79], drug dosing, and manipulations with added substrates [80,81] to shorten treatment time. Other changes in practice, such as the elimination of intensive-care monitoring also are being considered as workers gain more comfort with the use of lytic agents and therapy [82].

Although initial luminal recanalization and clinical improvement are achieved in a large majority of patients, there are contradictory opinions on the contribution of thrombolytic therapy to the long-term patency achieved in the lower extremity [60]. At the time of this writing, new information is emerging on the reduction of mortality in surgical patients who have undergone initial thrombolytic therapy [20]. The effect of that reduction has recently been analyzed in medical-economic terms [83]. This preliminary analysis suggests that thrombolytic therapy prior to surgery is potentially the most cost-effective treatment for patients with limb ischemia resulting from PAO [83]. Further research and controversy definitely are to be expected in this area.

References

1. McNicol GB, et al. Treatment of peripheral arterial occlusions by streptokinase perfusion. Br Med J 1963; 1:1508–1512.
2. Boyles PW, et al. Comparative effectiveness of IV and IA fibrinolysin therapy. Am J Cardiol 1960; 6:439–445.
3. Dotter CT, et al. Streptokinase treatment of thromboembolic disease. Radiology 1972; 102:283–290.
4. Dotter CT, Rosch J, Seaman AJ. Selective clot lysis with low-dose streptokinase. Radiology 1974; 111:31–37.
5. Katzen BT, van Breda A. Low-dose streptokinase in the treatment of arterial occlusions. AJR 1981; 136:1171–1178.
6. Hess H, et al. Local low-dose thrombolytic therapy of peripheral arterial occlusions. N Engl J Med 1982; 307:1627–1630.
7. McNamara TO, Fischer JR. Thrombolysis in peripheral arterial and graft occlusions: Improved results using high dose urokinase. AJR 1985; 144:764–775.
8. Graor RA, et al. Thrombolysis of peripheral arterial bypass grafts: surgical thrombectomy compared with thrombolysis. J Vasc Surg 1988; 7:347–355.
9. Bowles CR, et al. Diffuse arterial narrowing as a result of intimal proliferation: a delayed complication of embolectomy with the Fogarty balloon catheter. J Vasc Surg 1988; 7:487–494.
10. McNamara TO, Bomberger RA. Factors affecting initial and six month patency rates after intra-arterial thrombolysis with high dose urokinase. Am J Surg 1986; 152:709–712.
11. Luppatelli L, et al. Selective thrombolysis with low-dose urokinase in chronic arteriosclerotic occlusions. Cardiovasc Intervent Radiol 1988; 11:123–126.
12. Yeager RA, et al. Surgical management of severe acute lower extremity ischemia. J Vasc Surg 1992; 15:385–393.
13. Gardiner GA, et al. Thrombolysis of occluded femoropopliteal grafts. AJR 1986; 147:621–626.
14. Sullivan KL, et al. Efficacy of thrombolysis in infrainguinal bypass grafts. Circulation 1991; 83:[Suppl I]:I-99–I-105.
15. Motarjeme A. Thrombolytic therapy in arterial occlusion and graft thrombosis. Seminars in Vascular Surgery 1989; 2:155–178.
16. Traughber PD, et al. Intraarterial fibrinolytic therapy for popliteal and tibial artery obstruction: comparison of streptokinase to urokinase. AJR 1987; 149:543–456.
17. Lambiase RE, et al. Extensive thromboembolic disease of the hand and forearm: treatment with thrombolytic therapy. JVIR 1991; 2:210–208.
18. Brunner MC, et al. Ultrarapid urokinase in hemodialysis access occlusion. JVIR 1991; 2:503–506.
19. Kumpe DA, Cohen MAH, Durham JD. Treatment of failing and failed hemodialysis access sites: comparison of surgical treatment with thrombolysis/angioplasty. Semin Vasc Surgery 1992; 5:118–127.
20. Ouriel K. Thrombolysis versus operation in acute peripheral arterial occlusion. Presented at: The Twentieth Annual Symposium on Current Critical Problems and New Techniques in Vascular Surgery, November 1993. New York.
21. Belkin M, et al. Intra-arterial fibrinolytic therapy. Arch Surg 1986; 121:769–773.
22. McNamara TO. Thrombolysis as an alternative initial therapy for the acutely ischemic limb. Seminars Vasc Surg 1992; 5:89–98.
23. Graor RA, et al. Efficacy and safety of intraarterial local infusion of streptokinase, urokinase, or tissue plasminogen activator for peripheral arterial occlusion: a retrospective review. J Vasc Med Biol 1990; 2:310–315.
24. Holden RW. Plasminogen activators: pharmacology and therapy. Radiology 1990; 174:993–1001.
25. Woo KS, White HD. Comparative tolerability profiles of thrombolytic agents: a review. Drug Safety 1993; 8:19–29.
26. Anderson JL, et al. Older age and elevated blood pressure are risk factors for intracerebral hemorrhage after thrombolysis. Am J Cardiol 1991; 68:166–170.
27. Van Breda A. Thrombolytic therapy of peripheral vascular occlusions. In D Kim, DE Orron, eds. Peripheral Vascular Imaging and Intervention, St. Louis: Mosby, 1992. Pp 429–439.
28. Paulson EK, Miller FJ. Embolization of cardiac mural thrombolysis: complication of intraarterial fibrinolysis. Radiology 1988; 168:95–96.

29. Stratton JR. Embolic risk due to left ventricular thrombi. Card Board Rev 1988; 5:81–91.
30. McNamara TO, Goodwin SC, Kandarpa K. Complications associated with thrombolysis. Seminars in Interventional Radiology 1994; 11:134–144.
31. Kremer P, et al. Lysis of left ventricular thrombi with urokinase. Circulation 1985; 72:112–118.
32. Carpenter JP, et al. Popliteal artery aneurysms: improved results with thrombolytic therapy. Presented at North American Chapter ISCVS and SVS Annual Meeting, June 1993. Washington, D.C.
33. Leen VH, et al. Thrombolysis of thrombosed popliteal aneurysms. JVIR 1994; 5:46.
34. Haimovici H. Arterial embolism with acute massive ischemic myopathy and myoglobinuria. Surgery 1960; 47:739–747.
35. Fisher DR, Fogarty TJ, Morrow AG. Clinical and biochemical observations of the effect of transient femoral occlusion in man. Surgery 1970; 68:323–328.
36. Beyersdorf F, et al. Avoiding reperfusion injury after revascularization: experimental observations and recommendations for clinical application. J Vasc Surg 1989; 9:757–766.
37. Lang EK. Streptokinase Therapy: Complications of intra-arterial use. Radiology 1985; 154:75–77.
38. Gardiner GA, Sullivan KL. Complications of regional thrombolytic therapy. In S Kadir, ed. Current Practice of Interventional Radiology. Philadelphia: Decker, 1991. Pp 87–91.
39. Marder VJ. Relevance of changes in blood fibrinolytic and coagulation parameters during thrombolytic therapy. Am J Med 1987; 83(2A0):15–19.
40. Sullivan KL, et al. Acceleration of thrombolysis with a high-dose transthrombus bolus technique. Radiology 1989; 173: 805–808.
41. Kandarpa K, et al. Intraarterial thrombolysis of lower extremity occlusions: a prospective, randomized comparison of forced periodic infusion and conventional slow continuous infusion. Radiology 1993; 188:861–867.
42. Mewissen MW, et al. Symptomatic native arterial occlusions: early experience with "over-the-wire" thrombolysis. JVIR 1990; 1:43–47.
43. Valji K, et al. Pulsed-spray thrombolysis of arterial and bypass graft occlusions. AJR 1991; 156:617–621.
44. Fuster V, et al. Atherosclerotic plaque rupture and thrombosis: evolving concepts. Circulation 1990; 82[Suppl II]:II-47–II-59.
45. Rath B, Bennett DH. Monitoring the effect of heparin by measurement of activated clotting time during and after PTCA. Br Heart J 1990; 63:18–21.
46. LeBlang SD, et al. Low-dose urokinase regimen for the treatment of lower extremity arterial and graft occlusions: experience in 132 cases. JVIR 1992; 3:475–483.
47. Ogilby JD, et al. Variability of effective anticoagulation for PTCA is dependent upon heparin potency. Circulation 1991; 84[Suppl II]:2352.
48. Ogilby JD, et al. Adequate heparinization during PTCA: assessment using activated clotting times. Cath and Cardiovasc Diag 1989; 18:206–209.
49. Van Breda A, et al. Relative cost-effectiveness of urokinase versus streptokinase in the treatment of peripheral vascular disease. JVIR 1991; 2:77–87.
50. Graor RA, et al. Efficacy and safety of intraarterial local infusion of streptokinase, urokinase, or tissue plasminogen activator for peripheral arterial occlusion: a retrospective review. J Vasc Med Biol 1990; 2:310–315.
51. Graor RA, et al. Thrombolysis with recombinant human tissue-type plasminogen activator in patients with peripheral artery and bypass graft occlusions. Circulation 1986; 74[Suppl I]:I-15–I-20.
52. Clouse ME, et al. Percutaneous intraarterial thrombolysis: analysis of factors affecting outcome. JVIR 1994; 5:93–100.
53. Van Breda A, Katzen BT, Deutsch AS. Urokinase versus streptokinase in local thrombolysis. Radiology 1987; 165: 109–111.
54. Marder V, Sherry S. Thrombolytic therapy: current status. N Engl J Med 1988; 318:1512–1520.
55. Janosik JE, et al. Therapeutic alternatives for subacute peripheral arterial occlusion: comparison by outcome, length of stay, and hospital charges. Invest Radiol 1991; 26:921–925.
56. Meyerovitz MF, et al., Recombinant tissue-type plasminogen activator versus urokinase in peripheral arterial and graft occlusions: A Randomized Trial. Radiology 1990; 175:75–78.
57. Vaitkus PT, et al. Stroke complicating acute myocardial infarction. Arch Intern Med 1992; 152:2020–2024.
58. Durham JD, Rutherford RB. Assessment of long-term efficacy of fibrinolytic therapy in the ischemic extremity. Semin Intervent Radiol 1992; 9:166–173.
59. Cohen JR, et al. Recognition and management of impending graft failure. Arch Surg 1986; 121:758–759.
60. Lammer J, et al. Intraarterial fibrinolysis: long-term results. Radiology 1986; 161:159–163.
61. Belkin M, et al. Observations on the use of thrombolytic agents for thrombotic occlusion of infrainguinal vein grafts. J Vasc Surg 1990; 11:289–296.
62. Faggioli GL, et al. Failure of thrombolytic therapy to improve long-term vascular patency. J Vasc Surg 1994; 19:289–297.
63. Cragg AH, et al. Two urokinase dose regimens in native arterial and graft occlusions: initial results of prospective, randomized clinical trial. Radiology 1991; 178:681–686.
64. Valji K, Bookstein JJ. Fibrinolysis with intrathrombic injection of urokinase and tissue-type plasminogen activator: results in a new model of subacute venous thrombosis. Invest Radiol 1987; 22:23–27.
65. Kandarpa K, et al. Forceful pulsatile local infusion of enzyme accelerates thrombolysis: *in vivo* evaluation of a new delivery system. Radiology 1988; 168:739–744.
66. Valji K, et al. Occluded peripheral arteries and bypass grafts: lytic stagnation as an end point for pulse-spray pharmacomechanical thrombolysis. Radiology 1993; 188:389–394.
67. McNamara TO. The use of lytic therapy with endovascular "repair" for the failed infrainguinal graft. Seminars in Vascular Surgery 1990; 3:56–65.
68. Arnout J, et al. Correlation between level of heparinization and patency of the infarct-related coronary artery after treatment of acute myocardial infarction with alteplase (rt-PA). J Am Coll Cardiol 1992; 20:513–519.
69. Owen J, et al. Thrombolytic therapy with tissue plasminogen activator and streptokinase induces transient thrombin activity. Blood 1988; 72:616–620.
70. Fitzgerald DJ, et al. Marked platelet activation in vivo after intravenous streptokinase in patients with AMI. Circulation 1988; 77:142–150.
71. Baglin TP, et al. Thrombin generation and myocardial infarction during infusion of tissue-plasminogen activator. The Lancet 1993; 341:504–505.
72. Hirshberg A, et al. Errors and pitfalls in intraarterial thrombolytic therapy. J Vasc Surg 1989; 10:612–616.
73. Palaskas C, Totty WG, Gilula LA. Complications of local intraarterial fibrinolytic therapy. Semin Intervent Radiol 1985; 2:396–404.
74. Becker GJ, Holden RW, Rabe FE. Contrast extravasation from a gore-tex graft: a complication of thrombolytic therapy. AJR 1984; 142:573–574.
75. Eskridge JM, et al. Catheter-related thrombosis and fibrinolytic therapy. Radiology 1983; 149:429–432.

76. Eisenberg RL, Bank WO, Hedgkock MW. Renal failure after major angiography can be avoided with hydration. AJR 1981; 136:855–861.
77. Lambert GW, et al. Spontaneous splenic rupture associated with thrombolytic therapy and/or concomitant heparin anticoagulation. Cardiovasc Intervent Radiol 1992; 15:177–179.
78. Tachibana K. Enhancement of fibrinolysis with ultrasound energy. JVIR 1992; 3:299–303.
79. Starck EE, et al. Percutaneous aspiration thromboembolectomy. Radiology 1985; 156:61–66.
80. Stoughton J, et al. Plasminogen acceleration of urokinase thrombolysis. J Vasc Surg 1994; 19:298–305.
81. Pernes JM, et al. Acute peripheral arterial and graft occlusions: treatment with selective infusion of urokinase and lys-plasminogen. Radiology 1986; 158:481–485.
82. Routh WD, et al. Urokinase infusion: feasibility of monitoring for complications in a non-intensive care setting. JVIR 1991; 2:69–72.
83. Kollassa M. Economic issues in thrombolytic intervention. Presented at Advances in the Treatment of Lower Extremity Vascular Disease, April 1994. New York.

V

Specific Disorders

A

Arterial Disorders

33

Cerebrovascular Disease

Frances E. Jensen

Stroke remains the third leading cause of death in the United States, and there are approximately 500,000 cases each year [1,2]. The term **stroke** encompasses both hypoxic and ischemic brain infarction as well as a variety of hemorrhagic conditions, including hypertensive cerebral hemorrhage, subarachnoid hemorrhagic (SAH), and hemorrhage related to arteriovenous malformation (AVM) rupture.

Cerebrovascular disease can be broadly classified into several categories. The most common form is atherothrombotic stroke, which includes lacunar disease in addition to large-vessel disease (Tables 33-1 and 33-2). Transient ischemic attacks (TIA) occur almost as frequently, followed by cerebral embolism. Hemorrhagic disease accounts for the majority of the remainder of cases, including intracerebral hemorrhage and SAH.

The differential diagnosis of stroke and TIA encompasses all entities that may cause acute onset of a focal neurologic deficit or alteration of consciousness. These entities include syncope, seizure, classic migraine, brain tumor, metabolic encephalopathy, vestibular vertigo, drug intoxication, and conversion reaction.

Risk Factors

Over the last two decades, stroke incidence has been declining, largely due to the treatment of underlying disease (Table 33-3). Many of the risk factors are the same as those for atherosclerotic coronary vascular disease. According to the Framingham Study, the most prominent risk factor is hypertension [3], which affects both sexes and raises the risk of stroke by 3.1 in men and 2.9 in women. Borderline hypertension has a relative risk of 1.5. The relative contribution of systolic versus diastolic pressure remains controversial. Isolated systolic hypertension significantly increases stroke risk [4,5], and stroke risk is directly related to systolic pressure at any given diastolic value. The role of diastolic pressure is less clear, and there is little evidence that diastolic pressure has a primary role [6,7].

Coronary heart disease and myocardial infarction (MI) increase stroke risk by means of arterial embolism from a cardiac source. Anterior-wall MI carries a higher risk for thrombus formation and subsequent cardioembolic stroke than transmural MI [8]. Both symptomatic and silent MI carry an increased risk of stroke. A major risk factor for cerebral embolism is atrial fibrillation (AF), either isolated or associated with valvular disease. Chronic AF represents a 5.6 increased incidence of stroke, which increases with age and is the etiology of 36 percent of all strokes by the ninth decade [9]. When AF occurs in the absence of other coronary disease (**lone atrial fibrillators**), the risk is much lower, less than 0.5 percent [10]. In contrast, if AF is accompanied by rheumatic heart disease, the relative risk rises to 17 compared to the control population [11].

Diabetes is another major risk factor and raises the risk of stroke 1.8–4.0 times [12,13]. Diabetes also contributes to the progression of other diseases that represent independent risks, such as atherosclerosis and coronary artery disease.

Cigarette smoking recently has been demonstrated as an independent factor in both ischemic and hemorrhagic stroke. Smoking raises the risk by 1.56 in men and 1.86 in women. The risk is directly related to the number of cigarettes smoked per day, with patients smoking 40 cigarettes per day having approximately two times the risk of stroke than those smoking 10 per day [14].

The relationship between elevated serum lipids and stroke is less clear than for coronary artery disease. In fact, cholesterol and triglyceride levels have not been directly related to an increase in ischemic stroke. However, a low serum cholesterol has been related to intracerebral hemorrhage, especially in the setting of an elevated diastolic blood pressure [15].

Other risk factors for stroke include obesity, elevated hematocrit, and elevated fibrinogen. Oral contraceptive use raises stroke risk, which is further increased by con-

Table 33-1. Classification of stroke

Classification
Atherothrombotic brain infarction
Large-vessel thrombosis
Lacunar disease
Transient monocular blindness
Cerebral embolism
Artery-artery
Cardiogenic
TIA
Hemorrhagic
Subarachnoid hemorrhage
Intracerebral hemorrhage
Hypertensive
Amyloid angiopathy
Other
Coagulopathies
Vasculopathies
Migraine
Dissection
Venous occlusive disease

Table 33-2. Relative incidence of stroke subtypes

Stroke subtype	Relative incidence (%)
Atherothrombotic brain infarction (large vessel and lacunes)	44
TIA	21
Cerebral embolism	21
Subarachnoid hemorrhage	12
Intracerebral hemorrhage	5

Source: The Framingham Study.

Table 33-3. Risk factors for stroke

Risk factors
Cardiovascular
Hypertension
Coronary artery disease
Myocardial infarction
Atrial fibrillation
Paradoxical emboli (atrial or ventricular septal defect)
Diabetes
Cigarette Smoking
Obesity
Oral-contraceptive use
Hematologic risk factors
Elevated hematocrit (primary or secondary)
Sickle cell disease
Elevated fibrinogen
Disseminated intravascular coagulation
Antithrombin III deficiency
Protein S or C deficiency
Homocystenemia
Connective-tissue or autoimmune disease
Systemic lupus erythematosis (including antiphospholipid syndrome)
Temporal arteritis
Polyarteritis
Thrombocytopenic purpura
Wegener's granulomatosis
Takayasu's arteritis
Mitochondrial disorders
Mitochondrial encephalomyelopathy and stroke syndrome (MELAS)
Leigh's disease

comitant cigarette smoking [16]. The risk of stroke also increases with use of oral contraceptives containing high levels of estrogen.

Stroke can occur as a complication of systemic disease, including autoimmune diseases such as systemic lupus and antiphospholipid antibody syndrome, temporal arteritis, polyarteritis, and Wegener's granulomatosis. Coagulopathies such as TTP, antithrombin III deficiency, and protein S and C deficiencies are rarer causes of stroke, and are especially a consideration in younger patients. Other causes of stroke in the young include paradoxical cardiac emboli from a right-to-left shunt; complicated migraine; ischemic or hemorrhagic events associated with sympathomimetic drug use, such as occurs with cocaine; and ruptured arteriovenous malformations.

TIA

A TIA is defined as an episode of neurologic deficit lasting less than 24 hours. The term **reversible ischemic neurologic deficit,** or RIND, has been abandoned and presumed to be indistinguishable from a small stroke. The vast majority of TIAs last less than 30–60 minutes, usually less than 10 minutes. TIAs can occur in thrombotic, lacunar, and embolic disease, although they are usually associated with thrombotic disease. Embolic TIAs have been reported to be of longer duration than thrombotic [17].

TIAs can occur in all vascular territories. When transient ischemia occurs in the retinal arteries as a complication of carotid artery disease, vision is temporarily obscured and the phenomenon is termed **transient monocular blindness** (TMB), or amaurosis fugax. The classic description is one of a shade descending monocularly, but often the patient simply describes blurred, foggy, or hazy vision. In fact, positive symptoms such as bright lights or flashes can also occur as a manifestation of transient retinal ischemia. While hemispheric strokes are not common following TMB, that entity should be evaluated with as equal thoroughness as a TIA. TIAs carry a relative risk of subsequent stroke of 5 percent per year and 35 percent over 5 years [3,18]. The risk of coronary heart disease, however, remains greater than stroke in this population.

Ischemic Stroke

CAROTID DISEASE

Anatomy and Clinical Presentation. Stenosis of the extracranial common and internal carotid arteries is a major cause of both hemispheric TIAs and strokes. Large-vessel disease of the carotid artery can affect territory in its middle cerebral artery (MCA) and anterior cerebral artery (ACA) divisions (Fig. 33-1). The posterior cerebral artery (PCA) distribution usually is spared, since it is supplied primarily by the vertebrobasilar circulation. The major mecha-

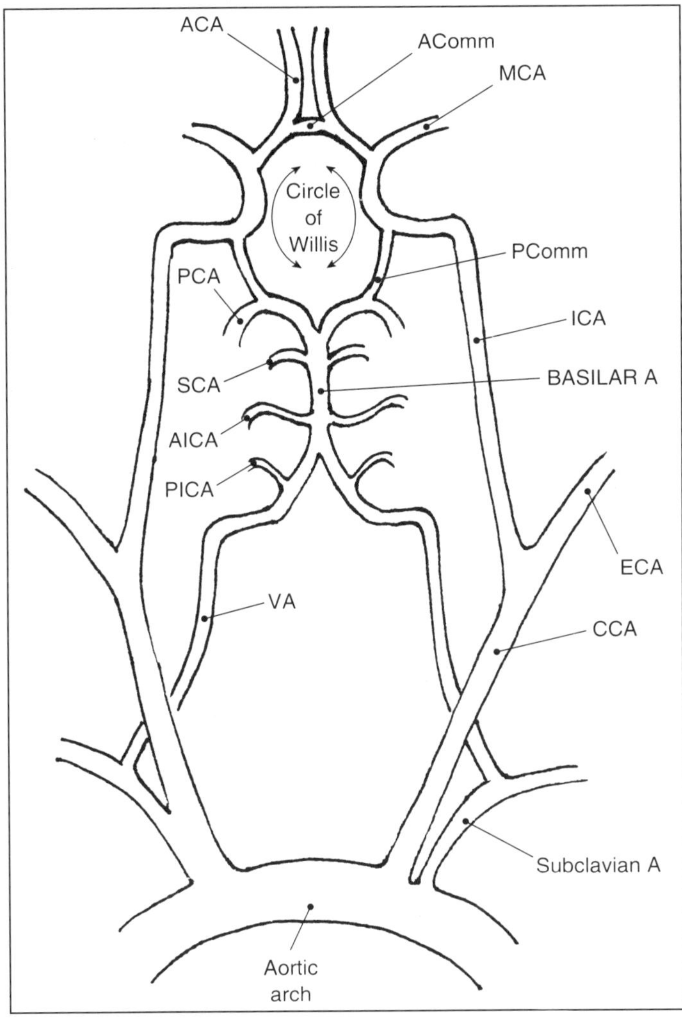

Fig. 33-1. Intracranial vascular anatomy and the circle of Willis. The anterior intracranial circulation is supplied by the carotid artery. The carotid artery bifurcates extracranially into the internal and external branches. The internal carotid artery (ICA) extends intracranially through the carotid canal, and makes an S-shaped curve as the carotid siphon. The ophthalmic artery originates at the siphon, and more distally the ICA gives rise to the anterior choroidal artery and the posterior communicating artery. The ICA then terminates into two major branches, the middle cerebral artery (MCA) and the anterior cerebral artery (ACA). A small communicating artery, the anterior communicating artery (AComm) joins the anterior cerebral circulations of the two hemispheres, constituting the anterior portion of the circle of Willis. The posterior circulation originates in the two vertebral arteries (VA), which are the first branches of the subclavian arteries. These two vessels course intracranially via the foramen magnum before joining together to form a single basilar artery. Each VA gives off posterior and anterior spinal artery branches, and then the posterior inferior cerebellar artery (PICA). The basilar artery gives rise to the anterior inferior cerebellar artery (AICA) and the superior cerebellar arteries (SCA) before finally bifurcating in to the right and left PCAs. The posterior circulation anastomoses with the anterior circulation via the posterior communicating (PComm) arteries.

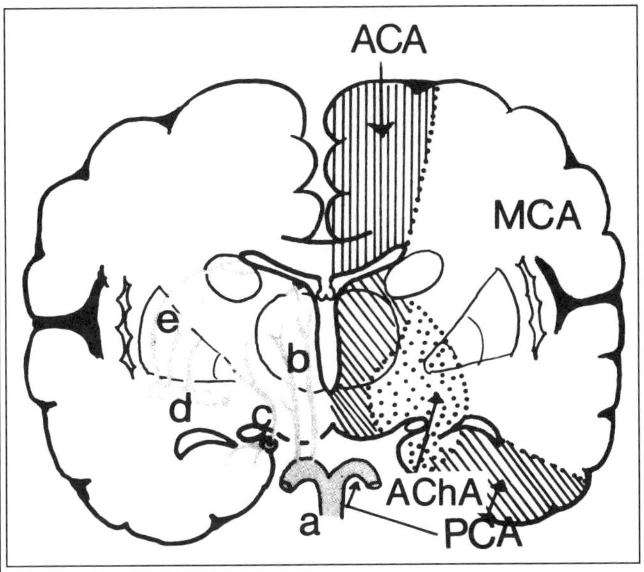

Fig. 33-2. Vascular territories of the cerebrum. The anterior cerebral artery (ACA) supplies the medial aspects of the cerebrum and the cortex. The anterior choroidal artery (AChA) supplies parts of the optic tract, hippocampus, and posterior internal capsule, while the middle cerebral artery (MCA) supplies basal ganglia, dorsal internal capsule, and the parietotemporal cortex. The posterior cerebral artery (PCA) originates as a bifurcation of the basilar artery to supply the occipital cortex and more proximally sends perforating arteries to the thalamus. (Reprinted with permission from LR Caplan. Stroke. A Clinical Approach. Boston: Butterworth-Heineman, 1993. P. 34.)

nisms of ischemic injury are reduced distal flow secondary to a proximal stenosis and artery-to-artery embolization from a proximal atherosclerotic plaque. Clinical deficits often are less severe in patients with distal artery insufficiency compared to those occurring as a result of embolism. Clinical syndromes relate to disruption of function subserved by tissue in a given vascular territory. In ACA occlusion, medial frontoparietal ischemia causes weakness and sensory deficits in the contralateral lower extremities, and other frontal lobe symptoms can occur, including incontinence and abulia. With MCA occlusion, the more lateral aspects of the frontoparietal and temporal lobes can be affected (Fig. 33-2). Those regions subserve strength and sensation in the contralateral face and upper extremities and language (dominant hemisphere), and deficits can occur in those functions. In nondominant-hemisphere ischemia, a severe neglect syndrome can result from parietal ischemia, in addition to contralateral weakness and sensory loss. Visual loss in the contralateral hemifield can occur as a result of ischemia to the radiating visual fibers coursing through the parietal-temporal region to the occipital lobes.

Artery-to-artery emboli most frequently originate in the proximal carotid circulation, usually from an atherosclerotic plaque. However, more proximal sources can be responsible for stroke. Atherothrombotic lesions of the aortic arch may give rise to emboli, which is particularly relevant to the setting of cardiothoracic surgery requiring aortic cross-clamping.

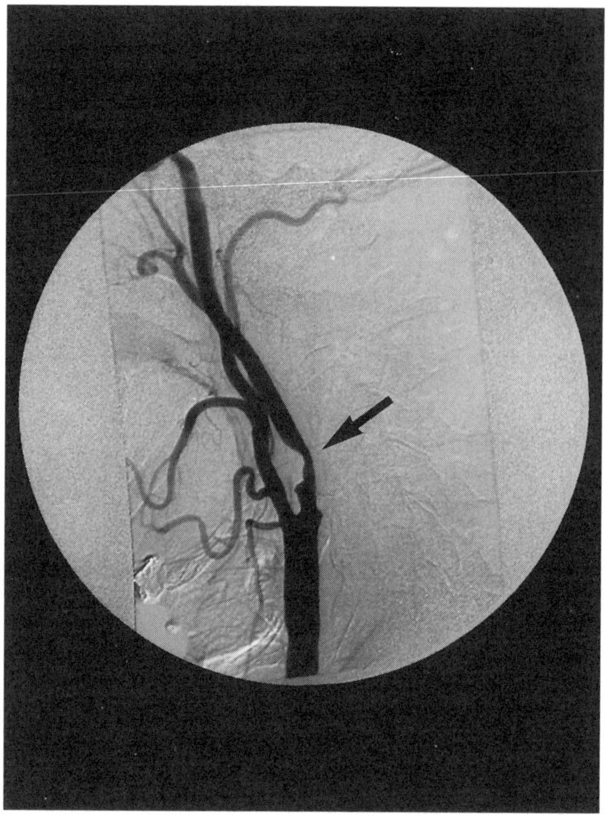

Fig. 33-3. The origin of the internal carotid artery (ICA) is the most common site for atherosclerotic plaque formation. Angiography demonstrates a stenosis and plaque in the proximal portion of the ICA (arrow).

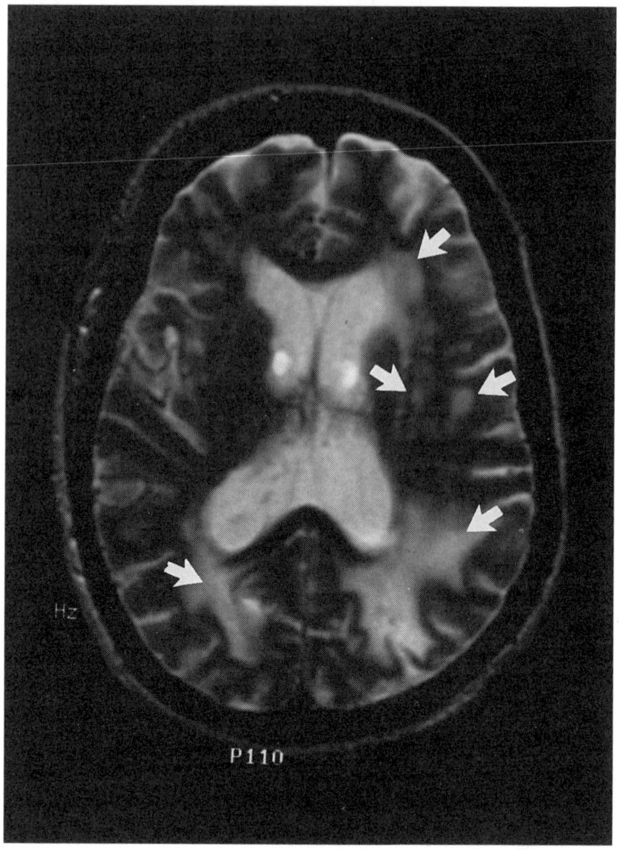

Fig. 33-4. Multiple lacunes in the periventricular white matter due to small-vessel disease. MRI reveals increased signal intensity in multiple loci with T2-weighted imaging (arrows).

Distal insufficiency can occur with high-grade proximal carotid-artery stenosis with or without superimposed systemic hypotension. In the case of severe systemic hypotension, watershed infarcts occur in the end-circulation border zones of the MCA and ACA territories. That results in a frontoparietal lesion, causing weakness and sensory loss in the contralateral leg or arm. With dominant hemisphere lesions, a transcortical aphasia also can occur.

Atherosclerotic lesions occur most commonly at the origin of the internal carotid artery in the neck (Fig. 33-3). Common intracranial sites include the carotid siphon and at the stems of the MCA and ACA. In whites, the extracranial circulation is affected more than intracranial sites, but in other races (blacks and Asians), intracranial MCA disease is more common than extracranial disease [19].

Carotid Dissection. Carotid dissection occurs as a result of traumatic or spontaneous tearing of the arterial wall, with subsequent hematoma formation and partial or total occlusion of the vascular lumen. Spontaneous dissection has been reported in younger patients [20] and can be associated with fibromuscular dysplasia (FMD). FMD primarily affects the extracranial carotid and vertebrobasilar arteries but can affect intracranial vessels [21,22]; it is bilateral in most cases [23] and can also be associated with dysplasia of the renal arteries. A characteristic pattern of a stringlike appearance interrupted by beading can be seen on the angiogram as the vessel wall narrows and dilates [24].

LACUNAR STROKE

The risk of small-vessel disease increases with age, hypertension, diabetes, smoking, hypercoagulable state, and hyperlipidemia. Lacunes are small areas of infarction in the distribution of penetrating arteries in the brain. The small-vessel occlusion has been attributed to microatheromatous deposits [25,26]. Lipohyalinosis, fibrinoid necrosis, and microemboli are less common etiologies for lacunes. Laboratory evaluation reveals punctate, hypodense lesions on CT scan or areas of increased T2 signal on MRI (Fig. 33-4). MRI is the imaging modality of choice, given its high resolution and the small size of the lesions. Common locations of lacunes are the subcortical white matter, basal ganglia, thalamus, and brain stem [25]. Strokes in those locations result in specific syndromes of subtotal deficits (Table 33-4). Frequently, patients have multiple lacunar lesions that have occurred over a protracted period of time. The cumulative effect of multiple lacunes is referred to as a **lacunar state.** The course of this syndrome is one of stuttering, stepwise deterioration.

Table 33-4. Common lacunar syndromes in vertebrobasilar disease

Syndrome	Location
Dysarthria–clumsy hand	Contralateral pons
Pure motor hemiplegia	Contralateral cerebral peduncle, pons, or medulla
Pure hemisensory deficit	Contralateral ventral thalamus
Ataxic hemiparesis	Contralateral pons or ventral thalamus
Contralateral motor and sensory deficit	Ventral thalamus and adcent internal capsule
Wallenberg	Lateral medulla

The multilacune state is distinctly different from Binswanger's disease, which describes diffuse white-matter abnormalities, termed **leukoariosis** [27]. In that syndrome, there is progressive rarefaction of the subcortical white matter, and CT or MRI reveal large, confluent areas of damage around the ventricles, with ventricular enlargement due to atrophy (Fig. 33-5). The incidence of the syndrome increases with age and hypertension. A subcortical dementia may be present in more severely affected individuals. The exact pathophysiology of the disease is unknown but may relate to the chronic effects of hypertension, because arterioles are seen to be thickened in areas of white-matter pallor [28].

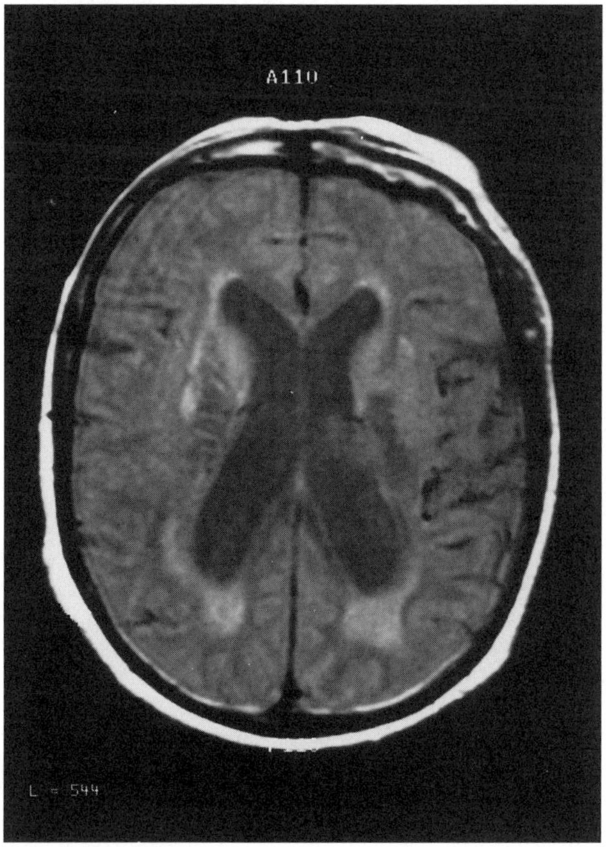

Fig. 33-5. MRI showing confluent periventricular lesions consistent with the diagnosis of Binswanger's disease. On T2-weighted imaging, the white matter surrounding the ventricles is enhanced diffusely.

VERTEBROBASILAR DISEASE

Like the carotid system, the vertebrobasilar circulation can be affected by atherosclerosis, lacunes, embolic occlusion, vasculopathy, and dissection. Extracranial vertebral artery disease is more common in whites and more common in men than in women [19]. Symptoms vary dramatically based on small changes in the location of ischemia, because much of the territory is the brain stem. The two vertebral arteries supply the cerebellum, medulla, and caudal pons before joining together to form the basilar artery. The two most common sites of infarction in the vertebral circulation are the cerebellum and the lateral medulla. Cerebellar infarction can result in ipsilateral limb ataxia and dysmetria. Occlusion of the posterior inferior cerebellar artery (PICA) results in the lateral medullary syndrome (Wallenberg's syndrome), which is a distinct constellation of symptoms occurring from medullary ischemia, including vertigo, nystagmus, ataxia, ipsilateral Horner's syndrome, facial numbness and mild weakness, contralateral pain and temperature loss, and hoarseness and dysarthria due to ipsilateral weakness of the vocal cords and palate (see Table 33-4) (Fig. 33-6). Basilar-artery occlusion can result in subtotal deficits due to partial ischemia in the pons and the medulla, but complete occlusion of the basilar in that region causes a "locked-in" syndrome. Occlusion of the "top of the basilar" causes ischemia in the thalamus, which can lead to a loss of consciousness or decreased flow to both PICAs, also resulting in visual loss due to occipital-lobe ischemia.

Lacunes occur commonly in the vertebrobasilar circulation since there is an abundance of small penetrating vessels in the brain stem and the thalamus. Stereotypical syndromes have been described, including pure motor hemiplegia, pure sensory stroke, dysarthria–clumsy hand syndrome, ataxic hemiparesis, and sensorimotor stroke (see Table 33-4).

CARDIOEMBOLIC STROKE

Cardiovascular disease accounts for 15–20 percent of all ischemic strokes [29–31]. Embolic occlusion occurs most frequently at sites of arterial branching. The most common site is the MCA, with emboli less frequently going to the ACA or the vertebrobasilar system (Fig. 33-7). Complications of cardiac-source emboli include hemorrhagic transformation and distal migration of the embolic fragments. Hemorrhage occurs secondarily in some cases, usually around 72 hours after the onset of embolic stroke.

The most common cardiac conditions associated with embolism have been described by the Cerebral Embolism Task Force [30,31]. These conditions include atrial fibrillation, acute myocardial infarction, left ventricular aneurysm, atrial myxoma, and other left-sided sources, as discussed above (Table 33-5). Paradoxical emboli originating from a right-to-left shunt can occur with a patent foramen ovale, an atrial septal defect, or, rarely, a pulmo-

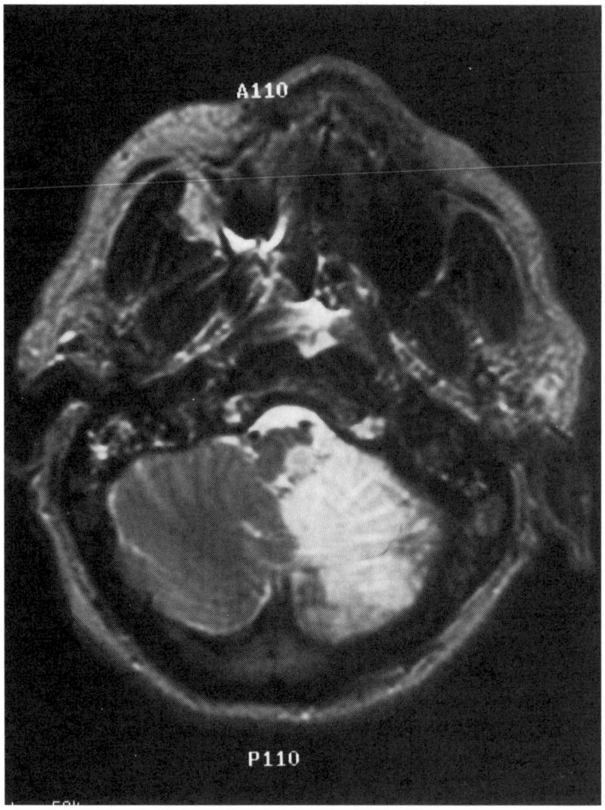

Fig. 33-6. MRI of a lateral medullary stroke associated with an ipsilateral cerebellar hemisphere stroke. Infarcted tissue is imaged as high-intensity lesions on T2-weighted MRI and is due to occlusion of the post inferior cerebellar artery (PICA).

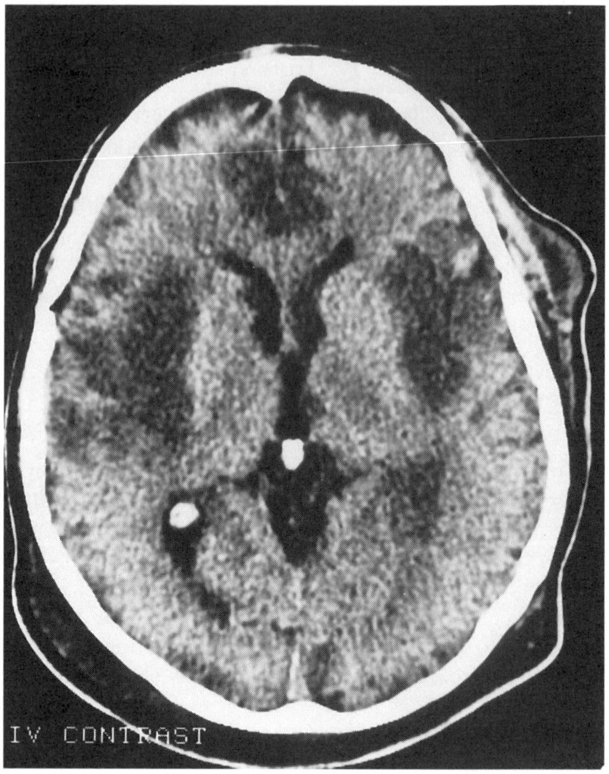

Fig. 33-7. CT scan demonstrating multiple areas of low attenuation consistent with multiple embolic infarctions. Infarctions are of similar attenuation, suggesting their simultaneous occurrence 72 hours prior to this CT scan as a complication of atrial fibrillation. Embolic infarcts most commonly involve cortical areas supplied by distal arterioles.

nary arteriovenous fistula [32,33]. Septic emboli may arise from an infected valve and in the past occurred as a superinfection of valves damaged by rheumatic heart disease. However, since rheumatic heart disease has been declining, subacute bacterial endocarditis is now encountered in individuals with prosthetic valves [34] and those with a history of intravenous drug abuse but otherwise normal valves. The organism associated with the highest rate of septic embolization is *Staphylococcus aureus*. Mycotic aneurysms and secondary hemorrhagic events are uncommon.

Table 33-5. Cardiogenic embolism

Embolism	Percent of all emboli
Nonvalvular AF	45
Acute MI	15
Ventricular aneurysm	10
Rheumatic heart disesae	10
Prosthetic valve	10
Other (i.e., paradoxical, myxoma, cardiomyopathy)	10

Source: Cerebral Embolism Task Force.

COLLAGEN VASCULAR DISEASE AND HYPERCOAGULABLE STATES

Stroke Due to Collagen Vascular Disease of Extracranial and Large Vessels. Temporal arteritis (giant-cell arteritis) affects extracranial vessels [35] and rarely involves the intracranial vasculature. The incidence of the disease is greater in women than in men and increases with age. Systemic involvement results in the syndrome of polymyalgia rheumatica, which often precedes the neurologic symptoms [36]. Headache is largely attributable to inflammation of the temporal arteries. The erythrocyte sedimentation rate (ESR) often is markedly elevated, but a normal value does not preclude the diagnosis of temporal arteritis. The ophthalmic artery becomes involved, leading to visual loss from ischemic optic neuropathy and retinal artery occlusion. Visual loss is reported in up to 50 percent of cases, and in most the loss is monocular [36]. Stroke due to giant-cell arteritis is more common in the vertebrobasilar system than in the carotid territory [37]. Biopsy of the temporal artery reveals a granulomatous, giant-cell arteritis. Treatment consists of corticosteroid suppression of symptoms. Efficacy of therapy can be monitored by following a reduction in the ESR. Takayasu's arteritis has a predilection for involvement of the aortic arch vessels but also can affect the extracranial carotid and vertebral circulation [38]. Takayasu's arteritis typically occurs in young women and is more common in Asians. Symptoms include general malaise and fever, with strokes and TIAs occurring as a result of proximal-vessel occlusion or embolic events. Subclavian steal syndrome can occur if the subclavian artery is occluded. The symptoms are accompanied by a high ESR, and angiography reveals stenosis of large vessels; the pathologic process is a granulomatous angiitis. Treatment consists of corticosteroids and cytotoxic agents, such as cyclophosphamide, and bypass surgery on major aortic branches.

Stroke Due to Collagen Vascular Disease of Intracranial and Small Vessels. Several arteritic conditions involve intracranial vessels rather than the proximal carotid or vertebral arteries. Arteritis can accompany a bacterial meningitis, as vessels become occluded as they course through the meningeal covering of the brain. Isolated granulomatous angiitis affects small arterioles and veins and causes multifocal strokes [39,40]. Constitutional symptoms such as headache, fever, and malaise are common and are not correlated with the ESR, which is low or normal in some cases. The cerebrospinal fluid (CSF) reveals a moderate pleocytosis but an elevated protein concentration (>100 mg%). Angiography does not reliably demonstrate abnormalities but can show a beading pattern, and CT scan or MRI reveals multiple strokes and hemorrhage. Treatment with corticosteroids and cyclophosphamide may result in improvement, but the progression of disease can be refractory to therapy. Polyarteritis nodosa is another condition that affects small and medium-size vessels in the brain. In polyarteritis, CNS involvement occurs usually when the systemic disease is well advanced [41,42]. Symptoms include headache, fever, seizures, and ischemic strokes, while hemorrhagic strokes are less common. Serologic testing reveals an elevated antinuclear antibody (ANA), while CSF may show only moderate abnormalities. Arteritis can be documented by biopsy of affected tissue, such as peripheral nerve. The vasculitis is necrotizing, and angiography may demonstrate aneurysmal dilation of the involved vessels. Treatment consists of corticosteroids and cyclophosphamide.

Systemic lupus erythematosis (SLE) can be associated with stroke from a variety of mechanisms [43]. A vasculopathy affecting small and medium intracranial vessels is present in some cases; this is not a vasculitis, but rather an inflammatory infiltrate in the perivascular space. More common causes of stroke in SLE are cardioemboli from Libman-Sacks endocarditis or hypercoagulability and from associated thrombotic thrombocytopenic purpura (TTP) or antiphospholipid antibody syndrome [44,45]. Involvement of intracranial vessels in SLE can result in ischemic infarcts, hemorrhages, and, rarely, venous thrombosis. Treatment is the same as for the systemic disease, and corticosteroids in combination with other immunosuppressants and cytotoxic agents are used. Wegener's granulomatosis causes a necrotizing vasculitis in medium-sized intracranial vessels as well as venous thrombophlebitis and thrombosis and secondary intraparenchymal hemorrhages [46]. The intracranial disease occurs in the setting of glomerulonephritis and systemic vasculitis, particularly in the respiratory tract. Granuloma formation can occur systemically as well as intracranially. Laboratory testing reveals an elevated ANA, and treatment with corticosteroids and cyclophosphamide is effective. Other less common inflammatory conditions causing strokelike events are arterial narrowing following an episode of Herpes zoster ophthalmicus or in patients with Sjögren's syndrome or rheumatoid arthritis. Behçet's disease is an inflammatory syndrome characterized by oral and genital ulcers, uveitis, and arthritis. The disease also causes an endarteritis in the brain and leptomeninges, and strokelike events can occur in the setting of an aseptic meningitis. CSF evaluation reveals a moderate pleocytosis and increased protein concentration, and MRI may reveal areas of increased signal intensity in the grey and white matter. Treatment for Behçet's disease consists of corticosteroids in combination with cytotoxic agents such as cyclophosphamide.

Stroke Due to Hypercoagulable States. Hypercoagulability can occur in some collagen vascular disease as well as other hematologic conditions (see Table 33-3). The two main conditions associated with SLE that can increase coagulability are the presence of antiphospholipids (lupus anticoagulant, anticardiolipin antibodies) and TTP. The antiphospholipid antibody syndrome can occur in patients with or without SLE [47]. Migrainelike headaches are a prominent symptom, and recurrent TIAs, strokes, and encephalopathy can occur. In women, the antiphospholipid antibody syndrome is associated with a high incidence of spontaneous abortion. Laboratory evaluation reveals the presence of antiphospholipid antibodies. CT or MRI reveals primarily cortical infarcts, and angiography has shown stenosis in intracranial vessels as well as the extracranial carotid and vertebrobasilar circulation. Patients also have been shown to have cardiac abnormalities on echocardiography, including valvular abnormalities and thrombi. Treatment begins with antiplatelet agents, but cases with recurrent symptoms require corticosteroids, immunosuppressants, and anticoagulation. In TTP, microangiopathic changes consisting of arterial and capillary thrombi cause a range of symptoms, including headache, encephalopathy, seizures, and strokelike events. Similar symptoms are observed in cryoglobulinemia, in which extra- and intracranial vessels may become occluded. Deficiencies of the anticoagulant proteins antithrombin III, protein S, and protein C occur as hereditary conditions or may be acquired. Hypercoagulable states can be acquired as a result of intercurrent malignancy or infection, in the perioperative period, and in pregnancy. Those conditions also may activate clotting factors such as factor-V, -VII, and -VIII coagulant activity. Elevated homocysteine levels in blood or urine usually occur as a result of an inborn error of metabolism and may predispose to stroke and premature atherosclerosis in young adulthood. Polycythemia and sickle cell disease both cause stroke by means of decreasing blood flow and should be included in the differential diagnosis of stroke etiology.

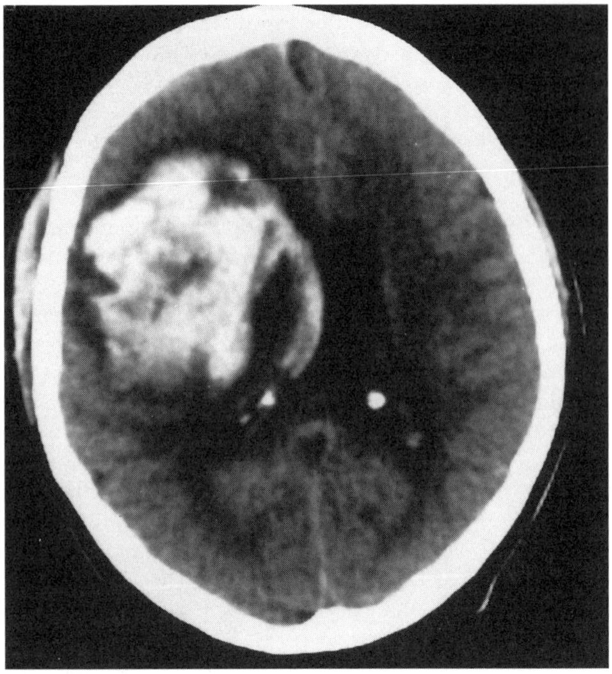

Fig. 33-8. CT scan showing an intracerebral hemorrhage in the basal ganglia and thalamus. CT scanning readily detects blood as increased density. In this scan, mass effect is evidenced by subfalcine herniation across the midline into the contralateral lateral ventricle. Basal ganglia and putaminal hemorrhages are seen most commonly in hypertensive patients.

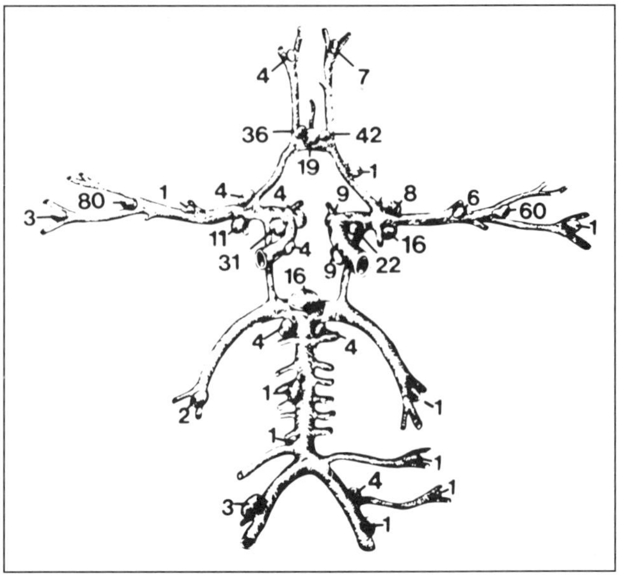

Fig. 33-9. Site of occurrence of saccular aneurysms, numbered in order of frequency in a population of 316 patients. Most aneurysms occur in the anterior circulation, and 12–31 percent are bilateral. (Reprinted with permission from F. McCormick. Vascular diseases. In: RN Rosenberg, ed. The Clinical Neurosciences. Vol. 3. New York: Churchill Livingston. P. 38.)

Hemorrhagic Stroke

Hemorrhage can occur in the brain parenchyma or in subarachnoid, subdural, or epidural spaces. Intraparenchymal or intracerebral hemorrhage (ICH) can occur secondarily as a complication of an ischemic infarct or as a primary event. Primary ICH is seen as a complication of severe hypertension, and the location is typically in the basal ganglia (putamen), thalamus, deep hemisphere (lobar) (Fig. 33-8), or pons. The source of bleeding is believed to be due to the rupture of Charcot-Bouchard aneurysms related to chronic hypertension. Nonhypertensive causes of bleeding include cerebral amyloid angiopathy, which causes smaller hemorrhages primarily located in the cortex and seen almost exclusively in elderly patients. Rupture of arteriovenous malformations (AVMs) can occur at any age and can at times result in large intraparenchymal hemorrhages with high morbidity and mortality. ICH may occur in the setting of anticoagulant or thrombolytic therapy, sympathomimetic drug use, or alcohol abuse and as a complication of a brain neoplasm.

SAH has an annual incidence of 4 to 10 per 100,000 and has a high mortality. SAH is due to the rupture of saccular aneurysms of cerebral vessels. Most aneurysms are in the ACA and MCA distributions, and multiple aneurysms are seen in up to 30 percent of cases [48] (Fig. 33-9). The risk of SAH increases with the size of the aneurysm and history of prior SAH. Prior to hemorrhage, patients may have premonitory headaches that are thought to represent leaking from the unstable aneurysm (**sentinel bleed**). A sudden, severe headache heralds the SAH and is often accompanied by loss of consciousness. Stroke can occur in the distribution of the ruptured artery. Other delayed complications include hydrocephalus from occlusion of CSF flow in the arachnoid villi beginning after the first 24 hours and ischemia from vasospasm in the first 2 weeks. Recurrent rupture occurs in 20 percent of cases in the first 2 weeks, 33 percent in the first month, and 50 percent in the first year [49–51]. The annual risk of rebleeding in survivors is 3 percent [52].

Stroke in Young People

Stroke in young people can be a significant diagnostic challenge (Table 33-6). Although most strokes are ischemic, there is a higher rate of hemorrhagic stroke compared to the older population. In studies including adults under 40–45 years, the most common causes of ischemic stroke have been found to be dissection and cardioembolism [29,53,54]. Cardiac sources include not only left-sided disease but also paradoxical emboli from a patent foramen ovale or other septal defect. Atherosclerosis occurs in this population but at a lower frequency. Another common cause of stroke is migraine, and the risk of ischemic stroke is increased further if there is concurrent use of oral contraceptives [16]. Other causes of ischemic stroke include hypercoagulable states, venous thrombosis, collagen vascular disease, and homocystinuria. Another recently elucidated entity is the group of related diseases caused by mitochondrial-gene deletions, resulting in defects in cellular respiration. When neurons are affected, a strokelike syndrome can occur. The best-known subtype is the mitochondrial encephalomyelopathy, lactic acidosis, and

Table 33-6. Causes of stroke in young adults

Ischemic stroke
Cardiogenic embolism (including paradoxical from PFO or ASD)
Arterial dissection
Migraine stroke
Reversible cerebral angiopathies (toxic, eclampsia)
Coagulopathy (e.g., autoimmune, paraneoplastic, sickle cell, thrombocytosis)
Atherosclerosis (accounts for less than 20%)
Cerebral venous thrombosis (pregnancy)
Fibromuscular dysplasia
Metabolic disorders (e.g., homocystinuria, MELAS)
Hemorrhagic stroke
AVM
Hypertension
Sympathomimetic agents
Anticoagulant therapy

strokelike episodes (MELAS) [55]. The disorder is maternally inherited and may present with extensive pedigrees of recurrent strokes, migraines, and seizures in multiple family members. Diagnosis is made by lactate levels, muscle biopsy (to examine tissue for ragged red fibers), and blood and urine screening for the genetic defect [55,56]. Hemorrhagic stroke in young adults can occur as a result of rupture of AVMs or aneurysms and use of sympathomimetic agents [54]. Hypertension is less common in this age group.

Laboratory Diagnosis of Stroke

Multiple modalities now exist for the localization of stroke and determination of its etiologic source. Imaging of the infarct may be carried out by CT scan, MRI, and single-photon-emission tomography (SPECT) scanning. CT scans detect acute blood in first 48 hours more easily than MRI. In addition, CT scan is the optimal technique for imaging blood over the brain convexities due to SAH, and a diagnostic lumbar puncture often can be avoided. An ischemic infarct appears as a hypodense area on CT scan. Unless the infarct is very large, CT scans do not reliably show the lesion until 24 to 48 hours (Fig. 33-10A). The CT image of an ischemic infarct can actually become less discrete during the interval between 48 hours and 2 weeks due to masking by intercurrent edema, which begins to peak at 72 hours. Later, the subacute or chronic infarct appears as a well-demarcated area of hypodensity. CT scanning with contrast is not useful for imaging ischemic infarcts or hemorrhages but is necessary for the identification of AVMs and other vascular anomalies.

Both T1- and T2-weighted MRI imaging is available in most centers. MRI can reveal areas of infarction earlier than CT scan, within the first 24 hours (Fig. 33-10B). In addition, because of their high resolution, MRI scans are more useful in the detection of small lesions, especially lacunar and brain-stem infarcts. By T1-weighted imaging, the stroke appears hypodense, while it is hyperdense with T2-weighted imaging. MRI scanning also picks up medium-size and large (>4 mm) vascular lesions, such as

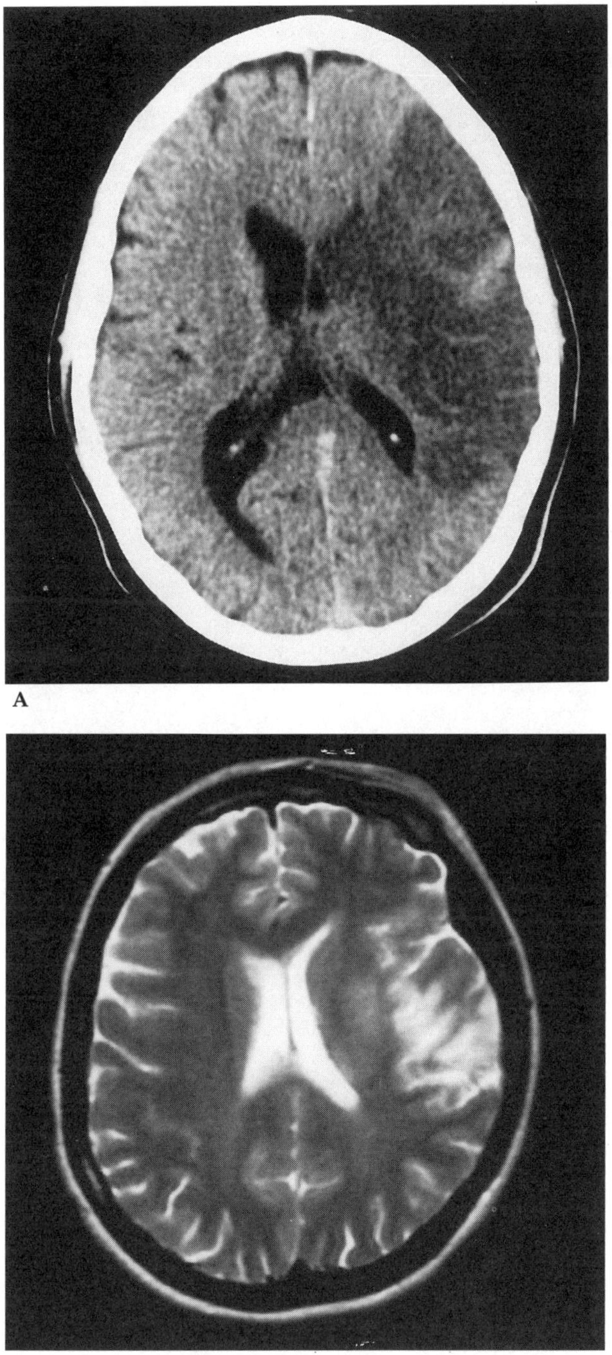

A

B

Fig. 33-10. Left hemispheric infarction involving the entire middle cerebral artery terrritory. **A.** With CT scanning, the infarction appears hypodense and was not fully apparent until 24–48 hours after onset. **B.** T2-weighted MRI taken within 24 hours of onset already shows increased signal in the area of the infarction.

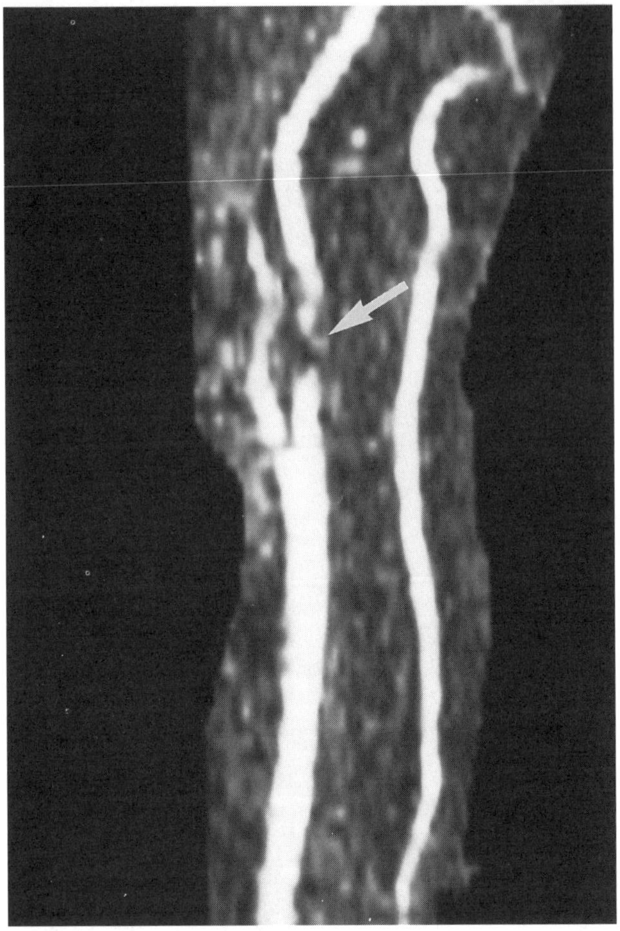

Fig. 33-11. MR angiogram of internal carotid-artery stenosis showing a region of narrowing proximally (arrow).

aneurysms and AVMs. MR angiography increasingly is used to determine extracranial stenoses, as well as intracranial vascular pathology (Fig. 33-11). Contrast angiography is the technique of choice for evaluation of aneurysms, AVMs, and intrinsic intracranial vascular disease. MRI scans can detect infarction as early as 6 hours, but cannot reliably detect infarcts until 24 hours. SPECT scanning can reveal hypoperfusion in the early hours of acute stroke, often before CT or MRI, but it cannot differentiate between ischemia and hemorrhage. Blood flow can be noninvasively documented by duplex ultrasonography of the carotid and extracranial vertebral arteries, transcranial Doppler (TCD) of the intracranial vessels, and MR angiography for both intracranial and neck vessels. TCD can be useful in detecting reduced flow in large- and medium-size intracranial vessels. Angiography is still the test of choice if high resolution is required to visualize the local vascular lesions and small caliber vessels extracranially.

For suspected cardioembolic strokes, cardiac arrhythmias are identified by electrocardiography and 24-hour monitoring. To isolate a source of cardiac embolus, echocardiography is appropriate to identify valvular or wall abnormalities. For determining paradoxical emboli, transthoracic echocardiography with a bubble study is indicated, often requiring a provocative stimulus such as cough or the Valsalva maneuver, and transesophageal echocardiography has even higher accuracy in detecting small right-to-left shunts.

Treatment of Stroke

PREVENTIVE TREATMENT

For all atherothrombotic stroke, a mainstay of therapy is to reduce concurrent risk factors. Adequate treatment of hypertension, diabetes, hypercholesterolemia, hyperlipidemia, and hypercoagulable states and discouragement of smoking and alcohol intake are all important in the chronic management of patients at risk for a primary or secondary stroke.

Symptomatic Carotid Artery Disease. In patients with strokes or TIAs referable to the hemisphere or eye ipsilateral to a stenotic carotid artery, treatment is determined by the severity of the stenosis. The North American Symptom Carotid Endarterectomy Trial (NASCET) Study revealed that endarterectomy significantly improved long-term outcome compared to medical therapy (ASA) in patients with high-grade (70%) stenosis [57]. The European Cooperative Study also has evaluated patients with moderate (30–69%) and low-grade (<30%) stenoses [58]. While no benefit of surgical therapy has been demonstrated in the low-grade group, the role of carotid endarterectomy in patients with moderate grade (30–69%) stenosis is still under study. It is important to note that carotid endarterectomy may result in significant complications, including stroke secondary to embolism, local hypoperfusion, carotid occlusion, cranial nerve damage, and death. In those studies, which demonstrated a benefit of endarterectomy over medical therapy, the surgical risk of major stroke and death was low, in the range of 2.0–2.5 percent. Hence, the assessment of surgical morbidity and mortality statistics is an integral part of determining management at a given institution.

Prophylactic medical therapy of carotid disease in cases where operative therapy is not indicated largely consists of antiplatelet agents or anticoagulation. Aspirin has been the mainstay of therapy and is usually the first-line agent used. Aspirin prevents platelet aggregation and has been shown in several large studies to reduce the risk of primary and secondary stroke related to carotid disease [59–65]. The dose used varied between 30 and 1,500 mg/day. Overall, the risk reduction in those studies ranged from 50- to 20-percent reduction for stroke and death, respectively. The optimal dose has been controversial, and 325 mg/day is used by most groups. The Dutch TIA Trial Study [59] randomized 3,131 patients to high-dosage aspirin (283 mg/day) versus low-dosage aspirin (30 mg/day) and followed patients for an average of 2.6 years. In the group randomized to 30 mg of aspirin, there was a 14.7-percent incidence of cardiovascular events; in the group randomized to high-dosage aspirin, there was a 15.2-percent incidence of events. The difference between the two groups was not significant. There were slightly fewer complications and fewer gastrointestinal symptoms in the patients randomized to low-dosage aspirin, and the study concluded that low-dosage aspirin is no less effective than high-dosage aspirin in patients with a history of TIA or stroke, but low-dosage aspirin has fewer side effects. The NASCET study is currently evaluating the relative risk reduction of secondary stroke in postendarterectomy patients taking aspirin at doses of 325 versus 1,300 mg/day.

Other agents that decrease platelet aggregation include dipyridamole (Persantine) [60], sulfinpyrazone [62,66], and suloctidil [67]. However, clinical trials and meta-analyses have shown no benefit of those agents either alone or in combination with aspirin [68]. In contrast, recent clinical trials have shown that ticlopidine, which inhibits adenosine diphosphate (ADP)–dependent platelet activation and release, effectively prevents both primary and secondary stroke [69–72]. The usual dosage of ticlopidine is 250 mg bid. Side effects of ticlopidine are more prominent than those of aspirin and can include diarrhea, rash, and neutropenia. The neutropenia has been reported in 1 percent of patients using ticlopidine but is reversible on discontinuing the drug.

Anticoagulation is used in the treatment of acute stroke as well as in appropriate nonsurgical candidates who have failed aspirin and ticlopidine. In addition, anticoagulation significantly reduces the risk of recurrent stroke in the setting of a known cardioembolic source. Heparin generally is reserved for the acute induction of anticoagulation, usually in the management of a new ischemic stroke of any etiology or acute arterial occlusion. Heparin also is used for chronic anticoagulation when it is necessary during pregnancy, because warfarin is teratogenic. Warfarin is the anticoagulant of choice for outpatient prophylaxis in patients who have failed antiplatelet therapy and are not surgical candidates. The warfarin dose should be adjusted to maintain a prothrombin time (PT) in the range of an international normalized ratio (INR) of 2.0 to 3.0 [73,74].

Asymptomatic Carotid Stenosis. Given the accuracy and the availability of carotid duplex technology, the documentation of internal carotid-artery stenosis has been increasing. Asymptomatic bruit in the neck is a relatively common finding, occurring in 4–5 percent of persons between the ages of 45 and 80 years [75,76]. The frequency of this finding is even higher in patients with known peripheral vascular disease [77]. Like TIAs, the presence of a carotid bruit has been reported to carry anywhere from a 1- to 15-percent risk of stroke over a 2- to 7-year period [78–80]. Asymptomatic carotid-artery occlusion has been reported to carry an annual risk of stroke of 2–5 percent, but that includes strokes in all vascular territories; thus, the risk is general rather than specific to the stenotic carotid artery [81–84].

The effect of endarterectomy in patients with asymptomatic carotid stenosis has been the subject of much study. The Veterans Administration Cooperative Study randomized patients with stenosis greater than 70 percent to medical or surgical treatment and evaluated the outcome risks of TIA, stroke, and endpoint of stroke and death [85]. In medically treated patients, 11.1 percent experienced either TIA or TMB versus 3.3 percent in the surgical group. Stroke occurred in 9.4 percent of the medically treated patients and 4.7 percent of the surgically treated patients. These results were not significant, most likely due to inadequate statistical power. In addition, the combined endpoint of TIA and stroke occurred less frequently in the group treated with carotid endarterectomy, but this was not significant [86]. An earlier study, the Carotid Surgery versus Medical Therapy in Asymptomatic Carotid Stenosis, or CASANOVA, Study also has reported negative results [87]. However, in 1994, the Asymptomatic Carotid Artery Study (ACAS) reported preliminary results from a multicenter trial examining the effect of carotid endarterectomy versus nonsurgical therapy in patients with asymptomatic stenosis greater than 60 percent. Of the 1,662 eligible patients in the trial, 828 were randomized to receive endarterectomy and 834 medical treatment, with an average follow-up of 2.7 years. In patients randomized to surgery, the risk of stroke or death was 4.8 percent, compared to 10.6 percent in the medically treated group, with a relative risk reduction of 55 percent ($p = 0.004$) [88].

TREATMENT OF CARDIOEMBOLIC STROKE

A number of studies have evaluated risk reduction of stroke in atrial fibrillation with the use of antiplatelet agents and anticoagulants. It generally is agreed that patients with valvular atrial fibrillation are candidates for anticoagulant therapy. The Veterans Affairs Stroke Prevention in Nonrheumatic Atrial Fibrillation Study examined the efficacy of warfarin versus placebo in patients with nonrheumatic atrial fibrillation. Warfarin significantly reduced the probability of stroke, with stroke occurring in 19 of 265 placebo patients versus 4 of 260 warfarin-treated patients ($p < 0.001$) [89]. In a study of patients with nonvalvular atrial fibrillation, the Stroke Prevention in Atrial Fibrillation (SPAF) Trial randomized patients to either aspirin or warfarin [90]. The results suggest that warfarin may be more useful in older patients. Similar findings were obtained in the Boston Area Trial [91] and the Copenhagen Study [92], with warfarin statistically reducing the risk of stroke as well as that of death from other causes. The acceptable range for the INR on warfarin therapy should be between 2 and 3.

Warfarin and aspirin both are used in the prevention of stroke following myocardial infarction, and a meta-analysis combining several studies concluded that warfarin is superior [68]. However, aspirin still had a role in reducing the risk of complications from peripheral vascular disease other than stroke. Neither aspirin nor anticoagulation are indicated in the case of emboli due to subacute bacterial endocarditis, because of the high risk of recurrent embolization and secondary hemorrhage [34,93]. Repeat angiography performed after antibiotic therapy is useful in identifying residual aneurysms in patients such as those with prosthetic valves in whom chronic anticoagulation is indicated [34].

TREATMENT OF ACUTE ISCHEMIC STROKE

Patients presenting with a new stroke should undergo immediate imaging to determine whether there is associated hemorrhage. The CT scan is preferable for initial screening, since it can be obtained rapidly in most centers and readily visualizes acute hemorrhage. MRI sequences are in development to image acute hemorrhage, but current T1- and T2-weighted studies are inferior to CT scans for that purpose. If the patient has a mild to moderate subtotal stroke in a branch of a major intracranial artery, then acute anticoagulation should be considered. If the carotid territory is suspected, then duplex ultrasonography and MR angiography should be obtained to determine whether there is a stenosis greater than 70 percent. If a high-grade ipsilateral stenosis is seen, the patient should be considered for emergent carotid endarterectomy. The timing of carotid endarterectomy depends on the patient's clinical presentation. In patients presenting with a small, nonhemorrhagic stroke and mild clinical deficit, immediate endarterectomy should be considered if a significant stenosis can be documented by duplex, MRI angiogram, or contrast angiography. However, in cases of infarcts complicated by hemorrhage or infarcts resulting from total or near-total intracranial branch occlusion, it is necessary to delay surgery until the acute lesion has resolved. In cases where no hemorrhage is demonstrated, anticoagulation may be used to prevent recurrent strokes in the interim before surgery. In nonsurgical patients with a large stroke involving all territory within a major branch of the intracranial carotid, appropriate measures to minimize edema should be taken, including fluid restriction and elevation of the head of the bed to 30 degrees. More aggressive measures, such as mannitol, may be used if edema progresses. Edema is maximal at 48–72 hours following stroke onset. Anticoagulation is deferred for at least 48 hours in the case of a large stroke, because that is the period of greatest risk for hemorrhagic transformation of the infarct. Likewise, in the case of a hemorrhagic infarct, anticoagulation is deferred for that period of time or longer, depending on the size of the hematoma.

TREATMENT OF HEMORRHAGIC STROKE

Intracerebral Hemorrhage. Intracerebral hemorrhage (ICH) frequently can be a life-threatening event. If the patient has altered consciousness, the airway should be protected and the patient intubated if necessary. The main complication is increased intracranial pressure from an enlarging hematoma or from ensuing secondary edema. CT or MRI scans must be performed serially if the patient is suspected of herniation across the midline or infratentorially, and scans should be repeated with any significant clinical deterioration. Judicious fluid restriction and elevation of the head of the bed are minimal steps necessary in a mild hemorrhage without significant neurologic deficit. However, with larger hemorrhages, hyperventilation can be used as the first step in lowering intracranial pressure, followed by mannitol if necessary. Underlying bleeding disorders should be promptly evaluated and treated. Hypertension should be cautiously corrected, since significant decreases in blood pressure in the setting of increased intracranial pressure may lower cerebral perfusion. Cerebral angiography usually is unrevealing in the acute setting of ICH, because it often is obscured by the hematomata. The decision to surgically evacuate a hematoma is made if the bleed is easily accessible and if the procedure is considered life saving; otherwise, conservative therapy is elected. A common indication for surgery is the occurrence of a cerebellar hemorrhage, where enlargement can cause compression of the brain stem and hydrocephalus from compression of the fourth ventricle.

AVMs may be diagnosed during a workup for a focal neurologic deficit or seizures, and the decision to resect them is made depending on their location and size. In addition to surgical resection, AVMs also can be reduced in size by stereotactic radiosurgery. In the case of very large AVMs, invasive neuroradiologic procedures such as embolization are performed prior to surgical resection to debulk the mass.

Subarachnoid Hemorrhage. The acute management of SAH is directed at controlling blood pressure, suppressing vasospasm, and preventing seizures that may increase blood pressure and cause rebleeding. In addition, the patient must be monitored for the development of hyponatremia and syndrome of inappropriate antidiuretic hormone (SIADH). Blood pressure can be reduced with agents such as sodium nitroprusside, and the calcium-channel blocker nimodipine is used to prevent vasospasm and reduce the risk of secondary stroke. If vasospasm occurs, blood pressure may be increased to maintain cerebral blood flow. Cerebral blood flow may be monitored with TCD, and anticonvulsants are administered as seizure prophylaxis. In most centers today, patients undergo contrast angiography acutely; if an operable aneurysm is detected, surgical resection is performed as early as possible. Recent evidence indicates that early timing of surgery improves outcome.

Future Directions in Stroke Therapy

A number of new directions in stroke therapy are experimental or undergoing clinical trials. Thrombolytic agents such as intravenous or intra-arterial tissue plasminogen activator (t-PA), urokinase, and prourokinase are being tested in the setting of acute intracranial arterial occlusion. Treatment must be conducted in the hyperacute phase of stroke, often within the first 2–4 hours of onset of symptoms. A recent study using t-PA showed that treatment of an ischemic stroke with this fibrinolytic agent within 3 hours of the onset of symptoms reduced the risk of permanent significant neurologic deficits by 31% [94].

The pathophysiology of neuronal death under conditions of stroke has been studied intensively over the past 10 years. A major breakthrough has been the demonstration that neuronal cells die during stroke because of overactivation of excitatory neurotransmitter receptors. The excess activity at these synapses, termed **excitotoxicity,** leads to a cascade of events beginning with excessive influx of calcium intracellularly, subsequent activation of kinases, generation of free radicals, and finally lipid peroxidation and membrane breakdown [95]. Many strategies are being investigated for blockade at each step of this excitotoxic sequence. Notably, it has been determined that the process of infarction continues up to 24 hours after the onset of symptoms, revealing a window of opportunity for therapy. These experimental treatments include pharmacologic blockers of the excitatory neurotransmitter receptors, calcium-channel blockers, free-radical scavengers, and inhibitors of lipid peroxidation [96,97]. Many studies still are at the level of animal trials, but increasing numbers are entering phase I and II clinical trials.

Given these advancements in both conventional and experimental therapies, it is imperative that public awareness be directed at the need to obtain prompt treatment and evaluation at the onset of stroke. Prompt evaluation by emergency personnel and primary caregivers should be performed as expeditiously as for a patient presenting with an acute myocardial infarction. Even with currently available diagnostic techniques and treatment modalities, morbidity and mortality, as well as duration of hospital stay, could be improved with more rapid referral of symptomatic patients for evaluation and therapy.

References

1. Broderick JP, Phillips SJ, Whisnant JP. Incidence rates of stroke in the eighties: the end of the decline on stroke? Stroke 1989; 20:577–582.
2. American Heart Association. 1991 Heart and Stroke Facts, 1991.
3. Wolf PA, et al. Probability of stroke: a risk profile from the Framingham Study. Stroke 1991; 22:312–318.
4. Colandrea MA, Friedman GD, Nichaman MZ. Systolic hypertension in the elderly: an epidemiologic assessment. Circulation 1970; 41:239–245.
5. Kannel WB, Wolf PA, McGee DL. Systolic blood pressure, arterial rigidity, and risk of stroke: the Framingham Study. JAMA 1981; 245:1225–1229.
6. Rutan GH, McDonald RH, Kuller LH. A historical perspective of elevated systolic vs diastolic blood pressure from an epidemiology and clinical trial viewpoint. J Clin Epidemiol 1989; 42:663–673.
7. Fisher CM. The ascendancy of diastolic blood pressure over systolic. Lancet 1985; 2:1349.
8. Stratton JR, Resnick AD. Increased embolic risk in patients with left ventricular thrombi. Circulation 1987; 75:1004–1011.
9. Wolf PA, Abbott RD, Kannel WB. Atrial fibrillation: a major contributor to stroke in the elderly: the Framingham Study. Arch Interna Med 1987; 147:1561–1564.
10. Kopecky SL, Gerah BJ, McGoon MD. The natural history of lone atrial fibrillation. N Engl J Med 1987; 317:669–674.
11. Wolf PA, et al. Epidemiologic assessment of chronic atrial fibrillation and risk of stroke: the Framingham study. Neurology 1978; 28:973–977.
12. Barrett-Connor E, Khaw K. Diabetes mellitus: an independent risk factor for stroke. Am J Epidemiol 1988; 128:116–123.
13. Kuller LH, Dorman JS, Wolf PA. Cerebrovascular diseases and diabetes. National Diabetes Data Group: Diabetes in America, Diabetes Data Compiled for 1984, 1985; 18:1.
14. Shinton R, Beevers G. Meta-analysis of relation between cigarette smoking and stroke. Br Med J 1989; 298:789–794.
15. Iso H, Jacobs DR, Wentworth D. Serum cholesterol levels and six-year mortality from stroke in 350,977 men screened for the multiple risk factor intervention trial. N Engl J Med 1989; 320:904–910.
16. Collaborative Group for the Study of Stroke in Young Women: Oral contraception and stroke in young women: associated risk factors. JAMA 1975; 231:718.
17. Pessin MS, et al. Clinical and angiographic features of carotid transient ischemic attacks. N Engl J Med 1977; 296:358–362.
18. Wolf PA, Abbott RD, Kannel WB. Atrial fibrillation: a major contributor to stroke in the elderly. The Framingham study. Arch Intern Med 1987; 147:1561–1564.
19. Caplan LR, Gorelick PB, Hier DB. Race, sex, and occlusive cerebrovascular disease: a review. Stroke 1986; 17:648–655.
20. Fisher CM, Ojemann R, Roberson G. Spontaneous dissection of cervico-cerebral arteries. J Can Sci Neurology 1978; 5:9–19.
21. Stanley JC, Gewertz BL, Bove EL. Arterial fibrodysplsia: histopathologic character and current etiologic concepts. Arch Surgery 1975; 110:561–566.
22. Ringel S, Harrison S, Norenberg M. Fibromuscular dysplasia: multiple "spontaneous" dissecting aneurysms of the major cranial arteries. Ann Neurology 1977; 1:301–304.
23. Luscher TF, Stanson AW, Hauser OW. Arterial fibromuscular dysplasia. Mayo Clinic Proceedings 1987; 62:931–952.
24. Osborne AG, Anderson RE. Angiographic spectrum of cervical and intracranial fibromuscular dysplasia. Stroke 1977; 8:617–626.
25. Fisher CM. Lacunar strokes and infarcts. Neurology (New York) 1982; 32:871.
26. Fisher CM. Capsular infarcts. Arch Neurology 1979; 36:65–73.
27. Hachinski VC, Potter P, Merksey H. Leukoariosis. Archives of Neurology 1987; 44:21–23.
28. Nichols FTI, Mohr JP. Binswanger's subacute arteriosclerotic encephalopathy, stroke: pathophysiology. In HJM Barnett et al., eds, Diagnosis and Management. New York: Churchill-Livingstone, 1986. P. 875.
29. Bogousslavsky J, Van Melle G, Regli F. The Laussane Stroke Registry: analysis of 1000 consecutive patients with first stroke. Stroke 1988; 19:1083.
30. Cerebral Embolism Task Force: Cardiogenic brain embolism. Arch Neurology 1986; 43:71–84.
31. Cerebral Embolism Task Force: Cardiogenic brain embolism. The second report of the cerebral embolism task force. Arch Neurol 1989; 46:727–743.
32. Loscalzo J. Paradoxical embolism: clinical presentation, diagnositic strategies, and therapeutic options. Am Heart J 1986; 112:141–145.
33. Jones HR Jr., et al. Cerebral emboli of paradoxical origin. Ann Neurol 1983; 13:314–319.
34. Davenport J, Hart RG. Prosthetic valve endocarditis 1976–1987: antiobiotics, anticoagulation, and stroke. Stroke 1990; 21:993–999.
35. Machado EDV, Michet CJ, Ballard DJ. Trends in incidence and clinical presentation of temporal arteritis in Olmsted County, Minnesota, 1950–1985. Arthritis Rheum 1988; 31:745–749.
36. Huston KA, Hunder GG, Lie JT. Temporal arteritis: a 25-year-epidemiologic, clinical and pathologic study. Ann Intern Med 1978; 88:162–167.
37. Missen GA. Involvement of the vertebrocarotid arterial system in giant cell arteritis. J Pathol 1972; 106:P2–3.
38. Hall S, Barr W, Lie JT. Takayasu arteritis: a study of 32 American patients. Medicine 1985; 64:89–99.
39. Calabrese LH, Mallek JA. Primary angiitis of the central nervous system: report of 8 new cases, review of the literature, and proposal for diagnosis. Medicine (Baltimore) 1988; 67:20–39.
40. Moore PM. Diagnosis and management of isolated angiitis of the nervous system. Neurology 1989; 39:167–173.
41. Ford RG, Siekert RG. Central nervous system manifestations of polyarteritis nodosa. Neurology 1965; 15:114.
42. Travers RL, et al. Polyarteritis nodosa: a clinical and angiographic analysis of 17 cases. Semin Arthritis Rheumatol 1979; 8:184–199.
43. Futrell N, Millikan C. Frequency, etiology, and prevention of stroke in patients with systemic lupus erythematosus. Stroke 1989; 20:583–591.
44. Devinsky O, Petito CK, Alonso DR. Clinical and neuropathological findings in systemic lupus erythematosis: the role of

vasculitis, heart emboli, and thrombolitic thrombocytopenic purpura. Ann Neurol 1988; 23:380–384.

45. Futrell N, Millikan C. Frequency, etiology, and prevention of stroke in patients with systemic lupus erythematosis. Stroke 1989; 20:583–591.
46. Fauci AS, et al. Wegener's granulomatosis: prospective clinical and therapeutic experience with 85 patients for 21 years. Ann Int Med 1983; 98:76–85.
47. Asherson RA, Khamashta MA, Ordi-Ros J. The "primary" antiphospholipid syndrome: major clinical and serological features. Medicine (Baltimore) 1989; 68:366–374.
48. Ostergaard JR, Hog E. Incidence of multiple intracranial aneurysms: influence of arterial hypertension and gender. J Neurosurg 1985; 63:49–55.
49. Rosenorn J, Eskesen V, Schmidt K. The risk of rebleeding from ruptured intracranial aneurysms. J Neurosurgery 1987; 67:329–332.
50. Kassell NF, Torner JC. The International Cooperative Study on Timing of Aneurysm Surgery—an update. Stroke 1984; 15:566–570.
51. Locksley HB. Report on the Cooperative Study of Intracranial Aneurysms and Subarachnoid Hemorrhage. Section V, Part I: Natural history of subarachnoid hemorrhage, intracranial aneurysms and arteriovenous malformations: based on 6368 cases in the Cooperative Study. J Neurosurgery 1966; 25: 219–239.
52. Jane JA, Kassell NF, Torner JC. The natural history of aneurysms and arteriovenous malformations. J Neurosurgery 1985; 62:321–323.
53. Gautier JC, Pradat-Diehl P, Loron P. Accidents vasculaires cerebraux des sujets jeunes: une etude de 133 patients ages de 9 a 45 ans. Rev Neurol 1989; 145:437–442.
54. Bogousslavsky J, Regli F. Ischemic stroke in adults younger than 30 years of age: cause and prognosis. Arch Neurol 1987; 44:479–482.
55. De Vivo DC. The expanding clinical spectrum of mitochondrial diseases. Brain and Development 1993; 15(1):1–22.
56. Ciafaloni E, et al. MELAS: Clinical features, biochemistry, and molecular genetics. Annals of Neurology 1992; 31:391–398.
57. North American Symptomatic Carotid Endarterectomy Trial Collaborators: Beneficial effect of carotid endarterectomy in symptomatic patients with high grade carotid stenosis. N Engl J Med 1990; 323:1505–1511.
58. European Carotid Surgery Trialists' Collaborative Group: MRC European carotid surgery trial: interim results from symptomatic patients with severe (70–90%) or mild (0–29%) carotid stenosis. Lancet 1991; 337:1235–1243.
59. The Dutch TIA Trial Study Group: A comparison of two doses of aspirin (30 mg vs. 283 mg a day) in patients after a transient ischemic stroke. N Engl J Med 1991; 325:1261–1266.
60. The American-Canadian Co-operative Study Group: Persantine aspirin trial in cerebral ischemia. Part II. Endpoint results. Stroke 1985; 16:406–415.
61. Antiplatelet Trialist's Collaboration: Collaborative overview of randomised trials of antiplatelet therapy—I: Prevention of death, myocardial infarction, and stroke by prolonged antiplatelet therapy in various categories of patients. British Medical Journal 1994; 308:81–106.
62. The Canadian Cooperative Study Group: A randomized trial of aspirin and sulfinpyrazone in threatened stroke. NEJM 1978; 299:53–59.
63. Sorensen PS, et al. Acetylsalicylic acid in the prevention of stroke in patients with reversible cerebral ischemic attacks. Stroke 1983; 14:15–22.
64. The SALT Cooperative Group: Swedish Aspirin Low-dose Trials (SALT) of 75 mg aspirin as secondary prophylaxis after cerebrovascular ischemic events. Lancet 1991; 338:1345–1349.
65. Farrell B, et al. The United Kingdom transient ischemic attack (UK-TIA) aspirin trial: final results. J Neurol Neurosurg Psychiatry 1991; 54:1044–1054.
66. Candelise L, et al. A randomized trial of aspirin and sulfinpyrazone in patients with TIA. Stroke 1982; 13:175–179.
67. Gent M, et al. A secondary prevention, randomized trial of suloctidil in patients with a recent history of thromboembolic stroke. Stroke 1985; 16:416–424.
68. Matchar DB, et al. Medical treatment for stroke prevention. Ann Intern Med 1994; 121:41–53.
69. Gent M, et al. The Canadian American Ticlopidine Study (CATS) in thromboembolic stroke. Lancet 1989; 1:1215–1220.
70. Hass WK, et al. A randomized trial comparing ticlopidine hydrochloride with aspirin for the prevention of stroke in high risk patients. N Engl J Med 1989; 321:501–507.
71. Harbison JW. Ticlopidine versus aspirin for the prevention of recurrent stroke. Analysis of patients with minor stroke from the Ticlopidine Aspirin Stroke Study. Stroke 1992; 23:1723–1727.
72. Grotta JC, Norris JW, Kamm B. Prevention of stroke with ticlopidine: who benefits most? TAAS Baseline and Angiographic Data Subgroup. Neurology 1992; 42:111–115.
73. Hirsh J, Poller L, Deykin D. Optimal therapeutic range for oral anticoagulants. Chest 1989; 95[Suppl 5]:S1–S11.
74. Poller L. The effect of low-dose warfarin on the risk of stroke in patients with nonrheumatic atrial fibrillation. N Engl J Med 1991; 325:129–130.
75. Heyman A, Wilkinson WE, Heyden S. Risk of stroke in asymptomatic persons with cervical arterial bruits. N Engl J Med 1980; 302:838–841.
76. Wolf PA, et al. Asymptomatic carotid bruit and the risk of stroke. JAMA 1981; 245:1442–1445.
77. Treiman RL, et al. Carotid bruit. Arch Surgery 1973; 106: 803–805.
78. Kartchner MM, McRae LP. Noninvasive evaluation and management of the "asymptomatic" carotid bruit. Surgery 1977; 82:840–847.
79. Cooperman M, Martin EW, Evans WE. Significance of asymptomatic carotid bruits. Arch Surg 1978; 113:1239–1240.
80. Kagan A, Popper J, Rhoads GG. Epidemiologic studies on coronary artery disease and stroke in Japanese men living in Japan, Hawaii, and California: prevalence of stroke. In P Scheinberg, ed. Cerebrovascular Diseases. New York: Raven, 1976. P. 267.
81. Furlan AJ, Whisnant JP. Long-term prognosis after carotid artery occlusion. Neurology (Minneapolis) 1980; 30:986–988.
82. Sacquegna T, DeCarolis P, Pazzaglia P. The clinical course and prognosis of carotid artery occlusion. J Neurol Neurosurg Psychiatry 1982; 45:1037–1039.
83. Bernstein NM, Norris JW. Benign outcome of carotid occlusion. Neurology (New York) 1989; 39:6.
84. Cote R, Barnett HJM, Taylor DW. Internal carotid occlusion: a prospective study. Stroke 1983; 14:898–902.
85. Mayberg MR, et al. for the Veterans Affairs Cooperative Studies Program 309 Trialist Group. Carotid endarterectomy and prevention of cerebral ischemia in symptomatic carotid stenosis. JAMA 1991; 266:3289–3294.
86. Hobson RW, et al. for the Veterans Affairs Cooperative Study Group. N Engl J Med 1991; 328:221–227.
87. CASANOVA Study Group. Carotid surgery versus medical therapy in asymptomatic carotid stenosis. Stroke 1994; 22:1229–1235.
88. The Asymptomatic Cartoid Atherosclerosis Study Group. Study design for randomized prospective trial of carotid endarterectomy for asymptomatic atherosclerosis. Stroke 1989;

20:844–849; and National Institiute of Neurological Disorders and Stroke Clinical Advisory on Carotid Endarterectomy for Patients with Asymptomatic Internal Carotid Artery Stenosis, 1994.
89. Ezekowitz, MD, et al., for the Veterans Affairs Stroke Prevention in Nonrheumatic Atrial Fibrillation Investigators. N Engl J Med 1992; 327:1406–1412.
90. Stroke Prevention in Atrial Fibrillation Investigators. Stroke Prevention in Atrial Fibrillation Study. Final Results. Circulation 1991; 84:527–539.
91. The Boston Area Anticoagulation Trial Fibrillation Investigators: The effect of low-dose warfarin on the risk of stroke in patients with nonrheumatic atrial fibrillation. N Engl J Med 1990; 323:1505–1511.
92. Petersen P, et al. Placebo-controlled, randomised trial of warfarin and aspirin for prevention of thromboembolic complications in chronic atrial fibrillation. The Copenhagen AFASAK Study. Lancet 1989; 1:175–179.
93. Hart RG, et al. Stroke in infective endocarditis. Stroke 1990; 21:695–750.
94. National Institute of Neurological Disorders and Stroke rt-PA Stroke Study Group: Tissue plasminogen activator for acute ischemic stroke. N Engl J Med 1995; 333:1581–1588.
95. Choi DW. Excitatory cell death. Journal of Neurobiology 1992; 23:1261–1276.
96. Ginsberg MD. Emerging strategies for the treatment of ischemic brain injury, Molecular and Cellular Approaches in the Treatment of Neurological Disease, SG Waxman, ed. New York: Research Publications, 1993; 71:207–237.
97. Lipton SA, Rosenberg PA. Excitatory amino acids as a final common pathway for neurological disorders. NEJM 1994; 330(9):613–622.

Coronary Artery Disease

Thomas C. Andrews
Gilbert H. Mudge, Jr.

Coronary artery disease accounts for the primary mortality and morbidity in the United States. As many as 1,500,000 Americans, half under 65 years of age, will suffer a myocardial infarction in 1994, and about one-third of those infarctions will be fatal. Moreover, over 6 million individuals carry the diagnosis of coronary disease, with varying degrees of morbidity and subsequent disability. Hence, coronary artery disease generates a tremendous economic loss in industrialized nations, estimated in the United States in 1994 to be 56 billion dollars in direct health care expenditures and lost productivity [1].

Pathogenic Mechanisms of Myocardial Ischemia

Once atherosclerosis has developed in the coronary arteries, approximately a 50-percent stenosis is required before coronary blood flow becomes limited during conditions of hyperemia, with a 90-percent stenosis required to limit blood flow under resting conditions (Fig. 34-1) [2]. Coronary angiography is useful in defining the presence and severity of these coronary stenoses and provides useful information when revascularization is contemplated. However, the severity of fixed atherosclerotic disease alone is not adequate in predicting the clinical course of patients, since superimposed thrombus formation and varying degrees of coronary vasospasm may abruptly transform a minimal stenosis into a critical one. In the past two decades, the importance of the vascular endothelium in these processes has become apparent, because endothelial dysfunction contributes to the growth of the fixed atherosclerotic plaque and renders it prothrombotic and prone to vasoconstriction.

ROLE OF THE VASCULAR ENDOTHELIUM

As recently as 20 years ago, the endothelium was considered a passive lining of the vascular wall that functioned only as a selective permeability barrier. Research over the last two decades has shown that these cells collectively are more appropriately viewed as the largest paracrine organ in the body, demonstrating important regulatory functions in health and contributing substantially to the pathogenesis of coronary atherosclerosis and ultimately to myocardial infarction and cardiac death. In health, the endothelial product endothelium-derived relaxing factor (EDRF) promotes vasodilation, inhibits platelet adhesion and aggregation, and also may inhibit smooth muscle-cell and mesangial-cell proliferation. Although other endothelial products, such as the endothelins, are vasoconstrictor, procoagulant, or both, the net effect in health is vasodilatory and anticoagulant [3]. In animal models [4] as well as in human coronary arteries [5], hypercholesterolemia is associated with a blunting of the actions of EDRF, and an imbalance between that vasoconstrictor and the vasodilator substances leads to an overall shift to a procoagulant, vasoconstrictor state and possibly to further stimulation of smooth muscle-cell proliferation in the process of atherogenesis.

Once atherosclerosis is established, the exact mechanism involved in the transition between chronic stable, and often subclinical, coronary artery disease and acute myocardial ischemia remains unclear, although the endothelium probably plays a major role. In patients with established atherosclerosis, the endothelium manifests a marked tendency to promote vasoconstriction [6]. In addition, plasma levels of endothelin are elevated in patients with acute myocardial infarction [7], as well as in experimental models of hypoxia [8] or thrombosis [9]. Ongoing research will determine whether treatment of risk factors early in the process of atherogenesis can lead to normalization of endothelial function and retard the development of fixed atherosclerosis. Similarly, once atherosclerosis has developed, risk-factor modification may lead to plaque stabilization and prevent the progression to acute ischemia.

ROLE OF SMOOTH MUSCLE PROLIFERATION

Endothelial dysfunction ultimately may be responsible for the smooth muscle proliferation that plays an important role in atherogenesis. Based on specimens obtained by coronary atherectomy, preliminary evidence suggests that smooth muscle-cell proliferation is associated with both unstable angina and restenosis following angioplasty but not with the syndrome of chronic stable angina. In addition, compared with atherectomy samples from patients with stable angina, samples from patients with unstable angina or restenosis express high levels of acidic and basic fibroblast growth factor, both known to be mediators of smooth muscle-cell migration and proliferation. Those observations suggest a mechanism of the transition from chronic stable angina to unstable angina, that is, smooth muscle-cell proliferation may lead to gradual plaque expansion and subsequent luminal narrowing without plaque rupture or thrombosis [10].

ROLE OF ABNORMAL CORONARY VASOMOTION

With the increasing recognition of the importance of endothelial-cell function in vascular responses, a potential pathogenic mechanism of myocardial ischemia is that of abnormal coronary artery vasomotion. For some time, coronary artery spasm has been documented as the etiologic factor of variant or Prinzmetal's angina [11], and recent experimental evidence suggests that the vasoactive substances endothelin-1 and serotonin may play etiologic roles [12,13]. Although this clinical syndrome of chest pain and ST-segment elevation remains relatively rare, more recent studies suggest that coronary artery vasomo-

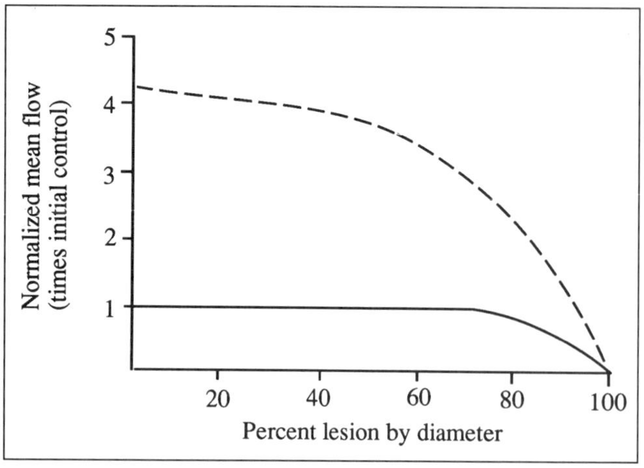

Fig. 34-1. Effect of progressive constriction on resting flow in the left circumflex artery (solid line) and hyperemic response (dashed line) to intracoronary injection of Hypaque in a single dog. (Adapted from K Gould, K Lipscomb, G Hamilton. Physiologic basis for assessing critical coronary stenosis. Instantaneous flow response and regional distribution during coronary hyperemia as measures of coronary flow reserve. Am J Cardiol 1974; 33:87.)

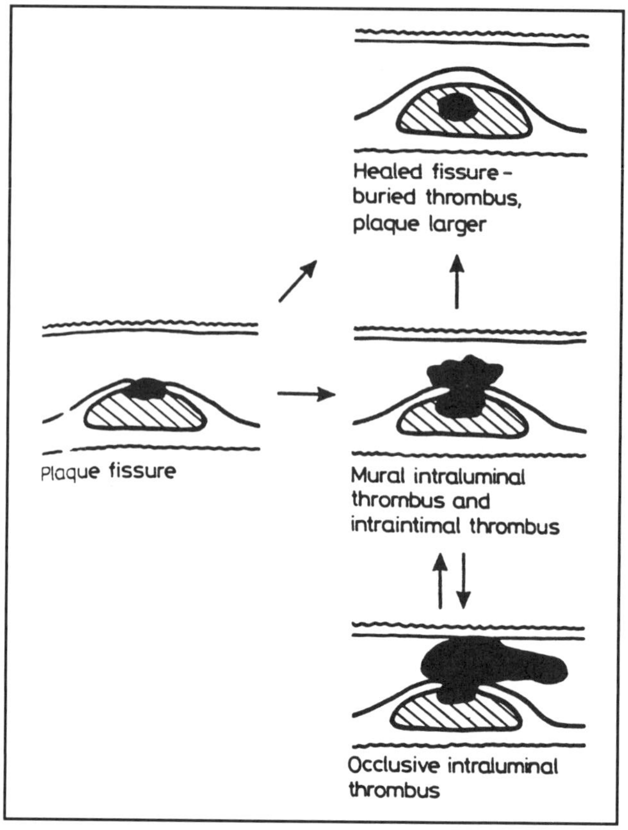

Fig. 34-2. Diagrammatic representation of the evolution of a plaque fissure either to reseal and stabilize or to progress to thrombotic occlusion. (Reproduced with permission from M Davies, A Thomas. Plaque fissuring—the cause of acute myocardial ischemia, sudden ischemic death, and crescendo angina. Br Heart J 1985; 53:363.)

tion is instrumental in the much more common syndromes of stable and unstable angina [14,15]. There is ample clinical evidence to suggest that the coronary circulation can respond to physiologic vasoconstrictor stimuli. Cold exposure, exercise, mental stress, and cigarette smoking all have been shown to produce decrements in coronary artery blood flow [16–19]. Damaged endothelium loses its ability to initiate appropriate dilatation of the coronary bed, and inappropriate vasoconstriction is elicited by serotonin [20], catecholamines [21], and acetylcholine [6], which in health are coronary vasodilators. In addition, the coronary arteries lose their ability to dilate in response to increased blood flow, further limiting the ability to adapt to increased metabolic demands [22]. Those minor changes in physiologic tone may be adequate to transform a subcritical lesion into a critical one and, hence, lead to more readily provoked ischemia with increases in myocardial oxygen demand.

ROLE OF THROMBOSIS

Since the pioneering work of DeWood and co-workers, there is now much evidence to incriminate thrombosis as a major pathogenic factor in acute ischemic syndromes [23]. There is little doubt that acute coronary artery thrombosis is the final pathogenic mechanism of acute myocardial infarction and sudden cardiac death [23,24], concluding a complex interplay among fixed coronary atherosclerosis, endothelial injury and dysfunction, vasospasm, smooth muscle proliferation, and platelet activation [25,26]. Angiographic studies also have implicated thrombosis in the pathogenesis of unstable angina, with filling defects on the coronary angiograms not visualized in patients with a stable anginal pattern [27–29]. There is evidence that, compared with newer methods, angiography is relatively insensitive in the detection of thrombus [27,28,30]. For example, with direct angioscopic visualization during coronary artery bypass surgery, thrombi are uniformly seen superimposed on atherosclerotic lesions in patients with unstable symptomatology, but they are not visualized in patients with chronic stable angina [28]. The ruptured atherosclerotic plaque acts as a nidus for thrombosis and is felt to be one potential pathogenetic link between stable and unstable ischemic syndromes. Some have theorized that thrombosis in the setting of a mildly obstructing fixed atherosclerotic plaque results simply in further narrowing of the plaque, whereas thrombosis associated with a more severely obstructing plaque may result in total thrombotic occlusion of the vessel (Fig. 34-2) [24,31–33]. In addition to plaque morphology, other investigators have implicated abnormal platelets in the genesis of thrombosis. For example, markers of platelet hyperactivity have been shown to predict future coronary events and mortality in low-risk survivors of myocardial infarction not treated with aspirin [34]. Thrombosis may be the single most important factor in the acute progression of atherosclerosis, culminating in worsening of anginal symptoms, myocardial infarction, or sudden death.

Recent work by a number of investigators suggests that

thrombosis may be important in the early stages of atherogenesis, as well. For example, platelets may serve as a lipid source in the development of the fatty streak [35], as well as encourage the mitogenic response to injury of the vessel wall [36]. The roles of thrombin, fibrin degradation fragments, and the fibrinolytic enzymes in atherogenesis are less well established.

Understanding the interplay among fixed atherosclerosis, thrombosis, smooth muscle proliferation, and vasomotion in acute ischemic syndromes requires further extensive studies at the cellular and clinical levels. The need for such correlation is highlighted by early clinical evidence to suggest that addressing each of these pathogenic mechanisms may substantially alter the natural history of coronary artery disease [37–40].

Prognosis and Natural History of Coronary Artery Disease

Current prognosis of coronary artery disease with modern therapeutic modalities is difficult to estimate from the natural history studies. The Framingham Heart Study suggests an annual mortality rate of 4 percent per year [41], whereas other studies report higher mortality in certain patient groups [42]. These long-term studies involved heterogeneous patient populations, with variable representation of risk factors known to affect prognosis adversely. Adverse prognostic factors included severity of anginal symptoms, abnormal resting electrocardiograms, history of myocardial infarction, hypertension, cigarette smoking, cardiomegaly on chest x-ray, evidence of congestive heart failure on physical examination, and the presence of associated comorbidities, including peripheral and cerebrovascular disease [43,44]. However, longitudinal epidemiologic studies have revealed important trends in the natural history of coronary artery disease, analysis of which provides insight into the effectiveness of the medical community in preventing coronary artery disease, improving patient education, and increasing public awareness of coronary disease risk factors.

CHANGING PATTERNS IN THE NATURAL HISTORY

The mortality rate of coronary artery disease rose dramatically through the first half of the twentieth century to peak in the late 1960s [45]. Since then, the mortality from ischemic heart disease has fallen by as much as 30 percent in the United States and some European countries [46]. That decline applies particularly to sudden death, but it also has been noted in the incidences of angina and acute myocardial infarction [47,48]. For example, Pell and Fayerweather reported a 28.2-percent decline in the incidence of first myocardial infarction among employees of the DuPont Company from 1957 to 1983, as well as a marked drop in the 30-day case-fatality rate [49]. In a more recent case series from Worcester, Massachusetts, the age-specific incidence of initial myocardial infarction fell approximately 25 percent between 1975 and 1988 in both men and women, with out-of-hospital coronary deaths decreasing by more than 60 percent [50]. The explanation for that decline in cardiovascular morbidity and mortality is multifactorial and undoubtedly includes improvements in diagnosis and therapy of chronic ischemic heart disease, risk stratification, and aggressive treatment of coronary risk factors, including lipid-lowering therapy [51] and smoking cessation [46,51–54]. In recognition of the limitations of retrospective analysis, it has been suggested that high-technology medical care has had minimal impact on the overall change in mortality and that medical therapy accounts for only about 40 percent of the decline in mortality in the American male population [54].

PROGNOSTIC FACTORS IN PATIENTS WITH ESTABLISHED CORONARY ARTERY DISEASE

The decline in cardiovascular mortality after myocardial infarction in the Minneapolis–St. Paul area between 1970 and 1980 is of particular interest. The survival in men with definite myocardial infarction improved 35 percent over that 10-year period, with 70 percent of the survival gain attributable to the hospitalization period. However, the improvement in survival extended to those discharged alive, and, hence, the authors concluded that factors affecting survival must extend to the recovery period, as well [53]. The explanation for this phenomenon is not readily apparent, but it is reasonable to speculate that in the 1980s we had a far better clinical appreciation for the primary determinants of survival after myocardial infarction, leading to a more aggressive treatment approach in high-risk patients in the months shortly after their sentinel events. Besides the angiographic predictors of prognosis, other major determinants of survival in patients with coronary artery disease include left ventricular function, symptomatic or functional status, and evidence of ischemia on noninvasive testing.

Left Ventricular Function. Left ventricular function has emerged as perhaps the most important determinant of long-term survival in patients with coronary artery disease. A number of randomized studies in patients with stable and unstable angina, including the Combined Veterans Administration Study [55], the Coronary Artery Surgery Study (CASS) [56–58], and the Veterans Study of Unstable Angina [55,59], came to the same conclusion: Poor left ventricular function, rather than the extent of coronary artery disease, portends a particularly adverse prognosis for patients who receive long-term medical therapy (Fig. 34-3). Medically treated patients with an ejection fraction below 36 percent have a 5-year mortality that may approach 60 percent [60]. A similar correlation between left ventricular dysfunction and mortality exists in patients initially surviving acute myocardial infarction, with the presence of cardiomegaly or pulmonary congestion on chest x-ray and the presence of widespread Q waves on the electrocardiogram carrying a particularly dire prognosis [61]. Hence, it is reasonable to suggest that all patients with coronary artery disease have noninvasive assessment of left ventricular function to help direct management in an effort to improve long-term outcome.

Angiographic Criteria. Coronary angiography frequently is utilized to provide prognostic information in patients with coronary artery disease, particularly when revascularization is contemplated. It is clear, however, that the extent and the severity of disease are imperfect predictors of

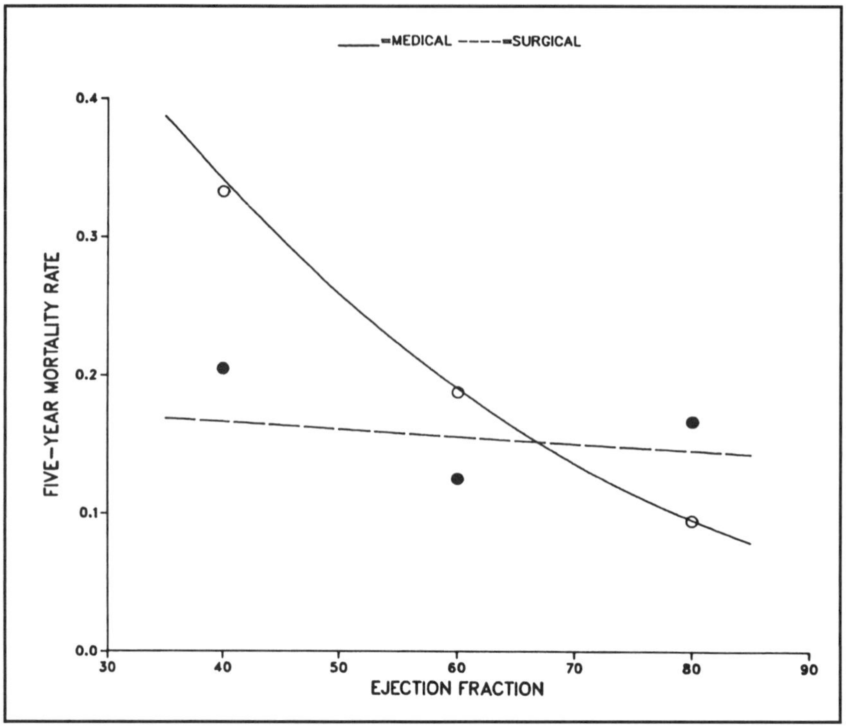

Fig. 34-3. Plot of mortality for medical and surgical patients using ejection fraction as a continuous variable. In this analysis, mortality was correlated with left ventricular function for medically treated patients with unstable angina, whereas no such relationship was seen with similar patients surgically treated. (Reproduced with permission of the American Heart Association from A Parisi et al. Medical compared with surgical management of unstable angina. 5-year mortality and morbidity in the Veterans Administration Study. Circulation 1989; 80:1176.)

the clinical course of individual patients. For example, approximately 11 percent of patients have minimal coronary artery disease on angiography 7 to 10 days after an acute myocardial infarction, but such patients continue to be at high risk for future cardiac events despite their "benign" coronary anatomy (Fig. 34-4) [30]. Furthermore, in patients undergoing serial angiograms before and after myocardial infarction, the infarct-related artery is infrequently involved with a high-grade stenosis on the preinfarction angiogram [62]. Another limitation of coronary arteriography is that visual estimation of lesion severity is often quite inaccurate in estimating the true severity of the lesion as judged by quantitative angiography [63].

Despite those shortcomings, the angiographic extent of disease can provide useful prognostic information to the clinician caring for symptomatic patients. Varying anatomic locations of stenoses can predict different clinical outcomes. For example, a high-grade lesion of the proximal left anterior descending coronary artery before the first septal perforator carries a mortality rate of approximately 10 percent per year compared to more distal lesions of the artery, which have a mortality rate of approximately 2 percent per year [64]. Patients with significant stenoses of the right coronary artery, which on a statistical basis supplies less jeopardized myocardium, have a better long-term survival rate than patients with disease of the left anterior descending [64]. The presence of a high-grade stenosis of the left main coronary artery carries a particularly dire prognosis, with 3-year survival approximating 50 percent with medical therapy [65]. Multivessel coronary artery disease is associated with a lower survival rate with medical therapy than is single-vessel disease [66]. Excluding patients studied after acute myocardial infarction, the finding of normal coronary arteries or minimal coronary artery disease portends a good prognosis [67]. Finally, in patients who have received thrombolytic therapy for acute myocardial infarction, the presence of multivessel coronary artery disease may be the strongest predictor of short-term prognosis [68] and the severity of residual stenosis the best predictor of 3-month patency of the infarct-related artery [69].

The presence of an ulcerated plaque may be more important than the absolute luminal narrowing when angiography is utilized to predict the clinical course of patients with established coronary artery disease. Patients with smoothly tapered or diffusely irregular atherosclerotic lesions generally have a stable clinical course, despite angina that may be provoked by minimal exercise [27]. In contrast, patients who have eccentric plaques with evidence of ulceration often experience a very unstable clinical course with associated escalating symptoms of angina, frequently culminating in acute myocardial necrosis (Fig. 34-5) [31–33,37,70–72]. Interestingly, these ulcerated lesions often progress rapidly to cause unstable symptoms, despite insignificant absolute luminal narrowing [27]. It has been suggested that plaque composition may be more

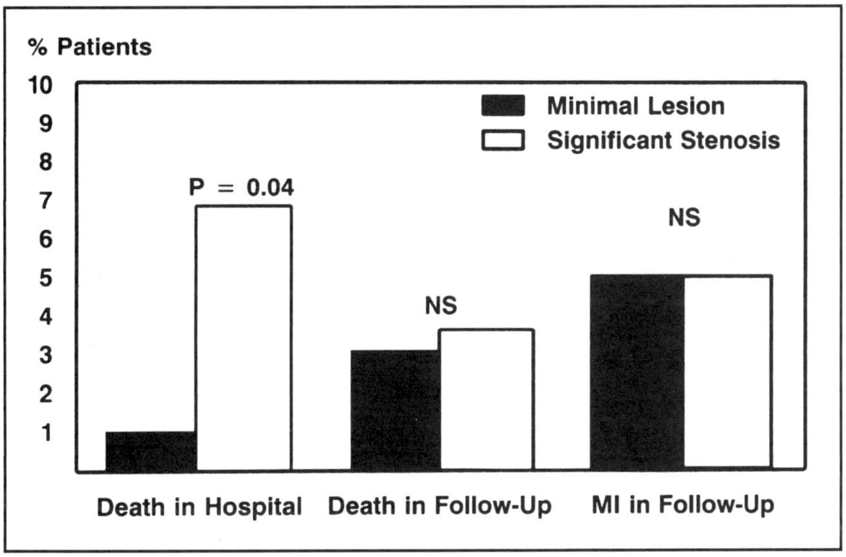

Fig. 34-4. In-hospital mortality rate and long-term follow-up study in patients with a minimal coronary lesion and those with significant stenosis after successful intravenous thrombolytic therapy for acute myocardial infarction. (Reproduced with permission from D Kereiakes et al. Myocardial infarction with minimal coronary atherosclerosis in the era of thrombolytic reperfusion. The Thrombolysis and Angioplasty in Myocardial Infarction (TAMI) Study Group. J Am Coll Cardiol 1991; 17:304.)

important than plaque size (degree of luminal narrowing) with soft, lipid-rich plaques more prone to rupture, causing clinical events [70].

Symptomatic and Functional Status. Despite the limitation that the symptomatic status of a patient with coronary artery disease may vary greatly with level of activity, the severity of anginal symptoms has emerged as an important prognostic indicator. For example, comparing subsets of patients treated with medical therapy or bypass surgery, surgical benefit is greatest in patients with the most severe symptoms without stratifying for angiographic extent of disease [73]. However, when coronary disease patients with and without symptoms are stratified by the presence or absence of ST-segment depression on treadmill testing, those with ischemia have a much worse prognosis than those without ischemia, regardless of the presence or absence of symptoms (Fig. 34-6) [74]. Indeed, although only a small fraction of coronary patients are completely asymptomatic, most patients with coronary disease have asymptomatic episodes of ST-segment depression on Holter monitoring during daily life. While it is clear that the presence of these episodes of asymptomatic ischemia portends a poor prognosis in patients with stable [75–77] or unstable angina [78], patients undergoing surgery for peripheral vascular disease [79–81], and patients surviving myocardial infarction [82], it is unclear whether specific treatment of asymptomatic ischemia can have a favorable effect on this poor prognosis. In summary, symptoms are a marker of ischemia: Those patients with severe symptoms are more likely to demonstrate severe ischemia and, consequently, to benefit from aggressive anti-ischemic therapy. However, the converse is not true: The absence of symptoms is not necessarily indicative of the absence of severe ischemia, and certain subgroups of patients with predominantly asymptomatic ischemia will benefit from aggressive therapy, including bypass surgery.

Because of substantial subjective variability in the assessment of symptoms, objective measures of functional status are more reliable for risk stratification in patients with otherwise stable coronary artery disease. The most commonly utilized measure of functional capacity is the conventional exercise treadmill test alone or in concert with various imaging modalities. Exercise capacity is more reliable than the magnitude of ST-segment depression in predicting long-term prognosis [83]. For example, one study using conventional exercise electrocardiography showed that, regardless of the angiographic extent of disease, patients able to exercise into stage IV of a standard Bruce protocol are at low risk for adverse cardiac events despite an ischemic ST-segment response, with an 8-year survival rate of 93 percent. In contrast, a group of patients with a similar ischemic ST-segment response unable to complete stage I of a standard Bruce protocol have an 8-year survival rate of 45 percent (Fig. 34-7) [84]. In a CASS database study, among patients with triple-vessel disease and preserved left ventricular function, 4-year survival was 53 percent for patients able to achieve only stage I or II of a standard Bruce protocol, compared with 100-percent survival in patients able to achieve stage V [85]. Other investigators have shown that preserved functional capacity also predicts an excellent short-term prognosis in patients undergoing surgery for peripheral vascular disease [86].

Noninvasive Evidence of Ischemia. Reversible ischemia with exercise or pharmacologic stress provides prognostic in-

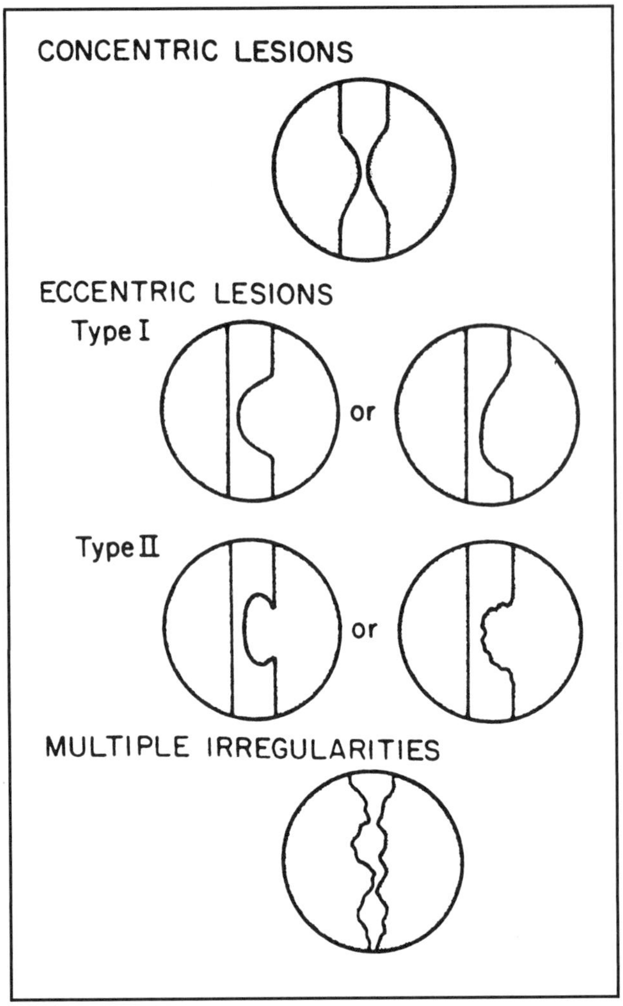

Fig. 34-5. Schematic drawings of the different configurations of stenotic lesions in coronary artery disease. Concentric lesions are symmetric and usually smooth. Type 1 eccentric lesions are asymmetric and smooth. Type II eccentric lesions are either smooth with a narrow neck or have irregular borders. Type II eccentric lesions, probably representing ulcerated plaques, are found to be much more frequently associated with lesion progression at repeat angiography and with symptoms of unstable angina than are concentric lesions or type I eccentric lesions. (Reproduced with permission from J Ambrose et al. Angiographic evolution of coronary artery morphology in unstable angina. J Am Coll Cardiol 1986; 7:472.)

formation that is additive to the measures of functional status. This ischemia can be documented by reversible ST-segment depression on the exercise electrocardiogram or Holter monitor, perfusion defects using radionuclides techniques, or reversible wall-motion abnormalities on echocardiography or radionuclide ventriculography with either exercise or pharmacologic stress.

A well-described relationship exists between the degree of exercise-induced ST-segment depression and angiographic severity of coronary artery disease [87], and patients with ST-segment depression beginning in stage I of a standard Bruce protocol represent a subgroup at high risk for adverse cardiac events [88,89]. Thallium or sestamibi scintigraphic techniques also may be helpful in assessing ischemia in patients with uninterpretable electrocardiograms, such as left bundle branch block, Wolff-Parkinson-White syndrome, or severe resting ST-segment abnormalities [90]. Large or multiple thallium-perfusion abnormalities, abnormal lung uptake, and delayed tracer redistribution correlate well with multivessel coronary disease on arteriography [91,92]. Advanced imaging techniques such as single-photon-emission computed tomographic (SPECT) imaging with thallium may add marginally to the prognostic information obtainable from conventional exercise testing at a substantial increase in cost [93]. Thallium scintigraphy after pharmacologic stress with dipyridamole [94], adenosine [95], or dobutamine [96] aids in the diagnosis of coronary artery disease and may provide prognostic information in patients unable to exercise [97]. In patients with chest pain, a normal thallium exercise test portends an excellent prognosis, similar to that of patients with normal coronary arteries [98].

The prognostic value of exercise radionuclide angiography is consistent with the recognized importance of left ventricular function in predicting the clinical course of individuals with coronary artery disease. A fall in exercise left ventricular ejection fraction or a lack of an appropriate increase predicts an adverse long-term prognosis [83,99–102]. Similar prognostic information can be garnered from exercise echocardiography, with the development of exercise-induced new or worsened wall-motion abnormalities predictive of future cardiac events [103], although the additive value of such specialized exercise studies to conventional exercise testing and assessment of resting left ventricular function continues to be questioned.

Diagnosis of Coronary Artery Disease

The diagnosis of coronary artery disease early in its natural course often is overlooked as perhaps the most important aspect of the long-term successful management of a patient. Once the diagnosis has been established, patients can be properly instructed in risk-factor modification, appropriate exercise limitations, and warning signs and symptoms that might signify impending infarction. Patient education may have as much impact on the long-term management of this chronic disease as initiating medical therapy. The patient who is not educated to the disease process, its precipitating causes, and its therapy continues to be at high risk despite all medical efforts.

HISTORY

The most important clinical clue to the diagnosis of coronary artery disease is the presence of anginal discomfort. Heberden's original description of the discomfort of anterior chest pressure associated with a sensation of strangulation and anxiety has withstood the test of time [104]. Although the exertional discomfort usually is retrosternal, radiation down the ulnar aspect of the left arm is common. Radiation to the right arm is less frequent, and jaw discomfort, throat pain, and neck discomfort occasionally are reported. Anginal discomfort is rarely manifested as sen-

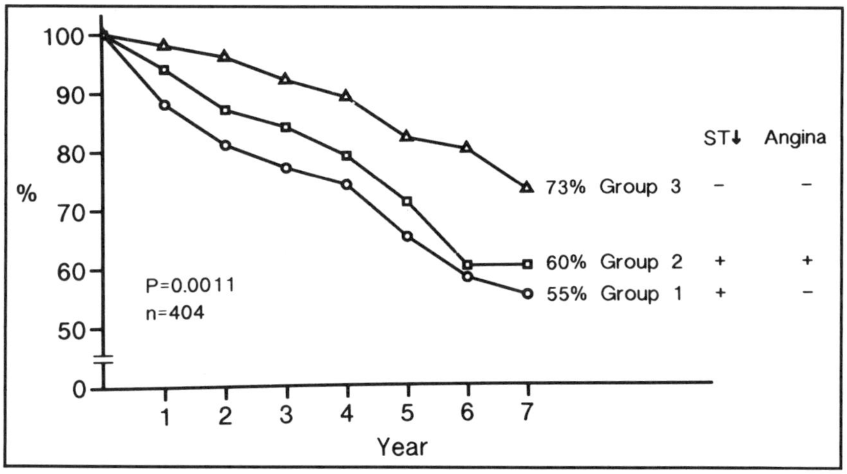

Fig. 34-6. Cumulative survival for patients with abnormal left ventricular function with silent ischemia (group 1), symptomatic ischemia (group 2), and no ischemia (group 3). The 7-year survival was similar for patients with silent or symptomatic ischemia. (Reproduced with permission from D Weiner et al. The role of exercise-induced silent myocardial ischemia in patients with abnormal left ventricular function. A report from the Coronary Artery Surgery Study (CASS) registry. Am Heart J 1989; 118:649.)

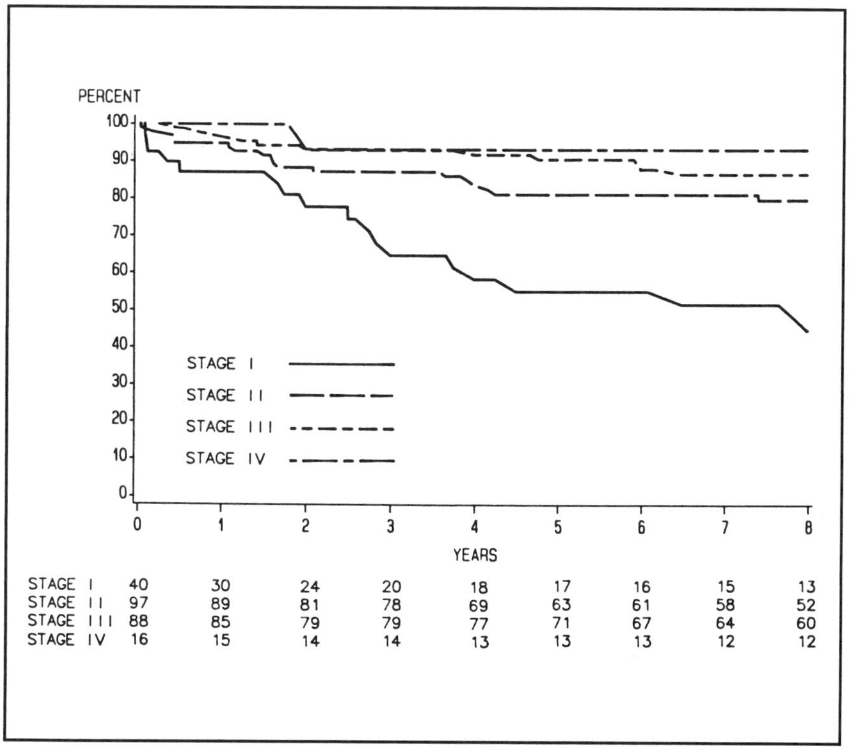

Fig. 34-7. Survival rates for 241 patients with strongly positive exercise tests by stage of termination on exercise testing. All patients developed at least 2 mm of ST-segment depression and had coronary artery disease documented by angiography. (Reproduced with permission from P Bogaty et al. Prognosis of patients with a strongly positive exercise electrocardiogram. Am J Cardiol 1989; 64:1284.)

Table 34-1. Differential diagnosis of chest discomfort

Angina pectoris
Pleurisy
Pericarditis
Costochondritis
Cervical radiculitis
Pulmonary embolism
Pulmonary hypertension
Pneumothorax
Biliary colic
Hiatus hernia
Esophageal spasm
Peptic ulcer disease
Aortic dissection
Esophageal rupture

sations above the jaw or below the diaphragm. It is usually of a crescendo-decrescendo quality, precipitated by exertion and dissipating with rest, rarely lasting less than 5 seconds. Discomfort greater than 20 to 30 minutes either represents myocardial infarction or is of noncardiac origin. Subtle precipitating factors of classic anginal pain include arm exercise, the postprandial state, emotional excitement, and secondary illnesses that alter myocardial oxygen delivery or requirements such as anemia, thyrotoxicosis, and fever. Whatever the primary pathogenic mechanism of myocardial ischemia—be it the result of increased myocardial oxygen demand, intracoronary thrombosis, or inappropriate coronary artery vasomotion—the quality of the discomfort is usually quite similar for any given patient. The precipitating factors of angina may vary somewhat for an individual patient, perhaps reflecting the dynamic pathogenic mechanisms. Anginal threshold may be quite variable, with more discomfort occurring during colder weather, in early morning hours, or following meals. Nocturnal or rest discomfort suggests a possible thrombotic or vasoconstrictor mechanism. Relief with nitrates may be helpful but not definitive in establishing the diagnosis of transient myocardial ischemia. It is important to remember that other clinical manifestations of ischemia, such as left ventricular dysfunction, may present as exertional dyspnea, near syncope, or fatigue.

Descriptions of nonischemic pain include pleuritic or positional discomfort, pain exacerbated by swallowing or relieved by food, focal discomfort over the anterior chest, or discomfort precipitated by thoracic motion. Moreover, the predictable precipitating causes of typical anginal pain often are absent from nonischemic chest pain. The differential diagnosis of such discomfort is extensive, and appropriate historic features may aid in making the proper diagnosis (Table 34-1). Aortic dissection is an important differential to emphasize, because the associated cardiovascular collapse may be identical to that of acute myocardial infarction; retrograde dissection of a coronary artery may confound the diagnosis; and (inappropriate) treatment with thrombolytic therapy may lead to a catastrophic outcome. Anginalike discomfort associated with normal coronary arteries has been reported extensively in the literature, with varying nomenclature that includes neurocirculatory asthenia, DaCosta's syndrome, psychogenic chest pain, and syndrome X. It may be impossible to differentiate this discomfort from that of classic myocardial ischemia on clinical grounds. Most of these patients display minimal objective evidence of transient ischemia (they do not have classic ST-segment depression on stress testing), have normal perfusion images on thallium studies and normal left ventricular function by echocardiography, and do not have ST-segment shifts on ambulatory monitoring during chest pain. Although the precise etiology of such discomfort is unknown, endothelial dysfunction with defective vasodilator reserve has been suggested as a possible mechanism [105–109], with abnormal lactate metabolism during stress and a reduction of left ventricular functional reserve described [110]. It should be emphasized that, in general, this syndrome has an excellent long-term prognosis, with a 96-percent 7-year survival [67]. However, such patients manifesting left bundle branch block at rest or with exercise may represent a higher-risk subgroup, with progressive deterioration in left ventricular performance over a period of several years [110].

PHYSICAL EXAMINATION

The general physical examination of patients suspected of coronary artery disease should be directed primarily toward assessing peripheral manifestations of atherosclerosis; searching for evidence of left ventricular dysfunction, valvular heart disease, or both; and excluding noncardiac causes of chest pain. Blood pressure must be carefully assessed in both upper extremities. Examination of the skin is important to detect manifestations of hypercholesterolemia, including arcus senilis, xanthelasmas, and tendinous xanthomas. The ophthalmologic examination may be helpful in gauging the extent of vascular pathology from diabetes mellitus and hypertension. The thyroid should be palpated to search for clues of thyrotoxicosis. Musculoskeletal examination may uncover an unrecognized, noncardiac cause of chest pain.

A brief vascular examination must be included. The carotid and peripheral vascular examinations are useful in establishing the extent of extracardiac vascular disease, the former also important to estimate cardiac output by the volume of carotid upstroke. The abdominal aorta deserves particular attention in the elderly patient and should be studied noninvasively if aneurysmal dilatation is suspected. The lost art of examination of the peripheral venous system may provide clues to left ventricular dysfunction.

The cardiac examination is important in patients with suspected anginal discomfort to evaluate left ventricular function, as well as to exclude valvular and subvalvular causes for such pain. Paradoxic precordial motion, right ventricular heave or thrust, and left ventricular enlargement are all important signs of left ventricular dysfunction. A fourth heart sound is not pathognomonic of coronary artery disease and may be found in normal individuals, but the development of a new presystolic sound may be of diagnostic significance when associated with chest discomfort. An S3 gallop occurring in concert with chest discomfort indicates significant ischemia-induced left ventricular dysfunction. Auscultation and associated diagnostic maneuvers should exclude aortic valve pathology as well as (dynamic) subvalvular stenosis. A murmur of mitral regurgitation may vary during an anginal episode, suggesting ischemia-induced papillary muscle dysfunction. Extracardiac diastolic-systolic murmurs suggest arteriovenous malformation, which may generate a high-output state sufficient to provoke myocardial ischemia.

LABORATORY TESTS

Easily obtained clinical laboratory studies often are overlooked in the evaluation of patients suspected of having coronary artery disease. Hemogloblin and thyroid function should be measured to determine possible exacerbating factors of chest pain, and serum cholesterol (including high density lipoprotein [HDL] and low density lipoprotein [LDL]) and fasting glucose measured in a search for risk factors of atherosclerosis. Renal function should be assessed to rule out comorbidities of coronary artery disease or end-organ damage due to prolonged hypertension.

NONINVASIVE EVALUATION

A supporting noninvasive evaluation is necessary not only to confirm a suspected clinical diagnosis of coronary artery disease but also to aid in risk stratification. The clinician has an ever increasing selection of noninvasive tests from which to choose, including the resting electrocardiogram, exercise testing with or without thallium or scotamibi scintigraphy, exercise radionuclide angiography and echocardiography, and Holter monitoring.

Resting Electrocardiography. Approximately one-half of patients with chronic stable coronary artery disease have normal electrocardiograms. A normal tracing does not predict the extent and severity of obstructive coronary artery disease. Pathologic Q waves are certainly the most specific marker of coronary artery disease and can be of further help in assessing the degree of left ventricular dysfunction, with Q waves in the anterior and inferior leads indicating extensive areas of left ventricular dyssynergy [111]. Electrocardiographic evidence of left ventricular hypertrophy in an individual with chronic stable angina should alert the clinician to the possibility of a valvular or hypertensive etiology of ischemia. Hypertrophic subaortic stenosis may be suspected, on the basis of the magnitude of QRS excursion and associated pseudoinfarction Q waves. In patients with clinical evidence of coronary artery disease, the presence of left bundle branch block is a marker of severe impairment of left ventricular function and carries an adverse prognosis [112]. Minor ST and T wave abnormalities on the resting electrocardiogram commonly are seen in patients with coronary artery disease but are not at all specific and must be interpreted in clinical context [113].

Exercise Electrocardiography. The accuracy of exercise testing in the diagnosis of coronary artery disease is highly variable, with reports of specificity ranging from 17 to 100 percent and sensitivity ranging from 23 to 100 percent. In accordance with Bayes' theorem, the positive predictive

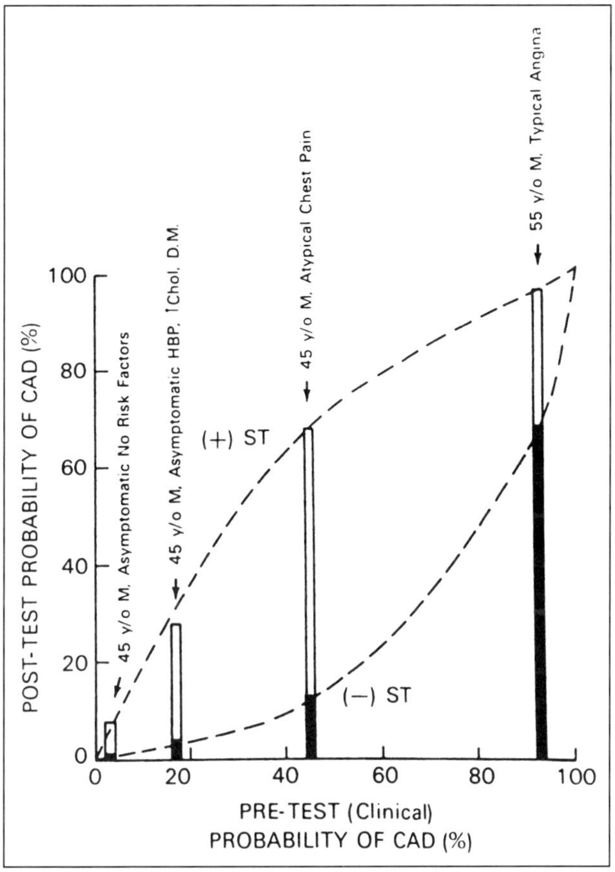

Fig. 34-8. Use of Bayes' theorem to calculate the probability of coronary artery disease from results of exercise testing. Although an exercise ECG positive for ST-segment depression always increased the probability of coronary disease, the posttest probability of coronary disease increased dramatically when the clinical history suggested a higher pretest probability of disease. (Reproduced with permission from R Patterson, S Horowitz. Importance of epidemiology and biostatistics in deciding clinical strategies for using diagnostic tests: a simplified approach using examples from coronary artery disease. J Am Coll Cardiol 1989; 13:1653.)

value of reversible ST-segment depression on exercise testing depends on the pretest probability of disease. Hence, in a population of patients with multiple risk factors for coronary artery disease or classic angina, an abnormal ST-segment response to exercise has a high predictive value. However, in patients not suspected of having coronary artery disease, for example, those undergoing evaluation for atypical chest pain, "diagnostic" ST-segment depression must be interpreted with caution (Fig. 34-8) [114,115]. Moreover, to maximize the sensitivity of this test, the subject must exercise to 85 percent or more of maximally predicted heart rate, which often is difficult for the elderly or the debilitated to achieve. The presence of typical anginal chest discomfort associated with the stress test in and of itself is highly predictive of ischemic heart disease [116]. It is quite helpful, however, to have confirmatory objective evidence of ischemia by ST-segment depression in evaluating a symptom complex of an individual patient. The classic positive ischemic response is horizontal or downsloping ST-segment depression occurring 0.08 second after the termination of the QRS complex. While 1 mm of ST-segment depression is the standard gauge of a "positive test," more severe degrees of ST-segment depression increase the specificity of the test for the diagnosis of coronary artery disease [117]. A combination of exercise variables such as time at onset of ST-segment depression, duration of ST-segment depression during recovery, number of leads involved, and severity of ST-segment depression can be combined to identify patients with severe coronary artery disease. For example, individuals who have ST-segment depression within the first 3 minutes of exercise, who have more than five leads with ST-segment depression, and who show greater than 8 minutes of ST-segment depression following termination of exercise should be suspected of having left main coronary artery disease or critical three-vessel disease [87].

In addition to the electrocardiographic response to exercise, the physiologic response is equally important in assessing severity of coronary disease. The failure to achieve 85 percent of the predicted maximal heart rate combined with ST-segment depression occurring at a low heart rate is an important predictor of severe coronary artery disease [118]. Exercise-induced hypotension or the failure to increase blood pressure by at least 20 mm Hg suggests that there is exercise-induced left ventricular dysfunction, and those outcomes are predictors of three-vessel disease, left main coronary artery disease, or substantial left ventricular damage [119].

The prognostic and diagnostic value of the exercise test may be limited by antianginal medication. Beta-adrenergic blocking therapy may limit exercise capacity, the patient stopping with fatigue before appropriate tachycardia, hypertension, and, hence, myocardial ischemia can be elicited [120]. The decision to continue or withdraw antianginal medication during stress electrocardiography should be determined by the indications for the test. If the stress test is intended to make the diagnosis of coronary artery disease, it probably should be performed after all antianginal medication has been withdrawn. A stress test performed in this fashion would provide the most useful diagnostic and prognostic information, and exercise-induced angina can be treated easily with sublingual nitroglycerin. If, however, the purpose of the test is to judge the efficacy of medical therapy or to guide in rehabilitation plans for the patient with known coronary artery disease, it should be performed with full medical therapy so as to define appropriate limitations of activity.

Thallium Scintigraphy. The addition of thallium-201 scintigraphy or other radionuclide imaging techniques, such as technicium sestamibi, to conventional exercise testing may increase the sensitivity and specificity of conventional stress electrocardiography [121, 122]. Hence, this test may be a useful diagnostic adjunct in many clinical situations, such as in patients whose resting electrocardiogram makes interpretation of ST-segment changes impossible or those with left bundle branch block [90]. In patients with atypical chest pain, the combination of a negative stress electrocardiogram and a negative stress thallium study nearly excludes significant coronary artery disease, and such patients have an excellent prognosis [123]. In patients with typical angina and negative exercise electrocardiography, reversible thallium perfusion defects with exercise select a subgroup with a much higher cardiac event rate than those without such defects [124]. As previously discussed, multiple global perfusion defects usually signify severe three-vessel coronary artery disease or left main stenosis, and the presence of pulmonary uptake or delayed tracer redistribution is indicative of extensive left ventricular dysfunction [91,92]. In patients unable to exercise, thallium imaging can be combined with pharmacologic stress with dipyridamole [125], adenosine [95,126] or dobutamine [96] to confirm the diagnosis of coronary artery disease.

Exercise Radionuclide Angiography and Echocardiography. Exercise radionuclide angiography and exercise echocardiography have emerged as sensitive and specific tests for the diagnosis of coronary artery disease [102,127–129]. In the past several years, there has been growing interest in exercise echocardiography because of the relative ease of imaging and the absence of radiation exposure. The addition of echocardiographic imaging to standard exercise testing may increase the sensitivity of the test without changing specificity in patients with suspected coronary disease [122]. The value of a negative exercise echocardiogram often is clinically useful as well: Even in patients with abnormal exercise electrocardiograms, a normal exercise echocardiogram carries an excellent long-term prognosis [130]. In patients unable to exercise, dobutamine echocardiography can be utilized as an alternative to dipyridamole-thallium imaging [131].

Ambulatory (Holter) Monitoring. Asymptomatic myocardial ischemia ("silent ischemia") has received much clinical attention in the past 5 years. Approximately 40 percent of all patients with otherwise stable coronary artery disease also display asymptomatic ischemia on ambulatory monitoring; in those patients, approximately 75 percent of all episodes of ambulatory ischemia are asymptomatic [132]. Despite the frequency with which ambulatory ischemia can be detected in patients with documented coronary artery disease, it is rare in patients with negative exercise electrocardiograms; hence, ambulatory monitoring cannot be recommended for the diagnosis of coronary artery disease [133]. Moreover, since it has not been proved that specific treatment of asymptomatic ischemia changes short- or long-term prognosis, screening patients with documented coronary disease with ambulatory monitoring is not justified at this time. As discussed earlier, the major utility of ambulatory monitoring may be to provide prognostic information in specific clinical situations, such as patients undergoing surgery for peripheral vascular disease [79–81].

Coronary Angiography. Although some might argue that cardiac catheterization with coronary angiography is the most direct method to define the presence and extent of coronary artery disease, it does not necessarily define the short- or long-term prognosis of an individual patient nor the physiologic significance of angiographic pathology. Although modern techniques have decreased the incidence of complications from the procedure, coronary angiography still carries a small risk of stroke, myocardial infarction, and death. Considerable research has led to advances in noninvasive assessment of coronary anatomy. For example, magnetic resonance techniques have advanced sufficiently that the proximal segments of major epicardial vessels can be imaged with reasonable accuracy [134]. Angiography remains the "gold-standard" imaging technique, but it must be limited to patients in whom the diagnosis of coronary disease remains a distinct possibility after a reasonable noninvasive evaluation or to patients in whom revascularization is contemplated.

The decision to refer a patient for angiography and possible revascularization must be considered with the realization that coronary artery disease is a chronic disease process, and revascularization procedures that have inherent morbidity and mortality are, at best, palliative. As discussed in more detail below, coronary angioplasty and the newer intracoronary devices used for revascularization suffer from a clinical recurrence rate of approximately 33 percent at the site of intervention, notwithstanding the rate of development of new lesions over time. Coronary surgery can be considered merely palliative as well, with a closure rate of saphenous vein grafts of approximately 5 percent per year. With growing concerns over health care resources, revascularization procedures, particularly repeat procedures, may become tightly regulated. Consequently, it is the responsibility of the clinician to refer patients with clear indications for planned procedures. Inasmuch as coronary artery disease is a chronic disease process, it may be as much an error to intervene prematurely as it is to delay appropriate therapy.

There are several clinical scenarios in which coronary angiography and revascularization clearly are indicated. For example, for the patient with unstable angina refractory to medical therapy, prompt cardiac catheterization clearly is justified since additional noninvasive tests may be dangerous and this clinical syndrome carries a high rate of cardiovascular events if not aggressively treated. Likewise, the patient who has suffered a non-Q wave myocardial infarction in the anterior distribution has a significant amount of myocardium at risk and a high rate of fatal or nonfatal reinfarction in the short term: Most cardiologists would refer such a patient to angiography and revascularization. Since abnormal left ventricular function portends a poor prognosis, patients with exertional angina and an ejection fraction between 25 and 40 percent should undergo coronary angiography to define the extent of vascular pathology, and those with three-vessel disease or left main stenosis should be considered for bypass surgery. Stable-angina patients with preserved left ventricular function and noninvasive testing that suggests the presence of severe coronary disease also deserve angiography to identify the subset who might enjoy a survival benefit from bypass surgery. Finally, patients with severe angina that is poorly controlled with medical therapy and that is life-style limiting should be considered for revascularization to facilitate a return to productivity. In summary, coronary angiography should be considered in patients with documented chronic ischemic heart disease only when a change in the therapeutic plan is contemplated.

Management of Coronary Artery Disease

The management of patients with coronary artery disease has two primary goals: to prolong life and to improve the quality of life. To prolong life, an attempt should be made to identify patients at high risk who may derive a survival benefit from surgical revascularization. Medical therapy should be instituted promptly, with special consideration of aspirin, beta blockers, and angiotensin converting enzyme (ACE) inhibitors; aspirin is effective in primary and secondary prevention of myocardial infarction, and beta blockers and ACE inhibitors are effective in prolonging survival after myocardial infarction in certain patient populations. In an effort to improve quality of life, attention should be directed toward relieving symptoms of coronary artery disease, with possible therapeutic options, including life-style modification, the use of antianginal medication, and coronary revascularization.

The management of ischemic heart disease begins with a thorough discussion with the patient of the disease process and the precipitating factors of ischemia during daily life. Potential modifications of life-style should be explicitly addressed, particularly smoking cessation [135], weight loss [136], and adherence to an exercise program [137,138]. In that context, patient performance on stress testing emerges as a particularly useful objective guideline for both the physician and the patient, since the heart rate at which ischemia is induced with supervised exercise on medical therapy can be related to normal daily activities. Patients should be advised to eat smaller meals and to avoid sudden bursts of physical activity and sudden exposure to cold. The prophylactic use of nitroglycerin before activities that involve a sudden increase in myocardial oxygen demand may dramatically improve the lifestyle of an individual patient.

Research in the last decade suggests that modification of serum lipids with intensive medical therapy can lead to regression of atherosclerosis and a decline in the incidence of cardiovascular morbidity and mortality. Considerable evidence points to the development of atherosclerotic lesions early in life [139], and those observations have led to treatment strategies aimed at modifying lipids in higher-risk asymptomatic populations. Data from the Helsinki Heart Study suggested that the modification of lipids with gemfibrozil in middle-aged, asymptomatic, dyslipidemic men led to a 34-percent reduction in coronary endpoints [140]. In a landmark study, Brown and coworkers showed that in men with elevated apolipoprotein B levels and a family history of coronary artery disease, lipid lowering with combination therapy with lovastatin and niacin or clofibrate resulted in less angiographic progression and more regression than the conventional therapy group. Moreover, clinical events (death, myocardial infarction, coronary revascularization) oc-

Table 34-2. Determinants of myocardial oxygen consumption

Major determinants
Myocardial-wall stress Contractile state of the myocardium Heart rate
Minor determinants
Maintenance of cell viability in the basal state Depolarization Activation Maintenance of the active state Direct metabolic effect of catecholamines Fatty acid uptake

Source: Adapted from E Braunwald et al. Coronary Blood Flow and Myocardial Ischemia. In E Braunwald ed. Heart Disease. Philadelphia: Saunders, 1988. Pp. 1191–1222.

Table 34-3. Antianginal mechanisms of nitroglycerin

Decreased myocardial oxygen requirements
Venous vasodilatation with decreased preload (low doses) Arterial vasodilatation with decreased afterload (higher doses)
Increased myocardial oxygen supply (coronary artery vasodilatation)
Relief of coronary-artery spasm Decreased normal physiologic coronary tone Dilatation of coronary-artery collateral vessels

curred in 19 percent of the conventional therapy group compared with 5 percent of those who received more aggressive therapy [40]. Ample evidence points to the benefits of lipid lowering as secondary prevention: In survivors of myocardial infarction, a 10-percent reduction in serum cholesterol is associated with an approximate 12-percent reduction in fatal myocardial reinfarction and a 19-percent reduction in nonfatal reinfarction [141]. The results of these and other studies have led to the recent recommendation that serum LDL levels be lowered to less than 100 mg/dl in patients with established coronary artery disease [142].

Medical Therapy of Coronary Artery Disease

The pathogenic mechanisms of myocardial ischemia and the transition from chronic, stable coronary artery disease to acute coronary syndromes involve a complex interplay among the fixed atherosclerotic plaque, intermittent thrombosis with complete obstruction of coronary blood flow, coronary artery vasomotion with episodic reductions in myocardial oxygen supply, and intimal hemorrhage that generates dynamic changes in the atherosclerotic lesion itself. If each of these pathogenic mechanisms is addressed therapeutically, there is reason to believe not only that the symptomatic status of the patient will improve but that the natural history of coronary artery disease may be altered, as well. It is important to remember that myocardial ischemia always results from an imbalance between myocardial oxygen demand and myocardial oxygen supply [143,144]. The determinants of myocardial oxygen demand are shown in Table 34-2. The minor determinants are of biochemical and physiologic importance, but they cannot be addressed by conventional therapeutic regimens and thus are not discussed here further. The major determinants of oxygen consumption—contractility, heart rate, and left ventricular wall stress—deserve brief description. Left ventricular wall stress, a variable describing the relationship among ventricular pressure, wall thickness, and chamber size, is the most important determinant of oxygen consumption [145]. By the LaPlace relationship, an increase in ventricular volume increases wall tension and, therefore, myocardial oxygen consumption. Heart rate is nearly as important a determinant of oxygen consumption; not only are oxygen requirements increased because of contraction frequency, but shortened diastolic periods reduce coronary blood flow. Changes in myocardial contractility are of less importance and more difficult to predict clinically, since they invariably are associated with changes in ventricular pressure and volume and, as a result, wall tension [145]. A useful framework for selecting medical therapy for coronary artery disease includes consideration of which determinants of myocardial oxygen demand are influenced by various therapeutic interventions.

NITRATE THERAPY

Nitroglycerin, the oldest form of treatment for anginal discomfort, remains the therapy of choice for an acute anginal attack. There is little evidence that nitrate administration prolongs survival in patients with chronic ischemic heart disease [146], and information regarding nitrate tolerance raises doubts about the role of nitrates in long-term prophylaxis of ischemia. However, little question remains that nitrates should be prescribed to all patients for treatment of episodic angina. Moreover, acute and chronic congestive heart failure are effectively treated with both sublingual nitroglycerin and long-acting nitrates via effects on venodilatation, which may be particularly advantageous for the patient with ischemia-induced mitral regurgitation or left ventricular dysfunction. Hence, nitrates continue to play a central role in the treatment of patients with coronary artery disease.

Pharmacologic Considerations. The combined venous and arterial vasodilator effect of nitrates accounts for the complexity of their antianginal effect (Table 34-3). At low plasma concentrations, nitrates are primarily venodilators, arterial vasodilatation becoming the primary pharmacologic effect at high plasma concentrations [147]. Systemic venous and arterial vasodilatation has a multiplicity of effects that act to improve the myocardial oxygen supply-demand ratio in patients with coronary artery disease. Systemic venodilatation leads to a reduction in left ventricular end-diastolic volume, reducing wall stress and myocardial oxygen consumption. The reduction in left ventricular end-diastolic volume is reflected in a reduction in end-diastolic pressure, leading to an increase in coronary blood flow to the subendocardium. Under certain physiologic conditions, reduced venous return may lower cardiac output and reduce blood pressure and, therefore, wall stress and myocardial oxygen consumption [147,148]. Systemic arterial vasodilatation at the arterial and arteriolar levels generates a reduction in systemic blood pressure and myocardial oxygen consumption. At high doses, nitrates may have a substantial effect on the coronary artery conductance vessels [149]. Ischemia may be reduced by relief of inappropriate coronary artery spasm, reduction of normal physiologic tone in the coronaries, dilation of coronary artery collaterals [150,151], or direct inhibition of platelet function [152,153]. The magnitude of the vasodilator response in venous, arterial, and coronary circulations depends on the dose given, with maximum pharmacologic response at high doses and with acute, rather than chronic, drug administration. Routes of administration include sublingual tablets or an oral aerosol spray. When nitrates are initially prescribed, the patient should be carefully instructed in their use and warned of potential hypotension, perhaps receiving the first dose under physician supervision. Moreover, the patient should be instructed to limit use to three or four tablets or sprays, each separated by 5 minutes, in an attempt to relieve discomfort before reporting to an emergency room, to exclude myocardial infarction. Patients need to be carefully counseled on the shelf life of nitroglycerin, replacing it every 6 months. Patients who have predictable effort-induced angina should be encouraged to use short-acting nitrates prophylactically, using either the spray or the sublingual tablet immediately prior to engaging in activity known to provoke anginal discomfort.

Many studies have shown long-acting nitrates to be effective therapy for the prevention of exertional anginal discomfort. Sublingual nitrate consumption is reduced, anginal frequency lessened, and overall exercise capacity improved with oral, buccal, and topical nitrates. If long-acting nitrate preparations are chosen as a primary antianginal therapy, a common clinical mistake is lack of adequate dosage. Low or moderate dosage is often employed, with little subsequent pharmacologic effect. The dosage should be increased carefully, noting variability in patient sensitivity. An arbitrary dosage regimen, universally applied, is of limited clinical value [147]. Clinical data suggest that nitrates administered 4 times daily are associated with the development of tolerance, although not when given 2 to 3 times daily with at least one 12-hour nitrate-free period daily [154].

Individual Nitrate Preparations. Sublingual nitroglycerin tablets are available in four dosages, ranging from 0.15 to 0.60 mg. Relief of exertional discomfort usually is achieved within 4 minutes of administration, as the venous and arterial vasodilating effects become apparent. The aerosol spray delivers a metered dose of 0.4 mg (200 doses per canister); in this preparation, nitroglycerin retains its potency for at least 3 years.

Sublingual isosorbide dinitrate is quite effective in relieving individual episodes of exertional discomfort but is not nearly as rapid as sublingual nitroglycerin or nitroglycerin spray in its pharmacologic effect. The usual dose is 2.5 to 5.0 mg, and 10 mg is feasible if hypotension is not provoked at lower dosage. The side-effect profile is similar to that of sublingual nitroglycerin, the medication often provoking dizziness, headache, or throbbing; and sublingual isosorbide dinitrate preparation is stable [155].

Buccal or transmucosal nitroglycerin administers nitroglycerin in an inert methylcellulose polymer matrix. Placed between the upper teeth and lip, it releases nitroglycerin into the capillary bed rapidly, generating prompt hemodynamic effects and symptomatic relief. Because a gel quickly forms around the tablet, keeping it in place, this route of administration also provides a sustained release of nitroglycerin for as long as the tablet remains in contact with the buccal mucosa. Dissolution may not occur for up to 6 hours [156].

A number of oral nitrate preparations are available, including those with sustained release. Such formulations are usually effective if sufficient dosage is prescribed. It should be reemphasized that oral dosing 2 to 3 times a day with meals usually is optimal for most patients with classic exertional discomfort. Moreover, the sustained-release preparation is usually associated with lower peak plasma concentrations than the same dosage of medication in the standard oral formulation. Although adequate dosage must be prescribed to relieve angina, the smallest effective dosage always should be used in the hope that nitrate tolerance can be avoided [155]. Recently, isosorbide mononitrate, the major active metabolite of isosorbide dinitrate, has been released for clinical use. Unfortunately, this compound also suffers from problems of nitrate tolerance and must be dosed with a nitrate-free interval.

The transcutaneous nitroglycerin ointment formulations are effective antianginal medications but often are logistically difficult to use. The ointment often is an excellent formulation for the hospitalized patient. Transdermal nitroglycerin disks have been well received by patients and physicians, but there continues to be concern about the efficacy of this particular formulation: It has been difficult to demonstrate that large doses do, indeed, have a sustained 24-hour antianginal effect, and the commonly used lower doses probably are not effective at all [157].

Intravenous nitroglycerin is the most effective formulation of nitrates for the hospitalized patient with unstable angina. By beginning with an infusion of 10 to 20 μg/minute and increasing the dose by the same amount every 10 to 15 minutes, chest pain usually can be controlled. A decline in blood pressure is usually not abrupt or precipitous, with adequate time available to readjust dosage. At higher dosages, intravenous nitroglycerin often is associated with a reflex tachycardia, which can be abolished with the concomitant use of beta-blocker therapy. Once the patient is stabilized, oral nitrates can be administered as the intravenous infusion is tapered off.

Nitrate Side Effects. The primary side effects of nitrate administration are related to its vasodilatory actions, including dizziness, near-syncope or syncope, nausea, and headache. Headaches are particularly common in patients with a history of migraine, and they may be so severe in some patients as to require either chronic acetaminophen administration or discontinuation of the medication. With

Table 34-4. Beta-adrenergic blocking agents available in the United States

Nonselective agents
Propranolol
Timolol
Nadolol
Perbutolol
Selective agents
Atenolol
Metoprolol
Betaxolol
Agents with intrinsic sympathomimetic activity
Pindolol
Acebutolol
Carteolol
Ultra-short-acting agent
Esmolol
Agent with additional alpha-adrenergic blocking effects
Labetolol
Agent with significant membrane-stabilizing effects
Sotalol*

*Investigational.

chronic nitrate therapy, however, most side effects disappear or become well tolerated.

BETA-ADRENERGIC BLOCKING THERAPY

If nitroglycerin is the mainstay of therapy for acute episodes of exertional anginal discomfort, beta-adrenergic blocking agents have emerged as the cornerstone of therapy for chronic coronary artery disease. These agents act as competitive inhibitors of circulating catecholamines at the beta-adrenergic receptor. The number of beta receptors is in a constant state of flux [158,159], which leads to alterations in tissue sensitivity to drug action. With chronic administration of beta-adrenergic receptor antagonists, the density of beta receptors increases, leading to potential catecholamine hypersensitivity when beta blockers are withdrawn. Consequently, abrupt discontinuation may exacerbate myocardial ischemia [158]. The number of beta receptors also varies with different clinical states. For example, the number of adrenergic binding sites increases with hyperthyroidism, and the converse occurs with hypothyroidism. Acute alcohol withdrawal also may increase beta-adrenergic receptors. The concentration of beta receptors may decrease with age, perhaps explaining progressive insensitivity to beta blockade [159]. Beta-adrenergic-receptor density is also reduced in patients with chronic congestive heart failure, perhaps owing to prolonged exposure to high circulating-catecholamine levels [160,161].

Pharmacologic Considerations. Many beta-adrenergic blocking agents are available for clinical usage (Table 34-4). There are four major differences among these agents: variation in the degree of selectivity between the beta-1 and beta-2 receptors, variations in intrinsic sympathomimetic activity, differences in the ancillary pharmacologic properties of the various agents, and major differences in pharmacokinetics.

Beta-1 and Beta-2 Selectivity. Beta-adrenergic blocking agents are considered nonselective or selective, depending on their relative potency as beta-1 and beta-2 receptor antagonists at low dosage. In higher dosages, the "selective" beta blockers produce general beta-adrenergic blockade of both types of beta receptors [162,163]. Selective beta-1 blocking agents block increases in heart rate, AV nodal conduction, and myocardial contractility; in noncardiac tissue, they prevent the release of renin from juxtaglomerular cells and inhibit lipolysis. Selective beta-1 agents in low dosages have minimal impact on bronchial and peripheral vascular beta-2 adrenergic receptors. Any cardioselective effect of these agents is reduced as dosage is increased, and many patients on moderate to high doses of selective beta blockers experience side effects similar to those of nonselective beta-blocking agents [162]. Hence, when patients with reactive airway disease are prescribed selective beta-adrenergic blocking agents, the lowest effective dosage should be used.

Intrinsic Sympathomimetic Activity. When beta-adrenergic blocking agents with intrinsic sympathomimetic activity bind to the beta receptor, a small degree of activation is induced while the receptor is blocked from more powerful beta-agonists; hence, these agents are termed **partial agonists** [164]. The stimulating effects of these particular agents are far less than those of epinephrine or isoproterenol. The net effect of these agents on resting heart rate, contractility, or blood pressure is minimal, but the catecholamine-driven increases in myocardial oxygen consumption occurring with exercise are substantially blocked. In the treatment of chronic coronary artery disease, however, it is unclear whether this particular pharmacologic property is advantageous. In survivors of myocardial infarction, these agents may not be as effective at secondary prevention as agents without intrinsic sympathomimetic activity [165–170].

Ancillary Pharmacologic Properties. At high dosage, certain beta-adrenergic blocking agents display a quinidinelike effect, reducing the spontaneous depolarization of cardiac muscle. For the conventional agents, this membrane-stabilizing effect is not acknowledged to be of clinical importance. Sotalol, a newly released agent, has potent class II antiarrhythmic properties and plays a unique role in the therapy of ventricular and supraventricular arrhythmias. Labetalol has additional alpha-adrenergic blocking activity, with resultant reduction in systemic vascular resistance and concomitant slowing of the heart rate through beta-adrenergic blockade, and is a useful agent in the treatment of severe hypertension [171].

Pharmacokinetics. One of the most important differences in the various beta-adrenergic blocking agents is in their pharmacokinetic properties. Various aromatic-ring structures alter the water lipid partition coefficient of the agents, accounting for marked differences in gastrointestinal absorption, lipid solubility, protein binding, body distribution, and CNS penetration [172,173]. In addition, differences in hepatic metabolism and renal clearance also account for great pharmacologic variability. Propranolol and metoprolol, which are primarily lipid soluble, are metabolized by the liver with relatively short plasma half-lives and variable bioavailability. Beta blockers that are more water soluble, such as atenolol, are slowly absorbed through the gut and eliminated unchanged by the kidney. Because plasma half-life is longer, the water-soluble beta-blockers often can be administered once a day, which may substantially improve patient compliance [174]. Esmolol is an ultra-short-acting beta blocker with an effective half-life of only a few minutes owing to its rapid metabolism by hepatic esterases; consequently, this agent enjoys a unique clinical niche as a continuous, titratable intravenous infusion in patients who may be at risk for beta-blocker side effects [175].

Despite the pharmacologic differences among them, most of the beta-adrenergic blocking agents have similar therapeutic efficacy in the treatment of chronic ischemic heart disease and can be considered the same generic group of drugs. If one beta blocker in adequate dosage is unsuccessful in controlling symptoms of myocardial ischemia, the substitution of a second beta blocker likely will be unsuccessful, as well [173]. The side effects may vary slightly from one agent to another, but there is substantial interpatient variability. The more serious side effects, including bronchospasm and acute left ventricular dysfunction, can be seen with any of the beta-blocking agents, including the beta-1 selective agents.

Antianginal Effects. The beta-adrenergic blocking agents protect the potentially ischemic myocardium from sudden increases in myocardial oxygen demand imposed by increases in catecholamines. Their primary impact on the determinants of myocardial oxygen consumption is to blunt increases in heart rate, contractility, and blood pressure due to exercise. Because of a lower heart rate and prolonged diastolic filling time, there may be an increase in left ventricular volume, but this has minimal impact on left ventricular wall stress in patients without resting left ventricular dysfunction. Contractility is minimally reduced in the resting state, but the increase in contractility with exercise is substantially blunted. Reduction in heart rate and blood pressure may significantly limit the necessary increases in cardiac output with exercise; hence, symptoms of fatigue and reduced exercise capacity in patients taking beta blockers may be due to fixed cardiac output rather than CNS side effects [174].

The patient with left ventricular decompensation can have exacerbation of anginal symptoms with beta-adrenergic blockade. Slowing the heart rate may increase left ventricular volume and pressure, with a corresponding increase in left ventricular wall stress. Increases in left ventricular end-diastolic pressure also may compromise subendocardial coronary artery perfusion. Thus, any potential benefit from beta-blocking agents in reducing heart rate is negated by their deleterious impact on left ventricular wall stress. It is for these reasons that beta-adrenergic blocking agents should be avoided in patients with unstable angina and left ventricular dysfunction until the ventricular dysfunction has been addressed by other therapeutic maneuvers.

Beta-adrenergic blocking agents also may have modest impact on the other pathogenic mechanisms of transient myocardial ischemia. It has been hypothesized that beta-adrenergic blocking agents may improve myocardial oxygen supply by increasing blood flow and prolonging the time for coronary flow during diastole [176], but this is probably of minimal clinical relevance. Beta-adrenergic blocking agents do have the potential for reducing coronary artery blood flow [14], particularly in patients whose primary pathogenic mechanism of ischemia is coronary artery spasm [177]. Although the pathogenic mechanism of this clinical observation is unclear, it has been suggested that nonspecific blockade of beta-2 receptors may leave coronary artery vasoconstriction unopposed [177]; such patients with coronary spasm are best treated with calcium-channel blocking agents [178].

Beta-adrenergic blocking therapy also may affect platelet activation and thrombus formation. There is in-vitro evidence to suggest that propranolol inhibits platelet aggregation [179]. Patients with coronary artery disease have been reported to have enhanced platelet aggregability that is normalized with propranolol administration [180]. The mechanism of this phenomenon is unknown, since only alpha-adrenergic receptors are found on platelet membranes. Moreover, not all beta blockers have antiplatelet effects [179], yet they have been shown to be equally effective in controlling symptoms of myocardial ischemia. Hence, the role of beta-adrenergic blocking agents in addressing the thrombotic component of transient ischemia remains to be further elucidated. One final property of beta-adrenergic blocking agents worth mentioning is their undesirable effects on serum lipids. These agents lower HDL while raising serum triglycerides and, thus, may accelerate the process of atherosclerosis [181]. Despite this theoretical disadvantage, a wealth of clinical data supports the routine use of this class of agents in patients with coronary artery disease, particularly in patients recovering from myocardial infarction.

Impact on Natural History of Coronary Artery Disease. To date, approximately 55 trials have investigated beta-adrenergic blockers in myocardial infarction, and pooled results suggest a 25-percent reduction in long-term mortality, with a similar reduction in nonfatal reinfarction [168–170,182–184]. The beneficial effects of beta blockade after infarction are detectable by the first 7 days [185] and are maintained for as long as 6 years after infarction [186]. There has been no prospective, direct comparison between placebo and beta blocker restricted to patients with non-Q wave infarction, but in the absence of contraindications, it is reasonable to utilize these medications for their proven benefit for preventing reinfarction. The early benefit of these agents following infarction may be to decrease cardiac rupture [187], while late benefit likely is due to preventing ventricular fibrillation. In addition to the proven benefit in patients recovering from myocardial infarction, there is also evidence that beta blockers may be effective in the primary prevention of myocardial infarction and cardiac death among patients with hypertension [188]. It has been suggested that beta-adrenergic blocking therapy accounts for approximately 18 to 20 percent of the overall 30-percent decline in mortality seen in the last two decades [54]. This contribution is probably greater than any other single form of therapy in reducing the mortality of established coronary artery disease.

Side Effects. The adverse side effects of beta-adrenergic blocking agents are related primarily to blockade of the beta receptor in selected organ systems: bronchoconstriction, symptoms of congestive heart failure, depression, psychosis, sexual dysfunction, and hypoglycemia [163]. Limited cardiac output with exercise may be responsible for lethargy and fatigue. Atrioventricular (AV) nodal block may be intensified. Claudication may be exacerbated, although a recent meta-analysis suggests that these agents do not adversely affect walking capacity or symptoms of claudication in patients with mild to moderate peripheral arterial disease [189]. No matter what the pharmacologic properties of a beta-blocking agent, be it cardioselective or with favorable pharmacokinetics, no such agent is free of all side effects. Thus, it is reasonable to suggest to the clinician that two or three beta-adrenergic blocking agents be chosen for routine use, based primarily on clinical experience and familiarity.

CALCIUM-CHANNEL ANTAGONIST THERAPY

The addition of calcium-channel blocking therapy to the treatment of chronic ischemic heart disease in the 1980s has had substantial impact on the therapy of myocardial ischemia, although probably little impact on the natural history of the disease. These agents all act as coronary vasodilators, but have varying effects on peripheral vascular tone and AV nodal conduction. Excitation and contraction of cardiac and vascular smooth muscle are intricately related to the regulation of intracellular calcium, which in turn is regulated by calcium channels. By altering calcium influx into the cell, the calcium-channel antagonists overall are associated with a reduction in the inotropic state of the myocardium, reduced spontaneous depolarization of the sinus and AV nodes, and vasodilation of the systemic, pulmonary, and coronary arteries. In contrast to nitrates, calcium-channel blocking agents have minimal venous vasodilatory effects. There is marked variation in the structure of the calcium-channel blocking agents, which may partially explain their different pharmacologic effects. Diltiazem and verapamil slow sinus-node depolarization and increase AV-nodal refractoriness but have little effect on peripheral vascular resistance. In contrast, nifedipine and the calcium-channel blocking agents of the dihydropyridine group are potent arterial vasodilators [190], with little or no effect on sinus or AV-nodal function. Two newer dihydropyridine preparations, extended-release nifedipine and amlodipine, are longer acting but do not induce reflex tachycardia characteristic of other agents in this group (Table 34-5). The lack of reflex tachycardia may explain why these agents are more effective anti-ischemic agents when prescribed as monotherapy [191]. Amlodipine is the most promising of the new dihydropyridine derivatives, because it can be given once daily, has minimal variation in blood levels, does not induce reflex tachycardia, and is the only calcium-channel antagonist without negative inotropic effects [192]. In summary, there are important differences in the pharmacology of the various calcium-channel antagonists; unlike the beta-adrenergic blocking agents, it never should be assumed that calcium-channel antagonists are interchangeable.

Table 34-5. Calcium-channel antagonists of the dihydropyridine class

Nifedipine
Nifedipine extended release[a,b]
Nicardipine
Nicardipine hydrochloride (sustained release)
Isradipine[c]
Amlodipine[a,b,d]
Felodipine[c]

[a] No reflex tachycardia.
[b] Once-daily dosing.
[c] Not currently approved for angina.
[d] No significant negative inotropic effects.

Side Effects. The adverse effects of the calcium-channel blocking agents are related primarily to their pharmacologic effect. As a potent peripheral vasodilator, nifedipine is associated with lightheadedness, dizziness, and headache. Peripheral edema occasionally can require discontinuation of the drug. Side effects with long-acting nifedipine preparations seem to be less frequent than with the conventional agent, because early peaking of blood levels is avoided. Diltiazem has minimal side effects in low dosage, developing a similar side effect profile to nifedipine when given in dosages above 360 mg per day. However, its negative chronotropic effect may be exacerbated by combined administration with beta-adrenergic blocking agents. Verapamil's hypotensive side effects resemble those of nifedipine and diltiazem, often also causing constipation or nausea. The side effects of all the agents are dosage related, and modification of dosage is usually successful in controlling them.

Impact on Natural History of Coronary Artery Disease. There has been a great deal of investigation of the various calcium-channel antagonists in attempts to show survival benefit in postinfarction patients prescribed these agents. Verapamil has proved to be of marginal benefit for this purpose in a large study considering the combined end-point of death or nonfatal reinfarction. While there was initial enthusiasm regarding the use of diltiazem in secondary prevention [193], long-term studies have not demonstrated long-term survival benefits [194]. Several studies have shown no benefit or frank adverse outcomes from routine administration of nifedipine to postinfarction patients [195–197]. Hence, while these agents are effective antianginals, they probably do not alter the natural history of coronary artery disease.

Combination Therapy with Beta-Adrenergic Blocking Agents. The addition of a calcium-channel antagonist to beta-adrenergic blockade reduces myocardial oxygen consumption more effectively than either agent alone; these agents routinely are used in combination in the management of patients with chronic ischemic heart disease. Several studies have demonstrated the beneficial effect of nifedipine when added to beta-adrenergic blocking therapy in controlling stable angina, with parallel improvement in performance on exercise tests [191,198,199]. The combination usually is well tolerated, because nifedipine has little effect on heart rate and beta blockers have little effect on peripheral vascular resistance. By gradually increasing dosages of one or the other medication, blood pressure and heart rate can be regulated to decrease myocardial oxygen consumption without the side effects sometimes seen when either medication is given in large dosages. With the newer longer-acting formulations, satisfactory anginal control may be achieved for many patients with once-a-day doses of each medication, for example, 50–100 mg of atenolol and 60–90 mg of long-acting nifedipine taken upon waking. In patients with severe left ventricular dysfunction, caution must be advised when combining the negative inotropic effect of calcium-channel blocking agents with the negative inotropic effect of beta-adrenergic blocking therapy.

Diltiazem also is often used in combination with beta-adrenergic blocking agents for control of angina, but caution must be advised, owing to the negative chronotropic effects of both drugs. To avoid the well-described adverse effects of excessive sinus bradycardia, sinus arrest, or AV block [200,201], these agents should be introduced at low dosages and patients monitored frequently. Despite the negative inotropic effects of both agents, in selected patients with normal left ventricular function, verapamil can be safely added to beta-blocker therapy to control exertional angina, with improvement in exercise duration [202]. However, since verapamil has even more negative chronotropic effects than diltiazem, extreme caution must be advised when prescribing verapamil in combination with beta blockers, since profound bradycardia, often refractory to atropine or isoproterenol infusion, may ensue [203,204].

ANTIPLATELET AND ANTICOAGULANT THERAPY

As discussed earlier, thrombus formation on the surface of disrupted atherosclerotic plaques may be the most important pathophysiologic mechanism by which stable coronary artery disease is transformed to unstable angina, acute myocardial infarction, or sudden cardiac death. Antiplatelet therapy with aspirin has been shown to decrease the incidence of those cardiovascular endpoints when prescribed as either primary [38] or secondary [205–211] prevention. The antiplatelet agent ticlopidine, which interferes with adenosine diphosphate (ADP)–mediated platelet activation as well as with the platelet fibrinogen receptor, decreases cardiovascular events when added to conventional therapy for unstable angina [212]. Beta-adrenergic blockers [179], calcium-channel antagonists [213], and nitrates [214] all have antiplatelet activity of unknown clinical relevance. It is possible that the beneficial effect on mortality seen with beta blockers may be mediated to some extent by this antiplatelet effect. Oral anticoagulation with warfarin sodium has been shown to be effective as secondary prevention when given to postinfarction patients [215,216], but it probably is no better than aspirin and is associated with more bleeding complications [216]. Intravenous heparin is effective in the treatment of unstable angina [217] and is necessary adjunctive therapy in patients receiving thrombolytic therapy [218]. Of all the agents with antiplatelet or anticoagulant effects, it has been aspirin therapy that has substantially altered the natural history of coronary artery disease.

At low dosages, aspirin inhibits platelet cyclooxygenase by irreversibly acetylating the enzyme, thus inhibiting thromboxane A_2 formation and platelet aggregation. For platelet function to normalize, new platelets must be produced by the bone marrow. At higher doses, aspirin also inhibits endothelial-cell cyclo-oxygenase. Endothelial-cell cyclo-oxygenase activity normally leads to prostacyclin production, which is a potent inhibitor of platelet function. Thus, low dosages of aspirin (80–325 mg/day) are commonly used in patients with coronary artery disease for the theoretical purpose of selectively inhibiting thromboxane A_2 production. As demonstrated by the aspirin arm of the Physician's Health study, when given to healthy male physicians, aspirin reduced the incidence of myocardial infarction by 44 percent compared with placebo. Of note, these effects were apparent only in physicians 50 years of age or older. In addition, there was a small but significant increase in cerebral hemorrhage and peptic ulcer disease in the group of patients treated with aspirin [38]. Hence, in the absence of contraindications, particularly in patients with risk factors for atherosclerosis, aspirin should be prescribed to most patients aged at least 50 years for primary prevention.

Aspirin is also of proven benefit in patients with unstable angina or acute myocardial infarction. When given to patients presenting with unstable angina, aspirin decreases the incidence of myocardial infarction by 75 percent during the first week of therapy [219]. The Veterans Administration Cooperative Study showed that unstable angina patients who received 324 mg/day aspirin had a 51-percent reduction in death or nonfatal infarction after 12 weeks of therapy compared with placebo-treated patients [220]. Finally, in the Canadian Multicenter Trial, patients were treated for up to 2 years after presentation with unstable angina with aspirin or placebo, and there was a 51-percent reduction in death or nonfatal infarction [221]. The role of aspirin in the routine therapy of acute myocardial infarction was proven by the ISIS 2 Trial, which showed that aspirin therapy alone was as effective as streptokinase in reducing 35-day mortality from suspected acute myocardial infarction [222].

At least seven different trials have investigated the use of aspirin or aspirin with dipyridamole as secondary treatment for myocardial infarction [205–211]. Although none of these trials individually showed a significant reduction in mortality, when data were pooled using the technique of meta-analysis, aspirin therapy was associated with a 13-percent reduction in cardiovascular mortality and a 31-percent reduction in nonfatal reinfarction. The follow-up of these seven trials ranged from 9 to 36 months [223].

OTHER TREATMENT AGENTS

Intravenous thrombolytic agents have become the standard of care for patients presenting early in the course of acute myocardial infarction, and these agents are discussed elsewhere [224]. Bepridil, a newer calcium-channel antagonist with type I antiarrhythmic properties, has been shown to be an effective antianginal agent, although exacerbation of ventricular arrhythmia occurs in approximately 1 percent of patients due to effects on ventricular repolarization [225]. Theophylline has been shown to display a significant antianginal effect, perhaps by redistribution of blood flow from nonischemic to ischemic myocardium [226–228]. The ACE inhibitor captopril has been shown to decrease significantly recurrent myocardial infarction, hospitalizations for congestive heart failure, and total mortality when prescribed after moderate-sized anterior infarctions to patients without symptomatic heart failure or severe angina.

PERCUTANEOUS TRANSLUMINAL CORONARY ANGIOPLASTY AND NEWER INTRACORONARY DEVICES

In the past few years, the field of interventional cardiology has burgeoned, with increasing numbers of procedures performed and several previously investigational devices released for general use. Conventional percutaneous transluminal coronary angioplasty (PTCA) remains the catheter-based procedure of choice for the majority of patients, while the new technologies occupy specific clinical niches. Directional coronary atherectomy (DCA) involves removal of atheromatous plaque with a rotational cutting tool and has a role in eccentric stenoses, aorto-ostial stenoses, lesions in saphenous vein grafts, and perhaps lesions in the proximal left anterior descending coronary artery [229–231]. Excimer laser–facilitated angioplasty is useful in the dilation of long stenoses, and perhaps in aorto-ostial lesions, as well [232]. Intracoronary stents have been released by the Food and Drug Administration (FDA) for use with abrupt vessel closure after conventional angioplasty and may significantly reduce the need for emergency bypass surgery [233]. In addition to these new devices, balloon and wire technology continues to evolve, allowing more complex stenoses to be approached with conventional balloon angioplasty. With yet more new devices due to be released by the FDA, clinicians must struggle with how to incorporate the new technologies into their practice of cardiology. The situation is somewhat analogous to the confusion regarding indications for bypass surgery before the results of the major randomized trials of medical versus surgical therapy became available in the mid-1980s. It is clear that catheter-based revascularization procedures have a role in the treatment of patients with coronary artery disease, but until these procedures are adequately evaluated in clinical trials, good clinical judgment must guide their application.

When PTCA or a newer intracoronary device to be used for revascularization is being considered, the critical question is not which technique to use but whether any technique should be used for an individual patient. There is yet to be a clinical trial to demonstrate a survival benefit from angioplasty in any patient population. However, the results of several clinical trials may help select patients likely to benefit from these procedures. The Angioplasty Compared to Medicine (ACME) trial randomized patients with single- or double-vessel coronary artery disease to medical therapy versus angioplasty. At six months, patients in the angioplasty group had significantly less angina and improved performance on exercise testing. There was no difference in coronary events, although the trial did not enroll sufficient numbers to compare survival in the two groups [234]. Several trials are underway or have been recently completed comparing angioplasty to bypass surgery in patients with multivessel coronary artery disease [235]. Data from the Randomised Intervention Treatment of Angina (RITA) trial suggest that patients undergoing bypass surgery have less angina 6 months after revascularization compared with patients treated with initial angioplasty. At 2 years of follow-up, patients treated with angioplasty were more likely to have undergone repeat angioplasty, but there was no difference in the rate of death or myocardial infarction between the two groups [236]. Unpublished results of several other trials support the findings of the RITA investigators. Longer-term follow-up will be necessary to compare the two revascularization strategies adequately.

Several recent trials have demonstrated that PTCA is a highly effective alternative to thrombolytic therapy in patients presenting early in the course of acute myocardial infarction. Those trials show that angioplasty is highly effective at reestablishing normal flow in occluded arteries and that the patients have less recurrent ischemia than similar patients treated with thrombolytic agents [237–239]. PTCA also is highly effective in patients with unstable angina [240], a clinical presentation associated with a high rate of myocardial infarction in the ensuing months. There are no trials comparing medical therapy with PTCA in unstable angina, and there would likely be difficulty in recruiting patients for such a trial, since PTCA has become the standard of care in patients with one- or two-vessel coronary artery disease.

Indications for angioplasty and other catheter-based revascularization techniques in patients with stable angina are less clear. The American College of Cardiology and the American Heart Association recently have published guidelines outlining indications for angioplasty [241]. The guidelines are relatively broad, allowing the clinician significant options in recommending the procedure. While these procedures have become increasingly safe, there remains a significant rate of major complications, including myocardial infarction, emergency bypass surgery, and procedure-related death [241]. Estimates of major complications for single-vessel disease include approximately 3 percent of patients requiring emergency bypass surgery, overall infarction rate of 2 to 4 percent, and 0.1 to 1 percent procedural mortality [242,243]. The best centers report only slightly higher complication rates with multivessel angioplasty, with Q-wave infarction in 1.4 percent, urgent coronary bypass surgery in 1 percent, and death in 1 percent of patients [244]. The complications must be balanced against the severity of symptoms experienced by an individual patient, as well as side effects from antianginal medications. The characteristics of coronary stenoses provide additional information regarding the risk of major complication and acute success in the dilation of an individual stenosis and may aid the clinician's choice

Table 34-6. Characteristics of type A, B, and C lesions and the procedural risks and success rates of angioplasty

Type A lesions
High procedural success rate (> 85%), low procedural risk
Discrete (< 10 mm in length)
Concentric
Readily accessible
Nonangulated segment, < 45 degrees
Smooth contour
Little or no calcification
Less than totally occlusive
Not ostial in location
No major branch involvement
Absence of thrombus
Type B lesions
Moderate procedural success rate (60–85%), moderate procedural risk
Tubular (10–20 mm in length)
Eccentric
Moderate tortuosity of proximal segment
Irregular contour
Moderate to heavy calcification
Total occlusions < 3 months old
Ostial in location
Bifurcation lesions requiring double guidewires
Some thrombus present
Type C lesions
Low procedural success rate (< 60%), high procedural risk
Diffuse (> 2 cm in length)
Excessive tortuosity of proximal segment
Extremely angulated segments > 90 degrees
Total occlusion > 3 months old
Inability to protect major side branches
Degenerated vein grafts with friable lesions

Source: Adapted from T Ryan et al. Guideline for percutaneous transluminal coronary angioplasty. J Am Coll Cardiol 1988; 12:529.

of therapeutic strategy (Table 34-6). In addition, patient-related variables aid in estimation of procedural risk, with increased complications in females, the elderly, and patients with unstable angina, congestive heart failure, chronic renal failure, or diabetes [241]. In the end, the choice among catheter-based revascularization, medical therapy, and coronary bypass surgery must be individualized. Patient preference often aids in the decision, as does the relative skill of the interventional cardiologist or cardiac surgeon.

Restenosis continues to occur in approximately 30 to 40 percent of lesions treated with PTCA [245,246], and no clinically useful, patient-related variables have been consistently found to predict such an outcome [247]. Moreover, the initial hope that the use of directional coronary atherectomy [229–231, 248] or laser-facilitated angioplasty [232,249] may be associated with less restenosis has proven unfounded. The long-term restenosis rate for lesions treated with intracoronary stents is not yet determined. The utility of treatment of patients with omega-3 fatty acids to prevent restenosis is controversial [250–252], and no other medical therapy has been proved to inhibit the process. Restenosis following angioplasty probably is related directly to endothelial injury, with an associated exaggerated response to such injury in the subset of patients developing restenosis. Acutely, endothelial injury results in platelet aggregation and activation of macrophages. Later in the process, smooth muscle proliferation occurs in response to growth factors and chemoattractants [246]. It seems that no matter how the endothelium is damaged—be it by balloon injury, laser vaporization, or intracoronary removal of plaque by atherectomy—restenosis is a predictable outcome in at least one-third of patients. Repeat angioplasty can always be performed with a similar degree of primary success and low risk, but such a procedure serves to increase the overall morbidity and cost of this treatment approach.

For all those reasons, the role of angioplasty in the treatment of chronic ischemic heart disease still is in flux. Most clinicians would recommend PTCA to a young male with single-vessel coronary artery disease and persistent troublesome symptoms of angina despite reasonable medical therapy. On the other end of the spectrum, an older patient with multivessel disease and comorbidity, compromised left ventricular function, and angiographic markers of high procedural risk is not an ideal candidate for the procedure and should be considered for surgical or continued medical therapy. In the end, therapy must be individualized and the experience of the potential operator considered. Perhaps an ideal decision-making practice is to allow the invasive cardiologist to provide an estimation of procedural risk and potential success of PTCA for an individual patient with a particular stenosis, allowing the primary care cardiologist to make a more objective therapeutic recommendation based on the patient's symptomatic status and other treatment options.

CORONARY ARTERY BYPASS SURGERY

Surgical therapy for coronary artery disease has been available for almost four decades, now with over 400,000 procedures performed annually in the United States [1]. Pericardial irritation and internal mammary artery implantation into myocardium represented the earliest efforts at improving myocardial oxygen supply. It was not until the use of saphenous-vein bypass grafting by Favaloro in 1967 that surgical revascularization became an accepted therapy for coronary artery disease. At present, most surgeons utilize at least one internal mammary artery, usually placed to the left anterior descending coronary artery. The internal mammary artery approximates the diameter of the left anterior descending coronary artery, with a much higher patency rate than that of saphenous-vein grafts: 80 to 95 percent at 10 years [253]. Additional evidence suggests that 10-year survival may be improved in patients who receive internal mammary-artery grafting compared with those receiving conventional saphenous grafts [254]. As surgical techniques have been refined, the critical issue has progressed from "how" to "when or if" surgery should be performed. There is no question that surgical improvement in coronary-artery blood flow can relieve symptoms of angina, improve exercise capacity, and allow partial or full withdrawal of medical therapy [255]. Hence, bypass surgery provides an important therapeutic option for the patient who remains symptomatic from coronary artery disease despite aggressive medical therapy [256].

Despite symptomatic improvement enjoyed by most patients undergoing bypass surgery, the impact of surgical revascularization on longevity is limited to only a subset of patients, a fact that may become more important as social and political forces increasingly dictate allocation of finite resources [257]. Although mortality from this operation has declined, combined data from all types of centers suggest that in-hospital mortality ranges from 2–4 percent in university hospitals to over 6 percent in community hospitals [258]. In addition, there continues to be substantial periprocedural morbidity, with perioperative myocardial infarction in approximately 2–6 percent of all surgical revascularization patients [66,259,260]. Furthermore, nonfocal neurologic damage, manifested as confusion or reduced cognitive function, and cerebrovascular accidents occur frequently [260]. In addition, saphenous-vein grafts have a limited patency rate, with a substantial early occlusion rate of up to 20 percent in the first year after surgery and approximately 2–4 percent per year thereafter [261–263]. Consequently, the recommendation for surgical revascularization must be considered carefully, with particular weight given to possible survival benefit to be gained by an individual patient. It generally is agreed that coronary artery bypass surgery improves the long-term prognosis of patients with stenoses of the left main coronary artery of 50 percent or more. Patients with left main stenosis who undergo revascularization have a 5-year survival rate approximating 85 percent, compared to those receiving medical therapy whose 5-year survival is less than 50 percent [256,264]. The Veterans Administration (VA) Cooperative Study and the CASS concluded that surgical revascularization may have a substantial impact on the longevity of patients with left ventricular dysfunction and three-vessel coronary artery disease. The VA study noted a significant difference in longevity at 5, 7, and 11 years following randomization [265], and the CASS investigators reported survival benefit at 7 and 10 years after randomization [56,58]. In contrast, revascularization probably has minimal impact on the long-term survival of patients with chronic stable angina and single- or double-vessel coronary artery disease when left ventricular function is preserved [266–270], although controversy exists about possible improvement in survival of the subgroup of patients with two-vessel coronary artery disease and involvement of the proximal left anterior descending coronary artery [269,270].

There is some controversy regarding the impact of surgical therapy on longevity in patients with three-vessel coronary artery disease and preserved left ventricular function. The European Coronary Surgical Study concluded that in those with preserved left ventricular function, patients with three-vessel coronary artery disease had an improved survival rate with surgical therapy after 12 years [268,269,271]. The CASS addressed a different study population, almost 75 percent of whom had left ventricular ejection fraction less than 50 percent, and came to different conclusions: There was no improved survival for patients with normal left ventricular function and three-vessel coronary artery disease who received initial surgical intervention rather than medical intervention [66]. The conclusion of the CASS investigators is consistent with the findings of the VA Cooperative Study, a study often criticized for an unacceptably high surgical mortality rate of 5.8 percent [265].

Recent changes in medical management strategies are reason to reexamine the conclusions of the surgical trials in patients with stable angina. Aspirin therapy and beta blockers are routinely used in the medical regimens of nearly all angina patients. The Survival and Ventricular Enlargement (SAVE) study reported a 19-percent reduction in mortality and a 25-percent reduction in recurrent myocardial infarction in patients with moderate left ventricular dysfunction when the ACE inhibitor captopril was added to the medical regimen [272]. If such therapy had been administered to the medical cohort, the favorable benefit of surgery for left ventricular dysfunction noted in both the VA Cooperative Study and the CASS might not have been so marked. Given limitations of health care resources, comparison of more modern medical regimens and more advanced surgical techniques may be justified.

In patients with unstable angina and single- or double-vessel disease, there is no evidence that immediate surgical revascularization is better than initiating medical therapy. Although survival probably is improved with initial surgery in patients with triple-vessel disease, the patient population with most improved survival resulting from immediate revascularization are those with left ventricular dysfunction [55,59]. A reasonable approach to the patient with unstable angina is to initiate medical therapy with aspirin, heparin, nitrates, beta-adrenergic blocking therapy, and perhaps calcium-channel blocking therapy. The patient who continues to have unstable anginal pain despite reasonable medical therapy should be considered a candidate for revascularization with bypass surgery or catheter-based techniques such as PTCA, because such continued symptoms justify aggressive intervention. In addition, patients with significant myocardium at risk, for example, those whose surface electrocardiogram suggests involvement of the left anterior descending or who present with pulmonary edema or hypotension, should be referred for coronary angiography to provide additional prognostic data and help guide therapy. For the remainder of patients, noninvasive risk stratification should help guide subsequent decisions regarding surgical intervention or angioplasty. This particular strategy seems most consistent with the dynamic nature of the mechanisms of ischemia in patients with unstable angina.

In summary, collective analysis of the randomized studies suggests the following guidelines for surgical intervention for coronary artery disease. In patients with chronic stable angina, coronary artery surgery improves the long-term survival of those with significant left main stenosis and of those with three-vessel coronary artery disease associated with left ventricular dysfunction. Patients with chronic stable angina and single- or double-vessel coronary artery disease may have improved symptomatic status with bypass surgery, but there is no evidence to suggest that longevity is altered. Patients with symptomatic three-vessel disease and preserved left ventricular function may have symptomatic improvement, but it is unclear whether survival is increased by surgery. Finally, in patients with unstable angina, there is no evidence to support the early surgical therapy of unstable angina in patients with one- or two-vessel disease, although patients with three-vessel disease may benefit from early surgical intervention.

Besides those considerations, the clinician must weigh additional factors when contemplating a recommendation of surgical revascularization for an individual patient. The success of revascularization may be related, in large part, to the extent of distal coronary artery disease. Saphenous-vein graft patency is threatened by any distal coronary artery bed when there is poor arterial flow, and vessels less than 1.5 mm in diameter may have a particularly poor patency rate [261]. Females have consistently poorer results with bypass surgery than do males, with higher operative mortality and lower angina-free survival, probably due to smaller epicardial coronary arteries [260]. Lack of adequate surgical conduits may limit surgical options; for example, vein use may be limited if there has been prior stripping. Mobilization of the left internal mammary artery should be carefully considered in patients with previous left radical mastectomy, because this procedure may compromise blood flow to the anterior chest wall. Associated surgical procedures at the time of bypass surgery also may substantially alter long-term prognosis. Concomitant left ventricular aneurysmectomy [273] or mitral valve replacement [274] with coronary artery revascularization carries a much higher perioperative mortality than bypass alone. The presence of carotid bruits increases the likelihood of stroke during artery surgery, but that increased risk is similar to the risk of stroke during carotid endarterectomy as performed in most centers [275]. There are as yet no well-designed randomized trials to guide therapy of the patient with combined carotid and coronary artery disease, and decisions regarding combined coronary bypass and carotid endarterectomy must be based on individualized factors such as the severity of carotid disease, history of previous stroke or transient ischemic attack in the carotid distribution, and the skill of the vascular surgeon performing the endarterectomy. In most institutions and for most patients, prophylactic carotid surgery is not indicated.

Despite successful coronary revascularization, long-term management of patients with coronary artery disease must continue. Patients should be encouraged to cease smoking and alter their diet to establish an ideal body weight [276]. Blood pressure must be controlled and hypercholesterolemia corrected [277]. It is hoped that such measures will retard or reverse atherosclerosis in native coronary arteries as well as venous bypass grafts. Antiplatelet agents should be prescribed to help maintain long-term patency of saphenous grafts [278,279], as well as for primary and secondary prevention.

References

1. American Heart Association. Heart and Stroke Facts: 1994 Statistical Supplement. Dallas: American Heart Association, 1993. P. 22.
2. Gould K, Lipscomb K, Hamilton G. Physiologic basis for assessing critical coronary stenosis. Instantaneous flow response and regional distribution during coronary hyperemia as measures of coronary flow reserve. Am J Cardiol 1974; 33:87.
3. Lerman A, Burnett J. Intact and altered endothelium in regulation of vasomotion. Circulation 1992; 86[Suppl III]:III-12.
4. Cohen R, et al. Loss of selective endothelial cell vasoactive functions caused by hypercholesterolemia in pig coronary arteries. Circ Res 1988; 63:903.
5. Vita J, et al. The coronary vasomotor response to acetylcholine relates to risk factors for coronary artery disease. Circulation 1990; 81:491.
6. Ludmer P, et al. Paradoxical vasoconstriction induced by acetylcholine in atherosclerotic coronary arteries. N Engl J Med 1986; 315:1046.
7. Stewart D, et al. Increased plasma endothelin-1 in the early hours of acute myocardial infarction. J Am Coll Cardiol 1991; 18:38.
8. Kourembanas S, et al. Hypoxia induces endothelin gene expression and secretion in cultured human endothelium. J Clin Invest 1991; 88:1054.
9. Lerman A, et al. Activation of endothelin during arterial thrombosis and thrombolysis (Abstract). J Am Coll Cardiol 1991; 17:27.
10. Flugelman M, et al. Smooth muscle cell abundance and fibroblast growth factors in coronary lesions of patients with nonfatal unstable angina. A clue to the mechanism of transformation from the stable to the unstable clinical state. Circulation 1993; 88:2493.
11. Oliva P, Potts D, Pluss R. Coronary arterial spasm in Prinzmetal angina. Documentation by coronary arteriography. N Engl J Med 1973; 288:745.
12. Toyo-oka T, et al. Increased plasma level of endothelin-1 and coronary spasm induction in patients with vasospastic angina pectoris. Circulation 1991; 83:476.
13. McFadden E, et al. Effect of intracoronary serotonin on coronary vessels in patients with stable angina and patients with variant angina. N Engl J Med 1991; 324:648.
14. Andrews T, et al. Subsets of ambulatory myocardial ischemia based on heart rate activity: Circadian distribution and response to anti-ischemic medication. Circulation 1993; 88:92.
15. Maseri A, et al. Coronary vasospasm in angina pectoris. Lancet 1977; 1:713.
16. Mudge GJ, et al. Reflex increase in coronary vascular resistance in patients with ischemic heart disease. N Engl J Med 1976; 295:1333.
17. Mudge GJ, et al. Comparison of metabolic and vasoconstrictor stimuli on coronary vascular resistance in man. Circulation 1979; 59:544.
18. Deanfield J, et al. Transient ST-segment depression as a marker of myocardial ischemia during daily life. Am J Cardiol 1984; 54:1195.
19. Yeung A, et al. The effect of atherosclerosis on the vasomotor response to coronary arteries to mental stress. N Engl J Med 1991; 325:1151.
20. Golino P, et al. Divergent effects of serotonin on coronary-artery dimensions and blood flow in patients with coronary atherosclerosis and control patients. N Engl J Med 1991; 324:641.
21. Vita J, et al. Patients with evidence of coronary endothelial dysfunction as assessed by acetylcholine infusion demonstrate marked increase in sensitivity to constrictor effects of catecholamines. Circulation 1992; 85:1390.
22. Nabel E, Selwyn A, Ganz P. Mechanisms of flow-mediated vasodilation in human epicardial coronary arteries: Impairment by atherosclerosis. J Am Coll Cardiol 1990; 16:349.

23. DeWood M, et al. Prevalence of total coronary occlusion during the early hours of transmural myocardial infarction. N Engl J Med 1980; 303:897.
24. Davies M, Thomas A. Thrombosis and acute coronary-artery lesions in sudden cardiac ischemic death. N Engl J Med 1984; 310:1137.
25. Aiken J, Gorman R, Shebuski R. Prevention of blockage of partially obstructed coronary arteries with prostacyclin correlates with inhibition of platelet aggregation. Prostaglandins 1979; 17:483.
26. Epstein S, Palmeri S. Mechanisms contributing to precipitation of unstable angina and acute myocardial infarction: Implications regarding therapy. Am J Cardiol 1984; 54:1245.
27. Ambrose J, et al. Angiographic evolution of coronary artery morphology in unstable angina. J Am Coll Cardiol 1986; 7:472.
28. Sherman C, et al. Coronary angioscopy in patients with unstable angina pectoris. N Engl J Med 1986; 315:913.
29. Rehr R, et al. Angiographic morphology of coronary artery stenoses in prolonged rest angina: evidence of introcoronary thrombus. J Am Coll Cardiol 1989; 14:1429.
30. Kereiakes D, et al. Myocardial infarction with minimal coronary atherosclerosis in the era of thrombolytic reperfusion. The Thrombolysis and Angioplasty in Myocardial Infarction (TAMI) Study Group. J Am Coll Cardiol 1991; 17:304.
31. Falk E. Plaque rupture with severe pre-existing stenosis precipitating thrombosis: Characteristics of coronary atherosclerotic plaque underlying fatal occlusion thrombi. Br Heart J 1983; 50:127.
32. Falk E. Unstable angina with fatal outcome: dynamic coronary thrombosis leading to infarction and/or sudden death. Circulation 1985; 71:699.
33. Davies M, Thomas A. Plaque fissuring—the cause of acute myocardial ischemia, sudden ischemic death, and crescendo angina. Br Heart J 1985; 53:363.
34. Trip M, et al. Platelet hyperreactivity and prognosis in survivors of myocardial infarction. N Engl J Med 1990; 322:1549.
35. Chandler A, Hand R. Phagocytized platelets: A source of lipids in human thrombi and atherosclerotic plaques. Science 1961; 134:946.
36. Friedman R, et al. The effect of thrombocytopenia on experimental atherosclerotic lesion formation in rabbits. J Clin Invest 1977; 60:1191.
37. Falk E. Morphologic features of unstable atherothrombotic plaques underlying acute coronary syndromes. Am J Cardiol 1989; 63:114.
38. Steering Committee of the Physicians' Health Study Research Group. Final report on the aspirin component of the ongoing Physician's Health Study. N Engl J Med 1989; 321:129.
39. Harrison D, et al. Restoration of endothelium-dependent relaxation by dietary treatment of atherosclerosis. J Clin Invest 1987; 80:1808.
40. Brown G, et al. Regression of coronary artery disease as a result of intensive lipid-lowering therapy in men with high levels of apolipoprotein B. N Engl J Med 1990; 323:1289.
41. Kannel W, Feinlieb M. Natural history of angina pectoris in the Framingham study: Progress and survival. Am J Cardiol 1972; 29:154.
42. Kaiser G, et al. Survival following coronary artery bypass grafting in patients with severe angina pectoris (CASS). J Thorac Cardiovasc Surg 1985; 89:513.
43. Detre K, et al. Effect of bypass surgery on survival in patients with low and high-risk groups dilineated by the use of simple clinical variables. Circulation 1981; 63:1329.
44. Rutherford J, Braunwald E, Cohn P. Chronic ischemic heart disease. In E Braunwald, ed. Heart Disease. Third ed. Philadelphia: Saunders, 1988. P. 1314.
45. Elveback L, Connolly D, Melton L. Coronary heart disease in residents of Rochester, Minnesota. VII. Incidence, 1950 through 1982. Mayo Clin Proc 1986; 61:896.
46. Marmot M. Interpretation of trends in coronary heart disease mortality. Acta Med Scan 1985; 701[Suppl]:58.
47. Elveback L, Connolly D. Coronary heart disease in residents of Rochester, Minnesota. V. Prognosis of patients with coronary heart disease based on initial manifestation. Mayo Clin Proc 1985; 60:305.
48. Elveback L, Connolly D, Kurland L. Coronary heart disease in residents of Rochester, Minnesota, 1950–1975. II. Mortality, incidence, and survival. Mayo Clin Proc 1985; 56:665.
49. Pell S, Fayerweather W. Trends in the incidence of myocardial infarction and in associated mortality and morbidity in a large employed population. 1957–1983. N Engl J Med 1985; 312:1005.
50. Goldberg R, et al. A community-wide perspective of sex differences and temporal trends in the incidence and survival rates after acute myocardial infarction and out-of-hospital deaths caused by coronary heart disease. Circulation 1993; 87:1947.
51. Burke G, et al. Trends in serum cholesterol levels from 1980 to 1987. N Engl J Med 1991; 324:941.
52. Sytkowski P, Kannel W, D'Agostino R. Changes in risk factors and the decline in mortality from cardiovascular disease. N Engl J Med 1990; 322:1635.
53. Gomez-Marin O, et al. Improvement in long-term survival among patients hospitalized with acute myocardial infarction, 1970 to 1980. N Engl J Med 1987; 316:1353.
54. Goldman L, Cook E. The decline in ischemic heart disease mortality rates. An analysis of the comparative effects of medical interventions and changes in lifestyle. Ann Intern Med 1984; 101:825.
55. Luchi R, et al. Comparison of medical and surgical treatment for unstable angina pectoris. N Engl J Med 1987; 316:977.
56. Alderman E, et al. Ten-year follow-up of survival and myocardial infarction in the randomized coronary artery surgery study. Circulation 1990; 82:1629.
57. Killip T, et al. Coronary artery surgery study (CASS): A randomized trial of coronary bypass surgery. Eight-year follow-up and survival in patients with reduced ejection fraction. Circulation 1985; 72[Suppl V]:102.
58. Chaitman B, et al. Coronary Artery Surgery Study (CASS): Comparability of 10 year survival in randomized and randomizable patients. J Am Coll Cardiol 1990; 16:1071.
59. Parisi A, et al. Medical compared with surgical management of unstable angina. 5-year mortality and morbidity in the Veterans Administration Study. Circulation 1989; 80:1176.
60. Alderman E, et al. Results of coronary artery surgery in patients with poor left ventriuclar function (CASS). Circulation 1983; 68:785.
61. Merrilees M, Scott P, Norris R. Prognosis after myocardial infarction. Results of 15-year follow-up. Br Med J 1984; 288:356.
62. Hackett D, et al. Coronary stenoses before and after acute myocardial infarction. Am J Cardiol 1989; 63:1517.
63. Hermiller J, et al. Quantitative and qualitative coronary angiographic analysis: Review of methods, utility, and limitations. Cath Cardiovasc Diag 1992; 25:110.
64. Califf R, et al. Outcome in one-vessel coronary artery disease. Circulation 1983; 67:283.
65. Demots H, et al. Left main coronary artery disease. Am J Cardiol 1975; 36:136.
66. CASS Principal Investigators and their Associates. A ran-

domized trial of coronary artery bypass surgery. Survival data. Circulation 1983; 68:939.
67. Kemp H, et al. Seven-year survival of patients with normal or near normal coronary arteriograms: A CASS Registry study. J Am Coll Cardiol 1986; 7:479.
68. Muller D, et al. Multivessel coronary artery disease: A key predictor of short-term prognosis after reperfusion therapy for acute myocardial infarction. Am Heart J 1991; 121:1042.
69. Veen G, et al. Culprit lesion morphology and stenosis severity in the prediction of reocclusion after coronary thrombolysis: angiographic results of the APRICOT study. J Am Coll Cardiol 1993; 22:1755.
70. Falk E. Why do plaques rupture? Circulation 1992; 86[Suppl III]:III-3.
71. Davies S, et al. Coronary lesion morphology in acute myocardial infarction: demonstration of early remodeling after streptokinase treatment. J Am Coll Cardiol 1990; 16:1079.
72. Bugiardini R, et al. Angiographic morphology in unstable angina and its relation to transient myocardial ischemia and hospital outcome. Am J Cardiol 1991; 67:460.
73. Bounous E, et al. Surgical survival benefits for coronary disease patients with left ventricular dysfunction. Circulation 1988; 78[Suppl I]:I-151.
74. Weiner D, et al. The role of exercise-induced silent myocardial ischemia in patients with abnormal left ventricular function. A report from the Coronary Artery Surgery Study (CASS) registry. Am Heart J 1989; 118:649.
75. Rocco M, et al. Prognostic importance of myocardial ischemia detected by ambulatory monitoring in patients with stable coronary artery disease. Circulation 1988; 78:877.
76. Yeung A, et al. Effects of asymptomatic ischemia on long-term prognosis in chronic stable coronary disease. Circulation 1991; 83:1598.
77. Deedwania P, Carbajal E. Usefulness of ambulatory silent myocardial ischemia added to the prognostic value of exercise test parameters in predicting risk of cardiac death in patients with stable angina pectoris and exercise-induced myocardial ischemia. Am J Cardiol 1991; 68:1279.
78. Gottlieb S, et al. Silent ischemia as a marker for early unfavorable outcomes in patients with unstable angina. N Engl J Med 1986; 314:1214.
79. Raby K, et al. Detection and significance of intraoperative and postoperative ischemia in peripheral vascular surgery. JAMA 1992; 268:222.
80. Raby K, et al. Long-term prognosis of myocardial ischemia detected by holter monitoring in peripheral vascular disease. Am J Cardiol 1990; 66:1309.
81. Raby K, et al. Correlation between preoperative ischemia and major cardiac events after peripheral vascular surgery. N Engl J Med 1989; 321:1296.
82. Gottlieb S, et al. Silent ischemia on Holter monitoring predicts mortality in high-risk postinfarction patients. JAMA 1988; 259:1030.
83. Dagenais G, et al. Survival of patients with a strongly positive exercise electrocardiogram. Circulation 1982; 65:452.
84. Bogaty P, et al. Prognosis of patients with a strongly positive exercise electrocardiogram. Am J Cardiol 1989; 64:1284.
85. Weiner D, et al. Prognostic importance of a clinical profile and exercise test in medically treated patients with coronary artery disease. J Am Coll Cardiol 1984; 3:772.
86. McPhail N, et al. The use of preoperative exercise testing to predict cardiac complications after arterial reconstruction. J Vasc Surg 1988; 7:60.
87. Weiner D, McCabe C, Ryan T. Identification of patients with left main and three-vessel coronary artery disease with clinical and exercise test variables. Am J Cardiol 1980; 46:21.
88. Shub C. Stable angina pectoris: 2. Cardiac evaluation and diagnostic testing. Mayo Clin Proc 1990; 65:243.
89. Ellestad M, Wan M. Predictive implications of stress testing: follow-up of 2700 subjects after maximum treadmill stress testing. Circulation 1975; 51:363.
90. Meyers D, et al. The effect of baseline electrocardiographic abnormalities on the diagnostic accuracy of exercise-induced ST segment changes. Am Heart J 1990; 119:272.
91. Kaul S, et al. Regional variability in the myocardial clearance of thallium-201 and its importance in determining the presence or absence of coronary artery disease. J Am Coll Cardiol 1986; 8:95.
92. Boucher C, et al. Increased lung uptake of thallium-201 during exercise myocardial imaging: Hemodynamic and angiographic implications of patients with coronary artery disease. Am J Cardiol 1980; 46:189.
93. Iskandrian A, et al. Independent and incremental prognostic value of exercise single-photon emission computed tomographic (SPECT) thallium imaging in coronary artery disease. J Am Coll Cardiol 1993; 22:665.
94. Younis L, et al. Prognostic value of intravenous dipyridamole thallium scintigraphy after an acute myocardial ischemic event. Am J Cardiol 1989; 64:161.
95. O'Keefe JJ, Bateman T, Barnhart C. Adenosine thallium-201 is superior to exercise thallium-201 for detecting coronary artery disease in patients with left bundle branch block. J Am Coll Cardiol 1993; 21:1332.
96. Fung A, Gallagher K, Buda A. The physiologic basis of dobutamine as compared with dipyridamole stress interventions in the assessment of critical coronary stenosis. Circulation 1987; 76:943.
97. Younis L, et al. Prognostic importance of silent myocardial ischemia detected by intravenous dipyridamole thallium myocardial imaging in asymptomatic patients with coronary artery disease. J Am Coll Cardiol 1989; 14:1635.
98. Pamelia F, et al. Prognosis with chest pain and normal thallium-201 exercise scintigrams. Am J Cardiol 1985; 55:920.
99. Bonow R, et al. Exercise-induced ischemia in mildly symptomatic patients with coronary artery disease and preserved left ventricular function. N Engl J Med 1984; 311:1339.
100. Jones R, et al. The role of radionuclide angiography in the perioperative prediction of pain relief and prolonged survival following coronary artery bypass grafting. Ann Surg 1983; 197:743.
101. Roig E, et al. Prognostic value of exercise radionuclide angiography in low risk acute myocardial infarction survivors. Eur Heart J 1993; 14:213.
102. Miller T, et al. Risk stratification of single or double vessel coronary artery disease and impaired left ventricular function using exercise radionuclide angiography. Am J Cardiol 1990; 65:1317.
103. Krivokapich J, et al. Prognostic usefulness of positive or negative exercise stress echocardiography for predicting coronary events in ensuing twelve months. Am J Cardiol 1993; 71:646.
104. Heberden W. Some account of a disorder of the breast. Med Trans Coll Physicians (London) 1772; 2:59.
105. Geltman E, et al. Increased myocardial perfusion at rest and diminished perfusion reserve in patients with angina and angiographically normal coronary arteries. J Am Coll Cardiol 1990; 16:586.
106. Cannon R, et al. Chest pain and "normal" coronary arteries—role of small coronary arteries. Am J Cardiol 1985; 55:50.
107. Quyygumi AA, et al. Endothelial dysfunction in patients with chest pain and normal coronary arteries. Circulation 1992; 86:1864-1871.

108. Cannon RO 3rd, Camici PG, Epstein SE. Pathophysiology of Syndrome X. Circulation 1992; 85:883-892.
109. Cannon RO 3rd. Chest pain with normal coronary arteriograms. N Engl J Med 1993; 328:1706-1708.
110. Opherk D, et al. Four-year follow-up study in patients with angina pectoris and normal coronary arteriograms ("syndrome X"). Circulation 1989; 80:1610.
111. Miller R, et al. Electrocardiographic and cineangiographic correlations in assessment of the location, nature and extent of abnormal left ventricular segmental contraction in coronary artery disease. Circulation 1974; 49:447.
112. Hamby R, et al. Left bundle branch block: A predictor of poor left ventricular function in coronary artery disease. Am Heart J 1983; 106:471.
113. Levine H. Non-specificity of the electrocardiogram associated with coronary artery disease. Am J Med 1953; 15:344.
114. Patterson R, Horowitz S. Importance of epidemiology and biostatistics in deciding clinical strategies for using diagnostic tests: a simplified approach using examples from coronary artery disease. J Am Coll Cardiol 1989; 13:1653.
115. Goldman L, et al. Incremental value of the exercise test for diagnosing the presence or absence of coronary artery disease. Circulation 1982; 66:945.
116. Weiner D, et al. The predictive value of anginal chest pain as an indicator of coronary disease during exercise testing. Am Heart J 1978; 96:458.
117. Cohn P, Vokonas P, Herman M. Postexercise electrocardiogram in patients with abnormal resting electrocardiograms. Circulation 1971; 43:648.
118. Kligfield P, Ameisen O, Okin P. Heart rate adjustment of ST segment depression for improved detection of coronary artery disease. Circulation 1989; 79:245.
119. Weiner D, et al. Decrease in systolic blood pressure during exercise testing: Reproducibility, response to coronary artery bypass surgery, and prognostic significance. Am J Cardiol 1982; 49:1627.
120. Ho S, McComish M, Taylor R. Effect of beta-adrenergic blockade on the results of exercise testing related to the extent of coronary artery disease. Am J Cardiol 1985; 55:258.
121. Mahmarian J, et al. Quantitative exercise thallium-201 single photon emission computed tomography for the enhanced diagnosis of ischemic heart disease. J Am Coll Cardiol 1990; 15:318.
122. Hoffman R, et al. Comparative evaluation of bicycle and dobutamine stress echocardiography with perfusion scintigraphy and bicycle electrocardiogram for identification of coronary artery disease. Am J Cardiol 1993; 72:555.
123. Wackers F, et al. Prognostic significance of normal quantitative planar thallium-201 stress scintigraphy in patients with chest pain. J Am Coll Cardiol 1985; 6:27.
124. Bairey C, et al. Exercise thallium-201 scintigraphy and prognosis in typical angina pectoris and negative exercise electrocardiography. Am J Cardiol 1989; 64:282.
125. Josephson M, et al. Noninvasive detection and localization of coronary stenoses in patients: comparison of resting dipyridamole and exercise thallium-201 myocardial perfusion imaging. Am Heart J 1982; 103:1008.
126. Verani M, et al. Diagnosis of coronary artery disease by controlled coronary vasodilation with adenosine and Thallium-201 scintigraphy in patients unable to exercise. Circulation 1990; 82:80.
127. Marwick T, et al. Accuracy and limitations of exercise echocardiography in a routine clinical setting. J Am Coll Cardiol 1992; 19:74.
128. Caldwell J, et al. The detection of coronary artery disease with radionuclide techniques: A comparison of rest-exercise thallium imaging and ejection fraction response. Circulation 1980; 61:610.
129. Armstrong W, et al. Complementary value of two-dimensional exercise echocardiography to routine treadmill exercise testing. Ann Int Med 1986; 105:829.
130. Sawada S, et al. Prognostic value of a normal exercise echocardiogram. Am Heart J 1990; 120:49.
131. Sawada S, et al. Echocardiographic detection of coronary artery disease during dobutamine infusion. Circulation 1991; 83:1605.
132. Cohn P. Silent myocardial ischemia. Ann Intern Med 1988; 109:312.
133. Mulcahy D, et al. Ischemia in the ambulatory setting—the total ischemic burden: relation to exercise testing and investigative and therapeutic implications. J Am Coll Cardiol 1989; 14:1166.
134. Manning W, et al. Fat-suppressed breath-hold magnetic resonance coronary angiography. Circulation 1993; 87:94.
135. Rosenberg L, et al. The risk of myocardial infarction after quitting smoking in men under 55 years of age. N Engl J Med 1985; 313:1511.
136. Manson J, et al. A prospective study of obesity and risk of coronary heart disease in women. N Engl J Med 1990; 322:882.
137. Hambrecht R, et al. Various intensities of leisure time physical activity in patients with coronary artery disease: Effects on cardiorespiratory fitness and progression of coronary atherosclerotic lesions. J Am Coll Cardiol 1993; 22:468.
138. Ekelund L-G, et al. Physical fitness as a predictor of cardiovascular mortality in asymptomatic North American men. N Engl J Med 1988; 319:1379.
139. Newman W, et al. Relation of serum lipoprotein levels and systolic blood pressure to early atherosclerosis. N Engl J Med 1986; 314:138.
140. Frick M, et al. Helsinki Heart Study: Primary-prevention trial with gemfibrozil in middle-aged men with dyslipidemia. N Engl J Med 1987; 317:1237.
141. Rossouw J, Lewis B, Rifkind B. The value of lowering cholesterol after myocardial infarction. N Engl J Med 1990; 323:1112.
142. Expert Panel on Detection and Treatment of High Blood Cholesterol in Adults. Summary of the second report of the national cholesterol education program (NCEP) Expert Panel on Detection, Evaluation, and Treatment of High Blood Cholesterol in Adults (Adult Treatment Panel II). JAMA 1993; 269:3015.
143. Hillis L, Braunwald E. Myocardial ischemia. N Engl J Med 1977; 296:971.
144. Kirk E, Sonnenblick E. Newer concepts in the pathophysiology of ischemic heart disease. Am Heart J 1982; 103:756.
145. Braunwald E, Sobel B. Coronary blood flow and myocardial ischemia. In E Braunwald, ed. Heart Disease. Third ed. Philadelphia: Saunders, 1988. P. 1191.
146. Rapaport E, Remedios P. The high risk patient after recovery from myocardial infarction: Recognition and managment. J Am Coll Cardiol 1983; 1:391.
147. Frishman W. Pharmacology of the nitrates in angina pectoris. Am J Cardiol 1985; 56:8.
148. Williams JJ, Glick G, Braunwald E. Studies on cardiac dimensions in intact unanesthetized man. V. Effects of nitroglycerin. Circulation 1965; 32:767.
149. DeCoster P, et al. Combined effects of nitrates on the coronary and peripheral circulation in exercise-induced ischemia. Circulation 1990; 81:1881.
150. Brown G, et al. The mechanisms of nitroglycerin action. Stenosis vasodilation as a major component of drug response. Circulation 1981; 64:1089.

151. Feldman R, Conti C. Editorial: Relief of myocardial ischemia with nitroglycerin: What is the mechanism? Circulation 1981; 64:1098.
152. Stamler J, Loscalzo J. The antiplatelet effects of organic nitrates and nitroso-derivatives and their importance in cardiomuscular disorders. J Am Coll Cardiol 1991; 18:1529.
153. Folts J, Stamler J, Loscalzo J. Intravenous nitroglycerin infusion inhibits periodic platelet thrombus formation in stenosed dog coronary arteries. Circulation 1991; 83:2122.
154. Parker J, et al. Effect of intervals between doses on the development of tolerance to isosorbide dinitrate. N Engl J Med 1987; 316:1440.
155. Abrams J. The use of nitroglycerin and long-acting nitrates in angina pectoris. In D Weiner, W Frishman, eds. Therapy of Angina Pectoris. New York: Marcel Dekker, 1986: 53. (Denolin H, Swan H, ed. Basic and Clinical Cardiology; vol 8.)
156. Abrams J. Buccal nitroglycerin. Am Heart J 1983; 105:848.
157. Abrams J. Pharmacology of nitroglycerin and long-acting nitrate esters. Am J Cardiol 1985; 56:12.
158. Motulsky H, Insel P. Adrenergic receptors in man: Direct identification, physiologic regulations, and clinical alterations. N Engl J Med 1982; 307:18.
159. Lefkowitz R. Direct binding studies of adrenergic receptors: Biochemical, physiologic, and clinical implications. Ann Intern Med 1979; 91:450.
160. Colucci S, et al. Decreased lymphocyte beta-adrenergic receptor density in patients with heart failure and tolerance to the beta-adrenergic agonist perbuterol. N Engl J Med 1981; 305:185.
161. Bristow M, et al. Decreased catecholamine sensitivity and beta-adrenergic receptor density in failing human hearts. N Engl J Med 1982; 307:205.
162. Koch-Weser J. Metoprolol. N Engl J Med 1979; 301:698.
163. Frishman W. Beta-adrenoceptor antagonists: New drugs and new indications. N Engl J Med 1981; 305:500.
164. Frishman W. Pindolol: A new beta-adrenoceptor antagonist with partial agonist activity. N Engl J Med 1983; 308:940.
165. European Infarction Study Group. European Infarction Study. Secondary prevention study with slow-release oxprenolol after myocardial infarction: Morbidity and mortality. Eur Heart J 1984; 5:189.
166. Taylor S, et al. A long-term prevention study with oxprenolol in coronary heart disease. N Engl J Med 1982; 307:1293.
167. Australian and Swedish Pindolol Study Group. The effects of pindolol on the two years mortality after complicated myocardial infarction. Eur Heart J 1983; 4:367.
168. Yusuf S, et al. Beta blockade during and after myocardial infarction: An overview of the randomized trials. Prog Cardiovasc Dis 1985; 27:335.
169. Yusuf S, Wittes J, Firedman L. Overview of results of randomized clinical trials in heart disease. 1. Treatments following myocardial infarction. JAMA 1988; 260:2088.
170. Boissel J, et al. Secondary prevention after high-risk acute myocardial infarction with low-dose acebutolol. Am J Cardiol 1990; 66:251.
171. Michelson E, Frishman W. Labetolol: An alpha and beta-adrenoceptor blocking drug. Ann Intern Med 1981; 99:553.
172. Frishman W. Clinical pharmacology of the new beta-adrenergic blocking drugs. Part 1. Pharmacokinetic and pharmacodynamic properties. Am Heart J 1979; 98:663.
173. Frishman W, Silverman R. Clinical pharmacology of the new beta-adrenergic blocking drugs. Part 3. Comparative clinical experience and new therapeutic applications. Am Heart J 1979; 98:119.
174. Frishman W. Beta-adrenergic blockade for the treatment of angina pectoris. In D Weiner, W Frishman, eds. Therapy of Angina Pectoris. New York: Marcel Dekker, 1986. P. 83.
175. Gorczyski R, et al. Pharmacology of ASL-8052, a novel beta-adrenergic receptor antagonist with an ultra-short duration of action. J Cardiovasc Pharmacol 1983; 5:668.
176. Boudoulas H, et al. Increased diastolic time: A possible important factor in the beneficial effect of propranolol in patients with coronary artery disease. J Cardiovasc Pharmacol 1979; 1:503.
177. Robertson R, et al. Exacerbation of vasotonic angina pectoris due to coronary artery spasm. Circulation 1982; 65:281.
178. Gunther S, et al. Therapy of coronary vasoconstriction in patients with coronary artery disease. Am J Cardiol 1981; 47:157.
179. Weksler B, Gillick M, Pink J. Effect of propranolol on platelet function. Blood 1977; 49:185.
180. Frishman W, et al. Reversal of abnormal platelet aggregability and changes in exercise tolerance in patients with angina pectoris following oral propranolol. Circulation 1974; 50:887.
181. Leren P, et al. Effects of propranolol and prazosin on blood lipids. The Oslo Study. Lancet 1980; 2:4.
182. Teo K, Yusuf S, Furberg C. Effects of prophylactic antiarrhythmic drug therapy in acute myocardial infarction. JAMA 1993; 270:1589.
183. May G, et al. Secondary prevention after myocardial infarction: a review of long-term trials. Prog Cardiovasc Dis 1982; 24:331.
184. Beta-Blocker Pooling Project Research Group. Beta-Blocker Pooling Project. Subgroup findings from randomized trials in post infarction patients. Eur Heart J 1988; 9:8.
185. ISIS-1 Collaborative Group. Randomized trial of intravenous atenolol among 16,027 cases of suspected acute myocardial infarction: ISIS-1. Lancet 1986; 2:57.
186. Pedersen T, The Norwegian Multicenter Study Group. Six-year follow-up of the Norwegian multicenter study on timolol after acute myocardial infarction. N Engl J Med 1985; 313:1055.
187. ISIS-1 Collaborative Group. Mechanisms for the early mortality reduction produced by beta-blockade started early in acute myocardial infarction. Lancet 1988; 1:921.
188. Wikstrand J, et al. Primary prevention with metoprolol in patients with hypertension: mortality results from the MAPHY study. JAMA 1988; 259:1976.
189. Radack K, Deck C. Beta-adrenergic blocker therapy does not worsen intermittent claudication in subjects with peripheral arterial disease. A meta-analysis of randomized controlled trials. Arch Intern Med 1991; 151:1769.
190. Stone P, et al. Calcium channel blocking agents in the treatment of cardiovascular disorders. Part II: Hemodynamic effects and clinical applications. Ann Intern Med 1980; 93:886.
191. Parmley W, et al. Attenuation of the circadian patterns of myocardial ischemia with nifedipine GITS in patients with chronic stable angina. J Am Coll Cardiol 1992; 19:1380.
192. Bainbridge A, et al. A comparative assessment of amlodipine and felodipine ER: pharmacokinetic and pharmacodynamic indices. Eur J Clin Pharmacol 1993; 45:425.
193. Gibson R, et al. Diltiazem and reinfarction in patients with non-Q wave myocardial infarction: results of a double-blind, randomized multicenter trial. N Engl J Med 1986; 315:423.
194. Multicenter Diltiazem Postinfarction Trial Research Group. The effect of diltiazem on mortality and reinfarction after myocardial infarction. N Engl J Med 1988; 319:385.
195. SPRINT Study Group. The secondary prevention re-infarction Israeli nifedipine trial (SPRINT) II: design and methods, results. Eur Heart J 1988; 9[Suppl 1]:350.
196. The Israeli Sprint Study Group. Secondary Prevention Reinfarction Israeli Nifedipine Trial (SPRINT). A randomized

intervention trial of nifedipine in patients with acute myocardial infarction. Eur Heart J 1988; 9:354.
197. Goldbourt U, et al. Early administration of nifedipine in suspected acute myocardial infarction. Arch Intern Med 1993; 153:345.
198. Strauss W, Parisi A. Combined use of calcium-channel and beta-adrenergic blockers for the treatment of chronic stable angina. Ann Intern Med 1988; 109:570.
199. Lynch P, et al. Objective assessment of antianginal treatment: a double-blind comparison of propranolol, nifedipine, and their combination. Br Med J 1980; 280:184.
200. Boden W, et al. Beneficial effects of diltiazem and propranolol, alone and in combination, in patients with persistent effort angina on beta-blockers and nitrates: a randomized, double-blind, placebo-controlled cross-over study. Circulation 1985; 71:1197.
201. Hung J, et al. The effect of diltiazem and propranolol, alone and in combination, on exercise performance and left ventricular function in patients with stable effort angina: a double-blind, randomized, and placebo-controlled study. Circulation 1983; 68:560.
202. Winniford M, Huxley R, Hillis L. Randomized, double-blind comparison of propranolol alone and a propranolol-verapamil combination in patients with severe angina of effort. J Am Coll Cardiol 1983; 1:492.
203. Wayne V, et al. Adverse interaction between beta-adrenergic blocking drugs and verapamil: report of three cases. Aust NZ J Med 1982; 12:285.
204. Findlay I, et al. A double blind placebo controlled comparison of verapamil, atenolol, and their combination. Br Heart J 1987; 57:336.
205. Krol W, The Persantine-Aspirin Reinfarction Study Group. Persantine and aspirin in coronary heart disease. Circulation 1980; 62:449.
206. Elwood P, et al. A randomized controlled trial of acetylsalicyclic acid in the secondary prevention of mortality from myocardial infarction. Br Med J 1974; 1:436.
207. Elwood P, Sweetnam P. Aspirin and secondary mortality after myocardial infarction. Lancet 1979; 2:1313.
208. Coronary Drug Project Group. Aspirin in coronary heart disease. J Chronic Dis 1976; 29:625.
209. Breddin K, et al. The German-Austrian Aspirin Trial: a comparison of acetylsalicyclic acid, placebo and phenprocoumon in secondary prevention of myocardial infarction. Circulation 1980; 62[Suppl V]:V63.
210. Aspirin Myocardial Infarction Study Research Group. A randomized, controlled trial of aspirin in persons recovered from myocardial infarction. JAMA 1980; 243:661.
211. Klimt C, et al. Part II. Secondary coronary prevention with Persantine and aspirin. J Am Coll Cardiol 1986; 7:251.
212. Balsano F, et al. Antiplatelet treatment with ticlopidine in unstable angina. Circulation 1990; 82:17.
213. Mehta J. Influence of calcium-channel blockers on platelet function and arachidonic acid metabolism. Am J Cardiol 1985; 55:158.
214. Diodati J, et al. Effects of nitroglycerin at therapeutic doses on platelet aggregation in unstable angina pectoris and acute myocardial infarction. Am J Cardiol 1990; 66:683.
215. Smith P, Arnesen H, Holme I. The effect of warfarin on mortality and reinfarction after myocardial infarction. N Engl J Med 1990; 323:147.
216. The E.S.P.I.N Research Group. A controlled comparison of aspirin and oral anticoagulants in prevention of death after myocardial infarction. N Engl J Med 1982; 307:701.
217. Theroux P, et al. Aspirin versus heparin to prevent myocardial infarction during the acute phase of unstable angina. Circulation 1993; 88:2045.
218. The GUSTO Investigators. An international randomized trial comparing four thrombolytic strategies for acute myocardial infarction. N Engl J Med 1993; 329:673.
219. Theroux P, et al. Aspirin, heparin, or both to treat acute unstable angina. N Engl J Med 1988; 319:1105.
220. Lewis H, et al. Protective effects of aspirin against acute myocardial infarction and death in men with unstable angina. N Engl J Med 1983; 309:396.
221. Cairns J, et al. Aspirin, sulfinpyrazone, or both in unstable angina. Results of a Canadian multicenter trial. N Engl J Med 1985; 313:1369.
222. ISIS 2 Collaborative Group. Randomized trial of intravenous streptokinase, oral aspirin, both, or neither among 17,187 cases of suspected acute myocardial infarction: ISIS 2. Lancet 1988; 2:349.
223. Acheson J, et al. Anti-platelet trialists collaboration: Secondary prevention of vascular disease by prolonged anti-platelet therapy. Br Med J 1988; 296:320.
224. Anderson H, Willerson J. Current concepts: thrombolysis in acute myocardial infarction. N Engl J Med 1993; 329:703.
225. DiBianco R. Bepridil treatment of chronic stable angina: a review of comparative studies versus placebo, nifedipine, and diltiazem. Am J Cardiol 1992; 69:56.
226. Crea F, et al. Comparative effects of theophylline and isosorbide dinitrate on exercise capacity in stable angina pectoris, and their mechanism of action. Am J Cardiol 1989; 64:1098.
227. Crea F, et al. Effects of theophylline, atenolol, and their combination on myocardial ischemia in stable angina pectoris. Am J Cardiol 1990; 66:1157.
228. Gaspardone A, et al. Bamiphylline improves exercise-induced myocardial ischemia through a novel mechanism of action. Circulation 1993; 88:502.
229. Adelman A, et al. A comparison of directional atherectomy with balloon angioplasty for lesions of the left anterior descending coronary artery. N Engl J Med 1993; 329:228.
230. Bittl J. Directional coronary atherectomy versus balloon angioplasty. N Engl J Med 1993; 329:273.
231. Topol E, et al. A comparison of directional atherectomy with coronary angioplasty in patients with coronary artery disease. N Engl J Med 1993; 329:221.
232. Bittl J, Sanborn T. Excimer laser-facilitated coronary angioplasty: relative risk analysis of acute and follow-up results in 200 patients. Circulation 1992; 86:71.
233. Lincoff A, et al. Intracoronary stenting compared with conventional therapy for abrupt vessel closure complicating coronary angioplasty: A matched case-control study. J Am Coll Cardiol 1993; 21:866.
234. Parisi A, Folland E, Hartigan P. A comparison of angioplasty with medical therapy in the treatment of single-vessel coronary artery disaese: Veterans Affairs ACME Investigators. N Engl J Med 1992; 326:10.
235. Lembo N, King SI. Randomized trials of percutaneous transluminal coronary angioplasty, coronary artery bypass grafting surgery, or medical therapy in patients with coronary artery disease. Cor Art Dis 1990; 1:449.
236. RITA Trial Participants. Coronary angioplasty versus coronary artery bypass surgery: the Randomised Intervention Treatment of Angina (RITA) trial. Lancet 1993; 341:573.
237. Gibbons R, et al. Immediate angioplasty compared with the administration of a thrombolytic agent followed by conservative treatment for myocardial infarction. N Engl J Med 1993; 328:685.
238. Zijlstra F, et al. A comparison of immediate coronary angioplasty with intravenous streptokinase in acute myocardial infarction. N Engl J Med 1993; 328:680.
239. Grines C, et al. A comparison of immediate angioplasty with

thrombolytic therapy for acute myocardial infarction. N Engl J Med 1993; 328:673.
240. Myler R, et al. Unstable angina and coronary angioplasty. Circulation 1990; 82[Suppl II]:II88.
241. ACC/AHA Task Force on Assessment of Diagnostic and Therapeutic Cardiovascular Procedures (Committee on Percutaneous Transluminal Coronary Angioplasty). Guidelines for Percutaneous Transluminal Coronary Angioplasty. J Am Coll Cardiol 1993; 22:2033.
242. Bredlau C, et al. In-hospital morbidity and mortality in patients undergoing elective coronary angioplasty. Circulation 1985; 72:1044.
243. Detre K, et al. Percutaneous transluminal coronary angioplasty in 1985–1986 and 1977–1981. The National Heart, Lung, and Blood Institute Registry. N Engl J Med 1988; 318:265.
244. O'Keefe J, et al. Multivessel coronary angioplasty from 1980 to 1989: Procedural results and long-term outcome. J Am Coll Cardiol 1990; 16:1097.
245. Leimgruber P, et al. Restenosis after successful coronary angioplasty in patients with single-vessel disease. Circulation 1986; 73:710.
246. McBride W, Lange R, Hillis L. Restenosis after successful coronary angioplasty. N Engl J Med 1988; 318:1734.
247. Macdonald R, et al. Patient-related variables and restenosis after percutaenous transluminal coronary angioplasty—a report from the M-HEART study. Am J Cardiol 1990; 66:926.
248. Garratt K, et al. Restenosis after directional atherectomy: differences between primary atheromatous and restenosis lesions and influence of subintimal tissue resection. J Am Coll Cardiol 1990; 16:1665.
249. Sanborn T, et al. Percutaneous coronary excimer laser-assisted balloon angioplasty: initial clinical and quantitative angiographic results in 50 patients. J Am Coll Cardiol 1991; 17:94.
250. Dehmer G, et al. Reduction in the rate of early restenosis after coronary angioplasty by a diet supplemented with n-3 fatty acids. N Engl J Med 1988; 319:733.
251. Grigg L, et al. Determinants of restenosis and lack of effect of dietary supplementation with eicosapentaenoic acid on the incidence of coronary artery restenosis after angioplasty. J Am Coll Cardiol 1989; 13:665.
252. Reis G, et al. Randomized trial of fish oil for prevention of restenosis after coronary angioplasty. Lancet 1989; 2:177.
253. Barnes H, Standevan J, Reese J. Twelve-year experience with internal mammary artery for coronary grafts. J Thorac Cardiovasc Surg 1985; 90:668.
254. Loop F, et al. Influence of the internal-mammary-artery graft on 10 year survival and other cardiac events. N Engl J Med 1986; 314:1.
255. Rogers W, et al. Ten-year follow-up of quality of life in patients randomized to receive medical therapy of coronary artery bypass graft surgery. The Coronary Artery Surgery Study (CASS). Circulation 1990; 82:1647.
256. Pigott J, et al. Late results of surgical and medical therapy for patients with coronary artery disease and depressed left ventricular function. J Am Coll Cardiol 1985; 5:1036.
257. Wittels E, Hay J, Gotto A. Medical costs of coronary artery disease in the United States. Am J Cardiol 1990; 65:432.
258. Kirklin J, et al. Summary of a consensus concerning death and ischemic events after coronary artery bypass grafting. Circulation 1989; 79[Suppl I]:81.
259. Daily P. Early and 5-year results for coronary artery bypass grafting. A benchmark for percutaneous transluminal coronary angioplasty. J Thorac Cardiovasc Surg 1989; 96:67.
260. Loop F, et al. Coronary artery surgery in women compared with men: Analyses of risks and long-term results. J Am Coll Cardiol 1983; 1:383.
261. Lesperance J, et al. Aorta to coronary artery saphenous vein grafts. Preoperative angiographic criteria for successful surgery. Am J Cardiol 1972; 30:459.
262. Grondin C, et al. Coronary artery bypass grafting with saphenous vein. Circulation 1989; 79[SupplI]:24.
263. Campeau L, et al. Atherosclerosis and late closure of aortocoronary saphenous vein grafts: Sequential angiographic studies at 2 weeks, 1 year, 5 to 7 years, and 10 to 12 years after surgery. Circulation 1983; 68[SupplI]:1.
264. Chaitman B, Fisher L, Bourssa M. Effect of coronary artery bypass surgery on survival patterns in subsets of patients with left main coronary artery disease. Report of the Collaborative Study in Coronary Artery Surgery (CASS). Am J Cardiol 1981; 48:765.
265. Veterans Administration Coronary Artery Bypass Surgery Cooperative Study Group. Eleven-year survival in the Veterans' Administration randomized trial of coronary bypass surgery for stable angina. N Engl J Med 1984; 311:1333.
266. Takaro T, et al. The Veterans Administration Cooperative Study of stable angina: Current status. Circulation 1982; 65[Suppl II]:II60.
267. Detre K, et al. Long-term mortality and morbidity results of the Veterans Administration randomized trial of coronary artery bypass surgery. Circulation 1985; 72[Suppl V]:V84.
268. European Coronary Surgery Study Group. Coronary artery bypass surgery in stable angina pectoris: Survival at two years. Lancet 1979; 1:889.
269. European Coronary Surgery Study Group. Long-term results of prospective randomized study of cornary artery bypass surgery in stable angina pectoris. Lancet 1982; 2:1173.
270. Varnauskas E. Twelve-year follow-up of survival in the randomized European Coronary Surgery Study. N Engl J Med 1988; 319:332.
271. European Coronary Surgery Study Group. Prospective randomized study of coronary artery bypass surgery in stable angina pectoris: a progress report on survival. Circulation 1982; 65[Suppl II]:II67.
272. Pfeffer M, et al. Effect of captopril on mortality and morbidity in patients with left ventricular dysfunction after myocardial infarction. N Engl J Med 1992; 327:669.
273. Couper G, et al. Relative risks of left ventricular aneurysmectomy in patients with akinetic scars versus true dyskinetic aneurysms. Circulation 1990; 82[Suppl IV]:248.
274. Karp R, Mills N, Edmunds L. Coronary artery bypass grafting in the presence of valvular disease. Circulation 1989; 79[Suppl I]:I-182.
275. Babu S, et al. Coexisting carotid stenosis in patients undergoing cardiac surgery: Indications and guidelines for simultaneous operations. Am J Surg 1985; 150:207.
276. Solymoss B, et al. Late thrombosis of saphenous vein bypass grafts related to risk factors. Circulation 1988; 78[SuppII]:140.
277. Blankenhorn D, et al. Beneficial effects of combined colestipol-niacin therapy on coronary atherosclerosis and coronary venous bypass grafts. JAMA 1987; 257:3233.
278. Chesebro J, et al. Effect of dipyridamole and aspirin on late vein-graft patency after coronary bypass operations. N Engl J Med 1984; 310:209.
279. Henderson W, et al. Antiplatelet or anticoagulant therapy after coronary artery bypass surgery. A meta-analysis of clinical trials. Ann Intern Med 1989; 111:743.

Arterial Obstructive Diseases of the Extremities

Jonathan L. Halperin
Mark A. Creager

Epidemiology

INCIDENCE AND PREVALENCE

The most widely recognized peripheral vascular disease in adults is obstructive atherosclerosis of the extremities. The term **arteriosclerosis obliterans** rather archaically denotes the distinction between the normal aging process by which the arteries increase in diameter, rigidity, and calcium content [1,2] and the development of obstructive lesions, since the histopathology is identical to atherosclerosis that affects the aorta and its branches, including the coronary, visceral, cervical, and cerebral arteries. The disease was defined in 1958 by a committee of the World Health Organization as a "variable combination of changes of the intima of arteries (as distinguished from arterioles) consisting of the focal accumulation of lipids, complex carbohydrates, blood and blood products, fibrous tissue and calcium deposits, and associated with medial changes" [3]. The prevalence of chronic atherosclerotic disease of the lower limbs has been underestimated in the general population, because the process may exist undetected in subclinical form for many years before symptoms of ischemia arise. Indeed, by the time the initial symptoms of obstructive arterial disease develop, there is usually at least 50-percent narrowing of the vascular lumen with attendant morbidity and the associated mortality related to manifestations of coronary or cerebrovascular insufficiency. Fatty streaks occur in most of the general population from the age of 3 years, and aortic calcification has been identified in 10 percent of 40-year-old executives. At autopsy, the incidence of atherosclerosis is considerably higher.

Estimates of the prevalence of claudication in populations aged 45 to 70 years range from approximately 1 to 5 percent in men and from 1 to 2 percent in women [4–7]. In the 26-year longitudinal surveillance of the Framingham Heart Study cohort of 5,209 subjects, the annual incidence of symptomatic ischemic arterial obstructive disease was 2.6 per 1,000 men and 1.2 per 1,000 women [8]. In that population, the incidence increased with age until age 75 years, with about a twofold male predominance at all ages (Fig. 35-1). The peak incidence of symptomatic limb arterial obstructive disease occurred in males in the sixth and seventh decades of life. Like atherosclerosis in general, prevalence was related to hypertension, hypercholesterolemia, diabetes mellitus, and tobacco smoking, factors that modify the inexorable effects of age, gender, and heredity. In Framingham, fewer than 10 percent of nondiabetic cases younger than 60 years were female; beyond menopause, the incidence in women rose quickly toward that in men.

The overall prevalence of peripheral arterial obstructive disease increases substantially with age and greatly exceeds that estimated by symptoms of claudication. Indeed, the aged population frequently develops gangrene as the initial symptom rather than intermittent (exertional) claudication, in part because coexisting conditions such as arthritis, cardiopulmonary disease, and cerebrovascular disorders may limit ambulation.

As determined by noninvasive measurements, the prevalence of peripheral arterial obstructive disease is less than 3 percent in those under age 60 years but rises to greater than 20 percent in those older than age 75 years [4,9,10]. The relation of age to the prevalence of peripheral atherosclerosis has been confirmed by a number of studies. In women over 65 years, the prevalence is 5.5 percent, whereas in elderly men it is approximately 25 percent [11,12]. Examination of 261 elderly patients in Belgium (mean age 81 years) hospitalized for nonvascular conditions found a disease prevalence of 58 percent [13]. In an elderly population of 60 patients in a nursing home, the incidence of severe obstructive arterial disease was approximately 50 percent [14]. In another study of 75 patients aged 90 years or older, the second most common surgical operation was lower-extremity amputation for limb arterial disease or gangrene [15].

ASSOCIATED FACTORS

Epidemiologic factors associated with the development of atherosclerotic disease were identified well before results of the population-based Framingham Heart Study became available, but that project confirmed the independent risk contributed by age, gender, and family history and the relation to diabetes mellitus, hypertension, hyperlipidemia, cigarette smoking, obesity, and physical inactivity. It is sometimes difficult to separate data pertaining to atherosclerotic disease in the peripheral circulation from that on coronary circulation and to limit extrapolation from observations of coronary artery disease to the peripheral bed, but there is little reason to suspect a substantial difference in the impact of the various risk factors on the basis of the anatomic site of involvement [8,16].

In the absence of recognized etiologic agents, the epidemiologic concept of risk factors has emerged, but that should not imply causation. Specific risk factors for the development of atherosclerosis appear synergistic and better predict relative risk than absolute risk. Since the disease is heterogeneous in its clinical expression, the evaluation of epidemiologic data must take into account the method of diagnosis and the demographics of the population examined. Overall, a risk profile made up of the major cardiovascular risk factors better predicts intermittent claudication than do clinical manifestations of coronary heart disease.

Hyperlipidemia. A relation between dietary cholesterol and the development of atherosclerosis has been demon-

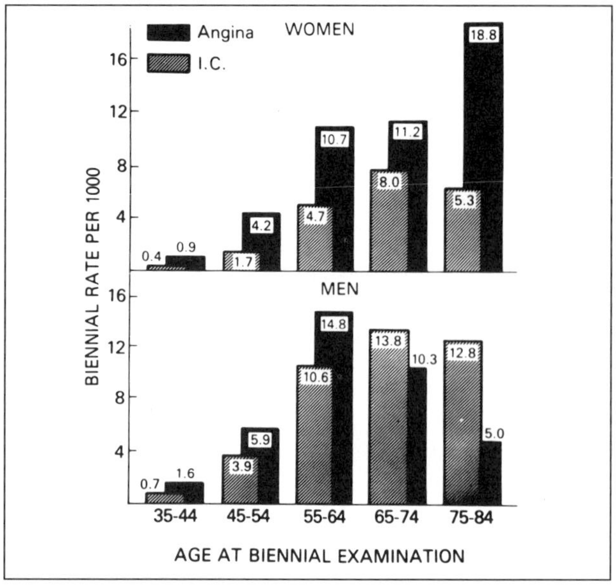

Fig. 35-1. The incidence of intermittent claudication (I.C.) observed during 26 years of longitudinal surveillance of the Framingham Heart Study cohort. Comparison is made with the incidence of angina pectoris. (Reproduced with permission from WB Kannel and DL McGee. Update on some epidemiologic features of intermittent claudication: the Framingham Study. J Am Geriatr Soc 1985; 33:13–18.)

strated in a number of animal species, but the biology of the disease in those models is not entirely identical to that in human beings. The association of hypercholesterolemia with atherosclerosis of the lower extremities has been known for over half a century [17]. The incidence of claudication in patients with serum cholesterol levels over 270 mg/dl averages over twice that in those without lipid elevations [8]. The relation of lipoprotein fractions to peripheral atherosclerosis has not been as convincingly demonstrated as that of coronary atherosclerosis, but patients with the most common forms of hyperlipoproteinemia, Frederickson types II and IV, are at increased risk of developing ischemic complications in the limbs [18,19]. In patients with type III hyperlipoproteinemia the increased incidence of premature atherosclerotic disease is even more pronounced in the vessels of the extremities than in the coronary circulation. This may be related to the presence of a specific apolipoprotein-E in these patients, which is not recognized by LDL-receptors on the surfaces of fibroblasts, smooth muscle cells, and parenchymal hepatic cells and that is responsible for lipid accumulation.

Diabetes Mellitus. Patients with diabetes mellitus develop more extensive and more rapidly progressive vascular disease than do nondiabetic individuals. A number of coexisting factors may contribute to atherogenesis in diabetes including dyslipidemia, hyperinsulinemia, protein glycation, and oxidant stresses. Yet, vascular disease in diabetics is both morphologically and physiologically distinguished from nondiabetic atherosclerosis. In practical terms, diabetes is associated with a high prevalence of distal arterial disease, a propensity to earlier calcification, increased thrombogenicity, an important interaction of ischemic tissues with the fundamental metabolic deficiency of the diabetic state, and generally poor prognosis. Coexisting sensory and autonomic neuropathy contributes to the clinical presentation of ischemic complications in diabetics and may produce ulcerative lesions even in the presence of a relatively normal arterial system. There is a particular predilection for the tibial and peroneal arteries, for which revascularization procedures often are more difficult [20–22]. The incidence of femoropopliteal arterial obstructive disease is similar to that in the nondiabetic population, and aortoiliac occlusive disease may actually occur less frequently in diabetics. The cumulative risk of amputation in individuals with diabetes approximates 11 percent over a 25-year period [23]. Patients with non-insulin-dependent diabetes mellitus have a 12-fold greater risk of below-knee amputation than nondiabetics [23].

The concept of diabetic vascular disease has been intertwined with the notion of microangiopathy because of the frequency with which diabetic patients seem to develop ischemic ulceration and gangrene despite the presence of relatively normal arterial pulses in the involved limbs. A specific small-vessel disease appears to contribute to the retinal, renal, and perhaps myocardial manifestations of diabetes, and periodic acid-Schiff staining material has been demonstrated in arteriolar lumens of amputation specimens obtained from diabetic patients [24]. Subsequent studies involving blinded histologic interpretation and more precise documentation of diabetic status failed to confirm those light microscopic observations, however, and the hyperemic responses to papaverine of the distal vascular beds of diabetic patients with limb atherosclerosis have demonstrated no impairment of arteriolar vasodilatation [20,25,26]. Hence, neither histologic nor physiologic studies have confirmed the occurrence of an occlusive microvascular disease in diabetics. Similarly, the notion that endothelial hyperplasia of the arterial intima develops in diabetics along the lines of a proliferative vasculopathy has not been supported in studies of either macroscopic branches or the capillary system [20,27,28]. Thickening of capillary basement membranes in skeletal muscle beds above the average normal value of 1,100 Å to about 1,400 Å in the latent phase of diabetes and 2,400 Å in overt diabetes was observed in over 90 percent of quadriceps biopsy specimens in one study. The abnormality of basement-membrane thickness might interfere with metabolic exchange at the level of the microcirculation in the skeletal muscle of diabetic patients. Meticulous control of blood glucose with insulin has been shown to decrease basement-membrane thickness [29]. In contrast to the observations in muscle tissue, capillary basement-membrane thickening has not been consistently demonstrated in skin biopsies [30,31]. Capillary hypertension and abnormal vascular permeability may account for the unique cutaneous manifestations of vascular disease in diabetics [32–37].

Peripheral neuropathy plays an important part in the development of foot complications in patients with diabetes as a result of involvement of myelinated nerve fibers of small diameter and unmyelinated nerve fibers [38,39].

Loss of both sensory and inflammatory function of unmyelinated nociceptive C fibers, as assessed by laser-Doppler flowmetry during axon reflex vasodilation has been demonstrated in patients with diabetic foot ulcers [40]. Lack of reflex hyperemia in the cutaneous vascular bed may contribute to the development of trophic lesions that occur in cases of small-fiber neuropathies, along with loss of pain sensation, autonomic dysfunction, and abnormal degrees of arteriovenous shunting [41–45].

Hypertension. Hypertensive patients show an increased incidence of atherosclerotic disease and its peripheral, coronary and cerebral complications [46–48]. Autopsy studies have demonstrated that hypertensive men have more extensive atherosclerosis of the aortoiliac arteries than age-matched normotensive controls [49]. In the Framingham Study, hypertension increased the risk of developing claudication over twofold in men and fourfold in women [8]. Hypertension is more frequently encountered in male patients with symptomatic aortoiliac and femoropopliteal atherosclerosis than in asymptomatic age-matched control patients [50].

The importance of hemodynamic forces in atherogenesis has been emphasized by some authors, and the theory has been invoked to explain the frequent occurrence of atherosclerotic lesions in Hunter's adductor canal and at the aortoiliac bifurcation [51–53]. Support for the concept that hypertension contributes directly to atherosclerotic obstruction of the extremity vasculature may be gleaned from reports based on angiographic examinations of operated limbs with peripheral arterial obstructive disease in which correction of proximal arterial stenoses accelerates the progression of distal disease [54]. The mechanism by which hypertension accelerates the atherosclerotic process is unknown, but thrombotic, metabolic, and vasomotor factors are thought to play roles. Vessels subjected to altered shear stress and elevated intraluminal pressure undergo changes in expression of adhesion molecules [55] and release a number of mitogens, which may stimulate proliferation of the vascular smooth muscle layer and alter the composition of the intercellular matrix.

Tobacco Smoking. The strong association between the use of tobacco, particularly cigarettes, and atherosclerosis of the extremities has been known for decades. Tobacco smoking contributes to the progression of the atherosclerotic process and the emergence of symptoms of ischemia. The Framingham Heart Study found a relation between the number of cigarettes smoked and the incidence of intermittent claudication [56], and multivariate analysis finds tobacco smoking the strongest single risk factor for development of symptomatic obstructive arterial disease regardless of gender. The occurrence of intermittent claudication is twice as frequent in smokers as in nonsmokers. In males with symptomatic atherosclerotic disease of the limb vessels, the majority report smoking cigarettes at the onset of the clinical phase of the disease. In women who smoke more than 20 cigarettes per day, the relative risk of developing aortic atherosclerosis is 2.3 [57]. Seventy-three to 90 percent of patients with limb arterial disease are smokers, such that it is distinctly rare to encounter a young female with the disease who does not smoke cigarettes. Clinical prognosis for those with arterial obstructive disease of the extremities also seems related to tobacco use. Observation of patients over a period of 5 years found that 11.4 percent of those who continued to smoke required amputation, while this fate befell none of those who quit [50].

Several components of tobacco smoke have been implicated in acceleration of the progression of atherosclerotic disease. Pathophysiologic mechanisms involve vasoconstrictor factors, effects on lipid metabolism, and thrombogenic effects [58]. Vasomotor effects are largely reproduced by intravenous administration of nicotine, in doses comparable to those delivered by use of most tobacco products. Sufficient absorption occurs, not only through inhalation of tobacco smoke but also across the oropharyngeal mucosa [59,60], to cause cutaneous vasoconstriction through stimulation of the sympathetic nervous system in chronic smokers, nonsmokers [61–64], and patients with arterial obstructive disease [65,66]. Carbon monoxide, another major component of tobacco smoke, increases the permeability of arterial endothelium for cholesterol [67]. Cigarette smoking may also increase serum lipid concentrations [68]. Adverse effects of tobacco smoking on endothelium-derived relaxing factor, prostaglandin metabolism, platelet aggregation, and thrombosis also have been reported [69].

Tobacco exposure has a specific etiologic role in the syndrome of **thromboangiitis obliterans** (Buerger's disease), which may be confused with atherosclerosis (see Chap. 44).

Heredity. Familial factors appear to increase the risk of atherosclerosis. Certain specific hereditary disorders are associated with ischemic complications in the limbs. Among these are homocysteinuria [70], oxalosis, inhibitors of von Willebrand factor, and inherited states associated with increased thrombogenicity, although the last more often cause venous than arterial disease.

Histopathology

Histologically, atherosclerotic disease of the arteries supplying the extremities resembles atheromatous disease affecting other parts of the body. The basic lesion is the atherosclerotic plaque, which consists mainly of fibrous tissue, smooth muscle cells, cholesterol, microphages, and platelets, producing localized stenosis of the lumen with or without areas of complete arterial obstruction. Deposition of thrombus and subsequently progressive fibrosis occur in eccentric layers. Fragmentation of the internal elastic lamina typically occurs along with the areas of intraplaque hemorrhage and calcification that characterize the advanced atherosclerotic lesion.

Segmental lesions usually produce stenosis or occlusion of large and medium-sized arteries. After the thoracoabdominal aorta, the coronary arteries are most commonly affected, followed in order of decreasing frequency by the iliofemoral, carotid, renal and mesenteric, vertebrobasilar, tibioperoneal, subclavian, brachial, radial, and ulnar arteries. Smaller arteries of the digits generally are spared even in advanced cases, though these may become obstructed by thrombus when there is atherosclerotic disease of more proximal segments. In patients with intermittent claudication, segmental involvement is not necessarily mutually exclusive, and patients may have disease at multiple arterial levels. In most cases (around 80 percent), femoropopliteal disease is present; approximately 30 percent of symptomatic patients have lesions at the aortoiliac level, and up to 40 percent have tibioperoneal obstruction. Involvement of the distal vessels is most frequent in diabetics and in elderly individuals. The peak age of occurrence of aortoiliac disease is in the sixth decade, earlier than that of femoropopliteal disease, which peaks in the seventh decade.

Natural History and Prognosis

The atherosclerotic lesion is characterized by wide variability in structure, biochemistry, progression, and regression. The clinical courses of patients with this disease also differ markedly, and the processes that mediate abrupt vascular occlusion in some cases and more favorable outcomes in others are incompletely understood. The segmental nature of atherosclerosis affecting the lower extremities leads to a syndromic approach to patient management, in part because the location of the stenotic segment bears a direct relationship to prognosis. In patients with aortoiliac disease, symptoms develop gradually, and a rather copious collateral circulation tends to develop. The prognosis generally is more favorable in terms of the outcome of the limbs in those patients. Patients with more distal tibioperoneal disease most often are diabetic, have a distinctly poorer outcome, and more frequently require amputation. The annual rate of amputation in patients with symptomatic arterial obstructive disease of the lower extremities treated without surgery is approximately 1.4 percent [71].

Followed without surgical intervention, the yearly mortality of these patients averages over 5 percent, and death is usually due to coronary or cerebral atherosclerotic disease. In the Framingham Heart Study, the relative mortality risk imposed by symptomatic peripheral arterial disease without cardiovascular comorbidity was 1.3 for men and 2.1 for women; the total mortality ratios were 2.2 and 4.1, respectively [16]. Hertzer et al. reported that the rate of coronary heart disease in patients with severely symptomatic peripheral arterial obstructive disease was nearly 90 percent, the disease defined angiographically in patients as more than 70-percent stenosis of at least one coronary vessel; about 50 percent of patients had decreased left ventricular function [72]. Epidemiologic studies have documented that patients with intermittent claudication or other clinical evidence of peripheral arterial occlusive disease carry a two- to threefold increased risk of cardiovascular mortality in comparison with age-matched controls without symptomatic limb arterial disease followed over a number of years [73–77].

Remissions of intermittent claudication are not uncommon. Among the patients in the Framingham Study followed 4 or more years from the onset of symptoms, 45 percent had disappearance of symptoms for at least 4 years [78]. In nondiabetic patients followed at the Mayo Clinic with obstructive disease of the superficial femoral artery, 24 percent improved and another 69 percent had no progression of symptoms; clinical deterioration occurred in only 7 percent [79]. Others have found the course similar, with 79 percent of patients stable after 2.5 years regardless of the severity of symptoms at outset [71]. Each year, approximately 5 percent of all patients with intermittent claudication develop severe ischemia or require surgery [80]. In some cases, a salutary outcome may be a matter of adopting a more sedentary life within the bounds of vascular reserve, a lack of vitality imposed by associated cardiovascular disease, or compensatory development of collateral circulation in the affected limbs; in other cases, regression of the atherosclerotic lesions may occur.

Clinical Presentation

INTERMITTENT CLAUDICATION

The primary symptom of obstructive arterial disease in the lower extremities is intermittent claudication. Typically, patients describe calf pain, since the gastrocnemius musculature has the highest oxygen consumption of any muscle group in the leg during activity of ambulation and tends to develop symptomatic ischemia earliest. Rather than pain, however, some patients report vague aching discomfort, heaviness, fatigue, or numbness when walking, but, regardless of form, distress is usually relieved within a few minutes of rest. Patients with distal tibial or peroneal arterial obstruction, often diabetics, may describe ankle or foot pain while walking, but it is difficult in such cases to distinguish the symptom of muscular ischemia from the ischemic neuropathy that frequently occurs in this setting. In cases of more proximal obstruction, such as that which occurs in aortoiliac occlusive disease, thigh, hip or buttock claudication may develop, or even low back pain while walking, but this usually has been preceded by calf pain. Proximal symptoms of claudication, impotency and global atrophy of the lower extremities characterize a classic presentation of aortoiliac obstructive disease, designated **Leriche syndrome.**

Multiple factors contribute to the onset of leg discomfort during exercise in patients with arterial occlusive disease. Hemodynamically significant stenosis of a limb artery may reduce pressure and flow minimally at rest. During exercise, however, a stenosis attenuates flow augmentation and the pressure gradient across the stenosis increases. Normally, increased blood flow, such as what occurs in response to exercise, results in dilation of conduit vessels. This is thought to be produced by release of endothelium-derived vasodilator substances [81,82]. In atherosclerotic vessels, however, flow-mediated vasodilation does not occur [83]. This may further blunt flow augmentation during exercise in the limbs of patients with arterial obstructive disease. Decline in distal vascular resistance mediated by the action of catecholamines on regional beta-adrenergic receptors and by autoregulatory processes further reduces perfusion pressure. These autoregulatory mechanisms are not well defined but probably involve adenosine, endothelium-derived relaxing and hyperpolarizing factors, prostaglandins, local acidemia, and hypoxemia. Furthermore, extravascular compressive forces in the closed compartments of the limb imposed by exercis-

Table 35-1. Causes of limb artery obstruction

Atherosclerosis
Acute arterial occlusion
Thrombus
Embolism
Dissection
Trauma
Fibromuscular dysplasia
Vasculitis
Thromboangiitis obliterans
Takayasu arteritis
Giant-cell arteritis
Arterial entrapment
Adventitial cysts or tumors

Table 35-2. Causes of exertional leg pain

Atherosclerotic arterial occlusive disease
Nonatherosclerotic arterial occlusive disease
Arterial embolism
Vasculitis
Thromboangiitis obliterans
Giant-cell arteritis
Fibromuscular dysplasia
Extravascular compressive lesion
Arterial entrapment syndrome
Adventitial cysts, tumors
Skeletal disorders
Lumbosacral radiculopathy (neurogenic pseudoclaudication)
Spinal stenosis; herniated disk
Arthritis of hips, knees
Muscular disorders
Myositis
McArdle syndrome
Venous claudication
Chronic venous insufficiency

ing muscle further depress leg blood flow. The discomfort that ensues may be related to activation of local sensory receptors due to accumulation of lactate or other metabolites.

Initial and absolute claudication thresholds involve time as well as distance and are best expressed in terms of pace and incline. Ambient environmental conditions such as temperature and wind seem to affect exercise performance. Training effect and recruitment of muscle groups in less ischemic zones improve walking capacity. Activities other than ambulation, such as swimming, bicycling, or mounting stairs, call on other muscle groups of the lower extremities, which may be differentially affected by proximal obstructive arterial lesions, producing substantial differences in functional capacity. These factors are important not only in clinical assessment, they also have therapeutic implications in maintaining overall cardiovascular conditioning in patients beset by atherosclerotic disease affecting isolated body parts.

Obstructive arterial diseases other than atherosclerosis that may produce intermittent claudication are discussed later in this chapter and are listed in Table 35-1. These diseases include arterial occlusion caused by thrombus or emboli, thromboangiitis obliterans and various other arteritides (see Chaps. 43 and 44), arterial entrapment syndromes (most commonly caused by the gastrocnemius or pectoralis muscles), fibromuscular dysplasia, adventitial cysts and tumors, and extravascular compressive lesions.

Exertional calf pain also may be produced by conditions unrelated to the arterial circulation (Table 35-2). Among these is neurogenic pseudoclaudication, actually a form of lumbosacral radiculopathy akin to sciatica, in which ambulation provokes nerve root irritation with pain referred to the posterior aspect of the lower extremity; either the calf alone or the foot, heel, ankle, thigh, hip, or buttock may be involved [84,85]. In the clinical history, a clue may be the occurrence of pain when walking rather short distances, such as between rooms of a home or even just a few steps, without progression to ischemic pain at rest, ulceration, or gangrene; or if pain occurs simply on standing without walking, which is unusual in true ischemic disease in the absence of tissue compromise. Relief of discomfort on hyperextending the low back is also suggestive of this diagnosis, particularly when associated with spinal stenosis. Physical examination may point to neurogenic pseudoclaudication when symptoms are reproduced by straight leg raising or manual pressure over the sciatic notch of the iliac crest, whether or not there is an arterial pulse deficit.

Venous claudication is of interest mainly because it illustrates the role of venous pressure as a factor in regional circulatory resistance. This syndrome of exertional leg pain (manifest especially near the medial aspect of the leg above the ankle) results when there is incompetence of deep venous valves with insufficiency of the musculovenous pumping mechanism. This mechanism normally produces a substantial decline in distal venous pressure during ambulation, but in cases of deep venous insufficiency venous pressure may become strikingly elevated instead. Venous hypertension then becomes an important factor contributing to local vascular resistance, and exertional ischemia may result. The syndrome of venous claudication is neither common nor subtle, and a component of arterial insufficiency is usually present simultaneously in these patients [86].

McArdle syndrome of skeletal muscle phosphorylase deficiency points out the importance of accumulation of certain tissue metabolites in evoking the symptoms responsible for exercise intolerance even in the absence of an anatomic substrate capable of producing ischemia [87]. It is believed that similar metabolites, including but not limited to lactic acid, develop in cases of obstructive arterial disease and are responsible for the pain of intermittent claudication.

ISCHEMIA AT REST

When perfusion is reduced sufficiently that it fails to meet even the minimal nutritional requirements of resting skin, muscle, nerves, and bone, then ischemic rest pain, ulceration, and gangrene ensue. Clinically, ischemia in the limb at rest generally is manifested first in the cutaneous tissues of the foot. The factors regulating cutaneous circulation differ from the processes governing muscle perfusion in the calf. Reflexive sympathetically mediated vasoconstrictor activity may further reduce foot blood flow even under conditions of ischemia.

As tissue necrosis develops, there typically is severe pain in the region of skin breakdown, worse at night with limb elevation and gravitationally improved on standing. In the setting of advanced neuropathy, even ulceration and gangrene may produce little or no pain, though there may be a vaguely described urge to maintain the limb dependent with reference to the level of the heart. Patients not infrequently spend nights sitting on the edge of the bed, dangling the legs below to alleviate pain. Other symptoms of ischemia at rest include hypesthesia, cold sensitivity, muscular weakness, joint stiffness, and contracture.

Severe ischemia of this kind usually demands angiographic examination with a view toward revascularization using either angioplasty or surgical techniques. When such therapy is not feasible, gangrene commonly ensues, leading either to spontaneous or surgical amputation, though remission has been described even at this advanced stage of disease [88].

Physical Findings. Examination begins with inspection of the limbs for trophic signs of chronic low-grade ischemia (subcutaneous atrophy, brittle toenails, hair loss, pallor, coolness, or dependent rubor), sympathetic denervation (absence of regional sweating and disorganization of the hair pattern due to piloerector involvement), and signs of sensorimotor neuropathy (impaired perception of vibration and fine touch and diminished deep tendon reflexes). Severe tissue ischemia produces petechiae, regional edema, tenderness, ulceration, and gangrene. Palpation of the femoral, popliteal, posterior tibial, and dorsalis pedis pulses allows estimation of the level of arterial obstruction when taken in conjunction with auscultation of the abdomen and groins for arterial bruits. These regional systolic murmurs denote the presence of turbulent flow and imply arterial disease but do not necessarily indicate that stenosis is hemodynamically significant.

Cutaneous perfusion pressure may be estimated by assessing the color and temperature of the feet during elevation above the level of the heart, at rest and following gastrocnemius muscle exercise. Standardized observations correlate fairly closely with objective measurements of distal pressure made in the laboratory. Next, collateral perfusion can be gauged on dependency by timing the hyperemic return of color to the skin of the foot and the development of venous refilling (unless the latter is accelerated by concomitant venous insufficiency). This provides a rather crude but dependable index of flow in physiologic terms along the dimensions of blood volume, tissue mass, and time.

When collateral perfusion is inadequate to meet minimal tissue perfusion requirements, cutaneous ulceration is a frequent finding [83]. Ulcers caused by arterial disease typically are painful, especially with elevation, and tend to be more bothersome at night than during the daytime.

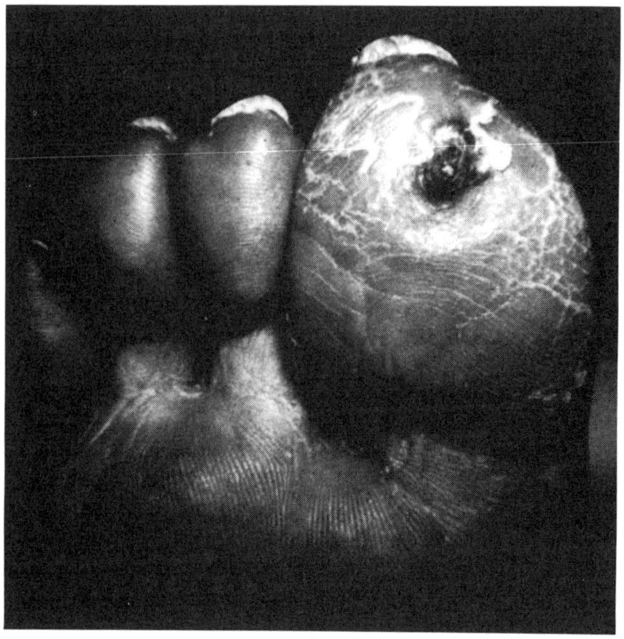

Fig. 35-2. Arterial ulcer on volar aspect of great toe in a patient with severe peripheral atherosclerotic occlusive disease.

The ulcers usually involve the tips of the toes or the heel of the foot, unless pressure necrosis plays a contributory role. Arterial ulcers often are as small as 3 to 5 mm in diameter, with irregular borders and a pale base. The clinical course of these ulcers is often one of rapid progression to more extensive gangrene (Fig. 35-2).

CATEGORIZATION OF LIMB ISCHEMIA

The severity of limb ischemia varies considerably among patients with peripheral arterial occlusive disease. Categorization of the clinical manifestations of limb ischemia enables communication among professionals caring for patients and provides a framework for defining indications for therapeutic interventions and assessing response to treatment. A classic categorization was described by Fontaine, but its utility is limited in contemporary management of patients with limb ischemia (Table 35-3). Patients were categorized into four stages, ranging from the asymptomatic patients to the patients with tissue necrosis. Rutherford has proposed a more descriptive and practical classification, which has been adopted by a number of

Table 35-3. Fontaine classification

Stage	Symptoms
I	Asymptomatic
II	Intermittent claudication
IIa	Pain-free, claudication walking > 200 m
IIb	Pain-free, claudication walking < 200 m
III	Rest and nocturnal pain
IV	Necrosis, gangrene

Table 35-4. Clinical categories of chronic limb ischemia

Grade	Category	Clinical description
	0	Asymptomatic, not hemodynamically correct
I	1	Mild claudication
	2	Moderate claudication
	3	Severe claudication
II	4	Ischemic rest pain
	5	Minor tissue loss: nonhealing ulcer, focal gangrene with diffuse pedal ischemia
III	6	Major tissue loss extending above transmetatarsal level, functional foot no longer salvageable

Adapted from Rutherford RB, et al. Suggested standards for reports dealing with lower extremity ischemia. J Vasc Surg 1986; 4:80–94.

Table 35-5. Sources of cardioembolism

Cause	Frequency (%)
Rheumatic heart disease	10
Prosthetic cardiac valves	10
Nonvalvular atrial fibrillation	45
Left ventricular aneurysm	10
Acute myocardial infarction	15
Other	10

professional vascular societies [89,90]. Symptoms, physical findings, perfusion pressure, pulse-volume recordings, and exercise capacity all contribute to the assignment to one of four grades in seven categories, which include: asymptomatic; mild, moderate, and severe claudication; rest pain; and minor and major tissue loss (Table 35-4).

Acute Arterial Occlusion

Acute arterial occlusion often presents as the sudden onset of severe limb ischemia. Its causes include thrombosis, embolism, dissection, and trauma. Thrombosis *in situ* typically develops in vessels already affected by atherosclerosis, a situation not unlike that which causes myocardial infarction in patients with coronary atherosclerosis. Acute thrombus formation also occurs in bypass grafts, typically at sites where flow is disrupted, including anastomoses, strictures, and retained valve cusps. Less frequently, procoagulant disorders may precipitate thrombus in an otherwise normal vessel. These disorders include heparin-induced thrombocytopenia; homocysteinuria; antiphospholipid antibody syndrome; and protein C, protein S, and antithrombin III deficiency. The last three are more likely to cause venous thrombosis. The severity of limb ischemia depends, in part, on the presence of collateral vessels. If thrombus were to occur in a stenosed atherosclerotic vessel, it is likely that adequate collateral vessels would be present to maintain blood flow and prevent severe ischemia.

Arterial embolism from a proximal source is the most common cause of acute arterial occlusion. Nearly 85 percent of systemic arterial emboli arise from thrombi in the chambers of the left side of the heart (Table 35-5). Atrial fibrillation accounts for about half of the cases, including patients with valvular heart disease, congestive heart failure, hypertension, and coronary artery disease. Infective endocarditis and prosthetic heart valves are additional sources of cardiac thromboembolism. Left ventricular thrombus, occurring after acute myocardial infarction or following aneurysm formation, also is a relatively common cause of arterial embolism. Cardiac tumors, usually left atrial myxomas, infrequently are a cause of embolism. A "paradoxical" embolus, originating from venous thrombosis, may enter the systemic circulation via a patent foramen ovale or an atrial or ventricular septal defect and occlude a limb artery. Noncardiac sources of thromboembolism include aneurysms in the aorta and the iliac, femoral, popliteal, and subclavian arteries. Acute arterial occlusion caused by embolism frequently occurs at branch points, where vessels narrow in size. The most common site of arterial embolism is the femoral bifurcation, followed by the popliteal trifurcation and the aortic and iliac bifurcations. Since collateral vessels typically are not present, the abrupt cessation of blood flow to the extremity is likely to produce severe limb ischemia. Emboli from atherosclerotic plaque usually affect small branch vessels and not major arteries and are discussed in the following section on atheroembolism.

Aortic dissection may obstruct branch vessels to the upper and lower extremities, as discussed in Chap. 40. Arterial dissection also may occur during diagnostic and interventional catheterization procedures. Penetrating injuries resulting from gunshot wounds or stabbings may lacerate the vessel, providing a nidus for thrombus formation. Vessel injury also may occur following fractures. Blunt trauma may disrupt the vessel, inducing endothelial injury or altering flow dynamics sufficient to incite thrombus formation.

The clinical presentation of severe limb ischemia resulting from acute arterial occlusion includes pain, pallor, pulselessness, paresthesias, and paralysis, the so-called **five Ps.** Not all these symptoms are necessarily present. Most often, patients will experience pain in the affected extremity below the level of occlusion. Pallor is evident to the examiner, and a reduction in skin temperature can be appreciated by palpation. The color and temperature changes occur distal to the level of obstruction. The location of pulselessness provides insight into the site of occlusion; proximal to the occlusion, the pulse may be bounding. With severe ischemia, the patient complains of paresthesias and has impaired sensation to light touch and position, which may progress to complete anesthesia. With prolonged severe ischemia, motor function deteriorates and paralysis develops. The skin becomes white or marbled. Ultimately, skin breakdown, ulceration, and gangrene ensue.

The diagnosis usually is established from the clinical presentation. Angiography may not be necessary to con-

Table 35-6. Clinical categories of acute limb ischemia

Category	Description	Capillary return	Muscle weakness	Sensory loss
Viable	Not immediately threatened	Intact	None	None
Threatened	Salvageable if promptly treated	Intact, slow	Mild, partial	Mild, incomplete
Irreversible	Major tissue loss, amputation regardless of treatment	Absent (marbling)	Profound, paralysis (rigor)	Profound, anesthetic

Adapted from Rutherford RB, et al. Suggested standards for reports dealing with lower extremity ischemia. J Vasc Surg 1986; 4:80–94.

firm acute arterial occlusion and may result in delay of treatment. If the diagnosis is unclear, arteriography will demonstrate the site and the nature of the acute arterial occlusion and often may distinguish thrombosis in situ from arterial embolism. The former typically has occurred in an atherosclerotic vessel, while the latter tends to be present at bifurcation sites and is characterized by an abrupt cutoff of radiocontrast in an otherwise normal vessel. Multiple filling defects may be evident following an embolism.

It is important to assess the severity of limb ischemia as rapidly as possible and institute restorative interventions. Rutherford *et al.* have proposed clinical categories of acute limb ischemia to distinguish a viable limb from one that is threatened but salvageable from one that is irreversibly damaged [89,90] (see Table 35-6). A limb that is threatened yet viable requires urgent treatment. Irreversible changes may occur as early as 4 to 6 hours after acute arterial occlusion. Revascularization for severe limb ischemia, if delayed 8 to 12 hours, is less likely to result in limb salvage.

Acute limb ischemia requires urgent revascularization. For arterial emboli, this is usually accomplished with a Fogarty embolectomy catheter (as discussed later in this chapter), by surgical revascularization (see Chap. 29), or on occasion by intra-arterial thrombolysis (see Chap. 32).

Atheroembolism

Microembolism of atherosclerotic debris consisting of lipid and thrombotic material may originate from the aorta or more distal arteries and lead to occlusion of small distal limb arteries (Fig. 35-3). The source may involve either aneurysmal disease or irregular ulceration of diffusely atherosclerotic vessels that are not dilated. The ischemic syndrome produced may be analogous to transient cerebral ischemic attacks involving the brain, which arise from microembolism of atherothrombotic material from the internal carotid arteries.

The clinical picture is often called **blue-toe syndrome** and is characterized by unilaterally or bilaterally painful, cyanotic toes in the presence of palpable pedal pulses [91] (Fig. 35-4). The lateral and plantar aspects of the feet

Fig. 35-3. Segment of abdominal aorta excised at autopsy in a patient who had atheroemboli. Note the characteristic appearance of atherosclerosis. Friable areas consisting of fatty deposits and fibrinous debris are apparent.

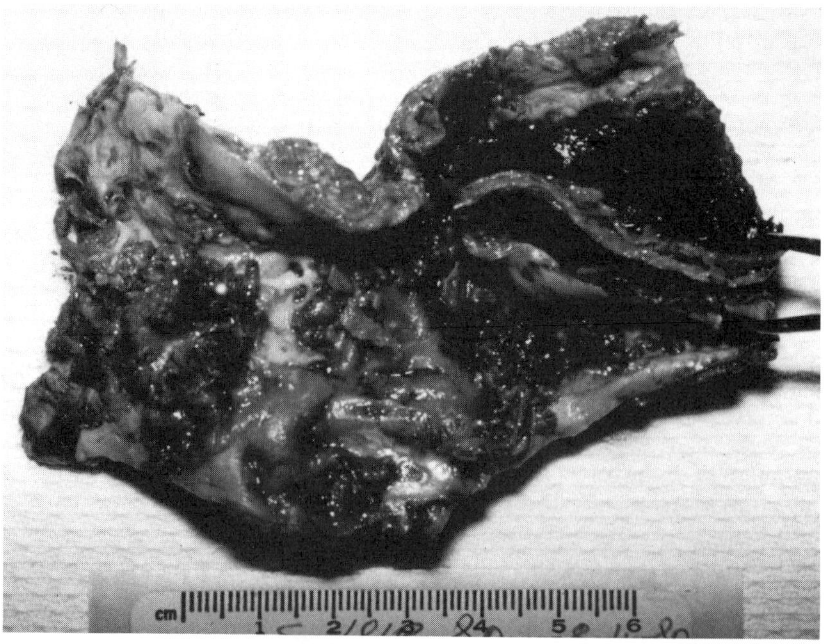

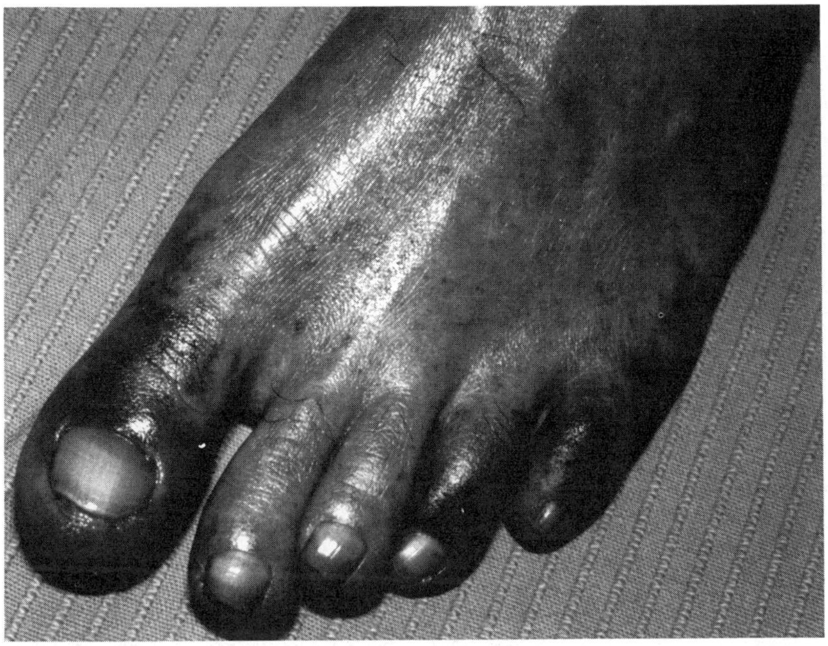

Fig. 35-4. Atheroemboli resulting in ischemic damage to several toes. There are multiple petechiae. Note the area of livedo reticularis along the lateral aspect of the foot.

frequently are involved, associated with livedo reticularis and petechiae on the feet and legs. The violet-colored parts generally blanch with pressure, and the surrounding skin may appear normally perfused. Calf pain and gastrocnemius-muscle tenderness often are present as a result of embolic occlusion of small intramuscular vessels. Fever, eosinophilia, and acceleration of the erythrocyte sedimentation rate may signal an inflammatory reaction to microembolization; in those cases, it may be difficult to distinguish the syndrome from acute vasculitis, such as polyarteritis nodosum.

Most cases of recognized atheroembolism involve male patients over 50 years of age. Often clinical embolic ischemia is provoked by arterial catheterization, which may be transient or recurrent and persistent. Definitive diagnosis requires skin or muscle biopsy, but the toes themselves should be avoided for that purpose because of the risk of creating nonhealing ulcers. The skin of more proximal portions of the limb or gastrocnemius muscle often is chosen to demonstrate the characteristic elongated, needle-shaped clefts in small arteries that are associated with inflammatory infiltration, intimal thickening, perivascular fibrosis, and lipid-laden giant cells.

The occurrence of atheroembolism implies a physically unstable proximal atherosclerotic lesion, and the risk of acute thrombotic arterial occlusion is relatively high in those cases. Antithrombotic therapy should be given in the form of platelet-inhibitor or anticoagulant medication [91–93], although it is not established that these treatments are effective in preventing recurrent atheroemboli. In patients already receiving warfarin, it may be necessary to distinguish the disorder from the cutaneous necrosis syndrome, which sometimes occurs in patients with protein C deficiency who are given that agent. It is not known whether thrombolytic medication will reduce or aggravate the embolic process. Although angioplasty has been reported effective, the intravascular catheterization also may provoke embolic phenomena, and the most definitive approach is to remove or exclude the source from the circulation [94–96]. When the lower limbs are ischemic, that approach often requires aortobifemoral bypass, but an alternative is axillobifemoral extra-anatomic bypass with ligation of the external iliac arteries proximal to the point of anastomosis. When renal emboli occur, more proximal aortic reconstruction may be necessary, the risks of which are considerable, particularly when there is severe atherosclerosis of the entire length of the aorta accompanied by a malignant syndrome of cerebral, mesenteric, and limb ischemia [92].

Fibromuscular Dysplasia

Fibromuscular dysplasia is a hyperplastic disorder that primarily involves medium-sized and small arteries, usually affecting white females. The renal and carotid arteries most frequently are involved, but fibromuscular dysplasia also has been described in the mesenteric, coronary, subclavian, and iliac arteries. Three histologic varieties—intimal, medial, and periadventitial dysplasia—have been delineated based on which layer of the arterial wall displays the predominant features of the process, with medial fibroplasia the most common type [97]. Histologically, there may be extensive hyperplasia of the media with or without fibrosis or effacement of the elastic membrane. Medial fibroplasia is characterized angiographically by a "string-of-beads" appearance, in which multiple thickened fibromuscular ridges alternate with areas in which

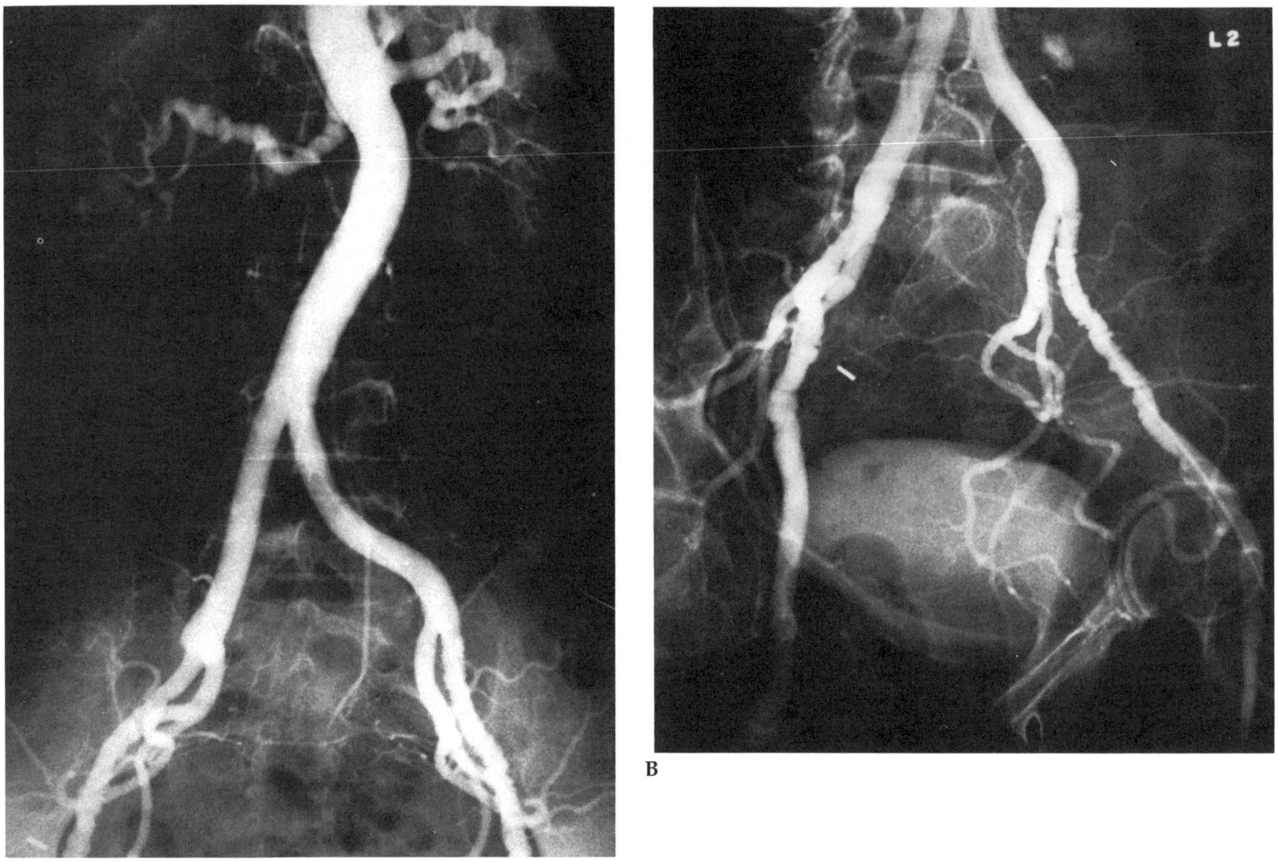

A B

Fig. 35-5. Angiograms demonstrating fibromuscular dysplasia affecting the renal arteries **(A)** and the external iliac arteries **(B)** in a 40-year-old woman. Note the "string-of-beads" appearance that is characteristic of this disorder.

the arterial wall is thin (Fig. 35-5). In adults, fibromuscular dysplasia of the intima is angiographically indistinguishable from the medial type, although in younger patients intimal lesions tend to produce longer, more tubular stenosis compared with the short, beaded configuration of medial fibroplasia. Histologically, intimal fibroplasia is distinguished from other arterial diseases by the preservation of the internal elastic lamina and the absence of inflammation or lipid accumulation unless there is superimposed atherosclerosis. Periadventitial fibroplasia is distinctly rare, characterized by collagenous encasement of the outer surface of the arterial wall and adhesion to surrounding tissues, which may be accompanied by infiltration of lymphocytes or plasma cells.

The etiology of fibromuscular dysplasia is unknown, but pathogenetic concepts include influence of female sex hormones, vascular microtrauma, ischemia of the vessel wall, and genetic factors [98]. The natural history of the disorder is less well defined in limb arteries than in the renal and carotid arteries, where progression of stenosis occurs in at least one-third of cases followed for 5 years [99] but where regression has been occasionally observed [100]. The development of superimposed atherosclerotic changes may be an important factor contributing to prognosis.

Clinical manifestations are similar to those of atherosclerosis, with intermittent claudication, rest pain, coldness and cyanosis of the limb, and even features suggestive of microembolism [101,102]. Surgical reconstruction and percutaneous angioplasty have been employed for management of fibromuscular dysplasia. Balloon dilatation has been successfully accomplished in the renal arteries, with relatively low inflation pressures in cases of beaded medial fibroplasia, whereas focal fibromuscular stenoses of the intimal or periadventitial varieties reportedly are more resistant to that approach [103,104]. There has been little experience with such an approach in the management of fibroplastic stenoses of the iliac or subclavian arteries.

Popliteal-Artery Entrapment

Popliteal-artery entrapment results from the congenital anomaly in which the medial head of the gastrocnemius muscle displaces or compresses (or both) the popliteal artery. Normally, the popliteal artery descends alongside the popliteal vein between the medial and lateral heads of the gastrocnemius muscle. Popliteal-artery entrapment can occur if that relationship is altered such that the artery passes medial and beneath the insertion of the medial head of the gastrocnemius muscle. Occasionally, the popliteal artery is entrapped by the popliteus muscle or by fibrous bands.

Popliteal-artery entrapment should be considered in the differential diagnosis of a young patient who presents with symptoms of intermittent claudication. In one series, 5 of 1,200 patients presenting with symptoms of claudication had popliteal-artery entrapment [105]. An important note is that those 5 were among a group of only 12 patients under the age of 30. Popliteal-artery entrapment affects males to a much greater extent than females and is unilateral in two-thirds of cases [106]. The majority of patients present with symptoms of claudication. Other presenting symptoms include paresthesias or rest pain; the presentation may suggest acute arterial embolism.

A number of noninvasive diagnostic tests provide supporting evidence for the diagnosis. Both passive dorsiflexion of the ankle or plantar flexion against resistance causes the gastrocnemius muscle to compress the popliteal artery. This can be demonstrated either by ankle pressure measurements or a pulse-volume recording obtained during the maneuvers. Duplex ultrasonography is useful for demonstrating compression of the popliteal artery and cessation of flow during those maneuvers. Angiography is used to demonstrate the altered course of the popliteal artery and may demonstrate popliteal-artery thrombosis as well as poststenotic dilatation. Once identified, popliteal-artery entrapment should be treated surgically. The operation is designed to eliminate compression of the artery and usually involves transection of the medial head of the gastrocnemius muscle or, if indicated, the popliteus muscle or a fibrous band. Occasionally, thrombectomy or bypass with a vein graft is indicated.

Noninvasive Laboratory Evaluation

A comprehensive discussion of noninvasive testing for evaluation of arterial obstructive disease is presented in Chap. 19. Salient aspects applicable to clinical assessment of patients are briefly reviewed here.

BEDSIDE INSTRUMENTATION

The clinical examination is readily supplemented by Doppler-velocity stethoscopy and sphygmomanometry, which have become standard parts of the initial examination of the vascular-disease patient at the bedside. The Doppler-ultrasound stethoscope is employed in conjunction with a standard brachial-sized sphygmomanometric cuff for determination of the ankle-to-arm systolic blood pressure index. The cuff is placed around the ankle, and the Doppler stethoscope is used to detect pulsatile arterial blood flow over the dorsalis pedis or posterior tibial arteries or beneath the plantar arterial arch. The cuff then is inflated to the point at which arterial pulsations become obliterated; that point is registered as the systolic arterial pressure at the level of cuff application (not at the level of flow detection with the Doppler probe). Here, the Doppler device serves principally as a flow detector; its use is largely obviated if arterial pulses are palpable or if sounds

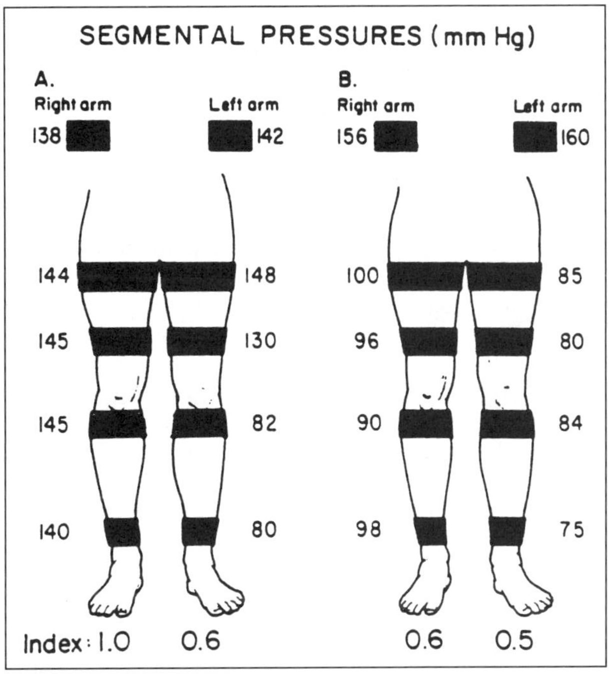

Fig. 35-6. Serial placement of pneumatic cuffs along the lower extremities is used to measure systolic pressure over multiple segments.

of Korotkoff can be identified by auscultation with the conventional stethoscope.

Normally, systolic arterial pressure at the ankle equals or exceeds that obtained by the same method over the brachial artery, because both systolic pressure and pulse pressure tend to increase as the pulse wave propagates from the heart. An ankle-to-arm systolic pressure ratio (tibial-brachial index) less than unity at rest indicates hemodynamically significant arterial obstruction proximal to the leg cuff. Advanced, calcific atherosclerotic changes in vessels directly beneath the pneumatic cuff may resist compression, producing overestimation of regional perfusion pressure. This constitutes the major limitation of sphygmomanometry and may lead to falsely elevated tibial-brachial pressure indices. The physician must be particularly alert to this possibility in patients with diabetes mellitus, even when glucose intolerance is comparatively mild; patients with chronic renal failure also are prone to arterial calcification.

SEGMENTAL PRESSURE MEASUREMENT

To localize one or more segmental arterial lesions, pneumatic cuffs are applied to various points on the limb to determine systolic pressure at several levels (Fig. 35-6). The principle is that obstruction must be proximal to the level at which pressure drops. In most laboratories, a pulse sensor is employed in conjunction with automatically inflatable segmental pressure cuffs for that purpose. Segmental pressure measurements typically are obtained in both lower extremities along with pulse-volume recordings. Pressure is determined at the site of the proximal occluding cuff when its pressure obliterates the pulse detected with the distal sensor. Data may be interpreted in terms of the pressure gradient between two adjacent sites in an extremity, by comparing the values in opposite limbs, or by calculating of the pressure ratio with reference to brachial systolic readings. After resting values have been obtained, the patient can exercise by walking on a treadmill, following which the cuffs are quickly reconnected to the inflation system and the recorder.

In general, segmental pressure measurements made in this fashion are subject to the same limitations as Doppler sphygmomanometry at the ankle. In addition, it is important to recognize that thigh pressure measurements may underestimate pressure in the common femoral artery, falsely suggesting arterial obstruction at aortoiliac level. In such cases, Doppler velocity waveforms obtained from the femoral artery at the groin appear normal. On the other hand, normal pressures at the level of the thigh cuff do not exclude significant stenosis in either the profunda femoris or the superficial femoral arteries. In general, ankle-to-arm systolic pressure indices over 0.85 may occur in individuals with obstructive disease in the absence of symptoms; values between 0.5 and 0.8 are typical at rest in patients with intermittent claudication, and values below 0.5 frequently are associated with ischemic rest pain, ulceration, and gangrene threatening the viability of the limb. In part because of arterial rigidity, systolic ankle pressures may be high in patients with diabetes mellitus even when limb loss is threatened.

Just as arterial pulses may remain palpable distally in patients with severe proximal arterial obstructive lesions, so the systolic pressure and the tibial-brachial index may appear in the normal range at rest. The single most sensitive test for hemodynamically significant arterial stenosis is a decline in the pressure index following exercise of the calf muscles, which usually remains below the baseline (resting) value for several minutes. Indeed, with the exception of cases of vascular noncompressibility, this test stands as one of the simplest, most effective means of screening for hemodynamically significant arterial obstructive disease. Postexercise systolic pressure readings below 90 mm Hg are typical of patients with intermittent claudication, and values below 60 mm Hg usually are encountered in patients with ulcerative ischemia at rest.

PULSE-VOLUME RECORDINGS

The quantitative segmental pneumatic plethysmograph is widely employed in conjunction with pressure measurements to monitor arterial wall motion indirectly. The amplitude of the pulse-volume recording reflects local arterial pressure, vascular wall compliance, the number of arterial vessels beneath the cuff, and the severity of atherosclerotic disease. The normal pulse is characterized by a sharp systolic upstroke, rises rapidly to a peak, and then drops off more slowly toward the baseline. The downslope is curved toward the baseline and usually contains a more or less prominent dicrotic notch and secondary wave about midway between the peak and the baseline. This dicrotic wave apparently is caused by the reflection of the arterial pulse from the periphery. The pulse recorded distal to an arterial obstruction differs in several ways: the general shape is more rounded, the anacrotic slope is reduced, the crest is delayed, the catacrotic limb descends more gradually, and the dicrotic (reflected diastolic) wave is lost.

Segmental compression cuffs combined with the Doppler-ultrasound device, photoplethysmograph, or other flow detector are subject to error related to arterial rigidity, but the pulse-volume recorder, using either pneumatic cuffs or mercury-in-Silastic strain gauges to reflect arterial wall motion, has the advantage of revealing distortions in pulse-wave contour even in patients with vascular calcification. The pulse waveforms appear depressed and altered even when arteries are noncompressible. The pulsatility index, which represents the ratio of pulse amplitude to mean volume obtained by integration of the deflection, is abnormally low even when systolic pressure readings are falsely elevated [91].

PLETHYSMOGRAPHY

Venous occlusion plethysmography using either volume-displacement or segmental strain-gauge apparatus has been in use longer than most other methods currently employed in clinical vascular diagnostic laboratories, and the technique remains the standard for measurement of perfusion in a portion of a limb. Nevertheless, its major application is in physiologic studies of vasomotor activity, since isolated measurements of resting blood flow are not helpful in distinguishing normal limbs from those with significant obstructive lesions. Flow measurements become depressed at rest only when ischemia is fairly advanced and vasodilator reserve has been exhausted [107]. Recovery of perfusion after exercise and postischemic reactive hyperemia approximate maximum vasodilatation and effectively differentiate normal from impaired circulation [108]. The methodology is cumbersome and used mainly to assess collateral resistance and hemorrheologic variables affecting treatment.

DOPPLER VELOCITY SPECTROSCOPY

Instead of pulse-volume recordings, some laboratories employ Doppler velocity analysis. In this method, a probe is placed along the course of the common femoral, superficial femoral, popliteal, peroneal, anterior tibial, and posterior tibial arteries, and the velocity of blood flow is graphically displayed. Normal arterial vessels show a triphasic velocity signal. Rapid acceleration to peak systolic velocity occurs along a narrow frequency spectrum. End-systolic deceleration culminates in protodiastolic reversal of flow, the amplitude of which is inversely proportional to the dynamic peripheral resistance, including rheologic factors. Antegrade flow resumes in middiastole as a consequence of the windkessel recoil effect in the proximal aorta. Peak systolic velocities diminish with advancing age but are not significantly different in males than females, despite smaller arterial diameters in women [109]. Arterial obstruction proximal to the probe transforms the morphology of the waveform, first by loss of the reversed flow component and later by attenuation of all parts of the velocity spectrum with delayed upstroke and decreased amplitude.

ULTRASOUND IMAGING

Duplex ultrasound scanning provides a direct, noninvasive test of functional and anatomic characteristics of arterial obstructive lesions. The methodology combines B-mode ultrasound imaging and pulsed Doppler velocity analysis to examine arterial configuration and localized velocity information at sites of stenosis. The pulsed Doppler sample volume detector is guided by the ultrasound image to specific arterial locations. The angle of incidence of the Doppler beam with the vessel axis is measured and used to derive velocity information, which is recorded graphically as a function of time. The amplitude of the velocity signal is indicated by shades of gray, or with directional vectors when color flow imaging is available. Flow through a stenosis is accelerated, and turbulence related to the configuration of the obstruction is detected as spectral broadening of the band of particulate velocities, instead of the narrow band seen with normal laminar flow.

Application of this technique to lower-extremity arteries was delayed by technical limitations involving transducer design. High-frequency apparatus proved satisfactory for relatively superficial arteries but could not be used for deeper structures, which required lower transducer frequencies. Both the focal point of the flow detector and the sampling volume had to be adjustable to accommodate vessels of varying diameters lying at different depths and that, in the abdomen, vary with respiration. These capabilities now coexist with fast Fourier transformations of the velocity spectrum and microprocessor-based systems for calculation of actual blood cell velocities, allowing precise estimation of instantaneous pressure gradients and degrees of stenosis [110].

The ultrasound-imaging procedure is performed with the patient supine, the lower extremities slightly rotated externally. The aorta is imaged in the midline just below the level of the xiphoid and traced distally to the level of the iliac bifurcation; each iliac artery can be examined to the groin. The common, deep, and superficial femoral arteries are imaged in the adductor canal. The patient is positioned prone for examination of the popliteal fossae, with the feet elevated about 30 degrees. The origins of the tibial arteries usually can be identified, but detailed examination of the distal tibioperoneal arteries is technically difficult. Waveforms are recorded from each accessible arterial segment, and detailed analysis is performed for each area in which disturbed flow is detected.

Duplex scanning is becoming an effective means of localizing and classifying peripheral arterial stenoses. It has particular advantages over other noninvasive methods for the evaluation of aortoiliac disease. Stenoses potentially amenable to angioplasty may be identified in patients who are less than optimal candidates for angiography. No other noninvasive method is as useful for distinguishing critical stenosis from occlusion, which may have direct bearing on the angioplasty technique selected. Duplex scanning is more sensitive and more specific than segmental blood pressure measurements for detection of restenosis, which can be detected by the ultrasound method even before pressure drops.

Ultrasound tissue-characterization techniques are currently under development that may allow precise descriptions of the atherosclerotic lesions themselves as fibrotic, lipoid, thrombotic, hyperplastic, or calcific, for example, and lead to more rational understanding of the impact of various interventions on this diversity of tissue types [111]. In excised aortic and iliac arterial segments, at least four histologic categories have been acoustically differentiated (normal, fatty, fibrous, and calcific), and ultrasound reflectance changes related to blood coagulation, temperature, and flow velocity have been documented both in vitro and in vivo [112,113]. In the future, we may look to the ultrasound probe for initial evaluation of patients for morphologic analysis of arterial lesions. This technology will compete, however, with advances in the fields of positron-emission tomography of the atherosclerotic lesions and magnetic resonance imaging.

RADIONUCLIDE LABELING METHODS

Radionuclide imaging is used to evaluate patients with arterial obstructive diseases of the limbs. Microspheres amenable to radionuclide labeling are commercially available, and medical diagnostic use is based on the assumption that distribution of particulate material injected into the arterial circulation is identical to that of blood flowing to the capillary microcirculation. There are four specific requirements of practical importance in application of this method for study of the limb circulation: (1) biocompatibility, (2) prompt, uniform dispersion of the particles in arterial blood, (3) distribution at arterial branch points in proportion to blood flow, and (4) complete first-pass extraction at the level of the microcirculation. The greatest material success at lower-extremity perfusion imaging has been achieved with technetium-99m-labeled microaggregated albumin. In patients with atherosclerosis studied at the time of translumbar aortography, blood-flow distribution in the lower extremities was indistinguishable from that in normal individuals [114]. During reactive hyperemia following relief of ischemia, however, variations in distribution of radioactive microspheres correlated with arteriographic findings and subjective symptoms in 83 percent of cases [115]. Similar applications have validated predictive value for spontaneous healing of ischemic ulcers [116]. In general, however, radioactive microsphere distribution techniques have not been clinically valuable, since peripheral arterial injection provides nonquantitative information about flow distribution. Radionuclide angiography using technetium-labeled autologous erythrocytes provides insufficient image quality for therapeutically directed assessment of atherosclerotic lesions [117].

The local clearance of isotopes has proved simpler and provides reliable quantitative data related to regional blood flow. In that method, a small volume of a solution of radioactive tracer, typically xenon in saline, is injected locally into tissue such as tibialis or gastrocnemius muscle, and the rate of disappearance is extrapolated to blood flow, assuming a monoexponential function. At rest, results obtained in patients with arterial disease often are in the normal range; again, hyperemic methods are recruited to enhance diagnostic value. The technique has the advantage of reproducibility, and one intriguing observation has been that exercise training of patients with claudication, although it improves walking tolerance, does not increase the rate of xenon clearance from calf skeletal muscle. The major limitation is that perfusion is gauged in a very small region of tissue, and local perfusion imbalance may drastically influence results; larger volumes of injectate, though, may induce direct changes in blood flow.

Thallium-201 imaging of lower-limb musculature at rest in comparison with exercise also has been of limited value in verifying areas of relative ischemia, but it depends too heavily on heterogeneity of perfusion to be of much practical benefit. Fruitful areas in the upcoming years seems to be tracer-labeled lipoprotein imaging of atherosclerotic lesions or indium-111-labeled platelet imaging. Those methods examine the dynamic roles of platelet-mediated thrombosis and lipid sequestration in the development of atherosclerotic disease, and therapeutic response to specific interventions such as angioplasty, which involve some degree of immediate tissue injury.

The future clearly promises more specific metabolically based isotope selection and positron-emission tomography for assessment of vascular disease, but current data are insufficient for comprehensive evaluation.

Clinical Interpretation

The value of various modalities employed in the vascular noninvasive laboratory sometimes can be enhanced by inclusion of measurements made after hemodynamic changes have been induced by exercise, reactive hyperemia, and vasodilator drugs. Exercise testing, in particular, is useful in evaluating patients with intermittent claudication. First, the test provides a quantitative estimate of functional capacity. Second, it is useful in distinguishing patients with claudication due to arterial disease from other disorders producing similar symptoms. In patients with arterial obstructive disease, the ankle-to-arm pressure index declines following exercise, which does not occur in such disorders as spinal stenosis. Third, the relative limitation imposed by coexisting coronary artery disease can be identified.

Assessment of limb perfusion on release of ischemia provides an index of flow during a state of maximum vasodilation. During reactive hyperemia in patients with arterial occlusive disease, there is a protracted decline in the ankle-to-arm pressure index, and the blood flow response also is attenuated. This test can be used in cases where exercise cannot be performed to estimate the functional severity of ischemia. Similarly, administration of vasodilator drugs such as phentolamine or papaverine can be used to help determine the relative hemodynamic significance of disease at various anatomic levels and the potential role of vasodilator therapy in cases of combined obstructive and vasospastic disease.

The modern clinical noninvasive vascular laboratory is subject to misconceptions that predispose to misuse. Among those misconceptions is that laboratory findings can establish the indications for specific therapeutic procedures. Such clinical decisions are best made on the basis of symptoms and the physical appearance of involved tissues. The laboratory does provide information, however, that may be helpful in judging the severity of ischemia, the contribution of obstructive arterial factors to symptoms, and the absolute and relative hemodynamic significance of lesions at various points along the course of the arterial circulation. Currently available noninvasive technology furnishes an objective perspective along anatomic and functional as well as hemodynamic lines, a perspective that has become virtually essential to clinical practice.

We may anticipate that, in the future, noninvasive tests will better help select potential candidates for certain forms of therapy prior to or without the need for contrast angiography. In that respect, the vascular laboratory holds the promise of identifying patients with conditions suitable for intervention so that the ticket to clinical decision making no longer will carry the cost of an invasive procedure without direct therapeutic potential. Beyond the horizon, the noninvasive vascular laboratory offers not only to enhance the clinical and angiographic principles on which standards of diagnosis and the evaluation of treatment are based but also to advance our understanding of the mechanisms of clinical success and failure.

ANGIOGRAPHY

Magnetic Resonance Angiography. Magnetic resonance imaging of flowing blood, that is, magnetic resonance angiography, is a noninvasive means to assess the patency of peripheral arteries and does not require the injection of contrast (see Chap. 20).

As its technology advances, magnetic resonance angiography increasingly is able to discriminate critical stenoses and occlusions of peripheral arteries [118]. Furthermore, magnetic resonance angiography may be even more sensitive than contrast angiography in identifying patent arteries that are distal to an occluded segment [119,120].

Contrast Angiography. The diagnosis of arterial obstructive disease generally does not require invasive techniques, and most patients with intermittent claudication do not need angiographic examination. Contrast angiography usually is indicated for mapping the extent and the location of arterial pathology prior to a revascularization procedure (Figs. 35-7, 35-8). Contrast angiography, therefore, should be reserved for those patients in which diagnosis is somehow in doubt and as a prelude to thrombolysis, surgery, or angioplasty, when more conservative approaches to management are not satisfactory. Such patients would include those with ischemic symptoms at rest, those whose limbs are in jeopardy on the basis of severe ischemia, and those with unacceptably limiting or progressive symptoms. An important clinical decision is the choice of method for angiographic examination, to ensure that adequate visualization of the involved arterial segments is provided without undue risk related to catheter manipulation or toxicity from contrast agents. Aortic injection of contrast material is indicated in patients with aortoiliac occlusive disease, which can be accomplished in some cases by retrograde transfemoral catheterization. In patients with occlusion of the aorta or the iliac arteries, the aorta can be cannulated by the translumbar approach or by transaxillary catheterization. Aortic injection of contrast material provides visualization of the aorta and proximal limb vessels; definition of the circulation distal to

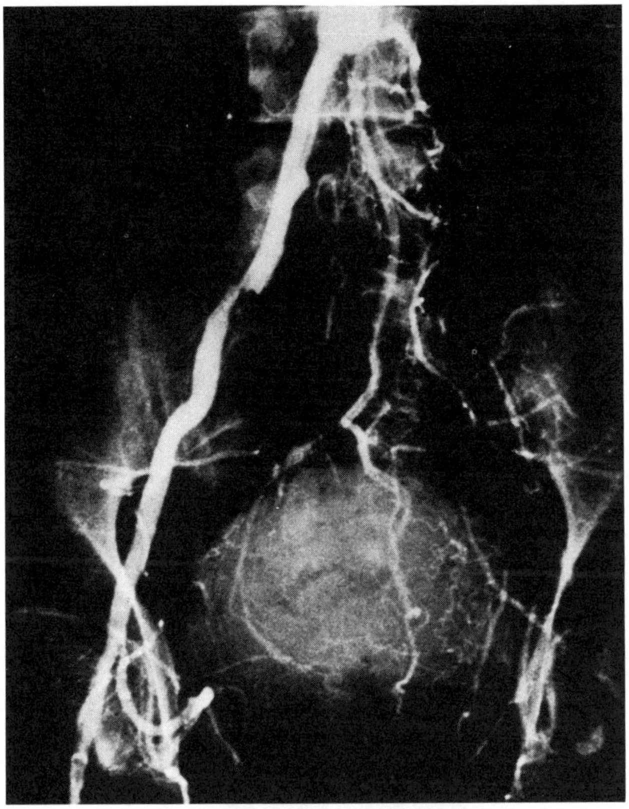

Fig. 35-7. Angiogram depicting a total occlusion of the left common iliac artery and a high-grade stenosis of the right external iliac artery.

the popliteal trifurcations may be compromised by the dilution of proximally injected contrast. In patients with femoropopliteal obstructive disease, angiography often can be confined to the involved extremity with fine definition of the distal vasculature.

Digital Subtraction Angiography. Digital subtraction angiography is a computer-enhanced angiographic study that often is useful in patients with localized obstructive lesions and in patients in whom the volume of contrast material injected must be kept to a minimum. Also, it can be used to improve resolution in cases of difficult interpretation of angiographic images. The technique can be used with either intravenous or intra-arterial contrast injection, although the latter provides enhanced resolution. It is a particularly useful modality for postoperative examination of anastomotic segments, but it is not effective as a means of visualizing large regions of the arterial tree.

Intravascular Imaging. Fiberoptic angioscopy is an innovative technique that allows direct visualization of the arterial intima using a percutaneous fiberoptic catheter. The method has been coupled with interventional devices to enhance the matching of therapeutic techniques with lesion morphology, but results are not yet sufficient to define fully the role of this form of endoluminal vascular imaging. Catheter-mounted ultrasound transducer crystals have made possible intravascular sonography, which has been well tolerated by patients in testing that involves iliofemoral vessels [121–123]. Areas of plaque narrowing and calcification are readily identified by this technique, and its use in conjunction with balloon, laser, atherectomy, or other forms of angioplasty may permit more accurate estimation of the impact on the various components of the arterial wall and associated atheromatous lesions, such that catheter systems of the future may incorporate several of those modalities in a single device. Information about the status of the vascular media and adventitia obtained through application of this technology may enhance outcome by reducing the potential for arterial dissection, aneurysm formation, and occlusion.

Medical Therapy

The general principles of patient management involve measures directed at protection of affected tissues, preservation of functional capacity, prevention of disease progression or acute arterial thrombosis, and improvement of blood flow. These principles can be categorized as local measures, treatment of associated factors, exercise training, avoidance of vasoconstrictor stimuli, and drug therapy.

LOCAL MEASURES

Local measures are interventions used to reduce the likelihood of skin breakdown and infection. Such measures are particularly important in diabetics with vascular disease and in patients with severe impairment of perfusion. The feet should be kept clean. Moisturizing cream should be applied to prevent drying and fissuring, but it must be carefully selected to avoid direct irritant effects. Well-fitted shoes should be worn to reduce the likelihood of pressure-induced necrosis, and stockings made of natural, absorbent fibers are recommended. The patient is advised to inspect the skin of the feet frequently so that minor abrasions can be tended promptly. Elastic support stockings generally should be avoided because they may restrict cutaneous blood flow. In patients with ischemia at rest, conservative measures include placing the affected limb in a dependent position below heart level to increase perfusion pressure and oxygen tension in ischemic tissues. In cases where edema, which may impair healing, is present, the limb should be kept horizontal instead. Sheepskin should be placed beneath the heels of the feet, since pressure against bed sheets accounts for the frequent occurrence of skin breakdown at those sites. A footboard should be used to cradle the blankets over the feet in a fashion that minimizes frictional trauma. Wisps of cotton inserted between the toes for separation help protect the digits from intertriginous friction and moisture. Unless infectious purulence is present, dryness is preferred to soaks, except in a limited fashion to permit intermittent cleansing. Gentle warmth is recommended to minimize vasoconstriction, but excessive heat should be avoided. Fungal onycholysis should be treated with appropriate antimicrobial preparations to reduce the likelihood of cutaneous breakdown leading to bacterial superinfection. In general, caution must be exercised in the use of topical medica-

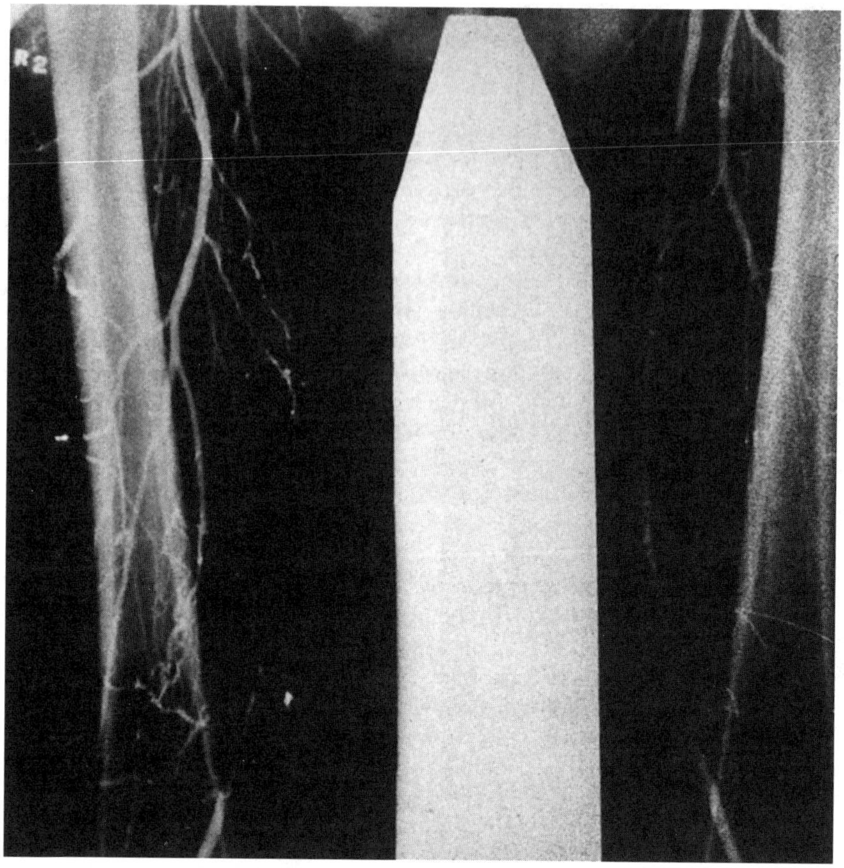

Fig. 35-8. Angiogram illustrating total occlusion of the right superficial femoral artery and diffuse atherosclerotic involvement of left superficial femoral artery.

ments because of the possibility of local inflammatory reactions. Open sores should be kept clean, and cultures should be obtained for surveillance, but antibiotic medication is not always effective, in part because of impaired delivery to ischemic tissue. Plain roentgenographic examinations of underlying bone may be helpful in assessing the possibility of osteomyelitis, for which antibiotic therapy generally is given. Passive physical therapy may proceed to progressive weight bearing and ambulation but must be accompanied by careful attention to foot care, the use of absorbent, natural-fiber (preferably cotton) stockings, and soft, nonconstrictive, properly fitted shoes.

TREATMENT OF ASSOCIATED RISK FACTORS

Modification of associated risk factors may reduce the likelihood of progression of atherosclerotic disease, and there has been considerable speculation that regression of obstructive lesions also might be achieved through those means. Accordingly, attention should be directed toward reduction of hyperlipidemia, control of hypertension, cessation of cigarette smoking, weight reduction in instances of obesity, and treatment of diabetes.

Studies in patients with coronary artery disease support the contention that reduction of high serum concentrations of cholesterol may retard the progression of atherosclerotic disease and potentially induce regression. In hyperlipidemic patients with peripheral arterial obstructive disease, two angiographic studies found that lipid-lowering therapy also attenuated progression of peripheral atherosclerosis [124,125]. Treatment of patients with type III hyperlipidemia sufficient to reduce serum cholesterol and triglyceride levels increased the blood flow response to reactive hyperemia in the limb [126], which implies improvement in either the effective luminal diameter or in vasodilator reserve. More sensitive studies are in progress using digitized videodensitometry to assess the impact of lipid-lowering therapy on the course of peripheral atherosclerosis. According to the National Cholesterol Program Adult Treatment Panel II, patients with atherosclerosis should reduce fasting low density lipoprotein (LDL)–cholesterol concentration below 100 mg/dl through dietary modulation and, if necessary, with the addition of lipid-lowering medication [127].

Although hypertension is a recognized risk factor for the development and progression of atherosclerosis, treatment should take into consideration the following concerns: (1) Certain antihypertensive medications, particularly beta-adrenergic inhibitors, may cause reflex peripheral cutaneous vasoconstriction, and (2) reduction of systemic arterial pressure to the normotensive range may reduce perfusion pressure in an ischemic extremity and aggravate symptoms. It remains to be proved on the basis of prospective clinical trials whether treatment of hypertension, once atherosclerotic peripheral vascular disease is manifest, improves prognosis.

The varied prognosis for patients with overt limb arterial obstructive disease based on continuation or cessation of tobacco smoking already has been cited. The likelihood of patients with intermittent claudication developing ischemic rest pain, ulcers, or gangrene is substantially higher in active smokers than in those who quit smoking [50,128]. Prognosis following surgical revascularization also is affected adversely by continued cigarette use. In a study of patients with aortofemoral bypass grafts, the occlusion rate was 25 percent among patients who continued to smoke more than five cigarettes daily, compared with 10 percent for those who smoked fewer [129]. In patients with femoropopliteal bypass grafts, the difference was even more striking, with the occlusion rate 40 percent among the heavier smokers and 10 percent in nonsmokers. In general, there was a direct relation between cigarette consumption and graft occlusion rates irrespective of age or gender; among those who quit smoking, the occlusion rates promptly paralleled those of nonsmokers.

EXERCISE TRAINING

Exercise training has been demonstrated to improve walking capacity among patients with obstructive arterial disease [130–135]. A number of factors may account for that improvement, including increased blood flow, more efficient skeletal muscle and metabolic function, and changes in ergonomics. Most studies have not identified consistent improvement in measured indices of perfusion [130,131,134], although studies in animals in which arterial obstructions have been created support the view that regular muscular exercise increases collateral development [136,137]. In a randomized study of supervised treadmill walking 1 hour a day, 3 days a week, for 12 weeks with progressive increments in speed and grade as tolerated, exercised subjects increased claudication-free walking time, exercise capacity, and peak oxygen consumption [138]. Although plethysmographically measured peak calf blood flow increased, it did not correlate with the improvement in peak walking time. In contrast, there was a significant inverse correlation between walking time and the concentration of plasma short-chain acylcarnitine, suggesting that exercise training was associated with improved oxidative metabolism in skeletal muscle [138].

Exercise training programs should be individualized for each patient, but supervised settings provide structure, guidance, and encouragement that often result in substantial improvements in claudication distance. One example of a supervised 3-month program would include 1-hour training periods 3 times a week, with each period consisting of a 5-minute warm-up, 50 minutes of intermittent exercise on a treadmill, and a 5-minute cool-down [138]. The treadmill exercise would begin with a low workload, for example, 0-percent grade at 2 mph. The patient would discontinue exercise when moderate to severe claudication developed and resume walking when the discomfort resolved. The workload in ensuing sessions can be increased gradually by raising the grade by 1–2 percent or by increasing the treadmill speed by 0.5 mph. Participants also should be encouraged to train, that is, walk independently, outside the supervised program.

Exercise training compares favorably to other forms of treatment for claudication. For example, pentoxifylline conferred no additional benefit to exercise capacity than training alone [139]. In one randomized trial, exercise training improved maximum walking distance significantly more than percutaneous transluminal angioplasty, despite the fact that ankle pressure increased following angioplasty but not with exercise training [140]. In contrast, another randomized trial in patients with intermittent claudication suggested that training was less effective in improving walking capacity than vascular surgery [141].

DRUG THERAPY AIMED AT REDUCING ISCHEMIA

Vasodilator Drugs. Based on the success of vasodilator-drug therapy for angina pectoris, it is tempting to assume that treatment with medication that reduces arteriolar resistance also might be effective for patients with atherosclerotic obstruction of limb arteries. Unfortunately, vasodilator-drug therapy has been disappointing for relief of intermittent claudication. The major action of such agents in treatment of coronary artery disease is to reduce myocardial workload through actions on the peripheral arterial and venous circulation, thereby improving the balance of oxygen supply and demand, although many agents also operate to reduce coronary vasomotor tone and directly increase myocardial blood flow in patients with coronary spasm. In patients with limb ischemia, however, the goal is to increase the work capacity of exercising muscle. Blood supply is limited when an obstructive arterial lesion produces critical stenosis, and distal perfusion pressure is reduced. Intramuscular arterioles normally dilate in response to the metabolic demands of exercise, but flow augmentation is blunted in patients with proximal stenotic disease. Also, distal pressure falls during exercise, leading to accumulation of the ischemic metabolites thought to mediate claudication. Those substances potentiate local vasodilatation, and perfusion pressure falls, no longer balancing the extravascular compressive force exerted by exercising muscle within the tissue compartment. The distal vasculature virtually collapses under those circumstances, and this mechanism cannot be mitigated by arteriolar vasodilator therapy of any sort.

The history of limb arterial disease therapeutics is replete with therapeutic agents widely advertised to physicians and the lay public alike, which achieve popularity for a while before falling into disrepute and disuse when adequate studies confirm ineffectiveness. Vasodilator drugs, including beta-adrenergic agonists (isoproterenol, nylidrin), alpha-adrenergic antagonists (reserpine, guanethidine, tolazoline), calcium-channel blockers, nitrates, and others (isoxsuprine, cyclandelate) have been evaluated in such clinical trials. None increases blood flow in exercising skeletal muscle subtended by significant arterial obstructive lesions, nor does any one improve symptoms of intermittent claudication or objective measures of exercise capacity [142,143].

Pharmacologic Enhancement of Collateral Flow. An alternative tactic is to attempt augmentation of collateral perfusion in patients with obstructive disease of major limb arteries. That is the rationale behind the use of the serotonin (S-2) antagonist, ketanserin, which in one study increased collateral blood flow in patients with obstructive lesions [144]. In a multicenter trial of ketanserin in patients with intermittent claudication, however, treadmill exercise performance was not significantly better after treatment for a year with ketanserin than with placebo [145]. Since the hypotensive effect of ketanserin might balance collateral vasodilatation, resulting in no net gain in terms of perfusion, further exploration of other agents exerting an action on collateral vasculature still seems warranted [146].

Hemorrheologic Agents. Application of hemorrheologic concepts to the management of patients with obstructive forms of cardiovascular disease is appealing, in part because of the failure of other forms of pharmacologic therapy, particularly vasodilator and antithrombotic agents, to improve symptoms related to impaired blood flow [147]. Abnormal rheology is present in many patients with atherosclerotic disease and its associated conditions. Based on salutary results in several, but not all, clinical trials, oral pentoxifylline is in clinical use to improve the walking capacity of patients with intermittent claudication related to obstructive arterial disease [148–154]. Abnormally reduced erythrocyte flexibility *in vitro* of blood obtained from patients with claudication is partially corrected [155,156], and skeletal-muscle oxygen tension has been reported to rise at rest following treatment with pentoxifylline [157], supporting a hemorrheologic mechanism of action. Improved blood fluidity in vivo has not been demonstrated conclusively, however, in patients with claudication during ischemia produced by leg exercise or arterial occlusion [158]. Minimum limb vascular resistance during reactive hyperemia, as determined by venous-occlusion plethysmography, showed no improvement after administration of pentoxifylline compared with placebo in a study of patients with stable intermittent claudication, suggesting that hemorrheologic effects of the drug, if they occurred at all, were not sufficient to reduce impedance to blood flow [159]. It seems that there may be subsets of patients with reduced indices of rheologic performance who could benefit from treatment with pentoxifylline, but suitable methods of case selection have not been developed [160].

Chelation Therapy. Intravenous administration of fluids containing metal-chelating compounds such as ethylenediaminetetraacetate (EDTA) have been advocated for treatment of advanced atherosclerosis based on the premise that calcium salts leached from the vascular lesions might potentiate regression of the disease [161,162]. A prospective evaluation of chelation therapy in patients with intermittent claudication found no advantage in comparison with placebo [163]. This treatment is most often a last resort for patients who have become disenchanted with standard therapeutic approaches. Because objective documentation of its effectiveness is lacking and because of its nephrotoxic effects, chelation therapy with EDTA has been compared with the defrocked anticancer cure laetrile.

Metabolic Agents. An alternative to increasing the oxygen supply to exercising skeletal muscle is enhancing cellular energetics to increase the efficiency of substrate utilization. This is the mechanism by which use of L-carnitine has been advocated for treatment of intermittent claudication. L-carnitine reportedly facilitates transfer of acetylated compounds and fatty acids across mitochondrial membranes, which leads to enhanced energy storage [164]. One study found that treatment with L-carnitine improved exercise capacity in patients with intermittent claudication, but confirmatory studies are lacking, making the effectiveness of this type of therapy an unresolved issue [165]. Derivatives of L-carnitine as well as other drugs that affect metabolic pathways are under investigation. In a recent study, propionyl-L-carnitine, an analog of L-carnitine, was found to increase maximal walking distance to a greater extent than placebo [166].

Prostaglandins. The mechanism by which the vasodilator and antithrombotic prostaglandins PGE_1 and PGI_2 might relieve ischemic rest pain and promote healing of ulcers remains controversial. A number of randomized trials have been conducted to determine whether parenteral administration of vasodilator prostanoids, including PGI_1, PGI_2, and iloprost, have been conducted in patients with severe limb ischemia [167]. Short-term (3–4 days) parenteral administration of vasodilator prostanoids (intra-arterial or intravenous administration) generally has not proved beneficial in alleviating pain or healing ulcers [168–177]. Long-term administration (2–6 weeks), however, has been shown to reduce pain and facilitate ulcer healing [173–175]. The potential roles of vasodilator prostaglandins for treatment of intermittent claudication is under investigation. Intravenous PGE_1 administered for four weeks, plus exercise training, *was reported* to improve walking distance more than exercise training alone [176].

Antithrombotic Therapy. Antithrombotic therapy may be considered for the management of peripheral arterial obstructive disease at various stages. In chronic disease, the goal is to prevent progression of the obliterative process that leads to thrombotic occlusion of arteries. After revascularization procedures, the objective is to prevent thrombotic complications and preserve the patency of reconstruction. In cases of acute arterial occlusion resulting from embolism or thrombosis, therapy is directed toward prevention of thrombus propagation and reduction of the likelihood of recurrence. Available approaches include anticoagulant, platelet-inhibitor, and thrombolytic drugs.

There is no conclusive evidence that antithrombotic therapy alters the clinical course of vascular insufficiency related to arteriosclerosis obliterans, although occasional reports have suggested a benefit of anticoagulant or platelet-inhibitor agents along those lines [177–179]. Among the individuals participating in the Physician's Health Study, primary prevention with aspirin reduced the risk of requiring surgical revascularization for peripheral arterial disease [180]. In two studies, serial angiography revealed less progression of arterial disease in patients randomly assigned to take platelet-inhibitor medication than in those given a matched placebo [178,179]. The role of platelet-inhibitor medication in retarding progression of atherosclerotic plaque also was demonstrated in patients with coronary artery disease, and it seems reasonable to extrapolate those results to the peripheral circulation [181]. There is limited information regarding the efficacy of platelet inhibition on symptoms such as leg claudication. Several studies, however, did find that ticlopidine, compared to placebo, improved walking distance in patients with claudication [182–184].

Although intermittent claudication is itself comparatively benign, it carries important prognostic weight in terms of other atherosclerotic cardiovascular events, such as myocardial infarction and stroke. An enlarging body of evidence supports the prophylactic use of aspirin for prevention of those complications in patients with atherosclerosis, as emphasized by the results of a pooled analysis of 145 randomized trials of platelet-inhibitor therapy involving over 51,000 patients [185]. The rate of nonfatal myocardial infarction was reduced 34 percent and cardiovascular mortality was reduced 17 percent, although the limitations inherent in retrospective meta-analyses of this sort should be noted. Whether patients at increased risk of morbid cardiovascular events (identified on the basis of intermittent claudication or other features of obstructive atherosclerosis affecting the limb circulation) specifically benefit from prophylactic administration of antithrombotic medication is an issue currently under investigation, but that line of reasoning increasingly characterizes clinical practice.

INTERVENTIONAL ANGIOGRAPHY

Percutaneous Transluminal Angioplasty. After Dotter introduced the technique of recanalization of occluded vascular segments using comparatively simple intravascular devices similar to angiographic guide wires, Gruentzig popularized the use of expandable plastic balloons, achieving greater rates of lasting patency. The mechanism of transluminal dilatation of stenotic arteries involves stretching the vessel wall, leading to longitudinal splits and fractures of the intima often extending into the medial layer [186,187]. (Details of the apparatus, technique, and results are discussed in Chap. 31.) Considerable success has attended the use of this methodology for correction of iliac arterial stenoses, but patency rates seem somewhat lower in the femoral and popliteal arteries. Percutaneous transluminal angioplasty (PTA) of iliac arteries is associated with an initial success rate of 90 percent and 1-, 3-, and 5-year patency rates approximating 80, 70, and 60 percent, respectively [188,189]. Preliminary studies have indicated that patency rates may be even greater following implantation of a stent. PTA of femoral and popliteal arteries has a lower initial success rate than that of iliac arteries and is associated with an average of 1-, 3-, and 5-year patency rates of approximately 65, 50, and 40 percent, respectively [190,191]. Patency rate is better in patients with good runoff, that is, open distal vessels and when PTA is performed for relief of claudication rather than for limb salvage. Experience with obstructions distal to the popliteal trifurcation has been limited and initially rather disappointing, but introduction of improved "steerable" devices drawn from the coronary catheterization laboratory may be expected to enhance the outcome in properly selected cases [192–194].

One randomized trial has compared PTA to bypass surgery in patients with either iliac or femoral artery lesions [195,196]. Patients had to have stenoses greater than 80 percent and that were amenable to PTA. After a median follow-up of 4 years, leg perfusion pressures and limb salvage rates were similar in each group.

Initial and long-term success is related to the acuity of ischemic symptoms as well as to a variety of morphologic features of the atherosclerotic segment, particularly the length of obstruction, its relation to anatomic branch points, and condition of the distal artery [197]. Antithrombotic therapy is advocated in conjunction with balloon angioplasty procedures; it is begun prior to catheter intervention to reduce thrombus formation and the associated risk of occlusion of the dilated site. Current practice tends toward the preprocedural administration of aspirin, alone or in addition to dipyridamole; intraprocedural administration of heparin; and postprocedural use of aspirin. In the absence of contraindications, maintenance therapy with aspirin is continued on a lasting basis. As for patients with intermittent claudication in general, the need for peripheral angioplasty for relief of ischemia related to atherosclerotic disease identifies a group of patients at ongoing risk of thromboembolic complications of cardiovascular disease, for which antithrombotic therapy of this sort appears to confer prophylactic benefit.

Laser Angioplasty. A variety of alternative recanalization tools have been developed in the wake of the success of balloon angioplasty and in view of the limitation of dilatation techniques. Use of optical laser energy has involved a number of different designs, including the Nd:YAG laser, the excimer laser, and photoluminescent degradation instruments (see Chap. 31). The potential advantages of laser techniques over balloon dilatation are related mostly to the greater feasibility of recanalizing completely occluded arteries, a task more frequently required in the management of patients with peripheral than coronary atherosclerotic lesions. Unlike the heart, where myocardial necrosis often follows quickly when arterial occlusion develops, the limbs remain viable for longer periods of time and may not be jeopardized at all even when large arteries become completely obstructed, since tissue oxygen consumption may be reduced to very low levels at rest. Arterial occlusions several centimeters long are, therefore, commonly encountered in patients with intermittent claudication and even more often in patients with more severe forms of limb ischemia, for which angioplasty may be appropriate. It has not been shown, however, that laser angioplasty produces longer-lasting patency of recanalized vessels than balloon dilatation.

Percutaneous Atherectomy. Directional and rotational atherectomy are discussed in detail in Chap. 31. Extraction of obstructive atherosclerotic material using a rotating blade device or a similar apparatus removes atheromatous material and leaves the remaining surface smooth. Methods involving abrasion and pulverization have been developed, but the most promising techniques entail either directional or coaxial slicing blades in a housing designed for positioning the probe and extracting obstructive material [198–200]. Atherectomy devices have the advantage over ablative methods of delivering specimens of extracted tissue for histopathologic examination. To date, trials of atherectomy have yielded results that appear to be comparable but not superior to those addressed with PTA [201]. For stenoses predominantly at the femoropopliteal level, technical and angiographic success is achieved in 87 to 93 percent of the lesions [202]. Symptoms recurred in 31 percent of patients during 6 months of clinical follow-up in one study [199]. Unlike other methods of angioplasty, atherectomy appears particularly well suited to arteries with atherosclerotic lesions that are eccentric and somewhat calcified [202].

Embolectomy. Introduction of the Fogarty catheter in 1963 reduced the mortality associated with embolic occlusion of limb arteries by nearly 50 percent and the need for amputation by approximately 35 percent [203,204]. So successful has this intervention been that prompt removal of thrombotic material after the appearance of acute limb ischemia due to systemic embolism is indicated in nearly every case, unless the patient is moribund or gangrene has progressed beyond the point of potential limb salvage. In patients with underlying obstructive arterial disease and satisfactory collateral blood supply, acute arterial occlusion may produce subacute ischemia, and more definitive revascularization using either surgical or percutaneous angioplasty techniques may be preferred over or in addition to catheter thrombectomy. Antithrombotic therapy is necessary in virtually every case of thrombotic arterial occlusion unless absolute contraindications are present and specific measures are taken to remove the source of embolism or provide sufficient arterial reconstruction to reduce the risk of reocclusion.

Intra-arterial Thrombolysis. The use of thrombolytic therapy for treatment of peripheral arterial occlusive disease is discussed in detail in Chap. 32. Local administration of streptokinase near the site of an occlusive arterial thrombus was introduced by Dotter in 1974; it carries a relatively low complication rate when small doses are given. Subsequently, there have been numerous reports of successful arterial thrombolytic therapy using streptokinase or urokinase in doses ranging from 1,000 to 250,000 units per hour for continuous periods ranging from several hours up to 2 weeks (Fig. 35-9). A typical regimen for administration of urokinase employs an initial bolus of 150,000–250,000 units followed by a 2-hour infusion at 240,000 units per hour, 120,000 units per hour for 2 hours, and 60,000 units for up to 24 hours or more.

Recombinant human tissue plasminogen activator (t-PA) when used for lysis of thrombotic occlusions of peripheral arteries and bypass grafts can be infused intra-arterially in doses of 0.05–0.10 mg/kg/hour for periods between 1 and 6 hours following an initial bolus of 0.10 mg/kg [205–207]. Mean time to lysis of thrombi is 3–4 hours. Higher doses are associated with greater systemic fibrinolysis and higher clinical rates of bleeding. A randomized trial comparing t-PA to urokinase in peripheral arterial and graft occlusions in 32 patients found more rapid thrombolysis, with 50 percent success at achieving more than 95-percent lysis and restitution of antegrade flow using t-PA, which was not significantly different from the 38-percent success after 24 hours with urokinase [208]. Verification of a difference in hemorrhagic complications (31 percent with t-PA and 13 percent with urokinase) will require larger trials and a close examination of dosage considerations and the severity of bleeding.

Although the rate of successful reperfusion (50–80%) is somewhat higher with local than with systemic (intravenous) thrombolytic therapy, there are other advantages and disadvantages. Local infusions allow concurrent angiographic definition of the measure's effectiveness as well as the morphology of associated regional vascular disease so that additional measures, such as angioplasty, may be incorporated to prevent reocclusion after successful thrombolysis. Protracted periods of indwelling arterial catheterization may be complicated by bleeding or thromboembolism in up to 20 percent of cases [209].

Intra-arterial thrombolysis is often effective in restoring patency in native arteries and bypass grafts that follow acute arterial occlusion [207,208,210]. Thrombolysis compared favorably to operative revascularization in a randomized trial of patients with acute peripheral arterial occlusion [211]. Thrombolytic therapy dissolved the occluding thrombus in 70 percent of patients and resulted in cumulative limb salvage of 82 percent at 1 year, similar to results in the surgical group [211]. Cumulative survival rate was greater in the thrombolytic group. Chronic atherothrombotic occlusions appear less responsive than acute thromboembolic occlusions, usually requiring adjunctive angioplasty or surgery to prevent reocclusion. Antecedent use of thrombolytic agents still may be useful in patients with chronic atherosclerotic disease complicated by acute arterial thrombosis, however, to allow greater visualization of the involved arterial segment and thereby facilitate angioplasty or to improve the arterial runoff distal to the site of surgical revascularization. Thrombolytic therapy may be particularly useful in severe ischemia related to acute thrombotic distal arterial occlusion in the forearm, hand, ankle, or foot, which may be surgically inaccessible.

Surgical Therapy

INDICATIONS

The most pressing indication for surgical revascularization in a patient with arterial obstructive disease of the lower extremities is ischemic rest pain, ulceration, or gangrene amenable to arterial reconstruction when more limited measures, including angioplasty, are insufficient,

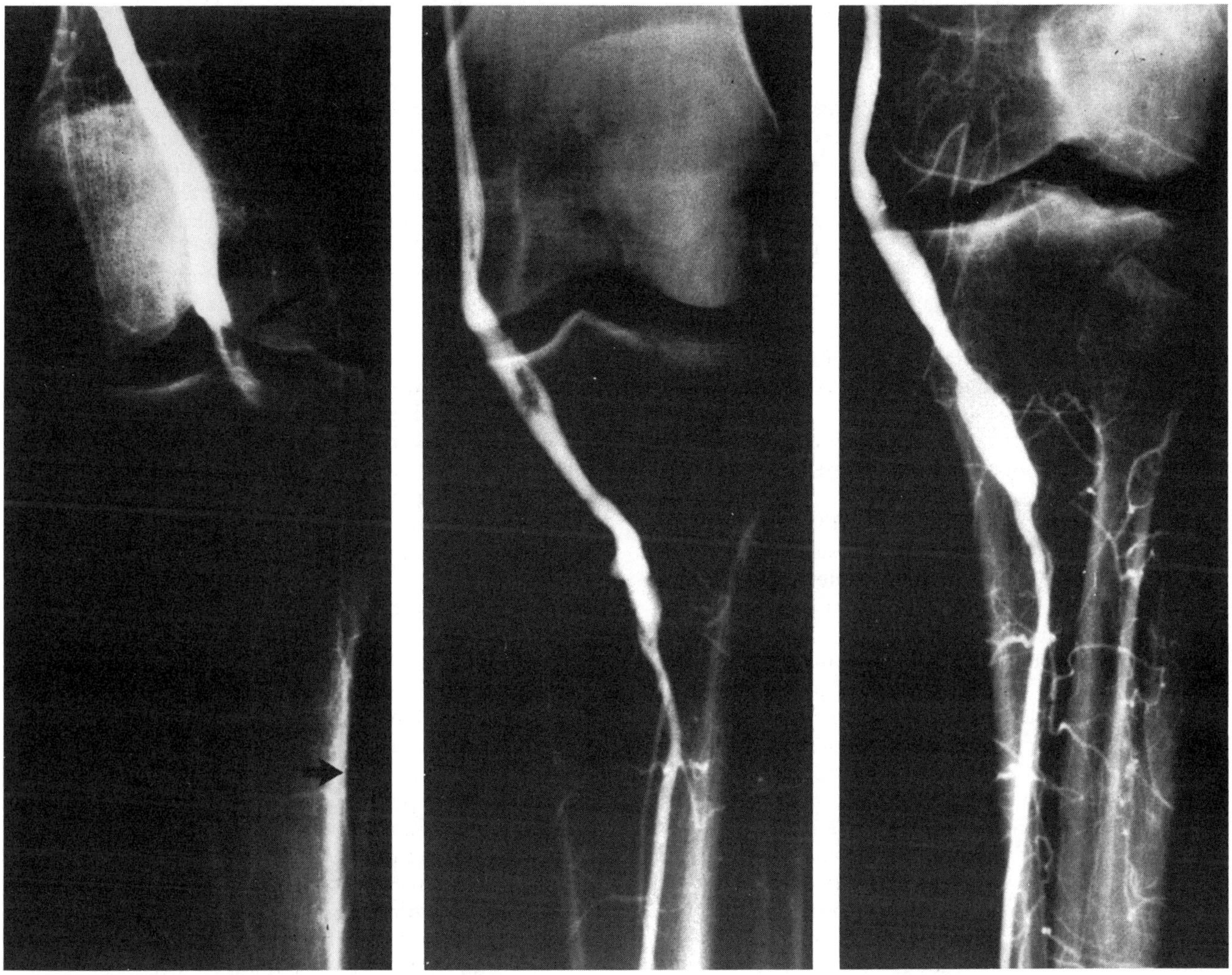

A B C

Fig. 35-9. **A.** A thrombus is apparent in the distal segment of the saphenous vein graft proximal to its anastomosis to the posterior tibial artery. The extent of the thrombus is indicated by the arrows. **B.** After an intra-arterial infusion of streptokinase, most of the thrombus has been lysed. **C.** The thrombus is completely dissolved. The anastomotic site is easily visualized and patent.

unsafe, or not feasible. Since the majority of patients whose symptoms are limited to intermittent claudication remain stable or improve with time, surgical revascularization becomes an appropriate basis for surgical intervention only when severely debilitating in individual circumstances or when progressive. When bedside examination demonstrates a marginal collateral circulation, surgical therapy may be offered more liberally than when that avenue of accessory blood supply is adequate to meet resting tissue nutritional requirements.

Beyond the severity of ischemia and associated symptoms, the anatomic pathology becomes an important consideration in deciding whether surgery should be undertaken. In general, the syndromic approach to disease classification reflects the success of surgical bypass procedures, with patency rates greatest for reconstructions of the aortoiliac segment, intermediate for femoropopliteal operations, and poorest for tibioperoneal revascularization. These results should be interpreted in the context of the patient's overall medical condition, with particular reference to risk imposed by associated coronary or cerebrovascular disease.

OPERATIVE PROCEDURES

Endarterectomy. The patency of endarterectomy compares favorably with prosthetic vascular grafts in arterial beds of wide diameter, specifically the aortoiliac vessels, obviating implantation of synthetic material but still entailing major intra-abdominal surgery. The procedure is employed most often for treatment of relatively short-segment stenosis of the distal aorta in young individuals, since more extensive endarterectomy may be complicated by pelvic autonomic denervation, resulting in impotence or loss of sphincter control. Focal atherosclerotic lesions distal to the aortoiliac bifurcation are today more frequently addressed with percutaneous transluminal angioplasty.

Aortoiliac Revascularization. The standard method of aortoiliac reconstruction is aortobifemoral bypass using a bifurcated Dacron prosthetic graft. The comparative advantages of end-to-end versus end-to-side anastomosis for aortoiliac reconstruction, means of maintaining internal iliac (hypogastric) arterial perfusion, and related details of surgical technique are discussed in Chap. 29. These operations require general anesthesia and cardiopulmonary monitoring and generally entail retroperitoneal exposure through an intraperitoneal approach, with infrarenal cross-clamping of the aorta. Although the short-term morbidity is substantial, success in terms of long-term patency and relief of ischemic symptoms in some series exceeds 85 percent over 10 years [212–214].

Extra-anatomic Bypass. As an alternative to major intra-abdominal aortoiliac reconstructive surgery, techniques of extra-anatomic bypass have been developed. That approach may be highly successful for purposes of limb salvage and relief of severe ischemic symptoms with lower risk of morbidity and mortality in the perioperative period, but there is some sacrifice of long-term patency [215]. Whether that limitation might be mitigated by the use of regimens of antithrombotic medication remains to be determined on the basis of randomized trials. Femorofemoral bypass can be carried out under regional anesthesia and may be appropriate in cases of unilateral iliac artery obstruction. Axillofemoral bypass avoids intra-abdominal operation when the contralateral femoral pulse is weak; indeed, the procedure is best combined with femorofemoral bypass (axillobifemoral bypass) to achieve revascularization of both lower limbs. The patency rate is enhanced when the inflow graft is bifurcated at the inguinal level to supply both extremities than when unilateral or bilateral axillofemoral grafts are employed. This observation indicates the importance of outflow considerations in determining the success of and planned approach to proximal revascularization.

Femoropopliteal Reconstruction. The results of surgical procedures for treatment of infrainguinal arterial disease have been generally less successful than those for proximal revascularization, leading to more restrictive indications for those procedures. Recent improvements in techniques, however, may broaden the availability of the procedures for the majority of patients with intermittent claudication whose symptoms derive from obstruction of the superficial femoral artery. The standard procedure, introduced in 1948, involves femoropopliteal bypass using a segment of reversed autologous saphenous vein. An alternative approach leaves the saphenous vein in situ, removes obstructing venous valves via a valvulotomy, and connects the vein to proximal and distal sites of the femoral and popliteal (or infrapopliteal) artery (see Chap. 29). These procedures can be performed under general or regional anesthesia and are most successful when the distal anastomosis can be constructed proximal to the knee. Five-year patency rates, adjusted to account for grafts that undergo revision, approximate 80–85 percent [216–218]. Patency rates decline proportionately when the distal anastomosis is performed more distally below the knee. Because the duration of the surgical procedure may be reduced through the use of synthetic graft material, which eliminates the need for phlebectomy and preparation of the saphenous vein, polytetrafluoroethylene (PTFE, Gore-Tex) gained popularity, particularly for cases in which above-knee distal anastomosis was feasible. It has become clear that the patency of prosthetic grafts is inferior to those composed of biologic tissue, particularly because of early postoperative thrombotic occlusion. Fibrous intimal hyperplasia is a later cause of vein graft failure, most often encountered between 6 and 18 months postoperatively. The pathophysiology of this hyperplasia is not well understood, but its prevention by means of antithrombotic medication or other measures represents one of the major challenges facing vascular surgeons over the next decade. In some cases, atherosclerotic involvement of vein grafts is a third mechanism of late graft failure, prevention of which is directly related to control of such risk factors as hyperlipidemia, cigarette smoking, and hypertension.

Tibioperoneal Revascularization: In-Situ Saphenous Vein Grafts. For patients with tibioperoneal disease, the success of revascularization techniques was previously so poor as to make any surgical intervention a reluctant undertaking, and prosthetic graft material has been virtually abandoned for this type of surgery. In recent years, however, the in-situ vein-graft operation has been refined. Long-term patency rates for infrapopliteal artery reconstruction are approximately 60 percent [219]. As a result, femorotibial bypass procedures are increasingly effective in achieving salvage of ischemic limbs of diabetics. In the future, we may anticipate a role for intraoperative angioplasty techniques alone or in conjunction with bypass surgery to achieve optimum revascularization of ischemic limbs.

Lumbar Sympathectomy. When direct revascularization is not feasible, lumbar sympathectomy has been employed in the hope of reducing alpha-adrenergic vasoconstrictor innervation, which may impair cutaneous perfusion of the foot. Since most patients in those circumstances are diabetics and many of them suffer some degree of autonomic neuropathy, there is valid reason for concern that the sympathectomy procedure will serve only to transect nonfunctioning nerve tissue to no avail in terms of enhancing perfusion. Among other potential limitations are the fact that sympathetic denervation is not expected to improve intermittent claudication, because the calf muscle vasculature is mainly under beta-adrenergic vasodilator control. Even in the cutaneous circulation of the foot, moreover, ischemia often provides so potent a vasodilator stimulus that sympathetic denervation is not capable of reducing vascular resistance further. That and the other caveats against the use of vasodilator drugs cited earlier make it difficult to place the procedure into proper clinical context, although up to 50 percent of desperate cases have been reported to respond to lumbar sympathectomy in some reports. Relative success may be related to case selection: Patients in whom active sympathetic tone is demonstrated in response to thermal stimuli may have a more favorable outcome with surgery. Even in those cases, intrinsic vasoconstrictor tone may be restored a year or more postoperatively.

Amputation. As a last resort and often to alleviate severe suffering, amputation may present a final alternative for the patient with advanced ischemic gangrene. Since the process of ischemic autoamputation invariably spares more tissue than the surgeon's blade, there is often considerable advantage to delaying surgical amputation until pain becomes unbearable or infection or a systemic toxic state threatens. Following acute arterial occlusion, it may take several weeks for collateral circulation to develop and for the level of ischemia to become clearly demarcated, but progressive gangrene with superimposed infection may force an earlier amputation procedure. Selection of the optimum amputation level requires careful assessment of the status of residual perfusion and appreciation of the patient's general condition as well as physiatric considerations. Each limb joint preserved contributes immeasurably to functional mobility and ease of rehabilitation: Transphalangeal amputation of one or more toes generally is followed by only transient disability largely related to phantom pains and the difficulty of emotional adjustment. Transmetatarsal amputation of the forefoot produces temporary problems of balance, which usually are overcome without much delay. Syme's amputation of the foot at the ankle with removal of the malleoli, which preserves calcarial weight bearing, is rarely feasible. When successful, however, it allows earlier ambulation than below-knee amputation of the lower leg, though it brings special problems of prosthesis management.

The advantage of below-knee amputation over above-knee amputation is borne out by measurements of the energy expenditure of ambulation. Even below-knee amputation requires about 10 to 40 percent more energy expenditure than normal for walking on a horizontal surface at a standard pace. Unilateral above-knee amputation requires about 65 percent more energy than normal, and the increment in energy expenditure for bilateral above-knee amputees is more than 100 percent above normal. Above-knee amputation also carries considerable in-hospital mortality, approaching 50 percent, mainly because of the severity of associated diseases in those cases, since the surgical procedure itself usually is remarkably well tolerated.

Discussion of the perioperative management and postoperative rehabilitation of the amputation patient is beyond the scope of this text, but a few general points demand mention. Because of the devastating psychologic impact of amputation for most patients, aggressive supportive efforts are needed. Unless systemic infection or toxicity threaten, a principal advantage to delaying amputation is to allow for the psychologic preparation of the patient, so that doubt does not later become confused with regret. In cases of chronic "dry" gangrene, there is much to be said for letting the patient come to the conclusion that it is time to be rid of the "rotten" foot and to get on with life. Early postoperative analgesia and sedation should be intensive, for relief of both physical pain and psychologic turmoil. Phantom limb pains should be anticipated, and tricyclic antidepressant medication has been advocated when problems of that sort persist. Ambulation training should begin in the first few days postoperatively. In the case of below-knee amputation, quadriceps-setting exercises should be encouraged to avoid the tendency to flexion contracture. Partial weight bearing may begin in the first week postoperatively, after the first surgical dressing change has confirmed the integrity of the wound. Most patients are dismissed from the hospital and must wait several weeks while a prosthesis is prepared. During that interval, they should become as facile as possible with crutches or other aids that allow mobility on one limb so that they need never fully depend on a prosthesis that may occasionally need adjustment or repair. Rehabilitation of the patient with above-knee amputation is considerably more challenging; many require the use of an ambulation aid such as a walker on a permanent basis. Advances in rehabilitation medicine make patients with extensive amputations increasingly functional, and society must adapt quickly to remove the architectural and other less tangible barriers that stand in the way of full recovery for these veterans of vascular disease.

References

1. Wilens SL. The nature of diffuse intimal thickening of arteries. Am J Pathol 1951; 27:825.
2. Movat HZ, More RH, Haust MD. The diffuse intimal thickening of the human aorta with aging. Am J Pathol 1958; 34:1023.
3. World Health Organization Study Group. Classification of atherosclerotic lesions: report of a study group. WHO Tech Rep Ser 1958; 143:1.
4. Criqui MH, et al. The prevalence of peripheral arterial disease in a defined population. Circulation 1985; 71:510–515.
5. De Backer G, et al. Intermittent claudication—epidemiology and natural history. Acta Cardiol 1979; 34:115–124.
6. Hughson WG, Mann JI, Garrod A. Intermittent claudication: prevalence and risk factors. Br Med J 1978; 1:1379–1381.
7. Reunanen A, Takkunen H, Aromaa A. Prevalence of intermittent claudication and its effect on mortality. Acta Med Scand 1982; 211:249–256.
8. Kannel WB, McGee DL. Update on some epidemiologic features of intermittent claudication: the Framingham Study. J Am Geriatr Soc 1985; 33:13–18.
9. Mathiesen FR, Mune O. Arterial insufficiency in the lower extremities of elderly patients. Acta Chir Scand[Suppl] 1966; 357:78–81.
10. Lombardi G, et al. Prevalence of asymptomatic peripheral vascular disease in a group of patients older than 50 (Letter). J Am Geriatr Soc 1986; 34:551–552.
11. Vogt MT, et al. Decreased ankle/arm blood pressure index and mortality in elderly women. JAMA 1993; 270:465–469.
12. Newman AB, et al. Morbidity and mortality in hypertensive adults with a low ankle/arm blood pressure index. JAMA 1993; 270:487–489.
13. Petermans J. Prevalence of disease of the large arteries in an elderly Belgian population: relationship with some metabolic factors. Acta Cardiol 1984; 39:365–372.
14. Paris BEC, et al. The prevalence and one-year outcome of limb arterial obstructive disease in a nursing home population. J Am Geriatr Soc 1988; 36:607–612.
15. Adkins RB Jr, Scott HW Jr. Surgical procedures in patients aged ninety years and older. South Med J 1984; 77:1357–1364.

16. Kannel WB, et al. Intermittent claudication: incidence in the Framingham Study. Circulation 1970; 41:875–883.
17. Aschoff L. Observations concerning the relationship between cholesterol metabolism and vascular disease. Br Med J 1932; 2:1131.
18. Davignon J, et al. Plasma lipids and lipoprotein patterns in angiographically graded atherosclerosis in the legs and in coronary heart disease. Can Med Assoc J 1977; 116:1245.
19. Greenhalgh RM, et al. Serum lipids and lipoproteins in peripheral vascular disease. Lancet 1971; 2:947–950.
20. Logerfo FW, Coffman JD. Vascular and microvascular disease of the foot in diabetes. Implications for foot care. N Engl J Med 1984; 311:1615–1619.
21. Ruderman NB, Haudenschild C. Diabetes as an atherogenic factor. Prog Cardiovasc Dis 1984; 26:373.
22. Reiber GE, Pecoraro RE, Koepsell TD. Risk factors for amputation in patients with diabetes mellitus. Ann Intern Med 1992; 117:97–105.
23. Humphrey LL, et al. The contribution of non-insulin dependent diabetes mellitus to lower extremity amputation in the community. Arch Intern Med 1994; 154:885–892.
24. Goldenberg SG, et al. Nonatheromatous peripheral vascular disease of the lower extremity in diabetes mellitus. Diabetes 1959; 12:261.
25. Strandness DE Jr, Priest RE, Gibbon GE. Combined clinical and pathologic study of diabetic and nondiabetic peripheral arterial disease. Diabetes 1964; 13:366.
26. Barner HB, Kaiser GC, Willman VL. Blood flow in the diabetic leg. Circulation 1971; 43:391–394.
27. Conrad MC. Large and small artery occlusion in diabetics and nondiabetics with severe vascular disease. Circulation 1967; 36:83–91.
28. Banson BB, Lacy PE. Diabetic microangiopathy in human toes: with emphasis on the ultrastructural change in dermal capillaries. Am J Pathol 1964; 45:41–58.
29. Raskin P, et al. The effect of diabetic control on the width of skeletal-muscle capillary basement membrane in patients with type I diabetes mellitus. N Engl J Med 1983; 309:1546–1550.
30. Vracko R, Strandness DE Jr. Basal lamina of abdominal skeletal muscle capillaries in diabetics and nondiabetics. Circulation 1967; 35:690–700.
31. Siperstein MD, Unger RH, Madison LL. Studies of muscle capillary basement membranes in normal subjects, diabetic and prediabetic patients. J Clin Invest 1968; 47:1973–1999.
32. Parving HH, Rasmussen SM. Transcapillary escape rate of albumin and plasma volume in short- and long-term juvenile diabetics. Scand J Clin Lab Invest 1973; 32:81–87.
33. Chavers B, Etzwiler D, Michael AF. Albumin deposition in dermal capillary basement membrane in insulin-dependent diabetes mellitus: a preliminary report. Diabetes 1981; 30:275–278.
34. Alpert JS, et al. Capillary permeability and blood flow in skeletal muscle of patients with diabetes mellitus and genetic prediabetics. N Engl J Med 1972; 286:454–460.
35. Handelsman MB, Morrione TG, Ghitman B. Skin vascular alterations in diabetes mellitus. Arch Intern Med 1962; 110:70–91.
36. Tooke JE. The microcirculation in diabetes. Diabetic Med 1987; 4:189–196.
37. Sandeman DD, Shore AC, Tooke JE. Relation of skin capillary pressure in patients with insulin-dependent diabetes mellitus to complications and metabolic control. N Engl J Med 1992; 327:760–764.
38. Said G, Slama G, Selva J. Progressive centripetal degeneration of axons in small fibre diabetic polyneuropathy: a clinical and pathological study. Brain 1983; 106:791–807.
39. Caputo GM, et al. Assessment and management of foot disease in patients with diabetes. N Engl J Med 1994; 331:854–859.
40. Parkhouse N, LeQuesne PM. Impaired neurogenic vascular response in patients with diabetes and neuropathic foot lesions. N Engl J Med 1988; 318:1306–1309.
41. Delbridge L, et al. The aetiology of diabetic neuropathic ulceration of the foot. Br J Surg 1985; 72:1–6.
42. Deanfield JE, Daggett PR, Harrison MJG. The role of autonomic neuropathy in diabetic foot ulceration. J Neurol Sci 1980; 47:203.
43. Ahmed ME, Delbridge L, LeQuesne LP. The role of autonomic neuropathy in diabetic foot ulceration. J Neurol Neurosurg Psychiatr 1986; 49:1002–1006.
44. Edmonds ME, Roberts VC, Watkins PJ. Blood flow in the diabetic neuropathic foot. Diabetologia 1982; 22:9–15.
45. Boulton AJM, Scarpello JHB, Ward JD. Venous oxygenation in the diabetic neuropathic foot: evidence of arteriovenous shunting? Diabetologia 1982; 22:6–8.
46. Kannel WB, Gordon T, Schwartz MJ. Systolic versus diastolic blood pressure and risk of coronary heart disease. Am J Cardiol 1971; 27:335–346.
47. Kannel WB, et al. Epidemiologic assessment of the role of blood pressure in stroke. JAMA 1970; 214:301–310.
48. Fowkes FG, et al. Smoking, lipids, glucose intolerance, and blood pressure as risk factors for peripheral atherosclerosis compared with ischemic heart disease in the Edinburgh Artery Study. Am J Epidemiol 1992; 135:331–340.
49. Wilkins RW, et al. Circulation 1959; 20:527.
50. Juergens JL, Barker NW, Hines EA Jr. Arteriosclerosis obliterans: review of 250 cases with special reference to pathogenic and prognostic factors. Circulation 1960; 21:188.
51. Chilvers AS, Thomas ML, Browse NL. The progression of arteriosclerosis: a radiological study. Circulation 1974; 50:402–408.
52. Glagov S, et al. Hemodynamics and atherosclerosis. Insights and perspectives gained from studies of human arteries. Arch Pathol Lab Med 1988; 112:1018–1031.
53. Bassiouny HS, Zarins CK, Kadowaki MH. Hemodynamic stress and experimental aortoiliac atherosclerosis. J Vasc Surg 1994; 19:426–434.
54. Morris PE, et al. Surgery and the progression of the occlusive process in patients with peripheral vascular disease. Radiology 1977; 124:343–348.
55. Nagel T, et al. Shear stress selectively upregulates intercellular adhesion molecule-1 expression in cultured human vascular endothelial cells. J Clin Invest 1994; 94:885–891.
56. Kannel WB, McGee D, Gordon T. A general cardiovascular risk profile: the Framingham Study. Am J Cardiol 1976; 38:46–51.
57. Witteman JC, et al. Cigarette smoking and the development and progression of aortic atherosclerosis. A 9-year population-based follow-up study in women. Circulation 1993; 88:2156–2162.
58. Coffman JD, Javett SL. Blood flow in the human calf during tobacco smoking. Circulation 1963; 28:932.
59. Larson PS. Absorption of nicotine under various conditions of tobacco use. Ann NY Acad Sci 1960; 90:31.
60. Armitage AK, Turner DM. Absorption of cigarette and cigar smoke through the oral mucosa. Nature 1970; 226:1231–1232.
61. Lampson RS. Quantitative state of vasoconstriction induced by smoking. JAMA 1935; 104:1963.
62. Coffman JD. The attenuation by reserpine or guanethidine of the cutaneous vasoconstriction caused by tobacco smoking. Am Heart J 1967; 74:229–239.
63. Eckstein JW, Wood JE, Wilkins RW. Comparative vasoconstrictor effects of inhaling tobacco smoke in warm and cool

environments before and after abstinence from tobacco. Am Heart J 1957; 53:455.
64. Roth GM, Schick RM. Effect of smoking on the cardiovascular system of man. Circulation 1958; 18:177.
65. Coffman JD, Wood JE, Wilkens RW. Effect of cooling and of smoking tobacco upon the blood flow of reactive hyperemia of the foot. Circulation 1958; 18:177.
66. Redisch W, et al. Evaluation of vascular responses to cigarette smoking. Angiology 1968; 19:232–237.
67. Astrup P, Kjeldsen K. Carbon monoxide, smoking and atherosclerosis. Med Clin N Am 1974; 58:323–350.
68. Craig WY, Palomaki GE, Haddow JE. Cigarette smoking and serum lipid and lipoprotein concentrations: an analysis of published data. BMJ 1989; 298:784–788.
69. Celermajer DS, et al. Cigarette smoking is associated with dose-related and potentially reversible impairment of endothelium-dependent dilation in healthy young adults. Circulation 1993; 88:2149–2155.
70. Malinow MR. Hyperhomocyst(e)inemia. A common and easily reversible risk factor for occlusive atherosclerosis. Circulation 1990; 81:2004–2006.
71. Imparato AM, et al. Intermittent claudication: its natural course. Surgery 1975; 78:795–799.
72. Hertzer NR, et al. Routine coronary angiography prior to elective aortic reconstruction. Arch Surg 1979; 114:1336–1344.
73. Reunanen A, Takkunen H, Aromaa A. Prevalence of intermittent claudication and its effect on mortality. Acta Med Scand 1982; 211:249–256.
74. Jelnes R, et al. Fate in claudication: outcome and risk factors. Br Med J 1986; 293:1137–1140.
75. Davey Smith G, Shipley MJ, Rose G. Intermittent claudication, heart disease risk factors and mortality: The Whitehall Study. Circulation 1990; 82:1925–1931.
76. Criqui MH, Coughlin SS, Fronek A. Noninvasively diagnosed peripheral arterial occlusive disease as a predictor of mortality: Results from a prospective population-based study. Circulation 1985; 72:768–773.
77. Criqui MH, et al. Mortality over a period of 10 years in patients with peripheral arterial disease. N Engl J Med 1992; 326:381–386.
78. The Framingham Study: An Epidemiologic Investigation of Cardiovascular Disease. Bethesda, Md.: U.S. Dept of Health, Education, and Welfare; National Institute of Health; Government Printing Office, Section 25, 1970.
79. Schadt DC, et al. Chronic atherosclerotic occlusion of the femoral artery. JAMA 1961; 175:937.
80. McDaniel MD, Cronenwett JL. Basic date related to the natural history of intermittent claudication. Ann Vasc Surg 1989; 3:273–277.
81. Rubanyi GM, Romero JC, Vanhoutte PM. Flow-induced release of endothelium-derived relaxing factor. Am J Physiol 1986; 250:H1145–H1149.
82. Joannides R, et al. Nitric oxide is responsible for flow-dependent dilatation of human peripheral conduit arteries in vivo. Circulation 1995; 91:1314–1319.
83. Liao JK, et al. Differential impairment and vasodilation responsiveness of peripheral resistance and conduit vessels in humans with atherosclerosis. Circ Res 1991; 68:1027–1034.
84. Verbiest H. A radicular syndrome from developmental narrowing of the lumbar vertebral canal. J Bone Joint Surg 1954; 36B:230.
85. Blau JN, Logue V. Intermittent claudication of the cauda equina: an unusual syndrome resulting from central protrusion of a lumbar intervertebral disc. Lancet 1961; 1:1081.
86. Bjordal RI. Intermittent venous claudication. Acta Chir Scand 1970; 136:641.
87. McArdle B. Myopathy due to a defect in muscular glycogen breakdown. Clin Sci 1951; 10:13.
88. Gupta SK, et al. Spontaneous resolution of popliteal artery thrombosis. Arch Surg 1981; 116:480–481.
89. Rutherford RB, et al. Suggested standards for reports dealing with lower extremity ischemia. J Vasc Surg 1986; 4:80–94.
90. Rutherford RR. Standards for evaluating results of interventional therapy for peripheral vascular disease. Circulation 1991; 83:I6–I11.
91. Coffman JD. Clinical forum: atheroembolism after cardiac surgery. J Vasc Med Biol 1989; 1:37–41.
92. Brewer MI, et al. Blue toe syndrome: treatment with anticoagulants and delayed percutaneous transluminal angioplasty. Radiology 1988; 166:31–36.
93. Morris-Jones W, Preston FE, Greeney M. Gangrene of the toes with palpable pulses: response to platelet suppressive therapy. Ann Surg 1981; 193:462–466.
94. Kumpe DA, Zwerdlinger S, Griffin DJ. Blue digit syndrome: treatment with percutaneous transluminal angioplasty. Radiology 1988; 166:37–44.
95. Lee BY, et al. Blue digit syndrome: urgent indication for digital salvage. Am J Surg 1984; 147:418–422.
96. Comerford JA, et al. Digital ischaemia and palpable pedal pulses. Br J Surg 1987; 74:493–495.
97. Stanley JC, et al. Arterial fibrodysplasia: histopathologic character and current etiologic concepts. Arch Surg 1975; 110:561–566.
98. Luscher TF, et al. Arterial fibromuscular dysplasia. Mayo Clin Proc 1987; 62:931–952.
99. Sheps SG, Kincaid OW, Hunt JC. Serial renal function and angiographic observations in idiopathic fibrous and fibromuscular stenoses of the renal arteries. Am J Cardiol 1972; 30:55–60.
100. Siegler RL, et al. Spontaneous reversal of hypertension caused by fibromuscular dysplasia. J Pediatr 1982; 100:83–85.
101. Najafi H. Fibromuscular hyperplasia of the external iliac arteries: an unusual cause of intermittent claudication. Arch Surg 1966; 92:394–396.
102. Mehigan JT, Stoney RJ. Arterial microemboli and fibromuscular dysplasia of the external iliac arteries. Surgery 1977; 81:484–486.
103. Houston C, et al. Fibromuscular dysplasia of the external iliac arteries: surgical treatment by graduated internal dilatation technique. Surgery 1979; 85:713–715.
104. Sos TA, et al. Technical aspects of percutaneous transluminal angioplasty in renovascular disease. Nephron 1986; 44[Suppl I]:45–50.
105. Hamming JJ, Vink M. Obstruction of the popliteal artery at early age. J Cardiovasc Surg 1965; 6:516.
106. Persky JM, Kempczinski RF, Fowl RJ. Entrapment of the popliteal artery. Surg Gynecol Obstet 1991; 173:84.
107. Bernstein EF. How does a vascular laboratory influence management of arterial disease? In RM Greenhalgh, CW Jamieson, AN Nicolaides, eds. Vascular Surgery: Issues in Current Practice. London: Grune & Stratton, 1986. Pp. 101–105.
108. Hillestad LK. The peripheral blood flow in intermittent claudication. V: Plethysmographic studies. The significance of the calf blood flow at rest and in response to timed arrest of the circulation. Acta Med Scand 1963; 174:23–41.
109. Halperin JL. Noninvasive vascular laboratory evaluation: applications for laser angioplasty. In TA Sanborn, ed. Laser Angioplasty. New York: Liss, 1989.
110. Bronez MA, et al. Measurement of ultrasound velocity in tissues utilizing a computer-based system. IEEE Trans Biomed Eng 1985; 32:723–726.
111. Shung KK, Fei DY, Ballard JO 3d. Further studies on ultra-

sonic properties of blood clots. J Clin Ultrasound 1986; 14:269–275.
112. Green SE, et al. In vivo ultrasonic tissue characterization of human intracardiac masses. Am J Cardiol 1983; 51:231–236.
113. Sigel B, et al. Variable ultrasound echogenicity in flowing blood. Science 1982; 218:1321–1323.
114. Siegel ME, et al. Peripheral vascular perfusion scanning: correlation with the arteriogram and clinical assessment in the patient with peripheral vascular disease. Am J Radiol 1975; 125:628–633.
115. Siegel ME, et al. Effect of reactive hyperemia on the distribution of radioactive microspheres in patients with peripheral vascular disease. Am J Radiol 1973; 118:814–819.
116. Siegel ME, et al. Perfusion of ischemic ulcers of the extremity: a prognostic indicator of healing. Arch Surg 1976; 110:265–268.
117. Lassen NA, Holstein P. Use of radioisotopes in assessment of distal blood flow and distal blood pressure in arterial insufficiency. Surg Clin N Am 1974; 54:39–55.
118. Owen RS, et al. Magnetic resonance imaging of angiographically occult runoff vessels in peripheral arterial occlusive disease. N Engl J Med 1992; 326:1577–1581.
119. Owen RS, et al. Symptomatic peripheral vascular disease: selection of imaging parameters and clinical evaluation with MR angiography. Radiology 1993; 187:627–635.
120. McCauley TR, et al. Peripheral vascular occlusive disease: accuracy and reliability of time-of-flight MR angiography. Radiology 1994; 192:351–357.
121. Pandian NG, et al. Ultrasound angioscopy: real-time, two-dimensional, intraluminal imaging of blood vessels. Am J Cardiol 1988; 62:493–494.
122. Roelandt JR, et al. Intravascular high-resolution real-time cross-sectional echocardiography. Echocardiography 1989; 6:1.
123. Rosenfield K, et al. Three-dimensional reconstruction of human coronary and peripheral arteries from images recorded during two-dimensional intravascular ultrasound examination. Circulation 1991; 84:1938–1956.
124. Barndt R Jr, et al. Regression and progression of early femoral atherosclerosis in treated hyperlipoproteinemic patients. Ann Intern Med 1977; 86:139–146.
125. Buchwald H, et al. Changes in sequential coronary arteriograms and subsequent coronary events. Surgical Control of the Hyperlipidemias (POSCH) Group. JAMA 1992; 268:1429–1433.
126. Zelis R, et al. Effects of hyperlipoproteinemias and their treatment on the peripheral circulation. J Clin Invest 1970; 49:1007–1015.
127. National Cholesterol Education Program. Second report of the expert panel on detection, evaluation, and treatment of high blood cholesterol in adults (Adult Treatment Panel II). NIH Publication No. 93-3095. September 1993.
128. Jonason T, Bergstrom R. Cessation of smoking in patients with intermittent claudication. Effects of the risk of peripheral vascular complications, myocardial infarction and mortality. Acta Med Scand 1987; 221:253–260.
129. Robicsek F, et al. The effect of continued cigarette smoking on the patency of synthetic vascular grafts in Leriche syndrome. J Thorac Cardiovasc Surg 1975; 70:107–113.
130. Larsen OA, Lassen NA. Effect of daily muscular exercise in patients with intermittent claudication. Lancet 1966; 2:1093–1096.
131. Ekroth R, et al. Physical training of patients with intermittent claudication: indications, methods and results. Surgery 1978; 84:640–643.
132. Jonason T, et al. Effect of physical training on different categories of patients with intermittent claudication. Acta Med Scand 1979; 206:253–258.
133. Skinner JS, Strandness DE Jr. Exercise and intermittent claudication. II: Effect of physical training. Circulation 1967; 36:23–29.
134. Sorlie D, Myhre K. Effects of physical training in intermittent claudication. Scand J Clin Lab Invest 1978; 38:217–222.
135. Gardner AW, Poehlman ET. Exercise rehabilitation programs for the treatment of claudication pain. A meta-analysis. JAMA 1995; 274:975–980.
136. Conrad MC. Effects of therapy on maximum walking time following femoral ligation in the rat. Circ Res 1977; 41:775–778.
137. Coffman JD. Peripheral collateral blood flow and vascular reactivity in the dog. J Clin Invest 1966; 45:923–931.
138. Hiatt WR, et al. Benefit of exercise conditioning for patients with peripheral arterial disease. Circulation 1990; 81:602–609.
139. Scheffler P, et al. Intensive vascular training in stage IIb of peripheral arterial occlusive disease. The additive effects of intravenous pentoxifylline during training. Circulation 1994; 90:818–822.
140. Creasy TS, et al. Is percutaneous transluminal angioplasty better than exercise for claudication? Preliminary results from a prospective randomized trial. Eur J Vasc Surg 1990; 4:135–140.
141. Lundgren F, et al. Intermittent claudication—Surgical reconstruction or physical training? Ann Surg 1989; 209:346–355.
142. Coffman JD, Mannick JA. Failure of vasodilator drugs in arteriosclerosis obliterans. Ann Intern Med 1972; 76:35–39.
143. Coffman JD. Intermittent claudication and rest pain: physiological concepts and therapeutic approaches. Prog Cardiovasc Dis 1979; 22:53–72.
144. Janicek MJ, Hollenberg NK. Responses to ketanserin in patients with peripheral vascular disease: implications of collateral arterial function. Circulation 1988; 78:II-404.
145. PACK Claudication Substudy Investigators. Randomized placebo-controlled, double-blind trial of ketanserin in claudicants: changes in claudication distance and ankle systolic pressure. Circulation 1989; 80:1544–1548.
146. Creager MA. Can claudication be treated medically? J Vasc Med Biol 1989; 1:269–271.
147. Spittell JA. Pentoxifylline and intermittent claudication (Editorial). Ann Intern Med 1985; 102:126–127.
148. Buckert D, Harwart D. Trials of 3,7-dimethyl-1-(5-oxohexyl) xanthine (BL-191) in double-blind tests. Farmaco 1976; 31:264–274.
149. Schubotz R. Double-blind trial of pentoxifylline in diabetics with peripheral vascular disorders. Pharmatherapeutica 1976; 1:172–179.
150. Angelkort B. Influence of pentoxifylline on microcirculation, poststenotic blood pressure and walking capacity in patients with chronic occlusive arterial disease. IRCS Med Sci 1977; 5:370–374.
151. Bollinger A, Frei C. Double-blind study of pentoxifylline against placebo in patients with intermittent claudication. Pharmatherapeutica 1977; 1:557–562.
152. Porter JM, et al. Pentoxifylline efficacy in the treatment of intermittent claudication: multicenter controlled double-blind trial with objective assessment of chronic occlusive arterial disease patients. Am Heart J 1982; 104:66–72.
153. Stergachis A, et al. Medical care and cost outcomes after pentoxifylline treatment for peripheral arterial occlusive disease. Arch Intern Med 1992; 152:1220–1224.
154. Lindgarder F, et al. Conservative drug treatment in patients with moderately severe chronic occlusive peripheral arterial disease. Circulation 1989; 80:1549–1556.

155. Dormandy JA, et al. Clinical, haemodynamic, rheological and biochemical findings in 126 patients with intermittent claudication. Br Med J 1973; 4:576–581.
156. Reid HL, et al. Impaired red cell deformability in peripheral vascular disease. Lancet 1976; 1:666–668.
157. Ehrly AM. The effect of pentoxifylline on the deformability of erythrocytes and on the muscular oxygen pressure in patients with chronic arterial disease. J Med 1979; 10:331–338.
158. Buzzi A, Canaveris G, Cibeira JB. Modifications of muscle blood flow produced by pentoxifylline in peripheral arterial occlusive disease. Pharmatherapeutica 1976; 1:234–240.
159. Halperin JL, Rothlauf EB, vonPolnitz A. Limb hemodynamic effects of pentoxifylline in patients with intermittent claudication. J Vasc Med Biol 1989; 1:294–299.
160. Lindgarde F, et al. Conservative drug treatment in patients with moderately severe chronic occlusive peripheral arterial disease. Circulation 1989; 80:1549–1556.
161. Lamar CP. Chelation endarterectomy for occlusive atherosclerosis. J Am Geriatr Soc 1966; 14(3):272–294.
162. Kitchell JR, Meltzer LE, Seven MJ. Potential uses of chelation methods in the treatment of cardiovascular diseases. Prog Cardiovasc Dis 1961; 14:798.
163. van Rij AM, et al. Chelation therapy for intermittent claudication. A double-blind, randomized, controlled trial. Circulation 1994; 90:1194–1199.
164. Bremer J. Carnitine: metabolism and functions. Physiol Rev 1983; 63:1420–1480.
165. Brevetti G, et al. Increases in walking distance in patients with peripheral vascular disease treated with L-carnitine: a double-blind, cross-over study. Ther Prev 1988; 77:767–773.
166. Bruetti G, et al. Propionyl-L-carnitine in intermittent claudication. Double-blind, placebo-controlled, dose titration, multicenter study. J Am Coll Cardiol 1995; 26:1411–1416.
167. European Working Group on Critical Leg Ischemia. Second European consensus document on critical leg ischemia. Circulation 1991; 84:IV-1–IV-22.
168. Nizankowski R, et al. Prostacyclin for ischemic ulcers in peripheral arterial disease: a random-assignment, placebo-controlled study. Thromb Res 1985; 37:21–28.
169. Negus D, Irving JD, Friedgood A. Intra-arterial prostacyclin compared to praxilene in the management of severe lower limb ischemia: a double-blind trial. J Cardiovasc Surg 1987; 28:196–199.
170. Schuler JJ, et al. Efficacy of prostaglandin E_1 in the treatment of lower extremity ischemic ulcers secondary to peripheral vascular occlusive disease. J Vasc Surg 1984; 1:160–170.
171. Belch JJF, et al. Epoprostenol (prostacyclin) and severe arterial disease. A double-blind trial. Lancet 1983; i:315–317.
172. Cronenwett JL, Zelenock GB, Whitehouse WM. Prostacyclin treatment of ischemic ulcers and rest pain in unreconstructible peripheral arterial occlusive disease. Surgery 1986; 100:369–375.
173. Sakaguchi S. Prostaglandin E_1 intra-arterial infusion therapy in patients with ischemic ulcer of the extremities. Int Angiol 1984; 3:39–42.
174. Trübestein G, et al. Prostaglandin E_1 in advanced occlusive arterial disease: results of a multicentre study. Vasa 1987; 17:39–43.
175. Norgren L, et al. A stable prostacyclin analogue (iloprost) in the treatment of ischaemic ulcers of the lower limb: A Scandinavian-Polish placebo-controlled, randomised multicenter study. Eur J Vasc Surg 1990; 4:463–467.
176. Scheffler P, et al. Intensive vascular training in stage IIb of peripheral arterial occlusive disease. The additive effects of intravenous prostaglandin E_1 or intravenous pentoxifylline during training. Circulation 1994; 90:818–822.
177. Verhaeghe R. Prophylactic antiplatelet therapy in peripheral arterial disease. Drugs 1991; 42[Suppl 5]:51–57.
178. Schoop W, et al. Experimentelle und klinische Studien zu der sekundären Prävention der peripheren Arteriosklerose. In A Bolinger, K Rhyner, eds., Thrombozytenfunktionshemmer. Stuttgart: George Thieme, 1983. Pp. 49–58.
179. Hess H, Mietaschk A, Deichsel G. Drug-induced inhibition of platelet function delays progression of peripheral occlusive arterial disease: a prospective double-blind arteriographically controlled trial. Lancet 1985; 1:415–419.
180. Goldhaber SZ, et al. Low-dose aspirin and subsequent peripheral arterial surgery in the Physicians' Health Study. Lancet 1992; 340:143–145.
181. Chesebro JH, et al. Antiplatelet therapy in coronary disease progression: reduced infarction and new lesion formation. Circulation 1989; 80:II-226–II-266.
182. Arcan JC, Panak E. Ticlopidine in the treatment of peripheral occlusive arterial disease. Semin Thromb Haemostas 1989; 15:167–170.
183. Balsano F, et al. Ticlopidine in the treatment of intermittent claudication: a 21-month double blind trial. J Lab Clin Med 1989; 114:84–91.
184. Boissel JP, Peyrieux JC, Destors JM. Is it possible to reduce the risk of cardiovascular events in subjects suffering from intermittent claudication of the lower limbs? Thromb Haemostasis 1989; 62:681–685.
185. Antiplatelet Trialists' Collaboration. Collaborative overview of randomised trials of antiplatelet therapy—I. Prevention of death, myocardial infarction, and stroke by prolonged antiplatelet therapy in various categories of patients. BMJ 1994; 308:81–106.
186. Isner JM, Rosenfield K. Redefining the treatment of peripheral artery disease. Role of percutaneous revascularization. Circulation 1993; 88:1534–1557.
187. Pentacost MJ, et al. Guidelines for peripheral percutaneous transluminal angioplasty of the abdominal aorta and lower extremity vessels. A statement for health professionals from a special writing group of the Councils on Cardiovascular Radiology, Arteriosclerosis, Cardio-thoracic and Vascular Surgery, Clinical Cardiology, and Epidemiology and Prevention, the American Heart Association. Circulation 1994; 89:511–531.
188. Tegtmeyer CJ, et al. Results and complications of angioplasty in aortoiliac disease. Circulation 1991; 83:I53–I60.
189. Johnston KW. Iliac arteries: Reanalysis of results of balloon angioplasty. Radiology 1993; 186:207–212.
190. Johnston KW. Femoral and popliteal arteries: Reanalysis of results of balloon angioplasty. Radiology 1992; 183:767–771.
191. Capek P, Mclean GK, Berdowitz HD. Femoropopliteal angioplasty. Factors influencing long-term success. Circulation 1991; 83:I70–I80.
192. Schwarten DE. Clinical and anatomical considerations for nonoperative therapy in tibial disease and the results of angioplasty. Circulation 1991; 83:I86–90.
193. Horvath W, Oertle M, Haidinger D. Percutaneous transluminal angioplasty of crural arteries. Radiology 1990; 177:565–569.
194. Bakal CW, Sprayregen S, Scheinbaum K. Percutaneous transluminal angioplasty of the infrapopliteal arteries: results in 53 patients. AJR 1990; 154:171–174.
195. Wilson SE, Wolf GE, Cross AP. Percutaneous transluminal angioplasty versus operation for peripheral arteriosclerosis. J Vasc Surg 1989; 9:1–9.
196. Wolf GL, et al. Surgery or balloon angioplasty for peripheral vascular disease. JVIR 1993; 4:639–648.
197. Johnston KW, et al. 5-year results of a prospective study of

percutaneous transluminal angioplasty. Ann Surg 1987; 206:403–413.
198. Vallbracht C, et al. Results of low speed rotational angioplasty for chronic peripheral occlusions. Am J Cardiol 1988; 62:935–940.
199. Zacca NM, et al. Treatment of symptomatic peripheral atherosclerotic disease with a rotational atherectomy device. Am J Cardiol 1989; 63:77–80.
200. Hinohara T, et al. Directional atherectomy. New approaches for treatment of obstructive coronary and peripheral vascular disease. Circulation 1990; 81:IV79–IV91.
201. vonPolnitz A, et al. Percutaneous peripheral atherectomy: angiographic and clinical follow-up of 60 patients. J Am Coll Cardiol 1990; 15:682.
202. Hofling B, et al. Percutaneous removal of atheromatous plaque in peripheral arteries. Lancet 1988; 1:384–386.
203. Fogarty TJ, et al. Experience with balloon catheter technic for arterial embolectomy. Am J Surg 1971; 122:231–237.
204. Elliott JP Jr, et al. Arterial embolization: problems of source, multiplicity, recurrence, and delayed treatments. Surgery 1980; 88:833–845.
205. Risius B, et al. Recombinant human tissue-type plasminogen activator for thrombolysis in peripheral arteries and bypass grafts. Radiology 1986; 160:183–188.
206. Risius B, et al. Thrombolytic therapy with recombinant tissue-type plasminogen activator: a comparison of two doses. Radiology 1987; 164:465–468.
207. Verstraete M, et al. Femoro-popliteal artery thrombolysis with intra-arterial infusion of recombinant tissue-type plasminogen activator: report of a pilot trial. Eur J Vasc Surg 1988; 2:155–159.
208. Meyerovitz MF, et al. Recombinant tissue-type plasminogen activator versus urokinase in peripheral arterial and graft occlusions: a randomized trial. Radiology 1990; 175:75–78.
209. Ricotta JJ, Green RM, DeWeese JA. Use and limitations of thrombolytic therapy in the treatment of peripheral arterial ischemia: results of a multi-institutional questionnaire. J Vasc Surg 1987; 6:45–50.
210. Sullivan KL, et al. Efficacy of thrombolysis in infrainguinal bypass grafts. Circulation 1991; 83:I99–I105.
211. Ouriel K, et al. A comparison of thrombolytic therapy with operative revascularization in the initial treatment of acute peripheral arterial ischemia. J Vasc Surg 1994; 19:1021–1030.
212. Szilagyi DE, et al. A thirty-year survey of reconstructive surgical treatment of aortoiliac occlusive disease. J Vasc Surg 1986; 3:421–436.
213. Crawford ES, et al. Aortoiliac occlusive disease: factors influencing survival and function following reconstructive operations over a twenty-five year period. Surgery 1981; 90:1055.
214. Brewster DC. Clinical and anatomical considerations for surgery in aortoiliac disease and the results of surgical treatment. Circulation 1991; 83:I42–I52.
215. LoGerfo FW, et al. A comparison of the late patency rates of axillobilateral femoral and axillounilateral femoral grafts. Surgery 1977; 81:33–40.
216. Taylor LM Jr., Edwards JM, Porter JM. Present status of reversed vein bypass grafting: Five year results of a modern series. J Vasc Surg 1990; 11:193–206.
217. Donaldson MC, Mannick JA, Whittemore AD. Femoral-distal bypass *in situ* greater saphenous vein. Ann Surg 1991; 213:457–465.
218. Bergamini TM, et al. Experience with in situ saphenous vein bypass as during 1981 to 1989: Determinant factors of long-term patency. J Vasc Surg 1991; 13:137–149.
219. Mannick JA, Whittemore AD, Donaldson MC. Clinical and anatomic considerations for surgery in tibial disease and the results of surgery. Circulation 1991; 83:I81–I85.

Renovascular Hypertension

Thomas G. Pickering

Occlusive disease of the renal arteries is an important diagnosis to make, first, because it is the most common curable form of hypertension at any age and, second, because it is one of the few potentially reversible causes of chronic renal failure. The demonstration of a renal artery stenosis in a hypertensive patient does not necessarily establish a diagnosis of renovascular hypertension, however, because essential hypertension may accelerate the development of atheromatous plaques, which may occur in the renal arteries and elsewhere. Ideally, it is necessary to demonstrate that there is also renal ischemia, since that is thought to be the stimulus that raises the blood pressure, acting mainly via the renin-angiotensin system. There are two main causes of renal vascular disease: the fibromuscular dysplasias in younger patients and atheroma in older ones. In contrast to fibromuscular disease, atherosclerosis is a diffuse process, involving not only one or both renal arteries but also other regional arterial beds. The temporal sequence of atherosclerotic renal arterial disease and its major consequences is outlined in Fig. 36-1. The major cardiovascular risk factors (smoking, hyperlipidemia, and hypertension) are presumed to accelerate the development of atherosclerotic plaques in the renal arteries as elsewhere. The distribution of the lesions is rarely symmetrical, and atherosclerotic renal arterial disease almost always starts out being functionally unilateral.

The major consequence of unilateral renal-artery stenosis is renovascular hypertension. In the case of atherosclerotic stenoses, it is important to recognize that the hypertension may be of mixed origin—a renovascular component superimposed on essential hypertension. That explains why the cure rate of the hypertension following successful revascularization is less for atheromatous disease than for fibromuscular disease.

The resulting hypertension may further accelerate the development of atheroma, such that functionally significant bilateral renal artery stenoses develop. That leads to the second major consequence of the disease process, which is a progressive impairment of renal function, commonly referred to as **ischemic nephropathy**. A third consequence, which occurs in a subset of patients with bilateral renal arterial disease, is the occurrence of **recurrent pulmonary edema**.

Pathophysiology of Occlusive Renal Arterial Disease

The demonstration of a renal-artery stenosis in a hypertensive patient does not necessarily establish a diagnosis of renovascular hypertension, because essential hypertension may accelerate the development of atheromatous plaques, which do not necessarily have any functional significance. Ideally, it is necessary to demonstrate that there is also renal ischemia, since this is thought to be the stimulus that raises the blood pressure, leading to a decline of renal function.

The role of the renin-angiotensin system in the development of renovascular hypertension is paramount and is outlined in Fig. 36-2. In experimental animals, two distinct models of renovascular hypertension can be produced [1–4]. In the first model, called the one-clip two-kidney model (analogous to unilateral renal-artery stenosis in humans), the hypertension is renin dependent. In the second, the one-clip one-kidney model (analogous to renal-artery stenosis in a solitary kidney or possibly to bilateral renal-artery stenosis in humans), the hypertension is sodium and volume dependent, and blockade of the renin-angiotensin system has little effect on blood pressure [2], unless the animal has been sodium depleted [5].

PATHOPHYSIOLOGIC DIFFERENCES BETWEEN UNILATERAL AND BILATERAL STENOSES

An important question is whether the pathophysiology of the two common human patterns can be equated with the two animal models. The resemblance between unilateral human renal-artery stenosis and the one-clip two-kidney model is close, since both clearly are dependent on increased secretion of renin by the ischemic kidney. What is much less clear is what occurs with bilateral stenoses. Relatively little information is available concerning peripheral renin levels, although two studies have reported that renin may be high in patients with both unilateral and bilateral disease [6,7]. Consistent with that finding, patients with bilateral renal-artery stenosis are just as likely to show a decrease of blood pressure when given converting enzyme inhibitors [7]. The pattern of renal-vein renin secretion is also indistinguishable, and in patients with bilateral renal-artery stenosis, the renins tend to lateralize to the most ischemic kidney [8].

In addition to the evidence of hypersecretion of renin in patients with bilateral renovascular disease, several pieces of circumstantial evidence suggest that there also may be an increased effective blood volume. First, in patients with bilateral disease, the cardiac output is usually higher than in patients with unilateral disease [9]. Second, as described in more detail below, we have found that recurrent pulmonary edema is more common in patients with bilateral than unilateral disease [10]. Third, successful revascularization by angioplasty in a patient with bilateral renal-artery stenosis or a solitary kidney frequently is followed by diuresis, which is not seen in patients with unilateral disease (Fig. 36-3) [11].

Thus, the overall picture in patients with bilateral renal-artery stenosis is a mixed one, with both renin and volume factors typically being involved (Table 36-1). In that respect, it differs from the one-kidney animal model, which is more highly dependent on volume factors. The most likely reason for that is that bilateral disease almost never develops symmetrically in the two kidneys, as witnessed

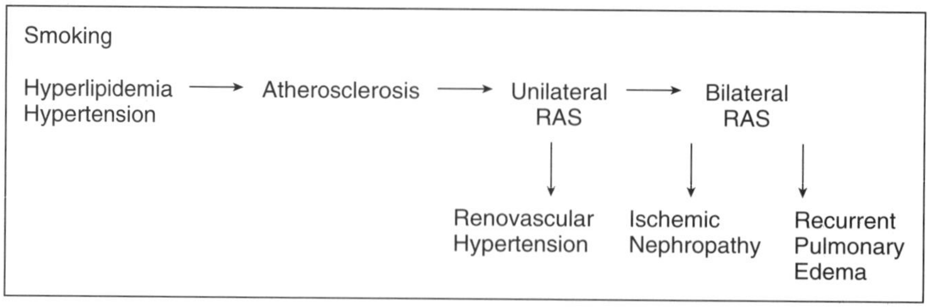

Fig. 36-1. Temporal sequence of progression of atherosclerotic renal-artery occlusive disease. RAS = renal artery stenosis.

by the common finding of unequal kidney sizes and asymmetrical renal-vein renin patterns. All bilateral cases presumably start out with unilateral disease. During the early stages of unilateral involvement, there may well be parenchymal disease developing in the contralateral kidney, which would impair the pressure natriuresis by which the contralateral kidney normally maintains the classic high renin–normal volume pattern of unilateral renal-artery stenosis. That volume retention would be exacerbated when the second stenosis developed in the contralateral renal artery.

Plasma catecholamines usually are normal in human renovascular hypertension [12], unless there is azotemia [13]. The ischemic kidney produces increased amounts of prostaglandins (particularly E_2) as well as renin, and both may be suppressed by nonsteroidal anti-inflammatory drugs such as aspirin [14]. Those agents may lower blood pressure in patients with renovascular hypertension, whereas they tend to raise blood pressure in essential hypertensives.

THE RENIN-ANGIOTENSIN SYSTEM AND THE CONTROL OF INTRARENAL HEMODYNAMICS

The clinical observation that converting-enzyme inhibitors may cause a deterioration of renal function in some patients with renovascular hypertension can be accounted for by animal studies that have demonstrated the important effects of angiotensin on intrarenal hemodynamics [15]. One of the most important intrarenal effects of angiotensin II is a decrease of renal blood flow, with a smaller decrease of glomerular filtration rate (GFR). Hence, filtration fraction increases [16]. It has been proposed that those changes are brought about by a vasoconstriction of both afferent and efferent arterioles, with the predominant effect being on the latter (Fig. 36-4). Thus, in the normal kidney, particularly when renin levels are high, angiotensin blockade increases renal blood flow, with less consistent changes of GFR [17]. In the ischemic kidney, GFR is maintained by angiotensin II–mediated efferent vasoconstriction, so that angiotensin blockade lowers it. This effect provides the rationale for captopril renography.

Fig. 36-2. The effects of renal ischemia on the renin-angiotensin-aldosterone system in renovascular hypertension.

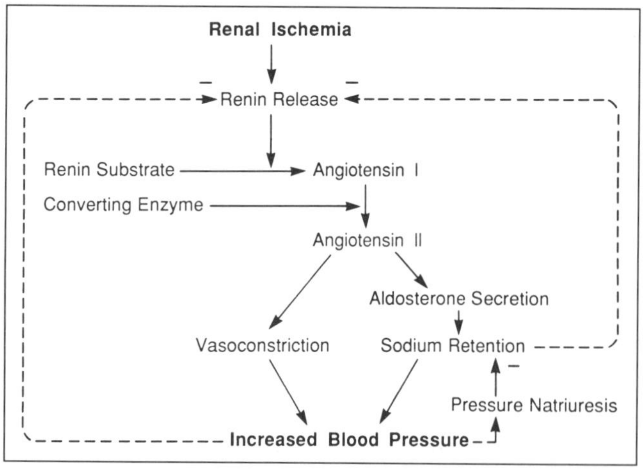

GLOMERULAR PRESSURE: A DETERMINANT OF RENAL VASCULAR DAMAGE

It is well recognized that in the one-clip two-kidney model of renovascular hypertension, the unclipped kidney suf-

Fig. 36-3. The effects of renal angioplasty in a patient with bilateral renal-artery stenosis, showing an improvement in serum creatinine and a diuresis.

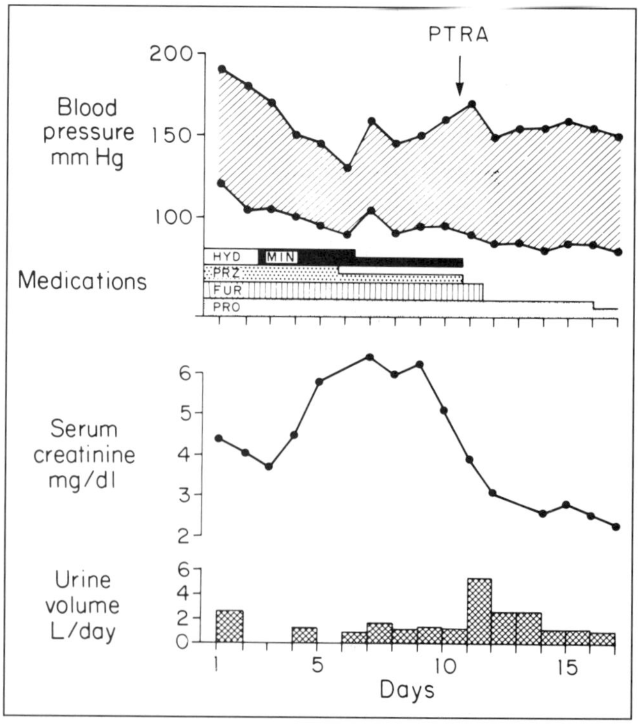

Table 36-1. Comparison of animal and human models of renovascular hypertension

	Renin	Plasma volume	BP response to ACE inhibitor
Animal model			
Two-kidney one-clip	High	Normal	Decrease
One-kidney one-clip	Normal	High	No change
Human model			
Unilateral stenosis	High	Normal	Decrease
Bilateral stenosis	Normal/high	High (?)	Decrease

fers a greater degree of vascular and glomerular damage than the clipped kidney [18]. Whether it is a direct hemodynamic effect of the blood pressure or due to the mitogenic and hypertrophic effects of hormones such as angiotensin II is not clear. Eng et al. [19] studied rats with one-clip two-kidney angiotensin-dependent hypertension and showed that the unclipped kidney, which was exposed to high blood pressure, developed significant glomerular and tubulointerstitial injury, tubulointerstitial-cell proliferation, and collagen deposition. The unclipped kidney, which was protected from hypertension but exposed to angiotensin, showed minimal damage, suggesting that the blood pressure was responsible.

The role of glomerular pressure is further suggested by studies comparing the effects of different types of antihypertensive drugs. In rats with renovascular hypertension, Wenzel et al. [20,21] found that the calcium-channel blocker nitrendipine aggravated glomerular damage if the blood pressure was not reduced. Treatment with enalapril did lower blood pressure without exacerbating renal damage, and combined treatment lowered blood pressure further and prevented the renal damage [21]. Those findings can be explained by the different effects of the two agents on intrarenal hemodynamics: Calcium channel blockers preferentially dilate the afferent glomerular arteriole [21], while angiotensin converting enzyme (ACE) inhibitors have a greater effect on the efferent arteriole [22,23]. Thus, if nitrendipine fails to lower the systemic pressure, its vasodilator action on the afferent arteriole actually could raise the glomerular pressure and, hence, exacerbate the damage. That would not occur with an ACE inhibitor.

Fig. 36-4. Hypothetical effects of angiotensin (ANG II), ACE inhibitors (ACEI),and calcium antagonists in renovascular hypertension. P_A = blood pressure in renal artery proximal and distal ($P_{A'}$) to a stenosis; R_a and R_e = afferent and efferent arteriolar resistance.

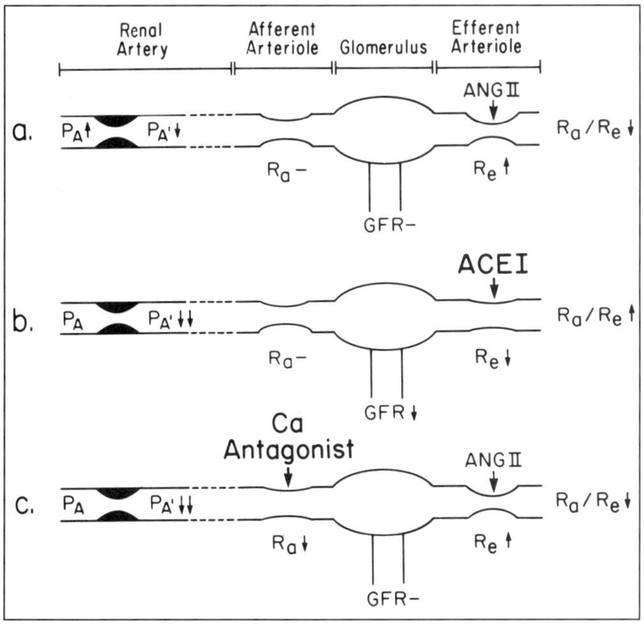

Consequences of Occlusive Renal Arterial Disease

RENOVASCULAR HYPERTENSION

The prevalence of renovascular hypertension is unknown, but it is probably anywhere between 0.2 and 5.0 percent of the general hypertensive population [24–27]; in patients with more severe hypertension, it may be much higher. In patients with accelerated or malignant hypertension (grade III or IV retinopathy), a prevalence of 43 percent in white patients and 7 percent in blacks has been reported [28]. Other studies also have reported a lower prevalence in blacks than in whites [29].

Those results were all based on clinical studies that, with one exception [28], did not utilize arteriography in all patients; therefore, the prevalence rates are almost certainly an underestimate. The situation is complicated by the fact that the demonstration of an anatomical stenosis in the renal artery of a hypertensive patient does not imply that the lesion is causing the hypertension, since renal-artery stenosis not infrequently has been reported in normotensive subjects [30,31]. In patients undergoing coronary angiography, a significant and previously unsuspected renal-artery stenosis was reported in 17 percent of hypertensives but was equally common in normotensives (Fig. 36-5) [31]. In patients referred for investigation of peripheral vascular disease, 59 percent had stenosis (of 50% or more) of at least one renal artery [32]. Again, the presence or absence of a stenosis was unrelated to hypertension. Those studies emphasize the importance of establishing the functional significance of a renal-artery stenosis before proceeding to revascularization.

RENAL FAILURE; ISCHEMIC NEPHROPATHY

Occlusive renal arterial disease that is either bilateral or present when there is a solitary kidney is becoming increasingly recognized as an important and potentially

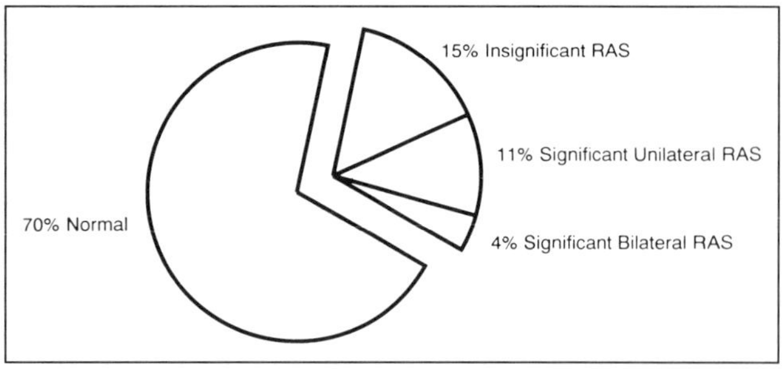

Fig. 36-5. Prevalence of previously unsuspected renal-artery stenosis in patients undergoing coronary angiography. (Data from MB Harding et al. Renal artery stenosis: prevalence and associated risk factors in patients undergoing routine cardiac catheterization. J Am Soc Nephrol 1992; 2:1608–1616.)

reversible cause of renal failure and is termed **ischemic nephropathy** [33]. In a recently reported surgical series, 72 percent of operations for renal revascularization were undertaken primarily for the salvage of renal function [34]; most of those cases had atheromatous renal arterial disease.

A striking and unexplained epidemiologic trend has been the sixfold increase over the past 10 years in the proportion of new cases of end-stage renal disease (ESRD) attributable to hypertension, at a time when the medical treatment of hypertension has become not only more effective but also more widely utilized [35]. The degree to which ischemic nephropathy has contributed to that increased rate is uncertain, although it has been estimated to be present in approximately 15 percent of new cases of ESRD [36].

There are several clinical manifestations of ischemic nephropathy. One clue to its presence may be a sudden deterioration of renal function that follows the introduction of an ACE inhibitor to a patient's antihypertensive regimen. As already discussed, this has been attributed to the abolition of angiotensin-mediated vasoconstriction of the efferent glomerular arterioles, which helps to maintain glomerular filtration in this condition. It should be pointed out, however, that the finding that renal function deteriorates with ACE inhibitors does not always indicate a diagnosis of ischemic nephropathy [37], and other antihypertensives can induce it in patients who do have ischemic nephropathy [38].

Ischemic nephropathy also may be suspected in azotemic patients who have evidence of atherosclerosis elsewhere in the body. In a small series of patients aged from 45 to 75 years and with serum creatinines above 2 mg/dl, ischemic nephropathy was detected in 15 percent [39]. Finally, in patients with known renovascular disease, particularly when they are treated medically, progression of azotemia may also occur when ischemic nephropathy evolves.

RECURRENT PULMONARY EDEMA

We have been impressed by the relatively frequent occurrence of pulmonary edema in patients with advanced renovascular hypertension [10]. In a series of 55 consecutive cases who were also azotemic, pulmonary edema had occurred in 13 (23%). In the majority of those cases (92%), the renal-artery stenosis was bilateral, or there was a solitary kidney with a stenosed artery. Successful revascularization of even one of the ischemic kidneys prevented further occurrence of the pulmonary edema. The occurrence of pulmonary edema was not related to the severity of the hypertension or renal failure. While it was more common in patients who had associated coronary heart disease, it also occurred in patients with normal coronary arteries. Others have reported similar cases [40,41].

Another series of 17 cases reported by Messina et al. [42] consisted of 8.9 percent of their patients undergoing surgical revascularization. All had severe hypertension and azotemia (mean serum creatinine 3.8 mg/dl), and 94 percent had bilateral renal artery disease. Renal revascularization was uniformly effective in controlling the episodes of pulmonary edema over an average follow-up period of 2.4 years.

The pathophysiology of pulmonary edema appears to be related to a number of factors. The common features are severe hypertension, bilateral renal artery disease, azotemia, and a generally excellent blood pressure response to revascularization, which may indicate that the hypertension is truly renovascular. In an analogy with the one-clip one-kidney animal model of renovascular hypertension, hypervolemia may be considered to be a factor. Hypervolemia is one of the physiologic features that distinguishes the condition from unilateral renal-artery stenosis. When the disease is unilateral, hypervolemia may be prevented by a pressure natriuresis operating via the normally functioning contralateral kidney; when it is bilateral, no renal tissue is exposed to the systemic level of blood pressure, so the natriuresis will be less.

The heart also may contribute to the pathogenesis. Although coronary artery disease is often present (in keeping with the advanced atherosclerosis typical of such patients), it usually is not severe and in some cases may be absent. Systolic function is good, as might be expected from the very high blood pressure levels that are frequently generated. The most consistent finding is marked left ventricular hypertrophy, and it may be presumed that the accompanying diminution of diastolic compliance also contributes to the increased pulmonary capillary pressure, which results in pulmonary edema.

Pathology of Renal Arteries

ATHEROMATOUS LESIONS

Atheromatous plaques occur most commonly in the proximal third of the renal artery, and in many cases plaques in the wall of the aorta may encroach on the ostium of the renal artery. Differentiation between proximal and ostial lesions is important because of their different responses to renal angioplasty (see below). If atheromatous lesions are left untreated, there is a high probability of progression to complete occlusion: In one series, the average rate of progression of the percentage of transluminal diameter stenosed was estimated to be about 1.5 percent a month [43]. It has been estimated that 15 percent of patients with ESRD have renovascular disease as the primary cause [36].

FIBROMUSCULAR DYSPLASIA

Fibromuscular dysplasia of the renal arteries is the most common cause of renovascular hypertension in younger patients and has been classified into four types according to the pathologic differences in the lesions [44]. **Medial fibroplasia** is the most common variety in adults (accounting for at least 70% of cases) but is rare in children. It produces the classic beaded appearance on angiography due to areas of thickening of the media, interspersed by areas of aneurysmal dilatation. This type of lesion also may occur in the carotid and cerebral arteries. Progression of the lesions to complete occlusion almost never occurs [45].

ARTERITIS

Takayasu's arteritis is a rare disease that affects mainly young women. It can cause discrete stenosis of the aorta and major arteries, including the renal arteries [44].

CHOLESTEROL EMBOLI

In patients who have diffuse atheroma, fragments of plaque may break off and cause embolization in the kidneys and other vascular beds. This may occur spontaneously or following aortic surgery and renal arteriography [46]. Pathologically, the lesions are characterized by microemboli of cholesterol crystals and amorphous debris, which are later replaced by foreign-body giant cells and fibrosis. Clinically, the emboli are manifested by a deterioration of renal function and an exacerbation of the hypertension [47]. Other features include symptoms of mesenteric vascular insufficiency, acute pancreatitis, and gangrene or livedo reticularis in the feet. The diagnosis may be suspected if the manifestations develop after an invasive procedure in a patient with known atheromatous disease but can only be established with certainty if the microemboli are visualized on a tissue biopsy.

Clinical Features of Renovascular Hypertension

CLINICAL SIGNS AND SYMPTOMS

Clues to the presence of renal artery stenosis may be derived from the history and clinical examination. Table 36-2 lists some of the most important features that distinguish renovascular hypertension from essential hypertension and the differences between the two most common types, atheroma and fibromuscular dysplasia.

In younger patients, particularly in women, fibromuscular disease is the most common cause, but it is relatively rare in blacks. A family history of hypertension is less likely to be present than in cases of essential hypertension, although a familial occurrence of fibromuscular dysplasia has occasionally been described [48]. Thus, in a young white woman with a recent onset of hypertension and a negative family history, there should be a very high index of suspicion for fibromuscular disease. Women with fibromuscular dysplasia tend to be taller than those with essential hypertension or atheromatous renal-artery stenosis [49].

Conversely, the finding of hypertension in a middle-aged man with other evidence of atheromatous disease such as coronary heart disease should raise the possibility of atheromatous renovascular hypertension. A history of smoking is another potential clue to the presence of renovascular hypertension. In our own series of patients with atheromatous renal-artery stenosis, 88 percent were smokers, compared to only 42 percent of patients with essential hypertension [50]. Smoking also may be a risk factor for fibromuscular disease [50,51].

Abdominal bruits are present in about 40 percent of patients and usually signify the presence of renal-artery stenosis, although they may originate from other vessels. Such bruits are, of course, most likely to be heard in thin patients.

Retinopathy may be particularly pronounced in patients with renovascular hypertension, perhaps because of its more brief and stormy course. Pulmonary edema in a hypertensive patient should raise consideration of bilateral renal-artery stenosis.

LABORATORY INVESTIGATIONS

Evidence of impaired renal function on routine biochemical tests, such as an elevated BUN or creatinine, suggests that there is either parenchymal disease, or that if there is renovascular disease, it is bilateral. In the U.S. Cooperative Study, 15 percent of patients with atheromatous renal-artery stenosis had an elevated serum creatinine, compared with 11 percent of patients with essential hypertension and only 2 percent of patients with fibromuscular dysplasia [48].

A low serum potassium is an occasional marker of renovascular disease: In the U.S. Cooperative Study, about 15 percent of patients had a potassium level below 3.4 mEq/liter. This occurs as a result of hyperreninemia stimulating angiotensin and aldosterone.

Urinalysis may show a slightly increased incidence of bacteriuria. Proteinuria is not uncommon [52], and may occasionally be sufficiently pronounced to present as a nephrotic syndrome [53]. In our own experience proteinuria in excess of 500 mg per 24 hours usually signifies complete occlusion of a renal artery in patients with renovascular hypertension [54]. This proteinuria may be reversed by surgery or angioplasty.

RENAL SEGMENTAL INFARCTION

In occasional patients who present with acute accelerated hypertension, the underlying abnormality may be renal segmental infarction [55]. Clinically, it is characterized by abdominal or flank pain sometimes associated with nausea, vomiting, and fever. Hematuria and proteinuria also may occur. Although there may be very high blood pressure with retinopathy, both the ECG and renal function may be normal. Investigations show hyperreninemia with lateralizing renal-vein renins. IVP and renal scans may demonstrate a decreased kidney size on one side, but the diagnosis is confirmed by arteriography, which shows characteristic defects in the nephrogram phase. The patients typically are young (e.g., 30 to 50 years old), and the underlying pathology usually is fibromuscular dysplasia with thrombosis occurring in an aneurysm. The hypertension is renin dependent and may respond dramatically to treatment with ACE inhibitors; therefore, surgery may not be necessary.

Table 36-2. Clinical characteristics of renovascular hypertension

	Percentage of patients		
	Essential hypertension	Renovascular atheroma	Hypertension FMD
Race (black)	29	7	10
Family history	67	58	41
Age at onset			
<20 years	12	2	16
>50 years	7	39	13
Duration >1 year	10	23	19
Obese	38	17	11
Abdominal bruit	7	41	57
High renin profile	15	80	80
Hypokalemia (K < 3.4 mEq/liter)	7	14	17
Smoking	42	88	71

Sources: MH Maxwell et al. Cooperative study of renovascular hypertension. Demographic analysis of the study. JAMA 1972; 220:1195–1204. AG Goldman, PD Varady, SS Franklin. Body habitus and serum cholesterol in essential hypertension and renovascular hypertension. Cooperative study of renovascular hypertension. JAMA 1972; 221:378–383. JP Nicholson et al. Cigarette smoking and renovascular hypertension. Lancet 1983; 2:765–766.

RENOVASCULAR HYPERTENSION IN CHILDREN

Fibromuscular dysplasia is the most common cause of renovascular hypertension in children and is usually of the intimal or perimedial type [56,57]. In contrast to adults, medial fibroplasia is rare. The lesions commonly are ostial and bilateral and may be associated with neurofibromatosis or coarctation of the abdominal aorta.

Diagnosis of Renovascular Hypertension

Renovascular hypertension is almost certainly underdiagnosed in clinical practice. Extensive screening of all hypertensive patients is impractical, but a number of clinical clues should increase the clinician's suspicion of its presence. Some of those clues are listed in Table 36-3.

There is no perfect screening test for the detection of renovascular hypertension. A large number of tests have been proposed, which can be classified into two categories. First are those tests that can be done in the physician's office—they are relatively simple to perform and inexpensive but do not indicate which kidney is involved. Measurement of peripheral plasma renin activity and the captopril test are in the first category. In the second category are tests that provide anatomical or functional information about each kidney. Ideally, one or more of these tests should be done following the first-stage test.

PERIPHERAL PLASMA RENIN ACTIVITY

A high plasma renin activity (PRA) level, measured in the morning with the patient in the seated position and indexed against sodium excretion, is present in about 75 percent of patients with proven renovascular hypertension [58,59]. Its predictive value in the absence of clinical clues of renovascular hypertension, however, is low. PRA is normal in some patients with renovascular hypertension but rarely, if ever, low.

Table 36-3. Testing for renovascular hypertension: clinical index of suspicion as a guide to selecting patients for work-up

INDEX OF CLINICAL SUSPICION
Low (should not be tested)
Borderline, mild, or moderate hypertension, in the absence of clinical clues
Moderate (noninvasive tests recommended)
Severe hypertension (diastolic blood pressure greater than 120 mm Hg)
Hypertension refractory to standard therapy
Abrupt onset of sustained moderate to severe hypertension at age < 20 or > 50 years
Hypertension with a suggestive abdominal bruit (long, high-pitched and localized to the region of the renal artery)
Moderate hypertension (diastolic blood pressure exceeding 105 mm Hg) in a smoker, a patient with evidence of occlusive vascular disease (cerebrovascular, coronary, peripheral vascular), or a patient with unexplained but stable elevation of serum creatinine
Normalization of blood pressure by an ACE inhibitor in a patient with moderate or severe hypertension (particularly in a smoker or patient with recent onset of hypertension)
High (may consider proceeding directly to arteriography)
Severe hypertension (diastolic blood pressure greater than 120 mm Hg) with either progressive renal insufficiency or refractoriness to aggressive treatment (particularly in a patient who has been a smoker or has other evidence of occlusive arterial disease)
Accelerated or malignant hypertension (grade III or IV retinopathy)
Hypertension with recent elevation of serum creatinine, either unexplained or reversibly induced by an ACE inhibitor
Moderate to severe hypertension with incidentally detected asymmetry of renal size

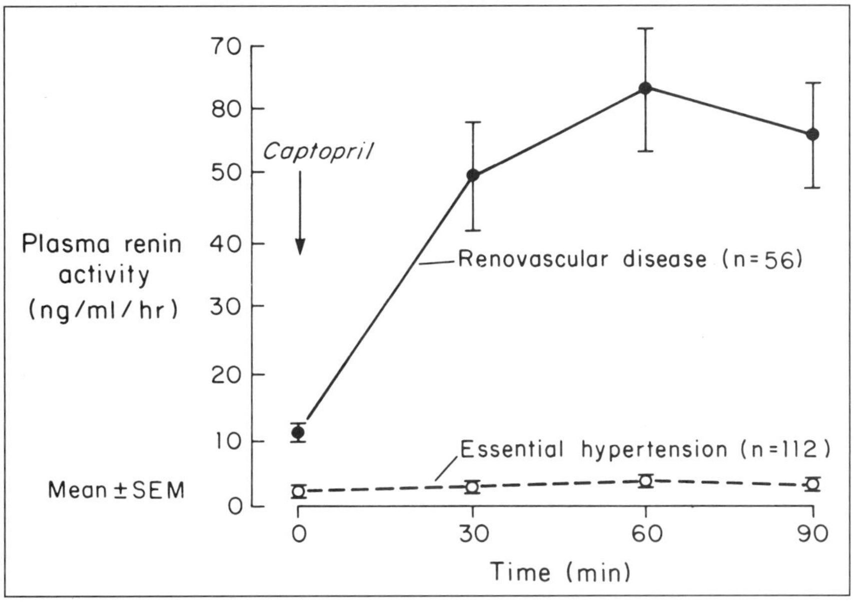

Fig. 36-6. Comparison of effects of a single oral dose of captopril on plasma renin activity in patients with essential hypertension and renovascular hypertension. (From DB Case, JH Laragh. Reactive hyperreninemia in renovascular hypertension after angiotensin blockade with saralasin or converting enzyme inhibitor. Ann Intern Med 1979; 91:153–160.)

CAPTOPRIL TEST

Case and Laragh [60] were the first to show that the reactive rise of renin following administration of captopril is greater in patients with renovascular hypertension than in those with essential hypertension (Fig. 36-6). The criteria found to be the most reliable for distinguishing patients with renovascular hypertension are shown in a postcaptopril renin of more than 12 ng/ml/hour, an absolute increase of 10 ng/ml/hour or more and a percent increase of 150 percent or more (400% if the baseline renin is below 3) [61].

Subsequent studies have confirmed the value of the captopril test [62–69]. The overall sensitivity is approximately 74 percent, and specificity is 89 percent. Differences in the reported accuracy of the test may be attributed to a number of factors, including the assay used, varying criteria for defining renovascular hypertension, and the position of the patient during the test.

Most investigators have found the test to be less reliable in patients who are azotemic, and it does not discriminate between patients with unilateral versus bilateral disease.

RENAL-VEIN RENIN DETERMINATIONS

In patients with unilateral renal-artery stenosis, the ischemic kidney typically secretes an increased amount of renin, causing an elevation in the systemic levels and suppression of renin secretion by the contralateral kidney. That results in a marked asymmetry in PRA in the two renal veins, which can be expressed either as the ratio of PRA in the two renal veins (with an upper limit of normal, or 1.5 : 1 or 2 : 1), or as a comparison of the increment of PRA between the renal vein (V) and the renal artery (A) separately on each side, expressed as (V − A)/A [58]. In practice, the PRA measured in the inferior vena cava distal to the renal veins can be substituted for the arterial level. The normal increment is 25 percent; in patients with renovascular hypertension, it typically is 50 percent or more in the ischemic kidney and zero in the contralateral kidney.

In patients with stenoses of both renal arteries, the pattern of renal-vein renins often shows the same degree of asymmetry as in patients with unilateral stenosis and usually lateralizes to the kidney that shows the greatest degree of stenosis on the arteriogram [8] (Fig. 36-7). The most marked asymmetry is seen in patients who have complete occlusion of one renal artery. Extreme elevations of renal-vein renin may represent low flow through the kidney rather than hypersecretion of renin.

RENAL SCINTIGRAPHY

The use of renal scintigraphy (isotope renography) was based on the finding that I-131 hippuran is selectively taken up by the kidney, and the technique has been used to measure both renal size and blood flow. Another isotope that has been used is technetium diethylene triamine penta-acetic acid (DTPA), which measures GFR. However, because the test has an unacceptably high rate of both false positives and false negatives [70], it is not recommended unless captopril is given first.

CAPTOPRIL RENOGRAPHY

Comparison of renograms obtained before and after a single dose of captopril may improve their diagnostic accuracy. The rationale is that the GFR and the renal blood flow of an ischemic kidney depend on the effects of angiotensin on the efferent glomerular arterioles and, hence, fall markedly with converting enzyme inhibition. Thus, the characteristic effect of captopril in a kidney with

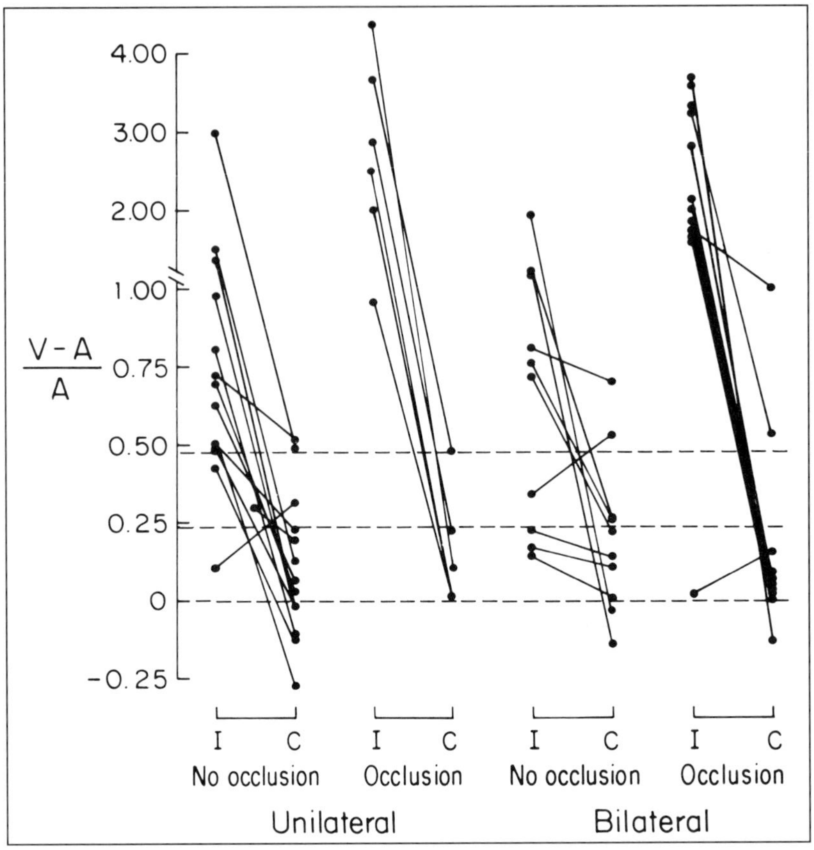

Fig. 36-7. Renal-vein renin patterns in patients with unilateral versus bilateral renal-artery stenosis. I = ischemic kidney; C = contralateral kidney. (Reproduced from TG Pickering et al. Comparison of renal vein renin activity in hypertensive patients with stenosis of one or both renal arteries. J Hypertension 1985; 3[Suppl 3]:S291–S293.)

a renal-artery stenosis is to cause a decrease of DTPA or hippuran uptake [71,72].

Captopril renography has been found to have a high sensitivity (92 percent) and specificity (93 percent), which has led to its becoming one of the most popular noninvasive diagnostic tests [62,72–76]. The test has been performed with two main isotopes, DTPA and hippuran, but more recently, technetium-99m-mercapto-acetyltriglycine (Mag_3) has become popular [77–79].

Several different diagnostic criteria have been proposed for evaluating captopril renography. Two different approaches have been used: comparison of the two kidneys in the postcaptopril scintigrams and examination of the effects of captopril on each kidney individually by comparing the pre- and postcaptopril scintigrams. The uptake of isotope is usually maximal 1.5–2.5 minutes following injection, and an asymmetry of uptake of more than 60:40 percent is a commonly used criterion for defining an abnormality (Fig. 36-8). A second criterion is the time to peak activity, which may be delayed in the presence of a renal-artery stenosis; a third criterion is the percentage of the peak activity that remains at 15 or 20 minutes following injection. When the stenosis is mild, a delayed excretion of isotope may be the only renographic abnormality.

The changes induced by captopril, when present, are highly specific for renovascular disease and are very helpful in distinguishing it from unilateral renal parenchymal disease. Their sensitivity, however, is relatively low (43–80%), and they may be difficult to detect when the stenosis is severe, because the uptake of isotope already may be low on the precaptopril scintigram [73]. It may be more appropriate to perform a single postcaptopril scintigram, which of course greatly reduces the cost.

INTRAVENOUS PYELOGRAM

The sensitivity of the IVP for detecting renovascular hypertension is around 75 percent and the specificity 85 percent [80]. The IVP is unreliable for detecting either branch stenoses or bilateral stenoses, and its low level of accuracy, together with the high doses of dye and radiation it necessitates, has rendered it obsolete as a routine screening test.

INTRAVENOUS DIGITAL SUBTRACTION ANGIOGRAPHY

When it was first introduced, intravenous digital subtraction angiography (DSA) was regarded as a great step forward, since it enabled direct visualization of the renal arteries, while avoiding many of the hazards of arteriography [81–83]. Today, however, it is little used, for several reasons. First, it requires a relatively large dye load, which must be injected centrally. That reduces its convenience

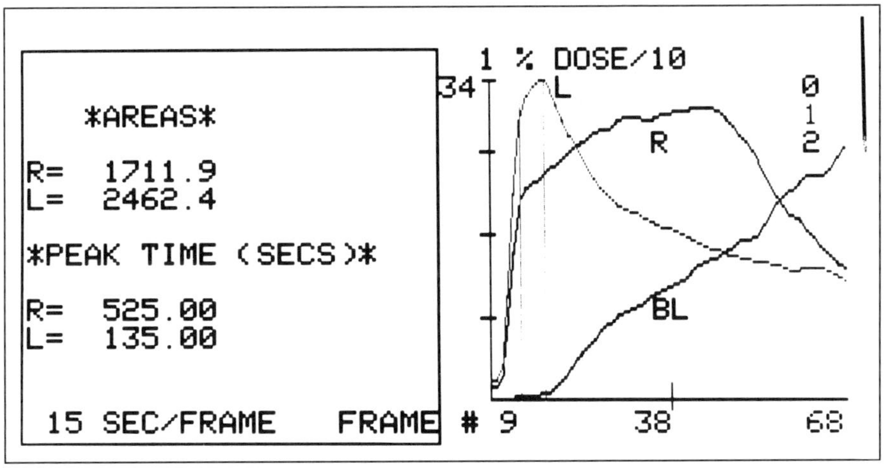

Fig. 36-8. DTPA renogram obtained after captopril administration, demonstrating a normal time-activity curve for the left kidney (L) and an abnormal curve resulting from stenosis of the renal artery in the right kidney (R). The normal curve (L) is characterized by a rapid initial uptake phase, a function of blood flow, with continued accumulation of radioactive counts until, at the peak, excretion begins to exceed uptake. The area under the curve for the uptake at 1.5 to 2.5 minutes (hatched bar) is represented numerically by the counts displayed to the left of the figure and correlates well with GFR. The time to peak, also displayed to the left of the figure, and the percent of the peak uptake retained at 15 minutes are derived from the time-activity. In the abnormal curve (R), uptake at 1.5 to 2.5 minutes is reduced, and, because of reduced excretion, total counts continue to increase, resulting in a delayed peak. The curve labeled BL is a measure of bladder uptake. (Reproduced with permission from SJ Mann et al. Captopril renography in the diagnosis of renal artery stenosis: accuracy and limitations. Am J Med 1991; 90:30–40.)

and poses hazards for patients with impaired renal function. Second, its resolution is significantly less than that obtained with arteriography; proximal stenoses may be obscured by overlapping mesenteric vessels, and branch stenoses may be missed. The resolution also may be impaired in obese patients or in the presence of impaired cardiac function. It has a sensitivity of about 88 percent and a specificity of 90 percent [84].

MAGNETIC RESONANCE ANGIOGRAPHY

Magnetic resonance angiography is a new technique that permits noninvasive visualization of the arteries. In one recent study of its use for diagnosing renovascular hypertension, eight out of nine renal-artery stenoses were detected [85]. There were no false positives, and the single false negative was a failure to detect a branch stenosis. Magnetic resonance angiography may exaggerate the severity of a stenosis, so given its high cost and questionable accuracy, it cannot be recommended for routine use at the present time.

ULTRASOUND SCANS

Another relatively new technique is the use of Doppler ultrasound scanning to record velocity profiles from the renal arteries [86,87]. In patients with renal-artery stenosis, the flow profile is abnormal, with an acceleration of flow across the stenosis.

Several problems with the technique have so far limited its widespread adoption as a routine diagnostic procedure. The number of reported studies is still relatively small; while some authors have claimed to be able to visualize the renal artery in 80 to 90 percent of cases [88,89], others give a figure of only 60 percent [90]. Problems may occur because of obesity, bowel gas, recent surgery, and the presence of multiple renal arteries. The technique cannot reliably detect branch-renal-artery stenoses. One area where ultrasound finds greater application is in the detection of transplant renal-artery stenoses, where the superficial location of the artery to the transplanted kidney may make it easier to detect [91].

ARTERIOGRAPHY

To cause renal ischemia and hypertension, a stenosis must occlude at least 75 percent of the arterial lumen, but the correlation between the arteriographic appearance and the degree of ischemia is poor [92,93]. Recent advances in arteriographic techniques have led to considerable improvements in the safety and convenience of arteriography. Digital subtraction technology enables the acquisition of high-resolution pictures with significantly reduced dye loads [94], and the use of smaller lumen catheters has helped to reduce the problems associated with the arterial puncture and cholesterol emboli [95]. In uncomplicated cases, arteriography can be done as an outpatient procedure.

DETECTION OF PATIENTS WITH RENOVASCULAR HYPERTENSION

The low prevalence of renovascular hypertension in the general population of hypertensive individuals, together with the cost and imperfect accuracy of the available screening tests for its diagnosis, means that universal

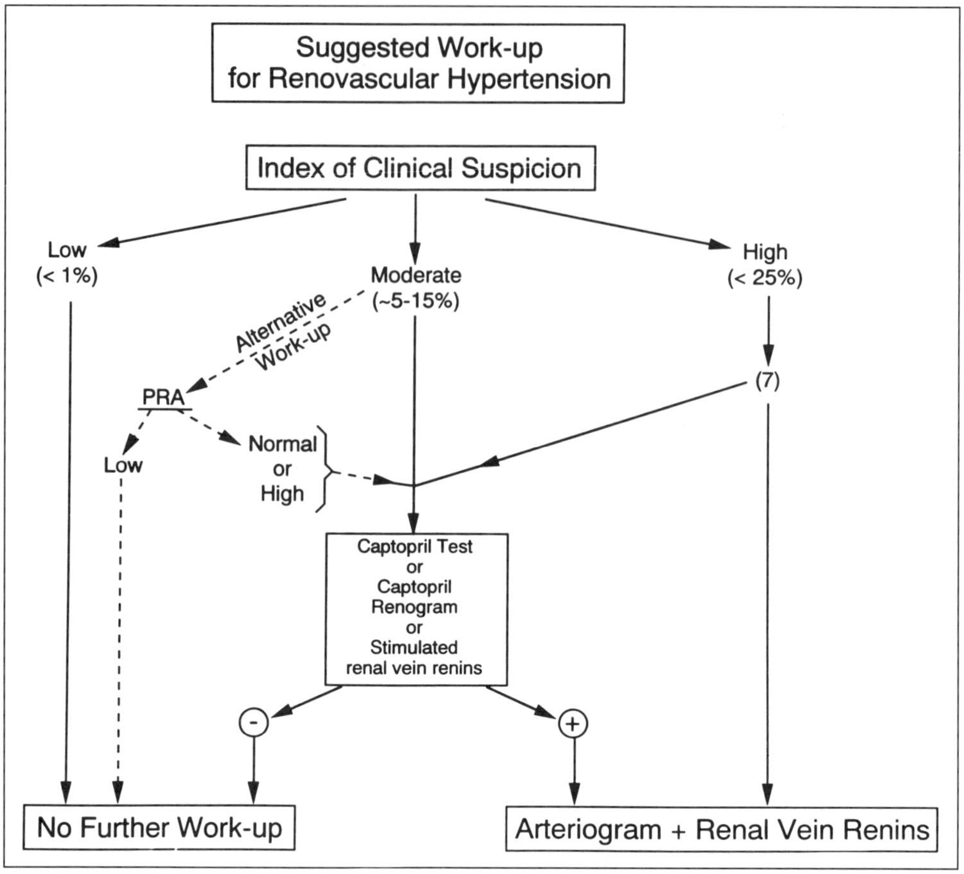

Fig. 36-9. Suggested work-up for patients with suspected renovascular hypertension.

screening of all hypertensive patients is inappropriate. That raises the question of when it is appropriate to perform the diagnostic tests. We suggest a triage approach, based on the level of clinical suspicion [96], as summarized in Table 36-3.

For patients with a low index of suspicion, no further evaluation is needed (Fig. 36-9). These would include the majority of patients with mild or borderline hypertension in whom clinical clues favoring the presence of renovascular disease are absent and patients with low-renin hypertension. In such cases, the prevalence of renovascular disease is likely to be less than 1 percent, and most of the positive test results will turn out to be false positives.

For patients with a moderate index of suspicion, that is, those in whom clinical clues are present, but the evidence for renovascular disease is not overwhelming, the prevalence is likely to be between 5 and 15 percent. In such cases, the predictive value of a negative result of a diagnostic test with a sensitivity and specificity of 90 percent would exceed 98 percent, and the predictive value of a positive result would be 32 percent, which would justify proceeding to an arteriogram.

Finally, there is a third group of patients in whom the index of suspicion is so high that an arteriogram would be justified even if the noninvasive diagnostic tests turned out to be negative. Examples would be patients with severe hypertension whose renal function deteriorates when treated with an ACE inhibitor and patients with accelerated hypertension; such patients have been reported to have a prevalence of renovascular disease of more than 30 percent. Because the presence of azotemia may impair the reliability of the noninvasive tests, it may be appropriate to proceed directly to arteriography.

Treatment of Renovascular Hypertension

There are in principle three modes of treatment for renovascular hypertension: medical, surgical, and angioplasty. Since renal-artery stenoses tend to lead to impairment of renal function as well as hypertension, some type of revascularization is preferred. While surgery is the traditional treatment of choice, angioplasty has gained popularity over the past few years and is now often attempted in preference to surgery.

SURGERY

The first curative treatment of renovascular hypertension was unilateral nephrectomy, which today is rarely performed except when there is no prospect of the preservation of renal function by revascularization, usually because the kidney is atrophic. The role of surgical revascularization was first established by the U.S. Cooperative Study, the results of which were published 20 years ago [97,98].

The blood pressure response to surgery (or angioplasty) is usually classified as cured (a diastolic pressure below 90 mm Hg without medication), improved (a decrease of

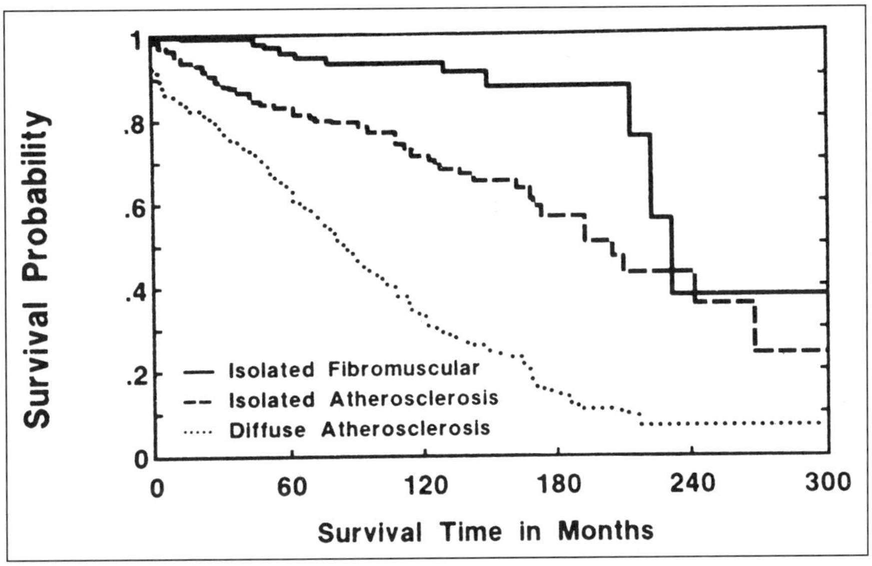

Fig. 36-10. Survival probablity (Kaplan-Meier curves) of patients following surgery for renovascular hypertension according to preoperative diagnosis. (Reproduced with permission from GM Lawrie et al. Renovascular reconstruction: factors affecting long-term prognosis in 919 patients followed up to 31 years. Am J Cardiol 1989; 63:1085–1092.)

at least 15% but still requiring medication), or failed (a decrease of less than 15%), according to the criteria originally developed for the U.S. Cooperative Study of surgery for renovascular hypertension. By today's standards, the results were not very good, but since then a number of large series have been reported with much better results [99–103]. Lawrie et al. [103] described a series of 919 patients followed for up to 31 years. Most had atherosclerotic disease and were treated with a dacron bypass or endarterectomy. The combined cure and improvement rate was 82 percent and the mortality 1.1 percent.

The major determinant of the results of surgical revascularization is the underlying diagnosis. In patients with fibromuscular dysplasia, the cure rate is as high as 80 percent and the morbidity very low. While those results are excellent, they are not significantly better than what can be achieved by renal angioplasty at less cost and inconvenience. However, there are some situations where surgery is clearly preferable, for example, when there is a fusiform stenosis from intimal hyperplasia, which may be resistant to angioplasty. And some lesions may be quite complex, with multiple branch stenoses and aneurysmal areas distal to the stenosis, which may preclude the use of angioplasty.

In patients with atherosclerotic renal-artery stenosis, the results are less good (Fig. 36-10), for three main reasons: First, in contrast to fibromuscular diseases, there is less certainty that the renal-artery stenosis is the cause of the hypertension, and second, the prognosis may be determined more by the extent of atherosclerosis elsewhere in the body. The third potential problem is the release of cholesterol emboli during the operation. In Lawrie's series, the 10-year survival rate was approximately 90 percent in patients with fibromuscular dysplasia, 70 percent in those with isolated atherosclerosis, and 30 percent when there was diffuse atherosclerosis [103]. It is noteworthy that the majority of deaths were due to the consequences of atheroma elsewhere in the body, for example, from myocardial infarction.

Several studies have demonstrated that neither age nor impaired renal function need exclude the possibility of surgical revascularization. In one series [104] of patients over the age of 60, surgical mortality was 2.8 percent and was not significantly higher in those with a baseline creatinine above 1.4 mg/dl.

RENAL ANGIOPLASTY

There are now several published series of clinical results obtained with angioplasty [105–109], but, as with surgery, it is appropriate to consider the results with atheroma and fibromuscular dysplasia separately.

The results with the fibromuscular patients are uniformly good (about 58% cured, 35% improved, and 7% failed) and comparable to those obtained with surgery. Restenosis is uncommon in these patients, and follow-up angiograms (up to 5 years after angioplasty) often show no trace of any stenosis at all.

When the stenosis is caused by atheroma, the results of revascularization are not as good (22% cured, 57% improved, and 21% failed), whichever modality (angioplasty or surgery) is used. Furthermore, in patients with diffuse atheromatous disease, the complication rate with both surgery and angioplasty is relatively high, and medical therapy may be preferred.

In those patients in whom the procedure is technically successful, there is usually a prompt fall of blood pressure. In the atheromatous patients with unilateral stenoses in our series, the eventual benefit rate (defined as an improvement or cure of the hypertension 3 months after angioplasty) was 87 percent and in the fibromuscular pa-

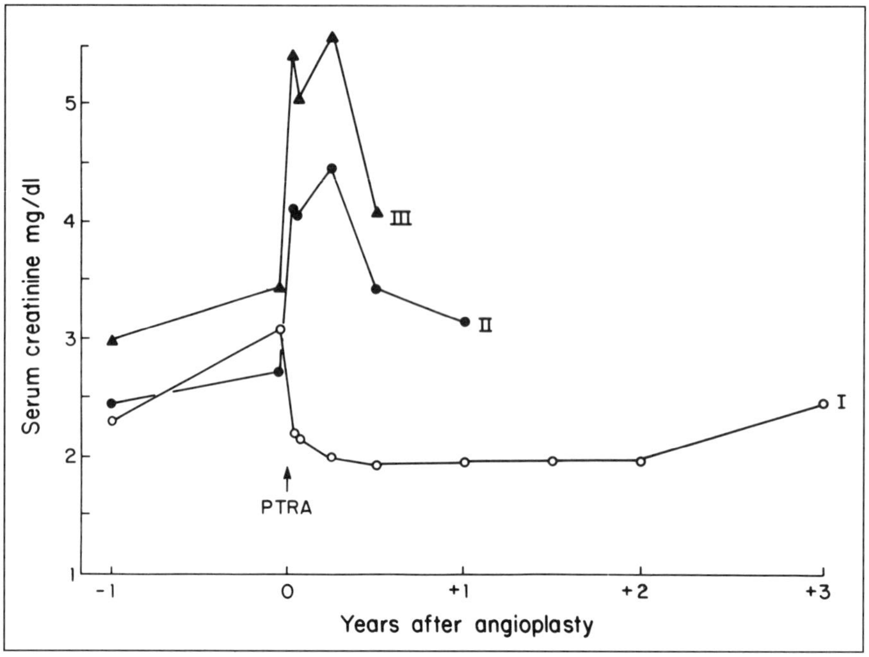

Fig. 36-11. Effects of renal angioplasty in azotemic patients. Patients were divided into three groups: group I—angioplasty successful, with improved creatinine at three months; group II—successful angioplasty but no improvement in renal function; group III—angioplasty unsuccessful. (Data from TG Pickering et al. Renal angioplasty in patients with azotemia and renovascular hypertension. J Hypertens 1986; 4[Suppl 6]:S667–S669.)

tients 92 percent [105]. The rate of restenosis in patients with atheromatous disease has been reported to be 19 percent after 9 months, 35 percent if the lesion was ostial [110]. The latter figure may be an underestimate. The use of stents for maintaining the patency of the artery, particularly if the stenosis is ostial, is being explored [111].

The complications of angioplasty, including hematoma at the puncture site, azotemia from the dye load, and cholesterol emboli, tend to be more common in older patients with diffuse atheromatous disease. Dissection or occlusion of the renal artery also may occur, but it is rare.

SURGERY AND ANGIOPLASTY

In patients with renal failure, both surgical revascularization and angioplasty can result in a significant improvement in renal function. We have seen this in patients who have a critical stenosis of a solitary kidney and in patients who have severe bilateral stenoses. Such patients are notoriously difficult to treat with medications, because a reduction of blood pressure is associated with a dramatic deterioration of renal function. This is most common when ACE inhibitors are used [112]. If angioplasty can be achieved, it is particularly rewarding, because it can both improve renal function and make the blood pressure easier to control (Fig. 36-11). However, we have seen other patients in whom renal function has not improved or has deteriorated despite a technically successful angioplasty. In our series of 57 patients, all of whom had baseline serum creatinines above 2 mg/dl, 43 (75%) could be successfully dilated; of those 43, 27 (63%) showed a decrease of creatinine, 5 (12%) no change, and 11 (26%) an increase [113].

Several studies reviewed by Rimmer and Gennari [36] have reported on the effects of surgical revascularization on renal function in azotemic patients. In many cases, the surgery involved aortic replacement as well as repair of the renal-artery stenosis. The mortality rate was 6 percent, and 55 percent had improved renal function postoperatively. Rimmer and Gennari compared the published results of surgery (eight studies) and angioplasty (six studies) performed in azotemic patients and concluded that improvement in renal function was seen in 55 percent of patients with surgery and in 43 percent with angioplasty [36].

Another advantage of angioplasty over surgery is that it can be undertaken in patients who would be turned down for surgery because of associated conditions such as coronary artery disease or cerebrovascular disease, both of which are common in patients with atheromatous renovascular hypertension.

MEDICAL MANAGEMENT

The two main concerns with medical treatment of patients who are judged to be ineligible for surgery or angioplasty are the progression of the renal-artery stenosis and the hemodynamic effects of blood pressure reduction on renal function. In 1974, Hunt et al. compared the results of medically and surgically treated patients and reported mortality over 7 to 14 years of 70 percent in the medically treated and 30 percent in the surgically treated patients [114]. Most of the deaths were due to complications of atheroma, such as myocardial infarction or stroke, with only a minority dying from uremia. In another series, Dean et al. followed 41 medically treated patients with atheromatous renovascular disease [115]. Twelve percent progressed to complete occlusion, and 41 percent had deterioration of renal function.

There have as yet been no randomized trials comparing medical and surgical treatment, but the studies by Hunt's group and Dean's group merely serve to underline the high probability of progression of atheromatous disease. Both studies were reported nearly 20 years ago, however, and it seems likely that, just as with coronary artery disease, the prognosis of medically treated patients with renal-artery disease should be better today. Introduction of the ACE inhibitors and calcium-channel blockers has greatly facilitated blood pressure control without seriously compromising patients' quality of life.

The long-term use of ACE inhibitors in patients with known renovascular disease is controversial. While animal experiments have indicated that atrophy of the ischemic kidney can be accelerated by ACE inhibitors [116–118], comparable data in humans are inconclusive. In patients with bilateral renal-artery stenosis or with a stenosed renal artery and a solitary kidney, treatment with ACE inhibitors may cause a dramatic increase in the serum creatinine and BUN [119] for the reasons described previously. Those acute changes generally are thought to be reversible. One retrospective analysis suggested a marginally significant association between the use of ACE inhibitors and the development of renal-artery occlusion [120], but another reported no adverse effects on creatinine clearance or kidney size in patients with unilateral renal-artery stenosis treated with captopril for 1 year [119].

In short-term studies, dihydropyridine calcium-channel blockers have been shown to lower blood pressure with less impairment of function of the ischemic kidney than ACE inhibitors [121,122]. The suggestion that that may have beneficial long-term effects remains uncertain [123]. The evidence from animal studies [20] that dihydropyridine calcium-channels blockers may exacerbate glomerular damage if they fail to lower blood pressure is of theoretical concern, but comparable human data are lacking.

References

1. Tobian L, Coffee K, and McCrea P. Contrasting exchangeable sodium in rats with different types of Goldblatt hypertension. Am J Physiol 1969; 217:458–460.
2. Brunner HR, et al. Hypertension of renal origin: evidence for two different mechanisms. Science 1971; 174:1344–1346.
3. Gavras H, et al. Angiotensin-sodium interaction in blood pressure maintenance of renal hypertensive and normotensive rats. Science 1973; 180:1369–1372.
4. Swales JD, et al. Dual mechanism for experimental hypertension. Lancet 1971; 2:1181–1183.
5. Gavras H, et al. Reciprocation of renin dependency in renal hypertension. Science 1979; 188:1316–1317.
6. Bianchi C, Bonadio M, Andriole VT. Influence of postural changes on the glomerular filtration rate in nephroptosis. Nephron 1976; 16:161–172.
7. Derkx RHM, et al. Captopril test for diagnosis of renal artery stenosis. In N Glorioso, et al., eds. Renovascular Hypertension. New York: Raven Press, 1917. Pp 295–315.
8. Pickering TG, et al. Comparison of renal vein renin activity in hypertensive patients with stenosis of one or both renal arteries. J Hypertension 1985; 3[Suppl 3]:S291–S293.
9. Vensel LA, et al. Cardiac structure and function in renovascular hypertension produced by unilateral and bilateral renal artery stenosis. Am J Cardiol 1986; 58:575–582.
10. Pickering TG, et al. Recurrent pulmonary edema as a manifestation of renovascular hypertension and its treatment by renal revascularization. Circulation 1987; 76[Suppl IV]:274.
11. Sutters M, et al. Diuresis and syncope after renal angioplasty in a patient with one functioning kidney. Br Med J 1987; 295:527–528.
12. Maslowski AH, et al. Mechanisms in human renovascular hypertension. Hypertension 1983; 5:597–602.
13. Lake CR, et al. Plasma catecholamine levels in normal subjects and in patients with secondary hypertension. Fed Proc 1984; 43:52–56.
14. Imanishi M, et al. Aspirin test for differentiation of unilateral renovascular hypertension from hyperreninemic essential hypertension. Am J Hypertens 1991; 4:761–768.
15. Navar LG, Rosivall L. Contribution of the renin-angiotensin system to the control of intrarenal hemodynamics. Kidney Int 1984; 25:857–868.
16. Lohmeier TE and Cowley AW. Hypertensive and renal effects of chronic low level intrarenal angiotensin infusion in the dog. Circ Res 1979; 44:154–160.
17. Hollenberg NK, et al. Increased glomerular filtration rate after converting-enzyme inhibition in essential hypertension. New Engl J Med 1979; 301:9.
18. Wilson C, Byrom FB. The vicious circle in Bright's disease. Experimental evidence from the hypertensive rat. Quart J Med 1940; 10:65–96.
19. Eng E, et al. Renal proliferative and phenotypic changes in rats with two-kidney, one-clip Goldblatt hypertension. Amer J Hypertens 1994; 7:177–185.
20. Wenzel UO, et al. Adverse effects of the calcium channel blocker nitrendipine on nephrosclerosis in rats with renovascular hypertension. Hypertension 1992; 20:233–241.
21. Wenzel UO, et al. Combination treatment of enalapril with nitrendipine in rats with renovascular hypertension. Hypertension 1994; 23:114–122.
22. Ploth DW, et al. Effects of verapamil and converting enzyme inhibition on bilateral renal function of two-kidney, one-clip hypertensive rats. Clin Sci 1987; 72:657–667.
23. Woods RL, Anderson WP, Korner PJ. Renal and systemic effects of enalapril in chronic one-kidney hypertension. Hypertension 1986; 8:109–116.
24. Gifford R. Evaluation of the hypertensive patient with emphasis on detecting curable causes. Millbank Mem Fund Q 1969; 47:170–186.
25. Lewin A, et al. Apparent prevalence of curable hypertension in the Hypertension Detection and Follow-Up Program. Arch Int Med 1985; 145:424–472.
26. Danielson M, Dammstrom BG. The prevalence of secondary and curable hypertension. Acta Med Scand 1981; 209:451–455.
27. Berglund G, Andersson O, Wilhelmsen L. Prevalence of primary and secondary hypertension: studies in a random population sample. Br Med J 1976; 2:554–556.
28. Davis BA, et al. Prevalence of renovascular hypertension in patients with Grade III or IV hypertensive retinopathy. N Engl J Med 1979; 301:1273–1276.
29. Keith TA. Renovascular hypertension in black patients. Hypertension 1982; 4:438–443.
30. Holley KE, et al. Renal artery stenosis. A clinical-pathologic study in normotensive and hypertensive patients. Am J Med 1964; 37:14–22.
31. Harding MB, et al. Renal artery stenosis: prevalence and associated risk factors in patients undergoing routine cardiac catheterization. J Am Soc Nephrol 1992; 2:1608–1616.

32. Choudri AH, et al. Unsuspected renal artery stenosis in peripheral vascular disease. Br Med J 1990; 301:1197–1198.
33. Jacobson HR. Ischemic renal disease: an overlooked clinical entity? Kidney Int 1988; 34:729–743.
34. Bredenberg CE, et al. Changing patterns in surgery for chronic renal artery occlusive diseases. J Vasc Surg 1992; 15:1018–1024.
35. Incidence and causes of treated ESRD. US Renal Data Systems, USRDS 1991 Annual Report. Bethesda, Maryland: The National Institutes of Health, National Institutes of Diabetes and Digestive and Kidney Diseases. August 1991:13–20.
36. Rimmer JM, Gennari FJ. Atherosclerotic renovascular disease and progressive renal failure. Ann Int Med 1993; 118:712–719.
37. Toto RD, et al. Reversible renal insufficiency due to angiotensin converting enzyme inhibitors in hypertensive nephrosclerosis. Ann Int Med 1991; 115:513–519.
38. Textor SC, et al. Critical perfusion pressure for renal function in patients with bilateral atherosclerotic renal vascular disease. Ann Int Med 1985; 302:308–314.
39. O'Neil EA, et al. Prevalence of ischemic nephropathy in patients with renal insufficiency. Ann Surg 1992; 58:485–490.
40. Diamond JR. Flash pulmonary edema and the diagnostic suspicion of occult renal artery stenosis. Am J Kid Dis 1993; 21:328–330.
41. Missouris CG, et al. Renal artery stenosis masquerading as congestive heart failure. Lancet 1993; 341:1521–1522.
42. Messina LM, et al. Renal revascularization for recurrent pulmonary edema in patients with poorly controlled hypertension and renal insufficiency: A distinct subgroup of patients with arteriosclerotic renal artery occlusive disease. J Vasc Surg 1992; 15:73–82.
43. Schreiber MJ, Pohl MA, Novick AC. The natural history of atherosclerotic and fibrous renal artery disease. Urol Clin N Amer 1984; 11:383–392.
44. Ratliff NB. Renal vascular disease: pathology of large blood vessel disease. In JG Porush, ed. Hypertension and the Kidney. Orlando: Grune & Stratton, 1985. Pp A93–A103.
45. Goncharenko V, et al. Progression of renal artery fibromuscular dysplasia in 42 patients as seen on angiography. Radiology 1981; 139:45–51.
46. Harrngton JT, Sommers SC, Kassirer JP. Atheromatous emboli with progressive renal failure. Renal arteriography as the probable inciting factor. Ann In Med 1968; 68:152–160.
47. Kassirer JP. Atheroembolic renal disease. New Engl J Med 1969; 280:812–817.
48. Maxwell MH, et al. Cooperative Study of Renovascular Hypertension. Demographic analysis of the study. JAMA 1972; 220:1195–1204.
49. Goldman AG, Varady PD, Franklin SS. Body habitus and serum cholesterol in essential hypertension and renovascular hypertension. Cooperative study of renovascular hypertension. JAMA 1972; 221:378–383.
50. Nicholson JP, et al. Cigarette smoking and renovascular hypertension. Lancet 1983; 2:765–766.
51. Sang CN, et al. Etiologic factors in renovascular fibromuscular dysplasia. A case-control study. Hypertension 1989; 14:472–479.
52. Simon N, et al. Clinical characteristics of renovacular hypertension. JAMA 1972; 220:1209–1218.
53. Berlyne GW, Tarill AS, Baker SBC. Renal artery stenosis and the nephrotic syndrome. Quart J Med 1964; 33:325–335.
54. Zimbler MS, et al. Proteinuria in renovascular hypertension and the effects of renal angioplasty. Ann J Cardiol 1987; 59:406–408.
55. Elkik F, et al. Renal segmental infarction: A cause of reversible malignant hypertension. J Hypertension 1984; 2:149–156.
56. Stanley JC, Fry WJ. Pediatric renal artery occlusive disease and renovascular hypertension. Etiology, diagnosis, and operative treatment. Arch Surg 1981; 116:669–676.
57. Novick AL, et al. Surgical treatment of renovascular hypertension in the pediatric patient. J Urol 1978; 119:794–799.
58. Vaughan ED, Jr., et al. Renovascular hypertension: renin measurements to indicate hypersecretion and contralateral suppression, estimate renal plasma flow, and score for surgical curability. Am J Med 1973; 55:402–414.
59. Vaughan ED Jr., et al. A physiologic definition of blood pressure response to renal revascularization in patients with renovascular hypertension. Kidney Int 1979; 15:S83–S92.
60. Case DB, Laragh JH. Reactive hyperreninemia in renovascular hypertension after angiotensin blockade with saralasin or converting enzyme inhibitor. Ann Intern Med 1979; 91:153–160.
61. Müller FB, et al. The Captopril test for identifying renovascular disease in hypertensive patients. Amer J Med 1986; 80:633–644.
62. Elliott WJ, Martin WB, Murphy MB. Comparison of two noninvasive screening tests for renovascular hypertension. Arch Int Med 1993; 153:755–764.
63. Frederickson ED, et al. A prospective evaluation of a simplified captopril test for the detection of renovascular hypertension. Arch Int Med 1990; 150:569–572.
64. Postma CT, et al. The captopril test in the detection of renovascular disease in hypertensive patients. Arch Int Med 1990; 150:625–628.
65. Mansen PD, Gardeal P, Fruergaard P. The captopril test for identification of renovascular hypertension: value and immediate adverse effects. J Intern Med 1990; 228:159–163.
66. Idrissi A, et al. The captopril challenge test as a screening test for renovascular hypertension. Kidney Int 1988 34[Suppl 25]:S138–S141.
67. Gosse P, et al. Captopril test in the detection of renovascular hypertension in a population with low prevalence of the disease. A prospective study. Am J Hypertens 1989; 2:191–193.
68. Svetkey LP, et al. Prospective analysis of strategies for diagnosing renovascular hypertension. Hypertension 1989; 145:217 257.
69. Kutkuhn B, et al. Validity of the captopril test for identifying correctable unilateral renovascular hypertension. Clin Exp Hyp 1991; A13:143–156.
70. Maxwell MH, Lupu AN, Taplin GV. Radioisotope renogram in renal arterial hypertension. J Urol 1968; 100:376–383.
71. Geyskes GG, et al. Unilateral renal failure after captopril in patients with renovascular hypertension. In N Glorioso, et al., ed. Renovascular Hypertension. New York: Raven Press, 1987. Pp 281–294.
72. Fommei E, et al. Renal scintigraphic captopril test in the diagnosis of renovascular hypertension. Hypertension 1987; 10:212–220.
73. Mann SJ, et al. Captopril renography in the diagnosis of renal artery stenosis: accuracy and limitations. Am J Med 1991; 90:30–40.
74. Chen CC, et al. Patients at high risk for renal artery stenosis: a simple method of scintigraphic analysis with TC-99M DPTA and captopril. Radiology 1990; 176:365–370.
75. Dondi M, et al. Evaluation of hypertensive patients by means of captopril enhanced renal scintigraphy with technetium-99m DTPA. J Nucl Med 1989; 30:615–621.
76. Dunnick AR, Sfakianakis GN. Screening for renovascular hypertension. Radiol Clin North Am 1991; 29:497–510.
77. Dondi M, et al. Use of technetium-99m-MAG_3 for renal scintigraphy after angiotensin-converting enzyme inhibition. J Nucl Med 1991; 32:424–428.

78. Russell DC, et al. Comparison of technetium-99m-MAG_3 with iodine-131 hippuran by a simultanous dual channel technique. J Nucl Med 198; 29:1189–1193.
79. Al-Nahhas AA, et al. Clinical experience with 99m Tc-MAG_3, mercaptoacetyltriglycine, and a comparison with 99m Tc-DTPA. Eur J Nuc Med 1988; 14:453–462.
80. Havey RJ, et al. Screening for renovascular hypertension. JAMA 1985; 254:388–393.
81. Buonocore E, et al. Digital subtraction angiography of the abdominal aorta and renal arteries. Radiology 1981; 139:281–286.
82. Clark RA, Alexander ES. Digital subtraction angiography of the renal arteries—prospective comparison with conventional arteriography. Invest Radiol 1983; 18:6–10.
83. Hillman BJ, et al. The potential impact of digital video subtraction angiography on screening for renovascular hypertension. Radiology 1982; 142:577–579.
84. Zabbo A, Novick AC. Digital subtraction angiography for noninvasive imaging of the renal artery. Urol Clin N Amer 1984; 11:3,409–416.
85. Debatin JF, et al. MR angiography: screening examination for renovascular hypertension? Am J Hypertens 1991; 4:38A.
86. Jenni R, et al. Combined two-dimensional ultrasound doppler technique. New possibilities for the screening of renovascular and parenchymatous hypertension? Nephron 1986; 44[Suppl 1]:2–4.
87. Kohler TR, et al. Noninvasive diagnosis of renal artery stenosis by ultrasonic duplex scaning. J Vasc Surg 1986; 4:450–456.
88. Hoffman V, et al. Role of duplex scanning for the detection of atherosclerotic renal artery disease. Kid Int 1991; 39:1232–1239.
89. Robertson R, Murphy A, Dubbins PA. Renal artery stenosis: the use of duplex ultrasound as a screening technique. Br J Radiol 1988; 61:196–201.
90. Lewis BD, James EM. Current applications of duplex and color doppler ultrasound imaging: Abdomen. Mayo Clinic Proc 1984; 643:1158–1169.
91. Taylor KJ, et al. Vascular complications in renal allografts. Detection and Duplex Doppler US. Radiology 1987; 162:31–38.
92. Shipley RE, Gregg DE. The effect of external constriction of a blood vessel on blood flow. Am J Physiol 1944; 141:289–296.
93. Levin DC, Beckmann CF, Serur JR. Vascular resistance changes distal to progressive arterial stenosis: A critical reevaluation of the concept of vasodilator reverse. Invest Radiol 1980; 14:120–128.
94. Talierco CP, et al. Risks for renal dysfunction with cardiac angiography. Ann Int Med 1986; 104:501–504.
95. Saint-Georges G, Aube M. Safety of outpatient angiography: a prospective study. AJR 1985; 144:235–236.
96. Mann SJ, Pickering TG. Detection of renovascular hypertension. State of the Art: 1992. Ann Int Med 1992; 117:845–853.
97. Franklin SS, et al. Operative morbidity and mortality in renovascular disease. JAMA 1975; 231:1148–1153.
98. Foster JH, et al. Renovascular occlusive disease: results of operative treatment. JAMA 1975; 231:1043.
99. Novick AC, et al. Diminished operative morbidity and mortality in renal revascularization. JAMA 1981; 246:749.
100. Novick AC, et al. Revascularization to preserve renal function in patients with atherosclerotic renovascular disease. Urol Clin N Amer 1984; 11:477.
101. Thevenet A, Mary H, Boennec M. Results following surgical correction of renovascular hypertension. J Cardiovasc Surg 1980; 21:517.
102. Ying CY, et al. Renal revascularization in the azotemic hypertensive patient resistant to therapy. New Engl J Med 1984; 311:1070.
103. Lawrie GM, et al. Renovascular reconstruction: factors affecting long-term prognosis in 919 patients followed up to 31 years. Am J Cardiol 1989; 63:1085–1092.
104. Bedoya L, et al. Baseline renal function and surgical revascularization in atherosclerotic renal arterial disease in the elderly. Cleve Clin J Med 1989; 56:415–421.
105. Sos TA, et al. Percutaneous transluminal renal angioplasty in renovascular hypertension due to atheroma or fibromuscular dysplasia. N Engl J Med 1983; 309:274.
106. Tegtmeyer CJ, Elson J, Glass TA. Percutaneous transluminal angioplasty: The treatment of choice for renovascular hypertension due to fibromuscular dysplasia. Radiology 1982; 143:631.
107. Martin ED, Mattern RF, Baer L. Renal angioplasty for hypertension: Predictive factors for long-term success. Amer J Radiol 1981; 128:951.
108. Grim CE, Luft FC, Yune HY. Percutaneous transluminal dilatation in the treatment of renal vascular hypertension. Ann Int Med 1981; 95:439.
109. Tegtmyer CG, Dyer R, Teates CD. Percutaneous transluminal dilatation of renal arteries. Radiology 1980; 135:589.
110. Plouin P-F, et al. Restenosis after a first percutaneous transluminal renal angioplasty. Hypertension 1993; 21:89–96.
111. Rees CR, et al. Palmaz stent in atherosclerotic stenoses involving the ostia of the renal arteries: preliminary report of a multicenter study. Radiology 1991; 181:507–514.
112. Hricik DE, et al. Captopril-induced functional renal insufficiency in patients with bilateral renal-artery stenoses or renal-artery stenosis in a solitary kidney. New Engl J Med 1983; 308:373.
113. Pickering TG, et al. Renal angioplasty in patients with azotemia and renovascular hypertension. J Hypertens 1986; 4[Suppl 6]:S667–S669.
114. Hunt JC, et al. Renal and renovascular hypertension: A reasoned approach to diagnosis and management. Arch Int Med 1974; 133:988.
115. Dean RH, et al. Renovascular hypertension. Anatomic and renal functional changes during drug therapy. Arch Surg 1981; 116:1408.
116. Michel JB, et al. Effects of antihypertensive treatment in one-clip, two kidney hypertension in rats. Kidney Int 1986; 29:1011–1020.
117. Jackson B, et al. Pharmacologic nephrectomy with chronic angiotensin converting enzyme inhibitor treatment in renovascular hypertension in the rat. J Lab Clin Med 1990; 115:21–27.
118. Grone HJ, Helmchen U. Impairment and recovery of the clipped kidney in two kidney, one clip hypertensive rats during and after antihypertensive therapy. Lab Invest 1986; 54:645–655.
119. Arzilli F, et al. ACE-inhibition vs surgical treatment in the outcome of ischemic kidney of renovascular patients: a one year follow-up. High Blood Press 1992; 1:47–50.
120. Postma CT, et al. Occlusion of unilateral stenosed renal arteries—relation to medical treatment. J Human Hypertens 1989; 3:185–190.
121. Ribstein J, Mourad G, Mimran A. Contrasting acute effects of captopril and nifedipine on renal function in renovascular hypertension. Amer J Hypertens 1988; 1:239–244.
122. Miyamori I, et al. Comparative effects of captopril and nifedipine on split renal function in renovascular hypertension. Amer J Hypertens 1988; 1:359–363.
123. Epstein M. Calcium antagonists and renal protection. Current status and future perspectives. Arch Intern Med 1992; 152:1572–1584.

Visceral Ischemic Syndromes

Kimberley J. Hansen
Stephen P. Murray
Ronald J. Stoney

Visceral ischemic syndromes embody a wide variety of clinical diseases that challenge the skills of both physician and surgeon. If allowed to proceed undiagnosed and untreated, visceral ischemic syndromes cause intestinal infarction and death [1–9].

Although they share the same disastrous endpoint, acute and chronic visceral ischemia differ in several other respects. Acute visceral ischemia presents as a medical and surgical emergency. Even vigorous treatment of acute visceral ischemia is associated with unacceptably high mortality rates [10]. In contrast to acute ischemia, chronic visceral ischemia often poses a diagnostic dilemma. Arterial reconstruction of the mesenteric circulation in chronic visceral ischemia reliably relieves abdominal symptoms and, most important, eliminates the risk of intestinal infarction [6,11].

This chapter reviews the historic evolution of current diagnostic and therapeutic strategies in management of visceral ischemic syndromes. For both acute and chronic visceral ischemia, features of clinical presentation, current theories of pathophysiology, diagnostic evaluation, and nonoperative and operative management are discussed (Table 37-1).

Historic Background

ACUTE VISCERAL ISCHEMIA

Elliott reported the clinical features of acute visceral ischemia complicated by gangrene in 1895 [12]. He proposed surgical intervention when physical findings consistent with peritonitis were present. Elliott and the surgeons who followed for the next 50 years emphasized intestinal resection of gangrenous segments as the sole surgical treatment for acute visceral ischemia. For the unfortunate patients of that era, almost certain death accompanied resectional therapy alone [13]. Contemporary surgical management of acute visceral ischemia began in 1951 with a report by Klass [14]. Klass described the distinguishing clinical and intraoperative features of mesenteric embolization and performed the first superior mesenteric–artery embolectomy. Despite his patient's death from cardiac complications 2 days after surgery, Klass shifted the surgical emphasis from intestinal resection to intestinal revascularization. Intestinal revascularization was applied successfully 7 years later, in 1958, when Shaw and Rutledge described the first superior mesenteric artery embolectomy without simultaneous bowel resection [15]. Shaw and Rutledge also contributed the concept of **second-look** laparotomy to contemporary management. Five years later, in 1963, preoperative recognition and successful intestinal revascularization of acute superior mesenteric–artery thrombosis was reported by Brittain and Earley [16].

In 1977, Boley and co-workers emphasized the necessity for early radiographic diagnosis and treatment of the reactive mesenteric vasospasm that occurs in response to acute visceral ischemia [10]. They reported the results of patients diagnosed with emergency mesenteric arteriography and managed with selective intra-arterial papaverine and surgical exploration. Utilizing a decision tree that combined aggressive and serial mesenteric arteriography with prompt laparotomy and intestinal revascularization, Boley reported improved patient survival with a diminished need for intestinal resection.

Because early information concerning acute visceral ischemia was drawn from autopsy series complicated by postmortem thrombosis, mesenteric-vein occlusion leading to intestinal infarction was recognized much later than its arterial counterpart. Mesenteric-vein occlusion leading to intestinal gangrene was first described by Warren and Eberhard in 1935 [17]. The clinical and pathologic features that distinguish it from arterial occlusive disease were reviewed 5 years later by Johnson, who identified a wide variety of underlying systemic disorders predisposing to venous infarction [18]. Berry and Bongas described "agnogenic," or idiopathic, mesenteric venous occlusion in the absence of predisposing disease states in 1950 [19]. By the mid-1960s, surgeons had come to accept mesenteric-vein occlusion with subsequent intestinal infarction as a vascular entity distinct from arterial ischemic infarction. The diagnosis requires early recognition, resectional therapy, and postoperative anticoagulation [20,21].

The existence of nonobstructive mesenteric ischemia and intestinal infarction has been recognized since 1958. In that year, Eude described acute visceral ischemia resulting from presumed splanchnic vasoconstriction [22]. A low perfusion state seemed to be the common denominator among several predisposing conditions. Current widespread use of diagnostic arteriography and sophisticated cardiac monitoring indicates that the proportion of mesenteric ischemia resulting from that nonobstructive mechanism is significant.

CHRONIC VISCERAL ISCHEMIA

The evolution of modern management of chronic visceral ischemia began nearly a century ago, when Councilman reported three cases of chronic superior mesenteric–artery occlusion associated with abdominal pain [23]. He suggested that gradual occlusion of the major mesenteric arteries could be responsible for intestinal ischemia, thus causing abdominal pain. That reasoning seemed flawed to many, however, since autopsy evidence demonstrated that chronic stenosis or even occlusion of all three major mesenteric arteries frequently could occur without abdominal symptoms [24]. In fact, Osler maintained that

Table 37-1. Visceral ischemic syndromes

- Acute visceral ischemia
  - Mesenteric-artery occlusion
    - Embolus
    - Thrombus
  - Mesenteric-vein occlusion
  - Nonobstructive mesenteric occlusion
- Chronic visceral ischemia

abdominal pain occurring in conjunction with diffuse atherosclerosis that included the mesenteric circulation was a manifestation of coronary artery disease and subsequent myocardial ischemia.

Despite Osler's rejection of intestinal ischemia as a cause for abdominal pain, proponents of the theory persisted, and Bacelli in 1918 was credited by Goodman [25] as being the first to suggest the term **angina abdominus** to characterize the condition. In the United States, it was Mikkelson [26] who coined the term **intestinal angina**, which has since been the prevailing descriptor. Klein [27], in 1921, described three possible patterns that may result from the gradual occlusion of the visceral vessels: (1) no symptoms, due to adequate collateral development; (2) a spectrum of intestinal infarction; and (3) visceral perfusion adequate for viability but not function (i.e., intestinal angina). He cited authors from Europe [28,29] who, 30 years earlier, had described patients with classic visceral ischemic symptoms, one of whom had mesenteric occlusive disease confirmed at autopsy.

The modern era of the pursuit and treatment of this disease was punctuated by Dunphy's description of premorbid symptoms of postprandial abdominal pains, weight loss, and altered intestinal motility occurring in 7 of 12 patients dying of mesenteric infarction [30].

The first reported attempt at revascularizing a patient suffering from acute intestinal ischemia was by Shaw and Rutledge in 1957 [31]. The following year, Shaw and Maynard [32] reported successful treatment of a patient with intestinal angina, without infarcted bowel, with a superior mesenteric artery thromboembolectomy. Soon to follow was Derrick's [33] report of a successful bypass to both the celiac and the superior mesenteric artery with an autologous iliac artery graft originating from the supraceliac aorta. As synthetic grafts became more widely available, a rapid proliferation of techniques were reported.

In 1962, Morris and associates described retrograde Dacron bypass grafting from the infrarenal aorta to the mesenteric arteries [34]. In 1966, Stoney and Wylie introduced antegrade aortovisceral bypass and transaortic visceral thromboendarterectomy [35]. Theoretical considerations and long-term clinical results seem to favor the latter two methods [6,11].

This historic review emphasizes the contemporary diagnostic and therapeutic features of acute and chronic visceral ischemia. In both acute and chronic ischemia, early surgical intervention prior to intestinal gangrene is essential. Obviously, the preoperative diagnostic evaluation for chronic visceral ischemia can be more deliberate than that for acute visceral ischemia; nevertheless, both acute and chronic ischemia ultimately require arteriographic evaluation and vascular reconstruction. Patients who are allowed to progress to intestinal infarction undergo crippling intestinal resection or ultimately die of septic complications. Clearly, prompt clinical recognition of the visceral ischemic syndromes is a prerequisite for successful treatment.

INCIDENCE

Complete data are lacking to support firm conclusions concerning the incidence of acute visceral ischemia. Boley and his associates have a special interest in acute mesenteric vascular disease, but they estimate that only one in every 1,000 patients is admitted to their hospital with that diagnosis [10], a rate equivalent to about 50 new patients per year in a 1,300-bed medical center.

Three main types of acute mesenteric ischemia affect the small bowel: (1) mesenteric-artery occlusion resulting from either embolus or thrombus, (2) mesenteric-vein occlusion, and (3) nonobstructive mesenteric ischemia (see Table 37-1).

When the three types of acute mesenteric ischemia are considered together, approximately half are secondary to mesenteric-artery occlusion. The remaining half are equally divided between mesenteric-vein occlusion and nonobstructive mesenteric ischemia. Arterial embolism and thrombosis seem to occur with equal frequency in most series [3,4], but Bergan and colleagues have reported that embolism accounted for two-thirds of their occlusive series [36]. Following the introduction of routine arteriography in the management of those acute visceral ischemia syndromes, the incidence of nonobstructive mesenteric ischemia seemed to be increasing. It is the clinical impression of the authors and others that this condition actually may be on the decrease [37]. Besides signaling improved cardiac management of critically ill patients, this apparent decreased incidence may reflect the widespread medical management of hypertension and ischemic heart disease with medications that cause direct arterial smooth muscle relaxation.

As in acute visceral ischemia, the incidence of symptomatic chronic visceral ischemia is unknown [5–8,11]. Although mesenteric atherosclerosis causing arterial stenosis or occlusion is common, symptoms of intestinal angina are infrequent [24]. Blood delivered through collateral pathways around major arterial occlusions is largely responsible for the infrequent occurrence of intestinal angina.

Etiology and Pathophysiology

Perfusion of the viscera obviously is as dependent on the state of the general circulation as any other organ system. However, diminished central pumping capacity due to hypovolemic or cardiogenic shock leads to a disproportionate loss of perfusion to the viscera, while other, more vital organs are preserved. In addition to the blood-carrying capacity of the three named visceral arteries, major congenital and acquired collateral pathways are critical. Beyond those are the autonomic and humoral influences, which vary depending on the relative state of

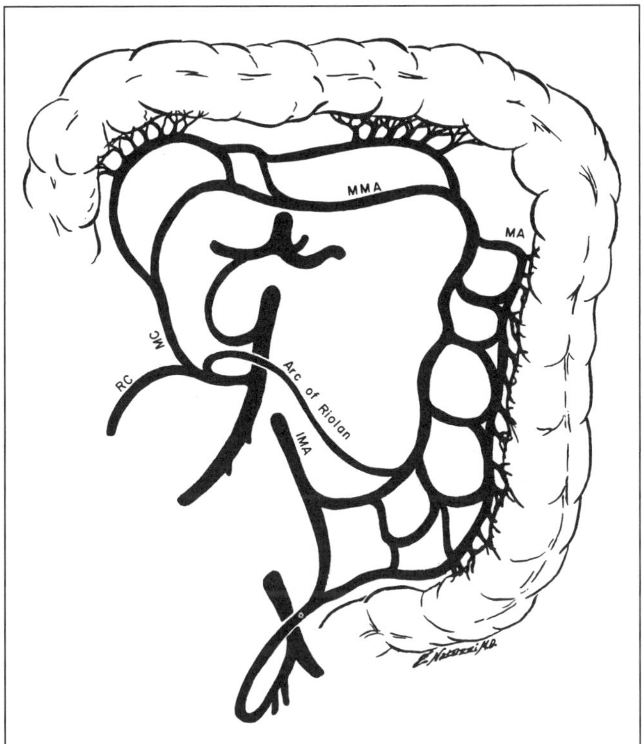

Fig. 37-1. Schematic drawing of major visceral arteries and collateral pathways. (RC = right colic, MMA = meandering mesenteric artery, MA = marginal artery, IMA = inferior mesenteric artery.)

perfusion and the functional demands of the gut. Investigators seeking to understand the confusing interplay of physiology are further hampered by the lack of an acceptable animal model, due to significant interspecies variations. In spite of that, many advances into the understanding of the elements of visceral ischemic syndromes have been made in the last 20 years.

The three major visceral arteries (celiac, superior mesenteric, and inferior mesenteric) that supply the mesenteric circulation are arranged in parallel fashion (Fig. 37-1). Despite the parallel arrangement, three major collateral pathways may develop to bypass proximal obstruction in the mesenteric arteries. First, the celiac and superior mesenteric arteries may communicate through the pancreaticoduodenal arteries. Similarly, the superior and inferior mesenteric arteries may communicate through the "meandering" mesenteric artery or a variably present Arc of Riolan that lies in the transverse mesocolon in an area generally known to be free of major blood vessels. Finally, the inferior mesenteric and internal iliac arteries may communicate through sigmoidal and hemorrhoidal arteries. Of those three collateral pathways, the demonstration of the meandering mesenteric artery is pathognomonic of significant obstruction to the major visceral branches. The meandering mesenteric artery is located deep in the colonic mesentery. It is different from the marginal artery of Drummond, which is located close to the colonic wall, and gives rise to penetrating arterioles.

Normally the three major arteries or their collaterals carry 25 percent of the total cardiac output [38]. The mesenteric venous system may harbor an additional 30 percent of the circulating blood volume. Those figures reflect the high metabolic demands of the gastrointestinal organs and the capacitance of the mesenteric venous system [39].

Blood flow through the major mesenteric arteries is controlled by the resistance of the vascular bed within the intestinal wall. This microcirculation consists of arteriae rectae that penetrate the muscular layer of the intestine to supply a rich bed of collaterals in the submucosal layer. There, arterioles lose their muscular coat as they enter the individual villi and penetrate to the tip of each villus. There they arborize into a dense capillary network, and blood makes the return trip to the base of the villus. This architectural arrangement has been likened to that in the nephron of the kidney, and a similar countercurrent exchange mechanism has been postulated [40–42]. Such an arrangement can, during ischemia, lead to shunting of oxygen and nutrients away from the distal villus (intestinal mucosa) as elements move preferentially across permeable vessels and interstitium closer to the base of the villus [43]. Such a situation could occur only as a result of a severe perfusion deficit, since regulatory elements control mesenteric perfusion so that the small intestine receives twice the blood flow per unit weight as the colon or the stomach receives [44].

The regulatory elements consist of autonomic, humoral, and local factors. The sympathetic nervous system is responsible for maintaining resting splanchnic arteriolar tone, while circulating cathecholamines play a lesser role. The primary regulation of mesenteric blood flow, however, occurs within the venous capacitance vessels of the postcapillary venules [45].

The severe vasospasm commonly seen with both obstructive and nonobstructive visceral ischemia is caused primarily by angiotensin II. When systemic hypotension occurs as an outcome of visceral ischemia, renin release from the hypoperfused kidney stimulates the creation of angiotensin II. The vasoconstrictor has a more pronounced effect in the visceral vessels than elsewhere [46,47].

Local factors also can affect the vascular tone of the splanchnic bed, including prostaglandins, leukotrienes [48], potassium [49], osmolality, oxygen tension, pH, and, to a minor degree, gastrointestinal hormones [50].

ACUTE VISCERAL ISCHEMIA

As major arterial branches of the upper abdominal aorta, the mesenteric arteries may be acutely occluded by emboli. In fact, the superior mesenteric artery is the recipient vessel for 3–4 percent of all arterioarterial emboli [51]. As with peripheral emboli in general, the embolic phenomenon reflects serious underlying cardiac disease in the vast majority of patients. Transmural myocardial infarction with mural thrombus and mitral stenosis with left atrial thrombus and atrial fibrillation are most frequently encountered. Less common sources also should be considered, including proximal aortic atheroma, left atrial myxoma, and paradoxic emboli from the venous circulation.

Superior mesenteric–artery thrombosis is most commonly superimposed on mesenteric atherosclerosis [15,16,52]. The anatomic pattern is usually an atheroma of the anterior aortic wall encroaching on the ostium of the superior mesenteric artery and occasionally extending 2–4 cm distally. The exact mechanism that precipitates acute thrombosis on this atheroma is poorly understood. It is interesting and important to recognize that half the patients presenting with acute mesenteric thrombosis have antecedent symptoms compatible with intestinal angina [53]. Infrequently, rheumatoid arthritis, polyarteritis nodosa, or systemic lupus erythematosus may predispose to mesenteric-artery thrombosis. Fibromuscular dysplasia also has been reported to cause celiac- and superior mesenteric–artery thrombosis as well as intestinal angina [54].

In mesenteric-vein occlusion, an underlying disorder can be identified in approximately half the cases. The remaining cases fail to demonstrate any predisposing factors and have been termed **agnogenic** [19]. Intraperitoneal sepsis resulting from appendicitis or diverticulitis is the most frequent predisposing disease process. Presumably, those intra-abdominal infections seed the portal system, causing pyelophlebitis and subsequent mesenteric venous thrombosis [18]. Additional underlying conditions that may lead to mesenteric-vein occlusion include a variety of hypercoagulable states. Polycythemia vera and postsplenectomy thrombocytosis have been associated with mesenteric-vein occlusion [55]. Antithrombin III deficiency is being recognized with increasing frequency among such patients [56]. Oral contraceptives have been associated with a variety of venous and arterial thrombotic events, and a clear association with mesenteric-vein thrombosis has been reported by several authors [57,58].

Reactive splanchnic vasoconstriction is responsible for nonobstructive mesenteric ischemia. Central to the pathogenesis of that entity are underlying disorders that lead to systemic hypoperfusion [10]. The majority of cases are associated with either severe congestive heart failure with low cardiac output or disease states resulting in dehydration. Digitalis overdose has been implicated in several cases of nonobstructive mesenteric ischemia. Although digitalis might be expected to improve intestinal perfusion through its myocardial ionotropic effects, the drug is a powerful vasoconstrictor of the mesenteric circulation [59–61].

Injury that occurs as a result of acute intestinal ischemia has been attributed to many causes [62–65]. Damage occurs both during the period of ischemia and during the period following restoration of blood flow. Reactive oxygen metabolites are produced primarily as ischemic tissue is reperfused, with the enzyme xanthine oxidase playing a lead role in this process [65]. Reactive toxic products of oxygen metabolism called **oxygen-free radicals** may mediate intestinal injury during the reperfusion period [66]. During reperfusion, both superoxide and hydroxyl free radicals are formed; they can destroy cell membranes directly or mediate damage through complement activation. Experimentally, oxygen radical scavengers administered prior to reperfusion after short periods of ischemia seem to protect the intestinal microcirculation [67]. Long periods of ischemia, however, are associated with widespread microcirculatory thrombosis and irreversible damage independent of oxygen-free radicals.

Nonocclusive mesenteric ischemia reflects mesenteric vasospasm in response to systemic hypoperfusion. That process represents an attempt to shunt blood from the gut to the central circulation to maintain cerebral and cardiac perfusion. The vasospastic response is mediated primarily through vasopressin and the renin-angiotensin axis [68]. Although vasopressin induces vasoconstriction in a number of circulatory beds, the effect is the greatest in the mesenteric circulation [46]. In a similar manner, an amplified vasoactive response in the mesenteric circulation is seen with angiotensin II. The splanchnic smooth muscle appears to have increased angiotensin II receptors compared to other circulatory beds. When vasopressin and angiotensin II are released in response to hypoperfusion states, they induce a powerful mesenteric vasoconstriction that is not reversed by local metabolic or myogenic reflexes. Even when systemic hypoperfusion is corrected, mesenteric vasospasm may persist, prompting intestinal infarction.

Studies have demonstrated that, prior to complete infarction (and certainly following it), bacterial translocation occurs as a result of perturbation of the mucosal integrity [69–72]. Also associated with ischemia is a change in the overall distribution and type of bacterial flora in the gut due to changes in the reduction-oxidation potential and lumenal pH [50]. Although normally anaerobic bacteria predominate in the colon, insults can lead to proliferation of those species in more proximal locations. Sepsis and associated multiorgan failure are the unfortunate result of such extralumenal migration of bacteria.

While both obstructive and nonobstructive visceral ischemia can lead to sepsis and its attendant complications, the opposite also is true. Sepsis itself can lead to ischemia of the abdominal viscera, especially the liver and the gastrointestinal tract. The effect appears to be due, in general, to both a decrease in oxygen delivery to and an increased oxygen demand by the splanchnic bed. Those competitive elements lead to mucosal cellular hypoxia, the release of numerous previously mentioned local factors, and, ultimately, nonocclusive mesenteric ischemia (vasospasm) [73].

CHRONIC VISCERAL ISCHEMIA

In chronic visceral ischemia, atherosclerosis is responsible for mesenteric-artery occlusion in over 95 percent of cases. As in mesenteric-artery thrombosis, these ostial lesions represent atherosclerosis of the anterior aortic wall that encroaches on the mesenteric lumen [33]. The proximal location of major visceral-artery atherosclerotic occlusion allows a protective collateral network to develop, preventing intestinal infarction in most cases. Chiene recognized the efficiency of the collateral network over a century ago when he described occlusion of all three major mesenteric arteries without infarction [24]. It is widely believed that at least two of the three major mesenteric vessels must be involved before symptoms of chronic visceral ischemia present [5–11].

Blood flow for that collateral network is provided by nonischemic parallel segments. The medium-sized mesenteric arteries do not limit flow; therefore, without decreasing their distal perfusion, the normal segments also can supply the ischemic segments. Reduced resistance in the ischemic segment favors its perfusion. Experimental data have shown that the resistance of the nonischemic segments remains unchanged, suggesting that vasoactive drugs given systematically might actually disrupt the protective collateral mechanism [74]. That is in contrast to the selective intra-arterial infusion of vasodilators, which may overcome local mesenteric vasospasm in response to circulating vasopressin and angiotensin II.

Mechanical compression of the celiac axis by the median arcuate ligament is another possible cause of visceral ischemic symptoms [75], although that view is controversial [76–80]. Clearly, celiac compression can be present in asymptomatic individuals. Symptoms attributed to this condition are varied in the literature, and a large percentage of patients present with past histories of prior abdominal surgery, alcohol abuse, and psychiatric disorders [81]. Nevertheless, celiac-axis compression is seen in patients with typical symptoms of chronic mesenteric ischemia and no other discernable cause. Furthermore, long-term relief can be gained following surgical decompression and arterial dilation or bypass.

Mechanical compression of the celiac axis is most commonly due to impingement by the overlying median arcuate ligament. With prolonged constriction, intimal fibrosis and poststenotic dilation have been observed. At times, the superior mesenteric artery is involved, though involvement of both visceral arteries is rare. When, as is most common, only the celiac artery is involved and typical symptoms of postprandial pain, altered intestinal motility, and weight loss are present, the cause is presumed to be inadequacy of collateral supply or some type of steal phenomenon. Curiously, the generous collateral network that develops in association with atherosclerotic occlusions is infrequently present.

Patients who present with this phenomenon typically are women in their fourth to fifth decade of life. About one-third present with postprandial symptoms, and one-quarter of those are only when lying supine after a meal. Weight loss is not as pronounced and occurs in only two-thirds of this population [81]. Careful physical exam can detect the classic finding of an epigastric bruit that is characteristically louder on expiration. Definitive diagnosis depends on imaging of the celiac axis by biplaner aortography. Occasionally, inspiration and expiration lateral views will demonstrate the compression.

We feel that surgery should be offered to those patients who present with classic symptoms and lateral aortography demonstrating celiac-axis compression. Patients not meeting those criteria should be observed until more overt symptoms develop or other conditions become manifest. It is important that other disease processes that can mimic these symptoms are first ruled out by careful evaluation.

The most recent report from our institution [81] studied the results of surgery on 51 patients followed an average of 9 years after operation to correct celiac-axis compression. The best results were obtained in women between 40 and 60 years of age, with typical postprandial pain and weight loss greater than 15 percent of body weight. The surgical procedure of choice was decompression followed by celiac-artery dilation or reconstruction. Success in relieving symptoms at long-term follow-up was 76 percent in this group compared with 53 percent in those undergoing only decompression. That finding is corroborated by Evans [77], who noted only 41 percent of 59 patients treated with decompression alone to be asymptomatic at late follow-up. External compression of the celiac axis also can be secondary to neurofibrotic encasement, as can be seen in von Recklinghausen's disease [82–84].

Rather than involving the ostia of the major mesenteric branches, atherosclerosis may produce a localized obstruction of the suprarenal aorta, where it has been termed a **coral reef** atheroma [85]. These lesions may diminish perfusion or embolize to the visceral, renal, or lower-extremity circulation. About one-fourth of these patients present with visceral ischemia, while the majority present with renovascular hypertension and lower-extremity ischemia.

In addition to the celiac-axis compression syndrome and the coral reef atheroma, spontaneous intimal dissection of the superior mesenteric artery has been reported as a rare cause of chronic visceral ischemia [86]. The celiac axis and the superior mesenteric artery also are affected by fibromuscular dysplasia, but the disease is rarely responsible for intestinal angina [54,87]. Visceral ischemic syndromes also have been described as a consequence of vasculitis secondary to rheumatoid arthritis, systemic lupus erythematosus, and external beam irradiation.

Although an ischemic basis for intestinal angina is widely accepted, the pathophysiologic mechanism that mediates the syndrome is poorly understood. Since severe pain occurs only with food intake in this syndrome, the pain seems secondary to a discrepancy between increased postprandial oxygen demands and the failure of the collateral system to provide adequate compensation. Most patients experience pain 15 to 20 minutes after food intake—well before the food bolus has reached the small intestine. Researchers have suggested that food ingestion increases demand for gastric blood flow, thereby creating a gastric steal from the remaining gastrointestinal tract [88]. Subsequent small-intestinal acidosis may mediate the characteristic abdominal pain.

Clinical Presentation and Diagnosis

ACUTE VISCERAL ISCHEMIA

Successful treatment of acute visceral ischemia requires prompt diagnosis, immediate arteriography, and appropriate surgical intervention [1–4,10]. An increase in patient mortality is the direct result of any delay in diagnosis and treatment. Under ideal circumstances, a patient with acute visceral ischemia who undergoes prompt treatment can expect a 40- to 50-percent rate of mortality [2]. When extensive intestinal gangrene results prior to treatment of acute visceral ischemia, the mortality rate approaches 95 percent.

Prompt diagnosis of acute visceral ischemia requires an awareness of the population at risk (Table 37-2). Acute ischemia occurs most commonly in patients over 50 years of age; in one large series, 75 percent of patients exceeded

Table 37-2. Patient risk factors for acute visceral ischemia

Any unexplained abdominal pain
Age greater than 50 years
Congestive heart failure
Digitalis therapy (especially with persistent heart failure)
Recent myocardial infarction
Cardiac dysrhythmia (especially with recent onset or recent infarction)
Previous arterioarterial emboli
Hypercoagulable states
Any disease state associated with hypovolemia

70 years of age [36]. Ottinger reported a mean age of 70 years for all three types of visceral ischemia and a mean age of 60 years for patients suffering embolic occlusion [89]. This patient population also is characterized by a high incidence of cardiac disease. Many patients present with long-standing congestive heart failure poorly controlled with digitalis and diuretics [22]. Patients with a past history of cardiac arrhythmias, recent transmural myocardial infarction, or previous peripheral arterioarterial embolization are at increased risk for mesenteric-artery embolus. Any disease process that leads to external or third-space fluid losses with hypovolemia and hypoperfusion predispose to acute mesenteric ischemia in this elderly population. As described earlier, a variety of hypercoagulable states also may lead to arterial or venous mesenteric thrombosis [55–58].

Abdominal pain is the clinical hallmark of acute visceral ischemia and is present in 75 to 98 percent of cases [1–4,10,21,35]. Mesenteric-artery occlusion typically produces sudden onset of severe periumbilical pain, which initially is poorly localized and visceral in quality. As the ischemia progresses, the pain becomes increasingly severe out of proportion to objective physical findings. Vomiting (56%) and diarrhea (29%) reflect forceful gut emptying in response to continuing ischemia. Severe abdominal pain followed by forceful gut emptying in the absence of significant physical findings strongly suggests acute arterial occlusion [1,2,4,89].

Embolic arterial occlusion produces a distinct clinical syndrome [4]. The patient often demonstrates one or more of the cardiac risk factors described above and usually does not have a history of weight loss or intestinal angina. One-third of the patients have suffered previous peripheral arterioarterial embolic episodes [36,51]. Simultaneous with mesenteric embolization, the patient experiences the sudden onset of severe abdominal pain. Shortly thereafter, forceful gut emptying occurs. If the ischemia progresses without intervention, abdominal distention, signs of peritoneal irritation, and gastrointestinal bleeding occur in three-fourths of patients [90].

In contrast to mesenteric embolization, mesenteric-artery thrombosis usually follows a more insidious course. Thrombotic occlusion is characterized by history of intestinal angina in one-half of cases and significant peripheral atherosclerotic disease in one-third [6]. Superimposed on the intermittent postprandial pain of chronic visceral ischemia, constant abdominal pain reflects thrombosis with continuous ischemia [53]. The pain may progress steadily until intestinal gangrene occurs, accompanied by the physical findings of peritonitis.

Like mesenteric thrombosis, acute mesenteric-vein occlusion and nonobstructive mesenteric ischemia frequently are characterized by vague abdominal findings and a subacute clinical course [20,21]. The clinical course of this abdominal discomfort may be protracted, lasting for weeks. Unexplained abdominal distention or gastrointestinal bleeding may be the only indication of these two varieties of visceral ischemia. In both groups of patients, the ill-defined abdominal complaints usually progress to colicky abdominal pain. Finally, frank intestinal gangrene may develop, with its usual symptoms and physical findings.

In summary, acute mesenteric ischemia presents with a marked disparity between severe symptoms of abdominal pain and a paucity of physical findings. The chance for patient survival is greatest when the bowel is ischemic rather than infarcted.

Laboratory findings are often characteristic for acute visceral ischemia but are never diagnostic. A leukocytosis is present in 90 percent of patients; in nearly half, it exceeds 20,000 cells/mm^3. A predominance of immature cells is characteristic, which in the elderly, occurs frequently without leukocytosis [89,90]. Approximately half the patients are found to have a significant uncorrected metabolic acidosis. A mild hyperamylasemia is found in 25 to 50 percent of patients [89]. Intestinal infarction routinely elevates the serum transaminases. None of these laboratory tests, however, are either sensitive or specific for the diagnosis of intestinal ischemia. Unfortunately, when leukocytosis and acidosis are recognized, it is relatively late, and the ischemic bowel has progressed to infarction.

Almost all patients who are evaluated for acute or subacute abdominal pain have plain abdominal roentgenography [91–94]. In the case of acute visceral ischemia, plain abdominal films are useful to exclude other more common causes of acute abdominal pain. Plain films may demonstrate the presence or absence of small-bowel obstruction, renal or biliary calculi, chronic calcific pancreatitis, or a perforated viscus. Retrospective evaluation of abdominal plain-film accuracy in the diagnosis of acute visceral ischemia ranges from 19 to 28 percent [92,93]. Roentgenographic findings range from "thumbprinting," which represents intramural edema or hemorrhage, to pneumatosis or portal-vein gas, which represents bowel infarction and bacterial invasion [94]. Nearly half of patients with acute visceral ischemia (40%) present with a pattern consistent with mechanical small-bowel obstruction [90,92,93].

Once the diagnosis of acute mesenteric ischemia is considered, emergency arteriography should be performed immediately [1]. Resuscitative therapy for acute visceral ischemia should begin while preparations are made for the arteriogram. Anteroposterior and lateral midstream aortograms are obtained to delineate concomitant aortic disease and to evaluate the collateral circulation. The aortogram usually is followed by selective catheterization of the superior mesenteric artery to diagnose an embolus, a

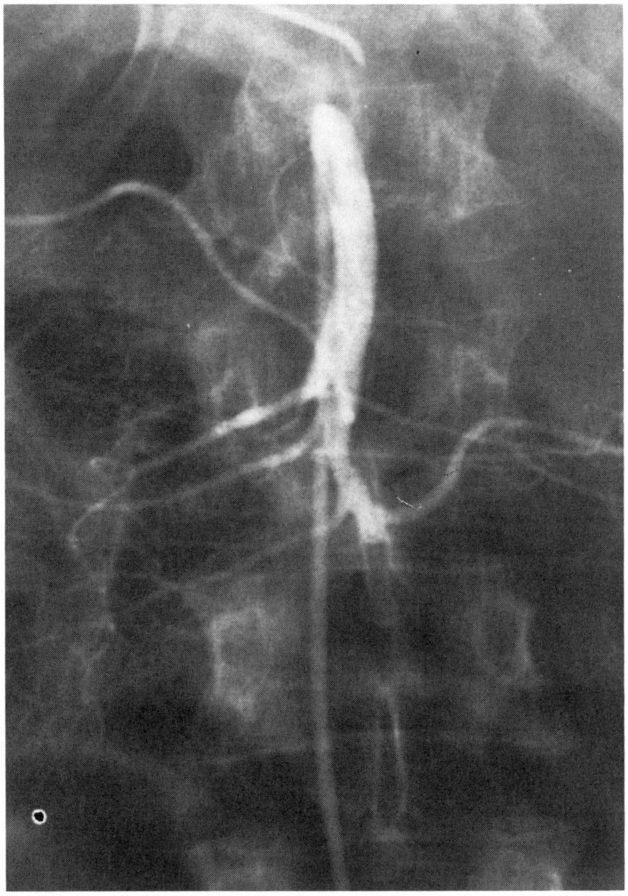

Fig. 37-2. Arteriogram demonstrating embolic occlusion of the superior mesenteric artery. Note the filling of the middle colic artery just proximal to the occlusion.

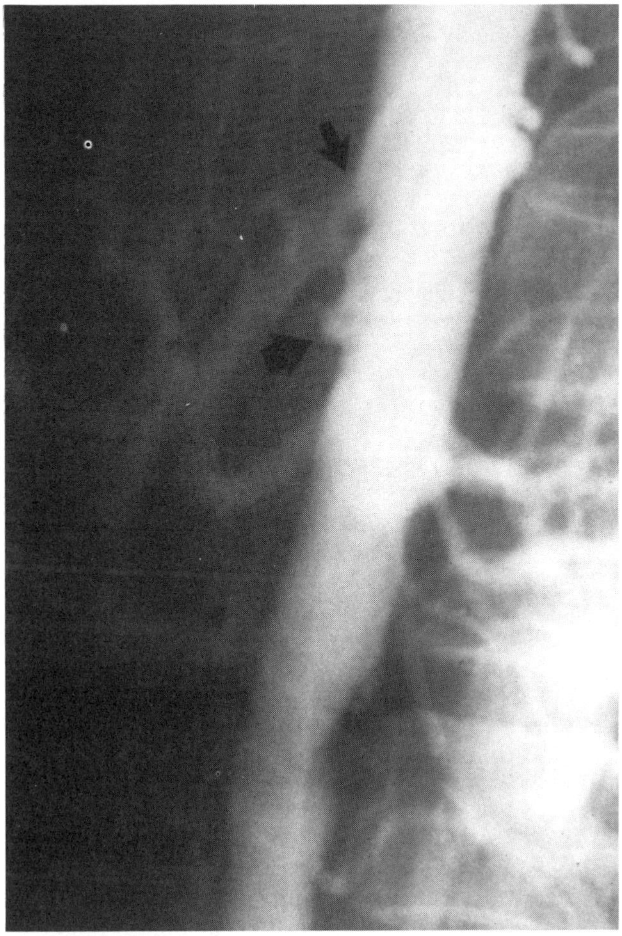

Fig. 37-3. Lateral aortogram demonstrating thrombosis of the superior mesenteric artery (large arrow). Note the stenosis (upper arrow) of celiac axis.

thrombus, or a nonobstructive visceral ischemia. Arteriography also may prove therapeutic by direct injection of vasodilators or thrombolytic agents through the arterial cannulae [1,10,95].

Anecdotal reports of treatment of acute ischemia by percutaneous dilation techniques alone have been made by several authors [96–98].

The use of papavarine has been strongly advocated for both occlusive and nonocclusive conditions, since the former condition is always complicated by the latter one, and improved survival rates have been attributed to the liberal use of papavarine. Systemic effects are abated by the high metabolism of the drug during the first pass through the liver [99].

A "meniscus" sign located 4 to 6 cm from the origin of the superior mesenteric artery is the classic arteriographic finding in mesenteric-artery occlusion resulting from an embolus [90,100] (Fig. 37-2). Emboli typically lodge just distal to the origins of either the middle colic artery or the first jejunal branch of the superior mesenteric artery. Proximal jejunal branches rapidly fill on the arteriogram, but the distal jejunal and ileal branches do not. These arteriographic findings are in contrast to the characteristic arteriogram in superior mesenteric–artery thrombosis (Fig. 37-3). Characteristically, a sharp cutoff in the proximal 3 cm of the superior mesenteric artery is seen without jejunal-branch sparing. Extensive collateral circulation from the celiac or inferior mesenteric artery often is seen in patients with thrombotic mesenteric-artery occlusion.

Nonobstructive mesenteric ischemia can be distinguished from embolic or thrombotic vascular disease because all the major mesenteric branches are easily visualized without proximal arterial obstruction. The abnormalities encountered in such patients may include generalized arterial narrowing with slow filling of distal branches, regular abrupt tapering of arterial branches, and diffuse arterial spasm [92,94]. When nonobstructive disease is present, intra-arterial infusion of vasodilators is begun with the hope of relieving regional mesenteric-artery vasospasm. Intra-arterial bolus injection of tolazoline and continuous infusions of papaverine have been successful in relieving local vasospasm. Papaverine infusion also has been useful preoperatively to prevent vasospasm distal to a mechanical occlusion while preparations for surgery are made.

A visceral arteriogram should be performed immediately whenever the diagnosis of acute visceral ischemia is considered. Arteriography is the gold standard for defining the patterns of occlusion in visceral branches and the adjacent aorta and collateral patterns. It may offer an option to treat certain patients with pharmacologic agents. It often requires transport of a critically ill patient with severe underlying cardiac disease to a remote radiology suite. Despite that unappealing scenario, immediate arteriography is mandatory to diagnose acute visceral ischemia. The three types of acute visceral ischemia usually are differentiated, thereby permitting appropriate surgical and nonsurgical management. Emergency visceral arteriography has decreased death from acute visceral ischemia in most reported series [1,2,10,90].

CHRONIC VISCERAL ISCHEMIA

As in acute visceral ischemia secondary to mesenteric-artery occlusion, chronic visceral ischemia produces a well-defined clinical syndrome in symptomatic patients. Likewise, successful treatment requires recognition of that clinical syndrome, confirmation of the diagnosis with arteriography, and appropriate visceral revascularization before severe nutritional depletion or intestinal infarction occurs with lethal sequelae. When recognized before the onset of those complications, chronic visceral ischemia can be treated successfully by visceral-artery reconstructions, with nearly all patients receiving long-lasting benefit [6,11].

The pain of chronic visceral ischemia usually is gnawing and dull in quality and either periumbilical or epigastric in location. Intestinal angina has its onset 15 to 30 minutes after meals and may persist from 1 to 4 hours. As the occlusive disease progresses, smaller amounts of food result in more severe and persistent abdominal discomfort. Finally, the patient develops food avoidance ("food fear"), which leads to significant weight loss (15% of ideal body weight in 79% of patients) [6].

On evaluation, patients often exhibit the signs of weight loss, with the severity paralleling the duration of symptoms. Examination of the abdomen reveals an epigastric bruit in the majority of patients (86%) [11]. Evidence of peripheral vascular disease (73%) and coronary artery disease (34%) is frequently present [6].

As with all visceral ischemic syndromes, diagnosis of chronic visceral ischemia depends on a high index of suspicion in any patient who demonstrates the triad of postprandial abdominal pain, food aversion, and weight loss. Currently, there are no definitive physiologic tests to establish the diagnosis. Some have attempted to extrapolate data from malabsorption tests (D-xylose) [101], while others have applied the hemodilution indocyanine green method of determining visceral blood flow [102]. Those older tests are, unfortunately, of little clinical use due to being nonspecific, cumbersome and technically demanding [99].

Definitive diagnosis of chronic visceral ischemia requires aortography performed in both anteroposterior and lateral projections [6,11,35]. The anteroposterior view best demonstrates the visceral collateral pathways (Fig. 37-4). The lateral projection demonstrates the proximal visceral artery stenosis or occlusion (Fig. 37-5). Intra-arterial digital subtraction arteriography may be performed with a very small amount of contrast agent in patients with preexisting renal dysfunction or contrast hypersensitivity. Selective visceral arteriography also provides the rare opportunity for percutaneous transluminal angioplasty in patients with distal mesenteric artery lesions [103,104]. In general, intravenous digital subtraction arteriography has been inadequate to define the mesenteric-artery anatomy necessary for diagnosis and planning of a surgical strategy. The volume of contrast agent required for an intravenous digital subtraction arteriogram may equal or exceed that for a routine intra-arterial study [105].

Most commonly, aortography and visceral arteriography reveal obstructive lesions of both the celiac axis and the superior mesenteric artery (94%) [6,11,35]. Half those patients have significant occlusive disease involving the inferior mesenteric artery as well. Additional atherosclerotic stenosis of one or both renal arteries is present in one-third of patients, and one-fourth have significant infrarenal aortic aneurysmal or occlusive disease [6].

ALTERNATIVES TO DIAGNOSIS OF VISCERAL ISCHEMIC SYNDROMES

Biplaner aortography represents the definitive diagnostic study in patients presenting with a visceral ischemic syndrome. Newer procedures, however, may prove useful in the future both as screening tests and as adjunctive means of diagnosis.

Magnetic resonance imaging is a powerful tool for defining soft-tissue anatomy. Tissue contrast is obtained without ionizing radiation or injection of contrast agents, and MRI can delineate between vessels containing thrombus and those with free-flowing blood. Because of the limitations of 24-hour availability and the period of time necessary for a completely arterial evaluation, MRI probably will not contribute to diagnosis of acute visceral ischemia. A future role for MRI seems most probable in some areas of evaluation for chronic visceral ischemia. For example, phase contrast cine magnetic resonance has been used to gather information about flow velocities in the mesenteric arteries of pre- and postprandial patients that can aid in determining the hemodynamic significance of established lesions [106]. Duplex ultrasound also has been used for the same purpose, but with a strong reliance on an experienced technician in a patient with an ideal body habitus.

A new generation of computed tomography known as cine-CT provides rapid scanning with multiple simultaneous tomographic sections. The images of cine-CT scanners can be reconstructed and played in series to provide calculations of mesenteric blood flow and total blood volume. Cine-CT scanning has had wide application in cardiac imaging and may prove useful in the future evaluation of both acute and chronic visceral ischemia.

Duplex assessment of the visceral vessels was first reported in 1984 by the Seattle group [107]. That initial experience was followed by others from the same investigators and others, the latest of which has yielded some impressive accuracy, compared with biplanner angiography [108,109]. Other investigators have not been as assert-

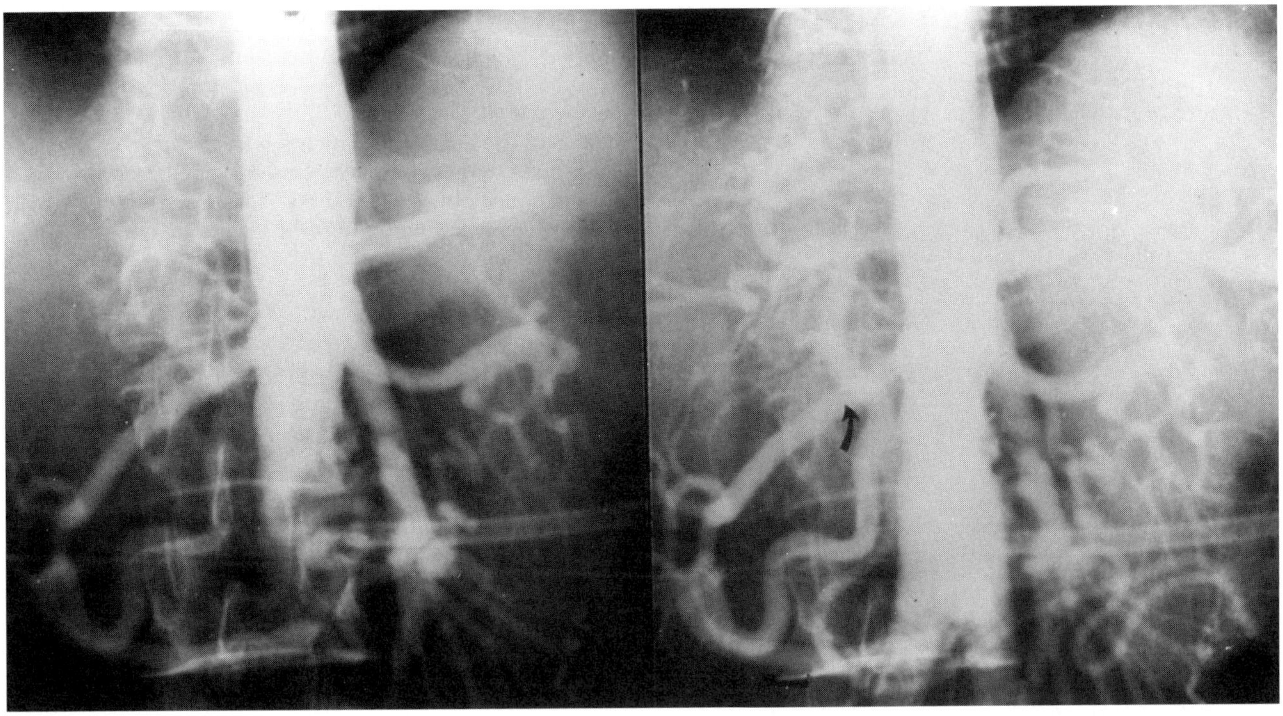

Fig. 37-4. Anteroposterior aortogram showing enlarged gastric duodenal collateral connecting superior mesenteric artery with celiac arterial system.

ive in recommending the method [110]. The difficulties in ultrasound imaging are attributed to (1) an inability to obtain accurate B-mode images with the low-frequency probes necessary to image those deep vessels, which leads to uncertainty as to which vessel is being insonated; (2) truncal obesity and the presence of bowel gas; (3) the tortuosity of the vessels results in difficulty in maintaining the requisite 70-degree angle of interrogation; and, most important, (4) technician inexperience. Current recommendations from centers with demonstrated expertise in the technique are that the study be used to screen patients referred for evaluation of possible intestinal angina. If the studies are normal, there is no need to proceed with angiography. Abnormal or equivocal results, though, will lead to biplaner visceral angiography. It is important to appreciate that the presence of hemodynamically significant lesions does not by itself make the diagnosis of chronic visceral ischemia, since there have been several instances of patients with occlusion of most or all of their visceral vessels who were asymptomatic [111,24].

Tonometry, first used by Bergovsky [112], is a means of measuring intraluminal gut pH. It is useful in evaluating patients with possible intestinal ischemia for the following reasons. As tissue oxygen demand exceeds its supply, there is a corresponding decline in intracellular pH. It has been demonstrated that the drop in intracellular pH translates into an intramural drop in pH and an associated drop in intraluminal pH as well [113,114]. The tonometer consists of a semipermeable balloon attached to a thin silastic catheter that can be introduced through the patient's mouth and with an endoscope placed into the small intestine. Saline is introduced into the balloon and, after equilibration with the lumen, is withdrawn and its carbon dioxide content determined. Use of the Hendersen-Hasselbalch equation then allows determination of the intraluminal pH and hence the intramural pH. Tonometry, therefore, is useful for indirectly monitoring cellular metabolism and implying the adequacy of oxygen delivery. It has been used with good success clinically in determining the likelihood of significant colonic ischemia after aortic operations based on the lumenal pH of the sigmoid during the operation [115]. Similarly, it has been used in the pre- and postprandial gut to diagnose the inadequacy of oxygen delivery (mesenteric perfusion) to the mucosa, as determined by a drop in the lumenal pH after a meal. In one case, that finding was reversed after the patient had visceral revascularization [116]. The future may hold some bright prospects for using tonometry to screen patients suspected of having visceral ischemic syndromes.

Phosphorus nuclear magnetic resonance (PNMR) spectroscopy has been used to study the metabolic responses to ischemia in a variety of tissues [117]. Characteristic changes in concentrations of phosphorylated metabolites occur with ischemia, which are reversible on recovery. These findings have led to investigation of its use for determining the adequacy of perfusion of the intestine in animal models [118,119]. PNMR spectroscopy also may prove of use clinically in the near future.

Via established endoscopic techniques, a laser can be introduced into the gut lumen and its light transmitted into the intestinal mucosa with a probe. The reflectance of the light off the mucosal-tissue red blood cells can be

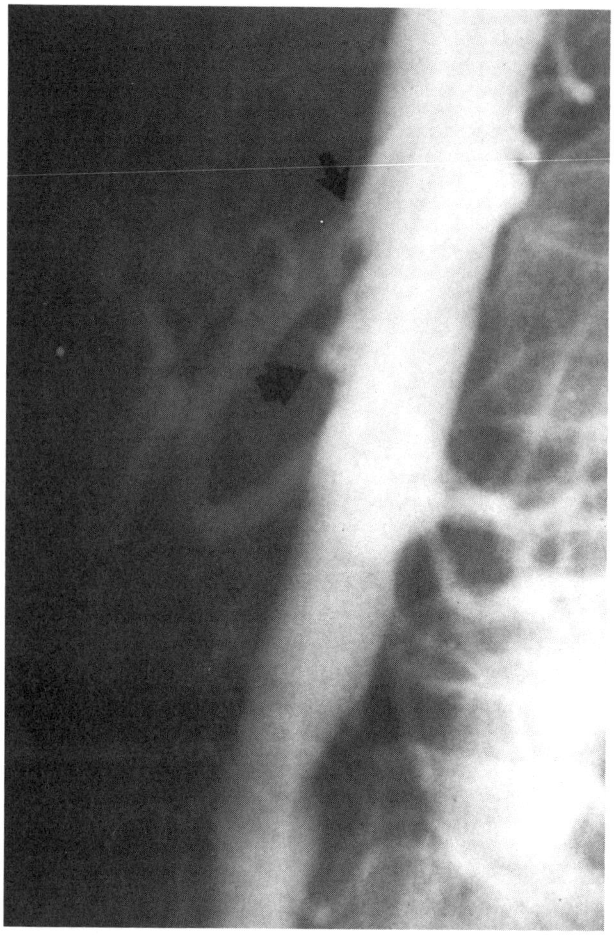

Fig. 37-5. Lateral aortogram showing celiac and superior mesenteric artery stenoses.

measured along with the wavelength shift. Using established principles of spectral analysis and the Doppler shift, mucosal blood flow can be measured. Because several confounding variables can influence the accuracy of this technique, more study is necessary before it can be applied clinically [120].

Reflectance spectrophotometry is a method of assessing mucosal blood flow and has the advantage that it can be used at the patient's bedside. The device makes use of an intraluminal intestinal probe attached to a spectrophotometer, which, through computerized measurement of reflected light and through a series of complicated equations, can determine oxygen saturation (ISO_2) and hemoglobin concentration (IHB) in the intestinal mucosa [121]. Distinct patterns of ISO_2 and IHB are associated with different types of intestinal ischemia. Although not yet available clinically, this method is also a promising new technology.

A number of experimental reports have studied radioisotope imaging to screen for acute mesenteric ischemia. These studies have included technetium-99m pyrophosphate imaging, technetium sulfur colloid–labeled autologous leukocytes, technetium-methylene-diphosphate scanning, and xenon clearance [122–126]. Although promising in experimental models, radioisotope imaging has not yet undergone comparative clinical trials.

Treatment

The goal of therapy in patients who suffer from visceral ischemia is the restoration of mesenteric blood flow and maintenance of bowel viability. The urgency with which that is accomplished varies with the mode of onset of the patient's symptoms.

ACUTE VISCERAL ISCHEMIA

Patients who develop acute visceral ischemia require expedient evaluation and institution of therapy if there is any hope of a successful outcome. **Embolic occlusion** of the visceral arteries produces the most dramatic onset of symptoms, because the collateral blood vessels have not developed sufficiently to avoid intestinal infarction. In such an individual, the goal of therapy is expeditious resuscitation and a timely operation. Throughout the course of the patient's initial evaluation (including arteriography), resuscitation and monitoring are established to optimize multiorgan function. Specific attention should be given to improving cardiac output, controlling cardiac dysrhythmias, and eliminating agents known to exacerbate mesenteric ischemia. Appropriate volume resuscitation is critical, and it should be realized that large volumes of fluid may be sequestered in the ischemic gut.

Abdominal exploration is carried out, usually through a midline incision. The operative findings depend on the site and the duration of the occlusion. Most emboli lodge 5 to 7 cm from the origin of the superior mesenteric artery at a point distal to the first jejunal branches. That location spares the duodenum and the first several centimeters of the jejunum, while the remainder of the small bowel and right colon show evidence of ischemia. The earliest signs of intestinal ischemia are vigorous bowel contraction and a pale to bluish white appearance. With longer ischemic periods the bowel begins to manifest evidence of hemorrhagic infarction, with bowel edema, dilation, and hemorrhage into the mesentery. Despite those otherwise ominous findings, restoration of mesenteric blood flow will allow normal color and contractility to return to the revascularized bowel.

The exposure of the superior mesenteric artery is begun by elevating the transverse colon and incising the base of the transverse mesocolon overlying the superior mesenteric artery. The point of obstruction can be identified by palpating the pulse at the origin of the superior mesenteric artery and noting its disappearance distal to the embolic occlusion. A transverse arteriotomy is made distal to the middle colic artery; bidirectional catheter thromboembolectomy is then completed, and the vessel is flushed with heparin and saline. The arteriotomy is closed with fine interrupted sutures and the bowel returned to its normal anatomic position for observation. Viability is reassessed after a period of observation, and areas of obvious gangrene are resected. When there is a question as to bowel viability, assessment may be aided by a Doppler flow probe coupled to the antimesenteric border to detect normal arterial flow signals [127] or by inspection of the bowel wall after fluorescein injection (10 mg/kg), utilizing ultraviolet light [128]. Primary intestinal anastomosis should be safe in the absence of extensive intra-abdominal contamination. Prior to the completion of the procedure, a decision should be made regarding the advisability of a second-look operation. Once a second-look procedure is planned, the subsequent clinical course should not alter that decision.

Thrombotic occlusion of the visceral vessels may have a more insidious onset: As the bowel ischemia becomes more severe, it can produce what may best be described as a "shocked bowel obstruction." Arteriography usually shows extensive occlusive disease involving the visceral vessels, and lateral aortography is required to evaluate the origins of the celiac and superior mesenteric arteries. Having established the diagnosis, the patient is prepared for the operation with continued volume replacement and correction of the associated metabolic acidosis. Exploration usually is accomplished through a midline incision. Attention is directed first at defining the extent of the vessel occlusion. The disease process begins as an aortic wall atheromatous plaque, which may involve only the anterior aortic wall or may produce a circumferential aortic atheroma. The atheromatous process then extends into the orifice of the visceral vessels. The superior mesenteric artery frequently has extensive arterial wall plaque, but the celiac artery may have only a short-segment orifice occlusion. Once the vascular anatomy is defined, autogenous reconstruction utilizing transvisceral or transaortic endarterectomy or an appropriate antegrade bypass from the supraceliac aorta is performed. Before completion of the reconstruction, balloon catheter embolectomy is performed to clear the distal mesenteric or celiac arterial tree of propagated thrombus. If a bypass procedure is required, the preferred vascular conduit is autogenous tissue (reversed saphenous vein), unless there is no evidence of intra-abdominal contamination, in which case a synthetic graft may be utilized [11]. Following revascularization, the bowel is observed and resected as indicated.

Nonocclusive mesenteric ischemia may have a clinical presentation similar to that of embolic and thrombotic visceral ischemia and must be distinguished from both. In the appropriate clinical setting, consideration of this disease process should lead to careful evaluation, reduction, or elimination of vasoconstricting agents and angiography to exclude obstruction of the visceral vessels. Although the critical angiographic findings are the exclusion of obstructing lesions, additional supportive evidence for nonocclusive visceral ischemia may be obtained by noting beading of the visceral vessels, poor peripheral perfusion, and proximal arterial dilation [95]. The diagnosis of nonocclusive mesenteric ischemia having been established, a catheter is inserted into the superior mesenteric artery to provide a route for selective intra-arterial vasodilators (papaverine, tolazoline). Selective intra-arterial papaverine infusion has been shown to interrupt splanchnic vasoconstriction and should be utilized [10]. Surgical intervention depends on the patient's response to medical management and is reserved for resection of nonviable bowel only.

Therapy for **mesenteric venous thrombosis** is directed

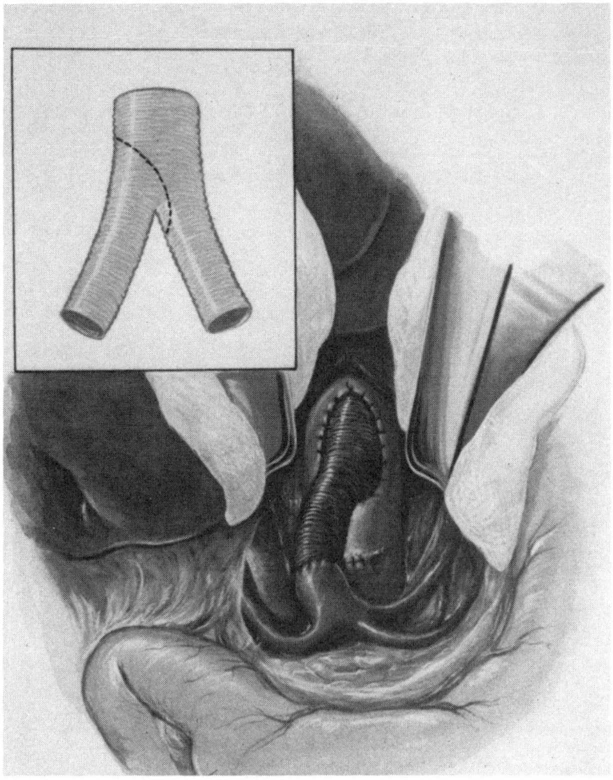

Fig. 37-6. Illustration of flanged prosthetic graft obtained from bifurcated prosthesis (inset) and inserted as an antegrade aortoceliac bypass. (Source: EJ Wylie, RJ Stoney, WK Ehrenfeld. Manual of Vascular Surgery, vol. 1. New York: Springer, 1980. Pp. 210–217.)

primarily toward treating the underlying cause leading to the thrombotic event. Phlebotomy and anticoagulation and antiplatelet agents have been utilized to reduce the hypercoagulable states associated with this disease. Surgical intervention is reserved for those patients who show evidence of peritonitis and require exploration in anticipation of bowel resection. Venous thrombectomy has been attempted, but rethrombosis of the mesenteric veins has caused that procedure to be abandoned.

Mortality rates from recent series for treatment of acute visceral ischemia range between 40 and 93 percent, with the average being 72 percent [129]. Boley and his group at Montefiore are staunch advocates of the use of papavarine once the diagnosis of visceral ischemia is made, regardless of whether it is from occlusive or nonocclusive means [99]. With that approach, they have reported mortalities of 45 percent with 70–90 percent of survivors losing less than 1 m of intestine.

CHRONIC VISCERAL ISCHEMIA

A patient with chronic visceral ischemic symptoms does not require the same urgency of diagnosis nor enormity of resuscitation as a patient with acute visceral ischemia. Prior to elective visceral reconstruction, however, nutritional repletion may be necessary, and intravenous alimentation may be required. It is important to anticipate

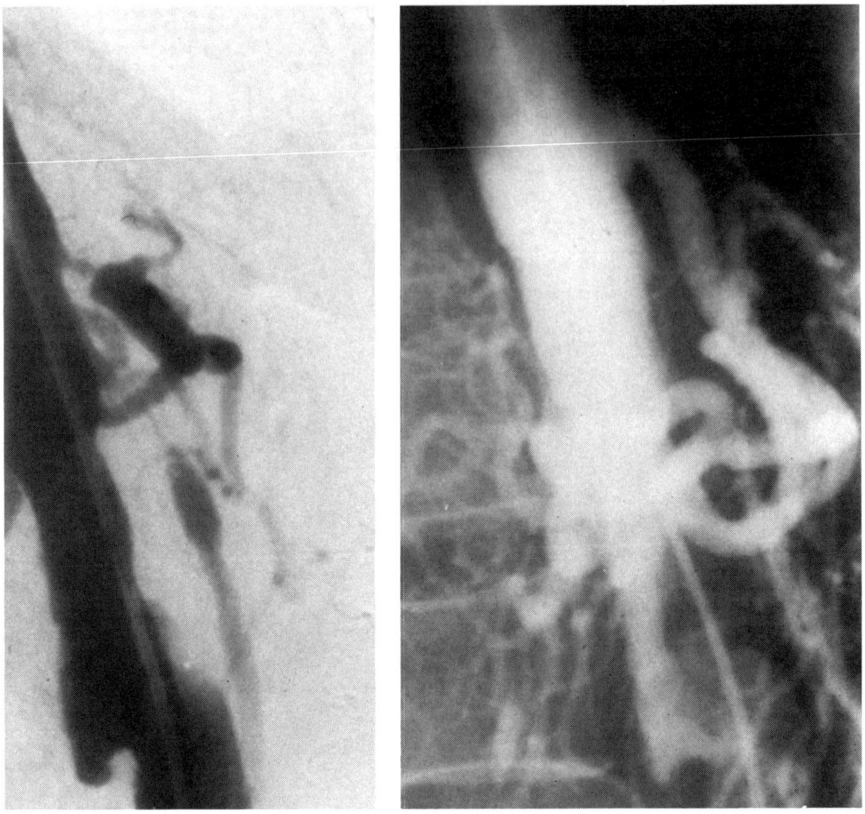

Fig. 37-7. Lateral aortogram: (left) preoperative showing severe celiac and superior mesenteric artery stenosis; (right) postoperative showing patent aortoceliac bypass graft. (Source: EJ Wylie, RJ Stoney, WK Ehrenfeld. Manual of Vascular Surgery, vol. 1. New York: Springer, 1980. Pp. 210–217.)

and avoid situations that can lead to dehydration to minimize the risk of a thrombotic occlusion and the precipitation of an acute ischemic event. Selection of the most appropriate operation for these patients depends on the pattern of the disease, the presence of associated arterial lesions, and the severity of associated systemic illness.

Our early operative experience treating chronic visceral ischemia included reimplantation, transarterial endarterectomy, and aortovisceral bypass using saphenous vein or arterial autograft. Late failures associated with these procedures (transmesenteric arterial thromboendarterectomy, 22%; saphenous-vein bypass, 83%; arterial autograft, 50%) led to our development of transaortic thromboendarterectomy (TA-TEA) and antegrade prosthetic aortovisceral bypass, which we have used exclusively in the past two decades.

The durability of such revascularizations supports their continued use in patients with symptomatic chronic visceral ischemia. In a series that now extends over 30 years in which 88 patients underwent primary repair for chronic visceral ischemia, 77 of those patients had TA-TEA (51 patients) or antegrade prosthetic aortovisceral bypass grafting (26 patients). Follow-up was available for 97.3 percent. There were 10 perioperative deaths. The cumulative percentage of patients who were asymptomatic following aortovisceral endarterectomy or antegrade bypass grafting was nearly identical at 1- and 5-year follow-up intervals [130,131]. Ninety percent of patients remained symptom free.

AORTOVISCERAL BYPASS GRAFTING

Autogenous or prosthetic grafts have been used to bypass obstructive lesions of the main visceral arteries. Grafts can be constructed to provide antegrade or retrograde blood flow. Early reports describe a retrograde orientation of the grafts, which originate along the ventral surface of the infrarenal aorta. The grafts are then attached to the side of the main visceral arteries beyond the site of obstructing disease to reestablish blood flow to the intestinal tract. Disadvantages inherent with that technique include turbulent flow from the retrograde orientation, inflow obstruction from the progressive nature of infrarenal atheromatous disease, and conduit kinking or buckling from the awkward course of the grafts. These inherent problems contribute to the late failures associated with this type of grafting procedure.

Autogenous reversed saphenous-vein grafts have been used for both renal and mesenteric arterial reconstruction. Progressive dilation or stricture formation in aortorenal saphenous-vein grafts has resulted in stenosis or vessel occlusion and failed procedures [132,133]. The internal iliac artery, which is an excellent conduit for renal-artery reconstruction, overcomes those objections, but it provides important collateral blood flow to the intestinal tract and therefore should not be sacrificed for visceral reconstruction.

Prosthetic conduits are ideal for aortovisceral bypass. They can be oriented in an antegrade fashion by attaching the proximal end to the undiseased supraceliac aorta and the distal end to the divided visceral vessel. That technique ensures antegrade flow and provides a short, unrestricted inflow to the mesenteric artery, the celiac artery, or both (Fig. 37-6, p. 879). Flanged knitted Dacron prostheses are preferred for single-vessel bypasses, and bifurcated grafts are utilized when both vessels are reconstructed.

The operation is conducted through a midline incision. The celiac artery and the supraceliac aorta are exposed through the lesser omentum. The abdominal viscera are retracted laterally and the crus of the diaphragm divided to provide circumferential control of the supraceliac aorta. Ganglionic tissue is excised from around the celiac and superior mesenteric arteries. A bifurcated prosthetic graft is anastomosed to the supraceliac aorta and the graft limbs individually anastomosed to the divided ends of the celiac and superior mesenteric arteries [134]. When extensive disease exists in the distal superior mesenteric artery, it may be sufficient to revascularize the celiac artery alone. Intraoperative duplex scanning is used to visualize the reconstruction and confirm adequacy of visceral blood flow [135]. Before the patient is discharged from the hospital, arteriography is obtained to confirm patency of the reconstruction (Fig. 37-7).

VISCERAL ENDARTERECTOMY

Endarterectomy was the first procedure used to relieve symptomatic obstruction of the superior mesenteric artery [32]. The original procedure was performed in a retrograde manner from the superior mesenteric artery into the aorta. Although the procedure successfully relieves the obstruction to flow, it fails to remove the aortic atheroma effectively, which progresses and is responsible for late failures. Transaortic visceral endarterectomy allows for the removal of both the aortic atheroma and the orifice disease that causes the obstruction to splanchnic blood flow.

The surgical approach to the region of the visceral vessels is best accomplished using left medial visceral rotation of the viscera, in a plane posterior to the pancreas and anterior to Gerota's fascia [136]. Using that approach, complete exposure of the involved upper-abdominal aortic segment and its four major branches may be obtained. A left lateral aortotomy is performed in a trapdoor fashion (Fig. 37-8), and the aortic and orifice atheroma contained in the ventral aorta are removed using extraction endarterectomy [137]. The visceral vessels are allowed to backbleed and then are flushed with a heparin-saline solution to confirm their patency. The aortotomy is closed with a running suture, and aortic continuity and flow are restored. If the atheromatous obstruction in the superior mesenteric artery has already progressed to occlusion, the distal propagated thrombus at the level of the reentry collateral may not be completely extracted through the aortotomy. A separate longitudinal arteriotomy is placed

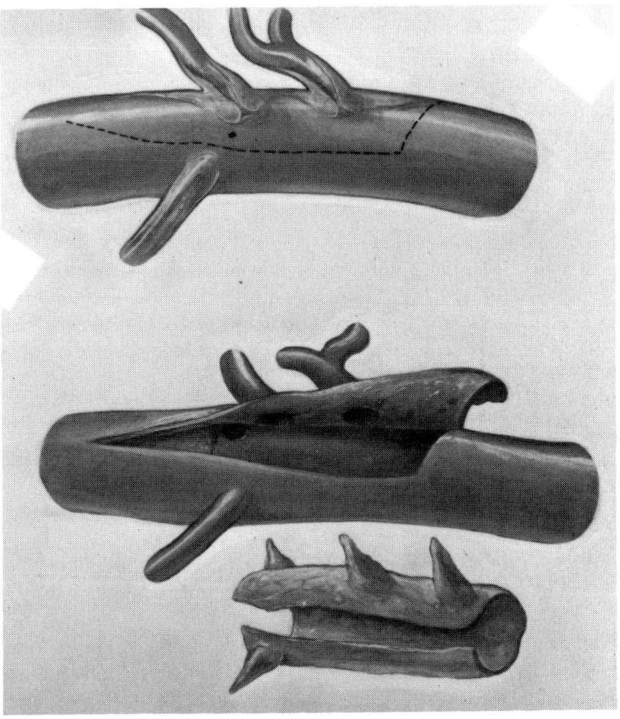

Fig. 37-8. Illustration of thoracoabdominal aortic exposure with outline of aortic incision for transaortic visceral endarterectomy (top). The aortic lumen after endarterectomy showing patent orifice of celiac superior mesenteric and left renal artery (middle). The specimen is a cylinder of aortic atheroma with projecting orifice lesions in both visceral and renal orifices (bottom). (Source: EJ Wylie, RJ Stoney, WK Ehrenfeld. Manual of Vascular Surgery, vol. 1. New York: Springer, 1980. Pp. 210–217.)

distally in the superior mesenteric artery, and the remaining thrombus is removed under direct visualization; the vessel is closed with a vein patch to prevent narrowing. Intraoperative patency is confirmed with duplex scanning of the endarterectomized upper-abdominal aorta and its branches.

Summary

Visceral ischemic syndromes constitute a spectrum of disease that may, if not detected and treated, culminate in fatal intestinal gangrene. Acute visceral ischemia is an emergency both in its diagnosis and in its treatment, whereas symptomatic chronic visceral ischemia may run a prolonged course before diagnosis and effective surgical revascularization.

The general physician plays an important role for all patients with visceral ischemic syndromes. He or she is usually the first physician to evaluate the patients and often can effectively and unerringly direct the efforts to diagnose the problem. An awareness of the disease and a high index of suspicion lead to the confirmatory arteriogram, after which appropriate consultation ensures appropriate treatment.

References

1. Boley SJ. Early diagnosis of acute mesenteric ischemia. Hosp Prac 1981; 8:63.
2. Boley SJ, et al. Acute mesenteric vascular occlusion. Contemp Surg 1983; 23:125.
3. Sachs SM, Morten JH, Schwartz SI. Acute mesenteric ischemia. Surgery 1982; 92:646.
4. Bergan JJ, Yao JST. Acute intestinal ischemia. In RB Rutherford, ed. Vascular Surgery, 2nd ed. Philadelphia: Saunders, 1984. Pp. 948–963.
5. Baur GM, et al. Treatment of chronic visceral ischemia. Am J Surg 1984; 148:138.
6. Hansen KJ, Stoney RJ. Antegrade bypass for chronic visceral ischemia. In JJ Bergan, JST Yao, eds. Vascular Surgery. New York: Grune & Stratton, 1987. Pp. 377–387.
7. Hertzer MR, Beven ER, Humpries AW. Chronic intestinal ischemia. Surg Gynecol Obstet 1977; 145:321.
8. Rogers DM, et al. Mesenteric vascular problems: a 26-year experience. Ann Surg 1982; 195:554.
9. Stanton PE, et al. Chronic intestinal ischemia: diagnosis and therapy. J Vasc Surg 1986; 4:338.
10. Boley SJ, et al. Initial results from an aggressive angiographic and surgical approach to acute mesenteric ischemia. Surgery 1977; 82:848.
11. Rapp JH, et al. Durability of endarterectomy and antegrade grafts in the treatment of chronic visceral ischemia. J Vasc Surg 1986; 3:799.
12. Elliott JW. Operative relief of gangrene of the intestine due to occlusion of the mesenteric vessels. Ann Surg 1895; 73:128.
13. Ficarra BJ. Mesenteric vascular occlusion; presentation of 15 cases. Am J Surg 1944; 66:168.
14. Klass AA. Embolectomy in acute mesenteric occlusion. Ann Surg 1951; 134:913.
15. Shaw RS, Rutledge RH. Superior mesenteric artery embolectomy in treatment of massive mesenteric infarction. N Engl J Med 1957; 257:595.
16. Brittain RS, Earley TK. Emergency thromboendarterectomy of the superior mesenteric artery: report of four cases. Ann Surg 1963; 158:138.
17. Warren S, Eberhard TP. Mesenteric venous thrombosis. Surg Gynecol Obstet 1935; 61:102.
18. Johnson MJ. Mesenteric venous occlusion: a clinical entity. Am J Surg 1940; 49:242.
19. Berry FB, Bongas JA. Agnogenic venous mesenteric thrombosis. Ann Surg 1950; 132:459.
20. Fontaine R, et al. Intestinal mesenteric infarction of venous origin: the place of thrombectomy in treatment. J Circ 1969; 97:145.
21. Inahara T. Acute superior mesenteric venous thrombosis: treatment by thrombectomy. Ann Surg 1971; 174:956.
22. Eude N. Infarction of the bowel in cardiac failure. N Engl J Med 1958; 258:879.
23. Councilman WT. Three cases of occlusion of the superior mesenteric artery. Boston Med Surg J 1894; 130:4.
24. Chiene J. Complete obliteration of the celiac and mesenteric arteries. J Anat Physiol 1869; 3:65.
25. Goodman EH. Angina abdominis. Amer J Med Sci 1918; 155:524.
26. Mikkelson W. Abdominal pain of vascular origin. Am J Surg 1957; 94:262.
27. Klein E. Embolism and thrombosis of the superior mesenteric artery. SGO 1921; 33:385.
28. Schnitzler F. Zur Symptomatik des Darmarterien-verschlusses. Wien Med Wchnschr 1901; 11/12:506.
29. Warburg E. Uber dyspragia intermittens angiosclerotica intestinalis. München med. Wchnschr 1905; 52:1174.
30. Dunphy J. Abdominal pain of vascular origin. Am J Med Sci 1936; 192:109.
31. Shaw R, Rutledge R. Superior mesenteric artery embolectomy in the treatment of massive infarction. New Eng J Med 1957; 257:596.
32. Shaw R, Maynard EI. Acute and chronic thrombosis of mesenteric arteries associated with malabsorption. Report of two cases successfully treated by thromboendartectomy. New Eng J Med 1958; 258:874.
33. Derrick JR, Pollard HS, Moore RM. The pattern of arteriosclerotic narrowing of the celiac and superior mesenteric arteries. Ann Surg 1959; 149:684.
34. Morris GC, et al. Revascularization of the celiac and superior mesenteric arteries. Arch Surg 1962; 84:95.
35. Stoney RJ, Wylie EJ. Recognition and surgical management of visceral ischemic syndromes. Ann Surg 1966; 164:714.
36. Bergan JJ, et al. Revascularization in treatment of mesenteric infarction. Ann Surg 1975; 182:430.
37. Bergan JJ, in discussion of Sachs FM, Morten JH, Schwartz SI: Acute mesenteric ischemia. Surgery 1982; 92:646.
38. Guyton AC. Textbook of Medical Physiology, 6th ed. Philadelphia: Saunders, 1981. P. 349.
39. Teppermen BL, Jacobson ED. Mesenteric circulation. In LR Johnson, ed. Physiology of the Gastrointestinal Tract. New York: Raven, 1981. P. 1317.
40. Hallback D, et al. Evidence for the existence of a countercurrent exchanger in the small intestine in man. Gastroenterology 1978; 74:683–690.
41. Lundgren O. Studies on blood flow distribution and counter-current exchange in the small intestine. Acta Physiol Scand[Suppl] 1967; 303:1–42.
42. Lundgren O. The circulation of the small bowel mucosa. Gut 1974; 15:1005–1013.
43. Kampp M, Lundgren O, Nilsson N. Extravascular shunting of oxygen in the small intestine of the cat. Acta Physiol Scand 1968; 72:396–403.
44. Folkow B. Regional adjustments of intestinal blood flow. Gastroenterology 1967; 52:423–432.
45. Rothe C. Reflex control of veins and vascular capacitance. Physiol Rev 1983; 63:1281–1342.
46. McNeill J, Stark R, Greenway C. Intestinal vasoconstriction after hemorrhage: role of vasopressin and angiotensin. Am J Physiol 1970; 219:1342.
47. Bulkley G, et al. Collateral blood flow in segmental intestinal ischemia: effects of vasoactive agents. Surgery 1986; 100: 157–165.
48. Hernandez R, Meyers I. Prostacyclin regulates splanchnic blood flow during early hemorrhage/reperfusion injury. Prostaglandins Leukotrienes and Essential Fatty Acids 1992; 48:401–405.
49. Boley S, et al. Experimental evaluation of thiazides and potassium as a cause of small bowel ulcers. JAMA 1965; 192:763–766.
50. Patel A, Kaleya R, Smmartano R. Pathophysiology of mesenteric ischemia. Surg Clin N A 1992; 72:31–42.
51. Darling RC, Austen WG, Linton RR. Arterial embolism. Surg Gynecol Obstet 1967; 124:106.
52. Pierce GE, Brockenbrough EC. The spectrum of mesenteric infarction. Am J Surg 1970; 119:233.
53. Dunphy JE. Abdominal pain of vascular origin. Am J Med Sci 1936; 192:102.
54. Ripley HR, Levin SM. Abdominal angina associated with fibromuscular dysplasia of the celiac and superior mesenteric arteries. Angiology 1966; 17:297.
55. Collins GJ Jr, et al. Hypercoagulability in mesenteric venous occlusion. Am J Surg 1976; 132:390.
56. Peters TG, et al. Anti-thrombin III deficiency causing post-

splenectomy mesenteric venous thrombosis coincident with thrombocytopenia. Ann Surg 1977; 185:229.
57. Nesbit RJ Jr, DeWeese JA. Mesenteric venous thrombosis and oral contraceptives. Southern Med J 1977; 70:360.
58. Lescher TJ, Bombeck CT. Mesenteric vascular occlusion associated with oral contraceptive use. Arch Surg 1977; 112:1231.
59. Pawlik W, Jacobson ED. Effects of digoxin on the mesenteric circulation. Cardiovasc Res Ctr Bull 1974; 12:80.
60. Danford RO. The splanchnic vasoconstrictive effect of digoxin and its reversal by glucagon. In SJ Boley, SS Schwartz, L Williams, eds. Vascular Disorders of the Intestine. New York: Appleton-Century-Crofts, 1971. Pp. 421–428.
61. Ferrer MI, et al. The effect of digoxin in the splanchnic circulation in ventricular failure. Circulation 1965; 32:524.
62. Horton J, Walker P. Oxygen radicals, lipid peroxidation, and permeability changes after intestinal ischemia and reperfusion. J Appl Physiol 1993; 74:1515–1520.
63. Boros M, Kaszaki J, Nagy S. Oxygen free radical-induced histamine release during intestinal ischemia and reperfusion. Eur Surg Res 1989; 21:297–304.
64. Montgomery A, Borgstrom A, Haglund U. Pancreatic proteases and intestinal mucosal injury after ischemia and reperfusion in the pig. Gastroent 1992; 102:216–222.
65. van der Vliet A, Bast A. Role of reactive oxygen species in intestinal diseases. Free Radical Biol and Med 1992; 12:499–513.
66. Parks DA, et al. Ischemic injury to the cat small intestine: role of superoxide radicals. Gastroenterology 1982; 82:4.
67. Parks DA, Bulkley GB, Granger DN. Role of oxygen-derived free radicals in digestive tract diseases. Surgery 1983; 94:415.
68. Said SI. Vasoactive peptides: state of the art review. Hypertension 1983; 5[Suppl 1]:17.
69. Parks D, Grogaard B, Granger D. Comparison of partial and complete arterial occlusion models for studying intestinal ischemia. Surgery 1982; 92:896–901.
70. Crissenger K, Granger D. Mucosal injury induced by ischemia and reperfusion in the piglet intestine: Influence of the age and feeding. Gastroenterology 1989; 97:920–926.
71. Tabata T, deSerres S, Meyer A. Antibody synthesis to peptidoglycan polysaccharide after ischemic injury of the intestine. J Trauma 1993; 35:598–603.
72. Deitch EA, Bridges RM. Effect of stress and trauma on bacterial translocation from the gut. J Surg Res 1987; 42:536–542.
73. Benjamin E, Oropello J, Iberti T. Acute mesenteric ischemia: pathophysiology, diagnosis, and treatment. Dis a Month 1993; 34(March 1993):1–210.
74. Bulkley GB, et al. Quantitative characterization of segmental collateral blood flow in the canine small intestines. Fed Proc 1984; 43:311.
75. Dunbar J, et al. Compression of the celiac trunk and abdominal angina: preliminary report of 15 cases. Am J Roenten 1965; 95:731.
76. Dunbar JD, et al. Compression of the celiac trunk and abdominal angina: preliminary report of 15 cases. Am J Roentgen 1965; 95:731.
77. Evans E. Long-term evaluation of the celiac band syndrome. Surgery 1974; 76:867–871.
78. Brandt IJ, Boley SJ. Celiac axis compression. A critical review. Am J Dig Dis 1978; 23:633.
79. Szilagyi DE, et al. The celiac axis compression syndrome. Does it exist? Surgery 1972; 72:849.
80. Reilly LM, et al. Late results following operative repair for celiac artery compression syndrome. J Vasc Surg 1985; 2:79.
81. Reilly LM, et. al. Late results following operative repair for celiac artery compression syndrome. J Vasc Surg 1985; 2:79–91.
82. Snyder MA, Mahoney EB, Rob CG. Symptomatic celiac artery stenosis due to constriction by the neurofibrous tissue of the celiac ganglion. Surgery 1967; 61:372.
83. Harjola P. A rare obstruction of the celiac artery. Ann Chir et Gynaec Fenniae 1963; 2:547–550.
84. Snyder MA, Mahoney EB, Rob CG. Symptomatic celiac artery stenosis due to constriction by the neurofibrous tissue of the celiac ganglion. Surgery 1967; 61:372–376.
85. Qvarfordt PG, et al. "Coral reef" atherosclerosis of the suprarenal aorta: a unique clinical entity. J Vasc Surg 1984; 1:903.
86. Krupski WC, Effeney DJ, Ehrenfeld WK. Spontaneous dissection of the superior mesenteric artery. J Vasc Surg 1985; 2:731.
87. Pallubinskas AJ, Ripley HR. Fibromuscular hyperplasia in extra-renal arteries. Radiology 1964; 82:451.
88. Poole JW, Sammartano BS, Boley SJ. Hemodynamic basis of the pain of chronic mesenteric ischemia. Am J Surg 1987; 153:171.
89. Ottinger LW. The surgical management of acute occlusion of the superior mesenteric artery. Ann Surg 1978; 188:721.
90. Boley SJ, et al. New concepts in the management of emboli of the superior mesenteric artery. Surg Gynecol Obstet 1981; 153:561.
91. Rendick RA, Harrington LA. Roentgenologic observations in mesenteric thrombosis. Am J Roentgen 1944; 52:317.
92. Wittenburg J, et al. A radiologic approach to the patient with acute extensive bowel ischemia. Radiology 1973; 106:13.
93. Tomchik FS, Wittenburg J, Ottinger LW. The roentgenographic spectrum of bowel infarction. Radiology 1970; 96:249.
94. Rigler LG, Pogue WL. Roentgen signs of intestinal neurosis. Am J Roentgen 1965; 94:402.
95. Siegleman SS, Sprayregan S, Boley SJ. Angiographic diagnosis of mesenteric arterial vasoconstriction. Radiology 1974; 112:533.
96. Simonetti G, et al. Interventional radiology in the treatment of acute and chronic mesenteric ischemia. Radiologia Medica 1992; 84:98–105.
97. VanDeinse W, Zawacki J, Phillips D. Treatment of acute mesenteric ischemia by percutaneous transluminal angioplasty. Gastroenterology 1986; 91:475.
98. Levy P, Haskell L, Gordon R. Percutaneous transluminal angioplasty of splanchnic arteries: and alternative method to elective revascularisation in chronic ischaemia. Eur J Rad 1987; 7:239–242.
99. Boley S, et al. Ischemic disorders of the intestines. Current Prob Surg 1978; 15:1.
100. Kaufman SL, Harrington DP, Siegleman SS. Superior mesenteric artery embolization: an angiographic emergency. Radiology 1977; 124:625.
101. Stanley JC, Brink BE, Fry WJ. Experimental intestinal ischemia: Provocative absorption studies following gradual celiac and superior mesenteric artery occlusion. J Surg Res 1973; 14:133–138.
102. Hansen HJ, et al. Splanchnic blood flow in patients with abdominal angina before and after arterial reconstruction. A proposal for a diagnostic test. Ann Surg 1977; (186):216–220.
103. Crotch-Harvey M, Gould D. Case report: percutaneous transluminal angioplasty of the inferior mesenteric artery in the treatment of chronic mesenteric ischaemia. Clin Rad 1992; 46:408–409.
104. McShane M, et al. Mesenteric angioplasty for chronic intestinal ischaemia. Eur J Vasc Surg 1992; 6:333–336.
105. Bounoire E, et al. Digital subtraction angiography of the abdominal aorta and renal arteries: comparison with conventional aortography. Radiology 1981; 139(2):281.
106. Li K, et al. Chronic mesenteric ischemia: evaluation with phase contrast cine MR imaging. Rad 1994; 190:175–179.

107. Jäger K, et al. Non-invasive diagnosis of intestinal angina. J Clin Ultrasound 1984; 12:588–591.
108. Moneta G, et al. Mesenteric duplex scanning: a blinded prospective study. J Vasc Surg 1993; 17:79–84.
109. Harward T, Smith S, Seeger J. Detection of celiac asis and superior mesenteric artery occlusive disease with the use of abdominal duplex scanning. J Vasc Surg 1993; 17:738–745.
110. Healy D, et al. Evaluation of celiac and mesenteric vascular disease with duplex ultrasonography. J of Ultrasound in Medicine 1992; 11:481–485.
111. Rob C, Owen K. Ligation of both the celiac axis and superior mesenteric artery with survival of the patient. Brit J Surg 1956; 44:247.
112. Bergovsky E. Determination of tissue oxygen tensions by hollow-visceral tonometers: effect of breathing enriched oxygen mixtures. J Clin Invest 1964; 43:193–200.
113. Grum C. Tissue oxygenation in low flow states and during hypoxemia. Crit Care Med 1993; 21[Suppl]:S44–S49.
114. Grum C, et al. Adequacy of tissue oxygenation in the intact dog intestine. J Appl Physiol 1984; 5:1065–1069.
115. Fiddian-Green R. A sensitive and specific diagnostic test for intestinal ischemia using Sliastic tonometers. Eur Surg Res 1984; 16:32.
116. Boley S, et al. A new provocative test for chronic mesenteric ischemia. Am J Gastroent 1991; 86:888–891.
117. Whitman G, Harkin A. Applications of nuclear magnetic resonance to surgical disease: a collective review. J Surg Res 1985; 38:187–199.
118. Blum H, et al. Acute intestinal ischemia studies by phosphorus nuclear magnetic resonance spectroscopy. Ann Surg 1986; 204:83–88.
119. Temes R, Kauten R, Schwartz M. Nuclear magnetic resonance as a noninvasive method of diagnosing intestinal ischemia: technique and preliminary results. J Ped Surg 1991; 26:775–779.
120. Perbeck L, et al. Correlation between fluorescein flowmetry and laser Doppler flowmetry. Scand J Gastroenterol 1990; 25:520–524.
121. Leung F, et al. Reflectance spectrophotometry for the assessment of gastroduodenal mucosal perfusion. Am J Physiol 1987; 252:G797–G804.
122. Schemmel DH, Moss AA, Hoffer PB. Radionuclide imaging of intestinal infarction in dogs. Invest Radiol 1976; 11:277.
123. Kressel HY, et al. Radionuclide imaging of bowel infarction complicating small bowel intussusception in dogs. Invest Radiol 1978; 13:127.
124. Bardfeld PA, et al. Scintigraphic diagnosis of ischemic intestine with 99m Tc sulfur colloid-labeled leukocytes. Radiology 1977; 124:439.
125. Frantzides CT, et al. Radionuclide visualization of acute occlusive and nonocclusive intestinal ischemia. Ann Surg 1986; 203:295.
126. Gharagozloo F, et al. The use of intraperitoneal xenon for early diagnosis of acute mesenteric ischemia. Surgery 1984; 95:404.
127. Wright CB, Hobson RW. Prediction of intestinal viability using Doppler ultrasound technique. Am J Surg 1975; 129:642.
128. Marfuggi RA, Greenspan M. Reliable intraoperative prediction of intestinal viability using a fluorescent indicator. Surg Gynecol Obstet 1980; 152:33.
129. Kalyea R, Sammartano R, Boley S. Aggressive approach to acute mesenteric ischemia. Surg Clin N A 1992; 72:157–182.
130. Cunningham C, et al. Chronic visceral ischemia: three decades of progress. Ann Surg 1991; 214:276.
131. Rapp JH, et al. Durability of endarterectomy and antegrade grafts in the treatment of chronic visceral ischemia. J Vasc Surg 1986; 3(5):799–806.
132. Dean RH, Wilson JP, Burko H. Saphenous vein aortorenal bypass grafts: serial arteriographic study. Ann Surg 1974; 180:469.
133. Stanley JC, Ernst CB, Fry WJ. Fate of 100 aortorenal vein grafts: characteristics of late graft expansion, aneurysmal dilatation, and stenosis. Surgery 1973; 74:931.
134. Stoney RJ, Ehrenfeld WK, Wylie EJ. Revascularization methods in chronic visceral ischemia caused by atherosclerosis. Ann Surg 1977; 186:468.
135. Okuhn SP, et al. Intraoperative assessment of renal and visceral artery reconstruction: the role of duplex scanning and spectral analysis. J Vasc Surg 1984; 5:137.
136. Stoney R, Effeney D. Thoracoabdominal aorta and its branches. In EJ Wylie. Atlas of Vascular Surgery, vol 5. Philadelphia: Lippincott, 1992.
137. Wylie EJ, Stoney RJ, Ehrenfeld WK. Manual of Vascular Surgery, vol. 1. New York: Springer, 1980. Pp. 210–217.

Vasculogenic Impotence

Irwin Goldstein

Impotence, the persistent inability to attain and maintain an erection adequate to permit satisfactory sexual performance, has been found in a recent epidemiologic study to afflict 52 percent of noninstitutionalized, free-living, community-based men between the ages of 40 and 70 years [1]. There are approximately 36 million men in the United States between the ages of 40 and 70, based on the 1990 U.S. population census. It thus can be predicted that impotence affects at least 18 million American men. Considering there are additional contributions from impotent men younger than 40 years (in particular, those who would be most interested in this topic) and impotent men older than 70 years, there is a potential population approaching 30 million impotent American men.

The most frequent cause of organic impotence is vascular impairment, that is, alterations in the inflow (cavernosal artery insufficiency, arteriogenic impotence, failure to fill) and outflow (corporal veno-occlusive dysfunction, venous leak, failure to store) of blood to and from the penis [2]. It is the intent of this chapter to review the emerging field of vasculogenic impotence. This work will detail the epidemiology of impotence; the physiology of penile erection, with emphasis on hemodynamic mechanisms; the pathophysiology of vasculogenic impotence, highlighting the new understanding of the trabecular smooth muscle cell and its role in trabecular extracellular matrix synthesis; the diagnostic tests for vasculogenic dysfunction, with a discussion of the modern principles for evaluation of erections during trabecular smooth muscle relaxation; and the treatment for hemodynamic alterations, including conservative, reconstructive, and prosthetic options.

Epidemiology

Impairment of erectile function, while nominally a benign disorder, has a profound impact on the well-being of many men. The National Center for Health Statistics data from the National Ambulatory Medical Care Survey showed that in 1985 in the United States impotence accounted for over 400,000 outpatient physician visits, over 30,000 hospital admissions, and a total cost of $146 million [2]. Epidemiologic studies on the prevalence of impotence and its possible physical and psychological correlates have been limited in purpose and in scope. The methods for obtaining study populations differed, the criteria for defining impotence varied, the reports of impotence were not stratified by age, and none examined physiological correlates. This lack of scientific information, especially of the prevalence in the general population and the relationship of impotence to intervening variables of physiologic and psychological concern, has hindered the true health significance of the field. Recently, the Massachusetts Male Aging Study (MMAS), the first large epidemiologic study on sexual function in a general population, provided current normative data on impotence, defining its prevalence and identifying physiologic and psychological correlates [1,3,4].

The MMAS was a cross-sectional, community-based, random-sample multidisciplinary epidemiologic survey of health and aging in men aged 40–70 years. The study was conducted between 1987 and 1989 in 11 randomly selected cities and towns in the Boston area. Of the 1,709 MMAS subjects, 1,290 (75.5%) provided complete responses to all the questions of the sexual function instrument and represented the study sample [1,3,4]. The sample size is considerably larger than any similar health research in aging to date and the largest sexual function survey since Kinsey's work in 1948.

More than half the men (657 of the 1,290) had some degree of erectile dysfunction. The largest category comprised 322 moderately impotent (25%), followed by 210 minimally impotent (17%) and 125 completely impotent (10%) men. The prevalence of impotence in the MMAS sample was 52 percent. The cross-sectional trend between ages 40 and 70 years for complete impotence was tripled; the probability of moderate as well as the overall impotence doubled, while the probability of minimal impotence remained almost constant. Over that age range, the probabilities of minimal, moderate, and complete impotence were 16.5, 17.4, and 4.9 percent, respectively, at the age of 40 and 18, 34, and 15 percent, respectively, at the age of 70. The overall probability of impotence at ages 40 and 70 years was 38.9 percent and 67.1 percent, respectively [1,3,4].

Treated diabetes, heart disease, and hypertension, as well as untreated ulcer, arthritis, and allergy, were the medical conditions associated with impotence. The impotence probability values referenced all have been age adjusted. Treated diabetes was associated with probability of impotence. Overall impotence increased by 11 percent. Those results imply that diabetes exacerbates minimal impotence to complete, over and above the higher probabilities of overall impotence of the treated diabetics. In terms of smoking, the data seem to imply that patients with heart disease and moderate impotence could have complete impotence if they were smokers. Treated heart disease is associated with 78-percent overall impotence in nonsmokers and 94.3 percent in smokers. In nonsmoking men with treated hypertension, no significant differences from the study sample as a whole were noted. Untreated ulcer was associated with 17.6-percent probability of complete impotence, compared to 9.5 percent of those without the disease [1,3,4].

In the MMAS, two impotence probability patterns were identified regarding high density lipoprotein (HDL) cholesterol. The first pattern represents changes in younger men, aged 38–55 years, and the second changes in older men, aged 56–70 years. Study findings implied that men in the younger range, with minimal impotence, may become moderately impotent if their levels of HDL drop from 90 to 30 mg/dl. For the older men, no one with complete impotence was identified (0% probability of complete impotence) in those with HDL values more than 90 mg/dl. Those data, together with the finding that total serum cholesterol was not correlated with impotence probabilities, support HDL levels as a strong determinant of impotence [1,3,4].

In the MMAS, one hormone was significantly predictive of the pattern of impotence probabilities: the adrenal androgen metabolite dihydroepiandrosterone sulfate (DHEAS). DHEAS levels of 0.5 mg/ml were associated with 16-percent probability of complete impotence, comparing to 6.5- and 3.4-percent probability of complete impotence when the DHEAS levels were 5 and 10 mg/ml, respectively. Testosterone—free, albumin-bound, or total—was not correlated with impotence to any statistical significance [1,3,4].

Impotence was statistically associated with vasodilators, antihypertensive, cardiac, and hypoglycemic medications. No correlation was found between impotence and the use of sympathetic drugs.

Impotence probabilities did not differ significantly between current smokers and nonsmokers or between subjects who reported exposure to cigarette smoke at home or at work and those who reported none. Among current smokers, impotence probabilities showed no dependence on dosage (packs per day) or on lifetime pack-years smoked. Cigarette smoking, however, had dramatic exacerbating effects in certain subgroups, namely, those reported being treated for heart disease and those reported being treated for hypertension.

In the MMAS, depression, anger (either expressed outward or kept inward), and low levels of dominance were psychologic factors found to be strongly associated with impotence [1,3,4].

Physiology of Erection

During erection, the penis accumulates blood under pressure. This function depends on the dilation of the resistance arterial bed of the penis and the relaxation of the trabecular smooth muscle of the corpora cavernosa [2]. The helicine arteries, which branch off the cavernosal artery and open directly into the lacunar spaces, have a crucial role in regulating the state of penile tumescence because they act as resistance vessels, controlling blood inflow and pressure to the cavernosal bodies. When the helicine arteries are constricted, there is a high resistance to arterial inflow and an associated large pressure gradient between the systemic circulation and the lacunar spaces, contributing to the maintenance of penile flaccidity. Dilation of the cavernosal and helicine arteries greatly increases blood flow to the corpora cavernosa with transmission of systemic blood pressure to the lacunar spaces. In addition, there is increased blood inflow into the lacunar spaces from 3–5 ml/minute in the flaccid state to 30–50 ml/minute at the onset of erection. The speed with which an erection develops and the pressure that may exist in the lacunar space at steady-state equilibrium conditions is directly related to the inflow and perfusion-pressure capabilities, respectively, of the cavernosal artery, assuming relaxation of the helicine arteries. The role of the cavernosal artery, therefore, is twofold: to increase the arterial inflow during sexual stimulation and to supply a perfusion pressure approximately equal to the mean systemic arterial perfusion pressure.

Entrapment of blood in the cavernosal bodies is also necessary for penile erection.The microscopic subtunical venules, located in the subtunical space between the periphery of the erectile tissue and the tunica albuginea, are the crucial vessels that provide venous outflow from the corpora via the peripheral lacunae. In the subtunical space, subtunical venules coalesce to form larger-sized emissary veins that pierce the tunica albuginea and drain into extratunical penile veins. Studies of the penile vasculature, utilizing casts, have shown that the restriction of venous outflow from the cavernosal bodies is due to the compression of subtunical venules by the expansion of the trabecular structures against the tunica. That mechanism, known as the **corporal veno-occlusive mechanism**, is regulated, in part, by the tone of the trabecular smooth muscle. When the smooth muscle is contracted, there is low resistance to venous outflow. That allows for the easy evacuation of the cavernosal bodies and may contribute to the maintenance of penile flaccidity. When the smooth muscle relaxes, the resistance to venous outflow from the cavernosal bodies greatly increases due to the elongation and compression of the subtunical venules. The ability to create a high venous-outflow resistance enables the corpora to act as a capacitor, store pressure energy and establish penile rigidity [5,6].

MECHANISMS REGULATING HELICINE ARTERIOLAR SMOOTH MUSCLE TONE

Despite their crucial role in penile erection, little is known about the physiologic mechanisms that regulate dilation of the cavernosal and helicine arteries. A recent study has shown that a nonadrenergic, noncholinergic neurotransmitter mediates dilation of those blood vessels [7]. The dilator responses elicited by nerve stimulation are inhibited by analogs of L-arginine, which inhibit the synthesis of nitric oxide, suggesting that the L-arginine–nitric oxide pathway is involved in the response. Another study has confirmed the role of nitric oxide in the dilator responses of the helicine arteriole [8]. That research has further shown that the helicine arterioles have a functional adrenergic innervation that mainly activates constrictory alpha-1 adrenoceptors. There is further evidence that nitric oxide release during relaxation occurs via blockade of alpha-2 adrenergic receptors. The neurogenic inhibitory responses and the endothelium-dependent relaxations to acetylcholine and bradykinin were only partly inhibited in the presence of an inhibitor of nitric oxide synthase. Thus, the relaxant mechanisms of penile resistance arteries seem to be different from those observed in the trabecular smooth muscle.

MECHANISMS REGULATING TRABECULAR SMOOTH MUSCLE TONE

The physiologic mechanisms regulating the tone of the trabecular smooth muscle have been the subject of many studies and are, therefore, better known [9,10,11]. As in blood vessels, it is now widely accepted that autonomic nerves as well as substances released by the endothelium lining the lacunar spaces control trabecular smooth muscle tone.

The vascular endothelium, when activated by chemical stimuli (i.e., acetylcholine, bradykinin) or physical stimuli (i.e., shear stress), releases an endothelium-derived relaxing factor (EDRF) that diffuses to the underlying smooth muscle, causing its relaxation. This paracrine mechanism for the control of vascular smooth muscle tone was first described in blood vessels by Furchgott and Zawadski and also has been demonstrated in the corpus cavernosum vascular bed [10,13,14,15]. The mechanical or chemical disruption of the endothelium lining the lacunar spaces completely eliminates the dilator effects of acetylcholine or bradykinin, two well-characterized endothelium-dependent dilators. In corpus cavernosum tissue, the EDRF released in response to acetylcholine has the chemical properties of nitric oxide [10,11,14], which also has been proposed to be the EDRF in other vascular beds [16,17]. Endothelium-derived nitric oxide diffuses into the smooth muscle, where it stimulates the production of cyclic guanosine monophosphate (cGMP), which, in turn, leads to smooth muscle relaxation.

The principal neurotransmitter mediating trabecular smooth muscle relaxation is resistant to adrenergic and cholinergic blockade and, therefore, is characterized as a nonadenergic, noncholinergic (NANC) neurotransmitter. Ignarro et al. demonstrated that electrical stimulation of dilator nerves in rabbit corpus cavernosum was associated with the release of a nitric oxide–like substance and the accumulation of cGMP [18]. Those observations have been extended to human corpus cavernosum. In the presence of muscarinic and adrenergic blockade, transmural electrical stimulation of corpus cavernosum tissue in which the endothelium has been mechanically or chemically disrupted elicits NANC neurogenic relaxation [9]. That response is significantly attenuated or blocked by substances that interfere with the synthesis or the effects of nitric oxide [9]. Nitric oxide also has been described as a putative NANC-inhibitory neurotransmitter in the peripheral nervous system in other organs [19]. Further, nitric oxide synthase has been localized with immunohistochemistry in the peripheral autonomic nerves innervating vascular and nonvascular smooth muscle [20]. Those findings strongly support the hypothesis that nitric oxide is the NANC dilator neurotransmitter in corpus cavernosum.

The transduction mechanisms mediating nitric oxide–induced relaxation of the trabecular smooth muscle appear to involve activation of guanylate cyclase with accumulation of cGMP and possibly activation of the sodium potassium adenosinetriphosphatase (ATPase) pump. The synthesis of nitric oxide is regulated by the local concentration of oxygen [11]. The involvement of the other neurotransmitters, such as vasoactive intestinal polypeptide, is possible but has yet to be demonstrated. Vasoactive intestinal polypeptide–mediated relaxation would involve the activation of adenylate cyclase with the accumulation of cyclic adenosine monophosphate (cAMP).

In a continuing search for mechanisms that might modulate corporal smooth muscle tone, the contribution of intercellular communication through gap junctions to the integration of corporal smooth muscle responses has been studied extensively. The anatomic substrate for cell-to-cell communication in the corpora and many other tissues is provided by gap junctions, which are aqueous intercellular channels that transverse the extracellular space to provide a conduit for partial cytoplasmic continuity between adjacent cells [21]. Gap junctions serve manifold functional roles in diverse vascular tissues, including corpus cavernosum, with connexin 43 being the predominant gap-junction protein present between human corpus cavernosum smooth muscle cells. More recently, computer modeling studies have evaluated the boundary conditions for and the physiologic relevance of junctional communication to the modulation of corporal smooth muscle activity [22].

Adrenergic nerves release norepinephrine that, through alpha-1 adrenergic receptors, causes contraction of trabecular smooth muscle [2]. Alpha-1A and alpha-1C are the alpha-1 receptor subtypes that are most abundantly expressed in this muscle [23]. Adrenergic nerves are thought to have a crucial role in the return of the erect penis to the flaccid state. The involvement of the adrenergic neuroeffector system in maintaining the state of flaccidity is not clear. Endothelin [24] and constrictor prostanoids [9] that are synthesized by the endothelium and possibly by the muscle itself may provide the sustained smooth muscle tone that is necessary to maintain penile flaccidity.

PHYSIOLOGY OF CORPORAL VENO-OCCLUSION

Recent animal and human studies have demonstrated that the tone of the trabecular smooth muscle regulates the venous-outflow resistance in the corpora [6]. When the trabecular smooth muscle was contracted in the animal model by adrenergic agonists, venous-outflow resistance was 50 to 200 times lower than the venous-outflow resistance recorded with the trabecular smooth muscle relaxed. Low resistance to venous outflow in the presence of contracted trabecular smooth muscle is theorized to permit the easy evacuation of the corporal bodies and probably contributes to some degree to the maintenance of penile flaccidity. The tone of the trabecular smooth muscle also was found to regulate the relationship of venous-outflow resistance and intracavernosal pressure. When the trabecular smooth muscle was under high tone (contracted), outflow resistance appeared dependent on intracavernosal pressure only.

In the presence of complete trabecular smooth muscle relaxation, venous-outflow resistance appeared constant and independent of intracavernosal pressure [6]. The low venous outflow from the corpora cavernosa following smooth muscle relaxation suggested that the inflow rate to the lacunar spaces determined the rate of filling of the corporal bodies and that a relatively small inflow rate was required to maintain penile erection. Thus, arterial perfusion pressure rather than arterial inflow appeared to govern penile rigidity under physiologic conditions. When the trabecular smooth muscle was fully relaxed, the intracavernosal pressure was dependent on several factors, including (1) the cavernosal arterial perfusion pressure, (2) the tissue properties of the relaxed smooth muscle fibers, and (3) the tissue properties of the fibroelastic elements in the trabeculae and the tunica albuginea.

Soft tissue typically displays nonlinear elastic properties. In the animal model, low intracavernosal pressure values of 30–60 mm Hg, which distort the tissue in its linear range, were associated with the erectile-tissue stiffness being relatively minimal and the capacitance (compliance) values maximally elevated [6]. As intracavernosal pressures increased, there was a decrease in capacitance. Because capacitance is inversely proportional to tissue stiffness, that may reflect the progressive stiffness of the tissue with increasing intracavernosal pressures. When the stiffness limit for the fibroelastic elements is reached, any increases in corpora cavernosa volume, associated with an increase in the length of the fibroelastic elements, requires progressively more force.

In summary, the role of the two constituents of the trabeculae, the trabecular smooth muscle and the fibroelastic frame, differ in their contributions to overall corporal veno-occlusive function. The contribution of the trabecular smooth muscle is variable and dependent on neurogenic and endothelium-dependent mechanisms that induce relaxation or contraction. The contribution of the fibroelastic frame is fixed and dependent on intrinsic structural characteristics.

THE TRABECULAR SMOOTH MUSCLE CELL AND EXTRACELLULAR MATRIX SYNTHESIS

The major role of vascular smooth muscle is to maintain tone in the vessels. Smooth muscle cells also have been reported to have synthetic capabilities; they are able to synthesize the connective tissue immediately surrounding them [25]. Pulmonary-artery smooth muscle cells have been demonstrated to synthesize both a 1(I) procollagen mRNA and type I collagen [26]. It has been suggested by Pease [27] that smooth muscle cells are the predominant cell type of the medial layer of muscular arteries. Smooth muscle cells may change phenotype from a contractile to a synthetic state, performing both roles as a multifunctional mesenchyme [28,29]. In the normal corpora cavernosa, the trabecular smooth muscle is the major mesenchymal cell type. These cells have been shown to synthesize extracellular matrix (collagen and other proteins) surrounding the individual smooth muscle cells and thus provide the structural integrity of the corpora. The normal processes of remodeling and deposition of that extracellular matrix as well as the events leading to excess matrix accumulation are virtually unknown in this tissue.

Cytokines and growth factors are thought to play key roles in the regulation of synthesis and the assembly of connective tissue proteins [28–36]. Transforming growth factor-beta 1 (TGF-β1) is a pleotrophic cytokine that induces extracellular matrix expression and inhibits growth of vascular smooth muscle cells [37,38], the two main phenotypic changes observed in corpus cavernosum fibrosis. TGF-β1 alters the composition of extracellular matrix by inducing expression of collagens, fibronectin, and proteoglycans, while inhibiting the activity and expression of collagenases and other proteases. That results in a net collagen accumulation in the extracellular matrix. In studies on pulmonary, hepatic, and renal fibrosis, severity of disease was correlated with increased expression of TGF-β1 [32,39,40]. In the vasculature, increased expression of TGF-β1 has been correlated with diffuse intimal thickenings in human coronary arteries and human restenosis lesions. Recent studies are available showing that this cytokine plays a role in extracellular matrix deposition in human corpus cavernosum [41]. In addition, in-situ hybridization studies in human corpora cavernosa, using two markers of connective-tissue synthesis, a 1(I) procollagen and fibronectin, have revealed increased sites of mRNA synthesis, with some occuring in recognizable trabecular smooth muscle cells [28,29].

It is thus hypothesized that increased collagen synthesis by the trabecular smooth muscle cell is the result of phenotypic changes from the contractile to the synthetic state. That would represent an accelerated endpoint of the trabecular smooth muscle cell change similarly found in other patients with vasculogenic impotence. A better understanding of the life cycle and molecular biology of the trabecular smooth muscle cell is key to an understanding of the disorder of vasculogenic impotence.

Pathophysiology of Vasculogenic Impotence

CAVERNOSAL-ARTERY INSUFFICIENCY

Cavernosal-artery insufficiency, either atherosclerotic or traumatic in origin, can (1) diminish the cavernosal arterial inflow to the lacunar spaces and (2) decrease the perfusion pressure in the cavernosal artery. The clinical consequences of the hemodynamic changes are (1) prolonged time to maximum erection and (2) lowered rigidity of the erect penis [42,43].

Atherosclerotic vascular disease is the most common cause of cavernosal-artery insufficiency. This vascular disease induces diffuse hemodynamic lesions in the hypogastric-cavernous arterial bed and is associated with adverse affects in the corporal smooth muscle, lacunar-space endothelium, and corporal microvasculature [43–45]. It has been found that erectile dysfunction develops when arterial occlusive disease occludes more than 50 percent of the luminal diameter of the arterial supply to the penis [43]. The risk factors for atherosclerotic disease include hypertension, hypercholesterolemia, cigarette smoking, diabetes, and heart disease. The main cause of cavernosal-artery insufficiency in young patients without vascular risk factors is arterial disease associated with blunt trauma [46,47]. Blunt pelvic, perineal, and penile trauma have characteristic patterns of arteriographically demonstrated occlusive disease in the distal hypogastric-cavernous arterial bed consistent with the site of the traumatic injury [46].

BLUNT TRAUMA–INDUCED ARTERIAL VASCULOPATHY

It has been documented that arterial occlusive disease can be caused by blunt trauma to specific locations within the entire arterial system [46,48]. Examples of site-specific arterial disease with their respective trauma include the occluded axillary artery from the use of crutches, the occluded brachial artery from objects striking the antecubital fossa, the occluded common femoral artery from motorcycle accidents, and the occluded superficial palmar arch from repeated use of the hand as a hammer.

Blunt Pelvic Trauma. Blunt pelvic trauma from pelvic fractures or crush injuries has been associated with a 23- to 80-percent incidence of impotence [49–52]. Levine et al. reviewed the findings of selective internal pudendal arteriograms in a group of impotent patients in which 7 had blunt pelvic trauma and 20 had blunt perineal trauma [46]. Those with impotence immediately following blunt pelvic trauma were found to have significantly different patterns of arteriographically demonstrated occlusive disease from those of patients who incurred blunt perineal trauma. In the 7 with pelvic injury, there was a higher incidence (92%) of arterial lesions in the distal internal pudendal or common penile artery than in the 20 patients with blunt perineal trauma (35%).

The mechanisms of arterial injuries in the distal hypogastric-cavernous arterial bed after pelvic fractures have been proposed to be the same as those described for urethral injuries following similar trauma. The most common mechanism for urethral injury [49,50] is an upward displacement of the symphysis, causing rupture of the puboprostatic ligaments stretching the urethra to the point of its rupture from the urogenital diaphragm. Such stretching in the area of the urogenital diaphragm could also lead to damage of the arteries that pierce and lie within it, that is, the common penile, cavernosal, and dorsal arteries. A second mechanism of urethral injury involves bilateral fractures of the superior and inferior pubic rami with posteroinferior displacement of the fractured segment. That causes a sudden retrocession of the urogenital diaphragm against the membraneous urethra, with the diaphragm acting as a guillotine and severing the urethra. The same guillotine action also could sever the arteries that pierce the urogenital diaphragm. A third mechanism of urethral injury, diastasis of the symphysis with rupture of one puboprostatic ligament, causes the urogenital diaphragm to be torn from its attachment to the contralateral pubic bone. That causes a shearing effect on the urethra as the urogenital diaphragm is pulled in the opposite direction. The shearing also could injure those arteries piercing the urogenital diaphragm. Finally, direct injury from a bony spicule may directly injure the urethra as well as an artery in close proximity. The internal pudendal and penile arteries lie in close apposition to the ischial and pubic rami.

Blunt Perineal Trauma. Blunt perineal trauma also can cause arteriogenic impotence, such as in cases of straddle injuries and kicks to or falls on the perineum [53,54]. Using penile Doppler ultrasonography, Kerstein [54] reported that 20 potent men, after sitting on an unpadded bicycle seat for 5 minutes, exhibited a decrease of normal penile blood pressure values to levels consistent with arterial vasculogenic impotence. In a case of impotence following perineal trauma in a basketball game, St. Louis [53] documented arterial injuries consisting of bilateral total occlusion of the cavernosal and dorsal penile arteries. In Levine's study [46], the incidence of a solitary arterial lesion in the cavernosal artery, without any proximal disease in the hypogastric-cavernous arterial bed, was found to be significantly higher in patients with blunt perineal trauma (48%) than in patients with blunt pelvic trauma (8%), thus confirming that the arteriographic locations were related to the site of the blunt trauma.

The mechanism of the arterial injury after blunt perineal trauma can be explained by anatomical considerations. The common penile artery lies medial to the inferior pubic ramus and bifurcates into the cavernosal and dorsal arteries just below the pubic symphysis. With such anatomical position, the arteries may be crushed between the object and the pubic bones. Such trauma has been reported to devitalize or sever the urethra. Proximal arterial occlusive pathology in the internal pudendal artery is infrequent, because the more proximal internal pudendal artery would be protected from blunt perineal injury by virtue of its position superiorly and laterally in Alcock's canal. Urethral injuries in impotent patients after perineal trauma usually are not present, which may be explained by the fact that a blunt perineal injury of lesser severity may result in arterial rather than urethral injury. Arterial injury can result more readily since the mechanism of arterial occlusive pathology depends on endothelial damage and not on a severing of the artery. Alternatively, the main force of the blunt perineal trauma may be directed in a location more specifically related to the ischiopubic ramus and lateral to the urethra, thus causing arterial but avoiding urethral injury. It is also possible that other mechanisms interplay in blunt perineal trauma. The distal common penile and cavernosal arteries are both smaller and in closer proximity to the ischiopubic ramus, the rigid bony structure, than the proximal urethra. Such factors may allow clinically relevant arterial injury to occur independent of urethral injury.

Blunt Trauma and Delayed Impotence. Is blunt perineal trauma a risk factor for arteriogenic impotence? The pattern of arterial injury in patients who had previous perineal trauma and delayed impotence was reported to be similar to the pattern seen in patients with perineal trauma and immediate impotence. Such observation may indicate that blunt perineal trauma, even if it does not result in immediate arterial occlusion, may still hasten its occurrence. The mechanism of such delayed arterial occlusive pathology is hypothesized to be intimal smooth muscle hyperplasia combined with fibrin, elastin, and lipid deposition secondary to increased endothelial and intimal permeability [55]. It may, therefore, be hypothesized that at the time of perineal trauma there is an injury to the artery not severe enough to cause an immediate arterial occlusion. The injury, however, may itself or in combination with other vascular risk factors progress to plaque formation, leading to an arteriographically demonstrated occlusion. Patterns of arterial injury after perineal trauma and immediate impotence were also similar to the patterns of patients with no obvious perineal trauma and no vascular risk factors [55]. Such an observation may suggest that those men had perineal trauma in the past, perhaps during childhood, but it was not remembered. Bicycle accidents, falls or kicks to the perineum, or possibly several lesser incidents of repeated perineal trauma conceivably could have caused arterial endothelial damage to the hypogastric-cavernous beds and could be a factor in inducing arterial occlusive lesions in such patients with idiopathic impotence.

Blunt Penile Trauma. The penis is also vulnerable to blunt injury in the erect state [56–60]. High pressures in the corpora cavernosa during erection play the major role in such injuries. Injury to the penis can occur during intercourse when the erect penis slips out of the vagina and is subsequently thrust against the partner's perineum or pubic bone, commonly with the partner in the superior position. Penile injury also has been reported following accidents and self-inflicted, abnormal bending of the penis during masturbation. Penson et al. [60] reported on 19 patients with a history of impotence following blunt trauma to the erect penis during intercourse, during masturbation, or after an accident. Cavernosal-artery insufficiency was found in 37 percent of the patients. A focal midshaft cavernosal-artery occlusion was demonstrated in 28 percent of the patients.

The mechanism of site-specific injury of the cavernosal arteries after blunt trauma of the erect penis is unknown. In the human penis, the internal stress during erection is borne not only by the tunica albuginea but by the intracavernous framework of fibromuscular columns that penetrate the corpora and attach to the intracavernosal vasculature [60]. Injury is hypothesized to result from short-term marked increases in intracavernosal pressures that approximate or exceed the tunica tensile strength. These supraphysiologic pressures result from the redistribution of corporal blood to nonloaded portions of the erect penile shaft. Such pressure elevations cause a spectrum of arterial injuries, including indirect trauma to the cavernosal arteries by means of a shearing action that might follow the excessive stresses on the fibrous columns, which attach to the tunica and to the intracavernosal neurovascular bundles. Such shearing action may be the consequence of the corporal circumference increase in the nonloaded portion of the penile shaft. Such a shearing action at excessive supraphysiologic pressures may result in focal bleeding, arterial occlusion, or both [60].

CORPORAL VENO-OCCLUSIVE DYSFUNCTION

Pathological alterations in the physiologic mechanisms that regulate the autonomic dilator nerves or the endothelium and the release of EDRFs can result in impaired trabecular smooth muscle relaxation [44,45]. The hemodynamic consequence of incomplete smooth muscle relaxation would be, predictively, the need for higher arterial inflow to maintain intracavernosal pressures.

Structural changes in the fibers of collagen and elastin may occur secondary to nonenzymatic glycosylation of the proteins associated with aging, diabetes mellitus, and collagen vascular diseases [2]. Such changes may result in increased tissue stiffness with reduced capacitance. An increase in stiffness of the fibroelastic frame may impede a normal corporal veno-occlusive mechanism and thus result in venous leakage impotence, or corporal veno-occlusive dysfunction [61].

The following theory concerns the pathophysiology of corporal veno-occlusive dysfunction. The corpora cavernosa consists of endothelial-lined lacunar spaces, trabecular contractile (smooth muscle), and trabecular structural (collagen/elastin) components. The lacunar-space endothelial cell may have a key role in the paracrine maintenance of normal corporal vascular homeostasis, with respect to the abluminal side in terms of vasodilation and erectile-tissue compliance as well as to the luminal side in terms of vascular thrombosis. The central hypothesis is that corporal veno-occlusive dysfunction begins with exposure to vascular insults, which subsequently induces abnormal lacunar-space endothelial-cell function. That leads to abnormal paracrine regulation of the trabecular smooth muscle tone and production of collagen/elastin, the initiation of abnormal corporal capacitor function, and ultimately to the development of clinical corporal veno-occlusive dysfunction [29].

In humans, lacunar-space endothelial cells undergo repetitive lifelong challenges in their pivotal position in the vascular wall of the corporal erectile tissue. Those endothelial cells may be exposed to hyperglycemia, hypercholesterolemia, episodes of ischemia or hypoxia especially during prolonged penile flaccidity, toxic radicals in cigarette smoke, oxygen-derived free radicals, and oxidized lipids and proteins, as well as increased physical stresses associated with systemic hypertension. Each of those vascular insults may be an important risk factor for vascular disease of the penis and the ultimate development of corporal veno-occlusive dysfunction. The cumulative success with which the lacunar-space endothelial cells respond to those challenges will determine the rate of progression of vascular disease to the point at which the clinical complication of corporal veno-occlusive dysfunction occurs. The lacunar-space endothelial cell may respond to vascular insults by elaborating short-lived vasoactive substances and platelet inhibitors and expressing proteins that may be vasoactive, thrombogenic, adhesion molecules, or growth controlling [9–11,41]. Having undergone those phenotypic changes, the lacunar-space endothelial cell may stop being entirely protective and begin to contribute to the progression of structural vascular disease in the corpora cavernosa. For instance, the endothelium in situ and in culture when exposed to hypoxia, oxygen-derived free radicals, hypertension, or hyperglycemia responds by expressing proteins such as growth factors, cytokines, permeability factors, and endothelin, which mediate increased vascular growth, permeability, abnormal compliance, and vasoconstriction. Decreased production of endothelium-derived nitric oxide [44,45] and increased production of vasoconstrictor prostanoids may contribute to the vasoconstriction and to the abnormal expression of proteins. Thus, the lacunar-space endothelial cell may undergo a myriad of phenotypic changes that are deleterious to corporal vascular function and that can lead to the complications of corporal veno-occlusive dysfunction.

In summary, veno-occlusive dysfunction can result from (1) functional inability to completely relax trabecular smooth muscle tone and (2) alterations in the fibroelastic structure, as has been described in patients with vascular risk factors. Impairment of the latter may be the consequence of arterial insufficiency and hypoxia to the lacunar endothelial cell.

Diagnosis of Vasculogenic Impotence

The evaluation of the impotent patient begins with a sexual, psychosocial, and medical history, a physical examination, and routine laboratory tests [2]. The initial evaluation will help in the determination of the disorder, particularly in the differentiation of psychogenic from organic impotence; however, the initial impressions should be corroborated by a series of examinations, including vascular testing. There is as yet no universally agreed-on diagnostic algorithm for the evaluation of all impotent patients. Furthermore, many of the tests are in evolution, and their reliability have not been fully determined.

SCREENING TESTS

Evaluation of penile arteries can be performed in the flaccid state and in the dynamic state following intracavernosal vasoactive-agent administration. In the flaccid state, the penile arteries are evaluated by determining penile-artery systolic blood pressure utilizing either a continuous-wave Doppler ultrasound probe or penile plethysmography. A shortcoming of those techniques is their inability to consistently measure blood pressure or flow in the cavernosal artery. Furthermore, testing in the flaccid state, as opposed to the dynamic state, does not address the ability of the cavernosal artery to dilate and increase blood flow [2].

The most commonly utilized test for vasculogenic impotence is an office intracavernosal injection test, in which the erectile response is observed following intracavernosal injection of vasoactive agents [62]. A normal rigid erection should develop promptly within 5–10 minutes and last approximately 1 hour or require injection with an adrenergic agonist to achieve detumescence. When such an erection develops in an impotent patient, it implies normal veno-occlusive function and a threshold value of arterial perfusion pressure. Arterial disease (as determined by a large pressure gradient between the systemic and cavernosal-artery perfusion pressures) has been reported to occur in 20 percent of patients who respond to injections with a rigid erectile response [62]. Typically, such patients develop their rigid erections more slowly. If a prompt rigid erection response occurs following intracavernosal injection, neurologic, endothelial, or psychological factors should be considered. If only a partial, short-lived, or absent erection results, then hemodynamic impairment may be suspected; however, failure to produce an erection in this setting may be due to excessive adrenergic constrictor tone secondary to anxiety. Thus, a negative result from a single injection is inconclusive. At present, there is no standardized approach as to pharmacologic agent, dose, or method of monitoring the erectile response. To reduce adverse psychological influences and to facilitate maximal smooth muscle relaxation, the intracavernosal injection test has been performed in conjunction with manual, vibratory, or audio-visual sexual stimulation. Such testing is useful as a screening procedure and provides a preliminary assessment of the responsiveness of the patient to treatment by intracavernosal self-injection of vasoactive drugs. In general, this form of testing should precede other, more invasive diagnostic techniques.

DUPLEX DOPPLER ULTRASOUND

Because there are shortcomings with the screening tests for vasculogenic impotence, methodologies such as duplex Doppler ultrasound have been developed. In 1985, Lue [63] introduced duplex ultrasonography, the combination of high-frequency, high-resolution ultrasonography with quantitative pulsed Doppler spectrum analysis for the improved evaluation of vasculogenic impotence. Duplex ultrasonography was developed to be utilized in conjunction with intracavernosal vasoactive-agent administration, similar to the office injection test. In addition, duplex Doppler ultrasonography had the capability of assessing changes in the cavernosal-artery diameter and in blood velocity. Refined by numerous investigators [64], pulsed duplex ultrasonography is currently an important initial, minimally invasive means of (1) improving the diagnostic yield of injection testing, (2) documenting the dynamic changes of blood velocity in the cavernosal arteries during pharmacologic erection, and (3) providing a preliminary assessment of responsiveness to intracavernosal self-injection of vasoactive-drug treatment.

Cavernosal-arterial pulsations are visualized on real-time imaging, and good symmetrical pulsations should be observed. The presence of thickened cavernosal arterial walls or little change in the cavernosal-artery diameter following injection of vasoactive agents may suggest arterial disease. Benson and Vickers [65] reported that the response of the cavernosal arteries to papaverine was not an accurate measure of arterial function and stated that cavernosal-artery peak systolic velocity is the best indicator of arterial function. They further suggested that the diagnosis of arterial dysfunction is suggested by a combination of clinical observations of the erectile quality and ultrasonographic findings of cavernosal-artery peak systolic velocity. Other reviews have shown that the cavernosal-artery peak systolic velocity is a better parameter to evaluate arterial function than cavernosal-arterial diameter changes alone. Schwartz et al. [66] studied normal male volunteers with duplex cavernosography following injection of intracavernosal vasoactive agents and reported a cavernosal-artery peak systolic velocity of 30–40 cm/second. Lue, when subjectively grading the erectile response, stated that patients with moderate to good responses to vasoactive agents had a cavernosal-artery peak systolic velocity of more than 25 cm/second, while none of the patients with a poor erectile response had a peak systolic velocity greater than 25 cm/second [67]. Similarly, Benson and Vickers [65] subdivided patients into three groups based on their cavernosal-artery peak systolic velocity. Patients with a cavernosal-artery peak systolic velocity greater than 47 cm/second were normal. The group with average peak systolic velocities of 35 cm/second had mild to moderate arterial dysfunction. Those with an average cavernosal-artery peak systolic velocity of 7 cm/second had severe arterial disease.

Several studies have evaluated impotent patients with

pelvic arteriography and duplex ultrasonography. Quam et al. [68] examined 12 impotent patients with suspected arterial disease by pelvic arteriography and duplex ultrasonography. They found that in all patients with demonstrable arteriographic disease (5 of the 12), the cavernosal-artery peak systolic velocity was less than 25 cm/second. Rajfer et al. [69] reported that the critical value of cavernosal-artery peak systolic velocity greater than 30 cm/second was an index of normal arterial function. Their studies yielded an 83-percent sensitivity of detecting arterial stenoses compared to pelvic angiography. To obtain a higher yield of sensitivity in detecting cavernosal-arterial disease, those authors recommended simultaneously recording cavernosal-artery-diameter changes. A 75-percent increase in the arterial diameter was considered an index of normal arterial compliance, along with a cavernosal-artery peak systolic velocity greater than 30 cm/second. Valji et al. [70], in their review of 30 patients, challenged the validity of a cavernosal-artery peak systolic velocity greater than 25 cm/second. They found that more than 50 percent of the patients diagnosed by arteriography to have significant arterial disease had a cavernosal-artery peak systolic velocity greater than 25 cm/second.

Additional indices may increase the sensitivity of detecting arterial disease. Cavernosal-artery accleration values are defined by the peak velocity over the pulse rise time (centimeters per second squared). In a study of 30 patients, cavernosal-artery accleration values were found to be more sensitive predictors of arterial insufficiency than cavernosal-artery peak systolic velocity alone [70]. In a study evaluating carotid-arterial insufficiency, a slower rate of rise of the transmitted pulse pressure revealed lower accleration values in patients with proximal carotid arterial disease. Other authors have noted that similar results of accleration values are able to define a more accurate correlation with results of arteriography than with cavernosal-artery peak systolic velocity values alone [69].

Since the volume of blood inflow is related to both vessel diameter and flow velocity, it is probable that reliance on a single variable, such as cavernosal-artery peak systolic velocity value, may not detect arterial disease in all patients. It is likely that multiple factors, such as the spectral waveform pattern, changes in the slope of flow velocities, changes in vessel diameter (compliance), and the quality of erectile response under conditions of smooth muscle relaxation, will provide the best hemodynamic information. Currently, normal arterial function is indicated by the indices of cavernosal-artery peak systolic velocity greater than 30 cm/second, an increase in the vessel diameter greater than 75 percent, and a normal spectral waveform. Arteriogenic dysfunction is diagnosed by the indices of cavernosal-artery peak systolic velocity less than 25 cm/second, poor arterial compliance, and poor progression of peak systolic velocities on the spectral waveform.

The duplex Doppler ultrasound can be utilized to gain an insight into the integrity of corporal veno-occlusive function. Physiologically, veno-occlusion and venous-outflow resistance are the result of subtunical venule luminal narrowing from elongation and compression during erection. In normal veno-occlusion, following complete trabecular smooth muscle relaxation, the outflow from the corporal bodies is minimal and has been recorded as 3–5 ml/min [2]. Under such conditions, the corpora are virtual closed spaces that allow for only arterial inflow during cardiac systole. Thus, the duplex ultrasound study during normal corporal veno-occlusion should reveal absent end-diastolic velocity. Suspicion of veno-occlusive dysfunction arises when there is evidence of end-diastolic velocity values after complete trabecular smooth muscle relaxation has occurred. While hemodynamic conditions of complete trabecular smooth muscle relaxation have been defined during pharmacocavernosometry, such conditions have not yet been defined during duplex Doppler ultrasonography. Until methodology is available to define the condition of complete trabecular smooth muscle relaxation during duplex ultrasonography, redosing with pharmacologic agents is an attractive and practical alternative. The accurate diagnosis of veno-occlusive dysfunction remains difficult with duplex Doppler ultrasonography.

DYNAMIC-INFUSION PHARMACOCAVERNOSOMETRY AND PHARMACOCAVERNOSOGRAPHY

To clinically test for corporal veno-occlusive function, the study must be able to discriminate between the structural and the functional components of corporal veno-occlusion. To date, that is possible only during dynamic-infusion pharmacocavernosometry.

Saenz de Tejada et al. [6] studied the flow-to-maintain and venous-outflow responses during pharmacocavernosometry in an animal model in the completely relaxed state (no added Ca^{2+}-papaverine combination) and in the fully contracted state (high K^{+}-norepinephrine combination). They found that in the presence of trabecular smooth muscle contraction, flow-to-maintain values were of a high magnitude and were nonlinear in their relation to intracavernosal pressures. Venous-outflow resistances, on the other hand, were of low magnitude and were nonconstant in their relation to pressure. In the presence of trabecular smooth muscle relaxation, however, flow-to-maintain values were found to be of low magnitude and were linear with intracavernosal pressures, while venous-outflow resistances were of high magnitude and were constant over the range of pressures studied.

Experience with the in-vitro isolated corporal animal model demonstrated that completely contracted trabecular smooth muscle could be reversibly induced to undergo complete trabecular smooth muscle relaxation by a relaxing infusion solution. In similar fashion, patients who demonstrated a nonlinear flow-pressure relation and variable venous-outflow resistance (consistent with incomplete trabecular smooth muscle relaxation) were found to convert to linear flow-pressure relations and constant venous-outflow resistance (consistent with complete trabecular smooth muscle relaxation) by using cumulative doses of vasodilatators. In a recent study of that methodology, a single dose of vasoactive-agent administration resulted in linear flow-pressure relations consistent with complete smooth muscle relaxation in only 17 percent of patients [71]. That finding underscored the high risks of invalid interpretation of hemodynamic events associated with single-dose testing, the technique most often utilized by practitioners. Such clinicians often have relied on the use of concomitant supplementary vibratory, visual, or manual sexual stimulation to aid in the development of trabecular smooth muscle relaxation. Multiple redosing with vasoactive agents, however, independent of supplementary erotic stimulation, successfully relaxed the trabecular smooth muscle in 91 percent of the cases.

Using the above research findings, a modified four-phase pharmacocavernosometry procedure has been proposed. Following intracavernosal administration of vasoactive agents, multiple parameters are documented in phase 1: penile circumference, penile length, the steady-state intracavernosal equilibrium pressure achieved, the buckling pressure (weight in kilograms applied axially to the erect penis that induces penile-shaft deformation) achieved, and the time to achieve the steady-state equilibrium pressure. Organic vascular pathology is suspected when, under conditions of complete smooth muscle relaxation, the intracavernosal pressure response is lower than the mean systemic arterial blood pressure [2,70].

The second phase assesses (1) the trabecular smooth muscle status and (2) the corporal veno-occlusive function by determining flow-to-maintain values at different intracavernosal pressures, typically chosen as 30, 60, 90, 120, and 150 mm Hg and by calculating the venous-outflow resistance values. A linear relation between flow-to-maintain values and intracavernosal pressure values and constant venous-outflow resistance implies the achievement of complete trabecular smooth muscle relaxation. If a nonlinear flow-pressure relation and variable venous-outflow resistance are found, the study should be repeated with additional doses of vasoactive agents, because that pattern is characteristic of inadequate trabecular smooth muscle relaxation. Under conditions consistent with complete trabecular smooth muscle relaxation, normal veno-occlusion is consistent with flow-to-maintain values of 3 ml/min or less.

Corporal veno-occlusive function also may be studied by determining the capacitor function or energy-storage capability of the erectile chambers. Capacitor function is estimated by recording intracavernosal pressure decay over time following termination of the infusion from suprasystolic intracavernosal pressure. In clinical assessment, the intracavernosal pressure decay may be recorded from a suprasystolic pressure of 150 mm Hg over a 30-second period. Normal corporal veno-occlusive function has been found associated with an intracavernosal pressure decay of less than 45 mm Hg in a period of 30 seconds. This test, performed after achieving complete trabecular smooth muscle relaxation, confirms the previous assessment of corporal veno-occlusive function. While flow-to-maintain tests record venous-outflow resistance, pressure-decay testing reflects both corporal capacitance and venous-outflow resistance.

Phase 3 of the pharmacocavernosometry procedure involves determination of cavernosal-artery perfusion pressure in the dynamic state. That determination is obtained by recording the intracavernosal pressure and simultaneously monitoring the pulsatile flow of the cavernosal artery utilizing a continuous-wave Doppler ultrasound probe. The intracavernosal pressure is raised by infusion of heparinized saline until the cavernosal-artery Doppler signal disappears. When saline infusion is terminated, the intracavernosal pressure will diminish below the cavernosal-artery systolic pressure with the resultant reappearance of cavernosal-artery pulsatile flow. The intracavernosal pressure at which cavernosal-artery pulsations return is defined as the effective cavernosal-artery systolic pressure, implying the maximal arterial pressure that can be delivered to the lacunar space during erection. The brachial-artery systolic pressure is simultaneously recorded, and a normal study exists when the two pressures are similar. A gradient between the cavernosal and brachial arteries of less than 35 mm Hg has been defined as normal, based on individuals with normal intracavernosal pressure responses to intracavernosal pharmacologic agents as controls. In one study, the sensitivity of cavernosal-artery systolic occlusion pressure was 77 percent in predicting arterial occlusive disease as diagnosed by arteriography. Since the test records perfusion pressure, it is the only test that can predict the maximum intracavernosal pressure obtained in a penile erection at equilibrium. Cavernosal-artery systolic occlusion pressures can be monitored on a multichannel recorder, in which heparinized saline flow, intracavernosal pressure, systemic blood pressure, and continuous-wave Doppler ultrasound of the cavernosal artery can be displayed simultaneously. The study is, however, usually performed during a simultaneous evaluation of corporal veno-occlusive function and, as such, requires indwelling intracavernosal needles. It is, therefore, more invasive than pulsed Doppler ultrasonography. Since the test records cavernosal-artery perfusion pressure, it is less subject to the adverse effects of dynamic studies, that is, the corporal smooth muscle vasoconstrictive effects of anxiety.

In phase 4, pharmacocavernosography is performed at a steady-state intracavernosal pressure of 90 mm Hg to confirm the findings of pharmacocavernosometry and to provide anatomical information of corporal veno-occlusive dysfunction. Phase 4 need not be performed, at the discretion of the physician, if indices of corporal veno-occlusive function are normal.

Those impotent patients who are consistently unable to achieve rigid sustained erections, who undergo pharmacocavernosometry under conditions of complete smooth muscle relaxation, and who (1) demonstrate an abnormal value of steady-state-equilibrium intracavernosal pressure, (2) abnormal flow-to-maintain various intracavernosal pressures, and (3) abnormal pressure-decay studies and an abnormal pharmacocavernosogram revealing visualization of veins draining the corporal bodies have corporal veno-occlusive dysfunction. Those patients who also have (1) a site-specific location of the abnormal drainage or, by corollary, do not have multiple sites of abnormal drainage on pharmacocavernosography, especially involving the corpus spongiosum, and (2) no evidence of arterial insufficiency are potential candidates for surgery for correction of corporal veno-occlusive dysfunction.

OTHER TESTS

Selective internal pudendal pharmacoarteriography usually is reserved for those patients being considered for arterial reconstructive surgery [2,42,46,47,52,60,69,70]. The study is performed under local anesthesia and intravenous sedation. Intracavernosal and intra-arterial vasoactive agents allow for optimal visualization of the penile arterial tree in the dynamic state. The study is expensive and has potential complications, including bleeding, thrombosis, or aneurysm formation of the femoral artery, as well as embolism of the distal peripheral arteries. Because the arteriogram is an anatomical study, its interpretation must be corroborated with the results of other erectile function studies of arterial integrity. Selective internal pudendal arteriography also may be utilized to diagnose and subsequently treat, via embolization, patients suspected of arterial priapism.

Newer studies of cavernosal-artery perfusion have been performed. Intracavernosal-arterial blood flow can be said to "percolate" through the lacunar spaces, in much the same fashion that blood flow traverses the placenta. It is for that reason that arteriographic studies, which require laminar flow for visualization, rarely record flow through the lacunar spaces. Nuclear magnetic resonance (NMR), using gadolinium diethylene triamine penta-acetic acid (DTPA) as the contrast medium, has the ability to enhance the proton density of such specialized vascular regions. In dynamic NMR with gadolinium-DTPA, a time-related enhancement of the corpora cavernosa and corpus spongiosum can be achieved. Such studies have the capability of observing blood flow through the erectile tissue. Preliminary studies with time-enhancement dynamic-NMR studies in normal penile erections have demonstrated a homogeneous distribution pattern requiring several minutes to fill the entire corporal chamber [72]. In atherosclerotic occlusive disease, a patchy distribution of contrast is seen, suggesting the possibility of multiple localized regions of arteriolar disease. Dynamic NMR has an obvious potential use as a measure of cavernosal-artery perfusion to determine the efficacy of vascular reconstructive surgery.

Another new study for arterial perfusion of the erectile tissue measures the intracavernosal blood oxygen partial pressure (Po_2) level following pharmacologic stimulation. In one study [73], the mean cavernosal blood Po_2 determinations at 0, 1, 5, 10, and 15 minutes following intracavernosal vasoactive-agent administration were 36.2, 88.0, 92.7, 97.3, and 95.5 mm Hg, respectively, in eight potent control patients. In contrast, in 19 patients with arteriogenic impotence, the mean Po_2 values at similar times were 30.5, 72.2, 77.2, 79.8, and 80.5 mm Hg, respectively. Statistical significance was obtained at the 1-, 5-, 10-, and 15-minute measurements. This technique of determining cavernous Po_2 levels in response to vasoactive medications may have ultimate use in documenting the functional existence of arteriogenic impotence as well as postoperative changes in cavernosal tissue perfusion following vascular reconstructive procedures.

Treatment for Vasculogenic Impotence

Therapeutic options available for the treatment of erectile dysfunction will be discussed under two broad categories: conservative, nonsurgical treatments and surgical. Conservative, nonsurgical treatments include psychologic therapy, noninjection pharmacologic (oral, intraurethral, sublingual, and topical agents), penile self-injection therapy, and vacuum erection devices. Surgical therapies include surgical procedures directed toward the amelioration of arterial insufficiency and corporal veno-occlusive dysfunction and the implantation of penile prostheses.

CONSERVATIVE, NONSURGICAL TREATMENT OPTIONS

Psychologic Therapy. The role of the psychotherapist in treating impotent patients is not confined to psychogenic impotence. Impotent men receiving medical or surgical treatment for vasculogenic impotence should, if necessary, receive psychological counseling before and after such treatments to reduce anxiety, sexual inhibition, and relationship conflict. The goals of sex therapy are primarily to decrease performance anxiety that may interfere with erectile development and to promote an adequate level of stimulation by increasing the repertoire of sexual activities that do not depend on achieving or maintaining an erection sufficient for intercourse [74]. When repeated attempts at coitus fail, men become anxious, preoccupied with fears of failure, and apprehensive about their partner's reactions. Whenever possible, psychosexual therapy involves the sexual partners together. That approach is preferable for both evaluation and treatment. One component of therapy is sensate-focus exercises, which are designed to progressively and slowly return potency and decrease anxiety and guilt by the couple's mutual enjoyment of noncoital activity. When erectile function returns, the couple continue the exercises until coitus is possible [74].

Noninjection Pharmacologic Agents. The most widely used oral medication has been yohimbine hydrochloride, an alpha-2 adrenergic blocking agent [75,76]. A new medication, delequamine hydrochloride, is an alpha-2 adrenoceptor antagonist 100 times more selective than yohimbine. The central mechanism of action of such agents is postulated to increase the level of norepinephrine. The presynaptic alpha-2 receptor on adrenergic sympathetic nerves normally is activated by norepinephrine release, which acts to reduce norepinephrine release in a negative feedback system. Blockade of the alpha-2 receptor is associated with increased release of norepinephrine and increased sexual activity in animals and, in recent preliminary studies, in humans. The peripheral mechanisms of action of such agents may involve the pressor effect of increased norepinephrine release and the increased release of nitric oxide from the helicine arterioles. Large clinical trials with delequamine in impotent men are underway. Clinical trials with yohimbine were performed approximately 10 years ago [75,76]. In a prospective double-blind placebo-controlled study in patients with predominantly organic disease, yohimbine did not show a statistically significant response rate over placebo control, although 21 percent of patients did receive a complete response when given yohimbine. A similarly designed study performed in patients with psychogenic impotence demonstrated that yohimbine provided a statistically significant response rate (31%) over the placebo control (5.3%).

Dopaminergic and serotonergic agonists have been utilized [77]. The positive erectile effect of dopaminergic agonists were first noted in patients treated with L-dopa. In addition, subcutaneously administered apomorphine, a dopaminergic agonist, has been shown to enhance erectile responses in humans. Laboratory investigations in rats and monkeys have corroborated that observation. A recent study [78] has shown that a dopaminergic compound that mimics the action of apomorphine and lengthens the duration of clinical response (methylenedioxy-n-propyl-norapophrine) was found to induce penile erections when given orally in the rat model. Studies are underway to use apomorphine sublingually to avoid the nausea associated with oral use.

Trazadone, a drug used clinically for depression, has been reported to be associated with priapism [79]. Meta-chlorophenylpiperazine (MCPP), a serotonergic agonist and metabolite of trazadone has been shown to induce erections in rats and monkeys [80]. A recent case report showing the beneficial qualities of trazadone in the treatment of organic erectile dysfunction has been published [81]. A recent study [82] in which six potent subjects were treated with oral trazadone, trimiprimine (a tricyclic antidepressant), and placebo demonstrated a statistically significant increase in nocturnal erectile activity with trazadone compared to the other two agents. In-vitro studies suggest that the potential mechanism for prolonging erectile activity is blockade of sympathetic-mediated detumescence.

Nitroglycerin, a smooth muscle relaxant, has been used widely in paste form for transcutaneous delivery in the treatment of angina. It also has been used in a similar manner for the treatment of impotence [83]. In a study of 30 patients, 1 cm of nitroglycerin paste or of placebo paste was placed on the penis, and patients then were shown visual sexual stimulation [84]. It was found that the group receiving nitroglycerin paste developed erections of better quality than those receiving placebo paste. That study obviously is limited and was performed in a clinical laboratory.

Penile Self-Injection Therapy. One of the most important advances in the treatment of impotence over the past decade has been the self-administered intracavernosal injection of various vasoactive agents. These vasoactive agents have been administered by intracavernosal injection either to directly relax the corporal smooth musculature or to block adrenergic tone and thus produce an erection.

The pioneering work in this area involved the use of papaverine hydrochloride [85], a direct smooth muscle relaxant, and phenoxybenzamine [86] or phentolamine mesylate [87], both alpha blocking agents. Use of these agents has become more clinically widespread. Papaverine alone was found not as effective as the combination of papaverine and phentolamine when injected together. Several years later, the synthetic prostanoid prostaglandin E_1 [88], a direct smooth muscle relaxant, was used successfully when injected intracavernosally to restore potency. A variety of solutions containing the above agents are currently being used in clinical practice: papaverine alone, papaverine and phentolamine, prostaglandin E_1 alone, phentolamine and prostaglandin E_1, or a mixture of all three agents. The mechanism of action of papaverine hydrochloride and prostaglandin E_1 is direct smooth muscle relaxation. Therefore, when injected intracavernosally, they will maximize arterial inflow as well as corporal veno-occlusion by relaxation of both arterial and trabecular smooth musculature, respectively. Phentolamine, on the other hand, blocks adrenergically induced muscle tone and therefore does not alone initiate erections.

Pharmaceutic industry-sponsored multi-institutional, placebo-controlled, double-blind studies have been performed in impotent men with the use of alprostadil sterile powder (Caverject). This new formulation of prostaglandin E_1 consists of 20 μg lyophilized alprostadil, 193.8 mg lactose, and 0.053 mg sodium citrate. It is expected that this investigational drug will be FDA approved for the treatment of erectile dysfunction in 1995. Satisfactory sexual activity was reported by patients and their partners after 87 percent and 86 percent of injections, respectively.

Impotent patients with vasculogenic dysfunction secondary to arterial insufficiency may respond by virtue of the long-acting nature of the pharmacologically induced smooth muscle relaxation that is being provided. Impotent patients with vasculogenic dysfunction secondary to significant corporal veno-occlusive dysfunction, however, would be the least likely to respond to this form of therapy. Those with poor manual dexterity, poor visual acuity, or morbid obesity or those in whom a transient hypotensive episode may have a deleterious effect (e.g., unstable cardiovascular disease and transient ischemic attacks) should be considered carefully prior to being offered this therapeutic option. Patients with significant psychiatric disease or potential for misuse or abuse of the therapy should be excluded from treatment. Once offered intracavernosal pharmacotherapy, the patient should be informed of its risks and complications. This form of therapy usually will not affect orgasm or ejaculation and is solely used for restoration of erectile capabilities. The usual therapeutic goal is to be able to create a rigid enough erection satisfactory for vaginal penetration that lasts between 30 minutes and 1 hour.

Reported side effects with penile self-injection therapy have included hematomas, burning pain after injection, urethral damage, cavernositis or local infections, fibrotic changes of the corpora cavernosa, curvature, and prolonged erections, or priapism. Cavernositis or infection due to injections has been an extremely rare event. Burning pain at the time of injection has been seen most commonly with prostaglandin E_1 and appears to be less of a problem when prostaglandin E_1 is mixed with other agents. Hematomas were noted in a small percentage of patients undergoing autoinjection therapy and usually resolve within a few days without any permanent sequelae.

The two most important complications are prolonged erections and localized fibrotic changes of the corpora cavernosum. Prolonged erections usually are encountered during the dosage-determination phase and have been reported in 2.3 to 15.0 percent of patients treated. Patients must be cautioned to call their physician if an erection persists for 4 hours or longer. Although the majority of these prolonged erections will detumesce on their own, some will require an intracavernosal injection of an alpha agonist to produce detumescence. Alpha agonists that have been used for that purpose include epinephrine, phenylephrine, and metaraminol. An initial intracavernosal injection of 200 μg of phenylephrine is the most commonly utilized and may be repeated as necessary until detumescence. Following the dosage-determination phase, the complication of prolonged erection is quite rare and is seen in less than 1 percent of injections. If treated by the protocol presented above, there should not be any permanent sequelae from this side effect.

Vacuum Constriction Devices. A variety of external penile appliances have been used for the management of vasculogenic impotence for many years [89,90]. Although many different devices are now manufactured, the majority have three common components: a vacuum chamber, a vacuum pump that creates negative pressure in the chamber, and a constrictor or tension band that is applied to the base of the penis after erection is achieved. The impotent patient, while standing, places his penis in a preformed, suitably sized chamber that is attached to a pump mechanism able to achieve negative pressure in the chamber. Prior to pump activation and creation of a vacuum, a correct airtight fit of the chamber is required. When the vacuum pump is activated, a vacuum or negative pressure is created in the chamber, thereby drawing blood into the penis to produce an erectionlike state. This usually requires 5 to 7 minutes of pump activation. At the point of achieving adequate tumescence and rigidity, a constrictor band at the base of the chamber is transferred to the base of the penis, thereby "trapping" blood in the penis.

A vacuum-induced erection is significantly different from a physiologically induced erection. The latter type is achieved by the initial relaxation of the corporal smooth musculature, thus allowing for engorgement of blood into the lacunar spaces. In a vacuum-induced erection, corporal smooth muscle relaxation does not occur initially, and blood is simply trapped in both the intra- and extracorporeal compartments of the penis. Distal to the constricting band that is placed at the base of the penis, one sees venous stasis and decreased arterial inflow, which may result in penile distension, edema, and cyanosis if the device is used for too long. In most cases, manufacturers recommend that the vacuum-induced erection be maintained for less than 30 minutes. Second, physiologically induced erection will cause rigidity along the entire length of the corpora, in contradistinction to a vacuum-induced erection, which causes rigidity only distal to the constricting band, allowing the penis to pivot at its base.

In monkeys, increases in cross-sectional corporal area secondary to vacuum-induced erections were found to be only 50 percent of cross-sectional area changes induced by intracavernosal papaverine [91]. This may be secondary to the continued smooth muscle contraction of the corpora, limiting corporal expansion. In humans, vacuum constrictive devices may induce a penile diameter equal to or greater than that attained during a physiologically induced erection, presumably secondary to blood trapped in extracorporeal tissues. In addition, cavernosography before and after application of a vacuum constrictor device demonstrated the disappearance of previously opacified glans penis, corpus spongiosum, and dorsal vein. Venous drainage from the corpora proximal to the constrictor device was not altered.

To date, the complications from the use of vacuum devices have been minor and self-limited. They have included difficulty with ejaculation, penile pain, ecchymoses, hematomas, and petechiae. Patients taking aspirin or coumadin are more likely to develop vascular complications. Many of the devices manufactured have a valve that limits the vacuum pressure (less than 250 mm Hg), which might aid in decreasing the complication rate. Patient acceptance and satisfaction with vacuum constrictive devices have been reported to be 68 percent to 83 percent [89,90]. The reasons for discontinuing treatment have included premature loss of penile tumescence and rigidity, penile pain, pain during ejaculation, and inconvenience. It can be concluded that vacuum constrictive devices are a viable therapeutic option for patients with vasculogenic erectile dysfunction by virtue of their lack of significant complications and high degree of acceptance in patients who elect to use this therapy.

SURGICAL TREATMENT OPTIONS

Microvascular Arterial Bypass Surgery. The goal of penile microvascular arterial bypass surgery is similar to that of other arterial bypass procedures, that is, to provide an arterial pathway circumventing the arterial occlusive lesions. This bypass surgery aims to increase the arterial blood perfusion and inflow to the erectile tissue, thus enabling a more rigid, spontaneous penile erection [42].

Young impotent patients without vascular risk factors or other health status concerns who have arteriogenic impotence without concomitant corporal veno-occlusive dysfunction, neurologic, or endocrinologic factors should consider microvascular arterial bypass surgery as a rational treatment option. Such young patients often have a history characterized by a consistent reduction in the erectile rigidity during sexual activity. They have poorly spontaneous erections, often taking much effort and excessive time to achieve a poorly rigid erectile response. They often lose the partial erection during preparatory sexual stimulation prior to penetration or soon after penetration. They characteristically possess an ability to achieve a more rigid, long-lasting erection on awakening in the morning. Hemodynamic information is needed in those patients to obtain a more precise diagnosis of the etiology of their erectile insufficiency and thus facilitate selection of therapy. This hemodynamic information is best obtained via pharmacocavernosometry performed under conditions consistent with complete relaxation of the trabecular smooth muscle of the corpora cavernosa [71]. Under such status, hemodynamic testing is comparable and reproducible. Duplex Doppler ultrasonography has become a widely utilized modality for diagnosing arterial insufficiency [64]. The major drawback to this form of invasive vascular testing is the inability of the Duplex ultrasonography test to assess the status of the trabecular smooth muscle tone [42].

Short-term successes with such surgery have varied from 38 to 86 percent. Further interpretation is difficult because the selection criteria, technical aspects of the procedure, as well as the criteria for success or improvement vary from one study to the next. Moreover, long-term results are limited. The multiplicity of surgical approaches to penile arterial bypass surgery would suggest that no one procedure is effective in all instances. The anatomic pattern of arterial occlusive disease on pharmacoarteriography will lead the surgeon to select the appropriate microvascular surgical procedure. According to the anatomy, increased arterial blood flow to the lacunar spaces may be accomplished in several ways. The first way is to increase the flow in the cavernosal arteries through their communications with the proximal dorsal arteries. Second, increased inflow to the lacunar spaces may occur by "arterialization" of the deep dorsal vein, retrograde through the plexus of emissary and subtunical veins.

An anatomically oriented approach for penile microvascular arterial bypass surgery, based on the identification and the description of four common types of pharmacoarteriographic patterns of penile arterial occlusive disease has been recently described. It should be noted that each of the four patterns has more than one selection option for the type of bypass. Based on the experience in other vascular beds, arterial grafts are superior to vein grafts in terms of longevity, and in-situ vein grafts are preferable to reversed vein grafts.

The vascular principles utilized in microvascular arterial bypass surgery for impotence are similar to those vascular and microvascular principles utilized in arterial bypass procedures for occlusive disease in other vascular beds. Long-term bypass patency is based on four microvascular principles: (1) prevention of ischemic, mechanical, or thermal injury to the vascular endothelium of the donor or recipient vascular structures; (2) transmission of systolic neo-arterial inflow pressures and flow; (3) technically accurate arterial anastomoses; and (4) low recipient vascular-outflow resistances.

Recent studies at our institution have revealed results elucidating those vascular principles. The first study documents the role of prevention of endothelial injury during surgical preparation using technically sound "no touch" techniques [92]. The second study examined the quality of the donor and recipient vessels prior to the anastomoses [55]. The integrity of those vessels are of paramount concern, since the donor vessels provide transmission of the systemic blood pressure and the recipient vessels provide low-resistance outflow runoff.

Vein grafts have been proposed as optimal conduits for small-vessel arterial occlusive disease, because they possess native endothelium with intrinsic biologic properties that modulate the blood-graft interface and foster maintenance of vascular patency. In-situ "arterialization" of the deep dorsal vein graft is a commonly performed procedure, especially in patients with bilateral cavernosal artery occlusions and absent dorsal-cavernosal arterial communications. However, vein grafts utilized in coronary or peripheral artery bypass surgery have been reported to develop late occlusion on the basis of myointimal proliferative lesions in the arterialized vein wall. Such lesions have been shown to be caused by injury to the vein-graft endothelium. The mechanism of endothelial injury in vein grafts remains controversial: Is the endothelial injury the result of ischemic, mechanical, or thermal insults during surgical preparation of the vein graft, or is the endothelial injury the consequence of exposure of the vein wall to arterial blood flow and pressures? Histomorphometric study of tissue sections from the same deep dorsal vein prior to and 10 months following microvascular arterialization of an in-situ deep dorsal vein graft were studied [92]. Extensive histomorphometric analysis revealed that the native architecture in the arterialized graft segment was preserved and that no myointimal proliferative lesions were noted 10 months later. That implied that exposure of the normal, healthy deep dorsal vein bypass graft to systemic arterial blood pressures and flow for 10 months did not result in histologic alterations. Furthermore, iatrogenic ischemic, thermal, or mechanical trauma was not inflicted on the vein graft during surgery. Such observations strongly imply that the use of "no-touch" endothelium-preserving vascular techniques will improve long-term vascular patency. Such techniques already have yielded improved clinical results in other vascular beds.

The second study explored possible preexisting pathology of the donor and recipient vessels prior to anastomosis [55]. Histomorphologic analyses revealed that preexisting atherosclerotic lesions existed in over 50 percent of the dorsal arteries studied. Although present, such preexisting lesions rarely were identified in the inferior epigastric artery and the deep dorsal vein. Vascular risk factors did not per se predict the quality of the vessels. Those data reinforce the use of the inferior epigastric artery as the neoarterial pathway. In addition, they support the concept of using multiple pathways to revascularize the corpora cavernosa.

Our experience with microvascular arterial bypass surgery for the treatment of arteriogenic impotence in over 500 cases has led us to identify three basic clinical principles:

1. **Strict selection criteria.** Erectile hemodynamics differ from those of other vascular organs in that function is dependent not only on arterial inflow but also on the development of venous outflow resistance. The surgery should be restricted to those patients with arteriogenic impotence with normal corporal veno-occlusion. In a recent clinical study that considered failures after penile microvascular arterial bypass surgery, we found that patients with coexisting corporal veno-occlusive dysfunction failed due to persistent venous leakage despite concomitant venous ligation surgery. That included those young patients with site-specific arterial occlusive pathology following blunt pelvic or perineal trauma.
2. **Anatomically oriented arterial bypasses.** Reconstruction should be based on the arteriographic pattern of arterial occlusive disease. There should not be one procedure universally applied.

3. **Endothelium-preserving microvascular technique.** The surgical technique should consist of modern endothelium-sparing vascular and microvascular surgical principles similar to those applied for occlusive disease in other peripheral vascular beds.

Penile Prosthesis Insertion. In the early 1970s, the urologic subspeciality of erectile dysfunction developed following the introduction of an intracorporeal penile prosthesis. It was the availability of such a device that made it necessary for urologists to evaluate patients with erectile dysfunction to determine etiology (i.e., psychogenic versus organic). Through the 1970s and early 1980s, the development of penile prostheses proceeded along two distinct lines: the malleable or rigid prosthesis and the multicomponent inflatable prosthesis. Modifications of the three-piece inflatable device have led to the introduction of a two-piece inflatable device. Second- and third-generation prostheses have attempted to increase aesthetic results, at times provide increased girth, decrease the likelihood for component failure, and, where possible, increase the ease of implantation.

With the advent of newer treatments for vasculogenic impotence, implantation of penile prosthesis has become in the minds of many physicians, as well as patients, the last treatment option to be considered after attempting therapy with other modalities. If a patient with vasculogenic impotence does not choose one of the conservative treatments or if those options do not result in an appropriate erectile response, then he is considered for prosthetic surgery. Appropriate counseling of a patient before the implantation of a prosthesis is essential to the success of the surgery. Expectations by a patient that a penile prosthesis will improve a deteriorating relationship are usually unreasonable. The purpose of the prosthesis is only to simulate an erection by providing penile rigidity sufficient for intercourse. The ability to ejaculate and have an orgasm is not altered by the implantation of a prosthesis but in some cases may be restored. In addition, a patient undergoing the surgery should be informed of the potential complications of prosthetic surgery as well as their frequencies and sequelae.

The postoperative complications of penile-implant surgery usually are relegated to those of component failure, postoperative infection, or device erosion. Probably the most significant complication of prosthetic surgery is infection. The best defense against infection is prophylaxis. The incidence of infections following penile prosthetic surgery have varied between 1 and 9 percent [2]. Following implantation, the time frame for the presentation of infection will vary depending on the organism involved. Infections with more virulent and aggressive bacteria usually will present in the first few postoperative days, with fever, pain, and swelling overlying the prosthesis accompanied by purulent wound drainage. There are patients, however, who will complain of prolonged pain overlying the device without any obvious purulent drainage from the wound. Prolonged pain, fixation of the pump or tubing to the overlying scrotal skin, and elevated white blood cell count and sedimentation rate may all be helpful in diagnosing a possible infection by less virulent organisms. When infection of that sort is highly suspected, wound exploration is mandatory. At the time of exploration, if no obvious purulence is demonstrated, a gram stain of the fluid surrounding the prosthesis should be made. Obviously, if no apparent infection is seen, the wound may be closed without further therapy. The reoperative rate for penile prosthetic surgery has been reported to be between 14 and 44 percent, with newer series showing a decreased need for reoperation. Patient and physician acceptance of penile prostheses has virtually become worldwide, with over 90 percent of patients reporting satisfaction after prosthetic surgery [93].

Summary

While great progress has been made in the investigation of vasculogenic impotence, much work needs to be performed. A wider appreciation for epidemiology is needed to better appreciate the influence of para-aging phenomena. Physiologic understanding needs to be more detailed to enable a better comprehension of the pathophysiology and to gain insights into a broader and more effective clinical pharmacologic intervention. Diagnostic studies and treatment outcomes need to be recorded in prospective studies so that data can be available to patients for knowledgeable treatment selections.

References

1. Feldman HA, et al. Impotence and its medical and psychosocial correlates: results of the Massachusetts male aging study. J Urol 1994; 151:54–61.
2. Krane RJ, Goldstein I, Saenz de Tejada I. Impotence. N Engl J Med 1989; 321:1648–1659.
3. Feldman HA, et al. Construction of a surrogate variable for impotence in the Massachusetts male aging study. J Clin Epidemiol 1994; 47:457–467.
4. Goldstein I, Hatzichristou DG. Epidemiology of impotence. In AH Bennett, ed. Impotence: Diagnosis and Management of Erectile Dysfunction. Philadelphia: Saunders, 1994. Pp. 1–17.
5. Lue TF, Tanagho EA. Physiology of erection and pharmacological management of impotence. J Urol 1987; 137:829–836.
6. Saenz de Tejada I, et al. The trabecular smooth muscle modulates the capacitor function of the penis. Studies on a rabbit model. Am J Physiol 1991; 260 (Heart Circ Physiol):H1590–H1593.
7. Seftel AD, Saenz de Tejada I. Physiologic control of penile arteries. Abstract presented at the 6th Annual Meeting of the Society for Basic Urologic Research, Washington, DC, May, 1992.
8. Simonsen U, Saenz de Tejada I, Carcia-Sacristan, A. Involvement of nitric oxide in the non-adrenergic non-cholinergic neurotransmission of horse deep penile arteries—role of charybdotoxin-sensitive K+ channels. Brit J Pharm 1995. In press.
9. Kim N, et al. A nitric oxide-like factor mediates non-adrenergic, non-cholinergic neurogenic relaxation of penile corpus cavernosum smooth muscle. J Clin Invest 1991; 88:112–118.
10. Azadzoi KM, et al. Endothelium-derived nitric oxide and cyclooxygenase products modulate corpus cavernosum smooth muscle tone. J Urol 1992; 147:220–225.
11. Kim N, et al. Oxygen tension regulates the nitric oxide pathway. J Clin Invest 1993; 91:437–442.
12. Furchgott RF, Zawadski JV. The obligatory role of endothelial cells in the relaxation of arterial smooth muscle to acetycholine. Nature 1980; 288:373–376.

13. Saenz de Tejada I, et al. Cholinergic neurotransmission in human corpus cavernosum. I. Responses of isolated tissue. Am J Physiol 1988; 254:H459–H467.
14. Knispel HH, Goessl C, Beckmann R. Basal and acetylcholine-stimulated nitric oxide formation mediates relaxation of rabbit cavernous smooth muscle. J Urol 1991; 146:1429–1433.
15. Kimoto Y, Kessler R, Constantinou CE. Endothelium dependent relaxation of human corpus cavernosum by bradykinin. J Urol 1990; 144:1015–1017.
16. Palmer RMJ, Ferrige AG, Moncada S. Nitric oxide release accounts for the biological activity of endothelium-derived relaxing factor. Nature (Lond) 1987; 327:524–526.
17. Ignarro LJ, Buga GM, Wood KS. Endothelium-derived relaxing factor produced and released from artery and vein is nitric oxide. Proc Natl Acad Sci USA 1987; 84:9265–9269.
18. Ignarro LJ, et al. Nitric oxide and cyclic GMP formation upon electrical stimulation cause relaxation of corpus cavernosum smooth muscle. Biochem Biophys Res Commun 1990; 170:843–850.
19. Bult H, et al. Nitric oxide as an inhibitory non-adrenergic non-cholinergic neurotransmitter. Nature (Lond) 1990; 345: 346–347.
20. Bredt DS, Hwang PM, Snyder SH. Localization of nitric oxide synthase indicating a neural role for nitric oxide. Nature (Lond) 1990; 347:768–770.
21. Lerner S, Melman A, Christ GJ. A review of erectile dysfunction: New insights and more questions. J Urol 1993; 149:1246–1255.
22. Christ GJ, Spray DC, Brink PR. Characterization of K^+ currents in cultured human corporal smooth muscle cells. J Andrology 1993; 14:319.
23. Abdul Sattar M, Johns EJ. Alpha 1-adrenoceptor subtypes mediating adrenergic vasoconstriction in kidney, one-clip Goldblatt and deoxycorticosterone acetate-salt hypertensive rats. J Cardiovasc Pharmacol 1994; 24:420–428.
24. Saenz de Tejada I, et al. Endothelin: location, synthesis, activity and receptor types in the human penis. Am J Physiol 1991; 261(Heart Circ Physiol 30):H1078–H1085.
25. Chamley-Campbell J, Campbell G, Ross R. The smooth muscle cell in culture. Physiol Rev 1979; 59:1.
26. Botney MD, et al. Active collagen synthesis by pulmonary arteries in human primary pulmonary hypertension. Am J Pathol 1993; 143:121.
27. Pease DC, Paule WJ. Electron microscopy of elastic arteries. The thoracic aorta of the rat. J Ultrastruct Res 1960; 3:469.
28. Moreland RB, et al. PGE1 suppresses the induction of collagen synthesis by transforming growth factor-β1 in human corpus cavernosum smooth muscle. J Urol 1995; 153:826–834.
29. Nehra A, et al. A case report of systemic sclerosis and impotence: a clinicopathologic correlation. J Urol 1995; 153:1140–1146.
30. Massague J. The transforming growth factor-β family. Annual Review of Cell Biology 1990; 6:597–641.
31. Sporn MB, Roberts AB. Transforming growth factor-β: Recent progress and new challenges. J Cell Biol 1992; 119:1017–1021.
32. Border WA, Ruoslahti E. Transforming growth factor-β in disease: the dark side of tissue repair. J Clin Inv 1992; 90:1–7.
33. Majack RA, Cook SC, Bornstein P. Platelet-derived growth factor and heparin-like glycosaminoglycans regulate thrombospondin synthesis and deposition in the matrix by smooth muscle cells. J Cell Bio 1985; 101:1059–1070.
34. Majack RA, Goodman LV, Dixit VM. Cell surface thrombospondin is functionally essential for vascular smooth muscle proliferation. J Cell Bio 1988; 106:415–422.
35. Takasaki I, et al. Effect of hypertension on fibronectin expression in the rat aorta. J Biol Chem 1990; 265:21935–21939.
36. Takasaki I, Chobanian AV, Brecher P. Biosynthesis of fibronectin in the rabbit aorta. J Biol Chem 1991; 266:17686–17694.
37. Edwards DR, et al. Transforming growth factor-β modulates the expression of collagenase and metalloproteinase inhibitor. EMBO J 1987; 6:1899–1904.
38. Overall CM, Wrana JF, Sodek J. Independent regulation of collagenase, 72-kDa progelatinase, and metalloendoproteinase inhibitor expression in human fibroblasts by transforming growth factor-β. J Biol Chem 1989; 264:1860–1869.
39. Raghow R, Irush P, Kang AH. Coordinate regulation of transforming growth factor β gene expression and cell proliferation in hamster lungs undergoing bleomycin-induced pulmonary fibrosis. J Clin Inv 1989; 84:1836–1842.
40. Castilla A, Prieto J, Fausto N. Transforming growth factor β1 and α in chronic liver disease. Effects of interferon alfa therapy. N Engl J Med 1991; 324:933–940.
41. Vane JR, Anggard EE, Botting RM. Regulatory functions of the endothelium. N Engl J Med 1990; 323:27–36.
42. Hatzichristou DG, Goldstein I. Arterial bypass surgery for impotence. Current Opinion in Urology 1992; 1:114.
43. Azadzoi KM, Goldstein I. Erectile dysfunction due to atherosclerotic vascular disease: the development of an animal model. J Urol 1992; 147:1675–1681.
44. Azadzoi KM, Saenz de Tejada I. Hypercholesterolemia impairs endothelium-dependent relaxation of rabbit corpus cavernosum smooth muscle. J Urol 1990; 146:238–240.
45. Azadzoi KM, Saenz de Tejada I. Diabetes mellitus impairs neurogenic and endothelium-dependent relaxation of rabbit corpus cavernosum smooth muscle. J Urol 1992; 148:1587–1591.
46. Levine FJ, Greenfield AJ, Goldstein I. Arteriographically-determined occlusive disease within the hypogastric-cavernous bed in impotent patients following blunt perineal and pelvic trauma. J Urol 1990; 144:1147–1153.
47. Rosen MP, et al. Arteriogenic impotence: findings in 195 impotent men examined with selective internal pudendal angiography. Radiology 1990; 174:1043–1048.
48. Rich NM, Spencer FC. Vascular Trauma. Philadelphia: Saunders, 1978.
49. Chambers HL, Balfour J. The incidence of impotence following pelvic fracture with associated urinary tract injury. J Urol 1963; 89:702.
50. Gibson J, Geoffrey R. Urological management and complications of fractured pelvis and ruptured urethra. J Urol 1974; 111:353–355.
51. King J. Impotence after fracture of the pelvis. J Bone Joint Surgery 1975; 57:1107–1109.
52. Sharlip ID. Penile arteriography in impotence after pelvic trauma. J Urol 1981; 126:477–481.
53. St. Louis EL, et al. Basketball-related impotence. N Engl J Med 1983; 308:595–596.
54. Kerstein MD, et al. Perineal trauma and vasculogenic impotence. J Urol 1982; 127:57.
55. Hatzichristou DG, Goldstein I, Quist W. Pre-existing vascular disease in donor and recipient vessels in microvascular arterial bypass surgery for impotence. J Urol 1994; 151:1217–1224.
56. Creecy AA, Beazlie FS Jr. Fracture of the penis: traumatic rupture of corpora cavernosa. J Urol 1957; 78:620.
57. Dever DP, et al. Penile fracture: operative management and cavernosography. Urology 1983; 22:394–396.
58. Kalash SS, Young JD Jr. Fracture of penis: controversy of surgical versus conservative treatment. Urology 1984; 24:21–24.
59. Godec CJ, Reiser R, Logush AZ. The erect penis: injury prone organ. J Trauma 1988; 28:124–126.
60. Penson DF, et al. The hemodynamic pathophysiology of im-

potence following blunt trauma to the erect penis. J Urol 1992; 148:1171–1180.
61. Azadzoi KM, Goldstein I. Atherosclerosis induced corporal leakage impotence. Surgical Forum 1987; 38:647.
62. Pescatori ES, et al. A positive intracavernosal injection test implies normal veno-occlusive but not necessarily normal arterial function: a hemodynamic study. J Urol 1994; 151:1209–1216.
63. Lue TF, et al. Vasculogenic impotence evaluated by high-resolution ultrasonography and pulsed Doppler spectrum analysis. Radiology 1985; 155:777–781.
64. Herbener TE, et al. Penile ultrasound. Sem Urol 1994; 12: 320–332.
65. Benson CB, Vickers MA. Sexual impotence caused by vascular disease: diagnosis with duplex ultrasonography. Am J Radiol 1989; 153:1149–1153.
66. Schwartz AN, Wang KY, Mack LA. Evaluation of normal erectile function with color Doppler sonography. Am J Radiol 1989; 153:1155–1160.
67. Aboseif SR, Lue TF. Hemodynamics of penile erection. Urol Clin N A 1988; 15:1–7.
68. Quam JP, King BF, James EM. Duplex and color Doppler sonographic evaluation of vasculogenic impotence. Am J Radiol 1989; 153:1141–1147.
69. Rajfer J, et al. Correlation between penile angiography and duplex scanning of cavernous arteries in impotent men. J Urol 1990; 143:1128–1130.
70. Valji K, Bookstein JJ, Parsons L. Pharmacoarteriography in the evaluation of impotence. J Urol 1987; 137:333–337.
71. Hatzichristou DG, et al. In vivo assessment of trabecular smooth muscle tone, its application in pharmaco-cavernosometry, and analysis of intracavernosal pressure determinants. J Urol 1995; 153:1126–1135.
72. Austoni E, et al. Use of dynamic NMR in the diagnostic evaluation of penile pathology. Int J Impotence Res 1990; 2[Suppl 2]:161.
73. Vardi Y, Lidgi S, Levin DR. Intracavernous pO2 response to vasoactive drugs as an indicator of corporal vascular dysfunction. Int J Impotence Res 1990; 2[Suppl 2]:242.
74. Smith AD. Psychologic factors in the multidisciplinary evaluation and treatment of erectile dysfunction. Urol Clin North Am 1988; 15:41–51.
75. Morales A, et al. Is yohimbine effective in the treatment of organic impotence? Results of a controlled trial. J Urol 1987; 137:1168–1172.
76. Morales A, et al. Oral and transcutaneous pharmacologic agents in the treatment of impotence. In RJ Krane, ed. Urologic clinics of North America. Philadelphia: Saunders, 1988. P. 87.
77. Foreman MM, Wernicke JF. Approaches for the development of oral drug therapies for erectile dysfunction. Seminars in Urology 1990; 8(2):107–112.
78. Heaton JPW, et al. Preliminary studies showing erectogenic activity in an oral agent. Int J Impotence Res 1990; 2[Suppl 2]:285.
79. Scher M, Krieger J, Juergens S. Trazodone and priapism. Am J Psychiat 1983; 140:1362–1363.
80. Szele FG, Murphy DL, Garrick NA. Fenfluramine, m-chlorophenylpiperazine and other serotonin re-uptake agonists and antagonists on penile erections in non-human primates. Life Sci 1988; 43:1297–1303.
81. Lal S, Rios O, Thavundayil JX. Treatment of impotence with trazodone: a case report. J Urol 1990; 143:819–820.
82. Saenz de Tejada I, et al. Pathophysiology of prolonged penile erection associated with trazodone use. J Urol 1991; 145:60–64.
83. Claes H, Baert L. Transcutaneous nitroglycerin therapy in the treatment of impotence. Urol Int 1989; 44:309–312.
84. Morales A, Heaton JPW. The medical treatment of impotence: an update. World J Urol 1990; 8:80–83.
85. Virag R. Intracavernous injection of papaverine for erectile failure. Lancet 1982; 1:938.
86. Brindley GS. Pilot experiments on the actions of drugs injected into the human corpus cavernosum penis. Br J Pharmacol 1986; 87:495–500.
87. Zorgniotti AW, Lefleur RS. Auto-injection of the corpus cavernosum with a vasoactive drug combination for vasculogenic impotence. J Urol 1985; 133:39–41.
88. Stackl W, Hasun R, Marberger M. Intracavernous injection of prostaglandin El in impotent men. J Urol 1988; 140:66–68.
89. Nadig PW, Ware JC, Blumoff R. Noninvasive device to produce and maintain an erection-like state. Urol 1986; 27: 126–131.
90. Wintherington R. Vacuum constriction device for management of erectile impotence. J Urol 1989; 141:320–322.
91. Diederichs W, et al. The effect of subatmospheric pressure on the simian penis. J Urol 1989; 142:1087–1089.
92. Hatzichristou DG, et al. The native venous architecture is preserved in an arterialized deep dorsal vein graft for arteriogenic impotence: a case report. J Urol 1993; 149:851–855.
93. Goldstein I, et al. Early experience with the first pre-connected three-piece inflatable penile prosthesis: The Mentor Alpha-1. J Urol 1993; 150:1814–1818.

Aneurysmal Disease of the Aorta and Its Branches

Mark A. Creager
Jonathan L. Halperin
Anthony D. Whittemore

The Normal Aorta

ANATOMY

The aorta is the body's major conductance vessel, through which all oxygenated blood passes in its course from the left ventricle to the organs and tissues. It has thoracic and abdominal portions. The thoracic aorta may be subdesignated into ascending, transverse (arch), and descending thoracic segments. The ascending aorta is approximately 5 cm in length with a maximum diameter of about 3 cm. The great artery begins at the base of the left ventricle at approximately the level of the third costal cartilage behind the left side of the sternum. The ascending portion terminates near the upper border of the second right costal cartilage. At the root of the ascending aorta are three aortic valve cusps that delineate the sinuses of Valsalva. The right and left coronary arteries arise from the anterior and left posterior sinuses. Along the anterior border of the ascending aorta lie the infundibulum of the right ventricle, the proximal trunk of the pulmonary arteries, and the right atrium. As the aorta ascends, structures anterior to it include the pericardium, the pleura, and the anterior margin of the right lung. Posteriorly sit the left atrium, right pulmonary artery, and right mainstem bronchus. The right border consists of the superior vena cava and right atrium, and the left side is bounded by the left atrium and the pulmonary vascular trunk.

The aortic arch is approximately 4 cm long. Its maximum diameter ranges from 2.5 to 3.5 cm, depending on body surface area and age. It begins behind the manubrium at the level of the second right sternocostal articulation. From there the conduit traverses superior, posterior, and toward the left as it passes in front of the trachea and arches farther to the left to terminate near the second left sternocostal junction. There it is bounded anteriorly and to the left by the pleura of the left lung, the left phrenic nerve, the trunk of the left vagus nerve and its lower cervical cardiac branches, and the superior cervical cardiac branch of the left stellate sympathetic nerve. Posteriorly and to the right are the trachea, esophagus, thoracic duct, vertebral column, deep cardiac plexus, and left recurrent laryngeal nerve. Beneath the arch are the bifurcation of the pulmonary trunk, the left mainstem bronchus, and the ligamentum arteriosus. Superiorly, the aortic arch gives rise to the brachiocephalic, left common carotid, and left subclavian arteries.

As the thoracic aorta descends in the posterior mediastinum, approximately 20 cm from the arch, its diameter tapers slightly, from an average of 2.3 cm to 2 cm. The descending thoracic aorta begins to the left of the midline at the lower border of the fourth thoracic vertebra and terminates anterior to the twelfth. In front lie the hilum of the left lung, the pericardium, left atrium, esophagus, and diaphragm. Adjacent posteriorly are the vertebral column and hemiazygos veins. To the right are the azygos vein and thoracic duct; to the left are the left lung and its pleura. From that segment arise pericardial, bronchial, and esophageal arteries and posterior intercostal branch arteries.

The abdominal aorta begins in the median plane at the aortic hiatus of the diaphragm, descends approximately 15 cm in front of the vertebral column to the level of the fourth lumbar vertebra, and then divides into two common iliac arteries. Along that course, its diameter narrows from 2.0–2.6 cm to a low of 1.7–1.9 cm, averaging 2 mm larger in males than in females. Anteriorly, the abdominal aorta is bounded by the body of the pancreas, horizontal segment of the duodenum, posterior parietal peritoneum, celiac plexus, lesser omentum, transverse colon, and para-aortic plexus of sympathetic nerves. Behind, it is bounded by the upper four lumbar vertebrae. To the right is the inferior vena cava; to the left is the left sympathetic trunk. From this segment of the aorta arise the celiac artery; superior and inferior mesenteric arteries; pairs of suprarenal, renal, and testicular or ovarian arteries; and the lumbar and median sacral arteries.

HISTOLOGY

General features of arterial histology are described elsewhere in this book. The aorta is categorized as an elastic artery. Its wall consists of three layers: the tunica intima, tunica media, and tunica adventitia. The innermost component of the tunica intima is the endothelium, a single layer of cells that rests on a thin basal lamina. The subendothelial tissue comprises fibroblasts, collagen fibers, elastic fibers, and mucoid ground substance. (More about the composition and properties of the subendothelial layer can be found in Chap. 2.) The internal elastic membrane forms the outer lining of the tunica intima. The tunica media is approximately 1 mm thick, comprising elastin, smooth muscle cells, collagen, and ground substance. It is the predominance of elastic fibers in the aortic wall and their arrangement as circumferential lamellae that distinguish this elastic artery from the smaller muscular arteries. A lamellar unit comprises two concentric elastic lamellae and the smooth muscle cells, collagen, and ground substance contained within [1,2]. The thoracic aorta incorporates 35 to 56 lamellar units and the abdominal aorta about 28 units [3]. Surrounding the tunica media is the tunica adventitia, which is composed of loose connective tissue, including fibroblasts, and relatively small amounts of collagen fibers, elastin, and ground substance. Within the tunica adventitia lie the nervi vasorum and vasa vasorum. The arteries arising along the course of the aorta give rise to the vasa vasorum, which develop into a capillary network that supplies the adventitia and media of the thoracic aorta. Vasa vasorum do not supply the media of the abdominal aorta [4].

PHYSIOLOGY

Ejection of blood from the left ventricle creates a pressure wave that traverses the aorta. The radial expansion and contraction of the arterial walls occur with passage of the pressure wave [5]. Potential energy derived from the force of left ventricular contraction is stored in the aortic wall during systole. During diastole, the aortic wall recoils, transforming potential energy to kinetic energy, thereby driving blood into the peripheral vessels during diastole [5,6]. The pressure wave is conducted along the aorta at a velocity of approximately 5 m/second [6]. As the wave of pressure travels distally, its configuration changes, steepening and increasing in amplitude [5]. Systolic pressure becomes higher as the pressure wave moves along the aorta. The incisura, present in the proximal portion of the thoracic aorta, gradually disappears and is generally absent in the abdominal aorta [7]. Forward flow in the aorta begins when the aortic valve opens. The velocity of flow rises rapidly to a peak and then gradually decreases. With aortic valve closure, there is a transient period of backward flow. Forward flow again occurs, particularly in the descending thoracic and abdominal aorta during diastole, albeit at a velocity considerably less than occurs during systole.

AGING

Each of the four components of the aortic wall—elastic tissue, collagen fibers, smooth muscle cells and mucoid ground substance—changes with age. Elastic fibers fragment, collagen becomes more prominent at the expense of smooth muscle cells, and glycosaminoglycans progressively accumulate [4,8–11]. As a result, the aorta becomes less distensible with aging, and its ability to absorb the forces derived from left ventricular contraction is diminished [11]. Thereafter, the aortic wall may weaken, leading to dilation of the lumen as well as elongation and uncoiling of the aortic arch, which collectively constitute the process of ectasia [12,13].

Classification of Aortic Aneurysms

The term aneurysm originates from a Greek word *aneurysma,* referring to dilation. The pathologic concept of an aortic aneurysm should be distinguished from ectasia, which might be defined as a modest generalized dilation of the aorta that occurs with aging [14]. Aneurysms can be classified according to morphology, etiology, or location. The gross morphologic classification distinguishes true aneurysms of the aorta as fusiform or saccular. A **fusiform aneurysm** is cylindrical and affects the entire circumference of the aorta; a **saccular aneurysm** is an outpouching of only a portion of the aortic wall (Figs. 39-1, 39-2; see also Fig. 22-3). Frequently, a small neck provides continuity between the aortic lumen and the saccular aneurysm. Fusiform aneurysms are more common than the saccular type. Infrarenal abdominal aortic aneurysms are almost exclusively fusiform. Thoracic aortic aneurysms are occasionally saccular with a relatively narrow commu-

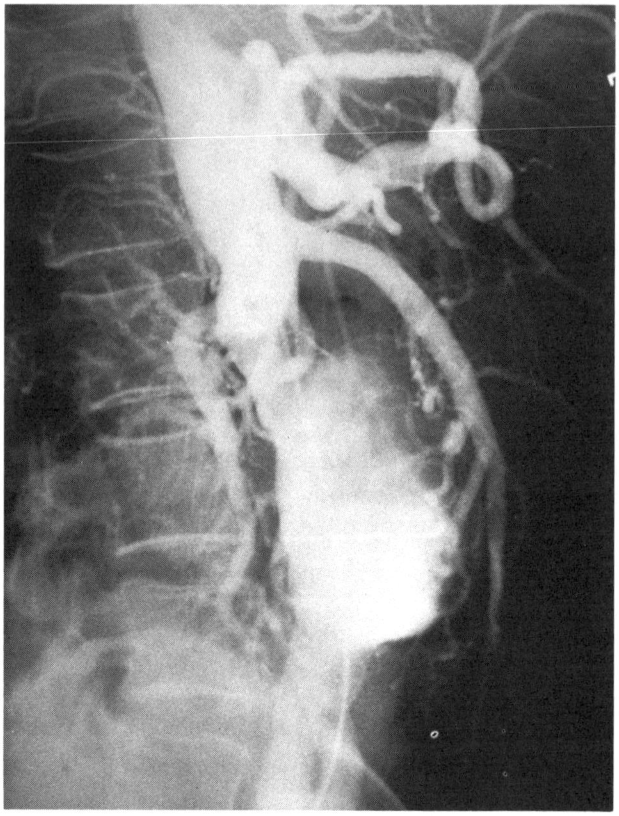

Fig. 39-1. Abdominal aortogram demonstrating an infrarenal fusiform abdominal aortic aneurysm.

nication between the cavity of the aneurysm and the aortic lumen. The limited orifice may protect the thin wall of the aneurysm from the force of intra-aortic pressure and reduce the risk of rupture, in contrast to fusiform aneurysms, in which the entire circumference of the dilated segment is exposed to the pulsatile distending forces from the cardiac systole.

Beyond gross morphology, aneurysms of the aorta also can be classified according to the segment involved. That practice simplifies the understanding of aortic aneurysms because the pathogenesis, clinical presentation, natural history, and treatment of such aneurysms depend in large measure on their location. Using this scheme, aortic aneurysms can be classified as thoracic, thoracoabdominal, or abdominal. Aneurysms also occur in other arteries, including the main branches of the aorta (iliac, subclavian, and mesenteric arteries) and more peripherally (femoral and popliteal arteries).

A **pseudoaneurysm**, or false aneurysm, is essentially a contained aortic rupture, in which the wall of the aneurysm is not the original wall of the aorta but rather a mass of connective tissue and structures surrounding extravasated blood. Pseudoaneurysms may resemble saccular true aneurysms by virtue of the relatively narrow communication that connects the sac to the main lumen. Aortic dissections have been designated, somewhat erroneously, as dissecting aneurysms. In this text, dissection of the aorta is considered as a separate entity (Chap. 40).

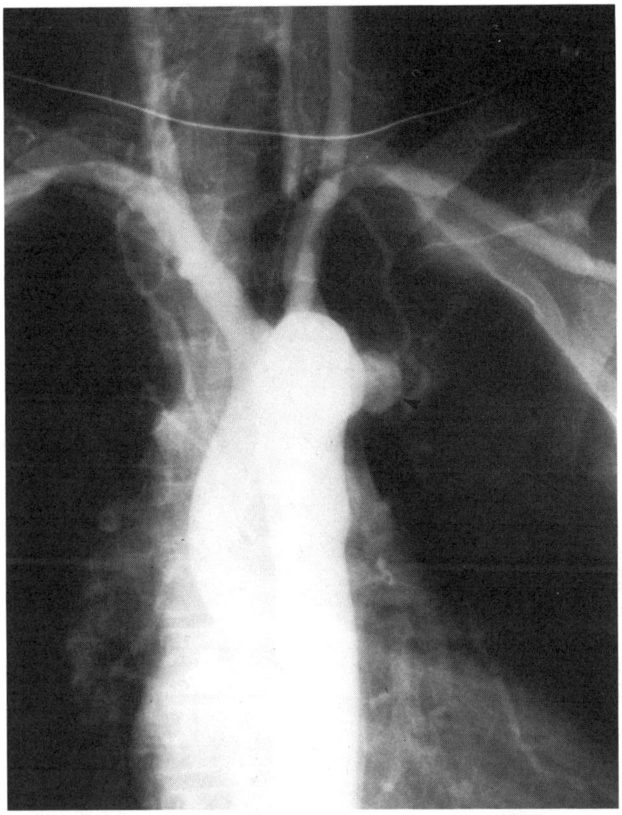

Fig. 39-2. Aortogram illustrating a saccular aneurysm affecting the arch of the thoracic aorta.

ETIOLOGY OF AORTIC ANEURYSMS

Dilatation of the aorta may occur as a consequence of aging, as well as of atherosclerosis, infection, inflammation, trauma, congenital anomalies, and medial degeneration (Table 39-1). The pathologic changes that accompany those conditions cause the aorta to thicken, thin, bulge, tear, rupture, stenose, dissect, or be altered by combinations of those conditions. When there is disease of the medial layer, tension on the aortic wall leads to progressive dilatation and increasing shear stress. That process is accelerated when hypertension is present and particularly when pulsatile forces are high. In conditions of increased peripheral vascular resistance, there is a reflected wave that has an impact additive to that of antegrade pulsatile flow.

Table 39-1. Causes of aortic aneurysms

Atherosclerosis
Cystic medial necrosis
Primary
Marfan syndrome
Ehlers-Danlos syndrome
Vasculitis
Takayasu arteritis
Giant cell arteritis
Ankylosing spondylitis
Rheumatoid arthritis
Reiter's syndrome
Relapsing polychondritis
Infectious aortitis
Syphilis
Tuberculosis
Mycotic
Staphylococcus, Streptococcus, Salmonella, Pseudomonas
Congenital
Trauma

Atherosclerosis. Fatty streaks are commonly found in the descending aortas of individuals younger than 10 years even in the absence of hypercholesterolemia. Fibrosis and complicated atherosclerotic lesions in young individuals develop mainly when total serum cholesterol exceeds 200 mg/dl [14]. Beyond the age of 20 years, atherosclerotic plaques occur more extensively in the abdominal aorta than in any other arterial area. (The histology and pathogenesis of atherosclerosis are discussed in Chaps. 11 to 13.) At first, the lesions affect only the intima, but as extracellular lipid accumulates, fibrocalcific degeneration leads to secondary atrophy of the underlying medial layer. The tubular portion of the ascending aorta generally is spared until the most advanced stages of atherosclerosis, except in patients with type II hyperlipoproteinemia, particularly of the homozygous variety [14]. Although ascending aortic atherosclerosis may develop in patients with diabetes mellitus, progression of the disease still lags behind that in the descending portion of the aorta. In cases of advanced syphilitic aortitis, secondary atherosclerotic degeneration also may affect the ascending aorta disproportionately in comparison with more distal areas.

The principal consequences of atherosclerosis in the aorta are aneurysmal dilatation and stenotic obstruction. The former process is considerably more widespread, potentially affecting almost the entire length of the aorta, whereas obstruction tends to involve only the abdominal portion of the aorta. In addition, atherosclerotic disease may compromise the lumens of branch arteries arising from virtually any level of the aorta. The most proximal aspects of the thoracic aorta rarely are sites of atherosclerotic aneurysm formation unless there is independent disease of the media. When the arch and descending portions become aneurysmal, there is usually aneurysmal involvement of the abdominal aorta as well. Indeed, the most common site of aneurysm formation is the abdominal aorta.

Cystic Medial Necrosis. Cystic medial necrosis of the aorta was first described by Gsell and shortly afterward by Erdheim [15,16]. Histologic evidence of severe elastic-fiber degeneration, necrosis of muscle cells, and cystic spaces filled with mucoid material most often are encountered in the ascending aorta from the region of the valve to the brachiocephalic artery, although similar changes may be seen in the remainder of the aorta as well (Fig. 39-3). Aneurysms in those cases almost invariably are fusiform. Because of the dilatation of the aortic root, aortic regurgitation may be a secondary feature, although the valve leaflets themselves are histologically unaffected.

One clinical entity frequently associated with cystic me-

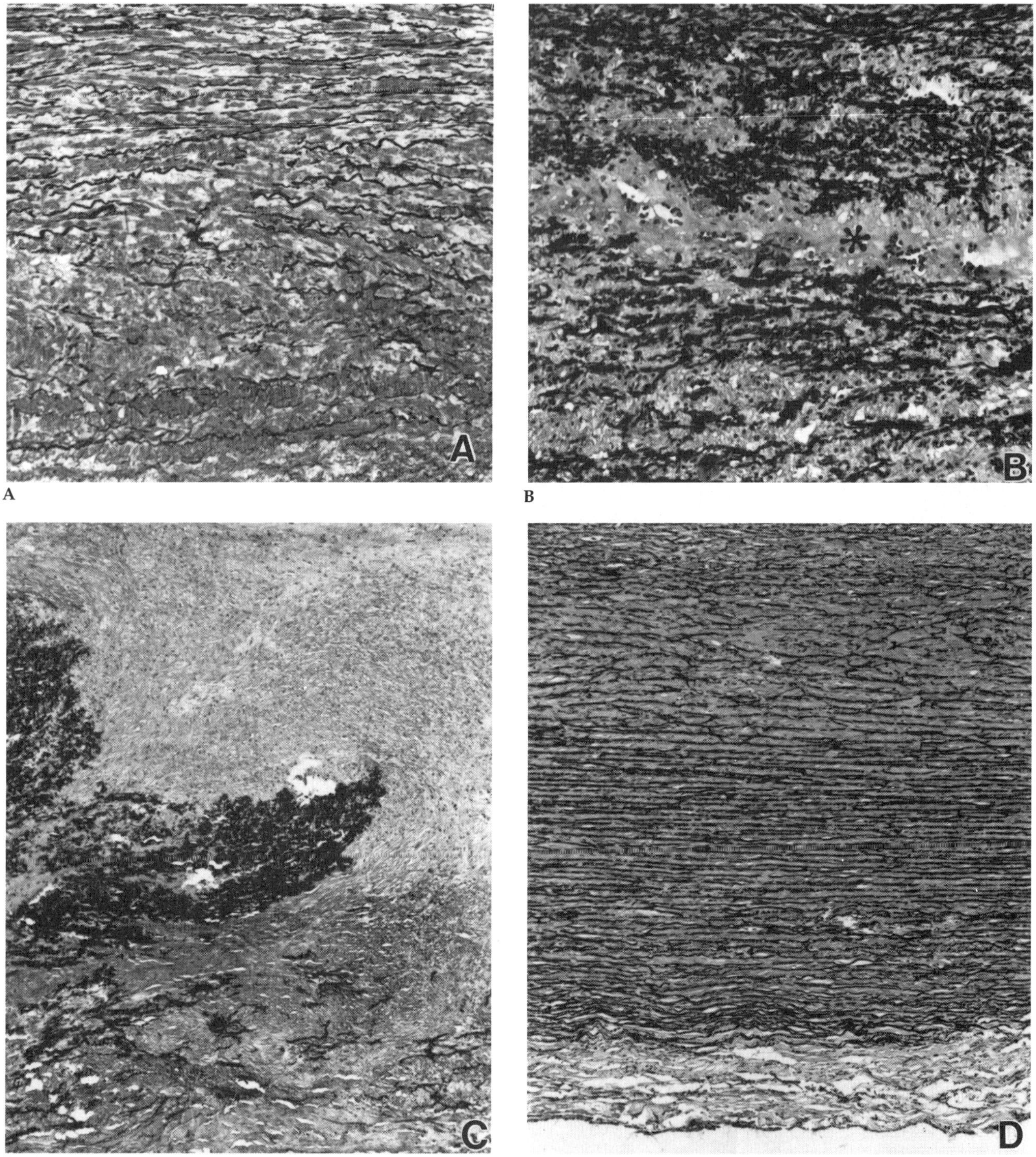

A B C D

Fig. 39-3. Histologic findings of medial degeneration progressing to those of cystic medial necrosis. **A.** Mild aortic lesion characterized by elastic tissue fragmentation in patient with Marfan syndrome. **B.** Higher-power photomicrograph of aorta from another patient demonstrating "cyst" formation (*), with elastic-tissue depletion, and focal loss of medial smooth muscle cells with mucopolysaccharide accumulation. **C.** Advanced cystic medial necrosis, with gross elastic-tissue deficiency. **D.** Normal aorta for comparison. All stained for elastic tissue, which appears black. (Reproduced with permission from FJ Schoen, Interventional and Surgical Cardiovascular Pathology, Philadelphia: Saunders, 1989.)

dial necrosis of the thoracic aorta is **Marfan syndrome**. This inherited disorder, described in 1896, is characterized by dolichostenomelia, ligamentous redundancy, ectopia lentis, ascending aortic dilatation, and incompetency of either aortic or mitral valves (or both) of the heart [17]. In cases of Marfan syndrome, there is a mutation in the gene regulating synthesis of fibrillin, a large lipoprotein essential to the structural integrity of the aortic wall. The mutation in chromosone 15 is linked to the rate of aortic disease as a familial trait but also may occur sporadically without a family history of Marfan syndrome. A mutation of chromosome 5 also has been identified in patients with Marfan syndrome and can arise spontaneously; in some cases, there may be concurrent mutations in both chromosomes 5 and 15. The variability in fibrillin-gene mutations accounts for the broad spectrum of aortic disease severity in patients with Marfan syndrome and may explain the occurrence of cystic medial necrosis of the aorta in patients with congenitally bicuspid aortic valves, in whom proximal aortic dilatation is a frequent finding. What is not clear is whether those mutations lead to a qualitative or quantitative defect of elastin, or both, but certainly there is a link between the pathology of the aortic media and the identification of specific genetic mutations of the two chromosomes [18,19].

In patients with Marfan syndrome, the aortic root tends to enlarge in fusiform fashion associated with aortic valvular regurgitation, and about half have mitral insufficiency as well. The aneurysms involve the sinuses of Valsalva and the tubular portion of the aorta, producing annuloaortic ectasia characterized by degeneration of elastic fibers and accumulation of mucoid material in the medial layer of the aortic wall. According to some pathologists but not others, neither cysts nor necrotic tissue characterize the histologic changes in the aorta that occur in Marfan syndrome, yet the gross pathology resembles that of cystic medial necrosis [15].As discussed more fully in Chap. 40, dissection is relatively common and may involve the entire length of the aorta, with or without other histologic features of the syndrome or aortic valvular incompetence. In fact, in Marfan syndrome true dissection tends not to develop in cases where fusiform aneurysm formation is present, such that there are two patterns of presentation: dissection and aneurysmal degeneration.

Increasingly recognized is the association of proximal aortic dilation with congenital bicuspid aortic valve with or without hemodynamically significant valvular stenosis or regurgitation [20]. Whether that is mediated by cystic medial necrosis of the aorta in all or some cases is not yet clear, although the prognosis appears better than in aortic aneurysm associated with other features of Marfan syndrome.

Vasculitides Associated with Aortic Aneurysm

TAKAYASU ARTERITIS. Takayasu arteritis, also designated **pulseless disease** or **idiopathic medial aortopathy**, is a chronic form of vasculitis of unknown etiology, with a predilection for the aorta and its primary branches [21–23]. Up to 90 percent of cases are female, with onset usually between the ages of 10 and 30 years. Although the highest incidence is in Asia, the disease has been reported in patients from many parts of the world. Identification of antiaortic antibodies and elevated serum concentrations of immunoglobulin in many cases suggest an autoimmune mechanism. The acute inflammatory phase of the disease typically subsides with or without antiinflammatory therapy and is replaced later in life by an obliterative ("pulseless") phase, although aneurysmal degeneration of the aorta and its proximal branches may appear in either stage. Hypertension occurs rather frequently in this disorder as a result of secondary aortic coarctation or renal-artery obstruction and may hasten the course of aneurysm development. Symptoms usually reflect systemic inflammation during the early stage and regional ischemia in the later stage, when upper- or lower-limb claudication, transient cerebral ischemia, mesenteric vascular insufficiency, and occasionally even coronary syndromes may develop. Aneurysms may be associated with thromboembolic phenomena, but rupture is uncommon. Surgical repair is more often required to address ischemic symptoms of obstructive arterial complications than the formation of aneurysms.

GIANT CELL ARTERITIS. Like Takayasu arteritis, giant cell arteritis may cause aneurysms of the aortic arch and descending thoracic aorta [24,25]. In giant cell arteritis, the onset of the inflammatory syndrome occurs generally later in life, and associated anemia is often more severe. It is generally encountered in individuals over 55 years of age and is twice as frequent among women than men. The predominant symptom is usually headache, and the most dreaded complication is blindness. Tender, prominent, inflamed temporal arteries may be identified on physical examination. More distal arteries of the upper half of the body are usually more involved than in arteritis of the Takayasu type, and aortic aneurysmal complications are, accordingly, less frequently encountered. Extensive involvement of the aorta and its branches may result in occlusion of the arteries derived from the aortic arch, dilatation or saccular aneurysm of the aorta, or aortic dissection [26,27]. Diagnosis may be suggested by angiography but is typically confirmed through temporal artery biopsy. Systemic administration of corticosteroid medication is the principal therapeutic approach; surgical experience is limited.

ANKYLOSING SPONDYLITIS. Among the seronegative spondyloarthropathies, ankylosing spondylitis has been associated with a number of cardioaortic anomalies, including aortic regurgitation, dilatation, and dissection. Abnormalities of the proximal aorta associated with ankylosing spondylitis include dilatation of the aortic valve annulus; fibrous thickening and focal inflammation of the aortic valve cusps, which may prolapse into the left ventricular cavity; dilatation of the sinus of Valsalva; and degenerative changes of the elastic tissue of the medial layer of the aortic wall. The lesions resemble those of luetic aortitis except for their proximity to the valve ring. Spondylitis of the axial skeleton may be accompanied by fever and accelerated erythrocyte sedimentation rate, but the serologic abnormalities typical of rheumatoid arthritis are absent; it is important to emphasize that cardiovascular manifestations may precede articular findings. Major complications involving the cardiovascular system more often are related to complete heart block or aortic regurgitation than to aortic dissection, which is comparatively rare in patients with ankylosing spondylitis [28].

Rheumatoid arthritis, relapsing polychondritis, and Reiter's syndrome have each been associated with dilatation of the aorta, usually the ascending aorta, and are sometimes accompanied by valvular aortic regurgitation [29].

Infectious Aortitis

SYPHILITIC AORTITIS. Aneurysms of the aorta resulting from cardiovascular syphilis follow interruption of the elastic fibers as a result of periaortitis and mesoaortitis, which thicken but weaken the aortic wall. Luetic aneurysms typically are saccular and involve the ascending aorta, whether or not the transverse and descending portions are also affected. Rupture is the major complication, but the enlarging aneurysm also may compress or erode adjacent structures of the mediastinum. Since the inflammatory process tends to interrupt the medial layer by transverse scars, dissection is distinctly uncommon. Approximately 40 percent of syphilitic aneurysms are located in the ascending aorta [30,31]. They may be associated with aortic valvular incompetence or coronary ostial stenosis; only a century ago, syphilis was more common than coronary atherosclerosis as a cause of angina pectoris. The aortic sinuses usually are not involved [32,33]. Approximately 50 percent of syphilitic aneurysms affect the arch [30]. The remainder occur in the descending thoracic aorta and abdominal aorta. Linear calcification of the wall of the ascending aorta may appear on roentgenography of the chest; that finding is not typically encountered in other types of aneurysmal disease of the ascending aorta. Although the prognosis for patients with uncomplicated syphilitic aortitis is comparable to that of the general population, the outlook is poor when syphilitic aneurysms of the aorta are large enough to produce symptoms [31,34,35]. Adequate antimicrobial therapy of early syphilis is the most important preventive measure. Aneurysmal disease caused by syphilis is subject to the same surgical considerations as aneurysms due to other causes.

Tuberculous Aortitis. Tuberculous involvement of the aorta may result in a true aneurysm, a false aneurysm, or stenosing aortoarteritis [36–38]. Aneurysmal dilatation and constricting lesions may coexist. The thoracic and abdominal aorta each may be affected.

Tuberculous aneurysms result usually from direct extension of infection from hilar lymph nodes or contiguous abscesses or from bacterial seeding. Granulomatous destruction of the medial layer leads to loss of aortic-wall elasticity. The posterior or posterolateral aortic wall is often the site of aneurysm formation in those cases. True aneurysms are saccular in appearance. A caseous granuloma may extend through the aortic wall, causing a perforation [36]. If that occurs, a thrombus or perivascular fibrosis may contain the rupture, prevent exsanguination, and produce a false aneurysm.

The stenotic form of tuberculous aortitis also is characterized by granulomatous lesions in the medial layer of the aortic wall and perivascular fibrosis [37]. The diagnosis of a tuberculous thoracic aortic aneurysm is suggested by other clinical evidence of the disease, including a characteristic chest x-ray demonstrating lymphadenopathy, cavitary lesions, apical scarring, or pleural effusions [36]. Often, a diffuse miliary pattern is evident. The aneurysm may appear as a mediastinal mass; it is rarely calcified. A tuberculous abdominal aortic aneurysm may present as an abdominal mass, possibly related to tuberculous spondylitis [36].

Mycotic Aneurysms. Primary mycotic aneurysms may occur as a consequence of infection with *Staphylococcus*, *Streptococcus*, *Salmonella*, *Pseudomonas*, and other gram-negative organisms, as well as fungi [39,40]. Bacterial infection of preexisting (usually atherosclerotic) aneurysms also occurs. Many cases arise as complications of infective endocarditis or arterial catheterization. An intrinsically abnormal aorta, however, may become infected as a consequence of bacteremia from any cause. Such infection produces suppurative aortitis, leading to weakness of a portion of the aortic wall. In those cases, aneurysms are typically saccular, and there is a comparatively high propensity to rupture (see Fig. 29-31).

Congenital Aneurysms. Congenital aortic aneurysms may be primary (idiopathic) or associated with other congenital anomalies such as a bicuspid aortic valve, coarctation of the aorta, and aneurysms of the sinuses of Valsalva [41–43]. They also occur in patients with inherited disorders of connective tissue such as Marfan syndrome and Ehlers-Danlos syndrome and in patients with tuberous sclerosis [44–48].

Idiopathic congenital aortic aneurysms may affect the thoracic or abdominal aorta. The aneurysms may be isolated or occur in association with additional aneurysms of the peripheral and visceral arteries [49]. Histologic examination often reveals intimal hyperplasia with fibrous caps, subendothelial lipid-laden foam cells, histiocytic giant cells, and degeneration of the media with fragmentation of the elastic fibers [49,50]. Cystic media necrosis is not characteristic of the disorder. Congenital aortic aneurysms that are associated with other anomalies or systemic disorders frequently affect the thoracic aorta and should be considered if clinical features characteristic of those disorders are present. Other causes of aortic aneurysms in childhood include trauma, bacterial infection, Takayasu arteritis, and Kawasaki disease [51–54].

Traumatic Aneurysms. Most common in the descending thoracic aorta just beyond the origin of the left subclavian artery, aneurysms may develop following penetrating or nonpenetrating chest trauma. Aneurysms may develop relatively late following aortic tear or transection of either the ascending or descending thoracic aorta. When the inciting injury involves blunt nonpenetrating trauma, pseudoaneurysms as well as true aneurysms may form [55]. Aortic injuries are relatively common consequences of severe blunt chest trauma and sudden deceleration. In one series of fatal automobile accidents, rupture of the thoracic aorta was found in over 15 percent of victims [28]. Similar damage may occur and lead to aortic rupture after falls from heights or from blast injuries. Thoracic aortic aneurysms resulting from sudden horizontal deceleration injury most commonly involve the relatively immobile isthmus just distal to the origin of the left subclavian artery, adjacent to the attachment of the ligamentum arteriosus. Vertical deceleration injuries more commonly produce rupture or aneurysm of the ascending aorta, often in its supravalvular portion or at the origin of the innominate artery. Surgical repair usually is advised, even when traumatic aneurysms are identified remote from the inciting injury because of the unpredictable course of the lesions, but clinical decision in a given case requires careful consideration of operative risk [56].

THORACIC AORTIC ANEURYSM

Aneurysms of the thoracic aorta can be divided into those involving the ascending thoracic aorta, the aortic arch, and the descending thoracic aorta. The etiology of the aneurysm, clinical manifestations, natural history, and surgical treatment differ, depending on its location in the thoracic aorta.

Etiology. The most common cause of ascending aortic aneurysm is cystic medial necrosis [15,16,57]. Although cystic medial necrosis occurs in patients with Marfan syndrome, it may occur in the absence of any clinical stigmata of that disorder. Aneurysms caused by cystic medial necrosis usually are fusiform and may involve the sinuses of Valsalva. Syphilis remains a common cause of aneurysm of the ascending aorta, although its frequency is considerably less than in the preantibiotic era [58]. Atherosclerosis is an unusual cause of ascending aortic aneurysms; when it is the etiology, there usually is evidence of atherosclerosis elsewhere. Atherosclerotic aneurysms are fusiform and typically extend into the arch. Mycotic aneurysms in that location are caused most frequently by infective endocarditis or infected angiographic catheters. Aortitis resulting from rheumatoid disorders is a relatively rare cause of ascending aortic aneurysms.

Aneurysms of the aortic arch occur more frequently in men than in women [59]. Their etiology is usually syphilis or atherosclerosis. They are often contiguous to aneurysms located in the ascending aorta; more frequently, however, atherosclerotic aneurysms affect the distal aspect of the arch and descending thoracic aorta [60]. As in the case of ascending aortic aneurysms, arch aneurysms caused by atherosclerosis usually are part of a more diffuse atherosclerotic process. Less frequent causes are cystic medial necrosis and bacterial or fungal infection. Mycotic aneurysms of the transverse arch most commonly are caused by tuberculosis as a result of direct extension from infected hilar nodes [58].

The majority of aneurysms of the descending thoracic aorta are caused by atherosclerosis [61–63] and may extend to the level of the abdominal aorta (see "Thoracoabdominal Aortic Aneurysm," later in this chapter). Typically, these aneurysms are fusiform and often begin distal to the origin of the left subclavian artery [64]. Syphilis is an unusual cause of descending thoracic aortic aneurysms, as are mycotic aneurysms secondary to bacterial infection, tuberculosis, or fungi [30]. Trauma may cause a descending thoracic aortic aneurysm. Descending thoracic aneurysms may also occur in patients with aortic coarctation [65].

Natural History and Prognosis. Etiology, size, and location of thoracic aortic aneurysms all contribute to their natural history. Syphilitic aneurysms, for example, tend to expand and rupture more frequently than atherosclerotic aneurysms [30]. Symptomatic patients have a much poorer prognosis than those who are asymptomatic, which may mean that symptoms indeed herald vascular catastrophe [31,32]. The overall rate of rupture approximates 40 to 50 percent [66,67]. In one autopsy series, the risk of rupture of aneurysms of the ascending aorta correlated with their diameter: rupture occurred in 2.3 percent of those aneurysms less than 5 cm, 11.5 percent of those 5 to 10 cm, and 44.4 percent of those greater than 10 cm in diameter [68].

Joyce and associates reviewed the natural history of 107 cases of untreated thoracic aortic aneurysms, most located in the descending aorta and due to atherosclerosis [62]. The prognosis was worse when the aneurysm was greater than 6 cm in diameter. Approximately one-third of deaths were attributed to aneurysm rupture, and nearly half to other associated cardiovascular disease, particularly coronary atherosclerosis. The 5-year mortality rate was 27 percent for patients with symptomatic aneurysms and 58 percent for the asymptomatic. In another study, 44 percent of patients with atherosclerotic aneurysms of the arch died of rupture [67]. The prognosis may be worse for patients with aneurysms of the arch than for those with aneurysms of other segments of the aorta [31].

Clinical Manifestations. Aneurysms of the thoracic aorta typically produce no symptoms, but a variety of symptom complexes may arise, related to the size of the aneurysm and its location within the thorax.

Patients with aneurysmal dilatation of the ascending aorta may develop clinical manifestations of congestive heart failure as a consequence of aortic valvular regurgitation. Enlargement of the sinuses of Valsalva may cause myocardial ischemia or infarction due to direct compression of the coronary arteries or coronary arterial thromboembolism [69]. Right ventricular outflow tract obstruction and tricuspid regurgitation may result from aneurysmal deformation of the noncoronary sinus [69]. Aneurysms of the sinuses of Valsalva may rupture directly into the right ventricular cavity, right atrium, or pulmonary artery, causing heart failure associated with a continuous murmur [70,71]. Chest pain may occur when the aneurysm compresses surrounding structures or erodes into adjacent bone, such as the ribs or sternum. Compression of the superior vena cava may produce venous congestion of the head, neck, and upper extremities. As noted, symptoms frequently are a harbinger of rupture or death. Rupture may occur into the left pleural space, pericardium, pulmonary artery, or superior vena cava [30,57,64].

Aneurysms of the aortic arch may produce symptoms by compression of contiguous structures, but most are asymptomatic. Dyspnea or cough may be caused by compression of the trachea or mainstem bronchi, dysphagia by compression of the esophagus, or hoarseness secondary to

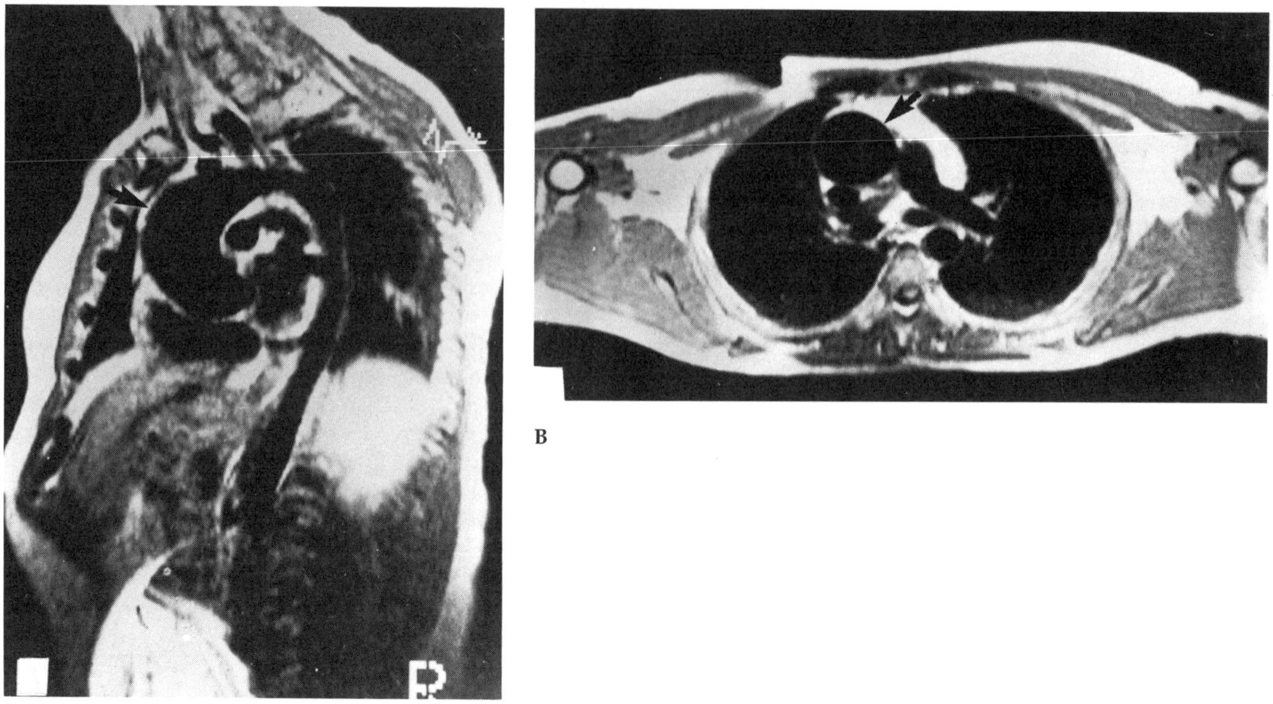

Fig. 39-4. Magnetic resonance image demonstrating a fusiform aneurysm (arrow) of the ascending thoracic aorta. **A.** Sagittal view. **B.** Transverse view.

left vocal cord paralysis related to compression of the left recurrent laryngeal nerve [72]. The superior vena cava syndrome and pulmonary artery stenosis result when those vessels are compressed [73–75]. Chest pain, related either to compression of adjacent structures or to erosion of ribs or vertebrae, typically is positional. Physical examination may demonstrate right sternoclavicular lift or tracheal deviation. Aneurysms of the aortic arch may rupture into the mediastinum, pleural space, tracheobronchial tree (causing hemoptysis), or esophagus (causing hematemesis). Arteriovenous fistulas may result from rupture into the superior vena cava or pulmonary artery.

Symptoms of descending thoracic aortic aneurysms include chest pain from compression of surrounding soft tissues or erosion of vertebrae. Irritation of the recurrent laryngeal nerve may produce hoarseness [65]. Dyspnea may result from bronchial compression, and hemoptysis from direct erosion into the lung parenchyma [76]. Dysphagia and hematemesis are features of esophageal compression or erosion. Rupture may occur into the mediastinum or left pleural space.

Diagnosis. Chest roentgenography is useful for evaluating aneurysms of the thoracic aorta and frequently is the first test to suggest the diagnosis in asymptomatic patients. Aneurysms of the ascending aorta usually are evident on the right side of the mediastinum. Aneurysms of the aortic arch widen the mediastinal shadow and may project more toward the left. These aneurysms may displace or compress the trachea or left mainstem bronchus. Descending thoracic aortic aneurysms typically appear as mediastinal masses extending into the left hemithorax. Adequate assessment of the aorta by chest roentgenography requires both posteroanterior and lateral projections. Failure to detect an ascending thoracic aortic aneurysm roentgenographically does not exclude the diagnosis, since aneurysms may not become apparent until considerable dilatation has occurred.

Two-dimensional ultrasound imaging can be used to assess the proximal ascending aorta and detect an ascending thoracic aortic aneurysm. Contrast-enhanced computed tomography is a sensitive and specific test for assessent of aneurysms of the thoracic aorta [77]. Magnetic resonance imaging is increasingly favored as a noninvasive method for diagnosis of aneurysms of the thoracic aorta [78,79] (Fig. 39-4). MRI can demonstrate the size and extent of a thoracic aortic aneurysm as well as its relationship to the vessels of the aortic arch.

Contrast aortography is the principal diagnostic test for confirming an aneurysm of the thoracic aorta and for determining its length and diameter (Fig. 39-5). Although the noninvasive diagnostic procedures discussed above may be adequate to establish the diagnosis, aortography is required preoperatively to address the length of the aneurysm and involvement of branch vessels.

Treatment. Medical therapy of patients with aneurysms of the thoracic aorta is directed at control of hypertension and other measures designed to reduce the circulatory forces that tend to lead to expansion. The magnitude of

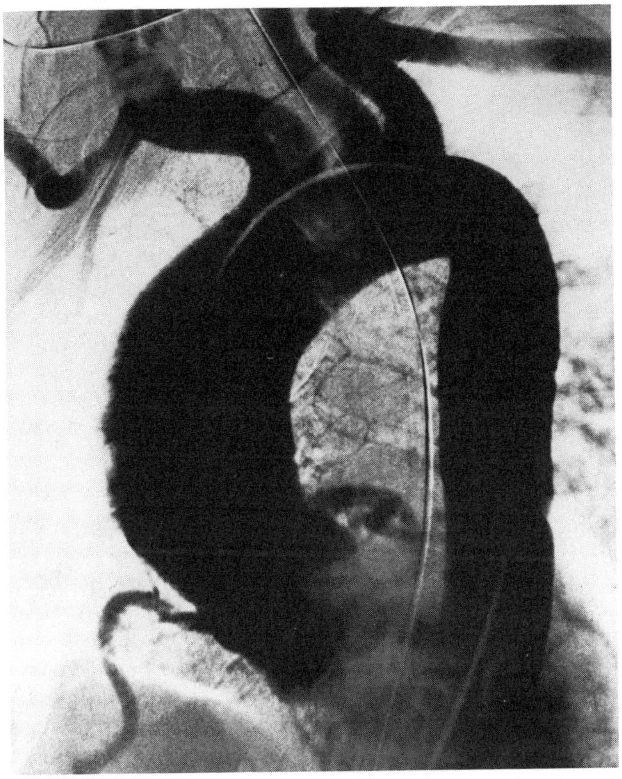

Fig. 39-5. Aortogram demonstrating a fusiform aneurysm of the ascending thoracic aorta in a patient with Marfan syndrome.

the aortic impulse is related not only to the level of systolic blood pressure but also to the rate of rise of pressure during that phase of the cardiac cycle (dP/dt). Agents that reduce arterial wall stress, such as the beta-adrenergic antagonists, may be favored; a controlled trial found that propranolol slowed the progression of aortic dilatation and reduced the development of clinical complications in patients with Marfan syndrome [80]. Whether that benefit applies to patients with other forms of aortic aneurysmal disease remains to be determined.

Timing of surgical intervention is controversial in the asymptomatic patient and depends on the location and etiology of the aneurysm and the age and general condition of the patient. Fusiform aneuryms of the thoracic aorta 5 cm or larger in patients with Marfan syndrome generally are considered appropriate for repair; in non-Marfan patients, it is usually safe to withhold surgical intervention until the aneurysm reaches 6 cm or larger [81]. Symptomatic aneurysms have a relatively high rate of rupture, and such cases typically are referred for surgery, as are those associated with severe aortic-valve insufficiency [19].

The surgical approach to the repair of thoracic aortic aneurysms consists of replacement of the diseased portion of the vessel, with technical variations depending on the segment involved. Thus, it is useful to consider repair of aneurysms of the ascending aorta, transverse arch, and descending aorta separately [82]. Surgical repair of aneurysms of the proximal ascending aorta is approached through a median sternotomy and routinely employs extracorporeal bypass. The aorta is clamped just proximal to the origin of the brachiocephalic artery and the aneurysm sac opened longitudinally along its anterolateral aspect between the ostia of the coronary arteries. Aneurysms without associated valvular insufficiency can be replaced with a simple tube graft. More commonly, however, ascending aortic aneurysms dilate the aortic annulus or coronary sinus sufficiently to warrant replacement of both the valve and the ascending aorta with a composite valve graft [83]. In such cases, the valve end of the graft is sutured to the aortic valvular annulus following excision of the native cusps. Elliptical patches of graft are excised adjacent to the ostia of the two coronary vessels, which subsequently are directly reimplanted. Finally, the distal end of the graft is sutured to the distal ascending arch just proximal to the brachiocephalic vessel. The distal aortic suture line frequently is reinforced with an outer strip of Teflon to prevent sutures from tearing out of attenuated aortic tissue. Thirty-day operative survival using those methods is now anticipated to exceed 90 percent [82,84]. In patients with thoracic aneurysms secondary to cystic medial necrosis, survival at 1, 3, and 5 years following surgery approximates 72, 64, and 57 percent, respectively [85].

Aneurysms of the transverse arch often are divided into two subgroups [82,86]. Those involving the distal arch can be repaired without the use of cardiopulmonary bypass by placing the proximal clamp just distal to the origin of the brachiocephalic vessel and using pharmacologic means to reduce afterload. If the aneurysm involves less than 50 percent of the circumference of the vessel, a simple elliptical patch graft can be used, as opposed to tube replacement, for a more expeditious repair. Aneurysms involving more than 50 percent of the circumference, however, are best repaired with a tube graft anastomosed distally first, then proximally. The left subclavian and left common carotid arteries may be directly reimplanted on the graft through separate ostia, through a common ostium, or reperfused using side-limb grafts. The second group of more extensive lesions involves the proximal arch and, therefore, the innominate artery and requires cardiac arrest with extracorporeal bypass. The distal aorta is cross-clamped, the aneurysm opened longitudinally throughout the anterolateral surface of the arch, and the distal anastomosis constructed using standard technique. An elliptical patch of Dacron on its superior aspect is excised, to which is anastomosed a contiguous elliptical section of aorta containing the ostia of the three brachiocephalic vessels. Finally, the proximal anastomosis is constructed to the ascending aorta or, in the case of more extensive aneurysmal disease, to a composite valve conduit, as described above. The 30-day operative mortality associated with repair of aneurysms of the aortic arch has been reduced substantially during the past decade. Utilizing the approaches outlined here, it is anticipated that operative survival will consistently exceed 90 percent [82].

Aneurysms involving the more distal descending thoracic aorta are best repaired through a posterolateral or thoracoabdominal incision [87]. Isolated descending tho-

Table 39-2. Classification of thoracoabdominal aneurysm

Group	Involvement
I	Thoracic and abdominal aorta without involvement of visceral vessels
II	Thoracic and abdominal aorta with visceral vessels
III	Distal thoracic and abdominal visceral vessels
IV	Abdominal aorta with visceral vessels

racic aneurysms are repaired with a simple tube graft and do not require cardiopulmonary bypass. Aneurysms involving both the arch and the distal descending thoracic aorta are best approached in two separate stages. The initial proximal repair is carried out through a median sternotomy and, a few months later, repair of the distal segment. Thirty-day operative survival for repair of descending thoracic aortic aneurysms, either atherosclerotic in origin or resulting from chronic dissection, also exceeds 90 percent. The incidence of paraplegia and paraparesis is less than 5 percent overall. Repair of acute aortic dissections involving the descending aorta, however, is still associated with a much lower (40–50%) 30-day survival and a slightly higher incidence (8%) of paraplegia [82].

Transluminal placement of endovascular stent grafts is undergoing investigation as a less invasive means to repair thoracic aortic aneurysms. The stent graft comprises two balloon-expandable stents, situated at each end of a Dacron graft. The stents are deployed proximally and distally to the aneurysm, resulting in exclusion and thrombosis of the aneurysmal sac. The stent graft is inserted via surgical cutdown and arteriotomy of the femoral artery while the patient is under general anesthesia and advanced under fluoroscopic guidance to the level of the aneurysm. In a recent report, custom-designed endovascular stent grafts were deployed successfully in 13 selected patients with thoracic aneurysms [88]. The aneurysm surrounding the graft thrombosed in 12 of the patients. There were no deaths and no complications such as paraplegia or embolization.

THORACOABDOMINAL AORTIC ANEURYSM

As suggested by the nomenclature, thoracoabdominal aortic aneurysms have features of both thoracic and abdominal aortic aneurysms. Although thoracoabdominal aneurysms constitute only about 3 percent of all aortic aneurysms, they are considered as a separate class, because of the diffuse and extensive aortic involvement and special considerations for surgical repair, which may entail reimplantation of the origins of visceral arteries [68]. Among the various proposed classification schemes, Crawford and colleagues delineated four types of thoracoabdominal aortic aneurysms according to the segment and extent of aorta involved [89] (Table 39-2; see also Fig. 29-29). In keeping with the notion that thoracoabdominal aortic aneurysms essentially represent a diffusely atherosclerotic and ectatic aorta with one or more aneurysmal segments of variable length, two types that are essentially confined to the abdominal aorta are included. The principal clinical implication is that surgical repair may require reimplantation or reconstruction of the origins of major branch arteries, which entails risks of ischemic-tissue injury greater than those associated with aneurysmectomy alone.

Etiology. Atherosclerosis is now the most common etiology of thoracoabdominal aortic aneurysms, but syphilis previously accounted for a larger proportion [90,91]. Other types, including those related to cystic medial necrosis, tuberculosis, mycosis, and trauma occur less often [92–96]. Thoracoabdominal aneurysms occur more frequently in males than in females, at least in the Western hemisphere.

Natural History. Because they occur infrequently, compared with discrete aneurysms of the aorta, relatively little information is available regarding the natural history of thoracoabdominal aneurysms. The etiologic factors and clinical presentation are more comparable to aneurysms of the abdominal than the thoracic aorta; thus, it has been speculated that the risk of rupture is similar to that of abdominal aortic aneurysms of equivalent diameter. In an autopsy series involving 7,642 cases between 1935 and 1954, Fomon and co-workers found 7 thoracoabdominal aneurysms, 4 of which had ruptured [68]. The patients manifested diffuse atherosclerosis, and mortality might have been a consequence of concomitant coronary or cerebral vascular disease.

Clinical Presentation. Although most patients with thoracoabdominal aortic aneurysms are asymptomatic, discomfort occasionally develops in the epigastrium or left upper quadrant of the abdomen. Back or flank pain may occur when the patient lies in the left lateral decubitus position. Erosion of the anterior surfaces of the vertebral bodies may occur, leading to radiculopathy [9,97,98]. Visceral artery occlusion may occur, but frank ischemia and infarction are infrequent [68]. Patients who complain of claudication also may have occlusive atherosclerotic disease of the aorta, iliac, or more distal arteries. Because mural thrombosis is so common in atherosclerotic aneurysms, they may be the source of peripheral atheroembolism, causing occlusion of distal vessels [99,100]. Rupture of the thoracic component of the aneurysms generally occurs into the left pleural space, producing a hemothorax; the abdominal component may rupture into the retroperitoneum, inferior vena cava, or duodenum.

Diagnosis. Thoracoabdominal aortic aneurysm may be suspected when there is prominent widening of the epigastric pulsation. The hands of the examiner should be placed along the lateral aspects of the pulsatile mass and systolic separation estimated. There may not be the palpable superior shelflike contour that is often encountered with abdominal aortic aneurysms. An epigastric bruit is a nonspecific finding that is not necessarily diagnostic of aneurysm. Other findings on physical examination that reflect coexisting atherosclerosis include diminished or absent arterial pulses and vascular bruits elsewhere. There also may be evidence of peripheral aneurysmal disease,

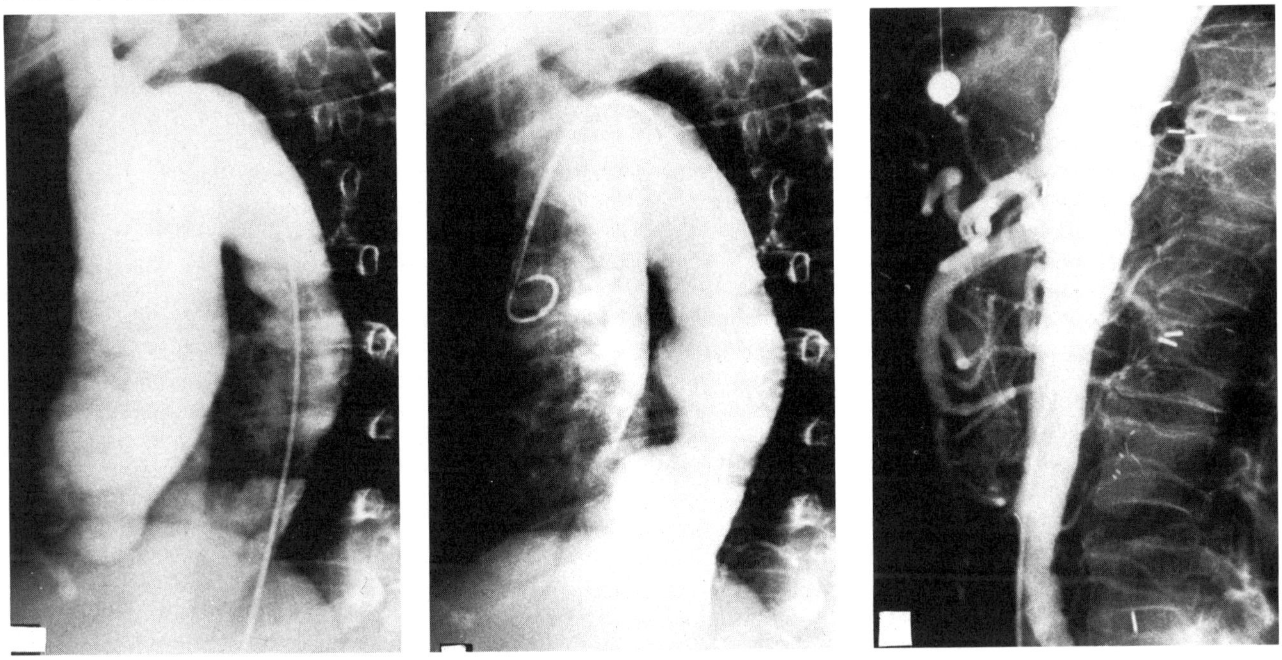

A B C

Fig. 39-6. Aortogram demonstrating an extensive thoracoabdominal aortic aneurysm. **A.** Ascending thoracic aorta. **B.** Descending thoracic aorta. **C.** Abdominal aorta.

particularly that involving the femoral or popliteal arteries.

Anteroposterior and "across-table" lateral abdominal roentgenograms may reveal evidence of a thoracoabdominal aortic aneurysm when there is calcification in the opposing walls of the aorta. Abdominal ultrasonography helps confirm the diagnosis and detect extension of the aneurysm proximal to the renal or even the mesenteric arteries. Ultrasound examination provides a reliable estimate of the diameter of the aneurysm in the abdomen and may demonstrate thrombus formation on the intimal surface extending into the lumen of the aneurysm.

Computed tomography is particularly useful for outlining the length as well as the diameter and shape of thoracoabdominal aortic aneurysms. The accuracy of CT is enhanced by injection of intravenous contrast material, which is usually necessary to define the relationship of the aneurysm to the mesenteric and renal arteries [77,101,102]. RI is another imaging technique to aid diagnosis of thoracoabdominal aneurysms [78,103].

Unlike routine cases of abdominal aortic aneurysm, aortography is required prior to operative correction of thoracoabdominal aneurysms, since the relationship of aneurysm to adjacent vascular structures, including branch arteries, must be carefully defined (Fig. 39-6). This modality also provides useful information about concomitant distal arterial occlusive disease and incidental anomalies of the urinary tract, such as an overriding horseshoe kidney, that could influence the surgical approach.

Treatment. Operative technique has evolved over the past three decades and is influenced by the location of the aneurysm. In 1955, Ellis and colleagues repaired an abdominal aortic aneurysm that involved the origin of the right renal artery using a side-arm aortic homograft [104]. Shortly thereafter, repair of an upper abdominal aortic aneurysm was reported by Etheredge and colleagues in which temporary bypass of the aorta was achieved with a polyethylene tube, and the celiac and superior mesenteric arteries were anastomosed directly to an aortic homograft [97]. DeBakey and co-workers performed a series of thoracoabdominal aortic reconstruction procedures using a temporary shunt and aortic homograft, and his group ultimately introduced the technique of aortic bypass through a Dacron conduit to which the visceral arteries were attached [100]. The mortality rate associated with such a procedure was about 25 percent.

Currently, most surgeons use a modification of the method advanced by Crawford and colleagues [89] (see Fig. 29-28). Abdominal aortic aneurysms extending proximal to the renal arteries can be approached through a midline incision in the anterior abdominal wall. The more extensive aneurysms involving the descending thoracic aortic segment require a left thoracoabdominal incision. Exposure is gained by retracting the stomach, spleen, pancreatic tail, left kidney, and descending colon, and the diaphragm is incised. Following minimal dissection of the aorta just beyond the proximal and distal margins of the aneurysm, the aorta is cross-clamped. The increased myocardial afterload imposed at this stage is reduced with the administration of vasodilator medication such as sodium nitroprusside, and the renal arteries may be perfused with a chilled, pH-balanced, saline solution. The left lateral aspect of the aorta is incised, and a woven Dacron graft is inserted into the aneurysmal sac and anastomosed to the less diseased portion of the aortic wall. Intercostal and visceral arterial ostia are incorporated into the graft. After the distal anastomosis has been completed, the clamps are gradually released. Blood pressure and cardiac filling pressures are monitored, and fluids are administered to restore hemodynamic stability. The sac of the aneurysm then is wrapped around the outside of the prosthetic graft, to protect the overlying viscera from erosion.

Thoracoabdominal aneurysm repair currently carries a mortality rate between 5 and 10 percent [85,105–107]. Ischemic injury to the spinal cord (paraplegia or paraparesis) appears after 9 to 16 percent of all such procedures and most often (13–30%) after repair of the more extensive type II cases [107,108]. It appears that the risk of spinal-cord injury may be minimized by limiting aortic cross-clamp time and by providing both spinal-fluid drainage and distal aortic perfusion with either preliminary axillofemoral bypass graft or intraoperative atriofemoral bypass [107]. Efforts to preserve intercostal and lumbar arterial blood supply to the spinal cord are made in an attempt to reduce the occurrence of this feared complication. Among the more common major adverse consequences of thoracoabdominal aortic aneurysm repair is renal insufficiency in approximately 9 percent of patients, often transient but sometimes sufficient to require long-term hemodialysis. Myocardial infarction may occur because associated coronary atherosclerosis tends to be severe. Other morbid events include congestive heart failure, pneumonia, respiratory insufficiency, and infection. Crawford's group reported that the 5-year survival rate for patients surviving thoracoabdominal aortic aneurysm repair approximates 60 percent [105]. That rate compares favorably with the outcome in patients who have undergone abdominal aortic aneurysm repair.

ABDOMINAL AORTIC ANEURYSM

The designation *abdominal aortic aneurysm* implies that the diameter of the infrarenal segment of the aorta is at least one-and-a-half times the diameter measured at the level of the renal arteries [108]. It has been suggested that the term *aneurysm* be restricted to situations where the diameter of the aorta exceeds 3 cm [108]. In over 90 percent of cases, the superior margins of abdominal aortic aneurysms are below the level of the renal arteries [109–111].

Aneurysms of the abdominal aorta account for approximately 15,000 deaths annually in the United States [112]. The incidence of abdominal aortic aneurysms in autopsy series have ranged from 1.8 to 6.6 percent of cases, leading to an estimated occurrence rate of 15 to 37 cases per 100,000 patient-years [113–123]. The incidence increases with age, ranging from less than 2.1 per 100,000 patient-years between the ages of 40 and 49 to more than 280 per 100,000 patient-years among individuals older than 80 [124,125]. Abdominal aortic aneurysms occur two to five times more frequently in males than in females, and more often in whites than in blacks [124,125]. One autopsy series reported an incidence of 4.2 percent among white males compared with 1.5 percent among black males [117]. The prevalence of abdominal aortic aneurysms is higher in patients with clinical evidence of atherosclerosis. In patients with coronary artery disease, for instance, the prevalence of abdominal aneurysms is approximately 5 percent, and nearly 10 percent of patients with atherosclerotic peripheral arterial obstructive disease have associated aortic aneurysms in the abdomen [116,124–126].

Etiology. Atherosclerosis has been held responsible for at least 90 percent of all abdominal aortic aneurysms, although some authors have suggested that atherosclerosis may be a secondary phenomenon in aneurysmal disease [108,127–130]. Aneurysmal atherosclerotic disease seems to differ from stenotic disease in that there frequently is generalized arteriomegaly, epithelial neoplasia, and an increased incidence of inguinal hernias in patients with aneurysms [130–133]. Several reports of familial clustering of abdominal aortic aneurysm have appeared, and decreased type 3 collagen and elastin content of the aortic wall as well as increased collagenase activity have been identified in some familial cases [115,118,134–141]. Whether atherosclerosis is the inciting cause of abdominal aortic aneurysms or a cofactor in otherwise predisposed individuals remains to be determined [142,143]. Cigarette smoking and hypertension have been implicated as related causal factors [144,145]. It has been proposed that atherosclerosis may represent a secondary response to vascular injury resulting from primary changes in elastin and collagen in patients predisposed to abdominal aortic aneurysm [146].

Cystic medial necrosis is an infrequent cause of abdominal aortic aneurysms. If the abdominal aorta is involved in patients with Marfan syndrome or Ehlers-Danlos syndrome, it usually is part of a thoracoabdominal aneurysm. Mycotic aneurysms, particularly those due to *Salmonella* species, when confined to the abdomen, often occur at the site of a preexisting atherosclerotic lesion [108,130]. Syphilitic aneurysms usually are located in the thoracic aorta but do occur occasionally in the abdomen. The vasculitides, such as Takayasu arteritis, may lead to abdominal aortic aneurysms during either the early systemic inflammatory stage or the later degenerative stage; this disease is more frequently the cause of abdominal aneurysms than is giant cell arteritis [147].

Natural History. Survival is limited in patients with abdominal aortic aneurysms because of the potential for aortic rupture and the prevalence of coronary artery disease (Fig. 39-7). In 1950, Estes reported the prognosis of 102 patients with abdominal aortic aneurysms identified on physical examination or roentgenography, almost all of which were atherosclerotic [148]. Survival at 1 year was 67 percent, at 3 years 49 percent, and at 5 years 19 percent. Of the fatalities, 63 percent were related to rupture of the aneurysm. Similar statistics have been reported by others [149–151]. Several investigators have examined the relation between the diameter of the aneurysm and risk of rupture. Darling and associates reviewed 24,000 consecutive autopsies over a 23-year period and found 591 cases of abdominal aortic aneurysm, of which 118 had ruptured. Rupture occurred in 9.5 percent of aneurysms smaller than 4 cm in maximum diameter, 25 percent of those 4 to 7 cm, 45 percent of those 7 to 10 cm, and 60 percent

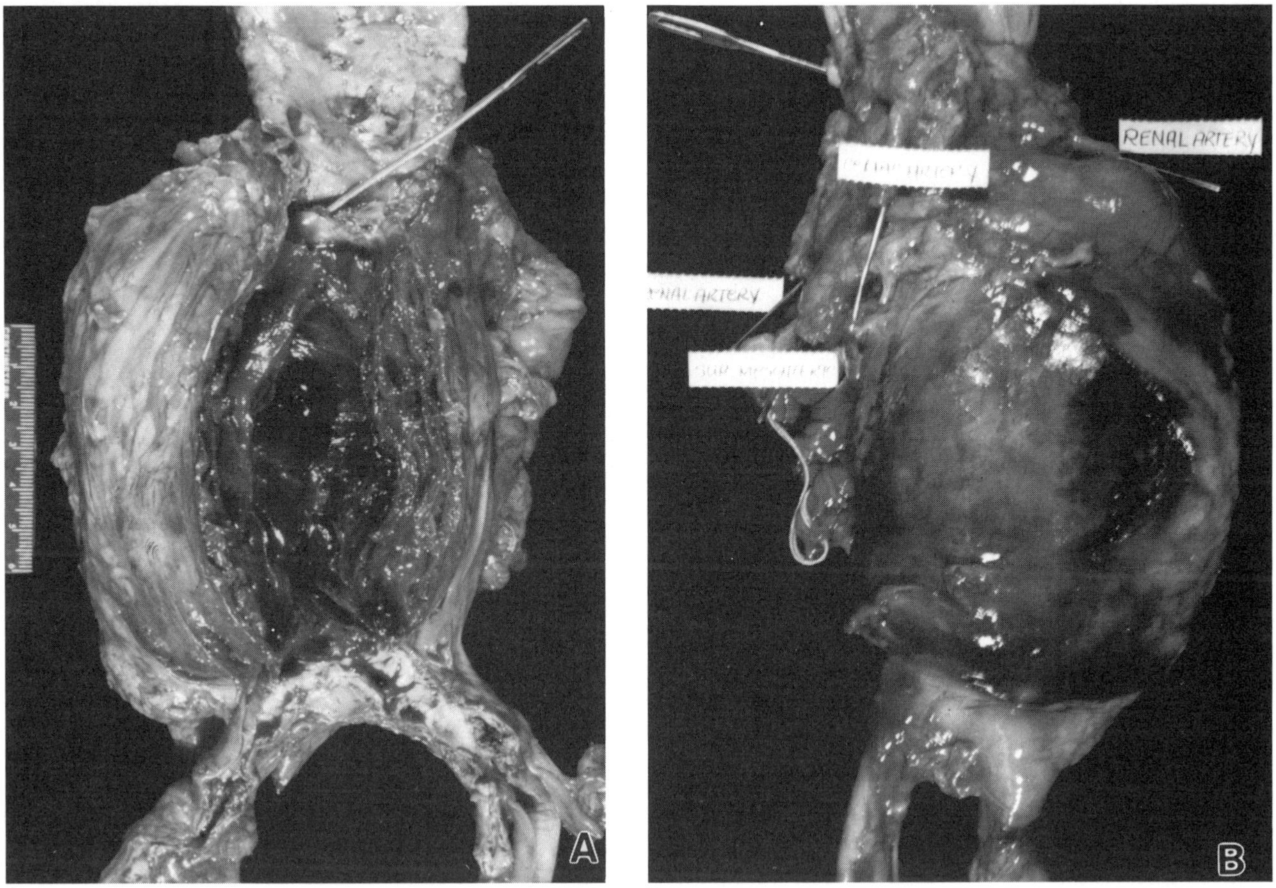

A B

Fig. 39-7. Abdominal aortic aneurysm complicated by fatal rupture. **A.** Open view demonstrating near-complete thrombosis. **B.** Closed, anterior view. The site of rupture is the darkened crescent-shaped area at 3 o'clock. (Reproduced with permission from FJ Schoen, Interventional and Surgical Cardiovascular Pathology. Philadelphia: Saunders, 1989.)

of aneurysms larger than 10 cm in diameter [117]. Szilagyi and co-workers compared survival rates in patients with abdominal aortic aneurysms less than and greater than 6 cm in diameter [152]. Survival rate for those with the smaller aneurysms was 75 percent after 1 year, 68 percent after 3 years, and 48 percent after 5 years. For those with aneurysms larger than 6 cm, the first-year survival rate was 48 percent, at 3 years 12 percent, and at 5 years 6 percent. Those authors later reported follow-up of 127 patients deemed medically unfit for surgery (predominantly because of severe coexisting coronary artery disease). Over a follow-up period of up to 20 years, 71 percent of the patients had died, 28 percent because of rupture [153]. Bickerstaff and colleagues followed patients with abdominal aneurysm over a 30-year period and recorded rupture in 20.3 percent of the patients, most with aneurysms over 5 cm in diameter [154]. Foster and colleagues reported the following survival rates in patients with untreated abdominal aortic aneurysms: 62 percent after 1 year, 32 percent after 3 years, and 19 percent after 5 years. Thirty-eight percent of the patients in that series died as a consequence of rupture; 55 percent of those with aneurysms larger than 6 cm died of rupture compared with 16 percent of those with aneurysms smaller than 6 cm in diameter [155]. Bernstein and Chan followed patients whose aneurysms were initially 3 to 6 cm in diameter; in those, the mean expansion rate was 0.4 cm per year [156]. More recently, Nevitt and associates reported an average rate of expansion of 0.21 cm per year; 24 percent expanded at a rate faster than 0.4 cm per year. In that series, there were no cases of rupture over a period of 5 years among patients with aneurysms less than 5 cm in diameter, while 25 percent of those with aneurysms greater than 5 cm in diameter suffered that complication [157]. The validity of those observations have been questioned, however, because patients with leakage within 48 hours of ultrasound examination were excluded from analysis [146].

The pathophysiologic processes that underlie aneurysmal expansion have not been clearly defined, but they appear to involve elastolysis and collagenolysis, promoted by inflammatory changes in the aortic wall, accelerated by hypertension [158]. Despite the greater risk of rupture with large aneurysms, it has been difficult to establish a clear correlation between the rate of aneurysm expansion and the risk of rupture. The problem may be one of observational methodology, however, and there is little reason to doubt that rapid expansion is a harbinger of rupture [159]. The clinician's dictum that expansion of abdominal aortic aneurysm at a rate in excess of 1 cm annually is predictive of rupture within 2 years is probably more true for atherosclerotic aneurysms over 5 cm in diameter than for others. It is also widely believed but difficult to prove that symptomatic aneurysms or those that generate a local or systemic inflammatory response show an earlier propensity to rupture.

Clinical Presentation. The prevalence of abdominal aortic aneurysm increases with age, occurring more frequently in patients aged 60 to 70 years than in younger individuals, although affected individuals range in age from 30 to over 90 years [111,129,160,161]. Coronary artery disease, peripheral arterial occlusive disease, and other manifestations of systemic atherosclerosis occur frequently in patients with abdominal aortic aneurysms, and hypertension often coexists [110,130,148,162]. Whether hypertension correlates with the risk of rupture is controversial [109,154,163].

Most patients with abdominal aortic aneurysms are asymptomatic, yet symptoms may take the form of abdominal discomfort or back pain, and some patients become aware of abdominal pulsation [110,164,165]. Less frequently, pain may occur in the legs, chest, or groin; anorexia, nausea, vomiting, constipation, or dyspnea may develop [148,149]. Compression of the left iliac vein may cause left leg swelling, just as compression of the left ureter may cause hydronephrosis or compression of testicular veins may cause varicocele. As the aneurysm expands and compresses vertebrae and lumbar nerve roots, pain may develop in the lower back and may radiate to the posterior aspects of the legs. Flank pain radiating to the anterior left thigh or scrotum may reflect compression of the left genitofemoral nerve. Nausea and vomiting may occur as the aneurysm compresses the duodenum. Bladder compression may cause urinary frequency or urgency.

The key physical finding is a pulsatile abdominal mass. Typically, aneurysms larger than 4 cm in diameter are palpable, except those occurring in obese individuals or in cases where adequate examination is made difficult by guarding. The patient should be positioned supine with the knees flexed. A pulsatile epigastric or periumbilical mass may be visible as well as palpable. To distinguish an abdominal aortic aneurysm from para-aortic masses requires that the examiner's hands address the lateral borders. An aneurysm expands laterally with each systole. This technique also permits estimation of the transverse diameter of the aneurysm [166]. Auscultation may reveal a bruit over the mass, but abdominal bruits are not specific for aneurysm formation, and only about 40 percent of such aneurysms are associated with bruits. The finding of a pulsatile mass in the groin, suggesting an iliac-artery aneurysm, or in the popliteal fossa, suggesting a popliteal-artery aneurysm, further raises the index of suspicion that an abdominal aortic aneurysm may be present, since multiple aneurysms often coexist. Physical signs may reflect atherosclerosis of other vessels, including carotid bruits or diminished arterial pulses in the lower extremities.

Rupture of an abdominal aortic aneurysm usually produces the clinical picture of extreme distress as a result of abdominal catastrophe. Despite surgical advances, mortality is still the rule because of the abrupt nature of circulatory collapse, which prevents timely intervention in most cases. Patients frequently have severe abdominal or back pain, but the pattern of pain varies considerably and may be either persistent or intermittent, sharp or dull, constricting or burning. The aneurysm may rupture into the retroperitoneum or into the peritoneal or pleural cavities. Patients may develop hypotension, tachycardia, pallor, diaphoresis, or deep shock, depending on the extent of rupture and associated blood loss into the extravascular space. On occasion, rupture occurs directly into the duodenum, causing an aortoduodenal fistula and acute gastrointestinal bleeding. That possibility should be considered when gastrointestinal bleeding is evident along with signs of an aneurysm on physical examination. Rupture also may occur into the inferior vena cava or iliac veins, producing an arteriovenous fistula; that is suggested by rapid development of leg swelling or "high-output" congestive heart failure in the presence of an abdominal aortic aneurysm.

Diagnosis. Several diagnostic procedures are available to confirm the presence of an abdominal aortic aneurysm and provide information regarding its diameter and length. Plain roentgenography frequently discloses an unsuspected aneurysm [110]. Anteroposterior and lateral views may disclose a curvilinear rim of calcification in the wall of the aneurysm, and the diameter of the aneurysm can be estimated when such calcification is visible in two opposing walls [110,167–170] (Fig. 39-8). In 25 to 50 percent of suspected cases, however, the walls of the aneurysm are not sufficiently calcified to permit radiographic identification [110,167–169,171–173]. Furthermore, it may underestimate anteroposterior aneurysm size by 15 percent [166].

The most useful noninvasive technique to assess abdominal aortic aneurysms is real-time ultrasound imaging, which offers a sensitivity approaching 100 percent [174]. Details of vascular sonography are discussed in Chap. 19 (see Fig. 19-9). The abdominal aorta is subject to anteroposterior, transverse, and longitudinal evaluation. Sonographic classification of abdominal aortic aneurysms begins when the maximum diameter exceeds 3 cm, in either anteroposterior or transverse dimensions. Care must be taken to image the aorta perpendicular to its longitudinal axis to avoid eccentricity, which may lead to overestimation of the true diameter. Thrombus frequently is identified in the lumen, and echodense calcification may be present in or adjacent to the aortic wall. Beyond determining the size of an aneurysm, ultrasound imaging may help define the relation of major arterial branches and adjacent organs. Certain ultrasound characteristics have potential value in predicting rupture. Intramural hematoma, appearing as a hypoechoic soft-tissue mass surrounding the aorta, which may silhouette the psoas muscle, appears to represent such a sign. It may be indistinguishable from periaortic fibrosis, which ultrasound examination shows as a hypoechoic mantle sur-

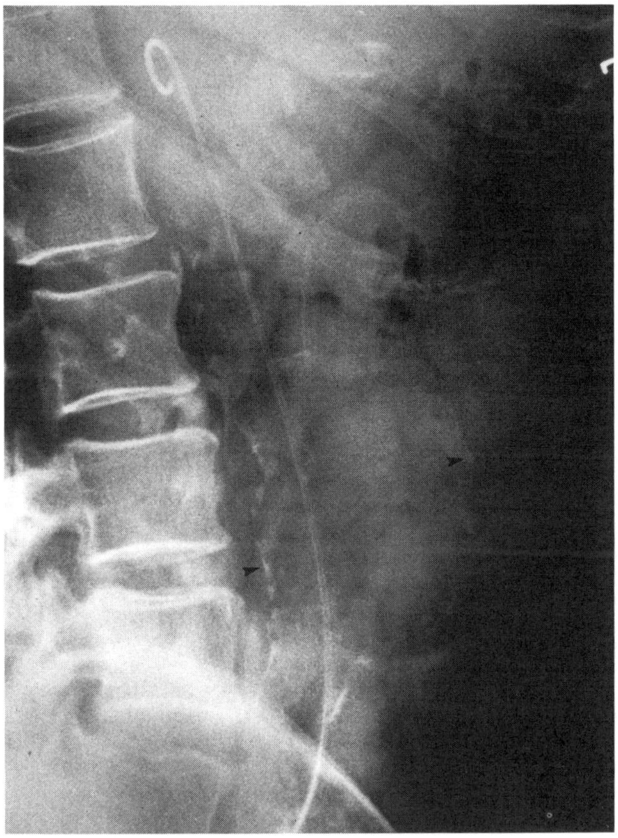

Fig. 39-8. Calcified anterior and posterior walls of an abdominal aortic aneurysm are illustrated on this lateral abdominal roentgenogram.

rounding the aortic wall in patients with inflammatory aortic aneurysms.

CT is an accurate test for determining aneurysm dimensions and the relation of major visceral branches and for detection of intraluminal mural thrombi [175,177] (Figs. 39-9, 39-10; see also Fig. 23-5). Calcification and inflammatory thickening of the aortic wall may be identified. A low-density para-aortic hematoma formation may indicate contained rupture. The false lumen of aortic dissection can be demonstrated using contrast enhancement and distinguished from the inferior vena cava, renal veins, and ureters [178]. In cases of ruptured abdominal aortic aneurysm, CT may disclose high-density blood collection in the retroperitoneal space [179–181].

MRI is not yet in widespread clinical use for evaluation of patients with abdominal aortic aneurysms. MRI holds promise as a means of more closely examining changes in the aortic wall that may reflect the potential for such rupture, compression of extraaortic structures, or thromboembolic complications. Because air in the overlying lung limits the utility of ultrasound for imaging of the descending thoracic aorta throughout its length, MRI has acquired a wider scope in the evaluation of thoracoabdominal aortic aneurysms than those confined to the abdomen.

Aortic angiography is not as essential a diagnostic procedure for the diagnosis of abdominal aortic aneurysms as might be imagined because the noninvasive tests discussed above generally are accurate. The procedure is performed to define associated vascular pathoanatomy, particularly when there are unusual features or prior to a more extensive reconstructive surgical procedure (see Fig. 39-1). The apparent lumen filled with contrast may substantially underestimate the true size of the aneurysm, because laminar thrombus often is present within the aneurysm. Aortography is most useful for studying associated renal, mesenteric, or spinal arterial occlusive disease or for determining whether there is atherosclerotic narrowing of the iliofemoral arteries. Angiography can delineate the superior and inferior margins of the aneurysmal segment and may suggest additional aneurysms proximal or distal to the abdominal aorta [172,182–184]. The risks of angiography, which include hematoma formation, atheroembolism, allergic reactions, and renal insufficiency, must be considered when deciding whether to undertake the procedure preoperatively.

A controversial area is the role of population-based screening programs for abdominal aortic aneurysm to provide selective surgical intervention before rupture occurs. The cost effectiveness of that strategy is based on the ratio of the expense of screening tests to the value of lives saved. Although such a model requires a number of assumptions and generalizations, selective screening may be cost effective when focused on a population at high risk, such as patients between 55 and 80 years old, and those with hypertension, aneurysms involving other parts of the arterial system, or a family history of abdominal aortic aneurysm [187,188].

Treatment. Since the first resection of abdominal aortic aneurysm was reported by Dubost and colleagues in 1952, impressive advances have taken place in the technique and outcome of surgical treatment [185]. In experienced hands, the in-hospital perioperative mortality rate has declined from a range of 3–9 percent to 1–2 percent over the past two decades [190–197]. The improvement in operative statistics and the increased knowledge of the natural history of abdominal aortic aneurysms have led to the targeting of patients for elective surgical intervention at earlier stages of the disease. Currently, elective repair is recommended for patients with aneurysms larger than 5 cm in diameter, as measured by B-mode ultrasound or CT imaging. In selected cases in which the operative risk is excessive due to severe cardiac or pulmonary disease, renal insufficiency, or other comorbidity, surgery might be deferred. If the prognosis from those other medical conditions is such that survival beyond 2 years is anticipated, it might then be appropriate to proceed with aneurysmectomy when the maximum diameter of the aorta reaches 5–6 cm. Serial noninvasive examinations are advised in asymptomatic patients to detect enlargement, since the rate of aneurysm expansion prior to rupture may be erratic. The autopsy study by Darling and colleagues argued for surgical repair of some abdominal aortic aneurysms at a diameter of 4 cm. While that is certainly appropriate for patients who are symptomatic, the management of aortic aneurysms less than 5 cm in diameter remains

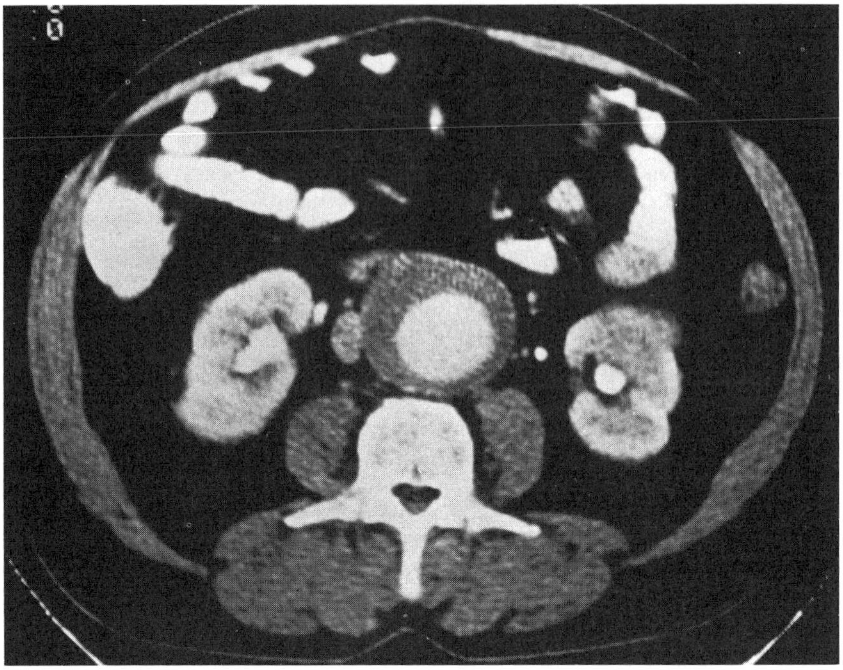

Fig. 39-9. CT scan of an abdominal aortic aneurysm performed with contrast. Note the aneurysm, just anterior to the vertebral body, consisting of a lumen, highlighted by contrast, surrounded by thrombus.

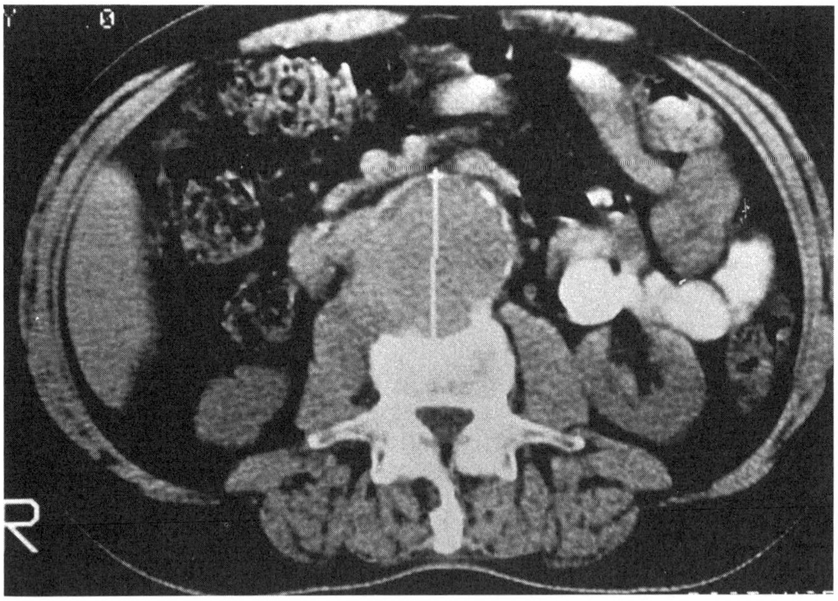

Fig. 39-10. CT scan of an abdominal aortic aneurysm that has been eroding the vertebral body.

controversial [116,184–195]. Emergency surgery is required as a life-saving procedure in patients presenting with aneurysm rupture.

The principles of aneurysm surgery are described in Chapter 29 (see Fig. 29-27). In general, the graft-inclusion technique originally described by Javid and co-workers and Creech is employed [198,199]. Following midline incision and retroperitoneal exposure, periaortic dissection is limited to minimize intraoperative blood loss and postoperative sequestration of fluid. The anterior and lateral aspects of the neck of the aneurysm and iliac arteries are exposed. Heparin (5,000–10,000 units) is administered intravascularly; arterial clamps are applied, and the aneurysm is opened longitudinally. Laminar thrombus is evacuated, and the orifices of the inferior mesenteric and lumbar vessels are suture ligated. A Dacron tube or bifurcation graft of appropriate diameter is sutured end to end to the inside of the proximal aorta at the neck of the aneurysm. The aneurysm sac is left intact to minimize dissection with attendant blood loss and third-space sequestration. For tube grafts, a similar anastomosis is constructed distally. Otherwise, the iliac orifices are oversewn, and each limb of the bifurcated graft is anastomosed to the iliac or common femoral arteries. Operative outcome is enhanced by identifying high-risk patients, such as those with severe coronary artery disease, congestive heart failure, respiratory insufficiency, or chronic renal disease preoperatively, and addressing those problems vigorously through optimum use of medication; more aggressive measures are implemented when necessary. Hemodynamic measurements derived from right heart and arterial catheterization guide drug administration and volume replacement and facilitate patient management [196,200]. Aortic cross-clamping compromises distal perfusion, resulting in ischemic vasodilation. Removal of the clamp is accompanied by reduced venous return from the lower extremities, followed by hypotension, which can be prevented by timely volume replacement dictated by monitoring blood pressure and right- and left-heart filling pressures. The immediate postoperative period is characterized by central and systemic shunting and by an uneven pattern of diuresis. Attention to cardiac filling pressures and the blood chemistry profile aids judgment about intravenous administration of fluid and electrolytes and determines the need for inotropic or vasodilator agents. Reabsorption of fluid from the extravascular compartment on the second or third postoperative day may produce a rather abrupt rise in cardiac filling pressures, requiring judicious use of diuretic therapy to avert the development of congestive heart failure. In the absence of respiratory insufficiency, most patients can be weaned from a mechanical ventilator and extubated within 24 hours of surgery.

Electrocardiography in the early postoperative period frequently can detect active myocardial ischemia. Serum assays of myocardial enzymes may be difficult to interpret because of associated surgical trauma, and unless quantitative analysis of various isoenzyme components is available, the diagnosis of myocardial infarction may prove challenging. Renal function and urine output should be measured repeatedly, because a decline in glomerular filtration rate and oliguria may result from reduced cardiac output, hypotension, or renal ischemia related to surgery. Those possibilities must be distinguished from one another so that appropriate and specific therapy can be initiated. In cases complicated by acute renal failure, hemodialysis is indicated even before frank uremia develops, to control volume status and improve the metabolic milieu for tissue healing and for general recovery.

Although there have been no well-controlled trials comparing surgical and nonsurgical management of patients with abdominal aortic aneurysms, retrospective analyses that are available with historic controls certainly suggest improved survivorship after successful aneurysm repair. The 5-year survival rate in patients with untreated aneurysms larger than 5 to 6 cm in diameter ranges between 5 and 10 percent, whereas the survival rate for patients who have had surgery is in the range of 50 to 70 percent [192,201–205]. After recovery from surgical repair, long-term survival is limited principally by concomitant coronary or cerebrovascular disease. Early or late postoperative complications occur in approximately 8 to 10 percent of patients and include embolism, graft infection, pseudoaneurysm, graft occlusion, aortoenteric fistula formation, renal insufficiency, and neurologic deficits [206].

Several studies have verified that coronary artery disease is the most important risk factor for cardiac events and death in patients undergoing aneurysm surgery [207–209]. Since operative mortality is related mainly to myocardial ischemia, it has been suggested that coronary revascularization be performed in certain patients prior to abdominal aortic aneurysm resection [210–213]. No well-designed studies are available that compare the outcome of serial myocardial revascularization and abdominal aortic aneurysm repair with aneurysm surgery alone. An effort should be made to identify preoperatively those patients at highest cardiac risk using one or more of the noninvasive diagnostic methods, including treadmill exercise testing for those able to ambulate freely, arm ergometry for those capable only of upper-body exercise, thallium myocardial perfusion imaging in conjunction with intravenous administration of dipyridamole for those unable to exercise sufficiently because of associated disorders, or ambulatory (Holter) electrocardiographic monitoring for those with intermediate functional limitation [207–209,214–216]. Abnormal findings indicative of extensive myocardial ischemia may prompt the clinician to recommend cardiac catheterization with coronary angiography to determine the nature of coronary artery disease and left ventricular function. Thereafter, decisions regarding coronary revascularization must be made individually based on symptoms, angiographic findings, and other elements of risk. Based on the results of large multicenter trials in patients with stable coronary artery disease, it is reasonable to consider coronary revascularization prior to aneurysm surgery in patients with left main coronary artery disease, in patients with stenosis greater than 70 percent in each of the three major coronary arteries in the presence of impaired left ventricular function, and in those with severe or unstable angina pectoris.

Endovascular stent grafts are under study as an alternative, less invasive means to treat abdominal aortic aneurysms [217–219]. The experience with the technique is limited, but early reports involving highly selected patients have been encouraging [217,218].

ILIAC-ARTERY ANEURYSMS

Aneurysms of the iliac arteries and their branches are usually caused by atherosclerosis or vascular trauma. Patients typically are males in the sixth or seventh decade of life [220,221]. Two-thirds have multiple aneurysms that may involve the abdominal aorta, contralateral iliac artery, or femoropopliteal arteries. Almost one-half of the patients are asymptomatic at the time of diagnosis. The

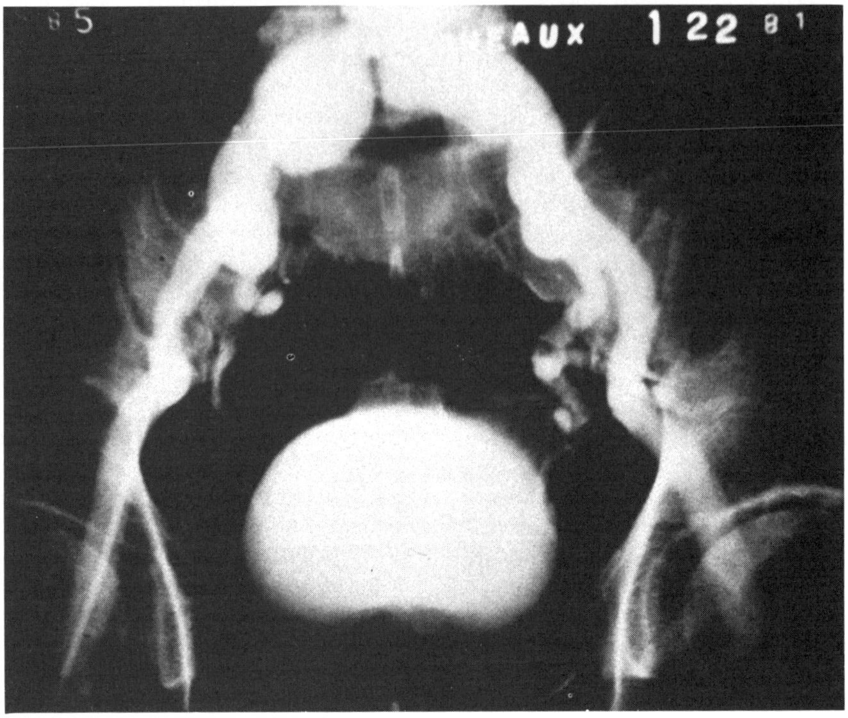

Fig. 39-11. Angiogram demonstrating bilateral iliac artery aneurysms.

remainder may have abdominal discomfort or pain caused by encroachment on contiguous nerves. Ureteral obstruction may occur. The aneurysm may be detected as a pulsating mass on abdominal, rectal, or vaginal examination. Diagnosis is confirmed by B-mode ultrasonography, computed tomography, or angiography (Fig. 39-11).

The risk of rupture is not known, since long-term studies examining natural history are not available; many iliac aneurysms are detected only at the time of surgery or postmortem examination. Anecdotal reports have suggested that one-third of patients with iliac artery aneurysm present with rupture [220,221]. As with aneurysms of the aorta, the risk of rupture appears proportional to the diameter of the aneurysm. Iliac artery aneurysms may be a source of thromboembolism, causing acute occlusion of distal vessels and resulting in leg ischemia.

TREATMENT. The isolated iliac aneurysm is approached through a lower-quadrant oblique flank incision and retroperitoneal exposure [220,222,223]. Bilateral iliac aneurysms or extensive involvement of a common iliac artery may require a formal transabdominal incision for adequate exposure to secure proximal aortic control. Simple ligation with exclusion of the aneurysm, often advocated in the past, is applicable only to the small internal iliac-artery aneurysm. Excision of the entire aneurysm is often hazardous to the adjacent pelvic structures. The current approach for most patients incorporates restoration of external iliac arterial continuity after exclusion of the proximal aneurysm sac. Dissection is limited to that required for adequate control of the vessels involved in an effort to minimize injury to adjacent structures, which often are densely adherent to the aneurysm.

If a common iliac-artery aneurysm involves the distal aortic bifurcation such that normal proximal iliac artery is not available, aortic control is required. The aneurysm sac is then opened longitudinally and the proximal anastomosis constructed end to end at that level. More often, however, the proximal iliac artery is ectatic or heavily calcified, precluding a technically satisfactory anastomosis. The proximal common iliac is oversewn and arterial continuity reestablished using the aorta or contralateral iliac artery as the donor vessel. The distal anastomosis is then constructed at the bifurcation of the common iliac artery from within the aneurysm sac or to the external iliac vessel with an end-to-side anastomosis.

Bilateral common iliac aneurysms require aorto-bi-iliac reconstruction with an end-to-end anastomosis proximally. The distal anastomoses are then constructed end to end to the bifurcations of the distal common iliac vessels. If that approach is not technically feasible, the limbs of the bifurcated prosthesis may be extended to the external iliac or femoral arteries, allowing the proximal aneurysm sacs to thrombose passively. Ideally, either antegrade or retrograde perfusion of at least one hypogastric artery should be maintained. When restoration of hypogastric flow is not possible, every effort should be made to preserve flow through the inferior mesenteric artery, since deprivation of inferior mesenteric artery and bilateral hypogastric artery flow may be associated with ischemic colonic complications.

Following occlusion of the common and external iliac arteries, the aneurysm is opened, and backbleeding branches are oversewn from inside the sac with nonresorbable suture material. Providing that the origin of the internal iliac artery is not involved, simple ligation of the proximal vessel should suffice for control. Frequently, however, the distal bifurcation of the common iliac artery and the proximal aspect of the internal iliac artery are involved, necessitating restoration of common to external iliac continuity, usually with a short-interposition prosthetic graft.

Small aneurysms limited to the external iliac artery may be excluded with proximal and distal ligation. Arterial continuity is restored with a prosthetic graft originating from the common iliac artery as an end-to-side anastomosis and extending to the external iliac or common femoral vessel distally. Larger external iliac aneurysms are best approached from within the sac and reconstructed with prosthetic material using end-to-end anastomosis proximally and distally, with subsequent incorporation of the graft within the aneurysm as the sac is reapproximated.

Operative mortality associated with elective repair of iliac aneurysms is less than 10 percent, in stark contrast to the 45 percent mortality associated with emergent repair [220]. Increased awareness of isolated iliac aneurysms in our aging population should facilitate earlier detection and reduced overall mortality.

FEMORAL- AND POPLITEAL-ARTERY ANEURYSMS

Like iliac-artery aneurysms, femoral and popliteal aneurysms are usually atherosclerotic. Men are affected far more often than women, in a ratio of about 30 : 1 [224–231]. The majority of patients have multiple aneurysms involving either the aorta or arteries of the lower extremities [227,229–238]. Concurrent aneurysms of the abdominal aorta occur in approximately 60 percent, and those of the iliac artery and femoral arteries occur in 35 to 40 percent of patients with popliteal artery aneurysms [239]. Bilateral lesions occur in 55 to 70 percent of patients [115,230].

Most femoral or popliteal aneurysms produce no symptoms [232]. Patients may notice a mass in the groin or behind the knee, sometimes with regional pain. Thrombosis rather than rupture is the most frequent complication of these aneurysms, occurring in approximately 25 percent of patients [239]. Then, claudication or rest pain and gangrene may arise. The potential prophylactic value of antithrombotic medication has not been studied. Reports variously indicate that 11 to 77 percent of patients with popliteal aneurysms require amputation during follow-up, unless surgical reconstruction is undertaken [225,228,230–234]. Rupture occasionally occurs, but that is unusual compared with aneurysms of the aorta and iliac arteries. Popliteal aneurysms may be detected on physical examination by palpation, particularly in patients with aortic aneurysms; those smaller than 3 cm seldom are detected in this fashion [229]. Bruits are audible in no more than half the cases. Diagnosis is most easily confirmed by B-mode ultrasonography. Angiography may be appropriate to identify associated atherosclerotic obstructive disease prior to surgical reconstruction (see Fig. 29-30).

Treatment. In the absence of extenuating circumstances, femoral and popliteal aneurysms should be repaired as soon as the diagnosis is established, irrespective of size, due to their propensity for acute thrombosis and subsequent limb loss [237,240–242]. Femoral artery aneurysms are repaired with a prosthetic graft of appropriate caliber interposed between the distal external iliac artery and the distal common femoral bifurcation. The repair usually is carried out under regional anesthesia through a vertical groin incision and is rarely complicated by significant morbidity or mortality [240].

Popliteal aneurysms are most frequently repaired with exclusion and standard femoropopliteal reconstruction utilizing a saphenous vein graft through medial thigh and calf incision. Results are excellent, with 85 percent of the repairs remaining patent after 5 years [237,241,242]. Direct exposure and repair with interposition technique, as described above, is fraught with injury to adjacent nerve and venous structures and compromises stability of the knee joint. Since rupture of aneurysms at this level accounts for fewer than 10 percent of the complications, it is notable that no trials of antithrombotic therapy as an alternative to surgical repair have been carried out.

ANEURYSMS OF UPPER-EXTREMITY ARTERIES

Aneurysms of the axillary, brachiocephalic, or subclavian arteries more often are a consequence of trauma than degenerative arteriopathy such as atherosclerosis. Penetrating injury may be iatrogenic, as a complication of attempted subclavian- or internal jugular-vein cannulation or axillary arterial catheterization. Chronic nonpenetrating trauma occurs in the vascular compression syndromes of the thoracic outlet, particularly the costoclavicular syndrome, associated with axillosubclavian arterial aneurysm formation. This is also relevant to axillary aneurysms resulting from incorrect compressive use of crutches. Mycotic aneurysms develop in cases of infective endocarditis. Patients with Ehlers-Danlos syndrome are prone to development of axillosubclavian aneurysms. Other etiologies include Takayasu arteritis and giant cell arteritis. Aneurysms of the brachial, radial, and ulnar arteries or of the arteries of the hand are usually traumatic, though vasculitis occasionally may produce those lesions. Mural thrombus generation may lead to unilateral emboli and limb ischemia as the mode of clinical presentation.

VISCERAL-ARTERY ANEURYSMS

Intra-abdominal visceral-artery aneurysms usually involve the celiac, mesenteric, and renal arteries and their branches. Aneurysms are uncommon lesions in those locations and usually are identified accidentally on radiographic examinations. Splenic-artery aneurysms are the most frequent and, unlike other types of visceral aneurysms, are found more often in women than in men. Autopsy series have suggested that the incidence of splenic-artery aneurysms ranges from 0.01 to 0.20 percent [243–248]. Splenic-artery aneurysms have a propensity to rupture during pregnancy in multiparous women [249–251]. They also occur with greater frequency in patients with portal hypertension. Atherosclerosis may be a secondary rather than a primary phenomenon in the wall of the aneurysm. Splenic-artery aneurysm may cause left-upper-quadrant abdominal pain, which may be difficult to distinguish from pathology involving the splenic flexure of the colon. Physical examination usually fails to disclose the aneurysm, although a pulsatile mass or localized abdominal bruit may be found in some cases. Ringlike calcification on plain roentgenograms of the abdomen can suggest the diagnosis. Ultrasonography, CT, or MRI provides additional information, but angiography is appropriate prior to elective surgical intervention (see Fig. 29-31). Up to 10 percent of splenic artery aneurysms rupture, prior to which there may be no symptoms [249]. Rupture tends to produce intracapsular or intra-abdominal hemorrhage, requiring urgent surgical intervention.

Hepatic-artery aneurysms have been described most often among patients in the fourth or fifth decades of life. Right upper-quadrant pain may arise, and when that occurs in association with jaundice and gastrointestinal bleeding, rupture of a hepatic-artery aneurysm into the biliary tract, the duodenum, or the stomach should be considered as a site [252]. When rupture does occur, surgical repair is challenging, and the mortality rate exceeds 50 percent.

Renal-artery aneurysms occur as a result of fibromuscular dysplasia, arterial dissection, arteritis, atherosclerosis, or idiopathic disease of the renal arteries. Rupture has been reported at a rate of 1 to 3 percent [253,254]. There may be an association with polycystic kidney disease. Hypertension is a common cofactor, but it is usually difficult to attribute hypertension to renal artery aneurysm in the absence of associated renal artery stenosis. Because of the risk of nephrectomy in the repair of distal or poorly accessible renal-artery aneurysms, the indications for surgical repair are poorly defined.

References

1. Glagov S, Wolinsky H. New concepts of the relation of structure to function in the arterial wall. Proc Inst Med Chic 1968; 27:106.
2. Wolinsky H, Glagov S. Comparison of abdominal and thoracic aortic medial structure in mammals: deviation of man from the usual pattern. Circ Res 1969; 25:677–686.
3. Wolinsky H, Glagov S. A lamellar unit of aortic medial structure and function in mammals. Circ Res 1967; 20:99.
4. Movat HZ, More RH, Haust MD. The diffuse internal thickening of the human aorta with aging. Am J Pathol 1958; 34:1023–1031.
5. Caro CG, et al. The Mechanics of the Circulation. New York: Oxford University Press, 1978.
6. Eagle KA, DeSanctis RW. Diseases of the aorta. In E Braunwald, ed. Heart Disease, vol 2. Philadelphia: Saunders, 1992. Pp. 1528–1557.
7. Nichols WW, O'Rourke MF. Contours of pressure and flow waves in arteries. In McDonald's Blood Flow in Arteries. Philadelphia: Lea and Febiger, 1990. Pp. 216–250.
8. Lakatta EG, et al. Human aging: changes in structure and function. J Amer Coll Cardiol 1987; 10:42A–47A.
9. Carlson RG, Lillehei CW, Edwards J. Cystic medial necrosis of the ascending aorta in relation to age and hypertension. Am J Cardiol 1970; 25:411–415.
10. Nichols WW, O'Rourke MF. Aging, high blood pressure and disease. In McDonald's Blood Flow in Arteries. Philadelphia: Lea and Febiger, 1990. Pp. 398–420.
11. Avolio AP, et al. Effects of aging on changing arterial compliance and left ventricular load in a northern Chinese urban community. Circulation 1983; 68:50–58.
12. Virmani R, McAllister HA Jr. Pathology of the aorta and major arteries. In A Lande, YM Berkmen, HA McAllister Jr, eds. Aortitis: Clinical, Pathologic, and Radiographic Aspects. New York: Raven, 1986. Pp. 7–53.
13. Becker AE. Medionecrosis aortae. Pathol Microbiol 1975; 43:124.
14. Roberts WC. The aorta: its acquired diseases and their consequences as viewed from a morphologic perspective. In J Lindsay, JW Hurst, eds. The Aorta. New York: Grune & Stratton, 1979. Pp. 51–117.
15. Gsell O. Wandnekrosen der Aorta als selbstandige Erkrankung und Ihre beziehung zur Spontanruptur. Virchows Arch Pathol Anat 1928; 270:1.
16. Erdheim J. Medionecrosis aortae idiopathica. Virchows Arch Pathol Anat 1929; 273:454.
17. Marfan AB. Un cas de deformation congenitale des quatre membres, plus prononcée des extremités, caracterisée par l'allongement des coeur avec un certain degré d'amincissement. Bull Mem Soc Med Hop Paris 1896; 13:220–226.
18. Francke U, Furthmayr H. Marfan's syndrome and other disorders of fibrillin. N Engl J Med 1994; 330:1384–1385.
19. Fuster V, Halperin JL. Aortic dissection: a medical perspective. J Card Surg 1994; 9:713–728.
20. Hahn RT, et al. Association of aortic dilation with regurgitant, stenotic and functionally normal bicuspid aortic valves. J Am Coll Cardiol 1992; 19:283–288.
21. Subramanyan R, Joy J, Balakrishnan KG. Natural history of aortoarteritis (Takayasu's disease). Circulation 1989; 80: 429–437.
22. Lupi-Herrera E, et al. Takayasu's arteritis: clinical study of 107 cases. Am Heart J 1977; 93:94–103.
23. Kerr GS, et al. Takayasu arteritis. Ann Intern Med 1994; 120:919–929.
24. Evans JM, O'Fallon WM, Hunder GG. Increased incidence of aortic aneurysm and dissection in giant cell (temporal) arteritis. A population-based study. Ann Intern Med 1995; 122:502–507.
25. Evans JM, et al. Thoracic aortic aneurysm and rupture in giant cell arteritis. A descriptive study of 41 cases. Arthritis Rheum 1994; 37:1539–1547.
26. Hunder GG, Ward LE, Burbank MK. Giant-cell arteritis producing an aortic arch syndrome. Ann Intern Med 1967; 66:578–582.
27. Klein RG, et al. Large artery involvement in giant cell (temporal) arteritis. Ann Intern Med 1975; 83:806–812.
28. Halperin JL. Collagen diseases and the heart. In WW Parmley, K Chatterjee, eds. Cardiology. Philadelphia: Lippincott, 1987. Pp. 1–23.
29. Lande A, Berkman YM. Aortitis: pathologic, clinical and arteriographic review. Radiol Clin N Am 1976; 14:219–240.
30. Cranley JJ, Herrmann LG, Preuninger RMK. Natural history of aneurysms of the aorta. Arch Surg 1954; 69:185.
31. Kampmeier RH. Saccular aneurysms of the thoracic aorta: a clinical study of 633 cases. Ann Intern Med 1938; 12:624–651.
32. Heggtveit HA. Syphilitic aortitis. Circulation 1964; 29:176–181.
33. Merten CW, Finby N, Steinberg I. Antemortem diagnosis of syphilitic aneurysms of the aortic sinuses. Am J Med 1956; 20:345–360.
34. Rich C Jr, Webster B. The natural history of uncomplicated syphilitic aortitis. Am Heart J 1952; 43:321–332.
35. Irvine RE. Outcome of uncomplicated syphilitic aortitis. Br Med J 1956; 1:832–834.
36. Felson B, et al. Mycotic tuberculous aneurysm of the thoracic aorta. JAMA 1977; 237:1104–1108.
37. Gajaraj A, Victor S. Tuberculous aortoarteritis. Clin Radiol 1981; 32:461–466.

38. Mally A, et al. Pulmonary tuberculosis with multiple saccular aneurysms of the aorta—a rare case report. Angiology 1990; 41:333–336.
39. Oskoui R, Davis WA, Gomes MN. Salmonella aortitis. A report of a successfully treated case with a comprehensive review of the literature. Arch Intern Med 1993; 153:517–525.
40. Feigl D, Feigl A, Edwards JE. Mycotic aneurysm of the aortic root. A pathologic study of 20 cases. Chest 1986; 90:553–557.
41. Fricker FJ, et al. Aneurysm of the aorta in children. Chest 1979; 76:305–309.
42. Chen S, et al. Aortic aneurysm in childhood: report of six instances. J Pediatr 1976; 89:231–234.
43. Skandalakis JE, et al. Coarctation of the aorta with aneurysm. Surg Gynecol Obstet 1960; 111:307–326.
44. Hardin CA. Ruptured abdominal aneurysm occurring in Marfan syndrome. N Engl J Med 1959; 260:821–822.
45. Hunter GC, et al. Vascular manifestations in patients with Ehlers-Danlos syndrome. Arch Surg 1982; 117:495–498.
46. Mirza FH, Smith PL, Lina WN. Multiple aneurysms in a patient with Ehlers-Danlos syndrome: angiography without sequelae. Am J Radiol 1979; 132:993–995.
47. Dutton RV, Singleton EB. Tuberous sclerosis: a case report with aortic aneurysm and unusual rib changes. Pediatr Radiol 1975; 3:184–186.
48. Hagood CO Jr, et al. Abdominal aortic aneurysm and renal hematoma in an infant with tuberous sclerosis. Surgery 1976; 79:713–715.
49. Sterpetti AV, Hunter WJ, Schultz RD. Congenital abdominal aortic aneurysms in the young: case report and review of the literature. J Vasc Surg 1988; 7:763–769.
50. Darden WA, et al. Congenital abdominal aortic aneurysms: report of a case and review of the literature. Surgery 1984; 96:567–573.
51. Rabin E, Vye MV, Farrell EE. Umbilical artery catheterization complicated by multiple mycotic aortic aneurysms. Arch Pathol Lab Med 1986; 110:442–444.
52. Klein RL. Abdominal aortic aneurysm in infancy subsequent to perinephric abscess. J Pediatr Surg 1986; 21:451–453.
53. Canter CE, Bower RJ, Strauss AW. Atypical Kawasaki disease with aortic aneurysm. Pediatrics 1981; 68:885–888.
54. Gelfand M. Giant cell arteritis with aneurysmal formation in an infant. Br Heart J 1955; 17:264–266.
55. Squire A, et al. Femoral pseudoaneurysm following nonpenetrating trauma in a patient with aortic insufficiency. Am J Med 1985; 78:719–720.
56. Spittell JA, McGoon DC. Acquired diseases of the thoracic aorta. In RO Brandenburg, et al., eds. Cardiology: Fundamentals and Practice. Chicago: Year Book, 1987. Pp. 1718–1731.
57. Campbell CD. Aneurysms of the ascending aorta. In CD Campbell, ed. Aortic Aneurysms: Surgical Therapy. Mount Kisco, NY: Futura, 1981. Pp. 19–46.
58. DeBakey ME, et al. Surgery of acquired cardiovascular disease. In WH Cole, RM Zollinger, eds. Textbook of Surgery, 9th ed. New York: Appleton-Century-Crofts, 1970. P. 997.
59. Noon GP, Short D. Aneurysms of the aortic arch. In AD Campbell, ed. Aortic Aneurysms: Surgical Therapy. Mount Kisco, NY: Futura, 1981. Pp. 79–100.
60. Morse DE. Embryology, anatomy and histology of the aorta. In J Lindsay, JW Hurst, eds. The Aorta. New York: Grune & Stratton, 1979. Pp. 15–37.
61. DeBakey ME, Noon GP. Aneurysms of the thoracic aorta. Mod Concepts Cardiovasc Dis 1975; 44:53–58.
62. Joyce JW, et al. Aneurysms of the thoracic aorta. Circulation 1964; 29:176–181.
63. Dillon ML, Young WG, Sealy WC. Aneurysms of the descending thoracic aorta. Ann Thorac Surg 1967; 3:430–438.
64. Lindsay J Jr. Thoracic aneurysms. In J Lindsay, JW Hurst, eds. The Aorta. New York: Grune & Stratton, 1979. Pp. 121–130.
65. Edwards JE. Aneurysm of the thoracic aorta complicating coarctation. Circulation 1973; 48:195–201.
66. Bickerstaff LK, et al. Thoracic aortic aneurysms: a population-based study. Surgery 1982; 92:1103–1108.
67. Pressler V, McNamara JJ. Thoracic aortic aneurysm: natural history and treatment. J Thorac Cardiovasc Surg 1980; 79:489–498.
68. Fomon JJ, Kurzweg FT, Broadaway RK. Aneurysms of the aorta: a review. Ann Surg 1967; 165:557–563.
69. Bulkley BH, Hutchins GM, Ross RS. Aortic sinus of Valsalva aneurysms simulating primary right sided valvular heart disease. Circulation 1975; 52:696–699.
70. Blieden LC, Edwards JE. Anomalies of the thoracic aorta: pathologic considerations. Prog Cardiovasc Dis 1973; 16:25–41.
71. Davies GJ, Watt J, Muir JR. Ruptured sinus of Valsalva aneurysm with aortic-left atrial fistula. Eur J Cardiol 1975; 3:213–218.
72. Birnholz JC, Fenucci JT, Wyman SM. Roentgen features of dysphagia aortica. Radiology 1974; 111:93–96.
73. Seymour J, Emanuel R, Pattinson N. Acquired pulmonary stenosis. Br Heart J 1968; 30:776–785.
74. Drachler DH, Willis PW III. Acquired right ventricular outflow tract obstruction. Am Heart J 1971; 82:536–540.
75. Banker VP, Maddison FE. Superior vena cava syndrome secondary to aortic disease. Dis Chest 1967; 51:656–666.
76. Varkey B, Tristani FE. Compression of pulmonary artery and bronchus by descending thoracic aortic aneurysm. Am J Cardiol 1974; 34:610–614.
77. White RD, et al. Noninvasive evaluation of suspected thoracic aortic disease by contrast-enhanced computed tomography. Am J Cardiol 1986; 57:282–290.
78. Dinsmore RE, et al. Magnetic resonance imaging of the thoracic aortic aneurysms: comparison with other imaging methods. Am J Roentgenol 1986; 146:309–314.
79. Glazer HS, et al. The thoracic aorta studied by MR imaging. Radiology 1985; 157:149–155.
80. Finkbohner R, et al. Marfan syndrome. Long-term survival and complications after aortic aneurysm repair. Circulation 1995; 91:728–733.
81. Shores J, et al. Progression of aortic dilatation and the benefit of long-term beta-adrenergic blockade in Marfan's syndrome. N Engl J Med 1994; 330:1335–1341.
82. Crawford ES, Stowe CL. True aneurysms of the aorta and iliac arteries. In WS Moore, ed. Vascular Surgery—A Comprehensive Review. Orlando, FL: Grune & Stratton, 1986.
83. Bentall H, Debono A. A technique for complete replacement of the ascending aorta. Thorax 1968; 23:338.
84. Gott VL, et al. Surgical treatment of aneurysms of the ascending aorta in the Marfan syndrome: results of composite-graft repair in 50 patients. N Engl J Med 1986; 314:1070–1074.
85. Marsalese DL, et al. Cystic medial necrosis of the aorta in patients without Marfan's syndrome: surgical outcome and long-term follow-up. J Am Coll Cardiol 1990; 16:68–73.
86. Crawford ES, Snyder DM. Treatment of aneurysms of the aortic arch: a progress report. J Thorac Cardiovasc Surg 1983; 85:237–246.
87. Crawford ES, et al. Graft replacement of aneurysm in descending thoracic aorta: results without bypass or shunting. Surgery 1981; 89:73–85.
88. Dake MD, et al. Transluminal placement of endovascular stent-grafts for the treatment of descending thoracic aortic aneurysms. N Engl J Med 1994; 331:1729–1734.
89. Crawford ES, et al. Progress in treatment of thoracoabdominal and abdominal aortic aneurysms involving celiac, su-

perior mesenteric and renal arteries. Ann Surg 1978; 188: 404–422.
90. DeBakey ME, Creech O Jr, Morris GC Jr. Aneurysm of thoracoabdominal aorta involving the celiac, superior mesenteric and renal arteries. Report of four cases treated by resection and homograft replacement. Ann Surg 1956; 144:549–573.
91. Crawford ES. Thoracoabdominal and abdominal aortic aneurysms involving renal, superior mesenteric, celiac arteries. Ann Surg 1974; 179:763–772.
92. Peyton RW. Surgical correction of tuberculous pseudoaneurysm of upper abdominal aorta: first reported case. Ann Surg 1965; 162:1069–1074.
93. Pierce WS, et al. Coarctation of the abdominal aorta with multiple aneurysms. Ann Thorac Surg 1975; 20:687–693.
94. James EC, Gillespie JT. Aortic mycotic abdominal aneurysm involving all visceral branches: excision and Dacron graft replacement. J Cardiovasc Surg 1977; 18:141–146.
95. Bennett DE, Cherry JK. The natural history of traumatic aneurysms of the aorta. Surgery 1967; 61:516–523.
96. Munda R, et al. The use of an external Dacron shunt in repair of a supraceliac abdominal aorta traumatic aneurysm. J Cardiovasc Surg 1977; 18:141–146.
97. Etheredge SN, et al. Successful resection of a large aneurysm of the upper abdominal aorta and replacement with homograft. Surgery 1955; 38:1071–1081.
98. Hardy JD, et al. Thoracoabdominal aortic aneurysm: simplified surgical management with case report. Ann Surg 1967; 166:1008–1011.
99. Heyde MN van der, Zwaveling A. Resection of an abdominal aortic aneurysm in a patient with Marfan's syndrome. J Cardiovasc Surg 1961; 2:359–366.
100. DeBakey ME, et al. Surgical considerations in the treatment of aneurysms of the thoracoabdominal aorta. Ann Surg 1965; 162:650–662.
101. Dixon AK, et al. Computed tomography of abdominal aortic aneurysms: determination of longitudinal extent. Br J Surg 1981; 68:47–50.
102. Gomes MN, Choyke PL. Pre-operative evaluation of abdominal aortic aneurysms: ultrasound or computed tomography? J Cardiovasc Surg (Torino) 1987; 28:159–166.
103. Amparo EG, et al. Comparison of magnetic resonance imaging and ultrasonography in the evaluation of abdominal aortic aneurysms. Radiology 1985; 154:451–456.
104. Ellis FH Jr, Helden RA, Hines EA Jr. Aneurysm of the abdominal aorta involving the right renal artery: report of case with preservation of renal function after resection and grafting. Ann Surg 1955; 142:992.
105. Crawford ES, et al. Thoracoabdominal aortic aneurysms: preoperative and intraoperative factors determining immediate and long-term results of operations in 605 patients. J Vasc Surg 1986; 3:389–404.
106. Svensson LG, et al. Experience with 1509 patients undergoing thoracoabdominal aortic operations. J Vasc Surg 1993; 17:357–370.
107. Safi HJ, et al. Neurologic deficit in patients at high risk with thoracoabdominal aortic aneurysms: The role of cerebral spinal fluid drainage and distal aortic perfusion. J Vasc Surg 1994; 20:434–443.
108. Weintraub AM, Gomes MN. Clinical manifestations of abdominal aortic aneurysm and thoracoabdominal aneurysm. In J Lindsay Jr, JW Hurst, eds. The Aorta. New York: Grune & Stratton, 1979. Pp. 131–168.
109. Sommerville RL, All EV, Edwards JE. Bland and infected arteriosclerotic abdominal aortic aneurysms: a clinicopathologic study. Medicine 1959; 38:207–221.
110. Friedman SA, et al. Abdominal aortic aneurysms. Clinical status and results of surgery in 100 consecutive cases. JAMA 1967; 200:1147–1151.
111. Gliedman ML, Ayers WB, Vestal BL. Aneurysms of the abdominal aorta and its branches. Ann Surg 1957; 146:207.
112. Silverberg E, Luvera J. Cancer Statistics, 1983. New York: American Cancer Society, 1983.
113. Auerbach O, Garfinkel L. Atherosclerosis and aneurysm of the aorta in relation to smoking habits and age. Chest 1980; 78:805–809.
114. Carlsson J, Sternby N. Aortic aneurysms. Acta Chir Scand 1964; 127:466–473.
115. Cole C, Barber GG. Abdominal aortic aneurysm: the consequences of a positive family history. Can J Surg 1989; 32:117–120.
116. Allardice JT, et al. High prevalence of abdominal aortic aneurysm in men with peripheral vascular disease: screening by ultrasonography. Br J Surg 1988; 75:240–242.
117. Darling RC, et al. Autopsy study of unoperated abdominal aortic aneurysms. The case for early resection. Circulation 1977; 56[Suppl 2]:II-161–164.
118. Johansen K, Koepsell T. Familial tendency for abdominal aortic aneurysm. JAMA 1986; 256:1934–1936.
119. Johnson G Jr, et al. Aneurysms of the abdominal aorta: incidence in blacks and whites in North Carolina. Arch Surg 1985; 120:1138–1140.
120. Leopold GR, Goldberger LE, Bernstein EF. Ultrasonic detection and evaluation of abdominal aortic aneurysms. Surgery 1972; 72:939–945.
121. Scott RAP. Ultrasound screening in the management of abdominal aortic aneurysms. Int Angiol 1986; 5:263–267.
122. Bickerstaff LK, et al. Abdominal aortic aneurysms: the changing natural history. J Vasc Surg 1984; 1:6–12.
123. Bowers D, Cave WS. Aneurysms of the abdominal aorta: a twenty-year study. J R Soc Med 1985; 78:812.
124. Cabellon S Jr, et al. Incidence of abdominal aortic aneurysms in patients with atheromatous arterial disease. Am J Surg 1983; 146:575–576.
125. Graham M, Chan A. Ultrasound screening for clinically occult abdominal aortic aneurysm. Can Med Assoc J 1988; 138:627–629.
126. Thurmond AS, Semler HJ. Abdominal aortic aneurysm: incidence in a population at risk. J Cardiovasc Surg 1986; 27:457–460.
127. Zarins CK, et al. Aneurysm formation in experimental atherosclerosis: relationship to plaque evolution. J Vasc Surg 1990; 12:246–256.
128. Schatz IJ, Fairbairn II JF, Juergens JL. Abdominal aortic aneurysms, a reappraisal. Circulation 1962; 26:200–205.
129. DeBakey ME, et al. Aneurysm of abdominal aorta—analysis of graft replacement therapy 1 to 11 years after operation. Ann Surg 1964; 160:622–639.
130. Reilly JM, Tilson MD. Incidence and etiology of abdominal aortic aneurysms. Surg Clin N Am 1989; 69:705–711.
131. Cannon D, Read R. Blood elastolytic activity in patients with aortic aneurysms. Ann Thorac Surg 1982; 34:10–15.
132. Tilson M. Histochemistry of aortic elastin in patients with nonspecific AAA disease. Arch Surg 1988; 123:503–505.
133. Tilson M, Fieg P, Harvey M. Malignant neoplasia in patients with abdominal aortic aneurysms. Arch Surg 1984; 119:792–794.
134. Norrgard O, Rais O, Angquist K. Familial occurrence of abdominal aortic aneurysms. Surgery 1984; 95:650–656.
135. Tilson M, Seashore M. Human genetics of the abdominal aortic aneurysm. Surg Gynecol Obstet 1984; 158:129–132.
136. Tilson M, Seashore M. Fifty families with abdominal aortic aneurysms in two or more first-order relatives. Am J Surg 1984; 147:551–553.

137. Darling RC et al. Are familial abdominal aortic aneurysms different? J Vasc Surg 1989; 10:39–43.
138. Busuttil R, Abou-Zamzam A, Machleder H. Collagenase activity of the human aorta: a comparison of patients with and without abdominal aortic aneurysms. Arch Surg 1980; 115: 1373–1378.
139. Menashi S, et al. Collagen in abdominal aortic aneurysm: typing, content, and degradation. J Vasc Surg 1987; 6:578–582.
140. Sumner D, Hokanson D, Strandness D. Stress-strain characteristics and collagen-elastin content of abdominal aortic aneurysms. Surg Gynecol Obstet 1970; 130:459–466.
141. Black PH, Kunz LJ, Swatz MN. Salmonellosis—a review of some unusual aspects. N Engl J Med 1960; 262:811–817.
142. Kuivanieri H, Tromp G, Prockup DJ. Genetic causes of aortic aneurysms. J Clin Invest 1991; 88:1441–1444.
143. Reed D, et al. Are aortic aneurysms caused by atherosclerosis. Circulation 1992; 85:205–211.
144. MacSweeney STR, Powell JT, Greenhalgh. Pathogenesis of abdominal aortic aneurysm. Br J Surg 1994; 81:935–941.
145. Strachan DP. Predictors of death from aortic aneurysm among middle-aged men. The Whitehall study. Br J Surg 1991; 78:401–404.
146. Ernst CB. Abdominal aortic aneurysm. N Engl J Med 1993; 328:1167–1172.
147. Marquis Y, et al. Idiopathic medial aortopathy and arteriopathy. Am J Med 1968; 44:939–954.
148. Estes JE Jr. Abdominal aortic aneurysm: a study of one hundred and two cases. Circulation 1950; 2:258–264.
149. Wright IS, Urdaneta E, Wright B. Re-opening the case of the abdominal aortic aneurysm. Circulation 1956; 13:754–768.
150. Blakemore AH, Voorhees AB Jr. Aneurysm of the aorta: a review of 365 cases. Angiology 1954; 5:209–231.
151. Kampmeier RH. Aneurysm of the abdominal aorta: a study of 73 cases. Am J Med Sci 1936; 192:97–109.
152. Szilagyi DE, et al. Contribution of abdominal aortic aneurysmectomy to prolongation of life. Ann Surg 1966; 164:678–699.
153. Szilagyi DE, Elliott JP, Smith RF. Clinical fate of the patient with asymptomatic abdominal aortic aneurysm and unfit for surgical treatment. Arch Surg 1972; 104:600–606.
154. Bickerstaff LK, et al. Abdominal aortic aneurysms: the changing natural history. J Vasc Surg 1984; 1:6–12.
155. Foster JH, et al. Comparative study of elective resection and expectant treatment of abdominal aortic aneurysm. Surg Gynecol Obstet 1969; 129:1–9.
156. Bernstein EF, Chan EL. Abdominal aortic aneurysm in high-risk patients: outcome of selective management based on size and expansion rate. Ann Surg 1984; 200:255–623.
157. Nevitt MP, Ballard DJ, Hallett JW Jr. Prognosis of abdominal aortic aneurysms: a population-based study. N Engl J Med 1989; 321:1009–1014.
158. Anidjar S, Dobrin PB, Chejfec G, Michel JB. Experimental study of determinants of aneurysmal expansion of the abdominal aorta. Ann Vasc Surg 1994; 8:127–136.
159. Cronenwett JL, et al. Actuarial analysis of variables associated with rupture of small abdominal aortic aneurysms. Surgery 1985; 98:472–483.
160. Stokes J, Butcher HR Jr. Abdominal aortic aneurysms. Factors influencing operative mortality and criteria of operability. Arch Surg 1973; 107:297–302.
161. Gore I, Hirst AE. Arteriosclerotic aneurysms of the abdominal aorta: a review. Prog Cardiovasc Dis 1973; 17:113–149.
162. Hall AD, et al. Surgical treatment of aortic aneurysm in the aged. Arch Surg 1970; 100:455–460.
163. Hammond EC, Garfinkel L. Coronary heart disease, stroke, and aortic aneurysm. Arch Environ Health 1969; 19:167–182.
164. Barrat-Boyes BG. Symptomatology and prognosis of abdominal aortic aneurysm. Lancet 1957; 2:716–720.
165. Tallgren LG, von Bonsdorff CH. Symptomatology and prognosis of abdominal aortic aneurysm. Acta Med Scand 1964; 175[Suppl 412]:287.
166. Brewster DC, et al. Assessment of abdominal aortic aneurysm size. Circulation 1977; 56:II164–II169.
167. Winsberg F, Cole-Beuglet C, Mulder DS. Continuous ultrasound "B" scanning of abdominal aortic aneurysms. Am J Roentgen 1974; 121:626–633.
168. Janower ML. Ruptured aneurysms of abdominal aorta. N Engl J Med 1961; 265:12–15.
169. Boyd DP, McCann JC. Abdominal aneurysm. Surg Clin N Am 1965; 45:675–687.
170. Smith RF, et al. Ultrasound evaluation of abdominal aortic aneurysms (Abstract). Circulation 1976; 53[Suppl 2]:11–12.
171. Retief PJ, Loubser JS. Diagnosis and treatment of abdominal aortic aneurysm: a report of 82 cases. S Afr Med J 1979; 56:67–69.
172. Steinberg I, Stein HL. Visualization of the abdominal aortic aneurysm. Am J Roentgen 1965; 95:684.
173. Gomes MN, Hufnagel CA. A new method for the diagnosis of abdominal aortic aneurysms. J Cardiovasc Surg 1979; 20:511–515.
174. LaRoy LL, et al. Imaging of abdominal aortic aneurysms. AJR Am J Roentgenol 1989; 152:785–792.
175. Machida K, Tasaka A. CT patterns of mural thrombus in aortic aneurysms. J Comput Assist Tomogr 1980; 4:840–842.
176. Kaufman JA, et al. MR imaging (including MR angiography) of abdominal arotic aneurysms: comparison with conventional angiography. AJR Am J Roentgenol 1994; 163:203–210.
177. Siegel CL, Cohan RH. CT of abdominal aortic aneurysms. AJR Am J Roentgenol 1994; 163:17–29.
178. Cullenward MJ, et al. Inflammatory aortic aneurysm (periaortic fibrosis) radiologic imaging. Radiology 1986; 159: 75–82.
179. Rosen A, et al. CT diagnosis of ruptured abdominal aortic aneurysm. Am J Roentgen 1984; 143:265–268.
180. Siegel CL, et al. Abdominal aortic aneurysm morphology: CT features in patients with ruptured and nonruptured aneurysms. Am J Roentgenol 1984; 163:1123–1129.
181. Mehard WB, Heiken JP, Sicard GA. High attenuating crescent in abdominal aortic aneurysm wall at CT: a sign of acute or impending rupture. Radiology 1994; 192:359–362.
182. Kwaan JH, et al. Value of arteriography before abdominal aortic aneurysmectomy. Am J Surg 1977; 134:108–114.
183. Brewster DC, et al. Angiography and the management of aneurysms of the abdominal aorta. N Engl J Med 1975; 292:822–825.
184. Robicsek F, et al. Value of angiography in diagnosis of unruptured aneurysms of the abdominal aorta. Ann Thorac Surg 1971; 11:538–550.
185. Cyr R, et al. Angiography: an essential diagnostic aid in asymptomatic aortic aneurysm. Can J Surg 1977; 20:57–59.
186. Baur GM, et al. The role of arteriography in abdominal aortic aneurysm. Am J Surg 1978; 136:184–189.
187. Webster MW, et al. Ultrasound screening of first-degree relatives of patients with an abdominal aortic aneurysm. J Vasc Surg 1991; 13:9–14.
188. Berridge DC, et al. Screening for clinically unsuspected abdominal aortic aneurysm in patients with peripheral vascular disease. Eur J Vasc Surg 1989; 3:421–422.
189. Dubost C. Resection of an aneurysm of the abdominal aorta—reestablishment of the continuity by a preserved human arterial graft with result after 5 months. Arch Surg 1952; 64:405–408.

190. Baker AG Jr, et al. Risk of excision of abdominal aortic aneurysm. Surgery 1970; 68:1129–1134.
191. Crawford ES, et al. Aortic aneurysm: current status of surgical treatment. Surg Clin N Am 1979; 59:597–636.
192. Scobie K, McPhail N, Hubbard C. Early and late results of resection of abdominal aortic aneurysms. Can Med Assoc J 1977; 117:147.
193. Hollier LH, Taylor LM, Ochsner J. Recommended indications for operative treatment of abdominal aortic aneurysms. J Vasc Surg 1992;6:1046–1056.
194. Cronenwett JL, et al. Variables that affect the expansion rate and outcome of small abdominal aortic aneurysms. J Vasc Surg 1990; 11:260–269.
195. Katz DA, Cronenwett JL. The cost-effectiveness of early surgery versus watchful waiting in the management of small abdominal aortic aneursyms. J Vasc Surg 1994; 19:980–981.
196. Whittemore AD, et al. Aortic aneurysm repair. Ann Surg 1980; 192:414–420.
197. Golden MA, et al. Selective evaluation and management of coronary artery disease in patients undergoing repair of abdominal aortic aneurysms. Ann Surg 1990; 212:415–420.
198. Javid M, et al. Complications of aortic aneurysm. Arch Surg 1962; 85:650–662.
199. Creech O Jr. Endo-aneurysmorrhaphy and treatment of aortic aneurysm. Ann Surg 1966; 164:935–946.
200. Attia RR, et al. Myocardial ischemia due to infrarenal aortic cross-clamping during aortic surgery in patients with severe coronary artery disease. Circulation 1976; 53:961–965.
201. Hertzer NR, Beven EG. Abdominal aortic aneurysm. Postgrad Med 1977; 61:72–80.
202. Fielding JWL, Black J, Ashton F, et al. Diagnosis and management of 528 abdominal aortic aneurysms. Br Med J 1981; 283:355–359.
203. Baker AG Jr, Roberts B. Long-term survival following abdominal aortic aneurysmectomy. JAMA 1970; 212:445–450.
204. DeWeese JA, et al. Optimal resources for vascular surgery. Circulation 1976; 53:A39-A50.
205. Soreide O, et al. Abdominal aortic aneurysms: survival analysis of four hundred thirty-four patients. Surgery 1982; 91:188–193.
206. Thompson WM, et al. Late complications of abdominal aortic reconstructive surgery: roentgen evaluation. Ann Surg 1977; 185:326–334.
207. Boucher CA, et al. Determination of cardiac risk by dipyridamole-thallium imaging before peripheral vascular surgery. N Engl J Med 1985; 312:389–394.
208. Leppo J, et al. Noninvasive evaluation of cardiac risk before elective vascular surgery. J Am Coll Cardiol 1987; 9:269–276.
209. Raby KE, et al. Correlation between preoperative ischemia and major cardiac events after peripheral vascular surgery. N Engl J Med 1989; 321:1296–1300.
210. Hertzer NR, et al. Coronary artery disease in peripheral vascular patients. Ann Surg 1984; 199:223–233.
211. Jamieson WRE, et al. Influence of ischemic heart disease on early and late mortality after surgery for peripheral occlusive vascular disease. Circulation 1982; 66:I92–I97.
212. Tomatis LA, Fierens EE, Verbrugge GP. Evaluation of surgical risk in peripheral vascular disease by coronary arteriography: a series of 100 cases. Surgery 1972; 71:429–435.
213. McCollum CH, et al. Myocardial revascularization prior to subsequent major surgery in patients with coronary artery disease. Surgery 1977; 81:302–304.
214. Fleisher LA, Rosenbaum SH, Barash PG. Preoperative silent ischemia is a predictor of postoperative cardiac events in patients undergoing elective noncardiac surgery. Soc Cardiovasc Anesthes 1990; 12:98.
215. Eagle KA, et al. Combining clinical and thallium data optimizes preoperative assessment of cardiac risk before major vascular surgery. Ann Intern Med 1989; 110:859–866.
216. McCabe CJ, et al. The value of electrocardiogram monitoring during treadmill testing for peripheral vascular disease. Surgery 1981; 89:183–186.
217. Parodi JC, et al. Endoluminal aortic aneurysm repair using a balloon-expandable stent-graft device: a progress report. Ann Vasc Surg 1994; 8:523–529.
218. May J, et al. Med J Aust 1994; 161:541–543.
219. Yusuf SW, et al. Tranfemoral endoluminal repair of abdominal aortic aneurysm with bifurcated graft. Lancet 1994; 344:650–651.
220. Richardson JW, Greenfield LJ. Natural history and management of iliac aneurysms. J Vasc Surg 1988; 8:165–171.
221. Bolin T, Lund K, Skau T. Isolated aneurysms of the iliac artery: what are the chances of rupture? Eur J Vasc Surg 1988; 2:214–215.
222. Lowry SF, Kraft RO. Isolated aneurysms of the iliac artery. Arch Surg 1978; 113:1289–1293.
223. Perdue GD, et al. Aneurysms of the internal iliac artery. Surgery 1983; 93:243–246.
224. Baird RJ, et al. Popliteal aneurysms: a review and analysis of 61 cases. Surgery 1966; 59:911–917.
225. Edmunds LH, Darling RC, Linton RR. Surgical management of popliteal aneurysms. Circulation 1965; 32:517–523.
226. Friesen G, Ivins JC, Janes JM. Popliteal aneurysms. Surgery 1962; 51:90–98.
227. Gaylis H. Popliteal artery aneurysms: a review and analysis of 55 cases. S Afr Med J 1974; 48:75–81.
228. Gifford RW, Hines EA, Janes JM. An analysis and follow-up of one hundred popliteal aneurysms. Surgery 1953; 33:284–293.
229. Inahara T, Toledo AC. Complications and treatment of popliteal aneurysms. Surgery 1978; 84:775–783.
230. Vermilion BD, et al. A review of 147 popliteal aneurysms with long-term follow-up. Surgery 1981; 90:1009–1014.
231. Wychulis AR, Spittell JA Jr, Wallace RB. Popliteal aneurysms. Surgery 1970; 68:942–952.
232. Dawson I, et al. Asymptomatic popliteal aneurysm: elective operation versus conservative follow-up. Br J Surg 1994; 81:1504–1507.
233. Varga ZA, Locke-Edmunds JC, Baird RN. A multicenter study of popliteal aneurysms. Joint Vascular Research Group. J Vasc Surg 1994; 20:171–177.
234. Carpenter JP, et al. Popliteal artery aneurysms: current management and outcome. J Vasc Surg 1994; 19:65–72.
235. Bouhoutsos J, Martin P. Popliteal aneurysm: a review of 116 cases. Br J Surg 1974; 61:469–475.
236. Dent TL, et al. Multiple arteriosclerotic arterial aneurysms. Arch Surg 1972; 105:338–344.
237. Szilagyi DE, Schwartz RL, Reddy DJ. Popliteal artery aneurysms. Arch Surg 1981; 116:724–728.
238. Tompkins WC Jr, et al. The atherosclerotic popliteal aneurysm—report of diagnosis and treatment in 26 cases. Am J Surg 1977; 134:813–816.
239. Whitehouse WM Jr, et al. Limb-threatening potential of arteriosclerotic popliteal artery aneurysms. Surgery 1983; 93:694–699.
240. Graham LM, et al. Clinical significance of arteriosclerotic femoral artery aneurysms. Arch Surg 1980; 115:502–507.
241. Anton GE, et al. Surgical management of popliteal aneurysms: trends in presentation treatment, and results from 1952 to 1984. J Vasc Surg 1986; 3:125–134.
242. Reilly MK, Abbott WM, Darling RC. Aggressive surgical management of popliteal artery aneurysms. Am J Surg 1983; 145:498–502.

243. Bedford PD, Lodge B. Aneurysm of the splenic artery. Gut 1960; 1:312–380.
244. Jones EL, Finnay GG. Splenic artery aneurysms: a reappraisal. Arch Surg 1968; 97:640.
245. Kreel L. The recognition and incidence of splenic artery aneurysm. A historical review. Aust Radiol 1972; 16:126–136.
246. Moore SW, Guida PM, Schumacher HW. Splenic artery aneurysms. Bull Soc Int Chir 1970; 29:210–218.
247. Saw EC, et al. Splenic artery aneurysms. Arch Surg 1973; 106:660–662.
248. Spittell JA, et al. Aneurysm of the splenic artery. JAMA 1961; 175:452–456.
249. Jorgensen BA. Visceral artery aneurysm: a review. Dan Med Bull 1985; 32:237–242.
250. Trastek VF, et al. Splenic artery aneurysms. Surgery 1982; 91:694–699.
251. Barrett JM, Van Hooydonk JE, Boehm FH. Pregnancy-related rupture of arterial aneurysms. Obstet Gynecol 1982; 37: 557–566.
252. Croom RD III, et al. Aneurysms of the hepatic artery. South Med J 1976; 69:1013–1016.
253. Stanley JC, et al. Renal artery aneurysms. Significance of macroaneurysms exclusive of dissections and fibrodysplastic mural dilations. Arch Surg 1975; 110:1327–1333.
254. Hageman JH, et al. Aneurysms of the renal artery: problems of prognosis and surgical management. Surgery 1978; 84:563–572.

Aortic Dissection

Patrick T. O'Gara
Roman W. DeSanctis

Aortic dissection is an uncommon clinical event albeit with potentially catastrophic consequences. It is estimated that approximately 2,000 cases occur spontaneously in the United States each year [1]. Aortic dissection may account for 3–5 percent of sudden deaths in humans [2]. Without treatment, the vast majority of patients with aortic dissection will not survive beyond 2 weeks [3]. Yet over the past three decades, significant advances in medical, surgical, and anesthetic treatment have resulted in a substantial decrease in the associated mortality rate. The key to survival lies in the prompt recognition of the condition and the institution of specific and aggressive treatment as soon as possible. Because dissection of the aorta can present with variable and sometimes puzzling clinical manifestations, the antemortem diagnosis is still not infrequently missed [4]. It therefore behooves the clinician to maintain a high index of suspicion for this disease, particularly in a hypertensive patient presenting with acute chest or back pain.

This chapter will review the pathogenesis, predisposing factors, salient clinical and laboratory features, diagnostic techniques, and current therapy for aortic dissection.

Historical Perspective

The first clear pathologic description of aortic dissection was that of Morgagni in 1761, who reported a case involving a tear in the ascending aorta with rupture into the pericardial space [5]. Laennec, in 1819, first used the term *aneurysme disseqūant* to describe the entity [6]; since then and until recently, the disease has been referred to as dissecting aneurysm of the aorta. However, the aorta is only rarely aneurysmal in this condition, and it is actually a hematoma that dissects. Thus, in recent years, the simple designation *aortic dissection* has emerged as the preferred term for this disease.

The first series of patients with aortic dissection was published in 1843 by Peacock [7], but it was not until 1856 that Swaine and Latham made the first antemortem diagnosis [8]. Historically, two classic reviews have provided important perspectives on the pathogenesis, manifestations, and natural history of aortic dissection: that of Shennan, who collected 300 cases in 1934 [9], and that of Hirst, Johns, and Kime, who reviewed 505 cases in 1958 [3].

Gurin and colleagues reported the first attempt at surgical therapy for aortic dissection in 1935 [10]. In 1955, DeBakey and colleagues published their landmark description of the modern surgical approach to the disease [11]. Their innovations, which included excision of the intimal tear, obliteration of the false channel, and reconstitution of the aorta, with or without the interposition of a prosthetic graft, remain the cornerstones of current operative therapy. Wheat and colleagues introduced the medical therapy of aortic dissection in 1965, emphasizing the dual objectives of lowering the blood pressure and diminishing its rate of rise [12]. Over the past 25 years, numerous reports have appeared that have further refined the indications for and results of medical and surgical therapy for aortic dissection [13–31].

The advances in therapy have been paralleled by equally impressive innovations in the diagnostic techniques available to the clinician for the evaluation of patients with suspected dissection. As a result, the recognition of aortic dissection can now be made quite promptly, thus allowing early institution of appropriate treatment.

Classification

There are two important aspects to the classification of aortic dissection: (1) the anatomic location and extent; and (2) the length of time between onset and presentation.

The anatomic classification of dissection is based on the site of the intimal tear and the extent of propagation of the hematoma. The most widely used classification system is that of DeBakey et al. (Fig. 40-1) [1]. In DeBakey types I and II dissections, the entry site is in the ascending aorta, usually within a few centimeters of the aortic valve. Type I dissections extend for variable distances beyond the ascending portion of the aorta, whereas Type II dissections are confined to it. Type III dissections originate in the descending thoracic aorta, most commonly just beyond the origin of the left subclavian artery. They almost always extend anterograde, stopping above (type IIIA) or propagating below (type IIIB) the level of the diaphragm. On rare occasions, the intimal tear is present in an unusual location, such as the aortic arch or the abdominal aorta. Because type I and II dissections tend to behave similarly, they frequently are referred to simply as **proximal** or **ascending** dissections, while type III dissections are termed **distal** or **descending** dissections, a terminology we shall use.

Dailey et al. have proposed a similar classification based on the presence or absence of involvement of the ascending aorta (Fig. 40-2) [32]. In their widely used scheme, type A refers to all dissections that involve the ascending aorta, regardless of the site of the primary intimal tear, and type B denotes those dissections that do not involve the ascending aorta.

Involvement of the ascending aorta by the dissecting hematoma is associated with a much less favorable outcome [3,13,22,26,33,34]. It is worth noting that in most necropsy series of aortic dissection, the majority of patients have a proximal origin of the dissection [3], whereas clinical series often contain a preponderance of patients with a distal origin [35]. That discrepancy likely reflects the less rapidly lethal nature of distal dissections, permit-

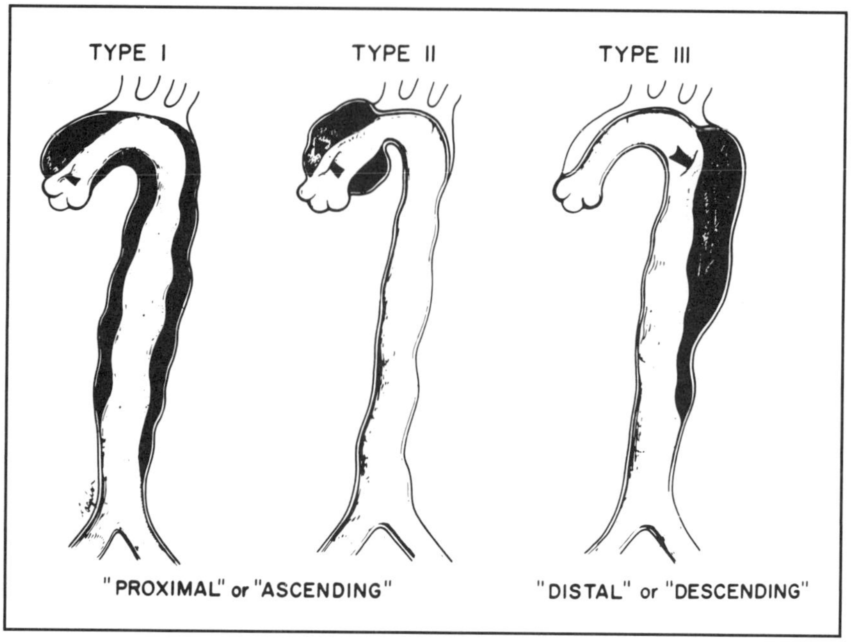

Fig. 40-1. The DeBakey classification system for aortic dissections. (Reproduced with permission from KA Eagle et al. The Practice of Cardiology, 2nd ed. Boston: Little, Brown, 1989. P. 1371.)

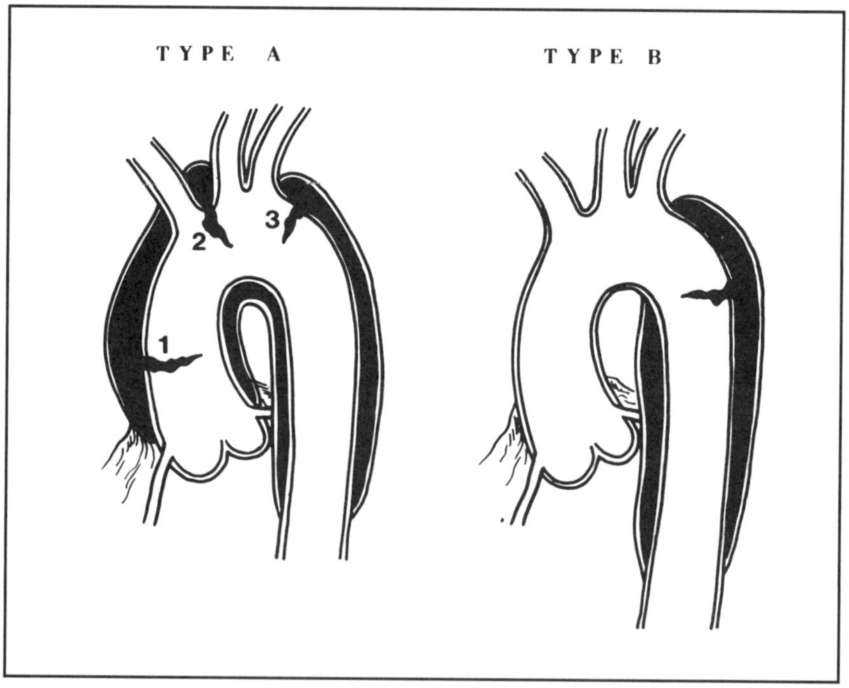

Fig. 40-2. The Stanford classification system for aortic dissections. Type A refers to all dissections that involve the ascending aorta, regardless of the site of origin. In this illustration, entry site 1 is in the ascending aorta, site 2 is in the arch, and site 3 is in the descending aorta. Type B dissections are those without ascending aortic involvement. (Reproduced with permission from DC Miller et al. Operative treatment of aortic dissection: experience of 125 patients over a 16-year period. J Thorac Cardiovasc Surg 1979; 78:365.)

ting a greater number of patients to survive long enough to reach hospital treatment centers.

Temporally, dissections are termed **acute** if presentation occurs within 2 weeks of onset and **chronic** if more than 2 weeks has elapsed. The importance of the temporal distinction derives from the fact that approximately 75 percent of patients with untreated dissection die within the first 2 weeks of onset [3].

Pathogenesis and Predisposing Factors

The signal event in aortic dissection is an intimal tear through which blood surges into the middle to outer third of the media, thereby separating the intima from the adventitia. Most commonly, dissections propagate in an anterograde direction owing to the propelling force of the column of blood; retrograde extension can occur, however, from a distal aortic entry site. Blood in the intramural false channel can reenter the true lumen anywhere along the length of the dissection. Alternatively, the hematoma can rupture, usually with catastrophic consequences. The site of external rupture is largely determined by the location of the primary intimal tear. Rupture into the pericardial space, the most common cause of death, is observed with proximal dissections. The second most common site of rupture is the left pleural space, usually in association with a distal dissection. Other less common sites of aortic rupture include the mediastinum, retroperitoneum and gastrointestinal tract.

In their 1958 review of 505 cases of aortic dissection, Hirst and colleagues reported that primary intimal tears were not found in 4 percent of autopsy specimens [3]. They postulated that dissections might arise from rupture of the aortic vasa vasorum with formation of an intramural hematoma that subsequently perforates through the intima. However, their data were derived mostly from previously published reports rather than from personal inspection of the gross specimens. In a more recent study in which 158 of 161 postmortem specimens were reviewed personally by the authors, an intimal tear was identified in every case [36]. Wheat succinctly summarized several compelling arguments against the vasa vasorum–rupture hypothesis [37]. He points out that the intraluminal aortic pressure is invariably higher than that in the vasa vasorum; that if dissections arose from vasa vasorum rupture, they should originate in the outer one-third to one-half of the media, which is not the case; that hydrodynamic data show that the site of greatest stress on the aortic wall is at the intima and inner third of the media; and that if dissections did arise in the outer third of the aortic wall, many more patients should die of aortic rupture at the very onset of the dissection than is actually the case [3]. Nevertheless, there has been a recent resurgence of interest in the vasa vasorum hypothesis based on the increasingly frequent identification of patients with aortic intramural hemorrhage in the absence of an intimal tear or oscillating flap, whether by cross-sectional imaging techniques or by direct inspection at operation [38–44]. By some estimates, spontaneous IMH may account for as many as 20% of cases of suspected aortic dissection [44].

As previously noted, aortic dissection begins most frequently in the ascending aorta, usually within a few centimeters of the aortic valve. The predilection for that site reflects the greater hemodynamic and torsional forces that operate on that portion of the aorta that is closest to the heart [37]. The second most common site of entry is in the descending thoracic aorta (the isthmus of the aorta) just distal to the insertion of the ligamentum arteriosum. That area of the aorta is situated at the junction between the relatively mobile arch and the fixed descending thoracic aorta and, by analogy to traumatic deceleration injuries, may be particularly susceptible to transverse tears [45]. Autopsy studies have demonstrated that the primary tear is located in the ascending aorta in approximately 60 percent of cases, in the descending aorta in approximately 30 percent, in the arch of the aorta in approximately 7 percent, and in the abdominal aorta in the remaining 3 percent of the cases [3].

Any major aortic branch vessel can be compromised by the propagating hematoma. Indeed, many of the clinical features of the disease process reflect hypoperfusion of critical vascular beds, including the coronary, brachiocephalic, mesenteric, renal, spinal, and iliac distributions. Reentry sites are identified far less commonly than primary tears but may be associated with an improved prognosis [46]. Presumably, reentry provides a mechanism for decompression of the hematoma, an action that may help to prevent aortic rupture and to restore flow in arteries whose origins are obstructed by the dissecting hematoma.

On rare occasions, an aortic dissection may spontaneously "heal," a process that leads to the formation of a double-lumen aorta. Pathologic examination in such cases usually reveals proximal entry and distal reentry sites. Interestingly, a highly cellular pseudointima forms along the dissection channel that is remarkably susceptible to accelerated atherogenesis [45,46]. Such double-lumen aortas may indeed become aneurysmal, particularly if the false lumen continues to expand against its weakened walls.

The competency of the aortic valve may be compromised by the dissection, a point that will be addressed more thoroughly later in this chapter. Patients with chronic proximal dissections may present with unexplained aortic regurgitation and congestive heart failure.

The tensile strength of the aortic wall derives primarily from the major supporting elements in its media, chiefly, the elastic tissue and smooth muscle cells. Certainly, any process leading to the destruction of those elements can predispose to dissection. In their review of 85 necropsy cases, Gore and Siewert found that elastic-tissue lesions predominated in those patients with aortic dissection under the age of 40 years [47], smooth muscle-cell abnormalities were more common among older patients. The bulk of accumulated pathologic evidence would indeed suggest that medial degenerative changes of a variety of types underlie many, if not most, cases of aortic dissection [48–51]. Perhaps the classic degenerative process is that of **cystic medial necrosis,** a term first employed by Gsell and Erdheim in their pathologic descriptions of the accumulation of mucoid substances, together with the disruption of the elastic and muscular components, found in patients with dissection or spontaneous aortic rupture [52,53]. It is important to note that such lesions are noninflammatory. More recent theory postulates that the cystic accumulations of mucopolysaccharide ground substances are a nonspecific response to the primary degeneration of elastic lamellar units, smooth muscle cells, or both. The simpler term **medial degeneration** may be more appropriate; cystic changes are not a universal feature of the several types of degenerative conditions observed in the aortic media [45].

The heritable disorders of connective tissue, most notably Marfan syndrome and Ehlers-Danlos syndrome, also are associated with degenerative changes in the medial elastic tissue and consequently a marked predisposition to aortic dissection and spontaneous rupture [54–60]. Indeed, changes consistent with medionecrosis of the aorta are often found in necropsy or operative specimens from such patients. The phenotypic features of Marfan syndrome may not always be obvious; they typically include a gracile habitus, arachnodactyly, lenticular dislocations, a high-arched palate, and various chest wall deformities (scoliosis, pectus excavatum). Cardiovascular abnormalities, such as annuloaortic ectasia, aortic insufficiency, and mitral valve prolapse, can occur in isolation, the so-called forme fruste of Marfan syndrome [61,62]. Ehlers-Danlos syndrome is characterized by hyperextensile skin ("India Rubber Man"), hypermobile joints, easy bruisability, and a bleeding diathesis. Those patients with a propensity to spontaneous gastrointestinal hemorrhage or aortic rupture [60] have a deficiency of type III collagen [63].

Aortic dissection can be induced experimentally in young rats fed meal made from the sweat pea (lathyrus odoratus) [64]. The active factor in the meal, beta-aminoproprionitrile [65], suppresses the activity of lysyl oxidase, an enzyme essential for elastin polymerization [66,70]. Analysis of necropsy specimens has revealed alterations in elastin concentration and amino acid composition [71].

Systemic hypertension is the most common major risk factor for the development of aortic dissection [2,33,69,70]. It is particularly prevalent among patients with distal dissection, being present in 90 percent of such cases [35]. Hypertension is present in 50 to 60 percent of patients with proximal dissections. In addition to the increased hydrostatic force associated with the elevated blood pressure, the process of gradual medial degeneration that occurs with aging is accelerated by hypertension [71,72].

Many other conditions have been associated with an increased risk of dissection. Although dissections predominate in males, with a ratio of 3:1 over females [1], an association with pregnancy, particularly the third trimester, has been observed [73]. Half of all dissections in women under the age of 40 occur in relationship to pregnancy [3,74]. Careful review of several cases during pregnancy frequently uncovers other potential causes for the dissection, such as hypertension or a connective-tissue disorder. Dissections have been observed in association with aortic-valve stenosis, particularly congenitally bicuspid or unicuspid valves [75–80], and with coarctation of the aorta [81–83]. Less commonly associated diseases have included Turner's syndrome (with or without coarctation) [84–86], Noonan's syndrome [87], giant cell aortitis [88–90], relapsing polychondritis [91], polycystic kidney disease [92], and systemic lupus erythematosus [93]. Mention should be made that aortic dissection is an extremely rare complication of syphilitic aortitis, perhaps because of the intense medial scarring that occurs in response to the initial spirochete-mediated injury [45,94]. Atherosclerosis generally is not regarded as a predisposing factor for aortic dissection. On the contrary, Roberts has argued that the most common cause of interruption of a propagating hematoma is "extensive atherosclerotic plaquing" [46]. However, we have noted dissections, especially of the distal aorta, arising by way of perforation through an atheromatous plaque [35].

External trauma is also an unusual cause of classic dissection (as opposed to a localized aortic transection), unless there exist other underlying predisposing factors. Iatrogenic dissections are rare but potentially catastrophic complications of cardiac surgery and cannulation or catheterization of the aorta [95]. Surgically related dissection can occur at locations where the aorta has been incised or cross-clamped. In particular, several dissections have been reported to originate at the site of incision of the aorta for the implantation of saphenous-vein bypass grafts [96] or for aortic-valve replacement [97]. Retrograde dissections that occur at the time of catheterization usually seal spontaneously without incident, but on rare occasion they may require surgical repair. Aortic dissection has been reported in association with cocaine use, probably as a result of the catecholamine surge and consequent hypertension that occur with its ingestion [98]. Specific aortic cocaine-related architectural changes, like those described in myocardium, have not been identified.

Clinical Presentation

Severe chest pain is the cardinal feature of aortic dissection and occurs in over 90 percent of patients [35]. In fact, pain is so nearly universal that its absence usually is associated with an impaired sensorium. The pain usually is excruciatingly severe and often accompanied by sweating. We have seen patients in whom the pain was so intense that they were knocked to the ground by it, writhing in agony. Nonetheless, painless dissection can occur [4,99]. A few features of the pain are typical for aortic dissection and deserve emphasis. In contrast to the crescendo or variable nature of the pain that is associated with acute myocardial infarction, the pain of a dissection is usually of abrupt onset and of maximal intensity at its inception. Not infrequently, patients may try to alleviate the discomfort by moving about, whereas patients with angina pectoris may tend to remain still. Patients with dissection often use such morbidly apt terms as "tearing" or "ripping" to describe the quality of their pain. An additional important distinguishing feature of the pain of aortic dissection is its tendency to migrate from its initial (entry) site to other locations (neck, back) as the hematoma spreads along the aorta. We found that to be present in 70 percent of our cases [35].

The location of the pain is of limited help in identifying the site of origin of the dissection. Anterior thoracic pain is more common with proximal than distal dissections, while posterior thoracic pain is noted more commonly with distal dissections. But there is much overlap, and pain felt simultaneously in both places is not uncommon with dissections beginning at either locus. However, the absence of posterior thoracic, interscapular pain is very much against a distal origin. It was present in over 90 percent of our patients with distal lesions [35]. The pain of aortic dissection also may be felt at peculiar sites. Those dissections originating in the aortic arch may cause pain in the neck, jaws, or hard palate.

Fifteen to 20 percent of patients with aortic dissection develop important neurologic abnormalities [35,100,101], which may be encountered when the patient presents. Syncope or sustained loss of consciousness can result from a stroke. In the absence of a stroke, we have found that syncope at the onset of a dissection is frequently indicative of cardiac tamponade following aortic rupture into the pericardial space [35]. Transient ischemic attacks or accomplished strokes may result from intermittent or sustained interruption of the circulation to either cerebral hemisphere or to the vertebrobasilar system and brain stem. A potentially catastrophic neurologic complication is that of paraparesis or paraplegia from the interruption of the circulation to the spinal cord, via the anterior spinal artery, the thoracic intercostals, or the artery of Adamkiewicz. An uncommon neurologic complication of aortic dissection is ischemic neuropathy, usually in either leg and resulting from an abrupt interruption of iliac-artery flow. Severe ischemia of the affected limb invariably is evident [102].

Rarely, patients may present with congestive heart failure due to acute, severe aortic insufficiency, the magnitude of which is often masked by the abrupt rise in left ventricular end diastolic pressure.

Aortic dissection may rarely (1% of cases) present with acute myocardial injury due to compromise of a coronary ostium with or without propagation along the right or left coronary artery [103]. The right coronary artery is involved more frequently than the left, probably because proximal aortic-entry tears occur more commonly along the right anterolateral aspect of the aorta, across from the valve orifice [45,79].

Patients who survive with chronic dissections usually present for medical attention because of unexplained aortic insufficiency and heart failure, in the case of a proximal event, or because of the incidental radiographic recognition of a descending thoracic aortic aneurysm, in the case of a distal process. We have encountered a small number of patients with the recent onset of aortic insufficiency who had a small localized dissection in the aorta confined to the region of the aortic annulus that rendered the aortic valve incompetent. Such small tears may occur without pain.

The diagnosis of dissection can be made with reasonable assurance at the bedside if certain physical findings are present. Despite their shocky appearance, patients with dissection very often are hypertensive [33]. That is particularly true for patients with distal dissection and most likely represents an exacerbation of their underlying, severe hypertension by the release of catecholamines in response to pain. Alternatively, the dissection may involve the origin of one or both renal arteries, leading to the development of severe, refractory hypertension due to renin release from renal hypoperfusion [104]. Hypotension can result from acute congestive heart failure or hypovolemia due to hemorrhage into the pleural, peritoneal, or pericardial spaces, the last with tamponade. Pseudohypotension can occur if there is luminal compromise of either or both subclavian arteries. Patients with aortic dissection often have a low-grade fever, that is, 100–101°F (39°C) [105].

An absent or diminished peripheral pulse is a major clue to the presence of a dissection. Pulse deficits are presented in roughly one-half of patients with proximal dissections and one-sixth of those with distal dissections [35]. Pulses may be lost either by compression of the arterial lumen by the dissecting hematoma or by occlusion of the ostium of the artery by a flap of dissected intima. Pulse deficits can occur anywhere along the arterial tree in patients with proximal dissection, whereas distal dissections usually involve the left subclavian and iliac arteries. The deficits may be transitory because they are influenced by the height of the blood pressure, the presence or absence of a distal reentry site, and the possible movement of the intimal flap toward or away from the arterial orifice. Thus, major peripheral pulses should be examined repeatedly in patients with suspected aortic dissection. Reduplication of pulses occasionally may be appreciated by palpation, a phenomenon that reflects the nonsimultaneous flow of blood through the true and false channels.

The recent onset of a diastolic murmur consistent with aortic insufficiency is another important clue to the presence of a proximal dissection; it is present in approximately two-thirds of such cases [33,35]. Aortic insufficiency can be produced by one of three mechanisms (Fig. 40-3): (1) critical widening of the aortic root by a circumferential hematoma that impairs leaflet coaptation; (2) displacement of one or more valve leaflets below the level of the valve annulus by asymmetric pressure from the hematoma; or (3) mechanical disruption of the annular support leading to a flail cusp [106]. The distinction is important because in the first two instances surgical decompression of the hematoma with resuspension of the native valve leaflets may restore valvular competence. However, with actual disruption of the annulus itself, aortic valve replacement usually is necessary.

The murmur of aortic insufficiency often has a peculiar musical quality in aortic dissection and may radiate better along the right than the left sternal border—a reflection of the widened aortic root, which is almost invariably present. Because the regurgitation may be dynamic, the murmur may wax and wane, paralleling rises and falls in aortic pressure. The murmur can be extremely difficult to appreciate in a critically ill patient lying supine on an emergency room stretcher. The prominence of the peripheral signs of aortic insufficiency depend on the severity and chronicity of the regurgitation and the presence or absence of congestive heart failure. Usually, the aortic incompetence is not very severe, but some exaggeration of peripheral arterial pulses and widening of the pulse pressure may be noted. However, if aortic regurgitation is severe enough to cause a marked increase in left ventricular end-diastolic pressure and congestive heart failure, the peripheral signs of aortic insufficiency may be attenu-

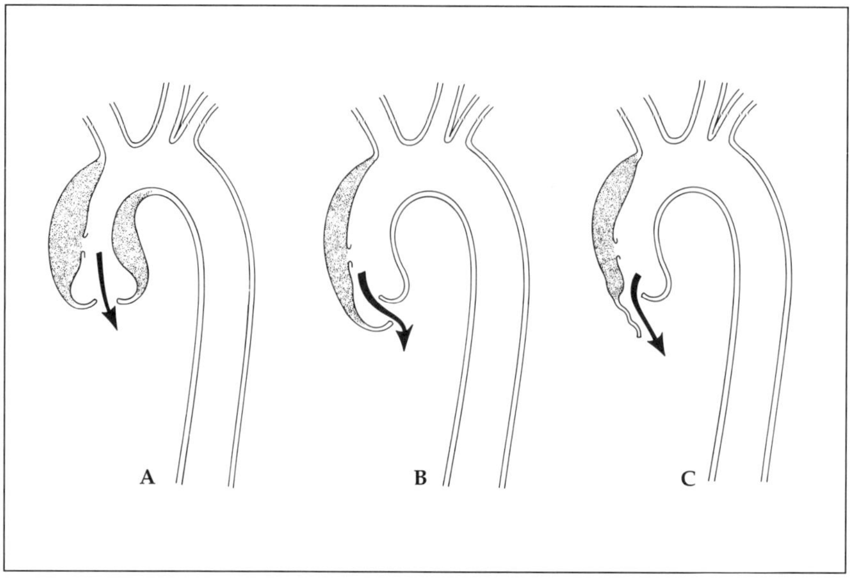

Fig. 40-3. Mechanisms of aortic regurgitation in proximal aortic dissection. **A.** A circumferential hematoma pulls the annulus apart and impairs leaflet coaptation. **B.** An asymmetric hematoma exerts pressure against one valve leaflet, depressing it below the level of valve closure. **C.** Annular support is disrupted, leading to a flail aortic leaflet and free regurgitation. (Reproduced with permission from KA Eagle et al. The Practice of Cardiology, 2nd ed. Boston: Little, Brown, 1989. P. 1375.)

ated. Nonetheless, in a few instances, we have been directed towards the correct diagnosis of aortic dissection in patients with disproportionately bounding peripheral pulses in the face of severe congestive heart failure, despite the absence of a murmur of aortic regurgitation.

Signs of possible pericardial involvement, the presence of which portend an ominous outcome, must be searched for carefully. Those signs include a pericardial friction rub, paradoxical pulse, venous distention, and a pericardial effusion as suggested by either chest radiograph or echocardiogram and electrocardiographic low voltage.

Many other interesting yet extremely uncommon manifestations of aortic dissection have been reported, including Horner's syndrome, due to compression of the superior cervical ganglion, vocal-cord paralysis due to pressure against the recurrent laryngeal nerve, sternoclavicular joint pulsation [107], superior vena cava syndrome from caval obstruction [108–112], aorticocaval [113] or aorticoright atrial fistula [114], hemoptysis due to rupture into a bronchus [115], hematemesis following extension into the esophagus [116], heart block due to extension of the dissection into the area of the atrioventricular (AV) node [117,118], signs of mesenteric infarction, and fever of undetermined source [105]. Rarely, aortic dissection presents only as a sudden loss of an arterial pulse, mimicking an arterial embolus.

Pleural effusions, predominantly left-sided, occur in approximately 10 percent of patients, most commonly in those with distal dissections. Quite often the fluid is not grossly sanguinous but straw-colored and may simply represent a nonspecific inflammatory response of the pleura to the intense tissue injury caused by the adjacent hematoma.

Laboratory Findings

In general, the routine laboratory findings in patients with aortic dissection are neither particularly striking nor helpful. The hemoglobin often is reduced owing to frank rupture or to sequestration of blood within the aortic false lumen. As the hematoma matures, some hemolysis ensues, leading to a mild increase in the level of lactic dehydrogenase and the indirect bilirubin fraction. Two-thirds of patients have a modest leukocytosis (>10,000 white cells/mm^3) [106]. Rarely, evidence for disseminated intravascular coagulation is present; that phenomenon has been attributed to the accelerated consumption of platelets and clotting factors on the surfaces of the dissection channel [119]. Microscopic hematuria may be found in cases involving the renal arteries.

The electrocardiogram and cardiac enzyme levels are helpful in a negative sense, that is, when they fail to disclose evidence of an acute myocardial infarction in a patient who presents with chest pain. However, as previously stated, acute myocardial infarction has been observed in a small subset of patients with proximal dissection due to involvement of the ostium of the right or left coronary artery.

Routine chest x-rays can provide important clues to the presence of aortic dissection, and will show abnormalities in 90 percent of cases [35,120]. If the patient's condition permits, careful posteroanterior, lateral, and oblique views of the chest should be obtained (Fig. 40-4). In particular, the posteroanterior view is important because the anteroposterior projection usually done in emergency rooms tends to exaggerate the width of the mediastinum. Although no single radiographic sign is specific for dissection, several are suggestive: (1) widening of the mediasti-

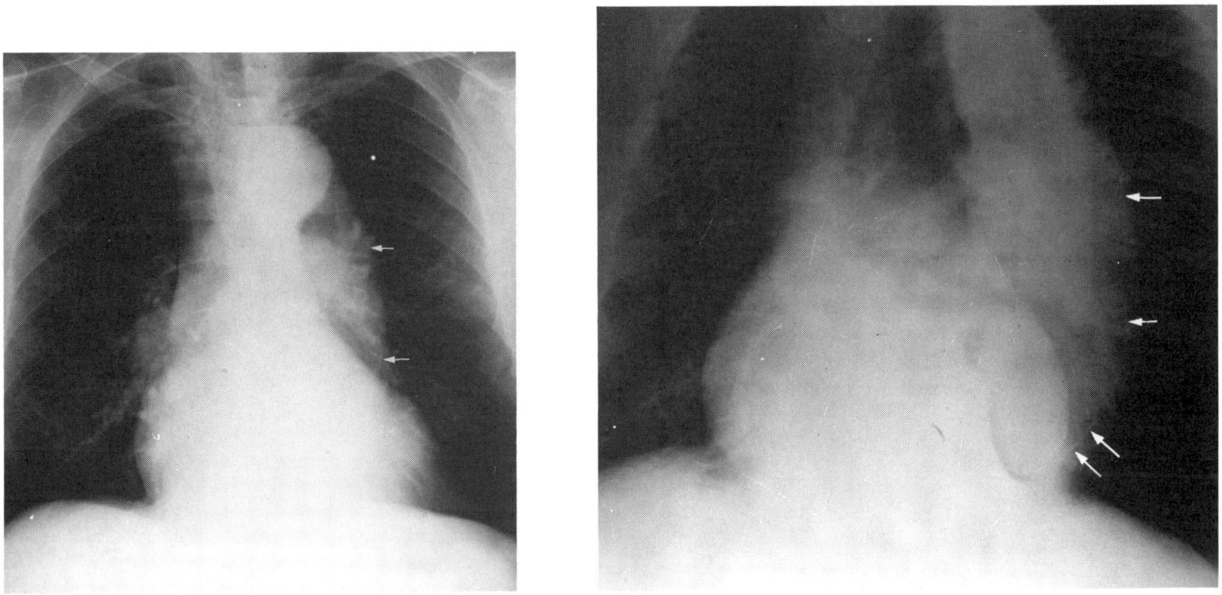

A B

Fig. 40-4. Posteroanterior **A.** and left oblique **B.** chest films of a 55-year-old man with an angiographically confirmed distal dissection. The posteroanterior film demonstrates an enlarged aortic knob (with tracheal deviation) and definite widening of the descending thoracic aorta. There are also faint linear calcifications, more easily seen on the left oblique film, that are clearly separated from the aortic soft-tissue border (arrows). (Courtesy of Robert Dinsmore, M.D., Massachusetts General Hospital, Boston.)

nal silhouette; (2) a disparity in caliber between the ascending and descending thoracic aorta [121,122]; (3) a localized bulge or angulation along the normally smooth aortic contour [123] (such a bulge usually indicates the point of origin of the dissection) (Fig. 40-5, see also Fig. 40-14); (4) separation of intimal calcification greater than 10 mm from the outer edge of the soft tissue border of the aorta, especially in the region of the aortic knob [124–126]; and (5) a double-density appearance of the aorta, which suggests the presence of true and false channels [121,123]. Pleural effusions are common, especially in the left pleural space, but right-sided effusions do occur. Small effusions usually are due to exudation from aortic inflammation around the dissection; larger effusions may reflect rupture of the dissection with hemothorax. Certainly, progressive changes in either the size or contour of the aorta as observed on serial radiographic studies would strongly imply that a dissection is present. It is possible, however, to have an entirely normal aortic shadow with a dissection (Fig. 40-6) [120].

Diagnostic Techniques

Extensive experience has accumulated in the application of noninvasive imaging techniques to the diagnosis of aortic dissection. The earliest of these techniques was M-mode ultrasonography, [114,127,128], followed by transthoracic echocardiography (TTE) and, more recently, transesophageal echocardiography (TEE) with color-flow Doppler mapping [129–135]. TTE criteria for the diagnosis of proximal aortic dissection include (1) an increase in the diameter of the aortic root to a width of 42 mm or more; (2) an anterior aortic wall measuring 16 mm or more in thickness, a posterior wall width of 10 mm or greater, or both; (3) maintenance of parallelism between the separated margins of either of the aortic walls; (4) normal aortic-valve-cusp movement within the aortic lumen; (5) oscillation of the intimal flap of the dissection; (6) demonstration of aortic regurgitation; and (7) premature aortic or mitral-valve closure, the latter, if present, a manifestation of significant aortic insufficiency [127,131] (Fig. 40-7). Advances in color Doppler techniques have allowed the skilled operator to provide comprehensive evaluations of flow dynamics within and possibly between the true and false lumens as well as quantitative estimates of the severity of any associated aortic regurgitation.

In clinical practice, the diagnosis of aortic dissection by ultrasound techniques hinges on the demonstration of an oscillating intimal flap with separation of the true and false lumens. TTE has a sensitivity of approximately 60 percent for the detection of aortic dissection [136]. For obvious reasons, its utility in cases of suspected distal aortic dissection is marginal. TTE also has inherent problems in delineating the extent of the dissection process and major aortic branch involvement, although it is quite sensitive for the detection of aortic regurgitation.

Transesophageal ultrasonic imaging provides significantly more accurate information regarding the thoracic aorta and is considered by many to be the noninvasive modality of choice for the study of patients with suspected acute dissection and in their longitudinal follow-up

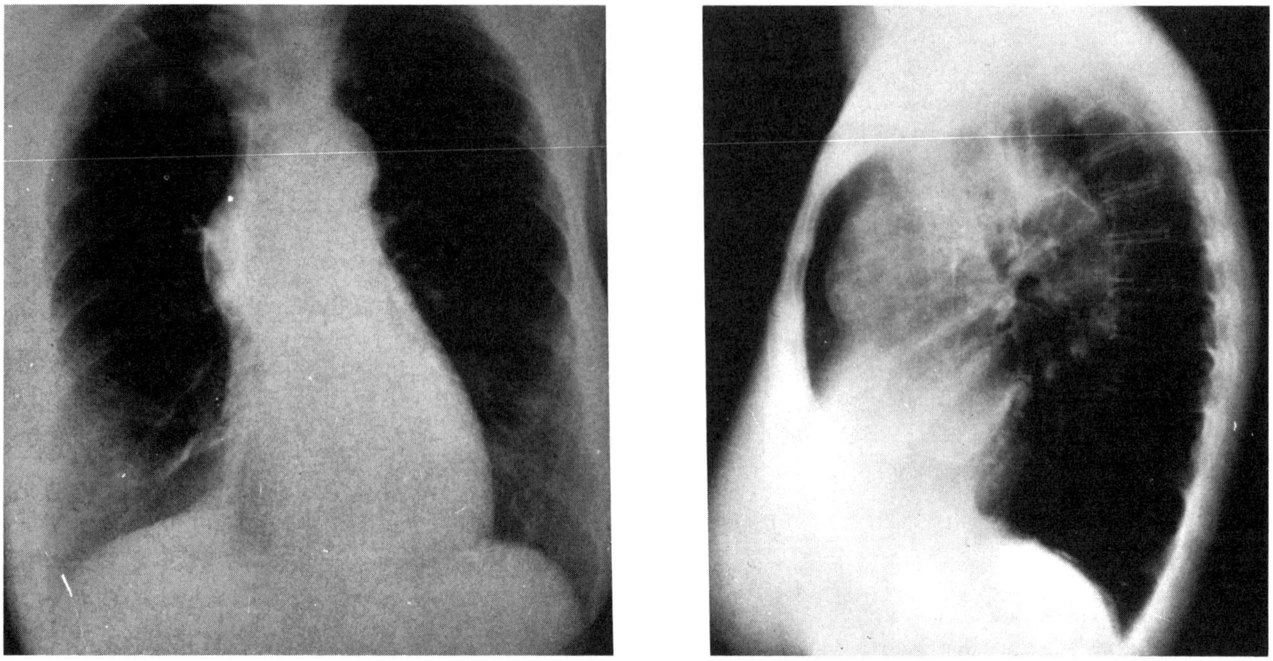

Fig. 40-5. PA (left) and lateral (right) chest x-rays of a 42-year-old woman with Marfan syndrome and an acute aortic dissection. The origin of the dissection was at the point of the bulge in the ascending aorta, and the dissection extended into the descending thoracic aorta.

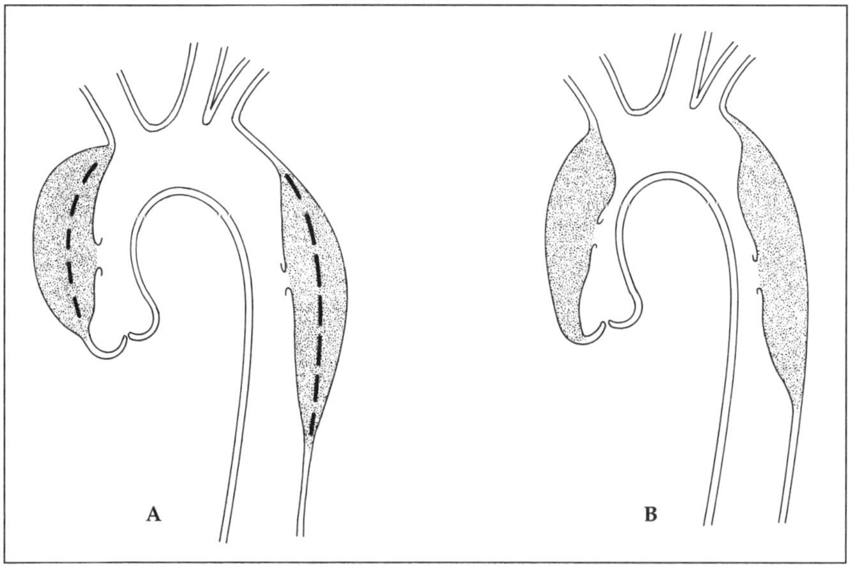

Fig. 40-6. The effect of the dissection on aortic size and contour. **A.** Proximal and distal hematomas that have expanded outward, resulting in abnormal enlargement of the ascending and descending aorta as well as prominent bulges along the aortic contour. **B.** Compression of the true lumen is more pronounced, without noticeable enlargement or bulging of the aorta. Accordingly, the chest film appearance of the aorta may be unremarkable.

[22,137,138]. Numerous reports have appeared attesting to the superior value of TEE, perhaps none more impressive than that of the European Cooperative Study Group's publication of a 99-percent sensitivity and 98-percent specificity in the diagnosis of acute aortic dissection in 164 consecutive patients [135]. The development of bi- and multiplane probes has circumvented many of the earlier pitfalls with single-plane probes [133,134], particularly the difficulty of adequately visualizing the upper portion of the ascending aorta and the transverse arch. A

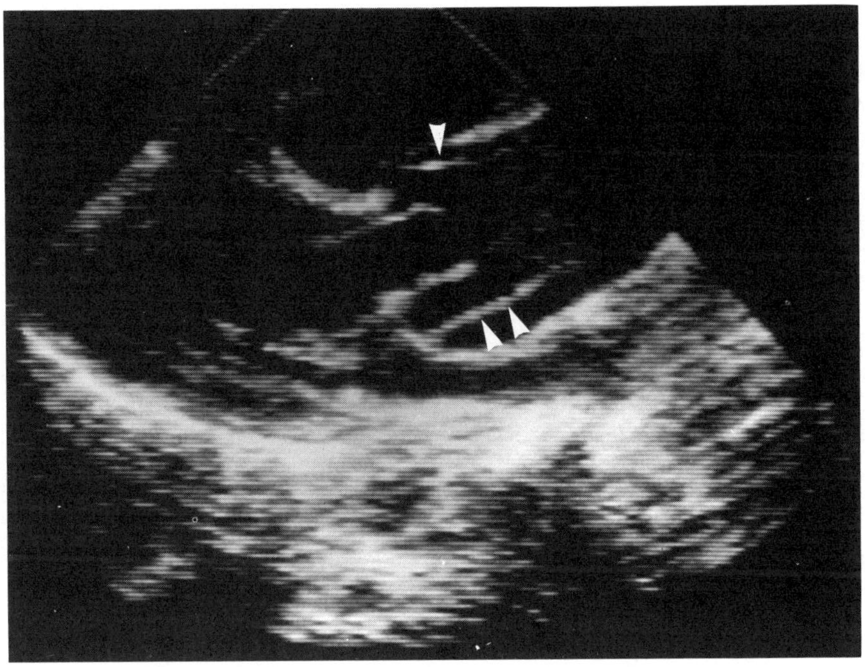

Fig. 40-7. Angulated parasternal long-axis image from a two-dimensional echocardiographic study of a 55-year-old woman with a proximal aortic dissection that extended to the bifurcation of the abdominal aorta. The separated components of the aortic wall are clearly seen in the dilated aortic root. The arrowheads point to the intimal flap. There was also a small pericardial effusion and pulsed Doppler evidence of aortic regurgitation. (Reproduced with permission from A Sanfilipo, AE Weyman. The role of echocardiography in managing critically ill patients. J Critical Illness 1988; 3:30.)

well-performed TEE with Doppler color-flow interrogation should allow identification of the site of entry, the oscillating intimal flap, differential luminal flow, brachiocephalic branch involvement, coexistent aortic regurgitation, the presence of pericardial fluid, and any associated ventricular wall motion abnormalities [139] (Fig. 40-8). Like TTE, TEE can be performed with little delay at the bedside with judicious sedation and appropriate suctioning. Abrupt surges in blood pressure with gagging must be avoided. One potential drawback is the inability of TEE to track the extent of the dissection into and beyond the abdominal aorta and its major branches. Many surgical centers now proceed directly to operation in appropriate cases following diagnostic TEE [139]. The intraoperative use of TEE can provide continued information regarding differential luminal flow following arterial cannulation and postrepair.

Several reports have appeared regarding the use of intravascular ultrasound imaging in the detection and delineation of aortic dissection, as well as in the depiction of the results of catheter-based techniques occasionally used to treat certain complications of the dissection process (e.g., stenting for the relief of limb or visceral ischemia) [140–142]. Its place among the several other diagnostic modalities has yet to be determined.

Contrast-enhanced CT also is a highly sensitive and specific imaging method in cases of suspected dissection [136,143–149]. Dynamic CT image processing may increase the diagnostic accuracy of the technique and provide even further information [150]. CT signs of aortic dissection include dilation of the aorta and the presence of an intimal flap, with demonstration of true and false lumens, often with differential rates of flow [151]. Using contrast-enhanced CT imaging, Moncada et al. reported the correct diagnosis of aortic dissection in 78 of 81 subsequently proven cases [152]. Nienaber et al. reported a sensitivity and specificity of 98 percent and 87 percent, respectively [136]. Figure 40-9 illustrates an example of an aortic dissection demonstrated by CT. Although CT imaging is a rapidly performed, valuable initial screening procedure for aortic dissection, the diagnosis and quantification of aortic regurgitation cannot be made on the basis of such studies alone, because the entry site is not effectively demonstrated nor is much information provided with respect to perfusion of the major aortic branches. On occasion, however, CT imaging has demonstrated dissections that were not shown on contrast aortography [153].

The rapidly accumulating experience with MR imaging in the detection of aortic dissection and in the long-term follow-up of patients after definitive repair has been very favorable [136,154–157]. Its wide field of view and superb resolution are unrivaled. Diagnostic sensitivity and specificity approach 100 percent in experienced centers [136]. MR imaging allows identification of the entry site, delineation of the intimal flap and its anatomic extent, and dem-

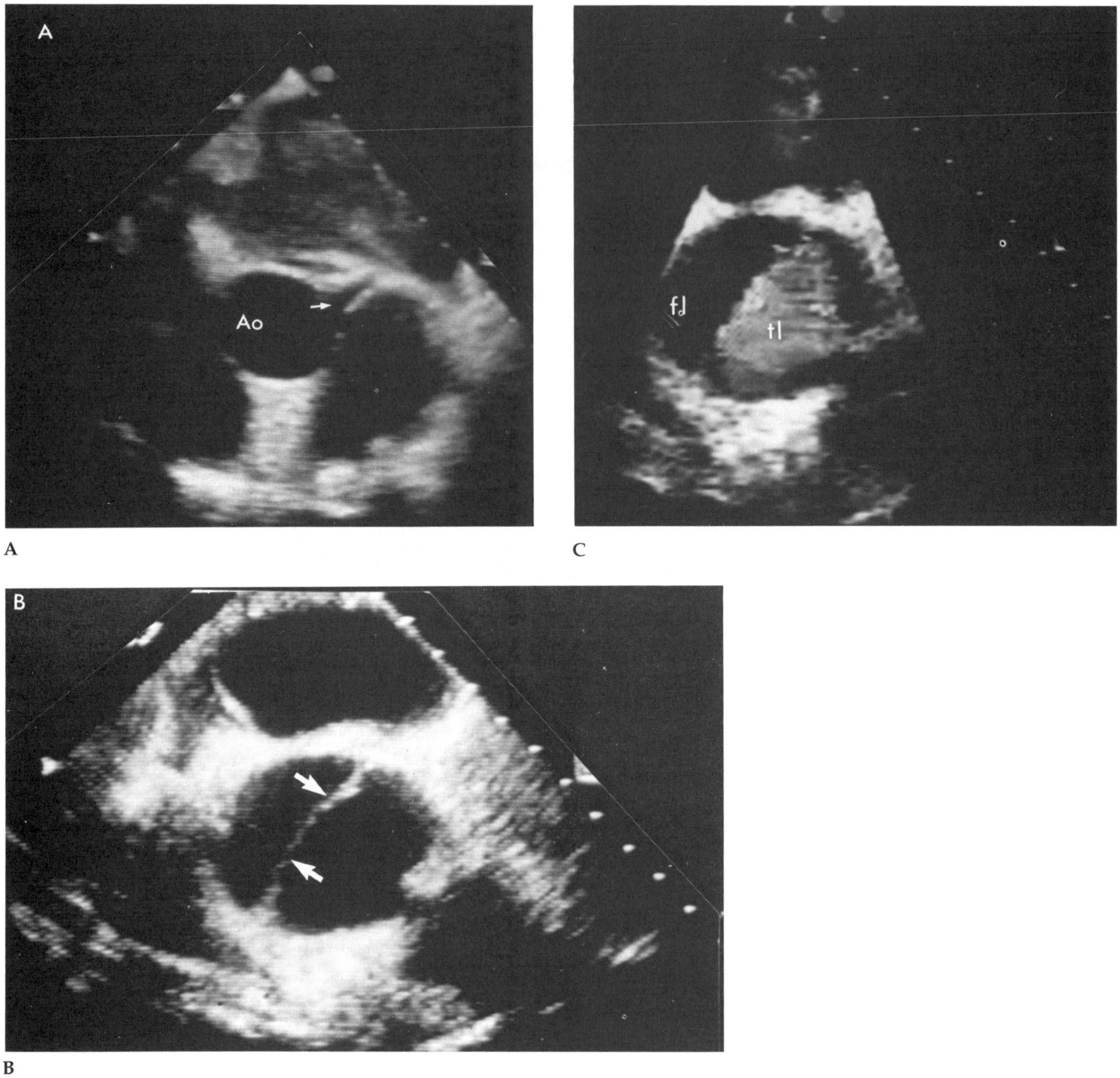

Fig. 40-8. **A.** Transesophageal echocardiographic image of short-axis view of the ascending aortic (Ao) at the level of the ostium of the left main coronary artery (arrow). **B.** Short-axis view of dissection of the ascending aorta. The intimal flap is noted by the arrows. **C.** Color flow map during systole of image in B. Normal flow in the true lumen (tl) is noted in blue. In this example, no flow is detected in the false lumen (fl). (Courtesy of Michael Picard, M.D., Massachusetts General Hospital, Boston.)

onstration of major branch involvement (Fig. 40-10). Velocity encoding, gating, and gradient-echo techniques can provide information regarding differential luminal-flow characteristics. The presence of pericardial or pleural effusions also can be easily appreciated. Finally, contrast substances are not necessary, and ionizing radiation is not employed.

There are several important limitations to the use of MR imaging in the acute setting. Careful imaging requires valuable time in a confining magnet that typically is located at a distance from the emergency department and operating suites. The patient may be claustrophobic or require special monitoring or infusion pumps that cannot be used in proximity to the magnet. A radiologist with expert knowledge of the appropriate acquisition algorithms must be present. For hemodynamically unstable or critically ill patients, MR imaging is not appropriate.

Despite recent advances in the imaging techniques

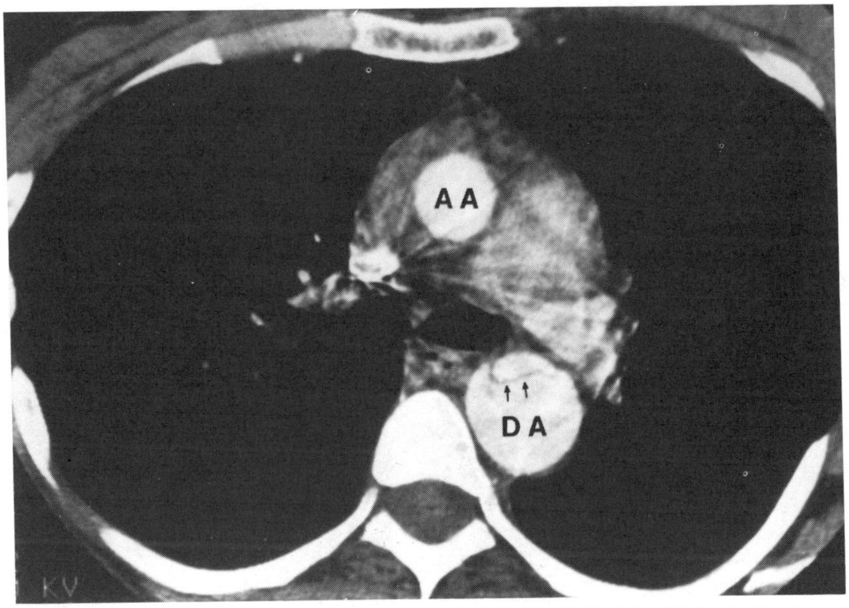

Fig. 40-9. CT scan with contrast showing an extensive aortic dissection in a 36-year-old woman with Marfan syndrome (see also Fig. 34-13). There is considerable hematoma surrounding the ascending aorta (AA). The descending thoracic aorta (DA) is significantly dilated. The black arrows point to the intimal flap that separates the large false lumen from the compressed true lumen. (Courtesy of Department of Radiology, Faulkner Hospital, Jamaica Plain, Mass.)

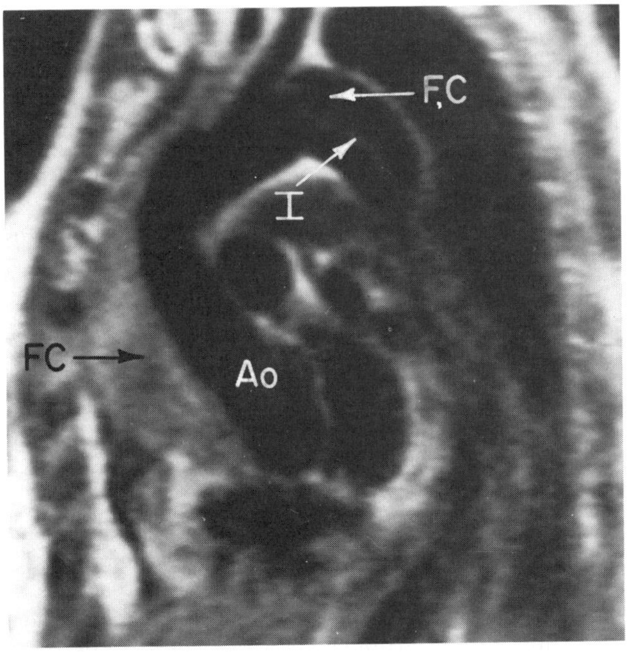

Fig. 40-10. Longitudinal MR image showing a proximal aortic dissection in a 55-year-old woman. The false channel (FC) is seen hugging the proximal aorta (Ao) and is noted again in the descending thoracic aorta. The intimal flap (I) is faintly seen.

available for the noninvasive assessment of the aorta, contrast aortography has retained its usefulness in the evaluation of patients with suspected dissection [35,158]. With skilled and experienced operators, it can be performed expeditiously and safely, even in the critically ill patient. The diagnostic accuracy of contrast aortography approaches 98 percent [105]. The procedure is still best accomplished following retrograde aortic catheterization, and, in general, only one radiographic projection, usually the right posterior oblique, is necessary (Figs. 40-11 and 40-12). In our laboratory, we prefer cut films, although some clinicians believe that more information is gained from cineaortography [159,160]. The critical features to be assessed include (1) the site of the entry tear, (2) the extent of the dissection, (3) the presence or absence of aortic valve involvement, and (4) the relation of the major aortic branch vessels to the dissection. All these features are of crucial importance for appropriate surgical planning. Rarely, the contrast aortogram may be falsely negative, either because the false channel is not thrown into proper relief and hence escapes detection by the x-ray beam or because the true and false lumens opacify simultaneously and to the same extent. Additionally, the dissection may be so well circumscribed and self-limited as to simply not be visible. Thrombosis of the false channel, such as might occur with a chronic dissection, also may prevent visualization of either an intimal flap or a double lumen. Clues to the presence of a dissection in such cases, however, would include the demonstration of extrinsic compression of the true aortic lumen, an abnormally thick aortic wall, an unexplained aortic branch abnormality, or a peculiar

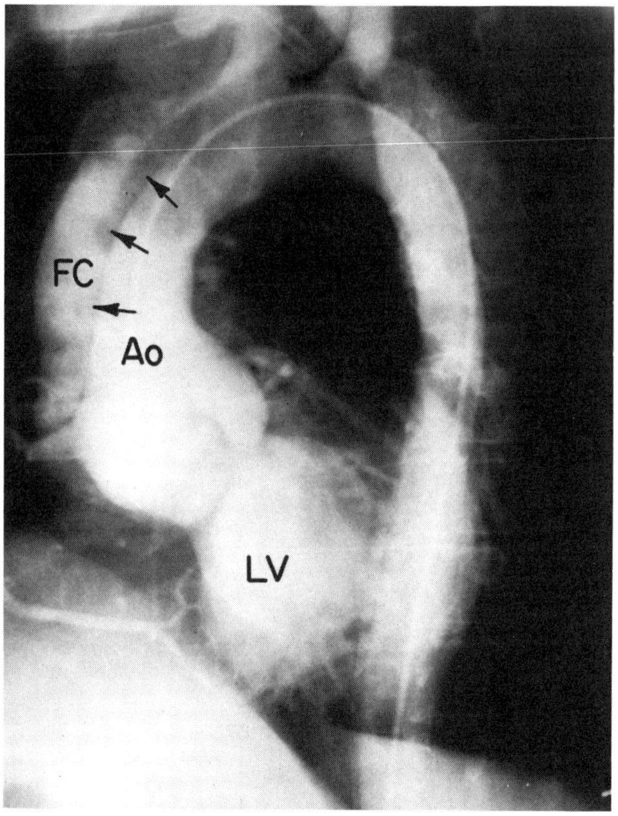

Fig. 40-11. Retrograde aortogram in a 59-year-old man with a proximal aortic dissection. The false channel (FC) fills faintly; there is considerable aortic regurgitation, which fills the left ventricle (LV) from the aorta (Ao). The arrows point to the intimal flap. The false channel extends into the descending thoracic aorta. (Courtesy of Robert Dinsmore M.D., Massachusetts General Hospital, Boston.)

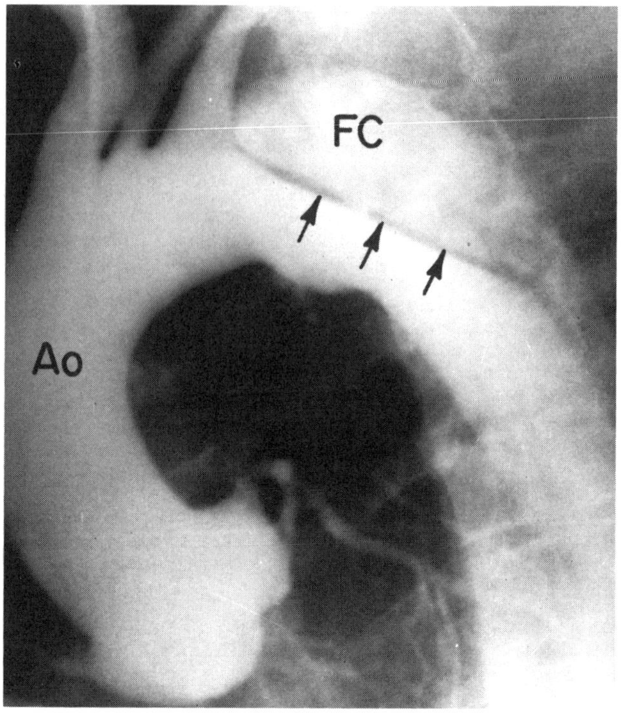

Fig. 40-12. Retrograde aortogram from the right brachial artery in a 63-year-old man showing a localized distal aortic dissection. The intimal flap is unusually well demonstrated (arrows). The false channel (FC) is confined to the proximal segment of the descending thoracic aorta (Ao). (Courtesy of Robert Dinsmore, M.D., Massachusetts General Hospital, Boston.)

position of the angiographic catheter [120]. Aortic dissection may be an unexpected finding during aortic cineangiography performed as part of an evaluation for aortic insufficiency.

The diagnosis of aortic dissection also can be confirmed by digital subtraction angiography [120] (Fig. 40-13). In general, however, that technique provides less resolution, particularly as regards aortic-branch detail, than standard contrast aortography. Videodensitometric analysis, though, can provide information regarding the relative rates of flow in the true and false channels.

Given all those choices, how should the clinician proceed to verify the diagnosis of acute dissection? Most institutions have developed diagnostic strategies that serve them best. An approach that has gained widespread acceptance includes the rapid performance of TTE, followed by expeditious TEE when the former proves inadequate. In those instances where uncertainty persists or the data are suboptimal, contrast aortography with multiplane imaging should be performed immediately. Certainly, any diagnostic strategy must accommodate the particular concerns of the individual surgeon who must undertake the operative repair. In institutions where TTE and TEE are not immediately available, contrast-enhanced CT scanning should suffice as the initial screening tool.

TEE, contrast-enhanced CT scanning, or MR imaging could be performed on any stable patient in whom the presence of dissection should be excluded when its likelihood is low. Any of those modalities should be adequate for the assessment of patients with suspected chronic dissection as well as for the long-term follow-up of treated survivors. We prefer MR imaging in those circumstances because of its superior performance characteristics.

DIFFERENTIAL DIAGNOSIS

The differential diagnosis of aortic dissection should include those conditions that are primarily associated with chest or back pain. The most frequently encountered conditions among patients recently reviewed by Eagle et al. from Massachusetts General Hospital were acute myocardial infarction, nondissecting thoracic aortic aneurysm, musculoskeletal pain, pericarditis, and mediastinal tumors [158]. Usually, patients with those conditions present with chest pain combined with one or more signs that suggest aortic dissection, such as a widened mediastinum on chest film, hypertension, or a murmur of aortic insufficiency. Mention has already been made of some of the features of the pain associated with dissection that may help to distinguish it from myocardial infarction. In addi-

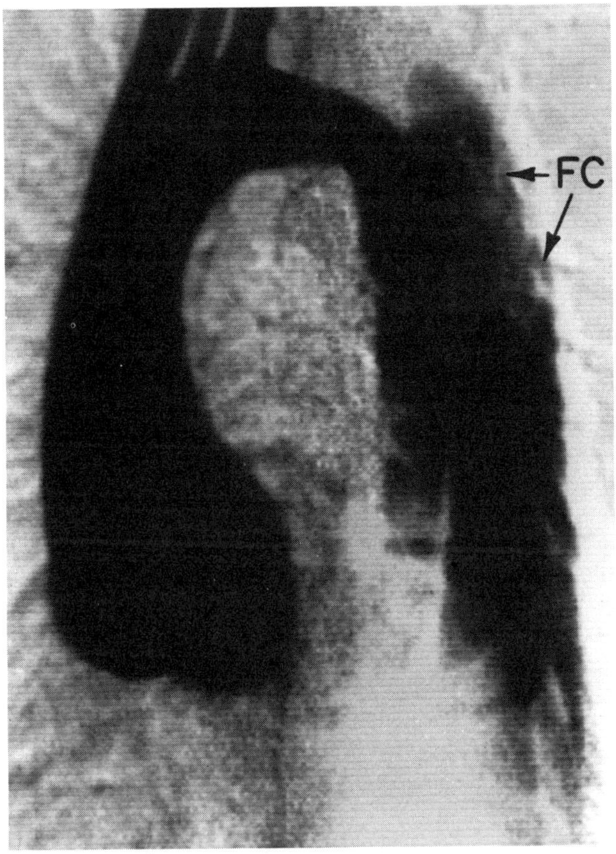

Fig. 40-13. Digital subtraction aortogram showing a distal aortic dissection in a 36-year-old woman with several phenotypic features of Marfan syndrome. The false channel (FC) is seen adjacent to the descending thoracic aorta. There is mild, asymmetric dilatation of the aortic root.

tion, a relatively short duration of symptoms, the presence of new aortic insufficiency, and the concomitant development of pulse deficits are helpful in identifying patients with dissection. Other conditions that can mimic some of the features of aortic dissection include pulmonary thromboembolism, pleuritis, acute cholecystitis, and systemic atherothrombotic embolism [158].

There are two important radiologic and pathologic variants of classic aortic dissection: penetrating aortic ulcer and intramural hemorrhage (IMH) without an intimal flap. Patients with either of these variants cannot be distinguished reliably from patients with dissection at presentation on clinical grounds alone. Chest or back pain on a background of chronic hypertension is a common theme. Penetrating aortic ulcers affect the mid-to-distal portion of the descending thoracic aorta in older individuals with a heavy burden of atherosclerotic disease. Medial hematoma formation occurs as a result of continuous erosion of the internal elastic membrane at the site of an atherosclerotic plaque and may lead to development of a false aneurysm or frank rupture [161–164]. Longitudinal spread of the hematoma with branch vessel compromise is not a feature of this process. The ulcers can be recognized by TEE, contrast CT, MR imaging, or contrast angiography. There is clear ulceration within the aortic wall beyond the intimal border with medical thickening, often a nipple-like projection, and surrounding adventitial reaction [163].

IMH without an intimal flap otherwise shares all of the clinical and radiologic features of classic aortic dissection [42,43]. Contrast angiography has proven relatively less sensitive than TEE, contrast CT scanning, or MR imaging for the detection of IMH. Indeed, in a recent study by Nienaber et al., digital angiography was falsely negative in 8 of 25 patients with aortic IMH [43]. Given the frequency of spontaneous IMH in a population of patients with suspected aortic dissection, the improved sensitivity of TEE and contrast CT scanning is yet another reason to choose one of these two diagnostic modalities as an initial screening tool [44]. Patients with aortic IMH should be managed along the same empirical guidelines that have been adopted successfully for patients with aortic dissection. This treatment strategy is predicated on the remarkable clinical similarities and natural histories of these two conditions.

Treatment

The modern era of therapy for aortic dissection began in the early 1950s with the landmark surgical approach developed by DeBakey and colleagues [11]. Although several modifications have been proposed over the subsequent three decades, the principal objectives of surgery remain the same—excision of the intimal tear whenever possible, obliteration of entry into the false channel both proximally and distally, and reconstitution of the aorta, usually with the interposition of a synthetic conduit. Simultaneously, significant aortic regurgitation must be eliminated, either by resuspension of the displaced aortic leaflets or by replacement of the aortic valve itself.

Not every center initially enjoyed the same promising early surgical results of DeBakey and his coworkers. In 1965, Wheat et al. reported the successful **medical** treatment of aortic dissection [12]. Using experimental models, the investigators were able to demonstrate that, in addition to intraluminal pressure per se, the rate of development of that pressure created a major stress on the aortic wall and served as an important force acting to initiate and propagate aortic dissections [165]. Thus, medical therapy was directed at two objectives: (1) lowering the arterial blood pressure and (2) reducing the rate of rise of pressure development (dP/dT).

Over the ensuing years, the treatment of aortic dissection has evolved largely by empiricism. There are no carefully controlled studies of comparable patients randomized to either medical or surgical therapy at the same institution. Nonetheless, the empirical approach has led to many areas of consensus among major centers, although some areas of disagreement do exist. Stated simply and summarily, it is generally agreed that, whenever possible, acute dissections of the proximal aorta should be treated surgically. Most centers favor medical therapy for stable uncomplicated acute dissections originating in the arch and distal thoracic aorta, although some groups favor surgical treatment of those as well. There is general agreement that chronic aortic dissections, regardless of anatomic location, should be treated medically unless surgery is mandated by the development of late complications, such as progressive aortic insufficiency, redissection, or the formation of a localized aneurysm.

There are two phases of the treatment of acute aortic dissection: initial emergency treatment and subsequent definitive treatment.

INITIAL EMERGENCY TREATMENT

Patients with suspected aortic dissection should be managed in an intensive care setting, with joint medical and surgical follow-up. We generally follow the blood pressure with an indwelling arterial cannula and monitor the electrocardiogram. If hypotension or congestive heart failure is present, a Swan-Ganz pulmonary arterial catheter also is advisable to determine left heart filling pressures. The urine output should be closely followed, with an indwelling urinary catheter if necessary, and maintained above 20 ml/hour. Patients who have experienced aortic rupture may require urgent blood transfusions. Sedation and relief of pain with opiates is important not only for patient comfort, but because pain and agitation contribute to hypertension. Because of the uncertainty of intestinal absorption in many ill patients, as well as the potential for surgical intervention, we prefer to give medications parenterally whenever possible and withhold all oral intake until the patient's condition has stabilized.

It cannot be emphasized too strongly that the **treatment of acute aortic dissections should begin as soon as possible after they occur.** Thus, in cases where there is a strong clinical suspicion of aortic dissection, we advise initiating treatment even before a definitive diagnosis has been established. Measures should be undertaken immediately to lower an elevated blood pressure, if it is present, and to reduce dP/dT. The drugs most widely used for those purposes are intravenous sodium nitroprusside combined with a beta adrenoreceptor antagonist.

Sodium nitroprusside is a powerful hypotensive agent with a rapid onset of action and an exceedingly short half-life that permits continual control of blood pressure. It is mixed as 50 mg in 250 ml of 5 percent dextrose and water. Because the drug is light sensitive, the solution must be made immediately prior to its use, and the bottle containing it should be wrapped in aluminum foil. The usual starting dose is 25–50 μg/minute. The dose can be escalated as necessary to lower the blood pressure. Doses of 100–300 μg/minute are common. We generally aim for a systolic blood pressure of 90 to 100 mm Hg or the lowest blood pressure compatible with the maintenance of adequate renal, cerebral, and cardiac perfusion. Side effects of sodium nitroprusside generally are minimal and include nausea, restlessness, somnolence, and—rarely—thiocyanate toxicity, which develops only after very high doses and rarely before 48 hours of continuous administration. Blood thiocyanate levels below 10 mg/dl usually are well tolerated. Signs of thiocyanate toxicity include confusion, hyperreflexia, and frank convulsions, associated with metabolic acidosis. Serious thiocyanate toxicity can be reversed with hydroxocobalamin. Rarely, methemoglobinemia occurs; hypoxemia may result from perfusion of poorly ventilated areas of lung. Although sodium nitroprusside appears to reduce platelet adhesiveness, this has not been of consequence clinically.

Used alone, sodium nitroprusside accelerates the heart rate and increases dP/dT. Appropriate concern has been expressed that it might therefore promote aortic dissection [166]. Thus, counteracting those effects with simultaneous beta-adrenergic blockade is mandatory. The drug that has been used most widely for that purpose in aortic dissection is propranolol. It is given as 0.5- to 2.0-mg intravenous bolus to a maximum dose of 0.15 mg/kg over approximately 30 minutes. In patients with a history of bronchial asthma or chronic obstructive lung disease, metoprolol, 5–10 mg intravenously given over 5 minutes, can be substituted. The initial dose of the beta blocker is repeated every 2–4 hours as needed. Esmolol, an ultrashort-acting cardioselective beta blocker, can be titrated by continuous intravenous infusion. It should be started as a bolus of 500 μg/kg and continued as an infusion at 50 μg/kg/minute and adjusted upward, much as is true for the treatment of supraventricular tachycardia. Repeat bolus doses can be given as necessary. The guidelines for beta-blocker administration are somewhat imprecise and should be directed by the patient's condition. In addition to lowering the blood pressure to the desired range, a pulse rate of approximately 60–70 beats per minute is a reasonable objective. However, in many seriously ill patients, a pulse rate that slow may be inappropriate, and the physician must let intuition serve as a guide to the appropriate dose of beta blocker. Labetalol, which has both alpha- and nonselective beta-adrenoreceptor blocking properties could be employed alone as an alternative approach. The drug is initiated as an intravenous bolus of 5–20 mg over a few minutes; repeat doses of as much as 20–40 mg can be given every 10–15 minutes until a satisfactory response is achieved or a total dose of 300 mg has been given. It then can be used as a constant intravenous infusion of 1–2 mg/minute, adjusting the dose as necessary.

Contraindications to beta blockade must always be kept in mind, including a sinus bradycardia of less than 50 beats/minute, marked first-, second-, or third-degree AV block, hypotension, congestive heart failure, and severe reactive airways disease.

Other drugs that can be employed to lower blood pressure rapidly include calcium channel antagonists, especially sublingually administered nifedipine [167]; angiotensin converting enzyme (ACE) inhibitors, such as the intravenous form of enalaparil (enalaprilat); and other direct vasodilators, such as intravenous hydralazine. Appropriate measures to counteract the associated increase in dP/dT must be taken. Trimethaphan camsylate, a ganglionic blocker, and reserpine are no longer in widespread use.

Because excessive fluid retention blunts the response to hypotensive medications, small doses of intravenous furosemide (10–20 mg) may help facilitate blood pressure control.

In normotensive patients with acute aortic dissection, beta-adrenergic blocking drugs can be given alone; alter-

Table 40-1. Guidelines for definitive surgical and medical therapy of aortic dissections

Surgical
All acute proximal dissections (Stanford type A)
Acute distal dissections (Stanford type B) complicated by the following:
Extension despite an adequate medical program
Compromise of perfusion to a vital organ or limb
Retrograde extension into the ascending aorta (becomes type A under the Stanford classification)
Evidence of leaking, rupture, or threatened rupture of the dissected aorta (e.g., rapid localized aortic enlargement)
Inability to control hypertension adequately
Any patient with Marfan syndrome
Arch dissection complicated by rupture or localized aneurysm formation
Chronic aortic dissections with complications that require surgical relief, i.e., progressive aortic insufficiency, localized aneurysm formation, or recurrent dissection
Medical
Uncomplicated acute distal dissection*
Chronic stable isolated arch dissections
Stable chronic dissection (uncomplicated dissection presenting 2 weeks or more after onset), regardless of its site of origin

*Some physicians prefer operative treatment of all distal as well as proximal dissections.

natively, a calcium-channel antagonist of the appropriate class can be used if beta blockers are contraindicated.

As soon as possible after the presence of an aortic dissection is suspected, a definitive diagnosis should be established by the imaging techniques outlined earlier. Once the dissection has been identified and characterized, the appropriate form of subsequent definitive therapy can be selected.

SUBSEQUENT DEFINITIVE THERAPY

The indications for definitive medical and surgical therapy of aortic dissection are outlined in Table 40-1. As has been previously stated, there is general agreement that all acute proximal dissections should be managed surgically whenever possible, provided the patient's overall condition so allows. Although major complications of dissection, such as an accomplished stroke or myocardial infarction increase the risk of operation, they do not serve as absolute contraindications to surgical intervention. A large, dense stroke or oligoanuric renal failure are two conditions that would mitigate against operation. The hospital mortality following surgical treatment of acute proximal aortic dissection is now 15–20 percent in most major medical centers with an interest in the treatment of aortic dissection [18–22,24,29,30,168,169]. Miller et al. reported a remarkably low mortality of only 7 percent in 31 cases of acute type A dissection who underwent operation at Stanford between 1977 and 1982 [18]. Those results have not been repeated, even at the same institution.

The definitive treatment of acute distal dissections is more controversial. In our experience, these patients more often exhibit the typical profile of patients with peripheral vascular disease than do those with proximal dissection: They are older, frequently are hypertensive, are heavy smokers with chronic pulmonary disease, and have generalized atherosclerosis, including coronary and renal artery disease [35]. All these factors serve to increase the operative risk [34]. In stable uncomplicated acute distal dissection, the hospital mortality in medically treated patients is approximately 15–20 percent—results that currently are comparable to or better than those with acute surgical therapy in many centers, including our own. Thus, we and others prefer to treat acute **stable** distal dissections medically [7,25,26,170]. Surgery is reserved for cases complicated by leaking or rupture of the dissection, rapid aortic expansion, compromise of a major arterial trunk sufficient to threaten the viability of an important organ or limb, refractory or recurrent severe pain, or extension of the dissection while on an adequate medical program. Inability to control hypertension adequately also is considered by some investigators to be an indication for surgery, but that is distinctly unusual with currently available medications, as well as endovascular techniques such as renal-artery angioplasty. On occasion we have found that a diagnostic thoracentesis may help in reaching a decision in the management of distal dissections if there is a sizable left pleural effusion. Frankly bloody fluid, as contrasted with serous or serosanguinous fluid, indicates leaking or rupture and points toward surgical intervention.

Counter to the policy of medical treatment for acute distal dissections is the previous experience of Miller et al., who reported an unusually low surgical mortality of 13 percent in a small number of cases of type B distal dissections [18]. They and other groups questioned whether surgery should be undertaken for **all** distal as well as proximal dissections [18,34,171]. A more recent analysis of the combined experiences at Stanford University and Duke University, however, again underscores the preference for medical therapy in the initial management of uncomplicated acute distal dissections [21].

One exception to the recommendation of medical therapy for distal dissections is that of patients with Marfan syndrome and other heritable connective-tissue disorders. Because they have such a high incidence of redissection and aortic rupture, there is agreement that for them surgery is the treatment of choice.

Acute dissections that originate in or extend into the aortic arch pose a substantial risk of neurologic impairment and increased bleeding following attempted surgical repair. Nevertheless, arch dissections with rupture or rapid localized aneurysm formation should be treated surgically. Kirklin and Kouchoukos also have advised that arch repair should be undertaken if the walls of the false channel are tenuous or fragmented [23].

A still unsettled point of contention is how to manage those rare dissections that begin in the descending thoracic aorta and propagate retrograde into the ascending aorta (see Figs. 40-9 and 40-13). Miller et al. have advocated that such dissections should be treated surgically, with the repair being directed at the ascending aorta so as to prevent rupture into the pericardial space, in contrast

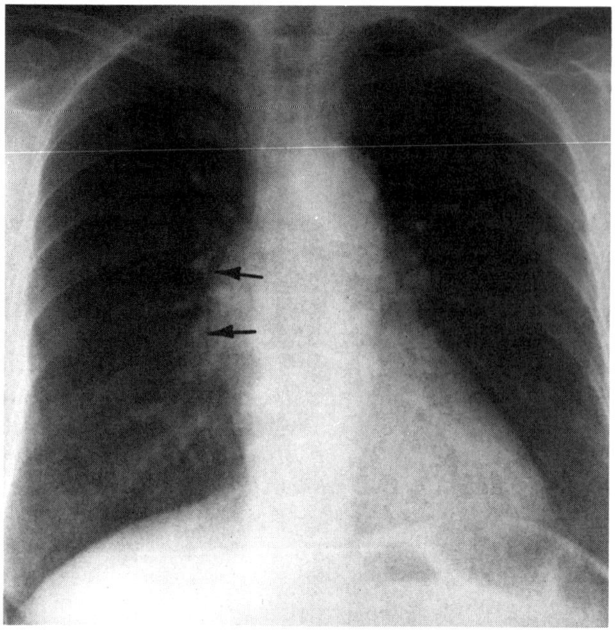

A

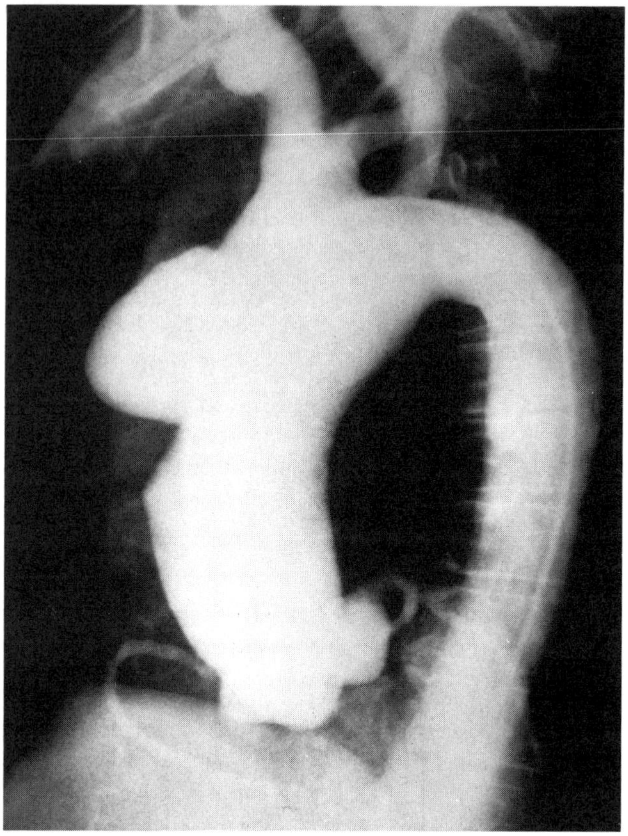

B

Fig. 40-14. Late development of a saccular aneurysm at the site of an aortic dissection. This 77-year-old hypertensive woman was referred for evaluation after a noncontrast chest CT scan, performed for the evaluation of pulmonary nodules, showed a dilated ascending aorta.
A. Prominence of the ascending aorta can be observed on the posteroanterior chest film (arrows).
B. The contrast aortogram showing an obvious saccular aneurysm in the ascending aorta. MR imaging provided clear demonstration of a chronic proximal dissection. (Reproduced with permission from E Braunwald, ed. Heart Disease: A Textbook of Cardiovascular Medicine, 3rd ed. Philadelphia: Saunders, 1988.)

to the traditional policy, which advocates surgery on the distal aorta aimed at excising the entry point [34]. His group has provided some evidence in support of that approach. Their long-term follow-up data have suggested that the inability to excise the intimal entry tear at the time of surgery may not adversely influence long-term prognosis [19].

Since patients presenting with chronic aortic dissections have survived the period of greatest mortality, they usually are treated medically unless complications warrant surgical repair. The most common of these are aortic insufficiency, localized aneurysm formation, and redissection (Fig. 40-14).

TECHNICAL SURGICAL CONSIDERATIONS

Dissections of the proximal aorta must be repaired using a median sternotomy approach and cardiopulmonary bypass. Arterial access is achieved via the femoral artery, and venous drainage usually is established via caval cannulae inserted through the right atrium. The entry site and as much of the dissected ascending aorta as possible are excised, stopping short of the innominate artery if the dissection does not extend further. The false channel is then obliterated by oversewing the ends of the transected aorta proximally and distally. The aorta is reconstituted, usually by the interposition of a graft made of synthetic material such as woven Dacron.

Careful attention must be directed to the relief of aortic insufficiency if it exists. In occasional patients, simple decompression of the aortic annulus by excision of the entry site and repair of the false channel may lead to resuspension of the aortic leaflets sufficient to restore aortic-valve competence. However, prosthetic aortic-valve replacement is often necessary. If there is any question at operation as to the degree to which aortic insufficiency has been alleviated by leaflet resuspension, most surgeons prefer replacement of the aortic valve at the time of the initial procedure to the less favorable approach of possible late

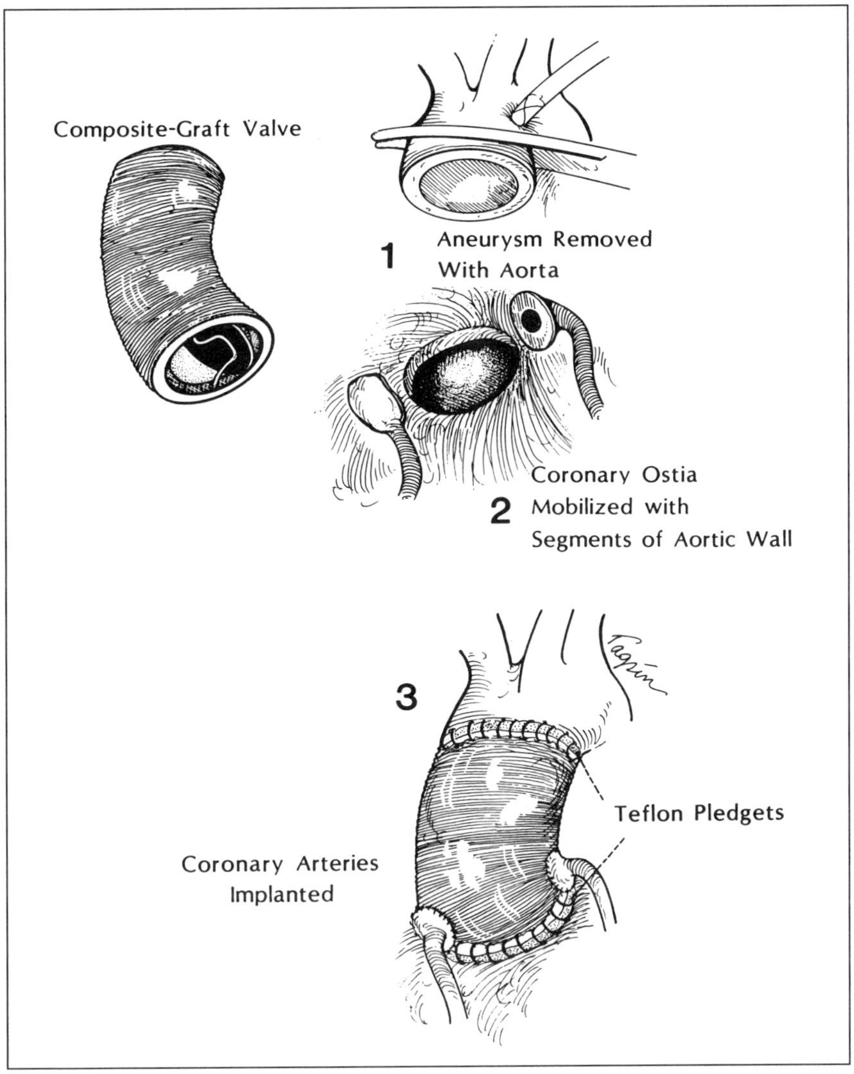

Fig. 40-15. Valve-graft conduit technique for the repair of a proximal aortic dissection with disruption of the aortic annulus and aortic regurgitation. A synthetic conduit is shown with a tilting disk prosthesis anchored to one end (upper left). **1, 2.** Excision of the dissected aorta, with mobilization of the coronary ostia, which are contained within buttons of the aortic wall. **3.** The conduit has been sewn in place using Teflon felt to reinforce the fragile aortic wall, and the ostia of the coronary arteries have been implanted onto the graft. (Reproduced with permission from E Braunwald, ed. Heart Disease: A Textbook of Cardiovascular Medicine, 3rd ed. Philadelphia: Saunders, 1988.)

aortic-valve replacement through a previously dissected aorta. For that reason, we also prefer a mechanical to bioprosthetic valve for aortic-valve replacement.

The modified composite valve-graft conduit technique, originally proposed by Bentall and DeBono [172], is frequently employed whenever significant aortic root pathology or distortion is encountered [27] (Fig. 40-15). The composite graft consists of a sleeve made of synthetic material, to which a prosthetic aortic valve has been attached at one end. The dissected ascending aorta is then excised proximal to the innominate artery if appropriate to the level of the aortic annulus. In the early experience, the dissected aorta often was left behind in situ; it is now more commonly excised. The composite graft is sewn to the repaired aorta distally and the aortic annulus proximally. The coronary arteries usually are excised, with a button of aorta around them, and are then reimplanted onto the graft. If the ostia of the coronary arteries are extensively damaged or if there is obstructive coronary artery disease, saphenous-vein bypasses can be constructed from the prosthesis to the distal coronary arteries. In a series of patients treated with that technique, which included 23 with chronic and 9 with acute dissections, Cabrol et al. reported an operative mortality of 4 percent [173]. Kouchoukos et al. reported two operative deaths among 12 patients with acute proximal dissections and 1 among 39 patients with chronic proximal dissections using that repair [174]. The composite graft technique has proved to be particularly effective in patients with Marfan syndrome, who often have marked annuloaortic ectasia and cephalad displacement of the coronary arteries [175,176]. A variation on the theme is the use of aortic valve/root homografts, as for the management of septic root pathology.

Repair of distal dissections proceeds via the same stages as those described for proximal dissection, that is, excision of the entry site, obliteration of the false channel, and the insertion of a synthetic conduit. Exposure is gained via a lateral thoracotomy. Knowledge of the distal vascular supply to vital organs is important, because on occasion major organs such as one or both kidneys may be perfused via the false channel. If that is the case, the surgeon usually does not close the false channel distally at the time of the operation. Many surgeons prefer to support the distal circulation either by the use of partial circulatory assistance or a shunt that carries blood around the excluded aortic segment while it is being repaired [177]. A heparinized-bonded conduit can be used to convey blood from the left ventricular apex to the left femoral artery or from the ascending to the descending aorta if the anatomy of the dissection permits [178]. Such a conduit has the advantage over circulatory assistance in that systemic heparinization is unnecessary, thus diminishing the risks of bleeding. Shunting of oxygenated blood from the left atrial appendage to the distal aorta via a centrifugal pump is also frequently employed. Others may try to perform the surgery as expeditiously as possible without a shunt if the anatomy is favorable. A devastating complication of surgery for distal dissection is ischemic spinal cord damage due largely to disruption of cord perfusion from the thoracic intercostal arteries and the artery of Adamkiewicz. There is some evidence that support of the distal circulation during the operative procedure may reduce the frequency of that complication and may also diminish the incidence of postoperative renal failure [179]. In general, the shorter the time period of aortic cross-clamping, the less frequently those complications occur.

Surgery of arch dissections usually is performed using profound hypothermia (15–16°C) and transient circulatory arrest [23,28,29,180–184]. Frist and co-workers reported good results with surgery and dissections involving the aortic arch using moderate systemic hypothermia and low-flow cardiopulmonary bypass (30–50 ml/kg body weight/minute) combined with selective perfusion of the brachiocephalic vessels [185]. Others have employed adjunctive retrograde superior vena caval perfusion to protect cerebral metabolism [186].

One of the most difficult technical problems for the surgeon at the time of operation is the extreme fragility of the acutely dissected aorta. A simple but major therapeutic advance in that regard is the use of Teflon felt to buttress the aortic suture lines, thus preventing the sutures from tearing through the dissected aorta.

In an attempt to make the surgery of aortic dissection simpler and safer, a number of innovative techniques have evolved over the last 10–15 years. Many groups have reported the use of an intraluminal prosthesis [187–192], which consists of a Dacron sleeve, to which rigid rings made of either metal or plastic are attached at each end. The aorta is incised, and the prosthesis is inserted into the lumen of the aorta such that the ends are proximal and distal to the point of origin of the dissection. Large tapes are then passed around the outside of the aorta and simply tied against the rings to fix the prosthesis in place. If necessary, major arterial trunks can be anastomosed to the prostheses. Bachet and co-workers reported the use of a glue made of gelatin, resorcinol, and formol to reinforce the fragile aortic tissue at the time of operation [193]. In an uncontrolled study, they found that patients in whom they used the glue had less blood loss, a reduced incidence of aortic-valve replacement, and a better operative and long-term survival then those in whom it was not employed. A fibrin glue also is available [194]. Tanabe et al. attempted to strengthen the wall of the dissected aorta by placing strips of Ivalon sponge in the false lumen [195]. The sponge strips promote thrombosis and organization of blood in the false channel. Limb or visceral ischemia has been managed by fenestration of the occluding intimal flap, a procedure that can now be accomplished percutaneously [196,197]. Obviously, this is palliative in scope. Catheter-based stenting procedures are under investigation [198].

In addition to the technical problems with the aorta at the time of operation, major surgical complications include bleeding, pulmonary infections, renal failure, and cerebrovascular accidents. Our surgical team, like others, frequently uses aprotinin, a serine protease inhibitor, to diminish the risk of early postoperative bleeding, thus far with favorable results. Using a mutlivariate analysis of the determinants of operative mortality, Miller et al. previously found that renal dysfunction, renal-visceral ischemia, the site of the intimal tear (ascending < descending < arch), cardiac tamponade, and pulmonary disease all increased the overall surgical mortality [18]. The surgical mortality of their type B dissections was increased by preoperative rupture and advanced age. They also found that their surgical mortality declined with increasing experience [18], an observation validated by the extensive experience of the late Dr. Crawford and co-workers [20].

The timing of surgery for aortic dissection was at one time a matter of some contention. Because the aortic tissues are so friable immediately at the time of dissection, some surgeons previously advocated a few days (if possible) of watchful waiting, treating the patient medically to allow time for the dissection to "stabilize." [15] However, we and most other groups believe that surgery in acute aortic dissection should be carried out as an emergency procedure and as soon as possible after the decision has been made to proceed with operation.

The surgery of chronic dissection is technically easier than that of acute dissection because the aortic tissues have had a chance to recover some of their tensile strength. The mortality risk for concomitant aortic-valve replacement in those patients is approximately 5 to 10 percent [17,18]. The mortality risk for resection and grafting of localized aneurysms depends on the site of the aneurysm and the age and general condition of the patient, but it is comparable to the mortality associated with resection of atherosclerotic aneurysms in similar locations.

CONSIDERATIONS IN DEFINITIVE MEDICAL TREATMENT

Patients with acute aortic dissections selected for definitive medical treatment are shifted within 48 to 72 hours from a program of parenteral to oral medications for long-term maintenance.

The core of long-term medical therapy is a beta-adrenoreceptor antagonist, provided there are no contraindications to its use. There is no real evidence that any single beta blocker is superior to any other, except that those with intrinsic sympathomimetic activity (e.g., pindolol and acebutalol) probably should be avoided. The choice of a beta-blocking drug should be left to the individual physician and be guided by such considerations as the need for cardioselectivity in patients with bronchospastic pulmonary disease, convenience of dosage schedules, potential side effects, and cost. Labetalol is available in oral form and can be used alternatively in doses of 200–400 mg bid.

Other antihypertensive medications are commonly required for long-term blood pressure control. A combination of a beta-adrenoreceptor antagonist and either an ACE inhibitor or a dihydropyridine calcium-channel antagonist (nifedipine, nicardipine, amlodipine) usually suffices. On rare occasion, drugs from all three classes (or a diuretic) are required. Again, the physician should be guided by the dual objectives of lowering the blood pressure as well as its rate of rise and by considerations of concomitant convenience and cost.

Acutely, the major side effects of medical therapy relate to overshoot hypotension; acute renal failure, particularly in patients with preexistent renal disease, may result. Hypotension may lead to inadequate perfusion of other vital organ beds and result in coronary insufficiency or transient ischemia in the cerebral or vertebrobasilar systems.

Medically treated patients are generally kept at bed rest for 2–3 days and then gradually ambulated. Postural hypotension is common when patients first begin to ambulate, and medication dosages may need to be readjusted at that time, particularly in older patients. After discharge, patients who have had an aortic dissection are advised against lifting more than 25 pounds for a period of at least 3 months. They should also be cautioned to wear seatbelts when driving, to prevent any steering wheel injury to the chest in the event of an automobile accident.

It is extremely important to emphasize that, in addition to those patients treated medically, **all patients who have undergone surgical treatment should be maintained on long-term medical therapy,** using the approach outlined above. In nonhypertensive patients, for example, those with Marfan syndrome, long-term maintenance therapy with a beta-adrenoreceptor antagonist is mandatory, unless it cannot be tolerated. A calcium-channel antagonist with negative inotropic and chronotropic properties, such as verapamil, might be a suitable alternative.

LONG TERM FOLLOW-UP

Hospital survivors of aortic dissection should be followed closely after discharge. The major aortic complications include progressive aortic insufficiency (rare, of course, in patients in whom the aortic valve has been replaced), the development of localized aneurysms anywhere along the course of the aorta, and redissection. Redissection is rare in patients who are treated adequately medically. Surgery may be necessary for these late complications. The frequency of serious complications of the aortic dissection that require late surgical intervention has varied. Over a mean follow-up period of 4 years, 3 of 119 patients in a series reported from our institution required reoperation: 1 for aortic regurgitation and 2 for localized aneurysms [17]. DeBakey et al., in one of the longest post-surgical follow-up evaluations (extending up to 20 years), found that 29.3 percent of all late deaths were due to the subsequent development and rupture of an aneurysm [15]. Haverich et al. reported an actuarial incidence of reoperation of 13 percent at 5 years and 23 percent at 10 years [19]. In Crawford's personal review of 690 patients who underwent surgery for aortic dissection between 1956 and 1989, the ten-year freedom from reoperation at the original surgical site was 78 percent [20]. Those data underscore the importance of the careful follow-up of survivors of acute dissection, regardless of whether they have been treated medically or surgically. We generally obtain routine chest x-rays every 3 months for the first-year follow-up and at least once or twice annually thereafter. As noted, aneurysms may form anywhere along the course of the dissected aorta. Aneurysms of the descending thoracic aorta usually are visible on chest x-rays. However, we have encountered a number of patients who have developed abdominal aortic aneurysms as a result of dissections extending into the abdominal aorta.

Noninvasive imaging techniques, particularly contrast-enhanced CT and MR scanning, are extremely valuable in the assessment of patients in whom the development of late aneurysms is suspected. Those techniques allow careful examination of the aorta throughout its length. Particular attention should be paid to patients who are at unusually high risk for the formation of late aneurysms, for example, those with Marfan syndrome. In such individuals, a contrast-enhanced CT or MR scan of the aorta is advisable at least annually.

Current estimates for long-term survival of patients with treated aortic dissection are encouraging, particularly when compared with the dismal outcomes observed in the pretreatment era. Analysis of the large autopsy study compiled by Hirst et al. would suggest that of patients with untreated acute dissection 3 percent die immediately from rupture. The untreated mortality then rises to 21 percent at 24 hours, 37 percent by 48 hours, 74 percent at 2 weeks, and 90 percent at 3 months [3]. By comparison, the present 10-year actuarial survival of all treated patients is in the range of 40 percent; it approaches 60 percent for those patients who survive to hospital discharge [17,19,20,199] (Fig. 40-16). This long-term survival is not dependent on the site of origin of the dissection, its acuity, or the type of therapy initially applied. In the earlier Stanford series, stroke, remote myocardial infarction, renal dysfunction, and operation during the early years of their surgical experience were the factors identified by multivariate analysis as independent, negative predictors for late survival [19]. Continued advances in the surgical, medical, and anesthetic care of patients with

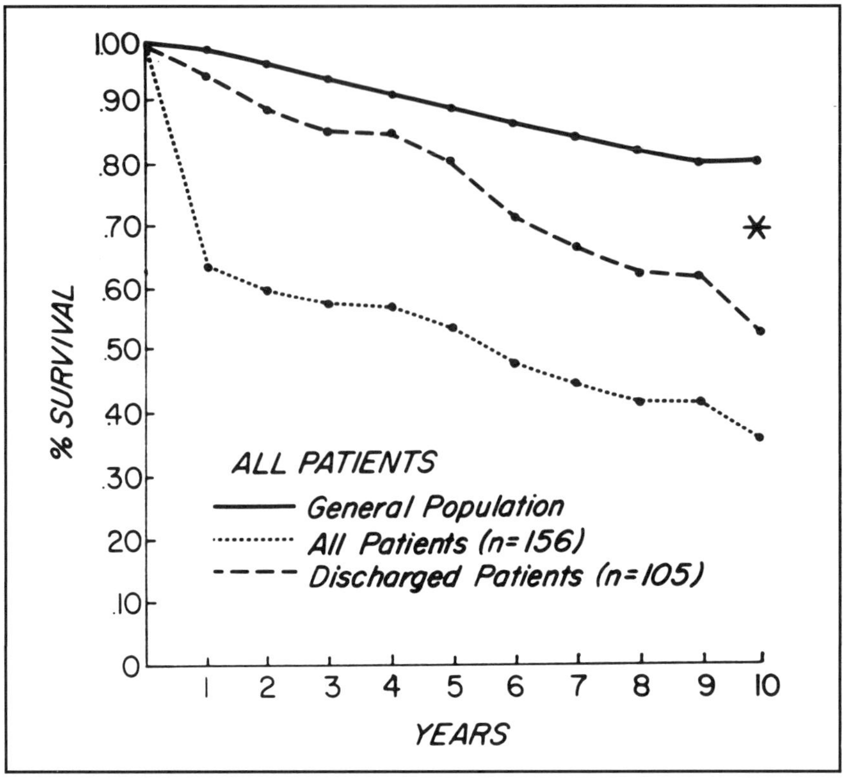

Fig. 40-16. Actuarial survival curves for 156 patients with aortic dissection treated at Massachusetts General Hospital from 1963–1978. The mean duration of follow-up was 48 months. * = significant difference in survival. (Reproduced from RM Doraghazi et al. Long-term survival of patients with treated aortic dissection. J Am Coll Cardiol 1984; 3:1026–1034. With permission from the American College of Cardiology.)

dissection, coupled with its earlier clinical recognition, should lead to even further improvements in long-term survival.

Patients with Marfan syndrome pose a particular problem because of the extraordinarily high incidence of redissection, aneurysm formation, and rupture. Accordingly, Gott et al. have recommended close monitoring of the size of the proximal aorta in patients with Marfan syndrome and prophylactic resection and repair if the diameter of the ascending aorta reaches 6 cm or more [175].

Dinsmore et al. have suggested that patients in whom the false lumen fails to opacify angiographically at the time of the acute dissection may have a better long-term prognosis than those in whom flow in the dissected channel is identified [200]. The reason for that may be that failure to opacify could be indicative of thrombus formation in the false channel. Over a period of time, that may serve to organize and strengthen the wall of the dissected aorta. Late follow-up suggests that that may be the case. We now have had the opportunity to evaluate two patients at postmortem examination who died 13 and 16 years after an acute aortic dissection, and in neither case did the false lumen opacify at the time of the original aortogram. Both were treated medically. Death was unrelated to the dissection, and at the time of autopsy, the dissections in both patients had healed to the point where they could have been easily missed if the aorta had not been specifically examined with the knowledge of a prior aortic dissection. Similar observations have been made with TEE [22].

References

1. Anagnostocopoulos CE. Acute Aortic Dissection. Baltimore: University Park Press, 1975.
2. Ponraj P, Pepper J. Aortic dissection. Br J Clin Pract 1992; 46(2):127–131.
3. Hirst AE Jr, Johns VJ Jr, Kime SW Jr. Dissecting aneurysm of the aorta: a review of 505 cases. Medicine 1958; 37:217.
4. Spittell PC, et al. Clinical features and differential diagnosis of aortic dissection: experience with 236 cases (1980–1990). May Clin Proc 1993; 68:642–651.
5. Morgagni GB. DeSedibus et Causis Morborum per Anatomen Indagatis Libri Quinique. Padua: Benetiis, 1761.
6. Laennec RTH. Ce l'Auscultations Mediate, ou Traite du Diagnostic des Maladies des Pourmons et du Coeur, Fonde Principalemente sur ce Nouveau Moyen d'Exploration. Paris: JA Brosson et JS Chaude, 1819.
7. Peacock TB. Cases of dissecting aneurysm, or that form of aneurysmal affection in which the sac is situated between the coats of the vessel. Edinburgh Med Surg J 1843; 60:276.
8. Swaine K, Latham PM. A case of dissecting aneurysm of the aorta. Trans Pathol Soc Lond 1855–1856; 7:106.
9. Shennan T. Dissecting Aneurysms. Special Report, Series No. 193, Medical Research Council, London, His Majesty's Stationery, 1934.
10. Gurin D, Bulmer JW, Derby R. Dissecting aneurysm of the

aorta. Diagnosis and operative relief of arterial obstruction due to this cause. NY State J Med 1935; 35:1200.
11. DeBakey ME, Cooley DA, Creech O Jr. Surgical considerations of dissecting aneurysm of the aorta. Ann Surg 1955; 142:586.
12. Wheat MW Jr, et al. Treatment of dissecting aneurysms of the aorta without surgery. J Thorac Cardiovasc Surg 1965; 50:364.
13. Applebaum A, Karp RB, Kirkline, JW. Ascending vs. descending aortic dissections. Ann Surg 1976; 183:296.
14. Miller DC, et al. Operative treatment of aortic dissection: experience of 125 patients over a 16-year period. J Thorac Cardiovasc Surg 1979; 78:365.
15. DeBakey ME, et al. Dissection and dissecting aneurysms of the aorta: twenty-year follow-up of five hundred twenty-seven patients treated surgically. Surgery 1982; 92:1118–1134.
16. Stephens DB, Killen DA, Reed WA. Operative experience with 50 thoracic aortic dissections. South Med J 1982; 75:1467–1470.
17. Doroghazi RM, et al. Long-term survival of patients with treated aortic dissection. J Am Coll Cardiol 1984; 3:1026–1034.
18. Miller DC, et al. Independent determinants of operative mortality for patients with aortic dissections. Circ 1984; 70[Suppl 1]:153–164.
19. Haverich A, et al. Acute and chronic aortic dissections—determinants of long-term outcome for operative survivors. Circ 1985; 72[Suppl 2]:22–34.
20. Svensson LG, et al. Dissection of the aorta and dissecting aortic aneurysms. Improving early and long-term surgical results. Circ 1990; 82[Suppl IV]:24–38.
21. Glower DD, et al. Comparison of medical and surgical therapy for uncomplicated descending aortic dissection. Circ 1990; 82[Suppl IV]:39–46.
22. Erbel R, et al. Effect of medical and surgical therapy on aortic dissection evaluated by transesophageal echocardiography. Implications for prognosis and therapy. The European Cooperative Study Group on Echocardiography. Circ 1993; 87:1604–1615.
23. Kirklin JW, Kouchoukos NT. When and how to include arch repair in patients with acute dissection involving the ascending aorta. Semin Thorac Cardiovasc Surg 1993; 5:27–32.
24. Miller DC. The continuing dilemma concerning medical versus surgical management of patients with acute type B dissections. Semin Thorac Cardiovasc Surg 1993; 5:33–46.
25. Neya K, et al. Outcome of Stanford type B acute aortic dissection. Circ 1992; 86:(II)1–7.
26. Mawda Y, et al. Prognosis of patients with medically treated aortic dissections. Circ 1991; 85:III:7–13.
27. Tamiguchi K, et al. Long-term survival and complications after composite graft replacement for ascending aortic aneurysm associated with aortic regurgitation. Circ 1991; 84:III:31–39.
28. Heinemann M, et al. Surgery extended into the aortic arch in acute type A dissection. Indications, techniques, and results. Circ 1991; 84:III:25–30.
29. Yun KL, et al. Aortic dissection resulting from tear of transverse arch: is concomitant arch repair warranted? J Thorac Cardiovasc Surg 1991; 102:355–368.
30. Faun JI, et al. Preservation of aortic valve in type A aortic dissection complicated by aortic regurgitation. J Thorac Cardiovasc Surg 1991; 102:62–73.
31. DeBakey ME, et al. Surgical management of dissecting aneurysms of the aorta. J Thorac Surg 1965; 49:130.
32. Daily PO, et al. Management of acute aortic dissections. Ann Thorac Surg 1970; 10:237.
33. Lindsay J Jr, Hurst JW. Clinical features and prognosis in dissecting aneurysms of the aorta: A re-appraisal. Circ 1967; 35:880.
34. Miller, DC. Surgical management of aortic dissection: indications, perioperative management and long-term results. In RM Doroghazi, EE Slater, eds. Aortic Dissection. New York: McGraw-Hill, 1983. Pp. 193–243.
35. Slater EE, DeSanctis RW. The clinical recognition of dissecting aortic aneurysms. Am J Med 1976; 60:625.
36. Larson EW, Edwards WD. Risk factors for aortic dissection: a necropsy study of 161 cases. Am J Cardiol 1984; 53:849–855.
37. Wheat MW. Pathogenesis of aortic dissection. In RM Doroghazi, EE Slater, eds. Aortic Dissection. New York: McGraw-Hill, 1983. P. 55.
38. Yamada T, Tada S, Harada J. Aortic dissection without intimal rupture: diagnosis with MR imaging and CT. Radiology 1988; 168:347–352.
39. Wolff KA, et al. Aortic dissection: atypical patterns seen at MR imaging. Radiology 1991; 181:489–495.
40. Mohr-Kahaly S, et al. Aortic intramural hemorrhage visualized by transesophageal echocardiography: findings and prognostic implications. J Am Coll Cardiol 1994; 23:658–664.
41. Lui RC, Menkis AH, McKenzie FN. Aortic dissection without intimal rupture: diagnosis and management. Ann Thorac Surg 1992; 53:886–888.
42. Robbins RC, et al. Management of patients with intramural hematoma of the thoracic aorta. Circulation 1993; 88[Suppl II]:II-1–II-10.
43. Nienaber CA, et al. Intramural hemorrhage of the aorta: diagnostic and therapeutic implications. Circulation 1995; 92:1465–1472.
44. Bansal RC, et al. Frequency and explanation of false negative diagnosis of aortic dissection by aortography and transesophageal echocardiography. J Am Coll Cardiol 1995; 25:1393–1401.
45. Hirst AE, Gore I. The etiology and pathology of aortic dissection. In RM Doroghazi, EE Slater, eds. Aortic Dissection. New York: McGraw-Hill, 1983. Pp. 13–53.
46. Roberts WC. Aortic Dissection: anatomy, consequences and causes. Am Heart J 1981; 101:195.
47. Gore I, Seiwert VJ. Dissecting aneurysm of the aorta: pathological aspects of eighty-five fatal cases. Arch Pathol Lab Med 1952; 53:121.
48. Tiessen IM, Roach MR. Factors in the initiation and propagation of the aortic dissections in human autopsy aortae. J Biomech Eng 1993; 115:123–125.
49. Berry CL, Sosa-Melgarejo JA, Greenwald SE. The relationship between wall tension, lamellar thickness, and intercellular junctions in the fetal and adult aorta: its relevance to the pathology of dissecting aneurysm. J Pathol 1993; 169:15–20.
50. Gutierrez PS, et al. Decrease in sulphated glycosaminoglycans in aortic dissection—possible role in pathogeneis. Cardiovasc Res 1991; 25:742–748.
51. Sariola H, Viljarren T, Luosto RT. Histological patterns and changes in extracellular matrix in aortic dissection. J Clin Pathol 1986; 39:1074–1081.
52. Gsell O. Wandnerkrosen der Aorta als selbstandige Erkrankung und ihre Beziehung sur Spontanruptur. Virchows Arc (Pathol Anat) 1928; 270:1.
53. Erdheim J. Medionecrosis aortae idiopathica. Virchows Arc (Pathol Anat) 1929; 273:454.
54. McKusick VA. The cardiovascular aspects of marfan's syndrome: A hereditable disorder of connective tissue. Circ 1955; 11:321–342.
55. McKusick VA. Hereditable disorders of connective tissue. 4th Ed. St Louis: Mosby, 1972. P. 329.
56. Murdoch JL, et al. Life expectancy and causes of death in the Marfan syndrome. N Engl J Med 1972; 286:804–808.

57. Pyeritz RE, McKusick VA. The Marfan syndrome: diagnosis and management. N Engl J Med 1979; 300:772–777.
58. Priest RE, Moinuddin JF, Priest JH. Collagen of Marfan's syndrome is abnormally soluble. Nature 1973; 245:264.
59. Boucek RJ, et al. The Marfan syndrome: a deficiency in chemically stable collagen cross-links. N Engl J Med 1981; 305:988.
60. McFarland W, Fuller D. Mortality in Ehlers-Danlos syndrome due to spontaneous rupture of large arteries. N Engl J Med 1964; 271:1309–1310.
61. Layman TE, Wang V. Idiopathic cystic medionecrosis and aneurysmal dilatation of the ascending aorta. Med Clin North Am 1968; 52:1145.
62. Emanuel R, et al. Forme frustes of Marfan's syndrome presenting with severe aortic regurgitation. Clinicogenetic study of 18 families. Br Heart J 1979; 39:190–197.
63. Bauer EA, Vitto J. Collagen in cutaneous disease. Int J Dermatol 1978; 18:251.
64. Ponseti IV, Baird WA. Scoliosis and dissecting aneurysm of the aorta in rats fed with lathyrus odoratus seeds. Am J Pathol 1952; 28:1059–1078.
65. Schilling ED, Strong FM. Isolation, structure, and synthesis of a lathyrus factor from L. odoratus. Am J Chem Soc 1954; 76:2848.
66. Harris ED, Rayton JK, Groot JE. Critical role for copper in aortic elasain structure and synthesis. Adv Exp Med Biol 1977; 79:543.
67. Nakashino Y, Sueishi K. Alteration of elastic architecture in lathymitic rat aorta implies the pathogenesis of aortic dissecting aneurysm. Am J Pathol 1992; 140:959–969.
68. Cottell MA, Haselton PS, Anderson JC. Increased elastic content and decreased elastin concentrations may be predisposing factors in dissecting aneurysms of human thoracic aorta. Cardiovasc Res 1993; 27:176–181.
69. Leonard JC, Rayton JK, Groot JE. Dissecting aortic aneurysms: Clinicopathological study. I. Clinical and gross pathological findings. QJ Med 1979; 48:55.
70. Wilson SK, Hutchins GM. Aortic dissecting aneurysms: causative factors in 204 cases. Arch Pathol Lab Med 1982; 106:175–180.
71. Schlatmann TJM, Becker AE. Histologic changes in the normal aging aorta: implications for dissecting aortic aneurysm. Am J Cardiol 1977; 39:13–20.
72. Schlatmann TJM, Becker AE. Pathogenesis of dissecting aneurysm of aorta: comparative histopathologic study of significance of medical changes. Am J Cardiol 1977; 39:21–26.
73. Pedowitz P, Perell A. Aneurysms complicated by pregnancy. I. Aneurysms of the aorta and its major branches. Am J Obstet Gynecol 1957; 73:720.
74. Mandel W, Evans EW, Walford RL. Dissecting aneurysms during pregnancy. N Engl J Med 1954; 251:1059.
75. Gore I. Dissecting aneurysm of the aorta in persons under forty years of age. Arch Pathol 1953; 55:1.
76. McKusick VA, Logue RB, Bahnson HT. Association of aortic valvular disease and cystic medionecrosis of ascending aorta: report of four instances. Circ 1957; 16:188.
77. McKusick VA. Association of congenital bicuspid aortic valve and Erdheim's cystic medial necrosis. Lancet 1972; 1:1026.
78. Edwards WD, Leaf DS, Edwards JE. Dissecting aortic aneurysm associated with congenital bicuspid aortic valve. Circ 1978; 57:1022–1025.
79. Edwards, JE. Manifestations of acquired and congenital disease of the aorta. Curr Prob Cardiol 1979; 3:1.
80. Roberts CS, Roberts WC. Dissection of the aorta associated with congenital malformation of the aortic valve. J Am Coll Cardiol 1991; 17:712–716.
81. Abbott ME. Coarctation of the aorta of the adult type. Am Heart J 1928; 3:574.
82. Reifenstein GH, Levine SA, Gross RE. Coarctation of the aorta: review of 104 cases of the adult type 2 years of age or older. Am Heart J 1947; 33:146–168.
83. Fikar CR, et al. Dissecting aortic aneurysm in childhood and adolescence. Clin Ped 1981; 20:578.
84. Nora JJ, et al. Characteristic cardiovascular anomalies of X0 Turner syndrome, XX and XY phenotype and X0/XX Turner mosaic. Am J Cardiol 1970; 25:639.
85. Lie JT. Aortic dissection in Turner's syndrome. Am Heart J 1982; 103:1077.
86. Price WH, Wilson J. Dissection of the aorta in Turner's syndrome. J Med Gen 1983; 20:61–63.
87. Schacter N, Perloff JK, Mulder DG. Aortic dissection in Noonan's syndrome (46 XA Turner). Am J Cardiol 1984; 54:464–465.
88. Garret R. Chronic diffuse giant cell mesoaortitis with dissecting aneurysm and rupture. Am J Clin Pathol 1962; 38:406–414.
89. Harris M. Dissecting aneurysm of the aorta due to giant cell aortitis. Br Heart J 1968; 30:840.
90. Save-Soderrberg J, et al. Giant cell arteritis as a cause of death: report of nine cases. J Am Med Assoc 1986; 255:493–496.
91. Hainer JW, Hamilton GW. Aortic abnormalities in relapsing polychrondritis. Report of a case with dissecting aortic aneurysm. N Engl J Med 1969; 280:1166.
92. Biagini A, et al. Familial clustering of aortic dissection in polycystic kidney disease. Am J Cardiol 1993; 72:741–742.
93. Walts AE, Dubois EL. Acute dissecting aneurysm of the aorta as the fatal event in systemic lupus erythematosus. Am Heart J 1977; 93:378.
94. Roberts WC. The aorta: its acquired diseases and their consequences as viewed from a morphologic perspective. In J Lindsay, JW Hurst, eds. The Aorta. New York: Grune & Stratton, 1979.
95. Kantrowitz A, et al. Intraaortic balloon pumping 1967 through 1982: analysis of complications in 733 patients. Am J Cardiol 1986; 57:976.
96. Murphy DA, et al. Recognition and management of ascending aortic dissection complicating cardiac surgical operations. J Thorac Cardiovasc Surg 1983; 85:247–256.
97. Muna WF, et al. Aortic dissection after aortic valve replacement in patients with valvular aortic stenosis. J Thorac Cardiovasc Surg 1979; 74:65–69.
98. Adhins MS, et al. Chronic type A aortic dissection: an unusual complication of cocaine inhalation. Ann Thorac Surg 1993; 56:997–999.
99. Cohen S, Littman D. Painless dissecting aneurysm of the aorta. N Engl J Med 1964; 271:143–145.
100. Weisman AD, Abramss RD. The neurologic complication of dissecting aortic aneurysm. Brain 1944; 67:69–92.
101. Prendes JL. Neurovascular syndromes of aortic dissection. AFP 1981; 23:175.
102. Young JR, Kramer J, Humphries AW. The ischemic leg: a clue to dissecting aneurysm. Cardiovasc Clin 1975; 7:201.
103. Statler LF, et al. Aortic dissection masquerading as acute myocardial infarction: implication for thrombotic therapy without cardiac catheterization. Am J Cardiol 1984; 54:1134–1135.
104. Noda Y, Fukiyama K, Omae T. Renin dependent hypertension by dissecting aortic aneurysm. A case report. Jp Heart J 1981; 22:281.
105. Murray HW, et al. Fever with dissecting aneurysm of the aorta. Am J Med 1976; 61:140.
106. Slater EE. Aortic dissection: presentation and diagnosis. In

RM Doroghazi, EE Slater, eds. Aortic Dissection. New York: McGraw-Hill, 1983. Pp. 61–70.
107. Logue RB, Sikes C. New sign in dissecting aneurysms of the aorta: pulsation of sternoclavicular joint. J Am Med Assoc 1952; 14:1209.
108. Banker VP, Maddison FE. Superior vena cava syndrome secondary to aortic disease. Report of two cases and review of the literature. Dis Chest 1967; 51:656–662.
109. Strax TE, Ryviker JJ, Elguezabal A. Superior vena caval syndrome due to a mediastinal hemota secondary to dissecting aortic aneurysms. Dis Chest 1969; 55:338–341.
110. Spitzer S, et al. Superior vena cava syndrome and dissecting aortic aneurysm. J Am Med Assoc 1975; 233:164.
111. Riley DJ, Lui RT, Saxanoff S. Aortic dissection: a rare cause of the superior vena cava syndrome. J Med Soc NJ 1981; 78:187.
112. Kahn S, et al. Superior vena caval obstruction secondary to acute dissecting aneurysm of the aorta. Am Heart J 1986; 111:606–608.
113. Calendar DG, Uricchio JF. Superior vena cava syndrome. Differentiation between simple obstruction and aortico-caval communication. Arch Int Med 1953; 91:800–807.
114. Millward DK, Robinson JJ, Craige E. Dissecting aortic aneurysm diagnosed by echocardiography in a patient with rupture of the aneurysm into the right atrium. Am J Cardiol 1972; 30:427.
115. McCarthy C, et al. Aortic dissection with rupture through ductus arteriosus into pulmonary artery. Br Heart J 1972; 34:428.
116. Roth JA, Parekh MA. Dissecting aneurysms perforating esophagus. N Engl J Med 1978; 299:776.
117. Yacoub MH, Schottenfeld M, Kittle CF. Hematoma of the interatrial septum with heart block secondary to dissecting aneurysm of the aorta. A clinicopathologic entity. Circ 1972; 46:537.
118. Thiene G, Rossi L, Becker AE. The atrioventricular conduction system in dissecting aneurysm of the aorta. Am Heart J 1979; 98:447.
119. Tencate JW, Timmens H, Becker AE. Coagulopathy in ruptured or dissecting aortic aneurysms. Am J Med 1971; 59:171.
120. Smith DC, Jang GC. Radiological diagnosis of aortic dissection. In RM Doroghazi, EE Slater, eds. Aortic Dissection. New York: McGraw-Hill, 1983. Pp. 71–132.
121. Eyler WR, Clark MD. Dissecting aneurysms of the aorta: roentgen manifestations including a comparison with other types of aneurysms. Radiology 1965; 85:1047.
122. Beachley MC, Ranniger K, Roth F. Roentgenographic evaluation of dissecting aneurysms of the aorta. Am J Roentgenol 1974; 121:617.
123. Earnest F IV, Muhm FR, Sheedy PF II. Roentgenographic findings in thoracic aortic dissection. Mayo Clin Proc 1979; 54:43.
124. Galbraith BT, Norman SL. Dissecting aneurysm of the aorta: a diagnostic approach. N Engl J Med 1954; 250:670.
125. Holesh S. Dissecting aneurysm of the aorta. Br J Radiol 1960; 33:302.
126. Dow J, Roebuck EJ, Cole F. Dissecting aneurysms of the aorta. Br J Radiol 1966; 39:915.
127. Nanda NC, Gramiak R, Sham PM. Diagnosis of aortic root dissection by echocardiography. Circ 1973; 48:506.
128. Brown OR, Poppo RL, Kloster FE. Echocardiographic criteria for aortic root dissection. Am J Cardiol 1975; 36:17.
129. Matthew T, Nanda NC. Two dimensional and Doppler echocardiographic evaluation of aortic aneurysm and dissection. Am J Cardiol 1985; 54:379–385.
130. Granato JF, Dee P, Gibson RS. Utility of two-dimensional echocardiography in suspected ascending aortic dissection. Am J Cardiol 1985; 56:123–129.
131. Smuckler AL, et al. Echocardiographic diagnosis of aortic root dissection by M-mode and two-dimensional techniques. Am Heart J 1982; 103:897.
132. Iliceto S, et al. Color Doppler evaluation of aortic dissection. Circ 1987; 75:758–765.
133. Adachi H, et al. Early diagnosis and surgical intervention of acute aortic dissection by transesophageal color flow mapping. Circ 1990; 82[Suppl IV]:19–23.
134. Matsuzaki M, Toma Y, Kusukawa R. Clinical applications of transesophageal echocardiography. Circ 1990; 82:709–722.
135. Erbel R, et al. European cooperative study group for echocardiography: echocardiography in the diagnosis of aortic dissection. Lancet 1989; 1:457–460.
136. Nienaber CA, et al. The diagnosis of thoracic aortic dissection by non-invasive imaging procedures. N Engl J Med 1993; 328:1–9.
137. Erbel R. Role of transesophageal echocardiography in dissection of the aorta and evaluation of degenerative aortic disease. Cardiol Clin 1993; 11:461–473.
138. Cigarroa JE, et al. Diagnostic imaging in the evaluation of suspected aortic dissection. Old standards and new directions. N Engl J Med 1993; 328:35–43.
139. Simon P, et al. Transesophageal echocardiography in the emergency surgical management of patients with aortic dissection. J Thorac Cardiovasc Surg 1992; 103:113–117.
140. Pandian NG, et al. Intravascular high-frequency two dimensional ultrasound detection of arterial disssection and intimal flaps. Am J Cardiol 1990; 65:1278–1280.
141. Paride A, et al. Intravascular ultrasound for diagnosis of aortic dissection. Am J Cardiol 1991; 67:662–663.
142. Weintraub AR, et al. Intravascular ultrasound imaging in acute aortic dissection. J Am Coll Cardiol 1994; 24:495–503.
143. Landtman M, et al. Computed tomography in pre- and postoperative evaluation of aortic dissection. Acta Radiol (Diagn) (Stockh) 1986; 27:273–278.
144. Gross SC, et al. Computed tomography in dissection of the thoracic aorta. Radiology 1980; 136:135.
145. Heiberg E, et al. CT findings in thoracic aortic dissection. Am J Roentgenol 1981; 136:13.
146. Godwin JD, et al. Computed tomography for follow-up of chronic aortic dissections. Radiology 1981; 139:655.
147. Oudkerk M, Overbosch E, Dee P. CT recognition of acute aortic dissection. Am J Roentgenol 1983; 141:671–676.
148. Thorsen MK, et al. Dissecting aortic aneurysms: accuracy of computed tomographic diagnosis. Radiology 1983; 148: 773–777.
149. White RD, et al. Noninvasive evaluation of suspected thoracic aortic disease by contrast-enhanced computed tomography. Am J Cardiol 1986; 57:282–290.
150. Godwin JD, et al. Evaluation of dissections and aneurysms of the thoracic aorta by conventional and dynamic CT scanning. Radiology 1980; 136:125.
151. Perez JE. Noninvasive diagnosis: computed tomography and ultrasound. In RM Doroghazi, EE Slater, eds. Aortic Dissection. New York: McGraw-Hill, 1983. Pp. 133–164.
152. Moncada R, Demos TC, Churchill R. Detecting disease of the aorta by computed tomography. J Cardiovasc Med 1983; 8:186.
153. Singh H, Fitzgerald E, Ruttley MS. Computed tomography: The investigation of choice for aortic dissection? Br Heart J 1986; 56:171–175.
154. Amparao EG, et al. Aortic dissection: magnetic resonance imaging. Radiology 1985; 155:399–406.
155. Geisinger MA, et al. Thoracic aortic dissections: magnetic resonance imaging. Radiology 1985; 155:407–412.
156. Goldman AP, et al. The complimentary role of magnetic resonance imaging, Doppler, echocardiography and com-

puted tomography in the diagnosis of dissecting thoracic aneurysms. Am Heart J 1986; 111:970–981.
157. Dinsmore RE, et al. Magnetic resonance imaging of thoracic aortic aneurysms: comparison with other diagnostic techniques. Am J Radiol 1986; 146:309.
158. Eagle KA, et al. Spectrum of conditions initially suggesting aortic dissection but with negative aortograms. Am J Cardiol 1986; 57:322–326.
159. Gutierrez FR, et al. Cineangiography in the diagnosis and evaluation of aortic dissection. Radiology 1980; 135:759.
160. Arcinegar JG, et al. Cineangiography in the diagnosis of aortic dissection. Am J Cardiol 1981; 47:890–894.
161. Cooke JP, Kazmier FJ, Orsulak TA. The penetrating aortic ulcer: pathologic manifestations, diagnosis, and management. Mayo Clin Proc 1988; 63:718–725.
162. Hussain S, et al. Penetrating atherosclerotic ulcers of the thoracic aorta. J Vasc Surg 1989; 9:710–717.
163. Kazerooni EA, Bree RL, Williams DM. Penetrating atherosclerotic ulcers of the descending thoracic aorta: evaluation with CT and distinction from aortic dissection. Radiology 1992; 183:759–765.
164. Mohr-Kahaly E, et al. Aortic intramural hemorrhage visualized by transesophageal echocardiography: findings and prognostic implications. J Am Coll Cardiol 1994; 23:658–664.
165. Prokop EK, Palmer RF, Wheat MW. Hydrodynamic forces in dissecting aneurysm: in vitro studies in a tygon model and in dog aortas. Circ Res 1970; 27:121.
166. Palmer RF, Lassitor KC. Nitroprusside and aortic dissecting aneurysm (Letter). N Engl J Med 1976; 294:1403.
167. White SR, Hall JB. Control of hypertension with nifedipine in the setting of aortic dissection. Chest 1985; 88:780–781.
168. Cachera JP, et al. Surgical management of acute dissections involving the ascending aorta. J Thorac Cardiovasc Surg 1981; 82:576.
169. Wolfe WG, et al. Surgical treatment of acute ascending aortic dissection. Ann Surg 1983; 197:738–742.
170. Wheat WG. Intensive drug therapy. In RM Doroghazi, EE Slater, eds. Aortic Dissection. New York: McGraw-Hill, 1983. Pp. 165–191.
171. Ergin MA, et al. Acute dissection of the aorta: current surgical treatment. Surg Clin North Am 1985; 65:721–741.
172. Bentall H, DeBono A. A technique for complete replacement of the ascending aorta. Thorax 1968; 23:338–339.
173. Cabrol C, et al. Long-term results with total replacement of the ascending aorta and reimplantation of the coronary arteries. J Thorac Cardiovasc Surg 1986; 91:17.
174. Kouchoukos NT, Marshall WG Jr, Wedige-Stecher TA. Eleven-year experience with composite graft replacement of the ascending aorta and aortic valve. J Thorac Cardiovasc Surg 1986; 92:691–705.
175. Gott VL, et al. Surgical treatment of aneurysms of the ascending aorta in the Marfan syndrome. Results of composite-graft repair in 50 patients. N Engl J Med 1986; 314:1070–1074.
176. Crawford ES. Marfan's syndrome: broad spectral surgical treatment of cardiovascular manifestation. Ann Surg 1983; 198:487–505.
177. Carpentier A, et al. New surgical approach to aortic dissection: flow reversal and thromboexclusion. J Thorac Cardiovas Surg 1981; 81:659.
178. Donahoe JE, Brawley RK, Gott VC. The heparin-coated vascular shunt for thoracic aorta and great vessel procedures. Ten year experience. Ann Thorac Surg 1977; 23:507.
179. Jex RK, et al. Early and late results following repair of dissection of the descending thoracic aorta. J Vasc Surg 1986; 3:336–337.
180. Galloway AC, et al. Surgical repair of type A aortic dissection by the circulatory arrest-graft inclusion technique in sixty-six patients. J Thorac Cardiovasc Surg 1993; 105:781–788.
181. Tabayashi K, et al. Replacement of the transverse aortic arch for type A acute aortic dissection. Ann Thorac Surg 1993; 55:864–867.
182. Carrel T, et al. Retrograde ascending aortic dissection: a diagnostic and therapeutic challenge. Eur J Cardiovasc Surg 1993; 7:146–150.
183. Miller DC. Concomitant arch repair in acute type A aortic dissection. J Thorac Cardiovasc Surg 1992; 104:206–208.
184. Laar J, et al. Advances in aortic arch surgery. Ann Thorac Surg 1992; 53:227–232.
185. Frist WH, et al. A reconsideration of cerebral perfusion in aortic arch replacement. Ann Thorac Surg 1986; 42:273–281.
186. Yasuura K, et al. Clinical application of total body retrograde perfusion to operation for aortic dissection. Ann Thorac Surg 1992; 53:655–658.
187. Leomole GM, et al. Improved results for dissecting aneurysms: intraluminal sutureless prosthesis. J Thorac Cardiovasc Surg 1982; 83:249–255.
188. Krause AH, et al. Early experience with the intraluminal graft prosthesis. Am J Surg 1983; 145:619–622.
189. Berger RL, et al. Graft replacement of the thoracic aorta with a sutureless technique. Ann Thorac Surg 1983; 35:231–239.
190. Spagna PM, et al. Rigid intraluminal prosthesis for replacement of thoracic and abdominal aorta. Ann Thorac Surg 1985; 39:47–52.
191. Koyamada K, Ishikawa S, Kakihata H. Surgical treatment for dissecting aneurysm of the aorta using a double ringed graft. J Cardiovasc Surg (Torino) 1985; 26:448–491.
192. Berger RL, et al. Replacement of the thoracic aorta with intraluminal autorelease prosthesis. Ann Thorac Surg 1992; 53:920–927.
193. Bachet J, et al. Quatre ans d'experience clinique de la colle gelatine-resorcine-formal dans lens dissections aigues de l'aorte ascendente. Arch Mal Coeur 1983; 76:87–94.
194. S'eguin JR, et al. Fibrin sealant improves surgical results of type A acute aortic dissections. Ann Thorac Surg 1991; 52:745–748.
195. Tanabe T, et al. Surgical treatment of aortic dissection: application of Ivalon sponge to the dissected lumen. Ann Thor Surg 1986; 41:169–175.
196. Walher PJ, et al. The use of endovascular techniques for the treatment of complications of aortic dissection. J Vasc Surg 1993; 18:1042–1051.
197. Williams DM, et al. Creation of reentry tears in aortic dissection by means of percutaneous balloon fenestration: gross anatomic and histologic considerations. J Vasc Interv Radiol 1993; 4:75–83.
198. Moon MR, et al. Intravascular stenting of acute experimental type B dissections. J Surg Res 1993; 54:381–388.
199. Elefteriader JA, et al. Long term experience with descending aortic dissection: the complication specific approach. Ann Thorac Surg 1992; 53:11–20.
200. Dinsmore RE, Willerson JT, Buckley MJ. Dissecting aneurysm of the aorta: aortographic features affecting prognosis. Radiology 1972; 105:567.

Pulmonary Hypertension

Lewis J. Rubin
Harold I. Palevsky
Alfred Fishman

The Normal Pulmonary Circulation

The normal pulmonary circulation is a high-flow, low-resistance circuit interposed between the systemic veins and the left heart. It differs from the circulation to other organs in that it is a largely passive circuit that lacks elaborate mechanisms for regulating regional blood pressure. The normal pulmonary circulation can accommodate large increases in cardiac output with only slight increments in pulmonary artery pressure (for example during maximal exercise) by its ability both to dilate existing vasculature and to recruit unused segments of the circulation.

Although low, the pulsatile pulmonary arterial pressure suffices to overcome pulmonary vascular impedance, thereby filling the left atrium adequately at end-diastole and maintaining pulmonary blood flow at a level equal to systemic blood flow. At sea level, the normal pulmonary blood flow is accomplished by an average mean pressure drop of only 5 to 10 mm Hg between the pulmonary artery and the left atrium (Table 41-1). Even during the increase in cardiac output with exercise, the upper limit of mean pulmonary-artery pressure at sea level for normal subjects under the age of 40 years is 30 mm Hg. In well-trained athletes with cardiac outputs greater than 20 liters per minute, mean pulmonary-artery pressures may be higher [1].

The definition of pulmonary hypertension depends on altitude because of the contribution of hypoxemia to resting pulmonary hemodynamics. At sea level, a mean pulmonary-artery pressure greater than 20 mm Hg is considered abnormal; at an altitude of 15,000 feet, the normal range for mean pulmonary-artery pressure extends to 25 mm Hg. Those pressures are important only in terms of the burden they impose on the right ventricle: Mild elevations in pulmonary-artery pressure are not clinically significant because they can be well tolerated by the right ventricle for indefinite periods. However, mild resting pulmonary hypertension in an individual residing at sea level generally signifies either a curtailment of the pulmonary vascular tree, an abnormally high pulmonary blood flow or volume, or a combination of the two. As a rule, in such individuals the barely abnormal pulmonary-arterial pressures increase inordinately when either vascular tone or blood flow increase, for example, during acute hypoxia or exertion.

Pulmonary hypertension frequently goes undetected until an explanation is sought for unexplained dyspnea or clinical signs of right-heart failure. The normal right ventricle can acutely generate systolic pressures up to about 50 mm Hg in response to an afterload. It can generate substantially higher pressures, even up to systemic arterial-pressure levels, if the afterload is applied gradually so that the right ventricle has time to adapt with hypertrophy. If the afterload is too severe, however, as in the case of protracted pulmonary hypertension approaching systemic levels, the ventricle ultimately decompensates and fails.

It has become customary to relate the pressure drop across the pulmonary circulation to the pulmonary blood flow (cardiac output) using an equation analogous to Ohm's law:

$$\text{Pulmonary vascular resistance, units} = \frac{\left(\begin{array}{c}\text{Mean pulmonary-}\\ \text{artery pressure,}\\ \text{mm Hg}\end{array}\right) - \left(\begin{array}{c}\text{Pulmonary-artery}\\ \text{wedge pressure,}\\ \text{mm Hg}\end{array}\right)}{\text{Pulmonary blood flow, liters/min}}$$

Expressed in this manner, the normal pulmonary vascular resistance is approximately 1 unit. Resistance also can be expressed in dynes/second/cm^{-5} by multiplying the numerator of the equation by 79.9; expressed in that way, normal pulmonary vascular resistance is approximately 100 dyne/second/cm^{-5}.

The calculation of pulmonary vascular resistance is an adaptation of Poiseuille's law, which is based on linear flow of a Newtonian fluid through rigid tubes, and hardly applies to the pulmonary circulation. The normal pulmonary vascular bed is composed of elastic, distensible vessels that change in caliber with changes in pulmonary blood volume, flow, and pressure [2]. Additionally, pulmonary blood flow is pulsatile and turbulent rather than laminar. The pulmonary blood volume can be altered by changes in blood flow, transthoracic pressures, and position. Both neurohumoral and chemical changes occur with different conditions, such as the start of exercise, that independently affect pulmonary vascular resistance. Because blood is a non-Newtonian fluid, its viscosity changes with flow velocity. Poiseuille's law may, therefore, be more directly applicable to the abnormal pulmonary circulation, in which vessel walls thickened by disease become more rigid.

Those factors complicate interpretation of calculated values for pulmonary vascular resistance, especially in evaluating the effect on the pulmonary circulation of a therapeutic intervention. Since the relation between pressure and flow in the normal pulmonary circulation is not linear, resistance varies with the flow through the system, the pressure drop across the pulmonary circulation, and with the other factors noted above. Thus, a change in resistance resulting from changes in flow or pressures does not necessarily indicate that active vasoconstriction or vasodilation has occurred in the resistance vessels [2]. One way to address the difficulty in interpretation of changes in vascular resistance following an intervention is to compare the values before and after the interven-

Table 41-1. Representative hemodynamic values for normal adult males at rest and moderate exercise

	Rest	Exercise
Cardiac output (liters/min)	6	16
Heart rate (beats/min)	80	130
Right atrial pressure (mm Hg)	4–6	6–8
Pulmonary artery pressure (mm Hg)		
Systolic	20–25	30–35
Diastolic	10–12	11–14
Mean	14–18	20–25
Pulmonary wedge pressure (mm Hg)	6–9	10–12
Systemic arterial pressure (mm Hg)	120/180	150/95
Mean	90–100	110–120
Pulmonary vascular resistance (units)	0.70–0.95	0.60–0.90

tion at either the same cardiac output or vascular pressures.

Clinical shortcuts in the use of the resistance equation, such as the substitution of mean pulmonary arterial pressure for the pressure drop between pulmonary artery and left atrium in the numerator, deprive the calculation of any physiologic meaning. Also, since the calculated value for resistance is based on a ratio, translating the result of the calculation in terms of clinical benefit can be uncertain, especially when data from different individuals are pooled. For example, a decrease in calculated pulmonary vascular resistance due to a drop in pulmonary arterial pressure in conjunction with an increased cardiac output and an unchanged heart rate is a more desirable clinical response than is an equivalent decrease in resistance due to a greater increase in cardiac output, an unchanged pulmonary arterial pressure, and tachycardia.

Overview of Pulmonary Hypertension

Pulmonary-artery hypertension is a consequence of a variety of etiologies and pathogenic sequences in which the common outcome is an increase in pulmonary vascular resistance. The causes of pulmonary hypertension are shown in Table 41-2. Six broad categories generally are recognized: (1) **passive**, or postcapillary, due to impaired pulmonary venous outflow caused by disorders such as fibrosing mediastinitis, mitral stenosis, or left-heart failure; (2) **hyperkinetic**, due to high flow states such as left-to-right shunts; (3) **obstructive**, as in pulmonary embolism or vasculitis; (4) **obliterative**, as in pulmonary parenchymal disease; (5) **vasoconstrictive**, as occurs during acute hypoxia or in some patients with scleroderma; and (6) **idiopathic**, if no etiology for the pulmonary hypertension can be identified. In each category, a substantial decrease in the extent or the distensibility (or both) of the pulmonary vascular bed and in its ability to accommodate increments in pulmonary blood flow without substantial increases in pressure is a prerequisite for the development of symptoms and signs of pulmonary hypertension.

Because the pulmonary circulation has the ability to accept large increments in pulmonary blood flow without a large change in pulmonary arterial pressure, widespread pulmonary vascular disease must be present before symptoms develop [2]. Symptoms occur first during exertion, often in the form of dyspnea, chest pain, dizziness, or syncope. Right-heart failure manifests itself by peripheral edema or ascites, early satiety, or epigastric or right-upper-quadrant pain.

Table 41-2. Causes of pulmonary hypertension

Passive (pulmonary venous hypertension)
Left ventricular failure
Mitral stenosis
Left atrial myxoma
Fibrosing mediastinitis
Hyperkinetic
Intracardiac shunts
Pulmonary arteriovenous malformations
Obstructive
Pulmonary embolic disease (thrombus, tumor)
Pulmonary intravascular thrombosis (hemoglobinopathies)
Obliterative
Pulmonary vasculitis (connective-tissue diseases)
Parenchymal lung disease (obstructive and restrictive)
Schistosomiasis
Vasoconstrictive
Hypoxia (acute and chronic)
Cocaine use
Idiopathic
Primary pulmonary hypertension
Persistent fetal circulation
Drug-induced pulmonary hypertension (anorexic agents, L-tryptophan)
Portal pulmonary hypertension syndrome
HIV infection

Physical examination is often unremarkable, particularly early in the course of the disease, unless the examiner has been alerted to the possibility of pulmonary hypertension. The difficulty in making an early diagnosis is compounded by the lack of widespread availability of noninvasive screening techniques for pulmonary hypertension. As a consequence, suspicion of the presence of pulmonary hypertension often is delayed until abnormalities in the chest radiograph, electrocardiogram, or echocardiogram are present and the suspicion confirmed by right heart catheterization [1].

SYMPTOMS

There are no symptoms that are specific for pulmonary hypertension [3,4]. Accordingly, there is often a substantial delay between the onset of symptoms and the establishment of a diagnosis [5]. The earliest and most consistent symptom of pulmonary hypertension is exertional dyspnea. As in the case of easy fatiguability, dyspnea due to pulmonary hypertension often is attributed to anxiety or deconditioning. Several explanations for the dyspnea of pulmonary hypertension have been proposed, including firing of peripheral chemoreceptors by hypoxemia, stimulation of irritant receptors in the pulmonary interstitial space or of stretch receptors in large pulmonary arteries, and failure of cardiac output to keep pace with metabolic needs.

Exertional dizziness or syncope are common and ominous symptoms of pulmonary hypertension. They tend to occur in patients with the greatest degree of hemodynamic compromise at rest [6] and are attributable either to an inability to increase the cardiac output during exertion coupled with exercise-induced systemic vasodilation or to an arrhythmia, such as vagally mediated bradycardia.

Chest pain occurs in approximately one-half of patients with advanced pulmonary hypertension [7]. This pain resembles typical angina pectoris and is probably due to right ventricular ischemia. Hemoptysis can occur in all forms of pulmonary hypertension. In postcapillary pulmonary vascular disorders, the source may be the engorged bronchial submucosal veins. In some forms of precapillary pulmonary hypertension, rupture of alveolar capillary aneurysms or arteriosclerotic pulmonary arteries can cause bleeding.

Hoarseness, due to compression of the left recurrent laryngeal nerve between the aorta and a dilated left pulmonary artery resulting in paralysis of the left vocal cord, may complicate severe pulmonary hypertension. Early satiety and epigastric or right-upper-quadrant pain may develop as a consequence of hepatic distension and congestion once right-heart dysfunction reaches the stage of elevated systemic venous pressure.

SIGNS

The physical signs of pulmonary hypertension are similar regardless of the underlying etiology or pathogenesis [8]. Early in the course of the disease, the jugular venous pressure contour is dominated by a large a wave. As pulmonary hypertension progresses to the development of right-heart failure with tricuspid regurgitation, the amplitude of the a wave diminishes and the v wave becomes more prominent. The right ventricular impulse becomes palpable near the left sternal border, and pulmonary arterial valve closure may be palpable in the second left intercostal space.

On auscultation, the second heart sound often is closely split, and the pulmonic component is accentuated [9]. A sharp systolic ejection click is often heard over the region of the pulmonary artery, and a right atrial gallop usually is present. A murmur of tricuspid insufficiency, sometimes accompanied by a thrill, frequently is heard at the left sternal border. Because of the large pressure gradient across the incompetent tricuspid valve during systole, the high-pitched murmur is quite different from the low-pitched, blowing tricuspid insufficiency murmur associated with organic disease of the valve. The murmur of pulmonic insufficiency also may be present. Patients with chronic thromboembolic pulmonary hypertension may have bruits audible on lung auscultation at sites that are partially obstructed by intraluminal organized clot. Patients with right-heart failure may manifest peripheral edema or, in advanced states, ascites. Peripheral cyanosis accompanies low cardiac-output states, while central cyanosis generally is observed in patients with congenital heart disease with Eisenmenger's syndrome. Digital clubbing is a feature of congenital heart disease, chronic parenchymal lung disease, and portal hypertension with concomitant pulmonary vascular disease.

DIAGNOSTIC STUDIES

With the exception of cardiac catheterization, available diagnostic techniques are not useful in detecting pulmonary hypertension early in its course [3]. The finding of right ventricular hypertrophy on the electrocardiogram [3,10] or right-heart enlargement and prominence of the central pulmonary arteries on the chest radiograph [11,12] should raise concern about the presence of moderate to severe pulmonary hypertension and prompt further investigation (Fig. 41-1).

Diagnostic tests that may help clarify the etiology of the pulmonary vascular disorder (Table 41-3) include the blood count, the profile of blood coagulation parameters, liver function tests, and tests for collagen vascular disease. Those tests may reveal unsuspected polycythemia, which raises the prospect of chronic hypoxia or hemoglobinopathy, hypercoagulable states suggestive of accelerated thrombosis, the coexistence of pulmonary hypertension and portal hypertension, or presence of a systemic connective-tissue disorder.

Chest radiographs and pulmonary function tests are useful in uncovering diffuse parenchymal lung disease or abnormalities of the mediastinum. A ventilation-perfusion lung scan is indispensable in identifying thromboembolic pulmonary vascular disease that would otherwise appear to be consistent with primary pulmonary hypertension [13,14]. Pulmonary angiography generally is reserved for patients with a strong clinical history or a lung scan suggestive of pulmonary thromboembolism. An echocardiogram is essential for demonstrating structural cardiac abnormalities, such as left atrial myxoma, mitral stenosis, or congenital defects. Flattening of the interventricular septum, resulting from elevation in right ventricular systolic pressure, is the earliest and most consistent echocardiographic finding of pulmonary hypertension. Intravascular ultrasound recently has been used to identify intravascular thrombi and medial hypertrophy. Right-heart catheterization is the gold standard for establishing the presence and degree of pulmonary hypertension, for excluding intracardiac structural anomalies, and for evaluating the responses to pharmacologic agents.

Secondary Pulmonary Hypertension

Pulmonary hypertension that results from an identifiable disease process occurs more frequently than primary (unexplained or idiopathic) pulmonary hypertension and is usually the result of coexistent cardiac or pulmonary disease. The mechanisms by which those conditions cause pulmonary hypertension differ markedly (see Table 41-2). Heart disease usually exerts its effects by increasing pulmonary venous pressure or by increasing pulmonary blood flow, whereas lung diseases and thromboembolic disease cause pulmonary hypertension by obliteration or obstruction of large portions of the pulmonary vascular bed.

CARDIAC DISEASE

Acquired disorders of the left side of the heart and certain types of congenital heart disease may cause pulmonary hypertension.

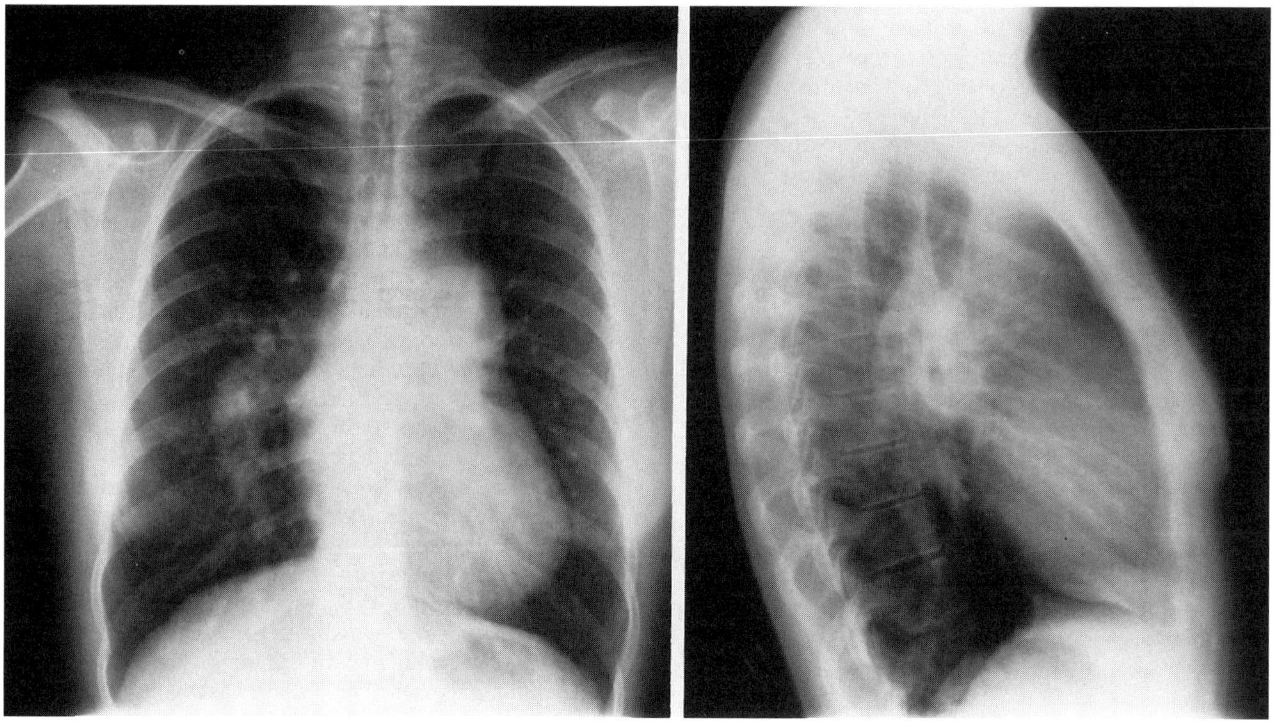

Fig. 41-1. Posteroanterior and lateral chest radiographs from a patient with primary pulmonary hypertension demonstrating enlarged central pulmonary vessels and right ventricular prominence.

Acquired Disorders of the Left Side of the Heart. Pulmonary hypertension occurs as a consequence of an increase in the downstream pressure in the pulmonary circulation, for example, from the elevated left ventricular end-diastolic pressure in congestive heart failure or from the increase in left atrial pressure that is a feature of mitral valve disease or left atrial myxoma. In time, a reactive (vasoconstrictive) process supplements the passive component, thereby increasing the level of pulmonary hypertension [15].

Left ventricular failure is both a common cause of pulmonary hypertension and the most common cause of right ventricular failure. However, the level of pulmonary hypertension observed rarely is sufficient to account for the clinical syndrome of right-heart failure. The discrepancy between the load on the right ventricle and the development of right-heart failure is unexplained, but it may be due in part to involvement of the right ventricle, particularly the interventricular septum, by the pathologic process that is primarily affecting the left ventricle.

Lesions of the mitral and aortic valves also are common causes of pulmonary hypertension. Far less common are other causes of high end-diastolic pressure in the left ventricle, such as constrictive pericarditis. All cause pulmonary arterial hypertension by evoking an increase in pulmonary venous pressure, which in turn prompts a reactive increase in pulmonary arterial pressure that is sufficient to maintain forward flow. In time, structural changes occur in both the pulmonary venous and arterial beds. Among those changes are (1) occlusive changes in the intima and medial hypertrophy and fibrosis of the pulmonary muscular arteries and arterioles that form after antecedent changes in the pulmonary veins and venules; (2) perivascular interstitial edema, most marked in the dependent parts of the lungs, which not only contributes to the increased pulmonary vascular resistance but also stimulates perivascular fibrosis; and (3) occlusion of small pulmonary vessels by thrombi, especially when pulmonary blood flow slows or if the pulmonary endothelium of the resistance vessels is damaged. Surgical relief of the mechanical cause of the pulmonary venous hypertension reduces pulmonary venous and arterial pressures and promotes regression of the reversible components of the vascular changes [15].

Congenital Heart Disease. Congenital cardiac defects that are associated with persistent left-to-right shunting within the heart or between the great vessels often cause pulmonary hypertension [16,17]. Because an acute left-to-right shunt does not by itself cause appreciable pulmonary hypertension in normal lungs unless the flow is markedly increased (at least three times normal), factors other than the level of pulmonary blood flow have been invoked to account for the pulmonary hypertension that accompanies chronic left-to-right shunts. Those factors include the duration of the hemodynamic abnormalities, secondary obstructive vascular lesions, reflex pulmonary vasoconstriction induced by distention of the pulmonary veins or left atrium, and coexisting hypoxemia. Depending on the congenital cardiac defect and whether increased pulmonary blood pressure or blood flow is the cause, the intima or the media may be primarily affected. As the hemody-

Table 41-3. Evaluation of unexplained pulmonary hypertension

Test	Objective
SCREENING	
History and physical exam, chest radiograph, electrocardiogram	To determine pressure and sensitivity of pulmonary vascular disease and to exclude lung disease, congenital heart disease (CHD), other cardiac diseases, pulmonary veno-occlusive disease
DIAGNOSIS	
Echocardiogram	To estimate pulmonary artery pressure, assess chamber size and valves, search for intracardiac shunts
Lung scan	To exclude thromboembolic disease
Pulmonary function tests	To exclude significant parenchymal lung disease
Arterial blood gases	To exclude hypoventilation, assess gas exchange
Polysomnography*	To exclude sleep-disorder breathing
Serologies	To exclude connective-tissue disease, vasculitis
CONFIRMATION	
Catheterization	To complete hemodynamic profile and exclude other cardiac disease
Angiography*	To exclude thromboembolic disease, vasculitis
Lung biopsy*	To exclude parenchymal lung disease, vasculitis

* Not required in every patient

namic abnormalities persist, anatomic changes in the pulmonary resistance vessels supervene and may become the dominant mechanism for sustaining the pulmonary hypertension and for determining its reversibility.

PULMONARY VENOUS DISEASE

Obstruction of the large pulmonary veins as they course through the mediastinum may result from metastatic neoplasm (e.g., breast or lung), lymphoma, infection (e.g., tuberculosis or histoplasmosis), miscellaneous inflammatory processes that affect lymph nodes (e.g., sarcoidosis) or may be of uncertain etiology (e.g., fibrosing mediastinitis). Pulmonary venous obstruction characteristically causes a "passive" form of pulmonary-artery hypertension. Although obstruction of the large pulmonary veins due to a definable cause often is referred to as **pulmonary veno-occlusive disease**, it should be distinguished from unexplained (idiopathic) pulmonary veno-occlusive disease, in which the small pulmonary veins and venules are affected by an inflammatory process or fibrosis. Although small-vessel pulmonary veno-occlusive disease is often included in classification of primary (unexplained) pulmonary hypertension, it appears to differ in etiology and pathogenesis as well as in the site of predominant injury.

PULMONARY PARENCHYMAL DISEASE

Pulmonary disorders, either restrictive or obstructive, can mechanically elicit pulmonary hypertension. Thus, interstitial fibrosis or inflammation (or both) in the vicinity of the pulmonary capillaries and resistance vessels can entrap and obliterate segments of the pulmonary vascular bed or encroach on vascular lumens, limiting their distensibility. Obstructive airways disease also can distort or occlude large portions of the pulmonary vascular bed. Alveolar hypoxia, arterial hypoxemia, and acidosis caused by pulmonary disease can contribute to pulmonary hypertension by producing vasoconstriction of the pulmonary resistance vessels.

Interstitial Lung Disease. Interstitial lung disease can result from a wide variety of diffuse processes, such as sarcoidosis, asbestosis, radiation pneumonitis, and collagen vascular disease, or it can be idiopathic. Common to these disorders is a restrictive ventilatory defect, with diminished lung volumes and relatively preserved airflow. An interstitial inflammatory infiltrate that entraps and eventually destroys the septal arterioles reduces the pulmonary vascular-bed surface area, limits distensibility of the remaining open vessels, and increases pulmonary vascular resistance. In time, those limitations, coupled with closure of peripheral airways by the peribronchiolar inflammatory process, result in arterial hypoxemia, aggravate the pulmonary hypertension, and lead to right ventricular failure. At that stage, hypocapnia gives way to eucapnia and thence to hypercapnia, which promotes further degrees of pulmonary vasoconstriction.

The clinical picture of diffuse interstitial disease usually is dominated by dyspnea and tachypnea; cough is occasionally a prominent feature. The chest radiograph or high-resolution CT scan often are diagnostic in disclosing a widespread pattern that is consistent with interstitial fibrosis, infiltration, or both. Corticosteroids or other immunosuppressive agents are usually the main approach to treatment, often in conjunction with supplemental oxygen therapy.

Obstructive Airways Disease. Chronic obstructive pulmonary disease (COPD) is the leading cause of pulmonary hypertension and is primarily a consequence of destruction of lung tissue, hyperinflation with compression of the vasculature, and arterial hypoxemia resulting from alterations in ventilation-perfusion relationships. In general, pulmonary hypertension is encountered in two different settings: acutely, in the "pink puffer," during an acute respiratory infection, and chronically, in the "blue bloater," with periodic exacerbations during an acute respiratory infection. In the blue bloater, the course of the pulmonary hypertension is gradual, but inexorably progressive. It is noteworthy that in the patient first seen during a bout of respiratory failure, clinical distinction between chronic bronchitis (blue bloater) and emphysema (pink puffer) often is difficult.

Even though chronic bronchitis and emphysema generally coexist, it is the chronic bronchitis that is predominantly responsible for the alveolar hypoxia and the low arterial oxygen partial pressure (P_{O_2}), high carbon dioxide partial pressure (P_{CO_2}), and resultant low pH that lead to pulmonary hypertension. Emphysema *per se* probably does predispose to pulmonary hypertension by destroying segments of the pulmonary vascular bed. But emphysema usually does not cause clinically significant pulmonary hypertension, even when involvement of the lungs is extensive, because the ventilation-perfusion relationships are not as severely deranged as in chronic bronchitis.

The usual findings and signs of pulmonary hypertension may be difficult to evaluate in the patient with severe obstructive airways disease. Right ventricular enlargement may be overlooked because of hyperinflation and clockwise rotation of the heart. Electrocardiographic findings may be difficult to interpret because of rotation and displacement of the heart, increased distances between electrodes and the cardiac surface, and a predominance of dilation over hypertrophy in the cardiac enlargement.

Because of those limitations, it is not surprising that standard electrocardiographic criteria for right ventricular enlargement apply to about only one-third of patients with chronic bronchitis and emphysema who have right ventricular hypertrophy at autopsy. Consecutive changes in the electrocardiogram are often more useful than a single electrocardiogram in detecting sustained or increasing right ventricular overload due to pulmonary hypertension. As the arterial Po_2 drops, T waves tend to become inverted, biphasic, or flat in the right precordial leads (V_1 to V_3); the mean electrical axis of the QRS shifts to the right of the patient's usual axis; ST segments become depressed in leads II, III, and aVF; and right bundle branch block (incomplete or complete) often appears. In addition, peaked p waves may be seen in the inferior limb or right precordial leads (*p pulmonale*) [18]. Those changes tend to reverse as systemic arterial oxygenation improves and the degree of pulmonary hypertension lessens.

Once suspected, the role of obstructive airways disease and ventilation-perfusion abnormalities in the genesis of right ventricular hypertrophy and failure can be confirmed by arterial blood gas sampling: Arterial hypoxemia, hypercapnia, and respiratory acidosis are the characteristic findings. That picture is distinctly uncommon in left-heart failure except when frank pulmonary edema is present.

Treatment at this point is directed at both the etiology of the exacerbation (i.e., infection, bronchospasm) and toward relieving the arterial hypoxemia. The judicious use of supplemental oxygen generally suffices to relieve the arterial hypoxemia and may return the pulmonary arterial pressures toward normal. Long-term studies have shown that continued oxygen therapy can decrease the level of pulmonary hypertension and prolong survival in hypoxemic chronic obstructive airways disease [19].

ALVEOLAR HYPOVENTILATION IN PATIENTS WITH NORMAL LUNGS

Pulmonary hypertension may develop in individuals with alveolar hypoventilation even though their lungs are normal. As in those patients with ventilation-perfusion abnormalities, the pathogenetic factors are alveolar hypoxia, arterial hypoxemia, and hypercapnia, generally accompanied by a partially compensated respiratory acidosis. The alveolar hypoventilation in patients with normal lungs usually originates in either an inadequate ventilatory drive or an ineffective respiratory-muscle system. Disorders associated with alveolar hypoventilation include the sleep apnea syndromes, neuromuscular disorders (e.g., myasthenia gravis, Guillain-Barré syndrome, and many of the muscular dystrophies), central-respiratory-drive impairment (e.g., after a cerebrovascular accident, Ondine's curse), kyphoscoliosis, and extreme obesity.

The clinical manifestations are determined by the etiology and the pathogenesis of the alveolar hypoventilation. In neuromuscular disorders and kyphoscoliosis, arterial hypoxemia (and hypercapnia) may appear initially only during exertion, that is, when ventilation fails to keep pace with metabolic demand. That pattern differs from those of the sleep apnea syndromes, in which arterial hypoxemia and hypercapnia often are manifested only during sleep. Treatment is directed toward the pathogenesis of the alveolar hypoventilation. In the neuromuscular disorders and kyphoscoliosis, some success has been achieved by resting the respiratory muscles at night using negative-pressure (cuirass-type) ventilators, which prevent chronic fatigue of the respiratory muscles and appear to minimize alveolar hypoventilation, even during daytime. In the obstructive sleep apnea syndromes, preventing obstruction through use of nasal continuous positive airway pressure (CPAP) or a tracheostomy eliminates the arterial hypoxemia and its cardiopulmonary consequences. In other conditions where specific therapies are not available, the use of supplemental oxygen to prevent arterial hypoxemia often is of benefit.

CONNECTIVE-TISSUE DISEASES

Pulmonary vascular disease is an important component of many connective-tissue diseases and can be a consequence of pulmonary vasculitis, interstitial inflammation, and interstitial fibrosis [20–23]. Although pulmonary hypertension occurs in many connective-tissue diseases, systemic lupus erythematosus and progressive systemic sclerosis (scleroderma) and its variant syndromes have received the most attention. In some patients who manifest the clinical picture of connective-tissue disease and pulmonary hypertension, the interstitium appears to be uninvolved, and the abnormalities in the pulmonary vessels resemble those of primary pulmonary hypertension. That coincidence has raised the hypothesis that primary pulmonary hypertension represents a variant of collagen vascular disease that is confined to the pulmonary vasculature. The possibility is supported by similarities in pulmonary vascular histology, the high incidence of positive serologic tests for antinuclear antibodies, the occurrence of Raynaud's phenomenon, and the predominance of collagen vascular disease in women [24]. It has been proposed that the coincidence of pulmonary hypertension and Raynaud's phenomenon represents a generalized vasoconstrictive disorder affecting both the systemic and pulmonary vascular beds. It is possible to demonstrate a pulmonary vasoconstrictor response in some patients with pulmonary hypertension due to connective-tissue disease who are exposed to stimuli such as cold. That response most often is seen in those patients who also report intense digital vasoconstriction on exposure to cold [25].

Systemic lupus erythematosus is a multisystem disease of unknown etiology that is characterized by autoantibodies and circulating immune complexes; inflammatory changes occur in the connective tissues, blood vessels, and serosal surfaces. The lungs and pleura are involved more frequently in lupus than in other connective-tissue diseases, with a reported incidence up to 70 percent. In recent years, attention has been called to the high incidence of pulmonary hypertension in lupus erythematosus and the common occurrence of steady progression from pulmonary hypertension to right-heart failure. Published reports indicate a 10-to-1 female-to-male predominance in cases of pulmonary hypertension associated with systemic lupus erythematosus; most of these patients also exhibit Raynaud's phenomenon [21].

The histopathologic lesions in such patients resemble those of primary pulmonary hypertension; vasculitis and extensive immune complex deposition are rare. The development of pulmonary hypertension in these patients has been attributed to microthrombi that are related to the hypercoagulable state that accompanies the presence of lupus anticoagulant in the blood. Another mechanism that has been invoked in some instances is a generalized vasoconstriction, as evidenced by the occurrence of Raynaud's phenomenon. Unfortunately, treatment of pulmonary hypertension associated with systemic lupus erythematosus using either anticoagulants or pulmonary vasodilators has had only modest success. In contrast, patients with active pulmonary vasculitis may experience either improvement or a stabilization in their vascular disease with immunosuppressive agents.

In progressive systemic sclerosis (scleroderma) and its variants, such as the CREST syndrome (calcinosis, Raynaud's syndrome, esophageal involvement, sclerodactyly, and telangiectasias) and in overlap syndromes (e.g., mixed connective-tissue disease), the incidence of pulmonary vascular disease is high, and the resultant pulmonary hypertension is responsible for considerable morbidity and mortality [23,26]. When first described, the CREST syndrome variant of scleroderma was thought to be relatively benign, with little visceral involvement. However, long-term follow-up has since shown a considerable incidence of pulmonary vascular disease in those patients. In a prospective study involving cardiac catheterization of patients with progressive systemic sclerosis or the CREST syndrome variant, pulmonary hypertension, either as an isolated finding or in association with pulmonary parenchymal or cardiac disease, was found in up to one-third of patients with progressive systemic sclerosis and in up to one-half of patients with the CREST syndrome [26]. The pulmonary vascular disease may be independent of pulmonary or other visceral disease, and its occurrence is associated with a marked reduction in survival [23]. As in the case of lupus erythematosus, the pathology of the lesions is often indistinguishable from that of primary pulmonary hypertension. The overlap of findings in patients with pulmonary hypertension and a scleroderma variant on the one hand and of primary pulmonary hypertension on the other (Raynaud's phenomenon, pulmonary vascular histology, high incidence of positive antinuclear antibodies in the blood) reinforces the ideas that a subset of patients with so-called primary pulmonary hypertension actually represents a scleroderma variant confined to the lungs. Even though it has been suspected that pulmonary vasoconstriction may contribute to the pulmonary hypertension of such patients, vasodilator therapy has not been highly effective.

PULMONARY THROMBOEMBOLIC DISEASE

Pulmonary hypertension occurs as a consequence of both acute and chronic unresolved pulmonary thromboembolism. Chronic thromboembolic occlusion of the pulmonary arterial tree remains one of the more misunderstood and overlooked causes of chronic pulmonary hypertension. Under this single descriptor appear to be two separate syndromes with quite distinct patterns of vascular involvement, different pathogenetic mechanisms, and unique therapeutic options [27]. The first is thrombotic occlusion of small pulmonary arteries; the second is chronic, unresolved thromboembolic occlusion of large pulmonary arteries.

Thrombotic Occlusion of Small Pulmonary Arteries and Arterioles. Thrombotic and recanalized lesions of the small muscular pulmonary arteries and pulmonary arterioles have been seen in biopsy and autopsy specimens from patients with a wide variety of causes of pulmonary hypertension. They also constitute one category of microvascular lesions observed in patients with primary pulmonary hypertension (Table 41-4). The microvascular lesions are found in the absence of a detectable source of embolization and in the absence of emboli in the larger pulmonary vessels. Such thrombotic and recanalized lesions were attributed not long ago to one or more showers of microemboli. Now they are widely held to be the result of in-situ thrombosis rather than the result of multiple pulmonary emboli. To account for in-situ thrombosis, attention has shifted to widespread injury to the endothelium of the distal arterial tree of the lungs, to upsets in the local balance between coagulation and fibrinolysis, and to platelet aggregation in the pulmonary microcirculation.

The pattern of vascular lesions in most types of pulmonary hypertension seems to be a function of the nature of the insult, its severity and duration, and the duration and severity of the resultant increase in pulmonary arterial pressure. That these patterns represent the limited ways in which the distal ramifications of the pulmonary arterial tree can respond to vascular injury is supported by recent studies of familial primary pulmonary hypertension. In those families, in which kindred members presumably underwent similar pathogenetic sequences, the pulmonary vascular lesions varied considerably, although microthrombi in the pulmonary arterial tree were the most frequent lesions [28].

Histologic proof of the presence of microthrombi in the pulmonary vascular bed does not appear to be of much practical use in management. The workup detailed in Table 41-3 is designed to exclude treatable etiologies of pulmonary hypertension. A ventilation-perfusion lung scan is necessary to exclude chronic proximal pulmonary thromboembolism. Patients with microthromboemboli demonstrate patchy inhomogeneity in their perfusion pat-

Table 41-4. Histologic classification of pulmonary arteriopathy associated with pulmonary hypertension

Classification	Intimal lesions	Medial lesions
Medial hypertrophy	Minimal proliferation	Extension of smooth muscle into arterioles, arterial medial hypertrophy
Intimal fibrosis	Eccentric or concentric initial proliferation	Medial hypertrophy may be present
Plexogenic arteriopathy	Fibrinoid degeneration, dilatation, and plexiform lesions	Fibrosis of smooth muscle
Thromboembolic arteriopathy	Thrombus or nonthrombotic embolism, may be recanalized, colander lesions	Fibrosis of smooth muscle
Arteritis	Small vessel arteritis, may be necrotizing	Fibrosis of smooth muscle
Capillary hemangiomatosis		Medial hypertrophy, extension of smooth muscle into arterioles

tern without defects that correspond to anatomic segments or subsegments. In that setting, pulmonary angiography generally is unrewarding. Treatment consists of long-term anticoagulation with warfarin-type agents, the administration of antiplatelet agents, or both. Vasodilators have no role in this condition since it is characterized by vascular obstruction rather than constriction.

Chronic Proximal Pulmonary Thromboembolism. This clinical syndrome results in pulmonary hypertension by occluding major portions of the proximal pulmonary arterial tree. By the time the diagnosis has been made, the obstructing material in the major branches of the pulmonary artery has become organized and fibrotic and no longer resembles a thrombus. It is unclear whether the obstruction is due to recurrent, unrecognized pulmonary emboli occurring over years or to a single shower of large emboli that, instead of lysing, propagate and organize. Most likely, the initial event is a pulmonary embolus from a deep leg vein or pelvic vein source. For unknown reasons, the embolic event is unrecognized clinically and may even be asymptomatic. Failure of local fibrinolytic mechanisms allows the clot to propagate antegrade and retrograde, to obstruct portions of the pulmonary vascular bed, and to decrease the compliance of the central pulmonary vessels.

It is important to recognize this cause of pulmonary hypertension because it is amenable to surgical treatment [29]. Ventilation-perfusion lung scanning is the cornerstone of diagnosis, and all patients with pulmonary hypertension of uncertain etiology should undergo the test (Fig. 41-2); perfusion defects that are segmental or larger call for pulmonary angiography, since perfusion lung scans underestimate both the number and the extent of thromboembolic lesions; moreover, identification of the precise location and extent of the organized clot is necessary prior to consideration of surgical removal (Fig. 41-3). Although contrast pulmonary angiography carries some risk in patients with pulmonary hypertension, use of selective or subselective injections of small contrast volumes minimizes the risk [30]. Fiberoptic angioscopy and magnetic resonance imaging are both under active investigation as modalities that may be helpful in defining the extent of lesions in thromboembolic pulmonary hypertension [31,32].

Surgery should be considered for patients with pulmonary hypertension who have persistent clot in lobar or more proximal pulmonary arteries after at least 6 months of anticoagulation (Fig. 41-4). Thromboendarterectomy generally is done via a median sternotomy, using deep hypothermic cardiopulmonary bypass with intermittent periods of circulatory arrest [33,34]. Hemodynamic improvement is usually quite dramatic, and the patients generally improve symptomatically by at least two classes, according to the New York Heart Association classification [29]. Surgical mortality, originally reported to exceed 15 percent, has been reduced to approximately 6 percent [33]. Patients require lifetime anticoagulation after the procedure, and most also should have a filter inserted into the inferior vena cava to further reduce the chance of recurrence.

PRIMARY PULMONARY HYPERTENSION

Primary pulmonary hypertension is a clinical syndrome characterized by pulmonary hypertension in the absence of a demonstrable cause [5,7,35]. The clinical diagnosis usually is based on three different types of evidence: (1) clinical, radiographic, and electrocardiographic or echocardiographic manifestations of pulmonary hypertension; (2) demonstration by right-heart catheterization of the typical hemodynamic constellation of abnormally high pulmonary arterial pressures and pulmonary vascular resistance in association with a normal pulmonary wedge pressure; and (3) inability to find a cause for the pulmonary hypertension in the heart, lungs, systemic circulation, or systemic disease. However, published reports that rely solely on those clinical criteria suffer the disadvantage that multiple etiologies can produce the same clinical syndrome [36].

Primary pulmonary hypertension is an uncommon disorder. Although the onset may occur at any age, symptoms are usually first manifested in early adulthood. The mean age at the time of diagnosis is usually between 30 and 36 years, although 9 percent of patients are over the age of 60 [5]. In some series, usually in those that represent special populations, the mean age of onset is less (e.g., 23 years) [36]. The sex incidence is approximately equal in childhood, but females predominate after puberty. In adults, the female-to-male ratio has ranged between 1.7 : 1 and 5 : 1 in different studies; the female-to-male predominance is higher among blacks [5]. In the epidemic of pri-

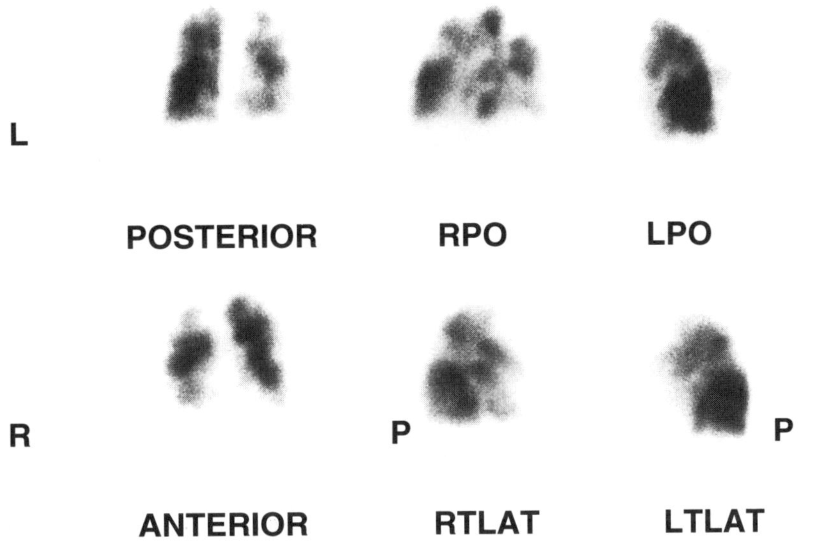

Fig. 41-2. Ventilation perfusion lung scan from a patient with chronic thromboembolic pulmonary hypertension demonstrating multiple large perfusion defects.

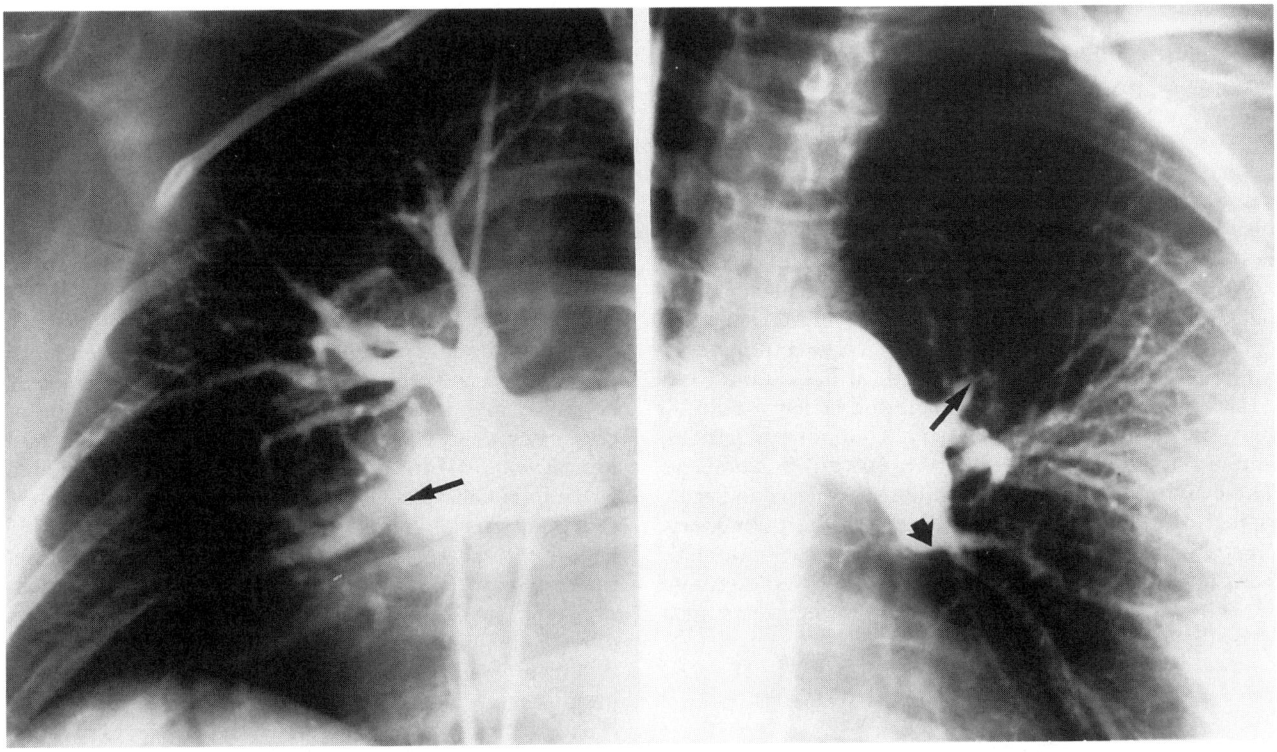

Fig. 41-3. Pulmonary angiogram from a patient with chronic thromboembolic pulmonary hypertension demonstrating large areas of avascularity. The arrows denote lobar vessels with complete occlusion due to organized thrombus.

mary pulmonary hypertension attributed to the ingestion of the anorectic agent aminorex fumarate, the female-to-male ratio was 9:1. The time delay from onset of first symptoms, generally dyspnea and fatigue, to the diagnosis of pulmonary hypertension, is about 2 years.

The clinical syndrome of primary pulmonary hypertension is identical to that of pulmonary hypertension originating from any type of obliterative pulmonary disease of the distal arterial tree (small muscular arteries and arterioles). The paradigm is a young woman, often dys-

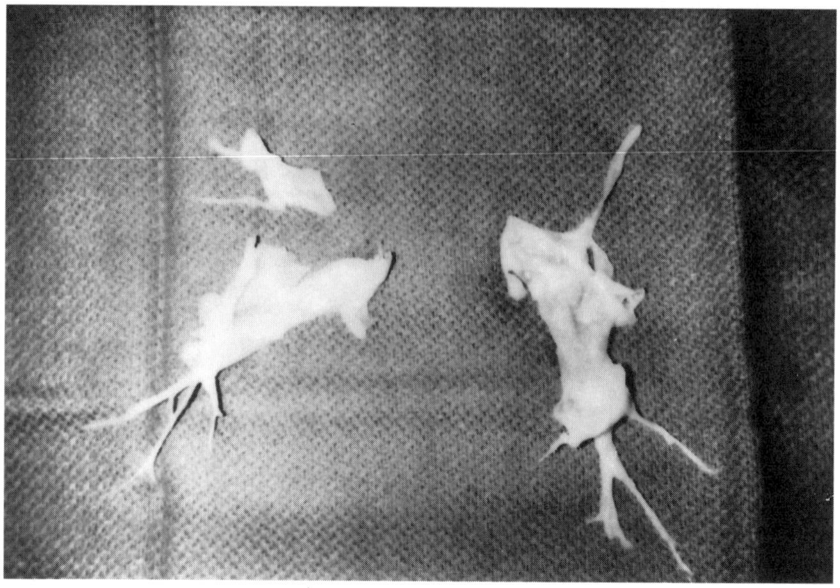

Fig. 41-4. Surgical specimen of chronic organized thrombus removed from a patient with chronic thromboembolic pulmonary hypertension at the time of thromboendarterectomy.

pneic and readily fatigable, sometimes with Raynaud's syndrome, who runs a rapidly progressive downhill course after the clinical manifestations set in, that is, 1 to 2 years.

The heterogeneity of the patient population and late diagnosis complicate the understanding of the natural history of primary pulmonary hypertension [5,37]. However, neither the age at which the disorder is recognized nor the level of pulmonary arterial pressure alone correlates with survival. Survival is most closely related to a combination of factors, including the levels of pulmonary-artery and right atrial pressures and cardiac output [38].

The vascular lesions responsible for primary pulmonary hypertension are in the small pulmonary arteries and arterioles, on the order of 50 to 500 μm in diameter. These precapillary, muscular pulmonary arteries and arterioles are the major site of resistance in the pulmonary circulation. Several histologic patterns have been identified in patients with primary pulmonary hypertension (Table 41-5; see also Table 41-4). Until a few years ago, the lesions were interpreted in terms of pathogenetic mechanisms. However, it now seems clear that a variety of histologic patterns can occur in a single patient and that certain lesions, instead of representing a specific injury, represent different stages in the morphologic expression of a single insult, differences in the rapidity of application and in the intensity of the pulmonary vascular injury, and differences in the duration of the pulmonary hypertension [28,39].

The mechanisms responsible for the development of primary pulmonary hypertension are not completely understood. Recent studies have suggested that there may be an imbalance between production or degradation of circulating vasoactive agents, such as thromboxane and prostacyclin [40] and that local production of endothelin, an endothelial-derived constricting factor and mitogen, may be enhanced in this disorder [41]. Impaired endothelial-dependent relaxation also has been observed in vessel rings from patients with primary pulmonary hypertension who have undergone transplantation. Presumably, those factors promote vasoconstriction in the lung circulation in predisposed individuals, leading to a cascade of progressive remodeling and obstructive vasculopathy.

Several therapeutic options now exist for patients with primary pulmonary hypertension, although there is no cure for the disease [35]. Anticoagulation has been advocated because of the prevalence of microthrombotic lesions in biopsies and in samples taken at autopsy [28,36,39] and the increased risk of a fatal embolic event in sedentary patients who have venous stasis and pulmonary vascular beds that no longer possess the capability of vascular distention or recruitment in the face of further vascular obstruction. Anticoagulation appears to prolong life in patients with primary pulmonary hypertension [42,43], although there is a risk of life-threatening compli-

Table 41-5. Histologic classification of other vasculopathic lesions associated with pulmonary hypertension

Classification	Findings
Pulmonary veno-occlusive disease (PVOD)	Intimal fibrosis and thrombus in pulmonary veins and venules, with medial hypertrophy of arteries
Pulmonary capillary hemangiomatosis (PCH)	Microvascular proliferation, infiltrating interstitium, pleura, lung parenchyma, and pulmonary veins with luminal obliteration

Table 41-6. Commonly used agents for vasodilator testing and treatment in primary pulmonary hypertension

	Acute testing	Maintenance therapy
Prostacyclin (PGI_2)	1–2 ng/kg/min, increasing by 2 ng/kg/min every 15 min to a maximal dose of 12 ng/kg/min (higher doses may be used in children)	Nifedipine (sustained-release) up to 240 mg/day; diltiazem up to 900 mg/day
		PGI_2 continuous infusion, 2–150 ng/kg/min
Nitric oxide (NO)	10–40 ppm inhaled	—
Adenosine	1 μg/kg/min IV, increasing every 10 min to a maximum of 50 μg/kg/min	—
Acetylcholine	1 mg/min IV, increasing every 15 min to a maximum of 10–15 mg/min	—
Prostaglandin E_1 (PGE_1)	5–30 μg/kg/min IV	—
Nifedipine or diltiazem	Hourly dosing PO until response or adverse effects	—

cations, particularly hemoptysis. Additionally, the presence of hepatic congestion due to right-sided heart failure may make adjusting the degree of anticoagulation difficult. In general, warfarin is administered to maintain the International Normalized Ratio (INR) at 2.0 to 3.0. Oxygen therapy to prevent arterial hypoxemia and to avoid hypoxic pulmonary vasoconstriction, especially during exercise, should be considered in patients with either resting hypoxemia or evidence of arterial desaturation with exercise. Arterial oxygenation may not improve with supplemental oxygen in patients with hypoxemia that results from right-to-left shunting through a patent foramen ovale; management of those patients is particularly difficult and should include oxygen therapy and diuretics to reduce right atrial pressure, thereby diminishing the interatrial pressure gradient, which promotes shunting.

Vasodilator therapy has been tried repeatedly for more than 30 years in an attempt to dilate the pulmonary resistance vessels and to arrest and even reverse the pulmonary vascular changes and to decrease right ventricular afterload. Most of those tests have been acute and limited by the uncertain long-term implications of an acute favorable response [44,45]. Also, it is not known if a nonresponder will experience vasodilation if therapy is prolonged. Moreover, vasodilator testing is potentially hazardous. The vasodilator agents currently used to test for responsiveness in patients with primary pulmonary hypertension are listed in Table 41-6. A calcium-channel blocker, generally nifedipine or diltiazem, often is included in the testing sequence during cardiac catheterization, because such agents are available for chronic oral administration, they evoke the fewest side effects, and their dosages can be tailored to the tolerance of the responsive patient.

The optimal vasodilator response to the administration of an acute vasodilator agent is a reduction in pulmonary arterial pressure accompanied by an increase in cardiac output, with minimal decrease in systemic arterial blood pressure. In practice, however, the most common response has proved to be an increase in cardiac output in association with relatively unchanged pulmonary-artery pressures. This combination of hemodynamic events results in a decrease in the calculated pulmonary vascular resistance; the increase in cardiac output generally is accompanied by improvement in exercise tolerance. Despite the increase in pulmonary blood flow (cardiac output), however, and the improved sense of well-being, the sustained high pulmonary arterial pressure and the increase in cardiac output, often in conjunction with an increase in heart rate, cause an increase in the work of the right ventricle. For that reason, clinical improvement may be short-lived unless the pulmonary arterial pressure falls.

Unfortunately, vasodilating agents often affect the systemic vascular bed more than the pulmonary vascular bed. If vasodilation should affect primarily the systemic circulation without an adequate increase in cardiac output, systemic hypotension results, which may be difficult to manage. Vasopressors administered in the hope of causing systemic vasoconstriction sometimes worsen the pulmonary hypertension, thereby increasing the right ventricular afterload. Systemic hypotension also runs the risk of decreasing coronary arterial perfusion and of producing myocardial ischemia, which can either precipitate or exaggerate right ventricular failure. Worsening hypoxemia, due either to increased perfusion to poorly ventilated lung units or to increased intracardiac shunting through the foramen ovale, also can complicate vasodilator therapy. In that setting, tissue oxygen delivery may remain unchanged or even decline, even if cardiac output increases significantly.

To avoid the untoward consequences of an unwanted systemic vasodilator response, attention has focused on the use of relatively short-acting vasodilators as potential screening agents for pulmonary vascular reactivity. Prostacyclin (PGI_2) is currently the most effective agent for that purpose [46]. It is available only for intravenous use. Prostacyclin has been approved by the Food and Drug Administration for the treatment of severe pulmonary hypertension. Alternatives to PGI_2 that have been used as acute testing agents include adenosine, prostaglandin E_1, and inhaled nitric oxide (NO). NO has the distinct advantage of being a highly selective pulmonary vasodilator when inhaled, since it becomes bound to hemoglobin and is inactivated in the pulmonary capillary network [47].

Despite the initial enthusiasm for vasodilator therapy, only approximately one-third of all patients who receive vasodilator therapy can be stabilized or improved with oral agents. Calcium-channel blockers, notably nifedipine or diltiazem, have met with most success, but occasionally other vasodilator agents, used singly or in combination, have proved effective. As a rule, patients are given the maximum tolerated dosage, which, with the calcium-channel blockers, can vary greatly from patient to patient [43,48]. Rich and colleagues have demonstrated that responders to calcium channel–blocking agents, defined as those patients who experience a substantial fall in pulmonary-artery pressure concomitant with an increased cardiac output, manifest sustained hemodynamic improvement as well as prolonged survival [43].

Since only one-third of patients are responders to oral vasodilator therapy, attention recently has been focused on developing strategies to treat the majority of patients with the disease who are nonresponders. Recent experience suggests that PGI_2 administered by continuous intravenous infusion using a portable infusion pump to deliver the drug through an implanted central venous catheter may improve hemodynamics, exercise tolerance, and survival in patients who are refractory to conventional therapy [49]. Using that approach, PGI_2 can be used either as a bridge to transplantation or as a primary mode of therapy in highly responsive patients.

Combined heart-lung transplantation was first performed for severe pulmonary hypertension with modest success. The limited availability of organs suitable for transplantation and the risks of rejection of either or both thoracic organs have tempered enthusiasm for the procedure. The demonstration that right ventricular function can be restored to normal or near-normal levels in patients with chronic thrombotic pulmonary hypertension undergoing thromboendarterectomy [29] led to the concept that lung transplantation alone may be a suitable procedure for nonthrombotic pulmonary hypertension, as long as a noncorrectable cardiac defect is not present. Single- or double-lung transplantation is now considered by many as the operation of choice for this disease. Pulmonary-artery pressure and right-heart function improve dramatically after surgery [50], although allograft rejection and opportunistic infections remain serious factors limiting long-term survival after the procedure. Although the availability of lungs for transplantation is greater than combined heart-lung blocs, many patients must wait for a year or longer before organs become available for transplantation, and many severely ill patients die awaiting transplantation.

DIETARY PULMONARY HYPERTENSION

Pulmonary hypertension with the histologic features of primary pulmonary hypertension has occurred in humans after the ingestion of certain substances, such as aminorex fumarate. That observation, coupled with the experimental production of pulmonary hypertension in animals by feeding monocrotaline, a pyrrolidine alkaloid contained in the shrub of *Crotolaria* species, has raised questions about the roles of ingested materials and of the liver in the pathogenesis of some instances of primary pulmonary hypertension [51].

Pulmonary hypertension attributed to aminorex fumarate, an appetite suppressant, has generated great interest not only because of its presumed etiology but also because of its potential reversibility. Introduced in Switzerland, Austria, and Germany in 1965, aminorex was related on epidemiologic grounds to the outbreak of "primary" pulmonary hypertension that occurred in those countries in 1966. After aminorex was withdrawn from over-the-counter sales in 1968, the epidemic subsided. Attempts to duplicate the phenomenon in animals were consistently unsuccessful. Nonetheless, the epidemic and its subsidence carried several important messages: (1) Pulmonary hypertension developed after aminorex fumarate ingestion in only a minute fraction of all those who ingested the medication, raising the prospect of genetic predisposition; (2) the incidence of pulmonary hypertension could not be related either to total dosage or to duration of use; and (3) in some who stopped the medication, the pulmonary hypertension subsided [52]. Pulmonary hypertension also has been observed in individuals who have taken related medications currently available in the United States, and, as with aminorex, the disease may be reversible on discontinuation of their use.

TOXIC OIL SYNDROME

A syndrome characterized by scleroderma-like features was observed in Spain a decade ago that was due to the ingestion of contaminated rapeseed oil used for cooking. In a minority of patients, pulmonary vascular disease developed as part of that illness and was fatal in some patients [53]. The contaminants responsible for the pathogenesis of toxic oil syndrome (TOS) have not been conclusively identified. A similar illness in the United States was associated with the ingestion of contaminated L-tryptophan. That disease, termed eosinophilia-myalgia syndrome (EMS), was characterized by myositis, pulmonary fibrosis or pulmonary hypertension, neuropathy, and cognitive functional alterations and pronounced blood eosinophilia in the early stages [54].

PULMONARY HYPERTENSION IN ASSOCIATION WITH PORTAL HYPERTENSION

Pulmonary hypertension with histologic features identical to those of primary pulmonary hypertension also occurs in conjunction with portal hypertension of diverse etiology [55–57]. The incidence of that association is at least five to six times that of primary pulmonary hypertension in the general population. The morphologic features are those of either primary pulmonary arteriopathy with plexiform lesions or primary pulmonary arteriopathy with thrombotic lesions (see Table 41-4). Originally, the pulmonary hypertension was believed to originate in emboli from thrombi in the portal venous system. It now seems, however, that pulmonary microthrombi occur without thrombosis in the portal system. As in the case of dietary pulmonary hypertension, the liver is suspect, possibly operating either by failing to inactivate a vasoconstrictor substance or by producing a metabolic intermediate that damages endothelium. An alternative hypothesis is that a vasodilator substance normally produced in the liver is no longer made, due to the hepatic injury. For the present, the etiology of concurrent pulmonary and portal hypertension remains speculative.

There is little to offer therapeutically to these patients. Vasodilators have been ineffective, and the patients generally are not considered candidates for transplantation because of coexistent hepatic disease.

PULMONARY HYPERTENSION ASSOCIATED WITH HIV INFECTION

Pulmonary vascular disease that is pathologically similar to primary pulmonary hypertension recently has been seen in some patients infected with the human immunodeficiency virus (HIV) [58]. The mechanism responsible for pulmonary vascular disease in that setting is unknown, although the virus is known to possess mitogenic properties that may stimulate vascular growth and proliferation. One histologic study did not find HIV infection in the vascular endothelium by electron microscopy, immunohistochemistry, DNA in-situ hybridization, and polymerase chain-reaction techniques. On electron microscopy, tubuloreticular structures were found, suggesting that HIV infection may be contributing to the pathogenesis of those cases of primary pulmonary hypertension through release of mediators such as interferon alpha and beta rather than by direct endothelial infection [59].

References

1. Palevsky HI. Exercise and the pulmonary circulation. In A Leff, ed. Cardiopulmonary Exercise Testing. Orlando, FL: Grune & Stratton, 1986. Pp. 89–106.
2. Fishman AP. Pulmonary circulation. In AP Fishman, ed. Handbook of Physiology—The Respiratory System. Bethesda, MD: American Physiologic Society, 1985. Pp. 93–165.
3. Reeves JT, Groves BM. Approach to the patient with pulmonary hypertension. In EK Weir, JT Reeves, eds. Pulmonary Hypertension. Mount Kisco, NY: Futura, 1984. Pp. 1–44.
4. Rubin LJ. Clinical evaluation. In LJ Rubin, ed. Pulmonary Heart Disease. Boston: Martinus Nijhoff, 1984. Pp. 107–115.
5. Rich S, et al. Primary pulmonary hypertension: a national prospective study. Ann Int Med 1987; 107:216–223.
6. Hughes JD, Rubin LJ. Primary pulmonary hypertension—An analysis of 28 cases and a review of the literature. Medicine 1986; 65:56–72.
7. Voelkel NF, Reeves JT. Primary pulmonary hypertension. In K Moser, ed. Pulmonary Vascular Disease. New York, NY: Marcel Dekker, 1979. Pp. 573–628.
8. Wood P. Pulmonary hypertension. In P Wood, Diseases of the Heart and Circulation, 3d ed. Philadelphia, PA: Lippincott, 1968. Pp. 964–985.
9. Perloff JK. Auscultatory and phonocardiographic manifestations of pulmonary hypertension. Prog Cardiovasc Dis 1967; 9:303–340.
10. Kanemoto N. Electrocardiogram in primary pulmonary hypertension. Eur J Cardiol 1980; 12:181–193.
11. Lupi E, et al. A radiologic index of pulmonary arterial hypertension. Chest 1975; 68:28–31.
12. Kanemoto N, et al. Chest roentgenograms in primary pulmonary hypertension. Chest 1979; 76:45–49.
13. Powe JE, et al. Usefulness of lung scanning in the evaluation of patients with pulmonary arterial hypertension. Radiology 1987; 164:727–730.
14. Moser KM, et al. Perfusion lung scans provide a guide to which patients with apparent primary pulmonary hypertension merit angiography. West J Med 1988; 148:167–170.
15. Dexter L. Pulmonary vascular disease in acquired heart disease. In KM Moser, ed. Pulmonary Vascular Diseases. New York, NY: Marcel Dekker, 1979. Pp. 427–487.
16. Perloff JK. Congenital heart disease and pulmonary hypertension. In KM Moser, ed. Pulmonary Vascular Diseases. New York, NY: Marcel Dekker, 1979. Pp. 489–526.
17. Edwards JE. Congenital pulmonary vascular disorders. In KM Moser, ed. Pulmonary Vascular Diseases. New York, NY: Marcel Dekker, 1979. Pp. 527–571.
18. Behar JV, et al. The performance of new criteria for right ventricular hypertrophy and myocardial infarction in patients with right ventricular hypertrophy due to cor pulmonale and mitral stenosis. J of Electrocardiography 1991; 24:231–237.
19. Fulmer JD, Snider GL. ACCP-NHLBI National Conference on Oxygen Therapy. Chest 1984; 86:234–247.
20. Kobayashi H, et al. Mixed connective tissue disease with fatal pulmonary hypertension. Acta Pathol Jpn 1982; 32:1121–1129.
21. Asherson RA, Oakley CM. Pulmonary hypertension and systemic lupus erythematosus. J Rheum 1986; 13:1–5.
22. Bunch TW, Tancredi RG, Lie JT. Pulmonary hypertension in polymyositis. Chest 1981; 79:105–107.
23. Stupi AM, et al. Pulmonary hypertension in CREST syndrome variant of systemic sclerosis (scleroderma). Arth Rheum 1986; 29:515–524.
24. Rich S, et al. Antinuclear antibodies in primary pulmonary hypertension. J Am Coll Cardiol 1986; 8:1307–1311.
25. Fahey PJ, et al. Raynaud's phenomenon of the lung. Am J Med 1984; 76:263–269.
26. Ungerer RG, et al. Prevalence and clinical correlates of pulmonary arterial hypertension in progressive systemic sclerosis. Am J Med 1983; 75:65–74.
27. Rich S, Levitsky S, Brundage BH. Pulmonary hypertension from chronic pulmonary thromboembolism. Ann Int Med 1988; 108:425–434.
28. Loyd JE, et al. Heterogeneity of pathologic lesions in familial primary pulmonary hypertension. Am Rev Respir Dis 1988; 138:952–957.
29. Moser KM, et al. Thromboendarterectomy for chronic, major vessel thromboembolic pulmonary hypertension: immediate and long-term results in 42 patients. Ann Int Med 1987; 107:560–565.
30. Nicod P, et al. Pulmonary angiography in severe chronic pulmonary hypertension. Ann Int Med 1987; 107:565–568.
31. Shure D, Gregoratos G, Moser KM. Fiberoptic angioscopy: role in the diagnosis of chronic pulmonary arterial obstruction. Ann Intern Med 1985; 103:844–850.
32. Gefter WB, et al. Identification of chronic thromboembolic pulmonary hypertension with MR imaging. Radiology 1988; 169:218.
33. Daily PO, et al. Risk factors for pulmonary thromboendarterectomy. J Thorac Cardiovasc Surg 1990; 9:670–678.
34. Moser KM, Auger WR, Fedullo PF. Chronic major-vessel thromboembolic pulmonary hypertension. Circulation 1990; 81:1735–1743.
35. Rubin LJ, et al. ACCP Consensus Statement: Primary pulmonary hypertension. Chest 1993; 104:236–250.
36. Wagenvoort CA, Wagenvoort N. Primary pulmonary hypertension: a pathologic study of the lung vessels in 156 clinically diagnosed cases. Circulation 1970; 42:1163–1184.
37. Glanville AR, et al. Primary pulmonary hypertension: length of survival in patients referred from heart-lung transplantation. Chest 1987; 91:675–681.
38. D'Alonzo GG, et al. Survival in patients with primary pulmo-

nary hypertension: Results from a national prospective registry. Ann Intern Med 1991; 115:343–349.
39. Palevsky HI, et al. Primary pulmonary hypertension: vascular structure, morphometry and responsiveness to vasodilator agents. Circulation 1989; 30:1207–1221.
40. Christman BW, et al. An imbalance between the excretion of thromboxane and prostacyclin metabolites in pulmonary hypertension. N Eng J Med 1992; 327:70–75.
41. Giaid A, et al. Expression of endothelin-1 in the lungs of patients with pulmonary hypertension. N Eng J Med 1993; 328:1732–1736.
42. Fuster V, et al. Primary pulmonary hypertension: Natural history and the importance of thrombosis. Circulation 1984; 70:580–587.
43. Rich S, et al. The effect of high doses of calcium channel blockers on survival in primary pulmonary hypertension. N Eng J Med 1992; 327:76–81.
44. Reeves JT, Groves BM, Turkevich D. The case for treatment of selected patients with primary pulmonary hypertension. Am Rev Respir Dis 1986; 134:342–346.
45. Weir EK, et al. The acute administration of vasodilators in primary pulmonary hypertension: experience from the NIH Registry on PPH. Am Rev Respir Dis 1989; 140:1623–1630.
46. Rubin LJ, et al. Prostacyclin-induced pulmonary vasodilation in primary pulmonary hypertension. Circulation 1982; 66:334–338.
47. Pepke-Zaba J, et al. Inhaled nitric oxide as a cause of selective pulmonary vasodilation in pulmonary hypertension. Lancet 1991; 338:1173–1174.
48. Rich S, Brundage BH. High-dose calcium channel-blocking therapy for primary pulmonary hypertension: evidence for long-term reduction in pulmonary arterial pressure and regression of right ventricular hypertrophy. Circulation 1987; 76:134–141.
49. Barst RJ, et al. Survival in primary pulmonary hypertension with long-term continuous intravenous prostacyclin. Ann Intern Med 1994; 121:409–415.
50. Pasque MK, et al. Single lung transplantation for pulmonary hypertension: three month hemodynamic follow-up. Circulation 1991; 84:2275–2279.
51. Fishman AP. Dietary pulmonary hypertension. Circ Res 1974; 35:657–660.
52. Gurtner HP. Aminorex pulmonary hypertension. In AP Fishman, ed. The Pulmonary Circulation: Normal and Abnormal. Mechanisms, Management and the National Registry. Philadelphia: University of Pennsylvania Press, 1990. Pp. 397–411.
53. Gomez-Sanchez MA et al. Clinical and pathological manifestations of pulmonary vascular disease in the toxic oil syndrome. J Amer Coll Cardiol 1992; 18:1539–1545.
54. Cotton CK, et al. Pulmonary involvement in the eosinophilia myalgia syndrome. Chest 1991; 99:327–329.
55. Edwards BS, et al. Coexistent pulmonary and portal hypertension: morphologic and clinical features. J Am Coll Cardiol 1987; 10:1233–1238.
56. Robalino BD, Moodie DS. Association between primary pulmonary hypertension and portal hypertension: analysis of its pathophysiology and clinical, laboratory and hemodynamic manifestations. J Am Coll Cardiol 1991; 17:492–498.
57. Hadengue A, et al. Pulmonary hypertension complicating portal hypertension: prevalence and relation to splanchnic hemodynamics. Gastroenterology 1991; 100:520–528.
58. Speich R, et al. Primary pulmonary hypertension in HIV infection. Chest 1991; 100:1268–1271.
59. Mette SA, et al. Primary pulmonary hypertension in association with Human Immunodeficiency Virus infection: A possible viral etiology for some forms of hypertensive pulmonary arteriopathy. Am Rev Respir Dis 1992; 145:1196–1200.

B

Vasospastic Disorders and Vasculitis

42

Raynaud's Phenomenon and Other Vascular Disorders Related to Temperature

Mark A. Creager
Jonathan L. Halperin
Jay D. Coffman

Raynaud's Phenomenon

In its simplest form, local syncope is a condition perfectly compatible with health. Persons who are attacked with it are ordinarily females. Under the least stimulus, sometimes without appreciable cause, one or many fingers become pale and cold all at once; in many cases, it is the same finger which is always first attacked; the others become dead successively and in the same order. It is the phenomenon known as "dead finger." The attack is indolent, the duration varies from a few minutes to many hours. The determining cause is often the impression of cold; but that which is only commonly produced under the influence of the most severe cold, appears in the subjects of whom I speak on the occasion of the least lowering of temperatures; sometimes even a simple mental emotion is enough . . . the skin of the affected parts assumes a dead white or sometimes a yellow colour; it appears completely exsanguine. The cutaneous sensibility becomes blunted, then annihilated; the fingers become like foreign bodies to the subject . . . the slight importance of this local abolition of the circulation is probably due to the fact that it is so transient . . . the attack is followed by a period of reaction, which is often very painful, and which gives place to a sensation quite analogous to that of being numbed by cold . . . and in the more pronounced cases, which the patients compared to tingling from cold, or to the stinging of nettles. . . . Finally, a patch of deep red is formed on the extremities of the fingers. This patch gives place to the normal pink colour, and then the skin is found to have entirely returned to the primitive condition (*Maurice Raynaud*). [1]

Episodic vasospastic ischemia of the digits was first described by Maurice Raynaud [1]. Raynaud's phenomenon comprises the sequential development of digital blanching, cyanosis, and rubor following cold exposure and subsequent rewarming [2] (Fig. 42-1). Emotional stress also may precipitate Raynaud's phenomenon. The color changes are episodic, usually well demarcated, and primarily confined to the fingers or toes. The blanching, or pallor, occurs during the ischemic phase of the phenomenon and is secondary to digital vasospasm. During ischemia, arterioles, capillaries, and venules dilate. Cyanosis results from the deoxygenated blood in those vessels. Cold, numbness, or paresthesias of the digits often accompanies the phases of pallor and cyanosis. With rewarming, the digital vasospasm resolves, and blood flow dramatically increases into the dilated arterioles and capillaries. This "reactive hyperemia" imparts a bright red color to the digits. In addition to rubor and warmth, patients often experience a throbbing sensation during the hyperemic phase. Thereafter, the color of the digits gradually returns to normal. Although the triphasic color response is typical of Raynaud's phenomenon, some patients may develop only pallor and cyanosis; others may experience only cyanosis.

The diagnosis of Raynaud's phenomenon is made from historic criteria. Rarely does a patient enter a physician's office during an episode of digital vasospasm. Furthermore, it usually is difficult to reproduce an episode of Raynaud's phenomenon in the examination room, even by placing the patient's hand in ice water. The inability to precipitate an attack, therefore, does not exclude the diagnosis. The physical findings in patients with Raynaud's phenomenon may be entirely normal or may reflect an associated systemic disorder that is associated with Raynaud's phenomenon. The severity of Raynaud's phenomenon ranges widely from those patients who experience mild infrequent "attacks" to those with frequently recurrent, prolonged episodes of ischemia. In the latter, digital ulcers, infection, gangrene, and autoamputation may occur (Fig. 42-2).

The classification of Raynaud's phenomenon is broadly separated into two categories: the idiopathic variety,

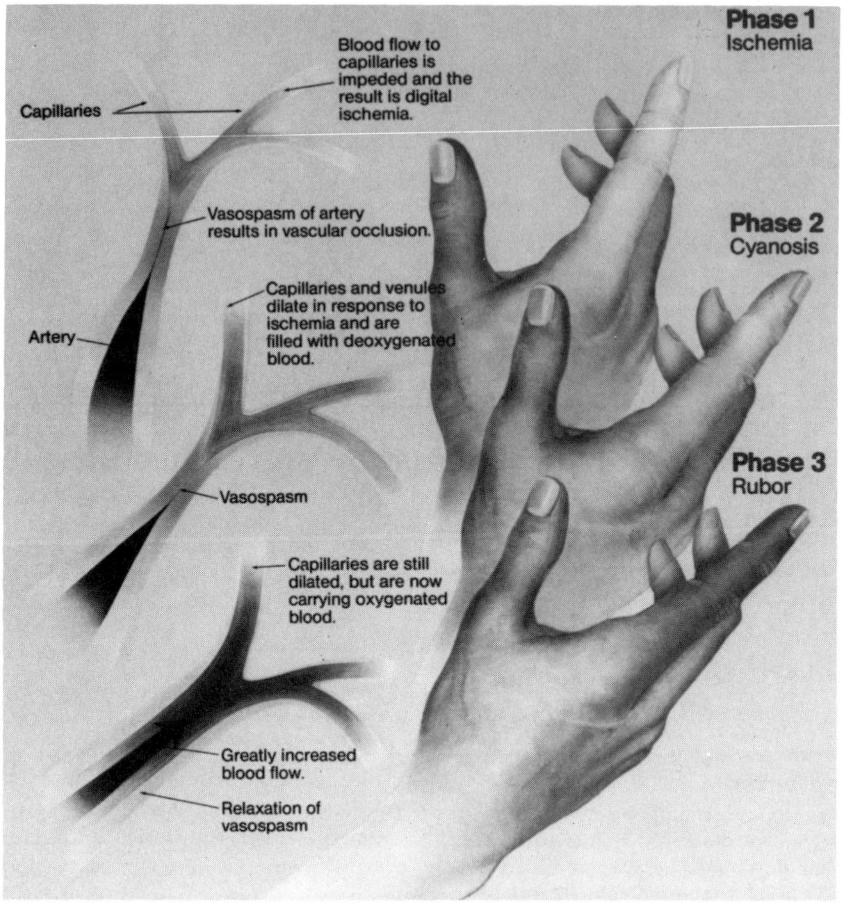

Fig. 42-1. Raynaud's phenomenon may have three color phases: blanching, cyanosis, and rubor. (Reproduced with permission from MA Creager, Raynaud's phenomenon. Illustrated Medicine 1983; 2:84).

termed primary Raynaud's phenomenon, and the secondary variety, which is associated with other disease states or known causes of vasospasm. The secondary causes of Raynaud's phenomenon include connective tissue diseases, arterial occlusive disease, thoracic outlet syndrome, several neurologic disorders, blood dyscrasias, trauma, and several drugs.

PATHOPHYSIOLOGY

The precise cause of Raynaud's phenomenon has not been clearly identified. It is quite likely that a variety of physiologic and pathologic conditions may contribute to or cause digital vasospasm [2–4].

Normally, the regulation of peripheral blood flow depends on several factors, including the intrinsic vascular tone, sympathetic nervous system activity, hemorheologic properties such as blood viscosity, and a variety of circulating hormonal substances. In contrast to other regional circulations that are supplied by both vasoconstrictor and vasodilator sympathetic fibers, the cutaneous vessels of the fingers and toes are innervated only by sympathetic adrenergic vasoconstrictor fibers. In those vascular beds, neurogenic vasodilation occurs by withdrawal of a sympathetic stimulus. Cooling evokes reflex sympathetic mediated vasoconstriction in the fingers and toes via neurons originating in cutaneous receptors. Environmental cooling or cooling of specific body parts such as the head, neck, or trunk normally causes a reduction in digital blood flow. Local digital cooling also induces vasoconstriction; however, digital vasoconstriction caused by local cooling is not mediated by the sympathetic nervous system. Thus, digital vasoconstriction may be a physiologic response to local cooling or to reflex activation of the sympathetic nervous system by environmental cold exposure or emotional stress.

Raynaud's phenomenon is not a normal physiologic response but rather an episode of digital artery vasospasm causing cessation of blood flow to the digits (Fig. 42-3). The term vasospasm must be distinguished from that of vasoconstriction. **Vasoconstriction** can be defined as the expected reduction in vessel lumen size as a result of endogenous neural, hormonal, or metabolic factors that cause smooth muscle contraction. **Vasospasm** implies an excessive vasoconstrictor response to stimuli that would normally cause modest smooth muscle contraction but that instead result in obliteration of the vascular lumen.

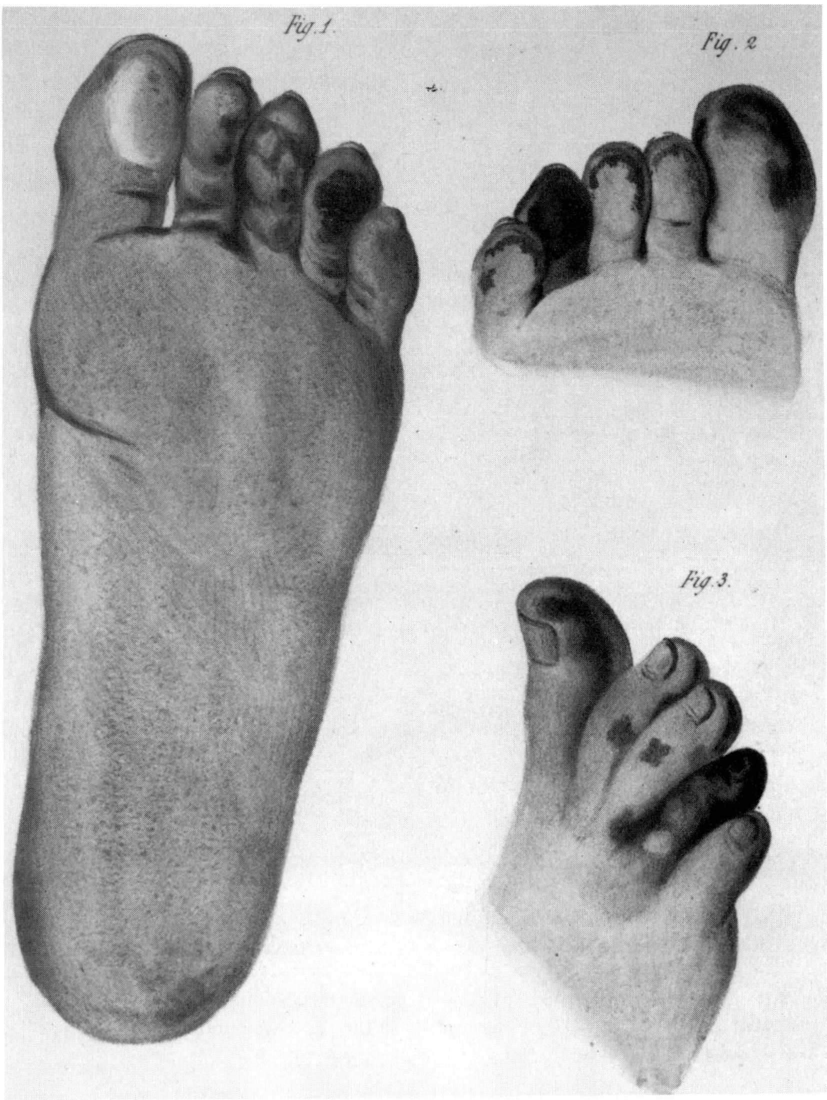

Fig. 42-2. A patient with Raynaud's phenomenon. (Reproduced from M. Raynaud, Local asphyxia and symmetrical gangrene of the extremities. New Sydenham Society, 1862. Courtesy of Boston Medical Library in the Francis A. Countway Library of Medicine.)

The patency of the digital artery depends on a favorable balance between the contractile forces of the muscular wall of the digital artery and its intraluminal pressure. Thus, a situation in which there is excessive vasoconstrictive force or decreased intravascular pressure upsets that balance and results in vasospasm. With these rather simple concepts, several theories have been proposed to explain the episodic digital vasospasm that defines Raynaud's phenomenon (Table 42-1).

Increased Vasoconstrictive Stimuli. Several theories implicate excessive vasoconstrictive stimuli as a cause of Raynaud's phenomenon. Postulated causes include increased sympathetic nervous system activity; elevated levels of vasoconstrictor hormones, such as angiotensin II, serotonin, and thromboxane A_2; as well as exogenously administered agents such as ergot alkaloids and sympathomimetic drugs.

INCREASED SYMPATHETIC NERVOUS SYSTEM ACTIVITY. The concept of excessive sympathetic nervous system activity as a cause of episodic digital vasospasm was first suggested by Maurice Raynaud in his seminal treatise entitled "New Researches on the Nature and Treatment of Local Asphyxia of the Extremities" [1]. In that monograph, Raynaud states, ". . . the marked symmetry of the lesions ought to suggest that they originate in a discharge either spontaneous or reflex, starting from the cord and radiating thence to the vascular nerves of the extremities."

Although appealing as a potential mechanism for digital vasospasm, the concept of exaggerated reflex sympathetic vasoconstrictor responses to a cold environment has not been convincingly demonstrated. Peacock re-

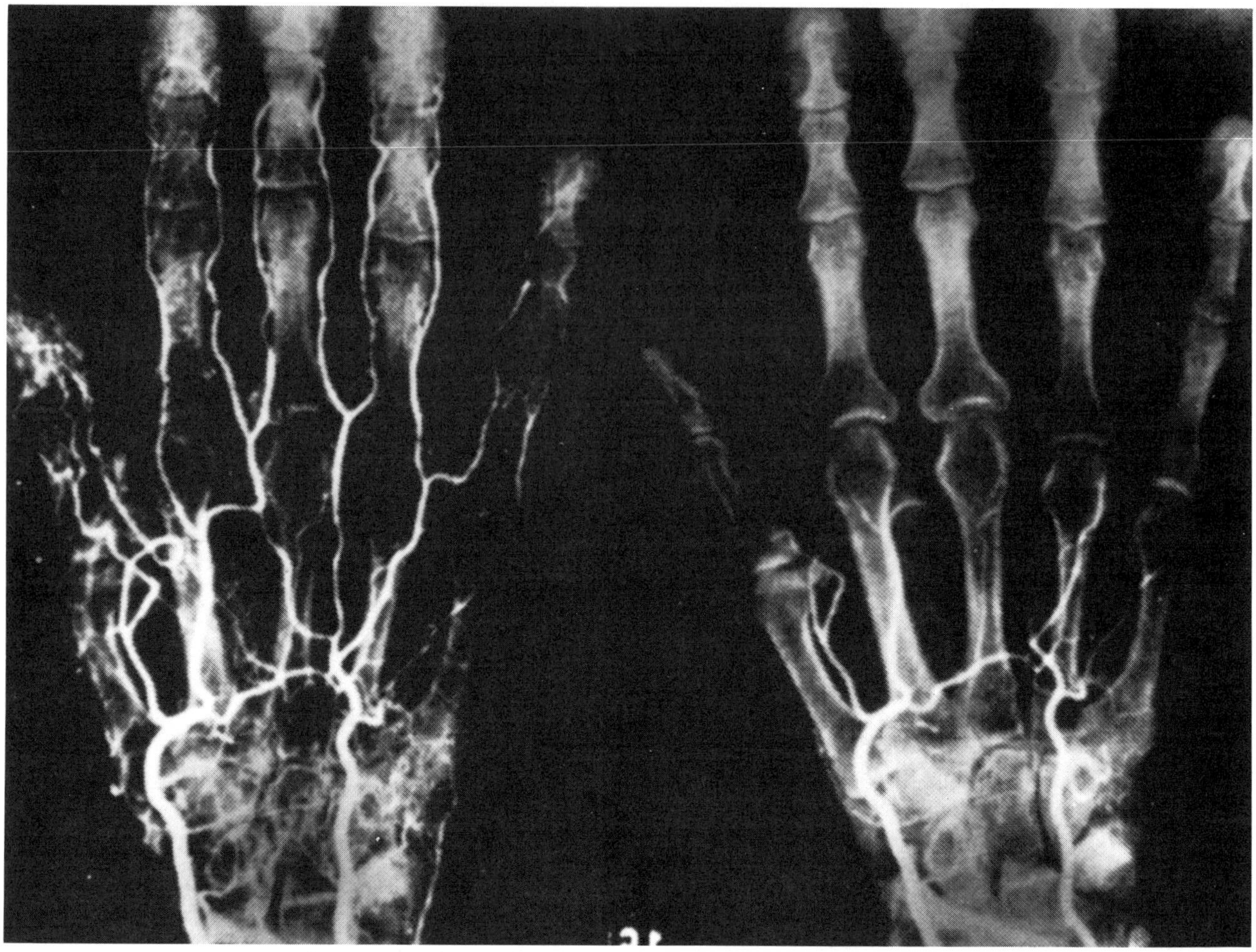

Fig. 42-3. Angiograms demonstrating the effect of local cold exposure on digital vessels. The angiogram on the left displays normal digital arteries. The angiogram on the right was obtained after cold-water immersion and demonstrates diffuse digital vasospasm.

ported that the concentrations of epinephrine and norepinephrine in the peripheral venous blood at the wrist was higher in patients with primary Raynaud's phenomenon than in normal subjects [5]. Furthermore, the norepinephrine values during cold stimulation appeared to be related to the clinical severity of the disease, being lowest in the mild cases and highest in the most severe cases in his series. One might speculate that the norepinephrine levels were raised by excessive reflex sympathetic nervous system activity. Peacock suggested that there was an abnormality of catecholamine metabolism following release from peripheral sympathetic nerve endings in the walls of the digital arteries. In his study, hand blood flow generally was lower in patients with primary Raynaud's phenomenon than in normal subjects; therefore, a reduction in arterial inflow may have been responsible for the increased catecholamine concentrations. Alternatively, the lower hand temperature in the patients with Raynaud's phenomenon may have limited catecholamine metabolism. Kontos and Wasserman found normal local levels of norepinephrine in brachial arterial and venous blood samples from patients with primary Raynaud's phenomenon [6]. They also reported that the reflex vasoconstrictor response of the hand to a cold stimulus was similar to that in a control group of subjects. There were comparable vasoconstrictor responses to the intra-arterial infusion of tyramine, a drug that causes vasoconstriction by releasing norepinephrine from sympathetic nerve terminals. Downey and Frewin also presented data opposing the concept of sympathetic overactivity. Although their patients with Raynaud's phenomenon had lower hand blood flow than did normal subjects, the vasoconstrictor response to cooling did not differ between the two groups [7]. In a separate study, Downey and colleagues reported that central thermoregulatory control of skin temperature was comparable in normal individuals and patients with primary Raynaud's phenomenon [8].

To examine further the possibility of excessive sympathetic nervous system activity, Coffman and Cohen measured total and capillary fingertip blood flow in patients with Raynaud's phenomenon and normal subjects in a warm environment and during reflex sympathetic nerve

Table 42-1. Pathophysiology of Raynaud's phenomenon: possible mechanisms

Vasoconstrictive stimuli
- Increased sympathetic nervous system activity
- Digital vascular hyperreactivity to sympathetic stimuli ("local fault") (e.g., cold potentiation of $alpha_2$ adrenoceptors)
- Beta-adrenoceptor blockade (loss of digital vasodilator mechanism vs. unopposed alpha adrenoceptors)
- Circulating vasoactive hormones
  - Angiotensin II
  - Serotonin
  - Thromboxane A_2
- Exogenous administration of vasoconstrictor
  - Ergot alkaloids
  - Sympathomimetic drugs

Decreased intravascular pressure
- Low systemic blood pressure
- Arterial occlusive disorder (e.g., atherosclerosis, thromboangiitis obliterans)
- Digital arterial occlusions (e.g., systemic sclerosis, rheumatoid arthritis, thromboembolism)
- Loss of potential energy (e.g., hyperviscosity syndrome, cold agglutinin disease, cryoglobulinemia)

stimulation caused by environmental cooling [9]. Both total fingertip blood flow and capillary blood flow were lower in patients with Raynaud's phenomenon than in normal subjects when studied in a warm (28.3°C) environment as well as in a cold (20°C) environment. Total fingertip blood flow, measured by venous occlusion plethysmography, decreased in both groups during cold exposure. In contrast, only patients with Raynaud's phenomenon showed a decrease in capillary flow, as determined by radioisotope clearance in the cold environment. Those results, however, neither prove nor disprove the possibility that excessive sympathetic nervous system activity is a cause of Raynaud's phenomenon. The decline in capillary blood flow during cold exposure in the patients with Raynaud's phenomenon could be due to excessive sympathetic nervous system activity. However, total fingertip blood flow and capillary blood flow were less in the patients with Raynaud's phenomenon in both warm and cool environments. Comparable levels of sympathetically mediated vasoconstriction during cold exposure would result in a smaller vascular lumen if the vessel wall was thickened in patients with Raynaud's phenomenon.

LOCAL VASCULAR HYPERREACTIVITY TO SYMPATHETIC STIMULI. The observation that episodic digital vasospasm occurs during cold exposure has led several investigators to consider the possibility that Raynaud's phenomenon occurs as a result of an increased sensitivity of digital vessels to sympathetic stimuli. In 1929, Sir Thomas Lewis observed that following exposure of the finger to cold, vasospasm could be produced even after nerve blockade or sympathectomy [10]. His work has not been widely accepted because many of the patients had Raynaud's phenomenon secondary to other diseases, and the observed vasoconstrictive attacks may have been related to structural vascular disease rather than cold sensitivity. Mendlowitz and Naftchi were unable to demonstrate increased sensitivity to intravenously administered norepinephrine in patients with primary Raynaud's phenomenon [11]. Lewis's theory, however, has gained support in a more recent study in which vasospastic attacks were induced in 80 percent of patients with primary Raynaud's phenomenon and Raynaud's phenomenon secondary to scleroderma by a combination of environmental and local cooling [12]. With that type of stimulus, vasospastic episodes continued to occur after digital-nerve block, indicating that the vasospastic response of Raynaud's phenomenon may occur in the absence of efferent digital nerves.

The possibility of local vascular hyperactivity was examined by Jamieson and co-workers [13]. They compared the magnitude of reflex vasoconstriction in each hand following application of ice to the neck while one hand was kept at 26°C and the other at 36°C. At 36°C, the reflex vasoconstrictor response was comparable in the normal subjects and patients with primary Raynaud's phenomenon. In the hand cooled to 26°C, however, the reflex vasoconstriction was exaggerated in the patients with Raynaud's disease. That response led the investigators to hypothesize that digital alpha adrenoceptors were sensitized by cold exposure. A series of studies by Vanhoutte and colleagues have supported the hypothesis that cooling potentiates the vascular response to sympathetic nerve activation [14–19]. Cooling increases further the constriction of canine cutaneous blood vessels to sympathetic nerve stimulation [14]. Vasoconstriction, in response to exogenous norepinephrine, also is increased by cooling. Augmentation of adrenergic-mediated vasoconstriction by cooling occurs despite generalized depression of the contractile machinery and diminished release of norepinephrine from sympathetic nerve endings in the vessel wall [15]. Membrane permeability to calcium is reduced during cooling, and contractions to depolarizing solutions of potassium, which are entirely dependent on entry of extracellular calcium, are inhibited [20]. Furthermore, cooling attenuates the action of high-energy phosphate compounds in vascular smooth muscle [16].

Two hypotheses have been offered to explain the augmented response of cutaneous blood vessels to sympathetic nervous system stimuli during moderate cooling. One is that the disposition of norepinephrine is depressed with cooling [17]. This could potentiate adrenergic responses by reducing norepinephrine metabolism and increasing the concentration of endogenous norepinephrine in the neuromuscular junction in the vicinity of the alpha adrenoceptors of the vascular smooth muscle cells. That possibility, however, has been discounted, in part, because inhibitors of catechol-O-methyltransferase and monoamine oxidase do not affect cold-induced potentiation of adrenergic responses in isolated vessels [18]. The second, and more likely, hypothesis is that cold causes changes at the level of the adrenoceptor, such as an increase in the affinity for norepinephrine or greater efficacy of the agonist-receptor complex. Vanhoutte and colleagues have reported that $alpha_2$ adrenoceptors are more sensitive than $alpha_1$ adrenoceptors to changes in temperature [19,21]. Whereas cooling slightly depresses $alpha_1$

adrenergic-mediated vasoconstriction, it markedly augments $alpha_2$ adrenergic-mediated responses. Conversely, warming augments $alpha_1$ and depresses $alpha_2$ adrenergic vasoconstriction [21].

Those experimental observations may have important implications regarding the pathophysiology of Raynaud's phenomenon. Flavahan and colleagues examined the distribution of $alpha_1$ and $alpha_2$ adrenoceptors in arteries of human limbs [22]. They obtained tissue from amputated limbs of patients who did not have vascular disease. They reported that $alpha_2$ adrenoceptors were more predominant in digital arteries. In support of that finding, Coffman and Cohen reported that $alpha_2$ adrenoceptors were more important than $alpha_1$ adrenoceptors in mediating sympathetic nerve-induced vasoconstriction in the fingers [23]. They administered the $alpha_1$ antagonist prazosin and the $alpha_2$ antagonist yohimbine to normal subjects during reflex sympathetic vasoconstriction caused by body cooling. Whereas prazosin caused no significant change in finger blood flow or finger vascular resistance, yohimbine significantly increased finger blood flow and decreased finger vascular resistance. Their study confirmed that postjunctional $alpha_2$ adrenoceptors are present in human digits and strongly suggested that those receptors contribute to digital vasoconstriction during cooling in normal subjects. Thereafter, Coffman and Cohen [24] demonstrated that patients with Raynaud's phenomenon, compared to normal subjects, are hypersensitive to the vasoconstrictor effects of clonidine, an $alpha_2$-adrenoceptor agonist but not to phenylephrine, an $alpha_1$-adrenoceptor agonist. Also, Keenan and Porter observed that the density of $alpha_2$ adrenoceptors is increased in platelets from patients with primary Raynaud's phenomenon [25]. Recently, Freedman and colleagues reported that intra-arterial administration of yohimbine decreased cold-induced digital vasospasm, more so than prazosin, in patients with Raynaud's phenomenon [26]. Taken together, these studies suggest that episodic digital vasospasm may be secondary to a predominance of postjunctional $alpha_2$ adrenoceptors in digits of patients with Raynaud's disease.

BETA-ADRENERGIC BLOCKADE. Raynaud's phenomenon is observed frequently in individuals treated with beta-adrenoceptor antagonists [27–29]. It may be inferred from such observation that beta-adrenergic vasodilation normally attenuates digital vasoconstrictor tone. Alternatively, blockade of beta adrenoceptors could potentiate vasoconstriction by unopposed alpha adrenoceptors.

Whether beta adrenoceptors actively cause digital vasodilation, however, has been difficult to demonstrate. Whereas intra-arterial isoproterenol causes marked vasodilation in the forearm skeletal muscle vasculature, its effects in the skin vessels of the hand and foot are comparatively mild and transient [30]. Cohen and Coffman examined the effect of isoproterenol and propranolol on fingertip blood flow after vasoconstriction had been induced by a brachial-artery infusion of norepinephrine or angiotensin or reflexively by environmental cooling [31]. Intra-arterial isoproterenol administration increased fingertip blood flow during the infusions of norepinephrine and angiotensin but not during reflex sympathetic vasoconstriction. Conversely, propranolol served to potentiate vasoconstriction caused by intra-arterial norepinephrine but not that caused by reflex sympathetic vasoconstriction. The investigators concluded that a beta-adrenergic vasodilator mechanism may be active in human digits but does not modulate sympathetic vasoconstriction. In the absence of pharmacologic blockade of beta adrenoceptors, there is no evidence supporting the contention that decreased sensitivity or number of beta adrenoceptors contributes to the pathophysiology of Raynaud's phenomenon.

VASOCONSTRICTION CAUSED BY CIRCULATING VASCULAR SMOOTH MUSCLE AGONISTS. A variety of neurotransmitters, hormones, and substances released by endothelial cells, platelets, and leukocytes are capable of constricting vascular smooth muscle and causing digital vasoconstriction, including angiotensin II, serotonin, thromboxane A_2, endothelin, and free radicals. It would be difficult to attribute all causes of Raynaud's phenomenon to excessive levels of those vasoconstrictor agents, but in some secondary causes of Raynaud's phenomenon, any one might contribute to vasoconstriction.

Serotonin (5-hydroxytryptamine, or 5-HT) is a neurotransmitter that is synthesized and released by selective neurons and enterochromaffin cells. It is metabolized by the liver and by endothelial cells and is taken up by platelets. Serotonin can cause vasoconstriction by directly activating serotonergic receptors on the smooth muscle cells [32]. Vasoconstriction also may be caused by direct activation of alpha adrenoceptors on smooth muscle cells or indirectly by facilitating the release of norepinephrine from adrenergic nerve terminals [32]. In preconstricted vessels, serotonin may cause vasodilation, most likely via release of endothelium-derived relaxing factor [33]. When infused into the brachial artery of normal individuals, serotonin decreases forearm, hand, and finger blood flow [34,35]. With prolonged infusion, finger temperature falls, and digital cyanosis occurs. The release of serotonin during platelet aggregation has been shown to constrict digital arteries [36].

Evidence is available that implicates but does not establish a role for serotonin in the pathophysiology of Raynaud's phenomenon. It is controversial whether plasma or platelet levels of serotonin (or both) are elevated in Raynaud's phenomenon [37–40]. The vasoconstrictive effects of serotonin are potentiated at lower temperatures [14]. Cutaneous vessel strips isolated from patients with scleroderma demonstrate hypersensitivity to serotonin [41]. Coffman and Cohen [35] demonstrated that S_2-serotonergic receptors are present in human fingers and play a role in vasoconstriction of the finger caused by body cooling. They also found that patients with Raynaud's phenomenon were hypersensitive to the digital vasoconstrictor effects of intra-arterial infusion of serotonin compared to normal subjects [24]. Halpern and colleagues infused serotonin into the brachial arteries of normal human subjects and patients with Raynaud's phenomenon [42]. Serotonin precipitated digital ischemia and a decreased digital temperature in both groups, but the duration of ischemia was more prolonged in the patients with

Raynaud's phenomenon. Concurrent administration of a serotonin antagonist attenuated the digital ischemia.

Serotonin antagonists have been used as pharmacologic probes to examine the contribution of serotonin to Raynaud's phenomenon [43–45]. Ketanserin is a drug that antagonizes serotonergic (5-HT_2) receptors on vascular smooth muscle cells; it also has some alpha-adrenoceptor blocking properties [46–48]. Ketanserin facilitates recovery of digital temperature and blood flow following hand immersion in cold water and increases finger blood flow in normal subjects during reflex sympathetic vasoconstriction [35,49]. Studies examining ketanserin in patients with Raynaud's phenomenon, however, have yielded inconsistent results. When administered intravenously, ketanserin increased digital blood flow in some studies but not in others [45,50,51]. Chronic administration of ketanserin has been variably reported to cause improvement or have no significant effect in the symptoms of patients with Raynaud's phenomenon [43–45,52,53]. Thus, the contribution of serotonin to digital vasospasm remains speculative.

The possibility that vasoconstrictors released during platelet aggregation may be pertinent to the pathophysiology of Raynaud's phenomenon has been further evaluated by studies that have either measured levels of thromboxane or administered a thromboxane synthetase inhibitor [54–60]. In patients with Raynaud's phenomenon secondary to systemic sclerosis, the urinary excretion of the thromboxane A_2 metabolite 2,3-dinor thromboxane B_2 is elevated [55]. Coffman and Rasmussen compared the thromboxane synthetase inhibitor dazoxiben to placebo in patients with either primary or secondary Raynaud's phenomenon [56]. Dazoxiben did not affect total fingertip blood flow or fingertip capillary blood flow, whether measured in a warm (28.3°C) or cool (20°C) environment. With chronic treatment, there was a small decrease in the frequency of vasospastic episodes in the patients with primary Raynaud's phenomenon. Similarly, studies by other investigators have been unable to establish that dazoxiben improves fingertip blood flow or that it relieves symptomatic digital vasospasm in patients with Raynaud's phenomenon [57,60]. Gresele and co-workers administered both a thromboxane-receptor antagonist and a thromboxane-synthase inhibitor to patients with Raynaud's phenomenon [38]. Although those drugs depressed thromboxane B_2 levels in serum by 95 percent, they did not affect cold-induced vasoconstriction. To date, there is insufficient evidence to support a role for thromboxane A_2 in digital vasospasm.

The plasma concentration of the potent vasoconstrictor angiotensin II is rarely elevated in patients with Raynaud's phenomenon. Therefore, this hormone is unlikely to contribute to the pathophysiology of digital vasospasm in most patients. Captopril, an angiotensin converting enzyme (ACE) inhibitor, has been reported, in uncontrolled studies, to improve digital blood flow in patients with primary Raynaud's phenomenon [61–63]. Captopril decreased the frequency of Raynaud's phenomenon in two patients with scleroderma when they were treated for malignant hypertension [64]. The efficacy of this drug in other patients who have scleroderma and Raynaud's phenomenon is not well established, and reports have been inconsistent [61,62,64]. The digital vessels in patients with scleroderma often are diseased and potentially hypersensitive to vasoactive stimuli. Thus, in this subgroup of patients, high circulating levels of angiotensin II conceivably could promote intense digital vasoconstriction.

Endothelial damage and dysfunction could contribute to the development of vasospastic attacks by affecting local release of vasodilator and vasoconstrictor substances. Lau et al. [65] found that the severity of Raynaud's phenomenon correlated with von Willebrand's factor antigen levels, a marker of endothelial damage. Marasini et al. [39] found high plasma levels of von Willebrand's factor and tissue plasminogen activator in systemic sclerosis but not in patients with primary Raynaud's phenomenon. Increased polymorphonuclear-cell activity and increased levels of malondiadehyde, an indication of free radical activity, also have been reported in patients with primary and secondary Raynaud's phenomenon [66]. Endothelin-1 is a potent, long-acting vasoconstrictor substance released from endothelial cells. Endothelin-1 levels are reported to be elevated in the plasma of patients with Raynaud's phenomenon [67,68] and to rise during provocation by a local cold stimulus [69]. Endothelin-1 levels are higher in diffuse scleroderma compared to limited scleroderma. Until an antagonist of endothelin-1 is developed for human use, its role in vasospastic attacks cannot be determined. There has been speculation, but no data, to support decreased release of the endothelium-derived relaxing factor nitric oxide as a cause of Raynaud's phenomenon. Indeed, the vasodilative response to a cholinergic agonist, a stimulus for endothelium-derived nitric oxide is increased in patients with Raynaud's phenomenon [70].

Exogenous administration of vasoconstrictor agents also have been reported to cause digital vasospasm. Ergot alkaloids have been used to treat migraine headaches and induce labor and may cause digital ischemia if large doses are taken [71–76]. The use of sympathomimetic drugs in critical care situations also are associated with digital ischemia if large doses are given or when extravasation of an infusion occurs.

Decreased Intravascular Pressure. The patency of a blood vessel requires the balance between the tension in the arterial wall (favoring closure of the vessel) and the intravascular distending pressure [77,78]. Landis measured intravascular pressure in patients with Raynaud's phenomenon by introducing a micropipette into a large digital capillary [79]. During cyanosis, capillary pressure fell to approximately 5 mm Hg, and flow ceased. These findings suggested that the site of closure was proximal to the capillaries at the arterial level. It is, therefore, of interest that Thulesius reported that brachial artery blood pressure in patients with primary Raynaud's phenomenon was significantly lower than that in a normal control population [80]. Cohen and Coffman also measured systolic blood pressure at the brachial artery as well as at the proximal and distal digital arteries of normal subjects and patients with primary Raynaud's phenomenon [81]. Blood pressure measured at these locations was significantly lower in the patients, averaging 18 mm Hg less than in the normal digits. It is of further interest that the centrifugal force generated by swinging the arms can relieve an episode of Raynaud's phenomenon, perhaps by increasing intravascular pressure [82].

A low digital artery pressure may occur in a variety of disorders associated with Raynaud's phenomenon, such as large-vessel arterial occlusive disease secondary to atherosclerosis, embolism, or thoracic outlet syndrome. When extrinsic vasoconstrictor force is applied, these vessels may collapse and cause digital ischemia. Distal vascular occlusions secondary to thromboangiitis obliterans, vasculitis, or vibration injury may also reduce digital arterial pressure distal to the diseased vascular segment. Lewis obtained digital arteries postmortem from a series of patients who experienced Raynaud's phenomenon during life [83]. The digits of patients who had experienced only mild episodes of Raynaud's phenomenon were indistinguishable from those of people of similar age who had not experienced a digital vasospasm. Thrombi were found, however, in the digital arteries of individuals who had more severe cases of Raynaud's phenomenon. Dabich and colleagues examined the arteriograms of patients with scleroderma and reported that 26 of 27 patients had digital arterial occlusions [84]. These findings were supported by a study by Rosch and colleagues, who found digital vascular obstruction in the majority of patients with Raynaud's phenomenon secondary to connective tissue disorders [85]. Kirstensen measured systolic blood pressure in the upper-arm and digital vessels of normal individuals and patients with Raynaud's phenomenon secondary to scleroderma [86]. The pressure gradient was greater in the patients with scleroderma, as indicated by decreased digital vascular pressure.

Hyperviscosity may cause a loss of potential energy in the digital vessels, leading to a decrease in intravascular pressure. Indeed, Raynaud's phenomenon occurs in patients with hyperviscosity caused by polycythemia vera or Waldenström's macroglobulinemia [87,88]. In patients with Raynaud's phenomenon secondary to disorders such as cryoglobulinemia and cold agglutinin disease, hyperviscosity caused by cooling may contribute to digital vasospasm [89–93]. Indeed, cooling has been shown to abolish hand blood flow in patients with cold agglutinins, possibly because the vessels become occluded by agglutinated red cells [93]. The data invoking hyperviscosity as a cause of Raynaud's phenomenon in patients who do not have an established blood dyscrasia is less compelling. Some investigators have found that whole blood or plasma viscosity is elevated when measured at varying shear rates in patients with primary Raynaud's phenomenon [94–97]. Goyle and Dormandy reported that the viscosity of whole blood cooled to 27°C was increased in patients with primary Raynaud's phenomenon [98]. Pringle and associates reported that patients with Raynaud's phenomenon had elevated levels of plasma fibrinogen, which contributed to an abnormally high blood viscosity [99]. In contrast, in multiple studies, it has been impossible to distinguish whole blood or plasma viscosities in patients with primary Raynaud's phenomenon from those hemorheologic properties in normal individuals, despite cooling the blood to 10°C [94,100–103].

Table 42-2. Classification of Raynaud's phenomenon

Raynaud's disease, or primary Raynaud's phenomenon
Raynaud's phenomenon, secondarily caused by:
Collagen vascular diseases
Systemic sclerosis (scleroderma)
Systemic lupus erythematosus
Rheumatoid arthritis
Dermatomyositis and polymyositis
Mixed connective-tissue disease
Sjögren's syndrome
Necrotizing vasculitis
Arterial occlusive disease
Atherosclerosis of the extremities
Thromboangiitis obliterans (Buerger's disease)
Thromboembolism
Thoracic outlet syndrome
Neurologic disorders
Carpal tunnel syndrome
Reflex sympathetic dystrophy
Stroke
Intervertebral disk disease
Syringomyelia
Poliomyelitis
Blood dyscrasias
Hyperviscosity syndrome
Cold agglutinin disease
Cryoglobulinemia
Cryofibrinogenemia
Myeloproliferative diseases
Trauma
Exposure to vibrating tools (vibration white finger)
Electric shock injury
Thermal injury
Percussive injury
Hypothenar hammer syndrome
Drugs and toxins
Ergot alkaloids
Methysergide
Vinblastine
Bleomycin
Beta-adrenoceptor antagonists
Polyvinyl chloride
Miscellaneous causes
Hypothyroidism
Arteriovenous fistula
Pulmonary hypertension

PRIMARY RAYNAUD'S PHENOMENON

Primary Raynaud's phenomenon, or idiopathic episodic digital vasospasm, also called Raynaud's disease, is the most common diagnosis of patients who present with Raynaud's phenomenon [2,104]. This entity is distinguished from the multiple secondary disorders associated with Raynaud's phenomenon discussed later in this chapter (Table 42-2). The diagnosis of primary Raynaud's phenomenon is based on criteria originally established by Allen and Brown from careful observations of a group of 150 cases at the Mayo Clinic [105]. The criteria include (1) intermittent attacks of ischemic discoloration of the extremities; (2) absence of organic arterial occlusion; (3) bilateral distribution; (4) trophic changes, when present, limited to the skin and never consisting of gross gangrene; (5) absence of any symptoms or signs of systemic disease that might account for the occurrence of Raynaud's phenomenon; and (6) duration of the symptoms for 2 years or longer. Additional findings that support the diagnosis of primary Raynaud's phenomenon include normal nailfold capillaries, normal erythrocyte sedimentation rate, and negative antinuclear antibody test [2,106].

Women are affected approximately three to five times more frequently than men [107–110]. One of the most comprehensive analyses of patients with Raynaud's phenomenon was presented by Gifford and Hines, who reviewed 756 female patients suspected of having primary Raynaud's phenomenon at the Mayo Clinic [111]; in approximately 50 percent, the diagnosis was made according to the criteria of Allen and Brown. Much of our knowledge about the clinical presentation and natural history of patients with primary Raynaud's phenomenon has been obtained from that review. The average age of onset of Raynaud's phenomenon was 31 years; 78 percent of the patients were younger than 40 years old when symptoms began. The onset of symptoms in women usually occurs between menarche and menopause. Primary Raynaud's phenomenon also occurs in young children [112,113]. The prevalence of Raynaud's phenomenon in a specific population depends on the climate. The prevalence is 5 percent in Charleston County, South Carolina (mean temperature 8.8°C in January, 26.9°C in July), but 16.8 percent in Tarentaise, Savoie, France (mean temperature −0.4°C in January, 17.7°C in July) [107].

There is no established genetic predisposition to primary Raynaud's phenomenon. Approximately 5 percent of patients may know of one or more relatives who have Raynaud's phenomenon [111]. However, the relative frequency of Raynaud's phenomenon in the general population may be sufficient to explain the rather frequent occurrence in family members.

In the vast majority of patients, the fingers are the initial site of involvement [2,104]. At first, blanching or cyanosis may involve only one or two fingers (Fig. 42-4). Later, color changes may develop in additional fingers, and symptoms occur bilaterally. In approximately 40 percent of patients, Raynaud's phenomenon involves the toes as well as the fingers. Isolated Raynaud's phenomenon of the toes occurs in only 1 to 2 percent of patients. Rarely, the earlobes, the tip of the nose, or the tongue is affected.

Episodes of Raynaud's phenomenon usually are precipitated by exposure to a cool environment or by direct exposure of the extremities to low temperatures. Some patients may experience Raynaud's phenomenon during either cold exposure or emotional stress. Infrequently, emotional stress may be the only precipitating factor. The duration, frequency, and severity of Raynaud's phenomenon increase during the cold months. The classic description of Raynaud's phenomenon involves three phases of color change, including pallor, cyanosis, and rubor. Many patients describe a triphasic color response, but the majority may experience only two colors or even just one phase of color change, such as pallor or cyanosis [108,110,111].

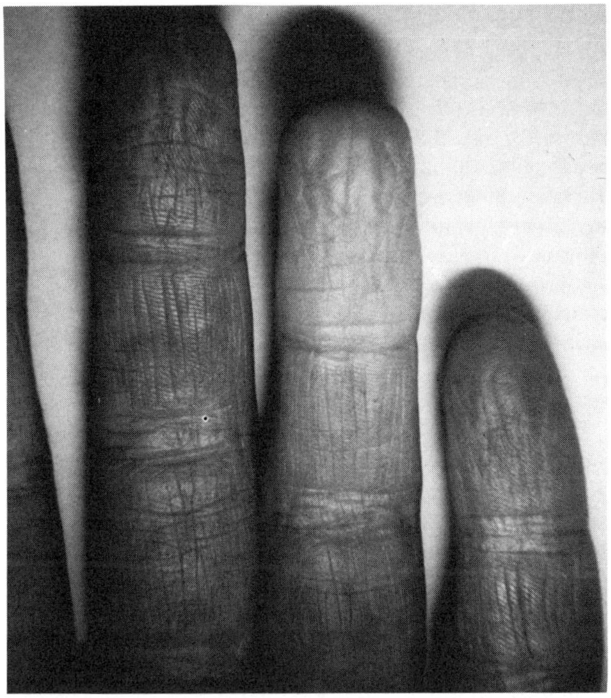

Fig. 42-4. Raynaud's phenomenon presenting as blanching of one finger.

The use of the term primary Raynaud's phenomenon as an appellation for idiopathic episodic digital vasospasm implies that there is no known etiology. Nonetheless, several studies have correlated Raynaud's phenomenon with migraine headaches and variant angina, suggesting a common mechanism for vasospasm. Miller and colleagues reported that Raynaud's phenomenon occurred in 15 of 62 patients undergoing catheterization for variant angina but in only 2 of 62 patients who had other causes of chest pain [114]. Furthermore, 16 of the 62 patients with variant angina had migraine headaches, compared with 4 of 62 in the control group. Similarly, Zahavi et al. [115] and O'Keeffe et al. [116] reported an increased prevalence of migraine headaches in patients with primary Raynaud's phenomenon. Krumholz and Goldberger [117] described a family with three generations of systemic arterial vasospastic diseases involving Raynaud's phenomenon, variant angina, and migraine headaches. Renal [118], myocardial [119], pulmonary [120], and retinal capillary [121] vasospasm have been described in patients with primary or secondary Raynaud's phenomenon. However, differences in the reactivity of the cerebral, myocardial, and digital vasculature and in responses to pharmacologic intervention makes the hypothesis of a common mechanism less convincing [122]. Propranolol has been successfully used to prevent migraine headaches [123,124]. In contrast, beta-adrenoceptor blockers are not beneficial in variant angina and may cause Raynaud's phenomenon [125,126]. Similarly, nitrates are used for variant angina but are not beneficial in Raynaud's phenomenon and often cause headaches. Ergot alkaloids are effective for treating migraine headaches but can cause coronary and digital vasospasm [72–76,127–129].

The physical examination of patients with primary Raynaud's phenomenon is often entirely normal. Sometimes, the fingers and toes are cool and may perspire excessively. The pulse examination is normal. The radial, ulnar, and pedal pulses should be easily palpable. Sclerodactyly, or thickening and tightening of the digital subcutaneous tissue, develops in approximately 10 percent of patients. Clubbing and deformity of the nails and shortening of the terminal phalanges may be observed. Trophic changes occur in approximately 5 percent of patients with primary Raynaud's phenomenon. The physical examination is important to exclude secondary causes of Raynaud's phenomenon.

Of all the forms of Raynaud's phenomenon, primary Raynaud's phenomenon has the most benign prognosis. In the group of patients identified by Gifford and Hines, followed for a period of 1 to 32 years, averaging 12 years, 16 percent reported worsening of their symptoms, whereas 10, 36, and 38 percent reported disappearance of, improvement of, or no change in their symptoms, respectively [111]. Sclerodactyly or trophic changes of the digits may occur in approximately 3 percent of patients during the follow-up, and less than 1 percent of patients lose part of a digit. In some patients, scleroderma may develop after Raynaud's phenomenon has been present as the only symptom for more than 20 years. Wollersheim et al. reported that measuring antinuclear antibodies by immunofluorescence and immunoblotting had a positive predictive value of 65 percent and 71 percent and a negative predictive value of 93 percent and 83 percent, respectively, for the development of a connective-tissue disease in patients with Raynaud's phenomenon [130].

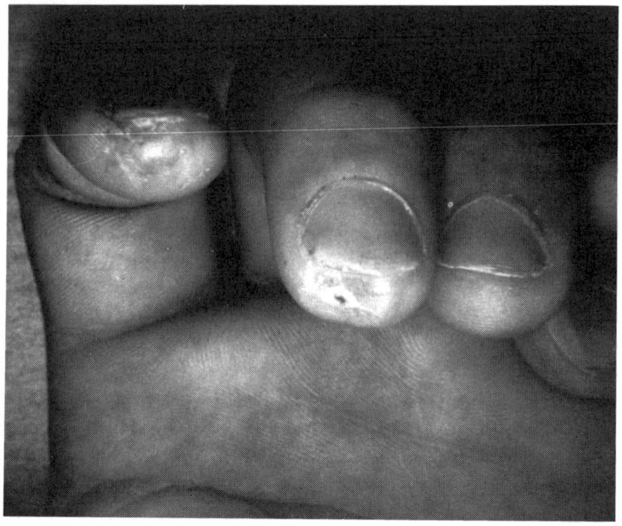

Fig. 42-5. Digital ulcerations in a patient with systemic sclerosis.

SECONDARY CAUSES OF RAYNAUD'S PHENOMENON

The secondary causes of Raynaud's phenomenon include connective tissue diseases, arterial occlusive disorders, thoracic outlet syndrome, several neurologic disorders, blood dyscrasias, and trauma, as well as several drugs (see Table 42-2).

Connective-Tissue Diseases.

SYSTEMIC SCLEROSIS (SCLERODERMA). Raynaud's phenomenon occurs in 80 to 90 percent of patients with systemic sclerosis. It may be the presenting symptom in approximately 33 percent of patients. In some patients, scleroderma may develop after Raynaud's phenomenon has been present as the only symptom for many years.

The frequency and severity of Raynaud's phenomenon in patients with systemic sclerosis is often worse than that observed in patients with primary Raynaud's phenomenon. The incidence of digital ulceration and gangrene is increased, possibly leading to amputation (Fig. 42-5). The diagnosis of systemic sclerosis is suggested by the appearance of typical sclerotic skin changes. These include tightness, thickening, and nonpitting induration involving the extremities, face, neck, or trunk. When present in the digits, those abnormalities produce changes in the contour of the fingers and toes, referred to as sclerodactyly. Other manifestations of systemic sclerosis include pitting scars of the tips of the digits, abnormal skin pigmentation, and telangiectasia. Visceral manifestations include pulmonary fibrosis, esophageal dysmotility, and colonic sacculation. The kidney and the heart also may be involved. As the disease progresses, the skin and subcutaneous tissue of the fingers become stiffer, the joints become immobile, and contractures develop. The American Rheumatism Association has suggested several clinical criteria for the diagnosis of systemic sclerosis [131]. The single major criterion is the presence of proximal scleroderma. Minor criteria include sclerodactyly, digital pitting scars, and basilar pulmonary fibrosis. A variant of systemic sclerosis is the CREST syndrome (calcinosis, Raynaud's phenomenon, esophageal dysmotility, sclerodactyly, and telangiectasia) in the absence of internal-organ involvement.

Histologically, the cutaneous vessels are sparse in patients with systemic sclerosis [132]. The intima of the small arteries of most organs is thickened, and thrombus may be present in the medium-sized digital arteries [83,133–135].

Several serologic studies are consistent with the diagnosis of scleroderma. The erythrocyte sedimentation rate may be elevated. Antinuclear antibodies are present in the majority of individuals with the disorder; patients may have antibodies to nucleolar antigens, nuclear ribonucleoprotein, and to the centromeric region of metaphase chromosomes. Increased plasma levels of von Willebrand factor and antigen have been reported in patients with scleroderma and may indicate endothelial cell abnormalities [136].

Tests in the noninvasive vascular laboratory are not specific for scleroderma. Digital vascular obstructive lesions are suggested by an abnormal pulse volume contour and decreased digital systolic blood pressures. In patients with systemic sclerosis and Raynaud's phenomenon, capillary microscopy often demonstrates enlarged and deformed capillary loops surrounded by relatively avascular areas, particularly in the nailfolds [137,138] (Plate 10).

Angiography frequently demonstrates digital and ulnar-artery obstruction [84].

SYSTEMIC LUPUS ERYTHEMATOSUS. Raynaud's phenomenon occurs in approximately 10 to 35 percent of patients with systemic lupus erythematosus. Persistent digital vasospasm, often due to proliferative endarteritis of the small digital vessels, also occurs and may result in gangrene. Diagnosis of systemic lupus erythematosus is based on the presence of at least 4 of the following 11 criteria: malar rash; discoid rash; photosensitivity; oral ulcers; arthritis; serositis, including pleuritis or pericarditis; renal disorders, including persistent proteinuria or cellular casts; neurologic disorders, such as seizures and psychosis; hematologic disorders, including hemolytic anemia, leukopenia, lymphopenia, or thrombocytopenia; immunologic disorders; and abnormal titers of antinuclear antibody, especially anti-DNA [139].

RHEUMATOID ARTHRITIS. Raynaud's phenomenon also occurs in patients with rheumatoid arthritis. These patients may have vasculitis of medium-sized vessels as well as proliferative endarteritis of small vessels [140]. Crops of small brown spots may be observed in the nail beds and digital pulp. Digital blood flow often is reduced in patients with rheumatoid arthritis, and angiography frequently reveals occlusions of one or more digital arteries [141,142]. The diagnosis is suggested in patients who meet the criteria of the American Rheumatism Association [143]. At least five or six of the following criteria must be present: morning joint stiffness, joint pain or tenderness on motion, joint swelling, subcutaneous nodules, radiologic changes typical of rheumatoid arthritis, the presence of rheumatoid factor in the serum, and characteristic histologic changes in the synovium and skin nodules.

DERMATOMYOSITIS AND POLYMYOSITIS. Thirty percent of patients with dermatomyositis or polymyositis have associated Raynaud's phenomenon [2,104]. Muscular manifestations include weakness of the proximal girdle muscles, particularly those involving the lower extremity. Patients may also experience aching in the buttocks, thighs, and calves. Some patients complain of dysphagia or dyspnea. Myocarditis develops in approximately one-third of individuals. The dermatologic abnormalities in dermatomyositis include localized or diffuse erythema, a maculopapular rash, and eczematoid dermatitis. A purplish (heliotrope) rash may develop on the upper eyelids, face, chest, limbs, or around the nail beds. Laboratory diagnosis of dermatomyositis and polymyositis is based on elevated serum levels of the skeletal-muscle enzymes, including creatine kinase, aldolase, serum glutamic oxaloacetic transaminase, and lactic acid dehydrogenase. There may be myoglobinuria. The erythrocyte sedimentation rate often is elevated. The electromyogram (EMG) reveals evidence of a myopathy.

Arterial Occlusive Disease. Occlusive disease of arteries that are proximal to the digital vessels is often associated with Raynaud's phenomenon. Proximal arterial occlusive disease may decrease intravascular pressure and upset the balance between tension in the arterial wall and intravascular distending pressure, which may make the vessel more prone to vasospasm when subjected to sympathetic nervous system stimuli.

Atherosclerosis of the extremities tends to occur most frequently in males greater than 50 years and females greater than 60 years old. When Raynaud's phenomenon occurs in those individuals, it tends to be unilateral and related to the affected extremity. Usually only one or two digits are involved. The diagnosis is suggested by the clinical history and physical examination. Symptoms of claudication or findings that would suggest atherosclerosis elsewhere, such as in the coronary or cerebral vasculature, often indicate the underlying disorder. Physical findings are noteworthy for decreased or absent pulses in the involved extremity. Such abnormalities can be confirmed by noninvasive vascular testing. Severe ischemia may be manifested as persistent digital pallor or cyanosis and must be distinguished from the episodic digital vasospasm of Raynaud's phenomenon.

Thromboangiitis obliterans (Buerger's disease) is an inflammatory occlusive vascular disorder involving small and medium-sized arteries and veins (see Chap. 44). It was first described by von Winiwarter in 1879 [144]. Buerger coined the term **thromboangiitis obliterans** in 1908 when he reviewed the clinical and pathologic features of this disorder [145]. The syndrome develops most frequently in males younger than 40 years. Its prevalence is greatest in Asians and in individuals whose lineage originates in Eastern Europe. The cause of thromboangiitis obliterans is not known. There is a definite relation to tobacco use. Individuals with this disorder have an increased incidence of human leukocyte antigens A9 and B5 [146]. Some patients have an increased cellular immune response to collagen types I and III [147]. In addition, anticollagen antibodies and antielastin antibodies develop in some patients.

The pathologic features of thromboangiitis obliterans include a polymorphonuclear leukocytic infiltrate throughout all layers of the blood vessel wall [148,149]. A thrombus, also containing polymorphonuclear leukocytes, frequently occludes the lumen of the vessel. The internal elastic lamina is preserved, and there is no necrosis of the media. In the subacute phase, mononuclear and giant cells replace the neutrophils. The chronic phase is characterized by perivascular fibrosis and thrombus recanalization. Prominent vasa vasorum may be present at the chronic stage. The distal vessels of the upper and lower extremities are most often affected [150]. Cerebral, visceral, and coronary vessels also may be involved [151–153].

In addition to Raynaud's phenomenon, clinical features of thromboangiitis obliterans include claudication of the affected extremity and migratory superficial vein thrombosis. In the presence of severe digital ischemia, painful ulcerations and gangrene may develop at the tips of the fingers. Arteriography may be helpful in making the diagnosis [150]. Smooth tapering segmental lesions are found in the more distal vessels. Numerous "tree-root" collaterals surround occluded vessels. Vessels may appear normal between the sites of occlusion. A diagnosis is confirmed by excisional biopsy and pathologic examination of an involved vessel. There is no specific treatment for the disorder, but the prognosis is worse in individuals who continue to smoke. Arterial bypass of larger vessels may be used in selected individuals, depending on the severity of ischemia. Anticoagulants, corticosteroids, and immunosuppressive drugs are not helpful.

Thoracic Outlet Syndrome. Compression of the neurovascular bundle as it courses through the neck and shoulder can result in a symptom complex that includes Raynaud's phenomenon as well as shoulder and arm pain, weakness, paresthesias, and claudication of the affected upper extremity. Cervical ribs, abnormalities of the scalenus anticus muscle, the proximity of the clavicle to the first rib, or abnormal insertion of the pectoralis minor muscle may compress the subclavian artery and brachial plexus as those structures pass from the thorax to the arm. Raynaud's phenomenon may result from the decreased intravascular pressure caused by extrinsic compression of the subclavian artery. It is not known whether compression of the brachial plexus alters sympathetic nervous system activity.

The examination of these patients is often normal unless provocative maneuvers are performed. Occasionally, however, distal pulses are decreased or absent, and digital cyanosis and ischemia may be present. Tenderness may be elicited in the supraclavicular fossa. Several maneuvers are useful to confirm the diagnosis and suggest the location of the abnormality, including the scalenus, costoclavicular, and hyperabduction maneuvers, which cause subclavian bruits and loss of arm pulses [2]. It is important that these maneuvers also reproduce symptoms or a pale hand. The scalenus anticus maneuver (Adson's maneuver) involves extending the neck fully with the chin turned toward the side being examined while a deep breath is held. The costoclavicular maneuver is performed by pulling the shoulders backward and downward into an exaggerated military position. In the hyperabduction maneuvers, the arm is raised above the head and rotated slightly away from the body. A chest x-ray indicates the presence of cervical ribs. Electromyography or nerve conduction velocities may be abnormal if the brachial plexus is involved.

Management generally is conservative. Patients should be advised to avoid positions that precipitate symptoms. Often patients benefit from exercises that focus on the shoulder girdle. At times, it may be necessary to remove the first rib or the scalenus anticus muscle to relieve symptoms or treat ischemia.

Neurologic Disorders. A variety of neurologic conditions, particularly those causing disuse of the limb, may be associated with disorders of circulatory vasomotion. These conditions include stroke, syringomyelia, intervertebral disk disease, spinal cord tumors, and poliomyelitis. The affected limb, including the hand or foot in addition to the digits, may be cool and cyanotic. In contrast to the episodic nature of Raynaud's phenomena, the changes tend to be persistent.

Raynaud's phenomenon has been reported in approximately 10 percent of patients with carpal tunnel syndrome [154–156]. This entrapment neuropathy is caused by compression of the median nerve as it passes through the carpal tunnel. It may result from a localized tenosynovitis, trauma, hypothyroidism, amyloidosis, or activities associated with repeated motion of the wrist. It is common during pregnancy and is an occupational disease of keyboard operators. Patients usually experience paresthesias or weakness in the distribution of the median nerve. The diagnosis is suggested when symptoms are reproduced by tapping the volar surface of the wrist (Tinel's sign) or by maintaining flexion of the wrist (Phalen's maneuver). Nerve conduction tests usually demonstrate abnormalities of the median nerve at the wrist. Supportive treatment includes splints and anti-inflammatory drugs. With severe persistent symptoms, surgical incision of the carpal ligament may be beneficial.

Reflex sympathetic dystrophy or causalgia (see Chap. 53), another neurologic disorder associated with cyanotic extremities, involves pain and tenderness of a distal extremity with accompanying vasomotor instability.

Blood Dyscrasias. Hyperviscosity syndromes, cold-precipitable plasma proteins, abnormalities of red cell agglutination, and certain myeloproliferative disorders are associated with Raynaud's phenomenon as well as with persistent digital ischemia.

Patients with cold agglutinins occasionally develop Raynaud's phenomenon [157–160]. It is generally thought that Raynaud's phenomenon develops when proteins precipitate or red blood cells agglutinate in the digital vessel during exposure to cold. Prolonged exposure may cause thrombosis and subsequent digital gangrene. Cold agglutinin disease usually involves IgM antibodies that are reactive with I or i antigen [161]. The antibody titer is high at 4°C and low at 37°C. Those antibodies also may cause cold-induced hemolysis. Agglutination usually does not occur in temperatures above 32°C. Cold agglutinins may arise spontaneously or occur in patients with mycoplasma pneumonia, infectious mononucleosis, or lymphoproliferative disorders. Cold agglutinin disease may be short-lived in patients with infectious causes but is often persistent in patients with lymphoproliferative disease.

Cryoglobulins are a group of proteins that precipitate in cold serum and may cause Raynaud's phenomenon. Cryoglobulins are associated with monoclonal and polyclonal gammopathies in disorders such as Waldenström's macroglobulinemia, systemic lupus erythematosus, and rheumatoid arthritis. Cryoglobulinemia has been categorized into three subtypes. Type 1 cryoglobulins include monoclonal immunoglobulins of a single class usually associated with lymphoproliferative disorders, such as multiple myeloma. Type 2 encompasses mixed cryoglobulins containing monoclonal IgM or rheumatoid factor and polyclonal IgG, which may occur in patients with Waldenström's macroglobulinemia or chronic active hepatitis. In patients with Waldenström's macroglobulinemia, about 10 percent of macroglobulins are cryoglobulins [162]. Type 3 cryoglobulinemia includes polyclonal IgM and IgG immunoglobulins, as may occur in systemic lupus erythematosus [163]. Indeed, approximately 80 percent of patients with lupus have cold-insoluble precipitates [164]. In those patients, there is a significantly higher level of cryoprecipitating IgM-class rheumatoid factors than in other patients. Horowitz and co-workers reported that 11 of 20 North African Jews with Raynaud's phenomenon had cryoglobulinemia, and 10 of those 11 had hepatitis-B surface markers, thereby suggesting an association between the two disorders [165, 166].

Cryofibrinogenemia is a rare condition that may be associated with digital vasospasm [167]. The plasma—but not the serum—of patients with cryofibrinogenemia forms a gelatinous precipitate at 4°C. Disorders associated with cryofibrinogenemia include disseminated intravascular coagulation, connective tissue diseases, thromboembolism, and diabetes mellitus [167,168].

Trauma. A variety of traumatic injuries are associated with Raynaud's phenomenon and have been designated **traumatic vasospastic diseases.** Causes of traumatic vasospastic disease include electric shock injury, thermal injuries such as frostbite, and mechanical percussive injury associated with piano playing and typing. The most common traumatic cause of Raynaud's phenomenon is repeated exposure to vibrating tools. Occasionally referred to as vibration white-finger syndrome, it has been reported in lumberjacks and chainsaw users, stonecutters who use air hammers, operators of pneumatic handgrinders and impact wrenches in the engine manufacturing industry, and road drillers [169–172]. The prevalence of Raynaud's phenomenon induced by vibration ranges from 30 to 50 percent among members of populations at risk [172–174]. It has been suggested that the combination of vibration and cold exposure in many of those workers is responsible for the development of Raynaud's phenomenon [175,176].

Pathophysiologic changes may involve both the vascular and neurologic systems in those individuals and may contribute to digital vasospasm. Intimal thickening of peripheral arteries has been reported in animals exposed to repeated vibration, but pathologic changes of the blood vessels have not been demonstrated consistently in humans [177]. Medial muscular hypertrophy and subintimal fibrosis have been found in biopsy specimens of digital arteries of patients in one study but not in others [178,179]. Nail-bed capillaroscopy has shown a reduction in the number of capillaries [180,181]. Arteriograms of patients have shown arterial occlusions of the distal radial and ulnar arteries and frequently of the palmar arch [182].

Neurophysiologic abnormalities have not been consistently demonstrated in patients with Raynaud's phenomenon secondary to vibration. Although some investigators have found a high incidence of abnormal electromyograms, others have found that episodes of Raynaud's phenomenon occur independently of electromyographic abnormalities [183,184]. Peripheral nerve conduction velocities often are abnormal in vibrating-tool operators, and pathologic changes also have been reported in the nerves of patients with vibration white finger, including axonal degeneration, demyelination, and collagenization of perineurium and endoperineurium [185–187]. Thus, the precise pathophysiology of Raynaud's phenomenon in patients repeatedly exposed to vibratory stimuli is unclear. Some have suggested that overexcitation of the Pacinian corpuscles causes reflex efferent sympathetic-nerve activity [188]. Others have suggested that following vibration, cutaneous vessels become more reactive to sympathetic stimuli [189,190].

Another trauma-induced cause of Raynaud's phenomenon is the hypothenar hammer syndrome. Patients develop an ulnar artery thrombosis after hammering with the palms of their hands or practicing karate [191–193]. Raynaud's phenomenon may be unilateral. The most frequently affected fingers are the third, fourth, and fifth. Angiography usually reveals thrombosis and often aneurysmal enlargement of the ulnar artery near the hamate bone. Occlusions of the palmar arch and digital arteries also may occur.

Drugs and Toxins. A variety of drugs have been implicated in producing Raynaud's phenomenon or digital vasospasm (see Table 42-2). Although some of the drugs act by directly causing vasoconstriction, the mechanism whereby others cause Raynaud's phenomenon is not known. Ergot derivatives cause vasospasm, primarily by stimulating alpha adrenoceptors [73,74]. Ergotamine may stimulate serotonergic receptors as well [74]. Vasospasm usually occurs when excessive doses of the drugs have been administered [194]. Spasm may affect digital vessels as well as the coronary, carotid, femoral, and splanchnic arteries [195,196]. Bromocriptine mesylate, an ergot derivative with dopamine agonist activity used to treat Parkinson's disease, hyperprolactinemia, and acromegaly, has been associated with Raynaud's phenomenon. Methysergide, used to treat migraine headaches, is another ergot derivative that has been associated with digital ischemia [197]. The tricyclic antidepressant imipramine and the amphetamines also have been reported to cause arterial spasm [198,199].

Raynaud's phenomenon also has been associated with the use of two chemotherapeutic agents, vinblastine and bleomycin [200–202]. It is not known how these compounds cause Raynaud's phenomenon, although it has been reported that bleomycin causes pathologic changes in small blood vessels [203]. Vinblastine can induce a peripheral neuropathy and perhaps interfere with the autonomic reflexes. Industrial exposure to vinyl chloride polymerization processes may cause acro-osteolysis of the distal phalanges of the fingers, changes that are occasionally associated with Raynaud's phenomenon [204–207].

Beta adrenoceptor–blocking drugs may cause Raynaud's phenomenon. Although the mechanism of action is not known, possibilities include unopposed stimulation of vascular alpha adrenoceptors or reflex sympathetic vasoconstriction initiated by the central cardiovascular depressant effect of beta-adrenergic blockade [208–211]. It remains controversial whether cardioselective beta adrenoceptor–blocking drugs cause Raynaud's phenomenon less frequently than nonselective drugs, and whether there is less digital vasospasm with drugs that also have alpha adrenoceptor–blocking properties or intrinsic sympathetic activity [209–220].

Most studies reporting Raynaud's phenomenon with beta-adrenoceptor blockers involved patients with hyper-

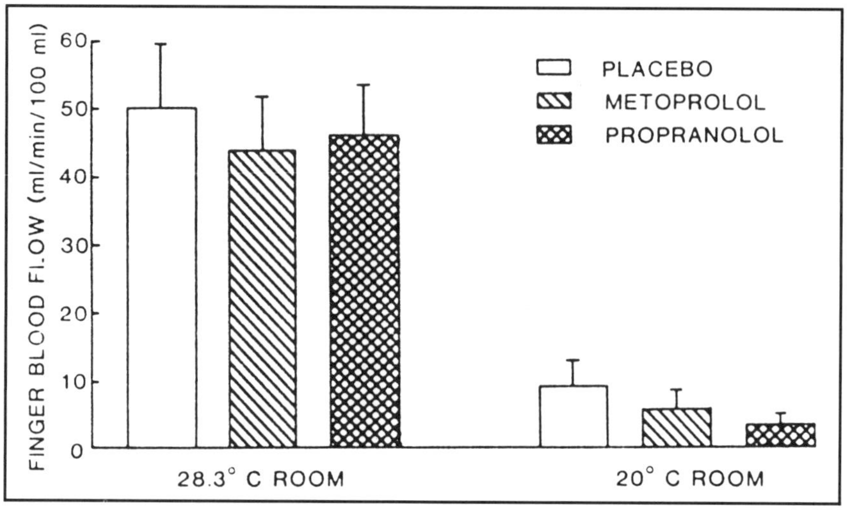

Fig. 42-6. Total finger blood flow in warm and cool environments in 16 patients with Raynaud's phenomenon during treatment with placebo, metoprolol, and propranolol. Data are means ± SEM. There were no significant differences between drug and placebo periods or between the two drug periods in the warm or the cool room. (Reproduced from JD Coffman, HM Rasmussen. Effects of beta-adrenoreceptor-blocking drugs in patients with Raynaud's phenomenon. Circulation 1985; 72:466–470. By permission of the American Heart Association, Inc.)

tension. Digital arterial tone during cooling is greater in hypertensive than normotensive individuals [221]. Also, it has been suggested that hypertension itself may predispose to vasospastic reactions [215]. Vasospastic phenomena have been recorded in nonhypertensive patients treated with beta blockers [210]. One placebo-controlled study recently examined both cardioselective and nonselective beta-adrenoceptor blockers in patients with Raynaud's phenomenon [222]. Compared to placebo, neither metoprolol nor propranolol decreased fingertip blood flow, despite exposure to a cool environment (Fig. 42-6). Furthermore, chronic treatment did not increase the number of vasospastic attacks in patients receiving either drug compared to placebo. One might conclude from those observations that beta adrenoceptor–blocking drugs may cause Raynaud's phenomenon in some individuals, but those drugs do not seem to affect the frequency of vasospastic attacks adversely, nor do they decrease finger blood flow in patients with Raynaud's phenomenon.

Miscellaneous Causes. Hypothyroidism may be associated with Raynaud's phenomenon [223,224]. In such cases, thyroid replacement alleviates the episodes of digital vasospasm. Although the mechanism is not known, peripheral vasoconstriction may occur in hypothyroid patients to conserve heat. Alternatively, thickening of the vascular wall could predispose to vessel closure during normal sympathetic stimuli.

Patients with arteriovenous fistula may develop Raynaud's phenomenon and is particularly prevalent in patients undergoing hemodialysis [225,226]. It may be secondary to decreased blood flow and blood pressure in the digits of the limb with the fistula.

Pulmonary hypertension and Raynaud's phenomenon may occur in the same patients [227–229]. Some of them may have a connective-tissue disorder such as scleroderma. In a study by Fuster and colleagues, approximately 10 percent of women with primary pulmonary hypertension had Raynaud's phenomenon [230]. That frequency is not different from the rate that occurs in the general population. Therefore, it is not clear whether the association of primary pulmonary hypertension and Raynaud's phenomenon is coincidence or related to a common neurohumoral mechanism.

DIAGNOSTIC TESTS

Noninvasive vascular tests can be used to evaluate patients with Raynaud's phenomenon (see Chap. 19), even though determination of digital blood flow or systolic pressure by plethysmographic or radioisotope clearance techniques has limited diagnostic utility (Fig. 42-7; Table 42-3). Many patients with Raynaud's phenomenon have low digital blood flow or low digital systolic pressure, but considerable overlap exists between individuals with and without Raynaud's phenomenon [9,231,232]. The most reliable diagnostic test is the measurement of digital systolic blood pressure during ischemic cooling of a digit while the body is being cooled [78,233–237]. However, it is a difficult, time-consuming procedure and, therefore, not suitable as a routine diagnostic test. The digital systolic blood pressure is measured after the proximal digit is cooled in 5°C decrements from 20°C to 5° C for 5-minute intervals. The finger is made ischemic at each temperature for 5 minutes so that it may cool to the external temperature. The room is cooled to 18°C [237]. Patients with Raynaud's phenomenon have a greater reduction or actually a loss of finger systolic pressure at a higher temperature than normal subjects, although color changes may not occur. Allen et al. [238] reported that they could grade the severity of the Raynaud's phenomenon by using different

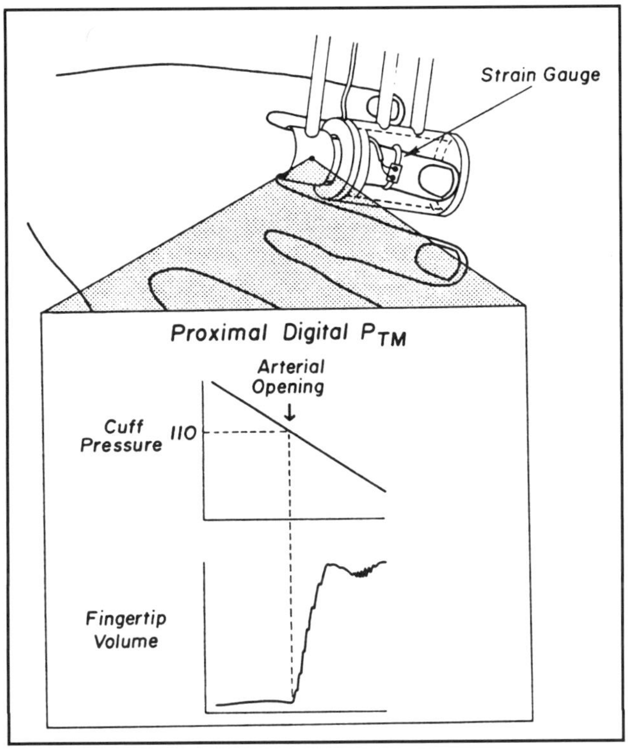

Fig. 42-7. Measurement of the proximal finger systolic blood pressure using a strain gauge to detect the increase in fingertip volume (P_{TM}) as the proximal cuff is slowly deflated from suprasystolic pressure. FIngertip pulsations and the volume increase are not detected until the cuff pressure deflates to 110 mm Hg, the point of digital artery opening. (Reproduced with permission from JD Coffman. Raynaud's Phenomenon. New York: Oxford University Press, 1989.)

finger and room temperatures, with and without arterial occlusion, to study the level at which finger systolic pressure disappeared. Other investigators [239] found that test to be of low sensitivity and incapable of grading the severity of the phenomenon. The test does not differentiate primary from secondary Raynaud's phenomenon.

The pulse volume waveform may distinguish patients with Raynaud's phenomenon who have digital ischemia secondary to vascular occlusive lesions. During local digital heating, the vessel walls become dilated. The pulse waveform usually is normal during warming in patients with Raynaud's phenomenon if obstructive lesions are not present. It may be abnormal if atherosclerosis, thromboangiitis obliterans, or other fixed obstructive digital vascular pathology impairs digital blood flow.

A variety of serologic studies are useful to screen for secondary causes of Raynaud's phenomenon, such as connective tissue disorders or blood dyscrasias. These tests include the erythrocyte sedimentation rate, assays for antinuclear antibody, rheumatoid factor, cryoglobulins and cold agglutinins, and serum protein electrophoresis. Indications for those and other serologic studies usually are suggested by the history and physical examination. Nailfold capillary microscopy may be used to detect the deformed capillary loops and avascular areas typical of connective tissue disorders [137,138] (see Plate 10). Roentgenography of the cervical spine is used to detect cervical ribs.

Table 42-3. Diagnostic tests in Raynaud's phenomenon

Digital hemodynamic measurements
Digital systolic pressure
Digital pulse volume recordings
Digital blood flow
Nailfold capillary microscopy
Serologic studies
Erythrocyte sedimentation rate
Antinuclear antibody
Rheumatoid factor
Cryoglobulins
Serum protein electrophoresis
Radiographic studies
Roentgenogram of cervical spine
Angiography

Note: This is a partial list of tests employed to evaluate patients with Raynaud's phenomenon. Not every test is indicated in each patient. The clinical presentation determines which test is most likely to be useful.

Angiography rarely is indicated, since Raynaud's phenomenon is a diagnosis based primarily on history. Angiography may be indicated, however, in patients with persistent digital ischemia secondary to atherosclerosis, thromboangiitis obliterans, hypothenar hammer syndrome or emboli from a subclavian-artery aneurysm, to plan revascularization procedures (Fig. 42-8).

TREATMENT

Treatment programs must be individualized and designed according to the underlying cause of Raynaud's phenomenon and the severity of the symptoms. Therapy directed specifically at the symptoms of Raynaud's phenomenon can be categorized as follows: (1) conservative measures, (2) pharmacologic intervention, and (3) surgical sympathectomy (Table 42-4). In individuals with well-defined secondary causes of Raynaud's phenomenon, treatment also should be directed specifically at the underlying cause. For example, if a patient has been taking a vasoactive medication, such as an ergot alkaloid, or has been treated with a beta adrenergic–blocking drug for hypertension, removal of the offending agent may reduce or eliminate the Raynaud's phenomenon. Similarly, specific treatment may be directed at other secondary causes, such as arterial occlusive disorders, connective tissue diseases, and blood dyscrasias. The following discussion focuses on treatment designed to palliate Raynaud's phenomenon.

Conservative Measures. Patients with primary Raynaud's phenomenon often benefit from reassurance. An explanation describing the frequency of primary Raynaud's phenomenon in the general population, its precipitating factors, and its benign prognosis is reassuring and allays fears of amputation. Patients should avoid unnecessary cold exposure and should wear loose and warm clothing. In addition to gloves and adequate foot protection, the

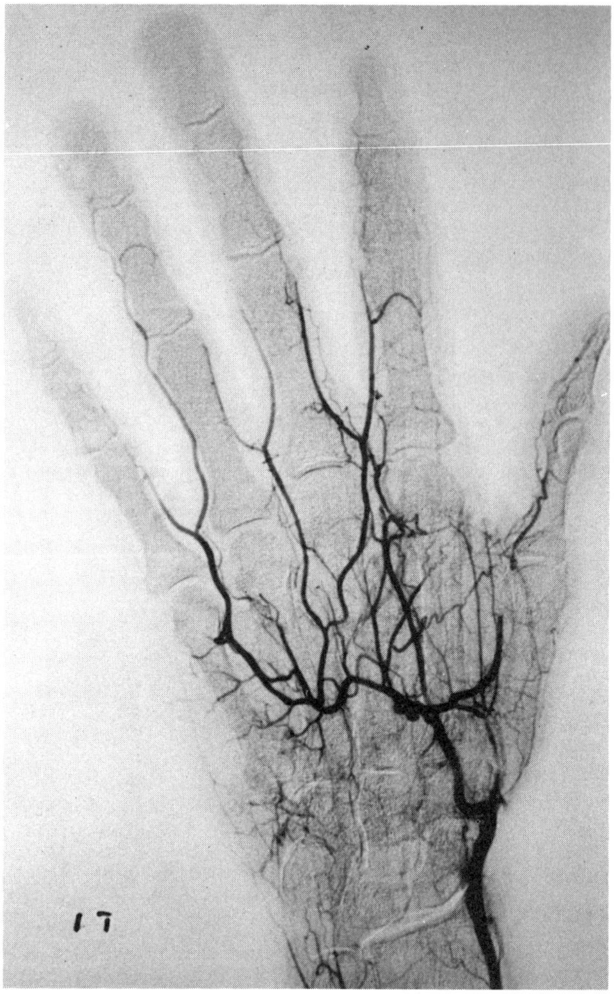

Fig. 42-8. Angiogram from a young woman with persistent digital ischemia. There are multiple areas demonstrating digital vascular occlusion. A blood vessel biopsy was performed to make the diagnosis of necrotizing vasculitis.

Table 42-4. Treatment of Raynaud's phenomenon

Conservative measures
Warm clothing
Avoidance of cold exposure
Abstinence from nicotine
Removal of offending drug (if present)
Behavioral therapy
Pharmacologic interventions
Sympathetic nervous system inhibitors
Reserpine
Prazosin
Guanethidine
Phenoxybenzamine
Yohimbine
Calcium-channel blockers
Nifedipine
Diltiazem
Serotonin antagonists
Ketanserin
Classes of drugs with unproven efficacy
Thromboxane inhibitors
ACE inhibitors
Organic nitrates
Vasodilator prostaglandins
Sympathectomy
Stellate ganglionectomy
Lumbar sympathectomy
Digital sympathectomy

trunk and head should be kept warm to avoid reflex vasoconstriction. Moving to a warmer climate is rarely feasible; furthermore, vasospasm may be induced after a move by even small changes in environmental temperature. Patients should use a moisturizing cream on their digits to prevent drying and cracking. Cigarette smoking should be avoided since nicotine causes cutaneous vasoconstriction [240]. If cold exposure cannot be avoided, chemically heated bags or electrically heated gloves and socks that operate by battery pack can be used.

Since the sympathetic nervous system mediates the vasoconstrictor response to cold and emotional distress, behavioral therapy has been proposed as a nonpharmacologic and nonsurgical means of ameliorating the symptoms of Raynaud's phenomenon. Studies have been reported both supporting and refuting the efficacy of biofeedback training in this disorder [241–247]. The techniques used for biofeedback training in most of these studies were different. Furthermore, objective means of assessing responses varied from determination of digital temperature during cold exposure to queries regarding symptomatic improvement. Several uncontrolled studies indicated that following biofeedback training, patients were able to increase digital temperature and possibly decrease the frequency of vasospastic attacks [241–245]. Patients usually were trained to increase their digital temperature during either local or environmental cold exposure. In one controlled study, there was no significant effect of biofeedback training on the frequency of Raynaud's phenomenon [246]. Another form of behavioral therapy, Pavlovian conditioning, has been shown to increase digital temperature during cold exposure [248]. Though behavioral therapy may be effective in some individuals, there are insufficient data to support its routine use for patients with Raynaud's phenomenon.

Pharmacologic Intervention. Two classes of drugs are effective for treatment of Raynaud's phenomenon: calcium channel blockers and sympathetic nervous system inhibitors. Other classes of drugs for which efficacy has not been firmly established include serotonin antagonists, ACE inhibitors, and direct-acting smooth muscle relaxants, such as nitrates and vasodilator prostaglandins.

CALCIUM CHANNEL BLOCKERS. Several calcium channel blocking drugs are effective in patients with Raynaud's phenomenon. Most of the evidence accumulated to date involves nifedipine, which interferes with vascular smooth muscle contraction by antagonizing calcium influx [249–250]. This drug decreases digital vascular resistance in patients with Raynaud's phenomenon during environmental cold exposure and increases digital systolic blood pressure and digital skin temperature during local cold exposure [251,252]. In multiple placebo-controlled trials, nifedipine decreased the frequency and severity of Raynaud's phenomenon [253–256]. Although nifedipine is not effective in all patients, symptoms improve in at least 50 percent of individuals. Furthermore, benefit occurs in patients with primary Raynaud's phenomenon, including children, as well as those with Raynaud's phenomenon secondary to other disorders such as scleroderma [257,258]. The starting dose of nifedipine is 10 mg orally tid. The usual effective dose is 20 mg orally tid. Side effects include hypotension, lightheadedness, indigestion, and peripheral edema. The extended-release forms of nifedipine may produce fewer side effects and be as effective as the short-acting preparation.

Less information is available about the other calcium channel–blocking drugs. Diltiazem, however, has been reported in several studies to improve symptoms of Raynaud's phenomenon [259,260]. One preliminary report also indicated that it was effective in patients with Raynaud's phenomenon secondary to vibration injury [261]. Reports on the therapeutic benefit of nicardipine have been contradictory; the largest study of 65 patients with primary Raynaud's phenomenon showed a small decrease in the frequency but not the severity of attacks [262]. Felodipine has been reported as beneficial [263,264]; in one study, it was of comparable benefit to nifedipine. Leppert et al., reported that isradipine improved 10 patients with primary Raynaud's phenomenon by subjective and objective criteria and there were fewer side effects than with nifedipine [265]. However, that was a single-blind study. Verapamil has not been shown to be effective in patients with Raynaud's phenomenon. Verapamil decreased the frequency of Raynaud's phenomenon in only 1 of 16 patients with scleroderma in one series [266].

INHIBITORS OF THE SYMPATHETIC NERVOUS SYSTEM. The vasoconstrictor response to cold exposure or emotional stress is mediated via the sympathetic nervous system. Sympathetic nervous system inhibitors that have been used to treat Raynaud's phenomenon include reserpine, prazosin, guanethidine, phenoxybenzamine, methyldopa, and tolazoline. Reserpine is an alkaloid isolated from *Rauwolfia serpentina* that depletes norepinephrine from nerve terminals and may have a brief direct vasodilator action [267]. Reserpine increases fingertip capillary blood flow in patients exposed to a cold environment [9] (Fig. 42-9). Furthermore, the vasoconstrictor responses to the application of ice to the forehead and to intra-arterial tyramine, a drug that releases norepinephrine from adrenergic-nerve terminals, are reduced following reserpine [6]. Improvement in Raynaud's phenomenon has been reported following administration of reserpine when given in doses of 0.25 to 0.50 mg [6,9,268]. Not all patients, however, achieve long-term benefit from this medication, and its use is associated with side effects that include nasal congestion, nausea, lethargy, depression, and peptic ulceration. Intra-arterial administration of reserpine has been advocated by some investigators to promote healing of digital ulcerations, but that benefit has not been confirmed by others [269–270].

Prazosin hydrochloride is an alpha$_1$-adrenoceptor blocker. Since postsynaptic alpha$_1$ adrenoceptors are found on digital vessels, clinical improvement following administration of this drug might be anticipated. However, one study reported only modest increases in digital blood flow during intra-arterial infusion of prazosin [23]. Uncontrolled observations have suggested that prazosin is effective in approximately 50 percent of patients with Raynaud's phenomenon [271]. A placebo-controlled double-blind study in a small number of patients suggested that prazosin in doses ranging from 1–4 mg bid reduced the frequency of Raynaud's phenomenon [272]. Tachyphylaxis may occur with prazosin, often necessitating dosage increments up to 10 mg tid. Side effects of prazosin include hypotension, particularly after the first dose, leading to lightheadedness or syncope. In addition, patients may develop headache, drowsiness, or fatigue. It is likely, though not proven, that longer-acting preparations, such as terazosin and doxazosin, would have actions similar to prazosin.

Guanethidine, like reserpine, decreases norepinephrine release from nerve terminals. In one study, guanethidine increased fingertip capillary blood flow in patients with Raynaud's phenomenon secondary to scleroderma [273]. Long-term studies that assess symptomatic responses are lacking. The dosage of guanethidine is 30–50 mg orally each day. Its utility is significantly limited because of important adverse effects, particularly orthostatic hypotension. Methyldopa is a central adrenergic antagonist that interferes with the formation of dihydroxyphenylethylamine, a precursor of norepinephrine, and inhibits the conversion of 5-hydroxytryptophane to serotonin. Although one group of investigators suggested that methyldopa was beneficial in Raynaud's phenomenon, no controlled studies attest to its efficacy [274]. Side effects include postural hypotension, lethargy, and impotence. In addition, it may cause fever, hemolytic anemia, and hepatic dysfunction. Tolazoline is an alpha adrenergic–blocking drug that causes cutaneous vasodilation. In doses of 75–100 mg orally, it improves skin blood flow in vasoconstricted normal subjects [275]. The efficacy of tolazoline in Raynaud's phenomenon has not been established in well-controlled studies. Furthermore, it is no longer marketed in the United States. Phenoxybenzamine is another adrenergic-blocking drug. Several uncontrolled studies have reported favorable results with this drug in patients with Raynaud's phenomenon [276]. The suggested dosage of phenoxybenzamine is 10–30 mg once daily. Side effects include postural hypotension, lightheadedness, edema, and ejaculatory dysfunction.

SEROTONIN ANTAGONISTS. Serotonin, as discussed earlier, may be pertinent to the pathophysiology of Raynaud's phenomenon. For that reason, ketanserin, a serotonin (5-HT$_2$) receptor antagonist with some alpha adrenoceptor–blocking activity, has been evaluated in patients with Raynaud's phenomenon. When given to normal subjects, ketanserin attenuates the digital vasoconstrictor response to local cold exposure [49]. When administered intravenously to patients with Raynaud's phenomenon, ketanserin increased digital blood flow in some studies but not in others [44,45,50]. The results of trials that assess the

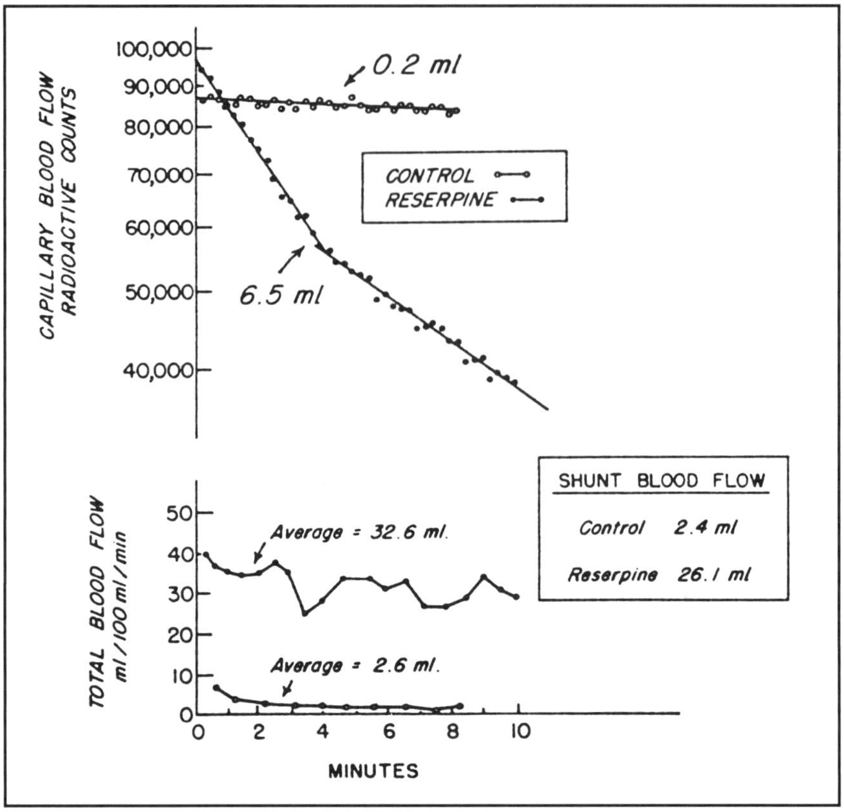

Fig. 42-9. Fingertip total, AV shunt, and capillary flow in a 20°C room before and during reserpine treatment. Shunt flow is calculated from total flow minus capillary flow. During reserpine treatment, total capillary and shunt flow also increased. (Reproduced from JD Coffman, AS Cohen. Total and capillary fingertip blood flow in Raynaud's phenomenon. N Engl J Med 1971; 285:259. By permission of N Engl J Med.)

effect of chronic oral therapy have been conflicting; improvement in symptoms was observed in some but not in others [44,45,50–53,277]. A large placebo-controlled trial involved 222 patients, 50 percent of whom had primary Raynaud's phenomenon and the rest of whom had Raynaud's phenomenon secondary to connective-tissue disorders [43]. Ketanserin decreased the frequency but not the duration or the severity of digital vasospastic attacks (Fig. 42-10). Digital blood flow measurements were obtained in a subgroup of that study population. Despite symptomatic improvement, there was no evidence that ketanserin improved digital blood flow during exposure to either a warm or a cool environment.

THROMBOXANE INHIBITORS. Thromboxane A_2 causes platelet aggregation and vasoconstriction and conceivably could contribute to digital vasospasm in some patients with Raynaud's phenomenon. Dazoxiben is a thromboxane-synthetase inhibitor that attenuates the forearm vasoconstrictor response to cold in normal subjects [57]. Dazoxiben decreases thromboxane A_2 levels and improves symptoms in some patients with Raynaud's phenomenon [278,279]. However, several placebo-controlled trials have failed to show that this drug reduces symptoms [55,56]. Furthermore, a combination of a thromboxane-receptor antagonist and a thromboxane-synthase inhibitor did not affect the response of patients with Raynaud's phenomenon to a cold challenge [38].

INHIBITION OF THE RENIN-ANGIOTENSIN SYSTEM. It is very unlikely that angiotensin II mediates digital vasospasm in most patients with Raynaud's phenomenon. If this hormone is elevated due to other pathologic conditions, it conceivably could contribute to digital vasospasm in patients already predisposed to Raynaud's phenomenon. One such population is patients with systemic sclerosis and malignant hypertension. One report described two patients with systemic sclerosis, malignant hypertension, renal failure, and digital ischemia who were treated with the ACE inhibitor captopril. Hypertension, renal insufficiency, and digital ischemia all improved following drug administration [64]. However, Tosi and co-workers reported that captopril decreased vasospastic attacks in patients with primary Raynaud's phenomenon but not in patients with Raynaud's phenomenon secondary to scleroderma [62]. Other uncontrolled studies have suggested that captopril reduces symptoms in primary Raynaud's phenomenon [61,63].

DIRECT VASCULAR SMOOTH MUSCLE RELAXANTS. The problem with most vasodilators is that they cause a general reduction in vascular resistance and may actually divert blood flow from the affected digits. As a result, patients

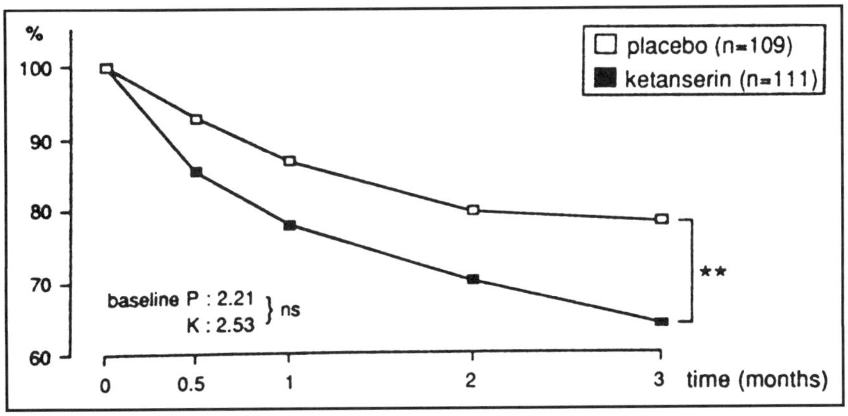

Fig. 42-10. Frequency of vasospastic episodes during ketanserin (K) and placebo (P) treatment in patients with Raynaud's phenomenon. On the ordinate axis is the percent reduction of frequency of vasospastic episodes from baseline. The 34% reduction in episodes with ketanserin therapy is significantly greater than the 18% decrease with placebo therapy (**$p < 0.011$). (Reproduced with permission from JD Coffman et al. International study of ketanserin in Raynaud's phenomenon. Am J Med 1989; 87:264.)

often experience adverse side effects, including hypotension, without deriving any benefit for the Raynaud's phenomenon.

Organic nitrate preparations have received some attention in patients with Raynaud's phenomenon. These agents are effective in coronary vasospastic disorders. Ammunition workers exposed to nitroglycerin may experience Raynaud's phenomenon during periods of nitrate withdrawal [280]. One study reported that topical glyceryl trinitrate is an effective adjunctive therapy for patients with primary Raynaud's phenomenon [281]. Nitroprusside has been used in the treatment of severe vasospasm caused by ergotism [282,283]. There is no other convincing evidence that chronic treatment with nitrate preparations ameliorates Raynaud's phenomenon.

Several uncontrolled studies have suggested that intravenous infusion of prostaglandin E_1 promotes healing of digital ulcers in patients with scleroderma [284,285]. In a placebo-controlled, multicenter study, however, intravenous PGE_1 was no more effective than placebo in reducing symptoms of Raynaud's phenomenon or healing digital ulcers [286]. Several placebo-controlled studies, however, have reported long-term benefit in the treatment of severe Raynaud's phenomenon with intravenous iloprost, a prostacyclin analogue, for 3 to 5 days, or with prostacyclin for 3 weeks [287–290]. There were significant decreases in the frequency, duration, and severity of vasospastic attacks and increases in indices of finger blood flow for up to 9 weeks. In one study [291] comparing intravenous iloprost with oral nifedipine, both drugs were of benefit subjectively, while parameters of finger blood flow were increased only with iloprost. In a recent study, oral iloprost or placebo was administered for 10 days [292]. Two weeks after drug cessation, there was a trend toward shorter and less severe vasospastic attacks in the iloprost group, but this did not achieve statistical significance. Side effects of iloprost depend on the dosage and include headaches, flushing, nausea, and vomiting. If an effective oral prostacyclin analogue is developed, it may be of value in the therapeutic armamentarium for Raynaud's phenomenon.

TRIIODOTHYROXINE. When patients did not respond to reserpine, Peacock added 20 μg of triiodothyroxine as a second drug to increase the patient's heat production [268]. Only 5 of 33 patients had no response to that regimen. Dessein et al. treated 18 patients with secondary Raynaud's phenomenon with 60–80 μg of triiodothyroxine daily [293]. In that double-blind, placebo-controlled, crossover trial, the active drug decreased the frequency, duration, and severity of vasospastic attacks compared to placebo. Skin temperatures and skin-temperature-recovery times after cold exposure improved. However, one-third of patients had episodic palpitations. Significant increases in pulse rate and pulse pressure also occurred. The adverse consequences of hyperthyroidism should preclude triiodothyroxine as a treatment alternative for patients with Raynaud's phenomenon.

Sympathectomy. The preganglionic sympathetic innervation of the upper limbs arises in the T1 to T10 segments of the spinal cord. These preganglionic fibers traverse anterior nerve roots and synapse in the middle cervical, stellate, and second thoracic ganglia. Postganglionic fibers travel in the branchial plexus and are distributed to the upper extremity. Sympathectomy of the upper extremities often is performed via a transaxillary or anterior approach and includes resection of the lower half of the stellate ganglion [294]. The upper half of the stellate ganglion is preserved to prevent the development of Horner's syndrome. Sympathetic innervation in the lower limbs originates from segments T10 to L2 of the spinal cord. Those fibers pass via anterior nerve roots and synapses in ganglia opposite to nerve roots of the femoral, obturator, and sciatic nerves, where they are distributed to the lower extremities. Sympathectomy of the lower limb is achieved by excision of the second and third lumbar ganglia [295–299].

The success rate of sympathectomy for episodic digital vasospasm of the upper extremities is not as good as might be anticipated. Raynaud's phenomenon recurs in approximately 50 percent of patients [300,301]. Successful relief of digital ischemia is less in patients with secondary forms of Raynaud's phenomenon than in patients with primary Raynaud's phenomenon [297–301]. In contrast, the majority of patients experience improvement in symptoms in their lower extremities following lumbar sympathectomy [299,301]. Possibly, lumbar sympathectomy is more complete than thoracodorsal sympathectomy, in which residual sympathetic pathways may develop following surgery.

Digital sympathectomy and radical microarteriolysis have been advocated by some surgeons for treatment of digital ischemia, particularly that secondary to severe Raynaud's phenomenon. Results indicate that these techniques may improve digital blood flow and allow healing of digital ulcerations [301–304].

Acrocyanosis

Acrocyanosis is a condition, first described by Crocq in 1896, in which there is persistent bluish discoloration of the digits of the hands, and less frequently, the feet [305]. This disorder has conventionally been distinguished from Raynaud's phenomenon on the basis of persistent rather than episodic discoloration, relative absence of blanching, and proximal extension beyond the digits to involve the hands or feet and even the wrists or ankles [306,307]. Occasionally, the elbows, knees, nose, cheeks, forehead, or earlobes may be affected. Though the vasospasm of acrocyanosis is persistent rather than episodic, cyanosis may intensify during cold exposure, and rubor may appear on warming. The incidence of acrocyanosis has not been studied. There is no gender predominance. It affects men and women, usually between the ages of 20 and 45 years.

CLINICAL PRESENTATION

The examination is noteworthy for peripheral cyanosis involving the digits and occasionally the hands and feet (Plate 11). The condition must be distinguished from central cyanosis, in which the sublingual mucosa also appear blue. Classically, cyanosis lessens or acral pallor occurs with limb elevation, and with dependency discoloration becomes more ruborous [305–307]. The involved areas are cool and often hyperhidrotic. The digits may appear puffy, but sclerodactyly does not occur. Occasionally, there may be decreased sensation in the digits. Trophic changes usually do not occur, and digital ulcerations are rare. Patients have normal peripheral pulses. Decreased arterial oxygen saturation indicates cardiac or pulmonary disease and is not a feature of idiopathic acrocyanosis.

PATHOPHYSIOLOGY

It has been proposed that vasospasm occurs in the small cutaneous arteries and arterioles, causing compensatory dilation of the capillaries and subpapillary venules. Decreased blood flow would result in increased oxygen extraction in the involved tissue, producing cyanosis. In 1930, Lewis and Landis [306] suggested a "local fault" in the small vessels of the extremities that were excessively sensitive to cold. They surmised that there was no venous obstruction since limb elevation produced pallor of the cyanotic extremity, and the pallor induced by pressure disappeared spontaneously. With body heating, the temperature of the fingers reached that of the forehead, and reactive hyperemia of the fingers was normal. Ulnar nerve block relieved the cyanosis of the fifth finger, and vasoconstrictor agents produced a normal response in acrocyanotic hands. That indirect evidence for arteriolar vasospasm was confirmed by the studies of Mendlowitz [308], Eliot and co-workers [309], and Lambie and Morson [310]. Peacock [311,312] reported that his patients with acrocyanosis had hand blood flow in the normal range during local warming to 42°C but low hand blood flow and skin temperature at 32°C. Evidence for an abnormal vasomotor response of central origin and against a local sensitivity of the blood vessels to cold was presented by Day and Klingman [313]. They described a young girl whose intensely cyanotic hands and forearms became warm and red during sleep, with a rise in finger and hand temperature. Cooling and cyanosis occurred on awakening. During barbiturate-induced sleep, the hand responded in a similar manner as the rest of the body to cold and heat exposures. Thus, most studies support either a local or central abnormality causing peripheral arteriolar vasoconstriction and are incompatible with a structural vascular lesion.

In patients with acrocyanosis, there are abnormalities in nailfold capillary loops and in capillary blood flow. Whether those changes are primary or secondary is not known. Jacobs and co-workers [314] described a decreased number of capillaries and larger capillary loops in patients with acrocyanosis compared with normal subjects and patients with primary Raynaud's phenomenon. According to Bollinger et al. [315], capillary blood flow is not homogenous; some capillaries show intermittent blood flow but are adjacent to capillaries with continuous flow. Delayed and asynchronous arrival of fluorescein sodium in different capillaries supports that finding [316].

PATHOLOGY

There are few histologic studies of acrocyanosis, but minimal hypertrophy of the media of cutaneous arterioles, local edema, fibrosis of skin, and dilation of the superficial capillaries has been reported [317,318]. Capillary elongation and widening also has been described [314].

The overall prognosis is good in that loss of digital tissue is uncommon in patients with the idiopathic disorder. Patients are advised not only to wear gloves but to dress warmly to avoid reflex sympathetic vasoconstriction during body cooling. Pharmacologic intervention usually is not necessary, but adrenergic-blocking drugs, such as reserpine or prazosin, may be tried. Calcium channel blockers, such as nifedipine, have not been tested in acrocyanosis.

Livedo Reticularis

Livedo reticularis is a mottled discoloration of the skin in a reticular, fishnet, or lacelike pattern, with primary and secondary forms. The primary form may be a benign skin finding or occur with ulcerations. The secondary form results from an underlying disease or drug treatment. Benign livedo reticularis also has been called cutis marmorata [319], idiopathic livedo reticularis, sympathetic livedo reticularis, livedo racemosa, livedo annularis, and asphyxia reticularis. Livedo reticularis with ulceration has been termed atrophie blanche en plaque [320], livedo vasculitis, and livedoid vasculitis.

Benign livedo reticularis is more frequent in women than men. The age of onset is approximately 20 to 40 years. One study reported that 30 percent of cases were associated with hypertension, and that 50 percent of patients exhibited "nervous instability" [321]. It may occur in patients who have Raynaud's phenomenon. Livedo reticularis with ulceration is rare and also more common in women [322]. The age of onset is usually 20 to 45 years of age but has been reported in patients from 9 to 80 years of age. It probably is due to a vasculitis or thrombosis of small blood vessels.

Secondary livedo reticularis may occur as a consequence of atheromatous emboli, polyarteritis nodosa, systemic lupus erythematosus, other vasculitides, hyperviscosity syndromes, cryoglobulinemia, infections, thrombocythemia, endocrine disorders, and neurogenic diseases. Anticardiolipin antibodies may be detected in patients with systemic lupus erythematosus and livedo reticularis [323,324]. Sneddon described a syndrome of livedo reticularis with cerebrovascular lesions causing transient ischemic attacks or stroke [325]. Cerebral angiograms have shown thromboses or no disease [326]. In that syndrome, anticardiolipin antibodies are not present. Amantadine hydrochloride, a drug used in patients with Parkinson's disease, also causes livedo reticularis (see below).

PATHOPHYSIOLOGY

The pathophysiology of livedo reticularis is not well established. The benign form probably is caused by vasospasm of the small perpendicular arterioles that perforate the deeper layers of skin [2,104,319]. Decreased blood flow in the distal, horizontally arranged venous plexi leads to oxygen desaturation and cyanosis, which causes the red to blue periphery of each web of the net. The color pattern is attenuated with warming, implicating increased sympathetic nervous system activity as a cause of the vasospasm. Also, livedo reticularis often is associated with Raynaud's phenomenon, and sympathetic blocking agents can reverse the color change. Increased sympathetic nervous activity also may be the mechanism whereby amantadine causes livedo reticularis. That drug releases norepinephrine from central- and peripheral-nerve terminals, inhibits the reuptake of dopamine and norepinephrine, and reduces limb blood flow and skin temperature [327,328].

There are two postulated causes of livedo reticularis with ulceration: vasculitis [322] and thromboses of arterioles [329]. IgM and FgA deposits, complement factors, and fibrin have been demonstrated in vessel walls, findings consistent with an immune complex pathogenesis [322]. Reports of decreased fibrinolytic activity [329] and abnormalities of platelet aggregation [330,331] support a thrombotic diathesis leading to occlusion of dermal vessels.

PATHOLOGY

In the benign form of livedo reticularis, skin biopsies are nonspecific or show an increased number of dilated capillaries [321]. In livedo reticularis with ulceration, a subsegmental hyalinizing vasculitis affecting the vessels of the middle dermis occurs [321,326,332–334]. There is hyaline degeneration of the vessels and focal thrombosis of arterioles. The vessel walls are thickened and occasionally surrounded by lymphocytes. New-vessel proliferation and hemorrhage may occur. Papillary and deeper dermal vessels may be affected.

CLINICAL PRESENTATION

Benign livedo reticularis is a common and mild condition consisting often of no more than a cosmetic blemish. The webs of the fishnet are a rose, red, violet, or blue color with normal or pale skin in the center. Usually the skin over the extremities is affected; occasionally, the trunk is involved. The skin may be cool; numbness and pain are rare [321]. The discoloration intensifies with cold exposure and often resolves completely with rewarming. Physical examination is otherwise unremarkable, and laboratory studies are normal.

Livedo reticularis with ulceration typically has a more widespread body distribution. Discoloration is persistent, yet may intensify following cold exposure. Rewarming is less effective than in the benign form. Purpuric macular lesions and cutaneous nodules appear and progress to ulcers, bordered by inflammation and often covered with eschars. Ulcers are most common during the winter, but some patients develop them during summer [333]. They usually occur on the lower parts of the legs and on the feet. The ulcers are painful and usually take months to heal. Following healing, ulcers leave a smooth ivory-white plaque of atrophic skin surrounded by telangiectatic blood vessels and hyperpigmented borders. The healed ulcers have been termed **atrophie blanche en plaque.** Edema of the legs also may be present, often before ulceration develops. Except for skin lesions, the physical examination is normal, as are laboratory tests.

In secondary livedo reticularis, there may or may not be ulcers. Symptoms, signs, and laboratory studies reflect the underlying disease. Amantadine hydrochloride causes a benign form, primarily affecting the legs, and is often accompanied by pedal edema. The skin manifestations usually disappear 2 to 6 weeks following drug cessation [335]. Atheromatous debris and cholesterol crystals originating in lesions of proximal vessels may embolize distally to occlude small arteries in the muscle and skin of the extremities. Pain, cyanosis, petechiae, localized erythematous plaques in the skin, muscle tenderness, and reticular discoloration typical of livedo reticularis occur [336].

TREATMENT

The benign type of livedo reticularis usually needs no treatment. Dressing warmly and avoiding cold exposure may decrease the discoloration. Small doses of reserpine (0.125–0.250 mg daily) may lessen the lacelike pattern.

Saline soaks and analgesic ointments are used to treat ulcers associated with livedo reticularis. The ulcers usually are unresponsive to other forms of treatment. Antiplatelet and fibrinolysis-promoting agents have been used, but not all patients benefit, and controlled studies are not available [330,331,337,338]. Vasodilator drugs and a variety of other agents have been tried [2,322,339]. Sympathectomy is not beneficial [321].

Pernio (Chilblains)

Pernio is a vasculitic disorder associated with cold exposure. Acute and chronic forms of pernio have been described. The term pernio is usually given to the acute form, in which raised red to blue lesions develop on the lower parts of the legs, frequently the shins, following cold exposure (Plate 12). The lesions often are associated with a pruritic and burning sensation and may blister and ulcerate. They resolve in 7 to 10 days, frequently leaving a residual pigmented area [340]. Pernio affects young women more commonly than men; it first occurs between the ages of 15 and 30. It is much more common in the United Kingdom than in the United States.

Chronic pernio is designated **chilblains** and typically presents as raised erythematous patches, ranging in size from 2 to 10 mm that develop on the lower extremity in an area that has been repeatedly exposed to cold. Thus, it may occur more frequently in women who wear skirts, leaving their legs unprotected. Multiple lesions usually develop at one time. Lesions akin to those seen in acute pernio gradually blister and ulcerate and often are painful. The base of the blister may appear blue, violet, or hemorrhagic. Areas of scarring and pigmentation usually remain after the ulcers heal.

The pathologic features of both pernio and chilblains are principally those of a vasculitis characterized by intimal proliferation and perivascular infiltration of mononuclear and polymorphonuclear leukocytes. Giant cells may be present in the subcutaneous tissue.

Treatment focuses on avoidance of cold exposure. Patients should dress warmly, and the limbs should be covered. Some have suggested that patients move to a warmer climate [340]. Although the disorder is related to environmental cold, there seems to be little contribution of the sympathetic nervous system. Therefore, sympathetic blocking drugs and sympathectomy usually are not effective. One blinded placebo-controlled study reported that nifedipine (20–60 mg daily) reduced the time to resolution of existing lesions and prevented the development of new lesions [341].

Immersion Foot (Trench Foot)

Immersion foot is due to prolonged exposure of the extremities to water. Immobility, constricting garments, body chilling, dehydration, trauma, or exhaustion also may contribute to the condition. Immersion foot has been common in shipwrecks and in most wars [342]. It is now being seen in homeless men and women [343]. The clinical presentation depends on whether the exposure is to cold or warm water (15–32°C). The combination of wetness and cold temperature produces the most serious syndrome and occurs in trench warfare or in persons rescued from the sea [342]. Warm-water immersion foot usually is a more benign condition; however, a more severe type has been described and termed tropical immersion foot or paddyfield foot [344,345].

PATHOPHYSIOLOGY AND PATHOLOGY

In cold-water immersion foot, there is a decreased blood flow due to vasoconstriction [342]. Cellular damage from local hypoxia leads to tissue necrosis and capillary-wall injury. Plasma leaks into the interstitial tissue, causing tense edema. Increased viscosity of the blood leads to stasis and occlusion of small blood vessels. There also may be Wallerian degeneration of the nerves. In the late stages of cold immersion foot, the pathologic picture includes vascular occlusions, desquamation of skin, deep fibrosis, and superficial gangrene. Fibrosis of blood vessel walls occurs, and nerves may be embedded in fibrous tissue scars.

Warm-water immersion foot probably is due to swelling of the stratum corneum with water and abrasion from footwear [345]. The thick skin on the soles of the feet has a greater susceptibility than thin skin. Typically, warm-water immersion foot includes only hyperhydration of the plantar stratum corneum. In the more severe tropical type, however, lymphocytic infiltration, diapedesis of red blood cells, and swelling and proliferation of the capillary endothelium in the dermis are seen. Tropical immersion foot may be caused by water entering the dermis of the skin. *Pseudomonas aeruginosa* is often cultured from the involved area, but its role in the disease is unknown [343].

CLINICAL PRESENTATION

Cold-water immersion foot is characterized by cold, numb feet with a stocking distribution of hypesthesia or anesthesia [342]. Pulses often are absent. As soon as the footwear is removed, edema, paresthesias, itching, and severe pain occur. The skin then becomes mottled yellow, blue, or black, and discoloration can last a few hours to days. Thereafter, a hyperemic phase occurs, with red, hot, dry feet, burning paresthesias, and shooting pains. Pulses become bounding and edema with blisters may occur. In severe cases, superficial gangrene and ulcerations may develop. The necrotic skin exfoliates, leaving healthy skin beneath. Depending on the severity of the injury, the hyperemic stage may last 1 to 10 weeks. The posthyperemic stage is characterized by a return of normal skin color and temperature. Some patients have late sequelae of cold sensitivity, hyperhidrosis, paresthesias, contracted toes, or even painful ulcers.

Warm-water immersion foot is characterized by very painful, tender feet with convoluted, white skin on the plantar surfaces; maceration of tissue may occur [345] (Fig. 42-11). In the more severe cases, there is redness and edema of the ankles and dorsal aspects of the feet [344]. Even without infection, fever and inguinal lymphadenopathy may occur. Diffuse ecchymoses, small blisters, and a maculopapular rash may be seen in the healing phase.

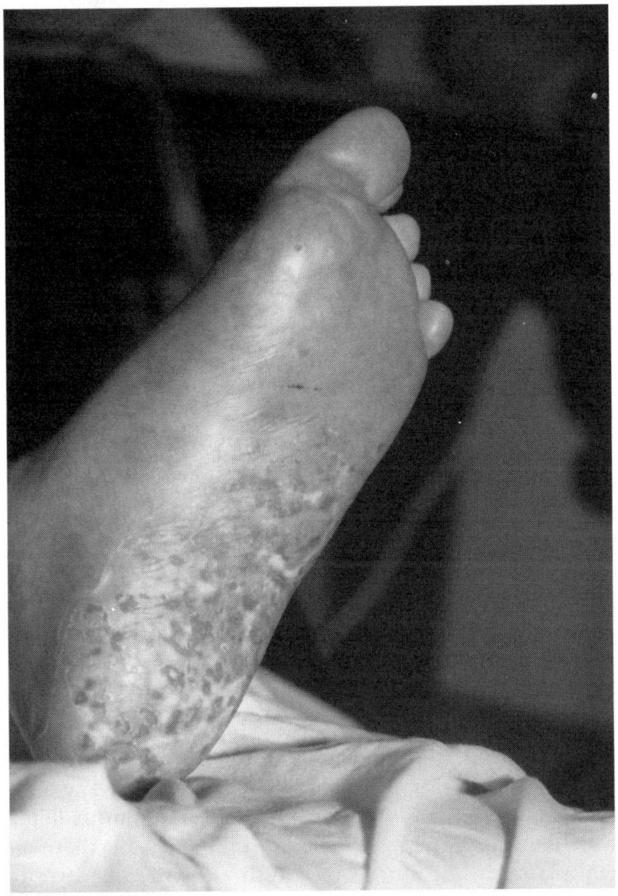

Fig. 42-11. Immersion foot. This patient with erythromelalgia (see also Plate 13) developed immersion feet because she chronically soaked her feet in a basin of water. Note the blistering and macerated tissue.

TREATMENT

The treatment of cold-water immersion foot in the prehyperemic phase comprises bed rest and body, but not local, warming. The limb should be kept at heart level until pulses are present and then elevated to prevent edema. During the hyperemic phase, air cooling of the foot may help control pain and edema. Affected tissues should be cleansed gently only if necessary; no tissue should be removed. Analgesics may be necessary. Antibiotics have not been proved efficacious, even when fever or lymphadenopathy is present. Ambulation is allowed when edema does not occur on dependency. Treatment may be necessary for several weeks. Sympathectomy may help the late sequelae of chronic painful ulcers, hyperhidrosis, or persistent vasospasm during cold exposure [346].

The treatment of warm-water immersion foot is bed rest with elevation of the limb above heart level. The foot should be kept dry by exposure to room temperature. Massage is contraindicated. Nonsteroid anti-inflammatory drugs or narcotics may be needed for pain relief. Treatment is continued until edema and pain subside. Symptoms and signs usually abate in 1 to 7 days.

Drying of the feet overnight is the only method to prevent immersion foot. Silicone grease has protective effects [347]. Frequent rest periods and several changes of clothes and boots during exposure may help.

Frostbite

Frostbite is defined as tissue damage resulting from severe cold exposure [348]. Freezing of tissues may injure skin, muscle, blood vessels, and nerves. Usually, injury is restricted to the extremities or parts of the face, such as the nose, chin, cheeks, and ears. Exposure to temperatures below 20°F (−6.5°C) can cause frostbite. The severity of injury is related to the intensity and the duration of cold exposure. Frostbite occurs more quickly and at higher temperatures when individuals are also exposed to high winds, dampness, altitude, or hypoxia. Additional predisposing factors include poor conditioning, inadequate protective clothing, fatigue, and malnutrition. Frostbite also may result from direct contact with a very cold object. Touching a cold metal object with wet hands "cements" the skin to the metal and quickly freezes the underlying tissue. Frostbite is most likely to occur in extremities already affected by arterial occlusive disease, Raynaud's phenomenon, or previous cold injury.

PATHOPHYSIOLOGY AND PATHOLOGY

The pathophysiology of frostbite involves direct damage to the tissue as a consequence of freezing as well as decreased blood flow resulting from vasoconstriction [349]. As discussed previously, vasoconstriction may be a direct response to local cold exposure or a reflex response to environmental cooling. Freezing may cause extracellular formation of ice crystals leading to intracellular loss of water and cellular damage. The process is exacerbated by the reduced blood supply caused by vasoconstriction and formation of arterial thrombi. Injury to the capillary walls may increase permeability and cause edema.

Depending on the extent of damage, frostbite can be categorized as superficial or deep. Superficial frostbite involves the skin and immediately subjacent tissue. The pathology depends on the severity of the frostbite. The endothelial cells, especially of the arterioles, show the first sign of injury in animal models [350]. Initially, there is an inflammatory response in the affected tissue as well as low-grade vasculitis [349]. The skin may become keratinized. Necrosis is evident in muscle, and neuronal degeneration occurs. Thrombi are seen in arterioles and capillaries. Deep frostbite extends beneath the subcutaneous tissue to involve muscle, deep blood vessels, and nerves.

CLINICAL PRESENTATION

The patient may note pain or numbness at the site of injury. The skin appears white or sallow and somewhat "waxy." With rewarming, there is local cyanosis or erythema, possibly wheal and flare formation, and edema [348]. Superficial blisters appear in 1 to 2 days. Within several weeks, superficial necrosis occurs. Gradually, the edema resolves.

Deep frostbite extends beneath the subcutaneous tissue to involve muscle, deeper blood vessels, and nerves. There often is considerable edema, perhaps involving the entire

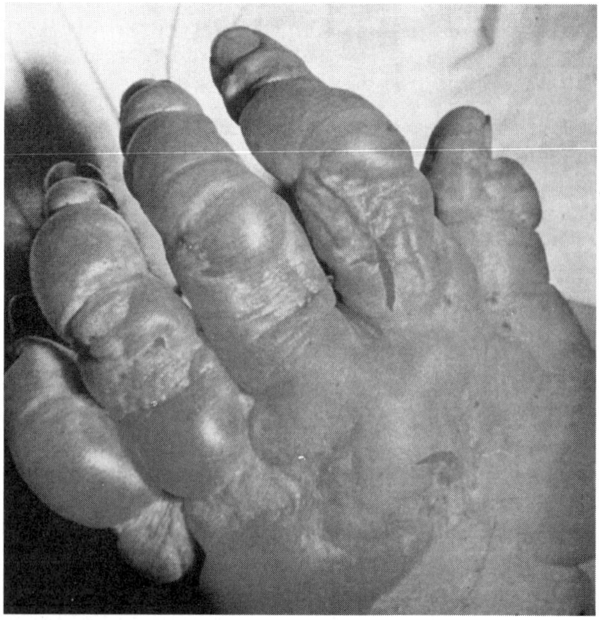

Fig. 42-12. Severe frostbite occurred in the hands of this patient after prolonged cold exposure. The fingers are markedly swollen and blisters are present. Gangrene has developed at the tips of several of the digits. (Reproduced with permission from B Washburn. Frostbite: what is it—how to prevent it—emergency treatment. N Engl J Med 1962; 266:974–989.)

hand or foot (Fig. 42-12). Vesicles and bullae develop; tissue necrosis and gangrene may ensue. Excessive perspiration or pruritis may persist long after the initial injury. Often the affected extremity exhibits increased sensitivity to cold.

TREATMENT

Treatment for frostbite is rewarming. Frostbite can be treated immediately by placing warm parts of the body on the frostbitten areas. For example, hands can be placed in the axilla or warmed on a partner's torso. A warm environment should be sought as soon as possible. The patient should not be reexposed to freezing conditions, because reexposure to cold following thawing can severely increase the degree of tissue damage. Rewarming can be accomplished by immersing the affected area in a waterbath at temperatures from 104° to 111°F (40° to 44°C). After rewarming in the bath for approximately 20 minutes, the affected area should be exposed to room air at a temperature of approximately 70° to 78°F (21° to 26°C). Analgesics often are required during the rewarming. Massage, application of ice water or snow, or exposure to excessively high temperatures are all contraindicated and likely to worsen the injury. The injured area should be cleansed with a mild soap or antiseptic. Vesicles and bullae should not be disturbed. Eschars should not be removed, since the extent of tissue damage often cannot be determined for several weeks [348]. Sterile dressings should be applied over blisters. Antibiotics may be administered if there is evidence of infection. It is not known whether sympathetic blocking drugs are effective, although regional sympathectomy may conserve tissue and reduce pain if performed within 24 to 48 hours after frostbite occurs [351].

PROGNOSIS

The prognosis of patients with superficial frostbite usually is good. Following recovery, there is often normal tissue. Even large eschars may separate in time, leaving normal tissue underneath. Paresthesias and sensitivity to cold may persist. With severe cases of frostbite, extensive tissue damage may lead to fibrosis and contractures, reducing effective use of the limb. The development of gangrene may require amputation.

PROPHYLAXIS

Frostbite can be prevented by adequate education about protection from cold exposure. Loose-fitting, dry clothing should be worn at all times. Exercise helps prevent frostbite. Wet gloves or boots should be removed as soon as possible. Colleagues should observe each other for signs of frostbite.

Erythromelalgia

Erythromelalgia (erythermalgia) is a disorder characterized by burning pain, increased temperature, and erythema of the extremities. The appellation erythromelalgia was first suggested by Mitchell in 1872 [352]. Erythermalgia is a term introduced by Smith and Allen in 1938 to emphasize that increased skin temperature is an important feature of this clinical syndrome [353].

Erythromelalgia can be categorized as primary or secondary. Primary erythromelalgia usually occurs spontaneously and may present at any age, but it is most common in middle age. Males are affected more than females. A kindred with 29 persons afflicted with the syndrome has been described; an autosomal dominant mode of transmission was suggested through five generations [354]. In the family, most of the affected members were females.

Secondary erythromelalgia occurs primarily in myeloproliferative disorders, particularly polycythemia vera and essential thrombocythemia [355–357]. Michiels et al. reported that 26 of 40 patients with thrombocythemia presented with symptoms of the syndrome [355]. Of those 26, 50 percent had essential thrombocythemia, and 50 percent had polycythemia. The diagnosis of the underlying myeloproliferative disorder may not be apparent for several years (median 2.5 years) [357]. The true incidence or prevalence of erythromelalgia in myeloproliferative disease is unknown; estimates have varied from 3 to 65 percent [355–357]. The disorder also has been reported in patients with hypertension, diabetes mellitus, systemic lupus erythematosus [358], and pox viruses [359] and in patients receiving calcium blocking agents [360–362] or bromocriptine [363]. An association of Raynaud's phenomenon and erythromelalgia has been reported [364]. Patients have typical vasospastic attacks but at other times have burning pain in bright red, warm or hot fingers.

PATHOPHYSIOLOGY

The pathophysiology of primary erythromelalgia is not well established. The skin may be very sensitive to temperature elevation. Erythema and vasodilation are important characteristics of the disorder but most likely are secondary events resulting from the increase in temperature [365]. Indeed, symptoms can be produced by increasing skin temperature while preventing any increase in flow by inflation of a sphygmomanometric cuff on the extremity to suprasystolic pressure [365].

There is indirect evidence that prostaglandins may be involved in secondary erythromelalgia associated with thrombocythemia. Both aspirin and indomethacin may reduce symptoms remarkably, implying that a platelet-mediated prostaglandin mechanism is active [355]. Aspirin causes relief for several days but indomethacin for less than 24 hours, perhaps because the former produces irreversible inactivation of cyclo-oxygenase while the latter's action is reversible. Antiplatelet agents that do not inhibit cyclo-oxygenase do not relieve symptoms. One patient has been reported to respond to piroxicam, a drug that may inhibit biosynthesis of prostaglandins [366]. The cause of the syndrome in other disease states listed above is unknown.

PATHOLOGY

Skin biopsy samples in patients with erythromelalgia secondary to myeloproliferative disease demonstrate lesions in the arterioles [357]. The venules, capillaries, and nerves do not appear to be involved. The endothelial cells are vacuolized and swollen. There is intimal proliferation, splitting of the internal elastic membrane, and proliferation of vascular smooth muscle cells. Some arterioles are occluded by thrombi. Priollet et al. [367] described one patient who showed no arteriolar pathology by skin biopsy.

CLINICAL PRESENTATION

Typically, the patient complains of burning pain and redness in the distal parts of the extremities, although the toes may not be involved. About two-thirds of patients have involvement of the lower extremities alone; in others, erythromelalgia may be confined to the upper extremities or affect all limbs. Bilateral involvement occurs in over 90 percent of the patients with primary erythromelalgia. In secondary erythromelalgia, asymmetric involvement of the extremities is more frequent than in primary cases. The symptoms usually are precipitated by environmental or local warmth and relieved by exposing the extremity to cool air, cold floors, or water. The duration of attacks lasts minutes to hours. Symptoms may be ameliorated with elevation of the extremity and potentiated by dependency of the extremity or exercise. Sometimes erythromelalgia is so severe and disabling that the patient spends most of the day and night lying down with the legs elevated and using some cooling device.

Examination of the patient during an attack reveals erythema and warmth of the affected extremities, usually the feet, less commonly the hands (Plate 13). There may be subcutaneous atrophy. The pulse examination is normal, and there should be no clinical evidence of a peripheral neuropathy. Approximately one-third of patients with thrombocytosis develop necrosis of the distal aspects of a digit. There may be blisters or ulcers secondary to self-applied treatments, such as ice water, used to relieve the pain.

DIAGNOSIS

Erythromelalgia can be precipitated by increasing the environmental temperature or by direct application of heat to the involved extremity. Dependency of the extremity or venous congestion may help induce attacks. Lewis indicated that raising the environmental temperature to a "critical point" could precipitate symptoms [365]. The specific temperature varies from person to person but usually exceeds 32°C.

Erythromelalgia should be distinguished from other disorders that cause painful (and) red extremities, such as arterial occlusive disease and peripheral neuropathies. Severe impairment of blood flow in patients with arterial occlusive disorders, such as atherosclerosis, thromboangiitis obliterans, or arterial emboli may cause cyanosis, dependent rubor, and severe pain, but the foot is cold, pulses are absent, and pallor of the foot occurs with leg elevation. The trophic skin changes often are present. Painful paresthesias and erythema also occur in patients with peripheral neuropathy. A careful neurologic examination to assess sensation, motor performance, and deep tendon reflexes usually is sufficient to identify these individuals.

TREATMENT

There is no specific treatment for primary erythromelalgia. Patients should be advised to avoid environmental temperatures that precipitate symptoms. An air-conditioned environment may reduce distress, especially at night. Vasoconstrictor agents, vasodilator drugs, and propranolol [368] have been reported to benefit some patients but usually are not of value. Baths, using heat below the threshold for pain, may give temporary relief. Section or alcohol injection of peripheral nerves and sympathectomy have been used in some patients, usually without success. Aspirin is not beneficial in the primary disorder. In secondary erythromelalgia due to thrombocytosis, aspirin has been shown to relieve symptoms for several days. Indomethacin can be used in aspirin-intolerant patients but produces relief for less than 24 hours. Successful treatment of the underlying disorder may alleviate symptoms in other causes of secondary erythromelalgia. Analgesics and sedatives may be necessary, but narcotics should be avoided in this chronic condition.

PROGNOSIS

The severe pain of primary erythromelalgia may cause disability. Some patients undergo spontaneous remissions. Prognosis in secondary erythromelalgia depends on the success of treating the underlying cause. Symptoms and signs may remit with treatment of the thrombocythemia in myeloproliferative disorders; hydroxyurea often is successful in lowering the platelet count. Digital necrosis will usually heal with treatment of the thrombocythemia.

References

1. Raynaud M. L'Asphyxie Locale et de la Gangrene Symmetrique des Extremities. Trans. Thomas Barlow. London: New Sydenham Society, 1862.
2. Coffman JD, ed. Raynaud's Phenomenon. New York: Oxford University Press, 1989.
3. Halperin JL, Coffman JD. Pathophysiology of Raynaud's disease. Arch Intern Med 1979; 139:89–92.
4. Cohen RA, Coffman JD. Digital vasospasm: the pathophysiology of Raynaud's phenomenon. Int Angiology 1984; 3: 47–55.
5. Peacock JH. Peripheral venous blood concentrations of epinephrine and norepinephrine in primary Raynaud's disease. Circ Res 1959; 7:821–827.
6. Kontos HA, Wasserman AJ. Effect of reserpine in Raynaud's phenomenon. Circulation 1969; 39:259–266.
7. Downey JA, Frewin DB. The effect of cold on blood flow in the hand of patients with Raynaud's phenomenon. Clin Sci 1973; 44:279–289.
8. Downey JA, et al. Thermoregulation and Raynaud's phenomenon. Clin Sci 1971; 40:211–219.
9. Coffman JD, Cohen AS. Total and capillary fingertip blood flow in Raynaud's phenomenon. N Engl J Med 1971; 285:259–263.
10. Lewis T. Experiments relating to the peripheral mechanism involved in spasmodic arrest of the circulation in the fingers, a variety of Raynaud's disease. Heart 1929; 15:7–12.
11. Mendlowitz M, Naftchi N. The digital circulation in Raynaud's disease. Am J Cardiol 1959; 4:580–584.
12. Freedman RR, Mayes MD, Sabharwal SC. Induction of vasospastic attacks despite digital nerve block in Raynaud's disease and phenomenon. Circulation 1989; 80:859–862.
13. Jamieson GG, Ludbrook J, Wilson A. Cold hypersensitivity in Raynaud's phenomenon. Circulation 1971; 44:254–264.
14. Vanhoutte PM, Shepherd JT. Effect of temperature on reactivity of isolated cutaneous veins of the dog. Am J Physiol 1970; 218:187–190.
15. Rusch NJ, Shepherd JT, Vanhoutte PM. The effect of profound cooling on adrenergic neurotransmission in canine cutaneous veins. J Physiol 1981; 311:57–65.
16. Vanhoutte PM, Lorenz RR. Effect of temperature on reactivity of saphenous, mesenteric, and femoral veins of the dog. Am J Physiol 1970; 218:1746–1750.
17. Janssens WJ, Vanhoutte PM. Effect of cooling on efflux of ^{3}H-noradrenaline in canine cutaneous veins. Br J Pharmacol 1979; 66:148P.
18. Janssens WJ, Vanhoutte PM. Effect of cooling on COMT-activity in canine saphenous vein homogenates determined by a micro-radioenzymatic assay. Arch Int Pharmacodyn Ther 1978; 236:305–306.
19. Vanhoutte PM, et al. Modulation of postjunctional alpha-adrenergic responsiveness by local changes in temperature. Clin Sci 1985; 68:121s–123s.
20. Somlyo AP. Sarcoplasmic reticulum and the temperature-dependent contraction of smooth muscle in calcium-free solutions. J Cell Biol 1971; 51:722–741.
21. Cooke JP, Shepherd JT, Vanhoutte PM. The effect of warming on adrenergic neurotransmission in canine cutaneous vein. Circ Res 1984; 54:547–553.
22. Flavahan NA, et al. Human postjunctional alpha-1 and alpha-2 adrenoceptors: differential distribution in arteries of the limbs. J Pharmacol Exp Ther 1987; 241:361–365.
23. Coffman JD, Cohen RA. Role of alpha-adrenoceptor subtypes mediating sympathetic vasoconstriction in human digits. Eur J Clin Invest 1988; 18:309–313.
24. Coffman JD, Cohen RA. Alpha-adrenergic and 5-HT_2 receptor hypersensitivity in Raynaud's phenomenon. J Vasc Med Biol 1990; 2:100–106.
25. Keenan EJ, Porter JM. Alpha$_2$-adrenergic receptors in platelets from patients with Raynaud's syndrome. Surgery 1983; 94:204–209.
26. Freedman RR, Baer RP, Mayes MD. Blockade of vasospastic attacks by alpha$_2$-adrenergic but not alpha$_1$-adrenergic antagonists in idiopathic Raynaud's disease. Circulation 1995; 2:1448–1451.
27. Greenblatt DJ, Koch-Weser J. Adverse reactions to β-adrenergic receptor blocking drugs. A report from the Boston Collaborative Drug Surveillance Program. Drugs 1974; 7:118–129.
28. Marshall AJ, Roberts CJC, Barritt DW. Raynaud's phenomenon as side effect of beta-blockers in hypertension. Br Med J 1976; 1:1498–1499.
29. Eliasson K, Lins LE, Sundqvist K. Peripheral vasospasm during β-receptor blockade—a comparison between metoprolol and pindolol. Acta Med Scand Suppl 1982; 665:109–112.
30. Cobbold AF, Ginsburg J, Paton A. Circulatory, respiratory, and metabolic responses to isopropylnoradrenaline in man. J Physiol (Lond) 1960; 151:539.
31. Cohen RA, Coffman JD. β-adrenergic vasodilator mechanism in the finger. Circ Res 1981; 49:1196–1201.
32. Vanhoutte PM. 5-Hydroxytryptamine and vascular disease. Fed Proc 1983; 42:233–237.
33. Cohen RA, Shepherd JT, Vanhoutte PM. 5-Hydroxytryptamine can mediate endothelium-dependent relaxation of coronary arteries. Am J Physiol 1983; 245:H1077–H1080.
34. Roddie IC, Shepherd JT, Whelan RF. The action of 5-hydroxytryptamine on the blood vessels of the human hand and forearm. Br J Pharmacol Chemother 1955; 10:445–450.
35. Coffman JD, Cohen RA. Serotonergic vasoconstriction in human fingers during reflex sympathetic response to cooling. Am J Physiol 1988; 254(Heart Circ Physiol):H889–H893.
36. Moulds RFW, Iwanov V, Medcalf RL. The effects of platelet-derived contractile agents on human digital arteries. Clin Sci 1984; 66:443–451.
37. Biondi ML, et al. Plasma free and intraplatelet serotonin on patients with Raynaud's phenomenon. Int J Cardiol 1988; 19:335–339.
38. Gresele P, et al. Thromboxane does not play a significant role in acute cold-induced vasoconstriction in Raynaud's phenomenon. Thromb Res 1992; 66:259–264.
39. Marasini B, et al. Tissue-type plasminogen activator and von Willebrand factor plasma levels as markers of endothelial involvement in patients with Raynaud's phenomenon. Int J Microcirc Clin Exp 1992; 11:375–382.
40. Coffman JD, Cohen RA. Plasma levels of 5-hydroxytryptamine during sympathetic stimulation and in Raynaud's phenomenon. Clin Sci 1994; 86:269–273.
41. Winkelmann RK, Goldyne ME, Linscheid RL. Hypersensitivity of scleroderma cutaneous vascular smooth muscle to 5-hydroxytryptamine. Br J Dermatol 1976; 95:51–56.
42. Halpern A, et al. Raynaud's disease, Raynaud's phenomenon, and serotonin. Angiology 1960; 11:151–167.
43. Coffman JD, et al. International study of ketanserin in Raynaud's phenomenon. Am J Med 1989; 87:264–268.
44. Seibold JR, Jageneau HM. Treatment of Raynaud's phenomenon with ketanserin, a selective antagonist of the serotonin$_2$ (5-HT_2) receptor. Arthritis Rheum 1984; 27:139–146.
45. Stranden E, Roald OK, Krohg K. Treatment of Raynaud's phenomenon with the 5-HT_2-receptor antagonist ketanserin. Br Med J 1982; 285:1069–1071.
46. Vanhoutte PM, et al. Antihypertensive properties of ketanserin (R 41 468). Fed Proc 1983; 42:182–185.
47. Reimann IW, Frolich JC. Mechanism of antihypertensive action of ketanserin in man. Br Med J 1983; 287:381–383.

48. Zabludowski JR, Ball SG, Robertson JIS. Ketanserin and alpha$_1$-adrenergic antagonism in humans. J Cardiovasc Pharmacol 1985; 7:S123–S125.
49. Hechtman DH, Jageneau A. Inhibition of cold-induced vasoconstriction with ketanserin. Microvasc Res 1985; 30:56–62.
50. Seibold JR, Terregino CA. Selective antagonism of S$_2$-serotonergic receptors relieves but does not prevent cold induced vasoconstriction in primary Raynaud's phenomenon. J Rheumatol 1986; 13:337–340.
51. Baart De la Faille H, et al. Cold-induced Raynaud's phenomenon ameliorated by intravenous administration of ketanserin: a double-blind cross-over study. Arch Dermatol Res 1986; 279:3–7.
52. Roald OK, Seem E. Treatment of Raynaud's phenomenon with ketanserin in patients with connective tissue disorders. Br Med J 1984; 289:577–579.
53. Lukac J, et al. Effect of ketanserin on Raynaud's phenomenon in progressive systemic sclerosis: a double-blind trial. Drugs Exp Clin Res 1985; 11:659–663.
54. Horrobin DF, Jenkins K, Manku MS. Raynaud's phenomenon, histamine, and prostaglandins. Lancet 1983; 2:747–748.
55. Reilly IAG, Roy L, Fitzgerald GA. Biosynthesis of thromboxane in patients with systemic sclerosis and Raynaud's phenomenon. Br Med J 1986; 292:1037–1039.
56. Coffman JD, Rasmussen HM. Effect of thromboxane synthetase inhibition in Raynaud's phenomenon. Clin Pharmacol Ther 1984; 36:369–373.
57. Ettinger WH, et al. Controlled double-blind trial of dazoxiben and nifedipine in the treatment of Raynaud's phenomenon. Am J Med 1984; 77:451–456.
58. Jones EW, Hawkey CJ. A thromboxane synthetase inhibitor in Raynaud's phenomenon. Prostalandins Leukot Med 1983; 12:67–71.
59. Luderer JR, et al. Dazoxiben, a thromboxane synthetase inhibitor in Raynaud's phenomenon. Clin Pharmacol Ther 1984; 36:105–115.
60. Tindall H, et al. Effect of dazoxiben, a thromboxane synthetase inhibitor on skin blood flow following cold challenge in patients with Raynaud's phenomenon. Eur J Clin Invest 1985; 15:20–23.
61. Trubestein G, et al. Behandling des Raynaud-syndroms mit captopril. Dtsch Med Wochenschr 1984; 109:857–860.
62. Tosi S, et al. Treatment of Raynaud's phenomenon with captopril. Drugs Exp Clin Res 1987; 13:37–42.
63. Miyazaki S, et al. Relief of digital vasospasm by treatment with captopril and its complete inhibition by serine proteinase inhibitors in Raynaud's phenomenon. Br Med J 1982; 284:310–311.
64. Lopez-Ovejero JA, et al. Reversal of vascular and renal crisis of scleroderma by oral angiotensin-converting enzyme blockade. N Engl J Med 1979; 300:1417–1419.
65. Lau CS, McLaren M, Belch JJF. Factor VIII von Willebrand factor antigen levels correlate with symptom severity in patients with Raynaud's phenomenon. Br J Rheumatol 1991; 30:433–436.
66. Lau CS, et al. Further evidence of increased polymorphonuclear cell activity in patients with Raynaud's phenomenon. Br J Rheumatol 1992; 31:375–380.
67. Biondi ML, et al. Increased plasma endothelin levels in patients with Raynaud's phenomenon. N Engl J Med 1991; 324:1139–1140.
68. Yamane K, et al. Significance of plasma endothelin-1 levels in patients with systemic sclerosis. J Rheumatol 1992; 19:1566–1571.
69. Kanno K, et al. Endothelin and Raynaud's phenomenon. Am J Med 1991; 90:130–132.
70. Kahn F, Coffman JD. Enhanced cholinergic vasodilation in Raynaud's phenomenon. Circulation 1994; 89:1183–1188.
71. Innes IR. Identification of the smooth muscle excitatory receptor for ergot alkaloids. Br J Pharmacol 1962; 19:120.
72. Bluntschli HJ, Goetz RH. The effect of ergot derivatives on the circulation in man with special reference to two new hydrogenated compounds (dihydroergotamine and dihydroergocornine). Am Heart J 1948; 35:873.
73. Cameron EA, French EB. St. Anthony's fire rekindled: gangrene due to therapeutic dose of ergotamine. Br Med J 1960; 2:28.
74. Muller-Schweinitzer E. Responsiveness of isolated canine cerebral and peripheral arteries to ergotamine. Naunyn Schmiedebergs Arch Pharmacol 1976; 292:113–118.
75. Henry LG, et al. Ergotism. Arch Surg 1975; 110:929–932.
76. Herlache J, Hoskins P, Schmidt CM. Ergotism. Angiology 1973; 24:369–373.
77. Burton AC. The physical equilibrium of the small blood vessels. Am J Physiol 1951; 164:319.
78. Krahenbuhl B, Nielsen SL, Lassen NA. Closure of digital arteries in high vascular tone states as demonstrated by measurement of systolic blood pressure in the finger. Scand J Clin Lab Invest 1977; 37:71–76.
79. Landis EM. Micro-injection studies of capillary blood pressure in Raynaud's disease. Heart 1930; 15:247–255.
80. Thulesius O. Methods for evaluation of peripheral vascular function in the upper extremities. Acta Chir Scand 1976; [Suppl]465:53–54.
81. Cohen RA, Coffman JD. Reduced fingertip arterial pressure in Raynaud's disease. J Vasc Med Biol 1989; 1:21–26.
82. McIntyre DR. A maneuver to reverse Raynaud's phenomenon of the finger. JAMA 1978; 240:2760.
83. Lewis T. The pathological changes in the arteries supplying the fingers in warm-handed people and in cases of so-called Raynaud's disease. Clin Sci 1938; 3:287–319.
84. Dabich L, et al. Digital arteries in patients with scleroderma. Arch Intern Med 1972; 130:708–714.
85. Rosch J, Porter JM, Gralino BJ. Cryodynamic hand angiography in the diagnosis and management of Raynaud's syndrome. Circulation 1977; 55:807–814.
86. Kristensen JK. Blood flow in fingers in generalized scleroderma with Raynaud's phenomenon: influence of arterial blood pressure reduction and proximal vasodilation. J Invest Dermatol 1981; 77:373–376.
87. Brown GE, Griffin HZ. Peripheral arterial disease in polycythemia vera. Arch Intern Med 1930; 46:705.
88. Imhof JW, Boars H, Verloop MC. Clinical haematologic aspects of macroglobulinaemia Waldenström. Acta Med Scand 1959; 163:349.
89. Jager BV. Cryofibrinogenemia. N Engl J Med 1962; 266:579.
90. Marshal RJ, Shepherd JT, Thompson ID. Vascular responses in patients with high serum titres of cold agglutinins. Clin Sci 1953; 12:255.
91. McGrath MA, Penny R. Blood hyperviscosity in cryoglobulinemia: temperature sensitivity and correlation with reduced skin blood flow. Aust J Exp Biol Med Sci 1978; 56:127–137.
92. Invernizzi F, et al. Secondary and essential cryoglobulinemias. Acta Haematol 1983; 70:73–82.
93. Hillestad LK. The peripheral circulation during exposure to cold in normals and in patients with the syndrome of high-titre cold haemagglutination. Acta Med Scand 1959; 164:211.
94. Jahnsen T, Nielsen SL, Skovborg F. Blood viscosity and local response to cold in primary Raynaud's phenomenon. Lancet 1977; 2:1001–1002.
95. Walder DN. Blood viscosity and Raynaud's disease. J R Coll Surg Edinb 1973; 18:277–280.
96. Blunt RJ, et al. Hyperviscosity and thrombotic changes in

idiopathic and secondary Raynaud's phenomenon. Br J Hematol 1980; 45:651–658.
97. Creager MA, Coffman JD. Plasma and blood viscosity in Raynaud's phenomenon. Clin Res 1977; 25:214A.
98. Goyle KB, Dormandy JA. Abnormal blood viscosity in Raynaud's phenomenon. Lancet 1976; 1:1317–1318.
99. Pringle R, Walder DN, Weaver JPA. Blood viscosity and Raynaud's disease. Lancet 1965; 1:1086–1089.
100. McGrath MA, Peek R, Penny R. Raynaud's disease: reduced hand blood flows with normal blood viscosity. Aust NZ J Med 1978; 8:126–131.
101. Ayres ML, Jarrett PEM, Browse NL. Blood viscosity, Raynaud's phenomenon and the effect of fibrinolytic enhancement. Br J Surg 1981; 68:51–54.
102. Sergio G, et al. Emoreologia e sindromi acrali neurovascolari. Ric Clin Lab 1983; 13[Suppl 3]:481–485.
103. Sandhagen B, Wegener T. Blood viscosity and finger systolic pressure in primary and traumatic vasospastic disease. Ups J Med Sci 1985; 90:55–59.
104. Coffman JD, Davies WT. Vasospastic diseases: a review. Prog Cardiovasc Dis 1975; 18:123–146.
105. Allen EV, Brown GE. Raynaud's disease: a critical review of minimal requisites for diagnosis. Am J Med Sci 1932; 183:187–200.
106. LeRoy EC, Medsger TA Jr. Raynaud's phenomenon: a proposal for classification. Clin Exper Rheumatol 1991; 10:485.
107. Maricq HR, et al. Geographic variation in prevalence of Raynaud's phenomenon. Charleston, SC, USA vs Tarentaise, Savoie France. J Rheumatol 1993; 20:70–76.
108. Hines EA, Christensen NA. Raynaud's disease among men. JAMA 1945; 129:1–4.
109. Blain A, Coller FA, Carver GB. Raynaud's disease: a study of criteria for prognosis. Surgery 1951; 29:387–397.
110. Maricq HR, et al. Prevalence of Raynaud's phenomenon in the general population. J Chronic Dis 1986; 38:423–427.
111. Gifford RW, Hines EA. Raynaud's disease among women and girls. Circulation 1957; 16:1012–1021.
112. Olsen N, Nielsen SL. Prevalence of primary Raynaud phenomena in young females. Scand J Clin Lab Invest 1978; 32:761–764.
113. Guntheroth WG, et al. Raynaud's disease in children. Circulation 1967; 36:724–729.
114. Miller D, et al. Is variant angina the coronary manifestation of a generalized vasospastic disorder? N Engl J Med 1981; 304:763–766.
115. Zahavi I, et al. Prevalence of Raynaud's phenomenon in patients with migraine. Arch Intern Med 1984; 144:742–744.
116. O'Keeffe ST, Tsapatsaris NP, Beetham WP Jr. Increased prevalence of migraine and chest pain in patients with primary Raynaud disease. Ann Intern Med 1992; 116:985–989.
117. Krumholz HM, Goldberger AL. Systemic arterial vasospastic syndrome: familial occurrence with variant angina. Am J Med 1992; 92:344–345.
118. Cannon PJ, et al. The relationship of hypertension and renal failure in scleroderma (progressive systemic sclerosis) to structural and functional abnormalities of the renal cortical circulation. Medicine 1974; 53:1–46.
119. Ellis WW, et al. Left ventricular dysfunction induced by cold exposure in patients with systemic sclerosis. Am J Med 1986; 80:385–392.
120. Vergnon J-M, et al. Raynaud's phenomenon of the lung. Chest 1992; 101:1312–1317.
121. Salmenson BD, et al. Macular capillary hemodynamic changes associated with Raynaud's phenomenon. Ophthalmology 1992; 99:914–919.
122. Coffman JD, Cohen RA. Vasospasm-ubiquitous? N Engl J Med 1981; 304:780–782.
123. Weber RB, Reinmuth OM. The treatment of migraine with propranolol. Neurology (Minneap) 1972; 22:366–369.
124. Tokola R, Hokkanen E. Propranolol for acute migraine. Br Med J 1978; 2:1089.
125. Yasue H, et al. Role of autonomic nervous system in the pathogenesis of Prinzmetal's variant form of angina. Circulation 1974; 50:534–539.
126. Marshal AJ, Roberts CJC, Barritt DW. Raynaud's phenomenon as side effect of beta-blockers in hypertension. Br Med J 1976; 1:1498–1499.
127. Schroeder JS, et al. Provocation of coronary spasm with ergonovine maleate: new test with results in fifty-seven patients undergoing coronary arteriography. Am J Cardiol 1977; 40:487–491.
128. Curry RC Jr, et al. Effects of ergonovine in patients with and without coronary artery disease. Circulation 1977; 56: 803–809.
129. Waters DD, et al. Comparative sensitivity of exercise, cold pressor and ergonovine testing in provoking attacks of variant angina in patients with active disease. Circulation 1983; 67:310–315.
130. Wollersheim H, et al. The diagnostic valve of several immunological tests for anti-nuclear antibody in predicting the development of connective tissue disease in patients presenting with Raynaud's phenomenon. Eur J Clin Invest 1989; 19:535–541.
131. Subcommittee for Scleroderma Criteria of the American Rheumatism Association Diagnostic and Therapeutic Criteria Committee. Preliminary criteria for the classification of systemic sclerosis (scleroderma). Arthritis Rheum 1980; 23:581–590.
132. Matsui S. Anatomic pathologique et pathogenie de la sclerodermie generalisée. Presse Med 1924; 32:142.
133. Sackner MA. Scleroderma in Modern Medical Monographs. New York: Grune & Stratton, 1966.
134. Laws JW, El Sallab RA, Scott JT. An arteriographic and histologic study of digital arteries. Br J Radiol 1967; 40:740–747.
135. Norton WL, Nardo JM. Vascular disease in progressive systemic sclerosis (scleroderma). Ann Intern Med 1970; 73: 317–324.
136. Kahaleh MB, Osborn I, LeRoy EC. Increased factor VIII/von Willebrand factor antigen and von Willebrand factor activity in scleroderma and in Raynaud's phenomenon. Ann Intern Med 1981; 94(Part 1):482–484.
137. Thompson RP. Nailfold biopsy in scleroderma and related disorders. Arthritis Rheum 1984; 27:97–103.
138. Maricq HR, Spencer-Green G, LeRoy EC. Skin capillary abnormalities as indicators of organ involvement in scleroderma (systemic sclerosis), Raynaud's syndrome and dermatomyositis. Am J Med 1976; 61:862–870.
139. Tan EM, et al. The 1982 revised criteria for the classification of systemic lupus erythematosus. Arthritis Rheum 1982; 25:1271–1277.
140. Glass D, Soter NA, Schur PH. Rheumatoid vasculitis. Arthritis Rheum 1976; 19:950–952.
141. Fischer M, et al. Generalized vasculopathy and finger blood flow abnormalities in rheumatoid arthritis. J Rheum 1984; 11:33–37.
142. Laws JW, Lillie JG, Scott JT. Arteriographic appearance in rheumatoid arthritis and other disorders. Br J Radiol 1963; 36:477.
143. Mitchell DM, Fries JF. An analysis of the American Rheumatism Association criteria for rheumatoid arthritis. Arthritis Rheum 1982; 25:481–487.
144. von Winiwarter F. Ueber eine eigenthumlich Form von Endarteris und Endophlebitis mit Gangran des Fusses. Arch Klin Chir 1879; 23:202.

145. Buerger L. Thromboangiitis obliterans: a study of the vascular lesions leading to presenile spontaneous gangrene. Am J Med Sci 1908; 136:567.
146. McLoughlin GA, et al. Association of HLA-A9 and HLA-B5 with Buerger's disease. Br Med J 1976; 2:1165–1166.
147. Adar R, et al. Cellular sensitivity to collagen in thromboangiitis obliterans. N Engl J Med 1983; 308:1113–1116.
148. Buerger L. Recent studies in the pathology of thrombo-angiitis obliterans. J Med Res 1914–15; 26:181.
149. McKusick VA, et al. Buerger's disease—a distinct clinical and pathologic entity. JAMA 1962; 181:5.
150. Lambeth JT, Yong WK. Arteriographic findings in thromboangiitis obliterans with emphasis on femoropopliteal involvement. Am J Roentgenol Radium Ther Nucl Med 1970; 109:553–562.
151. Fischer CM. Cerebral thromboangiitis obliterans. Medicine (Baltimore) 1957; 36:169.
152. Deitch EA, Sikkema WW. Intestinal manifestation of Buerger's disease: case report and literature review. Am J Surg 1981; 47:326.
153. Ohno H, et al. Acute myocardial infarction in Buerger's disease. Am J Cardiol 1986; 57:690–691.
154. Loebe M, Heidrich H. The carpal tunnel syndrome—a disease underlying Raynaud's phenomenon? Angiology 1988; 39(10):891–901.
155. Coffman JD. Evaluation of the patient with Raynaud's phenomenon. Postgrad Med 1985; 78(2):175–180.
156. Waller DG, Dathan JR. Raynaud's syndrome and carpal tunnel syndrome. Postgrad Med J 1985; 61(712):161–162.
157. Iwai S, Mei-Sai N. Etiology of Raynaud's diseases. Jap Med World 1926; 6:345.
158. Hansen PF, Faber M. Raynaud's syndrome originating from reversible precipitation of protein. Acta Med Scand 1947; 129:81.
159. Marshall RJ, Shepherd JT, Thompson ID. Vascular responses in patients with high serum titres of cold agglutinins. Clin Sci 1953; 12:255–264.
160. Erf LA. A note on the stability of cold haemagglutinins. Am J Clin Pathol 1945; 15:210.
161. Rosse W, Bunn HF. Hemolytic anemias. In E Braunwald, et al., eds. Harrison's Principles of Internal Medicine. New York: McGraw-Hill, 1994.
162. Longo DL. Plasma cell disorders. In E Braunwald, et al., eds. Harrison's Principles of Internal Medicine. New York: McGraw-Hill, 1994.
163. Winfield JB. Cryoglobulinemia. Hum Pathol 1983; 14(4): 350–354.
164. Gripenberg M, et al. Autoantibody activity of cryoglobulins and sera in systemic lupus erythematosus. Association of IgM class rheumatoid factors with Raynaud's syndrome. Scand J Rheumatol 1988; 17(4):249–254.
165. Horowitz J, Klein M, Sukenik S. Cryoglobulinemia and hepatitis B markers in North African Jews with Raynaud's disease. Arthritis Rheum 1986; 29:1026–1028.
166. Franklin EC. The role of cryoglobulins and immune complexes in vasculitis. J Allergy Clin Immunol 1980; 66(4): 269–273.
167. Ritzmann SE, Levin WC. Cryopathies: a review. Arch Intern Med 1961; 107:186.
168. Heinrich RA, Vonder Heide EC, Climie ARW. Cryofibrinogen: formation and inhibition in heparinized plasma. Am J Physiol 1963; 204:419.
169. Taylor W, et al. Effect of the air hammer on the hands of stonecutters. The limestone quarries of Bedford, Indiana, revisited. Br J Ind Med 1984; 41:289–295.
170. Litherland HK. Assessment of vibration white finger syndrome. Can J Surg 1986; 29:336–338.
171. Laroche GP. Traumatic vasospastic disease in chain-saw operators. Can Med Assoc J 1976; 115:1217–1221.
172. Theriault G, et al. Raynaud's phenomenon in forestry workers in Quebec. Can Med Assoc J 1982; 126:1404–1408.
173. Bovenzi M. Vibration white finger, digital blood pressure, and some biochemical findings on workers operating vibrating tools in the engine manufacturing industry. Am J Ind Med 1988; 14:575–584.
174. Brubaker RL, et al. Vibration white finger disease among tree fellers in British Columbia. J Occup Med 1983; 25:403–408.
175. Davies TAL, Glaser EM, Collins CP. Absence of Raynaud's phenomenon in workers using vibratory tools in warm climate. Lancet 1957; 1:1014.
176. Christophers AJ. Occupational aspects of Raynaud's disease: a critical historical survey. Med J Aust 1972; 2:730–733.
177. Okada A, Inaba R, Furuno T. Occurrence of intimal thickening of the peripheral arteries in response to local vibration. Br J Ind Med 1987; 44:470–475.
178. Ashe WF, Cook WT, Old JW. Raynaud's phenomenon of occupational origin. Arch Environ Health 1962; 5:333.
179. Gurdjian ES, Walker LW. Traumatic vasospastic disease of the hand (white fingers). JAMA 1945; 129:668.
180. Vayssairat M, et al. Raynaud's phenomenon in chain saw users. Hot and cold finger systolic pressures and nailfold capillary findings. Eur Heart J 1987; 8:417–422.
181. Patri B, et al. Raynaud's syndrome in lumberjacks using chain saws. Epidemiology, clinical and capillaroscopic findings. J Mal Vasc 1985; 10:259–263.
182. Schatz IJ. Occlusive arterial disease in the hands due to occupational trauma. N Engl J Med 1963; 268:281.
183. Okada A, et al. Studies on the diagnosis and pathogenesis of Raynaud's phenomenon of occupational origin. Br J Industr Med 1971; 28:353–357.
184. Katsunuma H, Suzuki T, Hasegawa T. Electromyographical studies of pneumatic tool diseases. Jap J Industr Health 1963; 5:453.
185. Hisanaga H. Studies of peripheral nerve conduction velocities in vibrating tool operators. Sangyo Igaku 1982; 24: 284–293.
186. Hashimoto K, Craig RS. Acrosclerosis associated with vibration: an electron microscopic study. J Cutan Pathol 1980; 7:373–386.
187. Takeuchi T, Takeya M, Imanishi H. Ultrastructural changes in peripheral nerves of the fingers of three vibration-exposed persons with Raynaud's phenomenon. Scand J Work Environ Health 1988; 14:31–35.
188. Hyvarinen J, Pyykko I, Sundberg S. Vibration frequencies and amplitudes in the aetiology of traumatic vasospastic disease. Lancet 1973; 1:791–794.
189. Azuma T, Ohhashi T, Sakaguchi M. Vibration-induced hyperresponsiveness of arterial smooth muscle to noradrenaline with special reference to Raynaud's phenomenon in vibration disease. Cardiovasc Res 1978; 12:758–764.
190. Azuma T, Ohhashi T, Sakaguchi M. An approach to the pathogenesis of "white finger" induced by vibratory stimulation: acute but sustained changes in vascular responsiveness of canine hindlimb to noradrenaline. Cardiovasc Res 1980; 14:725–730.
191. Little JM, Ferguson DA. The incidence of the hypothenar hammer syndrome. Arch Surg 1972; 105:684–685.
192. Millender LH, Nalebuff EA, Kasdon E. Aneurysms and thromboses of the ulnar artery in the hand. Arch Surg 1972; 105:686–690.
193. Vayssairat M, et al. Does karate injure blood vessels of the hand? Lancet 1984; 2:529.
194. Aellig WH. Influence of ergot compounds on compliance of

superficial hand veins in man. Postgrad Med J 1976; 52[Suppl 1]:21–23.
195. Greene FL, Ariynam S, Stansel HC Jr. Mesenteric and peripheral vascular ischemia secondary to ergotism. Surgery 1977; 81:176–179.
196. Kempczinski RF, Buckley CJ, Darling RC. Vascular insufficiency secondary to ergotism. Surgery 1976; 79:597–600.
197. Graham JR. Methysergide for prevention of headache. N Engl J Med 1964; 270:67.
198. Appelbaum PS, Kapoor W. Imipramine-induced vasospasm: a case report. Am J Psychiatry 1983; 140:913–915.
199. Bowen JS, et al. Diffuse vascular spasm associated with 4-bromo-2.5 dimethoxyamphetamine ingestion. JAMA 1983; 249:1477–1479.
200. Scheulen ME, Schmidt CG. Raynaud's phenomenon and cancer chemotherapy. Ann Intern Med 1982; 96:256–257.
201. Vogelzang NJ, Bosl GJ, Johnson K. Raynaud's phenomenon: a common toxicity after combination chemotherapy for testicular cancer. Ann Intern Med 1981; 95:288–292.
202. Rothberg H. Raynaud's phenomenon after vinblastine-bleomycin chemotherapy. Cancer Treat Rep 1978; 62:569–570.
203. Cohen IS, et al. Cutaneous toxicity of bleomycin therapy. Arch Dermatol 1973; 107:553–555.
204. Harris DK, Adams WGF. Acro-osteolysis occurring in men engaged in the polymerization of vinyl chloride. Br Med J 1967; 3:712–714.
205. Johnston ENM. Vinyl chloride disease. Br J Dermatol 1978; 978:45.
206. Falappa P, et al. Angiographic study of digital arteries in workers exposed to vinyl chloride. Br J Industr Med 1982; 39:169–172.
207. Maricq HR, et al. Capillary abnormalities in polyvinyl chloride production workers. JAMA 1976; 236:1368–1371.
208. White C de B, Udwadia BP. β-adrenoceptors in the human dorsal hand vein, and the effects of propranolol and practolol on venous sensitivity to noradrenaline. Br J Clin Pharmacol 1979; 2:99–105.
209. Marshall AJ, Roberts CJC, Barritt DW. Raynaud's phenomenon as side effect of beta-blockers in hypertension. Br Med J 1976; 1:1498–1499.
210. Eliasson K, Lins LE, Sundqvist K. Vasospastic phenomena in patients treated with beta-adrenoceptor blocking agents. Acta Med Scand Suppl 1979; [Suppl]628:39–46.
211. Eliasson K, et al. Raynaud's phenomenon caused by beta-receptor blocking drugs. Acta Med Scand 1984; 215:333–339.
212. Eliasson K, Lins L, Sundqvist K. Peripheral vasospasm during beta-receptor blockade—a comparison between metoprolol and pindolol. Acta Med Scand Suppl 1982; 665: 109–112.
213. Heck I, Trubestein G, Stumpe KO. Effects of combined beta and alpha receptor blockade on peripheral circulation in essential hypertension. Clin Sci 1981; 61:429s–432s.
214. Steiner JA, et al. Vascular symptoms in patients with primary Raynaud's phenomenon are not exacerbated by propranolol or labetalol. Br J Clin Pharmacol 1979; 7:401–403.
215. Bolli P, et al. Treatment of hypertension with labetalol. NZ Med J 1977; 86:557–563.
216. Feleke E, et al. Complaints of cold extremities among patients on antihypertensive treatment. Acta Med Scand 1983; 213:381–385.
217. Nielson PE, Nielsen SL. Digital arterial tone in hypertensive subjects treated with cardioselective and non-selective beta-adrenoreceptor blocking agents. Dan Med Bull 1981; 28:76–78.
218. Erb RJ, Plachetka JR. Thermographic evaluation of the peripheral vascular effects of labetalol and propranolol. Curr Thes Res 1985; 38.
219. Lenders JWM, et al. The influence of intrinsic sympathomimetic and beta-1 receptor selectivity on the recovery of finger skin temperature after finger cooling in normotensive subjects. Clin Pharmacol Ther 1986; 39:353–357.
220. McSorley PD, Warren DJ. Effects of propranolol and metoprolol on the peripheral circulation. Br Med J 1978; 2:1598–1600.
221. Nielsen SL, Olsen N, Nielsen PE. Increased digital arterial tone in hypertensive subjects indicated by local cooling and propranolol treatment. Clin Physiol 1981; 1:21.
222. Coffman JD, Rasmussen HM. Effects of beta-adrenoreceptor-blocking drugs in patients with Raynaud's phenomenon. Circulation 1985; 72:466–470.
223. Shagan BP, Friedman SA. Raynaud's phenomenon and thyroid deficiency. Arch Intern Med 1980; 140:832–833.
224. Nielsen SL, Parving H-H, Hansen JEM. Myxoedema and Raynaud's phenomenon. Acta Endocrinol (Copenh) 1989; 101:32–34.
225. Lappchen J, et al. Raynaud-Phänomen bei Dialysepatienten. Dtsch Med Wochenschr 1977; 102:521–525.
226. Nielsen SL, Lokkegaard H. Cold hypersensitivity and finger systolic blood pressure in hemodialysis patients. Scand J Urol Nephrol 1981; 15:319–322.
227. Smith WM, Kroop IG. Raynaud's disease in primary pulmonary hypertension. JAMA 1957; 165:1245.
228. Celoria GC, Friedell GH, Sommers SC. Raynaud's disease and primary pulmonary hypertension. Circulation 1960; 22:1055.
229. Winters WL, Joseph RR, Learner N. "Primary" pulmonary hypertension and Raynaud's phenomenon. Arch Intern Med 1964; 114:821.
230. Fuster V, et al. Primary pulmonary hypertension: natural history and the importance of thrombosis. Circulation 1984; 70:580–587.
231. Goetz RH. Raynaud's disease and Raynaud's phenomenon. In Samuels SS, ed. Diagnosis and Treatment of Vascular Disorders. Baltimore: Williams & Wilkins, 1956. Pp. 349–383.
232. Bollinger A, Schlumpf M. Finger blood flow in healthy subjects of different age and sex and in patients with primary Raynaud's disease. Acta Chir Scand 1976; 465[Suppl]:42–47.
233. Nielsen SL, Lassen NA. Measurement of digital blood pressure after local cooling. J Appl Physiol 1977; 43:907–910.
234. Nielsen SL, Sorensen CJ, Olsen N. Thermostatted measurement of systolic blood pressure on cooled fingers. Scand J Clin Lab Invest 1980; 40:683–687.
235. Hoare M, et al. The effect of local cooling on digital systolic pressure in patients with Raynaud's syndrome. Br J Surg 1982; 69[Suppl]:S27–S28.
236. Corbin DOC, Wood DA, Housley E. An evaluation of finger systolic-pressure response to local cooling in the diagnosis of primary Raynaud's phenomenon. Clin Physiol 1985; 5:383–392.
237. Carter SA, Dean E, Kroeger EA. Apparent finger systolic pressures during cooling in patients with Raynaud's syndrome. Circulation 1988; 77:988.
238. Allen JA, et al. An objective test for the diagnosis and grading of vasospasm in patients with Raynaud's syndrome. Clin Sci 1992; 82:529–534.
239. Leppert J. Limitation of finger systolic pressure measurement as a diagnostic test for primary Raynaud's phenomenon in a female population. Clin Physiol 1989; 9:457–465.
240. Coffman JD. Effect of propranolol on blood pressure and skin blood flow during cigarette smoking. J Clin Pharmacol J New Drugs 1969; 9(1):39–44.
241. Keefe FJ, Surwit RS, Pilon RN. A 1-year follow-up of Raynaud's patients treated with behavioral therapy techniques. J Behav Med 1979; 2:385–391.

242. Keefe FJ, Surwit RS, Pilon RN. Biofeedback, autogenic training, and progressive relaxation in the treatment of Raynaud's disease: a comparative study. J Appl Behav Anal 1980; 13:3–11.
243. Freedman RR, et al. Biofeedback treatment of Raynaud's disease and phenomenon. Biofeedback Self Regul 1981; 6:355–365.
244. Yocum DE, et al. Use of biofeedback training in treatment of Raynaud's disease and phenomenon. J Rheumatol 1985; 12:90–93.
245. Stambrook M, Hamel ER, Carter SA. Training to vasodilate in a cooling environment: a valid treatment for Raynaud's phenomenon? Biofeedback Self Regul 1988; 13:9–23.
246. Guglielmi RS, Roberts AH, Patterson R. Skin temperature biofeedback for Raynaud's disease: a double-blind study. Biofeedback Self Regul 1982; 7:99–120.
247. Freedman RR, Ianni P, Wenig P. Behavioral treatment of Raynaud's phenomenon in scleroderma. J Behav Med 1984; 7:343–353.
248. Jobe JB, et al. Induced vasodilation as treatment for Raynaud's disease. Ann Intern Med 1982; 97:706–709.
249. Antman EM, et al. Calcium channel blocking agents in the treatment of cardiovascular disorders. I: Basic and clinical electrophysiologic effects. Ann Intern Med 1980; 93:875–885.
250. Stone PH, et al. Calcium channel blocking agents in the treatment of cardiovascular disorders. II: Hemodynamic effects and clinical applications. Ann Intern Med 1980; 93:886–904.
251. Creager MA, et al. Nifedipine-induced fingertip vasodilation in patients with Raynaud's phenomenon. Am Heart J 1984; 108:370–373.
252. Nilsson H, et al. The effect of the calcium-entry blocker nifedipine on cold-induced digital vasospasm. Acta Med Scand 1987; 221:53–60.
253. Winston EL, et al. Nifedipine as a therapeutic modality for Raynaud's phenomenon. Arthritis Rheum 1983; 26:1177–1180.
254. Rodeheffer RJ, et al. Controlled double-blind trial of nifedipine in the treatment of Raynaud's phenomenon. N Engl J Med 1983; 4:880–883.
255. Smith CD, McKendry RJ. Controlled trial of nifedipine in the treatment of Raynaud's phenomenon. Lancet 1982; 2:1299–1301.
256. Smith CR, Rodeheffer RJ. Raynaud's phenomenon: pathophysiologic features and treatment with calcium-channel blockers. Am J Cardiol 1985; 55:154B–157B.
257. Kahan A, et al. Nifedipine in digital ulceration in scleroderma. Arthritis Rheum 1983; 26:809.
258. Matucci Cerinic M, et al. Nifedipine treatment of Raynaud's phenomenon in a paediatric age. Int J Clin Pharm Res 1985; 5:67–69.
259. Kahan A, Amor B, Menkes CJ. A randomised double-blind trial of diltiazem in the treatment of Raynaud's phenomenon. Ann Rheum Dis 1985; 44:30–33.
260. Rhedda A, et al. A double blind placebo controlled crossover randomized trial of diltiazem in Raynaud's phenomenon. J Rheumatol 1985; 12:724–727.
261. Matoba T, Chiba M. Effects of diltiazem on occupational Raynaud's syndrome (vibration disease). Angiology 1985; 36:850–856.
262. French Cooperative Multicenter Group for Raynaud's Phenomenon. Controlled multicenter double-blind trial of nicardipine in the treatment of primary Raynaud's phenomenon. Am Heart J 1991; 122:352–355.
263. Schmidt JF, Valentin N, Nielsen SL. The clinical effect of felodipine and nifedipine in Raynaud's phenomenon. Eur J Clin Pharmacol 1989; 37:191–192.
264. Kallenberg CGM, et al. Once daily felodipine in patients with primary Raynaud's phenomenon. Eur J Clin Pharmacol 1991; 40:313–315.
265. Leppert J, et al. The effect of isradipine, a new calcium-channel antagonist in patients with primary Raynaud's phenomenon: a single-blind dose-response study. Cardiovasc Drugs Ther 1989; 3:397–401.
266. Kinney EL, et al. The treatment of severe Raynaud's phenomenon with verapamil. J Clin Pharmacol 1982; 22:74–76.
267. Parks VJ, et al. The mechanism of the vasodilator action of reserpine in man. Clin Sci 1961; 20:289–295.
268. Peacock JH. The treatment of primary Raynaud's disease of the upper limb. Lancet 1960; 2:65.
269. Willerson JT, et al. Reserpine in Raynaud's disease and phenomenon. Ann Intern Med 1970; 72:17–27.
270. McFadyen IJ, Housley E, MacPherson AIS. Intraarterial reserpine administration in Raynaud syndrome. Arch Intern Med 1973; 132:526–528.
271. Waldo R. Prazosin relieves Raynaud's vasospasm. JAMA 1979; 241:1037.
272. Nielsen SL, Vitting K, Rasmussen K. Prazosin treatment of primary Raynaud's phenomenon. Eur J Clin Pharmacol 1983; 24:421–423.
273. LeRoy EC, Downey JA, Cannon PJ. Skin capillary blood flow in scleroderma. J Clin Invest 1971; 50:930–939.
274. Varadi DP, Lawrence AM. Suppression of Raynaud's phenomenon by methyldopa. Arch Intern Med 1969; 124:13–18.
275. Coffman JD. Effect of vasodilator drugs in vasoconstricted normal subjects. J Clin Pharmacol J New Drugs 1968; 8:302–308.
276. Carter SA. Finger systolic pressures and skin temperatures in severe Raynaud's syndrome: the relationship to healing of skin lesions and the use of oral phenoxybenzamine. Angiology 1981; 32:298–310.
277. Bounameaux HM, et al. Ketanserin ($5HT_2$-antagonist) in secondary Raynaud's phenomenon. J Cardiol Pharmacol 1984; 6:975–976.
278. Cowley AJ, Jones EW, Hanley SP. Effects of dazoxiben, an inhibitor of thromboxane synthetase on forearm vasoconstriction in response to cold stimulation, and on human blood vessel prostacyclin production. Br J Clin Pharmacol 1983; 15:107s–112s.
279. Belch JJF, et al. Dazoxiben, a thromboxane synthetase inhibitor in the treatment of Raynaud's syndrome: a double blind trial. Br J Clin Pharmacol 1983; 15:113s–116s.
280. Lange RL, et al. Nonatheromatous ischemic heart disease following withdrawal from chronic industrial nitroglycerin exposure. Circulation 1972; 46:666–678.
281. Franks AG Jr. Topical glyceryl trinitrate as adjunctive treatment in Raynaud's disease. Lancet 1982; 1:76–77.
282. Carliner N, et al. Sodium nitroprusside treatment of ergotamine-induced peripheral ischemia. JAMA 1974; 227:308–309.
283. Andersen PK, et al. Sodium nitroprusside and epidural blockade in the treatment of ergotism. Med Intell 1977; 296:1271–1273.
284. Baron M, et al. Prostaglandin E_1 therapy for digital ulcers in scleroderma. Can Med Assoc J 1982; 126:42–45.
285. Clifford PC, et al. Treatment of vasospastic disease with prostaglandin E_1. Br Med J 1980; 281:1031–1034.
286. Mohrland JS, et al. A multiclinic, placebo-controlled, double-blind study of prostaglandin E_2 in Raynaud's syndrome. Ann Rheum Dis 1984; 44:756–760.
287. McHugh NJ, et al. Infusion of Iloprost, a prostacyclin analogue, for treatment of Raynaud's phenomenon in systemic sclerosis. Ann Rheum Dis 1988; 47:43–47.
288. Yardumian DA, et al. Successful treatment of Raynaud's

syndrome with Iloprost, a chemically stable prostacyclin analogue. Br J Rheumatol 1988; 27:220–226.
289. Belch JJF, et al. Intermittent epoprostenol (prostacyclin) infusion in patients with Raynaud's phenomenon. Lancet 1983; 1:313–315.
290. Wigley FM, et al. Intravenous iloprost infusion in patients with Raynaud's phenomenon secondary to systemic sclerosis. Ann Intern Med 1994; 120:199–206.
291. Belch JJ, et al. Oral iloprost as a treatment for Raynaud's syndrome: a double-blind multicentre placebo controlled study. Ann Rheum Dis 1995; 54:197–202.
292. Rademaker M, et al. Comparison of intravenous infusions of iloprost and oral nifedipine in treatment of Raynaud's phenomenon in patients with systemic sclerosis: a double blind randomized study. Br Med J 1989; 298:561–564.
293. Dessein PH, et al. Triiodothyronine treatment for Raynaud's phenomenon: a controlled trial. J Rheumatol 1990; 17:1025–1028.
294. Manart FD, et al. Upper dorsal sympathectomy. Am J Surg 1985; 150:762–766.
295. Janoff KA, Phinney ES, Porter JM. Lumbar sympathectomy for lower extremity vasospasm. Am J Surg 1985; 150:147–152.
296. Welch E, Geary J. Current status of thoracic dorsal sympathectomy. J Vasc Surg 1984; 1:202–214.
297. van de Wal HJ, et al. Thoracic sympathectomy as a therapy for upper extremity ischemia. A long-term follow-up study. Thorac Cardiovasc Surg 1985; 33:181–187.
298. de Takats G, Fowler EF. Raynaud's phenomenon. JAMA 1962; 179:99–106.
299. Johnston ENM, Summerly R, Birnstingl M. Prognosis in Raynaud's phenomenon after sympathectomy. Br Med J 1965; 1:962–964.
300. Tsur N, et al. Upper thoracic sympathectomy. Israel J Med Sci 1973; 9:53–58.
301. Gifford RW, Hines EA, Craig WM. Sympathectomy for Raynaud's phenomenon. Circulation 1958; 17:5.
302. Flatt AE. Digital artery sympathectomy. J Hand Surg 1980; 5:550–556.
303. Jones NF, et al. Surgery for scleroderma of the hand. J Hand Surg 1987; 12:391–400.
304. O'Brien BM, et al. Radical microarteriolysis in the treatment of vasospastic disorder of the hand, especially scleroderma. J Hand Surg (Br) 1992; 17:447–452.
305. Crocq C. De l'acrocyanose. Sem Med 1896; 16:297.
306. Lewis T, Landis EM. Observations upon the vascular mechanism in acrocyanosis. Heart 1930; 15:229.
307. Cassirer R. Die vasomotorisch-trophischen Neurosen, 2d ed. Berlin: S. Karger, AG, 1912. Pp. 182–274.
308. Mendlowitz M. The Digital Circulation. New York: Grune & Stratton, 1954.
309. Eliot AH, Evans RD, Stone CS. Acrocyanosis: a study of the circulatory fault. Am Heart J 1936; 11:431.
310. Lambie CG, Morson SM. Acrocyanosis. Med J Aust 1937; 2:1070.
311. Peacock JH. Vasodilation in the human hand: observations on primary Raynaud's disease and acrocyanosis of the upper extremities. Clin Sci 1957; 17:575.
312. Peacock JH. A comparative study of the digital cutaneous temperatures and hand blood flows in the normal hand, primary Raynaud's disease and primary acrocyanosis. Clin Sci 1959; 18:25–33.
313. Day R, Klingman W. Effect of sleep on skin temperature reactions in case of acrocyanosis. J Clin Invest 1939; 18:271.
314. Jacobs MJH, et al. Nomenclature of Raynaud's phenomenon: a capillary microscopic and hemorheologic study. Surgery 1987; 101:136–145.
315. Bollinger A, Mahler F, Meier B. Velocity patterns in nailfold capillaries of normal subjects and patients with Raynaud's disease and acrocyanosis. Bibl Anat 1977; 16:142–145.
316. Franzeck UK, et al. Vidiodensitometric pattern recognition of Na-fluorescein diffusion in nailfold capillary areas of patients with acrocyanosis, primary vasospastic and secondary Raynaud's phenomenon. Int Angiol 1983; 2:143.
317. Stern ES. The aetiology and pathology of acrocyanosis. Br J Dermatol Syph 1937; 49:100.
318. Boas E. Capillaries of extremities in acrocyanosis. JAMA 1942; 79:1404.
319. Williams C, Goodman H. Livedo reticularis. JAMA 1925; 85:955.
320. Milian G. Les atrophies cutanees syphilitiques. Bull Soc Fr Dermatol Syphigr 1929; 36:865.
321. Barker NW, Hines EA Jr, Craig WM. Livedo reticularis: a peripheral arteriolar disease. Am Heart J 1941; 21:592.
322. Winkelmann RK, et al. Clinical studies of livedoid vasculitis (segmental hyalinizing vasculitis). Mayo Clinic Proc 1974; 49:746–750.
323. McHugh NJ, et al. Anticardiolipin antibodies, livedo reticularis, and major cerebrovascular and renal disease in systemic lupus erythematosus. Ann Rheum Dis 1988; 47:110–115.
324. Weinstein C, et al. Livedo reticularis associated with increased titers of anticardiolipin antibodies in systemic lupus erythematosus. Arch Dermatol 1987; 123:596–600.
325. Sneddon IB. Cerebrovascular lesions and livedo reticularis. Br J Dermatol 1965; 77:180.
326. Rebollo M, et al. Livedo reticularis and cerebrovascular lesions (Sneddon's syndrome). Brain 1983; 106:965–979.
327. Heimans RLH, Rand MH, Fennessy MR. Some actions of amantadine on peripheral tissues. J Pharm Pharmacol 1972; 24:869–874.
328. Pearch LA, Waterbury LD, Green HD. Amantadine hydrochloride: alteration in peripheral circulation. Neurology 1974; 24:46–48.
329. Cunliffe WJ, Menon IS. The association between cutaneous vasculitis and decreased blood fibrinolytic activity. Br J Dermatol 1971; 84:99–105.
330. Drucker CR, Duncan WC. Antiplatelet therapy in atrophie blanche and livedo vasculitis. J Am Acad Dermatol 1982; 7:359–363.
331. Yamamoto M, et al. Antithrombotic treatment in livedo vasculitis. J Am Acad Dermatol 1988; 18:57–62.
332. Cabbabe EB, Clift SD. Leg ulcerations in livedoid vasculitis. Plast Reconstr Surg 1985; 75:888–891.
333. Feldaker M, Hines EAJ, Kierland RR. Livedo reticularis with ulcerations. Circulation 1956; 13:196.
334. Schroeter AL, et al. Livedo vasculitis (the vasculitis of atrophie blanche). Arch Dermatol 1975; 111:188–193.
335. Silver DE, Sahs AL. Livedo reticularis in Parkinson's disease patients treated with amantadine hydrochloride. Neurology 1972; 22:665–669.
336. Coffman JD. Clinical forum: atheroembolism after cardiac surgery. J Vasc Med Biol 1989; 1:37–41.
337. Gilliam J, Herndon JH, Prystowsky SD. Fibrinolytic therapy for vasculitis of atrophie blanche. Arch Dermatol 1974; 109:664–667.
338. Milstone LM, et al. Classification and therapy of atrophie blanche. Arch Dermatol 1983; 119:963–969.
339. Purcell SM, Hayes TJ. Nifedipine treatment of idiopathic atrophie blanche. J Am Acad Dermatol 1986; 14:851–854.
340. Spittell JA Jr. Diseases of the vascular system related to temperature. In JF Fairbairn II, JL Juergens, JA Spittell Jr, eds. Peripheral Vascular Diseases. Philadelphia: Saunders, 1972.
341. Rustin MH, et al. The treatment of chilblains with nifedipine: the results of a pilot study, a double-blind placebo-controlled

randomized study and a long-term open trial. Br J Dermatol 1989; 120:267–275.
342. White JC. Vascular and neurologic lesions in survivors of shipwreck. N Engl J Med 1943; 228:211.
343. Wrenn K. Immersion foot. A problem of the homeless in the 1990s. Arch Intern Med 1991; 151:785–788.
344. Akers WA. Paddy foot: a warm water immersion foot syndrome variant. Milit Med 1974; 139:605–618.
345. Allen AM, Taplin D. Tropical immersion foot. Lancet 1973; 2:1185–1188.
346. Kyösola K. Clinical experiences in the management of cold injuries: A study of 110 cases. J Trauma 1974; 14:32–36.
347. Douglas JS Jr, Eby CS. Silicone for immersion foot prophylaxis: where and how much to use. Milit Med 1972; 137:386–387.
348. Washburn B. Frostbite: what is it—how to prevent it—emergency treatment. N Engl J Med 1962; 266:974–989.
349. Meryman HT. Tissue freezing and local cold injury. Physiol Rev 1957; 37:233–251.
350. Marzella L, et al. Morphologic characterization of acute injury to vascular endothelium of skin after frostbite. Plastic Reconstr Surg 1989; 83:67–76.
351. Golding M, et al. The role of sympathectomy in frostbite, with review of 68 cases. Surgery 1965; 57:774.
352. Mitchell SW. Clinical lecture on certain painful affections of the feet. Phila Med Times 1872; 3:81–113.
353. Smith JL, Allen T. Syndrome of burning, painful extremities. Arch Intern Med 1938; 15:121.
354. Finley WH, et al. Autosomol dominant erythromelalgia. Am J Med Genetics 1992; 42:310–315.
355. Michiels JJ, et al. Erythromelalgia caused by platelet-mediated arteriolar inflammation and thrombosis in thrombocythemia. Ann Intern Med 1985; 102:466–471.
356. Redding KG. Thrombocythemia as a cause of erythromalgia. Arch Dermatol 1977; 113:468–471.
357. Kurzrock R, Cohen PR. Erythromelalgia and myeloproliferative disorders. Arch Intern Med 1989; 149:105–109.
358. Alarcon-Segovia D, Diaz-Jouanen E. Case report: erythromelalgia in systemic lupus erythematosus. Am J Med Sci 1973; 266:149–151.
359. Zheng ZM, et al. Poxviruses isolated from epidemic erythromelalgia in China. Lancet 1988; 1:296.
360. Drenth JPH. Erythromelalgia induced by nicardipine. Br Med J 1989; 298:1582.
361. Brodmerkel GJ Jr. Nifedipine and erythromelalgia. Ann Intern Med 1983; 98:671.
362. Drenth JPH, et al. Verapamil-induced secondary erythermalgia. Br J Dermatol 1992; 127:292–294.
363. Eisler T, et al. Erythromelalgia-like eruption in Parkinsonian patients treated with bromocriptine. Neurology (NY) 1981; 31:1368–1370.
364. Lazareth I, Priollet P. Coexistence of Raynaud's syndrome and erythromelalgia. Lancet 1990; 335:1286.
365. Lewis T. Clinical observations and experiments relating to burning pain in the extremities, and to so-called "erythromelalgia" in particular. Clin Sci 1933; 1:175.
366. Calderone DC, Finzi E. Treatment of primary erythromelalgia with piroxicam. J Am Acad Dermatol 1991; 24:145–146.
367. Priollet P, et al. Erythromelalgia without arteriolar changes. Ann Intern Med 1985; 103:639.
368. Bada JL. Treatment of erythromelalgia with propranolol. Lancet 1977; 2:412.

The Clinical Spectrum of Vasculitis

Sheldon M. Wolff
Kenneth M. Pariser

Systemic Vasculitis

The vasculitic syndromes are heterogeneous in their pathologic and clinical features. Their single constant pathologic feature is inflammation of the vessel wall, often accompanied by necrosis. Although that finding is invariable in vasculitis, it also can be a consequence of a contiguous process. For example, there is dramatic blood vessel inflammatory infiltration and necrosis in the delayed-type hypersensitivity reaction of skin-contact sensitivity [1]. Inflammation and necrosis are not, therefore, pathognomonic of a primary vessel wall disorder. Such findings must be interpreted in light of the clinical situation.

Historically, the size, type, and location of the inflamed blood vessel as well as the type of inflammatory cell infiltrating the vessel were the major criteria for Zeek's classification of the vasculitic syndromes [2,3]. Overlap of the pathologic findings, however, makes it necessary for clinicians to integrate the clinical findings with the histology to create more workable classification schemes [4,5].

The schemata employed today by both clinicians and pathologists are in many ways revised versions of Zeek's original classification. They frequently group vasculitic syndromes on the basis of clinical findings, pathology, and prognosis. That practical approach assists in the diagnosis and management of patients. Still, the current classifications are hampered by the lack of established etiologies and the limited understanding of the pathophysiology of these diseases.

Table 43-1 is an adaptation of the classification presented by Fauci in 1978 [6]. Group I consists of the systemic necrotizing vasculitides. Those syndromes involve the major organ systems by destruction of medium-sized muscular arteries with an inflammatory infiltrate that often progresses to fibrinoid necrosis of the vessel wall [7]. In each condition, smaller vessels may be involved, mimicking the changes seen in the hypersensitivity vasculitides [8–11].

The hypersensitivity vasculitides, group II, are notable for the predominance of dermatologic findings with sporadic damage to the major organ systems, as seen in group I. The group II conditions commonly are either secondary to an underlying disease or a result of exposure to an environmental agent. The histologic picture is venulitis with leukocytoclasis, perivascular nuclear dust or debris (hence the term leukocytoclastic vasculitis), endothelial swelling, red blood cell extravasation, and fibrinoid necrosis.

Group III consists of two conditions with features that warrant a separate grouping. Although there are striking clinical and more subtle pathologic differences between Takayasu arteritis and temporal arteritis, both conditions demonstrate the distinct propensity for the large, elastic arteries. Infiltration of the vessel wall with giant cells and mononuclear cells and a segmental panarteritis, often with dramatic ischemic consequences, are characteristic of both disorders.

Several other entities are individually classified because of their particular clinical and pathologic findings, suggesting that they are separate diseases. Although the etiology and pathogenesis of those syndromes are not understood, the distinctions suggest that they are different processes.

The Diagnosis of Vasculitis

The relative infrequency of vasculitis often results in a delay in diagnosis. Given the low incidence, what clinical problems should alert the physician to the possibility that a systemic vasculitis is the diagnosis? First, the presence of a multisystem inflammatory condition is the classic situation suggesting a vasculitis (e.g., involvement of the skin, peripheral nerves, kidneys, and lungs).

Second, the final common pathway of tissue damage in vasculitis is often ischemia. Therefore, ischemic symptoms or events (1) in a person under 55 years of age, (2) involving organs or limbs in a distribution not typical of atherosclerotic peripheral vascular disease, or (3) occurring at an unusually accelerated rate should suggest vasculitis.

Within each organ system, certain problems may be more indicative of vasculitis than others. Table 43-2 lists signs that commonly occur in the first three vasculitic groups. The detection of palpable purpura, mononeuritis multiplex, migratory arthralgias and arthritis, muscle weakness and myalgias, active glomerulonephritis, and fleeting pulmonary infiltrates in conjunction with systemic symptoms of fatigue, malaise, anorexia, and weight loss suggests vasculitis. With those considerations in mind, the clinician cannot limit the physical examination to a single system but must be thorough, uncovering early signs of pathology to establish a diagnosis and prevent irreversible tissue damage.

LABORATORY EVALUATION

The clinical laboratory testing ordered for a patient with suspected vasculitis has two functions: to establish the diagnosis and to aid in management of the disease. For the first purpose, testing can range from routine evaluations—complete blood counts, urinalysis, blood cultures, liver-function tests, chest x-rays, and sedimentation rates—to more selected tests for partial characterization of the immunopathophysiology—serum complement components, autoantibodies, rheumatoid factors, antinuclear antibodies, antineutrophil cytoplasmic autoantibodies, cryoglobulins, serum or urine immunoelectrophoresis, immune complex assays, anti–hepatitis C virus, HBsAg, and anti-HBsAg. Ultimately, establishing a diagnosis depends on pathologic material or angiographic demonstration of a vasculopathy.

Table 43-1. The vasculitides[a]

GROUP I	
Systemic necrotizing vasculitides	
Polyarteritis nodosa	
Churg-Strauss Syndrome[b]	
Rheumatoid vasculitis[a]	
Wegener's granulomatosis[a,b]	
Essential cryoglobulinemia[a]	
GROUP II	
Hypersensitivity vasculitides	
Primary	
Microscopic polyarteritis nodosa[b]	
Henoch-Schönlein purpura	
Hypersensitivity vasculitis	
Erythema elevatum diutinum	
Secondary	
Mixed cryoglobulinemia	
Serum sickness	
Urticarial vasculitis (hypocomplementemic vasculitis)	
Vasculitis associated with infectious diseases, connective-tissue diseases, neoplasms, drugs, and other disorders (colitis, hepatitis, posttransplantation)	
GROUP III	
Giant cell arteritis	
Temporal arteritis	
Takayasu arteritis	
GROUP IV	
Miscellaneous	
Angiocentric immunoproliferative lesions	
Kawasaki syndrome	
Behçet's disease	
Cogan's syndrome	
Thromboangiitis obliterans	
Others	

[a] Syndrome may be present as either systemic necrotizing vasculitide or hypersensitivity vasculitide.
[b] Syndrome associated with antineutrophil cytoplasmic autoantibodies.
Source: Adapted from AS Fauci, BF Haynes, P Katz. The spectrum of vasculitis. Clinical, pathologic, immunologic, and therapeutic considerations. Ann Intern Med 1978; 89:660–676.

Two types of laboratory tests are used in conjunction with the history and physical examination to manage disease in vasculitic patients. The first type are tests that measure the inflammatory state, such as the erythrocyte sedimentation rate or C-reactive protein. Similarly, tests measuring circulating immune complexes, cryoglobulins, or autoantibodies have been used to monitor disease activity. Those tests aid in determining the overall activity of the vasculitis. Organ-specific measurements, documenting improvement or deterioration in the function of the kidneys, lungs, central and peripheral nervous system, and heart must be followed to determine the progress of treatment. Monitoring patients for adverse effects of the therapy is also a regular part of the patient's care. A review of selected tests most frequently used in diagnosing and managing patients with vasculitis follows.

Selected Tests

ERYTHROCYTE SEDIMENTATION RATE

An erythrocyte sedimentation rate is a useful test when there is a clear understanding of its limitations. The Westergren method for measuring red blood cell sedimentation is preferred. It must be interpreted with knowledge of the patient's age and sex. The normal rate of erythrocyte sedimentation increases with age at approximately 0.5 mm/hour/year [12]. In women, the usual rate of sedimentation is approximately 10 mm/hour faster than in men [12].

The erythrocyte sedimentation rate is determined predominantly by the degree to which erythrocytes align themselves in an aggregate that resembles a stack of coins, or rouleaux [13,14]. Increases in acute-phase plasma proteins, particularly fibrinogen and immunoglobulins, play the major role in aggregating red blood cells and facilitate rapid sedimentation [15]. Similarly, the shape and size of the red blood cells alter their ability to aggregate. Spherocytosis, acanthocytosis, poikilocytosis, and anisocytosis all reduce rouleaux formation [13]. Those alterations in the red blood cell may be sufficient to normalize an erythrocyte sedimentation rate even in the face of a considerable increase in acute-phase proteins.

The erythrocyte sedimentation rate does not offer any diagnostic specificity; instead, it imperfectly reflects the amount of tissue injury, inflammation, and plasma cell production of immunoglobulin. It can be falsely reassuring and normal even in the face of proven active vasculitis [16,17]. The erythrocyte sedimentation rate is most useful in assisting the clinician to evaluate the degree of inflammatory activity. It is more reliable with certain vasculitides, such as temporal arteritis, Wegener's granulomatosis, polyarteritis nodosa, and Takayasu arteritis [18–20]. It can be normal, however, despite active inflammation, in hypersensitivity vasculitis, isolated central nervous system vasculitis, and angiocentric immunoproliferative lesions [21–23]. In summary, the erythrocyte sedimentation rate is a marginally acceptable screening test and measure of disease activity. The test often can be misleading, so it cannot stand on its own in the diagnosis or management of vasculitis.

C-REACTIVE PROTEIN

C-reactive protein (CRP) is a pentameric protein weighing about 105,000 daltons that was originally detected in human serum because it precipitated the C-polysaccharide of the pneumococcus [24]. It has a wide range of physiologic functions in response to tissue injury and inflammation. The normal level of CRP varies from 0.05 to 0.20 mg/dl [25]. Within several hours of an inflammatory stimulus, there is a rapid increase in the serum concentration of CRP. The rise correlates with the degree of injury [26]. Measurement of CRP has been shown to be a useful method for following the response to therapy in patients with polyarteritis nodosa [27].

Increases of serum concentrations that do not exceed 1 mg/dl are usually considered minor elevations. Levels between 1 and 10 mg/dl reflect moderate amounts of inflammation or tissue damage. Increases above 10 mg/dl indicate severe inflammation [28]. Experience with this test in the management of vasculitides is limited, and it should be considered experimental, despite the fact that CRP was first described in 1930.

Table 43-2. Common signs of vasculitis

Organ	Group I	Group II	Group III
Skin	Palpable purpura, ulcers, digital ischemia	Purpura macules, bullae, urticaria, vesicles, Raynaud's phenomenon	Raynaud's phenomenon
Musculoskeletal system	Arthritis, myalgia, weakness	Arthralgia, mild symmetric arthritis, myalgia	Polymyalgia, mild arthritis
Central nervous system	Cerebrovascular accident, encephalopathy, myelopathy	Cerebrovascular accident	Cerebrovascular accident, visual loss, headache
Peripheral nervous system	Mononeuritis multiplex, polyneuropathy	Polyneuropathy	Carpal tunnel syndrome
GI tract	Ischemic bowel, pancreatitis, melena	Bleeding, colicky pain, intussusception	Ischemic bowel
Heart	Angina, myocardial infarction, congestive heart failure, heart block, pericarditis	Pericarditis, myocarditis	Angina, congestive heart failure, shortness of breath
Kidney	Hematuria, renal failure, nephrosis, hypertension	Hematuria, nephrosis	Renal artery stenosis, hematuria
Lung	Hemoptysis, cough, shortness of breath, wheezing, pleurisy	Hemoptysis	Cough, hemoptysis

COMPLETE BLOOD COUNT

Abnormalities in the complete blood count are the rule rather than the exception in patients with vasculitis. A moderate leukocytosis and neutrophilia are common. On the other hand, patients with vasculitis related to an underlying malignancy (e.g., hairy-cell leukemia), systemic lupus erythematosus, or vasculitis induced by acute hepatitis B are often leukopenic. Eosinophilia is nearly universal in patients with Churg-Strauss syndrome [29]. It also is found in some patients with hypersensitivity vasculitis and may, on occasion, be found in nearly any vasculitic syndrome.

Thrombocytosis is a typical finding in these inflammatory conditions. A normochromic, normocytic anemia also is commonly reported in the various vasculitides. Intravascular hemolytic anemia due to fragmentation of the red cells (microangiopathic hemolytic anemia) or blood loss from the gastrointestinal tract may accompany the more typical anemia of chronic disease.

COMPLEMENT ASSAYS

The complement cascade, a series of plasma proteins that, when triggered, mediate an inflammatory reaction, is frequently measured during the assessment of patients with vasculitis. The CH_{50} is a functional assay of the entire classic complement sequence. It quantifies the hemolysis of antibody-coated red blood cells [30]. It is a useful screening test for complement-deficiency states, whether inherited or acquired. The measurement of individual complement proteins usually is done by radial immunodiffusion or nephelometry [31], a type of assay most commonly used to measure C4 and C3, two early components of the complement cascade. The range of normal serum concentrations of the complement proteins is quite wide; the levels reflect the balance between production and utilization. Production of complement proteins is markedly increased in most inflammatory states [32].

The complement cascade can be triggered by circulating immune complexes as well as tissue-fixed immune complexes, both of which are sometimes found in vasculitis [22,33]. Despite the rapid utilization of complement, the assayed levels of complement in vasculitis often are not depressed [34]. The levels may, in fact, be lower than those found in inflammatory conditions not associated with chronic antigenemia or circulating immune complexes [35].

Low or falling levels of complement are found in certain active vasculitides, particularly essential mixed cryoglobulinemia, systemic lupus erythematosus, rheumatoid vasculitis, serum sickness, and urticarial vasculitis (hypocomplementemic vasculitis), and occasionally in polyarteritis nodosa. Normal or elevated levels are the rule in the granulomatous vasculitides (Wegener's granulomatosis, Churg-Strauss syndrome, angiocentric immunoproliferative lesions); the giant cell arteritides (temporal arteritis and Takayasu arteritis); Behçet's syndrome; isolated central nervous system vasculitis; and most cases of polyarteritis nodosa [22,33–36].

CIRCULATING IMMUNE COMPLEXES

Circulating immune complexes are a diverse group of noncovalently bound antigens and antibodies. The formation of these complexes usually is beneficial for the host, expediting the clearance of exogenous antigens by the fixed mononuclear phagocytic system. Soluble immune complexes, however, can deposit in vessel walls, the glomerular basement membranes, and the synovial membrane, resulting in vasculitis, glomerulitis, and arthritis [35].

Immune complexes have been detected in several vasculitides [37]. They have been detected in tissue specimens by electron microscopy and by specific immunohistochemical staining. Their presence in serum has been demonstrated by physiochemical techniques and biologic and immunologic assays. Some of the most commonly used techniques are briefly reviewed here.

I_{125} C1q Binding Assay. This fluid-phase binding assay is most useful in detecting complexes containing IgG subclasses 1, 2, and 3 as well as IgM. Ethylenediaminetetraacetic acid (EDTA)–treated serum in the presence of 2.5-percent polyethylene glycol is mixed with a known amount of I_{125} C1q. The percent of I_{125} C1q precipitated correlates with the level of circulating immune complexes [38]. False-positive tests can be induced by aggregated immunoglobulins or heparin. False-negative results have been reported in some patients with circulating free DNA.

C1q Solid-Phase Assay. This assay is based on principles similar to those of the I_{125} C1q binding assay. This technique is likely to detect the same types of immune complexes as the fluid-phase assay [39]. C1q in this assay is attached to the sides of plastic tubes. Any immune complexes that bind to C1q are then detected with radiolabeled antihuman immunoglobulin. False-positive results can be induced with aggregated immunoglobulins and serum IgM rheumatoid factor.

Raji Cell Radioimmunassay. This test uses Raji cells, which are human lymphoblastoid cells with surface receptors for C1q, C3b, and C3bi. This assay can detect circulating immune complexes containing those complement components and IgG with radiolabeled anti-IgG antibody [40]. Serum with antilymphocyte antibodies, for instance, in patients with systemic lupus erythematosus, gives false-positive results.

Monoclonal Rheumatoid Factor Assays. These tests measure rheumatoid factors, which bind with a high affinity to the Fc portion of aggregated IgG. Monoclonal rheumatoid factors, derived from patients with lymphoproliferative diseases, can be standardized and used to detect circulating immune complexes that contain IgG. The rheumatoid factors usually are attached to a solid-phase matrix. The patient's serum is tested against a known amount of radiolabeled, aggregated IgG in a competitive assay. False-negative results are found in patients with high-titer rheumatoid factor in their own serum.

Interpretation of results of the complement assays is complicated: serum samples must be collected in a standardized fashion; serum factors may interfere with the assay; and the different sensitivities and specificities of the various methods may make comparison of techniques difficult. Assays that may be appropriate for one disease, such as technologies detecting IgA-containing circulating immune complexes in Henoch-Schönlein purpura, may not detect immune complexes found in other vasculitides [41]. These tests are not of diagnostic value, but in carefully controlled situations, they may be of value in the management of patients with vasculitis.

CRYOGLOBULINS

Cryoglobulins are immunoglobulins that, although soluble at 37°C, precipitate at reduced temperatures. They are classified into three types: Type I are single monoclonal immunoglobulins; Type II are monoclonal immunoglobulins with rheumatoid-factor activity complexed to polyclonal immunoglobulins; and type III are complexes of polyclonal immunoglobulins, some of which have rheumatoid activity [42].

Table 43-3. Disease associations with cryoglobulin type

Associated disease	Cryoglobulin type I	II	III
Multiple myeloma	+++	++	
Waldenstrom's macroglobulinemia	+++	+++	
Lymphoma	++	+++	+
Connective tissue diseases (systemic lupus erythematosus, rheumatoid arthritis, Sjögren's syndrome)		++	+++
Chronic infections (hepatitis C, subacute bacterial endocarditis, cytomegalovirus, Lyme disease, Epstein-Barr virus, toxoplasmosis, hepatitis B)		++	+++
Chronic inflammatory disease (sarcoidosis, ulcerative colitis)		+++	
Essential cryoglobulinemia		++	+++

Key: + = occasional; ++ = common; +++ = usual.

Cryoglobulins are detected in patients with infectious, rheumatic, and neoplastic diseases. Type I and II cryoglobulins often are associated with lymphoproliferative diseases. Type I cryoglobulins may have clinical manifestations of hyperviscosity as well as vasculitis. Types II and III more often produce vasculitic signs and symptoms than manifestations of hyperviscosity [42]. The cryoglobulins found in patients with essential mixed cryoglobulinemia are types II and III [43]. In addition to essential cryoglobulinemia, cryoglobulins can be found in other vasculitic syndromes, including polyarteritis nodosa and Henoch-Schönlein purpura and in autoimmune diseases, such as systemic lupus erythematosus and Sjögren's syndrome. They are also found in other nonviral infectious diseases, such as malaria and syphilis [43,44].

Collection of the sample for cryoglobulins must be done with care to avoid cooling before clotting and centrifugation are complete. Failure to observe that rule will result in loss of cryoprecipitable material. Samples should be held at 4°C for at least 72 hours to allow time for precipitation of the cryoglobulins [45]. Levels greater than 0.1 mg/dl usually are considered abnormal. After quantitation, patients with elevated levels of cryoglobulin should have that cryoglobulin characterized. As mentioned, lymphoproliferative diseases are seen in the majority of those patients with type I or II cryoglobulins (Table 43-3).

ANTINEUTROPHIL CYTOPLASM AUTOANTIBODIES

In 1982, eight patients with segmental glomerulonephritis were reported to have IgG antibodies directed against the cytoplasm of fixed neutrophils, or antineutrophil cytoplasm autoantibodies (ANCA) [46]. Subsequent descriptions of those antibodies found a high degree of specificity for Wegener's granulomatosis when an indirect immunofluorescence assay produced a diffuse granular cytoplasmic staining pattern (C-ANCA) [47]. Further characterization of the antibodies has indicated that they are directed at an enzyme, proteinase 3 [48]. Antibodies that produce a perinuclear pattern by indirect immunofluorescence (P-ANCA) appear to be directed at neutrophil myeloperoxidase and elastase. They are found in some patients with vasculitis and frequently in patients with necrotizing and crescentic pauci-immune glomerulonephritis [49,50].

The specificity for Wegener's granulomatosis of autoantibodies producing granular cytoplasmic staining approaches 93 percent [51–53]. The sensitivity correlates with the extent and activity of the disease. In active localized disease, two-thirds of patients have positive assays, compared with 90 percent of patients with active generalized Wegener's granulomatosis. There may be a correlation between rising titers of ANCA and a relapse of disease [53], although other studies find a poor predictive value of changing ANCA titers and clinical disease [54].

RHEUMATOID FACTORS

Rheumatoid factors are antibodies that bind to the Fc portion of IgG. Classically, the rheumatoid factor is an IgM immunoglobulin; however, rheumatoid activity may be found in all the other classes of immunoglobulin. Rheumatoid factors are seen in a large number of conditions besides rheumatoid arthritis [55]. It is reported in some patients in most of the vasculitic syndromes. The titer detected in those conditions is variable [23,56–58], and so it has little diagnostic value in patients with vasculitis.

QUANTITATIVE IMMUNOGLOBULIN LEVELS

Elevated levels of polyclonal immunoglobulins are a common finding in vasculitis. In certain syndromes, elevations of one class of immunoglobulins are characteristic; for instance, IgA is frequently elevated in Henoch-Schönlein purpura [59]. IgE is sometimes elevated in Churg-Strauss syndrome, in Kawasaki syndrome, and in some patients with polyarteritis nodosa [31,57,60,61]. Most reported series of vasculitis have described elevations of IgG in patients.

These findings are not specific or diagnostic but, like the sedimentation rate, are evidence of an inflammatory condition. Monoclonal elevation of a class of immunoglobulins, on the other hand, suggests an underlying lymphoproliferative disease, making immunoelectrophoresis a valuable test in that setting.

SEROLOGIC TESTS FOR HEPATITIS B AND C

Between 30 and 68 percent of patients with systemic necrotizing vasculitis have evidence of chronic hepatitis B infection. HBsAg, anti-HBC, or anti-HBsAg has been found in the serum, in circulatory complexes, or in inflamed vessel walls [62–66]. A hypersensitivity type of vasculitis is seen in acute and chronic hepatitis B [67]. In patients with that syndrome, HBsAg and circulating complexes of HBsAg-anti-HBsAg are found [67,68]. Mixed cryoglobulinemia is much less frequently associated with hepatitis B infection. Instead, most cases appear related to hepatitis C virus infection [69–71]. All patients with hypersensitivity vasculitis, systemic necrotizing vasculitis, or mixed cryoglobulinemia should be tested for hepatitis B and C infection.

SINUS RADIOGRAPHS

Wegener's granulomatosis classically involves the upper respiratory tract early in the disease, with over half the patients presenting with sinusitis or nasal obstruction [72]. Ultimately, clinical paranasal sinus disease is evident in over 90 percent of patients [56]. Plain radiographs and computer tomography demonstrate a range of findings from mucosal thickening to air fluid levels. In severe cases, erosion through the walls of the sinuses occurs. Destruction of the hard palate or erosion through the skin, however, should suggest other upper respiratory diseases, such as midline granuloma [73].

BLOOD CULTURES

Before a diagnosis of vasculitis is made, it is critical to exclude bacteremia. Subacute bacterial endocarditis (SBE), intravascular infections, and chronic meningococcemia all may be misdiagnosed as an idiopathic vasculitic syndrome, usually of the hypersensitivity type. Mycotic aneurysms, found in up to 15 percent of patients with SBE, can simulate the angiographic findings of polyarteritis nodosa [74]. Fungal endocarditis can result in large-vessel thrombosis and inflammation, suggesting an arteritis.

RENAL-FUNCTION TESTS

Abnormalities in renal-function tests are common in most vasculitis syndromes. The alterations range from hematuria and slight proteinuria to rapidly progressive glomerulonephritis, nephrotic syndrome, and acute renal failure. The hypersensitivity types of vasculitis are more likely to manifest minor changes in the urinalysis without a decrease in the glomerular filtration rate. Systemic necrotizing vasculitides commonly are associated with reduced renal function, as are Wegener's granulomatosis and mixed cryoglobulinemia.

VASCULAR IMAGING STUDIES

For diagnosis as well as evaluation of therapy, angiographic studies play an important role in the management of vasculitides. As a method of diagnosis, it has particular usefulness in polyarteritis nodosa, Takayasu arteritis, thromboangiitis obliterans (Buerger's disease), and some cases of isolated central nervous system angiitis.

Saccular aneurysms in the vessels of multiple organ systems commonly are found in polyarteritis nodosa [75]. Abnormalities in vessel caliber and fusiform aneurysms are detected as well. Normal arteriograms do not exclude the diagnosis of polyarteritis nodosa, since they are found in up to 20 percent of cases [75]. Conversely, aneurysms may be detected in medium-sized arteries in many other diseases [74,76].

The angiographic changes involving the aortic arch and its primary branches in Takayasu arteritis often are diagnostic [77]. Similar success with that diagnostic approach in thromboangiitis obliterans has been reported [78]. In contrast, angiographic studies in temporal arteritis in the elderly are not diagnostic, although such studies may direct the clinician to the best site for biopsy [79]. In isolated central nervous system vasculitis, the angiogram frequently is abnormal, showing beading and multifocal, segmental narrowing in leptomeningeal and intracranial vessels [80].

The arteriogram has been used to demonstrate aneurysmal healing in patients with polyarteritis nodosa [81]. Thus, serial imaging studies may be of use to the clinician in management of the patient with systemic necrotizing arteritis. Ultrasonography and MRI in conjunction with angiography have been shown to be useful in monitoring and diagnosing selected patients with Takayasu arteritis [82–84].

It is important in polyarteritis nodosa and Takayasu arteritis to obtain a thorough angiographic study. In the former, a celiac study and a renal study are necessary, because abnormalities may not be present in both circulations. In the latter, a full aortogram may detect unanticipated disease [85].

TISSUE BIOPSY

Pathologic evaluation of diseased tissue usually is the means by which a diagnosis of vasculitis is confirmed. The tissues may be the result of an emergent surgical procedure (e.g., resection of ischemic intestine or inflamed gallbladder) or, more frequently, an elective biopsy of a symptomatic site. The selection of the site for biopsy depends on the preoperative diagnosis, the evidence for clinical involvement, and the morbidity of the procedure.

The preoperative clinical diagnosis substantially influences the diagnostic yield of a biopsy. For example, a temporal-artery biopsy for giant cell arteritis in the elderly is extremely useful and has a low morbidity [86]. The same procedure is much less useful in polyarteritis nodosa, although reports of temporal-artery involvement in polyarteritis exist [87]. In Churg-Strauss syndrome, Wegener's granulomatosis, and angiocentric lymphoproliferative lesions, biopsies of the lung have a relatively high yield [29,56,88]. Renal and sinus biopsies often are not diagnostic in Wegener's granulomatosis [89].

Symptoms and signs play a critical role in the yield of a biopsy. In hypersensitivity vasculitis, an active, fresh skin lesion has the highest yield [90]. Blind biopsies of testicular tissue in systemic necrotizing arteritis have a relatively low yield [91]. Blind muscle biopsies are slightly more productive, since diagnostic findings are reported in one-third of cases [92]. These considerations, along with recognition of the risks of the procedure, dictate the selection of the site for pathologic examination.

Clinical Summaries

POLYARTERITIS NODOSA

First clearly defined pathologically by Kussmaul and Maier in 1866 and called periarteritis nodosa because of the numerous nodules found along the course of the muscular arteries, polyarteritis nodosa was renamed at the turn of the century when the true nature of the nodules was defined [93,94]. Polyarteritis nodosa is a necrotizing arteritis that can involve small and medium-sized arteries of most organs but especially the kidney, liver, intestine, peripheral nerve, skin, and muscle. The inflammatory lesions found at biopsy usually are at different stages of development, with fresh as well as healing lesions evident in the same specimen. Sparing of the pulmonary vessels is characteristic [2].

Clinical Features. Systemic manifestations of anorexia, weight loss, fever, and fatigue are seen in the majority of patients [95]. Patients not infrequently present with those or other nonspecific complaints [96]. More commonly, a patient presents with those systemic complaints, along with one or more organ-related symptoms such as abdominal pain, myalgias, arthralgias, or paresthesias. Conversely, a rare patient may present with involvement of a single-organ system (e.g., appendix or uterus) without evidence of systemic disease [90,97,98].

Gastrointestinal-tract involvement is exceedingly common and may manifest as abdominal pain, nausea, vomiting, or diarrhea, thus reflecting the potential for disease the entire length of the gastrointestinal tract. Intestinal involvement may produce a clinical picture ranging from steatorrhea and malabsorption to ischemic colitis or bowel infarction [99,100]. Vasculitis of the gallbladder, appendix, and pancreas produces symptoms similar to other inflammatory conditions involving those organs. The most serious gastroenterologic complications of polyarteritis nodosa are bleeding, perforation, and infarction. Bowel infarction is one of the leading causes of death [101,102]. Hepatic involvement frequently is evidenced only by abnormal liver-function tests.

Myalgias, arthralgias, and arthritis are found in over half the patients. The myalgias are the result of ischemia of the muscles, which can on occasion produce intermittent claudication [103]. A nondeforming polyarthritis involving the larger joints in the lower extremities is the most common joint manifestation [96].

A high percentage of patients complain of neuropathic symptoms even early in the course of the disease. The classic pattern of neuropathy is mononeuritis multiplex, but a **stocking-glove** type of peripheral sensory neuropathy and a distal sensorimotor polyneuropathy are frequent. Mononeuritis tends to develop rapidly with the onset of pain, paresthesias, or weakness. Recovery with treatment is slow and often incomplete. The distal polyneuropathy has a more subacute onset; recovery is variable [104]. Histologic studies demonstrate vasculitic involvement of the vasa nervorum.

Although found in far fewer patients than is peripheral neuropathy, central nervous system complications are the second most common cause of death in polyarteritis nodosa [104]. The most common clinical problems are focal or multifocal thrombotic and hemorrhagic cerebral vascular accidents. A more diffuse encephalopathy of insidious onset is the other common clinical finding. Seizures, spinal-cord lesions, and cranial-nerve abnormalities are less common [20,104]. Ocular manifestations may be the result of hypertensive changes or retinal, ciliary, or choroidal arterial occlusion and aneurysm.

Involvement of the kidney is of critical importance because it is (1) the most frequently involved organ and (2) responsible for the largest percentage of deaths [105]. When present, renal disease may be due to arteritis (70%) or to segmental glomerulonephritis (30%). Usually, involvement is asymptomatic, with only hypertension or hematuria seen in one-third to one-half of patients [105]. Occasionally, patients present with uremia or flank pain, hematuria, and shock secondary to rupture of an aneurysm.

Cardiac manifestations, evident in one-third of patients, reflect coronary-artery inflammation and are manifest as angina, infarction, or congestive heart failure. Less frequently, arrhythmias and pericarditis are found. Pathologically, cardiac involvement is found in two-thirds of the autopsies, suggesting that its presence implies a poor prognosis. In fact, heart disease is the third leading cause of death in polyarteritis nodosa [106].

Dermatologic findings are part of the clinical picture in 40 percent of patients. The signs are highly variable. Livedo reticularis, purpura, urticaria, and ulcers frequently are reported. Classic subcutaneous painful nodules on the lower extremities are found in less than 15 percent [107].

Laboratory. Frequent abnormalities are a high sedimentation rate (over 90%), leukocytosis (75%), anemia (66%), abnormal urinary sediment (66%), elevated platelet count (50%), hematuria (40%), positive titer for rheumatoid factor (30%), and cryoglobulins (20%) [20,96,108,109]. Highly variable percentages for the presence of hepatitis B surface antigen, immune complexes, and low complement-component values are reported. Elevated levels of transaminases, creatine kinase, increased cerebrospinal fluid protein, and ischemic electrocardiograms are found in significant percentages of patients and should be looked for in the appropriate clinical setting.

Pathology. Pathologic involvement is diffuse, with the most frequent involvement in the kidneys, heart, liver, and gastrointestinal tract. The small and medium-sized muscular arteries are segmentally involved, often at the bifurcations, or branching points. The inflammatory lesion is characterized by fibrinoid necrosis and a cellular infiltration of the full width of the vessel wall with polymorphonuclear leukocytes and occasional lymphocytes and eosinophils (Fig. 43-1). The vessel wall and elastic laminae are disrupted, which may result in aneurysmal dilatation and thrombosis (Fig. 43-2) [2]. Chronic inflammation and scar formation can eventually result in tissue infarction despite control of the inflammatory process.

Any biopsy specimen may show the entire spectrum of lesions. The earliest endothelial proliferation with immune complex deposition, which would be evident on immunofluorescent staining or electron microscopy, may be seen next to granulation tissue and healed, end-stage scar tissue.

Diagnosis. The diagnosis of polyarteritis nodosa is established through surgical biopsy specimens or angiographic studies in the appropriate clinical setting. The pathologic diagnosis is made by histologic demonstration of a necrotizing vasculitis in small and medium-sized arteries (see Figs. 43-1, 43-2). Biopsies of clinically involved tissues often are limited by sampling error; for example, blind testicular biopsies establish the diagnosis in only 20 percent of samples, but autopsy studies indicate that up to 85 percent of male patients have testicular involvement [91]. Biopsies of asymptomatic muscle have a higher yield, but there remains a false-negative result of nearly 65 percent [92]. Sural-nerve biopsies appear to be a valuable source for pathologic tissue if the nerve-conduction studies show abnormal conduction velocities [110]. Clinically relevant pathologic tissue may have to be pursued in more than one organ system to make the diagnosis.

Fig. 43-1. Polyarteritis nodosa. Low-magnification photomicrograph of a small artery showing intense necrotizing inflammation of upper half of wall with slight aneurysmal bulging and extension of inflammation and hemorrhage into surrounding tissue.

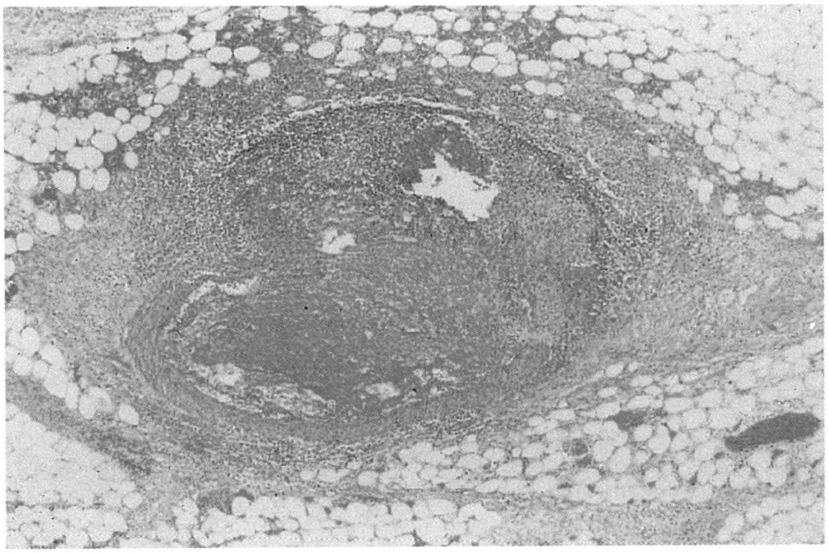

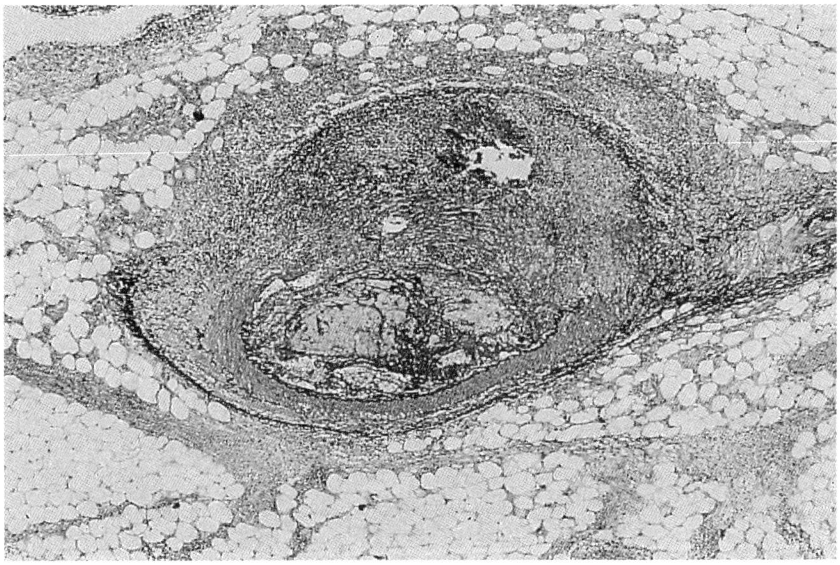

Fig. 43-2. Polyarteritis nodosa. Photomicrograph of elastic tissue stain of same artery as in Fig. 43-1, showing destruction of medial elastica in the area of necrosis.

The problem of sampling error in tissue biopsies has persuaded clinicians to make angiographic studies an important part of the diagnostic evaluation. The high frequency of saccular and fusiform aneurysms in the mesenteric, renal, and hepatic circulation makes angiographic studies diagnostic in up to 80 percent of patients with polyarteritis nodosa [75]. Angiographic studies are particularly useful when abdominal symptoms and signs are the sole manifestation of disease. Intraparenchymal aneurysms are not diagnostic of polyarteritis nodosa. They have been reported in other vasculitides, atrial myxomas, endocarditis, and fibromuscular dysplasia [76,111–113]. Angiography also may be useful in monitoring response to treatment as well as localizing a bleeding aneurysm [75,81].

It is important to keep in mind that there are conditions with an apparent causal relationship to polyarteritis nodosa. The most striking association is with hepatitis B infection. Up to 60 percent of patients with polyarteritis nodosa have evidence of hepatitis B infection [64–66]. Other associations include acute serous otitis media, human immunodeficiency virus (HIV) infection, hairy-cell leukemia, hyposensitization therapy, and amphetamine abuse [114–118]. Similarly, patients with connective tissue disease, such as systemic lupus erythematosus, rheumatoid arthritis, dermatomyositis, primary Sjögren's syndrome, and subacute bacterial endocarditis may develop symptoms, signs, and angiographic and pathologic findings essentially indistinguishable from primary polyarteritis nodosa.

Prognosis. Polyarteritis nodosa was a fatal disease prior to the availability of corticosteroids and immunosuppressives. Five-year survivals were less than 15 percent, with some studies having median survivals of 3 months from disease onset [106,108,109]. Adrenocorticosteroids markedly improved 5-year survival rates to 50 percent [109,119]. For patients with severe polyarteritis nodosa, the introduction of cytotoxic immunosuppressive drugs has further improved the survival rates. Recent studies suggest that over 80 percent of patients will survive past 5 years when those drugs are added to corticosteroids [109,120].

Prognosis and management are best understood if clinical subsets of patients are recognized; for instance, patients with single-organ disease (e.g., uterine or gallbladder) or only skin and muscle disease appear to have a better prognosis. Conversely, central nervous system, cardiac, and severe renal disease, as well as increasing age, are associated with a worse prognosis.

Treatment. Patients with systemic polyarteritis nodosa should be treated aggressively with high dosages of prednisone or a corticosteroid equivalent. Divided dosages given 3 times per day, with a total dosage of between 60 and 100 mg prednisone, should be administered. Patients who continue to deteriorate rapidly despite that therapy should be considered for intravenous pulse administration of 1,000 mg methylprednisolone for 3 consecutive days or for plasmapheresis in conjunction with corticosteroids and immunosuppressive agents. Proof that those two modalities are effective rests on small series and case reports and should be considered experimental [121–124]. Recent reports suggest that plasmapheresis may be beneficial when used in conjunction with steroids only in patients with severe renal disease [125].

Use of cytotoxic, immunosuppressive agents for long-term control of the disease and more rapid reduction of the dose of prednisone is indicated for patients with major organ involvement or steroid-resistant vasculitis [126]. Both azathioprine and cyclophosphamide in dosages of 2 mg/kg/day have been used for polyarteritis nodosa.

Higher dosages (3–4 mg/kg/day intravenously of cyclophosphamide for 3 to 4 days, followed by 2 mg/kg orally) have been used for patients with severe disease.

When the disease is controlled, the steroid dosage should be tapered and modified to an every-other-day schedule. Careful management includes control of hypertension—a frequent complication of renal involvement—and aggressive early therapy for any infectious complications of the immunosuppressives and corticosteroids. Reduction in the dosage of immunosuppressive agents simultaneously with the tapering of the corticosteroids frequently is required because of myelosuppression. Treatment should be continued for at least 1 year after all signs of active disease have been controlled. A gradual tapering off of the immunosuppressives while regularly following the patient allows a significant percentage of patients to be withdrawn from therapy [120].

The clinician should recognize that polyarteritis nodosa is frequently an explosive disease. The majority of deaths occur in the first 12 months. Immunosuppressive drugs frequently have been added relatively late, when patients have been thought to be steroid-treatment failures and significant organ damage has already occurred. The success or failure of those drugs may be due in part to those patient-selection factors. Earlier institution of immunosuppressive drugs may result in a better outcome.

CHURG-STRAUSS SYNDROME

Churg-Strauss syndrome is a systemic vasculitis characterized by eosinophilia and extravascular granulomas occurring in patients with a history of asthma, allergic rhinitis, or both. As initially described in 1951, the histologic criteria for the diagnosis are a necrotizing arteritis with eosinophilic infiltration along with extravascular granulomata [8]. However, those histologic findings are not always present in patients who fit the distinctive clinical pattern of disease [57]. Furthermore, the histologic findings of allergic angiitis and granulomatosis are found in patients without the clinical features of Churg-Strauss syndrome [127]. For those reasons, the clinician must be aware of the distinctive clinical pattern and incorporate the histologic findings to make the diagnosis of Churg-Strauss syndrome [57].

Clinical Features. Churg-Strauss syndrome is found in young people: the mean age of onset is 38, and there is a male predominance [57]. Churg-Strauss syndrome is often thought to have three phases. The initial phase is one of an allergic disease, which may last many years and is most typically manifested by either or both asthma and allergic rhinitis. Blood eosinophilia follows, with or without transient pulmonary infiltrates. A diagnosis of Löffler's syndrome commonly is entertained during this second stage. The final phase is the systemic vasculitis.

The time period between the onset of asthma and the occurrence of vasculitis varies from a few months to 30 years [29]. The asthma often remits during the onset of the vasculitis, only to recur later in the disease [57]. Three-fourths of patients with Churg-Strauss syndrome have pulmonary infiltrates. Radiographic findings are varied: Patchy peripheral infiltrates, hilar shadows, interstitial patterns, and massive pulmonary nodules have been reported [29]. The pathologic lung findings often progress from extensive eosinophilic infiltrates to a necrotizing arteritis with extravascular granulomas late in the disease [128].

Upper respiratory symptoms are common. Allergic rhinitis, polyposis, and radiologic evidence of sinusitis have been found in up to two-thirds of patients [129]. Equally common but occurring later than the rhinitis (usually at the onset of the vasculitic phase) are the cutaneous manifestations. Purpura or nodular lesions are typical lesions of the skin. The purpuric lesions are histologically leukocytoclastic vasculitis, and the nodules are frequently granulomatous.

Gastrointestinal involvement includes features of eosinophilic gastroenteritis and polyarteritis nodosa. Eosinophilic infiltration of the bowel wall can produce diarrhea, bleeding, and nodular masses with obstruction [130–132]. Serosal involvement can result in eosinophilic ascites. Vasculitis of the gastrointestinal tract can produce ischemia with bowel perforation, bleeding, or colitis [132,133]. Abdominal pain from ischemic cholecystitis also is seen. The pattern of eosinophilic gastroenteritis can evolve into or coincide with the vasculitis [131].

Mirroring the findings of polyarteritis nodosa, mononeuritis multiplex, symmetric peripheral neuropathy, ischemic optic neuritis, cranial-nerve palsies, confusion, coma, and cerebral hemorrhage or infarction can be found in nearly two-thirds of patients with Churg-Strauss syndrome [8,57,134]. Vasculitis of the vasa nervorum and perineural eosinophilic infiltrate are two known mechanisms of the peripheral neuropathy [8]. The central nervous system disease appears to be ischemic secondary to vasculitis [134].

Other manifestations include fever, arthritis, myalgias, pericarditis, myocardial infarction, focal segmental glomerulonephritis, and granulomatous prostatitis [57]. Cardiac and urinary-tract involvement are frequent and significantly contribute to the morbidity and mortality of the disease. Kidney involvement is milder and less frequent than in polyarteritis nodosa, but the lower urinary tract is frequently diseased, producing hematuria or obstruction [29]. Cardiac disease results in nearly one-half of the deaths. Evidence of cardiac involvement is found in 60 percent of autopsies [57]. Coronary-artery inflammation, pericarditis, myocardial eosinophilic infiltrates and granulomas, and endomyocardial fibrosis similar to that seen in hypereosinophilic syndrome have been found [8,57,133].

Laboratory. Although considered a characteristic of Churg-Strauss syndrome, peripheral blood eosinophilia occasionally may be transient or absent. Fluctuating levels of eosinophils is a true hallmark of this disease. There is often a good correlation between disease activity and the eosinophil count [57]. Peak eosinophil counts may exceed 5×10^9 per liter but are not as high as those seen in the hypereosinophilic syndrome [135]. An increase in IgE level is seen and appears to mirror the activity of the vasculitis [136]. Antibodies to myeloperoxidase with positive C-ANCA assays frequently are found [137]. Other laboratory findings are similar to polyarteritis nodosa, with anemia, leukocytosis, elevated erythrocyte sedimentation rate, and a positive rheumatoid factor. Unlike polyarteritis nodosa, however, the frequency of hepatitis B antigenemia is not greater than that found in normal populations.

Pathology. The histologic findings of Churg-Strauss syndrome are widely distributed. Lesions typically are found at different phases of evolution [133]. Churg and Strauss suggested that the development of the characteristic lesion begins with eosinophilic infiltration of the tissues, followed by the introduction of macrophages with ultimate granuloma formation [8]. Extravascular granulomas are most common in the lung, heart, liver, skin, and spleen [138].

The vasculitis of Churg-Strauss syndrome involves predominantly small but also medium-sized vessels [132]. Unlike polyarteritis nodosa, there is a striking involvement of veins as well as arteries [138]. Eosinophils and granulomatous involvement around the vessels evolving to a panmural necrotizing vasculitis identical to polyarteritis nodosa can be found. Vessel involvement is segmental. Fibrinoid necrosis, aneurysm formation, and vessel thrombosis are seen less frequently than in polyarteritis nodosa. Healed fibrotic lesions are found often.

Diagnosis. Although the clinician often can make the diagnosis of Churg-Strauss syndrome, pathologic specimens for confirmation should be obtained. Chest radiographs provide valuable evidence for the diagnosis. Angiographic studies have proved helpful in some patients when arteritis as well as aneurysms are found [57,75]. Antimyeloperoxidase antibodies may provide additional evidence in support of the diagnosis in the proper clinical setting.

The differential diagnosis of diseases with granulomas and eosinophilia is wide. Allergic bronchopulmonary aspergillosis has eosinophilia and asthma as well as pulmonary infiltrates, but a vasculopathy is not found. Wegener's granulomatosis has a more destructive upper-airway component, and asthma is not a characteristic feature. The hypereosinophilic syndromes, Löffler's syndrome, the syndrome of pulmonary infiltrates with eosinophilia, and eosinophilic gastroenteritis also may be difficult to differentiate from Churg-Strauss syndrome, especially since the pathologic findings of true angiitis or granulomas have been reported in some patients [127,139]. Occasional cases of sarcoidosis are associated with eosinophilia, although asthma is rare. Ultimately, the typical clinical picture along with the pathologic findings make the diagnosis.

Prognosis. Churg-Strauss syndrome appears to respond well to corticosteroids. Median survival of more than 9 years in one series and a more recent report of 14 out of 16 patients entering remission with corticosteroids alone suggest that the prognosis for this disease is far better than for polyarteritis nodosa [29,57]. The primary causes of deaths in most series are pulmonary and cardiac failure. Some patients with fulminating vasculitis have responded to immunosuppressive drugs when corticosteroids have failed [126,140].

HYPERSENSITIVITY VASCULITIS

The hypersensitivity vasculitides are a group of diseases that have been reported under a variety of names, including allergic vasculitis, leukocytoclastic vasculitis, and cutaneous necrotizing angiitis. The characteristic, although not universal, features of this group of diseases are (1) inflammation of small vessels, particularly venules but also arterioles and capillaries; (2) the presence of leukocytoclasis (nuclear debris) in the biopsy; and (3) involvement of the skin. Within this group, several clinical syndromes are recognized, such as Henoch-Schönlein purpura, serum sickness, drug hypersensitivity reactions, mixed cryoglobulinemia, and urticarial vasculitis (hypocomplementemic vasculitis).

Some of these patients have an underlying related disease or have been exposed to an environmental agent that triggered the hypersensitivity vasculitis (Table 43-4). In some series, up to one-third of cases are associated with an infection [141]. Those associations signify that the detection of leukocytoclastic vasculitis requires the clinician to search for an associated illness or precipitating agent or drug.

Pathology. The characteristic biopsy finding is acute necrotizing inflammation of vessels less than 1 mm in diameter, with infiltrating polymorphonuclear cells or, less frequently, lymphocytes (Figs. 43-3, 43-4). Lymphocytic infiltration of cutaneous blood vessels has been associated with normal serum complement in one series, whereas an infiltrate of neutrophils is accompanied by complement activation [142]. Other investigators suggest that a lymphocytic infiltrate is more suggestive of a chronic process [143]. Leukocytoclasis, extravasated red blood cells, endothelial swelling, and fibrinoid necrosis frequently are seen. Immunofluorescent staining of an early lesion usually demonstrates IgM, IgG, and C3 [44]. IgA also is deposited, especially in Henoch-Schönlein purpura [144].

The fact that the skin is the most frequently involved organ in hypersensitivity vasculitis should not obscure the possibility of similar infiltrative processes in other tissues. Although usually less destructive than the systemic necrotizing arteritides, complications of internal-organ involvement by hypersensitivity vasculitis can be fatal.

Clinical Features. Hypersensitivity vasculitis usually is self-limited, occurring in all age groups and in men and women in nearly equal percentages. It frequently has an abrupt onset. A chronic or recurrent course is not uncommon [145]. Systemic symptoms of fever and weight loss occur in a minority of cases. Such symptoms commonly are seen in patients whose vasculitis is a manifestation of another disorder such as an infection, colitis, or serum sickness [141,145,146].

Cutaneous signs of hypersensitivity vasculitis are varied. Palpable purpura is the classic finding. Petechiae, vesicles and bullae, urticaria, papules, pustules, necrotic ulcerations, and nodules are less common [44]. The lesions

Table 43-4. Hypersensitivity vasculitis

Possible etiologic agents of hypersensitivity vasculitis		
Infections	Drugs	Chemicals
Streptococcal	Penicillins	Insecticides
Staphylococcal	Sulfonamides	Pesticides
Subacute bacterial endocarditis	Iodides	Petroleum products
Meningococcal	Phenothiazines	Miscellaneous
Gonococcal	Quinidine	Influenza vaccine
Leprosy	Phenytoin	Insect bites
Malaria	Allopurinol	Hyposensitization injections
Mycobacterial	Aspirin	
Hepatitis B	Propylthiouracil	
Influenza	Tetracycline	
Cytomegalovirus	Phenylbutazone	
Epstein-Barr virus	Cimetidine	
HIV	Zidovudine	
Rubella		

Underlying diseases associated with hypersensitivity vasculitis	
Connective-tissue diseases	Other diseases
Dermatomyositis	Chronic active hepatitis
Rheumatoid arthritis	Primary biliary cirrhosis
Scleroderma	Inflammatory bowel disease
Sjögren's syndrome	Intestinal bypass surgery
Other vasculitides	Neoplasms
Churg-Strauss syndrome	Macroglobulinemia
Wegener's granulomatosis	Cryoglobulinemia
Polyarteritis nodosa	

tend to appear in crops, symmetrically manifest on dependent areas. Mucosal and facial lesions are unusual. A minority of patients complain of pruritus or burning with the rash. An accompanying dependent edema frequently is seen [10]. Resolution of the lesions may take up to 4 weeks. Hyperpigmentation or scars sometimes persist.

Arthralgias or arthritis is present in the majority of cases, but deforming or destructive lesions are found only when the vasculitis is a manifestation of a systemic arthritis [147]. The knees most frequently are afflicted, followed by ankles, wrists, and elbows. Significant peripheral nerve or muscle disease involvement also is more commonly

Fig. 43-3. Leukocytoclastic vasculitis. Low-magnification photomicrograph of skin showing intense inflammation of dermal capillaries and venules.

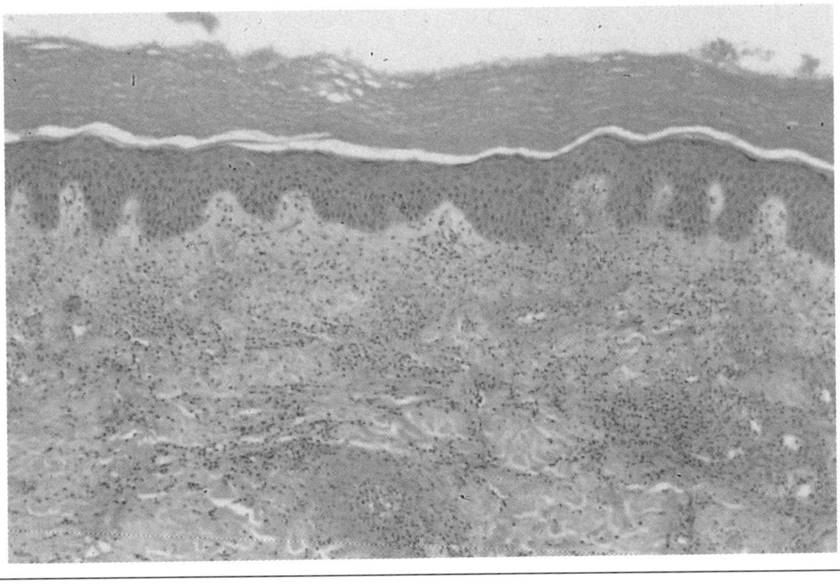

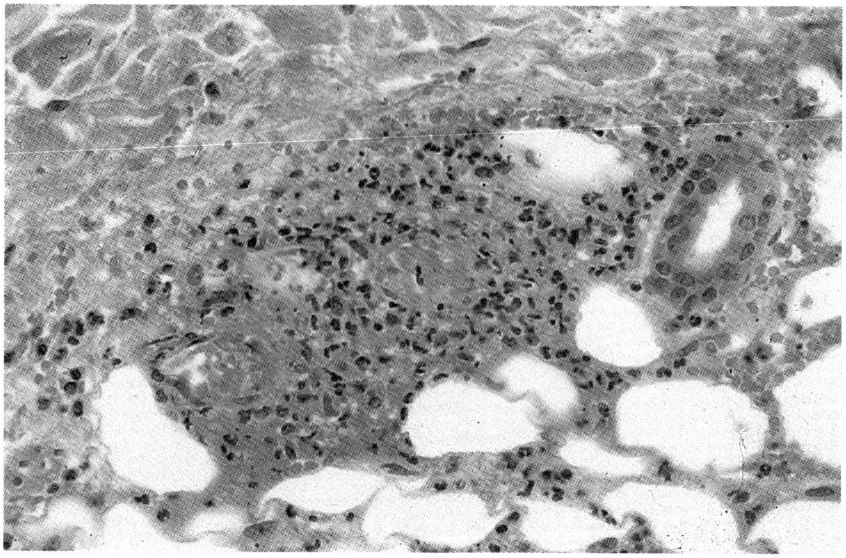

Fig. 43-4. Leukocytoclastic vasculitis. Higher-magnification photomicrograph of skin deep in the dermis showing necrotizing inflammation of venules with thrombosis, intense neutrophilic infiltration, and hemorrhage. Note the extensive fragmentation of leukocytes.

seen in patients with connective-tissue diseases or cryoglobulinemia [147–149].

Renal manifestations span a range from asymptomatic hematuria in 25 percent of patients to the less frequent finding of nephrosis or renal failure. The latter is found most commonly in essential cryoglobulinemia or Henoch-Schönlein purpura and is a major cause of death in those patients. Gastrointestinal symptoms suggest Henoch-Schönlein purpura or vasculitis associated with inflammatory bowel disease. Colicky pain, melena, hematemesis, or perforation is seen in a small number of patients with any of the hypersensitivity vasculitides. Reports of pericarditis and cerebrovascular events are unusual [148].

Laboratory. Abnormalities reflect both the vasculitis and the inciting condition. An elevation of the erythrocyte sedimentation rate along with a leukocytosis generally is noted [90]. Eosinophilia, anemia, guaiac-positive stools, hematuria, proteinuria, cryoglobulinemia, hypocomplementemia, abnormal liver- and renal-function tests, as well as antiglobulin and antinuclear antibodies are present in a significant number of patients [10,44]. IgA-containing immune complexes are found primarily in Henoch-Schönlein purpura [150]. Those tests and others may lead the clinician to a diagnosis of the underlying systemic disease.

Diagnosis. The diagnosis usually is established by the presence of a leukocytoclastic pattern in the small vessels at the site of a dermal lesion. Occasionally, the diagnosis is made through the histologic evaluation of another organ, such as kidney or muscle. Having established the diagnosis of a hypersensitivity vasculitis, the clinician must evaluate the patient carefully for an underlying systemic illness or exposure to an agent or drug (see Table 43-4).

Therapy. Hypersensitivity vasculitis represents a large group of disorders, the prognosis and therapy of which vary significantly. Spontaneous resolution is common [151–153]. Vasculitis due to an infection or medication frequently resolves with treatment or withdrawal of the drug. Therapy of the systemic illness, such as colitis, may be effective. Chronic or recurrent vasculitis or patients with significant organ disease, such as Henoch-Schönlein purpura with abdominal involvement, may require corticosteroids for control of the disease. Immunosuppressive drugs have been used with some effectiveness in patients with severe unresponsive disease.

CLINICAL SYNDROMES

Henoch-Schönlein Purpura. Henoch-Schönlein purpura (anaphylactoid purpura) is a syndrome defined by its clinical presentation of skin, joint, intestinal, and renal vasculitis. It is distinct because of its often self-limited course and its association with circulating IgA-immune complexes [21,154]. Occurring predominantly in male children after an upper respiratory infection in the spring, this syndrome is described in adults as a similar illness with possibly more joint disease and a slightly greater risk of serious renal disease [21]. Elevated serum IgA also is seen in one-half of the cases [59]. IgA is deposited in the glomerular mesangium and involved blood vessels of the skin [143,144,155].

The skin rash occurs predominantly on the extensor surfaces of the lower extremities, with 50 percent involving the buttocks [152]. The urticarial lesions become palpable purpura in a short time. Edema is often evident in the legs and feet. A transient arthritis can be clinically significant, although deformity is not seen. The abdominal symptoms of pain, nausea, blood loss, and, in children, nonreducible intussusception or perforation are manifestations of the intestinal vasculitis [156]. Pancreatitis also is reported. Renal involvement usually is limited to asymptomatic hematuria, although patients do develop nephrosis and renal failure [153]. Carditis, pleuritis, pneumonitis, and cerebrovascular accidents are rare.

The diagnosis is established by the combination of the characteristic clinical findings and a skin biopsy consistent with a leukocytoclastic vasculitis. Deposits of IgA help confirm the diagnosis. Treatment usually is conservative because of the excellent prognosis. Fewer than 8 percent of patients followed for more than 2 years develop significant azotemia [157]. However, those with nephrosis or decreased glomerular filtration rates during the initial phase of the disease have a 44-percent likelihood of developing chronic azotemia or hypertension. Patients may require corticosteroids to control the gastrointestinal manifestations, but the value of those drugs in patients with renal failure is disputed. In rare patients, cytotoxic drugs may be indicated.

Hypocomplementemic Vasculitis. The clinical hallmarks of this form of leukocytoclastic vasculitis are chronic or recurrent episodes of urticaria occurring on the face, trunk, and upper extremities in a young patient with arthralgias and abdominal pain [158,159]. The rash may be nonpruritic. The arthritis mimics that found in systemic lupus erythematosus, being nondeforming. A similar condition, called the systemic lupus erythematosus-related syndrome, is seen with abdominal pain and edema of the bowel wall during the episodes [160]. Mild membranoproliferative glomerulonephritis with hematuria, proteinuria, and red blood cell casts is seen but not usually accompanied by significant azotemia (although the latter may occur) [161]. Associations with chronic obstructive pulmonary disease and hereditary deficiencies of the complement components C1q and C2 have been reported [160,162].

Classic complement activation with marked depression of the early components of the complement pathway, a circulating C1q precipitant (7s), circulating immune complexes, deposition of immunoglobulin and complement in the glomerular basement membrane, low levels of circulating cryoglobulins, and skin biopsies demonstrating a necrotizing venulitis with leukocytoclasis—all suggest that this condition is an immune complex–induced process [142,161]. However, clinically identical patients with chronic urticaria may present without evidence of immune-complex disease or vasculitis [117]. Other immune-complex diseases, such as the vasculitis seen in acute hepatitis B infection or systemic lupus erythematosus, may manifest urticaria, making the clinical delineation of this distinct syndrome difficult at times.

Mixed Essential Cryoglobulinemia. Cryoglobulins are immunoglobulins that precipitate at temperatures below 37°C. The mixed cryoglobulins (type II and type III) usually described in patients with this syndrome are composed of a polyclonal IgG and a monoclonal (type II) or polyclonal (type III) IgM. The IgM usually possesses anti-Fc (rheumatoid factor) activity [42,45]. A majority of patients with this syndrome show evidence of hepatitis C infection in their serum and cryoprecipitate [70,71]. Hepatitis C virus antibodies and hepatitis C virus RNA have been found both in the serum and in concentrated amounts in the cryoprecipitate [70].

An episodic rash with some edema of the lower extremities is seen in over 90 percent of patients. The rash may be precipitated by prolonged standing or exposure to cold. Arthralgias are common. The clinical syndrome differs from typical hypersensitivity vasculitis in that there is a higher incidence of significant renal disease [163]. The glomerulonephritis seen may progress to renal failure or the nephrotic syndrome [43,164,165]. Mononeuritis multiplex, cerebrovascular events, and peripheral neuropathy also are frequently reported [148,166,167]. Involvement of the lungs, with hemoptysis, wheezing, and dyspnea as well as hepatosplenomegaly and coronary vasculitis do occur rarely [168]. Leg ulcers and Raynaud's phenomenon are seen in one-fourth of the patients [165].

With the arthralgias, peripheral edema, abdominal pain, and hematuria, this syndrome may be difficult to distinguish from Henoch-Schönlein purpura. The higher levels of cryoglobulins, positive rheumatoid factor, and low C1q and C4 seen in cryoglobulinemia help to distinguish the entities [169]. Anemia, mild leukocytosis, and an elevated sedimentation rate are common in both conditions.

Patients with type I cryoglobulinemia often present with symptoms of a nature different from that of essential mixed cryoglobulinemia. The symptoms and signs are similar to those of hyperviscosity syndrome [42]. Severe Raynaud's phenomenon with distal gangrene and ulcerations, arterial thromboses, and hemorrhage are seen with a high frequency in patients with an IgM type I cryoglobulin [170].

Diagnosing this condition and characterizing the type of cryoglobulin is important. Cryoglobulins are associated with many underlying diseases (see Table 43-3). The vasculitic syndrome can be the presenting manifestation. Knowing the type of cryoglobulin aids in determining the underlying disease [42]. The prognosis of the vasculitis of cryoglobulinemia depends to some extent on the underlying condition.

Differentiating essential mixed cryoglobulinemia from other forms of hypersensitivity vasculitis is important because its prognosis generally is less favorable [171,172]. Milder symptoms may respond to nonsteroidal anti-inflammatory agents or antihistamines. Corticosteroids alone appear to be marginally effective in the severely ill patient, who may respond to a combination of plasmapheresis, cytotoxic drugs, and steroids [148,164]. In type II mixed cryoglobulinemia associated with hepatitis C virus, interferon-alpha (IFNa) has been shown to reduce cryoglobulin levels, improve kidney function, and reduce purpura. Treatment for 3–6 months has resulted in remissions lasting as long as 40 months [173–176]. Treatment of cryoglobulinemic vasculitis in patients with type I cryoglobulinemia and hyperviscosity also may require emergency plasmapheresis. Poor prognosis is associated with the presence of renal disease. The major factors contributing to death are severe renal disease, central nervous system involvement, and infection [165].

Serum Sickness and Similar Syndromes. Originally described as a result of the parenteral administration of foreign serum, true serum sickness rarely is seen today, with the exception of patients treated with antilymphocyte antisera for transplant rejection. A similar syndrome with most of the features of classic serum sickness is reported occasionally after administration of medications, particularly penicillins, sulfonamides, iodides, and phenytoin [177,178].

Immune-complex deposition appears to be the pathogenetic process responsible for the vasculitic lesions, although detecting antibodies to the offending agent may be difficult. A leukocytoclastic venulitis is found as the pathologic basis of the dermal manifestations that are nearly universal in these patients. The rash frequently is present in dependent areas and spans the range of palpable purpura, urticaria, and macules [145]. Fever, arthralgias, arthritis, lymphadenopathy, and abdominal pain characterize the full-blown syndrome. Only rarely do patients develop impairment of a major organ system.

Leukocytosis, an elevated sedimentation rate, and eosinophilia are common laboratory manifestations. Occasionally, hematuria and mild proteinuria are seen. The diagnosis is made when the syndrome is recognized after recent exposure to an offending foreign antigen. Treatment consists of removal of the offending agent. Resolution may occur in 2 days or take as long as 2 weeks. Conservative management with antihistamines and aspirin usually suffices, although an occasional patient requires a short course of corticosteroids.

Wegener's Granulomatosis. Wegener's granulomatosis, a disease of unknown etiology, is a necrotizing granulomatous process of the respiratory tract, systemic vasculitis, and a glomerulonephritis. It is an uncommon disease, occurring predominantly in young and middle-aged persons, slightly more often in males [89]. Because it often begins with respiratory symptoms before evidence of a more widespread illness is noted, Wegener's was thought to be an infectious process. The reports of circulating immune complexes, glomerular subepithelial deposits, positive rheumatoid factors, and elevated immunoglobulin levels all suggest an immune pathogenesis [56,61,113].

PATHOLOGY. The pathologic findings consist of three components: a necrotizing vasculitis involving small arteries and veins; necrotizing granulomata, often in the vicinity of the vasculitis; and a glomerulonephritis [179,180]. Granulomata or vasculitis may be found in any organ, but there is a predilection for the upper and lower respiratory tracts, skin, central and peripheral nervous system, and heart. Like polyarteritis nodosa, the vascular lesions have fibrinoid necrosis, and vessels at different stages of inflammation and healing can be found in one specimen. Wegener's granulomatosis vasculitis is distinguished from polyarteritis nodosa by the predominant infiltration of mononuclear cells and the frequent involvement of small veins (Figs. 43-5, 43-6).

The perivascular areas have a wide zone with an inflammatory infiltrate. Within that zone, the necrotizing granulomas can be found with palisading fibroblasts, mononuclear cells, and occasional multinucleated giant cells, which help distinguish this syndrome from the other systemic vasculitides. Biopsies may demonstrate only the extravascular lesion without vascular lesions [179]. The renal lesion most typically is a focal segmental glomerulonephritis [180]. Diffuse proliferative lesions with crescents and severe interstitial nephritis also have been described. Vasculitis or granulomata are found in fewer than 10 percent of biopsies.

CLINICAL FEATURES. Presenting signs and symptoms span a broad range, but the earliest complaints usually are

Fig. 43-5. Wegener's granulomatosis. Photomicrograph of lung with obliteration of architecture by intense chronic inflammation with a central focus of necrosis surrounded by giant cells. Many giant cells are also seen throughout the tissue.

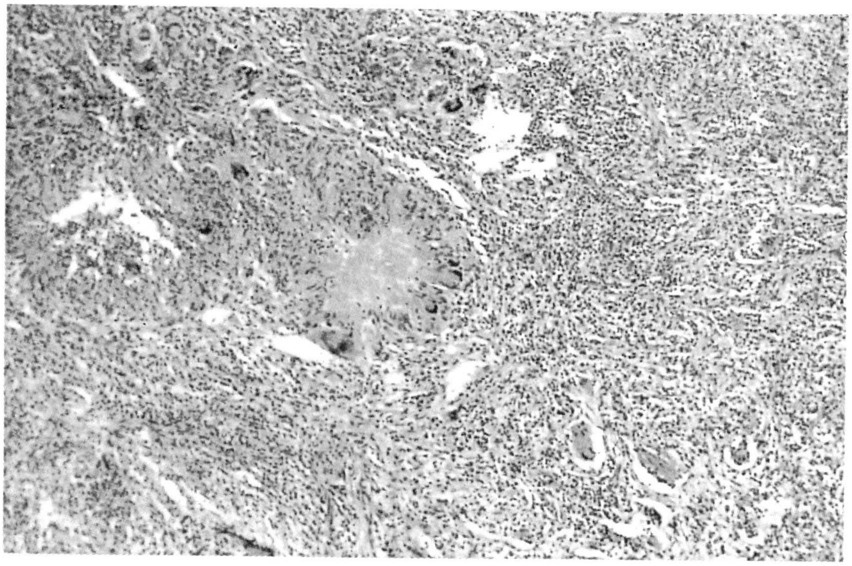

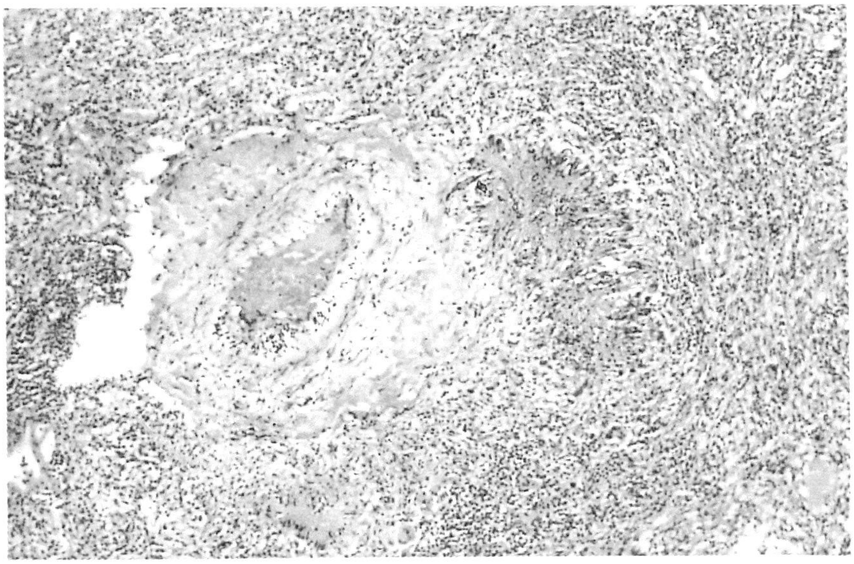

Fig. 43-6. Wegener's granulomatosis. Photomicrograph of lung showing chronic inflammation of an artery with subintimal and medial lymphocytic infiltration. Foci of necrosis surrounded by palisaded cells are present in the immediately surrounding tissue.

related to the upper respiratory tract (Table 43-5). Despite the high frequency of pulmonary infiltrates in this series, a surprising number are asymptomatic. Patients with azotemia at presentation are at significant risk (30%) for progression to end-stage renal failure [56].

Upper-airway disease ultimately is present in more than 90 percent of patients. Rhinitis, sinusitis, mucosal ulceration, gingivitis, and serous otitis media are the milder manifestations. More destructive processes, including cholesteatomas, suppurative otitis, erosion of sinus cavities, hearing loss, and saddle-nose deformities, do occur. Severe destruction with erosion through the hard palate and skin evident in idiopathic midline granuloma and neoplastic processes involving the upper airways are not seen in Wegener's granulomatosis [73].

Secondary infection of the sinus and nasal passages is seen in nearly every patient with significant upper-airway involvement. *Staphylococcus aureus* is the most common organism isolated. Not surprisingly, then, biopsy of the involved tissues frequently demonstrates nonspecific acute and chronic inflammation rather than granulomatous vasculitis [72].

The lower respiratory tract, like the upper passages, is involved in more than 90 percent of patients. The characteristic radiographic finding is bilateral nodular infiltrates with cavitation [56,89]. Nodules and infiltrates may spontaneously wane, while other manifestations exacerbate. Pleural effusions are not uncommon, but hilar and mediastinal adenopathy rarely is seen [10,181]. Endobronchial involvement can occur, leading to atelectasis or subglottal stenosis. Secondary infection complicates lung manifestations, as it does sinus disease. Lung biopsies frequently demonstrate the diagnostic findings of granulomatous vasculitis [56].

Renal disease usually does not produce early symp-

Table 43-5. Presenting signs or symptoms in Wegener's granulomatosis

	Patients*	
Sign or symptom	Number	Percent
Pulmonary infiltrate	60	71
Sinusitis	57	67
Arthralgia or arthritis	37	44
Fever	29	34
Otitis	21	25
Cough	29	34
Rhinitis or nasal symptoms	19	22
Hemoptysis	15	18
Ocular inflammation	14	16
Weight loss	14	16
Skin rash	11	13
Epistaxis	9	11
Renal failure	9	11
Chest discomfort	7	8
Anorexia or malaise	7	8
Proptosis	6	7
Shortness of breath	6	7
Oral ulcers	5	6
Hearing loss	5	6
Pleuritis or effusion	5	6
Headache	5	6

* 85 patients followed for 21 years.
Source: Reproduced with permission from AS Fauci, et al. Wegener's granulomatosis: prospective clinical and therapeutic experience with 85 patients for 21 years. Ann Intern Med 1983; 98:76–85.

toms. It is detected early by thorough urinalyses. In general, more than 80 percent of patients manifest renal disease. Unlike the pulmonary lesions, which can wax and wane, the glomerulonephritis of Wegener's granulomatosis is generally progressive and, before the advent of cytotoxic therapy, was usually fatal. Hypertension that complicates the renal involvement of polyarteritis nodosa is uncommon in Wegener's.

Up to one-half of patients with Wegener's granulomatosis have cutaneous lesions [56]. Purpura, ulcerations, papules, vesicles, and nodules are all well described [182]. Histologically, leukocytoclastic vasculitis or granulomatous vasculitis is found. Skin signs, although they mirror underlying disease activity, are usually a minor manifestation. Similarly, the arthralgia involving the large joints in a symmetric pattern parallels the disease activity and is found in over 50 percent of patients. Joint damage or deformity rarely occurs.

Ocular disease is reported in nearly two-thirds of patients [58]. It ranges from conjunctivitis and episcleritis to uveitis, vasculitis of the optic nerve, retinal-artery occlusion, and—the most common finding in some series—proptosis [183]. The proptosis is a result of retrobulbar inflammatory or granulomatous mass lesions. Patients with visual deterioration require CT imaging to determine the cause: vasculitis or a compressing mass lesion that might require surgical intervention [183].

Disease in the peripheral and central nervous system may be based on vasculitis or mass lesions. Peripheral and cranial neuropathies are the most common. As in polyarteritis nodosa, the peripheral neuropathy may be a symmetric polyneuropathy or mononeuritis multiplex and is the result of vasculitis-induced ischemia. Cranial nerves II, III, IV, and VI are the most frequently affected [184]. Those nerves may be damaged by arteritis or extension of granulomas from the upper respiratory passages to the middle and posterior fossa of the brain [185]. Other described complications include cerebrovascular accidents, meningitis, brachial plexitis, spinal cord compression, and diabetes insipidus [186]. A mild pleocytosis and elevated protein in the cerebrospinal fluid are common with central nervous system involvement. Response to therapy of all the neurologic manifestations is variable, and spontaneous improvement is not uncommon. Since the introduction of immunosuppressive therapy, there is a lower incidence of nervous system involvement, with fewer than one-fourth of patients having those complications [56].

Carditis, pericarditis, and coronary vasculitis are found in a limited number of patients [187]. Myositis, hepatic portal triaditis, and granulomatous masses in a variety of organs occasionally are seen. In addition to those widespread complications, a more limited form of Wegener's granulomatosis has been reported [188]. Such patients, with primarily lung, sinus, and cutaneous involvement, are remarkable for their apparent lack of renal disease and apparent response to corticosteroids [22]. Other investigators have described patients with similar patterns of disease, that is, prolonged courses but variable responses to therapeutic intervention [181,189]. Whether such a limited form exists or merely has yet to develop renal disease is an unanswered question [89].

LABORATORY. As in the other vasculitides, there is ample laboratory evidence of a chronic inflammatory process in Wegener's granulomatosis. An elevated erythrocyte sedimentation rate, leukocytosis, and thrombocytosis with an accompanying anemia of chronic disease are the usual pattern [89]. C-ANCA is found in up to 93 percent of patients with active generalized disease [51–53]. Significantly fewer patients with more localized or inactive disease have positive tests for ANCA. That diffuse cytoplasmic staining pattern correlates well in these patients with antibodies to proteinase-3. Over one-half of patients have a positive rheumatoid factor, and a polyclonal elevation of serum immunoglobulins is common. Complement component assays usually are normal, consistent with the rare identification of circulating immune complexes [190]. Antinuclear antibodies are not a feature of Wegener's granulomatosis.

Chest radiographs also detect abnormalities, often without corresponding clinical symptomatology. More common than the classical bilateral multiple nodules are pulmonary infiltrates, which can occur in any lobe and are notorious for their fleeting nature. Cavitation, both thick and thin walled, may occur in the nodules or infiltrates. Sinus films are abnormal in the majority of patients, and lesions vary from mucosal thickening to bony erosion. CT scans often clearly define bony thinning as well as delineate the retrobulbar disease [191].

DIAGNOSIS. A diagnosis is established by finding a granulomatous vasculitis in a patient with the appropriate clinical picture. A physician may find only the characteristic extravascular granuloma and still diagnose Wegener's granulomatosis in the appropriate clinical setting [188]. With clinical involvement, a nasopharyngeal biopsy has about a 40-percent likelihood of confirming a diagnosis of Wegener's granulomatosis. Similarly, a skin biopsy demonstrates granulomatous vasculitis in a minority of patients. More commonly, a leukocytoclastic vasculitis is found. Renal biopsies often demonstrate a focal glomerulonephritis. In the proper clinical setting, that suggests the diagnosis while excluding similar entities such as angiocentric immunoproliferative lesion and midline granuloma [192]. An open-lung biopsy has the highest yield for demonstrating the classic pathologic findings. Antineutrophil cytoplasm antibody studies have a high degree of both specificity and sensitivity for active generalized Wegener's granulomatosis [51–53]. In a classic clinical setting, a positive C-ANCA may be diagnostic, but most clinicians continue to rely on tissue pathology to make a diagnosis and institute treatment. During treatment, up to one-fourth of patients will have a rising titer of ANCA preceding a relapse [193]. In up to one-half of the patients in remission, the test becomes negative or the titer falls significantly [51,53,54].

The differential diagnosis, depending on the clinical manifestations, may be quite large. The granulomatous diseases (such as sarcoid and midline granuloma) and the infectious granulomatous diseases (tuberculosis, histoplasmosis, blastomycosis, and syphilis) need to be excluded. Patients with allergic angiitis and granulomatosis—Churg-Strauss syndrome—and angiocentric immunoproliferative lesion also may present with similar clinical findings, making a careful clinical and pathologic evaluation critical.

PROGNOSIS. Before treatment was available, the outlook for Wegener's granulomatosis was dismal [194]. Cyclophosphamide has been demonstrated to induce remissions in more than 70 to 90 percent of patients [56,195,196]. Chlorambucil, azathioprine and methotrexate have been used with mixed results [56,197,198]. Earlier reports had suggested that trimethoprim-sulfamethoxazole may be effective in limited Wegener's [199]. More recent studies are less enthusiastic [193]. The data to date suggest that patients with active Wegener's granulomatosis should be treated with a combination of corticosteroids and cyclophosphamide and that therapy should be continued for at least a year after the patient goes into remission. In those individuals in whom renal failure persists despite induction of remission, transplantation may be useful.

TEMPORAL ARTERITIS

Temporal arteritis, also known as giant cell arteritis, usually occurs in individuals over the age of 50. Its incidence rate climbs from 1.4 per 100,000 in those 50 to 59 years of age to 29.6 per 100,000 in those between 70 and 79 years old [200]. The condition usually occurs in whites, with the highest prevalence rates reported in populations of northern-European ancestry [201]. Reports from hospitals serving black populations demonstrate a considerably lower incidence [202].

Temporal arteritis predominantly involves those branches of arteries originating from the aortic arch. It rarely involves intracranial vessels, but giant-cell infiltration has been found in the arteries of nearly every organ, making temporal arteritis a misnomer [203].

Pathology. The inflammation of the arteries is patchy, with predominant involvement of the superficial temporal, vertebral, ophthalmic, and posterior ciliary arteries [204]. Other commonly affected arteries noted in postmortem studies are the carotid, subclavian, brachial, coronary, and aorta, with rare involvement of intracranial and abdominal vessels [201,205].

The earliest lesions have intimal thickening with lymphocyte infiltration of the elastic lamina. Progressive involvement of the entire arterial wall follows, with T helper cells and some fibroblasts [206]. Focal necrosis and granulomatous inflammation with multinucleated giant cells in the region of the fragmented internal elastic lamina are the classic findings in temporal arteritis [207]. Because of the notorious skip lesions, many hundreds of sections may have to be examined before the diagnosis is excluded [208]. Granulomatous myocarditis and hepatitis occasionally have been reported in this syndrome [209,210]. Portal triaditis is common.

Clinical Features. The mean age of onset is approximately 70 years. Women predominate, by a ratio of about 2:1 [200]. At presentation, there may be many symptoms. Headache is the most common, but visual symptoms, scalp tenderness, fever, malaise, and weight loss frequently are seen [200,207]. Although patients may present with a fever of unknown origin, most patients with temporal arteritis have claudicatory symptoms related to arterial involvement during their disease [211].

Headache is most commonly a severe, boring bilateral pain in the frontal-temporal region. Unilateral and occipital headaches are less common. When the scalp is tender, it is usually over the temporal arteries, but more diffuse tenderness occurs. Interruption of the blood vessels leading to the special sensory organs may result in dysfunction in taste, smell, hearing, and balance, along with the well-known visual complications.

Inflammation of the ophthalmic and posterior ciliary arteries results in ischemia to the optic nerve and loss of vision. The fundoscopic exam may reveal ischemic optic neuritis. Occasional patients have involvement of the occipital or retinal arteries, resulting in visual loss. Blindness may be the initial symptom, but a careful history usually reveals prior symptoms suggestive of giant cell arteritis as well as past transient visual disturbances. Unfortunately, once blindness develops, it is rarely reversible. Ischemia of the contralateral eye may follow shortly thereafter, making recognition of the underlying condition critical. Overall, nearly 20 percent of patients with giant cell arteritis develop permanent loss of vision in at least one eye [18].

A second common ischemic manifestation is muscle claudication. Although classically described in the masticatory muscles, the arms, legs, neck, and tongue also may be involved [203]. The diffuse claudication is further evidence that the inflammatory process is not located simply in the extracranial vessels. In fact, evidence of large-artery inflammation in the aorta, axillary, brachial, coronary, subclavian, and carotid arteries is found in about 15 percent of patients [203,212]. Such inflammation results in ischemic complications ranging from asymptomatic bruits to infarction (myocardial, tongue, and cerebral). Aortic-valve regurgitation, aortic dissection, and rupture have been reported [213].

The clinical syndrome of polymyalgia rheumatica—aching with morning stiffness in the neck, shoulders, and hip girdle muscles along with synovitis of the wrists and knees—is found in nearly half the patients with giant cell arteritis [214]. The syndrome may begin before or after giant cell arteritis. Although polymyalgia rheumatica is common in patients with proven giant cell arteritis, fewer than 15 percent of all patients with polymyalgia rheumatica have any evidence of temporal arteritis. The etiologic relationship between the two conditions is unclear.

Laboratory. As in other chronic inflammatory conditions, a normocytic, normochromic anemia usually is found. An elevated platelet count and a markedly elevated Westergren sedimentation rate are characteristic. It is important to recognize that biopsy-proven cases of temporal arteritis with sedimentation rates below 40 mm/hour have been described [17]. From 4 to 17 percent of patients with biopsy-proven temporal arteritis will have normal sedimentation rates [215]. The acute-phase reactants, alpha-2-globulins, complement, and fibrinogen are elevated, as would be expected. Other laboratory findings include an increased alkaline phosphatase (liver fraction) in one-third of patients. Abnormal renal function, elevated muscle enzymes, antinuclear antibodies, and rheumatoid

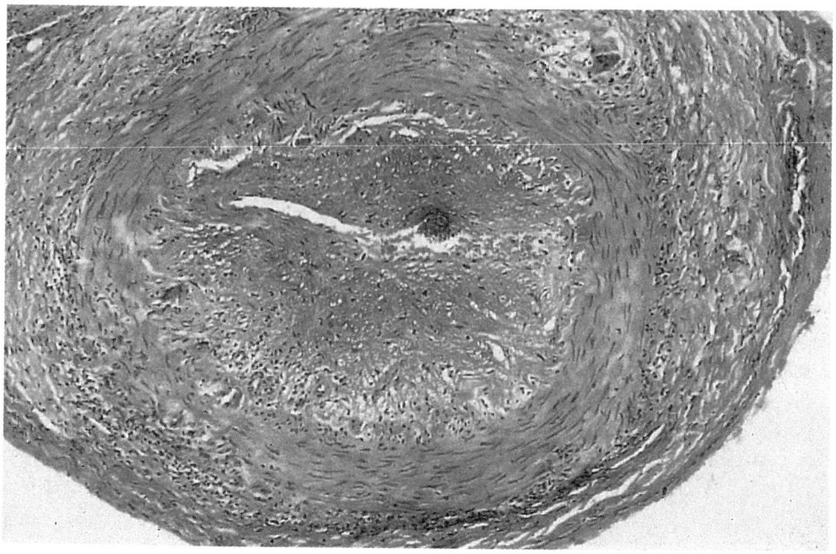

Fig. 43-7. Cranial arteritis. Low-magnification photomicrograph of temporal artery showing chronic inflammation of outer and inner media with near obliteration of lumen by proliferation of intimal fibrous tissue as well as extensive fibrosis of adventitia. Giant cells can be seen adjacent to internal and external elastic laminas.

factors are found no more often than in the normal population.

Diagnosis. Patients over the age of 50 with the onset of headache, visual loss, fever, and polymyalgia rheumatica with an elevated sedimentation rate are relatively easy to diagnose. Less classic presentations, including fever of unknown origin, weight loss, anorexia, dizziness, sore throat, cough, arm claudication, stroke, and myocardial infarction, make establishing the diagnosis more difficult [216–218]. In patients with those complaints, a careful review for coexistent symptoms suggestive of a systemic illness or local claudicatory manifestations is helpful.

If local signs of tenderness, decreased temporal-artery pulse, or temporal-artery nodules are present, a biopsy of that vessel of several centimeters' length should be done. In patients with features that strongly suggest temporal arteritis with no localizing arterial findings, the clinician should be prepared to biopsy both temporal arteries if the first biopsy is not diagnostic [208] (Figs. 43-7, 43-8).

In patients who present with symptoms of polymyalgia rheumatica and no claudicatory findings, a temporal-artery biopsy is not indicated, although patients with an associated fever of unknown origin are an exception to that rule [219]. Such patients need to be followed carefully for the onset of giant cell arteritis [219,220].

Differentiating giant cell arteritis from other vasculitides usually is not a problem. Although the temporal artery has been found to be inflamed in polyarteritis nodosa, both on pathologic and clinical grounds those conditions can be distinguished.

Prognosis and Treatment. Before corticosteroids were available for treatment, blindness developed in nearly 80 percent of patients [221]. Death is an unusual complication of giant cell arteritis, although several series document its occurrence [203,204,222]. A recent series documented nine deaths caused by persistent vasculitis. Five of the deaths were due to cerebral vascular accidents; there were two myocardial infarctions and two dissecting aortic aneurysms [222]. Death from vascular causes appears to be increased during the first 4 months after diagnosis [223]. With treatment, the survival rate does not appear to be reduced in patients with giant cell arteritis [224].

Treatment of giant cell arteritis with prednisone in dosages of 45 to 60 mg/day in divided doses is adequate to bring the disease under control in most patients. Within 2 weeks, the dose of steroids can be consolidated. After 4 weeks of treatment, the daily dose of prednisone can be tapered. Depending on the response of the individual patient, a gradual reduction of the daily dosage with careful clinical and laboratory monitoring allows most patients to be maintained on low dosages of daily steroids. Although exacerbations are not uncommon, many patients remit after 1 to 2 years of therapy [225].

TAKAYASU ARTERITIS

Takayasu arteritis involves the large arteries, primarily the aorta and its major branches, along with the pulmonary artery. Its occurrence appears to be most common in young women of Asian ancestry. Reports from North America and Europe suggest that it is a rare condition in whites, with a marked female predominance [226,227]. Takayasu arteritis also has been called pulseless disease, aortic arch syndrome, occlusive thromboaortopathy, and nonspecific aortoarteritis [85].

Pathology. Takayasu arteritis is an inflammatory and fibrotic disease. It involves the aorta and its main branches in a focal manner. The early stages show an inflammatory

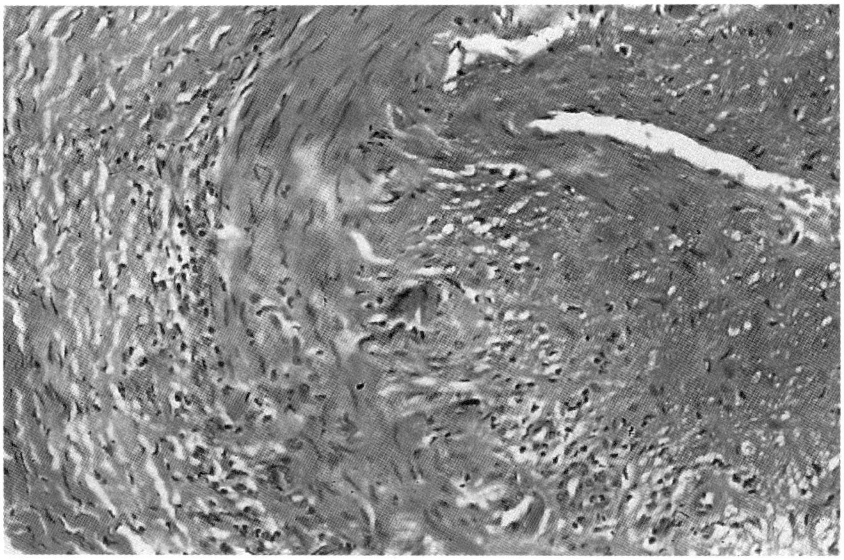

Fig. 43-8. Cranial arteritis. Higher-magnification photomicrograph of temporal artery showing lymphocytic infiltration of adventitia and inner media. Giant cells are seen near internal elastic lamina.

infiltrate of plasma cells and lymphocytes, predominantly in the adventitia and outer layer of the media. The process progresses to involve the entire media with neovascularization, diffuse inflammation, and occasional giant cells [228]. As in temporal arteritis, those cells appear most commonly at sites of disintegration of the elastic lamina.

The inflammatory process ultimately gives way to fibrosis beginning in the adventitia and extending into the media. Coexistent intimal proliferation is often extensive and may obliterate the lumen. Eventually, the inflammatory process subsides, and the muscular and elastic components of the vessel are entirely replaced by thickened fibrotic tissues [229]. The extent of involvement varies greatly throughout the aorta and large vessels. Severely scarred vessel may border on entirely normal artery. Lesions in different stages of inflammation and fibrosis often are found in the same patient.

Clinical Features. Takayasu arteritis is often divided into two stages. The first stage is characterized by systemic symptoms of fever, malaise, and weight loss. Arthralgias, myalgias, and pleurisy are common. A skin rash similar to erythema nodosum also is reported [230]. The initial phase may last for several months or even years. Not all patients experience early systemic symptoms prior to manifesting arterial obstruction [19]. The second stage consists of symptoms and signs of vascular insufficiency, often concomitantly with the continuing systemic features [231].

There are several proposed classifications of Takayasu arteritis, depending on the anatomic distribution of the vascular lesions [232,233]. An early classification scheme divided patients into types, depending on the presence or absence of aortic-arch involvement. Type I (Shimizu-Sano) has involvement of the arch and its branches. In Type II (Kimoto), the thoracic, descending, and abdominal aorta are involved, while the arch is spared. Type III (Inada) has features of both types I and II. A type IV, patients with pulmonary-artery involvement, was added later [232]. These early classifications provide little prognostic information. A subsequent scheme included natural history and included four groups, depending on the degree of involvement at presentation [19]. Group I had patients with narrowing or occlusion of the aorta or its branches but without complications. Group II had complications such as retinopathy, aneurysm, secondary hypertension, or claudication. That group was subdivided into mild or moderate complication, IIa, and severe, IIb. Group III had two or more complications. The value of any of the classifications is suspect given the erratic course of the disease [226].

The most common cardiovascular findings are bruits, which are present in over 90 percent of patients (Table 43-6). The typical locations for the bruits are over the carotid arteries and abdominal aorta [226,230]. Subclavian and femoral bruits also are common findings. Pulse deficits usually are found in the upper extremities. They do not correlate well with symptoms of claudication, since the gradual pace of obstruction frequently allows for the development of collateral circulation. Neurologic symptoms, on the other hand, varying from light-headedness and headache to syncope and stroke, correlate well with carotid- or vertebral-artery disease.

In most series, the finding of hypertension signals the presence of renal-artery stenosis [226,230,234]. Other potential causes of hypertension are coarctation of the aorta, decreased elasticity of the aorta, and aortic-valve incompetence [19]. Blood pressure elevation is usually moderate and is treated medically in most cases [234].

Abdominal aortitis commonly extends into the superior

Table 43-6. Clinical features of Takayasu arteritis from three series

Features	Number/ Total number cases	Percent
Bruits	145/161	90
Fatigue	115/161	71
Pulse deficit	138/161	86
Hypertension	91/139	65
Arthralgia	84/161	52
Headache	81/161	50
Arm claudication	54/161	34
Fever	34/116	29
Fundoscopic abnormalities	45/161	28
Weight loss	36/139	26
Syncopy	27/139	19
Angina/myocardial infarct	29/161	18
Hemiplegia	9/161	6

Sources: Data from A Fraga et al. Takayasu arteritis: frequency of systemic manifestations (study of 22 patients) and favorable response to maintenance steroid therapy with adrenocorticosteroids. Arthr Rheum 1972; 15:617–623. HE Lupi et al. Takayasu arteritis: clinical study of 107 cases. Am Heart J 1977; 93:94. S Hall et al. Takayasu arteritis. A study of 32 North American patients. Medicine 1985; 64:89–99.

and inferior mesenteric arteries, which may result in abdominal angina, although abundant collateral circulation frequently limits the symptomatic evidence of abdominal disease. Celiac arterial stenosis is rare. Glomerular disease, usually a mild mesangial proliferative or focal glomerulonephritis, has been reported in several patients [235].

Coronary-artery insufficiency is most frequently the result of ostial stenosis [236,237]. Obstructions in the proximal portions of the coronary arteries also are found. Symptoms of angina, palpitation, and congestive heart failure are found but are not necessarily the result of coronary-artery insufficiency. Aortic-valve incompetence, caused by dilatation of the aortic root as well as thickening of the valve cusps, also may result in those symptoms. Despite the frequency of aortic insufficiency, reported in up to one-fifth of patients, valve replacement is uncommon. Myocarditis and pericarditis are unusual [228].

Constriction of the aorta is a late complication of Takayasu arteritis. Similarly, dilatation or aneurysm formation at the site of previous constriction is a common late finding in Takayasu arteritis. Alternating lesions of stenosis and dilatation with intervening normal aorta is a pattern characteristic of Takayasu arteritis [229].

Pulmonary-artery involvement is reported in between one-fourth and one-half of patients [238]. Evidence for that complication often is obtained through the physical examination, chest radiograph, and electrocardiogram [232]. Vessels in the right lung are predominantly involved. Pulmonary hypertension develops frequently and may be due to pulmonary-artery stenosis, left ventricular failure, or both [232]. The angiographic pattern shows a marked decrement of pulmonary vessels, indicative of large pulmonary artery involvement [19,229]. Clinical manifestations of that problem are infrequent, with only an occasional report of hemoptysis.

Visual symptoms are a common complaint of patients with Takayasu arteritis [226]. Amaurosis may be transient or permanent and may be precipitated by postural changes or exercise [239]. Visual loss can be the result of retinal, optic-nerve, or cerebral ischemia. Retinal findings may be the result of either hypertensive or Takayasu retinopathy, the latter correlating well with severe carotid disease and retinal hypoperfusion.

Laboratory. An anemia, elevated erythrocyte sedimentation rate, and thrombocytosis characterize the laboratory findings in active Takayasu arteritis. The sedimentation rate is elevated in patients with active disease [226]. Control of symptoms as well as progression of inflammatory arterial involvement are not always mirrored by the erythrocyte sedimentation rate [226,230,240]. Hypergammaglobulinemia is common, but autoantibodies are not found more commonly than in the normal population. Suggestions that positive tuberculin skin tests are more common in this disease than in the population have not been borne out [234]. Certain radiographic findings may be found in this disease, including dilatation of the ascending aorta, segmental dystrophic calcifications, rib notching, cardiac enlargement, and irregularities of the descending aorta [233].

Diagnosis. The diagnosis is usually established by the finding of characteristic abnormalities on the angiograms, including stenoses, occlusions with collaterals, luminal irregularities, and aneurysms or ectasia (Fig. 43-9). The earliest lesions are localized irregularities, which progress to segmental circumferential narrowings. The narrowings may be short segments or long and diffuse. They may be clearly demarcated, irregular, smooth, or a gradually tapered lesion. Complete stenosis or dilatation and aneurysm ultimately may occur [233].

Multiple sites and types of involvement coexisting in the same patient are the usual pattern [233]. Although the aortic arch and brachiocephalic vessels are the most commonly involved vessels angiographically, disease limited solely to the distal aorta and its branches, the so-called Kimoto variety, is frequent enough, especially in younger patients, to warrant a full arteriographic study [241]. The increasing sensitivity of B-mode ultrasonography and MRI along with the ability to repeat such studies without exposing the patient to the risk of contrast dye and invasive angiography have increased the interest in those procedures for diagnosis and management of patients with Takayasu arteritis [242,243].

The differential diagnosis is limited to several infectious aortitides and a few rheumatic conditions. Among the former are syphilis, mycotic aneurysm, and tuberculous aortitis; the latter include the spondyloarthropathies with aortitis and resultant aortic insufficiency, rheumatic fever with aortitis, Buerger's disease, and relapsing polychondritis. Noninflammatory conditions, including Marfan syndrome, Ehlers-Danlos syndrome, osteogenesis imperfecta, and fibromuscular dysplasia may produce some-

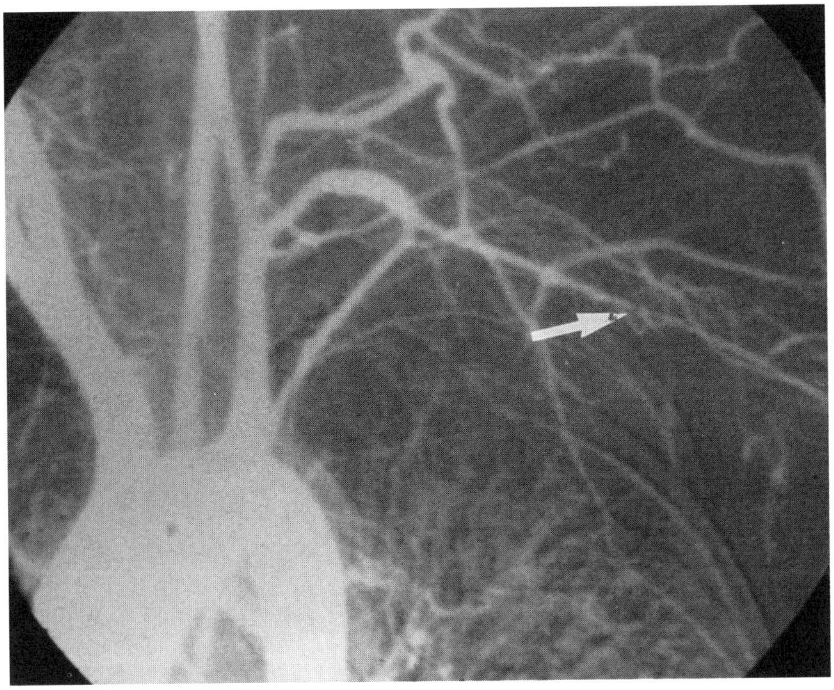

Fig. 43-9. Arteriogram of the aortic arch in a young woman with Takayasu arteritis who presented with left-arm claudication. There is narrowing of the proximal portion of the left common carotid artery. There is a total occlusion of the left subclavian artery (arrow). An extensive collateral network of vessels is providing blood flow to the arm distal to the occlusion.

what similar clinical and radiographic findings and should be considered [244–246].

Treatment and Prognosis. Several large retrospective studies are available for evaluation of prognostic factors [19,152,226,230,234,238]. Severe complications, such as retinopathy with microaneurysm and arteriovenous anastomoses, secondary hypertension, severe aortic regurgitation, and marked aneurysm formation, appear to compromise survival [238]. Without those complications, the 5-year survival is greater than 90 percent [208,238]. Patients with more than one severe complication have a survival rate of 74 percent at 5 years. Deaths most often are the result of congestive heart failure, cerebrovascular accident, and lethal arrhythmias [238].

Medical treatment with corticosteroids usually is instituted in initial doses ranging from 30–60 mg prednisone. Improvement in systemic symptoms and a fall in the erythrocyte sedimentation rate occur quickly after treatment is begun. A lower maintenance dosage of prednisone is sufficient to control the disease in many cases, and a substantial number of patients discontinue steroids after several years of therapy. Many patients have restoration of absent pulses after several months of treatment [152,247]. Some patients have responded to cytotoxic drugs when the inflammatory disease does not respond to steroids [226]. Low-dosage methotrexate (0.15–0.30 mg/kg) appears to be an effective steroid-sparing agent [248].

Surgical bypass procedures, endarterectomies, or aneurysm resections are performed in fewer than 10 percent of patients reported in the 1975 survey in Japan [249]. On the other hand, 12 out of 32 patients followed at the Mayo Clinic underwent surgical procedures. The end results of those procedures are adversely affected by ongoing inflammation [234,238]. Up to one-third of reconstructive procedures eventually reocclude [234]. Renal angioplasty has been shown to be effective in 70 to 83 percent of patients initially. Five-year patency rates are less impressive—33 percent [250]. Angioplasty of abdominal aortic coarctation has similar short-term value. Patients with coarctation and tight proximal renal-artery stenosis have the poorest long-term results [251].

ANGIOCENTRIC IMMUNOPROLIFERATIVE LESIONS

Originally described by Liebow and Carrington in 1972 as lymphomatoid granulomatosis, the disease of angiocentric immunoproliferative lesions has the characteristic histologic appearance of an angiocentric, angiodestructive polymorphic cellular infiltrate. The vessels of the lung, skin, and central nervous system are most commonly involved. The predominant infiltrating cells are T lymphocytes with morphologic characteristics ranging from atypia to lymphoma [22]. Epstein-Barr virus has been identified in the more malignant lesions and may play a role in the transformation of those lesions from atypia to neoplasia [252]. The lesion has characteristics of both a granulomatous and lymphoproliferative disease. Progression to frank lymphoma occurs in 13 to 47 percent of patients [88,253].

Most patients experience onset of disease in their third

to sixth decade. Occasionally, children and elderly are reported. There appears to be a slight male predominance. Patients present with constitutional symptoms, particularly fever, along with cough, chest pain, and dyspnea. Erythematous macular or plaquelike lesions are seen in 40 percent of patients and may precede other manifestations. Involvement of the brain and spinal cord, even at presentation, is not uncommon. Central nervous system disease presents as a mass lesion and results from extensive infiltration of the blood vessels and cerebral substance [253]. Peripheral nervous system disease is uncommon.

More unusual is involvement of the upper respiratory tract, liver, spleen, kidneys, and heart. The rarity of upper-respiratory-tract findings helps distinguish this condition clinically from Wegener's granulomatosis. The occasional report of focal glomerulonephritis may make the differential diagnosis difficult. Chest radiographic lesions are characteristically bilateral, peripheral, lower-lobe nodular infiltrates [22]. Diffuse infiltrates and pleural effusions also are seen. The laboratory findings are not specific. A mild anemia occurs in some patients, as do abnormalities of the leukocyte counts. The sedimentation rate may be normal in half the patients [254]. Hypergammaglobulinemia and autoantibodies do not usually accompany the condition.

Optimal drug therapy for this condition has not been found. Initial 4-year survival rates of 10 percent despite therapy with corticosteroids suggest a very poor prognosis [22]. Death usually is due to extensive central nervous system and pulmonary disease or progression to lymphoma [22,88,255]. Short-term response to steroids as well as spontaneous remissions make evaluation of therapeutic efficacy difficult. Katzenstein's large retrospective study had a 63.5 percent mortality rate with a median survival of 14 months. No clear survival advantage could be demonstrated by any treatment when compared with no treatment [88].

Other studies suggest that treatment with steroids and cyclophosphamide may be beneficial [225,256]. It has been suggested that early treatment with cyclophosphamide and corticosteroids induces remission, and prevention of lymphoma may be achieved [257].

KAWASAKI SYNDROME

Kawasaki syndrome (KS) is an acute febrile illness first described in Japan in 1967 and called acute febrile mucocutaneous lymph node syndrome [258]. The disease occurs in endemic or epidemic outbreaks and has been reported worldwide. The use of high-dosage intravenous gammaglobulin during the first 10 days of illness has reduced the number of coronary aneurysms and made the early diagnosis of KS critical [259].

The incidence of KS peaks at the age of 1 year in Japan. Children in the United States usually are slightly older, but there is a male predominance in both populations [260–262]. A sudden onset of fever, conjunctivitis, pharyngitis, dry erythematous lips, and a strawberry tongue characterize the illness. Cervical adenopathy and a diffuse erythematous rash appear within a few days. Erythema of the palms and soles followed by a diffuse swelling of the hands and feet occur early in the course of the disease.

Table 43-7. CDC case definition of Kawasaki syndrome

Fever of at least 5 days' duration
Presence of at least four of the five following conditions:
Bilateral nonexudative conjunctival injection
One of the following in the oropharynx:
injected or fissured lips
injected pharynx
strawberry tongue
One of the following:
erythema of the palms and soles
edema of hands or feet
periungual desquation
Nonvascular polynerphous rash
Acute nonsupportive cervical lymphadenopathy
Illness not explained by any other known disease

Source: Rauch A, Hurwitz E. Centers for Disease Control: case definition of Kawasaki syndrome. Pediatr Infect Dis J 1985; 4:702–703.

Those clinical findings make up the diagnostic criteria for Kawasaki syndrome [261] (Table 43-7). Unfortunately there is considerable overlap with known infectious diseases such as group A beta-hemolytic streptococcal infection and measles [261]. Oligoarticular arthritis and iridocyclitis frequently are seen [263].

The most feared complications are cardiovascular. Early in the course of the disease, up to 50 percent of patients may develop carditis, as evidenced by clinical, electrocardiographic, and echocardiographic studies [264]. Within 2 weeks, coronary-artery aneurysms are detected by two-dimensional echocardiography in 23 percent of patients treated with aspirin [259]. Despite those dramatic figures, the mortality rate is less than 2 percent. The usual cause of death is myocardial infarction secondary to coronary-artery thrombosis seen in patients with larger coronary aneurysms [265]. Ruptured coronary aneurysms with pericardial tamponade or fatal hemorrhage are unusual [266].

The aorta and coronary, carotid, celiac, subclavian, pulmonary, and iliac vessels may all be involved by a panangiitis [267,268]. A mononuclear infiltrate with disruption of the elastic lamina, vessel-wall necrosis, and endothelial-cell proliferation is seen in the coronary arteries at autopsy. Other vessels are more likely to have endothelial-cell proliferation alone [267]. The changes are similar to the findings of infantile polyarteritis nodosa, suggesting that infantile polyarteritis nodosa may be a severe form of KS [269].

The laboratory studies reveal anemia, marked neutrophilia, and an elevated platelet count during the acute phase of the disease. A high sedimentation rate and elevated serum IgG and IgE also are seen [263]. Occasional pyuria and proteinuria have been reported.

Treatment remains under investigation. Multicenter randomized trials have demonstrated that aspirin in dosages of 80–100 mg/kg/day for 2 weeks plus a single high-dose intravenous gammaglobulin infusion of 2 g/kg given within the first 10 days of illness significantly reduce the fever and the incidence of coronary aneurysms. When the patient is afebrile, the dose of salicylates may be reduced to platelet-inhibiting levels [259,270].

Patients with Kawasaki disease should undergo baseline echocardiography at diagnosis and again at 3 and 7 weeks. If the test is normal and there is no laboratory evidence of inflammation, salicylates may be discontinued. However, if the echocardiography is abnormal, aspirin plus regular monitoring should be continued for at least 1 year after the aneurysms have resolved. Patients failing medical treatment have successfully undergone coronary-artery bypass surgery [271].

BEHÇET'S SYNDROME

Behçet's syndrome is a chronic relapsing disorder defined by a triad of recurrent aphthous stomatitis, genital aphthous ulcers, and uveitis [272]. Three other manifestations occur with great regularity: cutaneous vasculitis, synovitis, and meningoencephalitis. The disease has its highest prevalence in the eastern Mediterranean region and Japan [273]. Most patients first develop symptoms in their third and fourth decades.

The etiology and pathogenesis of Behçet's syndrome remain unknown. Many patients with the condition demonstrate a host of immunologic abnormalities, including circulating antibody to and lymphocytotoxicity against mucosal cells, circulating immune complexes, elevated immunoglobulin levels, and decreased levels of secretory component of IgA [274–277]. In Behçet's syndrome, an increased frequency of the HLA antigen B-5 and split antigen HLA-B51 has been reported in Japanese, Turkish, and Israeli patients [278–281].

The most common manifestation of Behçet's disease are the aphthous ulcers. They usually are the initial manifestation, painful and recurrent. Genital ulcers are the second most frequent finding, present in 90 percent of patients. Like the oral ulcers, they are recurrent and painful. Uveitis, both anterior and posterior, is seen later in the course of the disease. Posterior-chamber involvement is more serious: It is often bilateral and is the major cause of blindness in Behçet's syndrome [282].

Cutaneous lesions span a large spectrum. Papules, pustules, and vesicles are the usual manifestations of the cutaneous vasculitis. Erythema nodosum–like lesions may, unlike erythema nodosum, ulcerate. They are a manifestation of superficial phlebitis [283]. Recurrent thrombophlebitis of both superficial and deep veins, sometimes occurring at the site of venipuncture and often associated with fever, is a common finding of Behçet's syndrome. Obstruction of the superior and inferior vena cava, cerebral sinus, hepatic veins, and right ventricular thrombi are common, major complications of Behçet's syndrome [284]. Phlebitis can be resistant to anticoagulant therapy [283]. Decreased fibrinolysis appears to be one of the mechanisms of that hypercoagulable state [275].

Aneurysms and occlusions of large arteries are potentially life-threatening complications of the condition [273]. Cerebrovascular accidents, renovascular hypertension, and limb claudication are seen as a result of the arteritis or thrombosis. Fatal rupture of pulmonary-artery aneurysms have been seen in Behçet's disease.

Neurologic involvement occurs in up to 45 percent of patients. Cerebral venous thrombosis occurs in 10 percent of patients and generally responds to treatment with anticoagulation and steroids [285]. The high morbidity and not infrequent mortality of the other neurologic manifestations of Behçet's have made them the most feared complications. Meningoencephalitis, presenting with fever, stiff neck, and focal neurologic signs, is the most common neurologic problem and may occur early in the disease course. Response to high-dosage steroids often is poor [286]. Other more focal central nervous system manifestations indicative of arterial occlusive disease are not uncommon.

Half the patients have a subacute synovitis usually involving the knees and ankles. A mild pericarditis and glomerulonephritis also are seen. Ulcers of the gastrointestinal tract may lead to perforation. Topical or systemic corticosteroids, depending on the severity of involvement, may improve the skin, joint, eye, and mucosal manifestations. Posterior uveitis and the central nervous system manifestations often are resistant to steroids and convey the worst prognosis. Treatment with immunosuppressive drugs have, in uncontrolled series, been successful [287]. Transfer factor, estradiol, dapsone, phenformin, colchicine, cyclosporin, and levamisole have all had mixed results in the therapy of Behçet's disease.

COGAN'S SYNDROME

A rare syndrome of nonsyphilitic interstitial keratitis and audiovestibular symptoms, Cogan's syndrome is associated with systemic manifestations, particularly vasculitis and aortitis, in up to one-sixth of patients [288]. Cogan's syndrome is a disease of young adults. Two-thirds of patients have a preceding upper respiratory infection [289]. Eye and ear manifestations are the initial findings in most patients. The ocular complaints of interstitial keratitis are redness, lacrimation, photophobia, and decreased visual acuity. The symptoms develop suddenly and may be evanescent, recurrent, and unilateral or bilateral. Other ocular manifestations are uveitis, scleritis, and optic neuritis. Multiple ophthalmologic examinations may be necessary to demonstrate keratitis. Sudden loss of hearing can be accompanied by vertigo, tinnitus, nausea, vomiting, ataxia, and nystagmus. Early audiograms may detect abnormalities before they are reported by the patient.

Up to one-half of patients have fever, myalgias, weight loss, or fatigue. Those findings are seen in patients with vasculitis or aortic insufficiency [290]. Similarly, abdominal discomfort, melena, cutaneous nodules, cranial neuropathies, mononeuritis multiplex, and lymphadenopathy are all more likely to be found in those patients who are ultimately found to have vasculitis.

The aortitis found in Cogan's syndrome involves the media and intima predominantly. A mixed infiltrate of neutrophils, mononuclear cells, and occasional giant cells is found in areas with disruption of the elastic lamina, necrosis, and scarring of the vessel wall [288]. Aortic insufficiency develops as well, due to inflammation of the cusps. Medium and small arteries as well as veins have been inflamed in some patients with the syndrome [290]. The infiltrate, necrosis, and scarring in those vessels is little different from those of the aorta.

Laboratory findings, as in other vasculitides, include elevated acute-phase reactants, anemia, thrombocytosis, and leukocytosis. The rarity of this condition and the not infrequent involvement of the eyes and ears in other systemic vasculitides make the diagnosis difficult to establish if the existence of interstitial keratitis is verified. In the absence of congenital syphilis, rubella, or mumps, nonulcerative stromal keratitis and audiovestibular findings strongly suggest Cogan's syndrome [290].

The prognosis in this syndrome is not benign. Deafness (66%), aortic insufficiency (11%), blindness (7%), and death (9%) were reported in one of the larger series [290]. Systemic corticosteroid treatment appears to ameliorate the eighth-nerve dysfunction and, with topically applied steroids, improves the ocular manifestations in most patients. With high dosages, glucocorticoids appear to control the aortitis and vasculitis in most patients. Experience with immunosuppressive agents is limited. Aortic-valve replacement is required occasionally and may prevent an otherwise fatal outcome [290].

THROMBOANGIITIS OBLITERANS

Thromboangiitis obliterans, also known as Buerger's disease, is discussed in detail in Chap. 44.

ISOLATED CENTRAL NERVOUS SYSTEM VASCULITIS

Isolated central nervous system vasculitis is an inflammatory disease involving predominantly the leptomeningeal and parenchymal small arteries, with less frequent involvement of larger arteries and veins of the central nervous system. The vessels are infiltrated by mononuclear cells with, in many cases, the development of a granulomatous reaction. The number of reported cases is quite small. There is a male-to-female ratio of 1:1. The condition appears to be associated with herpes zoster, Hodgkin's disease, and non-Hodgkin's lymphoma [291,292].

The most common presenting symptom is headache. Global dysfunction of the central nervous system, including memory loss, personality change, weakness, seizures, and loss of consciousness, is also a common presentation. Focal lesions are less frequent as an initial problem but develop eventually in over 90 percent of cases. Systemic symptoms such as malaise, arthralgias, myalgias, fever, and rash are uncommon [293]. Multiple focal neurologic abnormalities are found in most patients, including muscle weakness, pathologic reflexes, hemiplegia, ataxia, and myelopathy.

The laboratory studies are highly variable. The erythrocyte sedimentation rate, complete blood count, urinalysis, antinuclear antibodies, rheumatoid factor, and circulating immune complexes may all be normal or absent [6,294]. Cerebrospinal fluid often has a slightly elevated protein and a mild pleocytosis. Electroencephalograms are nonspecifically abnormal in most patients. Brain scans may be normal, and computed axial tomography is usually abnormal, although there is no diagnostic appearance [296].

Angiographic studies are diagnostically valuable in a majority of patients [6]. The most common finding is either an isolated or a multifocal symmetric narrowing and beading of the small and medium-sized cerebral and meningeal arteries [291,292]. Dilatation and aneurysm formation are less common [291]. In a sizable minority of pathologically proven cases, angiographic studies are normal [295]. Conversely, other diseases such as herpes zoster ophthalmicus, Hodgkin's disease, polyarteritis nodosa, Sjögren's syndrome, cryoglobulinemia, temporal arteritis, Takayasu arteritis, systemic lupus erythematosus, angiocentric immunoproliferative lesions, and Wegener's granulomatosis may be associated with central nervous system vasculitis. For those reasons, a careful search for other systemic diseases should be performed before the diagnosis of isolated central nervous system vasculitis is made [291].

As already noted, angiographic studies may be normal. Biopsies frequently are necessary to establish the diagnosis. Leptomeningeal vessels frequently appear to be involved. Intimal proliferation along with a mononuclear cell infiltrate, giant cells, and granulomas often are seen. The latter are most common in the vicinity of disrupted elastic lamella. Fibrosis is common. Involvement of the arteries is dramatically segmental, and veins may be involved [296]. Subcortical vessels are less frequently involved than leptomeningeal vessels. A biopsy of the cortex and leptomeninges is indicated if the arteriogram is nondiagnostic, although the segmental nature of that condition may result in a normal biopsy [166].

The early reported cases had a poor prognosis, with a mean survival of 45 days [291]. With more rapid diagnosis and institution of therapy with high-dosage steroids and cytotoxic agents (either azathioprine or cyclophosphamide), the outcome has improved.

MALIGNANCY AND VASCULITIS

Systemic necrotizing vasculitis, granulomatous vasculitis, and hypersensitivity vasculitis can all be rare manifestations of a coexisting malignant process. Most of the small reported series associate hematologic or lymphoreticular neoplastic conditions with these vasculitides [297].

A systemic necrotizing arteritis simulating polyarteritis nodosa has been seen in patients with hairy-cell leukemia [118,298–301]. The clinical findings in those patients were similar to those reported in polyarteritis nodosa except for the frequent involvement of the temporal artery, the presence of leukopenia (uncommon in polyarteritis nodosa), circulating "hairy cells," and infiltration of the vessel wall with leukemic cells. Polyarteritis nodosa–like lesions also have been described in patients with Hodgkin's disease. That association does not appear to be as frequent as the relation between Hodgkin's and granulomatous angiitis of the central nervous system [291].

Hypersensitivity vasculitis has been reported in association with many neoplastic diseases, including Hodgkin's and non-Hodgkin's lymphomas, solid tumors, multiple myeloma, myelodysplastic syndromes, and leukemia [297,302–304]. The presumed mechanism has been the deposition of circulating immune complexes. Circulating immune complexes are detected in up to one-third of cancer patients [40]. Tumor-associated antigen and antibody to that antigen has been demonstrated in circulation, yet the incidence of vasculitis in malignant diseases is quite small, and malignancy represents a very infrequent cause of hypersensitivity vasculitis [305]. B-cell neoplasms are associated with cryoglobulinemic vasculitis, hyperviscosity, amyloidosis, and lambda light-chain vasculopathy, which has a similar appearance to hypersensitivity or systemic vasculitis [306].

Although rare, systemic and hypersensitivity vasculitis does complicate malignant diseases. The manifestations of the vasculitis often predate the neoplastic process. The reverse also may occur, especially in hairy-cell leukemia [297,307]. Treatment of the underlying neoplastic condition is often but not always sufficient therapy for the vasculitis [307].

ANTIPHOSPHOLIPID ANTIBODY SYNDROME

Antiphospholipid antibody syndrome is defined by the clinical features of recurrent thromboembolism, recurrent fetal loss, and livedo reticularis in an individual who has elevated anticardiolipin antibody or lupus anticoagulant [308–311]. These patients commonly have thrombocytopenia and valvular heart disease [312].

Antiphospholipid antibody syndrome frequently is found in patients with systemic lupus erythematosus and occasionally in other connective-tissue diseases. It also exists as a primary disease. Antiphospholipid antibody can be induced by infectious agents (HIV, *Borrelia burgdorferi, Treponema pallidum*) and by drugs (chlorpromazine, procainamide, quinidine). Patients with induced antibody rarely manifest the clinical syndrome [313–315].

Anticardiolipin antibodies are measured routinely using an enzyme-linked immunosorbent assay (ELISA). International standards for measurement of IgG and IgM exist [316]. Lupus anticoagulants are discovered by detection of an abnormal activated partial thromboplastin time, Russell's viper venom time, or a kaolin clotting time, which is not corrected by addition of normal plasma. The mechanism by which anticardiolipin antibodies induce thromboembolic disease is unclear.

Clinical manifestation includes arterial thrombosis involving single vessels. Rarely, multiple vessels can be occluded in a crescendo manner with widespread infarctions [317]. Antiphospholipid antibody syndrome is responsible for up to one-third of new strokes in patients under 50 years of age [318]. Once having had a stroke, a patient with antiphospholipid antibody syndrome has nearly a 20-percent-per-year risk of recurrence [319]. Involvement of coronary, digital, and mesenteric vessels is reported.

Venous thrombosis with complications that include pulmonary emboli and Budd-Chiari syndrome occur at increased frequency in patients with antiphospholipid antibody syndrome. Thrombosis of veins of the upper extremity also occurs. In young patients with phlebitis and no overt risk factors, screening for anticardiolipin antibody may be reasonable [320].

Fetal loss is a third common manifestation of antiphospholipid antibody syndrome. A high titre of IgG anticardiolipin antibody or a lupus anticoagulant appears to confer increased risk of fetal loss [321]. It is less clear that lowering the level of anticardiolipin reduces the risk of recurrent second-trimester fetal death. The risk of recurrent fetal death appears to be highest in women with both anticardiolipin antibody and systemic lupus erythematosus [322].

Other manifestations, such as valvular heart disease with aortic and mitral-valve insufficiency and Libman-Sacks–type endocardial lesions, are found in antiphospholipid antibody syndrome [312]. Livido reticularis, skin ulcers and thrombocytopenia are found in both primary and secondary antiphospholipid antibody syndrome.

Treatment of most patients with antiphospholipid antibody syndrome requires anticoagulant or antiplatelet therapy rather than immunosuppression. The rare patients with acute widespread arterial occlusions may best be treated with combination of apheresis, anticoagulation, and high-dosage corticosteroids [317]. Intravenous gammaglobulin and cytotoxic agents also have been used. Although not confirmed by any prospective randomized studies, asymptomatic patients with isolated laboratory abnormalities probably do not require treatment [308, 309,311].

Management and Treatment. Proper management of a vasculitic syndrome requires establishment of the diagnosis along with the degree of organ damage induced by the vasculitic process. Vasculitides may be self-limited with minimal morbidity or progressive, persistent, fatal conditions, depending, to a large extent, on the size and type of vessels involved. It is also a function of the organs involved. The presence or absence of an offending antigen, drug, or infectious agent that can be isolated and then eliminated also affects the outcome.

Establishing a diagnosis and assessing the extent of the vasculitic process allows the clinician to determine the length and aggressiveness of treatment. That information also creates the database necessary to follow the disease's progression and therapeutic response. Thorough periodic reevaluation of the degree of organ dysfunction, along with measurement of inflammatory parameters, enables the physician to manage these conditions properly.

Approaches to therapy follow several principles: If a foreign substance that has induced the vasculitis can be identified, it should be eliminated, and the inflammation will typically recede. Although that option is available only in a minority of patients, it is most likely to occur in the hypersensitivity vasculitides. Control of an underlying systemic condition is the second principle in the treatment of vasculitis. Whether that means treatment of a known infection, resection of a tumor, or therapy for inflammatory bowel disease, the vasculitis usually disappears with such an approach. Occasionally, the damage induced by the vasculitis requires short, directed therapy for control concurrent with treatment of the systemic disease.

If the aforementioned options are not available, then the vasculitis, if not treated, is likely to induce continued organ damage, and direct intervention aimed at the vasculitic process is indicated. That may mean removal of circulating immune complexes (plasmapheresis), inhibition of the inflammatory response (aspirin, corticosteroids), or immune suppression (corticosteroids, azathioprine, cyclophosphamide).

The role of plasmapheresis remains controversial. Much of the literature in the treatment of vasculitis is anecdotal [121,323,324]. Relapse of the vasculitis associated with higher levels of circulating immune complexes has been a concern when plasma exchange has been used without immunosuppression [121,323]. A randomized study in polyarteritis nodosa and Churg-Strauss syndrome demonstrated no added benefit to plasmapheresis when added to prednisone [126,325]. There was some benefit to plasma exchange when used with prednisone and cytotoxic drugs in patients with severe renal disease in a separate randomized study [125]. Although not confirmed, the role of plasmapheresis in vasculitis may be limited to patients with rapidly progressive disease. Simultaneous immunosuppressives should be instituted.

Aspirin and other nonsteroidal anti-inflammatory drugs appear to have a limited role in vasculitis. In a mild hypersensitivity vasculitis with prominent arthralgias and myalgias, those drugs may be sufficient. Colchicine (0.6 mg bid) has been used to control chronic cutaneous leukocytoclastic vasculitis. Success rates of 65 percent with complete response have been reported [326].

Of the many glucocorticoids available, prednisone and prednisolone are used most frequently. Prednisolone is the bioactive metabolite of prednisone. Both agents have a relatively high anti-inflammatory and immunosuppressive activity in comparison with their sodium-retaining qualities. Prednisone has a short to intermediate half-life, making it suitable for alternate-day therapy. Detailed reviews of these medications are available [327,328].

Corticosteroids are the primary treatment for temporal arteritis, Takayasu arteritis, and severe hypersensitivity vasculitis. In the hypersensitivity syndromes, the dosages of prednisone depend on the organ involved and the extent of the damage. Doses of 10–20 mg/day may be sufficient for milder manifestations of skin, muscle, and joint disease. Renal disease or peripheral neuropathy, as is seen in essential cryoglobulinemia, may require doses of 1 mg/kg in divided daily dosages initially, to control the damage (2 weeks often is sufficient). Subsequently, a single daily dosage or alternate-day dosaging may be adequate to maintain control of the disease.

In systemic necrotizing and granulomatous vasculitis, the initial therapy is prednisone in doses of 1 mg/kg, often in conjunction with a cytotoxic agent. The objective is to taper the corticosteroid as soon as the cytotoxic medication has become effective. In practice, the initial divided daily dosage is unified to a daily dosage and then tapered to alternate-day dosaging.

In severe, rapidly progressive vasculitis, "pulse" prednisolone in doses of 1,000 mg intravenously over 1–3 hours has been given on 3 to 4 successive days. It then may be followed by a daily dosage of prednisone of 1 mg/kg and a cytotoxic agent. The effectiveness of that approach remains unproven.

In the treatment of severe vasculitis, daily corticosteroid therapy is often rapidly changed to alternate-day therapy when cytotoxic agents demonstrate effective control of the disease [120]. Alternate-day therapy results in less hypothalamic-pituitary-adrenal axis suppression and a lower risk of infection [329]. The dosage of corticosteroid given on an every-other-day basis should be approximately 2.5 times the daily dosage. It should not, however, exceed 80 mg prednisone. This method usually maintains significant anti-inflammatory and immunosuppressive effects.

Cytotoxic drugs used in low doses are both immunosuppressive and anti-inflammatory [330]. Azathioprine and cyclophosphamide are reported most frequently for the treatment of vasculitis. The former is an antimetabolite and the latter an alkylating agent. Both have significant toxic capabilities, and patients on these agents should be carefully monitored.

Azathioprine is a purine analogue that when metabolized to the ribonucleotide thioinosinic acid suppresses synthesis of adenine and guanine. Given in dosages of 2.0 to 2.5 mg/kg/day, it has been shown in retrospective studies to be effective in polyarteritis nodosa [109,331]. It also has demonstrated some usefulness in the treatment of Wegener's granulomatosis as an alternative to cyclophosphamide [56]. Monitoring for hematologic complications is critical during therapy with this agent; leukopenia is the most common effect.

Cyclophosphamide covalently links nucleophilic cellular material, leading to cross-linking of nucleic acids and interfering with a large number of cellular functions [332]. It markedly depresses lymphocyte survival and function [333]. The immunosuppressive effect of the agent correlates well with the total peripheral lymphocyte count.

Cyclophosphamide has been shown to be of considerable value in the treatment of systemic necrotizing vasculitis, Wegener's granulomatosis, and some patients with Takayasu arteritis [56,81,120]. It also has been used in patients with rheumatoid vasculitis [122]. The usual starting dosage is 2 mg/kg/day in a single morning dose. Severe cases may require initial treatment with dosages of 3–4 mg/kg/day for several days given intravenously, followed by daily oral dosage of 2 mg/kg. Pulses of monthly intravenous cyclophosphamide also have been used in the treatment of systemic necrotizing vasculitis and Wegener's granulomatosis with variable success [295,334].

The dosage administered during the induction and the maintenance period of therapy should not induce a total granulocyte count of less than 1,500/cu mm. Lower polymorphonuclear leukocyte counts are associated with an increased risk of infection [120]. Other adverse effects besides bacterial infections are alopecia, sterility, interstitial pneumonitis, herpes zoster, hemorrhagic cystitis, fibrosis of the bladder wall, bladder carcinoma, leukemia, and lymphoma [335,336].

It has been recommended that the duration of treatment with cytotoxic agents be extended for 1 year after remission has been induced [56]. Gradual tapering of cyclophosphamide is then instituted. Relapses during tapering are not uncommon. Control usually can be regained by increasing the dosage of cyclophosphamide and prednisone.

Other treatments include low-dosage methotrexate, which has had some success in temporal arteritis, Takayasu arteritis, and Wegener's granulomatosis [337,338]. Intravenous gammaglobulin has been used in Wegener's granulomatosis, Henoch-Schönlein purpura, and systemic vasculitis [339,340]. Cyclosporin has been effective in some patients with Behçet's syndrome and alpha interferon has shown promise in treatment of patients with essential mixed cryoglobulinemia [173–176].

Management of the patient with vasculitides requires thorough and frequent evaluations. Careful analysis of the inflammatory activity of the vasculitis, the complications induced by previous or ongoing organ damage, and the adverse effects of the medications, particularly infection, are the three major areas that must be assessed. A high percentage of patients treated with anti-inflammatory, immunosuppressive agents develop adverse effects; however, a growing number of patients are entering remission from these previously fatal conditions [196].

References

1. Greene MI, Schatten S, Bromberg JS. Delayed hypersensitivity. In WE Paul, ed. Fundamental Immunology. New York: Raven, 1984; Pp. 685–696.
2. Zeek PM, Smith CC, Weeter JC. Studies on periarteritis nodosa. III: The differentiation between vascular lesions of periarteritis nodosa and of hypersensitivity. Am J Pathol 1948; 24:889.
3. Zeek PM. Periarteritis: a critical review. Am J Clin Pathol 1952; 22:777.
4. Alareon-Segovia D, Brown AL Jr. Classification and etiologic aspects of necrotizing angiitides: analytic approach to a confused subject with a critical review of the evidence for hypersensitivity vasculitis in polyarteritis nodosa. Mayo Clin Proc 1964; 39:205.
5. Christian CL, Sergent JS. Vasculitis syndromes: clinical and experimental models. Am J Med 1976; 61:385.
6. Fauci AS, Haynes BF, Katz P. The spectrum of vasculitis. Clinical, pathologic, immunologic, and therapeutic considerations. Ann Intern Med 1978; 89:660–676.
7. Arkin A. A clinical and pathological study of periarteritis nodosa. A report of five cases, one histologically healed. Am J Pathol 1930; 6:401.
8. Churg J, Strauss L. Allergic granulomatosis, allergic angiitis and periarteritis nodosa. Am J Pathol 1951; 27:277.
9. DeShazo RD, Levinson AI, Lawless OJ. Systemic vasculitis with coexistent large and small vessel involvement. JAMA 1977; 238:1940–1942.
10. Fan PT. Clinical approach to systemic vasculitis. Semin Arthr Rheum 1980; 8:248–304.
11. Scott DGI. Systemic vasculitis in a district hospital 1972–1980: clinical and laboratory features, classification and prognosis of 80 cases. Q J Med 1982; 203:292–311.
12. Miller A, Green M, Robinson D. Simple rule for calculating normal erythrocyte sedimentation rate. Br Med J 1983; 286:266.
13. Lascari AD. The erythrocyte sedimentation rate. Ped Clin N Amer 1972; 19:1113.
14. Rovel A, L'Huillier JF, Vigneron C. Mechanisms of erythrocyte sedimentation. Biomedicine 1978; 28:248.
15. Talstad I, Haugen HF. The relationship between the erythrocyte sedimentation rate (ESR) and plasma proteins in clinical materials and models. Scand J Clin Lab Invest 1979; 39:519.
16. Biller J. Temporal arteritis associated with normal erythrocyte sedimentation rate. JAMA 1982; 247:486–487.
17. Wong RL, Korn JH. Temporal arteritis without an elevated sedimentation rate. Amer J Med 1986; 80:959–964.
18. Calamaria KT, Hunder GC. Clinical manifestations of giant cell (temporal) arteritis. Clin Rheum Dis 1980; 6:389–402.
19. Ishikawa K. Natural history and classification of occlusive thromboaortopathy (Takayasu's arteritis). Circulation 1978; 57:27.
20. Leib ES. Correlation of disease activity in systemic necrotizing vasculitis with immune complexes. J Rheum 1981; 8:258–265.
21. Cream JJ, Gumbel JM, Peachey DG. Schönlein-Henoch purpura in the adult. Quart J Med 1970; 39:461–484.
22. Liebow AS, Carrington CRB, Friedman PJ. Lymphomatoid granulomatosis. Hum Path 1972; 3:457.
23. Nurick S, Blackwood W, Mair GP. Giant cell granulomatous angiitis of the central nervous system. Brain 1972; 95:133–142.
24. Tillett WS, Francis T Jr. Serologic reactions in pneumonia with a nonprotein somatic fraction of pneumococcus. J Exp Med 1930; 52:561.
25. Claus DR, Osmand AP, Gewurz H. Radioimmunoassay of human C-reactive protein in normal sera. J Lab Clin Med 1976; 87:120.
26. Kushner I, Broder MI, Karp D. Control of the acute phase response: serum C-reactive protein kinetics after acute myocardial infarction. J Clin Invest 1978; 61:235.
27. Hind CRK. Objective monitoring of disease activity in polyarteritis by measurement of serum C-reactive protein concentrations. Br Med J 1984; 288:1027–1030.
28. Morley JJ, Kushner I. Serum C-reactive protein levels in disease. Ann NY Acad Sci 1982; 389:406.
29. Chumbley LC, Harrison EG, DeRemee RA. Allergic granulomatosis and angiitis (Churg-Strauss syndrome). Report and analysis of 30 cases. Mayo Clin Proc 1977; 52:477.
30. Mayer MM. Complement and complement fixation. In EA Kabat, MM Meyer, eds. Experimental Immunochemistry. Springfield IL.: Charles C. Thomas, 1961. P. 133.
31. Kohler PF, Muller-Eberhard HJ. Immunochemical quantitation of the third, fourth and fifth components of human complement: concentrations in the serum of healthy adults. J Immunol 1967; 99:1211–1216.
32. Colten HR. Biosynthesis of complement. Adv Immunol 1976; 22:67.
33. Imamura S, Yanase K. Demonstration of circulating and tissue fixed immune complexes in cutaneous necrotizing vasculitis. Acta Dermatovener (Stockholm) 1980; 60:389–392.
34. Conn DL. Immunologic mechanisms in systemic vasculitis. Mayo Clin Proc 1976; 51:511–518.
35. Kammer GM, Soter NA, Schur PH. Circulating immune complexes in patients with necrotizing vasculitis. Clin Immun Immunopath 1980; 15:658–672.
36. Reithmuller G. Serum complement levels in patients with mixed (IgG-IgM) cryoglobulinemia. Clin Exp Immunol 1966; 24:401.
37. Zubler RH, Lambert PH. Detection of immune complexes in human disease. Prog Allergy 1978; 24:1.
38. Zubler RH, et al. Detection of immune complexes in unheated sera by a modified ^{125}I C1q binding test. Effect of heating on the binding of C1q by immune complexes and application of the test to systemic lupus erythematosus. J Immunol 1976; 116:232–235.
39. Hay FC, Nineham LJ, Roitt IM. Routine assay for detection of immune complexes of known immunoglobulin class using solid phase C1q. Clin Exp Immunol 1976; 24:396–400.
40. Theophilopoulos AN, Wilson CB, Dixon FJ. The Raji cell radioimmune assay for detecting immune complexes in human sera. J Clin Invest 1976; 57:169–182.
41. Levinsky RJ, Barratt TM. IgA immune complexes in Henoch-Schönlein purpura. Lancet 1979; 2:1100.
42. Brouet JC, et al. Biologic and clinical significance of cryoglobulins. A report of 86 cases. Amer J Med 1974; 57:775–788.

43. Meltzer M, et al. Cryoglobulinemia—a clinical and laboratory study. Amer J Med 1966; 40:837–856.
44. Cream JJ. Clinical and immunological aspects of cutaneous vasculitis. Q J Med 1976; 45:255.
45. Grey HM, Kohler PF. Cryoimmunoglobulins. Semin Hematol 1973; 10:87.
46. Davies DJ, et al. Segmental necrotizing glomerulonephritis with antineutrophil antibody: possible arbovirus aetiology? Br Med J 1982; 285:606–608.
47. van der Woude, et al. Autoantibodies against neutrophils and monocytes: tool for diagnosis and marker of disease activity in Wegener's granulomatosis. Lancet 1985; 1:425–429.
48. Jennette JC, Hoidal JH, Falk RJ. Specificity of anti-neutrophil cytoplasmic autoantibodies for proteinase 3. Blood 1990; 78:2263–2264.
49. Falk RJ, Jennette JC. Anti-neutrophil cytoplasmic autoantibodies with specificity for myeloperoxidase in patients with systemic vasculitis and idiopathic necrotizing and crescentic glomerulonephritis. N Engl J Med 1988; 318:1651–1657.
50. Cohen Tervaert JW, et al. Autoantibodies against myeloid lysosomal enzymes in crescentic glomerulonephritis. Kidney Int 1990; 37:799–806.
51. Cohen Tervaert JW, et al. Association between active Wegener's granulomatosis and anticytoplasmic antibodies. Arch Intern Med 1989; 149:2461–2465.
52. Nolle B, et al. Anticytoplasmic autoantibodies: their immunodiagnostic value in Wegener's granulomatosis. Ann Intern Med 1989; 111:28–40.
53. Specks U, et al. Anticytoplasmic autoantibodies in the diagnosis and follow-up of Wegener's granulomatosis. Mayo Clin Proc 1989; 64:28–36.
54. Hagan EC, et al. Fundamental and clinical aspects of antineutrophil cytoplasmic antibodies. Autoimmunity 1992; 11: 199–207.
55. Bartfield H. Incidence and significance of seropositive tests for rheumatoid factor in non-rheumatic diseases. Ann Intern Med 1960; 52:1059.
56. Fauci AS, et al. Wegener's granulomatosis: prospective clinical and therapeutic experience with 85 patients for 21 years. Ann Intern Med 1983; 98:76–85.
57. Lanham JG, et al. Systemic vasculitis with asthma and eosinophilia: a clinical approach to the Churg-Strauss syndrome. Medicine 1984; 63:65–81.
58. Savage CS, et al. Microscopic polyarteritis: presentation, pathology and prognosis. Quart J Med 1985; 56:467–483.
59. Trygstand CW, Steihm ER. Elevated serum IgA globulin in anaphylactoid purpura. Pediatrics 1971; 47:1023.
60. Kusakawa S, Heiner DC. Elevated levels of immunoglobulin E in the acute febrile mucocutaneous lymph node syndrome. Pediatr Res 1976; 10:108.
61. Ronco P, et al. Immunopathological studies of polyarteritis nodosa and Wegener's granulomatosis: a report of 43 patients with 51 renal biopsies. Quart J Med 1983; 206:212–223.
62. Gocke DJ, et al. Association between polyarteritis and Australia antigen. Lancet 1970; 2:1149.
63. Prince AM. Role of immune complexes involving SH antigen in pathogenesis of chronic active hepatitis and polyarteritis nodosa. Lancet 1971; 1:1309.
64. Sergent JS, et al. Vasculitis with hepatitis B antigenemia: long term observations in nine patients. Medicine 1976; 55:1–18.
65. Duffy J, et al. Polyarthritis, polyarteritis and hepatitis B. Medicine 1976; 55:19.
66. Marcellin P, et al. Latent hepatitis B virus (HBV) infection in systemic necrotizing vasculitis. Clin Exp Rheumatol 1991; 9:23–28.
67. Popp JW, et al. Cutaneous vasculitis associated with acute and chronic hepatitis. Arch Intern Med 1981; 141:623.
68. Shumaker JB, et al. Arthritis and rash. Arch Intern Med 1974; 133:483.
69. Popp JW Jr, et al. Essential mixed cryoglobulinemia without evidence for hepatitis B virus infection. Ann Intern Med 1980; 92:379–383.
70. Agnello V, Chung RT, Kaplan LM. A role for hepatitis C virus infection in type II mixed cryoglobulinemia. N Engl J Med 1992; 327:1490–1495.
71. Misian R, et al. Hepatitis C virus infection in patients with essential mixed cryoglobulinemia. Ann Intern Med 1992; 117:577.
72. Kornblut AD, et al. Wegener's granulomatosis. Otolaryngol Clin North Am 1982; 15:673–684.
73. Fauci AS, Johnson RE, Wolff SM. Radiation therapy of midline granuloma. Ann Intern Med 1976; 84:140–147.
74. Clark RE, McNamara TO, Palubinskas AJ. Intrarenal mycotic aneurysm detected angiographically. Br J Radiology 1965; 45:66.
75. Travers RL, et al. Polyarteritis nodosa: a clinical and angiographic analysis of 17 cases. Semin Arthr Rheum 1979; 8:184.
76. Easterbrook JS. Renal and hepatic microaneurysms. Report of a new entity simulating polyarteritis nodosa. Radiology 1980; 137:629.
77. Lande A, Rossi P. The value of total aortography in the diagnosis of Takayasu's arteritis. Radiology 1975; 114:287.
78. Shinonoya S, et al. Pattern of arterial occlusion in Buerger's disease. Angiology 1982; 33:375–384.
79. Layfer LF, et al. Temporal arteriography. Analysis of 21 cases and a review of the literature. Arthr Rheum 1978; 21:780.
80. Lie JT. Primary (granulomatosus) angiitis of the central nervous system: a clinical pathologic analysis of 15 new cases and review of the literature. Human Pathol 1992; 23:164–171.
81. Fauci AS, Doppman JL, Wolff SM. Cyclophosphamide-induced remissions in advanced polyarteritis nodosa. Am J Med 1978; 64:890–894.
82. Buckley A, et al. The role of ultrasound in evaluation of Takayasu's arteritis. J Rheumatol 1991; 18:1073–1080.
83. Maeda B, et al. Carotid lesions detected by B mode ultrasonography in Takayasu's arteritis: "Macaroni sign" as an indicator of the disease. Ultrasound Med Biol 1991; 17:695–701.
84. Tannigawa K, et al. Magnetic resonance imaging detection of aortic and pulmonary artery wall thickening in the acute stage of Takayasu's arteritis: improvement of clinical and radiologic findings after steroid therapy. Arthritis Rheum 1992; 35:476–480.
85. Herrara EL, Seoane M. Takayasu's arteritis (nonspecific aortoarteritis). In A Lande, YM Berkman, HA McAllister, eds. Aortitis: Clinical, Pathologic and Radiographic Aspects. New York: Raven, 1986. Pp. 173–191.
86. Hall S, Hunder GG. Is temporal artery biopsy prudent? May Clin Proc 1984; 59:793–796.
87. Morgan GJ Jr, Harris ED Jr. Non-giant cell temporal arteritis: three cases and a review of the literature. Arthr Rheum 1978; 21:362.
88. Katzenstein AA, Carrington CB, Liebow AA. Lymphomatoid granulomatosis. A clinicopathologic study of 152 cases. Cancer 1979; 43:360.
89. Fauci AS, Wolff SM. Wegener's granulomatosis: studies in eighteen patients and a review of the literature. Medicine 1973; 52:535.
90. Winkelmann RK. The spectrum of cutaneous vasculitis. Clin Rheum Dis 1980; 6:413.
91. Dahl EV, Baggenstoss AH, DeWeerd JH. Testicular lesions

of periarteritis nodosa, with special reference to diagnosis. Am J Med 1960; 28:222.
92. Maxeiner SR, McDonald JR, Kirklin JW. Muscle biopsy in the diagnosis of periarteritis nodosa. An evaluation. Surg Clin N Amer 1952; 32:1225.
93. Kussmaul A, Maier R. Ueber eine bishir nicht beschriebene eigenthumliche arterienerkrankung (Periarteritis nodosa) die mit Morbus Brightii und rapid fortschreitender allgemeiner Muskellahmung einhergeht. Dtsch Arch Klin Med 1866; 1:484–517.
94. Dickson WEC. Polyarteritis acuta nodosa and periarteritis nodosa. J Path Bacteriol 1908; 12:31–57.
95. Rose GA, Spencer H. Polyarteritis nodosa. Q J Med 1957; 26:43.
96. Cohen RD, Conn DL, Ilstrup DM. Clinical features, prognosis and response to treatment in polyarteritis. Mayo Clin Proc 1980; 55:146.
97. Makota I, Sano K, Inaba H, et al. Localized necrotizing arteritis. Arch Pathol Lab Med 1991; 115:780–783.
98. Piette JC, et al. Systemic polyarteritis nodosa diagnosed at hysterectomy. Am J Med 1987; 82:836–838.
99. Nightengale EJ. The gastroenterological aspects of periarteritis nodosa. Am J Gastroenterol 1959; 31:152.
100. Carron DB, Douglas AP. Steatorrhea in vascular insufficiency of the small intestine. Five cases of polyarteritis nodosa and allied disorders. Q J Med 1965; 34:331.
101. Hans SY, Jander P, Laws HL. Polyarteritis nodosa causing severe intestinal bleeding. Gastrointest Radiol 1976; 1:285.
102. Camilleri M, et al. Gastrointestinal manifestations of systemic vasculitis. Q J Med 1983; 206:141–149.
103. Golding DN. Polyarteritis presenting with leg pains. Br Med J 1970; 1:277.
104. Moore PM, Fauci AS. Neurologic manifestations of systemic necrotizing arteritis: clinical and pathologic features in 24 cases. Am J Med 1981; 71:517–524.
105. Serra A, Carmeron JS. Clinical and pathological aspects of renal vasculitis. Sem Nephro 1985; 5:15–33.
106. Frohnert PP, Sheps SG. Long term follow-up study of periarteritis nodosa. Am J Med 1967; 43:8–14.
107. Lyell A, Church R. The cutaneous manifestations of polyarteritis nodosa. Br J Derm 1954; 66:335.
108. Rose GA. The natural history of polyarteritis. Br Med J 1957; 1:1148.
109. Leib ES, Restivo C, Paulus HE. Immunosuppressive and corticosteroid therapy of polyarteritis nodosa. Am J Med 1979; 67:941–947.
110. Wees SJ, Sunwoo IN, Joong S. Sural nerve biopsy in systemic necrotizing vasculitis. Am J Med 1981; 71:525–532.
111. Meyers DS, Grim CE, Keitzer WF. Fibromuscular dysplasia of the renal artery with medial dissection. A case simulating polyarteritis nodosa. Am J Med 1974; 56:412.
112. Leonhardt ETG, Kullenberg KPC. Bilateral atrial myxomas with multiple arterial aneurysms—a syndrome mimicking polyarteritis nodosa. Am J Med 1977; 62:792.
113. Baker SB, Robinson DR. Unusual renal manifestations of Wegener's granulomatosis. Report of two cases. Am J Med 1978; 64:883.
114. Halpern M, Citron BP. Necrotizing angiitis associated with drug abuse. Am J Roentgen Radiat Ther Nucl Med 1971; 111:663.
115. Sergent JS, Christian CL. Necrotizing vasculitis after acute serous otitis media. Ann Intern Med 1974; 81:195–199.
116. Elkon KB, Hughes GRV, Catovsky D. Hairy cell leukemia with polyarteritis nodosa. Lancet 1979; 2:280–282.
117. Phanuphak P, et al. Vasculitis in chronic urticaria. J Allergy Clin Immunol 1980; 65:436–444.
118. Valeriono-Marcet J, Ravichandrion L, Kerr LD. HIV associated systemic necrotizing vasculitis. J Rheumatol 1990; 17:1091–1093.
119. Lockshin MD. Letter. N Engl J Med 1979; 301:1123.
120. Fauci AS, et al. Cyclophosphamide therapy for severe systemic necrotizing vasculitis. N Engl J Med 1979; 301:235–238.
121. Scott DGI, et al. Plasma exchange in rheumatoid vasculitis. J Rheum 1981; 8:433–439.
122. Scott DGI, Bacon PA. Intravenous cyclophosphamide plus methylprednisolone in the treatment of systemic rheumatoid vasculitis. Am J Med 1984; 76:377–384.
123. Serra A, et al. Vasculitis affecting the kidney: presentation, histopathology and long-term outcome. Q J Med 1984; 53:181–207.
124. Chaplopin JM, et al. Immunological findings during successful treatment of HBsAg-associated polyarteritis nodosa by plasmapheresis alone. Br Med J 1980; 280:368.
125. Pusey CD, et al. Plasma exchange in focal necrotizing glomerulonephritis without anti-GBM antibodies. Kidney Int 1991; 40:757–763.
126. Guillevin L, et al. A long term follow-up after treatment of polyarteritis nodosa and Churg-Strauss angiitis with comparison of steroids, plasma exchange and cyclophosphanide to steroids and plasma exchange. J Rheumatol 1992; 18:567–574.
127. Suen KC, Burton JD. The spectrum of eosinophilic infiltration of the gastrointestinal tract and its relationship to other disorders of angiitis and granulomatosis. Hum Path 1979; 10:31.
128. Erlich JC, Romanoff A. Allergic granuloma of the lung. Arch Intern Med 1951; 87:259.
129. Olsen KD, et al. Nasal manifestations of allergic granulomatosis and angiitis (Churg-Strauss syndrome). Otolaryngol Head Neck Surg 1980; 88:85.
130. Abell MR, et al. Allergic granulomatosis with massive gastric involvement. N Engl J Med 1970; 282:665.
131. Heatley RV, Harris A, Atkinson M. Treatment of a patient with clinical features of both eosinophilic gastroenteritis and polyarteritis nodosa with oral sodium chromoglycate. Dig Dis Sci 1980; 25:470.
132. Modigliani R, et al. Allergic granulomatous vasculitis (Churg-Strauss syndrome). Report of a case with widespread digestive involvement. Dig Dis Sci 1981; 26:264.
133. Rosenberg TF, et al. Allergic granulomatous angiitis (Churg-Strauss syndrome). J Allergy Clin Immunol 1975; 55:56.
134. Kinsella DL, Simpson HN. Loeffler's pneumonia terminating in fatal periarteritis nodosa. JAMA 1967; 202:101.
135. Chusid MJ, et al. The hypereosinophilic syndrome: analysis of fourteen cases with review of the literature. Medicine 1975; 54:1.
136. Bush RK, et al. Response to corticosteroids in the hypereosinophilic syndrome. Arch Intern Med 1978; 138:1244.
137. Cohen Tervaert JW, et al. Detection of autoantibodies against myeloid lysosomal enzymes: a useful adjunct to classification of patients with biopsy proven necrotizing arteritis. Am J Med 1991; 91:59–66.
138. Churg J, Strauss L. Interstitial eosinophilic pneumonitis, pleuritis and angiitis (Letter). N Engl J Med 1981; 304:611.
139. Roberts WC, Liegler DG, Carbone PP. Endomyocardial disease and eosinophilia. Am J Med 1969; 46:28.
140. Cooper BJ, Bacal E, Patterson R. Allergic angiitis and granulomatosis. Prolonged remission induced by combined prednisone-azathioprine therapy. Arch Intern Med 1978; 138:367.
141. McCombs RP. Systemic allergic vasculitis. JAMA 1965; 194:1059.
142. Soter NA, et al. Two distinct cellular patterns in cutaneous necrotizing angiitis. J Invest Derm 1976; 66:334–350.
143. O'Duffy JD, et al. Necrotizing angiitis. I: a clinical review of twenty-seven autopsied cases. Cleve Clin Q 1965; 32:7–98.

144. Baart de La Faille-Kuyper EH, et al. IgA deposits in cutaneous blood vessel walls and mesangium in Henoch-Schönlein syndrome. Lancet 1973; 21:892.
145. Calabrese LH, Clough JD. Hypersensitivity vasculitis group. Cleve Clin Quart 1982; 49:17–42.
146. Gilliam JN, Smilery JD. Cutaneous necrotizing vasculitis and related disorders. Ann Allergy 1976; 37:328.
147. Conn DL, Hunder GG. Necrotizing vasculitis. In WN Kelley et al., eds. Textbook of Rheumatology. Philadelphia: Saunders, 1985. P. 1150.
148. Chad D, et al. The pathogenesis of cryoglobulinemic neuropathy. Neurol 1982; 32:725–729.
149. Molina R, Provost TT, Alexander EL. Peripheral inflammatory vascular disease in Sjögren's syndrome: association with nervous system complications. Arthr Rheum 1986; 29:1341–1347.
150. Piette WN, Stone MS. A cutaneous sign of IgA-associated small dismal leukocytoclastic vasculitis in adults (Henoch-Schönlein pupura). Arch Dermatol 1989; 125:53–56.
151. Sams WM Jr, et al. Leukocytoclastic vasculitis. Arch Dermatol 1976; 112:219–226.
152. Gairdner D. The Schönlein-Henoch syndrome (anaphylactoid purpura). Q J Med 1948; 17:95.
153. Roth DA, Wilz DR, Theil GB. Schönlein-Henoch syndrome in adults. Q J Med 1985; 55:145–152.
154. Kauffmann RH, et al. Circulating IgA-immune complexes in Henoch-Schönlein purpura. Am J Med 1980; 69:859–866.
155. Stevenson JA, et al. Henoch-Schönlein purpura. Simultaneous demonstration of IgA deposits in involved skin, intestine and kidney. Arch Path Lab Med 1982; 106:192.
156. Noussias M, Blandy AC, Ward-McQuaid N. Intussusception in Henoch-Schönlein purpura. Br J Surg 1969; 56:503.
157. Meadow SR. The prognosis of Henoch-Schönlein nephritis. Clin Nephrol 1978; 9:87.
158. McDuffie FC, et al. Hypocomplementemia with cutaneous vasculitis and arthritis: possible immune complex syndrome. Mayo Clin Proc 1970; 48:340–348.
159. Soter NA. Chronic urticaria as a manifestation of necrotizing venulitis. N Engl J Med 1977; 296:1440–1442.
160. Agnello V. Detection of immune complexes. J Invest Dermatol 1976; 67:339.
161. Zeiss CR, et al. A hypocomplementemic vasculitis urticarial syndrome. Report of four new cases and definition of the disease. Am J Med 1980; 68:867.
162. Schwartz HR, et al. Hypocomplementemic urticarial vasculitis: association with chronic obstructive pulmonary disease. Mayo Clin Proc 1982; 57:231.
163. Epstein W. Mixed cryoglobulinemia and glomerulonephritis. Ann Intern Med 1968; 69:1221.
164. Barnett EV, et al. Cryoglobulinemia and disease. Ann Intern Med 1970; 73:95–107.
165. Gorevic PD, et al. Mixed cryoglobulinemia: clinical aspects and long-term follow-up of 40 patients. Am J Med 1980; 69:287–308.
166. Case Records of the Massachusetts General Hospital. Case 35-1985. N Engl J Med 1985; 313:566–575.
167. Abramsky O, Slavin S. Neurologic manifestations in patients with mixed cryoglobulinemia. Neurology (Minneap) 1974; 24:245–249.
168. Bombardieri S, et al. Lung involvement in essential mixed cryoglobulinemia. Am J Med 1979; 66:748.
169. Garcia Fuentes M, et al. Serum complement components in Henoch Schönlein purpura. Arch Dis Child 1978; 53:417.
170. Pruzanski W, Watt JG. Serum viscosity and hyperviscosity syndrome in IgG multiple myeloma. Ann Intern Med 1972; 77:853.
171. Invernizzi F, et al. A long-term follow-up study in essential cryoglobulinemia. Acta Haematol 1979; 61:93.
172. Lightfoot RW Jr. Cryoglobulinemia and other dysproteinemias. In WN Kelley et al., eds. Textbook of Rheumatology. Philadelphia: Saunders, 1985. Pp. 1337–1350.
173. Knox TA, et al. Mixed cryoglobulinemia responsive to interferon treatment. Am J Med 1991; 91:554–555.
174. Casato M, et al. Long-term results of therapy with interferon treatment for type II essential mixed cryoglobulinemia. Blood 1991; 78:3142–3147.
175. Ferri C, et al. Interferon treatment in mixed cryoglobulinemia patients: a randomized, crossover-controlled trial. Blood 1993; 81:1132–1136.
176. Misiani R, et al. Interferon alfa-2a therapy in cryoglobulinemia associated with hepatitis C virus. N Engl J Med 1994; 330:751–756.
177. Curd JG, et al. Potassium iodide sensitivity in four patients with hypocomplementemic vasculitis. Ann Intern Med 1979; 91:853–857.
178. Mollick FG, et al. Drug-related vasculitis: Clinicopathological correlations in 30 patients. Hum Path 1979; 3:313–325.
179. Godman GC, Churg J. Wegener's granulomatosis. Pathology and review of the literature. Arch Pathol 1954; 58:533.
180. Wolff SM, et al. Wegener's granulomatosis. Ann Intern Med 1974; 81:513–525.
181. Israel HL, Patchefsky AS. Wegener's granulomatosis of lung. Diagnosis and treatment: experience with twelve cases. Ann Intern Med 1971; 74:881–891.
182. Cupps TR, Fauci AS. Wegener's granulomatosis. Int J Dermatol 1980; 19:76.
183. Haynes BF, et al. The ocular manifestations of Wegener's granulomatosis. Fifteen years experience and review of the literature. Am J Med 1977; 61:131.
184. Drachman DA. Neurological complications of Wegener's granulomatosis. Arch Neurol 1963; 8:145.
185. Anderson JM, Jamieson DG, Jefferson JM. Non-healing granuloma and the nervous system. Q J Med 1975; 44:309–323.
186. Moore PM, Cupps TR. Neurological complications of vasculitis. Ann Neurol 1983; 14:155–167.
187. Gatenby PA, et al. Myocardial infarction in Wegener's granulomatosis. Aust NZ J Med 1976; 6:336–340.
188. Fienberg R. The protracted superficial phenomenon in pathergic (Wegener's) granulomatosis. Hum Pathol 1981; 12: 458–467.
189. DeRemee RA, et al. Wegener's granulomatosis: anatomic correlates: a proposed classification. Mayo Clin Proc 1976; 51:777–781.
190. Howell SB, Epstein WV. Circulating immunoglobulin complexes in Wegener's granulomatosis. Am J Med 1976; 60:259–268.
191. Vermess M, et al. Computer assisted tomography of orbital lesions in Wegener's granulomatosis. J Comp Assist Tomog 1978; 2:45.
192. Horn RG, et al. Renal biopsy pathology in Wegener's granulomatosis. Hum Path 1974; 74:423.
193. Hoffman GC, et al. Wegener's granulomatosis: an analysis of 158 patients. Ann Intern Med 1992; 116:488–498.
194. Walton EW. Giant-cell granuloma of the respiratory tract (Wegener's granulomatosis). Br Med J 1958; 2:265.
195. Reza MJ, et al. Wegener's granulomatosis. Long-term followup of patients treated with cyclophosphamide. Arthr Rheum 1975; 18:501.
196. Weiner SR, Paulus HE. Treatment of Wegener's granulomatosis with cyclophosphamide: an outcome analysis. Arthr Rheum 1987; 30:S16.
197. Raitt JW. Wegener's granulomatosis: treatment with cyto-

toxic agents and adrenocorticoids. Ann Intern Med 1971; 74:344.

198. Hoffman GC, et al. Treatment of Wegener's granulomatosis with glucocorticoids and methotrexate. Arthritis Rheum 1992; 35:1322–1329.
199. DeRemee RA, MacDonald TJ, Weiland LH. Wegener's granulomatosis: observations on treatment with antimicrobial agents. Mayo Clin Proc 1985; 60:27–32.
200. Huston KA, et al. Temporal arteritis: a 25 year epidemiological, clinical and pathologic study. Ann Intern Med 1978; 88:162.
201. Ostberg G. Temporal arteritis in a large necropsy series. Ann Rheum Dis 1971; 30:224.
202. Love DC, et al. Temporal arteritis in blacks. Ann Intern Med 1986; 105:386–389.
203. Klein RG, et al. Large artery involvement in giant cell (temporal) arteritis. Ann Intern Med 1975; 83:806–812.
204. Wilkinson IMS, Russel RWR. Arteries of the head and neck in giant cell arteritis: a pathological study to show the pattern of artery involvement. Arch Neurol 1972; 27:378–391.
205. Cardell DS, Hanley T. A fatal case of giant cell or temporal arteritis. J Pathol Bacteriol 1951; 63:587.
206. Banks PM, et al. Immunohistological and cytochemical studies of temporal arteritis. Arth Rheum 1983; 26:120.
207. Hamilton CR Jr, Shelley WM, Tumulty PA. Giant cell arteritis: including temporal arteritis and polymyalgia rheumatica. Medicine 1971; 50:1.
208. Klein RG, et al. Skip lesions in temporal arteritis. Mayo Clin Proc 1976; 51:504.
209. Hamrin R, Johnson N, Hellsten S. "Polymyalgia rheumatica": further clinical and histopathological studies with a report of six autopsy cases. Ann Rheum Dis 1968; 27:397.
210. Long R, James O. Polymyalgia rheumatica and liver disease. Lancet 1974; 1:77.
211. Esposito AL, Gleckman RA. Fever of unknown origin in the elderly. J Amer Geriat Soc 1978; 26:498–505.
212. Hamrin B, Jonsson N, Landberg T. Involvement of large vessels in polymyalgia arteritica. Lancet 1965; 1:1193.
213. How J, Strachan RW. Aortic regurgitation as a manifestation of giant cell arteritis. Br Heart J 1978; 40:1052.
214. Chuang T-Y, et al. Polymyalgia rheumatica: A ten-year epidemiologic and clinical study. Ann Intern Med 1982; 97:672.
215. Jundt J, Mock D. Temporal arteritis with normal erythrocyte sedimentation rates presenting as occipital neuralgia. Arthritis Rheum 1991; 34:217–219.
216. Healey LA, Wilske KR. Presentation of occult giant cell arteritis. Arthr Rheum 1980; 23:641.
217. Sofferman RA. Cranial arteritis in otolaryngology. Ann Oto Rhinol Laryngol 1980; 89:215–219.
218. Larson TS, et al. Respiratory tract symptoms as a clue to giant cell arteritis. Ann Intern Med 1984; 101:594–597.
219. Spiera H, Davison S. Long term follow-up of polymyalgia rheumatica. Mt Sinai J Med 1978; 45:225–229.
220. Rynes RI, Mika P, Bartholomew LE. Development of giant cell (temporal) arteritis in a patient 'adequately' treated for polymyalgia rheumatica. Ann Rheum Dis 1977; 36:88.
221. Russell R. Giant cell arteritis. Q J Med 1959; 28:471.
222. Save-Soderbergh J, et al. Giant cell arteritis as a cause of death. JAMA 1986; 255:493–496.
223. Nordberg E, Benjtisson BA. Death rates and causes of death in 284 consecutive patients with giant cell arteritis confirmed by biopsy. BMJ 1989; 299:549–550.
224. Bengtsson BA, Mamvall BE. Prognosis of giant cell arteritis including temporal arteritis and polymyalgia rheumatica. Acta Med Scand 1981; 209:337–345.
225. Lundberg I, Hedfors E. Restricted dose and duration of corticosteroid treatment in patients with polymyalgia rheumatica and temporal arteritis. J Rheumatol 1990; 17:1340–1345.
226. Kerr GS, et al. Takayasu arteritis. Ann Int Med 1994; 120: 919–929.
227. Freissinger JN, et al. Maladie de Takayasu. Criteres diagnostiques. Nouv Prasse Med 1982; 11:583.
228. Nasu T. Pathology of pulseless disease: systemic study and critical review of twenty-one autopsy cases reported in Japan. Angiology 1963; 14:225–242.
229. Lande A, LaPorta A. Takayasu's arteritis, an arteriographic pathologic correlation. Arch Pathol 1976; 100:437–440.
230. Fraga A, et al. Takayasu's arteritis: frequency of systemic manifestations (study of 22 patients) and favorable response to maintenance steroid therapy with adrenocorticosteroids. Arthr Rheum 1972; 15:617–623.
231. Strachan RW. The natural history of Takayasu arteritis. Quart J Med 1964; 33:57.
232. Lupi HE, et al. Pulmonary artery involvement in Takayasu's arteritis. Chest 1975; 67:69.
233. Lande A, Berkman YM. Radiologic aspects of aortitis. In A Lande, YM Berkman, HA McAllister, eds. Aortitis: Clinical Pathologic and Radiographic Aspects. New York: Raven, 1986. Pp. 81–143.
234. Hall S, et al. Takayasu's arteritis. A study of 32 North American patients. Medicine 1985; 64:89–99.
235. Lai K, Chan K, Ho D. Glomerulonephritis associated with Takayasu's arteritis: report of three cases and review of the literature. Am J Kidney Dis 1986; 7:197–204.
236. Ishikawa K, et al. Pulmonary hypertension in occlusive thromboaortopathy (Takayasu's arteritis). Jpn Circ J 1976; 40:517.
237. Makino N, et al. Coronary arterial involvement in Takayasu's disease. Jpn Heart J 1982; 23:1007–1013.
238. Lupi HE, et al. Takayasu's arteritis: clinical study of 107 cases. Am Heart J 1977; 93:94.
239. Heinemann MH, Sigelman J. Ocular manifestations of Takayasu's disease. In A Lande, YM Berkman, HA McAllister, eds. Aortitis: Clinical Pathologic and Radiographic Aspects. New York: Raven, 1986. Pp. 233–242.
240. Gardner JD, Lee KR, Abdou NI. Takayasu's arteritis: reversal of pulse deficits after early treatment with corticosteroids. J Rheum 1984; 11:92–93.
241. Ueda H, et al. Clinical observations of 52 cases of aortitis syndrome. Jpn Heart J 1969; 10:277–288.
242. Yamada I, Numano R, Suzuki S. Takayasu arteritis: evaluation with MR imaging. Radiology 1993; 188:89–94.
243. Buckley A, et al. The role of ultrasound in evaluation of Takayasu's arteritis. J Rheumatol 1991; 18:1073–1080.
244. Whelan TJ Jr, Baugh JH. Non-atherosclerotic arterial lesions and their management. Parts I-IV. Curr Probl Surg 1967; Feb: 3–76, March: 1–47.
245. Tucker CR, et al. Aortitis in ankylosing spondylitis. Early detection of aortic root abnormalities with two dimensional echocardiography. Am J Cardiol 1982; 49:680–686.
246. Ferrans VJ, Boyce SW. Metabolic and familial diseases. In MD Silver, ed. Cardiovascular Pathology. New York: Churchill-Livingston, 1983. Pp. 945–1004.
247. Cipriano PR, et al. Coronary arterial narrowing in Takayasu's arteritis. Am J Cardiol 1977; 39:744.
248. Hoffman GS, et al. Treatment of glucocorticoid-resistant or relapsing Takayasu arteritis with methotrexate. Arthritis Rheum 1994; 37:578–582.
249. The aortitis syndrome research committee of Japan organized by the Ministry of Health and Welfare. (A report of the Survey of Aortitis in Japan in 1975.) Gifu, Japan: Ministry of Health and Welfare. 1976; 54.
250. Sharma S, et al. Renal artery stenosis caused by nonspecific

arteritis (Takayasu's disease): results of treatment with percutaneous transluminal angioplasty. Am J Roentgenol 1992; 158:417–422.
251. Fava MP, et al. Percutaneous transluminal angioplasty in patients with Takayasu arteritis: five year experience. J Vasc Intern Radiol 1993; 4:649–652.
252. Medeiros LJ, et al. Localization of Epstein-Barr viral genomes in angiocentric immunoproliferative lesions. Am J Surg Pathol 1992; 16:439–447.
253. Fauci AS, et al. Lymphomatoid granulomatosis: prospective clinical and therapeutic experience over 10 years. N Engl J Med 1982; 306:68–74.
254. Patton WF, Lynch JP. Lymphomatoid granulomatosis. Clinicopathologic study of four cases and literature review. Medicine 1982; 61:1–12.
255. Israel HL, Patchefsky AS, Saldana MJ. Wegener's granulomatosis, lymphomatoid granulomatosis, and benign lymphocytic angiitis and granulomatosis of lung: recognition and treatment. Ann Intern Med 1977; 87:691–699.
256. Lee SC, Roth LM, Brashear RE. Lymphomatoid granulomatosis: a clinicopathologic study of four cases. Cancer 1976; 38:846–853.
257. Lipford EH, et al. Angiocentric immunoproliferative lesions: a clinicopathologic spectrum of post-thymic T-cell proliferations. Blood 1988; 72:1674–1681.
258. Kawasaki T. Acute febrile mucocutaneous lymph node syndrome: clinical observations of 50 cases. Jpn J Allerg 1967; 16:178–222 (in Japanese).
259. Newburger JW, et al. The treatment of Kawasaki syndrome with intravenous gamma globulin. N Engl J Med 1986; 315:341–347.
260. Melish ME, Hicks RM, Larson EJ. Mucocutaneous lymph node syndrome in the United States. Am J Dis Child 1976; 130:599.
261. Burns JC, et al. Clinical and epidemiologic characteristics of possible Kawasaki disease. J Pediat 1991; 118:680–686.
262. Meade RH, Brandt L. Manifestations of Kawasaki's disease in New England outbreak of 1980. J Pediatrics 1982; 100:558.
263. Feigin RD, Scheien CL. Kawasaki's disease. In JS Remington, MN Swartz, eds. Current Clinical Topics in Infectious Diseases. New York: McGraw-Hill, 1983. Pp. 30–63.
264. Hiraishi S, et al. Clinical course of cardiovascular involvement in the mucocutaneous lymph node syndrome. Relation between clinical signs of carditis and development of coronary arterial aneurysm. Am J Cardiol 1981; 147:323.
265. Tatara K, Kusakawa A. Long term prognosis of giant coronary aneurysm in Kawasaki disease: an angiographic study. J Pediatr 1987; 111:705–710.
266. Kato H, et al. Fate of coronary aneurysms in Kawasaki's disease: serial coronary angiography and long-term follow-up study. Am J Cardiol 1982; 49:1758.
267. Amano S, Hazaama F, Hamashima Y. Pathology of Kawasaki disease. I: Pathology and morphogenesis of the vascular changes. Jpn Circ J 1979; 43:633.
268. Amano S, Hazaama F, Hamashima Y. Pathology of Kawasaki disease. II: Distribution and incidence of the vascular lesions. Jpn Circ J 1979; 43:741.
269. Landing BH, Larson EJ. Are infantile periarteritis nodosa with coronary artery involvement and fatal mucocutaneous lymph node syndrome the same? Comparison of 20 patients from North America with patients from Hawaii and Japan. Pediatrics 1977; 59:651.
270. Newburger JW, et al. A single intravenous infusion of gammaglobulin as compared with four infusions in the treatment of acute Kawasaki syndrome. N Eng J Med 1991; 324:1633–1639.
271. Sanford FM, Vargo TA, Shih JY. Successful triple coronary artery bypass in a child with multiple coronary aneurysms due to Kawasaki's disease. J Thorac Cardiovasc Surg 1980; 79:283.
272. Behçet H. Uber rezidivierende, apthose, durch ein Virus verursachte Geschwure am mund, am Auge und an den Genitalien. Derm Wschr 1937; 105:1152–1157.
273. Shimizu T, et al. Behçet disease (Behçet syndrome). Semin Arthr Rheum 1979; 8:223–260.
274. Lehner T. Behçet's syndrome and autoimmunity. Br Med J 1967; 1:465.
275. Abdou NI, et al. Behçet's disease: possible role of secretory component deficiency, synovial inclusions, and fibrinolytic abnormality in the various manifestations of the disease. J Lab Clin Med 1978; 91:409.
276. Gupta RC, et al. Circulating immune complexes in active Behçet's disease. Clin Exp Immunol 1978; 34:213.
277. Reimer G, et al. Lytic effect of cytotoxic lymphocytes on oral epithelial cells in Behçet's syndrome. Br J Dermatol 1982; 107:529.
278. Ohno S, et al. Specific histocompatibility antigens associated with Behçet's disease. Am J Ophthalmol 1975; 80:636.
279. O'Duffy JD, Taswell HF, Elveback LR. HL-A antigens in Behçet's disease. J Rheum 1976; 3:1–3.
280. Yazici H, et al. HLA antigens in Behçet's disease: a reappraisal by a comparative study of Turkish and British patients. Ann Rheum Dis 1980; 39:344.
281. Arber N, et al. Close association of HLA-B51 and HLA-B52 in Israeli patients with Behçet's syndrome. Ann Rheum Dis 1991; 50:351–353.
282. Colvard JM, Robertson DM, O'Duffy JD. The ocular manifestations of Behçet's disease. Arch Ophthalm 1977; 95:1813–1817.
283. Chajek T, Fainaru M. Behçet's disease. Report of 41 cases and a review of the literature. Medicine 1975; 54:179–196.
284. Koc Y, et al. Vascular involvement in Behçet's disease. J Rheumatol 1992; 19:402–410.
285. Wechsler B, Vidailhet M, Piette JC. Cerebral venous thrombosis in Behçet's disease: clinical study and long-term follow-up of 25 cases. Neurology 1992; 42:614–618.
286. O'Duffy JD, Goldstein NP. Neurologic involvement in seven patients with Behçet's disease. Am J Med 1976; 61:170.
287. O'Duffy JD, Robertson DM, Goldstein NP. Chlorambucil in the treatment of uveitis and meningoencephalitis. Am J Med 1984; 76:75.
288. Cheson BD, Bluming AZ, Alroy J. Cogan's syndrome: a systemic vasculitis. Am J Med 1976; 60:549.
289. Haynes BF, et al. Cogan syndrome: studies in thirteen patients, long-term follow-up, and a review of the literature. Medicine 1980; 59:426–441.
290. Vollertsen RS, et al. Cogan's syndrome: 18 cases and a review of the literature. Mayo Clin Proc 1986; 61:344–361.
291. Sigal LH. The neurologic presentation of vasculitic and rheumatologic syndromes. Medicine 1987; 66:157–180.
292. Lie JT. Primary (granulomatous) angiitis of the central nervous system: a cliniopathologic analysis of 15 new cases and a review of the literature. Hum Pathol 1992; 23:164–171.
293. Cupps TR, Moore PM, Fauci AS. Isolated angiitis of the central nervous system. Am J Med 1983; 74:97–105.
294. Bryant GL, et al. Cerebral vasculopathy: an analysis of sixteen cases. Sem Arth Rheum 1986; 15:297–302.
295. Harrison HL, et al. Bolus corticosteroids and cyclophosphamide for initial treatment of Wegener's granulomatosis. JAMA 1980; 244:1599–1600.
296. Jellinger K. Giant cell granulomatous angiitis of the central nervous system. J Neurol 1977; 215:175–190.
297. Greer JM, et al. Vasculitis associated with malignancy: expe-

rience with 13 patients and literature review. Medicine 1988; 67:222–230.
298. Pope A, et al. Hairy cell leukemia and vasculitis. J Rheum 1980; 7:895.
299. Goedert JJ, et al. Polyarteritis, hairy cell leukemia and splenosis. Am J Med 1981; 71:323–326.
300. LePogamp P, Ghandour C, Leprise PY. Hairy cell leukemia and polyarteritis nodosa. J Rheum 1982; 9:441.
301. Farcet JP, et al. Arch Intern Med 1987; 147:660–664.
302. Sams WM Jr, Harville DD, Winkelmann RK. Necrotising vasculitis associated with lethal reticuloendothelial diseases. Br J Derm 1968; 80:555–560.
303. Johnson PC, et al. Paraneoplastic vasculitis of nerve: a remote effect of cancer. Ann Neurol 1979; 5:437–444.
304. Castro M, et al. Rheumatic manifestations in myelodysplastic syndromes. J Rheumatol 1991; 18:721–727.
305. Costanza ME, et al. Carcinoembryonic antigen-antibody complexes in a patient with colon carcinoma and nephrotic syndrome. N Engl J Med 1973; 289:520.
306. Kois JM, Sexton M, Lookingbill DP. Cutaneous manifestations of multiple myeloma. Arch Dermatol 1991; 127:69–74.
307. Longley S, Caldwell JR, Panush RS. Paraneoplastic vasculitis—Unique syndrome of cutaneous angiitis and arthritis associated with myeloproliferative syndromes. Am J Med 1986; 80:1027–1030.
308. Alarcon-Segovia D, Sanchez-Guerrero J. Primary antiphospholipid syndrome. J Rheumatol 1989; 16:762.
309. Aserson RA, et al. The "primary" antiphospholipid antibody syndrome: Major clinical and serologic features. Medicine (Baltimore) 1989; 68:366.
310. Mackworth-Young C, Loizou S, Walport M. Primary antiphospholipid syndrome: Features of patients with raised anticardiolipin antibodies and no other disorder. Ann Rheum Dis 1989; 48:362.
311. Sammaritano LR, Gharavi AE, Lockshin MD. Antiphospholipid antibody syndrome: immunologic and clinical aspects. Semin Arthritis Rheum 1990; 20:81.
312. Khamashta MA, et al. Association of antibodies against phospholipids with heart valve disease in systemic lupus erythematosus. Lancet 1990; 335:1541.
313. Canoso RT, de Oliveira RM. Chlorpromazine-induced anticardiolipin antibodies and lupus anticoagulant: Absence of thrombosis. Am J Hemato 1988; 127:272.
314. Levy RA, et al. IgG antiphospholipid antibodies of patients with SLE and with syphilis differ. J Rheumatol 1990; 17:1036.
315. Lillicrap DP, et al. Heterogeneity of laboratory results for antiphospholipid antibodies in patients with chlorpromazine and other phenothiazines. Am J Clin Pathol 1990; 93:771.
316. Harris EN. The second international anticardiolipin antibody standardization workshop/the Kingston antiphospholipid antibody study (KAPS) group. Am J Clin Pathol 1990; 94:476.
317. Greisman SG, et al. Occlusive vasculopathy in systemic lupus erythematosus: association with anti-cardiolipin antibody. Arch Intern Med 1991; 151:389–392.
318. Kittner SJ, Gorelick PB. Antiphospholipid antibodies and stroke: An epidemiological perspective. Stroke 1992; 23[Suppl I]:19.
319. Levine SR, et al. Risk of recurrent thromboembolic events in patients with focal cerebral ischemia and antiphospholipid antibodies. Stroke 1992; 23[Suppl I]:29.
320. Rosove MH, Brewer PMC. Antiphospholipid thrombosis: Clinical course after the first thrombotic event in 70 patients. Ann Intern Med 1992; 117:303.
321. Lynch A, et al. Antiphospholipid antibodies in predicting adverse pregnancy outcome. Ann Intern Med 1994; 12: 470–475.
322. Out HG, et al. A prospective, controlled muticenter study on the obstetric risks of pregnant women with antiphospholipid antibodies. Am J Obstet Gynecol 1992; 167:26.
323. Cohen J, Lockwood CM, Calnan CD. Plasma exchange in treatment of leukocytoclastic vasculitis. J R Soc Med 1980; 73:457–460.
324. Leatherman JW, Davies SF, Hoidal JR. Alveolar hemorrhage syndromes: diffuse microvascular lung hemorrhage in immune and idiopathic disorders. Medicine 1984; 63:343–361.
325. Guillevin L, et al. Lack of superiority of steroids plus plasma exchange to steroids alone in the treatment of polyarteritis nodosa and Churg-Strauss syndrome: a prospective randomized trial in 78 patients. Arthritis Rheum 1992; 35:208–215.
326. Callen JP. Oral colchicine therapy is effective for chronic cutaneous leukocytoclastic vasculitis. Arth Rheum 1987; 30:S106.
327. Axelrod L. Glucocorticoid therapy. Medicine 1976; 55:39.
328. Meuleman J, Katz P. The immunologic effects, kinetics and use of glucocorticosteroids. Med Clin N Amer 1985; 69: 805–816.
329. Dale DC, Fauci AS, Wolff SM. Alternate-day prednisone. Leukocyte kinetics and susceptibility to infection. N Engl J Med 1974; 291:1154.
330. Stevens JE, Willoughby DA. The anti-inflammatory effect of some immunosuppressive agents. J Pathol 1969; 97:367–373.
331. Garges L, Beaulieu R, Bardana EJ. Combined azathioprine-steroid therapy in periarteritis nodosa. Clin Res 1973; 21:268.
332. Nashel DJ. Mechanisms of action and clinical applications of cytotoxic drugs in rheumatic disorders. Med Clin N Amer 1985; 69:817–840.
333. Balow JA, Parillo JE, Fauci AS. Characterization of the direct effects of cyclophosphamide on cell-mediated immunological responses. Immunology 1977; 32:899–904.
334. Hoffman GS, et al. Treatment of Wegener's granulomatosis with intermittent high-dose intravenous cyclophosphamide. Am J Med 1990; 89:399–402.
335. Calabresi P. Leukemia after cytotoxic chemotherapy—a Pyrrhic victory? N Engl J Med 1983; 309:1118–1119.
336. Gershwin ME, Goetzel EJ, Steinberg AD. Cyclophosphamide use in practice. Ann Intern Med 1974; 80:531–540.
337. Hoffman GS, et al. The treatment of Wegener's granulomatosis with glucocorticoids and methotrexate. Arthritis Rheum 1992; 35:1322–1329.
338. Hoffman GS, et al. Treatment of Glucocorticoid-resistant or relapsing Takayasu arteritis with methotrexate. Arthritis Rheum 1994; 37:578–582.
339. Rostoker G, et al. High dose immunoglobulin therapy for severe IgA Nephropathy and Henoch-Schönlein purpura. Ann Intern Med 1994; 120:476–484.
340. Jayne DR, et al. Treatment of systemic vasculitis with pooled intravenous immunoglobulin. Lancet 1991; 337:1137–1139.

Thromboangiitis Obliterans (Buerger's Disease)

Jeffrey W. Olin
J. T. Lie

Thromboangiitis obliterans (TAO) also known as Buerger's disease, is a nonatherosclerotic segmental inflammatory disease that most commonly affects the small and medium-sized arteries and veins in both the upper and lower extremities. In the early reports, TAO was exclusively a disease confined to men; recently, however, more women have been diagnosed with Buerger's disease. Virtually all patients are heavy users of tobacco, usually cigarette smoking.

In 1879, von Winiwater described a 57-year-old man who had complained of pains in his feet for the previous 12 years. In the pathologic specimen that was examined, there was intimal proliferation, thrombosis, and fibrosis. von Winiwater suggested that the endarteritis and endophlebitis that were present in the amputated specimen were distinct from atherosclerosis [1]. That report was the first description of TAO, which later became known as Buerger's disease. Twenty-nine years later, in 1908, Leo Buerger stated in his landmark paper, "There is an interesting group of cases characterized by typical symptoms which the Germans have described under the name 'Spontangangran'" [2]. Buerger provided a detailed and accurate description of the pathology of the endarteritis and endophlebitis in 11 amputated limbs [2]. Based on his pathologic examination, Buerger called the disease thromboangiitis obliterans. He made a point to differentiate the clinical and pathologic findings of TAO from atherosclerosis. However, in a subsequent monograph [3], it appears that many of the patients described with TAO in actuality may have had atherosclerosis instead.

Allen and Brown [4] studied 200 cases of TAO seen at the Mayo Clinic from 1922 to 1926. Most of their patients were Jewish males, and all patients smoked large amounts of tobacco. The clinical description of TAO provided by Allen and Brown was quite accurate [4]: "The disease first manifests itself by excessive fatigue in the extremities followed shortly by the pain of claudication . . . which is in turn followed by or associated with marked rubor when the extremities are dependent and excessive pallor when they are elevated. Trophic changes occur either in a minor form, such as excessive callosities in the weight bearing areas, or in the major form as gangrenous ulcers of the digits or gangrene involving the toes or the entire foot." The pathologic description in that report was virtually identical to Buerger's original description. Allen and Brown suggested that TAO was a disease of infectious origin. Their hypothesis has never been proved, and an infectious etiology currently is not thought to play a major role in the pathogenesis of Buerger's disease.

Epidemiology

Although Buerger's disease has a worldwide distribution, it is more prevalent in the Middle, Near, and Far East regions than in North America and Western Europe [5,6].

UNITED STATES AND EUROPE

The reported number of new patients with Buerger's disease in the United States and Europe has decreased mainly through the adoption of stricter diagnostic criteria. Before the late 1960s, overdiagnosis of Buerger's disease occurred even at Mount Sinai Hospital in New York City, where Buerger began his work on TAO: Of the 205 cases diagnosed as Buerger's disease at the hospital from 1933 through 1963, only 33 were later considered to be compatible with the correct diagnosis; the diagnosis was questionable in 28 cases and incorrect in 144 cases [7].

At the Mayo Clinic, over a 40-year period from 1947 to 1986, the annual patient registration has increased from 166,232 in 1947 to 221,000 in 1986, but the prevalence rate of patients with the diagnosis of Buerger's disease has declined steadily from 104 per 100,000 patient registrations in 1947 to 12.6 per 100,000 patient registrations in 1986 [6,8].

At the International Symposium on Buerger's disease in Badgastein, Austria, in 1986, Cachovan [9] reported the following prevalence rate of Buerger's disease in patients with peripheral arterial occlusive disease in Europe and other countries: 1–3% in Switzerland, 0.5–5.0 percent in West Germany, 1.2–5.6 percent in France, 4 percent in Belgium, 0.5 percent in Italy, 0.25 percent in the United Kingdom, 3.3 percent in Poland, 6.7 percent in East Germany, 11.5 percent in Czechoslovakia, 39 percent in Yugoslavia, 80 percent in Israel (Ashkenazim), 45–63 percent in India, and 16–66 percent in Korea and Japan. Those rates were calculated from selected series of patients treated at specialized institutions rather than from the general population as a whole.

ASIA

In Asia, a much higher proportion of patients with limb ischemia has been attributed to Buerger's disease than in the United States and Europe. In 1980, Nigam et al. [10] in Delhi reported that Buerger's disease accounted for 63 percent, arteriosclerosis obliterans for 15 percent, and miscellaneous causes for 22 percent out of 169 cases of limb ischemia during a 3-year period. At the Christian Medical College Hospital in Vellore, South India [11], in 1989, 186 (53%) of 352 cases of peripheral vascular disease were diagnosed as Buerger's disease and the remaining 166 (47%) as arteriosclerosis obliterans.

In 1931, reviewing the data of 50 cases of the disease in Korea, Ludlow [12] reported that the ratio of the number of patients with Buerger's disease to all inpatients was 1:400 and to male inpatients only 1 : 250. In 1961, McKusick and Harris [13] reported 28 cases of Buerger's disease reviewed at the Presbyterian Medical Center in Chonju, Korea: All patients were male and smokers. Twenty-three of the 28 patients were farmers or farm laborers, and all 23 were of the lowest socioeconomic status.

In 1973, Hill and colleagues (14) described an analysis of 106 patients with Buerger's disease in Java, Indonesia: All the patients were cigarette smokers, and only one was a woman. In general, the patients were from the lowest socioeconomic sector of the community, and there were no patients who could be judged middle class even by Indonesian standards. They concluded that the environmental factors of significance in the disease as it occurred in Java appeared to be tobacco, cold injury, and a past history of mycotic infection.

In 1931, Noble [15] described 15 cases (14 men and 1 woman) of Buerger's disease in Bangkok, Thailand. The majority of them had an outdoor job; all but one were heavy smokers, and the one exception was a woman who habitually chewed betel nut. In China, Whyte [16], a missionary surgeon in Swatow, reported the clinical features of two patients with Buerger's disease in 1917. Although it is well known that the disease occurs widely throughout Asia, to date no nationwide epidemiologic study has been carried out in all those countries.

In 1976, the Buerger's Disease Research Committee of the Ministry of Health and Welfare of Japan [17] analyzed 3,034 patients (2,930 men and 104 women) with the disease from all over Japan and estimated its incidence to be about 5 per 100,000 population. In 1986, the Epidemiology of Intractable Disease Research Committee of the Ministry of Health and Welfare of Japan [18] estimated that there were 8,858 patients with the disease who were treated at various medical institutions in Japan, also about 5 per 100,000 population, and there was no significantly greater prevalence among manual laborers. The number of new patients with Buerger's disease in Japan seems to be decreasing slightly, but the number of the patients under the care of a physician remains almost unchanged due to recurrences [19].

BUERGER'S DISEASE IN WOMEN

Buerger's disease was uncommon in women; the reported incidence was 1–2 percent in most published series of cases before 1970. Several recently published series showed a much higher prevalence of women with the disease. In Lie's report [8], 12 (11%) of 109 cases of the disease from 1981 to 1985 in Rochester, Minnesota, were female; 5 (19%) of 26 in 1987 in the Oregon study [20]; 48 (14%) of 355 from 1975 to 1984 in Yugoslavia [21]; 12 (23%) of 53 patients in a Swiss study [22]; and 26 (23%) of 112 patients from 1970 to 1987 from the Cleveland Clinic Foundation [23]. It is unclear whether the greater number of smokers among young women in recent years is solely responsible for the increased prevalence of Buerger's disease in women, or the reported incidence varied with the diagnostic criteria adopted. The prevalence of Buerger's disease in Japanese women remains relatively low compared to the increased number of female smokers [19].

Etiology and Pathogenesis

The etiology of Buerger's disease is unknown. Pathologically, TAO is a vasculitis [24]. Most vasculitides are believed to be immunologically mediated. TAO differs from most forms of vasculitis in that the usual immunologic markers—elevation of acute phase reactants such as Westergren sedimentation rate and C-reactive protein, presence of circulating immune complexes, and presence of commonly measured autoantibodies (antinuclear antibody, rheumatoid factor, complement levels, etc.)—usually are normal or negative.

There is an extremely strong association between heavy tobacco use and TAO [23,25]. It has been suggested that some patients may be abnormally sensitive or allergic to some component of tobacco and that that sensitivity in some way leads to small-vessel occlusive disease [26,27]. The incidence of TAO is higher in countries where the consumption of tobacco is large. In India, many patients who develop TAO are in a low socioeconomic class and smoke *bidis* (homemade cigarettes with raw tobacco). It has been suggested that that accounts for the higher incidence of TAO in the Indian population [28,29].

Kjeldsen and Mozes [30] have demonstrated that patients with TAO had higher tobacco consumption and carboxyhemoglobin levels than patients with atherosclerosis or a control group of patients. However, there have been occasional cases of TAO in nonsmokers [31] and in users of smokeless tobacco or snuff [32–34].

Whether cigarette smoking is causative or contributory to the development of TAO is unknown. What is clearly known is that tobacco use is a major factor in disease progression and continued symptoms associated with TAO. While passive smoking (secondary smoke) has not been shown to be associated with the onset of TAO, it may be an important factor in the continuation of symptoms in patients during the acute phase of Buerger's disease. Matsuhita and colleagues studied urinary cotinine measurements in patients with Buerger's disease [35]. In their study, cotinine, a major metabolite of nicotine, was used as a marker to determine if patients were actively smoking, being passively exposed to smoke, or not smoking at all. There was a close relationship between active smoking and an active course of Buerger's disease. The effect of passive smoking on the disease process was inconclusive in that study.

Lie described one case of pathologically proven Buerger's disease affecting the upper extremities of a 62-year-old man who "allegedly" had discontinued smoking 15 years earlier [36]. That report, however, did not contain urinary nicotine measurements, cotinine measurements, or carboxyhemoglobin levels. Therefore, it is possible that the man was still smoking.

Some investigators have suggested that purified tobacco glycoprotein (TGP) could be related to changes in vascular reactivity that may occur in cigarette smokers [37]. Papa and colleagues studied 13 patients with Buerger's disease, 16 healthy smokers, and 12 nonsmoking, healthy, young male subjects [38]. There was no difference in the humoral response among the three groups of patients. Patients with TAO and healthy smokers had the same cellular response to TGP antigen, whereas nonsmokers did not respond at all.

In summary, most investigators believe that tobacco is an important etiologic factor in patients who develop TAO. However, because only a small number of smokers worldwide eventually develop TAO, other factors must be involved in the pathogenesis of TAO.

Several studies suggest that there may be a genetic predisposition to developing TAO. There are considerable differences found in the human lymphocyte antigen (HLA) among patients from varied populations. In the United Kingdom, there was a preponderance of HLA-A9 and HLA-B5 antigens, whereas other HLA haplotypes were increased in patients with TAO from Japan, Austria, and Israel [25,39–42]. There is no consistent pattern in HLA haplotypes among patients with Buerger's disease. That may be based on genetic differences in various populations, as well as methodologic differences in each of the studies cited [25]. Mills and colleagues performed HLA testing in 11 patients with TAO and found no identifiable distinctive pattern [20].

Older reports had failed to identify a specific hypercoagulable state in patients with Buerger's disease [43]. Chaudhury and colleagues [44] showed that the level of urokinase-plasminogen activator was twofold higher and free plasminogen activator inhibitor I was 40 percent lower in patients with TAO compared to healthy volunteers. After venous occlusions, tissue plasminogen activator antigen was increased in both patients with Buerger's disease and healthy volunteers but was much more pronounced in the control group. That finding suggests that there is some form of endothelial derangement characterized by increased urokinase-plasminogen activator release and decreased plasminogen activator inhibitor 1 release in patients with Buerger's disease. It also has been shown by the same group of investigators that there is an increased platelet response to serotonin in patients with Buerger's disease [45]. There was one case report published of increased levels of antiphospholipid antibodies in a pregnant patient with Buerger's disease [46]. However, it is a possibility that that patient did not have TAO because both diseases (Buerger's disease and antiphospholipid antibody syndrome) can cause identical signs, symptoms, and arteriographic appearances. Since a biopsy was not performed in that case, there is no way to determine definitively whether or not that patient had TAO.

A number of studies have examined the immunologic mechanisms in patients with TAO. Adar and colleagues studied 39 patients with Buerger's disease and measured the cell-mediated sensitivity for type I and III collagen by an antigen-sensitive thymidine-incorporation assay [47]. They noted an increased cellular sensitivity to type I and III collagen (normal constituents of human arteries) in patients with TAO compared to patients with arteriosclerosis obliterans and to healthy male controls. In addition, 7 of 39 serum samples from patients with TAO demonstrated a low but significant level of anticollagen antibody, whereas that antibody was not detected in the control group of patients. Other investigators have found circulating immune complexes in the peripheral arteries of patients with TAO [48,49].

Based on the above information, there is no single etiologic mechanism present in all patients with TAO. Tobacco seems to play a central role in both the initiation and the continuance of the disease. Other etiologic factors such as genetic predisposition, autoimmune mechanisms, and abnormalities in coagulation may play a role in some patients.

Pathology

Buerger's disease is fundamentally an inflammatory thrombosis that affects both arteries and veins, and the histopathology of the involved blood vessels varies according to the chronologic age of the disease at which the tissue sample is obtained for examination. The histopathology is most likely to be diagnostic at the acute phase of the disease. It evolves to changes being consistent with or suggestive of the disease in the appropriate clinical setting at the immediate stage or subacute phase and becomes virtually indeterminate at end stage or chronic phase, when all that remains is organized thrombus and fibrosis of the blood vessels [2,7,50–53].

Dible [50], almost 30 years ago, acknowledged that the pathologic diagnosis of Buerger's disease was by no means always secure: "There is so much variation from case to case, depending upon the stage of the disease and the characteristic capriciousness of the lesions, that it is difficult to give a succinct account of the histology . . . ." Nevertheless, Dible [50] believed that the histologic distinction between Buerger's disease and arteriosclerosis obliterans was so clear-cut that a differentiation could be made with a high degree of accuracy by simply examining tissue sections containing digital arteries and veins, the small blood vessels that usually are not affected by arteriosclerosis in individuals under the age of 40.

ACUTE-PHASE LESIONS

The early-phase, or acute-phase, lesion is characterized by acute inflammation involving all coats of the vessel wall, especially of the veins, in association with occlusive thrombosis. Around the periphery of the thrombus are frequently what appear to be collections of polymorphonuclear leukocytes with karyorrhexis, the so-called microabscesses, in which one or more multinucleated giant cells may be present (Fig. 44-1). That histologic finding in thrombophlebitis is most characteristic of but may not be specific for Buerger's disease [54]. The striking inflammatory thrombotic lesion occurs with greater regularity in veins than in arteries (Fig. 44-2) and is infrequently seen when organization of the thrombus is well underway (Fig. 44-3).

Whether the vascular lesions of Buerger's disease are primarily thrombotic or primarily inflammatory never has been settled satisfactorily and probably never will be. In either event, the intense inflammatory infiltration and cellular proliferation seen in the acute stage lesions are peculiar and distinctive, especially when the veins are involved. If, by chance, the acute and often tender nodular subcutaneous phlebitic lesion is biopsied at an early stage, one may indeed observe in different segments of the same affected vein several coexisting lesions. Those lesions are acute phlebitis without thrombosis, acute phlebitis with thrombosis, and acute phlebitis with thrombus containing microabscesses and giant cells.

INTERMEDIATE-PHASE AND END-STAGE LESIONS

The intermediate (or subacute) phase is signified by progressive organization of the occlusive thrombus in the arteries and veins, which is usually accompanied by a prominent inflammatory cell infiltrate within the throm-

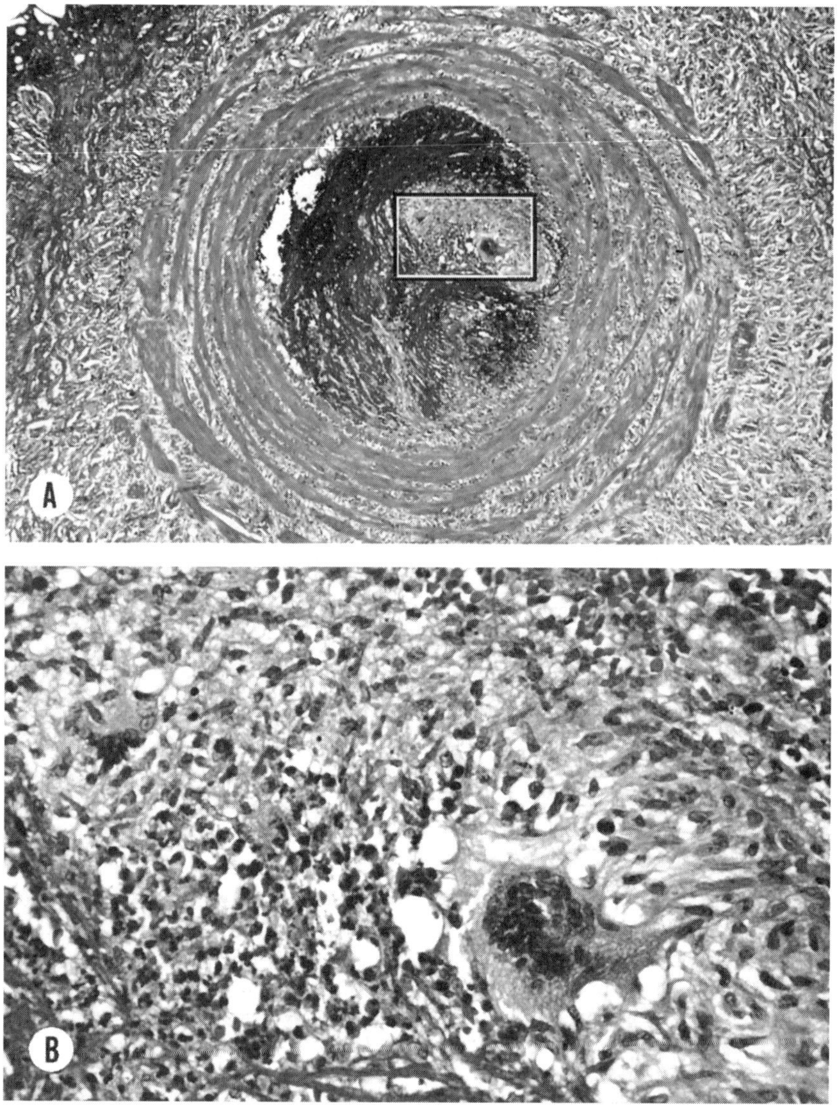

Fig. 44-1. **A.** Typical acute histologic lesion of Buerger's disease in a vein with intense thromboangiitis. **B.** Close up of a boxed area in **(A)**, showing microabscess in the thrombus and two multinucleated giant cells (H&E: **A.**, ×64; **B.**, ×400). (Reproduced with permission from JT Lie. Thromboangiitis obliterans (Buerger's disease) revisited. Pathol Annu 1988; 23(Part2):257–291.)

bus and less so in the vessel wall. The chronic phase or end stage is characterized by completed organization of the occlusive thrombus with extensive recanalization, prominent vascularization of the media, and adventitial and perivascular fibrosis (Fig. 44-4). In all three stages, the normal architecture of the vessel wall subjacent to the occlusive thrombus and including the internal elastic lamina remains essentially intact. These findings distinguish TAO from arteriosclerosis and from other systemic vasculitides, in which there usually is more striking disruption of the internal elastic lamina and the media, disproportional to those attributable to aging change.

Buerger's disease is segmental in distribution; "skip" areas of normal vessels between diseased ones are common, and the intensity of the periadventitial reaction may be quite variable in different segments of the same vessel. Bland arterial and venous thromboses with little or no cellular reaction often intermingle with inflammatory thrombosis in the vascular bed.

ADDITIONAL DIAGNOSTIC HISTOPATHOLOGIC FEATURES

Histologic diagnosis of Buerger's disease usually is inconclusive or tentative at best when only the amputated specimens or occluded arteries and veins are examined. The intermediate-phase and chronic-stage lesions have far fewer characteristic features and are seldom diagnostic. The intermediate lesions coincide with the early phase of organization of the occlusive thrombi in arteries and veins of all sizes. That process is characteristic, if not unique, to Buerger's disease, because of the marked cellular prolif-

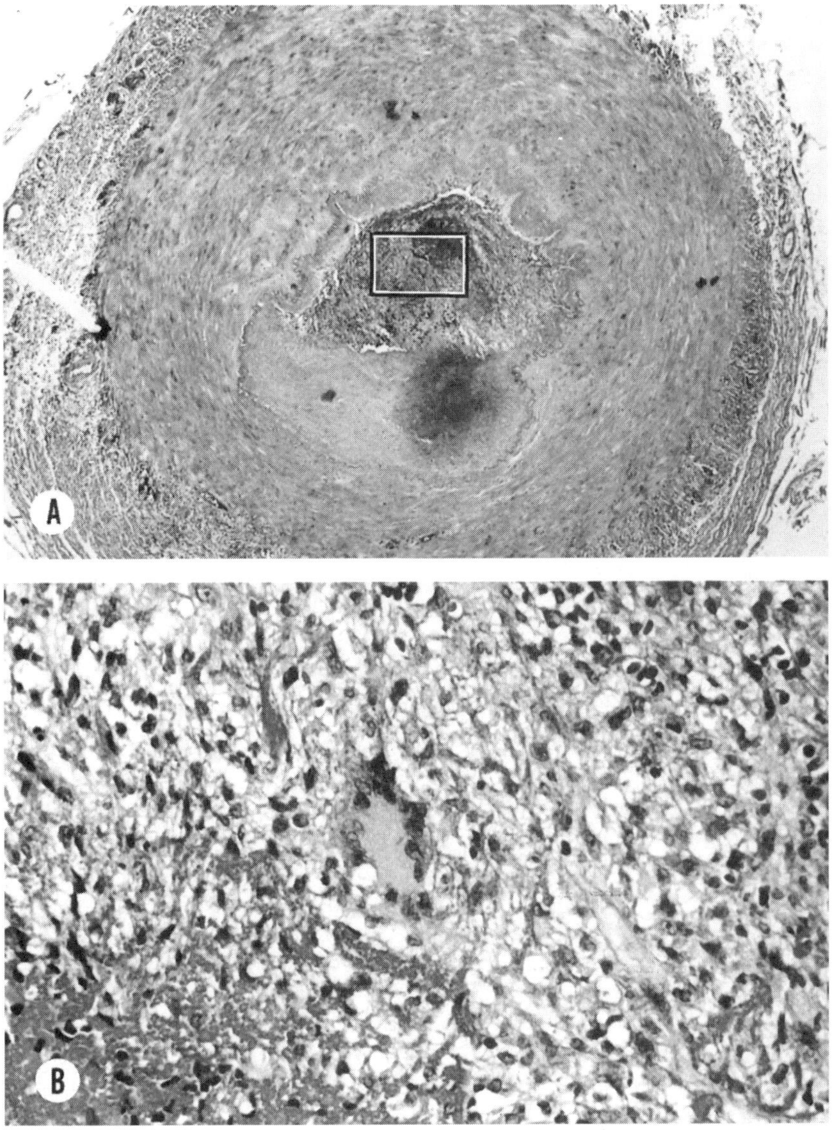

Fig. 44-2. **A.** Acute arterial lesion in Buerger's disease with inflammatory thrombosis and microabscess within the thrombus. **B.** Close-up view of the boxed area in **(A),** showing a giant cell and microabscess within the thrombus (H&E: **A.,** ×40; **B.,** ×400). (Reproduced with permission from JT Lie. Thromboangiitis obliterans (Buerger's disease) revisited. Pathol Annu 1988; 23(Part 2): 257–291.)

eration and inflammatory infiltrate, which rarely are seen in the organization of the ordinary, bland arterial and venous thrombi. Lymphohistiocytic cells and, to a much lesser extent, granulocytic leukocytes contribute to the inflammatory infiltrates. Eosinophils may be present but seldom in excess number. The elastic laminae usually remain essentially intact. Such changes frequently are observed in small digital blood vessels, which normally are not affected by arteriosclerosis or atherosclerosis.

The end-stage chronic lesions are understandably the least distinctive of the three morphologic stages of Buerger's disease. The lesions are characterized by occluded arteries and veins with organized and recanalized thrombi accompanied by fibrosis and neovascularization (see Fig. 44-4). As such, they represent the end products of vascular injury and occlusive thrombosis. The degree of perivascular fibrosis and lymphoid infiltration observed in the organized thrombi and vessel walls varies throughout the obliterated vascular segments. Focal residual inflammatory reaction of the organized thrombus still may be sufficiently characteristic to suggest Buerger's disease. Overall, those features are consistent with a disease process in which focal or segmental vasculitis, combined with thrombosis and endarteritic changes, affects a variable pattern of vascular obliteration that is quite distinct from arteriosclerosis with bland thrombosis. One hardly needs to be reminded that in some patients, especially those over the age of 40, both Buerger's disease and arterioscle-

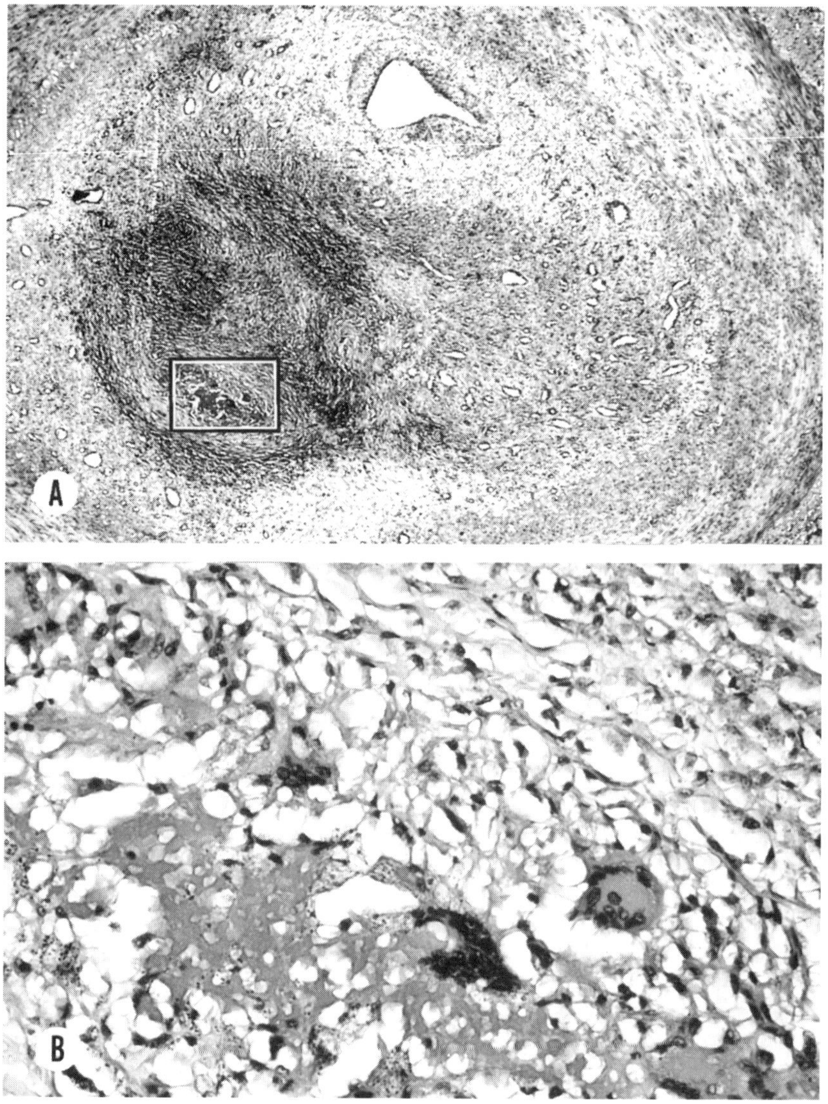

Fig. 44-3. **A.** Femoral artery in Buerger's disease with an organizing thrombus has a rarely seen microabscess (boxed area). **B.** Close-up view of boxed area in **(A)** to show several giant cells in the microabscess of an organizing thrombus (H&E: **A.**, ×64; **B.**, ×400).

rosis may coexist and thus create further diagnostic uncertainty and controversy. Buerger's disease does not confer an immunity to atherosclerosis or arteriosclerosis that is aging related.

IMMUNOCHEMISTRY

To date, there have been very few published studies focusing on the cytoskeleton and immunochemistry of the cellular elements in Buerger's disease [55,56].

Soon after the thrombus has occluded the vessel lumen, spindle cells begin to appear in the periphery of the thrombus. They originate in the media and pass through fenestrations along the internal elastic lamella into the intima and from there into the thrombus. These cells express vimentin and alpha-1-actin (monoclonal marker for smooth muscle actin) and are derived from smooth muscle cells of the media. Capillaries also appear in the marginal zones of the thrombus. The endothelial cells express factor VIII–related antigen and *Ulex europaeus* agglutinin.

In later stages of thrombus organization, the spindle cells in the thrombus lose their positivity staining for alpha-1-actin along with their differentiation into fibroblasts. The demonstration of the internal elastic lamella by collagen type IV markers (Dakopats C 4) confirms that the lamella is intact and that the media smooth muscle cells migrate inward through existing fenestrations to enter the intima. The newly formed capillaries within the thrombus are surrounded by a thin basement membrane mainly composed of type IV collagen produced by the endothelial cells.

In summary, the process of thrombus organization in TAO essentially is identical to that in ordinary thrombosis

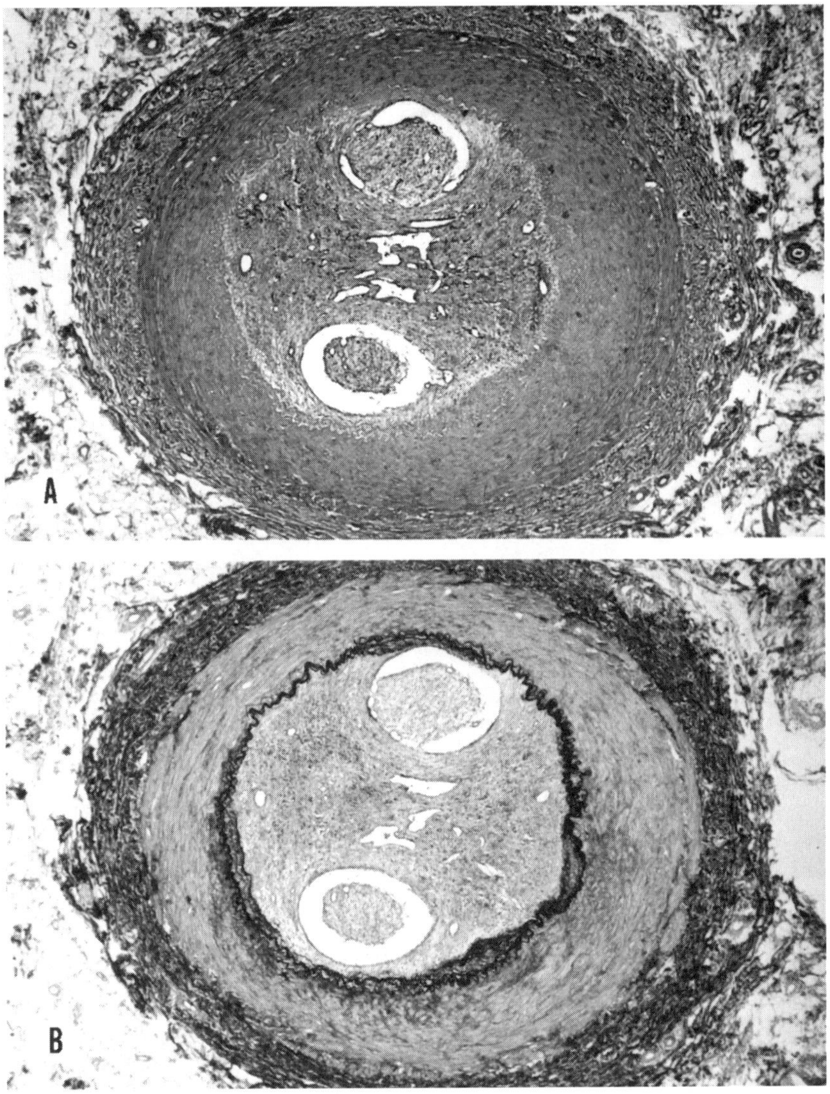

Fig. 44-4. Chronic phase of Buerger's disease with nonspecific organized occlusive arterial thrombus and a fairly intact internal elastic lamina (**A.**, H&E; **B.**, elastic stain, ×16).

but with an added inflammatory component. The invasion of organizing smooth muscle cells from the media of the blood vessel appears more intensified, resulting in a hypercellular thrombus with rapid organization. Prominent inflammatory cell infiltrate in thrombus organization is a hallmark of Buerger's disease. Initial preservation of the internal elastic lamina is another feature that distinguishes TAO from arteriosclerosis, atherosclerosis, and necrotizing vasculitis.

BUERGER'S DISEASE OF BLOOD VESSELS IN UNUSUAL LOCATIONS

Buerger's disease, as already noted, is almost exclusively a disease of the blood vessels in the lower and upper limbs. There have been only occasional reports, usually without adequate histologic proof, of involvement of large elastic arteries, such as the aorta, the pulmonary artery, and iliac arteries. Although Buerger [3] had noted that vascular obliteration could affect blood vessels other than those of the limbs, the involvement of the cerebral arteries, coronary arteries, renal arteries, and mesenteric arteries have been documented in only a handful of patients, almost all as single-case reports [7,57,58]. The most spectacular case of Buerger's disease with combined peripheral and visceral involvement was that of an 18-year-old male cigarette smoker who, in a span of 15 years, underwent bilateral lumbar and dorsal sympathectomies, two bowel resections, and 13 amputations, including bilateral above-elbow and above-knee amputations, before he succumbed at age 33 to another episode of bowel infarction from recurrent Buerger's disease of the mesenteric arteries and veins [59].

The histopathology of visceral TAO is identical to that observed in blood vessels of the limbs with involvement of both arteries and veins. Verging on being true pathologic curiosities are a unique case of Buerger's disease in a

Table 44-1. Presenting signs and symptoms of TAO

	Number (%)
Intermittent claudication	70 (63)
Rest pain	91 (81)
Ischemic ulcers	85 (76)
Upper extremity	24 (28)
Lower extremity	39 (46)
Both	22 (26)
Thrombophlebitis	43 (38)
Raynaud's phenomenon	49 (44)
Sensory findings	77 (69)
Abnormal Allen test	71 (63)
Abnormal pulses	
Brachial	0
Radial	22 (20)
Ulnar	46 (41)
Popliteal	25 (22)
Dorsalis pedis	87 (78)
Posterior tibial	73 (65)

Used with permission from Olin JW et al. The changing clinical spectrum of thromboangiitis obliterans (Buerger's disease). Circulation 1990; 82(Suppl IV):IV-3–IV-8.

saphenous-vein arterial graft [60] and the unusual examples of Buerger's disease in the temporal arteries of young smokers, in some preceded by peripheral ischemia ending in amputations [61]. Also not widely known is the occurrence of Buerger's disease in testicular and spermatic arteries and veins, as was originally described by Buerger [3].

Clinical Features

Classically, Buerger's disease presents in young, male heavy smokers who often have the onset of symptoms before the age of 45 years. As noted previously, recent reports have suggested an increased incidence of TAO in women [8,20,23]. The predominant clinical presentation is that of ischemia that begins distally and involves the small and medium-sized arteries and veins. Occasionally, large-artery involvement has been reported in TAO, but that is unusual and rarely occurs in the absence of small-vessel occlusive disease [62].

Initially, patients present with ischemia or claudication of foot, legs, and, occasionally, the hands. Foot or arch claudication may be the presenting manifestation. Foot claudication often is mistaken for an orthopedic problem, and there may be considerable delay before the correct diagnosis is made. Later in the course of the disease, patients may develop ischemic ulcerations in the distal portion of the toes, fingers, or both.

At the Cleveland Clinic Foundation, 112 patients with Buerger's disease were evaluated between 1970 and 1987 [23]. The presenting clinical signs and symptoms are listed in Table 44-1. Intermittent claudication occurred in 70 patients (63%). The initial location of claudication in many patients was the arch of the foot. As the disease progresses, claudication often moves proximally to cause typical calf claudication.

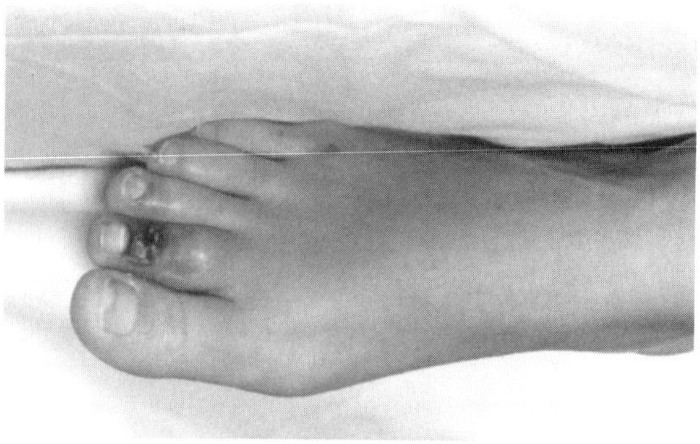

Fig. 44-5. Ischemic ulcer on the second toe in a young woman with TAO.

Seventy-six percent of patients had ischemic ulcerations at the time of presentation [23]. As stated earlier, with heightened awareness of the early manifestations of TAO (foot or arch claudication), many patients could be identified and treated before they ever develop ischemic ulcerations (Figs. 44-5, 44-6).

Two or more limbs almost always are involved in Buerger's disease [34]. Shionoya noted that two limbs were affected in 16 percent of patients, three limbs in 41 percent, and all four limbs in 43 percent of patients [63].

In patients with lower-extremity ulceration in whom Buerger's disease is a consideration, an Allen test should be performed to assess the circulation in the hands and fingers [64,65] (Fig. 44-7). An abnormal Allen test in a young smoker with lower-extremity ulcerations is highly suggestive of TAO, since it demonstrates small-vessel involvement in both the upper and lower extremities. In the Cleveland Clinic series, 63 percent of all patients demonstrated an abnormal Allen test. The distal nature of TAO and involvement of the lower and upper extremities helps to differentiate TAO from atherosclerosis. Except in patients with end-stage renal disease and diabetes,

Fig. 44-6. Ischemic ulcer of the index finger in a patient with Buerger's disease.

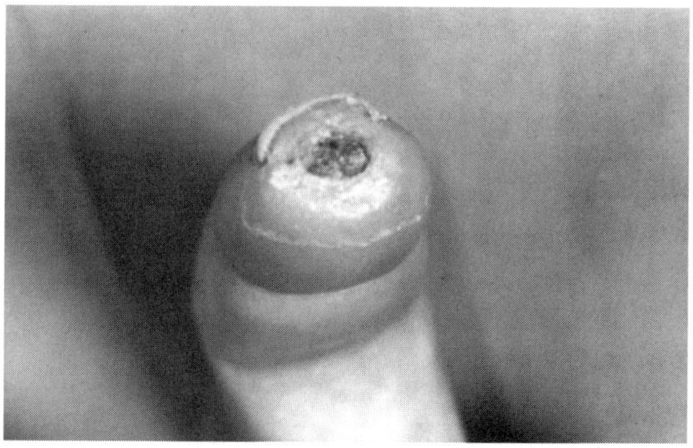

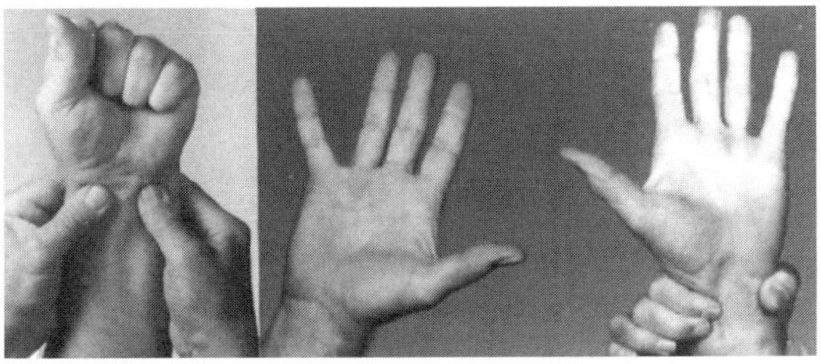

Fig. 44-7. Allen test with occlusion of the radial and ulnar pulse by compression (left photograph). The pressure on the ulnar pulse is released, while the radial is still compressed. The hand does not fill with blood; note the paleness of the hand on the right compared with the left, indicating occlusion of the ulnar artery (right photograph). Reproduced with permission from JW Olin, JT Lie. Thromboangiitis obliterans (Buerger's disease). In JP Cooke, ED Frohlich, eds. Current Management of Hypertension and Vascular Disease. St. Louis: Mosby-Yearbook, 1992. Pp. 265–271.)

atherosclerosis does not occur in the hand and rarely occurs distal to the subclavian artery.

Superficial thrombophlebitis occurs in approximately 40 percent of patients with TAO [23] (Fig. 44-8). The thrombophlebitis may be migratory and may parallel disease activity [25].

Cold sensitivity is common and may be one of the earliest manifestations of TAO [31]. It may be related to ischemia or to markedly increased muscle sympathetic-nerve activity, as has been demonstrated in patients with TAO compared to a control group [66]. Typical Raynaud's phenomenon has been reported in approximately 40 percent of patients. Juergens [31], however, noted that the extremities may be "abnormally red, particularly on dependency; occasionally they may be cyanotic." Kimura et al. [67] termed that discoloration "Buerger's colour." Using nailfold capillaroscopy, those investigators demonstrated an increase in the number and dilatation of capillary loops and correlated that increase with the cyanotic color change. They suggested that Buerger's color was due to an excessive congestion of venous blood in the subcapillary venous plexus. There have not been other reports demonstrating similar changes on capillaroscopy.

Sensory findings are common in TAO and occurred in

Fig. 44-8. Multiple ischemic ulcerations of the toes of both feet. Note the area of superficial thrombophlebitis on the dorsum of the right foot (arrow).

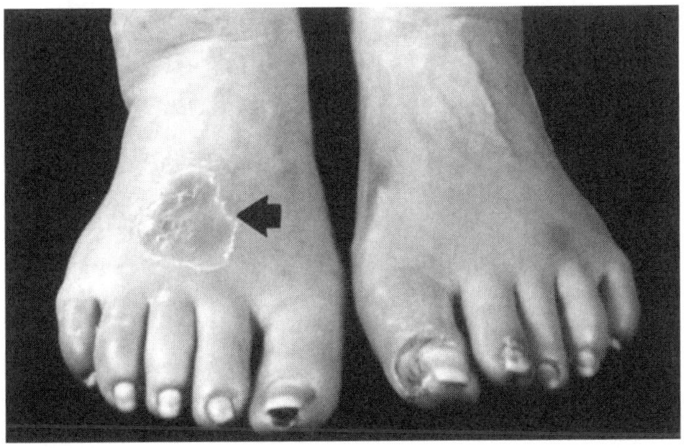

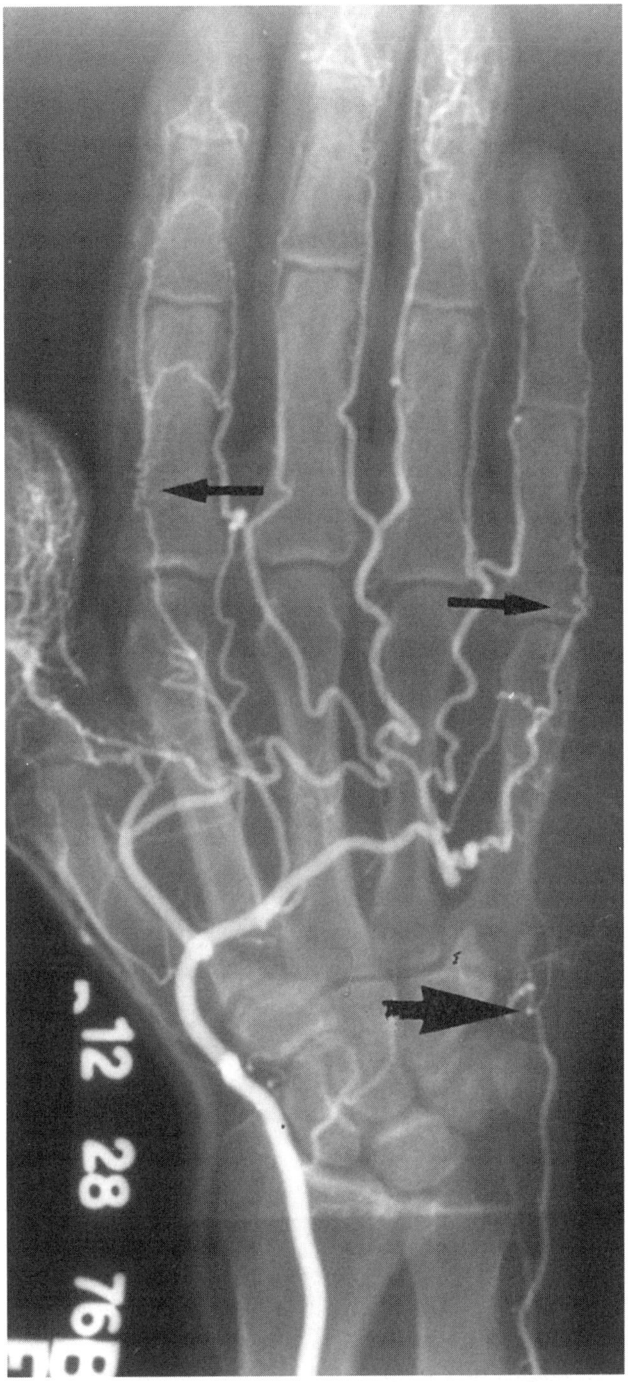

Fig. 44-9. Arteriogram of the hand demonstrating an extremely small ulnar artery, which eventually occludes distal to the wrist (arrow). Note multiple digital-artery occlusions and several areas of corkscrew collaterals (small arrows).

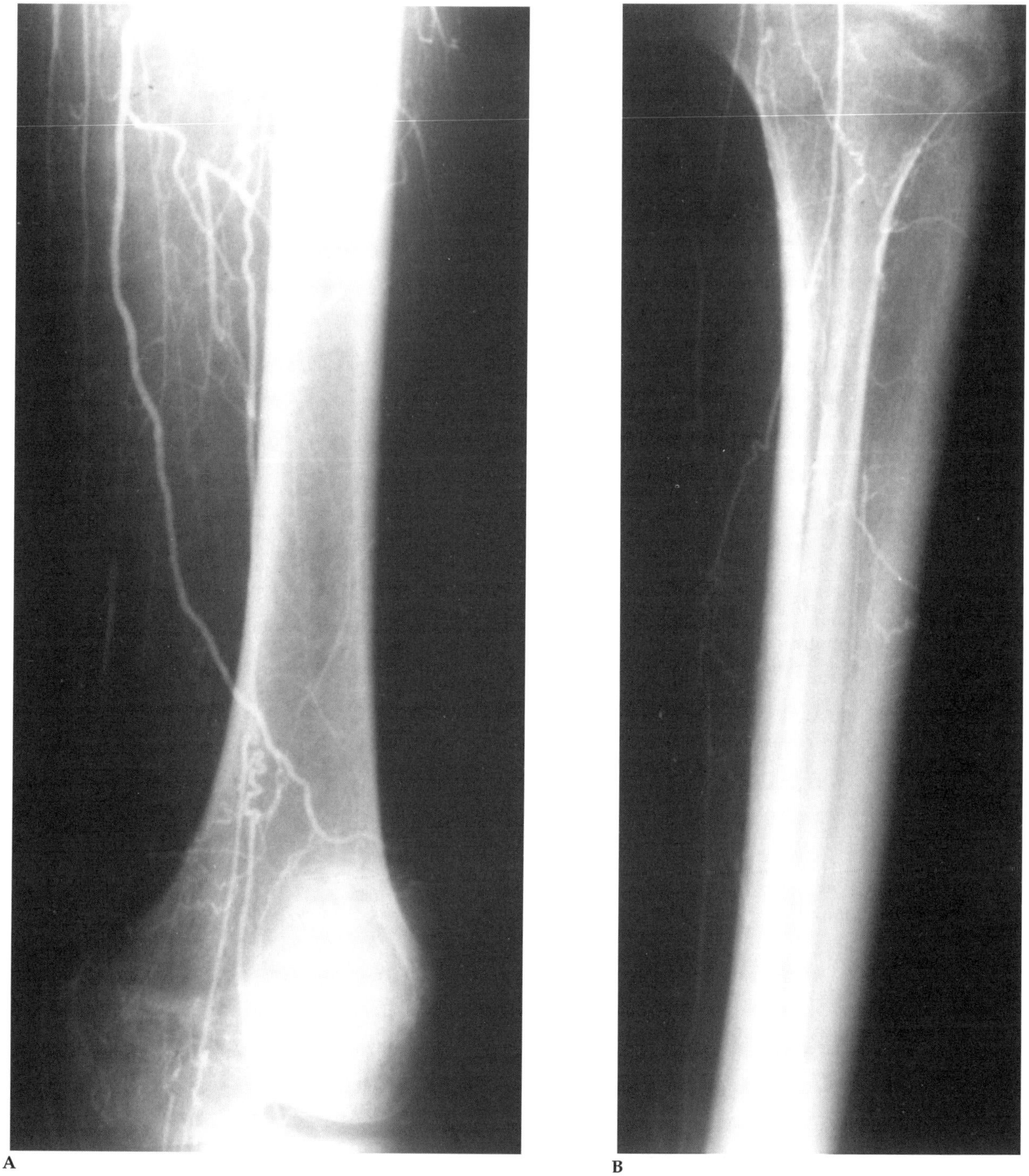

A B

Fig. 44-10. **A.** Occlusion of the superficial femoral artery. Note small collateral arteries. **B and C.** There is severe disease in the infrapopliteal vessels in patient with TAO. Note that no major vessels are seen. This patient eventually required an above-knee amputation.

69 percent of cases in the Cleveland Clinic series [23]. Many of the sensory abnormalities are due to ischemic neuropathy, which occurs late in the course of TAO. Some investigators also have suggested that the nerve fibers are encased with the inflammatory or fibrotic material that may occur in Buerger's disease, thus accounting for some of the sensory abnormalities.

Papa and Adar have proposed various clinical, angiographic, histopathologic, and exclusionary criteria for the diagnosis of TAO [25]. Mills and Porter have proposed major and minor diagnostic criteria for the diagnosis of Buerger's disease [32]. Their major criteria include the following: onset of distal-extremity ischemic symptoms before the age of 45 years, tobacco abuse, undiseased

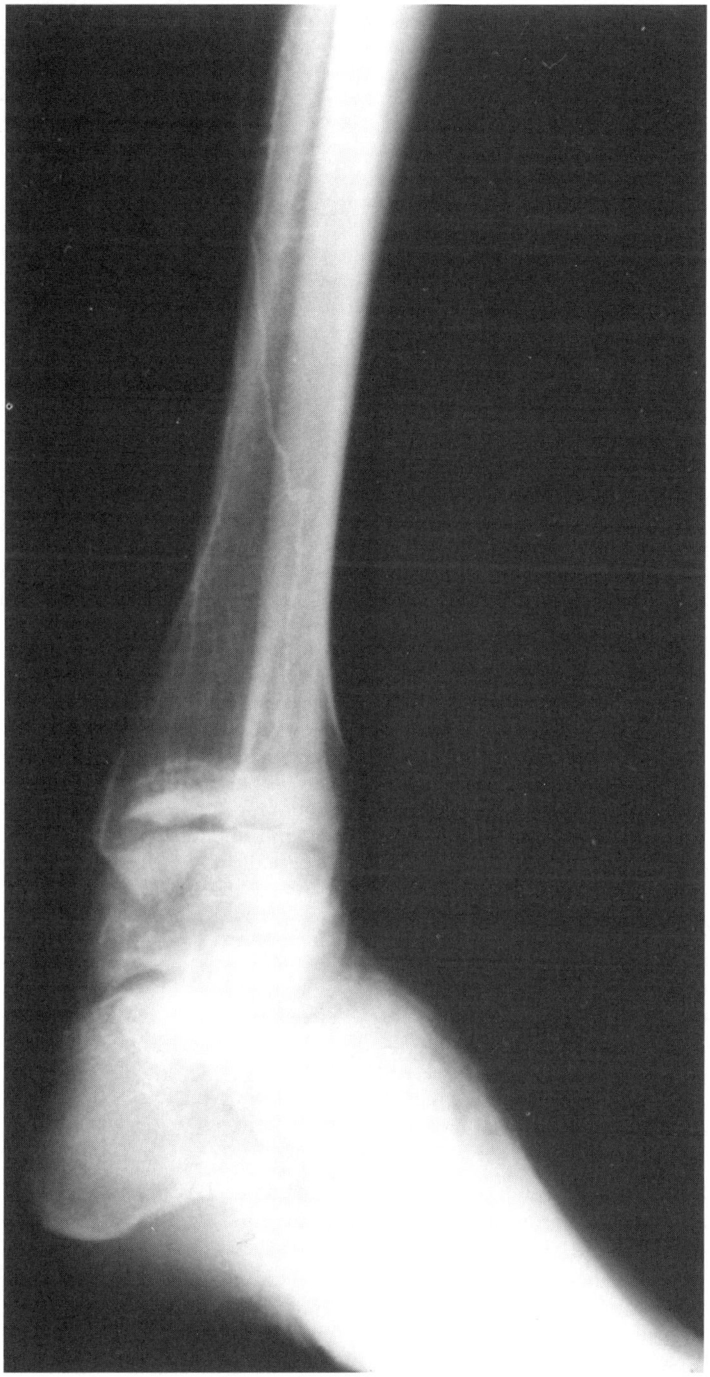

C

Fig. 44-10. (continued)

arteries proximal to the popliteal or brachial level, objective documentation of distal occlusive disease by four-limb plethysmography, arteriography or histopathology, and exclusion of proximal embolic sources, trauma and local lesions, autoimmune diseases, hypercoagulable states, atherosclerosis (diabetes, hyperlipidemia, renal failure, hypertension). Their minor criteria include migratory superficial phlebitis, Raynaud's syndrome, upper-extremity involvement, and instep claudication.

Classifying the criteria as major and minor serves no useful purpose. It does not help to diagnose TAO, nor is it helpful in understanding the pathophysiology or in formulating a treatment plan. In addition, an increasing number of individuals fulfill all the major criteria for TAO but also have the exclusionary criterion of hypertension or hyperlipidemia. Some of those individuals go on to develop typical atherosclerosis 15 or 20 years after the original diagnosis of TAO. Therefore, if patients meet the criteria of distal-extremity involvement, tobacco use, exclusion of a proximal source of emboli or atherosclerosis, in the absence of a definable hypercoagulable state, hyperlipidemia or hypertension should not be exclusionary for the diagnosis of thromboangiitis obliterans.

LABORATORY AND ARTERIOGRAPHIC FINDINGS

There are no specific laboratory tests to aid in the diagnosis of TAO. A complete serologic profile to exclude other diseases that can mimic TAO should be obtained, including complete blood count with differential, liver function, renal function, fasting blood sugar, urinalysis, acute-phase reactants (Westergren sedimentation rate and C-reactive protein), antinuclear antibody, rheumatoid factor, complement measurements, serologic markers for CREST syndrome (calcinosis cutis, Raynaud's phenomenon, esophageal dysfunction, sclerodactyly, telangiectasia) and scleroderma (anticentromere antibody and SCL-70), and a complete hypercoagulability screen to include antiphospholipid antibodies.

To exclude a proximal source of emboli, the patient may need to undergo echocardiography and arteriography. McKusick and colleagues have described in great detail the arteriographic features present in patients with TAO [68,69]. Other investigators further defined the arteriographic findings that may occur in patients with TAO [70,71]. While the arteriogram may be suggestive of TAO, there are no pathognomonic angiographic findings in TAO. Most patients in those series had clinical or arteriographic evidence of involvement of more than one limb.

Examples of typical arteriographic findings are demonstrated in Figs. 44-9, 44-10 and 44-11. Proximal arteries should be normal, demonstrating no evidence of atherosclerosis, aneurysm, or other source of proximal emboli. While the disease has been rarely reported in the proximal arteries [62], in most cases the proximal arteries should be normal. To diagnose Buerger's disease with proximal artery involvement, a pathologic specimen is necessary. The disease most often is confined to the distal circulation and is almost always infrapopliteal in the lower extremities and distal to the brachial artery in the upper extremities. There is small and medium-sized vessel involvement such as the digital arteries in the fingers and toes and the palmar and plantar arteries in the hand and foot, as well as the tibial, peroneal, radial, and ulnar arteries [68,69]. Isolated disease below the popliteal artery virtually never occurs in arteriosclerosis obliterans. Even the patient with diabetes mellitus often has multisegment disease with some evidence of proximal-artery involvement. However, because diabetes is exclusionary for the diagnosis of TAO (in the absence of a pathologic specimen), there should be no confusion between the two diseases.

Arteriographically, TAO is a segmental disorder, demonstrating areas of diseased vessels interspersed with normal blood vessel segments. There often is evidence of multiple vascular occlusions with collateralization around the obstructions (corkscrew collaterals) (see Fig. 44-9). Corkscrew collaterals are not pathognomonic of Buerger's disease, since they may be seen in any small-vessel occlusive disease. The arteriographic appearance of Buerger's disease may be identical to that seen in patients with

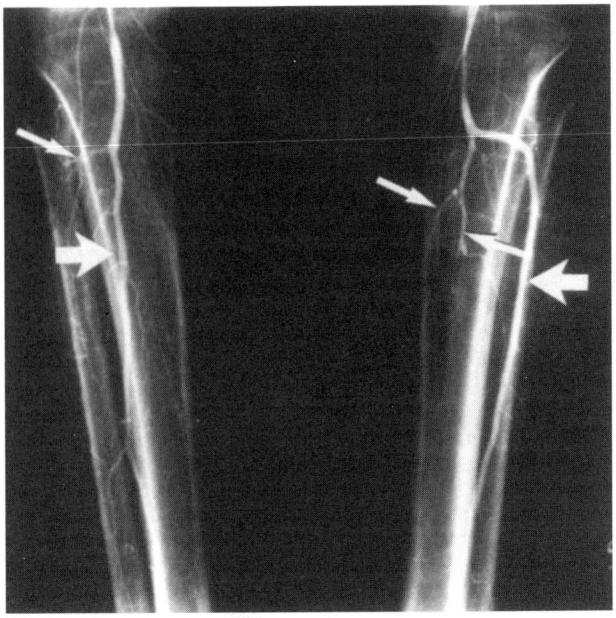

Fig. 44-11. Severe infrapopliteal disease in a patient with TAO. In the right leg, the anterior tibial artery (small arrows) and the posterior tibial artery are occluded at their origin. The peroneal is patent (large arrow). In the left leg, the anterior tibial is patent (large arrow), but the posterior tibial and peroneal arteries (small arrows) are occluded proximally. (Reproduced with permission from JW Olin, JT Lie. Thromboangiitis obliterans (Buerger's disease). In JP Cooke, ED Frohlich, eds. Current Management of Hypertension and Vascular Disease. St. Louis: Mosby-Yearbook, 1992. Pp. 265–271.)

scleroderma or CREST syndrome. However, the other clinical and serological manifestations of scleroderma and CREST syndrome should help to differentiate those diseases from TAO. Irregularity or calcification of the blood vessel wall should be exclusionary for the diagnosis of Buerger's disease [25]. A diagnostic alogrithm for the diagnosis of TAO is shown in Fig. 44-12.

DIFFERENTIAL DIAGNOSIS

The diagnosis of TAO should not be difficult if diseases that mimic TAO are excluded (Table 44-2). The most important diseases to exclude are atherosclerosis, emboli, and autoimmune diseases such as scleroderma and CREST syndrome. Under most circumstances, with the use of echocardiography and arteriography, atherosclerosis and emboli can be excluded with a high degree of clinical certainty.

The diagnosis in patients who have scleroderma or CREST syndrome is usually obvious from a clinical examination of the skin, a history of other systemic features that occur in those diseases, and the presence of serologic markers such as SCL-70 or anticentromere antibodies. Nailfold capillaroscopy usually is quite distinctive in patients with CREST syndrome or scleroderma.

Clinical evidence for features of systemic lupus erythematosus, rheumatoid arthritis, and other types of vasculi-

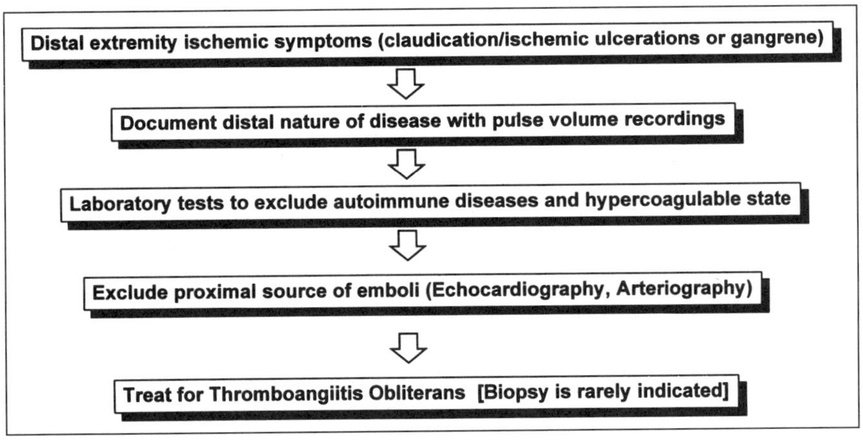

Fig. 44-12. Diagnostic algorithm for the diagnosis of TAO.

tides should be searched for. Serologic markers often help to eliminate the presence of such conditions. Patients with the antiphospholipid antibody syndrome may present with evidence of both arterial and venous thrombotic events. These patients usually have positive circulating "lupus-type" anticoagulants, the presence of high-titer anticardiolipin antibodies or both. Several cases of typical Buerger's disease with the presence of elevated anticardiolipin antibodies have been encountered at our institution (unpublished data). A pathologic specimen would clearly differentiate the two entities, since antiphospholipid antibody syndrome is in reality a vasculopathy (the presence of thrombus with no inflammatory components) as opposed to the typical pathologic findings in Buerger's disease.

Table 44-2. Thromboangiitis obliterans (differential diagnosis)

- Atherosclerosis
- Emboli
  - Cardiac
  - Aneurysms (thoracic, abdominal, femoral, popliteal; thoracic outlet syndrome)
- Connective-tissue disease and/or vasculitis
  - Systemic lupus erythematosus
  - Rheumatoid arthritis
  - Other leukocytoclastic vasculitis
  - Scleroderma
  - Polyarteritis nodosa
  - Giant cell or Takayasu arteritis
  - Antiphospholipid antibody syndrome
- Cystic adventitial disease
- Popliteal-artery entrapment syndrome
- Idiopathic arterial thrombosis
  - Cancer
  - Infection
- Blood dyscrasias
  - Polycythemia vera and other myeloproliferative diseases
- Ergotamine abuse
- Occupational hazards
  - Vibratory-tool use
  - Hypothenar hammer syndrome
- Thrombosis of aneurysms
- Ehlers-Danlos syndrome
- Pseudoxanthoma elasticum
- Calciphylaxis

Reproduced with permission from JW Olin, JT Lie. Thromboangiitis obliterans (Buerger's disease). In JP Cooke, ED Frohlich, eds. Current Management of Hypertension and Vascular Disease. St. Louis: Mosby-Yearbook, 1992. Pp. 265–271.

Patients with TAO present with distal extremity ischemia, whereas patients with Takayasu arteritis or giant cell arteritis present with proximal vascular involvement. The arteriographic features of Takayasu disease or giant cell arteritis are very distinctive. Many patients with Takayasu arteritis have elevations in the acute-phase reactants (erythrocyte sedimentation rate and C-reactive protein), but that finding is not invariable and may not correlate with disease activity [72].

In the presence of lower-extremity involvement, the possibility of popliteal-artery entrapment syndrome or cystic adventitial disease should be considered, both of which should be readily apparent on arteriography. An aneurysm of the popliteal artery should be easily diagnosed by physical examination.

A careful history should be taken for the possibility of ergotamine abuse, which can cause severe ischemia in multiple limbs. That, as well as TAO, may cause both lower- and upper-extremity ischemia. Even if the patient denies a history of migraine headaches or previous ergotamine use, ergotamine blood levels should be obtained to exclude the condition. If there is isolated involvement of the upper extremity, occupational hazards such as vibratory-tool use and hypothenar hammer syndrome should be considered.

Therapy

Various therapies available for the treatment of TAO are shown in Table 44-3. The cornerstone of any therapy is the complete discontinuation of cigarette smoking or the use of tobacco in any form. It has been demonstrated in many case reports and series that complete abstinence from tobacco is really the only way to halt the progression of Buerger's disease and to avoid future amputations

Table 44-3. Therapy for TAO

Cessation of smoking or use of tobacco in any form
Treatment of local ischemic ulcerations:
Foot Care
Lubrication of skin with lanolin-based cream
Lamb's wool between toes
Avoidance of trauma (heel protectors, bed cradle)
Trial of calcium-channel blockers, pentoxifylline, or both
Iloprost (not currently available in United States)
Sympathectomy
Treatment of cellulitis with antibiotics and superficial phlebitis with nonsteroidal antiinflammatory agents
Amputation when all else fails

Source: JW Olin, JT Lie. Thromboangiitis obliterans (Buerger's disease). In JP Cooke, ED Frohlich, eds. Current Management of Hypertension and Vascular Disease. St. Louis: Mosby-Yearbook, 1992. Pp. 265–271.

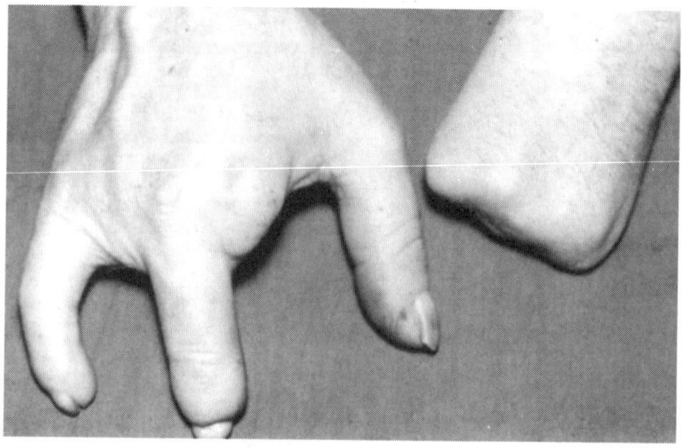

Fig. 44-14. Results of multiple amputations in patient with TAO who was unable to stop smoking.

[23,73,74]. Even one or two cigarettes a day are enough to keep the disease active. In patients with documented TAO, smokeless tobacco (chewing tobacco or snuff) also has been reported to cause Buerger's disease and to keep it active once it has already occurred [33,34]. Of the 112 patients with Buerger's disease studied at the Cleveland Clinic, adequate follow-up was obtained in 89 patients (Fig. 44-13) [23]. Thirty-seven patients (42%) discontinued cigarette smoking. If gangrene was not present at the time the patient discontinued smoking, amputations did not occur. Overall, 35 patients (95%) avoided amputation in the exsmoking group. In the 52 patients who continued smoking, 22 patients (42%) ended up with one or more amputations over a mean follow-up period of 91.6 ± 84 months (range, 1–460 months)(Figs. 44-14, 44-15). Using chi-square analysis, those data were highly significant [6].

Mills and Porter wrote [32], "In fact, it has been cynically stated that if a patient quits smoking cigarettes, he does not truly have the disease." In reality, patients with Buerger's disease may stop smoking more frequently than patients who have atherosclerosis. Olin and associates [23] reported that 42 percent of the patients with TAO were able to discontinue smoking long term. Matsushita and colleagues [35] used conicotine levels to determine whether a patient had discontinued cigarette smoking and demonstrated that approximately 50 percent of their patients had, in fact, stopped. Those data illustrate the importance of education and counseling on the part of the physician in trying to get the patients to discontinue tobacco use.

Some investigators have recommended using anecdotes or photographs of patients who had prior amputations or group meetings with other TAO patients as a means to get the patient to stop smoking [34]. Education is probably the most important aspect. Patients can be reassured that if they are able to discontinue tobacco use, the disease will remit and amputations will not occur as long as critical limb ischemia (gangrene and tissue loss) have not already occurred. However, if significant arterial segments are occluded, the patient may continue to have intermittent claudication, Raynaud's phenomenon, or both.

It is unclear whether involuntary smoking (secondary smoke) can cause TAO. We recommend that patients with active TAO avoid as much involuntary smoking as possible until the disease becomes quiescent.

Other than discontinuation of cigarette smoking, all

Fig. 44-13. Smoking status related to amputation in patients with TAO. (Adapted from JW Olin et al. The changing clinical spectrum of thromboangiitis obliterans (Buerger's disease). Circulation 1990; 82(Suppl IV):IV-3–IV-8).

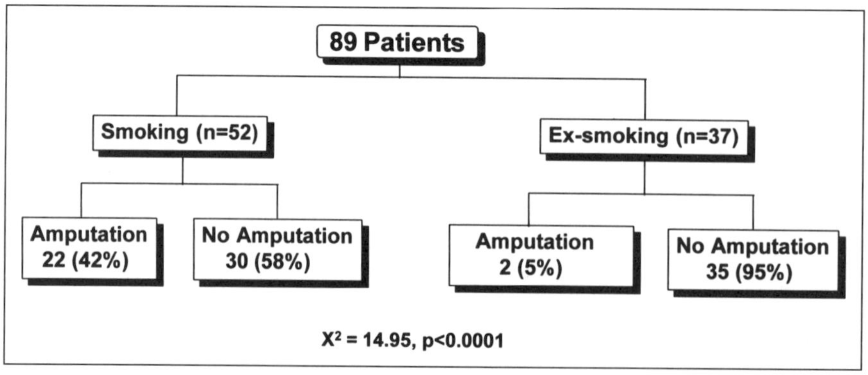

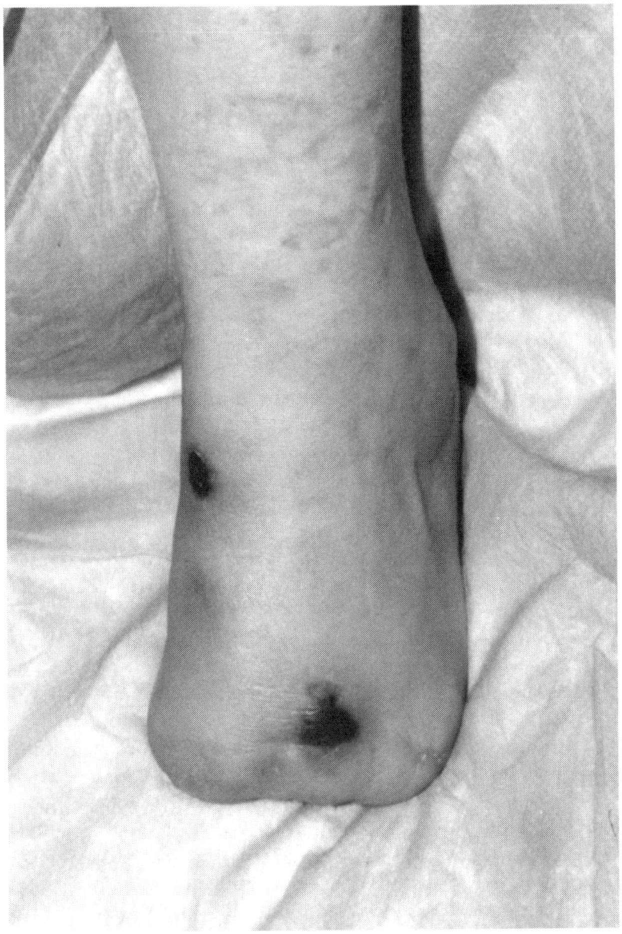

Fig. 44-15. This patient underwent a transmetatarsal amputation in the past. He continued to smoke and has developed several areas of ischemic ulceration on the foot.

Table 44-4. Aspirin versus Iloprost for critical limb ischemia in TAO

	Iloprost	Aspirin
At day 28	*n* = 68	*n* = 65
Responders	58 (85%)*	11 (17%)
Relief of rest pain	43 (63%)	18 (28%)
Ulcer healing	18/52 (35%)	6/46 (13%)
At 6 months	*n* = 51	*n* = 44
Responders	45 (88%)	12 (21%)
Amputations	3 (6%)	8 (18%)

*$P < 0.05$.
Source: JN Fiessinger et al. Trial of Iloprost vs. aspirin. Treatment for critical limb ischemia of thromboangiitis obliterans. Lancet 1990; 335:555.

other forms of therapy are palliative. Fiessinger and Schafer conducted a prospective randomized double-blind trial comparing a 6-hour daily infusion of Iloprost (a prostaglandin analog) to aspirin [75]. All patients entered into the study had critical limb ischemia defined as continuous ischemic rest pain in a limb for which continuous analgesics in the hospital were required for at least 7 days with or without tissue necrosis. Iloprost was superior to aspirin at 28 days in causing total relief of rest pain and complete healing of all trophic changes. In addition, at 6 months, 88 percent of the patients receiving Iloprost responded to therapy, compared to 21 percent of the aspirin group. Only 6 percent ended up with amputations, compared to 18 percent in the aspirin group (Table 44-4). It appears that Iloprost is a useful modality in helping patients with critical limb ischemia get through the early time period when they first discontinue cigarette smoking. Iloprost is not available for use in the United States, although it is available in several European countries.

There is no substitute for good general vascular care in the treatment of patients with severe ischemia. A reverse Trendelenburg's (vascular) position should be used in patients who have severe ischemic rest pain. Adequate narcotics should be made available during the time period of severe ischemia. Standard anticoagulation never has been demonstrated to be effective in TAO. However, if other options are not available, some investigators will use anticoagulants in an attempt to buy time and improve collateral flow in a severely ischemic limb. Good foot and hand care should be undertaken. If significant vasospasm is present, calcium channel–blocking agents such as nifedipine, nicardipine, or amlodipine should be used [64]. Pentoxifylline has not been formally or adequately studied in patients with TAO. Since pentoxifylline increases the red blood cell membrane flexibility and allows red blood cells to fit through a smaller vascular space, it is not unreasonable to try it in the severely ischemic patient.

The role of sympathectomy in preventing amputations or in treating pain is unclear. Twenty-three patients from the Cleveland Clinic underwent sympathectomy, and there was no difference in the amputation rate between those undergoing sympathectomy and those not [23]. Occasionally sympathectomy may help the healing of superficial ischemic ulcerations.

There is little information regarding the use of intra-arterial thrombolytic therapy as an adjunct for the treatment of Buerger's disease. In a recent series [76], selective low-dosage intra-arterial streptokinase (10,000-unit bolus followed by 5,000 units/hour) was administered to 11 patients with long-standing Buerger's disease who had gangrene or pregangrenous lesions of the toes or feet. Many of those patients had previous lumbar sympathectomies. The investigators report an overall success rate (defined as amputation being avoided or altered) of 58.3 percent. Our experience with the use of thrombolytic therapy has not been as successful as reported by Hussein and Dorri [76]. Thrombi in the superficial femoral artery has been successfully lysed, but the severe distal occlusive disease is resistant to thrombolysis (unpublished data). From a pathologic standpoint, a highly inflammatory thrombus quickly becomes encased with connective tissue and fibrous material. Therefore, it does not appear logical that thrombolytic therapy would offer a substantial improvement in many of those patients. However, if the patient is facing amputation, it is not unreasonable to give a short trial of thrombolytic therapy to see if the circulation can be improved enough to avoid amputation as long as no contraindications exist.

Surgical revascularization for Buerger's disease usually is not a viable alternative due to the diffuse segmental involvement and extreme distal nature of the disease. Usually, a distal blood vessel is not available for bypass surgery. However, if the patient is severely ischemic and has a distal infrapopliteal blood vessel available as a target, bypass surgery should be considered with the use of autogenous vein [32]. Inada et al [77] demonstrated that of 236 patients with Buerger's disease, only 11 (4.6%) patients had lesions that were amenable to surgical revascularization. In the 11 patients who underwent surgical revascularization, the bypass remained patent for 4 months to 7 years with a mean time of 2.8 years. Other investigators have reported an early success rate of arterial reconstruction in patients with TAO of 29 percent [78]. Sayin and colleagues [79] recently reported on the surgical treatment of 216 patients with Buerger's disease. That number represented 9.7 percent of all of the patients treated in the Department of Cardiovascular Surgery at Istanbul University Cerrahpasa Medical School from 1981 to 1991. Lumbar sympathectomy was performed in 183 of the 216 patients (85%). Twenty-one patients underwent direct arterial reconstruction consisting of thromboendarterectomy with patch angioplasty (five), aortofemoral or iliofemoral bypass grafting (five), femoropopliteal bypass grafting (six), and femoralcrual bypass grafting (five). Thirty-three patients underwent amputation. The authors noted that four of the five endarterectomized segments had occluded by the 7-year follow-up. One iliofemoral, three femoropopliteal, and two femorocrural bypasses also were occluded. The authors suggested that the long-term patency of those grafts were not good, but in many instances the short-term patency was sufficient to allow healing of the ulcerations associated with TAO. Other investigators have agreed with that indication for surgical revascularization [63].

Summary

TAO is a nonatherosclerotic segmental, inflammatory disease that affects the small and medium-sized arteries and veins in the lower and upper extremities. In some way, as of yet unexplained, it is causally related to tobacco use. Discontinuation of tobacco is the mainstay of treatment. In those patients who successfully stop smoking, amputation almost never occurs.

References

1. von Winiwater F. Ueber eine eigenthumliche Form von Endarteritis und Endophlebitis mit Gangran des Fusses. Arch Klin Chir 1879; 23:202–226.
2. Buerger L. Thromboangiitis obliterans: A study of the vascular lesions leading to presenile spontaneous gangrene. Am J Med Sci 1908; 136:567–580.
3. Buerger L. The circulatory disturbance of the extremities: Including gangrene, vasomotor and trophic disorders. Philadelphia: W.B. Saunders, 1924.
4. Allen EV, Brown GE. Thrombo-angiitis obliterans: A clinical study of 200 cases. Ann Intern Med 1928; 1: 535–549.
5. Lie JT. Thromboangiitis obliterans (Buerger's disease) revisited. Pathol Annu 1988; 23(Part 2):257–291.
6. Lie JT. The rise and fall and resurgence of thromboangiitis obliterans (Buerger's disease). Acta Pathol Jpn 1989; 39:153–158.
7. Herman BE. Buerger's syndrome. Angiology 1975; 26:713–716.
8. Lie JT. Thromboangiitis obliterans (Buerger's disease) in women. Medicine 1987; 64:65–72.
9. Cachovan M. Epidemiologie und geographisches Verteilungsmuster der Thromboangiitis obliterans. In H Heidrich, ed. Thromboangiitis Obliterans Morbus Winiwarter-Buerger. Stuttgart, New York: Georg Thieme, 1988. Pp. 31–36.
10. Nigam R, et al. Thromboangiitis obliterans and arteriosclerosis obliterans as cause of limb ischemia in Delhi. Ind J Surg 1980; 42:9–15.
11. Booshanam VM. Role of sympathectomy in Buerger's disease. Read at the 7th Congress of the Asian Surgical Association in Penang. Personal communication, 1989.
12. Ludlow AI. Thromboangiitis: A review and report of the disease in Koreans. China Med J 1931; 45:487–514.
13. McKusick VA, Harris WS. The Buerger syndrome in the Orient. Bull Johns Hopkins Hosp 1961; 109:241–291.
14. Hill GL, et al. The Buerger syndrome in Java: A description of the clinical syndrome and some aspects of its aetiology. Br J Surg 1973; 60:606–613.
15. Noble TP. Thromboangiitis obliterans in Siam. Lancet 1931; 220:288–291.
16. Whyte GD. Thromboangiitis obliterans. China Med J 1917; 31:371–378.
17. Annual Report of the Buerger's Disease Research Committee of Ministry of Health and Welfare of Japan. K. Ishikawa, ed. Tokyo, 1976. Pp. 3–15, 86–97.
18. Nishikimi N, et al. Result of national epidemiological study of Buerger's disease. J Jpn Coll Angiol 1987; 27:1125–1130.
19. Shionoya S. Buerger's disease. Pathology, diagnosis and treatment. Nagoya: The University of Nagoya Press, 1990. P. 261.
20. Mills JL, Taylor LM, Porter JK. Buerger's disease in the modern era. Am J Surg 1987; 154:123–154.
21. Pirnat L, Simic LJ. Epidemiologie und geographisches Verteilungsmuster der Endangiitis obliterans. In H. Heidrich, ed. Thromboangiitis Obliterans Morbus Winiwarter-Buerger. Stuttgart, New York: Georg Thieme. 1988. Pp. 36–38.
22. Leu HJ. Thromboangiitis obliterans Buerger. Pathologisch-anatomische Analyse von 53 Fallen. Schweiz med Wschr 1985; 115:1080–1086.
23. Olin JW, et al. The changing clinical spectrum of thromboangiitis obliterans (Buerger's disease). Circulation 1990; 82[Suppl IV]:3–8.
24. Lie JT. Diagnostic histopathology of major systemic and pulmonary vasculitic syndromes. Rheum Clin N Am 1990; 16:269–292.
25. Papa MZ and Adar R. A critical look at thromboangiitis obliterans (Buerger's disease). Vasc Surg 1992; 5:1–21.
26. Westcott FN, Wright IS. Tobacco allergy and thromboangiitis obliterans. J Allerg 1938; 9:555–564.
27. Harkavy J. Tobacco sensitivities in thromboangiitis obliterans, migratory phlebitis, and coronary artery disease. Bull NY Acad Med 1933; 9:318–322.
28. Grove WJ, Stansby GP. Buerger's disease and cigarette smoking in Bangladesh. Ann Roy Coll Surg Eng 1992; 74: 115–118.
29. Jindal RM and Patel SM. Buerger's disease and cigarette smoking in Bangladesh. Ann Roy Coll Surg Eng 1992; 74:436–437.
30. Kjeldsen K and Mozes M. Buerger's disease in Israel. Investigations on carboxyhemoglobin and serum cholesterol levels after smoking. Acta Chir Scand 1969; 135:495–498.
31. Juergens JL. Thromboangiitis obliterans (Buerger's disease, TAO). In JL Juergens, JA Spittell Jr, JF Fairborn II, eds. Periph-

eral Vascular Diseases. Philadelphia: WB Saunders Co, 1980. Pp. 467–491.
32. Mills JL, Porter JM. Buerger's disease: a review and update. Semin Vasc Surg 1993; 6:14–23.
33. Lie JT. Thromboangiitis obliterans (Buerger's disease) and smokeless tobacco. Arthritis Rheum 1988; 31:812–813.
34. Joyce JW. Buerger's disease (thromboangiitis obliterans). Rheum Dis Clin N Am 1990; 116:463–470.
35. Matsushita M, Shionoya S, Matsumoto T. Urinary cotinine measurements in patients with Buerger's disease—effects of active and passive smoking on the disease process. J Vasc Surg 1991; 14:53–58.
36. Lie JT. Thromboangiitis obliterans (Buerger's disease) in an elderly man after cessation of cigarette smoking—a case report. Angiology 1987; 38:864–867.
37. Becker CG, Dublin T, Wiedman A. Hypersensitivity to tobacco antigen. Proc Soc Nat Acad Sci USA 1976; 73:1712–1716.
38. Papa M, et al. Autoimmune mechanisms in thromboangiitis obliterans (Buerger's disease): The role of tobacco antigen and the major histocompatibility complex. Surgery 1992; 111:527–531.
39. McLoughlin GA, et al. Association of HLA-A9 and HLA-B5 with Buerger's disease. Br Med J 1976; 2:1165–1166.
40. Numano F, et al. HLA in Buerger's disease. Exp Clin Immunogenet 1986; 3:195–200.
41. Ohtawa T, et al. HLA antigen in thromboangiitis obliterans. JAMA 1974; 230:1126.
42. Smolen JS, et al. Auto immunological aspects of thromboangiitis obliterans (Buerger's disease). Clin Immunol Immunopathol 1978; 11:168–177.
43. Craven JL, Cotton RC. Haematological differences between thromboangiitis obliterans and atherosclerosis. Br J Surg 1967; 54:862–867.
44. Chaudhury NA, et al. Plasminogen activators and plasminogen activator inhibitor 1 before and after venous occlusion of the upper limb in thromboangiitis obliterans (Buerger's disease). Thromb Res 1992; 66:321–329.
45. Pietraszek MH, et al. Enhanced platelet response to serotonin in Buerger's disease. Thromb Res 1990; 60:241–246.
46. Casellas M, Perez A, Cabero L. Buerger's disease and antiphospholipid antibodies in pregnancy. Ann Rheum Dis 1993; 52:247–248.
47. Adar R, et al. Cellular sensitivity to collagen and thromboangiitis obliterans. N Engl J Med 1983; 308:1113–1116.
48. De Albuquerque RR, et al. Circulating immune complexes in Buerger's disease-endarteritis obliterans in young men. J Cardiovasc Surg 1989; 30:821–825.
49. Gulati SM, et al. Significance of circulating immune complexes in thromboangiitis obliterans (Buerger's disease). Angiology 1984; 35:276–281.
50. Dible JH. The pathology of the limb ischaemia. Edinburgh: Oliver & Boyd, 1966. Pp. 79–96.
51. Williams G. Recent view on Buerger's disease. J Clin Pathol 1969; 22:573–578.
52. Leu HJ. Early inflammatory changes in thromboangiitis obliterans. Pathol Microbiol 1975; 43:151–156.
53. Leu HJ. Thromboangiitis obliterans Buerger. Schweiz Med Wschr 1985; 115:1080–1086.
54. Leu HJ, Bollinger A. Phlebitis saltans sive migrans. Vasa 1978; 7:440–442.
55. Gulati SM, et al. Autoantibodies in thromboangiitis obliterans. Angiology 1982; 33:642–650.
56. Roncon A, et al. Circulating immune complexes in Buerger's disease. J Cardiovasc Surg 1989; 30:821–825.
57. Deitch EA, Sikkema WW. Intestinal manifestation of Buerger's disease. Am Surg 1981; 47:326–328.
58. Rosen N, Sommer I, Knobel B. Intestinal Buerger's disease. Arch Pathol Lab Med 1985; 109:962–963.
59. Cebezas-Moya R, Dragstedt LR III. An extreme example of Buerger's disease. Arch Surg 1970; 101:632–634.
60. Lie JT. Thromboangiitis obliterans (Buerger's disease) in a saphenous vein arterial graft. Hum Pathol 1987; 18:402–404.
61. Lie JT, Michet CJ Jr. Thromboangiitis obliterans with eosinophilia (Buerger's disease) of the temporal arteries. Hum Pathol 1988; 19:598–602.
62. Shionoya S, et al. Involvement of the iliac artery in Buerger's disease (pathogenesis and arterial reconstruction). J Cardiovasc Surg 1978; 19:69–76.
63. Shionoya S. Buerger's disease (thromboangiitis obliterans). In RB Rutherford, ed. Vascular Surgery. Philadelphia: WB Saunders, 1989. Pp. 207–217.
64. Olin JW, Lie JT. Thromboangiitis obliterans (Buerger's disease). In JP Cooke, ED Frohlich, eds. Current Management of Hypertension and Vascular Disease. St. Louis: Mosby Yearbook, 1992. Pp. 265–271.
65. Allen EV. Thromboangiitis obliterans. Methods of diagnosis of chronic occlusive arterial lesions distal to the wrist with illustrative cases. Am J Med Sci 1929; 178:237–244.
66. Yamamoto K, et al. Muscle sympathetic outflow in Buerger's disease. J Autonom Nerv Sys 1993; 44:67–76.
67. Kimura T, et al. Buerger's colour. Br J Surg 1990; 77:1299–1301.
68. McKusick VA, et al. The Buerger syndrome in the United States. Arteriographic observations with special reference to involvement of the upper extremities and the differentiation from atherosclerosis and embolism. Bull Johns Hopkins Hosp 1962; 110:145–176.
69. McKusick VA, et al. Buerger's disease: A distinct clinical and pathologic entity. JAMA 1962; 181:93–100.
70. Lambeth JT, Yong NK. Arteriographic findings in thromboangiitis obliterans with emphasis on femoropopliteal involvement. AJR 1970; 109:553–562.
71. Szilagi D, DeRusso FJ, Elliot JP. Thromboangiitis obliterans, clinico-angiographic correlations. Arch Surg 1964; 88:824–835.
72. Jaff M, Olin JW, Young JR. Failure of acute phase reactants to predict disease activity in Takayasu's arteritis. J Vasc Med Biol 1994; 4:223–227.
73. Gifford RW, Hines EA. Complete clinical remission in thromboangiitis obliterans during abstinence from tobacco: report of a case. Proc Staff Meetings Mayo Clinic 1951; 26:241–245.
74. Corelli F. Buerger's disease: Cigarette smoker disease may always be cured by medical therapy alone. Uselessness of operative treatment. J Cardiovasc Surg 1973; 14:28–36.
75. Fiessinger JN, Schafer M for the TAO Study. Trial of Iloprost vs. aspirin. Treatment for critical limb ischemia of thromboangiitis obliterans. Lancet 1990; 335:555–557.
76. Hussein EA, Dorri AE. Intra-arterial streptokinase as adjuvant therapy for complicated Buerger's disease: early trials. Internat Surg 1993; 78:54–58.
77. Inada K, et al. Non-atherosclerotic segmental arterial occlusion of the extremities. Arch Surg 1974; 108:663–667.
78. Mills JL, Porter JM. Buerger's disease (thromboangiitis obliterans). Ann Vasc Surg 1991; 5:570–572.
79. Sayin A, et al. Surgical treatment of Buerger's disease: experience with 216 patients. J Cardiovasc Surg 1993; 1(4):377–380.

C

Venous Thromboembolism and Chronic Venous Disorders

45

Venous Thrombosis

Russell D. Hull
Graham F. Pineo

Despite significant advances in the prevention and treatment of venous thromboembolism (venous thrombosis and pulmonary embolism), pulmonary embolism remains the most common preventable cause of hospital death [1] and is responsible for approximately 150,000 to 200,000 deaths per year in the United States [2,3]. Many patients who die from pulmonary embolism succumb suddenly or within 2 hours after the acute event, that is, before therapy can be initiated or take effect [4]. Effective and safe means of prophylaxis against venous thromboembolism are now available in most high-risk patients [5–7]. Although venous thromboembolism usually complicates the course of patients who are sick and hospitalized, it also may affect ambulatory and otherwise healthy individuals. It is vital, therefore, that efforts be made to continue to find more effective and safer means of managing venous thromboembolism. The use of prophylaxis is more effective for preventing death and morbidity from venous thromboembolism than is the treatment of established disease.

Etiology and Pathogenesis

Factors predisposing to the development of venous thrombosis include venous stasis, activation of blood coagulation, and vascular damage. Venous thrombi commonly form at sites of slow or disturbed flow and begin as a small deposit of platelets, fibrin, and red cells in the valve cusp pockets, intramuscular sinuses of the leg veins, or venous segments that have been exposed to direct trauma (e.g., in the femoral vein following total hip replacement). When the thrombus grows, it occludes the lumen of the vein, producing further venous stasis and then extending both proximally and distally as a thrombus composed largely of red blood cells with interspersed fibrin. The protective mechanisms counteracting thrombogenic stimuli include the inactivation of activated coagulation factors by natural inhibitors, clearance of activated coagulation factors and soluble fibrin polymer complexes by the reticuloendothelial system and the liver, and dissolution of fibrin by fibrinolytic enzymes derived from endothelial cells, plasma, and circulating leukocytes.

Clinical risk factors predisposing to the development of venous thromboembolism are shown in Table 45-1.

Deep-vein thrombosis (DVT) usually arises in the deep veins of the calf muscles or, less commonly, in the proximal deep veins of the leg. DVT that remains confined to the calf veins is associated with a low risk of clinically important pulmonary embolism [8–11]. Without treatment, however, approximately 20 percent of calf-vein thrombi extend into the proximal venous system [12,13], where they may pose a serious and potentially life-threatening disorder. Untreated proximal venous thrombosis is associated with a 10-percent risk of fatal pulmonary embolism and at least a 50-percent risk of pulmonary embolism or recurrent venous thrombosis [10,11,14]. Furthermore, the postphlebitic syndrome is associated with extensive proximal venous thrombosis and carries its own long-term morbidity.

Pulmonary emboli in most cases (90%) originate from thrombi in the deep venous system of the legs. Other less common sources of pulmonary embolism include the deep pelvic veins, renal veins, inferior vena cava, right heart, and occasionally axillary veins. It is now well established that clinically important pulmonary emboli arise from thrombi in the proximal deep veins of the legs [15–19]. The clinical significance of pulmonary embolism depends on the size of the embolus and the cardiorespiratory reserve of the patient.

It is widely accepted that venous thromboembolism is a single disorder [20–22]. Therefore, the diagnostic ap-

Table 45-1. Risk factors predisposing to the development of venous thromboembolism

CLINICAL RISK FACTORS
Surgical and nonsurgical trauma
Age (> 40)
Previous venous thromboembolism
Immobilization
Malignant disease
Heart failure
Myocardial infarction
Leg paralysis
Obesity
Varicose veins
Estrogens
Parturition
INHERITED ABNORMALITIES
Antithrombin III deficiency
Protein C deficiency
Protein S deficiency
Dysfibrinogenemia

Table 45-2. Alternative diagnoses in 87 consecutive patients with clinically suspected venous thrombosis and negative venograms

Diagnosis*	Patients (%)
Muscle strain	24
Direct twisting injury to leg	10
Leg swelling in paralyzed limb	9
Lymphangitis, lymphatic obstruction	7
Venous reflux	6
Muscle tear	5
Baker's cyst	3
Cellulitis	2
Internal abnormality of knee	1
Unknown	26

*The diagnosis was made once venous thrombosis had been excluded by the finding of a negative venogram.
Source: Reproduced with permission from RD Hull et al. Clinical validity of a negative venogram in patients with clinically suspected venous thrombosis. Circulation 1981; 64:622.

proach may be directed toward the legs or the lungs, starting with the least invasive testing and proceeding to more invasive tests. The treatment of venous thrombosis and pulmonary embolism is basically the same.

Clinical Features

Common clinical features of venous thrombosis include leg pain, tenderness, swelling, discoloration, venous distention and prominence of the superficial veins, and the presence of a palpable cord (a palpable thrombosed vessel). The clinical diagnosis of venous thrombosis is highly nonspecific because none of the symptoms or signs is unique and each may be caused by nonthrombotic disorders. In more than 50 percent of patients with a clinical suspicion of venous thrombosis, the diagnosis is not confirmed by objective testing [23]. Furthermore, patients with relatively minor symptoms and signs (or none at all) may be found to have extensive DVT with or without pulmonary embolism when the appropriate tests are performed. Thus, objective testing is mandatory to confirm or exclude a diagnosis of venous thrombosis. The rare exception may be the patient with phlegmasia cerulea dolens in whom the diagnosis of massive ileofemoral thrombosis usually is clinically obvious. That syndrome occurs in fewer than 1 percent of patients with symptomatic venous thrombosis, but it is important because treatment is required on an urgent basis.

Laboratory Features

A variety of laboratory abnormalities have been associated with venous thromboembolism, including increased levels of fibrinopeptide A and fibrinogen-degradation products, thrombin-antithrombin III complexes, prothrombin fragment 1.2, and D-dimer. Patients with venous thromboembolism frequently have other comorbid conditions, including recent surgery or trauma, cancer, infection, or inflammation, and many of the laboratory changes associated with venous thromboembolism are nonspecific.

The quest for a simple blood test to detect or eliminate venous thromboembolism continues. The only reasonable contender is measurement of the D-dimer using either an enzyme-linked immunosorbent assay (ELISA) or latex agglutination [24,25]. A cut-off value can be determined below which the sensitivity and negative predictive value of the tests are extremely high [24,25]. The specificity and positive predictive values, however, remain in the 50-percent range. A recent study reported in abstract form demonstrated that a rapid red cell agglutination assay (SIMPLIRED test) when performed in patients with suspected DVT in whom the diagnosis was confirmed by either compression ultrasonography or venography yielded a sensitivity of 89 percent and a negative predictive value of 95 percent for all DVT [26]. For proximal DVT, the sensitivity was 92 percent and the negative predictive value 96 percent. Because it can be performed in minutes, the SIMPLIRED test can be useful in making management decisions.

Differential Diagnosis

A number of clinical conditions can mimic DVT, as shown in Table 45-2. An alternative diagnosis frequently is not evident at presentation, and it is impossible to exclude venous thromboembolism without the use of objective tests. In a number of patients who do not have DVT, the cause of pain, tenderness, and swelling may remain uncertain even after careful follow-up.

Objective Tests for the Diagnosis of Venous Thromboembolism

In the diagnosis of venous thrombosis, objective tests include B-mode ultrasound, duplex ultrasound, ultrasonography and color flow ultrasonography, impedance plethysmography (IPG), and ascending venography.

ULTRASONOGRAPHY

Venous imaging using real-time B-mode ultrasound with or without Doppler assessment is becoming the standard technique for evaluating patients with clinically suspected DVT [27–31]. Prospective studies have shown that the single criterion of vein compressibility is highly sensitive and specific for proximal-vein thrombosis (sensitivity and specificity both greater than 95%) [27–31]. Other criteria such as echogenicity or change in venous diameter during a Valsalva's maneuver are less useful. The visualization of an echogenic band is highly sensitive but nonspecific (specificity 50%). The percentage change in venous diameter during a Valsalva's maneuver is both insensitive and nonspecific.

Real-time B-mode venous ultrasound and duplex ultrasonography are insensitive for isolated calf-vein thrombosis, and, like IPG, serial testing is required to detect proximal extension. B-mode venous ultrasound may fail to detect isolated iliac-vein thrombi. This is a practical clinical limitation in patient groups in whom isolated vein thrombosis is not uncommon, such as the pregnant patient with clinically suspected venous thrombosis. Color flow imaging and other technologic advances have improved the ability of B-mode venous imaging to detect isolated iliac-vein and calf-vein thrombi [32–40].

The Doppler ultrasound is highly sensitive and specific in the diagnosis of proximal-vein thrombosis in symptomatic patients. Doppler ultrasound is more sensitive than IPG for detection of symptomatic calf-vein thrombosis and is more reliable than IPG for detecting proximal-vein thrombosis in patients with increased central venous pressure or arterial insufficiency. The technique can be used in patients who have a leg in a plaster cast or external fixation, are in traction, or have had leg amputation.

Although the Doppler ultrasound is rapidly replacing venography in verifying the diagnosis of DVT in symptomatic patients, it lacks both sensitivity and specificity for the detection of asymptomatic venous thrombosis in postoperative patients [41–46]. Ultrasonography is now readily available and has replaced IPG as the most popular noninvasive test for the detection of venous thrombosis.

IMPEDANCE PLETHYSMOGRAPHY

IPG is sensitive and specific for proximal-vein thrombosis in symptomatic patients, but it is insensitive to calf-vein thrombosis [47–53]. In patients with clinically suspected venous thrombosis, positive IPG results can be used to make therapeutic decisions in the absence of clinical conditions known to produce false-positive results [50,53]. A normal result essentially excludes the diagnosis of proximal-vein thrombosis but does not exclude calf-vein thrombosis. That potential limitation can be overcome by performing serial IPG. The use of serial IPG is based on the concept now confirmed by clinical observation that calf-vein thrombi are clinically important only when extension into the proximal veins occurs, at which point detection with IPG is possible. The effectiveness and safety of IPG have been evaluated by prospective clinical trials in patients with clinically suspected venous thrombosis. Based on the data provided by those studies, the following recommendations can be made: (1) A positive result by IPG is highly predictive of acute proximal-vein thrombosis (positive predictive value greater than 90%), and (2) it is safe to withhold anticoagulant therapy in symptomatic patients who remain negative by serial IPG for 10 to 14 days.

Although the IPG has a high sensitivity and specificity for symptomatic venous thrombosis, it lacks sensitivity for the detection of asymptomatic venous thrombosis following surgery, such as total hip replacement, or in trauma patients [54,55]. In such circumstances, the only reliable method for detection of DVT is bilateral ascending venography.

IPG has certain limitations. False-positive results may occur with disorders that interfere with arterial inflow or venous outflow, including severe congestive heart failure, constrictive pericarditis, severe arterial insufficiency, hypotension, and external compression of veins. Most of those disorders are readily recognized on clinical grounds. False-positive results also may occur if the test is performed incorrectly or the patient is not relaxed. The test cannot be performed on some patients, for example, those who are in plaster casts or who cannot be adequately positioned because of immobilization or pain.

VENOGRAPHY

Until recently, venography has been accepted as the standard objective method for the diagnosis of venous thrombosis. Although the diagnosis of proximal venous thrombosis can now be established with noninvasive tests (i.e., ultrasonography and IPG), venography remains the only reliable test for making the diagnosis of DVT in asymptomatic patients, for example, following orthopedic surgery or trauma [56–58]. Venography is a difficult technique to perform well and requires considerable experience to execute adequately and interpret accurately. A number of venographic abnormalities have been defined as criteria for the diagnosis of acute DVT [23]. The most reliable criterion is the presence of an intraluminal filling defect that is constant in all films and is seen in a number of projections. Other venographic abnormalities, such as nonfilling of a segment of the deep venous system or nonfilling of the entire deep venous system above the knee, may be caused by technical artifacts, particularly if the dye is injected too far proximally into the dorsal foot vein. The artifacts may then be interpreted as either being caused by thrombus because the vein is not filled or as normal because a filling defect is not seen. The common femoral, external iliac, and common iliac veins may not be adequately filled by ascending venography, which can lead to an incorrect diagnosis based on inadequate venography. In the case of nonfilling of an entire segment of the deep venous system, the diagnosis of acute or recurrent venous thrombosis must depend on the use of other tests such as IPG or ultrasound [47]. A number of other problems are related to venography. Even in the best of circumstances, it may be impossible to cannulate a vein on the dorsum of the foot, making ascending venography impossible on one or both legs. If there is inadequate filling of the common femoral or iliac systems, a femoral venogram may be necessary.

Venography is associated with a number of clinically

troublesome side effects. Pain may occur in the foot while dye is being injected, or there may be delayed pain in the calf 1 or 2 days after injection. The procedure may be complicated by superficial phlebitis or even DVT in a small percentage of patients with normal venograms (1–2%) [47]. Other less common complications of venography include hypersensitivity to the radiopaque dye and local skin or tissue necrosis from extravasation of dye at the site of injection. Both nonionic and high-ionic contrast media may cause or aggravate renal insufficiency in patients at high risk for such complications, for example, patients with established renal disease, hypertension, heart failure, diabetes, or multiple myeloma [59,60]. The risks of venography must be carefully weighed in such circumstances and reviewed with the patient before venography is performed.

Diagnosis and Treatment of Pulmonary Embolism Based on Objective Testing for Proximal DVT

It is well established that at least 80 percent of patients with pulmonary embolism have thrombi originating in the lower-leg veins [8–10,61,62]. Because of the diagnostic inaccuracy of noninvasive tests for pulmonary embolism, particularly those with nondiagnostic lung-scan results, the concept of using objective tests for the detection of proximal venous thrombosis in the legs was developed in patients suspected of having pulmonary embolism [11,20–22,63,64]. That combined strategy for the diagnosis and treatment of pulmonary embolus or venous thrombosis (i.e., venous thromboembolism) has been applied in prospective clinical trials [11,63,64].

The noninvasive tests, such as IPG or B-mode venous ultrasound, have advantages because they are free of morbidity and readily repeatable. Proximal-vein thrombosis is revealed by IPG in 10 to 25 percent of patients with nondiagnostic ventilation-perfusion scans. That has important implications for management: Untreated or inadequately treated proximal-vein thrombosis is associated with a high risk (20–50%) of recurrent venous thromboembolism.

A positive result by venography or noninvasive testing is an indication for therapy; however, the venogram is negative in approximately 30 percent of patients with angiographically documented pulmonary embolism. There are two possible explanations for this finding. The first is that the pulmonary embolism may have originated from a source other than the deep veins of the legs. Alternatively, the embolism may have originated from the deep veins of the legs, but all or most of the thrombus embolized, leaving no residual thrombosis detectable at the time of presentation.

Patients with abnormal but nondiagnostic lung scans and negative objective tests for venous thrombosis require pulmonary angiography to confirm or exclude pulmonary embolism, which may be impractical or unavailable. In patients who do not have severely limited cardiac or respiratory reserve, serial objective testing for proximal-vein thrombosis is an alternative approach, based on the concept that clinically important recurrent pulmonary embolism is unlikely (<1%) in the absence of proximal-vein thrombosis. That concept is supported by the findings of studies of the natural history of venous thrombosis and by clinical trials of noninvasive testing in patients with symptoms or signs suggesting DVT [8,9,11]. Furthermore, recent prospective studies indicate that the use of serial objective testing for proximal-vein thrombosis is an effective and practical alternative to pulmonary angiography in patients with nondiagnostic lung scans who have adequate cardiorespiratory reserve [63,64].

Table 45-3. Features of ideal prophylactic method

Effective compared with placebo or active approaches
Safe
Good compliance with patient, nurses, and physicians
Ease of administration
No need for laboratory monitoring
Cost effective

Prevention of Venous Thromboembolism

In the absence of prophylaxis, the frequency of fatal pulmonary embolism ranges from 0.1–0.8 percent in patients undergoing elective general surgery [65–67], 2–3 percent in patients undergoing elective hip replacement [68], and 4–7 percent in patients undergoing surgery for fractured hip [69]. It is surprising that physicians and surgeons still do not comply with recommendations for prophylaxis of venous thromboembolism despite the fact that there is convincing evidence for the efficacy and safety of a number of agents [5–7,69,70,71]. In a recent retrospective audit of hospitals in Massachusetts, it was shown that prophylaxis of venous thromboembolism even in high-risk patients was grossly underutilized, particularly in nonteaching hospitals [72]. In orthopedic surgery, as was shown in surveys conducted in England and Sweden, some form of prophylaxis, usually in the form of drugs, is used in the majority of cases [73,74].

Two approaches can be taken to prevent fatal pulmonary embolism: (1) secondary prevention by the early detection and treatment of subclinical venous thrombosis by screening postoperative patients with objective tests that are sensitive for venous thrombosis and (2) primary prophylaxis, using either drugs or physical methods that are effective for preventing DVT. The latter approach of primary prophylaxis is preferred in most clinical circumstances. Furthermore, prevention of DVT and pulmonary embolism are more cost effective than treating the complications when they occur [75–79]. Secondary prevention by case-finding studies should never replace primary prophylaxis. It is reserved for patients in whom primary prophylaxis is either contraindicated or relatively ineffective.

The ideal primary prophylactic method is described in Table 45-3. The recommended primary prophylactic approach depends on the patient's risk category (Table 45-4) and the type of surgery. The prophylactic measures most commonly used are low-dose or adjusted-dose unfractionated heparin, low-molecular-weight heparin, oral anticoagulants (International Normalized Ratio, or INR,

Table 45-4. Risk of venous thromboembolism, as assessed by objective tests

Risk category	Calf-vein thrombosis	Proximal-vein thrombosis	Fatal pulmonary embolism
High risk	40–80%	10–30%	1–5%
Major orthopedic surgery of lower limbs			
General and urological surgery in patients over 40 years with recent history of DVT or pulmonary embolism			
Extensive pelvic or abdominal surgery for malignant disease			
Moderate risk	10–40%	2–10%	0.1–0.8%
General surgery in patients over 40 years lasting 30 minutes or more and in patients below 40 years on oral contraceptives			
Low risk	< 10%	< 1%	< 0.01%
Minor surgery (i.e., less than 30 minutes) in patients over 40 years without additional risk factors			
Uncomplicated surgery in patients under 40 years without additional risk factors			

Source: Reproduced with permission from AN Nicolaides et al. Prevention of venous thromboembolism. Int Angiol 1992; 11(3):151.

2.0–3.0), and intermittent pneumatic leg compression. Other less commonly used measures include aspirin and intravenous dextran.

Ideally, prophylaxis should be started before the operation and continued until the patient is fully ambulatory. No data are available to allow specific recommendations for continued prophylaxis in patients discharged from hospital.

SPECIFIC PROPHYLACTIC MEASURES

Low-Dose Heparin. Low-dosage subcutaneous heparin usually is given in a dose of 5,000 units 2 hours preoperatively and then postoperatively every 8 or 12 hours. The effectiveness of low-dosage heparin for preventing DVT has been established by multiple randomized clinical trials. Most of the patients in those trials underwent abdominothoracic surgery particularly for gastrointestinal disease, but also included were gynecologic and urologic surgery as well as some patients having mastectomy or vascular procedures. Pooled data from meta-analyses confirm that low-dosage heparin reduces the incidence of all DVT, proximal DVT, and all pulmonary emboli, including fatal pulmonary emboli [5–7,67,70]. The International Multicentre Trial also established the effectiveness of low-dosage heparin for preventing fatal pulmonary embolism, a clinically striking reduction from 0.7 percent to 0.1 percent [67].

Although individual clinical trials reported failure of low-dosage heparin to prevent thrombosis following total hip replacement surgery, one meta-analysis demonstrated a 68-percent risk reduction with no increased risk of bleeding [6]. That risk reduction is similar to the one seen with low-molecular-weight heparin, although low-molecular-weight heparin has been shown to be superior to low-dosage heparin in individual trials. The incidence of major bleeding complications is not increased by low-dosage heparin, but there is an increase in wound hematomas. The platelet count should be monitored regularly in all patients on low-dosage heparin to detect the rare but significant development of heparin-induced thrombocytopenia.

Low-dosage heparin has the advantages of being relatively inexpensive and easily administered, and it does not require anticoagulant monitoring.

Adjusted-Dosage Heparin. Adjusted-dosage subcutaneous heparin was shown to be an effective approach for prophylaxis when compared with low-dosage heparin in patients undergoing total hip replacement [80]. Adjusted-dosage heparin therapy decreased the incidence of DVT significantly (13% versus 39%) without any increase in the frequency of bleeding complications. In a more recent study by the same group, adjusted-dosage heparin was compared with low-molecular-weight heparin [81]. The decrease in the incidence of DVT was not as striking (16%), and there was a surprisingly high incidence of proximal-vein thrombosis (13%). Adjusted-dosage heparin has not become popular because of the time and expense required for laboratory monitoring.

Low-Molecular-Weight Heparin. Several low-molecular-weight (LMW) heparin fractions have been evaluated by randomized clinical trials in moderate-risk general surgical patients [82–89]. The heparin fractions that have been evaluated include fragmin, fraxiparine, enoxaparin, and logiparin. In randomized clinical trials comparing LMW heparin with unfractionated heparin, the LMW heparins given once or twice daily have been shown to be as effective or more effective in preventing thrombosis [82–89]. Most of the trials documented similarly low frequencies of bleeding for LMW heparin and low-dosage unfractionated heparin, although the incidence of bleeding was somewhat higher with unfractionated heparin when various bleeding endpoints were combined [82].

In the past 5 years, there have been several large randomized clinical trials in patients undergoing total joint replacements (hip ± knees) [90–102]. Different LMW heparins have been compared with either placebo, unfractionated heparin, adjusted-dosage heparin, dextran 40, or warfarin sodium. Compared with placebo, LMW heparin significantly decreased the rates of both distal and proximal DVT with no significant increase in bleeding rates [91,96,99,102]. LMW heparins were at least as effective as low-dosage unfractionated heparin given two to three times daily [92–94]. Bleeding rates were comparable in the unfractionated heparin and LMW heparin groups with the exception of one study [93] that used unfractionated heparin, 7,500 units twice daily. Studies comparing LMW heparin with dextran 70 showed a significant improvement in thrombosis rates for LMW heparin (6.5, 13% versus 21.6, 35%) with no significant differences in bleeding rates [97].

Two large multicenter studies compared the use of LMW heparin twice [100] or once [101] daily with warfarin sodium both started postoperatively in the prevention of DVT following total hip or total knee replacement. For patients undergoing hip replacement, both studies showed that LMW heparin was as effective as warfarin, but for those undergoing total knee replacements, LMW heparin was superior. When the data for patients undergoing hip or knee replacements were pooled, LMW heparin was statistically superior to warfarin. The incidence of major and minor bleeding and wound hematomas was higher in the LMW heparin group [101].

The LMW heparinoid ORG-10172 (lomoparin) effectively reduced the rates of DVT following total hip replacement when compared with placebo (15.5% versus 56.6%) [102]. It was evaluated in two clinical trials involving patients with hip fracture [103,104]. The DVT rates were significantly lower when compared with intravenous dextran [103] (13% versus 35%) and with low-intensity warfarin [104] (7% versus 21%). More blood transfusions were required in the dextran group [103].

In recent meta-analyses, LMW heparin has been shown to be more effective than unfractionated heparin in the prevention of venous thrombosis but with a slightly higher risk of bleeding [105]. The LMW heparins have the advantage that they can be given once a day at a constant dosage without any laboratory monitoring. Studies comparing the cost effectiveness of LMW heparin and either warfarin or unfractionated heparin currently are underway.

Oral Anticoagulants. Prophylaxis with oral anticoagulants can be commenced preoperatively, at the time of operation, or in the early postoperative period. Oral anticoagulants commenced at the time of surgery or early postoperatively may not prevent small venous thrombi that form during surgery or soon after surgery because the anticoagulant effect is not achieved until the third or fourth postoperative day. However, prophylaxis with oral anticoagulants is effective in inhibiting the extension of those thrombi and thereby preventing clinically important venous thromboembolism.

Warfarin started postoperatively has been compared with LMW heparin [100,101] or intermittent pneumatic compression with little or no difference in the incidence of postoperative venous thrombosis or bleeding [106–108]. Initiation of warfarin in small doses 7–10 days preoperatively to prolong the prothrombin time 1.5–3.0 seconds followed by less intense warfarin started the night of surgery yielded results similar to warfarin started postoperatively [106].

In patients suffering hip fractures, warfarin was compared with aspirin and placebo with the following rates of DVT: warfarin 20 percent, aspirin 40.9 percent, placebo 46 percent [109].

Very-low-dosage oral anticoagulants (warfarin 1 mg/day) when compared with placebo was shown to decrease postoperative thrombosis rate in patients undergoing gynecologic surgery or major general surgery [110] and to decrease the thrombosis rate in indwelling central line catheters [111]. There was no increase in bleeding rates. Very-low-dosage warfarin did not, however, provide protection against DVT following hip or knee replacement [112].

Intermittent Leg Compression. Intermittent pneumatic leg compression prevents venous thrombosis by enhancing blood flow in the deep veins of the legs, thereby preventing venous stasis. It also increases blood fibrinolytic activity, which may contribute to its antithrombotic properties. Intermittent pneumatic leg compression is effective for preventing venous thrombosis in moderate-risk general surgical patients [113] and in patients undergoing neurosurgery [114–116]. In patients undergoing hip surgery, intermittent pneumatic compression of the calf is effective for preventing calf-vein thrombosis, but it is relatively ineffective against proximal-vein thrombosis [117]. Sequential compression using calf and thigh cuffs produces greater acceleration of femoral venous blood flow than compression of the calf alone. Recent clinical trials indicate that sequential calf and thigh compression is effective for preventing venous thrombosis in patients undergoing elective total hip replacement, but the incidence of proximal venous thrombosis remains moderately high [106,117].

Intermittent pneumatic compression of the calf decreased distal venous thrombosis following knee replacement, but proximal thrombosis rates remained high [118]. Studies with calf and thigh compression significantly decreased the incidence of both distal and proximal thrombosis rates (6%, 10%, and 22%) [119].

Intermittent pneumatic leg compression is virtually free of clinically important side effects and offers a valuable alternative in patients who have a high risk of bleeding. It may produce discomfort in the occasional patient and should not be used in patients with overt evidence of leg ischemia caused by peripheral vascular disease. A variety of well-accepted, comfortable, and effective intermittent pneumatic devices are currently available that may be applied preoperatively, at the time of operation, or in the early postoperative period. Intermittent pneumatic compression should be continued for the entire period until the patient is fully ambulatory.

Graduated Compression Stockings. Graduated compression stockings reduce venous stasis in the limb by applying a graded degree of compression to the ankle and the calf, with greater pressure being applied more distally in the limb. Clinical trials have demonstrated graduated compression stockings to be effective for preventing postoperative venous thrombosis in low-risk general surgical patients [120–122] and in selected moderate-risk patients (neurosurgical) [114,116]. A recent meta-analysis confirmed the reduction of venous thrombosis following moderate-risk surgery with the use of graduated compression stockings [123]. However, there was inadequate information to verify whether the use of graduated compression stockings in combination with other forms of prophylaxis resulted in any further risk reduction [123]. The use of graduated compression stockings along with other prophylactic measures in patients undergoing high-risk surgery has not been adequately studied.

Other Agents. Although aspirin decreases the percent-odds reduction of venous thrombosis following general or orthopedic surgery, that reduction is significantly less than that seen with other agents. Aspirin, therefore, cannot be recommended for the prevention of venous thrombosis in high-risk patients [124]. Also, although intravenous dextran has been shown to be effective in the prevention of venous thrombosis following major orthopedic surgery, it is cumbersome, expensive, and associated with significant side effects and thus has been replaced by other agents.

SPECIFIC RECOMMENDATIONS

Low Risk Patients. Low risk patients may receive prophylaxis in certain circumstances [5,70,125]. It is clinical custom in some countries to use graduated compression stockings.

Moderate-Risk Patients

GENERAL ABDOMINAL, THORACIC, OR GYNECOLOGIC SURGERY. In all moderate-risk patients, the use of subcutaneous low-dosage heparin (5,000 units every 8 or 12 hours) or subcutaneous LMW heparin is recommended [5,70,125]. Subcutaneous LMW heparin is as effective as subcutaneous heparin prophylaxis and has the advantage of once-per-day injection. An alternative recommendation may be intermittent pneumatic compression used continuously until the patient is ambulatory. That method is indicated in patients with a high risk of bleeding. In some countries, it is routine clinical custom to combine pharmacologic methods with graduated compression stockings in selected patients.

NEUROSURGERY. Neurosurgery patients should receive intermittent pneumatic compression. In some countries, that approach is used in conjunction with graduated compression stockings [5,70,125].

HIGH-RISK PATIENTS. The optimal approach for high-risk patients remains uncertain because all approaches have not been directly compared in this patient category. The recommended approaches include oral anticoagulants, LMW heparin [5,70], intermittent pneumatic compression, subcutaneous low-dosage heparin using the every-8-hours regimen, adjusted-dosage subcutaneous heparin, or intravenous dextran. Primary prophylaxis also could be supplemented by postoperative screening to detect patients who break through prophylaxis.

ELECTIVE HIP REPLACEMENT. Several approaches have been evaluated and are effective. Prophylaxis with oral anticoagulants adjusted to maintain an INR of 2.0 to 3.0 is effective and is associated with a low risk of bleeding [5]. Subcutaneous LMW heparin given once or twice daily is effective and safe. Several such agents are approved for use in Europe, and one is available in North America [5,70,93]. Other effective approaches include adjusted-dosage subcutaneous heparin, intravenous dextran, and intravenous dextran combined with intermittent pneumatic leg compression [5].

FRACTURED HIP. Oral anticoagulant prophylaxis (INR 2.0 to 3.0) is the preferred approach [5]. Intravenous dextran is effective, but it is also inconvenient and relatively expensive.

MAJOR KNEE SURGERY. Intermittent pneumatic compression is the preferred approach [5].

Other Conditions

PREGNANCY. Subcutaneous low-dosage heparin is the prophylaxis of choice for pregnant patients at high risk of DVT and pulmonary embolism, although data of efficacy from controlled trials are lacking [70]. The benefits of prophylaxis are uncertain in patients undergoing cesarean section who have no additional risk factors [70]. Oral anticoagulants are contraindicated throughout pregnancy.

Medical Patients. Medical patients should be classified as low, moderate, or high risk for suffering venous thromboembolism. Low-risk patients should be considered for graduated pressure stockings. Moderate-risk patients should receive either subcutaneous low-dosage heparin, subcutaneous LMW heparin, or intermittent pneumatic leg compression (if at high risk of bleeding). High-risk patients should receive adjusted oral anticoagulants (INR 2.0 to 3.0) or subcutaneous LMW heparin [5,70].

Treatment of Venous Thrombosis

The classic anticoagulant therapy of venous thromboembolism (DVT, pulmonary embolism, or both) is a combination of continuous intravenous heparin and oral warfarin sodium [126,127]. The use of heparin and warfarin simultaneously has become clinical practice for all patients with venous thromboembolism who are medically stable [128,129]. Exceptions include patients who require immediate medical or surgical intervention, such as thrombolysis or insertion of a vena cava filter, patients in the intensive care unit with multiple invasive lines, and patients with conditions that predispose them to major bleeding. The length of the initial intravenous heparin therapy has been reduced to 5 days, thus shortening the hospital stay and leading to significant cost saving [128,129].

HEPARIN THERAPY

The anticoagulant activity of unfractionated heparin depends on a unique pentasaccharide that binds to antithrombin III (ATIII) and potentiates the inhibition of thrombin and activated factor X (X_a) by ATIII [130–133]. In addition, heparin catalyses the inactivation of thrombin by another plasma cofactor, heparin cofactor II, which acts independently of ATIII [134]. Heparin has a number of other effects, including the release of tissue-factor inhibitor; the binding to numerous plasma and platelet proteins, endothelial cells, and leukocytes; and increasing vascular permeability [135,136]. The last effect may explain some of the nonanticoagulant effects as well as the hemorrhagic effects of heparin and the variability in the action of heparin among individuals. It also may help explain why relative heparin resistance develops in some individuals [135]. The basic biochemistry, pharmacology, and pharmacokinetics of heparin recently have been reviewed [135]. The anticoagulant response to a standard dose of heparin varies widely among patients, making it necessary to monitor the anticoagulant response of heparin with either the activated partial thromboplastin time (APTT) or heparin levels and to titrate the dose to the individual patient [135,136].

APTT is the laboratory test most commonly used to monitor heparin therapy. A traditional and widely used approach has been to adjust the heparin infusion dosage to maintain the results of the APTT in a defined therapeutic range. Over the years, that therapeutic range has evolved, based on clinical custom, to the use of an upper and lower limit (an APTT ratio of 1.5 to 2.5 times control). The clinical practice of adjusting the heparin dose to maintain the APTT response in that range is based on two concepts: (1) Maintaining the APTT ratio above the lower limit of 1.5 will minimize recurrent venous thromboembolic events, and (2) maintaining the APTT ratio below the upper limit of 2.5 will minimize the risk of bleeding complications [137,138].

It has been established from experimental studies and clinical trials that the efficacy of heparin therapy is dependent on a critical therapeutic level of heparin being achieved within the first 24 hours of treatment. The critical therapeutic level of heparin as measured by the APTT is 1.5 times the mean of the control value or a heparin blood level of 0.2 to 0.4 units/ml by the protamine sulfate titration assay [139]. There is, however, wide variability in the APTT and heparin blood levels with different reagents and even with different batches of the same reagent. It is vital, therefore, for each laboratory to establish the minimal therapeutic level of heparin as measured by the APTT that will provide a heparin blood level of at least 0.2 units/mL by the protamine titration assay for each batch of thromboplastin reagent being used, particularly if the reagent is provided by a different manufacturer [139].

The observed variability in the APTT response to different heparin blood levels supports the need for an aggressive approach to heparin therapy to ensure that all patients achieve adequate therapy early in the course of their treatment. The use of LMW heparin eliminates that problem because laboratory monitoring is not required. However, until such agents are approved for use, the problem of APTT standardization will remain.

Data from three randomized clinical trials [138,140,141] provide firm support for the use of an APTT ratio of 1.5 as the lower limit of the therapeutic range. The first randomized trial evaluated the clinical outcomes in patients with proximal-vein thrombosis who were treated with either continuous intravenous heparin or intermittent subcutaneous heparin adjusted to prolong the APTT greater than 1.5 times the control [138]. The subcutaneous regimen resulted in an initial anticoagulant response below the lower limit in the majority (63%) of patients and a high frequency of recurrent venous thromboembolism (11 of 57 patients, or 19.3%), which was virtually confined to patients with a subtherapeutic anticoagulant response [138]. In contrast, continuous intravenous heparin resulted in an adequate anticoagulant response in the majority (71%) of patients and a low frequency of recurrent thromboembolic events (3 of 58 patients, or 5.2%); the recurrences in that group also were limited to patients with an initial subtherapeutic anticoagulant response [138]. Thus, 13 of 53 patients (24.5%) with an APTT response below the lower limit for 24 hours or more had recurrent venous thromboembolism, compared with only 1 of 62 patients (1.6%) in whom an APTT ratio of 1.5 or more was achieved ($p < 0.001$), a relative risk for recurrent venous thromboembolism of 15:1. Similar results were found when a weight-based heparin-dosaging nomogram (starting dose 90 units/kg bolus and 18 units/kg/hour infusion) was compared with a standard-care nomogram (starting dose 5,000-unit bolus and 1,000 units/hour infusion) [141]. Using the weight-based nomogram, 60 of 62 patients (97%) exceeded the therapeutic threshold within 24 hours, compared with 37 of 48 (77%) patients in the standard-care group ($p < 0.002$). Recurrent thromboembolism in the 3-month treatment period was more frequent in the standard-care group: relative risk 5.0 (95% confidence interval [CI] 1.1–21.9) [141].

The above findings are strongly supported by a recent randomized trial that compared intravenous heparin with oral anticoagulants alone for the initial treatment of patients with proximal-vein thrombosis [140]. The latter treatment group, by the nature of the treatment, have an inadequate APTT response for at least the first 48 hours, because the onset of the anticoagulant effect of oral anticoagulants is delayed. Recurrent venous thromboembolism occurred in 12 of 60 patients (20%) treated with oral anticoagulants alone over the subsequent 3 months, compared with 4 of 60 patients (6.7%) who received initial intravenous heparin plus oral anticoagulants ($p = 0.058$) [140]. In all those trials, recurrent thromboembolism typically occurred between 3 and 12 weeks. Thus, it may not be recognized that the recurrent clinical events relate to failure of initial therapy.

A recent randomized trial (level I) provides important new information about the upper limit of the therapeutic range for the APTT [137]. That study evaluated the clinical outcomes in patients with proximal-vein thrombosis who were randomized to receive initial treatment with either intravenous heparin alone or intravenous heparin with simultaneous warfarin sodium. Both regimens achieved adequate therapy in almost all patients, but the combined heparin and warfarin group received more intensive anticoagulation, with the majority of patients exceeding the predefined upper limit (APTT ratio 2.5) for sustained periods of time [137]. This was shown by the finding that 69 of 99 patients (69%) in the combined group had a supertherapeutic APTT value (ratio 2.5 or more) persisting for 24 hours or more, compared with 24 of 100 patients

(24%) receiving heparin alone ($p < 0.001$). Despite the more intense therapy in the combined group, bleeding complications occurred with similar frequency in the two groups: Nine of 99 patients in the combined group (9.1%) had bleeding complications, compared with 12 of 100 patients (12.0%) in the group given heparin alone [137]. An important result is that bleeding complications occurred in 8 of 93 patients (8.6%) with supertherapeutic APTT, compared with 13 of 106 patients (12.3%) without supertherapeutic APTT (relative risk 0.7, $p = 0.49$). Major bleeding occurred in 3 of 93 patients (3.2%) with supertherapeutic APTT, compared with 10 of 106 patients (9.4%) without supertherapeutic APTT (relative risk 0.3, $p = 0.09$) [137].

The above findings refute the finding of retrospective reviews [142] that suggest an association between a supertherapeutic APTT result (ratio 2.5 or more) and the risk of clinically important bleeding complications. The incidence of major bleeding correlated with the clinical risk of bleeding. Patients considered at low risk for bleeding and who received the higher heparin dosage had a low frequency of major bleeding (1%), whereas those considered at high risk of bleeding who received a lower dosage of heparin had a higher frequency of major bleeding (11%) ($p = 0.007$) [137].

Audits of heparin therapy suggest that administration of intravenous heparin is fraught with difficulty [143–146] and that the clinical practice of using an ad-hoc or intuitive approach to heparin dose-titration frequently results in inadequate therapy. For example, an audit of physician practices at three university-affiliated hospitals [145] documented that 60 percent of patients failed to achieve an adequate APTT response (ratio 1.5) during the initial 24 hours of therapy and, further, that 30 to 40 percent of patients remained subtherapeutic over the next 3 to 4 days. Several practices were identified that led to inadequate therapy. The common theme that explains those practices is clinicians' exaggerated fear of bleeding complications. Consequently, it has been common practice for many clinicians to start treatment with a low heparin dosage and to increase that dosage cautiously over several days to achieve the therapeutic range. The clinical trial data indicate that such practice is inappropriate and, indeed, dangerous because it places the patient at an unacceptably high risk for recurrent venous thromboembolism [138] and may induce the development of heparin resistance [147].

The use of a prescriptive approach or protocol for administering intravenous heparin therapy has been evaluated in two studies of patients with venous thromboembolism [137,141]. In a randomized clinical trial, patients were given either intravenous heparin alone followed by warfarin sodium or intravenous heparin and simultaneous warfarin in the treatment of proximal venous thrombosis [137]. The heparin nomogram we evaluated is summarized in Tables 45-5 and 45-6.

Only 2 percent and 1 percent of the patients were subtherapeutic for more than 24 hours in the heparin and warfarin group and in the heparin group, respectively [137]. Recurrent venous thromboembolism (objectively documented) occurred infrequently in both groups (7%) [137],

Table 45-5. Heparin protocol

1. Initial intravenous heparin bolus: 5,000 units.
2. Continuous intravenous heparin infusion: Commence at 42 ml/hour of 20,000 units (1,680 units/hour) in 500 ml of two-thirds dextrose and one-third saline (a 24-hour heparin dose of 40,320 units), except in the following patients, in whom heparin infusion will be commenced at a rate of 31 ml/hour (1,240 units/hour) (i.e., a 24-hour dose of 29,760 units):
   a. Patients who have undergone surgery within previous 2 weeks.
   b. Patients with a previous history of peptic ulcer disease or gastrointestinal or genitourinary bleeding.
   c. Patients with recent stroke (i.e., thrombotic stroke within previous 2 weeks).
   d. Patients with a platelet count $< 150 \times 10^9$/liter.
   e. Patients with miscellaneous reasons for a high risk of bleeding (e.g., hepatic failure, renal failure, or vitamin K deficiency).
3. Heparin dosage adjusted using the APTT. The APTT is performed in all patients as outlined below:
   a. 4–6 hours after commencing heparin; the heparin dose is then adjusted according to the nomogram shown below.
   b. 4–6 hours after implementing the first dosage adjustment.
   c. The APTT is then performed as indicated by the nomogram for the first 24 hours of therapy.
   d. Thereafter, the APTT will be performed once daily, unless the patient is subtherapeutic, in which case the APTT will be repeated 4–6 hours after increasing the heparin dose.

Source: Reproduced with permission from RD Hull et al. Optimal therapeutic level of heparin therapy in patients with venous thrombosis. Arch Int Med 1992; 152:1589.

rates similar to those previously reported [21,31,32]. Those findings demonstrated that subtherapy was avoided in most patients and that the heparin protocol resulted in effective delivery of heparin therapy in both groups. Further, because of the influence of warfarin on the APTT response, patients in the combined treatment group received less heparin per 24 hours than those in the group given heparin alone without an adverse outcome [34].

The frequencies of bleeding were 9 percent in the group treated with heparin and warfarin simultaneously and 12 percent in the group that received heparin alone [137]. Again, those frequencies are similar to previously reported rates of bleeding. The same heparin nomogram also was used in a randomized clinical trial comparing the use of fixed-dosage subcutaneous LMW heparin with continuous intravenous heparin in the initial treatment of proximal venous thrombosis [148]. Warfarin was started on day 2 in all patients. Use of the heparin nomogram in the 15 different treatment centers ensured that the vast majority of patients were within the therapeutic range within 24 hours. A review of the findings from one of the treatment centers indicated that 91 percent of patients were within the therapeutic range (APTT $> 1.5 \times$ control) within 24 hours, compared with 60 percent of the patients who were treated without the use of a heparin protocol [146].

Table 45-6. Intravenous heparin dosage-titration nomogram for APTT

IV INFUSION			
APTT	Rate change, ml/hour	Dose change, U/24 hour[a]	Additional action
≤ 45	+6	+5760	Repeated APTT[b] in 4–6 hours
46–54	+3	+2880	Repeated APTT in 4–6 hours
55–85	0	0	None[c]
86–110	−3	−2880	Stop heparin sodium treatment for 1 hour; repeated APTT 4–6 hours after restarting heparin treatment
> 110	−6	−5760	Stop heparin treatment for 1 hour; repeated APTT 4–6 hours after restarting heparin treatment

[a]Heparin sodium concentration 20,000 U in 500 ml = 40 U/ml.
[b]With the use of Actin-FS thromboplastin reagent (Dade, Mississauga, Ontario).
[c]During the first 24 hours, repeated APTT in 4 to 6 hours. Thereafter, the APTT will be determined once daily, unless subtherapeutic.
Source: Reproduced with permission from RD Hull et al. Optimal therapeutic level of heparin therapy in patients with venous thrombosis. Arch Int Med 1992; 152:1589.

In another randomized clinical trial, a weight-based heparin-dosaging nomogram was compared with a standard-care nomogram [141], as shown in Table 45-7. Patients treated according to the weight-adjusted heparin nomogram received a starting dose of 80 units/kg as a bolus and 18 units/kg/hour as an infusion. Patients on the standard-care nomogram received a bolus of 5,000 units followed by 1,000 units/hour by infusion. Heparin dosage was suggested to maintain an APTT of 1.5–2.3 times control. The primary outcomes were (1) the time to exceed the therapeutic threshold of an APTT greater than 1.5 times control and (2) the time to achieve the therapeutic range (APTT of 1.5–2.3 × control). Ninety-seven percent of patients in the weight-based heparin group exceeded the therapeutic threshold within 24 hours, compared with 77 percent in the standard-care group ($p = 0.082$) [141]. In the weight-adjusted group, 89 percent of patients achieved the therapeutic range within 24 hours, compared with 75 percent in the standard-care group [141]. The risk of recurrent thromboembolism was more frequent in the standard-care group. The study included patients with unstable angina and arterial thromboembolism in addition to venous thromboembolism, indicating that it may be possible to generalize the principles applied through a heparin nomogram for the treatment of venous thromboembolism to other clinical conditions.

Table 45-7. Weight-based nomogram

Initial dose	80 u/kg bolus, then 18 U/kg/hour
APTT < 35 seconds (< 1.2 × control)	80 u/kg bolus, then 4 U/kg/hour
APTT, 35–45 seconds (1.2–1.5 × control)	40 u/kg bolus, then 2 U/kg/hour
APTT, 46–70 seconds (1.5–2.3 × control)	No change
APTT, 71–90 seconds (2.3–3.0 × control)	Decrease infusion rate by 2 U/kg/hour
APTT > 90 seconds (> 3.0 × control)	Hold infusion 1 hour, then decrease infusion rate by 3 U/kg/hour

Source: Reproduced with permission from RA Raschke et al. The weight-based heparin dosing nomogram compared with a "standard care" nomogram. Ann Intern Med 1993; 119:874–881.

ORAL ANTICOAGULANT THERAPY

There are two distinct chemical groups of oral anticoagulants: the 4-hydroxy coumarin derivatives (e.g., warfarin sodium) and the indane-1, 3-dione derivatives (e.g., phenindione) [149]. The coumarin derivatives are the oral anticoagulants of choice because they are associated with fewer nonhemorrhagic side effects than are the indanedione derivatives.

Warfarin produces an anticoagulant effect by inhibiting the vitamin K–dependent gamma-carboxylation of coagulation factors II, VII, IX, and X [149–151], resulting in the synthesis of immunologically detectable but biologically inactive forms of those coagulation proteins. Warfarin also inhibits the vitamin K–dependent gamma-carboxylation of proteins C and S [152]. Protein C circulates as a proenzyme that is activated on endothelial cells by the thrombin-thrombomodulin complex to form activated protein C. Activated protein C inhibits activated factor VIII activity directly and, in the presence of protein S, also inhibits activated factor V [153]. Therefore, vitamin K antagonists such as warfarin create a biochemical paradox by producing an anticoagulant effect due to the inhibition of procoagulants (factors II, VII, IX, X) and a potentially thrombogenic effect by impairing the synthesis of naturally occurring inhibitors of coagulation (proteins C and S) [152]. Thus, heparin and warfarin treatment should be overlapped by 4 to 5 days when switching from heparin to warfarin treatment in patients with thrombotic disease [151].

The anticoagulant effect of the vitamin K antagonists is delayed until the normal clotting factors are cleared from the circulation, and the peak effect does not occur until 36 to 72 hours after drug administration [153]. During the first few days of warfarin therapy, the prothrombin time reflects primarily the depression of factor VII, which has a half-life of 5–7 hours. Equilibrium nadir levels of factors II, IX, and X are not reached until about 1 week after the initiation of therapy. The use of small initial daily doses (e.g., 10 mg) is the preferred approach for initiating warfarin treatment. The dosage-response relationship to warfarin therapy varies widely among individuals; therefore, the dosage must be carefully monitored to prevent overdosing or underdosing. There is some evidence that elderly subjects are more sensitive to the effects of warfarin, and greater caution is required in establishing maintenance dosages to prevent overanticoagulation of those patients [154].

A number of drugs interact with warfarin. Critical appraisal of the literature reporting such interactions indicates that the evidence substantiating many of the claims is limited [155]. Nonetheless, patients must be warned against taking any new drugs without the knowledge of their attending physician.

LABORATORY MONITORING AND THERAPEUTIC RANGE

The laboratory test most commonly used to measure the effects of warfarin is the one-stage prothrombin time, which is sensitive to reduced activity of factors II, VII, and X but insensitive to reduced activity of factor IX. Confusion about the appropriate therapeutic range has occurred because the different tissue thromboplastins used for measuring the prothrombin time vary considerably in sensitivity to the vitamin K–dependent clotting factors and in response to warfarin [151]. Rabbit-brain thromboplastin, which is widely used in North America, is less sensitive than standardized human-brain thromboplastin, which has been widely used in the United Kingdom and other parts of Europe. A prothrombin time ratio of 1.5 to 2.0 using rabbit-brain thromboplastin (i.e., the traditional therapeutic range in North America) is equivalent to a ratio of 4.0 to 6.0 using human-brain thromboplastin [27,36]. Conversely, a two- to threefold increase in the prothrombin time using standardized human-brain thromboplastin is equivalent to a 1.25- to 1.5-fold increase in the prothrombin time using a rabbit-brain thromboplastin such as Simplastin or Dade-C [151,156].

The optimal therapeutic range for warfarin therapy in patients with venous thrombosis has recently been established [151,156]. The findings of randomized trials indicate that venous thrombosis can be treated effectively and more safely with a therapeutic range of 1.25 to 1.5 times control using a rabbit-brain thromboplastin such as Simplastin or Dade-C, rather than the range of 1.5 to 2.0 times control conventionally recommended in North America [151,156].

To promote standardization of the prothrombin time for monitoring oral anticoagulant therapy, the World Health Organization (WHO) has developed an international reference thromboplastin from human brain tissue and has recommended that the prothrombin time ratio be expressed as the International Normalized Ratio (INR) [151]: the INR is the prothrombin time ratio obtained by testing a given sample using the WHO reference thromboplastin. For practical clinical purposes, the INR for a given plasma sample is equivalent to the prothrombin time ratio obtained using a standardized human-brain thromboplastin known as the Manchester Comparative Reagent, which has been widely used in the United Kingdom. The currently recommended therapeutic range of 1.25 to 1.5 times control using a rabbit-brain thromboplastin such as Simplastin or Dade-C corresponds to an INR of 2.0 to 3.0 [151].

In a survey of 53 hospital laboratories, only 21 percent reported prothrombin times as INR results, and 30 percent of hospitals could not provide data on the ISI (International Sensitivity Index) of the thromboplastin being used [157]. In a survey of 860 laboratories in Canada in 1992, 50.9 percent reported INR alone or with the prothrombin time ratio [158]. Only 42 percent of physicians requested INR results for anticoagulant control. Similar results were shown in a survey of laboratories in Utah [159]. Those studies indicate that the current recommendations regarding ISI and INR are being disregarded by many laboratories and that anticoagulant monitoring will, therefore, be substandard.

Warfarin is administered in an initial dosage of 10 mg/day for the first 2 days, and the daily dosage is then adjusted according to the INR. Heparin therapy is discontinued on the fourth or fifth day following initiation of warfarin therapy, provided the INR is prolonged into the therapeutic range (INR 2.0 to 3.0) [151]. The selection of the correct dosage of warfarin must be individualized, because some individuals are either fast or slow metabolizers of the drug. Therefore, frequent INR determinations are required initially to establish therapeutic anticoagulation.

Once the anticoagulant effect and the patient's warfarin dosage requirements are stable, the INR is monitored weekly throughout the course of warfarin therapy. However, if there are factors that may produce an unpredictable response to warfarin (e.g., concomitant drug therapy) [155], the INR should be monitored more frequently to minimize the risk of complications from poor anticoagulant control.

Attempts have been made to improve the control of warfarin while at the same time decreasing the risk of bleeding complications, including the use of warfarin protocols to predict dosaging requirements [160] and the use of a prothrombin home monitor device [161]. An alternative to the measurement of the INR is the use of an immunoassay to detect native prothrombin antigen [162].

LONG-TERM TREATMENT OF VENOUS THROMBOEMBOLISM

Clinical trial findings indicate that patients with established venous thrombosis or pulmonary embolism require long-term anticoagulant therapy to prevent recurrent thromboembolism [118]. Warfarin therapy is highly effective and is preferred in most patients. In patients with proximal-vein thrombosis (popliteal-, femoral-, or iliac-vein thrombosis), long-term therapy with warfarin reduces the frequency of objectively documented recurrent venous thromboembolism from 47 percent to 2 percent [118]. The less intense warfarin regimen (INR 2.0 to 3.0) markedly reduces the risk of bleeding (from 20% to 4%) without loss of effectiveness [156].

Long-term warfarin therapy is continued for 3 months in patients with a first episode of proximal venous thrombosis or pulmonary embolism. In the past, attempts were made to decrease the treatment period with warfarin in an attempt to decrease bleeding risks (approximately 20% with higher-intensity warfarin treatment, i.e., INR 3.0 to 4.5) [163–167]. Limited evidence from either the randomized clinical trials or the retrospective studies indicated that treatment with warfarin for 12 weeks was superior to treatment for 4 or 6 weeks, but all those studies had significant limitations. In the British Thoracic Society study that evaluated the optimal duration of less intense warfarin therapy for venous thromboembolism, patients were randomized to receive either 4 or 12 weeks of treatment [167]. There was a higher recurrence rate of venous thromboembolism in patients treated for 4 weeks (7.8%) as opposed to 12 weeks (4.0%) during an unspecified follow-up period. A post-hoc analysis suggested that patients being treated for postoperative venous thromboembolism had a low rate of recurrence regardless of the duration of warfarin therapy, whereas the recurrence rate of venous thromboembolism in medical patients was higher, particularly for those receiving only 4 weeks of treatment [167]. For the present, it is recommended that all patients with the first episode of venous thrombosis receive warfarin therapy for 12 weeks. If the findings of the above-mentioned studies are confirmed, it may be possible to shorten the length of therapy for patients with postoperative venous thrombosis to 4 weeks.

The recurrence rate following a 3-month period of treatment with less-intense warfarin for first-episode venous thromboembolism is 4–7 percent [138,156]. However, the long-term prognosis of patients treated for a first episode of venous thrombosis was shown to be poor, with a cumulative 3-year mortality rate of 30 percent in an audit of 16 short-stay hospitals in Massachusetts [3]. Also, in a prospective follow-up study of consecutive patients treated for 3 months with oral anticoagulants for first-episode DVT, the recurrence rate of venous thromboembolism was high (24% over 80 weeks) for patients with idiopathic venous thrombosis, compared with patients with a known risk factor such as surgery (4.8%) [168]. Therefore, although treatment with warfarin for 3 months may be adequate for most patients with first-episode DVT, there may be other patients, such as those with idiopathic venous thrombosis, who would benefit from a longer treatment period. Clinical trials are currently underway to test that hypothesis.

Treatment with warfarin for more than 3 months is indicated for patients with recurrent venous thromboembolism and for patients in whom there is a continuing risk factor operative for venous thromboembolism [151]. Discontinuation of warfarin therapy at 3 months in patients with recurrent venous thrombosis is associated with a 20-percent risk of recurrent venous thromboembolism during the following year and a 5-percent risk of fatal pulmonary embolism [3]. The recent consensus report on antithrombotic therapy of the American College of Chest Physicians recommends an indefinite period of warfarin treatment for patients with recurrent venous thrombosis, although that statement was not based on published data [125]. The optimum duration of therapy in patients with recurrent venous thromboembolism is the subject of clinical trials currently underway.

In patients with a continuing risk factor that is potentially reversible (e.g., prolonged bed rest), long-term therapy should be continued until the risk factor is reversed. Anticoagulant therapy probably should be continued indefinitely in patients with an irreversible risk factor, such as a deficiency of antithrombin III or protein C [125].

Although definitive evidence from clinical trials supports the use of long-term warfarin therapy for proximal venous thrombosis, the treatment of calf-vein thrombosis remains controversial. Without treatment, the likelihood of proximal extension of calf-vein thrombosis is approximately 20 percent, which usually occurs in the first 1 to 2 weeks following diagnosis. Proximal extension of calf-vein thrombosis can be detected by noninvasive testing with IPG or Doppler ultrasound [9,63,64]. Where those tests are readily available, it is safe to withhold anticoagulants, providing proximal extension of the thrombosis is not detected [9,63,64]. If facilities to monitor extension of calf-vein thrombosis are not available, those patients should be treated with heparin and warfarin in the usual fashion [13].

OTHER APPROACHES

LMW heparin has been shown to be effective in the treatment of proximal venous thrombosis. A number of studies used repeat venography 5–7 days after commencing therapy [169–175]. LMW heparin given intravenously or by once- or twice-daily subcutaneous injection was compared with subcutaneous or intravenous unfractionated heparin. Those studies showed equal or improved effectiveness of LMW heparin over unfractionated heparin with a similar bleeding risk [169–176].

Two multicenter randomized clinical trials using clinical end points compared the use of LMW heparin subcutaneously once or twice daily with continuous intravenous heparin with warfarin commenced at the beginning of the study [148] or after 10 days of treatment [173]. In the largest treatment trial to date [148], fixed-dosage subcutaneous low-molecular-weight heparin (logiparin, 175 X_a units/kg) once daily was compared with intravenous heparin by continuous infusion adjusted to maintain an APTT of 1.5–2.5 times the mean normal control value. All patients had venographically proven proximal-vein thrombosis and at the time of entry had ventilation-perfusion lung scans, chest radiographs, and IPG. Outcome events included objectively documented venous thromboembolism (recurrence or extension of DVT or pulmonary embolism), major or minor bleeding, thrombocytopenia, and death. New episodes of venous thromboembolism were seen in 6 of 213 patients receiving LMW heparin (2.8%) and in 15 of 219 patients receiving intravenous unfractionated heparin (6.9%; $p = 0.07$; 95% Cl for the difference = 0.02 to +8.1%) [148]. Major bleeding associated with initial therapy occurred in one patient receiving LMW heparin (0.5%) and in 11 patients receiving intravenous unfractionated heparin (5.0%), a reduction in risk of 95 percent ($p = 0.006$). During long-term warfarin therapy, major hemorrhage was seen in five patients who had received LMW heparin (2.3%) and in none of those receiving intravenous heparin ($p = 0.028$). Ten patients who received LMW heparin (4.7%) died, compared to 21 patients who received intravenous unfractionated heparin (9.6%), representing a risk reduction of 51% ($p = 0.049$). The most striking difference was in abrupt deaths in patients with metastatic carcinoma, and the majority of those deaths occurred within the first 3 weeks [148].

LMW heparin (CY216 fraxiparine) was compared with continuous intravenous unfractionated heparin in the treatment of patients with proximal venous thrombosis [173]. Either LMW heparin or intravenous heparin was continued for 10 days, followed by oral warfarin sodium treatment for 3 months. Patients in the LMW heparin groups received subcutaneous injections every 12 hours according to body weight (12,500 anti-X_a ICU for patients <55 kg; 15,000 anti-X_a ICU for patients between 55 and 80 kg; and 17,500 anti-X_a ICU for patients >80 kg). Patients in the adjusted-dosage intravenous heparin group received a continuous infusion to maintain the APTT within 1.5–2.0 times the mean normal control value. All patients had baseline perfusion lung scans and chest x-rays. In those studies as well, contrast venography was repeated on day 10 or earlier if new symptoms developed. The principal end point for the assessment of efficacy was symptomatic recurrent venous thrombosis or symptomatic pulmonary embolism. Secondary end points for efficacy assessment were changes between days 0 and 10 in the venograms and perfusion lung scans. The frequency of objectively diagnosed recurrent venous thromboembolism did not differ significantly between the unfractionated heparin and the LMW heparin groups (12 [14%] versus 6 [7%]; 95% Cl = −3 to +15%; p = 0.13). There was no significant difference in clinically evident bleeding between the two groups (3.5% for unfractionated heparin versus 1.1% for LMW heparin; $p > 0.2$). In the 6-month follow-up period, there were 12 deaths in the unfractionated heparin group versus 6 in the LMW heparin group; that difference was due largely to cancer deaths (8 of 18 in the unfractionated heparin group versus 1 of 15 in the LMW heparin group) [173].

When the results of the two studies were combined [148,173], the decrease in the mortality rate was even more striking, particularly in patients with metastatic carcinoma. The long-term use of LMW heparin has been shown to be safe in the long-term treatment of patients experiencing side effects on oral anticoagulants [177] and in small case series in pregnant patients [178,179]. Randomized clinical trials assessing the effectiveness of long-term use of LMW heparin are currently underway. LMW heparin is at least as effective and as safe as unfractionated heparin in the treatment of proximal venous thrombosis, and is more cost effective [147]. Furthermore, the drug can be given by a once-daily subcutaneous injection without laboratory monitoring, which will enable the use of out-of-hospital treatment. Once the LMW heparins become available for treatment, they rapidly will replace the use of unfractionated heparin in the treatment of venous thromboembolism.

Thrombolysis has a limited role in the treatment of proximal venous thrombosis. Randomized studies comparing the use of streptokinase with intravenous heparin show a higher degree of thrombolysis with streptokinase and a trend toward reduction in postthrombotic sequelae [180]. However, there is an increased risk of major bleeding with streptokinase compared with heparin, particularly in older subjects. Thrombolysis may be of benefit in younger patients with the recent onset of extensive iliofemoral thrombosis, particularly if there is threatened vascular insufficiency. The hope that the early use of thrombolytic therapy can decrease the incidence of postphlebitic changes has not been substantiated by randomized clinical trials.

VENOUS THROMBOSIS IN PREGNANCY

Pregnancy constitutes a significant risk for venous thrombosis particularly in patients who have had previous episodes of deep venous thrombosis or who have a deficiency of inhibitors of the coagulation system, for example, deficiency of protein C, protein S, or antithrombin III. The risk of thrombosis continues throughout pregnancy and into the postpartum period. Therefore, for either the prevention or the treatment of venous thrombosis, anticoagulants must be given for an extended period of time. Very few randomized clinical trials of sound methodology have been performed, so recommendations must be based on a meager database. Oral anticoagulants are contraindicated throughout pregnancy and, therefore, cannot be used [181]. Low-dosage heparin does not prevent embolism from prosthetic heart valves [182]. Therefore, subcutaneous heparin given twice daily and adjusted to maintain an APTT of 1.5 times control six hours after the injection has been recommended, based on that observation and the evidence that adjusted-dosage subcutaneous heparin is effective in the long-term treatment of venous thromboembolism in nonpregnant patients [183]. It has been recommended that twice-daily adjusted subcutaneous heparin be used both for the prevention of thrombosis of artificial heart valves and for the treatment of venous thromboembolism during pregnancy [184]. For patients with previous venous thromboembolism who are planning pregnancy or who become pregnant, heparin remains the agent of choice. Subcutaneous heparin may be given in a fixed dosage of 5,000 units 2–3 times a day or by adjusted dosage, but there are no good data to support either approach [184]. Clinical trials comparing the use of LMW heparin with adjusted-dosage subcutaneous heparin are awaited with interest.

References

1. Dismuke SE, Wagner EH. Pulmonary embolism as a cause of death. The changing mortality in hospitalized patients. JAMA 1986; 255:2039–2042.
2. Dalen JE, Alpert JS. Natural history of pulmonary embolism. Prog Card Dis 1975; 17:257–270.
3. Anderson FA, et al. A population-based perspective of the hospital incidence and case-fatality rates of deep vein thrombosis and pulmonary embolism. Arch Int Med 1991; 151:933–938.
4. Donaldson GA, et al. A reappraisal of the application of the Trendelenburg operation to massive fatal embolism. N Engl J Med 1963; 268:171.
5. Clagett GP, Reisch JS. Prevention of venous thromboembolism in general surgical patients. Results of meta-analysis. Ann Surg 1988; 208:227–240.
6. Collins R, et al. Reduction in fatal pulmonary embolism and venous thrombosis by perioperative administration of subcutaneous heparin. N Engl J Med 1988; 318:1162–1173.
7. Colditz GA, Tuden RL, Oster G. Rates of venous thrombosis after general surgery: combined results of randomized clinical trials. Lancet July 1986; 19:143–146.
8. Hull RD, et al. Diagnostic efficacy of impedance plethysmography for clinically suspected deep-vein thrombosis: a randomized trial. Ann Int Med 1985; 102:21–28.

9. Huisman MV, et al. Serial impedance plethysmography for suspected deep venous thrombosis in outpatients. The Amsterdam General Practitioner Study. N Engl J Med 1986; 314:823–828.
10. Moser KM, Le Moine JR. Is embolic risk conditioned by location of deep venous thrombosis? Ann Int Med 1981; 94:439–444.
11. Huisman MV, et al. Management of clinically suspected acute venous thrombosis in outpatients with serial impedance plethysmography in a community hospital setting. Arch Int Med 1989; 149:511–513.
12. Kakkar VV, et al. Natural history of post-operative deep-vein thrombosis. Lancet 1969; 2:230–233.
13. Lagerstedt CI, et al. Need for long-term anticoagulant treatment in symptomatic calf-vein thrombosis. Lancet 1985; 2:515–518.
14. Hull RD, et al. Warfarin sodium versus low-dose heparin in the long-term treatment of venous thrombosis. N Engl J Med 1979; 301:855–858.
15. Huisman MV, et al. Unexpected high prevalence of silent pulmonary embolism in patients with deep venous thrombosis. Chest 1989; 95:498–502.
16. Sevitt S, Gallagher N. Venous thrombosis and pulmonary embolism. A clinico-pathological study in injured and burned patients. Br J Surg 1961; 48:475–489.
17. Mavor GE, Galloway JMD. The iliofemoral venous segment as a source of pulmonary emboli. Lancet 1967; 1:871–874.
18. Hull RD, et al. Diagnostic value of ventilation-perfusion lung scanning in patients with suspected pulmonary embolism. Chest 1985; 88:819–828.
19. A collaborative study by the PIOPED Investigators. Value of the ventilation/perfusion scan in acute pulmonary embolism: results of the prospective investigation of pulmonary embolism diagnosis (PIOPED). JAMA 1990; 263:2753–2759.
20. Bone RC. Ventilation/perfusion scan in pulmonary embolism. 'The emperor is incompletely attired.' JAMA 1990; 263:2794–2795.
21. Secker-Walker RH. On purple emperors, pulmonary embolism, and venous thrombosis. Ann Int Med 1983; 98:1006–1008.
22. Stein PD, et al. Strategy for diagnosis of patients with suspected acute pulmonary embolism. Chest 1993; 103(5):1553–1559.
23. Rabinov K, Paulin S. Roentgen diagnosis of venous thrombosis in the leg. Arch Surg 1972; 104:134.
24. Ginsberg JS, et al. d-dimer in patients with clinically suspected pulmonary embolism. Chest 1993; 104(6):1679–1684.
25. Harrison KA, et al. Plasma d-dimer: a useful tool for evaluating suspected pulmonary embolus. J Nuc Med 1993; 34(6):896–898.
26. Wells PS, et al. A rapid d-dimer (DD) assay with high sensitivity and negative predictive value (NPV) in patients with suspected deep vein thrombosis (DVT). Blood 1993; 82(10):407a.
27. Cronan JJ, et al. Deep venous thrombosis: US assessment using vein compressibility. Radiology 1987; 162:191–194.
28. Lensing AWA, et al. Detection of deep-vein thrombosis by real-time B-mode ultrasonography. N Engl J Med 1989; 320:342–345.
29. Monreal M, et al. Real-time ultrasound for diagnosis of symptomatic venous thrombosis and for screening of patients at risk. Angiology 1989; 40:527–532.
30. Habscheid W, et al. Real-time ultrasound in the diagnosis of acute deep venous thrombosis of the lower extremity. Angiology 1990; 599–602.
31. Gudmundsen TE, Vinje B, Pedersen T. Deep vein thrombosis of lower extremities. Diagnosis by real-time ultrasonography. Acta Radiol 1990; 31:473–475.
32. Baxter GM, McKechnie S, Duffy P. Colour Doppler ultrasound in deep venous thrombosis: a comparison with venography. Clin Radiol 1990; 42:32–36.
33. Rose ST, et al. Symptomatic lower extremity deep venous thrombosis: accuracy, limitations, and role of colour duplex flow imaging in diagnosis. Radiology 1990; 175:639–644.
34. Mitchell DC, et al. Comparison of duplex ultrasonography and venography in the diagnosis of deep venous thrombosis. Br J Surg 1991; 78:611–613.
35. Quintavalla R, et al. Duplex ultrasound diagnosis of symptomatic proximal deep vein thrombosis of lower limbs. Eur J Radiol 1992; 15:32–36.
36. Schindler JM, et al. Colour coded duplex sonography in suspected deep vein thrombosis of the leg. Br Med J 1990; 301:1369–1370.
37. Mattos MA, et al. Color-flow duplex scanning for the surveillance and diagnosis of acute deep venous thrombosis. J Vasc Surg 1992; 15:366–376.
38. Vogel P, Laing FC, Jeffrey RB, et al. Deep venous thrombosis of the lower extremity: US evaluation. Radiology 1987; 163:747–751.
39. O'Leary DH, Kane RA, Chase BM. A prospective study of the efficacy of B-scan sonography in the detection of deep venous thrombosis in the lower extremities. J Clin Ult 1988; 16:1–4.
40. Mantoni M. Diagnosis of deep venous thrombosis by duplex sonography. Acta Radiol 1989; 30:575–579.
41. Ginsberg JS, et al. Venous thrombosis in patients who have undergone major hip or knee surgery: detection with compression US and impedance plethysmography. Radiology 1991; 181:651–654.
42. Borris LC, et al. Comparison of real-time B-mode ultrasonography and bilateral ascending phlebography for detection of postoperative deep vein thrombosis following elective hip surgery. Throm Haemost 1989; 61:363–365.
43. Barnes RW, et al. Perioperative asymptomatic venous thrombosis: role of duplex scanning versus venography. J Vas Surg 1989; 9:251–260.
44. Elliott GC, et al. Duplex ultrasonography for the detection of deep vein thrombi after total hip or knee arthroplasty. Angiology 1993; 44:26–33.
45. Davidson B, Elliott GC, Lensing AWA. Low accuracy of color Doppler ultrasound to detect proximal leg vein thrombosis during screening of asymptomatic high-risk patients. Ann Int Med 1992; 117:735–738.
46. Rose SC, et al. Insensitivity of color Doppler flow imaging for detection of acute calf deep venous thrombosis in asymptomatic postoperative patients. J Vasc Int Radiol 1993; 4:111–117.
47. Hull RD, et al. The diagnosis of acute recurrent deep-vein thrombosis: A diagnostic challenge. Circulation 1983; 67:901–906.
48. Richards KL, et al. Noninvasive diagnosis of deep venous thrombosis. Arch Int Med 1976; 136:1091–1096.
49. Hull RD, et al. Impedance plethysmography using the occlusive cuff technique in the diagnosis of venous thrombosis. Circulation 1976; 53:696.
50. Hull RD, et al. Combined use of leg scanning and impedance plethysmography in suspected venous thrombosis: an alternative to venography. N Engl J Med 1977; 296:1497–1500.
51. Hull RD, et al. Replacement of venography in suspected venous thrombosis by impedance plethysmography and ^{125}I-fibrinogen leg scanning: A less invasive approach. Ann Int Med 1981; 94:12–15.
52. Prandoni P, et al. A new computerized impedance plethys-

mograph: accuracy in the detection of proximal deep vein thrombosis in symptomatic outpatients. Throm Haemost 1991; 65:229–232.
53. Heijboer H, et al. Detection of deep vein thrombosis with impedance plethysmography and real-time compression ultrasonography in hospitalized patients. Arch Int Med 1992; 152:1901–1903.
54. Paiement G, et al. Surveillance of deep vein thrombosis in asymptomatic total hip replacement patients. Impedance plethysmography and fibrinogen scanning versus roentgenographic phlebography. Am J Surg 1988; 155:400–404.
55. Cruickshank MK, et al. An evaluation of impedance plethysmography and ^{125}I-fibrinogen leg scanning in patients following hip surgery. Throm Haemost 1989; 62:830–834.
56. Lensing AWA, et al. Lower extremity venography with iohexol: results and complications. Radiology 1990; 177: 503–505.
57. Lensing AWA, et al. Contrast venography, the gold standard for the diagnosis of deep vein thrombosis: improvement in observer agreement. Throm Haemost 1992; 67:8–12.
58. McLachlan MSF, et al. Observer variation in the interpretation of lower limb venograms. Am J Radiol 1979; 132: 227–229.
59. Parfrey PS, et al. Contrast material-induced renal failure in patients with diabetes mellitus, renal insufficiency or both. N Engl J Med 1989; 320:143–149.
60. Schwab SJ, et al. Contrast nephrotoxicity: a randomized controlled trial of a non-ionic and an ionic radiographic contrast agent. N Engl J Med 1989; 320:149–153.
61. Hull RD, et al. Clinical validity of a negative venogram in patients with clinically suspected venous thrombosis. Circulation 1981; 64:622–625.
62. Hull RD, et al. Impedance plethysmography: the relationship between venous filling and sensitivity and specificity for proximal-vein thrombosis. Circulation 1978; 58:898–902.
63. Hull RD, et al. A new non-invasive management strategy for patients with suspected pulmonary embolism. Arch Int Med 1989; 149:2549–2555.
64. Hull RD, et al. A noninvasive strategy for the treatment of patients with suspected pulmonary embolism. Arch Int Med 1994; 154:289–297.
65. Skinner DB, Salzman EW. Anticoagulant prophylaxis in surgical patients. Surg Gynecol Obstet 1967; 125:741–746.
66. Shephard RM, White HA, Shirkey AL. Anticoagulant prophylaxis of thromboembolism in post-surgical patients. Am J Surg 1966; 112:698–702.
67. International Multicentre Trial. Prevention of fatal postoperative pulmonary embolism by low doses of heparin. Lancet 1975, 2:45–51.
68. Coventry MB, Nolan DR, Beckenbaugh RD. "Delayed" prophylactic anticoagulation: a study of results and complications in 2,012 total hip arthroplasties. J Bone Joint Surg [Am] 1973; 55:1487–1492.
69. Eskeland G, Solheim K, Skhorten F. Anticoagulant prophylaxis, thromboembolism and mortality in elderly patients with hip fracture: a controlled clinical trial. Acta Chir Scand 1986; 131:16–29.
70. Nicolaides AN, et al. Prevention of venous thromboembolism. Int Ang 1992; 11(3):151–161.
71. Kakkar V, et al. Prophylaxis for post-operative deep-vein thrombosis. JAMA 1979; 241:39–42.
72. Anderson FA, et al. Physician practices in the prevention of venous thromboembolism. Ann Int Med 1991; 115:581–585.
73. Bergqvist D. Prevention of postoperative deep vein thrombosis in Sweden: results of a survey. World J Surg 1980; 4:489–495.
74. Laverick MD, Croak SA, Mollan RA. Orthopedic surgeons and thromboprophylaxis. Br Med J 1991; 303(6802):549–550.
75. Salzman EW, Davies GC. Prophylaxis of venous thromboembolism. Analysis of cost-effectiveness. Ann Surg 1980; 191:207.
76. Hull R, et al. Cost-effectiveness of primary and secondary prevention of fatal pulmonary embolism in high-risk surgical patients. Can Med Ass J 1982; 127:990–992.
77. Oster G, Tuden RL, Colditz GA. A cost-effectiveness analysis of prophylaxis against deep vein thrombosis in major orthopedic surgery. JAMA 1987; 257:203–208.
78. Bergqvist D, et al. The cost-effectiveness of prevention of post-operative thromboembolism. Acta Chir Scand Suppl 1990; 556:36–41.
79. Hauch O, Kyattar SC, Jorensen LN. Cost-benefit analysis of prophylaxis against deep vein thrombosis in surgery. Semin Thromb Hemost 1991; 17[Suppl 3]:280–283.
80. Leyvraz PF, et al. Adjusted versus fixed dose subcutaneous heparin in the prevention of deep-vein thrombosis after total hip replacement. N Engl J Med 1983; 309:954–958.
81. Leyvraz PF, et al. Prevention of deep vein thrombosis after hip replacement: randomised comparison between unfractionated heparin and low molecular weight heparin. Br Med J 1991; 303:543–548.
82. Kakkar VV, et al. Low molecular weight versus standard heparin for prevention of venous thromboembolism after major abdominal surgery. Lancet 1993; 341:259–265.
83. Kakkar VV, Murray WJG. Efficacy and safety of low-molecular-weight heparin (CY216) in preventing postoperative venous thromboembolism: a co-operative study. Br J Surg 1985; 72:786–791.
84. Bergqvist D, et al. Low-molecular-weight heparin given the evening before surgery compared with conventional low-dose heparin in prevention of thrombosis. Br J Surg 1988; 75:888–891.
85. Fricker JP, et al. Low dose heparin versus low molecular weight heparin Kabi 2165 in the prophylaxis of thromboembolic complications of abdominal oncological surgery. Eur J Clin Invest 1988; 18:561.
86. Samama M, et al. Low-molecular-weight heparin compared with unfractionated heparin in prevention of postoperative thrombosis. Br J Surg 1988; 75:128–131.
87. The European Fraxiparin Study Group. Comparison of a low-molecular-weight heparin and unfractionated heparin for the prevention of deep vein thrombosis in patients undergoing abdominal surgery. Br J Surg 1988; 75:1058–1063.
88. Caen JP. A randomized double-blind study between a low-molecular-weight heparin Kabi 2165 and standard heparin in the prevention of deep-vein thrombosis in general surgery. A French multicentre trial. Thromb Haemost 1988; 59:216–220.
89. Leizorovicz A, et al. Prevention of perioperative deep vein thrombosis in general surgery: a multicentre double-blind study comparing two doses of logiparin and standard heparin. Br J Surg 1991; 78:412.
90. Dechavanne M, et al. Randomized trial of a low-molecular-weight heparin (Kabi 2165) versus adjusted-dose subcutaneous standard heparin in the prophylaxis of deep-vein thrombosis after elective hip surgery. Haemostasis 1989; 1:5–12.
91. Turpie AGG, et al. A randomized controlled trial of a low-molecular-weight heparin (enoxaparin) to prevent deep-vein thrombosis in patients undergoing elective hip surgery. N Engl J Med 1986; 315:925–929.
92. Planes A, et al. Prevention of postoperative venous thrombosis: a randomized trial comparing unfractionated heparin with low-molecular-weight heparin in patients undergoing total hip replacement. Thromb Haemost 1988; 60:407–410.

93. Levine MN, et al. Prevention of deep vein thrombosis after elective hip surgery: a randomized trial comparing low molecular weight heparin with standard unfractionated heparin. Ann Int Med 1991; 114(7):545–551.
94. Eriksson BI, et al. Prevention of deep vein thrombosis and pulmonary embolism after total hip replacement. J Bone Joint Surg [Am] 1991; 73-A(4):484–493.
95. The Danish Enoxaparin Study Group. Low-molecular weight heparin (enoxaparin) vs dextran 70. Arch Int Med 1991; 151:1621–1624.
96. Tørholm C, et al. Thromboprophylaxis by low-molecular-weight heparin in elective hip surgery: a placebo controlled study. J Bone Joint Surg [Br] 1991; 73-B:434–438.
97. Lassen MR, et al. Prevention of thromboembolism in 190 hip arthroplasties. Acta Orth Scand 1991; 62(1):33–38.
98. Planes A, et al. Prevention of deep vein thrombosis after total hip replacement: the effect of low-molecular-weight heparin with spinal and general anesthesia. J Bone Joint Surg [Br] 1991; 73-B:418–422.
99. Leclerc JR, et al. Prevention of deep vein thrombosis after major knee surgery—a randomized, double-blind trial comparing a low-molecular-weight heparin fragment (enoxaparin) to placebo. Thromb Haemost 1992; 67(4):417–423.
100. Heit J, et al. Efficacy and safety of RD heparin (a LMWH) versus warfarin for prevention of deep-vein thrombosis after hip or knee replacement. Blood 1991; 78(10)[Suppl]:739.
101. Hull RD, et al. A comparison of subcutaneous low-molecular-weight heparin with warfarin sodium for prophylaxis against deep-vein thrombosis after hip or knee implantation. N Engl J Med 1993; 329:1370–1376.
102. Hoek J, et al. Prevention of deep vein thrombosis following total hip replacement by a low-molecular-weight heparinoid. Thromb Haemost Suppl 1989; 62:1637.
103. Bergqvist D, et al. Thromboprophylaxis in hip fracture patients—a prospective randomized comparative study between ORG 10172 and dextran. Surgery 1991; 109:617–622.
104. Gerhart TN, et al. Low-molecular-weight heparinoid compared with warfarin for prophylaxis of deep vein thrombosis in patients who are operated on for fracture of the hip. A prospective, randomized trial. J Bone Joint Surg 1991; 73-A(4).494–502.
105. Nurmohamed MT, et al. Low molecular weight heparin in the prophylaxis of venous thrombosis: a meta-analysis. Lancet 1992; 340:152–156.
106. Francis CW, et al. Comparison of warfarin and external pneumatic compression in prevention of venous thrombosis after total hip replacement. JAMA 1992; 267(21):2911–2915.
107. Paiement F, et al. Low-dose warfarin versus external pneumatic compression for prophylaxis against venous thromboembolism following total hip replacement. J Arth 1987; 2:23–26.
108. Kaempffe FA, Lifeso RM, Meinking C. Intermittent pneumatic compression versus Coumadin: prevention of deep vein thrombosis in lower-extremity total joint arthroplasty. Clin Orth 1991; 269:89–97.
109. Powers PJ, et al. A randomized trial of less intense postoperative warfarin or aspirin therapy in the prevention of venous thromboembolism after surgery for fractured hip. Arch Int Med 1989; 149:771–774.
110. Poller L, et al. Fixed minidose warfarin: a new approach to prophylaxis against venous thrombosis after major surgery. Br Med J 1987; 285:1309–1312.
111. Bern MM, et al. Very low doses of warfarin can prevent thrombosis in central venous catheters. Ann of Int Med 1990; 112:423–428.
112. Dale C, et al. Prevention of venous thrombosis with minidose warfarin after joint replacement. Br Med J 1991; 303:224.
113. Roberts VC, et al. The effect of intermittently applied external pressure on the hemodynamics of the lower limb in man. Br J Surg 1972; 59:233–236.
114. Turpie AGG, et al. Prevention of venous thrombosis in patients with intracranial disease by intermittent pneumatic compression of the calf. Neurology 1977; 27:435–438.
115. Turpie AG, et al. Prevention of venous thrombosis by intermittent sequential calf compression in patients with intracranial disease. Thromb Res 1979; 16:611–616.
116. Skillman JJ, et al. Prevention of deep vein thrombosis in neurosurgical patients: a controlled, randomized trial of external pneumatic compression boots. Surgery 1978; 83: 354–358.
117. Hull RD, et al. Effectiveness of intermittent pneumatic leg compression for preventing deep vein thrombosis after total hip replacement. JAMA 1990; 263:2313–2317.
118. Hull RD, et al. Effectiveness of intermittent pulsatile elastic stockings for the prevention of calf and thigh vein thrombosis in patients undergoing elective knee surgery. Thromb Res 1979; 16:37–45.
119. Mckenna R, et al. Prevention of venous thromboembolism after total knee replacement by high-dose aspirin or intermittent calf and thigh compression. Br Med J 1980; 1:514–517.
120. Turner GM, Cole SE, Brooks JH. The efficacy of graduated compression stockings in the prevention of deep vein thrombosis after major gynaecological surgery. Br J Obstet Gynaecol 1984; 91:588–591.
121. Ishak MA, Moreley KD. Deep venous thrombosis after total hip arthroplasty: a prospective controlled study to determine the prophylactic effect of graded pressure stockings. Br J Surg 1981; 68:429–432.
122. Allan A, et al. The use of graduated compression stockings in the prevention of postoperative deep vein thrombosis. Br J Surg 1983; 70:172–174.
123. Wells PS, Lensing AWA, Hirsh J. Graduated compression stockings in the prevention of postoperative venous thromboembolism. Arch Int Med 1994; 154:67–72.
124. Antiplatelet Trialists' Collaboration. Collaborative overview of randomized trials of antiplatelet therapy—III: Reduction in venous thrombosis and pulmonary embolism by antiplatelet prophylaxis among surgical and medical patients. Br Med J 1994; 308:235–246.
125. Hyers TM, Hull RD, Weg J. Antithrombotic therapy for venous thromboembolic disease. Chest 1992; 102:408S–425S.
126. Moser KM. Venous thromboembolism. Am Rev Respir Dis 1990; 141:235–249.
127. Salzman EW, et al. Management of heparin therapy: controlled prospective trial. N Engl J Med 1976; 292:1046–1050.
128. Gallus A, et al. Safety and efficacy of warfarin started early after submassive venous thrombosis or pulmonary embolism. Lancet 1986; 2:1293–1296.
129. Hull RD, et al. Heparin for 5 days as compared with 10 days in the initial treatment of proximal venous thrombosis. N Engl J Med 1990; 322:1260–1264.
130. Bjork I, Lindahl U. Mechanism of the anticoagulant action of heparin. Mol Cell Biochem 1982; 48:161–182.
131. Lindahl U, et al. Structure of the antithrombin-binding site of heparin. Proc Natl Acad Sci USA 1979; 76:3198–3202.
132. Rosenberg RD, Damus PS. The purification and mechanism of action of human antithrombin-heparin co-factor. J Biol Chem 1973; 248:6490–6506.
133. Rosenberg RD, Lam L. Correlation between structure and function of heparin. Proc Natl Acad Sci USA 1979; 76:1218–1222.
134. Tollefsen DM, Majerus DW, Blank MK. Heparin co-factor II: purification and properties of thrombin in human plasma. J Biol Chem 1982; 257:2162–2169.

135. Hirsh J, et al. Heparin: mechanism of action, pharmacokinetics, dosing consideration, monitoring, efficacy, and safety. Chest 1992; 102(4):337S–351S.
136. Levine MN, et al. A randomized trial comparing activated thromboplastin time with heparin assay in patients with acute venous thromboembolism requiring large daily doses of heparin. Arch Int Med 1994; 154:49–56.
137. Hull RD, et al. Optimal therapeutic level of heparin therapy in patients with venous thrombosis. Arch Int Med 1992; 152:1589–1595.
138. Hull RD, et al. Continuous intravenous heparin compared with intermittent subcutaneous heparin in the initial treatment of proximal-vein thrombosis. N Engl J Med 1986; 315:1109–1114.
139. Brill-Edwards P, et al. Establishing a therapeutic range for heparin therapy. Ann Int Med 1993; 119:104–109.
140. Brandjes DPM, et al. Acenocoumarol and heparin compared with acenocoumarol alone in the initial treatment of proximal-vein thrombosis. N Engl J Med 1992; 327:1485–1489.
141. Raschke RA, et al. The weight-based heparin dosing nomogram compared with a "standard care" nomogram. Ann Int Med 1993; 119:874–881.
142. Levine MN, Hirsh J, Kelton JG. Heparin-induced bleeding. In DA Lane, U Lindahl, eds. Heparin, Chemical and Biological Properties, Clinical Applications. CRC Press, Inc., 1989. Pp. 517–531.
143. Cruickshank MK, et al. A standard nomogram for the management of heparin therapy. Arch Int Med 1991; 151:333–337.
144. Fennerty A, et al. Audit of control of heparin treatment. Br Med J 1985; 290:27–28.
145. Wheeler AP, Jaquiss RD, Newman JH. Physician practices in the treatment of pulmonary embolism and deep-venous thrombosis. Arch Int Med 1988; 148:1321–1325.
146. Elliott GC, et al. Physician guided treatment compared with a heparin protocol for deep vein thrombosis. Arch Int Med 1994; 154(9):999–1004.
147. Hull RD, et al. Heparin (H) resistance as a predictor of recurrent venous thromboembolism (RVTE). Blood 1993; 82;10[Suppl 1]:1613.
148. Hull RD, et al. Subcutaneous low-molecular weight heparin compared with continuous intravenous heparin in the treatment of proximal-vein thrombosis. N Eng J Med 1992; 326:975–982.
149. Freedman MD. Oral anticoagulants: pharmacodynamics, clinical indications and adverse effects. J Clin Pharm 1992; 32:196–209.
150. Furie B, Furie BC. Molecular basis of vitamin K-dependent gamma-carboxylation. Blood 1990; 75:1753–1762.
151. Hirsh J, et al. Oral anticoagulants; mechanism of action, clinical effectiveness, and optimal therapeutic range. Chest 1992; 102(4)[Suppl]:312S–326S.
152. Clouse LH, Comp PC. The regulation of haemostasis: The protein C system. N Engl J Med 1986; 314:1298–1304.
153. O'Reilly RA, Aggeler PM. Studies on coumarin anticoagulant drugs: initiation of warfarin therapy without a loading dose. Circulation 1968; 38:169–176.
154. Gurwitz JH, et al. Aging and the anticoagulant response to warfarin therapy. Ann of Int Med 1992; 116:901–904.
155. Wells PS, et al. Warfarin and its drug/food interactions; a critical appraisal of the literature. Throm Haemost 1993; 69(6):1133.
156. Hull R, et al. Different intensities of oral anticoagulant therapy in the treatment of proximal-vein thrombosis. N Engl J Med 1982; 307:1676–1681.
157. Bussey HI, et al. Reliance on prothrombin time ratios causes significant errors in anticoagulation therapy. Arch Int Med 1992; 152:278–282.
158. Turpie AGG (on behalf of Thrombosis Interest Group). Control of anticoagulant therapy: a cross Canada survey. Thromb Haemost 1993; 69(6):677.
159. Garr SB, Rodgers GM. Laboratory monitoring of warfarin therapy in Utah. Am J Hem 1994; 45:85–87.
160. Ovesen L, Lyduch S, Ott P. A simple technique for predicting maintenance dosage of warfarin—is it better than empirical dosing? Eur J Clin Pharm 1989; 37:573–576.
161. White RH, et al. Home prothrombin time monitoring after the initiation of warfarin therapy. Ann Int Med 1989; 111:730–737.
162. Furie B, et al. Comparison of the native prothrombin antigen and the prothrombin time for monitoring oral anticoagulant therapy. Blood 1984; 64:445–451.
163. Holmgren K, et al. One-month versus six-month therapy with oral anticoagulants after symptomatic deep-vein thrombosis. Acta Med Scand 1985; 218:279–284.
164. O'Sullivan EF. Duration of anticoagulant therapy in venous thromboembolism. Med J Aust 1972; 2:1104–1107.
165. Petitti DB, Strom BL, Melmon KL. Duration of warfarin anticoagulant therapy and the probabilities of recurrent thromboembolism and hemorrhage. Am J Med 1986; 81:255–259.
166. Schulman S, Lockner D, Juhlin-Dannfelt A. The duration of oral anticoagulants after deep-vein thrombosis: a randomized study. Acta Med Scand 1985; 217:547–552.
167. Research Committee of the British Thoracic Society. Optimum duration of anticoagulation for deep-vein thrombosis and pulmonary embolism. Lancet 1992; 340:873–876.
168. Prandoni P, et al. Deep-vein thrombosis and the incidence of subsequent symptomatic cancer. N Engl J Med 1992; 327:1128–1133.
169. Bratt G, et al. A comparison between low molecular weight heparin (KABI 2165) and standard heparin in the intravenous treatment of deep venous thrombosis. Thromb Haemost 1985; 54:813–817.
170. Bratt G, et al. Two daily subcutaneous injections of Fragmin as compared with intravenous standard heparin in the treatment of deep venous thrombosis (DVT). Throm Haemost 1990; 64:506–510.
171. Holm HA, et al. Subcutaneous heparin treatment of deep venous thrombosis: a comparison of unfractionated and low molecular weight heparin. Haemostasis 1986; 16:30–37.
172. Albada J, Nieuwenhuis HK, Sixma JJ. Treatment of acute venous thromboembolism with low molecular weight heparin (Fragmin). Results of a double-blind randomized study. Circulation 1989; 80:935–940.
173. Prandoni P, et al. Comparison of subcutaneous low-molecular-weight heparin with intravenous standard heparin in proximal deep-vein thrombosis. Lancet 1992; 339:441–445.
174. Huet Y, et al. Treatment of established venous thromboembolism with Enoxaparin: preliminary report. Acta Chir Scand Suppl 1990; 556:116–120.
175. Siegbahn A, et al. Subcutaneous treatment of deep venous thrombosis with low molecular weight heparin. A dose finding study with LMWH-Novo. Thromb Res 1989; 55:767–778.
176. Simonneau G, et al. Subcutaneous low-molecular-weight heparin compared with continuous intravenous unfractionated heparin in the treatment of proximal deep vein thrombosis. Arch Int Med 1993; 153:1541–1546.
177. Harenberg J, et al. Long term anticoagulation with low molecular weight heparin in outpatients with side effects on oral anticoagulants. Nouv Rev Fr Hematol 1989; 31:363–369.
178. Melissari E, et al. Use of low molecular weight heparin in pregnancy. Throm Haemost 1992; 68(6):652–656.
179. Forestier F, et al. Absence of transplacental passage of Fragmin (Kabi) during the second and the third trimesters of pregnancy. Throm Haemost 1992; 67(1):180–181.

180. Goldhaber SZ. Pooled analyses of randomized trials of streptokinase and heparin in phlebographically documented acute deep venous thrombosis. Am J Med 1984; 76: 393–397.
181. Pineo GF, Hull RD. Adverse effects of coumarin anticoagulants. Drug Safety 1993; 9(4):263–271.
182. Wang RYC, et al. Efficacy of low dose, subcutaneously administered heparin in treatment of pregnant women with artificial heart valves. Med J Aust 1983; 2:126–128.
183. Hull R, et al. Adjusted subcutaneous heparin versus warfarin sodium in the long-term treatment of venous thrombosis. N Engl J Med 1982; 306:189–194.
184. Ginsberg JS, Hirsh J. Use of antithrombotic agents during pregnancy. Chest 1992; 102(4)[Suppl]:385S–390S.

Pulmonary Embolism

Samuel Z. Goldhaber

Pulmonary embolism (PE) and deep venous thrombosis (DVT) constitute an interdisciplinary illness managed by primary physicians, cardiologists, pulmonologists, hematologists, vascular surgeons, and specialists in vascular medicine. PE and DVT together account for more than 250,000 hospitalizations per year in the United States and, therefore, constitute a very common medical problem [1]. Since most cases of venous thrombosis are not recognized clinically, estimates of hospitalization rates understate the true frequency of the condition.

Epidemiology

PE causes or contributes to between 30,000 and 50,000 deaths per year in the United States, a rate that probably has remained constant for the past three decades [2]. Whereas postoperative PE is the most commonly recognized in-hospital setting for this potentially catastrophic disease, PE also can strike young, otherwise healthy individuals as well as those with concomitant medical illnesses. PE is also the most common cause of maternal mortality in the United States [3].

Approximate annual charges for the diagnosis and treatment of venous thrombosis in the United States exceed $2.8 billion [4]. Those charges do not include the cost of time lost from work, discomfort from chronic pulmonary hypertension due to PE, and the value placed on the loss of life. During the past decade, important advances in prevention, diagnosis, and treatment strategies have made possible a future decrease in the mortality, morbidity, and cost of venous thrombosis.

In the 1990s, emphasis has focused on prevention of venous thrombosis. In the United States, there are about 400,000 elective total hip or knee replacements annually as well as about 400,000 coronary artery bypass operations per year. Those types of surgery, in particular, continue to be associated with high rates of venous thrombosis. It is estimated that for every 1,000,000 patients undergoing general, orthopedic, or urologic surgery, preventive measures can improve patient outcomes and reduce total health care costs by about $60 million [4].

Patients suspected of PE should be evaluated for the presence of risk factors for venous thrombosis (Table 46-1). Many patients with an underlying hypercoagulable state will not manifest venous thrombosis unless there is underlying cancer (often occult) or an obvious precipitant such as recent immobilization or surgery.

Some patients have a genetic predisposition to PE. Therefore, a family history of venous thrombosis should be sought in all patients diagnosed or suspected of venous thrombosis. Young patients, especially those with recurrences, should be worked up with blood tests to detect a hypercoagulable state (Table 46-2). Ordinarily, such testing is best in the outpatient setting because the results of in-hospital work-ups can be misleading. For example, consumption coagulopathy due to acute PE may be misdiagnosed as either antithrombin III or protein C deficiency. Heparin administration can depress antithrombin III levels, and use of warfarin ordinarily will cause a mild protein C or S deficiency.

In one study, 50 percent of heterozygotes for a mutation in the protein C gene and 10 percent of normal relatives can be expected to have an episode of venous thrombosis by age 45. About half of those thrombotic events appear to be precipitated by immobilization or surgery [5].

A poor anticoagulant response to activated protein C (Fig. 46-1) is the most exciting and far-reaching discovery in the field of prethrombotic markers [6]. Normally, one can add a known amount of activated protein C to plasma and observe prolongation of the activated partial thromboplastin time (PTT). However, if the PTT prolongation is less than twice control, patients have a poor anticoagulant response. In one cohort, that abnormality was detected in 21 percent of unselected consecutive patients (< 70 years old) with venous thrombosis and only among 5 percent of controls [7]. The anticoagulant cofactor that corrects inherited activated protein C resistance is thought to be unactivated factor V [8].

Dr. Goldhaber receives support from the National Heart, Lung, and Blood Institute Academic Award in Systemic and Pulmonary Vascular Medicine.

Pathophysiology

Pulmonary embolism can have the following pathophysiologic effects: (1) **increased pulmonary vascular resistance**, owing to vascular obstruction, neurohumoral agents, pulmonary-artery baroreceptors, or increased pulmonary artery pressure; (2) **impaired gas exchange**, owing to increased alveolar dead space from vascular obstruction and hypoxemia from alveolar hypoventilation, low V-Q units, and right-to-left shunting, as well as impaired carbon monoxide transfer owing to loss of gas exchange surface; (3) **alveolar hyperventilation**, owing to reflex stimulation of irritant receptors; (4) **increased airway resistance**, owing to bronchoconstriction; and (5) **decreased pulmonary compliance**, owing to lung edema, lung hemorrhage, and loss of surfactant [9].

Prevention

PE is easier and less expensive to prevent than to diagnose or treat [10]. Virtually all patients hospitalized for more than a day or two should receive prophylactic measures against venous thromboembolism [11–14]. Each patient's level of risk for PE should be assessed to determine whether to use mechanical, pharmacologic, or combined mechanical and pharmacologic prevention modalities (Table 46-3). In general, the type of prophylaxis strategy selected should match the level of risk for developing venous thrombosis.

Table 46-1. Common risk factors for venous thrombosis

Immobilization, trauma, surgery
Obesity
Increasing age
Oral contraceptives, pregnancy, postpartum
Cancer, especially adenocarcinoma
Stroke, spinal cord injury
Indwelling central venous catheter
Prior venous thrombosis

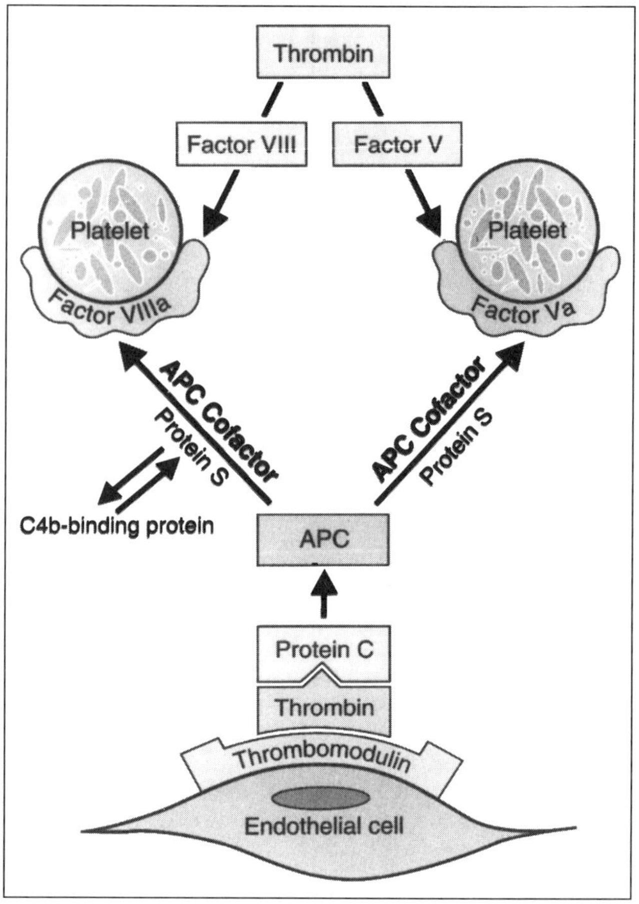

Fig. 46-1. Thrombin converts factors VIII and V to their activated forms, factors VIIIa and Va. A complex of thrombin with the endothelial-cell receptor thrombomodulin activates protein C. Activated protein C inactivates factors VIIIa and Va on the platelet surface. That reaction is accelerated by APC cofactor, which is thought to be unactivated factor V, as well as by free protein S. (Reprinted with permission from KA Bauer. Hypercoagulability—a new cofactor in the protein C anticoagulant pathway. N Engl J Med 1994; 330:566–567.)

In a Swedish autopsy study, a surprisingly large proportion of postoperative patients succumbed to PE more than 2 weeks postoperatively [15]. One-quarter of those patients died between the fifteenth and thirtieth postoperative day, and 15 percent died of PE more than 30 days postoperatively (Fig. 46-2). A separate study of general abdominal surgery patients showed that as many as 30 percent of postoperative PEs may occur as late as one month after discharge from the hospital [16]. Because the risk of PE continues after discharge from the hospital, prophylaxis should be continued at home among those patients at moderate or high risk for venous thromboembolism.

Despite the availability of effective measures to curb venous thromboembolism, prophylaxis continues to be underutilized, even among high-risk hospitalized patients. In a survey of 16 short-stay hospitals in central Massachusetts [17], only 32 percent of patients at high risk for venous thrombosis received prophylaxis. The rates of prophylaxis varied widely, from 9 percent to 56 percent at the different hospitals. Patients received prophylaxis at teaching hospitals more often than at nonteaching hospitals. Fixed low-dosage subcutaneous heparin was utilized in about four-fifths of patients who did receive preventive measures.

Venous thrombosis is almost certainly a problem among hospitalized medical patients as well as those who undergo surgery. In a survey [18] of 152 patients in our medical intensive care unit, we found that prophylaxis against venous thromboembolism was administered in only 33 percent of cases. There was also an average delay of 2 days prior to institution of preventive measures. Of the 152 patients, 88 percent had at least one risk factor, and 53 percent had multiple risk factors for venous thrombosis.

We believe that prevention programs should be established at all hospitals, with nurses and physicians collaborating to establish protocols that are streamlined and standardized [19]. Prevention options are broad (see Table 46-3). The mental discipline of assessing all patients for some type of prophylaxis is far more important than the specific modality that is selected.

Table 46-2. Hypercoagulable states associated with venous thrombosis

Genetic predisposition or family history
Poor anticoagulant response to activated protein C
Protein C or S deficiency
Antithrombin III deficiency
Presence of lupus anticoagulant
Elevated level of anticardiolipin antibodies

Graduated compression stockings (GCS) and intermittent pneumatic compression (IPC) have complementary mechanisms. GCS provide continuous stimulation of blood flow and prevent perioperative venodilation of the legs. They are inexpensive, simple, and free of serious complications, such as hemorrhage. In randomized trials evaluating GCS for prevention of venous thrombosis after nonorthopedic surgery (general surgery, gynecologic surgery, and neurosurgery), there is an overall reduction of 72 percent in the likelihood of having a DVT [20]. IPC devices compress the veins more forcefully than GCS but for a relatively brief period; they also stimulate the endogenous fibrinolytic system [21].

Table 46-3. Prevention options

MECHANICAL
Graduated compression stockings (GCS)
Intermittent pneumatic compression (IPC)
Combined GCS and IPC
Inferior vena caval filter
PHARMACOLOGIC
Unfractionated heparin (low dosage, fixed dosage)
Low-molecular-weight heparin (low dosage, fixed dosage)
Dextran 500 ml/24 hours as continuous infusion
Warfarin (adjusted to a target INR of 2.0–3.0 in orthopedic surgery)
COMBINED MECHANICAL AND PHARMACOLOGIC
GCS plus heparin
IPC plus heparin
IPC plus warfarin

Subcutaneous administration of unfractionated heparin has become the standard pharmacologic prophylaxis measure during the past two decades. Collins and colleagues pooled the data from 78 randomized controlled unfractionated-heparin trials with 15,598 patients undergoing surgery [22]. There was a 40-percent reduction in nonfatal PE and a 64-percent reduction in fatal PE among patients treated prophylactically with heparin. Patients assigned to heparin had about one-third as many DVTs as control patients, regardless of whether they had undergone general, urologic, elective orthopedic, or trauma surgery. Although there was no significant difference in fatal hemorrhage between the heparin group and the control group, an absolute excess in important bleeding of about 2 percent occurred among patients assigned to heparin, especially those who underwent urologic procedures.

Low-molecular-weight (LMW) heparin, approved by the Food and Drug Administration (FDA) in 1993, is the most recent innovation in pharmacologic prophylaxis against venous thrombosis. LMW heparins exhibit less binding to plasma proteins and to endothelial cells than unfractionated heparin. Consequently, they tend to have a more predictable dosage response, more dosage-independent mechanism of clearance, and longer plasma half-life than unfractionated heparin. In most prevention trials, LMW heparins are administered as once- or twice-daily subcutaneous injections in fixed or weight-adjusted dosages, without laboratory monitoring or dosage adjustment. For prophylaxis in elective hip surgery, LMW heparins have consistently performed well compared with other prevention modalities [23]. Only one LMW heparin, enoxaparin, is FDA approved; the indication for administering enoxaparin is prophylaxis against venous thrombosis among patients undergoing elective total hip replacement [24]. The approved dosage is 30 mg subcutaneously twice daily for 10–14 days.

Fig. 46-2. The interval between operation and death in autopsied patients with major pulmonary embolism. (Reprinted with permission from D Bergqvist, B Lindblad. A 30-year survey of pulmonary embolism verified at autopsy: an analysis of 1274 surgical patients. Br J Surg 1985; 72:105–108.)

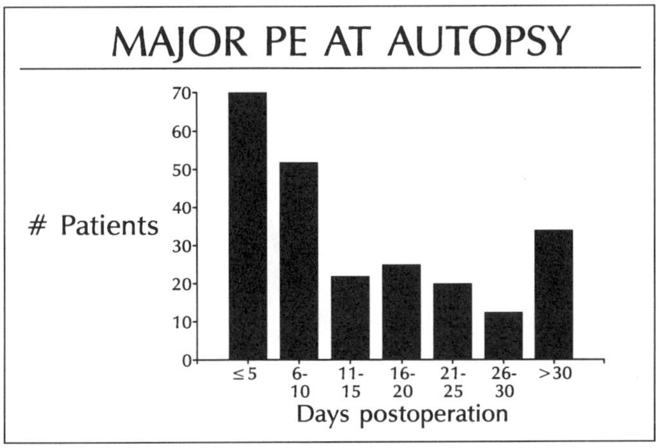

Most North American orthopedic centers currently use adjusted-dosage warfarin, with a target International Normalized Ratio (INR) of 2.0–3.0, to help prevent venous thrombosis in elective total hip replacement. At Brigham and Women's Hospital in Boston, we begin warfarin and an IPC device simultaneously because it takes 3–5 days for the warfarin to become effective. We continue adjusted-dosage warfarin for approximately 4 to 6 weeks [25].

An even more protracted prevention strategy after hospital discharge was recently reported in 268 patients undergoing total hip replacement who received adjusted-dosage warfarin for 12 weeks [26]. The target INR was approximately 2.0. In that cohort, two patients suffered nonfatal pulmonary embolism, and the major bleeding rate was 4 percent.

Warfarin and LMW heparin were compared in a randomized trial [27] to prevent venous thrombosis among 1,207 patients undergoing elective total hip or total knee replacement. Disappointingly, both strategies resulted in surprisingly high rates of venographically proven DVT. Although the rate of isolated calf-vein thrombosis was slightly higher in the warfarin-treated patients, the major bleeding complication rate was three times higher among those who received LMW heparin.

PE is no longer considered a rare complication of coronary artery bypass grafting (CABG). In a review of 819 consecutive patients undergoing CABG (without other concomitant cardiac surgery) [28], 4 percent were found to have suffered postoperative PE according to autopsy, angiography, or high-probability lung scanning. The majority were identified during the second postoperative week. Of those with PE, 19 percent died, compared with an operative mortality of 3 percent among those without PE. In a case series of 29 patients who had undergone uncomplicated CABG at Brigham and Women's Hospital, leg ultrasonography was obtained prior to hospital discharge [29]. Although none had postoperative signs or symptoms suggestive of DVT, ultrasonography detected DVT in 48 percent. In all but one, the DVT was limited to the calf veins. Unexpectedly, half of the venous thrombi occurred in the leg contralateral to the saphenous-vein harvest site.

Table 46-4. Electrocardiographic findings in pulmonary embolism

Incomplete or complete right bundle branch block
S in lead I and aVL > 1.5 millimeter
Transition zone shift to V5
Qs in leads III and aVF, but not in lead II
QRS axis > 90 degrees or indeterminate axis
Low limb lead voltage
T wave inversion in leads III and aVF or in leads V1-V4

Source: Adapted with permission from N Sreeram et al. Value of the 12-lead electrocardiogram at hospital admission in the diagnosis of pulmonary embolism. Am J Cardiol 1994; 73:298–303.

Diagnosis

PE can be quite difficult to diagnose, despite the availability of lung scanning and pulmonary angiography. Thus, appreciation of the clinical setting and maintenance of a high degree of clinical suspicion for possible PE are of paramount importance. The most common symptoms and signs are nonspecific: dyspnea, tachypnea, chest pain, and tachycardia. Usually, patients who present with severe chest pain or with hemoptysis have anatomically small PE near the periphery of the lung, where nerve innervation is greatest and where pulmonary infarction is most likely to occur because of poor collateral circulation. Ironically, patients with lifethreatening PE often have a painless presentation characterized by dyspnea, syncope, or cyanosis.

PE should be suspected in hypotensive patients when (1) there is evidence of or predisposing factors for venous thrombosis; (2) there is clinical evidence of acute cor pulmonale (acute right ventricular failure), such as distended neck veins, an S3 gallop, a right ventricular heave, tachycardia, or tachypnea; and, especially, (3) there is electrocardiographic evidence of acute cor pulmonale manifested by a new S1 Q3 T3 pattern, new incomplete right bundle branch block, or right ventricular ischemia [12].

IMAGING AND LABORATORY TESTS

Enlargement of a central pulmonary artery, especially with progressive enlargement on serial radiographs, is a cardinal plain-chest radiographic sign of pulmonary embolism [30]. The chest x-ray also can help exclude diseases, such as lobar pneumonia or pneumothorax, that can have similar clinical presentations (although patients with those illnesses also can have concomitant PE).

The electrocardiogram is useful to help exclude acute myocardial infarction. In addition, among patients with large PE, at least several electrocardiographic manifestations of right heart strain (Table 46-4) often can be detected [31].

Unfortunately, neither room-air arterial blood gases (Fig. 46-3) nor calculation of the alveolar-arterial oxygen gradient (Fig. 46-4) helps to differentiate patients with a confirmed PE at angiography from those with a normal pulmonary angiogram [32]. Therefore, arterial blood gases should not be obtained as a screening test in patients suspected of PE.

The most promising blood test for screening is an abnormally elevated level of plasma D-dimer (> 500 ng/ml) performed with a quantitative enzyme-linked immunosorbent assay (ELISA) (Fig. 46-5), which has a more than 90-percent sensitivity for angiographically proven PE [33]. D-dimer is a specific proteolytic degradation product released into the circulation by endogenous fibrinolysis of a cross-linked fibrin clot. In 908 patients suspected of PE from nine trials (prevalence of PE 38%), elevation of the plasma D-dimer by ELISA had a 97-percent sensitivity and a 45-percent specificity for PE [34].

Fig. 46-3. Distribution of partial pressure of oxygen in arterial blood (PO_2), while breathing room air, among 88 patients with angiographically proven PE and no preexisting cardiac or pulmonary disease and 202 patients in whom PE was excluded with normal pulmonary angiograms. (Reprinted with permission from PD Stein et al. Clinical, laboratory, roentgenographic, and electrocardiographic findings in patients with acute pulmonary embolism and no pre-existing cardiac or pulmonary disease. Chest 1991; 100:598–603.)

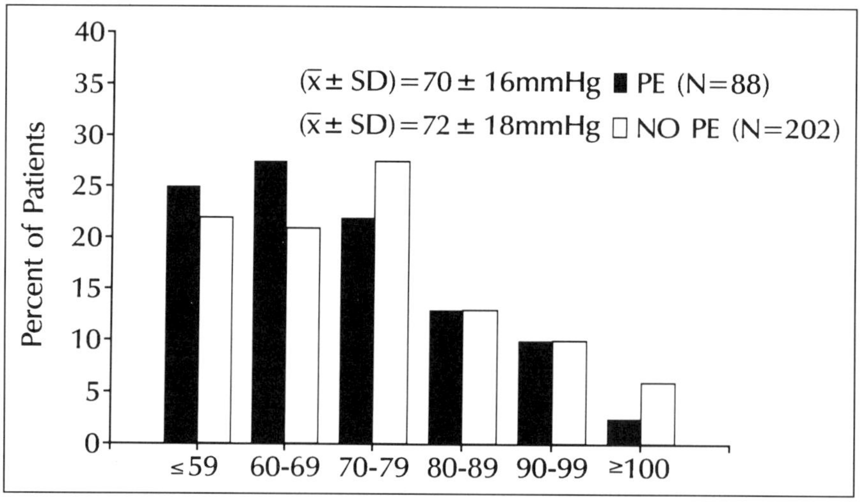

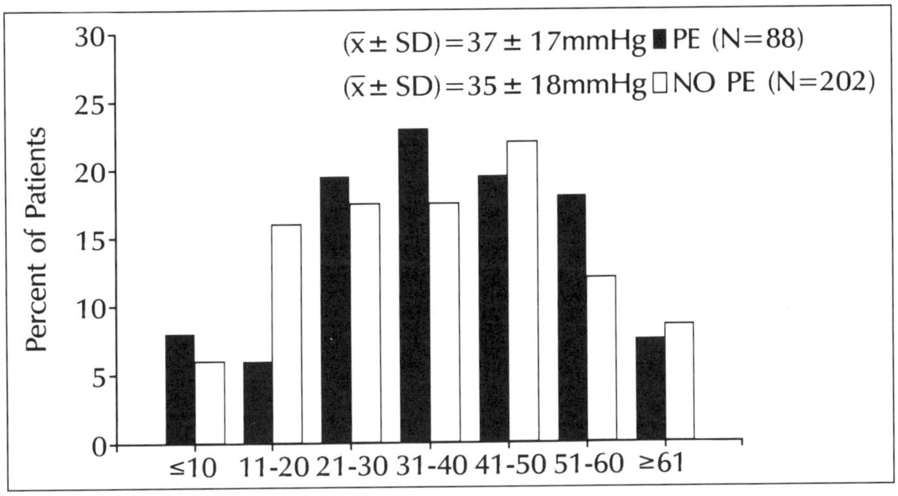

Fig. 46-4. Distribution of alveolar-arterial oxygen gradient among 88 patients with angiographically proven PE and no preexisting cardiac or pulmonary disease and 202 patients in whom PE was excluded with normal pulmonary angiograms. (Reprinted with permission from PD Stein et al. Clinical, laboratory, roentgenographic, and electrocardiographic findings in patients with acute pulmonary embolism and no pre-existing cardiac or pulmonary disease. Chest 1991; 100:598–603.)

Ventilation-perfusion (V-Q) lung scanning should be the principal diagnostic test when PE is being seriously considered (Fig. 46-6) [35]. The V-Q scan is most useful if it is clearly normal or if it demonstrates a pattern suggestive of a high probability for PE. Intermediate-probability scans or low-probability scans with high clinical suspicion do not exclude PE [35] (Table 46-5). Patients in the latter categories may require pulmonary angiography. When the clinician strongly suspects PE, the diagnostic workup should not necessarily cease as a consequence of a low-probability lung scan [36].

A constant intraluminal-filling defect seen in more than

Fig. 46-5. Distribution of plasma D-dimer ELISA levels, sorted according to angiographic findings, among 173 patients with suspected acute pulmonary embolism. (Reprinted with permission from SZ Goldhaber et al. Quantitative plasma D-dimer levels among patients undergoing pulmonary angiography for suspected pulmonary embolism. JAMA 1993; 270:2819–2822.)

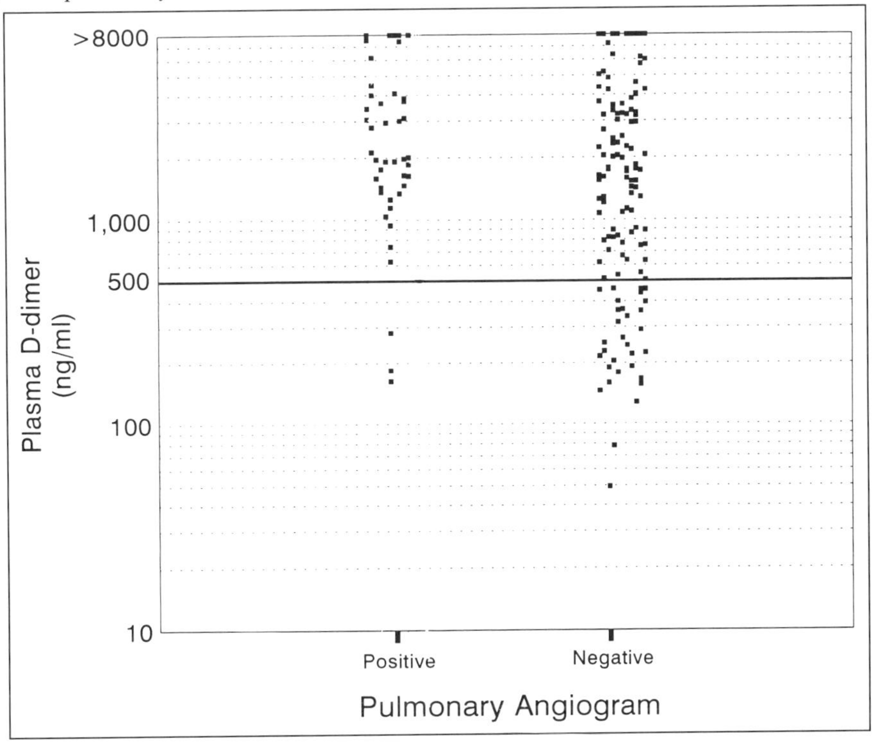

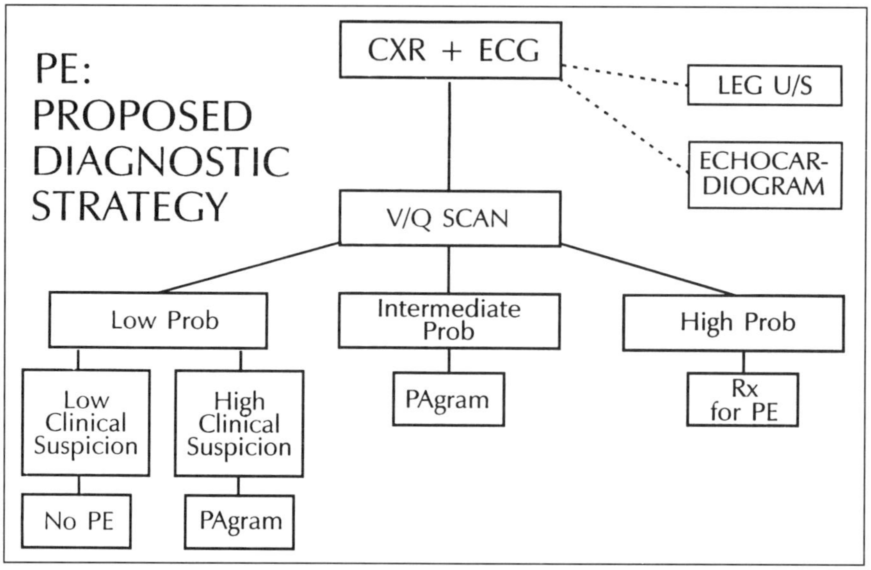

Fig. 46-6. Suggested diagnostic strategy for investigation of suspected pulmonary embolism. (Reprinted with permission from SZ Goldhaber. Recognition and management of pulmonary embolism. Heart Disease and Stroke 1993; 2:142–146.)

one projection is the most reliable feature for the diagnosis of PE among patients undergoing pulmonary angiography. This procedure almost always can be accomplished safely if these guidelines are followed: (1) Selective angiography is performed, with the perfusion lung scan serving as a road map to the angiographer; (2) soft flexible catheters with side holes are used, rather than stiff catheters with end holes; and (3) a low-osmolar contrast agent is utilized to minimize the transient hypotension and the transient heat and coughing sensation that often occur with conventional radiocontrast agents [12].

Ultrasonography of the leg veins is usually accurate in diagnosing proximal leg DVT in symptomatic outpatients and may sometimes serve as a useful surrogate for PE. However, even high-resolution compression ultrasonography of the legs with color Doppler imaging may be insensitive for DVT diagnosis among asymptomatic inpatients, especially those who have undergone recent total hip or total knee replacement [37]. Overall, one-third to one-half of PE patients have no ultrasound or venogram evidence of leg DVT. Therefore, if clinical suspicion of PE is high, patients without clinical or imaging evidence of DVT still should be worked up for PE.

A recent decision model combined the measurement of plasma D-dimer ELISA and leg ultrasonography among patients with intermediate-probability lung scans and intermediate clinical suspicion of PE. The results suggested that the combination of D-dimer and leg ultrasonography might reduce by one-third the requirement for pulmonary angiography [38].

Among hemodynamically unstable patients, bedside echocardiography may suggest PE (Fig. 46-7) if the following constellation of findings is present: right ventricular dilatation and hypokinesis, bowing of the interventricular septum into the left ventricle, tricuspid regurgitation, and preserved left ventricular function. Echocardiography in that setting also can help to exclude other life-threatening conditions, such as ventricular septal rupture, aortic dis-

Table 46-5. PIOPED: pulmonary embolism status

	Clinical probability (%)			
Lung scan category	80–100 No. PE cases/ no. patients (%)	20–79 No. PE cases/ no. patients (%)	0–19 No. PE cases/ no. patients (%)	0–100 No. PE cases/ no. patients (%)
High	28/29 (96)	70/80 (88)	5/9 (56)	103/118 (87)
Intermediate	27/41 (66)	66/236 (28)	11/68 (16)	104/345 (30)
Low	6/16 (40)	30/191 (16)	4/90 (4)	40/296 (14)
Very low	0/5 (0)	4/62 (6)	1/61 (2)	5/128 (4)
Total	61/90 (68)	170/569 (30)	21/228 (9)	252/887 (28)

Source: Adapted with permission from PIOPED Investigators. Value of the ventilation/perfusion scan in acute pulmonary embolism. JAMA 1990; 263:2757.

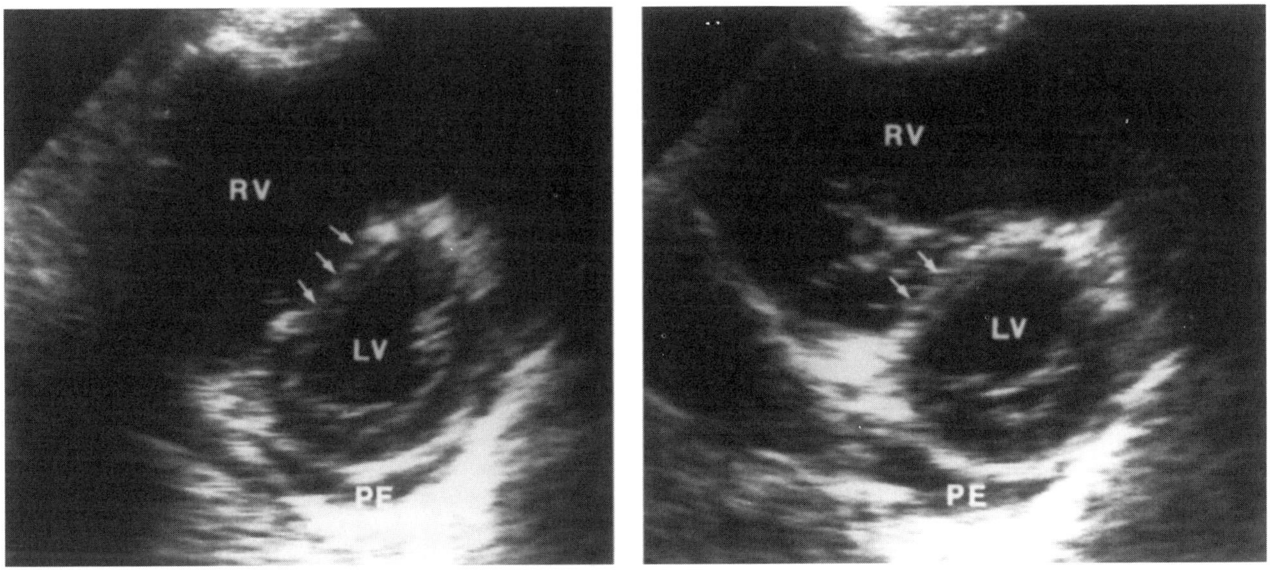

Fig. 46-7. Parasternal short-axis views of the right ventricle (RV) and left ventricle (LV) in diastole (*left*) and systole (*right*). There is diastolic and systolic bowing of the interventricular septum (*arrows*) into the left ventricle compatible with right ventricular volume and pressure overloads, respectively. The right ventricle is appreciably dilated and markedly hypokinetic, with little change in apparent right ventricular area from diastole to systole. PE = small pericardial effusion. (Reprinted with permission from PC Come. Echocardiographic evaluation of pulmonary embolism and its response to therapeutic interventions. Chest 1992; 101:151S–162S.)

section, and pericardial tamponade. Nevertheless, patients can have a normal echocardiogram despite an anatomically extensive PE. Therefore, echocardiography should be considered an ancillary rather than a principal diagnostic test.

A new diagnostic approach to be considered is intravascular ultrasound [39]. Once a femoral sheath is in place, an experienced operator can introduce the intravascular ultrasound catheter and advance it to the pulmonary arteries within several minutes.

Therapy

When PE is strongly suspected on clinical grounds, heparin should be initiated with a bolus of 5,000–10,000 units followed by a continuous intravenous infusion of approximately 1,250 units/hour while the diagnostic work-up is pursued. The PTT should be targeted to 1.5 to 2.5 times control. Failure to use heparin in adequate dosages can prolong the hospital stay, predispose to recurrent PE, and increase the costs of medical care. There is a much stronger relationship between subtherapeutic heparin administration and recurrent thrombosis than between supertherapeutic concentrations of heparin and bleeding complications.

Oral anticoagulation with warfarin (Coumadin) can be started as soon as the PTT is within the therapeutic range. Patients should receive at least 5 days of heparin while an adequate level of oral anticoagulation is established. The prothrombin time, utilized to adjust the dose of oral anticoagulation, should be reported according to the INR, not the prothrombin time ratio or the prothrombin time expressed in seconds.

The INR is essentially a "corrected" prothrombin time that adjusts for the several dozen assays used in North America and Europe. For example, in North America, a prothrombin time of 18 seconds and prothrombin time ratio of 1.5 at one laboratory could be equivalent to a prothrombin time of 22 seconds and prothrombin time ratio of 1.8 at another laboratory. The same blood specimen in some European laboratories might yield a prothrombin time of 30 seconds and prothrombin time ratio of 2.5. The INR for the same blood sample would be 3.0 at all three laboratories, despite the markedly different prothrombin time ratios and prothrombin times given in this example [12].

For PE patients, I use a target INR of 3.0 to 4.0 and usually prescribe warfarin for 12 months. Lifelong anticoagulation may be required in patients with persistent risk factors, such as massive obesity or cancer.

THROMBOLYTIC THERAPY

Thrombolytic therapy can be a useful adjunct to heparin in patients who have either hemodynamic instability or a normal systemic arterial pressure with echocardiographic evidence of right ventricular dysfunction (Fig. 46-8). Contraindications to thrombolysis (such as intracranial disease, recent surgery, or trauma) preclude its use in some patients who can receive heparin alone safely.

To test whether thrombolysis followed by heparin more rapidly reverses right ventricular dysfunction and restores pulmonary-tissue perfusion than heparin alone, our multicentered Pulmonary Embolism Research Group randomized 101 hemodynamically stable patients to rt-PA 100 mg over 2 hours followed by intravenous heparin or heparin

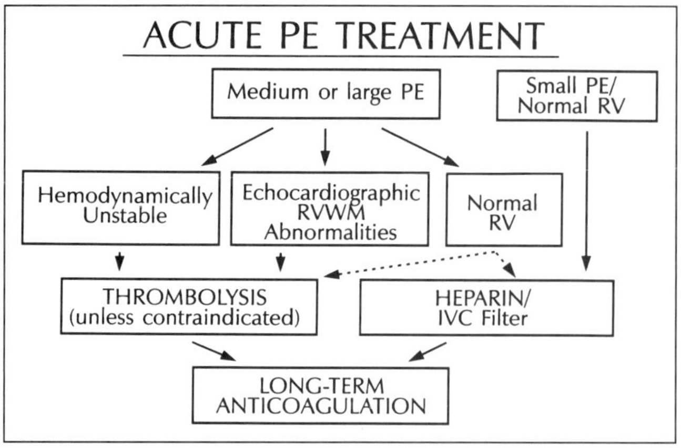

Fig. 46-8. Suggested management strategy for pulmonary embolism. (Reprinted with permission from MW Wolfe, LK Skibo, SZ Goldhaber. Pulmonary embolic disease: diagnosis, pathophysiologic aspects, and treatment with thrombolytic therapy. Curr Probl in Cardiol 1993; 18:585–636.)

alone [40]. The initial systolic arterial pressure was at least 90 mm Hg in every patient we studied. Only 20 percent of the patients underwent diagnostic pulmonary angiography; the others were enrolled on the basis of high-probability lung scans. Serial echocardiograms were obtained at baseline, 3 hours, and 24 hours. Pulmonary perfusion scans were obtained at baseline and 24 hours.

At entry into the trial, about half the patients with PE had entirely normal right ventricular function. Qualitative assessment of right ventricular wall motion at baseline versus 24 hours (Fig. 46-9) demonstrated that 39 percent of the rt-PA patients improved and 2.4 percent worsened, compared with 17-percent improvement and 17-percent worsening among those who received heparin alone ($p = 0.005$). Quantitative assessment showed that rt-PA patients had a significant decrease in right-ventricular end-diastolic area during the 24 hours after randomization compared with none among those allocated to heparin alone ($p = 0.01$). rt-PA patients also had an absolute improvement in pulmonary perfusion of 14.6 percent at 24 hours, compared with 1.5-percent improvement among heparin-alone patients ($p < 0.0001$).

Most important, no clinical episodes of recurrent PE occurred among rt-PA patients, but there were five (two fatal and three nonfatal) clinically suspected recurrent PEs within 14 days in patients randomized to heparin alone ($p = 0.06$). All five presented initially with right ventricular hypokinesis on echocardiogram. The latter observation suggests that echocardiography may help identify a subgroup of PE patients at high risk of adverse clinical outcomes if treated with heparin alone. Such patients, in particular, would appear to be excellent candidates for thrombolytic therapy in the absence of contraindications. Our findings suggest but do not prove that rapid improvement of right ventricular function and pulmonary perfusion, accomplished with thrombolytic therapy followed

Fig. 46-9. Echocardiograms (four-chamber view) in a 53-year-old previously healthy ophthalmologist with a high-probability lung scan for PE. **Left Panel.** Right ventricular enlargement before treatment. The right-ventricular end-diastolic area was 42.9 sq cm, and the interventricular septum (arrow) was displaced toward the left ventricle. The Echocardiogram Panel, which was not aware of the timing of the echocardiogram or of the patient's assignment to rt-PA therapy, graded this examination as showing moderately severe right ventricular hypokinesis. **Right Panel.** Three hours after initiating rt-PA therapy, the right ventricle normalized in size (with a planimetered area of 25.7 sq cm), and the interventricular septum resumed its normal configuration. The Echocardiogram Panel, which was not aware of the timing of the echocardiogram or of the patient's assignment to rt-PA therapy, graded this examination as showing normal right ventricular wall motion.

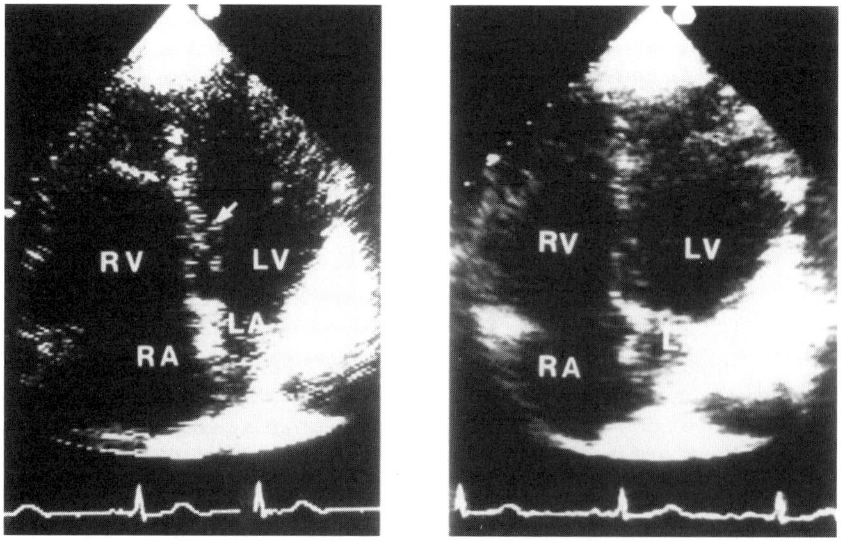

Table 46-6. FDA-approved thrombolytic regimens for PE

Streptokinase: 250,000 IU as a loading dose over 30 minutes, followed by 100,000 U/hour for 24 hours; approved in 1977.

Urokinase: 2,000 IU/lb as a loading dose over 10 minutes, followed by 2,000 IU/lb/hour for 12–24 hours; approved in 1978.

rt-PA: 100 mg as a continuous peripheral intravenous infusion administered over 2 hours; approved in 1990.

by heparin, may lead to a lower rate of death and recurrent PE, especially among patients who present with right ventricular hypokinesis.

Currently, there are three FDA-approved thrombolytic regimens from which to choose (Table 46-6). Heparin is not administered concomitantly and is simply restarted without a bolus at the conclusion of fibrinolytic therapy administration. Because thrombolysis dosaging regimens are fixed, no coagulation tests need be obtained during the thrombolytic infusion. We recently have learned how to make thrombolytic therapy safer, more streamlined, and more economical (Table 46-7).

INFERIOR VENA CAVAL FILTER

The two major indications for placement of an inferior vena caval (IVC) filter are (1) **venous thrombosis** in the setting of active, clinically important **bleeding** that prohibits the use of heparin and (2) **recurrent PE** despite adequate heparin therapy. An IVC filter is also useful in hemodynamically compromised patients who cannot be treated with thrombolytic therapy. It should be kept in mind, however, that an IVC filter prevents PE, not DVT. Therefore, anticoagulation also should be utilized, if possible, to prevent propagation of the venous thrombus. Despite placement of an IVC filter, there is a small possibility of recurrent PE through collateral venous channels that may develop. Recently, a removable IVC filter has been tested with an infusion port that can be used to deliver thrombolytic therapy. In a case series of 69 patients, the efficacy appeared promising, and the complication rate was low [41].

Table 46-7. New concepts in PE thrombolysis

Variable	Old concept	New concept
Diagnosis	Mandatory pulmonary angiogram	High-probability lung scan or suggestive echocardiogram (if hypotensive) or angiogram
Indications	Hypotension; hemodynamic instability	Hypotension or normotension with accompanying right ventricular hypokinesis
Time window	5 days or less	14 days or less
Agents	Streptokinase (SK) or urokinase (UK)	rt-PA, SK, or UK
Dosaging regimens	24 hours SK or 12–24 hours UK	100 mg/2 hours rt-PA (FDA approved), 3,000,000 U/2 hours UK (not FDA approved), or 1,500,000 U/1 hour SK (not FDA approved)
Route	Via pulmonary-artery catheter	Via peripheral vein
Coagulation tests	DIC screen every 4–6 hours during infusion	PTT at conclusion of thrombolysis
Location	Intensive care unit	Intermediate care unit

Key: DIC = disseminated intravascular coagulation.

SURGERY OR CATHETER-BASED INTERVENTION

Occasionally, a patient with an acute, massive PE may not respond to thrombolytic therapy or may have absolute contraindications to its use. Such individuals should be evaluated for acute surgical pulmonary embolectomy [42], suction catheter embolectomy [43], or mechanical fragmentation of thrombus with a pulmonary-artery catheter [44].

A device called "the Thrombolizer" is undergoing clinical testing. It consists of a 5 French teflon catheter whose distal tip is divided into four 15-mm bends. The high-speed mechanical rotation of the catheter (about 100,000 revolutions/minute) causes centrifugal force to open the distal bends and form a soft, flexible helical spiral that can pulverize thrombus into microscopic particles in a few seconds [45].

Patients with chronic pulmonary hypertension due to prior PE may be virtually bedridden with breathlessness from high pulmonary arterial pressures. They should be considered for pulmonary thromboendarterectomy, which, if successful, can reduce and at times even cure pulmonary hypertension [46]. The operation involves a median sternotomy incision, institution of cardiopulmonary bypass, and deep hypothermia with circulatory arrest periods. Incisions are made in both pulmonary arteries into the lower-lobe branches. Pulmonary thromboendarterectomy is always bilateral, with removal of both organized thrombus and an endarterectomy plane from all involved vessels. At the University of Southern California at San Diego, the most recent 150 cases (performed over a 29-month period) were associated with a mortality rate of 9 percent. The average pulmonary-artery systolic pressure declined from 79 mm Hg preoperatively to 47 mm Hg on the second or third postoperative day [47]. Thus, at selected centers, pulmonary thromboendarterectomy can be performed with good results and at an acceptable risk among patients debilitated from chronic pulmonary hypertension due to PE.

EMOTIONAL SUPPORT

Although PE can be as devastating emotionally as myocardial infarction, the burden on PE patients may be greater because the general public does not have as good an understanding of PE, particularly regarding the possibility of long-term disability and incomplete recovery. Young patients with PE repeatedly voice a common theme: Although they appear healthy, they often have difficulty expressing their fears and feelings about their potentially life-threatening illness to family and friends.

Virtually all patients with PE will wonder why they were stricken with the illness and whether they have an underlying coagulopathy or "bad genes" that predisposed them to PE. They may become especially anxious if no specific hypercoagulable state can be identified. When anticoagulation is discontinued after an "adequate" course of therapy, patients will fear recurrent PE and may resist attempts to be weaned from warfarin.

By taking the time to discuss the implications of the illness with the patient and the patient's family, we may be able to ease the emotional burden of PE. In 1993, we began a Pulmonary Embolism Support Group, which is led by a nurse-physician team. Although the sessions have an educational component, the major emphasis is discussing the anxieties and living difficulties that occur in the aftermath of PE.

References

1. Anderson FA Jr, et al. A population-based perspective of the hospital incidence and case-fatality rates of venous thrombosis and pulmonary embolism: The Worcester DVT Study. Arch Intern Med 1991; 151:933–938.
2. Lilienfeld DE, et al. Mortality from pulmonary embolism in the United States: 1962 to 1984. Chest 1990; 98:1067–1072.
3. Koonin LM, et al. Maternal Mortality Surveillance, United States, 1979–1986. CDC Surveillance Summaries. MMWR 1991; 40:1–13.
4. Landefeld CS, Hanus P. Economic burden of venous thromboembolism. In SZ Goldhaber, ed. Prevention of Venous Thromboembolism. New York: Marcel Dekker, Inc., 1993. Pp. 69–85.
5. Allaart CF, et al. Increased risk of venous thrombosis in carriers of hereditary protein C deficiency defect. Lancet 1993; 341:134–138.
6. Bauer KA. Hypercoagulability—a new cofactor in the protein C anticoagulant pathway. N Engl J Med 1994; 330:566–567.
7. Köster T, et al. Venous thrombosis due to poor anticoagulant response to activated protein C: Leiden Thrombophilia Study. Lancet 1993; 342:1503–1506.
8. Dahlbäck B, Hildebrand B. Inherited resistance to activated protein C is corrected by anticoagulant cofactor activity found to be a property of factor V. Proc Natl Acad Sci USA 1994; 91:1396–1400.
9. Elliott CG. Pulmonary physiology during pulmonary embolism. Chest 1992; 101:163S–171S.
10. Goldhaber SZ. Practical aspects of venous thromboembolism prevention: an overview. In SZ Goldhaber, ed. Prevention of Venous Thromboembolism. New York: Marcel Dekker, 1993. Pp. 129–144.
11. National Institutes of Health Consensus Conference. Prevention of venous thrombosis and pulmonary embolism. JAMA 1986; 256:744–749.
12. Goldhaber SZ, Morpurgo M, for the WHO/ISFC Task Force on Pulmonary Embolism. Diagnosis, treatment, and prevention of pulmonary embolism. Report of the WHO/International Society and Federation of Cardiology Task Force. JAMA 1992; 268:1727–1733.
13. European Consensus Statement. Prevention of Venous Thromboembolism. International Angiology 1992; 11:151–159.
14. Thromboembolic Risk Factors (THRIFT) Consensus Group. Risk of and prophylaxis for venous thromboembolism in hospital patients. BMJ 1992; 305:567–574.
15. Bergqvist D, Lindblad B. A 30-year survey of pulmonary embolism verified at autopsy: an analysis of 1274 surgical patients. Br J Surg 1985; 72:105–108.
16. Huber O, et al. Postoperative pulmonary embolism after hospital discharge. An underestimated risk. Arch Surg 1992; 127:310–313.
17. Anderson FA Jr, et al. Physician practices in the prevention of venous thromboembolism. Ann Intern Med 1991; 115: 591–595.
18. Keane MG, Ingenito EP, Goldhaber SZ. Utilization of venous thromboembolism prophylaxis in the Medical Intensive Care Unit. Chest 1994; 106:13–14.
19. Morrison RB. Nurse and physician collaborative responsibility. In SZ Goldhaber, ed. Prevention of Venous Thromboembolism. New York: Marcel Dekker, Inc., 1993. Pp. 577–582.
20. Wells PS, Lensing AWA, Hirsh J. Graduated compression stockings in the prevention of postoperative venous thromboembolism. A meta-analysis. Arch Intern Med 1994; 154:67–72.
21. Allenby F, et al. Effects of external pneumatic intermittent compression on fibrinolysis in man. Lancet 1973; 2:1412–1414.
22. Collins R, et al. Reduction in fatal pulmonary embolism and venous thrombosis by perioperative administration of subcutaneous heparin. Overview of results of randomized trials in general, orthopedic, and urologic surgery. N Engl J Med 1988; 318:1162–1173.
23. Mohr DN, et al. Prophylactic agents for venous thrombosis in elective hip surgery. Meta-analysis of studies using venographic assessment. Arch Intern Med 1993; 153:2221–2228.
24. Enoxaparin—a low-molecular-weight heparin. Medical Letter 1993; 35:75–78.
25. Reis SE, et al. Program for the prevention of venous thromboembolism in high-risk orthopaedic patients. J Arthroplasty 1991; 6:S11–S16.
26. Paiement GD, et al. Routine use of adjusted low-dose warfarin to prevent venous thromboembolism after total hip replacement. J Bone and Joint Surg 1993; 75A:893–898.
27. Hull R, et al. A comparison of subcutaneous low-molecular-weight heparin with warfarin sodium for prophylaxis against deep-vein thrombosis after hip or knee implantation. N Engl J Med 1993; 329:1370–1376.
28. Josa M, et al. Pulmonary embolism after cardiac surgery. J Am Coll Cardiol 1993; 21:990–996.
29. Reis SE, et al. Frequency of deep venous thrombosis in asymptomatic patients with coronary artery bypass grafts. Am Heart J 1991; 122:478–482.
30. Skibo L, Goldhaber SZ. Diagnosis of acute pulmonary embolism. In SZ Goldhaber, ed. Cardiopulmonary Disorders and Cardiac Tumors, Vol III. Atlas of Heart Diseases (E. Braunwald, ed.), 1995. Pp. 2.1–2.31.
31. Sreeram N, et al. Value of the 12-lead electrocardiogram at hospital admission in the diagnosis of pulmonary embolism. Am J Cardiol 1994; 73:298–303.
32. Stein PD, et al. Clinical, laboratory, roentgenographic, and electrocardiographic findings in patients with acute pulmonary embolism and no pre-existing cardiac or pulmonary disease. Chest 1991; 100:598.
33. Goldhaber SZ, et al. Quantitative plasma D-dimer levels among patients undergoing pulmonary angiography for suspected pulmonary embolism. JAMA 1993; 270:2819–2822.
34. Bounameaux H, et al. Plasma measurements of D-dimer as a diagnostic aid in suspected venous thromboembolism: an overview. Thrombosis and Haemostasis 1994; 71:1–6.
35. PIOPED Investigators. Value of the ventilation/perfusion scan in acute pulmonary embolism. Results of the Prospective Investigation of Pulmonary Embolism Diagnosis (PIOPED). JAMA 1990; 263:2753.

36. Bone RC. The low-probability lung scan. A potentially lethal reading. Arch Intern Med 1993; 153:2621–2622.
37. Davidson BL, Elliott CG, Lensing AWA for the RD Heparin Arthroplasty Group. Low accuracy of color Doppler ultrasound in the detection of proximal leg vein thrombosis in asymptomatic high-risk patients. Ann Intern Med 1992; 117:735–738.
38. Perrier A, et al. Contribution of D-dimer plasma measurement and lower-limb venous ultrasound to the diagnosis of pulmonary embolism: a decision analysis model. Am Heart J 1994; 127:624–635.
39. Tapson VF, et al. Rapid visualization of massive pulmonary emboli utilizing intravascular ultrasound. Chest 1994; 105:888–890.
40. Goldhaber SZ, et al. Alteplase versus heparin in acute pulmonary embolism: randomised trial assessing right ventricular function and pulmonary perfusion. Lancet 1993; 341:507–511.
41. Dievart F, et al. New infusion removable inferior vena caval filter catheter (Filcard RF 02) for protected thrombolytic treatment in deep venous thrombosis (DVT) and pulmonary embolism (PE): results of an international multicentric study. J Am Coll Cardiol 1994; 95A (abstract).
42. Meyer G, et al. Pulmonary embolectomy: A 20-year experience at one center. Ann Thorac Surg 1991; 51:232–236.
43. Timsit J-F, et al. Pulmonary embolectomy by catheter device in massive pulmonary embolism. Chest 1991; 100:655–658.
44. Brady AJB, Crake T, Oakley CM. Percutaneous catheter fragmentation and distal dispersion of proximal pulmonary embolus. Lancet 1991; 338:1186–1189.
45. Dievart F, et al. Treatment of severe pulmonary embolism by means of a high speed rotational catheter (Angiocor Thrombolizer): first experience of mechanical thrombolysis in human beings. J Am Coll Cardiol 1994; 474A (abstract).
46. Moser KM, Auger WR, Fedullo PF. Chronic major-vessel thromboembolic pulmonary hypertension. Circulation 1990; 81:1735–1743.
47. Jamieson SW, et al. Experience and results with 150 pulmonary thromboendarterectomy operations over a 29-month period. J Thorac Cardiovasc Surg 1993; 106:116–127.

Chronic Venous Disorders

Magruder C. Donaldson

Chronic venous disease, although not an immediate threat to life or limb, accounts for suffering and disability in large numbers of individuals. Significant superficial varicose veins have been estimated to occur in about 12 percent of the adult population [1]. Cutaneous manifestations of deep venous insufficiency of the lower extremities were found in approximately 20 percent of employees in one study, with severe changes in approximately 9 percent and a history of ulceration in 1.3 percent [2]. Venous obstruction of the upper extremities is recognized as a cause of disabling chronic symptoms [3,4]. Gradual improvements in the understanding of the pathogenesis, diagnosis, and treatment have allowed more effective management of these syndromes.

Normal Venous Anatomy and Physiology

ANATOMY

Venous anatomy is more variable than that of adjacent peripheral arteries and nerves. Veins situated superficial to the deep fascia are of concern mainly in the **lower extremity** (Fig. 47-1). The greater (long, internal) saphenous vein usually is identifiable on the dorsal surface of the foot; it passes immediately anterior to the medial malleolus at the ankle and immediately posterior to the medial femoral condyle at the knee en route to the groin. There it joins the common femoral vein at the fossa ovalis, approximately two fingerbreadths lateral and two fingerbreadths inferior to the pubic tubercle. Afferent tributaries join the greater saphenous vein from the foot, calf, thigh, groin, and lower abdomen. Two of the thigh branches, termed the lateral and medial accessory saphenous veins, are particularly large and notable when varicose. Efferent communicating (perforating) veins leave both the main saphenous and its larger branches to penetrate the deep fascia and join the deep venous system. The clinically most important communicating veins are relatively constant, with several located in the ankle and the calf and one or two in the thigh [5] (Fig. 47-2). Several of the lowest medial calf and ankle communicators commonly connect with a tributary of the greater saphenous vein rather than with the saphenous itself. That vein, sometimes termed the accessory saphenous or posterior arch vein, joins the greater saphenous in the region of the knee. The saphenous nerve follows the superficial femoral artery and vein through the adductor canal in the thigh, emerging at the level of the knee and closely accompanying the saphenous vein in the calf and the ankle.

The lesser (short, external) saphenous vein is located posterior to the lateral malleolus of the ankle, running proximally posterolaterally up the calf, piercing the fascia and joining the popliteal vein immediately below the knee joint in 57 percent of cases [6]. In 10 percent of cases, the lesser saphenous joins the deep veins below the level of the popliteal. In another 12 percent, the vein passes posteriorly up the thigh, turns medially, and joins the greater saphenous vein below the saphenofemoral junction. In the remaining 21 percent, there is a direct connection to the popliteal vein but with a posterior thigh component draining into the connection. Collateral branches run between the greater and lesser saphenous veins.

Bicuspid valves are located along the superficial venous systems, most commonly immediately distal to branches. There is a constant valve in the greater saphenous vein immediately below the saphenofemoral junction. In most limbs, one or, rarely, more valves are located proximal to this level in the common femoral or external iliac veins, but in up to 25 percent of limbs there are no proximal valves [7–9]; thus, the saphenofemoral junction is exposed to pressures transmitted from above. The valve cusps are attached to the superficial and deep walls of the vein, so the commissure of the valve is in the same plane as the skin.

Valves in the communicating veins normally guide unidirectional flow from the superficial toward the deep systems, except in the foot, where deep venous blood is transmitted superficially to the branches of the saphenous veins. The superficial veins function mainly to collect blood from the subcutaneous tissues and to carry it to the closest communicator for rapid transit through the deep veins back to the heart. Approximately 15 percent of the venous blood volume in the leg is contained in the superficial veins, with the remaining 85 percent in the deep system [10].

In the **upper extremity,** valved, superficial veins drain the subcutaneous tissues, connecting at intervals through communicators with the subfascial system. In the forearm, the cephalic and basilic veins run laterally and medially, respectively, interconnecting in the antecubital fossa. The cephalic vein continues laterally up the arm into the deltopectoral groove at the shoulder and ends in the axillary vein near the clavicle. The larger basilic vein pursues a deep medial course and ends in the axillary vein.

The anatomy of the veins deep to the muscular fascia follows that of the arterial trees to both upper and lower extremities. In the **leg** (see Fig. 47-1), two veins accompany each tibial artery, and the popliteal vein also is usually double below the knee joint but more often single as it enters the adductor canal and becomes the superficial femoral vein. The profunda femoris vein joins the superficial femoral to form the common femoral, which becomes the external iliac and then the common iliac after the internal iliac joins on the way to the inferior vena cava. Bicuspid valves are present at intervals throughout the deep system, with the most proximal valve being in the common femoral vein in about 55 percent of limbs and in the external iliac vein in 10 percent of limbs [8,9]. In the **arm,** deep veins also are doubled and accompany the major arteries to the level of the axilla. There the basilic vein merges with the brachial vena comitantes to form the axillary vein, which becomes the subclavian vein at

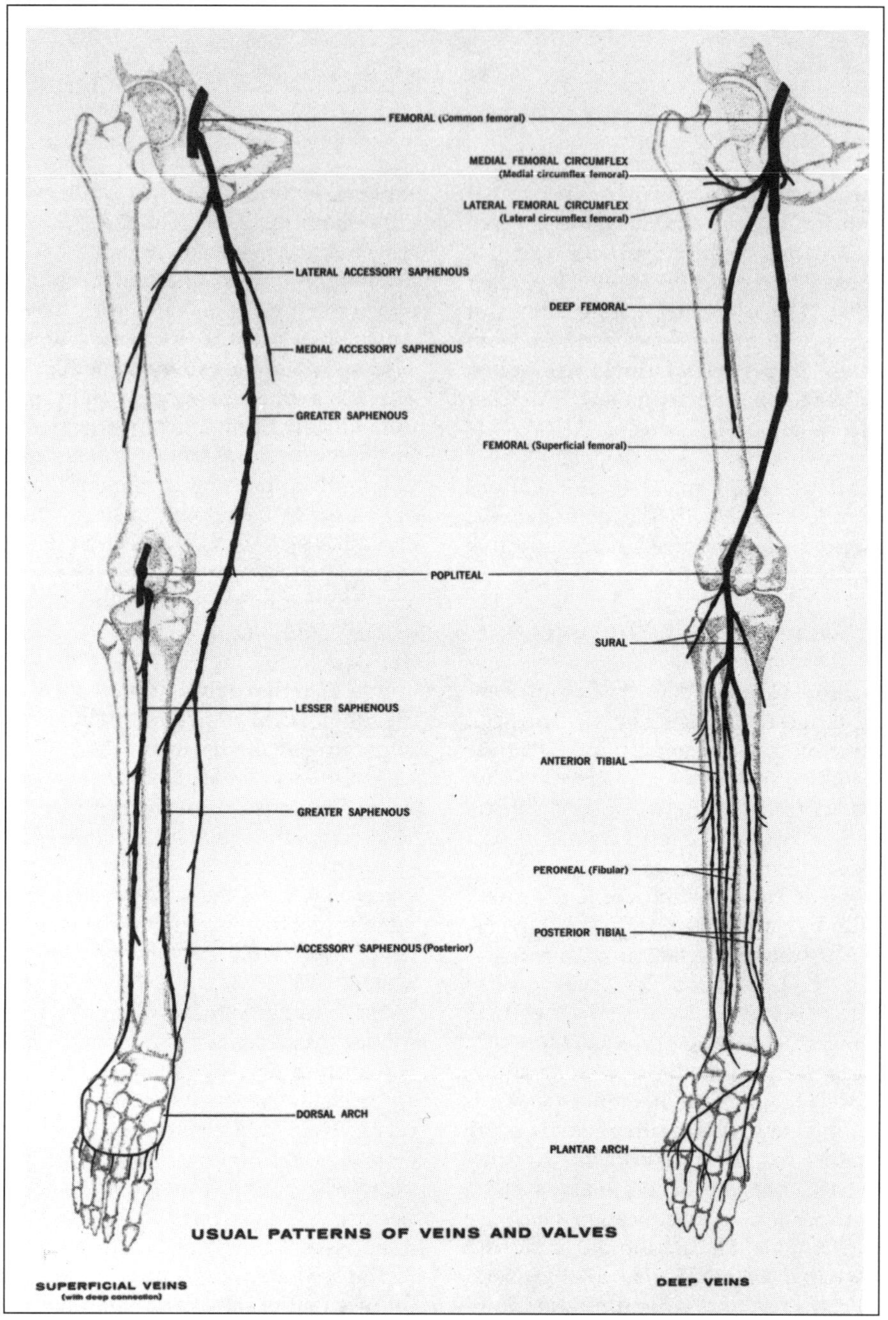

Fig. 47-1. Anatomy of superficial and deep veins of the leg. Note slight enlargement at common sites of valves. (Reprinted courtesy of Eastman Kodak Company and JA DeWeese, University of Rochester School of Medicine and Dentistry, Rochester, NY.)

the lateral border of the first rib. The internal jugular joins to form the innominate (brachiocephalic) vein, which then joins the opposite innominate to form the superior vena cava. Valves are rarely present proximal to the axillary vein.

PHYSIOLOGY

The **volume** of blood in the venous system is 65 to 75 percent of the total blood volume, or about three times the volume of blood in the arterial system. The veins are capacitance vessels that constrict in response to systemic hypovolemia and act to moderate the effects of gravitational shifts in blood during changes in posture. Normally, assuming a standing position increases leg blood volume promptly by about 500 cc [11]. During prolonged quiet standing, the uninterrupted elevation of hydrostatic pressure in excess of opposing oncotic pressure and tissue pressure causes a gradual increase in interstitial fluid volume that may approach 15 percent of circulating blood volume. Increasing tissue pressure by use of elastic com-

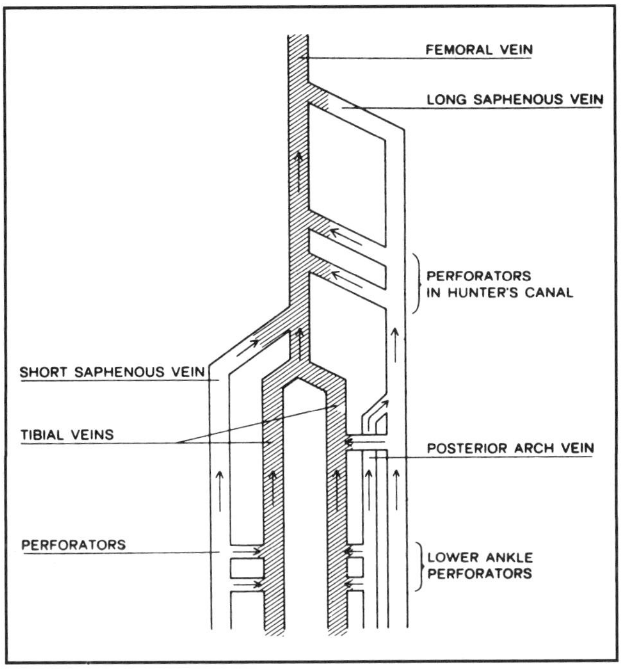

Fig. 47-2. Diagrammatic representation of flow from superficial veins (clear) through perforators into the deep system (shaded). (Reproduced with permission from K Haeger. The anatomy of the veins of the leg. In JT Hobbs. The Treatment of Venous Disorders. Philadelphia: Lippincott, 1977. P. 19.)

pression decreases that fluid sequestration. Activation of muscle contraction causes venous volume in the extremities to fall dramatically.

Pressure at any particular location in the venous system is a composite of static filling pressure, hydrostatic pressure, and cardiogenic pressure [12]. Static filling pressure is determined by the elasic recoil of the vein wall, extravascular tissue pressure, and atmospheric pressure and is normally less than 2 cm of water. Hydrostatic pressure is determined by the vertical distance of the vein from the right atrium. Cardiogenic pressure is determined by the pumping and siphoning actions of the heart. Hydrostatic pressure changes dramatically with posture, varying at the ankle from about 10 mm Hg recumbent, to 50–60 mm Hg sitting, to 80–100 mm Hg standing [13]. Hydrostatic-pressure changes are equal in neighboring arteries and veins, with no impact on the cardiogenic arteriovenous pressure gradient in dependent limbs. Because veins are collapsible, elevation of a limb causes near closure of its veins. With limb elevation arterial hydrostatic pressure also decreases, and, since venous hydrostatic pressure can go no lower than zero, the arteriovenous pressure gradient decreases. If venous valves are normal, contraction of the muscles in the deep compartments reduces pressure in the distal venous tree, with values below 30 mm Hg in the distal parts of the lower extremity (Fig. 47-3). Intermittent muscle contraction has no persistent effect on arterial pressure; therefore, the overall arteriovenous pressure gradient is increased during exercise, enhancing flow across the capillary bed.

Flow of venous blood centripetally toward the heart is driven by energy and pressure gradients that are determined by cardiac contraction, peripheral muscle contraction, respiratory action, and posture [12]. Heart pumping maintains a pressure gradient of about 15 mm Hg from the venule level to the right atrium. Muscle contraction in the extremities in the presence of normal venous valves provides a strong propulsive force for venous blood, supplying as much as 30 percent of the energy driving overall circulation during strenuous exercise [14]. The function of that so-called muscle pump, centered in the gastrocnemius and soleus muscles in the lower limbs, is analogous to the action of the heart on the arterial side of the circulation (Fig. 47-4). During muscle contraction (systole), valves in the communicating veins close to prevent flow back into the superficial system, as antegrade flow is augmented in both deep and superficial veins. During muscle relaxation (diastole), the valves of the deep system close, minimizing retrograde flow and allowing the deep system to refill from the superficial veins and the capillary bed. Some degree of valvular reflux or leakage occurs in normal asymptomatic subjects [15–17]. Respiration cyclically alters extravascular pressure in the thorax and abdomen, influencing flow in the veins within those cavities. The Valsalva maneuver can stop flow in both upper and lower limbs by greatly increasing intracavitary pressure and collapsing the trunk veins.

Chronic Disorders of Superficial Veins of the Lower Limb

Varicose veins are pathologically enlarged subcutaneous venous channels, variably involving partially or entirely the greater and lesser saphenous systems or their tributaries. It has been estimated that 12 percent of the adult population harbors significant varicose veins for which symptomatic relief might be sought at one time or another [1]. Adding small veins of strictly cosmetic importance increases the overall incidence. In **primary** varicose veins, the problem originates in the superficial system, with no involvement of the deep subfascial veins. In the case of **secondary** varicose veins, superficial veins become enlarged as a result of disease originating in the deep system and communicating veins. Among a large number of patients presenting for therapy at the Mayo Clinic, 72 percent were thought to have primary varicose veins and 28 percent to have secondary veins. The greater saphenous system was involved five to six times more often than the lesser saphenous [18].

PATHOGENESIS AND PATHOPHYSIOLOGY

Patients seeking therapy for varicose veins most commonly are beyond their third decade of life, with advancing age clearly associated with increasing incidence and severity of varicose veins [18]. Suggested mechanisms of pathogenesis of primary varicose veins include defective structure and function of valves in the saphenous vein, intrinsic weakness of the vein walls, and the presence of tiny arteriovenous connections that gradually lead to venous engorgement. More than 50 percent of individuals with primary varicose veins have a family history [18], suggesting that there is an inherited defect in vein struc-

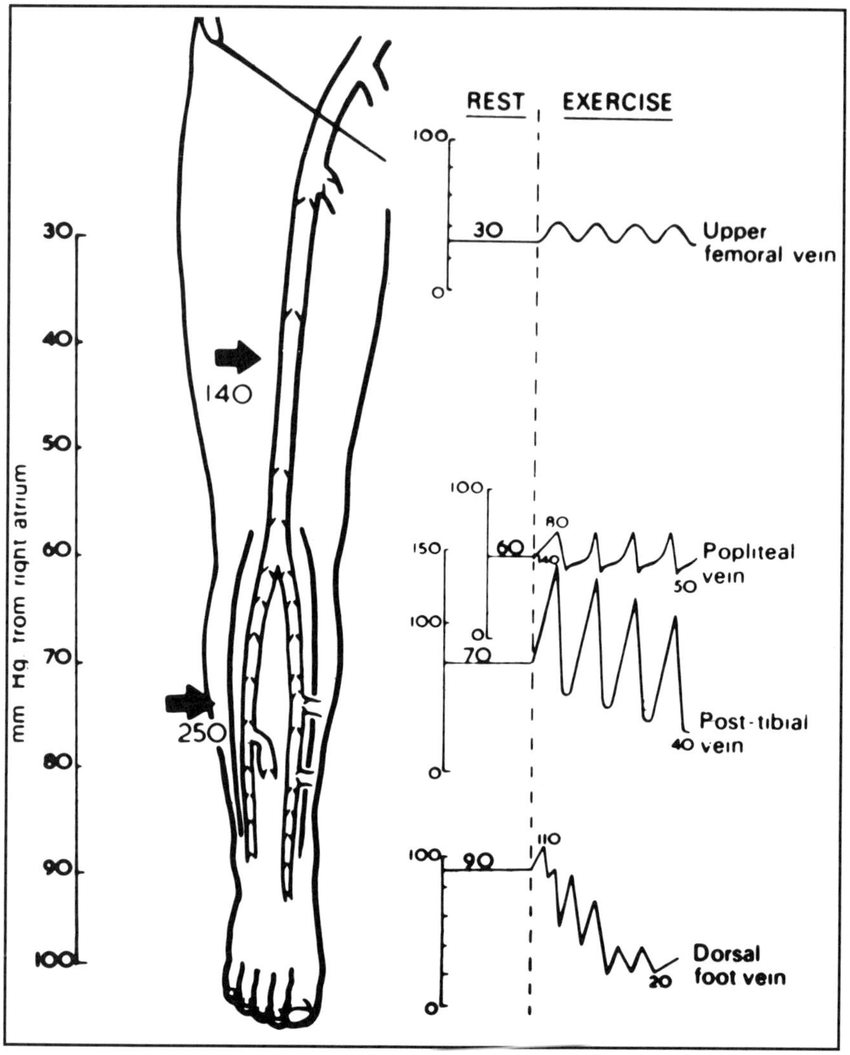

Fig. 47 3. Pressure changes in the normal dependent leg at rest and with exercise. Hydrostatic pressure is highest in the distal leg at rest, lowest in the distal leg with exercise if deep valves are intact. (Reproduced with permission from D Negus. Perforating vein interruption in the postphlebitic syndrome. In JJ Bergan, JST Yao. Surgery of the Veins. Orlando: Saunders, 1985. P. 193.)

ture or function that predisposes to varicosity. In one study, saphenofemoral reflux detected by Doppler ultrasound was twice as common in children of parents with varicose veins as in children of parents without varicosities [19]. Attenuation and disorganization of connective tissue and smooth muscle components in varicose veins have been noted [20,21], as well as increased collagen content and reduced elastin content and elasticity [22,23], suggesting that a cellular synthetic defect may predispose toward varicosity, perhaps on a familial basis. Events during pregnancy include increased intravascular volume, elevated pressure on the intra-abdominal and pelvic veins, and perhaps softening of vein walls along with many other connective-tissue elements, which helps to explain the 2 : 1 female-to-male prevalence ratio of significant varicose veins [24].

A number of observers have noted the high level of oxygen saturation in blood obtained from varicose veins [25,26]. Anatomic study [27,28] and careful survey using Doppler ultrasound [29] have found evidence of minute arteriovenous fistulas connecting to the varicose system. It is unclear whether those fistulas are causative or arise at a later stage of development of the lesions, and the contribution of those connections to typical varicose veins remains somewhat controversial. Fistulas do not occur in the Klippel-Trenaunay syndrome, where large superficial varicosities occur on a congenital basis, associated with cutaneous nevi and bone and soft-tissue hypertrophy [30,31].

By definition, secondary varicose veins arise as a result of disease of the deep veins. Most often, deep-vein thrombosis (DVT) is the inciting factor, resulting in deep valvular incompetence leading to communicator incompetence or in deep-vein occlusion leading to enlargement of superficial veins as collateral channels. In a minority of patients, primary valvular reflux in the deep veins or communicat-

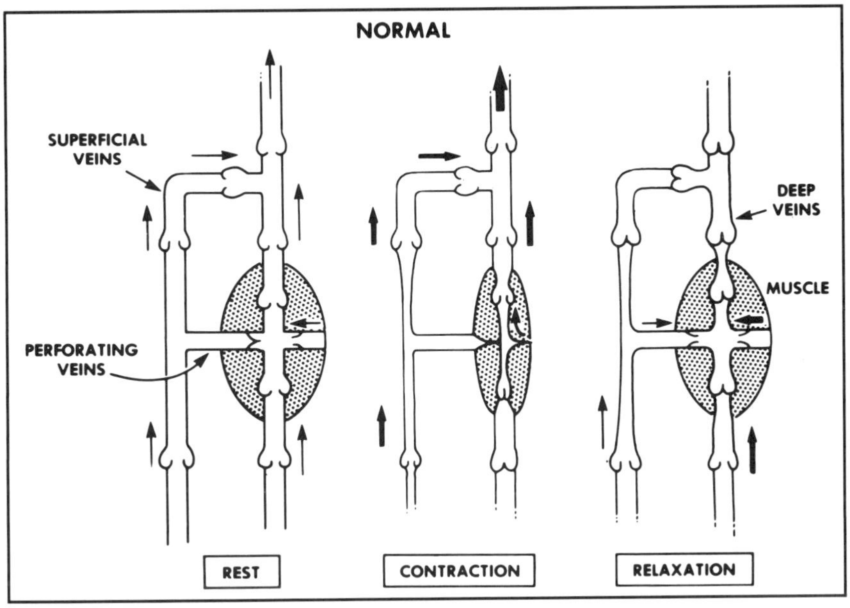

Fig. 47-4. Normal action of the "muscle pump." Blood flows up the deep veins with systolic muscle contraction against competent distal and perforator valves. Flow through open distal valves into the empty pump occurs during diastole. (Reproduced with permission from DS Sumner. Venous dynamics-varicosities. Clin Obstet Gynecol 1981; 24:743–760.)

ing veins gives rise to secondary varicosities without prior DVT [32].

Regardless of the original cause of varicose veins, the resulting abnormality is enlargement of normal veins. Valvular incompetence is present in the varicosities and, as blood refluxes, further venous enlargement pulls the valve leaflets apart, causing more valvular incompetence in sections of the adjacent distal vein and branches. As the segment of engorged vein becomes longer, the hydrostatic pressure exerted by the uninterrupted column of blood increases. Furthermore, with exercise, pressures fail to decrease normally because effective valves are absent [33] (Fig. 47-5). Eventually, communicating veins may become involved when they are exposed to high pressures below an incompetent valve in the main channel [34]. When communicator incompetence is present, activation of the muscle pump forcefully ejects blood outward into the superficial system, greatly increasing pressures on the subcutaneous tissues. With return to the deep system through adjacent competent communicators, ineffective circus motion of venous blood occurs with each muscle contraction. With high pressures and inefficient emptying of the leg, edema and microscopic extravasation of cellular elements of blood can occur, with a secondary inflammatory reaction in the subcutaneous tissues. Although it is much more common with deep venous insufficiency, that process confined solely to primary superficial varicosities can lead to eczema and ulceration of the skin, particularly in the more severe cases involving secondary communicator incompetency [35–37].

The presence of varicose veins is associated epidemiologically with a two- to fourfold increased risk of DVT [38]. Much of this statistical risk is due to the presence of secondary varicosities, where there is also deep venous disease increasing the risk of recurrent thrombosis. Superficial phlebitis also occurs, typically with abrupt onset of red, painful induration along the course of the vein. Recent reports suggest that about 20 percent of instances of superficial phlebitis are associated with DVT, presumably via connections at communicating veins or the saphenofemoral junction, and more commonly with thigh-segment than calf-segment phlebitis [39,40]. Phlebitis of the superficial veins alone presents no significant threat of postphlebitic syndrome or pulmonary embolism. It is also important to note that patients with repetitive attacks of superficial phlebitis may be harboring a malignancy.

CLINICAL MANIFESTATIONS

History. The most common complaint of patients with varicose veins concerns the cosmetic appearance of their legs. Often a relatively small cluster of veins becomes visible in a young woman with a family history, and there is concern about arresting the process before it becomes unmanageable. Many patients are also concerned about the possibility of developing dangerous blood clots in the veins. Most patients with involvement of a long segment of vein that extends across the knee or ankle joint have some discomfort. The typical syndrome involves a dull ache, heaviness, or pressure sensation in the area of the vein, particularly after a period of standing, with relief on elevation of the leg. In women, those complaints usually are more noticeable immediately prior to the menses and become dramatically worse during pregnancy. Superficial phlebitis occurs episodically in some patients. A small percentage of patients with extensive primary varicose veins develop eczema and ulceration at the level of the ankle [35–37]. Finally, some extremely superficial varicose veins may be subject to rupture with a startling

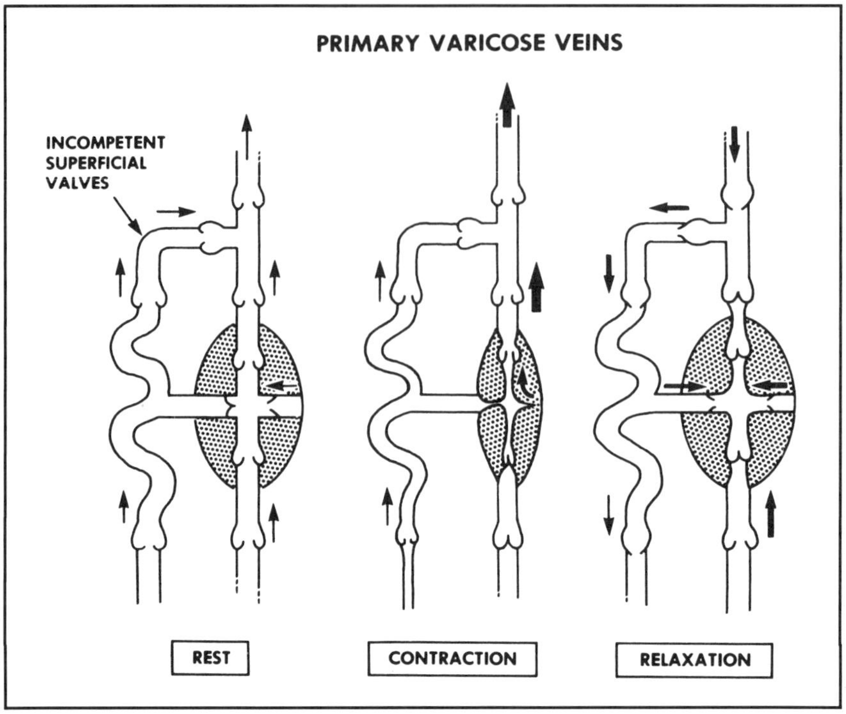

Fig. 47-5. Abnormal "muscle pump" with primary varicose veins. Significant reflux of blood down the incompetent superficial system occurs, with filling of pump from proximal veins, resulting in inefficient circular flow of blood and impaired reduction in distal venous pressure. (Reproduced with permission from DS Sumner. Venous dynamics-varicosities. Clin Obstet Gynecol 1981; 24:743–760.)

amount of bleeding, which can be dangerous because it is painless and therefore can go unnoticed.

Physical Findings. Simple examination of the legs demonstrates most varicosities, which are more easily seen over the calf and ankle than over the thigh. The dependent position with oblique lighting enhances visibility (Figs. 47-6, 47-7). If the subcutaneous tissue is thick, veins are not as evident, in which case palpation is helpful. Enlarged veins generally can be balloted, particularly with the leg in the dependent position. Percussion of a distal portion of a vein transmits a fluid wave proximally, proving continuity. When valvular competence is in question, percussion of a vein proximally transmits a fluid wave distally when the valves are not functional. The wave is dampened by a competent valve. Similar abnormal retrograde-pulse transmission can be elicited by coughing when all proximal valves are incompetent.

Primary and secondary varicosities can be differentiated by the Brodie-Trendelenburg test [41,42] (Fig. 47-8). The leg is raised and a tourniquet is placed above the knee to obstruct the flow of blood through the superficial veins. The leg is then lowered to a dependent position while the examiner monitors filling of the varicosities over the calf and ankle. If the varicosities fill promptly, there must be reflux of blood through incompetent communicators from an incompetent deep venous system, which makes the varicose veins secondary. On the other hand, if filling with a tourniquet in place takes more than 20 seconds with prompt filling only after removal of the tourniquet, the source of reflux is likely to be the superficial system, making those varicose veins primary. In some patients, both deep-communicator and superficial incompetence are identified by the Brodie Trendelenburg test.

Perthes' test can be used to elicit the presence of deep-vein valvular incompetence or occlusion of hemodynamic importance with consequent secondary varicosities [43] (Fig. 47-9). A tourniquet is placed on the elevated leg at midthigh or proximal calf level to obstruct the superficial veins, and the patient is asked to walk. With deep valvular reflux, varicosities below the tourniquet enlarge as blood is forced retrograde through incompetent communicators to the superficial system. If significant obstruction is present in the deep system, typical venous claudication accompanies exercise. Under that circumstance, the secondary varicose veins are critical collateral channels and should not be interrupted or removed. Other occasional findings of significance are the presence of thickened cords over chronically occluded veins and changes consistent with chronic venous hypertension such as induration and hyperpigmentation.

Laboratory. Laboratory study of varicose veins rarely is necessary. On occasion, however, certain techniques may be helpful to supplement the physical examination, particularly when there is a question about the status of the deep venous system. Using Doppler ultrasound to detect flow, the percussion tests can be performed with greater

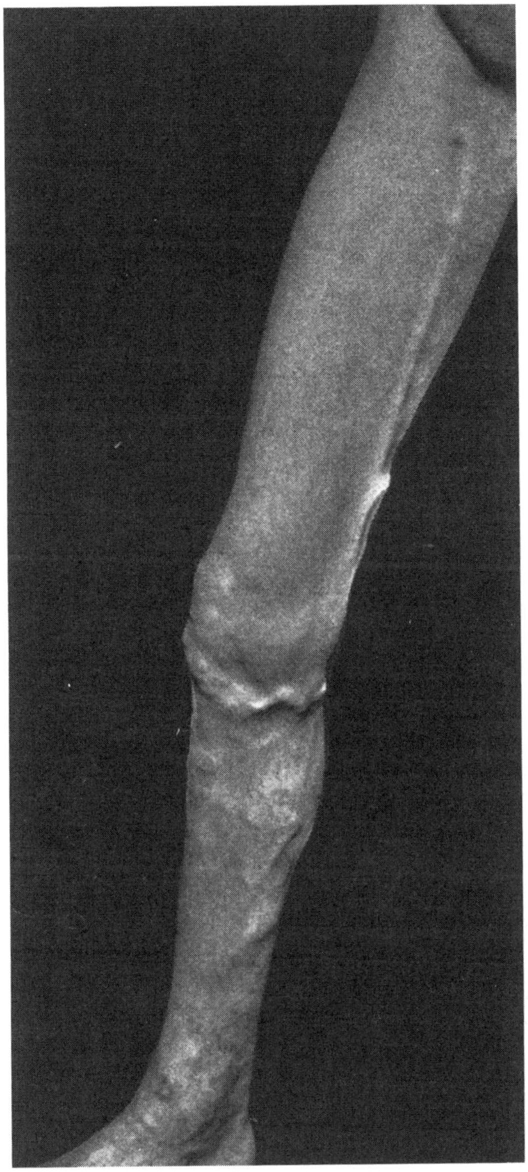

Fig. 47-6. Primary varicose veins involving the greater saphenous vein and calf tributaries. (Reproduced with permission from H Dodd, FB Cockett. The Pathology and Surgery of the Veins of the Lower Limb. Edinburgh: Livingstone, 1976. P. 91.)

precision. The presence of venous occlusions also can be detected in both superficial and deep systems, and communicating veins can be located with the Doppler probe [44].

A variant of the Brodie-Trendelenburg test can be performed using the photoplethysmograph, which detects blood volume in the subcutaneous capillary bed [45,46]. After a baseline reading is obtained at the ankle level, ankle flexion several times in succession normally decreases blood volume in the veins, reducing the baseline tracing dramatically. Refilling of the veins after exercise normally takes more than 20 seconds. In the presence of valvular reflux, emptying with ankle flexion is less efficient, and venous refill time after exercise occurs in less than 20 seconds. Placement of a tourniquet immediately below the knee normalizes refill time if reflux involves the superficial veins (primary varicosities). If refill time remains shortened with the tourniquet in place, reflux must involve incompetent communicating veins from a diseased deep venous system (secondary varicosities). Impedance plethysmography, phleborheography, and venous ultrasound imaging are useful mainly to help document patency of the large proximal veins of the deep system.

Ascending venography is a precise means of defining venous anatomy [47] and is rarely, if ever, indicated in evaluating varicose veins. Radiographic dye is introduced into a foot vein, and, with a tourniquet placed at the level of the ankle, the dye is forced to flow into the deep system outlining the deep veins. If incompetent communicators are present, reflux into the superficial system is detected. With no ankle tourniquet, dye introduced at the level of the foot remains largely superficial, outlining the saphenous vein and associated varicosities. Venography by direct puncture of a varicosity is sometimes useful to outline unusual vein patterns.

MANAGEMENT

Conservative Measures. An important aspect of the management of varicose veins is patient education about natural history, emphasizing the small potential for major impact on health. It is particularly helpful to differentiate between venous disease and the more ominous course of arterial disease and between superficial and deep venous disease, especially with regard to the potential for thrombosis and pulmonary embolism. An understanding of the pathophysiology of varicose veins encourages compliance with conservative measures by which to reduce symptoms and retard progression of vein enlargement.

Among those measures, elastic support is most useful. Numerous brands of pantyhose or styled stocking are commercially available for both men and women. To be effective, stockings must fit firmly with diminishing compression as the garment ascends the leg, avoiding a proximal constricting band [48]. Graduated external compression should provide a counterbalance to the graduated hydrostatic pressure within the superficial veins. The most precise physiologic control is afforded by prescription stockings measured to fit properly and available either off the shelf or by custom tailoring. Prescription stockings can be designed to provide compression pressures at the ankle ranging from 20 to 60 mm Hg. Compression at the ankle of 20 to 30 mm Hg is sufficient for most patients with primary varicose veins. Knee-length hose are quite satisfactory, although name-brand thigh-length or pantyhose-style stockings with sufficient elasticity are often preferred by women. Special maternity brands are advisable during the last trimester of pregnancy. Trial and error of various types may be necessary to balance efficacy against comfort, cost, and appearance. Stockings lose their elasticity with wear and washing, and patients should be aware that new garments will be needed every few months.

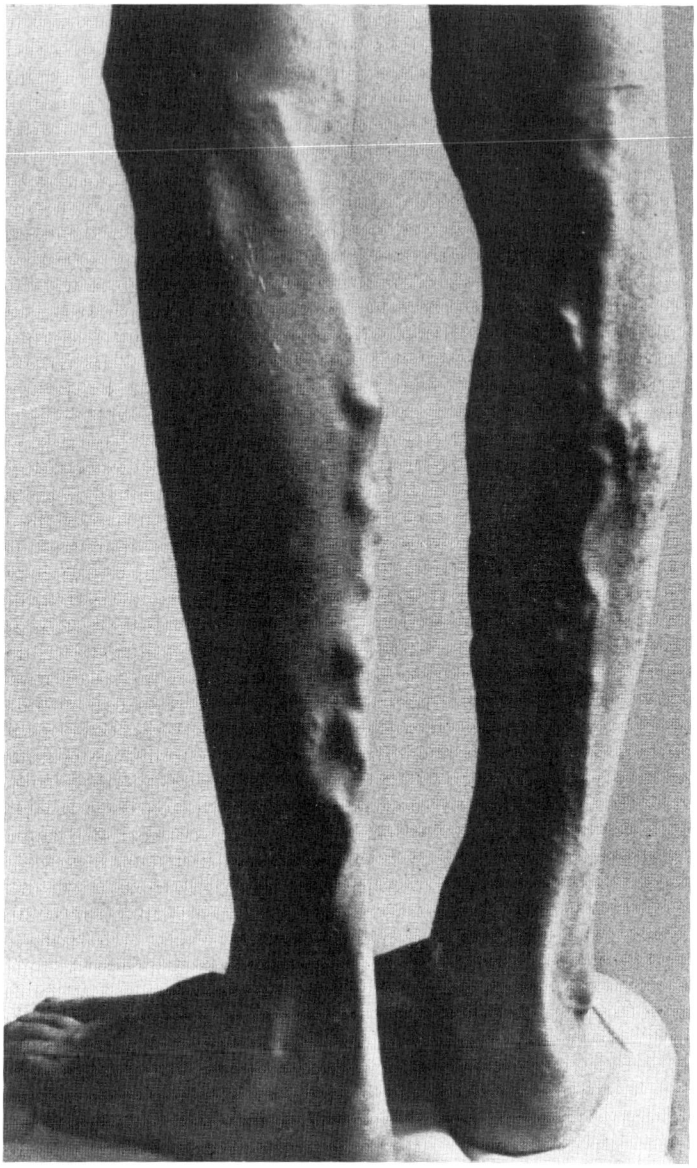

Fig. 47-7. Bilateral primary lesser saphenous varicose veins, seen best in indirect light. (Reproduced with permission from H Dodd, FB Cockett. The Pathology and Surgery of the Veins of the Lower Limb. Edinburgh: Livingstone, 1976. P. 94.)

Ablative Measures. If symptoms warrant, ablation of varicose veins is possible with minimal morbidity. Sclerotherapy has been used extensively in Europe and is gaining popularity in North America; it has the major advantage of avoiding hospital costs since it is easily performed in the office setting. The principle of therapy is to inject a material into the varicosities that induces inflammation and scarring sufficient to close the lumen. Various methods employ different sclerosing liquids (e.g., 50% glucose; hydroxypolyethoxidodecaine, 0.5–3.0%; sodium tetradecyl sulfate, 1–3%) and different regimens of compression and activity to optimize efficacy [49–52]. In general, after careful mapping of the involved veins, a small-gauge needle on a syringe containing the sclerosant is inserted into the vein with the leg in a dependent position. The syringe is taped to the leg while two or three other veins are punctured. The leg is then elevated to empty the veins, and 0.5 cc of the sclerosant is slowly injected into the vein at each site. Compression with a gauze pad and tape is applied over the vein as the needle is withdrawn. At the completion of the injections, with the leg still elevated, a firm elastic bandage is wrapped carefully from the foot to six inches above the most proximal injection site. Patients are instructed to maintain their usual activities, to avoid prolonged sitting or standing, and to leave the bandage in place for several days. Some physicians recommend continuous compression for as long as 6 weeks [49], but others [51] indicate that the inconvenience is probably

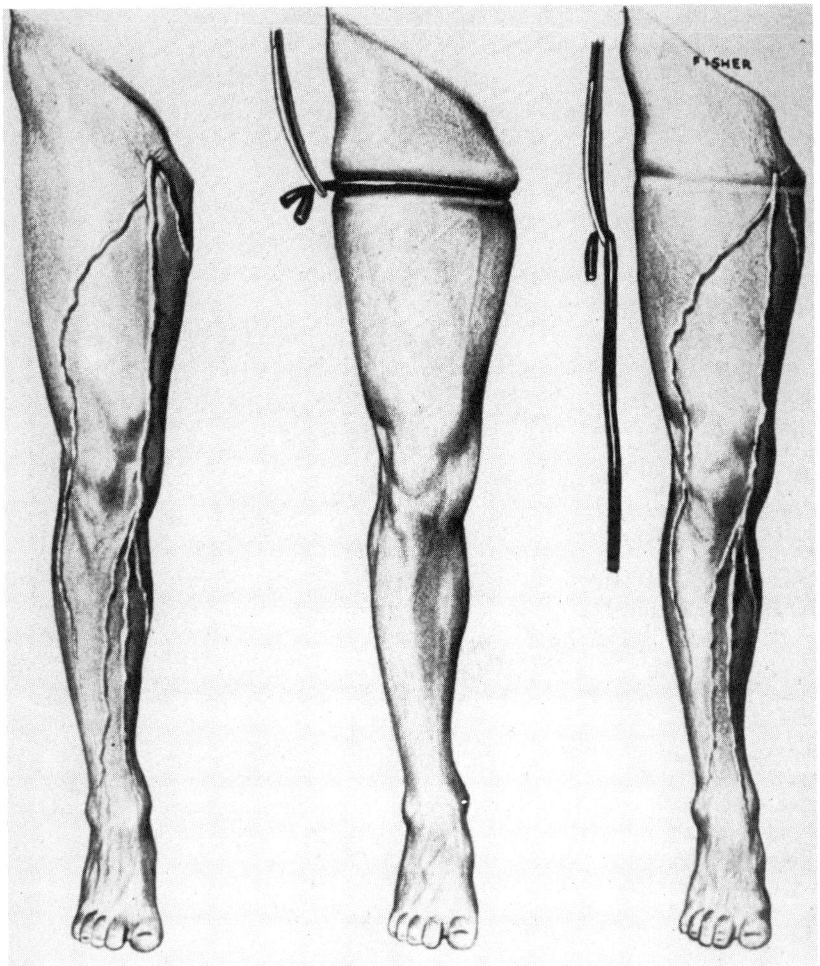

Fig. 47-8. Brodie-Trendelenburg test demonstrating primary varicosity of the greater saphenous vein. Vein fills with leg dependency and no tourniquet (left). After elevation to empty the vein, tourniquet is applied that obstructs abnormal retrograde filling of the varicosity with dependency (center). Release of the tourniquet allows prompt reflux to fill varicose system (right). (Reproduced with permission from H Dodd, FB Cockett. The Pathology and Surgery of the Veins of the Lower Limb. Edinburgh: Livingstone, 1976. P. 82.)

unnecessary and that equivalent results may be obtained with periods as short as 8 hours [50]. The patient returns to the office for removal of the bandages and inspection of the early results. Further injections can be performed at that visit, and the cycle repeated until all troublesome veins are eliminated. The occluded veins are palpable as sclerotic cords and may be faintly visible after sclerosis.

Severe complications from sclerotherapy have been estimated to occur in about 0.1 percent of patients [52], with mild local reactions in up to 10 percent [51]. Occasionally, there is extravasation of sclerosant from the injection site, which can cause subcutaneous inflammation or even sloughing of a small disk of skin. Hyperpigmentation over the course of the injected vein occurs in some patients. Very rarely, a systemic reaction results from the injection, or the sclerotic process extends to the deep veins [53].

Early results (the first 1 to 3 years) generally are excellent in over 80 percent of patients [49,51]. In smaller superficial veins or lower-leg communicating veins, the recurrence rate at 5 years was 19 percent in one careful study by Hobbs [52,54]. The 5-year recurrence rate in the large main venous trunks, however, was 69 percent, presumably owing to the continued presence of the causative valvular defect in the main saphenous or communicating vein. Such large saphenous varicosities are treated more effectively with surgery in most instances.

Surgical therapy is directed at ligating the varicose system at its origin and removing the varicosities to prevent persistent filling by capillary inflow and collateral routes. Early efforts employed ligation alone, often with only a temporary decrease in vein size [55]. Many surgeons then began to use extensive ligation and stripping of both greater and lesser saphenous veins in attempts to ablate the entire superficial system. Most recently, particularly with recognition of the value of the saphenous vein as a conduit for arterial bypass, efforts have been made to use

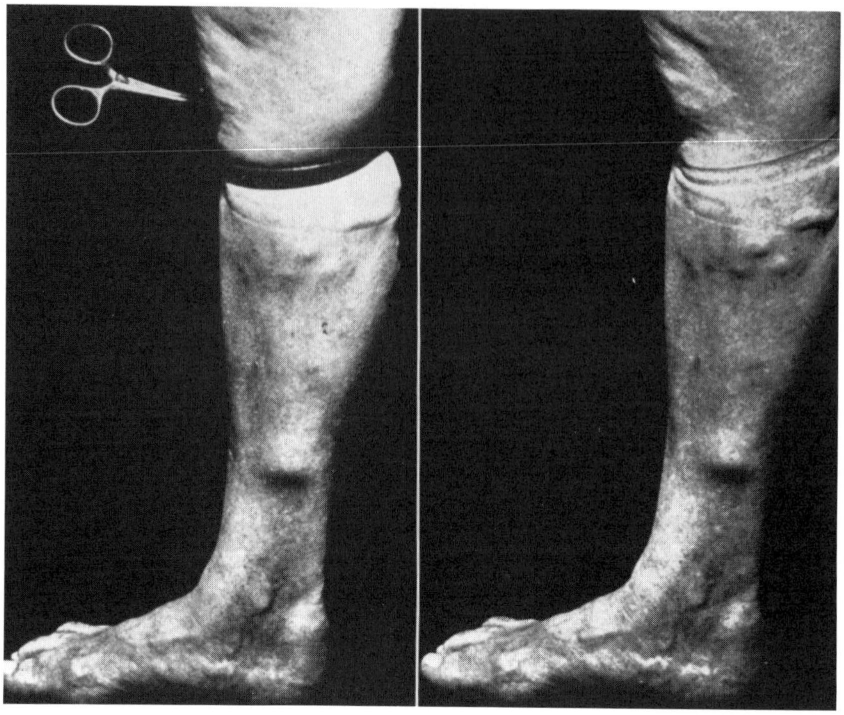

Fig. 47-9. Perthes' test, demonstrating secondary varicosity of calf veins. After elevation of leg to empty varicosities, tourniquet is applied to obstruct retrograde flow down the superficial system, and leg dependency is restored. At rest, varicosities may enlarge promptly due to reflux down incompetent deep veins and out incompetent communicators. With exercise (left), muscle-pump action accentuates abnormal flow through perforators into the varicosities, particularly if proximal deep-vein obstruction is present, with no augmentation of varicose filling from above after tourniquet is released (right). (Reproduced with permission from H Dodd, FB Cockett. The Pathology and Surgery of the Veins of the Lower Limb. Edinburgh: Livingstone, 1976. P. 84.)

surgery more selectively, directed at specific segments and branches of the main veins [56].

The procedure generally requires at least a spinal or epidural anesthetic but usually can be performed without overnight hospitalization. Typically, after careful preoperative mapping, a small incision is placed at the distal end of the involved vein, near the medial malleolus in the case of the greater saphenous. An internal vein stripper is advanced proximally, a counterincision is made over the saphenofemoral junction, and the stripper secured. The ends of the vein are ligated, leaving the proximal saphenous vein flush with the common femoral vein. The stripper is then used to pull the vein out and downward toward the foot, with less likelihood of traumatic saphenous neuropathy than when the vein is pulled upward [57]. Side branches are avulsed during the process, and any significant residual branches can be removed separately with an internal or external stripper or simply ligated through a series of several small incisions. An alternative method uses a series of small punctures placed over the course of branches of the varicose system, employing a small hook to pull the veins out for removal and enabling preservation of much of the main saphenous trunk [58].

Postoperatively, the leg is wrapped with an elastic bandage, and ambulation held to a minimum for 8 to 12 hours. There is receding postoperative pain for a few days, as well as ecchymosis and edema over the track of the vein, which resolve within 2 to 3 weeks. Return to many activities is possible within a week, with the use of compression for comfort. Occasional hemorrhage, infection, and local neuropathy occur, but DVT and other significant morbidity and mortality are rare [59]. With a thorough surgical approach to saphenous varicosities, at least 85 percent of patients remain free of recurrences at 5 years [60]. Hobbs, in a randomized trial of surgery and sclerotherapy, found a 12-percent incidence of recurrence at 5 years among patients treated surgically for large saphenous-system veins [52]. On the other hand, the 5-year recurrence rate of lower-limb communicating veins and superficial small veins treated surgically was approximately 56 percent, suggesting that the less tractable smaller veins may be treated more cost effectively by primary sclerotherapy. Optimal ablative therapy of varicose veins combines surgery and sclerotherapy, depending on the presenting pathology [59].

SPIDER VEINS

Clusters of small cutaneous veins occur frequently, particularly in women after childbirth and as middle age approaches. The lesions often appear to arise from a single feeding vein with a caput medusa pattern of serpiginous branches. This arrangement has led to the names **venous telangiectasia, spider hemangioma,** and **spider vein.** Alternatively, the veins may take on a linear pattern. Their distribution varies from a few isolated locations in the thigh or calf to diffuse involvement throughout the legs, most heavily around the ankles and feet. Self-consciousness about the appearance of the legs is the only usual complaint.

Therapy emphasizes education about the veins and their benign natural history. Hose and makeup are effective ways of covering the veins in many instances. Alternatively, sclerotherapy using a 30-gauge needle, magnification, and a suitable sclerosant solution is possible. Patients should be warned that a blemish as bad or worse than the venous abnormality itself could result should there be extravasation at the site of injection. Lasers [61] and electrocautery [62] also have been used to obliterate spider veins.

Chronic Disorders of Deep Veins of the Lower Limb

The general term **venous insufficiency** refers to the physiologic consequence of either deep-vein obstruction, valvular incompetence, or a combination of both lesions. The terms **postphlebitic** and **postthrombotic** are commonly used to describe the pathologic and clinical features of venous insufficiency arising from DVT, the most common etiology of deep venous disorders. Modern prospective analysis has demonstrated that within 5 years after DVT, up to 80 percent of patients have signs, symptoms, or laboratory findings of venous insufficiency [63–68]. From an epidemiologic standpoint, cutaneous manifestations of deep venous insufficiency of the lower extremities were found in about 20 percent of employees in one study, with severe changes in 9 percent and a history of ulceration in 1.3 percent [2]. The prevalence of severe venous insufficiency has been estimated at about 0.5 percent of the population of England and Wales [69]. The discussion that follows focuses on the mechanisms of obstruction and valvular incompetence separately, though they often are simultaneously operative in a given patient.

PATHOGENESIS AND PATHOPHYSIOLOGY

Valvular Incompetence. The most important cause of chronic venous insufficiency in the lower extremities is valvular incompetence of the deep veins [70]. In most instances, that condition arises after DVT, when the majority of veins eventually become partially or totally recanalized [64,71,72]. In the process of phlebitic inflammation, the extremely delicate valve leaflets become thickened, shortened, or embedded in the scarred vein wall, rendering them incapable of promoting antegrade flow and of halting retrograde flow of blood [73]. Rather than a fine, reactive unidirectional channel, the vein becomes a rigid, thick-walled tube with remnants of ineffectual valves and fibrous synechiae strung across its lumen. Secondary valvular incompetence arises in areas distal to either chronic obstruction or significant reflux, where high pressures distend the vein, causing the leaflets to elongate, separate, and leak [70]. There is some evidence that rapid clearance of acute DVT with fibrinolytic agents may protect valve leaflets from damage sufficiently to diminish the impact of postphlebitic sequelae [73,74–77].

Floppy valves with redundant, leaky cusps may occur as a primary disorder without previous DVT; they have been studied in some detail [32,78]. Valvular reflux occurs in normal, asymptomatic subjects [15,17]; therefore, pathologic incompetence simply may be an accentuation of a physiologic phenomenon. More severe degrees of primary reflux can lead to symptoms and secondary communicator involvement with varicose veins. Reduced numbers of valves and rare congenital absence [79,80] of venous valves have been recognized.

Valvular reflux to the popliteal and tibial levels is more damaging than is isolated reflux at more proximal levels [81–83]. In the presence of valvular incompetence, efficient directional flow of blood and emptying of the deep veins cannot occur (Fig. 47-10). With activation of the muscle pump, blood is driven partially in retrograde directions determined by the pattern of valve damage. Pressure in the distal venous tree and deep tissues fails to decrease normally during muscle activity [33,84]. Secondary communicating-vein and superficial-system engorgement and valvular failure occur, subjecting the subcutaneous tissues to high pressures, particularly during muscle contraction [85–87].

Muscle biopsies from patients with valvular incompetence reveal atrophic changes and enlargement and fibrosis of the interstitial space [88]. There is an increase in the number of capillaries in the subcutaneous tissue, with abnormally high levels of fibrinogen and fibrin in the interstitial space [89]. Macrophages and other inflammatory cells appear, leading to pericapillary fibrosis manifested as subcutaneous thickening and induration. Hemosiderin deposits result from erythrocyte lysis, causing brown pigmentation. Recurring episodes of barotrauma and persistent venous capillary hypertension, interstitial edema, and inflammation cause local hypoxia [90] and malnutrition. Fat necrosis and liposclerosis occur, followed by loss of skin integrity with consequent eczema and ulceration. At that stage, secondary bacterial colonization and invasion can occur, with cellulitis greatly aggravating the process. Secondary lymphatic insufficiency occurs with progressive sclerosis of lymph channels in the face of increased demands for clearance of interstitial fluid. With chronicity, tissue fibrosis causes relative fixation of the ankle joint, with subsequent disuse atrophy of the involved muscular apparatus. In a small number of long-standing chronic ulcers, malignant degeneration occurs to form a Marjolin's ulcer.

Obstruction. In the lower extremity, DVT accounts for the bulk of chronic partial or total vein obstruction. Although the majority of veins recanalize after thrombosis, large proximal veins are more likely to remain occluded than are distal ones [91]. Other rare causes of intrinsic obstruction are recognized, including venous aplastic lesions [92,93], webs in the vena cava [94], and primary venous tumors, seen most frequently in the vena cava [95]. Extrinsic obstruction of the left common iliac vein may occur

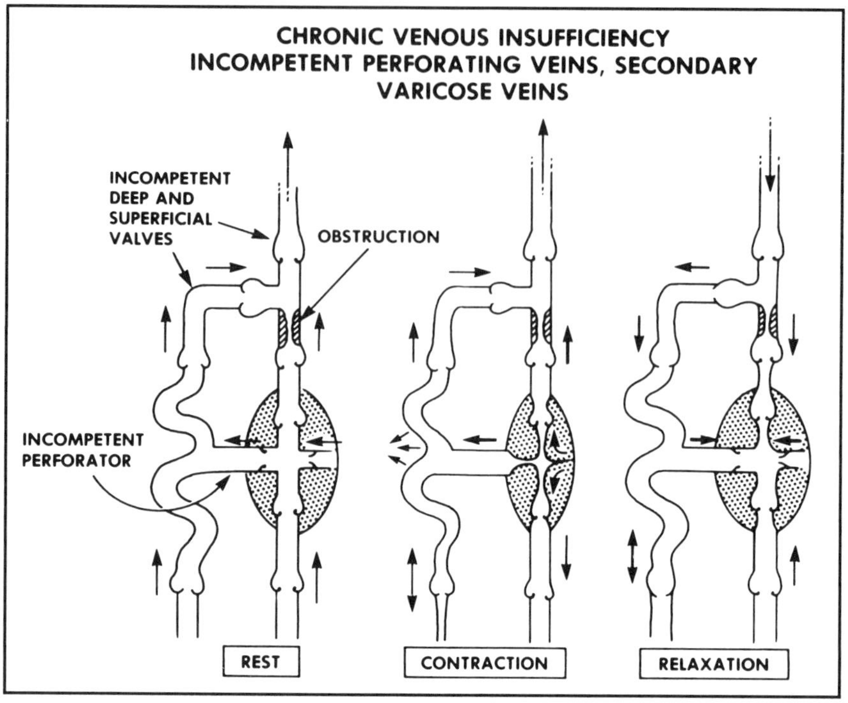

Fig. 47-10. Abnormal "muscle pump" with deep venous insufficiency and secondary varicose veins. Muscle contraction with some proximal obstruction and incompetent deep, communicating, and superficial veins causes retrograde flow in all veins, resulting in high pressures in distal leg. (Reprinted with permission from DS Sumner. Venous dynamics-varicosities. Clin Obstet Gynecol 1981; 24:743–760.)

as the right common iliac artery crosses anterior to the vein [96]. Other examples of extrinsic compression include fibrous bands across the iliac veins [97], tumor masses, and aneurysms arising in arteries such as the femoral or popliteal, which are adjacent to major veins. Important veins occasionally are ligated or removed by surgery or become obstructed in association with trauma. For years, vena cava and femoral vein ligations were carried out to prevent pulmonary embolism. The more modern nonocclusive caval filtering devices lead to caval occlusion in 4 to 5 percent of patients [98].

Isolated obstructions in smaller veins of the lower extremity, such as those below the knee, produce little hemodynamic impact on the limb as a whole. Obstruction at levels at or above the popliteal vein compromises venous flow, with physiologic and clinical impact depending on the availability of collaterals [99]. The effects of obstruction are most marked acutely after an abrupt occlusion of a major vein. In acute experiments on dogs [100], ligation of the common femoral vein causes an abrupt decrease in femoral artery flow to 50 percent of baseline values, with a slow recovery to 80 percent of baseline after a few hours. The clinical parallel to that experiment would be acute iliofemoral thrombosis, producing phlegmasia alba dolens with arterial spasm and insufficiency, followed within a short time by phlegmasia cerulea dolens with plethora and venous congestion from virtual cessation of venous flow in the entire limb.

As acute obstruction becomes chronic, increased distal venous pressure causes increased flow through all available collateral channels that lead to the lower-pressure proximal venous tree. Increased flow gradually enlarges those preexisting channels, beginning within moments of occlusion and continuing over a period of weeks. With sufficient enlargement of vein caliber to produce valvular insufficiency, communicating veins become incompetent, resulting in collateral secondary varicosities in the superficial veins. Chronic communicator incompetence below the level of obstruction promotes stasis changes in the overlying subcutaneous tissues.

Even in the presence of extensive collaterals, venous volume and pressure may remain elevated when measured in resting recumbency [91]. With exercise, arterial flow into the limb dramatically increases, with a consequent increased demand on the venous system to return blood to the vena cava. In the face of significant obstruction and fixed resistance of the collateral bed, distal venous volume and pressure increase [91] (Fig. 47-11). A combination of increased deep-compartment pressure causing stretching of fascial envelopes and decreased capillary inflow of nutrients and clearance of metabolic byproducts results in pain termed **venous claudication.** With cessation of exercise, the severe physiologic aberrations recede, and pain is relieved.

CLINICAL MANIFESTATIONS

History. Although venous insufficiency most frequently is the result of DVT, there often is no supporting history, since many episodes of DVT are asymptomatic. If there is a story suggesting past DVT, it is helpful to obtain as

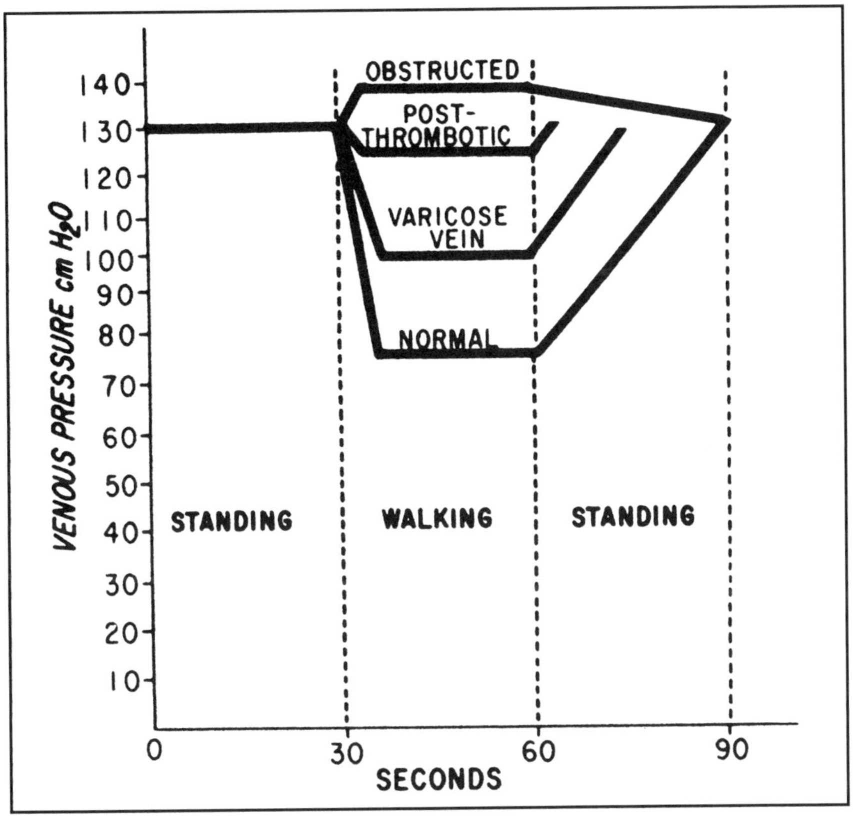

Fig. 47-11. Ambulatory pedal venous pressure curves (diagrammatic). Pressure is greatly reduced in normal system with gradual return to baseline after exercise. Presence of varicose veins decreases efficiency of muscle pump, with more impairment in presence of deep-vein incompetence, causing less pressure reduction and prompt return to baseline due to passive reflux. Obstructed proximal veins may actually cause pressure to increase. (Reproduced with permission from JA DeWeese. Venous and lymphatic disease. In SI Schwarz et al. (eds.). Principles of Surgery (4th ed.). New York: McGraw-Hill, 1983. P. 975.)

much documentation as possible, particularly laboratory evidence of the location and extent of involvement. A careful history of previous surgery or trauma is important, and historic clues may reveal the presence of a pelvic malignancy or other cause for extrinsic compression of a major vein.

As mentioned above, valvular incompetence and obstruction often are present simultaneously. When **valvular incompetence** predominates, early symptoms consist of a dull, bursting pressure in the lower leg with dependency, perhaps associated after more prolonged periods with edema of the foot and ankle. The symptoms are relieved with elevation. With time, secondary superficial varicosities may become evident, usually over the medial aspect of the leg and ankle, where communicating veins emerging from the deep system are most abundant. Pain, itching, and eczema involve those same areas, and foci of hyperpigmentation gradually appear in the subcutaneous tissues. Eventually, weeping of serum or overt skin ulceration arises spontaneously or after trivial injury. Subcutaneous inflammation may become prominent with varying degrees of cellulitis.

If significant total or partial **venous obstruction** predominates, its contribution to symptoms may be relatively mild at rest when collateral channels more easily decompress the lower limb. Pressure symptoms are worse with prolonged dependency. Exercise elicits the most important symptoms of obstruction, including deep, intense pressure in the distal leg relieved by rest. The pattern of such venous claudication generally is stereotypic in each patient. Although cutaneous manifestations are not prominent in cases of pure obstruction, skin breakdown and ulceration may occur in conjunction with secondary incompetence of communicating veins.

Physical Findings. Leg circumference is usually increased, with peripheral edema and tightness of muscle compartments evident when the legs are balloted and compressed. Cyanosis and plethora of the feet are often evident with dependency. Secondary varicose veins are generally present, and in cases of predominant obstruction, the location of visible superficial collaterals over the leg or lower abdomen indicates the site of obstruction. Brawny induration is obvious under healed skin lesions and surrounding other sites of old minor trauma or inflammation (Fig. 47-12). Most of those lesions are distributed medially over the ankle and lower leg, with the highest frequency just above the medial malleolus. Untreated ulcerations usually

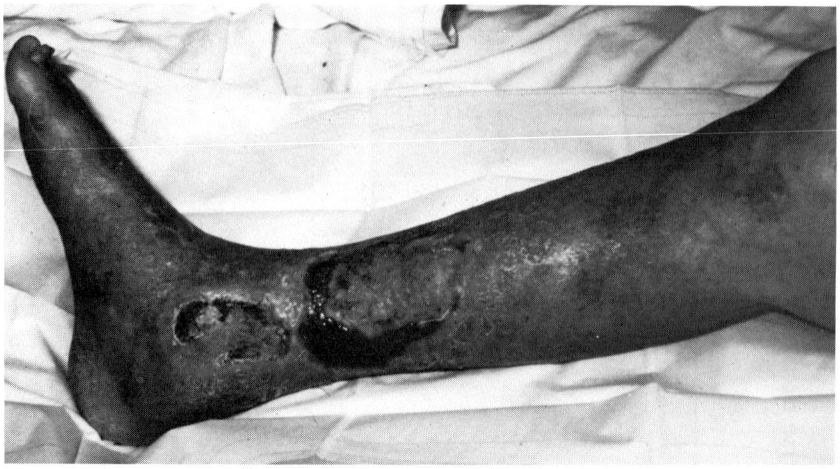

Fig. 47-12. Chronic venous stasis changes in leg. Note hyperpigmentation of skin, ulcers above medial malleolus, muscular atrophy.

are punched out and necrotic, with copious drainage from the open bed. There frequently are signs of surrounding cellulitis, occasionally ascending up the leg with lymphangitic involvement. Chronicity usually results in stiffening of the ankle joint and loss of proximal muscle bulk and strength.

Laboratory. The noninvasive vascular laboratory has developed into a valuable adjunct in understanding and managing deep venous disease. Improved diagnostic methods have been helpful in differentiating deep venous disease from other conditions; they also provide an objective baseline for following the natural history of the disease and for later reference when symptoms of recurrent acute DVT overlap those of the postphlebitic syndrome. Finally, although initial management usually is unchanged by laboratory findings, noninvasive screening is an important means of detecting potential candidates for further evaluation by venography prior to the application of more interventional approaches to treatment.

In cases of predominant deep-vein valvular incompetence, reflux of blood down the leg is evident by either continuous-wave or duplex ultrasound imaging. Duplex ultrasound increasingly is being used as a screening test to characterize abnormalities in vein-wall and valve morphology as well as to quantitate flow and reflux [101,102]. Testing using photoplethysmography or air plethysmography can be used to demonstrate abnormal venous filling time or poor emptying of the distal veins [45,103,104]. Venography confirms the presence of scarred, patent proximal veins, often with scattered branch occlusions or stenoses. Valvular reflux through incompetent communicating veins is evident on ascending venography when the superficial system is visualized above the level of an occluding tourniquet. Communicating branches often can be located by Doppler or venography near, but not necessarily directly under, previous or current skin ulcers. Descending venography dramatically demonstrates valvular function, with dye cascading down the leg after the fluoroscopy table is tilted [16,32,105]. All degrees of valvular dysfunction can be characterized, ranging from total reflux through a valve that is all but invisible to minimal reflux evident only during the Valsalva maneuver through a leaflet that may be slightly scarred or redundant (Fig. 47-13).

In cases of venous obstruction, continuous-wave Doppler ultrasound evaluation in practiced hands allows accurate indirect localization of the obstructed vein segment. Duplex ultrasound scanning, particularly with color-flow assistance, can accurately visualize obstructions in the involved veins [106]. Collateral patterns can be mapped, typically involving the saphenous system in the case of superficial-femoral-vein occlusion and cross-pudendal routes in the case of iliac-vein occlusion. Plethysmography by one of the available techniques also can document in most instances the hemodynamic abnormality caused by proximal-vein obstruction, although the test can be normal at rest in the presence of large collaterals. Venous-pressure studies can be performed, puncturing a foot vein and comparing the involved limb with the normal leg or arm to demonstrate increased pressures occasionally at rest and typically with exercise or reactive hyperemia [91,107]. Ascending venography accurately outlines occluded veins, provided the radiographic dye has been presented properly to the deep system by appropriate tourniquets. The iliac veins frequently are poorly visualized by a dye injection at the level of the foot, and techniques using femoral or brachiocephalic venous access may be necessary.

MANAGEMENT

Conservative Measures. Therapy of venous insufficiency, whether caused by total or partial obstruction, valvular reflux, or a combination of both lesions, is directed at countering the damaging effects of peripheral venous hypertension. Thorough education of the patient about the underlying problem and the pathophysiology involved is essential, with counseling about beneficial changes in

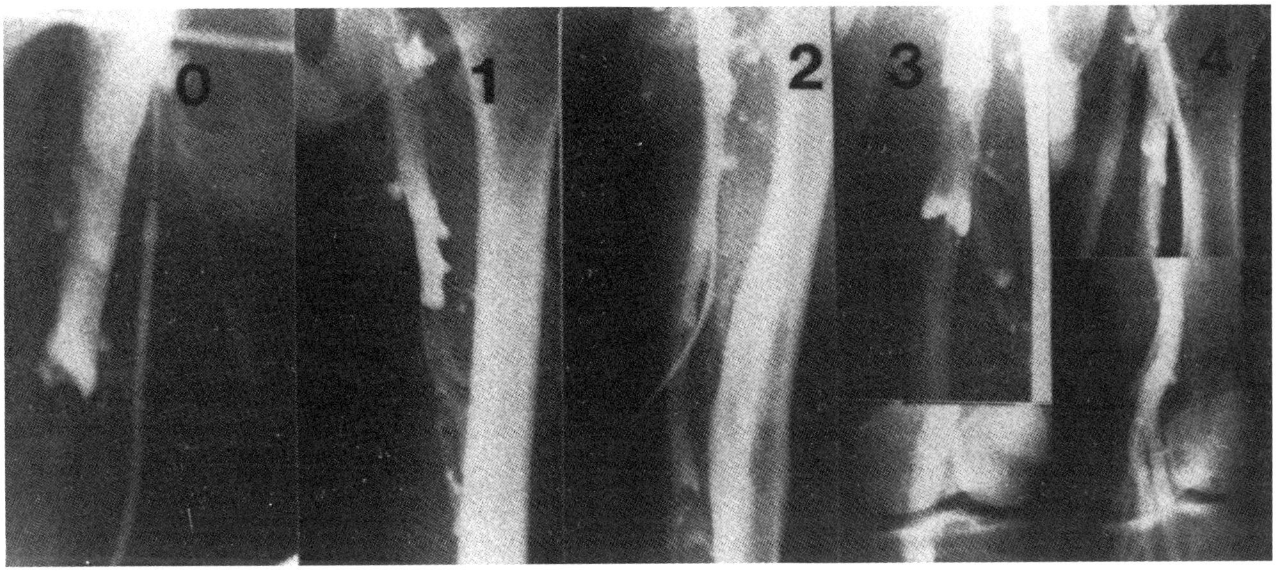

Fig. 47-13. Descending venography, demonstrating degrees of valvular incompetence in leg ranging from none (0) to minimal (1) in the presence of healthy valves, to free retrograde flow (4), to calf level with gross valvular damage. (Reproduced with permission from RL Kistner et al. A method of performing descending venography. J Vasc Surg 1986; 4:464.)

life-style. Prolonged standing or sitting promotes stasis and sustained hypertension in the lower leg. Prescription graduated compression stockings with 30–40 mm Hg pressure at the ankle should be obtained and worn during the day, to help control edema; they also may reduce valvular reflux [108,109]. Gentle exercise and usual ambulatory activities are recommended to enlarge and maintain venous collaterals, provided adequate stocking support is employed. Jogging or other types of exercise that involve cyclic dependent thrusting of the legs should be replaced by sports such as rowing or swimming. Moderate tipping of the bed into a head-down position promotes mobilization of edema and relief of muscle compartment tension at night. All these measures help to protect patent veins from recurrent DVT. The noninvasive laboratory should be used to advantage whenever repeated episodes of thrombosis or further deterioration are suspected.

When eczema and skin ulceration supervene, efforts to reduce venous hypertension must be increased, and other measures must be directed at the skin itself. Enforced temporary bed rest combined with careful hygiene and gentle protective dressings of nonadherent gauze usually control eczema. If bacterial cellulitis or lymphangitis is suspected, antibiotics should be directed initially against staphylococcal and streptococcal skin colonizers, modified later by cultures that can yield a wide variety of organisms. Open ulcers should be treated with a gentle debriding regimen of dressing changes 2 to 4 times a day using wet-to-dry normal saline on coarse mesh cloth gauze. A dilute antibiotic solution (bacitracin, neomycin) or other preparation (Burow's solution, dilute boric acid) can be substituted for saline. Once the ulcer is clean and cellulitis appears controlled, less frequent dressing changes must be combined with continued firm compression over the region to achieve healing [110]. Use of several hours of intermittent pneumatic compression per day has been shown to accelerate healing [111]. Representative of various regimens is Unna's paste boot [112–114], which combines support to combat venous hypertension and edema with a mixture of zinc oxide, calamine, and gelatin to provide gentle medication of the open ulcer. The patient is able to maintain most normal activities, and essentially no care is required, with changes of the boot every 1 to 4 weeks. Sclerotherapy of adjacent feeding veins in conjunction with the application of Unna's boot reduces healing time [115]. Occasionally, dermatitis occurs under the boot, and because cellulitis may be exacerbated if the ulcer is infected, the boot must be used only on relatively clean ulcers. If the ulcer is large or persistent, split-thickness skin grafts can be applied to ulcers after sufficient preparation.

Surgical Measures. Conservative measures allow up to 70-percent cumulative success over 5 years, with lack of compliance the most important determinant of failure [116]. In instances of failure, it is appropriate to consider surgical measures directed at the underlying causes of venous hypertension [117].

Interruption of appropriate incompetent communicating veins reduces barotrauma to the subcutaneous tissues. Optimally, any ulcer should be healed or small and free of cellulitis prior to surgery, and preoperative imaging is helpful to demonstrate communicator anatomy. In general, the procedure should be directed at all communicating veins in the region of the ulcer and not specifically at the single vein that may appear to be nearest to the base of the ulcer. Collateral channels connected to adjacent communicators from a severely diseased deep system may predispose to recurrent ulceration if the surgical approach is too limited. The most definitive surgery, as advocated by Linton [118], involves an incision from the ankle to the proximal calf with subfascial ligation of all communicating veins. Modifications of the Linton flap generally employ a somewhat less extensive incision in the leg [119,120]. Ulcer recurrence at 5 years varies widely, with rates of 2 to 55 percent in reported series [119–122]. Results appear to be best when the extent of underlying deep-vein disease is limited and when long-term postoperative use is made of support stockings. Sloughing of the skin edge, infection, DVT, hemorrhage, inadvertent nerve injury, and delayed contracture of the ankle joint all occur, with variable combined morbidity rates of 4 to 30 percent in published series [122].

Because of relatively high recurrence rates with subfascial ligation of communicating veins in patients with extensive valvular dysfunction, methods to correct underlying deep-vein valve reflux have been sought. Linton adopted selective ligation of the superficial femoral vein to halt venous reflux [121]. Kistner developed a valvuloplasty operation that can be applied to patients with primary valvular reflux due to redundancy and laxity of the valve leaflets [78]. After careful documentation of reflux and valve anatomy by descending venography, the valve is exposed and opened between the valve leaflets. Fine sutures are used to reef the lax leaflets, restoring competency (Fig. 47-14). A recent modification allows performance of the procedure without opening the vein, using angioscopic visualization [123].

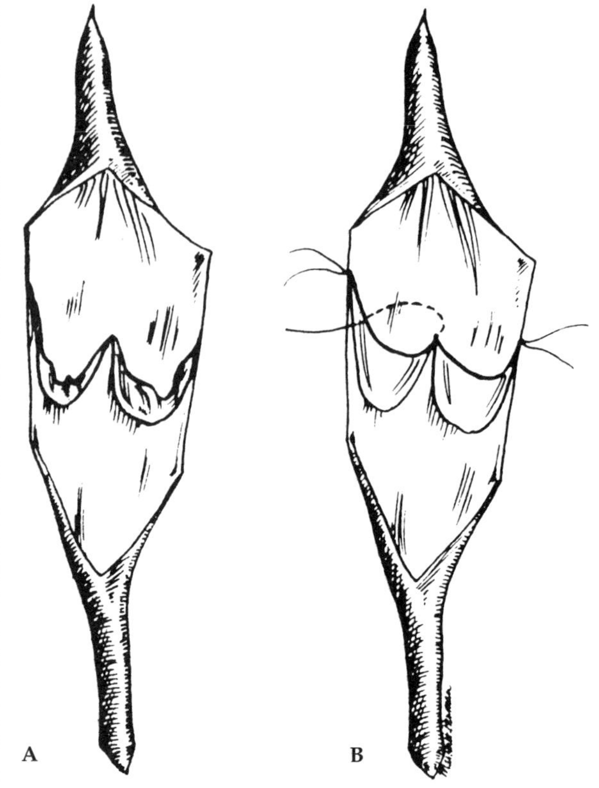

Fig. 47-14. Valvuloplasty to repair floppy valve causing reflux. **A.** Vein opened through valve commissure during surgery, showing redundant leaky valve leaflets. **B.** Fine sutures placed at valve corners to correct redundancy by reefing leaflets. (Reproduced with permission from RL Kistner, Transvenous repair of the incompetent femoral vein valve. In JJ Bergan, JST Yao. Venous Problems. Chicago: Year Book, 1978. P. 503.)

When valves are too damaged to be repaired, a new competent valve may be juxtaposed into the incompetent system. If the superficial femoral vein is involved and the saphenous vein is normal, end-to-end transposition of the competent proximal saphenous vein into the distal femoral vein introduces a valve into the system (Fig. 47-15). Alternatively, the profunda femoris vein can be transposed into the superficial femoral vein [124]. When no normal valve is available nearby, a segment of the axillary vein containing a competent valve may be transplanted into the femoral or popliteal vein [125,126]. Finally, a sling of Silastic has been constructed between the hamstring muscles to cause impingement on the popliteal vein during knee flexion to reduce reflux of blood [127].

All these valvular reconstructive procedures are somewhat investigational and at best are applicable only to a relatively small number of patients who have been found by careful evaluation to have appropriate pathophysiology and a favorable anatomic situation. Experience is still small, but it appears that about 80 percent of selected patients are improved for variable periods after surgery [124,125,128,129]. Interestingly, it sometimes has been difficult to demonstrate dramatic improvement in objective measures of venous physiology commensurate with apparent clinical improvement [129]. Evidence suggests that restoration of a single competent valve in an extensively diseased femoral vein may not be sufficient to control ulceration, with deterioration in laboratory findings and clinical status within 2 years following surgery [130]. When valvular reflux is extensive, it is advisable to combine communicator interruption with antireflux valve repair to obtain the best results [128,130]. Controversy continues about the proper balance of surgical approaches to valvular reflux.

Restoration of the patency of veins occluded by thrombus is practicable only in the acute phase. Surgical thrombectomy or fibrinolytic therapy has been used with inconsistent success [63,75,76,131]. With chronic thrombotic occlusion, veins become fibrotic, and attempts to open them are almost always unsuccessful. On the other hand, if external compression or a discrete intraluminal web is present, efforts to relieve the obstruction may be helpful occasionally. In rare instances of iliac-vein compression by the crossing iliac artery, a bridgelike prosthesis has actually been devised to lift the iliac artery off the caval bifurcation [132].

Surgical bypass of venous occlusions has been employed in selected instances for some 30 years. Palma and Esperon [133] and then Dale and Harris [134] described a procedure in which the contralateral saphenous vein is mobilized and tunneled across the pubis to the femoral vein to direct flow from the leg away from an obstructed iliac system (Fig. 47-16). This procedure has been used successfully in palliating disabling symptoms in patients

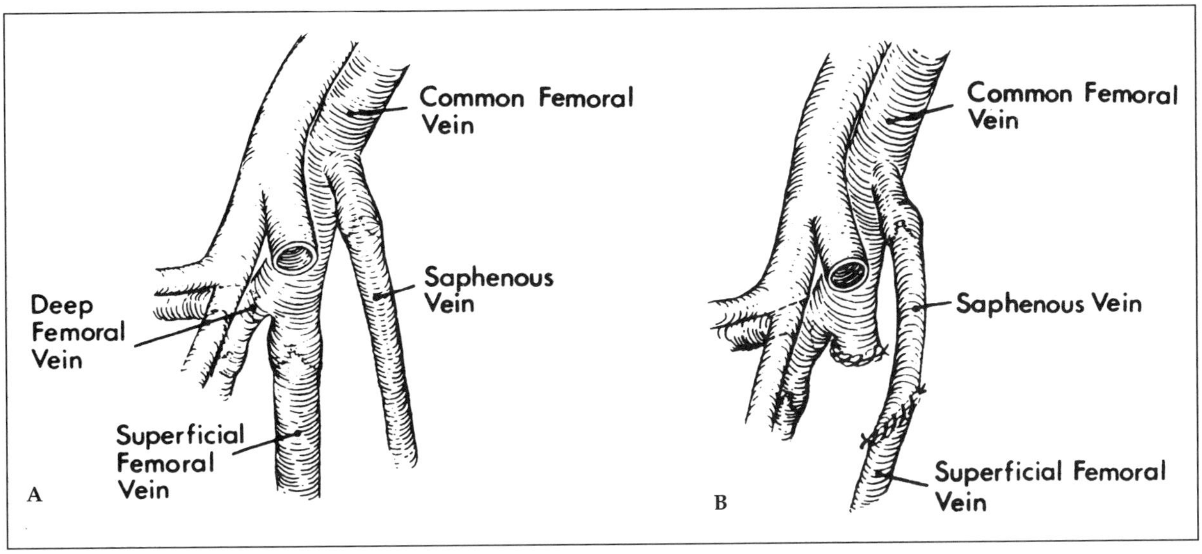

Fig. 47-15. Vein transposition. **A.** Anatomy of proximal femoral region, with incompetent valves in superficial femoral vein. **B.** Restoration of superficial femoral competence by transposition below normal valve in saphenous vein. (Reproduced with permission from LA Queral et al. Surgical correction of chronic deep venous insufficiency by valvular transposition. Surgery 1980; 87:688.)

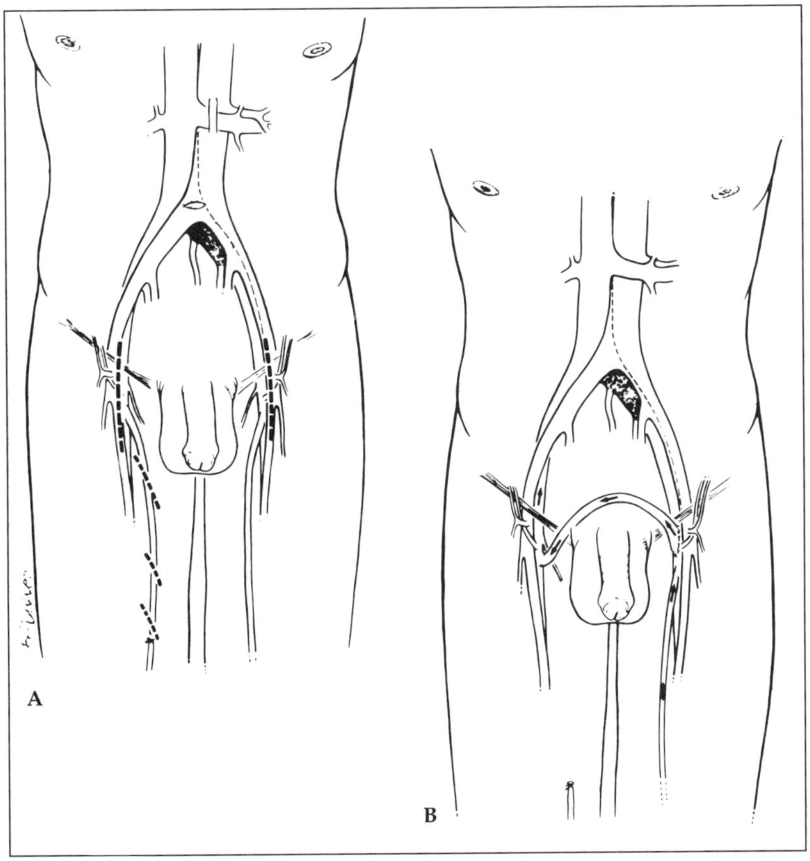

Fig. 47-16. Palma-Dale cross-pubic bypass, using mobilized saphenous vein **A.** to drain contralateral femoral system through a subcutaneous tunnel **B.** to relieve symptoms from iliac vein obstruction. (Reproduced with permission from JJ Bergan et al. Surgical treatment of venous obstruction and insufficiency. J Vasc Surg 1986; 3:174–181.)

with pelvic malignancy. Another operation makes use of the ipsilateral saphenous vein connected to the popliteal vein to provide a collateral channel around obstruction or incompetence limited to the superficial femoral and proximal popliteal veins [135].

Prosthetic grafts have been used from time to time in the femoral, cross-femoral, and iliocaval positions [136,137]. Experimental work suggests that externally supported polytetrafluoroethylene is the preferred prosthetic among those currently available, because it appears to be least thrombogenic and resists collapse under pressure from surrounding tissues [138,139]. Endothelial seeding of such grafts appears to improve patency only slightly in the canine experimental model [139]. A complementary temporary arteriovenous fistula (AVF) probably improves long-term patency of venous bypass grafts, particularly prosthetics. An AVF increases flow velocity and reduces platelet deposition on the graft surface [140] and augments the capacity of autogenous collateral channels. It has been suggested that a primary temporary AVF might be a reasonable means of enlarging collaterals, with improvement in venous hemodynamics after closure of the fistula [141].

Surgical reconstructions have good results when assessed by symptom relief, physiologic improvement, or bypass patency. In a compilation of the largest published series of procedures designed to relieve obstruction, clinical improvement occurred in about 80 percent of patients at varied postoperative intervals [129,135,142]. Graft patency does not appear to be as durable as symptomatic relief [143]. Some surgeons recommend a period of anticoagulation with coumarin after surgery, although there are no data clearly indicating that bypass patency is improved. Overall surgical morbidity is low, with a surprising lack of thromboembolic complications. Recent experience suggests a role for percutaneous balloon angioplasty and intraluminal stent placement in selected cases of lower- and upper-extremity venous occlusion [144].

Chronic Disorders of Veins of the Upper Extremity

PATHOGENESIS AND PATHOPHYSIOLOGY

Valvular incompetence is of no consequence in veins of the upper extremity, but chronic proximal obstruction can be an important clinical problem. The most common cause of proximal occlusion of the subclavian veins is thrombus forming around the wide variety of central-access catheters currently in use [145,146] and, to a much smaller extent, around pacemaker wires. Primary spontaneous axillary- or subclavian-vein thrombosis also occurs, usually in association with fibrous bands, muscular hypertrophy, or bony compression. Intermittent subclavian-vein occlusion has been detected rarely as a precursor to thrombosis [147] and has been reported in 1.5 to 3.5 percent of patients with thoracic outlet syndrome [4,148]. Vigorous arm activity can precipitate so-called effort thrombosis (Paget-von Schroetter syndrome), seen most commonly in athletes such as swimmers and baseball players in whom extreme abduction and extension of the shoulder apparently traumatizes the axillary and subclavian veins [146,149]. Finally, extrinsic compression by mediastinal fibrosis or malignancy can cause obstruction of the superior vena cava, with compromised venous drainage of the brachiocephalic regions.

Acute axillary- or subclavian-vein thrombosis may be quite dramatic, but it is rarely severe enough to threaten the arm [150]; it is associated with clinically important pulmonary embolism in 4 to 12 percent of patients [4,151]. Recanalization of proximal-arm thrombosis probably occurs in a majority of cases, particularly those caused by intravascular catheters that have been removed. If the cause of thrombosis persists, as in the thoracic outlet syndrome, restoration of an adequate venous channel is less likely. With residual chronic obstruction, a rich collateral network develops around the shoulder and upper chest, but hemodynamic impairment is sufficient to produce symptoms long-term in 40 to 85 percent of patients [3,4,146]. In one series, 39 percent of subjects were forced to change occupation to accommodate arm disability [3].

CLINICAL MANIFESTATIONS

History. Symptoms are most impressive in the acute stage of thrombosis, with sudden onset of tightness and bursting pain, which is worse with dependency and exercise. As the course becomes chronic and collaterals develop, resting symptoms become less prominent than venous claudication induced by exercise, or the limb may be largely asymptomatic. If thoracic outlet compression is the cause of venous occlusion, symptoms of associated arterial or neurologic compression may be prominent [148]. If venous compression is intermittent, without thrombosis, symptoms of temporary obstruction of the subclavian vein are evident only during certain arm activities.

Physical Findings. Physical findings are absent or subtle in many patients with proximal segmental occlusions located in the axillary or subclavian veins. Large subcutaneous collateral veins around the shoulder usually are evident on inspection. In more severe cases, increased arm circumference, tightness of muscle compartments, cyanosis, and venous engorgement are evident. In the presence of thoracic outlet syndrome, there may be tenderness over the brachial plexus, findings of ulnar neuropathy, or aggravation of symptoms and loss of the radial pulse with hyperextension and abduction of the arm.

Laboratory. The noninvasive vascular laboratory can be used to gather confirmatory evidence of venous occlusion [152]. Ultrasound is capable of detecting occlusion in the arm and interference with normal flow dynamics caused by more proximal occlusion. Phleborheography and other forms of plethysmography are also helpful. Resting venous pressure measured in a forearm vein is elevated compared to the contralateral normal arm [147]. With intermittent subclavian-vein compression, pressure gradients can be measured across the point of impingement at the thoracic outlet [153]. Although experience with noninvasive techniques is evolving, venography remains the most valuable diagnostic method.

MANAGEMENT

Thrombosis around central venous catheters responds well in most instances to removal of the catheter and a short course of anticoagulation, when possible. Spontaneous thrombosis is more difficult to manage, with a higher likelihood of long-term sequelae [4,146]. Surgical thrombectomy has a role if used within a few days of thrombosis, but there is a substantial incidence of recurrent clotting [148,154]. Systemic or local fibrinolytic therapy is often applicable and has gained popularity as a means of opening veins acutely, with satisfactory long-term patency provided extrinsic causes of thrombosis also are promptly addressed [155]. That most often means decompression of the thoracic outlet by a combination of first-rib resection, scalenectomy, and lysis of fibrous bands [156] followed by anticoagulation for several months [4].

In the chronic situation, therapy is almost exclusively conservative because there are few good alternatives. Careful patient education is critical, with counseling about possible changes in occupation to decrease stress on the involved arm. Gentle exercise should be encouraged to enlarge and maintain collaterals. Compression sleeves may be necessary in some instances to control symptoms and swelling. If venous obstruction is intermittent, thoracic outlet decompression should be performed to prevent thrombosis. Experience with direct surgical approaches to chronically occluded veins is limited. In selected patients with segmental proximal subclavian obstruction, the ipsilateral jugular vein can be used to provide a bypass around the obstruction [157,158]. Superior vena cava reconstruction is possible using autogenous spiral vein grafts or prosthetic substitutes [137].

References

1. Coon WW, Willis PW III, Keller JB. Venous thromboembolism and other venous disease in the Tecumseh Community Health Study. Circulation 1973; 48:839.
2. DaSilva A, et al. Varicose veins and chronic venous insufficiency. Vasa 1974; 3:118.
3. Tilney NL, Griffiths HJ, Edwards EA. Natural history of major venous thrombosis of the upper extremity. Arch Surg 1970; 101:792.
4. Gloviczki P, Kazmier FJ, Hollier LH. Axillary-subclavian venous occlusion: the morbidity of a nonlethal disease. J Vasc Surg 1986; 4:333.
5. Dodd H, Cockett FB. The Pathology and Surgery of the Veins of the Lower Limb. Edinburgh: Livingstone, 1976. Pp. 18–49.
6. Kosinski C. Superficial venous system of the lower extremity. J Anat 1926; 60:131.
7. Nicholson BB. Varicose veins: etiology and treatment. Arch Surg 1927; 15:351.
8. Eger SA, Casper SL. Etiology of varicose veins from an anatomic aspect, based on a dissection of thirty-eight adult cadavers. JAMA 1943; 123:148.
9. Powell T, Lynn RB. The valves of the external iliac, femoral and upper third of the popliteal veins. Surg Gynecol Obstet 1951; 92:453.
10. Shepherd JT. Role of the veins in the circulation. Circulation 1966; 33:484.
11. Rushmer RF. Cardiovascular Dynamics. Philadelphia: Saunders, 1970. Pp. 192–219.
12. Strandness DE, Sumner DS. Hemodynamics for Surgeons. New York: Grune & Stratton, 1975. P. 120.
13. Pollack AA, Wood EH. Venous pressure in the saphenous vein at the ankle in man during exercise and changes in posture. J Appl Physiol 1949; 1:649.
14. Stegall HF. Muscle pumping in the dependent leg. Circ Res 1966; 19:180.
15. Luke JC. The deep vein valves: a venographic study in normal and postphlebitic states. Surgery 1951; 29:381.
16. Ackroyd JS, Lea Thomas M, Browse NC. Deep vein reflux: an assessment by descending phlebography. Br J Surg 1986; 73:31.
17. Bishara RA, et al. Deterioration of venous function in normal lower extremities during daily activity. J Vasc Surg 1986; 3:700.
18. Lofgren EP. Treatment of long saphenous varicosities and their recurrence: a long-term follow-up. In JJ Bergan, JST Yao, eds. Surgery of the Veins. New York: Grune & Stratton, 1985. P. 285.
19. Reagan B, Folse R. Lower limb venous dynamics in normal persons and children of patients with varicose veins. Surg Gynec Obstet 1971; 132:15.
20. Rose SS, Ahmed A. Some thoughts on the aetiology of varicose veins. J Cardiovasc Surg 1986; 27:534.
21. Staubesand J, Fischer N. The ultrastructural characteristics of abnormal collagen fibrils in various organs. Connect Tiss Res 1980; 7:213.
22. Clarke GH, et al. Venous wall function in the pathogenesis of varicose veins. Surgery 1992; 111:402.
23. Gandhi RH, et al. Analysis of the connective tissue matrix and proteolytic activity of primary varicose veins. J Vasc Surg 1993; 18:814.
24. Widmer LK, Mall T, Martin H. Epidemiology and sociomedical importance of peripheral venous disease. In JT Hobbs, ed. The Treatment of Venous Disorders. Philadelphia: Lippincott, 1977. Pp. 3–12.
25. Blumoff RL, Johnson G. Saphenous vein Ppo2 in patients with varicose veins. J Surg Res 1977; 23:35.
26. Baron HC, Cassaro S. The role of arteriovenous shunts in the pathogenesis of varicose veins. J Vasc Surg 1986; 4:124.
27. Piulachs P, Vidal-Barraquer F. Pathogenic study of varicose veins. Angiology 1953; 4:59–100.
28. Schalin L. Arteriovenous communications in varicose veins localized by thermography and identified by operative microscopy. Acta Chir Scand 1981; 147:409.
29. Haimovici H. Arteriovenous shunting in varicose veins: its diagnosis by Doppler ultrasound flow detector. J Vasc Surg 1985; 2:684.
30. Gloviczki P, et al. Surgical implications of Klippel-Trenaunay syndrome. Ann Surg 1983; 197:353.
31. Baskerville PA, Ackroyd JS, Browse NL. The etiology of the Klippel-Trenaunay syndrome. Ann Surg 1985; 202:624.
32. Almgren B, et al. Phlebographic evaluation of nonthrombotic deep venous incompetence: new anatomic and functional aspects. J Vasc Surg 1990; 11:389.
33. DeCamp PT, Ward JA, Ochsner A. Ambulatory venous pressure studies in postphlebitic and other disease states. Surgery 1951; 29:365.
34. Bjordal RI. Circulation patterns in the incompetent perforating veins in the calf and in the saphenous system in primary varicose veins. Acta Chir Scand 1972; 138:251.
35. Hoare MC, et al. The role of primary varicose veins in venous ulceration. Surgery 1982; 92:450.
36. Darke SG, Penfold C. Venous ulceration and saphenous ligation. Eur J Vasc Surg 1992; 6:4.
37. Shami SK, et al. Venous ulcers and the superficial venous system. J Vasc Surg 1993; 17:487.
38. Nicolaides AN, Irving D. Clinical factors and the risk of deep venous thrombosis. In AN Nicolaides, ed. Thromboembolism. Baltimore: University Park Press, 1975. Pp. 193–204.
39. Skillman JJ, et al. Simultaneous occurrence of superficial and

deep thrombophlebitis in the lower extremity. J Vasc Surg 1990; 11:818.
40. Jorgensen JO, et al. The incidence of deep venous thrombosis in patients with superficial thrombophlebitis of the lower limbs. J Vasc Surg 1993; 18:70.
41. Brodie B. Lectures Illustrative of Various Subjects in Pathology and Surgery, vol. VII. London: Longmans, Green, 1846.
42. Trendelenburg J. Uber die Unterbindung der Vena Saphena magna bei Unterschenkelvaricen. Beitr Klin Chir 1890–1891; 7:195.
43. Perthes G. Über die Operation der Unterschenkelvaricen noch Trendelenburg. Dtsch Med Wochenschr 1895; 21:253.
44. Tibbs DJ, Fletcher EWL. Direction of flow in superficial veins as a guide to venous disorders in lower limbs. Surgery 1983; 93:758.
45. Abramowitz HB, et al. The use of photoplethysmography in the assessment of venous insufficiency: a comparison to venous pressure measurements. Surgery 1979; 86:434.
46. Nicolaides AN, Miles C. Photoplethysmography in the assessment of venous insufficiency. J Vasc Surg 1987; 5:405.
47. Rabinov K, Paulin S. Roentgen diagnosis of venous thrombosis in the leg. Arch Surg 1972; 104:134.
48. Godin MS, Rice JC, Kerstein MD. Effect of commercially available pantyhose on venous return in the lower extremity. J Vasc Surg 1987; 5:844.
49. Fegan WG. Continuous compression technique of injecting varicose veins. Lancet 1963; II:109.
50. Raj TB, Makin GS. A random controlled trial of two forms of compression bandaging in outpatient sclerotherapy of varicose veins. J Surg Res 1981; 31:440.
51. Sladen JG. Compression sclerotherapy: preparation, technique, complications and results. Am J Surg 1983; 146:228.
52. Hobbs JT. Surgery and sclerotherapy in the treatment of varicose veins: a random trial. Arch Surg 1974; 109:793.
53. Williams RA, Wilson SE. Sclerosant treatment of varicose veins and deep vein thrombosis. Arch Surg 1984; 119:1283.
54. Hobbs JT. The management of varicose veins. Surg Annual 1980; 12:184.
55. McMullin GM, Coleridge-Smith PD, Scurr JH. Objective assessment of ligation without stripping the long saphenous vein. Br J Surg 1992; 78:1139.
56. Sarin S, Scurr JH, Coleridge-Smith PD. Assessment of stripping the long saphenous vein in the treatment of primary varicose veins. Br J Surg 1992; 79:889.
57. Cox SJ, Wellwood JM, Martin A. Saphenous nerve injury caused by stripping of the long saphenous vein. Brit Med J 1974; 1:415.
58. Large J. Surgical treatment of saphenous varices, with preservation of the main saphenous trunk. J Vasc Surg 1985; 2:886.
59. Neglen P. Treatment of varicosities of saphenous origin: Comparison of ligation, sclerotherapy, and selected stripping. In JJ Bergan, MP Goldman, eds. Varicose Veins & Telectasias: Diagnosis & Management. St. Louis: Quality Medical Publishing, 1993. Pp. 148–165.
60. Larson RH, et al. Long-term results after vein surgery: study of 1000 cases after 10 years. Mayo Clin Proc 1974; 49:114.
61. Arndt KA. Argon laser therapy of small cutaneous vascular lesions. Arch Dermatol 1982; 118:220.
62. Villavicencio JL, et al. Nonsurgical management of lower extremity venous problems. In JJ Bergan, JST Yao, eds. Surgery of the Veins. New York: Grune & Stratton, 1985. P. 323.
63. Kakkar VV, Lawrence D. Hemodynamic and clinical assessment after therapy for acute deep vein thrombosis: a prospective study. Am J Surg 1985; 150:54–62.
64. Bauer G. Roentgenological and clinical study of the sequelae of thrombosis. Acta Chir Scand 1942; 86[Suppl 74]:1–110.
65. Lindner DJ, et al. Long-term hemodynamic and clinical sequelae of lower extremity deep vein thrombosis. J Vasc Surg 1986; 4:436.
66. Negus D. The post-thrombotic syndrome. Ann R Coll Surg Engl 1970; 47:92–105.
67. Lawrence D, Kakkar VV. Post-phlebitic syndrome: a functional assessment. Br J Surg 1980; 67:686.
68. Strandness DE, et al. Long-term sequelae of acute venous thrombosis. JAMA 1983; 250:1289.
69. Boyd AM, et al. Logical management of chronic ulcers of the leg. Angiology 1952; 3:207.
70. Markel A, et al. Valvular reflux after deep vein thrombosis: Incidence and time of occurrence. J Vasc Surg 1992; 15:377.
71. Homans J. The late results of femoral thrombophlebitis and their treatment. N Engl J Med 1946; 235:259.
72. Havig O. Deep vein thrombosis and pulmonary embolism: an autopsy study with multiple regression analysis of possible risk factors. Acta Chir Scand 1977; 38[Suppl 478]:222.
73. Edwards EA, Edwards JE. The effect of thrombophlebitis on the venous valve. Surg Gynec Obstet 1937; 65:310.
74. Elliot MS, et al. A comparative randomized trial of heparin versus streptokinase in the treatment of acute proximal venous thrombosis. Br J Surg 1979; 66:838.
75. Albechtsson U, et al. Streptokinase treatment of deep vein thrombosis and the postthrombotic syndrome. Arch Surg 1981; 116:33.
76. Arnesen H, Hoiseth A, Ly B. Streptokinase or heparin in the treatment of deep vein thrombosis: follow-up results of a prospective study. Acta Med Scand 1982; 211:65.
77. Arnesen H. Heparin versus streptokinase in the treatment of deep venous thrombosis: Short- and long-term results. In AJ Comerota, ed. Thrombolytic Therapy. New York: Grune & Stratton, 1988. Pp. 41–50.
78. Kistner RL. Surgical repair of the incompetent femoral vein valve. Arch Surg 1975; 110:1336.
79. Plate G, et al. Physiologic and therapeutic aspects of congenital vein valve aplasia of the lower limb. Ann Surg 1983; 198:229.
80. Friedman EI, Taylor LM, Porter JM. Congenital venous valvular aplasia of the lower extremities. Surgery 1988; 103:24.
81. Moore DJ, Himmel PD, Sumner DS. Distribution of venous valvular incompetence in patients with the postphlebitic syndrome. J Vasc Surg 1986; 3:49–57.
82. Shull KC, et al. Significance of popliteal reflux in relation to ambulatory venous pressure and ulceration. Arch Surg 1979; 114:1304.
83. Gooley NA, Sumner DS. Relationship of venous reflux to the site of venous valvular incompetence: implications for venous reconstructive surgery. J Vasc Surg 1988; 7:50.
84. Arnoldi CC. Venous pressure in patients with valvular incompetence of the veins of the lower limb. Acta Chir Scand 1966; 132:628.
85. Burnand KG, et al. The relative importance of incompetent communicating veins in the production of varicose veins and venous ulcers. Surgery 1977; 82:9–14.
86. Christopoulos D, et al. Pathogenesis of venous ulceration in relation to the calf muscle pump function. Surgery 1989; 106:829.
87. Nicolaides AN, et al. The relation of venous ulceration with ambulatory venous pressure measurements. J Vasc Surg 1993; 17:414.
88. Taheri SA, et al. Muscle changes in venous insufficiency. Arch Surg 1984; 119:929.
89. Browse NL. The pathogenesis of venous ulceration. In JJ Bergan, JST Yao, eds. Surgery of the Veins. New York: Grune & Stratton, 1985. Pp. 25–31.
90. Clyne CAC, et al. Oxygen tension on the skin of the gaiter area of limbs with venous disease. Br J Surg 1985; 72:644.

91. Killewich LA, et al. Pathophysiology of venous claudication. J Vasc Surg 1984; 1:507.
92. Edwards EA. Clinical anatomy of lesser variations of the inferior vena cava and a proposal for classifying the anomalies of this vessel. Angiology 1951; 2:85–99.
93. Lea Thomas M, Posniak HV. Agenesis of the iliac veins. J Cardiovasc Surg 1984; 25:64.
94. Ono J, Sakoda K, Kawada T. Membranous obstruction of the inferior vena cava. Ann Surg 1983; 197:454.
95. Fischer MG, et al. Primary smooth muscle tumors of venous origin. Ann Surg 1982; 196:720.
96. Cockett FB, Thomas LM. The iliac compression syndrome. Br J Surg 1965; 52:816.
97. Connett MC. An anatomical basis for unilateral leg edema in adolescent girls. West J Med 1974; 121:324.
98. Symposium on Transvenous Vena Cava Interruption. J Vasc Surg 1984; 1:487–506.
99. Masuda EM, Kistner RL, Ferris EB. Long-term effects of superficial femoral vein ligation: thirteen-year follow-up. J Vasc Surg 1992; 16:741.
100. Hobson RW, et al. Hemodynamics of canine femoral venous ligation: significance in combined arterial and venous injuries. Surgery 1973; 74:824.
101. Weingarten MS, et al. Distribution and quantification of venous reflux in lower extremity chronic venous stasis disease with duplex scanning. J Vasc Surg 1993; 18:735.
102. Vasdekis SN, Clarke GH, Nicolaides AN. Quantification of venous reflux by means of duplex scanning. J Vasc Surg 1989; 10:670.
103. von Bemmelen PS, et al. Does air plethysmography correlate with duplex scanning in patients with chronic venous insufficiency? J Vasc Surg 1993; 18:796.
104. Welch HJ, et al. Comparison of descending phlebography with quantitative photoplethysmography, air plethysmography, and duplex quantitative valve closure time in assessing deep venous reflux. J Vasc Surg 1992; 16:913.
105. Kistner RL, et al. A method of performing descending venography. J Vasc Surg 1986; 4:464.
106. Mattos MA, et al. Color-flow duplex scanning for the surveillance and diagnosis of acute deep vein thrombosis. J Vasc Surg 1992; 15:366.
107. Raju S. New approaches to the diagnosis and treatment of venous obstruction. J Vasc Surg 1986; 4:42–54.
108. Nehler MR, et al. Perimalleolar subcutaneous tissue pressure effects of elastic compression stockings. J Vasc Surg 1993; 18:783.
109. Mayberry JC, et al. The influence of elastic compression stockings on deep venous hemodynamics. J Vasc Surg 1991; 13:91–100.
110. Blair SD, et al. Sustained compression and healing of chronic venous ulcers. Br Med J 1988; 297:1159.
111. Smith PC, et al. Sequential gradient pneumatic compression enhances venous ulcer healing: a randomized trial. Surgery 1990; 108:871.
112. Kikta MJ, et al. A prospective, randomized trial of Unna's boots versus hydroactive dressing in the treatment of venous stasis ulcers. J Vasc Surg 1988; 7:478.
113. Rubin JR, et al. Unna's boot vs polyurethane foam dressings for the treatment of venous ulceration: a randomized prospective study. Arch Surg 1990; 125:489.
114. Cordts PR, et al. A prospective, randomized trial of Unna's boot versus Duoderm CGF hydroactive dressing plus compression in the management of venous leg ulcers. J Vasc Surg 1992; 15:480.
115. Queral LA, et al. The role of sclerotherapy as an adjunct to Unna's boot for treating venous ulcers: a prospective study. J Vasc Surg 1990; 11:572.
116. Mayberry JC, et al. Fifteen-year results of ambulatory therapy for chronic venous ulcers. Surgery 1991; 109:575.
117. Bergan JJ, et al. Surgical treatment of venous obstruction and insufficiency. J Vasc Surg 1986; 3:174.
118. Linton RR. The communicating veins of the lower leg and the operative technic for their ligation. Ann Surg 1938; 197:582.
119. Blumenberg RM, Gelfand ML. The posterior stocking seam approach to radical subfascial clipping of perforating veins. Am J Surg 1978; 136:202.
120. DePalma RG. Surgical therapy for venous stasis: results of a modified Linton operation. Am J Surg 1979; 137:810.
121. Linton RR. The post-thrombotic ulceration of the lower extremity: its etiology and surgical therapy. Ann Surg 1953; 138:415.
122. Johnson WC, et al. Venous stasis ulceration: effectiveness of subfascial ligation. Arch Surg 1985; 120:797–800.
123. Gloviczki P, Merrell SW, Bower TC. Femoral vein valve repair under direct vision without venotomy: A modified technique with use of angioscopy. J Vasc Surg 1991; 14:645.
124. Queral LA, et al. Surgical correction of chronic deep venous insufficiency by valvular transposition. Surgery 1980; 87:688.
125. Raju S, Fredericks R. Valve reconstruction procedures for nonobstructive venous insufficiency: rationale, techniques, and results in 107 procedures with two- to eight-year followup. J Vasc Surg 1988; 7:301.
126. Taheri SA, et al. Vein valve transplant. Surgery 1982; 91:28–33.
127. Psathakis ND. The substitute "valve" operation by technique II in patients with postthrombotic syndrome. Surgery 1984; 95:542.
128. Ferris EB, Kistner RL. Femoral vein reconstruction in the management of chronic venous insufficiency. Arch Surg 1982; 117:1571.
129. O'Donnell TF, et al. Clinical, hemodynamic and anatomic follow-up of direct venous reconstruction. Arch Surg 1987; 122:474.
130. Johnson ND, et al. Late objective assessment of venous valve surgery. Arch Surg 1981; 116:1461.
131. Neglen P, et al. Iliofemoral venous thrombectomy followed by percutaneous closure of the temporary arteriovenous fistula. Surgery 1991; 110:493.
132. Trimble C, et al. A prosthetic bridging device to relieve iliac venous compression. Surg Forum 1972; 23:249–251.
133. Palma EC, Esperon R. Vein transplants and grafts in the surgical treatment of the post-phlebitic syndrome. J Cardiovasc Surg 1960; 1:94–102.
134. Dale WA, Harris J. Cross-over vein grafts for iliac and femoral venous occlusion. J Cardiovasc Surg 1969; 10:458.
135. Husni EA. In situ saphenopopliteal bypass graft for incompetence of the femoral and popliteal veins. Surg Gynec Obstet 1970; 130:1–6.
136. Dale WA, Harris J, Terry RB. Polytetrafluoroethylene reconstruction of the inferior vena cava. Surgery 1984; 95:625.
137. Gloviczki P, et al. Reconstruction of large veins for nonmalignant venous occlusive disease. J Vasc Surg 1992; 16:750.
138. Robison RJ, et al. Venous prostheses: improved patency with external stents. J Surg Res 1984; 36:306.
139. Herring M, et al. Patency in canine inferior vena cava grafting. Effects of graft material, size, and endothelial seeding. J Vasc Surg 1984; 1:877.
140. Plate G, et al. Overcoming failure of venous vascular prostheses. Surgery 1984; 96:503.
141. Sawchuk AP, et al. A temporary distal arteriovenous fistula improves venous hemodynamics in a model of venous occlusion. Surgery 1987; 102:256.
142. Dale WA. Reconstructive venous surgery. Arch Surg 1979; 114:1312.

143. Halliday P, Harris J, May J. Femoro-femoral crossover grafts (Palma operation): a long-term follow-up study. In JJ Bergan, JST Yao, eds. Surgery of the Veins. New York: Grune & Stratton, 1985. P. 241.
144. Elson JD, et al. Vena caval and central venous stenoses: Management with Palmaz balloon-expandable intraluminal stents. JVIR 1991; 2:215.
145. Warden GD, Wilmore DW, Pruitt BA. Central venous thrombosis: a hazard of medical progress. J Trauma 1973; 13:620.
146. Hill SL, Berry RE. Subclavian vein thrombosis: a continuing challenge. Surgery 1990; 108:1–9.
147. Adams JT, et al. Intermittent subclavian vein obstruction without thrombosis. Surgery 1968; 63:147.
148. Rutherford RB, Piotrowski JJ. Axillary-subclavian vein thrombosis. In RB Rutherford, ed. Vascular Surgery, 3rd ed. Philadelphia: Saunders, 1989. P. 883.
149. Adams JT, DeWeese JA. "Effort" thrombosis of the axillary and subclavian veins. J Trauma 1971; 11:923.
150. Smith BM, et al. Venous gangrene of the upper extremity. Ann Surg 1985; 201:511.
151. Adams JT, McEvoy RK, DeWeese JA. Primary deep venous thrombosis of the upper extremity. Arch Surg 1965; 91:29–42.
152. Sotturai VS, et al. Diagnosis of upper extremity deep venous thrombosis using noninvasive technique. Surgery 1982; 91:582.
153. Schubart PJ, Haeberlin JR, Porter JM. Intermittent subclavian venous obstruction: utility of venous pressure gradients. Surgery 1986; 99:365.
154. DeWeese JA, Adams JT, Gaiser DL. Subclavian venous thrombectomy. Circulation 1970; 41, 42[Suppl II]:158.
155. Machleder HI. Evaluation of a new treatment strategy for Paget-Schroetter syndrome: spontaneous thrombosis of the axillary-subclavian vein. J Vasc Surg 1993; 17:305.
156. Thompson RW, et al. Circumferential venolysis and paraclavicular thoracic outlet decompression for "effort thrombosis" of the subclavian vein. J Vasc Surg 1992; 16:723.
157. Inahara T. Surgical treatment of "effort" thrombosis of the axillary and subclavian veins. Am Surg 1968; 34:479.
158. Jacobson JH, Haimov M. Venous revascularization of the arm: Report of three cases. Surgery 1977; 81:599.

D

Miscellaneous Disorders of the Vasculature

48

Vascular Infection

Paul F. Kamitsuka

Vascular infection encompasses a number of different syndromes involving the heart as well as both the arterial and the venous sides of the circulatory system. The major syndromes include infective endocarditis, infective endarteritis, vascular graft infection, and suppurative thrombophlebitis (Table 48-1). In addition, small-vessel vasculitis occurs as part of infection due to rickettsial organisms such as *Rickettsia rickettsii,* the causal agent of Rocky Mountain spotted fever. The four major syndromes of vascular infection will be reviewed in this chapter.

Infective Endocarditis

DEFINITION

Infective endocarditis is a microbial infection of the endothelial lining of the heart and typically involves the valvular leaflets. Other sites may be involved, including the chordae tendineae, the atrial or ventricular endocardium, and septal defects. The characteristic lesion of endocarditis is a vegetation, consisting of platelets, fibrin, various host-derived proteins, and microorganisms. While extracardiac endothelium also may harbor infection as in coarctation of the aorta or patent ductus arteriosus, those infections are more accurately referred to as infective endarteritis [1,2].

RISK FACTORS AND RECENT EPIDEMIOLOGY

Each year, 10,000–15,000 cases of infective endocarditis occur in the United States [3]. The estimated incidence of endocarditis among adults in the United States is 1.7–4.9 cases per 100,000 person years [4–7], and is virtually unchanged since the preantibiotic era [8]. However, important changes have occurred in the populations at risk, the underlying valvular disorders, and the microorganisms involved.

Currently, major groups at risk for endocarditis include (1) patients with mitral valve prolapse with regurgitation [5,9–12] or those with echocardiographic findings of thickened and redundant valvular tissue [13,14]; (2) elderly persons with calcific valvular sclerosis, usually involving the aortic valve [15–17]; (3) persons with prosthetic cardiac valves; and (4) intravenous drug users. Rheumatic heart disease, predominantly affecting the left-sided valves with mitral more frequent than aortic, is decreasing in importance as a predisposing factor for endocarditis and currently is found in about 30 percent of cases [18–20]. Congenital cardiac lesions predisposing to endocarditis in adults include bicuspid aortic valves, Marfan's syndrome, syphilitic heart disease, and idiopathic hypertrophic subaortic stenosis [21–23]. In about one-quarter of patients with endocarditis, no underlying cardiac valvular abnormalities are identified [15].

An increase in the average age of endocarditis patients has occurred as a result of changes in the populations at risk for the infection [17,24,25]. The age increase is more apparent in community hospitals, compared with urban referral centers that treat a higher proportion of intravenous drug users. Moreover, the decline in rheumatic heart disease along with the increased prevalence of calcific aortic sclerosis and of intravenous drug use has led to a relative decline in mitral valve endocarditis and a relative increase in aortic and tricuspid valve endocarditis compared with previous decades [15].

Among children, congenital cardiac abnormalities, particularly those associated with cyanosis, are the major predisposing factors [26]. Thus, patent ductus arteriosus, ventricular septal defects, coarctation of the aorta, tetralogy of Fallot, transposition of the great arteries, and tricuspid and pulmonary atresia and stenosis all predispose to endocarditis. Isolated atrial septal defects in the absence of mitral regurgitation are low-risk lesions. While the incidence rate of endocarditis for specific congenital defects such as ventricular septal defect is lower among those

Table 48-1. Major syndromes of vascular infection

Infective endocarditis
Infective endarteritis
Vascular graft infection
Suppurative thrombophlebitis

undergoing surgical correction [27], an overall increase in the incidence of pediatric cases of endocarditis has been noted over the past few decades, from 0.55 to 0.78 case per 1,000 pediatric hospital admissions [1]. That increase has been attributed to several factors, including increased survival of children with cyanotic heart disease, the increased performance of cardiac surgery with the placement of prosthetic material, valves, conduits, and patch material, and intravenous drug use among children in older age groups.

The incidence of endocarditis among intravenous drug users is 2–5 percent per year [28,29], which exceeds by severalfold the estimated annual risk associated with rheumatic heart disease or valve prostheses [30]. That risk, while excessive, still seems astonishingly low considering the intensity of microbial challenge expected with the regular practice of injecting drugs [31]. The proportion of endocarditis associated with intravenous drug use has increased over the past few decades, particularly in urban areas [32–34]. Most recently, however, anecdotal reports from several urban centers suggest that the incidence of endocarditis may be declining in this population, perhaps as a result of reduced needle sharing and an increase in clean-needle use prompted by the AIDS epidemic [31].

Iatrogenic interventions are now a common precipitant of infective endocarditis, with a nosocomial source for endocarditis implicated in 10–29 percent of cases. Bacteremia secondary to intravascular devices is the most common cause [19,32,35–37]. Patients with nosocomial endocarditis are more likely than those with community-acquired disease to have underlying valvular abnormalities and less likely to be intravenous drug users.

Prosthetic-valve infection accounts for 12–33 percent of all cases of infective endocarditis [19,20,38–40]. The overall incidence of prosthetic-valve endocarditis (PVE) is 1–4 percent [41,42]. The risk of PVE is 1.4–3.1 percent in the first postoperative year, with highest rates within the first 6 months. The risk reduces to 0.5 percent or less per year thereafter [43–45]. Risk factors that have been identified for PVE include black race, male sex, aortic-valve replacement, multiple prosthesis insertion in the elderly, intravenous drug use, and prolonged cardiopulmonary bypass time [43,46].

PATHOGENESIS

Native-Valve Endocarditis. With the exception of early PVE due to intraoperative contamination, infective endocarditis appears to result from a dynamic interplay between (1) an antecedent focal abnormality of the endothelial surface and (2) bacteremia with organisms from a distant source, such as the oropharynx, skin, or gastrointestinal or genitourinary tract, that is able to adhere to and establish infection at that site [47–49].

Intact endocardium is exceedingly resistant to infection following bacteremia [50]. A key factor promoting initial attachment of organisms to valve surfaces is the occurrence of endothelial injury. Endothelial injury occurs when a high-velocity jet stream, resulting from a pressure gradient across a relatively narrow orifice separating a high- and a low-pressure chamber, passes over or strikes the endothelial surface [51–53]. Areas vulnerable to endothelial injury correspond to the typical sites of infective endocarditis. Those areas include the ventricular surface of an incompetent aortic valve, the atrial surfaces of incompetent mitral or tricuspid valves, the atrial wall opposite the mitral orifice in mitral regurgitation, and the papillary muscle of the left ventricle in aortic regurgitation. Alternatively, endothelial injury may occur iatrogenically from intracardiac catheters or at surgical sites.

Clumps of fibrin and platelets are deposited at sites of endothelial injury, forming sterile vegetations referred to as nonbacterial thrombotic endocarditis (NBTE). Sterile vegetations also may occur in patients with underlying illnesses, such as malignancy or collagen vascular disease. NBTE lesions may become seeded by bloodborne microorganisms, giving rise to an infected vegetation that is the pathologic hallmark of endocarditis [50].

The relative necessity of antecedent endothelial injury as a predisposing factor for endocarditis depends in part on the virulence of the organism. Certain virulent pathogens such as *Staphylococcus aureus* or *Streptococcus pneumoniae* appear able to cause endocarditis on previously normal valves. The mechanism by which endocarditis might occur in those instances is uncertain. One possibility, raised by recent studies that demonstrate phagocytosis of *S. aureus* or *Candida* by endothelial cells in tissue culture [54,55], is that intracellular multiplication may lead to endothelial-cell destruction, which in turn initiates platelet-fibrin deposition.

Pathogens that are the most frequent causes of endocarditis, such as the gram-positive cocci, are also those that are best able to adhere to the platelet and fibrin components of NBTE lesions and resist protective host factors in serum such as complement [56,57]. Once adherent to the platelet-fibrin clot, subsequent deposition of additional platelets and fibrin entrap the organisms and provide a protected focus, allowing the organisms to grow unimpeded to high titers (10^9–10^{10} organisms/gram of tissue).

The precise mechanisms by which pathogens adhere to endothelial cells or to platelet-fibrin aggregates have been the subject of intense investigation. Several strains of bacteria that cause endocarditis are known to bind specifically to certain host proteins such as laminin, a protein present in the subendothelial matrix [58], vitronectin [59], and fibrinogen [60]. Endocarditis-causing bacterial strains are also known to bind to and activate platelets in the presence of plasma proteins [61]. Gram-negative bacilli, which are uncommon causes of endocarditis, lack that activity.

Bacteria-induced platelet activation may promote further aggregation of platelets and fibrin, amplifying a process that ultimately may lead to an infected vegetation [62,63]. Herrmann et al. [64] found that adherence of radiolabeled *S. aureus* was extensively promoted (28-fold) by the presence of purified platelets coating the surface of polymethylmethacrylate (PMMA) cover slips when compared to binding to PMMA coverslips coated with albumin. Pretreatment of platelets with anti-GPIIb/IIIa monoclonal antibodies or inhibitors of platelet activation decreased plasma-enhanced adhesion, suggesting a role for platelet activation in *S. aureus* adhesion. In addition, plasma-enhanced adhesion was inhibited by thrombin antagonists, protease inhibitors, heparin, and antifibrinogen antibodies, suggesting that fibrinogen, fibrin, or both play a role in bridging between cellular receptors on adherent platelets and *S. aureus.* It has been suggested that integrins such as GPIIb/IIIa may serve as cellular receptors. *S. aureus* is known to possess binding sites for integrins found on platelet surfaces [65].

Much investigative interest also has focused on the plasma protein fibronectin, which is known to bind directly to pathogens such as *S. aureus*, viridans streptococci, *S. pneumoniae,* other streptococci, and *Candida,* but not to gram-negative organisms [66–72]. In the case of streptococci, lipoteichoic acid appears to be the fibronectin receptor [73]. Fibronectin is secreted by endothelial cells, platelets, and fibroblasts in response to vascular injury and is capable of binding simultaneously to fibrin, collagen, platelets, fibroblasts, and bacteria.

Intravenous Drug Use. The pathogenesis of endocarditis occurring among intravenous drug users, most of whom initially have no underlying valvular disease, is unclear. It has been suggested that particulate material contained in the injectate may traumatize valvular endothelium, giving rise to platelet-fibrin deposits to which pathogens subsequently adhere [31]. There also appears to be a difference in the relative risk of infection based on which drug is injected, with an increased risk associated with cocaine compared with heroin [74]. The reason for that distinction is not entirely clear, although it is possible that the practice of boiling heroin to dissolve it into solution prior to injection may confer some protection against infection.

Among intravenous drug users with endocarditis, the tricuspid valve alone is involved in about 54 percent, the aortic valve in 25 percent, and the mitral valve in 20 percent; mixed right- and left-sided involvement occurs in 6 percent [75]. When *S. aureus* is the pathogen, however, infection involves the right-sided valves, particularly the tricuspid valve, in 80–100 percent of patients [76–78]. Left-sided involvement, either alone or as part of bilateral involvement, occurs in 7–15 percent of patients [77–79]. Why tricuspid-valve involvement is so much more common than pulmonic-valve involvement remains unexplained [28,80].

Prosthetic-Valve Endocarditis. Primary adherence of coagulase-negative staphylococci to prosthetic devices is thought to be mediated by hydrophobic interactions between the cell wall and the surface of the prosthesis itself or of ligand-specific binding to host-derived factors such as fibronectin [81–85], fibrinogen [60,69,86–88], laminin [81,89,90], vitronectin [59], and thrombospondin [91], which coat the surface of the prosthesis. These proteins have been shown experimentally to promote staphylococcal adherence to polymer surfaces. As in the case of microbial adherence to denuded endothelial surfaces, platelets may play an important facilitatory role in adherence to intravascular prostheses. Wang et al. [92] recently showed that contact-activated platelets appear to mediate adherence of *Staphylococcus epidermidis* to the surface of hydrophobic biomedical polymer disks. They found that while platelets represented only 4 percent of the total exposed surface on the disk, 50 percent or less of adherent bacteria were bound to the platelets, suggesting a specific interaction between ligands on the bacterial surface and the platelets. In the case of nonencapsulated strains of *S. epidermidis,* binding appears to be mediated by lipoteichoic acid [63].

Once infecting pathogens become adherent, the surface of the prosthesis eventually becomes covered with a matrix, referred to as **biofilm** [93–95]. Biofilm consists of bacteria; extracellular polysaccharide; or slime, which is produced by certain strains of coagulase-negative staphylococci [96–100]; and host-derived matrix proteins. The biofilm may achieve a thickness of 140 μm [101] and interferes with the ability of antibiotics to kill the imbedded organisms [102].

Endocarditis involving mechanical prostheses usually begins in the tissue adjacent to the prosthesis at the sewing ring [103]. A partial or completely circumferential "ring abscess" forms, often leading to valvular dehiscence and paravalvular regurgitation. The paravalvular abscess may burrow into the myocardium, leading to fistulae, conduction-system abnormalities, coronary arteritis with thrombosis and infarction, or pericarditis. As in the case of native-valve endocarditis, such complications are more likely with valves in the aortic than in the mitral positions [104,105].

In contrast to mechanical-valve endocarditis, infective endocarditis involving bioprosthetic valves typically involves the valve tissue itself. Valvular involvement leads to tearing and perforation of the valve leaflet(s) and valvular incompetence. Less commonly, valvular obstruction due to bulky vegetations may occur [106–108].

Calderwood and associates [43] noted a difference in the timing of infective endocarditis occurring on mechanical versus bioprosthetic valves. In the early postoperative period, mechanical valves have a greater risk of infection, but the rate of bioprosthetic-valve infection steadily increases with time such that, by 5 years, the overall incidence of endocarditis is similar for both types of valves. A lack of difference in rates of infection for Bjork-Shiley mechanical versus porcine valves was likewise noted by Bloomfield et al. at 7 and 12 years following both mitral- and aortic-valve replacement [109].

MICROBIOLOGY

The importance of specific pathogens as causes of endocarditis varies with the clinical setting. When considering microbial etiology, patients with infective endocarditis may be classified as follows: (1) those with native valves who do not use intravenous drugs, (2) intravenous drug users, (3) those with prosthetic valves, (4) those with nosocomially acquired endocarditis, and (5) those with culture-negative endocarditis.

Native-Valve Endocarditis, No Intravenous Drug Use. Streptococci (50–70%), staphylococci (25%), and enterococci (10%) are the predominant causes of endocarditis on native valves of those who do not use intravenous drugs. Over half the streptococci that cause endocarditis in this population are the so-called viridans streptococci, which are part of the normal oropharyngeal flora [110] and include *Streptococcus sanguis, Streptococcus salivarius, Streptococcus mutans,* and *Streptococcus mitior.* Those organisms cause endocarditis primarily in patients with underlying valvular abnormalities, often in the wake of dental procedures. *Streptococcus bovis* endocarditis is primarily a disease of the elderly and has been associated with the presence of colonic polyps or malignancy [111–114]. Other streptococci account for fewer than 5 percent of cases of endocarditis in that population. Group A and group B streptococci may cause infection on previously normal valves. *S. pneumoniae* currently causes about 3 percent of all cases of infective endocarditis and typically behaves as an aggressive, destructive pathogen [115–117].

S. aureus is the predominant staphylococcal species causing native-valve endocarditis. *S. aureus* may attack normal valves on either the left or the right side of the heart and is typically associated with an aggressive clinical course.

Coagulase-negative staphylococci account for less than 10 percent of isolates in non-drug-using patients with native-valve endocarditis. *Staphylococcus epidermidis* causes about half of those cases, while other species such as *Staphylococcus warnerii, Staphylococcus cohnii, Staphylococcus saprophyticus, Staphylococcus hemolyticus,* and *Staphylococcus hominis* account for the rest [118,119]. Coagulase-negative staphylococcal endocarditis typically presents subacutely, affecting previously abnormal left-sided valves [118,119]. However, some strains may cause a destructive endocarditis that necessitates valve replacement and has high associated mortality [118–122].

Enterococci, including *Streptococcus faecalis* and *Streptococcus faecium,* may attack either normal or abnormal heart valves and generally are an infection of elderly men with a recent history of urinary-tract instrumentation, urinary-tract infection, or uro-obstructive disease. Occasionally, young women who have undergone abortion, pregnancy, or cesarean section may develop endocarditis due to these organisms [123].

Gram-negative bacilli account for only 5.7 percent of native-valve endocarditis among patients who do not use intravenous drugs. That low incidence is striking in view of the high incidence of gram-negative bacteremia associated with infection or instrumentation of the urinary and gastrointestinal tract and may be explained in part by deficits in adherence properties, as discussed above. Occasional causes of endocarditis on native valves include *Neisseria gonorrheae* [124,125] and *Pseudomonas aeruginosa* [126], both of which have the capacity to attack and destroy previously normal valves. Rare causes of endocarditis in this population include enteric gram-negative bacilli such as *Escherichia coli* [127,128] and *Salmonella* sp. [129].

Listeria [130,131], anaerobes [132,133], spirochetes such as *Spirillum minor* (a cause of rat-bite fever), and *Erysipelothrix rhusiopathiae* (the agent of erysipeloid) [134–136] occasionally cause endocarditis.

Intravenous Drug Use. The predominant cause of endocarditis among injecting drug users is *S. aureus,* accounting for 60 percent of cases overall and 80 percent of cases involving the right side of the heart [28,75]. Methicillin-resistant *S. aureus* (MRSA) infections have been reported among intravenous drug users in Detroit [76,77,137], Boston [138], New York [139], and San Francisco [140]. Risk factors for addict-related MRSA endocarditis include recent hospitalization [141], unauthorized use of antibiotics [141], and drug injection in shooting galleries [139,141]. Other gram-positive organisms, such as streptococci or enterococci, together account for 20 percent of cases in this population and usually involve the left side of the heart. There is a marked and unexplained regional variation in the incidence of gram-negative pathogens such as *P. aeruginosa* (common in Detroit, Chicago, and Cleveland but not in San Francisco) and *Serratia marcescens* (common in San Francisco during the 1970s but not since) [142–145]. Fungal organisms, especially non-*albicans Candida* sp., are cultured in a minority (about 14 percent) of patients and usually affect the left side of the heart, in particular the aortic valve [146]. Finally, polymicrobial infection occurs in about 5 percent of drug addicts with endocarditis, with addicts accounting for 70 percent of all patients with polymicrobial endocarditis [147].

The source of microorganisms causing endocarditis among intravenous drug users is unclear. At least in the case of *S. aureus,* the source of the organism appears to be the patient's own skin, although how, short of injecting through a cutaneous abscess, an inoculum of sufficient magnitude gains access to the bloodstream remains unexplained [31,148]. Attempts to recover *S. aureus* from samples of street drugs or from syringes have been largely unsuccessful [149]. However, reports of the same pathogen causing infection in drug users sharing injection paraphenalia support the role of contaminated syringes, at least in some cases [150–152].

Prosthetic-Valve Endocarditis. The spectrum of microbial agents causing PVE depends on the timing of the infection following surgery. Traditionally, PVE has been classified as "early" or "late," with 60 days being the point of separation [153]. A more pathophysiologically relevant point of separation would be between 6–12 months postoperatively [43]. The key distinction between early and late cases is that most early PVE results from intra- or perioperative contamination and, thus, is predominantly due to nosocomial or cutaneous flora [42,154,155]. In contrast, late PVE is due to bacteremic seeding of the valve and, thus, is caused by a spectrum of organisms more closely mimicking those of native-valve endocarditis [43,105,156–159]. Molecular typing has revealed that PVE caused by intra- or perioperative contamination with *S. epidermidis* may remain dormant for 6–12 months before becoming clinically apparent [154,160–162], accounting in part for the delay in conversion from early to late flora.

Early PVE is caused by methicillin-resistant nosocomial strains of *S. epidermidis* (25–30%), *S. aureus* (15–20%), gram-negative bacilli (about 20%), fungi such as *Candida* or *Aspergillus* (10–12%), streptococci and enterococci (5–10%), and diptheroids (5–10%). On the other hand, viridans streptococci are the organisms most frequently isolated in late PVE (25–30%), with other streptococci and enterococci (5–10%); *S. epidermidis*, which are predominantly methicillin-sensitive and community-acquired (23–28%); *S. aureus* (10–12%); gram-negative bacilli (10–12%); fungi (5–8%); and diptheroids (4–5%) accounting for the rest of the cases [43,163].

While coagulase-negative staphylococci generally are regarded as pathogens of low virulence, PVE due to those organisms, particularly cases occurring in the first postoperative year and involving an aortic prosthesis [164], frequently present as a locally invasive, destructive infection. Valve replacement is required in the majority of cases either during active infection or within 6 months. In the series of Karchmer et al., prosthetic-valve dysfunction, usually due to annular infection causing partial valve dehiscence and insufficiency, was noted in 38 of 55 patients [163]. Myocardial abscess was noted in 17 patients.

Nosocomial Endocarditis. Gram-positive organisms, including staphylococci, streptococci, and enterococci, are the predominant causes of nosocomial endocarditis [19,34,35,165]. Nosocomial endocarditis generally refers to endocarditis resulting from a hospital-based procedure performed in the 4 weeks prior to the onset of symptoms or when the onset of symptoms occurs at least 48 hours after admission. Over 75 percent of these cases are due to staphylococci, with an equal proportion due to coagulase-negative staphylococci and *S. aureus*. Despite the frequency of gram-negative bacteremia in the nosocomial setting, endocarditis due to those organisms is rare [35,165]. A definable source of infection was felt to be present in 97 percent of cases of nosocomial infective endocarditis in two series, with 46 percent secondary to an intravascular device (including peripheral and central lines, angiography, or pacemaker related) and 44 percent attributed to postsurgical procedures such as gastrointestinal or genitourinary instrumentation. The elderly are disproportionately affected by nosocomial endocarditis, and preexisting valvular abnormalities are present in the majority [118,119].

Culture-Negative Endocarditis. The overall frequency of negative cultures among patients with the classic infective endocarditis syndrome is around 9 percent, with somewhat lower frequencies among intravenous drug users or those with prosthetic valves. The most common cause of culture-negative endocarditis is antecedent antibiotic therapy [166–169]. In the absence of antibiotic therapy and with proper culture techniques, the proportion of endocarditis cases that are culture-negative should be less than 5 percent [170,171]. Other causes of culture-negative endocarditis include fastidious or slow-growing organisms with particular growth requirements such as nutritionally variant streptococci, the so-called HACEK organisms (*Haemophilus* sp., *Actinobacillus actinomycetemcomitans, Cardiobacterium hominis, Eikenella corrodens*, and *Kingella* sp.) [172–181], and *Brucella* sp. [182]. Other slow-growing organisms include corynebacteria (diptheroids) [183,184], lactobacilli [185], propionibacteria, and *Rothia dentocariosa*. Fungal endocarditis, particularly that due to species other than *Candida albicans*, often is associated with negative cultures [186–190]. In such cases, the diagnosis is determined at surgery for embolectomy or valve replacement or at autopsy. Other causes of culture-negative endocarditis are diagnosed serologically, including *Chlamydia psittaci* [191,192], and *Coxiella burnetii* (Q fever) [193–196]. Additional causes of culture-negative endocarditis include *Chlamydia trachomatis*, mycoplasma [197], *Legionella* [198], mycobacteria, *Nocardia* sp., L-forms of bacteria, and possibly viruses [166].

CLINICAL PRESENTATION OF PATIENTS WITH INFECTIVE ENDOCARDITIS

The clinical presentation of infective endocarditis depends in part on the etiologic agent, on whether left or right-sided valves are involved, and whether the patient has a valve prosthesis. Fever almost always is present in patients with endocarditis but may be absent in the very elderly, in debilitated patients, or in those with renal failure. Fever is typically low grade and remittent. However, endocarditis due to virulent pathogens such as *S. aureus* may be associated with high spiking fevers and frank rigors [79,199].

Pathologic cardiac murmurs are present in greater than 90 percent of patients with left-sided endocarditis but are absent in the majority of those with mural infection [200]. A new or changing murmur is described in 36–52 percent of patients with left-sided valvular endocarditis [20,36]. Among intravenous drug users with right-sided endocarditis, a pathologic murmur may not be appreciated initially in up to a half of patients but eventually becomes apparent in most cases [79,201].

Congestive heart failure is the most frequent complication of infective endocarditis, occurring in about a third of patients, and is the leading cause of death [202]. Acute congestive heart failure in native-valve endocarditis is usually due to left-sided valvular incompetence resulting from leaflet destruction and perforation. Heart failure also may result from bulky vegetations, chordae or papillary-muscle rupture, myocarditis or myocardial abscess, arrhythmias, infarct, sinus of Valsalva rupture, or worsening of antecedent valvular disease [32,203–205]. In patients with right-sided endocarditis, overt evidence of right-heart failure is uncommon.

Ring abscess, usually involving the aortic annulus, most commonly occurs in infection due to virulent organisms such as *S. aureus* and as a complication of endocarditis involving mechanical prostheses [206]. Annular abscess may be associated with persistent fever, conduction blocks, arrhythmias, and hemodynamic deterioration due to perivalvular leak and valve dehiscence if not urgently tended to surgically.

Peripheral stigmata of endocarditis include mucocutaneous lesions as well as retinal lesions. Mucocutaneous manifestations such as nonblanching petechiae, splinter hemorrhages, Osler's nodes, and Janeway lesions are seen most commonly in the setting of subacute endocarditis and in acute endocarditis due to *S. aureus*. In subacute endocarditis, the pathogenesis is thought to involve immune complex deposition, while in acute staphylococcal endocarditis, septic embolization is more likely [207]. Petechiae are most common on the conjunctivae, palate, buccal mucosa, and the extremities. Splinter hemorrhages are subungual, appear as linear dark red streaks, and are more suggestive of endocarditis if proximally located [208]. Osler's nodes are tender nodules found on the pads of the fingers or toes, postulated in the case of subacute endocarditis to be due to a necrotizing vasculitis of the glomus body [209,210]. Osler's nodes in the setting of *S. aureus* endocarditis appear to contain microabscesses in the papillary dermis with septic microemboli in small dermal arterioles, with cultures positive on aspiration [211]. Janeway lesions are flat, nontender, hemorrhagic lesions typically found on the palms and the soles [209]. Finally, clubbed fingers are present in 10–20 percent of patients with long-standing endocarditis. The pathogenesis of clubbing in this setting is unclear, and clubbing often resolves with treatment of the endocarditis [24].

Opthalmic stigmata of endocarditis include cotton wool spots, representing nerve-fiber-layer infarcts, retinal hemorrhages, and Roth spots. Roth spots are retinal hemorrhages with a pale center located near the optic disk and are highly suggestive of endocarditis in the appropriate clinical setting, although they also may be seen in patients with connective-tissue disease and hematologic disorders [212,213]. Emboli to the central retinal artery occur in about 2 percent of cases of infective endocarditis and present as sudden monocular blindness.

Splenomegaly is noted especially with infective endocarditis of long duration [214] and is thought to be associated with chronic immune stimulation. Patients with septic emboli to the spleen may develop splenic abscess.

Arthralgias and clinical arthritis have been noted retrospectively in 38 percent and 31 percent, respectively, of infective endocarditis cases [215]. The arthritis is usually migratory and culture negative and is thought be on an immune complex basis. Alternatively, frank septic arthritis may occur in 2–27 percent of patients, particularly with *S. aureus* infections [32,216,217]. About a third of patients with subacute endocarditis complain of backache, which improves with therapy, although occasionally that symptom is indicative of a focus of metastatic infection such as vertebral osteomyelitis. Myalgias are seen in 19 percent of patients and may represent focal myositis [215]. Musculoskeletal complaints are particularly prominent in intravenous drug users with endocarditis.

Embolic phenomena are the second most common life-threatening complication of endocarditis, after congestive heart failure [218]. Embolic complications have been reported in 15–35 percent of cases, though many more embolic lesions generally are found at autopsy than are clinically identified [207]. Septic emboli, along with immune complex phenomena, have been implicated in a variety of neurologic and systemic complications associated with endocarditis and with the development of mycotic aneurysms. Emboli to visceral arteries may be associated with acute abdominal pain, ileus, hematuria, or melena. Emboli to coronary arteries may result in myocardial infarction, myocarditis, or arrhythmias. Emboli to the extremities may result in acute vascular insufficiency. In drug users with right-sided endocarditis, septic pulmonary emboli may be associated with dyspnea, cough, pleuritic chest pain, and hemoptysis [75,78,79,219]. The majority (70–85%) of those with tricuspid endocarditis have radiographic evidence of septic pulmonary emboli, typically presenting as peripheral nodular infiltrates with or without cavitation [77–79,220]. Pleural effusions also are common but usually are uncomplicated and resolve with antibiotics alone.

The neurologic complications of endocarditis have recently been summarized by Salgado et al. [221], who found a 37-percent incidence among 113 patients with native- or prosthetic-valve endocarditis seen over a 12-year period. Lesions noted included emboli, meningitis, encephalopathy, and neuropathy. Intracranial emboli usually involve the middle cerebral artery and its branches and give rise to cerebral infarcts, abscesses, arteritis, and mycotic aneurysms. Meningitis usually is sterile in the case of subacute endocarditis. Purulent meningitis may occur, particularly in the setting of *S. aureus* infection [222]. Encephalopathy due to diffuse microemboli [223], and neuropathy resulting from emboli to vessels supplying peripheral nerves also may occur [224].

Infective endarteritis with aneurysmal dilatation (mycotic aneurysm) has been found in 5–10 percent of infective endocarditis cases at autopsy [222], although that figure likely overestimates the current incidence of the complication. The topic of infective endarteritis is reviewed later in this chapter.

The most common cause of renal insufficiency in patients with infective endocarditis is congestive heart failure. However, a number of other renal complications may occur, such as petechiae and embolic sequelae, including infarcts, endarteritis, and abscess. Immune complex glomerulonephritis, either focal or diffuse, may occur, as may interstitial inflammation [225]. Diffuse glomerulonephritis may be of either an acute proliferative or a membranoproliferative variant [226,227]. Renal insufficiency due to glomerulonephritis usually responds to antibiotics [228].

In terms of laboratory abnormalities, the white blood cell count often is normal, although the differential may be left-shifted [53]. Normochromic normocytic anemia is present in 70–90 percent of cases of infective endocarditis with subacute or chronic presentations. The erythrocyte sedimentation rate almost always is elevated except in the presence of heart or renal failure. Rheumatoid factor is positive in 50 percent of patients with subacute presentations, and nonspecific generalized hypergammaglobulinemia is seen in at least one-quarter of patients. An abnormal urinalysis, with hematuria or findings consistent with glomerulonephritis, commonly is found.

DIAGNOSIS OF INFECTIVE ENDOCARDITIS

The strict case definition of von Reyn et al [20] categorized endocarditis cases as "definite," "probable," "possible," and "rejected," with definite endocarditis reserved for cases with direct evidence of infective endocarditis by histopathologic or microbiologic examination of surgical or autopsy specimens of valvular vegetation or peripheral embolus. That definition gained widespread acceptance, but it has been criticized for being too restrictive, with only a minority of cases fulfilling "definite" criteria. In addition, the von Reyn criteria were devised prior to the availability of two-dimensional or transesophageal echocardiography, diagnostic tools that have become an integral part of the clinical evaluation of patients with suspected endocarditis.

The reported sensitivity of transthoracic echocardiography (TTE) in detecting valvular vegetations is about 70–80 percent [140,229–231], while transesophageal echocardiography (TEE) has a sensitivity in the range of 90 percent or greater [206,230,232–234]. TEE has the additional benefit of a high level of sensitivity for detecting intracardiac abscesses [206,235,236]. Thus, while echocardiography alone can never be used to definitively diagnose endocarditis, the high sensitivity of TEE imparts significant negative predictive value to a negative study by this modality. Occasional false-positive results occur with both TTE and TEE, however. Nodular thickening, tumor, and rupture of a valve leaflet or of chordae tendiniae all may mimic a valvular vegetation.

Revised diagnostic criteria that incorporate modern echocardiography have been developed by the Duke Endocarditis Service [170,237]. That definition is modeled after the Jones criteria for rheumatic fever, with both major and minor clinical criteria for the diagnosis of endocarditis. **Definite** endocarditis is diagnosed if (1) there is direct pathologic evidence of endocarditis or (2) in the absence of pathologic evidence, two major, one major and three minor, or five minor clinical criteria are fulfilled. Major clinical criteria include (1) documentation of bacteremia due to organisms commonly associated with endocarditis or the demonstration by persistently positive blood cultures of continuous bacteremia highly suggestive of intravascular infection and (2) echocardiographic findings that are considered highly suggestive of endocarditis. Minor criteria include the presence of predisposing cardiac conditions or intravenous drug use, fever, vascular phenomena, immunologic phenomena, blood culture positivity not meeting the criteria cited above, serologic evidence of infection, and echocardiographic findings consistent with but not highly suggestive of endocarditis.

Early experience with the Duke criteria has been favorable. Bayer and associates applied the criteria to the study of 63 prospectively enrolled adult patients with suspected endocarditis at an urban medical center [238]. Each of 10 pathologically confirmed cases of infective endocarditis would have been designated by the Duke clinical criteria as definite, while the von Reyn criteria would have rejected half of those cases. The inclusion of two-dimensional echocardiographic data in the Duke criteria enabled significantly more cases of suspected endocarditis to be classified as definite and fewer cases to be rejected, compared to the von Reyn criteria. The Duke criteria currently are undergoing further validation with a variety of patient populations.

Strict definitions aside, the diagnosis of endocarditis should be suspected in (1) patients with heart murmur and unexplained fever; (2) persons with a sudden neurologic event, particularly if they are young; (3) all febrile intravenous drug users; and (4) patients with prosthetic valves with fever or valvular dysfunction.

Blood cultures remain the most important diagnostic test. The hallmark of bacteremia associated with endocarditis, as mentioned above, is that it is continuous [169]. Thus, in cases of suspected endocarditis, one should not wait for a fever spike to draw the cultures. Rather, blood cultures should be spaced at least 30 minutes apart to prove that the bacteremia is, in fact, continuous [239]. Three sets of blood cultures, drawn prior to the initiation of antibiotic therapy, should have a sensitivity in the range of 95 percent. An exception to the rule of continuous bacteremia is in patients with prosthetic-valve endocarditis where the infection is located in the subvalvular ring [42]. In such cases, the bloodstream may be intermittently seeded with microorganisms.

In patients with suspected endocarditis where blood cultures remain negative after 2 or 3 days, several additional interventions may be taken to optimize the chance of recovering the pathogen. First, blood cultures should be held for at least 3 weeks, since the isolation of some slow-growing or fastidious organisms may be delayed. The microbiology laboratory should be alerted to look for fastidious organisms such as nutritionally variant streptococci, which may require cysteine- or pyridoxine-supplemented media [171,240–242]. Other pathogens for which special attention is required include the HACEK organisms, where subculture onto chocolate agar with incubation under conditions of increased ambient carbon dioxide enhances recovery. Recovery of brucella and *Neisseria* sp. is facilitated by the use of special media in biphasic Castaneda bottles with prolonged incubation in carbon dioxide–enriched atmosphere [167]. Charcoal-yeast-extract agar is used for *Legionella* culture. For fungal cultures, the use of the lysis-centrifugation blood culture technique may increase yield, particularly for species other than *C. albicans*.

Other diagnostic modalities include serology, which is most useful in cases of Q fever (*C. burnetii*), brucellosis, and psittacosis. Bone-marrow stain and culture can be helpful in diagnosing fungal endocarditis, particularly when due to non-*albicans Candida*, which may not grow as readily as *C. albicans* in routine culture. Bone-marrow biopsy also may be helpful to diagnose brucella and mycobacterial endocarditis [167]. Finally, buffy-coat gram stains occasionally are positive for intraleukocytic bacteria and can provide an early diagnostic clue [243,244].

TREATMENT OF ENDOCARDITIS: GENERAL PRINCIPLES

In general, prolonged therapy with antibiotic regimens that are microbicidal and not merely inhibitory is essential for successful therapy of infective endocarditis. The minimum bactericidal concentration (MBC) is the minimum concentration of antibiotic that achieves a 99.9-percent decrease in numbers of bacteria at 24 hours *in vitro;* the minimal inhibitory concentration (MIC) is the minimum concentration of antibiotic that inhibits growth *in vitro.* Agents for which the MBC is equal to or within one dilution of the MIC are considered to be bactericidal [245]. Those agents for which the difference between MIC and

MBC is 16 dilutions or fewer are considered to be bacteriostatic.

Some organisms display a property known as **tolerance.** Tolerance is said to occur when there is a large gap between MIC and MBC (e.g., MBC-MIC ratio $\geq$ 32) for an antibiotic that normally is bactericidal. Simply put, it takes far higher concentrations of antibiotic to kill tolerant organisms than simply to inhibit their growth. A number of organisms, including some streptotocci and most enterococci [246–248], display tolerance in response to therapy with normally bactericidal cell wall–active agents such as penicillin, ampicillin, and vancomycin. In such cases, an aminoglycoside such as gentamicin or streptomycin is added to the cell wall–active agent to achieve reliable killing through the synergistic activity of the two drugs. In the case of enterococci, relapse rates in the range of 50 percent are expected if aminoglycosides are not added [249], compared with rates of around 15 percent with combination therapy [239,249,250].

Antimicrobial resistance has emerged as a major impediment to the therapy of endocarditis. MRSA is an increasingly common cause of endocarditis both among intravenous drug users and in the nosocomial setting and generally requires the use of vancomycin for therapy. There recently has been an alarming and explosive increase in clinical isolates of enterococci, both *S. faecalis* and, especially, *S. faecium,* which are resistant not only to cell wall–active agents such as penicillin, ampicillin, and vancomycin but also to high levels of gentamicin and streptomycin [251–253]. No bactericidal regimens currently are available to treat such multiresistant strains [248,254], and high rates of treatment failure are expected for endocarditis due to those strains.

In addition to antimicrobial resistance, a variety of other factors impair the ability of antibiotics to reach and kill microorganisms imbedded in vegetations [245,255].

1. **Serum drug level and degree of protein binding.** Because only unbound antibiotic is free to diffuse into vegetations, the extent of protein binding is a major determinant of the level of antibiotic actually available *in vivo.* On the other hand, MICs determined by the laboratory are based on total rather than free drug levels.
2. **Antibiotic penetration into vegetations.** Antibiotics vary in their ability to penetrate platelet-fibrin vegetations [256–259]. For example, small molecules such as the penicillins and aminoglycosides are able to penetrate to the core, while bulky molecules such as teicoplanin, which is similar in structure to vancomycin, penetrate only the periphery [259,260]. In addition, biofilm produced by *S. epidermidis* in the setting of prosthetic valve endocarditis may pose a permeability barrier for antibiotics as well [102].
3. **Microbial density and antibiotic-inactivating factors in vegetations.** High densities of microorganisms may be associated with high concentrations of enzymes such as beta-lactamase, which may inactivate antibiotics. Furthermore, organisms in the stationary phase of growth exhibit reduced susceptibility to cell wall–active agents such as beta-lactams, which are most active against actively dividing organisms [261,262].

In addition to MIC and MBC determinations for pathogens that cause infective endocarditis, the **serum bactericidal test** can be performed to determine the ability of the antibiotic regimen present in the patient's serum to inhibit or kill the infecting organism. Because of lack of standardization and questions regarding its predictive value, routine use of this test is discouraged [245,255]. However, determination of serum bactericidal level may be helpful when response to therapy is suboptimal, when endocarditis is due to an unusual organism, or when unconventional treatment is used [56]. The American Heart Association recommends that a peak bactericidal titer be maintained at 1 : 8 or higher in the treatment of streptococcal endocarditis [56].

TREATMENT OF ENDOCARDITIS: ANTIBIOTIC REGIMENS

Native-Valve Endocarditis, No Intravenous Drug Use. For patients with suspected native-valve endocarditis who are not intravenous drug users (Table 48-2), initial empiric antibiotics should be directed against streptococci and enterococci; thus, the combination of high-dosage penicillin G plus low-dosage gentamicin (for synergy) is recommended pending culture results. With an acute presentation, *S. aureus* should be targeted, so a semisynthetic penicillin such as nafcillin (or oxacillin) is substituted for penicillin G and gentamicin is retained for synergy.

Once blood culture results are known, the antibiotic regimen may be modified. Streptococci vary in their susceptibility to penicillin and whether or not they display tolerance. Those factors influence the choice and duration of the antibiotic regimen used. As a guide to therapy, therefore, MIC and MBC should be determined. Suggested regimens for the various levels of penicillin resistance (MIC $\leq$ 0.1 μg/ml, MIC $>$ 0.1 and $<$ 0.5 μg/ml, and MIC $\geq$ 0.5 μg/ml) are listed in Table 48-2. For patients with penicillin-susceptible streptococcal endocarditis, either a 4-week course of penicillin alone, or a 2-week course of penicillin plus gentamicin are accepted therapies [263]. Use of the short-course regimen should be reserved for younger patients with normal renal function with uncomplicated endocarditis and a short duration of symptoms prior to initiation of therapy. Streptococcal strains that display tolerance should be treated with the regimen cited for resistant (MIC $\geq$ 0.5 μg/ml) streptococci.

Ceftriaxone, a third-generation cephalosporin, has emerged as an alternative therapy for selected patients with penicillin-susceptible streptococci [264–266]. Because this agent has a serum half-life of 6–9 hours, enabling once-a-day dosaging, it is a convenient agent for outpatient intravenous therapy. To be considered for ceftriaxone therapy, the patient should be (1) reliable and compliant; (2) without evidence for heart failure or for echocardiographic findings that portend an increased risk of heart failure such as premature mitral valve closure, torn aortic cusps, or large vegetations; (3) infected with a susceptible, nontolerant streptococcal isolate; and (4) clinically stable during an initial inpatient course (1–2 weeks) of antibiotic therapy [264,267]. Trials are under-

Table 48-2. Suggested antibiotic therapy for native-valve endocarditis in persons who do not use intravenous drugs

Cause of infection	Therapy[a]
Empiric therapy pending cultures	Subacute presentation: Penicillin G 20 million U daily plus gentamicin 1 mg/kg (maximum 80 mg, peak level 3 μg/ml) q8h IV. Substitute vancomycin 1 gram q12h IV for penicillin if penicillin allergic.
	Acute presentation: Nafcillin or oxacillin 2 g IV q4h plus gentamicin 1 mg/kg (maximum 80 mg, peak 3 μg/ml) q8 hours IV. Substitute vancomycin 1 g q12h IV for nafcillin (or oxacillin) if patient is penicillin allergic or known to harbor methicillin-resistant *S. aureus* (MRSA).
Penicillin-susceptible streptococci (MIC ≤ 0.1 μg/ml)	Penicillin G 10–20 million U daily for 4 weeks. Substitute cefazolin 1 g IV q8h or vancomycin 1 g IV q12 hours for 4 weeks if penicillin allergic.
	Penicillin G 10–20 million U daily plus gentamicin 1 mg/kg (maximum 80 mg, peak 3 μg/ml) q8h IV for 2 weeks.[b]
	Ceftriaxone 2 g IV daily for 4 weeks.[b]
Relatively resistant streptococci (MIC > 0.1 and < 0.5 μg/ml)	Penicillin G 20 million U daily for 4 weeks plus gentamicin 1 mg/kg (maximum 80 mg, peak 3 μg/ml) q8h IV for the first 2 weeks.
Streptococci with penicillin MIC ≥ 0.5	Penicillin G 20–30 million U daily plus gentamicin 1 mg/kg q8h IV (maximum 80 mg, peak 3 μg/ml) for 4–6 weeks. Consider penicillin desensitization or substitute vancomycin for penicillin if penicillin allergic.
Enterococci	**Beta-lactam susceptible:** Ampicillin 2 g IV q4h plus either gentamicin 1 mg/kg q8h IV (peak 3 μg/ml) or streptomycin 7.5 mg/kg q12h IM (maximum 500 mg, peak level 20 μg/ml) for 4–6 weeks. Check for high-level aminoglycoside resistance.[b]
	Beta-lactam resistant: Vancomycin 1 g q12h IV plus either gentamicin or streptomycin (if not high-level resistant) for 4–6 weeks.
	Beta-lactam and vancomycin-resistant: No reliably bactericidal therapy currently available.[b]
Staphylococci	**Methicillin sensitive:** Nafcillin or oxacillin 2 g q4h IV for 4–6 weeks, with the optional addition of gentamicin 1 mg/kg q8h IV (maximum 80 mg, peak 3 μg/ml) for the first 3–5 days. Substitute cefazolin 2 g q8h IV or cephalothin 2 g q4h IV or vancomycin 1 g q12h IV if penicillin allergic.
	Methicillin resistant: Vancomycin 1 gram q12h IV for 4–6 weeks.
HACEK organism	Ampicillin 2 g q4h IV or ceftriaxone 1 g q12h IV plus gentamicin 1.7 mg/kg q8h IV for 4 weeks.[b]
Enteric gram-negative bacillus	Ceftriaxone 1 g q12h IV (or other third-generation cephalosporin, or aztreonam 2 g q6h IV) plus gentamicin 1.7 mg/kg q8h IV for 4–6 weeks.
Pseudomonas aeruginosa	Ceftazidime 2 g q8h IV (or piperacillin 3 g q4h IV or aztreonam 2 g q6h IV or imipenem 500 mg q6h IV) plus tobramycin 1.7 mg/kg q8h IV for 6 weeks.
Fungi	Amphotericin B 1 mg/kg daily IV plus valve replacement.[b]

[a]Adult dosages for persons with normal renal function.
[b]See text.

way to evaluate the efficacy of a 14-day regimen of ceftriaxone combined with an aminoglycoside, both administered as a once-a-day dosage, for the treatment of streptococcal endocarditis [268].

Enterococci are intrinsically more resistant to cell wall–active antibiotics than streptococci [254] and often display the property of tolerance, which was discussed earlier. Thus, a combination regimen of a cell wall–active agent plus an aminoglycoside is required for the entire duration of therapy to achieve reliable bactericidal activity. Enterococcal isolates should be tested routinely for resistance to high levels (2,000 μg/ml) of both gentamicin and streptomycin, since 30–50 percent of high-level gentamicin-resistant isolates may remain susceptible to high levels of streptomycin [248]. Isolates that are susceptible to penicillins and that are not high-level aminoglycoside-resistant should be treated with a penicillin (e.g., ampicillin)–aminoglycoside combination. Vancomycin is substituted for a penicillin if the isolate is penicillin resistant, or if the patient is penicillin allergic. In either case, a low dosage of aminoglycoside (e.g., aiming for a peak level of 3 $\mu g/ml$ in the cases of gentamicin) should be used to reduce the risk of nephro- and ototoxicity, while maintaining synergistic benefit. If the enterococcus is high-level resistant to both gentamicin and streptomycin, no benefit of synergy is achieved by adding the aminoglycoside. Such isolates are treated with a cell wall–active agent alone, and in such cases prolonged therapy (e.g., 8 weeks) is suggested. Because a high risk of relapse is expected, these patients require close clinical follow-up during and following treatment. For endocarditis due to multiply resistant enterococcal isolates, that is, isolates that are resistant to cell wall–active agents (penicillins and vancomycin) **and** to high levels of aminoglycosides, reliable therapeutic options currently do not exist.

Staphylococci that are methicillin-susceptible generally are treated with a semisynthetic penicillin such as nafcillin or oxacillin. Limited data suggest that the addition of gentamicin results in more rapid clearance of bacteremia, although that is accomplished at the expense of an increased rate of renal insufficiency with no demonstrated difference in clinical outcome [269,270]. For that reason, many experts recommend the initial use of gentamicin (at low dosages) to promptly sterilize the bloodstream, with discontinuation after 3–5 days to avoid a significant risk of aminoglycoside-associated nephrotoxicity. For endocarditis due to MRSA, vancomycin is the drug of choice.

Antibiotic therapy of gram-negative endocarditis involves a combination of a beta-lactam agent and an aminoglycoside, with aminoglycosides given at full systemic dosages. Monotherapy with a third-generation cephalosporin (e.g., ceftriaxone or cefotaxime) has been used with success in the treatment of endocarditis due to the HACEK organisms and may emerge as the regimen of choice. The role of quinolone agents such as ciprofloxacin in the treatment of endocarditis remains to be defined, but there are theoretical reasons to believe that they would be quite favorable in this setting [255,271]. HACEK organisms are generally amenable to medical therapy, although bulky vegetations and emboli are not uncommon complications [172,272]. In contrast, treatment of endocarditis due to enteric gram-negative bacilli or *P. aeruginosa* often is complicated, with the frequent requirement for surgical intervention [271].

Empiric therapy of fungal endocarditis, most commonly due to *Candida* or *Aspergillus* sp., is with amphotericin B [273]. However, amphotericin penetrates vegetations poorly [146], and some *Candida* isolates, such as *Candida lusitaniae*, are resistant to amphotericin B *in vitro*. Determination of ideal therapy for such isolates is complicated by limited published experience and the fact that antifungal testing is neither routinely available nor standardized. Dismal experience with medical therapy for fungal endocarditis has led most authors to consider valve replacement to be mandatory. A minimum total dose of 40 to 50 mg/kg of amphotericin should be given, and some authors advocate the addition of flucytosine if *in-vitro* synergy is demonstrated for these two agents. The role of the azole antifungals, including fluconazole and itraconazole, in the treatment of fungal endocarditis remains to be defined.

Intravenous Drug Use. Thirteen percent of febrile intravenous drug users presenting to urban emergency rooms have infective endocarditis [3]. Suggested empiric therapy pending culture results and further evaluation is the combination of vancomycin plus full-dosage gentamicin to cover *S. aureus* (including MRSA), the predominant pathogen, as well as streptococci, enterococci, and gram-negative bacilli (Table 48-3). Recent concerns have been raised regarding the delayed response of *S. aureus* bacteremia to vancomycin [140,201,274–276]. Thus, in locales where MRSA is known not to be prevalent in this population, nafcillin or oxacillin may be substituted for vancomycin. In addition, if antimicrobial susceptibility testing indicates that the isolate is methicillin sensitive, either nafcillin or oxacillin should be used in preference to vancomycin for those who are not penicillin allergic. The regimens suggested above for left-sided endocarditis in patients who do not use injectable drugs also are appropriate for the treatment of left-sided or bilateral endocarditis in intravenous drug users, with the exception that outpatient ceftriaxone therapy (with maintenance of an indwelling vascular catheter) should not be used.

For *S. aureus* endocarditis confined to the right-side valves, two potential therapeutic options include (1) nafcillin (or oxacillin or vancomycin for penicillin-allergic patients or for MRSA) intravenously for 4 weeks or (2) the combination of nafcillin (or oxacillin) plus low-dosage gentamicin intravenously for 2 weeks. The short-course regimen is useful because these patients often fail to comply with extended therapy. However, short-course therapy is appropriate only for patients who fulfill the following criteria: (1) HIV-negative; (2) uncomplicated endocarditis (without heart failure, empyema, abscess, multiple cavitary lung lesions, or metastatic site(s) of infection); (3) methicillin-susceptible isolate; and (4) endocarditis confined to the right side of the heart [277]. Overall, about 50 percent of *S. aureus* endocarditis among injecting drug users will be suitable for 2-week combination therapy. Finally, limited experience with a predominantly orally administered regimen of ciprofloxacin and rifampin has been published [278], although such regimens still must be considered experimental. The early development of resistance to both drugs has unfortunately been reported with this therapy [279].

Prosthetic-Valve Endocarditis. Suggested therapy for endocarditis in patients with prosthetic valves is listed in Table 48-4. The combination of vancomycin and gentamicin is suggested as empiric therapy pending culture results, because of the predominance of staphylococci, which may be methicillin-resistant, as causative agents. Major differences in the therapeutic approach to PVE compared with native-valve endocarditis include the following:

1. The routine use of combination therapy including a cell wall–active agent plus an aminoglycoside for synergy is advocated for the treatment of gram-positive organisms. The further addition of rifampin in the case of *S. epidermidis* infection is recommended, based on both animal model data as well as limited clinical evidence [56,163,280,281].

Table 48-3. Suggested antibiotic therapy for infective endocarditis in intravenous drug users

Cause of infection	Therapy
Empiric therapy pending cultures	Vancomycin 1 g q12h IV plus gentamicin 1.7 mg/kg q8h IV.
Staphylococcus aureus	**Methicillin sensitive:** **Right-sided endocarditis.** Nafcillin (or oxacillin) 2 g q4h IV for 4 weeks. Alternatively, for selected candidates (see text), nafcillin (or oxacillin) 2 g q4h IV plus gentamicin 1 mg/kg (maximum 80 mg, peak 3 μg/ml) q8h IV for 2 weeks. **Left-sided or bilateral endocarditis or endocarditis with extrapulmonary metastatic septic foci.** Nafcillin (or oxacillin) 2 g q4h IV for 4–6 weeks with the optional addition of gentamicin 1 mg/kg q8h IV for the first 3–5 days. **Methicillin resistant:** Vancomycin 1 g q12h IV for 4–6 weeks.

Table 48-4. Suggested antibiotic therapy for prosthetic-valve endocarditis

Cause of infection	Therapy*
Empiric therapy pending cultures	Vancomycin 1 g q12h IV plus gentamicin 1 mg/kg q8h IV (maximum 80 mg, peak 3 μg/ml)
Streptococci	**Penicillin sensitive (MIC ≤ 0.1 μg/ml):** Penicillin G 20 million U daily for 6 weeks plus gentamicin 1 mg/kg q8h IV for 2 weeks. **Relatively resistant (MIC > 0.1, < 0.5):** Penicillin G 20 million U daily for 6 weeks plus gentamicin 1 mg/kg q8h IV for 6 weeks. **Resistant streptococci (MIC ≥ 0.5 μg/ml).** Penicillin G 20 million U daily for 6–8 weeks plus gentamicin 1 mg/kg q8h IV for 6–8 weeks.
Staphylococcus aureus	**Methicillin sensitive:** Nafcillin (or oxacillin) 2 g q4h IV for 6–8 weeks plus gentamicin 1 mg/kg q8h IV for the first 2 weeks. **Methicillin resistant:** Vancomycin 1 g q12h IV for 6–8 weeks plus gentamicin 1 mg/kg q8h IV for the first 2 weeks.
Staphylococcus epidermidis	Vancomycin 1 g q12h IV for 6–8 weeks plus rifampin 300 mg q8h PO for 6–8 weeks plus gentamicin 1 mg/kg q8h IV for the initial 2 weeks.
Enterococci	Treat as for native-valve endocarditis, except extend therapy to 6–8 weeks.
HACEK organisms	Treat as for native-valve endocarditis, except extend therapy to 6 weeks.
Enteric gram-negative bacilli	Treat as for native-valve endocarditis, except extend therapy to 6–8 weeks.
Diphtheroids	Penicillin G 20 million U daily plus gentamicin 1 mg/kg q8h IV for 6 weeks. Alternatively, vancomycin 1 g q12h IV alone for 6 weeks if penicillin allergic.
Fungi	Treat as for native-valve endocarditis.

*Adult dosages for persons with normal renal function.

2. A longer course of antibiotic therapy, generally 6–8 weeks, should be given.
3. A much higher proportion of patients, in the range of 50–65 percent, will require valve replacement to eliminate infection and to restore effective valve function [106,164].

THERAPY OF LESS COMMON CAUSES OF ENDOCARDITIS

C. burnetii (Q fever). Optimal therapy of Q-fever endocarditis has not been defined. The absence of available bactericidal therapy against this organism and its intracellular location make its eradication exceedingly difficult, with valve cultures remaining positive even after 2 or more years of therapy [282–284]. Mortality rates remain in the range of 34–65 percent [282]. The combination of doxycycline plus either trimethoprim-sulfamethoxazole [193,196,283,285,286] or doxycycline plus a flouroquinolone such as ofloxacin [282,285] has been recommended, with suggested duration of therapy ranging from a year to lifetime. The value of following anti–phase I antibody titers to *C. burnetii* is unclear, since the titers may remain quite elevated for years [196,282]. For native-valve disease, cardiac-valve replacement should be reserved for cardiac failure attributable to valve dysfunction. In the case of an infected prosthesis, the likelihood of eradicating infection short of valve replacement is remote [2,87].

Brucella sp. Combination therapy with a tetracycline such as doxycycline and another agent such as an aminoglycoside, rifampin, or trimethoprim-sulfamethoxazole is generally given to treat brucella endocarditis [182,288–291]. Initial employment of doxycycline plus gentamicin is favored by many authors [285], with a change to doxycycline plus either trimethoprim-sulfamethoxazole or rifampin after 4–6 weeks. The latter regimen is continued for up to 10 months, depending on the clinical course. Titers of antibrucella antibody, as determined by the 2-mercaptoethanol modification of the standard tube agglutinin (STA) assay should progressively fall with effective therapy [292]. Unfortunately, only a minority of patients with definite brucella endocarditis have been cured without cardiac-valve replacement [293]. Indications for surgery include congestive heart failure, abscess, persistent fever, and prosthetic-valve infection [290].

Chlamydia. Chlamydia are rare causes of endocarditis, with most of the reported cases due to *C. psittaci.* Optimal therapy has not been defined, but the combination of tetracycline plus rifampin for 6 weeks, followed in some cases by a prolonged course of doxycycline, has been used [294]. Chlamydia antibody titers are followed as a guide to therapy. Almost half of reported cases have required surgery, usually performed electively for valve-related heart failure after microbiologic cure was achieved.

Corynebacteria (Diptheroids). Group JK organisms are the most common diptheroid cause of PVE [294]. Persons with prosthetic valves, underlying heart disease, immunocompromise, and intravenous drug use are at risk for endocarditis due to these organisms. Recommended therapy is vancomycin plus an aminoglycoside for 6 weeks [294]. Mortality associated with corynebacterium endocarditis is in the range of 26 percent, while mortality may be as high as 83 percent for early prosthetic-valve endocarditis [183].

INDICATIONS FOR SURGICAL INTERVENTION

Native-Valve Endocarditis, No Intravenous Drug Use. Absolute indications, agreed on by most authorities, for valve replacement in patients with native-valve endocarditis include (1) class III or IV congestive heart failure, (2) valvular obstruction, (3) persistent bacteremia for more than 1 week of therapy in the absence of metastatic foci of infection, and (4) fungal endocarditis [295,296]. Relative indications include suppurative intracardiac disease such as periannular or myocardial abscess [297], recurrent emboli, and endocarditis due to aggressive pathogens such as *S. aureus* or gram-negative bacilli that are not responding promptly to antibiotic therapy [298,299].

Mortality among endocarditis patients who develop moderate to severe heart failure is in the range of 50–90 percent [300]. Several studies indicate that surgical intervention dramatically improves outcome, with mortality reduced to the range of 15–37 percent [301]. Surgery is recommended for patients with class III or IV heart failure or progressive heart failure due to valvular dysfunction, with the timing of surgery dictated by the patient's hemodynamic status [300,302].

Persistent fever in association with infective endocarditis often is associated with a complicated course. Lederman et al. [303] reviewed the duration of fever among 123 patients treated for infective endocarditis at University Hospitals of Cleveland during the period 1972–1984. Half the patients defervesced within 3 days of therapy, nearly three quarters after 1 week, and nearly 90 percent after 2 weeks. Prolonged fever was associated with infective endocarditis due to *S. aureus,* gram-negative bacilli, or culture-negative endocarditis. By multivariate analysis, microvascular phenomena and major-vessel embolization were found to be independently associated with longer duration of fever. Patients with fever for more than 1 week following institution of antibiotic therapy experienced a higher mortality (18% versus 2%, $p < 0.002$) than those who promptly defervesced.

Blumberg et al. [304] compared the clinical courses of 26 patients with endocarditis and fever lasting 2 weeks or longer (median duration, 35 days) despite appropriate antibiotic therapy with other age-matched endocarditis patients without prolonged fever. Causes of persistent fever included myocardial abscess (27%), drug fever (19%), nosocomially acquired infection (19%), persistent bacteremia (12%), a cardiac focus as suggested by resolution of fever following valve replacement (12%), postpericardiotomy syndrome (4%), splenic abscess (4%), and unknown (3%). Sixteen of 26 persistently febrile patients required cardiac surgery, seven on an emergent basis, compared with only two of the controls ($p < 0.001$). Based on their experience, the authors recommend an extensive diagnostic evaluation for any patient with infective endocarditis and fever lasting more than one week. Evaluation should include TEE to look for myocardial abscess or other cardiac source, which may require surgical intervention, as well as abdominal CT scan and bone scanning to look for metastatic foci of infection. In the absence of positive findings with those tests, the possibility of drug fever should be assessed by changing medications if possible.

A highly controversial issue is whether certain echocardiographic findings are predictive of an increased risk of emboli, therefore indicating the need for surgical intervention. Mugge and associates found that patients with mitral valve vegetations of less than 10 mm in size were significantly more likely to suffer major emboli, and they recommend surgery for such patients [230]. In a retrospective review by Sanfilippo et al. of endocarditis patients seen at Massachusetts General Hospital between 1982 and 1987, vegetation size, extent, and mobility emerged as predictors of complications, including embolic events, by multivariate analysis [305]. In contrast, Steckelberg et al. [306] noted in-hospital clinical embolic events in 38 percent of patients with definite vegetations, 40 percent of those without detectable vegetations, and 22 percent of those with indeterminate findings. Other authors similarly have failed to find an association between echocardiographically apparent vegetations and embolic events [307,308].

While embolic events may occur at any time during the course of endocarditis, several studies suggest that most occur either before admission (i.e., as the event precipitating admission) or during the first several days of antibiotic therapy [306,307,309,310]. Hart et al. [310] observed that 74 percent of CNS embolic events had occurred by the time of initial presentation, and 87 percent occurred within 48 hours of the diagnosis. Similarly, Steckelberg and colleagues found that the incidence of emboli fell from 13 per 1,000 patient-days during the first week of antibiotics to fewer than 1.2 per 1,000 patient-days after 2 weeks of therapy [306].

It is clear that a prospective study with adequate sample size and blinded echocardiographic interpretation, which takes into account both the timing of antibiotic therapy and of any embolic events that occur, will be needed to resolve whether the size and characteristics of vegetations should influence decisions regarding surgical intervention. Based on existing data, however, many authors do not recommend surgery to prevent embolic complications based on echocardiographic findings alone [311].

Intravenous Drug Use. Right-sided endocarditis due to *S. aureus* among intravenous drug users almost always responds to antibiotic therapy alone [312–314]. Several authors have suggested that the echocardiographic finding of vegetations greater than 1.0 cm, especially when accompanied by prolonged fever, may identify a group of patients likely to require surgical intervention [314–317]. However, the study by Hecht and Berger [312] does not support that contention. Those authors reviewed the clinical courses of 121 intravenous drug users with evidence of 132 episodes of endocarditis, all of whose two-dimensional echocardiograms revealed right-sided valvular vegetations as determined by an observer blinded to clinical information. *S. aureus* was the infecting organism in 82 percent of cases. Vegetations greater than 1.0 cm were present in the majority of cases (80%). Despite a mean vegetation size of 1.5 cm, the vast majority (91%) of their patients were cured with medical therapy. Moreover, 92 percent of episodes in which fever persisted for more than 3 weeks ultimately responded to medical therapy.

The indications for surgery among intravenous drug users with endocarditis are controversial, since recurrent endocarditis associated with continued drug use occurs in 20–40 percent of cases [318,319]. In general, for left-sided disease, the same criteria used for non–drug users apply, with congestive heart failure due to valve dysfunction, uncontrolled sepsis, and fungal infection being the major indications. Surgery in patients with right-sided endocarditis should be reserved for patients who fail to clear bacteremia despite a week of optimal antibiotic therapy, those with severe right-heart failure, and those with fungal infection. Valve debridement or resection, without the placement of a prosthesis, is usually favored [315]. About 20 percent of patients with tricuspid endocarditis who have valvulectomy eventially require tricuspid-valve replacement (TVR) because of right-heart failure [320,321].

Prosthetic-Valve Endocarditis. Fifty to 65 percent of patients with PVE will require valve replacement to eliminate infection and restore effective valve function [106,164]. Indications for surgery include (1) increasing or refractory congestive heart failure secondary to valve dysfunction; (2) evidence of perivalvular abscess with valve dehiscence, paravalvular regurgitation seen on echocardiography, or new electrocardiographic conduction abnormalities; (3) persistent bacteremia despite 1 week of antibiotic therapy; (4) recurrent systemic embolization; (5) fungal infection; and (6) relapse after optimal therapy [295]. Congestive heart failure is the key predictor of mortality. While patients with PVE and mild or no heart failure have a mortality of 20–35 percent, those with moderate to severe heart failure have a mortality of 60–85 percent, and surgical therapy clearly improves survival in the latter population (e.g., 51% survival with surgery compared with 0% survival without) [322].

The risk that PVE will relapse after surgical replacement of an actively infected prosthetic valve is in the range of 15–25 percent [323,324]. If clinically feasible, 7 days of antibiotic therapy preceding surgery is desirable to gain initial control over active infection. However, surgery should not be postponed if there is severe hemodynamic compromise or clinical evidence of progression of infection.

RELAPSES AND REINFECTIONS

Relapse is defined as failure of therapy, that is, recurrence of symptoms and bacteremia due to the same organism. Most relapses occur within 2 months and generally within 2–4 weeks of completing antibiotic therapy. The most important cause of relapse is failure to administer bactericidal therapy for an adequate length of time. In the case of certain organisms such as multiresistent enterococci, fungi, or *C. burnetii,* no bactericidal therapy currently exists, and high relapse rates are expected. Likewise, for aggressive organisms like *S. aureus,* relapse rates of up to 40 percent are reported [199,325]. In contrast, for drug-sensitive pathogens such as viridans streptococci, relapse rates of less than 10 percent are expected with appropriate therapy [326]. Another factor possibly associated with an increased risk of relapse is a duration of endocarditis for greater than 3 months prior to the initiation of therapy [327]. Because the risk of relapse is not insignificant, follow-up blood cultures should be drawn 1–2 weeks following completion of therapy, and for any episode of fever occurring in the subsequent two months.

Resolution of clinical findings associated with endocarditis may take a long while to subside, and their continued presence should not raise concern, in the absence of fever, of persistent bacteremia. Splenomegaly may persist for months after cure, as may anemia, hematuria, and peripheral stigmata such as Osler's nodes or petechiae [326].

The management of patients with relapsing endocarditis has been reviewed by Wilson et al. [328]. For first relapses due to virulent organisms such as *S. aureus* or enteric gram-negative bacilli or for refractory organisms such as *C. burnetii,* valve replacement is suggested. For other organisms, a second course of medical therapy is suggested, with surgery reserved for standard indications such as heart failure or persistent sepsis. For patients with a second episode of relapse, surgical intervention is recommended for most patients except those with uncomplicated infection due to drug-sensitive organisms such as viridans streptococci, in which case, surgery is reserved for a third relapse.

One or more episodes of recurrent endocarditis due to a different organism may occur in 5–8 percent of patients with a prior history of endocarditis [319,329,330]. Other risk factors for reinfection include intravenous drug use and the presence of periodontitis [319,331].

PREVENTION OF ENDOCARDITIS

Most cases of endocarditis, unfortunately, are not preventable. Episodes of transient bacteremia that could potentially seed a focus of NBTE occur on a daily basis, in association with activities as trivial as brushing teeth. A history of an antecedent dental or surgical procedure or of instrumentation (e.g., endoscopy, bladder catheterization) in the preceding 3–6 months is found in only a quarter of patients with viridans streptococcal endocarditis and in 40 percent of those with enterococcal endocarditis [332].

Preventative efforts are focused on (1) encouraging patients to maintain a high level of dental hygiene and (2) providing patients who have cardiac lesions at high risk for bacteremic seeding with prophylactic antibiotics during procedures associated with sustained bacteremia. The antibiotic(s) chosen are those effective against pathogens most likely to adhere to abnormal endothelial foci during the episode of bacteremia, including viridans streptococci for oral or upper respiratory procedures and enterococci for genitourinary or gastrointestinal procedures.

The underlying cardiac conditions and the dental or surgical procedures for which prophylaxis is not recommended by the American Heart Association (AHA) are listed in Table 48-5 [333]. The table lists selected conditions and procedures but is not meant to be all-inclusive. Additional caveats include the following:

1. Although endocarditis prophylaxis is recommended for mitral valve prolapse (MVP) patients with evidence of valvular regurgitation, prophylaxis also should be considered in persons with MVP associated with thickening or redundancy of the valve leaflets, particularly for men 45 years of age and older.
2. In addition to providing standard prophylaxis for persons with underlying cardiac-risk lesions who are undergoing genitourinary procedures, the antibiotics given also should cover any pathogens that might be causing active infection at the time of the procedure. Obviously, elective procedures should be postponed until after active infection has resolved.
3. In persons with prosthetic heart valves, a previous history of endocarditis, or surgically constructed systemic-pulmonary shunts or conduits, the clinician may elect to provide antibiotic prophylaxis even for low-risk dental or surgical procedures.

Suggested prophylactic antibiotic regimens (adult dosages) are listed in Table 48-6. While the AHA guidelines suggest 3 g of amoxicillin for standard dental and upper respiratory prophylaxis, a recent paper by Dajani et al. suggests that a 2-g dose may be given with similar expected efficacy but with fewer side effects [334].

Infective Endarteritis (Mycotic Aneurysm)

Infective endarteritis is defined as inflammation involving the arterial wall secondary to microbial infection, which may occur with or without aneurysmal dilatation. Traditionally, the lesions have been referred to as **mycotic aneurysms,** a term coined in the last century by William Osler. The term mycotic strictly refers to fungal infection. Thus, the more general term of **infective endarteritis** is preferred. For the sake of simplicity, however, the terms will be used interchangeably in this discussion.

A pathogenic classification of infective endarteritis is cited in Table 48-7. In the preantibiotic era, most (90%) cases occurred as a result of emboli in patients with infective endocarditis [335], with other causes including syphilis and tuberculosis. Currently, most cases of infective endarteritis occur secondary to bacteremic seeding of atherosclerotic arteries, where the source of bacteremia may be unknown (cryptogenic) or a defined focus of infection such as osteomyelitis, cellulitis, pneumonia, or urinary-tract infection [336]. Trauma, either accidental, inadvertent (iatrogenic), or self-inflicted (intravenous drug use), is another important cause of infective endarteritis. While published reports from 2 decades ago suggested that this complication occurred in up to 15 percent of patients with endocarditis [337,338], the current rate probably is much lower.

PATHOGENESIS AND CLINICAL PRESENTATION

Infective endarteritis secondary to endocarditis is thought in most cases to be due to septic emboli to vaso vasora [311]. Less commonly, endarteritis results from emboli to the lumen of narrow-caliber arteries or at points of arterial bifurcation. In most cases, the involved vessels are thought to be normal prior to infection. Infective endarteritis due to septic emboli tend to be saccular and rapidly enlarging, compared to the fusiform nature of aneurysms resulting from seeding of atherosclerotic vessels. Most lesions become manifest within 2–3 weeks of the diagnosis of endocarditis, although a diagnostic delay of up to 6 months may occur [339]. Persistent fever, symptoms related to enlargement or leakage, and frank rupture are the usual presentations.

Mycotic aneurysms complicating infective endocarditis involve, in descending frequency, the aorta, the cerebral arteries, the visceral arteries, and the arteries of the lower and upper extremities [311]. Multiple lesions may be present. Mycotic aneurysm may involve the sinus of Valsalva or the coronary arteries. The lesions may be complicated by the development of vascular shunts and rupture into the right ventricle or coronary-artery occlusion. Lesions of the aortic root may lead to pericardial tamponade and atrioventricular conduction block [340]. Mycotic aneurysms of the pulmonary arteries may occur in patients with right-sided endocarditis.

Intracranial mycotic aneurysms are characteristically located in the peripheral middle cerebral-artery distribution [223,338,339,341]. The lesions usually are clinically silent and most often present as catastrophic hemorrhage

Table 48-5. American Heart Association recommendations for endocarditis prophylaxis

CARDIAC CONDITIONS FOR WHICH ENDOCARDITIS PROPHYLAXIS IS RECOMMENDED
Prosthetic cardiac valves, including bioprosthetic and homograft valves
Previous bacterial endocarditis, even in the absence of heart disease
Most congenital cardiac malformations
Rheumatic and other acquired valvular dysfunction, even after valvular surgery
Hypertrophic cardiomyopathy
Mitral valve prolapse with valvular regurgitation
CARDIAC CONDITIONS FOR WHICH ENDOCARDITIS PROPHYLAXIS NOT RECOMMENDED
Isolated secundum atrial septal defect
Surgical repair without residua beyond 6 months of secundum atrial septal defect, ventricular septal defect, or patent ductus arteriosus
Previous coronary artery bypass graft surgery
Mitral valve prolapse without valvular regurgitation*
Physiologic, functional, or innocent heart murmurs
Previous Kawasaki disease without valvular dysfunction
Previous rheumatic fever without valvular dysfunction
Cardiac pacemakers and implanted defibrillators
DENTAL OR SURGICAL PROCEDURES FOR WHICH ENDOCARDITIS PROPHYLAXIS IS RECOMMENDED
Dental procedures known to induce gingival or mucosal bleeding, including professional cleaning
Tonsillectomy or adenoidectomy
Surgical operations that involve intestinal or respiratory mucosa
Bronchoscopy with rigid bronchoscope
Sclerotherapy for esophageal varices
Esophageal dilatation
Gallbladder surgery
Cystoscopy
Urethral dilatation
Urethral catheterization if urinary-tract infection is present*
Urinary-tract surgery if urinary-tract infection is present*
Prostatic surgery
Incision and drainage of infected tissue
Vaginal hysterectomy
Vaginal delivery in the presence of infection*
DENTAL OR SURGICAL PROCEDURES FOR WHICH ENDOCARDITIS PROPHYLAXIS NOT RECOMMENDED*
Dental procedures not likely to induce gingival bleeding, such as simple adjustment of orthodontic appliances or fillings above the gum line
Injection of local intraoral anesthetic (except infraligamentary injections)
Shedding of primary teeth
Tympanostomy tube insertion
Endotracheal intubation
Bronchoscopy with a flexible bronchoscope, with or without biopsy
Cardiac catheterization
Endoscopy with or without gastrointestinal biopsy
Cesarean section
In the absence of infection for urethral catheterization, dilatation and currettage, uncomplicated vaginal delivery, therapeutic abortion, sterilization procedures, or insertion or removal of intrauterine devices

*See text.
Source: Adapted with permission from Dajani et al.

associated with headache and deterioration in the level of consciousness. A herald bleed, presenting as a sudden headache with focal neurologic deficit, occurs in fewer than a quarter of cases and should trigger prompt evaluation by CT or MRI and angiography [221].

Many aortic and visceral mycotic aneurysms are clinically silent until catastrophic rupture occurs. Some aortic mycotic aneurysms may present as a tender pulsatile mass. Surgical therapy of such lesions generally includes excision of all infected tissue, if feasible, and arterial recon-

Table 48-6. Recommended regimens for endocarditis prophylaxis (Adult Doses)*

STANDARD PROPHYLACTIC REGIMEN FOR DENTAL, ORAL, OR UPPER-RESPIRATORY-TRACT PROCEDURES IN PATIENTS AT RISK, INCLUDING THOSE WITH PROSTHETIC HEART VALVES
Amoxicillin 3.0 g or 2.0 g* PO 1h before procedure, then 1.5 g 6h after initial dose
For patients who are penicillin allergic
Erythromycin ethylsuccinate 800 mg or erythromycin stearate 1.0 g PO 2h before procedure, then half the dose 6h after initial dose
or
Clindamycin 300 mg PO 1h before procedure and 150 mg 6h after initial dose
ALTERNATIVE PROPHYLACTIC REGIMENS FOR DENTAL, ORAL, OR UPPER-RESPIRATORY-TRACT PROCEDURES IN PATIENTS WHO ARE AT RISK
For patients unable to take oral medications:
Ampicillin 2.0 grams IV/IM 30 minutes before procedure, then 1.0 g IV/IM 6h after initial dose
or
Clindamycin 300 mg IV 30 min. before procedure and 150 mg IV 6h after initial dose (for penicillin-allergic patients)
For patients considered high risk and not candidates for the standard regimen:
Ampicillin 2.0 g IV/IM plus gentamicin 1.5 mg/kg (not to exceed 80 mg) 30 minutes before procedure, followed by amoxicillin 1.5 g PO 6h after initial dose (alternatively, the parenteral regimen may be repeated 8h after initial dose)
or, for penicillin-allergic patients,
Vancomycin 1.0 g IV over 1h starting 1h before procedure; no repeated dose necessary
REGIMENS FOR GENITOURINARY AND GASTROINTESTINAL PROCEDURES
Standard regimen:
Ampicillin 2.0 g IV/IM plus gentamicin 1.5 mg/kg (not to exceed 80 mg) 30 minutes before procedure, followed by amoxicillin 1.5 g orally 6h after initial dose (alternatively, parenteral regimen may be repeated once 8h after initial dose)
or, for penicillin-allergic patients,
Vancomycin 1.0 g IV over 1h, plus gentamicin 1.5 mg/kg (not to exceed 80 mg) IV/IM 1h before procedure; may be repeated once 8h after initial dose
Alternative regimen for low-risk patients:
Amoxicillin 3.0 g orally 1h before procedure, then 1.5 g 6h after initial dose

*See text.
Source: Adapted with permission from Dajani et al.

struction through noninfected tissue planes with autogenous graft whenever possible, along with prolonged antibiotic therapy. Mycotic aneurysm complicating infective endocarditis may involve the superior mesenteric, celiac, hepatic, renal, and, rarely, splenic arteries [336,342–

Table 48-7. Pathogenic classification of infective endarteritis with or without associated (mycotic) aneurysm

Secondary to infective endocarditis
Secondary to bacteremic seeding of diseased aorta (atherosclerosis, congenital lesion, syphilitis) in the absence of infective endoarteritis
Infective endarteritis and infected pseudoaneurysm secondary to trauma—accidental, iatrogenic (arterial puncture), or due to intravenous drug use
Secondary to direct arterial invasion by a contiguous septic focus (e.g., pancreatitis, vertebral osteomyelitis)
Aortoenteric fistula (duodenal, colonic)

344]. Hepatic-artery aneurysms may present as biliary colic, hemobilia, gastrointestinal bleeding, or jaundice and are diagnosed by celiac angiography [336]. Occasionally, renal-artery aneurysms may present with hypertension and hematuria [311].

The second and currently most common pathogenic category of infective endarteritis (see Table 48-7) is that caused by microbial seeding of arteries that are diseased as a result of atherosclerosis or, less commonly, syphilic aortitis or congenital abnormality. The usual sites of involvement correlate with common sites of atherosclerosis, including the distal aorta, superior mesenteric, common iliac, femoral, and popliteal arteries and less commonly the brachial, splenic, or distal arteries of the extremities. Aneurysms due to bacteremic seeding usually are large and fusiform and may be multiple. The classic clinical presentation is that of vascular insufficiency or disruption in the setting of fever, chills, continuous bacteremia that does not clear with antibiotic therapy, and a pulsatile mass. Other patients may present with back or abdominal pain. Rarely, patients will present with a gastrointestinal bleed secondary to an aortoenteric fistula that most commonly involves the third portion of the duodenum [345]. Most often, short periods of herald bleeding occur in such cases, but bleeding may be sudden and catastrophic. A draining cutaneous sinus rarely may be found. Finally, the patient may present with aneurysmal rupture with exsanguination.

While an extravascular source may be found on clinical evaluation, up to half of cases of infective endarteritis due to intimal seeding of a diseased vessel are cryptogenic [346]. The spectrum of microorganisms causing mycotic aneurysm in this setting differ from those associated with infective endocarditis. About 60 percent of these infections are due to gram-positive organisms, with staphylococci, mostly *S. aureus,* accounting for two-thirds [347]. Salmonellae, either *Salmonella typhimurium, Salmonella enteritidis* strains, or *Salmonella choleraesuis* (only rarely *S. typhi*) account for 20 percent of cases. A variety of other gram-negative and gram-positive organisms and, rarely, fungal pathogens account for the rest of cases.

Salmonella sp. have a special propensity to adhere to abnormal vascular surfaces. Blood cultures should be drawn in any patient with salmonella cultured from sputum or urine without adequate explanation. The diagnosis of salmonella mycotic aneurysm should be pursued in persons with positive blood cultures, especially if they are over the age of 50 years and have symptoms such as fever, back or abdominal pain, chest pain, or a pulsatile abdominal mass [348,349].

While infective endarteritis may occur secondary to intimal seeding by microorganisms of an aorta previously damaged by syphilis, syphilitic aortitis itself results from seeding of the vasa vasora of the adventitia by *Treponema pallidum*. Syphilitic aortitis most commonly involves the proximal aorta. Treponemes that lodge in the vasa vasora incite inflammatory changes that eventually lead to an obliterative endarteritis, adventitial scarring, and patchy medial necrosis with destruction of elastic fibers [350]. Diffuse atherosclerotic changes may follow in the intima, with characteristic "egg shell" calcification. Weakening of the aortic wall may lead to aortic root dilatation and aneurysm formation. Moreover, contraction of scar tissue may lead to aortic insufficiency and coronary ostial stenosis.

Infective endarteritis and infected pseudoaneurysm may occur secondary to accidental trauma [351], iatrogenic arterial puncture, or arterial puncture by injecting drug users [352]. Infected pseudoaneurysms due to contamination of sites of arterial injury are found predominantly in the extremities. Infected pseudoaneurysms present as a tender indurated mass that may be pulsatile and may be associated with an audible bruit, local pain, frank suppuration, and diminished distal pulses. An associated septic arthritis also may be present. Staphylococci, especially *S. aureus*, are the most common pathogen in the nosocomial setting. Among injecting drug users, *S. aureus* is the predominant pathogen (76%) with *P. aeruginosa* (18%) and a variety of other bacterial and fungal pathogens accounting for the rest [352].

Infective endarteritis also may occur secondary to direct arterial invasion by contiguous septic foci, such as vertebral osteomyelitis or pancreatitis [353]. Finally, the aortic wall may become infected secondary to erosion into a loop of bowel, a so-called aortoenteric fistula [354].

DIAGNOSIS OF INFECTIVE ENDARTERITIS

CT scan with contrast is the initial diagnostic procedure of choice, with ultrasound also useful for evaluating pseudoaneurysms in the groin. Findings that suggest aneurysmal infection include (1) the absence of intimal calcification; (2) a perianeurysmal collection of fluid or gas; (3) gas in the aortic wall, which is a rare but diagnostic finding; and (4) osteomyelitis in adjacent bones [355]. Nuclear scans, including gallium [356], indium-labeled WBC scan, or indium-labeled IgG scan, may corroborate the presence of inflammation at the aneurysmal site [357–360]. However, a negative scan does not exclude the diagnosis. Moreover, because gallium activity is found in the intestine and may confound the interpretation of intra-abdominal foci of activity, indium-labeled scans are preferred in cases of suspected aortic mycotic aneurysm. Angiography is performed to delineate the extent of infection and to plan the surgical approach.

In the absence of bacteremia, aortic mycotic aneurysms may be difficult to distinguish from the entity of inflammatory abdominal aortic aneurysm [361–363]. Inflammatory abdominal aortic aneurysms are usually infrarenal, often tender to palpation, and often associated with dense fibrosis surrounding the vessel. Fibrosis may be difficult to distinguish from fluid on CT scan, and MRI may be better able to accurately distinguish the two [364].

THERAPY OF INFECTIVE ENDARTERITIS

Intracranial mycotic aneurysms that have bled should be surgically resected. The distal location of most of these lesions allows ligation and excision with fewer complications compared to resection of more proximal aneurysms. The therapeutic approach to intracranial mycotic aneurysms that have not bled is controversial [338,339,365]. Serial angiography may be used to follow the lesions and to look for evidence of new lesions. Alternatively, Ahmadi et al. have suggested that the lesions may be followed by serial thin-section CT or MRI scans after their location and size have been initially defined by angiography [366]. Aneurysms that appear to be expanding should be resected [366–368]. About 50 percent of cerebral mycotic aneurysms in the series reported by Bingham resolved with antibiotic therapy alone [365]. Anticoagulation should be avoided in patients with known or suspected intracranial mycotic aneurysms.

The time-honored approach to the therapy of mycotic aneurysm involving the aorta is extra-anatomic bypass grafting followed by aneurysm resection, extensive debridement, and prolonged (6–8 weeks) antibiotic therapy [369]. *In-situ* grafting may be necessary, however, when the patient is *in extremis* and an expedient operation is mandatory, or when the aneurysm is at or above the level of the renal arteries [370,371]. The overall mortality associated with infected atherosclerotic aneurysms can exceed 90 percent [372,373].

Recently, several authors have suggested that *in-situ* reconstruction for elective therapy of infrarenal aneurysms may be feasible under certain circumstances [374]. Based on a review of the literature and of 21 cases performed at their hospital, Fichelle and coworkers suggest that *in-situ* reconstruction can be performed safely if the following conditions are met: (1) the resection is as complete as possible, with removal of the infected aorta and neighboring retroperitoneal tissues; (2) the anastamosis is done on healthy uninfected tissue; (3) a pediculated omental flap covers the prosthesis and all sutures; and (4) prolonged antibiotic therapy (e.g., 6 weeks) is administered with regular postoperative follow-up, including serial CT scans. Other authors have recommended lifelong antibiotic therapy if *in-situ* grafting is performed [370]. Fichelle et al. believe that extra-anatomic bypass is preferable only if an extremely diffuse retroperitoneal infection with abscess is apparent on CT scan. Further studies are awaited to assess the validity of that controversial approach.

Surgical resection of visceral mycotic aneurysms should be performed immediately because of the risk of rupture and exsanguination. Peripheral mycotic aneurysms generally are treated by ligation and excision, with vascular bypass performed if needed, preferably with the use of autogenous graft.

Vascular Graft Infection

The incidence of aortic graft infection ranges from 0.77–2.6 percent [375,376]. In the largest series of vascular grafts, that of Szilagyi et al. [377], an infection rate of 1.5 percent was reported, a rate similar to the 1.7-percent infection rate noted for clean operations in Cruse's survey of 23,649 surgical wounds [378].

PATHOGENESIS

Vascular grafts generally become infected by one of three routes: (1) perioperative contamination, (2) hematogenous seeding; and (3) secondary to enteric erosion or fistula. Perioperative graft contamination is believed to occur most commonly as a result of breaks in surgical technique [379]. Known or occult bowel injury, perioperative wound infection [378], groin incision, local complications such as skin necrosis, hematoma, lymphocele [375], and reoperation for bleeding or graft thrombosis [380] also predispose to infection. There is little evidence that the performance of secondary procedures (e.g., cholecystectomy or appendectomy) as part of the same operation is associated with an increased risk of graft infection [381,382], although many authors discourage that practice [379,383].

The value of intraoperative cultures as a routine practice when vascular grafts are placed is controversial, with some authors suggesting that they are not useful [379,384–386], while others maintain that the cultures are imperative [387–390]. In cases where infective aortitis is suspected, gram stains and cultures of aneurysm contents and of the arterial wall always should be obtained. Cultures also should be obtained in cases of aneurysm rupture where hemorrhage may obscure intraoperative evaluation for evidence of infection or in patients undergoing vascular reoperation [380]. Positive cultures in those settings may be useful as a guide to the choice and duration of antibiotic therapy. On the other hand, if there is no preoperative suspicion of infection and the aneurysm is not ruptured, the value of intraoperative culture is questionable. Farkas et al. [391] retrospectively reviewed 500 cases of abdominal aortic aneurysm in which microbiologic examination of the thrombus, the aneurysm, or both was performed on specimens at the time of surgery. Of those 500 cases, 185 (37%) cultures were positive, with most isolates being members of normal skin flora. Of the 185 patients with positive culture, no patient developed infection due to the same organism after a mean follow-up of almost 3 years. Based on those findings, the authors conclude that in cases of asymptomatic unruptured aneurysm, routine culturing is not necessary.

Vascular grafts are vulnerable to bacteremic seeding particularly during the first several months following placement. The surfaces of synthetic implants in contact with the bloodstream are covered by a pseudointima, a layer of platelets and fibrin that forms in the first 4–6 weeks following graft placement [46,392]. Bacteria such as *S. epidermidis* may establish infection by binding directly to the graft surface [393], binding to the platelet component of pseudointima [92], or binding to host-derived factors such as fibronectin or fibrinogen, which in turn mediate attachment to the graft.

A decreasing incidence of graft infection with time on bacteremic challenge with *S. aureus* has been noted in animal models. While all grafts became infected when challenged within 2 weeks of placement, at the end of 1 year only 30 percent became infected [394]. Some resistance to infection probably is afforded by the presence of a pseudointima. However, breaks in the pseudointima, along with intrinsic properties of the pseudointima that afford less protection against microbial seeding than intact endothelium, may account for the continued (although decreased) susceptibility to late vascular graft infection. Most investigators believe that a true endothelial graft lining never develops on long grafts, since endothelialization progresses from the suture margins at variable rates depending on the type of graft and other ill-defined host factors [336].

Whether biomaterials used in vascular grafts differ in their propensity for infection *in vivo* is unclear. Greater bacterial adherence to velour-knitted Dacron grafts compared with woven Dacron grafts was demonstrated in one study, while expanded polytetraflouroethylene (PTFE) demonstrated the least adherence [395]. Recent studies suggest that endothelium-seeded PFTE grafts may be even more resistant to infection than their nonseeded counterparts [396,397].

TIMING OF VASCULAR GRAFT INFECTION

The timing of vascular graft infection following implantation has changed as surgical therapy has evolved. Earlier series, such as that of Szilagyi et al. in 1972 [377], reported that most infections present soon after implantation, with 65 percent of the infections presenting within 30 days. More recent series have indicated a more delayed onset [398]. Goldstone and Effeney [399] reported that the mean interval for graft infection was about 2 years postoperatively. Infections associated with aortofemoral grafts tend to present earlier than aortoiliac grafts, an observation that has been attributed to the more superficial location of the femoral limb [400].

MICROBIOLOGY

Prostheses underlying groin incisions become infected more frequently than those entirely within the abdomen. Organisms recovered from groin infection generally are gram-positive organisms such as *S. aureus* or *S. epidermidis*, while infection at other sites often is due to gram-negative organisms from an enteric or urinary source (e.g., *E. coli*, *Klebsiella* spp.). The sensitivity of culture may depend in part on the technique used to process the specimen. One study found enhanced recovery of *S. epidermidis* in the laboratory by sonic disruption in broth of biofilm material on the surface of the resected graft [401], while others have suggested submitting the graft fabric itself for culture [399].

S. aureus is the most common isolate causing graft infections, accounting for 24–43 percent in most series [377,398,402,403]. In recent years, coagulase-negative staphylococci such as *S. epidermidis* have emerged as increasingly common isolates, accounting for 15–42 percent of cases overall [377,402,404]. Other organisms commonly implicated in graft infection include streptococci (5–51%), gram-negative bacilli such as *E. coli* (9–23%), *Proteus mira-*

bilis (1–20%), and *P. aeruginosa* (2–33%) [377,398,402–404]. Brook was able to culture anaerobes from 13 of 16 (82%) aortofemoral graft specimens [405], although the clinical significance of that finding is uncertain.

CLINICAL PRESENTATION

Over three-quarters of graft infections occur in the groin. Infected grafts located in that region usually present as an inguinal mass accompanied by signs of erythema, pain, and fever [383]. Frank drainage is present in almost half of cases [403], with a sinus tract apparent in about 9 percent. A false aneurysm will be present in about 10 percent of patients, while graft occlusion, hemorrhage, and septic emboli occur less commonly. Infections involving the intra-abdominal segment of aortic grafts generally present as smoldering processes with or without fever, chills, or leukocytosis. Localizing findings usually are absent, although back pain may be present. Graft-enteric fistulae generally present with upper gastrointestinal bleeding, which may be massive if they involve the aortic anastamosis. If the anastamosis of the graft is not involved, bleeding is more commonly of low volume and usually is secondary to irritation of the intestinal wall [354,398].

DIAGNOSIS

Four diagnostic modalities available to the clinician include (1) an imaging procedure, such as CT scan, ultrasound (of the groin), or MRI to look for fluid or air around a graft and to detect pseudoaneurysms; (2) nuclear scans, such as an indium-labeled WBC or indium-labeled immunoglobulin scans; (3) a sinogram, performed under antibiotic coverage, to evaluate a sinus tract in the groin; and (4) aspiration of a fluid collection under CT or ultrasound guidance, for gram stain and culture. Angiography generally is used to assist in planning the surgical approach, but it is of limited utility for the diagnosis of graft infection.

While fluid or air around a graft may be found postoperatively under normal circumstances, the presence of either beyond 3 months is highly suggestive of infection [355,406–408]. CT scan is highly sensitive in detecting fluid or air. However, the relatively poor soft-tissue contrast of CT makes it difficult to distinguish postoperative changes such as fibrosis from inflammation; thus, MRI may be preferred [364]. Indium scans (either labeled WBC or Ig) [409–412] can be used to verify the presence of an active inflammatory focus, as long as they are performed no earlier than 3–4 months postoperatively, since normal postoperative inflammation may give a false-positive scan if performed before then [413]. Unfortunately, recent reports have documented a number of other causes for false-positive in WBC scans, including uninfected pseudoaneurysm, lymphocele, perigraft inflammation after surgery, wound infection without graft involvement, diverticular abscess, and pancreatic necrosis [364,414]. Other potential causes of false positives include gut activity from inflammation secondary to multiple enemas, colonic carcinoma, swallowed leukocytes in patients with pneumonia, and ischemic bowel. Because of those uncertainties, fine-needle aspiration of any accessible perigraft fluid discovered by either CT or MRI more than 3 months after graft implantation is recommended [415].

Initial reports suggested that indium scans are exceedingly sensitive, so that a negative scan could be used to exclude the presence of infection. It is now known that false-negative scans do occur in the setting of a chronic, smoldering infection, particularly if a course of antibiotics has been given [410]. Thus, a negative indium scan does not rule out the diagnosis of graft infection.

THERAPY

The time-honored approach to the surgical therapy of vascular graft infections is complete excision of the graft and revascularization through a clean tissue bed with an extra anatomic bypass. For infected aortic grafts, recent studies have suggested better survival in selected patients if extra-anatomic bypass is performed prior to graft excision [401,416], with graft resection and oversewing of the aorta performed several days later. Gram stains and cultures of the proximal aortic stump should be obtained. A prolonged (6–8 weeks) course of postoperative antibiotics should be given, with the choice of antibiotics guided by preoperative blood and intraoperative stump culture and sensitivity results. For more limited infections, such as superficial wound infections involving exposed but patent grafts without involvement of the anastamosis, several authors have reported successful graft preservation with intravenous and topical antibiotic therapy followed by tissue coverage [402,417]. If the anastamosis is involved, removal of the infected limb of the graft is mandatory, and the decision to remove the contralateral limb or the aortic shaft must be based on intraoperative findings [400].

Mortality rates are highest when the proximal portion of aortic grafts are infected, ranging from 14–85 percent [400]. On the other hand, amputation rates are highest for peripheral graft infections (13–75%) [400,418].

PREVENTION

Perhaps the most important measure to prevent vascular graft infection is careful attention to surgical and aseptic technique. Several studies suggest that the use of prophylactic antibiotics perioperatively reduces the incidence of graft infection [419–421]. Cefazolin, infused 1 hour prior to skin incision and continued for 24 hours postoperatively generally is used, although vancomycin should be substituted for cefazolin in patients known to harbor MRSA.

Topical antibiotic irrigation of the surgical wound has yet to be shown in a randomized controlled study to be beneficial. Whether antibiotic bonding to graft material leads to reduced infection rates also is unknown. A practical problem is that of rapid leaching of antibiotics from the graft *in vivo*, generally within 24 hours of graft placement [397,422,423].

Some authors have suggested that careful division and ligation of groin lymphatics may be helpful in preventing graft infection. The stated rationale is to reduce the risk of lymphatic seeding of the graft by bacteria that may be present in lymphatic drainage from the extremities [424]. The utility of that practice is unproved.

Suppurative Thrombophlebitis

Suppurative thrombophlebitis is an infection involving the walls of a vein, often associated with thrombosis and bacteremia. Suppurative thrombophlebitis can be classified into four different forms: (1) the superficial form, usually a complication of an intravenous catheter; (2) the central form, including both suppurative thrombophlebitis of the thoracic central veins secondary to central venous catheters and septic pelvic-vein thrombophlebitis; (3) suppurative thrombosis involving a cerebral venous sinus; and (4) infection of the portal vein [425]. The first two forms, more common by far than the others, will be discussed here.

SUPERFICIAL SUPPURATIVE THROMBOPHLEBITIS

Three groups at particular risk for superficial suppurative thrombophlebitis are (1) burn patients, where it occurs in 4–8 percent of patients and is a common cause of death due to infection [426–429]; (2) hospitalized patients with indwelling vascular catheters [430,431]; and (3) intravenous drug users [432]. While patients with suppurative thrombophlebitis in each of those settings may present with fever, signs of sepsis, a high incidence of bacteremia (80–90%), and pulmonary findings consistent with septic emboli, noteworthy differences in clinical presentation exist among the three groups. For example, superficial septic thrombophlebitis in burn patients most commonly occurs in the lower extremities, associated with the common practice of placing intravenous catheters in that location [427,429]. Local signs of infection such as warmth, erythema, tenderness, swelling, and lymphangitis are apparent in only about a third of those patients. In contrast, most other hospitalized patients with suppurative thrombophlebitis have involvement of the upper extremities, and local signs of inflammation are present in the majority of cases [432].

The use of cutdowns, the type of cannula placed, and the duration of cannulation have been identified as risk factors for suppurative thrombophlebitis. Plastic cannulas are associated with an approximately 40-fold increased risk (8%) compared with steel "scalp vein" cannulas (0.2%); the risk is also greater with polyethylene catheters compared with Teflon or Silastic catheters [425]. Duration of cannulation beyond 48–72 hours is associated with an increased risk of suppurative thrombophlebitis [431,433].

The pathogenesis of superficial suppurative thrombophlebitis has not been precisely defined. Infection may occur as a result of (1) ingress of cutaneous microorganisms along the outer surface of the catheter; (2) hematogenous seeding of the fibrin sheath surrounding the catheter from a distant source; and (3) infusion of contaminated fluids. In burn patients, the favored mode of pathogenesis is seeding of the fibrin sleeve surrounding the catheter by bloodborne pathogens, in a fashion analagous to bacteremic seeding of platelet-fibrin aggregates in the case of endocarditis [426]. In support of that contention are the facts that the predominant organism in burn wounds, *P. aeruginosa,* is a rare cause of suppurative thrombophlebitis and that suppurative thrombophlebitis typically occurs days to weeks after cutdown incisions are healed [426,428].

The diagnosis of superficial suppurative thrombophlebitis is suggested by the presence of fever and bacteremia along with either local signs of infection or pulmonary infiltrates consistent with septic emboli. Simple needle aspiration of the suspected vein may be diagnostic. In burn patients, where local signs of infection are absent in the majority of patients, the late onset of pneumonia or sepsis mandates surgical exploration of all previously catheterized veins, beginning with the most recent, looking for intraluminal purulence. Suppurative thrombophlebitis may extend for long distances both proximally and distally from the site of catheterization, and multiple segments of intraluminal infection may be present proximal to areas that grossly appear normal [427].

A combination of antibiotics and surgical excision is generally required for cure of superficial suppurative thrombophlebitis. Of 14 burn patients treated without surgery in one series, all died either directly from suppurative thrombophlebitis with sustained bacteremia or secondary to metastatic complications [428]. In contrast, of 10 patients who underwent surgical exploration, 7 survived with only 1 of the 3 deaths attributed to suppurative thrombophlebitis. Since *S. aureus* and enteric gram-negatives such as *Klebsiella* and *Enterobacter* are the most commonly implicated pathogens, antibiotic therapy should begin with a semisynthetic penicillin (e.g., nafcillin) or vancomycin (if MRSA is suspected) along with an aminoglycoside. In burn patients, complete excision of the infected vein is recommended up to the point where the vein becomes a tributary to the next higher order of veins or until the wall is unequivocally normal with brisk retrograde flow of unaltered blood from the more proximal segment. The venotomy wound site is left open and loosely packed and is subsequently closed secondarily or with a skin graft after all signs of infection have resolved [434].

The role of less radical surgery for nonburn patients with suppurative thrombophlebitis has not been systematically studied. In a recent report, six of eight pediatric patients with infection due to gram-negative bacilli or *Candida* sp. were cured by antibiotic therapy in combination with local incision and drainage [435].

The optimal duration of antibiotic therapy following surgical intervention has not been defined and should be dictated by clinical response and whether metastatic or adjacent foci of infection (e.g., endocarditis, osteomyelitis) are present. In the latter instance, at least 6 weeks of antibiotics is suggested. The treatment of superficial septic thrombophlebitis due to *Candida* is controversial [436,437], although many authors favor the combination of vein excision and a short course (e.g., 200-mg total dose) of amphotericin B [425].

CENTRAL SUPPURATIVE THROMBOPHLEBITIS

Central suppurative thrombophlebitis may occur as a complication of central venous cannulation, particularly in critically ill hospitalized patients [438–440]; as a complication of intravenous drug use [441]; or as a complication of parturition, abortion, gynecologic surgery, or pelvic abscess in the case of pelvic-vein involvement [442].

Suppurative thrombophlebitis of a central thoracic vein should be suspected in any patient if bacteremia or fungemia fails to resolve despite removal of the catheter and appropriate antibiotic therapy. The diagnosis may not be immediately apparent, because local signs of inflammation are present in only a minority of cases, and the onset is often insidious. However, full-blown suppurative thrombophlebitis usually is associated with spiking fever, septic shock, and metastatic foci of infection [443]. Septic pulmonary emboli, which occur in about 40 percent of patients, often are the first diagnostic clue.

The diagnosis may be established by CT scan with contrast enhancement that demonstrates the presence of an intravascular thrombus or alternatively by venography. Experience with other diagnostic tests such as MRI or indium-labeled WBC scanning is limited. Needle aspiration of the suspected vein may prove diagnostic. Moreover, the diagnosis is suggested by the finding of confluent growth after venous catheter segments are rolled across the surface of culture plates using the semiquantitative technique of Maki et al. [444].

Therapy should include catheter removal, antibiotic directed against *S. aureus* and gram-negative bacilli, and anticoagulation with heparin [445,446]. In many cases, surgical intervention will not be required, although the response to medical therapy may be slow [440]. However, in cases where the vein is infected secondary to infection and abscess in the surrounding tissue, surgery usually is required. For infection due to *Candida,* a full course of amphotericin B ($\geq$ 22 mg/kg) should be given. 5-flourocytosine therapy (100–150 mg/day in four divided doses) may be added, especially if *in-vitro* synergy with amphotericin is demonstrated for the pathogen isolated [447].

Suppurative thrombophlebitis of the pelvic veins typically develops 1–2 weeks following birth, abortion, or pelvic surgery. Patients present with high fever, chills, anorexia, nausea, vomiting, abdominal pain, and abdominal tenderness, which is usually right-sided [442]. Although any component of the venous system draining the pelvis may be involved, the most common are veins draining the uterus, including the ovarian veins and the inferior vena cava [448,449]. The predominance of right-sided involvement has been attributed to compression of the right ovarian vein at the pelvic brim by the enlarged uterus, with thrombus formation resulting from stasis of blood flow in the setting of pregnancy-associated hypercoagulability. Presumably, the thrombus becomes seeded by vaginal or perineal flora via the bloodstream, regional lymphatics, or both [425].

In contrast to suppurative thrombophlebitis of the central thoracic veins, bacteremia is present in only 20–30 percent of patients with suppurative pelvic-vein thrombophlebitis [442,449,450]. As in the case of suppurative thrombophlebitis at other sites, however, septic pulmonary emboli and metastatic abscesses are common.

The diagnosis of suppurative pelvic-vein thrombophlebitis is indicated by the finding on CT scan of an area within the pelvic vein of low attenuation associated with contrast enhancement [451,452]. Ultrasound also can be used to determine the location and extent of the thrombus. The roles of MRI, indium-labeled WBC scanning, pelvic venography, and transuterine phlebography have yet to be defined, although initial evidence suggests that MRI may be even more sensitive than CT and provide information regarding the age of the thrombus present [453].

Both the microbiology and the therapy of suppurative pelvic-vein thrombophlebitis are poorly defined. Since blood cultures are positive in only a minority of cases, and since adequate anaerobic-culture techniques have not been used in most series, the precise spectrum and frequency of organisms involved are uncertain. Existing data indicate that anaerobic flora (*Bacteroides* sp., microaerophilic or anaerobic streptococci) predominate, with enteric gram-negatives and beta-hemolytic streptococci accounting for the rest. Thus, the combination of clindamycin plus an aminoglycoside or broad-spectrum agents such as ampicillin-sulbactam or imipenem are suggested. Most clinicians would also add heparin therapy, although its use in this setting has not been systematically studied [442,450]. Patients who fail to respond to medical therapy will require surgery for drainage of abscesses and ligation of the implicated venous system.

References

1. Harris S. Definitions and demographic characteristics. In D Kaye, ed. Infective Endocarditis. Second ed. New York: Raven, 1992. Pp. 1–18.
2. Durack D. Infective and noninfective endocarditis. In J Hurst, R Schlant, eds. The Heart Arteries and Veins. 7th ed. New York: McGraw-Hill, 1990. Pp. 1230–1255.
3. Bayer A. Infective endocarditis. Clin Infect Dis 1993; 17: 313–322.
4. King J, Nguyen V. Results of a prospective statewide reporting system for infective endocarditis. Am J Med Sci 1988; (295):517–527.
5. Hickey A, MacMahon S, Wilcken D. Mitral valve prolapse and bacterial endocarditis: when is antibiotic prophylaxis necessary. Am Heart J 1985; 109:431–435.
6. Griffin M, et al. Infective endocarditis, Olmsted County Minnesota. JAMA 1985; 254:1199–1202.
7. Steckelberg J, Melton L, Ilstrup D. Influence of referral bias on the apparent clinical spectrum of infective endocarditis. Am J Med 1990; 88:582–588.
8. Gray I. Infective endocarditis. Br Heart J 1987; 57:211.
9. Clemens J, Horwitz R, Jaffe C. A controlled evaluation of the risk of bacterial endocarditis in persons with mitral valve prolapse. N Engl J Med 1982; 307:776–781.
10. MacMahon S, Roberts J, Kramer-Fox R. Mitral valve prolapse and infective endocarditis. Am Heart J 1987; 113:1291–1298.
11. MacMahon S, Hickey A, Wilcken D. Risk of infective endocarditis in mitral valve prolapse with and without precordial murmurs. Am J Cardiol 1986; 58:105–108.
12. Nagger C, Forgacs P. Infective endocarditis: a challenging disease. Med Clin North Am 1986; 70:1279.
13. Marks A, Choong C, Sanfilippo A. Identification of high-risk and low-risk subgroups of patients with mitral valve prolapse. N Engl J Med 1989; 320:1031–1036.
14. Nishimura R, McGoon M, Shub C. Echocardiographically documented mitral valve prolapse. Long-term follow-up of 237 patients. N Engl J Med 1985; 313:1305–1309.
15. McKinsey D, Ratts T, Bisno A. Underlying cardiac lesions in adults with infective endocarditis: the changing spectrum. Am J Med 1987; 82:681–688.
16. Thell R, Martin F, Edwards J. Bacterial endocarditis in subjects 60 years of age and older. Circulation 1975; 51:174–182.
17. Weinberger I, Rotenber Z, Zacharovitch D. Native valve infective endocarditis in the 1970's versus the 1980's: underlying cardiac lesions and infecting organisms. Cardiovasc Dis 1990; 22:193.
18. Moulsdale M, Eykyn S, Phillips I. Infective endocarditis,

1970–79. A study of culture-positive cases in St. Thomas Hospital. J Med 1980; 49:315.
19. Venezio F, Wedenfelder G, Cook F. Infective endocarditis in a community hospital. Arch Intern Med 1982; 142:789–792.
20. von Reyn C, Levy B, Arbeit R. Infective endocarditis: an analysis based on strict case definitions. Ann Intern Med 1981; 94:505–518.
21. Alessandri N, Pannarale G, del Monte F. A report of seven cases and a review of the literature. Eur Heart J 1990; 11:1041–1048.
22. Chagnac A, Rudniki C, Loebel H. Infectious endocarditis in idiopathic hypertrophic subaortic stenosis. Report of three cases and review of the literature. Chest 1982; 81:346–349.
23. Wang K, Gobel F, Gleason D. Bacterial endocarditis in idiopathic hypertrophic subaortic stenosis. Am Heart J 1973; 89:359.
24. Lerner P, Weinstein L. Infective endocarditis in the antibiotic era. N Engl J Med 1966; 274:199–206, 259–266, 323–331, 388–393.
25. Rabinovich S, et al. A long term view of bacterial endocarditis. Ann Intern Med 1965; 63:185–198.
26. Geva T, Frand M. Infective endocarditis in children with congenital heart disease; the changing spectrum. Eur Heart J 1988; 9:1244–1249.
27. Gersony W, Hayes C. Bacterial endocarditis in patients with pulmonary stenosis, aortic stenosis or ventricular septal defect. Circulation 1977; 56(1):I-84–I-87.
28. Banks T, Fletcher R, Ali N. Infective endocarditis in heroin addicts. Am J Med 1973; 55:444–451.
29. Simberkoff M. Narcotic-associated infective endocarditis. In E Kaplan, A Taranta, eds. Infective Endocarditis. Dallas: American Heart Association, 1977. Pp. 46–50.
30. Ransey R, Gunnar R, Tobin J. Endocarditis in the drug addict. Am J Cardiol 1970; 25:608–618.
31. Sande M, Lee B, Mills J, Chambers H. Endocarditis in intravenous drug users. In D Kaye, ed. Infective Endocarditis. Second ed. New York: Raven, 1992. Pp. 345–359.
32. Pelletier L, Petersdorf R. Infective endocarditis: a review of 125 cases from the University of Washington Hospital, 1963–72. Medicine 1977; 56:287–313.
33. Cherubin C, Neu H. Infective endocarditis at the Presbyterian Hospital in New York City from 1938–1967. Am J Med 1971; 51:83–96.
34. Garvey G, Neu H. Infective endocarditis—an evolving disease: a review of endocarditis at the Columbia-Presbyterian Medical Center, 1968–1973. Medicine 1978; 57:105–127.
35. Friedland G, Von Reys C, Levy B. Nosocomial endocarditis. Infect Control 1984; 5:284–288.
36. Terpenning M, Buggy B, Kauffman C. Infective endocarditis: clinical features in young and elderly patients. Am J Med 1987; 83:626–634.
37. Greene J, Fitzwater J, Clemmer T. Septic endocarditis and indwelling pulmonary artery catheters. JAMA 1975; 233:891–897.
38. Kaye D. Changing pattern of endocarditis. Am J Med 1985; 78(6B):157–162.
39. Quenzer R, Edwards L, Levin S. A comparative study of 48 host valve and 24 prosthetic valve endocarditis cases. Am Heart J 1976; 92:15–22.
40. Richardson J, et al. Treatment of infective endocarditis: a 10-year comparative analysis. Circulation 1978; 58:589–597.
41. Cowgill L, et al. Prosthetic valve endocarditis. Curr Probl Cardiol 1986; 11:617–664.
42. Heimberger T, Duma R. Infections of prosthetic heart valves and cardiac pacemakers. Infect Dis Clin North Am 1989; 3:221–245.
43. Calderwood S, et al. Risk factors for the development of prosthetic valve endocarditis. Circulation 1985; 72:31–37.
44. Ivert T, Dismukes W, Cobbs C. Prosthetic valve endocarditis. Circulation 1984; 69:223–232.
45. Rutledge R, Kim B, Applebaum R. Actuarial analysis of the risk of PVE in 1,598 patients with mechanical and bioprosthetic valves. Arch Surg 1985; 120:469–472.
46. Schoen F. Interventional and Surgical Cardiovascular Pathology. Philadelphia: Saunders, 1989. Pp. 141–143.
47. Everett E, Hirschmann J. Transient bacteremia and endocarditis prophylaxis: a review. Medicine 1977; 56:61–77.
48. Sipes J, Thompson R, Hook E. Prophylaxis of infective endocarditis: a re-evaluation. Ann Rev Med 1977; 28:371–391.
49. Lowy F, Steigbel N. Infective endocarditis. Part III. Prevention of bacterial endocarditis. Am Heart J 1977; 96:689–695.
50. Baddour L, et al. Pathogenesis of experimental endocarditis. III. Production and progress of the disease in rabbits. Br J Exp Pathol 1973; 54:142–151.
51. Lepeschkin E. On the relation between the site of valvular involvement in endocarditis and the blood pressure resting on the valve. Am J Med Sci 1952; 224:316–319.
52. Rodbard S. Blood velocity and endocarditis. Circulation 1963; 27:18.
53. Weinstein L, Rubin R. Infective endocarditis—1973. Prog Cardiovasc Dis 1973; 26:239.
54. Hammill R, Vann J, Proctor R. Phagocytosis of *Staphylococcus aureus* by cultured bovine aortic endothelial cells: model for post-adherence events in the endovascular infections. Infect Immun 1986; 54:833–836.
55. Rotrosen D, Edwards J, Gibson T. Adherence of candida to cultured vascular endothelial cells: mechanisms of attachment and endothelial penetration. J Infect Dis 1985; 152:1264–1274.
56. Bisno A, Dismukes W, Durack D. Antimicrobial treatment of infective endocarditis due to viridans streptococci, enterococci and staphylococci. JAMA 1989; 261:1471–1477.
57. Sullam P, Valone J, Mills J. Mechanisms of platelet aggregation by viridans group streptococci. Infect Immun 1987; 55:1743–1750.
58. Switalski L, Murchison H, Timpl R. Binding of laminin to oral and endocarditis strains of viridans streptococci. J Bacteriol 1987; 169:1095.
59. Chatwai G, et al. Specific binding of the human S protein (vitronectin) to streptococci, *Staphylococcus aureus,* and *Escherichia coli.* Infect Immun 1987; 55:1878–1883.
60. Hawiger J, et al. Identification of a region of human fibrinogen interacting with the staphylococcal clumping factor. Biochemistry 1982; 21:1407–1413.
61. Clawson C, White J. Platelet interaction with bacteria I. Reaction phases and effects of inhibitors. Am J Pathol 1971; 65(2):367–380.
62. Johnson C. Adherence events in the pathogenesis of infective endocarditis. Infect Dis Clin NA 1993; 7(1):21–36.
63. Chugh T, et al. Adherence of *Staphylococcus epidermidis* to fibrin-platelet clots in vitro mediated by lipoteichoic acid. Infect Immun 1990; 58:315–319.
64. Herrmann M, et al. Adhesion of *Staphylococcus aureus* to surface-bound platelets: Role of fibrinogen/fibrin and platelet integrins. The Journal of Infectious Diseases 1993; 167:312–322.
65. Ginsberg M, Loftus J, Plow E. Platelets and the adhesion receptor superfamily. Prog Clin Biol Res 1988; 283:171–195.
66. Kuusela P. Fibronectin binds to *Staphylococcus aureus.* Nature 1978; 276:718–720.
67. Proctor R, Mosher D, Olbrantz P. Fibronectin binding to *Staphylococcus aureus.* J Biol Chem 1982; 257:14788–14794.
68. Abraham S, Beachey E, Simpson W. Adherence of *Streptococ-*

cus pyogenes, Escherichia coli and *Pseudomonas aeruginosa* to fibronectin-coated and uncoated epithelial cells. Infect Immun 1983; 41:1261–1268.
69. Kuusela P, et al. Attachment of staphylococci and streptococci on fibronectin, fibronectin fragments, and fibrinogen bound to a solid phase. Infect Immun 1985; 50:77–81.
70. Myhre E, Kuusela P. Binding of human fibronectin to groups A, C, and G streptococci. Infect Immun 1983; 40:29–34.
71. Skerl K, Calerone R, Segal E. In vitro binding of *Candida albicans* yeast cells to human fibronectin. Can J Microbiol 1984; 30:221–227.
72. Lowrance J, Baddour L, Simpson W. The role of fibronectin binding in the rat model of experimental endocarditis caused by *Streptococcus sanguis*. J Clin Invest 1990; 86:7–13.
73. Nealon T, et al. Release of fibronectin-lipoteichoic acid complexes from group a streptococci with penicillin. Infect Immun 1986; 51:529–535.
74. Chambers H, et al. Cocaine use and the risk for endocarditis in intravenous drug users. Ann Intern Med 1987; 106:833–836.
75. Reisberg B. Infective endocarditis in the narcotic addict. Prog Cardiovasc Dis 1979; 22:193.
76. Levine D, et al. Community-acquired methicillin-resistant *Staphylococcus* aureus endocarditis in the Detroit Medical Center. Ann Intern Med 1982; 97:330–338.
77. Levine D, Crane L, Zervos M. Bacteremia in narcotic addicts at the Detroit Medical Center. II. Infectious endocarditis: a prospective comparative study. Rev Infect Dis 1986; 8:374–396.
78. Sklaver A, Hoffmann T, Greenman R. Staphylococcal endocarditis in addicts. South Med J 1978; 71:638–641.
79. Chambers H, Korzeniowski O, Sande M. *Staphylococcus aureus* endocarditis: clinical manifestations in addicts and nonaddicts. Medicine 1983; 62:170.
80. Menda K, Gorbach S. Favorable experience with bacterial endocarditis in heroin addicts. Ann Intern Med 1973; 78:25–32.
81. Herrmann M, Vaudaux P, Didier P. Fibronectin, fibrinogen, and laminin act as mediators of adherence of clinical staphylococcal isolates to foreign material. J Infect Dis 1988; 158:693–701.
82. Vaudaux P, Lew D, Waldvogel F. Host factors predisposing to foreign body infections. In A Bisno, F Waldvogel, eds. Infections Associated With Indwelling Medical Devices. Washington: American Society for Microbiology, 1989. Pp. 3–26.
83. Vaudaux P, Pittet D, Haeberli A. Host factors selectively increase staphylococcal adherence on inserted catheters: a role for fibronectin and fibrinogen or fibrin. J Infect Dis 1989b; 160:865–875.
84. Toy P, et al. Effect of fibronectin on adherence of *Staphylococcus aureus* to fibrin thrombi in vitro. Infect Immun 1985; 48:83–86.
85. Vaudaux P, Yasuda H, Velazco M. Role of host and bacterial factors in modulating staphylococcal adhesion to implanted polymer surfaces. J Biomater Appl 1990; 5:134–153.
86. Cheung A, Fischett V. The role of fibrinogen in staphylococcal adherence to catheters in vitro. J Infect Dis 1990; 161:1177–1186.
87. Strong D, et al. Isolation, characterization, and synthesis of peptides from human fibrinogen that block the staphylococcal clumping reaction and construction of a synthetic clumping peptide. Biochemistry 1982; 21:1414–1420.
88. Boden M, Flock J. Fibrinogen-binding protein/clumping factor from Staphylococcus aureus. Infect Immun 1989; 57:2358–2363.
89. Vercellotti G, et al. Extracellular matrix proteins (fibronectin, laminin, and type IV collagen) bind and aggregate bacteria. Am J Pathol 1985; 120:13–21.
90. Lopes J, dos Reis M, Brentani R. Presence of laminin receptors in *Staphylococcus aureus*. Science 1985; 229:275–277.
91. Herrmann M, et al. Thrombospondin binds *Staphylococcus aureus* and promotes staphylococcal adherence to surfaces. Infect Immun 1991; 59:279–288.
92. Wang I, Anderson J, Marchant R. *Staphylococcus epidermidis* adhesion to hydrophobic biomedical polymer is mediated by platelets. J Infect Dis 1993; 167:329–336.
93. Gristina A, Hobgood C, Barth E. Biomaterial specificity, molecular mechanisms and clinical relevance of *S. epidermidis* and *S. aureus* infections in surgery. Zentralbl Bakteriol Mikrobiol Hyg 1987; 1(16):143–157.
94. Gristina A, et al. Adhesive colonization of biomaterials and antibiotic resistance. Biomaterials 1987b; 8:423–426.
95. Gristina A. Biomaterial-centered infection: microbial adhesion versus tissue integration. Science 1987c; 237:1588–1595.
96. Christensen G, et al. Adherence of slime-producing strains of *Staphylococcus epidermidis* to smooth surfaces. Infect Immun 1982; 37:318–326.
97. Christensen G, et al. Characterization of clinically significant strains of coagulase-negative staphylococci. J Clin Microbiol 1983; 18:258–269.
98. Christensen G, Simpson W, Beachey E. Experimental foreign body infection in mice challenged with slime-producing *Staphylococcus epidermidis*. Infect Immun 1983b; 40:407–410.
99. Christensen G, Simpson W, Younger J. Adherence of coagulase-negative staphylococci to plastic tissue culture plates: a quantitative model for the adherence of staphylococci to medical devices. J Clin Microbiol 1985; 22:996–1006.
100. Christensen G, et al. Microbial and foreign body factors in the pathogenesis of medical device infections. In AL Bisno, FA Waldvogel, eds. Infections Associated With Indwelling Medical Devices. Washington: American Society for Microbiology, 1989. Pp. 27–59.
101. Peters G, et al. Biology of *S. epidermidis* extracellular slime. Bakteriol Mikrobiol 1987; 16:15–32.
102. Dunne M, Mason E, Sheldon K. Diffusion of rifampin and vancomycin through a *Staphylococcus epidermidis* biofilm. Antimicrob Agents Chemother 1993; 37(12):2522–2526.
103. Schoen F, Hobson C. Anatomic analysis of removed prosthetic heart valves: causes of failure of 33 mechanical valves and 58 bioprostheses, 1980–1983. Hum Pathol 1985; 16: 549–559.
104. Watanakunakorn C. Prosthetic valve infective endocarditis. Prog Cardiovasc Dis 1979; 22:181–192.
105. Arnett E, Roberts W. Prosthetic valve endocarditis: clinicopathologic analysis of 22 necropsy patients with comparison of observations in 74 necropsy patients with active infective endocarditis involving natural left-sided cardiac valves. Am J Cardiol 1976; 38:281–292.
106. Karchmer A, Bisno A. Infections of prosthetic heart valves and vascular grafts. In A Bisno, F Waldvogel, eds. Infections Associated With Indwelling Medical Devices. Washington: American Society for Microbiology, 1989. Pp. 129–160.
107. Cortina J, Martinell J, Artiz V. Surgical treatment of active prosthetic valve endocarditis: results in 66 patients. Thorac Cardiovasc Surg 1987; 35:209.
108. Ferrans V, et al. Infection of glutaraldehyde-preserved porcine valve heterografts. Am J Cardiol 1979; 43:1123–1136.
109. Bloomfield P, Wheatley D, Prescott R, Miller H. Twelve-year comparison of a Bjork-Shiley mechanical heart valve with porcine bioprostheses. N Engl J Med 1991; 324:573–579.
110. Parker M, Ball L. Streptococci and aerococci associated with systemic infection in man. J Med Microbiol 1976; 9:275–302.

111. Leport C, et al. Incidence of colonic lesions in *Streptococcus bovis* and enterococcal endocarditis. Lancet 1987; 1:748.
112. Emiliani V, Chodos J, Comer G. Streptococcus bovis brain abscess associated with an occult colonic villous adenoma. Am J Gastroenterol 1990; 85:78.
113. Klein R, et al. Association of *Streptococcus bovis* with carcinoma of the colon. N Engl J Med 1977; 297:800–802.
114. Steinberg D, Naggar C. *Streptococcus bovis* endocarditis with carcinoma of the colon. N Engl J Med 1977; 297:1354–1355.
115. Ugolini V, et al. Pneumococcal endocarditis update: analysis of 10 cases diagnosed between 1974 and 1984. Am Heart J 1986; 112:813–819.
116. Powderly W, Stanley S, Medoff G. Pneumococcal endocarditis: report of a series and review of the literature. Rev Infect Dis 1986; 8:786–791.
117. Bruyn G, Thompson J, Van der Meer J. Pneumococcal endocarditis in adult patients. A report of five cases and review of the literature. Q J Med 1990; 74:33–40.
118. Etienne J, Eykyn S. Increase in native valve endocarditis caused by coagulase-negative staphylococci: an Anglo-French clinical and microbiological study. Br Heart J 1990; 64:381–384.
119. Caputo G, Archer G, Calderwood S. Native valve endocarditis due to coagulase-negative staphylococci: clinical and microbiologic features. Am J Med 1987; 83:619–625.
120. Vandenesch F, et al. Endocarditis due to *Staphylococcus lugdunensis:* report of 11 cases and review. Clin Infect Dis 1993; 17:871–876.
121. Baddour L, Phillips T, Bisno A. Coagulase-negative staphylococcal endocarditis. Occurrence in patients with mitral valve prolapse. Arch Intern Med 1986; 146:119–121.
122. Harris L, O'Shields H. Coagulase-negative staphylococcal endocarditis: a view from the community hospital. South Med J 1986; 79:1379–1384.
123. Mandell G, et al. Enterococcal endocarditis. An analysis of 38 patients observed at The New York Hospital-Cornell Medical Center. Arch Intern Med 1970; 125:258–264.
124. Wall T, Peyton R, Cory G. Gonococcal endocarditis: a new look at an old disease. Medicine 1989; 68:375–380.
125. Jurica J, Bomzer C, England A. Gonococcal endocarditis: a case report and review of the literature. Sex Transm Dis 1987; 14:231–233.
126. Wieland M, Lederman M, Kline-King C. Left-sided endocarditis due to *Pseudomonas aeruginosa.* A report of 10 cases and review of the literature. Medicine 1986; 65:180–189.
127. Geraci J, Wilson W. Endocarditis due to gram-negative bacteria. Report of 56 cases. Clin Proc 1982; 57:145–148.
128. Carruthers M. Endocarditis due to enteric bacilli other than *Salmonellae:* case reports and literature review. Am J Med Sci 1977; 273:203–211.
129. Schneider P, Nernoff J, Gold J. *Salmonella* endocarditis: report of a case and review. Arch Intern Med 1967; 120:478–482.
130. Gallagher PCW. *Listeria monocytogenes* endocarditis: a review of the literature 1950–1986. Scand J Infect Dis 1988; 20:359–368.
131. Carvajal A, Frederiksen W. Fatal endocarditis due to *Listeria monocytogenes.* Rev Infect Dis 1988; 10:616–623.
132. Felner J, Dowell V. Anaerobic bacterial endocarditis. N Engl J Med 1979; 283:1188–1192.
133. Nastro L, Finegold S. Endocarditis due to anaerobic gram-negative bacilli. Am J Med 1979; 54:482–496.
134. Gorby G, Peacock J. *Erysipelothrix rhusiopathiae* endocarditis: microbiologic, epidemiologic, and clinical features of an occupational disease. Rev Infect Dis 1988; 10:317–325.
135. Schuster M, Brennan P. Persistent bacteremia with *Erysipelothrix rhusiopathiae* in a hospitalized patient. Clin Infect Dis 1993; 17:783–784.
136. Procter W. Subacute bacterial endocarditis due to *Erysipelothrix rhusiopathiae:* report of a case and review of the literature. Am J Med 1965; 38:820–824.
137. Saravolatz L, Pohlod D, Arking L. Community-acquired methicillin-resistant *Staphylococcus* aureus infections: a new source for nosocomial outbreaks. Ann Intern Med 1982; 97:325–329.
138. Craven D, et al. Methicillin-resistant *Staphylococcus aureus* bacteremia linked to intravenous drug abusers using a "shooting gallery." Am J Med 1986; 80:770–776.
139. Berman D, et al. *Staphylococcus aureus* colonization in intravenous drug abusers, dialysis patients, and diabetics. J Infect Dis 1987; 155:829–831.
140. Small P, Chambers H. Vancomycin for *Staphylococcus aureus* endocarditis in intravenous drug abusers. Antimicrob Agents Chemother 1990; 34:1227–1231.
141. Crane L, et al. Bacteremia in narcotic addicts at the Detroit Medical Center. I. Microbiology, epidemiology, risk factors, and empiric therapy. Rev Infect Dis 1986; 8:364–373.
142. Reyes M, Palutke W, Wylin R. Pseudomonas endocarditis in the Detroit Medical Center—1969–1972. Medicine 1973; 52:173–194.
143. Reyes M, Brown W, Lerner A. Treatment of patients with *Pseudomonas* endocarditis with high-dose aminoglycoside and carbenicillin therapy. Medicine 1978; 57:57–67.
144. Shekar R, et al. Outbreak of endocarditis caused by *Pseudomonas aeruginosa* serotype 011 among pentazocine and tripelenamine abusers in Chicago. J Infect Dis 1985; 151:203–208.
145. Mills J, Drew D. *Serratia marcescens* endocarditis: a regional illness associated with intravenous drug abuse. Ann Intern Med 1976; 84:29–35.
146. Rubenstein E, et al. Tissue penetration of amphotericin B in Candida endocarditis. Chest 1974; 66:376–377.
147. Baddour L, Meyer J, Henry B. Polymicrobial infective endocarditis in the 1980s. Rev Infect Dis 1991; 13:963–970.
148. Tuazon C, Sheagren J. Staphylococcal endocarditis in parenteral drug abusers: source of the organism. Ann Intern Med 1975; 82:788–790.
149. Tuazon C, Hill R, Sheagren J. Microbiologic study of street heroin and injection paraphernalia. J Infect Dis 1974; 129:327–329.
150. Hall R, Bayer A, Mayer W. Infective endocarditis following human-to-human enterococal transmission: a complication of intravenous narcotic abuse. Arch Intern Med 1976; 136:1173–1174.
151. Scalcini M, Sanders C. Endocarditis from human-to-human transmission of *Staphylococcus aureus.* Arch Intern Med 1980; 140:111–112.
152. Cooper R, Mills J. *Serratia* endocarditis. A follow-up report. Arch Intern Med 1980; 140:199–202.
153. Dismukes W, Karchmer A, Buckley M. Prosthetic valve endocarditis: analysis of 38 cases. Circulation 1973; 48:365–377.
154. Boyce J, et al. A common-source outbreak of *Staphylococcus epidermidis* infections among patients undergoing cardiac surgery. J Infect Dis 1990; 161:493–499.
155. Blakemore W, McGarrity G, Thurer R. Infection by airborne bacteria with cardiopulmonary bypass. Surgery 1971; 70: 830–838.
156. Petheram I, Boyce M. Prosthetic valve endocarditis: a review of 24 cases. Thorax 1977; 32:478–485.
157. Moore-Gillon J, Eykyn S, Phillips I. Prosthetic valve endocarditis. Br Med J 1983; 287:739–741.
158. Slaughter L, Morris J, Starr A. Prosthetic valvular endocarditis: a 12-year review. Circulation 1973; 47:1319–1326.
159. Shafer R, Hall W. Bacterial endocarditis following open heart surgery. Am J Cardiol 1970; 25:602–607.
160. Archer G, Vishniavsky N, Stiver H. Plasmid pattern analysis

of *Staphylococus epidermidis* isolates from patients with prosthetic valve endocarditis. Infect Immun 1982; 35:627–632.
161. van den Broek P, et al. Epidemic of prosthetic valve endocarditis caused by *Staphylococcus epidermidis.* Br Med J 1985; 291:949–950.
162. Mickelsen P, et al. Instability of antibiotic resistance in a strain of *Staphylococcus epidermidis* isolated from an outbreak of prosthetic valve endocarditis. J Infect Dis 1985; 152:50–58.
163. Karchmer A, Archer G, Dismukes W. *Staphylococcus epidermidis* causing prosthetic valve endocarditis: microbiologic and clinical observations as guides to therapy. Ann Intern Med 1983; 98:447–455.
164. Calderwood S, et al. Prosthetic valve endocarditis: analysis of factors affecting outcome of therapy. J Thorac Cardiovasc Surg 1986; 92:776–783.
165. Terpenning M, Buggy B, Kauffman C. Hospital-acquired infective endocarditis. Arch Intern Med 1988; 148:1601–1603.
166. Tunkel A, Kaye D. Endocarditis with negative blood cultures. N Engl J Med 1992b; 326:1215.
167. Van Scoy R. Culture-negative endocarditis. Mayo Clin Proc 1982; 57:149–154.
168. Pesanti E. Infective endocarditis with negative blood cultures, an analysis of 52 cases. Am J Med 1979; 66:43–50.
169. Werner A, et al. Studies on the bacteremia of bacterial endocarditis. JAMA 1967; 202:199–203.
170. Lukes A, Bright D, Durack D. Diagnosis of infective endocarditis. Infect Dis Clin NA 1993; 7(1):1–8.
171. Kaye K, Kaye D. Laboratory findings including blood cultures. In D Kaye, ed. Infective Endocarditis. Second ed. New York: Raven, 1992. Pp. 117–124.
172. Ellner J, et al. Infective endocarditis caused by slow-growing, fastidious, gram-negative bacteria. Medicine 1979; 58: 145–158.
173. Elster S, et al. *Hemophilus aphrophilus* endocarditis: review of 23 cases. Am J Cardiol 1975; 35:72–79.
174. Parker S, Apicella M, Fuller C. *Hemophilus* endocarditis. Two patients with complications. Arch Intern Med 1983; 143:48–51.
175. Raucher B, et al. Occult polymicrobial endocarditis with *Haemophilus parainfluenzae* in intravenous drug abusers. Am J Med 1989; 86:169–172.
176. Lynn D, Kane J, Parker R. *Haemophilus parainfluenzae* and *influenzae* endocarditis: a review of forty cases. Medicine 1977; 56:115–128.
177. Decker M, et al. Endocarditis and infections of intravascular devices due to *Eikenella corrodens.* Am J Med Sci 1986; 292:209–212.
178. Jenny D, Letendre P, Iverson G. Endocarditis caused by *Kingella indologenes.* Rev Infec Dis 1987; 9:787–789.
179. Jenny D, Letendre P, Iverson G. Endocarditis due to *Kingella* species. Rev Infect Dis 1988; 10:1065–1066.
180. Bieger R, Brewer N, Washington J. *Haemophilus aphrophilus:* a microbiologic and clinical review and report of 42 cases. Medicine 1978; 57(4):345–355.
181. Chen Y, Chang S, Luh K. *Actinobacillus actinomycetemcomitans* endocarditis: a report of four cases and review of the literature. Q J Med 1992; 81:871–878.
182. Jacobs F, et al. *Brucella* endocarditis: the role of combined medical and surgical approach. Rev Infect Dis 1990; 12:740–744.
183. Gerry J, Greenough W. Diphtheroid endocarditis. Report of nine cases and review of the literature. Johns Hopkins Med J 1976; 139:61–68.
184. Vanbosterhaut B, et al. *Corynebacterium jeikeium* (group JK diphtheroids) endocarditis. A report of five cases. Diagn Microbiol Infect Dis 1989; 1989:265–268.
185. Sussman J, et al. Clinical manifestations and therapy of *Lactobacillus* endocarditis: report of a case and review of the literature. Rev Infect Dis 1986; 8:771–776.
186. Seelig M, et al. Patterns of candida endocarditis following cardiac surgery: importance of early diagnosis and therapy (an analysis of 91 cases). Prog Cardiovasc Dis 1974; 17:125–160.
187. Blair T. *Histoplasma capsulatum* endocarditis. Chest 1981; 79(6):620.
188. Goodwin R, et al. Disseminated histoplasmosis: clinical and pathological correlations. Medicine 1980; 59:1–33.
189. Harford C. Postoperative fungal endocarditis: fungemia, embolism, and therapy. Arch Intern Med 1974; 134:116–120.
190. Rubinstein E, et al. Fungal endocarditis: analysis of 24 cases and review of the literature. Medicine 1975; 54:331–344.
191. Jones R, Priest J, Kuo C. Subacute chlamydial endocarditis. JAMA 1982; 247:655.
192. van der Bel-Kahn J, Watanakunakorn C, Menefee M. Chlamydia trachomatis endocarditis. Am Heart J 1978; 95:627.
193. Tobin M, Cahill G, Gearty G. Q fever endocarditis. Am J Med 1982; 72:396.
194. Kimbrough R, Ormsbee R, Peacock M. Q fever endocarditis in the United States. Ann Intern Med 1979; 91:400.
195. Sawyer L, Fishbein D, McDade J. Q fever: current concepts. Rev Infect Dis 1987; 9:935.
196. Varma M, Adgey A, Connolly J. Chronic Q fever endocarditis. Br Heart J 1980; 43:695.
197. Cohen J, Sloss L, Kundsin R. Prosthetic valve endocarditis caused by *Mycoplasma hominis.* Am J Med 1989; 86:819–821.
198. Tompkins L, Roessier B, Redd S. Legionella prosthetic-valve endocarditis. N Engl J Med 1988; 318:530.
199. Bayer A. Staphylococcal bacteremia and endocarditis. State of the art. Arch Intern Med 1982; 142:1169–1176.
200. Bush L, Johnson CC. Clinical syndrome and diagnosis. In D Kaye, ed. Infective Endocarditis. Second ed. New York: Raven, 1992. Pp. 99–115.
201. Chambers H, Miller R, Newman M. Right-sided *Staphylococcus aureus* endocarditis in intravenous drug abusers: two-week combination therapy. Ann Intern Med 1988; 109:619–624.
202. Mills J, Utley J, Abbott J. Heart failure in infective endocarditis: predisposing factors, course and treatment. Chest 1974; 66:151–157.
203. Atkinson J, Virmani R. Infective endocarditis: changing trends and general approach for examination. Hum Pathol 1987; 18:603–608.
204. Edwards W. Surgical pathology of the aortic valve. In BF Waller, ed. Pathology of the Heart and Great Vessels. New York: Churchill-Livingstone, 1988. Pp. 43–100.
205. Waller B. Etiology of mitral stenosis and pure mitral regurgitation. In B Waller, ed. Pathology of the Heart and Great Vessels. New York: Churchill-Livingstone, 1988. Pp. 101–189.
206. Daniel W, Muggs A, Martin R. Improvement in the diagnosis of abscesses associated with endocarditis by transesophageal echocardiography. N Engl J Med 1991; 324:795–800.
207. McFarland M. Pathology of infective endocarditis. In D Kaye, ed. Infective Endocarditis. Second ed. New York: Raven, 1992. Pp. 57–83.
208. Kilpatrick Z, Greensberg P, Sanford J. Splinter hemorrhages—their clinical significance. Arch Intern Med 1965; 115:730–735.
209. Farrior J, Silverman M. A consideration of the differences between a Janeway's lesion and an Osler's node in infectious endocarditis. Chest 1976; 70:239–243.
210. Von Gemmingen G, Winkelmann R. Osler's node of subacute bacterial endocarditis: focal necrotizing vaculitis (*sic*) of the glomus body. Arch Derm 1967; 95:91–94.

211. Alpert J, et al. Pathogenesis of Osler's nodes. Ann Intern Med 1976; 85:471–473.
212. Silverberg H. Roth's spots. Mt Sinai J Med 1970; 37:77–79.
213. Kennedy J, Wise G. Clinicopathological correlation of retinal lesions: subacute bacterial endocarditis. Arch Opthalmol 1965; 74:658–662.
214. Freedman L. Consequences of intravascular infection. In L Freedman, ed. Infective Endocarditis and Other Intravascular Infections. New York: Plenum, 1982. Pp. 77–124.
215. Churchill M, Geraci J, Hunder G. Musculoskeletal manifestations of bacterial endocarditis. Ann Intern Med 1977; 87:754–759.
216. Thadepalli H, Francis C. Diagnostic clues in metastatic lesions of endocarditis in addicts. West J Med 1978; 128:1–5.
217. Good A, Hague J, Kauffman C. Streptococcal endocarditis initially seen as septic arthritis. Arch Intern Med 1978; 138:805–806.
218. Weinstein L. Life-threatening complications of infective endocarditis and their management. Arch Intern Med 1986; 146:953–957.
219. Julander I. Staphylococcal septicaemia and endocarditis in 80 drug addicts. Scand J Infect Dis 1983; 41:49–54.
220. Neufeld G, Branson C, Marshall L. Infective endocarditis as a complication of heroin use. South Med J 1976; 69:1148–1151.
221. Salgado A, Furlan A, Keys T. Mycotic aneurysm, subarachnoid hemorrhage, and indications for cerebral angiography in infective endocarditis. Stroke 1987; 18:1057–1060.
222. Weinstein L, Schlesinger J. Pathoanatomic, pathophysiologic and clinical correlations in endocarditis (two parts). N Engl J Med 1974; 291:1122–1126.
223. Pruitt A, Rubin R, Karchmer A. Neurologic complications of bacterial endocarditis. Medicine 1978; 57:329.
224. Pamphlett R, Walsh J. Infective endocarditis with inflammatory lesions in the peripheral nervous system. Acta Neuropathol 1989; 78:101–104.
225. McKinsey D, McMurray T, Flynn J. Immune complex glomerulonephritis associated with *Staphycococcus aureus* bacteremia: response to corticosteroid therapy. Rev Infect Dis 1990; 12:125.
226. Feinstein E, Eknoyan G, Lister B. Renal complications of bacterial endocarditis. Am J Nephrol 1985; 5:457–469.
227. Morel-Maroger L, et al. Kidney in subacute endocarditis: pathological and immunofluorescence findings. Arch Pathol 1972; 94:205–213.
228. Neugarten J, Baldwin D. Glomerulonephritis in bacterial endocarditis. Am J Med 1984; 77:297.
229. Jaffe W, Morgan D, Pearlman A. Infective endocarditis, 1983–1988: echocardiographic findings and factors influencing morbidity and mortality. J Am Coll Cardiol 1990; 15:1227.
230. Mugge A, et al. Echocardiography in infective endocarditis: reassessment of prognostic implications of vegetation size determined by the transthoracic and the transesophageal approach. J Am Coll Cardiol. 1989; 14:631–638.
231. Popp R. Echocardiography and infectious endocarditis. In J Remington, M Swartz, eds. Current Clinical Topics in Infectious Diseases. 4th ed. New York: McGraw-Hill, 1983. P. 98.
232. Shapiro S, Bayer A. Transesophageal and doppler echocardiography in the diagnosis and management of infective endocarditis. Chest 1991; 100:1125.
233. Daniel W, Schroder E, Mugge A. Transesophageal echocardiography in infective endocarditis. Am J Card Imaging 1988; 2:78.
234. Erbel R, Rohmann S, Drexler M. Improved diagnostic value of echocardiography in patients with infective endocarditis by transesophageal approach: a prospective study. Eur Heart J 1988; 1:43.
235. Taams M, et al. Enhanced morphological diagnosis in infective endocarditis by transesophageal echocardiography. Br Heart J 1990; 63:109–113.
236. Zeineddin M, Stewart JA. Echocardiographic detection of non-valve-ring myocardial abscess complicating aortic valve endocarditis. Am J Med Sci 1988; 85:97.
237. Durack D, Lukes A, Bright D. New criteria for diagnosis of infective endocarditis: utilization of specific echocardiographic findings. Am J Med 1994; 96:200–209.
238. Bayer A, et al. Evaluation of new clinical criteria for the diagnosis of infective endocarditis. Am J Med 1994; 96: 211–219.
239. Rice L, Calderwood S, Eliopoulos G. Enterococcal endocarditis: a comparison of prosthetic and native valve disease. Rev Infect Dis 1991; 13:1.
240. Washington J, Ilstrup D. Blood cultures: issues and controversies. Rev Infect Dis 1986; 8:792–802.
241. Auckenthaler R. Laboratory diagnosis of infective endocarditis. Eur Heart J 1984; 5:49–51.
242. Carey R, Gross K, Roberts R. Vitamin B6-dependent *Streptococcus mitior* (*mitis*) isolated from patients with systemic infections. J Infect Dis 1975; 131:722–726.
243. Powers D, Mandell G. Intraleukocytic bacteria in endocarditis patients. JAMA 1974; 227:312–313.
244. Whitcomb D. Bugs in the blood: acute staphylococcal septicemia and endocarditis diagnosed by staining the buffy coat. N C Med J 1974; 47:293–295.
245. Baldassarre J, Kaye D. Principles and overview of antibiotic therapy. In D Kaye, ed. Infective Endocarditis. Second ed. New York: Raven, 1992. Pp. 169–190.
246. Fontana R, et al. Mechanisms of resistance of enterococci to beta-lactam antibiotics. Eur J Clin Microbiol Infect Dis 1990; 9:103–105.
247. Eliopoulos G. Enterococcal endocarditis. In D Kaye, ed. Infective Endocarditis. Second ed. New York: Raven, 1992. Pp. 209–223.
248. Eliopoulos G. Aminoglycoside resistant enterococcal endocarditis. Infect Dis Clin NA 1993; 7(1):117–134.
249. Geraci J, Martin W. Antibiotic therapy of bacterial endocarditis: VI. subacute enterococcal endocarditis: clinical, pathologic, and therapeutic consideration of 33 cases. Circulation 1954; 10:173.
250. Eliopoulos G, Eliopoulos C. Therapy of enterococcal infections. Eur J Clin Microbiol Infect Dis 1990; 9:118.
251. Frieden T, Munsiff S, Low D. Emergence of vancomycin-resistant enterococci in New York City. Lancet 1993; 342: 76–79.
252. Handwerger S, et al. Nosocomial outbreak due to *Enterococcus faecium* highly resistant to vancomycin, penicillin, and gentamicin. Clin Infect Dis 1993; 16:750–755.
253. Goldman D. Vancomycin-resistant *Enterococcus faecium:* headline news. Infect Control Hosp Epidemiol 1992; 13:695–699.
254. Eliopoulos G. Increasing problems in the therapy of enterococcal infections. Eur J Clin Microbiol Infect Dis 1993b; 12:409–412.
255. Levison M. In vitro assays. In D Kaye, ed. Infective Endocarditis. Second ed. New York: Raven, 1992. Pp. 151–167.
256. Bayer A, Crowell D, Nast C. Intravegetation antimicrobial distribution in aortic endocarditis analyzed by computer-generated model. Chest 1990; 97:611–617.
257. Cremieux AC, Maziere B, Vallois JM. Evaluation of antibiotic diffusion into cardiac vegetations by quantitative autoradiography. J Infect Dis 1989; 159:938–944.
258. Cremieux A, Maziere B, Vallois J. Ceftriaxone diffusion into cardiac fibrin vegetation. Qualitative and quantitative evaluation by autoradiography. Fundam Clin Pharmacol 1991; 5:53–60.

259. Cremieux A, Saleh-Mghir A, Vallois J. Autoradiographic pattern of diffusion of C-daptomycin throughout infected cardiac vegetations in rabbits. Programs and Abstracts of the 32nd International Conference on Antimicrobial Agents and Chemotherapy. Anaheim, CA, 1992.
260. Mortara L, Bayer A. *Staphylococcus aureus* bacteremia and endocarditis: new diagnostic and therapeutic concepts. Infect Dis Clin NA 1993; 7(1):53–68.
261. Durack D, Beeson P. Experimental bacterial endocarditis. I. Colonization of a sterile vegetation. Br J Exp Pathol 1972; 53:44–49.
262. Durack D, Beeson P. Experimental bacterial endocarditis II. Survival of bacteria in endocardial vegetations. Br J Exp Pathol 1972b; 53:50.
263. Roberts R. Streptococcal endocarditis: the viridans and beta hemolytic streptococci. In D Kaye, ed. Infective Endocarditis. Second ed. New York: Raven, 1992. Pp. 191–208.
264. Francioli P. Ceftriaxone and outpatient treatment of infective endocarditis. Infect Dis Clin NA 1993; 7(1):97–116.
265. Francioli P, Etienne J, Hoigne R. Treatment of streptococcal endocarditis with a single daily dose of ceftriaxone for 4 weeks: efficacy and out-patient treatment feasibility. JAMA 1992; 267:264.
266. Stamboulian D, Bonvehi P, Arevalo C. Antibiotic management of outpatients with endocarditis due to penicillin-susceptible streptococci. Rev Infect Dis 1991; 13(2):S160.
267. Wilson W. Ceftriaxone sodium therapy of penicillin G-susceptible streptococcal endocarditis. JAMA 1992; 267(2):279–280.
268. Stamboulian D, Francioli P. Two-week treatment of streptococcal endocarditis with single daily dose of ceftriaxone plus netilmicin. ECCMID Oslo, 1991.
269. Korzeniowski O, Sande M. Combination antimicrobial therapy for *Staphylococus aureus* endocarditis in patients addicted to parenteral drugs and in nonaddicts: a prospective study. Ann Intern Med 1982; 97:496–503.
270. Watanakunaknorn C. Changing epidemiology and newer aspects of infective endocarditis. Adv Intern Med 1977; 22:21–47.
271. Hessen M, Abrutyn E. Gram-negative bacterial endocarditis. In D Kaye, ed. Infective Endocarditis. Second ed. New York: Raven, 1992. Pp. 251–264.
272. Meyer D, Gerding D. Favorable prognosis of patients with prosthetic valve endocarditis causd by gram-negative bacilli of the HACEK group. Am J Med 1988; 85:104–107.
273. Moyer D, Edwards J. Fungal endocarditis. In D Kaye, ed. Infective Endocarditis. Second ed. New York: Raven, 1992. Pp. 299–312.
274. Levine D, Fromm B, Reddy B. Delayed response to vancomycin or vancomycin plus rifampin therapy among patients with methicillin-resistant *Staphylococcus aureus* endocarditis. Ann Intern Med 1991; 115:674–680.
275. Markowitz N, Quinn E, Saravolatz L. Trimethoprim-sulfamethoxazole compared to vancomycin for the treatment of *Staphylococcus aureus* infection. Ann Intern Med 1992; 117:390.
276. Hartstein A, Mulligan M, Morthland V. Recurrent *Staphylococcus aureus* bacteremia. J Clin Microbiol 1992; 30:670.
277. Chambers H. Short-course combination and oral therapies of *Staphylococcus aureus* endocarditis. Infect Dis Clin NA 1993; 7(1):69–80.
278. Dworkin R, Lee B, Sande M. Treatment of right-sided *Staphylococcus aureus* endocarditis in intravenous drug users with ciprofloxacin and rifampin. Lancet 1989; 2:1071–1073.
279. Tebas P, et al. Early resistance to rifampin and ciprofloxacin in the treatment of right-sided Staphylococcus aureus endocarditis. J Infect Dis 1991; 163:204–205.
280. Kobasa W, Kaye K, Shapiro T. Therapy for experimental endocarditis due to *Staphylococcus epidermidis.* Rev Infect Dis 1983; 5:5533–5537.
281. Karchmer A, Archer G. Methicillin-resistant *Staphylococcus epidermidis* prosthetic valve endocarditis: a therapeutic trial (abstract 476). Abstracts of the 24th Interscience Conference of Antimicrobial Agents and Chemotherapy, Washington, DC. American Society for Microbiology, 1984.
282. Levy P, Draancourt M, Etienne J. Comparison of different antibiotic regimens for therapy of 32 cases of Q fever endocarditis. Antimicrob Agents Chemother 1991; 35:533.
283. Haldane E, Marrie T, Faulkner R. Q fever endocarditis in Nova Scotia. Experience with five patients in 1981–1982. J Infect Dis 1983; 148:978.
284. Turck W, Howitt G, Turnberg L. Chronic Q fever. Q J Med 1976; 45:193.
285. Fernandez-Guerrero M. Zoonotic endocarditis. Infect Dis Clin NA 1993; 7(1):135–152.
286. Appelfeld M, Billingsley L, Tucaker J. Q fever endocarditis—a case occurring in the United States. Am Heart J 1977; 93:669–670.
287. Fernandez-Guerrero M, Muelas J, Aguado J. Q fever endocarditis on porcine bioprosthetic valves. Ann Intern Med 1988; 108:209.
288. Montejo J, et al. Open randomized therapeutic trial of six antimicrobial regimens in the treatment of human brucellosis. Clinical Infectious Diseases 1991; 16:671–676.
289. Al-Kasab S, Al-Fagih M, Al-Youset R. Brucella infective endocarditis. Thorac Cardiovasc Surg 1988; 95:862–867.
290. Fernandez-Guerrero M, Martinell J, Aguado J. Prosthetic valve endocarditis caused by *Brucella melitensis.* Arch Intern Med 1987; 147:1141.
291. Jeroudi M, Halim M, Harder E. Brucella endocarditis. Br Heart J 1987; 58:279.
292. Buchanan T, Faber L. 2-Mercaptoethanol brucella agglutination test: usefulness for predicting recovery from brucellosis. J Clin Microbiol 1980; 11:691–693.
293. Cisneros J, Pachon J, Cuello J. *Brucella* endocarditis cured by medical treatment. J Infect Dis 1989; 160(5):907.
294. Siller K, Johnson W. Unusual bacterial causes of endocarditis. In D Kaye, ed. Infective Endocarditis. Second ed. New York: Raven, 1992. Pp. 265–297.
295. Alsip S, et al. Indications for cardiac surgery in patients with active infective endocarditis. Am J Med 1985; 78:138–148.
296. DiNubile M. Surgery in active endocarditis. Ann Intern Med 1982; 96:650.
297. Murphy J, Foster-Smith K. Management of complications of infective endocarditis with emphasis on echocardiographic findings. Infect Dis Clin NA 1993; 7(1):153–166.
298. Mullany C, et al. The surgical treatment of infective endocarditis. World J Surg 1989; 13:132–136.
299. D'Agostino R, Miller D, Stenson E. Valve replacements in patients with native valve endocarditis: what really determines operative outcome. Ann Thorac Surg 1985; 40:429–438.
300. Douglas J, Dismukes W. Surgical therapy of infective endocarditis on natural valves. In D Kaye, ed. Infective Endocarditis. Second ed. New York: Raven, 1992b. Pp. 397–411.
301. Croft C, et al. Analysis of surgical vs. medical therapy in active complicated native valve endocarditis. Am J Cardiol 1983; 51:1650–1655.
302. Abdelnoor M, Nitter-Hauge S, Trettli S. Relative survival of patients after heart valve replacement. Eur Heart J 1990; 11:23–28.
303. Lederman M, et al. Duration of fever during treatment of infective endocarditis. Medicine 1992; 71(1):52–57.
304. Blumberg E, et al. Persistent fever in association with infective endocarditis. Clin Infect Dis 1992; 15:983–990.

305. Sanfilippo A, Picard M, Newell J. Echocardiographic assessment of patients with infectious endocarditis: prediction of risk for complications. J Am Coll Cardiol 1991; 18:1191.
306. Steckelberg J, Melton J, Ilstrup D. Emboli in infective endocarditis: the prognostic value of echocardiography. Ann Intern Med 1991; 114:635.
307. Salgado A, et al. Neurologic complications of endocarditis: a 12 year experience. Neurology 1989; 39:173–178.
308. Lutas E, Roberts R, Devreus R. Relation between the presence of echocardiographic vegetations and the complication rate in infective endocarditis. Am Heart J 1986; 112:107.
309. Paschalis C, Pugsley WEJ. Rate of cerebral embolic events in relation to antibiotic and anticoagulant therapy in patients with bacterial endocarditis. Eur Neurol 1990; 30:87.
310. Hart R, et al. Stroke in infective endocarditis. Stroke 1990; 21:695–700.
311. Steckelberg J, Murphy J, Wilson W. Management of complications of infective endocarditis. In D Kaye, ed. Infective Endocarditis. Second ed. New York: Raven, 1992. Pp. 435–453.
312. Hecht S, Berger M. Right-sided endocarditis in intravenous drug users—prognostic features in 102 episodes. Ann Intern Med 1992; 117:560.
313. DiNubile M. Endocarditis related to intravenous drug use. Current Opinion In Infectious Diseases 1991; 4:603–608.
314. Bayer A, et al. Tricuspid valve endocarditis due to *Staphylococcus aureus.* Correlation of two-dimensional echocardiograpy with clinical outcome. Chest 1988; 93:247–253.
315. Robbins J, et al. Right-sided valvular endocarditis: etiology, diagnosis, and an approach to therapy. Am Heart 1986; 11:128–135.
316. Wong D, et al. Clinical implications of large vegetations in infectious endocarditis. Arch Intern Med. 1983; 143:1874–1877.
317. Ginzton L, Siegel R, Criley J. Natural history of tricuspid valve endocarditis: a two dimensional echocardiographic study. Am J Cardiol 1982; 49:1853–1859.
318. Hubbell G, Rapaport E. Presentation, management, and follow-up evaluation of infective endocarditis in drug addicts. Am Heart J 1981; 102:85–94.
319. Welton D, Young J, Gentry W. Recurrent infective endocarditis. Analysis of predisposing factors and clinical features. Am J Med 1979; 66:932–938.
320. Barbour D, Roberts W. Valve excision only versus valve excision plus replacement for active infective endocarditis involving the tricuspid valve. Am J Cardiol 1986; 57:475–478.
321. Arbulu A, Asfaw I. Tricuspid valvulectomy without prosthetic replacement. Ten years of clinical experience. J Thorac Cardiovasc Surg 1981; 82:684–691.
322. Whitener C, et al. Endocarditis due to coagulase-negative staphylococci: microbiologic, epidemiologic, and clinical considerations. Infect Dis Clin NA 1993; 7(1):81–96.
323. Baumgartner W, Miller D, Reitz B. Surgical treatment of prosthetic valve endocarditis. Ann Thorac Surg 1983; 38:87–104.
324. Karchmer A, et al. Late prosthetic valve endocarditis: clinical features influencing therapy. Am J Med 1978; 64:199–206.
325. Watanakunakorn C, Tan J, Phair J. Some salient features of *Staphylococcus aureus* endocarditis. Am J Med 1973; 54:473–481.
326. Santoro J, Ingerman M. Response to therapy: relapses and reinfections. In D Kaye, ed. Infective Endocarditis. Second ed. New York: Raven, 1992. Pp. 423–433.
327. Malacoff R, Frank E, Andriole V. Streptococcal endocarditis (nonenterococcal, non group A). Single vs. combination therapy. JAMA 1979; 241:1807–1810.
328. Wilson W, et al. Management of complications of infective endocarditis. Mayo Clin Proc 1982b; 57:152–170.
329. Gold M. Cure rates and long-term prognosis. In D Kaye, ed. Infective Endocarditis. Second ed. New York: Raven, 1992. Pp. 455–464.
330. Levison M, Kaye D, Mandell G. Characteristics of patients with multiple episodes of bacterial endocarditis. JAMA 1970; 211:1355–1357.
331. Baddour L. Twelve-year review of recurrent native-valve infective endocarditis: a disease of the modern antibiotic era. Rev Infect Dis 1988; 10:1163–1170.
332. Kaye D, Abrutyn E. Prevention of infective endocarditis. Ann Intern Med 1991; 114:803–804.
333. Dajani A, Bisno A, Chung K. Prevention of bacterial endocarditis: recommendations by the American Heart Association. JAMA 1990; 264:2919–2922.
334. Dajani A, Bawdon R, Berry M. Oral amoxicillin as prophylaxis for endocarditis: what is the optimal dose. Clinical Infectious Diseases 1994; 18:157–160.
335. Stengel A, Wolferth C. Mycotic (bacterial) aneurysms of intravascular origin. Arch Intern Med 1923; 31:527.
336. Wilson S, Wagenen P, Passaro E Jr. Arterial infection. Curr Probl Surg 1978; 15(9):1–89.
337. Anderson C, Butcher H, Ballinger W. Mycotic aneurysms. Arch Surg 1974; 109:712–717.
338. Bohmfalk G, Story J, Wissenger J. Bacterial intracranial aneurysm. Neurosurg 1978; 48:369–382.
339. Frazee J, Cahan L, Winter J. Bacterial intracranial aneurysms. J Neurosurg 1980; 53:633.
340. Feigel D, Feigl A, Edward J. Mycotic aneurysms of the aortic root. A pathologic study of 20 cases. Chest 1986; 90:553–557.
341. Bullock R, Van Dellen J, Van den Heever C. Intracranial mycotic aneurysms. A review of 9 cases. S Afr Med J 1981; 60:970–973.
342. Jarrett F, Darling R, Mundth E. The management of infected arterial aneurysms. J Cardiovasc Surg 1977; 18:361.
343. Friedman S, Pogo G, Moccio C. Mycotic aneurysm of the superior mesenteric artery. J Vasc Surg 1987; 6:87–90.
344. Sukerkar A, Dulay C, Anandappa E. Mycotic aneurysm of the hepatic artery. Radiology 1977; 124:444.
345. Morrow C, Safi H, Beall A. Primary aortoduodenal fistula caused by *Salmonella* aortitis. J Vasc Surg 1987; 6:415–418.
346. Bennett D, Cherry J. Bacterial infection of aortic aneurysms. A clinicopathologic study. Am J Surg 1967; 113:321–326.
347. Jarrett F, Darling C, Mundth E. Experience with infected aneurysms of the abdominal aorta. Arch Surg 1975; 110:1281.
348. Oskoui R, Davis W, Gomes M. Salmonella aortitis. Arch Intern Med 1993; 153:517–525.
349. Goldberg M, Rubin R. The spectrum of Salmonella infection. Infect Dis Clin NA 1988; 2:571–598.
350. Jackman J, Radolf J. Cardiovascular syphilis. Am J Med 1989; 87:425–433.
351. Patel S, Johnston K. Classification and management of mycotic aneurysms. Surg Gynecol Obstet 1977; 144:691.
352. Johnson J, Ledgerwood A, Lucas C. Mycotic aneurysm. New concepts in therapy. Arch Surg 1983; 118:577.
353. McHenry M, et al. Vertebral osteomyelitis and aortic lesions: case report and review. Rev Infect Dis 1991; 13:1184–1194.
354. Champion M, Sullivan S. Aortoenteric fistula. Incidence, presentation, recognition, management. Ann Surg 1982; 195:314–317.
355. Vogelzang R, Sohaey R. Infected aortic aneurysms: CT appearance. J Comput Assist Tomogr 1988; 12:109–112.
356. Rivera J, Blanco G, Perez M. Gallium-67 localization in a mycotic aneurysm of the throacic aorta. Clin Nucl Med 1985; 10:814–816.

357. Blumoff R, et al. Diagnosis of mycotic abdominal aortic aneurysm using 67-gallium citrate. Am Surg 1982; 48:601–603.
358. Ben-Haim S, et al. Leukocyte scintigraphy in the diagnosis of mycotic aneurysm. J Nucl Med 1992; 33:1486–1493.
359. Junewick J, Beckerman C. Complementary imaging modalities in the diagnosis of a mycotic aneurysm. Clin Nucl Med 1991; 16:874–875.
360. Moriarty J, Edelman R, Tumeh S. CT and MRI of mycotic aneurysms of the abdominal aorta. J Comput Assist Tomogr 1992; 16:941–943.
361. Plate G, Forsley N, Stigsson L. Management of inflammatory abdominal aortic aneurysm. Acta Chir Scand 1988; 154:19–24.
362. Pennell R, Hollier L, Lie J. Inflammatory abdominal aortic aneurysms: a thirty year review. J Vasc Surg 1985; 2:859–869.
363. Bourekas E, Tapler R, Turbiner E. Indium-111 imaging of an inflammatory abdominal aortic aneurysm. J Nucl Med 1992; 33:1553–1555.
364. Hansen M, Waltman A. STIR imaging of synthetic vascular graft infection. Cardiovasc Intervent Radiol 1993; 16:30–36.
365. Bingham W. Treatment of mycotic intracranial aneurysms. J Neurosurg 1977; 46:428–437.
366. Ahmadi J, et al. Monitoring of infectious intracranial aneurysms by sequential computed tomographic/magnetic resonance imaging studies. Neurosurg 1993; 32:45–50.
367. Rodesch G, Noterman J, Thys J. Treatment of intracranial mycotic aneurysm: surgery or not. Acta Neurochir 1987; 85:63–68.
368. Leipzig M, Brown F. Treatment of mycotic aneurysms. Surg Neurol 1985; 23:403–407.
369. Taylor L, Deitz D, McConnell D. Treatment of infected abdominal aneurysms by extra-anatomic bypass, aneurysm excision, and drainage. Am J Surg 1988; 155:655–658.
370. Cull D, et al. Mycotic aneurysm of the suprarenal abdominal aorta. J Cardiovasc Surg 1992; 33:181–184.
371. Bitseff E, et al. Infected abdominal aortic aneurysms. Southern Med J 1987; 80:309–312.
372. Cohen J, Bartlett J, Corey G. Extra-intestinal manifestations of Salmonella infections. Medicine 1987; 66:349–388.
373. Johansen K, Devin J. Mycotic aortic aneurysms. A reappraisal. Arch Surg 1983; 118:583.
374. Fichelle J, et al. Infected infrarenal aortic aneurysms: when is in situ reconstruction safe? J Vasc Surg 1993; 17:635–645.
375. Lorentzen J, Nielsen O, Arendrup H. Vascular graft infection: an analysis of sixty-two graft infections in 2411 consecutively implanted synthetic vascular grafts. Surgery 1985; 98:81–86.
376. O'Hara P, Hertzer N, Beven E. Surgical management of infected abdominal aortic grafts: review of a 25-year experience. J Vasc Surg 1986; 3:725–731.
377. Szilagyi D, Smith D, Elliot J. Infection in arterial reconstruction with synthetic grafts. Ann Surg 1972; 176:321–333.
378. Cruse P, Foord R. A five-year prospective study of 23,649 surgical wounds. Arch Surg 1973; 107:206–210.
379. Golan J. Vascular graft infection. Infect Dis Clin NA 1989; 3(2):247–258.
380. Durham J, Malone J, Bernhard V. The impact of multiple operations on the importance of arterial wall cultures. J Vasc Surg 1987; 5(1):160.
381. Ouriel E, Ricotta J, Adams J. Management of cholelithiasis in patients with abdominal aortic aneurysm. Ann Surg 1983; 198:717–719.
382. Ochsner J, Cooley D, DeBakey M. Associated intra-abdominal lesions encountered during resection of aortic aneurysms: surgical considerations. Dis Colon Rectum 1966; 3:485–490.
383. Edwards W, Martin R, Jenkins J. Primary graft infections. J Vasc Surg 1987; 6:235–239.
384. McAuley C, Steed D, Webster M. Bacterial presence in aortic thrombus at elective aneurysm resection: is it clinically significant? Am J Surg 1984; 147:322–324.
385. Eriksson I, et al. Significance of positive bacterial cultures from aortic aneurysms. Acta Chir Scand 1983; 149:33–35.
386. Scobie K, et al. Bacteriologic monitoring in abdominal aortic surgery. Can J Surg 1979; 22:368–371.
387. Ernst C, Campbell H, Daugherty M. Incidence and significance of intraoperative bacterial cultures during abdominal aortic aneurysmectomy. Ann Surg 1977; 185:626–633.
388. Ilgenfritz F, Jordan F. Microbiological monitoring of aortic aneurysm wall and contents during aneurysmectomy. Arch Surg 1988; 123:504–508.
389. Buckels J, et al. Significance of positive bacterial cultures from aortic aneurysm contents. Br J Surg 1985; 72:440–442.
390. Schwartz J, Powell T, Burnham S. Culture of abdominal aortic aneurysm contents: an additional series. Arch Surg 1987; 122:777–780.
391. Farkas J-C, et al. Long-term follow-up of positive cultures in 500 abdominal aortic aneurysms. Arch Surg 1993; 128:284–288.
392. Didisheim P, Olsen D, Farrar D. Infections and thromboembolism with implantable cardiovascular devices. ASAIO Trans 1989; 35:54–70.
393. Dankert J, Hogt A, Jeijen J. Biomedical polymers: bacterial adhesion, colonization and infection. CRC Crit Rev Biocompatibility 1986; 2:219–301.
394. Malone J, Moore W, Goldstone J. Proceedings: the natural history of aorto-bifemoral bypass grafts for lower extremity ischemia. J Cardiovasc Surg 1976; 17:83.
395. Schmitt D, Bandyk D, Pequet A. Bacterial adherence to vascular prostheses. J Vasc Surg 1986; 3:732–740.
396. Keller J, Falk J, Bjornson H. Bacterial infectability of chemically implanted endothelial cell-seeded expanded polytetrafluoroethylene vascular grafts. J Vasc Surg 1988; 7(4):524.
397. Birinyi L, Douville E, Lewis S. Increased resistance to bacteremic graft infection after endothelial cell-seeding. J Vasc Surg 1987; 5(1):193–197.
398. Bunt T. Synthetic vascular graft infections. I. graft infections. Surgery 1983; 93:733–746.
399. Goldstone J, Effeney D. Prevention of arterial graft infections. In V Bernhard, J Towne, eds. Complications in Vascular Surgery. 2nd ed. New York: Grune & Stratton, 1985. Pp. 487–498.
400. O'Donnell T, Jr, Nitzberg R. Vascular graft infections. In SL Mandell et al., eds. Infectious Diseases. Philadelphia: Harcourt Brace Jovanovich, Inc., 1992. Pp. 557–565.
401. Trout H, Kozloff L, Giordano J. Priority of revascularization in patients with graft enteric fistulas, infected arteries, or infected arterial prostheses. Ann Surg 1984; 199:669–683.
402. Calligaro K, Veith F, Gupta S. A modified method for management of prosthetic grafts involving an anastomosis to the common femoral artery. J Vasc Surg 1990; 11:485–492.
403. Liekweg W, Greenfield L. Vascular prosthetic infections: collected experience and results of treatment. Surgery 1977; 81:335–342.
404. Bandyk D, Berni G, Thiele B. Aortofemoral graft infection due to *Staphylococcus epidermidis*. Arch Surg 1984; 119:102–108.
405. Brook I. Role of anaerobic bacteria in aortofemoral graft infection. Surgery 1988; 104(5):843.
406. Johnson K, et al. Diagnosis of synthetic vascular graft infection: comparison of CT and gallium scans. American Journal of Radiology 1990; 154:405–409.
407. O'Hara P, Borkowski G, Hertzer N. Natural history of periprosthetic air on computerized axial tomographic examina-

tion of the abdomen following abdominal aortic aneurysm repair. J Vasc Surg 1984; 1:429–433.
408. Quarfordt P, Reilly L, Mark A. Computerized tomographic assessment of graft incorporation after aortic reconstruction. Am J Surg 1985; 150:227–231.
409. Chung C, et al. Indium-111-labeled leukocyte scan in detection of synthetic vascular graft infection: the effect of antibiotic treatment. J Nucl Med 1991; 32:13–15.
410. LaMuraglia G. Chronic prosthetic vascular graft infection visualization with gallium-67. J Nucl Med 1991; 32(7):1427–1428.
411. Brunner M, Mitchell R, Baldwin J. Prosthetic graft infection: limitations of indium white blood cell scanning. J Vasc Surg 1986; 3:42–48.
412. Williamson M, et al. 111-In labeled leukocytes in the detection of prosthetic vascular graft infections. AJR 1986; 147:173.
413. Sedwitz M, et al. Indium 111-labeled white blood cell (WBC) scans after vascular prosthetic reconstruction. J Vasc Surg 1987; 6(5):476.
414. Chung C, et al. Uptake of In-111 labeled leukocytes by lymphocele. A cause of false-positive vascular graft infection. Clin Nucl Med 1992; 17(5):368–370.
415. Reilly L, Goldstone J. The infected aortic graft. In J Bergan, J Yao, eds. Reoperative Arterial Surgery. Orlando: Grune & Stratton, 1986. Pp. 231–253.
416. Reilly L, Stoney R, Goldstone J. Improved management of aortic graft infection: the influence of operation sequence and staging. J Vasc Surg 1987; 5:421–431.
417. Kwaan J, Connolly J. Successful management of prosthetic graft infection with continuous povidone-iodine irrigation. Arch Surg 1981; 116:716.
418. Greco R, Harvey R, Henry R. Prevention of graft infection by antibiotic bonding. Surg Forum 1980; 31:29.
419. Pitt H, Postier R, MacGowan W. Prophylactic antibiotics in vascular surgery: topical, systemic, or both. Ann Surg 1980; 192:356–364.
420. Kaiser A, Clayson K, Mulherin J. Antibiotic prophylaxis in vascular surgery. Ann Surg 1978; 188:283–289.
421. Moore W, Rosson C, Hall A. Effect of prophylactic antibiotics in preventing bacteremic infection of vascular prostheses. Surgery 1971; 69:825–828.
422. Greco R, Harvey R. The biochemical bonding of cefoxitin to a microporous polytetrafluoroethylene surface. J Surg Res 1984; 36:237–243.
423. Prahlad A, Harvey R, Greco R. Diffusion of antibiotics from a polytetrafluoroethylene-benzalkonium surface. Am Surg 1981; 47:516–518.
424. Rubin J, Malone J, Goldstone J. The role of the lymphatic system in acute arterial prosthetic graft infections. J Vasc Surg 1985; 2:92.
425. Scheld W, Sande M. Endocarditis and intravascular infections. In G Mandell, R Douglas, J Bennett, eds. Principles and Practice of Infectious Diseases. New York: Churchill-Livingstone, 1990. Pp. 670–706.
426. Pruitt B, McManus W, Kim S. Diagnosis and treatment of cannula related intravenous sepsis in burn patients. Arch Surg 1980; 191:546.
427. Pruitt B, Stein J, Foley F. Intravenous therapy in burn patients. Suppurative thrombophlebitis and other life-threatening complications. Arch Surg 1970; 100:399.
428. Stein J, Pruitt B. Suppurative thrombophlebitis: a lethal iatrogenic disease. N Engl J Med 1970; 282:1452.
429. O'Neill J, Pruitt B, Foley F. Suppurative thrombophlebitis—a lethal complication of intravenous therapy. J Trauma 1968; 8:256.
430. Sacks-Berg A, Strampfer M, Cunha B. Suppurative thrombophlebitis caused by intravenous line sepsis. Heart Lung 1987; 16:318–320.
431. Garrison R, Richardson J, Fry DE. Catheter-associated septic thrombophlebitis. South Med J 1982; 75:917.
432. Baker C, Peterson S, Sheldon G. Septic phlebitis: a neglected disease. Am J Surg 1979; 138:97–103.
433. Missavage A, McManus W, Pruitt B Jr. Suppurative thrombophlebitis. In C Ernst, J Stanley, eds. Current Therapy and Vascular Surgery. Philadelphia: BC Decker, 1987. Pp. 450–453.
434. Pruitt B Jr, McManus W, Kim S. Burns. In S Gorbach, J Bartlett, N Blacklow, eds. Infectious Diseases. Philadelphia: Saunders, 1992. P. 786.
435. Berkowitz F, Argent A, Baise T. Suppurative thrombophlebitis: a serious nosocomial infection. Pediatr Infect Dis 1987; 6:64–67.
436. Walsh T, Bustamente C, Vlahov D. Candidal suppurative peripheral thrombophlebitis: recognition, prevention, and management. Infect Control 1986; 7:16–22.
437. Torres-Rojas J, Stratton C, Sanders C. Candidal suppurative peripheral thrombophlebitis. Ann Intern Med 1982; 96:431.
438. Slagle D, Gates R. Unusual case of central vein thrombosis and sepsis. Am J Med 1986; 81:351–354.
439. Kaufman J, Demas C, Stark K. Catheter-related septic central venous thrombosis-current therapeutic options. West J Med 1986; 145:200–203.
440. Verghese A, Wildrich W, Arbeit R. Central venous septic thrombophlebitis—the role of medical therapy. Medicine 1985; 64:394–400.
441. Lisse J, Thurmond-Anderle M, Davis C. Deep venous thrombosis in intravenous cocaine abuse mimicking septic arthritis of the shoulder. South Med J 1991; 84(2):278–279.
442. Josey W, Cook C. Septic pelvic thrombophlebitis. Report of 17 patients treated with heparin. Obstet Gynecol 1970; 35:891.
443. de Marie S, et al. Suppurative thrombophlebitis of the superior vena cava. Scand J Infect Dis 1989; 21:107–111.
444. Maki D, Weise C, Sarafin H. A semiquantitative culture method for identifying intravenous-catheter related infection. N Engl J Med 1977; 296:1305.
445. Ang A, Brown O. Septic deep vein thrombosis. Journal of Vascular Surgery 1986; 4:563–566.
446. Topiel M, Bryan R, Kessler C. Treatment of silastic catheter-induced central vein septic thrombophlebitis. Am J Med Sci 1986; 291:425–428.
447. Strinden W, Helgerson R, Maki D. *Candida* septic thrombosis of the great central veins associated with central catheters. Ann Surg 1985; 202:653–658.
448. Collins C. Suppurative pelvic thrombophlebitis. A study of 202 cases in which the disease was treated by ligation of the vena cava and ovarian vein. Am J Obstet Gynecol 1970; 108:681–687.
449. Collins C, MacCallum E, Nelson E. Suppurative pelvic thrombophlebitis. I. Incidence, pathology, and etiology. Surgery 1951; 30:298.
450. Josey W, Staggers S. Heparin therapy in septic pelvic thrombophlebitis: a study of 46 cases. Am J Obstet Gynecol 1974; 120:228.
451. Angel J, Knuppel R. Computed tomography in diagnosis of puerperal ovarian vein thrombosis. Obstet Gynecol 1984; 63:61–64.
452. Isada N, Landy H, Larson J. Postabortal septic pelvic thrombophlebitis diagnosed with computed tomography. J Reprod Med 1987; 32:866–868.
453. Martin B, Molopulos G, Bryan P. MRI of puerperal ovarian vein thrombosis. AJR 1986; 147:291–292.

Lymphedema

John P. Cooke
Thom W. Rooke

When lymphatic flow from the extremities is impeded, interstitial fluid accumulates and the extremity becomes swollen. Depending on the chronicity of the condition, variable degrees of subcutaneous fibrosis and hypertrophy may occur. This disorder of the lymphatic circulation is known as lymphedema. Large gaps in our understanding of this entity have limited treatment, but recent advances in imaging and therapeutic modalities, as well as insights gained from physiologic studies, hold promise of more definitive therapy.

Anatomy of the Lymphatic Circulation

Recognition and understanding of the lymphatic system came relatively late to the medical and scientific communities. Although a number of early anatomists and physicians made oblique references to various aspects of the lymphatic circulation, it was not until the seventeenth century that Gasparo Aselli recognized the lymphatics as a distinct anatomic entity [1]. The gifted professor of anatomy and surgery from Milan was frequently asked by friends and colleagues to perform his elegant vivisections, and on July 23, 1622, he intended to demonstrate to them the action and innervation of the canine diaphragm.

> While I was attempting this, and for that purpose had opened the abdomen and was pulling down with my hand the intestines and stomach . . . I suddenly beheld a great number of cords, as it were, exceedingly thin and beautifully white, scattered over the whole of the mesentery and the intestine, and starting from almost innumerable beginnings. . . . I noticed that the nerves belonging to the intestine were distinct from these cords, and wholly unlike them, and besides, were distributed quite separately from them. Wherefore struck by the novelty of the thing, I stood for some time silent. . . . When I gathered my wits together for the sake of the experiment, having laid hold of a very sharp scalpel, I pricked one of these cords and indeed one of the largest of them. I had hardly touched it, when I saw a white liquid like milk or cream forthwith gush out. Seeing this, I could hardly restrain my delight. [1]

The chylous return from the intestine of the recently fed animal allowed Aselli to recognize the lymphatics; when he repeated the demonstration several days later, no vessels were to be seen. Aselli eventually realized the relation between feedings and the visibility of the mesenteric lymphatics and duplicated the work in several species (Fig. 49-1). Over the following half century, Aselli's work was extended by Pecquet, Bartholinus, and Rudbeck, who defined the gross anatomy of the lymphatic system in toto [1]. By the eighteenth century, smaller lymphatic channels were visualized by Anton Nuck using mercury injections. Using those techniques, Sappey observed and recorded the human lymphatic system in exquisite detail (Fig. 49-2). Even greater resolution of the anatomy was provided by von Recklinghausen in 1862 with his discovery that the lymphatic endothelium stained darkly with silver nitrate. Using that technique, von Recklinghausen differentiated the lymphatic capillaries from the blood vessel capillaries.

We now know that lymphatic capillaries are blind-ended tubes formed by a single layer of endothelial cells. Endothelial cells from lymphatic capillaries closely resemble those of blood vessels and have a common embryonic origin [2]. Like vascular endothelium, lymphatic endothelial cells in culture form confluent "cobblestone" monolayers, which "sprout" to form tubules and which demonstrate identical histologic markers (von Willebrand factor, F-actin, fibronectin, and Weibel-Palade bodies). Unlike systemic capillaries, the basement membrane of lymphatic capillaries is absent or widely fenestrated, allowing greater access to interstitial proteins and particles.

The capillaries join to form larger vessels (100–200 μ), which are invested with smooth muscle and capable of vasomotion. Those vessels in turn merge to form larger conduits composed of three distinct layers: intima, media, and adventitia. Those conduits possess intraluminal valves that are usually tricuspid, are located a few millimeters to centimeters apart, and ensure that the flow of interstitial fluid (now called lymph) is directed centrally [3,4].

In the lower limbs, the larger conduits form a system of lymphatic return that is divided into superficial and deep components. The superficial component comprises medial and lateral channels, the medial channel originating on the dorsum of the foot and along the course of the saphenous vein, the lateral channel beginning on the lateral aspect of the foot and ascending to the midleg, where the tributaries cross anteriorly to the medial side to follow the course of the medial lymphatics up to the inguinal nodes. Deep lymphatics do not usually communicate with the superficial system except through the popliteal and inguinal lymph nodes. Those vessels originate subcutaneously, follow the course of the deep blood vessels, and eventually pass through the inguinal nodes.

Small and medium-sized lymphatic vessels empty into main channels, of which the thoracic duct is the largest. That vessel, roughly 2 mm wide and 45 cm long, ascends from the abdomen through the lower chest just to the right of and anterior to the vertebral column. At approximately the level of the fifth thoracic vertebra, it crosses to the left of the spine, where it continues to ascend through the superior mediastinum to the base of the neck and eventually empties into the left brachiocephalic vein. Other large right- and left-sided lymphatic ducts may exist, although their arrangement, size, and course are highly variable. Those vessels join with the main thoracic duct or empty directly into great veins; they provide im-

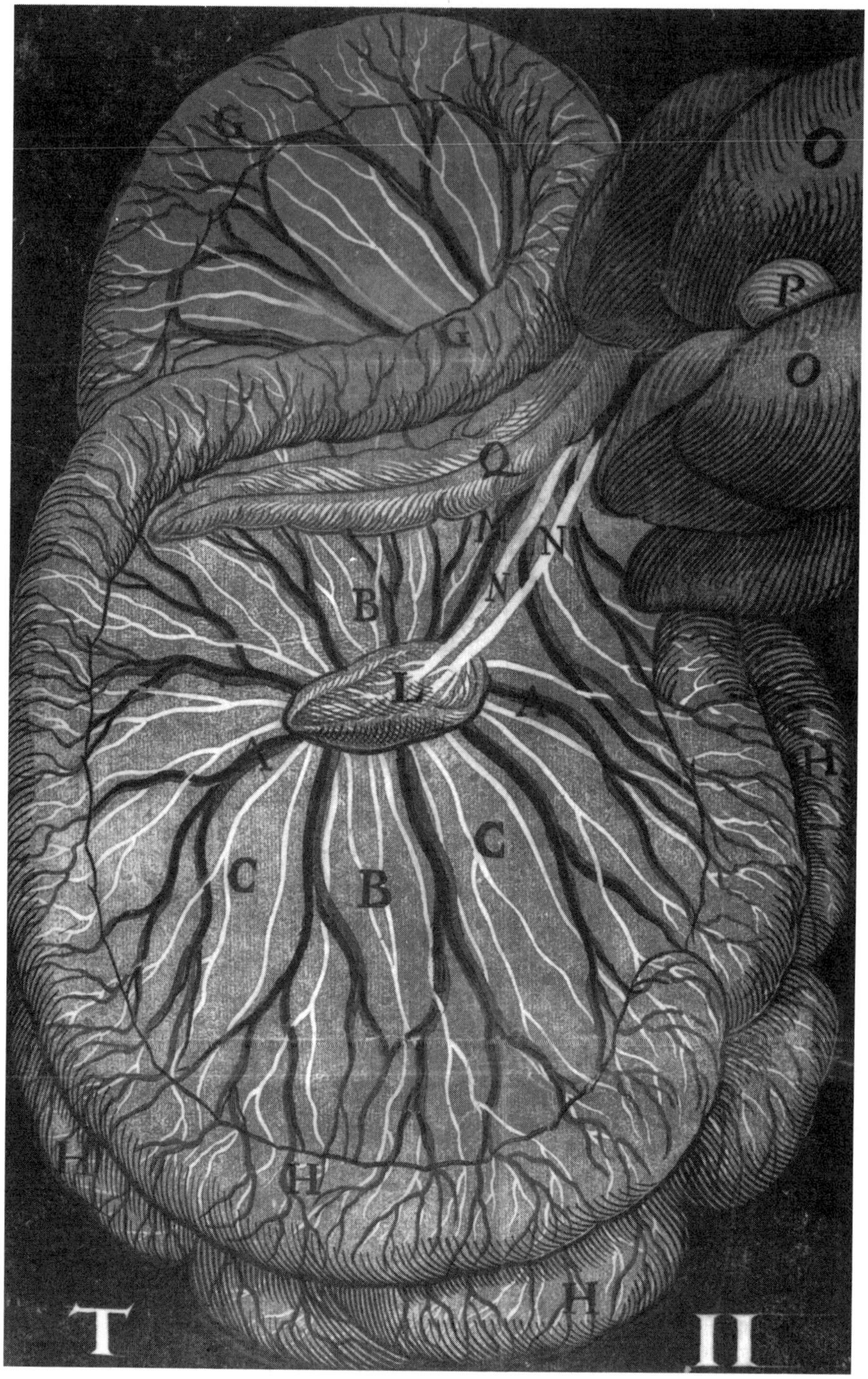

Fig. 49-1. Photograph of a woodcut from the monograph *De Lactibus Sive Lacteis Venis . . .* , by Gasparo Aselli. The book details Aselli's discovery of the mesenteric lymphatics and contains the first representation of them. (Courtesy of Mr. Richard Wolfe, Rare Books Section, Francis A. Countway Library of Medicine, Harvard University.)

portant collateral conduits should the thoracic duct become obstructed.

Physiology of the Lymphatic Circulation

In 1786, William Hunter and two of his pupils, William Cruikshank and William Hewson, published the results of their work, laying a foundation for the physiology of the lymphatic system [1]. They correctly inferred from clinical observation that the lymphatics were involved in the response to infection as well as in the absorption of interstitial fluid. A century later, their theories received experimental support from the physiologic studies of Karl

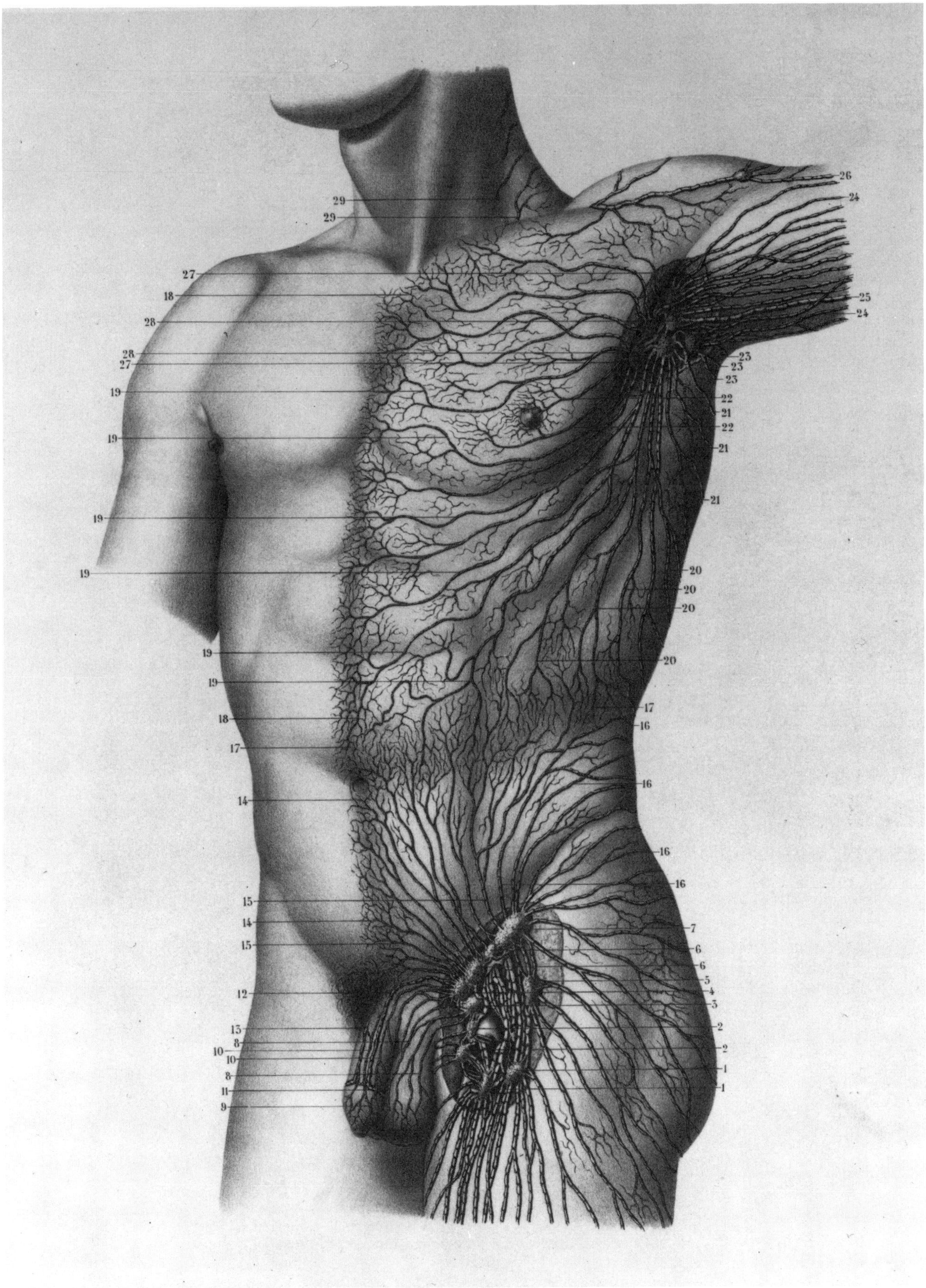

Fig. 49-2. From the text *Anatomie, Physiologie, Pathologie des Vaisseaux Lymphatiques,* by PC Sappey (1874). His detailed drawings of the lymphatic system remain unequalled today; he also contributed a description of the lymphatic valves. (Courtesy of Mr. Richard Wolfe, Rare Books Section, Francis A. Countway Library of Medicine, Harvard University.)

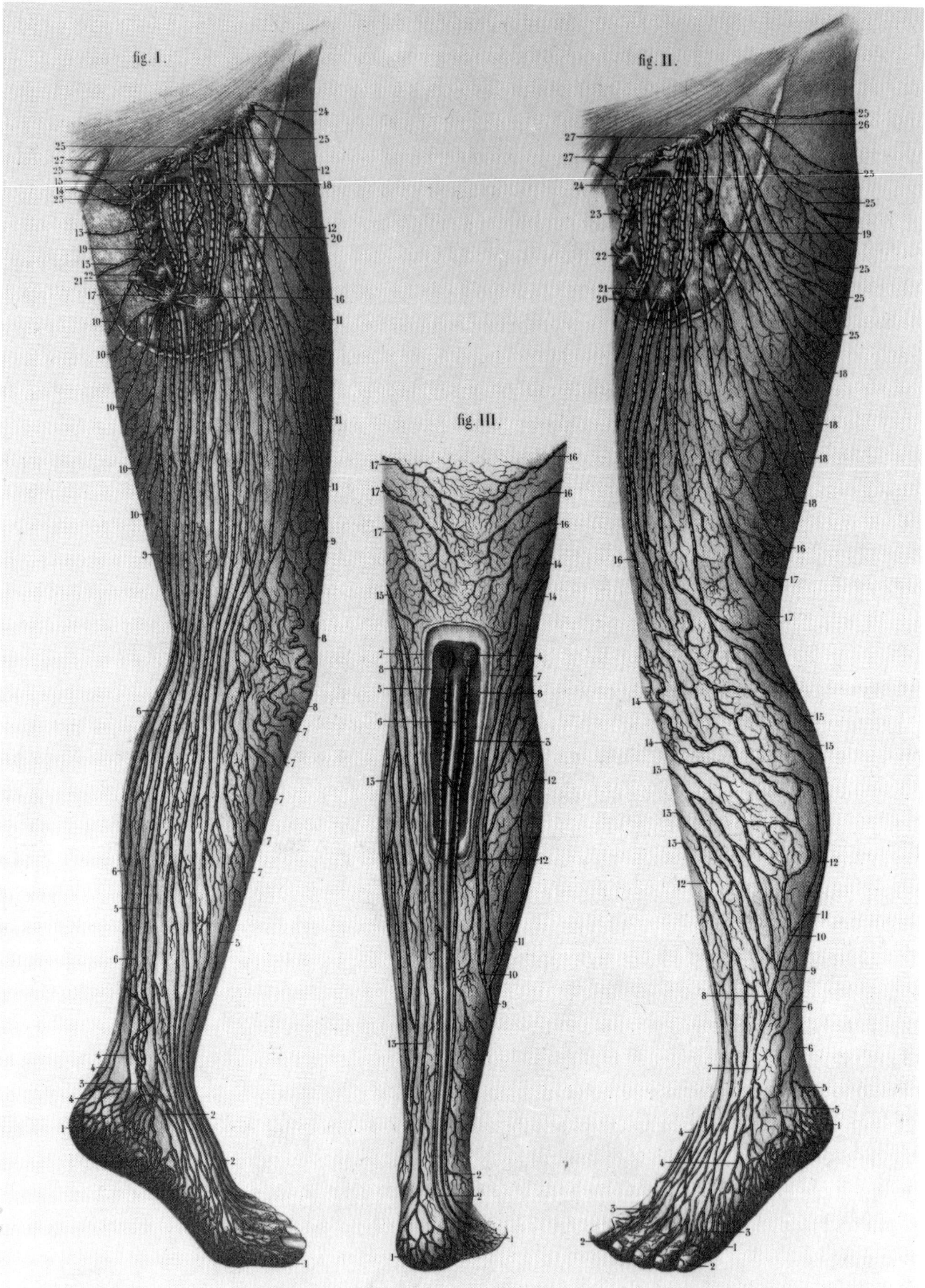

Fig. 49-2 (continued)

Ludwig and Ernest Starling. Ludwig cannulated lymph vessels, collected and analyzed the lymph, and proposed that it was a filtrate of plasma. Starling elucidated the forces governing fluid transfer from the blood capillaries to the interstitial space and offered evidence that the same forces apply to the lymphatic capillaries. He proposed that an imbalance in those forces could give rise to edema formation [5]:

> In health, therefore, the two processes of lymph-production and absorption are exactly proportional. Dropsy depends on a loss of balance between these two processes—on an excess of lymph-production over lymph-absorption. A scientific investigation of the causation of dropsy will therefore involve, in the first place, an examination of the factors which determine the extent of these two processes and, so far as is possible, the manner in which these processes are carried out.

As first enunciated by Starling, interstitial fluid is largely an ultrafiltrate of blood. Its rate of production reflects the balance between factors that favor filtration out of capillaries (capillary hydrostatic pressure and tissue oncotic pressure) and those that favor reabsorption (interstitial hydrostatic pressure and capillary oncotic pressure) [6]. Under normal conditions, filtration exceeds reabsorption at a rate sufficient to create 2 to 4 liters of interstitial fluid per day. There is a net filtration of protein (primarily albumin) from the vasculature into the interstitium; approximately 100 g of circulating protein may escape into the interstitial space daily [3]. The interstitial fluid also receives the waste products of cellular metabolism, as well as foreign matter or microbes that enter through breaks in the skin or by hematogenous routes.

The volume and the composition of the interstitial fluid are kept in balance by the lymphatic system. The functions of that system include (1) transport of excess fluid, protein, and waste products from the interstitial space to the blood stream; (2) distribution of immune cells and substances from the lymphoid tissues to the systemic circulation; and (3) filtration and removal of foreign material from the interstitial fluid.

Several forces drive fluid through the lymphatic system. The lymphatic vessels in skeletal muscle are compressed by extrinsic muscular contractions that propel the fluid centrally through the unidirectional valves. In other tissues, such as the splanchnic and cutaneous systems, it is primarily contractions of lymphatic smooth muscle that generate the driving force [7,8]. These contractions are increased in frequency and amplitude by elevated filling pressure, sympathetic nerve activity, and shock, and they may be modulated by circulating hormones and prostanoids [9–13]. Considerable force can be generated by those contractions; experimentally induced obstruction of the popliteal lymphatic system augments the strength and frequency of contraction, generating pressures of up to 50 mm Hg [14]. Other factors that may contribute to lymphatic flow include intermittent compression from arterial pulsations and gastrointestinal peristalsis. Once lymph enters the thorax, negative intrathoracic pressure generated during inspiration aspirates fluid into the thoracic duct (the "respiratory pump") [14].

Pathophysiology

PATHOGENESIS OF EDEMA

Edema develops when the production of interstitial fluid (lymph) exceeds its transport through the lymphatic system. Thus, an overproduction of lymph or a decreased ability to remove fluid from the interstitium may result in edema. Conditions associated with overproduction of lymph include elevated venous pressures, increased capillary permeability, and hypoproteinemia. Elevated hydrostatic pressure in the veins results in increased filtration of plasma from venules and blood capillaries (as seen in right-sided congestive heart failure, tricuspid regurgitation, and deep-vein thrombosis). Conversely, local inflammation increases capillary permeability, accelerating the loss of protein and fluid to the interstitium despite a normal capillary hydrostatic pressure. That causes lymph production to increase up to 10- to 20-fold, exceeding lymphatic transport and resulting in marked edema [15]. Hypoproteinemia also may lead to marked edema, in which case hydrostatic pressure and capillary permeability are normal, but capillary oncotic pressure is reduced, favoring osmotic flow to the interstitium. Although secondary to the accumulation of excess lymph, the edema seen with those conditions is not commonly referred to as lymphedema; the term lymphedema is reserved to describe edema that results from impaired removal of lymph from the interstitium.

PATHOGENESIS OF LYMPHEDEMA

Lymphedema occurs whenever lymphatic vessels are absent, underdeveloped, or obstructed. Impedance to lymphatic flow may be due to an inborn defect (primary lymphedema) or an acquired loss of lymphatic patency (secondary lymphedema).

Primary Lymphedema. Primary lymphedema occurs in approximately 1 in 10,000 persons less than 20 years of age, with females being affected more frequently than males [16]. It can be divided into three clinical subtypes:

1. Congenital lymphedema, which appears at or near birth
2. Lymphedema that has its onset around the time of puberty, also known as lymphedema praecox, a term used by Allen in 1934 [17]
3. Lymphedema that begins after the age of 35, also known as lymphedema tarda

In a minority of cases, there is a family history of lymphedema; the term **Milroy's disease** is applied to the congenital form and **Meige's disease** to the praecox form [18].* These disorders most often are inherited in an autosomal

* In 1892, Milroy described "heredity edema" affecting 22 individuals of one family over six generations [19]. The condition he described was likely primary lymphedema and was present from birth in all but one of the affected family members. Sir William Osler first designated the entity Milroy's disease. In 1898, Henry Meige described a similar familial affliction first presenting at puberty; in France, that condition became known as Meige's disease. It is evident from Milroy's review in 1928 that he considered the congenital, praecox, and tarda forms of primary lymphedema as variants of the disease that bears his name, and it could be argued that all forms of familial lymphedema be termed Milroy's disease [20].

dominant manner with variable penetrance; autosomal or sex-linked recessive forms occur less commonly [21–23]. Primary lymphedema may be associated with Turner's syndrome, Noonan's syndrome, yellow nail syndrome, intestinal lymphangiectasia, lymphangiomyomatosis, and arteriovenous malformation [24–29]. The association of lymphedema with vascular anomalies belies the common anlage of the lymph and blood vessels [2].

Wolfe has classified primary lymphedema by its lymphographic appearance [21]. Lymphograms obtained in 372 patients with primary lymphedema revealed four patterns: (1) hypoplasia (or obstruction) of lymphatic vessels distal to the inguinal nodes; (2) obstruction of pelvic vessels, with or without obliteration of distal vessels; (3) hyperplasia of the lymphatic vessels; and (4) incompetent dilated lymphatic channels (megalymphatics).

Approximately one-third of all cases are secondary to agenesis, hypoplasia, or obstruction of the **distal** lymphatic vessels, with relatively normal proximal vessels [17,21]. In those cases, the swelling usually is bilateral and mild and affects females much more frequently than males. The prognosis in such cases is good. Generally, after the first year of symptoms, there is little extension in the same limb or to uninvolved extremities. Although the extent of involvement is established early in the disease in about 40 percent of patients, the girth of the limb continues to increase.

In over half of cases, the defect primarily involves obstruction of the **proximal** lymphatics or nodes, with initially uninvolved distal lymphatic vessels. Surgical biopsy of lymph nodes in this group typically shows an intranodal fibrotic process that cannot be attributed historically to cellulitis [18]. In those cases, the swelling tends to be unilateral and severe; there may be a slight predominance of females in this group [17,21]. In patients with proximal involvement, the extent and degree of the abnormality is more likely to progress and to require surgical intervention. Initially uninvolved distal lymphatic vessels may become obliterated with time.

A minority of patients have a pattern of bilateral hyperplasia of the lymphatic channels or tortuous dilated megalymphatics. In those less common forms of primary lymphedema, there is a slight male predominance. Megalymphatics are associated with a greater extent of involvement and a worse prognosis.

Secondary Lymphedema. Secondary lymphedema is an acquired condition resulting from loss or obstruction of previously normal lymphatic channels. A wide variety of pathologic processes may lead to such lymphatic obliteration.

1. **Infection.** Recurrent episodes of bacterial lymphangitis lead to thrombosis and fibrosis of the lymphatic channels and are one of the most common causes of lymphedema [30]. The responsible bacteria are almost always streptococci, which tend to enter through breaks in the skin or fissures induced by trichophytosis. Recurrent bacterial lymphangitis is also a frequent complicating factor of lymphedema from any cause.
2. **Tumor.** Malignancies are another common cause of secondary lymphedema. Tumor cells may obstruct lymphatic vessels, inducing lymphedema directly or predisposing the patient to bacterial lymphangitis. In males, the most common neoplastic etiology is prostate cancer; in females it is lymphoma [4]. Therapy directed against the tumor also may be pathogenetic. Radical mastectomy for breast carcinoma (in which axillary or chest-wall nodes are resected and lymphatics disrupted) and radiation therapy are capable of producing arm and chest swelling. Although it is unclear whether lymphedema is more likely to be caused by surgery or radiation therapy, it is evident that those treated with both modalities are especially susceptible [31,32]. The incidence of postsurgical lymphedema has declined, however, as modified procedures have replaced the radical mastectomy.
3. **Filariasis.** Worldwide, filarial disease is the most frequent etiology for secondary lymphedema. The World Health Organization estimates that 90 million people may be affected by filarial infections; in India alone, there are up to 14 million symptomatic cases [33,34]. Common tropical filaria include *Wuchereria bancrofti* and *Brugia malayi* or *timori* [35,36]. Other *Brugia* species are found in North America and occasionally cause lymphatic obstruction [37–39].

   The microfilaria are transmitted by a mosquito vector and induce recurrent lymphangitis and eventual fibrosis of lymph nodes [40]. It is unclear whether filaria themselves produce the lymphangitis or simply predispose those afflicted to recurrent episodes of bacterial lymphangitis. The filaria also can be identified in blood specimens of tissue obtained by fine-needle biopsy of the affected areas, and eosinophilia is a common local and systemic feature [38]. Diethylcarbamazine remains the most popular drug for treating filariasis, although side effects are frequent [36,41]. Ivermectin is a new antifilarial agent that may replace diethylcarbamazine; it is less toxic, and a single oral dose (25 $\mu g/kg$) appears to be as efficacious as a 2-week course of diethylcarbamazine [42].
4. **Other Causes.** Other conditions leading to or associated with obstruction of lymphatic channels include trauma, tuberculosis, contact dermatitis, rheumatoid arthritis, and pregnancy [29,43–45]. Autoimmune destruction of the lymphatics remains an interesting but unproven etiology [46]. Factitious lymphedema (oedema bleu) also occurs; that condition usually affects the hand or arm or both, is unilateral, and is induced by applications of tourniquets, self-inflicted cellulitis, or maintenance of the limb in an immobile and dependent state [47]. Chronic subcutaneous injections of drugs (most notably, pentazocine hydrochloride, or Talwin) also may lead to lymphatic sclerosis and obstruction.

PATHOLOGY OF LYMPHEDEMA

In chronic lymphedema, the skin is rough and thickened, having the texture of pigskin with little pitting edema. On cut section of the gross specimen, the dermis is firm and gray, as is the deep fascia [48]. The intervening subcutaneous fat is abundant and septated by prominent fibrous strands. In some specimens, compression causes lymph to

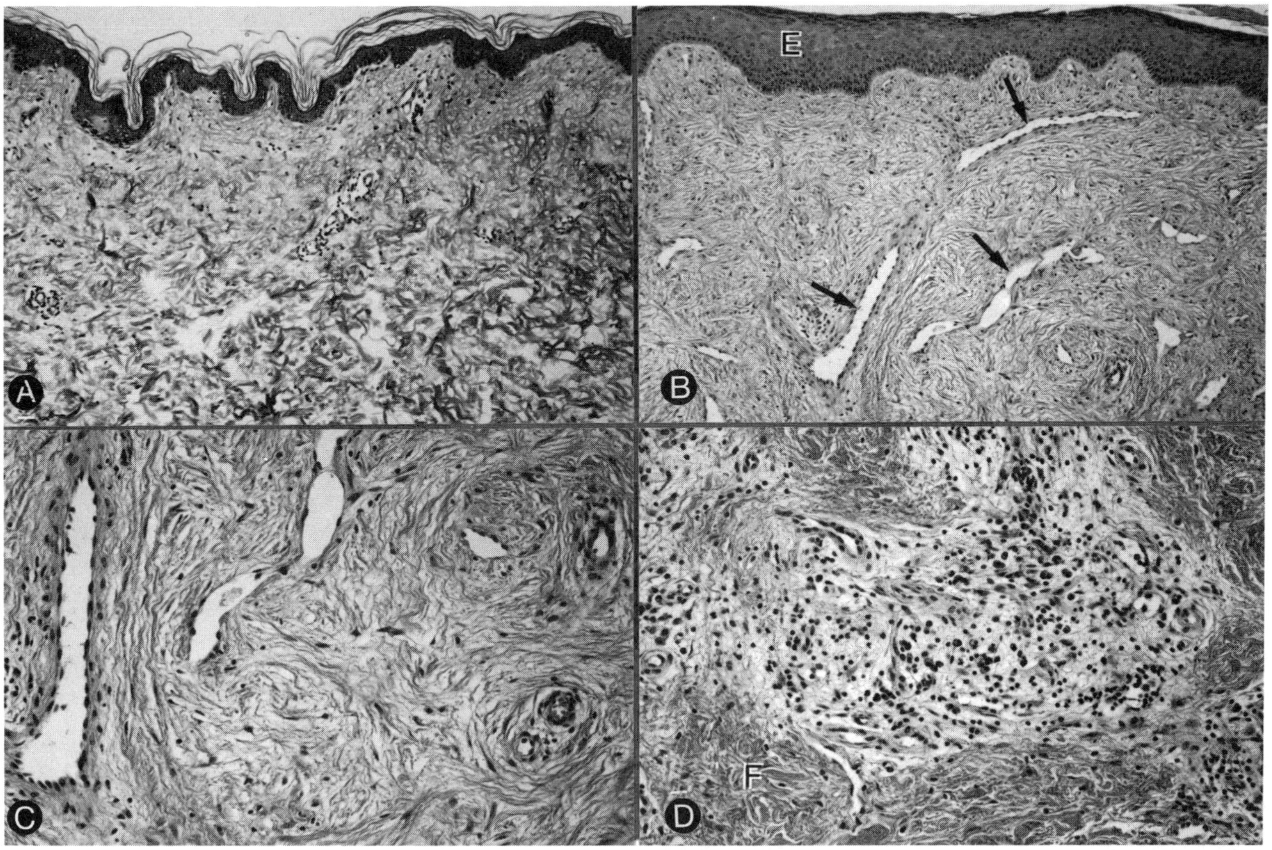

Fig. 49-3. Photomicrograph of skin biopsies. **A.** Normal skin, for comparison. **B–D.** Lymphedematous skin from the lower extremity of a 41-year-old man with the congenital disorder. **B.** Epidermis (E) is thickened, and dermal lymphatics (arrows) are dilated. **C.** Dilated dermal lymphatics. **D.** Dermal fibrosis (F) and chronic perivascular inflammation. (Hematoxylin and eosin stain; **(A)** and **(B)** × 90; **(C)** and **(D)** × 180.) (Courtesy of William D. Edwards, M.D., Division of Pathology, Mayo Clinic.)

exude from the dermis and subcutaneous tissue, although that is not a prominent feature. Microscopic examination reveals epidermal atrophy with prominent dermal fibrosis as well as variable degrees of dermal edema [48] (Fig. 49-3). Abundant subcutaneous fat with prominent fibrous septa is apparent in all cases. Often, perivascular inflammatory cells (lymphocytes, plasma cells, and occasionally eosinophils) can be seen. The lymphatic vessels often are difficult to visualize and may be obliterated or thrombosed by previous inflammatory episodes or may be congenitally absent or hypoplastic. In a small percentage of cases, dilatation of the lymphatics (lymphangiectasia) may be seen.

CLINICAL PRESENTATION

Clinical signs and symptoms of lymphedema depend on the duration and the severity of the disease. Initially, there is a simple volume and protein overload of the interstitial space, and the swelling produced by that fluid collection typically is soft, pits easily with pressure ("pitting edema"), and may decrease or disappear with elevation of the limb. In the lower extremities, the edema may extend to the very end of the feet, resulting in the typical "square toes" seen in this condition. Over a period of years, the limb may take on a woody texture as the surrounding tissue becomes indurated and fibrotic (Fig. 49-4). At that stage, pitting edema is no longer a major component, and limb elevation or external compression is much less successful at reducing the girth of the extremity. Proliferation of subcutaneous connective and adipose tissue leads to thickening of the skin and loss of flexibility; the affected limb is grossly enlarged, and a mossy or cobblestone skin texture may develop.

The hypertrophied limb with thickened skin seen in **chronic** lymphedema has little similarity to the edematous limb of deep venous insufficiency. In the latter case, a soft pitting edema is prominent and seen in association with stasis dermatitis, hemosiderin deposition, and superficial venous varicosities. The history and examination easily differentiate chronic lymphedema from venous disorders and other causes of limb swelling (see Fig. 49-4). Earlier in the presentation, however, it may be more difficult to distinguish lymphedema from venous disease, reflex sympathetic dystrophy, or other causes of limb swelling.

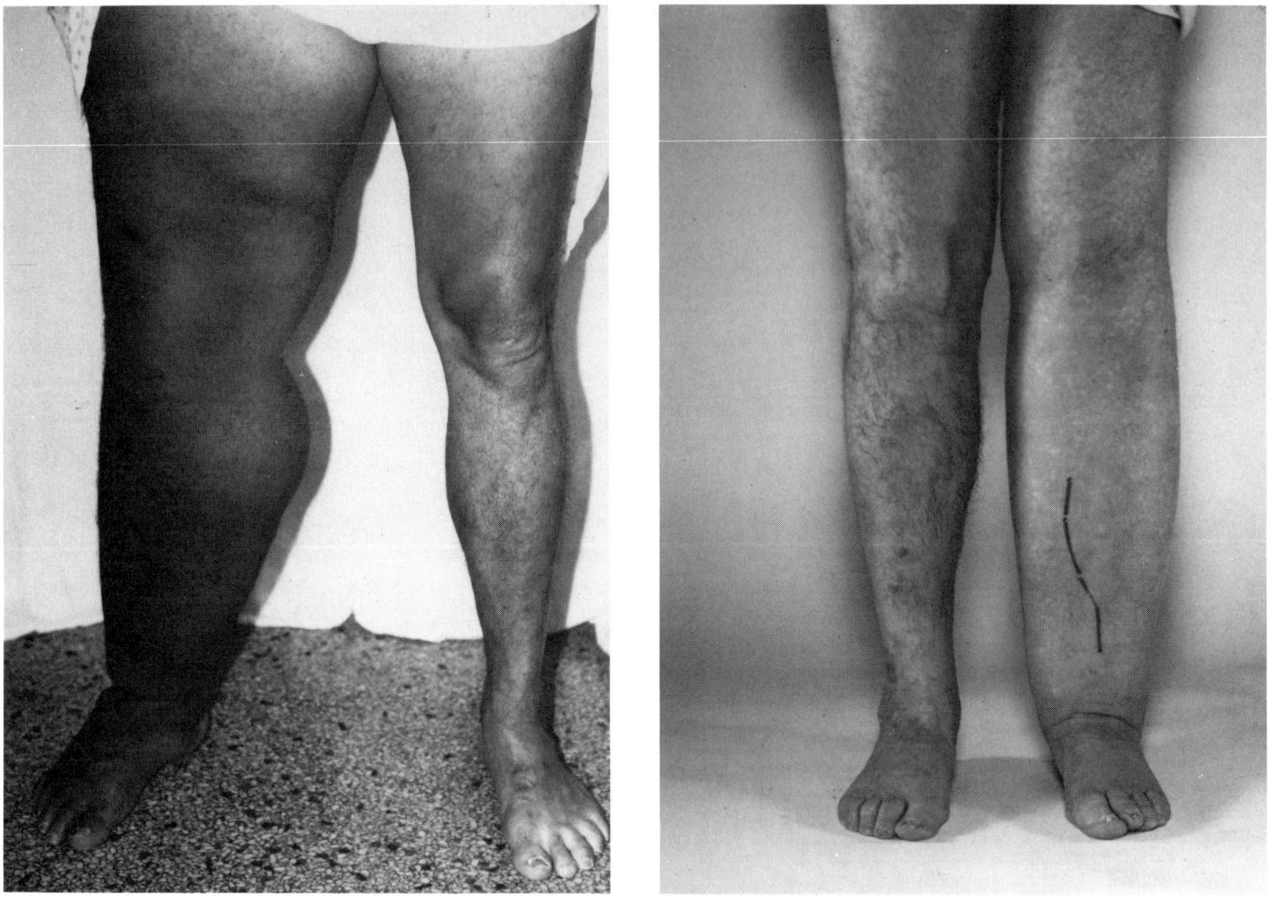

Fig. 49-4. Photographs of two cases of severe, unilateral lymphedema affecting the lower extremity. (Courtesy of Peter Gloviczki, M.D., Division of Vascular Surgery, Mayo Clinic.)

In such cases, studies of the lymphatic system may be necessary to confirm obstructive disease.

Diagnostic Modalities

It is sometimes necessary to obtain more information about the nature and degree of lymphatic involvement when (1) the etiology of a swollen limb remains uncertain, (2) the diagnosis is evident but the etiology is unclear, or (3) a surgical drainage procedure is being considered.

LYMPHANGIOGRAPHY

The human lymphatics were first visualized in vivo by Hudack and McMaster at the Rockefeller Institute in 1933 [1]. They used each other as subjects to demonstrate superficial lymphatic plexuses along the forearm and inner thigh using subcutaneous injections of vital dyes. In 1948, Glenn cannulated a lymphatic vessel in the dog hind limb and injected contrast media to produce a lymphangiogram in the canine leg and groin. Subsequently, Servelle and Deysson visualized the lymphatics in patients with elephantiasis using retrograde injection. Visualization of the dilated lymph channels, however, depended on partial or complete valvular incompetence. Lymphangiography as it is performed today was developed by Kinmonth and co-workers in 1952 [49]. The technique involves identification of a distal vessel made visible by an intradermal injection of a vital dye into the metatarsal web spaces. The vessel is isolated and cannulated, and iodinated contrast material is injected. Following the injection, the contrast material is visualized radiographically as it progresses proximally through lymphatic channels (Fig. 49-5).

There are several drawbacks to the procedure, including frequent requirements for cut-downs in the edematous limb, microsurgical techniques to achieve direct cannulation, and occasionally a need for general anesthesia [17]. More important, the irritation caused by the contrast agent results in lymphangitis in one-third of the studies and potentially can worsen the lymphedema [50].

LYMPHOSCINTIGRAPHY

Lymphoscintigraphy involves the injection of technetium-containing colloids into the subcutaneous tissue of the distal aspect of the affected extremity (e.g., the dorsum of the foot). The progress of the radionuclide through the lymphatic system is followed by a radioscintigraphic camera. In primary lymphedema, channels are obliterated or absent; in 10 percent of cases, they are ectatic and

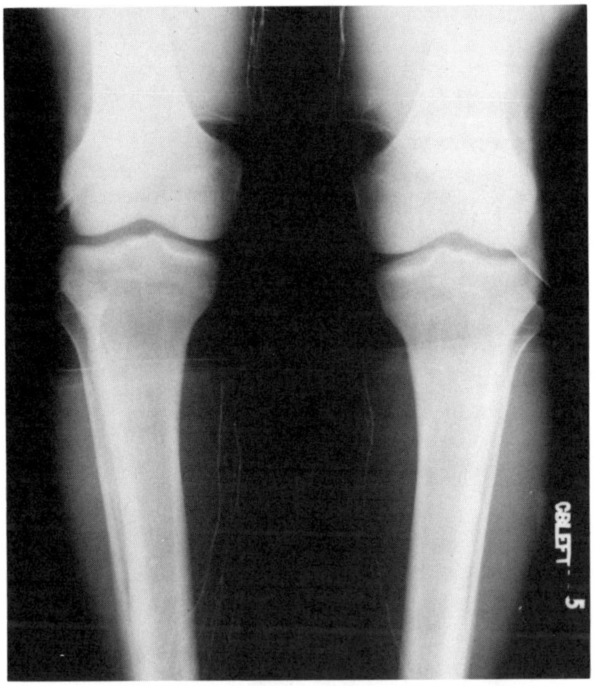

A

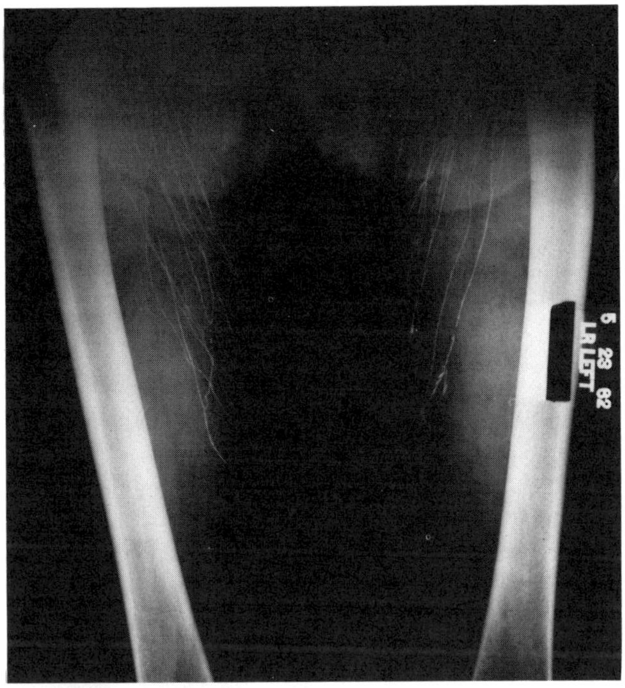

B

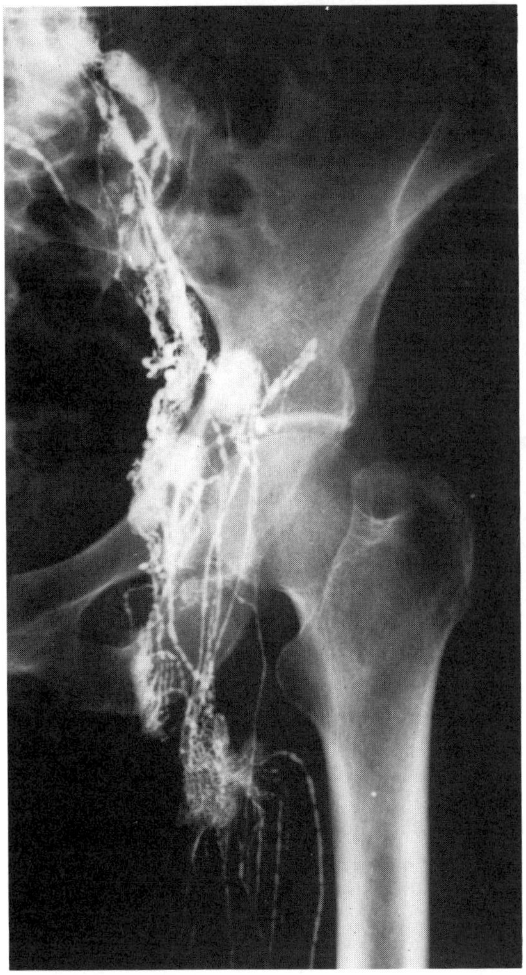

C

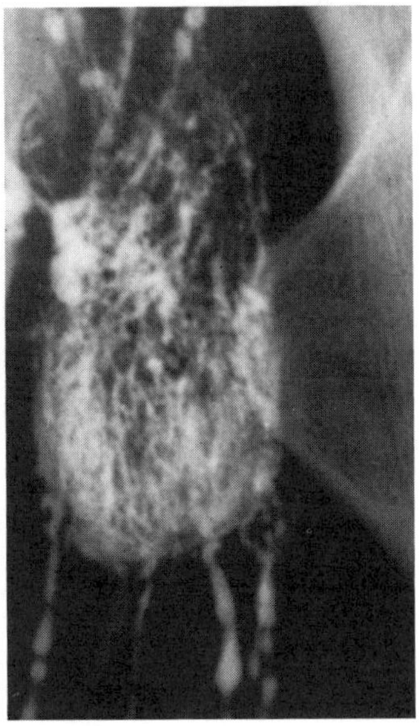

D

Fig. 49-5. **A–C.** Lymphangiograms showing normal leg and pelvic lymphatic vessels. **D.** Close-up view of a normal inguinal lymph node. Note the fine reticular network formed by the branching lymphatic vessels as they cross the node. (Courtesy of W. E. Miller, M.D.)

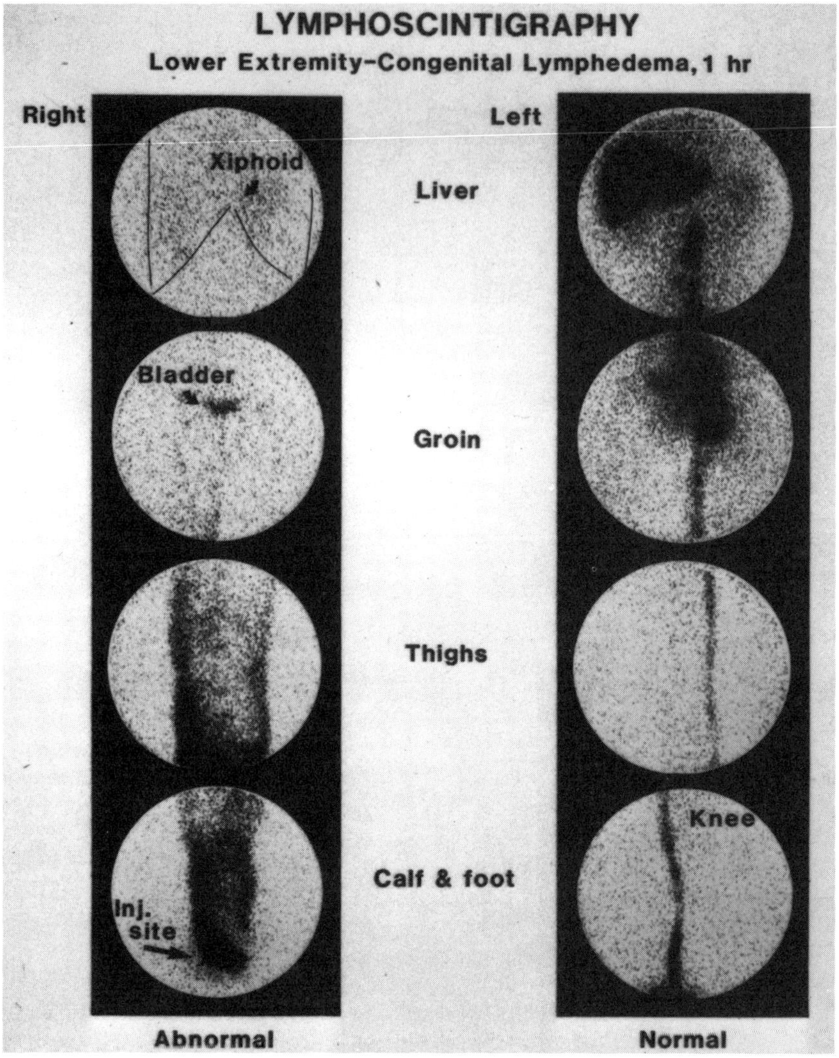

Fig. 49-6. Lymphoscintigram showing an abnormal radioisotope uptake pattern in the right leg of a patient with unilateral congenital lymphedema. One hour after injection into the dorsum of the foot, radioisotope has been taken up and distributed in a *dermal backflow pattern*, reflecting loss or obstruction of lymphatic vessels. In addition, the lymphedematous right limb demonstrates little transport of radiolabeled material into the thigh, pelvis, and abdomen during the hour following injection. In contrast, the lymphoscintigram of the normal left limb (performed the following day) shows lymphatic patency throughout the limb and more rapid transport of radiolabel. (Courtesy of H. Wahner, M.D.)

incompetent. In secondary lymphedema, the channels can be seen to be dilated, and the level of obstruction can be determined [51]. In lymphedema of any cause, the proximal progression of the radionuclide is delayed, and its accumulation distally in the dilated channels of the dermis is manifested as a "dermal backflow" pattern (Fig. 49-6). Lymphoscintigraphy is easier to perform than lymphangiography and is not reported to cause lymphangitis. Compared to lymphangiography, it may lack some spatial resolution; resolution is maximized by reducing the swelling of the extremity as much as possible prior to the study (reducing dilution of the radionuclide in stagnant lymph). Lymphoscintigraphy increasingly is replacing lymphangiography in practice.

COMPUTED TOMOGRAPHY

CT scans of a lymphedematous limb are characterized by a honeycomb pattern in the affected area [52]. CT cannot localize the level of obstruction or differentiate lymphedema that is surgically correctable from that which is not [53]. Its greatest usefulness is in determining the cause of secondary lymphedema (e.g., lymphoma, pelvic tumor).

Treatment

MEDICAL THERAPY

Successful treatment of lymphedema requires close collaboration between the patient and the physician. To that end, the physician should (1) carefully instruct the patient in the details of the medical program and (2) attend to the psychological impact of the disease. Associated emotional problems are not uncommon and are often neglected by physicians [18]. The need to address the psychological aspects of long-term disfigurement, especially with adolescent patients, cannot be overemphasized. In discussing these issues with the patient, the physician should be realistic about the possibility of progression but should emphasize the patient's ability to modulate the course of the disease by careful attention to the details of the medical program.

Without guidance from the physician, some patients become sedentary in response to uncomfortable or heavy sensations in the affected limb. Reduced physical activity at work and at home leads to apathy and malaise; that consequence can be averted by encouraging **physical activity** with proper support hose. Regular exercise appears to reduce lymphedema as long as elastic support (or hydrostatic pressure) is applied [54]. Swimming is a particularly good physical activity for these patients, because the hydrostatic pressure of the surrounding water negates the need for compressive support.

Elastic support hose should be fitted to the patient's limb after the edema in the extremity has been maximally reduced by compression and elevation [30,54]. This is an important detail. The stocking does not reduce the size of the leg but only maintains the circumference to which it is fitted. If the limb is fitted for a stocking while in a swollen state, it will be maintained by the stocking in a swollen state. To reduce the diameter of the extremity to a minimum may take several days of **elevation** and bandaging unless a pneumatic device is utilized. **Pneumatic devices** are available that intermittently compress the limb; techniques that employ sequential graduated compression (in which the cuffs are inflated sequentially from distal to proximal sites with a pressure gradient from the most distal cuff to the most proximal) are most effective [55,56]. The patient should be fitted for a compressive garment (to maintain pressures of approximately 40–50 mm Hg in the limb) and should be instructed to place the garment on the extremity when first arising in the morning. The garment needs to be replaced every 3 months because it loses elasticity over time. These compressive therapies are the mainstay of lymphedema treatment. By reducing the volume of edema fluid, recurrent infections can be avoided and progression of the disease reduced. A new form of compressive garment, the Reid sleeve, is under investigation at Stanford. The Reid sleeve is a foam-filled cylinder with velcro straps, which is generally worn at night. Preliminary studies have been encouraging, with reduction in limb edema of 30–40 percent.

Manual lymph drainage (MLD) is a method of massage promoted by some therapists as an adjunctive therapeutic modality. MLD differs from other massage therapies in that it focuses on subcutaneous tissue rather than muscle. It takes advantage of the fact that the lymphatic tributaries include not only the limb but also the quadrant in which the lymphatic plexus resides. For example, the tissue drained by the axillary lymph nodes includes the arm and the ipsilateral quadrant of the trunk. According to Foldi, the quadrants are separated by "lymphatic watersheds," over which bridging collateral vessels allow lymph to drain into adjacent quadrants. The first step in MLD treatment is to stimulate lymphokinesis in the normal lymphatics of the contralateral quadrant; that promotes drainage across the lymphatic watershed. The second step is to gently massage the edema fluid from the affected quadrant to the normal, contralateral quadrant. In some individuals, MLD therapy appears to be useful, is easily learned by the patient, and can supplement their therapeutic program.

Recurrent cellulitis and local infections pose a constant threat of exacerbation. **Skin hygiene** is essential. An emollient should be applied twice daily to prevent drying and fissuring of the skin. Trauma must be avoided (when ambulatory, the feet should be covered by slippers or shoes; a podiatrist should attend to nail care as needed). Fungal infections should be aggressively treated with topical **antifungal agents**. The patient should be instructed to take antibiotics at the earliest sign of cellulitis and should be given a prescription for a course of an oral semisynthetic penicillin or (for penicillin-sensitive patients) erythromycin. We occasionally have observed an indolent form of lymphangitis that is characterized by pitting edema refractory to the usual measures, slight tenderness to palpation of the affected limb, and hyperemia of the extremity in a dependent position. There may be a slight increase in the white blood cell count with a left shift, and a minor elevation of the erythrocyte sedimentation rate. After a course of antibiotics, the edema responds to compressive therapy, and the tenderness resolves. In those patients and in patients with lymphangitis refractory to the usual antibiotic regimen, we have observed good responses to azithromycin (10-day course), which is particularly effective in penetrating subcutaneous tissue.

An understanding of the mechanisms inducing the proliferation of subcutaneous connective tissue and lymphedema may lead to more definitive treatment. Agents might then be designed to alter the relationship between the deposition and lysis of collagen fibers such that lysis is favored, thereby reducing fibrosis [3,57]. Benzopyrones are a new class of agents that reduce the volume of edema in the affected limb, probably by stimulating tissue macrophages, which in turn increase interstitial proteolysis. That reduces the oncotic pressure of interstitial fluid, facilitating its reabsorption. A recent randomized, double-blind, placebo-controlled cross-over trial demonstrated that 5,6-benzopyrone (400 mg daily) effectively reduced limb girth and favorably affected skin texture and temperature [58]. An important question left unanswered by that study is whether that agent is additive in its effects to the usual compressive measures. The agent is not yet approved by the FDA for use in the United States. Another experimental therapy is intralymphatic injections of steroids, which may help by inhibiting the proliferation of connective tissue [59]. The development of angiogenic steroids that have some tissue specificity could make this a feasible approach.

Although it is not necessary to burden the patient about the possibility of **malignancy**, the patient should be alerted to report any changes in the appearance of the limb. Neoplastic transformation of the blood or lymph vessels can develop in long-standing lymphedema of any cause, including primary or secondary lymphedema [3,60–62]. Angiosarcomas or lymphangiosarcomas are potentially devastating but fortunately uncommon complications of long-standing lymphedema, occurring in fewer than 1 percent of cases [63,64]. Early detection and amputation can be life-saving, but recognition of the condition often is delayed by a lack of awareness on the part of the patient and the physician. Other malignancies, including lymphoma, Kaposi's sarcoma, squamous cell cancer, and malignant melanoma, have been reported in association with chronic lymphedema [65–68].

SURGICAL TREATMENT

When the limb becomes so grossly enlarged that function is significantly impaired, surgical reduction of the limb may be considered. When the lymphatic obstruction is of a proximal type and the lymphatic channels distal to the obstruction are of adequate diameter, a drainage procedure is occasionally feasible under certain well-defined circumstances. Surgery is not curative, but it can make the disorder more manageable by conservative measures [69].

Reduction procedures generally are reserved for limbs that have become so bulky or unsightly that they constitute a significant impairment to daily living. The procedure is a last resort, and itself results in a limb that is scarred and disfigured, albeit more mobile. The procedures involve resecting a portion of the skin and subcutaneous tissue and subsequent closure of the wound to reduce the limb diameter [17,70,71]. Overall, patient satisfaction with reduction surgery is good, and only 20 percent report poor outcomes from surgery [18,48]. Acute complications include wound infection or necrosis of the skin flaps; late complications include recurrent cellulitis or verrucous hyperplasia of the skin grafts. Swelling of the extremity is more likely to progress if recurrent bouts of cellulitis are not adequately controlled, or if adequate compressive support is not provided postoperatively (the procedure does not correct the obstruction to lymph efflux). These limbs require lifelong compressive support and, because of their vulnerability to infection, fastidious atention to hygiene.

A variety of **drainage procedures** have been attempted. In the 1800s, surgical treatment of lymphedema consisted of puncturing the skin at several sites and allowing interstitial fluid to drain [71]. Such therapy usually failed to produce significant improvement; after the turn of the century, it became popular to implant a network of subcutaneous threads (originally, silk), which served as drainage channels. A beneficial effect on lymph efflux occasionally persisted after the threads were removed.

More recently, flaps of tissue rich in lymphatics have been implanted into the edematous region [71]. In theory, if the lymphatic vessels in the flap remain functional, they eventually may anastomose with the surrounding lymphatics and provide an alternative pathway for drainage from the edematous area. The myocutaneous flap (using latissimus dorsi) has been useful for the upper extremity, and the intestinal flap (interomesenteric bridge) may improve drainage in the lower extremity [72,73].

Direct microsurgical anastomotic procedures also have been used. Lymphovenous anastomoses can be made between lymphatic vessels distal to an obstruction in nearby small veins; that allows lymph from the obstructed region to flow directly into the venous system [71]. Anastomoses also can be made from the lymph nodes to the adjacent vein. One of the latest techniques involves harvesting normal autogenous lymphatic vessels for use as bypass grafts around a lymphatic obstruction. All these microsurgical techniques require the presence of dilated lymphatic vessels distal to the obstruction [71,74]. These operations obviously are of no value when the lymphatic obstruction is at the level of the smaller distal vessels. The argument can be made, however, that lymphatic bypass operations should be performed as soon as possible after the onset of obstruction to avoid the cutaneous changes of chronic lymphedema as well as the gradual destruction of the distal lymphatic channels [75]. An appropriate candidate for such surgery would be an individual with a recent onset of lymphedema secondary to trauma and with an otherwise normal lymphatic system proximal and distal to the area of obstruction. However, even with appropriate patient selection and a technically skilled vascular surgeon, 2-year patency rates are less than 50 percent [76].

Currently, medical therapy is directed at preventing complications and retarding progression of the disorder, whereas surgery is palliative. More definitive therapy for lymphedema awaits a greater understanding of the abnormalities in development underlying congenital lymphedema and the pathophysiologic processes set in motion by obstruction of the lymphatic channels.

References

1. Kanter MA. The lymphatic system: an historical perspective. Plast Reconstr Surg 1987; 79:131–139.
2. Witte MH, Witte CL. Lymphatics and blood vessels, lymphangiogenesis and hemangiogenesis: from cell biology to clinical medicine. Lymphology 1987; 20:257–266.
3. Kobayashi MR, Miller TA. Lymphedema. Clin Plast Surg 1987; 14:303–313.
4. Merli GJ. Lymphedema. Clin Podiatry 1984; 1:36372.
5. Starling EH. Classics in lymphology. Lymphology 1984; 17:83–88.
6. Sparks HV, Rooke TW. Essentials of Cardiovascular Physiology. Minneapolis: University of Minnesota Press, 1987.
7. Johnston MG, Elias R. The regulation of lymphatic pumping. Lymphology 1987; 20:215–218.
8. Olszewski WL, Engeset A. Intrinsic contractility of prenodal lymph vessels and lymph flow in the human leg. Am J Physiol 1980; 239:H775–783.
9. Pippard C, Roddie IC. Comparison of fluid transport systems in lymphatics and veins. Lymphology 1987; 20:224–229.
10. McHale NG, Roddie IC, Thornsbury KD. Nervous modulation of spontaneous contractions in bovine mesenteric lymphatics. J Physiol 1980; 309:461–472.
11. McHale NG, Roddie IC. The effect of intravenous adrenaline and noradrenaline infusions on peripheral lymph flow in the sheep. J Physiol 1983; 341:517–526.
12. Hayashi A, et al. Increased intrinsic pumping activity of intestinal lymphatics following hemorrhage in anesthetized sheep. Circ Res 1987; 60:265–272.
13. Sinzinger H, Kallman J, Manheimer E. Regulation of human

lymph contractility by prostaglandins and thromboxame. Lymphology 1984; 17:43–45.
14. Hall JL, Morris B, Wooley L. Intrinsic rhythmic propulsion of lymph in anesthetized sheep. J Physiol 1965; 180:336–349.
15. Sarnuels LD. Lymphoscintigraphy. Lymphology 1987; 20:4.
16. Browse NL. The diagnosis and management of primary lymphedema. Vasc Surg 1986; 3:181–184.
17. Allen EV. Lymphedema of the extremities: classification, etiology and differential diagnosis: a study of three hundred cases. Arch lntern Med 1934; 54:606–624.
18. Smeltzer DM, Stickler GB, Schirger A. Primary lymphedema in children and adolescents: a followup study and review. Pediatrics 1985; 76:206–218.
19. Milroy WF. An undescribed variety of hereditary edema. NY Med J 1892; 56:505–508.
20. Milroy WF. Chronic hereditary edema: Milroy's disease. JAMA 1928; 91:1172–1174.
21. Wolfe JHN. The prognosis and possible cause of severe primary lymphoedema. Ann R Coli Surg Eng 1984; 66:251.
22. Lewis JM, Wald ER. Lymphedema praecox. J Pediatr 1984; 104:641–648.
23. Kahlberg PJ, et al. Autosomal or x-linked recessive syndrome of congenital lymphedema, hypoparathyroidism, nephropathy, prolapsing mitral valve, and brachytelephalangy. Am J Med Genet 1983; 16:99.
24. Mucke J, et al. Early onset lymphoedema, recessive form—a new form of genetic lymphoedema syndrome. Eur J Pediatr 1986; 145:195.
25. Henriksen HM. Turner's syndrome associated with lymphoedema, diagnosed in the newborns. Z Geburtshilfe Perinatol 1980; 184:313–315.
26. White SW. Lymphedema in Noonan's syndrome. Int J Dermatol 1984; 23:656–657.
27. Venencie PY, Dicken CH. Yellow nail syndrome: report of five cases. J Am Acad Dermatol 1984; 10:187–192.
28. Wheeler ES, et al. Familial lymphedema praecox: Meige's disease. Plast Reconstr Surg 1981; 67:362–364.
29. Abe R, et al. Retroperitoneal lymphangiomyomatosis with lymphedema of the legs. Lymphology 1980; 13:62.
30. Schirger A. Lymphedema. Cardiovasc Clin 1983; 13:293–305.
31. Kissin MW, et al. Risk of lymphoedema following the treatment of breast cancer. Br J Surg 1986; 73:580–584.
32. Yeoh EK, et al. Primary breast cancer. Complications of axillary management. Acta Radiol (Oncol) 1986; 25:105–108.
33. Lymphatic filariasis—tropical medicine's origin will not go away. Lancet (Editorial) 1987; 1:1409.
34. Dandapat MC, Mahapatro SK, Dash DM. Management of chronic manifestations of filariasis. J Indian Med Assoc 1986; 84:219.
35. Tan TJ, Kosin E, Tan TH. Lymphographic abnormalities in patients with Brugia malayi filariasis and "idiopathic tropical eosinophilia." Lymphology 1985; 18:169.
36. Ottesen EA. Efficacy of diethylcarbamazine in eradicating infection with lymphatic-dwelling filariae in humas. Rev Infect Dis 1985; 4:341.
37. Baird JK, et al. North American Brugian filariasis: report of nine infections of humans. Am J Trop Med Hyg 1980; 35:1205–1209.
38. Clark WR, Lieber MM. Genital filariasis in Minnesota. Urology 1986; 28:518.
39. Leonard JC, Humphrey GB, Basamakjian G. Lymphedema secondary to filariasis. Clin Nucl Med 1985; 10:203.
40. Jayaram G. Microfilariae in fine needle aspirates from epididyrnal lesions. Acta Cytol (Baltimore) 1987; 31:59.
41. Partono F. Treatment of elephantiasis in a community with timorian filariasis. Trans R Soc Trop Med Hyg 1985; 79:44–46.
42. Kumaraswami V, et al. Ivermectin for the treatment of Wuchereria bancrofti filariasis: efficacy and adverse reactions. JAMA 1988; 259:3150–3153.
43. Lynde CW, Mitchell JC. Unusual complication of allergic contact dermatitis of the hands—recurrent lymphangitis and persistent lymphoedema. Contact Dermatitis 1982; 8:279–280.
44. Kyle VM, DeSilva M, Hurst G. Rheumatoid lymphoedema. Clin Rheumatol 1982; 1:126.
45. Reed BR, et al. Lymphedema of the lower abdominal wall in pregnancy. J Am Acad Dermatol 1985; 12:930–932.
46. Majeski J. Lymphedema tarda. Cutis 1985; 38:105–107.
47. Brunning J, Gibson AG, Perry M. Oedema bleu: a reappraisal. Lancet 1980; 1:810–812.
48. Sakulsky SB. Lymphedema: results of surgical treatment in 64 patients [1936–1984]. Lymphology 1977; 10:15–26.
49. Klinmonth JB, Taylor GW, Harper RK. Lymphangiography: a technique for its clinical use in the lower limb. Br Med J 1955; 1:940–942.
50. O'Brien BM, et al. Effect of lymphangiography on lymphedema. Plast Reconstr Surg 1981; 68:922–926.
51. Vaqueiro M, et al. Lymphoscintigraphy in lymphedema: an aid to microsurgery. J Nucl Med 1986; 27:1125–1130.
52. Hadjis NS, et al. The role of CT in the diagnosis of primary lymphedema of the lower limb. Am J Roentgen 1985; 144:361–364.
53. Gamba JL, et al. Primary lower extremity lymphedema: CT diagnosis. Radiology 1983; 149:218.
54. Schirger A, Peterson LFA. Lymphedema. In JL Jergens, JA Spittell, JF Fairbairn II, eds. Peripheral Vascular Diseases. Philadelphia: Saunders, 1980. Pp. 823–851.
55. Zanolla R, et al. Evaluation of the results of three different methods of postmastectomy lymphedema treatment. J Surg Oncol 1984; 26:210.
56. Compression for lymphoedema. Lancet (Editorial) 1986; 1:896.
57. Piller NB. Lymphoedema, macrophages and benzopyrones. Lymphology 1980; 13:109–119.
58. Casley-Smith JR, et al. Treatment of lymphedema of the arms and legs with 5,6-benzopyrone. N Engl J Med 1993; 329(16):1158–1163.
59. Fyfe NC, et al. Intralymphatic steroid therapy for lymphoedema: preliminary studies. Lymphology 1982; 15:23–28.
60. Muller R, Hajdu SI, Brennan MF. Lymphangiosarcoma associated with chronic filarial lymphedema. Cancer 1987; 59:179–183.
61. Alessi E, Sala F, Berti E. Angiosarcoma in lymphedematous limbs. Am J Dermatopathol 1986; 8:371–378.
62. Benda JA, Al Jurf AS, Benson AB III. Angiosarcoma of the breast following segmental mastectomy complicated by lymphedema. Am J Clin Pathol 1987; 87:651–655.
63. Servelle M. Surgical treatment of lymphedema: a report on 652 cases. Surgery 1987; 101:485–495.
64. Schmitz-Rixen T, et al. Angiosarcoma in primary lymphedema of the lower extremity—Stewart-Treves syndrome. Lymphology 1984; 17:50–53.
65. Tatnall FM, Mann BS. Non-Hodgkin's lymphoma of kin associated with chronic limb lymphoedema. Br J Dermatol 1985; 113:751–756.
66. Ruocco V, et al. Kaposi's sarcoma in a lymphedematous immunocompromised limb. Int J Dermatol 1984; 23:56.
67. Epstein JI, Mendelsohn G. Squamous carcinoma of the foot arising in association with long-standing verrucous hyperplasia in a patient with congenital lymphedema. Cancer 1984; 1:943–947.
68. Bart AH, Pinsky CM. Malignant melanoma appearing in a postmastectomy lymphedematous arm: a novel association of double primary tumors. J Surg Oncol 1985; 30:316–318.
69. Zelilovski A, Haddad M, Reiss R. Non-operative therapy com-

bined with limited surgery in management of peripheral lymphedema. Lymphology 1986; 19:106.
70. Miller TA. Surgical approach to lymphedema of the arm after mastectomy. Am J Surg 1984; 148:152–156.
71. Savage RC. The surgical management of lymphedema. Surg Gynecol Obstet 1984; 160:283–290.
72. Medgyesi S. A successful operation for lymphoedema using myocutaneous flap as a "wick." Br J Plast Surg 1983; 36:64–66.
73. Hurst PAE, et al. Long-term results of the enteromesenteric bridge operation in the treatment of primary lymphoedema. Br J Surg 1985; 72:272–274.
74. Ho LCY, Lai MF, Kennedy PJ. Micro-lymphatic bypass in the treatment of obstructive lymphoedema of the arm: case report of a new technique. Br J Plast Surg 1983; 36:350–357.
75. Fyfe NC, Wolfe JH, Kinmonth JB. "Die-back" in primary lymphedema—lymphographic and clinical correlatioms. Lymphology 1982; 15:66–69.
76. Glovicski P. Personal communication. Mayo Clinic, Rochester, MN. 1994.

Vascular Trauma

James O. Menzoian • Nancy L. Cantelmo
J. Gordon Wright • Michael Belkin
Jeanne E. Doyle

The management of patients with vascular injuries has been enhanced by the pioneering studies of DeBakey and Simeone reporting on their experience in World War II [1], Hughes reporting on the experience from the Korean Conflict [2], and Rich and Hughes reporting on the experience from the Vietnam Conflict [3–6]. Although the severity and complications of military injuries are usually greater than those incurred from civilian trauma, management principles gleaned from wartime experiences have greatly benefited our treatment of these complex injuries. Rapid triage, adequate resuscitation, control of bleeding, management of fractures and soft tissue, and principles of surgical repair utilized in the management of civilian vascular injuries are based on lessons learned from extensive military experience.

The following pages detail the epidemiology, pathophysiology, evaluation, and treatment of patients with vascular injuries incurred from blunt, penetrating, and iatrogenic trauma.

EPIDEMIOLOGY OF CIVILIAN VASCULAR TRAUMA

Etiology and Incidence

The etiology of civilian vascular trauma is either blunt or penetrating injury. Most series, including our own from Boston University [7,8], report a 10- to 15-percent incidence of blunt injuries, mostly from motor vehicle accidents. The remaining injuries are of a penetrating nature, with about 50 percent firearm injury and 30 to 40 percent from sharp instruments, such as knives or glass. In our experience, arterial injuries are most common (66%), with isolated venous injuries being the least common (10%) [7]. A venous injury is more likely to occur in combination with arterial injury (23%). The larger the vein, the greater the chance of an isolated injury.

The extremities are the most common location for vascular injury (accounting for 75% of most series), with lower-extremity injuries being slightly more common than upper-extremity injuries. Other sites of arterial trauma, in order of decreasing frequency, are cervical, visceral, and aortic injuries.

Most series report young males to be the most frequent victims of vascular trauma, as with other types of trauma. In our series, 90 percent of patients were male, and 65 percent were between 15 and 30 years of age. The majority, therefore, have few, if any, other significant health problems. The major exception is drug abuse, which may either be the etiology of vascular injury or affect the availability of vein for possible reconstruction of other injuries. In the elderly patient, the preexistence of atherosclerotic disease, particularly peripheral vascular disease, is important in the assessment of the magnitude of injury and the consideration for repair.

Pathophysiology of Vascular Trauma

Knowledge of the mechanism of injury can be especially helpful in patient assessment. With vascular trauma resulting from violence, details about the traumatic event often are unavailable. With penetrating injuries, it is helpful to know the type of weapon, angle of entry, and depth of penetration, but that information often is unknown.

Vascular injuries caused by blunt trauma are increasing as traffic and the number of roadways increase and the size of vehicles decreases. The vector of the blunt force may directly traumatize a vascular structure (Fig. 50-1). Another type of blunt injury is caused by the shearing force of rapid deceleration on a fixed point in a blood vessel. This injury most commonly occurs in the thoracic aorta distal to the left subclavian artery at the attachment of the ligamentum arteriosum. Vehicular accidents often cause multiple injuries, and frequently an associated fracture or dislocation causes vascular damage. The popliteal artery and vein, for example, are likely to be traumatized by a posterior dislocation of the knee.

With penetrating wounds from sharp instruments and low-velocity bullets, the damage usually is limited to the wound tract (see Fig. 50-1). The energy carried in higher-velocity missiles is transmitted to the surrounding tissues, outside the wound tract. This "blast effect" can cause vessel damage, even if the bullet itself does not strike the vascular structures. Severe concomitant soft-tissue injury can occur with high-velocity missiles, as well as with close-range but lower-velocity gunshot wounds.

Vascular injuries resulting from diagnostic and therapeutic intervention, as well as intravenous drug abuse, are increasingly common. Iatrogenic vascular injuries are discussed in further detail later in this chapter.

Penetrating injuries result in punctures, lacerations, and transections of blood vessels. Indirect bullet injury may cause an intimal disruption, although the outer layers of the arterial wall remain intact. Similar intimal injury also may result from blunt trauma, which may crack the intima, raising a flap that protrudes into the lumen, or denude the endothelial surface, providing a nidus for thrombosis (Fig. 50-2).

The puncture site of an artery may form a false aneurysm, which may be detected at the time of puncture or at a later date. False aneurysms are prone to infection or rupture. A fistula between an artery and a vein may result from injury to both structures. It may develop at the time of initial injury or later at the site of initial thrombus. Embolization of arterial wall or missile fragments from the entry site to a distant location is a rare but reported occurrence. A dissection of the arterial wall, forming a false lumen, occasionally may result from blunt or penetrating trauma. It is most often seen, however, in iatrogenic catheter injury.

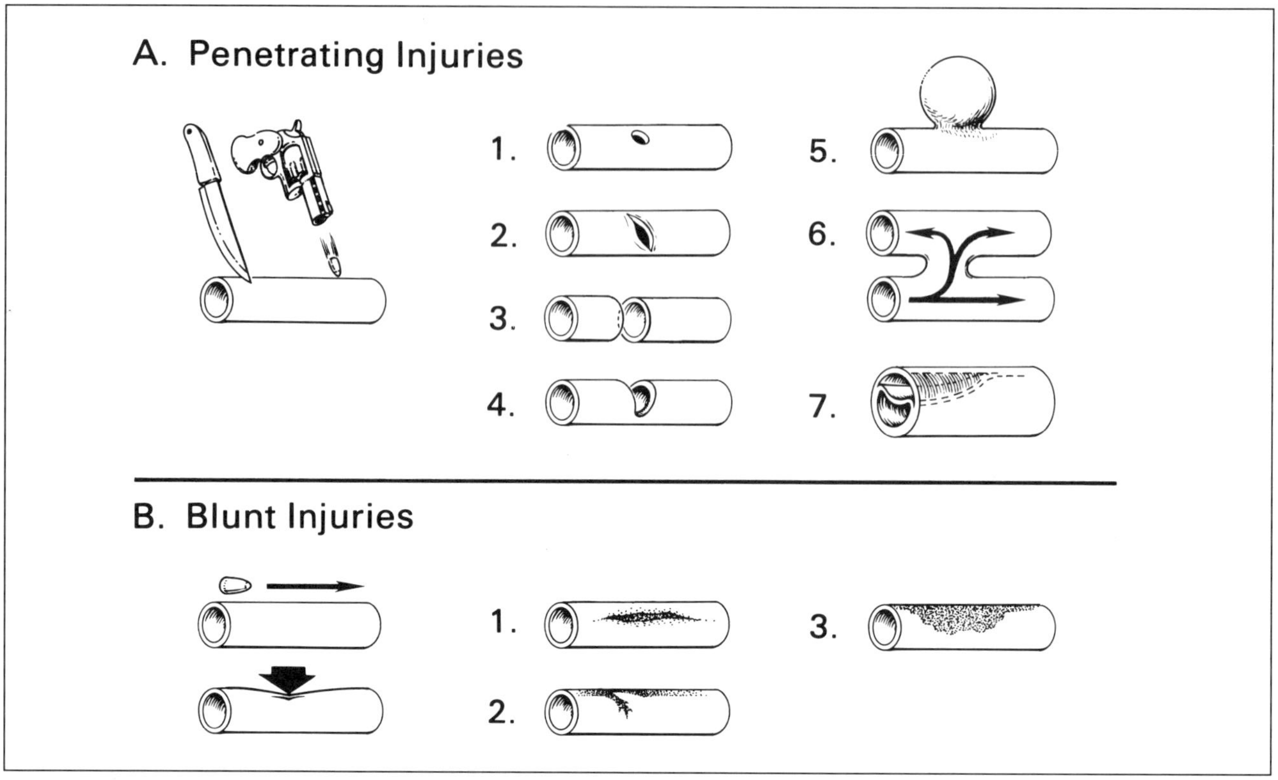

Fig. 50-1. Mechanisms of vascular injury. **A.** Penetrating injury: (1) puncture, (2) laceration, (3) complete transection, (4) partial transection, (5) aneurysm, (6) arteriovenous fistula, (7) dissection. **B.** Nonpenetrating injury (external compression or blast effect): (1) intimal contusion, (2) intimal flap, (3) intimal injury with thrombosis.

The structure of the artery and vein walls influence the outcome of vascular injury. The more muscular medial layer of the artery permits an injured artery to contract and thrombose more readily than the thin-walled vein. The intact intima of the artery and vein has numerous mechanisms to prevent thrombosis, whereas the underlying medial and adventitial layers are actually thrombogenic. Therefore, endothelial injury promotes intravascular thrombosis.

The anatomic proximity of nerves to arteries and veins is important in the recognition of vascular injury. A neurologic deficit may alert the astute physician to the possibility of an arterial or venous injury that otherwise may not be readily apparent. In a report from our institution, compression neuropathies of the brachial plexus were the first sign of traumatic pseudoaneurysms of the axillary artery [9].

A compartment syndrome may result from vascular injury, or it may cause extrinsic vascular compression and thrombosis. This syndrome occurs when increased pressure in the noncompliant fascia compromises circulation and neuromuscular function in that anatomic space. Major soft-tissue injury, arterial or venous bleeding, prolonged ischemia, and intra-arterial injection of drugs are the more common causes of compartment syndrome. Regardless of the etiology, increased pressure within the compartment further compromises circulation, leading to increased edema, higher compartment pressures, and a progressively worsening situation. If left untreated, the syndrome causes permanent destruction of the neurovascular structures in the compartment itself. Systemic manifestations of advanced compartment syndrome also are seen. The toxic effects of severe ischemic muscle catabolism lead to systemic acidosis, hyperkalemia, and hypovolemia, which may result in multisystem failure and sometimes death.

CLINICAL DIAGNOSIS

The evaluation and assessment of patients with possible vascular injury is often obvious, but in selected patients it may prove to be quite difficult [10]. Brink has suggested a classification of patients with vascular injuries into three categories. Category I includes patients with obvious life-threatening vascular injuries; category II includes patients with obvious vascular injuries that may be limb threatening or organ threatening but not life threatening; category III includes patients with injuries near major blood vessels but with no obvious direct vascular injury. Evaluation and treatment of patients in category I represent no significant clinical problem in that urgent surgery is indicated. Patients in categories II and III warrant further clinical assessment and judgment relevant to the need for continued observation, further diagnostic evaluation, or surgery.

History. Any history of preexisting vascular disease, for example, intermittent claudication or rest pain, obviously

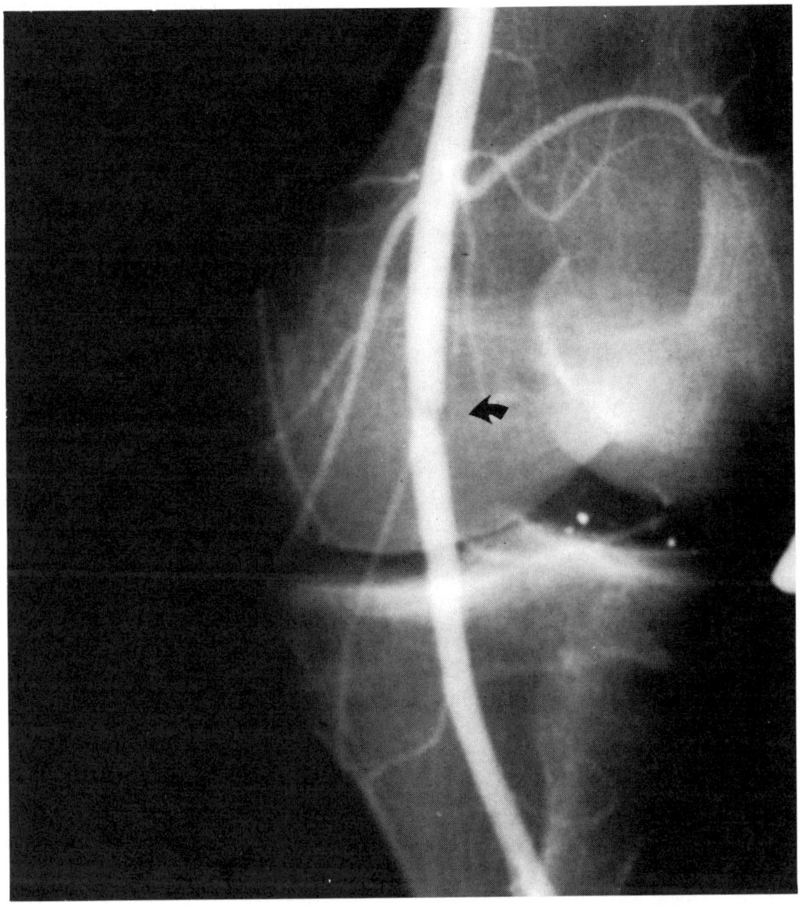

Fig. 50-2. A gunshot wound of the popliteal fossa. Patient had intact pulses. An angiogram was performed for proximity and showed intimal disruption. At surgery the artery was thrombosed.

would be extremely helpful in evaluating patients with suspected vascular injury. That is especially true in elderly patients in whom absent pulses could be related to long-standing atherosclerosis and not to vascular trauma.

An understanding of the mechanism of injury likewise can be extremely helpful in patient evaluation. Patients with blunt trauma of sufficient force may suffer significant soft-tissue injury resulting in compartment syndromes, which must be quickly recognized and treated before permanent damage results.

Patients suffering motor vehicle accidents or falls deserve special consideration relevant to deceleration vascular injuries, which occur most commonly in the thoracic aorta. Deceleration injuries in that area can result in intimal disruption of the thoracic aorta just distal to the left subclavian artery.

Injuries of the lower extremity should be evaluated for the possibility of knee dislocation or supracondylar fractures of the femur. The popliteal artery is firmly attached by the overlying muscle and the geniculate arteries. Any disruption of the knee by fracture or dislocation can result in stretching, contusion, and thrombosis of the popliteal artery at that level [11].

Bullet injuries differ according to the caliber, velocity, and trajectory of the bullet. High-velocity bullets can result in significant soft-tissue injury due to the so-called cavitation effect created by the missile. Shotgun injuries result in a large amount of soft-tissue necrosis related to the blast effect. The injuries must be constantly evaluated for the possibility of ischemic necrosis of the soft tissue.

Physical Assessment. Evaluation of a patient with possible vascular injury should encompass the usual physical parameters, including blood pressure, pulse, and signs of orthostatic hypotension. In extremity injuries, the limb should be evaluated by palpation for the presence of pulses, skin temperature of the extremity, and presence of a sensory deficit and by auscultation for the presence of a bruit. We have found an excellent correlation between certain physical findings and the confirmation of a significant vascular injury at the time of surgical exploration. The presence of a bruit or thrill (100%), signs of distal ischemia (100%), absent pulses (90%), active hemorrhage (82%), neurologic deficit (80%), and hematoma (50%) correlated strongly with positive findings at surgery [7]. Earlier in our experience, we advocated surgical exploration in patients with extremity injuries in proximity to a major vessel, even in the absence of those findings, with 20 percent found to have a significant vascular injury. Recently we have abandoned that routine in favor of selective angiography [12].

Diagnostic Testing

NONINVASIVE EVALUATION. Doppler assessment of an injured extremity is especially helpful in patients with absent distal pulses. The quality of the Doppler sound as well as a Doppler ankle-to-brachial index pressure determination is helpful in diagnosing an arterial injury, as well as providing a baseline that can be followed during the course of therapy. A decreased ankle-to-brachial index and abnormal arterial waveform analysis should raise suspicion of a significant arterial injury.

Duplex ultrasonography has recently been advocated in diagnosing arterial injuries [13–16]. Its advantages are that it is noninvasive, it can be promptly obtained even in the emergency room setting, and it eliminates the risks of invasive arteriography. Recent studies have reported excellent sensitivity and specificity in comparisons of the results of duplex scanning with arteriography in the management of vascular trauma. It may be that in those centers in which duplex imaging is available on a 24-hour basis that modality could replace conventional angiography. As usual with any new modality, it is suggested that each center assess the sensitivity and specificity of duplex ultrasonography compared with conventional angiography and surgical exploration.

X-RAYS. Plain films of the injured area should be obtained to confirm obvious bone injuries. Additionally, the chest x-ray may demonstrate mediastinal widening or capping of the apical pleura in patients with significant mediastinal vascular or thoracic outlet injuries. Abdominal films may demonstrate obliteration of the psoas muscle margin, suggesting retroperitoneal hematoma.

ARTERIOGRAPHY. The liberal yet judicious use of arteriography has been extremely helpful in evaluating patients with possible vascular injuries [17,18]. In extremity injuries, if time permits, we recommend arteriography to specifically localize the injury (Fig. 50-3). If the patient or the extremity is at risk due to active bleeding or severe ischemia, we proceed directly with surgical exploration. In selected instances, arteriography can be performed in the operating room.

In patients with injuries in proximity to major vessels, even in the absence of any obvious physical findings of an arterial injury, we have previously recommended arteriography [19,20]. In our experience, approximately 12 percent of such patients show a significant finding on angiography that was not suspected after clinical assessment (Fig. 50-4) [7]. Recent data, however, have suggested that that approach may be less fruitful than expected and that proximity angiography may not be indicated in all instances [21–28].

Arteriography is essential in patients with a widened mediastinum or first-rib fractures and the possibility of thoracic outlet injury. Patients with hematuria and suspected renal-artery injuries, large retroperitoneal hematomas, and pelvic fractures with significant blood loss also should undergo arteriography. Although each patient must be evaluated individually, we stress that we have been extremely pleased and rewarded by arteriography and strongly recommend its judicious use.

We have recently been utilizing intra-arterial digital subtraction angiography (DSA) and find it very helpful in evaluating patients with vascular injuries. We have, however, been dissatisfied with the quality of venous DSA. Arterial DSA does have some distinct advantages to conventional angiography (CA), including the following:

1. DSA can be done faster.
2. A smaller dose of contrast can be used in a single area of study.
3. DSA has increased contrast sensitivity for better visualization of poorly perfused vessels.
4. A smaller catheter can be used for DSA, permitting the use of contrast material of lesser viscosity.
5. DSA is less expensive because of the need for a smaller number of films with less expensive film material.

There are, however, some disadvantages to DSA, which include the following:

1. More complicated equipment and demanding technical assistance are required.
2. In studies involving a large area, the moving table in CA permits one complete study with a smaller amount of contrast than that used in the repeated injections required for each station of DSA. A moving table cannot be used with DSA because the technique does not allow for any motion.
3. Diminished resolution of DSA (two line-pairs) compared with CA (eight line-pairs) may limit intimal detail.
4. Increased sensitivity to movement makes resolution of the arch aorta suboptimal. A noncompliant patient also yields a poor-quality study because of motion artifact.

ASSOCIATED INJURIES. In the complete evaluation of a traumatically injured patient, an awareness of associated injuries is essential in evaluating the possibility of a significant vascular injury. Specific examples are detailed later in this chapter, but the association of vascular injuries with pelvic fractures, knee dislocation, supracondylar fractures of the femur, first-rib fractures, and tibial fractures is well known. If any of those injuries is present, further evaluation of the patient must be undertaken, even in the absence of overt signs of significant vascular injury. The use of arteriography is especially helpful in such instances.

GENERAL ASPECTS OF TREATMENT

Priorities

Resuscitation of the patient is the first priority in patients with significant injuries. Once an airway has been established, active hemorrhage has been controlled, and large-bore intravenous catheters have been placed, patients can be further evaluated for the possibility of a vascular injury. In the presence of active bleeding, direct pressure is the preferred method of control. Exploration of wounds in the emergency room for control of bleeding vessels is not

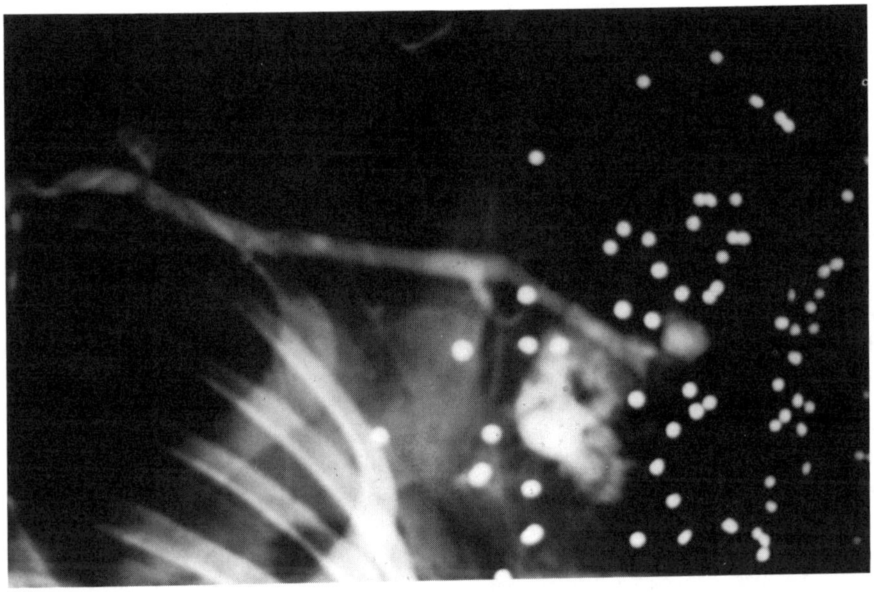

Fig. 50-3. This angiogram was obtained to localize the clinically evident arterial injury. The massive amount of soft-tissue injury precluded accurate clinical localization of the arterial injury.

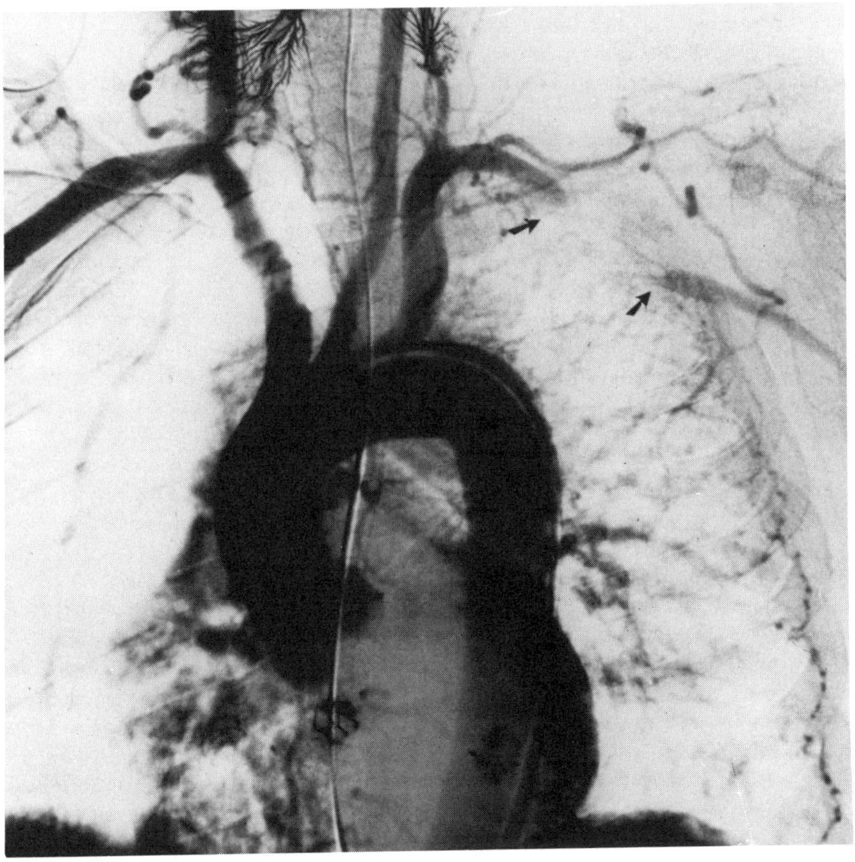

Fig. 50-4. Patient with a fractured left clavicle from blunt trauma had a diminished radial artery pulse. Angiogram reveals a thrombosed axillary artery secondary to direct trauma with arterial contusion and thrombosis.

recommended because it is not possible to get adequate vessel exposure, and the possibility of further injuring the vessels and associated nerves is high. A firm compression bandage over the site of bleeding should be attempted first. If that is unsuccessful, direct digital pressure is achieved by inserting a gloved finger in the wound. Manual pressure should not be released until the patient is in the operating room, where the surgeon can gain proximal and distal control of the injured vessel. That often requires prepping the patient while maintaining vascular control into the operative field [29]. The use of a tourniquet to control hemorrhage generally is contraindicated, since it can cause significant soft-tissue ischemia. We have, however, used a tourniquet in the operating room in select circumstances to achieve temporary control of active bleeding from an injured extremity until the time of surgical exploration.

In patients with significant chest trauma and the potential of superior vena cava, inferior vena cava, or subclavian vein injuries, intravenous lines should not be placed in the injured extremity, because the resuscitative fluids could be infused into the thoracic cavity. In cases of abdominal and pelvic trauma with hemodynamic instability, the use of military antishock trousers (MAST suit) can be helpful in tamponading active bleeding.

Obvious fractures should be stabilized in the emergency room since, in many instances, that controls bleeding and enhances perfusion of the injured extremity.

In patients with active bleeding who fall into Brink's category I, direct transfer to the operating room is essential. There further resuscitative measures can be undertaken, and prompt surgical exploration for the control of bleeding can be completed. Patients in Brink's category II, who have obvious vascular injury to an organ or a limb that is not life threatening, can undergo further stabilization and evaluation in the emergency room, but urgent surgical exploration should follow. Patients in Brink's category III, who have injuries near major vessels without obvious signs of vascular trauma, can undergo further resuscitative efforts and diagnostic evaluation.

Preoperative Preparation

In patients requiring urgent surgery, preoperative preparation should include chest x-ray, ECG, baseline blood chemistries, evaluation of hemoglobin and hematocrit, and a coagulation profile. Baseline blood gases are also helpful. Additionally, in these critically ill patients we insert an indwelling Foley catheter into the bladder to assess urine production adequately.

We routinely use preoperative antibiotics, especially in penetrating injuries, because in some instances repair of the vascular injury may require the placement of a prosthetic graft [30]. We prefer first-generation cephalosporins, which should be continued for a total of no more than 24 hours.

Preoperative anticoagulants generally are contraindicated in patients with vascular injuries because of the high risk of hemorrhage. There are, however, some limited exceptions. In patients with acute arterial occlusion, such as with a posterior dislocation of the knee and subsequent contusion and thrombosis of the popliteal artery, we often judiciously use intravenous heparin to prevent clot propagation (away from the area of injury), which might occlude collateral blood supply to the injured extremity. These patients require vigilant observation for the possibility of hemorrhage into the injured soft tissue.

Anesthesia

The type of anesthesia used for operative intervention should depend on the preference and expertise of the anesthesiologist. For many patients, regional anesthesia such as axillary or intrascalene block for the upper extremity or spinal or epidural anesthesia for abdominal, pelvic, and lower-extremity injuries is safe and effective. For others, however, general inhalation anesthesia can be administered more promptly and is the technique of choice. Regardless of the type of anesthesia utilized, close monitoring of the patient during any operation for vascular injuries is critical. In patients in whom a significant blood loss is anticipated, the placement of a central venous- or pulmonary-artery (Swan-Ganz) catheter is helpful in monitoring hemodynamics and cardiac function. Intraoperatively, close monitoring of cardiac output, blood pressure, and urine production is critical, since vascular repairs often are tedious and lengthy. Close assessment of blood loss and replacement with blood, fresh frozen plasma, platelets, and calcium after multiple transfusions is critical. In patients with isolated vascular injuries, the use of cell-saver autotransfusion systems have been extremely helpful.

Arterial, Venous, and Orthopedic Injuries

In extremity trauma with combined vascular and orthopedic injuries, consideration must be given to the priority of handling those multiple insults. Although traditional teaching advocates orthopedic stabilization followed by vascular repair, we and others often deviate from that plan when reperfusion of the injured extremity must be done promptly [31–33]. Fasciotomy is performed first, followed by repair of arterial and venous injuries and finally by orthopedic stabilization. A critical amount of time can be lost if orthopedic stabilization is attempted first. In many instances, an awareness of the need for fasciotomy is critical, since tissue perfusion suffers if a compartment syndrome exists. Once fasciotomy and vascular repair have been completed, close observation of the repaired vessels is necessary to ensure that there is no tension on the repair nor injury to it during the period of orthopedic stabilization.

In patients with extensive soft-tissue trauma in association with vascular and orthopedic injuries, we have come to prefer external fixation of the fracture. An external fixation device allows for adequate postoperative monitoring of the soft-tissue injury as well as arterial flow and neurologic function without obstruction from a cast. In some patients, the device is removed and replaced with internal fixation once the soft tissue has healed or skin grafting has been performed.

In the presence of an arterial injury, temporary indwelling synthetic shunts can be used to bridge the gap in the injured vessel and provide perfusion while other injuries are attended to [34]. We do not recommend the routine use of shunts because their replacement requires heparin to prevent thrombosis and they can further traumatize the artery.

There are numerous methods of repairing arterial injuries, including simple suturing of lacerations, end-to-end anastomosis of transected vessels, and interposition bypass grafts when the extent of the arterial defect precludes end-to-end repair. Our conduit of choice is autogenous vein, preferably the saphenous vein from the noninjured extremity. If saphenous vein is not available, our next preference is cephalic or basilic vein from the upper extremity. When none of those is available, we use synthetic-prosthetic graft materials such as polytetrafluoroethylene (PTFE, Gore-Tex). We do not recommend the routine use of synthetic materials, however, because of the greater potential for graft thrombosis and infection. PTFE has been shown to be far superior to Dacron in traumatic vascular repair [35].

Once the arterial repair is complete, we recommend completion angiography in all instances. In our experience and that of others, angiography delineates any technical problems as well as residual distal thrombosis that may not be clinically evident [36,37]. Once identified, such problems can be corrected easily, thus precluding the necessity of returning the patient to the operating room and minimizing the risk of subsequent graft thrombosis.

Significant venous injuries always should be repaired if the patient's general condition allows. In some instances, venous ligation is necessary because of other multiple complex injuries [38]. Rich and others have shown that when injured veins are repaired there is less resultant soft-tissue edema and improved limb perfusion [39–42]. That is especially true when there are combined arterial and venous injuries [43]. Major veins can be repaired by lateral suture techniques, end-to-end anastomosis, and, in some instances, interposition vein grafts. In a recent analysis of 191 major venous injuries by Sharma [44], a treatment algorithm was offered to help decide whether major venous injuries should be repaired or ligated. Considerations included hemodynamic stability, extent and location of injury, and clinical measurement of venous hypertension. In hemodynamically stable patients, major venous injuries were repaired. If the patient was hemodynamically unstable, an assessment of venous pressure either by direct stump-pressure measurement or by clinical assessment was undertaken. If markedly engorged veins suggested venous hypertension, venous repair was undertaken.

Any devitalized soft tissue should be aggressively debrided. In patients with a large tissue defect or a fasciotomy, every effort should be made to cover the area of vascular repair with living tissue. The subcutaneous layer can be left open and subsequently repaired by delayed primary closure or split-thickness skin grafting.

FASCIOTOMY

In patients with significant ischemia or blunt trauma, edema of skeletal muscle can result. If the swelling is excessive, limb perfusion decreases, especially in areas where the muscle is contained in compartments with strong fascial investiture. As outlined above, fasciotomy often is required prior to any attempt at arterial or venous repair. In patients in whom there is no obvious need for fasciotomy as judged by clinical evaluation or direct compartmental-pressure measurements, close observation is needed for the subsequent development of edema following arterial reconstruction. Signs and symptoms of increasing compartmental pressure include numbness in the extremity, loss of pulses, and a decreased Doppler perfusion pressure. If a compartment syndrome is suspected, pressure measurements can be obtained by previously described techniques. If the pressures exceed 40 mm Hg or if there is obvious muscle bulging, fasciotomy should be performed promptly. When tissue edema has subsided (usually after 48–72 hours), delayed primary closure or split-thickness skin grafting can be performed [45–47].

Postoperative Management

Following vascular repair, the patient must be closely monitored for the possibility of continued bleeding, failure of the arterial repair, signs of progressive ischemia, developing compartment syndrome, and hemorrhage. We do not routinely use anticoagulants following the repair of vascular injuries. In many instances, anticoagulation is contraindicated because of significant concomitant soft-tissue and orthopedic injuries. The rare exception is those patients with isolated vascular injury undergoing venous repair who receive heparin to prevent local venous thrombosis. Heparin is continued for a limited time in the postoperative period. Long-term anticoagulation is not recommended. In addition to that short course of heparin, we recommend the use of external pneumatic compression, which minimizes edema, augments venous flow, and diminishes the incidence of venous thrombosis [48].

Prophylactic antibiotic therapy is continued for a total of 24 hours in the perioperative period in patients with a penetrating injury and in those with a prosthetic vascular graft. If autogenous vein is used for vascular repair in the absence of a penetrating injury, we do not continue the antibiotics in the postoperative period.

Reperfusion edema can occur following repair of an extremity vascular injury. It is manifest by pitting edema that develops rather precipitously and likely is related to a loss of capillary integrity during the ischemic period. If significant edema does develop, we recommend noninvasive evaluation of the extremity to assess for deep-vein thrombosis.

Reperfusion edema usually is short-lived and disappears within a week to 10 days. Postoperative deep-vein thrombosis is well known following vascular injury and is probably related to immobility and venous stasis in the injured extremity. In some patients, however, debilitating edema can persist. In those patients we recommend the use of compression-gradient elastic stockings. If there is evidence of deep-vein thrombosis, anticoagulant therapy should be initiated with intravenous heparin followed by oral warfarin sodium (Coumadin) for the usual period of time.

Postoperative physical therapy is essential for patients with injured extremities and should be pursued as aggressively as possible given the individual patient's capabilities and injuries. Physical therapy has been shown to increase blood flow, decrease venous stasis and edema, and result in enhanced earlier mobility.

COMPLICATIONS OF VASCULAR TRAUMA

Complications of vascular trauma may be broadly divided into perioperative and late groups. Although these complications are similar to those encountered in vascular surgery in general, several problems characteristically occur in the setting of trauma.

Perioperative Complications

GENERAL

In the early postoperative period after vascular trauma, patients must be monitored closely. That requires both serial physical examination and, when necessary, Doppler examinations. Two of the more commonly encountered early complications are thrombosis of the repaired vessel and hemorrhage. In a series of 207 arterial repairs for vascular trauma, Perry and associates had 19 (9.2%) early occlusions and 4 (1.9%) cases of bleeding that required return to the operating room [49]. Numerous factors contribute to these early problems. Perioperative use of heparin and systemic coagulopathies in transfused patients as well as those with severe multisystem injury can contribute to hemorrhage. Most often, however, a discrete bleeding point is encountered.

The coexistence of extensive soft-tissue injury as well as long-bone fractures may contribute to early occlusion. Those same factors may promote vascular spasm, which may be particularly severe in the young trauma patient with otherwise normal vessels. Although vascular spasm frequently is encountered, in general, ischemia in the early postoperative period should not be attributed to spasm without an arteriogram that demonstrates vascular patency.

REPERFUSION SYNDROME

When perfusion is restored to an ischemic extremity, a variety of local and systemic effects occur that can threaten both the limb and the life of the patient (Fig. 50-5). One of the most serious and preventable local complications is acute compartment syndrome. When blood flow is restored to an ischemic extremity, a reactive hyperemia occurs. The increased flow, coupled with increased vascular permeability, contributes to massive intracellular and extracellular edema. When the swelling occurs in the confines of an enclosed osseofascial compartment, an acute increase in compartmental pressure occurs. As pressure reaches and exceeds venous pressure, nutrient flow to the tissues in the compartment ceases. The resultant added ischemia to the already compromised limb can lead to irreversible neural and muscular injury. Although compartment syndrome can occur in numerous areas of the upper and lower extremity, the four calf compartments are at greatest risk. Furthermore, the anterior compartment of the calf, which contains the deep peroneal nerve, almost always is involved when compartment syndrome affects the leg.

The most important factor in preventing morbidity from compartment syndrome is early diagnosis and treatment. Early diagnosis depends on a high index of suspicion and careful examination. Compartment syndrome should be anticipated in the setting of delayed vascular repair (more than 6 hours), combined arterial and venous injuries, and associated soft-tissue injuries. Serial examination should focus on the perfusion to the skin, the patient's mobility of the calf and toes, calf rigidity, swelling, and sensation. Sensation in the great toe web space, which is innervated by the deep peroneal nerve, is particularly important. Presence of palpable arterial pulses is of no value in ruling out compartment syndrome, since they may persist long after capillary pressure is exceeded and nutrient flow has stopped. Excessive calf pain should increase the clinician's suspicion of increased compartment pressure. The adjunctive measurement of compartment pressure may be employed to diagnose and monitor for elevated compartment pressure. A variety of techniques have been described, including manometric, wick catheter, and slow continuous infusion [46–51]. Compartmental pressures normally are below 10 mm Hg, with pressures above 20 mm Hg being abnormal and pressures above 40 mm Hg requiring surgical decompression [52].

Prompt surgical treatment of compartment syndrome is essential to prevent functional disability and limb loss. Standard treatment is wide decompression of the four calf compartments. A variety of techniques have been employed, including fibulectomy and parafibular fasciotomy. The most direct and simple approach, however, is two-incision, four-compartment decompression. A medial longitudinal incision is made parallel and 2 cm posterior to the tibia, through which the superficial and deep posterior compartments are decompressed by incising the fascia overlying each compartment. An anterolateral incision between the tibia and the fibula is made; then the anterior and lateral compartments are decompressed in a similar fashion. When compartment syndrome is anticipated (as in the settings outlined above), experienced surgeons perform prophylactic fasciotomy at the time of the original vascular repair.

In addition to acute compartment syndrome, it has become clear that other detrimental effects can occur locally in the ischemic limb at the time perfusion is restored. Pathologic and experimental studies have documented that a significant degree of ischemic injury occurs with reperfusion of ischemic tissue [53]. This reperfusion injury is believed to be mediated by oxygen-derived free radicals, which are generated by cellular enzymes when oxygen is reintroduced. The resultant superoxide, peroxide, and hydroxyl radicals are believed to damage cell membranes through peroxidation of phospholipids. Membrane-bound organelles, such as lysosomes and mitochondria, also are disrupted. The pathologic significance of these free oxygen radicals and the potential therapeutic benefits of free-radical scavengers (such as superoxide dismutase and mannitol) have been demonstrated in a variety of tissues, including skeletal muscle [54].

The perioperative complications discussed to this point represent local problems that may significantly compro-

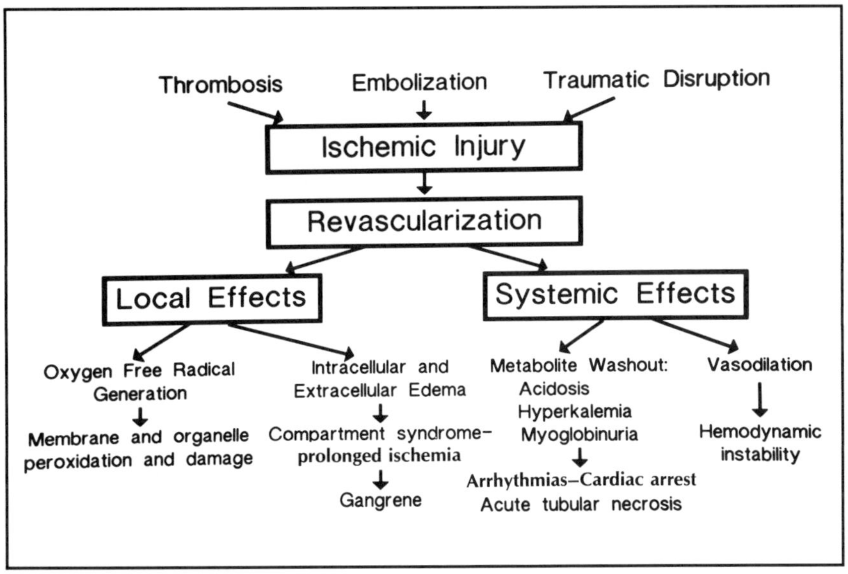

Fig. 50-5. Revascularization syndrome. Combined local and systemic effects of reperfusion of ischemic muscle.

mise the salvage of the injured extremity. Reperfusion of a traumatized, ischemic limb may have a profound systemic impact as well, leading to a cascade of complications that may ultimately threaten the patient's life. Haimovici described the systemic metabolic effects of reperfusion syndrome in 1959 [55]. The syndrome is also well recognized immediately following thromboembolectomy of the acutely ischemic extremity [56]. When perfusion is restored to the limb that has suffered ischemic myonecrosis, acidic metabolites and potassium are washed out into the systemic circulation, resulting in acidosis and hyperkalemia. Resultant arrhythmias and vasomotor instability may cause significant morbidity and mortality.

Rhabdomyolysis also results in the release of myoglobin, which is washed into the general circulation. Within a few hours, the myoglobin appears in the urine, where acidic conditions lead to precipitation in the renal tubules. Oliguria with progression to acute tubular necrosis may result if prompt recognition and therapy do not take place. Recognition is based on observation of the characteristic cherry-red urine discoloration as well as urine chemistries detecting myoglobin. Treatment consists of alkalinization of the urine and the maintenance of a brisk osmotic diuresis with mannitol. Aggressive fluid replacement to maintain intravascular volume is essential. When prolonged ischemia in the traumatized limb has resulted in a large necrotic muscle mass, the risk of morbid systemic effects in the face of a negligible chance of limb salvage may necessitate primary amputation.

Late Complications of Vascular Trauma

The vast majority of late complications of vascular trauma are directly related to circumstances surrounding the vascular repair or injuries that were missed or underestimated. A wide variety of late complications have been reported. The most common and troublesome include graft infections, false-aneurysm formation, arteriovenous fistulas, and posttraumatic pain syndrome.

GRAFT INFECTIONS

Infection of prosthetic vascular grafts represents one of the most dreaded complications in vascular surgery. Under the ideal circumstances of clean, elective vascular procedures with appropriate prophylactic antibiotics, graft infection rates from 1.34 to 6 percent have been reported [57–59]. Infection generally presents months to years after the original surgery and can be a significant source of morbidity and mortality [58]. The infection generally is related to direct contamination at the time of surgery, and the incidence is increased in grafts involving groin anastomoses, contaminated wounds, and prolonged or emergent procedures. The infection may result in thrombosis or in infected false aneurysms when an anastomosis is involved or simply persistent sepsis when the graft is involved away from an anastomosis. Successful management of an infected graft is one of the greatest challenges in vascular surgery and depends on prompt recognition. The principles of treatment include removal of the infected graft, debridement of the infected tissue, effective antibiotic coverage, and revascularization through uninfected tissue planes.

The superior patency and resistance to infection of autogenous graft (such as saphenous vein) has led to its preferential use. That has been especially true in the setting of vascular trauma, where the emergent nature of the surgery and contaminated wounds are felt to predispose to infection of prosthetic graft material. Rich and Hughes reported their experience with prosthetic grafts in 26 patients who suffered vascular trauma during the Vietnam War. There were 20 major complications, including 9 graft infections, in those patients [60]. Military wounds, however, generally involve more contamination and soft-tissue injury than those encountered in civilian trauma, and some authors have continued to employ prosthetic grafts in selected cases. Feliciano and associates recently reported on the use of 236 PTFE grafts in vascular wounds [61]. Although their long-term follow-up is limited, they found an acceptable patency (5.8% early arterial occlusion) and no graft infections in the absence of exposure of the graft or osteomyelitis. Advantages of PTFE grafts cited by those authors include immediate availability in a variety of sizes and maintenance of structural integrity in the setting of infection (where autogenous vein grafts may weaken and rupture).

Regardless of the conduit ultimately chosen for vascular repair, successful avoidance of infection depends on adhering to several basic principles. Those principles include the use of perioperative antibiotics, extensive debridement of devitalized and contaminated tissue, copious local irrigation with local antibiotic solution, and prompt revascularization of the ischemic tissue.

TRAUMATIC ANEURYSMS

Chronic traumatic aneurysms generally arise from missed arterial injuries. In most instances, localized arterial disruption leads to a perivascular hematoma, which goes on to form a pseudoaneurysm. In some cases, however, arterial injury (usually blunt) leads to arterial-wall weakening and true aneurysm formation. Traumatic aneurysms are not unusual injuries. Rich and associates identified 296 cases in the Vietnam Vascular Registry [62]. These lesions most commonly occur in the extremities and usually arise from penetrating injuries and long-bone fractures.

Traumatic aneurysms generally present as painless expanding pulsatile masses in patients with previous histories of trauma. Distal ischemia is relatively unusual but may occur in the setting of secondary thrombosis. Symptoms of neural compression may occur. Abdominal and thoracic aneurysms may go unrecognized until a complication develops. Diagnostic work-up is based on complete angiographic evaluation. In some cases, ultrasound, CT scanning, and venography may be useful.

Because of numerous possible complications, including rupture, thrombosis, and compression syndromes, operative management is recommended in low-risk patients. Small distal aneurysms can be managed by simple ligation. Larger, more proximal aneurysms require more formal repair. The initial step in such repair always includes proximal and distal vascular control. In many cases, once vascular control has been established, the aneurysm can be directly entered and the vessel repaired from within. In other cases where the artery is significantly damaged or distorted, resection of the aneurysm with repair by an interposition graft may be necessary. The results of these repairs usually are excellent.

An increasingly common and difficult problem is mycotic-pseudoaneurysm formation in drug abusers. The pseudoaneurysms occur at a variety of sites, but the femoral and brachial arteries are most commonly involved (Fig. 50-6). They usually result from direct arterial injury from contaminated needles, although secondary bacterial seeding from endocarditis is not unusual. *Staphylococcus aureus* accounts for the majority of these infections [63].

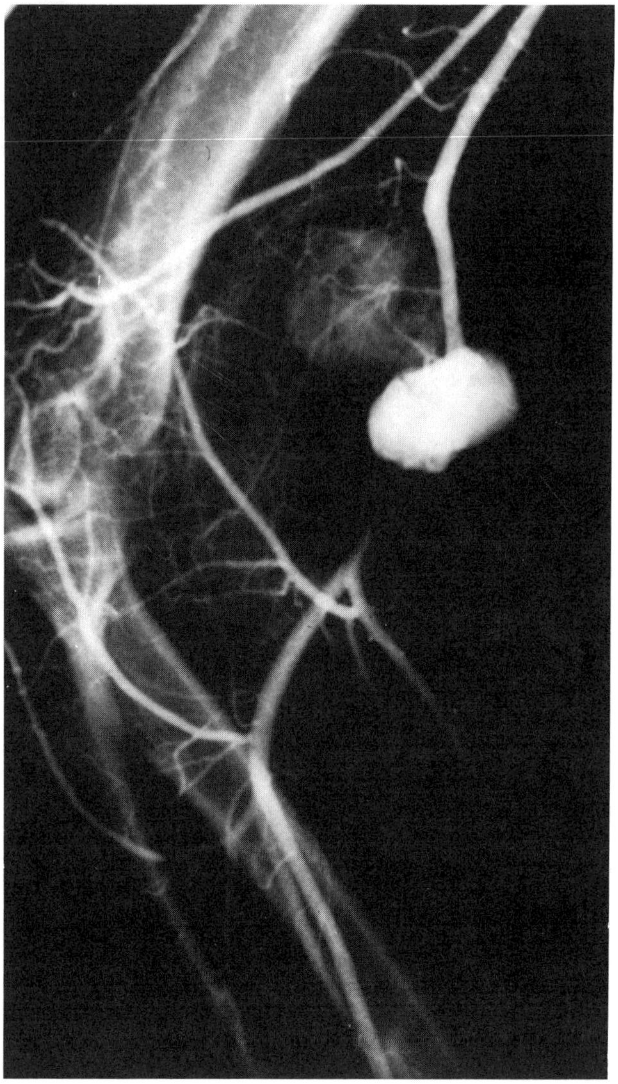

Fig. 50-6. Brachial-artery mycotic pseudoaneurysm secondary to drug abuse.

Patients often present late, after secondary complications have developed. Management generally involves wide excision, debridement, and aggressive antibiotic coverage. Vascular reconstruction is best reserved for cases demonstrating limb-threatening ischemia. The reconstructions usually require more complicated, extra-anatomic bypass to avoid infection. Other vascular complications encountered in drug abusers include chemical arteritis, particulate embolization, and septic thrombophlebitis.

CHRONIC TRAUMATIC ARTERIOVENOUS FISTULAS

Traumatic arteriovenous fistulas generally result from penetrating injuries to contiguous arteries and veins. They may be associated with traumatic aneurysms and tend to occur in the extremities (Fig. 50-7, 50-8). Like traumatic aneurysms, however, they may appear anywhere in the body. The presenting symptoms depend on the size of the fistula. The patient may note a pulsating mass or a

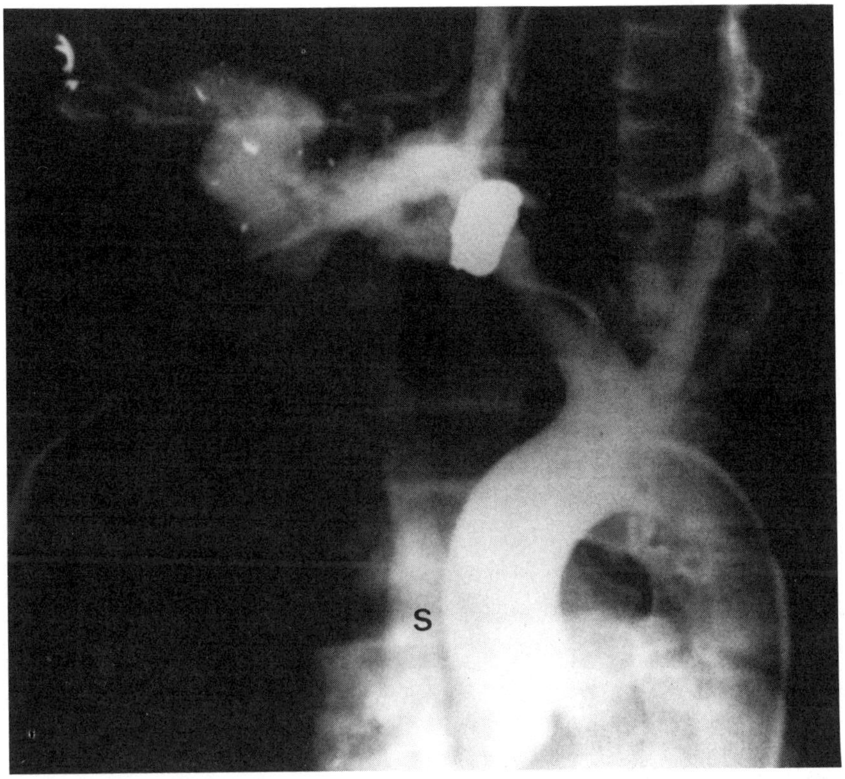

Fig. 50-7. A traumatic arteriovenous fistula of the right subclavian artery and vein caused by a gunshot wound. Note the prompt filling of the superior vena cava (S).

thrill in the region of previous penetrating trauma. Large extremity fistulas may have warmth of the overlying skin, which contrasts with distal coolness. There may be signs of venous hypertension, including varicosities, and chronic venous insufficiency. Large fistulas may impose significant hemodynamic stresses, leading to high-output cardiac failure.

The natural history of traumatic arteriovenous fistulas is gradual enlargement. The enlargement leads to increasingly severe hemodynamic, venous, and arterial insufficiency problems. Operative repair is therefore recommended in low-risk patients. Preoperative evaluation should include complete angiographic studies to assess the size and location of the fistula. In some cases, angiographic embolization may be sufficient to obliterate smaller distal fistulas. As with traumatic aneurysms, the type of repair depends on the location and size of the fistula. Small distal fistulas can be treated effectively by simple ligation of the involved artery and vein proximal and distal to the fistula. In general however, larger and more proximal fistula repair should include restoration of continuity of both the artery and the vein. Proximal and distal vascular control of both the artery and the vein are essential to safe, precise repair. Well-established fistulas may be divided and the artery and vein repaired. In most instances, however, a portion of the artery and vein is resected along with the fistula. If mobilization is satisfactory, the vessels can be repaired end to end, but often an interposition graft may be necessary. Successful repair generally leads to prompt hemodynamic and peripheral vascular improvement.

POSTTRAUMATIC PAIN SYMDROMES

Although poorly understood, the posttraumatic syndrome of causalgia is a well-recognized and difficult problem. Causalgia occurs in both the upper and the lower extremities following trauma. The trauma may or may not involve peripheral nerves. Although there are a variety of manifestations, the salient features include severe pain, sympathetic dysfunction, hyperhidrosis, delayed functional recovery, and trophic changes [64]. Burning pain occurs in the distal extremity and may be accompanied by a severe cutaneous dysesthesia. The sympathetic dysfunction may lead to either vasodilatation or vasoconstriction. Surgical sympathectomy is the most effective treatment of this disabling pain syndrome. Although most patients are relieved of their pain, many have some residual symptoms. A sympathetic nerve block may be useful in confirming the diagnosis and in predicting the response to surgical sympathectomy. Chemical sympathectomy following sympathetic-nerve block may be an alternative useful form of sympathetic ablation in some cases.

Specific Aspects of Diagnosis and Treatment

INJURIES OF THE HEART

Trauma to the heart may cause injury to the pericardium, free cardiac wall, cardiac septum, valves, or coronary ar-

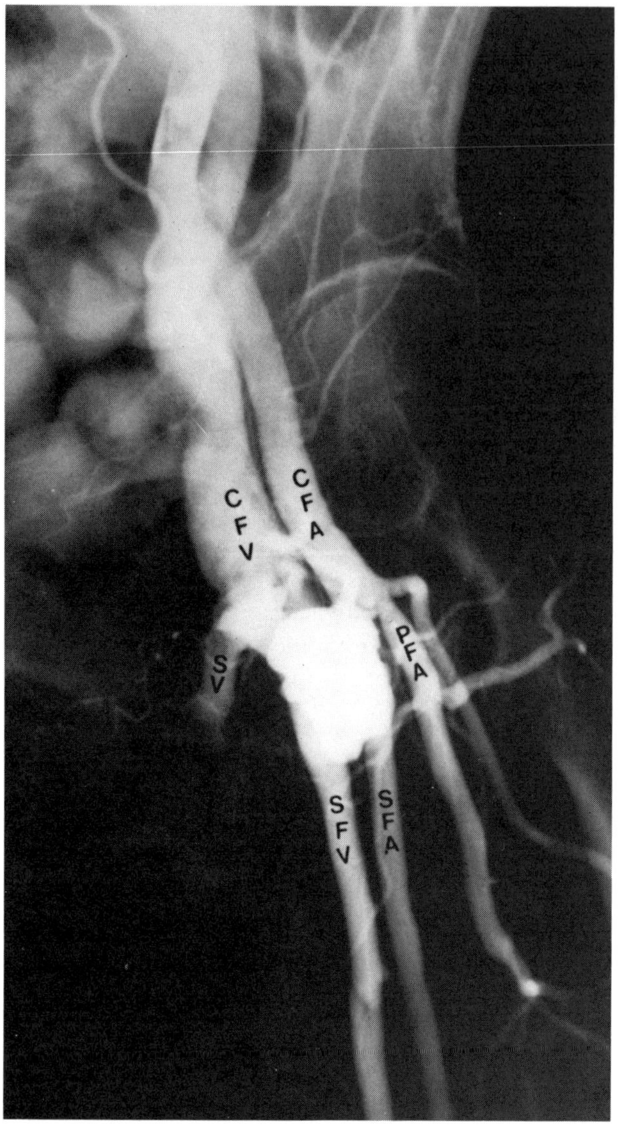

Fig. 50-8. Combined arteriovenous fistula and pseudoaneurysm secondary to stab wound to the groin. Note the early venous filling. (CFA = common femoral artery, PFA = profunda femoris artery, SFA = superficial femoral artery, CFV = common femoral vein, SFV = superficial femoral vein, SV = saphenous vein.)

teries. The right ventricle is the most frequently injured chamber, owing to its anterior presentation, followed by the left ventricle, the right atrium, and the left atrium. Penetrating wounds of the heart can be caused by missiles, knives, ribs, or sternal fragments. They are frequently seen with precordial injury but also may be associated with injury to the neck, lateral thorax, back, or abdomen. The clinical course and presentation following penetrating heart injuries depend on the size of the hole in the heart, the associated coronary and intracardiac injury, and whether the pericardium remains open or fills with clot. The various signs and symptoms that may accompany penetrating cardiac injury include hemothorax, hemoperitoneum, hemorrhage, or cardiac tamponade. The physical signs of cardiac tamponade may include hypotension, paradoxical pulse, narrow pulse pressure, a hypodynamic and rapid pulse, distant heart tones, and elevated central venous pressure (CVP). If cardiac tamponade is suspected, our preference is to perform an immediate thoracotomy. In the stable patient who is suspected of having a hemopericardium, a cardiac echo can be very helpful. We would emphasize that all precordial penetrating injuries occurring between the nipple lines laterally, the clavicles superiorly, and the epigastrium inferiorly should, until they are ruled out, be assumed to involve the heart. Furthermore, all gunshot injuries with entrance and exit wounds that, when connected by a straight line, cross the mediastinum should, until they are ruled out, be assumed to involve the heart. We have recently seen such an injury (entrance site in the left sixth intercostal space, midaxillary line, exit in right flank) that presented with no pneumothorax and no signs of tamponade but had a superficial wound of the apex of the right ventricle. Apparently, the bullet followed an extrapleural tract and entered the extrapleural mediastinum, penetrated the pericardium and the heart, then exited via the central tendon of the diaphragm. If hemothorax is present, a thoracostomy tube should be placed, and the collected blood can be autotransfused.

If anesthesia is required, the patient should be prepped and draped prior to induction of anesthesia. A median sternotomy incision is made. The pericardium is opened parallel to the phrenic nerves, and all intrapericardial blood is quickly evacuated. Bleeding from the heart, if present, is controlled digitally, and the heart is inspected for other injuries and to assess its performance. The cardiac wound then is repaired primarily, if possible. On rare occasions, an injury to the free wall cannot be repaired primarily, or an associated intracardiac injury might require cardiopulmonary bypass, with repair carried out with or without the use of a prosthesis.

Most intracardiac wounds are of such a magnitude that the patient does not survive the preoperative preparation and resuscitative stage. If a patient does make it to the operating room with an intracardiac injury, it usually is small enough to be managed surgically at a later date, following repair of the free cardiac wall injury and subsequent cardiac catheterization. Wounds of small, terminal branches of the coronary arteries are ligated, whereas all other wounds of the coronaries should be repaired by saphenous-vein bypass graft.

INJURIES OF THE NECK

Penetrating Trauma to Carotid Artery. The most common cause of carotid arterial injury is penetrating trauma, which may manifest with pulsatile hematomas, pulsatile bleeding, or carotid-artery thrombosis. Occasionally, blunt trauma to the head may result in carotid-jugular arteriovenous fistula. Depending on the details of the injury, various neurologic deficits may result from the injuries [65].

Blunt Trauma. Blunt trauma to the internal carotid artery often results in intimal tears in the distal internal carotid artery. The thrombosis that eventually occurs is especially difficult to treat because of its distal location, and neurologic deficits may be delayed in appearance. Patients with major head trauma may present with carotid cavernous fistulas, which are best treated by balloon occlusion of the fistula. Under ideal conditions, a balloon can be placed such that it occludes the fistula and still maintains patency of the internal carotid artery [66].

Zones of Injury. Patients with physical findings of injury in zone II of the neck (from the sternal notch to the angle of the mandible) [67] are best approached through an oblique cervical incision along the anterior border of the sternocleidomastoid muscle. Hemodynamically and neurologically stable patients with injury in zone I (below the sternal notch) or zone III (above the angle of the mandible) usually undergo arch aortography to diagnose or define the presence and location of injury in those anatomically complex areas. Injuries in zone I generally require a median sternotomy for adequate exposure and often require an extension of the incision obliquely into the neck, similar to the incision used for zone II. Zone III injuries are best approached by lateral mandibulotomy [68] or subluxation of the temporomandibular joint followed by the application of arch bars and intermaxillary wires or the simple application of a towel clip in the mandible to use as a retractor to maintain that position [69].

CAROTID-ARTERY LIGATION. The major clinical dilemma involving patients with injuries to the common or internal carotid artery is whether to ligate or repair the vessels of patients who have developed a major stroke or frank coma early after their injury. The classic argument against revascularization is that acute reperfusion of the ischemic brain converts an ischemic infarct into a hemorrhagic infarct. The documentation of the phenomenon, however, is seriously lacking. Autopsy studies of patients dying after acute reperfusion have demonstrated that cerebral edema (not hemorrhagic infarct) was the most common cause of death [70]. Our general approach to the dilemma is to repair the carotid artery if some prograde flow is present at the time of operative exploration and if the neurologic deficit is of short duration. When the neurologic deficit has been present for a long time (as is common after blunt trauma) or if the carotid artery is thrombosed and has no prograde flow, revascularization is probably of no benefit, and the carotid artery should be ligated to control bleeding [71]. Most injuries of the intracranial internal carotid artery can be treated nonoperatively, but all such injuries should be fully evaluated by a vascular surgeon, a neurosurgeon, and a neurologist [66].

EXTRACRANIAL-INTRACRANIAL BYPASS. On rare occasions, extracranial-intracranial (EC-IC) bypass may be beneficial after an injury to the distal carotid artery has required ligation and a neurologic deficit develops shortly thereafter [72].

Vertebral Artery. Vertebral-artery injuries are being seen with increasing frequency in recent years, probably because of the widespread availability of safe carotid angiography [73]. The first portion of the vertebral artery can be exposed easily through a supraclavicular incision. Exposure of the second portion (in the bony canal of the transverse vertebral processes) or the third portion (posterior to the atlas) is a difficult operative procedure [74]. If the contralateral vertebral artery is normal, and if no major branches to the spinal cord arise from the injured vertebral artery, ligation of the vertebral artery or placement of an occlusive balloon catheter at the site of injury is appropriate treatment.

Jugular Vein. Lateral venorrhaphy is preferred for repair of the simply injured jugular vein, but ligation usually is performed if a unilateral injury is extensive. A single internal jugular vein may be ligated with impunity, but if bilateral ligation is required, transient cerebral edema and airway problems may result. The internal jugular vein is exposed by a standard oblique cervical incision.

THORAX AND THORACIC OUTLET

Penetrating Injury. Penetrating wounds to the thoracic aorta are rarely seen clinically, since most patients exsanguinate before they arrive at the hospital emergency room. If a precordial wound is present and the patient is in shock or cardiac arrest, and if any report from witnesses at the scene or from the transport personnel suggests that the vital signs were at one time better than they are on arrival, then a left or bilateral anterolateral thoracotomy just below the nipple in the male or the retracted breasts in a female should be performed immediately. Wounds of the ascending or descending thoracic aorta often can be controlled with the application of partially occluding clamps in young trauma victims, but wounds of the transverse arch must be controlled with finger pressure while primary repair is undertaken.

TREATMENT. Occasionally, the patient with a penetrating wound to the thorax may present hemodynamically stable, with a hematoma or a "proximity" injury alone. In the patient with an expanding hematoma and hypotension, however, with or without an associated hemothorax, immediate thoracotomy is necessary. With an anterior stab wound, the ascending or transverse aortic arch is likely to be injured, and a median sternotomy can be considered if clamping of the descending thoracic aorta will not be necessary. For that reason, gunshot wounds, which may create posterior, descending thoracic perforations, are best approached through a bilateral anterolateral thoracotomy incision. In a stable patient with a small, nonexpanding hematoma or a proximity wound, retrograde arch aortography is indicated if it can be obtained expeditiously.

Blunt Injury

DIAGNOSIS. Blunt trauma to the thoracic aorta often occurs following deceleration injury in motor vehicle accidents and falls from heights. Even though 85 percent of patients with rupture of the thoracic aorta exsanguinate at the scene, the remaining 15 percent survive long enough to reach the hospital. Once in the hospital, the mortality of untreated patients is approximately 1 percent per hour; therefore, early diagnosis and treatment are mandatory [75,76]. The history, as previously noted, is often so suggestive that aortography is decided on even before a physical examination is performed. In unconscious patients, a deceleration accident coupled with the appearance of precordial contusions (especially the classic imprint of the hub of the steering wheel), strongly suggests the need for further emergent studies. In stable patients without vertebral or spinal cord injury, an anteroposterior chest x-ray is obtained while the patient is sitting up and leaning forward approximately 115 degrees, with the x-ray cassette placed behind the patient's chest (Ayella maneuver). Widening of the superior mediastinum or observation of the aortic knob on such a portable chest x-ray film in the emergency room confirms the need for immediate aortography [77]. It should be emphasized that routine, supine chest x-rays are inadequate for this type of evaluation. Other radiographic findings on the chest x-ray that suggest the need for aortography include fractures of the first or multiple ribs or sternum and fracture dislocation of lower thoracic vertebrae. Occasionally, findings such as a left apical cap, depression of the left main-stem bronchus, an associated left hemothorax, or deviation of a nasogastric tube to the right may help indicate the need for aortography. As with penetrating wounds, aortography is not indicated in hypotensive patients with marked widening of the superior mediastinum; those patients require emergent operative intervention.

LOCATION OF THE INJURY. Retrograde femoral aortography can be safely performed by an experienced angiographer, even when complete disruption of the descending thoracic aorta is present. Aortography avoids unnecessary thoracotomy in patients with mediastinal widening from venous bleeding and no aortic injury. When an aortogram is positive, it localizes the site of injury or even the presence of a second tear in the aorta. The most common site of injury is in the descending thoracic aorta at the insertion of the ligamentum arteriosum just distal to the left subclavian artery (Fig. 50-9). In patients who have fallen from a height, the tear may occur in the ascending aorta above the cusp of the aortic valve. On rare occasions, the aortic tear is in the distal descending thoracic aorta adjacent to a fracture or dislocation in the lower thoracic spine.

TREATMENT. The classic tear in the proximal descending thoracic aorta is approached through a left posterolateral thoracotomy at the fourth intercostal space after the insertion of a double-lumen endobronchial tube. Techniques of repair include (1) simple cross-clamping of the aorta ("clamp/repair") without shunt or bypass; (2) left-sided heart or aortic bypass using heparin-bonded shunts or external pumps and systemic heparinization; and (3) partial or complete cardiopulmonary bypass using an oxygenator and systemic heparinization. These techniques have been retrospectively compared in innumerable articles, usually with regard to operative mortality and postoperative paraplegia. A recent report from the Ben Taub General Hospital (Houston, Texas) summarizes many of those journal articles and emphasizes the preferred approach of clamp/repair [78]. Another recent report has emphasized the monitoring of somatosensory-evoked potentials and distal aortic pressure in preventing ischemic damage to the spinal cord, but the practical role of those measurements remains unclear [79].

Once proximal and distal control have been obtained, the aortic hematoma is opened. The adventitia may be intact at the site of the tear (60%), or all three aortic layers may be disrupted (40%). Repair is usually by insertion of a woven Dacron graft, although primary repair occasionally is possible. Mortality with clamp/repair or shunt techniques is 10 to 15 percent, and postoperative paraplegia rates range from 8 to 10 percent.

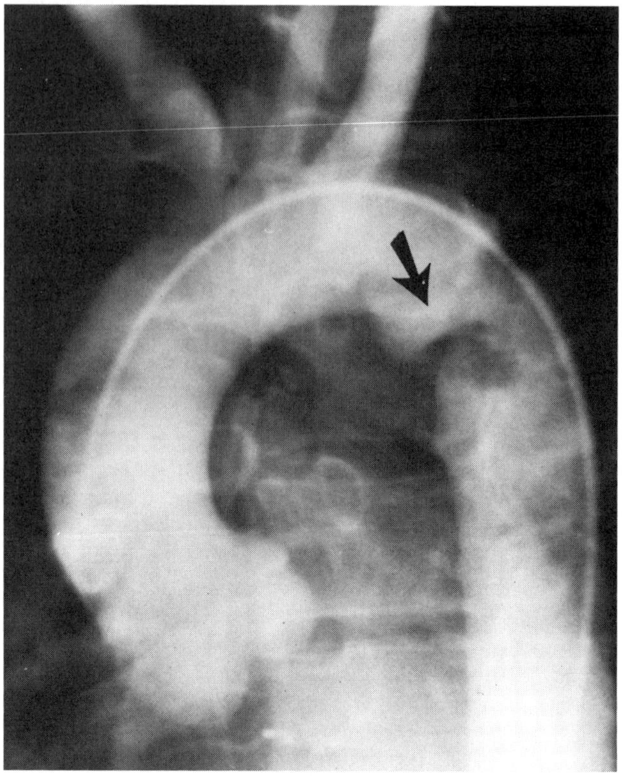

Fig. 50-9. An example of blunt chest trauma and rapid deceleration causing a shearing force in the thoracic aorta just distal to the left subclavian artery, where the aorta is fixed by the attachment of the ligamentum arteriosum.

INNOMINATE, COMMON CAROTID, AND SUBCLAVIAN ARTERIES

Patients with penetrating wounds to the innominate, common carotid, and subclavian arteries present in a manner similar to that described concerning penetrating wounds to the thoracic aorta; that is, they are either profoundly hypotensive and may require an emergency room thoracotomy, or they are stable enough to be transported to the operating room or to an angiographic suite. In patients with exsanguinating hemorrhage into the ipsilateral pleural cavity from an injury to the subclavian artery, a high anterolateral thoracotomy with transpleural apical packing on the right or clamping of the intrapleural proximal left subclavian artery may be life-saving.

Blunt Trauma. Blunt trauma to the subclavian and common carotid arteries is rare, but blunt disruption of the innominate artery at the origin of the aortic arch is not rare in trauma centers where victims of deceleration injury commonly are seen. Many of these individuals have a peculiar "pointed" appearance to the right side of the widened superior mediastinum.

OPERATIVE MANAGEMENT. In the operating room, a median sternotomy followed by mobilization of the left innominate vein allows for adequate exposure of the proximal innominate artery and left common carotid artery (as well as the superior vena cava). A right cervical or supraclavicular extension with or without resection of the clavicle allows for proximal exposure of the right common carotid or right subclavian artery, respectively. The same extensions on the left allow for distal exposure of the left common carotid artery or the second and third portions of the left subclavian artery, respectively. The intrapleural proximal left subclavian artery, which is rarely injured, is approached through a left anterolateral thoracotomy in the third intercostal space.

PERFUSION DURING REPAIR. A variety of techniques, including cardiopulmonary bypass, moderate or profound hypothermia, and shunts for perfusion of the right common carotid artery, have been utilized in the past for repair of injuries to the innominate artery [80]. In the absence of profound intraoperative hypotension or the need to simultaneously occlude the left common carotid artery and the innominate artery, none of these adjuncts is necessary in the young trauma patient. When those conditions are present, however, an internal shunt for carotid perfusion should be considered. In the patient with a blunt tear to the innominate artery at its origin, an 8- to 12-mm prosthetic graft generally is sewn to the side of the ascending aorta prior to entering the hematoma. Once proximal and distal control of the injured vessel have been obtained, the injured segment is resected, the origin of the innominate artery is oversewn, and the prosthetic graft is sewn to the distal innominate artery proximal to its bifurcation.

EXPOSURE OF THORACIC (NONMEDIASTINAL) INJURIES. Exposure for injuries to the second and third nonmediastinal portion of either subclavian artery is enhanced by resection of the clavicle through the supraclavicular incision [81]. Resection or division can be performed in a subperiosteal plane if time is available, or the clavicle simply can be divided completely. If the latter approach is chosen, great care must be taken to avoid injury to the underlying and adherent subclavian vein. No morbidity results from resection of the clavicle. If division only is used, the clavicle can be approximated using either a dynamic compression plate or Kirschner wires.

RESULTS. In series in which penetrating wounds predominated, a survival rate of 85 to 95 percent can be expected with wounds to the innominate or subclavian arteries when the patient has not suffered a cardiac arrest either in the field or shortly after arrival in the emergency center [82,83].

UPPER EXTREMITY

Axillary-Artery Injuries. Axillary-artery injuries frequently are associated with benign-appearing wounds when first seen clinically. Associated brachial- or subclavian-vessel injuries (or both) (34%) and concomitant brachial-plexus injuries (35%) have been noted in recent civilian series [84], the latter accounting for the majority of the long-term morbidity. Progressive signs of brachial-plexus injury by an adjacent hematoma is the most common indication for exploration of axillary-artery injuries in stable patients who do not have rapidly expanding hematomas (Fig. 50-10). Preservation of collateral vessels is essential in operative exposure and repair. The approach to the axillary artery is made via an infraclavicular incision that easily can be extended down the medial aspect of the arm if exposure of the brachial artery is needed. The axillary artery then is exposed by separation of the pectoralis-major muscle fibers and lateral retraction of the pectoralis-minor tendon. Interposition bypass grafting with 6- or 8-mm expanded PTFE is the most commonly used means of repair. However, the details of the type of injury, its location, associated findings, and the general condition of the patient might suggest another type of treatment.

Brachial-Artery Injuries. Like axillary injuries, the major morbidity of brachial-artery injuries arises primarily from associated nerve and soft-tissue injury [85]. Almost half of patients who present with major nerve injury will have neurologically dysfunctional limbs after long-term follow-up. Associated fractures in the arm usually are repaired prior to vascular repair. Most brachial-artery injuries can be successfully repaired by primary repair, with interposition grafting reserved for cases with extensive loss of arterial tissue. Ligation of the brachial artery may lead to amputation in approximately 35 percent of the cases [86].

Radial- and Ulnar-Artery Injuries. Although there is general agreement that all major brachial-artery injuries should be repaired, reconstruction of minor arteries (brachial profunda, radial, and ulnar) is felt by some investigators to be warranted only in cases of complete or nearly complete severance of the upper extremity, when signs of severe ischemia are present, or when both the radial and ulnar arteries are injured [2,87]. Johnson and associates [88] reported that the patency following repair of radial and ulnar arteries was approximately 50 percent. Later hand symptoms, if they developed, related to nerve or tendon damage but not to arterial patency. The authors' recommendation was that, in the absence of acute hand ischemia, ligation of the radial or ulnar artery was appropriate. Smith and co-workers demonstrated that no postoperative functional deficit occurred after ligation of most upper-extremity injuries, including brachial arteries [87]. Nevertheless, given the current state of the art, it seems reasonable to attempt repair of injured forearm vessels to obtain the best possible result, as long as the patient's general condition permits.

ABDOMINAL VASCULAR INJURIES

Penetrating Injuries. Patients with penetrating abdominal vascular injuries often present with exsanguinating hemorrhage or contained hematomas [89]. The sequence of vascular repair versus repair of the bowel is determined by the presentation. All intra-abdominal hematomas, including supramesocolic, inframesocolic, perirenal, pelvic, portal, and mesenteric, are opened in cases of penetrating trauma.

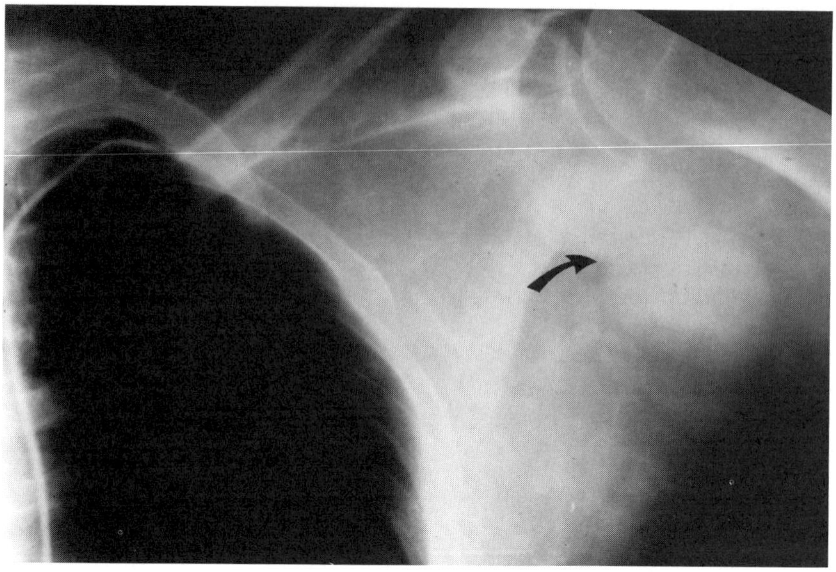

Fig. 50-10. This patient presented with signs of a brachial plexus injury. Three months previously he had a stab wound to the axilla with no clinical findings of a vascular injury. Note the large pseudoaneurysm of the axillary artery (arrow).

Blunt Trauma. Patients who have suffered blunt trauma occasionally hemorrhage from avulsed mesenteric vessels, partially avulsed renal veins, or other pelvic vessels associated with adjacent fractures. Direct injury to the abdominal aorta from blunt trauma is reported, although it is a relatively unusual occurrence [90]. After blunt injury, midline supramesocolic, inframesocolic, portal, and mesenteric hematomas are opened. In the presence of a normal preoperative intravenous pyelogram or CT of the kidney, lateral perirenal hematomas are not ordinarily opened in this group of patients. When pelvic hematomas from fractures are not rapidly expanding at the time of celiotomy, they too are not ordinarily opened.

MANAGEMENT OF SPECIFIC INJURIES

Supramesocolic Hematoma. A midline supramesocolic hematoma or active hemorrhage from that area generally is best approached laterally, unless the site of hemorrhage can be easily visualized in the lesser sac. If hemorrhage is rapid, an aortic-compression device or an assistant's hand can be used to occlude the aorta at the diaphragmatic hiatus prior to formal dissection and clamping. The left colon, left kidney, spleen, tail of the pancreas, and gastric fundus are then rapidly mobilized past the midline by a combination of sharp and blunt dissection. Occasionally, a partial left radial phrenotomy further improves the exposure. Once the aorta is palpated and exposed, a long DeBakey aortic clamp is used to occlude it. Dissection then proceeds distally so that the actual bleeding site in the aorta or one of the visceral branches is exposed and distal vascular control obtained.

Inframesocolic Hematoma. The inframesocolic hematoma or active hemorrhage from that area is best approached directly in the midline just below the mesocolon, just as one would approach an infrarenal abdominal aortic aneurysm.

Direct Aortic Injury. Stab wounds or small-caliber gunshot wounds of the abdominal aorta can be repaired with a running suture of 4-0 or 5-0 polypropylene. If excessive narrowing results, a patch aortoplasty utilizing expanded PTFE can then be performed to improve blood flow. When the aorta suffers extensive destruction, as can occur in seatbelt-associated blunt abdominal aortic trauma [91], an appropriately sized prosthetic interposition graft is inserted. Extensive experience with aortic prostheses in the face of enteric or fecal contamination from penetrating wounds has clearly demonstrated that this is, surprisingly, a relatively safe approach [92,93].

Celiac-Artery Injury. Unless a small injury is present at the origin of the celiac axis, we typically ligate this vessel, since little morbidity results in young trauma patients due to a generous collateral circulation via the superior mesenteric artery.

Injury to Superior Mesenteric Artery. Extensive wounds requiring ligation of the superior mesenteric artery at its origin or distal to the midcolic artery or inferior pancreaticoduodenal artery lead to ischemia of the entire midgut. Retrograde bypass grafting from the distal infrarenal abdominal aorta to the superior mesenteric artery will be necessary if such a patient is to survive [94].

Renal-Artery Injury. When life-threatening hemorrhage necessitates ligation of the renal artery, a nephrectomy should be performed. On rare occasions in stable patients with penetrating renal-artery injury, bypass grafting from the infrarenal abdominal aorta to the distal renal artery may be justified. When renal-artery thrombosis secondary to an intimal contusion from blunt trauma is recognized soon after it occurs, resection of the renal artery with an end-to-end anastomosis is preferred [95,96]. As soon as the abdomen is entered, the affected kidney is packed in ice and flushed with cold Collins solution. If the warm ischemia time is longer than 6 hours, nephrectomy is preferred.

Exposure of Inferior Vena Cava and Its Visceral Branches. The infrahepatic inferior vena cava and both renal veins may be exposed by mobilizing the right colon and hepatic flexure past the midline and performing a Kocher maneuver. The retrohepatic vena cava is exposed, dividing the triangular and anterior and posterior coronary ligaments of the hepatic lobe and mobilizing the lobe to the midline.

Control of the Infrarenal Vena Cava. Vascular control of the infrarenal vena cava usually can be obtained by applying sponge sticks or vascular clamps both proximally and distally around the perforations. With injuries at the level of the renal veins, both renal veins should be encircled with Silastic vessel loops and clamped, and the vena cava should be controlled below that level and as it passes beneath the liver.

Injury to Retrohepatic Vena Cava. The rare injury to the retrohepatic vena cava can be approached in several ways. In the hemodynamically stable patient, simultaneous cross-clamping of the portal triad, suprahepatic (intra-abdominal) vena cava, and suprarenal vena cava (below the liver) occasionally may slow bleeding enough to allow for the placement of sutures [97]. If that maneuver fails or if the patient is unstable, a sternotomy incision is added to the celiotomy incision and an atriocaval shunt is placed. Umbilical tape tourniquets around the vena cava are pulled tight on the shunt, thus excluding the area of injury and allowing direct repair [98]. Occasionally, in the patient with an extensive hepatic injury, a deep hepatotomy without the aid of a shunt may be used to approach the perforation directly [99].

Repair of Major Venous Injuries. The vena cava is repaired using a running suture of 4-0 or 5-0 polypropylene. Extensive infrarenal injuries can be ligated as long as the patient's lower extremities are tightly wrapped and elevated for the first 1 to 2 weeks after operation. Extensive suprarenal injuries below the liver should be treated by patch venoplasty or the insertion of an externally supported PTFE conduit of appropriate size. The right renal vein and left renal vein near the left kidney are repaired by lateral venorrhaphy, and the left renal vein at the midline can be ligated.

Exposure and Control of Iliac Vessels. Injuries to the iliac arteries and veins present with lateral pelvic hemorrhage or hematomas. Proximal vascular control is obtained by exposing the infrarenal abdominal aorta and vena cava in the midline. Distal control is obtained by dividing the peritoneum over the external iliac vessels just proximal to the inguinal ligament as the vessels come out of the pelvis. Full exposure of the right iliac vessels usually necessitates mobilization of the cecum and right colon. On the left, the sigmoid colon must be mobilized for complete exposure.

Repair Versus Ligation. Destructive injuries to the common or external iliac arteries in the presence of extensive enteric or fecal contamination are best treated by ligation rather than insertion of a vascular conduit, because infection and blowout may occur. In such a patient, a fasciotomy in the ipsilateral leg probably is necessary. The extremity may develop significant ischemia, requiring an extra-anatomic crossover femorofemoral graft. Extensive injuries to the internal iliac vessels or iliac veins should be ligated. Appropriate precautions, such as extremity elevation and wrapping, must be taken in the postoperative period [100].

LOWER-EXTREMITY INJURIES

Techniques of exposure and basic principles of repair are well described in other publications [8,101] and previously in this chapter. Careful handling of small vessels; use of small vascular clamps, bulldog clamps, and vascular loops; and an open anastomosis technique are keys to the successful completion of an end-to-end anastomosis or insertion of a vascular conduit in an extremity [12]. Distal clot always should be removed with an embolectomy catheter once vascular control has been achieved. Regional heparin then should be injected to prevent thrombosis of distal collateral vessels during the period of vascular occlusion. Completion arteriography is mandatory. Postoperative care includes the use of intravenous antibiotics, monitoring of arterial pulses, wound assessment, and elevation and wrapping for all major venous ligations.

Common and Profunda Femoral Artery. Common femoral and profunda femoris arterial injuries often can be repaired primarily, although interposition bypass grafting or patch angioplasty with autogenous or prosthetic material also is frequently employed. During World War II, ligation of injuries to the common femoral artery carried an 81-percent amputation rate [1]; therefore, we attempt to repair all common-femoral-artery injuries unless operative repair seems to jeopardize the patient's life. Ligation of distal branches of the profunda femoris artery can be performed safely. The approach to the common and proximal profunda femoris artery is made via a standard vertical groin incision, exactly like that used for elective femoral-popliteal reconstructive procedures. The incision easily can be extended proximally for retroperitoneal exposure of the iliac system, if necessary.

Superficial Femoral Artery. The proximal superficial femoral artery can be exposed through the vertical groin incision described previously. For injuries in the more distal aspects of the femoral artery, an appropriately positioned incision can be made on the medial aspect of the thigh, reflecting the sartorius muscle laterally. Associated femoral venous trauma should be repaired if the patient is stable. The seminal work by Rich and associates from the Vietnam Vascular Registry [102] and the clinical [103] and experimental [104] observations of Hobson and colleagues have made repair of concomitant venous injuries the standard of good surgical care.

Popliteal Artery. Injury to the popliteal artery carries the highest amputation rate of all arterial injuries to the lower extremity. Some recent civilian series have reported amputation rates as high as 42 percent [105]. Blunt injury to the knee with resultant popliteal artery injury is an especially difficult problem to manage. Blunt injury sufficient enough to disrupt the stabilization of the knee often causes direct injury to the popliteal artery. Diagnosis and management of those injuries is difficult and likewise have a high amputation rate [106]. The relatively high failure rate with popliteal-artery injuries results from the popliteal artery being smaller and therefore technically harder to repair than the more proximal vessels. The vessel also does not have the collateral supply of the tibial vessels and is functionally an "end artery" to the lower leg.

The approach to the popliteal artery can be through a standard incision in the medial aspect of the knee or through a posterior approach, making a horizontal S-shaped incision through the popliteal space, with the horizontal portion of the incision parallel to the skin crease in the knee. If the injury is isolated to the popliteal artery (as it often is), a pneumatic tourniquet placed around the midthigh can be life-saving because it allows immediate proximal control during the prepping, draping, and surgical exposure of the artery.

Associated venous injury is common in popliteal-artery injury, and on occasion, an isolated popliteal venous injury is encountered during exploration of the injured knee for other reasons. As with femoral venous injuries, we routinely repair all popliteal venous injuries for the reason outlined above. The postoperative patency of repaired veins in the extremities can be improved with the use of intermittent pneumatic compression devices applied distally, because such devices increase the rate of blood flow across the venous repair site and prevent stagnation, with its attendant thrombosis [48].

Tibial and Peroneal Artery. Injuries to the tibial or peroneal arteries (collectively referred to as the tibial arteries) present a special problem because in most cases they do not cause severe ischemia unless two of the three vessels are interrupted. Arteriographic survey of these patients is essential to determine if indeed there is a significant problem. That is especially true in a patient who has multiple wounds as the result of a shotgun blast. In a patient who has penetrating trauma to the lower leg resulting in occlusion of one tibial artery without bleeding or open fracture, the injury can be accepted without arterial repair. Such patients should be observed with serial circulatory assessment rather than direct operation. Surgical exploration of a single tibial artery injury customarily is performed only if the artery is bleeding or if an arteriovenous fistula or false aneurysm is seen on the arteriogram. In contrast, patients with injuries of two tibial arteries should have one of those vessels repaired to ensure adequate function of the extremity [107–109]. We have on occasion accepted only one patent tibial artery with no adverse effects. A recent article by Padberg et al. [110] reports that ischemic symptoms were worse in blunt tibial injuries when compared with penetrating tibial injuries. In patients with a single arterial injury, a plan of observation or ligation resulted in no amputations. Some patients with two tibial vessels injured did not have ischemic complications except if the single remaining tibial vessel was the peroneal artery. The authors' recommendation based on their experience is that if the only remaining tibial vessel is the peroneal artery, then one of the other tibial vessels should be repaired.

IATROGENIC VASCULAR INJURIES

As diagnostic and therapeutic techniques have become more advanced and invasive, the incidence of iatrogenic complications has increased. The nature of invasive procedures places the vascular system at high risk for iatrogenic injury. The injuries sustained in that setting often are less dramatic than those suffered in penetrating or blunt injuries and therefore are underemphasized in the surgical literature. Many early reports of the vascular-trauma experience from large centers fail even to mention iatrogenic injuries [49,111]. Unfortunately, the compromised health of patients undergoing diagnostic or therapeutic invasive procedures makes them ill suited to contend with hemorrhagic, thrombotic, and embolic iatrogenic complications.

Operations for iatrogenic vascular complications constitute 10 to 29 percent of all surgery for civilian vascular trauma [112]. Ninety percent of those operations are for arterial trauma, whereas 10 percent are for venous injuries [113]. The experience with surgery for iatrogenic vascular injuries at the Walter Reed Army Medical Center has been extensively reviewed [113,114]. The reports find that approximately 30 percent of such injuries are related to cardiac catheterization; 30 percent to angiography, including percutaneous transluminal angioplasty (PTA); 30 percent to various surgical complications, including injuries secondary to intra-aortic balloon counterpulsation; and 10 percent to miscellaneous procedures (central venous, arterial, and pulmonary arterial catheter complications). Since many of the vascular complications of the miscellaneous procedures do not require surgical intervention, their incidence is underestimated.

The most common iatrogenically injured artery is the femoral artery (42%), followed by the brachial (17%), axillary (14%), and iliac arteries (11%) and the aorta (4%). Most injuries can be repaired by vascular suture or simple thrombectomy, but approximately 20 percent require complex vascular reconstruction [113,114].

The most important factor in limiting mortality and morbidity of iatrogenic vascular injuries is prompt recognition and treatment. In one series, a delay in repair of an iatrogenic vascular injury was an important factor in six of eight permanent functional disabilities and three of four amputations [115]. Other important factors include attention to details of technique, judicious management of anticoagulants, a sound knowledge of anatomy, and a recognition of when the risks of continued intervention outweigh the benefits.

Vascular Complications of Angiography. Angiography has become a standard diagnostic modality that is available in nearly every general and tertiary-care hospital. Its broad application has resulted in a significant amount of iatrogenic vascular injury. Hessel and associates conducted a national survey of hospitals to determine the incidence of angiography-related complications [116]. They found that the incidence of complications, including vascular injuries, was highly dependent on the site of cannulation. The more common transfemoral approach had a 1.73-percent incidence of complications, whereas the translumbar and the transaxillary routes had a 2.89- and 3.29-percent incidence, respectively. There were 30 deaths out of 118,591 examinations. At least 10 of those deaths were related to vascular injuries, including aortic dissection or aneurysm rupture (eight cases), aortic occlusion (one case), and bowel infarction (one case). An inverse relationship was found between the complication rate and the annual number of arteriograms performed.

The major types of arterial injuries are related to vessel cannulation and guidewire manipulation. Those injuries include (in descending order) vessel perforation and hemorrhage, thrombosis, embolism, pseudoaneurysm formation, arterial dissection, and arteriovenous fistula. Special problems with the axillary approach are well recognized and are related to the location, small size, and relative mobility of that artery. These factors make hemostasis difficult and predispose to brachial plexus–compression injuries as well as cerebral emboli [9,117].

Catheter-induced vessel thrombosis is influenced by the relationship of catheter size to the vessel being cannulated. That factor explains the relatively high incidence of thrombosis in the axillary artery and in children who are subjected to angiography [118].

The risks of cerebral angiography warrant special consideration. The risk of neurologic deficits is approximately 1 percent with the transfemoral approach [116,119]. The majority of those deficits are transient, however, with the incidence of completed stroke being somewhat lower. Cerebral emboli account for the majority of neurologic events. Neurotoxic effects of contrast agents, however, may play a role in some cases.

Iatrogenic complications of coronary angiography can be a source of significant morbidity and mortality. As with peripheral angiography, the rate of complications seems to vary with the cannulation site. The reported incidence of myocardial infarction, cerebrovascular accidents, and death varies, with some studies showing the superiority of the transfemoral route and others demonstrating the superiority of the transbrachial route [120,121]. As with peripheral angiography, however, the incidence of peripheral vascular complications is higher when the transbrachial route is employed [122]. In the Coronary Artery Surgery Study, the complications of 7,551 coronary angiograms were reviewed [121]. The rates of arterial embolization, thrombosis, and dissection were each higher for the transbrachial route, and the overall vascular complication rate was 2.85 percent versus 0.45 percent for the transfemoral route. The brachial-artery route has been found to be especially dangerous in women undergoing coronary angiography [122]. One study demonstrated a relative risk of a vascular complication of 11.6 for females compared to males with this approach [123]. Patients undergoing coronary angiography often are highly compromised. Fortunately, the brachial artery often has excellent collateral flow, and observation may be warranted after brachial-artery thrombosis when the hand is not compromised [124].

Vascular complications appear to occur more frequently when coronary angioplasty is performed [125]. The most frequent complications of diagnostic angiography are the development of false aneurysms and arteriovenous fistulas. The management of those two specific injuries is the subject of some debate. It may be that small arteriovenous fistulas and small pseudoaneurysms may resolve on their own. The question of which can be observed and which will require repair is as of yet unresolved. It is apparent that a number of these types of vascular injuries will resolve [126–129]. Management of false aneurysms and arteriovenous fistulas can be treated with ultrasound-guided compression repair. Ultrasonography is used to identify the neck of the false aneurysm or the arteriovenous fistula, then a downward compression is applied with the transducer until flow in the false aneurysm or arteriovenous fistula is eliminated. Some potential problems of this approach are discomfort associated with the compression and the possibility of thrombosis of the compressed vessel. The utilization of this modality has been reported by various authors and with variable success rates [128,130,131].

Peripheral venous angiography generally does not carry the same risk of major hemorrhage and peripheral embolization that arterial studies do. Postvenography venous thrombosis is a major concern, however, and thrombosis rates as high as 26 percent have been reported [132]. Another uncommon but significant problem is contrast-induced thrombophlebitis, which has occurred in 0.7 percent of studies [116].

Percutaneous Transluminal Balloon and Laser Angioplasty. Percutaneous transluminal angioplasty (PTA) of the iliac, femoral, and popliteal arteries has gained widespread acceptance. That acceptance may be attributed to several factors, including an acceptable safety record, cost effectiveness, and initial results comparable to those of reconstructive surgery. Nonetheless, overall complication rates ranging between 2 and 25 percent have been reported, with many of those complications representing vascular injuries. Weibull and associates collectively reviewed the literature to determine the complication rate of PTA [133]. In 2,043 percutaneous angioplasties, there was an 8.6-percent overall complication rate. Vascular complications requiring surgical intervention included distal embolization (2.0%), vessel thrombosis (1.8%), groin hematoma (0.25%), retroperitoneal hemorrhage (0.1%), pseudoaneurysm (0.1%), and intimal injury (0.1%). Other complications that did not require surgery included groin hematoma (2.0%), subintimal dissection (0.75%) guidewire perforation of the vessel (0.25%), and arteriovenous fistula (0.25%). The incidence of complications was inversely related to the angiographer's experience.

A report of 4,988 coronary PTA procedures revealed a

complication rate of 1 percent. Pseudoaneurysm was the most frequent complication, followed by arteriovenous fistula and hemorrhage at the puncture site. Age, female gender, thrombolytic therapy, and anticoagulation correlated with the risk of complications [134].

Recently, significant enthusiasm has been generated for the use of lasers, both alone and in combination with balloon angioplasty, for the management of atherosclerotic occlusive disease. These techniques are subject not only to the risks of vessel cannulation but also to the additional risk of laser-induced vessel perforation. That problem has been fairly common in series where laser energy is applied directly to the plaque. Ginsburg and associates, for example, had three perforations in 16 cases using a bare-tipped argon laser [135]. More recently, a metal-tipped laser probe has been employed to vaporize plaque with thermal energy. Early results at our institution with that approach showed an 83-percent clinical success rate and no perforations in 13 patients [136]. Subsequent procedures in patients with limb-threatening ischemia did result in some perforation and puncture-site hematomas [137]. When perforations and puncture-site hematomas do occur, they generally are manageable with external compression and cause minimal clinical sequelae in previously occluded vessels.

Vascular Complications of Surgical Procedures. Complications of surgical procedures constitute approximately 30 percent of iatrogenic vascular injuries [113,114]. Because of the wide variety of surgical operations, such injuries have involved nearly every artery in every imaginable location. The wide range of potential injuries has been reflected in numerous case reports as well as in large surgical series of iatrogenic vascular injuries [138]. Furthermore, the complications have occurred in nearly every surgical discipline, including general surgery, orthopedics, urology, neurosurgery, obstetrics, and gynecology.

Despite the wide variety of complications, several interesting generalizations can be drawn. Youkey and associates, for example, found that 4 of 6 gynecologic complications, 10 of 11 urologic complications, and the single general-surgery vascular complication in their series all occurred during difficult dissections for retroperitoneal tumor [114]. The radical nature of those operations, the proximity of major vessels, and the disruption of normal anatomic planes by tumor all contributed to the injuries.

Other well-described vascular injuries include iliac-artery and -vein injury during lumbar-disk surgery, vascular injury during trocar insertion for laparoscopy, inadvertent arterial injury during venous stripping, iliofemoral injuries related to cardiac bypass, and femoral artery and vein injuries with inguinal hernia repair [113,114,138,139].

A variety of vascular injuries have been reported with orthopedic surgery, including direct vascular trauma related to open reduction and internal fixation, total joint arthroplasty, and acute compartment syndromes induced by constricting casts.

Complications of Intra-aortic Balloon Counterpulsation. The insertion and operation of intra-aortic balloon pumps (IABP) are a major source of surgically induced iatrogenic vascular injury. These injuries accounted for 15 percent of all iatrogenic vascular injuries in one series, and complication rates as high as 36 percent have been reported [112,140]. The 8.8-percent vascular complication rate noted by Perler and associates in their series is more typical [141]. Those complications included ischemic injuries (4.5%), arterial injury (2.5%), and hemorrhagic complications (0.9%), as well as septic complications. The limb ischemia was due to either thromboembolism or arterial obstruction by the large intraluminal balloon catheter. That usually necessitated movement of the balloon to the contralateral leg, embolectomy of the femoral vessel, or both. In a series of 1,454 patients treated with intra-aortic balloon counterpulsation, Friedell and associates report the use of femorofemoral crossover grafting to treat limb-threatening ischemia in 80 (5%) patients [142]. The arterial injuries included both local injuries at the insertion site and dissection of the iliac arteries and the aorta. The local injuries were easily managed with simple repair. The arterial dissections were devastating, however, with five of six patients dying from bowel infarction or aortic occlusion. Complications appear to correlate with a history of peripheral vascular disease, diabetes, and female gender [143,144]. A recent report by Barnett [145] on vascular complications in 72 patients shows that a history of peripheral vascular disease, female gender, history of cigarette smoking, and postoperative insertion were independent predictors of vascular complications. However, the most risk for vascular complications could not be explained by those factors alone. There appear to be conflicting reports on the complication rates comparing operative and percutaneous placement of IABPs, with Iverson et al. reporting a decrease in the complication rate with the percutaneous approach [146] and Gottlieb et al. reporting a bigger complication rate with the percutaneous technique [143]. The recent report by Barnett showed no difference in complication rate when comparing percutaneous placement and open techniques for the placement of IABP. There are several important factors in the prevention of IABP complications. Most important is careful selection of the insertion site based on physical examination and, if necessary, preinsertion angiography. Selection of the appropriate size of balloon catheter, careful insertion, and movement to the contralateral side when the balloon does not pass easily are other important factors. Recent studies show that the overall incidence of vascular complications related to IABP have not changed and that the severity of the complications has decreased [145].

Vascular Complications of Invasive Monitoring. Sophisticated hemodynamic monitoring techniques have had a major impact in complementing the clinician's surveillance techniques. Unfortunately, the invasive nature of these techniques has resulted in a variety of complications, including iatrogenic vascular injuries.

One of the more common invasive procedures performed is central-vein cannulation. (In addition to hemodynamic monitoring, this technique is useful for a variety of purposes, including fluid resuscitation, parenteral nutrition, and hemodialysis access.) A wide variety of complications have been reported with both the subclavian and internal jugular approach. The major vascular complications are arterial puncture of the carotid or subclavian vessels, which occur in 3.3 to 6.7 percent of cases, depending on the experience of the physician and the condition of the patient [147]. Those injuries may result in significant hematomas as well as hemothoraces. Hemorrhage from the subclavian artery is particularly troublesome, because it cannot be directly tamponaded. Other complications of central venous lines include catheter-induced venous thrombosis and catheter embolization. Venous thrombosis has been reported in 6 percent of central venous cannulations and may result in pulmonary emboli [148].

Flow-directed pulmonary artery catheterization is subject to the same complications as central venous cannulation as well as several additional vascular injuries. One of the most serious of those is catheter-induced pulmonary-artery perforation, which occurred in 4 of 6,245 cases in one large series [149]. Barash and associates reviewed six such cases and identified pulmonary hypertension, anticoagulation, and hypothermia as significant risk factors [150]. The major causes identified included catheter-tip erosion through the pulmonary artery, eccentric balloon inflation, and balloon overinflation. The authors stress several factors in preventing those complications, including avoidance of overinsertion of the catheter, avoidance of overinflating the balloon, and a reliance on pulmonary artery diastolic pressures whenever possible.

Another important vascular complication of pulmonary-artery catheterization is pulmonary infarction, resulting when the balloon remains inflated or the catheter floats into the wedged position [151]. Other more unusual complications include cardiac-valve and -wall damage and intravascular knotting of the catheter [152].

Indwelling arterial catheters allow continuous monitoring of blood pressure and facilitate frequent blood sampling. In most instances, the radial artery is the site of choice. The major risk associated with radial-artery cannulation is radial-artery thrombosis with secondary vascular insufficiency of the hand and digits [153]. Fortunately, although radial-artery thrombosis is common, ischemic damage is rather unusual. In a series of 1,699 consecutive short-term percutaneous radial-artery cannulations, Slogoff and colleagues found that the radial artery was occluded or partially occluded in 25 percent of cases [154]. Despite that finding, no ischemic damage or hand disability occurred in any patient. It is generally held that documentation of collateral flow from the ulnar artery with an Allen test is an important factor in preventing ischemic complications. The authors, however, did not find the Allen test to be a useful predictor of ischemia, with 16 patients having an uncomplicated radial-artery cannulation despite a positive test. When percutaneous insertion is not possible and radial-artery cutdown is necessary, the incidence of complications increases to 50 percent [155]. In that situation, it may be prudent to switch to a percutaneous femoral approach rather than a radial cutdown. Two prospective studies have compared percutaneous radial- and femoral-artery cannulation and found that the complication rates are similar and that the femoral catheters are more durable [155,156]. Due to the relative sizes of the catheter and the vessel, arterial occlusion is unusual in the femoral artery. When there is preexisting peripheral vascular disease, however, the complication rate of femoral-artery cannulation increases significantly, so that route should be avoided, if possible [155].

PEDIATRIC VASCULAR TRAUMA

Principles of evaluation and treatment of vascular injuries in the pediatric population are similar to those in adults. There are, however, some differences that need to be considered. Spasm of blood vessels is a major factor in pediatric vascular injuries, both in iatrogenic injuries and in traumatic injuries. Because of the small size of a child's vessels, spasm can result in thrombosis and permanent occlusion. In pediatric patients in which spasm is felt to be the cause of the arterial insufficiency, intravenous heparin is indicated with a defined period of observation prior to deciding to surgically intervene. Depending on the condition of the injured extremity, that period of observation can be as short as 6 hours, as suggested by Flanigan et al. [157], or as long as 48 hours, as suggested by Klein et al. [158], prior to taking the patient to the operating room.

Another major consideration in the pediatric population that is different than in adults is the issue of altered limb growth. It is well documented that in pediatric patients with vascular injuries retardation of limb growth can occur if there is an interruption in blood flow for any significant period of time. That retardation of limb growth can occur when the vascular occlusion is not recognized, which can easily occur in the infant population. It also can occur if the vascular injury is not promptly recognized and the patient has a late repair of the vascular injury. Because of the possibility of altered limb growth in the pediatric population, special awareness of the possibility of a vascular injury becomes even more critical [159,160]. Signs of vascular insufficiency may not be as clear as they would be in an adult; thus, the likelihood of a missed vascular injury is much greater in this population. All authors of articles concerning pediatric vascular trauma clearly point out the need for thorough evaluation of the injured extremity; a heightened awareness of the possibility of vascular injury; prompt recognition and diagnosis of vascular injury by a combination of physical examination, Doppler examination, and arteriography; and the immediate institution of appropriate therapy to repair the injury [161–163].

Principles of repair in the pediatric population generally are similar to those in adults. However, there have been some recommendations that more liberal use of gentle vessel dilatation with heparinized papaverine solutions may be important [164]. Other technical considerations, including long spatulation of the anastomoses using interrupted sutures for the repair to allow the anastomosis to grow with the child, may be important. In addition, there have been some suggestions of the possibility of using absorbable sutures [164,165]. The choice of conduit in the pediatric population probably is similar to that in adults in that the saphenous vein is a very good conduit because of the matched size, because it contains endothelium, and because it has the potential to grow with the child. Issues of aneurysmal dilatation in the pediatric population have been raised, since those grafts must last for the entire life of the young patient. Because of that, some authors have suggested the use of autografts using the hypogastric artery. That is appropriate only when a relatively short graft is available; it also has the disadvantage of requiring an abdominal incision. General use of the hypogastric artery probably is appropriate in a limited number of circumstances [164]. Postoperative management of such patients has special considerations, again because of the relatively small size of the repaired vessel. Many authors feel that continued use of heparin and low-molecular-weight dextran, if possible, may be appropriate to prevent postoperative thrombosis [165]. As in adults, pediatric patients with knee dislocations pose special problems because of the high likelihood of direct injury to the popliteal artery. In a series of 37 knee dislocations in 35 patients reported by Kendall [166], **all** patients with a popliteal-artery injury had a pulse deficit, signs of peripheral ischemia, or both. Angiography was used only in selected cases.

ENDOVASCULAR REPAIR OF VASCULAR INJURIES

The use of an endovascular prosthesis to repair an arteriovenous fistula involving the left superficial femoral artery and vein has been reported by Marin [167]. That type of approach is an extension of a similar technique used to repair abdominal aortic aneurysms that was first reported by Parodi [168,169]. The repair of a 5-cm false aneurysm of the right subclavian artery using an intraluminal graft stent device placed through the brachial artery also has been reported [169]. It is difficult to assess how successful these techniques will be, but certainly early limited experience seems to suggest that this technique may become a tool for management of vascular injuries in the future [167].

ARTERIAL INJURIES: TO REPAIR OR NOT TO REPAIR?

There appears to be a growing movement in adopting a less aggressive approach to vascular injuries. There was a time when all penetrating extremity injuries were surgically explored due to the possibility of there being a significant vascular injury. That approach was subsequently modified whereby certain physical findings, noninvasive evaluations, and arteriographic findings could be used to assess the need for surgical exploration. That was further modified to the point where it was felt that in the absence of any hard findings on physical examination or Doppler evaluation further evaluation of the possibility of vascular injury need not be undertaken. Simultaneously, some authors reported that minor vascular injuries such as small pseudoaneurysms, small arteriovenous fistulas, and certain intimal defects need not undergo surgical repair since they were insignificant injuries and did not result in permanent harm to the patient. A recent article by Perry [170] cautions about the morbidity of missed arterial injuries and suggests that further analyses are necessary before we continue in this relatively unaggressive approach to vascular injuries. It is further pointed out that the natural history of iatrogenic injuries occurring under controlled circumstances may be different from injuries from blunt and penetrating trauma.

The natural history of vascular injuries is currently the subject of investigation by a number of authors, and they certainly merit our attention [171–173].

References

1. DeBakey ME, Simeone FA. Battle injuries of arteries in World War II: an analysis of 2,471 cases. Ann Surg 1946; 123:534–579.
2. Hughes CW. Arterial repair during the Korean War. Ann Surg 1958; 147:555–561.
3. Rich NM, Hughes CW. Vietnam Vascular Registry: a preliminary report. Surgery 1969; 65:218–226.
4. Rich NM, Manion WC, Hughes CW. Surgical and pathological evaluation of vascular injuries in Vietnam. J Trauma 1969; 9:279–291.
5. Rich NM, Baugh JH, Hughes CW. Acute arterial injuries in Vietnam: 1,000 cases. J Trauma 1970; 10:359–369.
6. Rich NM, Baugh JH, Hughes CW. Significance of complications associated with vascular repairs performed in Vietnam. Arch Surg 1970; 100:646–651.
7. Menzoian JO, et al. Evaluation and management of vascular injuries of the extremities. Arch Surg 1983; 118:93–96.
8. Perry MO. The Management of Acute Vascular Injuries. Baltimore: Williams & Wilkins, 1981. Pp. 1–148.
9. Gallen J, et al. Traumatic pseudoaneurysm of the axillary artery. Report of three cases and literature review. J Trauma 1984; 24:350–353.
10. Brink BE. Vascular trauma. Surg Clin N Amer 1977; 57: 189–196.
11. Brewster DC, ed. Common Problems in Vascular Surgery. Chicago: Year Book, 1989.
12. Menzoian JO, et al. A comprehensive approach to extremity vascular trauma. Arch Surg 1985; 120:801–804.
13. Meissner M, Paun M, Johansen K. Duplex scanning for arterial trauma. Am J Surg 1991; 161:552–555.
14. Bynoe RP, et al. Non-invasive diagnosis of vascular trauma by duplex ultrasonography. J Vasc Surg 1991; 14:346–352.
15. Bergstein JM, et al. Pitfalls in the use of color-flow duplex ultrasound for screening of suspected arterial injuries in penetrated extremities. J Trauma 1992; 33:395–402.
16. Fry WR, et al. The success of duplex ultrasonographic scanning in diagnosis of extremity vascular proximity trauma. Archives of Surgery 1993; 128:1368–1372.
17. Sclafani SJ, et al. Arterial trauma: diagnostic and therapeutic angiography. Radiol 1986; 161:165–168.
18. Rose SC, Moore EE. Emergency trauma angiography: accuracy, safety, and pitfalls. Am J Radiol 1987; 148:1243–1247.
19. Feliciano DV, et al. Delayed diagnosis of arterial injury. Am J Surg 1987; 154:579–584.
20. Geuder JW, et al. The role of contrast angiography in suspected arterial injuries of the extremities. Am Surg 1985; 51:89–93.
21. Tohmeh AG, Perler BA. Angiography in the evaluation of proximal arterial injury. Surg Gynecol Obstet 1990; 170: 117–120.
22. Reid JDS, et al. Wounds of the extremities in proximity to major arteries: value of angiography in the detection of arterial injury. Am J Roentgen 1984; 151:1035–1039.
23. Anderson RH, et al. Penetrating extremity trauma: identification of patients at high-risk requiring arteriography. J Vasc Surg 1990; 11:544–547.
24. Dennis JW, et al. New perspectives on the management of penetrating trauma in proximity to major limb arteries. J Vasc Surg 1990; 11:85–93.
25. Weaver FA, et al. Is arterial proximity a valid indication for

arteriography in penetrating extremity trauma? Arch Surg 1990; 125:1256–1260.
26. Kaufman JA, et al. Arteriography for proximity of injury in penetrating extremity trauma. JVIR 1992; 3:719–723.
27. Gillespie DL, et al. Role of arteriography for blunt or penetrating injuries in proximity to major vascular structures: an evolution in management. Annal of Vasc Surg 1993; 7: 145–149.
28. Schwartz MR, et al. Redefining the indications for arteriography in penetrating extremity trauma: a prospective analysis. J Vasc Surg 1993; 17:116–124.
29. Rich NM. Vascular trauma. Surg Clinic N Amer 1973; 53:1367–1392.
30. Kaiser AB, et al. Antibiotic prophylaxis in vascular surgery. Ann Surg 1978; 188:283–286.
31. Menzoian JO, et al. Management of vascular injuries to the leg. Am J Surg 1983; 144:231–234.
32. Howe HR Jr, et al. Salvage of lower extremities following combined orthopedic and vascular trauma: a predictive salvage index. Am Surg 1987; 53:205–208.
33. Modrall JG, Weaver FA, Yellin AE. Vascular considerations in extremity trauma. Orthop Clin North Am 1993; 24:557–563.
34. Nichols JC, Sanborn JA, Parks SN. Use of temporary intraluminal shunts in selected peripheral arterial injuries. J Trauma 1986; 26:1094–1098.
35. Shah DM, et al. Polytetrafluoroethylene grafts in the rapid reconstruction of acute contaminated vascular injuries. Am J Surg 1984; 148:229–232.
36. Liebman PR, et al. Intraoperative arteriography in femoropopliteal and femorotibial bypass grafts. Arch Surg 1981; 116:1019–1022.
37. Pasch AR, et al. Optimal limb salvage in penetrating civilian vascular trauma. J Vasc Surg 1986; 3:189–192.
38. Timberlake GA, O'Connell RC, Kerstein MD. Venous injury: to repair or ligate, the dilemma. J Vasc Surg 1986; 4:553–557.
39. Rich NM. Principles and indications for the primary venous repair. Surgery 1982; 91:492–496.
40. Phifer TJ, et al. Long-term patency of venous repairs demonstrated by venography. J Trauma 1985; 25:342–346.
41. Borman KR, Jones GH, Snyder WH III. A decade of lower extremity venous trauma: patency and outcome. Am J Surg 1987; 154:608–612.
42. Phifer TJ, et al. Amputation risk factors in concomitant superficial femoral artery and vein injuries. Ann Surg 1984; 199:241–244.
43. Posner MP, Alty CG, Lee HM. Cross-femoral bypass graft for combined arterial venous injury. Annals of Vascular Surgery 1991; 5:286–290.
44. Sharma PV, et al. Central and regional hemodynamics determine optimal management of major venous injuries. J Vasc Surg 1992; 16:887–894.
45. Matsen F. Compartmental syndrome: a unified concept. Clin Orth 1975; 113:8–10.
46. Mubarak SJ, et al. Acute compartment syndrome; diagnosis and treatment with the aid of the wick catheter. J Bone Joint Surg (Am) 1978; 60:1091–1095.
47. Patman RD, Thompson JE. Fasciotomy and peripheral vascular surgery: report of 164 patients. Arch Surg 1970; 101:663–672.
48. Hobson RW II, Lee BC, Lynch TG. Use of intermittent pneumatic calf compression in femoral venous reconstruction. Surg Gynecol Obstet 1983; 130:225–228.
49. Perry MO, Thal DR, Shires GT. Management of arterial injuries. Ann Surg 1971; 172:403–406.
50. Whitesides TE, et al. Tissue pressure measurement as a determinant for the need for fasciotomy. Clin Orthop 1975; 113:43–51.
51. Matsen FA, Winquist RA, Krugmire RB. Diagnosis and management of compartmental syndromes. J Bone Joint Surg (Am) 1980; 62:286–290.
52. Rutherford RB. Nutrient bed protection during lower extremity arterial reconstruction. J Vasc Surg 1987; 5:529–534.
53. Bulkley GB. Pathophysiology of free radical mediated reperfusion injury. J Vasc Surg 1987; 5:512–516.
54. Walker PM, et al. Salvage of skeletal muscle with free radical scavengers. J Vasc Surg 1987; 5:68–75.
55. Haimovici H. Late arterial embolectomy. Surg 1959; 46: 775–778.
56. Blaisdell FW, Steele M, Allen RE. Management of acute lower extremity ischemia due to embolism and thrombosis. Surg 1978; 84:822–826.
57. Fry WJ, Lindenauer SM. Infection complicating the use of plastic arterial implants. Arch Surg 1967; 94:600–605.
58. Szilagyi DE, et al. Infection in arterial reconstruction with synthetic grafts. Ann Surg 1972; 176:321–324.
59. Huffert PW, Gensler S, Haimovici H. Infection complicating arterial grafts. Personal experience with 12 cases and review of the literature. Arch Surg 1965; 90:427–431.
60. Rich NM, Hughes CW. The fate of prosthetic material used to repair vascular injuries in contaminated wounds. J Trauma 1972; 12:459–463.
61. Feliciano DV, et al. Five-year experience with PTFE grafts in vascular wounds. J Trauma 1985; 25:71–82.
62. Rich NM, et al. Traumatic arteriovenous fistulas and false aneurysms: a review of 558 lesions. Surg 1975; 78:817–828.
63. Johnson JR, Ledgerwood AM, Lucas CE. Mycotic aneurysm: new concepts in therapy. Arch Surg 1983; 118:577–582.
64. Patman RD, Thompson JE, Persson AV. Management of post-traumatic pain syndromes: report of 113 cases. Ann Surg 1973; 117:780–783.
65. Brown MF, et al. Carotid artery injuries. Am J Surg 1982; 144:748–751.
66. Welling RE, et al. Management of blunt injury to the internal carotid artery. J Trauma 1987; 27(11):1221–1226.
67. Saletta JD, et al. Penetrating trauma of the neck. J Trauma 1976; 16:579–582.
68. Dichtel WJ, et al. Lateral mandibulotomy: a technique of exposure for penetrating injuries of the internal carotid artery at the base of the skull. Laryngoscope 1984; 94:1140–1143.
69. Fry RE, Fry WJ. Extracranial carotid artery injuries. Surgery 1980; 88:581–584.
70. Ledgerwood AM, Mullins RJ, Lucas CE. Primary repair versus ligation for carotid artery injuries. Arch Surg 1980; 115:488–491.
71. Chandler WF. Penetrating injuries of the carotid artery. In WF Chandler. Carotid Artery Injuries. New York: Futura, 1982. Pp. 77–106.
72. Gewertz BL, et al. Management of penetrating injuries of the internal carotid artery at the base of the skull utilizing extracranial-intracranial bypass. J Trauma 1980; 20:365–369.
73. Meier DE, Brink BE, Fry WJ. Vertebral artery trauma: acute recognition and treatment. Arch Surg 1981; 116:236–239.
74. Quatromoni JC, Johnson JM, Wood M. Vertebral arteriovenous fistulas. Am J Surg 1979; 138:907–910.
75. Parmley LF, et al. Nonpenetrating traumatic injury of the aorta. Circulation 1958; 17:1086–1089.
76. Hudson HM II, Woodson J, Hirsch E. The management of traumatic aortic tear in the multiply-injured patient. Annals of Vasc Surg 1991; 5:381–384.
77. Marsh DG, Sturm JT. Traumatic aortic rupture: roentgenographic indications for aortography. Ann Thorac Surg 1976; 21:337–340.

78. Mattox KL, et al. Clamp/repair: a safe technique for treatment of blunt injury to the descending thoracic aorta. Ann Thor Surg 1985; 40(5):456–460.
79. Cunningham JN, et al. Measurement of spinal cord ischemia during operations upon the thoracic aorta. Initial clinical experience. Ann Surg 1982; 196:285–288.
80. Graham JM, et al. Innominate vascular injury. J Trauma 1982; 22:647–651.
81. Elkin DC, Cooper FW Jr. Resection of the clavicle in vascular injuries. J Trauma 1980; 20:537–540.
82. Graham JM, et al. Management of subclavian vascular injuries. J Trauma 1980; 20:537-540.
83. Johnston RH Jr, Wall MJ Jr, Mattrox KL. Innominate artery trauma: A thirty-year experience. J Vasc Surg 1993; 17: 134–139.
84. Graham JM, et al. Vascular injuries of the axilla. Ann Surg 1982; 195(2):232–238.
85. Saide R, et al. Management of peripheral vascular trauma. Am Surg 1981; 47(10):429–432.
86. Rich NE, Spencer FC. Vascular Trauma. Philadelphia: Saunders, 1978.
87. Smith LL, Foran R, Gaspar MR. Acute arterial injuries of the upper extremity. Am J Surg 1963; 106:1144–1148.
88. Johnson M, Ford M, Johansen K. Radial or ulnar artery laceration. Repair of ligate? Archives of Surgery 1993; 128:971–974.
89. Jackson MR, et al. Abdominal vascular trauma: a review of 106 injuries. Am Surg 1992; 58:622–626.
90. Pisters PWT, Heslin MJ, Riles TS. Abdominal aortic pseudoaneurysm after blunt trauma. J Vasc Surg 1993; 18:307–309.
91. Randhawa MPS, Menzoian JO. Seat belt aorta. Ann Vasc Surg 1990; 4:370–377.
92. Mattox KL, et al. Management of upper abdominal vascular trauma. Am J Surg 1974; 128:823–826.
93. Buchness MP, LoGerfo FW, Mason GR. Gunshot wound of the suprarenal abdominal aorta. Am Surg 1976; 42:1–7.
94. Accola KD, et al. Management of injuries to the suprarenal aorta. Am J Surg 1987; 154(6):613–617.
95. Brown MF, et al. Renovascular trauma. Am J Surg 1980; 140:802–806.
96. Spirnak JP, Resnick MI. Revascularization of traumatic thrombosis of the renal artery. Surg Gynecol Obstet 1987; 164:22–26.
97. Yellin AE, Chafee CB, Donovan AJ. Vascular isolation in treatment of juxtahepatic venous injuries. Arch Surg 1971; 102:566–569.
98. Schrock T, Blaisdell FW, Mathewson C Jr. Management of blunt trauma to the liver and hepatic veins. Arch Surg 1968; 96:698–704.
99. Pachter HL, et al. The management of juxtahepatic venous injuries without an atriocaval shunt: preliminary clinical observations. Surgery 1986; 99:569–573.
100. Mullins RJ, Lucas CE, Ledgerwood AM. The injuries of the axilla. Ann Surg 1982; 195(2):232–238.
101. Van Way CW III, Rutherford RB. Peripheral vascular injuries. In GD Zuidema, RB Rutherford, WF Ballinger, eds. The Management of Trauma. Philadelphia: Saunders, 1985. P. 631.
102. Rich NM, Hughes CW, Baugh JH. Management of venous injuries. Ann Surg 1970; 171:724–727.
103. Hobson RW II, et al. Femoral venous trauma: techniques for surgical management and early results. Am J Surg 1983; 146:220–224.
104. Hobson RW II, et al. Hemodynamics of canine femoral venous ligation: significance in combined arterial and venous injuries. Surgery 1973; 74:824–827.
105. Orcutt MB, et al. The continuing challenge of popliteal vascular injuries. Am J Surg 1983; 146:758–762.
106. van Wijngaarden M, et al. Management of blunt vascular trauma to the extremities. SG&O 1993; 177(1):41–48.
107. Lange RH, et al. Open tibial fractures with associated vascular injuries: prognosis for limb salvage. J Trauma 1985; 25:203–206.
108. Segal D, Brenner M, Gorczyca J. Tibial fractures with infrapopliteal arterial injuries. J Orthop Trauma 1987; 1:160–169.
109. Shah DM, et al. Optimal management of tibial arterial trauma. J Trauma 1988; 28(2):228–234.
110. Padberg FT Jr, et al. Infrapopliteal arterial injury: prompt revascularization affords optimal limb salvage. J Vasc Surg 1992; 16:877–885.
111. Drapanas T, et al. Civilian vascular injuries: a critical appraisal of two decades of management. Ann Surg 1970; 172:251–254.
112. Orcutt MB, et al. Iatrogenic vascular injury. A reducible problem. Arch Surg 1985; 120:384–385.
113. Rich NM, Hobson RW II, Fedde CW. Vascular trauma secondary to diagnostic and therapeutic procedures. Arch Surg 1974; 128:715–721.
114. Youkey JR, et al. Vascular trauma secondary to diagnostic and therapeutic procedures: 1974 through 1982. A comparative review. Arch Surg 1983; 146:788–791.
115. Mills JL, et al. Minimizing mortality and morbidity from iatrogenic arterial injuries: the need for early recognition and prompt repair. J Vasc Surg 1986; 4:22–27.
116. Hessel SJ, Adams DF, Abrams HL. Complications of angiography. Radiology 1981; 138:273–281.
117. Molnar W, Paul DJ. Complications of axillary arteriotomies: an analysis of 1762 consecutive studies. Radiology 1972; 104:269–276.
118. Franklin EA, Girod A, Sequcira FW. Femoral artery spasm in children: catheter size is the principal cause. AJR 1982; 138:295–298.
119. Maini RL, Eiserberg RL, McDonald EJ Jr. Complications of catheter cerebral arteriography: analysis of 5000 procedures. I, II, and III. Am J Roentgen 1978; 131:861, 867, 871.
120. Chahine RA, Raizner AE, Miller RR. The lesson from complications of coronary angiography. Chest 1979; 75:5–6.
121. Davis K, et al. Complications of coronary angiography from the collaborative study of coronary artery surgery (CASS). Circulation 1979; 59:1105–1111.
122. McCollum CH, Mavor E. Brachial artery injury after cardiac catheterization. J Vasc Surg 1986; 4:355–359.
123. Harris JM. Coronary angiography and its complications, the search for risk factors. Arch Int Med 1984; 144:337–341.
124. Menzoian JO, et al. Management of the upper extremity with absent pulses following cardiac catheterization. Am J Surg 1978; 135:484–488.
125. Ricci MA, Trevisani GT, Pilcher DB. Vascular complications of cardiac catheterization. Am J Surg 1994; 167:375–378.
126. Rivers SP, et al. Successful conservative management of iatrogenic femoral arterial trauma. Annals of Vascular Surgery 1992; 6:45–49.
127. Kent KC, et al. A prospective study of the clinical outcome of femoral pseudoaneurysms and arteriovenous fistulas induced by arterial puncture. J Vasc Surg 1993; 17:125–133.
128. McCann RL, Schwartz LB, Pieper KS. Vascular complications of cardiac catheterization. J Vasc Surg 1991; 14:375–381.
129. Kotval RS, et al. Doppler sonographic demonstration of the progressive spontaneous thrombosis of pseudoaneurysms. J Ultrasound Med 1990; 9:185–190.
130. Fellmeth BD, Roberts AC, Bookstein JJ. Postangiographic femoral artery injuries: Non-surgical repair with US-guided compression. Radiology 1991; 178:671–675.
131. Dorfman GS, Cronan JJ. Postcatheterization femoral artery

injuries: is there a role for non-surgical treatment? Radiology 1991; 178:629–630.
132. Laerum F, Holm H. Post phlebographic thrombosis, a double blind study with methylglucamine metrizoate and metrizamide. Radiology 1981; 140:651–655.
133. Weibull H, et al. Complications after percutaneous transluminal angioplasty in the iliac, femoral, and popliteal arteries. J Vasc Surg 1987; 5:681–686.
134. Oweida SW, et al. Postcatheterization vascular complications associated with percutaneous transluminal coronary angioplasty. J Vasc Surg 1990; 12:310–314.
135. Ginsburg R, et al. Percutaneous transluminal angioplasty for treatment of peripheral vascular disease: clinical experience with 16 patients. Radiology 1985; 156:619–622.
136. Sanborn TA, et al. Human percutaneous and intraoperative laser thermal angioplasty: initial clinical results as an adjunct to balloon angioplasty. J Vasc Surg 1987; 5:83–90.
137. Wright JG, et al. Laser angioplasty for limb salvage: observations on early results. J Vasc Surg 1989; 10:29–33.
138. Natali J, Benhamou AC. Iatrogenic vascular injuries. A review of 125 cases (excluding angiographic injuries). J Cardiovasc Surg 1979; 20:169–176.
139. McDonald PT, et al. Vascular trauma secondary to diagnostic and therapeutic procedures: laparoscopy. Arch Surg 1978; 135:651–655.
140. Alpert J, et al. Vascular complications of intra-aortic balloon pumping. Arch Surg 1976; 111:1190–1195.
141. Perler BA, et al. Vascular complications of intra-aortic balloon counterpulsation. Arch Surg 1983; 118:957–962.
142. Friedell ML, et al. Femorofemoral grafts for lower limb ischemia caused by intraaortic balloon pump. J Vasc Surg 1987; 5:180–186.
143. Gottlieb SO, et al. Identification of patients at high risk for complications of intraaortic balloon counterpulsation: a multivariate risk factor analysis. Am J Cardiol 1984; 1:53, 8:1135–1139.
144. Kantrowitza A, et al. Intraaortic balloon pumping 1967 through 1982: analysis of complications in 733 patients. Am J Cardiol 1986; 15:57, 11:976–980.
145. Barnett MG, et al. Vascular complications of intraaortic balloons: risk analysis. J Vasc Surg 1994; 19:81–89.
146. Iverson LI, et al. Vascular complications of intraaortic balloon counterpulsation. Am J Surg 1987; 154:99–103.
147. Sznajder JI, et al. Central vein catheterization: failure and complication rates by three percutaneous approaches. Arch Int Med 1986; 146:259–261.
148. Borrow M, Crowley JG. Prevention of thrombosis of central venous catheters. J Cardiovasc Surg 1986; 27:571–574.
149. Shah KB, et al. A review of pulmonary artery catheterization in 6,245 patients. Anesthesiol 1984; 61:271–275.
150. Barash PG, et al. Catheter induced pulmonary artery perforation: mechanisms, management, and modifications. J Thorac Cardiovasc Surg 1981; 82:5–12.
151. Foote GA, Schabel SI, Hodges M. Pulmonary complications of the flow-directed balloon-tipped catheter. N Engl J Med 1974; 290:927–930.
152. Duncan JW, Powner DJ. Complications associated with the use of pulmonary artery catheters. Arizona Med 1982; 39:433–435.
153. Baker RJ, Chunprapaph B, Nyhus LM. Severe ischemia of the hand following radial artery catheterization. Surg 1976; 80:449–457.
154. Slogoff S, Keats AS, Arlund C. On the safety of radial artery cannulation. Anesthesiol 1983; 59:42–47.
155. Russell R, et al. Prospective evaluation of radial and femoral artery catheterization sites in critically ill patients. Crit Care Med 1983; 3:10–18.
156. Soderstrom CA, Wasserman DH, Dunham CM. Superiority of the femoral artery for monitoring: a prospective study. Am J Surg 1982; 144:309–313.
157. Flanigan DP, et al. Experience with iatrogenic pediatric vascular injuries: incidence, etiology, management and results. Ann Surg 1983; 198:430–442.
158. Klein MD, et al. Management of iatrogenic arterial injuries in infants and children. J Ped Surg 1982; 17:933–939.
159. Schnitzer JJ, Fitzgerald D. Peripheral vascular injuries from plastic bullets in children. Surg Gynecol Obstet 1993; 176(2):172–174.
160. Bloom JD, et al. Defective limb growth as a complication of catheterization of the femoral artery. Surg Gynecol Obstetrics 1974; 138:524–526.
161. Evans WE, King DR, Hayes JP. Arterial trauma in children: diagnosis and management. Annals of Vasc Surg 1988; 2(3):268–270.
162. Navarre JR, et al. Vascular trauma in children and adolescents. Am J Surg 1982; 143:229–231.
163. Meagher DP Jr, et al. Vascular trauma in infants and children. J Trauma 1979; 19:532–536.
164. McNeil JW, et al. Penetrating thermal vascular injury in child: a case report. Journal of Vascular Surgery 1993; 18(6):1060–1063.
165. Shaker IJ, et al. Special problems of vascular injuries in children. J Trauma 1976; 16:863–866.
166. Kendall RW, et al. The role of arteriography in assessing vascular injuries associated with dislocations of the knee. J Trauma 1993; 35(6):875–879.
167. Marin ML, et al. Percutaneous transfemoral insertion of a stented graft to repair a traumatic femoral arteriovenous fistula. J Vasc Surg 1993; 18:299–302.
168. Parodi JC, Palmaz JC, Barone HD. Transfemoral intraluminal graft implantation for abdominal aortic aneurysms. Annals of Vascular Surgery 1991; 5:491–499.
169. May J, et al. Transluminal placement of a prosthetic graft-stent device for treatment of subclavian artery aneurysm. J Vasc Surg 1993; 18:1056–1059.
170. Perry MO. Complications of missed arterial injuries. Journal of Vasc Surg 1993; 17:399–407.
171. Panetta TF, et al. Natural history, duplex characteristics, and histopathologic correlation of arterial injuries in a canine model. J Vasc Surg 1992; 16:876–880.
172. Neville RF, et al. The arterial wall response to intimal injury in an experimental model. Annals of Vascular Surgery 1992; 6:50–54.
173. Sawchuk AP, Eldrup-Jorgensen J, Tober C. The natural history of intimal flaps in a canine model. Archives of Surgery 1990; 125:1614–1616.

Vascular Ulcers

Pedal Ulcers of Arterial or Diabetic Origin Ronald L. Dalman • Christopher K. Zarins
Venous Ulcers E. John Harris, Jr. • Christopher K. Zarins

Chronic or nonhealing ulcerations of the lower extremities may be due to a number of etiologies, including neuropathic, infectious, traumatic, neoplastic, and vascular. Vascular insufficiency should be considered as a possible primary or contributing cause to all nonhealing lower-extremity ulcerations. This chapter reviews the pathophysiology, diagnosis, and treatment of both arterial and venous ulcerations of the lower extremity.

Pedal Ulcers of Arterial or Diabetic Origin

Pedal and lower-extremity ulcerations may be due to venous, arterial, or nonvascular etiologies. Patients with diabetes mellitus are particularly vulnerable to such lesions regardless of their cause (Table 51-1). Although costly and debilitating [1,2], recent insights into the pathophysiology of the lesions have contributed to dramatically improved outcomes. This section discusses the pathophysiology, assessment, and treatment of inframalleolar skin ulcers due to arterial insufficiency with or without coexistant diabetes mellitus. The natural history of intervention and nonintervention will be reviewed. Lower-extremity ulcers due primarily to venous etiologies are discussed in the next section.

ARTERIAL VERSUS VENOUS INSUFFICIENCY

Approximately 1 percent of Europeans have chronic nonhealing ulcerations of the lower extremity [3]. The majority of those ulcerations are due to venous valvular insufficiency and venous hypertension. Although a traditional distinction has been made between inframalleolar ulcers (arterial) and lower-leg ulcers (venous), in practice some overlap frequently exists between the two etiologies. The distinction has evolved into a more sophisticated appreciation of the causes of leg ulceration.

Fully 10 percent of patients in a population-based study of lower-leg ulcers had significant arterial ischemia at rest, and an additional 30 percent were found to have an abnormal arterial exam based on Doppler-determined ankle arterial pressures. The likelihood of arterial involvement was not sex specific, but it was highly age related in this study: Under the age of 40, few ulcerated lower extremities demonstrated arterial ischemia. By the patient's ninth decade, however, the probability of arterial involvement increased to 50 percent [3] (Fig. 51-1). In the elderly patient with type II diabetes mellitus, the possibility of arterial ischemia must be considered whenever a patient presents with lower-extremity ulceration, regardless of the location of the ulcers.

DIABETES MELLITUS AND ARTERIAL INSUFFICIENCY

The prevalence of diabetes mellitus in North America is estimated to be 2–6 percent of the population (at least 5,000,000 patients). Within a diabetic cohort, an active leg ulcer is present in 3.5 percent of patients [4]. Thus, hundreds of thousands of patients have pedal ulceration associated with their diabetes. Frequently, arterial ischemia also is present [5]. The risk of peripheral vascular occlusive disease associated with diabetes rises significantly with the patient's age and the duration of diabetes. Eight percent of patients with diabetes have evidence of peripheral vascular disease at the time of diagnosis, increasing to 45 percent 20 years later [6].

Arterial insufficiency is present and felt to be contributory in at least half of all ulcerated legs in diabetic patients and may be the dominant cause in as many as one-third. Diabetic neuropathy alone is responsible for a much smaller fraction (15%) of isolated foot ulcers in this population [4]. Even in the setting of advanced diabetes mellitus, arterial ischemia plays a dominant role in the etiology and morbidity associated with pedal ulcers. Therefore, the possibility of arterial insufficiency must be considered in all diabetic patients who present with pedal ulceration, regardless of the location or severity of the lesion.

ISCHEMIA, DIABETES, AND THE DEVELOPMENT OF PEDAL ULCERS

Nail, cuticle, and callus care can prevent many of the complications of ischemia before ulcers develop. Once started, however, their clinical course is marked by intrasigence and chronicity. Diminished tissue perfusion hinders normal reparative processes after trivial injuries to the forefoot or the shear forces associated with ambulation.

Diabetic neuropathy and retinopathy prevent many patients with advanced diabetes from recognizing minor injuries to their feet at an early stage. Severe retinopathy hinders preventative foot care in even the most motivated patient. The relative role of sensory impairment in the etiology of diabetic foot lesions is uncertain, but indirect evidence suggests it is very important. When the effects are minimized by aggressive preventative foot care, outcome is improved. Aggressive preventative foot care has been shown to shorten lesion duration, prevent reoccurrence, decrease length of inpatient time, and lower the major and minor amputation rate in a population of patients prospectively identified as having feet at risk [7].

The relationship between ulcers of the leg above the ankle and arterial ischemia is less direct. Arterial insufficiency, if present, hinders reparative processes after injury or ulceration occurs. While not directly responsible for the ulcer itself, ischemia can greatly complicate its care, especially if it is not appreciated.

PATHOPHYSIOLOGY OF CHRONIC LOWER-LIMB ISCHEMIA

Many clinical data exist regarding the sequela of ischemic pedal ulceration and potential precipitating factors. The basic pathophysiology of the process remains much less

Table 51-1. Etiologies of pedal and lower-extremity ulcerations

NONVASCULAR ETIOLOGIES OF DIABETIC FOOT LESIONS
Trauma
Fungal dermatophytosis
Eczema
Psoriasis
Bacterial skin infections
Necrobiosis lipodica diabeticorum
Mal perforans ulcers
Other neuropathic pressure sores
CHRONIC ARTERIAL OBSTRUCTION CAUSING DIABETIC FOOT LESIONS
Inflow obstruction (proximal to the inguinal ligament)
Outflow obstruction (distal to the inguinal ligament)
Intrinsic arterial disease within the foot
CHRONIC VENOUS ETIOLOGIES OF DIABETIC FOOT LESIONS
Deep venous insufficiency
Valvular incompetence
Superficial venous insufficiency
Incompetent perforating veins

certain. The ankle-brachial pressure index (ABI) (Fig. 51-2), while of considerable clinical value in identifying patients with arterial ischemia, is a crude estimator of limb and foot perfusion. The inability to assess tissue perfusion and limb blood flow in a direct, noninvasive fashion has hindered the recognition of the metabolic adaptation of the lower limb to chronic ischemia.

What is the volume flow present at the ankle, the mixed venous oxygen saturation of the effluent blood, or the volume of tissue perfusion in cubic centimeters per gram of tissue per minute in the ischemic versus the reperfused limb? Newer techniques of blood-flow measurement and tissue perfusion hold great promise in understanding those adaptations. MRI sequences demonstrate pedal blood-flow volume in normal and ischemic limbs with great accuracy in animal models as well as in volunteers and patients.

Mean pedal blood flow (as determined by a summation of all visualized vessels at the level of the ankle) at room temperature in normal volunteers after 30 minutes rest is 80–90 ml/minute. Significantly less flow is present in ischemic, ulcerated feet (as low as 10 ml/minute). Using an uninvolved limb as an internal control, flow is consistently less in the ulcerated foot (mean 27.6 ml/minute versus 48.9 ml/minute) [8]. Future investigations using magnetic resonance flow data promise additional information regarding the physiologic effects of low perfusion, the relative increments of perfusion present after revascularization, and important data regarding pedal metabolism.

ASSOCIATED DIABETIC COMPLICATIONS

In the diabetic patient with a chronic pedal ulcer, complex etiologies other than ischemia alone frequently are responsible for the recalcitrant nature of the wound. Neuropathy, with associated abnormal pressure loading and functional microcirculatory disorders, and increased susceptibility to infection (Plate 14) constitute additional major pathogenetic factors in the diabetic foot. However, as in the patient without diabetes, the presence and severity of significant arterial obstruction proximal to the ankle or in named vessels in the foot represent the major determinant of clinical outcome [9].

Neuropathic and Endothelial Microcirculatory Disorders. The exact pathophysiology of diabetic neuropathy remains unknown. While some patients experience painful paresthesias, the majority of patients with diabetic peripheral neuropathy in our practice manifest diminished sensation to light touch in a "stocking" distribution. As previously noted, such insensitivity plays a considerable role in the pathogenesis of diabetic foot ulceration. Diminished pe-

Fig. 51-1. Age and sex distribution among leg-ulcer patients (n = 827). (Used with permission from O Nelzen, A Lindhagen, T Hallbook. Chronic leg ulcers: an underestimated problem in primary health care. J Epi Comm Health 1991; 45:185.)

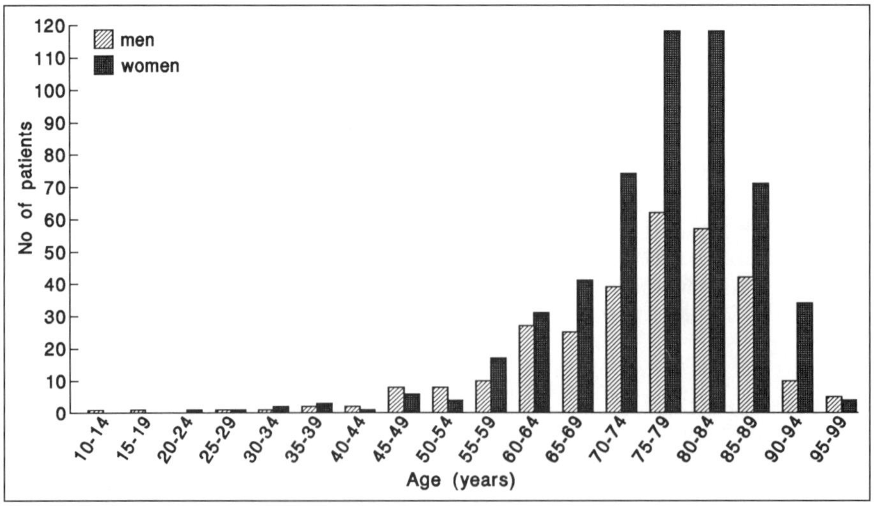

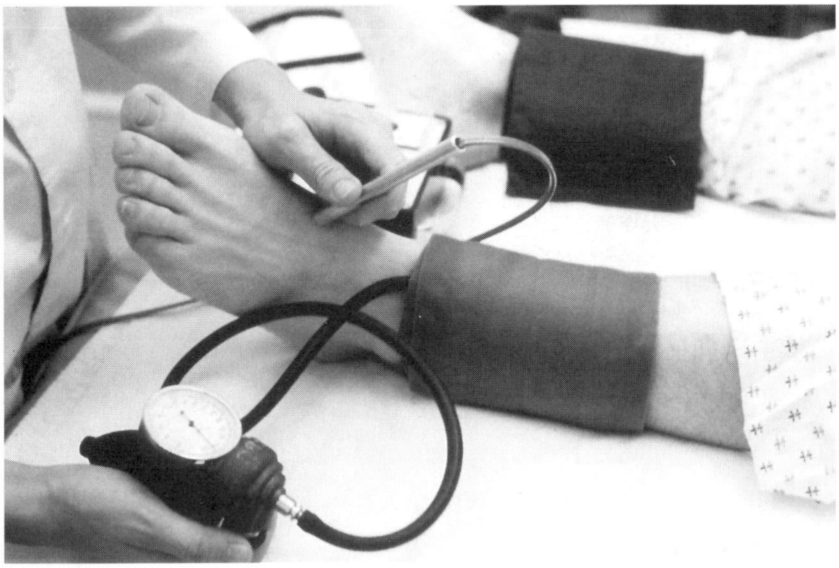

Fig. 51-2. The ankle-brachial index (ABI) is the most accurate and reproducible method of assessing the severity of pedal ischemia and should be obtained whenever pedal pulses are absent.

ripheral motor nerve function also may be present, which promotes postural deformity, thus affecting pressure distribution and balance in the foot.

Recent investigations suggest an important role for autonomic nerve dysfunction in the formation of pedal ulcers in the diabetic patient [10]. Peripheral autonomic neuropathy impairs the normal functional responses of the microcirculation of the foot, which may render diabetic feet more susceptible to trauma. Functional microangiopathy is distinguished from occlusive microangiopathy, which is demonstrated on histiologic examination [11,12].

Autonomic denervation impairs microcirculatory homeostasis. Impaired autonomic neurogenic control mechanisms include increased arteriovenous shunting [13–15], altered distribution between capillary perfusion and shunted blood, impaired postural vasoconstriction [16,17], leading to postural capillary hypertension, injury and edema formation, and impaired cutaneous hyperemic response to injury [18,19].

Unlike other peripheral neuropathic manifestations, the functional microcirculatory abnormalities associated with autonomic impairment respond favorably to tight control of serum glucose levels. Acute and chronic control of hyperglycemia restores the balance between nutritive flow and arteriovenous shunting in the skin [20,21]. The clinical significance of these observations remains unknown, but the possibility exists that careful diabetes management may favorably affect ulcer outcome through that mechanism.

Independent of autonomic nervous dysfunction, changes in arteriolar and capillary endothelial cells also contribute to the loss of peripheral vascular autoregulation in diabetic patients. Patients without proximal vascular occlusive disease demonstrate increased limb, arteriolar, and capillary flow with increasing duration of impaired serum glucose control, due to decreased precapillary resistance. The change in precapillary resistance may be due to diminished endothelial-cell production of vasoactive factors such as endothelial derived relaxing factor (EDRF) (Fig. 51-3). Changes in shear stress due to increased plasma viscosity, increased erythrocyte aggregability, and reduced erythrocyte deformability also may affect endothelial regulation of vasomotor tone [22,23]. With increased duration of diabetes, reactive hyperemic responses are lost, which may impair the response to injury [24].

Medial arteriolar calcification is more frequent in patients with diabetes mellitus and is reported to be associated with diabetic peripheral somatosensory and autonomic neuropathy. Interestingly, the total amount of pedal medial arteriolar calcification is closely correlated to the length and severity of diabetic neuropathy. Total calcification is higher in neuropathic patients with current or previous ulcers than in neuropathic patients without a history of ulcers. The amount of calcification is closely related to the length of diabetes, regardless of age of the patient.

The development of medial arterial calcification is believed to be due to autonomic denervation of the intima and media of the small muscular arteries of the foot. Increased medial arterial calcification has been reported following sympathectomy. Medial calcification increases as nonneuropathic patients move through neuropathy toward neuropathic-associated ulceration [25]. While a marker of autonomic and sensory dysfunction, the role of medial calcification in the development of pedal and plantar ulcers remains to be determined.

Occlusive microangiopathy may not constitute a significant etiologic factor specific to patients with diabetes. Amputation specimens demonstrate a similar degree of arteriolar occlusion in diabetic and nondiabetic subjects

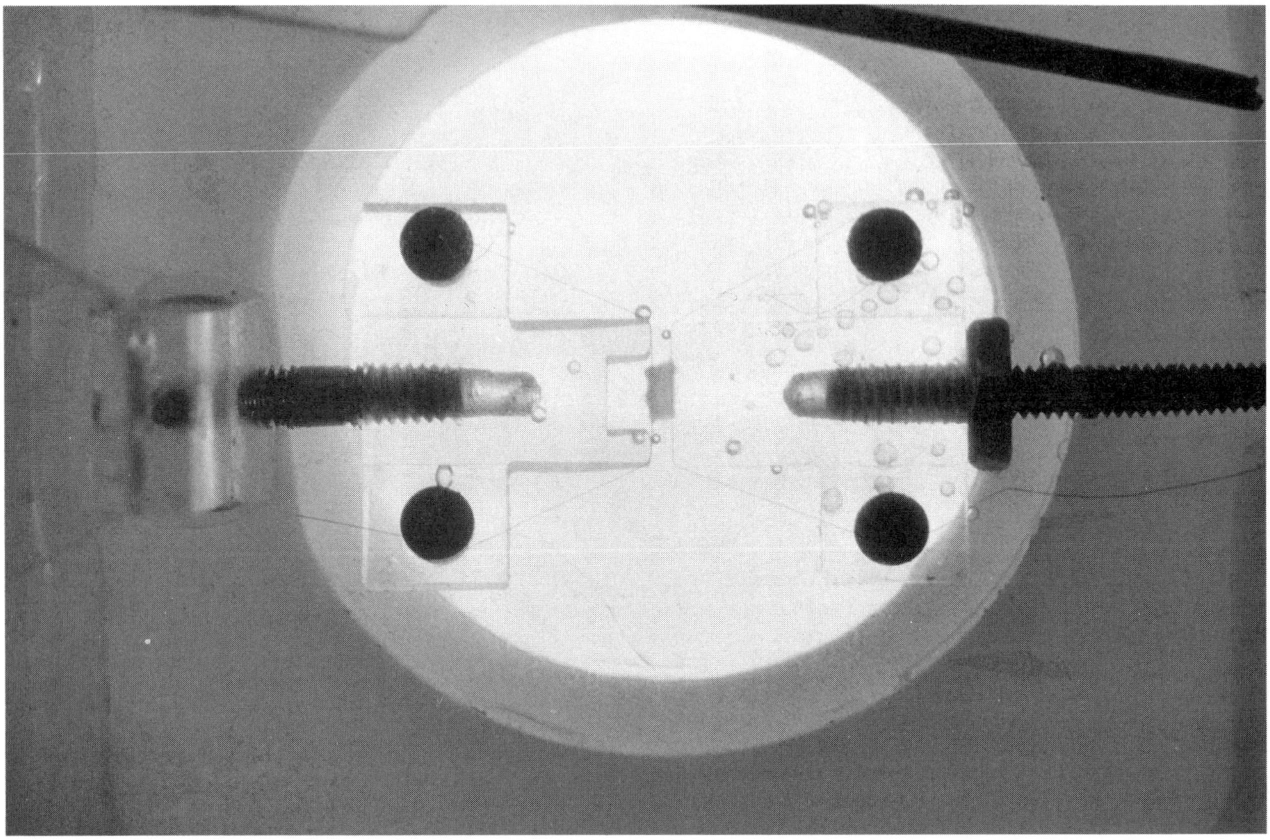

Fig. 51-3. Arteriole (600 μm diameter) suspended in a myograph. This preparation is used to determine changes in isometric tone induced by agonists and antagonists such as nitric oxide (EDRF) in the setting of diabetes and other diseases that can influence vascular smooth muscle tone.

with ischemic and neuropathic foot ulcers. Capillary-basement-membrane thickening is a late marker of microvascular disease in the diabetic patient. Basement-membrane thickening probably represents a proliferative response of the vascular endothelium to nonspecific chronic injury and is not directly responsible for tissue ischemia and ulceration [24].

Infection. Superimposed bacterial tissue penetration and infection frequently complicate diabetic pedal and leg ulcers. The bacteriologic milieu of severe diabetic foot infections is polymicrobial (average 2.6–4.8 organisms cultured per wound), usually demonstrating anerobic and gram-negative aerobic growth [26–29]. The number of bacterial isolates identified has been suggested by one investigator to correlate with the severity of clinical infection [26]. In patients with fulminant, severe infections, the major amputation rate may run as high as 26 percent [26]. Such acute situations usually require aggressive surgical assessment in the operating room, with soft-tissue debridement, toe and ray amputation, and plantar fascia excision performed when appropriate.

In the chronic-ulcer setting, standard techniques of wound culture are important in identifying the pathogenic organisms present. Recent advances in antimicrobial therapy, including less toxic, gram-negative–specific, broad-spectrum agents, have greatly simplified initial therapy for such lesions. With the development of affective, relatively nontoxic agents, the importance of the infectious process in the pathogenesis of such lesions has become less clear. Superimposed infection clearly is an integral component of the development and progression of diabetic and ischemic ulcers, but the relative role of infection in the development of most such ulcers is uncertain.

The diagnosis of osteomyelitis involving phalanges, metatarsal, sesamoid, and tarsal bones, as well as deep infection of the tendons and sheaths continues to be problematic. Despite widespread use of radiolabeled white cell scans and technetium-99m bone scans, including newer "three phase" bone scans, frequently a distinction cannot be made among deep soft-tissue infection, periosteal inflammation, and osteomyelitis. Shults and co-authors recently described their experience with foot radiographs, bone scans, and wound cultures and concluded that none should be used as the sole criterion for determining the use of antibiotic therapy or amputation in diabetic patients with foot ulcers [30]. In our own experience, once ulcers have penetrated through the plantar fascia and underlying bony or cartilaginous structures are exposed, the possibility of osteomyelitis can no longer be reliably excluded and has to be presumed to exist. Aggressive pedal revascularization where indicated, followed by operative ulcer debridement and wound closure, generally is pursued in such patients regardless of the results of foot radiographs or bone scans. In addition, the diagnosis of osteomyelitis is virtually unobtainable short of bone biopsy and culture in the setting of suggestive radiographic periosteal and bony changes following previous partial foot amputation. That is also true in the patient with acute Charcot degeneration of the foot and dependant ulceration. We currently are unsure of the role of bone scans or extensive radiographic evaluation in patients with chronic diabetic ulceration, preferring operative assessment when the question of bony involvement exists.

Following a cohort of diabetic patients initially identified with intact limbs, Pecoraro and Reiber described 23 unique causative pathways to lower-extremity amputation among 80 consecutive cases [31]. Since more than 80 percent of diabetes-related leg amputations are proceeded by unsuccessful management of a pedal ulcer, examining the causes of such failure can be very illustrative. Of the 23 separate pathways identified, all but one (ischemia) were multifactorial. The authors calculated the proportions of amputations attributed to each specific cause. Infection played a significant role in two-thirds of the cases but accounted for the dominant or final component of each pathway in less than half those described. The authors concluded that infection is a frequent complication of the prolongation or failure of cutaneous wound healing in patients with diabetes but that it was not usually the major indication for limb amputation.

Table 51-2. Proposed classification of ulcers and arterial ischemia

1. Infection
   a. Cellulitis
      i. Complicating an obvious ulcer
      ii. No obvious associated ulcer
      iii. Associated with preexisting gangrene
      iv. Caused by trauma
   b. Osteomyelitis
      i. Complicating an obvious ulcer
      ii. No obvious associated ulcer
      iii. Associated with preexisting gangrene
2. Ischemia
   a. Symptomatic ischemia without an ulcer
      i. Claudication
      ii. Rest pain
   b. Painless scabbed lesions of the skin
      i. Single
      ii. Multiple
   c. Gangrene
      i. Of the digits
      ii. Of the forefoot
   d. Persistent unhealing ischemic lesions
      i. Neuroischemic ulcers
      ii. Following surgery
      iii. Following other trauma
      iv. With no known cause
   e. Ischemic heel ulcers
      i. Small
      ii. Large
      iii. Painful cracks
   f. Blisters (epidermis intact)
      i. Caused by definable trauma
      ii. No known cause
3. Neuropathy
   a. Ulcers with surrounding callus over an area of increased pressure
      i. Under metatarsal head
      ii. On toe
      iii. Complicating Charcot deformity
      iv. Complication of surgery
      v. Complicating other deformity
   b. Neuropathic ulcers under the calcaneum
   c. Ulcers caused by unnoticed trauma
   d. Acutely evolving Charcot deformity

ASSESSMENT AND CLASSIFICATION OF ULCERS AND ARTERIAL ISCHEMIA

Outcome analysis of diabetic ulcer management is central to a rational comparison of various methods of treatment. A ranking system similar to that which exists for wounds such as pressure ulcers or open fractures would greatly facilitate research and outcome analysis. Several severity scores based on depth of penetration or involvement of subdermal structures have been proposed, but no one system has come into common use. The Wagner classification is the most widely used [32].

The Wagner classification relies on depth of penetration (0 = intact, 1 = superficial, 2 = deep but clean), with complexity modifiers for superimposed infection (3 = deep and infected) or gangrene (4 = localized, 5 = widespread). The score is simple and reproducible and thus of great utility because of its ease of use. However, the imprecision inherent in a 1–5 scale, without a distinction made for the presence or absence of osteomyelitis, often prevents meaningful outcome analysis. Recent investigations confirm the value of recognizing differences among healing rates for diabetic ulcers based on depth of penetration. Superficial or deep dermal ulcers heal more quickly than deeper ulcers involved with abscesses, fasciitis, or osteomyelitis. Location on the foot is a much less significant indicator of the rate of healing [33].

Jeffcoate and associates recently reviewed the shortcomings of current classification systems and proposed new clinical determinants of primary management [34]. Based on the presence or absence of infection, the degree of arterial perfusion, and an assessment of neuropathic involvement, they proposed a new system incorporating the pathophysiology of ulcer development as well as the depth of penetration (Table 51-2) [1]. Widespread application of such a system to reporting standards on terminology and classification will greatly facilitate outcome analysis and the comparison of results.

Until such time as the Jeffcoate or some similar system is in widespread use, ulcers ideally should be photographed for serial examination. Narrative descriptions of lesions should address the depth of ulcer penetration, the involvement of fascial or bony structures, the presence or degree of bacterial penetration, the presence or severity of neuropathic sensory disorders, and the presence or absence of a palpable pedal pulse (with an ABI documented if the pulse is absent or diminished).

Interest is increasing in the preventative assessment of the presence or severity of lower-extremity ischemia in diabetic patients with intact feet. The American Heart Association (AHA) and the American Diabetes Association (ADA) recommend annual lower-extremity vascular examinations in diabetic patients, regardless of the presence or absence of ulcers or symptomatic vascular disease [35]. The screening program is similar in scope and purpose to the diabetic retinopathy program, to identify and treat complications at an early stage.

Traditional subjective screening techniques (such as the Rose questionnaire) for peripheral vascular occlusive disease consistently underestimate the severity of disease present in diabetic patients. Only 20 percent of patients with objective evidence of peripheral vascular occlusive disease (as determined by a low ABI) report symptoms of claudication [35]. Palpable pulse deficits also have a low predictive value when examined in larger series [35]. The AHA and the ADA suggest that those discrepancies are due to the limited, distal nature of early diabetic and atherosclerotic peripheral vascular occlusive disease. Diabetes-associated vascular disease may affect only one or two tibial vessels.

Individual tibial-artery involvement will not precipitate claudication or affect the ABI. While asymptomatic, this early stage of disease has significant prognostic importance regarding overall survival. Isolated posterior tibial-artery stenosis or occlusion in a patient with diabetes mellitus carries a threefold risk of all-cause mortality and a fourfold risk of coronary heart disease mortality, in addition to its influence on the development of pedal ulceration [35]. Thus, accurate identification of early stages of peripheral vascular occlusive disease in the diabetic patient is important.

Determination of both the posterior tibial and dorsal pedal ABI assesses the presence and severity of lower-extremity ischemia. The prevalence of abnormal ABIs suggestive of occlusive disease (< 0.90) increases with both patient age and diabetes duration. While concern exists regarding the diagnosis of occlusive disease in the patient with medial calcification and incompressibility, in practice only a small minority of patients and examinations are compromised by that problem. The toe systolic blood pressure (TSBP) [36] can provide an accurate and reproducible estimation of pedal perfusion pressure in the setting of medial calcification of the more proximal tibial and pedal vessels. The examination is useful because the digital arteries commonly are spared from the process of medial calcification.

The TSBP can be of great prognostic value. A TSBP of 30 mm Hg or more is predictive of a healing rate of toe and forefoot ulcers in greater than 90 percent of patients assessed in a large, representative clinical series. A TSBP of less than 20 mm Hg is associated with only a 29-percent primary healing rate. Two-thirds of limbs with a TSBP of less than 30 mm Hg in that same series eventually went on to amputation, as opposed to none with a TSBP of 30 mm Hg or higher [37].

Many other indirect methods predict lower-extremity wound healing [38]. In practice, none is as accurate as the ABI or the TSBP. Pecoraro and associates at the Seattle Veterans Affairs Medical Center claim reproducible success with their technique using transcutaneous oxygen tension (TcO_2) and carbon dioxide tension ($TcCO_2$) as predictors of wound healing [31]. TcO_2 determinations require careful instrument calibration and dedicated diagnostic facilities, which are not widely available. Perhaps due to those limitations, the general experience with periwound oxygen and carbon dioxide determination has been less successful [35]. Evaluation of velocity-waveform patterns (loss of normal triphasic or biphasic waveform, spectral broadening, and increasing peak systolic velocity ($>100\%$) between segments) in the Vascular Laboratory has shown good reproducibility and reliability in assessing the degree and significance of inflow disease in the lower extremity and, by inference, the likelihood of ulcer healing [35].

THERAPY

Treatment for ischemic or diabetic lesions differs greatly from therapy directed toward venous ulcers whereas the venous ulcer responds to compression. Compression is ineffectual and potentially harmful in the patient with symptomatic arterial ischemia. Effective therapy for ischemic and diabetic ulcers relies on accurate and rapid assessment of limb perfusion, directed specifically at the arterial examination.

New patients with pedal abscesses, plantar fasciitis, ulceration with lymphangiitis, or other forms of supporative infections require operative drainage and debridement as their initial intervention. Frequently, those patients are examined, drained, and debrided in the operating room to optimize patient safety and comfort. Once the local infection is addressed, assessment of the arterial inflow status is obtained. Therapy is then determined by the presence or absence of palpable pulses. The presence of palpable pulses is reassurance that careful attention to wound management and antibiosis will result in ulcer resolution and limb salvage.

Very occasionally, patients present with advanced infections unresponsive to optimal medical and surgical therapy, requiring emergency amputation despite palpable pulses. Such a situation arises when most or all of the foot is involved or necrotic. In such circumstances, emergency guillotine amputation is indicated to save as much limb length as possible. Happily, that degree of tissue destruction is rarely present. Emergency foot or leg amputation should be considered only when insufficient surface area remains on the foot to bear weight.

Pulseless, ulcerated feet need objective estimation of arterial perfusion (ABI or TSBP) once local sepsis has been addressed. Contrast arteriography may be necessary if the ABI is compromised by medial calcification and the hallux is involved or absent. Hemodynamically significant inflow stenosis proximal to the ankle needs to be corrected. Our experience mirrors that of LoGerfo [5], Taylor [39], and many others: Restoration of pulsatile blood flow

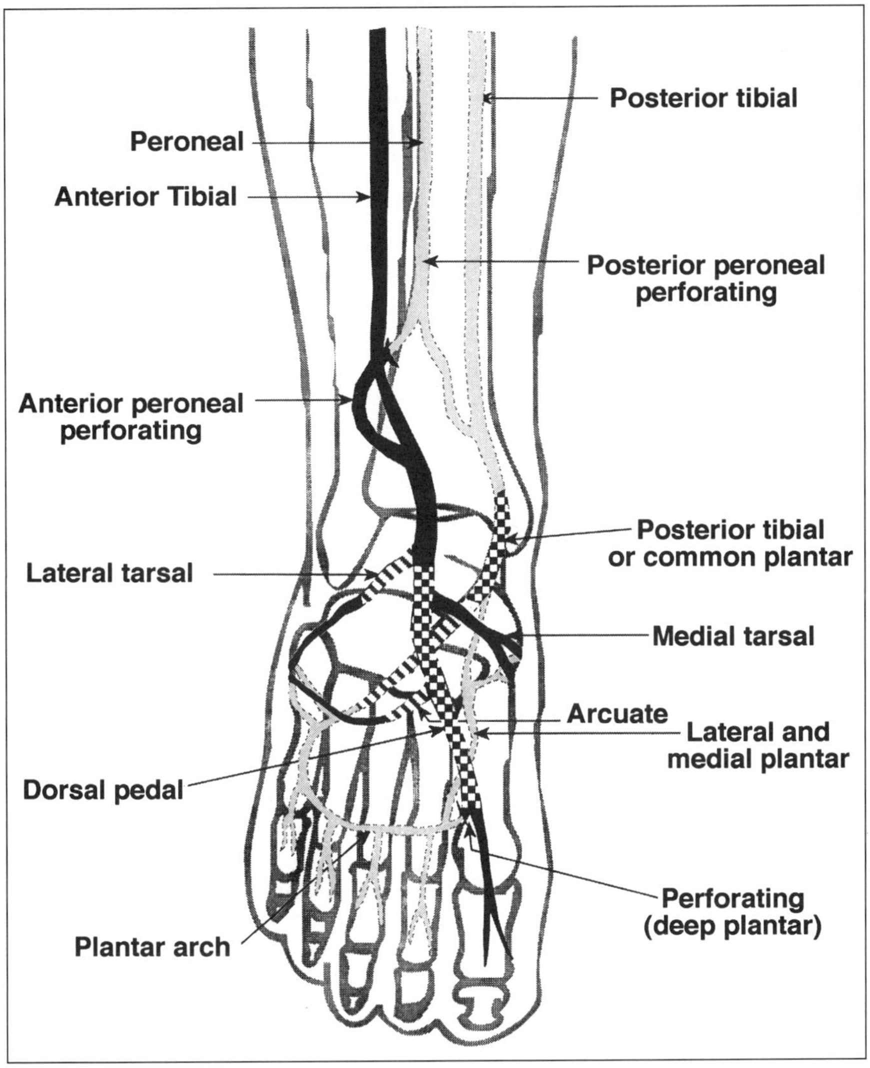

Fig. 51-4. Likely pedal-artery bypass targets based on a series of 60 consecutive pedal arteriograms. Used with permission from EV Lang, RL Dalman, EJ Harris. Impact of anatomic criteria on feasibility of inframallelolar bypass surgery: optimization of pedal arteriography. Radiology. In press.

to the ulcerated, ischemic foot is critical to the healing process.

In our own practice, ischemic feet with stable, chronic ulcers are revascularized as the initial intervention. Debridement and toe or forefoot amputation in patients without suppurative, necrotizing infections are performed later during the same hospitalization. The procedures are performed with an ankle-block anesthetic a few days after revascularization. The timing allows for demarcation of viable tissue. We have found that allowing a few days to separate revascularization from amputation frequently preserves the maximum amount of forefoot tissue. If definitive debridement or closure is accomplished at this sitting, the patient frequently can be discharged the following day.

The dorsalis pedis artery is frequently preserved in the diabetic foot and is of great utility as a bypass target [5,40] (Fig. 51-4). Our experience suggests that the durability of inframalleolar grafts compares with those to the more proximal tibial vessels. Healing of pedal incisions has not been particularly morbid if the incisions are placed directly over the bypass target. Our operative technique uses reversed or nonreversed autogenous vein and is described elsewhere [41].

Once inflow is established, the perfused foot is debrided. Operative exploration is the most reliable method of determining the integrity of underlying bone and connective tissue. Callus is trimmed to eliminate pressure points. Granulation tissue is debrided. Ray amputations are performed well proximal to the area of involvement. Foot incisions are made on non-weight-bearing surfaces whenever possible. Phalanx amputations are made through keyhole-type vertical incisions to draw the remaining toes together.

We spare as much soft tissue as possible during wound debridement and closure, leaving all viable tissue. Once

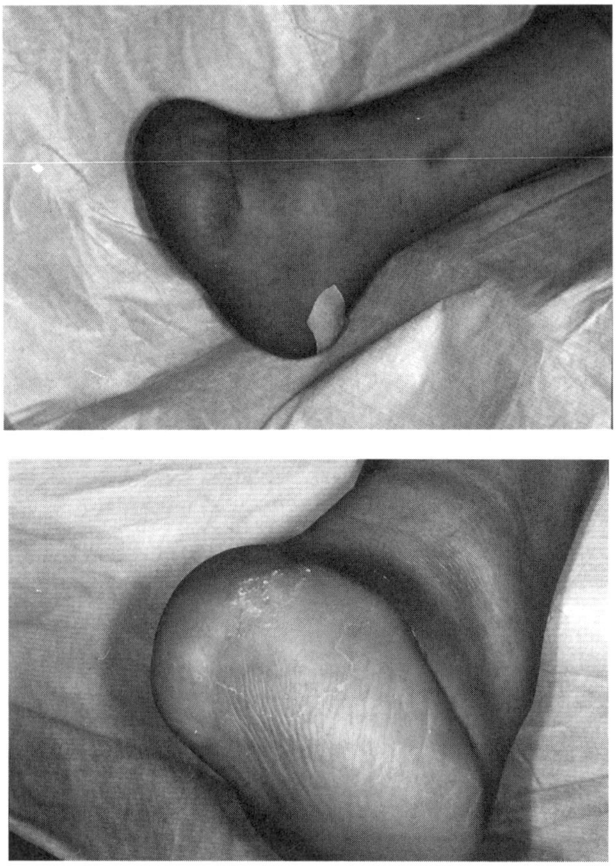

Fig. 51-5. Partial foot amputation retaining maximal amount of functional, weight-bearing foot.

healing has begun, full-thickness skin flaps can be used to cover exposed periosteum and connective tissue. First-metatarsal head ulcers usually are treated by first metatarsal head and sesamoid removal through a medial incision, with debridement of the ulcer and Penrose drain placement through the residual plantar defect. The medial incision is generally closed.

In chronic stable ulcers, most commonly the wound is debrided and closed at the same operation. Closure is most commonly accomplished by widely spaced, monofilament suture placed in a mattressed fashion. Potential areas of dead space are minimized by the mattress action of the percutaneous suture. No suture is placed in subcutaneous layers unless a considerable amount of dead space is otherwise inevitable. The technique minimizes potentially infective foreign material within the wound and allows some drainage between the sutures. If acute infection predominates, closure is followed sometime after drainage and revascularization.

To the greatest extent possible, the foot is preserved as the weight-bearing platform (Fig. 51-5). In our practice, a Syme amputation has not been well tolerated by diabetics with moderate or severe neuropathy. Exposed and involved os calsus may not necessarily prompt complete amputation of the foot. Recent advances in free-flap technology and an evolving interest in limb salvage on the part of plastic surgeons are improving chances for limb salvage even in patients with advanced hind-limb lesions. Casting is rarely employed in any patient other than the diabetic with acute Charcot degeneration, which may not be accompanied by an ulcer.

Debridement and closure are followed by a prolonged period of non-weight bearing, which may last 4 to 6 weeks and is facilitated by crutch walking, use of a walker or wheelchair, or a short stay in a skilled nursing facility, depending on the overall health, strength, and ambulatory status of the patient. During this period, the patient's wound is examined on a weekly or biweekly basis. A prolonged course of oral antibiotic therapy is continued during this aspect of the healing phase in diabetic patients [5]. Overgrowth of resistent or nonbacterial pathogens may limit the length or utility of antibiotic therapy. After revascularization and debridement, autogenous bypass grafts are evaluated at regular intervals in the vascular laboratory using published criteria [42] to maintain long-term patency.

RESULTS OF THERAPY

Aggressive revascularization is a recent development in the treatment of diabetic foot ulcers. Prolonged periods of bedrest, antibiotics, and local wound care have long been the norm. Rivers and colleagues described a contemporary policy of nonoperative therapy for severely ischemic patients judged to be noncandidates for operative revascularization based on excessive operative risk [43]. Seventy-one percent (10 out of 14) of this patient population suffered diabetes. Management consisted of bed rest, simple saline soaks, occasional gentle debridement, and antibiotics when indicated. Only half (7 patients) healed their wounds following this treatment regimen, between 4 weeks and 18 months. The remainder (3 patients) remained stable or eventually required bypass surgery, which was successful in 1 patient. The costs of such a policy were not addressed by the authors but obviously were considerable, especially when wound care stretched out over several months.

Gibbons and co-authors described the impact on their practice of a switch to aggressive revascularization from prolonged wound care as solo therapy in the ulcerated foot [44]. That shift occurred between 1984 and 1990. They noted a significant decrease in the number of amputations performed, improved outcome for all patients, and lower overall cost per wound healed following the implementation of that type of practice. By comparison, the patients described by Rivers and Veith required much longer hospital stays and had less satisfactory outcomes. While cost issues are not comparable between the two groups, a considerable savings can be attributed to accelerated wound healing.

The role of primary amputation in the treatment of limb-threatening ischemia and pedal ulcers has recently been reviewed by the Oregon group [45]. Their conclusion, based on 10 years' experience with a uniform reconstructive policy strongly supports aggressive revascularization. As demonstrated by those investigators, nonrevascularization can significantly prolong resolution of lesions and carries substantial intercurrent morbidity associated with permanent immobility.

Patients with Charcot degeneration of the foot and neuropathic ulcers with normal pedal arterial perfusion present a special clinical problem. Protective shoe inserts, custom deep-box shoes, serial casting techniques, and prolonged non-weight-bearing status all play important roles in patient management. The benefit of metatarsal head amputation for treatment of mal perforans ulcers remains uncertain. Griffiths and Wieman described their recent experience with 25 diabetic patients who underwent 34 metatarsal head amputations for neuropathic ulcers. The authors note uniform lesion healing following removal of the underlying pressure point, after uniform failure of prolonged conservative wound care prior to surgery [46]. Long-term follow-up was not reported.

We perform many metatarsal head resections in patients with mal perforans ulcers. In general, the procedure is very successful at achieving initial healing. Less certain are the long-term consequences of such amputations. A few patients with healed neuropathic lesions return with recurrent ulcers despite protective prosthetic design. If weight is simply shifted between metatarsal heads, further ulceration may be inevitable. Some experienced clinicians suggest transmetatarsal amputations as the initial procedure for mal perforans ulcers. While we do not follow that policy, we are concerned about recurrent mal perforans ulcers following ray amputation. This procedure is definitely contraindicated during the unstable phase of Charcot degeneration.

Immune compromise and the lack of protective sensation that characterize diabetes may preclude successful resolution of neuropathic ulcers even with prolonged non-weight-bearing and antibiotic therapy. The question of underlying bony infection or structural abnormalities frequently are a complicating issue. The participation of an experienced orthotist and podiatrist in such patients' care dramatically improves outcome in difficult situations such as these. We rely heavily on multidisciplinary interactions to maximize outcome during the treatment of these lesions.

Finally, in the age of cost containment and managed care, outcome analysis is the essential standard of benefit. Several regional models now exist of multidisciplinary clinics that are dedicated to treatment of threatened limbs. The presumption has been that those clinics will improve limb salvage and prolong ambulatory status, but the documentation to justify the efforts is only now developing. Griffiths and Wieman compared the number of lesions, length to time healed, length of inpatient stay, and number of major amputations required to achieve wound healing between a group of patients regularly followed in their preventative care clinic and a larger group referred only for intervention for more advanced lesions [47]. That study suggests a model that similar clinical efforts will have to follow in documenting outcome. In the cost-sensitive environment of modern health care, establishing the utility of aggressive educational and screening programs designed to prevent pedal ulceration in diabetes is crucial to the widespread implementation of those programs and ultimate attempts at improved limb salvage.

Pedal ulceration remains a morbid complication of peripheral vascular disease and diabetes. Although other etiologies commonly are involved, arterial ischemia is the most common denominator. Accurate, rapid assessment of arterial inflow, followed by revascularization, debridement, wound care, antimicrobial therapy and prevention of further injury represent the state of the art in treatment of such lesions. Further advances in preventative care and promoting healing events at the cellular level will be required to lower the morbidity and cost associated with contemporary treatment of these lesions.

Venous Ulcers

Chronic venous insufficiency is a common yet often misunderstood condition. In its most severe form, chronic venous insufficiency may lead to venous ulceration. Venous ulceration accounts for as much as 50 percent of lower-extremity ulceration in the United States [48]. Several epidemiologic studies in the United States suggest as many as 400,000 to 600,000 new venous ulcers develop each year [49,50], figures that are quite similar to prevalence data outside the United States. Despite a well-recognized prevalence, little progress has been made in the treatment of venous ulceration since its first clinical description by the early Greeks and Romans. Successful treatments all have employed some form of compression therapy with leg elevation. Failure to identify progress in the treatment of chronic venous insufficiency reflects the incomplete understanding of the pathophysiology of chronic venous insufficiency and venous ulceration.

John Homans identified varicose veins adjacent to sites of ulceration and proposed that "stagnation" of that blood under pressure would readily lead to the development of open sores [51]. That concept is the origin for the term **stasis ulceration**. The concept remained largely unchallenged for more than 60 years. More recent investigations into the pathophysiology of venous ulceration discount the concept of stasis. Current investigations are focused on the macro- and microcirculatory hemodynamics associated with chronic venous insufficiency, as well as the cellular and humoral changes of chronic venous insufficiency and their influence on the skin and subcutaneous tissues.

VENOUS HEMODYNAMICS

The lower-extremity venous system is composed of three components: superficial veins, perforating or communicating veins, and deep veins. The superficial venous system is composed of the greater and lesser saphenous veins (Fig. 51-6). Connecting the superficial veins to the deep veins are the perforating veins, which perforate the fascial compartments of the leg. The perforating veins have valves that open only toward the deep system. Under normal conditions, blood from the skin and subcutaneous tissues is collected in the superficial veins, then directed through the perforating veins to the deep veins and then cephalad to the heart. The deep venous system follows the major arterial tree of the lower extremity. In the foot, venae comitantes of the lateral plantar artery empty into

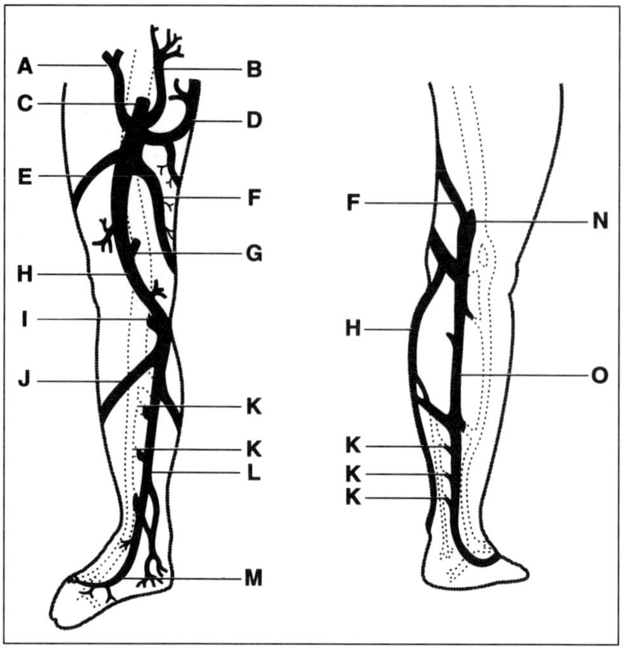

Fig. 51-6. General relationship of the greater (left) and lesser (right) saphenous veins to the deep venous system (dotted lines) via the communicating veins. A = superficial circumflex iliac vein; B = superior epigastric vein; C = saphenofemoral bulb; D = superior external pudendal; E = anterolateral thigh vein; F = posteromedial thigh vein; G = Hunterian communicating vein; H = greater saphenous vein; I = Boyd's communicating vein; J = anterior saphenous vein; K = Cockett's communicating veins; L = posterior arch vein; M = dorsal arch; N = saphenopopliteal junction; O = lesser saphenous vein.

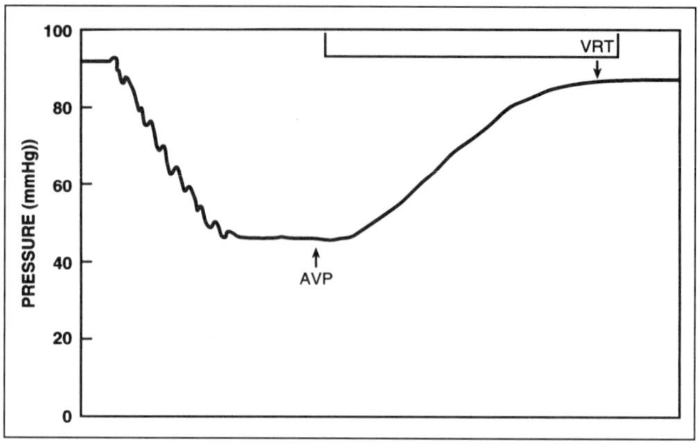

Fig. 51-7. A normal plethysmographic tracing approximating dorsal foot venous pressure. The tracing begins with the patient standing and the ankle pressure of 90 mmHg. After 10 toe-up exercises, the pressure drops to 35 mmHg and is termed the ambulatory venous pressure (AVP). The pressure then slowly returns to baseline. The time required for the dorsal foot venous pressure to return to 90 percent of baseline from the AVP value is termed the venous recovery time (VRT). Normal VRT is greater than 16–20 seconds; abnormal VRTs are shorter.

the posterior tibial venae comitantes. The tibial veins are paired structures, with all three uniting at the popliteal fossa to form the single popliteal vein. At the adductor canal, the popliteal vein becomes the superficial femoral vein, which continues cephalad to join the profunda femoris vein as the common femoral vein. The deep veins have valves, yet fewer valves than are present in either the superficial or the perforating venous system.

Venous intravascular pressure is defined by the summation of dynamic pressure produced by the contracting left ventricle, hydrostatic pressure produced by the weight of the column of blood, and static filling pressure that is related to the elasticity of the venous wall. In most circumstances, static filling pressures are neglible in the venous system. Although the hydrostatic pressure at the ankle in a standing patient may reach 100 mm Hg, it usually is canceled by gravitational potential energy. The driving force for venous return from the lower extremities to the heart is the dynamic pressure, which can reach 15–20 mm Hg in the venules, allowing flow along the energy gradient to the heart with atrial pressures of 0–6 mm Hg [52]. In the upright position, without muscle contraction, the baseline dorsal foot vein pressure is 80–90 mm Hg [53,54].

Ambulatory venous pressures (AVP) are obtained by cannulating a dorsal vein of the foot in a standing position, exercising the calf muscles, and obtaining a new baseline pressure. With the onset of calf-muscle contraction, venous pressure may initially rise, but then it steadily decreases as the calf veins are emptied, usually to a value below 40 mm Hg in normal subjects [55] (Fig. 51-7). Nicoliades has correlated abnormal ambulatory venous pressure with an increased incidence of venous ulcer. Ulcers seldom develop in limbs with ambulatory venous pressures 45 mm Hg or less. With increasing ambulatory venous pressure, the incidence of ulcer formation increases sharply; 15 percent of patients with AVP between 50 and 59 mm Hg, 50 percent of patients with AVP between 60 and 69 mm Hg, and 80 percent of patients with AVP greater than 80 mm Hg will develop venous ulcers [56].

A more recently defined component of lower-extremity venous return is the venous "footpump" proposed by Gardner [57]. The abnormally large venae comitantes of the lateral plantar artery have been confirmed by video phlebography. This plantar venous pump is activated by simple weight bearing, with stretching of the venous plexus rather than extrinsic compression causing venous ejection [58]. The plantar venous pump has a stroke volume of 20–30 ml and can generate enough force to dislocate blood against a pressure gradient of 100 mm Hg.

With venous insufficiency, the normal decrease in standing venous pressures during ambulation is not observed. The pressure may stay the same as before ambulation or fall minimally, a situation somewhat erroneously termed **venous hypertension**. There are at least four possible mechanisms for the development of venous hypertension. Ultimately, venous hypertension results in valvular damage, reflux, and retrograde flow of venous blood from the deep to the superficial systems. Retrograde flow can occur because of (1) traumatic or congenital damage to the valves of the superficial or communicating

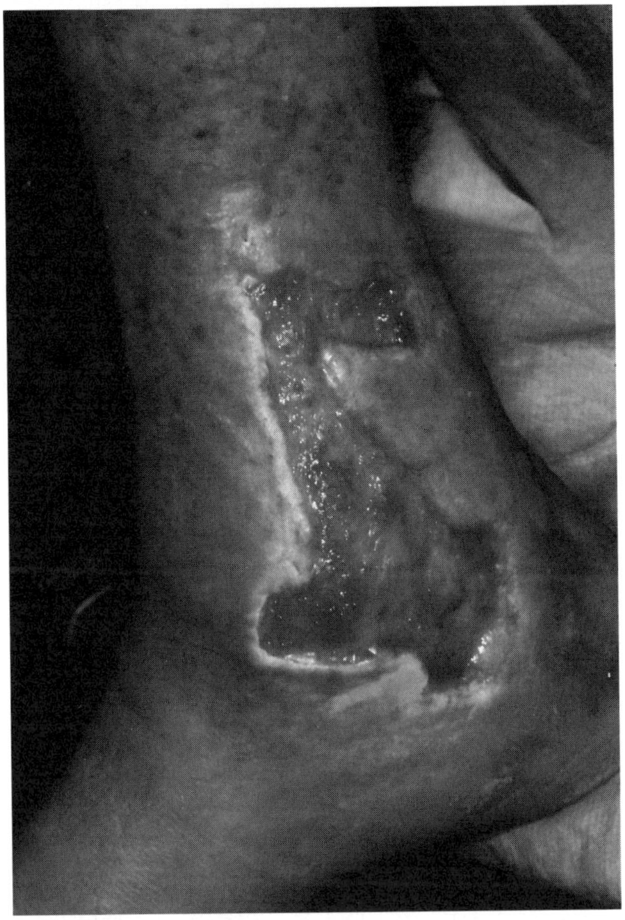

Fig. 51-8. Typical appearance and location for venous ulceration.

veins; (2) traumatic or congenital damage to the valves of the deep veins, with secondary incompetence of the communicating or superficial vein valves; (3) obstruction of the deep venous system, with secondary incompetence of the valves of the communicating or superficial veins; or (4) traumatic or congenital failure of the venous pumps, calf muscle, or foot.

Most current investigation into the pathophysiology of venous ulcers is centered on the effects of venous hypertension on the skin and subcutaneous tissues and the secondary cellular and humoral changes observed in that environment. Most venous ulcers are identified in the "gaiter" region of the lower leg, that region inferior to the tapering of the calf muscles posteriorly and superior to the talocalcaneal joint (Fig. 51-8). The largest hydrostatic and ambulatory venous pressures are located in that gaiter region. It is believed that the abnormally increased venous pressure transmitted from the macro- to the microcirculation is the driving force behind the development of venous ulceration.

PATHOGENESIS

The oxygenation of venous blood in varicose veins was historically thought to be important in the development of venous ulceration. It was hypothesized that the superficial venous blood was hypoxic, rendering local tissue hypoxemia and subsequent ulceration. It is now clear that in supine and standing positions, hemoglobin saturation of the blood in varicose veins is higher than and equal to that in normal veins, respectively [59,60]. The increase in supine venous oxygen saturation in varicose veins led some to suspect occult arteriovenous communications, although specific investigation of the skin of patients with venous disease failed to detect any such communications [61,62].

Browse and Burnand have shown in animal models and in humans that increased capillary pressure as a consequence of venous hypertension allows an increased leak of plasma proteins into the pericapillary dermis. The proteins extravasated into the dermis include fibrinogen, which subsequently polymerizes and forms the "fibrin cuffs" that may be seen around the dermal capillaries by both histochemical and immunohistochemical techniques [63,64]. Others have shown pericapillary fibrin in skin adjacent to venous ulcers, and those patients have increased plasma fibrinogen levels and reduced plasma fibrinolytic activity [65]. Most recently, the pericapillary fibrin deposits in patients with venous ulceration have been characterized, and the fibrin is mostly undegraded [66]. Proponents of the fibrin-cuff theory of venous ulceration believe those fibrin cuffs diminish oxygen diffusion in the skin of affected areas [61]. In spite of innovative tests to define the oxygen tension in skin of patients with venous insufficiency and ulceration, there is no conclusive evidence to prove that fibrin cuffs provide a diffusion barrier for tissue oxygenation [67]. Yet certain aspects of the fibrin-cuff theory are undeniable. Fibrin deposits are observable in a dermal pericapillary distribution in patients with chronic venous insufficiency and appear to be a histologic marker for venous ulceration. To date, there remains no convincing evidence that pericapillary fibrin cuffs are essential to the development of venous ulcers.

The most recent theory concerning the pathogenesis of venous ulceration from chronic venous insufficiency is the white blood cell–trapping theory. That theory is based on the presumption that white blood cell trapping in the microcirculation of the skin of limbs with venous hypertension leads to congestion and subsequent thrombosis. White blood cells then migrate into the interstitial tissues and release their lysosomal enzymes, which become activated and begin tissue degradation and necrosis. The impetus for that theory came from observations by Moyses et al., who compared the hematologic parameters in blood samples from the dependent limbs of normal patients after their legs remained dependent for a period of 40 minutes [68] with samples obtained from the same limb in a supine position. They found that the hematocrit and red blood cell count increased in parallel, but that the white cell count remained unchanged, despite the increasing hematocrit. White blood cells appeared to be lost from the circulation, with the loss calculated at 20 percent. Differential white blood cell counts identified monocytes as the predominant cell type lost. Others have shown a more exaggerated "trapping" of white blood cells in patients with chronic venous insufficiency [69,70].

Based on those observations, Coleridge Smith et al. examined nonulcerated perimalleolar skin in patients with video microscopy and documented the number of visible capillary loops per unit area [71]. Capillary microscopy of perimalleolar skin and samples of femoral-vein blood were obtained in normal patients, patients with varicose veins, and patients with lipodermatosclerosis supine and after 30 minutes of limb dependency. They found fewer capillary loops in patients with lipodermatosclerosis and a decrease in the white blood cell counts obtained from the femoral-vein sample in the dependent position compared to the supine position. Those observations did not hold true in the other two groups. Further evidence for white blood cell trapping comes from skin-punch biopsies performed in patients with healed venous ulcers. Skin-punch biopsies from perimalleolar skin were obtained in control patients and patients with lipodermatosclerosis and a history of ulceration. There were significantly more white blood cells per cubic millimeter in the venous insufficiency group than in the control group (217 versus 6.2 cells/cu mm) [72]. Yet as with the fibrin cuffs, the presence of white blood cell trapping in chronic venous insufficiency does not prove that the phenomenon causes ulceration. To date, there is no conclusive evidence that white blood cell trapping causes diminished microcirculation and cellular malnutrition leading to ulceration. White blood cell trapping remains another marker of chronic venous insufficiency.

TREATMENT OF VENOUS ULCERS

The essential components of treatment of venous ulcers are leg elevation and compression therapy to help decrease leg edema and venous hypertension [73]. Bed rest is impractical in most situations, so leg compression assumes increased importance. There are three choices of compression therapy, all with their advocates. Leg pumps or sequential compression devices have shown efficacy in the treatment of chronic venous ulcers, especially in patients who will not tolerate graduated compression stockings or with dysfunctional muscle pumps [77]. While those systems are expensive and often cumbersome, they can be very useful and cost effective for recalcitrant ulcers. The remaining choices for compression therapy are elastic or nonelastic bandaging, both of which are effective. Some believe topical agents improve the effects of compression [75], while others have failed to identify any benefits of specific dressing types on wound healing [76]. Similarly, occlusive dressings with hydrocolloid require adjunctive compression therapy to effectively heal venous ulcers and offer no advantages over traditional compression therapy [77,78].

We currently favor local wound care and ambulation with elastic compression stockings. Local wound care for the ulcer consists of cleansing the wound with soap and water several times a day, application of a sterile dry dressing, and a custom-fit compression stocking, usually a 30–40 mm Hg below-knee variety. Additional localized pressure may be applied over the ulcer by adding extra layers of dressings under the stocking.

Newer therapies with fibrinolytic agents and hemorrheologic agents have been reported, yet those therapies require adjunctive compression therapy for successful healing. A randomized, crossover trial of the fibrinolytic agent stanozolol compared with placebo, with both groups receiving compression therapy, showed no difference in ulcer healing [79]. A newer antithrombotic and profibrinolytic agent, defibrotide, has shown promising results in venous ulcer healing, when combined with adjunctive compression therapy [80]. Pentoxifylline, whose properties include reduction in white blood cell aggregation and activation, has recently been shown to be efficacious as an adjunctive agent to compression therapy for refractory venous ulcers [81].

Summary

Venous ulceration is a common problem whose treatment has remained largely unchanged for centuries. Currently there is no satisfactory macro- or microvascular concept able to wholly explain the occurrence of venous ulceration in chronic venous insufficiency. Although the several theories presented have alternatively gained and lost favor over time, no one concept adequately accounts for all the anatomic and physiologic abnormalities identified with venous ulcers. Venous hypertension from whatever mechanism is closely related to the development of venous ulcers. In spite of recent interest in fibrinolytic and leukocyte-inhibiting agents, to date the mainstay of treatment for venous ulcers remains compression therapy.

References

1. Gibbons GW. The diabetic foot: amputations and drainage of infection. J Vasc Surg 1987; 5:791–793.
2. Review of charges for fiscal year 1993 for CPT and IDCM-9 codes pertinent to diabetic and ischemic pedal ulcerations at Stanford University Hospital, Stanford, California, by R. Dalman.
3. Callam MJ, et al. Arterial disease in chronic leg ulceration: an underestimated hazard? Lothian and Forth Valley leg ulcer study. British Med J 1987; 294:929–931.
4. Nelzen O, Dergqvist D, Lindhagen A. High prevalence of diabetes in chronic leg ulcer patients: a cross-sectional population study. Diabetic Medicine 1993; 10:345–350.
5. LoGerfo FW, et al. Trends in the care of the diabetic foot. Arch Surg 1992; 127:617–621.
6. Melton LJ 3d, et al. Incidence and prevalence of clinical peripheral vascular disease in a population-based cohort of diabetic patients. Diabetes Care 1980; 3:650–654.
7. Griffiths GD, Wieman TJ. Meticulous attention to foot care improves the prognosis in diabetic ulceration of the foot. Surg Gyn and Obst 1992; 174:49–51.
8. Debatin JF, et al. Phase contrast MRI assessment of pedal blood flow. Eur Radiol 1955; 5:36–42.
9. Edmonds ME, Blundell P, Morris ME. Improved survival of the diabetic foot: the role of the specialised foot clinic. Q J Med 1986; 232:763–771.
10. Edmonds ME, Nicoliades KH, Watkins PJ. Autonomic neuropathy and diabetic foot ulceration. Diab Med 1986; 3:56–59.
11. LoGerfo FW, Coffman JD. Vascular and microvascular disease of the foot in diabetes. Implications for foot care. NEJM 1984; 311:1615–1619.
12. Blumenthal HT. More on microvascular disease of the foot in diabetes. NEJM 1985; 313:696–697.
13. Boulton AJM, Scarpello JHB, Ward JD. Venous oxygenation in the diabetic neuropathic foot. Diabetologia 1982; 22:6–8.

14. Archer AG, Roberts VC, Watkins PJ. Blood flow patterns in painful diabetic neuropathy. Diabetologia 1984; 27:563–567.
15. Edmonds ME, Roberts VC, Watkins PJ. Blood flow in the diabetic neuropathic foot. Diabetologia 1982; 22:9–15.
16. Flynn MD, et al. Direct measurement of capillary blood flow in the diabetic neuropathic foot. Diabetologia 1988; 31:652–656.
17. Ward JD. The diabetic leg. Diabetologia 1982; 22:141–147.
18. Rayman G, et al. Impaired microvascular hyperaemic response to minor skin trauma in type I diabetes. Br Med J 1986; 292:1295–1298.
19. Walmsley D, Wales JK, Wiles PG. Reduced hyperaemia following skin trauma: evidence for an impaired microvascular response to injury in the diabetic foot. Diabetologia 1989; 32:736–739.
20. Flynn ME, Tooke JE. Microcirculation and the diabetic foot. VMR 1990; 1:121–138.
21. Tymms DJ, Tooke JE. The effect of continuous subcutaneous insulin infusion on microvascular blood flow in diabetes mellitus. Int J Microcirc Clin Exp 1988; 7:347–356.
22. McMillen DE. The effects of diabetes on blood flow properties. Diabetes 1983; 32[Suppl 2]:56–63.
23. Barnes AJ. Rheology of diabetes mellitus. In GDL Lowe, ed. Clinical Blood Rheology, vol II. Boca Raton: CRC Press, 1988. Pp. 163–187.
24. Flynn MD, Tooke JE. Aetiology of diabetic foot ulceration: a role for the microcirculation? Diab Med 1992; 8:320–329.
25. Young MJ, Boulton AJM, Cavanagh PR. Medial arterial calcification in the feet of diabetic patients and diabetic and nondiabetic control subjects. Diabetologia 1993; 36:615–621.
26. Criado E, et al. The course of severe foot infections in patients with diabetes. SGO 1992; 175:135–140.
27. Wheat LJ, et al. Diabetic foot infections. Bacteriologic analysis. Arch Int Med 1986; 146:1935–1940.
28. Sharp CS, et al. Microbiology of superficial and deep tissues in infected diabetic gangrene. SGO 1979; 149:217–219.
29. Sapico FL, et al. The infected foot in the diabetic patient: quantitative microbiology and analysis of clinical features. Rev Inf Dis 1984; [Suppl 1]6:171–176.
30. Shults DW, et al. Value of radiographs and bone scans in determining the need for therapy in diabetic patients with foot ulcers. Am J Surg 1989; 158:525–530.
31. Pecoraro RE, Reiber GE, Burgess EM. Pathways to diabetic limb amputation. Diabetes Care 1990; 13:513–521.
32. Wagner FW. The dysvascular foot: a system for diagnosis and treatment. Foot and Ankle 1981; 2:64–122.
33. Apelqvist J, et al. Wound classification is more important than site of ulceration in the outcome of diabetic foot ulcers. Diabetic Medicine 1993; 10:526–529.
34. Jeffcoate WJ, MacFarlane RM, Fletcher EM. The description and classification of diabetic foot lesions. Diabetic Medicine 1993; 10:676–679.
35. Orchard TJ, et al. Assessment of Peripheral Vascular Disease in Diabetes. Report and Recommendations of an International Workshop Sponsored by the American Diabetes Association and the American Heart Association. Circulation 1993; 88:819–827.
36. Strandness DE, Bell JW. Peripheral vascular disease: diagnosis and objective evaluation using a mercury strain gauge. Ann Surg 1965; 161:3–35.
37. Holstein P. The distal blood pressure predicts healing of amputations on the feet. Acta Orthop Scand 1984; 55:227–233.
38. Defrang RF, Taylor LM, Porter JM. Basic data related to amputations. Ann Vasc Surg 1991; 5(2):202–207.
39. Taylor LM Jr, Porter JM. The clinical course of diabetics who require emergent foot surgery because of infection or ischemia. J Vasc Surg 1987; 6:454–459.
40. Dalman RL, Taylor LM. Basic data related to lower extremity revascularization. Ann Vasc Surg 1990; 4(3):309–312.
41. Dalman RL, Taylor LM, Porter JM. Technique of reversed vein bypass to distal leg arteries. In JB Chang, ed. Modern Vascular Surgery, Volume 5. New York: Springer, 1992.
42. Yao JST. Noninvasive studies of peripheral vascular disease. In FJ Veith, ed. Vascular Surgery: Principles and Practice. Second Edition. New York: McGraw-Hill, 1994.
43. Rivers SP, et al. Successful conservative therapy of severe limb-threatening ischemia: the value of nonsympathectomy. Surgery 1986; 99:759–762.
44. Gibbons GW, et al. Improved quality of diabetic foot care, 1984 vs. 1990. Arch Surg 1993; 128:576–581.
45. Taylor LM, et al. Limb salvage vs. amputation for critical ischemia: the role of vascular surgery. Arch Surg 1991; 126:1251–1258.
46. Griffiths GD, Wieman TJ. Metatarsal head resection for diabetic foot ulcers. Arch Surg 1990; 125:832–835.
47. Griffiths GD, Wieman TJ. Meticulous attention to foot care improves the prognosis in diabetic ulceration of the foot. SGO 1992; 174:49–51.
48. Falanga V. Venous ulceration. J Dermatol Surg Oncol 1993; 19:764–771.
49. Coon WW, Willis PW, Keller JB. Venous thromboembolism and other venous disease in the Tecumseh Community Health Study. Circulation 1973; 48:839–845.
50. Falanga V, Eagelstein WH. A therapeutic approach to venous ulcers. J Am Acad Dermatol 1986; 14:777–784.
51. Homans J. The etiology and treatment of varicose ulcers of the leg. Surg Gynecol Obstet 1917; 24:300–315.
52. Sumner DS. Hemodynamics and pathophysiology of venous disease. In RB Rutherford, ed. Vascular Surgery. 3rd Edition. Philadelphia: Saunders, 1989. Pp. 1483–1504.
53. Pollack AA, Wood EH. Venous pressure in the saphenous vein at the ankle in man during exercise and changes in posture. J Appl Physiol 1949; 1:649–662.
54. Hojensgard IC, Sturup H. Static and dynamic pressures in the superficial and deep veins of the lower extremity in man. Acta Physiol Scand 1952; 27:49–67.
55. Porter JM, et al. Reporting standards in venous disease. J Vasc Surg 1988; 8:172–181.
56. Nicoliades AN, Zukowski AJ. The value of dynamic pressure measurements. World J Surg 1986; 10:919–923.
57. Gardner AMN, Fox RH. The venous footpump: influence on tissue perfusion and prevention of venous thrombosis. Ann Rheum Dis 1992; 51:1173–1178.
58. Gardner AMN, et al. Reduction of post-traumatic swelling and compartment pressure by impulse compression of the foot. J Bone Joint Surg [Br] 1990; 72-B:810–815.
59. Blumhoff RL, Johnson G. Saphenous vein PO2 in patients with varicose veins. J Surg Res 1977; 23:35–36.
60. Scott HJ, et al. A reappraisal of the oxygenation of the venous blood of varicose veins. Br J Surg 1990; 77:934–936.
61. Brewer AC. Arteriovenous shunts. Br Med J 1950; 2:270.
62. Lindmayr W, et al. Arteriovenous shunts in primary varicosis: a critical essay. Vasc Surg 1972; 6:9–14.
63. Browse NL, Burnand KG. The cause of venous ulceration. Lancet 1982; 2:243–245.
64. Burnand KG, et al. The effect of sustained venous hypertension on the skin capillaries of the canine hind limb. Br J Surg 1982; 69:41–44.
65. Falanga V, et al. Dermal pericapillary fibrin in venous disease and venous ulceration. Arch Dermatol 1987; 123:620–623.
66. Claudy AL, et al. Detection of undegraded fibrin and tumor necrosis factor-alpha in venous leg ulcers. J Am Acad Dermatol 1991; 25:623–627.
67. Nehler MR, Moneta GL, Porter JM. The lower extremity ve-

nous system: Part II; the pathophysiology of chronic venous insufficiency. In J Goldstone, ed. Perspectives in Vascular Surgery 1992; 5:81–97.
68. Moyses C, Cederholm-Williams SA, Michel CC. Haemoconcentration and accumulation of white cells in the feet during venous stasis. Int J Microcirc Clin Exp 1987; 5:311–320.
69. Thomas PR, Nash GB, Dormandy JA. Increased white cell trapping in the dependent limbs of patients with chronic venous insufficiency. J Mal Vasc 1990; 15:35–37.
70. Thomas PR, Nash GB, Dormandy JA. White cell accumulation in dependent legs of patients with venous hypertension: a possible mechanism for trophic changes in the skin. Br Med J 1988; 290:1693–1695.
71. Coleridge Smith PD, et al. Causes of venous ulceration: a new hypothesis. Br Med J 1988; 296:1726–1727.
72. Scott HJ, Coleridge Smith PD, Scurr JH. Histologic study of white blood cells and their association with lipodermatosclerosis and venous ulceration. Br J Surg 1991; 78:210–211.
73. Mayberry JC, et al. The influence of elastic compression stockings on deep venous hemodynamics. J Vasc Surg 1991; 13:91–99.
74. Coleridge Smith P, et al. Sequential gradient pneumatic compression enhances venous ulcer healing: a randomized trial. Surgery 1990; 108:871–875.
75. Ormiston MC, et al. Controlled trial of Iodosorb in chronic venous ulcers. Br Med J 1985; 291:308–310.
76. Backhouse CM, et al. Controlled trial of occlusive dressings in healing chronic venous ulcers. Br J Surg 1987; 74:626–627.
77. Kitka MJ, et al. A prospective randomized trial of Unna's boot versus hydroactive dressing in the treatment of venous stasis ulcers. J Vasc Surg 1988; 7:478–483.
78. Partsch H. Compression therapy of the legs: A review. J Dermatol Surg Oncol 1991; 17:799–808.
79. Layer GT, Stacey MC, Burnand KG. Stanozolol and the treatment of venous ulceration—an interim report. Phlebology 1986; 1:197–203.
80. Belcaro G, Marelli C. Treatment of venous lipodermatosclerosis and ulceration in venous hypertension by elastic compression and fibrinolytic enhancement with defibrotide. Phlebology 1989; 4:91–106.
81. Colgan MP, et al. Oxypentifylline treatment of venous ulcers of the leg. Br Med J 1990; 300:972–975.

Neurovascular Compression Syndromes of the Thoracic Outlet

Herbert I. Machleder

The region generally referred to as the thoracic outlet is characterized by a number of unique embryologic and developmental features that have particular and often dramatic effects on the neurovascular structures. The boundaries of the clavical above and the first rib below form an unyielding yet mobile passage for the axillosubclavian artery, vein, and brachial plexus as they traverse the intersection of neck and chest, to upper arm. The scalenus anticus and scalenus medius muscles form the interscalene triangle, an additional anatomical passage for artery and nerve not encountered elsewhere in the body. An understanding of neurovascular compression at the thoracic outlet is perhaps best developed in the context of the historic evolution of etiologic concepts, and the unique anatomic characteristics that underlie the varied clinical manifestations (Fig. 52-1).

In 1986, the neurologist W. S. Fields wrote [1]:

All shoulder girdle compression syndromes have one common feature, namely, compression of the brachial plexus, the subclavian artery, and subclavian vein, usually between the first rib and the clavicle. With elevation of the upper limb, there is a scissorlike approximation of the clavicle superiorly and the first rib inferiorly. Grouping the various conditions under the single heading of thoracic outlet syndrome has resulted in more correct diagnoses and improved therapy. This syndrome should be considered in all neurologic and vascular complaints of the arm previously reported as scalenus anticus, hyperabduction, costoclavicular, cervical rib, fractured clavicle, cervicobrachial compression, pneumatic hammer, effort vein thrombosis, subcoracoid pectoralis minor, and first thoracic rib syndromes.

Development of Anatomic Concepts

THE CERVICAL RIB

In the spring of 1861, a 26-year-old servant woman was admitted to St. Bartholomew's Hospital in London with a painful, dysesthetic, and somewhat ischemic left arm. It was noted on examination that she had a walnut-sized pulsation above the left clavicle, and a clinical diagnosis was made of cervical rib displacing the subclavian artery and brachial plexus. It was noted that the patient had pain in her arm, particularly the elbow, and decreased sensation in her fingers. She dropped objects from her left hand. On March 30 (8 days after admission), Mr. Holmes Coote proceeded with operation to remove the cervical rib. His operative comments, as recorded in the *Lancet*, remain instructive and reiterate some of the anatomic features. "The region was not a pleasant one for any proceeding demanding the use of the knife. The subclavian artery and vein were in front; the axillary plexus of nerves lay spread out above; below, the apex of the lung, covered by the pleura, rose up in dangerous proximity; on the scalenus was the phrenic nerve; while towards the mesial line were the important vessels and nerves passing to the head, together with the vertebral vessels and thoracic duct. You can understand, therefore, why I was cautious in what I did." Despite the technical challenge, the patient had return of the radial pulse and was discharged improved, with an optimistic prognosis [2].

A similar case was seen in Charing Cross Hospital several months previously. Mary O., a 21-year-old woman, had been admitted to Dr. W. H. Wilshire's service, and a pulsatile supraclavicular mass was noted and cervical rib diagnosed. The striking difference was that the young woman had been admitted for the treatment of anemia, her arms presumably asymptomatic, and the pulsatile mass and cervical rib were of no demonstrable clinical significance [3].

As with other diseases, it is perhaps axiomatic that an underlying anomaly is only a predisposing factor in a complex interaction of events that lead to the manifestations of a clinical disorder.

THE FIRST RIB

After Coote's successful case, cervical rib and its syndrome were increasingly encountered, particularly after 1900, when recognition was facilitated by the growing use of roentgenography. A number of subsequent surgical reports appeared in the literature, and cervical-rib excision became an accepted therapeutic approach for upper-extremity radicular neurovascular symptoms.

Paradoxically, patients were increasingly recognized with seemingly identical symptoms but without a demonstrable cervical rib. Some were found to have a rudimentary cervical rib manifest by an enlarged C7 transverse process and a radiologically undetected fibrocartilagenous band that compressed the brachial plexus [4]. Other patients, however, had no discernible bony abnormality. Particularly in the industrial regions of England and Australia, physicians reported patients with neurogenic and vasomotor symptoms of the "cervical-rib syndrome" without radiologic evidence of a cervical rib or enlarged C7 transverse process.

Those reports proved to be an important milestone in the development of a more generalized concept of upper-extremity neurovascular compression. In a landmark clinical and anatomic study of a large number of men, women, and children, T. Wingate Todd concluded in 1912 that "symptoms of 'cervical rib' may be caused by an apparently normal first dorsal rib, and may be cured by its removal." He concluded from his studies that, "in consequence of the action of these forces, pressure symptoms on the lowest brachial trunk are most likely to occur in women at the commencement of adult age." Those observations, derived from anatomic measurements of postnatal shoulder development, would foretell the actual clinical prevalence reported over the next 80 years [5].

Todd expanded his observations by noting that the upper limb develops at the level of the seventh cervical segment, and consequently the first and second thoracic nerves must travel upward until they have crossed the

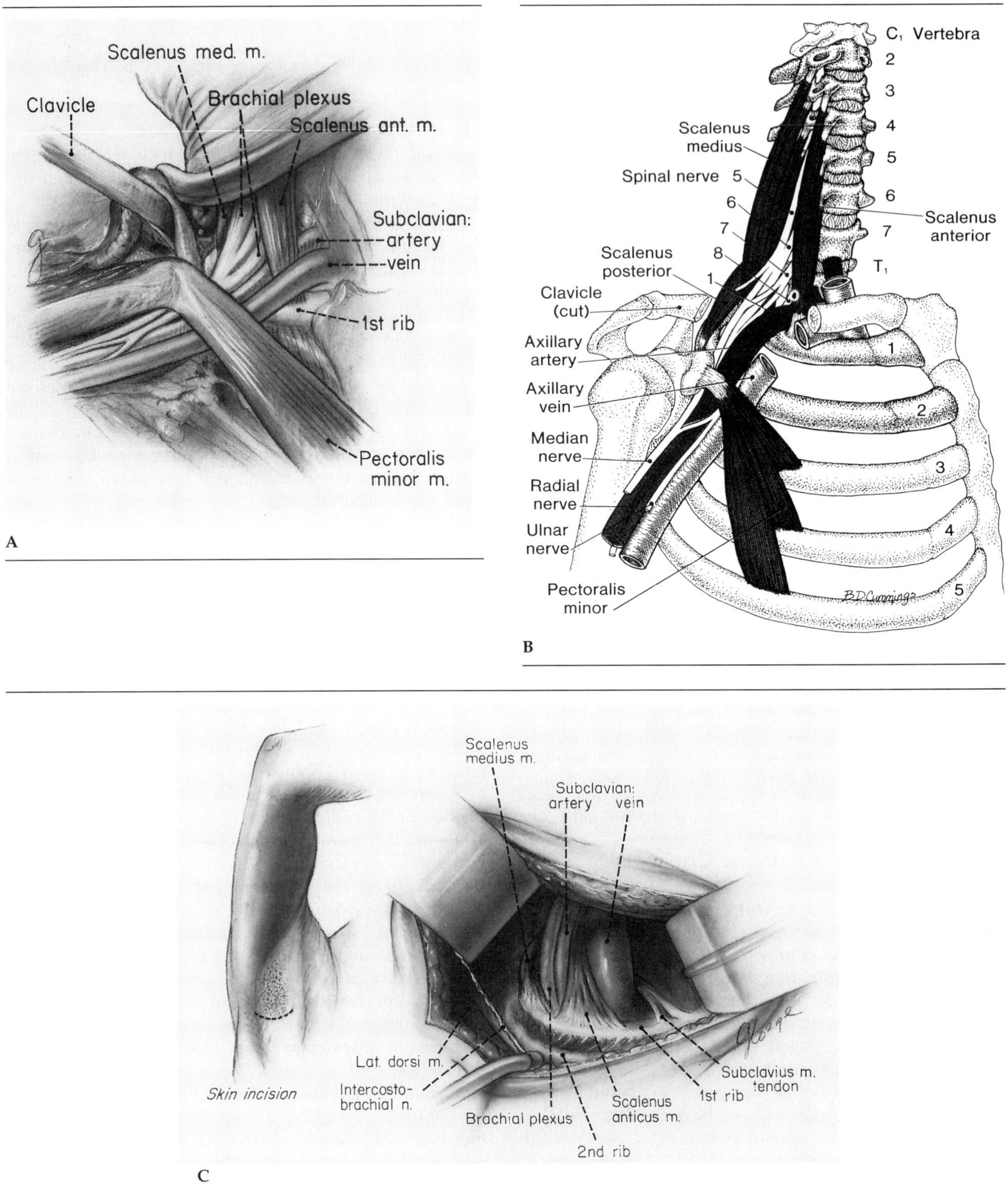

Fig. 52-1. **A.** Anatomic dissection showing the anatomy at the thoracic outlet. Cadaver head is turned to the left and clavicle is reflected laterally. (From HI Machleder. Vascular Disorders of the Upper Extremity. 2nd ed. Mt. Kisco, N.Y.: Futura, 1989.) **B.** Diagram of interscalene triangle showing passage of brachial plexus and axillosubclavian artery. (From JG Travell, DG Simons. Myofascial Pain and Dysfunction. Baltimore: William & Wilkins 1983.) **C.** Thoracic outlet anatomy as seen from the transaxillary surgical approach. (From HI Machleder. Vascular Disorders of the Upper Extremity. 2nd ed. Mt. Kisco, N.Y.: Futura, 1989.)

uppermost rib and then angulate downward to enter the arm. Because of that configuration, any elevation of the rib or depression of the shoulder must stretch the lower connections with the brachial plexus. Todd had shown additionally that in the course of normal skeletal development there is a gradual descent of the shoulder with advancing years. That tendency, he noted, is exaggerated when the individual carries a heavy weight and is reduced when the weight is taken off the arm by supporting the elbow in a sling or on the arm of a chair. "It is just these maneuvers which frequently result in exacerbation or relief of symptoms."

In 1920, Stopford and Telford reported a group of clinical cases seen in Manchester, England, where the lower trunk of the brachial plexus was compressed by the first thoracic rib rather than a supernumerary cervical rib. They described the essential characteristics of these cases of neurovascular compression [6]. As Todd had predicted, the symptoms were predominantly in the sensory and motor distribution of the lower trunk of the brachial plexus. The patients complained of loss of grip strength, fatigue of the hand with exercise, weakness of the intrinsic muscles, loss of sensation in the distribution of the lower trunk (of brachial plexus), and vasomotor instability with episodes of cyanosis and coolness. They noted that after removal of the impinging portion of the first rib there was rapid resolution of the vasomotor and sensory changes and slow resolution of atrophic and motor changes.

In succeeding years, abnormalities in development of the first thoracic rib would be recognized and, as with the cervical rib, be associated with radicular neurovascular symptoms [7,8].

THE ANTERIOR SCALENE MUSCLE

At about the time of Stopford and Telford's report, the large neurosurgical clinics in the United States were encountering similar perplexing cases of "cervical rib syndrome without cervical rib." At the Mayo Clinic, Adson had begun to treat cervical rib patients by scalenectomy alone [9]. His work, which emphasized the compressive role of the anterior scalene muscle, directed attention in the United States to soft-tissue abnormalities, whereas in Great Britain research and treatment continued to focus on the normal and abnormal first rib.

It is not surprising that in the United States, scalenectomy would be applied to this new group of patients with cervical rib–type symptoms of radicular neurovascular compression. Adson's discovery inaugurated a remarkable intensity of clinical work involving university departments and large private clinics in all parts of the United States.

Naffziger, chief of neurosurgery at the University of California, considered the anterior scalene muscle to be the key to the neurovascular compressive abnormalities and used the term **scalenus syndrome** [10,11]. Ochsner and colleagues first published that term in a landmark paper entitled "Scalenus anticus (Naffziger) syndrome," giving credit to Naffziger, even though their paper antedated his by 3 years [12]. The concept began to flourish with dramatic cures and failures.

During the 1930s and 1940s, before the widespread recognition of patients with carpal tunnel syndrome, cervical-disk disease, and neuroforamenal compression, the application of scalenotomy was certain to lead to failures, particularly when applied to patients with predominantly upper-plexus or median-nerve distribution symptoms.

Despite considerable interest in scalenotomy in the United States, it was likely applied too broadly. There were failures, partly due to diagnostic imprecision during the gradual recognition of other overlapping neurogenic syndromes and partly due to incomplete decompression of the neurovascular structures. As a consequence, scalenotomy did not entirely live up to expectations.

THORACIC OUTLET COMPRESSION SYNDROME

It seems evident that sometime in the 1950s the term **thoracic outlet syndrome** (TOS) crept into general usage as well as first appeared in the medical and surgical literature. The term was used to describe both the arterial and neurogenic presentations and recognized the commonality of etiology and frequent overlap of vascular and neurogenic symptoms [13,14]. The "Mayo Clinic Number" of the 1946 Surgical Clinics of North America was devoted to a symposium on pain in the shoulder and arm [15]. Eaton, the consultant in neurology, described what he would regularly refer to, 10 years later (in 1956), as the "thoracic outlet syndrome" [16]:

> Almost always the patient seeks relief from pain and paresthesia of the upper extremity. The patient most often complains of a dragging sensation through the shoulders and pain distributed over the deltoid area to the elbow. When the condition is more severe, pain and paresthesia occur in the ulnar aspect of the forearm and hand, and in the fourth and fifth digits. At times, it spreads to the radial aspect of the forearm, hand and digits, and to the neck, scapular and pectoral regions. Sometimes, the patient may complain of pain in the head and face on the same side. There is a decided tendency for the symptoms to become worse at night while the patient is lying down. At this time paresthesia may be particularly intense and may involve the whole upper extremity. The patient may be awakened several times and find relief by lying prone and swinging the arm over the side of the bed. However, when the syndrome is well developed, symptoms also occur at other times. They may be aggravated by the use of the arms and particularly by use which depresses the shoulder girdle, such as the carrying of heavy objects or the maintenance for long periods of the position of the arms required in holding a book to be read.

THE DECLINE OF SCALENOTOMY

O.T. Clagett, chief of the section of thoracic surgery at the Mayo Clinic, became interested in the new syndrome of thoracic outlet compression. He noted the very frequent cases of residual and recurrent symptoms from the scalenotomy era of his surgical predecessor Adson. Drawing from his experience with thoracoplasty and a rediscovery of the English literature, he inaugurated the new era of first-rib removal [17]. Clagett described a posterior approach to first-rib removal that was, for most surgeons, a difficult operation that had been devised primarily for the treatment of tuberculosis by thoracoplasty. Although Clagett's article had considerable impact, delivered as the presidential address to the American Thoracic Society, there was relatively limited further clinical application.

CURRENT CONCEPTS

A major milestone occurred in 1966 when Roos reported a series of 15 patients treated by removal of the first thoracic rib through a transaxillary approach [18,19]. The dramatic superiority of that technique was readily appreciated and became widely accepted. The combination of the improved ability to identify patients with carpal tunnel syndrome and cervical-disk disease with an effective operative approach to TOS led to renewed interest in the treatment of **thoracic outlet compression syndrome**. Roos's superb ability in communicating the critical elements in the clinical work-up as well as the operative details proved to be one of the keys to acceptance in every country with modern surgical practice. The transaxillary procedure became the standard operation for removal of the first thoracic rib.

Recognition that cumulative-trauma disorders (due to performance of repetitive tasks) account for extensive upper-extremity disability has been increasing in all industrialized countries. These musculoskeletal disorders make up more than 50 percent of all occupational illnesses in the United States today [20]. In emerging industrial countries, the same experience is being reported. In a large hand service in Shanghai, for example, 20 percent of cases of upper-extremity neurovascular symptoms were attributed to compression at the thoracic outlet [21].

The acceptance of soft-tissue abnormalities in thoracic outlet compression syndromes parallels, in many regards, the evolution of thinking about carpal tunnel syndrome. In reviewing the history of that entity at the Mayo Clinic, Amadio had the following to say: "Initially, treatment was limited to those patients with the most severe neuropathies and derangement of wrist anatomy. As confidence with the diagnosis and therapy increased, progressively less severe anatomic deformities and then progressively less severe neurologic impairments were considered for surgical management" [22].

In the early years, during the 1920s, many centers began experimenting with decompression of the median nerve by removing bony deformity. There was a progressive building on previous operations that eventually led to the understanding of the soft-tissue abnormality. Until the late 1940s, the condition was known by a variety of names. Diagnosis was entertained only "when a severe and obvious distal median neuropathy was present." In 1947, the eminent British neurologist Sir Russell Brain proposed that less severe neuropathies characterized by intermittent paresthesias, pain, and weakness might be part of the same spectrum and might, in fact, be fairly common [23].

Pathologic Anatomy

Anatomic variation at the region of the thoracic outlet has intrigued surgical anatomists from the early descriptions of supernumerary ribs to modern studies of ultrastructural changes in the scalene muscles [24,25]. During transaxillary resections of the first rib for arterial, venous, or brachial plexus compression at the thoracic outlet, a spectrum of changes representing intermediate developmental variation can be recognized in addition to the discreet abnormalities, such as cervical ribs, cervical fibrocartilagenous bands, and supernumerary scalene muscles [26,27].

Working in Paris, Milliez emphasized that anomalies at the thoracic outlet rarely exist in isolation, that there is interaction in development of the different elements [28]. The anatomist J. C. White and his colleagues clarified that concept in describing cervical ribs and congenital malformations of first thoracic ribs as linked to errors of bodily segmentation in early embryonic development, where variation in the formation of the brachial plexus appears before bony-skeleton development. Cervical-rib development, for example, is determined by the formation of the spinal nerve roots. The regression of the C5 through C7 ribs is occasioned by the rapid development of the enlarging roots of the brachial plexus in the region of the limb bud. In cases of a cervical C7 rib, there generally is a prefixed plexus with only a small neural contribution from the T1 nerve root. The inhibition to rib development at that level is lost or reduced, and the size of the cervical rib then is related to the extent of contribution of the T1 root to the brachial plexus. As a corollary, in the postfixed plexus where there is a contribution of the T2 root to the brachial plexus, the first thoracic rib is often rudimentary, having been inhibited in its development by the unusual nerve growth [29]. This embryologically determined morphologic interdependence is evident with other structural relationships at the thoracic outlet.

A series of 200 consecutive cases reported from the University of California at Los Angeles (UCLA) gives an idea of the relative frequency of the three forms of TOS as well as the anatomic variations that can be seen from the transaxillary exposure [30]. Forty cases (20%) in that series presented with problems related to venous obstruction or to arterial insufficiency and embolization. Twenty-six cases (65%) of this vascular subgroup had additional neurogenic symptoms associated with abnormal sensory-evoked responses in the affected extremity. In the entire group, of 200 symptomatic extremities, 153 (76.5%) exhibited signs of arterial compression in stress positions on clinical examination or with digital photoplethysmography.

In 68 cases (34%), there was no structural abnormality discernible from the transaxillary surgical approach. Seventeen cases (8.5%) had a cervical rib articulating with the first rib directly or by fibrocartilagenous extension. Twenty (10%) had a scalenus minimus muscle inserting either on the first rib or Sibsons fascia. Thirty-nine patients (19.5%) had an anomaly of the subclavius tendon or its insertion tubercle. Eighty-six cases (43%) had an anomaly of scalene-muscle development or insertion. In 15 cases (7.5%), there were other categories of anomalies that could not be related to specific developmental characteristics. Those categories included ligamentous or fibrous structures that did not correspond to regression residua of recognized embryologic structures. More than one abnormality was recognized in 22.5 percent of the cases, and 32 percent of 25 patients undergoing bilateral procedures had similar anomalies on both sides.

There was only one clinical setting that could be correlated with a characteristic anatomic abnormality. Of 33 patients presenting with spontaneous axillosubclavian-vein thrombosis (Paget-Schroetter syndrome), 18 (55%) had hypertrophy of the subclavius tendon associated with enlargement of the insertion tubercle. Among male patients with Paget-Schroetter syndrome 14 out of 20 (70%) had that anomaly [31].

EMBRYOLOGIC DEVELOPMENT

The abdominal, thoracic, and cervical musculature develops from the hypomeric portion of the paraxial and epaxial mesoderm, with the scalene and prevertebral muscles in the neck corresponding to the intercostal and ventrolateral abdominal muscles in the thorax and abdomen, respectively [32]. In the embryo, plates of axially running muscle segments differentiate into the discrete muscle groups seen in the adult.

The subclavian artery, which is the artery of the seventh cervical segment, and the spinal nerves from C5 to T1 pierce the muscle plates in the cervical segment much the same as the intercostal nerve and artery do in the thoracic segments. The growth of the limb bud and development of the pectoral girdle then lead to the particular structural changes seen in that region, particularly the segmentation of the scalenic muscle mass into discrete muscles.

FIRST-RIB AND CERVICAL-RIB ANOMALIES

During development, the C7 rib forms and then regresses to the C7 transverse process. Various stages in that evolution range from a complete C7 rib to rudimentary forms associated with a fibrocartilagenous band [33,34]. The only radiologic indication of this residual band may be an enlarged C7 transverse process.

Anomalies of the first or cervical rib are encountered in about 10 percent of modern series of patients with TOS. The incidence of those autosomal dominant abnormalities in the general population can be estimated from the medical literature. Adson reports that Galen and Vesalius both described cervical ribs in their anatomical dissections [35,36].

In a study of 40,000 consecutive chest x-rays in American army recruits, Etter encountered 68 complete articulated cervical ribs (0.17%) and 31 anomalous and 67 rudimentary first ribs (0.25%). He additionally recognized 77 synostoses of first and second ribs and 16 bifid first ribs [37]. In 1947, Adson reviewed his experience with cervical ribs citing a Mayo Clinic radiologic study prior to 1927 that identified an incidence of 0.563%, or 5.6 patients per 1,000, with cervical rib. Twenty-eight percent were males and 72 percent were females; 47 percent of the cervical ribs were bilateral. The right side was involved in 23 percent and the left side in 30 percent. Forty-five percent of the group were symptomatic [38]. Adson quotes a review by Haven of 5,000 routine roentgenograms of the thorax in which he found 38 first-rib abnormalities and 37 cervical ribs, an incidence of 0.74 percent or 7.4 persons per 1,000. Adson subscribed to the concept linking formation of cervical ribs to a failure of rudimentary rib regression as the nerve roots form [39].

In the Soviet Union, Firsov reported fluorographic examination of 510,893 people, observing 1,379 cervical ribs, for an incidence of 0.27 percent. Women accounted for 76.8 percent and men for 23.2 percent; 33.3 percent were bilateral [40]. A cervical rib or the C7 rib most often is associated with a prefixed type of brachial plexus where there is a minor contribution to the brachial plexus from the T1 nerve root and a major contribution from C4. When the C7 rib is incomplete, there is often a rudimentary band in place of the regressed portion of the rib.

Cervical rib clearly represents one of the predisposing abnormalities for development of thoracic outlet compression syndrome. The significantly higher incidence of these recognized congenital abnormalities in women compared with men also may be reflected in the higher incidence of thoracic outlet nerve compression symptoms in women.

The symptom characteristics associated with the presence of cervical ribs have been addressed by several authors. In 205 patients treated for cervical rib or TOS at Montefiore Medical Center (New York City), 12 patients had arterial lesions (5.9%) [41]. Halsted reported that in 716 cases of cervical rib he had reviewed, there were 27 cases of subclavian artery dilatation (3.7%). He indicated that of 360 symptomatic clinical cases, 235 (65.3%) had nerve symptoms alone, 106 (29.4%) had nerve and vascular symptoms, and 19 (5.3%) had vascular symptoms alone [42]. Brown and Charlesworth performed 23 cervical rib excisions and reported that 15 (65%) had predominantly neurologic symptoms, and 8 (35%) had vascular symptoms [43].

Telford and Mottershead encountered anomalous fibrous bands from rudimentary cervical ribs in 12 and complete cervical ribs in 70 of 105 surgical cases. Telford writing with Stopford attributed the vascular complications of cervical rib to stimulation of the sympathetic innervation through the lowest two nerve roots, a view that prevailed for many years. In their otherwise excellent discussion, they seemed to have neglected the possibility of arterial embolism [44]. Fibrocartilagenous bands extending from the end of incompletely formed cervical ribs are best thought of as an anomaly of cervical-rib formation. Those abnormalities have been referred to as type 1 and type 2 bands by Roos [27,51] (Fig. 52-2).

SCALENE-MUSCLE ANOMALIES

Milliez in his recent studies of scalene muscle in a 2.5-cm embryo emphasized the influence of neurovascular structure development on the ultimate configuration of the scalene-muscle mass. He recognized a confluent scalene muscle distinguished only by a groove at the site of anterior and middle scalene differentiation. Actual separation into two muscles occurred at the points where the muscle mass was traversed by the roots of the brachial plexus. Rather than the scalenus minimus forming as a separate muscle entity, it represents one form of segmentation of the scalenic mass. Milliez quotes Poitevin's studies of 1988, which indicated that the scalenic mass is differentiated into specific muscle groups only by the traversing of the neurovascular bundle. The persistence of certain muscle inclusions in the brachial plexus, as well as muscle groups that traverse various elements of the brachial plexus, is related to the original mass of the scalene variously segmented by the passage of those advanc-

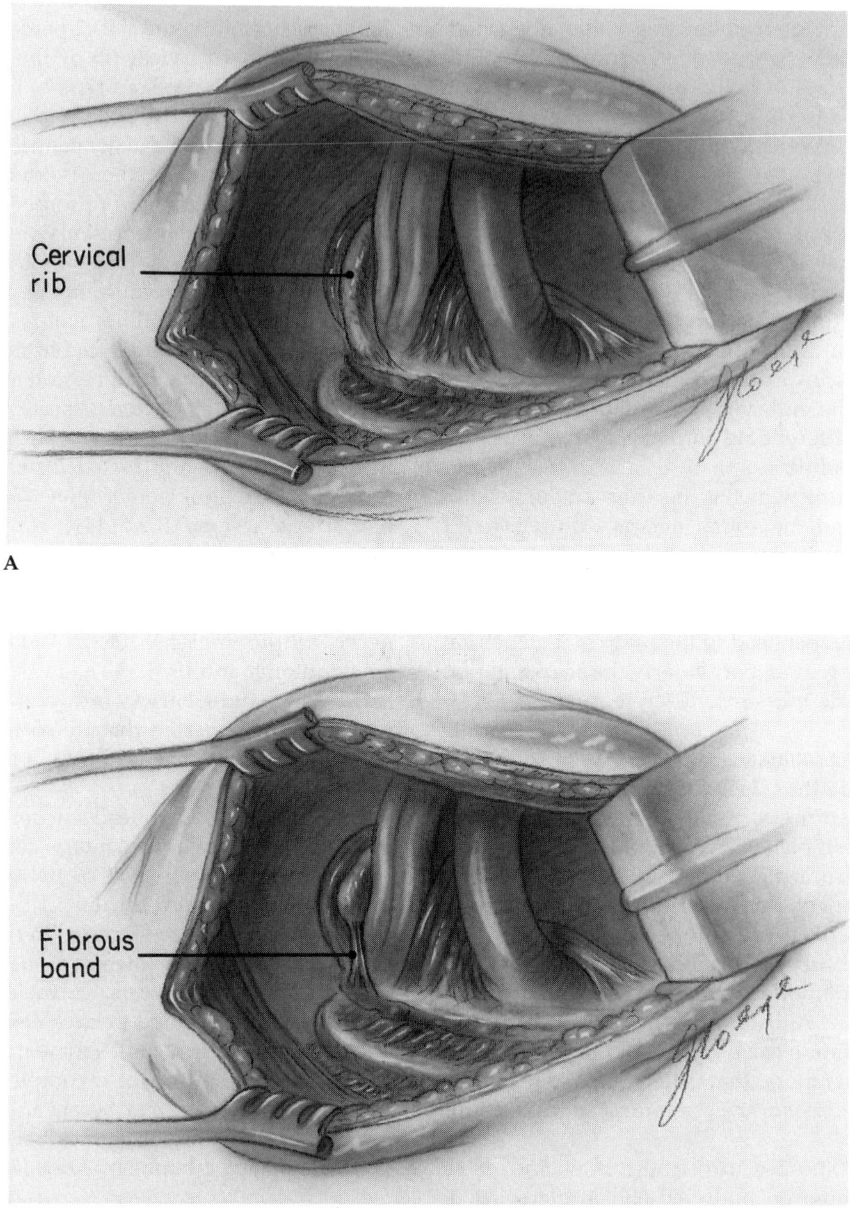

A

B

Fig. 52-2. **A.** Appearance of cervical rib from the transaxillary approach. **B.** Fibrocartilagenous band as described by Gilliat. This lesion has been implicated in the "wasted hand." (Both illustrations from RG Makhoul, HI Machleder. Developmental anomalies at the thoracic outlet. J Vasc Surg 1992; 16:534–545.)

ing structures as the limb bud develops. Milliez does acknowledge, however, an alternative opinion that accessory scalene muscles may be representations of phylogenetic recapitulation wherein muscles persist that ordinarily would regress either completely or to a small tendon.

That separation of muscle bundles interdigitating between the neurovascular structures accounts for the muscular bridges seen between the middle and anterior scalene that often penetrate the brachial plexus. Roos and Sanders demonstrated in their recent anatomic dissections that these abnormalities of scalene segmentation are seen quite frequently in the adult [45]. Although not pathologic in their own right, those fibers may result in neurogenic symptoms as a consequence of later abnormal growth, peculiarities of occupational or recreational use, or post-traumatic changes.

Adson, Ochsner, Naffziger, and their coworkers made the initial observations of scalene-muscle involvement in neurovascular compression at the thoracic outlet [46,47]. Recent ultrastructural studies have helped to clarify the fiber type and hypertrophic changes that underlie the gross morphologic observations.

In addition to metabolic changes and the discrete anomalies previously described, there is wide variation in "normal" scalene-muscle anatomy. Those variations may well explain differing sequelae in individual patients after comparable trauma or in comparable work situations. In a series of methodical dissections, Lang described the range of scalene-muscle insertions and configurations of the interscalene triangle. The variations govern the available passage space for artery and brachial plexus through the interscalene triangle.

Telford and Mottershead found the ventral attachment of the anterior scalene to vary from 2.4 to 6.0 cm from the chondrosternal junction, and the width of the anterior scalene insertion to vary from 0.4 to 2.5 cm with the interscalene interval varying from 0 to 2.4 cm. They encountered crossing of the insertions of the anterior and middle scalene muscles in 8 of 105 operative cases and in 15 (15%) of 102 cadaver dissections [48]. Sunderland and Bedbrook encountered that crossing of the scalene insertions in 15 percent of 35 cadaver dissections [49]. That abnormality (which in the extreme is a slinglike crossing of the scalene muscles described by some as a V-shaped deformity) traps the subclavian artery and brachial plexus. It corresponds to the type 4 band described by Roos and has been called intercostalization by Makhoul and Machleder, to reflect the embryonic derivation of those muscles (first recognized by Todd) [50]. Roos subdivided the crossing bands into an eighth and ninth abnormality in 1980: Type 8 represents a band from the middle scalene to the costochondral junction, and type 9 a fascial band in the concave curve of the first rib [51].

Unique configurations of scalene-muscle insertion that tend to compress the neurovascular structures in the interscalene triangle accounted for 43 percent of the congenital variations seen in the series reported from UCLA [30]. The scalenus minimus muscle, present in 20 of the University of California at Los Angeles cases (10%) can be represented by a residual ligament that variously has been called the **costovertebral** or **pleurospinal** ligament when the muscle has regressed. Roos described those ligaments as type 5 or type 6 bands, depending on the site of insertion to rib or apical pleura [52].

Sanders and Roos, studying the anatomy of the interscalene triangle, found interdigitating fibers between the scalene muscles through the brachial plexus in 75 percent of dissections in TOS patients and in 40 percent of 60 cadaver dissections. In 45 percent of cadaver dissections, the C5,C6 nerve roots emerged between fibers of the anterior scalene muscle rather than between the anterior and middle scalene muscles (Fig. 52-3).

SUBCLAVIUS ANOMALIES

Telford and Mottershead noted in anatomical dissections that during movements of abduction or retraction of the shoulder, the tendon of the subclavius muscle compressed the subclavian vein against the first rib. In the Paget-Schroetter type–deformity, Sampson emphasized the striking hypertrophy of the subclavius tendon, with those observations later corroborated by Aziz et al. and Kunkle et al. [53,54]. That particular manifestation of compression at the thoracic outlet is related to progressive enlargement of the subclavius muscle system with repetitive compressive trauma to the subclavian vein followed by fibrosis, stricture, and thrombosis. An abnormality of this type was found in 19.5 percent of the UCLA cases, with 15.5 percent having an exostosis at the subclavius tubercle.

Despite the congenital nature of these deformities, the onset of symptoms in early to middle adult life has been recorded by virtually all physicians treating the clinical disorders. The delay in onset most likely is related to postnatal development. The chest widens and the clavicle continues its growth to approximately age 22 or 25, after which the pectoral girdle begins to descend. Still later, with loss of strength or tone in the supporting musculature of the thoracic girdle, there is further traction on the neurovascular structures at the thoracic outlet.

The Clinical Syndromes

ARTERIAL COMPRESSION

From the extensive literature discussing symptomatic cervical ribs came the recognition that ischemic symptoms of the hand could follow as a consequence of thoracic outlet compression. Initial explanations focused on sympathetic innervation of the arm via the C8-T1 nerve roots, postulating that compression of those roots as they rest on the first rib leads to sympathetic induction of vasospasm and Raynaud's symptoms [55]. It was subsequently recognized that the subclavian artery can be compressed, either against a cervical rib by the anterior scalene muscle or between the normal first thoracic rib and overlying clavicle. At the site of compression, a spectrum of changes can be observed, ranging from mild intimal injury and irregularity, which can give rise to mural thrombus and subsequent embolization, to poststenotic dilatation and small-aneurysm formation [56]. Repetitive episodes of embolization with progressive obliteration of the distal vessels account for the attacks of Raynaud's symptoms, which in some cases are followed by ischemia and digital gangrene (Fig. 52-4).

The angiographic appearance may underestimate the pathologic changes by disclosing only very subtle luminal abnormalities, particularly when the patient is supine. That disparity between the angiographic appearance and operative findings reflects the similar underestimation of the magnitude of mural thrombus, propagating clot, and poststenotic dilatation. On occasion, minor areas of irregularity with associated thrombus may be more demonstrable on CT or MRI scan. The CT scan is often difficult to interpret, since the subclavian-artery course is such that in the sagittal sections it moves in and out of the field. The coronal sections of the MRI provide a better picture for interpretation. Often, no bony abnormality is encountered, and posttraumatic changes in the anterior scalene muscle may account for the compression.

In 1958, Rob and Standeven reported 10 cases of arterial occlusion as a complication of what they termed "thoracic outlet compression syndrome." They remarked at the often delayed diagnosis of thoracic outlet problems, suspecting that the subtle early manifestations of arterial compression often were masked by formation of collateral vessels. They further observed that "Three cases have been recorded in the literature in which proximal spread

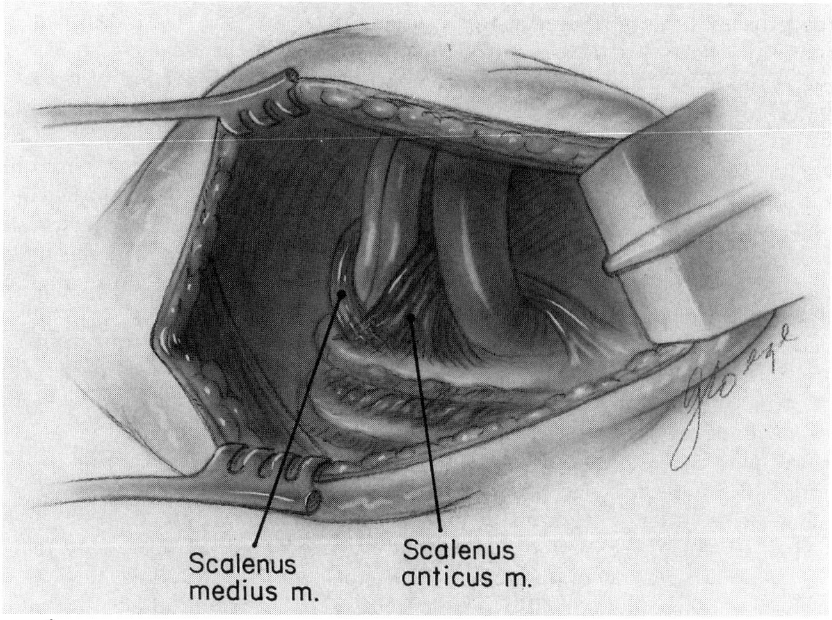

A

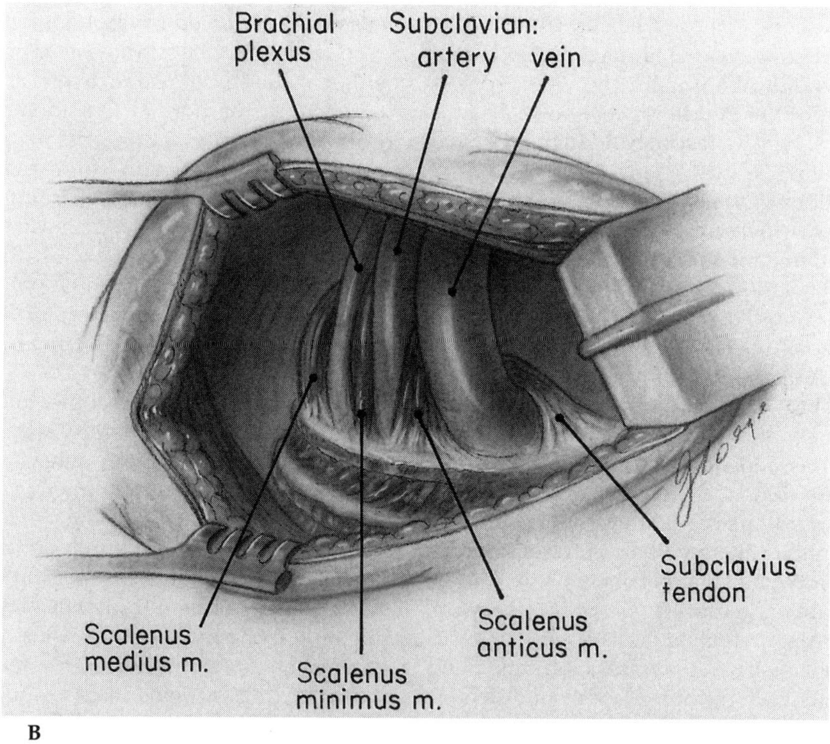

B

Fig. 52-3. **A.** Crossing of the insertions of anterior and middle scalene muscles. **B.** Appearance of the scalenus minimus abnormality. (Both illustrations from RG Makhoul, HI Machleder. Developmental anomalies at the thoracic outlet. J Vasc Surg 1992; 16:534–545.)

of arterial thrombosis had reached the bifurcation of the innominate artery and caused hemiplegia.''

Almost three decades later, major league pitcher J. R. Richards suffered the identical consequence during a playoff game for the World Series. He developed a sudden left-sided hemiparesis. The neurologist W. S. Fields recognized that the preceeding cramping pain in the arm had been considered tendonitis, when in reality the pitcher had subclavian-artery occlusion from thoracic outlet compression syndrome. As the clot propagated in a retrograde

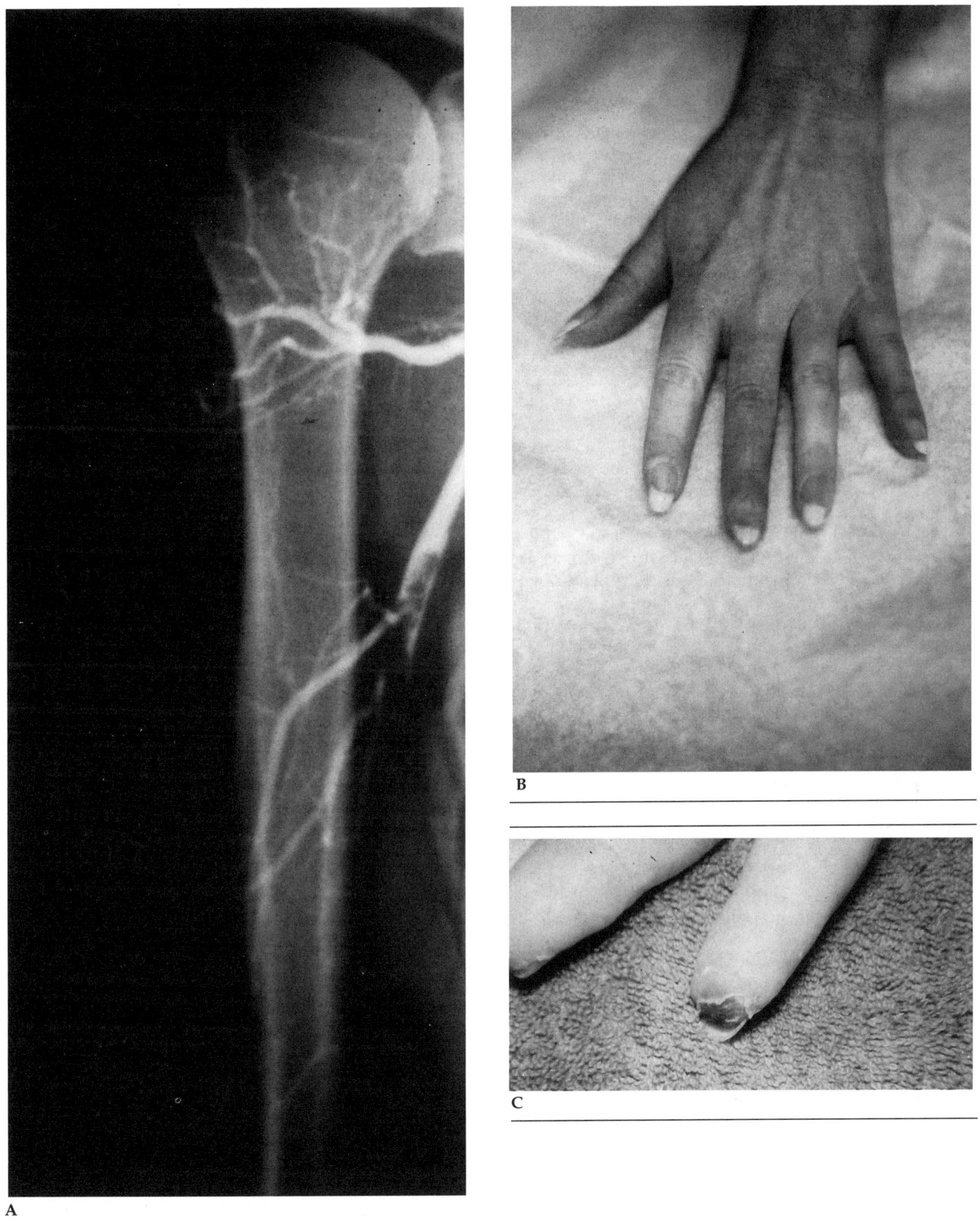

Fig. 52-4. **A.** Embolus in brachial artery from thoracic outlet compression of the axillosubclavian artery. **B.** Episode of Raynaud's vasospasm in patient with arterial TOS. **C.** Digital ischemic ulcer from embolizing poststenotic subclavian artery from TOS. (From HI Machleder. Vaso-occlusive disorders of the upper extremity. Curr Probl Surg 1988; 25(1):1–67.)

fashion, the tail reached the innominate artery and subsequently embolized up the right carotid system. Both Rob in 1958 and Fields in 1986 decried the lack of diagnostic awareness when physicians encountered such neurovascular compression disorders.

Presenting History and Physical Signs. Patients with arterial compression may, in the early stages, have symptoms suggestive of autonomic dysfunction such as unilateral cold hypersensitivity, Raynaud's phenomenon, episodes of rubor, and recurrent mild edema. The disorder often may be attributed erroneously to a collagen vascular disease. The unilaterality of the symptoms, however, are an indication that it is more likely an embolic or neurovascular compressive process.

As the disorder progresses, there will be episodes of cold-induced ischemia, fingertip pain, and frank punctate ischemic ulcers at the paronichial area. Examination occasionally will show splinter hemorrhages in the nailbeds. Digital plethysmography often will show dampened waveform shapes in the affected fingers with evidence of digital-artery occlusion. Once again, the unilaterality must suggest to the examiner the possibility of an axillosubclavian-artery lesion or central embolizing source.

Alternatively, in the face of complete occlusion, patients will complain of aching of the hand and arm with exercise, usually associated with cold hypersensitivity or cold intolerance in the hand and fingers. Although a misnomer, the symptom often is referred to as "arm claudication" because of its similarity to the exercise-induced lower-extremity symptoms of arterial insufficiency. At this stage, Doppler-derived segmental arterial pressures of the upper extremities will be clearly abnormal.

Arteriography almost invariably is required, with recognition of the problems of interpretation discussed previously. The studies should be done with the arm in the neutral position and then with the arm placed in abduction, at a right angle to the thorax. Failure to utilize stress positions will result in many false-negative or incomplete studies (Fig. 52-5).

Treatment. Treatment of arterial compression should be prompt surgical repair, to avoid progressive loss of the outflow vessels from repetitive embolization. Our standard approach has been removal of the first thoracic rib, to decompress the thoracic outlet and facilitate a normal anatomic reconstruction. When there is poststenotic dilatation of the axillosubclavian artery, aneurysmal formation, or complete obstruction, resection and direct repair or interposition graft will provide a durable correction of the abnormality. In patients who have developed severe autonomic changes or reflex sympathetic dystrophy, cervicothoracic sympathectomy will provide additional relief of symptoms when coupled with vascular reconstruction.

BRACHIAL PLEXUS COMPRESSION

Physical Examination. Patients with neurogenic TOS often incur symptoms in the overhead position (abduction and external rotation, or AER), typically developing numbness of the fourth and fifth fingers and ulnar aspect of the forearm. They rapidly note impairment in strength and endurance with exercise in AER. When fatigue occurs in that position, a bruit often can be auscultated inferior to the lateral third of the clavicle over the axillary artery. This positional neurovascular compression affects mechanics, painters, stone masons, electricians, and others who work with arms in abduction. The symptom characteristics can be replicated on physical examination by having the patient clench and unclench the fingers with arms elevated in the so-called elevated arm stress test (EAST). The EAST and the AER maneuver have been studied in industrial workers in Sweden and found to correlate both with symptoms at work and with the presence of nocturnal dysesthesias [57]. During elevated-arm exercise, the hand often will become pale and show reactive hyperemia on resuming the neutral position.

Characteristically, there is tenderness over the anterior scalene muscle and hypersensitivity to clavicular percussion on the affected side. That hypersensitivity very often is associated with a positive Tinnel's sign at the brachial plexus. In addition, fine finger movement and grip strength become progressively impaired as patients develop difficulty performing tasks both in the AER position and with their arms in neutral positions. That accounts for the disabilities seen in many patients from industrial and white-collar repetitive-motion occupations.

The loss of tactile ability and fine-motor coordination is a consequence of impairment in the C8-T1 nerve-root contribution to both median and ulnar nerves. Median nerve–innervated muscles such as the opponens pollicis and the lumbricalis-interossei on the radial side are supplied completely by the C8-T1 roots. The flexor pollicis longus and brevis as well as the abductor pollicis brevis derive substantial innervation from C8-T1, as does flexor digitorum profundus and sublimis.

Most of the ulnar-innervated muscles derive their entire innervation from C8-T1. Those muscles include the flexor digitorum profundus (fingers 3 and 4), adductor pollicis, dorsal interossei, palmar interossei, and abductor digiti quinti. The motor innervation of the fifth finger, opponens digiti quinti and flexor digiti quinti, is predominantly from the inferior trunk of brachial plexus (C8-T1)

It is essential to evaluate the patient for the possibility of cervical-disk or neuroforaminal disease, as well as for peripheral-nerve entrapment. In that regard, the motor and sensory examination augments the clinical history in establishing the diagnosis. Additionally, the deep tendon reflexes have characteristic patterns in the different disorders.

The sensory and motor changes in neurogenic thoracic outlet compression explain the various complaints and disabilities described by patients in a variety of occupational and daily life situations. They also emphasize the necessity for differentiating compression of the inferior trunk of brachial plexus from isolated median-nerve compression at the wrist and ulnar-nerve compression at the cubital tunnel or Guyon's tunnel. In that regard, the clinical evaluation is enhanced by careful electrophysiologic assessment.

Particular care must be exercised in patients who may have the "double-crush" syndrome of multiple sites of

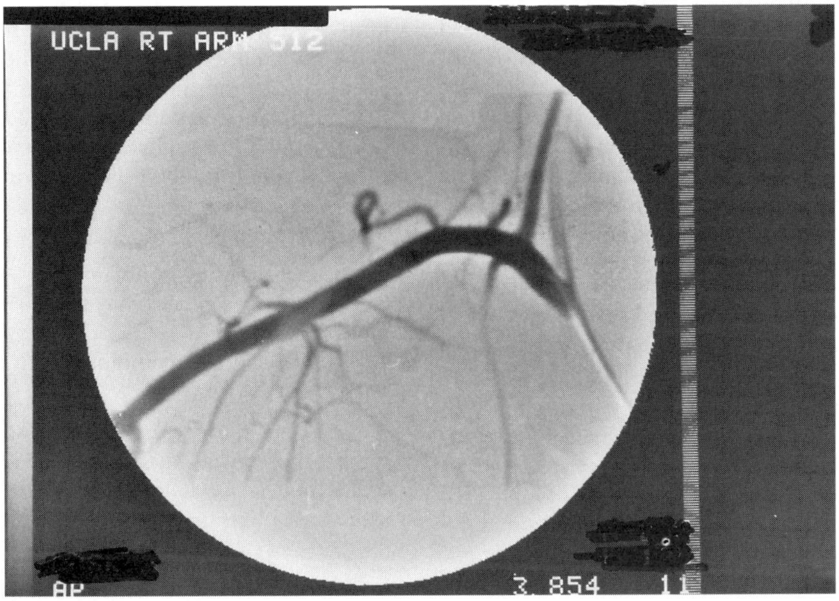

A

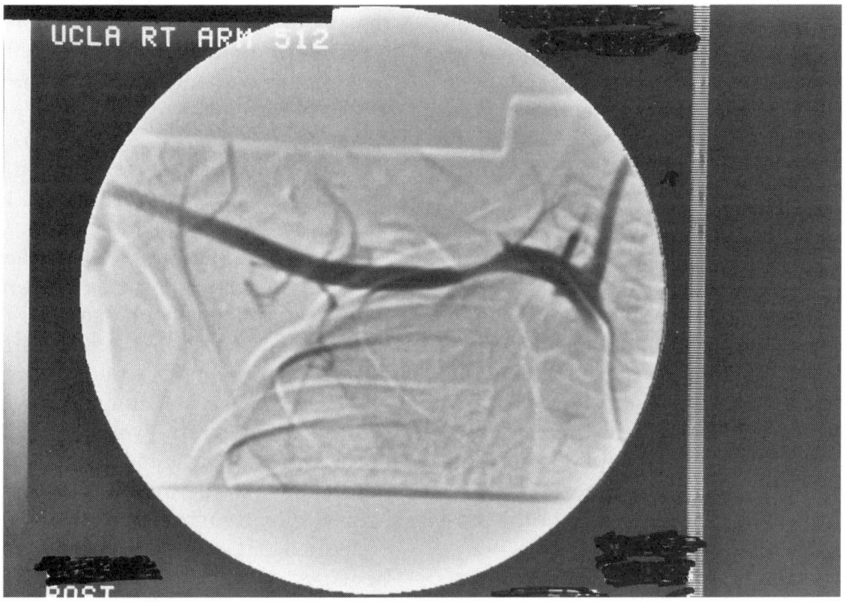

B

Fig. 52-5. **A.** Axillosubclavian artery in neutral position. **B.** Area of thoracic outlet compression demonstrated in the abducted position.

peripheral-nerve compression. Compression at the thoracic outlet often can be seen concurrently with carpal tunnel syndrome and tardy ulnar palsy [58]. Patients who fail to achieve symptomatic relief after median-nerve decompression or ulnar nerve translocation often have an unrecognized site of brachial plexus compression at the thoracic outlet. The converse also can be seen with residual focal neuropathic symptoms after otherwise successful correction of thoracic outlet compression.

Electrophysiologic Examination. In advanced stages, the neurogenic symptom complexes of TOS can be associated with characteristic electrophysiologic changes. At the outset, it is important to recognize the limitations of electrophysiologic evaluation. Pain and dysesthesias are the predominant early symptoms of patients presenting with brachial plexus compression at the thoracic outlet, particularly when those symptoms are positionally enhanced. The pain is considered to be mediated by the smaller myelinated or unmyelinated nerve fibers. The integrity or function of those fibers is not tested by the standard electrophysiologic techniques. In advanced cases of brachial plexus compression (similar to the findings with carpal tunnel compression of the median nerve), in which weakness and atrophy are evident on clinical examination, there generally will be concomitant abnormalities on electromyography and nerve-conduction studies.

A more sensitive method for determining abnormalities in the larger fibers would be by the use of electrical tests in the symptomatic positions. Although that is feasible for carpal tunnel compression of the median nerve, the parameters have not been established for the brachial plexus. It is likewise important to recognize that there are substantial variations in normal nerve conduction that tend to limit sensitivity and specificity. Consequently, the electrophysiologic findings frequently must be interpreted in light of the presenting signs and symptoms.

Nerve conduction, electromyography, and F-wave determinations often are normal in patients with neurogenic thoracic outlet compression. In more advanced stages of compression, there may be evidence of denervation in the distribution of the inferior trunk of the brachial plexus. In those cases, the ulnar-nerve F-wave response likewise may be abnormal. A more sensitive evaluation of the brachial plexus may be accomplished by measuring somato-sensory evoked responses for median and ulnar nerves in neutral and stress positions. In neurogenic thoracic outlet compression, there may be a characteristic loss of amplitude at the brachial plexus (or Erb's point) potential. Occasionally, there will be an increase in latency. Those changes have been documented in the literature with pre- and postoperative studies [59–61].

Radiologic Studies. Chest and cervical spine x-rays should be obtained regularly in patients with brachial plexus compression, particularly those in the third decade of life and older. Neither the CT nor MRI scan has demonstrated any particular usefulness in evaluating the thoracic outlet compression syndromes. Their current application is confined to research protocols. The three-dimensional MRI reconstructions, as done by Collins, appear to be the most promising of the new imaging studies.

Arteriography and venography are used in the particular settings where arterial insufficiency or venous obstruction are prominent components of the clinical picture. Those tests should be performed with the arms in neutral position (at the sides) and again with the arm abducted (humerus at right angles to the chest). It has been demonstrated additionally that arteriography should be done in the erect position to be most useful in documenting positional, nonocclusive compression [62].

Conservative Management. The initial physiotherapy management program described by Peet at the Mayo Clinic has been added to and modified [13]. In France, Aligne and Barral reviewed the general principles of physical therapy as improving and strengthening the muscle groups they consider "openers" of the thoracic outlet area. Those openers are the middle and superior segments of the trapezius, the levator scapulae, and the sternocleidomastoid muscles. Such physical therapy is done concomitantly with relaxation of the muscle group called "closers," the anterior and middle scalene, subclavius, pectoralis minor, and pectoralis major. They recognized that moderate to severe cases should be referred for surgical treatment but reported a 70-percent success rate with physical therapy when the following criteria were met:

1. Early entrance into the physical therapy program
2. Absence of bony abnormalities
3. Neurologic symptoms only, without vascular compromise
4. Physical therapy combined with exercises at home

Aligne and Barral recognized poor outcomes in cases where there was antecedent cervical trauma, and with what they termed "moderate-to-average severity, combining vascular and neurological involvement" [63].

VENOUS COMPRESSION: THE PAGET-SCHROETTER VARIANT OF THORACIC OUTLET COMPRESSION

Spontaneous or effort-related thrombosis of the axillosubclavian vein is a disabling thoracic-outlet disorder affecting young, otherwise healthy individuals. The first two cases were published independently over 100 years ago by Paget in England and Von Schroetter in Germany. In 1949, Hughes analyzed 320 cases of spontaneous upper-extremity venous thrombosis collected from the medical literature and recognized that they represented a unique disorder by naming the entity the **Paget-Schroetter syndrome** [64].

At the time of Hughes's report, the primary therapy was surgical thrombectomy in an attempt to restore normal upper-extremity venous hemodynamics. In fact, despite increasing recognition of early rethrombosis, primary surgical therapy remained the standard approach until the early 1980s, when techniques for local catheter-directed thrombolytic therapy were popularized.

A number of authors had studied and reported on the natural history of the disorder, providing a yardstick against which therapeutic advances could be measured. Untreated patients with Paget-Schroetter syndrome can be expected to have varying degrees of disability as a consequence of chronic venous hypertension or recurrent episodes of venous thrombosis. The disability incidence ranges from a low of 25 percent reported by Linblad from Sweden to 40 percent reported by Gloviczki from the Mayo Clinic, to 47 percent reported by Donayre, and to 74 percent by Tilney [65,66]. In addition, there is a small incidence of pulmonary embolism [67].

The underlying cause of Paget-Schroetter syndrome is now recognized to be a mechanical abnormality at the costoclavicular portion of the axillosubclavian vein, with superimposed thrombosis resulting in the complexity of the clinical manifestations. The acute thrombosis almost invariably is in an area of chronic compression and stricture of the axillosubclavian vein at the thoracic outlet. The vein is compressed between a hypertrophied scalene or subclavius tendon and the first rib. A large exostosis often is found at the costoclavicular junction (Fig. 52-6).

Presenting History and Physical Signs. Patients, who very often are tradesmen or competitive athletes, suddenly notice severe and uniform swelling of one upper extremity, which usually occurs in the absence of any recognizable trauma. In addition to edema, the arm has a slight rubor or cyanosis, often erroneously suggesting a cellulitis but without fever or any other systemic signs or symptoms. The patient may notice prominence of the upper-extremity veins or be aware of collateral veins appearing around the shoulder or lateral pectoral region. Ordinarily, there is minimal pain except in the axilla, where pain and tenderness may occur over the course of the axillary vein.

If untreated, the swelling will often resolve in a few days to several weeks and the patient will be remarkably asymptomatic at rest. Symptoms of swelling, tightness, heaviness, and easy fatigue, occasionally associated with vasomotor changes of pallor and sweating, will occur with various levels of upper-extremity activity. Those symptoms are exacerbated in warm weather or other situation stimulating vasodilation in the upper trunk and arms.

A group of 50 consecutive patients studied at UCLA gives an accurate description of the contemporary demographic characteristics in the disorder. There were 31 men, with a mean age of 24 years and a range of 14 to 50 years, and 19 women with a mean age of 38 and a range of 23 to 51 years. The women as a group were significantly older ($p < 0.0001$). Forty-seven (94%) of the patients were right-hand dominant, and in 33 patients (66%), the dominant hand was the symptomatic side.

All but one of the men had been engaged in vigorous physical activity at the time of the episode of swelling and cyanosis, including 10 who were student athletes. Eleven women were engaged in relatively sedentary occupations, while eight were working in activities involving upper-extremity effort, including three who were student athletes. (The student athletes, male and female, included five weightlifters, three baseball players, two swimmers, and one each tennis, volleyball, and rowing crew competitors.) As a group then, 38 (76%) of the patients had an episode associated with effort, and 12 (24%) were sedentary. As a good characterization of their customary activities, 15 patients were engaged in competitive sports, 18 were laborers, and 17 were white-collar workers.

The physical examination will vary, depending on the interval between occurrence and examination. In patients who have had an acute episode of thrombosis, the characteristics outlined above will be readily evident to the examiner. In patients who have an established thrombus with collateral venous development, there may be surprisingly few physical findings during the interval periods, and the examiner may need to examine the patient after exercise. A series of push-ups, particularly in a warm room, often will disclose the underlying difference between the two arms. The edema may be quite minimal under those circumstances, although a general duskiness will be evident as well as increased prominence of the collateral veins. With further exercise, the patient often will complain of pain in the collateral veins, particularly in the supraclavicular, pectoral, or axillary region. In addition, those veins may be tender. The rapid resolution after rest will discount the impression of phlebitis.

It should be recognized that a tradesperson normally will have a 1- to 1.5-cm increase in circumference at the biceps in the dominant compared to the nondominant arm, and a 0.5- to 1-cm asymmetry at the forearm. Measurements, if made, should be done before and after exercise.

Because of extensive and progressive collateral development, the disparity between symptoms and signs will increase with time. In most patients, however, the resistance in the collaterals will be such that symptoms almost invariably will increase with increasing work of the arm. In a characteristic remarkably similar to that of patients with other forms of thoracic outlet compression syndrome, individuals with Paget-Schroetter syndrome will complain of severe exacerbation when the arm is used in the outstretched or overhead position. That position leads to rapid fatigue and typical dysesthesias in the C8-T1 dermatomal distribution. Signs of sympathetic hyperreactivity also will be present to a variable degree, though true causalgia is uncommon in this disorder.

Diagnosis. Patients presenting with a swollen arm, without an obvious etiology such as cellulitis, insect bite, or trauma, should undergo axillosubclavian venography. Venography preferentially is performed in two supine positions: with the arm at the patient's side and with the humerus at a right angle to the chest wall. Unfortunately, duplex ultrasound scanning and magnetic resonance angiography are reported to be inaccurate for venous assessment in the area of the retroclavicular space [68–70].

Thrombolytic and Anticoagulant Therapy. Immediately after verification of the diagnosis, patients should be treated by catheter-directed fibrinolytic therapy into the thrombus, when available. Heparin is administered concomitantly and continued until therapeutic anticoagulation with warfarin sodium (Coumadin) can be accomplished [71]. Although streptokinase had been used successfully in axillosubclavian-vein thrombosis, much of the prior reported experience suggests the superiority of urokinase for this disorder: Consequently the latter drug generally is considered to be the preferred agent [72–74].

This approach is based on the effectiveness of thrombolytic therapy as reported by Zimmerman in 1981. The case reports of Taylor and Porter (1985), then of Perler and Mitchel (1986) added surgical treatment of the underlying anatomic abnormality and the use of selective transluminal angioplasty to this new therapeutic design [75–77].

In 1989, Kunkle reported the results of a definitive, staged, multidisciplinary approach to the problem that had been initiated at UCLA. The results of that approach in a series of 50 consecutive patients was published in 1993 [78,79].

To avoid rethrombosis, surgical therapy is delayed following successful thrombolysis and anticoagulation. Drawing from experience with lower-extremity venous thrombosis and studies of upper-extremity venous endothelium, a 1- to 3-month period of anticoagulation with warfarin sodium is preferable prior to definitive treatment of the underlying structural abnormality [80].

Although initial thrombolytic therapy and the staged

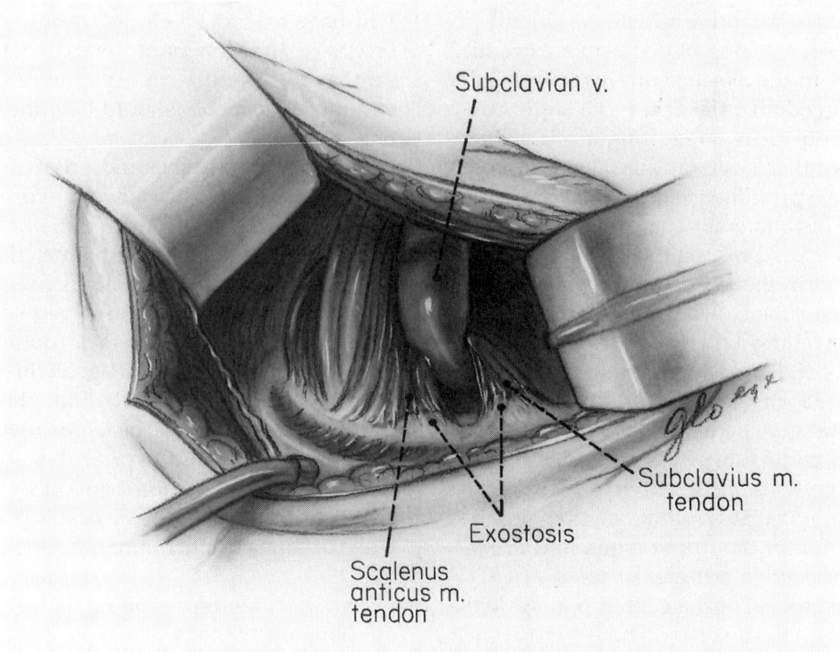

A

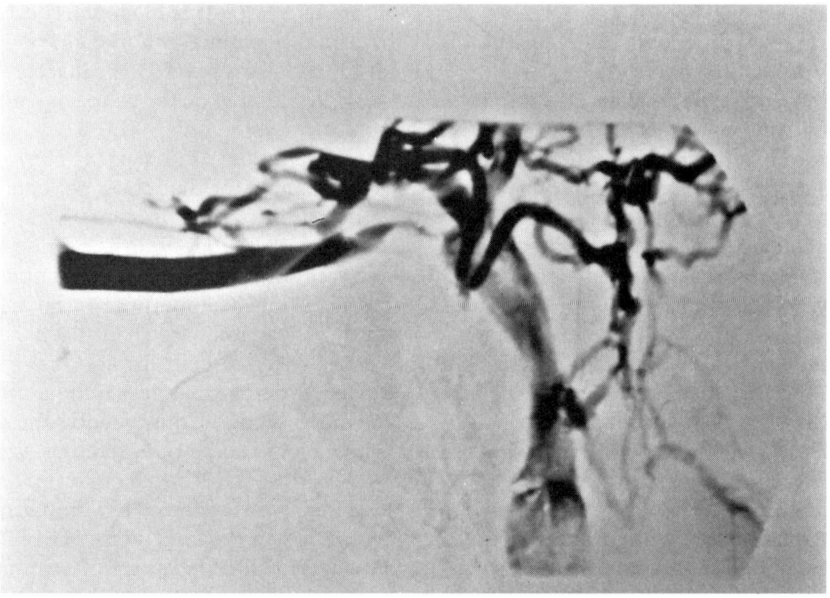

B

Fig. 52-6. **A.** Typical Paget-Schroetter abnormality, seen from the transaxillary view. Note compression of the axillosubclavian vein. (From JM Kunkel, HI Machleder. Treatment of Paget-Schroetter syndrome: a staged, multidisciplinary approach. Arch Surg. 1989; 124:1153–1158.) **B.** Radiologic appearance of compressed area. (From HI Machleder. Evaluation of a new treatment strategy for Paget-Schroetter syndrome: spontaneous thrombosis of the axillary-subclavian vein. J Vasc Surg 1993; 17:305–317.) **C.** Venogram immediately following an episode of effort-induced axillosubclavian-vein thrombosis. **D.** Appearance of vein following use of successful catheter-directed urokinase. Note clearance of thrombus and visualization of underlying compressive abnormality. (Do not dilate this lesion.)

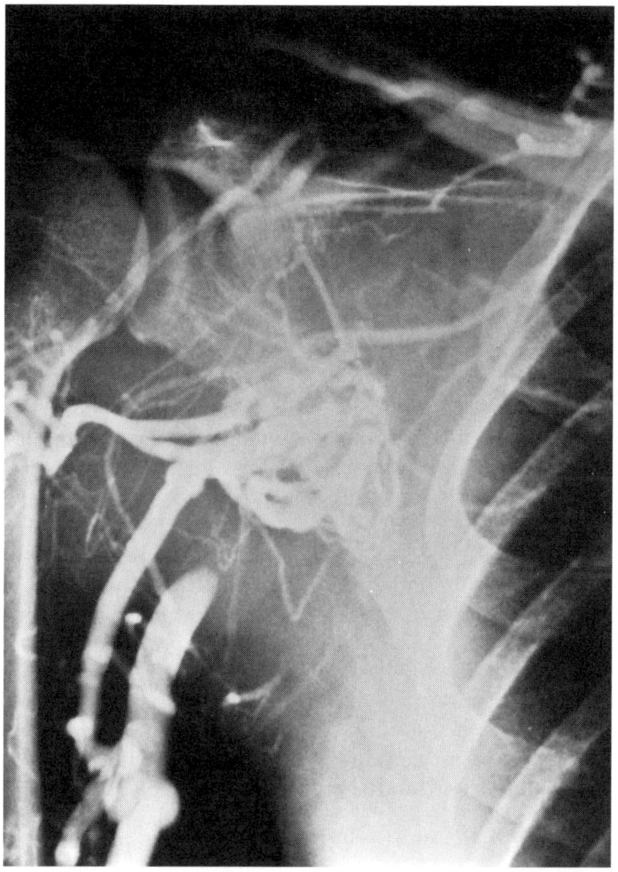

C

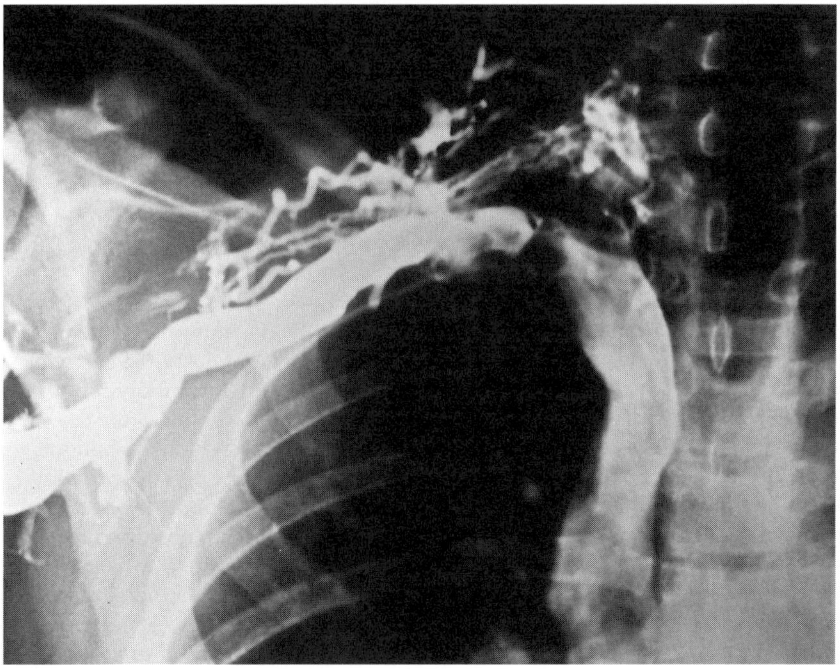

D

Fig. 52-6 (continued)

approach have been gaining wider acceptance, there remain proponents of early surgical thrombectomy as well as initial surgical repair [81,82]. Nevertheless, surgical intervention at the time when the vein is most thrombogenic has considerable theoretical disadvantages. This variation on the staged approach remains to be validated by appropriate follow-up studies [83,84]. Several authors have additionally suggested treating the thrombotic process alone without addressing the underlying anatomic abnormality. The rational for that approach is neither supported by these authors' published data nor by our own experience [85].

It must be appreciated that there are substantial differences between the spontaneous, effort-related axillosubclavian-vein thrombosis and the secondary thrombosis that results from indwelling lines and other iatrogenic trauma. A number of studies have documented those essential differences in pathophysiology and outcome [86–89].

Surgical Treatment. Surgical treatment is recommended if one of the following is true:

1. An underlying compressive abnormality is demonstrated venographically, following restoration of vein patency.
2. A symptomatic patient with an occluded vein demonstrated obstruction of the venous collaterals with abduction of the arm.

Transaxillary first-rib resection is considered the procedure of choice in this situation, based on the extensive literature documenting long-term results, effectiveness of decompression, and the excellent anatomic visualization of the area [90,91].

Transluminal Balloon Venoplasty. Postoperative transluminal angioplasty can be employed when the subclavian vein does not return to a normal configuration if a residual stricture is demonstrated on postoperative venogram. The continued presence of collateral venous channels following operation generally signifies that the stricture is hemodynamically significant.

Recurrent episodes of thrombosis characterize this group of patients if the underlying anatomic abnormality is not corrected. Prior to definitive therapy, 34 percent had multiple venographically verified recurrent episodes of thrombosis. The contralateral vein was studied venographically in 34 patients (68%). Five of those patients (15%) had an episode of thrombosis of the contralateral axillosubclavian vein, and 18 (53%) had evidence of 50-percent or greater diameter compression. The vein was normal in 11 patients and not studied in 16 patients. One patient had a clinically diagnosed and angiographically proven pulmonary embolus associated with the initial thrombotic event.

Results of Treatment. At the time of final clinical evaluation, 88 percent of the patients had resumed their usual occupations and full activity. Forty patients (80%) either were completely asymptomatic (31) or had minimal symptoms (9). Ten patients (20%) were symptomatic (4 working, but with symptoms, and 6 disabled for their usual occupations). Nine of the 10 symptomatic patients were laborers, and those nine represented 50 percent (9/18) of that working group. This was a significantly higher percentage of symptomatic patients than in the athlete or white-collar worker groups (1/32 or 3%; $p = 0.0002$).

In a final analysis of results, patients who underwent first rib resection had a significantly higher percentage of patent veins at the conclusion of the study than those not treated surgically ($p = 0.05$). The objectives for correcting the underlying disorder are as follows:

1. Relief of the venous hypertension
2. Correction of compression of both the axillary-subclavian and the collateral veins
3. Prevention of further episodes of thrombosis

These objectives have been achieved with first-rib and subclavius-tendon resection. After surgical decompression of the costoclavicular space, no patient experienced a recurrent episode of thrombosis. Viewed from another perspective, 29 of 35 patients (83%) who underwent transaxillary first-rib resection were asymptomatic at the conclusion of the study. Twenty-two of those had a patent and normal appearing vein, with 13 patients having residual occlusion. The three patients who remained symptomatic postoperatively all had residual venous occlusion.

The most significant determinant of ultimate vein patency was establishment of patency at the outset with medical therapy ($p = 0.0003$). Nevertheless, recanalization has been observed, even in chronically occluded veins, when the external compression is relieved.

In the group of patients who remained symptomatic or disabled, there was a significantly higher incidence of contralateral vein occlusion ($p = 0.05$) and inability to open the ipsilateral vein by initial medical therapy ($p = 0.03$). Of 35 patients who underwent first-rib resection, 30 (86%) were essentially symptom free (25 completely, 5 with minimal symptoms) and engaged in unrestricted normal activity. Five patients had residual symptoms, and two of those remained disabled for their usual occupations.

Angioplasty. Twenty-one patients underwent percutaneous balloon venoplasty. Twelve were done preoperatively after successful thrombolytic therapy, with seven veins occluding immediately after the procedure. The five uncomplicated preoperative balloon angioplasties had no effect on the extrinsic compressive abnormality. With long-term follow-up, three of the occluded veins had restoration of patency postoperatively, with four remaining occluded. The failure of preoperative balloon angioplasty had a significantly adverse association with long-term patency of the vein ($p = 0.02$). Conversely, in patients with uncomplicated balloon angioplasty following successful thrombolysis, there was no additional benefit in terms of long-term patency over those veins treated with thrombolytic therapy alone ($p = 0.99$). Nine angioplasties were attempted postoperatively for residual stricture. Of seven immediately successful cases, one required redilation due

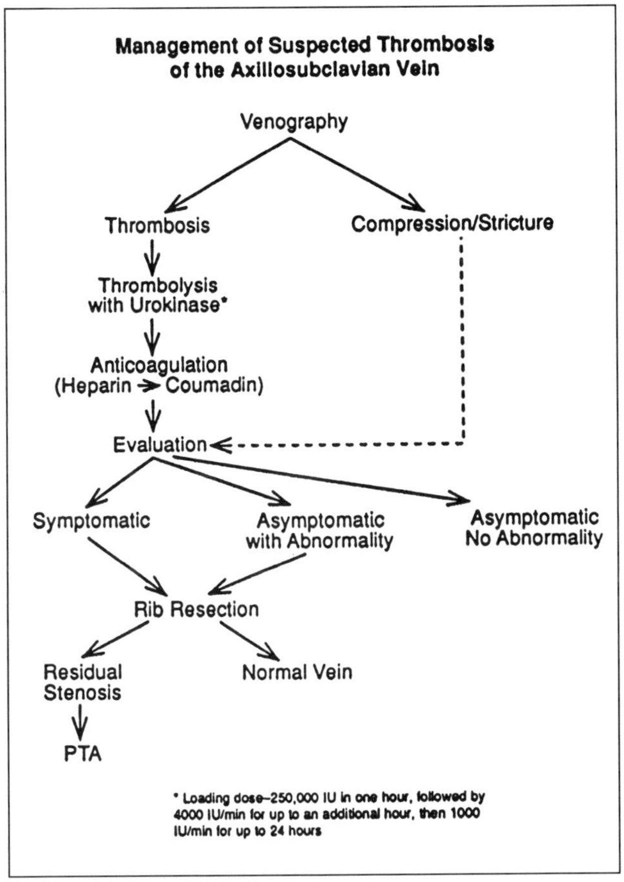

Fig. 52-7. Algorithm for management.

to an inadequate initial result with an undersized balloon. The remainder were uncomplicated. At long-term venographic follow-up (of the entire group of postoperative venoplasties), two remained occluded, and seven were patent.

Summary. In the natural history of Paget-Schroetter syndrome, resumption of normal activity after a period of recuperation (following an episode of thrombosis) frequently leads to symptoms of upper-extremity venous hypertension exacerbated by using the arms in the overhead position. That position can be demonstrated venographically to further occlude collateral vessels in the thoracic outlet. A number of patients develop more extensive symptoms of neurogenic TOS accompanied by positional numbness and dysesthesias.

Anticoagulation may protect the collateral vessels and interrupt the period of active clot propagation, producing a better functional result than would be expected from the natural history of the thrombotic event (Fig. 52-7). A summary of our experience follows:

1. Local urokinase was the most effective means for reestablishing venous patency.
2. With clot dissolution, the underlying compression of the vein at the thoracic outlet can be demonstrated.
3. Balloon angioplasty should not be undertaken in the acute setting or prior to relieving the musculotendinous compression.
4. The acute phlebitic process should resolve under the protection of warfarin sodium for one to three months. At that time it can be determined more effectively which patients require additional therapy. If lytic treatment has been prompt, and vein patency restored within 24 to 36 hours, surgical therapy can be undertaken in four weeks.
5. Removal of the first rib will decompress the axillosubclavian vein and the thoracic outlet collaterals, permitting the vein to regain its normal configuration (particularly in younger patients with more acute onset of compression).
6. Postoperative transluminal balloon venoplasty can be used in those patients with more chronic compression where the vein has become stenotic. Improvement of the luminal configuration has been accomplished without the necessity for venous reconstructive procedures.

Patients with Paget-Schroetter syndrome have a symptom complex that often reflects more extensive neurovascular compression at the thoracic outlet than that which might result from venous hypertension alone. Although thrombolytic therapy can restore patency of the axillosubclavian vein, first-rib resection is necessary to relieve the external compression. The procedure was very effective in patients who had restoration of subclavian-vein patency and to a lesser degree in those with residual occlusion.

Operative Management of TOS

There are three main surgical approaches to relief of thoracic outlet compression: transcervical, posterior, and transaxillary. In the hands of skilled surgeons who recognize the underlying bony and soft-tissue abnormalities that cause compression of the neurovascular structures, the surgical approach is not of particular significance. Each approach is capable of accomplishing the same end and tends to vary by surgical training and skill, concepts about the underlying pathophysiology, and inclination.

The anterior approach has the historic advantage of being the primary exposure and being the vantage point from which the anatomy has always been exposed and studied. There have been many variations of operative technique, from simple excision of a cervical rib, to division of the anterior scalene muscle or middle scalene muscle, to excision of the scalene muscle and resection of the first rib.

The anterior approach this suffered from a high incidence of failures during the "scalenous anticus syndrome" era, when the operation was applied to patients who had radicular symptoms predominantly in the upper plexus or median-nerve distribution. That era antedated the understanding of cervical-disk and neuroforaminal disease as well as an understanding of carpal-ligament compression of the median nerve. The failures were attributed to faulty diagnosis as well as inadequacies of the procedure. The primary technical failure was reattachment of the severed end of the scalene muscle to the deep cervical fascia with subsequent reappearance of neurocompressive symptoms. That procedural deficiency has

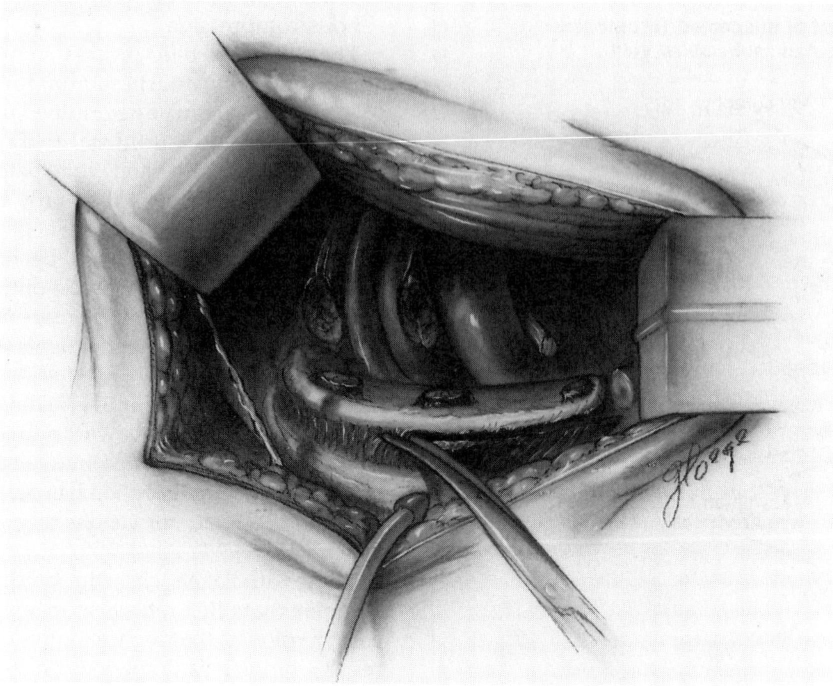

A

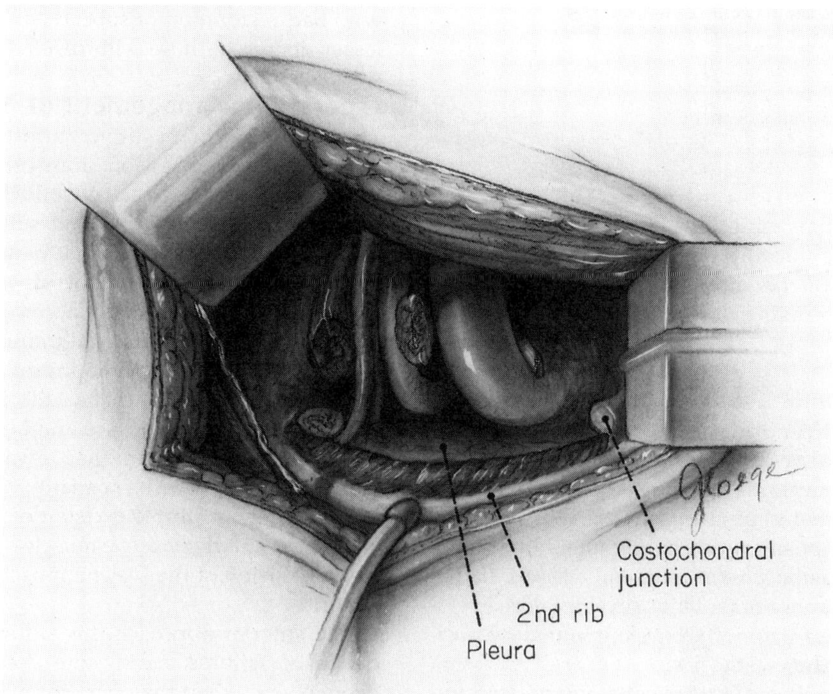

B

Fig. 52-8. **A.** Transaxillary removal of first rib. **B.** Appearance of thoracic outlet after decompression from transaxillary approach and correction of soft-tissue compressing elements. Note effective decompression of vein, artery, and inferior trunk of brachial plexus. (From HI Machleder. Transaxillary operative management of thoracic outlet syndrome. In CB Ernst, JC Stanley, eds. Current Therapy in Vascular Surgery II. Philadelphia: Decker, 1994.)

been corrected by scalenectomy, in which the entire portion of the anterior scalene muscle that overlies the brachial plexus is removed.

The importance of soft-tissue abnormalities has been emphasized by many authors and has encouraged some to reconsider the anterior supraclavicular approach [92–94]. In an attempt to incorporate the advantages of both the supraclavicular and transaxillary approaches, Stoney and colleagues reported on the combined surgical approach [95]. Sanders and Pearce emphasized similar results with three different operative approaches that were performed in a setting of considerable expertise and operative experience: transaxillary-rib resection, scalenectomy, and supraclavicular-rib resection. In that study, there were 80-percent good results at 1–2 years and 70-percent good results at 5–10 years of follow-up evaluations [96].

In summary, then, it has become evident that operative effectiveness depends more on recognition of anomalies and the compressing elements than on the particular route chosen for surgical exposure of the thoracic outlet.

Despite diagnostic and therapeutic concerns, excellent success rates in the 90-percent range are reported from many countries with the transaxillary approach [97]. Safe performance of first-rib resection by that route has been emphasized by Roos and Machleder [98,99]. The posterior approach proposed by Clagget and furthered by others largely has been abandoned except for complex recurrent problems [100,101] (Fig. 52-8).

Follow-Up Care

Follow-up evaluations by the surgical team have been a reliable indicator of the response to operation. Lindgren and co-workers from Sweden had the following to say: "The outcome of surgery as evaluated by the surgeon correlated well with the record of sick-leave from the regional social insurance offices." They further stated, "A long pre-operative period of sick-leave due to symptoms of TOS did not exclude the possibility of a successful operation" [102].

Although excellent relief of neurovascular compressive symptoms can be expected from surgical correction, some patients are troubled by residual regional muscle pains referred to as **fibrositis** or the more generalized condition of **fibromyalgia**. It is perhaps most important that these patients be returned to some regular activity despite continued symptoms. There are growing proponents of progressive activity rather than rest to treat TOS [103,104]. As with carpal tunnel syndrome and neuroforaminal or disk disease, a good therapeutic result depends on careful rehabilitative measures.

Summary

In their most obvious manifestations, the congenital and acquired abnormalities recognized in association with the thoracic outlet compression syndromes are considered discreet anomalies. However, they should more properly be viewed as part of a continuum of developmental variation. The particular spectrum of developmental variations seen may be significant as predisposing elements when complicated by either increased functional requirements or a change in muscle-fiber type (or isoforms of myosin) consequent to trauma.

Greater resilience of the arterial and venous systems seems to result in relatively innocuous symptoms until compression reaches levels of hemodynamic significance or structural damage. It is evident that the threshold for neurogenic symptoms from the brachial plexus is lower than that of the vascular system.

Coincident with the range and the continuum of developmental abnormalities, there are a range and a continuum of compression of the normal structures that traverse the thoracic outlet area. Symptoms associated with the extremes of the compressive abnormalities are easy to distinguish because they represent the following classic cases:

1. Paget Schroetter axillosubclavian vein occlusion
2. Hand ischemia from thrombosis or embolization from the compressed or aneurysmal subclavian artery
3. The "wasted hand" of cervical-band compression of the brachial plexus.

In addition to those end-stage conditions, it is important to recognize the full spectrum of symptoms that can arise from neurovascular compression at the thoracic outlet. The lesser degrees of compression often will be disabling in settings of specific physical or occupational requirements.

References

1. Fields WS, Lemak NA, Ben-Menachem Y. Thoracic outlet syndrome: review and reference to stroke in a major league pitcher. AJNR 1986; 7:73–78.
2. Coote H. Exostosis of the left transverse process of the seventh cervical vertebrae, surrounded by blood vessels and nerves, successful removal. Lancet 1861; 1:360–361.
3. Wilshire WH. Supernumerary first rib: clinical records. Lancet 1860; 2:633.
4. Gilliat RW, et al. Wasting of the hand associated with a cervical rib or band. J Neurol Neurosurg Psychiatry 1970; 33:615–624.
5. Todd TW. The descent of the shoulder after birth. Its significance in the production of pressure-symptoms on the lowest brachial trunk. Anat Anz Bd 1912; 41:385–395.
6. Stopford JSB, Telford ED. Compression of the lower trunk of the brachial plexus by a first dorsal rib. Br J Surg 1919; 7:168–177.
7. White JC, Poppel MH, Adams R. Congenital malformations of the first thoracic rib. SG&O 1945; 81:643–659.
8. Edwards PR, Moody AP, Harris PL. First rib abnormalities in association with cervical ribs: a cause for postoperative failure in the thoracic outlet syndrome. Eur J Vasc Surg 1992; 6:677–681.
9. Adson AW, Coffey JR. Cervical rib: a method of anterior approach for relief of symptoms by division of the scalenus anticus. Ann Surg 1927; 85:839–853.
10. Naffziger HC. The scalenus syndrome. Surg Gyn Obstet 1937; 64:119–120.
11. Naffziger HC, Grant WT. Neuritis of the brachial plexus, mechanical in origin: the scalenus syndrome. Surg Gyn Obstet 1938; 67:722–730.
12. Ochsner A, Gage M, DeBakey M. Scalenus anticus (Naffziger) syndrome. Am J Surg 1935; 28:669–695.
13. Peet RM, et al. Thoracic-outlet syndrome: evaluation of a

therapeutic exercise program. Proc Mayo Clinic 1956; 31: 281–287.
14. Rob CG, Standeven A. Arterial occlusion complicating thoracic outlet compression syndrome. Brit Med J 1958; 2: 709–719.
15. Eaton LM. Neurologic causes of pain in the upper extremities; with particular reference to syndromes of protruded intervertebral disk in the cervical region and mechanical compression of the brachial plexus. Surg Clin North America 1946; 4–6:810–832.
16. Eaton LM. In discussion of Peet et al. Proc Mayo Clinic 1956; 312:81–87.
17. Clagett OT. Research and prosearch. J Thorac Cardiovasc Surg 1962; 44:153–166.
18. Roos DB. Transaxillary approach for first rib resection to relieve thoracic outlet syndrome. Ann Surg 1966; 163: 354–358.
19. Roos DB. Experience with first rib resection for thoracic outlet syndrome. Ann Surg 1971; 173:429–442.
20. Rempel DM, Harrison RJ, Barnhard S. Work-related cumulative trauma disorders of the upper extremity. JAMA 1992; 267:838–842.
21. Gu YD, et al. Thoracic outlet syndrome. Clin Med Jour 1988; 101:689–694.
22. Amadio PC. The Mayo Clinic and carpal tunnel syndrome. Mayo Clin Proc 1992; 67:42–48.
23. Brain WR, Wright AD, Wilkinson M. Spontaneous compression of both median nerves in the carpal tunnel: six cases treated surgically. Lancet 1947; 1:277–282.
24. Machleder HI, Moll F, Verity A. The anterior scalene muscle in thoracic outlet compression syndrome: histochemical and morphometric studies. Arch Surg 1986; 121:1141–1144.
25. Sanders RJ, et al. Scalene muscle abnormalities in traumatic thoracic outlet syndrome. Am J Surg 1990; 159:231–236.
26. Law AA. Adventitious ligaments simulating cervical ribs. Ann Surg 1920; 72:497–499.
27. Roos DB. Congenital anomalies associated with thoracic outlet syndrome. Am J Surg 1976; 132:771–778.
28. Milliez PY. Contribution A L'Etude De L'Ontogenese Des Muscles Scalenes (Reconstruction D'Un Embryon De 2.5 cm). June 28, 1991 Universite Paris 1 Pantheon-Sorbonne Musee De L'Homme, Museum D'Histoire Naturelle.
29. White JC, Poppel MH, Adams R. Congenital malformations of the first thoracic rib; a cause of brachial neuralgia which simulates the cervical rib syndrome. Surg Gyn Obst 1945; 81:643–659.
30. Makhoul RG, Machleder HI. Developmental anomalies at the thoracic outlet: an analysis of 200 consecutive cases. J Vasc Surg 1992; 16:534–545.
31. Kunkel JM, Machleder HI. Treatment of Paget-Schroetter syndrome: a staged multidisciplinary approach. Arch Surg 1989; 124:1153–1158.
32. Hamilton, Boyd, Massman. Human Embryology, Third Edition. Cambridge 1952. Pp. 548–559.
33. Todd TW. The relations of the thoracic operculum considered in reference to the anatomy of cervical ribs of surgical importance. J Anat Physiol 1911; 45:293–304.
34. Gruber W. Uber die Halsrippen des Menschen mit vergleichend-anatomischen Bemerkungen. Mem Acad Imper Sci. St Petersburg 1869; 7 ser 13, No 2.
35. Adson AW, Coffee JR. Cervical rib. Ann Surg 1927; 85: 839–857.
36. Schapera J. Autosomal dominant inheritance of cervical ribs. Clinical Genetics 1987; 31:386–388.
37. Etter LE. Osseous abnormalities of the thoracic cage seen in forty thousand consecutive chest photoroentgenograms. Am J Roentgenol 1944; 51:359–363.
38. Adson WA. Surgical treatment for symptoms produced by cervical ribs and the scalenus anticus muscle. Surg Gyn Obstet 1947; 85:687–700.
39. Adson AW. Cervical ribs: symptoms, differential diagnosis, and indication for section of the insertion of scalenous anticus muscle. J Int Coll Surgeons 1951; 16:546–559.
40. Firsov GI. Cervical ribs and their distinction from underdeveloped first ribs. Arkhiv Anatomii, Gistologii i Embriologii 1974; 67:101–103.
41. Scher LA, et al. Staging of arterial complications of cervical rib: guidelines for surgical management. Surgery 1984; 95:644–649.
42. Halsted WS. An experimental study of circumscribed dilation of an artery immediately distal to a partially occluding band, and its bearing on the dilation of the subclavian artery observed in certain cases of cervical rib. J Exper Med 1916; 24:271–279.
43. Charlesworth D, Brown SCW. Results of excision of a cervical rib in patients with the thoracic outlet syndrome. Brit J Surg 1988; 75:431–433.
44. Telford EC, Stopford JSB. The vascular complications of cervical rib. Brit J Surg 1931; 18:557–564.
45. Sanders RJ, Roos DB. The surgical anatomy of the scalene triangle. Contem Surg 1989; 35:11–16.
46. Ochsner A, Gage M, De Bakey M. Scalenus Anticus (Naffziger) Syndrome. Am J Surg 1935; 28:669–695.
47. Naffziger HC, Grant WT. Neuritis of the brachial plexus mechanical in origin: the Scalenus Syndrome. Surg Gynec & Obst 1938; 67:722–730.
48. Telford ED, Mottershead S. Pressure at the cervico-brachial junction (an operative and anatomical study). J Bone and Joint Surg 1948; 30B:249–263.
49. Sunderland S, Bedbrook GM. Narrowing of the second part of the subclavian artery. Anat Record 1949; 104:299–307.
50. Todd TW. Cervical rib: factors controlling its presence and its size, its bearing on the morphology of the shoulder, with four cases. J Anat & Physiol 1911–1912; 45:293–304. Figure 5A, 10.
51. Roos DB. Pathophysiology of congenital anomalies in thoracic outlet syndrome. Acta Chir Belgica 1980; 79:353–361.
52. Lang J. Topographische anatomie des plexus brachialis und thoracic-outlet syndrom. Berlin: Walter de Gruyter, 1985.
53. Sampson JJ. In Medico-Surgical Tribute to Harold Brunn. Berkeley: University of California Press, 1942. Pp. 453–471.
54. Aziz S, Straehley CJ, Whelan TJ. Effort-related axillosubclavian vein thrombosis: a new theory of pathogenesis and a plea for direct surgical intervention. Am J Surg 1986; 152:57–61.
55. Telford ED, Stopford JSB. The vascular compression of cervical rib. Br J Surg 1931; 18:557.
56. Falconer MA, Weddell G. Costoclavicular compression of the subclavian artery and vein: relation to the scalenus anticus syndrome. Lancet 1943; 2:539–544.
57. Toomingas A, et al. Outcome of the abduction external rotation test among manual and office workers. Am J Indust Med 1991; 19:215–227.
58. Wood VE, Biondi J. Double-crush nerve compression in thoracic outlet syndrome. J Bone Joint Surg 1990; 72:85–87.
59. Siivola J, Sulg I, Pokela R. Somatosensory evoked responses as diagnostic aid in thoracic outlet syndrome. Acta Chir Scand 1982; 148:647–652.
60. Yiannikas C, Walsh JC. Somatosensory evoked responses in the diagnosis of thoracic outlet syndrome. J Neurol Neurosurg Psychiatry 1983; 46:234–240.
61. Machleder HI, et al. Somatosensory evoked potentials in the assessment of thoracic outlet compression syndrome. J Vasc Surg 1987; 6:177–184.

62. Benzian SR, Mainzer F. Erect arteriography: its use in the thoracic outlet syndrome. Radiology 1974; 111:275–277.
63. Aligne C, Barral X. Rehabilitation of patients with thoracic outlet syndrome. Ann Vasc Surg 1992; 6:381–389.
64. Hughes ESR. Venous obstruction in the upper extremity (Paget-Schroetter's syndrome). Int Abstr Surg 1949; 88: 89–127.
65. Tilney NL, Griffiths HJG, Edwards EA. Natural history of major venous thrombosis of the upper extremity. Arch Surg 1970; 101:792–796.
66. Linblad B, et al. Venous haemodynamics of the upper extremity after subclavian vein thrombosis. Vasa 1990; 19: 218–222.
67. Harley DP, et al. Pulmonary embolism secondary to venous thrombosis of the arm. Am J Surg 1984; 147:221–224.
68. Haire WD, et al. Utility of duplex ultrasound in the diagnosis of asymptomatic catheter-induced subclavian vein thrombosis. J Ultrasound Med 1991; 10:493–496.
69. Haire WD, et al. Limitations of magnetic resonance imaging and ultrasound-directed (duplex) scanning in the diagnosis of subclavian vein thrombosis. J Vasc Surg 1991; 13:391–397.
70. Baxter GM, et al. Comparison of colour Doppler ultrasound with venography in the diagnosis of axillary and subclavian vein thrombosis. Br J Radiol 1991; 64:777–781.
71. Machleder HI. Upper extremity venous thrombosis. Seminars in Vascular Surgery 1990; 3:219–226.
72. Druy EM, et al. Lytic therapy in the treatment of axillary and subclavian vein thrombosis. J Vas Surg 1985; 2:821–827.
73. Steed DL, et al. Streptokinase in the treatment of subclavian vein thrombosis. J Vasc Surg 1986; 4:28–32.
74. Landercasper J, et al. Thrombolytic therapy of axillary-subclavian venous thrombosis. Arch Surg 1987; 122:1072–1075.
75. Zimmerman R, et al. Urokinase therapy of subclavian-axillary vein thrombosis. Klin Wochenschr 1981; 59:851–856.
76. Taylor LM, et al. Thrombolytic therapy followed by first rib resection for spontaneous ("effort") subclavian vein thrombosis. Am J Surg 1985; 149:644–647.
77. Perler BA, Mitchel SE. Percutaneous transluminal angioplasty and transaxillary first rib resection: A multidisciplinary approach to the thoracic outlet compression syndrome. Amer Surg 1986; 52:485–487.
78. Kunkel JM, Machleder HI. Treatment of Paget-Schroetter syndrome: a staged, multidisciplinary approach. Arch Surg 1989; 124:1153–1158.
79. Machleder HI. Evaluation of a new therapeutic strategy for treatment of Paget-Schroetter Syndrome: axillary-subclavian vein thrombosis. J Vasc Surg 1993; 17:305–317.
80. Sundqvist SB, et al. Deep venous thrombosis of the arm: a study of coagulation and fibrinolysis. Acta Chir Scand 1972; 138:313–319.
81. Deweese JA. Results of surgical treatment of axillary-subclavian venous thrombosis. In JJ Bergan, JST Yao, eds. Venous Disorders. Philadelphia: Saunders, 1991. Pp. 421–433.
82. Aziz S, Staehley CJ, Whelan TJ. Effort-related axillosubclavian thrombosis. A new theory of pathogenesis and a plea for direct surgical intervention. Am J Surg 1986; 152:57–61.
83. Molina JE. Surgery for effort thrombosis of the subclavian vein. J Thorac Cardiovasc Surg 1992; 103:341–346.
84. Urschel HC, Razzuk MA. Improved management of the Paget-Schroetter syndrome secondary to thoracic outlet compression. Ann Thorac Surg 1991; 52:1217–1221.
85. Wilson JJ, Zahn CA, Newman H. Fibrinolytic therapy for idiopathic subclavian-axillary vein thrombosis. Am J Surg 1990; 159:208–211.
86. Tilney NL, Griffiths MB, Edwards EA. Natural history of major venous thrombosis of the upper extremity. Arch Surg 1970; 101:792–796.
87. Donayre CE, et al. Pathogenesis determines late morbidity of axillosubclavian vein thrombosis. Am J Surg 1986; 152:179–184.
88. Gloviczki P, Kazmier FJ, Hollier LH. Axillary-subclavian venous occlusion: the morbidity of a nonlethal disease. J Vasc Surg 1986; 4:333–337.
89. AbuRahma AF, et al. Conventional versus thrombolytic therapy in spontaneous (effort) axillary-subclavian vein thrombosis. Am J Surg 1991; 161:459–465.
90. Roos DB. Thoracic outlet syndromes: update 1987. Am J Surg 1987; 154:568–573.
91. Pittam MR, Darke SG. The place of first rib resection in the management of axillary-subclavian vein thrombosis. Eur J Vasc Surg 1987; 1:5–10.
92. Stallworth JM, Quinn GJ, Aiken AF. Is rib resection necessary for relief of thoracic outlet syndrome? Ann Surg 1979; 185:581–592.
93. Reilly LM, Stoney RJ. Supraclavicular approach for thoracic outlet decompression. J Vasc Surg 1988; 8:329–334.
94. Sanders RJ, Raymer S. The supraclavicular approach to scalenectomy and first rib resection: description of technique. J Vasc Surg 1985; 2:751–763.
95. Qvarfordt PG, Ehrenfeld WK, Stoney RJ. Supraclavicular radical scalenectomy and transaxillary first rib resection for the thoracic outlet syndrome. A combined approach. Am J Surg 1984; 148:111–116.
96. Sanders RJ, Pearce WH. The treatment of thoracic outlet syndrome: a comparison of different operations. J Vasc Surg 1989; 10:626–634.
97. Carty NJ, Carpenter R, Webster JHH. Continuing experience with transaxillary excision of the first rib for thoracic outlet syndrome. Br J Surg 1992; 79:761–762.
98. Roos DB. Essentials and safeguards of surgery for thoracic outlet syndrome. Angiol 1981; 32:187–193.
99. Machleder HI. Transaxillary operative management of thoracic outlet syndrome. In CB Ernst, JC Stanley, eds. Current therapy in vascular surgery. 2nd ed. Philadelphia: BC Decker, Inc. 1991. Pp. 227–230.
100. Martinez NS. Posterior first rib resection for total thoracic outlet syndrome decompression. Contemp Surg 1979; 15: 13–21.
101. Kline DG, Judice DJ. Management of selected brachail plexus lesions. J Neurosurg 1983; 58:631–649.
102. Lindgren SHS, Ribbe EB, Norgren EH. Two year follow-up of patients operated on for thoracic outlet syndrome. Effects on sick-leave incidence. Eur J Vasc Surg 1989; 3:411–415.
103. Nies KM. Treatment of the fibromyalgia syndrome. J Musculoskel Med 1992; 9:20–26.
104. Wolfe F, et al. The American College of Rheumatology 1990 Criteria for the Classification of Fibromyalgia. Report of the Multicenter Criteria Committee. Arthritis Rheum 1990; 33:160–172.

Reflex Sympathetic Dystrophy

Robert J. Schwartzman

Reflex sympathetic dystrophy (RSD) was first clinically described in 1864 [1]. It is a progressive illness that usually is initiated by peripheral trauma to a nerve plexus or soft tissue [2–4]. It has five major components: (1) pain, (2) swelling, or edema, (3) autonomic dysfunction, (4) movement disorder, and (5) trophic changes [2,5–7]. In general, pain, swelling, and autonomic dysfunction dominate the first phase of the illness, while the movement disorder, trophic changes, and autoimmune phenomenon become apparent in stages II and III of the disease [8–10]. It is a significant problem worldwide in and of itself and complicates many other pain syndromes [8].

Pain

The pain of RSD is its most disabling feature. It is burning, intense, and out of proportion to the initial injury [2,3,10]. It is felt diffusely, deeply, and distally as well as superficially, with palmar or plantar predominance [11]. It respects neither a nerve nor a dermatomal distribution and is exacerbated by movement, dependent posture, and emotional upset [11–15]. It may spread in a mirror distribution and may envelop the entire body [2,3]. Spontaneous episodes of pain are frequent, and some patients suffer a deep ache in addition to pain [2,11,15]. A few patients obtain relief by packing the affected extremity in ice [16,17]. Most patients shield the affected part from all stimuli [1,2]. Hyperalgesia (lowered pain threshold and enhanced pain perception) and allodynia (pain from innocuous mechanical or thermal stimuli) frequently are seen [18,19]. Early in the course of the illness, the pain is sympathetically maintained, but in stages II and III of the disease, it frequently becomes sympathetically independent [20–22].

Clinical studies of RSD patients, utilizing quantitative sensory threshold testing, differential nerve blocks, pharmacologic manipulation, intraneural microstimulation, and recording, provide some insight into the pain mechanisms of this disorder [23–43].

Microneurographic stimulation studies in human sensory nerves reveal that the perception of the quality, localization, and magnitude of a sensation can be achieved from the input of a single primary somatosensory unit [44]. A specific modality of sensation is dependent on the receptor that is stimulated [45]. Pain occurs following activation of A-delta or C-nociceptor units [44,46–48]. A-delta fibers carry sharp, well-localized first pain, and unmyelinated C-fibers transmit second pain [49–51]. During natural and tissue-destructive stimulation, there is coactivation of different receptors. Their summated activity produces a blended perception [52–55]. Thus, burning or cold pain is a combination of activation of specific A-δ cold receptors and C-fiber nociceptors. Some patients with RSD and hyperalgesia following peripheral-nerve injury demonstrate C-nociceptor receptor sensitization to thermal and mechanical stimuli [11,56]. A-delta nociceptors also may be sensitized to heat and contribute to thermal hyperalgesia in those patients [11]. Cross-modality threshold sensitization at the receptor level has been clearly demonstrated in a subset of RSD patients [16]. Such patients relieve pain by packing the affected part in ice [16]. Their polymodal C-nociceptors discharge to touch when their skin is warm but not when it is cold [20]. Other patients complain of increased pain when their skin is cold [21]. Clearly, sympathetic blockade will increase the pain of the first group (by raising skin temperature) and reduce that of the second [16]. In many RSD patients, there is a graded perception of pain or hyperalgesia in the injured area. That may be due to inhomogeneous receptor sensitization of polymodal C-nociceptors that occurs following the release of algogenic agents or inflammatory mediators from damaged tissue [56,57]. The intensity of perceived pain is related to the frequency of discharge in specific groups of nociceptors [23]. In an area affected by RSD, the state of the receptor may determine if hypoalgesia (receptor fatigue) or hyperalgesia (receptor sensitization) occurs after a particular stimulus [23].

In some RSD patients, allodynia to touch and cold is maintained by alpha$_1$ responsive receptors and A-beta fibers (large myelinated fibers) [34,58,59]. In other patients, it is sustained by sensitized C-fibers [17,60]. A pressure block of a peripheral nerve causes specific perceptual loss related to fiber size [27]. The larger fibers are the most sensitive to pressure. The first sensation lost with cuff-pressure block is touch, followed by cold, warmth, and pain [25]. After release of a pressure block in RSD patients, allodynia to cold and tactile stimuli returned concomitantly with touch and cold sensibility [34]. Allodynia to heat persisted when touch and cold sensation were lost during the compression block and therefore must have been mediated by the C-fibers, which were still conducting [34,38].

Evidence for the role of large myelinated fibers in the pain of RSD has been obtained from differential nerve-fiber-stimulation studies of patients with paresthesias. Postischemic paresthesias occur from ectopic firing in myelinated fibers [55,61,62]. In control subjects, they are reported as tingling, pricking, and squeezing sensations. In two RSD patients, induced postischemic paresthesias were extremely painful and must have been transmitted by large myelinated fibers [34]. Intraneural microstimulation studies of the median nerve in normal subjects evokes a tactile sensation at the threshold of perception in 80 percent of control subjects and pain in 20 percent [31]. In two patients with RSD and allodynia to touch, pain was noted at the threshold of sensation [34]. The pain increased with high frequencies of stimulation and decayed slowly. In normal subjects, there is a rapid decrement of pain after high-frequency stimulation, which is characteristic of unmyelinated axons [23]. Because only myelinated fibers can follow high-frequency stimulation, they therefore were involved in production of the pain experienced by these patients.

The sympathetic innervation and the alpha adrenoreceptor clearly are involved in the early stages of RSD pain [63,64]. The strongest evidence for that is the relief of pain by sympathetic blockade [28,29]. However, microneurographic recordings from sympathetic efferents in four RSD patients revealed normal responses to activity and mental stress but no overall increase in sympathetic discharge [34]. The role of the alpha adrenoreceptor in RSD can be demonstrated by the effect of its activation or blockade. Injection of noradrenaline into the asymptomatic limb of a former RSD patient (cured by sympathectomy) reproduced the original pain within 30 minutes [34,37]. The intravenous phentolamine test (alpha-receptor antagonist) is successfully utilized to correlate the relationship of experienced pain to adrenoreceptor activation [58]. If a patient's pain is significantly reduced by alpha-receptor blockade, it is sympathetically maintained [58].

Possible mechanisms that underlie the painful phenomena seen in RSD patients have been suggested by recent investigations in newly developed experimental models of causalgiform and neuropathic pain [65–71].

In the experimental neuroma model, the sprout of a regenerating afferent axon fires spontaneously [72]. Ectopic discharge from sprouts can be elicited by local and systemic noradrenaline administration and is blocked by the alpha-receptor antagonist phentolamine [72–76]. Activation of sympathetic efferents by electrical stimulation of preganglionic-nerve fibers excite afferents from the neuroma [75]. The noradrenaline released from sympathetic efferent fibers in the neuroma activates ectopic midnerve-sprout afferent adrenergic receptors to produce local depolarization and repetitive spike discharge [76]. Afferents in the neuroma that are discharging from a prolonged noxious stimulus can be excited further by sympathetic stimulation [77]. Sympathetic stimulation does not excite nociceptors in normal skin [78–80]. New evidence from recent experiments in a rabbit model of mixed peripheral-nerve injury shed light on the suspected peripheral somatosympathetic link in RSD. In that model, a subset of C-nociceptive units increase their discharge to sympathetic stimulation [67]. Those effects are seen days after the injury in intact sensory fibers that have maintained their connectivity and are mediated by alpha$_1$ adrenergic–like receptors [67]. It is postulated that there is an accumulation of ectopic alpha-adrenergic binding sites on the terminals of intact nociceptive axons in the damaged nerve. Those sites are activated by released noradrenaline from efferent sympathetic activity caused by the nociceptive-afferent barrage from the partially damaged nerve [67]. Stretching a nerve also causes those neurophysiologic changes [67]. That type of injury to soft tissue, root, and plexus commonly initiates RSD [2]. The peripheral linkage may be maintained and expanded by somatosympathetic reflexes, whereby nociceptive spinal-cord afferent input evokes sympathetic efferent activity over multiple spinal segmental levels [81,82].

The spontaneous pain seen following partial nerve injury may be caused by several mechanisms acting separately or in concert. In the damaged nerve or its terminals, there may be ectopic impulse activity, supersensitivity of regenerating axon sprouts to circulating catecholamines, or sensitization and increased firing of nociceptive receptors activated by algesic substances released at the site of the injury [67,83–90].

The importance of spinal mechanisms in the physiology of RSD pain is now clear [91]. The superficial dorsal-horn neurons of Rexed layers I and II have small, well-defined peripheral receptive fields that respond to noxious and near tissue-destructive stimuli transmitted by C-fiber and A-delta fiber afferents [92]. The small primary sensory neurons of the dorsal-root ganglion (the cells of origin of C- and A-nociceptive afferents) synthesize neuropeptides, which are transported to both their peripheral and central terminals [93–95]. Specific neuropeptides may be associated with separate aspects of sensation [96,97]. Stimulation of C-fibers signal temperature-release somatostatin (SOM), whereas stimulation of mechanonociceptive-specific fibers release substance P (SP) [96,97]. A population of C unmyelinated pain afferents utilizes glutamate as the neurotransmitter in the dorsal horn [98–100]. Recent work supports an interaction between excitatory amino acids (EAAs) and neuropeptides in the DH [101–103]. The rapid time course of EAA action suggests their role in fast synaptic transmission, whereas neuropeptides are more likely to effect excitability or transmission for prolonged periods of time [104].

The receptive fields of superficial dorsal-horn neurons enlarge and their excitability increases under varying physiologic and pathologic conditions [105,106]. Concomitant with that physiologic plasticity are changes in the neuropeptide content of the DH [65,95,107–109]. In the Bennett and Xie model, (sciatic-nerve ligature in the rat), there is a decrease of SP, calcitonin gene-related peptide (CGRP), and fluoride-resistant acid phosphatase (FRAP) in primary afferent terminal arbors primarily in lamina I–III, while an increase in galinin, neuropeptide Y (NPY), vasointestinal peptide (VIP), and dynorphin occurs in the DH [95]. In models of chronic inflammation and painful peripheral neuropathy, the marked increase of dynorphin peptides and their mRNA is localized to intrinsic DH neurons [110,111]. Specific neuropeptide release and their regulation may determine the functional physiology of the cord [96,97]. As an example of this interaction, recent utilization of cDNA-hybridization techniques has demonstrated differential activation of spinal-cord dynorphin and enkephalin neurons in a chronic-inflammation model in which mechanical and thermal hyperalgesia are present [111]. The interaction of dynorphin and enkephalin peptides with opioid receptors in the DH appears important for pain modulation [111,112]. The enlargement of peripheral receptive fields of lamina I neurons, as well as a decrease in their firing threshold following nerve injury, may be a reflection of the increased level of spinal-cord dynorphin, because it enhances the excitability of those neurons and would expand their receptive fields [111]. The correlation of spinal-cord neuropeptide levels to hyperalgesia, allodynia, hyperpathia, and other aspects of RSD pain awaits further experimentation [102,113].

Recent studies in the painful peripheral neuropathy model demonstrate that excess or prolonged depolarization may injure and destroy neurons [95,114]. Smaller neurons may be more susceptible to that type of injury [95]. The small dark neurons seen in lamina I–III after peripheral-nerve injury demonstrate changes of transsynaptic degeneration [95]. The afferent nociceptive discharge produced by nerve and tissue injury releases EAAs and neuropeptides that induce prolonged cellular depolarization in their terminal arborizations, which may differentially injure the small inhibitory interneurons of the DH [95,102,114,115]. Afferent-induced excitotoxicity is attractive as a mechanism for the progressive refractoriness of RSD pain. In stage II and III disease, patients frequently no longer respond to either sympathetic blockade or large doses of oral narcotics [2,11]. At those stages of the illness, DH inhibitory mechanisms may be irreversibly lost or altered.

The critical role of low-threshold mechanoreceptors (LTM) and central DH mechanisms in the pain of RSD was reemphasized by Roberts [91]. His hypothesis rests on the thesis that peripheral trauma activates nociceptive afferents that sensitize DH wide-dynamic-range (WDR) neurons [91,116]. Those neurons receive convergent excitatory input from both low- and high-threshold primary afferents [116,117]. In anesthetized cats, WDR neurons are activated by electrical stimulation of sympathetic efferent fibers and are inhibited from firing by alpha adrenergic–blocking agents [116]. Nociceptor-specific (NS) spinal neurons are not activated by sympathetic stimulation [116,118]. It is postulated that in RSD peripheral sympathetic stimulation activates low-threshold mechanoreceptors, which would discharge those sensitized WDR neurons and cause touch-evoked pain. Evidence against sensitization of the WDR neuron as the pathogenic mechanism for the pain of RSD has come from clinical studies [119]. In patients suffering sympathetically maintained pain, noxious heat pulses, innocuous mechanical stimuli, and transcutaneous electrical nerve stimulation reveal the coexistence of A-beta–evoked pain, normal heat-evoked pain, and normal heat-pain summation [119]. If the WDR neurons were sensitized, the response to heat-evoked pain also would be abnormal, because the neurons respond to both stimuli. Dorsal-column stimulation also should exacerbate pain in patients with RSD by preferential stimulation of low-threshold mechanoafferents, but the reverse is the case [120].

Central nervous system control of sympathetic efferent activity is important in RSD, because almost all patients demonstrate exacerbation of sympathetic mediated pain (SMP) under stressful conditions [2,3]. The preganglionic sympathetic intermediolateral-column neurons are modulated by projections from multiple supraspinal nuclei, including the nucleus Magnus Raphus (NMR) of the medulla [121–126]. The NMR exerts tonic central inhibitory control of spinal nociceptive neurons and possibly those of the intermediolateral column [127–129]. Intrathecal morphine may be effective in relieving refractory RSD pain by increasing NMR inhibition of sympathetic outflow in addition to its inhibitory effects on nociceptive neurons [130].

The demonstration that nociceptive-afferent input can induce central sensitization in pain-projecting neurons of the DH suggests a mechanism that may be operative in RSD patients [102,131,132]. The neurophysiologic manifestations of central sensitization are (1) enlarged cutaneous receptive fields, (2) a lowered threshold to fire, (3) a greater response per stimulus, and (4) afterdischarge. Those parameters correlate with hyperalgesia and persisting pain after injury in patients and an enhanced flexion-withdrawal reflex in animals [133].

The early stage of central sensitization appears to be related to the "windup" phenomenon of central pain-projecting (CPP) neurons of the DH [134]. After conditioning stimuli of C-fibers, CPP neurons increase their action-potential discharges incrementally to successive stimuli. The mechanism underlying that response is the release of EAAs and neuropeptides by afferent nociceptive volleys that produce long-lasting excitatory postsynaptic potentials [101]. Those potentials summate and depolarize a population of DH interneurons whose afferent discharge decreases the voltage-dependent Mg^{++} block of the N-methyl D-aspartate (NMDA) ion-channel complex of the CPP neuron. The consequent increased inward current causes depolarization and increases the security of synaptic transmission of the CPP [134]. The exciting implication is that reversal of central sensitization, by manipulation of NMDA mechanisms, may be effective in treating sympathetic independent pain [70,134–136].

Current evidence suggests that both peripheral sensitization of receptors and central sensitization of pain-projecting neurons of the DH contribute to the pathologic pain of RSD [17,58,102,133]. The contribution of LTM and myelinated A-beta fibers to hyperalgesia and touch-evoked pain is supported by experimental evidence [59,65]. The sympathetic-nervous-system modulation of nociceptive afferents in a partially damaged peripheral nerve and the maintenance and spread of that interaction by somatosympathetic reflexes in the spinal cord suggest mechanisms for the observed importance of sympathetic activation in stage I disease [63,67]. The appearance of small dark neurons in the DH may be the morphologic marker for the centralization of that evolving process and its refractoriness to current treatment [95,107,108].

Edema

A major component of RSD in its early stages is edema [2,3,15]. The plasma extravasation is seen at the site of injury, distal to it, and at times over major areas of the body [3]. Recent studies of the axon reflex suggest a mechanism for that phenomenon that may be of importance in RSD [137,138]. The small bipolar cells of the dorsal-root ganglia (cells of origin of C-nociceptors) manufacture and colocalize neuropeptides that are transported to, stored, and released at their peripheral and central terminals [137,139–142]. Their central arborizations project to the dorsal, ventral, and intermediolateral zones of the spinal cord. Stimulation of a cutaneous nerve mechanically or electrically releases neuropeptides from the peripheral terminals of the unmyelinated C-nociceptors [143–145]. The released neuropeptide SP increases capillary permeability directly and potentiates that effect by also releasing histamine from mast cells [146–150]. CGRP, which is colocalized and released from the same small unmyelinated terminals as SP, causes vasodilatation by relaxing vascular smooth muscle [151]. That increases local blood flow and enhances plasma extravasation to produce a subcutaneous wheal [152,153]. The tachykinins, neurokinin A and B (NKA and NKB) also are found in the axons of small-diameter unmyelinated afferents of small dorsal root ganglia (DRG) neurons and are released by C-fiber afferent depolarization [146,147]. They are volume conductors (they act over a distance) and produce both vasodilation and increased vascular permeability, which further promote neurogenic edema [146]. The flare seen following C-fiber stimulation is a reflection of vasodilatation caused by histamine release from mast cells induced by released SP [149,154]. The process spreads locally through the terminal arborizations of the stimulated C-unmyelinated afferents [149].

A series of investigations has demonstrated the role of the peripheral and sympathetic nervous system in mediating swelling and hyperalgesia at sites remote from an original injury [155]. That phenomenon has been termed **reflex neurogenic inflammation** [156,157].

A small quantity of saline injected daily for 3 days into the hind paw of a rat induces swelling and a decrease in mechanical nociceptive threshold ipsilaterally as well as in the contralateral hind limb [155]. Bilateral neurectomy, sympathectomy, and destruction of C-polymodal afferents in either sciatic nerve diminish the contralateral response [155,158,159]. A ligature around the saphenous vein draining the ipsilateral paw does not alter the phenomenon. That demonstrates that there is no humoral component to the response, which had been suggested by earlier studies [159–161]. The process appears to be mediated segmentally at a spinal-cord level. Adjuvant-induced arthritis and direct inflammation of a joint are profoundly influenced neurogenically [16,155,159]. C-nociceptive afferent release of neuropeptides into the joint space has been suggested as a mechanism [159].

SP has multiple inflammatory and immune modulating functions that may be operative in RSD. It interacts with leukocyte receptors, degranulates mast cells, causes pavementing of leukocytes in venules, and releases inflammatory mediators from lymphocytes and macrophages [158,162–164]. Its immunologic functions include (1) stimulation, synthesis, and release of monocyte derived cytokines; (2) modulation of chemotaxis of mononuclear and polymorpholeukocytes; and (3) stimulation of human T lymphocytes [165–172]. SP enhances the proliferation of smooth muscle cells, endothelial cells, and fibroblasts [169,170]. In a joint, it activates synoviocytes to secrete prostaglandin E_2 and collagenase, which mediate tissue destruction [173]. The experimental use of the neurotoxin capsaicin (8-methyl-N-vanillyl-6-nonenamide) has strengthened the evidence for the role of C-unmyelinated fibers and their neuropeptides in inflammation and RSD [163,164,173,174]. The compound is effective if administered neonatally or after inflammation has been produced [163,175,176]. When administered to neonatal rats (50 mg/kg SC), it destroys up to 95 percent of C-unmyelinated fibers and the small, type B dorsal-root ganglion cells [177]. Its action is seen within 24 hours and lasts for days [177]. It depletes SP in primary DRG sensory neurons, their CNS terminals in the dorsal horn, and their peripheral-nerve-terminal arborizations [163,175–179]. When given to adult rats, capsaicin treatment depletes SP in similar areas that are affected by neonatal administration [180,181]. Its effect on inflammation has the same time course as its effect on SP in the saphenous nerve or hindpaw skin. It blocks C-fiber–mediated neurogenic edema and vascular extravasation produced from antidromic nerve stimulation [182–184]. The reduction in edema is parallel to its block of chemical pain [181]. If administered on days 2–10 of neonatal life, the neurogenic inflammatory response is permanently blocked [179]. Intracisternal capsaicin blocks pain sensibility in the adult rat but does not alter neurogenic edema, which suggests independent function of the peripheral and central end of the sensory B neuron of the DRG [185].

Morphine and its agonists inhibit neurogenic plasma extravasation by blocking the release of SP from C-unmyelinated terminals [186,187]. The effect is reversed with naloxone and is not dependent on blood flow [186]. In those patients who have undergone implantation of a morphine pump for generalized stage III RSD, a decrease in generalized edema may be seen 24–48 hours prior to pain relief, which suggests that SP has a role both in the pain and the edema of RSD [188].

The evidence that neuropeptides, C-unmyelinated afferents, and the sympathetic nervous system modulate tissue swelling, pain, joint pathology, and changes in the integument of adjuvant-induced arthritis is compelling [163,189,190]. Those same phenomena are seen in stage II and III RSD and suggest that RSD is the human counterpart of reflex neurogenic inflammation [2,3,155].

Autonomic Dysfunction

Autonomic dysfunction is evident in all stages of RSD [3,11,191–193]. In general, early in the illness, the involved extremity may be warm, suffused, red, and dry but with time becomes cool, pale, hyperhidrotic, and cyanotic [2,11]. In a high percentage of patients, mottling, cyanosis, and livedo reticularis will be seen in the contralateral uninvolved extremity [3]. The generalized dysfunction of the skin circulation can be measured in all fingers and toes of the affected extremity compared to the unaffected side [11]. Jänig and Blumberg demonstrated that the reflex discharge patterns of postganglionic sympathetic neurons to arterial baroreceptor, cutaneous nociceptive and arterial chemoreceptive stimuli could be altered following nerve injury [194–196]. In their experimental paradigm (anastomosis of the central portion of a motor nerve to the distal portion of a cutaneous nerve), the reflex pattern of discharge in many postganglionic sympathetic cutaneous vasoconstrictor neurons changed to a pattern more characteristic of muscle vasoconstrictor neurons [196]. Those changes also were noted in a contiguous, intact cutaneous nerve. Noxious cutaneous stimuli in control animals inhibit cutaneous postganglionic sympathetic ganglia neurons. That inhibition of cutaneous vasoconstrictor neurons was lost following nerve injury [196,197]. Deafferentation of the extremity and reanastomosis of a severed cutaneous nerve did not change the reflex discharge pattern of the sympathetic vasoconstrictor neurons. Those results suggest altered reflex control of vasoconstrictive neurons at the spinal level [196].

A clear sympathetic defect has been demonstrated at some stage in almost all patients with RSD [2,192,193,196]. Recent studies have shown that this defect is partly central in origin [198,199].

In RSD patients, cutaneous blood flow responds differently to both peripheral and central autonomic nervous system stimuli than it does in normal controls [198]. In control patients, significant decreases in extremity blood flow are seen in response to the Valsalva maneuver and cold pressor test [200,201]. Rosen demonstrated that the cold pressor test caused an average 37.5-percent blood-flow decrease in the skin microvasculature of the extremities in controls but a decrease of only 0–8 percent in RSD patients [202,203]. A recent study utilizing the cold pressor test, Valsalva maneuver, hyperventilation, and exercise demonstrated that cutaneous blood flow was increased in both the affected and the unaffected extremity [199]. The increased bilateral extremity blood flow in RSD patients under those varying conditions suggests a loss of differential control of extremity blood flow that occurs at a central level [199,203]. Recent clinical investigations in RSD patients under generalized thermal stress support earlier findings of abnormal reflex control of arterial-skin blood flow in the affected extremity [204]. The entire distal extremity (more than the involved spinal segment) responded abnormally to whole-body cooling. That finding was interpreted as a demonstration of abnormal reflex excitability of spinal intermediolateral-column vasoconstrictor neurons [11,204].

In general, resting temperature and blood flow in RSD-affected extremities varies with the stage of the disease [2,3,11,205]. In the experimental painful peripheral neuropathy model, hyperthermia is seen at earlier stages, while hypothermia is observed later [206–208]. In those animals that had abnormally cold hind paws on the nerve-damaged side, immediate warming of their extremities followed complete nerve section [206]. That suggests that the hypothermia is maintained through active vasoconstriction caused by afferent-induced efferent sympathetic outflow. A possible mechanism for that phenomenon is that damage to a nerve causes the rapid onset of spontaneous firing (20–40 Hz) of myelinated A-delta nociceptive afferents at the site of injury and from the dorsal root [209,210]. Such a barrage would increase sympathetic efferent activity [79,81]. In normal control subjects, intraneural microstimulation produces vasoconstriction and extremity cooling by overriding neurogenic vasodilatation evoked by topical capsaicin administration [211]. That would correlate with the later stages of the nerve-injury model. In those RSD patients with warm suffused extremities, angry backfiring C-nociceptors may elicit neurogenic vasodilatation that predominates over vasoconstrictive sympathetic activity [16]. In the nerve-injury model, temperature of the hind paw did not correlate with the adrenergic innervation of the vasculature. At 1 month post–nerve injury, there is almost total loss of arterial adrenergic innervation [212,213]. Examination at that time revealed that some rats with abnormally hot hind paws had normal adrenergic innervation, while other animals with no temperature abnormality demonstrated no detectable adrenergic innervation in the hind-paw vasculature [206]. Striking variability of temperature was noted over hours in some animals. The short-lived temperature variability seen in those animals could be the result of the interplay of released neuropeptides, somatosympathetic vasoconstrictive reflexes, and the effects of substances released from the vascular endothelial wall [206,211]. The same temperature variability has been clearly demonstrated in RSD patients [2,3,11]. The cold limbs noted at later periods in the animal model may represent a combination of adrenergic denervation hypersensitivity of the vasculature to circulating catecholamines or active vasoconstriction [206].

Vascular physiologists have described spontaneous changes of arteriolar diameter in cutaneous vessels under physiologic conditions [214,215]. Those rhythmic variations can be blocked by anesthetic medications [216]. RSD patients do not demonstrate such rhythmic variations in cutaneous blood flow [199].

Blumberg suggests that the pain and swelling of RSD are secondary to activation of peripheral nociceptors caused by dysregulation of peripheral blood flow [11]. The hypothesis posits that a peripheral traumatic event initiates a barrage of nociceptive input to the DH that disrupts the discharge patterns of sympathetic neurons so that there would be a greater outflow to venous capacitance vessels than to arterial resistance vessels. That imbalance would cause increased capillary filtration pressure and consequent edema formation. The resultant higher tissue interstitial pressure would discharge peripheral nociceptors and further excite preganglionic sympathetic neurons by means of somatosympathetic reflexes [204]. Central preganglionic sympathetic vulnerability at the time of the injury is required to initiate the process [11,204]. No direct experimental data support an imbalance between arterial and venous vasoconstrictor tone in RSD patients, although Ficat and Arlet have reported increased bone pressure with diminished venous return in RSD patients [217]. Those authors suggest that the frequent finding of hypothermia in all fingertips or toetips in an affected RSD extremity is an indication of disturbance in the spinal vasoconstrictor system and that the deep bone pain of RSD is secondary to activation of bone nociceptors by increased interstitial pressure [204,217].

Peripheral autonomic neurons contain several neuropeptides [207,208,218]. The axons that innervate blood vessels store NPY in large vesicles that may be released in concert with noradrenalin [219]. NPY is a potent vascular constrictor in some vascular beds and is released preferentially at high frequencies of sympathetic stimulation [220,221]. In specific vessels, it may enhance vascular constriction produced by noradrenalin and sympathetic-nerve stimulation [221]. NPY-induced contractions of blood vessels are slower in onset and longer lasting than those produced by noradrenaline [222–224]. In the painful peripheral-nerve-injury model, there is a dramatic decrease of both NPY and dopamine-beta-hydroxylase (DBH) (synthesizing enzyme marker for norepinephrine [NE]) in the arterial wall by 30 days, which may affect vessel contractibility [209]. In RSD patients, venous mottling and cool skin frequently are seen in all stages of the disease, which may be a reflection of abnormal reactivity of the cutaneous vasculature [2,3,217]. As reviewed earlier, neurogenic vasodilatation is caused by the release of SP, CGRP, and NKA from polymodal nociceptors that directly dilate or release mediators that dilate cutaneous blood vessels [225]. It has been postulated that peptidergic afferents may counterbalance spontaneous release of adrenergic mediators from sympathetic efferents under physiologic conditions [225]. That that balance may be disordered in RSD is suggested by the striking livedo reticularis of the skin in the affected extremities of such patients [2,3].

Movement Disorder

The movement disorder of RSD is well described [226–232]. It consists of an inability to initiate movement, weakness, tremor, muscle spasm, dystonia, and increased reflexes. The motor manifestations may precede pain, appear suddenly, and are frequently noted in a "mirror distribution" on the contralateral side of the body [226]. The manifestations are always present in stage II and III disease in association with the severe pain and dystrophic and atrophic phenomena suffered by RSD patients. Early, the motor manifestations may be alleviated by intense sympathetic blockade or sympathectomy, but with time they escape sympathetic modulation and may be permanent [226].

The sympathetic nervous system has profound physiologic and pharmacologic effects on skeletal-muscle contraction, neuromuscular transmission, anterior-horn-cell function, and spinal-cord reflexes [233–237]. The effects of catecholamines are complex and dose dependent [238–243]. B_2-adrenergic stimulation in type II (fast-contracting) skeletal-muscle membrane enhances and prolongs isometric twitch tension while inhibiting the same parameters in type I (slow-contracting) muscle [235,244]. Sympathetic stimulation of fatigued mammalian type II muscle increases isometric twitch tension (Orbelli effect) [245].

Brain-stem noradrenergic nuclei innervate the dorsal and ventral horns of the spinal cord [246,247]. Sympathetic projections have been traced to bag and chain intrafusal fibers of the muscle spindle, the intrafusal fibers themselves, and ventral efferent fibers [248,249]. Sympathetic-nerve stimulation increases firing of muscle-spindle afferents that increase muscle tension in parallel with an increase in spindle firing rate [250,251]. That effect is mediated by $alpha_1$ and $alpha_2$ adrenoreceptors and is proportional to the number of spindles stimulated [250,251]. The increased firing of muscle-spindle afferents has been shown to modulate deep-tendon reflexes in decerebrate and spinal cats [233,234]. Sympathetic stimulation modifies some nociceptor and mechanoreceptor receptors directly [252,253]. Their axons project to reticular formation neurons that effect muscle tone through the gamma loop [254,255]. Thus, the increase in muscle tone, reflexes, and spasms seen in RSD patients may be partially spindle mediated via an interaction with the sympathetic system.

Postural and movement-related tremors as well as involuntary jerks frequently are seen in RSD patients [226,227]. A recent study of 21 patients suffering from unilateral upper-extremity RSD and tremor demonstrated the following: (1) There is no relation of the tremor to any specific symptom of RSD; (2) the frequency of the tremor but not its electromyogram (EMG) synchronization can be reduced by weight loading; (3) the tremor is both postural and related to voluntary movement; and (4) the tremor ceases with sympathetic block and with recovery from RSD [256]. Synchronization of anterior-horn-cell discharge from peripheral or central inputs initiates tremors and increases their amplitude [257]. Increased proprioceptive reflex input to the spinal cord has been proposed as a cause of synchronization and tremor [255]. The authors of that proposal suggest that the tremor of RSD is an enhanced physiologic tremor due to sensitization of muscle spindles through the B_2 receptor [256]. Alternatively, neuropeptide mechanisms may be primary or act concomitantly with the sympathetic innervation to initiate and maintain the motor manifestation of RSD. SP and related peptides (tachykinins) have a profound effect on motor-neuron function [258,259]. Immunohistochemical studies have localized SP to the dorsal, ventral, and intermediolateral columns of the spinal cord [260]. Those peptides produce prolonged depolarization of anterior-horn cells in vitro [258,259]. The depolarization follows a long latent period after application and causes afterdischarge [258]. It is blocked in the rat spinal cord by the gamma-aminobutyric acid (GABA) derivative baclofen [261]. Intrathecal administration of SP enhances flexion withdrawal to nociceptive stimuli [262]. Somatosympathetic reflexes may be the physiologic expression of the neuroanatomical network that links nociceptive and mechanoreceptive fibers to both intrinsic spinal-cord sympathetic neurons and their prevertebral ganglia [263]. It is postulated that the combined action of the sympathetic nervous system and SP initiates and sustains the intense and prolonged depolarization of anterior-horn cells that may underlie the dystonia of RSD [264,265]. The physiologic effects of sympathetic stimulation on peripheral receptors, muscle spindles, the reticular formation, and the muscle itself seem critical to the motor manifestations of RSD. Central sensitization of anterior-horn cells through NMDA mechanisms may be more important in latter stages of the illness [131,132].

Summary

Converging lines of research suggest that RSD is a form of reflex neurogenic inflammation. Early on in the course of the disease, the sympathetic nervous system appears to have an initiating and sustaining role. In later states of the illness, structural changes at the DH level seem to correlate with centralization of the process. Neuropeptides and EAAs released from thin or unmyelinated nociceptive afferents may produce both the inflammation and the suspected central sensitization of the DH neurons seen in later stages of the disease. Effective treatment of RSD will follow a clearer understanding of the physiology of each stage of the disease.

References

1. Mitchell SW, Morehouse GR, Keen WW. Gunshot wounds and injuries of nerves. New York: Lippincott, 1864.
2. Schwartzman RJ, McLellan TL. Reflex sympathetic dystrophy, a review. Arch Neurol 1987; 44:555–561.
3. Schwartzman RJ. Reflex sympathetic dystrophy. In HL Frank, ed. Spinal Cord Trauma. Amsterdam: Elsevier, 1992.
4. Gellman H, et al. Reflex sympathetic dystrophy in brain-injured patients. Pain 1992; 51:307–311.
5. Levine JD, Goetzl EJ, Basbaum AI. Contribution of the nervous system to the pathophysiology of rheumatoid arthritis and polyarthritis. Rheumatoid Clinics of North America 1987; 13:369–383.
6. Stanton-Hicks M, et al. Reflex sympathetic dystrophy: changing concepts and taxonomy. Pain 1995; 63:127–133.
7. Webster GF, et al. Reflex sympathetic dystrophy: occurrence of chronic edema and non-immune bulbous skin lesions. Archives Am Acad Dermatol 1992; 28:29–32.
8. Abram SH. Incidence and epidemiology. In M Stanton-Hicks, W Jänig, RA Boas, eds. Reflex Sympathetic Dystrophy. Boston: Kluwer Academic Publishers, 1990.
9. DeTakats G. Reflex dystrophy of the extremities. Arch Surg 1937; 34:939.
10. Bonica JJ. The Management of Pain. Philadelphia: Lea and Febiger, 1953.
11. Blumberg H. Development and treatment of the pain syndrome of reflex sympathetic dystrophy: clinical picture, experimental investigations and new pathological considerations. Der Schmerz 1988; 2:125–143.
12. Livingston WK. Pain mechanisms; a physiological interpretation of causalgia and its related states. New York: Macmillan, 1943.
13. Bonica JJ. Causalgia and other reflex sympathetic dystrophies. In JJ Bonica, JC Liebeskind, DG Albe-Fessard, eds. Advances in Pain Research and Therapy, vol. 3. New York: Raven, 1979. Pp. 141–166.
14. Nathan PW. On the pathogenesis of causalgia in peripheral nerve injuries. Brain 1947; 70:145.
15. Blumberg H, Griesser HJ, Hornyak ME. Mechanisms and role of peripheral blood flow dysregulation in pain sensation and edema in reflex sympathetic dystrophy. In M Stanton-Hicks, W Jänig, RA Boas, eds. Reflex Sympathetic Dystrophy. Boston: Kluwer Academic Publishers, 1990.
16. Ochoa J. The newly recognized painful ABC syndrome: thermographic aspects. Thermology 1986; 2:65–107.
17. Cline MA, Ochoa J, Torebjörk AE. Chronic hyperalgesia and skin warming caused by sensitized C nociceptors. Brain 1990; 112:621–647.
18. Lindblom U, et al. Pain terms: a current list with definition and notes on usage. Pain 1986; 3:5215–5221.
19. Willis WD. Hyperalgesia and allodynia. Summary and overview. In ED Willis, ed. Hyperalgesia and allodynia. New York: Raven, 1992. Pp. 1–13.
20. Campbell JN, Raja SN, Meyer RA. Painful sequelae of nerve injury. In R Dubner, GF Gebhart, MR Bond, eds. Pain Research and Clinical Management. Amsterdam: Elsevier, 1988.
21. Frost SA, et al. Does hyperalgesia to cooling stimuli characterize patients with sympathetically maintained pain (reflex sympathetic dystrophy)? In R Dubner, GF Gebhart, MR Bond, eds. Pain Research and Clinical Management. Amsterdam: Elsevier, 1988.
22. Campbell JN, et al. Sympathetically maintained pain: a unifying hypothesis. In WD Willis Jr, ed. New York: Raven, 1992. Pp. 141–151.
23. Torebjörk EH, Lamotte RH, Robinson CJ. Peripheral neural correlates of magnitude of cutaneous pain and hyperalgesia: simultaneous recordings in humans of sensory judgements of pain and evoked responses in nociceptors with C-fibers. J Neurophysiol 1984; 2:325–339.
24. Robinson CJ, Torebjörk HE, LaMotte RH. Psychophysical detection and pain ratings of incremental thermal stimuli: a comparison with nociceptor responses in humans. Brain Res 1983; 247:87–106.
25. Machenzie RA, et al. Fiber function and perception during cutaneous nerve block. J Neurol Neurosurg Psychiat 1975; 38:865–873.
26. Collins WF, Nielsen FE, Randt CT. Relation of peripheral nerve fiber size and sensation in man. Arch Neurol 1960; 3:381–385.
27. Torebjörk HE, Hallin RG. Perceptual changes accompanying controlled preferential blocking of A and C fiber responses in intact human skin nerves. Exper Brain Res 1973; 16:321–332.
28. Wang JK, Johnson KE, Ilstrup DM. Sympathetic blocks for reflex sympathetic dystrophy. Pain 1985; 23:13–17.
29. Betcher AM, Bean G, Casten DG. Continuous procaine block of paravertebral sympathetic ganglions. Observations on one hundred patients. J Amer Med Assoc 1953; 151:288–292.
30. Jurna I. Neuropharmacological aspects of reflex sympathetic dystrophy. In M Stanton-Hicks, W Jänig, RA Boas, eds. Reflex Sympathetic Dystrophy. Boston: Kluwer Academic Press, 1990.
31. Schady WJL, Torebjörk HE, Ochoa JL. Peripheral projections of nerve fibers in the human median nerve. Brain Res 1983; 277:249–261.
32. Torebjörk HE, Schady W, Ochoa JL. A new method for demonstration of central effects of analgesic agents in man. J Neurol Neurosurg Psychiat 1984; 47:862–869.
33. Ochoa JL, Torebjörk HE. Paresthesia from ectopic impulse generation in human sensory nerves. Brain 1980; 103: 835–853.
34. Torebjörk E. Clinical and neurophysiological observations relating to pathophysiological mechanisms in reflex sympathetic dystrophy. In M Stanton-Hicks, W Jänig, RA Boas, eds. Reflex Sympathetic Dystrophy. Boston: Kluwer Academic Press, 1990.
35. Hallin RG, Torebjörk HE. Studies on cutaneous A and C fiber afferents, skin nerve blocks and perception. In Y Zotterman, ed. Sensory Functions of the Skin in Primates with Special Reference to Man. Oxford: Pergamon Press, 1976.
36. Torebjörk HE, Hallin RG. Activity in C fibers correlated to perception in man. In C Hirsch, Y Zotterman, eds. Cervical Pain. Oxford: Pergamon Press, 1972.
37. Wallin G, Torebjörk HE, Hallin RG. Preliminary observations in the pathophysiology of hyperalgesia in the causalgic pain syndrome. In Y Zotterman, ed. Sensory Function of the Skin in Primates with Special Reference to Man. Oxford: Pergamon Press, 1976. Pp. 489–502.
38. Torebjörk HE, Wallin G. Sensitization of polymodal C-nociceptor fibers in man. Proc Int Union Physiol Sci 1977; 13:758.
39. Koltzenburg M, Lundberg LER, Torebjörk HE. Dynamic and static components of mechanical hyperalgesia in human hairy skin. Pain 1992; 51:207–219.
40. Lamotte RH. Neurophysiological mechanisms of cutaneous secondary hyperalgesia in the primate. In WD Willis Jr, ed. Hyperalgesia and Allodynia. New York: Raven, 1992. Pp. 175–187.
41. LaMotte RH, et al. Neurogenic hyperalgesia, psychophysical studies on underlying mechanisms. J Neurophysiol 1991; 66:190–211.
42. Price DD, Long S, Hui HC. Sensory testing of pathophysiological mechanisms of pain in patients with reflex sympathetic dystrophy. Pain 1992; 49:163–173.

43. Kress M, et al. Responsiveness and functions attributes of electrically localized terminals of cutaneous C-fibers in vivo and in vitro. J Neurophysiol 1992; 68:581–595.
44. Ochoa J, Torebjörk E. Sensations evoked by intraneural microstimulation of single mechanoreceptor units innervating the human hand. J Physiol 1983; 633–654.
45. Valbo AB. Sensations evoked from the glabrous skin of the human hand by electrical stimulation of unitary mechanosensitive afferents. Brain Res 1981; 215:359–363.
46. Hallin RG, Torebjörk HE. Afferent and efferent C units recorded from human skin nerves in situ. Acta Soc Med Opsal 1970; 75:277–281.
47. Torebjörk HE, Hallin RG. Identification of afferent C units in intact human skin nerves. Brain Res 1974; 67:387–403.
48. Van Hees J. Human C-fiber input during painful and nonpainful skin stimulation with radiant heat. In JJ Bonica, D Albe-Fessard, ed. Advances in Pain Research and Therapy. New York: Raven, 1976.
49. Adriaensen H, et al. Response properties of thin myelinated (A-δ) fibers in human skin nerves. J Neurophysiol 1983; 49:111–122.
50. Van Hees J, Gybels JC. Nociceptive activity in human nerve during painful and nonpainful skin stimulation. J Neurol Neurosurg Psychiatry 1981; 44:600–607.
51. Campbell JN, et al. Peripheral mechanisms of nociception. In PD Wall, R Melzak, eds. Textbook of Pain. Edinburgh: Churchill-Livingstone, 1989.
52. Torebjörk HE. Nociceptor activation and pain. Philos Trans R Soc Lond (Biol) 1985; 308:227–234.
53. Ochoa J, Torebjörk E, Culp W. Determinants of subjective attributes of normal cutaneous sensation and of paresthesia from ectopic nerve impulse generation. In K Von Euler, et al., eds. Somatosensory Mechanisms. London: MacMillan, 1984. Pp. 377–387.
54. Yarnitsky D, Ochoa JL. Release of cold-induced burning pain by block of cold-specific afferent input. ISR Brain 1990; 113/4:893–902.
55. Merrington WR, Nathan PW. A study of post-ischaemic parasthesiae. J Neurol Neurosurg Psychiat 1949; 12:1–18.
56. Handwerker HO, et al. Nociceptor function in intact skin and ın neurogenic or non-neurogenic inflammation. Acta Physiol Hung 1987; 69:333–342.
57. Konietzny F, Hensel H. The effect of capsaicin on the response characteristic of human C-polymodal nociceptors. J Therm Biol 1983; 8:213–215.
58. Treede RD, et al. Evidence that alpha adrenergic receptors mediate sympathetically maintained pain (reflex sympathetic dystrophy). Pain (Abstr) 1990; 5:S487.
59. Campbell JN, et al. Myelinated afferents signal the hyperalgesia associated with nerve injury. Pain 1988; 32:89–94.
60. Gracely RH, Lynch SA, Bennett GJ. Painful neuropathy: altered central processing maintained dynamically by peripheral input. Pain 1992; 51:175–194.
61. Ochoa JL, Torebjörk AE. Paraesthesiae from ectopic impulse generation in human sensory nerve. Brain 1980; 103:835–853.
62. Ochoa J, et al. Abnormal spontaneous activity in single sensory nerve fibers in humans. Muscle and Nerve 1982; 5:574–577.
63. Bennett GJ. The role of sympathetic nervous sytem in painful peripheral neuropathy. Pain 1991; 45:221–223.
64. Treede RD, et al. The plasticity of cutaneous hyperalgesia during sympathetic ganglionic blockade in patients with neurogenic pain. Brain 1992; 115:607–621.
65. Bennett GJ, Xie YK. A peripheral mononeuropathy in rat that produces disorders of pain sensation like those seen in man. Pain 1988; 33:87–107.
66. Woolf CJ. Evidence for a central component of post-injury pain hypersensitivity. Nature 1983; 306:686–688.
67. Sato J, Perl ER. Adrenergic excitation of cutaneous pain receptors induced by peripheral nerve injury. Science 1991; 251:1608–1610.
68. Seltzer Z, Dubner R, Shir Y. A novel behavioral model of neuropathic pain disorders produced in rats by partial sciatic nerve injury. Pain 1990; 43:205–218.
69. Shir Y, Seltzer Z. Effects of sympathectomy in a model of causaliform pain produced by partial sciatic nerve injury. Pain 1991; 45:309–320.
70. Dubner R. Pain and hyperalgesia following tissue injury: new mechanisms and treatments. Pain 1991; 44:213–214.
71. Shir Y, Seltzer Z. A-fibers mediate mechanical hyperesthesia and allodynia and C-fibers mediate thermal hyperalgesia in a new model of causalgiform pain disorders in rats. Neurosc Letters 1990; 115:62–67.
72. Devor M. The pathophysiology of damaged peripheral nerves. In PD Wall, R Melzack, eds. Textbook of Pain, 2nd edition. Edinburgh: Churchill-Livingstone, 1989.
73. Torebjörk HE, Ochoa JL, McCann FV. Paresthesiae: Abnormal impulse generation in sensory nerve fibers in man. Acta Physiol Scand 1979; 105:518–520.
74. Devor M. Nerve pathophysiology and mechanisms of pain in causalgia. J Auton Nerv Syst 1983; 7:371–384.
75. Devor M, Jänig W. Activation of myelinated afferents ending in a neuroma by stimulation of the sympathetic supply in the rat. Neurosci Letters 1981; 24:43–47.
76. Wall PD, Gutnick M. Ongoing activity in peripheral nerves: the physiology and pharmacology of impulses originating from a neuroma. Exp Neurol 1974; 43:580–593.
77. Hu S, Zhu J. Sympathetic facilitation of sustained discharges of polymodal nociceptors. Pain 1989; 38:85–90.
78. Shea UK, Perl ER. Failure of sympathetic stimulation to effect responsiveness of rabbit polymodal nociceptors. J Neurophysiol 1985; 54:513–520.
79. Barasi S, Lynn B. Effects of sympathetic afferent units from the rabbit pinna. Brain Res 1986; 328:21–27.
80. Roberts WJ, Elardo SM. Sympathetic activation of A-delta nociceptors. Somatosens Res 1985; 3:33–44.
81. Beacham WS, Perl ER. Characteristics of a spinal sympathetic reflex. J Physiol 1964; 173:431–448.
82. Blinn G, Heinz G, Jurna I. Effects of substantia nigra stimulation on suralis evoked spinal reflex activity: comparison with the effects of morphine and stimulation in the periaqueductal gray matter. Neuropharmacology 1980; 19:75–85.
83. Devor M, Wall PD, Catalon N. Systemic lidocaine silences ectopic neuroma and DRG discharge without blocking nerve conduction. Pain 1992; 48:261–268.
84. Koltzenburg M, McMahon SB. The enigmatic role of the sympathetic nervous system in chronic pain. Trends Pharmacol Sci 1991; 12:399–402.
85. Cunha FQ, et al. Interleukin-8 as a mediator of sympathetic pain. Br J Pharmacol 19911; 104:765–767.
86. Kajander KC, Bennett GJ. Onset of a painful peripheral neuropathy in rat: a partial and differential and spontaneous discharge in Aβ and Aδ primary afferent neurons. J Neurophysiology 1992; 68:734–744.
87. Kajander KC, Wakisak S, Bennett GJ. Spontaneous discharge originates in the dorsal root ganglion at the onset of a painful peripheral neuropathy in the rat. Neurosci Lett 1992; 138: 225–228.
88. Marchettine P, et al. Lidocaine test in neuralgia. Pain 1992; 48:377–382.
89. Laird JMA, Bennett GJ. Dorsal root potentials and afferent input to the spinal cord in rats with an experimental peripheral neuropathy. Brain Res 1992; 548:181–190.

90. Schwartzman RJ. Reflex sympathetic dystrophy. Current Opinions in Neurology and Neurosurgery 1993; 6:531–536.
91. Roberts WJ. A hypothesis on the physiological basis for causalgia and related pains. Pain 1986; 24:297–341.
92. Laird J, Cervero F. A comparison of the receptive field plasticity of nocireceptive and multireceptive dorsal horn neurones following noxious mechanical stimulation. In F Cervero, GJ Bennett, PM Headley, eds. Processing of Sensory Information in the Superficial Dorsal Horn of the Spinal Cord. New York: Plenum, 1989. Pp. 473–476.
93. Hökfelt T, et al. Peptidergic neurons. Nature (Lond) 1980; 284:515–521.
94. Hökfelt T, et al. Immunohistochemical evidence for separate populations of somatostatin containing and substance P-containing primary afferent neurons in the rat. Neurosc 1976; 1:131–136.
95. Bennett GJ, et al. Neurochemical and anatomical changes in the dorsal horn of rats with an experimental painful peripheral neuropathy. In F Cervero, GJ Bennett, PM Headley, eds. The Superficial Dorsal Horn of the Spinal Cord. New York: Plenum.
96. Wiesenfeld-Hallin Z. Substance P and somatostatin modulate spinal excitability via physiologically different sensory pathways. Brain Res 1986; 372:172–175.
97. Kuraishi Y, et al. Evidence that substance P and somatostatin transmit separate information related to pain in the spinal dorsal horn. Brain Res 1985; 325:294–298.
98. Watkins JC, et al. Recent advances in the pharmacology of excitatory amino acids. In TP Hicks, D Lodge, H McLennan, eds. Excitatory Amino Acid Transmission. New York: Liss, 1987.
99. Watkins JC. Excitatory amino acids and central synaptic transmission. Trends Pharm Sci 1984; 5:373–376.
100. Curtis DR, Johnston GAR. Amino acid transmitters in the mammalian central nervous system. Ergebn Physiol 1974; 69:97–188.
101. Dougherty PM, Willis WD. Long-lasting enhancement of excitability of spinothalamic tract neurons following combined application of excitatory amino acids (EAA) and substance P in anesthetized macaques. J Physiol (Lond) 1990; 222:1415.
102. Bennett GJ. Evidence from animal models on the pathogensis of painful peripheral neuropathy: relevance for pharmacotherapy. In AI Basbaum, JM Beeson, eds. Toward a New Pharmacotherapy. Philadelphia: Wiley, 1991.
103. Davar G, et al. MK-801 blocks the development of thermal hyperalgesia in a rat model of experimental painful neuropathy. Brain Research 1991; 553(2):327–330.
104. Murase K, Randic M. Actions of substance P on rat spinal cord and dorsal horn neurons. J Physiol (Lond) 1984; 346: 203–217.
105. Cook AJ, et al. Dynamic receptive field plasticity in rat spinal cord dorsal horn following C-primary afferent input. Nature 1987; 325:151–153.
106. Hylden JLK, et al. Expansion of receptive fields of spinal I projection neurons in rats with unilateral adjuvant-induced inflammation: the contribution of dorsal horn mechanisms. Pain 1989; 37:229–243.
107. Ruda MA, Bennett GJ, Dubner R. Neurochemistry and neural circuity in the dorsal horn. In PC Emson, MN Roosor, M Tohyama, eds. Peptides and Neurological Disease/Progress in Brain Research. Amsterdam: Elsevier, 1986; 66:219–268.
108. Ruda MA, et al. In situ hybridization histochemistry and immunocytochemistry reveal an increase in spinal dynorphin biosynthesis in a rat model of peripheral inflammation and hyperalgesia. Proceedings of the National Academy of Sciences (USA) 1988; 85:622–626.
109. Shebab SAS, Atkinson ME. Vasoactive intestinal polypeptide (VIP) increases in the spinal cord after peripheral axotomy of the sciatic nerve originates from primary afferent neurons. Brain Res 1986; 372:37–44.
110. Iadarola MJ, et al. Enhancement of dynorphin gene expression in spinal cord following experimental inflammation: stimulus specificity, behavioral parameters and opiod receptor binding. Pain 1988; 35:313–326.
111. Iadarola MJ, et al. Differential activation of spinal cord dynorphin and enkephalin neurons during hyperalgesia: evidence using cDNA hybridization. Brain Res 1988; 455:205–212.
112. Corbett AD, et al. Dynorphin-g and dynorphin-q are ligands for the K-subtype of opiate receptor. Nature (Lond) 1982; 299:79–81.
113. Dubner R, Ruda MA. Activity dependent neuronal plasticity following tissue injury and inflammation. Trends Neurosci 1992; 15:96–102.
114. Sugimoto T, Bennett GJ, Kajander KC. Strychnine enhanced transsynaptic degeneration of dorsal horn neurons in rats with an experimental painful peripheral neuropathy. Neurosci Lett 1989; 98:139–143.
115. Sugimoto T, Bennett GJ, Kajander KC. Transsynaptic degeneration in the superficial dorsal horn after sciatic nerve injury: effects of a chronic constriction injury, transection and strychnine. Pain 1990; 205–213.
116. Roberts WJ, Fogelsong MEI. Spinal recordings indicate that wide-dynamic range neurons mediate sympathetically maintained pain. Pain 1988; 34:289–304.
117. Roberts WJ. Identification of afferents contributing to sympathectically evoked activity in wide-dynamic range neurons. Pain 1988; 34:305–314.
118. Besson JM, Chaouch A. Peripheral and spinal mechanisms of nociception. Physiol Rev 1987; 67:67–153.
119. Price DD, Bennett GJ, Rafii A. Psychophysical observations on patients with neuropathic pain relieved by a sympathetic block. Pain 1988; 36:273–288.
120. Barolat G, Schwartzman RJ, Woo R. Epidural spinal cord stimulation in the management of reflex sympathetic dystrophy. Steriotac and Func Neurosurg 1989; 53:29–39.
121. Dembowsky KP. Factors contributing to the control of sympathetic nervous activity. In AI Basbaum, JM Besson, eds. Towards a New Pharmacotherapy of Pain. Philadelphia: Wiley, 1991.
122. Laskey W, Polosa C. Characteristics of the sympathetic preganglionic neuron and its synaptic input. Prog Neurobiol 1988; 31:47–84.
123. Strack AM, et al. A general pattern of CNS innervation of the sympathetic out flow demonstrated by transneuronal pseudorabies viral infections. Brain Res 1989; 49:156–162.
124. Coote JH. The organization of cardiovascular neurons in the spinal cord. Rev Physiol Biochem Pharmacol 1988; 110:147–285.
125. Siddal PJ, Dampney RAL. Relationship between cardiovascular neurones and descending antinociceptive pathways in the rostral ventrolateral medulla of the cat. Pain 1989; 37:347–355.
126. Skagerberg G, Jorkland B. Topographic principles in the spinal projections of serotonergic and non-serotonergic brainstem neurons in the rat. Neurosci 1985; 15:445–480.
127. Fields HL, Besson JM, eds. Pain Modulation. Prog Brain Res, vol. 77, 1988.
128. Basbaum AI, Clanton CH, Fields HL. Three bulbospinal pathways from the rostral medulla of the cat: an autoradiographic study of pain modulating systems. J Comp Neurol 1978; 1:209–224.

129. Basbaum AI, Fields HL. Endogenous pain control systems. Annu Rev Neurosci 1984; 7:309–338.
130. Karoum FJ, Commissiong J, Wyatt RJ. Effects of morphine on norepinephrine turnover in various functional regions of rat spinal cord. Biochem Pharmacol 1982; 31:3141–3143.
131. Woolf CJ, Thompson SWN. The induction of maintenance of central sensitization is dependent on N-methyl-D-aspartic acid receptor activation; implications for the treatment of post-injury pain hypersensitivity states. Pain 1991; 44: 293–299.
132. Thompson SWN, King AE, Woolf CJ. Activity-dependent changes in rat ventral horn neurons in vitro; summation of prolonged afferent evoked postsynaptic depolarizations produce a d-APN sensitive windup. Eur J Neurosci 1990; 2:638–649.
133. Woolf CJ. Evidence for a central component of post-injury pain hypersensitivity. Nature 1983; 306:686–688.
134. Davies SH, Lodge D. Evidence for involvement of N- methyl-aspartate receptors in "wind-up" of class 2 neurons in the dorsal horn of the rat. Brain Res 1987; 424:402–406.
135. Mao J, et al. Differential roles of NMDA and non-NMDA receptor activation in induction and maintenance of thermal hyperalgesia in rats with painful peripheral mononeuropathy. Brain Res 1992; 598:271–278.
136. Mao J, et al. Intracthecal MK-801 and local nerve anesthesia synergistically reduce nociceptive behaviors in rats with experimental peripheral mononeuropathy. Brain Res 1992; 576:254–262.
137. Kruger L. Morphological features of thin sensory afferent fibers: a new interpretation of nociceptor function. In W Hamann, A Iggo, eds. Progress in Brain Research. New York: Elsevier, 1988.
138. Kennins P. Identification of the unmyelinated sensory nerves which evoke extravasation in response to antidromic stimulation. Neurosci Letts 1981; 25:137–141.
139. Lembeck F, Holzer P. Substance P as neurogenic mediator of antidromic vasodilatation and neurogenic plasma extravasation. Naunyn-Schmiedebergs Arch Pharmacol 1979; 310: 175–183.
140. Chahl A. Effect of putative peptide neurotransmitters and cutaneous vascular permeability in the rat. Naunyn-Schmeidebergs Arch Pharmacol 1979; 309:159–163.
141. Brain SD, Williams TJ. Inflammatory oedema induced by synergism between calcitonin gene-related peptide (CGRP) and mediators of increased vascular permeability. Br J Pharmacol 1985; 86:855–860.
142. Mendell LM. Physiological properties of unmyelinated fiber projections to the spinal cord. Exp Neurol 1966; 16:316–332.
143. Fuller RW, et al. Sensory neuropeptide effects in human skin. Br J Pharma 1987; 92:781–788.
144. Dalsgaard CJ, et al. Localization of substance P immunoreactive nerve fibers in the human digital skin. Experimentia 1983; 39:1018–1020.
145. Hagermark O, Hökfelt T, Pernow B. Flare and itch induced by substance P in human skin. J Invest Dermatol 1978; 71:233–235.
146. Foreman JC, et al. Structure-activity relationships for some substance P related peptides that cause wheal and flare reactions in human skin. J Physiol 1983; 335:449–465.
147. Pernow B. Role of tachykinins in neurogenic inflammation. J Immunol 1985; 135:812–815.
148. Laufer R, et al. Neurokinin B is a preferred agonist for a neuronal substance P receptor and its action is antagonized by enkephalin. Proc Natl Acad Sci USA 1985; 82:7444–7448.
149. Fewtrell CMS, et al. The effects of substance P on histamine and 5-hydroxytrypamine release in rat. J Physiol Lond 1982; 330:393–411.
150. Foreman J, Jordan C. Histamine release and vascular changes induced by neuropeptides. Agents and Actions 1983; 13:2/3:105–116.
151. Brain SD, et al. Calcitonin gene-related peptide is a potent vasodilator. Nature 1985; 313:54.
152. Bernstein JE, et al. Inhibition of axon reflex vasodilatation by topically applied capsaicin. J Invest Derm 1981; 76:394–395.
153. Wharton J, et al. Capsaicin induces a depletion of calcitonin gene-related peptide (CGRP) immunoreactive nerves in the cardiovascular system of the guinea pig. J Autonom Nerv Sys 1986; 16:289.
154. McEwan JR, et al. Vasodilatation by calcitonin gene-related peptide and by substance P: a comparison of their effects on resistance and capacitane vessels of human forearms. Circulation 1958; 77:1072–1080.
155. Chahl LA, Ladd RJ. Local edema and general excitation of cutaneous sensory receptors produced by electrical stimulation of the saphenous nerve in the rat. Pain 1976; 2:25.
156. Szolcanyi J. Capsaicin-sensitive chemoceptive neural system with dual sensory efferent function. In A Chahl, J Szolcanyi, F Lembeck, eds. Neurogenic inflammation and antidromic vasodilatation. Budapest: Akademia Kiado 1984. Pp. 27–55.
157. Levine JD, et al. Reflex neurogenic inflammation. I. Contribution of the peripheral nervous system to spatially remote inflammatory responses that follow injury. J Neurosci 1985; 3:1380.
158. Levine JD, et al. Contribution of sensory afferents and sympathetic efferents to joint injury in experimental arthritis. J Neurosci 1986; 6:3423.
159. Levine JD, Goetzl EJ, Basbaum AI. Contribution of the nervous system to the pathophysiology of rheumatoid arthritis and other polyarthritides. Rheum Dis Clin North Am 1987; 13:369–383.
160. Colpaert FC, Donnerer J, Lembeck F. Effects of capsaicin on inflammation and on substance P content of nervous tissues in rats with adjuvant arthritis. Life Sci 1983; 32:1825–1827.
161. Fitzgerald M. The spread of sensitization of polymodal nociceptors in the rabbit from nearby injury by antidromic stimulation. J Physiol (London) 1979; 297:207.
162. Lembeck F, Gamse R, Juan H. Substance P and sensory nerve endings. In US VonEuler, B Pernow, eds. Substance P. 37th Nobel Symposium, Stockholm 1976. New York: Raven, 1977.
163. Bar-shavi Z, et al. Enhancement of phagocytosis—a newly found activity of substance P residing in its N-terminal tetrapeptide sequence. Biochem Biophys Res Commun 1980; 94:1445–1451.
164. Fitzgerald M. Capsaicin and sensory neurones—a review. Pain 1983; 15:109.
165. Goetzl EJ, Chernov-Rogan T, Furuichi K. Neuromodulation of mast cell and basophil function. In AD BeFus, J Bienenstock, JA Denberg, eds. Mast Cell Differentiation and Heterogeneity. New York: Raven, 1986.
166. Payan DG, McGillis JP, Goetzl EJ. Neuroimmunology. In FJ Dickson, et al., eds. Advances in Immunology. Orlando, FL: Academic, 1986.
167. Stanisz AM, Befus D, Bienenstock J. Differential effects of vasoactive intestinal peptide, substance P, and somatostatin on immunoglobulin synthesis and proliferation by lymphnodes and spleen. J Immunol 1986; 136:152.
168. Payan DG, Brewster EJ, Goetzl EJ. Stereospecific receptor for substance P on cultured human IM-9 lymphoblasts. J Immunol 1984; 133:3260.
169. Nilsson J, VonEuler AM, Dalsgaard CJ. Stimulation of connective tissue cell growth by substance P and substance K. Nature 1985; 315:61.
170. Payan DG. Receptor-mediated mitogenic effects of substance

P on cultured smooth muscle cells. Biochem Biophys Res Commun 1985; 130:104.

171. Lotz M, Vaughan JH, Carson DA. Effects of neuropeptide on production of inflammatory cytokines by human monocytes. Science 1988; 241:1218–1221.
172. Kimball ES, Perisco FJ, Vaughan JH. Substance P, neurokinin A and neurokinin B induce generation of IL-1-like activity in P388 D1 cells. J Immunology 1988; 141:3564–3569.
173. Lotz M, Carson DA, Vaughan JH. Substance P activation of rheumatoid synoviocytes: neural pathway in pathogenesis of arthritis. Science 1987; 235:893–896.
174. Jansco G, Kiraly E, Jansco-Gabor A. Pharmacologically induced selective degeneration of chemosensitive primary sensory neurones. Nature (Lond) 1977; 270:741–743.
175. Nagy JL, et al. Biochemical and anatomical observations in the degeneration of peptide-containing primary afferent neurons after neonatal capsaicin. Neuroscience 1981; 6:1923–1934.
176. Levine J, et al. Intraneuronal substance P contributes to the severity of experimental arthritis. Science 1984; 226:542–549.
177. Lawson SN, Nickels SM. The use of morphometric techniques to analyse the effect of neonatal capsaicin treatment of rat dorsal root ganglia and dorsal roots. Proc Phys Soc February 1980; P19.
178. Nagy JI, et al. Neurotoxic action of capsaicin on spinal substance P neurones. Brain Res 1980; 186:435–444.
179. Levine JD, Moskowitz MA, Basbaum AI. The contribution of neurogenic inflammation in experimental arthritis. J Immunol 1985; 135:843s–847s.
180. Jansco G, Kiraly E, Jansco-Gabor A. Chemosensitive pain fibers and inflammation. Int J Tiss Reac 1980; 2:57–66.
181. Gamse R, et al. Differential effects of capsaicin on the content of somatostatin, substance P and neurotensin in the nervous system of the rat. NS Arch Pharmacol 1981; 317:140–148.
182. Gamse R, Holzer P, Lembeck F. Decrease of substance P in primary afferent neurones and impairment of neurogenic plasma extravastation by capsaicin. Brit J Pharmacol 1980; 68:207–213.
183. Jancso N, Jancso-Baro A, Szolcsany J. Direct evidence for neurogenic inflammation and its prevention by denervation and by pretreatment with capsaicin. Brit J Pharmacol Chemother 1967; 31:138.
184. Lembeck F, Donnerer J. Time course of capsaicin induced functional impairments in comparison with changes in neuronal substance P content. NS Arch Pharmacol 1981; 316:240–243.
185. Jancso G. Intracisternal capsaicin: selective degeneration of chemosensitive primary sensory afferents in the adult rat. Neurosci Lett 1981; 27:41–45.
186. Bartho L, Szolcsany J. Opiate agonists inhibit neurogenic plasma extravasation in the rat. European Journal of Pharmacology 1981; 73:101–104.
187. Yaksh TL, et al. Intrathecal morphine inhibits substance P release from mammalian spinal cord in vivo. Nature (Lond) 1980; 284:155.
188. Barolat G, Schwartzman RJ, Arias L. Chronic intrathecal morphine infusion for intractable pain in reflex sympathetic dystrophy. 11th meeting of the European Society for Sterotactic and Functional Neurosurgery. Budapest June 1–3, 1988.
189. Lembeck F, Donnerer J, Colpaert FC. Neuropeptides. 1981; 1:175–180.
190. Lembeck F, Gamse R. Substance P in the peripheral sensory process. In R Porter, M O'Connor, eds. Substance P in the Nervous System. Ciba Foundation Symposium 91. London: Pitman Books Ltd., 1982.
191. Schott GD. Mechanisms of causalgia and related clinical conditions. Brain 1986; 109:717–738.
192. Schumacker HB. Causalgia III: a general discussion. Surgery 1948; 24:485–504.
193. Schumacker HB, Speigel IJ, Upjohn RH. Causalgia II: the signs and symptoms with particular reference to vasomotor disturbance. Surg Gynecol Obstet 1948; 86:452–460.
194. Blumberg H, Jänig W. Neurophysiological analysis of afferent and efferent (sympathetic) fibers in skin nerves with experimentally produced neuromata. In J Siegfried, Zimmerman, eds. Phantom and Stump Pain. New York: Springer, 1981.
195. Blumberg H, Jänig W. Changes of reflexes in vasoconstrictor neurons supplying the cat hindlimb following chronic nerve lesions: a model for studying mechanisms of reflex sympathetic dystrophy? J Auton Nerv Syst 1983; 7:399.
196. Blumberg H, Jänig W. Reflex patterns in post ganglionic vasoconstrictor neurons following chronic nerve lesions. J Aut Nerv Syst 1985; 14:157.
197. Jänig W. Causalgia and reflex sympathetic dystrophy: in which way is the sympathetic nervous system involved? Trends in Neurosci 1987; 8:471–477.
198. Jänig W. Pathobiology of reflex sympathetic dystrophy: Some general considerations. In M Stanton-Hicks, W Janig, RA Boos, eds. Reflex Sympathetic Dystrophy. Boston: Kluwer, 1990. Pp. 41–54.
199. Bej MD, Schwartzman RJ. Abnormalities of cutaneous blood flow regulation in patients with reflex sympathetic dystrophy as measured by laser Doppler fluxmetry. Arch Neurol 1991; 48:912–915.
200. Low PA, et al. Evaluation of skin vasomotor reflexes by using laser Doppler volocimetry. Mayo Clin Proc 1983; 58:583–592.
201. Bannister R, Mathias R. Testing autonomic reflexes. In R Bannister, ed. Autonomic Failure: a Textbook of Clinical Disorders of the Autonomic Nervous System, 2nd ed. Oxford: Oxford University Press, 1988.
202. Rosen L, et al. Skin microvasculature circulation in the sympathetic dystrophies evaluated by videophotometric capillaroscopy and laser Doppler fluxmetry. Eur J Clin Invest 1988; 18:305–308.
203. Rosen L, et al. Bilateral involvement and the effect of sympathetic blockade on skin microcirculation in the sympathetic dystrophies. Microvasc Res 1989; 37:289–297.
204. Blumberg H, Griesser HJ, Hornyak ME. Mechanisms and role of peripheral blood flow dysregulation in pain sensation and in reflex sympathetic dystrophy. In M Stanton-Hicks, W Janig, RA Boas, eds. Reflex Sympathetic Dystrophy. Boston: Kluwer Academic Publishers, 1990.
205. Tahmoush AJ, Malley J, Jennings JR. Skin conductance, temperature, and blood flow in causalgia. Neurology 1983; 33:1483–1486.
206. Bennett GJ, Ochoa JL. Themographic observations on rats with experimental neuropathic pain. Pain 1991; 45:61–67.
207. Morris JL, et al. Co-localization of neuropeptide Γ, vasoactive intestinal polypeptide and dynorphin in non-noradrenergic axons of the guinea pig uterine artery. Neurosci Lett 1985; 62:31–37.
208. Fried G, et al. Evidence for differential localization of noradrenaline and neuropeptide Γ in neuronal storage vesicles isolated from rat vas deferens. J Neurosci 1985; 5:450–458.
209. Kajander KC, Bennett GJ. Analysis of the activity of primary afferent neurons in a model of neuropathic pain in the rat. Soc Neurosci Abst 1988; 14:912.
210. Kajander KC, Wakisaka S, Bennett GJ. Early ectopic discharges are generated at the dorsal root ganglion in rats with a painful peripheral neuropathy. Soc Neurosci Abst 1989; 15:816.

211. Ochoa J, et al. Antidromic vasodilatation overridden by somatosympathetic reflexes in man. Intraneural stimulation and thermography. Soc Neurosci Abst 1990; 16:1280.
212. Wakisaka S, Kajander KC, Bennett GJ. An abnormality of the cutaneous temperature and its relation to the sympathetic innervation in rats with an experimental peripheral neuropathy. Pain 1990; 5:5417.
213. Wakisaka S, Kajander KC, Bennett, GJ. Abnormal skin temperature and abnormal sympathetic vasomotor innervation in an experimental painful peripheral neuropathy. Pain 1991; 46(3):299–313.
214. Chambers R, Zweifach VW. The topography and function of the mesenteric capillary circulation. Am J Anat 1944; 75:173–205.
215. Clark ER, Clark EL. Observations on living arteriovenous anastomoses as seen in transparent chambers introduced into the rabbit's ear. Am J Anat 1934; 54:229–286.
216. Salerud EG, et al. Rhythmical variations in human skin blood flow. Int J Microcirc Clin Exp 1983; 2:91–102.
217. Ficat RP, Arlet J. Ischemia and necroses of bone (translated from the French by DS Hungerford). Baltimore: Williams & Wilkins, 1980.
218. Morris JL, Gibbons IL. Neuronal colocalization of peptides, catecholamines and catechoamine-synthesizing enzymes in guinea pig paracervical ganglia. J Neurosci 1987; 7:3117–3130.
219. Fried G, Lundberg JM, Theordorsson-Norheim E. Subcellular storage and axonal transport of neuropeptide Γ (NPY) in relation to catecholamines in the cat. Acta Physiol Scan 1985; 125:145–154.
220. Lundberg JM, et al. Corelease of neuropeptide Γ and catecholamines during physical exercise in man. Biochem Biophys Res Commun 1985; 133:30–36.
221. Lundberg JM, et al. Neuropeptide Γ and sympathetic vascular control in man. Rogul Pept 1985; 13:41–52.
222. Wahlestedt C, et al. Neuropeptide Γ potentiates noradrenaline evoked vasoconstriction mode of action. J Pharmacol Exp Ther 1985; 234:735–741.
223. Lundberg JM, Tatemoto K. Pancreatic polypeptide family (APP, BPP, NPY and PYY) in relation to sympathetic vasoconstriction resistant to α-adrenoceptor blockade. Acta Physiol Scan 1982; 1167:393–402.
224. Morris JL, Murphy R. Evidence that neuropeptide Γ released from noradrenergic axons causes prolonged contraction of the guinea-pig uterine artery. J Auton Nerv Syst 1988; 24:241–249.
225. Sann H, et al. Peptidergic afferents might contribute to the regulation of skin blood flow. Agents and Actions 1988; 3:14–15.
226. Schwartzman RJ, Kerrigan J. The movement disorder of reflex sympathetic dystrophy. Neurology 1990; 40:57–61.
227. Jankovic J, VanDerlinder C. Dystonia and tremor induced by peripheral trauma: predisposing factors. J Neurol Neurosurg Psychiatry 1988; 51:1512–1519.
228. Schott GD. The relationship of peripheral trauma and pain to dystonia. J Neurol Neurosurg Psychiatry 1985; 48: 698–701.
229. Schott GD. Induction of involuntary movements by peripheral trauma: an analogy with causalgia. Lancet 1986; 2:712–716.
230. Scherokman B, et al. Peripheral dystonia. Arch Neurol 1986; 48:830–832.
231. Marsden CD, et al. Muscle spasms associated with Sudek's atrophy after injury. Br Med J 1984; 228:173–176.
232. Mitchell SW. Injuries of nerves and their consequences. New York: Dover Publications, 1977. Pp. 363–368.
233. Grassi C, Passatore M. Action of the sympathetic system on skeletal muscle. Ital J Neurol Sci 1988; 9:23–28.
234. Francini F, Peruzzi P, Staderine G. Effects of sympathetic lumbar trunk stimulation on the myotatic reflex activity on the quadriceps muscle in decerebrate cat. Boll Soc Ital Biol Sper 1978; 54:1353–1356.
235. Bowman WC, Goldberg AA, Raper C. A comparison between the effects of a tetanous and the effects of sympatheomimetic amines on fast-and-slow-contracting mammalian muscle. Brit J Pharmacol 1962; 19:464–484.
236. Snider RM, Gerald MC. Studies on the mechanisms of (+)−amphetamine enhancement of neuromuscular transmission: muscle contraction, electrophysiological and biochemical results. J Pharmacol Exp Ther 1982; 221:14–21.
237. Kuba K. Effects of catecholamines on the neuromuscular junction in the rat diaphragm. J Physiolog (Lond) 1970; 211:551–570.
238. Dun NJ, Karczmar AG. Actions of substance P on sympathetic neurons. Neuropharmacology 1979; 215–218.
239. Bowman WC. Effects of adrenergic activators and inhibitors. In L Szekeres, ed. Handbook of Experimental Pharmacology. Adrenergic Activators and Inhibitors. New York: Springer, 1981.
240. Holmberg E, Waldeck B. Analysis of the B-receptor mediated effect of fast contracting skeletal muscle in vitro. Naunyn-Schmiedbergs Arch Pharmacol 1977; 301:109–113.
241. Osada E, et al. Pharmacological studies of mabuterol, a new selective B_2 stimulant. Arzneimittel Forschung 1984; 34:1652–1658.
242. Wislicki Z, Rosenblum I. The effects of propranalol on normal and denervated muscle. Arch Int Pharmacoldyn 1967; 170:117–123.
243. Hedberg A, Mattsson H. Beta adrenoceptor interaction of full and partial agonists in the cat heart and soleus muscle. J Pharmacol and Exp Ther 1981; 219:798–807.
244. Bowman WC, Zaimis E. The effects of adrenaline, noradrenaline and isoprenaline on skeletal muscle contractions in the cat. J Physiol (Lond) 1958; 144:92–107.
245. Bulbring E, Burn JH. Blood flow during muscle contraction and the Orbeli phenomenon in the dog. J Physiol (Lond) 1939; 95:203–225.
246. Hökfelt T, et al. Immunohistochemical evidence for the existence of adrenaline neurons in the rat brain. Brain Res 1974; 66:235–251.
247. Ljungdahl A, et al. Distribution of substance P-like immunoreactivity in the central nervous system of the rat II-light microscopic localization in relation to catecholamine containing neurons. Neurosci 1978; 3:945–976.
248. Barker D, Saito M. Autonomic innervation of receptos and muscle fibers in cat skeletal muscle. Proc Roy Soc Lond B 1981; 212:317–332.
249. Santini M, Ibata Y. The fine structure of unmyelinated axons within muscle spindles. Brain Res 1971; 33:289–302.
250. Grassi C, Filippi GM, Passatore M. Tension development in lumbrical muscles and concomitant increase of activity in alpha and beta afferents during sympathetic stimulation in the cat. Brain Res 1987; 435:15–23.
251. Eldred E, Schnitzlein HN, Buchwald J. Response of muscle spindles to stimulation of the sympathetic trunk. Exp Neurol 1960; 2:13–25.
252. Hallin RG, Wiesenfeld-Hallin Z. Does sympathetic activity modify afferent inflow at the receptor level in man? J Auton Nerve Sys 1983; 7:391–397.
253. Roberts WJ, Elardo SM. Sympathetic activation of unmyelinated mechanoreceptors in cat skin. Brain Res 1985; 339: 123–125.
254. McIntyre AK. Proske U, Tracey DJ. Fusimotor responses

to volleys in joint and interosseous afferents in the cat's hindlimbs. Neurosci Letters 1978; 10:287–292.

255. Stein RB, Lee RG. Tremor and clonus. In VK Brooks, ed. Handbook of Physiology, The Nervous System. Bethesda: American Physiology Society 1982.
256. Peuschl G, Blumberg H, Lucking CH. Tremor in reflex sympathetic dystrophy. Arch Neurol 1991; 48:1247–1252.
257. Logigian EL, et al. Motor unit synchronization in physiologic, enhanced physiologic and voluntary tremor in man. Ann Neurol 1988; 23:242–250.
258. Akagi H, et al. The role of substance P as a neurotransmitter in the reflexes of slow time courses in the neonatal rat spinal cord. Br J Pharmac 1985; 84:666–673.
259. Takahaski T, et al. Identification of the motorneuron depolarizing peptide in bovine dorsal root as hypothalamic substance P. Brain Res 1974; 73:59–69.
260. Hökfelt T, et al. Experimental immunohistochemical studies on the localization and distribution of substance P in cat primary sensory neurons. Brain Res 1975; 100:235–252.
261. Saito K, Onishi S, Otsuka M. Antagonism between lioresal and substance P in rat spinal cord. Brain Res 1975; 97: 117–180.
262. Woolf C, Wiesenfeld-Hallin Z. Substance P and calcitonin gene related peptide synergistically modulate the gain of the nociceptive flexor withdrawal reflex in the rat. Neurosci Letters 1986; 66:226–230.
263. Koizumi K, et al. Contributions of unmyelinated afferent excitation to sympathetic reflexes. Brain Res 1970; 20: 99–106.
264. Jan LY, Jan YN. Peptidergic transmission in sympathetic ganglia of the frog. J Physiol (Lond) 1982; 327:219–246.
265. Urban L, Randic M. Slow excitatory transmission in rat dorsal horn: possible mediation by peptides. Brain Res 1984; 290:336–342.

Congenital Malformations of the Vasculature

Renu Virmani
Allen P. Burke

VASCULAR MALFORMATIONS WITHIN THE HEART

Anomalous Venous Connections

Anomalous venous connections are abnormal connections of a systemic or pulmonary vein to another venous structure or directly to the left or right atrium. The connections arise from failed development of normal embryologic venous communications or persistence, lack of regression of normal embryologic venous communications, or both.

ANOMALOUS PULMONARY VENOUS CONNECTIONS

Anomalous pulmonary venous connection refers to the absence of one or more pulmonary venous connections to the left atrium without reference to the subsequent drainage of the anomalously disconnected pulmonary vein(s). **Total anomalous pulmonary venous connection** (TAPVC) usually refers to the bilateral absence of a connection of both pulmonary veins of each lung to the left atrium. The pulmonary veins connect directly into the right atrium or into one of its tributaries. TAPVC almost always is associated with some type of atrial septal defect (ASD) in order for life to be sustained beyond the newborn period [1–4]. **Partial anomalous pulmonary venous connection** (PAPVC) is the lack of connection of one or more—but not all—pulmonary veins to the right atrium or one of its tributaries. TAPVC is found in about 2 percent of autopsied cases with congenital heart disease and has a male predominance. PAPVCs constitute about 0.6 percent of autopsied cases of congenital heart disease [1–4].

Embryology. In the human embryo, the lung buds and their pulmonary veins connect to the veins of the foregut, the splanchnic plexus. With growth, a new pulmonary venous channel—the primary pulmonary vein—grows as a bulging of the left atrium. At the same time, the intrapulmonary veins lose their connections with the splanchnic plexus and fuse with the primary pulmonary vein. The intrapulmonary veins eventually form the four pulmonary veins and are absorbed into the left atrium. The failure to sever the connection between the intrapulmonary and splanchnic veins results in the anomalous pulmonary venous connections, which may be total, partial, bilateral, or unilateral. The drainage site of pulmonary veins may be supradiaphragmatic or infradiaphragmatic.

When drainage is supradiaphragmatic, both lungs may drain into a confluence, which may then drain into the left innominate vein and the superior vena cava (SVC), or the supradiaphragmatic drainage may be directly into the left SVC or, indirectly, to the SVC via azygos or hemiazygos veins (Fig. 54-1) [2,3].

Total Anomalous Pulmonary Venous Connection. TAPVC is best classified by Darling and colleagues, as follows: type I, anomalous connection at the supracardiac level; type II, anomalous connection at the cardiac level; type III, anomalous connection at the infracardiac level; and type IV, anomalous connection at two or more of those levels [5]. The common forms of TAPVC are illustrated in Fig. 54-2. The frequency from two separate studies is 26 percent to left innominate vein (LIV), 18 percent to coronary sinus, 8 percent to right atrium, 15 percent to right SVC, 24 percent to the portal system, 5 percent to multiple sites, and 4 percent to unknown or other sites [4,6]. In one-third of the patients with TAPVC, there are other major cardiac malformations; in the other two-thirds, TAPVC exists as an isolated anomaly.

The presence of obstructive lesions determines the hemodynamic state, clinical features, and survival in infants with TAPVC. The obstruction may be at the interatrial septum and, when small, results in inadequate flow to the left atrium. The size of the ASD has been shown to relate to longevity in TAPVC; the larger the ASD, the longer the survival. There may be obstruction in the anomalous venous channel, which may result from intrinsic narrowing of the wall of the channel or by extrinsic compression [6]. The individual pulmonary-vein size at diagnosis also is a strong, independent predictor of survival in patients with TAPVC [7].

Associated cardiac anomalies are transposition of the great arteries (TGA), pulmonary atresia (PA), coarctation of the aorta (COA), and anomalies of systemic veins. There is a high frequency of TAPVC in patients with congenital heart disease and asplenia. In 25 to 30 percent of the cases, there also may be major extracardiac malformations, such as malrotation of the intestine, asplenia, polysphenia, endocrine abnormalities, and cystic disease of the kidneys.

PHYSIOLOGY. The right atrium serves as a mixing chamber for the pulmonary venous blood and the systemic circuits. The physiologic features of TAPVC depend on the distribution of the mixed venous blood between the pulmonary and systemic circuits and the state of the interatrial septum. If the ASD is small, the volume of blood reaching the left atrium is small, and the systemic cardiac output is reduced. The right atrial pressure is increased, which is reflected in elevation of pressure in both venous circuits.

In patients with a widely patent foraman ovale or ASD, which allows free communication between the two atria and mixing of the venous blood, the flow of blood depends on the resistance in the pulmonary and systemic arterial

From the Department of Cardiovascular Pathology, Armed Forces Institute of Pathology, Washington, D.C.

The opinions and assertions contained herein are the private views of the authors and are not to be construed as official or reflecting the views of the Department of the Army, Air Force, or the Department of Defense.

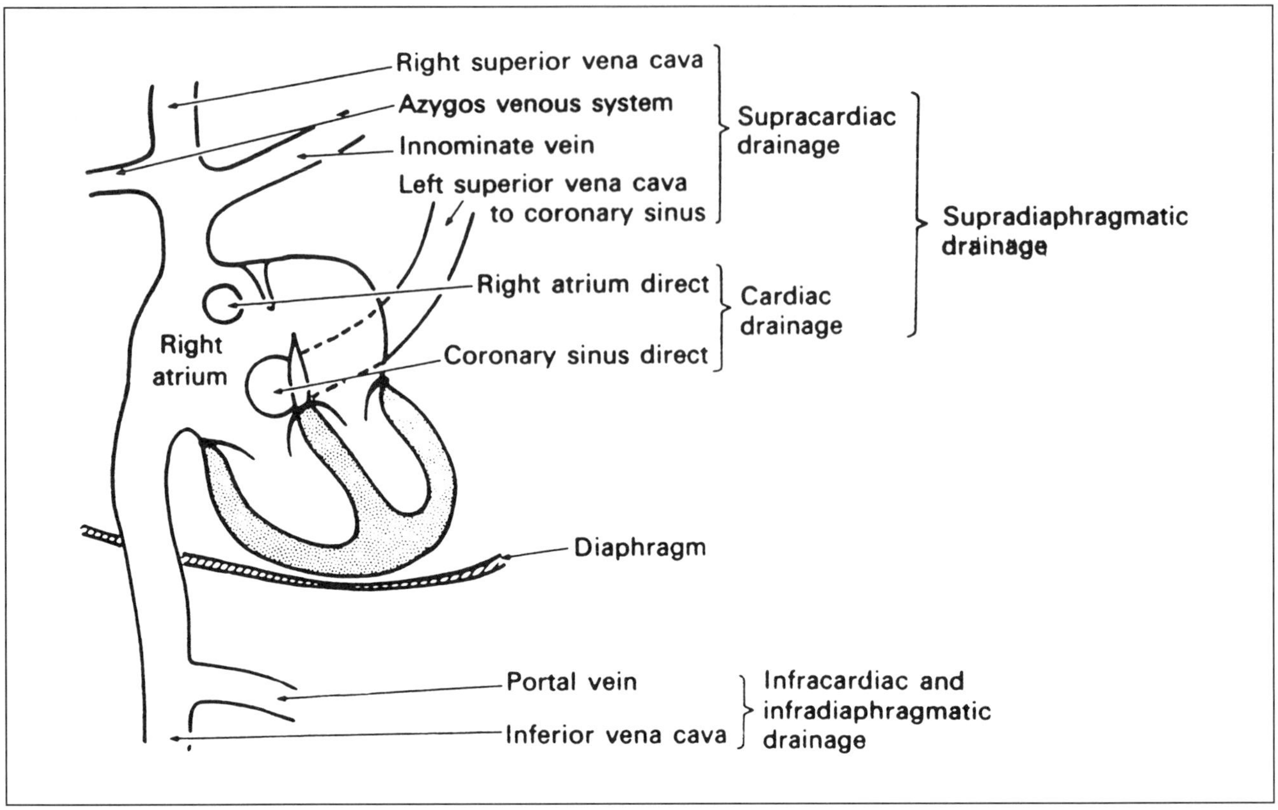

Fig. 54-1. Possible sites of drainage for anomalous pulmonary venous connections into the systemic venous system. (Reproduced with permission from AE Becker, RH Anderson. Pathology of Congenital Heart Disease. London: Butterworths, 1981. Pp. 47–66, 333.)

circuits. In cases without pulmonary venous obstruction, the resistance at birth is equal; therefore, the distribution of blood is equal between the pulmonary and the systemic circuits. However, within a few weeks of birth, the pulmonary resistance decreases, and a larger proportion of the mixed venous blood returns to the pulmonary circuit, resulting in a nearly three to five times greater pulmonary to systemic flow ratio of 3:1 to 5:1 and an equalization of oxygen saturation between the right and the left heart. In the presence of pulmonary venous obstruction, there is elevated pulmonary venous pressure, which results in pulmonary edema, a decrease in pulmonary flow, pulmonary hypertension, right ventricular hypertrophy, and ultimately right heart failure.

The signs and symptoms, therefore, depend on the underlying hemodynamics, that is, presence or absence of pulmonary venous obstruction and the extent of the mixing of blood between the right and left atrium. If interatrial mixing is inadequate, symptoms occur at birth or shortly thereafter. In TAPVC without pulmonary venous obstruction, the patients usually are asymptomatic at birth; however, at least 50 percent become symptomatic within 1 month of life and the remainder within the first year. Of the patients with obstruction, at least 70 percent became symptomatic within 1 month of life but usually not in the first 12 hours of life. Once symptoms appear, however, they are rapidly progressive. Diagnosis may be established by angiography, echocardiography, or T1-weighted spin-echo magnetic resonance [8].

NATURAL HISTORY. Infants with TAPVC have an unfavorable prognosis, with only 20 percent surviving the first year of life. Surgical repair of TAPVC was associated with a high mortality until recently. Overall, early mortality from 14 centers is 18 percent to 20 percent for infants less than 1 month of age. Many factors have been implicated in poor survival in patients with TAPVC, including the type of anatomic connection, year of operation, sex, age at operation, intraatrial communication size, pulmonary venous obstruction, pulmonary hypertension, arterial oxygen saturation, and heart volume [9].

Partial Anomalous Pulmonary Venous Connection. PAPVC is defined when one or more, but not all, pulmonary veins are connected to the right atrium or to a systemic vein. Usually, only one lung or part of a lung is involved. The right pulmonary veins are six times more commonly involved than the left pulmonary veins, and the upper lobes of the lung are more commonly involved than the lower [2].

The left-sided pulmonary veins usually connect to the derivatives of the left cardinal system, that is, the coronary sinus and the LIV. The right pulmonary veins connect to the derivatives of the right cardinal system, that is, the SVC and the inferior vena cava (IVC) or the right atrium.

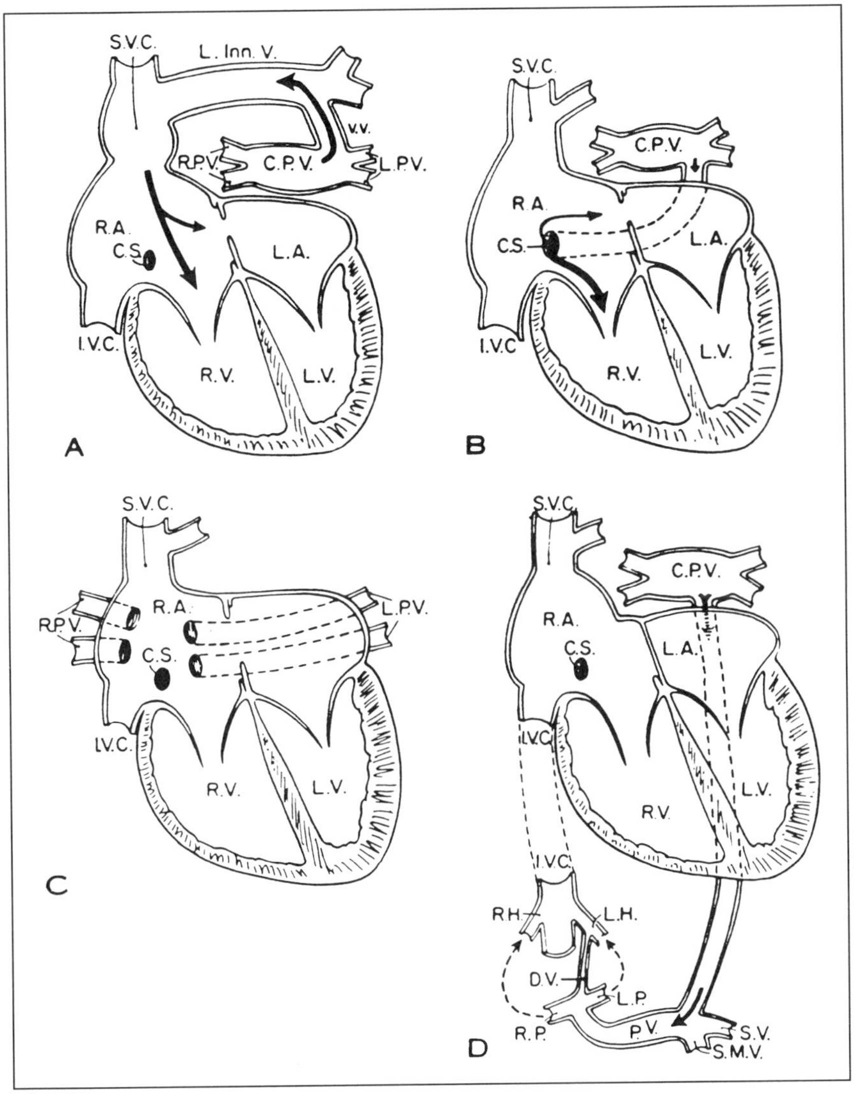

Fig. 54-2. The most common patterns of circulation in total anomalous pulmonary connection (TAPVC). **A.** TAPVC to the left innominate vein by way of a vertical vein. **B.** TAPVC to coronary sinus. **C.** TAPVC to right atrium. The right and left pulmonary veins usually enter the right atrium separately. **D.** TAPVC to the portal vein. Key: C.P.V. = common pulmonary vein, C.S. = coronary sinus, D.V. = ductus venosus, I.V.C. = inferior vena cava, L.A. = left atrium, L.H. = left hepatic vein, L. Inn. V. = left innominate vein, L.P. = left portal vein, L.P.V. = left pulmonary vein, L.V. = left ventricle, P.V. = portal vein, R.A. = right atrium, R.H. = right hepatic vein, R.P. = right portal vein, R.P.V. = right pulmonary vein, R.V. = right ventricle, S.M.V. = superior mesenteric vein, S.V. = splenic veins, S.V.C. = superior vena cava, v.v. = vertical vein. (Reproduced with permission from RV Lucas, RA Krabill. Anomalous venous connections, pulmonary and systemic. In FH Adams, GC Emmanouilides, eds. Moss' Heart Disease in Infants, Children and Adolescents, 4th ed. Baltimore: Williams & Wilkins, 1989. P. 580.)

The most common connections are right pulmonary veins to SVC, right pulmonary veins to the right atrium, veins of the right lung to the IVC, and left pulmonary veins to LIV. The heart usually exhibits mild dilatation and hypertrophy of right atrium and ventricle with dilatation of pulmonary artery. The left-sided chambers are normal. Usually, ASD accompanies PAPVC. Nine percent of cases of ASD have PAPVC [2].

In the case of the right pulmonary vein connecting to the SVC, the right upper and middle lobe veins connect to the SVC. The vein of the right lower lobe usually enters the left atrium but may connect to the right atrium. The lower part of the SVC, below the azygos vein and above the right atrium, is dilated approximately twice the normal size. Most cases have associated ASD of the sinus venosus type, but occasionally a secundum or, rarely, a primum ASD may occur (Fig. 54-3).

When the right pulmonary veins connect to the IVC, all right pulmonary veins or veins draining the right middle and lower lobes enter the IVC, either above or below

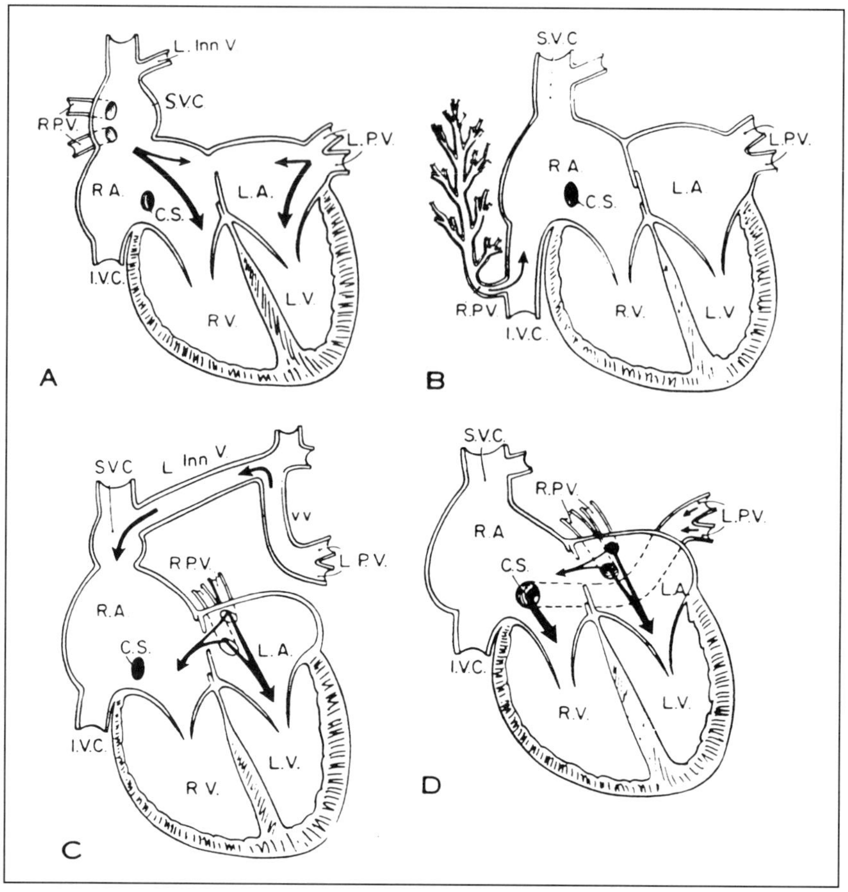

Fig. 54-3. The most common patterns of circulation in partial anomalous pulmonary venous connection (PAPVC). **A.** Anomalous connection of the right pulmonary veins to superior vena cava. **B.** Anomalous connections of the right pulmonary veins to the inferior vena cava in the presence of an intact atrial septum. **C.** Anomalous connection of the left pulmonary veins to the left innominate by way of a vertical vein. **D.** Anomalous connection of the left pulmonary veins to coronary sinus. Key: C.S. = coronary sinus, I.V.C. = inferior vena cava, L.A. = left atrium, L. Inn. V. = left innominate vein, L.P.V. = left pulmonary vein, L.V. = left ventricle, R.A. = right atrium, R.P.V. = right pulmonary vein, R.V. = right ventricle, S.V.C. = superior vena cava, v.v. = vertical vein. (Reproduced with permission from RV Lucas, RA Krabill. Anomalous venous connections, pulmonary and systemic. In FH Adams, GC Emmanouilides, eds. Moss' Heart Disease in Infants, Children and Adolescents, 4th ed. Baltimore: Williams & Wilkins, 1989. P. 580.)

the diaphragm. The pattern of the pulmonary veins is altered, giving a "fir-tree" appearance (Fig. 54-3). The atrial septum is intact, and this malformation is called "Scimitar syndrome," which is associated with right-lung anomalies, dextrocardia of the heart, hypoplasia of the right pulmonary artery, and anomalous connection between aorta and right lung. In the connection of the left pulmonary veins to the LIV, the veins of the left upper lobe or the whole left lung connect to the LIV via the vertical vein. ASD of the secundum type usually is present, and the septum rarely is intact (Fig. 54-3). Other sites of PAPVC are the left pulmonary veins draining into the coronary sinus, IVC, right SVC, right atrium, or left subclavian vein. In rare cases, veins of both lungs drain anomalously, but a small segment of the pulmonary venous system drains normally. That condition has been termed by Edwards as **subtotal anomalous pulmonary venous connection**.

The hemodynamic consequences of PAPVC connection depend on the number of anomalously connected veins, the site of the anomalous connections, the presence or absence of an interatrial communication, the size and location of the interatrial communication, and associated cardiac and extracardiac abnormalities. If there is no interatrial communication, there is no right-to-left shunting and, therefore, no pulmonary hypertension. If there is an ASD, the hemodynamics and clinical course are those of a large ASD [1–4].

In PAPVC, major cardiac anomalies are found in about 20 percent of cases and include tetralogy of Fallot, ventricular septal defect, single ventricle, CA, TGA, and hypoplastic left heart syndrome.

NATURAL HISTORY. PAPVC was found in 0.6 percent of 801 anatomic dissections, but clinical studies indicate a much lower incidence, which may be the result of PAPVC not being recognized. In untreated patients, there is paucity of information regarding the prognosis, but overall, if one pulmonary vein is anomalously connected and there is no ASD, the prognosis is excellent. However, in patients with high pulmonary flow, surgical repair is associated with dramatic reduction in symptoms and a normal longevity. The prognosis may not be so favorable if pulmonary hypertension is present.

ATRESIA OF COMMON PULMONARY VEIN. In this rare anomaly, the pulmonary veins unite into a blind pouch posterior to the left atrium and have no communication with the left atrium or with any other cardiac chamber or systemic veins.

Physiologically, there is severe obstruction to pulmonary venous flow, and the patients usually become cyanotic and die within a few days of birth [6].

STENOSIS OF COMMON PULMONARY VEIN. Cor triatriatum is a relatively rare cardiac anomaly (0.4% of autopsied cases with congenital heart disease, ratio of males to females 1.5 : 1). In this condition, the pulmonary veins enter an accessory chamber lying posterior to the left atrium and joining the left atrium through a narrow opening [6]. The following broad classification has been suggested by a number of authors [6]:

1. Accessory atrial chamber that receives all pulmonary veins and communicates with the left atrium; no other connections (classic cor triatriatum)
2. Accessory atrial chamber that receives part of pulmonary veins and does not communicate with left atrium
3. Subtotal cor triatriatum:
   a. Accessory atrial chamber that receives part of the pulmonary veins and connects to the left atrium
   b. Accessory atrial chamber that receives part of the pulmonary veins and connects to the right atrium

Physiologically, when the blood from the accessory atrial chamber drains into the right atrium, the hemodynamic features are those of TAPVC. A stenotic opening between the accessory atrium and the left atrium, however, results in features of severe pulmonary obstruction. In subtotal cor triatriatum when obstruction affects only one lung, the result is reflex pulmonary arterial obstruction with decreased flow through that portion of the lung. The rest of the unobstructed lung receives increased flow, but there is no elevation in pulmonary arterial pressure [6].

The classic cor triatriatum patients have onset of symptoms in the first few years of life. Some patients, however, are asymptomatic until the second or third decade of life. Patients usually have history of breathlessness and frequent respiratory infections. Right-heart failure usually is present, along with signs of pulmonary hypertension. Diagnosis is established noninvasively by echocardiography. On cardiac catheterization, there is a delay between opacification of the accessory left atrial chamber and the opacification of the true left atrium and ventricle.

Prognosis of cor triatriatum is related to the size of the orifice in the obstructing membrane with survival of 3.3 months if the opening is less than 3 mm and 16 years if the opening is greater than 3 mm. When pulmonary edema and right-heart failure occur, the survival is just a few months. Surgical repair is curative with excellent prognosis.

CONGENITAL STENOSIS OF PULMONARY VEINS. There are two types of stenosis of pulmonary veins: One is localized stenosis of the pulmonary veins at the junction of the left atrium, which may involve one or more pulmonary veins; the other is characterized by narrowing of the lumen of the pulmonary vein, either intra- or extrapulmonary in location, and is called **hypoplasia of the pulmonary veins**. The latter type is occasionally present in patients with pulmonary artery atresia or hypoplastic left-heart syndrome. Clinically, patients have a history of respiratory symptoms, which may progress to right-heart failure. The localized stenosis of pulmonary veins at the junction of the left atrium is best visualized by echocardiography, whereas the distal stenosis of pulmonary veins is seen angiographically, revealing prolongation of transit time of the dye through the lung. Because of poor surgical results, balloon angioplasty and stenting currently are being tried [1–4].

ANOMALOUS SYSTEMIC VENOUS CONNECTIONS

Anomalous systemic venous connections usually are asymptomatic and are of little functional significance because systemic venous flow to the right atrium is not impaired. However, if they are not recognized, systemic venous anomalies may be accidentally severed during cardiac surgery [1–3]. A classification based on embryologic principles includes anomalies of the cardinal venous system, anomalies of the IVC, and anomalies of the valves of the sinus venosus.

Anomalies of the cardinal venous system include persistent left SVC; persistent left SVC connecting to the right or left atrium with and without failure of development of coronary sinus [6]; right SVC connected to the left atrium; and anomalies of the coronary sinus. Anomalies of the IVC include double IVC, left IVC, and many lesser anomalies, which usually are of no clinical significance except that they may present problems to the surgeon [10,11]. Infrahepatic interruption of the IVC with drainage via the enlarged azygous vein to the SVC has been found to occur in 2.9 percent of congenital heart defects [1–3]. Anomalies of the valves of the sinus venosus involve the eustachian and thebesian valves and crista terminalis. Minor abnormal persistence results in larger valves and Chiari's network [6]. Large outgrowth of the valve of the sinus venosus may result in complete or partial subdivision of the right atrium [6].

Embryology. The early embryonic vascular plexus forms three sets of paired venous systems, which return venous blood to the sinus venosus at the atrial end of the embryonic heart. The umbilical veins are the most medial veins in the caudal aspect of the embryo and conduct oxygenated blood from the chorionic villi to the sinus venosus. Just lateral to the umbilical veins are the vitelline veins, which conduct caudal venous blood from the yolk sac to the sinus venosus. The third and most lateral veins are the posterior cardinal veins, which also drain the caudal region of the embryo. The anterior cardinal veins drain the cranial region of the embryo into the sinus venosus.

After the formation of the posterior cardinal vein, the paired subcardinal veins form to drain the developing midline urogenital system. Next is the formation of the intersubcardinal anastomosis between the subcardinal veins. Hepatocardinal channels form venous connections between the hepatic sinusoids and the proximal portions of the vitelline veins. Normally, the left anterior cardinal vein regresses in the sixth fetal month, leading to the formation of the innominate vein and its connection across the midline to the right SVC. The paired precursors of the IVC coalesce into a single IVC, which may persist as paired IVCs. These are not uncommon but are usually incidental and not functionally significant [1–3].

Persistence of the left anterior cardinal vein results in a persistent left SVC, which usually drains via the coronary sinus into the right atrium and rarely directly into the left atrium, or via the coronary sinus into the left atrium. Persistent left SVC is found in about 0.3 percent of all autopsies and up to 5 percent of autopsied congenital heart disease cases, particularly in conditions with cyanosis [1–3].

Coronary-Artery Anomalies

Coronary-artery anomalies are a rare occurrence [12,13]. The incidence in the general population is unknown. In patients undergoing coronary angiography, the incidence varies from 0.9 to 1.55 percent; in the autopsy population, it is much less, 54 among 18,950 (0.29%) cases [14,15].

Many classifications of coronary-artery anomalies have been used. By far the most extensive and descriptive classification was recently published by Roberts [16,17]. The four major groups are as follows:

1. Origin of one or more coronary arteries from the pulmonary trunk and one or more arteries from the aorta
2. Origin of one or more coronary arteries from the pulmonary trunk without origin of a coronary artery from the aorta
3. Anomalous origin of one or more coronary arteries from the aorta
4. Origin of only one coronary artery from the aorta without origin of a coronary artery from the pulmonary trunk (single coronary ostium) [16]

Table 54-1. Classification of coronary-artery anomalies

- I. Origin of one or more coronary arteries (CAs) from the pulmonary trunk (PT)
  - A. Both CAs from PT
  - B. Left main (LM) from PT
  - C. Right (R) from PT
  - D. Left anterior descending (LAD) from PT
  - E. Accessory CA from PT
- II. Anomalous origin of one or more CAs from the aorta
  - A. LM and RCA from the right aortic sinus
    - 1. LAD courses between the Aorta (Ao) and PT
    - 2. LM anterior to PT
    - 3. LM posterior to Ao
    - 4. LM courses posterior to right ventricular outflow tract within the ventricular septum
  - B. LM and RCA from the left aortic sinus
  - C. Anomalous origin of left circumflex (Cx) from the right aortic sinus or from the RCA
    - 1. double ostium from right aortic sinus
    - 2. single ostium from right aortic sinus
  - D. Anomalous origin of CAs from the posterior aortic sinus
    - 1. R from posterior aortic sinus
    - 2. LM from posterior aortic sinus
    - 3. R and LM from posterior aortic sinus
  - E. Right and LAD from the right aortic sinus
    - 1. LAD from RCA
    - 2. LAD from right aortic sinus
- III. Single coronary artery ostium from the aorta
  - A. Single right coronary ostium and LM coursing posterior to the Ao
  - B. Single right coronary ostium and LM coursing between Ao and PT
  - C. Single right coronary ostium and LM coursing anterior to PT
  - D. Single right coronary ostium and Cx continuing as right
  - E. Single left coronary ostium and R coursing between Ao and PT
- IV. Left anterior descending and left Cx coronary arteries from a separate ostium in the left aortic sinus
- V. Congenital hypoplastic coronary arteries
- VI. Coronary artery fistula

Source: Reproduced with permission from R Virmani, K Rogan, MD Cheitlin. Congenital coronary artery anomalies: pathologic aspects. In R Virmani, MB Forman, eds. Non-atherosclerotic Ischemic Heart Disease. New York: Raven, 1989.

The groups have been subdivided, depending on the course of the coronary artery, for example, anterior to the pulmonary trunk, between the aorta and pulmonary trunk, posterior to the right ventricular outflow tract (within the ventricular septum), or posterior to the aorta. We have chosen to simplify the vast maze of possibilities into six main groups, as shown in Tables 54-1 and 54-2 and Figs. 54-4 through 54-8, based on our experience at the Armed Forces Institute of Pathology (AFIP) from a study of 256 autopsy hearts and records of isolated coronary-artery anomalies in the absence of major congenital heart disease [18].

CORONARY ARTERIES ARISING FROM PULMONARY TRUNK

Total anomalous origin of coronary arteries from a pulmonary artery (TCAPA) is extremely rare, with only 25 cases having been reported [19]. Of the 25 cases, we personally have observed this anomaly in 4. However, most of the patients have had other major congenital anomalies of the heart in conjunction with the coronary-artery anomalies. Only 11 cases had minor congenital heart anomalies that would not have caused the demise of the patient [8]. Most became symptomatic before 3 days of age. The majority of the patients were 2 to 7 days old at the time of their death. Five patients survived longer. The reason for that, in the absence of other cardiovascular defect, is uncertain but may be related to a delay in the physiologic decrease in pulmonary vascular resistance.

TCAPA is incompatible with life, and at least two cases have been recognized preoperatively. Surgical correction has been attempted but has failed, probably due to preexisting severe myocardial damage. Increased awareness of the condition may alter the dismal prognosis.

Table 54-2. Distribution of 232 autopsy patients with isolated coronary-artery anomalies and the frequency of cardiac death

Coronary-artery anomalies	Number of patients	Age range (mean)	Sex ratio (F:M)	Number of cardiac deaths
I. Origin of CAs from PT				
A. Both CAs from PT	3	7 hr– 7d	1:2	3/3 (100%)
B. LM from PT	36	3 d–17 yr (0.5)	12:24	36/36 (100%)
C. R from PT	1	34 yr	0:1	1/1 (100%)
D. LAD from PT	1	32 yr	0:1	1/1 (100%)
E. Accessory from PT	2	1 d–50 yr	1:1	0/2 (0%)
II. Anomalous origin of one or more CAs from Ao				
A. LM and R from R sinus	49	2–87 yr (30)	5:44	36/49 (73%)
B. R and LM from L sinus	52	0–82 yr (39)	4:48	15/52 (29%)
C. Cx and R from R sinus	21	20–82 yr (49)	4:17	8/21 (38%)
D. R and/or LM from post sinus	17	1–67 yr (39)	3:14	9/17 (53%)
E. R and LAD from R sinus	1	20 yr	0:1	1/1 (100%)
III. Single CA ostium from Ao	44	1–80 yr (47)	8:36	19/44 (43%)
IV. LAD and Cx ostium from Ao	12	24–80 yr (52)	1:11	6/12 (50%)
V. Hypoplastic CAs	13	1–69 yr (20)	2:11	9/13 (69%)
VI. Coronary-artery fistula	4	1–7 d (2 d)	1:3	4/4 (100%)
Total	256	0–87 yr	42:214	148/256 (58%)

Ao = aorta; CAs = coronary arteries; Cx = left circumflex; d = days; LAD = left anterior descending; LM = left main; PT = pulmonary trunk; R = right.

Origin of Left Main Coronary Arteries from Pulmonary Trunk. The origin of the left coronary artery from the pulmonary trunk occurs more frequently (over 140 reported cases) than both coronary arteries arising from the pulmonary trunk [20]. The incidence of left coronary artery origin from the pulmonary trunk ranges from 1 in 50,000 [24] to 1 in 300,000 [15] and accounts for 0.25 to 0.50 percent of congenital heart disease [21,22]. The majority of patients are seen in the first year of life. The usual presentation consists of paroxysmal attacks of acute distress precipitated by the exertion of nursing, and the episodes are accompanied by pallor and cold sweats. The attacks occur

Fig. 54-4. Diagram illustrating origin of one or more coronary arteries from the pulmonary trunk. Key: Ao = aorta, CA = coronary artery, LAD = left anterior descending, LC = left circumflex, LM = left main, LOM = left obtuse marginal, PT = pulmonary trunk, R = right coronary artery. (Reproduced with permission from R Virmani, K Rogan, MD Cheitlin. Congenital coronary artery anomalies: pathologic aspects. In R Virmani, MB Forman, eds. Non-atherosclerotic Ischemic Heart Disease. New York: Raven, 1989. Pp. 153–183.)

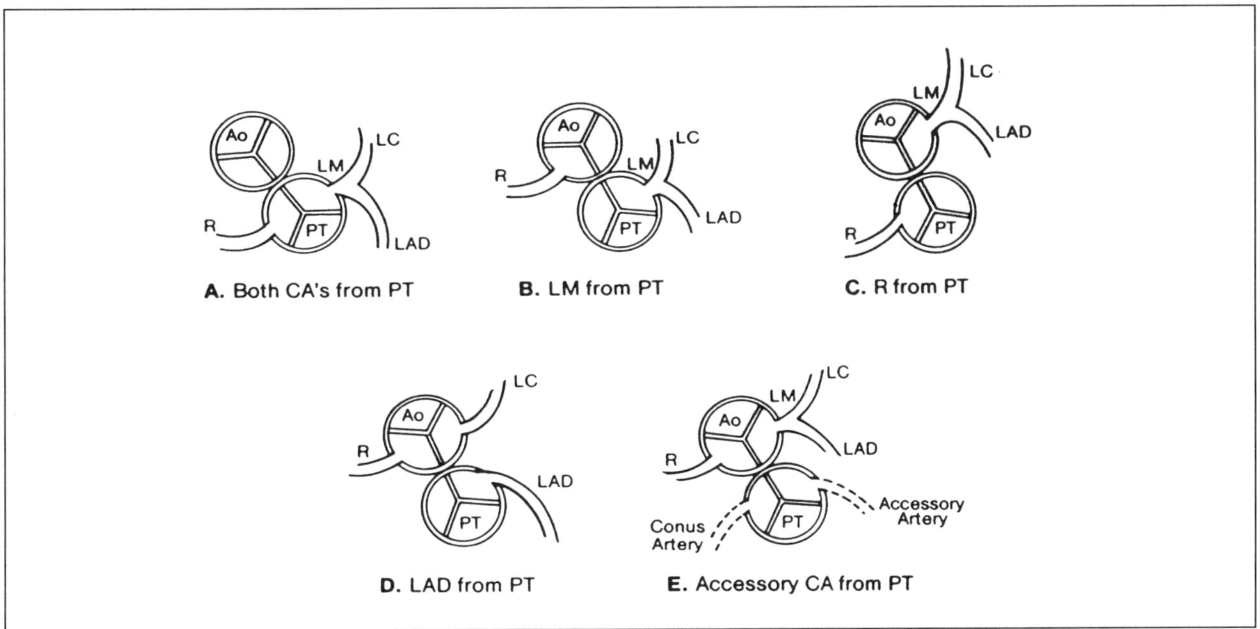

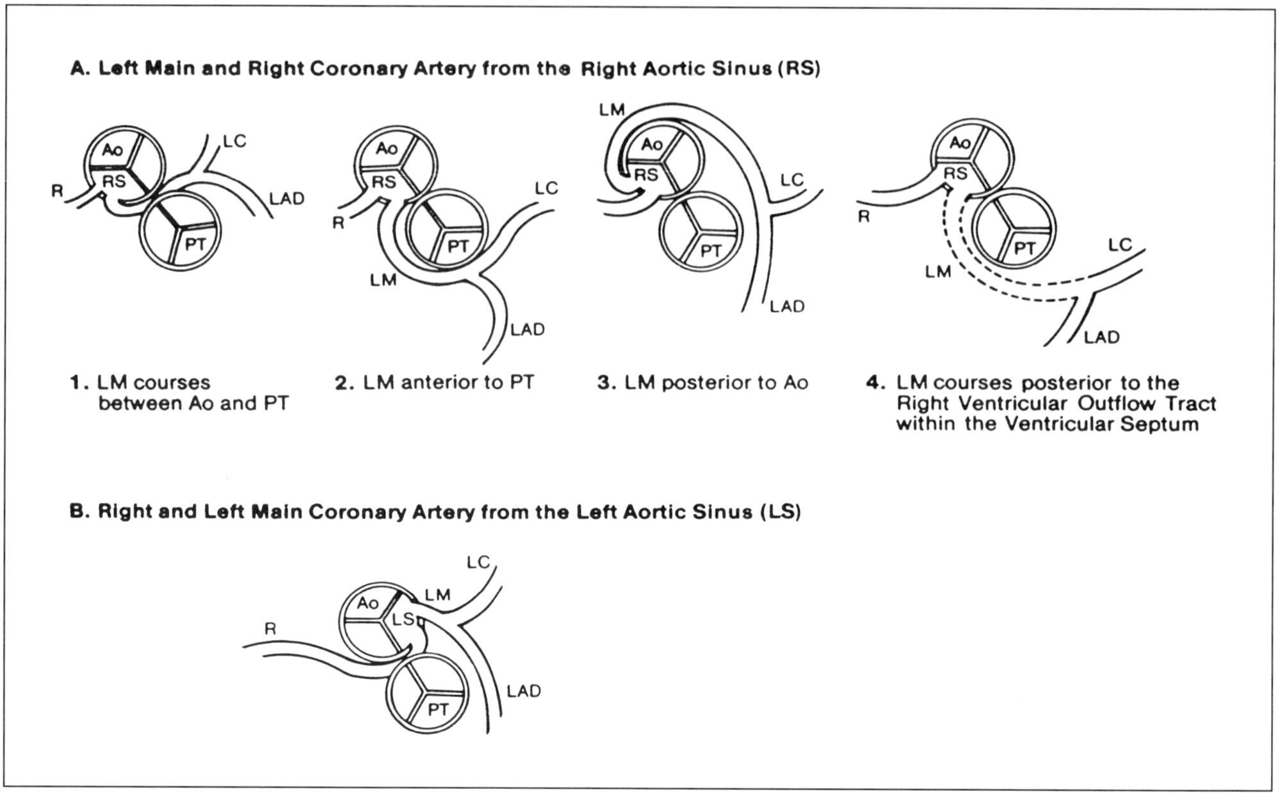

Fig. 54-5. Diagram illustrating anomalous origin of one or more coronary arteries from the aorta, with both coronary arteries arising from the right aortic sinus or from the left aortic sinus. (Reproduced with permission from R Virmani, K Rogan, MD Cheitlin. Congenital coronary artery anomalies: pathologic aspects. In R Virmani, MB Forman, eds. Non-atherosclerotic Ischemic Heart Disease. New York: Raven, 1989. Pp. 153–183.)

with increasing frequency and are followed by chronic dyspnea and heart failure. When heart failure develops, most infants succumb within a few weeks. A few cases have been reported in the teens and adult life and usually have a precordial murmur, often continuous. Electrocardiogram shows ischemic changes, and others present as sudden death. The adult survivors develop collaterals between the right and left coronary arteries. All patients died a cardiac death, and 50 percent died suddenly.

The left coronary artery arises from the pulmonary trunk, usually from the left pulmonary sinus (95%). The wall of the artery is thinner than normal and appears veinlike. The right coronary artery usually is normal in location, and there may be many collateral vessels present over the surface of the heart, thus connecting the right and left coronary arteries.

The heart is enlarged for the age of the patient, and there usually is extensive scarring and thinning of the anterolateral wall of the left ventricle, including the papillary muscle. The posterobasal portion of the left ventricle is hypertrophied as a compensatory mechanism. The endocardium in children is invariably thickened, showing marked fibroelastosis. The operative treatment used should be ligation of the left main coronary artery near its attachment to the pulmonary trunk and insertion of saphenous vein graft to proximal left anterior descending. However, Vouhie et al. report an 84-percent late surgical success with direct aortic reimplantation of the anomalous artery [23]. The severity of preoperative left ventricular function was the only predictor of mortality: 31-percent mortality rate in patients with left ventricular shortening fraction (LVSF) of less than 0.20 versus 0 percent among patients with LVSF of 0.20 or greater [23].

Right Coronary Artery from Pulmonary Trunk. This anomaly is far less common than the left coronary artery arising from the pulmonary trunk. It has been found in 0.003 percent of patients undergoing coronary arteriography [24]. In 1979, Lerberg et al. reported 14 patients with origin of right coronary from the pulmonary trunk, while 140 patients had origin of left main coronary from the pulmonary trunk [25]. The right coronary artery usually is thin-walled and larger, whereas the left is dilated and tortuous and may show varying degrees of atherosclerosis, depending on the presence of risk factors. The heart is not hypertrophied, and there is no fibrosis and necrosis. Although the majority of patients reported are free of cardiac symptoms, angina pectoris has been reported on rare occasions with this anomaly. Surgical correction consists of transection of the right coronary from the pulmonary trunk and direct anastomosis to the aorta [26].

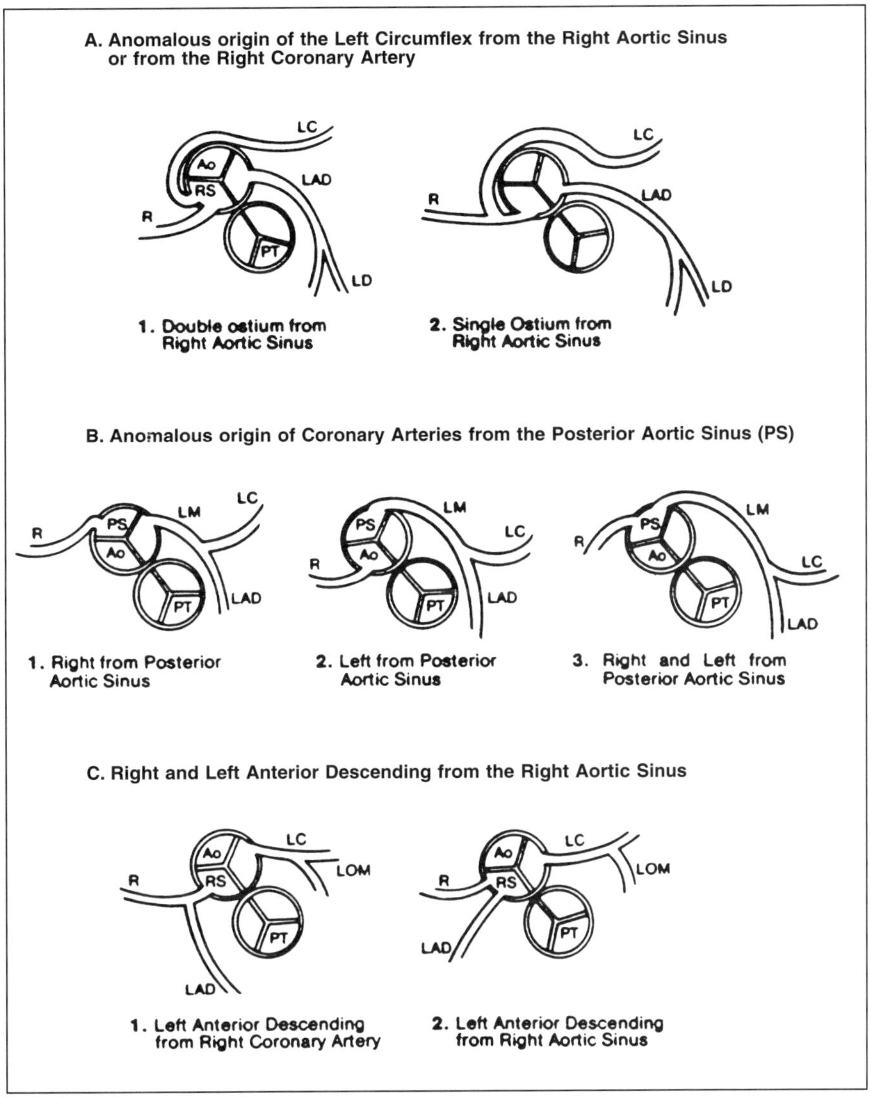

Fig. 54-6. Diagram illustrating: **A.** origin of the left circumflex from the right aortic sinus or from the right coronary artery; **B.** anomalous origin of coronary arteries from the posterior aortic sinus; and **C.** right and left anterior descending from the right aortic sinus or the left anterior descending from the right coronary sinus (E). (Reproduced with permission from R Virmani, K Rogan, MD Cheitlin. Congenital coronary artery anomalies: pathologic aspects. In R Virmani, MB Forman, eds. Non-atherosclerotic Ischemic Heart Disease. New York: Raven, 1989. Pp. 153–183.)

Left Anterior Descending Coronary Artery from Pulmonary Trunk. The anomalous origin of the left anterior descending (LAD) coronary artery from the pulmonary artery, with the right coronary and the left circumflex arising from the aorta, is extremely rare. Most have symptomatic heart disease.

A total of 15 patients have been reported. Ten presented with angina, myocardial infarction, congestive heart failure, or all three [27]; the other 5 were free of symptoms but had a heart murmur. In only two cases was treadmill exercise performed: In one case, the results were normal; the other case showed a horizontal ST-T depression. The right and left circumflex arteries are dilated, thin walled, and tortuous, and the LAD is filled by extensive collaterals. Three different types of revascularization procedures have been performed: (1) simple ligation of the LAD, (2) reimplantation of the LAD to aorta, and (3) combined ligation of the LAD and coronary-artery bypass with vein graft or internal mammary-artery graft [27].

The left circumflex coronary artery may arise from the pulmonary trunk and the right and LAD coronary artery from the aorta. Although this anomaly has been reported by others [28], we have not observed it in our series.

Accessory Coronary Artery from Pulmonary Trunk. Origin of a small coronary artery from the pulmonary trunk with the right and left main coronary arteries arising from the aorta is of no functional significance.

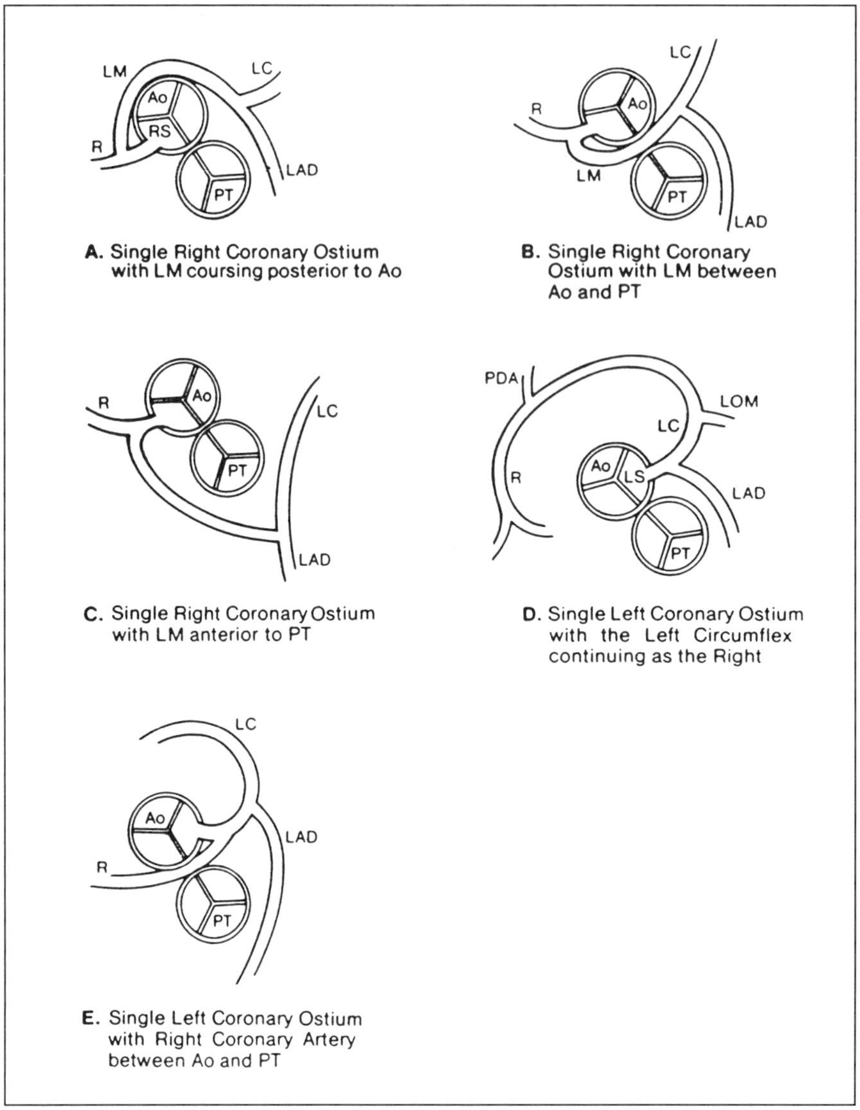

Fig. 54-7. Diagram illustrating single coronary artery ostium from the aorta and the most common course taken by the main coronary artery branch. (Reproduced with permission from R Virmani, K Rogan, MD Cheitlin. Congenital coronary artery anomalies: pathologic aspects. In R Virmani, MB Forman, eds. Non-atherosclerotic Ischemic Heart Disease. New York: Raven, 1989. Pp. 153–183.)

ORIGIN OF CORONARY ARTERIES FROM AORTA

Left Main and Right Coronary Artery from Right Aortic Sinus. This anomaly is further classified according to the course of the left main coronary artery after its origin from the right aortic sinus:

1. Left main between aorta and pulmonary trunk
2. Left main anterior to the pulmonary trunk
3. Left main posterior to the aorta
4. Left main posterior to the right ventricular outflow tract and within the ventricular septum (see Tables 54-1 and 54-2, Fig. 54-5).

Review of the recent literature revealed a total of 48 patients with this anomaly [15,16]. The ages ranged from 1 to 87 years, and the majority were men (male-to-female ratio 43 : 5). Sudden death occurred in 22 (46%); of those 22, death occurred during or soon after exercise in 19 (86%). The majority of the patients (19 of 22) who died suddenly were less than 20 years of age. At autopsy, only 5 of the 22 had evidence of myocardial necrosis or fibrosis. We have recently published on the occurrence of sudden death in patients with isolated congenital coronary artery anomalies [29]. Of 49 patients (2 to 87 years, mean age 30; 5 females and 44 males) with left main coronary artery arising from the right coronary sinus or as a first branch of right coronary artery, 28 (57%) died suddenly; of those, 18 (64%) died during or soon after exercise. Sudden death was particularly common when the left coronary artery coursed between the aorta and the pulmonary trunk. Twenty-three (82%) of the 28 patients with this anomaly died suddenly.

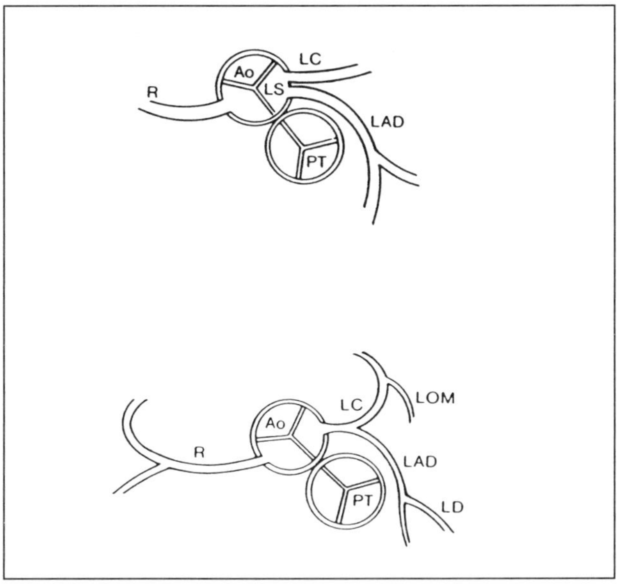

Fig. 54-8. Diagram illustrating the origin of the left anterior descending and left circumflex coronary arteries from a separate ostium in the left aortic sinus (**top**) and congenital hypoplastic coronary arteries (**bottom**). (Reproduced with permission from R Virmani, K Rogan, MD Cheitlin. Congenital coronary artery anomalies: pathologic aspects. In R Virmani, MB Forman, eds. Non-atherosclerotic Ischemic Heart Disease. New York: Raven, 1989. Pp. 153–183.)

The mechanism by which this coronary anomaly causes deaths is unknown. It has been postulated that compression of the left coronary artery occurs between the aorta and the pulmonary artery. We believe that when the coronary artery travels within the aortic wall, it is much more likely to be subjected to compression than when it is free of the aortic wall immediately after take-off. As the aortic wall lengthens during diastole, it compresses the coronary artery, especially during exercise, as the demand on the myocardium is increased. It is unclear, however, why some patients survive into adulthood without any symptoms from the anomaly. It is possible that the degree to which the coronary artery travels within the aorta is variable. Therefore, if the coronary artery is minimally attached to the aortic wall, it does not result in sudden compression and death.

Right and Left Main Coronary Arteries from Left Aortic Sinus. Until recently, this anomaly was considered to be a minor congenital anomaly with no clinical cardiac consequences (see Fig. 54-5). Roberts and associates [30] described 10 patients (aged 17–51 years, mean age 34 years; 8 males, 2 females) with both arteries arising from the left aortic sinus and the right coronary artery passing between the aorta and the pulmonary trunk. In three patients, all of whom died suddenly, the only significant abnormality to account for the patients' demise was the presence of this anomaly. A total of 40 patients have been reported at necropsy; over one-half were males. Only five died suddenly; of those five, three deaths were associated with exercise. In our files at the AFIP, anomalous origin of the right coronary artery from the left coronary sinus was the second most frequently observed anomaly, with sudden death occurring in 13 (25%) of 52 cases [29]. The mechanism by which this anomaly causes dysfunction is unclear. Again, it is most likely that, similar to the left coronary artery origin from the right aortic sinus, there is acute angulation of the right coronary artery at its origin. When it traverses the aortic wall, compression of the coronary artery may occur during diastole, or the vessel may be compressed between the aorta and the pulmonary trunk.

Anomalous Origin of Left Circumflex Coronary Artery from Right Aortic Sinus or from Right Coronary Artery. White and Edwards, in 1948, reported origin of the left circumflex coronary artery from the right aortic sinus or right coronary artery in 4 of 600 hearts examined from men 30 to 89 years of age [31]. Alexander and Griffith described 5 cases with this anomaly among 18,950 autopsies during a 10-year period; all 5 died from nontraumatic causes [24]. By angiography, Page and associates recognized this anomaly in 20 of 2,996 patients, an incidence of 0.67 percent [32]. In our files at the AFIP, we have seen this anomaly in 21 cases; of those, 2 died suddenly. In one case, the death was believed to be due to severe atherosclerosis; in the other, death was attributed to dilated cardiomyopathy with congestive heart failure.

The only clinical significance of this anomaly is that if the patient undergoes cardiac surgery, perfusion of the left circumflex artery may be missed during coronary bypass. Roberts reported compression of the left circumflex artery between the prosthetic valve rings in the mitral and tricuspid positions, resulting in focal acute myocardial necrosis in the ventricular septum [16].

Right or Left Main Artery from Posterior Aortic Sinus. These anomalies are extremely rare (see Fig. 54-6). We have observed the origin of the right or left coronary artery (or both) from the posterior sinus in 17 cases, 5 with both the right and the left main from the posterior aortic sinus. Only one patient, a 29-year-old man, died a sudden cardiac death during exercise. Voldaver and colleagues have reported this anomaly in two patients: a 70-year-old man who died with terminal carcinoma of the prostate and a 72-year-old man who died from atherosclerotic coronary heart disease [33,34]. Roberts described this anomaly in a 19-year-old boy who died suddenly while playing basketball and attributed the cause of death to the anomaly [16,17].

Anomalous Origin of Right and Left Anterior Descending Artery from the Right Aortic Sinus. This anomaly is also a rare occurrence (see Fig. 54-6). We have seen it in only one patient, a 20-year-old man who died suddenly at rest. At autopsy, he had a bicuspid aortic valve that appeared incompetent. Russo et al. described a 51-year-old woman with exertional angina pectoris with this anomaly with the LAD coursing in front of the pulmonary artery and was free of any disease. The cause of ischemia could not be identified [35]. This anomaly usually occurs in the presence of other congenital anomalies, especially in tetralogy of Fallot and TGA.

SINGLE CORONARY OSTIUM FROM AORTA

The incidence of single coronary artery, as described by Sharbaugh and White is 0.04 percent, but that includes cases with and without congenital heart disease [36]. Hillestad and Eie report an incidence of 0.3 percent (3 in 1,056 cases) [37], whereas Lipton and co-workers found single coronary artery in 10 of 4,382 (0.4%) coronary arteriograms [38]. Recently, Desmet et al. reported a frequency of 0.066% of a single coronary artery among 50,000 consecutive coronary angiograms performed in adults from March 1973 to August 1991 [39]. Lipton et al. proposed a classification for single coronary artery. In group I, the single coronary artery follows the course of either a normal right or left coronary artery (see Fig. 54-7) arising from either right or left sinus, respectively. In group II, the single artery arises from the right or left sinus and then gives rise to the normal contralateral artery near its origin. Lipton and co-workers subclassified group II into anterior to the right ventricle or the pulmonary trunk (A), traversing between the aorta and the pulmonary trunk (B), or coursing posterior to the aorta (P). The group was further divided into right (R) and left (L) if the single artery arose from the right or left coronary sinus. Group III has a single coronary artery arising from the right coronary sinus and then giving rise to two separate branches, first the left circumflex and then the LAD and the left circumflex continuing as the right. Bicuspid aortic valve and cardiomyopathy have been associated with a single coronary artery [38,40,41].

We have chosen to classify single coronary artery into five types: (1) single coronary artery from the right coronary sinus with left main coursing posterior to the aorta; (2) single coronary artery from the right sinus with the left main coursing between the aorta and the pulmonary trunk; (3) single coronary artery from the right sinus with the left main coursing anterior to the pulmonary trunk; (4) single coronary artery from the left sinus with the left circumflex continuing as the right, and (5) single coronary artery from the left sinus and the right arising as the first branch and coursing between the aorta and the pulmonary trunk (see Fig. 54-7). However, a single coronary artery may arise from the posterior aortic sinus also. We studied 22 patients (1–72 years old, mean age 48; 19 males, 3 females) in whom single coronary artery arose from the right sinus. Eight of the 22 died a cardiac death, and of those, 5 died suddenly. In 2 patients (13 and 19 years old) with sudden death, death occurred during or soon after exercise. The left main coronary artery traversed between the aorta and the pulmonary trunk. Roberts described five adult patients with single coronary ostium; none of the patients was symptomatic from the coronary anomalies [16,17]. However, when the coronary artery courses between the aorta and the pulmonary trunk, there is a potential for symptomatic heart disease due to compression of the coronary artery or to acute angulation and valvelike ridge.

ORIGIN OF LEFT CIRCUMFLEX AND LEFT ANTERIOR DESCENDING CORONARY ARTERIES AS SEPARATE OSTIUM IN THE LEFT AORTIC SINUS

This is the most common artery anomaly and is reported to occur in 0.2 to 1 percent of autopsy cases [42,43] (see Fig. 54-8). We have observed this anomaly in 12 patients aged 24 to 80 years (mean age 52 years; 11 males and 1 female). Six of the patients died from severe atherosclerotic heart disease; the rest died of noncardiac causes, and the anomaly was an incidental finding. The total number of cases in our collection is small because most pathologists regard this anomaly as a normal variant; therefore, it is underreported in our series. However, this anomaly is of great significance at the time of cardiopulmonary bypass, since perfusion of only one ostium would result in inadequate oxygenation of the myocardium.

HYPOPLASTIC CORONARY ARTERIES

This anomaly is rarely reported in the literature, probably because of the difficulty in defining a hypoplastic coronary artery. Hypoplasia of the coronary artery may involve the left circumflex or the right coronary artery (see Fig. 54-8). An area of the myocardium is relatively ischemic, that is, there is a disproportion between the demand and the supply. We have observed this anomaly in 13 patients (1–69 years old, mean age 29; 11 males, 2 females). Four patients (aged 16, 18, 27, and 35 years) died suddenly; death occurred during exercise in three (16, 18, and 27 years) and in one at rest. Another four patients died a cardiac death; three had severe coronary atherosclerotic heart disease, and one patient had severe aortic-valve stenosis. Hypoplastic coronary artery as a cause of death has been reported by Maron and co-workers in a young, highly trained 17-year-old female athlete who ran 30 miles per week and collapsed after a 3-mile race [44]. Hypoplastic coronary arteries have been well described and illustrated by McClellan and Jokl in a 16-year-old boy who died suddenly while playing basketball [45].

HIGH TAKE-OFF CORONARY ARTERY

High take-off of coronary artery is said to occur when the coronary arteries arise above the sinotubular junction. We have chosen not to include this entity in our classification because of the frequency of its occurrence. We consider a high take-off to be a variant of normal and not an anomaly.

Coronary-Artery Fistulas

Coronary-artery fistula consists of a direct communication between one or more of the coronary arteries and a cardiac chamber or vein. This anomaly is one of the most common major congenital malformations that permit adult survival [46]. A coronary arteriovenous fistula may be an incidental finding in 0.13 to 0.66 percent of adults undergoing coronary angiography for the evaluation of coronary disease, chest pain syndromes, and rheumatic heart disease [46–49]. Most patients are less than 20 years of age and at least 50 percent of patients are asymptomatic and the rest develop congestive heart failure, infective endocarditis, myocardial ischemia, or rupture of an aneurysmal fistula [48,49]. Patients become symptomatic when there is a large left-to-right shunt with a decreased coronary blood flow. Asymptomatic patients are often referred because of a cardiac murmur that is loud, continuous, and with maximum intensity at the site of drainage of the fistula. Drainage occurs in the right ventricle in 41 percent, the right atrium in 26 percent, the pulmonary artery in 17 percent, the left ventricle in 3 percent, and the SVC in 1 percent [46–49]. The fistula involved the right coronary artery or its branches in 55 percent of cases, the left coronary artery in 35 percent, and both arteries in 5 percent [48,49]. The fistulous coronary artery is dilated and tortuous and may even have focal aneurysmal dilatations and calcification. Rarely the coronary-artery fistula may be normal. Contrast echocardiography is considered superior to angiography for the demonstration of right-ventricle drainage. Doppler echocardiography, especially in large shunts, shows turbulent flow distal to the point of drainage [50–52].

In the past, surgical treatment was recommended; however, the reported mortality is 2.2 to 4 percent [50]. Today, transcatheter embolization is the preferred treatment using detachable balloon, platinum microcoils, or a combination of the two [50].

Coronary-Artery Aneurysms

Coronary aneurysms are rare, saccular or fusiform dilatations of one or more coronary arteries. By definition, the minimum diameter of an aneurysm is at least one and one-half times that of the proximal normal segment of the artery from which the aneurysm arises [53]. A congenital coronary-artery aneurysm without fistula develops from a congenital weakness in the arterial media that may not become aneurysmally dilated until later in life, perhaps in adulthood [47]. Too few cases of congenital coronary-artery aneurysms have been studied in detail to determine whether they occur familially or sporadically. Most congenital coronary-artery aneurysms involve the right artery and are usually single, whereas acquired aneurysms in adults affect the left coronary artery and usually are secondary to atherosclerosis, may be single or multiple, and are often associated with peripheral atherosclerosis [47,54].

The cause of the medial weakening is unknown. Aneurysm without a fistula should be diagnosed as congenital in origin only after elimination of other possibilities, such as atherosclerosis, inflammation (Kawasaki's disease, bacterial endocarditis, polyarteritis nodosa, and syphilis), or trauma. Because of the rarity of the entity, there is a paucity of data on the histologic features of congenital isolated coronary-artery aneurysms. At the time of surgery or autopsy, the wall of the aneurysm usually shows dense fibrosis and an absence of the orderly arrangement of smooth muscle cells and elastic fibers seen in a normal arterial wall. The fibrosis is prominent, with giant congenital coronary-artery aneurysms that may exceed 15 cm in diameter [47,53]. Larger aneurysms often have luminal thrombus, with varying degrees of organization and secondary mural calcification and mild atherosclerosis in the absence of atherosclerosis in any other arteries [47,53–60]. Lie and Berg have reported spontaneous coronary-artery dissection and aneurysm formation in a 24-year-old man with isolated fibromuscular dysplasia of the artery [61]. These data may encourage more interest in histologic evaluation of the aneurysm wall for the presence of fibromuscular dysplasia or other abnormalities in the arrangement of the different components. Clues to the etiology of congenital coronary-artery aneurysm may come from the study of analogous congenital aneurysms in other arteries. In the cerebral circulation, congenital arterial aneurysms often arise from defects in the media at branch point, causing inherent weakness and progressive aneurysm formation [62].

In Ehlers-Danlos syndrome, a hereditary disease involving abnormal connective tissue with decreased tensile strength, coronary-artery aneurysms have been found in association with multiple peripheral- and visceral-artery aneurysms. Routine microscopic examination usually reveals no histologic abnormalities [63]. Patients with atherosclerotic abdominal aortic aneurysms frequently do not have concomitant occlusive disease of the peripheral arteries. The patients seem to have an independent tendency to form aneurysms not related to serum concentrations of triglyceride, cholesterol, high density lipoprotein (HDL) cholesterol, and very low density lipoprotein (VLDL) and low density lipoprotein (LDL) cholesterol [64]. Deficiencies in the copper metalloenzyme lysyl oxidase have been detected in the skin from patients with abdominal aortic aneurysms. This enzyme is necessary for lysyl-derived cross-linkages in collagen and elastin; its absence results in weakness in arterial-wall structure not apparent in routine microscopic examination [65]. Familial studies have shown increased prevalence of abdominal aortic aneurysms in families of patients with those aneurysms [66]. Intracranial aneurysms also tend to be familial. Large thrombosed congenital coronary aneurysms have been treated successfully with aortocoronary bypass grafts [55,57,58,67,68].

MALFORMATIONS AFFECTING THE GREAT VESSELS

Coarctation of the Aorta

Coarctation of the aorta (COA) occurs as a congenital narrowing of the aortic arch, either as a discrete narrowing or one of some length that is usually located adjacent to the junction of the ductus arteriosus [69]. The obstruction may be in the form of uniform tubular narrowing of some part of the aortic arch system, usually the isthmus (which lies between the left subclavian artery and the ductus arteriosus) or as a shelflike coarctation within the arch (Table 54-3). The latter is the more common of the two lesions. The narrowing may vary in severity but becomes significant only when there is a pressure gradient across the area of narrowing. That usually occurs when there is greater than 50-percent cross-sectional area reduction, but there may be lesser narrowing for tubular coarctation.

More than 200 years ago, Morgagni described the anatomy of coarctation, and Wernicke, in 1875, outlined the physical findings [70–74]. The classification of coarctation into adult (postductal) and infantile (preductal) types by Bonnett [75] is now generally accepted as being inadequate. The first extensive review of 200 autopsy cases (mean age 30 years) was published by Abbot in 1928 [76]. All patients were older than 3 years; the oldest was a 92-year-old man and is probably the longest recorded survival. Bicuspid aortic valve was present in 24 percent of patients with coarctation and bacterial endocarditis in 10 percent. Reifenstein and co-workers described another 104 autopsy cases; all were older than 3 years [77]. Bicus-

Table 54-3. Classification of coarctation of aorta

I. Discrete coarctation of aorta
  A. Coarctation distal to ductus arteriosus
    1. with closed ductus
    2. with patent ductus
  B. Coarctation proximal to ductus arteriosus
    1. with closed ductus
    2. with patent ductus
  C. Coarctation with anomalies of subclavian arteries or aortic arches
    1. atresia or stenosis of left subclavian artery
    2. stenosis of right subclavian artery
    3. anomalous origin of right subclavian artery
      a. distal to coarctation
      b. proximal to coarctation
    4. double aortic arch with stenosis of right and coarctation of the left
  D. Coarctation of unusual locations
    1. proximal to left subclavian artery
      a. with normal branches
      b. with anomalous origin of right subclavian artery
    2. at multiple sites
    3. of lower thoracic
II. Tubular hypoplasia (isolated or coexistent with discrete COA)
  A. Involving aorta beyond the origin of innominate to the origin of ductus arteriosus
  B. Involving only part of the segment of the aorta

Source: Modified from JE Edwards. Congenital malformations of the heart and great vessel. H. Malformations of the thoracic aorta. In SE Gould, ed. Pathology of the Heart and Blood Vessels, 3rd ed. Springfield, Ill.: Thomas, 1968. Pp. 391–454.

pid aortic valve was seen twice as frequently [43%], and the incidence of bacterial endocarditis was higher. In the early series, it was believed that when COA occurred as an isolated malformation it rarely caused death. That concept has changed only since 1950, when several authors reported that isolated COA could cause death in infancy [78,79].

INCIDENCE

Isolated COA is the fifth or sixth most common anomaly of all the congenital heart diseases [73]. Among the New England regional study of congenital heart defects, COA accounts for 7.5 percent of infants less than 1 year of age [80]. That may be an underestimation, since COA in newborn infants may not be detected because of similar blood pressure in the upper and lower extremities [4]. The male-to-female ratio is 1.74:1 [81]. In older patients with isolated COA, the incidence also is higher in males. There is no evidence of a Mendelian pattern of inheritance in the majority of patients with COA [73]. COA is the most common cardiovascular defect found with Turner's syndrome. Noncardiac abnormalities that have been reported with COA are hypospadias, clubfoot, and ocular defects [81].

PATHOLOGY

The severity of luminal narrowing in the region of the coarctation at autopsy reveals 42 percent severe (pinhole) stenosis, 25 percent atresia, and 33 percent moderate narrowing in individuals 2 years of age and older [77]. In cases of COA containing a contraductal shelf, there is an infolding of the aortic media into the lumen located opposite the ductus arteriosus, marked on the adventitial side by a localized indentation like a waist in the aortic wall [82]. The aorta distal to the coarctation shows poststenotic dilatation and the wall of the aorta is thicker, whereas proximally, where the pressure is higher, the wall is thinner. The shelf of the coarctation may be pre- or postductal, but most often it is juxtaductal [83]. Flow patterns in the fetus with various congenital defects determine the development of the aortic isthmus. In a normal fetus, the level of blood flow across the aortic isthmus is lower (25% of the combined total ventricular output) than after birth; therefore, the aortic isthmus at birth is narrower than the descending thoracic aorta [83]. In congenital heart disease with reduced pulmonary arterial flow (pulmonary stenosis), the diameter of the isthmus is wider than normal because it carries greater flow in the fetus, and coarctation is virtually unknown. In lesions interfering with left ventricular outflow (mitral and aortic stenosis), the aortic isthmus is underdeveloped. When localized juxtaductal coarctation is present, aortic obstruction is not present during fetal life, but when the ductus arteriosus begins to close at birth, obstruction will appear after birth [84]. The ductus closes from the pulmonary end; obstruction of the aortic end and a gradient across the coarctation may be delayed.

The ductal tissue itself plays an important role in the mechanism of coarctation formation. Normally, ductal tissue, composed mostly of smooth muscle cells, extends only partially around the circumference of the aorta. In a patient with left-sided obstruction, there is right-to-left flow through the ductus in utero. That results in migration of ductal tissue into the adjacent aortic wall, resulting in a circumferential distribution [83]. Ho and Anderson, using a serial-section technique, have confirmed that ductal tissue completely surrounds the juxtaductal aorta such that "the ductal and descending aorta form a common channel of structural continuity, and the isthmus enters this channel" rather than the ductus entering the isthmus descending aortic region [85,86].

COLLATERAL CIRCULATION

Olney and Stephens and Bahn et al. have reported that collateral circulation in infants that die with coarctation is poorly developed [87,88] (Fig. 54-9). Bahn et al. noted that this depends on the location of the coarctation in relation to the ductus arteriosus; if the blood from the ductus enters the aorta proximal to the coarctation (preductal), then collateral circulation will develop [88] (Fig. 54-10). If the ductal blood flow enters below the coarctation (postductal), however, there is little stimulation during fetal life for development of collateral circulation. In that situation, postnatal closure of the ductus results in obstructive hypertension and hypovolemia, which together result in left ventricular failure.

The collateral circulation in COA between the proximal aorta and the distal aorta usually is present to some extent at birth but develops further as the patient ages. Collateral

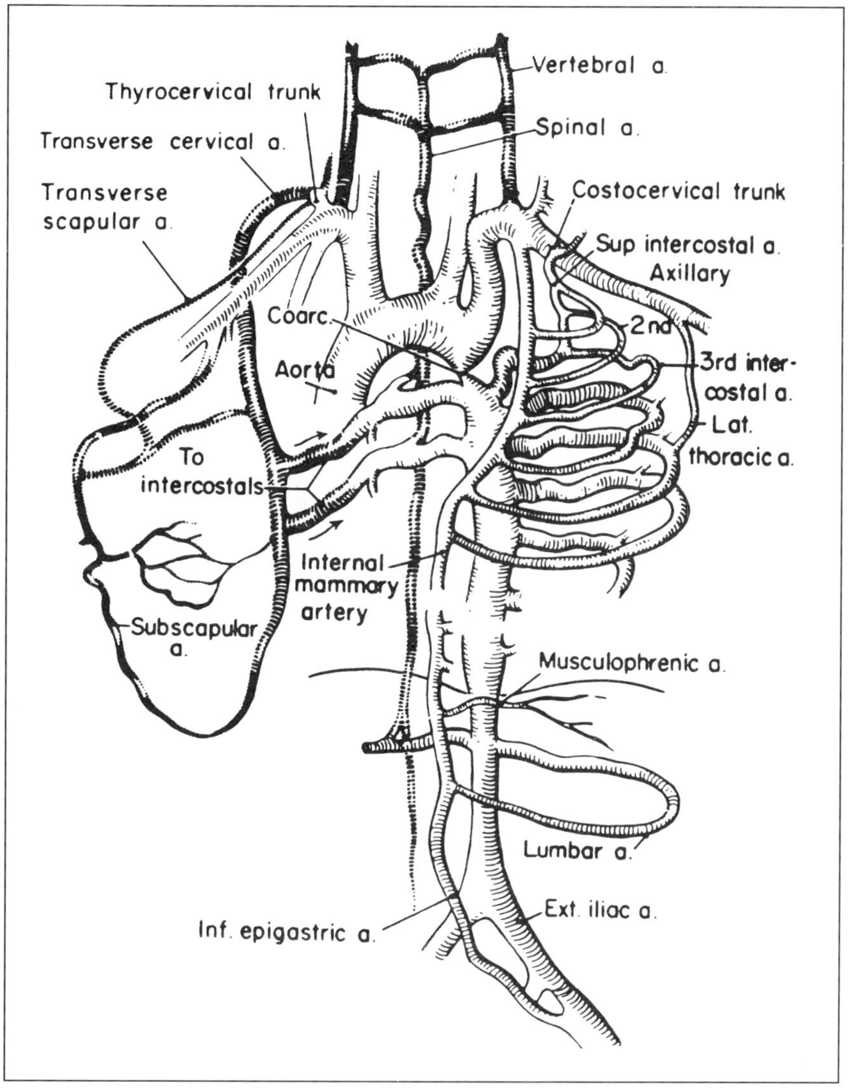

Fig. 54-9. Collateral circulation in coarctation of aorta. On the right side, the internal mammary artery connects to the epigastric arteries for supply to the lower limbs. On the left, the vessels arise from the subclavian artery and supply the scapula. They communicate via the intercostal arteries with the descending aorta to supply blood to the abdominal organs. The anterior spinal artery enlarges to supply additional collateral channels through communication to the abdominal aorta. (Reproduced with permission from JE Edwards et al. Pathologic considerations in coarctation of the aorta. Proc Staff Meet Mayo Clin 1948; 23:324.)

circulation involves primarily branches of both subclavian arteries, especially the internal mammary, vertebral, costocervical, and thyrocervical trunks, which carry blood to the lower limbs, usually through third and fourth intercostal arteries and the subscapular arteries. The subclavian arterial branches become greatly enlarged and are responsible for the classic signs of coarctation, such as rib notching and parascapular pulsations [69,72,89]. Collateral circulation also reaches the lower limbs through the internal mammary to the superior epigastric, which in turn connects with the inferior epigastric and joins the iliac arteries. The anterior spinal artery may provide additional collateral channels through its communication with the vertebral arteries above the coarctation and with intercostal and vertebral arteries below the coarctation [69,72]. Development of good collateral circulation and clinical manifestations vary, depending on the presence of stenosis of the left subclavian artery, which is an important source of collateral circulation; rib notching is seen only on the right side. If the right subclavian artery arises as a fourth branch and is distal to the coarctation, it is not a source of collateral flow, and rib notching occurs only on the left side [73].

ASSOCIATED CONDITIONS

As stated earlier, COA commonly is associated with bicuspid aortic valve, but the exact incidence remains speculative (27 to 46%) [86,90]. Among 250 patients with COA

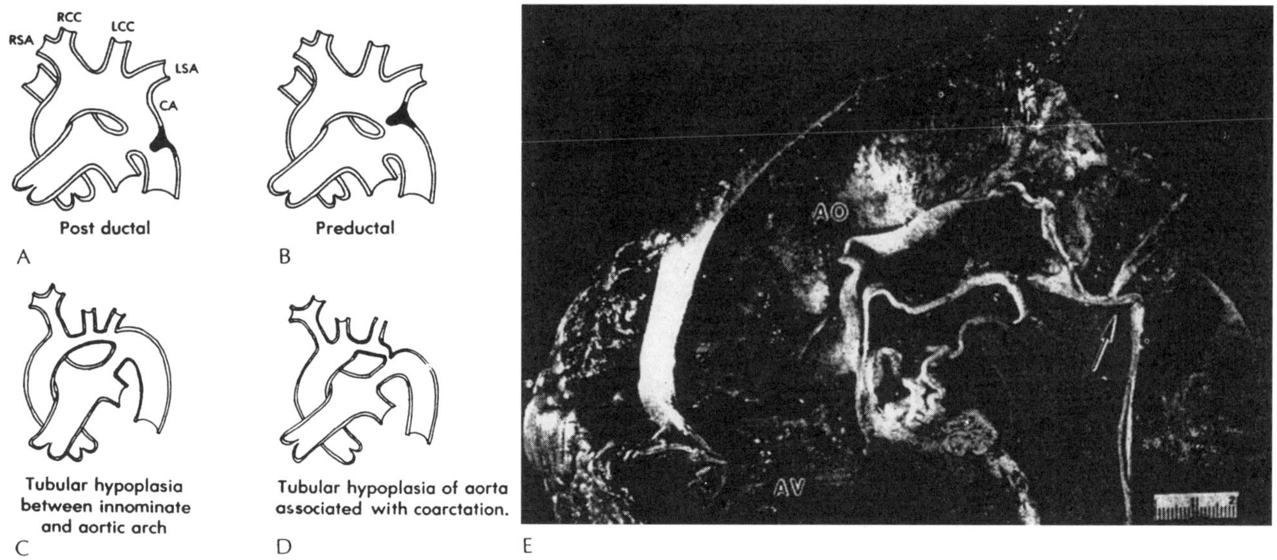

Fig. 54-10. Coarctation of aorta in the upper panel. **A.** Postductal and **B.** preductal, with patent ductus arteriosus. **C.** Tubular hypoplasia of aortic arch between innominate and subclavian artery with patent ductus arteriosus. **D.** Tubular hypoplasia (between common carotid and left subclavian) associated with coarctation of the aorta. **E.** Gross photograph of heart and aorta from a 76-year-old man with postductal coarctation of aorta (arrow). Note dilated and thinned aorta both proximally and distally to the COA. He also had a heavily calcified congenital bicuspid aortic valve. Key: AO = aorta, AV = aortic valve. (A–D modified from JH Moller, K Amplatz, JE Edwards. Congenital Heart Disease. Kalamazoo, Mich.: Upjohn, 1974. Pp. 46–51.)

studied by Tawes and associates [90], bicuspid valve disease was present in 32 (13%). The most common lesion is stenosis and, unusually, incompetence, which occurs on the basis of bicuspid valve with persistent hypertension [74].

There is a high incidence (85%) of major cardiac defects associated with COA in neonates [91]; in infants aged 1 to 11 months, however, the incidence drops to 52 percent. After 1 year of age, the incidence drops further to 40 percent (excluding bicuspid valve), as reported by Kirklin and Barratt-Boyes [74]. Infants undergoing operation in the first 3 months of life have a 60-percent incidence of other congenital cardiac anomalies, compared to 25 percent of those between 6 and 12 months [74].

Patent ductus arteriosus is present in virtually all neonates and is considered part of the coarctation complex [74]. Ventricular septal defect (VSD) occurs in 30 to 36 percent of cases of COA [72,73]. COA in TGA occurs in 10 percent, ASD in 6 to 7 percent [92]. Mitral-valve disease, which causes mitral stenosis and regurgitation, is present in fewer than 10 percent [92].

COMPLICATIONS

Aortic rupture usually occurs in the second or third decade and normally involves the ascending aorta, with resultant tamponade. Aortic rupture also may occur distal to the coarctation, where the aorta is thin and dilated (poststenotic dilatation) [74]. Some of the ruptures may be accompanied by dissecting aneurysms [74].

Cerebrovascular accidents, as reported by Liberthson and colleagues, usually occur in older patients: over 40 years, 21 percent; 11 to 39 years, 8 percent; and patients under 11 years, less than 1 percent [92]. The main cause usually is rupture of a congenital berry aneurysm in the circle of Willis and is secondary to the presence of hypertension [6]. Other causes are atherosclerosis in older patients and emboli from bacterial endocarditis. Infective endocarditis normally involves the bicuspid aortic valve and, rarely, the mitral valve, at the site of VSD, or at sites of jet lesion in the aortic wall.

TREATMENT

Surgical treatment of COA has been available for over 35 years [93,94]. Surgical repair early in life (ages 2 to 4 years for elective, earlier in the presence of severe hypertension) has become safer due to improvement in surgical technique [73,74]. The technique of operation consists of subclavian flap aortaplasty in neonates and infants, subclavian flap aortoplasty or end-to-end anastomosis in children up to 10 years of age, and end-to-end anastomosis in adolescents and adults [73,74]. There is increased mortality in patients with associated major cardiac anomalies [74]. Balloon angioplasty has been utilized as an alternative to surgery, but the procedure is controversial because its success rate is lower than that reported for surgical repair. The poor outcome from balloon angioplasty is due to persistent stenosis or to aneurysm formation; however, surgical repair is safe and effective after unsuccessful balloon angioplasty [95].

Table 54-4. Aortic-arch malformations

I. Vascular rings
  A. Double aortic arch
  B. Right aortic arch
    1. without retroesophageal component
    2. with retroesophageal component
  C. Left aortic arch
    1. aberrant right subclavian artery
    2. ductus arteriosus sling
II. Cervical aorta
III. Complete interruption of the aortic arch

Aortic-Arch Anomalies

Malformations of the aortic arch are a complex group of lesions first described in the eighteenth century. A classification of the aortic-arch malformations is presented in Table 54-4. Observations of the basic development of the aortic arches and their derivatives, reviewed and summarized by Congdon in 1922 [96], were of little use to clinicians until the 1940s, when Gross pioneered the first surgical repairs of vascular rings [97]. **Vascular ring** is the broad term used to describe an aortic-arch malformation in which the trachea and the esophagus are compressed. The first clinical description of tracheal and esophageal compression by a double aortic arch is credited to Wolman in 1939 [98].

INCIDENCE

The true incidence of aortic-arch malformations and vascular rings is difficult to determine because so many lesions are asymptomatic. The incidence of vascular rings is thought to be approximately 1 percent of congenital heart disease. In 1948, Edwards proposed the hypothetical double-aortic-arch model to conceptualize all the known and possible aortic-arch malformations (Fig. 54-11) [99]. The scheme was elaborated on by Kirklin and Clagett in 1950 [100]. All known aortic-arch malformations can be explained by the regression of a part of the arch that normally remains patent or by persistence of a structure that regresses in normal development.

Morphology. Aortic-arch anomalies (vascular rings) are anomalies of the great arteries that compress the trachea, the esophagus, or both [101].

DOUBLE AORTIC ARCH

The double aortic arch is the most frequent type of aortic-arch malformation to result in a vascular ring. The double aortic arch represents a failure of regression of the right eighth dorsal aortic segment; it is formed as the ascending aorta leaves the pericardium and divides into right and left aortic arches. From each arch arises a carotid artery and a subclavian artery (Fig. 54-12). The arches pass behind the trachea and esophagus and unite to form a single descending aorta, thus a vascular ring. The arches usually are not equal in size: One arch, often the right, is larger. One arch may be represented by an atretic segment only; in that case, the right arch usually persists. It is theoretically possible, using the double-aortic-arch model, that the ductus arteriosus could be bilateral or on the right or left side only. No case of functional double arch with bilateral ducti arteriosus has been reported. The descending aorta may be on the right, on the left, or, occasionally, in the midline [99,101–103]. Associated cardiac anomalies usually are not seen but include tetralogy of Fallot and TGA [102].

Fig. 54-11. The hypothetical double-aortic-arch system proposed by Edwards as the mechanism underlying vascular rings. (Reproduced with permission from AE Becker, RH Anderson. Pathology of Congenital Heart Disease. London: Butterworths, 1981. Pp. 47–66, 333.)

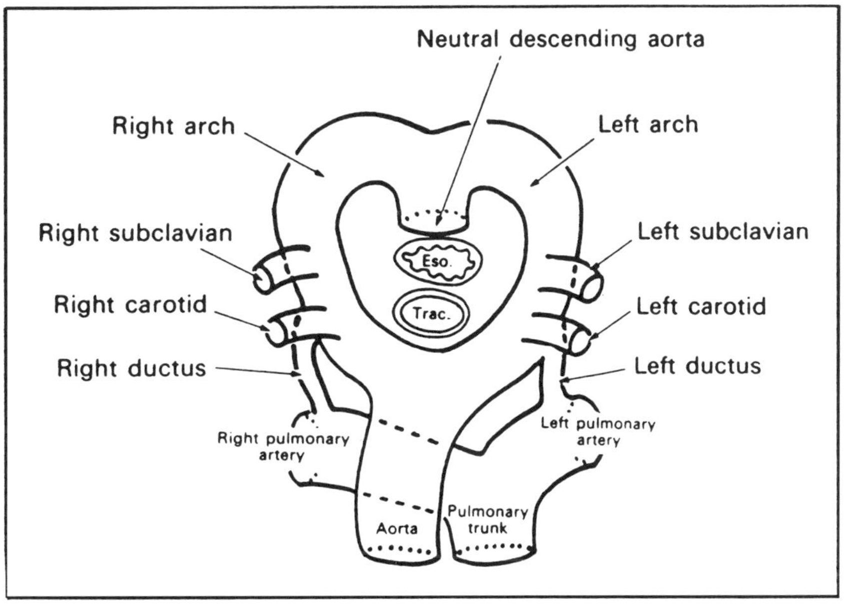

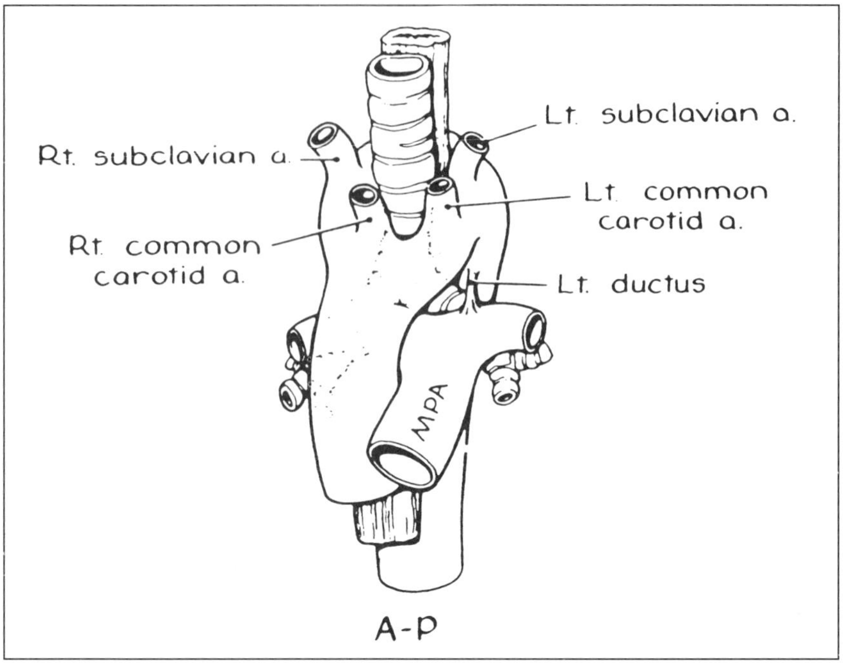

Fig. 54-12. Anatomy of a double aortic arch from an anteroposterior (A-P) view. From each arch arises a carotid and a subclavian artery. The right and left arches unite behind the trachea and esophagus to form a vascular ring. MPA = main pulmonary artery. (Reproduced with permission from JR Stewart, OW Kincaid, JE Edwards. An Atlas of Vascular Rings and Related Malformations of the Aortic Arch System. Springfield: Thomas, 1964.)

RIGHT AORTIC ARCH

A right aortic arch is present when the ascending aorta and arch pass anterior to the right main-stem bronchus. There are two main types of right aortic arch: without a retroesophageal component (mirror-image branching) and with a retroesophageal component.

Right Aortic Arch without Retroesophageal Component. In the usual right aortic arch, there is mirror-image branching of the arch vessels compared to the normal left arch. The first vessel is a left innominate artery, the second and third are the right common carotid and right subclavian arteries (Fig. 54-13). The majority of patients have a left ductus arteriosus arising from the left pulmonary artery and inserting into the left subclavian artery. Bilateral ducti are associated with congenital cardiac anomalies, usually tetralogy of Fallot or truncus arteriosus [103]. Right aortic arch without retroesophageal component does not produce a vascular ring (see Fig. 54-13). The abnormality does not produce symptoms but may be picked up radiographically.

Right Aortic Arch with Retroesophageal Component. A vascular ring usually is present in the right aortic arch with retroesophageal component. The right aortic arch extends to the left, behind the esophagus, in the form of a diverticulum. The vascular ring is formed by the right arch and a left-sided ductus arteriosus arising from the left pulmonary artery and extending to the upper descending thoracic aorta. This group of abnormalities also includes anomalous retroesophageal left subclavian artery. The vascular ring is completed by the left ductus arteriosus extending from the left pulmonary artery to the retroesophageal left subclavian artery or aorta. Right aortic arch with retroesophageal component is rarely associated with cardiac abnormalities [101,103].

LEFT AORTIC ARCH

A vascular ring is frequently associated with left aortic arch.

Aberrant Right Subclavian Artery. The most common left-arch abnormality is aberrant right subclavian artery. The right subclavian artery arises as the fourth branch of the aortic arch, distal to the left subclavian artery. This anomaly results from the regression of the fourth aortic arch and persistent patency of the eighth right segment. Aberrant right subclavian artery does not result in a vascular ring unless there is a right ductus arteriosus extending from the right pulmonary artery to the right subclavian (Fig. 54-14). This anomaly is of importance because of its frequent association with tetralogy of Fallot and the difficulty of using this vessel for the Blalock-Taussig anastomosis [104]. Aberrant right subclavian artery also is associated with COA [102]. Compression of the esophagus by the aberrant right subclavian was once thought to induce dysphagia lusoria [105]. That view is disputed, and the anomaly is generally thought not to be a cause of major symptoms [103].

DUCTUS ARTERIOSUS SLING

An aberrant ductus arteriosus extending from the right pulmonary artery between the trachea and the esophagus

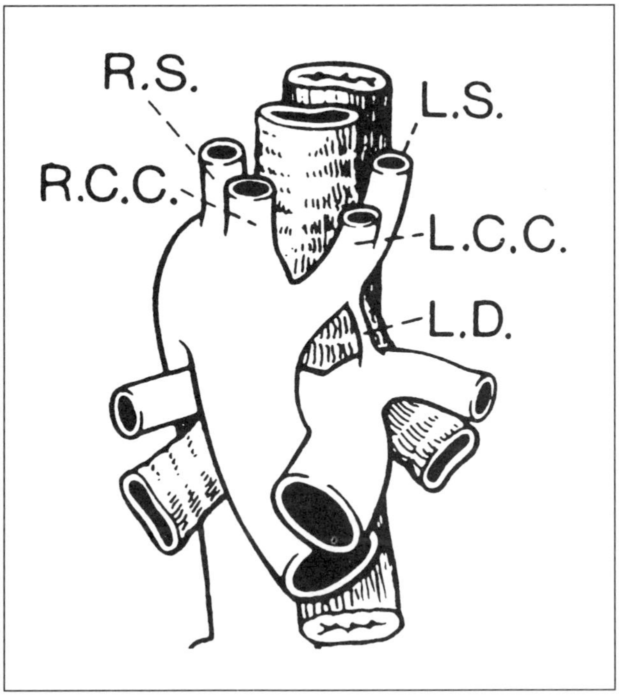

Fig. 54-13. Right aortic arch with mirror-image branching and left ductus arteriosus. Key: RS = right subclavian artery, RCC = right common carotid artery, LS = left subclavian artery, LCC = left common carotid artery, LD = left ductus arteriosus. (Reproduced with permission from H Bankl. Congenital malformations of the heart and great vessels. Synopsis of Pathology, Embryology and Natural History. Baltimore: Urban & Schwarzenberg, 1977. Pp. 159–166.)

to the aorta near the origin of an aberrant right subclavian artery has been reported [106]. The patient, a 7-week-old infant, had dyspnea and wheezing, which were relieved by surgical division of the vessel.

CERVICAL AORTIC ARCH

Cervical aortic arch results from the failure of the aortic arch to descend in the eighth fetal week [106]. The left arch crosses behind the esophagus, and the right patent ductus arteriosus or ligamentum is present and a vascular ring is formed. When the right arch gives rise to the aberrant left subclavian artery via an aortic diverticulum, a vascular ring is formed and is often situated in the cervical position [101,103]. Patients may present with a pulsating mass or aneurysm in the supraclavicular space. Some patients present with signs and symptoms of a vascular ring [103].

COMPLETE INTERRUPTION OF THE AORTIC ARCH

Complete interruption of the aortic arch is different from coarctation of the aortic arch in that there is no continuity of the aorta. Almost all cases have a patent ductus arteriosus and associated intracardiac anomalies such as VSD, subaortic stenosis, and truncus arteriosus. The symptoms of complete interruption of the aortic arch are severe right-to-left shunting. Treatment involves prostaglandin therapy to dilate the ductus arteriosus and surgery to restore the continuity of the arch, including the placement of aortic graft [101].

CLINICAL PRESENTATION AND DIAGNOSIS

Patients with vascular rings present within the first 6 months of life. The signs and symptoms of tracheal and esophageal compression vary with the severity of compression. Infants may present with stridor, wheeze, and recurrent respiratory infections. They often demonstrate poor feeding and dysphagia for solid foods [90]. The plain-film chest x-ray may be normal, or a right aortic arch may be detected. Esophagram is a very useful diagnostic tool, for example, for demonstrating right and left indentations in the esophagus when a double aortic arch is present [102].

Diagnostic procedures include chest roentgenography, barium swallow, aortography, and MRI techniques for adequate delineation of the vascular and tracheal anatomy. Echocardiography further helps in defining associated cardiac defects [107,108]. Surgery is indicated when esophageal- and tracheal-compression symptoms are severe. No operative or late deaths have occurred in isolated vascular rings since 1967 [107,109]. On long-term follow-up, 92 percent of patients are free of respiratory symptoms [109]. When symptoms are of borderline severity, they may disappear as the child grows [109].

Malformations of the Pulmonary Trunk and Arteries

Isolated pulmonary-artery abnormalities are rare and can be divided into those with anomalous arterial supply to one lung in the presence of separate aortic and pulmonary valves (and without inherent interposition of ductal tissue) and those with both lungs receiving normally connected pulmonary arteries.

ORIGIN OF RIGHT OR LEFT PULMONARY ARTERY FROM ASCENDING AORTA

When the right pulmonary artery arises from the aorta, it usually arises from the right or posterior aspect of the ascending aorta [110]. The origin usually is within 1 to 3 cm of the aortic valve, and the right pulmonary artery is larger than the left [110]. The pulmonary vascular bed of both lungs may be similar, especially in patients dying within 6 months of life [111]. In older patients, however, hypertensive vascular disease usually is present and usually is similar in its extent in both lungs [110]. This lesion is seen as an isolated defect in 20 percent of cases, but most often it is associated with patent ductus arteriosus (50%) [112,113]. Occasionally, the lesion coexists with (left) pulmonary-vein stenosis [110]. The pulmonary stenosis may be tubular or membraneous [110].

The origin of the left pulmonary artery from the ascending aorta is rarer than the right pulmonary artery from the aorta and usually is seen in association with right aortic arch [110]. This anomaly is isolated in 40 percent of cases, and the most commonly associated lesion is tetralogy of Fallot. Also, part of one lung may receive anomalous vascular supply, called **sequestration of the lung**. A distinct form of sequestration, **scimitar syndrome**, involves abnormal arterial supply as well as venous drain-

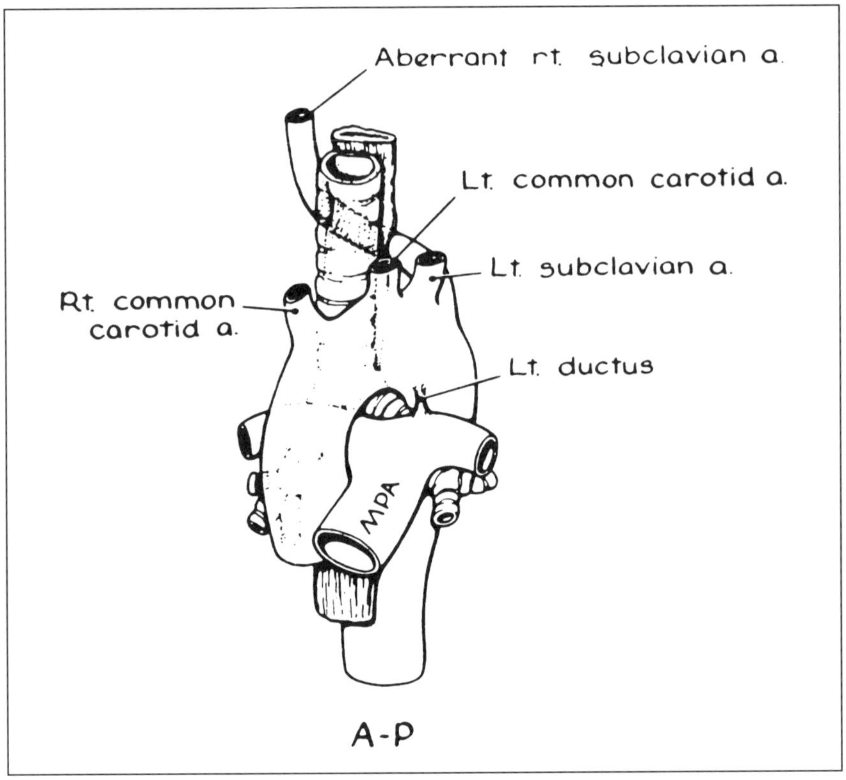

Fig. 54-14. Aberrant right subclavian artery from an anteroposterior (A-P) view. (Reproduced with permission from JR Stewart, OW Kincaid, JE Edwards. An Atlas of Vascular Rings and Related Malformations of the Aortic Arch System. Springfield: Thomas, 1964.)

age into the IVC [114]. The more severe type of sequestration occurs when one lung is supplied completely from a systemic source. Only one case has been reported where both the right and the left pulmonary arteries arose from the ascending aorta [110,115]. Much more common is absence of one pulmonary artery, either right or left [114].

Pulmonary arteries may arise from the pulmonary trunk, but the left artery connects to the right lung and vice versa [114]. This anomaly has been described in truncus arteriosus as well as when the pulmonary trunk is normally connected to the right ventricle [114].

AORTOPULMONARY COMMUNICATION

Aortopulmonary communication or window is a distinct anatomic lesion, with communication between the ascending aorta and the pulmonary trunk and the presence of separate aortic and pulmonary valves [116]. The defect is a true window with no length to the communication between the aorta and the pulmonary trunk. Usually the defect is single, large, and oval; infrequently ($<$ 10% of cases) the defect is small [117]. The communication usually is situated in the left lateral wall of the ascending aorta (close to the origin of the left coronary artery) in communication with the right wall of the pulmonary trunk (inferior to the origin of the right pulmonary artery) [117,118]. It is not surprising, therefore, that the right or, more rarely, the left coronary arteries may be seen arising from the pulmonary trunk. Rarely, the communication may be more downstream [117–119]. Because the defect usually is large, it is not surprising that pulmonary vascular disease may develop early, similar to that seen in VSDs and patent ductus arteriosus [116,117].

Aortopulmonary window is associated with other cardiovascular malformations, usually VSDs, tetralogy of Fallot, subaortic stenosis, and, infrequently, right aortic arch, ASD, or patent ductus arteriosus [117,120].

VASCULAR MALFORMATIONS

The classification of benign vascular proliferations is problematic. The term "hemangioma" has been used for all types of tumorlike lesions of vessels, including malformations and telangiectasias. The pathogenesis and true nature of many types of benign vascular lesions are yet unknown. Vascular malformations are diagnosed differently by clinicians, radiologists, and pathologists. Although a precise classification using histologic criteria has been adopted for many vascular tumors, it can be difficult to adapt the classification for one organ system to another [121–126]. The clinical relevance of the subclassification of vascular tumors is still uncertain for some organs, although the value of precise diagnosis is becoming more evident with currently available imaging techniques and the identification of clinical syndromes [127–129]. In this review, we will adopt a simplified classification of vascular malformations, but the reader should bear in mind that, at this time, there is no consensus on the issue.

Arteriovenous Malformation

Arteriovenous malformations (AVM) represent abnormal vascular communications between arteries and veins that occur without an intervening capillary bed and that result in the formation of a mass [130]. These malformations also are referred to as arteriovenous fistulas, arteriovenous hemangiomas, arteriovenous aneurysms, or racemose or cirsoid aneurysms.

CLINICAL FINDINGS AND DIAGNOSIS

Arteriovenous malformations may be present at birth, become apparent soon after birth, or be asymptomatic until adulthood [130,131]. Unlike capillary hemangiomas in infants, AVMs do not regress, but grow with the growth of the child. Although AVMs are described in almost every organ of the body [121–133], approximately 50 percent are located in the head and neck region. Other locations for AVMs include the central nervous system, extremities, heart, liver, and kidney. A specialized form of AVM that occurs in the gastric mucosa is termed Dieulafoy's disease and is prone to massive upper gastrointestinal hemorrhage. AVM of the pulmonary circulation deserves special mention and is discussed below.

The physical findings in AVM are closely related to the location and size of the lesion. Patients may present with swelling, pain, or hemorrhage. If located near the skin, the lesion is often a pulsatile mass with a thrill or bruit. There may be erythema or cyanosis distal to the lesion. Cutaneous or mucosal AVMs may ulcerate and bleed, or there may be thrombosis, cellulitis, or both superficially. Hypertrophy of an extremity can occur if a large shunt is present. Cardiomegaly in infancy occasionally is due to an unsuspected AVM, and large aneurysms, particularly in the brain or liver, may cause neonatal heart failure. Central nervous system AVM may present as repeated episodes of intracranial hemorrhage or as seizure disorders secondary to gliosis or atrophy of the adjacent cortex.

Angiographically, the lesions have multiple anomalous arterial branches and anastomoses with early filling of the venous system. Vessels are dilated, elongated, and tortuous. MRI also is capable of differentiating AVMs from other types of hemangiomas, both in the central nervous system as well as the skin and subcutaneous tissue [127,128].

PATHOLOGY

The pathologic diagnosis of AVM rests on the presence of communicating arteries and veins in a vascular lesion. In the larger AVM, the gross appearance of the specimen is one of multiple blood-filled spaces, often aneurysmally dilated. A smaller AVM removed for pathologic examination may require extensive sectioning to demonstrate the lesion, and ultimately the diagnosis may rest on radiologic correlation. Microscopically, AVM is marked by the presence of arteries and veins with little intervening tissue (Fig. 54-15). The direct communication between an artery and a vein may be difficult to locate. Vessels often are elongated and dilated, and the structure of the vessel walls in AVM usually is abnormal. Artery walls are thinned or may be hypertophied, with disruption and loss of elastic lamina and medial smooth muscle. The medial smooth muscle also may form nodules projecting into the vessel lumen. Vein walls become thickened, or arterialized, with the acquisition of internal elastic lamina. Elastic stains can be helpful, but it is not always possible in AVM to classify a vessel as an artery or a vein.

TREATMENT

Indications for the treatment of AVM include congestive heart failure, cosmetic deformity, hemorrhage, and ulceration [130,134,135]. The treatment of AVM is tailored to the particular location and size of the lesion. A variety of therapeutic modalities have been used to treat AVM, including radiation, surgery, and embolization techniques. Surgical treatment of AVM involves resection. Isolated ligation of the vessel is not curative, since collateral circulation can reestablish flow to the lesion [121,133,134]. AVM can recur if not completely excised [134]. The morbidity of surgery is related to hemorrhage, disseminated intravascular coagulation, and cosmetic deformity [133].

A variety of materials have been used for embolization, including autologous materials such as fat or muscle, hemostatic agents such as gelatin sponges and polyvinyl alcohol, and methyl methacrylate or silicon spheres. More recently, coils and balloons have been used. The amount of shunting and the diameter of the shunts determine the size of the embolization particles. Complications of embolization therapy include stroke, skin slough, and blindness [133,135].

PULMONARY ARTERIOVENOUS MALFORMATIONS

Pulmonary AVMs were first described at autopsy in the nineteenth century, but the first clinical diagnosis based on the triad of cyanosis, clubbing, and polycythemia was made in 1939 [136]. Pulmonary AVM causes a shunting of venous blood from the pulmonary arteries to the pulmonary veins, thus decreasing arterial oxygen saturation. Occasionally, a pulmonary AVM receives blood from a systemic artery in addition to a pulmonary artery [137]. Pulmonary AVM may be single or multiple, small or large enough to involve an entire lung (Fig. 54-16). Up to 36 percent of patients with solitary pulmonary AVM and 60 percent of patients with multiple pulmonary AVM have associated Osler-Weber-Rendu disease, which is described below [138,139].

Clinical Features and Diagnosis. Cyanosis is present from childhood, occasionally from birth. Neurologic symptoms may be due to brain abscesses resulting from a loss of the filtering function of the lung [137–140]. Decrease in arterial oxygen saturation occurs with pulmonary AVM, and pulmonary angiography demonstrates the malformation with early filling of the left atrium [139].

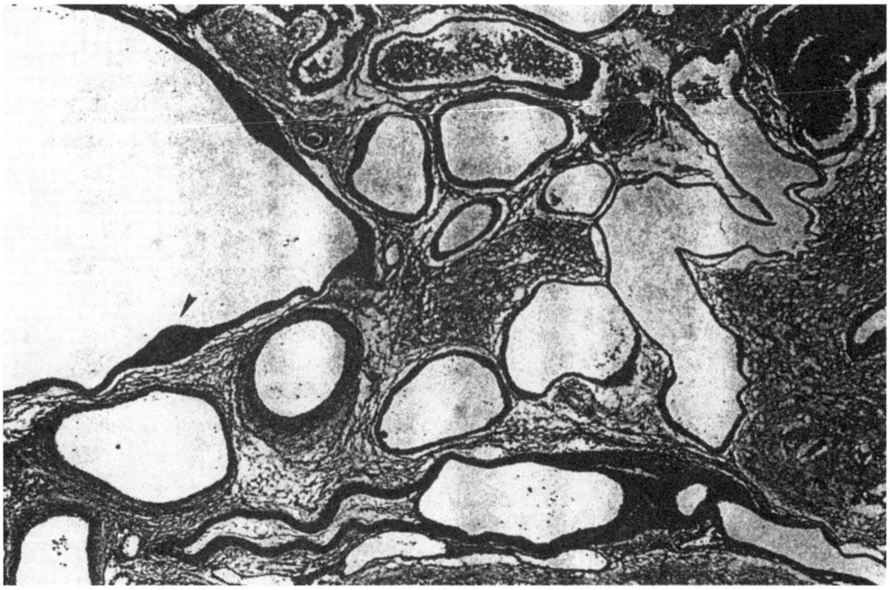

Fig. 54-15. Arteriovenous malformation from the occipital lobe of an 18-year-old woman. Note dilatation of multiple arterial and venous channels and medial smooth muscle nodule projecting into the vessel lumen (arrow) (Movat penachrome stain × 30).

Treatment. The frequency of fatal complications in pulmonary AVM is significant [139]. They include rupture, hemorrhage, endocarditis, and brain abscess. Surgery is indicated with segmental resection whenever possible to preserve the maximum amount of lung tissue, but lobectomy may be necessary [140].

Telangiectasias

Telangiectasias are localized dilatations of capillaries and venules that are presumed congenital and may form part of an inherited syndrome. Unlike hemangiomas, there is no proliferation of vessels, but rather an idiopathic dilatation of preexisting capillaries and venules. However, the term "hemangioma" is often used, especially clinically, for these lesions. Most forms of telangiectasias are present in the skin, but internal organs, including the brain, can be affected. There generally are few or no symptoms attributable to the telangiectasia itself, other than cosmetic problems when it involves the skin or hemorrhagic complications of gastrointestinal hemangiomas. In-

Fig. 54-16. Pulmonary arteriovenous malformation from a 4-day-old male infant born with low Apgar and cyanosis. The infant died in congestive heart failure. **A.** Autopsy revealed AVM of the left upper lobe of lung. **B.** Histologic section of the AVM showing multiple dilated vessels replacing pulmonary parenchyma (Movat pentachrome stain × 3).

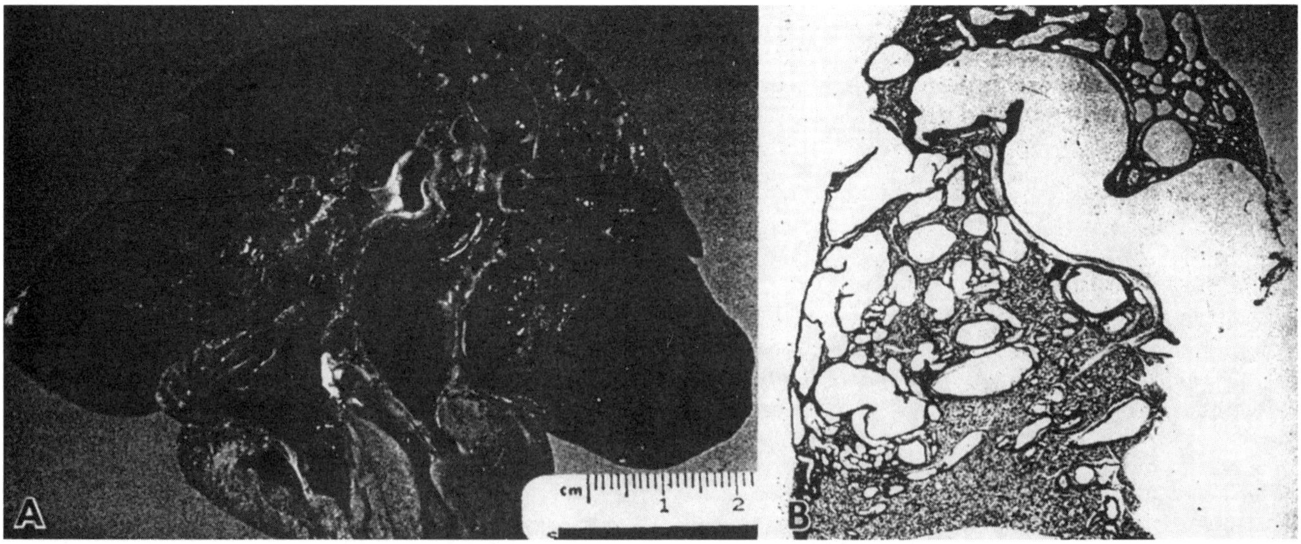

cidental telangiectasias of the brain are quite common in the pons and the cortex but only rarely have been reported to cause symptoms by bleeding.

CUTANEOUS TELANGIECTASIAS

The most common congenital cutaneous telangiectasia is the nevus flammeus, or ordinary birthmark. Nevus flammeus appears as mottled macular lesion on the head and neck and usually regresses. The nevus vinosus, or port-wine stain, is a specialized form of nevus flammeus that demonstrates no tendency to fade and often becomes elevated, reminiscent of a true hemangioma [141]. Unlike true hemangiomas, telangiectasias appear histologically as congested, normal vessels that are separated by intervening tissue. Indeed, in most cases, there is no detectable histopathologic abnormality after the tissue has been processed for examination.

There are at least three syndromes associated with port-wine stains. The **Sturge-Weber syndrome** is characterized by telangiectasias of the face in the distribution of the trigeminal nerve and ipsilateral vascular malformations of the leptomeninges or retina. Patients afflicted with the full-blown syndrome suffer from seizures, hemiplegia, and mental retardation. The **Klippel-Trenaunay syndrome** is characterized by port-wine stains of an extremity, usually one leg. The affected leg is hypertrophied, and there are severe venous varicosities and often an absence of deep veins by phlebography. A subset of patients with Klippel-Trenaunay syndrome have associated AVMs. Because of the difference in clinical symptoms, the term **Parke-Weber syndrome** usually is applied to these individuals, who may suffer from congestive heart failure [142].

HEREDITARY HEMORRHAGIC TELANGIECTASIA

Hereditary hemorrhagic telangiectasia, or Osler-Weber-Rendu disease (OWRD), is a disorder characterized by multiple skin and mucosal telangiectasias and pulmonary AVMs [143,144]. The disease is believed to have an autosomal dominant mode of transmission affecting the sexes equally. A small number of cases are sporadic.

Telangiectasias are found in the skin or mucosal surfaces of the gastrointestinal, respiratory, and urinary tracts. Nose bleeds and gastrointestinal- and urinary-tract bleeding are common clinical manifestations. Vascular lesions also may be present in other organs such as the liver and brain, where they usually are incidental autopsy findings. Patients with OWRD may present with hepatomegaly or neurologic symptoms. The hemorrhagic tendency in patients with OWRD appears to increase with age. OWRD is strongly associated with pulmonary AVM. In a review of 350 cases of pulmonary AVM, 36 percent of patients with solitary AVM and 57 percent of patients with multiple AVM had OWRD [137]. In a review of 91 members of a family with OWRD, 15 percent had pulmonary AVM [138].

ATAXIA TELANGIECTASIA

Ataxia telangiectasia is an autosomal dominant inherited disease that is characterized by the appearance in childhood of telangiectasias of the bulbar conjunctivae and skin of the face and extremities [145]. The vascular lesions are preceded by ataxia, which occurs in infancy. The patients generally succumb to an underlying immunologic abnormality that results in recurrent infections and the development of lymphoproliferative disorders. Histologic examination of the telangiectasias demonstrates the presence of dilated subpapillary venous channels. A chromosomal defect has recently been identified in the long arm of chromosome 11 [146].

CAVERNOUS MALFORMATIONS

Cavernous malformations, like AVMs, usually are considered to be malformations rather than neoplasms. For that reason, they have been termed cavernous malformations in the radiologic literature [127], although the term cavernous hemangioma is likely to persist. Histologically, cavernous malformations are composed of dilated vessels that lack smooth muscle or elastic tissue; the vessels form a tumorlike proliferation with little intervening tissue. A subgroup of lesions has been designated venous malformations [127,128]; those lesions have thicker walls with large amounts of smooth muscle more reminiscent of venous walls than seen in most cavernous hemangiomas. The distinction between the two entities is not always possible, and mixed lesions exist. Cavernous malformations of the central nervous system may be more likely to rupture than venous malformations, and there may be differences in imaging characteristics using computed tomography, magnetic resonance imaging, and angiography [127].

Cavernous malformations of the skin appear in infancy and are particularly common in the head, neck, and upper body. Because they do not regress spontaneously, and because they often involve deeper layers of the skin, they must be surgically removed.

There are several syndromes associated with cavernous malformations. **Kasabach-Merritt syndrome** is characterized by thrombocytopenia and usually complicates large solitary cavernous malformations of the extremity [147]. Kasabach-Merritt syndrome was originally described in patients with capillary hemangiomas and has been seen in other types of vascular lesions, including angiosarcoma. **Von Hippel Lindau syndrome** is an autosomal dominant phakomatosis characterized by cerebellar hemangioblastoma and cysts of long bones, pancreas, liver, spleen, kidneys, lungs, and other organs; occasionally, there are visceral cavernous malformations. **Blue rubber bleb nevus syndrome** [148], which may have an autosomal dominant mode of inheritance, is characterized by cutaneous cavernous malformations that look and feel like rubber nipples. Patients with blue rubber bleb syndrome also have gastrointestinal-tract hemangiomas. **Maffucci's syndrome** (dyschondroplasia with vascular hamartomas) is defined by the presence of multiple hemangiomas and enchondromas. The bone tumors may progress to chondrosarcomas. A number of vascular tumors have been described in these patients, including cavernous malformations, phlebectasias, and lymphangiomas [149].

Cavernous malformations are the second most common vascular malformation of the central nervous system, after AVM. Like AVMs, they have a propensity to bleed. However, the amount of hemorrhage is usually small, and the lesions are often clinically silent. One-half lie in the brain stem and, before the advent of MRI scans, often were misdiagnosed as multiple sclerosis. About 10 percent are multiple, and 5 percent familial. As mentioned above, they sometimes are divided into venous malformations and cavernous malformations, the latter having a higher likelihood of bleeding.

CAPILLARY HEMANGIOMAS

Capillary hemangiomas are common vascular proliferations that usually affect infants and occur on the skin. Although they commonly regress, they commonly are considered to be neoplasms, not malformations. Histologically, they are composed of a proliferation of capillarylike vessels that are quite cellular in infancy and that become more dilated as the patient reaches childhood.

Fibromuscular Dysplasia

Fibromuscular dysplasia (FMD) is a generic term for a group of structural abnormalities of one or more layers of medium-sized and large arteries that result in luminal narrowing by fibrous, smooth muscle cells or fibromuscular tissue with or without associated aneurysms and dissections of the media. The process usually is due to congenital malformation of the arterial structure, affecting young white women and involving most commonly the renal and carotid arteries. Classification is based on the histopathologic localization and pattern of the structural abnormalities, which affect the angiographic appearance [145–147]. Most often, the initial manifestations are hypertension, stroke, and abdominal pain, depending on the vascular bed involved.

The cause or causes of FMD remain obscure and may include estrogen exposure, mechanical factors, ischemic factors, environmental toxins such as cigarette smoke, and autoantibodies [150]. There is no doubt that there is an underlying genetic predisposition to the development of FMD. Whites are much more likely to develop FMD than blacks, and many cases are familial, with an autosomal dominant transmission with variable penetrance.

FMD can be discussed by the type of artery involved: renal arteries, aortic-arch vessels, and miscellaneous arteries.

FIBROMUSCULAR DYSPLASIA OF RENAL ARTERIES

FMD of the renal arteries is a common condition that accounts for approximately 25 percent of cases of renovascular hypertension and about 2 percent of all cases of hypertension [145–147]. The renal arteries are by far the most common site of symptomatic FMD, accounting for about 75 percent of cases. Multivessel FMD, which involves renal as well as other arteries, occurs in approximately 25 percent of patients with renal FMD.

Histologic Subtypes. The histologic classification of renal FMD generally is based on the layer of vessel involved [148] (Fig. 54-17). Although that classification is well established in the literature, we, as well as others [149], have not always found it useful and reproducible. A simplified classification based on the presence of smooth muscle hyperplasia recently has been proposed [149].

Classically, FMD has been divided into medial, intimal, and adventitial types. Medial FMD accounts for up to 95 percent of cases and has been further subdivided into medial fibroplasia, perimedial fibroplasia, and medial hyperplasia [151]. Intimal fibroplasia, medial fibroplasia, and perimedial hyperplasia impart the typical "beading" appearance on angiography.

Medial fibroplasia is characterized by fibromuscular ridges of hyperplastic smooth muscle cells and fibrous tissue that project into the lumen of the affected artery. Perimedial hyperplasia implies a predominance of fibrous tissue, and the proliferation is primarily in the outer layer of the media. Pure medial hypertrophy is quite rare and represents a concentric hypertrophy of the medial wall, which is relatively smooth, lacking fibrosis and causing severe stenosis. Angiographically and grossly, the stenosis usually is subtotal, sometimes tubular and smooth. Intimal hyperplasia, which represents fewer than 5 percent of lesions, is characterized by proliferation of fibrous tissue, including smooth muscle cells, within the intimal. There is no lipid deposition or inflammatory cell infiltrate, and the internal elastic lamina is preserved. Endarteritis secondary to inflammatory conditions or trauma may be associated with intimal fibroplasia in muscular arteries that may mimic the histologic picture of intimal fibroplasia. The morphologic appearance may be virtually indistinguishable from that of secondary or reactive intimal fibroplasia seen after endarterectomy or in the initial proliferative stage of atherosclerosis. Intimal fibroplasia also may occur concomitantly with medial fibromuscular dysplasia. In adventitial, or periarterial, fibroplasia, the primary lesion is a dense collagenous replacement of the loose fibrous tissue of the arterial adventitia. The fibrosis may extend into the surrounding adipose and connective tissues. The media and the intima are normal.

Clinical Findings. Patients with renal FMD are often young women. The diagnosis of FMD usually is made on investigation for unexplained hypertension. The right renal artery is involved more often than the left, and cases of bilateral involvement often are associated with extrarenal FMD. The distal two-thirds of the artery is typically involved, with frequent extension into the branch arteries. Complications of arterial occlusion and renal infarction may result from arterial dissection, embolization originating in the aneurysm, and aneurysmal thrombosis. Treatment includes medical management of hypertension, surgical vascular reconstruction, percutaneous transluminal angioplasty, and, in cases refractory to treatment, nephrectomy. Progression of disease is the rule without mechanical or surgical intervention, although rare cases may reverse with medical treatment [146].

FIBROMUSCULAR DYSPLASIA OF AORTIC-ARCH VESSELS

Pathology. FMD has been described involving the carotid, subclavian, and vertebral arteries [146,147,152]. The inter-

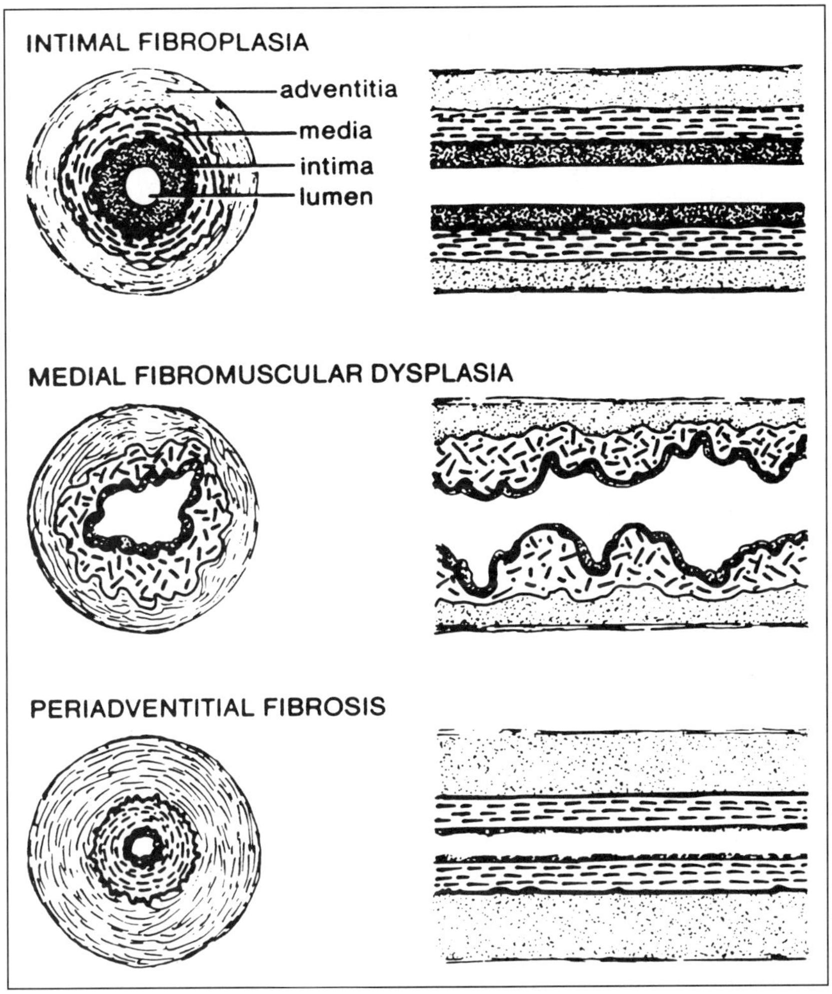

Fig. 54-17. Schematic showing transverse and longitudinal patterns of involvement of the arteries by the major types of fibromuscular dysplasia. (Modified from EG Harrison Jr, LJ McCormack. Pathologic classification of renal arterial disease in renovascular hypertension. Mayo Clin Proc 1971; 46:161–167. TF Luschner et al. Arterial fibromuscular dysplasia. Mayo Clin Proc 1987; 62:931–952.)

nal carotid artery is typically involved at the level of C-1 and C-2 and is usually "typical" medial FMD, resulting in the classic string-of-beads angiographic appearance. Subclavian and vertebral FMD is less likely to have a characteristic angiographic appearance and has been termed, on the basis of radiologic findings, as "atypical" FMD. Patients with cerebrovascular FMD have a high incidence of berry aneurysms of the circle of Willis, especially the intracranial internal carotid artery and the middle cerebral artery. Aneurysms in those locations are found more frequently in females with other vascular lesions such as FMD or other aneurysms. In contrast, aneurysms of the anterior cerebral artery are more likely to be sporadic and found in men.

Clinical Findings. Cerebrovascular FMD and FMD of the subclavian arteries are often asymptomatic and may be an incidental angiographic finding. The overall incidence of this disease and, therefore, the proportion of cases that are asymptomatic are unknown. Symptoms occur if there is stenosis of major cephalic arteries, embolization from thrombosed areas of FMD, or severe narrowing of the subclavian artery. Symptoms include transient ischemic attacks, strokes, subarachnoid hemorrhage from associated berry aneurysms of the circle of Willis, the subclavian steal syndrome, and weakness or claudication of the arms. Complications of cerebrovascular FMD include arterial dissections and carotid cavernous fistulas. FMD of the cerebrovascular circulation and subclavian arteries appears to be multifocal and bilateral more often than isolated renovascular FMD. Patients with subclavian FMD often have systemic FMD, including FMD of the renal arteries.

The natural history of cerebrovascular and subclavian FMD is relatively benign. Patients with ischemic cerebral symptoms and involvement of multiple vessels, however, have a poor prognosis. Treatment of cerebrovascular and subclavian FMD includes percutaneous transluminal angioplasty, graduated intraluminal dilatation, surgical resection with end-to-end anastomosis or interposition graft, and bypass grafts. Antiplatelet drugs and other anticoagulants are alternative medical therapies for patients with symptomatic FMD with or without dissections.

FIBROUS DYSPLASIA IN MISCELLANEOUS SITES

FMD has been described in the visceral arteries, iliac, axillary, brachial, and coronary arteries and the aorta [150,153–163]. Typical arteries involved in FMD of the visceral arteries are the celiac artery, mesenteric arteries, hepatic artery, and splenic artery. Symptoms related to stenotic lesions of the visceral arteries are rare due to well-developed collateral circulation. FMD of miscellaneous arteries is prone to similar complications of renal FMD and FMD of the aortic arch, including dissection and embolization.

References

1. Becker AE, Anderson RH. Pathology of Congenital Heart Disease. London: Butterworths, 1981. Pp. 47–66, 333.
2. Bankl H. Congenital Malformations of the Heart and Great Vessels. Synopsis of Pathology, Embryology, and Natural History. Munich: Urban and Schwarzenberg, 1977. Pp. 176–198.
3. Hudson RE. Cardiovascular Pathology. Baltimore: Williams & Wilkins, 1965. P. 1754.
4. Edwards JE. Anomalous pulmonary venous connection. In SE Gould, ed. Pathology of the Heart and Blood Vessels. 3rd ed. Springfield: Thomas, 1968. Pp. 455–478.
5. Darling RC, Rothney WB, Craig JM. Total pulmonary venous drainage into the right side of the heart. Report of 17 autopsied cases not associated with other major cardiovascular anomalies. Lab Invest 1957; 6:44–64.
6. Lucas RV, Krabill RA. Anomalous venous connections, pulmonary and systemic. In FH Adams, GC Emmanouilides, eds. Moss' Heart Disease in Infants, Children and Adolescents, 4th ed. Baltimore: Williams & Wilkins, 1989. P. 580.
7. Jenkins KJ, et al. Individual pulmonary vein size and survival in infants with totally anomalous pulmonary venous connection. J Am Coll Cardiol 1993; 22:201–206.
8. Masui T, et al. Abnormalities of the pulmonary veins: evaluation with MR imaging and comparison with cardiac angiography and echocardiography. Radiology 1991; 181:645–649.
9. Raisher BD, et al. Complete repair of total anomalous pulmonary venous connection in infancy. J Thorac Cardiovasc Surg 1992; 104:443–448.
10. Lincoln CR, et al. Surgical risk factors in total anomalous pulmonary venous connection. Am J Cardiol 1988; 61:608.
11. Yee ES, et al. Infant total anomalous pulmonary venous connection: Factors influencing timing of presentation of operative outcome. Circulation 1987; 76:III83.
12. Chin AJ, et al. Accuracy of subcostal two-dimensional echocardiography in prospective diagnosis of total anomalous pulmonary venous connections. Am Heart J 1987; 113:1153.
13. Baldridge ED Jr, Canos AJ. Venous anomalies encountered in aortoiliac surgery. Arch Surg 1987; 122:1184.
14. Baltaxe HA, Wixson D. The incidence of congenital anomalies of the coronary arteries in the adult population. Radiology 1977; 122:47–51.
15. Hobbs RE, et al. Congenital coronary artery anomalies: clinical and therapeutic implications. Cardiovasc Clin 1981; 12:43–58.
16. Roberts WC. Major anomalies of coronary arterial origin seen in adulthood. Am Heart J 1986; 111:941.
17. Roberts WC. Congenital coronary arterial anomalies unassociated with major anomalies of the heart or great vessels. In WC Roberts, ed. Congenital Heart Disease in Adults, 2nd ed. Philadelphia: Davis, 1986. Pp. 583–629.
18. Virmani R, Rogan K, Cheitlin MD. Congenital coronary artery anomalies: pathologic aspects. In R Virmani, MB Forman, eds. Non-atherosclerotic Ischemic Heart Disease. New York: Raven, 1989. Pp. 153–184.
19. Heifetz SA, et al. Total anomalous origin of the coronary arteries from the pulmonary vein. Ped Cardiol 1986; 7:11.
20. Ogden JA. Congenital variations of the coronary arteries. A clinicopathologic survey. Thesis presented to Faculty of the School of Medicine, Yale University, 1968.
21. Keith JD. Diseases of coronary arteries and aorta. In JD Keith, RD Rowe, P Vlad, eds. Heart Disease in Infancy and Childhood, 3rd ed. New York: Macmillan, 1978. P. 1014.
22. Neufeld HN, Schneeweiss A, eds. Coronary Artery Disease in Infants and Children. Philadelphia: Lea & Febiger, 1983. Pp. 1–30.
23. Vouhie PR, et al. Anomalous left coronary artery from pulmonary artery: results of isolated aortic reimplantation. Ann Thorac Surg 1992; 54:621–626.
24. Alexander RW, Griffith GC. Anomalies of the coronary arteries and their clinical significance. Circulation 1956; 14:800.
25. Lerberg DB, et al. Anomalous origin of the right coronary artery from pulmonary artery. Ann Thorac Surg 1979; 27:87–94.
26. Tinglestad JB, Lower RR, Eldredge WJ. Anomalous origin of the right coronary artery from the main pulmonary artery. Am J Cardiol 1972; 30:670–673.
27. Fu M, et al. Reversal of silent myocardial ischemia by surgery for isolated anomalous origin of the left anterior descending coronary artery from the pulmonary artery. Am Heart J 1992; 124:1369–1371.
28. Ott DA, et al. Anomalous origin of the left circumflex coronary artery from right pulmonary artery. Report of a rare anomaly. J Thorac Cardiovasc Surg 1978; 76:190.
29. Taylor AJ, Rogan KM, Virmani R. Sudden cardiac death associated with isolated congenital coronary artery anomalies. J Am Coll Cardiol 1992; 20:640–647.
30. Roberts WC, Siegel RJ, Zipes EG. Origin of the right coronary artery from the left sinus of Valsalva and its functional consequences: analysis of ten necropsy patients. Am J Cardiol 1982; 49:863.
31. White NK, Edwards JE. Anomalies of the coronary arteries. Report of four cases. Arch Pathol 1948; 45:766.
32. Page HL Jr, et al. Anomalous origin of the left circumflex coronary artery: recognition, angiographic demonstration and clinical significance. Circulation 1974; 50:287.
33. Vlodaver DP, et al. Coronary Heart Disease. Clinical Angiographic and Profiles. New York: Springer, 1976. P. 154.
34. Vlodaver DP, Neufeld HN, Edwards JE. Coronary Arterial Variations in the Normal Heart and in Congenital Heart Disease. New York: Academic, 1975. P. 171.
35. Russo G, et al. Isolated, anomalous origin of the left anterior descending coronary artery from the right coronary artery with angina pectoris. Eur Heart J 1992; 13:428–429.
36. Sharbaugh AH, White RS. Single coronary artery. Analysis of the anatomic variation, clinical importance and report of five cases. JAMA 1974; 23:243.
37. Hillestad L, Eie H. Single coronary artery: a report of three cases. ACTA Med Scand 1971; 189:409.
38. Lipton MJ, et al. Isolated single coronary artery: diagnosis, angiographic classification and clinical significance. Radiology 1979; 130:39–47.
39. Desmet W, et al. Isolated single coronary artery: a review of 50,000 consecutive coronary angiographies. Eur Heart J 1992; 13:1637–1640.

40. Fortuin NJ, Roberts WC. Congenital atresia of the left main coronary artery. Am J Med 1971; 50:385.
41. Sping DA, Thomsen JH. Severe atherosclerosis in the single coronary artery. Report of a previously undescribed pattern. Am J Cardiol 1973; 31:662.
42. Ogden JA. Anomalous aortic origin; circumflex anterior descending or left main coronary arteries. Arch Pathol 1969; 88:323.
43. Zechmeister A. Calcification of epicardial stretches of bridged coronary artery in man. J Ath Research 1969; 9:121.
44. Maron BJ, et al. Sudden death in young athletes. Circulation 1980; 62:218.
45. McClellan JT, Jokl E. Congenital anomalies of coronary arteries as a cause of sudden death associated with physical exertion. In E Jokl, ed. Medicine and Sports, vol. 5. Basel, Krager, 1971, p. 91.
46. Levine DC, Fellows KE, Abrams HL. Hemodynamically significant primary anomalies of the coronary arteries. Angiographic aspects. Circulation 1978; 58:25–34.
47. Case records of the Massachusetts General Hospital. Case 35-1980. N Engl J Med 1980; 303:571.
48. Liberthson RR, et al. Congenital coronary arteriovenous fistula: report of 13 patients, review of the literature, and delineation of management. Circulation 1979; 59:849–854.
49. Hobbs RE, et al. Coronary artery fistulae: a 10-year review. Cleve Clin J Med 1982; 49:191.
50. Reidy JF, et al. Transcatheter embolization in the treatment of coronary artery fistulas. J Am Coll Cardiol 1991; 18:187–192.
51. Cooper MJ, Bernstein D, Silverman NH. Recognition of left coronary artery fistula to left and right ventricles by contrast echocardiography. J Am Coll Cardiol 1985; 6:923–926.
52. Agatston AS, et al. Diagnosis of a right coronary artery—right atrial fistula using two-dimensional and Doppler echocardiography. Am J Cardiol 1984; 54:238–239.
53. Virmani R, et al. Acquired coronary arterial aneurysms. An autopsy study of 52 patients. Hum Pathol 1986; 17:575.
54. Wei J, Wang DJ. A giant congenital aneurysm of the right coronary artery. Ann Thorac Surg 1986; 41:322–324.
55. Wei J, Wang DJ. A giant congenital aneurysm of the right coronary artery. Ann Thorac Surg 1986; 41:322.
56. Seabra-Gomes R, et al. Congenital coronary artery aneurysms. Br Heart J 1974; 36:329.
57. Chahramani A, et al. Myocardial infarction due to congenital coronary arterial aneurysm with successful saphenous vein bypass graft. Am J Cardiol 1972; 29:863.
58. Lim CH, et al. Giant congenital aneurysm of the right coronary artery. Am J Cardiol 1977; 39:751.
59. Fujita S, et al. Congenital coronary arterial aneurysm without arteriovenous fistula resulting in myocardial infarction. Case report and review of the literature. Jpn Circ J 1983; 47:363.
60. Chen Y-T, Hwang C-L, Kan M-N. Large, isolated, congenital aneurysm of the anterior descending coronary artery. Br Heart J 1993; 70:274–275.
61. Lie JT, Berg KK. Isolated fibromuscular dysplasia of the coronary arteries with spontaneous dissection and myocardial infarction. Hum Pathol 1987; 18:654.
62. Lozano AM, Leblanc R. Familial intracranial aneurysms. J Neurosurg 1987; 66:522.
63. Haynes CD, et al. Multiple congenital aneurysms associated with spontaneous vascular rupture. Surgery 1982; 92:910.
64. Norrgard O, Angquist KA, Johnson O. Familial aortic aneurysms: serum concentrations of triglyceride, cholesterol, HDL-cholesterol and (VLDL + LDL)-cholesterol. Br J Surg 1985; 73(2):113.
65. Tilson MD, Davis G. Deficiencies of copper and a compound with ion-exchange characteristics of pyridinoline in skin from patients with abdominal aortic aneurysm. Surgery 1983; 94:134.
66. Johansen K. Familial tendency for abdominal aortic aneurysms. JAMA 1986; 94:134.
67. Mattern AL, et al. Congenital coronary aneurysms with angina pectoris and myocardial infarction treated with saphenous vein bypass graph. Am J Cardiol 1972; 30:906.
68. Tibbits P, et al. Congenital coronary aneurysms nine years following saphenous vein bypass graft surgery. Ann Thorac Surg 1981; 32:411.
69. Edwards JE. Congenital malformations of the heart and great vessel. H. Malformations of the thoracic aorta. In SE Gould, ed. Pathology of the Heart and Blood Vessels, 3rd ed. Springfield: Thomas, 1968. Pp. 391–454.
70. Edwards JE, et al. Pathologic considerations in coarctation of the aorta. Proc Staff Meet Mayo Clin 1948; 23:324.
71. Christenson NA. Coarctation of the aorta: historical review. Proc Staff Meet Mayo Clin 1948; 23:322.
72. Moller JH, Amplatz K, Edwards JE. Congenital Heart Disease. Kalamazoo: Upjohn, 1974. Pp. 46–51.
73. Gersony WM. Coarctation of the aorta. In FH Adams, GC Emmanouilides, eds. Moss' Heart Disease in Infants, Children and Adolescents. Baltimore: Williams & Wilkins, 1989. P. 243.
74. Kirklin JW, Barratt-Boyes BG. Coarctation of the aorta and interrupted aortic arch. In Cardiac Surgery, 2nd Edition. New York: Wiley, 1993. Pp. 1263–1326.
75. Bonnett LM. Sur la lesion dite stenose congenitale de l'aorte dans la region de l'isthme. Rev de Med 1903; 23:108–255, 335, 418, 481.
76. Abbot ME. Coarctation of the aorta of the adult type II. A statistical study and historical retrospect of 200 recorded cases with autopsy of stenosis or obliteration of the descending aorta in subjects over the age of two years. Am Heart J 1928; 3:574–618.
77. Reifenstein GH, Levine SA, Gross RE. Coarctation of the aorta: a review of 104 autopsied cases of the "adult type," 2 years of age or older. Am Heart J 1974; 33:339–368.
78. Calodney MM, Carson MJ. Coarctation of the aorta in early infancy. J Pediat 1950; 1:41–55.
79. Gross RN. Coarctation of aorta. Surgical treatment of 100 cases. Circulation 1950; 1:41–55.
80. Flyer DC, et al. The determinants of five year survival of infants with critical congenital heart disease. Cardiovasc Clin 1981; 11:393–405.
81. Campbell M, Polani PE. The etiology of coarctation of the aorta. Lancet 1961; 1:463.
82. Pellegrino A, et al. Aortic coarctation in the first three months of life. An anatomopathological study with respect to treatment. J Thorac Cardiovasc Surg 1985; 89:121.
83. Shinebourne EA, El Seed AM. Relation between fetal flow patterns, coarctation of the aorta and pulmonary blood flow. Br Heart J 1974; 36:492.
84. Rudolph AM, Heymann MA, Spitznas U. Hemodynamic considerations in the development of narrowing of the aorta. Am J Cardiol 1972; 30:514–525.
85. Ho SY, Anderson RH. Coarctation, tubular hypoplasia and the ductus arteriosus. Histological study of 35 specimens. Br Heart J 1979; 41:268.
86. Becker AE, Becker MJ, Edwards JE. Anomalies associated with coarctation of the aorta. Particular reference in infancy. Circulation 1970; 41:1067.
87. Olney MB, Stephens HB. Coarctation of the aorta in children: observations in fourteen cases. J Pediat 1950; 37:639.
88. Bahn RC, Edwards JE, DuShane JW. Coarctation of the aorta as cause of death in early infancy. Pediatrics 1951; 8:192–203.

89. Edwards JE, et al. Pathologic considerations in coarctation of the aorta. Proc Staff Meet Mayo Clin 1948; 23:324.
90. Tawes RL, Berry LL, Aberdeen E. Congenital bicuspid aortic valve associated with coarctation of the aorta in children. Br Heart J 1969; 31:127.
91. Shinebourne EA, et al. Coarctation of the aorta in infancy and childhood. Br Heart J 1976; 38:375.
92. Liberthson RR, et al. Coarctation of the aorta: review of 234 patients and clarification of management of problems. Am J Cardiol 1979; 43:835.
93. Crafoord C, Nylin G. Congenital coarctation of the aorta and its surgical treatment. J Thorac Surg 1945; 14:347.
94. Gross RE, Hufnagel CA. Coarctation of the aorta: experimental studies regarding its surgical correction. N Engl J Med 1945; 233:287.
95. Minich LL, et al. Surgical repair is safe and effective after unsuccessful balloon angioplasty of native coarctation of the aorta. J Am Coll Cardiol 1992; 19:389–393.
96. Barry A. The aortic derivatives in the human adult. Anat Rec 1948; III:221.
97. Gross RE. Surgical relief for tracheal obstruction from a vascular ring. N Engl J Med 1945; 233:586.
98. Wolman LJ. Syndrome of constricting double aortic arch in infancy: report of a case. J Pediatr 1939; 14:527.
99. Edwards JE. Anomalies of the derivatives of the aortic arch system. Med Clin N Amer (July) 1948; 6:925.
100. Kirklin JW, Clagett OT. Vascular rings producing respiratory obstruction in infants. Proc Mayo Clin 1950; 25:360.
101. Kirklin JW, Barratt-Boyes BG. Vascular rings and slings. In Cardiac Surgery. New York: Wiley, 1986. P. 1111.
102. Stewart JR, Kincaid OW, Edwards JE. An Atlas of Vascular Rings and Related Malformations of the Aortic Arch System. Springfield: Thomas, 1964.
103. Sissman NJ. Anomalies of the aortic arch complex. In FH Adams, GC Emmanouilides, eds. Moss' Heart Disease in Infants, Children and Adolescents. Baltimore: Williams & Wilkins, 1983. Pp. 199–215.
104. Taussig HB. Congenital Malformations of the Heart, 2nd ed. Vol 2. Cambridge, Mass.: Harvard University Press, 1960.
105. Lincoln JCR, et al. Vascular abnormalities compressing the esophagus and trachea. Thorax 1960; 24:295–306.
106. Binet JP, et al. Ductus arteriosus sling: report of a newly recognized anomaly and its surgical correction. Thorax 1978; 33:72.
107. Bankl H. Congenital malformations of the heart and great vessels. Synopsis of Pathology, Embryology and Natural History. Baltimore: Urban & Schwarzenberg, 1977. Pp. 159–166.
108. van Son JA, et al. Surgical treatment of vascular rings: the Mayo Clinic experience. Mayo Clin Proc 1993; 68:1056–1063.
109. Backer CL. Vascular rings, slings, and tracheal rings. Mayo Clin Proc 1993; 68:1131–1133.
110. Kirklin JW, Barrett-Boyes BG. Origin of the right or left pulmonary artery from the ascending aorta. In Cardiac Surgery, 2nd Edition. New York: Wiley, 1993. Pp. 1159–1166.
111. Keane JF, et al. Anomalous origin of one pulmonary artery from the aorta: diagnostic, physiologic and surgical considerations. Circulation 1974; 50:588.
112. Calder AL, et al. Variant of tetralogy of Fallot with absent pulmonary valve leaflets and origin of one pulmonary artery from the ascending aorta. Am J Cardiol 1980; 46:106.
113. Penkoske PA, et al. Origin of pulmonary artery branch from the ascending aorta. J Thorac Cardiovasc Surg 1983; 85:537.
114. Becker AE, Anderson RH. Malformations of the pulmonary trunk and arteries. In Pathology of Congenital Heart Disease. London: Butterworths, 1981. P. 339.
115. Beitzke A, Shinebourne EA. Single origin of right and left pulmonary arteries from ascending aorta, with main pulmonary artery from right ventricle. Br Heart J 1980; 43: 363.
116. Becker AE, Anderson RH. Aortopulmonary communications. In Pathology of Congenital Heart Disease. London: Butterworths, 1981. P. 345.
117. Kirklin JW, Barratt-Boyes BG. Aortopulmonary window. In Cardiac Surgery. 2nd Edition. New York: Wiley, 1993. Pp. 1153–1158.
118. Neufeld HN, et al. Aorticopulmonary septal defect. Am J Cardiol 1962; 9:12–25.
119. Luisi SV, et al. Anomalous origin of the right coronary artery with aortopulmonary window: functional and surgical considerations. Thorax 1980; 35:446.
120. Blieden LC, Moller JH. Aorticopulmonary septal defect. An experience with 17 patients. Br Heart J 1974; 36:630.
121. Persky MS. Congenital vascular lesions of the head and neck. Laryngoscope 1986; 96:1002.
122. Finn MC, Celowack J, Mulliken JB. Congenital vascular lesions: clinical application of a new classification. J Pediatr Surg 1983; 18:894–900.
123. Watson WL, McCarthy WD. Blood and lymph vessel tumors—a report of 1,056 cases. Surg Gynecol Obstet 1940; 71:569.
124. Jellinger K. Vascular malformations of the central nervous system: a morphologic overview. Neurosurg Rev 1986; 9:177–216.
125. Trout HH, et al. Vascular malformations. Surgery 1983; 97:36–41.
126. Neichajev IA, Clodius L. Diagnostic criteria of vascular lesions in the face. Ann Plast Surg 1993; 31:32–41.
127. Rak KM, et al. MR imaging of symptomatic peripheral vascular malformations. Am J Roentgenol 1992; 159:107–112.
128. Awad IA, et al. Mixed vascular malformations of the brain: clinical and pathogenetic considerations. Neurosurgery 1993; 33:179–188.
129. Baker LL, et al. Hemangiomas and vascular malformations of the head and neck: MR characterization. Am J Neuroradiol 1993; 14:307–314.
130. Jimenez MQ, Guillen FA. Arteriovenous fistulas. In FH Adams, GC Emmanouilides, eds. Moss' Heart Disease in Infants, Children and Adolescents. Baltimore: Williams & Wilkins, 1983. Pp. 491–500.
131. Garcia-Gonzalez R, Gonzalez-Palacios J, Maganto-Pavon E. Congenital renal arteriovenous fistula (cirsoid aneurysm). Urology 1984; 24:495.
132. Szikigyi DE, et al. Congenital arteriovenous anomalies of the limbs. Arch Surg 1976; 111:423.
133. Coleman CC. Diagnosis and treatment of congenital arteriovenous fistulas of the head and neck. Am J Surg 1973; 126:424.
134. Trout HH. Management of patients with hemangiomas and arteriovenous malformations. Surg Clin N Amer 1986; 66: 333.
135. Leikensohn JR, Epstein LI, Vasconez LO. Superselective embolization and surgery of noninvoluting hemangiomas and A-V malformations. Plast Reconstr Surg 1981; 68:143.
136. Smith HL, Horton BT. Arteriovenous fistula of the lung associated with polycythemia vera; report of a case in which the diagnosis was made clinically. Am Heart J 1939; 18:589.
137. Bosher LH, Blake A, Byrd BR. An analysis of the pathologic anatomy of pulmonary arteriovenous aneurysms with particular reference to the applicability of local excision. Surgery 1959; 45:91–104.
138. Hodgson C, et al. Hereditary hemorrhagic telangiectasia and

pulmonary arteriovenous fistula: survey of a large family. N Engl J Med 1959; 26:625.
139. Burke CM, et al. Pulmonary arteriovenous malformations: a critical update. Am Rev Respir Dis 1986; 134:334.
140. Chow LT, et al. Pulmonary arteriovenous malformation. Progressive enlargement with replacement of the entire right middle lobe in a patient with concomitant mitral stenosis. Med J Aust 1993; 158:632–634.
141. Finley JL, et al. Port wine stains. Morphologic variations and developmental lesions. Arch Dermatol 1984; 120:1253–1255.
142. Lindenauer SM. The Klippel-Trenaunay syndrome: varicosity, hypertrophy, and hemangioma with arteriovenous fistula. Ann Surg 1965; 162:303.
143. Guillen B, et al. Hereditary hemorrhagic telangiectasia: report of 15 affected cases in a Mexican family. Clin Genet 1991; 39:214–218.
144. Chu KM, Lai EC, Ng IO. Hereditary hemorrhagic telangiectasis involving the ampulla of Vater presented with recurrent gastrointestinal bleeding. Am J Gastroenterol 1993; 88:1116–1119.
145. Woods CG, Taylor AM. Ataxia telangiectasia in the British Isles: the clinical and laboratory features of 70 affected individuals. Q J Med 1992; 82:169–179.
146. Gatti RA, et al. Ataxia-telangiectasia: an interdisciplinary approach to pathogenesis. Medicine (Baltimore) 1991; 70:99–117.
147. El-Dessouky M, et al. Kasabach-Merritt syndrome. J Pediatr Surg 1988; 23:109–111.
148. Rice JS, Fischer DS. Blue rubber bleb nevus syndrome. Arch Dermatol 1962; 86:503–511.
149. Bean WB. Dyschondroplasia and hemangiomata (Maffucci's syndrome). Arch Intern Med 1958; 102:544–550.
150. Mandreoli M, Zuccala A, Zucchelli P. Fibromuscular dysplasia of the renal arteries associated with antiphospholipid autoantibodies: two case reports. Am J Kidney Dis 1992; 20:500–503.
151. Harrison EG Jr, McCormack LJ. Pathologic classification of renal arterial disease in renovascular hypertension. Mayo Clin Proc 1971; 46:161–167.
152. Luschner TF, et al. Arterial fibromuscular dysplasia. Mayo Clin Proc 1987; 62:931–952.
153. Perry MO. Fibromuscular dysplasia. Surg Gynecol Obstet 1974; 139:97–104.
154. Alimi Y, et al. Fibromuscular disease of the renal artery: a new histopathologic classification. Ann Vasc Surg 1992; 6:220–224.
155. Hata J, Hosoda Y. Perimedial fibroplasia of the renal artery. Arch Pathol Lab Med 1979; 103:220–223.
156. Sato S, Hata J. Fibromuscular dysplasia. Its occurrence with a dissecting aneurysm of the internal carotid artery. Arch Pathol Lab Med 1982; 106:332–335.
157. Thevenet A, Latil JL, Albat B. Fibromuscular disease of the external iliac artery. Ann Vasc Surg 1992; 6:199–204.
158. Gatalica Z, Gibas Z, Martinez-Hernandez A. Dissecting aortic aneurysm as a complication of generalized fibromuscular dysplasia. Hum Pathol 1992; 23:586–588.
159. Schneider PA, et al. Isolated thigh claudication as a result of fibromuscular dysplasia of the deep femoral artery. J Vasc Surg 1992; 15:657–660.
160. Insall RL, Chamberlain J, Loose HW. Fibromuscular dysplasia of visceral arteries. Eur J Vasc Surg 1992; 6:668–672.
161. Letsch R, et al. Arterial fibromuscular dysplasia. Report of a case with involvement of the aorta and review of the literature. Thorac Cardiovasc Surgeon 1980; 28:206–210.
162. Lie JT, Berg KK. Isolated fibromuscular dysplasia of the coronary arteries with spontaneous dissection and myocardial infarction. Hum Pathol 1987; 18:654–656.
163. Cheu HW, Mills JL. Digital artery embolization as a result of fibromuscular dysplasia of the brachial artery. J Vasc Surg 1991; 14:225–228.

Iatrogenic Vascular Injuries

Renu Virmani
Andrew Farb
Allen P. Burke

Although individual vascular procedures and interventions carry only a small risk of complication, the total number of patients with iatrogenic complications is not small. Because a large number of interventions and catheter placements are being performed today, complications of the procedure must be considered, especially in high-risk patients such as the elderly, female patients, diabetic individuals, immunocompromised patients, patients with bleeding diathesis, and patients with underlying pulmonary disease. As a result of a lack of awareness of certain iatrogenic vascular injuries, many complications are not recognized clinically, and it is only at autopsy that a complication is noted. In this chapter, vascular complications are considered in the following order: those involving diagnostic coronary catheterization, central venous line placement, coronary interventions, coronary revascularization surgery, and intra-aortic balloon pump placement.

Diagnostic Cardiac Catheterization

Cardiac catheterization is performed to evaluate coronary artery disease as a guide to medical or surgical therapy. Coronary angiography was first described by Sones and Shirley in 1959, using brachial-artery access; the femoral-artery approach, first described by Judkin, is more frequently used and results in comparable or reduced complication rates [1–5]. Today, angiography is performed in most general and tertiary-care hospitals, and the incidence of iatrogenic vascular injury, although low, may require surgical correction and rarely may result in death (0.14% to 0.51%) [3,6,7]. Complications include myocardial infarction, coronary dissection, serious arrhythmia, local puncture-site complications, thrombosis, false aneurysm, and cerebral ischemia [3,6,7]. The decreased complication rate during coronary angiography over time may be related to greater operator experience, the use of heparin, and shorter procedure time.

Davis et al. in 1979 reported complications occurring in 7,553 consecutive patients undergoing coronary angiography at 13 institutions and compared the complications in patients studied by brachial approach versus femoral artery approach. Although the incidences of death, myocardial infarction, cerebral ischemia, and local vascular complications were higher with the brachial than the femoral approach, there were no cases of dissection with either access site. The factors that increased the risk of complications were left main coronary artery disease, unstable angina, congestive heart failure, multiple premature ventricular contractions, and hypertension. A more recent extensive analysis of complications or coronary angiography among 222,553 patients from the Registry of the Society for Cardiac Angiography and Interventions showed death in 0.10 percent, myocardial infarction in 0.06 percent, stroke in 0.07 percent, serious arrhythmias in 0.47 percent, vascular complication in 0.46 percent, and unspecified contrast reactions in 0.23 percent [8]. The vascular complication rate was higher for the brachial than for the femoral approach, but no differences were noted for death, myocardial infarction, and stroke. The incidences of death and myocardial infarction were higher in patients with left main disease, triple-vessel disease, and ejection fraction less than 30 percent [3,7]. Possible mechanisms include coronary spasm, platelet or air emboli, and coronary dissection. Because surgery may be life-saving, prompt recognition and therapy of these major complications are imperative.

Catheter-induced coronary artery dissection is a rare complication of coronary arteriography; the reported incidence ranges from 0 percent to 0.46 percent, with decreasing incidence as operator experience increases. At least 50 cases have been reported in the literature. The patients' ages ranged from 21 to 72 years, without sex predominance [9–11]. Right coronary artery dissection is reported more frequently than the left (64% right, 36% left). Although most patients with dissection have underlying atherosclerotic disease of the involved artery, some dissections occur in angiographically normal arteries.

Various theories have been advanced for the possible mechanisms of dissection. Catheter-induced coronary-artery dissection has occurred with all types of catheters, including Sones or preformed types for percutaneous entry. Dissections have occurred before selective coronary cannulation (Fig. 55-1), as well as by the passage of a guidewire (Fig. 55-2). Most iatrogenic dissections start in close proximity to the catheter tip. Wedging of the catheter is most likely to occur in arteries with a short proximal horizontal segment. A jet of contrast agent introduced in an abnormally seated catheter with or without prior intimal damage may cause progression of the dissection. An atheromatous plaque in the proximal segment of the artery may be elevated during catheter placement and may lead to dissection. Most often, the atherosclerotic plaques have a necrotic core; the catheter traumatizes the plaque, and a contrast jet results in arterial dissection. Why dissections are not seen as frequently in the left coronary artery as in the right is poorly understood, although there is less likelihood of the left catheter to advance deeply into the left ostium and cause mechanical trauma compared to the right ostium. Morise et al. described three patients with catheter-related dissection, and all had medial necrosis of

From the Department of Cardiovascular Pathology, Armed Forces Institute of Pathology, Washington, D.C.
The opinions or assertions contained herein are the private views of the authors and are not to be construed as official or reflecting the views of the Department of the Army, the Department of the Air Force, or the Department of Defense.

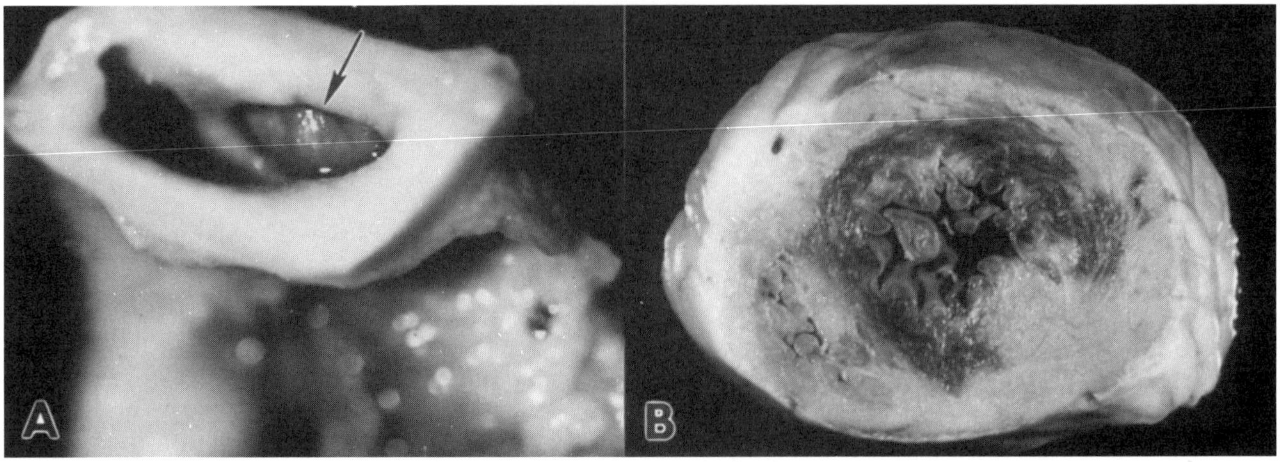

Fig. 55-1. **A.** Left main coronary ostium showing acute dissection (arrow) from a patient who died 24 hours after coronary catheterization. **B.** Bread-loaf slice of apical half of left ventricle showing subendocardial hemorrhagic infarct.

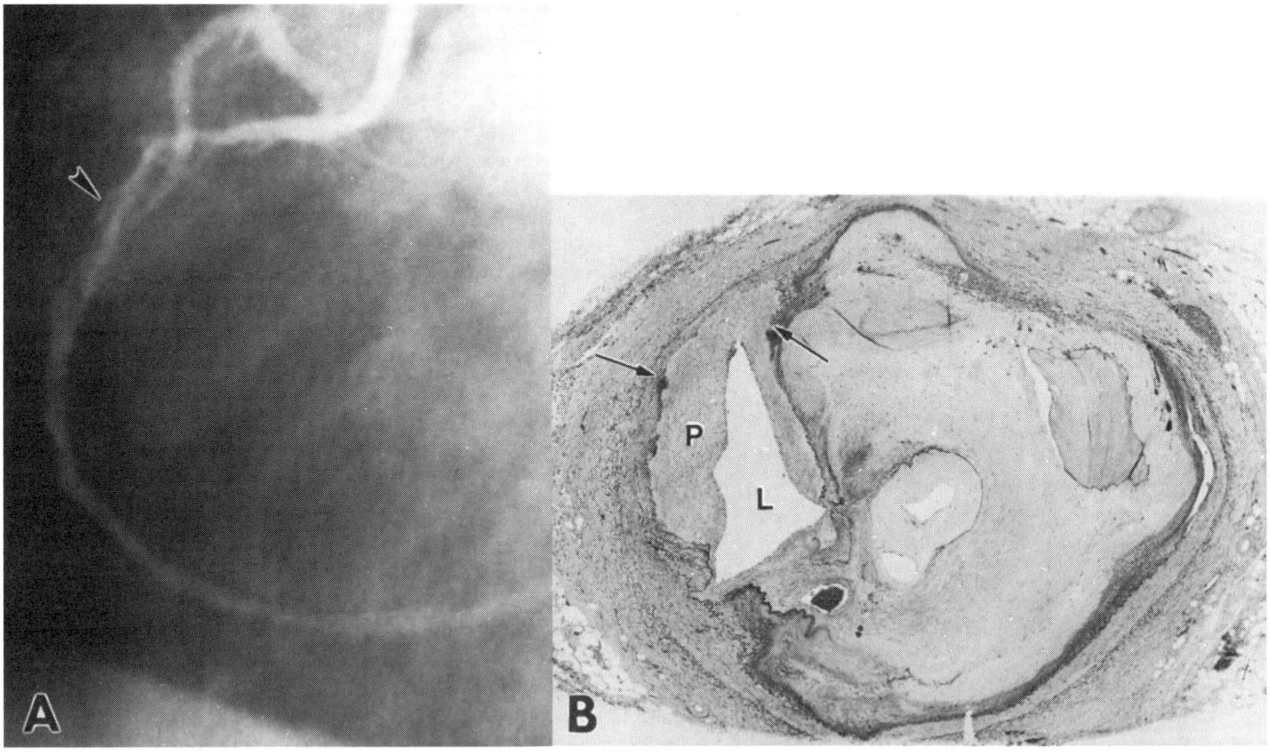

Fig. 55-2. **A.** Coronary angiogram of the right coronary artery performed in a 72-year-old man 7 weeks prior to death (left anterior oblique projection). After multiple attempts with various guidewires, there was short dissection (arrowhead) of the right coronary artery. **B.** Histologic section of the proximal right coronary artery at the site of angiographic dissection. Note disrupted segments of the internal elastic lamina (arrows) and fibrocellular proliferation (P) expanding the dissected media. (L = lumen.) (Reproduced with permission from A Farb et al. Percutaneous transluminal coronary angioplasty guidewire-induced coronary artery dissection without balloon inflation. Hum Pathol 1991; 22:97–98.)

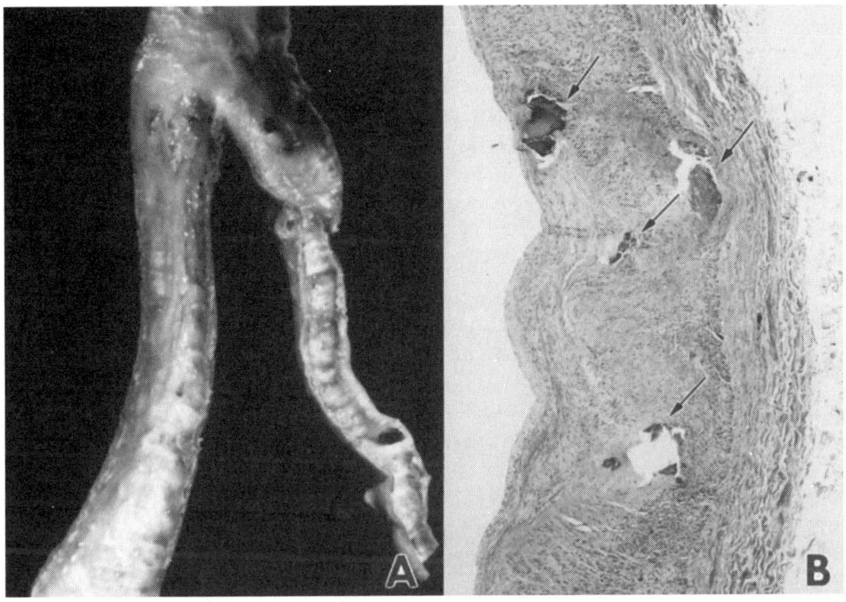

Fig. 55-3. A 79-year-old male who underwent cardiac catheterization for symptomatic coronary heart disease died 12 hours postprocedure from massive bleeding from puncture site. **A.** Gross photograph of the distal aorta and bifurcation of the iliac arteries; note thick, stiff walls with intimal rugal folds. **B.** Histologic section of the iliac artery showing marked medial calcification, which prevented arterial vasoconstriction.

the coronary artery at autopsy. Therefore, they postulated that the presence of medial necrosis may increase the risk of dissection. Our own experience in 16 patients with spontaneous coronary-artery dissection is that only two had medial necrosis [12,13]. Therefore, the presence of an abnormal vessel wall, that is, atheroma or medial necrosis is not a prerequisite for dissection.

Because catheter-induced coronary spasm is not uncommon during catheterization, it is important to clinically differentiate spasm from dissection. Coronary dissections can occur in atherosclerotic or normal arteries, there usually is an intimal flap, the contrast agent shows slow filling or washout in dissected vessels (or both), and dissections extend with repeat injections of dye. Conversely, spasm almost always occurs in areas of atherosclerosis, an intimal flap is absent, the contrast agent shows slow filling or washout only when there is underlying severe obstruction, and repeated injections of dye into the vessel do not cause progressive narrowing. In contrast to catheter-induced spasm, which rarely results in irreversible ischemia, dissections of coronary artery often result in myocardial infarction.

The local complications of catheterization in the brachial location include injury to the median nerve and hemorrhage during surgical arterial exposure. Dehiscence of arterial sutures, arteritis, fistulas, and cellulitis are delayed complications of brachial-artery catheterization. Complications related to the femoral-artery approach include hematoma with vascular and neural compression, arterial and venous thrombosis, distal embolization, false aneurysm, rupture of either the femoral or iliac arteries (Fig. 55-3), rupture of aortic aneurysm, aortic and iliac-artery dissection, arteriovenous fistula, and delayed hemorrhage. Hemorrhage may be related to anticoagulation, and patients often require blood transfusion.

Complications of Central Venous Catheters

Central venous catheters (CVCs) have become indispensable in the treatment of the critically ill patient. Long-term CVCs are being used extensively for chemotherapy, for parenteral nutrition and for hemodialysis. CVCs are also used as diagnostic tools in the differential diagnosis of cardiogenic versus noncardiogenic pulmonary edema, constrictive versus restrictive cardiomyopathy, and congestive heart failure versus chronic obstructive pulmonary disease [14–16]. CVCs routinely are used in intensive-care settings for hemodynamic monitoring of cardiogenic shock, adult respiratory distress syndrome, and septic shock [14]. There is, however, a lack of appreciation of the severity of complications that may accompany the use of CVCs. All CVC procedures may result in life-threatening complications: cardiac perforation, tamponade, hydrothorax, hemothorax, pneumothorax, chylothorax, and hydromediastinum. Other less serious complications include those related to positioning, such as mural thrombus, knotted catheters, cardiac arrhythmias, and infections. Specific indications for the use of CVCs must be thoroughly reviewed and the risk-benefit ratios determined to justify their placement.

For venous access of pulmonary-artery catheters, Seneff recommends the right internal jugular vein (IJV) or, alternatively, the subclavian vein (SV) [14]. For emergency transvenous pacing, the right IJV should be used because of the direct route to the right ventricle or, as a second choice, the subclavian vein. For total parenteral nutrition with hyperosmolar solutions, the SV is preferable (although the IJV may be used) because of the ease of catheter management and the patient's comfort [14]. In patients requiring preoperative CVC placement, the right IJV is the vein of choice, since there is less chance of pneumothorax [14].

There are no definite contraindications to CVCs in patients requiring their use; specific sites, however, may be contraindicated. For example, the IJV and the SV should not be used in patients with prolonged clotting times or platelet counts less than 50,000/cu mm, because it may be difficult to directly compress the SV or subclavian artery [1]. The SV should not be used in a patient with respiratory compromise because a pneumothorax is likely to be poorly tolerated acutely. Sites with previous surgery, trauma, infection, thrombosis, or an anatomic anomaly should not be used [17].

The most innocuous location for the catheter tip is in the distal innominate or proximal superior vena cava because the complications associated with those locations are minimal [18]. The catheter-tip position should be verified radiographically and regularly monitored. The right atrium is not an acceptable location because of the following complications: right atrial perforation with cardiac tamponade, supraventricular arrhythmias, and migration of the catheter tip to the inferior vena cava, hepatic veins, right ventricle, or pulmonary arteries [14,19]. The routes used for central venous catheters (Fig. 55-4) and specific complications of each site are discussed next.

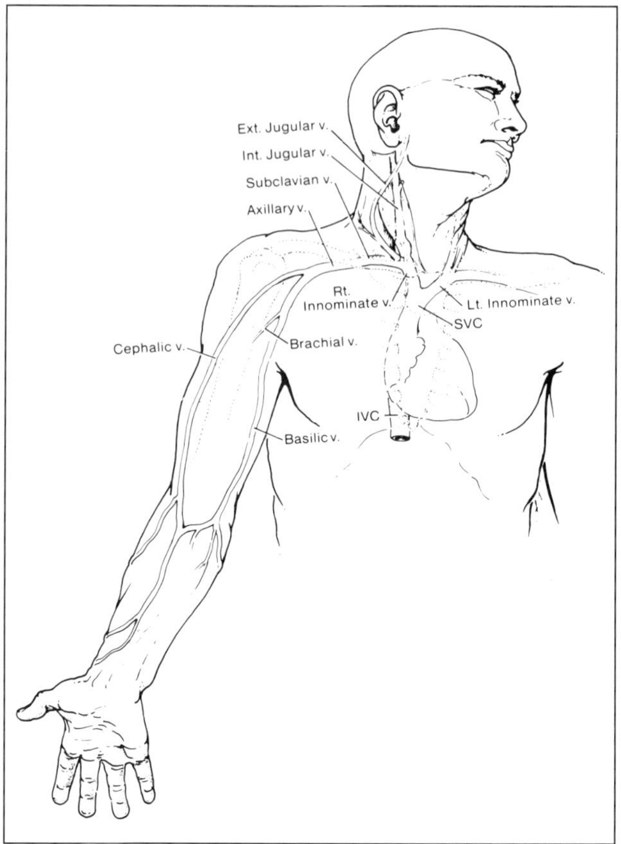

Fig. 55-4. Anatomy of the neck and arm veins used for central venous catheterization.

THE VEINS OF THE ANTECUBITAL FOSSA

The veins available for cannulation are the basilic (success rate 60–80% at first attempt), cephalic (30–50%), and brachial (which is difficult to cannulate by venipuncture). The advantage of those sites is the low incidence of major thoracic complications [14]. The sites also can be used in the presence of clotting abnormalities; however, catheter insertion is time consuming and the success rate is lower than that using SV or IJV access. The right arm should be chosen first, because the distance traversed by the catheter is shorter than it would be in the left arm [14].

Thrombotic complications can be of three types: local sterile phlebitis (5–15%), deep-vein thrombosis (1–2%), and pulmonary embolism (0.5%) [14]. Thrombotic complications are related to the length of the time the catheter has been in place, and the risk increases markedly after 48 to 72 hours. Infectious complications such as cellulitis, septic phlebitis, bacteremia, and septicemia occur in 1–2 percent of veins when catheter duration is less than 3 days. The infection rate increases dramatically after 3 days [15,20]. Other complications include catheter embolism, air embolism, perforation of the central veins, and pericardial tamponade [14].

EXTERNAL JUGULAR VEIN

Serious complications arising from the right external jugular vein approach are rare, and nearly all the complications are the result of catheter maintenance rather than venipuncture [14]. In 1–5 percent of patients, there will be a hematoma formed at the site of venipuncture. Other complications include right atrial or ventricular wall rupture with pericardial tamponade and catheter embolism [15]. Thrombus is detected clinically in 3–5 percent of patients and is dependent on the number of days the catheter has been in place. The reported infection rate is 1–2 percent for catheters in place for less than 3 days [14].

FEMORAL VEIN

Femoral-artery puncture is a frequent (4–6%) complication of attempted femoral venopuncture because of the proximity of the artery to the vein. Arterial punctures usually are inconsequential; however, a large hematoma may form in 1 percent of cases. Other reported complications include arteriovenous fistulas and pseudoaneurysms [14]. With systemic anticoagulation, vein puncture can cause scrotal bleeding or retroperitoneal bleeding, which may be massive and life threatening [14].

Because femoral vein catheterization occurs at a joint line, catheter breakage and embolization are significant risks. Venous thrombus is the most feared complication, and the incidence increases with the duration that the catheter is in place. Infectious complications have been reported in 1–2 percent of cases when the catheter has been in place for less than 24 hours. Thus, the femoral vein is a useful site for short-term catheterization only [14].

INTERNAL JUGULAR VEIN

The IJV is probably the safest site for a CVC; it has a high success rate and a low incidence of major complications

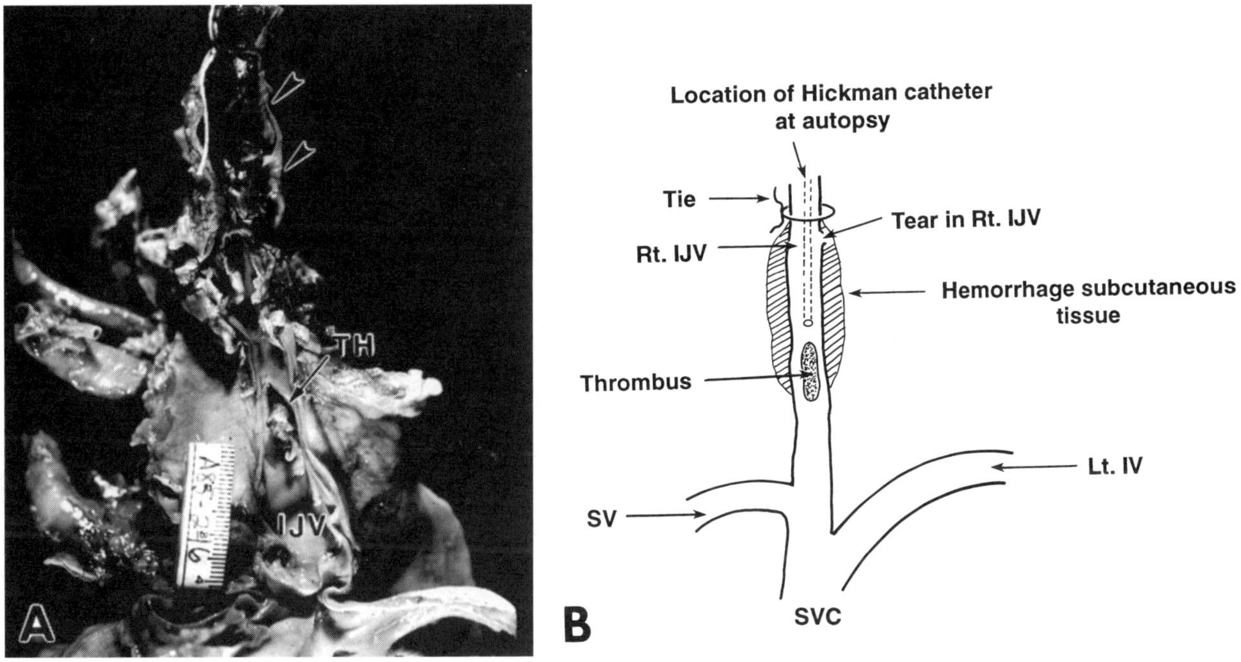

Fig. 55-5. A 67-year-old female with cholecyto-jejunostomy and duodenostomy had a Hickman catheter inserted via right jugular vein, which resulted in acute blood loss of 2,000 cc. Patient became hypotensive, bradycardic, and cyanotic. Resuscitation measures were successful, but patient remained unconscious without cerebral function. Five days later, the respirator was disconnected, and the patient died. At autopsy, there was extensive hemorrhage into the soft tissues of the neck, with adventitial hematoma involving the right carotid artery. A thrombus was present in the right jugular vein that extended into the right innominate and subclavian veins. **A.** Gross photograph of the veins of the right neck showing extensive hematoma (arrowheads) around the right internal jugular vein and presence of thrombus (TH, arrow). **B.** Line drawing of the specimen in A showing the various branches, catheter location, and tear in the right internal jugular vein (Rt IJV). (SV = subclavian vein, SVC = superior vena cava, Lt. IV = left innominate vein.)

[21]. It is the ideal site for Swan-Ganz catheters and temporary venous pacemakers. On the right side, the IJV and the SV form a straight path to the superior vena cava. On the left side, the IJV joins the left SV at right angles and the left innominate vein enters the superior vena cava at almost a right angle, thus forcing the catheter to make several sharp turns on its way toward the heart [21].

The complication rate for insertion of IJV catheters ranges in most reports from 0.1–4.2 percent. In three series, however, the incidence was greater than 8 percent [22]. Carotid-artery puncture represents 80–90 percent of all complications [22], and arterial puncture may result in arteriovenous fistulas and pseudoaneurysm [22]. However, the vast majority of complications are minor hematomas [22]. Infrequently, large hematomas form (Fig. 55-5) and may exert pressure, causing airway compromise and nerve compression requiring surgical evacuation [22].

Other complications that occur with IJV catheterization are pneumothorax, thrombosis, tracheal puncture, air embolism, catheter embolism, pericardial tamponade, and cerebrovascular accident [21]. Pneumothorax occurs in 0–0.2 percent of cases and is associated with punctures close to the clavicle or guidewire puncture through the IJV. Thrombosis is unlikely to occur with IJV catheterization because of the large diameter of the vein and the straight path of the vessel. Infectious complications occur in 1–3 percent of cases and are usually related to inexperience of the operator and long duration of catheter use [21].

SUBCLAVIAN VEIN

The SV is the vein of choice for long-term intravenous total parenteral nutrition (TPN) [21,22]. Subclavian catheterization is successful, usually at first attempt, in 90–95 percent of cases. Catheter malposition occurs in 5–20 percent of cases (Fig. 55-6), and the most frequent sites are the ipsilateral IJV and the contralateral SV. Major complications occur in 1–3 percent of cases, and the overall complication rate is 5 percent [23]. Complications occur most frequently from operator inexperience, multiple punctures, and catheterization under emergency situations [21]. Pneumothorax (1–2%), arterial puncture, thromboembolism, and infections [21] are the major complications. Pneumothorax usually results from puncture of the lung at the time of the procedure. Late pneumothorax also has been reported. Subclavian-artery puncture occurs in 0.5 percent of cases and can be controlled by local pres-

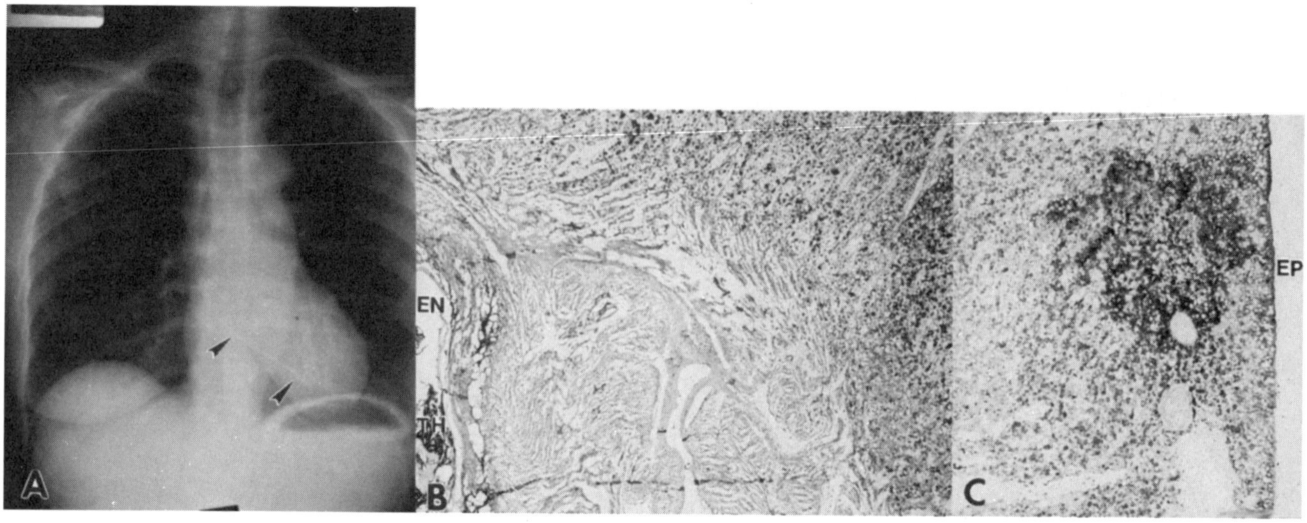

Fig. 55-6. A 54-year-old female had a hyperalimentation catheter placed 14 days after antrectomy and vagotomy. Cardiac arrest occurred 3 days later. **A.** X-ray demonstrated tip of catheter (arrowhead) in right ventricle; bradycardia and hypotension followed by cardiac arrest. Patient was resuscitated for 20 minutes and died in 3 days with anoxic encephalopathy. At autopsy, there were 100 cc of milky white fluid in the pericardial sac. A nodular lesion was noted in the epicardial surface of anterior right ventricle measuring 0.5 to 1.0 cm in diameter. **B, C.** Right ventricular endocardium had a thrombus, and the nodular lesion of the right ventricular wall had extensive fat globules (appearing as large black dots) that stained red with oil red O stain. (EN = endocardium; EP = epicardium, TH = thrombus.)

sure. Thrombosis usually is underdiagnosed clinically; the autopsy rate is 20–40 percent (Figs. 55-7, 55-8).

The incidence of clinically evident large vein thrombosis following TPN administration is 1–3 percent. However, phlebography demonstrates fibrin sleeves in 40–90 percent, nonocclusive mural thrombi in 5–10 percent, and occlusive thrombi in 5–10 percent of TPN catheters. Complications of thrombosis include superior vena cava syndrome and pulmonary embolism (Fig. 55-9). The infectious complication rate of TPN catheters is 1–3 percent; the infection rate is higher, however, when catheters are inserted in the critical-care setting and when they are maintained for more than 3 to 5 days [14]. It has been suggested that changing catheters every 3 days reduces the rate of infection. However, Cobb et al. demonstrated recently that replacement of CVC every 3 days does not prevent infections and that, in fact, exchanging catheters with guide wires increases the risk of infection [24].

Complications of Coronary-Artery Interventions

In the 1980s and 1990s, cardiac catheterization began to be used to treat cardiac disease with the aim of increasing myocardial blood flow [25,26]. Interventions included balloon dilatation catheters, lasers, atherectomy catheters, and endovascular stents [27–29]. Although those interventions generally are safe, none is free of complications [30–32]. Catheter-induced complications include arrhythmia, arterial embolization, thrombosis, vascular injury at the entry site and at the tip of the catheter, dissection, rupture, contrast-agent toxicity, and late complication of restenosis [30–36]. Balloon angioplasty results in the cracking of the atherosclerotic plaque as well as stretching and even rupture of the media and adventitia, with resultant enlargement of the vessel lumen and increased blood flow [17,37–41]. The use of larger balloons and high inflation pressures (10 to 20 atm) may be required in calcified, rigid lesions and may result in greater trauma to the vessel with subsequent increase in the complication rate [33,34]. Because the angiographer is unable to accurately assess lesion morphology, and because angioplasty results in uncontrolled injury, the probability of complications for an individual patient is unknown.

The complications associated with balloon angioplasty, atherectomy, lasers, and stents are essentially similar to those associated with diagnostic catheterization, but a few complications are seen with greater frequency with interventions. Abrupt closure is the major cause of morbidity and mortality and is seen in 3 to 8 percent of interventional procedures [42–48]. Coronary-artery dissection (Fig. 55-10) is the major cause of abrupt closure, and hypotension during or soon after angioplasty often precedes abrupt closure. The clinical and angiographic characteristics associated with abrupt closure are listed in Table 55-1 [49]. Although successful resolution can be achieved by use of autoperfusion catheters, atherectomy, and stenting, morbidity is high. Mortality ranges from 4 to 10 percent; 20 to 30 percent of patients require emergency bypass surgery; and 9 percent have Q-wave infarction [44,48,50]. Other complications of balloon angioplasty include embolization of atherosclerotic plaque or thrombus, coronary perforation, laceration, and rupture of coronary

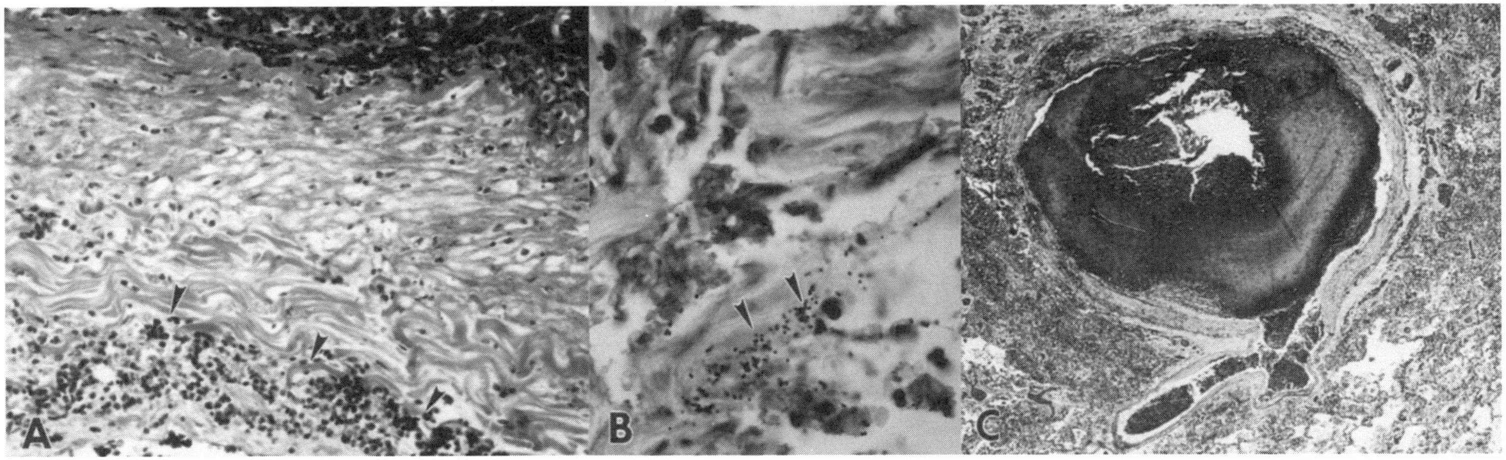

Fig. 55-7. A 52-year-old male with idiopathic dilated cardiomyopathy had Swan-Ganz catheter placed for hemodynamic monitoring through right subclavian vein. A subcutaneous abscess formed at the catheter site; culture grew *Staphylococcus aureus*. Patient died of multiple pulmonary emboli 7 days after Swan-Ganz catheter placement. **A.** Histologic section of the subcutaneous tissue showing collection of polymorphonuclear leukocytes (arrowheads). **B.** Brown and Hopps stain demonstrating gram positive cocci (arrowheads). **C.** Pulmonary embolus in a muscular pulmonary artery.

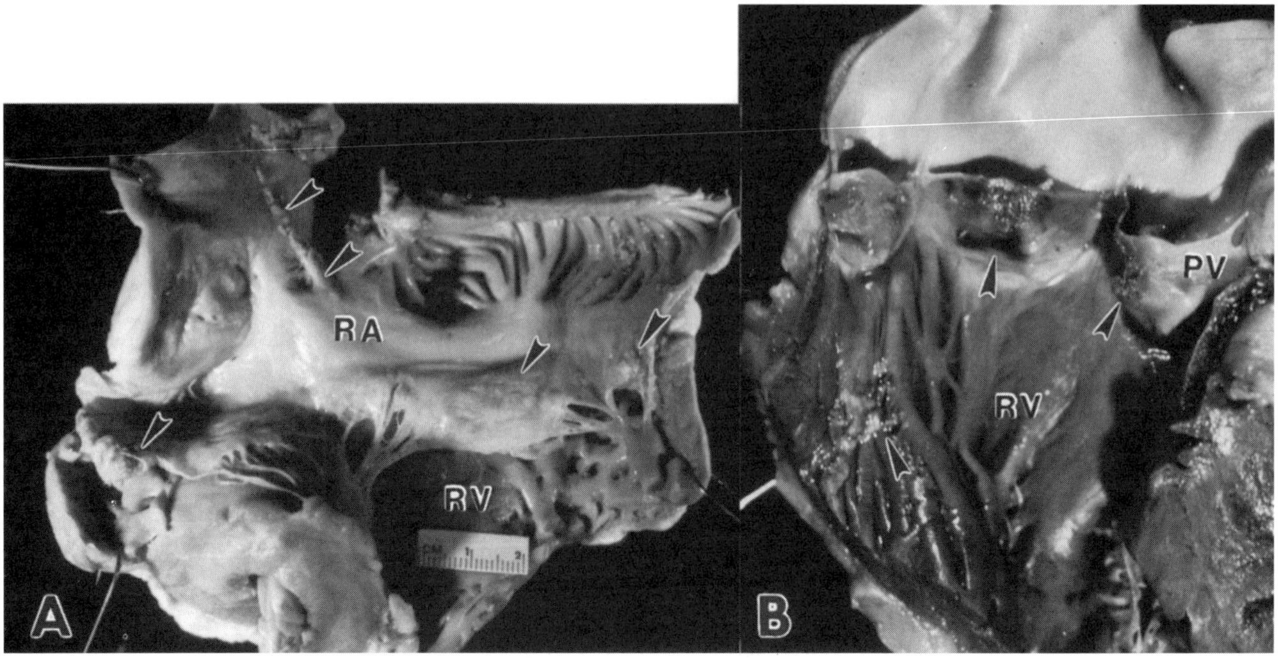

Fig. 55-8. **A.** A 39-year-old woman with metastatic breast carcinoma had a central catheter for hyperalimentation. Note marantic endocarditis of the superior vena cava and tricuspid valve (arrowheads). (RA = right atrium, RV = right ventricle.) **B.** A 63-year-old female with metastatic melanoma had a flow-directed pulmonary-artery catheter placed for hemodynamic monitoring 6 days before death. At autopsy, patient had marantic endocarditis involving the superior vena cava, tricuspid valve, right ventricular (RV) outflow tract, and pulmonary valve (PV). Photograph shows thrombi in right ventricular outflow tract and on two of three pulmonary valve leaflets (arrowheads).

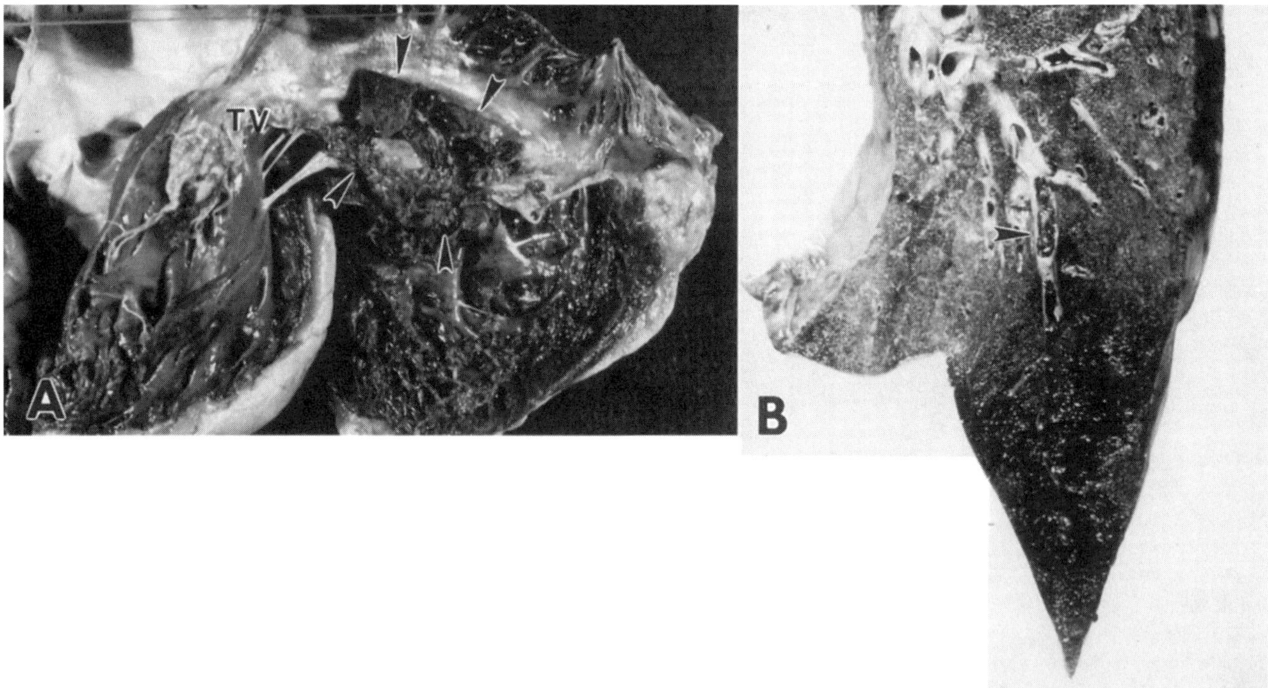

Fig. 55-9. A 31-year-old burn victim had Swan-Ganz catheter placement for hemodynamic monitoring 7 days prior to death. Blood cultures obtained 1 day before death grew fungal forms identified as *Candida albicans*. At autopsy, there were tricuspid valve endocarditis, **A,** and pulmonary emboli (arrow) with infarction of the left lower lobe, **B**.

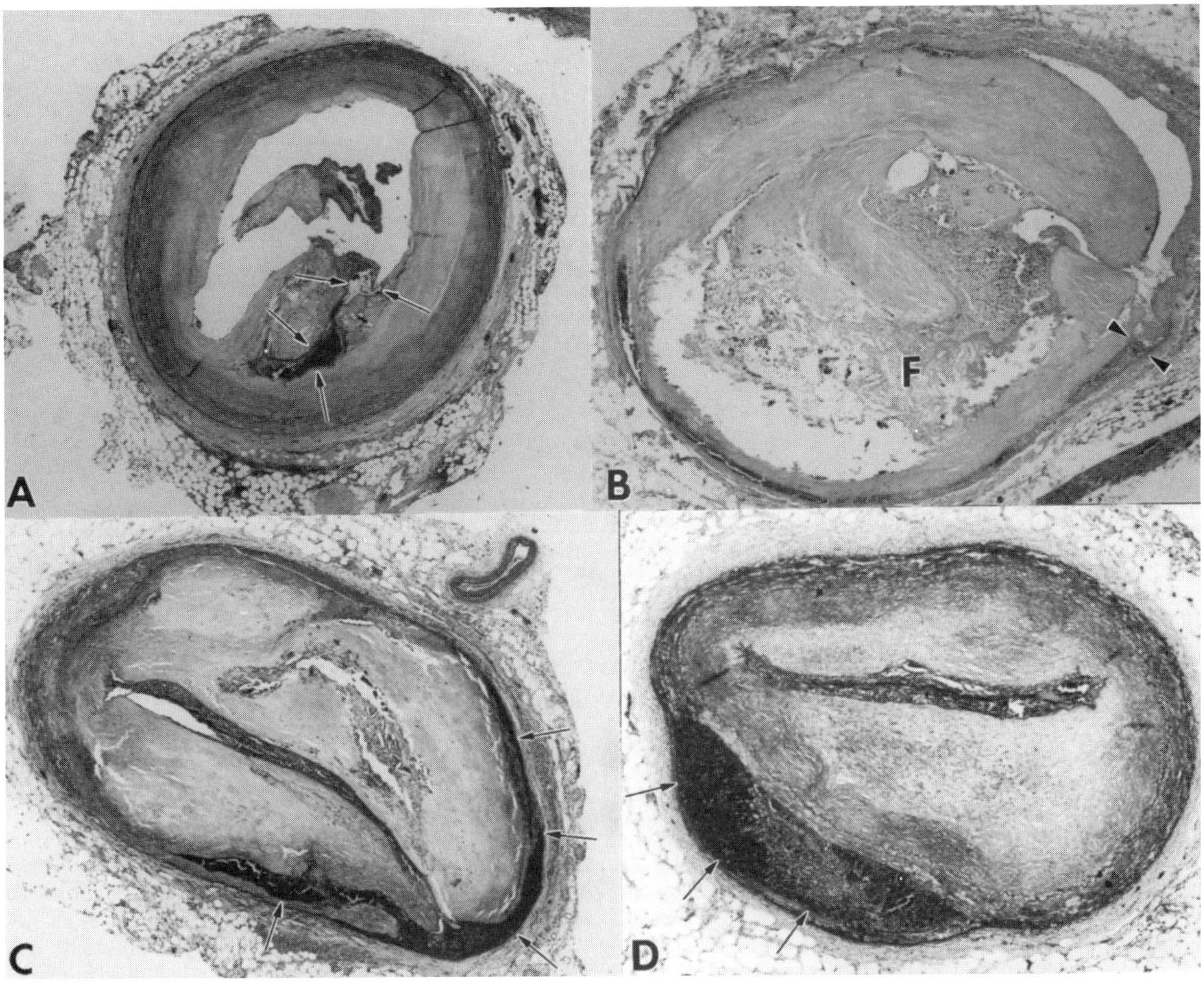

Fig. 55-10. Serial sections from a left anterior descending coronary artery from a patient who died 3 days after angioplasty, demonstrating proximal pathologic success but distal failure as a result of extensive longitudinal dissection. **A.** Note intimal cracks (arrows) (Movat stain, × 25). **B.** Intimal split extends into fibropultaceous debris (F) with an accompanying medial dissection (arrowheads) (hematoxylin-eosin stain, × 30). **C, D.** Note dissecting hematoma within the media and between the media and the adventitia (arrows), resulting in critical luminal compromise (C, Movat stain, × 15; D, Movat stain, × 20). (Reproduced with permission from A Farb et al. Plaque morphology and pathologic changes in arteries from patients dying after balloon angioplasty. J Am Coll Cardiol 1990; 16:1421–1429.)

artery with hemopericardium and tamponade. The incidence of atherosclerotic-plaque embolization (Fig. 55-11) following angioplasty is greater in saphenous-vein bypass graft atherosclerosis than in native coronary atherosclerosis. Saber et al. reported the rate of embolization to be as high as 81 percent after coronary balloon angioplasty or thrombolytic therapy [51]. In their study [51], emboli were composed of thrombus in 49 percent, atheromatous plaque in 29 percent, a mixture of thrombus and atheroma in 17 percent, and foreign material in 5 percent [51].

Coronary balloon angioplasty has been plagued since its inception by a high restenosis rate [52,53]. Using a definition of greater than 50-percent-diameter stenosis at follow-up angiography, the restenosis rate is 30–40 percent [54]. The pathogenesis of restenosis (neointimal proliferation) is not completely understood, but it involves organization of a thrombus at the site of injury and smooth muscle cell proliferation in a matrix rich in proteoglycans (Fig. 55-12) [39]. The pathologic features of restenosis are nonspecific, because all interventions are accompanied by trauma to the vessel, which will heal by a process of thrombosis, granulation tissue, and neointimal formation. Thus far, none of the randomized pharmacologic drug trials has shown that that process in humans can be reduced. A major determinant of long-term success, as suggested by Kuntz et al., is dependent on the creation of a

Table 55-1. Factors predictive of abrupt vessel closure

Factor
PREPROCEDURE
Clinical factors
Female sex
Unstable angina
Insulin-dependent diabetes mellitus
Inadequate antiplatelet therapy
Angiographic factors
Intracoronary thrombus
>90% stenosis
Stenosis length 2 or more luminal diameters
Stenosis at branch point
Stenosis on bend (45-degree angle)
Right coronary-artery stenosis
POSTPROCEDURE
Intimal dissection >10 mm
Residual stenosis >50%
Transient in-lab closure
Residual transstenotic gradient 20 mm Hg

Source: Reproduced with permission from Ryan et al. Guidelines for percutaneous transluminal coronary angioplasty. A report of the American Heart Association/American College of Cardiology Task Force on assessment of diagnostic and therapeutic cardiovascular procedures. (Committee on Percutaneous Transluminal Angioplasty). Circulation 1993; 88:2987–3007.

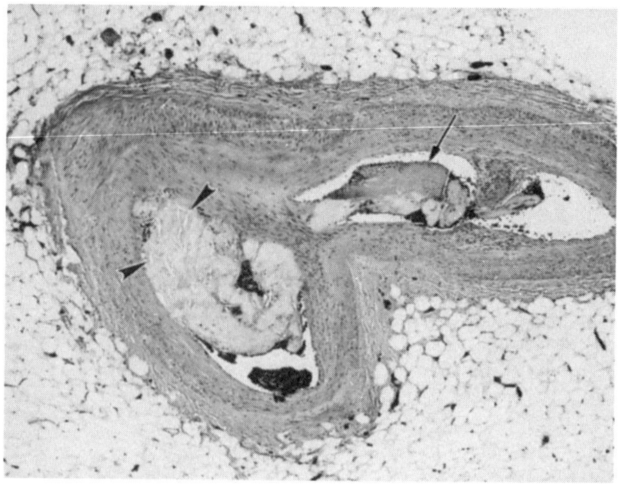

Fig. 55-11. Atheroembolus in a distal small epicardial coronary artery. The lumen shows presence of pultaceous debris, cholesterol clefts (arrowheads), and thrombus (arrow) (H&E × 40).

larger lumen at the time of balloon angioplasty, since the amount of neointimal proliferation is similar with different interventions [55].

The peripheral vascular complications of therapeutic coronary interventions are similar to those seen with diagnostic catheterization, the most frequent being false aneurysms and bleeding. Higher complication rates are seen with use of large guiding catheters, prolonged procedures, advanced age of the patients, and use of heparin or fibrinolytic agents prior to the procedure [56].

Vascular Complications of Cardiac Surgery

Coronary bypass surgery has proved to be efficacious in patients with triple-vessel disease and left main disease [57]. In 1987, approximately 230,000 coronary bypass operations were performed; the operative mortality at most major medical centers is 1 to 2 percent or less [58]. Mortality was associated with patient age greater than 60 years, diabetes mellitus, left ventricular hypertrophy, hypertension, poor left ventricular function, severe angina, and, in some series, female sex [59]. Operative death may result from myocardial necrosis (55%), miscellaneous operative and systemic complications (24%), nonanatomic causes (13%), and technical factors (8%) [60,61]. The vascular complications from bypass surgery can be early, intermediate, and late. They include graft thrombosis (8–12%), technical factors (excessive graft length and tension), atheroma at the arteriotomy site, poor runoff, coronary dissections, atheroemboli, accelerated intimal hyperplasia, and graft atherosclerosis [62–70].

Perioperative myocardial infarction occurs in about 5 percent of patients undergoing coronary bypass surgery. Graft thrombosis is an uncommon finding in patients dying with perioperative myocardial infarct. Although it previously was believed that incomplete revascularization was the underlying cause of perioperative infarcts, an association between prolonged bypass time and perioperative infarction has been demonstrated.

Rare causes of mortality are inadvertent cutting of a major vessel, excessive bleeding from surgical wounds, especially in patients undergoing reoperations, and perioperative coronary-artery dissection [71]. The etiology of the dissection may be related to blunt trauma, intraluminal damage from a cannula, and dissection at the site of incision into the artery for anastomosis. Dissections also may complicate aortic-valve replacement, especially with Starr-Edwards prostheses. In such cases, a combination of aortic-wall necrosis resulting from stretching by the rigid valve frame and isolated coronary arterial systolic hypertension contribute to coronary dissection [71].

EARLY GRAFT CLOSURE

Early graft closure can result from mechanical problems, including faulty surgical technique, inadequate size of the coronary vessels, and poor runoff [72]. Mechanical problems are rare and include taut grafts and twisting of the grafts [73].

Thrombosis is a universal result of venous-graft placement. A fine deposit of platelet, fibrin, erythrocytes, and polymorphonuclear leukocytes in the intima of the vein graft is seen consistently in patients who die shortly after operation. The incidence of a fine layer of fibrin thrombus on the intima of saphenous vein grafts has been reported to be 73 percent in patients who die within 24 hours of surgery [74]. Various blood elements can be seen in the intima of some patients, suggesting insudation of blood elements secondary to increased permeability of the endothelium, probably from high arterial pressure in the lumen [75]. In an experimental model of saphenous-vein grafts [76], it has been shown that the endothelium sloughs and platelet microthrombi form. That development may be related to vessel-wall injury caused by high flow or "jet"

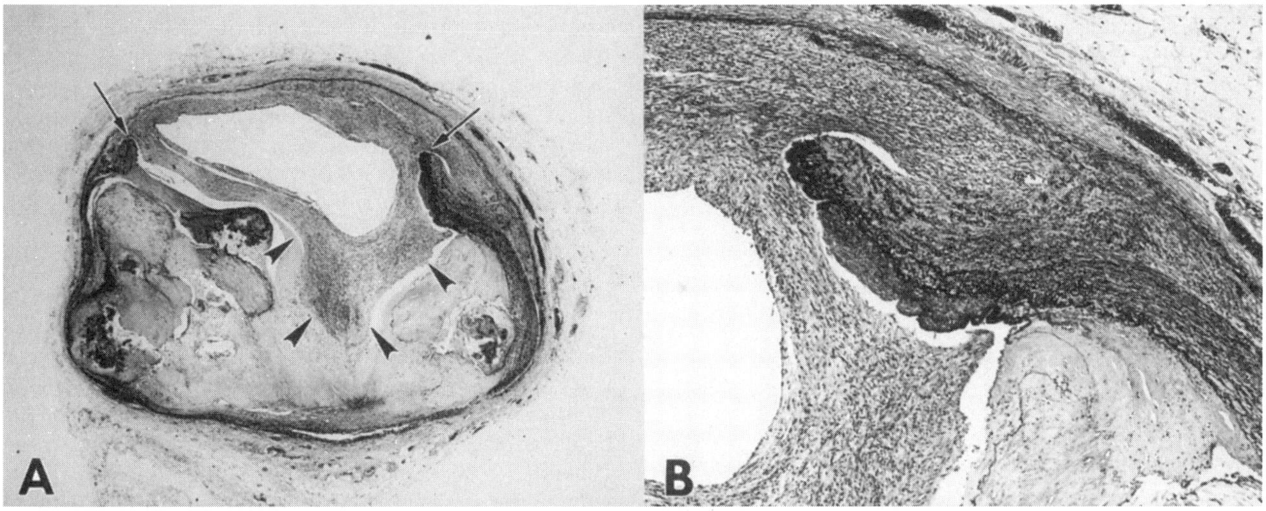

Fig. 55-12. Coronary-artery sections from 62-year-old man who underwent balloon angioplasty 20 months before his death. **A.** Note highly calcified fibrous plaque with eccentric lumen. Media is ruptured (arrows), and lumen immediately after angioplasty was markedly enlarged (acute lumen = final lumen + area of neointimal proliferation). Area of neointima is enclosed by arrowheads. **A, B.** Profuse proliferation of spindle-shaped smooth muscle cells in neointima occurred, which resulted in an 80-percent cross-sectional area luminal narrowing (Movat stain; A × 15, B × 50. (Reproduced with permission from R Virmani, A Farb, AP Burke. Coronary angioplasty from the perspective of atherosclerotic plaque: morphologic predictors of immediate success and restenosis. Am Heart J 1994; 127:163–179.)

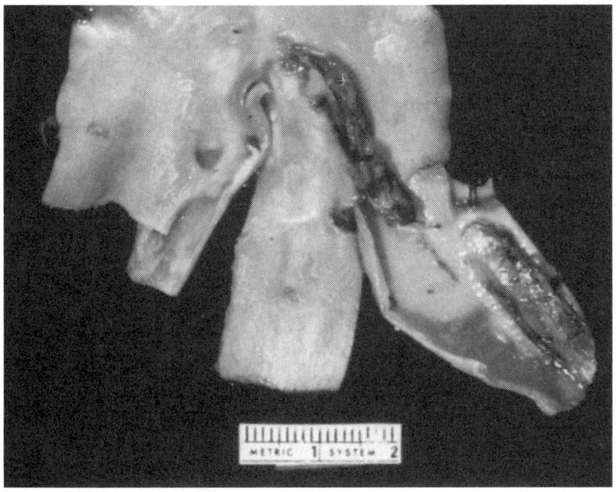

Fig. 55-13. Intimal surface of the abdominal aorta and common iliac arteries, showing thrombus in the left common iliac artery in a 50-year-old man. The thrombus was adherent to both the balloon device and the intima of the left common iliac artery. The balloon produced transient hemodynamic benefit for 2 days before refractory hypotension from hypertrophic cardiomyopathy developed. (Reproduced with permission from JM Isner et al. Complications of the intra-aortic balloon counter pulsation device: clinical and morphologic observations in 45 necropsy patients. Am J Cardiol 1980; 45:260–268.)

lesions. In humans, thrombus probably is a response to the endothelial injury that is probably an unavoidable consequence of manipulation and preparation of the graft [77,78].

Although small nonocclusive thrombi are common, occlusive thrombi rarely form within 24 hours of implantation. However, 33 percent of graft occlusions within 30 days of operation [79] are caused by thrombi, and the incidence of thrombus reaches 75 percent in patients who die more than 1 month after operation [79]. Patients treated with warfarin or dipyridamole and aspirin have a higher patency rate after coronary bypass surgery [80,81].

Another cause of early graft closure is compression, or loss of circumference of coronary artery when part of the native coronary wall is averted or compressed by suturing during construction of graft artery anastomosis [79]. Griffith and associates [79] have calculated the percent reduction in luminal area in coronary arteries secondary to eversion of the arterial wall. In a 2-mm artery, suture bites that are 0.5 mm or 1.0 mm back from the edge of the arteriotomy result in reduction of the cross-sectional area of the coronary lumen by 29 and 54 percent, respectively. In a 1-mm artery, on the other hand, the same two sutures will reduce the area by 52 and 89 percent, respectively.

An important factor in the development of thrombosis and graft closure is the presence of severe atherosclerotic plaque in the distal segment of the coronary artery. Plaque results in reduced internal circumference of the arterial wall available for anastomosis; plaque that is present distal to the anastomosis will reduce coronary flow, and, thereby, predispose to thrombosis [79]. If atherosclerotic

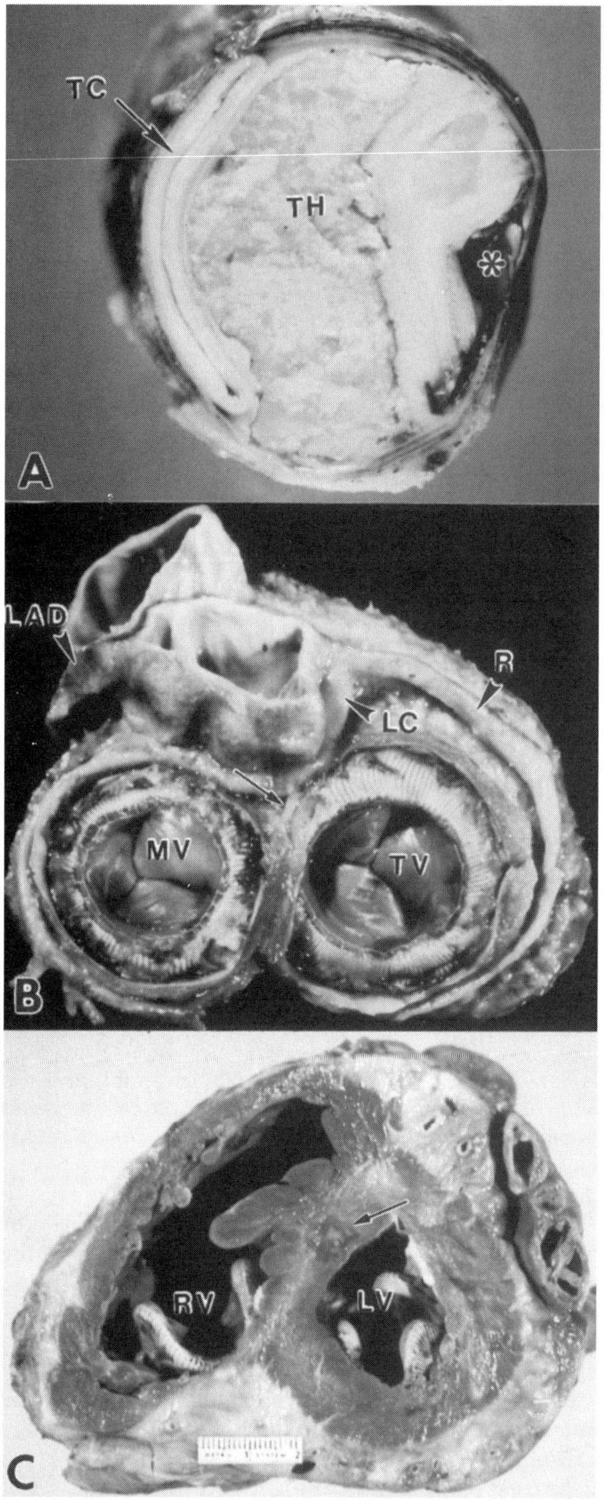

Fig. 55-14. Aorta and heart in a 65-year-old woman with aortic dissection at the time of insertion of IABAD. **A.** Intimal surface of abdominal aorta showed ulcerated atherosclerotic plaque where balloon catheter left the true lumen of the aorta and entered the medial wall of the aorta, producing a false channel filled with thrombus (TH) that compressed the true channel (TC), virtually closing it. The residual site of the balloon catheter is shown by an asterisk. **B.** The patient had the balloon inserted intraoperatively because she could not be weaned from cardiopulmonary bypass after replacement of the mitral valve (MV) and tricuspid valve (TV) with porcine prostheses. The balloon was removed on the third postoperative day, when she was in hemodynamically stable condition. (LAD = left anterior descending coronary artery; LC = left circumflex coronary artery, with anomalous origin from right coronary; R = right coronary artery.) Note compression of a branch of left circumflex artery between mitral and tricuspid prostheses (arrow). **C.** Note focal myocardial necrosis, ventricular septum (arrow) from compression of the branch of the left circumflex artery. (Reproduced with permission from JM Isner et al. Complications of the intra-aortic balloon counter pulsation device: clinical and morphologic observations in 45 necropsy patients. Am J Cardiol 1980; 45:260–268.)

plaque is present at the site of anastomosis, it may detach from the coronary wall and result in coronary-artery dissection at the level of the vein graft, as well as distal to the anastomosis. The length of the dissection, however, usually is short. Spray and Roberts [77] report a 17-percent incidence, and Griffith and co-workers report an 8-percent incidence of coronary-artery dissection at graft anastomoses [79]. Although the incidence of dissection is low, it is an important cause of lumen compression.

Complications of the Intra-aortic Balloon Assist Device

The intra-aortic balloon assist device (IABAD) has been in use for longer than three decades. Although the balloon device was initially developed for the treatment of patients with cardiogenic shock, its application has been expanded to include prophylactic management of patients with severe left ventricular dysfunction (with or without myocardial necrosis), intra- or postoperative open-heart surgery, high-risk or complicated coronary angioplasty, and end-stage cardiomyopathy.

Intra-aortic balloon counter pulsation can result in iatrogenic vascular injury. After the first decade of IABAD, the complication rate ranged from 0 to 36 percent, with an average of 12 percent [81]. More recently, the clinical incidence of complications has varied from 9 to 15 percent. The autopsy rate of complications is as high as 36 percent, because clinical recognition occurs only when there are catastrophic complications [82–84].

The most frequent complication of IABAD is dissection of the aorta, its distal branches, or both. Other less frequent complications include arterial perforation, thrombi, emboli, limb ischemia, and local wound infection [82–86]. A minority of complications (20%) are recognized clinically, and most occur during insertion of the device [83]. In one autopsy series describing 20 complications in 16 patients, there were 9 dissections of the aorta or its distal branches (Figs. 55-13–55-16), 3 arterial perforations, 3 arterial thrombi, 3 arterial emboli, 1 ischemic limb, and 1 local wound infection. None of the 9 cases of arterial dissection were diagnosed or suspected before autopsy. Of the 20 complications, only 4 (20%) were suspected before death. In other clinical series, the most frequent complications

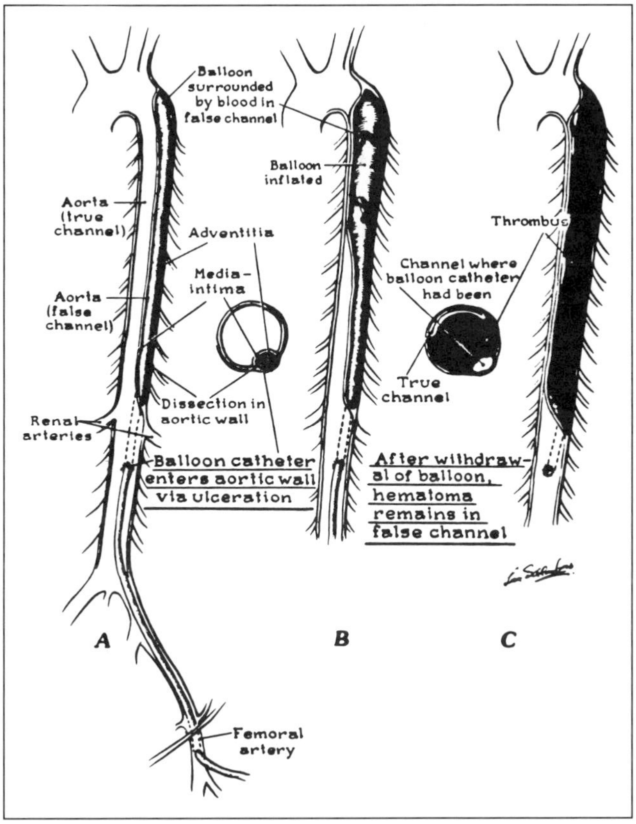

Fig. 55-15. Drawing of patient in Fig. 55-14 of the apparent manner in which dissection was produced. **A.** The catheter entered through an ulcerated atherosclerotic plaque in the abdominal aorta and functioned successfully for 3 days even though it was located in the false channel. **B.** After removal of the balloon, the patient survived for 28 days, during which time, **C,** organized thrombus filled the false channel. (Reproduced with permission from JM Isner et al. Complications of the intra-aortic balloon counter pulsation device: clinical and morphologic observations in 45 necropsy patients. Am J Cardiol 1980; 45:260–268.)

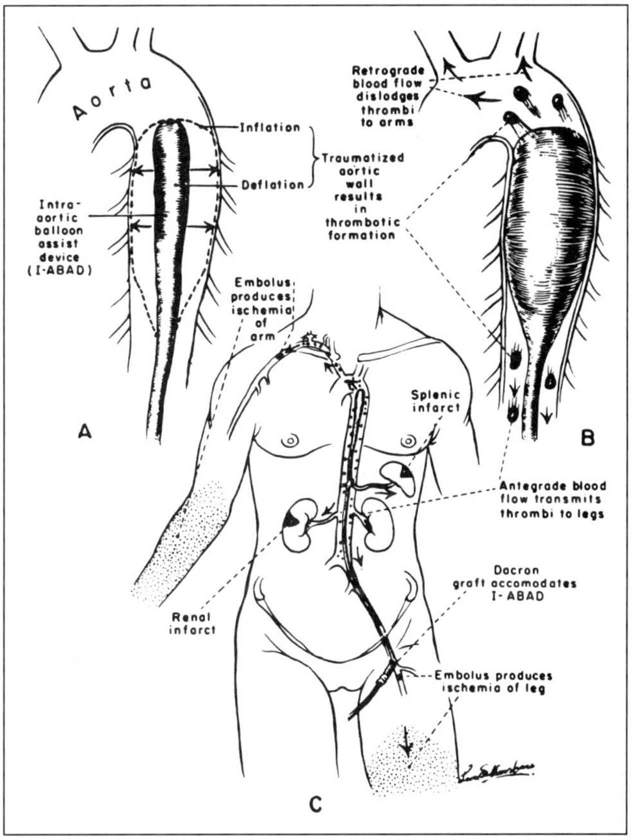

Fig. 55-16. Drawing of the presumed pathogenesis of limb ischemia resulting from use of IABAD in a 50-year-old woman with shock from acute myocardial infarction. **A.** During the 5 days that the device was in place, the patient had ischemia of the right arm and left leg. At necropsy, there were embolic infarcts of the spleen and right kidney and thrombi adherent to the intimal surface of the aorta along the path of the balloon catheter. (No thrombus was present in the heart.) **B.** Emboli from the balloon catheter–induced thrombus along the aortic wall appear to have resulted in right-arm ischemia from retrograde perfusion of the proximal arch arteries by the balloon during ventricular diastole. **C.** Distal (anterograde) emboli resulted in visceral and left leg ischemia. (Reproduced with permission from JM Isner et al. Complications of the intra-aortic balloon counter pulsation device: clinical and morphologic observations in 45 necropsy patients. Am J Cardiol 1980; 45:260–268.)

of IABAD were vascular, with lower-limb ischemia being the most common complication [87]. Other complications include embolization, thrombosis, cerebrovascular accidents, transient ischemic attacks, pseudoaneurysms, arteriovenous fistula, hemorrhage, laceration of femoral artery, balloon rupture, and infections [88,89]. The mortality and morbidity are greater with aortic than with femoral insertion [90]. There is a lower incidence of vascular complications using an unsheathed versus a sheathed intra-aortic balloon device [91].

Naunheim et al. have reported complications from IABAD insertion for perioperative cardiac failure from 1983 to 1990 [92]. Of 580 patients (374 men and 206 women, mean age 64 years) with IABAD, 419 had intraoperative insertion, 107 preoperative insertion, and 54 postoperative insertion. Operations included 376 coronary-artery bypass grafts, 100 mitral valve replacements, 72 aortic valve replacements, and 32 other procedures. The complication rate was 12.4 percent (72 patients); of those, 41 needed surgical intervention, including thrombectomy in 21, vascular repair in 13, fasciotomy in 2, aortic repair in 1, and amputation in 4. Operative mortality for patients on IABAD was 44 percent. The predictors of mortality were preoperative New York Heart Association class III and IV, transthoracic intra-aortic balloon insertion, preoperative administration of intravenous nitroglycerine, age, female sex, and preoperative balloon insertion [92]. Funk et al. report that long-term lower-limb ischemia is a frequent (18%) complication of IABAD. The risk factors for long-term ischemia include occurrence of acute limb ischemia and smoking [93].

References

1. Sones FM Jr, Shirey EK. Cine coronary angiography. Mod Concepts Cardiovasc Dis 1962; 31:735–738.

2. Judkins MP. Selective coronary angiography. A percutaneous transfemoral technic. Radiology 1967; 89:815–824.
3. Davis K, et al. Complications of coronary arteriography from the collaborative study of coronary arteriography from the collaborative study of coronary artery surgery (CASS). Circulation 1979; 59:1105–1112.
4. Hass JM, Peterson CR, Jones RC. Subintimal dissection of the coronary arteries. A complication of selective coronary arteriography and the transfemoral percutaneous approach. Circulation 1968; 38:678–683.
5. Hessel SJ, Adams DF, Abrams HL. Complications of angiography. Radiology 1981; 138:273–281.
6. Kennedy JW. Complications associated with cardiac catheterization and angiography. Cathet Cardiovasc Diagn 1982; 8:5–11.
7. Bourassa MG, Noble J. Complication rate of coronary arteriography. A review of 5250 cases studied by a percutaneous femoral technique. Circulation 1976; 53:106–114.
8. Johnson LW, et al. Coronary arteriography 1984–1987: a report of the Registry of the Society for Cardiac Angiography and interventions. I. Results and complications. Cathet Cardiovasc Diagn 1989; 17:5–10.
9. Virmani R, et al. Coronary artery dissections. Cardiol Clin 1984; 2:633–646.
10. MacAlpin RN. Mistaking catheter-induced coronary arterial dissection for coronary spasm. Am Heart J 1987; 114:671–686.
11. Morise AP, et al. Coronary artery dissection secondary to coronary arteriography. Presentation of three cases and review of the literature. Cathet Cardiovasc Diagn 1981; 7:283–296.
12. Robinowitz M, Virmani R, McAllister HA. Spontaneous coronary artery dissection and eosinophilic inflammation. A cause and effect relationship? Am J Med 1982; 72:923–928.
13. Virmani R, Forman MB. Coronary artery dissections. In R Virmani, MB Forman, eds. Non-atherosclerotic Ischemic Heart Disease. New York: Raven, 1989. Pp. 325–354.
14. Seneff MG. Central venous catheterization: a comprehensive review, Part I. J Intensive Care Med 1987; 2:163–175.
15. Robin ED. The cult of the Swan-Ganz catheter. Ann Intern Med 1985; 103:445–449.
16. Swan HJC, Ganz W. Hemodynamic measurements in clinical practice: a decade in review. J Am Coll Cardiol 1983; 1:103–113.
17. Sanborn TA, et al. The mechanism of transluminal angioplasty: evidence for formation of aneurysm in experimental atherosclerosis. Circulation 1983; 68:1136–1140.
18. Thomas TV. Location of catheter tip and its impact on central venous pressure. Chest 1972; 61:668–673.
19. Sheep RE, Guiney WB. Fatal cardiac tamponade occurrence with other complications after left internal jugular vein catheterization. JAMA 1982; 248:1632–1635.
20. Malatinsky J, et al. Surgical, infectious and thromboembolic complications of central venous catheterization. Resuscitation 1983; 10:271–281.
21. Seneff MG. Central venous catheterization: a comprehensive review, Part II. J Intensive Care Med 1987; 2:218–232.
22. Linos DA, Mucha P, Van Heerden JA. Subclavian vein—a golden route. Mayo Clin Proc 1980; 55:315–321.
23. Ecrola R, Kankinen L, Kankinen S. Analysis of 13,800 subclavian catheterizations. ACTA Anesthesiol Scan 1985; 29: 193–197.
24. Cobb DK, et al. A controlled trial of scheduled replacement of central venous and pulmonary artery catheters. N Engl J Med 1992; 327:1062–1068.
25. Gruntzig A, Kumpe DA. Technique of percutaneous transluminal angioplasty with the Gruntzig balloon catheter. Am J Radiol 1979; 132:547–552.
26. Gruntzig AR, Senning A, Siegenthaler WE. Non-operative dilatation of coronary artery stenosis—percutaneous transluminal coronary angioplasty. N Engl J Med 1979; 301:61–68.
27. Waller BF. "Crackers, breakers, stretchers, drillers, scrapers, shavers, burners, welders, and melters"—the future treatment of atherosclerotic coronary artery disease. A clinical-morphologic assessment. J Am Coll Cardiol 1989; 13:969–987.
28. Baim DS, Detre K, Kent K. Problems in the development of new devices of coronary intervention—possible role for a multicenter registry. J Am Coll Cardiol 1989; 14:1389–1391.
29. Topol EJ. Promises and pitfalls of new devices for coronary artery disease. Circulation 1991; 83:689–694.
30. Weibull H, et al. Complications after percutaneous transluminal angioplasty in the iliac, femoral, and popliteal arteries. J Vasc Surg 1987; 5:681–686.
31. Wyman RM, et al. Current complications of diagnostic and therapeutic cardiac catheterization. J Am Coll Cardiol 1988; 12:1400–1406.
32. Plante S, et al. Acute complications of percutaneous transluminal coronary angioplasty for total occlusion. Am Heart J 1991; 121:417–426.
33. Roubin GS, et al. Influence of balloon size on initial success, acute complications, and restenosis after percutaneous transluminal coronary angioplasty. A prospective randomized study. Circulation 1988; 78:557–565.
34. Saffitz JE, et al. Coronary artery rupture during coronary angioplasty. Am J Cardiol 1983; 51:902–904.
35. Oweida SW, et al. Post catheterization vascular complications associated with percutaneous transluminal coronary angioplasty. J Vasc Surg 1990; 12:310–315.
36. Black AJ, et al. Tear or dissection after coronary angioplasty—morphologic correlates of an ischemic complication. Circulation 1989; 79:1035–1042.
37. Essued CE, Van den Brand M, Becker AE. Transluminal coronary angioplasty and early restenosis: fibrocellular occlusion after wall laceration. Br Heart J 1983; 49:393–396.
38. Farb A, et al. Plaque morphology and pathologic changes in arteries from patients dying after balloon angioplasty. J Am Coll Cardiol 1990; 16:1421–1429.
39. Virmani R, Farb A, Burke AP. Coronary angioplasty from the perspective of atherosclerotic plaque: morphologic predictors of immediate success and restenosis. Am Heart J 1994; 127:163–179.
40. Beatt KJ, et al. Restenosis after coronary angioplasty: the paradox of increased luminal diameter and restenosis. J Am Coll Cardiol 1992; 19:258–266.
41. Kuntz RE, et al. Novel approach to the analysis of restenosis after the use of three new coronary devices. J Am Coll Cardiol 1992; 19:1493–1499.
42. Detre KM, et al. Incidence and consequences of periprocedural occlusion: the 1985–1986 National Heart, Lung, and Blood Institute Percutaneous Transluminal Coronary Angioplasty Registry. Circulation 1990; 82:739–750.
43. Ellis SG, et al. Angiographic and clinical predictors of acute closure after native vessel coronary angioplasty. Circulation 1988; 77:372–379.
44. de Feyter PJ, et al. Acute coronary artery occlusion during and after percutaneous transluminal coronary angioplasty: frequency, prediction, clinical course, management, and follow-up. Circulation 1991; 83:927–936.
45. Gaul G, et al. Acute occlusion in multiple lesion coronary angioplasty: frequency and management. J Am Coll Cardiol 1989; 13:283–288.
46. Kuntz RE, et al. Changing incidence and management of abrupt closure following coronary intervention in the new device era. Cathet Cardiovasc Diagn 1992; 27:183–190.
47. Simpfendorfer C, et al. Frequency, management, and follow-

up of patients with acute coronary occlusions after percutaneous transluminal coronary angioplasty. Am J Cardiol 1988; 11:211–216.
48. Ellis SG, et al. In-hospital cardiac mortality after acute closure after coronary angioplasty: analysis of risk factors from 8207 procedures. J Am Coll Cardiol 1988; 11:211–216.
49. Ryan TJ, et al. Guidelines for percutaneous transluminal coronary angioplasty. A report of the American Heart Association/American College of Cardiology Task Force on assessment of diagnostic and therapeutic cardiovascular procedures. (Committee on Percutaneous Transluminal Angioplasty). Circulation 1993; 88:2987–3007.
50. Lincoff AM, et al. Abrupt vessel closure complicating coronary angioplasty: clinical, angiographic, and therapeutic profile. J Am Coll Cardiol 1992; 19:926–935.
51. Saber RS, et al. Coronary embolization after balloon angioplasty or thrombolytic therapy: an autopsy study of 32 cases. J Am Coll Cardiol 1993; 22:1283–1288.
52. Califf RM, et al. Restenosis after coronary angioplasty: an overview. J Am Coll Cardiol 1991; 17:2B–13B.
53. Popma JJ, Topol EJ. Factors influencing restenosis after coronary angioplasty. Am J Med 1990; 88:16N–24N.
54. Ellis SG, Muller DW. Arterial injury and the enigma of coronary restenosis. J Am Coll Cardiol 1992; 19:275–277.
55. Kuntz RE, et al. Novel approach to the analysis of restenosis after the use of three new coronary devices. J Am Coll Cardiol 1992; 19:1493–1499.
56. Ryan TJ, Klocke FJ, Reynolds WA. Clinical competence in percutaneous transluminal coronary angioplasty: a statement for physicians from the ACP/ACC/AHA Task Force on Clinical Privileges in Cardiology. J Am Coll Cardiol 1990; 15:1469–1474.
57. Killip T. Twenty years of coronary bypass surgery. New Engl J Med 1988; 319:366–368.
58. Miller DC, et al. Discriminant analysis of the changing risks of coronary artery operations: 1971–1979. J Thorac Cardiovasc Surg 1983; 85:197–213.
59. Kirklin JW, Barratt-Boyes BG. Stenotic arteriosclerotic coronary artery disease. In JW Kirklin, BG Barratt-Boyes eds. Cardiac Surgery. New York: Wiley, 1986. Pp. 207–277.
60. Schoen FJ, Fallon JT. Pathologic findings in patients dying early following coronary artery bypass surgery. Lab Invest 1985; 52:60A.
61. Schoen FJ, ed. Interventional and surgical cardiovascular pathology. Clinical correlations and basic principles. Philadelphia: Saunders, 1989.
62. Spray TL, Roberts WC. Morphologic observations in biologic conduits between aorta and coronary artery. In S Rahimtoola, ed. Coronary Bypass Surgery. Philadelphia: FA Davis Co., 1977.
63. Campeau L, et al. Atherosclerosis and late closure or aortocoronary saphenous vein grafts. Sequential angiographic studies at 2 weeks, 1 year, 5 to 7 years, and 10 to 12 years after surgery. Circulation 1983; 68[Suppl II]:1–7.
64. Vlodaver Z, Edwards JE. Pathologic changes in aortic-coronary arterial saphenous vein grafts. Circulation 1971; 44: 719–728.
65. Atkinson JB, Forman MB, Virmani R. Correlation of saphenous vein bypass graft angiography with histologic changes at necropsy. Am J Cardiol 1985; 55:952–955.
66. Virmani R, Atkinson JB, Forman MB. Aortocoronary bypass grafts and extracardiac conduits. In MD Silver, ed. Cardiovascular Pathology. Second Edition. New York: Churchill-Livingstone, 1991. Pp. 1607–1647.
67. Rich NM, Hobson RW II, Fedde CW. Vascular trauma secondary to diagnostic and therapeutic procedures. Arch Surg 1974; 128:715–721.
68. Youkey JR, et al. Vascular trauma secondary to diagnostic and therapeutic procedures 1974 through 1982. A comparative review. Arch Surg 1983; 146:788–791.
69. Natali J, Benhamou AC. Iatrogenic vascular injuries. A review of 125 cases (excluding angiographic injuries). J Cardiovascular Surg 1979; 20:169–176.
70. Shelton ME, et al. A comparison of morphologic and angiographic findings in long-term internal mammary artery and saphenous vein bypass graft. J Am Coll Cardiol 1988; 11:297–307.
71. Bulkley BH, Roberts WC. Isolated coronary artery dissection. A complication of cardiac operations. J Thorac Cardiovasc Surg 1974; 67:148–151.
72. Campeau L, et al. The relation of risk factors to the development of atherosclerosis in saphenous-vein bypass grafts and the progression of disease in the native circulation. A study 10 years after aortocoronary bypass surgery. N Engl J Med 1984; 311:1329–1332.
73. Roberts WC, Lachman AS, Virmani R. Twisting of an aortocoronary bypass conduit. A complication of coronary surgery. J Thoracic Cardiovasc Surg 1978; 75:772–775.
74. Bulkley BH, Hutchins GM. Pathology of coronary artery bypass graft surgery. Arch Pathol Lab Med 1978; 102:273–280.
75. Unni KK, et al. Pathologic changes in aortocoronary saphenous vein grafts. Am J Cardiol 1974; 34:526–532.
76. Brody WR, Angell WW, Kosek JC. Histologic fate of the venous coronary artery bypass in dogs. Am J Pathol 1972; 66:111–130.
77. Spray TL, Roberts WC. Status of the grafts and the native coronary arteries proximal and distal to coronary anastomotic sites of aortocoronary bypass grafts. Circulation 1977; 55:741–749.
78. Bulkley BH. Pathology of coronary artery bypass graft surgery. Am Heart J 1979; 98:539–540.
79. Griffith LSC, et al. Occlusive changes at the coronary artery bypass graft anastomosis. Morphologic study of 95 grafts. J Thorac Cardiovasc Surg 1977; 73:668–679.
80. McEnany MT, et al. Effect of antithrombolytic therapy on aortocoronary vein graft patency rates. Circulation 1976; 54[Suppl II]:124.
81. Cheesbro JH, et al. Effect of dipyridamole and aspirin on late vein-graft patency after coronary bypass operations. N Engl J Med 1984; 310:209–214.
82. Orcutt MB, et al. Iatrogenic vascular injury. A reducible problem. Arch Surg 1985; 120:384–385.
83. Isner JM, et al. Complications of the intra-aortic balloon counter pulsation device: clinical and morphologic observations in 45 necropsy patients. Am J Cardiol 1980; 45:260–268.
84. Perler BA, et al. Vascular complications of intracardiac balloon counter pulsation. Arch Surg 1983; 118:957–962.
85. Friedell ML, et al. Femorofemoral grafts for lower limb ischemia caused by intra-aortic balloon pump. J Vasc Surg 1987; 5:180–186.
86. Alle KM, et al. Iatrogenic vascular trauma associated with intra-aortic balloon pumping: identification of risk factors. Am Surg 1993; 59:813–817.
87. Messina LM, et al. Clinical characteristics and surgical management of vascular complications in patients undergoing cardiac catheterization: interventional versus diagnostic procedures. J Vasc Surg 1991; 13:593–600.
88. Hazelrigg SR, Auer JE, Seifert PE. Experience in 100 transthoracic balloon pumps. Ann Thorac Surg 1992; 54:528–532.
89. Lazar JM, et al. Outcome and complications of prolonged intraaortic balloon counterpulsation in cardiac patients. Am J Cardiol 1992; 69:955–958.

90. Pinkard J, et al. Relative risk of aortic and femoral insertion of intraaortic balloon pump after coronary artery bypass grafting procedures. J Thorac Cardiovasc Surg 1993; 105:721–728.
91. Tatar H, et al. Vascular complications of intraaortic balloon pumping: unsheathed versus sheathed insertion. Ann Thorac Surg 1993; 55:1518–1521.
92. Naunheim KS, et al. Intraaortic balloon pumping in patients requiring cardiac operations. Risk analysis and long-term follow-up. J Thorac Cardiovasc Surg 1992; 104:1654–1660.
93. Funk M, et al. Frequency of long-term lower limb ischemia associated with intraaortic balloon pump use. Am J Cardiol 1992; 70:1195–1199.

Neoplastic Diseases of the Blood Vessels

Janina A. Longtine

Vascular tumors are a heterogeneous group of neoplasms encompassing a spectrum of tumors from extremely common benign hemangiomas, to intermediate-grade lesions that are locally aggressive but that infrequently metastasize, to the relatively rare highly malignant angiosarcomas. Vascular lesions also may present as congenital malformations, such as Sturge-Weber syndrome; as nonneoplastic inflammatory vascular proliferations, such as the oral pyogenic granuloma of pregnancy; or as tumorlike conditions that often are difficult to differentiate clinically and histologically from true neoplasms. For those reasons, neoplasms of the blood vessels have always presented complexities in clinical categorization and in histologic classification.

This chapter presents clinical and pathologic descriptions of vascular tumor and tumorlike conditions that are common, clinically important, or representative of entities whose nature has only recently been elucidated.

Vascular tumors are composed of cells that make up the vascular wall—endothelium, smooth muscle cells, and pericytes—most often singly but sometimes in combination. The vast majority of tumors are made up of proliferations of endothelial cells. Because the only differentiating histologic characteristic of an endothelial cell is its position as the lining of a vascular lumen, identification of endothelial tumors (when they are not sufficiently differentiated to form vascular lumina) requires either the immunocytochemical localization of specific endothelial antigens or electron-microscopic identification of the Weibel-Palade bodies [1]. Although specific for endothelial cells, the rod-shaped organelles are not easily demonstrated in all endothelial cells; therefore, their diagnostic usefulness is limited. The most commonly used immunohistochemical marker of endothelial cells is von Willebrand factor (vWF, formerly factor VIII-related antigen) [2], which can be localized by monoclonal or polyclonal antisera (Fig. 56-1). However, even vWF is not uniformly expressed in the endothelium of all vessels, and, not surprisingly, some tumors, especially the poorly differentiated ones, do not contain easily demonstrable vWF immunoreactivity. The human hematopoietic progenitor cell antigen, CD34, also is present in vascular endothelial cells. Immunohistochemical localization of CD34 in frozen or formalin-fixed tissue has proved to be a relatively sensitive marker for endothelial derivation. It is not entirely specific, however, because immunoreactivity is noted in other soft-tissue tumors such as epithelioid sarcomas, leiomyosarcomas, dermatofibrosarcoma protuberans, and neurofibromas [3–8]. CD31, platelet-endothelium cell-adhesion molecule (PECAM-1), appears to be a relatively specific and sensitive marker of endothelial cells and neoplasms in frozen or formalin-fixed tissue [8,9]. Another, less specific marker of endothelium is the lectin *Ulex europaeus L*, which binds an L-fucose glycoprotein found in endothelial cells [10,11]. Other monoclonal antibodies that mark endothelial cells include E92 [12], OKM5 (CD36) [13], EN3 [14], PAL-E [15], and BMA 120 (BW200) [16]. The use of these monoclonal antisera generally is restricted to frozen or specially fixed tissues, although the epitope for BMA 120 is preserved in formalin-fixed, paraffin-embedded tissue [17]. In general, it is most informative to use a combination of endothelial markers to optimize diagnosis of vascular tumors.

Vascular neoplasms are called either **benign** or **malignant** based on two major anatomic characteristics: (1) the degree to which the neoplasm is composed of well-formed vascular channels and (2) the abundance and regularity of endothelial-cell proliferation. In general, benign neoplasms are comprised of well-formed vessels lined by flattened, regular endothelial cells. Frankly malignant tumors are pleomorphic and anaplastic and produce scant numbers of abortive vascular channels. Table 56-1 is a current classification of vascular tumors.

Benign Tumors

HEMANGIOMAS

In this chapter, the term **hemangiomas** is used broadly as a designation for benign, nonreactive vascular lesions histologically characterized by increased numbers of vessels. It should be understood that the term encompasses both proliferative vasoformative tumors and vascular malformations that result from aberrant embryogenesis [18,19]. Although clinical features, such as presence at birth and commensurate growth with the child, may indicate that a vascular lesion is a malformation rather than a true neoplasm, histologic criteria cannot reliably distinguish between the pathogenic mechanisms.

Hemangiomas frequently are present at birth or develop during childhood. They most often occur in the skin or subcutaneous tissue but may involve internal organs, especially the liver. The tumors are benign and have no propensity to undergo malignant change.

Capillary Hemangiomas. Capillary hemangiomas are the largest subgroup of hemangiomas and occur primarily in the skin or subcutaneous tissue as small, red to blue, slightly elevated lesions. As their name implies, they consist of numerous, narrow, blood-filled, thin-walled vessels lined by flattened endothelium (Fig. 56-2). The vessels may be partially or completely occluded by thrombus with organization. There is scant intervening connective tissue. The lesions are circumscribed, but small projections may extend along stromal planes. The overlying epithelium is intact. Except for the juvenile hemangioma described below, these lesions do not regress; they persist but do not enlarge throughout life. Capillary hemangiomas are most common in women and may fluctuate in size with pregnancy, suggesting a response to circulating hormones.

One variant of the capillary hemangioma is the **juvenile** or **strawberry hemangioma**, which appears in the skin

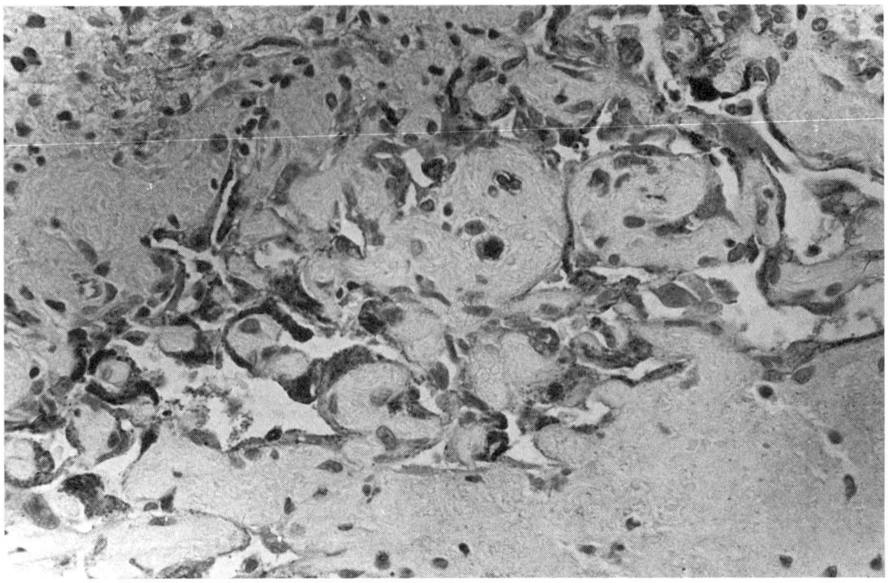

Fig. 56-1. Angiosarcoma with immunoreactivity for von Willebrand factor in neoplastic cells lining lumina. The majority of the tumor cells are positive.

shortly after birth, grows rapidly during infancy, and then regresses during childhood. At their peak, they are dome-shaped, red, soft, compressible lesions reminiscent of strawberries. With involution, they develop patchy whiteness of the surface with eventual fading, leaving a small, pigmented scar. Histologically, juvenile hemangiomas are characterized by vessels lined with plump endothelium and have inconspicuous lumina. With maturation, the tumor resembles the adult capillary hemangioma and finally is replaced by fibrosis on involution. Because these lesions spontaneously regress, no clinical intervention generally is required.

Senile angiomas (cherry angiomas) are bright-red papules appearing on the trunk and extremities of adults,

Table 56-1. Classification of vascular tumors

- Benign vascular lesions
  - Hemangiomas
    - Capillary hemangiomas
    - Cavernous hemangiomas
    - Deep soft tissue hemangiomas
  - Angiolymphoid hyperplasia with eosinophilia
  - Vascular malformations
  - Spindle-cell hemangioendothelioma
  - Glomus tumor
- Vascular tumors of intermediate grade
  - Epithelioid hemangioendothelioma
  - Retiform hemangioendothelioma
  - Malignant endovascular papillary angioendothelioma
  - Kaposi-like infantile hemangioendothelioma
- Malignant vascular tumors
  - Angiosarcoma
  - Kaposi's sarcoma
  - Hemangiopericytoma

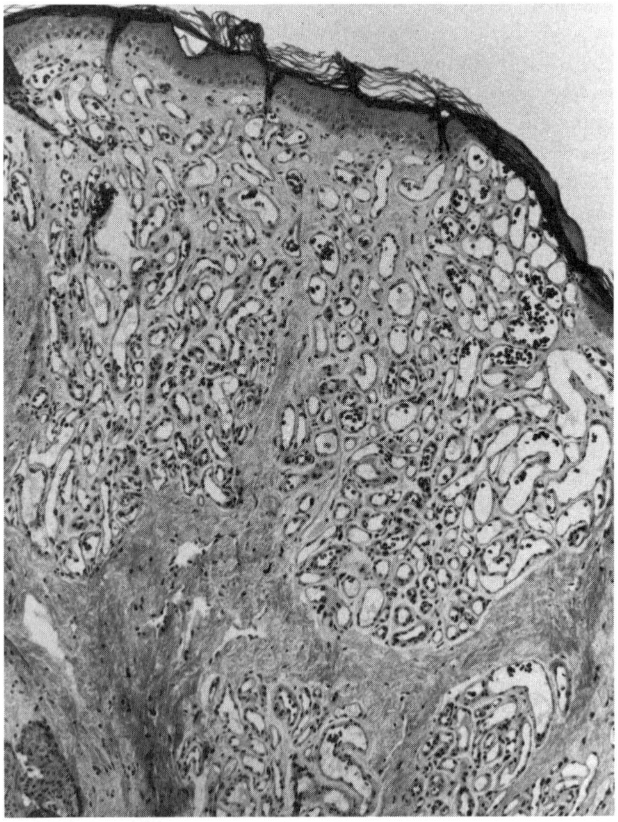

Fig. 56-2. Cutaneous capillary hemangioma consists of a lobular array of thin-walled vessels lined with flattened endothelium.

especially over the age of 50. Histologically, thin-walled dilated vessels are present in the superficial dermis. The lesions are insignificant and can be removed easily surgically or with electrocoagulation.

Pyogenic granulomas (lobular capillary hemangioma) occur on the skin and mucous membranes, usually the oral mucosa, face, or upper extremities. The oral lesions are common in pregnant women. The lesions are rapidly developing, polyploid, red, friable growths that are sometimes associated with a history of antecedent trauma and may ulcerate. Histologically, the pyogenic granuloma is an exophytic, lobulated mass of capillary-size vessels with a prominent inflammatory infiltrate in a loose stroma. The mass is at the end of a narrow stalk, with a surrounding collar of squamous epithelium. The resemblance of the lesion to granulation tissue prompted its epithet. Whether pyogenic granuloma is a reactive process or a neoplasm is still unclear. After removal, the lesion may recur, and in some cases, may recur as multiple, nonpedunculated satellite lesions [20]. Excision generally is curative.

Bacillary angiomatosis (epithelioid angiomatosis) is not a neoplasm but an infectious disease occurring primarily in immunocompromised individuals, particularly those seropositive for human immunodeficiency virus (HIV) [21,22]. It is mentioned in this chapter because clinically and pathologically it can resemble pyogenic granuloma or Kaposi's sarcoma (see below). The angiomatous skin lesions may be superficial, deep dermal, or subcutaneous. In all locations, there is a lobular pattern of vascular proliferation similar to the pyogenic granuloma. The vessels may be lined by plump endothelium, however, and are associated with neutrophils and neutrophil debris. In addition, there are interstitial clumps of bacilli that stain with the Warthin-Starry silver stain. Similar lesions may be present in bone, bronchial tree [23,24], lymph node, liver, and spleen. The liver and spleen involvement may appear as peliosis. Some patients have persistent fevers and bacteremia. The causative agent was first identified by amplification of a portion of eubacterial 16S rRNA from lesions using the polymerase chain reaction [25]. Sequence analysis identified a new rickettsia-like organism, *Rochalimaea henselae*. Subsequently, further DNA isolations and developed-culture methods have identified both *R. henselae* and the closely related *Rochalimaea quintana*, the louse-born agent of trench fever, in lesions of bacillary angiomatosis [26,27]. Epidemiologic data suggest that cat scratches or cat bites are strong risk factors for the disease [28]. The disease is easily treated with antibiotics.

Cavernous Hemangiomas. Cavernous hemangiomas are less common than the capillary type and occur in the skin and viscera, including liver, spleen, pancreas, and brain. The hemangiomas are present in childhood, with a tendency to locate on the head and neck. The dermal lesions frequently are larger and extend deeper than capillary hemangiomas. They appear as flat or rounded, violaceous, spongy, compressible lesions. Deep tumors may have no overlying skin changes but may be visualized by radiography highlighted by dystrophic calcification in the vessel wall or phleboliths. Histologically, these lesions are composed of large, dilated vessels with flattened endothelium (Fig. 56-3). The vessel walls occasionally may have adventitial fibrosis. Smaller, capillary-calibered vessels may be interspersed among the cavernous vessels, raising the possibility that these lesions are a mature or involuting phase of capillary hemangiomas. Alternatively, they may represent large-channel malformations or clinically distinct benign neoplasms. The lesions generally do not regress and may require surgical intervention for destructive compression of adjacent structures.

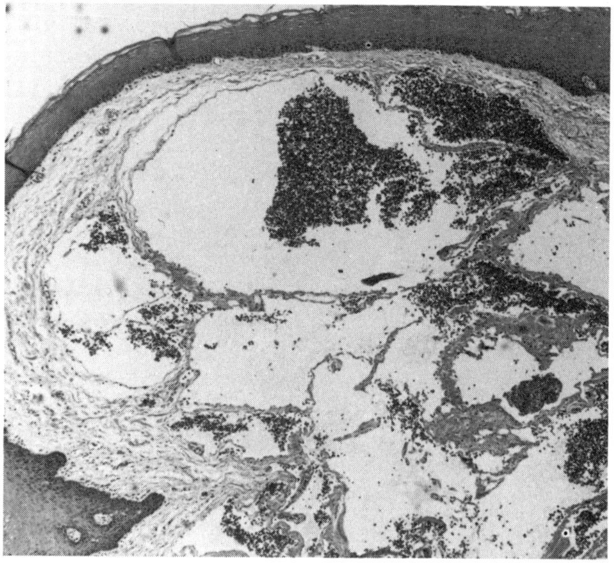

Fig. 56-3. Cutaneous cavernous hemangioma with large, dilated, blood-filled vessels and flattened endothelium.

Several clinical syndromes are associated with cavernous hemangiomas. Single or multiple giant hemangiomas complicated by thrombocytopenia characterize **Kasabach-Merritt syndrome**. Patients develop systemic petechiae and purpura and may have multiple bleeding episodes. The pathogenesis of the bleeding tendency is related to intravascular coagulation and platelet sequestration within the hemangiomas [29,30]. The syndrome, which is seen most commonly in children, has a high mortality rate secondary to bleeding complications. Excision or embolization of the hemangioma reverses the coagulopathy. If that is not feasible, medical therapy may be efficacious [31].

Von Hippel-Lindau (VHL) disease is a rare autosomal dominant disorder characterized by cavernous hemangiomas in the retina, cerebellum or brain stem, liver, kidney, and other organs. Patients also develop hemangioblastomas of the central nervous system and retina, renal-cell adenomas and carcinomas, and pheochromocytomas. The VHL tumor–suppressor gene has been mapped to chromosome 3p25-26 and encodes a novel protein that contains an acidic tandem repeat and that may be involved in signal transduction or cell adhesion [32].

Cavernous hemangiomas of the skin and gastrointestinal tract are the features of the **blue rubber bleb nevus syndrome**. The interesting appellation describes the blue, rubbery, cutaneous lesions, but most clinical complications arise from bleeding of the gastrointestinal hemangiomas. **Maffucci's syndrome** consists of multiple hemangiomas and enchondromas. Patients with this congenital syndrome have a high incidence of chondrosarcoma.

SPINDLE-CELL HEMANGIOENDOTHELIOMA. Spindle-cell hemangioendothelioma was first described as a clinicopathologic entity in 1986 by Weiss and Enzinger [33]. These painless vascular nodules have a predilection for the distal extremities, increase in size over months or years, and have a tendency to recur over a wide discontinuous area. The age of onset has a wide distribution with the majority in childhood or early adult life. Some patients have associated disease such as chronic lymphedema, Mafucci's syndrome, and Klippel-Trenaunay syndrome. The lesions are circumscribed, located in the dermis or superficial subcutis, and have features reminiscent of cavernous hemangioma and Kaposi's sarcoma. Thin-walled, cavernous vascular channels are intimately admixed with spindle cells arranged in fascicles or lining slit-like spaces. Plump epithelioid cells or vacuolated cells may be present focally within the spindle-cell areas. The dilated spaces often contain organized thrombi or phleboliths.

In Weiss and Enzinger's original description [33], 10 of 14 patients with follow-up developed new lesions in the vicinity of the original lesion over a 2- to 40-year period. One patient who was irradiated developed a high-grade angiosarcoma. Due to the multifocal, progressive growth pattern, the process was considered an intermediate-grade hemangioendothelioma. Subsequently, Fletcher [34] observed that the lesions often are associated with malformed vasculature similar to arteriovenous shunts and have smooth muscle components. Those features suggest that the spindle-cell hemangioendothelioma is a reactive vascular lesion arising in association with abnormal blood flow. The observed multiplicity of lesions is secondary to the wide distribution of the vascular malformation. Several other authors have confirmed that observation [35–37].

Deep-Soft-Tissue Hemangiomas. Hemangiomas of the deep soft tissues are much less common than their cutaneous counterparts. However, they are more likely to cause concern to the clinician and the pathologist.

INTRAMUSCULAR HEMANGIOMAS. Probably the most common of deep-soft-tissue hemangiomas, intramuscular hemangiomas present as a soft-tissue mass. There usually is no associated skin discoloration, pulsation, or bruit. A history of pain or recent trauma may be elicited. Radiographic demonstration of phleboliths or angiography may support the diagnosis. Allen and Enzinger's review [38] of 89 cases divides the intramuscular hemangiomas into three pathologic groups: small-vessel, large-vessel, and mixed. These groups morphologically mimic the cutaneous capillary, cavernous, and mixed hemangiomas, respectively. The lesions usually are seen in young adults (mid-20s), with the capillary hemangiomas most commonly involving the head and neck and the cavernous and mixed involving the lower limb. For the pathologist, capillary intramuscular hemangiomas offer the greater diagnostic challenge. Grossly, they are poorly circumscribed and yellow to tan or brown. Their vascular nature is not always readily apparent histologically. The plumpness of the endothelial cells and the cellularity of the proliferation may obscure the vascular lumina. Common features such as mitosis, intraluminal papillary projections of endothelial cells, and infiltration between muscle fibers and in nerve sheaths elicit trepidation in the inexperienced observer. True angiosarcomas of the skeletal muscle are extremely rare, however, and the malignant criteria of anastomosing channels lined by plump piles of bizarre, hyperchromatic cells are not fulfilled in this benign lesion. The cavernous and mixed intramuscular hemangiomas are easily recognized both grossly and microscopically. The cavernous subtype may have an admixture of adipose tissue, fibrous tissue, or even bone. Intravascular thrombi also are noted. The mixed variant has features of both the capillary and the cavernous hemangioma. Intramuscular hemangiomas may cause deformity or disability and are cured by surgical removal. They may sometimes recur but respond to reexcision.

SYNOVIAL HEMANGIOMAS. Synovial hemangiomas are rare, but they usually present as an intra-articular mass in the knee joint [39]. They may be palpated by physical exam, but routine x-rays are unrevealing. Histologically, they resemble cavernous hemangiomas covered by a reactive synovium. Not surprisingly, there is disagreement as to whether these vascular lesions represent a reactive process, a malformation, or a benign neoplasm. Symptoms from pedunculated lesions can be relieved by surgical excision. Diffuse lesions are more difficult to remove.

Other Hemangiomas. Hemangiomas can also be present in other sites, such as peripheral nerve or bone [40], especially vertebral, cranial, and facial bones. The neural lesions may be painful or associated with muscle weakness or wasting. The bony lesions usually are incidental findings on radiographic examination. Histologically, the lesions resemble their cutaneous counterparts. Therapy is conservative.

Hemangiomas also may occur in internal organs, such as liver, spleen, pancreas, and brain. The lesions usually are clinically insignificant unless confused with metastatic disease in the workup of an oncology patient or unless a brain angioma presents as intracranial hemorrhage, mass effect, or seizures [41]. Large liver hemangiomas may cause congestive heart failure in infants because of left-to-right shunting. These unusual cases may require radiation therapy, excision, or embolization [42]. Breast hemangiomas [43] are benign and clinically significant only in that they present as a mass.

Angiomatosis. A rare condition, angiomatosis is a diffuse hemangioma involving a segment of the body. It presents in childhood as swelling of the part, usually a lower limb. The lesions are distinguished from intramuscular hemangiomas by clinical involvement rather than pathologic criteria. Treatment is conservative and complicated by coagulopathy or problems associated with mass effect. A similar entity rarely may be seen in the female breast [44] and is benign.

ANGIOLYMPHOID HYPERPLASIA WITH EOSINOPHILIA

Angiolymphoid hyperplasia with eosinophilia (epithelioid hemangioma) [45] has been known as pseudo– or atypical pyogenic granuloma, inflammatory angiomatous nodule, and a host of other names. It presents as single or multiple, dull pink to red, often pruritic papules most commonly on the head and neck, especially around the ear. Patients range in age from teens to the elderly, with the majority in the third to fifth decade [46,47]. Occasional patients may have regional lymphadenopathy or peripheral eosinophilia, but the eosinophilia in the name refers to the microscopic appearance. Histologically, the tumor usually involves the subcutis or dermis and consists of a proliferation of vessels, both small-capillary and thick-walled, with intramural myxoid change. Admixed is an inflammatory infiltrate of lymphocytes, histiocytes, and especially eosinophils (Fig. 56-4A). Lymphoid aggregates or follicles may be present. The striking feature of this entity is the endothelial cell that lines the vessels [48] (Fig. 56-4B). This epithelioid or histiocytoid endothelial cell has a large, irregular, often indented vesicular nucleus with abundant acidophilic cytoplasm, which may be vacuolated. These cells may appear as compact nests or may narrow lumina as they line both small and larger vessels. Their endothelial origin is well documented. They have the ultrastructural features of endothelial cells, namely, microfilaments, pinocytotic vesicles, and Weibel-Palade bodies. Many of the cells contain the endothelial marker vWF, by immunoperoxidase techniques. However, these endothelial cells differ from normal capillary endothelial cells ultrastructurally and histochemically as well as histologically. Their fine structure is distinguished by the presence of extensive intercellular gaps, prominent cytoplasmic filaments, and occasional dense bodies. Histochemically, these cells have low levels of alkaline phosphatase and high levels of respiratory enzymes, the reverse of normal endothelium [49]. Endothelial cells with these morphologic features have been noted in reactive vascular proliferations and in vascular tumors.

There is debate as to whether this lesion represents a true neoplasm or a reactive process because of the accompanying inflammatory infiltrate [46,47]. An inflammatory infiltrate does not preclude malignant potential (e.g., Hodgkin's disease). The lesions usually persist if not excised, and they recur if excision is inadequate. They also may be locally destructive, although there is no strong evidence of metastatic potential. The lesions are probably best regarded clinically as benign neoplasms and treated with surgical excision.

Rosai and colleagues have included this neoplasm in the spectrum of **histiocytoid hemangiomas** [50], which includes entities of skin, soft tissue, large vessels, bone, and heart. These lesions are all characterized by a proliferation of histiocytoid endothelial cells, so called because of their morphologic similarity to histiocytes, but the lesions have diverse clinical features and natural histories [47].

GLOMUS TUMORS

Glomus tumors (glomangioma) are benign neoplasms that arise from specialized smooth muscle cells of the glomus body, a temperature-sensitive regulator of blood flow [51]. The glomus body is composed of a branching arteriovenous anastomosis surrounded by smooth muscle cells interspersed with round glomus cells. Glomus bodies are located in the dermis of the skin anywhere in the body, but they are most common in the extremities, especially the subungual regions. The tumors also are most common subungually, but they are also seen in the hands and feet and even in areas without glomus bodies, such as stomach, nose, and cervix. The tumors usually occur in adult life with equal frequency in both sexes, although the subungual lesions are more common in women. Clinically, glomus tumors are striking because of the exquisite pain associated with even the smallest of tumors. The pain is paroxysmal, burning, and radiating, and induced by temperature change or pressure. The tumor appears as a small, red to blue, firm, painful nodule. Subungual lesions may appear as small areas of red or bluish discoloration. Some cases of multiple glomus tumors have been reported and often are familial. Those patients present in childhood with numerous lesions that usually are not subungual and are asymptomatic.

Glomus tumors are composed of varying proportions of vessels, smooth muscle cells, and glomus cells. The subungual tumors are well-circumscribed proliferations of capillary-sized vessels surrounded by cuffs of regular, round glomus cells. The glomus cells have distinct nuclei, moderate amounts of eosinophilic cytoplasm, and distinct cell borders. Tumors in other sites may have dilated, cavernous vascular channels with clusters of glomus cells or have a component of mature smooth muscle cells. Ultrastructurally, glomus cells have features of smooth muscle cells, that is, investment by a basal lamina, abundant thin filaments associated with dense bodies, and pinocytotic vesicles [52,53].

These benign tumors are readily cured by surgical excision, which gives complete symptomatic relief.

VASCULAR ECTASIAS

Vascular ectasias (telangiectasias) are not neoplasms but localized dilatations or malformations of dermal vessels. Because they must be differentiated from true neoplasms, they are included in this chapter.

Nevus Flammeus. Most commonly, nevus flammeus are flat, macular, pink to red congenital lesions present unilaterally on the face and neck, especially over the eyelid, forehead, or nuchal area. They characteristically disappear with age.

A special subtype of nevus flammeus is the **port-wine stain**, which does not regress but grows commensurately with the child. Most commonly unilateral on the face or neck, the port-wine stain varies from pink to dark red, blanches with pressure, and intensifies in color with crying or exertion. It usually is smooth but may develop some nodularity. Histologically, port-wine stains are ectasias of the vessels in the superficial vascular plexus. Since there is no vascular proliferation, they may be due to local abnormal blood-flow regulation, perhaps neurogenic in origin [54]. They are unresponsive to most therapies and seem best treated cosmetically or with pulsed dye lasers [55,56]. Occasionally, port-wine stains may be associated with a deeper hemangioma [57].

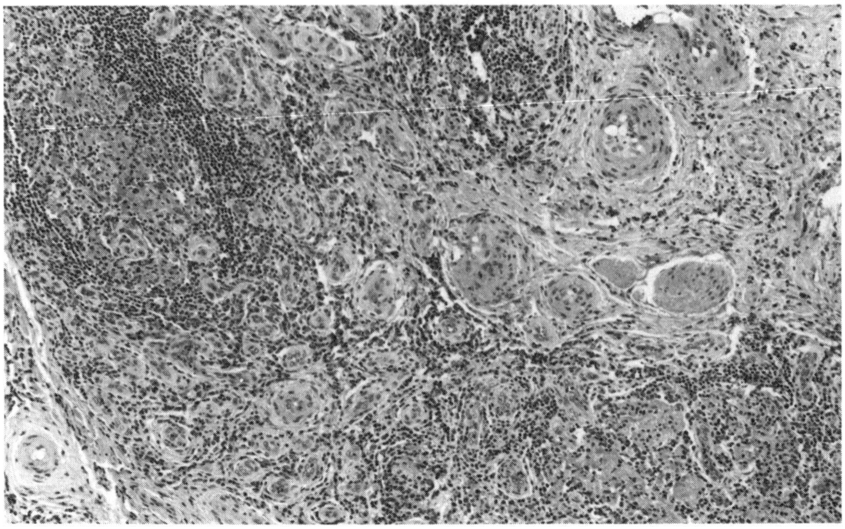

A

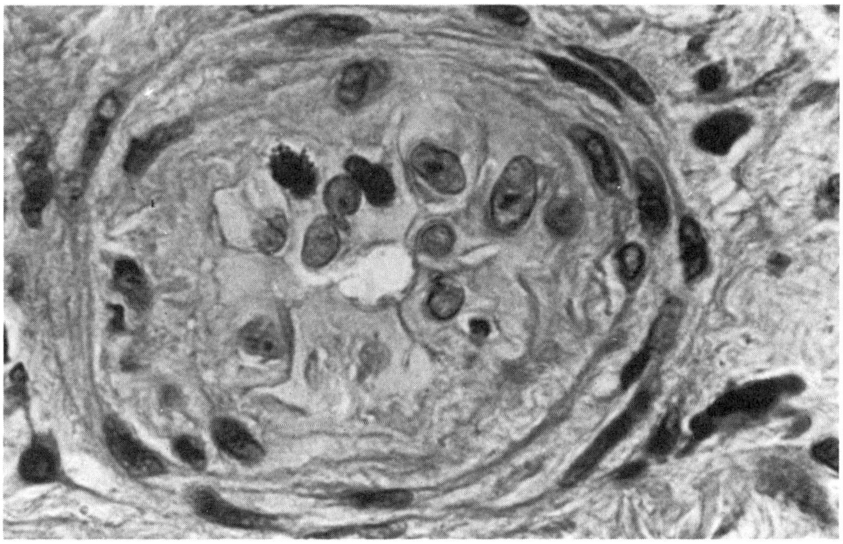

B

Fig. 56-4. **A.** Angiolymphoid hyperplasia composed of numerous small vessels admixed with inflammatory cells. **B.** Higher magnification of one of the vessels demonstrates the large epithelioid or histiocytoid endothelial cells with vesicular nuclei and abundant cytoplasm.

Some port-wine stains are associated with clinical syndromes. The **Sturge-Weber syndrome** is characterized by a port-wine stain in the distribution of the superior and middle branches of the trigeminal nerve, ipsilateral hemangiomas of the retina and leptomeninges, seizures, hemiparalysis, and mental retardation. Characteristic double-contoured radiopacities outline the cerebral cortex of the involved area. The rare **Klippel-Trenaunay syndrome** consists of port-wine stain of a lower extremity with associated absence or atresia of the deep venous system, superficial varicosities, and bony and soft-tissue hypertrophy. The hypertrophy is probably secondary to the increased blood flow through the region.

Spider Telangiectasia. Spider telangiectasias consist of a central superficial arteriole with radiating fine vessels producing a small, red, pulsatile, spiderlike, cutaneous lesion. These telangiectasias are most commonly found on the face, neck, or upper torso of pregnant women and patients with cirrhosis or other liver diseases. They are believed to be secondary to elevated estrogen levels. In pregnant women, the lesions resolve postpartum.

Intermediate-Grade Tumors

HEMANGIOENDOTHELIOMA

True neoplasms of vascular origin that cannot be accurately classified as to malignant potential by histologic

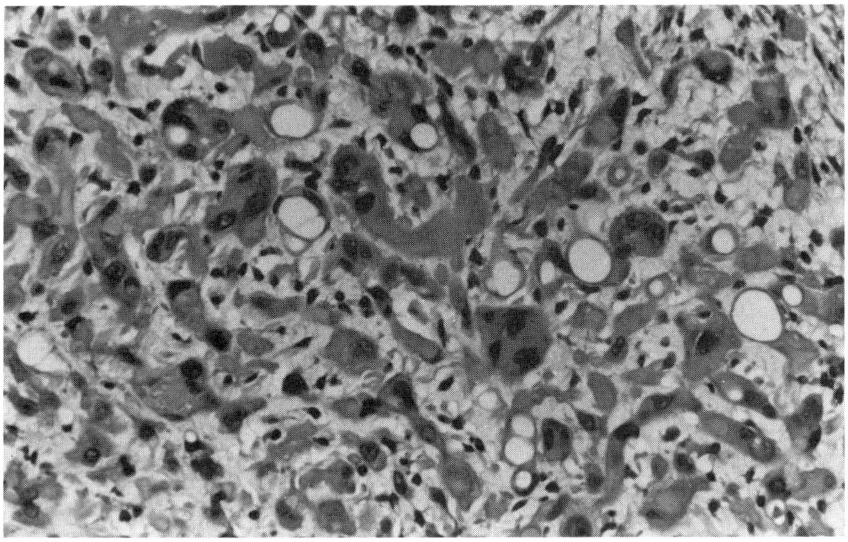

Fig. 56-5. Epithelioid hemangioendothelioma with characteristic epithelioid endothelial cells, showing prominent cytoplasmic vacuolization.

criteria fall into the category of hemangioendothelioma. These tumors are present in a distribution similar to that of benign hemangiomas, involving the skin or viscera. They differ in their histologic features, which suggest a more aggressive biologic potential. The tumors may have a more disorganized low-power architecture, larger, pleomorphic cells, or more mitoses than normally observed in benign hemangiomas. These histologic features in themselves are not sufficient for an intermediate-grade neoplasm—the clinical setting is an important consideration.

EPITHELIOID HEMANGIOENDOTHELIOMA

Epithelioid hemangioendothelioma is a unique vascular tumor of intermediate grade, containing plump, epithelioid endothelial cells [58]. The tumors occur most commonly in the soft tissues, subcutis, or muscle in the extremities of adults. Similar tumors also have been described in the head and neck [59], the liver, the mediastinum [60,62], and the lung [62] (see below, this section). Frequently, the neoplasm is associated with a vessel, usually a midsized or large vein. Presenting symptoms are nonspecific, usually a tender mass with additional symptoms, such as thrombophlebitis, depending on the site of involvement. Histologically, the tumor has nests or cords of plump endothelial cells in a basophilic, myxoid matrix. The tumor cells frequently contain large vacuoles or are present as small nests with inapparent lumina, features that recapitulate angiogenesis (Fig. 56-5). Well-formed vascular spaces are not easily found. These features may lead to a mistaken diagnosis of carcinoma. The associated midsized vessel may be centrifugally expanded by the tumor, which lines the vessel and extends through the wall into the adjacent soft tissue. The tumor cells are endothelial in origin, containing vWF immunoreactivity and characteristic ultrastructural features. Some of the tumor cells may be spindled, but the majority are the plump endothelial cells, with prominent cytofilaments encountered in angiolymphoid hyperplasia with eosinophilia (epithelioid hemangioma) and in "activated" endothelium.

These tumors may have features suggestive of a malignant potential, such as pleomorphism or an increased mitotic rate. Weiss and Enzinger [58,63] reviewed the Armed Forces Institute of Pathology's experience with this tumor and noted a local recurrence rate of 13 percent and a metastatic rate of 31 percent, prompting the classification of intermediate grade. They found, however, that no histologic criterion accurately predicts the malignant potential. They felt that the best predictor of biologic potential is the presence of mitotic figures (>1 per high-power field). Significant atypia, focal spindling of the cells, and necrosis also are associated with a more aggressive course.

The tumors are treated with surgical excision. The more benign-appearing lesions are excised with a margin of uninvolved tissue, the more malignant-appearing neoplasms with more extensive resection. Each tumor nonetheless must be considered individually with respect to anatomic location, morbidity of radical surgery, and the understanding that pathologic features are not predictive of biologic potential.

Histologically similar tumors have been described in the lung and liver. In 1975, Dail and Liebow described a rare lung tumor thought to be of epithelial origin and designated **intravascular bronchioloalveolar tumor** (IVBAT) [64]. It subsequently has been documented that these tumors are of endothelial origin based on vWF immunoreactivity [65] and ultrastructural studies [65–67] and that they are pulmonary epithelioid hemangioendotheliomas. The pulmonary tumors occur predominantly in females, often those under 30 years of age. Initially, the patient usually is asymptomatic, presenting with multiple small nodules on routine chest x-ray or perhaps with complaints of mild dyspnea on exertion. On biopsy, the tumor is histologically similar to the soft-tissue epithelioid hemangioendothelioma, with nests of plump tumor cells in a myxoid to hyaline stroma and focal intravascular extension. There are few cases with spread outside the thorax [68], but the tumors progress within the lungs, resulting in a progressive course of pulmonary insufficiency.

Epithelioid hemangioendothelioma of the liver [69] is identical histologically to that of the lung and the soft tissues; its endothelial origin has been demonstrated ultrastructurally and immunophenotypically. Several reported cases of the liver tumors have documented extrahepatic spread in lymph nodes, peritoneum, and distant sites, confirming the malignant potential of this group of endothelial tumors [70,71]. Patients with unresectable liver tumors have been treated with liver transplantation [71,72].

Epithelioid hemangioendothelioma of all sites is included under Rosai's rubric of histiocytoid hemangioma [50].

RETIFORM HEMANGIOENDOTHELIOMA

Retiform hemangioendothelioma is a recently recognized cutaneous vascular neoplasm of low or borderline malignant potential [73]. It typically occurs in the extremities and trunk of young to middle-aged adults as a slow growing exophytic or plaquelike mass. There is a high rate of local recurrence and infrequent lymph-node metastases. The dermis and subcutis are infiltrated by elongated thin-walled blood vessels in an arborizing pattern reminiscent of the rete testis. The vessels are lined by monomorphic, hobnail endothelial cells with minimal cytologic atypia. Occasionally, intraluminary papillary projections with hyalinized central cores are seen. A prominent lymphocytic infiltrate may be present. Other areas of the neoplasm have a more solid appearance with epithelioid or spindle cells. These tumors should be recognized as distinct from cutaneous angiosarcoma (see below), which has a much worse prognosis.

Malignant endovascular papillary angioendothelioma, described by Dabska in 1969, is a rare vascular tumor of low-grade malignancy [74–76]. The few reported cases occurred in the skin or subcutaneous tissue of infants or children, causing swelling or nodules. The tumors consist of vascular channels lined by prominent endothelial cells that pile into tuftlike projections with central hyaline cores, a characteristic feature. The tumors have a good prognosis, with cure by wide local excision even in cases of regional lymph-node metastases.

Another rare childhood vascular neoplasm is **Kaposi-like infantile hemangioendothelioma** [77,78]. The tumors involve the deep soft tissue, retroperitoneum or skin and are composed of nodules of spindle cells lining slit-like vascular spaces that contain red blood cells. The nodules are separated by fibrous septae. Some cases are associated with lymphangiomatosis or Kasabach-Merritt syndrome. The lesions may be locally aggressive, warranting the hemangioendothelioma designation.

Malignant Tumors

ANGIOSARCOMA

Angiosarcomas are rare malignant neoplasms of endothelial origin that have been described in the literature under a wide variety of terms, such as hemangioblastoma, hemangioendothelioma, and lymphangiosarcoma. These tumors have four different clinical presentations and courses, depending on the site and context of origin. Angiosarcomas involve (1) the skin of the head and neck in the elderly, (2) chronic lymphedematous skin, (3) the breast, and (4) the viscera. Histologically, the angiosarcomas of different sites are similar. The characteristic pattern is freely anastomosing thin vascular channels that dissect and invade surrounding tissues. The channels are lined by enlarged, hyperchromatic, or bizarre endothelial cells that may crowd and protrude into the lumen. Another histologic pattern encountered is fascicles of spindle cells without obvious lumen formation, but there may be slits or spaces between the spindle cells that suggest vascular lumina. A third and least diagnostic pattern is of sheets of undifferentiated, pleomorphic, polygonal cells with hyperchromatic nuclei (see below). Red blood cells are frequently present in all three histologic patterns. In any single angiosarcoma, only one histologic pattern may predominate with foci of the other patterns. Obviously, if biopsy yields only the undifferentiated pattern, definitive diagnosis would rely on the presence of more characteristic histologic features or special techniques. It must be stated, however, that the techniques of electron microscopy and immunoperoxidase may not be helpful in poorly differentiated tumors, since they may lack distinctive ultrastructural features and may not fully express antigens of differentiation. Although angiosarcomas are of endothelial origin, whether they are lymphatic or blood-vessel endothelial cells is still debated. Tumors arising in the background of chronic lymphedema have supported their lymphatic endothelial-cell origin. Other tumors have demonstrable Weibel-Palade bodies, a feature of blood vessel endothelial cells. It appears best at this time to consider these histologically similar lesions under the generic term of angiosarcoma.

A morphologically distinct variant of angiosarcoma, epithelioid angiosarcoma, has been described in the skin, thyroid, and deep soft tissue [79,80]. The tumors are composed of sheets of large, round epithelioid cells with abundant cytoplasm and prominent nucleoli. The epithelioid cells contain intracytoplasmic intermediate filaments and are immunoreactive for keratin proteins. Those features may lead to an incorrect diagnosis of carcinoma. The coexpression of endothelial antigens, such as vWF, and the focal intracytoplasmic lumina or vasoformative architecture confirms its endothelial origin.

Cutaneous Angiosarcoma of the Head and Neck. Angiosarcoma most commonly presents as a cutaneous tumor in elderly patients, with a tendency to locate in the head and neck, especially the scalp [80–82]. The tumor usually appears as an ill-defined, bluish, bruiselike macule or plaque or an erythematous nodule [82]. Ulceration and bleeding, spontaneously or secondary to mild trauma, are additional features. The prognosis of these tumors is poor,

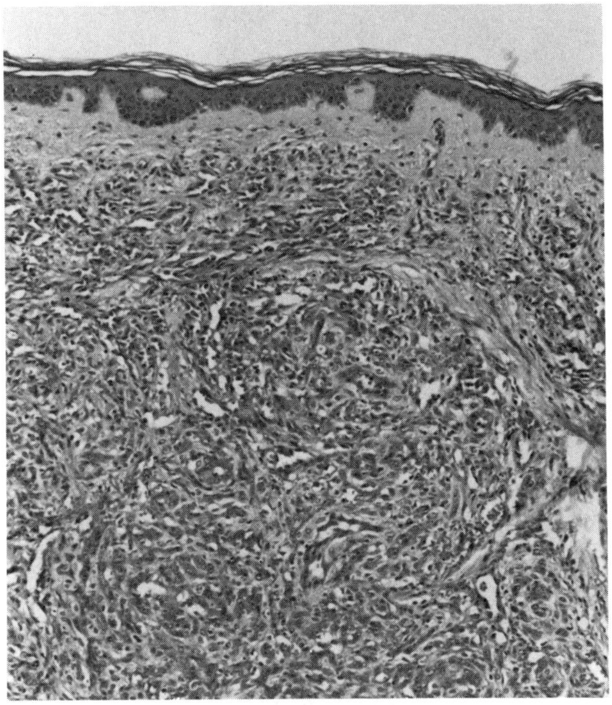

Fig. 56-6. Cutaneous angiosarcoma of the forehead in an elderly man. Numerous anastomosing vascular channels lined by plump, hyperchromatic endothelial cells dissect through dermis and subcutaneous tissue.

with over half of patients dying of the disease and few patients cured [81,83]. The poor outcome is due to several factors. Diagnosis often is delayed due to physicians' unawareness of the entity and patients' procrastination in seeking medical advice. The size of the tumor is an important determinant of response to therapy; therefore, early diagnosis is critical [81]. Important therapeutic characteristics of this tumor are a tendency to extend far beyond its gross borders and multicentricity. Those features make complete surgical excision difficult and recurrence after the initial therapy the norm. In addition to local recurrences, angiosarcomas may metastasize to regional lymph nodes and hematogenously to lung. Histologically, the tumor may appear as any of the types described above (Fig. 56-6). The clinically flat or plaquelike lesions are well or moderately differentiated tumors, and the nodular areas are poorly differentiated spindle-cell tumors. The histologic differentiation does not correlate with the clinical course of the neoplasm. Therapy providing complete remission of these tumors is unusual. The tumors are best treated with surgical removal with required reconstructive techniques as well as wide-field radiation therapy to eradicate the residual foci of tumor. That approach occasionally has been successful in eliminating the tumor from the primary site, but some patients have recurred with distant (pulmonary) metastases [83,84].

Angiosarcoma Arising in Chronic Lymphedema. A rare presentation of angiosarcoma is in the skin and soft tissue in settings of chronic lymphedema. Stewart and Treves first described these tumors in the arms of women who had chronic lymphedema secondary to radical mastectomy and lymph-node dissection [85]. Other etiologies of lymphedema, such as congenital forms, also have been implicated. The causal factors of the lymphedema in promoting the tumor are unclear. Suggestions include uncontrolled proliferation of lymphatic vessels and locally impaired cell-mediated immunity. The tumors appear within 10 years of mastectomy. Superficial lesions are bluish and palpable, whereas the deep lesions may appear only as skin discoloration superimposed on the edema. Although a lymphatic origin has been proposed for this tumor (lymphangiosarcoma), it is histologically similar to the other angiosarcomas. Electron microscopy [86,87], immunoperoxidase studies [86], and lectin binding [88] have confirmed that these tumors are of vascular origin and not recurrences of the primary breast malignancy. These angiosarcomas are highly aggressive and require radical surgery. The tumors are often multifocal and prone to local recurrence with late hematogenous metastases.

Angiosarcoma of the Breast. Angiosarcoma of the breast is a rare and lethal neoplasm occurring in women in the third and fourth decade [89–93]. The tumor most commonly presents as an enlarging, painless mass (Fig. 56-7A) and has great variability in histologic grade, from foci of well-differentiated vascular channels to sheets of spindle cells (Fig. 56-7B). Diagnosis may be delayed owing to the soft, blood-filled nature of the mass, negative mammography, and deceptively benign histology on biopsy. Therapy consists of surgical excision with wide margins, usually total mastectomy. Delayed diagnosis and subsequent tumor growth may compromise adequate treatment. The role of adjuvant radiation therapy and chemotherapy remain to be fully evaluated. Currently, prompt diagnosis and removal provides the best survival. Low-grade tumors composed of well-formed anastomosing vascular channels are associated with significantly better disease-free survival than are high-grade sarcomatous tumors. One study [94] revealed a median disease-free survival of greater than 15 years for low-grade tumors and 15 months for high-grade tumors. Metastases most commonly occur in bone, lung, and liver. Since the tumor occurs in women of reproductive age, even during pregnancy, and some cases have hormonal receptors, a hormonal influence on this tumor has been suggested but requires further investigation [90,95].

Angiosarcoma of the Liver. Angiosarcoma of the liver is an uncommon tumor. It is interesting because of its association with exposure to environmental agents, such as Thorotrast, arsenic (pesticides), vinyl chloride (plastics), androgenic-anabolic steroids, and oral contraceptives [96–98]; however, the majority of cases have had no known exposure to those agents. The latency period is long, approximately 20 years. Thorotrast, a radiologic contrast medium containing thorium, used until the 1940s and 1950s, is deposited for life in the reticuloendothelial system, including the Kupffer cells of the liver. Its carcinogenicity most likely is related to its radioactive emission

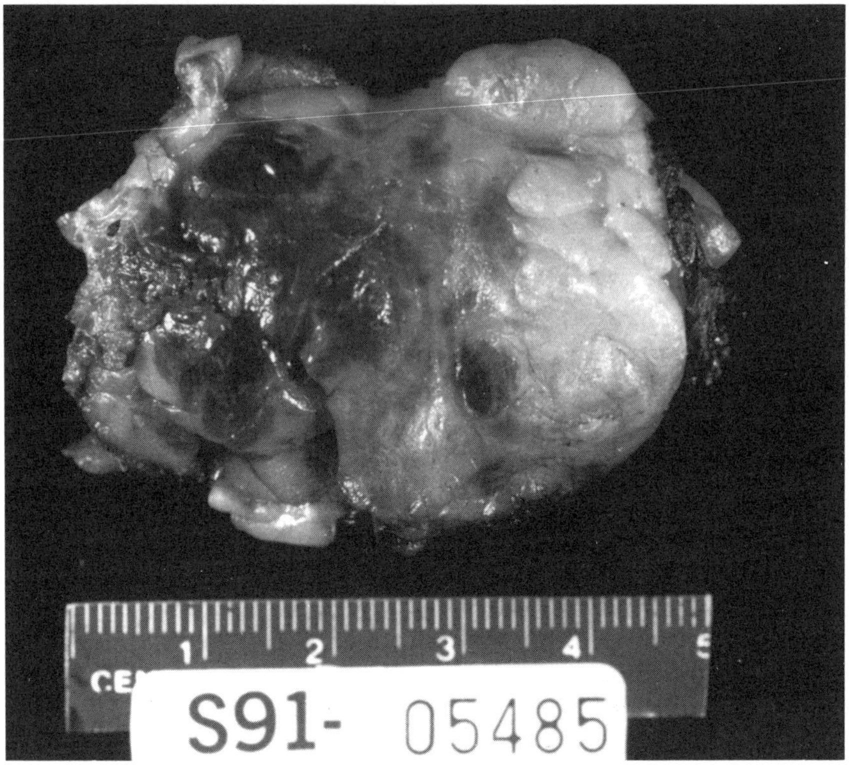

A

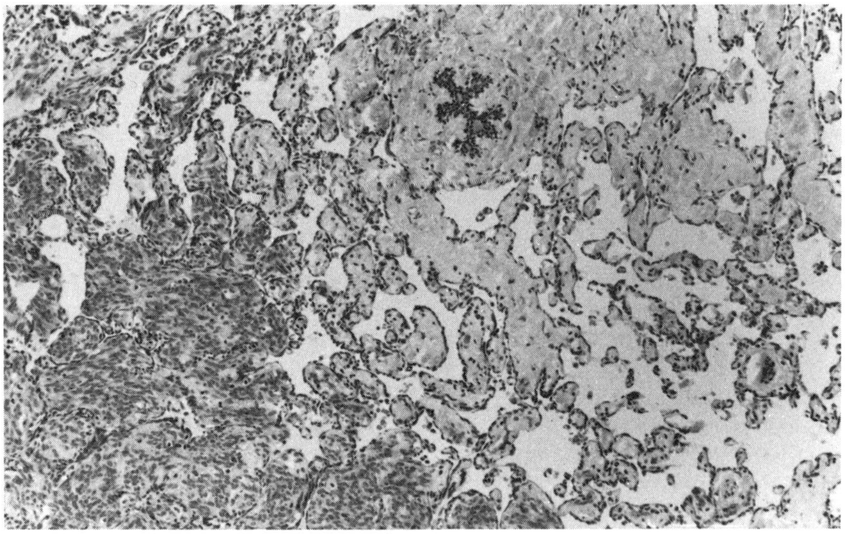

B

Fig. 56-7. **A.** Angiosarcoma of breast. An ill-defined, hemorrhagic mass containing blood-filled spaces is present in fatty breast tissue. **B.** Histologically, the tumor varies from well-differentiated vascular channels invading around a breast duct to poorly differentiated spindle cells.

of alpha particles and its long half-life. The Thorotrast-related angiosarcomas, as well as those related to occupational exposures to vinyl chloride and arsenic, should decrease in incidence now that the association has been exposed.

Liver angiosarcomas present as any liver neoplasm, with pain, weakness, anorexia, and weight loss. There also may be hemorrhagic complications. The tumors frequently are multicentric, and their endothelial origin has been confirmed by electron-microscopic and immunoperoxidase studies [99] for endothelial-specific features. There is no morphologic difference between the tumors of unknown etiologies and those related to specific agents. These angiosarcomas have a poor prognosis, with only 3 percent of patients living longer than 2 years. Death is secondary to widespread metastases, liver insufficiency, or, occasionally, hemoperitoneum.

HEMANGIOPERICYTOMA

Hemangiopericytoma is a tumor of pericyte origin occurring in adults with an equal sex distribution [100]. It is primarily a tumor of the deep, soft tissues of the lower extremity, pelvic fossa, and retroperitoneum, but it can involve any site, including the orbit [101], CNS [102], and viscera [103]. Clinical presentation is that of an enlarging mass. These highly vascular tumors are fairly well circumscribed and surrounded by a thin pseudocapsule. They consist of tightly packed cells with oval nuclei and ill-defined cellular borders lining a ramifying vascular network. The vascular channels are lined by continuous, flat endothelial cells and range from capillary size to dilated sinusoids. The vascular channels frequently have a characteristic "staghorn" pattern. Reticulin stain demonstrates that the tumor cells surround and are distinct from the endothelium-lined channels. This distinction is confirmed by electron microscopy. The tumor cells have few distinguishing ultrastructural features, however. They are surrounded by a basal lamina and have pinocytotic vesicles and sparse organelles. Hemangiopericytomas have a varied clinical behavior, which is difficult to predict by morphologic criteria. Generally, tumors with frequent mitoses (4 or more per 10 high-power fields), pleomorphism, and necrosis have a tendency to recur and metastasize [100]. Some tumors fall into an intermediate group in which biologic potential cannot be predicted. Malignant tumors metastasize to lung and bone, rarely lymph node [100]. The tumors are treated with surgical excision. Ligation of the afferent vessels or embolization of the tumor prior to removal reduces operative hemorrhage and facilitates surgery. There is no agreement as to the efficacy of radiation therapy and chemotherapy.

Infantile hemangiopericytomas are distinct from the adult form. They occur in the subcutis of infants and children as a multilobulated mass. The neoplasm has worrisome histologic features, such as increased mitoses and focal necrosis, but it usually has a benign course cured by local excision.

KAPOSI'S SARCOMA

Kaposi's sarcoma, first described in 1872 by Moritz Kaposi, is a vascular tumor with an intriguing epidemiology. Prior to the AIDS epidemic, Kaposi's sarcoma (KS) was seen in three populations: older men of Eastern European (especially Ashkenazic Jews) or Mediterranean descent (classic KS) [104], children and young adults in equatorial Africa (African endemic KS) [105,106], and the iatrogenically immunosuppressed, especially solid-organ-transplant recipients [107,108]. KS has been associated with the AIDS epidemic since its onset in 1981 and is an AIDS-defining condition. The association has sparked much interest in the pathophysiology of the neoplasm.

The clinical manifestations and courses differ in the four KS groups. Classic KS is a skin disease appearing as single or multiple red-purple or brown patches, plaques, or nodules primarily on the legs of older (50–70 years) men. The tumor is locally aggressive with an erratic course of relapses and remission, rarely causing death. Clinically similar cases occur in Africa, but in a younger male population (mean age 35 years) and with a higher prevalence [106,108]. A generalized form of the disease is also present there, occurring in young adults with cutaneous, nodal, and visceral involvement and in children with primarily lymph-node-based disease. These generalized forms have a poor prognosis. The iatrogenically immunosuppressed have a cutaneous or disseminated lymph-node- and visceral-based disease. Although KS has been described in patients on drug immunosuppression for various diseases, it is most commonly associated with solid-organ transplantation, in which there is a 400- to 500-fold increased incidence over the general population [109,110]. The average time to develop KS after transplantation is 16 months [107]. Regression may occur on withdrawal of immunosuppression. Iatrogenically immunosuppressed KS demonstrates the interplay of immune function and KS, which is further highlighted in AIDS KS.

AIDS KS is a generalized mucocutaneous, lymph node, and visceral disease [111,112]. The overall risk of KS in AIDS patients is more than 20,000 times that of the general population and 300 times that of other immunosuppressed patients [108]. But within the AIDS population, certain subgroups are more commonly affected [108,110]. Homosexual or bisexual men have a much higher incidence than hemophiliacs [108]. In Africa, where AIDS is most commonly spread by heterosexual contact, KS is seen more often in women [110]. Women who contract HIV from bisexual men rather than from heterosexual drug abusers are at an increased risk for AIDS KS [108,110]. AIDS KS is more common in homosexual men in certain urban centers [108]. Finally, classic KS has been reported in young homosexual, sexually active, HIV-negative men in the United States [110,113,114]. Those findings have prompted investigation into the role of a sexually transmitted infectious agent in KS [108,110]. Studies have focused on cytomegalovirus, human papilloma virus-16, herpes viruses, hepatitis A and B, and various sexual practices. No conclusive associations have been found to date.

Other studies on the pathophysiology of KS have focused on HIV and cytokines. Fifteen percent of the male offspring of transgenic mice that contain the HIV transactivating gene (Tat) develop dermal spindle-cell lesions that resemble KS [115]. In those mice, Tat is expressed in the skin but not in the tumor cells, suggesting a paracrine effect. Furthermore, Tat protein derived from the supernatant of HIV-infected cells promotes the growth of KS cell cultures [116]. That effect can be blocked by anti-Tat antibodies. Those studies point to a role of HIV regulatory proteins in KS cell transformation and growth. Studies of AIDS KS cells have shown cytokines and growth factors to be important in promoting KS cell growth. AIDS KS cells placed on chorioallantoic membranes of fertilized chick eggs induce extensive vascularization [117]. Human AIDS KS cells injected in nude mice induce a lesion of mouse origin that resembles early KS [117]. The lesions regress when the inoculated AIDS KS cells die. Those studies suggest that AIDS KS cells secrete factors that

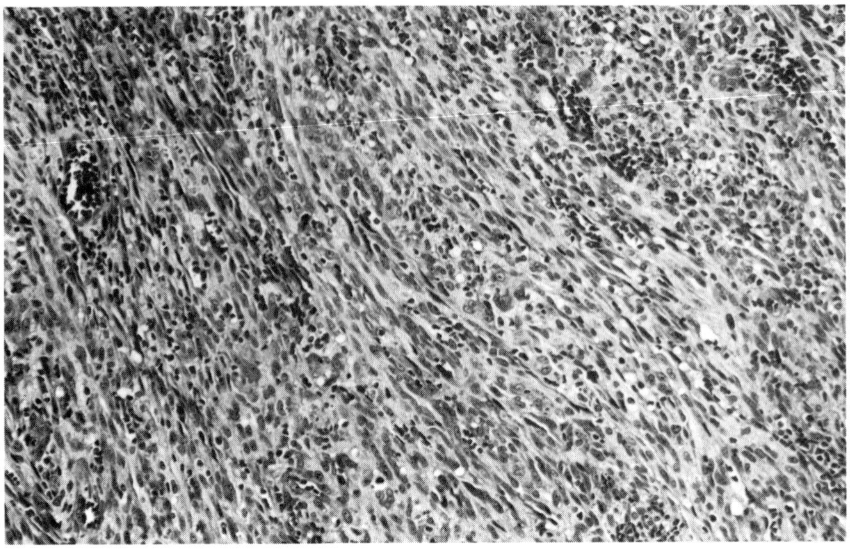

Fig. 56-8. Kaposi's sarcoma.

induce KS lesions. Further studies on cultured AIDS KS cells show that they produce basic fibroblast growth factor (bFGF), interleukin-1 beta (IL-1β), interleukin-6 (IL-6), platelet derived growth factor (PDGF), and other cytokines and growth factors that have both paracrine and autocrine growth effects [118,119]. Those cytokines can act synergistically with Tat in stimulating vascular cell growth [120]. Finally, the immune system also appears to play a role in the development of KS lesions. Conditioned media of chronically activated or retrovirally infected CD4+ T-cells support long-term AIDS KS cell cultures [120,121]. The T-cells produce cytokines, which support the KS cells [121]. In particular, oncostatin M has proven to be a potent mitogen for AIDS KS cells, acting directly and indirectly through IL-6 [122–124]. Those studies imply a complex interplay between HIV-Tat protein, cell transformation, growth factors, and cytokines in the development and progression of AIDS KS.

The different clinical manifestations of KS share similar histologic features. The early, or patch, stage of KS [125] is characterized by jagged, thin-walled, dilated vascular spaces in the upper dermis. The vessels are lined by thin endothelial cells and surrounded by an infiltrate of lymphocytes and plasma cells. This early lesion may be difficult to distinguish from a perivascular dermatitis. The more characteristic histopathologic features of KS are seen in the nodular lesions. Sheaves of spindle cells containing slitlike spaces with red blood cells are intertwined with vascular channels lined by recognizable endothelium (Fig. 56-8). The periphery contains dilated vascular channels. The plaque lesions have features of both patch and nodular lesions.

A variety of cell types, including Schwann cells, pericytes, smooth muscle cells, primitive mesenchymal cells, macrophage dendritic cells, and vascular and lymphatic endothelial cells, have been proposed as the cell of origin of KS [126–131], but the issue currently is unresolved.

The sporadic, non-AIDS-associated tumors in the United States have a good prognosis, with a long course and a 10- to 20-percent disease-related mortality. Radiation therapy is recommended for lesions of the extremities, and chemotherapy has been utilized in patients with nodal disease. Almost all patients with AIDS-associated KS develop disseminated disease. The survival appears related to the degree of immunosuppression and HIV infection rather than tumor burden. Therapy is palliative and includes surgery, radiation therapy, chemotherapy, or alpha-interferon with or without zidovudine [107,108].

TUMORS OF THE LARGE VESSELS

Neoplasms of the large vessels are exceedingly rare. Leiomyosarcomas—tumors of smooth muscle origin—are the best documented, arising most frequently in the inferior vena cava [132,133]. The inferior vena cava leiomyosarcomas occur most commonly in women in their mid- to late adult life, with symptoms related to the level of obstruction. Perihepatic tumors produce Budd-Chiari syndrome; midlevel tumors produce pain and possible renal dysfunction; tumors below the renal veins produce leg edema.

Vascular leiomyosarcomas have intersecting bundles of elongated cells with blunt-end nuclei and are histologically similar to the leiomyosarcomas of other sites. The vascular neoplasms are attached to the vessel wall and grow intraluminally as polyploid masses. The tumor may extend through the thin-walled vein into the surrounding tissue. Therapy of these tumors is directed at surgical removal, and success depends on the tumor location.

Neoplasms of the aorta and the pulmonary artery are mostly poorly differentiated or undifferentiated luminal sarcomas, termed "intimal" sarcomas [133]. The neoplastic spindle cells show little evidence of differentiation by histologic pattern or immunophenotype. The cells are immunoreactive for only vimentin and smooth muscle actin. The pulmonary-artery sarcomas generally are seen in younger patients (mean age 41.3 years) than the aortic sarcomas (mean age 62.3 years). Both groups most commonly present with embolic phenomena. These intimal sarcomas have a worse prognosis than the inferior vena cava leiomyosarcomas, with a mean survival of 23 months for pulmonary-artery sarcomas and 5 months for aortic sarcomas. Patients succumb to metastatic disease or local complications.

References

1. Carstens PHB. The Weibel-Palade body in the diagnosis of endothelial tumors. Ultrastructural Path 1981; 2:315–325.
2. Mukai K, Rosai J, Burgdorf WHC. Localization of factor VIII-related antigen in vascular endothelial cells using an immunoperoxidase method. Am J Clin Pathol 1980; 4: 273–276.
3. Traweek ST, et al. The human hematopoeitic progenitor cell antigen (CD34) in vascular neoplasia. Am J Clin Pathol 1991; 96:25–31.
4. Aiba S, et al. Dermatofibrosarcoma protuberans (DFSP) is a unique fibrohistiocytic tumour expressing CD34. Br J Dermatol 1992; 127:79–84.
5. Abenoza P, Lillemore T. CD34 and Factor XIIIa in the differential diagnosis of dermatofibroma and dermatofibrosarcoma protuberans. Am J Dermatopathol 1993; 15:429–434.
6. Cohen PR, Rapini RP, Farhood AI. Expression of the human hematopoietic progenitor cell antigen CD34 in vascular and spindle cell tumors. J Cutan Pathol 1993; 20:15–20.
7. Sirgi KE, Wick MR, Swanson PE. B72.3 and CD34 immunoreactivity in malignant epithelioid soft tissue tumors. Adjuncts in the recognition of endothelial neoplasms. Am J Surg Pathol 1993; 17:179–185.
8. Miettinen M, Lindenmayer AE, Chaubal A. Endothelial cell markers CD31, CD34, and BNH9 antibody to H- and Y-antigens—evaluation of their specificity and sensitivity in the diagnosis of vascular tumors and comparison with von Willebrand factor. Mod Pathol 1994; 7:82–90.
9. Parnums DV, et al. JC70: a new monoclonal antibody that detects vascular endothelium associated antigen on routinely processed tissue sections. J Clin Pathol 1990; 43: 752–757.
10. Miettinen M, et al. *Ulex europaeus I* lectin as a marker for tumors derived from endothelial cells. Am J Clin Pathol 1983; 79:32–36.
11. Ordonez NG, Batsakis JG. Comparison of *Ulex europaeus I* lectin and Factor VIII-related antigen in vascular lesions. Arch Pathol Lab Med 1984; 108:129–132.
12. Kaplan KL, et al. Monoclonal antibodies to E92, an endothelial cell surface antigen. Arteriosclerosis 1983; 3:403–412.
13. Knowles DM II, et al. Monoclonal anti-human monoclonal antibodies OKM1 and OKM5 possess distinctive tissue distributions including differential reactivity with vascular endothelium. J Immunol 1984; 142:2170–2173.
14. Cui YC, et al. A vascular endothelial cell antigen with restricted distribution in foetal, adult and malignant tissues. Immunology 1983; 49:183–189.
15. Schlingemann RO, et al. Monoclonal antibody PAL-E specific for endothelium. Lab Invest 1985; 52:71–76.
16. Alles JL, Bosslet K. Immunohistochemical and immunochemical characterization of a new endothelial cell-specific antigen. J Histochem Cytochem 1986; 34:209–214.
17. Alles JV, Bosslet K. Immunocytochemistry of angiosarcomas. A study of 19 cases with special emphasis on the applicability of endothelial specific markers to routinely prepared tissues. Am J Clin Pathol 1988; 89:463–471.
18. Mulliken JB, Glowacki J. Hemangiomas and vascular malformations of infants and children: a classification based on endothelial characteristics. Plast Reconstr Surg 1982; 69: 412–420.
19. Fishman SJ, Mulliken JB. Hemangiomas and vascular malformations of infancy and childhood. Pediatr Clin North Am 1993; 40:1177–1200.
20. Warner J, Wilson-Jones E. Pyogenic granuloma recurring with multiple satellites. A report of 11 cases. Br J Dermatol 1968; 80:218–227.
21. Leboit PE, et al. Bacillary angiomatosis. The histopathology and differential diagnosis of a pseudoneoplastic infection in patients with human immunodeficiency virus disease. Am J Surg Pathol 1989; 13:909–920.
22. Tappero JW, et al. Bacillary angiomatosis and bacillary splenitis in immunocompetent adults. Ann Int Med 1993; 118: 363–365.
23. Slater LN, Min KW. Polypoid endobronchial lesions. A manifestation of bacillary angiomatosis. Chest 1992; 102:972–974.
24. Foltzer MA, Guiney WB Jr, Wager GC. Bronchopulmonary bacillary angiomatosis. Chest 1993; 104:973–975.
25. Relman DA, et al. The agent of bacillary angiomatosis. An approach to the identification of uncultured pathogens. N Engl J Med 1990; 323:1573–1580.
26. Koehler JE, et al. Isolation of *Rochalimaea* species from cutaneous and osseus lesions of bacillary angiomatosis. N Engl J Med 1992; 327:1625–1631.
27. Berger TG, Koehler JE. Bacillary angiomatosis. AIDS Clin Rev 1993; 94:43–60.
28. Birtles RJ, Harrison TG, Taylor AG. Cat scratch disease and bacillary angiomatosis: aetological agents and the link with AIDS. Commun Dis Rep CDR Review 1993; 3R:107–110.
29. Warrell RP, Kempin SJ. Treatment of severe coagulopathy in the Kasabach-Merritt syndrome with aminocaproic acid and cryoprecipitate. N Engl J Med 1985; 313:309–312.
30. Warrell RP, et al. Intratumoral consumption of Indium-111 labeled platelets in a patient with hemangiomatosis and intravascular coagulation (Kasabach-Merritt syndrome). Cancer 1983; 52:2256–2260.
31. Larsen EC, et al. Kasabach-Merritt syndrome: therapeutic considerations. Pediatrics 1987; 79:971–980.
32. Latif F, et al. Identification of the von Hippel-Lindau disease tumor suppressor gene. Science 1993; 260:1317–1320.
33. Weiss SW, Enzinger FM. Spindle cell hemangioendothelioma. A low grade angiosarcoma resembling a cavernous hemangioma and Kaposi's sarcoma. Am J Surg Pathol 1986; 10:521–530.
34. Fletcher CDM, Beham A, Schmid C. Spindle cell hemangioendothelioma: a clinicopathological and immunohistochemical study indicative of a non-neoplastic lesion. Histopathology 1991; 18:291–301.
35. Ding J, et al. Spindle cell hemangioendothelioma: probably a benign vascular lesion not a low-grade angiosarcoma. A clinicopathological, ultrastructural and immunohistochemical study. Virchows Arch A Pathol Anat Histopathol 1992; 420:77–85.
36. Battocchio S, Facchetti F, Brisigotti M. Spindle cell hemangioendothelioma: further evidence against its proposed neoplastic nature. Histopathology (Letter) 1993; 22:296–298.
37. Perkin PL, Weiss SW. Spindle cell hemangioendothelioma: a clinicopathologic analysis of 77 cases. Mod Pathol (Abstr) 1994; 7:9A.
38. Allen PW, Enzinger FM. Hemangioma of skeletal muscle. Cancer 1972; 29:8–22.
39. Dwaney K, Vinh TN, Sweet DF. Synovial hemangioma: a report of 20 cases with differential diagnostic considerations. Hum Pathol 199; 24:737–745.
40. Wold LE, Swee RG, Sim FH. Vascular lesions of bone. In S

Sommers, PP Rosen, R Fechner, eds. Pathology Annual 1985, part 2. Norwalk, Conn.: Appleton-Century-Crofts, 1985. Pp. 101–137.

41. Simard JM, et al. Cavernous angioma: a review of 126 collected and 12 new clinical cases. Neurosurg 1986; 18:162–172.
42. Ehren H, Mahour GH, Isaacs H Jr. Benign liver tumors in infancy and childhood. Am J Surg 1983; 145:325–329.
43. Rosen PP, Jozefczyk MA, Boram LH. Vascular tumors of the breast. IV: The venous hemangioma. Am J Surg Pathol 1985; 9:659–665.
44. Rosen PP. Vascular tumors of the breast. III: Angiomatosis. Am J Surg Pathol 1985; 9:652–658.
45. Olsen TG, Helwig EB. Angiolymphoid hyperplasia with eosinophilia. A clinicopathologic study of 116 patients. J Am Acad Dermatol 1985; 12:781–796.
46. Fetsch JF, Weiss SW. Observations concerning the pathogenesis of epithelioid hemangioma (angiolymphoid hyperplasia). Mod Pathol 1991; 4:449–455.
47. Allen PW, Ramakrishna B, MacCormac LB. The histiocytoid hemangiomas and other controversies. Pathol Annu 1992; 27 Pt 2:51–87.
48. Rosai J. Angiolymphoid hyperplasia with eosinophilia of the skin. Its nosological position in the spectrum of histiocytoid hemangioma. Am J Dermatopath 1982; 4:175–184.
49. Eady RAJ, Jones EW. Pseudopyogenic granuloma. Enzyme histochemical and ultrastructural study. Hum Pathol 1977; 8:653–668.
50. Rosai J, Gold J, Landy R. The histiocytoid hemangiomas. A unifying concept embracing several previously described entities of skin, soft tissue, large vessels, bone and heart. Hum Pathol 1979; 10:707–730.
51. Enzinger FM, Weiss SW. Soft Tissue Tumors, 2nd ed. St. Louis: Mosby, 1988. Pp. 581–595.
52. Tsuneyoshi M, Enjoji M. Glomus tumor. A clinicopathologic and electron microscopic study. Cancer 1982; 50:1601–1607.
53. Venkatachalam MA, Greally JG. Fine structure of the glomus tumor. Similarity of glomus cells to smooth muscle. Cancer 1969; 23:1176–1184.
54. Smoller BR, Rosen S. Port wine stains. A disease of altered neural modulation of blood vessels? Arch Derm 1986; 122:177–179.
55. Garden JM, Bakus AD. Clinical efficacy of the pulsed dye laser in the treatment of vascular lesions. J Dermatol Surg Oncol 1993; 19:321–326.
56. Wheeland RG. Treatment of port-wine stains for the 1990s. J Dermatol Surg Oncol 1993; 19:348–356.
57. Finley JL, et al. Port-wine stains. Morphologic variations and developmental lesions. Arch Dermatol 1986; 122:177–179.
58. Weiss SW, Enzinger FM. Epithelioid hemangioendothelioma. A vascular tumor often mistaken for a carcinoma. Cancer 1982; 50:970–981.
59. Ellis GL, Kratochvil FJ. Epithelioid hemangioendothelioma of the head and neck: a clinicopathologic report of twelve cases. Oral Surg Oral Med Oral Pathol 1986; 61:61–68.
60. Lamovec J, et al. Epithelioid hemangioendothelioma of the anterior mediastinum with osteoclast-like giant cells. Light microscopic, immunohistochemical and electron microscopic study. Am J Clin Pathol 1990; 93:813–817.
61. Toursarkian B, O'Connor WN, Dillon ML. Mediastinal epithelioid hemangioendothelioma. Ann Thorac Surg 1990; 49:680–685.
62. Yousem SA, Hochholzer L. Unusual thoracic manifestations of epithelioid hemangioendothelioma. Arch Pathol Lab Med 1987; 111:459–463.
63. Weiss SW, et al. Epithelioid hemangioendothelioma and related lesions. Semin Diagn Pathol 1986; 3:259–287.
64. Dail D, Liebow AA. Intravascular bronchioloalveolar tumor. Am J Pathol (Abstract) 1975; 78:6a, 7a.
65. Bhagavan BS, et al. Intravascular bronchioloalveolar tumor (IVBAT). A low-grade sclerosing epithelioid angiosarcoma of lung. Am J Surg Pathol 1982; 6:41–52.
66. Corrin B, et al. Histogenesis of the so-called "intravascular bronchioloalveolar tumor." J Pathol 1978; 128:163–167.
67. Weldon-Linne CM, et al. Angiogenic nature of the "intravascular bronchioloalveolar tumor" of the lung. An electron microscopic study. Arch Path Lab Med 1981; 105:174–179.
68. Azumi N, Churg A. Intravascular sclerosing bronchioloalveolar tumor. Am J Surg Pathol 1981; 5:587–596.
69. Ishak KG, et al. Epithelioid hemangioendothelioma of the liver: a clinicopathologic and follow-up study of 32 cases. Hum Pathol 1984; 15:839–852.
70. Dean PJ, Haggitt RC, O'Hara CJ. Malignant hemangioendothelioma of the liver in young women. Am J Surg Pathol 1985; 9:695–704.
71. Kelleher MB, Iwatsuki S, Sheahan DG. Epithelioid hemangioendothelioma of liver. Clinicopathological correlation of 10 cases treated by orthotopic liver transplantation. Am J Surg Pathol 1989; 13:999–1008.
72. Marino IR, et al. Treatment of hepatic epithelioid hemangioendothelioma with liver transplantation. Cancer 1988; 62: 2079–2084.
73. Calonje E, et al. Retiform hemangioendothelioma. A distinctive form of low-grade angiosarcoma delineated in a series of 15 cases. Am J Surg Pathol 1994; 18:115–125.
74. Dabska M. Malignant endovascular papillary angioendothelioma of skin in childhood. Cancer 1969; 24:503–510.
75. Manivel JC, et al. Endovascular papillary angioendothelioma. A vascular lesion possibly characterized by "high" endothelial cell differentiation. Hum Pathol 1986; 17:1240–1244.
76. Patterson K, Chandra RS. Malignant endovascular papillary angioendothelioma. Cutaneous borderline tumor. Arch Pathol Lab Med 1985; 109:671–673.
77. Tsang WYW, Chan JKC. Kaposi-like infantile hemangioendothelioma. A distinctive vascular neoplasm of the retroperitoneum. Am J Surg Pathol 1991; 15:982–989.
78. Zukerberg LR, Nickoloff BJ, Weiss SW. Kaposiform hemangioendothelioma of infancy and childhood. An aggressive neoplasm associated with Kasabach-Merritt syndrome and lymphangiomatosis. Am J Surg Pathol 1993; 17:321–328.
79. Fletcher CDM, et al. Epithelioid angiosarcoma of deep soft tissue: a distinctive tumor readily mistaken for an epithelial neoplasm. Am J Surg Pathol 1991; 15:915–924.
80. Tsang WYW, Chan JKC, Fletcher CDM. Recently characterized vascular tumors of skin and soft tissues. Histopathology 1991; 19:489–501.
81. Hodgkinson DJ, Soule EH, Woods JE. Cutaneous angiosarcoma of the head and neck. Cancer 1979; 44:1106–1113.
82. Rosai J, et al. Angiosarcoma of the skin. A clinicopathologic and fine structural study. Hum Pathol 1976; 7:83–109.
83. Holden CA, Spittle MF, Jones EW. Angiosarcoma of the face and scalp, prognosis and treatment. Cancer 1987; 59:1046–1057.
84. Mark RJ, et al. Angiosarcoma of the head and neck. The UCLA experience 1955 through 1990. Arch Otolaryngol Head Neck Surg 1993; 119:973–978.
85. Stewart F, Treves N. Lymphangiosarcoma in postmastectomy lymphedema. Cancer 1949; 1:64–81.
86. Kanitakis J, et al. Stewart-Treves syndrome: a histogenic (ultrastructural and immunohistochemical) study. J Cutan Pathol 1986; 13:30–39.
87. Silverberg SG, Kay S, Koss LG. Post-mastectomy lymphan-

giosarcoma. Ultrastructural observation. Cancer 1971; 27: 100–108.
88. Miettinen M, Lehto V, Virtanen I. Postmastectomy angiosarcoma (Stewart-Treves syndrome). Light microscopic, immunohistochemical and ultrastructural characteristics of two cases. Am J Surg Pathol 1983; 7:329–339.
89. Antman KH, et al. Multimodality therapy in the management of angiosarcoma of the breast. Cancer 1982; 50:2000–2003.
90. Chen KTK, Kirkegaard DD, Bocian JJ. Angiosarcoma of the breast. Cancer 1980; 46:368–371.
91. Donnell RM, et al. Angiosarcoma and other vascular tumors of the breast. Am J Surg Pathol 1981; 5:629–642.
92. Hunter TB, et al. Angiosarcoma of the breast. Cancer 1985; 56:2099–2106.
93. Merino MJ, Berman M, Carter D. Angiosarcoma of the breast. Am J Surg Pathol 1983; 7:53–60.
94. Rosen PP, Kimmel M, Ernsberger D. Mammary angiosarcoma. The prognostic significance of tumor differentiation. Cancer 1988; 62:2145–2151.
95. Brentani MM, et al. Steroid receptors in angiosarcoma. Cancer 1983; 51:2105–2111.
96. Brady J, et al. Angiosarcoma of the liver: an epidemiologic survey. JNCI 1977; 59:1383–1385.
97. Falk H, et al. Epidemiology of Thorotrast induced hepatic angiosarcoma in the United States. Environmental Res 1979; 18:65–73.
98. Popper H, et al. Development of hepatic angiosarcoma in man induced by vinyl chloride, Thorotrast and arsenic. Comparisons with cases of unknown etiology. Am J Pathol 1978; 92:349–378.
99. Manning JT, Ordonez NG, Barton JH. Endothelial cell origin of thorium oxide-induced angiosarcoma of liver. Arch Pathol Lab Med 1983; 107:456–468.
100. Enzinger FM, Smith BH. Hemangiopericytoma. An analysis of 106 cases. Hum Pathol 1976; 7:61–82.
101. Croxotta JO, Font RL. Hemangiopericytoma of the orbit. A clinicopathologic study of 30 cases. Hum Pathol 1982; 13: 210–218.
102. Mena H, et al. Hemangiopericytoma of the central nervous system: a review of 94 cases. Hum Pathol 1991; 22:84–91.
103. Yousem SA, Hochholzer L. Primary pulmonary hemangiopericytoma. Cancer 1987; 59:549–555.
104. Laor Y, Schwartz RA. Epidemiologic aspects of American Kaposi's sarcoma. J Surg Onc 1979; 12:299–303.
105. Gomes D'Olivieira JJ, Oliveira Torres F. Kaposi's sarcoma in the Bantu of Mozambique. Cancer 1972; 30:553–561.
106. Taylor JF, et al. Kaposi's sarcoma in Uganda: a clinicopathological study. Int J Cancer 1971; 8:122–135.
107. Krigel RL, Freidman-Kien AE. Epidemic Kaposi's sarcoma. Semin Oncol 1990; 17:350–360.
108. Tappero JW, et al. Kaposi's sarcoma. Epidemiology, pathogenesis, histology, clinical spectrum, staging criteria and therapy. J Am Acad Dermatol 1993; 28:371–395.
109. Penn I. The changing pattern of posttransplant malignancies. Transplant Proc 1991; 23:1101–1103.
110. Levine A. AIDS-related malignancies: the emerging epidemic. J Natl Cancer Inst 1993; 85:1382–1397.
111. Freidman-Kien AE, et al. Disseminated Kaposi's sarcoma in homosexual men. Ann Int Med 1982; 96:693–699.
112. Gottlieb GJ, Ackerman AB. Kaposi's sarcoma. An extensively disseminated form in young homosexual men. Hum Pathol 1982; 13:882–892.
113. Afrasiabi R, Mitsuyasu R, Nashanian P. Characterization of a distinct subgroup of high risk persons with Kaposi's sarcoma and good prognosis who present with normal T4 cell numbers and T4:T8 ratio and negative HTLV-III/LAV serologic test results. Am J Med 1986; 81:969–973.
114. Freidman-Kien AE, et al. Kaposi's sarcoma in HIV-negative homosexual men. Lancet 1990; 335:168–169.
115. Vogel J, et al. The HIV tat gene induces dermal lesions resembling Kaposi's sarcoma in transgenic mice. Nature 1988; 335:606–611.
116. Ensoli B, et al. Tat protein of HIV-1 stimulates growth of cells derived from Kaposi's sarcoma lesions of AIDS patients. Nature 1990; 345:84–86.
117. Salahuddin SZ, et al. Angiogenic properties of Kaposi's sarcoma-derived cells after long-term culture in vitro. Science 1988; 242:430–433.
118. Ensoli B, et al. AIDS-Kaposi's sarcoma-derived cells express cytokines with autocrine and paracrine growth effects. Science 1989; 243:223–226.
119. Ensoli B, Barillari G, Gallo RC. Cytokines and growth-factors in the pathogenesis of AIDS-associated Kaposi's sarcoma. Immunol Rev 1992; 127:147–155.
120. Barillari G, et al. Effects of cytokines from activated immune cells on vascular cell growth and HIV-1 gene expression. Implications for AIDS-Kaposi's sarcoma pathogenesis. J Immunol 1992; 149:3727–3734.
121. Nakamura S, et al. Kaposi's sarcoma cells: long term culture with growth factor from retrovirus-infected $CD4^+$ T cells. Science 1988; 242:426–430.
122. Miles SA, et al. Oncostatin M as a potent mitogen for AIDS-Kaposi's sarcoma-derived cells. Science 1992; 255:1432–1434.
123. Nair BC, et al. Identification of a major growth factor for AIDS-Kaposi's sarcoma cells as Oncostatin M. Science 1992; 255:1430–1432.
124. Radka S, et al. Correlation of Oncostatin M secretion by human retrovirus-infected cells with potent growth stimulation of cultured spindle cells from AIDS-Kaposi's sarcoma. J Immunol 1993; 150:5195–5201.
125. Ackerman AB. Subtle clues to the diagnosis by conventional microscopy. The patch stage of Kaposi's sarcoma. Am J Dermatopath 1979; 1:165–172.
126. Burgdorf WHC, Mukai K, Rosai J. Immunohistochemical identification of factor VIII-related antigen on endothelial cells of cutaneous lesions of alleged vascular nature. Am J Clin Pathol 1981; 75:167–171.
127. Guarda LG, et al. Factor VIII in Kaposi's sarcoma. Am J Clin Pathol 1981; 76:197–200.
128. Nadji M, et al. Kaposi's sarcoma. Immunohistologic evidence for an endothelial origin. Arch Pathol Lab Med 1981; 105: 274–275.
129. Nickoloff BJ, Griffiths CEM. Factor XIIIa-expressing dermal dendrocytes in AIDS-associated cutaneous Kaposi's sarcomas. Science 1989; 243:1736–1737.
130. Nickoloff BJ, Griffiths CEM. The spindle-shaped cells in cutaneous Kaposi's sarcoma. Histologic simulators include Factor XIIIa dermal dendrocytes. Am J Pathol 1989; 135:793–800.
131. Zhang Y-M, et al. Vascular origin of Kaposi's sarcoma. Expression of leucocyte adhesion molecule-1, thrombomodulin and tissue factor. Am J Pathol 1994; 144:51–59.
132. Kevorkian J, Cento DP. Leiomyosarcoma of large arteries and veins. Surgery 1973; 73:390–400.
133. Burke AP, Virmani R. Sarcomas of the great vessels. A clinicopathologic study. Cancer 1993; 71:1761–1774.

Index

Abdominal aorta, 901
aneurysms, 403–404, 912–917
angiography, 496, 499, 500
noninvasive testing, 425–430
patient examination, 403–404
postoperative, computed tomography, 524, 530
pulse, 402
Abdominal arteries, computed tomography, 524, 531–532
Abdominal injuries
blunt, 1162
penetrating, 1161
Abdominal pain, in visceral ischemia, 874, 876
Abdominal vena cava, computed tomography, 524
Abduction and external rotation (AER), 1196
Accelerated hypertension, 632
ACE inhibitors. *See* Angiotensin-converting enzyme (ACE) inhibitors
Acetylcholine, 132, 370
adrenergic nerves and, 132
for atherosclerosis, 248–249
coronary vasospasm and, 374
endothelium and, 132
for pulmonary hypertension, 961
vascular smooth muscle and, 132
Acetylsalicylic acid (aspirin). *See* Aspirin
Acidic fibroblast growth factor (aFGF), 18
Acid mucopolysaccharides, 56
Acquired antithrombin III deficiency, 270
Acrocyanosis, 377, 984
Actin
myosin interaction, 95–96, 100
in smooth muscle contraction, 95–96, 103
Acyl coenzyme A:cholesterol acyltransferase (ACAT), 315
Adenosine, 77–78, 334
for pulmonary hypertension, 961
Adenosine diphosphatase (ADPase), 265
Adenosine diphosphate (ADP), 77, 168
in magnetic resonance imaging, 448
purinergic receptors and, 132–133
Adenosine triphosphate (ATP), 5, 76–77
force of contraction and, 96–99
in magnetic resonance imaging, 448
purinergic receptors and, 132–133
Adenovirus-mediated gene transfer, 667–668
Adenylyl cyclase, modulation of, 85, 86–87
Adhesion
flow rate and, 165–167
hematocrit and, 168
platelet, 161–162, 167–168, 207
vessel wall shear rate and, 172
Adhesion proteins, 5–6
Adipsin-acylation-stimulating protein (ASP) pathway, 593
ADP. *See* Adenosine diphosphate (ADP)
Adrenergic blocking therapy, beta-. *See* Beta-adrenergic blocking therapy
Adrenergic nerves, 131
acetylcholine and, 132
anatomy, 122
beta-adrenoceptors, 131
in digital vasospasm, 377–378
endings, 122–125
prejunctional alpha$_2$ inhibition, 131
serotonin and, 134
Adrenergic receptors
alpha-. *See* Alpha-adrenergic receptors
beta-. *See* Beta-adrenergic receptors
Adson maneuver, 408–409
Adventitia
in atherogenesis, 303
fibroplasia, 1246
in normal arteries, 289
Afferent renal sympathetic nerves, 356
aFGF (acidic fibroblast growth factor), 18
Age
arterial stiffness and, 190–192
as risk factor for peripheral arterial disease, 703
Aggrecan, 56, 57–60
Aggregation, platelet. *See* Platelets, aggregation
AIDS, Kaposi's sarcoma and, 1279–1280
Alcohol consumption
as risk factor for cardiovascular disease, 578
as risk factor for hypertension, 611, 624, 625
Aldosterone, 621
Aldosteronism, primary, 618, 621–622
Aliasing, 416
Allen test, 407
Allodynia, 1209
Allopurinol, for endothelial dysfunction, 249
Allysine, 45, 51
aldehydes of, 45
Alpha$_2$-adrenergic inhibition, prejunctional, 131
Alpha$_2$-plasmin inhibitor, 212–213
Alpha actinin, 100
Alpha-adrenergic receptors, 69–71
classification, 69–70
distribution and location, 70
heterogeneity, 71
mechanism of action, 70–71
postjunctional, 130–131
in Raynaud's phenomenon, 970
reflex sympathetic dystrophy and, 1210, 1214
vasomotion and, 369–370, 371
Alpha chains
collagens, 40, 42, 47, 49
integrins, 5–6
Alpha-tocopherol, 579–580
Alpha-Tocopherol Beta-Carotene Cancer Prevention Trial (ATBC Trial), 580
Alternative complement pathway, 387
Alveolar hypoventilation, 956
Amaurosis fugax, 782
Ambulatory blood pressure monitoring (ABPM), 614–615
Ambulatory (Holter) monitoring, 707–708, 710, 806
Ambulatory venous pressure (AVP), 1182
Aminorex fumarate, as cause of pulmonary hypertension, 962
Amlodipine, 812
Amputation
for arterial obstructive diseases of the extremities, 847
for pedal ulcers, 1177–1181
for thromboangiitis obliterans, 1046, 1047–1048
Anesthesia, for vascular trauma, 1152
Aneurysms, *See also* Aortic aneurysms; Pseudoaneurysms
abdominal aortic, 403–404, 912–917
angiography for, 499
aortic, 425–427, 901–920
abdominal, 403–404, 912–917
computed tomography, 526
noninvasive testing of, 425–427
arterial
peripheral, 698–699
surgery, 693–697
visceral, surgery, 698–699
cerebral, computed tomography, 549, 550
congenital, 906
coronary-artery, 1235
false, 1147
of Galen's vein, computed tomography, 552
hepatic artery, 698, 920
iliac artery, 406, 429, 917–919
inflammatory aortic
computed tomography, 528–530
noninvasive testing of, 427
intracranial vessels, computed tomography, 539–541
mesenteric artery, 698–699
mycotic (infective endarteritis), 906, 1116–1119
computed tomography, 529, 530
patient examination, 403–406
peripheral arterial, 698
popliteal artery, 404–405, 919
renal artery, 535–537, 699, 920
ruptured, computed tomography, 556
splenic artery, 698
surgery, 697–698, 910–912
traumatic, 906–907, 1156
visceral artery, 698–699, 919–920
Angina
coronary vasospasm and, 376–377
left ventricular function, 799
mortality, 799, 800
nitrate therapy, 808–810
percutaneous transluminal coronary angioplasty for, 814
stable, 337, 376
unstable, 341, 376
aspirin for, 647, 813
variant, 376–377
Angina abdominus, 870
Anginal discomfort, 802, 804
during stress test, 805
nitroglycerin for, 808–810
Angina Pectoris Aspirin Trial, 647

Angiocentric immunoproliferative lesions, 1019–1020
Angioendothelioma, malignant endovascular papillary, 1276
Angiogenesis, 16–20
 endothelial migration, 17
 endothelial proliferation, 17–20
 matrix degradation, 17
 role of, 17
Angiography, 493–516
 aorta, 496–499, 500
 approaches, 496
 cardiac, 511–512
 cerebral, 511
 complications, 1164–1165
 contrast, for peripheral arteries, 838–839
 coronary, 806–807
 digital subtraction, for peripheral arteries, 839
 embolectomy, for peripheral arteries, 844
 equipment
  catheters, 495–496, 724, 1077, 1165, 1255–1258
  contrast agents, 495
  guidewires, 495–496, 734, 742, 743, 745
  imaging equipment, 493–495
 history, 493
 intra-arterial thrombolysis, for peripheral arteries, 844
 intravascular imaging, for peripheral arteries, 839
 intravenous digital subtraction, 860–861
 lower-extremity, 504
 magnetic, for peripheral arteries, 838
 percutaneous transluminal, for peripheral arteries, 843
 in peripheral arterial occlusive disease, 499–504
 peripheral arteries, 495, 499–504, 838–839, 843, 844
 pulmonary, 514–516
 renal, 506–507
 upper-extremity, 505–516
 venography, 512–514
 visceral, 507–511
Angiolymphoid hyperplasia with eosinophilia, 1273
 histiocytoid hemangiomas, 1273
Angiomatosis, 1272
Angioplasty. *See* Laser angioplasty; Percutaneous transluminal angioplasty (PTA)
Angioplasty Compared to Medicine (ACME) trial, 814
Angiosarcoma, 1276–1279
 arising in chronic lymphedema, 1277
 of breast, 1277
 cutaneous, of the head and neck, 1276–1277
 epithelioid, 1276
 of liver, 1277–1279
 Thorotrast-related, 1278
Angiotensin I, 5, 136
 hypertension and, 351, 353
Angiotensin II, 72–73, 136
 classification, 72
 distribution and location, 72
 heterogeneity, 73
 hypertension and, 351, 353, 360–361, 363
 mechanism of action, 72–73
 PAI-1 release and, 254
 in Raynaud's phenomenon, 971
 role of, 370
Angiotensin III, 136
Angiotensin-converting enzyme (ACE), 5
 hypertension and, 351, 353
Angiotensin-converting enzyme (ACE) inhibitors
 for arterial stiffness, 198
 effects on myocardial infarction, 254–255
 hypertension and, 355, 360–361
 for renal vascular hypertension, 856, 864, 865
 smooth muscle proliferation and, 224–225
Angiotensinogen, hypertension and, 351
Ankle-brachial pressure index (ABI), 434, 1174, 1178
Ankylosing spondylitis, 905–906
Anomalous pulmonary venous connection, 1223–1227
 atresia of common pulmonary vein, 1227
 congenital stenosis of pulmonary veins, 1227
 defined, 1223
 embryology, 1223
 partial (PAPVC), 122–125, 1223
 stenosis of common pulmonary vein, 1227
 total (TAPVC), 1223–1224, 1225
Anoxia, 129, 333
Antecubital fossa veins, central venous catheterization complications, 1256
Anterior cerebral artery (ACA), 782–784, 785
Anterior choroidal artery (AChA), 783
Anterior communicating artery (AComm), 783
Anterior inferior cerebellar artery (AICA), 783
Anti-adrenergics, for hypertension, 630–631
Anticoagulants, 6–8, 639–643, *See also* Coagulation; Heparin; Warfarin
 antithrombin III, 7, 265, 269–271
 complications, 643
 for coronary artery disease, 813
 general clinical use, 639–641
 glycosaminoglycans, 7, 18, 56–63
 mechanisms of action, 639
 protease nexin, 7, 212
 protein C, 7, 265–266, 269, 270–271, 277, 278
 protein S, 7, 265, 266, 269, 270–271
 for pulmonary embolism, 1071, 1074–1075
 for pulmonary hypertension, 960–961
 specific clinical use, 641–643
 thrombomodulin, 6–7
 tissue factor pathway inhibitor (TFPI), 7–8, 265
 for venous compression, 1194–1202, 1203
 for venous thromboembolism, 1056, 1060–1061
Antifungal agents, for lymphedema, 1143
Antihemophilic factor (AHF), 209
Antihypertensive therapy, 623–634
 for aortic dissection, 945
 for arterial stiffness, 198
 drug interactions, 628
 drug summary, 630–633
 drug therapy, 625–629
 goals of, 623
 hypertensive crisis, 629, 632–633
 nonpharmacological, 623–625
 pharmacological, 625–629
 refractory hypertension, 633–634
Antimicrobial resistance, in infective endarteritis, 1110
Antineutrophil cytoplasmic autoantibodies (ANCAs), 391, 1002–1003
Antioxidants, 318–319
 dietary, coronary heart disease and, 579–580
 for endothelial vasomotor function, 251–252
Antiphospholipid antibody syndrome, 273, 1023
Antiplatelet agents, 643–655
 aspirin, 644–648
 cAMP and cGMP stimulation, 650
 for coronary artery disease, 813
 dipyridamole, 650–651
 fibrinolytic agents, 653–655
 nonsteroidal anti-inflammatory drugs (NSAIDs), 648
 omega-3 fatty acids, 648–649
 platelet activation and aggregation, 643–644
 platelet membrane glycoprotein antagonists, 652–653
 sulfinpyrazone, 651
 thromboxane-receptor antagonists, 649–650
 thromboxane-synthase inhibitors, 649–650
 ticlopidine, 651–652, 791, 813
Antiplatelet Trialists' Collaboration, 646, 648
Antithrombin III, 7, 265
 deficiency, 269–271
Antithrombotic therapy
 for acute arterial occlusion, 832–833
 for arterial obstructive diseases of the extremities, 842–843
 mechanisms, 265–268
Aorta
 abdominal, 901
 aging and, 190–192, 902
 anatomy, 901
 angiography, 496–499
 coarctation of, 618, 620, 1235–1238
 computed tomography, 525–531
 congenital anomalies, 525–526
 cystic medial necrosis of, 903–905
 histology, 901–902
 injury, 1162
 magnetic resonance imaging, 460, 463
 normal, 525, 901–902
 physiology, 902
 postoperative abdominal, 530
 radionuclide imaging, 486
 rupture, 1238
 sarcomas, 1280–1281
 thoracic, 901
 wall strength, 929
Aortic aneurysms, 901–920
 abdominal, 403–404, 912–917
 computed tomography, 526, 528–530
 dissecting, 902
 vs. ectasia, 902
 etiology, 903–907, 910, 912
  atherosclerosis, 903
  congenital aneurysms, 906
  cystic medial necrosis, 903–905
  infectious aortitis, 906
  mycotic aneurysms, 906
  traumatic aneurysms, 906–907

tuberculous aortitis, 906
vasculitides, 905–906
femoral-artery, 919
fusiform, 902
hypertension and, 632–633
iliac-artery, 917–919
inflammatory, 427, 528–530
noninvasive testing, 425–427
popliteal-artery, 919
pseudoaneurysms, 902
rupture of, 427, 526
saccular, 902
thoracic, 907–910
thoracoabdominal, 910–912
of upper-extremity arteries, 919
visceral-artery, 919–920
Aortic arch, 901, 944
anomalies, 1239–1241
cervical, 1241
clinical presentation and diagnosis, 1241
complete interruption, 1241
double, 1239
ductus arteriosus sling, 1240–1241
incidence, 1239
left, 1239–1240
right, 1239–1240
arteries, fibromuscular dysplasia of, 1246
narrowing of, in coarctation of the aorta, 1235–1238
therapy, 941, 944
Aortic dissection, 927–946
acute arterial occlusion and, 831
anginal pain and, 804
classification, 927–929
clinical presentation, 930–932
computed tomography, 527
defined, 927
diagnosis, 933–939
distal (descending), 927
history, 927
laboratory findings, 932–933
mortality, 927, 945
noninvasive testing of, 427–428
pathogenesis, 929–930
proximal (ascending), 927
spontaneous, angiography for, 498
treatment, 939–946
emergency, 940–941
long-term follow-up, 945–946
technical surgical considerations, 942–945
therapy, 941–942
Aortic graft
computed tomography, 532
infection, 1120–1121
Aortic insufficiency, aortic dissection and, 931, 942, 945
Aortic valve, aortic dissection and, 929
Aortitis
syphilitic, 906
tuberculous, 906
Aortobifemoral bypass graft, 682–685
computed tomography, 531
Aorto-coronary vein grafting, gene transfer and, 671
Aortography, retrograde femoral, 1160
Aortoiliac occlusive disease
bypass graft, 682 683
endarterectomy for, 682
in extremities, revascularization, 846
percutaneous transluminal angioplasty for, 722–729
surgery, 681–685
Aortopulmonary communication, 1242
Aortorenal bypass, 692
Aortovisceral bypass grafting, 880–881
Apical adhesion proteins, 5
Apolipoprotein E, 300
Apoproteins, 307, 308, 309, 311, 319
Apparent viscosity, 146
L-Arginine
EDRF action and, 250
effects of, 256
endothelium-derived relaxing factors (EDRFs) and, 127, 128
Arginine vasopressin (AVP), 370
Arterial aneurysms, *See also* Aneurysms; Aortic aneurysms
peripheral, 698–699
surgery, 693–699
visceral, 698–699
Arterial disorders
chronic obliterative arterial diseases, thrombosis in, 275
dissections, 498–499, 784, 935–938, 1251–1255, 1258
embolism, as cause of acute arterial occlusion, 831
insufficiency
diabetes mellitus and, 1173
in vascular ulcers, 1173
thromboembolism, 269
thrombosis, 269, 275–276
ulcers. *See* Pedal ulcers
vasculopathy, blunt trauma-induced, vasculogenic impotence and, 888–890
Arterial pressure-pulse contour, arterial stiffness and, 194–197
Arterial pulse, 194
Arterial stiffness, 185–197
aging effects, 190–191
defined, 185–188
disease effects, 193
drug effects, 192, 193–194
hypertension effects, 192–193
indices of, 186
measurements, 188–189
monitoring, 198–201
pulse wave effects, 187, 194–197
therapeutic strategies, 198
ventricular-vascular interaction and, 197–198
Arterial walls. *See* Vessel walls
Arteries, *See also* Carotid arteries; Cerebral arteries; Coronary arteries; Digital arteries; Femoral arteries; Iliac arteries; Mesenteric arteries; Pulmonary arteries; Renal arteries; Subclavian arteries; Vessels
adventitia, 289
bifurcation, 145
compliance, 186
compression, subclavian (thoracic outlet), 1193–1196
distensibility, 186–187, 189
elastic recoil, 50
functions of, 39, 185, 189–190
injuries, 1152–1153
intima, 289
mechanical properties of, 189–190
media, 289
narrowing, hypertension and, 231
normal, 289
pulses, 402–403
punctures, as catheterization complication, 1256–1257
structure of, 39–40, 189–190
Arteriography
for brachial plexus compression, 1198
digital subtraction, 861
for renal vascular hypertension, 861
for vascular trauma, 1150
Arterioles, structure, 39–40
Arteriosclerosis, benign, 231
Arteriosclerosis obliterans, 825
Arteriovenous fistula, Raynaud's phenomenon and, 978
Arteriovenous malformations (AVM), 1243–1244
clinical findings and diagnosis, 1243
computed tomography, 541–543, 551, 557
pathology, 1243
pulmonary, 1243
treatment, 1243
Arteritis
Takayasu, 786–787, 857, 905, 999, 1000, 1016–1019
temporal (giant cell), 905, 999, 1015–1016
Arthritis, in infective endocarditis, 1108
Arthus reaction, 387
Artificial materials, thrombogenic potential in circulating blood, 275
Aspirin, 644–648
as anticoagulant, 644–648
benefits of, 646–648
for carotid artery disease, 790–791
for coronary artery disease, 813
for ischemic stroke, 791
low-dose, 579, 645–646
for unstable angina, 647, 813
for vasculitis, 1024
for venous thromboembolism, 1057
Asymptomatic Carotid Artery Study (ACAS), 791
Asymptomatic ischemia, 801
ambulatory (Holter) monitoring of, 707–708, 710, 806
Asymptomatic lesions, treatment of, 676–677
Ataxia telangiectasis, 1245
Atherectomy
directional, 730–731
rotational, 731, 740
Atheroembolism, 832–833
Atherogenesis
cellular interactions during, 292–293
cholesterol and, 587–588
coronary vasospasm and, 377
early development of, 297–298
endothelial control of, 255–257
endothelial injury and, 290–291, 293–295
fatty acids and, 587–588
fatty streaks and, 290
fibrous plaque and, 290
lipoproteins and, 310–312
macrophages and, 291
platelets and, 291
risk factors, 587
thrombosis and, 798
Atherogenic dyslipoproteinemias, 587–601
Atheromatous gruel, 339
Atheromatous lesions, in renal arteries, 856
Atheronecrosis, 324
Atherosclerosis, 225–228
abnormal coronary vasomotion and, 797–798
aortic aneurysms caused by, 903
arterial stiffness and, 193

Atherosclerosis—(*continued*)
computed tomography, 525, 526
endothelium and, 245–257, 797
fatty spot (fatty streak) lesions, 225
fibrinolysis in, 254–255
insudation hypothesis of, 228
intimal cell masses, 225
LDL oxidation and, 318
lesions, 225–228
monoclonal hypothesis of, 230
mortality, 333
oxygen supply and, 333
pathogenesis, 289–295
cellular interactions, 297–303
lipid metabolism, 307–326
platelet hypothesis of, 228
Raynaud's phenomenon caused by, 975–976
renal-artery stenosis, 747–751
renovascular hypertension, 619, 620
replication in, 222–228
response-to-injury hypothesis of, 293–295
risk factors, 377
smooth muscle proliferation in, 225, 797
ultrasound imaging, 423–425
unifying hypothesis for, 230–231
Atherosclerosis obliterans
thrombolytic therapy, 765–775
complications, 773–775
monitoring and termination of infusion, 770–771
patient selection, 765–766
procedural considerations, 767–770
results, 772–773
techniques for shortening, 771–772, 775
Atherosclerotic lesions. *See* Lesions
ATP. *See* Adenosine triphosphate (ATP)
Atrial fibrillation, 342
as cause of acute arterial occlusion, 831
lone fibrillators, 781
pulmonary, 642, 643
Atrial natriuretic factor (ANF), 137
Atrial natriuretic peptide (ANP), 79, 371
Atrophie blanche en plaque, 985
Autocrine PDGF-A, 301
Autonomic denervation, in diabetes, 1175
Autonomic dysfunction, reflex sympathetic dystrophy and, 1212–1214
Autoregulation, 231
Axial dependence, platelets, abnormalities, 178
Axillary-artery injuries, 1161
Axillary-vein thrombosis, 1098
Axillobifemoral bypass graft, 684–685, 846
Axillofemoral bypass graft, 846
Azathioprine, for vasculitis, 1024

Bacillary (epithelioid) angiomatosis, 1271
Back projection, in magnetic resonance imaging, 451
Balloon angioplasty. *See* Percutaneous transluminal angioplasty (PTA)
Balloon-ultrasound-inflation catheter (BUIC), 724
Basal adhesive proteins (integrins), 5–6
Basement membrane collagen, 47–48
Basic fibroblast growth factor (bFGF), 17–18
Basilar-artery occlusion, 785
Behçet's syndrome, 1021
thrombosis in, 275
Benign arteriosclerosis, 231
Bepridil, for coronary artery disease, 814
Bernard-Soulier syndrome, 177, 207
Beta-adrenergic blocking therapy, 131
ancillary pharmacologic properties, 810
antianginal effects, 811
for aortic dissection, 940, 945
combined with calcium-channel antagonist therapy, 812–813
coronary artery disease and, 810–812
for hypertension, 131–132
intrinsic sympathomimetic activity, 810
pharmacokinetics, 810–811
postjunctional, 131
Raynaud's phenomenon and, 970, 977–978
for reducing cardiac risk, 711
selectivity, 810
side effects, 812
vasospasm and, 373
Beta-adrenergic receptors, 71–72, 131
classification, 71
distribution and location, 71–72
heterogeneity, 73
mechanism of action, 72
postjunctional, 131
in Raynaud's phenomenon, 970
vasomotion and, 370, 371
Beta-carotene, 579–580
Beta chains, integrins, 5–6
Beta index (β), 188
bFGF (basic fibroblast growth factor), 17–18
Big endothelin, 129
Biglycan, 60
Biofilm, 1105
Biplaner aortography, for visceral ischemia, 876
Bleeding, from anticoagulant use, 643, 644–645
Bleeding disorders
axial dependence abnormalities and, 178
fibrin formation and, 178–179
platelet diffusion abnormalities and, 177–178
platelet shear rate abnormalities and, 176–177
platelet-vessel wall interaction abnormalities and, 176–179
Bleomycin, Raynaud's phenomenon caused by, 977
Blood, *See also* Blood cells; Flow; Platelets; Red blood cells; Vessels
dyscrasias, Raynaud's phenomenon and, 976–977
hyperviscosity of, 276
islands, 219
leukocyte and platelet redistribution, 157–160
vasomotion effects, 371–372
velocity distribution, 146
Blood cells, *See also* Red blood cells; White blood cells
in annular vortex, 160–162
cell-cell collisions
aggregation due to, 152–155
red cells and platelets, 152–153
shear induced-platelet aggregation, 153–155
two-body collision model, 152
deformation, 151–152
in disturbed flow, 160–162
flow properties, 151–160
in Poiseuille flow, 151
rotation, 151–152
wall migration, 151–152
Blood flow. *See* Flow
Blood pressure
ankle-to-brachial, 434, 1174, 1178
autoregulation, 231
defined, 574
diastolic, 185
hypertension diagnosis, 349, 609–610, 612–615
intermediate phenotypes, 350
kidneys and, 352–357
load, 615
morbidity and mortality, 613
optimal, 574
peripheral resistance, 231
Raynaud's phenomenon and, 971–972
systolic
ankle-to-brachial index, 434
cardiovascular events and, 185
digital, 435–436
exercise testing, 432–433
extremity measurement, 432–433
variability, 613–615
varicose veins and, 1085
in venous system, 1083
Blood pressure measurement, 421–422, 613–614
ambulatory monitoring, 614–615
Doppler spectroscopy, 835
errors, 616
extremity, 432–433
home monitoring, 614
segmental pressure measurement, 835–836
systolic, for Raynaud's phenomenon, 978–979
Blood volume
pulmonary, 951
tracers, 473, 474, 476, 478
in venous system, 1082–1083
"Blue bloater," 955
Blue rubber bleb nevus syndrome, 1245, 1271–1272
Blue-toe syndrome, 681, 736, 832–833
Blunt trauma, 888–890, 1147
delayed impotence and, 889–890
pelvic, 889
penile, 891
perineal, 889
vasculogenic impotence and, 888–890
Bolusing, transthrombus, 770, 771
Boston Area Trial, 791
Boundary layer
defined, 142
in disturbed flow, 143–146
theory, 162–163
Bowel disease, ischemic, computed tomography, 542
Brachial artery, 402
injuries, 1161
Brachial plexus compression, thoracic outlet, 1196–1198
Bradykinin, 5, 136–137
classification, 76
distribution and location, 76
heterogeneity, 77
hypertension and, 361
mechanism of action, 76–77
nonapeptide, 209
Brain death, radionuclide imaging of, 480
Bramwell, J. C., 185
Bramwell-Hill equation, 187
Breast, angiosarcoma of, 1277, 1278
Bretylium tosylate, 123

Bright, Richard, 185
British Doctors' Study, 569
Brodie-Trendelenburg test, for varicose veins, 1086, 1089
Bromocriptine mesylate, as cause of Raynaud's phenomenon, 977
Brownian motion, 141
Brucella spp., as cause of infective endocarditis, 1114
Bruits, 338
 abdominal, in renal vascular hypertension, 857
 continuous, 407
 defined, 406
 epigastric, 407
 neck, asymptomatic, 791
 patient examination, 406–407
 supraclavicular, 407
Buccal nitroglycerin, 809
Budd-Chiari syndrome (hepatic-vein thrombosis), 274
 computed tomography, 545
Buerger's disease. *See* Thromboangiitis obliterans (Buerger's disease)
Bulk flow, 141
Bypass grafts
 angiography, 503
 aortobifemoral, 531, 682–685
 aorto-coronary vein, 671
 aortoiliac, 682–683
 aortovisceral, 880–881
 axillobifemoral, 684–685, 846
 axillofemoral, 846
 carotid artery, 680–681, 1159
 coronary, 531, 708–710, 815–817, 1262
 early closure, 1262–1264
 extra-anatomic, 846
 failure, duplex ultrasonography, 435
 femoropopliteal, 685–686
 infection, 1120–1121, 1155–1156
  clinical presentation, 1121
  diagnosis, 1121
  microbiology, 1120–1121
  pathogenesis, 1120
  prevention, 1121
  therapy, 1121
 microvascular, 896–897
 penile microvascular arterial, 896–898
 percutaneous revascularization and, 740–745
 for venous insufficiency, 1096–1098

Cadherins, 5
Calcified plaque, detected by intravascular ultrasound (IVUS), 718–722
Calcitonin gene-related peptide (CGRP), 137
Calcium
 beta-adrenergic receptors, 72
 cAMP and, 90, 121
 cGMP and, 90, 122
 coupling role of, 95–96
 endothelium-derived relaxing factor (EDRF) release and, 127
 excitation-contraction coupling and, 91–92
 hypertension and, 362, 624, 625
 messenger function, 90–91
 phosphoinositide hydrolysis and, 88, 89
 in smooth muscle proliferation, 104, 117
 sources of, 92–94
 stimulus-response coupling of vascular smooth muscle, 90–91
Calcium-channel blockers, 119–121
 for arterial stiffness, 198
 beta-adrenergic blocking agents and, 812–813
 binding sites, 119–120
 for coronary artery disease, 812–813
 coronary artery disease and, 812
 defined, 43
 heterogeneous response to, 120–121
 for hypertension, 630–631
 for occlusive renal artery disease, 855
 for pulmonary hypertension, 962
 for Raynaud's phenomenon, 980–981
 side effects, 812
 vascular smooth muscle contractile response and, 120
Calcium channels
 alpha-adrenergic receptors, 70
 angiotensin II, 72
 potential (voltage-operated), 91, 117, 121
 receptor-operated, 70, 71, 91, 117, 121
 voltage-operated channels, 70, 71
Calcium gene-related peptide (CGRP), 79
Caldesmon, 103
Calf pain, 828, 829
cAMP. *See* Cyclic adenosine monophosphate (cAMP)
Canadian-American Ticlopidine study, 652
Canadian Multicenter Trial, 813
Candida
 in infective endocarditis, 1104–1105
 suppurative thrombophlebitis due to, 1122, 1123
Candidate-gene approach, hypertension, 350, 351
Capacitive compliance, 186, 188
Capillaries
 functions, 39
 structure, 39–40
Capillary blockade, 475–476, 478
Capillary hemangiomas, 1246, 1269–1271
 bacillary (epithelioid) angiomatosis, 1271
 juvenile (strawberry), 1269–1270
 pyogenic granulomas (lobular), 1271
 senile (cherry) angiomas, 1270–1271
Captopril, 360
 for coronary artery disease, 814
 for hypertension, 236, 237
 in Raynaud's phenomenon, 971
 for renal vascular hypertension test, 859
 renography, 859–860
 scintigraphy, for renovascular hypertension, 620
Carbacyclin analogues, 650
Cardiac angiography, 511–512
Cardiac catheterization, 1253–1255
 complications of, 1253–1255, 1258
Cardiac imaging, 458–460
Cardiac surgery
 early graft closure, 1262–1264
 mortality, 1262
 peripheral vascular, risk, 703–713
 valve replacement, aspirin and, 648
 vascular complications, 1262–1264
Cardiovascular diseases
 cardioembolic stroke, 785–786, 791
 diastolic pressure and, 185
 gene therapy for, 665–672
 modifiable risk factors, 569–581
  alcohol consumption, 578
  diabetes mellitus, 575–576
  dietary antioxidants, 579–580
  hemostatic risk factors, 578–579
  high-density lipoproteins (HDL) and, 307
  hypertension, 574–575
  obesity, 577–578
  physical inactivity, 576
  postmenopausal estrogen therapy, 576–577
  prophylactic low-dose aspirin, 579
  psychological factors, 578
  serum cholesterol, 572–574
  smoking, 571–572
 oral contraceptives and, 273
 prevalence, 333
 risk indices, 704
 systolic blood pressure and, 185
Cardioversion, anticoagulants and, 642
L-Carnitine, for arterial obstructive diseases of the extremities, 842
Carotid arteries
 bilateral lesions, 680
 blunt trauma to, 1156–1157
 computed tomography, 532
 endarterectomy, 675–680
 extracranial-intracranial bypass, 1159
 internal carotid artery (ICA), 783
 ligation, 1159
 noninvasive testing of, 422–425
 penetrating trauma to, 1158
 pulse, 402
 trauma to, 1160–1161
Carotid artery disease, 343–344, 782–784
 asymptomatic carotid stenosis, 791
 carotid dissection, 784
 clinical presentation, 782–784
 symptomatic, 790–791
Carotid bifurcation, 145–146, 147
Carotid-cavernous fistula, computed tomography, 543, 553
Carotid-subclavian bypass, 680–681
Carotid Surgery versus Medical Therapy in Asymptomatic Carotid Stenosis (CASANOVA), 791
Case-control studies, of risk factors, 570
Case reports/series, of risk factors, 569
Catecholamines, 130–132
 adrenergic nerves, 131
 beta blockers and treatment of hypertension, 131–132
 endothelium, 131
 in Raynaud's phenomenon, 968
 tumors secreting, 622–623
 vascular smooth muscle, 130–131
Catheters
 angiography, 495–496
 balloon-ultrasound-inflation catheter (BUIC), 724
 central venous, 1255–1258
 complications
  central venous, 1255–1258
  coronary-artery, 1253–1255, 1258
  vessel-thrombosis, 1165
 pulmonary embolism therapy, 1077
 subclavian veins, 1255, 1257–1258
Causalgia. *See* Reflex sympathetic dystrophy (RSD) (causalgia)
Caval occlusive syndromes, patient examination, 411–412
Cavernosal-artery insufficiency, vasculogenic impotence and, 888
Cavernous hemangiomas, 1245–1246, 1271–1272
 blue rubber bleb nevus syndrome, 1271–1272
 Kasabach-Merritt syndrome, 1271

Cavernous hemangiomas—(*continued*)
 Maffucci's syndrome, 1272
 Von Hippel-Lindau (VHL) disease, 1271
CD31, 15, 1269
CD34, 1269
Ceftriaxone, for infective endarteritis, 1110–1111
Celiac arteries
 injury, 1162
 ultrasonography, 425
Celiac-axis compression, in chronic visceral ischemia, 873
Cell-mediated hypersensitivity, 387
Cell ploidy, 359–361
Cell-receptor proteins, 54
Cellular immune-mediated vasculitis, 390–391
Cellular interactions, *See also* Blood cells; Red blood cells
 in atherosclerosis, 297–303
 during atherogenesis, 292–293
  among smooth muscles, 301
  lipid mediators, 302–303
  macrophage-smooth muscle cell, 291, 299–300
  monocyte-endothelial, 297–298
  research directions, 303
  role of, 297
  T-cell, 301–302
 lipoproteins, 314–315
Central nervous system, hypertension and, 358–359
Central pain-projecting (CPP) neurons, 1211
Central venous catheterization
 antecubital fossa veins, 1256
 complications of, 1255–1258
 external jugular vein, 1256
 femoral vein, 1256
 internal jugular vein, 1255, 1256–1257
 subclavian vein, 1255, 1257–1258
 uses of, 1255
Cerebral angiography, 511
 iatrogenic complications of, 1165
Cerebral arteries
 aneurysms, 549, 550
 blood flow and ischemia, 335
 computed tomography, 551, 558, 559
 thrombotic microcirculation obstruction, 274
 vasospasm of, 369, 379–381
Cerebral hemorrhage
 computed tomography, 559
 hypertensive, computed tomography, 551, 558
 subarachnoid, 380–381
Cerebral ischemia
 acute, 342
 computed tomography, 545, 547
Cerebral perfusion, radionuclide imaging of, 480–481
Cerebral venous angiomas, computed tomography, 552
Cerebral venous occlusive disease, computed tomography, 552
Cerebrovascular accidents, in coarctation of the aorta, 1238
Cerebrovascular diseases, 781–793, *See also* Stroke
 categories, 781
 chronic ischemia, 337–338
 hemorrhagic stroke, 789
 ischemic stroke
  cardioembolic stroke, 785–786
  carotid disease, 782–784
  collagen vascular disease, 786–787
  hypercoagulable states, 786–787
  lacunar stroke, 784–785
  vertebrobasilar disease, 785
 magnetic resonance imaging, 456–457
 noninvasive testing, 422–425
 radionuclide imaging of, 480–481
 risk factors, 781–782
 stroke diagnosis, 789–790
 stroke treatment, 790–793
 stroke in young people, 788–789
 transient ischemic attacks, 338, 342, 545, 675–676, 781, 782, 931
Cervical aortic arch, 1241
Cervical ribs, anatomy, 1190–1191
Cervical rib syndrome, 1187–1189
cGMP. *See* Cyclic guanosine monophosphate (cGMP)
Characteristic impedance, 186, 188
Chelation therapy, 842
Chemokines, 16
Cherry (senile) angiomas, 1270–1271
Chest pain/discomfort
 in aortic dissection, 930–931
 in coronary artery disease, 802, 804
 nonischemic, 804
 in pulmonary hypertension, 953
Chest trauma, angiography for, 497
Chilblains (Pernio), 986
Chlamydia, as cause of infective endocarditis, 1114
Cholesterol, *See also* Lipoproteins
 atherogenesis and, 310
 cellular metabolism, 315
 dietary
  claudication and, 825–826
  hypertension and, 625
 drugs lowering, 574
 economy, in lesions, 300
 emboli, in renal arteries, 857
 flow of, 587–589
 HDL and, 310, 312, 320, 590
 intracellular, 317
 LDL and, 307, 310, 320
 loading, of macrophages, 316
 physical chemistry of, 319–320
 regulation of, 314–316
 removal from cells, 317–318
 reverse transport, 310, 311
Cholesterol Lowering Atherosclerosis Study (CLAS), 252
Cholesteryl ester, 588, 590, 591
Cholesteryl ester transfer protein (CETP), 311, 590, 591
Cholinergic fibers, 370
Chondronectin, 56
Chronic obstructive airways disease (COPD), 955–956
Churg-Strauss syndrome, 1007–1008
Chylomicrons, 307, 312, 587, 589
 defined, 587, 588
 in fatty-acid cycle, 587
 metabolism, 308
 remnants, 587
Chymase, 225
Cigarettes. *See* Smoking
Cine-CT scanning, for visceral ischemia, 876
Circulating immune complexes, in vasculitis, 1001–1002
Classic complement pathway, 387
Claudication
 arm, 1196
 beta-adrenergic blocking agents and, 812
 causes of, 399, 400
 defined, 397–398
 dietary cholesterol and, 825–826
 exercise and, 398
 incidence, 825
 intermittent, 338–339
  in aortoiliac occlusive disease, 681–682
  in arterial disease in lower extremities, 828–829
  in infrainguinal occlusive disease, 685–686
  prevalence, 333
  remissions, 828
 patient examination, 397–401
 percutaneous transluminal angioplasty for, 722, 724
 in peripheral arterial disease, 717
 quantification of, 398
 stable, 339
 variants of, 399–401
 vasospastic, 400
 venous, 400, 829
Clopidogrel, 651
Clot dissolution, fibrinolysis and, 210
CNS catastrophe, hypertension and, 632
Coagulation, *See also* Anticoagulants; Hemostasis
 common pathway of, 208
 extrinsic pathway of, 208–209
 factors, platelets and, 175–176
 fibrinolysis and, 210–214
 hemostasis, 207–210
 intravascular clotting, 213
 intrinsic pathway of, 208, 209
 physical factors affecting, 171–176
 platelet-induced, 178–179
 regulation of, 63
 thrombosis initiation and, 165
 wall shear rate and, 172
Coarctation of the aorta (COA), 618, 620, 1235–1238
 associated conditions, 1237–1238
 classification, 1236
 collateral circulation, 1236–1237
 complications, 1238
 incidence, 1236
 pathology, 1236
 treatment, 1238
Cocaine, vasoconstriction effects, 373
Cogan's syndrome, 1021–1022
Colchicine, for vasculitis, 1024
Cold pressor test, coronary vasospasm and, 376
Collagens
 alpha chains, 40, 42, 47, 49
 basement-membrane (type IV), 47–48
 biosynthesis of, 43–45
 endothelial cell-matrix interaction, 64–65
 extracellular maturation, 45–46
 FACIT (types IX, XII, and XIV), 49–50
 fibers, 189
 fibronectin binding, 54
 functions, 40
 interstitial, 42–43, 46–47
 metabolism, 43–45
 metalloproteinases, 46–47
 microfibrillar (type VI), 48–49
 minor, 47–50
 molecules, 40–42
 turnover, 46
 types, 39, 40–43
Collagen vascular diseases
 of extracranial and large vessels, 786–787

of intracranial and small vessels, 787
Collateral circulation, *See also* Flow
in coarctation of the aorta, 1236–1237
limb perfusion, 830
pharmacologic enhancement of, 842
role of, 343–344
Collision frequency, 152
Colony-stimulating factor, 319
Common pathway, of coagulation, 208
Communicating arteries, 783, 1242
Communicating veins, 1081
Compartment syndrome
diagnosis, 400
thrombolytic therapy and, 774
in vascular trauma, 1148, 1154
Complement
activation of, 387–388
assays, in vasculitis, 1001
binding to immune complexes, 387–388
defined, 387
pathways, 387–388
Complete blood count, in vasculitis, 1001
Compliance
arterial, 186
capacitive, 186, 188
oscillatory, 186, 188
Complicated lesions, 323
Compression
intermittent, 1056, 1081
for venous ulcers, 1184
Compression stockings
for lymphedema, 1143
for pulmonary embolism prevention, 1070
for varicose veins, 1087
for venous thromboembolism, 1056–1057
for venous ulcers, 1184
Compression syndromes of thoracic outlet, 1187–1205
anatomic concepts, 1187–1190
arterial compression, 1193–1196
brachial plexus compression, 1196–1198
follow-up care, 1205
operative management, 1203–1205
pathologic anatomy, 1190–1193
venous compression, 1198–1203
Computed tomography (CT), 519–563
abdominal arteries, 531–532
aorta, 525–531
contrast enhancement, 523, 935, 938
coronary arteries, 482–483, 532–535
defined, 519
in diagnosis, 525–563
dosimetry, 524–525
dynamic (rapid) scanning, 523
image characteristics, 523
intracranial perfusion, 553–555
intracranial vessels, 539–553
lymphedema, 1142
pulmonary arteries, 531
scanners, 519–523
stable xenon-enhanced, 555
stroke diagnosis, 788–789
for vascular graft infection, 1121
vena cava, 535–539
weaknesses of, 523–524
Congenital disorders, 1223–1248
aneurysms, 906
great vessels
aortic-arch anomalies, 1239–1241
coarctation of the aorta, 1235–1238
pulmonary trunk and arteries, 1241–1242
heart
anomalous venous connections, 1223–1228
coronary-artery anomalies, 1228–1234
coronary artery fistulas, 1234–1235
heart disease, 954–955
radionuclide imaging of, 487–488
vascular
arteriovenous malformation, 1243–1244
fibromuscular dysplasia, 1246–1248
telangiectasias, 1244–1246
Congestive heart failure
arterial stiffness and, 193
hypertension and, 632
in infective endocarditis, 1107
Connective tissue of subendothelium, 39–65
biological considerations, 63–65
collagen chemistry and structure, 40–43
collagen metabolism, 43–47
diseases, 956–957, 974–975
elastin, 50–53
fibronectin, 53–55
glycosaminoglycans, 56–63
laminin, 55–56
minor collagens, 47–50
Raynaud's phenomenon and, 974–975
variations in vasculature, 39–40
Continuous bruits, 407
Contractile proteins, 100
Contraction of vascular smooth muscle, 91–107, 117
calcium antagonists and, 120
calcium sources, 92–94
excitation-contraction coupling, 91–92
force generation, 94–103
force of, 94–103
proliferation, 103–107
regulatory mechanisms, 100–103
Contrast agents, for angiography, 495
Contrast angiography, for peripheral arteries, 838–839
Contrast aortography, for aortic dissection, 937
Contrast-enhanced computed tomography, 523, 935, 938
Contrast pulmonary angiography, 958
Convective-diffusive transport
classic theory of, 162–165
defined, 162
physical factors affecting, 165–171
Convective transport, 148–151, 162
Copenhagen Study, 791
Coral reef atheroma, 873
Core proteins, 60, 62
Coronary angiography, 799–801
complications of, 1253, 1254
iatrogenic complications of, 1165
value of, 806–807
Coronary angioplasty, 710
Coronary arteries, *See also* Arteries
anomalies, 1228–1234
aneurysms, 1235
classification, 1228
distribution, 1229
fistulas, 1234–1235
high take-off, 1234
hypoplastic, 1234
originating in aorta, 1232–1233
originating in left aortic sinus, 1234
originating in pulmonary trunk, 1228–1232
single ostium from aorta, 1234
catheterization complications, 373, 1251–1253, 1256, 1258–1262
computed tomography, 532–535
dissection
catheter-induced, 1253
as catheterization complication, 1258
medial necrosis and, 1255
revascularization, cardiac risk and, 708–710
vasospasm of, 374–377
Coronary artery disease (CAD), 797–817
angiographic criteria, 799–801
anticoagulant therapy, 813
antiplatelet therapy, 813
beta-adrenergic blocking therapy, 810–811
calcium-channel antagonist therapy, 812–813
catheterization complications, 1251–1253, 1256
diagnosis, 802–807
history, 802, 804
laboratory tests, 805
noninvasive evaluation, 805–807
physical examination, 804–805
intracoronary devices for, 814–815
left ventricular function, 799, 803
lipoprotein (a) and, 598
magnetic resonance imaging, 458–460
management, 807–808
medical therapy, 808–817
mortality and morbidity, 797, 799
multivessel, 800
nitrate therapy, 808–810
pathogenic mechanisms, 797–799
pathophysiology of myocardial ischemia in, 245–246
percutaneous transluminal coronary angioplasty for, 814–815
peripheral arterial surgery and, 703–704
prevalence, 333
prognosis and natural history of, 799–802
radionuclide imaging of, 481–485
Coronary Artery Study, 1165
Coronary Artery Surgery Study (CASS), 336
Coronary bypass grafting, 708–710, 815–817
complications, 1262
computed tomography, 531
Coronary heart disease (CHD)
acute coronary syndromes, 341–342
dietary antioxidants and, 579–580
gender factors, 576–577
HDL cholesterol and, 310–312
health care costs, 609
high-density lipoproteins (HDL) and, 307
mortality rates, 569
risk factors, 569
alcohol consumption, 578
diabetes mellitus, 575–576
estrogen therapy, 576–577
hemostatic, 578–579
high blood pressure, 574
hypertension, 574–575
obesity, 577–578
psychological, 578
serum cholesterol elevation and, 572–574
Coronary vasospasm, 374–377
coronary catheters and, 373
defined, 369
diagnosis, 374
Corporal veno-occlusion, 887–888
dysfunction, 890
mechanism, 886

Corticosteroids, for vasculitis, 1024
Cor triatriatum, 1227
Corynebacteria (diptheroids), as cause of infective endocarditis, 1114
Cost-benefit analyses, of risk factors, 571
Costoclavicular maneuvers, 408
Costovertebral ligament, 1193
Costs, health care. *See* Health care costs
Cranial vessels, magnetic resonance imaging, 457–458
C-reactive protein (CRP), in vasculitis, 1000
Creatinine kinase, 99
CREST syndrome, 957, 974
Cross-cultural studies, of risk factors, 569–570
Cross-femoral grafting, 724, 727
Cross-flow, 145
Cross-linking, elastin, 50, 51, 52
Cryofibrinogenemia, 977
Cryoglobulinemia, mixed essential, 1011–1012
Cryoglobulins, 1011
 in Raynaud's phenomenon, 976–977
 in vasculitis, 1002
c-sis, 221
Culture-negative endocarditis, 1107
Cumulative-trauma disorders, 1190
Cushing reflex, 359
Cushing's syndrome, 618, 620–621
 corticotropin-dependent, 620
 corticotropin-independent, 620
Cushions, 225
Cutaneous perfusion pressure, in limbs, 830
Cutaneous telangiectasis, 1245
Cyclic adenosine monophosphate (cAMP), 371, 644, 650
 cellular effects of, 121
 dopaminergic receptors and, 78
 formation of, 89
 histaminergic receptors and, 76
 junctional permeability and, 5
 muscarinic receptors and, 74
 penile erection and, 887
 platelet-derived growth factor (PDGF) and, 81, 104
 prostanoid receptors and, 80
 purinergic receptors and, 77
 signal transduction and, 84
 vascular smooth muscle activity and, 89–90
Cyclic guanosine monophosphate (cGMP), 371, 644, 650
 atrial natriuretic factor (ANF) and, 137
 cellular effects of, 121–122
 formation of, 122
 G-protein regulation of, 85
 histaminergic receptors and, 76
 muscarinic receptors and, 74
 opioid peptides and, 79
 penile erection and, 887
 prostanoid receptors and, 80
 signal transduction and, 84
 vascular smooth muscle activity and, 90
Cyclic nucleotides, 89–90
Cyclooxygenase-dependent endothelium-derived contracting factors, 128–130
Cyclooxygenase-independent endothelium-derived contracting factors, 128–130
Cyclophosphamide, for vasculitis, 1024
Cyclosporine-related hypertension, 623
Cystic medial necrosis, 193
 aortic aneurysms and, 903–905, 907
 aortic dissection and, 927, 929
Cytokines
 endothelium and, 4, 16
 monocyte adhesion and, 299
 synthesis of, 16
 in vasculitis, 390, 391
Cytoskeletal anchor proteins, 5–6
Cytotoxic drugs, for vasculitis, 1024

DAG. *See* 1,2-diacylglycerol (DAG)
Dazoxiben, for Raynaud's phenomenon, 971, 982
"Dead finger," 965
Deceleration injuries, angiography, 496, 497
Decorin, 60
Deep-soft-tissue hemangiomas, 1272
Deep-vein thrombosis (DVT), *See also* Thrombosis
 anticoagulants for, 641–642
 magnetic resonance imaging, 463
 noninvasive testing, 436–439
 patient examination, 410–411
 pulmonary embolism and, 1051
 radionuclide imaging for, 486
 varicose veins caused by, 1084–1085
 venous insufficiency and, 1092–1093
Deferoxamine, for endothelial dysfunction, 249
Defibrotide, for venous ulcers, 1184
Dehydroepiandrosterone sulfate (DHEAS), 886
Delequamine hydrochloride, for vasculogenic impotence, 894
Demographic analysis, for hypertension, 626, 627
Dendritic cells, in vasculitis, 391
Dense bands, 100
Dense bodies, 100
Dermatan sulfate (DS), 57, 60, 62, 63
Dermatomyositis, as cause of Raynaud's phenomenon, 975
Desamino-[Arg^8]-vasopressin, 9
Descemet's membrane, 42
Descriptive studies, of risk factors, 569–570
Diabetes Control and Complications Trial (CCT), 575
Diabetes mellitus
 arterial insufficiency and, 1173
 atherosclerosis of the extremities and, 826–827
 insulin-dependent (IDDM), 575–576
 lipoproteins and, 587, 598–599
 non-insulin-dependent (NIDDM), 575–576
 pedal ulcers and, 1173, 1174–1177
 as risk factor for cardiovascular disease, 575–576
 as risk factor for peripheral arterial disease, 703
 as risk factor for stroke, 781
 thrombosis in, 274
1,2-diacylglycerol (DAG), 84
 mechanism of action, 88, 89
 PDGF and, 104
Diastolic pressure, cardiovascular events and, 185
Diet
 antioxidants, 579–580
 calcium, 362
 cholesterol, 625, 825–826
 control of atherosclerotic lesions through, 326
 hypertension and, 361–363, 625, 962
 potassium, 362–363, 624, 625
 protein, 625
 saturated fat, 624, 625
 sodium, 354–357, 359, 361–362, 611, 624, 625
 starch, 625
Dietary Intervention Study in Hypertension, 575
Dietary pulmonary hypertension, 962
Dieulafoy's disease, 1243
Diffusible tracers, 476, 478
Diffusive transport, 148–151, 162–163, 164–165, 167–168
Digital angiography, 494, 505–506
Digital arteries
 in Raynaud's phenomenon, 966–967, 969–972
 sensitivity of, 969–970
 vasospasm of, 377–379
Digital ischemia, 274, 505–506
Digital pulse-volume contour, for Raynaud's phenomenon, 435
Digital subtraction angiography (DSA), 494–495
 for aortic dissection, 938
 intravenous, 860–861
 for peripheral arteries, 839
 for vascular trauma, 1150
Digital subtraction arteriography, for renal vascular hypertension, 861
Digital systolic pressure, 436
Diltiazem, 812, 813, 981
Diptheroids (corynebacteria), as cause of infective endocarditis, 1114
Dipyridamole, 650–651
 for coronary artery disease, 813
Dipyridamole thallium imaging, for ischemia, 706
Directional atherectomy, 730–731
 coronary (DCA), 814, 815
Direct lymphocyte-mediated vasculitis, 390–391
Dissections, *See also* Aortic dissection
 angiography for, 498–499
 aortic aneurysms, 902
 carotid, 784
 catheter-induced, 1251–1255
 coronary artery, 1253, 1255, 1258
 hematoma, computed tomography, 526–528
 magnetic resonance imaging for, 499, 935–937, 938
Dissector technique, for estimating cells in vessel walls, 235
Disseminated intravascular coagulation (DIC), 210, 272
Distensibility, 186–187, 189
Diuretics, for hypertension, 630–631
Dizziness, in pulmonary hypertension, 952–953
DNA, gene therapy, 665–669
Docosahexanoic acid (DHA), 649
Dopamine, 122
Dopaminergic agonists, 895
Dopaminergic receptors, 78
Doppler shift, 415–416
 blood flow velocity and, 430
 in cerebrovascular disease, 424
 waveform, 430–431
Doppler stethoscopy, 835
Doppler ultrasonography, 415–418
 for abdominal aorta diseases, 425–430
 aliasing, 416
 for aortic aneurysms, 427

for aortic dissection, 933
for arterial occlusive disease of the extremities, 430–433
bidirectional systems, 415
blood pressure measurement with, 422
for cerebrovascular disease, 422–425
color, 416–418
for abdominal aorta diseases, 424–425
advantages, 424
for cerebrovascular disease, 423–425
duplex, 434–435
for venous diseases, 438
continuous-wave systems, 415
for deep-vein thrombosis, 436, 437–439
duplex
for arterial obstructive diseases of the extremities, 836–837
for chronic venous disorders, 438–439
color-assisted, 434–435
for vascular trauma, 1150
for vasculogenic impotence, 891–892, 896–897
for venous diseases, 438
for venous insufficiency, 1094
for visceral ischemia, 876–877
pulse repetition frequency (PRF), 416
pulse wave systems, 415, 416
for renal vascular hypertension, 861
transcranial, 425
for vascular trauma, 1150
for venous insufficiency, 1094
for venous thromboembolism, 1053–1054
Doppler velocity spectroscopy, 836
Dorsalis pedal pulse, 403
Dosimetry, computed tomography, 524–525
"Double-crush" syndrome, 1196–1197
Ductus arteriosus
in coarctation of the aorta, 1236, 1238
sling, 1240–1241
Duplex Doppler ultrasonography
for arterial obstructive diseases of the extremities, 836–837
for chronic venous disorders, 438–439
color-assisted, 434–435
for vascular trauma, 1150
for vasculogenic impotence, 891–892, 896–897
for venous diseases, 438
for venous insufficiency, 1094
for visceral ischemia, 876–877
Dysbetalipoproteinemia, 308
Dysfibrinogenemia, 271
Dyslipidemia, as risk factor for hypertension, 611
Dyslipoproteinemias, 587–601
deep abdominal obesity and, 599
diabetes mellitus and, 598–599
familial defective apoB100 syndrome, 595–597
familial hypercholesterolemia, 595–597
familial hypertriglyceridemia (FHTG), 594–595
HDL deficiency (hypoalphalipoproteinemia), 594–595
hyperapoB100 (familial combined hyperlipidemia), 592–594
hyperlipoproteinemia, Type III, 597–598
hypothyroidism and, 599
lipoprotein (a), 598
medications and, 599
plasma profiles, 591–592
renal disease and, 599
therapy, 600–601
East Boston Elderly Cohort, 575
Echocardiography, 707
exercise, 806
for pulmonary embolism, 1074–1075, 1076
Edema
pathogenesis, 1137–1138
in reflex sympathetic dystrophy, 1211–1212
EDRF. *See* Endothelium-derived relaxing factor (EDRF)
Efferent renal sympathetic nerve activity (ERSNA), 357
Efferent renal sympathetic nerves, 356
Effort thrombosis, 275, 1098, *See also* Paget-Schroetter syndrome
Ehlers-Danlos syndrome, 930, 1235
Eicosanoids, 11
Eicosapentaenoic acid (EPA), 649
Ejection fraction, 707, 799, 800
Elastic fibers, 189, 190–192
Elastic modulus, 186
Elastin, 50–53
cross-links, 50, 51, 52
metabolism, 52–53
precursors, tropoelastin, 51–52
structure, 50
turnover, 53
Electrocardiography, 805–806
Electromagnetic flowmeter, 445
Electrophysiologic examination, for brachial plexus compression, 1197–1198
Elevated arm stress test (EAST), 409, 1196
Elevation-dependency testing, 407
Embolectomy, for peripheral arteries, 844
Embolism
acute peripheral ischemia and, 342
arterial occlusion, 874, 878
in infective endocarditis, 1108, 1114–1115
pulmonary, anticoagulants for, 641–642
of thrombus fragments during thrombolytic therapy, 774
Emotional support, for pulmonary embolism, 1077–1078
Endarterectomy
aortoiliac, 682
carotid, 675–680
extremities, 680, 845–846
visceral, 693, 881
EndoCAM, 15
Endocrine model, 297
Endocrinologic hypertension, 620–623
Cushing's syndrome, 618, 620–621
pheochromocytoma, 618, 622–623
primary (hyper)aldosteronism, 618, 621–622
Endocytosis, 312
Endoperoxides, 126
Endothelial cells, 125–130
acetylcholine and, 132
activation of circulating substances by, 125–126
adhesion functions, 5–6, 13–15, 297–298
angiogenesis, 16–20
anticoagulants, 6–8
barrier functions, 3–6
capillary, 64
catecholamines and, 131
cell-matrix interactions, 63–64
continuous, 3
cytokines and, 4, 16
cytoskeletal anchor proteins, 5–6
denudation, 222–223, 232
discontinuous, 3
dysfunction, 245–257, 374
embryonic development of, 219
fenestrated, 3
fibrinolysis, 10–11, 253–255
functions, 3, 4–5, 125, 245, 797
gamma interferon and, 301–302
hemostasis and, 6–10, 209–210
immunohistochemical markers, 1269, 1273
intimal growth regulation by, 255–257
leukocyte interactions, 13, 298–299
lumen caliber and, 226
lymphatic, 1133
matrix properties, 6, 17
metabolic functions, 4–5
microcirculatory disorders, diabetic, 1174–1176
migration, 17
monocyte interactions, 297–299
permeability of, 3–4
platelet regulation, 8, 246–253
procoagulant activities, 8–10
proliferation, 17–20, 106
protease treatment, 63
scavenger-receptor activity, 317
serotonin and, 134
smooth muscle cell interaction, 300–301
thrombosis regulation, 207, 253–255
vascular tone regulation, 11–12, 246–253
vasoconstrictor response, 343
vasomotor function, 250–253, 371, 372
Endothelial injury, 374, 376
atherogenesis and, 290–291, 293–295
atherosclerosis and, 293–295
cell response, 12–16
cerebral vasospasm and, 381
LDL oxidation and, 318
in Raynaud's phenomenon, 971
vasomotion and, 798
Endothelial leukocyte adhesion molecule (ELAM), 14, 298
Endothelin (ET), 11–12, 128–130, 371
coronary vasospasm and, 376
smooth muscle proliferation and, 106–107
Endotheliolopathy, 245
Endothelium-derived contracting factors, 11
cyclooxygenase-dependent, 128
cyclooxygenase-independent, 128–130
Endothelium-derived hyperpolarizing factor (EDHF), 11, 128, 132
release of, 246
as vasodilator, 371, 372
Endothelium-derived relaxing factor (EDRF), 11, 74, 126–128, 132, 236, 265, 300–301, 343, 370
bradykinin and, 137
coronary vasospasm and, 374
effects of, 254, 255–256, 797
impairment of, 246, 247–250, 257
nitric oxide (NO), 265
nonprostanoid, 126–128
penile erection and, 887
release, 246, 255
serotonin and, 134
as vasodilator, 371
Endotoxins, endothelium permeability and, 4
Endovascular repair, of vascular injuries, 1168
End-stage renal disease (ESRD), 856
En passant synapse, 123

Entactin, 56
Enterococci, in infective endocarditis, 1106–1107, 1111
Entrance length, 142
Eosinophilia, angiolymphoid hyperplasia with, 1273
Eosinophilia-myalgia syndrome (EMS), 962
Epidermal growth factor (EGF), 81, 211, 221–222, 291–292
Epigastric bruits, 407
Epinephrine, 72
  physiologic effects of, 130
  in Raynaud's phenomenon, 968
  role of, 371
  sources of, 130
Epithelioid (bacillary) angiomatosis, 1271
Epithelioid angiosarcoma, 1276
Epithelioid hemangioendothelioma, 1275–1276
Epithelioid hemangioma (angiolymphoid hyperplasia with eosinophilia), 1273
Erection physiology, penis, 886–888
Ergot drugs
  finger circulation effects, 378
  Raynaud's phenomenon caused by, 977
  vasospasm and, 373
Erythrocytes
  in annular vortex, 160
  dispersion induced by, 155–160
  sedimentation rate, in vasculitis, 1000
Erythromelalgia (erythermalgia), 274, 988–989
Esmolol, 811
Essential hypertension, 349–363
Estrogen therapy
  for endothelial vasomotor function, 252–253
  postmenopausal, as cardiovascular risk factor, 576–577
  thromboembolism and, 273
Ethylenediaminetetraacetate (EDTA), for arterial obstructive diseases of the extremities, 842
European Coronary Surgical Study, 816
European Working Party on Hypertension in the Elderly, 185
European Cooperative Study, 790
Evaluation of 7E3 for the Protection of Ischemic Complications (EPIC), 652
Examination procedures, 397–413
  arterial system, 397–409
    acute arterial occlusion, 401–409
    Allen test, 407
    aneurysms, 403–406
    bruits, 406–407
    chronic occlusive arterial disease, 397–401
    claudification, 397–401
    coronary artery disease, 804
    elevated arm test, 409
    elevation-dependency testing, 407–408
    exercise test, 407
    historic examination, 397
    ischemic neuropathy, 401
    outlet maneuvers, 408–409
    pulses, 402–403
    rest pain, 401
    skin, 409
  hypertension, 615–616
  lymphatic disease, 413
  venous system, 409–413
    caval occlusive syndrome, 411–412
    deep venous thrombosis, 410–411
    superficial phlebitis, 410
    varicose veins, 410
    venous insufficiency, 412–413
Excimer-laser angioplasty, 740, 743, 814, 815
Excitation-contraction coupling, in vascular smooth muscle, 91–92
Excitatory amino acids (EAAs), reflex sympathetic dystrophy and, 1210, 1211, 1214
Excitatory junction potential (EJP), 69–70
Excitotoxicity, 792
Exercise
  cardiovascular disease and, 576
  claudication and, 398, 828
  endothelial vasomotor function and, 253
  high-density lipoproteins and, 576
  hypertension and, 624
  low-density lipoproteins and, 576
Exercise echocardiography, 806
Exercise electrocardiography, 805–806
Exercise radionuclide angiography, 806
Exercise testing, 407, 705–706
  for arterial occlusive disease of the extremities, 433–434, 841
  cardiac, 705–706
  examination procedures, 407
  for long-term prognosis, 801, 803
  systolic blood pressure, 432–433
  treadmill, 421, 433–434, 705–706, 801
  value of, 805, 806
External iliac artery, pulse, 402
External jugular vein, central venous catheterization complications, 1256
Extra-anatomic bypass, 846
Extracellular matrix synthesis, 888
Extracranial cerebrovascular disease, surgery, 675–680
Extracranial tissue perfusion, computed tomography, 539
Extracranial vessels, magnetic resonance imaging, 457–458
Extremities, *See also* Limbs; Lower extremities; Upper extremities
  amputation, 847, 1046, 1047–1048, 1177–1181
  lower
    angiography, 504
    atherosclerosis in, 344
    chronic disorders of deep veins, 1091–1098
    chronic disorders of superficial veins, 1083–1091
    intermittent claudication in, 828–829
    vascular trauma, 1084–1090
    veins, 1081, 1082, 1083–1098
    venography, 512–514
    venous ulcers, 1173, 1174
  magnetic resonance imaging, 460
  noninvasive testing, 430–436
  occlusive diseases of, 430–436, 680–681, 825–847
  pressure measurement, 432–433
  radionuclide imaging of, 485
  upper
    angiography, 505–516
    aortic aneurysms, 919
    arterial injuries, 1161
    chronic venous disorders, 1098–1099
    occlusive disease of, 680–681
    swelling, in venous compression, 1199
    veins, 1081–1082, 1098–1099
Extrinsic pathway, 208–209

FACIT collagens, 49–50
Factor IX, 9
Factor V, 8
Factor VII, 8, 579
Factor VIIa, 8, 208–209
Factor VIII, 209
Factor X, 9
Factor Xa, 208, 209
Factor XIa, 209
Factor XIIa, 209
Factor XII deficiency, 271
False aneurysms, 1147, *See also* Pseudoaneurysms
False channel, in dissecting hematoma, 526
Familial Atherosclerosis Treatment Study (FATS), 251
Familial combined hyperlipidemia (FCH) (hyperapoB100), 592–594
Familial defective apoB100 syndrome, 595–597
Familial hypercholesterolemia (FH), 595–597, 601
Familial hypertriglyceridemia (FHTG), 594–595
Fasciotomy, 1153
Fatigue, of elastic fibers, 190–191
FATS trial, 600
Fatty acids
  cycle, 587–589
  impaired removal of, 593
  omega-3, 648–649
Fatty spots, 225, *See also* Fatty streaks
Fatty streaks
  cellular interactions during atherogenesis, 292
  characteristics, 322
  defined, 290, 312
  incidence, 825
  progression, 322, 336
  regression, 299
  response-to-injury hypothesis of atherosclerosis and, 293–295
  reversibility, 295
Felodipine, for Raynaud's phenomenon, 981
Femoral arteries
  aneurysms, 404–405, 919
  angiography, 499
  injuries, 1163
  percutaneous revascularization, 729–738
  stenotic and occlusive lesions, 736
Femoral Artery Stent Trial (FAST), 733, 739
Femoral veins
  anatomy, 1081
  central venous catheterization complications, 1256
Femoropopliteal bypass grafts
  for arterial obstructive diseases of the extremities, 846
  for infrainguinal occlusive disease, 685–686
Fenestrae, endothelium, 3
Fiber, dietary, hypertension and, 625
Fiberoptic angioscopy, 839
Fibril, 64
Fibrillation, atrial, 342, 642, 653, 781, 831
Fibrin
  cuffs, in venous ulcers, 1183
  formation of, 178–179, 207
  matrix, 10
Fibrinogen, 55
  coronary heart disease risk and, 579
  pregnancy levels, 273
  role of, 207
  thrombus formation and, 177

Fibrinoid necrosis, 232
Fibrinolysis, 10–11, 210–214
 agents, 653–655
 endothelial regulation of, 253–255
Fibrinolytic system, 265, 266–268, 653–655
 disorders, 271
 function of, 207
 in pregnancy, 273
 state of activation of, measurement of, 277–278
Fibrinopeptide (FPA), 172
 measurement of, 277
Fibroblast growth factor (FGF), 17–18, 219, 222, 292, 293
 smooth muscle proliferation and, 104–105, 223
Fibroblasts, 53, 56, 303
Fibrocan, 61
Fibrocellular proliferation, 325–326
Fibrolipid lesions, 319, 322–323
Fibromodulin, 60
Fibromuscular disease, 749
 as cause of renal vascular hypertension, 857
Fibromuscular dysplasia (FMD), 619, 784, 833–834, 857, 1246–1248
 of aortic-arch arteries, 1246–1247
 defined, 1246
 in miscellaneous sites, 1248
 of renal arteries, 1246
Fibromyalgia, 1205
Fibronectin, 53–55, 56
 functional domains, 54–55
 gene, 54
 structure, 53–54
Fibrositis, 1205
Fibrous cap, rupture of, 339
Fibrous plaque. *See* Plaque
Filamentous actin (F-actin), 100
Filamin, 103
Filariasis, 1138
Fingers, *See also* Digital arteries; Raynaud's phenomenon
 "dead," 965
 in Raynaud's phenomenon, 965, 973
Fish oils
 as antiplatelet agent, 648–649
 hypertension and, 625
Fistulas
 chronic traumatic arteriovenous, 1156–1157
 coronary-artery, 1234–1235
 varicose veins and, 1084
Fixed neurological deficits, treatment of, 677
Flow, 141–151, *See also* Blood; Transport
 in annular vortex, 160–162
 blood cell properties, 151–160
 Brownian motion, 141
 bulk, 141
 cerebral, 335
 convective-diffusive transport, 162–165
 coronary, 334
 cross-, 145
 determinants of, 333–336
 diffusion, 162–163
 digital, quantification of, 436
 disturbed, 143–146
  arterial wall injury and, 160
  defined, 143
  generation of, 143
  thrombogenesis and, 160–165
  vessel geometry and, 143–146
 Doppler ultrasonography, 430
 erythrocyte-induced dispersion, 155–157
 fluid convection, 162
 imaging, 452–455
 ischemia and, 334–335
 magnetic resonance imaging, 447–448, 452–455
 non-Newtonian properties, 146–148
 nourishment, 453
 particle deformation in, 155, 157
 peripheral, 335–336
 physiological parameters, 147
 platelet-vessel wall interactions and, 165–176
 Poiseuille, 141–142, 143
 pulsatile, 143
 rate of, 165–167
 reflex sympathetic dystrophy and, 1213
 separation, 143–146
 through circular tube, 141–142
 tubular, 163–165
 turbulent, 143
 in venous system, 1083
 void effect, in magnetic resonance imaging, 452
 volume tracers, 473, 474, 476, 478
Fluid convection, blood-vessel wall interaction and, 162
Fluid mechanics, 162
Fluids, ideal, 143, 144
Foam cells, 225, 289–290, 320, 325
Force of contraction, 94–103
Fracture, of elastic fibers, 190–191
Framingham Heart Study, 185, 198, 333, 573, 575, 579, 781, 799, 828
Free induction decay (FID), in magnetic resonance imaging, 447
Frostbite, 987–988
Fungal endocarditis, 1112
Fusiform aortic aneurysms, 902
Fusigenic-liposome mediated gene transfer, 668–669

Galen's vein, aneurysm of, computed tomography, 552
Gamma interferon, 301–302, 319
Gamma-receptor, 70
Gap junctions, 5, 887
Gastrointestinal bleeding, angiography for, 508
Gastrointestinal tract infarction, computed tomography, 535
G-CSF (granulocyte colony stimulating factor), 16
Gelatinous lesions, 322
Gene therapy, 665–672
Genetics. *See* Hereditary disorders
Gene transfer
 adenovirus-mediated, 667–668
 cardiovascular system techniques, lipid-mediated, 668
 defined, 665
 fusigenic-liposome mediated, 668–669
 retroviral mediated, 666–667
 techniques, 666–672
Germinal matrix hemorrhage, in low-birth-weight newborns, 552
Ghost cells, 155–159
Giant cell (temporal) arteritis, 905, 999, 1015–1016
Glidewire™, 734, 743, 745
Glomerular pressure, renal vascular damage and, 854–855
Glomus tumors (glomangioma), 1273
Glucagon, as vasodilator, 371
Glucocorticoids, for vasculitis, 1024
Glucose-6-phosphate dehydrogenase (G-6-PD), 225
Glu-plasminogen, 211
Glyceryltrinitrate, for Raynaud's phenomenon, 983
Glycosaminoglucuronoglycans, 56
Glycosaminoglycans (GAGs), 7, 56–63
 biological interactions of, 63
 cell-matrix interactions, 63–64
 collagen-platelet interaction, 64–65
 FGFs and, 18
 proteoglycans, 57–63
 structure and distribution of, 57
Glycosylation, of collagens, 44
Glypican, 61
GM-CSF (granulocyte-macrophage colony stimulating factor), 16
G proteins, 83, 84–87, 644
 cAMP and, 89
 cGMP and, 90
 endothelium-derived relaxing factors (EDRFs) and, 127
 functions, 86–87
 mechanism, 86
 structure, 85–86
Gradient echo, in magnetic resonance imaging, 451
Gradient recall, in magnetic resonance imaging, 451
Graduated compression stockings. *See* Compression stockings
Graft thrombosis, 1262
Gram-negative bacilli, in infective endocarditis, 1106
Granulocyte colony stimulating factor (G-CSF), 16
Granulocyte-macrophage colony stimulating factor (GM-CSF), 16
Granulomatosis, Wegener's, 1012–1015
Growth factors
 defined, 291–292
 embryonic development of blood vessels and, 219
 receptor-associated protein-tyrosine kinases (PTKs), 81–82
 response-to-injury hypothesis of atherosclerosis and, 293
 role in cellular interactions during atherogenesis, 293
 smooth muscle proliferation and, 221–226
 synthesis of, 16
GTP binding to G proteins, 86
Guanethidine, 123, 981
Guanosine diphosphate (GDP), 86
Guanylate cyclase, 122
Guidewires
 for angiography, 496, 734, 743, 745
 traversal test, 767
Guillain-Barré syndrome, 359
Gyromagnetic ratio, in magnetic resonance imaging, 446

HACEK organisms, for infective endocarditis, 1112
Hagen-Poiseuille law, 141
HAM-56, 290
Health care costs
 coronary heart disease, 609
 peripheral arterial disease (PAD), 749, 758–759
 pulmonary embolism, 1069
 renal-artery stenosis, 749
 risk factor cost-benefit analysis, 571
 stroke, 609

Health Professional Follow-up Study, 251–252
Heart
  acquired disorders of left side, 954
  chronic failure, gene transfer and, 671
  congenital malformations, 954–955, 1223–1235
    coronary artery, 1228–1234
    venous connections, 122–126
  trauma to, 1157–1158
Heart-lung transplantation, for pulmonary hypertension, 962
Helicine arteriolar smooth muscle tone, 886
Helsinki Heart Study, 807
Hemangioendothelioma, 1274–1275
  epithelioid, 1275–1276
  Kaposi-like infantile, 1276
  spindle-cell, 1272
Hemangiomas, 1269–1272
  capillary, 1246, 1269–1271
  cavernous, 1245–1246, 1271–1272
  deep-soft-tissue, 1272
  defined, 1269
Hemangiopericytoma, 1279
Hematocrit
  in annular vortex, 160
  platelet adhesion and, 168
  red cell flow behavior and, 155–160
Hematomas
  dissecting, computed tomography, 526–528
  inframesocolic, 1162
  noninvasive testing of, 427–428
  retroperitoneal, 773–774
  supramesocolic, 1162
Hemodialysis conduits, 751–759
Hemodynamics
  of hypertension and drug effects, 627–629
  monitoring, iatrogenic complications of, 1166–1167
Hemoglobin, vasomotion and, 372
Hemolytic uremic syndrome (HUS), 276
Hemorrhage
  computed tomography
    cerebral, 559
    hypertensive cerebral, 551, 558
    nontraumatic intracranial, 547–552
    subarachnoid, 380–381
  germinal matrix, 552
  intracerebral, 792
  intracranial, 547–552
  intramural, 939
  intraparenchymal, 788
  splinter, 1108
  subarachnoid, 380–381, 792
  telangiectasis, 1245
Hemorrhagic stroke, 788
Hemorrheologic agents, 842
Hemostasis, 6–10, 64, 207–210, *See also* Coagulation
  anticoagulants, 6–8
  components, 207
  functions, 207
  laboratory tests, 277
  platelet function inhibitors, 8
  primary, 209
  procoagulant activities, 8–10
  risk factors for cardiovascular disease, 578–579
  secondary, 209
Henoch-Schönlein purpura, 1010–1011
Heparan sulfates, 19, 60–61, 222–223, 303
Heparin, 19, 62, 63, 639–643
  adjusted-dosage, 1055
  antithrombin III and, 265
  for carotid artery disease, 791
  defined, 639
  fibronectin binding, 54–55
  in intra-arterial thrombolytic therapy, 770
  low-dose, 1055
  low-molecular-weight, 1055–1056
  mechanism of action, 639
  protein C/S deficiency and, 270
  for pulmonary embolism, 1071, 1075
  for venous thromboembolism, 1055–1056, 1057–1060, 1062–1063
Heparin-associated thrombocytopenia, 275
Heparin-associated thrombosis, 275
Heparin-binding epidermal growth factor (HB-EGF), 301
Heparin cofactor II, 265, 269
  deficiency, 270
Hepatic-artery aneurysms, 698, 920
Hepatic lipoproteins, 589–590
Hepatic-vein thrombosis (Budd-Chiari syndrome), 274
Hepatitis B serologic tests, in vasculitis, 1003
Hepatitis C serologic tests, in vasculitis, 1003
Hereditary disorders
  atherosclerosis of the extremities and, 827
  hemorrhage telangiectasis, 1245
  hypertension and, 349–352
12(R)HETE 12(r) (Hydroxyeicosatrienoic acid), 19
Heterogeneity-of-nephrons hypothesis, 354, 355
Heterogeneous reaction rate kinetics, 162
Heterozygous protein C deficiency, 278
HHF-35, 290
High blood pressure, 574, *See also* Hypertension
High-density lipoproteins (HDL), 300, 320
  alcohol consumption and, 578
  atherogenesis and, 310–312
  atherogenic dyslipoproteinemias, 592–601
  beta-adrenergic blocking agents and, 811
  binding sites, 317
  classification, 591
  coronary heart disease and, 307
  deficiency (hypoalphalipoproteinemia), 594–595
  defined, 590
  estrogen therapy and, 576–577
  exercise and, 576
  fish oils and, 649
  hypertension and, 611
  impotence and, 885–886
  serum cholesterol levels and, 572–574
High endothelial venules (HEV), 15
High-molecular weight (HMW) kininogen, 5, 209
High-molecular weight (HMW) urokinase, 212
High take-off coronary artery, 1234
Histamine, 134–136
  coronary vasospasm and, 376
  effects of, 135
Histamine-receptor antagonists, 134–135
Histaminergic receptors, 75–76
Histiocytoid hemangiomas, 1273
HMGCoA reductase, 601
Hoarseness, in pulmonary hypertension, 953
Holter (ambulatory) monitoring, 707–708, 710, 806
Home blood pressure monitoring, 614
Homing, lymphocyte, 15
Homocystinuria, 276
Hookean material, 187
Human immunodeficiency virus (HIV), pulmonary hypertension and, 963
Human leukocyte antigens (HLS), in vasculitis, 391
Hyaluronan, 56
Hydralazine, 236–237, 360
12(r) Hydroxyeicosatrienoic acid (12(R)HETE), 19
Hydroxylysine, 45
  aldehydes of, 45
3-Hydroxy-3-methylglutaryl-coenzyme (HMG-CoA), 315
3-Hydroxyproline, 44
5-Hydroxytryptamine (5HT) receptors, 74–75
Hyperabduction maneuver, 408
Hyperaldosteronism, 355, 618, 621–622
Hyperalgesia, 1209
HyperapoB100 (familial combined hyperlipidemia (FCH)), 592–594
Hyperbetalipoproteinemia, 274
Hypercholesterolemia, 325
  arterial stiffness and, 193
  endothelial dysfunction in, 246
  familial, 308, 310, 316
Hypercoagulable states, 268–276
  clinical approaches to patients, 279
  defined, 268
  laboratory tests, 276–278
  pathogenesis, 278
  primary, 268–271
  secondary, 268, 271–276
  stroke due to, 787
Hyperemia, reactive, 434
Hyperhomocysteinemia, 276
Hyperlipemia, 230
Hyperlipidemia, 274, 825–826
Hyperlipoproteinemia, type III, 597–598
Hypernatriuretic response, 355
Hyperpolarization, 72, 74, 118
Hypersensitivity, 390
  cell-mediated, 387
  defined, 387
  immune complex-mediated, 387
Hypersensitivity vasculitis, 999, 1008–1010
Hypertension, 349–363, 609–634, *See also* Antihypertensive therapy; Pulmonary hypertension
  accelerated, 632
  angiotensin II and, 136
  arterial stiffness and, 192–193
  atherosclerosis of the extremities and, 827
  baseline tests, 616
  blood pressure and, 349, 609–610, 612–615
  candidate-gene approach, 350, 351
  catecholamines and, 131
  central nervous system and, 357–358
  defined, 349, 574, 609
  diagnosis, 609–615, 619
  diet and, 361–363, 625
  genetics and, 349–352
  initial lesions, 231–237

J-curve phenomenon, 613
kidneys and, 352–357
linkage studies, 350–351
lipoproteins and, 587
malignant, 232
mass changes/replication relationship, 236–237
moderate, 232, 234
morbidity and mortality, 613
morphologic pathology, 231–232
nonmodulators, 350
patient evaluation, 615–623
patient history, 615
patient management, 359, 575, 623–634
beta blockers, 131–132
demographic analysis, 626
drug therapy, 233–234, 625–632
hemodynamics, 627–629
hypertensive crisis, 629, 632–633
individualized approach, 627
nonpharmacologic treatment
alcohol restriction, 624, 625
dietary changes, 625
exercise, 624
sodium restriction, 625
stress reduction, 625
weight reduction, 623–624
refractory hypertension, 633–634
renin-profile analysis, 626–627
stepped care, 626
treatment considerations, 840–841
treatment initiation, 612
treatment risks, 612–613
positional cloning, 351–352
prevalence, 609–610
radionuclide imaging for, 488
refractory, 633–634
relative-pair analysis, 350–351
renal vascular, 853–865
risks associated with, 574–575, 609, 610–613, 704
secondary
aortic coarctation, 618, 620
Cushing's syndrome, 618, 620–621
endocrinologic, 620–623
evaluation, 616–617
hyperthyroidism, 618, 623
overview, 618
pharmacologic, 618, 623
pheochromocytoma, 618, 622–623
prevalence, 616–617
primary (hyper)aldosteronism, 618, 621–622
renal parenchymal disease, 617–618
renovascular, 618–620
vascular, 618–620
serotonin and, 134
smooth muscle mass vs. smooth muscle cell number, 234–236
smooth muscle proliferation in, 232, 234, 358–361
sodium and, 354–357, 359, 361–362
system, aortic dissection and, 930
tunica media and, 221
vascular growth and, 359–361
Hypertensive cerebral hemorrhage, 551, 558
Hyperthyroidism, 618, 623
Hyperviscosity, 276, 972
Hypervolemia, 856
Hypoalphalipoproteinemia, 594–595
Hypocomplementemic vasculitis, 1011
Hypoplasia
of coronary arteries, 1234
of pulmonary veins, 1227
Hypothenar hammer syndrome, 977
Hypothermia, serotonin and, 75
Hypothyroidism
lipoprotein disorders and, 599
Raynaud's phenomenon and, 978
Hypoventilation, alveolar, 956
Hypoxemia, 333
Hypoxia, 333
Hypoxic injury, coronary vasospasm and, 374

Iatrogenic interventions, infective endocarditis and, 1104
Iatrogenic vascular injuries, 1164–1168, 1253–1265
angiography, 504, 1154–1155
cardiac catheterization complications, 1253–1255
cardiac surgery complications, 1262–1264
central venous catheter complications, 1255–1258
coronary artery catheter complications, 1258–1262
endovascular repair of, 1168
intra-aortic balloon device complications, 1166, 1264–1265
invasive monitoring complications, 1166–1167
laser angioplasty, 1165–1166
pediatric trauma, 1167–1168
percutaneous transluminal balloon angioplasty, 1165–1166
surgical complications, 1166
ICAM-1 (intercellular adhesion molecule-1), 14–15
ICAM-2 (intercellular adhesion molecule-2), 15
Ideal fluids, 143, 144
Idiopathic episodic digital vasospasm, 973, *See also* Raynaud's phenomenon
Idiopathic medial aortopathy, 905
Idiopathic venous thrombosis, 272
IGF (insulin-like growth factor) binding proteins, 19, 81, 221, 223
IL-6 (interleukin-6), 16
IL-8 (interleukin-8), 16, 19
Iliac arteries
aneurysms, 406, 429, 917–919
angiography, 499
injuries, 1163
noninvasive testing, 429
percutaneous transluminal angioplasty, 721, 722–729
Iloprost, 650, 983
Image-intensifier, for angiography, 494
Imaging, ultrasonic. *See* Ultrasonography
Imaging equipment, for angiography, 493–495
Immersion foot (trench foot), 986–987
Immobilization, thrombosis and, 275
Immune complexes
defined, 387
deposition on vessel walls, 388, 392
formation of, 387
in human diseases, 390
hypersensitivity, 387
models, 387
radionuclide imaging, 488
in vasculitis, 387–392, 1001–1002
Immunoglobulins, in vasculitis, 1003
Immunohistochemical markers, endothelial cells, 1269
Impedance, 186, 187–188
Impedance plethysmography (IPG)
for deep-vein thrombosis, 436–437
for venous thromboembolism, 1053
Impotence. *See* Vasculogenic impotence
Indicator dilution, 477–478
Inducible cell adhesion molecule (INCAM-110), 15
Infarction
Angiotensin-converting enzyme (ACE) inhibitors and, 254–255
gastrointestinal tract, 535
ischemia, 555
liver, 535, 541
micro-, 338
myocardial
anticoagulants for, 642
aspirin for prevention of, 647
mortality, 797
percutaneous transluminal coronary angioplasty for, 814
perioperative, 1262
radionuclide angiography, 484
smoking cessation and, 571
non-Q-wave, 341
renal, 540, 857
splenic artery, 535, 540
tissue, 532, 535
Infection
aortic graft, 1120–1121
bypass grafts, 1120–1121, 1155–1156
radionuclide imaging, 488
Infectious aortitis, aortic aneurysms caused by, 906
Infective endarteritis (mycotic aneurysm), 1116–1119
antibiotic regimes, 1110–1112
antimicrobial resistance, 1110
defined, 1116
diagnosis, 1119
in infective endocarditis, 1108
native-valve, 1110–1112
pathogenesis and clinical presentation, 1116–1119
therapy, 1119
Infective endocarditis, 1103–1116
clinical presentation, 1107–1108
culture-negative, 1107
defined, 1103
diagnosis, 1108–1109
epidemiology, 1103–1104
fungal, 1112
in intravenous drug users, 110, 1104, 1105, 1106
microbiology, 1105–1107
native-valve, 1104–1105, 1106
nosocomial, 1107
pathogenesis, 1104–1105
prevention, 1116
prosthetic-valve, 1104, 1105–1106
relapses and reinfections, 1115–1116
risk factors, 1103–1104
treatment
antibiotic regimes, 1110–1113
general principles, 1109–1110
of less common causes, 1113–1114
surgery, 1114–1115
Inferior cerebellar arteries, 783, 785
Inferior epigastric artery, pulse, 403
Inferior vena cava, 537, 543–545
filter, for pulmonary embolism, 1077
leiomyosarcomas, 1280, 1281
Inflammatory disorders
aortic aneurysms, 427, 528–530
monocyte-endothelial cell interactions, 297
radionuclide imaging of, 488

Infrainguinal occlusive disease, 685–687
Inframalleolar (arterial) ulcers, 1173
Inframesocolic hematoma, 1162
Infrapopliteal arteries, percutaneous revascularization of, 738–740
Injuries, *See also* Blunt trauma; Endothelial injury; Iatrogenic vascular injuries; Trauma, vascular; Vascular injuries
- abdominal, 1161, 1162
- aorta, 1162
- arterial, 160, 1152–1153, 1159, 1161–1164
- balloon, 224–225
- deceleration, 496, 497
- endothelial response to, 12–15
- endovascular repair of, 1168
- heart, 1157–1158
- hypoxic, 374
- integrated responses to, 12–16
- neck, 1158–1159
- orthopedic, 1152–1153
- penetrating, 1147
- response-to-injury hypothesis of atherosclerosis, 228, 293–295
- thoracic, 1159–1160
- venous, 1152–1153, 1163

Innominate arteries
- percutaneous revascularization of, 745–747
- trauma to, 1160–1161

Inositol 1,4,5-triphosphate (IP_3), 84
Inositol-lipid metabolism, 88–89
In-situ saphenous vein graft, 689–691
In-situ thrombosis, 342
Insudation hypothesis, of atherosclerosis, 228, 231
Insulin, 19, 371
Insulin-like growth factor (IGF), 19, 81, 221, 223
Integrins, 5–6, 54
Intercellular adhesion molecule-1 (ICAM-1), 14–15, 297, 298, 299
Intercellular adhesion molecule-2 (ICAM-2), 15
Interleukins, in vasculitis, 16, 19, 43, 390
Intermediate-density lipoproteins (IDL), 307, 308
- as atherogenic, 592
- defined, 589
- therapy, 600–601

Intermediate lesions, 319
Intermediate phenotypes, blood pressure, 350
Intermittent claudication, 338–339
- in aortoiliac occlusive disease, 681–682
- in arterial disease in lower extremities, 828–829
- in infrainguinal occlusive disease, 685–686
- prevalence, 333
- remissions, 828

Intermittent compression
- leg, for venous thromboembolism, 1056
- pneumatic (IPC), for pulmonary embolism prevention, 1070

Internal carotid artery (ICA), 783
Internal elastic lamina (IEL), 219, 221
Internal jugular vein
- central venous catheterization complications, 1255, 1256–1257
- thrombosis, computed tomography, 553

Internal mammary artery, 815
INTERSALT study, 362, 363, 611
Interstitial collagens, 42–43
- metabolic turnover, 46
- metalloproteinases, 46–47

Interstitial fluid, lymphatic system regulation of, 1137
Interstitial lung disease, 955
Intestinal angina, 870
Intima
- capillary formation in, 325
- cell masses, 225, 230, 231
- endothelial regulation of, 255–257
- fibrocellular proliferation and, 326
- fibroplasia, 1246
- normal artery, 289
- sarcomas, 1280–1281
- smooth muscle cells, 221, 290–291, 300

Intra-abdominal visceral-artery aneurysms, 919
Intra-aortic balloon assist device (IABAD), *See also* Percutaneous transluminal angioplasty (PTA)
- iatrogenic complications, 1166–1167, 1264–1265

Intra-arterial thrombolytic therapy (IATT), *See also* Thrombolytic therapy
- in atherosclerosis obliterans, 765–775
- complications, 773–774
- infusion techniques, 771–772, 775
- monitoring and termination of infusion, 770, 775
- patient selection, 765–766
- for peripheral arteries, 844
- preparation, 767
- purpose, 765
- results, 772–773
- technique, 767–770

Intracavernosal blood oxygen partial pressure, 894
Intracavernosal injection test, 891
Intracerebral hemorrhage (ICH), 788, 792
Intracoronary devices, for coronary artery disease, 814–815
Intracranial hemorrhage, nontraumatic, computed tomography, 547–552
Intracranial perfusion, computed tomography, 553–555
Intracranial vessels
- aneurysm, 539–541
- computed tomography, 539–553
- magnetic resonance imaging, 457–458

Intramural hemorrhage (IMH), aortic dissection and, 939
Intramuscular hemangiomas, 1272
Intraparenchymal (intracerebral) hemorrhage (ICH), 788, 792
Intravascular bronchioloalveolar tumor (IVBAT), 1275–1276
Intravascular pressure, Raynaud's phenomenon and, 971–972
Intravascular ultrasound (IVUS), 717, 718–722
- angioplasty mechanisms and, 718–719, 722
- for aortic dissection, 935
- lesion characterization by, 718

Intravenous digital subtraction angiography (DSA), 860–861
Intravenous drug use, infective endocarditis in, 113, 1104, 1105, 1106, 1112, 1115
Intravenous nitroglycerin, 809
Intravenous pyelogram, 860
Intrinsic pathway, 208, 209
Invaginated caveolae, 92, 93
Invasive monitoring, iatrogenic complications of, 1166–1167
In-vitro labeling, 473–475
In-vivo gene transfer, 665
In-vivo labeling, 473–475
Iodine-125 fibrinogen scanning, for deep-vein thrombosis, 437
Ion channels, regulation of, 87
Ion fluxes, in smooth muscle proliferation, 104
Ischemia, 333–344, *See also* Transient ischemic attacks (TIAs)
- asymptomatic, 801
  - Holter monitoring for, 707–708, 710
  - myocardial (silent), 806
- blood flow determinants, 333–336
- bowel disease, 542
- cerebral, acute, 342
- cerebrovascular, 337–338, 545, 547
- collateral circulation and, 343–344
- computed tomography, 542, 545, 547, 555
- defined, 333
- determinants, 333–336
- dipyridamole thallium imaging, 706
- heart disease
  - angioplasty for, 815
  - hypertension and, 632
  - management of, 807–808
- infarction, 555
- limb, 829–831, 1173–1174, 1177–1181, 1265
  - at rest, 829–830
  - intra-arterial thrombolytic therapy, 766
  - lower-, 339, 1173–1174, 1265
- noninvasive tests, 801–802
- pathophysiology, 336–339
- peripheral, acute, 342
- postoperative, 710
- reperfusion-caused, 1154
- skin, transcutaneous oximetry, 433
- spinal cord, 400
- stable angina, 337
- vasospasm and, 342–343

Ischemic nephropathy, 853, 855–856
Ischemic neuropathy, 401
Ischemic stroke
- cardioembolic stroke, 785–786
- carotid disease, 782–784
- collagen vascular disease and, 786–787
- hypercoagulable states, 786–787
- lacunar stroke, 784–785
- treatment, 791–792
- vertebrobasilar disease, 785

Isolated central nervous system vasculitis, 1020
Isosorbide dinitrate, arterial stiffness and, 194
Isotope imaging, 474
Isotope renography, 859

Janeway lesions, in infective endocarditis, 1108
J-curve phenomenon, in hypertension, 613
Jugular veins
- central venous catheterization complications, 1255, 1256–1257
- injuries, 1159
- thrombosis, computed tomography, 553

Jugular venous hum, 407
Juvenile (strawberry) hemangiomas, 1269–1270

K+ channels, 118, 128
Kallikrein, 209

Kaposi-like infantile hemangioendothelioma, 1276
Kaposi's sarcoma, 1279–1280
Kasabach-Merritt syndrome, 1245, 1271
Kawasaki disease, 275, 1020–1021
Ketanserin, for Raynaud's phenomenon, 981–982
Kidneys
 blood pressure and, 352–357
 magnetic resonance imaging, 460
 nerve fibers, 356
Kinase, myosin light-chain, 101, 103
Kininogens, 136–137
 high-molecular weight (HMW), 5
Kinin receptors, 76–77
 classification, 76
 distribution and location, 76
 heterogeneity, 77
 mechanism of action, 76–77
Klippel-Trenaunay syndrome, 1245, 1274
Kringles, 210, 211

Labetalol, 810, 940, 945
Lacunar state, 338, 784–785
Laminar flow, 142, 143
Laminin, 55–56, 61
Lanthanum, 92
LaPlace relationship, 808
Laser angioplasty, 731–732, 740, 743, 814, 815
 excimer-, 740, 743, 814, 815
 iatrogenic complications of, 1165–1166
 for peripheral arteries, 843–844
Laser Doppler flowmeter, 421
Latch state, of smooth muscle, 103
Lateral adhesive proteins, 5
Lateral geniculate artery, pulse, 403
Lateral medullary syndrome (Wallenberg's syndrome), 785
Lecithin:cholesterol acyltransferase (LCAT), 310, 311
Lectin *Ulex europaeus L*, 1269
Left heart, acquired disorders, 954
Left ventricle
 aneurysmectomy, 817
 arterial stiffness and, 197–198
 ejection fraction, 707
 failure, 954
 function, 197–198, 799, 803
 hypertrophy, 704
Leg compression, intermittent, for venous thromboembolism, 1056
Leg discomfort/pain, intermittent claudication and, 828–829
Legions of atherogenesis, cholesterol economy in, 300
Leg pumps, for venous ulcers, 1184
Leiomyomas, 229
Leiomyosarcomas, 1280
Leiotonin, 103
Leriche syndrome, 828
Lesion-prone endothelium
 altered shear stress characteristics, 298–299
 monocyte adherence to, 297–298
Lesions, 225–228, 289–291
 angiocentric immunoproliferative, 1019–1020
 angioplasty, 814–815
 assumptions, 230
 calcium deposition, 325
 capillary formation, 325
 clinical syndromes, 337–339
 complicated, 324
 development, 321–324
 in extremities, 827–828
 fatty streaks, 322
 features, 326
 fibrocellular proliferation, 325–326
 fibrolipid, 319, 323–324
 fibrous plaques, 321–322
 gelatinous, 323
 intermediate, 319
 intervention, 326
 lipid metabolism control at, 319
 lipid-rich core regions, 324–325, 326
 monoclonal antibody identification, 289–291
 monocytes and, 222
 in primary hypotension, 960
 in pulmonary hypertension, 957
 regression, 295
 smooth muscle proliferation and, 226
 stable, 333, 336–337
 in stable angina, 337
 T-cell interactions, 301–302
 in thromboangiitis obliterans, 1035–1036
 ulcerated, 675
 ultrasound imaging of, 424
 unstable, 333
Leukemia, 276
Leukoariosis, 785
Leukocytes
 adhesion molecule interactions tumor cells, 15–16
 cellular interactions during atherogenesis, 292
 endothelial interactions, 13, 297–299
 redistribution of, 157–160
 rolling, 13, 14
Leukotrienes, 81, 371–372
Libman-Sacks vegetations, 273
Life-style
 coronary artery diseases and, 807
 hypertension and, 626
Ligands
 fibronectin binding, 54
 gating, 87
 transmembrane signaling, 83, 84
Limbs, *See also* Extremities; Lower extremities; Upper extremities
 blood pressure measuring techniques, 422
 ischemia, 829–831, 1173–1174, 1177–1181, 1265
 perfusion, laser Doppler flowmeter measuring, 421
 plethysmographic volume measurement, 419–421
Linkage studies, hypertension, 350–351
Link protein, 60
Lipase, 587
Lipedema, 413
Lipid-lowering therapy, 226–227, 574
 for arterial obstructive diseases of the extremities, 840
 for coronary artery diseases, 807–808
 for endothelial vasomotor function, 250–251
Lipid-mediated gene transfer, 668
Lipid Research Clinics Coronary Prevention Trial, 579
Lipid-rich lesion core regions, 324–325, 326
Lipids, 307
 accumulation, 312–321
 core, 336
 mediators, 302
 metabolism, 307–326
 transport, 307, 308–310, 319–320
Lipoproteins, 307–326, 598, *See also* Cholesterol; High-density lipoproteins (HDL); Low-density lipoproteins (LDL); Very-low density lipoproteins (VLDL)
 abnormalities, coronary heart disease risk and, 572–574, 579
 accumulation in normal arteries, 313–314
 alternative receptors, 316–317
 apoproteins, 307, 308, 309
 atherogenesis and, 310–312
 cell interactions, 314–315
 cholesterol rich (LDL), 307, 310
 chylomicrons, 307, 310, 312, 587, 588, 589
 defined, 307
 flux, 314
 hemostatic risk factors and, 578–579
 hepatic, 589–590
 high-density (HDL), cardiovascular risk and, 307
 intermediate-density (IDL), 307, 308
 lipase, 63, 308
 metabolism, 308–310
 phenotyping system limitations, 591
 protein rich (HDL), 307, 310–312
 residence time, 314
 risk factor interactions, 587
 structure, apoproteins and, 307, 308
 transport, in normal arterial walls, 312–314
 triglyceride rich, 307, 310, 312, 587, 588, 589
 very low-density (VLDL), 307, 308
Livedo reticularis, 377, 984–986
Liver
 angiosarcoma, 1277–1279
 infarction, computed tomography, 535, 541
Lobular capillary hemangioma, 1271
Local faults, in digital arteries, 378
Local measures, for arterial obstructive diseases of the extremities, 839–840
Local syncope, 965
Lone atrial fibrillators, 781
Lovastatin, 315
Low-birth-weight newborns, germinal matrix hemorrhage, 552
Low-density lipoproteins (LDLs), 63, 300, 590–591
 accumulation in normal artery walls, 313–314
 atherogenesis and, 310
 as atherogenic, 592–601
 classification, 591
 EDRF action and, 248, 249
 endothelial cell activity and, 254
 estrogen therapy and, 576–577
 exercise and, 576
 fish oils and, 649
 impaired pathway function, 596
 lipoprotein transport, 313
 oxidation of, 318–319
 pathways, 320
 serum cholesterol levels and, 572–574
 small, dense, atherogenicity of, 591
 smooth muscle-cell proliferation and, 325–326
 therapy, 600–601
Lower extremities, *See also* Extremities; Limbs
 angiography, 504
 atherosclerosis in, 344

Lower extremities —(*continued*)
  chronic disorders of deep veins, 1091–1098
    venous insufficiency, 1091–1098
  chronic disorders of superficial veins, 1083–1091
    spider veins, 1090–1091
    varicose veins, 1084–1090
  intermittent claudication, 828–829
  intermittent leg compression, 1056
  ischemia, 1173–1174, 1177–1181, 1265
  leg discomfort/pain, 828–829
  leg pump, 1184
  vascular trauma, 1163–1164
  veins, 1081, 1082, 1083–1098
  venography, 512–514
  venous ulcers, 1173, 1174
Low-molecular weight (LMW) urokinase, 212
Low-osmolality agents, for angiography, 495
Low-threshold mechanoreceptors (LTM), 1211
Lumbar sympathectomy, 846–847
Lumen
  caliber, 226–227
  in dissecting hematoma, 526
  size, hypertension and, 231
Lung disease, interstitial, 955
Lupus anticoagulant, 273
Luxury perfusion, 479
Lymphangiography, for lymphedema, 1140, 1141
Lymphatic circulation
  anatomy, 1133–1134
  distal lymphatic vessels, 1138
  physiology of, 1134–1137
  proximal lymphatic vessels, 1138
Lymphatic disease, patient examination, 413
Lymphedema, 1133–1144
  chronic, angiosarcoma arising in, 1277
  clinical presentation, 1139–1140
  diagnosis, 1140–1142
  drainage procedures, 1144
  microsurgical anastomotic procedures, 1144
  pathogenesis, 1137–1138
  pathology, 1138–1139
  patient examination, 413
  primary, 1137–1138
  reduction procedures, 1144
  secondary, 1138
  treatment, 1142–1144
Lymphocyte homing, regulation of, 15
Lymphoscintigraphy, for lymphedema, 1140, 1142
Lysine, 44, 51
Lysolecithin, 319
Lys-plasminogen, 211
Lysyl hydroxylase, 44
Lytic therapy, 735

McArdle syndrome, 829
Macrophage-colony stimulating factor (M-CSF), 299–300
Macrophages, 225
  cell replication roll, 291
  cholesterol loading, 316
  fibrocellular proliferation and, 325
  in fibrous cap, 339
  LDL oxidation and, 318–319
  lipid-loading, 317
  proliferation, 293
  response-to-injury hypothesis of atherosclerosis and, 293
  scavenger receptors, 316, 319
  smooth muscle cell interactions, 299–300
  T-cells and, 302
Maffucci's syndrome, 1245, 1272
Magnesium, hypertension and, 625
Magnetic resonance imaging (MRI), 445–464
  applications
    aortic diseases, 460, 463
    aortic dissection, 935–937, 938
    cerebrovascular diseases, 456–457
    coronary artery disease, 458–459
    deep-vein thrombosis, 463
    dissections, 499, 935–937, 938
    extracranial vessels, 457–458
    extremities, 459
    intracranial vessels, 457–458
    mesenteric vessels, 460
    peripheral arteries, 838
    pulmonary embolism, 463
    pulmonary hypertension, 463
    renal vascular hypertension, 861
    renovascular disease, 460
    stroke diagnosis, 788–789
    vascular graft infection, 1121
    visceral ischemia, 876
  history, 445
  instrumentation
    flow imaging, 452–455
    image creation, 448–452
    metabolism, 111–112
    nonimaging, 445–448
    paramagnetic compounds, 456
  for vasculogenic impotence, 894
Mainstream, in disturbed flow, 143–146
Major histocompatibility complex (MHC) class II antigens, 391
Malignancy
  endovascular papillary angioendothelioma, 1276
  hypertension, smooth muscle replication in, 232
  lymphedema and, 1143–1144
  thrombosis incidence with, 272
Manual lymph drainage (MLD), 1143
Marfan syndrome, 905, 930, 941, 945
Massachusetts Male Aging Study (MMAS), 885–886
Mass transport
  boundary layer, 163
  simplifying assumptions, 164
  in tubular flow, 163–165
Mast cells, 303
Matrix adhesion, of endothelial cells, 6
Matrix metalloproteinases (MMPs), 17, 46–47
Maximum intensity projection (MIP) algorithm, 455
Mechanical stress, 12
Media
  arterial calcification, in diabetes, 1175
  degeneration, 930
  fibroplasia, 1246
  geniculate artery, pulse, 403
  necrosis, coronary-artery dissection and, 1255
  in normal artery, 289
Meige's disease, 1137
Membrane activation, myogenic tone, 82
Membrane-bounded calcium, 92
Mesenteric arteries, 235
  aneurysms, 698–699
  blood flow through, 871
  collateral pathways among, 871
  magnetic resonance imaging, 460
  occlusion, 869–870, 874
  radionuclide imaging, 485–486
  revascularization, 693, 869–870
  stenosis, 430
  superior
    injuries, 1162
    percutaneous transluminal angioplasty, 720
    thrombosis, 871–872
    ultrasonography, 425
  thrombosis, 871–872, 874
Mesenteric ischemia, *See also* Visceral ischemia
  nonobstructive, 869, 870, 872, 875
    nonocclusive, 879
Mesenteric veins
  magnetic resonance imaging, 460
  occlusion
    diagnosis, 874
    etiology, 872
    incidence, 870
    intestinal gangrene and, 869
  thrombosis, 879
Metabolism
  agents, for arterial obstructive diseases, 842
  magnetic resonance imaging of, 455–456
  radiopharmaceutical measurement of, 479–480
Metalloproteinases, 46–47
Methotrexate, 1024–1025
Methyldopa, 122, 981
α-methylnorepinephrine, 122
Methylxanthines, 132–133
Methysergide
  Raynaud's phenomenon caused by, 977
  vasospasm and, 373
Metoprolol, 811
Microfibrillar collagen, 48–49
Microinfarctions, 338
Microvascular arterial bypass surgery, 896–898
Microvascular resistance vessels, 235
Middle cerebral artery (MCA), 782–784
Migraine headaches
  Raynaud's phenomenon and, 973
  vasomotor instability and, 379–380
Migration studies, of risk factors, 570
Migratory superficial thrombophlebitis, 272
Milroy's disease, 1137
Minimum bactericidal concentration (MBC), 1109–1110
Minimum inhibitory concentration (MIC), 1109–1110
Mitochondria, calcium source regulation by, 94
Mitogens, smooth muscle proliferation and, 223–224
Mitral valve replacement, 817
Moens-Korteweg equation, 187
Molecular biology, gene therapy, 665–672
Monoclonal antibodies
  atherosclerosis "hypothesis," 230
  lesions of atherosclerosis identified with, 289–291
  platelet aggregation and, 652
Monocyte-chemoattractant protein-1 (MCP-1), 16, 298–299, 319

Monocytes
activated as macrophages, 291
cellular interactions during atherogenesis, 292
interactions with endothelial cells, 297–299
smooth muscle proliferation and, 222
Morphine, reflex sympathetic dystrophy and, 1212
Movement disorder
reflex sympathetic dystrophy, 1214
Mucocutaneous lesions, in infective endocarditis, 1107–1108
Mucocutaneous lymph node syndrome (Kawasaki disease), 275, 1020–1021
Mucosal addressin, 15
Multiple Risk Factor Intervention Study, 571
Mural thrombosis, 295, 339, 342
Murmurs
in aortic dissection, 931
defined, 407
in infective endocarditis, 1107
Muscarine receptors, 73–74, 132
Muscle relaxants, for Raynaud's phenomenon, 982–983
Mycotic aneurysms, 906, 1119, *See also* Infective endarteritis (mycotic aneurysm)
aortic aneurysms caused by, 906
computed tomography, 529, 530
Mycotic-pseudoaneurysms, 1156
Myeloproliferative disorders, 274
Myocardial autonomic innervation, 484
Myocardial infarction
acute
anticoagulants for, 642
percutaneous transluminal coronary angioplasty for, 814
aspirin for prevention of, 647
mortality, 797
perioperative, 1262
radionuclide angiography, 484
risk of, smoking cessation and, 571
Myocardial ischemia, 245–246, 797–799
Myocardial metabolism, 197, 483–485, 808
Myogenic tone, 82
Myosin
actin interaction, 95–96, 100
heavy-chain phosphorylation, 101–103
light-chain kinase, 101, 103
molecule diagram, 98
in smooth muscle contraction, 95–96, 99–103

National Cholesterol Education Program (NCEP), 572
Adult Treatment Panel (ATP), 574
National Health Interview Study, 576
National Health and Nutrition Examination Survey (NHANES-1), 362, 363, 575
Native-valve endocarditis, 1104–1105, 1106
in infective endarteritis
antibiotic regimes, 1110–1112
surgery, 112–113
Natriuretic response, 355
Neck, trauma to, 1158–1159
Neoplastic blood vessel diseases, 1269–1281
benign tumors, 1269–1274
intermediate-grade tumors, 1274–1276
malignant tumors, 1276–1281
Nephropathy, ischemic, 855–856
Nephrotic syndrome, 273
Nernst equilibrium potential, 118
Nerves
adrenergic, 122–125, 131, 132, 134, 231
afferent renal sympathetic, 356
efferent renal sympathetic, 356
Neuraminidase, 92
Neurogenic pseudoclaudication, 829
Neurohumoral mediators, 130–137
acetylcholine, 132
catecholamines, 130–132
histamine, 134–136
peptides, 136–137
purines, 132–133
serotonin, 133–134
Neurologic disorders, as cause of Raynaud's phenomenon, 976
Neuron
atherogenesis and, 303
death, in stroke, 792
Neuropathic disorders, diabetic, 1173, 1174–1176
Neuropeptides
reflex sympathetic dystrophy and, 1211–1212, 1214
Y (NPY), 78–79
Neutral endopeptidase (NEP), 5
Neutrophils, vasomotion and, 371
Nevus flammeus, 1273–1274
Klippel-Trenaunay syndrome, 1274
port-wine stain, 1273
Sturge-Weber syndrome, 1274
Nicardipine, for Raynaud's phenomenon, 981
Nicotinic acid, 601
Nicotinic receptors, 132
Nifedipine, 812
for Raynaud's phenomenon, 983
Ni-Hon-San study, 570
Nitrate therapy, 711–712, 808–810
Nitrendipine, for occlusive renal artery disease, 855
Nitric oxide (NO), 11, 122
antiproliferation effects of, 255–256
donors, 650
endothelium-derived relaxing factors (EDRFs) and, 127–128, 249
for pulmonary hypertension, 961
radical, 301
synthesis of, 246
as vasodilator, 371
Nitroglycerin
for anginal discomfort, 808
arterial stiffness and, 194
industrial, vasospasm and, 373
for vasculogenic impotence, 895
Nitroprusside, for Raynaud's phenomenon, 983
Nitrovasodilators, 122
Nonadrenergic, noncholinergic (NANC) neurogenic relaxation, 887
Nonapeptide bradykinin, 209
Nonbacterial thrombotic endocarditis (NBTE), 272
Noninvasive testing, 415–439, *See also specific test methods*
abdominal aorta diseases, 425–430
arterial obstructive disease
bedside instrumentation, 835
Doppler velocity spectroscopy, 836
plethysmography, 836
pulse-volume recordings, 836
radionuclide labeling methods, 837–838
segmental pressure measurement, 835–836
ultrasound imaging, 836–837
arterial occlusive disease of the extremities, 430–436
cardiac, 705–708
dipyridamole thallium imaging for ischemia, 706–707
exercise testing, 705–706
holter monitoring for asymptomatic ischemia, 707–708
left-ventricular ejection fraction assessment, 707
stress echocardiographic imaging, 707
cerebrovascular disease, 422–425
methods
blood pressure determination, 421–422
Doppler ultrasonography, 415–418
plethysmography, 419–421
ultrasonic imaging, 418–419
venous diseases, 436–439
venous insufficiency, 1094
Nonischemic chest pain, 804
Nonmodulators, 350
Nonocclusive mesenteric ischemia, 879
Nonprostanoid endothelium-derived relaxing factors (EDRFs), 126–128
Non-Q-wave infarction, 341
Nonspecialized surface membrane, 92
Nonsteroidal anti-inflammatory drugs (NSAIDs), 648
Nontraumatic intracranial hemorrhage, computed tomography, 547–552
Noradrenaline, reflex sympathetic dystrophy and, 1210
Norepinephrine, 72, 122–125, 357, 359
deamination of, 124
extraneuronal uptake of, 124–125
neuronal uptake of, 123–124
penile erection and, 887
physiologic effects of, 130
in Raynaud's phenomenon, 968, 969
relaxing effects of, endothelium and, 131
role of, 370
serotonin and, 134
sources of, 130
uptake of, 125
vasomotion and, 369–370
North American Symptom Carotid Endarterectomy Trial (NASCET), 790, 791
Nosocomial endocarditis, 1107
Nuclear magnetic resonance (NMR), 877–878, *See also* Magnetic resonance imaging (MRI)
Nuclear Magnus Raphus (NMR), reflex sympathetic dystrophy and, 1211
Nuclear medicine, 467–488
instrumentation, 468–473
planar imaging, 469–470
principles, 468
tomography, 470–473
measurement principles, 477–480
capillary blockade, 475–476, 478
diffusible tracers, 476, 478
indicator dilution, 477–478
metabolism, 479–480
organ uptake, 478–479
radionuclide imaging
for acute deep venous thrombosis, 486
for aortic diseases, 486
for cerebrovascular disease, 480–481
for chronic venous disorders, 486–487
for congenital disorders, 487–488

Nuclear medicine—(*continued*)
for coronary artery disease, 481–485
of extremities, 476
for hypertension, 488
for infectious diseases, 488
for inflammatory and immunologic disorders, 488
for mesenteric vascular disease, 485–486
for pulmonary embolism, 486
for renal vascular disease, 485
for vascular disorders, 480–486
for venous diseases, 486–487
radionuclides, 467–468
radiopharmaceuticals, 473–477
Nuclear regulatory proteins, 43
Nucleus tractus solitarius (NTS), 358
Nurses' Health Study, 252, 577

Obesity
as cardiovascular disease risk factor, 577–578
deep abdominal, lipoprotein disorders and, 599
defined, 577
hypertension and, 610–611, 624
Observational analytic studies, 570, 571
Obstructive airways disease, 955–956
Occipital artery, pulse, 403
Occlusive arterial disease, 274
acute, 831–832
categories, 832
defined, 401
localizing, 401–402
patient examination, 401–409
aortoiliac, 681–685
chronic, patient examination, 397–401
in extremities, 825–847
acute, 831–832
associated risk factors, 825–827, 840–841
atheroembolism, 832–833
clinical interpretation, 838–839
clinical presentation, 828–831
claudication, 828–829
ischemia at rest, 829–830
limb ischemia, 830–831
fibromuscular dysplasia, 833–834
histopathology, 827–828
incidence and prevalence, 825
local measures, 839–840
medical therapy, 839–844
natural history and prognosis, 828
noninvasive testing, 430–436, 835–838
popliteal-artery enlargement, 834–835
surgical therapy, 844–847
upper, surgery, 680–681
infrainguinal, 685–687
peripheral, angiography, 499–504
Raynaud's phenomenon and, 975–976
renal, 853–865
consequences, 855–856
pathophysiology, 853–855
Occlusive disease
peripheral vascular, 675–691
visceral vessel, 691–693
Occlusive venous disease
cerebral, computed tomography, 552
in upper extremities, 1098
venous insufficiency and, 1091–1092, 1093
Omega-3 fatty acids, 648–649
Onion skinning, 232
Opioid peptides, 79
Oral contraceptives
endothelial function and, 253
thrombosis and, 273
Organic nitrates, 650
for Raynaud's phenomenon, 983
Organ uptake, of radiopharmaceuticals, 478–479
Orthopedic injuries, 1152–1153
Oscillatory compliance, 186, 188
Osler's nodes, in infective endocarditis, 1108
Osler-Weber-Rendu disease (OWRD), 1245
Osteomyelitis, 1176–1177
Outlet maneuvers, 408–409
Oxidant-induced endothelial stress, 12–13, 249, 250, 252
Oxidized LDL (ox-LDL), 249, 250, 257, 318–319
Oxygen-free radicals, 872
Oxygen supply, ischemia and, 333
Oxytocin, 80

Paget-Schroetter syndrome, 275, 1098, 1198–1203
angioplasty, 1202–1203
cause, 1198
diagnosis, 1199
presenting history and signs, 1199
surgical treatment, 1202
therapy, 1199–1202, 1203
transluminal balloon venoplasty, 1202
Pain
abdominal, 874, 876
anginal, 804
calf, 828, 829
central pain-projecting (CPP) neurons, 1211
chest, 802, 804, 930–931, 953
leg, 828–829
posttraumatic syndromes, 1157
reflex sympathetic dystrophy, 1209–1211
rest, 401, 681–682
sympathetic mediated, 1211
Palmar xanthomas, 597
Paracrine model, 297
Paramagnetic compounds, in magnetic resonance imaging, 456
Parenchymal disease, pulmonary, 955
Parke-Weber syndrome, 1245
Paroxysmal nocturnal hemoglobinuria (PNH), 274
Partial agonists, 810
Partial anomalous pulmonary venous connection (PAPVC), 1223, 1224–1227
defined, 1223, 1224
natural history, 1226–1227
physiology, 122–124
PDGF. *See* Platelet-derived growth factor (PDGF)
PECAM, 15
Peclet number, 149, 150
Pedal ulcers, 1173–1181
arterial vs. venous insufficiency, 1173
assessment, 1177–1178
classification, 1177–1178
diabetes and, 1173, 1174–1177
etiology, 1174
limb amputation for, 1175–1179
therapy, 1178–1181
Pediatric vascular trauma, 1167–1168
Pelvic trauma, blunt, impotence and, 889
Penetrating aortic ulcer, aortic dissection and, 939
Penetrating atherosclerotic ulcers (PAU), computed tomography, 528
Penetrating injuries, 1147
Penicillin, for infective endocarditis, 1110–1111
Penile erection physiology, 886–888
corporal veno-occlusion, 887–888
extracellular matrix synthesis, 888
helicine arteriolar smooth muscle tone, 886
trabecular smooth muscle tone, 886–888
Penis
blunt trauma, 890
microvascular arterial bypass surgery, 896–898
prosthesis insertion, 898
self-injection therapy, 895–896
vacuum constriction devices, 896–897
Pentoxifylline
for arterial obstructive diseases, 842
for thromboangiitis obliterans, 1047
for venous ulcers, 1184
Peptides, 136–137
angiotensin II, 136
atrial natriuretic factor (ANF), 137
bradykinin, 136–137
calcitonin gene-related (CGRP), 137
receptors, 78–80
substance P, 137
vasoactive intestinal polypeptide (VIP), 137
vasoconstrictors, 106–107
vasopressin, 136
Percutaneous transluminal angioplasty (PTA), 717–759
aortoiliac disease, 722–729
atherectomy in, 844
balloon injury research, 224–225
bypass grafts and, 740–745
coarctation of the aorta, 1238
complications, 1258–1262
coronary (PTCA), 814–815
femoral arteries, 729–738
iatrogenic complications, 1165–1166
iliac artery, 721, 722–729
for impending vein graft failure, 740–745
infrapopliteal arteries, 738–740
innominate arteries, 745–747
limitations of, 718
for maintaining hemodialysis conduits, 752–756
mechanisms of, 718–722
partial, 717
in peripheral arterial disease, 717–759, 843, 844
popliteal arteries, 729–738
popularity of, 717–718
renal (PTRA), 863–864
for atherosclerotic renal-artery stenosis, 749–751
for fibromuscular disease, 749
lesion location and, 751
for peripheral arterial disease, 757–758
for renal-artery stenosis, 749
subclavian arteries, 745–747
superior mesenteric artery, 720
vasospasm and, 374
for venous compression, 1202–1203
Perfusion
cerebral, imaging, 480–481
coronary, 334
imaging, 481–483
defined, 333
extracranial tissue computed

tomography, 539
intracranial tissue computed tomography, 553–555
limb
collateral, 830
cutaneous pressure, 830
measuring, 421
luxury, 479
regional perfusion index, 433
Periaortic fibrosis, 427, 528–530
Perineal trauma, blunt, impotence and, 889
Perioperative cardiac failure, 1265
Perioperative hypertension, 633
Perioperative myocardial infarction, 1262
Peripheral arterial disease (PAD), 333
angiography, 495, 499–504
health care costs, 749, 758–759
intra-arterial thrombolytic therapy, 765–775
obstructive diseases of the extremities, 825–847
percutaneous transluminal angioplasty, 717–759
prevalence, 717
treatment, 756–759
Peripheral arteries
aneurysms, surgery, 698
blood flow and ischemia, 335–336
intravascular imaging, 839
Peripheral ischemia, acute, 342
Peripheral vascular resistance, 231, 359
Peripheral vascular surgery, 675–691
cardiac risk in, 703–713
high-risk patients, treatment options for, 708–712
noninvasive cardiac testing, 705–708
preoperative clinical evaluation, 703–705
Peripheral venous angiography, iatrogenic complications, 1165
Perlecan, 61
Pernio (chilblains), 986
Peroneal artery injuries, 1164
Peroxynitrous acid, 249
Perthes' test, for varicose veins, 1086, 1090
Pertussis toxin, endothelium-derived relaxing factors (EDRFs) and, 127
Pharmacoarteriography, 894
Pharmacocavernosography, 892–893
Pharmacocavernosometry, 892
Pharmacologic hypertension, 618, 623
Pharmacology, 117–137
effector systems, 117–130
adrenergic-nerve endings, 122–125
endothelium, 125–130
vascular smooth muscles, 117–122
neurohumoral mediators, 130–137
acetylcholine, 132
catecholamines, 130–132
histamine, 134–136
peptides, 136–137
purines, 132–133
serotonin, 133–134
Pharmacomechanical coupling, 70
Phenoxybenzamine, for Raynaud's phenomenon, 981
Phentolamine, reflex sympathetic dystrophy and, 1210
Phenylethylamine, migraine headaches and, 380
Pheochromocytoma, 618, 622–623
Phlebitis, superficial, patient examination, 410
Phosphoinositides, 87–89
Phospholipids, plasmalemma, 91
Phosphorus nuclear magnetic resonance (PNMR), 877–878
Phosphorylation, myosin heavy-chain, 101–103
Photoplethysmography
chronic venous disorders, 439
reactive hyperemia, 434
varicose veins, 1087
venous insufficiency, 1094
Phylactic coronary revascularization, 708
Physical inactivity, as risk factor, 576, 611
Physicians' Health Study, 252, 254, 579, 646, 647, 813
"Pink puffer," 955
Planar imaging, 469–470
Plaque
advanced, 336
assumptions, 230
calcified, 718–722
cellular interactions, 292, 293
characteristics, 321–322
composition, 342
defined, 290
developmental stages, 325
in extremities, 827
growth mechanisms, 336–337
initiation of, 336
monoclonal hypothesis, 228–230
morphology, 423
platelet hypothesis, 228
regression of, 295
response-to-injury hypothesis of atherosclerosis, 293
rupture, 339–341, 342, 798
rupture-mediated growth, 336
stable, 336
thrombus-mediated growth, 336
ulcerated, 675, 800–801
ultrasound imaging, 423–425, 718–722
unstable, 336
Plaque lipid, derivation of, 228
Plasma-D dimer ELISA, for pulmonary embolism, 1072, 1074
Plasmalemma phospholipids, 91
Plasma membrane, calcium source regulation by, 92–93
Plasmapheresis, for vasculitis, 1024
Plasma renin activity (PRA), peripheral, 858
Plasmin, 211–212, 266–267
Plasminogen, 10, 210–214
Plasminogen activator inhibitors (PAI), 10–11, 213, 214, 254, 257, 266
Plasminogen activators (PAs), 17, 266–268, 653–654, *See also* Tissue-type plasminogen activator (t-PA)
coronary heart disease risk and, 579
fibrinolytic disorders and, 271
single-chain urokinase-type (scu-PA), 210–214, 653
tissue-type (t-PA), 266
urokinaselike (u-PAs), 266
Platelet activating factor (PAF), 9–10
Platelet-derived growth factor (PDGF), 18–19, 81–82, 219
atherogenesis cellular interactions and, 293
endothelial-derived, 236, 291, 292, 300
functions, 65
hypertension and, 361
isoforms, 293, 300, 301
secretion of, 291
smooth muscle regulation by, 104–105, 221, 223–224, 230, 291, 301
Platelet factor 4 (PF4), 63, 278
Platelets
abnormalities
axial dependence, 178
in diabetes mellitus, 274
diffusion, 177–178
shear rate, 176–177
activation, 278, 643–644
adhesion, 207
in annular vortex, 161–162
collagen and, 64
inhibitors of, 8
shear rate and, 168, 172
aggregation, 151–155, 160–162, 207, 643–646
in annular vortex, 160–162
antiplatelet agents, 643–644
arterial wall injury and, 160
cell-cell collisions and, 152–155
collagen and, 64
conditions for, 151
inhibitors of, 8
monoclonal antibodies and, 652
in Poiseuille flow, 152–153
shear rate and, 153–155, 176
shear stress and, 153–155
thrombosis and, 146–148, 151
velocity gradient and, 151
aspirin and, 645–646
atherogenesis and, 228, 291
axial position, 169–170, 178
coagulation factors, 175–176, 178–179
collagen interactions, 64–65
concentration, 168–169, 173–175
coronary vasospasm and, 376
diffusivity, 167–168, 173–175, 177–178
endothelial control of, 246–253
fibrin formation and, 178–179
function of, 8
growth factors, 291–292
inhibitors of, 8
interaction, cohesion, 165, 178–179
membrane glycoprotein antagonists, 652–653
plug, 207
reactivity of, flow effects, 170–171
red cell collisions, 152–153
redistribution of, 157–160
release reaction, 278
thrombosis formation/growth and, 165, 173–175
vasomotion and, 372
vessel wall interactions
abnormalities, 176–179
deposits, 165–167
disorders related to, 176–180
flow and, 165–171
flow chambers, 164
intravascular, 165
in nonanticoagulated blood, 171–176
shear rate and, 178–179
transport processes affecting, 162–176
Plethysmography, 419–421, 836
air, 420
arterial stiffness, 201
chronic venous disorders, 439
impedance, 420
for deep-vein thrombosis, 436–437
for venous thromboembolism, 1053
reactive hyperemia, 434
strain-gauge, 419–420
for chronic venous disorders, 439
for reactive hyperemia, 434

Plethysmography—(*continued*)
venous insufficiency, 1094
venous-occlusion, 420
Pleural effusions, in aortic dissection, 932
Pleurospinal ligament, 1193
Ploidy, hypertension and, 234, 235, 236
Pneumatic devices, for lymphedema, 1143
Pneumothorax, as catheterization complication, 1257–1258
Poiseuille flow, 141–142, 143
aggregation in, 152–153
rotation and deformation in, 151–152
wall migration in, 151–152
Poiseuille's law, 421
exercise testing and, 433
pulmonary vascular resistance, 951
Polyarteritis nodosa, 1004–1007
Polycythemia, thrombosis and, 276
Polymyalgia rheumatica, 1015
Polymyositis, as cause of Raynaud's phenomenon, 975
Polytetrafluoroethylene (PTFE) grafts, 691
Popliteal artery
aneurysms, 404–405, 919
angiography, 499
entrapment, 834–835
injuries, 1163–1164
occlusion of, 733–737
percutaneous revascularization for, 729–738
pulse, 402
stenoses of, 729–733
Portal hypertension, 962–963
Port-wine stain, 1273
Positional cloning, hypertension, 351–352
Positron-emission tomography (PET), 472–473
Posterior arch vein, 1081
Posterior cerebral artery (PCA), 782–784
Posterior communicating arteries (PComm), 783
Posterior inferior cerebellar artery (PICA), 783, 785
Posterior tibial artery, pulse, 402–403
Postischemic paresthesias, 1209
Postjunctional alpha-adrenoceptors, 130–131
Postjunctional beta-adrenoceptors, 131
Postmenopausal estrogen therapy, as risk factor, 576–577
Postoperative abdominal aorta, computed tomography, 530
Postoperative ischemia, 710
Postoperative thromboembolism, 275
Postphlebitic venous insufficiency, 1091
Postthrombotic venous insufficiency, 1091
Posttraumatic pain syndromes, 1157
Potassium, dietary, hypertension and, 362–363, 624, 625
Potassium (K+) channels, 118
Potential-sensitive calcium channels, 91
Prazosin, for Raynaud's phenomenon, 970, 981
Prednisolone, for vasculitis, 1024
Prednisone, for vasculitis, 1024
Pregnancy
hypertension and, 633
thrombosis and, 272–273
venous thrombosis in, 1063
Prejunctional alpha-adrenergic inhibition, 131
Prejunctional receptors, 370
Pre-proendothelin, 129
Pressure-strain elastic modulus, 186
Pressure-wave analysis, 200
Primary hypercoagulable states, 268–271
Primary pulmonary hypertension, 958–962
Probucol Quantitative Regression Swedish Trial (PQRST), 252
Procoagulants, 8–10
Procollagen, 43, 45
Profunda femoris artery disease, angiography, 499
Program on Surgical Control of the Hyperlipidemias (POSCH), 600
Progressive systemic sclerosis, 957
Proliferating cell nuclear antigen (PCNA), 227
Prolonged immobilization, thrombosis and, 275
Prolyl hydroxylase, 43, 44
Prophylactic low-dose aspirin, 579, *See also* Aspirin
Prophylactic revascularization therapy, 708
Propionyl-L-carnitine, 842
Propranolol, 373, 810–811
Prospective cohort studies, risk factors, 570
Prostacyclins, 8, 11, 126, 265, 376, 650, 651
for pulmonary hypertension, 961–962
vasomotion and, 372
Prostaglandins, 8, 80–81, 842
for arterial obstructive diseases of the extremities, 842
for Raynaud's phenomenon, 983
Prostanoid receptors, 80–81
Prosthetic-valve endocarditis, 1104, 1105–1106
Protease nexin, 7, 212
Protein kinase
cAMP-dependent, 90
cGMP-dependent, 90
in smooth muscle proliferation, 104
Protein-rich lipoproteins, 307, 310–312
atherogenesis and, 310–312
lipolysis of, 310, 311
Proteins
adhesion, 5–6
cell-receptor, 54
in diet, 625
dietary, hypertension and, 625
G proteins, 83, 84–87, 89, 90, 127, 644
link, 60
protein C, 7, 265–266, 269
activate peptide (PCP), 277
deficiency, 270–271, 278
protein S, 7, 265, 266, 269
deficiency, 270–271
Protein-tyrosine kinases (PTKs), 81–82
Proteoglycans, 56, 57–63
biosynthesis, 62
degradation, 62–63
sulfated, 19
Prothrombin, 8, 172
Proximal pulmonary thromboembolism, chronic, 958
Pseudoaneurysms, 1156
angiography, 497, 504
aortic, 902
computed tomography, 530–531, 534
noninvasive testing of, 429–430
Pseudoclaudication, 400, 829
Psychological risk factors, 578
Psychologic counseling, for vasculogenic impotence, 894
Pulmonary arteries
abnormalities, 1241–1242
angiography, 514–516
blood volume, 951
circulation, 951–952
computed tomography, 531
malformations, 1243
sarcomas, 1280–1281
total anomalous origin of coronary arteries from (TCAPA), 1228–1232
Pulmonary edema, 632, 853
Pulmonary embolism, 1069–1078
anticoagulants for, 641–642
death from, 1051, 1054
diagnosis, 1054, 1072–1075
epidemiology, 1069
health costs, 1069
magnetic resonance imaging, 463
pathophysiology, 1069
prevention, 1069–1072
radionuclide imaging, 486, 488
therapy, 1054, 1075–1078
catheter-based intervention, 1077
emotional support, 1077–1078
inferior vena caval filter, 1077
surgery, 1077
thrombolytic, 1075–1077
Pulmonary hypertension, 951–963
categories, 952
computed tomography, 531
defined, 951
diagnostic studies, 953
magnetic resonance imaging, 463
primary, 958–962
Raynaud's phenomenon and, 978
secondary
acquired diseases of the left side of the heart, 954
alveolar hypoventilation, 956
cardiac disease, 953–954
chronic proximal pulmonary thromboembolism, 958
congenital heart disease, 954–955
connective-tissue diseases, 956–957
dietary pulmonary hypertension, 962
HIV association, 963
interstitial lung disease, 955
obstructive airways disease, 955–956
parenchymal disease, 955–956
portal hypertension association, 962–963
primary pulmonary hypertension, 958–962
pulmonary thromboembolic disease, 957–958
thrombotic occlusion, 957–958
toxic oil syndrome, 962
venous diseases, 955
signs, 952
symptoms, 951–952
Pulmonary parenchymal disease, 955–956
Pulmonary thromboembolic disease, 957–958
Pulmonary vascular disease, 955, 956–957
Pulmonary vascular resistance, 951–952
Pulmonary veins, 955, 1227
Pulmonary veno-occlusive disease, 955
Pulsatile flow, 143
Pulseless disease, 905
Pulses, 194
deficits, in aortic dissection, 931

patient examination, 402–403
repetition frequency (PRF), 416
volume recordings, 836, 979
Pulse waves
arterial stiffness effects on, 194–197
contour analysis, 200, 201
velocity
aging and, 190, 191
arterial stiffness and, 186, 187
measuring, 188
Pulsus tardus-parvus pattern, Doppler ultrasonography, 430
Purinergic receptors, 77–78, 132–133
Purines, 132–133
Pulse-volume recording, for arterial occlusive disease, 431–432
Pyelogram, intravenous, 860
Pyogenic granulomas (lobular capillary hemangioma), 1271

Q waves, 341, 805

Radial arteries
injuries, 1161
pulse, 402
Radiation doses, computed tomography, 524–525
Radioactive decay, types of, 467–468
Radionuclide imaging, 837–838, *See also* Nuclear medicine
acute deep venous thrombosis, 486
aortic diseases, 486
cerebrovascular disease, 480–481
chronic venous disorders, 486–487
congenital disorders, 487–488
coronary artery disease, 481–485
exercise, 806
extremities, 476
hypertension, 488
infectious diseases, 488
inflammatory and immunologic disorders, 488
mesenteric vascular disease, 485–486
pulmonary embolism, 486
renal vascular disease, 485
vascular disorders, 480–486
venous diseases, 486–487
Radionuclides, 467–468, *See also* Nuclear medicine
Radiopharmaceuticals, 473–477
binding of, 477, 479
blood-volume tracers, 473–476
capillary blockade, 475–476
in-vitro labeling, 473–475
in-vivo labeling, 473–475
organ uptake of, 478–479
Raised fibrolipids, 336
Randomized Intervention Treatment of Angina (RITA), 814
Randomized trials, risk factors, 571
Rarefaction, hypertension and, 231
Raynaud's disease, 972–974
digital vasospasm and, 377–378, 379
Raynaud's phenomenon, 373, 956, 957, 965–984
angiography, 505–506
classification, 965–966
defined, 965
diagnosis, 435–436, 965, 978–979
digital vasospasm and, 377, 378–379
digital vessel sensitivity and, 969–970
incidence, 973
pathophysiology, 966–972
primary, 972–974
secondary causes of
arterial occlusive disease, 975–976
blood dyscrasias, 976–977
connective-tissue disease, 974–975
drugs and toxins, 977–978
neurologic disorders, 976
thoracic outlet syndrome, 976
trauma, 977
sympathetic nervous system activity and, 967–969
treatment
calcium channel blockers, 980–981
conservative measures, 979–980
direct vascular smooth muscle relaxants, 982–983
renin-angiotensin system inhibition, 982
serotonin antagonists, 981–982
sympathectomy, 983–984
sympathetic nervous system inhibitors, 980–981
thromboxane inhibitors, 982
triiodothyroxine, 983
vasoconstriction and, 966–967, 969, 970–971
Reaction rate-controlled transport, 164–165
Reactive hyperemia, noninvasive testing, 434
Reactive oxygen intermediates (ROIs), 12–13
Real-time scanning, 418
Receptor-operated calcium channels, 70, 71, 91
Recombinant-DNA technology, 665
Recombinant peptide, 54
Recurrent migratory superficial thrombophlebitis, 272
Recurrent pulmonary edema, 853
Red blood cells, *See also* Blood; Blood cells; Flow
deformation of, 155, 157
flow at normal hematocrits, 155–160
platelet collisions, 152–153
platelet diffusivity and, 167–168
Reflectance spectrophotometry, for visceral ischemia, 878
Reflex neurogenic inflammation, 1212, 1214
Reflex sympathetic dystrophy (RSD) (causalgia), 378, 976, 1157, 1209–1214
autonomic dysfunction, 1212–1214
defined, 1209
edema, 1211–1212
movement disorder, 1214
pain, 1209–1211
Refractory hypertension, 633–634
Regional perfusion index, 433
Relative apparent viscosity, shear rate and, 150
Relaxation training, for hypertension, 625
Relaxation, of vascular smooth muscles, 117–122
cAMP, 121
cGMP, 121–122
hyperpolarization, 118
calcium inhibition, 119–121
Remodeling, of vessel walls, 226, 227, 235, 360
Renal angiography, 506–508
Renal angioplasty, 863–864
Renal arteries
aneurysms, 535–537, 699, 920
arteritis, 857
atheromatous lesions, 856
cholesterol emboli, 857
computed tomography, 535–537
fibromuscular dysplasia, 857, 1246
injuries, 1162–1163
insufficiency, in infective endocarditis, 1108
occlusive disease, 853–865
pathology, 856–857
stenosis
atherosclerotic, 749–751
fibromuscular disease, 749
health care costs, 749
hemodialysis conduits, 751–759
indications for therapy, 748–749
noninvasive testing, 429–430
prevalence, 747–749
in renovascular hypertension, 853
revascularization, 749
treatment, 751
unilateral vs. bilateral, 853–854
ultrasonography, 425–427
Renal disease
end-stage, 599
infarcts, computed tomography, 540
lipoprotein disorders and, 599
magnetic resonance imaging, 460
parenchymal, 540, 617–618
radionuclide imaging, 485
renal failure, 855–856
acute, 599, 617–618
chronic, 618
Renal-function curve
animal models, 354–357
hypertension and, 353–357
tests, in vasculitis, 1003
Renal scintigraphy, 859
Renal veins, renin determinations, 859
Renin
angiotensin-aldosterone system (RAS), 352–353
angiotensin system, 136
hypertension and, 351, 363
inhibitors, in Raynaud's phenomenon, 982
in occlusive renal artery disease, 853, 854
profile, in hypertension, 612, 626–627
renal-vein ratio, 859
Renography, captopril, 859–860
Renovascular hypertension, 618, 619–620, 853–865
in children, 858
clinical features, 857–858
detecting, 861–862
diagnosis, 858–862
index of clinical suspicion, 858
laboratory investigations, 857
prevalence, 855
renal segmental infarction, 857
signs and symptoms, 857
treatment, 862–865
medical management, 864–865
renal angioplasty, 863–864
surgery, 862–863
surgery and angioplasty, 864
Renovascular reconstruction, 691–693
Reperfusion syndrome, 766
edema, 1153
in vascular trauma, 1153, 1154–1155
Reserpine, for Raynaud's phenomenon, 981
Response-to-injury hypothesis of atherosclerosis, 228, 293–295
Restenosis, 738, 751, 752, 754, *See also* Stenosis
after angioplasty, 815

Restenosis—(*continued*)
after coronary balloon angioplasty, 1261–1262
after renal angioplasty, 864
replication in, 227–228
Resting electrocardiography, 805
Rest pain
in aortoiliac occlusive disease, 681–682
patient examination, 401
Rethrombosis, during thrombolytic therapy, 774
Retiform hemangioendothelioma, 1276
Retinopathy, 857, 1173
Retrograde femoral aortography, 1160
Retroperitoneal hematoma, 773–774
Retroviral mediated gene transfer, 666–667
Reverse cholesterol transport, 300
Reversed autogenous saphenous vein graft, 686–687
Reversible ischemic neurologic deficit (RIND), 782
Reynolds number
in annular vortex, 161
defined, 142
disturbed flow and, 143, 145
wall migration and, 151–152
Rhabdomyolysis, reperfusion-caused, 1155
Rheumatoid arthritis, as cause of Raynaud's phenomenon, 975
Rheumatoid factors, in vasculitis, 1002, 1003
Ribs
anatomy, 1190–1191
compression syndrome, 1187–1189
Ridogrel, 650
Ring abscess, in infective endocarditis, 1105, 1107
RISC (Risk of Myocardial Infarction or Death) study, 647
Risk-benefit analyses, 571
Risk factors, 279
atherogenesis, 587
atherosclerosis, 377
cardiac, 703–713
cardiovascular diseases, 307, 569–581
cerebrovascular, 781–782
coronary heart disease, 569, 575–579
cost-benefits analyses, 571
diabetes mellitus as, 575–576, 703, 781
dyslipoproteinemias, 587–601
epidemiology in, 569–571
hypertension, 574–575, 609, 610–613, 704
lipoprotein interaction, 587
occlusive arterial disease in extremities, 840–841
peripheral arterial disease, 703
reducing, 569–581
stroke, 781
studies, 569–571
surgery, 703–713
thrombosis, 254
venous thromboembolism, 1052, 1055
venous thrombosis, 1070
Rolling, 13, 14
Rotation, of blood cells in Poiseuille flow, 151
Rotational atherectomy, 731, 740
Roth spots, in infective endocarditis, 1108

Saccular aortic aneurysms, 902
Salmonella spp., in infective endarteritis, 1118–1119
Saphenous veins
anatomy, 1081
grafts, 846
autogenous reversed, 880–881
patency, 817
Saralasin, 136
Sarcoplasmic reticulum (SR), 92, 94–95
Saturated fat, dietary, hypertension and, 624, 625
Scalene muscle, 1189, 1191–1193
Scalenotomy, 1189
Scalenus syndrome, 1189
Scandinavian Simvastatin Survival Study, 574
Scanners, ultrasonic imaging, 418–419
Scatter factor (SF), 19
Scavenger receptors, 316, 319
Scimitar syndrome, 1226, 1241
Scintigraphy
captopril, 620
renal, 859
thallium, 806
Sclerodactyly, 973
Scleroderma
Raynaud's phenomenon and, 957, 974
thrombosis in, 275
Sclerotherapy
for spider veins, 1091
for varicose veins, 1088–1089
Secondary hypercoagulable states, 268, 271–276
Sector scanners, ultrasonic imaging, 418–419
Segmental pressure measurement, 835–836
L-Selectin, 15
P-Selectin, 13–14
E-Selectin, 14
Selective intra-arterial thrombolytic therapy, 765–775
Sendai virus (HV)/liposome gene transfer, 668, 670
Senile (cherry) angiomas, 1270–1271
Sepsis, acute visceral ischemia and, 872
Sequestration of the lungs, 1241
Serotonin, 133–134
adrenergic nerves and, 134
antagonists, 981–982
coronary occlusion and, 376
endothelium and, 134
Raynaud's phenomenon and, 970–971, 981–982
receptors, 75
vascular disease and, 134
vascular smooth muscle and, 133
as vasoconstrictor in finger circulation, 378
Serotoninergic receptors, 74–75
classification, 74–75
distribution and location, 75
heterogeneity, 75
mechanism of action, 74
Serum albumin, 3
Serum cholesterol, elevated
intervention strategies, 574
nonvascular mortality, 573–574
prevalence, 572
as risk factor for cardiovascular disease, 572–574
treatment risks, 573
Serum sickness, 387, 390, 1012
7E3, 652
Sex therapy, for impotence, 894
Shear rates
coagulation and, 175–176
defined, 141
fibrin formation and, 178–179
platelet aggregation and, 153–155, 176
platelet function abnormalities, 176–177
platelet reactivity and, 170–171
relative apparent viscosity and, 150
thrombosis and, 146, 148
vessel walls, 165–167, 168, 169, 172–173
Shear stress
blood cell behavior and, 151
defined, 141–142
endothelial cell response to, 12
in lesion-prone endothelium, 298–299
platelet aggregation and, 153–155
platelet reactivity and, 170–171
thrombosis and, 180
Shear-stress response element (SSRE), 12, 299
Shock, 148
Shocked bowel syndrome, 879
Sickle-cell disease, 276
Signal cascades, 83, 84
Signal transduction, in vascular smooth muscle, 83–91
calcium messenger system, 90–91
cyclic nucleotides, 89–90
G proteins, 83, 84–87
mechanisms of, 85
phosphoinositides, 87–89
Silent ischemia (asymptomatic myocardial ischemia), 806
Single-chain urokinase-type plasminogen activator (scu-PA), 210–214, 653
Single-photon-emission computed tomography (SPECT), 472, 788–789
Sinus radiographs, in vasculitis, 1003
Skin
ischemia, transcutaneous oximetry, 433
necrosis, from cutaneous microvascular thrombosis, 271
patient examination, 409
Smoking
atherosclerosis of the extremities and, 827
cardiovascular diseases and, 571–572
cessation, 571, 624
coronary heart disease risk and, 571
hypertension and, 611–612, 624
impotence and, 886
intervention strategies, 571–572
lipoproteins and, 587
prevalence, 571
renovascular hypertension and, 857
stroke and, 781
thromboangiitis obliterans and, 1033, 1034, 1046–1047
Smooth muscle, vascular
acetylcholine and, 132
calcium antagonists and, 120
catecholamines and, 130–131
cells, 69–107
endothelial regulation of, 300–301
gamma interferon and, 301–302
interactions among, 301
macrophage interactions, 299–300
migration, 230
PDGF regulation of, 230, 301
potassium and, 363
response process, 69
scavenger-receptor activity, 316–317
contraction, 91–107, 117
calcium sources, 92–94
excitation-contraction coupling, 91–92
force generation, 94–103
regulation, 70

function, 117
helicine arteriolar tone, 886
innervation, 370
membrane activation, 69–82
proliferation, 103–107
in atherosclerosis, 225, 226
cell number vs. organ mass, 234–236
control of, 209–212
fibrous plaque and, 293
in hypertension, 232, 234, 359–361
intima, 290–291
lipoprotein stimulation of, 325–326
macrophages and, 291
mass changes and, 236–237
research, 224–225
in restenosis, 227–228
role of, 797
theories of, 228–231
waves, 224
relaxation, 117–122, 126–128
serotonin and, 134
signal transduction, 83–91
calcium messenger system, 90–91
cyclic nucleotides, 89–90
G proteins, 84–87
phosphoinositides, 87–89
surface receptor systems
alpha-adrenergic receptors, 69–71
angiotensin II, 72–73
atrial natriuretic peptide, 79
beta-adrenergic receptors, 71–72
calcitonin, 79
dopaminergic receptors, 78
growth factor receptor-associated protein-tyrosine kinases (PTKs), 81–82
histaminergic receptors, 75–76
kinins, 76–77
muscarinic receptors, 73–74
neuropeptide Y, 78–79
opioid peptides, 79
oxytocin, 80
prostanoid receptors, 80–81
purinergic receptors, 77–78
serotoninergic receptors, 74–75
tachykinins, 79
vasoactive intestinal polypeptide, 79
vasopressin, 79–80
trabecular tone, 886–888
vessel wall properties, 189
Sodium, dietary, hypertension and, 354–357, 359, 361–362, 611, 624, 625
Sodium hydrogen antiporter system, 73
Sodium nitroprusside, for aortic dissection, 940
Sodium potassium ATPase pump, inhibitors of, 370–371
Soft-tissue trauma, 1152–1153
Somatomedin C, smooth muscle proliferation and, 221
Sotalol, 810
Sphygmomanometry, for monitoring arterial stiffness, 199
Spider veins (spider hemangioma, venous telangiectasia), 1090–1091, 1274
Spinal cord ischemia, 400
Spindle-cell hemangioendothelioma, 1272
Splenic artery
aneurysms, 698
infarcts, computed tomography, 535, 540
Splenomegaly, in infective endocarditis, 1108
Splinter hemorrhages, in infective endocarditis, 1108
"Square toes," 1139
Stable angina, 337, 376
Stable claudication, 339
Stable lesions, 333
Stable plaque, 336
Stable xenon-enhanced computed tomography, 555
Stanozolol, for venous ulcers, 1184
Staphylococci, in infective endocarditis, 1106–1107, 1110
Staphylococcus aureus, in infective endocarditis, 1104–1105, 1106
Starch, dietary, hypertension and, 625
Stasis ulceration, 1181
Stem-cell diseases, 274
Steno Hospital Study, 575
Stenosis, *See also* Restenosis
in atherosclerosis of the extremities, 827
blood pressure determination, 421
color Doppler analysis, 416, 418
grafts, 742–745
lesions, treatment of, 675–680
popliteal artery, 729–733
pulmonary veins, 1227
renal artery, 747–751
replication in, 227–228
severity, 245, 797
superficial femoral artery (SFA), 729–733
ultrasound imaging of, 423–424
vessel diameter changes, 374
Stepped care, for hypertension, 626
Steroids, sympathetic-nerve stimulation and, 125
Stethoscopy, Doppler, 835
Stiffness index, 186
Stimulus-response coupling, 103–104
Stockings. *See* Compression stockings
Stokes-Einstein equation, 149
Storage-pool disease, 177
Strawberry (juvenile) hemangiomas, 1269–1270
Streptococci, in infective endocarditis, 1104–1105, 1106–1107, 1110
Streptokinase (SK)
effects of, 653–655, 774
in intra-arterial thrombolytic therapy, 765, 772–773, 774
Stress
echocardiographic imaging, 707
integrated responses to, 12–16
mechanical, 12
reduction, for hypertension, 624, 625
as risk factor for hypertension, 612
testing, value of, 806
Stretch-dependent (myogenic) tone, 82
Stroke, 781–793, *See also* Cerebrovascular disease
anticoagulants for, 643
aortic dissection causing, 931
aspirin for prevention of, 647
cardioembolic, treatment, 791
defined, 781
health care costs, 609
hemorrhagic, 788
ischemic
cardioembolic stroke, 785
carotid artery disease, 782–784
collagen vascular disease, 786–787
hypercoagulable states, 786–787
lacunar, 784–785
treatment of, 791–792
vertebrobasilar disease, 785
laboratory diagnosis of, 789–790
mortality rates, 569
neuronal death in, 792
new therapy, 792–793
risk factors, 781–782
ticlopidine for, 651
transient ischemic, 781, 792
treatment, 790–792
types, 781
in young people, 809
Stroke Prevention in Atrial Fibrillation (SPAF) trial, 648, 791
ST-segment depression, 802
interpretation of, 805–806
Sturge-Weber syndrome, 1245, 1274
Subarachnoid hemorrhage, 380–381, 792
Subclavian arteries, 1191
compression of, 1193–1196
percutaneous revascularization of, 745–747
trauma to, 1160–1161
Subclavian pulse, 402
Subclavian veins
catheterization complications, 1255, 1257–1258
thrombosis, 1098
Subclavius muscle, 1193
Subendothelium, 39–65
biological considerations, 63–65
collagen chemistry and structure, 40–43
collagen metabolism, 43–47
elastin, 50–53
fibronectin, 53–55
functions of, 63, 69
glycosaminoglycans, 56–63
laminin, 55–56
minor collagens, 47–50
vasculature variations, 39–40
Sublingual isosorbide dinitrate, 809
Sublingual nitroglycerin, 809
Substance P, 137
Subtotal anomalous pulmonary venous connection, 1226
Sudden coronary death, 341
Sulfated proteoglycans, 19
Sulfation, in biosynthesis of proteoglycans, 62
Sulfinpyrazone, 651
Superficial femoral artery (SFA)
occlusion of, 722, 724, 733–737
stenosis of, 729–733
Superficial hypogastric artery, pulse, 403
Superficial phlebitis, patient examination, 410
Superior cerebellar arteries (SCA), 783
Superior mesenteric artery
injuries, 1162
percutaneous transluminal angioplasty, 720
thrombosis, 871–872
ultrasonography, 425
Superior vena cava (SVC) syndrome, 537, 539
Superoxide anion, EDRF action and, 249
Superoxide dismutases (SOD), 13
Suppurative thrombophlebitis, 1121–1123
central, 1122–1123
superficial, 1122
Supraclavicular bruits, 407
Supramesocolic hematoma, 1162
Surface couplings, 92, 93
Surgery, 675–699
for aortic dissection, 941
for aortoiliac occlusive disease, 681–685

Surgery—(*continued*)
for arterial aneurysm, 693–697
peripheral, 698–699
for arterial obstructive diseases of the extremities, 844–847
amputation, 847
aortoiliac revascularization, 846
endarterectomy, 845–846
extra-anatomic bypass, 846
femoropopliteal reconstruction, 846
lumbar sympathectomy, 846–847
tibioperoneal revascularization, 846
upper extremities, 680–681
cardiac, vascular complications, 1262–1264
for cerebrovascular disease, extracranial, 675–680
coronary artery bypass, 815–817
for infrainguinal occlusive disease, 685–687
mesenteric revascularization, 693
for peripheral vascular occlusive disease, 675–691, 703–713
for renovascular hypertension, 862–863, 864
renovascular reconstruction, 691–693
for thoracoabdominal aneurysms, 697–698
for varicose veins, 1089–1090
for vein graft failure, 687–691
for venous compression, 1202
for venous insufficiency, 1095–1098
for visceral arterial aneurysm, 698–699
for visceral vessel occlusive disease, 691–693
Surgery and Thrombolysis for Ischemia of the Lower Extremity (STILE) Trial, 735
Survival and Ventricular Enlargement (SAVE) study, 816
Swedish Aspirin Low-dose Trial (SALT), 647
Sympathectomy
for posttraumatic pain syndromes, 1157
for Raynaud's phenomenon, 983–984
for thromboangiitis obliterans, 1047
Sympathetic blockade, reflex sympathetic dystrophy and, 1209, 1210
Sympathetic mediated pain (SMP), 1211
Sympathetic nervous system, 369
inhibitors, 981
Raynaud's phenomenon and, 967–969, 981
reflex sympathetic dystrophy and, 1209–1214
Syncope
aortic dissection causing, 931
local, 965
in pulmonary hypertension, 952–953
Syndecan, 61
Synovial hemangiomas, 1272
Syphilitic aortitis, 906
Systemic hypertension, aortic dissection and, 930
Systemic lupus erythematosus (SLE), 787, 957
as cause of Raynaud's phenomenon, 975
thrombosis in, 275
Systemic sclerosis (scleroderma), 957
as cause of Raynaud's phenomenon, 974–975
Systolic blood pressure
ankle-to-brachial pressure index, 434
cardiovascular events and, 185
digital, 435–436
exercise testing, 432–433
extremity measurement, 432–433
measurement, for Raynaud's phenomenon, 978–979
Systolic Hypertension in the Elderly Project (SHEP), 185

T-200 monoclonal antibody, 290
Tachykinins, 79, 1212
Tachyphylaxis, 73
Takayasu arteritis, 786–787, 857, 905, 999, 1000, 1016–1019
T-cells, 228, 301–302
Telangiectasis, 1244–1246, 1273–1274
ataxia, 1245
capillary hemangiomas, 1246
cavernous hemangiomas, 1245–1246
cutaneous, 1245
hereditary hemorrhage, 1245
spider, 1274
Temperature, reflex sympathetic dystrophy, 1209, 1213
Temporal arteries, pulse, 403
Temporal arteritis (giant cell arteritis), 999, 1015–1016
Temporal trends studies, of risk factors, 569–570
Tendon xanthomas, 596
Tetrodotoxin, 123
TFPI, 266
Thallium scintigraphy, 806
Theophylline, for coronary artery disease, 814
Thoracic aorta, 901
aneurysms, 405–406, 907–910
angiography, 496, 497
Thoracic outlet
anatomic concepts, 1187–1190
arterial compression, 1193–1196
brachial plexus compression, 1196–1198
cervical rib, 1187–1189, 1190–1191
compression syndromes, 1187–1205
defined, 1187
first rib, 1187–1189
management and care, 1203–1205
pathologic anatomy, 1190–1193
scalenus muscle, 1189, 1191–1193
subclavius muscle, 1193
trauma to, 1159–1160
venous compression, 1198–1203
Thoracic outlet syndrome, 976, 1189–1190
Thoracic trauma, 1159–1160, 1161
Thoracoabdominal aneurysms, 697–698, 910–912
Thorotrast-related angiosarcomas, 1278
Thrombin, 207–208, 213–214, 653
formation, 172, 208, 209
function, 172
Thrombin-antithrombin complexes (T-AT), 277
Thromboangiitis obliterans (Buerger's disease), 399, 827, 1033–1048
as cause of Raynaud's phenomenon, 975
clinical features, 975–976, 1040–1045
epidemiology, 1033–1034
etiology and pathogenesis, 1034–1035
pathology, 1035–1040
therapy, 1045–1048
thrombosis in, 275
Thrombocytopenia, heparin-associated, 275
Thrombocytosis, 274
Thromboembolectomy, 765
Thromboembolism, 214
causes, 342
postoperative, 275
Thromboendarterectomy, for pulmonary hypertension, 958
Thrombogenesis
angiography catheters, 495–496
disturbed flow and, 160–165
factors affecting, 175–176, 340–341
Thrombolizer, 1077
Thrombolysis in Myocardial Infarction (TIMI), 652
Thrombolytic therapy, 735, *See also* Intra-arterial thrombolytic therapy (IATT)
agents, 654–655, 813–814
for atherosclerosis obliterans, 765–775
intra-arterial, for peripheral arteries, 844
for pulmonary embolism, 1075–1077
selective intra-arterial, 765–775
for thromboangiitis obliterans, 1047
for venous compression, 1194–1202
for venous thrombosis, 1063
Thrombomodulin, 6–7
Thrombophlebitis, suppurative, 1121–1123
Thrombosis, *See also* Deep-vein thrombosis (DVT)
abnormalities, 177
aggregation and, 146–148
antiphospholipid syndrome and, 273
antithrombin III deficiency and, 269–271
antithrombotic mechanisms, 265–268
atherosclerosis and, 798–799
blood hyperviscosity and, 276
blood vessel abnormalities and, 275–276
as catheterization complication, 1256–1258
clinical, 269–270, 279
deep venous, 410–411
defined, 213
diabetes mellitus and, 274
dysfibrinogenemia and, 281
"effort," 275
endothelial control of, 253–255
factor XII deficiency and, 281
fibrinolytic disorders and, 281
graft, 1262–1263
hemostasis and, 207
heparin-associated, 275
hypercoagulable states, 268–276
laboratory tests, 276–278
pathogenesis, 276–278
hyperlipidemia and, 274
inherited predisposition toward, 278
initiation of, 165
in-situ, 342
internal jugular vein, computed tomography, 553
location of, 180
lupus anticoagulant and, 273
malignancy and, 282
mesenteric venous, 879
mural, 339, 342
myeloproliferative disorders and, 274
nephrotic syndrome and, 273
oral contraceptives and, 273
paroxysmal nocturnal hemoglobinuria and, 274
pathophysiology of, 265–279
in patients with malignancies, 272
plaque rupture response, 339–341
platelet diffusivity and concentration and, 173–175

platelet-vessel wall interaction and, 176–180
pregnancy and, 272–273
process, 141
protein C and S deficiency and, 280–281
radionuclide venography, 480
risk factors for, 254
subarachnoid hemorrhage and, 380–381
superior mesenteric artery, 871–872
thrombotic thrombocytopenic purpura (TTP) and, 276
unstable ischemic syndromes and, 339–340
in upper extremity veins, 1098–1099
velocity gradient and, 151
of vena cava, 537
vessel wall shear rate and, 172–173
Thrombospondin (TSP), 9, 20
Thrombotic occlusion
of small pulmonary arteries and arterioles, 957–958
of visceral arteries, 879
Thrombotic thrombocytopenic purpura (TTP), 276
Thromboxane, 207, 278
biosynthesis, 278
inhibitors, for Raynaud's phenomenon, 982
receptor antagonists, 649–650
synthase inhibitors, 649–650
Tibial arteries, injuries, 1164
Tibioperoneal revascularization, for arterial obstructive diseases of the extremities, 846
Ticlopidine, 651–652, 791, 813
Ticlopidine versus Aspirin Stroke Study (TASS), 651
Time-of-flight loss, in magnetic resonance imaging, 452
Tissue biopsy, in vasculitis, 1004
Tissue factor (TF), 8, 208, 340
pathway inhibitor (TFPI), 7–8, 265
Tissue infarction, computed tomography, 532, 535
Tissue inhibitors of matrix metalloproteinases (TIMPs), 17
Tissue perfusion, computed tomography, 539, 553–555
Tissue-type plasminogen activator (t-PA), 10–11, 210–214, 254, 257, 266, 271, 653–654, 844, *See also* Plasminogen activators (PAs)
coronary heart disease risk and, 579
efficiency of, 774–775
risk factors associated with, 254
Tobacco glycoprotein (TGP), thromboangiitis obliterans and, 1034
Tobacco smoke, vasospasm and, 373
Toe systolic blood pressure (TSBP), 1178
Tolazoline, for Raynaud's phenomenon, 981
Tolerance, in infective endarteritis, 1110
Tomography
computed. *See* Computed tomography (CT)
technology, 470–473
Tonometry, for visceral ischemia, 877
Total anomalous origin of coronary arteries from a pulmonary artery (TCAPA), 1228–1232
Total anomalous pulmonary venous connection (TAPVC), 1223–1224, 1225
defined, 1223
natural history, 1224
physiology, 1223–1224
Total parenteral nutrition (TPN), complications of, 1257–1258
Toxic oil syndrome, 952
Trabecular smooth muscle tone, 886–888
Tracers, diffusible, 476, 478
Transcranial Doppler ultrasonography, 425
Transcutaneous nitroglycerin ointment, 809
Transcutaneous oximetry, 432–433
Transcytosis, 312
Transesophageal echocardiography (TEE)
for aortic dissection, 933–935, 938
for infective endocarditis, 1109
Transforming growth factor (TGF), 19–20, 43, 81, 291, 292, 294
hypertension and, 361
role of, 888
smooth muscle proliferation and, 105–106
Transient ischemic attacks (TIAs), 338, 342, 545, 781, 782
aortic dissection causing, 931
reversible ischemic neurologic deficit (RIND), 782
transient monocular blindness (TMB), 782
treatment of, 675–676
Transient monocular blindness (TMB), 782
Transluminal balloon venoplasty, for venous compression, 1202
Transmucosal nitroglycerin, 809
Transport, 141–151, *See also* Flow
basic concepts, 162–176
convective, 148–151
convective-diffusive, 162–165
diffusive, 148–151, 162–163, 164–165, 167–168
endothelial cells and, 4–5
in tubular flow, 163–165
Transthoracic echocardiography (TTE)
for aortic dissection, 933, 938
for infective endocarditis, 1109
Transthrombus bolusing, 770, 771
Trapping hypothesis, for atherosclerosis, 230
Trauma, vascular, 1147–1168
abdominal, 1161–1162
anesthesia for, 1152
angiography for, 503–504, 505
aorta, 930, 1162
arterial injuries, 1152–1153
blunt injuries, 1147
carotid arteries, 1160–1161
celiac-arteries, 1162
diagnosis, 1148–1150
endovascular repair of, 1168
etiology, 1147
fasciotomy, 1153
femoral arteries, 1163
heart injuries, 1157–1158
iatrogenic complications, 1164–1167
angiography, 1164–1165
intra-aortic balloon counterpulsation, 1166
invasive monitoring, 1166–1167
laser angioplasty, 1165–1166
percutaneous transluminal angioplasty, 1165–1166
surgery, 1166
iliac vessels, 1163
incidence, 1147
inferior vena cava, 1163
inframesocolic hematoma, 1162
infrarenal vena cava, 1163
innominate arteries, 1160–1161
jugular vein, 1159
late complications
chronic traumatic arteriovenous fistulas, 1156–1157
graft infections, 1155–1156
traumatic aneurysms, 906–907, 1156
lower-extremities, 1163–1164
management, 1152–1153
neck injuries, 1158–1159
orthopedic injuries, 1152–1153
pathophysiology, 1147–1150
pediatric, 1167–1168
penetrating injuries, 1147
perioperative complications, reperfusion syndrome, 1154–1155
peroneal arteries, 1164
physical assessment, 1149–1150
popliteal artery, 1163–1164
postoperative management, 1153–1154
preoperative preparation, 1152
Raynaud's phenomenon caused by, 977
renal artery, 1162–1163
repair decision, 1163, 1168
retrohepatic vena cava, 1163
subclavian arteries, 1160–1161
superior mesenteric artery, 1162
supramesocolic hematoma, 1162
thoracic injuries, 1159–1160
tibial arteries, 1164
treatment priorities, 1150–1152
upper extremity, 1161
venous injuries, 1152–1153, 1163
vertebral artery, 1159
Traumatic aneurysms, 906–907, 1156
Traumatic arteriovenous fistulas, chronic, 1156–1157
Traumatic vasospastic diseases, 977
Trazadone, for vasculogenic impotence, 895
Treadmill exercise testing, 421, 433–434, 705–706, 801
Trench foot (immersion foot), 986–987
Trendelenburg test, 410
Triglyceride-rich lipoproteins, 307, 310, 312
Triglycerides
defined, 587
flow of, 587–589
impaired clearance of, 593
Triiodothyroxine, for Raynaud's phenomenon, 983
Tropoelastin, 51–52, 53
Tropomyosin, 100, 103
Troponin, 100
Trousseau's syndrome, 272
TxS inhibitors, 649–650
Tuberculous aortitis, 906
Tuberous xanthomas, 597
Tubular flow, mass transport in, 163–165
Tumor necrosis factor alpha (TBF-α), 43
Tumors, vascular
benign, 1269–1274
angiolymphoid hyperplasia, 1273
glomus, 1273
hemangiomas, 1269–1272
spindle-cell hemangioendothelioma, 1272
vascular ectasias, 1273–1274
classification, 1269, 1270
composition, 1269
defined, 1269

Tumors, vascular—(*continued*)
intermediate-grade, 1274–1276
epithelioid hemangioendothelioma, 1275–1276
hemangioendothelioma, 1274–1275
Kaposi-like infantile hemangioendothelioma, 1276
malignant endovascular papillary angioendothelioma, 1276
retiform hemangioendothelioma, 1276
leukocyte adhesion molecule interactions, 15–16
malignant, 1269, 1276–1281
angiosarcoma, 1276–1279
hemangiopericytoma, 1279
Kaposi's sarcoma, 1279–1280
large vessel neoplasms, 1280–1281
Tunica adventitia, 39
Tunica intima, 39, 219, 221, 225
Tunica media, 39, 219, 221
Turbulent flow, 143

Ulcers, 1173–1184
lesions, 675
pedal (arterial), 1173–1181
assessment, 1177–1178
classification, 1177–1178
therapy, 1178–1181
penetrating atherosclerotic, computed tomography, 528
plaque, 800–801
venous, 1181–1184
hemodynamics, 1181–1183
pathogenesis, 1183–1184
treatment, 1184
Ulnar arteries
injuries, 1161
pulse, 402
Ultrasonography, 418–419, 836–837, *See also* Doppler ultrasonography
for cerebrovascular disease, 422–425
iatrogenic complications of, 1165
for monitoring arterial stiffness, 201
for pulmonary embolism, 1074
sound wave frequency, 419
for vascular trauma, 1150
for venous thromboembolism, 1053
Underhydroxylated procollagen, 43–44
Unmyelinated nociceptive afferents, 1209, 1212, 1214
Unna's paste boot, for venous insufficiency, 1095
Unstable angina, 341, 376
aspirin for, 647, 813
Unstable lesions, 333
Unstable plaque, 336
Upper extremities, *See also* Extremities; Limbs
angiography, 505–516
aortic aneurysms, 919
arterial injuries, 1161
chronic venous disorders, 1098–1099
occlusive disease of, 680–681
swelling, in venous compression, 1199
veins, 1081–1082, 1098–1099
Urokinase (uPA), 10, 17, 212, 653–655, 770
receptors (uPARs), 17
Urokinaselike plasminogen activators (u-PAs), 266

Vacuum constriction devices, for vasculogenic impotence, 896
Valve-graft conduit technique, for aortic dissection, 943–944
Valvular heart disease
anticoagulants for, 642, 643
as risk factor for peripheral arterial disease, 704
Valvular incompetence
deep veins, 1091
surgery for, 1096
upper extremities, 1098
venous insufficiency and, 1091, 1093
Valvular reflux, venous insufficiency and, 1091, 1094
Varicose veins, 1084–1090
arteriovenous fistulas and, 1084
clinical manifestations, 1085–1087
defined, 1083
management, 1087–1090
noninvasive testing, 439
pathogenesis and pathophysiology, 1083–1085
patient examination, 410
primary, 439, 1083
secondary, 439, 1083
Vasa vasorum, 295
Vascular addressins, 15
Vascular cell adhesion molecule-1 (VCAM-1), 15, 297–299, 318–319
Vascular ectasias (telangiectasis), 1273–1274
nevus flammeus, 1273–1274
spider telangiectasis, 1274
Vascular endothelial growth factor (VEGF), 18
Vascular hypertension, 618–620
aortic coarctation, 618, 620
renovascular, 618–619
Vascular-imaging studies, in vasculitis, 1003–1004
Vascular injuries, 219–237
atherosclerotic vascular disease, 225–231
hypertension, 231–236
recent research, 224–225
smooth muscle proliferation, 221–224
vessel wall cells, 219
vessel wall layers, 219, 221
Vascular malformations, 1242–1248
arteriovenous, 1243
fibromuscular dysplasia, 1246–1248
telangiectasias, 1244–1246
Vascular permeability factor (VPF), 18
Vascular rings, 1239–1241
Vascular surgery. *See* Surgery
Vascular system, defined, 39
Vascular tone
endothelial control of, 246–253
regulation of, 11–12
Vasculitides, aortic aneurysms and, 905–906
Vasculitis, 999–1025
angiocentric immunoproliferative lesions, 1019–1020
antiphospholipid antibody syndrome, 1023
Behçet's syndrome, 295, 1021
cellular immune-mediated, 390–391
Churg-Strauss syndrome, 1007–1008
classification of, 999, 1000
Cogan's syndrome, 1021–1022
defined, 388
diagnosis, 999–1004
direct lymphocyte-mediated, 390–391
Henoch-Schönlein purpura, 1010–1011
hypersensitivity, 999, 1008–1010
hypocomplementemic, 1011
immune complexes in, 387–392
immunogenetic factors in, 391
isolated central nervous system, 1020
Kawasaki syndrome, 1020–1021
malignant diseases and, 1022–1023
mixed essential cryoglobulinemia, 1011
pathogenic mechanisms, 391–392
pathophysiology of, 387–392
polyarteritis nodosa, 1004–1007
serum sickness, 1012
signs of, 1001
systemic necrotizing, 999
Takayasu arteritis, 999
temporal arteritis, 999, 1015–1016
thrombosis in, 275
treatment, 1023–1025
Wegener's granulomatosis, 1012–1015
Vasculogenic impotence, 885–898
causes, 885
defined, 885
delayed, blunt trauma and, 889–890
diagnosis, 891–894
duplex Doppler ultrasound, 891–892
intracavernosal blood oxygen partial pressure, 894
nuclear magnetic resonance (NMR), 894
pharmacoarteriography, 894
pharmacocavernosography, 892–893
pharmacocavernosometry, 892–893
screening tests, 891
epidemiology, 885–886
pathophysiology, 888–891
blunt-trauma-induced arterial vasculopathy, 888–890
cavernosal-artery insufficiency, 888
corporal veno-occlusive dysfunction, 890–891
physiology of erection, 886–888
corporal veno-occlusion, 887–888
extracellular matrix synthesis, 888
helicine arteriolar smooth muscle tone, 886
trabecular smooth muscle tone, 886–888
prevalence, 885
treatment, 894–898
microvascular arterial bypass surgery, 896–897
noninjection pharmacologic agents, 894–895
penile self-injection therapy, 895–896
psychologic therapy, 894
vacuum constriction devices, 896
Vasoactive intestinal polypeptide (VIP), 79, 137
Vasoconstriction, 343
atherosclerotic plaque site, 336
defined, 966
hypertension and, 359, 623
Raynaud's phenomenon and, 966–967, 969, 970–971
Vasoconstrictors, 11–12
bradykinin, 137
EDRF action and, 250
endothelial-derived contractile factors, 11
endothelin, 11–12, 129
in finger circulation, 378
histaminergic receptors, 76
kinin receptors, 76, 77
oxytocin, 80
peptide, 106–107
role of, 379
types of, 370–371
vasopressin, 80, 136

Vasodepression, endothelins and, 106
Vasodilation, 343
bradykinin and, 137
dopaminergic receptors and, 78
endothelin and, 129
histamine and, 136
histaminergic receptors and, 76
kinin receptors and, 76, 77
oxytocin and, 80
reactive hyperemia, 434
regulation of, 371–372
vasopressin and, 80, 136
Vasodilators, 11
eicosanoids, 11
endothelial-derived hyperpolarizing factor (EDHF), 11, 128, 132
endothelial-derived relaxing factor (EDRF), 11, 74, 126–128, 132, 236, 265, 300–301, 343, 370
for hypertension, 237, 630–631
for pulmonary hypertension, 961–962
for reducing ischemia in extremities, 841–842
role of, 379
types of, 371
Vasomotion
abnormal coronary, role of, 797–798
blood elements, 371–372
circulating vasoactive substances, 370–371
endothelium, 371
exogenous influences, 373–374
migraine headaches and, 379–380
neurogenic control, 369–370
physiology of, 369–374
Vasopressin, 79–80, 136
Vasospasm
cerebral arteries, 369, 379–381
coronary arteries, 369, 374–377
defined, 369, 966
digital arteries, 377–379
pathophysiology of, 369–381
Raynaud's phenomenon, 966, 973
role of, 342–343
vasomotion and, 369–374
in visceral ischemia, 871
Vasospastic claudication, 400
Vein grafts
failure, 687–691
in-situ saphenous, 689–691
reversed autogenous saphenous, 686–687
saphenous, 846
stenosis, 742–745
for vasculogenic impotence, 897
for venous insufficiency, 1096–1098
Veins
anatomy, 1081–1082
blood flow, 1083
blood pressure, 1083
blood volume, 1082–1083
communicating, 1081, 1224–1228
hemodynamics, 1181–1183
lower extremity
deep, 1091–1098
superficial, 1083–1091
physiology, 1082–1083
upper extremity, 1098–1099
valvular incompetence, 1091
venous "footpump," 1182
venous pressure, 1094, 1182
Velocity distribution
in small vessels, 146
thrombosis and, 148
Velocity gradient, thrombus formation and, 151
Velocity profile, hematocrit and, 155
Vena cava
abdominal, computed tomography, 524
computed tomography, 524, 535–539, 543–545
congenital anomalies, 537
exposure of, in trauma, 1163
inferior, 537, 543–545
filter, for pulmonary embolism, 1077
leiomyosarcomas, 1280, 1281
occlusion, 411–412
superior, 537, 539
thrombosis of, 537
ultrasonography, 425
Venography, 512–514
for brachial plexus compression, 1198
for venous insufficiency, 1094
for venous thromboembolism, 1053–1054
Venospasm, 369, 381
Venous claudication, 400, 829
Venous compression, 1198–1203
angioplasty, 1202–1203
anticoagulant therapy, 1198–1202, 1203
diagnosis, 1198
presenting history and signs, 1199
surgery, 1202
thrombolytic therapy, 1198–1202
transluminal balloon venoplasty, 1202
Venous disorders
chronic, 1081–1099
deep veins of lower limbs, 1091–1098
noninvasive testing for, 438–439
radionuclide imaging for, 486–487
superficial veins of lower limbs, 1083–1091
veins in upper extremity, 1098–1099
hypertension, 1182–1183
injuries, 1152–1153, 1163
insufficiency, 1091–1098, 1181
defined, 1091
management, 1094–1098
patient examination, 412–413
postphlebitic, 1091
postthrombotic, 1091
surgical measures, 1095–1098
valvular incompetence and, 1091, 1093
in vascular ulcers, 1173
venous obstruction and, 1091–1092, 1093
noninvasive testing, 436–439
radionuclide imaging of, 486–487
telangiectasia (spider veins), 1090–1091
venous hum, 407
Venous thromboembolism, 272
death from, 1051
defined, 1054–1057
diagnostic tests, 1052–1054
risk factors, 1052, 1055
treatment, 1057–1063
Venous thrombosis, 1051–1063
clinical features, 1052
diagnosis, 1052–1054
etiology and pathogenesis, 1051–1052
laboratory features, 1052
in pregnancy, 1063
risk factors, 1070
thromboembolism prevention, 1054–1057
treatment, 1057–1063
Venous ulcers, 1181–1184
hemodynamics, 1181–1183
pathogenesis, 1183–1184
treatment, 1184
Ventilation-perfusion lung scanning
for pulmonary embolism, 1073
for pulmonary hypertension, 958
Ventricular failure, left, 954
Ventricular-vascular interaction, 185, 197–198
arterial stiffness and, 197–198
Verapamil, 812, 813, 981
Versican, 56, 57
Vertebral arteries, 783, 1159
Vertebrobasilar disease, 785
Very low-density lipoproteins (VLDL), 63, 307, 308, 312, 589
in atherogenic dyslipoproteinemias, 592–601
classification, 591
heterogeneity, 590–591
Vessels, *See also* Arteries; Veins
abnormalities, thrombosis and, 275–276
endothelial cells, 3
geometry, disturbed flow and, 143–146
innervation, 122, 369
neoplastic diseases of, 1269–1281
benign tumors, 1269–1274
intermediate-grade tumors, 1274–1276
malignant tumors, 1276–1281
pharmacology of, 117–137
radius, arterial stiffness and, 187
rupture, angiography, 504
size, hypertension and, 235
types of, 39
velocity distribution, 146, 148
Vessel walls
adhesion, in annular vortex, 161–162
blood cell migration in Poiseuille flow, 151
calcium deposition, 325
capillary formation, 325
cells of, 219, 234–235
embryonic development, 219
injury, disturbed flow and, 160
layers, 219, 221, 230
mass
cell number and, 234–236
replication and, 236–237
normal
lipoprotein accumulation in, 313–314
lipoprotein transport in, 312–314
platelet interactions
abnormalities, 176–179
deposits, 165–167
disorders related to, 176–178
flow chambers, 164
influence of flow on, 165–171
intravascular, 165
in nonanticoagulated blood, 171–176
shear rate and, 178–179
transport processes affecting, 162–176
remodeling, 226, 227, 235, 360
shear rates, 165–167, 168, 169, 172–173
steroid effects on sympathetic-nerve stimulation, 125
thickness, hypertension and, 359
transport processes, 162–176, 219
Veterans Administration Cooperative Study, 791, 813, 816
Veterans Affairs Stroke Prevention in Nonrheumatic Atrial Fibrillation, 791
Vibration white-finger syndrome, 977
Vinblastine, Raynaud's phenomenon caused by, 977
Vinculin, 100
Viral-mediated gene transfer, 666–668

Visceral angiography, 508, 511
Visceral-artery aneurysms, 698–699, 919–920
Visceral endarterectomy, 881
Visceral ischemia, 869–891
acute
clinical presentation and diagnosis, 873–876
etiology and pathophysiology, 871–872
historic background, 869
treatment, 878–881
aortovisceral bypass grafting, 880–881
chronic
clinical presentation and diagnosis, 876
etiology and pathophysiology, 872–873
historic background, 869–870
treatment, 879–880
clinical presentation and diagnosis, 873–878
defined, 869
etiology and pathophysiology, 870–873
historic background, 869–870
incidence, 870
treatment, 878–881
visceral endarterectomy, 881
Visceral vessel occlusive disease, 691–693
Viscosity of blood
apparent, 146
relative apparent, shear rate and, 150
Vitamin E, coronary artery disease and, 251–252
Vitamin K antagonists, 639, 641
Vitronectin, 10
Voltage-operated channels (VOCs), 70, 71
Volume elastic modulus, 186
Volume expanders, hypertension and, 623
Von Hippel Lindau syndrome, 1245, 1271
Von Willebrand factor (vWF), 8–9, 207, 254, 276, 1269, 1270
atherosclerosis and, 254–255
coronary heart disease risk and, 579
Raynaud's phenomenon and, 971
Von Willebrand's disease (vWD), 9, 176–177, 207

Wall-active agents, for infective endocarditis, 1110–1112
Wallenberg's syndrome (lateral medullary syndrome), 785
Warfarin, 639–643
antithrombin II levels, 270–271
for carotid artery disease, 791
defined, 639
for ischemic stroke, 791
mechanism of action, 639
protein C/S deficiency and, 270–271
for pulmonary embolism, 1071, 1075
sodium, for coronary artery disease, 813
for venous compression, 1199
for venous thromboembolism, 1056, 1060–1062
Warfarin Reinfarction Study (WARIS), 642
Wegener's granulomatosis, 1012–1015
Weibel Palade bodies, 8–9
Weight
cardiovascular disease risk and, 577–578
hypertension and, 623–624
obesity, 577–578, 599, 610–611, 624
White blood cells
margination of, 160
trapping theory, of venous ulcers, 1183–1184
Wide-dynamic range (WDR) neurons, 1211
Women, postmenopausal estrogen therapy, 576–577

Xanthomas
palmar, 597
tendon, 596, 597
tuberous, 597
Xase complex, 209
X-rays
for brachial plexus compression, 1198
generator, for angiography, 494
multiple exposures, for computed tomography, 519
for vascular trauma, 1150

Yohimbine
for Raynaud's phenomenon, 970
for vasculogenic impotence, 894–895
Young's modulus of elasticity, 186

Zeumatography, 445